CORMAN'S COLON and RECTAL SURGERY

Sixth Edition

CORMAN'S COLON and RECTAL SURGERY

Sixth Edition

Editor:
Marvin L. Corman, MD, FASCRS, FACS
Professor of Surgery
Division of Colon and Rectal Surgery
Stony Brook University
Stony Brook, New York

Associate Editors:
Roberto C. M. Bergamaschi, MD, PhD, FRCS, FASCRS, FACS
Professor and Chief
Division of Colon and Rectal Surgery
Stony Brook University
Stony Brook, New York

R. John Nicholls, MD
Professor of Colorectal Surgery
Imperial College, London
Emeritus Consultant Surgeon
St. Mark's Hospital, London
United Kingdom

Victor W. Fazio, AO, MB, BS, MD, FRACS
Rupert B. Turnbull, Jr., MD Chair
Chairman, Digestive Disease Institute (Emeritus)
Cleveland Clinic Foundation
Cleveland, Ohio

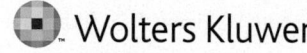 **Wolters Kluwer** | Lippincott Williams & Wilkins
Health

Philadelphia · Baltimore · New York · London
Buenos Aires · Hong Kong · Sydney · Tokyo

Acquisitions Editor: Brian Brown
Product Manager: Brendan Huffman
Production Manager: Alicia Jackson
Senior Manufacturing Manager: Benjamin Rivera
Marketing Manager: Lisa Lawrence
Design Coordinator: Doug Smock
Production Service: Absolute Service, Inc.

Printed in China

Library of Congress Cataloging-in-Publication Data

Corman's colon and rectal surgery / editor, Marvin L. Corman ; associate editors, Roberto C.M. Bergamaschi ... [et al.]. — 6th ed.
    p. ; cm.
  Colon and rectal surgery
  Rev. ed. of: Colon and rectal surgery / Marvin L. Corman. 5th ed. c2005.
  Includes bibliographical references and index.
  ISBN 978-1-4511-1114-9
  I. Corman, Marvin L., 1939- II. Corman, Marvin L., 1939- Colon and rectal surgery. III. Title: Colon and rectal surgery.
  [DNLM: 1. Rectal Diseases—surgery. 2. Colonic Diseases—surgery. 3. Postoperative Complications—prevention & control. WI 650]

  617.5'547—dc23

                                                                              2012027785

Care has been taken to confirm the accuracy of the information presented and to describe generally accepted practices. However, the authors, editors, and publisher are not responsible for errors or omissions or for any consequences from application of the information in this book and make no warranty, expressed or implied, with respect to the currency, completeness, or accuracy of the contents of the publication. Application of the information in a particular situation remains the professional responsibility of the practitioner.

The authors, editors, and publisher have exerted every effort to ensure that drug selection and dosage set forth in this text are in accordance with current recommendations and practice at the time of publication. However, in view of ongoing research, changes in government regulations, and the constant flow of information relating to drug therapy and drug reactions, the reader is urged to check the package insert for each drug for any change in indications and dosage and for added warnings and precautions. This is particularly important when the recommended agent is a new or infrequently employed drug.

Some drugs and medical devices presented in the publication have Food and Drug Administration (FDA) clearance for limited use in restricted research settings. It is the responsibility of the health care provider to ascertain the FDA status of each drug or device planned for use in their clinical practice.

To purchase additional copies of this book, call our customer service department at (800) 638-3030 or fax orders to (301) 223-2320. International customers should call (301) 223-2300.

Visit Lippincott Williams & Wilkins on the Internet at LWW.com. Lippincott Williams & Wilkins customer service representatives are available from 8:30 a.m. to 6:00 p.m., EST.

10 9 8 7 6 5 4 3 2 1

Contributors

Alan V. Abrams, MD
Clinical Assistant
Professor of Surgery
Section of Colon and Rectal Surgery
Weill Medical College of Cornell
    University
New York, New York

Salim Amrani, MD
Colon and Rectal Surgery
Carlsbad Medical Center
Carlsbad, New Mexico

Robert W. Beart, Jr., MD
Emeritus Professor of Surgery
USC Keck School of Medicine
Los Angeles, California
Medical Director, Colorectal Surgery
    Institute
Glendale, California

Roberto C. M. Bergamaschi, MD,
    PhD, FRCS, FASCRS, FACS
Professor and Chief
Division of Colon and Rectal Surgery
Stony Brook University
Stony Brook, New York

E. Leslie Bokey, AM, MBBS (USyd),
    MS (Syd)
Clinical Dean and Foundation
    Professor
University of Western Sydney
Professor of Colon and Rectal Surgery
    and Director of Surgery
Liverpool Hospital
Sydney, Australia

James M. Church, MB ChB
Victor W. Fazio Chair of Colorectal
    Surgery
Director, Sanford R. Weiss, MD Center
    for Hereditary Colorectal Neoplasia
Department of Colorectal Surgery
Digestive Disease Institute
Cleveland Clinic Foundation
Cleveland, Ohio

Marvin L. Corman, MD, FASCRS,
    FACS
Professor of Surgery
Division of Colon and Rectal Surgery
Stony Brook University
Stony Brook, New York

Eric J. Daniels, MD, MBA
Vice President, Marketing and Sales
Tensys Medical, Inc.
San Diego, California

Herbert M. Dean, MD
Oncology Consultant
University of Massachusetts
    Medical School
Worcester, Massachusetts

Paula I. Denoya, MD
Assistant Professor of Surgery
Division of Colon and Rectal Surgery
Stony Brook University Hospital
Stony Brook, New York

Jonathan E. Efron, MD
Associate Professor
The Mark M. Ravitch, MD
    Endowed Professorship in Surgery
Chief of the Ravitch Division
Johns Hopkins University
Baltimore, Maryland

Paula Erwin-Toth, MSN, RN, ET,
    CWOCN, CNS
Director Emerita WOC Nursing
    Education
Cleveland Clinic Foundation
Cleveland, Ohio

Victor W. Fazio, AO, MB, BS, MD,
    FRACS
Rupert B. Turnbull, Jr., MD Chair
Chairman, Digestive Disease
    Institute (Emeritus)
Cleveland Clinic Foundation
Cleveland, Ohio

Ana Garza, MD
Colorectal Surgeon
Colorectal Surgery Institute
Glendale, California

Anthony A. Goodman, MD, FACS
Adjunct Professor of Medicine
W.W.A.M.I. Medical Sciences
    Department
Montana State University
Bozeman, Montana
Affiliate Professor
Department of Biologic Structure
University of Washington School of
    Medicine
Seattle, Washington

Lester Gottesman, MD
Associate Professor of Surgery
Columbia University
New York, New York

Neil H. Hyman, MD
Samuel B. and Michelle D. Labow
    Professor of Colon and Rectal
    Surgery
Codirector, Digestive Disease Center
University of Vermont College of
    Medicine
Burlington, Vermont

Gerald A. Isenberg, MD
Professor of Surgery
Jefferson Medical College
Philadelphia, Pennsylvania

Sanjay P. Jobanputra, MD
Colon and Rectal Surgeon
Winthrop University Hospital
Mineola, New York

**Matthew F. Kalady, MD, FACS,
    FASCRS**
Assistant Professor of Surgery
Krause-Lieberman Chair in Colorectal
    Surgery
Department of Colorectal Surgery
Digestive Disease Institute
Cleveland Clinic Foundation
Cleveland, Ohio

Pranat Kumar, MD
Surgeon
Department of General Surgery
Saint Francis Hospital and Health
    Centers
Poughkeepsie, New York

Albert O. Kwon, MD
Division of Colon and Rectal Surgery
Stony Brook University
Stony Brook, New York

Alex Jenny Ky, MD
Associate Professor
Department of Surgery
Mount Sinai School of Medicine
Director of Surgical Specialty
    Downtown
New York, New York

Sergio W. Larach, MD
Program Director, Colon and Rectal
    Surgery
Florida Hospital
Associated Professor of Surgery
Florida State University
Tallahassee, Florida

Chris E. Lascarides
Assistant Professor of Medicine
Attending Gastroenterologist
Division of Gastroenterology
Stony Brook University
Stony Brook, New York

Marc A. Levitt, MD
Director, Colorectal Center for
    Children
Cincinnati Children's Hospital
Professor of Surgery
Department of Surgery
University of Cincinnati
Cincinnati, Ohio

Ian Lindsey, MBBS
Consultant Colorectal Surgeon and
    Lead for Pelvic Floor Surgery
Oxford Pelvic Floor Centre
Department of Colorectal Surgery
Oxford University Hospitals
Oxford, United Kingdom

Slawomir Marecik, MD
Attending Surgeon
Advocate Lutheran General Hospital
Park Ridge, Illinois
Assistant Professor of Surgery
University of Illinois at Chicago
Chicago, Illinois

R. John Nicholls, MD
Professor of Colorectal Surgery
Imperial College, London
Emeritus Consultant Surgeon
St. Mark's Hospital, London
United Kingdom

Alberto Peña, MD
Founding Director, Colorectal Center
Professor, Division of Pediatric
    Surgery
Cincinnati Children's Hospital
Cincinnati, Ohio

John L. Petrini, Jr., MD
Chief of Gastroenterology
Sansum Clinic
Santa Barbara, California

Alessio Pigazzi, MD, PhD
Associate Professor
Division of Colon and Rectal Surgery
University of California, Irvine
Orange, California

Michael H. Polcino, MD
Resident, Division of Surgery
Stony Brook University
Stony Brook, New York

Brett E. Ruffo, MD
Colorectal Surgeon
Peconic Bay Medical Center
Riverhead, New York
Stony Brook University Medical
    Center
Stony Brook, New York

Theodore J. Saclarides
Director of Colorectal Surgery
Loyola University Health System
Maywood, Illinois
Professor of Surgery
Loyola University Chicago Stritch
    School of Medicine
Chicago, Illinois

Dana R. Sands, MD
Director, Colorectal Physiology Center
Staff Surgeon
Department of Colorectal Surgery
Cleveland Clinic Florida
Weston, Florida

Emily Steinhagen, MD
General Surgery Resident
The Mount Sinai Medical Center
New York, New York

Elsa B. Valsdottir, MD
Associate Professor
Division of General Surgery
University Hospital of Iceland
Reykjavik, Iceland

George C. Velmahos, MD, PhD
John F. Burke Professor of Surgery
Harvard Medical School
Chief of Division of Trauma
Emergency Surgery and Surgical
    Critical Care
Massachusetts General Hospital
Boston, Massachusetts

Steven D. Wexner, MD
Chief Academic Officer and Emeritus
    Chief of Staff
Professor and Chair
Department of Colorectal Surgery
Cleveland Clinic Florida
Weston, Florida

Julia Zakhaleva, MD
Chief Surgical Resident
Department of General Surgery
State University of New York at
    Stony Brook
Stony Brook, New York

Foreword

Any author whose work has become a "standard text" in his or her field of expertise must feel challenged to not only keep its content current but also provide something unique for each new edition. Dr. Marvin L. Corman's fifth edition of *Colon and Rectal Surgery* was very well received nationally and internationally. Its success had to make consideration of writing a sixth edition even more intimidating than previously. Marvin must have wondered what he could possibly do to make the sixth edition distinctive and better than the preceding versions. His answer to this dilemma was to invite three colorectal surgeons to serve as coeditors. The three— Roberto C. M. Bergamaschi, R. John Nicholls, and Victor W. Fazio—are not your average colorectal surgeons. These three gentlemen bring an incredible depth of international colorectal surgical experience that no one, not even Marvin Corman, can claim alone. As I review the proofs of the new text, I am most struck by the manner in which Dr. Corman, as senior editor, has used the contributions of his coeditors and other guest authors to infuse the text with their cumulative wisdom and practical advice. The practicing surgeon will love this combination of colorectal surgical firepower coupled with outstanding and accurate medical illustrations, useful and clear photographs, accurate reproductions of imaging studies, and pleasing graphics and tables. Fortunately, Dr. Corman has retained a feature from prior editions that I especially enjoy. Short historical vignettes accompanied by a photograph of famous surgeons or scientists who influenced colorectal surgery are interspersed throughout the text. I find it great fun to read a section of text, turn the page, and unexpectedly find a photograph of Antonio Maria Valsalva (Valsalva maneuver) or John Houston (valves of Houston) or Heinrich Wilhelm Gottfried Von Waldeyer-Hartz (Waldeyer's fascia) or countless others whose names we use repeatedly in our professional lives usually without knowing much about them. The sixth edition of this now classic textbook continues the legacy of providing a highly practical, surgeon-friendly, "go-to" textbook for colorectal surgery.

David A. Rothenberger, MD
June 28, 2012

Foreword
to the Second Edition

I have reproduced the Foreword to the Second Edition of this text as a memorial to John Cedric Goligher, my mentor, my role model, and my treasured friend.

MLC
September 1, 2012

To be asked by a colleague to write a foreword for one of his literary works is always a considerable compliment and honor. But Marvin Corman's invitation to contribute such an introduction to the second edition of his *Colon and Rectal Surgery* has afforded me special pleasure for a very personal reason. I recognize full well that most of his surgical knowledge and expertise has been derived from his training at the University of Pennsylvania and The Harvard Surgical Service at Boston City Hospital, and from his years of practice at the Lahey Clinic in Boston and the Sansum Clinic in Santa Barbara. But I believe it would be fair to claim that his first really intensive exposure to colorectal surgery was obtained whilst he was doing a 12-month overseas assignment as an assistant with me in Leeds in 1968, and that that experience influenced him considerably in deciding subsequently to concentrate his efforts on this field of surgical endeavour. Naturally, therefore, it has been with much interest and no small measure of pride that I have followed the gradual evolution over the years of this talented young trainee into the present immensely experienced and successful colorectal surgeon, now in an extremely busy middle period of this career.

As I see it, the traditional role of an independent foreword is twofold—to say something by way of introduction about the author, especially when he happens to be relatively little known, and to offer some words of explanation and commendation about the book itself (all these remarks, needless to say, being couched in as favorable terms as possible). But on this occasion there can be little excuse for indulging in such ritual praises and platitudes, for Marvin Corman already enjoys a truly international reputation in colorectal surgery, and the uniformly favorable reviews accorded to the first edition of his book (including First Prize of The American Medical Writers Association) and the large readership that it has since acquired have established beyond question its great merits and rendered inappropriate any further exercises in unalloyed eulogy. What then can one say? Well, it might

be interesting and even useful to try to identify those factors that may have helped to secure the outstanding success of this work. Perhaps the best way to do so would be, first of all, to itemize the features that appear, at any rate to me, especially necessary in any text that aims to cover an area of surgical practice and to be available for consultation, not merely in hospital or medical school libraries, but also and more importantly in the surgeon's own office or study, and then to see how well Marvin Corman's book satisfies those postulated requirements.

I consider one of the most desirable attributes to be *really comprehensive coverage of the subject matter*, so that the readers can feel confident that in turning to it they will, as a rule, be able to obtain good advice and not too often encounter disconcerting hiatuses. To be able to offer such an assurance involves a thorough analysis of current knowledge, including an up-to-date review of the relevant literature. Naturally the author's own personal experience and his favored concepts on controversial issues and preferred methods of treatment of various conditions may receive some special attention, but this should not be at the expense of independent essays on selected subtopics, however authoritatively written and valuable for library reading, leaves too many gaps to be an adequate substitute for a well-integrated, relatively unbiased text as a personal reference volume.

An equally important requirement is a book of this kind is a *high quality of illustrations*. As is generally agreed, good illustrations are a considerable help in imparting knowledge on many subjects, but they become well-nigh indispensable when expounding on operative techniques. Indeed, trying to describe surgical operations without the aid of a good illustrative material is about as difficult as attempting to perform these very procedures with one arm tied behind one's back! A few well-executed sketches can enormously clarify and shorten accounts of operative maneuvers.

The *relative merits of single and multiple authorship* have been much debated. Multiple authorship has the advantage of making it possible to allocate to different writers subjects in which they have a special interest and experience. But, even with firm editorship, this arrangement affords a much less even literary format and incurs a greater risk of creating defects or overlaps in coverage. A single authorship has the great merit of presenting a uniform and more agreeable literary style. Moreover, I feel compelled to say that, when writing on a fairly limited theme, such as diseases of the colon and rectum, it ought in my opinion to be possible for one experienced and determined writer to circumscribe the whole field with adequate authority entirely by himself, with perhaps a little assistance from one or two colleagues on slightly more esoteric or specialized aspects of the subject.

Turning now to Marvin Corman's *Colon and Rectal Surgery*, I feel that it warrants high ratings on each of these three important points. It unquestionably provides good or very adequate coverage on all major issues. The illustrations, particularly those of operative techniques, are quite superb and represent one of the most attractive features of the works. The text is essentially by one author, insofar as Dr. Corman himself has been responsible for all of it except for that part pertaining to pediatric conditions, which are dealt with very effectively by the well-known pediatric surgeon, Dr. Alberto Peña. Dr. Corman writes clearly and attractively, making for easy reading and ready understanding, the outcome is a most handsome and helpful volume, which it is a pleasure to consult.

In conclusion and at the risk of exposing myself to a charge of conceit, I should like to point out that for most of the past three decades the need of surgeons for a comprehensive, consistently updated text, covering the whole field of colorectal surgery with some thoroughness, has been met mainly—and,

for a considerable part of that time, solely—by my *Surgery of the Anus, Rectum and Colon* (London: Baillière-Tindall, 1st ed, 1961; 5th ed, 1984 [editor's note: newly revised by Keighley and Williams in 1999]). But in more recent years several other books on this subject (or on selected parts of it) have emerged—and, if rumor is to be believed, two more are due to appear in the near future—so that a steadily increasing number of alternative texts is becoming available. Doubtless each of these volumes will suit different surgical tastes and needs. He would be a brave man who would attempt any sort of objective assessment of their relative merits, and certainly this is not the place in which to undertake such an adjudication. All I would like to say in this connection is that in my opinion one of these works, the second edition of Corman's *Colon and Rectal Surgery*, is certainly a very good substitute for mine, and I have no hesitation in recommending it strongly as a reliable guide to the sound practice of contemporary colorectal surgery.

John Goligher
Emeritus Professor of Surgery,
University of Leeds, England;
Consulting Surgeon,
St. Mark's Hospital for Diseases of the Rectum and Colon,
London, England
June 1, 1988

Preface

I have asked the question in different ways over these multiple revisions as to why someone elects to author a medical book? It has been said that writing and publishing may be the safest means for achieving fame or at least some level of eminence. The alternative avenues for comparable recognition were for me either impossible or unacceptable, such as becoming a surrealistic poet, dying in battle, facing capital punishment for apostasy, or going on an ill-fated expedition—just to name a few options. So I thought I would continue to rewrite this text. But it has never, ever been a labor of love. To quote that extraordinary statesman and prolific author, Winston Churchill, "A book is an unforgiving mistress." And in a not dissimilar vein, when asked by a reporter to describe the playwright's profession, the late Herb Gardner replied, "How do you ask a kamikaze pilot if his work is going well?"

I am fortunate again to have the opportunity of changing my mind, of clarifying confusion and my confused thinking, of correcting misstatements, as well as attempting to remain contemporary. I am doomed to the embarrassment of living with my previous inaccuracies. Still, it is better to recant than to be accused of having a pertinacious little mind.

But much more important, it is now long past the hour for one to move on and to advance the baton to the next generation. This incunabulum of time had its birth in 1976. David A. Rothenberger stated in the Foreword to this edition that I had a dilemma. What could I possibly accomplish that would be distinctive and perhaps even superior to that of prior versions? His answer was "to invite three colorectal surgeons to serve as coeditors." I am certain the readership will agree that Roberto C. M. Bergamaschi, R. John Nicholls and Victor W. Fazio are not your average colorectal surgeons. They do indeed bring an incredible depth of international colorectal surgical experience, a depth which I surely cannot claim for myself, alone. For all of their commitments, I am very grateful. I hope and I trust that the reader will concur that the efforts exerted have achieved substantive results and at least a modicum of success.

Yet, why should one revise a text approximately every 5 years? What is so special about this interval that motivates authors and publishers to rejuvenate their interest in such an endeavor? Laënnec encouraged one not to fear to repeat that which has already been said. "People need truth dinned into their ears many times from all sides." He wrote that the first rumor makes them prick up their ears, the second registers, and the third enters. But advances in the field of colon and rectal surgery have proceeded at such a pace that it makes one incredulous. Henry Bowditch stated in 1887 that the accumulated literature in medicine is already so enormous and is increasing at such a rapid rate that "any association or individual undertaking to contribute thereto should do so only under a sense of grave moral responsibility." His comment is even more applicable today.

Every chapter has been rewritten, new references added, and art expanded. Areas of management no longer considered applicable have been deleted. The fact is, as George Pickering implied, that within 30 to 40 years, 50 percent of medical writing will be wrong or obsolete. The question, of course, is "Which 50 percent?"

I am so pleased that my coeditors and contributors have strived to maintain the somewhat opinionated nature of the contents. Reasonable people have the right to disagree, but there should be no doubt as to one's position, especially where there are issues of controversy. Of course, there is an extensive literature that accompanies each chapter which, hopefully, will stimulate an individual to pursue additional reading.

I continue to be aware that my book has been inappropriately used as an "authoritative" treatise, at least in the United States, by members of the legal profession through our tort system. How one defines the word, authoritative, is of no mean consequence when one appears on the witness stand. I wish to state for the record that herein there are no sacred truths, no dicta, only personal opinion and the perspectives and reflections of clinical and laboratory investigators, especially those of highly experienced surgeons. One may rely on the integrity of the process, but clearly I do not agree with all of the comments and opinions that are expressed within these pages. Moreover, I acknowledge that every reasonable surgeon has the right to harbor heterodox beliefs.

Because of my particular interest in the history of medicine, specifically colon and rectal surgery, I have expanded the *biographic sketches* considerably. In *Ecclesiastes* it is said, "All these were honored in their generations and were the glory of their times." As important to the contemporary surgeon, however, is the result that one's failure to know our history causes us to lack any meaningful perspective as to where we are going. Accordingly, I have encouraged a number of students and residents in surgery to undertake the task of providing much of this additional material. Where these contributions appear the individuals are recognized. These wonderful people have been the greatest source of joy for me. As a surgeon who has the temerity to believe that I have actually devoted my life in no small part to that of teaching, I take great pride in their accomplishments.

Da Costa commented that to write a book is to reveal oneself. Such an endeavor is, in a sense, somewhat like an autobiography. Laënnec further stated that he risked his life, but he hoped that the book he was going to publish would be useful enough sooner or later to be worth the life of a man. Critical writing has never been more important to the health of the medical profession. I wish those that succeed me a successful voyage, an adventurous enterprise, one

that will give fulfillment beyond measure but will, I hope, liberate you from the mundane and the trivial as you with comfort and confidence achieve the exalted status of the "dear and the glorious physician." While I offer no apologia for the book's contents, I value the opinions, criticisms, and suggestions of the reader. After all, I am still in the process of learning.

Marvin L. Corman
September 2012
Stony Brook University

Acknowledgments

There are so many individuals whom I would like to thank for their help in the completion of this text. In addition to the contributors, whom I recognize individually in their chapters, I am, of course, indebted to Lois Barnes, a medical illustrator of international repute. She was required to provide illustrative consistency by rendering all of the art of the contributors. She did so with remarkable patience, grace, compulsivity, and her usual professionalism. I am certain that the reader will recognize the exceptional quality of her work. She continues to actively pursue her illustrative talents.

Although I risk omitting someone, I want to acknowledge a number of individuals who offered special help in the completion of this book: Herand Abcarian, Donato Altomare, Cornelius Baeten, Randolph Bailey, Clive Bartram, David Beck, Renato Bonardi, Philip Caushaj, John Coller, Herbert Dean, Alberto del Genio, Theodore Eisenstat, Abraham Fingerhut, James Fleshman, Robert Fry, Jules Garbus, Gary Gecelter, Stanley Goldberg, Anthony Goodman, Jose Guillem, Angelita Habr-Gama, Thorolf Hager, Paul Hartendorp, Jorge Hequera, John Hinchey, the late Barton Hoexter, David Hong, Andreas Kaiser, Joan Kavanaugh, Clifford Ko, Antonio Longo, Jeffrey Milsom, Deborah Morganelli, Basil Morson, Heidi Nelson, Per-Olaf Nystrom, Olival D'Oliveira, Bruce Orkin, Adrian Ortega, Lars Påhlman, Yves Panis, Dean Pappas, Elliot Prager, Aurora Pryor, Thomas Read, Maryann Reiss, John Ricotta, Basil Rigas, Todd Rosengart, David Rothenberger, Mario Salomon, Eugene Salvati, Cristina Sardinha, Anthony Senagore, David Schoetz, Richard Scriven, Francis Seow-Choen, Marc Sher, William Smithy, Selman Sokmen, Michael Stamos, Joan Stern, Deborah Thornton, Alan Thorson, Petr Tsarkov, Walter Weder, Bruce Wolff, the late Douglas Wong, Zehiel Ziv, and Oded Zmora. I want to express my sincerest appreciation to three dear and special friends: Elliot Prager, Edouard Seroussi, and David Wanicur. They were important counselors to me during this ordeal. Moreover, I want to express my appreciation to Ariana and Danielle Saunders for their help and their special facility with the computer. During the more than 1 year it took me to rewrite this little vade mecum, my wife, Claudia, had to endure my seclusion. She represents the epitome of patience, kindness, and generosity. My sons, John and Alex, and my daughters-in-law, Linnea Peterson and Charlotte Brownlee, as well as my wonderful grandchildren have always been there with smiles and encouragement. I adore them all.

I wish also to thank my publisher, Lippincott Williams & Wilkins, for its dedicated support and commitment to excellence through a relationship that now exceeds 45 years. These include my Product Manager Brendan Huffman, Editor Brian Brown, and Publisher Lisa McAllister. Additionally, I am most grateful to my manuscript editor, Keith Donnellan, and to my typesetter, Harold Medina at Absolute Service, Inc.

Many others have made contributions to the completion of this text. Please excuse my failure to acknowledge personally every one.

With sincere appreciation,
Marvin L. Corman
September 2012
Stony Brook University

Contents

Anatomy and Embryology of the Anus, Rectum, and Colon

Ana Garza and Robert W. Beart, Jr.

In anatomy,
it is better to have learned and lost
than never to have learned at all.
   —W. SOMERSET MAUGHAM: *Of Human Bondage*

Although the need for an understanding of colonic, anorectal, and pelvic anatomy is consistent with the objective of a comprehensive textbook on colon and rectal surgery, little emphasis is placed on these subjects in training programs today. The most extensive observations had been made as early as 1543 by Andreas Vesalius through anatomic dissections. Several aspects, however, remain controversial. Anatomy of this region, especially that of the rectum and anal canal, is so intrinsically related to its physiology that much can be appreciated only in the living. Therefore, it is a region in which the colorectal surgeon has an advantage over the anatomist through in vivo dissection, physiologic investigation, and endoscopic examination. More recently, the accumulated experience with diverse operative techniques such as the ileoanal procedure has added to advances in our understanding of continence and has demanded more in-depth knowledge of the anatomy and physiology of the large intestine.[33,51,52,57,121–123]

▶ EMBRYOLOGY

The primitive gut tube develops from the endodermal roof of the yolk sac. At the beginning of the third week of development, it can be divided into three regions: the foregut in the head fold; the hindgut with its ventral allantoic outgrowth

in the smaller tail fold; and, between these two portions, the midgut, which at this stage opens ventrally into the yolk sac (Figure 1-1). After the stages of physiologic herniation, return to the abdomen, and fixation, the midgut progresses below the major pancreatic papilla to form the small intestine, the ascending colon, and the proximal two-thirds of the transverse colon. This segment is supplied by the midgut (superior mesenteric) artery, with corresponding venous and lymphatic drainage.[106] The sympathetic innervation of the midgut and likewise the hindgut originates from T8 to L2 via splanchnic nerves and the autonomic abdominopelvic plexuses. The parasympathetic outflow to the midgut is derived from the 10th cranial nerve (vagus) with preganglionic cell bodies in the brain stem.

The distal colon (distal third of the transverse colon), the rectum, and the anal canal above the dentate line are all derived from the hindgut. Therefore, this segment is supplied by the hindgut (inferior mesenteric) artery with corresponding venous and lymphatic drainage. Its parasympathetic outflow comes from S2, S3, and S4 via splanchnic nerves.

The dentate line marks the fusion between endodermal and ectodermal tubes, where the terminal portion of the hindgut or cloaca fuses with the proctodeum, an ingrowth from the anal pit. The cloaca originates at the portion of the rectum below the pubococcygeal line, whereas the hindgut originates above it. Before the fifth week of development, the intestinal and urogenital tracts terminate in conjunction with the cloaca. At the sixth week, the urorectal septum migrates caudally, and the two tracts are separated. The cloacal part of the anal canal, which has both endodermal and ectodermal elements, forms the anal

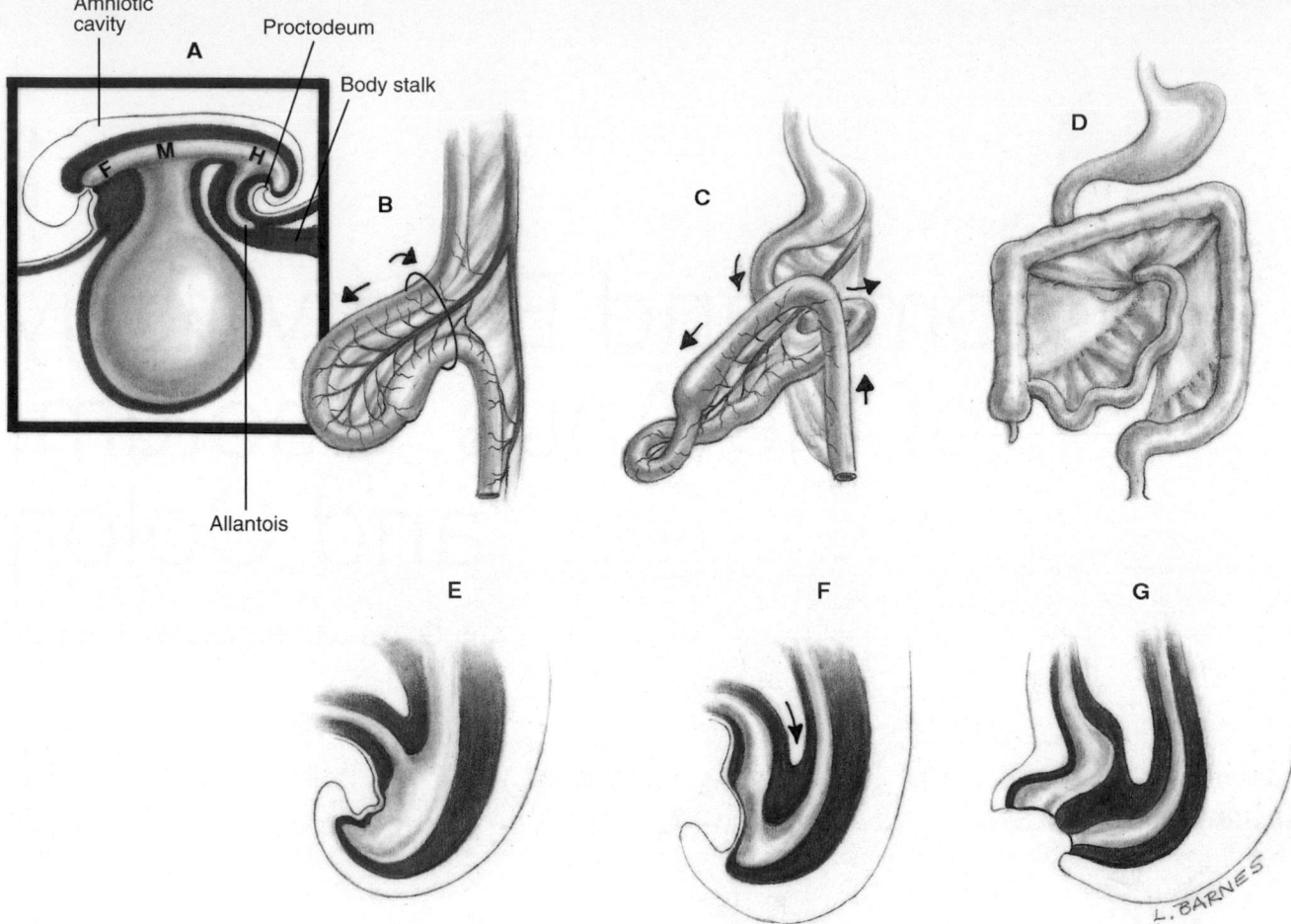

FIGURE 1-1. Embryology of the large intestine. **A:** At the third week of development, the primitive tube can be divided into three regions: the foregut in the head fold, the hindgut with its ventral allantoic outgrowth in the smaller tail fold, and the midgut between these two portions. Stages of development of the midgut are shown. **B:** Physiologic herniation. **C:** Return to the abdomen. **D:** Fixation. **E:** At the sixth week, the urogenital septum migrates caudally and separates the intestinal and urogenital tracts **(F, G).**

transitional zone after breakdown of the anal membrane.[106] During the 10th week, the anal tubercles, a pair of ectodermal swellings around the proctodeal pit, fuse dorsally to form a horseshoe-shaped structure and anteriorly to create the perineal body. The cloacal sphincter is separated by the perineal body into urogenital and anal portions (external anal sphincter [EAS]). The internal anal sphincter (IAS) is formed later (6th to 12th week) from enlarging fibers of the circular layer of the rectum.[66,87] The sphincters apparently migrate during their development; the external sphincter grows cephalad, and the internal sphincter moves caudally. Concomitantly, the longitudinal muscle descends into the intersphincteric plane.[66,127]

▶ ANATOMY OF THE COLON

The colon, so named from the Greek *koluein* ("to retard"), is a capacious tube described in humans to be somewhere between the short, straight type with a rudimentary cecum, such as that of the carnivores, and a long, sacculated colon with a capacious cecum, such as that of the herbivores. The colon roughly surrounds the loops of small intestine as an arch. Its length in the adult is variable, averaging approximately 150 cm, about one-fourth the length of the small intestine. Its diameter, which can be substantially augmented by distension, gradually decreases from 7.5 cm at the cecum to 2.5 cm at the sigmoid.

Anatomic differences between the small and large intestines include position; caliber; degree of fixation; and, in the colon, the presence of three distinct characteristics: the taeniae coli, the haustra, and the appendices epiploicae. The three taeniae coli, anterior (taenia libera), posteromedial (taenia mesocolica), and posterolateral (taenia omentalis), represent bands of the outer longitudinal coat of muscle that traverse the colon from the base of the appendix to the rectosigmoid junction where they merge. The muscular longitudinal layer is actually a complete coat around the colon, although it is considerably thicker at the taeniae.[35] The haustra or haustral sacculations are outpouchings of bowel wall between the taeniae; they are caused by the relative shortness of the taeniae, about one-sixth shorter than the length of bowel wall.[83] The haustra are separated by the plicae semilunares or crescentic folds of the bowel wall, which give the colon its characteristic radiographic appearance when filled with air or barium. The appendices epiploicae are small appendages of fat that protrude from the serosal aspect of the colon (Figure 1-2).

Cecum

The cecum is the segment of the large bowel that projects downward as a blind pouch (Latin *caecus*, "blind") below the entrance of the ileum. It is a sacculated organ of 6 to 8 cm in both length and breadth, usually situated in the right iliac fossa. The cecum is almost entirely, or at least in its lower

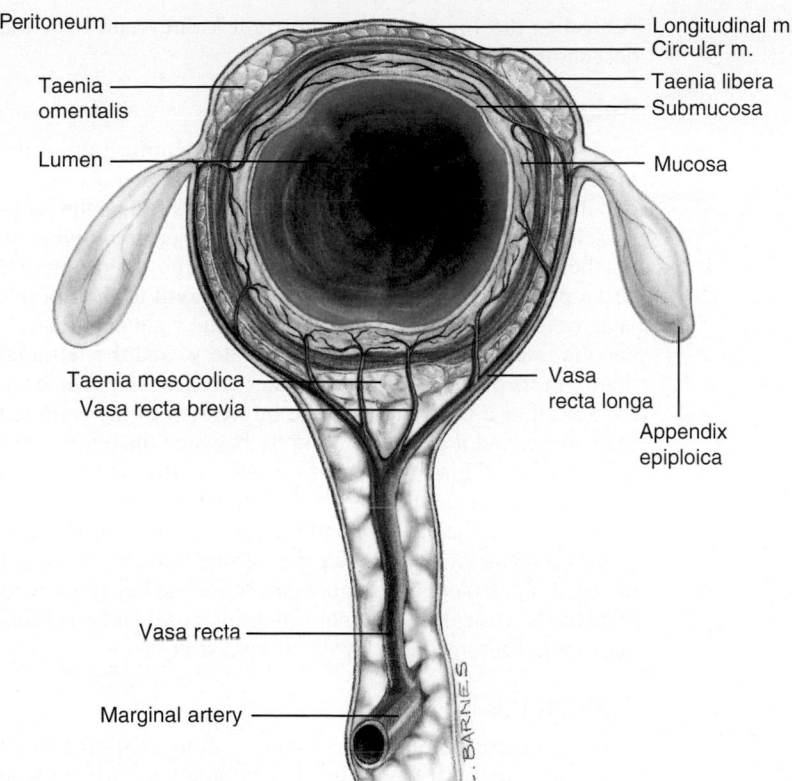

Peritoneum

Taenia
omentalis

Lumen

Taenia mesocolica
Vasa recta brevia

Vasa recta

Marginal artery

Longitudinal m.
Circular m.
Taenia libera
Submucosa

Mucosa

Vasa
recta longa

Appendix
epiploica

FIGURE 1-2. Cross section of the colon and mesocolon demonstrates the arrangement of the vasa recta and their branches.

half, invested with peritoneum. However, its mobility is usually limited by a small mesocecum. In approximately 5% of individuals, the peritoneal covering is absent posteriorly; it then rests directly on the iliacus and psoas major muscles.[41] Alternatively, an abnormally mobile cecum-ascending colon, resulting from an anomaly of fixation, can be found in 10% to 22% of individuals.[98] In this case, a long mesentery is present, and the cecum may assume varied positions. This lack of fixation may predispose to the development of volvulus (see Chapter 28).

The ileum terminates in the posteromedial aspect of the cecum; the angulation between these two structures is maintained by the superior and inferior ileocecal ligaments. These ligaments, along with the mesentery of the appendix, form three pericecal recesses or fossae: superior ileocecal, inferior ileocecal, and retrocecal (Figure 1-3). Viewed from the cecal lumen, the ileocecal junction is represented by a narrow, transversely situated, slitlike opening known as the ileocecal valve or the valve de Bauhin. At either end, the two prominent semilunar lips of the valve fuse and continue as a single frenulum of mucosa. A competent ileocecal valve is related to the critical closed-loop type of colonic obstruction. However, ileocecal competence is not always demonstrated on barium enema studies. Instead of preventing reflux of colonic contents into the ileum, the ileocecal valve regulates ileal emptying. The ileocecal valve seems to relax in response to the entrance of food into the stomach.[48]

As in the gastroesophageal junction, extrasphincteric factors apparently play a role in the prevention of reflux from the colon to the ileum. The ileocecal angulation has been emphasized by Kumar and Phillips.[61] They filled the ascending colon with saline solution in a retrograde fashion and found that the ileocecal junction was competent to pressures up to 80 mm Hg in 12 of 14 human autopsy specimens. In this group, removal of mucosa at the ileocecal junction or a strip of circular muscle did not impair

competence to pressures above 40 mm Hg, but division of the superior and inferior ileocecal ligaments rendered the junction incompetent in all specimens. Furthermore, surgical reconstruction of the ileocecal angle restored competence in four of them.

Appendix

The vermiform appendix is an elongated diverticulum that arises from the posteromedial aspect of the cecum about 3 cm below the ileocecal junction. Its length varies from 2 to 20 cm

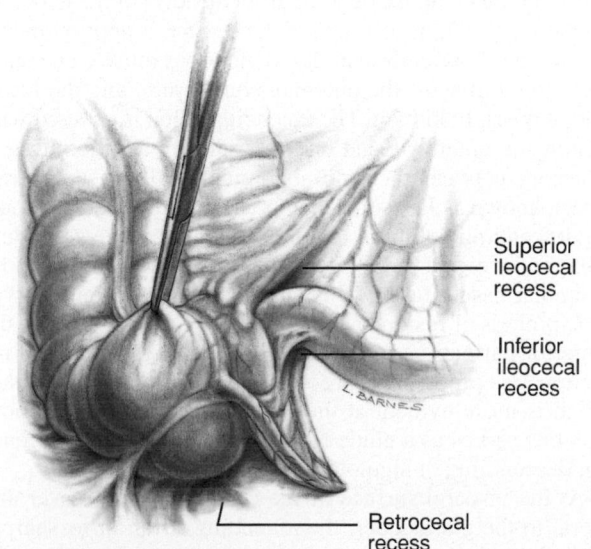

Superior
ileocecal
recess

Inferior
ileocecal
recess

Retrocecal
recess

FIGURE 1-3. Ileocecal region. The superior ileorectal, inferior ileocecal, and rectocecal recesses are shown.

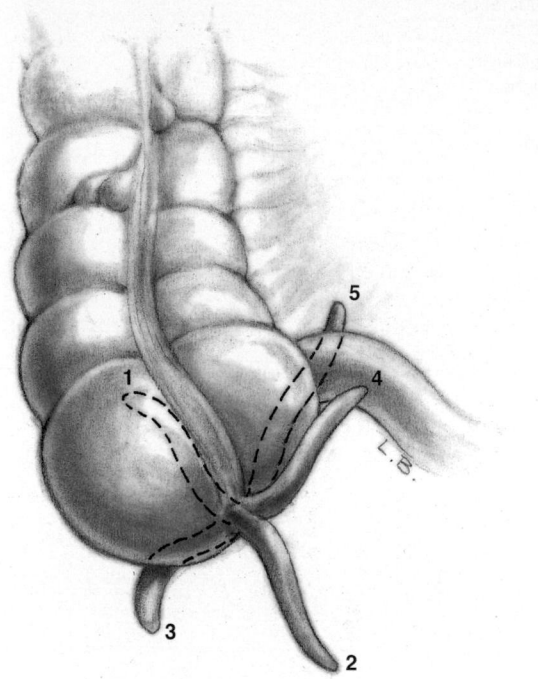

FIGURE 1-4. Vermiform appendix. The five most common variations in its position are shown in order of frequency.

ventral to the lower part of the right kidney and over the descending duodenum.

Relationship to Ureters

In resections of the right and left colon, identification of the ureters is usually necessary to avoid injury to their abdominal or pelvic portions.[74] On both sides, the ureters rest on the psoas muscle in their inferomedial course; they are crossed obliquely by the spermatic vessels anteriorly and the genitofemoral nerve posteriorly. The right ureter lies lateral to the inferior vena cava and is crossed anteriorly by the right colic and ileocolic arteries, the root of the mesentery, and the terminal ileum. In its pelvic portion, the ureter crosses the pelvic brim in front of or a little lateral to the bifurcation of the common iliac artery, and it descends abruptly between the peritoneum and the internal iliac artery. Before entering the bladder in the male, the vas deferens crosses lateromedially on its superior aspect. In the female, as the ureter traverses the posterior layer of the broad ligament and the parametrium close to the side of the neck of the uterus and upper part of the vagina, it is enveloped by the vesical and vaginal venous plexuses and is crossed above and lateromedially by the uterine artery.

Transverse Colon

The transverse colon is the longest segment of the large bowel (45 cm long). It crosses the abdomen, usually with an inferior curve immediately caudad to the greater curvature of the stomach. The transverse colon is relatively fixed at each flexure. In between, it is completely invested with peritoneum and suspended by a transverse mesocolon having an average width of 10 to 15 cm and providing variable mobility; the nadir of the transverse colon may reach the hypogastrium. The greater omentum is fused on the anterosuperior aspect of the transverse colon. Therefore, an intercoloepiploic dissection is necessary to mobilize this portion of the colon or to enter the lesser sac of the peritoneum. The left colic (splenic) flexure is situated beneath the lower angle of the spleen and firmly attached to the diaphragm by the phrenocolic ligament, which also forms a shelf to support the spleen (see Figure 23-49). Because of the risk for hemorrhage, mobilization of the splenic flexure should be approached with great care, preceded by dissection upward along the descending colon and medially to laterally along the transverse colon toward the splenic flexure (see Chapter 23). This flexure, when compared with the hepatic flexure, is more acute, higher, and more deeply situated.

Descending Colon

This segment of the large intestine courses downward from the splenic flexure to the brim of the true pelvis, a distance of approximately 25 cm. The segment of descending colon between the iliac crest and the brim of the true pelvis is also known as the iliac colon.[41] Like the ascending colon, the descending colon is covered by peritoneum only on its anterior and lateral aspects. Posteriorly, it rests directly against the left kidney and the quadratus lumborum and transversus abdominis muscles. However, the descending colon is narrower and more dorsally situated than the ascending colon.

Sigmoid Colon

The sigmoid colon, extending from the lower end of the descending colon at the pelvic brim to the proximal limit

(mean, 8 to 10 cm), and it is approximately 5 mm in diameter. The confluence of the three taeniae is a useful guide in locating the base of the appendix. The appendix, because of its great mobility, may occupy a variety of positions, possibly at different times in the same individual: retrocecal (65%), pelvic (31%), subcecal (2.3%), preileal (1.0%), and retroileal (0.4%) (Figure 1-4).[116] Some authors have found, however, that in 85% to 95% it lies posteromedial on the cecum toward the ileum.[106] The mesoappendix, a triangular fold attached to the posterior leaf of the mesentery of the terminal ileum, usually contains the appendicular vessels close to its free edge.

Ascending Colon

The ascending colon, extending from the level of the ileocecal junction to the right colic or hepatic flexure, is approximately 15 cm long. It ascends laterally to the psoas muscle and anteriorly to the iliacus, the quadratus lumborum, and the lower pole of the right kidney. The ascending colon is covered with peritoneum anteriorly and on both sides. In addition, fragile adhesions between the right abdominal wall and its anterior aspect, known as Jackson's membrane, may be present.[86] Like the descending colon on its posterior surface, the ascending colon is devoid of peritoneum, which is instead replaced by an areolar tissue (fascia of Toldt), resulting from an embryologic process of fusion or coalescence of the mesentery to the posterior parietal peritoneum.[106] In the lateral peritoneal reflection, this process is represented by the white line of Toldt, which is more evident at the descending sigmoid junction. This line serves as a guide for the surgeon when the ascending, descending, or sigmoid colon is mobilized.

At the visceral surface of the right lobe of the liver and lateral to the gallbladder, the ascending colon turns sharply medially and slightly caudad and ventrally to form the right colic (hepatic) flexure (see Figure 22-39). This flexure is supported by the nephrocolic ligament and lies immediately of the rectum, varies dramatically in length (15 to 50 cm; mean, 38 cm) and configuration. More commonly, the sigmoid colon is a mobile, ω-shaped loop completely invested by peritoneum. The mesosigmoid is attached to the pelvic walls in an inverted V shape, resting in a recess known as the intersigmoid fossa. The left ureter lies immediately underneath this fossa and is crossed on its anterior surface by the spermatic, left colic, and sigmoid vessels.

Rectosigmoid Junction

Both the anatomy and function of the rectosigmoid junction have been matters of substantial controversy. O'Beirne postulated that because the rectum is usually emptied and contracted, the sigmoid plays a role in continence as the fecal reservoir.[88] Subsequently, a thickening of the circular muscular layer between the rectum and sigmoid was described and diversely termed the sphincter ani tertius,[51] rectosigmoid sphincter,[73] and pylorus sigmoidorectalis,[16] and it has probably been mistaken for one of the transverse folds of the rectum.[53,91] Balli considered the rectosigmoid junction to be one of the functional sphincters of the colon.[5] The rectosigmoid junction has been considered, at least externally, an indistinct zone, a region that to some surgeons comprises the last 5 to 8 cm of sigmoid and the uppermost 5 cm of the rectum.[31,41] However, surgeons as well as anatomists have divergent opinions. Others have considered it a clearly defined segment because it is the narrowest portion of the large intestine; in fact, it is usually characterized endoscopically as a narrow and sharply angulated segment.[14,105] Stoss, in a study of 39 human cadavers, found the rectosigmoid junction situated 6 to 7 cm below the sacral promontory.[110] Macroscopically, it has been identified as the point where the taenia libera and the taenia omentalis fuse to form a single anterior taenia and where both haustra and mesocolon terminate. With microdissection, this segment is characterized by conspicuous strands of longitudinal muscle fibers that are more prominent than in the sigmoid and less so than in the rectum. Additionally, curved interconnecting fibers between the longitudinal and circular muscle layers have been noted, resulting in a delicate syncytium of smooth muscle that allows synergistic interplay between the two layers. Stoss concluded, based on the anatomic definition of a sphincter as "a band of thickened circular muscle that closes the lumen by contraction and of a longitudinal muscle that dilates it," that the rectosigmoid cannot be considered as such.[67,110] Still, this segment may be regarded as a functional sphincter because mechanisms of active dilation and passive "kinking" occlusion do exist.[108]

Rectum

The rectum is believed to be 12 to 15 cm in length, but both the proximal and distal limits are debatable (Figure 1-5).[127] For example, the rectosigmoid junction is considered to be

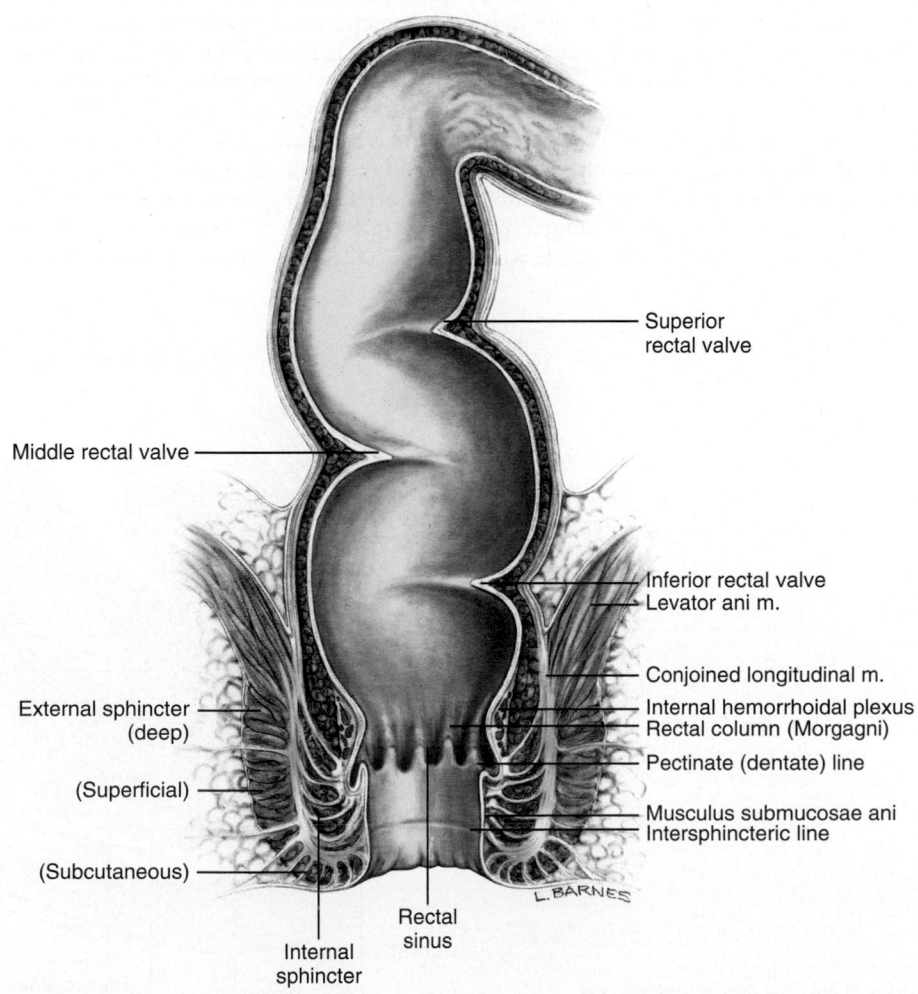

Superior
rectal valve

Middle rectal valve

Inferior rectal valve
Levator ani m.

Conjoined longitudinal m.
Internal hemorrhoidal plexus
Rectal column (Morgagni)
Pectinate (dentate) line

External sphincter
(deep)

(Superficial)

Musculus submucosae ani
Intersphincteric line

(Subcutaneous)

L. BARNES

Internal
sphincter

Rectal
sinus

FIGURE 1-5. Anorectal anatomy illustrating curves and valves.

JOHN HOUSTON (1802–1845)

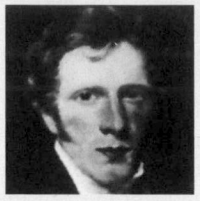

Born in the north of Ireland, Houston was adopted by a physician uncle. He attached himself to one of the first native Dublin anatomists and became a curator of the museum of the Royal College of Surgeons in Ireland in 1824. In 1826, he received his medical degree from Edinburgh University. On the establishment of the City of Dublin Hospital in 1832, Houston became one of its surgeons. He was regarded as an acute observer of disease and an excellent clinical surgeon. In 1830, he published the report in which he described the valves that bear his name. He died while lecturing, presumably of complications of an intracranial hemorrhage. (Houston J. Observations of the mucous membrane of the rectum. *Dublin Hosp Rep Communications Med Surg.* 1830;5:158–165.)

at the level of the third sacral vertebra by anatomists but at the coalescence of taeniae coli by surgeons. Likewise, the distal limit is regarded to be the muscular anorectal ring by surgeons and the dentate line by anatomists. The rectum occupies the sacral concavity and ends 2 to 3 cm anteroinferiorly from the tip of the coccyx. At this point, it angulates backward sharply to pass through the levators and becomes the anal canal. The median sacral vessels and the roots of the sacral nerve plexus lie posterior to the rectum. Anteriorly, in women, the rectum is closely related to the uterine cervix and posterior vaginal wall; in men, it lies behind the bladder, vas deferens, seminal vesicles, and prostate.

The nonmobilized rectum has three lateral curves: the upper and lower are convex to the right and the middle is convex to the left (Figure 1-5). These curves correspond intraluminally to the folds or valves of Houston.[2,53] The two left-sided folds are usually noted at 7 to 8 cm and at 12 to 13 cm, respectively, and the one on the right is generally at 9 to 11 cm. The middle valve is the most consistent in presence and location (also known as Kohlrausch's plica) and corresponds to the level of the anterior peritoneal reflection. The rectal valves do not contain all the muscle wall layers and do not have a specific function. However, from a clinical point of view, they are an excellent location for performing a rectal biopsy because they are readily accessible with minimal risk for perforation.[86] The valves of Houston must be negotiated during proctosigmoidoscopy. However, they are not present after mobilization of the rectum; this is attributed to the 5-cm length gained following complete surgical dissection.

The rectum is characterized by the absence of taeniae, epiploic appendices, haustra, or a well-defined mesentery. The prefix "meso," in gross anatomy, refers to two layers of peritoneum that suspend an organ. Normally, the rectum is not suspended but entirely extraperitoneal on its posterior aspect and close to the sacral hollow. Consequently, the term mesorectum is anatomically inappropriate.[18,81] An exception, however, is that a peritonealized mesorectum may be noted in patients with procidentia. Nonetheless, the term mesorectum has gained widespread popularity among surgeons to address the perirectal adipose tissue, which is thicker posteriorly, containing terminal branches of the inferior mesenteric artery, lymph nodes, and enclosed by the fascia propria (Figure 1-6).[17,52,59] The mesorectum may be a metastatic site for rectal cancer and is removed during surgery for rectal

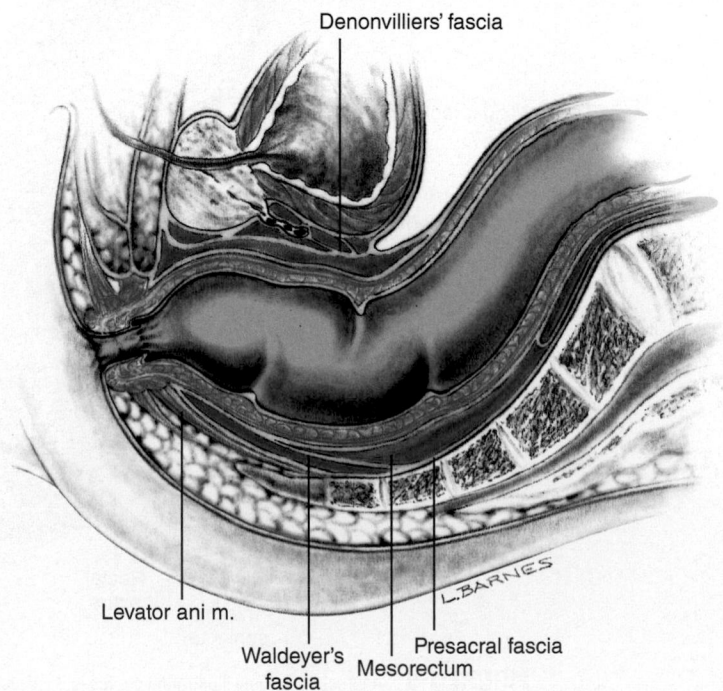

FIGURE 1-6. Lateral view of the male rectum illustrating the mesorectum and its relationship with other pelvic structures.

cancer (see Chapter 24). Its removal is undertaken without clinical sequelae because no functionally significant nerves pass through it.[52] Although it is quite variable, in classical descriptions, the upper third of the rectum is anteriorly and laterally invested by peritoneum; the middle third is covered by peritoneum on its anterior aspect only. Finally, the lower third of the rectum is entirely extraperitoneal because the anterior peritoneal reflection occurs at 9.0 to 7.0 cm from the anal verge in men and at 7.5 to 5.0 cm from the anal verge in women.

The rectum has a wide, easily distensible lumen. The rectal mucosa is smooth, pink, and transparent, which allows visualization of small and large submucosal vessels. This characteristic vascular pattern disappears in inflammatory conditions and in melanosis coli.

Fascial Relationship of the Rectum

The walls and floor of the pelvis are lined by the parietal *endopelvic fascia*, which continues on the internal organs as a visceral pelvic fascia. The fascia propria of the rectum is therefore an extension of the pelvic fascia, enclosing the rectum, fat, nerves, and the blood and lymphatic vessels. It is present mainly in the lateral and posterior extraperitoneal portion of the rectum. Distal condensations of this fascia form the lateral ligaments or lateral stalks of the rectum. These are described by Goligher as a roughly triangular structure with a base on the lateral pelvic wall and an apex attached to the lateral aspect of the rectum.[41] As pointed out by Church and colleagues, these ligaments have been the subject of anatomic confusion and misconception.[20]

One such misconception is that they are composed essentially of connective tissue and nerves, and that the middle rectal artery traverses the lateral stalks of the rectum. Minor branches of the middle rectal artery course through the lateral stalks in approximately 25% of cases.[13,126] Consequently, division of the lateral stalks during rectal mobilization is associated with a 25% risk for bleeding. Although the lateral stalks do not contain important structures, the middle rectal artery and the pelvic plexus are both closely related, coursing at different angles beneath them in various patients.[85] One theoretical concern in ligation of the stalks is leaving behind lateral mesorectal tissue, which may limit adequate lateral or mesorectal margins during cancer surgery (Figure 1-7).[17,52,97]

The *presacral fascia* is a thickened part of the parietal endopelvic fascia that covers the concavity of the sacrum and coccyx, nerves, the middle sacral artery, and presacral veins (Figure 1-8). Operative dissection deep to the presacral fascia may cause troublesome bleeding from the underlying presacral veins. The incidence of such hemorrhage has been cited to be as high as 4.6% to 7.0% of resections for rectal neoplasms.[57,118,128] These veins are avalvular and communicate via the basivertebral veins with the internal vertebral venous system (Figure 1-8). With the patient in the lithotomy position, this system can attain hydrostatic pressures of 17 to 23 cm H_2O, two to three times the normal pressure of the inferior vena cava.[118] The adventitia of the basivertebral veins adheres firmly to the sacral periosteum at the level of the ostia of the sacral foramina (mainly at the level of S3–4).[118] Despite its venous nature, presacral

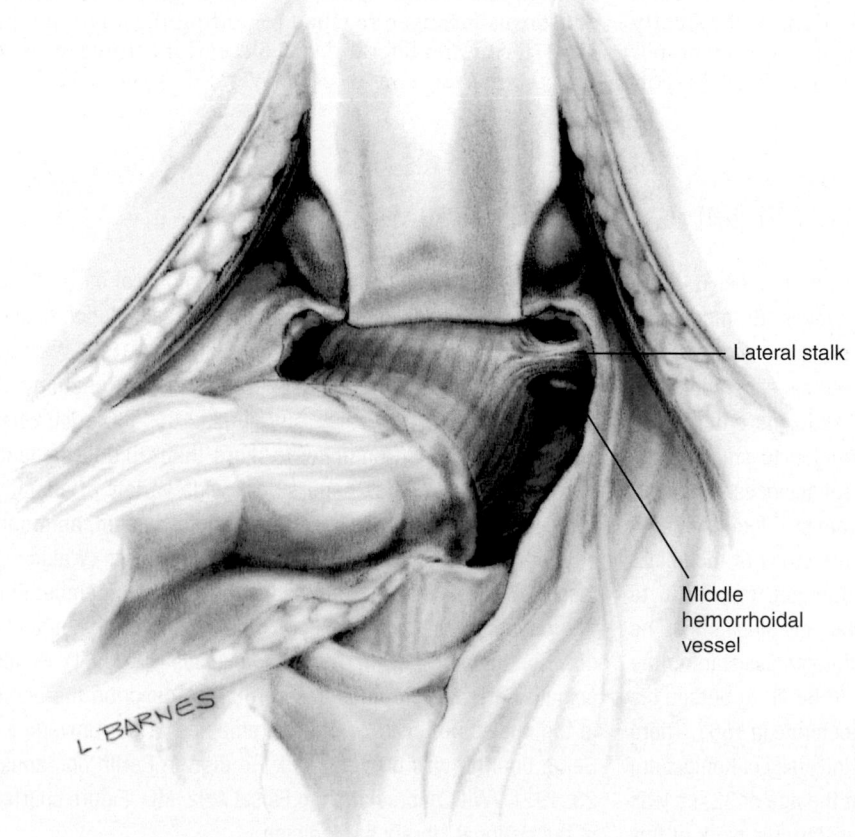

Lateral stalk

Middle hemorrhoidal vessel

L. BARNES

FIGURE 1-7. The right lateral stalk with associated middle hemorrhoidal artery is seen.

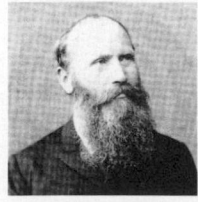

FIGURE 1-8. Sagittal section of the pelvis showing the fascial relationships of the rectum and the presacral and vertebral venous system.

hemorrhage can be life threatening. This is a consequence of the high hydrostatic pressure and the difficulty in securing control because of retraction of the vascular stump into the sacral foramen.

The *rectosacral fascia* is an anteroinferiorly directed thick fascial reflection from the presacral fascia at the S4 level to the fascia propria of the rectum just above the anorectal ring.[23] The rectosacral fascia, an important landmark during posterior rectal dissection, is classically known as the fascia of Waldeyer, but this is a misnomer because Wilhelm Waldeyer first described all of the pel-vic fascia, not particularly emphasizing the rectosacral fascia.[20,23] Anteriorly, the extraperitoneal rectum is separated from the prostate and seminal vesicles or vagina by a tough fascial investment, the visceral pelvic fascia of Denonvilliers.[114] Therefore, three structures lie between the anterior rectal wall and the seminal vesicles and prostate: the anterior mesorectum, the fascia propria of the rectum, and Denonvilliers' fascia (Figure 1-6). A general consensus has been reached regarding the anatomic plane of posterior and lateral rectal dissection. However, anteriorly the matter is more controversial. Most would accept

HEINRICH WILHELM GOTTFRIED VON WALDEYER-HARTZ (1836–1921)

Waldeyer was born on October 6, 1836 in Helen an der Weser, Germany, the son of an estate manager and a school teacher. He received his early education at Paderborn. In 1856, he entered the University of Göttingen to study mathematics and natural sciences. However, through his acquaintance with the anatomist Friedrich Henle, whose lectures he attended, he began the study of medicine. Waldeyer attended the University of Göttingen from 1856 to 1859. As a Prussian, he could not complete his studies, and he transferred to Greifswald, where he became an assistant in the Anatomical Institute. He then moved on to Berlin to pursue his great interest in anatomy, obtaining his doctorate in 1861. There followed a series of appointments to the University of Königsberg and the University of Breslau. In 1868, at the age of 32, he was appointed to the chair of pathology at Breslau. His work at this time was chiefly concentrated on the diagnosis of early cancer. In 1887, he was one of the German doctors called upon to diagnose Emperor Frederick III's vocal cord tumor. In 1872, Waldeyer went to the University of Strasbourg as chair of anatomy. He remained there for 11 years, returning in 1883 to Berlin, where he eventually taught anatomy to more than 20,000 students. He published numerous papers on a wide variety of anatomic subjects, including studies of the urogenital system, anthropology, and topographical observations of the pelvis (Waldeyer's fascia). Today, Wilhelm von Waldeyer-Hartz is remembered as the founder of the neuron theory, coining the term "neuron" to describe the cellular unit of the nervous system (1891). He also coined the term "chromosome" (1888) to describe the bodies in the nucleus of cells. Waldeyer remained at the University of Berlin until he was 80 years old. He died in Berlin on January 23, 1921. (With appreciation to Faisal Aziz, MD. Figure courtesy of the National Library of Medicine.)

CHARLES-PIERRE DENONVILLIERS (1808–1872)

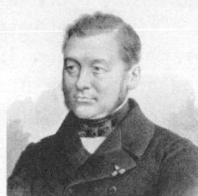

Son of a landlord, Denonvilliers was born in Paris on February 4, 1808. He studied medicine at the Paris Faculty, from which he graduated in 1835. His first post was that of surgeon to the Bureau Central (1840). In 1842, he became chief of the School of Practical Anatomy of the Hôtel-Dieu, and in 1856 he achieved the position as professor of surgery at the same institution. Denonvilliers' interests resided more in anatomy than in surgery. Through the years, he made numerous and varied contributions to the field, including a description of the fascia for which he achieved eponymous immortality. In 1836, Denonvilliers reported to the Société Anatomique concerning an "aponeurosis" as follows: "Behind the prostate and between the seminal vesicles and the rectum, there is a distinct membranous layer, which I call prostatoperitoneal." In 1858, Denonvilliers was awarded the important position of inspector general of Public Instruction for Medicine. Through this role, he has been credited with modernizing the French medical curriculum by the development of new concepts in the teaching of physiology, pathology, and surgery. His extensive work in the field of descriptive and surgical anatomy led to the publication of numerous articles and textbooks as well as to the elaboration of innovative surgical techniques, particularly in the field of reconstructive plastic surgery. His professional activity ceased in 1864 with the death of his prematurely born son, a tragedy from which he never fully recovered. Thought to be a great loss to the field of medical science by his contemporaries, Denonvilliers died of a stroke on July 5, 1872. (With appreciation to Keith P. Meslin, MD.)

the appropriateness of dissection in the plane between Denonvilliers' fascia and the fascia propria. The use of the terms close rectal, mesorectal, and extramesorectal have been suggested to describe the anterior planes.[69] The close rectal plane, also known as the perimuscular plane, lies immediately on the rectal musculature, inside the fascia propria of the rectum. However, it is more difficult to navigate, bloodier than the mesorectal plane, and consequently is not considered a true anatomic plane. The mesorectal plane represents the continuation of the same plane of posterior and lateral dissection of the rectum. It is the appropriate anterior plane for most rectal cancers, a natural anatomic plane that is familiar to colorectal surgeons. Finally, the extramesorectal plane involves resection of Denonvilliers' fascia, with exposure of the prostate and seminal vesicles. This plane is associated with a high risk of both parasympathetic and sympathetic injury to the periprostatic plexus. In addition, dissection in this plane generally predisposes to an increased risk of intraoperative hemorrhage.

Anal Canal

Although representing a relatively small segment of the digestive tract, the anal canal is anatomically unique, with a complex physiology that accounts for both its vital role in continence and its susceptibility to a variety of diseases. In the literature, two definitions are found to describe the anal canal. The "surgical" or "functional" anal canal extends for approximately 4 cm from the anal verge to the anorectal ring. This definition correlates with both digital and sonographic assessment, but it does not correspond to either the embryologic or histologic architecture of the anal canal. The "anatomic" or "embryologic" anal canal is shorter (2 cm), extending from the anal verge to the dentate line (see Figure 11-2). The latter is the level that corresponds to the proctodeal membrane.[87,127]

The anus or anal orifice is an anteroposterior cutaneous slit that, along with the anal canal, remains virtually closed at rest. This is the result of tonic circumferential contraction of both the sphincters and the anal cushions. Posteriorly, the anal canal is related to the coccyx and anteriorly to the urethra (in the male) and to the perineal body and the lowest part of the posterior vaginal wall (in the female). Laterally, the ischiorectal fossa is situated on either side. The fossa contains fat and the inferior rectal vessels and nerves, which cross it to enter the wall of the anal canal.

Epithelium

The lining of the anal canal consists of an upper mucosal and a lower cutaneous segment. The dentate (pectinate) line describes the "saw-toothed" junction of the ectoderm and the endoderm. It therefore represents an important landmark between two distinct origins of venous and lymphatic drainage, nerve supply, and epithelial lining.[125] Above the dentate line, the intestine is innervated by the sympathetic and parasympathetic systems, with venous, arterial, and lymphatic drainage to and from the hypogastric vessels. Distal to the dentate line, the anal canal is innervated by the somatic nervous system, with blood supply and drainage from the inferior hemorrhoidal system. These differences are important when the classification and treatment of hemorrhoids are considered.

The pectinate or dentate line corresponds to a line of anal valves that represent remnants of the proctodeal membrane. Above each valve, there is a little pocket known as an anal sinus or crypt. These crypts are connected to a variable number of glands, with an average of six (range, 3 to 12 crypts per patient [see Figures 25-1 and 25-2]).[43,68] The anal glands are more concentrated in the posterior quadrants. More than one gland may open into the same crypt, whereas half the crypts have no communication. The anal gland ducts enter the submucosa in an outward and downward route; two-thirds enter the IAS, and half of them terminate in the intersphincteric plane (see Figures 25-3 and 13-1).[68] The anal glands were first described by Chiari in 1878, but it was not until 1961 that Parks addressed their role in the pathogenesis of fistulous abscess[19,93] (see Chapters 13 and 14). Obstruction of these ducts, presumably by accumulation of foreign material in the crypts, may lead to abscesses and fistula.[93]

Cephalad to the dentate line, 8 to 14 longitudinal folds, known as the rectal columns (columns of Morgagni), have their bases connected in pairs to each valve at the dentate line (see Figure 11-2). At the lower end of the columns are the anal papillae. The mucosa in the area of the columns consists of several layers of cuboidal cells. The lining exhibits a deep purple color because of the underlying internal hemorrhoidal plexus. The 0.5- to 1.0-cm strip of mucosa above the dentate line is known as the anal transitional or cloacogenic zone and represents the site and source of certain anal tumors (see Chapter 25). Cephalad to this area, the epithelium changes to a single layer of columnar cells, macroscopically acquiring the characteristic pink color of the rectal mucosa.

The cutaneous part of the anal canal consists of modified squamous epithelium—thin, smooth, pale, stretched, and devoid of hair and glands. The terms *pecten* and *pecten band* have been used to define this segment.[1] However, as pointed out by Goligher, the round band of fibrous tissue called pecten band, which is divided in the case of anal fissure (pectenotomy), probably represents a spastic IAS.[41,42] The anal verge (anocutaneous line of Hilton; see Biography, Chapter 12) marks the lowermost edge of the anal canal and is sometimes the level of reference for measurements taken during colonoscopy or surgery.[30,32] Others favor the dentate line as a landmark because it is more precise.[14] The difference between the two can be as great as 1 to 2 cm. Distal to the anal verge, the lining becomes thicker and pigmented and is arranged in radiating folds around the anus. The epithelium then acquires hair follicles, glands (including apocrine glands), and other features of normal skin. For this reason, perianal hidradenitis suppurativa, inflammation of the apocrine glands, may be excised with preservation of the anal canal (see Chapter 9).

Anal Canal and Pelvic Floor Musculature

The muscles within the pelvis can be divided into three categories: the anal sphincter complex, the pelvic floor muscles, and the muscles that line the sidewalls of the osseous pelvis.[59] This

HANS CHIARI (1851–1916)

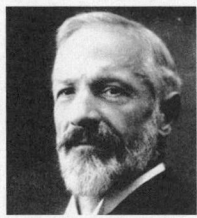

Hans Chiari was born in Vienna on September 4, 1851, ultimately studying medicine in that city. From 1874 to 1875, he served as assistant to the famous pathologist, Karl Freiherr von Rokitansky (1804–1878). His other influential mentor was Richard Ladislaus Heschl (1824–1881), for whom he served as assistant from 1876 until 1879. Chiari was appointed that year professor in pathologic anatomy at the German University of Prague and the following year became superintendent of the pathologic–anatomic museum. In 1906, he was appointed director of pathologic anatomy in Strasbourg, where he remained until his death in 1916. During the years 1876 to 1916, Chiari published more than 175 papers. The majority of his work concerned systematic postmortem examinations. He was in constant search of new and interesting material because of his academic interests but also for the museum. Out of his many investigations, his work on glands, neural deformities, large vessels, and the heart are considered of special importance. He first described the concept of autodigestion of the pancreas gland. In 1891, he reported the first case of herniation of the cerebellar hemispheres and the medulla oblongata into the spinal canal, now named Arnold–Chiari syndrome. He described additional cases and identified the distinction between deformities of the brain stem and the cerebellum. In 1898, he reported on liver infarction due to thrombosis of the hepatic veins, a condition now known by the eponym Budd–Chiari syndrome. Other work concerned atherosclerotic lesions of the carotid arteries wherein he suggested an association with cerebral emboli. (With appreciation to Udo Rudloff, MD.)

GIOVANNI BATTISTA MORGAGNI (1682–1771)

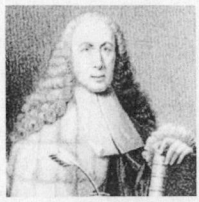

Giovanni Battista Morgagni was born in Bologna, Italy and studied medicine at the University of Bologna, graduating with degrees in philosophy and medicine at the age of 19. In 1706, he succeeded Valsalva in his position as anatomic demonstrator, and in 1715 he was appointed to the first chair of anatomy at the University of Padua, a tenure that he held with distinction for the rest of his life. His work, *Adversaria Anatomica* (1706–1719), is a series of researches into anatomy, an effort that secured his reputation. Morgagni's studies produced new information about the larynx, trachea, and glottal regions, the male urethra, and the female genitalia. He also described the fine vertical folds in the mucous membrane of the upper half of the rectum, still known as the columns of Morgagni. His most important work, *Seats and Causes of Disease Investigated by Means of Anatomy*, was published in 1761. In this work, one of the most fundamentally important works in the history of medicine, he reports in precise detail his findings in 640 autopsy dissections. He was the first to describe cerebral gumma, diseases of heart valves, heart block, Fallot's tetralogy, aortic coarctation, and pneumonia with consolidation. The Royal Society of England elected him a fellow in 1724, the Academy of Sciences of Paris made him a member in 1731, the Imperial Academy of St. Petersburg in 1735, and the Academy of Berlin in 1754. (Courtesy of University of Virginia Health Sciences Library and with appreciation to Yossef Yonatan Nasseri, MD.)

last category forms the external boundary of the pelvis and includes the obturator internus and piriform muscles. These muscles, compared with the other two groups, lack clinical relevance to anorectal diseases; however, they do provide open communication to allow pelvic infection to reach extrapelvic spaces. For example, infection from the deep postanal space originating from the posterior midline glands can track along the obturator internus fascia and reach the ischiorectal fossa.

The anal sphincter and pelvic floor muscles, based on phylogenetic studies, are derived from two embryonic cloaca groups, sphincter and lateral compressor, respectively.[120] The sphincteric group is present in almost all animals. In mammals, this group is divided into ventral (urogenital) and dorsal (anal) components.[92] In primates, the latter forms the EAS. The lateral compressor or pelvicaudal group connects the rudimentary pelvis to the caudal end of the vertebral column. This group is more differentiated and subdivided into lateral and medial compartments only in reptiles and mammals. The homologue of the lateral compartment is the ischiococcygeus, and of the medial pelvicaudal compartment, the pubococcygeus, and iliococcygeus. In addition, most primates possess a variably sized group of muscle fibers close to the inner border of the medial pelvicaudal muscle, which attaches the rectum to the pubis. In humans, the fibers are more distinct and are known as the puborectalis muscle.

Internal Anal Sphincter

The IAS represents the distal (2.5 to 4.0 cm) condensation of the circular muscle layer of the rectum (see Figure 11-2). As a smooth muscle in a state of continuous maximal contraction, the IAS is a natural barrier to the involuntary loss of stool and gas.[95] This is a consequence of both intrinsic myogenic and extrinsic autonomic neurogenic properties. The IAS is responsible for 50% to 85% of the resting tone, the EAS accounts for 25% to 30%, and the remaining 15% is attributed to expansion of the anal cushions.[36,40,65]

The lower rounded edge of the IAS can be felt on physical examination, about 1.2 cm distal to the dentate line. The groove between it and the EAS, the intersphincteric sulcus, can be visualized or easily palpated. The different echogenic patterns of the anal sphincters facilitate their visualization during endosonography (see Figure 7-17). The IAS is a 2- to 3-mm thick circular band exhibiting a uniform hypoechogenicity. The puborectalis and the EAS, despite their mixed linear echogenicity, are both predominantly hyperechogenic, with a mean thickness of 6 mm (range, 5 to 8 mm). Distinction is made by position, shape, and topography.[24,113] Both anal endosonography and endocoil magnetic resonance imaging have been used to detail the anal sphincter complex in living healthy subjects (Figure 1-9).[12,37,82,124] These tests provide a three-dimensional mapping of the anal sphincter; furthermore, they help to identify gender differences in the anatomic arrangement of the EAS as well as to uncover any sphincter disruption or defect during vaginal deliveries.

Conjoined Longitudinal Muscle

Whereas the inner circular layer of the rectum gives rise to the IAS, the outer longitudinal layer, at the level of the anorectal ring, mixes with fibers of the levator ani muscle to form the conjoined longitudinal muscle (CLM [see Figure 11-2]). This muscle descends between the IAS and the EAS, and ultimately some of its fibers (referred to as the

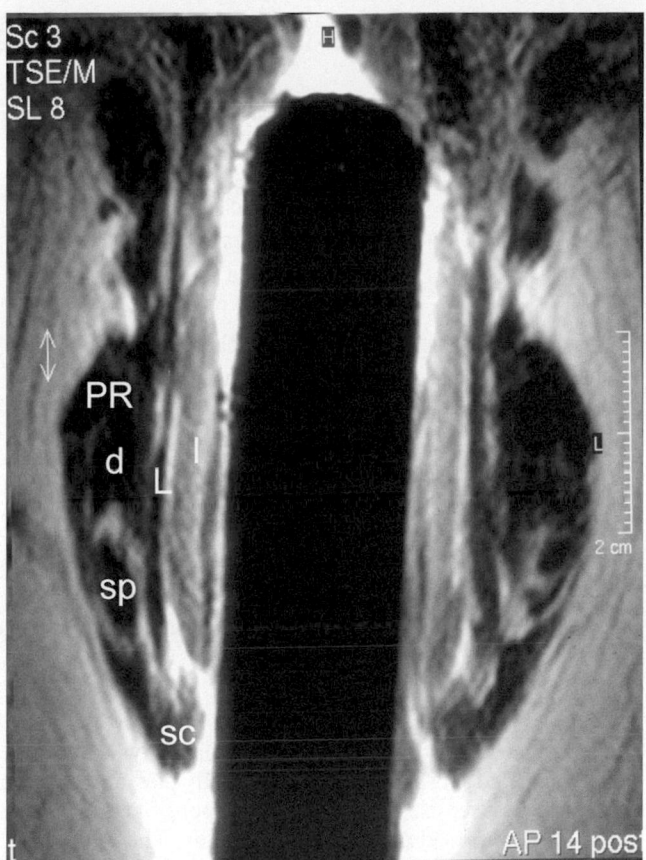

FIGURE 1-9. An endocoil magnetic resonance image of the anal canal in the coronal plane view. *I*, internal anal sphincter (moderate signal); *L*, longitudinal muscle (low signal); *PR*, puborectalis, with *d*, deep part of the external sphincter; *sp*, superficial part; and *sc*, subcutaneous part. All the striated muscle is of low signal. The high signal on either side of the longitudinal muscle indicates a thin layer of fat. (Courtesy of Professor Clive Bartram, clinical director of St. Mark's Hospital, Northwick Park, United Kingdom.)

corrugator cutis ani muscle) traverse the lowermost part of the EAS to insert into the perianal skin.

Lunniss and Phillips, in a comprehensive review of the CLM, explored the controversy and speculation of both the anatomy and physiology of this muscle.[72] Other sources for the striated component of the CLM include the puborectalis and deep EAS,[79] the pubococcygeus and top loop of the EAS,[103] and the lower fibers of the puborectalis.[63] In its descending course, the CLM may give rise to medial extensions that cross the IAS to contribute the smooth muscle of the submucosa (musculus canalis ani, sustentator tunicae mucosae, Treitz muscle, musculus submucosae ani).[99] Others describe outward filamentous extensions of the CLM crossing the whole length of the EAS to enter the fat of the ischiorectal fossa.[22] Possible functions of the CLM include attaching the anorectum to the pelvis and acting as a skeleton that supports and binds the IAS and EAS complex together.[22] Shafik considers only a minimal role for the CLM in the maintenance of continence, and that is specifically to potentiate the action of the base loop in maintaining an anal seal.[103] He ascribes its primary responsibility during defecation as causing shortening and widening of the anal canal as well as eversion of the anal orifice. Shafik has proposed the term, "evertor ani muscle," for the CLM. Haas and Fox consider that the meshwork formed by the CLM may minimize functional deterioration of the sphincters after surgical division and act as a support to

VACLEV TREITZ (1819–1872)

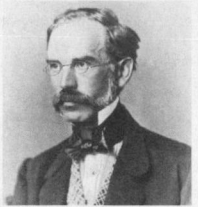

Treitz was born in Hostomice, Bohemia within the present-day Czech Republic. He attended the Piarist College in Benešov and studied medicine at Charles-Ferdinand University in Prague. He pursued postgraduate training in anatomy and pathology at the Pathological Institute of Allgemeines Krankenhaus ("Vienna General Hospital"). After a brief private practice stint in Prague, Treitz served as prosector for the Jagiellonian University in Kraków, Poland. Here he published *On a New Muscle in the Human Duodenum* in which he described what is now called the *ligament of Treitz*. He returned to Charles-Ferdinand University where he would spend the rest of his career lecturing medical students and elucidating new anatomic findings. Notable among these was "hernia retroperitonealis," in which he described an internal hernia occurring at the duodeno-jejunal junction (now known as a *Treitz hernia*) and offered 13 suggestions to prevent strangulation. Along with his close friend and colleague Johannes Purkinjě, Treitz actively championed the cause of Czech nationalism at a time when pro-German sentiment was robust and the European political climate volatile. His insistence on lecturing in Czech, as well as his strong Czech nationalist sentiment, made him a favorite among Czech medical students but placed him at odds with predominantly German-speaking colleagues. These conflicts prompted frequent public attacks on his integrity, which took an increasingly heavy toll on Treitz's physical and emotional health until he succumbed in 1872. He ingested potassium cyanide pills lamenting, "But I will still be pursued." (Reference: Fox RS, Fox CG, Graham WP III. Václav Treitz [1819–1872]: Czechoslovakian pathoanatomist and patriot. *World J Surg.* 1985;9(2):361–366.) (With appreciation to Merrit M. DeBartolo, MD.)

prevent hemorrhoidal and rectal prolapse.[49] Finally, the CLM and its extensions to the intersphincteric plane divide the adjacent tissues into subspaces and may actually play a role in the containment of sepsis.[72] They also are responsible for the septation of thrombosed external hemorrhoids. Therefore, cure of such a thrombus requires excision of this septated region rather than simply an incision between fibers of a single clot.

External Anal Sphincter

The EAS is the elliptical cylinder of striated muscle that envelops the entire length of the inner tube of smooth muscle, but it ends slightly more distal to the terminus of the IAS (see Figure 11-2). The EAS was initially described as encompassing three divisions: subcutaneous, superficial, and deep.[79] However, Goligher and colleagues described the EAS as a simple, continuous sheet that forms, along with the puborectalis and levator ani, one funnel-shaped skeletal muscle.[42] The deepest part of the EAS is intimately related with the puborectalis muscle; they opine that the latter is actually considered a component of both the levator ani and the EAS muscle complexes. Others consider the EAS as being composed of a deep compartment (deep sphincter and puborectalis) and a superficial compartment (subcutaneous and superficial sphincter).[38,86] Oh and Kark noted differences in the arrangement of the EAS between the sexes.[89] In the male, the upper half of the EAS is enveloped anteriorly by the CLM, whereas the lower half is crossed by it. In the female, the entire EAS is encapsulated by a mixture of fibers derived from both longitudinal and IAS muscles. Based on embryologic study, the EAS also seems to be subdivided into two parts, superficial and deep, neither having any connection with the puborectalis.[66] Shafik proposed the concept of a three-U–shaped loop system in which each loop is a separate sphincter with distinct attachments, muscle bundle directions, and innervations; each loop complements the others to help maintain continence (Figure 1-10).[101,104] However, clinical experience has not supported Shafik's three-part schema. The EAS is, in fact, more likely to be one muscle unit, attached by the anococcygeal ligament posteriorly to the coccyx and anteriorly to the perineal body, not divided into layers or laminae.[4] However, there is some degree of anatomic asymmetry of the EAS, which accounts for both radial and longitudinal functional asymmetry observed during anal manometry.[56]

The EAS, along with the pelvic floor muscles, unlike other skeletal muscles that are usually inactive at rest, maintains unconscious resting electrical tone through a reflex arc at the cauda equina level. Histologic studies have shown that the EAS, puborectalis, and levator ani muscles have a predominance of type I fibers, which are a peculiarity of skeletal muscles that produce tonic contractile activity.[112] In response to conditions of threatened incontinence, such as increased intra-abdominal pressure and rectal distension, the EAS and puborectalis reflexively or voluntarily contract further to prevent fecal leakage. Because of muscular fatigue, maximal voluntary contraction of the EAS can be sustained for only 30 to 60 seconds. The automatic continence mechanism is then formed by the resting tone, maintained by the IAS, and magnified by reflex EAS contraction.[58] Garavoglia and coworkers suggest three types of striated muscular function as the mechanism for continence: lateral compression from the pubococcygeus, circumferential closure from the deep EAS, and angulation from the puborectalis.[38]

Levator Ani

Figure 1-11 illustrates the male perineal muscle at three different levels. The levator ani muscle, or pelvic diaphragm, comprises the major component of the pelvic floor (Figure 1-11C). It is a pair of broad, symmetric sheets composed of three striated muscles: iliococcygeus, pubococcygeus, and puborectalis (Figure 1-12). A variable fourth component, the ischiococcygeus or coccygeus, is rudimentary in humans and represented by only a few muscle fibers on the surface of the sacrospinous ligament.[125] Iliococcygeus fibers arise from the ischial spine and posterior part of the obturator fascia and course inferiorly and medially. They insert into the lateral aspects of S3 and S4, the coccyx, and the anococcygeal raphe. The pubococcygeus arises from the posterior aspect of the pubis and the anterior part of the obturator fascia. It runs dorsally alongside the anorectal junction to decussate with fibers of the opposite side at the anococcygeal

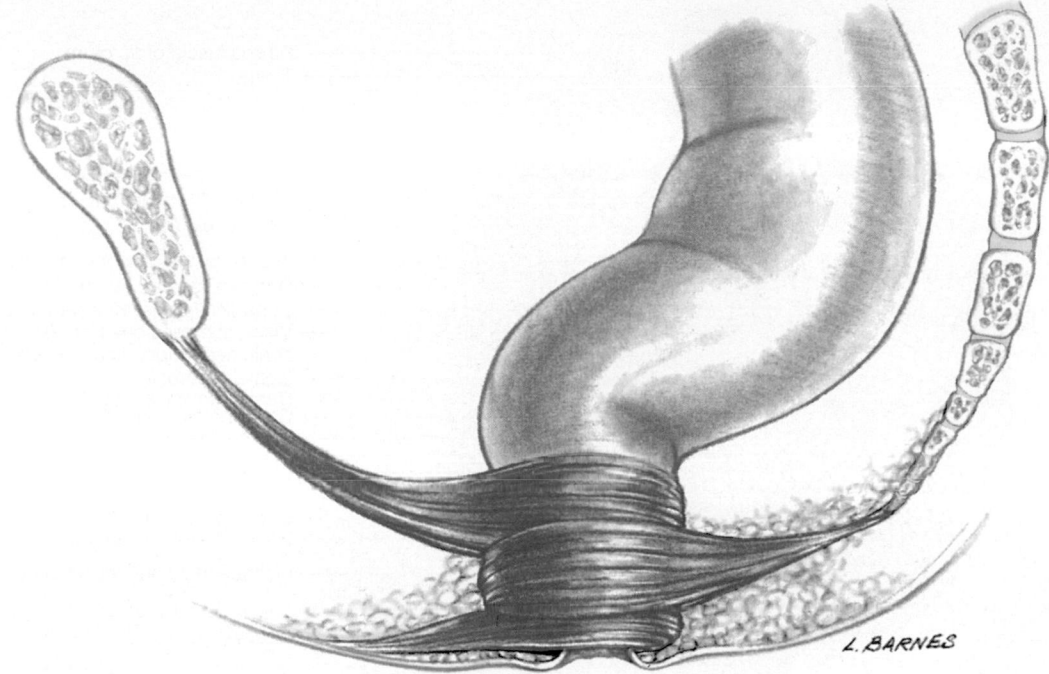

FIGURE 1-10. Triple-loop system of Shafik.[101] The top loop arises and inserts on the pubis and is made up of the deep external sphincter and puborectalis. The middle loop attaches to the coccyx (superficial external sphincter). The lower loop inserts in the anterior perianal skin (subcutaneous external sphincter).

raphe, inserting into the anterior surface of the fourth sacral and first coccygeal segments.

The pelvic floor is "defective" in the midline where the lower rectum, urethra, and either the dorsal vein of the penis in men, or the vagina in women, pass through it. This defect is called the levator hiatus; this consists of an elliptical space situated between the two pubococcygeus muscles.[100] The hiatal ligament, originating from the pelvic fascia, keeps the intrahiatal viscera together and prevents their constric-

tion during contraction of the levator ani. A dilator function has been attributed to the anococcygeal raphe because of its crisscross arrangement.[102]

The puborectalis muscle is a strong, U-shaped loop of striated muscle that slings the anorectal junction to the posterior aspect of the pubis. The puborectalis is the most medial portion of the levator ani muscle. It is situated immediately cephalad to the deep component of the external sphincter. Because the junction between the two muscles

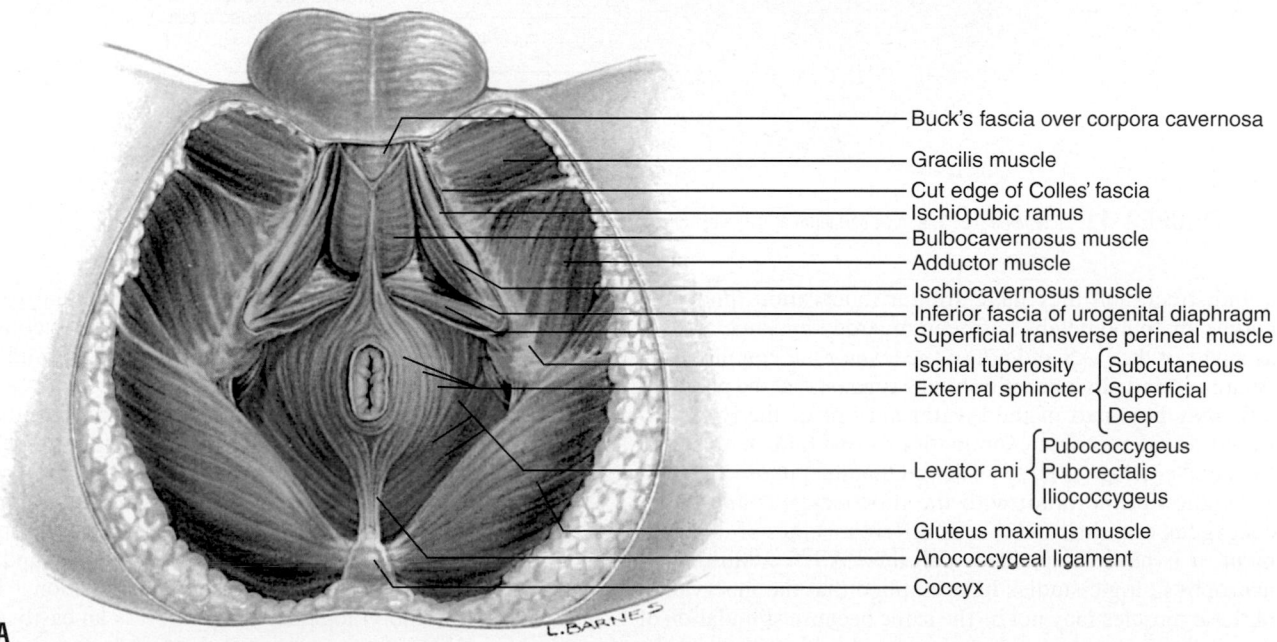

Buck's fascia over corpora cavernosa
Gracilis muscle
Cut edge of Colles' fascia
Ischiopubic ramus
Bulbocavernosus muscle
Adductor muscle
Ischiocavernosus muscle
Inferior fascia of urogenital diaphragm
Superficial transverse perineal muscle
Ischial tuberosity
External sphincter { Subcutaneous / Superficial / Deep }
Levator ani { Pubococcygeus / Puborectalis / Iliococcygeus }
Gluteus maximus muscle
Anococcygeal ligament
Coccyx

A

FIGURE 1-11. Male perineal musculature. **A:** Inferior view of the male perineum at a superficial level with the skin and subcutaneous tissue removed. *(continued)*

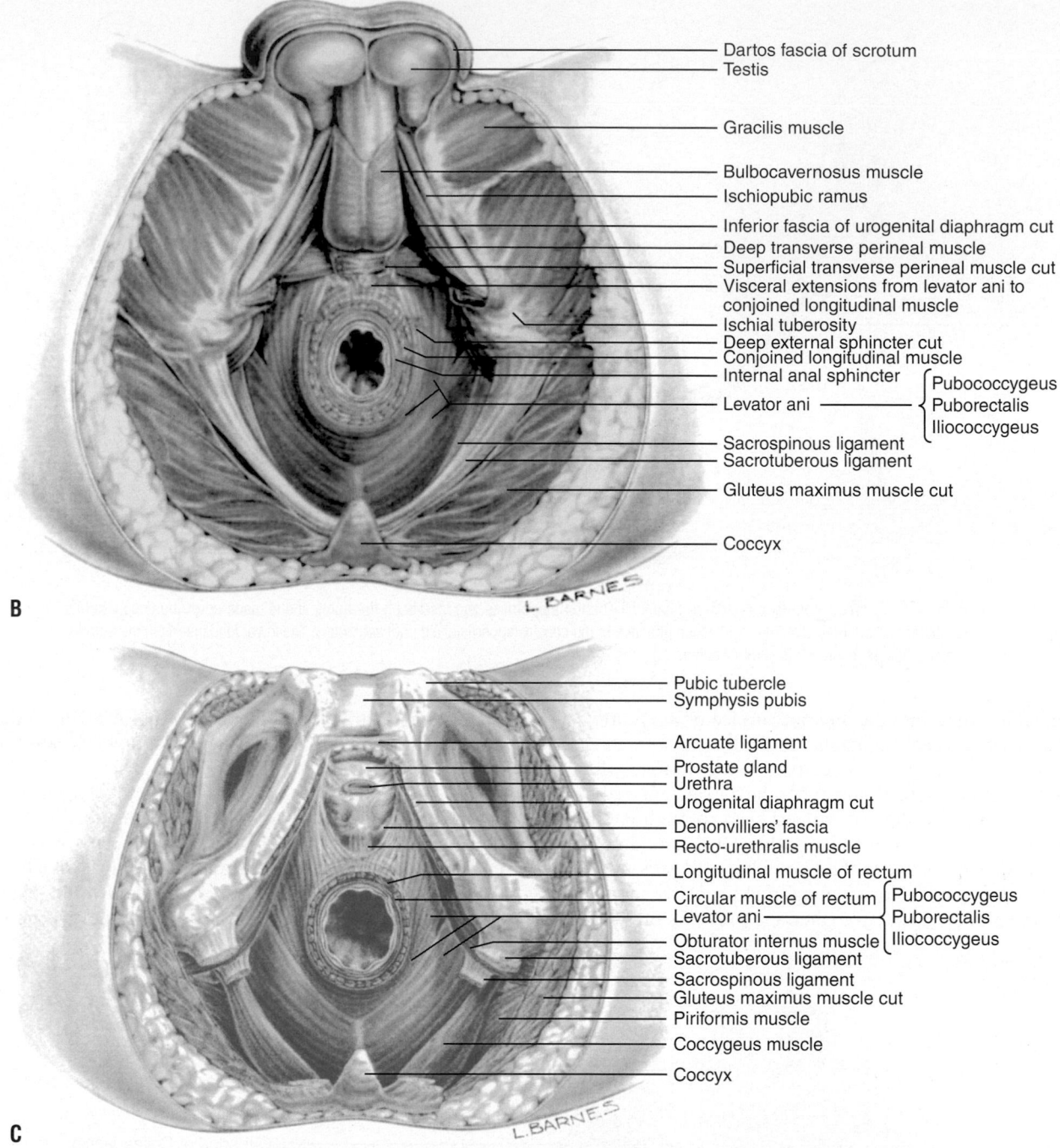

FIGURE 1-11. *(continued)* **B:** The male perineum at the level of the midanal canal. **C:** The male perineum at the level of the lower rectum.

is indistinct, and they have similar innervation (pudendal nerve), the puborectalis has been regarded by some authors as a part of the EAS and not of the levator ani complex.[89,102] Anatomic and phylogenetic studies suggest that the puborectalis may be a part of the levator ani[92] or of the EAS.[63,120] Based on microscopic examinations in 18 human embryos, Levi and colleagues have observed that the puborectalis has a common primordium with the iliococcygeus and pubococcygeus muscles, and that in different stages of development, it is never connected with the EAS.[66] Additionally, neurophysiologic studies have implied that the innervation of these muscles may not be the same because stimulation of the sacral nerves results in electromyographic activity in the ipsilateral puborectalis muscle but not in the EAS.[96] How-

ever, one can appreciate that this is a controversial issue, and as a consequence, the puborectalis is currently considered to belong to both muscular groups: the EAS and the levator ani.[100]

Two anatomic structures of the junction of the rectum and anal canal are related to the puborectalis muscle: the anorectal ring and the anorectal angle (Figure 1-13). The anorectal ring, a term coined by Milligan and Morgan (see Biographies, Chapter 11), is a strong muscular ring that represents the upper end of the sphincter (more precisely the puborectalis) and the upper border of the IAS around the anorectal junction.[79] Despite its lack of embryologic significance, it is an easily recognized boundary of the anal canal that can be appreciated on physical examination. It is of particular clinical relevance

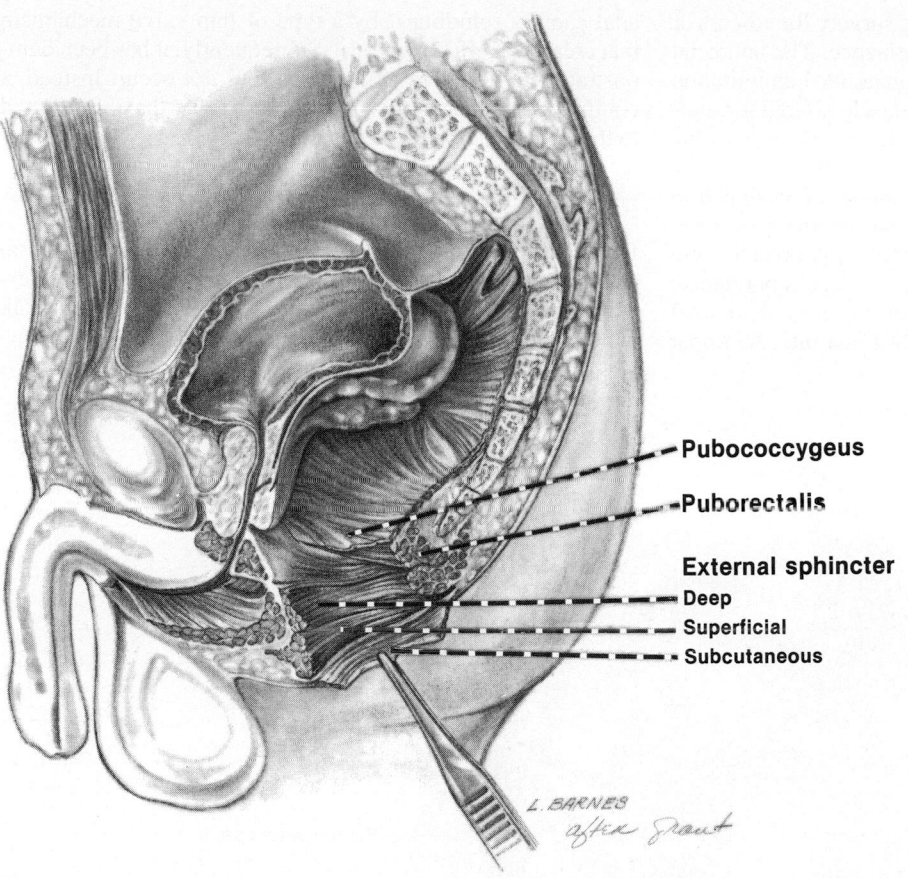

Pubococcygeus

Puborectalis

External sphincter

Deep

Superficial

Subcutaneous

L. BARNES
after grant

FIGURE 1-12. Muscles of the pelvic floor.

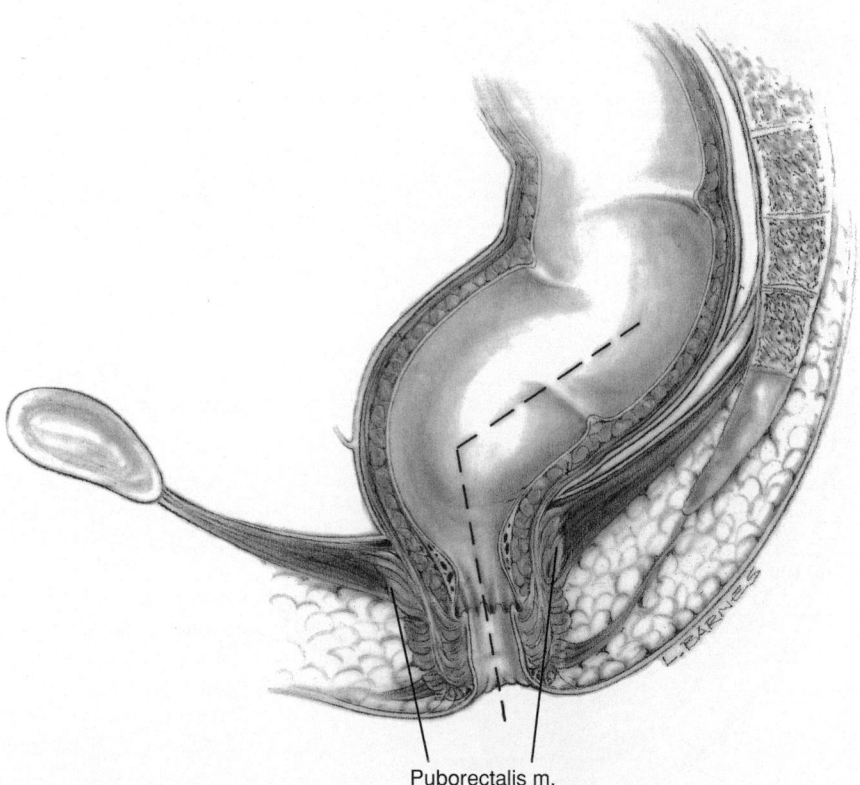

Puborectalis m.

FIGURE 1-13. The anteriorly directed pull of the puborectalis contributes to the angulation between the rectum and anal canal, the anorectal angle (*dashed line*).

because division of this structure during surgery for abscess or fistula inevitably results in fecal incontinence. The anorectal angle is thought to be the result of the anatomic configuration of the U-shaped sling of puborectalis muscle around the anorectal junction. Whereas the anal sphincters are responsible for closure of the anal canal to retain gas and liquid stool, the puborectalis muscle and the anorectal angle are designed to maintain gross fecal continence. Different theories have been postulated to explain the importance of the puborectalis and the anorectal angle in the maintenance of fecal continence. Parks and coworkers opined that increasing intra-abdominal pressure forces the anterior rectal wall down into the upper anal canal, occluding it by a type of flap valve mechanism that creates an effective seal.[94] Subsequently, it has been demonstrated that the flap mechanism does not occur. Instead, a continuous sphincteric occlusion-like activity that is attributed to the puborectalis has been observed.[7,8]

Para-Anal and Para-Rectal Spaces

Potential spaces of clinical significance in the anorectal region include the following: ischiorectal, perianal, intersphincteric, submucous, superficial postanal, deep postanal, supralevator, and retrorectal (Figure 1-14).

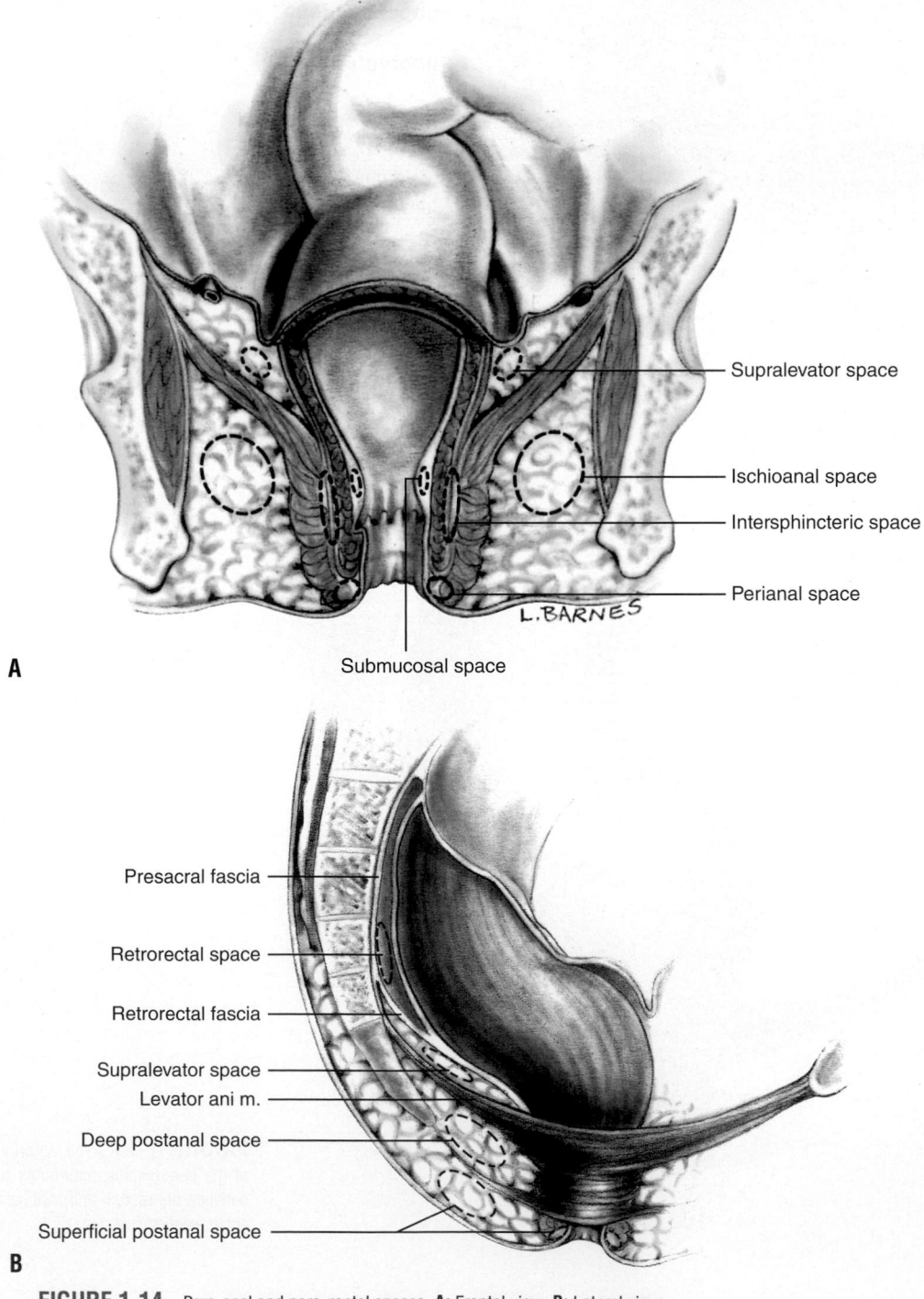

A

Supralevator space

Ischioanal space

Intersphincteric space

Perianal space

L. BARNES

Submucosal space

Presacral fascia

Retrorectal space

Retrorectal fascia

Supralevator space

Levator ani m.

Deep postanal space

Superficial postanal space

B

FIGURE 1-14. Para-anal and para-rectal spaces. **A:** Frontal view. **B:** Lateral view.

The ischiorectal fossa is subdivided by a thin horizontal fascia into two spaces: the perianal and ischiorectal. The ischiorectal space comprises the upper two-thirds of the ischiorectal fossa. It is pyramidal in shape and is situated on both sides between the anal canal and the lower part of the rectum medially and the sidewall of the pelvis laterally. Some authors consider the term ischiorectal fossa misleading and prefer to use the expression ischioanal fossa because its medial limit is at the level of the anal canal rather than the rectum.[59] The apex is at the origin of the levator ani muscle from the obturator fascia; the base is the perianal space. Anteriorly, the fossa is bounded by the urogenital diaphragm and the transversus perinei muscle. Posterior to the ischiorectal fossa is the sacrotuberous ligament and the inferior border of the gluteus maximus. On the superolateral wall, the pudendal nerve and the internal pudendal vessels run in the pudendal canal (Alcock's canal). The ischiorectal fossa contains fat and the inferior rectal vessels and nerves.

The perianal space surrounds the lower part of the anal canal. It is continuous with the subcutaneous fat of the buttocks laterally and extends into the intersphincteric space medially. The external hemorrhoidal plexus lies in the perianal space and communicates with the internal hemorrhoidal plexus at the dentate line. This space is the typical site of anal hematomas, perianal abscesses, and anal fistula tracts. The perianal space also encloses the subcutaneous part of the EAS, the lowest part of the IAS, and fibers of the longitudinal muscle. These fibers function as septa, dividing the space into a compact arrangement, which may account for the severe pain caused by a perianal hematoma or abscess.

The intersphincteric space is a potential space between the IAS and the EAS. It is important in the genesis of perianal abscess because most of the anal glands end in this space. The submucous space is situated between the IAS and the mucocutaneous lining of the anal canal. This space contains the internal hemorrhoidal plexus and the muscularis submucosae ani. Above, it is continuous with the submucous layer of the rectum, and inferiorly it ends at the level of the dentate line.

The superficial postanal space is interposed between the anococcygeal ligament and the skin. The deep postanal space, also known as the retrosphincteric space of Courtney, is situated between the anococcygeal ligament and the anococcygeal raphe.[21] Both postanal spaces communicate posteriorly with the ischiorectal fossa and are the sites of horseshoe abscesses.

The supralevator spaces are situated between the peritoneum superiorly and the levator ani inferiorly. Medially, these bilateral spaces are limited by the rectum and, laterally, by the obturator fascia. Supralevator abscesses may occur as a result of upward extension of a cryptoglandular infection or develop from a pelvic origin. The retrorectal space is located between the fascia propria of the rectum anteriorly and the presacral fascia posteriorly. Laterally are found the lateral rectal ligaments and inferiorly the rectosacral ligament; the space above is continuous with the retroperitoneum. The retrorectal space is a frequent site for embryologic remnants and rare presacral tumors (see Chapter 26).

Arterial Supply

Two of the three major gut vessels, the superior and inferior mesenteric arteries, nourish the entire large intestine (Figure 1-15). The limit between the two territories is the junction between the proximal two-thirds and the distal third of the transverse colon. This represents the embryologic division between the midgut and the hindgut. Collateral circulation between these two arteries is formed by a "continuous" communicating arcade along the mesenteric border of the colon, the marginal artery, from which the vasa recta supply the bowel. The colon is much less vascular and consequently more vulnerable to necrosis than is the small bowel because communications between both adjacent and opposite-sided vasa recta are few. The anorectum is, in addition, supplied by the internal iliac arteries.

Superior Mesenteric Artery

The superior mesenteric artery originates from the aorta behind the superior border of the pancreas at L1, supplying the cecum, appendix, ascending colon, and most of the transverse colon. Additionally, the superior mesenteric artery supplies the entire small bowel, the pancreas, and occasionally the liver. After passing behind the neck of the pancreas and anteromedial to the uncinate process, the superior mesenteric artery crosses the third part of the duodenum, continuing downward and to the right, along the base of the mesentery. From its left side arises a series of 12 to 20 jejunal and ileal branches. From its right side arise the colic branches: middle, right, and ileocolic arteries. The ileocolic is the most constant of these vessels, being present in all 600 specimens studied by Sonneland and coworkers.[107] It bifurcates into a superior or ascending branch, which communicates with the descending branch of the right colic artery, and an inferior or descending branch, which gives off the anterior cecal, posterior cecal, and appendicular divisions. Finally, it supplies the distal small bowel mesentery as the ileal branch.

The right colic artery may also arise from the ileocolic or middle colic arteries; it is absent in 2% to 18% of specimens.[77,107,109] This vessel supplies the ascending colon and hepatic flexure through its ascending and descending branches, both of which join with neighboring vessels to contribute to the marginal artery.

The middle colic artery is the highest of the three colic branches of the superior mesenteric artery, arising close to the inferior border of the pancreas. Its right branch supplies the right transverse colon and hepatic flexure, anastomosing with the ascending branch of the right colic artery. Its left branch supplies the distal half of the transverse colon. Anatomic variations of this artery include absence in 4% to 20% of cases and the presence of an accessory middle colic artery in 10%; the middle colic artery is the main supply to the splenic flexure in about one-third of individuals.[44,107]

Inferior Mesenteric Artery

The inferior mesenteric artery originates from the left anterior surface of the aorta, 3 to 4 cm above its bifurcation at the level of L2–3, and runs downward and to the left to enter the pelvis. Within the abdomen, the inferior mesenteric artery branches into the left colic artery and two to six sigmoidal arteries. After crossing the left common iliac artery, it acquires the name superior hemorrhoidal artery (superior rectal artery is generally not preferred [Figure 1-15]).

The left colic artery, the highest branch of the inferior mesenteric artery, bifurcates into an ascending branch, which runs upward to the splenic flexure to contribute to the arcade of Riolan, and a descending branch, which supplies most of the descending colon. The sigmoidal arteries form arcades within the sigmoid mesocolon, resembling the small bowel vasculature, and anastomose with branches of the left colic artery proximally and with the superior hemorrhoidal artery

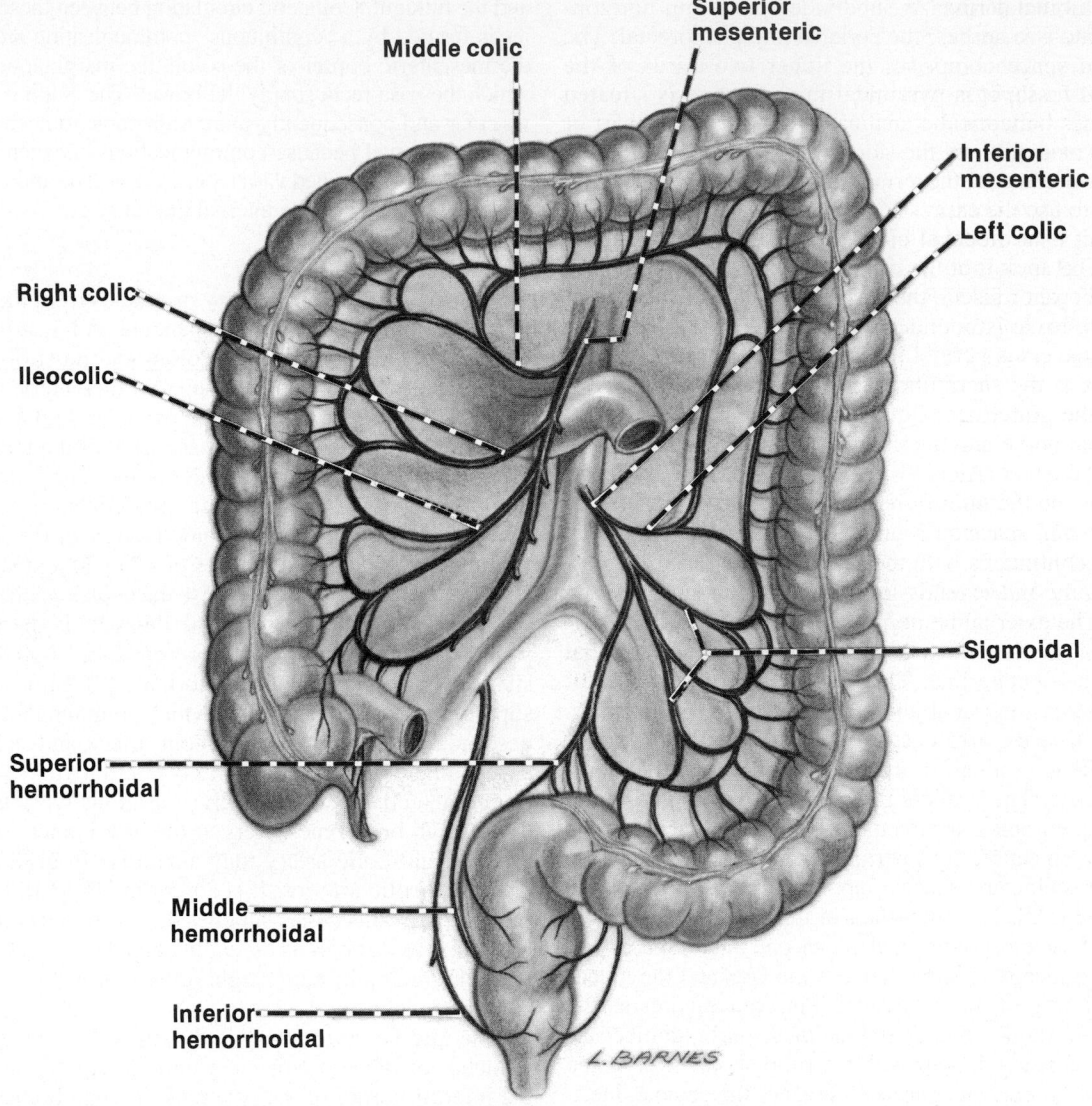

FIGURE 1-15. The blood supply to the colon originates from the superior and inferior mesenteric arteries.

distally. The marginal artery terminates within the arcade of sigmoidal arteries. The superior hemorrhoidal artery is the continuation of the inferior mesenteric artery once it crosses the left iliac vessels. The artery descends in the sigmoid mesocolon to the level of S3 and then to the posterior aspect of the rectum. In 80% of cases, it bifurcates into right (usually wider) and left terminal branches; multiple branches are present in 17% of patients.[77] These divisions, once within the submucosa of the rectum, run straight downward to supply the lower rectum and anal canal. The branches that reach the level of the rectal columns (approximately five) condensate in capillary plexuses, mostly at the right posterior, right anterior, and left lateral positions; these branches correspond to the location of the major internal hemorrhoid groups.

The major blood supply to the anorectum is represented by the superior and inferior hemorrhoidal arteries. The contribution of the middle hemorrhoidal artery varies with the size of the superior hemorrhoidal artery; this may explain its controversial anatomy. Some authors report absence of the middle hemorrhoidal artery in 40% to 88%,[3,27] whereas others identify it in 94% to 100% of specimen.[48,77] This vessel originates more commonly from the anterior division of

the internal iliac or the pudendal arteries and reaches the rectum. The middle hemorrhoidal artery reaches the lower third of the rectum anterolaterally, close to the level of the pelvic floor and deep to the levator fascia. Contrary to popular misconception, it therefore does not run in the lateral ligaments (inclined posterolaterally).[20,85] The middle hemorrhoidal artery is more prone to be injured during low anterior resection, when anterolateral dissection of the rectum is performed close to the pelvic floor, and the prostate and seminal vesicles or upper part of the vagina are being separated.[85] The anorectum has a profuse intramural anastomotic network, which probably accounts for the fact that division of both superior and middle hemorrhoidal arteries does not result in necrosis of the rectum. This tenet is fundamental to ileoanal reservoir surgery and restorative proctocolectomy.

The paired inferior hemorrhoidal arteries are branches of the internal pudendal artery, which, in turn, is a branch of the internal iliac artery. The inferior hemorrhoidal artery arises within the pudendal canal and is throughout its course entirely extrapelvic. It traverses the obturator fascia, the ischiorectal fossa, and the EAS to reach the submucosa of the anal canal, ultimately ascending in this plane. The inferior rectal artery needs to be ligated during the perineal stage of abdominoperineal resection. Klosterhalfen and coworkers performed postmortem angiographic, manual, and histologic evaluations, identifying two topographic variants of this vessel.[60] In the so-called type I, the most common type (85%), the posterior commissure was less well perfused than were the other sections of the anal canal. In addition, the blood supply could be jeopardized by contusion of the vessels passing vertically through the muscle fibers of the IAS when sphincter tone was increased. These authors postulated that in a pathogenetic model of primary anal fissure, the resulting decreased blood supply may lead to ischemia at the posterior commissure.

Collateral Circulation

In spite of the fact that prior to the 17th century, anatomy of the mesenteric circulation was a source of concern, this subject still has not been clarified in most textbooks. This, in part, may be attributed to the inherent confusion in the use of eponyms. A central anastomotic artery that connects all colonic mesenteric branches was initially described by Haller in 1786.[50] Later it became known as the marginal artery of Drummond, because it was he, in 1913, who first demonstrated its surgical significance. Drummond proved that the sigmoidal vessels could be filled with contrast material following injection of the ileocolic artery and ligation of the right, middle, and left colic arteries at their origin.[28,29] Subsequent examiners have demonstrated discontinuity of the marginal artery at the lower ascending colon and especially at the splenic flexure and sigmoid colon. This theoretically hypovascular area is a potential source of concern during colonic resection.[125] The splenic flexure comprises the watershed between midgut and hindgut blood supply (Griffiths' critical point); this anastomosis is of variable significance, and in fact, it may be absent in about 50% of cases.[76] For this reason, ischemic colitis usually affects or is most severe near the splenic flexure.[26] Despite this logic, a predilection for the right colon has been found by several investigators.[47,62,71] Sudeck's critical point, an area of discontinuity of the marginal artery between the distal sigmoid and the superior hemorrhoidal arteries, may be unnecessarily emphasized.[111] Surgical experience and radiologic studies have both demonstrated adequate communication between these vessels.[44,115] Furthermore, anastomosis between the superior and middle hemorrhoidal arteries, commonly observed with

DAVID DRUMMOND (1852–1932)

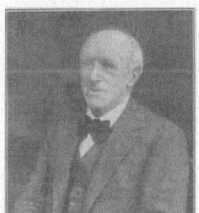

Drummond was born in Dublin and received his early education at private schools in Ireland and England. He studied medicine at Trinity College, Dublin, graduating in 1874. Following a period of additional education in Prague, Vienna, and Strasbourg, he achieved his MD degree and settled in Newcastle, England. He was soon appointed assistant physician to the Children's Hospital. In 1878, he was elected to the honorary staff of the Royal Victoria Infirmary as pathologist and assistant physician. For more than 50 years, he was closely associated with the University of Durham College of Medicine at Newcastle. He had been lecturer in physiology, in pathology, and in therapeutics, and from 1911 to 1924 was professor of the principles and practice of medicine. He also served as chancellor of the university and president of the College of Medicine. For his services in the first World War as physician to the Northumberland War Hospital, he was created CBE in 1920, and 3 years later received the honor of knighthood. As a physician/anatomist, Sir David Drummond devoted much time to the study of diseases of the brain and spinal cord, but his work ranged widely, and he was a pioneer in other fields of clinical medicine. As a keen observer and prosector, he formulated and clarified the vascular anatomy of the colon and achieved eponymous immortality through his description of the meandering artery. (Abstracted from Obituary in *Br Med J.* 1937;7:1(3722):865–866. Photograph, Courtesy of the *British Medical Journal*.)

PAUL HERMANN MARTIN SUDECK (1866–1945)

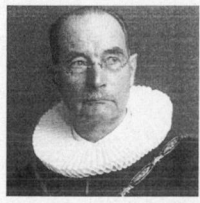

Paul Sudeck was born in 1866 in Pinneberg, Holstein, Germany, the son of an attorney. Despite his father's wishes, he entered the study of medicine at the Universities of Tübingen, Kiel, and Würzburg. In 1890, he earned his doctorate at the Pathological Institute of the University of Würzburg, after which he became an assistant at the Eppendorf Hospital in Hamburg. It was there that he spent his entire career. Sudeck became professor of surgery in 1919 and was named the first director and chairman of the department in 1923 at the new University of Hamburg. His primary contributions to medicine were in anesthesia and orthopedics. He was responsible for reintroducing inhalational anesthesia into Germany, using ether and chloroform. In 1901, he developed a new anesthetic mask (the Sudeck Inhalator), which contained an exhalation valve that avoided the accumulation of toxic gas. He recognized reflex sympathetic dystrophy, a debilitating soft tissue atrophy following bony fractures, which now bears his name (Sudeck's dystrophy). He emphasized that there is a failure of the marginal artery circulation between the lowest sigmoid artery and the branches of the superior hemorrhoidal artery (Sudeck's point). He had a strong interest in biomechanics and made many contributions to the rehabilitation of trauma victims. Sudeck died in Hamburg, September 28, 1945. (With appreciation to Ali Khoynezhad, MD and Udo Rudloff, MD.)

JEAN RIOLAN (1577–1657)

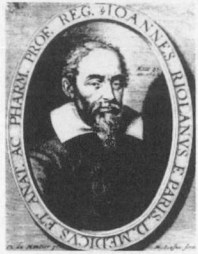

Riolan was born in Paris, France, the son of a physician and leading member of the Paris Medical Faculty. His mother's family also played a prominent role in Parisian medicine during the 16th and 17th centuries. He studied chiefly under his uncle and received his doctorate in medicine in 1604. Riolan was also named archdeacon of schools, a position that placed him in charge of the material for anatomy courses.

He became a trained anatomist and dissector and advocated active anatomic observation in preference to long reading and meditation. He was also a staunch defender of traditional medicine and considered himself an enemy of chemical healers. A violent adversary of Harvey, he maintained that if dissections no longer agreed with those of Galen, it should be attributed to the fact that nature had changed since Galen's time. He believed that one should never admit that Galen was incorrect. Despite his reactionary opinions, Riolan distinguished himself through a series of textbooks, including *Anthropographia* in 1626 and *Encheiridium* in 1648. From 1604 to 1640, he was professor of anatomy and botany at the University of Paris and professor of medicine at the College Royal, as well as dean of the Royal College from 1640 to 1657. Riolan also served as physician to Henry IV and Louis XIII. He died at the age of 77 in Paris. (With appreciation to the Galileo Project Files, Rice University, and Michael Eng, MD.)

aortography, may prevent gangrene of the pelvis and even the lower extremities, wherein the distal aorta is occluded. This can be attributed to the collateral network involving middle hemorrhoidal, internal iliac, and external iliac arteries.[45,70]

Jean Riolan (1580 to 1657) was the first to describe the communication between the superior and inferior mesenteric arteries, and the term arc of Riolan was vaguely defined in the author's original work. Later, the eponym, marginal artery of Drummond, confused the subject.[34] In 1964, Moskowitz and coworkers proposed another term, meandering mesenteric artery, and differentiated it from the marginal artery of Drummond.[84] The meandering mesenteric artery is a thick and tortuous vessel that makes a crucial communication between the middle colic artery and the ascending branch of the left colic artery, especially in advanced atherosclerotic disease. Fisher and Fry claimed that the meandering mesenteric artery could be easily recognized either preoperatively by arteriography (because of its size, tortuosity, and uniform caliber) or intraoperatively (by palpation because of its prominent arterial pulsations flow).[34] The presence of the meandering mesenteric artery indicates severe stenosis of either the superior mesenteric artery (retrograde flow) or inferior mesenteric artery (antegrade flow). If during a left colon operation the meandering mesenteric artery is divided, vascular compromise may ensue, depending on the direction of the flow. Necrosis of the right colon and entire small bowel may occur if the flow is retrograde, and necrosis of the sigmoid colon and upper rectum, as well as vascular insufficiency in the lower extremity, may occur if the flow is antegrade.

Venous Drainage

The venous drainage of the large intestine basically follows its arterial supply (Figure 1-16). Blood from the right colon, via the superior mesenteric vein, and from left colon

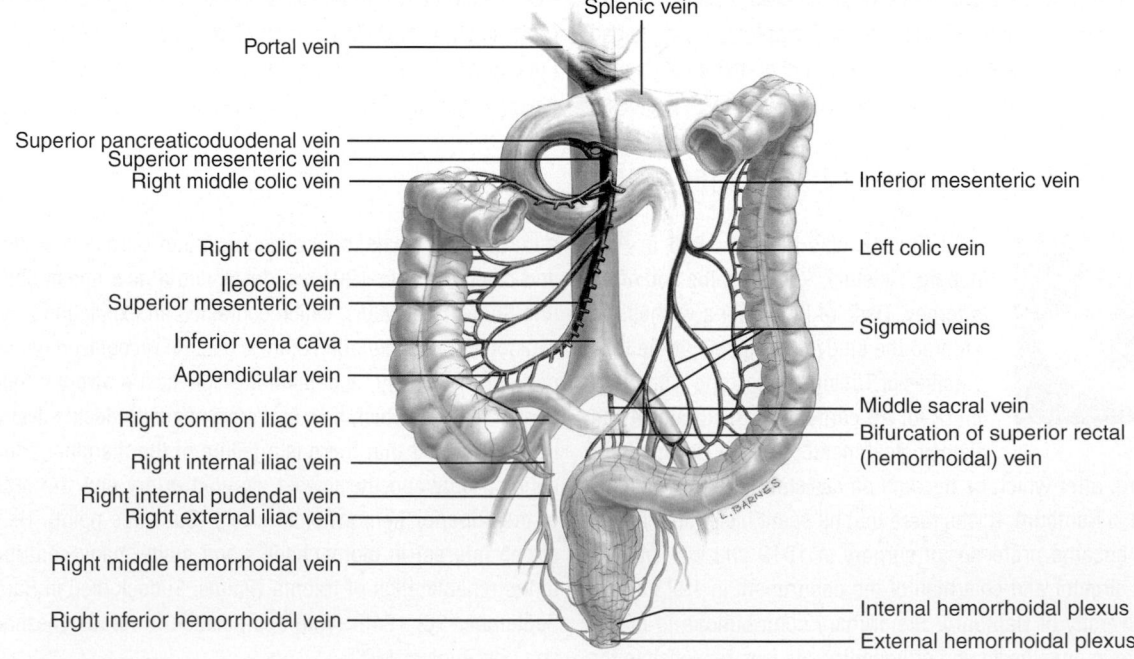

FIGURE 1-16. Venous drainage of the colon.

and rectum, via the inferior mesenteric vein, reaches the intrahepatic capillary bed through the portal vein. The anorectum also drains, via middle and inferior hemorrhoidal veins, to the internal iliac vein and then to the inferior vena cava. Although it is still a controversial subject, the presence of communications among these three venous systems may explain the lack of correlation between portal hypertension and hemorrhoids.[10]

The paired inferior and middle hemorrhoidal veins and the single superior hemorrhoidal vein originate from three anorectal arteriovenous plexuses (Figure 1-17). The external hemorrhoidal plexus, situated subcutaneously around the anal canal below the dentate line, constitutes the external hemorrhoids when it is dilated. The internal hemorrhoidal plexus is situated submucosally, around the upper anal canal and above the dentate line. The internal hemorrhoids originate from this plexus. The perirectal or perimuscular rectal plexus drains to the middle and inferior hemorrhoidal veins.

Lymphatic Drainage

The lymphatic drainage from all parts of the colon follows its vascular supply. The submucous and subserous layers of the colon and rectum have a rich network of lymphatic plexuses, which drain into an extramural system of lymph channels and nodes.[11] Colorectal lymph nodes are classically divided into four groups: epiploic, paracolic, intermediate, and principal (Figure 1-18).[55] The epicolic group lies on the bowel wall under the peritoneum and in the appendices epiploicae; they are more numerous in the sigmoid and are known in the rectum as the nodules of Gerota. The paracolic nodes are situated along the marginal artery and on the arcades; they are considered to have the most numerous filters. The intermediate nodes are situated on the primary colic vessels, and the main or principal nodes are situated on the superior and inferior mesenteric vessels. The lymph then drains to the cisterna chyli via the para-aortic chain of nodes. Colorectal carcinoma staging systems are based on the neoplastic involvement of these various lymph node groups.

Lymph from the upper two-thirds of the rectum drains exclusively upward to the inferior mesenteric nodes and then to the para-aortic nodes (Figure 1-19). Lymphatic drainage from the lower third of the rectum occurs, not only cephalad along the superior hemorrhoidal and inferior mesentery arteries but also laterally, along the middle hemorrhoidal vessels to the internal iliac nodes. Studies using

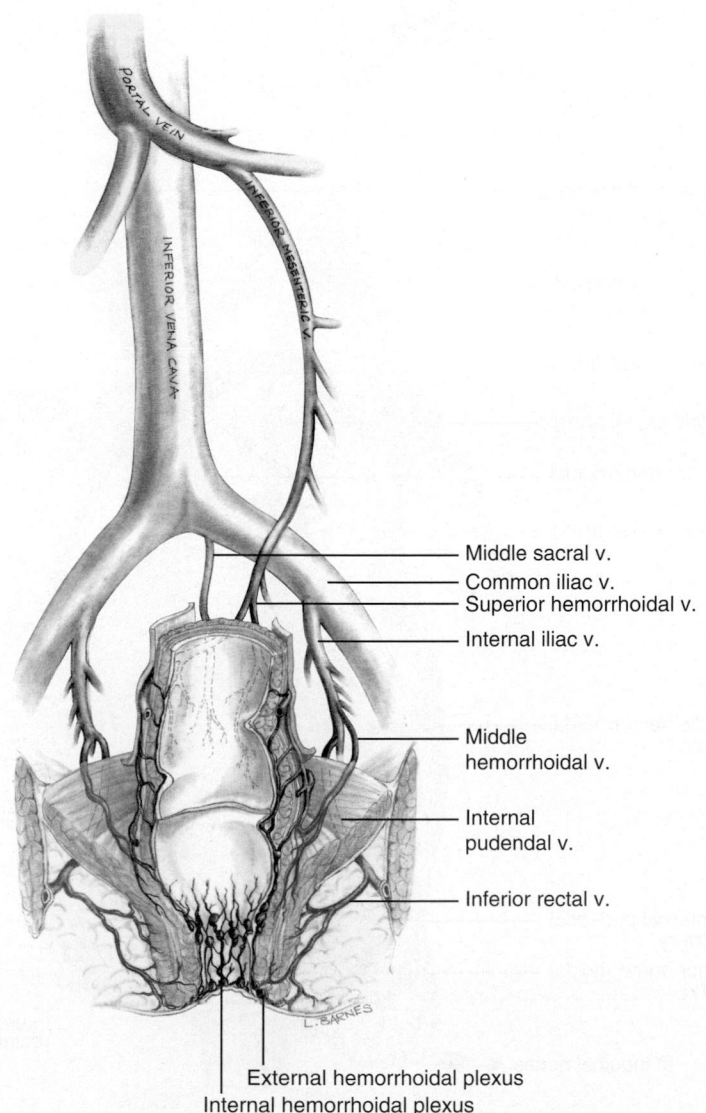

Middle sacral v.
Common iliac v.
Superior hemorrhoidal v.
Internal iliac v.

Middle hemorrhoidal v.

Internal pudendal v.

Inferior rectal v.

External hemorrhoidal plexus
Internal hemorrhoidal plexus

FIGURE 1-17. Venous drainage of the colon.

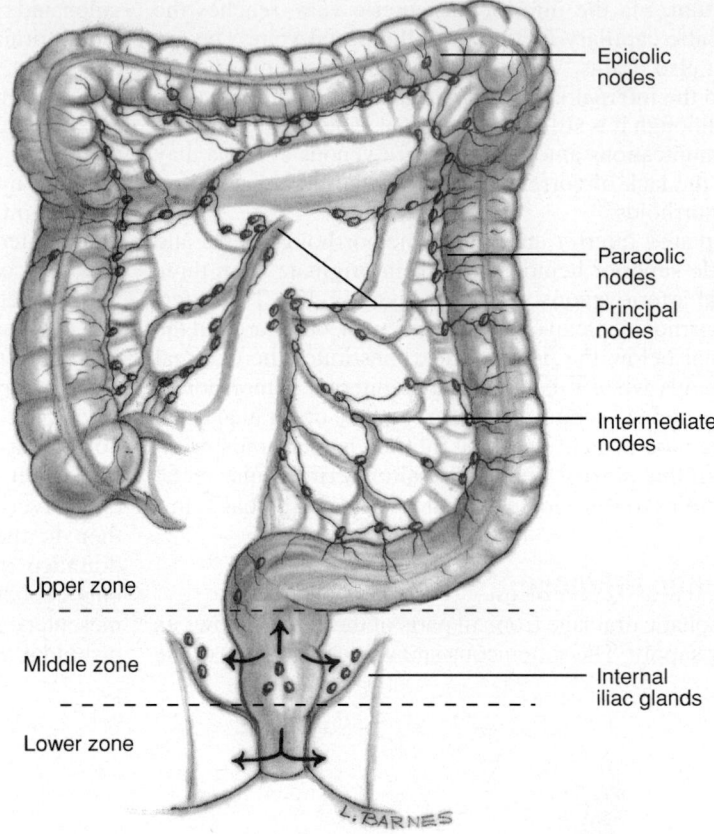

FIGURE 1-18. Lymphatic drainage of the colon.

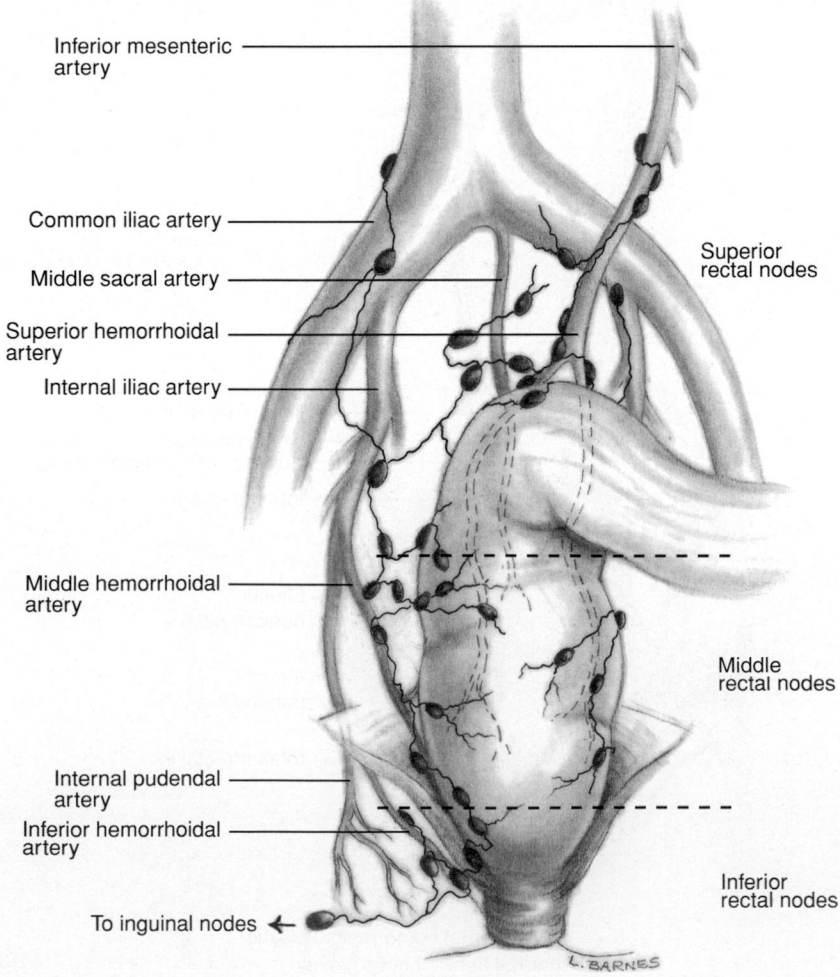

FIGURE 1-19. Lymphatic drainage of the colon.

lymphoscintigraphy have failed to demonstrate communications between inferior mesenteric and internal iliac lymphatics.[80] In the anal canal, the dentate line is the landmark for two different systems of lymphatic drainage: above, to the inferior mesenteric and internal iliac nodes, and below, along the inferior rectal lymphatics to the superficial inguinal nodes or less frequently along the inferior hemorrhoidal artery. Block and Enquist injected dye 5 cm above the anal verge in the female and demonstrated that lymphatic drainage may also spread to the posterior vaginal wall, uterus, cervix, broad ligament, fallopian tubes, ovaries, and cul-de-sac.[11] After injection of dye at 10 cm above the anal verge, spread occurred only to the broad ligament and cul-de-sac, and at the 15-cm level, no spread to the genitals was seen.

Innervation

The sympathetic and parasympathetic components of the autonomic innervation of the large intestine closely follow the blood supply.

Right Colon

The sympathetic supply originates from the lower six thoracic segments. These thoracic splanchnic nerves reach the celiac, preaortic, and superior mesenteric ganglia, where they synapse. The postganglionic fibers then course along the superior mesenteric artery to the small bowel and right colon. The parasympathetic supply comes from the right (posterior) vagus nerve and celiac plexus. The fibers travel along the superior mesenteric artery and finally synapse with cells in the autonomic plexuses within the bowel wall.

Left Colon and Rectum

The sympathetic supply arises from L1, L2, and L3. Preganglionic fibers, via lumbar sympathetic nerves, synapse in the preaortic plexus, and the postganglionic fibers follow the branches of the inferior mesenteric artery and superior rectal artery to the left colon and upper rectum. The lower rectum is innervated by the presacral nerves, which are formed by fusion of the aortic plexus and lumbar splanchnic nerves. Just below the sacral promontory, the presacral nerves form the hypogastric plexus (or superior hypogastric plexus). Two main hypogastric nerves, on either side of the rectum, carry sympathetic innervation from the hypogastric plexus to the pelvic plexus. The pelvic plexus lies on the lateral side of the pelvis at the level of the lower third of the rectum, adjacent to the lateral stalks. The term inferior hypogastric plexus has been used to mean the hypogastric nerves or the pelvic plexus; therefore, it is inaccurate.[20]

The parasympathetic supply derives from S2, S3, and S4 (Figure 1-20). These fibers emerge through the sacral foramen and are called the *nervi erigentes*. They pass laterally, forward, and upward to join the sympathetic hypogastric nerves at the pelvic plexus. From the pelvic plexus, combined postganglionic parasympathetic and sympathetic fibers are distributed to the left colon and upper rectum via the inferior mesenteric plexus and directly to the lower rectum and

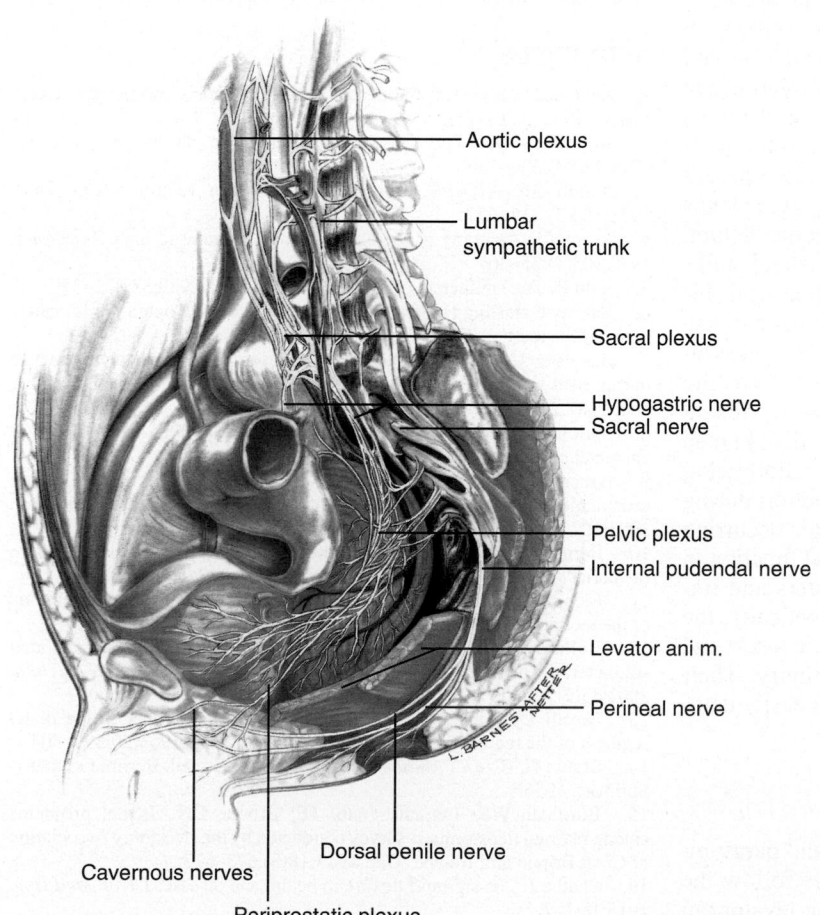

Aortic plexus

Lumbar sympathetic trunk

Sacral plexus

Hypogastric nerve
Sacral nerve

Pelvic plexus
Internal pudendal nerve

Levator ani m.

Perineal nerve

Cavernous nerves

Dorsal penile nerve

Periprostatic plexus

FIGURE 1-20. Innervation of the rectum and sphincters.

upper anal canal. The periprostatic plexus, a subdivision of the pelvic plexus situated on Denonvilliers' fascia, supplies the prostate, seminal vesicles, corpora cavernosa, vas deferens, urethra, ejaculatory ducts, and bulbourethral glands.

Sexual function is regulated by cerebrospinal, sympathetic, and parasympathetic components. Erection of the penis is mediated by both parasympathetic (arteriolar vasodilation) and sympathetic inflow (inhibition of vasoconstriction). Urinary and sexual dysfunctions are commonly seen after a variety of pelvic surgical procedures, including low anterior resection and abdominoperineal resection. Permanent bladder paresis occurs in 7% to 59% of patients after abdominoperineal resection of the rectum[39]; the incidence of impotence is reported to range from 15% to 45% and that of ejaculatory dysfunction from 32% to 42%.[90] The overall incidence of sexual dysfunction after proctectomy may reach 100% when the procedure is performed for malignant disease[6,25,119]; however, these rates are much lower for benign conditions, such as inflammatory bowel disease (0% to 6%).[6,9,25,117] This may be a consequence of the fact that dissections performed for benign conditions are undertaken closer to the bowel wall, thus reducing the possibility of nerve injury.[64] A more likely reason, however, is the age of the patient and the preoperative libido.

All pelvic nerves lie in the plane between the peritoneum and the endopelvic fascia and are in danger of injury during rectal dissection. Trauma to the autonomic nerves may occur at several points. During high ligation of the inferior mesenteric artery, close to the aorta, the sympathetic preaortic nerves may be injured. Division of both superior hypogastric plexus and hypogastric nerves may occur also during dissection at the level of the sacral promontory or in the presacral region. In such circumstances, sympathetic denervation with intact nervi erigentes results in retrograde ejaculation and bladder dysfunction. The nervi erigentes are located in the posterolateral aspect of the pelvis and at the point of fusion with the sympathetic nerves are closely related to the middle hemorrhoidal artery. An isolated injury to these nerves will completely abolish erectile function.[9] The pelvic plexus may be damaged either by excessive traction on the rectum, particularly laterally, or during division of the lateral stalks when this is performed close to the lateral pelvic wall. Finally, dissection near the seminal vesicles and prostate may damage the periprostatic plexus, leading to a mixed parasympathetic and sympathetic injury. This can result in erectile impotence as well as a flaccid, neurogenic bladder. Sexual complications after rectal surgery are readily evident in men but are probably underdiagnosed in women.[75] Following proctocolectomy in female patients, some discomfort during intercourse is reported in 30%,[15] with dyspareunia occurring in 10%.[46] Some investigators believe that sexual function in women is primarily mediated by cerebral centers and impulses carried by the pudendal nerves.[9] Parenthetically, the pudendal nerves are covered by dense endopelvic fascia and are therefore more protected from operative injury. Their function is completely independent of the more easily damaged nervi erigentes.

Anal Canal
Motor Innervation
The IAS is supplied by the sympathetic (L5) and parasympathetic nerves (S2, S3, and S4); these nerves follow the same route as those leading to the rectum. The levator ani is supplied by sacral roots on its pelvic surface (S2, S3, and S4) as well as the perineal branch of the pudendal nerve on its inferior surface. The puborectalis muscle receives additional innervation from the inferior rectal nerves. The EAS is innervated on each side by the inferior rectal branch of the pudendal nerve (S2 and S3) and by the perineal branch of S4. Despite the fact that the puborectalis and EAS have somewhat different innervations, these muscles seem to act as an indivisible unit.[101,102] After unilateral transection of a pudendal nerve, EAS function is still preserved because of the crossover of the fibers at the spinal cord level.

Sensory Innervation
The upper anal canal contains a rich profusion of both free and organized sensory nerve endings, especially in the vicinity of the anal valves.[30] Organized nerve endings include Meissner's corpuscles (touch), Krause's bulbs (cold), Golgi-Mazzoni bodies (pressure), and genital corpuscles (friction). Anal sensation is carried in the inferior rectal branch of the pudendal nerve and is thought to play a role in maintenance of fecal continence.[78]

▶ SUMMARY

In this chapter, one has attempted not merely to present a description of the anatomy of the colon, rectum, and anus but also to provide clinical correlation wherever appropriate or helpful. Knowledge of colon and rectal anatomy, blood supply, lymphatic drainage, innervation, and muscle function and distribution are all extremely important in order to minimize complications represented by the host of surgical challenges that are discussed in subsequent chapters.

References

1. Abel AL. The pectin: the pecten band: pectenosis and pectenectomy. *Lancet.* 1932;1:714–718.
2. Abramson DJ. The valves of Houston in adults. *Am J Surg.* 1978;136(3):334–336.
3. Ayoub SF. Arterial supply of the human rectum. *Acta Anat.* 1978;100(3):317–327.
4. Ayoub SF. Anatomy of the external anal sphincter in man. *Acta Anat.* 1979;105(1):25–36.
5. Balli R. The sphincters of the colon. *Radiology.* 1939;33:372–376.
6. Balslev I, Harling H. Sexual dysfunction following operation for carcinoma of the rectum. *Dis Colon Rectum.* 1983;26(12):785–788.
7. Bannister JJ, Gibbons C, Read NW. Preservation of faecal continence during rises in intra-abdominal pressure: is there a role for the flap valve? *Gut.* 1987;28(10):1242–1245.
8. Bartolo DC, Roe AM, Locke-Edmunds JC, et al. Flap-valve theory of anorectal continence. *Br J Surg.* 1986;73(12):1012–1014.
9. Bauer JJ, Gerlent IM, Salky B, et al. Sexual dysfunction following proctocolectomy for benign disease of the colon and rectum. *Ann Surg.* 1983;197(3):363–367.
10. Bernstein WC. What are hemorrhoids and what is their relationship to the portal venous system? *Dis Colon Rectum.* 1983;26(12):829–834.
11. Block IR, Enquist IF. Studies pertaining to local spread of carcinoma of the rectum in females. *Surg Gynecol Obstet.* 1961;112:41–46.
12. Bollard RC, Gardiner A, Lindow S, et al. Normal female anal sphincter: difficulties in interpretation explained. *Dis Colon Rectum.* 2002;45(2):171–175.
13. Boxall TA, Smart PJ, Griffiths JD. The blood-supply of the distal segment of the rectum in anterior resection. *Br J Surg.* 1963;50:399–404.
14. Brauss H, Elze C. *Anatomie des Menschen.* 3rd ed. Berlin, Germany: Springer; 1956.
15. Burnham WR, Lennard-Jones JE, Brooke BN. Sexual problems among married ileostomists: survey conducted by the Ileostomy Association of Great Britain and Ireland. *Gut.* 1977;18(8):673–677.
16. Cantlie J. The sigmoid flexure in health and disease. *J Trop Med Hyg.* 1915;18:1–7.

17. Cawthorn SJ, Parums DV, Gibbs NM, et al. Extent of mesorectal spread and involvement of lateral resection margin as prognostic factors after surgery for rectal cancer. *Lancet*. 1990;335(8697):1055–1059.

18. Chapuis P, Bokey L, Fahrer M, et al. Mobilization of the rectum: anatomic concepts and the bookshelf revisited. *Dis Colon Rectum*. 2002;45(1):1–8.

19. Chiari H. Über die Nalen Divertik Fel der Rectum-schleimhaut und Ihre Beziehung zu den anal fisteln. *Wien Med Press*. 1878;19:1482.

20. Church JM, Raudkivi PJ, Hill GL. The surgical anatomy of the rectum—a review with particular relevance to the hazards of rectal mobilisation. *Int J Colorectal Dis*. 1987;2(3):158–166.

21. Courtney H. The posterior subsphincteric space: its relation to posterior horseshoe fistula. *Surg Gynecol Obstet*. 1949;89(2):222–226.

22. Courtney H. Anatomy of the pelvic diaphragm and anorectal musculature as related to sphincter preservation in anorectal surgery. *Am J Surg*. 1950;79(1):155–173.

23. Crapp AR, Cuthbertson AM. William Waldeyer and the rectosacral fascia. *Surg Gynecol Obstet*. 1974;138(2):252–256.

24. Cuesta MA, Meijer S, Derksen EJ, et al. Anal sphincter imaging in fecal incontinence using endosonography. *Dis Colon Rectum*. 1992;35(1):59–63.

25. Danzi M, Ferulano GP, Abate S, et al. Male sexual function after abdominoperineal resection for rectal cancer. *Dis Colon Rectum*. 1983;26(10):665–668.

26. Dickstein G, Boley SJ. Colonic ischemia. In: Zuidema GD, ed. *Shackelford's Surgery of the Alimentary Tract*. Philadelphia, PA: WB Saunders; 1991:84–94.

27. Didio LJ, Diaz-Franco C, Schemainda R, et al. Morphology of the middle rectal arteries. A study of 30 cadaveric dissections. *Surg Radiol Anat*. 1986;8(4):229–236.

28. Drummond H. Some points relating to the surgical anatomy of the arterial supply of the large intestine. *Proc R Soc Med*. 1913;7(surg sect):185–193.

29. Drummond H. The arterial supply of the rectum and pelvic colon. *Br J Surg*. 1914;1:677–685.

30. Duthie HL, Gairns FW. Sensory nerve-endings and sensation in the anal region in man. *Br J Surg*. 1960;47(206):585–595.

31. Ewing MR. The significance of the level of the peritoneal reflection in the surgery of rectal cancer. *Br J Surg*. 1952;39(158):495–500.

32. Ewing MR. The white line of Hilton. *Proc R Soc Med*. 1954;47(7):525–530.

33. Farouk R, Duthie GS, Bartolo DC. Functional anorectal disorders and physiological evaluation. In: Beck DE, Wexner SD, eds. *Fundamentals of Anorectal Surgery*. New York, NY: McGraw-Hill; 1992:68–88.

34. Fisher DF Jr, Fry WJ. Collateral mesenteric circulation. *Surg Gynecol Obstet*. 1987;164(5):487–492.

35. Fraser ID, Condon RE, Schulte WJ, et al. Longitudinal muscle of muscularis externa in human and nonhuman primate colon. *Arch Surg*. 1981;116(1):61–63.

36. Frenckner B, Euler CV. Influence of pudendal block on the function of the anal sphincters. *Gut*. 1975;16(6):482–489.

37. Fritsch H, Brenner E, Lienemann A, et al. Anal sphincter complex: reinterpreted morphology and its clinical relevance. *Dis Colon Rectum*. 2002;45:188–194.

38. Garavoglia M, Borghi F, Levi AC. Arrangement of the anal striated musculature. *Dis Colon Rectum*. 1993;36(1):10–15.

39. Gerstenberg TC, Nielsen ML, Clausen S, et al. Bladder function after abdominoperineal resection of the rectum for anorectal cancer. Urodynamic investigation before and after operative in a consecutive series. *Am J Surg*. 1980;191(1):81–86.

40. Gibbons CP, Trowbridge EA, Bannister JJ, et al. Role of anal cushions in maintaining continence. *Lancet*. 1986;1(8486):886–888.

41. Goligher JC. *Surgery of the Anus, Rectum and Colon*. London, United Kingdom: Baillière Tindall; 1984:1–47.

42. Goligher JC, Leacock AG, Brossy JJ. The surgical anatomy of the anal canal. *Br J Surg*. 1955;43(177):51–61.

43. Gordon PH. Anorectal anatomy and physiology. *Gastroenterol Clin North Am*. 2001;30(1):1–13.

44. Griffiths JD. Surgical anatomy of the blood supply of the distal colon. *Ann R Coll Surg Engl*. 1956;19(4):241–256.

45. Griffiths JD. Extramural and intramural blood supply of the colon. *BMJ*. 1961;1(5222):322–326.

46. Grüner OP, Naas R, Fretheim B, et al. Marital status and sexual adjustment after colectomy. Results in 178 patients operated on for ulcerative colitis. *Scand J Gastroenterol*. 1977;12(2):193–197.

47. Guttormson NL, Bubrick MP. Mortality from ischemic colitis. *Dis Colon Rectum*. 1989;32(6):469–472.

48. Guyton AC, ed. *Textbook of Medical Physiology*. 7th ed. Philadelphia, PA: WB Saunders; 1986:754–769.

49. Haas PA, Fox TA Jr. The importance of the perianal connective tissue in the surgical anatomy and function of the anus. *Dis Colon Rectum*. 1977;20(4):303–313.

50. Haller A. The large intestine. In: Cullen W, ed. *First Lines of Physiology*. [Reprint of the 1786 edition.] Sources of Science 32. New York, NY: Johnson Reprint Corporation; 1966:139–140.

51. Harnsberger AM, Vernava AM III, Longo WE, et al. The utility of the anorectal physiology lab in influencing clinical decision making. *Dis Colon Rectum*. 1993;36:11–12.

52. Heald RJ, Husband EM, Ryall RD. The mesorectum in rectal cancer surgery—the clue to pelvic recurrence? *Br J Surg*. 1982;69(10):613–616.

53. Houston J. Observations on the mucous membrane of the rectum. *Dublin Hosp Rep Communications Med Surg*. 1830;5:158–165.

54. Hyrtl J. *Handbuch der topographischen Anatomie und ihrer praktisch medicinisch-chirurgischen Anwendungen*. Vol 2. 4th ed. Wien, Germany: Braumüller; 1860.

55. Jamieson JK, Dobson JF. The lymphatics of the colon. *Proc R Soc Med*. 1909;2(surg sect):149–174.

56. Jorge JM, Habr-Gama A. The value of sphincter asymmetry index in anal incontinence. *Int J Colorectal Dis*. 2000;15(5–6):303–310.

57. Jorge JM, Habr-Gama A, Souza AS Jr, et al. Rectal surgery complicated by massive presacral hemorrhage. *Arq Bras Circ Dig*. 1990;5:92–95.

58. Jorge JM, Wexner SD. Etiology and management of fecal incontinence. *Dis Colon Rectum*. 1993;36(1):77–97.

59. Kaiser AM, Ortega AE. Anorectal anatomy. *Surg Clin North Am*. 2002;82:1125–1138.

60. Klosterhalfen B, Vogel P, Rixen H, et al. Topography of the inferior rectal artery: a possible cause of chronic, primary anal fissure. *Dis Colon Rectum*. 1989;32(1):43–52.

61. Kumar D, Phillips SF. The contribution of external ligamentous attachments to function of the ileocecal junction. *Dis Colon Rectum*. 1987;30(6):410–416.

62. Landreneau RJ, Fry WJ. The right colon as a target organ of nonocclusive mesenteric ischemia. Case report and review of the literature. *Arch Surg*. 1990;125(5):591–594.

63. Lawson JO. Pelvic anatomy. II. Anal canal and associated sphincters. *Ann R Coll Surg Engl*. 1974;54(6):288–300.

64. Lee EC, Dowling BL. Perimuscular excision of the rectum for Crohn's disease and ulcerative colitis. A conservation technique. *Br J Surg*. 1972;59(1):29–32.

65. Lestar B, Penninckx F, Kerremans R. The composition of anal basal pressure. An in vivo and in vitro study in man. *Int J Colorectal Dis*. 1989;4(2):118–122.

66. Levi AC, Borghi F, Garavoglia M. Development of the anal canal muscles. *Dis Colon Rectum*. 1991;34(3):262–266.

67. Liebermann-Meffert D. Anatomie des gastrooesophagealen Verschluborgans. In: Blum AL, Siewert JR, eds. *Refluxtherapie*. New York, NY: Springer; 1981.

68. Lilius HG. Fistula-in-ano, an investigation of human foetal anal ducts and intramuscular glands and a clinical study of 150 patients. *Acta Chir Scand Suppl*. 1968;383:7–88.

69. Lindsey I, Guy RJ, Warren BF, et al. Anatomy of Denonvilliers' fascia and pelvic nerves, impotence, and implications for the colorectal surgeon. *Br J Surg*. 2000;87(10):1288–1299.

70. Lindstrom BL. The value of the collateral circulation from the inferior mesenteric artery in obliteration of the lower abdominal aorta. *Acta Chir Scand*. 1950;100(4):367–374.

71. Longo WE, Ballantyne GH, Gursberg RJ. Ischemic colitis: patterns and prognosis. *Dis Colon Rectum*. 1992;35(8):726–730.

72. Lunniss PJ, Phillips RK. Anatomy and function of the anal longitudinal muscle. *Br J Surg*. 1992;79:882–884.

73. Mayo WJ. A study of the rectosigmoid. *Surg Gynecol Obstet*. 1917;25:616–621.

74. McVay CB. *Anson and McVay Surgical Anatomy*. Philadelphia, PA: WB Saunders; 1984:565–777.

75. Metcalf AM, Dozois RR, Kelly KA. Sexual function in women after proctocolectomy. *Ann Surg*. 1986;204(6):624–627.

76. Meyers MA. Griffiths' point: critical anastomosis at the splenic flexure. Significance in ischemia of the colon. *AJR Am J Roentgenol*. 1976;126(1):77–94.

77. Michels NA, Siddharth P, Kornblith PL, et al. The variant blood supply to the small and large intestines: its importance in regional resections. A new anatomic study based on four hundred dissections with a complete review of the literature. *J Int Colorectal Surg*. 1963;39:127–170.

78. Miller R, Bartolo DC, Cervero F, et al. Anorectal sampling: a comparison of normal and incontinent patients. *Br J Surg*. 1988;75(1):44–47.

79. Milligan ET, Morgan CN. Surgical anatomy of the anal canal: with special reference to anorectal fistulae. *Lancet.* 1934;2:1150–1156.

80. Miscusi G, Masoni L, Dell'Anna A, et al. Normal lymphatic drainage of the rectum and the anal canal revealed by lymphoscintigraphy. *Coloproctology.* 1987;9:171–174.

81. Morgado PJ. Total mesorectal excision: a misnomer for a sound surgical approach. *Dis Colon Rectum.* 1998;41(1):120–121.

82. Morren GL, Beets-Tan RG, van Engelshoven JM. Anatomy of the anal canal and perianal structures as defined by phased-array magnetic resonance imaging. *Br J Surg.* 2001;88(11):1506–1512.

83. Morson BC, Dawson IM. *Gastrointestinal Pathology.* Oxford, United Kingdom: Blackwell Scientific Publications; 1972:603–606.

84. Moskowitz M, Zimmerman H, Felson H. The meandering mesenteric artery of the colon. *Am J Roentgenol Radium Ther Nucl Med.* 1964;92:1088–1099.

85. Nano M, Dal Corso HM, Lanfranco G, et al. Contribution to the surgical anatomy of the ligaments of the rectum. *Dis Colon Rectum.* 2000;43(11):1592–1597.

86. Nivatvongs S, Gordon PH. Surgical anatomy. In: Gordon PH, Nivatvongs S, eds. *Principle and Practice of Surgery for the Colon, Rectum and Anus.* St. Louis, MO: Quality Medical Publishing; 1992:3–37.

87. Nobles VP. The development of the human anal canal. *J Anat.* 1984;138:575.

88. O'Beirne J, ed. *New Views of the Process of Defecation and Their Application to the Pathology and Treatment of Diseases of the Stomach, Bowels and Other Organs.* Dublin, Ireland: Hodges and Smith; 1833.

89. Oh C, Kark AE. Anatomy of the external anal sphincter. *Br J Surg.* 1972;59(9):717–723.

90. Orkin BA. Rectal carcinoma: treatment. In: Beck DE, Wexner SD, eds. *Fundamentals of Anorectal Surgery.* New York, NY: McGraw-Hill; 1992:260–369.

91. Otis WJ. Some observations on the structure of the rectum. *J Anat Physiol.* 1897;32(pt 1):59–63.

92. Paramore RH. The Hunterian lectures on the evolution of the pelvic floor in non-mammalian vertebrates and pronograde mammals. *Lancet.* 1910;175(4526):1459–1467.

93. Parks AG. Pathogenesis and treatment of fistula-in-ano. *BMJ.* 1961;1(5224):463–469.

94. Parks AG, Porter NH, Hardcastle J. The syndrome of the descending perineum. *Proc R Soc Med.* 1966;59(6):477–482.

95. Pemberton JH. Anatomy and physiology of the anus and rectum. In: Zuidema GD, ed. *Shackelford's Surgery of the Alimentary Tract.* Philadelphia, PA: WB Saunders; 1991:242–273.

96. Percy JP, Swash M, Neill ME, et al. Electrophysiological study of motor nerve supply of pelvic floor. *Lancet.* 1981;1(8210):16–17.

97. Quirke P, Durdey P, Dixon MF, et al. Local recurrence of rectal adenocarcinoma due to inadequate surgical resection. Histopathological study of lateral tumour spread and surgical excision. *Lancet.* 1986;2(8514):996–999.

98. Romolo JL. Congenital lesions: intussusception and volvulus. In: Zuidema GD, ed. *Shackelford's Surgery of the Alimentary Tract.* Philadelphia, PA: WB Saunders; 1991:45–51.

99. Roux C. Contribution to the knowledge of the anal muscles in man. *Arch Mikr Anat.* 1881;19:721–723.

100. Russell KP. Anatomy of the pelvic floor, rectum and anal canal. In: Smith LE, ed. *Practical Guide to Anorectal Testing.* New York, NY: Igaku-Shoin Medical Publishers; 1991:744–747.

101. Shafik A. A new concept of the anatomy of the anal sphincter mechanism and the physiology of defecation. The external anal sphincter: a triple-loop system. *Invest Urol.* 1975;12(5):412–419.

102. Shafik A. A new concept of the anatomy of the anal sphincter mechanism and the physiology of defecation. II. Anatomy of the levator ani muscle with special reference to puborectalis. *Invest Urol.* 1975;13(3):175–182.

103. Shafik A. A new concept of the anatomy of the anal sphincter mechanism and the physiology of defecation. III. The longitudinal anal muscle: anatomy and role in sphincter mechanism. *Invest Urol.* 1976;13(4):271–277.

104. Shafik A. A concept of the anatomy of the anal sphincter mechanism and the physiology of defecation. *Dis Colon Rectum.* 1987;30(12):970–982.

105. Sieglbauer F. *Lehrbuch der normalen Anatomie des Menschen.* 9th ed. Wien, Germany: Urban und Schwartzenberg; 1963.

106. Skandalakis JE, Gray SW, Ricketts R. The colon and rectum. In: Skandalakis JE, Gray SW, eds. *Embryology for Surgeons: The Embryological Basis for the Treatment of Congenital Anomalies.* Baltimore, MD: Williams & Wilkins; 1994:242–281.

107. Sonneland J, Anson BJ, Beaton LE. Surgical anatomy of the arterial supply to the colon from the superior mesenteric artery based upon a study of 600 specimens. *Surg Gynecol Obstet.* 1958;106(4):385–398.

108. Stelzner F. Die Verschlubsysteme am Magen-Darm-Kanal und ihre chirurgische Bedeutung. *Acta Chir Aust.* 1987;19:565–569.

109. Steward JA, Rankin FW. Blood supply of the large intestine: its surgical considerations. *Arch Surg.* 1933;26(5):843–891.

110. Stoss F. Investigations of the muscular architecture of the rectosigmoid junction in humans. *Dis Colon Rectum.* 1990;33(5):378–383.

111. Sudeck P. Über die Gefassversorgung des Mastdarmes in Hinsicht auf die Operative Gangran. *Munch Med Wochenschr.* 1907;54:1314.

112. Swash M. Histopathology of pelvic floor muscles in pelvic floor disorders. In: Henry MM, Swash M, eds. *Coloproctology and the Pelvic Floor.* London, United Kingdom: Butterworth-Heinemann; 1992:173–183.

113. Tjandra JJ, Milsom JW, Stolfi VM, et al. Endoluminal ultrasound defines anatomy of the anal canal and pelvic floor. *Dis Colon Rectum.* 1992;35(5):465–470.

114. Tobin CE, Benjamin JA. Anatomical and surgical restudy of Denonvilliers' fascia. *Surg Gynecol Obstet.* 1945;80:373–388.

115. Torsoli A, Ramorino ML, Crucioli V. The relationships between anatomy and motor activity of the colon. *Am J Dig Dis.* 1968;13(5):462–467.

116. Wakeley CP. The position of the vermiform appendix as ascertained by an analysis of 10,000 cases. *J Anat.* 1983;67(pt 2):277–283.

117. Walsh PC, Schlegel PN. Radical pelvic surgery with preservation of sexual function. *Ann Surg.* 1988;208(4):391–400.

118. Wang Q, Shi W, Zhao Y, et al. New concepts in severe presacral hemorrhage during proctectomy. *Arch Surg.* 1985;120(9):1013–1020.

119. Weinstein M, Roberts M. Sexual potency following surgery for rectal carcinoma. A follow-up of 44 patients. *Ann Surg.* 1977;185(3):295–300.

120. Wendell-Smith CP. *Studies on the Morphology of the Pelvic Floor* [PhD thesis]. London, United Kingdom: University of London; 1967.

121. Wexner SD, Cheape JD, Jorge JM, et al. Prospective assessment of biofeedback for the treatment of paradoxical puborectalis contraction syndrome. *Dis Colon Rectum.* 1992;35(2):145–150.

122. Wexner SD, Daniel N, Jagelman DG. Colectomy for constipation: physiologic investigation is the key to success. *Dis Colon Rectum.* 1991;34(10):851–856.

123. Wexner SD, Jorge JM. Colorectal physiological tests: use or abuse of technology? *Eur J Surg.* 1994;160(3):167–174.

124. Williams AB, Bartram CI, Halligan S, et al. Endosonographic anatomy of the normal anal compared with endocoil magnetic resonance imaging. *Dis Colon Rectum.* 2002;45(2):176–183.

125. Williamson RCN, Mortensen NJMcC. Anatomy of the large intestine. In: Kirsner JB, Shorter RG, eds. *Diseases of the Colon, Rectum and Anal Canal.* Baltimore, MD: Williams & Wilkins; 1987:1–22.

126. Wilson PM. Anchoring mechanisms of the anorectal region. *S Afr Med J.* 1967;41:1138–1143.

127. Wood BA, Kelly AJ. Anatomy of the anal sphincters and pelvic floor. In: Henry MM, Swash M, eds. *Coloproctology and the Pelvic Floor.* London, United Kingdom: Butterworth-Heinemann; 1992:3–19.

128. Zama N, Fazio VW, Jagelman DG, et al. Efficacy of pelvic packing in maintaining hemostasis after rectal excision for cancer. *Dis Colon Rectum.* 1988;31(12):923–928.

2

Physiology of the Colon

Eric J. Daniels and Marvin L. Corman

Man and the animals are merely
a passage and channel for food,
a tomb for other animals,
a haven for the dead,
giving life by the death of others,
a coffer full of corruption.
—LEONARDO DA VINCI: *Codice Atlantico,* 76

The study of large bowel physiology has historically been overshadowed by concerted efforts to comprehend the workings of the stomach and small intestine. Despite this indifference, which is perhaps in part a consequence of the knowledge that human beings can thrive in the absence of a colon, we have become aware that the large intestine is responsible for maintaining important homeostatic functions. The primary physiologic purposes of the large bowel include the following: further breakdown of ingested materials by microfloral metabolism, absorption of water and electrolytes, secretion of electrolytes and mucus, storage of semisolid matter, and propulsion of feces toward the rectum and anus. These colonic functions act in concert to respond to the needs of the body while concomitantly producing fecal material suitable for evacuation. For example, although the digestive functions of the large bowel are dwarfed by the contributions of the small intestine, the absorptive and secretory capacities of the colonic mucosa are critical for regulating the intraluminal fluid volume and contributing to serum electrolyte balance. In addition, the role of the colon in intermittent storage and propulsion of semisolid matter is central to normal defecation and is the consequence of complex neural and hormonal interactions. The purpose of this chapter is to present a current, general view of normal large bowel physiology to facilitate the discussion of colonic pathophysiologic processes presented subsequently.

► FUNCTIONAL CLASSIFICATION

The large bowel is approximately 150 cm (5 ft) in length and consists of the vermiform appendix, cecum, colon (ascending, transverse, descending, sigmoid), and rectum. This somewhat arbitrary segmentation of the large bowel is not strictly anatomic because it is widely appreciated that the large intestine is a heterogeneous organ with regional, biochemical, pharmacologic, and thus functional differences.

Cecum and Ascending Colon (Right Colon)

Digested material entering the large intestine at the ileocecal junction remains in the cecum and right colon for an extended period. Here, the resting propulsion rate is only 1 cm/hour.[96] This retention and mixing of ileal effluent permit aerobic and anaerobic metabolism of residual carbohydrate and protein by the intestinal flora, thereby producing multiple by-products, most of which are then absorbed through the remaining colon. In addition to being the primary site for bacterial fermentation, the ascending colon (along with the transverse colon) is involved in regulating intraluminal fluid volume as well as sodium and water absorption.[37,38] The importance of these colonic functions can be appreciated by reviewing recorded motility patterns, which demonstrate frequent retropulsive waves extending from the transverse colon back toward the cecum.[15,96]

Transverse Colon

The transverse colon is generally believed to serve as a rapid conduit between the proximal (right) and distal (left) components of the large bowel. This belief is supported by the finding that the basal electrical rhythm and muscle-generated pressure waves in this segment occur with a greater frequency than is identified in the right colon. This observation suggests a rapid, propulsive function.[19,118,122] As mentioned previously, the transverse colon is also an important site for sodium and water absorption, a function that is critical to volume regulation.

Left Colon

The left colon is the site for final modulation of intraluminal contents before evacuation. The diminished rate of fluid and electrolyte transfer seen in the descending colon is ultimately a result of distinct protein ion channels in the luminal (apical) and serosal (basolateral) membranes of mucosal cells, which exhibit different biochemical and pharmacologic properties when compared with those of the ascending colon. The distal large intestine also is thought to exhibit a reservoir function or storage capacity, which some believe is important in maintaining anal continence. Although the concept is somewhat controversial, it theoretically relies on the physical barrier of the sigmoid angulations and myoelectrical differences between the sigmoid colon and rectum. This is discussed later. With respect to the rectum, in vitro studies have demonstrated that little or no net absorption occurs there.[37,38]

▶ DIGESTION

Digestion within the large bowel is an often overlooked issue, given the enormous capacity of the small intestine in this regard. However, despite its poorly recognized participation in the breakdown of foodstuffs to fulfill energy requirements, the healthy colon is capable of salvaging calories from poorly absorbed carbohydrates and proteins.

Flora of the Large Intestine

The digestive processes of the colon are a consequence of the microorganisms that colonize the bowel and thereby participate in a symbiotic relationship with the host. Whereas yeast and other fungi are normally present in very small numbers,[30] bacteria clearly dominate the lumen. In humans, the large intestine is the primary site of bacterial colonization, with more than 400 different species of bacteria identified.[46] Bacterial colonization begins in infancy and occurs predominantly in the cecum and right colon. Studies reveal up to 10^{12} bacteria per gram of wet feces.[103] Given this amount, it is not surprising that bacteria make up 40% to 55% of fecal solids in individuals consuming a typical Western diet.[113]

The primary tasks of gut flora can be divided into metabolic, trophic, and protective functions. Metabolic functions include fermentation of nondigestible dietary residue and endogenous mucus, production of short-chain fatty acids (SCFAs), and production of vitamin K. Trophic functions include controlling epithelial cell proliferation and differentiation as well as homoeostasis of the immune system. The protective activity of the colonic flora stems from the ability to serve as a barrier to colonization against pathogens. Although these functions are robust in healthy individuals, a breakdown of the dynamic relationship between the gut flora and its host may lead to disease states.

Guarner and Malagelada reviewed the role of gut flora in health and disease.[58] The authors note that a dysfunction in the barrier activity of gut flora can result in the translocation of many viable microorganisms, particularly the gram-negative aerobic genera. Once beyond the epithelial reef, the organisms can travel to extraintestinal organs via the lymphatic highway.[58] Dissemination of enteric bacteria can lead to sepsis, shock, multisystem organ failure, and ultimately death of the patient. The rates of positive blood cultures are significantly higher in individuals with conditions such as intestinal obstruction and inflammatory bowel disease.[74] O'Boyle and colleagues reported that bacterial translocation is associated with an increase in postoperative sepsis.[88] In addition to translocation of bacteria, gut flora have been implicated to play an active role in carcinogenesis and inflammatory bowel disease. Bacteria belonging to the *Bacteroides* and *Clostridium* genera have been shown to increase the incidence of tumor formation in laboratory animals.[65] In patients with Crohn's disease and ulcerative colitis, there is increased secretion of immunoglobulin G, a class of antibody that can damage intestinal mucosa through activation of the complement cascade.[12,77]

Within the complex ecosystem of the large intestine, certain groups of bacteria thrive over others. In principle, those able to transform variable amounts and types of substrate into energy are likely to be present in large proportions. Although *Bacteroides* organisms (gram-negative rods) are most commonly identified, the gram-positive *Eubacterium* and *Bifidobacterium* are also present in large numbers, along with several gram-positive cocci and *Clostridium* species.[30,46,84] It is axiomatic that the surgeon's knowledge of normal colonic flora is paramount to proper antibiotic management for both prophylactic and postoperative situations.

Substrates for Fermentation

Nondigestible Starch

To appreciate the end products of bacterial fermentation, one must first look at the substrate that passes through the ileocecal junction and is presented to the microorganisms. Quantitatively, the most important is nonhydrolyzed or resistant starch. Christl and colleagues performed breath hydrogen and methane studies using whole-body calorimetry to measure undigested polysaccharide reaching the large intestine.[23] The authors noted that starch is to some degree incompletely digested in the small bowel and is passed to the ascending colon. Others have confirmed this observation.[44,73] Generally, it is accepted that approximately 10% of ingested starch will elude small bowel digestion to reach the colon and be available for fermentation in individuals consuming a Western diet.[30]

Nonstarch Polysaccharides

Nonstarch polysaccharides represent another class of substrate available for bacterial metabolism. These molecules are the derivatives of plant material and include cellulose as well as noncellulose substrates. The degree of nonstarch polysaccharide metabolism is dependent on several physiologic circumstances. For example, the smaller and more hydrophilic the substrate, the more readily digestible it is.[62,112] This and other physiologic variables, such as transit time, ultimately determine the extent of cellulose and noncellulose breakdown by the resident flora. Topping and Clifton contrasted the role of resistant starch and nondigestible starch in human colonic function.[117] The authors viewed the actions of resistant starch and nondigestible starch in the context of a balance between luminal passage and fermentation. Fiber-rich foods, with a high content of insoluble nonstarch polysaccharides, are not as fermentable by microflora. As such, fiber-rich foods serve well as laxatives. On the other hand, most resistant starches are readily fermentable by large bowel microflora, giving rise to the SCFAs discussed later. Topping and Clifton state that the greatest difference between resistant starches and nonstarch polysaccharides lies in relation to cancer risk.[117] The authors report that whereas the protective effect of resistant starches to chemically induced cancers is inconsistent in small animals,[7,61] there exist strong epidemiologic data pointing to a negative relationship between total starch consumption and large bowel neoplasms.[111,116] However, evidence of a discrete benefit for fiber is not as strong, with several low-risk populations ingesting little fiber.[63,71,89] The authors conclude that although the protective effect of resistant starch is encouraging, the limitations of methodology and small animal models cannot justify a recommendation to increase dietary levels at this time.

Other Substrates

Although most of the substrate made available to the colonic bacteria consists of the starch and nonstarch polysaccharides mentioned earlier, other substances do pass into the cecum and are subsequently metabolized. For example, sugar and sugar alcohols, such as lactose, raffinose, lactulose, and sorbitol, are readily metabolized by the bowel microorganisms.[30,114] In addition to polysaccharides, various peptide substrates are made available for bacterial digestion. Poorly absorbed protein sources include elastin, collagen, and albumins, and most abundant are the pancreas-derived proteases.[30] In contrast, urea and ammonia are not generally available as nitrogen sources for the colonic flora.[48] Overall, the daily ileal effluent will make available 6 to 18 g of nitrogen-containing compounds for bacterial fermentation, compared with 8 to 40 g of carbohydrate.[30]

Products of Bacterial Metabolism

The principal products of microorganism fermentation of polysaccharides in the large bowel are SCFAs or volatile fatty acids. The production of SCFAs decreases from the proximal to the distal colon, an observation that can be most likely attributed to the different bacterial populations in these regions. These fatty acids contain from one to six carbons and are the predominant colonic anions. The three most abundant are acetate, propionate, and butyrate, with their production accounting for up to 95% of total SCFA generation.[30]

It has long been thought that dietary intake should have profound effects on fermentation products. However, several investigators have noted that variations in diet have only a minimal effect on SCFA production. Saunders and Wiggins employed three different sugars—mannitol, lactulose, and raffinose—and measured SCFA production.[107] They found no significant variability among the different sugar substrates. This finding has been confirmed by others through a variety of fermentation substrates, including wheat bran.[29] Based on these metabolic studies, it has been calculated that the conversion for the amount of SCFAs produced per unit weight of carbohydrate is 50%.

Short-Chain Fatty Acid Absorption

More than 90% of SCFAs produced by bacterial fermentation are taken up by the colonic mucosal cells.[81,95] In small animal models, approximately 60% of the uptake is by simple diffusion of protonated, neutral SCFA. The remainder of uptake (ionized SCFA) occurs by active, cellular uptake.[47] However, the mechanism for uptake by the colonic epithelium remains unresolved. It is clear, however, that the absorption mechanism differs from that of the long-chain fatty acids absorbed in the small intestine. For example, long-chain fatty acids require emulsification with bile salts.

Experimental models have been used to attempt to clarify the transport mechanisms involved. A large body of evidence exists pointing to the passive diffusion of these fatty acids toward the serosa.[24,105] As mentioned earlier, SCFAs are weak acids with negative logs of dissociation constant ranging from 4.75 to 4.87, and most of these molecules exist in their ionized form at a pH higher than 5. As charged species, the SCFAs would be unable to traverse the hydrophobic environment of the apical membrane. However, studies of the mammalian gastrointestinal tract have shown SCFAs to be absorbed rapidly at a pH of 7.[2] In light of this apparent contradiction, some investigators have pursued the possible protonization (binding of a hydrogen ion) of the anionic form of the SCFA, rendering the molecule neutral and thus better able to cross the lipophilic membrane. One proposed mechanism is that protons are generated from the conversion of carbon dioxide and water by intramucosal carbonic anhydrase. This would account for the accumulation of bicarbonate seen with SCFA absorption.[4,104] An additional source of protons may be found in the presence of a sodium ion-proton antiport (exchange), an idea supported by the fact that SCFA absorption has been reported to increase sodium and water absorption.[105] Using in situ perfusion of guinea pig colon, Oltmer and von Engelhardt reported that inhibition of the apical proton antiport and carbonic anhydrase systems resulted in decreased SCFA absorption.[90] Although neither of these mechanisms can completely explain SCFA absorption, their existence is consistent with the fact that SCFA transport is associated with increased luminal pH, increased bicarbonate ion concentration, and enhanced sodium absorption.[60]

Outside of the passive mechanisms discussed earlier, the presence of an apical, carrier-mediated anionic exchange involving SCFAs and bicarbonate ion has been suggested.[79,121] Harig and colleagues used human luminal vesicles to investigate the transport of N-butyrate.[60] The authors found that butyrate transport was minimal in the presence of an inward pH gradient but significantly increased by an outward bicarbonate ion gradient. Furthermore, the effects of sodium and chloride on transport were negligible. The authors concluded that the primary mechanism for butyrate transport appears to be through a bicarbonate-SCFA antiport system independent of sodium transport or bicarbonate-chloride anion exchange. As more becomes known about the mechanisms of SCFA transport, it is increasingly clear that this function is a heterogeneous one, with observed segmental differences.[86,110]

Additional investigations are being conducted on the transport mechanisms responsible for SCFA absorption. This interest is being stimulated by the potential utility of such knowledge in clinical situations, such as promoting caloric intake in patients with short-bowel syndrome, developing SCFA enemas for patients with ulcerative colitis, and understanding mechanisms underlying diarrhea and even colonic neoplasms.

Physiologic Actions of Short-Chain Fatty Acids

The SCFAs produced as a result of bacterial fermentation of poorly absorbed polysaccharides play several important roles in large bowel function. SCFAs are relatively weak acids. Therefore, higher concentrations of SCFAs lower the luminal pH. Lower pH values can alter the growth profiles of pH-sensitive pathogenic bacteria such as *Escherichia coli* and *Salmonella*.[20] As such, SCFAs have been shown to assist in the treatment of infectious diarrhea. Furthermore, elevation of fecal SCFAs has been shown to diminish the fluid loss and speed of remission during the active phase of cholera.[94]

These acids are readily absorbed by the columnar epithelium, as discussed earlier.[13,27,28] Once absorbed, the SCFAs have been reported to contribute up to 7% of the basal metabolic requirements of humans.[28] In fact, the colonic epithelium derives almost 75% of its energy needs from these fatty acids through metabolism to carbon dioxide, ketone bodies, and lipid precursors.[100,101] In addition to luminal nutrition, SCFAs have been investigated for their anti-inflammatory properties as well as their antitumor effects.[1] They have also been shown to increase regional blood flow and have a demonstrable effect upon gastrointestinal muscular activity. Rectal infusion of SCFA into human surgical patients leads to a 1.5- to 5-fold increase in splanchnic blood flow as well as to a decrease in gastric tone leading to volume expansion.[85,102] Additionally, the absorption of SCFAs is tied closely to the transport of bicarbonate, sodium, and water, thus providing a mechanism for the regulation of intraluminal volume.[82,108]

Other Products of Noncarbohydrate Fermentation

The fermentation of peptides by microorganisms results in substances such as SCFAs, branched-chain fatty acids, isobutyrate, and methylbutyrate. However, not all end products of peptide metabolism are of benefit to the organism. For example, the deamination of amino acids gives rise to ammonia, which has been demonstrated to have toxic effects on colonic epithelium by altering normal cell metabolism.[123,127] In addition, the catabolism of amino acids results in the production of phenols, indoles, and amines, which have been implicated in disease states such as hepatic coma and colorectal cancer.[39,40,91]

Conclusion

The digestive processes that take place in the large bowel are clearly focused on the activities of the colonic flora. The surgeon's interest in these normal metabolic processes is obvious because disruption of this otherwise stable community by either pathologic or surgical intervention may lead to disease states discussed later in this text.

▶ COLONIC ABSORPTION AND SECRETION

The absorption and secretion of water, mucus, and electrolytes, particularly sodium, are complex and central processes of normal colonic activity. These processes determine the electrolyte and volume content of feces. However, the capacity of the colon to absorb and digest material is not uniform, with the proximal mucosa exhibiting different properties from its distal counterpart. Although colonic epithelium does not participate in active glucose or amino acid absorption,[9] as occurs in the small intestine, the mechanistic and functional segmental differences of these cells are of importance to the surgeon because the diverse colonic resection procedures have various consequences. As with the evaluation of absorption and secretion in other organs, such as the small intestine and kidney, study of transport in the colon is directed toward an understanding of the epithelial phenomena.

Sodium Absorption

Animal studies have demonstrated that sodium movement across the colonic wall involves overcoming two opposing forces. First, a formidable concentration gradient opposes the movement of sodium. This is a consequence of the higher sodium concentration of plasma in comparison with the colonic lumen.[126] In addition to the uphill concentration gradient, measurement of the transmural potential differences reveals an electronegative lumen (5 to 15 mV), which serves to retard the movement of sodium across the membrane.[31] Despite these two forces, measurements of normal daily fecal water show 1 to 5 mEq of sodium, representing more than 90% absorption of the 200 mEq of sodium found in the ileal effluent.[95,108] One must conclude from these perfusion studies that sodium transport is an active process.

Transport Mechanisms
Electrogenic Transport

The movement of sodium across a membrane resulting in a separation of charge is a common method of sodium transport widely known to be active in small intestine and kidney epithelia. This type of transport has also been reported to be present in the distal human colon.[26,57] The mechanism involves the movement of sodium from the lumen into the mucosal cell down an electrochemical gradient. The sodium ions, unable to permeate the phospholipid membrane, pass through protein channels characterized by their sensitivity to amiloride, a sodium transport blocker and aldosterone antagonist.[125] These amiloride-sensitive epithelial sodium channels consist of three homologous subunits—α, β, and γ—with a small unitary conductance of approximately 5 picosiemens (pS).[75] The permeability of sodium across the apical membrane is dependent on several physiologic factors. One is the intracellular sodium concentration, shown to be inversely related to apical membrane sodium permeability.[120] In order to ensure an adequate concentration difference, this value must be kept relatively low compared with the luminal sodium concentration. This challenge is met by the sodium/potassium-adenosine triphosphatase (ATPase) located on the basolateral aspect of the colonic epithelial cells. Therefore, the net movement of sodium across the colonic wall through this active mechanism is a combination of both apical and basolateral membrane activities. Thus, regulation of this method of transport can be targeted to either apical or basolateral processes.

Electroneutral Absorption

Bulk transport of sodium chloride in colonic epithelium is secondary to electroneutral absorption. Several lines of experimental evidence support the belief that this electroneutral process occurs primarily through the coupling of parallel, apical sodium-hydrogen and chloride-bicarbonate ion exchanges.[11] For example, the addition of a carbonic anhydrase inhibitor blocks the net flux of sodium and chloride, presumably by inhibiting the intracellular production of necessary protons and bicarbonate ions.[10] Further studies have indicated the existence of several types of sodium-hydrogen as well as chloride-bicarbonate exchanges, all having an impact on the electroneutral absorption of sodium chloride and mucosal pH in the colonic epithelium.[70]

Effects of Aldosterone

For decades, aldosterone has been known to have marked effects on epithelial transport activities, including but not limited to acceleration of sodium absorption and sodium/potassium-ATPase rates.[18,51,119,124] These effects are believed to be brought about primarily through stimulation of sodium absorption by the electrogenic mechanism discussed earlier. This belief coincides well with the fact that aldosterone has been repeatedly shown to increase the colonic transpotential differences.[41] As a steroid hormone, aldosterone crosses the cell membrane and binds to an intracellular receptor. This ligand-receptor interaction eventually leads to the events seen empirically. In the distal colon of animals treated with mineralocorticoids, a large increase in the β and γ subunits of amiloride-sensitive sodium channels is observed.[75] This upregulation of electroneutral sodium absorption is paralleled by downregulation of electrogenic absorption, shedding light on why no significant electrogenic sodium absorption is seen in the proximal colon, despite the presence of aldosterone receptors. Although much emphasis has been placed on the ability of aldosterone to augment sodium permeability and to increase the rate of ATPase activity, the specific roles played by aldosterone in mammalian tissue remain undefined.[80]

Segmental Heterogeneity

As stressed earlier in this chapter, the colon is anatomically and functionally segmented. The aforementioned mechanisms of sodium absorption and the effects of aldosterone on these actions have been elucidated primarily from studies of mammalian distal bowel. Investigations focused on mammalian proximal colon reveal differing modes of transport and regulation. For instance, studies of rat proximal colocytes using voltage clamp techniques have demonstrated that sodium absorption is electroneutral, yet no net chloride movement is measured.[49] In addition, the application of aldosterone upregulates sodium chloride electroneutral absorption, in clear contrast to the electrogenic induction seen in the distal colon.[49] These unique features, along with distinct mechanisms of transport seen in the rabbit proximal colon,[109] naturally raise many unanswered questions and underscore the lack of definitive sodium transport characterization. Consequently, the continuing investigation of colonic (specifically cecal) sodium transport is undoubtedly warranted.

Chloride Ion Absorption

The mechanism of chloride ion transport across the human colonic apical membrane remains without clear definition, appearing to result from several processes. Chloride absorption in the colon is generally accepted to occur by means of an energy-independent, passive mechanism.[5] This process relies on the negative charge of the ion and the diffusion potential generated by electrogenic sodium absorption. The presence of the chloride ion in an environment where the gastrointestinal lumen is electronegative establishes a force driving chloride across the apical membrane. Davis and coworkers, investigating human colon in vivo, opined that upward of 75% of total chloride absorption occurs via this favorable electrochemical gradient.[32] These authors believe that the remaining 25% occurs through an active, apical chloride-bicarbonate antiport. Additional evidence for the existence of this active antiport comes from multiple investigative approaches. These include perfusion studies demonstrating that filling the luminal space with a chloride solution results in a decrease in chloride ion concentration, with a concomitant increase in luminal bicarbonate ion concentration.[8] Furthermore, Mahajan and colleagues used a rapid millipore filtration

system to study the uptake of $^{36}Cl^-$ in human proximal colonic apical vesicles.[78] They found that luminally directed bicarbonate gradients stimulated the uptake of chloride ions and concluded that an electroneutral chloride-bicarbonate transport contributes to the primary mechanism of sodium chloride absorption in the human proximal colon. In rat distal colon, Rajendran and Binder described two distinct ion exchanges (chloride-bicarbonate and chloride-hydroxyl) as the mechanism responsible for chloride uptake.[93] The authors postulated that these two ion channels possess unique functional features, with one involved in chloride transcellular transport and the other concerned with intracellular pH maintenance.[93] Additional studies are needed to explore the detailed mechanism, regulation, and relative contributions of both active and passive chloride transport.

With respect to colonic chloride secretion, the cystic fibrosis transmembrane conductance regulator (CFTR) (mutated in patients with CF) is primarily responsible.[1] Numerous studies have demonstrated that CFTR is the primary chloride channel in airways, sweat ducts, and the colon. As such, patients with CF have mutations in CFTR and have impaired secretion of chloride as well as diminished absorption of sodium in the colon through modulation of the sodium electroneutral absorption mechanism.

Water Movement

One of the central functions of the large intestine is to control the level of fecal water. Average ileocecal flow for a healthy individual is approximately 1,500 to 2,000 mL/day.[33] Of this amount, only 100 to 150 mL of water appears in the stool. The colon harbors a tremendous reserve transport capacity and is capable of absorbing as much as 5 to 6 L over a 24-hour period if challenged.[33] Whereas water absorption is affected by the volume and flow of luminal contents, it is generally believed to follow the osmotic gradient established by the absorption of electrolytes.[33] For example, if the gastrointestinal lumen is perfused with a hypertonic mannitol solution, water will flow into the lumen, lending support to its passive movement.[8] Evidence suggests that intestinal aquaporin channels, as well as CFTR, may play a role in colonic fluid absorption and fecal dehydration.[1,68] Ultimately, regulating the amount of water absorption is accomplished by any mediator of luminal flow, fluid composition, or net electrolyte transport. A basic appreciation of colonic water-absorbing capacity is fundamental to the understanding of the possible causes of diarrhea.[92]

Bicarbonate Transport

As previously indicated in the discussion of sodium and chloride absorption, transport of bicarbonate ion across the apical membrane of colonic epithelium is generally considered a secretory process involving a chloride-bicarbonate ion antiport. To appreciate the mechanism of this system, the transmural potential difference and charged nature of the ion species must be considered. However, the measured intraluminal bicarbonate ion concentration is higher than can be generated by the available electrochemical forces under physiologic conditions. This suggests an energy-requiring secretory process.[80] Evidence for this active transport mechanism comes from experiments in which a significant reduction of chloride within the gastrointestinal lumen results in a reduced rate of bicarbonate secretion.[54] Clearly, the most likely source of the intracellular bicarbonate ion is the conversion of carbon dioxide and water by carbonic anhydrase, whose levels have been found to be elevated in colonic mucosal cells.[17]

Potassium Transport

The mechanisms of colonic potassium transport have historically been poorly defined and confusing. For example, perfusion studies have pointed to the passive absorption and secretion of potassium,[36,56] whereas other in vivo reports using small intraluminal dialysis bags found evidence against diffusion and in support of active mechanisms. However, since the mid-1990s, numerous efforts have been successfully undertaken to elucidate better the mechanisms involved in the movement of potassium. As with other colonic functions, the transport mechanisms associated with potassium transport have been found to be segmental, with proximal mucosal cells behaving distinctly from their distal counterparts.[25] Binder and Sandle have used this point to explain the inconsistency of previous in vivo perfusion studies, postulating that experiments not targeted to specific segments of the colon can provide at best only limited data.[11]

Foster and coworkers, measuring potassium currents in isolated segments of proximal rat colon, demonstrated a net potassium secretion.[50] The authors found that this secretory mechanism was abolished by sodium removal, stimulated by aldosterone, not inhibited by amiloride, and probably electrogenic. Additional ion flux studies have shown potassium secretion to be abolished by the addition of ouabain, an inhibitor of the sodium/potassium-ATPase pump.[59,80] These results, and similar studies, point to a secretory mechanism in which energy is used to drive a basolateral sodium/potassium or sodium/potassium/chloride pump, which, in turn, promotes the diffusion of potassium ions down an electrochemical gradient into the lumen through apical, potassium-permeable ion channels. Other investigators have confirmed this mechanism.[34]

The same methods used to ascertain the mechanism for potassium secretion have been applied to discern the mechanisms for absorption. McCabe and colleagues measured ion fluxes in 16 pairs of rabbit descending colon tissue.[80] Through the addition of ouabain and 2,4-dinitrophenol, the authors found that the distal colon was able both to absorb and to secrete potassium. In a similar study by Halm and Frizzell, potassium absorption was inhibited by the addition of barium to the serosal surface.[59] The authors concluded that these findings were consistent with an energy-dependent apical uptake of potassium, with potassium exit occurring through a basolateral, barium-sensitive ion channel. Others have proposed a similar mechanism.[35] As a result of these and other studies, potassium absorption is believed to be predominantly a phenomenon of the distal colon that is electroneutral, sodium independent, and mediated through an apical potassium/hydrogen-ATPase and a basolateral potassium ion channel.

However, not all data are consistent with these findings.[25] Feldman and Ickes reported their experience using ion-specific electrodes to measure ion fluxes in segments of rat distal colon.[45] The authors applied various chemical mediators and were unable to correlate proton and potassium ion fluxes. The authors postulated that these currents occur through separate pathways. Because the maintenance of potassium levels is critical to proper cell and body function, continuing interest in colonic regulation of this ion is of obvious importance.

▶ COLONIC MOTILITY

The phenomenon of gastrointestinal motility integrates numerous complex tissue functions, including smooth muscle electrical activity, contractile activity, intraluminal pressure, and both extrinsic and intrinsic neural coordination. However, a clear understanding of the normal function, underlying motility, and regulatory patterns is often unappreciated.

The failure to comprehend the intricacies of colonic motility can be attributed to the following circumstances:

- Intermittent and irregular nature of activity
- Absence of a reliable, consistent animal model
- Lack of ready accessibility to the entire organ
- Heterogeneity of colonic function

In the face of these limitations, certain techniques have been employed to study colonic motility. Three methods of measurement have been employed—colonic manometry, radiographic observation (i.e., radiopaque markers, fluoroscopy, defecography), and scintigraphy.[53,99] Through these modalities, investigators have reported macroscopic patterns of motility that can be seen in numerous mammalian species. For the practicing surgeon, an understanding of basic patterns of motility can lead to an enhanced appreciation of the functional gastrointestinal disorders, including functional dyspepsia, irritable bowel syndrome, and constipation.

Patterns of Motility

It is well known that patterns of motility illustrate considerable variability from one segment of bowel to another. Early investigators, by using contrast radiography and by direct observation in animals, observed a unique antiperistaltic pattern of ring contractions in the right colon.[15,43] From these findings and other studies, it has been proposed that this retrograde movement serves to retard the progression of contents, in order to encourage thorough mixing, microbial metabolism, and absorption of substances.[96] Although investigations have shown that segmental movements of the ascending bowel promote mixing and absorption, the presence of a retrograde pattern of motility in the *human* proximal colon has not been definitively demonstrated.[42] Furthermore, Krevsky and colleagues, through the use of colonic transit scintigraphy in seven normal volunteers, showed that the cecum and ascending colon empty rapidly and suggested that the transverse colon may be the site of colonic storage.[69]

An additional pattern observed by early investigators[15,43] and confirmed by others[98] is described by intermittent, contractile waves that result in a segmented appearance of the colon. These tonic or rhythmic contractions have been observed to move luminal contents slowly in an aboral direction. In addition, these contractions propel material in a back-and-forth pattern over short distances, thereby encouraging mixing and kneading of fecal matter.

The smooth muscle wall of the large intestine has also been shown to generate strong, propulsive, contractile movements over a large area. These forceful waves of contraction have been termed *mass movement*. Because these waves are infrequent, it is only through recent technical developments, permitting prolonged recording of myoelectrical and contractile activity, that this phenomenon has been observed and studied.[6] Increased electrical activity and mass propulsion are initiated at the transverse colon and seem to occur primarily after awakening or following the intake of food.[52,64,97] Narducci and coworkers reported their experience with 14 healthy individuals in whom motor activity of the transverse, descending, and sigmoid colon was recorded for 24 hours by means of colonoscopically positioned catheters.[87] The authors reported that all but two of the patients demonstrated isolated, high-amplitude (200 mm Hg) contractions at 1 cm/second that propagated over long distances. In agreement with the findings of other investigations, the majority of these contractions occurred after awakening and were associated with the urge to defecate.

Regulation of Motility

Myogenic Regulation

Electrical slow waves are the result of the rhythmic alterations in smooth muscle membrane potentials as recorded on electromyogram studies. In the colon, these slow waves are of variable amplitude and frequency but do not necessarily correlate with the contraction of muscle fibers.[53] Contraction of the muscle occurs only with those slow waves that carry a strong initiating depolarization or spike. Christensen characterizes the slow wave as a mechanism to fix muscular contraction to a given time and place, and, as such, the slow wave regulates this contractility.[21] The cells responsible for production of slow waves are known as the *pacemaker cells of the colon*. Studies using mammalian models have demonstrated the origin of these pacemaker cells to be in the circular muscle layer of the colonic wall.[16] Using phase contrast microscopy and patch clamp techniques, which allow for the detailed study of electrical properties of isolated cell membranes, Langton and coworkers provided evidence that the interstitial cells of Cajal are the actual, spontaneous pacesetters of the colon.[72] The same authors propose that the mechanism for spontaneous depolarization appears to be sodium independent but does require calcium.[72] Camilleri, in his review of functional disorders, points out evidence that the interstitial cells of Cajal are involved in the pathophysiology underlying constipation, both in acquired slow-transit constipation without colonic dilatation to megacolon and in neonatal colonic pseudoobstruction.[14]

Electromyographic studies have been undertaken in several mammalian models, particularly the cat, to correlate the observed macroscopic patterns of contraction with the underlying myoelectrical activity. Investigations of this type have demonstrated a frequency gradient of slow waves generated by a single, variably placed pacemaker in the transverse colon.[22] In this model, slow waves propagated toward the cecum (away from the pacemaker), whereas migrating spike bursts moved toward the rectum.

Additional myoelectrical studies have been conducted in the human colon in an effort to discover similar patterns of muscle activity. In most of these investigations, slow-wave activity has been demonstrated to be intermittent. Some of these, through the use of both electrodes and intraluminal probes, have demonstrated the presence of contractile activity in the low-frequency range.[52,106] It has been suggested that this type of electrical activity produces the observed colonic segmentation that may be attributed to these short, bidirectional contractions.[66] Continued investigation of myoelectrical behavior in the human colon has revealed migrating bursts of contractions occurring over long lengths of colon that are likely associated with mass movements.[52,55] These studies have provided insight into in vivo colonic motility. Some authors, however, express caution regarding the interpretation of such studies because of a lack of in vitro evidence, variability of recording sites, and segmental heterogeneity of the colon.[21]

Neural Regulation

From numerous pharmacologic and histologic studies, four types of external nerves have been found to be active in colonic muscle.[21] They are cholinergic and noncholinergic *excitatory* nerves and adrenergic and nonadrenergic *inhibitory* nerves.[15] As with so many colonic functions, a clear understanding of the nerves involved and of their mechanisms of action is thus far an unattained ideal.

Cholinergic innervation of the large bowel is provided by the vagus and the sacral nerves. The main parasympathetic supply arises from the second and third sacral roots, innervating the distal colon and rectum. The vagus nerve, carrying cranial parasympathetic supply, is generally believed to innervate the ascending colon. An important component of this nerve carries the afferent supply from the colon. In fact, the afferent supply is reported to contain 10 times as many fibers as the efferent.[55] In addition, animal studies have shown that afferent fibers of the vagus nerve contain the following neuropeptides: substance P, somatostatin, gastrin, cholecystokinin, and vasoactive inhibitory peptide.[76]

Vagal innervation of the myenteric plexus, which controls the intrinsic neural regulation of motility, is believed to contain two types of neurons.[3] In addition to the well-characterized preganglionic cholinergic nerve, the vagus supply to the colon is believed to contain a preganglionic, noncholinergic, nonadrenergic neuron. This type of neuron is believed to synapse with inhibitory neurons of the myenteric plexus and use vasoactive inhibitory peptide as a neurotransmitter. It is worth mentioning that several pharmacologic agents have been reported to improve postoperative ileus by increasing parasympathetic activity.[115] The best known of these, cisapride, which promotes the release of acetylcholine at the mesenteric plexus, was removed from the United States market secondary to several instances of cardiac arrhythmias.[83]

Sympathetic innervation of the colon begins with cell bodies located in the dorsal horn of the lumbar spinal cord. The axons from these nerves course through several pathways to synapse with postganglionic adrenergic neurons found in the celiac, superior, and inferior mesenteric ganglia. Most of these fibers find their way to the array of ganglia making up the inferior mesenteric plexus.[55,67] Large numbers of postganglionic nerves arise from the inferior mesenteric ganglia and pass on to innervate the colon as the lumbar colonic nerves. Segmental organization of these nerves has been reported.[66] Cell bodies in T10–12 supply the proximal colon, those in L1–2 supply the distal colon, and cell bodies in T12 to L1 innervate the mid-colon.

The sympathetic nervous system is well known to exhibit an inhibitory influence on the colon, as evidenced by the fact that disruption of pelvic sympathetic flow results in colonic contraction. In addition to efferent adrenergic nerves, the sympathetic neurons of the inferior mesenteric ganglia receive input from neurons whose cell bodies are in the colon wall as well as in other abdominal viscera.[66] The neurotransmitters in these ganglion cells are the same neuropeptides seen mediating parasympathetic function as well as numerous other activities unrelated to motility. Continued interest in and study of these neuropeptides will undoubtedly reveal

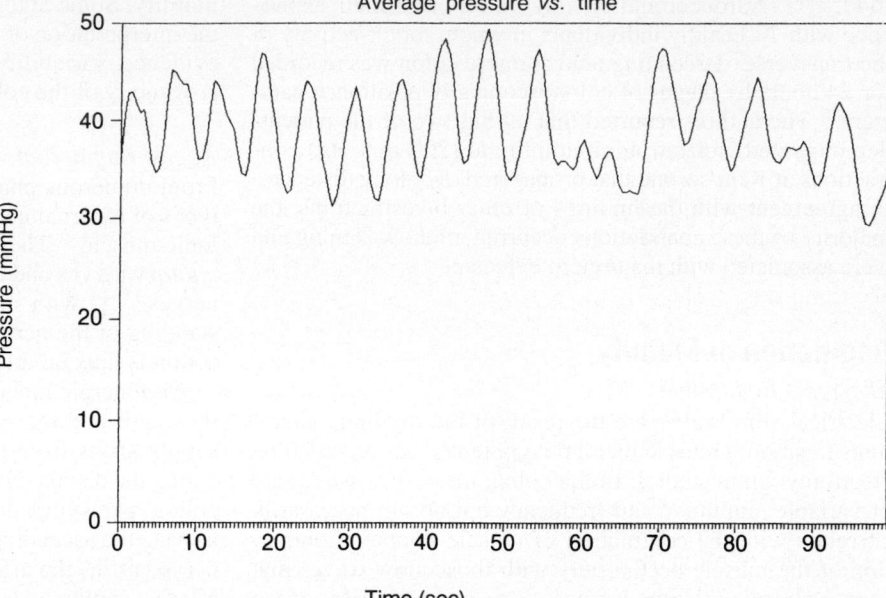

FIGURE 2-1. Evaluation of anal motility of a slow wave, which is usually found in the proximal portion of the anal sphincter. Typically, it has a frequency of approximately 10 to 14 cycles/minute and an average amplitude of 2 to 6 mm Hg. In this instance, an amplitude of 12 mm Hg has been recorded. (Courtesy of John A. Coller, MD.)

important new information regarding the mechanisms of colonic function.

The Defecation Process (See also Chapter 20)

The process of evacuation of feces consists of two stages. The first is involuntary, during which the contents are gradually propelled into the rectum. This is the total effect of short-duration, long-duration, and giant migrating contractions. The second stage is the act of defecation, during which feces are expelled (Figures 2-1 and 2-2)

Mechanical and physiologic retentive forces in the rectosigmoid normally maintain the distal rectum in an empty and collapsed state. The bends and folds of the rectosigmoid as well as the valves of Houston were originally believed

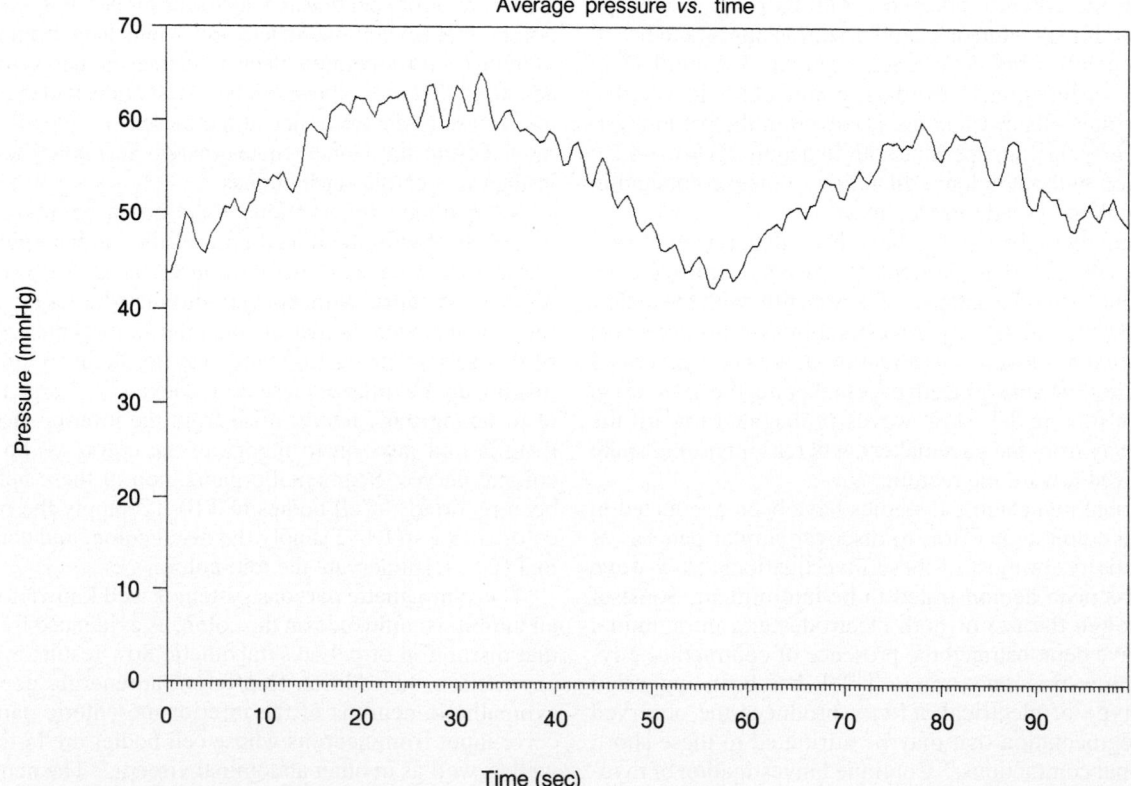

FIGURE 2-2. Evaluation of anal motility of an ultraslow wave, which usually has a frequency of one cycle every 50 to 70 seconds and an amplitude of 6 to 30 mm Hg. However, it may have an amplitude in excess of 60 mm Hg, and under such circumstances is often identified in the presence of sphincter hypertonia or obstructed defecation. (Courtesy of John A. Coller, MD.)

to retard the material from entry into the rectum, but it is doubtful whether such a hypothesis is valid. The maintenance of continence and the mechanism of defecation depend on the interaction of neurosensory and neuromotor impulses. As feces accumulate in the rectum, the bowel wall muscle relaxes, allowing distension and accommodation of the enlarging fecal mass. Sensory receptors within the anal canal determine the nature of the luminal contents, whether flatus, liquid, or solid stool. Threshold stimulation of the afferent nerve endings is reached, and involuntary precipitation of the anal reflex occurs, enabling the rectum to empty. Successive functional segments of colon coordinate their activity to produce a mass peristaltic wave above the fecal mass. Concomitantly, the distal part of the intestine and the internal sphincter relax, and the external sphincter contracts. If elimination is to proceed, voluntary inhibition of external sphincter contraction occurs.

With voluntary inhibition of external sphincter contraction during a mass peristaltic propulsion, defecation will occur without effort, or gas will be passed selectively. With contraction of the external sphincter, accommodation occurs by relaxation of the rectal wall muscle. This, in a matter of seconds will remove the urgency to defecate unless the volume is large or the individual has an impaired sphincter mechanism.

If a voluntary effort is required to defecate, intra-abdominal pressure is increased by closure of the glottis and by contraction of the muscles of the pelvic floor (resisting the forward movement of stool and closing the lumen distally). The diaphragm descends, and the voluntary muscles of the abdominal wall are contracted, creating a closed system. Relaxation of the pelvic muscles produces descent of the pelvic floor and straightening of the previously angulated rectum. Closure of the anal canal by the sphincters allows an increase of pressure within the rectum so that subsequent sphincteric inhibition results in expulsion of stool. The point at which complete inhibition of the external sphincter occurs can be demonstrated experimentally with an intrarectal balloon. When the volume reaches 150 to 200 mL of air, the intrarectal pressure achieves 45 to 55 mm Hg. At the end of defecation, when straining is discontinued, the pelvic floor rises to its normal position and again obliterates the lumen. A rebound contraction of the anal sphincter occurs; this has been termed the *closing reflex*.

▶ CONCLUSION

The three central functions of the normal, healthy colon are digestion, motility, and transport. All are important components of human physiology. Unfortunately, they have not only been poorly understood but also inadequately studied. This is changing, however. From the information provided in this chapter, one can appreciate that the mechanisms of colonic function are an active topic of research, which in time may lead to the introduction of new treatments for a host of conditions that affect the large bowel.

References

1. Andoh A, Tsujikawa T, Fujiyama Y. Role of dietary fiber and short-chain fatty acids in the colon. *Curr Pharm Des*. 2003;9(4):347–358.
2. Argenzio RA, Southworth M. Sites of organic acid production and absorption in the gastrointestinal tract of the pig. *Am J Physiol*. 1974;228(2):454–460.
3. Armstrong DN, Ballantyne GH. Physiology of the small and large intestines. In: Mazier WP, Levien DH, Luchtefeld MA, et al., eds. *Surgery of the Colon, Rectum, and Anus*. Philadelphia, PA: WB Saunders; 1995:40–65.
4. Ash RW, Dobson A. The effect of absorption on the acidity of rumen contents. *J Physiol*. 1963;169:39–61.
5. Barrett KE, Keely SJ. Chloride secretion by the intestinal epithelium: molecular basis and regulatory aspects. *Annu Rev Physiol*. 2000;62:535–572.
6. Bassotti G, Crowell MD, Whitehead WE. Contractile activity of the human colon: lessons from 24 hour studies. *Gut*. 1993;34(1):129–133.
7. Bauer HG, Asp NG, Dahlqvist A, et al. Effect of two kinds of pectin and guar gum on 1,2-dimethylhydrazine initiation of colon tumors and on fecal beta-glucoronidase activity in the rat. *Cancer Res*. 1981;41(6):2518–2523.
8. Billich CO, Levitan R. Effect of sodium concentration and osmolality on water and electrolyte absorption from the intact human colon. *J Clin Invest*. 1969;48(7):1336–1347.
9. Binder HJ. Amino acid absorption from the mammalian colon. *Biochim Biophys Acta*. 1970;219(2):503–506.
10. Binder HJ, Foster ES, Budinger ME, et al. Mechanism of electroneutral sodium chloride absorption in distal colon of the rat. *Gastroenterology*. 1987;93(3):449–455.
11. Binder HJ, Sandle GI. Electrolyte transport in the mammalian colon. In: Johnson LR, ed. *Physiology of the Gastrointestinal Tract*. 3rd ed. New York, NY: Raven Press; 1994:2133.
12. Brandtzaeg P, Halstensen TS, Kett K, et al. Immunobiology and immunopathology of human gut mucosa: humoral immunity and intraepithelial lymphocytes. *Gastroenterology*. 1989;97(6):1562–1584.
13. Bugaut M. Occurrence, absorption and metabolism of short chain fatty acids in the digestive tract of mammals. *Comp Biochem Physiol B*. 1987;86(3):439–472.
14. Camilleri M. Dyspepsia, irritable bowel syndrome, and constipation: review and what's new. *Rev Gastroenterol Disord*. 2001;1(1).2–17.
15. Cannon WB. The movements of the intestines studied by means of the roentgen rays. *Am J Physiol*. 1902;6:251–277.
16. Caprilli R, Onori L. Origin, transmission and ionic dependence of colonic electrical slow waves. *Scand J Gastroenterol*. 1972;7(1):65–74.
17. Carter MJ, Parsons DS. The isoenzymes of carbonic anhydrase: tissue, subcellular distribution and functional significance, with particular reference to the intestinal tract. *J Physiol*. 1971;215(1):71–94.
18. Charney AN, Kinsey MD, Myers L, et al. Na$^+$-K$^+$-activated adenosine triphosphate and intestinal electrolyte transport. Effect of adrenal steroids. *J Clin Invest*. 1975;56(3):653–660.
19. Chauve A, Devroede G, Bastin E. Intraluminal pressures during perfusion of the human colon in situ. *Gastroenterology*. 1976;70(3):336–340.
20. Cherrington CA, Hinton M, Pearson GR, et al. Short-chain organic acids at pH 5.0 kill *Escherichia coli* and *Salmonella* spp. without causing membrane perturbation. *J Appl Bacteriol*. 1991;70(2):161–165.
21. Christensen J. The motility of the colon. In: Johnson LR, ed. *Physiology of the Gastrointestinal Tract*. 3rd ed. New York, NY: Raven Press; 1994:991.
22. Christensen J, Anuras S, Hauser RL. Migrating spike bursts and electrical slow waves in the cat colon: effect of sectioning. *Gastroenterology*. 1974;66(2):240–247.
23. Christl SU, Murgatroyd PR, Gibson GR, et al. Production, metabolism, and excretion of hydrogen in the large intestine. *Gastroenterology*. 1992;102(4 pt 1):1269–1277.
24. Clarkson TW, Rothstein A, Cross A. Transport of monovalent anions by isolated small intestine of the rat. *Am J Physiol*. 1961;200:781–788.
25. Clauss W, Hörnicke H. Segmental differences in K-transport across rabbit proximal and distal colon in vivo and in vitro. *Comp Biochem Physiol A Comp Physiol*. 1984;79(2):267–269.
26. Cremaschi D, Ferguson DR, Hénin S, et al. Post-natal development of amiloride sensitive sodium transport in pig distal colon. *J Physiol*. 1979;292:481–494.
27. Cummings JH. Dietary fibre. *Br Med Bull*. 1981;37(1):65–70.
28. Cummings JH. Short chain fatty acids in the human colon. *Gut*. 1981;22(9):763–779.
29. Cummings JH, Hill MJ, Jenkins DJ, et al. Changes in fecal composition and colonic function due to cereal fiber. *Am J Clin Nutr*. 1976;29(12):1468–1473.
30. Cummings JH, Macfarlane GT. The control and consequences of bacterial fermentation in the human colon. *J Appl Bacteriol*. 1991;70(6):443–459.
31. Curran PF, Schwartz GF. Na, Cl, and water transport by rat colon. *J Gen Physiol*. 1960;43:555–571.
32. Davis G, Morawski SG, Santa Ana CA, et al. Evaluation of chloride/bicarbonate. Exchange in the human colon in vivo. *J Clin Invest*. 1983;71(2):201–207.

33. Debongnie JC, Phillips SF. Capacity of the human colon to absorb fluid. *Gastroenterology*. 1978;74(4):698–703.

34. Del Castillo JR, Sepúlveda FV. Activation of a $Na^+/K^+/2Cl^-$ cotransport system by phosphorylation in crypt cells isolated from guinea pig distal colon. *Gastroenterology*. 1995;109(2):387–396.

35. Del Castillo JR, Súlbaran-Carrasco MC, Burguillos L. K^+ transport in isolated guinea pig colonocytes: evidence for $Na(^+)$-independent ouabain-sensitive K^+ pump. *Am J Physiol*. 1994;266(6 pt 1):G1083–G1089.

36. Devroede GJ, Phillips SF. Conservation of sodium, chloride, and water by the human colon. *Gastroenterology*. 1969;56(1):101–109.

37. Devroede GJ, Phillips SF. Failure of the human rectum to absorb electrolyte and water. *Gut*. 1970;11(5):438–442.

38. Devroede GJ, Phillips SF, Code CF, et al. Regional differences in rates of insorption of sodium and water from the human large intestine. *Can J Physiol Pharmacol*. 1971;49(12):1023–1029.

39. Drasar BS, Hill MJ. *Human Intestinal Flora*. London, United Kingdom: Academic Press; 1974.

40. Dunning WF, Curtis MR, Maun ME. The effect of added dietary tryptophane on the occurrence of 2-acetylaminofluorescence-induced liver and bladder cancer in rats. *Cancer Res*. 1950;10(7):454–459.

41. Edmonds CJ, Marriott JC. The effect of aldosterone and adrenalectomy on the electrical potential difference of rat colon and on the transport of sodium, potassium, chloride and bicarbonate. *J Endocrinol*. 1967;39(4):517–531.

42. Edwards DA, Beck ER. Fecal flow, mixing and consistency. *Am J Dig Dis*. 1971;16(8):706–708.

43. Elliot TR. Antiperistalsis and other muscular activities of the colon. *J Physiol*. 1904;31(3–4):272–304.

44. Englyst HN, Cummings JH. Digestion of polysaccharides of potato in the small intestine of man. *Am J Clin Nutr*. 1987;45(2):423–431.

45. Feldman GM, Ickes JW Jr. Net H^+ and K^+ fluxes across the apical surface of rat distal colon. *Am J Physiol*. 1997;272(1 pt 1):G54–G62.

46. Finegold SM, Sutter VL, Mathisen GE. Normal indigenous intestinal flora. In: Hentges DJ, ed. *Human Intestinal Microflora in Heath and Disease*. London, United Kingdom: Academic Press; 1983:3–31.

47. Fleming SE, Choi SY, Fitch MD. Absorption of short-chain fatty acids from the rat cecum in vivo. *J Nutr*. 1991;121(11):1787–1797.

48. Florin TH, Neale G, Cummings JH. The effect of dietary nitrate on nitrate and nitrite excretion in man. *Br J Nutr*. 1990;64(2):387–397.

49. Foster ES, Budinger ME, Hayslett JP, et al. Ion transport in proximal colon of the rat. Sodium depletion stimulates neutral sodium chloride absorption. *J Clin Invest*. 1986;77(1):228–235.

50. Foster ES, Hayslett JP, Binder HJ. Mechanism of active potassium absorption and secretion in the rat colon. *Am J Physiol*. 1984;246(5 pt 1):G611–G617.

51. Foster ES, Zimmerman TW, Hayslett JP, et al. Corticosteroid alternation of active electrolyte transport in rat distal colon. *Am J Physiol*. 1983;245(5 pt 1):G668–G675.

52. Frexinos J, Bueno L, Fioramonti J. Diurnal changes in myoelectric spiking activity of the human colon. *Gastroenterology*. 1985;88(5 pt 1):1104–1110.

53. Frexinos J, Delvaux M. Colonic motility. In: Kumar D, Wingate D, eds. *An Illustrated Guide to Gastrointestinal Motility*. 2nd ed. New York, NY: Churchill Livingstone; 1993:427.

54. Frizzell RA, Koch MJ, Schultz SG. Ion transport by rabbit colon. I. Active and passive components. *J Membr Biol*. 1976;27(3):297–316.

55. Gabella G. *Structure of the Autonomic Nervous System*. New York, NY: John Wiley & Sons; 1976.

56. Giller J, Phillips SF. Electrolyte absorption and secretion in the human colon. *Am J Dig Dis*. 1972;17(11):1003–1011.

57. Grady GF, Duhamel RC, Moore EW. Active transport of sodium by human colon in vitro. *Gastroenterology*. 1970;59(4):583–588.

58. Guarner F, Malagelada JR. Gut flora in health and disease. *Lancet*. 2003;361(9356):512–519.

59. Halm DR, Frizzell RA. Active K transport across rabbit distal colon: relation to Na absorption and Cl secretion. *Am J Physiol*. 1986;251(2 pt 1):C252–C267.

60. Harig JM, Ng EK, Dudeja PK, et al. Transport of n-butyrate into human colonic luminal membrane vesicles. *Am J Physiol*. 1996;271(3 pt 1):G415–G422.

61. Heitman DW, Hardman WE, Cameron IL. Dietary supplementation with pectin and guar gum on 1,2-dimethylhydrazine-induced colon carcinogenesis in rats. *Carcinogenesis*. 1992;13(5):815–818.

62. Heller SN, Hackler LR, Rivers JM, et al. Dietary fiber: the effect of particle size of wheat bran on colonic function in young adult men. *Am J Clin Nutr*. 1980;33(8):1734–1744.

63. Hill MJ. Cereals, cereal fibre and colorectal cancer risk: a review of the epidemiological literature. *Eur J Cancer Prev*. 1997;6(3):219–225.

64. Holdstock DJ, Misiewicz JJ, Smith T, et al. Propulsion (mass movements) in the human colon and its relationship to meals and somatic activity. *Gut*. 1970;11(2):91–99.

65. Horie H, Kanazawa K, Okada M, et al. Effects of intestinal bacteria on the development of colonic neoplasm: an experimental study. *Eur J Cancer Prev*. 1999;8(3):237–245.

66. Huizinga JD, Daniel EE. Motor functions of the colon. In: Phillips SF, Pemberton JH, Shorter RG, eds. *The Large Intestine: Physiology, Pathophysiology, and Disease*. New York, NY: Raven Press; 1991:93–114.

67. Hultén L. Extrinsic nervous control of colonic motility and blood flow. An experimental study in the cat. *Acta Physiol Scand Suppl*. 1969;335:1–116.

68. Koyama Y, Yamamoto T, Tani T, et al. Expression and localization of aquaporins in rat gastrointestinal tract. *Am J Physiol*. 1999;276(3 pt 1):C621–C627.

69. Krevsky B, Malmud LS, D'Ercole F, et al. Colonic transit scintigraphy. A physiologic approach to the quantitative measurement of colonic transit in humans. *Gastroenterology*. 1986;91(5):1102–1112.

70. Kunzelmann K, Mall M. Electrolyte transport in the mammalian colon: mechanisms and implications for disease. *Physiol Rev*. 2002;82(1):245–289.

71. Kuratsune M, Honda T, Englyst HN, et al. Dietary fiber in the Japanese diet as investigated in connection with colon cancer risk. *Jpn J Cancer Res*. 1986;77(8):736–738.

72. Langton P, Ward SM, Carl A, et al. Spontaneous electrical activity of interstitial cells of Cajal isolated from canine proximal colon. *Proc Natl Acad Sci U S A*. 1989;86(19):7280–7284.

73. Levitt MD, Hirsch P, Fetzer CA, et al. H2 excretion after ingestion of complex carbohydrates. *Gastroenterology*. 1987;92(2):383–389.

74. Lichtman SM. Bacterial translocation in humans. *J Pediatr Gastroenterol Nutr*. 2001;33(1):1–10.

75. Lingueglia E, Voilley N, Lazdunski M, et al. Molecular biology of the amiloride-sensitive epithelial Na^+ channel. *Exp Physiol*. 1996;81(3):483–492.

76. Lundberg JM, Hökfelt T, Nilsson G, et al. Peptide neurons in the vagus, splanchnic and sciatic nerves. *Acta Physiol Scand*. 1978;104(4):499–501.

77. Macpherson A, Khoo UY, Forgacs I, et al. Mucosal antibodies in inflammatory bowel disease are directed against intestinal bacteria. *Gut*. 1996;38(3):365–375.

78. Mahajan RJ, Baldwin ML, Harig JM, et al. Chloride transport in human proximal colonic apical membrane vesicles. *Biochim Biophys Acta*. 1996;1280(1):12–18.

79. Mascolo N, Rajendran VM, Binder HJ. Mechanism of short-chain fatty acid uptake by apical membrane vesicles of rat distal colon. *Gastroenterology*. 1991;101(2):331–338.

80. McCabe R, Cooke HJ, Sullivan LP. Potassium transport by rabbit descending colon. *Am J Physiol*. 1982;242(1):C81–C86.

81. McNeil NI. Human large-intestinal absorption of SCFAs. In: Kasper H, Goebel H, eds. *Colon and Nutrition*. Boston, MA: MTP Press; 1982:55.

82. McNeil NI, Cummings JH, James WP. Rectal absorption of short chain fatty acids in the absence of chloride. *Gut*. 1979;20(5):400–403.

83. Miedema BW, Johnson JO. Methods for decreasing postoperative gut dysmotility. *Lancet Oncol*. 2003;4(6):365–372.

84. Moore WE, Holdeman LV. Human fecal flora: the normal flora of 20 Japanese-Hawaiians. *Appl Microbiol*. 1974;27(5):961–979.

85. Mortensen FV, Hessov I, Birke H, et al. Microcirculatory and trophic effects of short chain fatty acids in the human rectum after Hartmann's procedure. *Br J Surg*. 1991;78(10):1208–1211.

86. Mortensen PB, Clausen MR. Short-chain fatty acids in the human colon: relation to gastrointestinal health and disease. *Scand J Gastroenterol Suppl*. 1996;216:132–148.

87. Narducci F, Bassotti G, Gaburri M, et al. Twenty four hour manometric recording of colonic motor activity in healthy man. *Gut*. 1987;28(1):17–25.

88. O'Boyle CJ, MacFie J, Mitchell CJ, et al. Microbiology of bacterial translocation in humans. *Gut*. 1998;42(1):29–35.

89. O'Keefe SJ, Kidd M, Espitalier-Noel G, et al. Rarity of colon cancer in Africans is associated with low animal product consumption, not fiber. *Am J Gastroenterol*. 1999;94(5):1373–1380.

90. Oltmer S, von Engelhardt W. Absorption of short-chain fatty acids from the in-situ-perfused caecum and colon of the guinea pig. *Scand J Gastroenterol*. 1994;29(11):1009–1016.

91. Phear EA, Ruebner B. The in vitro production of ammonium and amines by intestinal bacteria in relation to nitrogen toxicity as a factor in hepatic coma. *Br J Exp Pathol*. 1956;37(3):253–262.

92. Phillips SF, Giller J. The contribution of the colon to electrolyte and water conservation in man. *J Lab Clin Med*. 1973;81(5):733–746.

93. Rajendran VM, Binder HJ. Cl-HCO₃ and Cl-OH exchanges mediate Cl uptake in apical membrane vesicles of rat distal colon. *Am J Physiol.* 1993;264(5 pt 1):G874–G879.

94. Ramakrishna BS, Venkataraman S, Srinivasan P, et al. Amylase-resistant starch plus oral rehydration solution for cholera. *N Engl J Med.* 2000;342(5):308–313.

95. Rechkemmer G, Rönnau K, von Engelhardt W. Fermentation of polysaccharides and absorption of short chain fatty acids in the mammalian hindgut. *Comp Biochem Physiol A Comp Physiol.* 1988;90(4):563–568.

96. Ritchie JA. Colonic motor activity and bowel function. I. Normal movement of contents. *Gut.* 1968;9(4):442–456.

97. Ritchie JA. Colonic motor activity and bowel function. II. Distribution and incidence of motor activity at rest and after food and carbachol. *Gut.* 1968;9(5):502–511.

98. Ritchie JA. Movement of segmental constrictions in the human colon. *Gut.* 1971;12(5):350–355.

99. Ritchie JA. Mass peristalsis in the human colon after contact with oxyphenisatin. *Gut.* 1972;13(3):211–219.

100. Roediger WE. Role of anaerobic bacteria in the metabolic welfare of the colonic mucosa in man. *Gut.* 1980;21(9):793–798.

101. Roediger WE. Short chain fatty acids as metabolic regulators of ion absorption in the colon. *Acta Vet Scand Suppl.* 1989;86:116–125.

102. Ropert A, Cherbut C, Rozé C, et al. Colonic fermentation and proximal gastric tone in humans. *Gastroenterology.* 1996;111(2):289–296.

103. Rosebury T. *Microorganisms Indigenous to Man.* New York, NY: McGraw-Hill; 1962:435.

104. Rübsamen K, Engelhardt WV. Bicarbonate secretion and solute absorption in forestomach of the llama. *Am J Physiol.* 1978;235(1):E1–E6.

105. Ruppin H, Bar-Meir S, Soergel KH, et al. Absorption of short-chain fatty acid by the colon. *Gastroenterology.* 1980;78(6):1500–1507.

106. Sarna SK. Colonic motor activity. *Surg Clin North Am.* 1993;73(6):1201–1223.

107. Saunders DR, Wiggins HS. Conservation of mannitol, lactulose, and raffinose by the human colon. *Am J Physiol.* 1981;241(5):G397–G402.

108. Schultz SG. Ion transport by mammalian large intestine. In: Johnson LR, ed. *Physiology of the Gastrointestinal Tract.* New York, NY: Raven Press; 1981:991.

109. Sellin JH, DeSoignie R. Rabbit proximal colon: a distinct transport epithelium. *Am J Physiol.* 1984;246(5 pt 1):G603–G610.

110. Sellin JH, DeSoignie R, Burlingame S. Segmental differences in short-chain fatty acid transport in rabbit colon: effect of pH and Na. *J Membr Biol.* 1993;136(2):147–158.

111. Steinmetz KA, Potter JD. Vegetables, fruit, and cancer. I. Epidemiology. *Cancer Causes Control.* 1991;2(5):325–357.

112. Stephens AM, Cummings JH. Water holding by dietary fibre in vitro and its relationship to faecal output in man. *Gut.* 1979;20(8):722–729.

113. Stephens AM, Cummings JH. The microbial contribution to human faecal mass. *J Med Microbiol.* 1980;13(1):45–56.

114. Tadesse K, Smith D, Eastwood MA. Breath hydrogen (H₂) and methane (CH₄) excretion patterns in normal man and in clinical practice. *Q J Exp Physiol.* 1980;65(2):85–97.

115. Thompson JS, Quigley EM. Prokinetic agents in the surgical patient. *Am J Surg.* 1999;177(6):508–514.

116. Thun MJ, Calle EE, Namboodiri MM, et al. Risk factors for fatal colon cancer in a large prospective study. *J Natl Cancer Inst.* 1992;84(19):1491–1500.

117. Topping DL, Clifton PM. Short-chain fatty acids and human colonic function: roles of resistant starch and nonstarch polysaccharides. *Physiol Rev.* 2001;81(3):1031–1064.

118. Torsoli A, Ramorino ML, Crucioli V. The relationships between anatomy and motor activity of the colon. *Am J Dig Dis.* 1968;13(5):462–467.

119. Turnamian SG, Binder HJ. Regulation of active sodium and potassium transport in the distal colon of the rat. Role of the aldosterone and glucocorticoid receptors. *J Clin Invest.* 1989;84(6):1924–1929.

120. Turnheim K, Thompson SM, Schultz SG. Relation between intracellular sodium and active sodium transport in rabbit colon: current-voltage relations of the apical sodium entry mechanism in the presence of varying luminal sodium concentrations. *J Membr Biol.* 1983;76(3):299–309.

121. Umesaki Y, Yajima T, Yokokura T, et al. Effect of organic acid absorption on bicarbonate transport in rat colon. *Pflugers Arch.* 1979;379(1):43–47.

122. Vanasin B, Ustach TJ, Schuster MM. Electrical and motor activity of human and dog colon in vitro. *Johns Hopkins Med J.* 1974;134(4):201–210.

123. Visek WJ. Diet and cell growth modulation by ammonia. *Am J Clin Nutr.* 1978;31(10 suppl):S216–S220.

124. Will PC, Lebowitz JL, Hopfer U. Induction of amiloride-sensitive sodium transport in the rat colon by mineralocorticoids. *Am J Physiol.* 1980;238(4):F261–F268.

125. Wills NK, Alles WP, Sandle GI, et al. Apical membrane properties and amiloride binding kinetics of the human descending colon. *Am J Physiol.* 1984;247(6 pt 1):G749–G757.

126. Wrong OM, Metcalfe-Gibson A, Morrison RB, et al. In vivo dialysis of faeces as a method of stool analysis. I. Technique and results in normal subjects. *Clin Sci.* 1965;28:357–375.

127. Wrong OM, Vince AJ, Waterlow JC. The contribution of endogenous urea to faecal ammonia in man, determined by 15N labeling of plasma urea. *Clin Sci (Lond).* 1985;68(2):193–199.

3
Pediatric Surgical Problems

Marc A. Levitt and Alberto Peña

We can say with some assurance that,
although children may be the victims
of fate, they will not be the victims of our neglect.
—JOHN F. KENNEDY

► HIRSCHSPRUNG'S DISEASE

Historical Review

In 1691, Frederick Ruysch reported the autopsy findings of a child who died with what appeared to be a congenital megacolon[52]; however, the name for this disease originated with Harold Hirschsprung, who, in 1886, at the Pediatric Congress in Berlin, described an infant with this condition.[41] The first reference relating to an absence of ganglion cells as the cause for the underlying disturbance is that of Tittle in 1901.[116] In 1940, Tiffin and coworkers described the disturbed peristalsis of the aganglionic intestine.[115] Robertson and Kernohan in 1938,[94] and Zuelzer and Wilson in 1948, were able to correlate the functional disturbances of the distal colon with aganglionosis.[123] Swenson and colleagues, in 1949, described the main principles for

HAROLD HIRSCHSPRUNG (1830–1916)

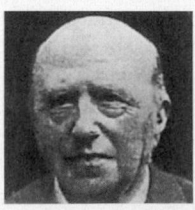

Hirschsprung was born in Copenhagen, Denmark. He passed his examinations in 1855 and was made a teacher in 1861. He was professor of pediatrics at the University of Copenhagen and head physician to the Queen Louise Children's Hospital. Hirschsprung is best known for his description of the disease that was named after him, perhaps because of his excellent account of the condition, given that this was not the original report. Parry actually described a case that is recorded in his collected papers in 1825. Levine of Chicago, in 1867, noted the first American case. In his paper, he does not identify the pathogenicity, nor does he offer a suggestion for treatment of aganglionic megacolon. Hirschsprung contributed extensively to the pediatric literature, publishing one of the first comprehensive reports on pyloric stenosis in 1888, and he was a pioneer in the use of hydrostatic pressure for the reduction of intussusception in 1905. Although theories abounded for 50 years, Lennander in 1900 was one of the first to suggest a neurogenic origin—there was so much confusion, and there were so many differences of opinion that it was not until the 1940s that the absence of ganglion cells was believed to be the etiologic factor. (Hirschsprung H. Stuhltrúgheit neugeborener in folge von dilatation und hypertrophie des colon. *Jahrb Kinderheilkd.* 1888;27:1.)

the radiologic diagnosis of this condition, observations that are still useful today.[112] The first surgical approach was reported by Swenson and Bill in 1948.[111] Modifications of this technique, such as the Duhamel approach[25] and the Soave operation,[104] were developed in order to avoid some of the complications seen with the Swenson method but were based on the same principles of repair. More recently, a laparoscopic approach has been used,[17,31,32,102] as well as a transanal operation.[20,51]

Pathophysiology and Embryology

Hirschsprung's disease is an anomaly characterized by partial or complete colonic obstruction associated with the absence

ORVAR SWENSON (1909–PRESENT)

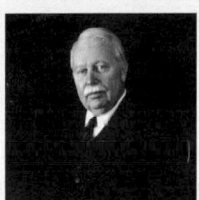

Orvar Swenson was born in Halsingborg, Sweden, on February 7, 1909, the son of a Mormon missionary father. The family returned to the United States and settled in Independence, Missouri. Swenson attended William Jewell College in Liberty, Kansas, and received his bachelor's degree in 1933. He then enrolled in Harvard Medical School, graduating in 1937. Following a year as an intern at Ohio State University Hospital, he returned to Boston and to the Peter Bent Brigham Hospital and the Boston Children's Hospital, where he completed training in general surgery and in pediatric surgery in 1945. Swenson remained on the staff of these two hospitals for 5 years, during which time he ascertained the etiology of and developed a surgical treatment for Hirschsprung's disease. In 1950, he took the position as surgeon-in-chief of the Boston Floating Hospital and professor of surgery at Tufts University School of Medicine. In 1960, he moved to Chicago to become surgeon-in-chief at Children's Memorial Hospital. In 1973, he moved on again, this time to the University of Miami, where he remained until his retirement in 1978. Swenson shared the second Mead Johnson Research Award in 1952 with Edward B. Neuhauser for their research on the elucidation, pathogenesis, and treatment of congenital megacolon. He later received the William Ladd Medal. He was recognized in 2009 in honor of his 100th birthday by a tribute in the *Journal of Pediatric Surgery*. (With appreciation to Avraham Belizon, MD; photograph courtesy of Keith E. Georgeson, MD.)

ALBERTO PEÑA (1938–PRESENT)

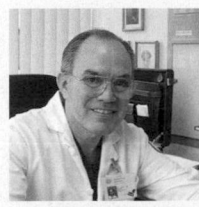

Alberto Peña was born August 16, 1938, in Mexico City, Mexico. He received his medical degree at the Military Medical School in Mexico City in 1962 and completed his general surgical training at the same institution in 1966. He then became interested in pediatric surgery and decided to do a Research Fellowship in Cardiovascular Surgery at Children's Hospital in Boston, Massachusetts. In pursuit of his pediatric surgery training, he continued at Children's Hospital for 2 additional years. Peña then returned to Mexico City to become the surgeon-in-chief and professor of pediatric surgery at the National Institute of Pediatrics, a position he occupied until 1985. He then accepted the post of chief of pediatric surgery and professor of surgery at the Schneider Children's Hospital in New Hyde Park, New York. In 2005, he moved with Dr. Marc Levitt to Cincinnati where they established the Colorectal Center for Children. He is currently professor of pediatric surgery at that institution. Peña has contributed to numerous areas in the field of pediatric surgery, including deformities of the chest wall, esophageal replacement, and pancreatectomy in the newborn. However, he is best known for his innovative approach to the management of congenital anorectal malformations. Peña has received numerous honors throughout the world, including recognition by the United Nations for his work with children in Africa, the Coe Medical from the Pacific Association of Pediatric Surgeons, and Honorary Fellowship of the Royal College of Surgeons of England. He continues to lecture and operate around the world and to teach pediatric surgeons his approach to the management of congenital anorectal malformations. (Courtesy of Avraham Belizon, MD.)

BERNARD GEORGES DUHAMEL (1917–1996)

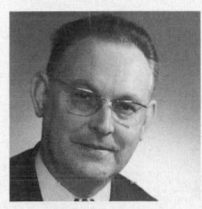

Bernard Duhamel was born in Paris, May 11, 1917. His father was a well-known author and a member of the Academie Française, and his mother was an artist. After completing his medical studies, he began his surgical training in 1939 in Paris. Following this, he undertook a fellowship in pediatric surgery at the Sick Children's Hospital of Paris (Hôpital des Enfants Malades). In 1954, he was appointed chairman of the Department of Pediatric Surgery at the Hôpital de Saint-Denis, and in 1955 he was elevated to professor of surgery. Duhamel made numerous contributions to neonatal surgery and wrote a number of books on surgical technique. He was elected president of the French Society of Pediatric Surgery in 1967 and was an influential member of the French Academy of Surgery. (With appreciation to Rolland F. Parc, MD.)

FRANCO SOAVE (1917–1984)

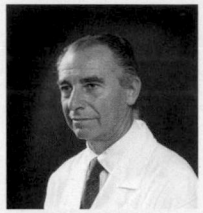

Born in Naples on June 14, 1917, Franco Soave completed his medical degree at the University of Genoa in 1943 and his surgical residency at the Clinica Chirurgica of the University of Turin in 1950. He returned to his alma mater in Genoa as assistant professor from 1951 to 1954 while serving in the medical corps. He later became surgeon-in-chief at the Gaslini Institute Hospital and professor and chair of pediatric surgery at the University of Genoa until his death. He published more than 160 papers and served on several editorial boards, including the *Journal of Pediatric Surgery*. He was awarded honorary membership in several international pediatric surgical societies and was president of the *Società Italiana di Pediatria* from 1970 to 1972. In 1984, he presented his milestone work on his alternative operation for Hirschsprung's disease at the American Pediatric Surgical Association and unfortunately died the same year. (Reference: Carachi R, Young DG, Buyukunal C. *F. Soave—A History of Surgical Pediatrics*. Toh Tuck Link, Singapore: World Scientific Publishing; 2009—with special appreciation to Ahmed Nasser, MD.)

of intramural ganglion cells.[43,69] The aganglionic portion of the colon is always located distally, but the length of the segment varies. This is the factor that determines the manifestations of the disease (Figure 3-1). The so-called typical and most frequent variation is the one in which the aganglionic segment includes the rectum and some of the sigmoid colon (Figure 3-1B), accounting for approximately two-thirds of all patients. The long-segment variety represents approximately 10% of presentations (Figure 3-1C).[101] In this manifestation, the aganglionic portion may extend to any level between the splenic flexure and the descending colon. Total colonic aganglionosis is a very serious condition in which the entire colon is aganglionic, frequently including a variable length of terminal ileum (Figure 3-1D). This type also represents approximately 10% of the entire group.[27] There is some debate about the existence of so-called ultrashort aganglionosis or short-segment Hirschsprung's disease (Figure 3-1E). It is frequently confused with idiopathic constipation.

Typically, the aganglionic portion of the colon appears narrow when compared with the distended, proximal part

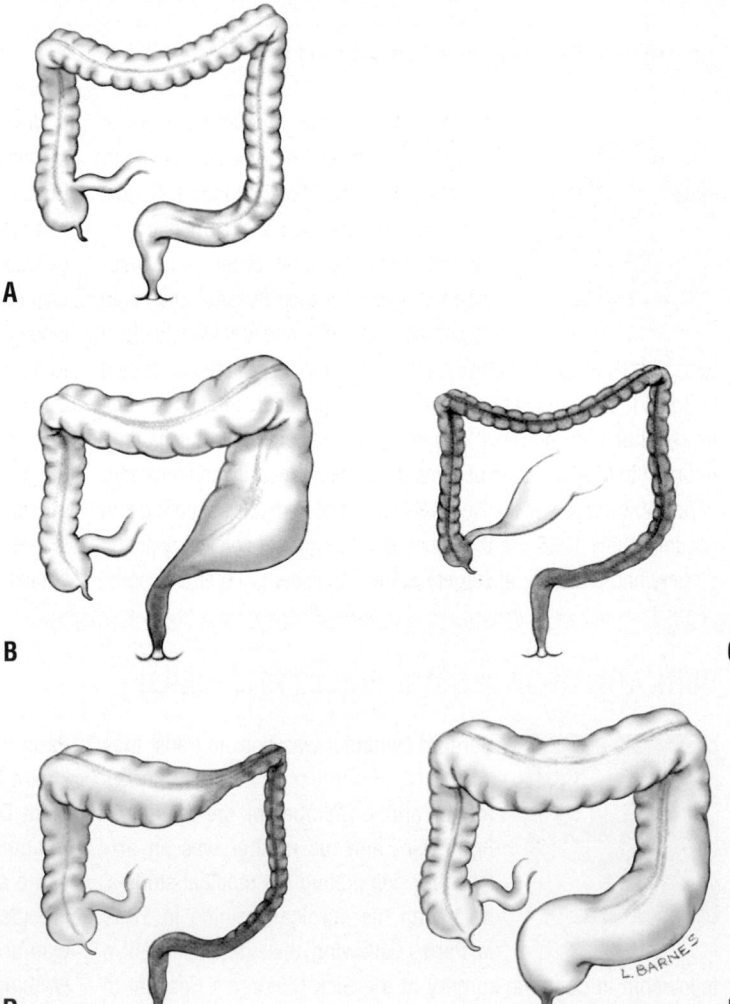

FIGURE 3-1. Different presentations of Hirschsprung's disease according to the length of the aganglionic segment. **A:** Normal bowel. **B:** Typical sigmoid involvement. **C:** Long-segment disease. **D:** Total colonic aganglionosis. **E:** Short-segment disease.

and has an absence of intramural, submucosal, and intermuscular ganglion cells. Increased size and prominence of nerve fibers are also seen in this area. The proximal, normally innervated portion of the colon is usually distended, and its wall is thickened because of muscle hypertrophy. Between these two areas is the "transition zone," a cone-shaped portion of colon that is hypoganglionic, with thickened nerve trunks. An increase in the enzyme acetylcholinesterase has been demonstrated in the aganglionic colon.[28,45,46] Acetylcholinesterase staining demonstrates a significant increase in the number of oversized nerve fibers located in the muscularis mucosa, the lamina propria, and the submucosa.

Hirschsprung's is believed to be a disease caused by the failure in the development of tissue derived from the neural crest. As such, there appears to be an arrest in the craniocaudal migration of the neuroenteric ganglion cells from the neural crest into the upper gastrointestinal tract, down through the vagal fibers and along the distal intestine.[75] As a consequence, ganglion cells are missing from Auerbach's myenteric plexus (located between the circular and longitudinal layers of bowel wall), Henle's plexus (located in the deep submucosa), and also Meissner's plexus in the superficial submucosa (Figures 3-2 and 3-3). Under normal circumstances, the ganglia appear to act as a final common pathway for both sympathetic and parasympathetic influences. Their absence produces the uncoordinated contractions of the affected bowel. Spasm, lack of propulsive peristalsis, and mass contraction of the

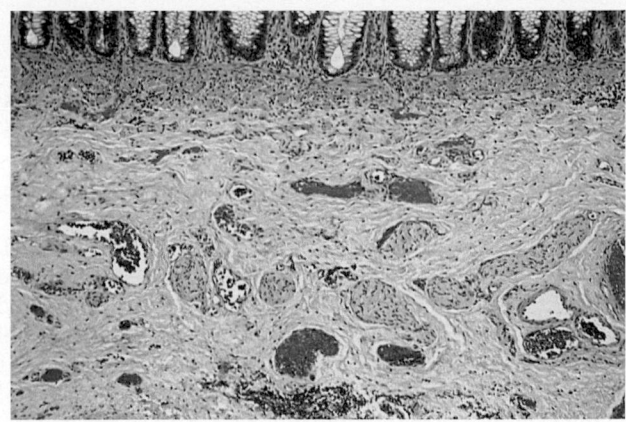

FIGURE 3-3. Histologic section including mucosa and submucosa of the rectum showing tortuous and hypertrophic nerve trunks of the submucosal plexus. There is no evidence of any ganglion cell present. This establishes the diagnosis of Hirschsprung's disease. (Courtesy of Hector L. Monforte-Muñoz, MD, Department of Pathology, Children's Hospital, Los Angeles, CA.)

aganglionic segment[40] have all been well documented, in addition to the lack of relaxation of the bowel and the spasm of the internal sphincter.[18,117] The clinical result of these pathophysiologic events is partial or total colonic obstruction.

There has been a special interest in the role of nitric oxide as a neurotransmitter responsible for the inhibitory action elicited by the intrinsic enteric nerves. A lack of nitric oxide synthase (the enzyme required for nitric oxide production) has been demonstrated in the myenteric plexus of the aganglionic segment.[5,76] The significance of this finding and the potential therapeutic implications are theoretically profound but have yet to be demonstrated.

Incidence and Associated Malformations

It is generally accepted that the incidence of Hirschsprung's disease is in the range of 1 in 5,000 births.[27] Although boys are much more frequently affected than girls, the long-segment manifestation is seen at least as often in female patients. Inheritance patterns seem to be multifactorial. The risk for a sibling sister of a male patient is 0.6%, whereas the risk for a brother of a female patient with long-segment disease is 18%.[5,29,72]

Approximately 5% to 21% of all individuals affected with Hirschsprung's disease have an associated congenital anomaly.[42] Hirschsprung's disease has been erroneously overdiagnosed in patients with anorectal malformations because many suffer some degree of constipation.[55] Another associated condition is Down's syndrome; this anomaly is found in 5% of these infants.[35]

There have been developments in determining the genetic defects associated with Hirschsprung's disease. A deletion in the long arm of chromosome 10 has been found.[66] More detailed evaluation indicates that the location of this mutation is between 10Q11.2 and Q21.2 2.[30,63] The deletion seems to overlap the region of the *RET* proto-oncogene. Patients with multiple endocrine neoplasia (MEN 2A) also have a deletion of this proto-oncogene. This genetic discovery is an important advance in the study of this complex disease, and the identification of the gene and the exact sequence of the DNA code is likely to be realized soon.[72]

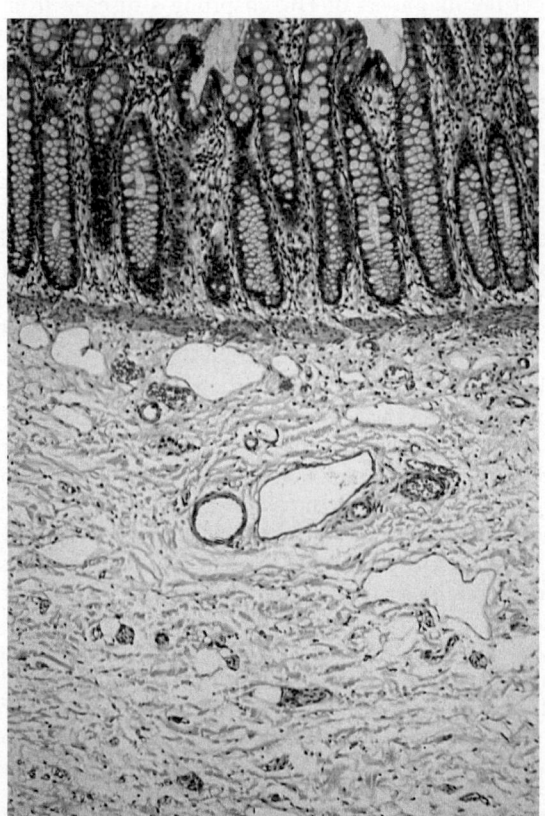

FIGURE 3-2. Histologic section including mucosa with submucosa of the rectum showing clusters of ganglion cells in the submucosal plexus. This excludes Hirschsprung's disease at this level. (Courtesy of Hector L. Monforte-Muñoz, MD, Department of Pathology, Children's Hospital, Los Angeles, CA.)

Clinical Manifestations and Differential Diagnosis

Infants suffering from Hirschsprung's disease usually become symptomatic during the first 24 to 48 hours of life. Occasionally, a child may have minimal or absent clinical manifestations during the first days or weeks and may exhibit moderate, intermittent bouts of symptoms at a later age (Figure 3-4).

Abdominal distension, delayed passage of meconium, and vomiting are the most frequent observations. This triad of symptoms may be followed by a spontaneous or induced explosive, massively deflating passage of liquid bowel movement and gas, which dramatically improves the baby's condition. This is followed by a period of hours or days of relative absence of symptoms followed by recurrence of the same manifestations. Stools are frequently liquid and foul smelling. When the abdomen is distended, the infant usually is very ill from sepsis, hypovolemia, and endotoxic shock. Ischemic enterocolitis with necrosis proximal to the aganglionic segment is the most serious complication. Other supervening problems are pneumatosis, intra-abdominal abscess, and cecal perforation.[105] There is a 25% to 30% mortality if the disease is unrecognized or untreated.[26,42]

Typically, rectal examination of an ill infant with Hirschsprung's disease produces an explosive bowel movement with immediate symptomatic improvement. The differential diagnosis includes any condition that causes intestinal obstruction in the newborn, probably the most frequent being *meconium-plug syndrome*. The expulsion of a plug of meconium with resolution of symptoms and the absence of other signs characteristic of Hirschsprung's disease help to establish this diagnosis. *Meconium ileus* is manifested by a clinical picture consistent with that of intestinal obstruction, and the child may exhibit respiratory symptoms due to association with cystic fibrosis.[24] The absence of air-fluid levels on an upright abdominal film and the "ground-glass" appearance of the lower abdomen are characteristic radiographic signs of

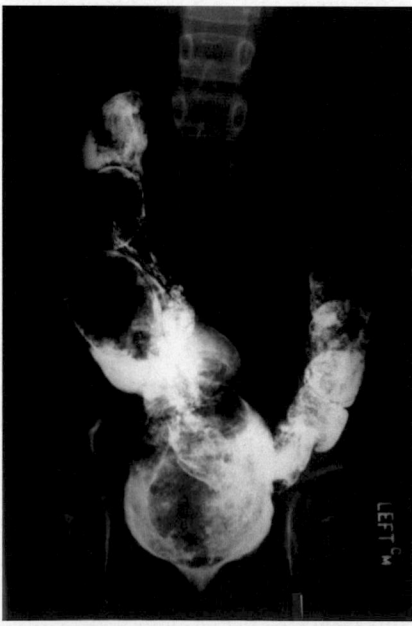

FIGURE 3-4. Contrast study of a young man with presumed short-segment Hirschsprung's disease with lifelong constipation. Note the dilated bowel with considerable fecal impaction.

this condition. Another disease that may lead to confusion is the *small left colon syndrome*. Contrast enema demonstrates a rather narrow left colon to the level of the splenic flexure but a normal caliber rectum. Symptoms usually improve following this study and resolve after several weeks. The mother is frequently diabetic. Other nonsurgical conditions that may be confused with Hirschsprung's disease include hypothyroidism, adrenal insufficiency, cerebral injury, opiate withdrawal, and magnesium sulfate intoxication.

Patients with Hirschsprung's who survive despite inadequate treatment or who have relatively mild symptoms ultimately develop the classic clinical picture initially described for this condition. Nowadays this is quite rare. These children suffer severe constipation with an enormously distended abdomen. The proximal colon is huge and full of inspissated fecal material (Figure 3-4). At this stage, the diagnosis may be confused with severe idiopathic constipation. In the latter condition, children usually become symptomatic after the sixth month of life; they neither vomit nor become seriously ill and often experience overflow incontinence or encopresis, a constant, chronic soiling. Rectal examination in such children reveals a fecal impaction just above the anal canal. Patients with Hirschsprung's disease may have an empty rectum, or examination may disclose only a small amount of feces.

Diagnosis

Radiologic Studies

It is very difficult to differentiate a distended colon from distended small bowel based on a plain abdominal film of a neonate with intestinal obstruction. Therefore, one can only suspect the diagnosis of Hirschsprung's disease from this study. The presence of air-fluid levels is evidence of obstruction, but it is nonspecific. An enema examination performed with water-soluble contrast material is the most valuable radiologic study for establishing the diagnosis.

No bowel preparation is required. The infant is placed in a lateral position, and a rectal tube is introduced to barely above the anal canal. Injection of contrast is optimally controlled by hand with a syringe. The introduction of a catheter beyond the limit of the anal canal will risk a misdiagnosis because the tip may reach the distended colon and result in injection above the aganglionic portion. The dye is instilled until it reaches the distended portion of the intestine.

This study may reveal a very distended proximal colon, the transition zone, and a narrowed distal rectosigmoid (Figure 3-5). The older the patient, the more obvious the size difference between the normal ganglionic intestine and the abnormal aganglionic bowel. Therefore, sometimes the typical changes are not very obvious during the neonatal period. A second contrast enema performed a few days or weeks later may show a much more dramatic appearance than that seen previously (Figure 3-5B). Generally, however, the transition zone is recognized in most newborns. Contrast enema is less accurate in infants with very short aganglionosis or when the entire colon is involved.[97] In instances of total colonic aganglionosis, contrast enema may reveal a rather short colon, with retraction of the hepatic and splenic flexures and straightening of the sigmoid.

Anorectal Manometry

Normally, when the rectum is distended with a balloon, pressure in the anal canal falls because of internal sphincter relaxation (the rectoanal inhibitory reflex). In infants with aganglionosis, this reflex is absent.[118] This abnormal response has been

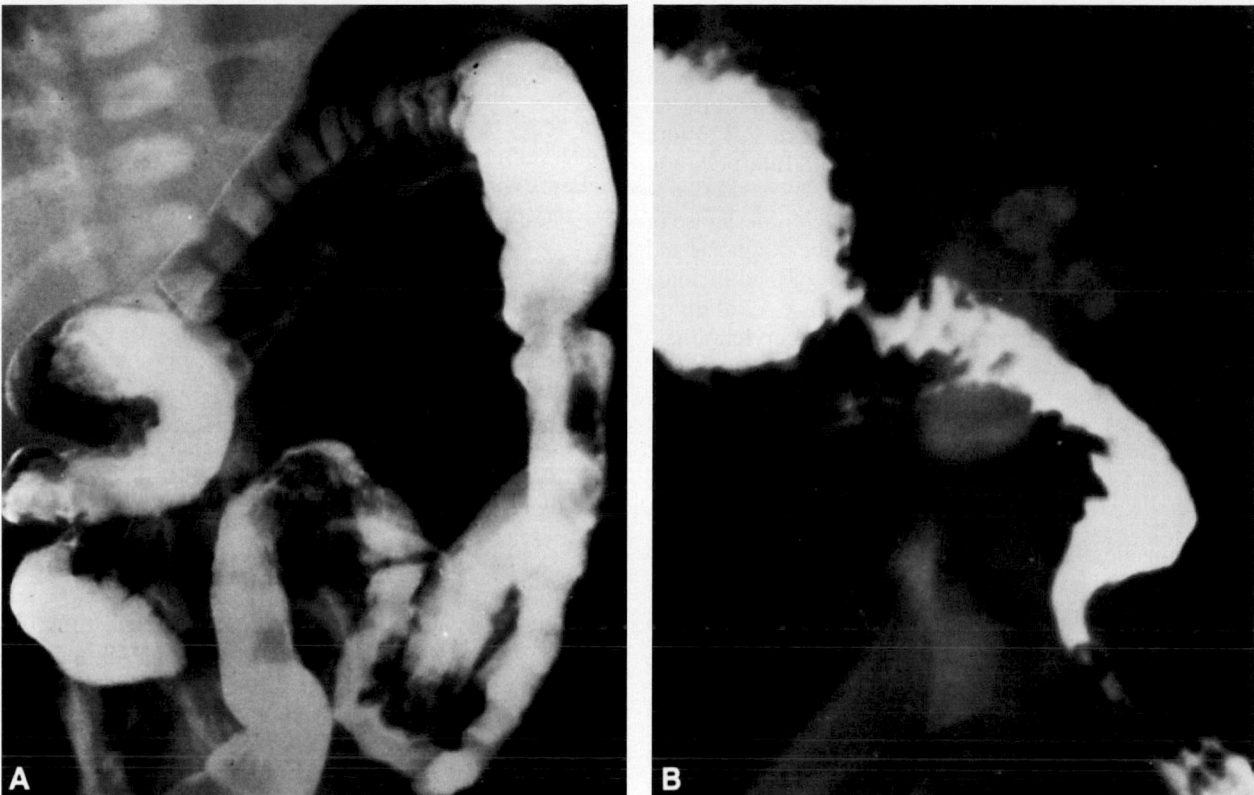

FIGURE 3-5. Hirschsprung's disease. **A:** Contrast enema performed in a newborn with Hirschsprung's disease. Often, classical changes are not obvious in the neonatal period. **B:** A later study demonstrates the typical megacolon, transition zone, and nondistended, aganglionic portion.

interpreted as diagnostic for this condition. However, this test has several limitations, the primary ones being the technical difficulty of evaluating the newborn and the mismatch of the manometry balloon to the wide variety of colonic luminal diameters. We, therefore, do not use this test in our clinical practice.

Rectal Biopsy

The confirmation of the diagnosis is based on the absence of ganglion cells and the presence of hypertrophic nerves in an adequate rectal biopsy (Figure 3-6). The specimen must be taken at least 1.5 cm above the pectinate line. The traditional

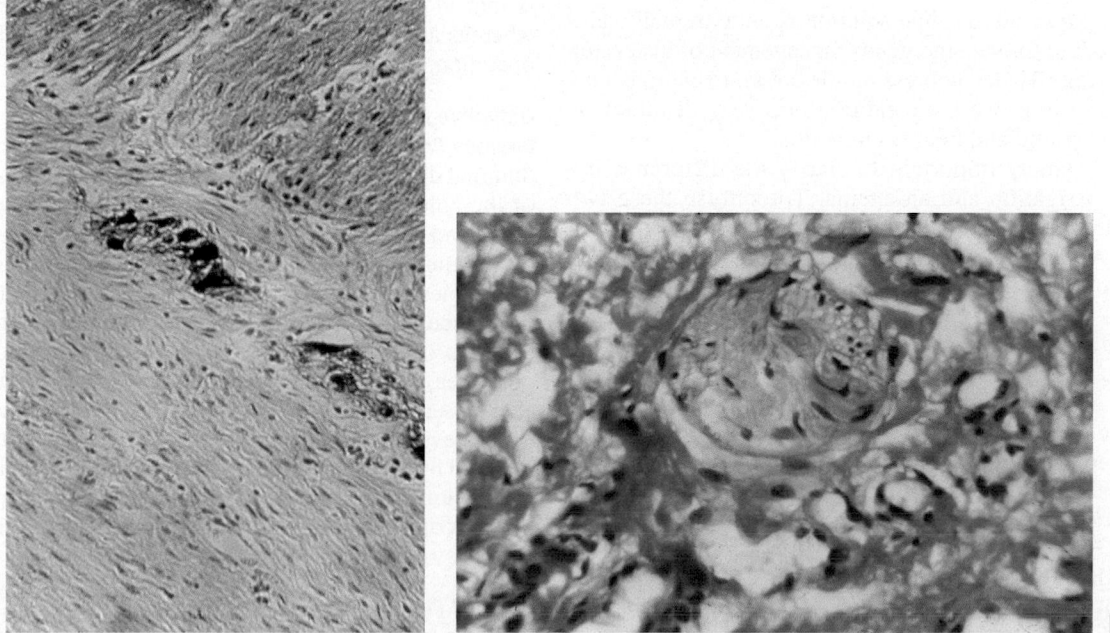

FIGURE 3-6. Diagnosis of Hirschsprung's disease is made by biopsy. **A:** Normal ganglion cells in the submucosa are stained for acetylcholinesterase. (Original magnification × 200.) **B:** The nerve trunk in the submucosa of the bowel without ganglion cells. (Original magnification × 600; courtesy of Rudolf Garret, MD.)

full-thickness rectal biopsy has obvious diagnostic value but requires good rectal exposure and a general anesthetic. Suction rectal biopsy is easily performed, is associated with virtually no risk of perforation, and does not require an anesthetic.[23,74] The specimen usually measures 1 × 3 mm and should include mucosa and submucosa. Interpretation requires expertise.

The presence of large amounts of acetylcholinesterase in the mucosa and submucosa helps to make the diagnosis and is used in many centers.[28,45,46,69] The absence of nicotinamide adenine dinucleotide phospate diaphorase–containing neurons and an increase in the amount of acetylcholinesterase-containing nerve bundles are all characteristic.[68,70] Furthermore, nitric oxide synthase is a candidate neurotransmitter responsible for relaxation of the internal anal sphincter.[70]

Opinion

There is considerable difference of opinion with respect to the reliability of the various diagnostic methods. It is our impression that the most important variable is the experience of the radiologist, physiologist, and pathologist. We have found the contrast enema to be the most valuable diagnostic test, with rectal suction biopsy a means for confirming the clinical and radiologic impression. Although biopsy may establish the diagnosis when the specimen is obtained through the rectum, it reveals nothing about the transition zone site. That valuable piece of information must be obtained radiologically, clinically, and with full-thickness biopsy analysis, guided by an experienced eye in the operating room during the definitive operation. The aganglionic segment is contracted; the transition zone is thick and leathery; and a normal caliber, smooth colon is found above the transition zone.

Management

Medical Treatment

Bowel irrigation with saline solution is an extremely valuable procedure for the emergency management of distension and vomiting. By decompressing the colon, irrigations may dramatically improve the condition of a very ill infant, as well as to prevent and treat enterocolitis.

It is extremely important to clarify the difference between an irrigation and an enema. To confuse these two terms may be dangerous for babies with Hirschsprung's disease. An enema is a procedure in which a determined amount of fluid is instilled into the rectum and colon. The fluid is expected to be spontaneously expelled. A rectal irrigation, conversely, is a procedure in which a large tube (e.g., 24F) is introduced through the rectum, and small amounts of saline solution are instilled through the tube in order to cleanse the bowel. The rectal and colonic content is expected to drain through the lumen of the tube. The tube is then rotated in different directions and moved in and out. The operator continues to instill small amounts of saline solution, allowing the evacuation of gas and liquid stool through the tube.

Patients with Hirschsprung's disease suffer from a very serious dysmotility disorder. An enema, as defined here, may worsen the problem because the patient does not have the capacity to expel the infused volume of fluid. With an irrigation, the patient benefits from the evacuation of the rectosigmoid contents through the lumen of the large tube. Essentially the tube overcomes the functional distal obstruction.

Surgical Treatment
General Principles

Patients with Hirschsprung's disease can usually undergo a primary procedure within the first few months of life.[11,13,15,103] The circumstances for performing the surgery are different from country to country, and there is often quite a bit of variability in the experience of surgeons and their access to resources.[90] In addition, the availability of fully trained, experienced clinical pathologists may be problematic. If one is to perform a primary neonatal pull-through procedure, the surgeon must rely on frozen-section analysis. For this, he or she must interact with an experienced pathologist. In the very ill, low-birth-weight newborn, one who suffers from associated defects or concomitant serious medical conditions, or in the absence of pathologic support, an initial fecal diversion may be required.

In addition to the issue of whether the performance of a colostomy is appropriate, there is a difference of opinion as to the type and the location of the stoma. In our experience, if diversion is to be considered, an ileostomy is an effective and safe method for decompressing the bowel in the vast majority of infants with this condition. By using this location, the risk of opening the stoma in an aganglionic area is much reduced. And, the sigmoid mesentery is unaffected by the diversion. It is a particularly useful option in the emergency situation, especially if the surgeon cannot rely on the radiologist, or if a pathologist capable of making the diagnosis based on frozen-section analysis is unavailable.

Many surgeons advocate the creation of the stoma just above the transition zone, a leveling colostomy, which requires confirmatory frozen-section analysis. This alternative obligates one to pull the colostomy down at the time of the definitive repair. Obviously, the advantage to this approach is that the child will require only a two-stage procedure, whereas an ileostomy commits the surgeon to a three-stage operation.

Definitive Operations

Swenson Procedure. Swenson and Bill described a transabdominal dissection with resection of the aganglionic portion of the colon, including that of the most dilated portion of the bowel (Figure 3-7A).[111] Typical Hirschsprung's disease may require only mobilization of the sigmoid arcade and sometimes the splenic flexure, but the long-segment type may necessitate mobilization of even the right colon in order to obtain sufficient length. Freeing of the aganglionic area below the peritoneal floor is carried out by precise dissection as close as possible to the rectal wall down to the level of the levators (Figure 3-7B). Anastomosis is effected by a transanal, hand-sewn technique (Figure 3-7C). The abdominal component nowadays is usually performed laparoscopically. The transanal dissection includes full-thickness rectal wall.

Duhamel Procedure. Duhamel's procedure[25,102] was devised in order to avoid the extensive pelvic dissection required of Swenson's operation. This is accomplished by preserving the aganglionic rectum and dividing the bowel at the peritoneal reflection as distally as possible (Figure 3-8A).

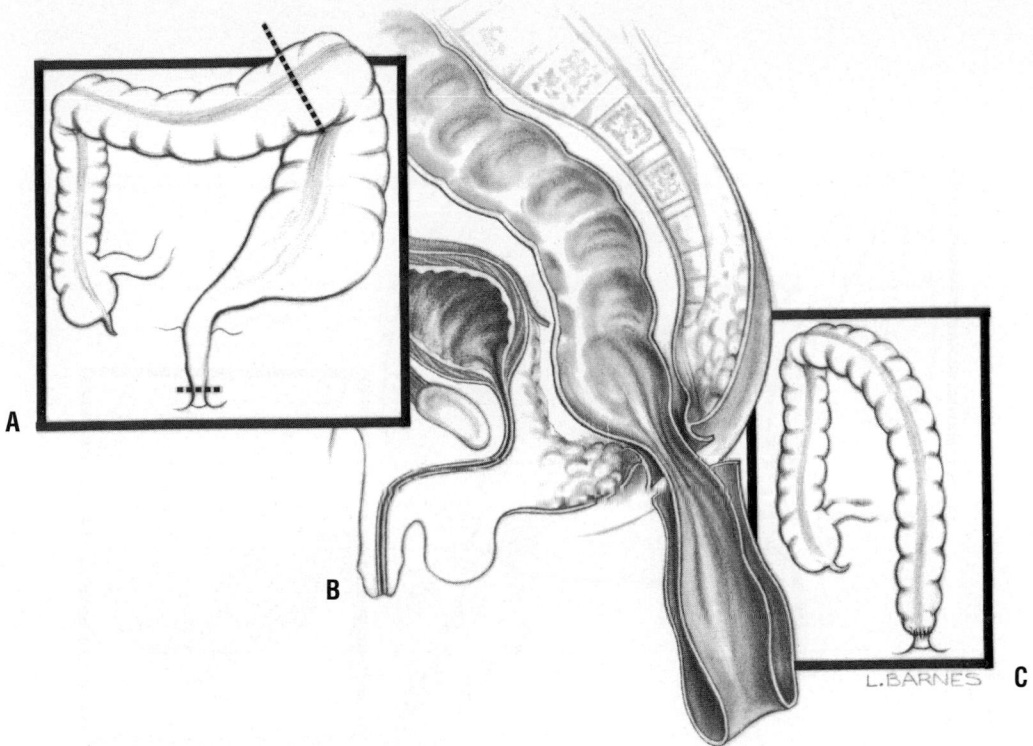

FIGURE 3-7. Swenson's procedure. **A:** Bowel resection including aganglionic and distended bowel. **B:** Pull-through of normally innervated colon. **C:** Anastomosis completed.

The rectal stump is then closed (Figure 3-8B). Normal (i.e., ganglionic) intestine, usually above the most dilated portion, is pulled through a presacral space that has been created by blunt dissection (Figure 3-8B,C). The posterior rectal wall is incised above the dentate line, entering the previously dissected retrorectal space (Figure 3-8D). The new, normally innervated colon is pulled through the rectal incision, and a gastrointestinal anastomotic stapler is used to effect the anastomosis to the aganglionic rectum (Figure 3-9A,B). The posterior wall of the colon is also sutured to the edge of the proctotomy (Figure 3-9C). The anastomosis between the colon and the aganglionic

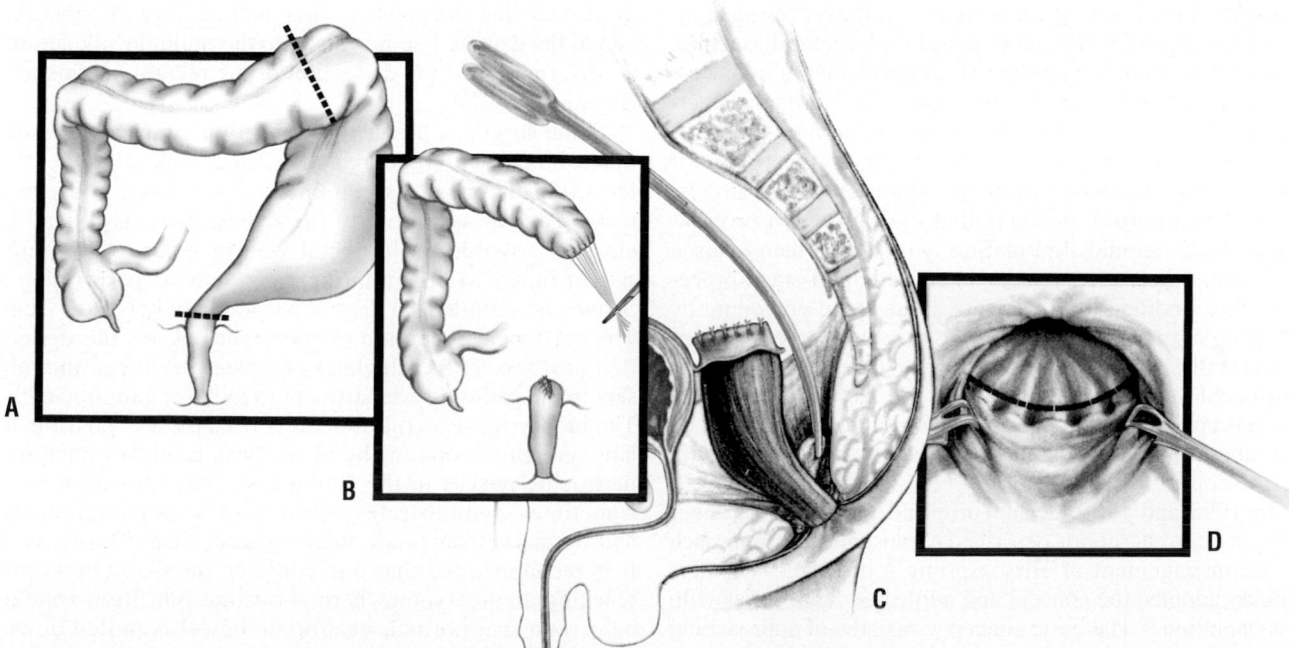

FIGURE 3-8. Duhamel's procedure. **A:** Colon resection leaving the aganglionic portion in place. **B:** Ganglionic bowel ready to be pulled down; the rectal stump has been closed. **C:** Presacral dissection. **D:** Posterior rectal wall incision.

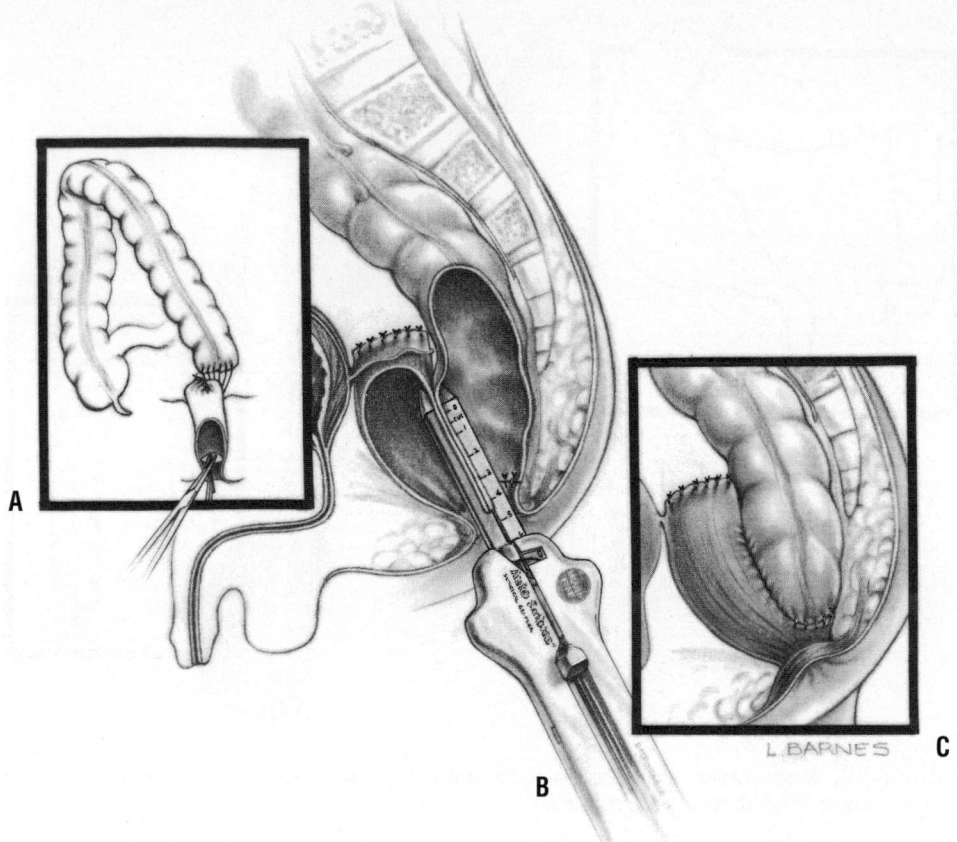

FIGURE 3-9. Duhamel's procedure. **A:** Retrorectal pull-through. **B:** Gastrointestinal anastomosis stapler used to join the colon to the aganglionic rectum. **C:** Completed reconstruction.

rectum must be created as wide as possible, and the rectal stump as small as possible.

Soave Procedure. The Soave procedure[104] removes the aganglionic rectosigmoid by a submucosal endorectal dissection, theoretically minimizing the risk to pelvic nerve injury associated with the Swenson procedure. The normally innervated colon is passed through a rectosigmoid muscular cuff. The cuff (outer wall of the rectum) that is aganglionic, if left too long, can cause obstructive symptoms.[54] Originally, Soave left a portion of the pulled-through colon protruding beyond the anal skin margin, which was then excised at a second operation 1 week later. This two-stage procedure was modified by Boley into a one-stage procedure by effecting a primary anastomosis to the anal verge.[8] The endorectal dissection is initiated usually 1 or 2 cm above the peritoneal reflection (Figure 3-10). The normal, ganglionic colon is anastomosed to the anorectal mucosa (Figure 3-11). The abdominal component here is also usually done with laparoscopy.[31,32]

In 1998 and 1999, de la Torre and Ortega and Langer et al. in different reports described a transanal-only approach to the management of Hirschsprung's disease.[20,51] Others quickly adopted the concept and published large series with this operation.[50] The basic concept consisted of approaching the disease through the anus. A Lone Star retractor is used (Figure 3-12). The circumferential traction exposes the anal canal, the pectinate line, and the rectal mucosa. Multiple fine

sutures are placed in the rectal mucosa in a circumferential manner in order to exert uniform traction to facilitate the dissection of this part of the bowel and to carefully preserve the dentate line. A circumferential incision about 1 cm proximal to the dentate line just distal to the multiple silk sutures is performed, and the dissection of the rectum commences (Figure 3-13A,B).

Some surgeons prefer to perform this transanal dissection submucosally (endorectally), (Soave-like) but we prefer a full-thickness dissection (Swenson-like). A specific recommendation in both of these dissections is to stay as close as possible to the rectal wall in order to minimize risk of injury to important pelvic nerves. If performing a Soave, the submucosal dissection should only be 1 to 2 cm. The peritoneal reflection is soon reached. As the dissection progresses, full-thickness biopsies are taken that are sent to the pathology department to look for ganglion cells. The biopsy must be full thickness because it is possible to have ganglion cells in the muscularis layer but have hypertrophic nerves in the submucosa. The transition zone sometimes demonstrates an area of hypoganglionosis, and the nerve trunks are thick (greater than 50 microns). It is recommended that one continue the dissection until reaching an area somewhere above the transition zone to be certain that normal, ganglionic bowel is pulled down. The surgeon looks for a smooth-walled nondilated segment of bowel. The normal, ganglionic bowel is transanally anastomosed to the anal canal 1 cm above the pectinate

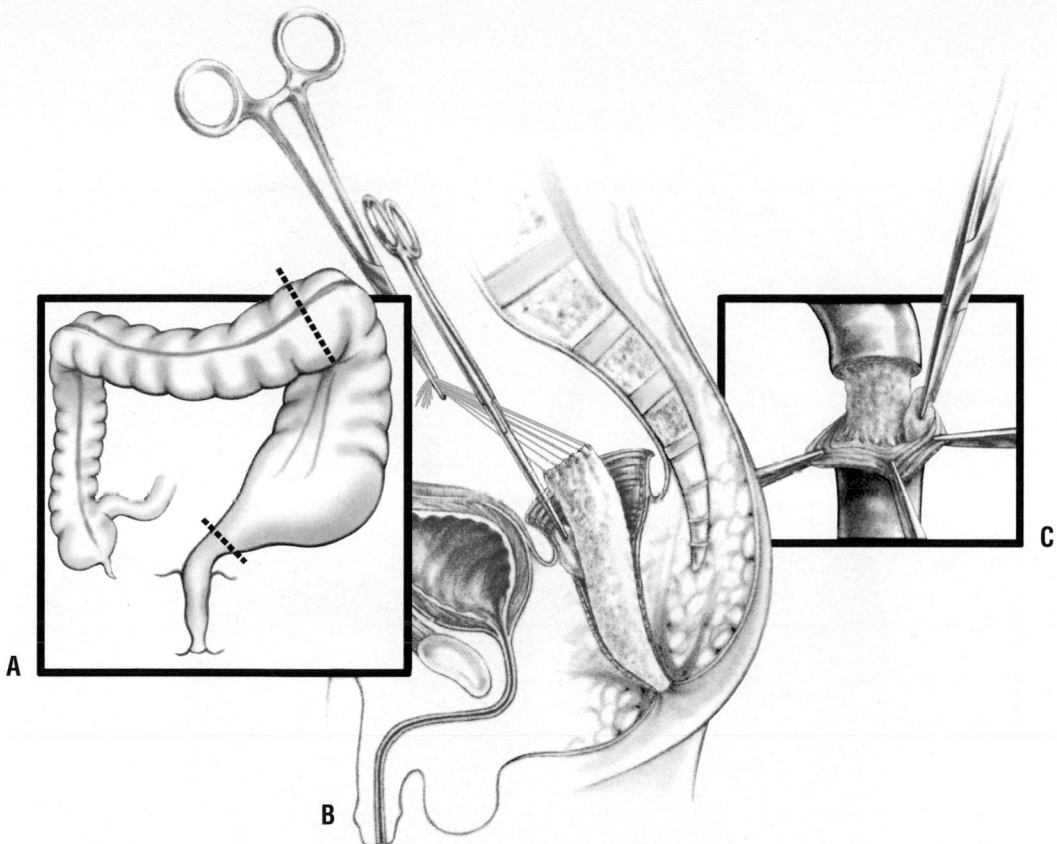

FIGURE 3-10. Soave's procedure. **A:** Resection of most dilated portion of the bowel. **B,C:** Endorectal dissection.

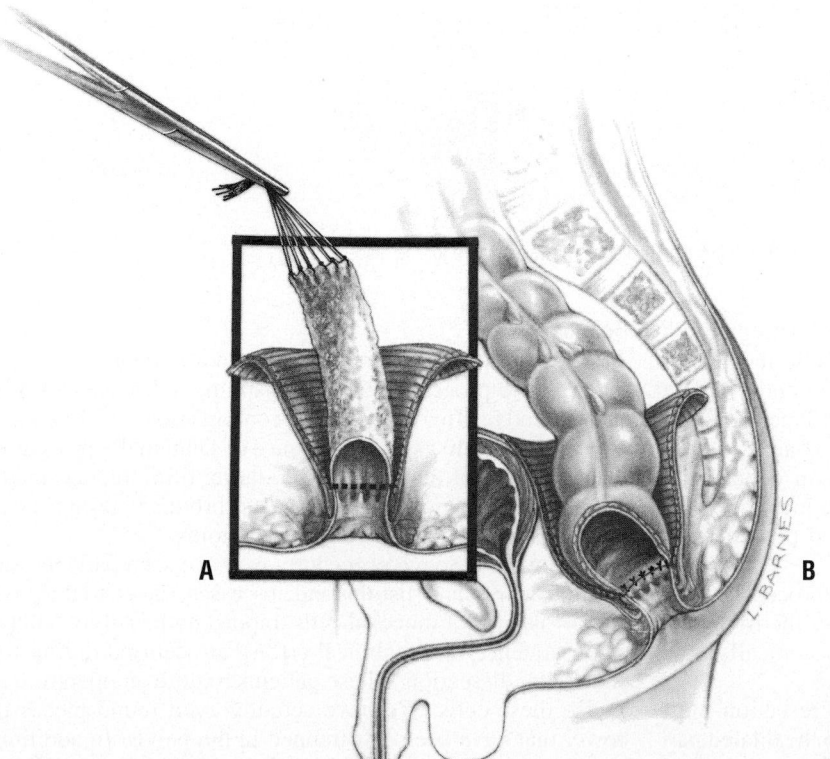

FIGURE 3-11. Soave's procedure. **A:** Endorectal dissection completed above the dentate line. **B:** Ganglionic bowel pulled through and anastomosis completed.

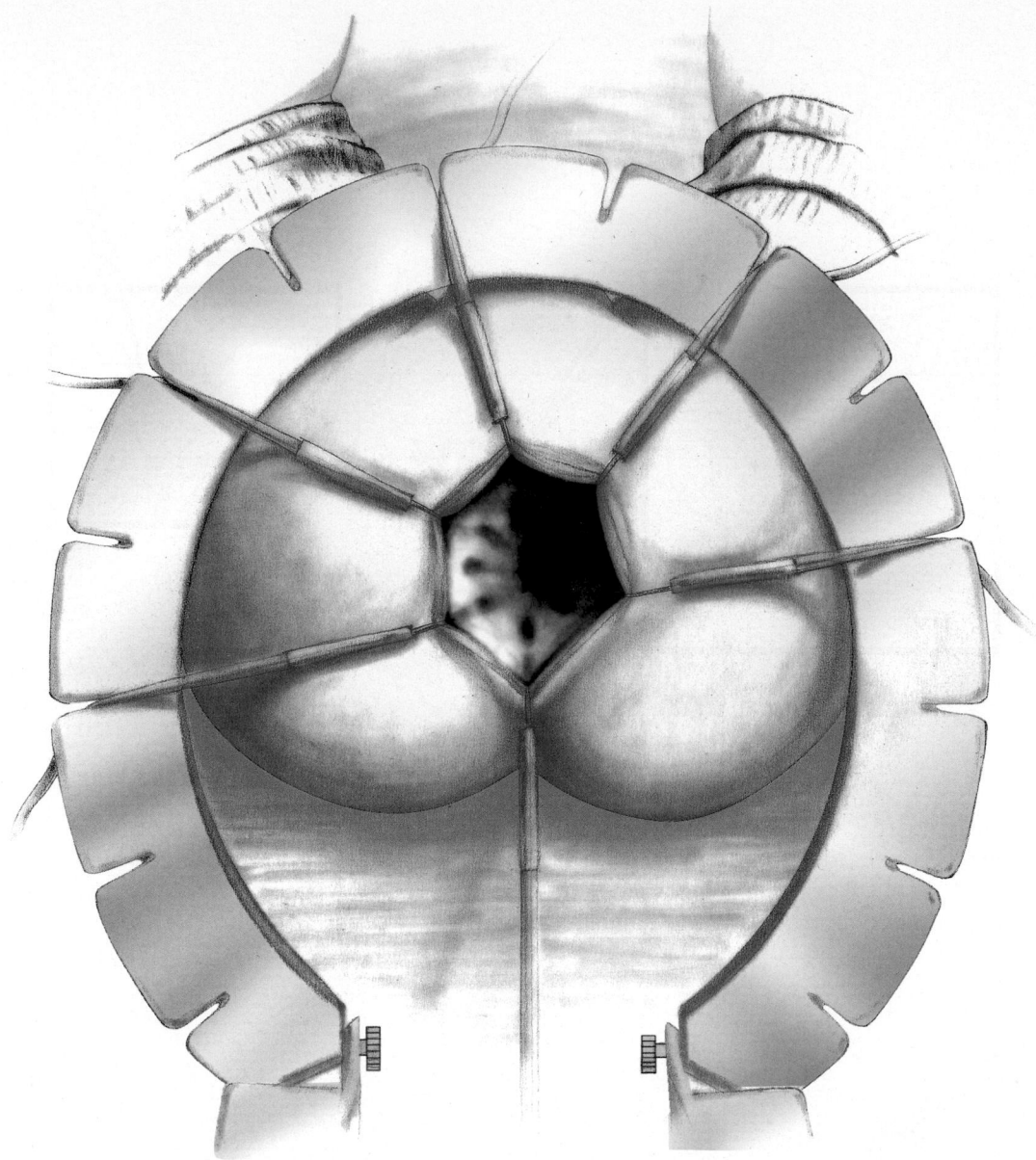

FIGURE 3-12. A Lone Star retractor in position with hooks in place to provide exposure for the dissection.

line (Figure 3-13C). Considering that most patients with Hirschsprung's disease have a transition zone in the sigmoid colon, it is often possible to repair the entire defect using only the transanal approach without a laparotomy or laparoscopy. However, when the transition zone is located higher, or the surgeon does not feel safe in conducting this dissection further from below, then one must open the abdomen or perform a laparoscopic-assisted procedure in order to mobilize the colon.

Some surgeons advocate commencing the procedure laparoscopically, performing a biopsy to identify the transition zone, mobilizing the sigmoid colon laparoscopically, and then dissecting transanally.

It is important to keep in mind that the resection must include not only the aganglionic part but also the dilated part of the bowel. Pulling down a very dilated segment of colon even though it may be ganglionic will result in severe constipation later in life because dilated bowel tends to lose its peristaltic ability.[54]

Opinion

At our institution, we are often referred patients who have undergone a procedure for Hirschsprung's disease and who subsequently suffer from serious complications.[54,85] The most common problem as a consequence of Duhamel's procedure is persistence of an aganglionic, large, blind rectal pouch. This tends to grow with time and to produce chronic fecal impaction with multiple related symptoms.

Following a Soave procedure, we have seen patients suffering from perianal fistulas and abscesses related to the presence of islands of mucosal cells trapped in the pelvis. This is a consequence of a technical error that occurred during the endorectal dissection. These patients require an operation to excise these cells. We have actually even found pieces of bowel that have been left trapped in the pelvis. In addition, an excessively long or a scarred Soave cuff can obstruct the ganglionic pull-through.[54]

A feared and unfortunately frequent complication is fecal incontinence. This is most likely related to injury to the

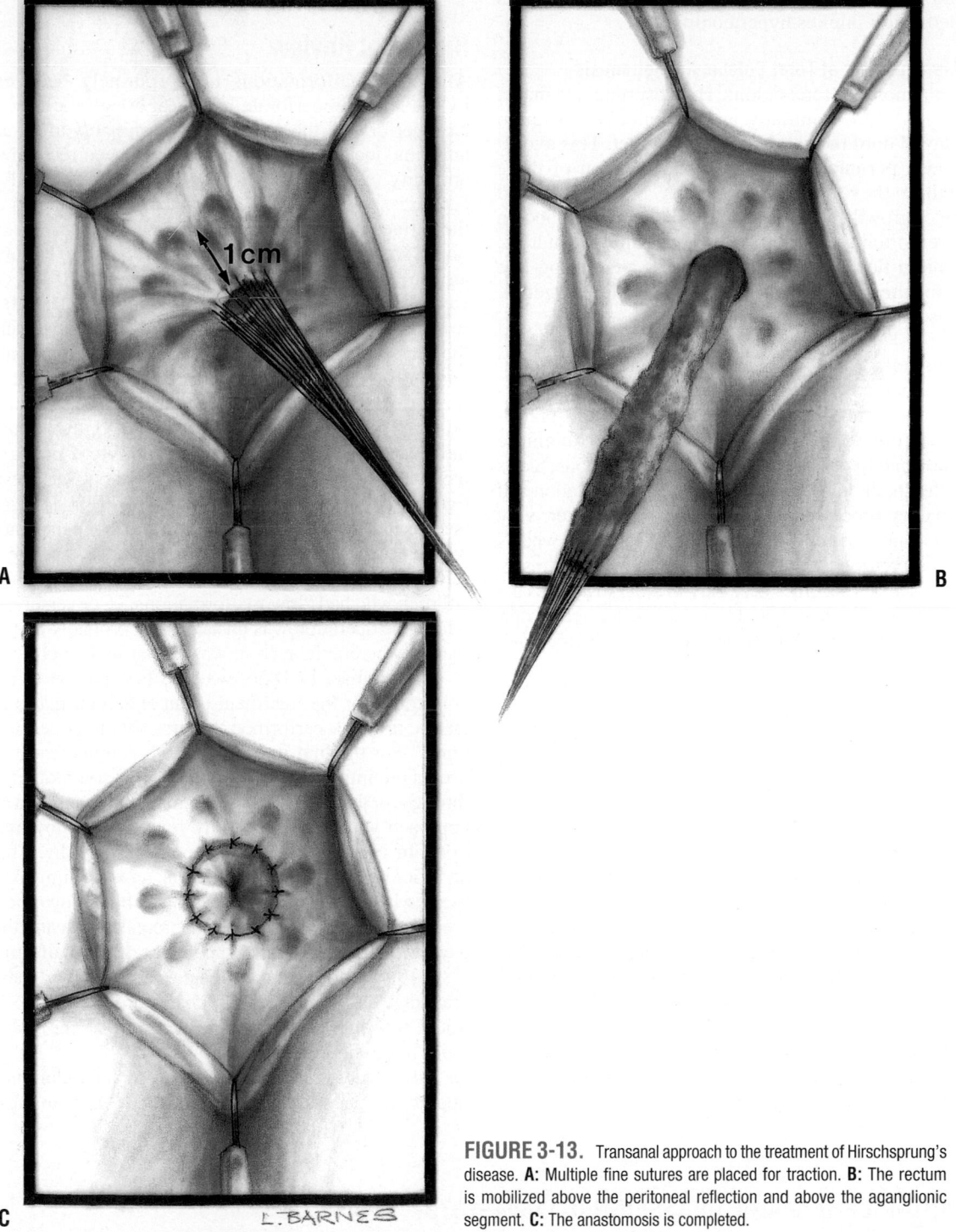

FIGURE 3-13. Transanal approach to the treatment of Hirschsprung's disease. **A:** Multiple fine sutures are placed for traction. **B:** The rectum is mobilized above the peritoneal reflection and above the aganglionic segment. **C:** The anastomosis is completed.

continence mechanism during one of these procedures.[57] The anal canal can be inadvertently resected or the sphincters can be damaged by overstretching. All operations for this condition are designed to prevent this from happening, provided the procedures are performed properly. Dehiscence, retraction, stricture, abscess, and fistula are all the result of technical errors.

A complication one understands poorly is enterocolitis. This problem is a true challenge for pediatric surgeons. Although the etiology is not known, it is believed that fecal stasis is a predisposing factor. Anatomic causes for obstruction such as a cuff or retained dilated segment can lead to enterocolitis.[54]

Constipation after surgery should be anticipated and aggressively managed. When a pull-through procedure leaves behind a portion of significantly dilated colon, these children will suffer from constipation. A dilated colon is almost as severe a pathologic entity as an aganglionic segment, and as previously mentioned, it should be resected at the time of the pull-through. Despite meticulous attention to surgical technique, constipation still occurs in approximately 15% of cases. Hypermotility resulting from resection of the rectosigmoid reservoir may also occur, but this is less common. A contrast enema helps differentiate between these two conditions; a dilated colon means constipation, whereas a nondilated colon implies hypermotility.

Surgical Management of Total Colonic Aganglionosis

When the diagnosis of total colonic Hirschsprung's is made, an ileostomy is required initially, and the definitive operation ideally delayed until the child can sit on a toilet. This avoids the often seen perianal excoriation. Management of these patients while they have an ileostomy requires careful monitoring of growth. Sodium loss is also a source of concern with children often requiring oral sodium supplementation. We perform an ileoanal pull-through using a Swenson-like technique for the definitive reconstruction. Many surgeons, however, use an ileo-Duhamel approach.

Opinion. Long-term follow-up of patients with total colon aganglionosis has demonstrated that the concept of integrating a portion of aganglionic colon with the normal ganglionic, pulled-through bowel (often employed in the past) in order to minimize stool retention and frequency has proved to be erroneous. Stasis of stool in the small bowel produces bacterial proliferation and an inflammatory process. Rather than absorbing water, very often the intestine secretes it into the lumen, producing what is essentially a secretory diarrhea. It is not uncommon that resection of these pouches becomes necessary in order to address the problems of malnutrition and fluid loss.[54,85] We, as well as others, believe that a straight ileorectal anastomosis is the preferred option because of the better long-term results.[113]

Total Intestinal Aganglionosis

Patients can have total (extending to the stomach) or near-total intestinal aganglionosis. Such children require an intestinal transplantation to survive.

Commentary

Hirschsprung's disease is a subject of active research and study. This has led to the production of a large number of publications causing one to hope that many of these children will soon realize the benefits. For example, considerable effort has been made in transplanting ganglion cells.[96] Moreover, advances in the field of genetics should ultimately allow us to predict which individuals are at risk for having children with this condition.[72] Additionally, genetic engineering could one day be used to prevent this condition, an exciting area of exploration indeed.

▶ ANORECTAL MALFORMATIONS

Historical Review

Anorectal malformations have routinely been classified by the term "imperforate anus"; although the vast majority are "perforate," the rectum just terminates in an abnormal anatomic location. The condition has been recognized since antiquity (e.g., by Paulus Aegineta of Greece).[1] For many centuries, physicians understood that by creating an orifice in the perineum many of the children with imperforate anus survived, some even with normal bowel function. Unfortunately, an anal stricture was often a consequence. If the condition went uncorrected, intestinal obstruction and death frequently resulted. Ancient operations consisted of making an incision in the perineum deep enough to open the rectal pouch and to obtain meconium. The surgeon packed the wound and changed the packing daily in an attempt to create a permanent perineal orifice. The primary concern was directed toward survival of the infant, and therefore, these operations took only a few minutes and were obviously undertaken without anesthesia, blood transfusion, or other adjunctive measures. In 1835, Amussat (see his biography, Chapter 24) was the first person not merely to open the rectal pouch, but also to suture it to the skin.[3] In retrospect, perhaps those who survived that operation were children who had "low malformations." Conversely, those for whom the operation was unsuccessful probably had a malformation wherein the rectum was higher in the pelvis.

Chassaignac, in 1856, was the first person to perform a colostomy for the treatment of an anorectal malformation.[14] Hadra, in 1886, performed the first abdominoperineal procedure.[37] For the first part of the 20th century, most surgeons used a preliminary colostomy and an abdominoperineal pull-through for the treatment of high malformations, and a perineal approach without a colostomy for so-called low malformations. In 1930, Wangensteen (see his biography, Chapter 23) and Rice described the invertogram, an x-ray film taken during the newborn period with the infant's head down, in order to measure the distance between the rectal pouch and the skin as a criterion for determining the height of the malformation.[122]

In 1948, Rhoads and colleagues reintroduced the neonatal one-stage abdominoperineal procedure.[93] In 1953, Stephens noted the importance of preservation of the puborectalis sling in maintaining fecal continence.[106,107,108] He proposed an initial sacral approach followed by an abdominoperineal operation, if necessary. Since 1980,[21,83] these malformations

---

EDOUARD-PIERRE-MARIE CHASSAIGNAC (1804–1879)

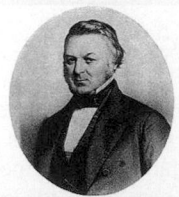

Edouard Chassaignac was born on December 24, 1804, in Nantes, France. He received his medical school education at the University in Nantes and graduated in 1835. His great forte was the design of new instruments, and he was an ingenious experimenter. For example, he perfected the use of the new product, rubber, for use as a fenestrated drain and developed the concept of the occlusive dressing for wounds. He became surgeon to the Lariboisiàre in 1852 and is recognized as the first surgeon to perform a colostomy for the management of an anorectal malformation. Other signal contributions included his classic dissertation on fractures of the femoral neck, his treatise on suppuration and surgical drainage, his classification of breast abscess, and his book (*The Subject of Surgical Anatomy and Pathology*) in which he relates his experiences in clinical surgery. He is also eponymously recognized for his description of the carotid (cervical) tubercle (Chassaignac's tubercle). In 1861, he was awarded the Legion of Honor, and in 1868 he was named a member of the Academy of Medicine. Chassaignac died in Versailles on August 26, 1879.

were found to be ideally approached through a posterior sagittal incision, using an electrical stimulator to identify the sphincter complex.[78,79,80,83] This technique was instrumental in revealing the very important anatomic area of the pelvis that, until 1980, was a matter mostly of speculation.

Incidence

Most authors report that 1 of every 5,000 newborns have an anorectal malformation.[10,98,120] Male infants seem to suffer from this condition more frequently than females. The most common type of malformation seen in boys is rectourethral fistula, and the most common type of anomaly in girls is rectovestibular fistula. There is an increased incidence of imperforate anus in children with Down's syndrome who frequently have a low-lying rectal pouch without a genitourinary or perineal fistula.[119]

Embryologic Considerations

Anorectal malformation defects develop during gestational weeks 4 to 12.[107] The urinary, genital, and rectal tracts empty into a common channel, the cloaca. Ultimately, they will be segregated by the urorectal septum during its craniocaudal descent, separating the cloaca into an anterior urogenital sinus and a posterior intestinal canal. Two lateral folds of the cloaca also move simultaneously toward the midline. The perineal mound appears to be the caudal extension of the urorectal septum, which develops into the perineal body. In the male, the inner and outer genital ridges meet to form the urethra. In the female, these ridges do not coalesce but form the labia minora and majora. Various types of failures in this process have been postulated to explain each of the anorectal malformations. The resulting defects constitute a spectrum that ranges from the most severe examples (e.g., caudal regression and persistent cloaca) to the more easily managed concerns (rectoperineal fistula).

Classification

In our experience, the posterior sagittal approach to these malformations has permitted the opportunity for directly

TABLE 3-1 Classification
Male
Rectoperineal fistula
Rectourethral fistula
Bulbar
Prostatic
Rectobladder neck fistula
Imperforate anus without fistula
Rectal atresia/rectal stenosis
Female
Rectoperineal fistula
Rectovestibular fistula
Imperforate anus without fistula
Rectal atresia/rectal stenosis
Cloaca
Complex malformations

exposing the anatomy of each of these defects. This has led to important therapeutic implications in addition to those of terminology and classification, making previous classifications now obsolete.[49,109,110]

With imperforate anus, one is dealing with a spectrum of malformations. Thus, in attempting to separate these groups of defects into categories, one risks being arbitrary. With this cautionary note, the classification shown in Table 3-1 is considered practical for therapeutic purposes.

Anatomy

The posterior sagittal approach used for the repair of anorectal malformations, in addition to the management of tumors, rectal trauma, and rectal prolapse, clarified the anatomic details of a normal male (Figure 3-14) and a normal female

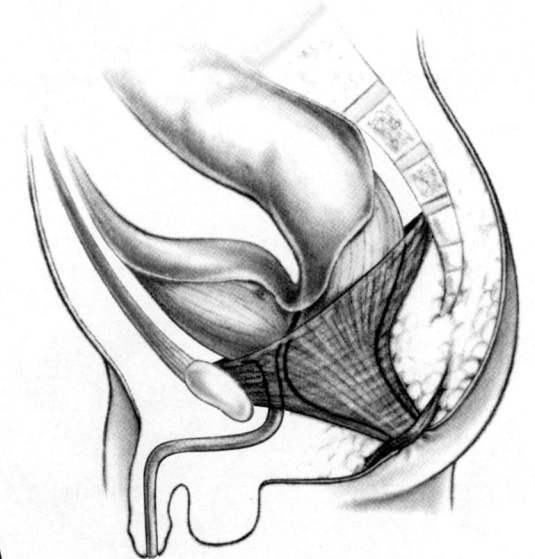
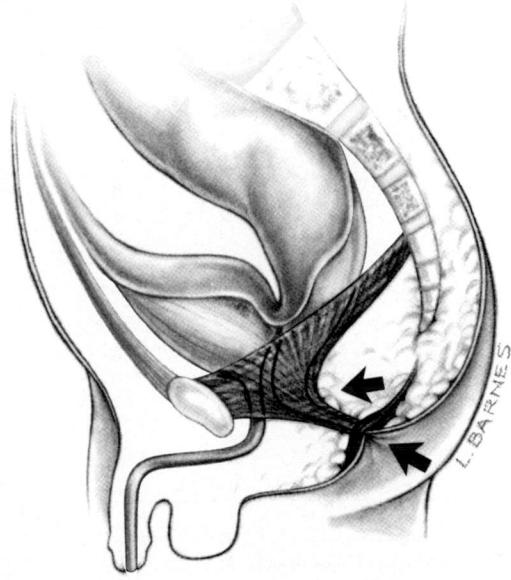

FIGURE 3-14. Normal male anatomy. **A:** During defecation. **B:** During sphincter contraction (i.e., retention).

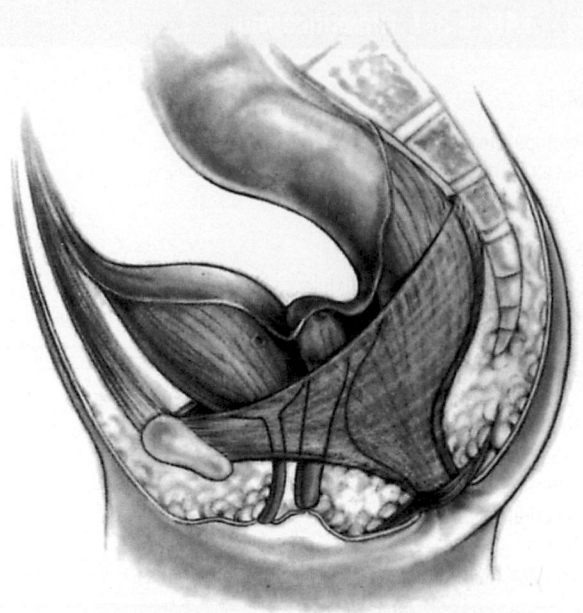

FIGURE 3-15. Normal female anatomy during defecation.

and push the rectum forward. In the lower part of the funnel (muscle complex), vertical fibers predominate and elevate the anus. Because the parasagittal fibers meet together in front of the anus as well as posterior to it, contraction occludes the anus. This gives the fibers a circular appearance.

The spectrum of anatomic defects in the male patient is shown in Figure 3-16.

Description of Specific Defects in the Male Patient

Rectoperineal Fistula

Rectoperineal fistula is the lowest malformation. In this anomaly, the rectum has passed normally through much of the sphincter mechanism; the lowest part of the rectum is anteriorly deviated and ends as a perineal fistula anterior to the center of sphincter mechanism (Figure 3-16A). Frequently, the fistula tract lies immediately below a very thin layer of skin, with the external opening found somewhere in the midline from the anus to the ventral portion of the penis. One often perceives beneath the midline skin, a black, or white ribbonlike structure resulting from meconium or mucous (Figure 3-17). The infant does not require further investigation and can undergo surgery without a colostomy as the rectum is reliably found 1 to 2 cm from the skin surface. Prognosis is excellent because the patient has all the necessary anatomic elements for bowel control.

In all anorectal malformations, the higher the defect, the less the likelihood will be of achieving bowel control. Conversely, the lower the malformation, the higher the incidence will be of constipation. Therefore, in treating an infant with a rectoperineal fistula, the surgeon should expect good bowel control but should anticipate constipation and be prepared to treat it effectively.[55]

(Figure 3-15). The sphincter complex is represented by a group of parasagittal muscle fibers, a muscle complex, and the levators, which form a funnel-shaped continuum of muscle. The portion of muscle located between the parasagittal fibers and the levator, integrated mainly by vertical fibers that run parallel to the rectum, is called the muscle complex. In the upper portion of the funnel, horizontal fibers predominate

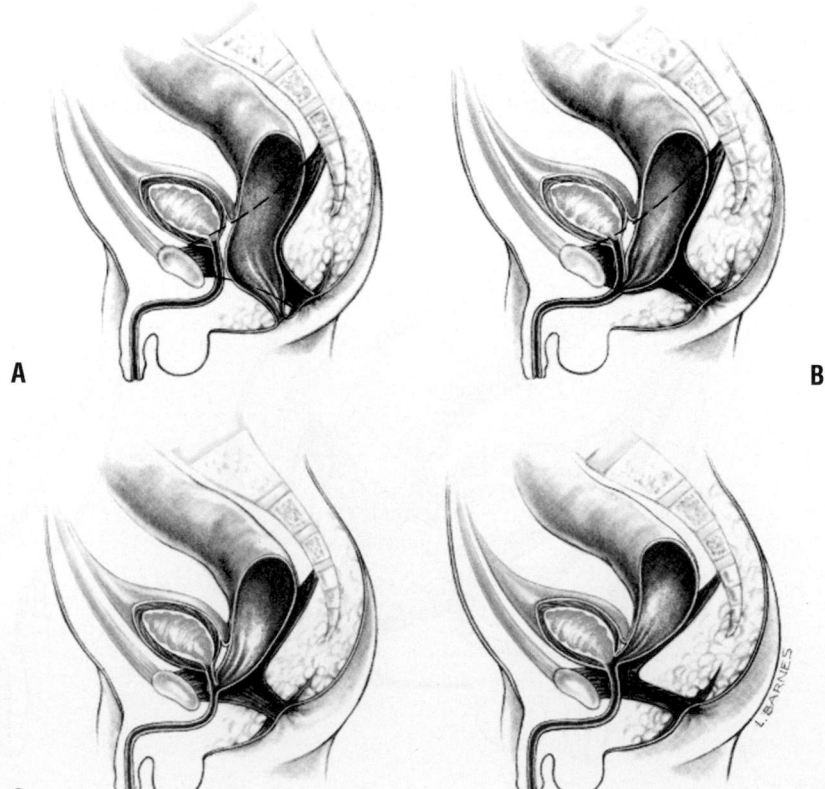

FIGURE 3-16. Spectrum of male defects. **A:** Rectoperineal fistula. **B:** Rectobulbar urethral fistula. **C:** Rectoprostatic urethral fistula. **D:** Rectobladder neck fistula.

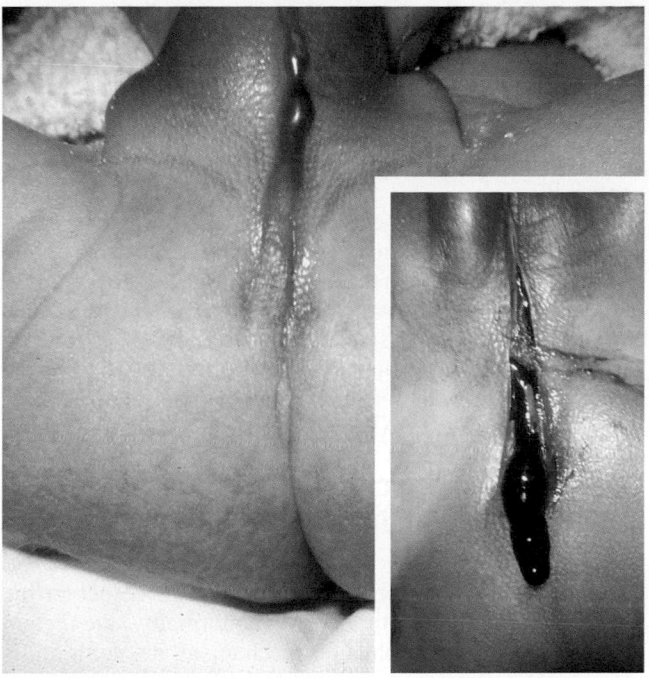

FIGURE 3-17. Rectoperineal fistula. Note the ribbonlike structure containing meconium. The tract is unroofed (*inset*).

Even when repair of a rectoperineal fistula is accomplished by means of a relatively minor operation, the surgeon must be mindful of the fact that the anterior wall of the rectum is intimately attached to the posterior wall of the urethra. Meticulous dissection is therefore required in order to separate the two structures and to prevent a urethral injury. One must always perform the operation with a Foley catheter in place.

Anal Stenosis and Rectal Atresia

Anal stenosis is another, rather benign defect that consists of a ring of fibrous tissue located at the anal verge. This causes a stricture that may result in varying degrees of functional abnormality, but the muscle structure is completely normal. From the external perspective, the anus also appears normal and is properly located within the sphincter mechanism. One must introduce a Hegar dilator to detect the malformation; digital rectal examination is impossible. The typical symptom is difficulty moving the bowels, with the parent describing a ribbonlike appearance to the feces. This malformation may be associated with a presacral mass.

Rectal atresia is the complete interruption of the rectal lumen between the anal canal and the rectum. The anal canal usually measures 1 to 2 cm in length and is rather narrow, whereas the rectum is usually quite distended. The distance between the rectal pouch and the anal canal in these patients is variable. One may see a very thin membrane separating both structures or a rather long fibrous space. These infants have all the necessary elements to achieve bowel control. Repair requires a PSARP (see later) with or without prior colostomy, and the normal anal canal is preserved. The posterior aspect of it is incised, and it becomes the anterior 180 degrees of the anoplasty. The posterior rectum is mobilized and becomes the posterior 180 degrees of the anoplasty. The results of treatment for this malformation are excellent. A presacral mass must be screened for.

Rectourethral Fistula

Rectourethral fistula is the most frequent malformation seen in the male patient. Congenitally, the rectum descends through a considerable portion of the funnel-shaped muscle structure, but at some point it deviates anteriorly and connects with the urethra. The most frequent site of the fistula is to the bulbar urethra (Figure 3-16B). However, significant numbers of urethral fistulas open at the prostatic urethra (Figure 3-16C). The quality of muscle in an infant with a rectourethral fistula is usually good. A patient with rectobulbar fistula usually has a better potential for continence because the rectum has already passed through much of the sphincter mechanism, the muscle quality is more satisfactory, and the sacrum is more normally developed. Higher malformations are more frequently associated with a poor sacrum; spinal anomalies; and, consequently, poor innervation with a poor quality of muscle. The perineum in patients with rectourethral bulbar fistula usually exhibits a well-developed midline groove and an easily recognized anal dimple (Figure 3-18). These signs are usually indicative of good muscle development.

Occasionally, however, a patient with a rectourethral fistula, usually *prostatic*, has a rather poor sacrum and a "flat" or "round bottom" with an absent anal dimple and a minimal midline groove (Figure 3-19). All of these signs usually imply that the patient has poor sphincter muscles. Patients with rectoprostatic fistula sometimes have a bifid scrotum. The center of the sphincter mechanism is sometimes located very close to the scrotum. These findings do not

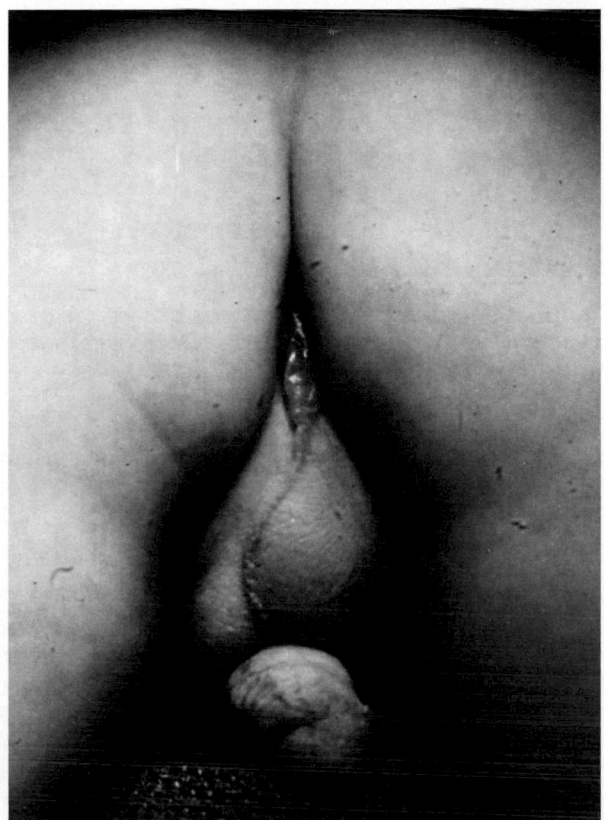

FIGURE 3-18. Perineum of a child with a rectourethral fistula. Note the prominent midline groove and a distinct anal dimple.

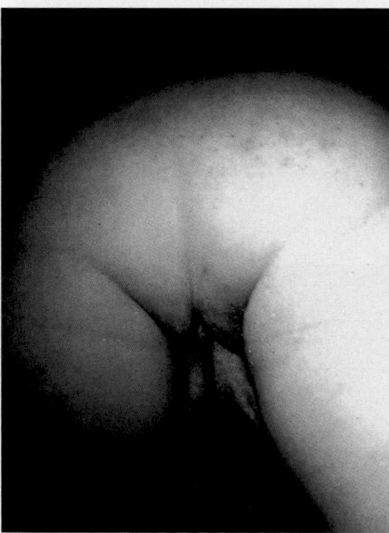

FIGURE 3-19. Perineum of a male and female child with poor muscles (flat bottom). (Reprinted from Peña A. *Atlas of Surgical Management of Anorectal Malformations*. New York, NY: Springer Verlag; 1989, with permission.)

occur as frequently in cases of rectourethral bulbar fistula. These infants ultimately require a posterior sagittal anorectoplasty (PSARP). A protective colostomy is performed in the first days of life.

Rectobladder Neck Fistula

In the case of Necka rectobladder neck fistula, the rectum opens at the level of the bladder neck (Figure 3-16D). The levators, muscle complex, and parasagittal fibers are frequently underdeveloped. The frequency of association with an abnormal sacrum, "flat bottom," and poor-looking perineum—all signs of poor prognosis for fecal continence—is very high. These infants must be treated with a colostomy in the newborn period, followed by a PSARP and a laparotomy or laparoscopy to reach a very high rectum. This group represents approximately 10% of cases.

Imperforate Anus without Fistula

Imperforate anus with no fistula represents 5% of all children with anorectal malformations, half of whom suffer from Down's syndrome. More than 90% of the patients with Down's syndrome with an anorectal malformation have this specific defect. Eighty percent will achieve voluntary bowel control.[119]

The rectum usually ends blindly, approximately 2 cm above the perineal skin at a similar level to that of the rectobulbar urethral defect. Even without a fistula, only a very thin layer separates rectum from urethra. These infants usually have good muscle quality and a well-developed sacrum, and the perineum exhibits signs implying a good prognosis for bowel control. Treatment consists of a colostomy followed by a PSARP.

Description of Specific Defects in the Female Patient

Rectoperineal Fistula

Perineal fistula represents the most benign defect in the female spectrum. As with the male abnormality, the rectum traverses most of the sphincter mechanism, deviating in its most distal portion to communicate with the skin through a fistula located a few millimeters anterior to the center of the sphincter. These infants have all the necessary elements for bowel control. The anterior rectal wall and the posterior vaginal wall are completely separated, as is seen during the surgical repair (Figure 3-20). A simple anoplasty (i.e., minimal PSARP) is sufficient to treat this type of malformation without the need for a colostomy. Treatment objectives are to make the anus an adequate size, place it in the center of the sphincter, and create a normal length perineal body.

Rectovestibular Fistula

Rectovestibular fistula is the malformation most frequently seen in females. The bowel is anteriorly deviated at a higher level, opening immediately behind the hymen into the vestibule. The rectum and the vagina are opposed, with only a very thin layer separating the two structures. The quality of muscle is usually excellent. Most patients have the potential for normal continence, a normal sacrum, and a good-looking perineum. However, as with boys, there are exceptions in which one can find a vestibular fistula associated with a rather poor muscle structure and sacrum.

This malformation can be misdiagnosed as a *rectovaginal fistula*. A true vaginal fistula is extremely rare. Meticulous examination of the genitalia of a newborn is required to localize the fistula site precisely.

When a girl is born with this anatomy, has no associated defects, and is otherwise well, she can be operated on within the first 48 hours without a colostomy (Figures 3-21 and 3-22). However, one must be mindful that a protective colostomy is still very valuable in a baby with an associated defect, in very poor clinical condition, and to avoid a perineal dehiscence.

This particular malformation is the one that we have seen most frequently managed incorrectly. Even when these children have an excellent potential for bowel control, a failed procedure requires a reoperation and negatively affects bowel control. A simple cut-back procedure, which does not include separating the vagina from the rectum, requires a secondary repair as a consequence of resulting incontinence and because of an inadequate perineal body.

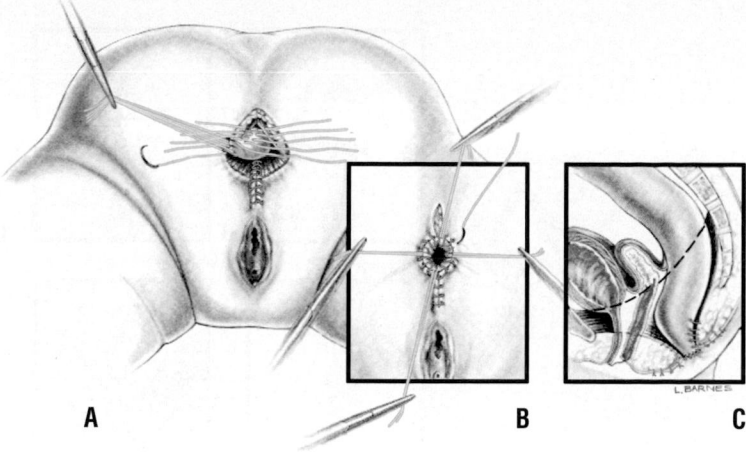

A **B** **C**

FIGURE 3-20. Repair of a rectoperineal fistula. **A:** The rectum has been dissected and the perineum reconstructed. Sutures are placed through the posterior edge of the muscle complex (behind the rectum) and include the bowel wall. **B:** Anoplasty by means of interrupted mucocutaneous sutures. **C:** Operation completed.

Rectovaginal Fistula

Rectovaginal fistula is a very unusual malformation in females. The rectum may open in the lower one-half of the vagina or, as an even more uncommon manifestation, in the upper portion (Figure 3-23). The higher the malformation, the shorter the common wall between the rectum and vagina. A low vaginal fistula is usually associated with absence of the posterior rim of the hymen. One cannot see the fistula orifice by inspection, and the meconium seems to come from within the vagina. The higher the fistula, the greater the likelihood for an abnormal sacrum and a poor-looking perineum. The potential for normal continence in these infants is generally less than one would expect with vestibular fistula. Treatment consists of a PSARP.

Imperforate Anus without Fistula

Imperforate anus without fistula is also an uncommon malformation in females. The rectum is usually located about 2 cm above the skin. The rectovaginal septum is rather thin, there is a good sphincter muscle, a good-looking perineum, and a well-developed sacrum. Half of these babies, like the boys, suffer from Down's syndrome, and they have the same good prognosis for bowel control.[7,119] In these babies, one can see gas in the most distal part of the rectum, below the coccyx, on a cross-table lateral film with the patient in prone position.[73] The surgeon can approach such a patient posterior sagittally and without a colostomy during the newborn period, provided he or she has experience with this operation. The creation of a

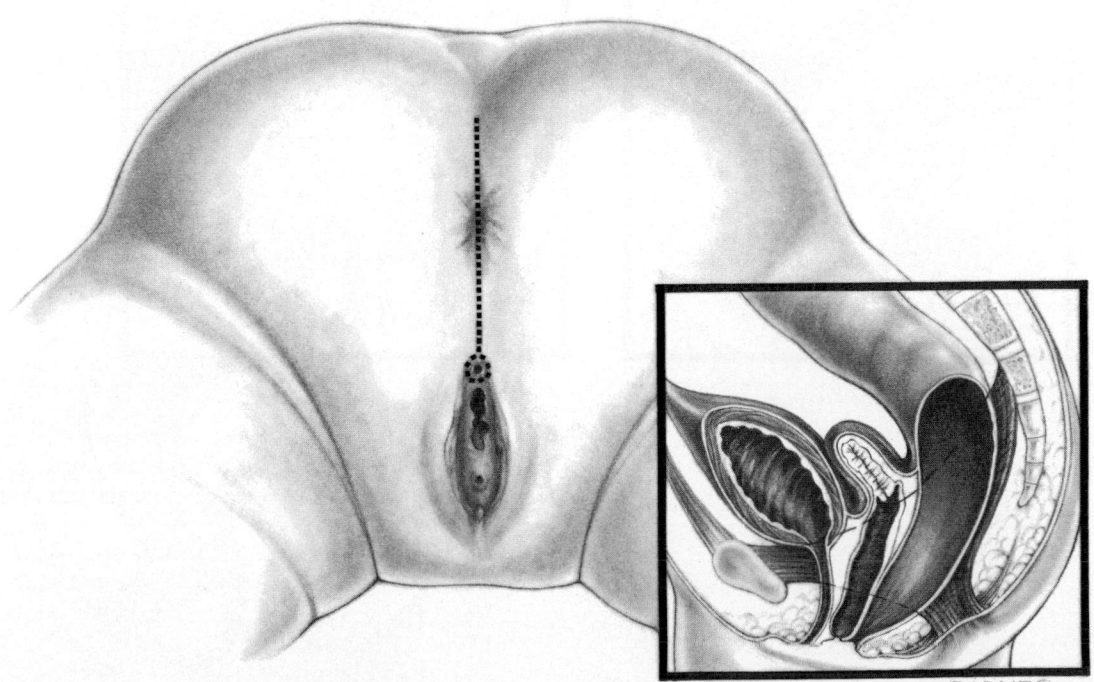

FIGURE 3-21. Surgical incision in a case of vestibular fistula. Sagittal appearance (*inset*). Note the common wall between rectum and vagina.

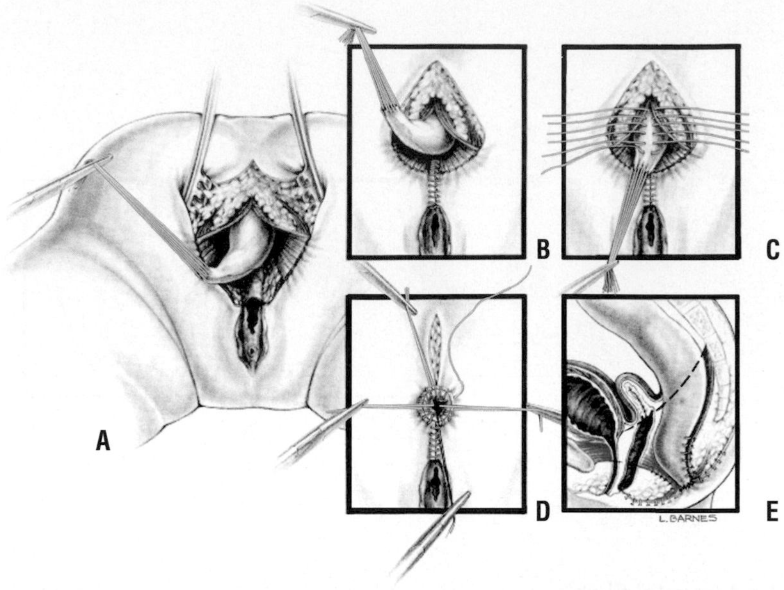

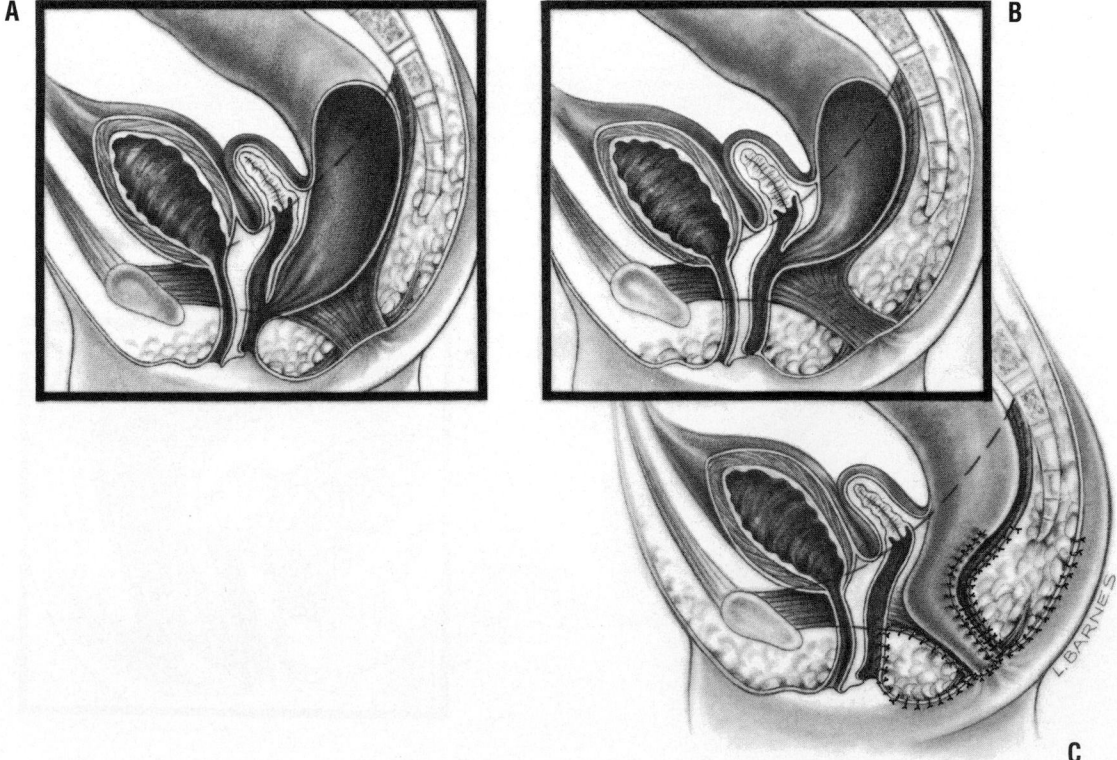

FIGURE 3-22. Repair of vestibular fistula. **A:** The rectum has been dissected, including meticulous separation from the vagina. **B:** The anterior perineum is reconstructed. The anterior edge of the muscle complex has been approximated anterior to the rectum. **C:** Sutures are placed through the posterior edges of the muscle complex including the back of the rectal wall. **D:** Anoplasty (mucocutaneous suture). **E:** Completed operation.

colostomy is still a reasonable alternative when the circumstances are not ideal.

Anal Stenosis and Rectal Atresia

As described for males, management for females is the same. Once again, a presacral mass must be screened for.

Persistent Cloaca

Persistent cloaca represents the extreme in the spectrum of complexity of female malformations. With this anomaly, the rectum, vagina, and urinary tract meet and fuse together into a single channel (Figure 3-24). Inspection of the perineum in these infants reveals rather small-looking external genitalia. Meticulous examination discloses a single orifice just under the clitoris with no evidence of a vagina or a rectum.

Persistent cloaca, itself, is represented by its own spectrum of defects. Many infants have a double or septated vagina, with different degrees of division of the uterus. Frequently, the vaginal opening into the cloaca is narrow, with a resultant hydrocolpos. The length of the common channel varies from 1 to 7 cm and is considered a very important indicator of the

FIGURE 3-23. Vaginal fistula. **A:** Low fistula. **B:** High fistula. **C:** Repaired malformation including tapering of the rectum.

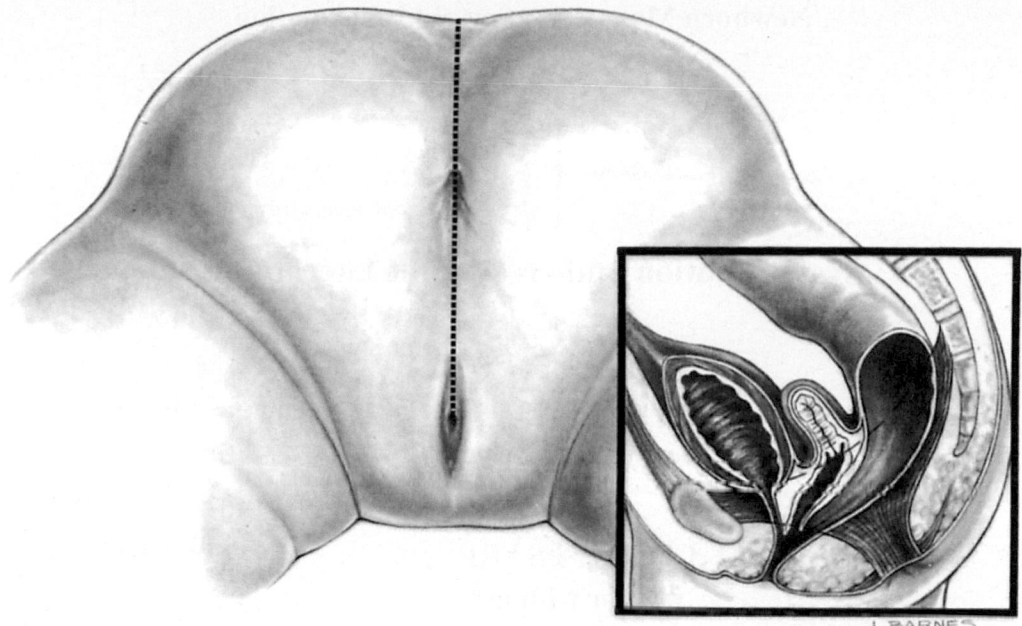

FIGURE 3-24. Persistent cloaca. Surgical incision; note the small-appearing labia. Sagittal appearance (*inset*); the rectum, vagina, and urinary tract form a common channel.

potential difficulty that the surgeon will encounter when attempting to repair the defect. Lower, short cloacae, with good muscle and sacrum, are easier to repair. Longer cloacae are frequently associated with poor muscles and hypodeveloped sacrum. These children require a complex reconstruction and are unlikely to achieve continence.[61]

In managing this malformation, one is focused on achieving normal bowel control, normal urinary continence, and normal sexual function, as well as childbearing potential. Success is more likely in children with a normal sacrum and spine and an adequate vagina. These malformations are frequently associated with an obstructive uropathy. They require a colostomy and often also need a vaginostomy for decompression of a hydrocolpos. On rare occasion, a vesicostomy is also required. At an appropriate interval, definitive reconstruction is achieved with a posterior sagittal anorectovaginourethroplasty.[38,61]

Associated Anomalies

Sacrum and Spine

In children with anorectal malformations, the sacrum is frequently hypodeveloped, and a hemisacrum is sometimes seen. It is generally accepted that the more severe the sacral defect, the less is the potential for bowel and urinary function.

Spinal ultrasound and magnetic resonance imaging[39] have permitted early detection and treatment of important associated defects, such as tethered cord, syringomyelia, and presacral masses (e.g., anterior meningocele, lipoma, dermoid, and teratoma).[77,91,95]

Urogenital Defects

Genital and urinary abnormalities are often associated with anorectal malformations. The frequency of this association varies from 20% to 54%.[6,108] This discrepancy is probably a reflection of the level of suspicion as well as the accuracy and thoroughness of the urologic and gynecologic workup.

Major urologic problems in children with imperforate anus are more common in those with higher malformations.

A patient with a persistent cloaca or rectobladder neck fistula has a 90% chance of an associated genital and urinary abnormality. Most of these are major, with the potential for significant morbidity if undiscovered and untreated. Conversely, children with a low fistula (i.e., rectoperineal) exhibit less than a 10% incidence of associated malformations.

The most common urinary anomalies encountered are vesicoureteral reflux, followed by unilateral renal agenesis. Other important associated defects include cryptorchidism, ureteral duplication, hypospadias, ectopic kidney, ectopic ureters, neurogenic bladder, renal dysplasia, megaureter, hydronephrosis, and ureterovesical obstruction.

A renal and bladder ultrasound must be performed on all children born with imperforate anus before creation of a colostomy or performance of a newborn repair. If the study discloses an abnormality, the surgeon should proceed with a more comprehensive urologic evaluation.

Algorithmic Approach to Decision Making

Figures 3-25 and 3-26 illustrate an algorithmic approach to decision making in the management of newborn infants with anorectal malformations.

Male Newborns

Ninety percent of the time, inspection of the perineum and a urinalysis will reveal whether the patient needs a colostomy. Usually, babies with anorectal malformations are not born with a distended abdomen. It takes at least 16 to 24 hours for this to develop. The distal rectum (the blind portion or the one connected to a fistula) is usually collapsed. Intraluminal pressure ultimately becomes sufficient to overcome the muscle tone of the sphincter mechanism to allow the meconium or the gas to reach the

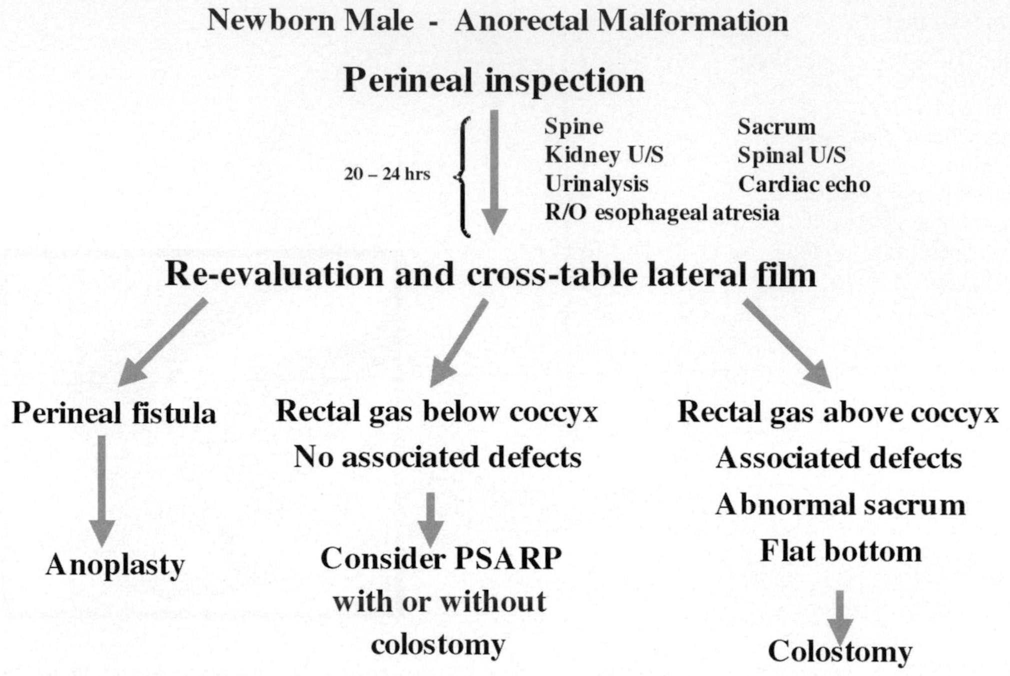

Newborn Male - Anorectal Malformation

Perineal inspection

20 – 24 hrs

Spine   Sacrum
Kidney U/S   Spinal U/S
Urinalysis   Cardiac echo
R/O esophageal atresia

Re-evaluation and cross-table lateral film

Perineal fistula

Rectal gas below coccyx
No associated defects

Rectal gas above coccyx
Associated defects
Abnormal sacrum
Flat bottom

Anoplasty

Consider PSARP
with or without
colostomy

Colostomy

FIGURE 3-25. Algorithm for the management of a newborn male with an anorectal malformation.

most distal part of the bowel, and to be forced through a tiny fistula orifice. This explains why studies to determine the height of the malformation and the location of the fistula performed prior to 16 to 24 hours can lead to an erroneous diagnosis of a "high" anorectal malformation. Diagnostic tests should, therefore, be performed after the baby is 16 to 24 hours old. However, during this first day, one should rule out associated conditions, such as cardiac, esophageal, and urologic disorders. The baby receives

intravenous fluids and antibiotics, and remains fasting. A nasogastric tube is inserted to avoid vomiting and the risk of aspiration.

The following studies are performed: abdominal and spinal ultrasound, x-ray of the lumbar and sacral spine, and echocardiogram. The infant is observed for symptoms and signs of esophageal obstruction. After 24 hours of observation, most of the time there is sufficient information to determine whether the baby requires a colostomy or whether a primary

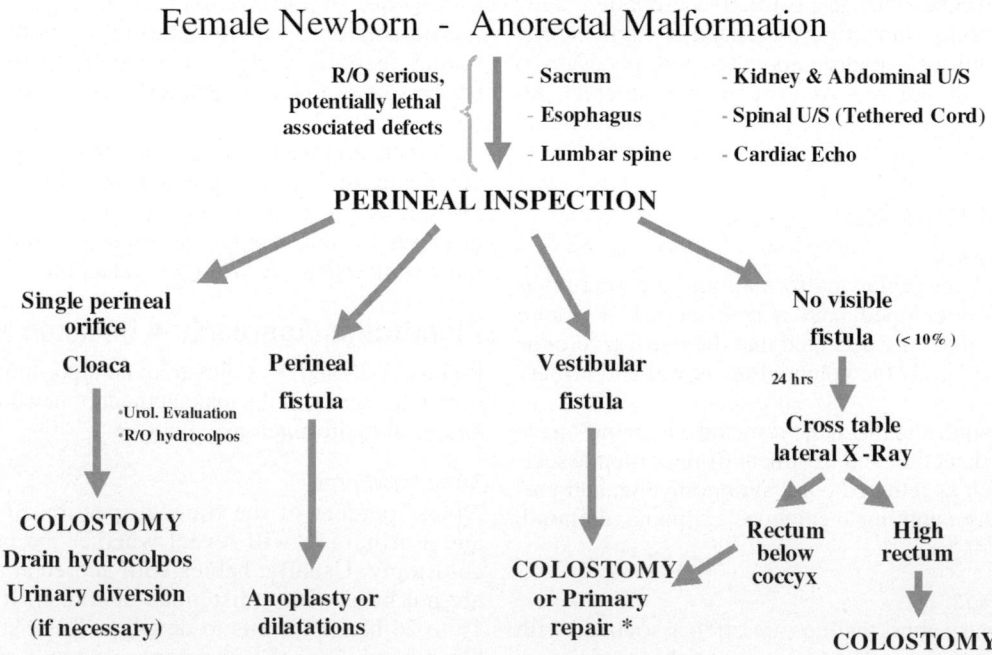

FIGURE 3-26. Algorithm for the management of a newborn female with an anorectal malformation.

repair of the anorectal malformation may be performed. For a small minority (10%) in whom the surgeon does not have adequate information for decision making, a cross-table lateral film is taken with the baby in the prone position. This will show the presence of gas in the distal rectum. The position of this bubble and its relationship to the coccyx are important for determining whether the surgeon can perform a reconstruction with or without a colostomy.

Sometimes the perineal fistula is a very obvious orifice that is located in the midline of the perineum between the genitalia and the anal dimple. One can observe meconium coming out through it. At other times, the orifice is so tiny that it is not seen on first inspection. It requires a significant amount of intraluminal bowel pressure to force the meconium through it. The presence of a rectoperineal fistula permits an anoplasty without a protective colostomy within the infant's first 48 hours, or the fistula can be dilated and the repair performed at 1 to 3 months of life.

If the baby does not pass meconium in the urine, does not demonstrate a perineal fistula, and does not have a flat bottom, a cross-table lateral film is taken. If the rectal gas is located below the coccyx and the baby is in good condition, with no significant associated defects, the surgeon should consider performing a primary posterior sagittal operation without a colostomy. This, as previously mentioned, will depend very much on the experience of the surgeon. Conversely, if the rectal gas is located well above the coccyx and if the baby has significant associated defects, an abnormal sacrum, a flat bottom, and/or meconium in the urine, it is advisable to create a colostomy and to avoid a primary approach to the perineum. Without evidence of the location of the rectum, this is a prudent policy in order to prevent injury to the urinary tract and other adjacent structures, such as the vas deferens, seminal vesicles, and prostate.

Female Newborns

Determination of the need for a colostomy is an easier decision in female infants because in the vast majority (>95%) the bowel opening is externally evident. The same rule concerning fecal diversion applies for females—that is, decisions concerning colostomy or primary repair should not be taken prior to 24 hours of life. The first day should be used, as mentioned for boys, to rule out the presence of potentially lethal conditions and to be certain that the baby does not have hydrocolpos, hydronephrosis, tethered cord, a cardiac malformation, esophageal atresia, or spinal defects. The presence of a rectoperineal fistula (Figure 3-27) is evidence of a low malformation that can be treated with a minimal PSARP without a colostomy. The operation can be performed in the newborn period or within the first months of life.

The presence of a vestibular fistula may be an indication for a colostomy or a primary approach, depending on the circumstances. If the surgeon is experienced, and the baby is full term and has no significant associated malformations, the operation can be accomplished primarily within the first few days of life. Conversely, if the baby is ill or has significant associated defects, or if the surgeon does not have the requisite experience, it is preferable to create a colostomy or to dilate the fistula, postponing the primary repair for a later date.

If the baby has a single perineal orifice, the diagnosis of a cloaca is established. This infant requires a complete urologic evaluation. The presence of hydrocolpos must be excluded. A colostomy is required, and it is mandatory to drain the hydrocolpos during the same operation. If the vagina is sufficiently capacious that it can reach the abdominal wall above the bladder, the patient can undergo a tubeless vaginostomy. Alternatively, if the vagina is dilated but does not reach above the bladder, a tube vaginostomy will be necessary. Occasionally, an infant with a cloaca may have

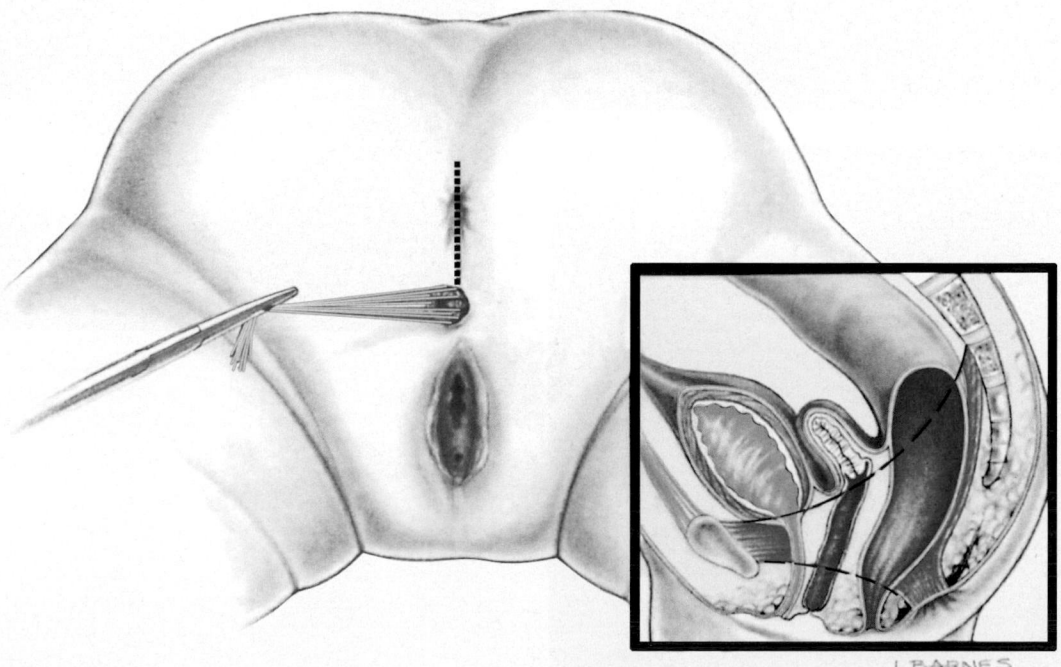

FIGURE 3-27. Rectoperineal fistula. Surgical incision. Sagittal appearance of the rectoperineal fistula (*inset*). Note the separation between the rectum and the vagina.

a near atresia of the urethra. Such an individual requires a temporary vesicostomy as well.[61]

If the baby does not have a visible fistula (5% of the cases), a cross-table lateral x-ray film is indicated with the infant in the prone position. When the gas in the rectum is seen below the coccyx, depending on the surgeon's experience, the patient can be repaired primarily using a posterior sagittal approach. If the gas is located much higher than the coccyx, it is advisable to create a colostomy.

Surgical Technique

Colostomy

A diverting colostomy is a very important step in the management of anorectal malformations. Still, a primary neonatal operation without a protective colostomy allows for fewer operations and avoids the potential morbidity associated with a colostomy.[2,34,71] This approach can be used for rectoperineal fistulas, vestibular fistulas, and imperforate anus without fistula.

The main limitation to primary repair without a colostomy is the lack of an accurate diagnostic test for delineating the precise anatomy of the malformation. The high-pressure distal colostogram is the most valuable tool for assessment in these patients because it allows one to precisely see the location of the rectum as well as the location of the fistula site (Figure 3-28).[36] A newborn infant should not be subjected to a procedure if the location of the rectum is unknown because this would be essentially a blind perineal exploration. Patients operated upon in this way frequently suffer serious consequences.[60] For example, the surgeon who is looking for a rectum that was located too high in the pelvis can cause injury to the urethra, vas deferens, seminal vesicles, prostate, and nerves affecting erection and bladder function.[44]

The ultimate functional result in these patients depends largely on preservation of whatever anatomic structures are present. A failed pull-through provokes severe scarring, fibrosis, and destruction of the original anatomy.[60] Thus, a diverting colostomy, specifically a left descending colostomy

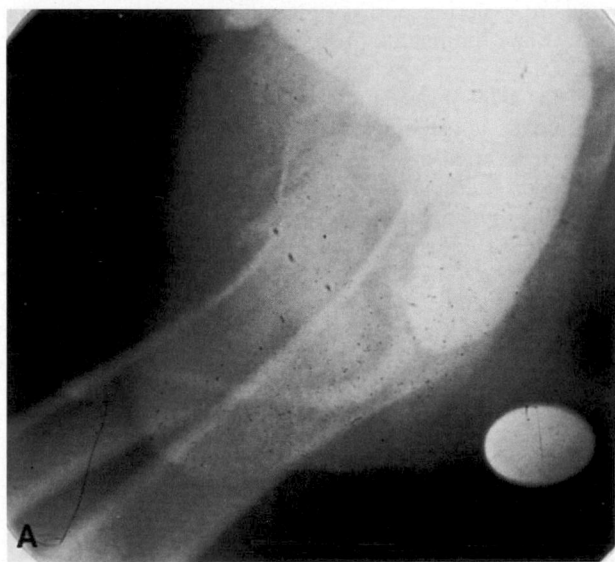

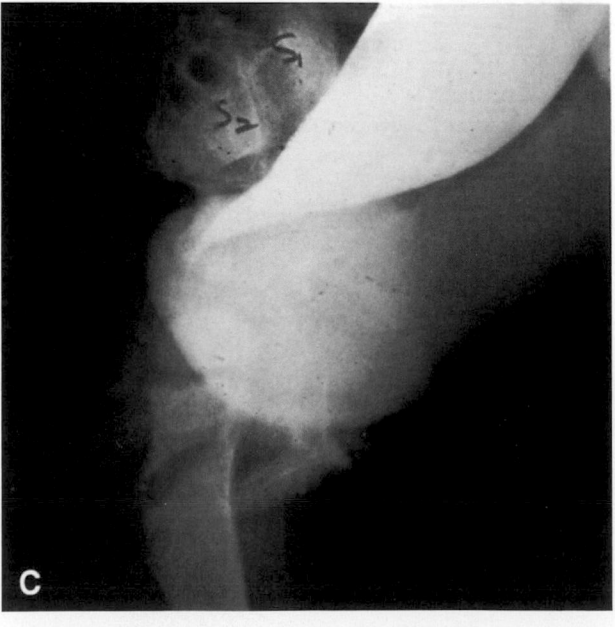

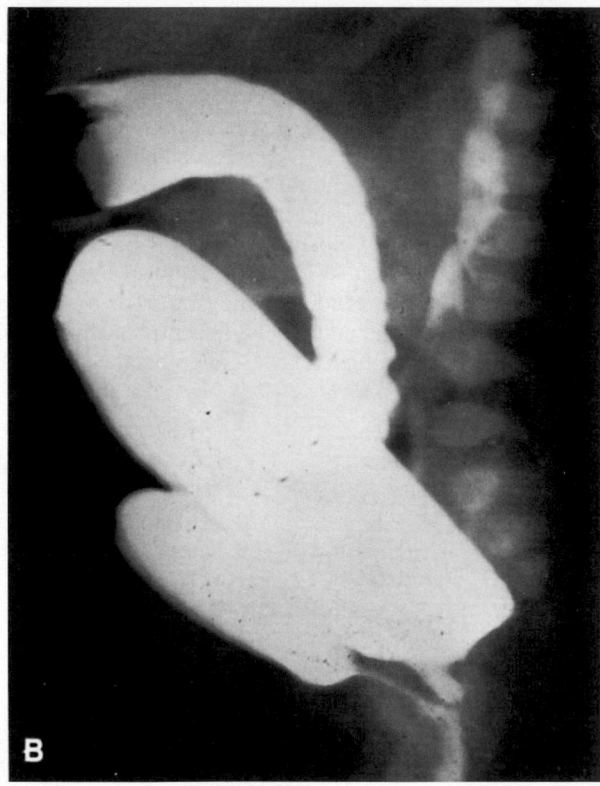

FIGURE 3-28. Distal colostograms. **A:** Bulbar-urethral fistula. **B:** Prostatic fistula. **C:** Bladder fistula.

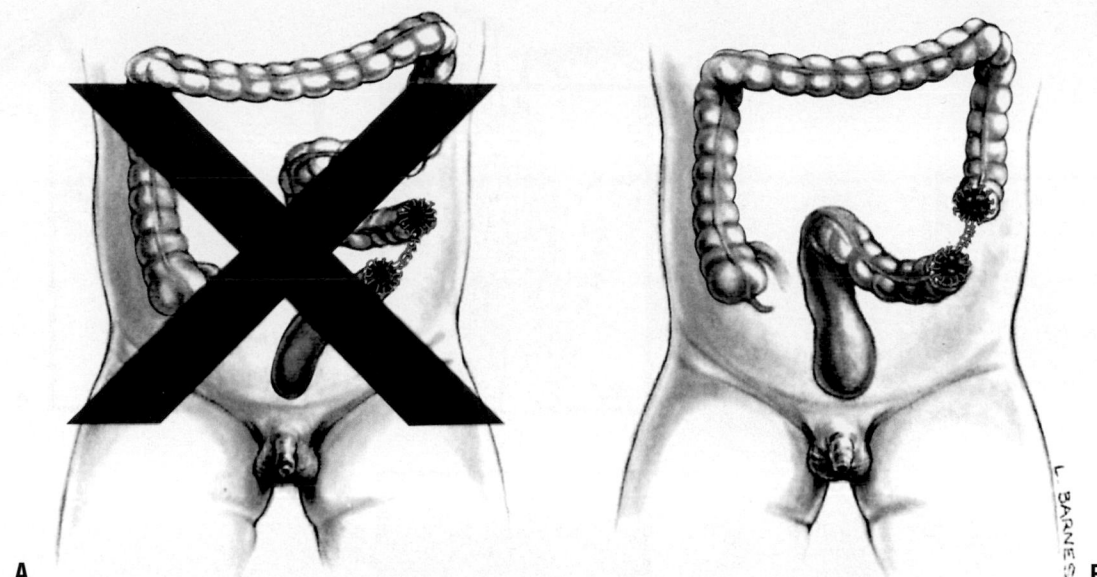

FIGURE 3-29. Possible colostomy alternatives. **A:** Inadequate colostomy; short distal bowel interferes with the subsequent pull-through. **B:** Recommended colostomy, located in the descending colon; redundant distal sigmoid permits subsequent pull-through. Note the separated stomas.

with separate stomas, still represents the safest method of treating these patients in the newborn period (Figure 3-29). An inadequately diverting loop colostomy allows for the passage of feces into the distal bowel and contamination of the urinary tract through the fistula.

Repair of Low Malformations in the Male Patient (Rectoperineal Fistula)

Low malformations represent the most benign type of male anorectal defect. No colostomy is required with the reconstruction. The primary characteristic of patients with this malformation is the location of the rectal fistula, immediately anterior to the center of the sphincter (see Figure 3-16A). The surgical technique used for repair is very similar to that described for perineal fistula in females. This technique will be described in the appropriate section.

In male patients, the most common and feared intraoperative complication is a urethral injury.[44] The surgeon must recognize that the anterior rectal wall is intimately attached to the posterior urethra. A Foley catheter must always be inserted before the operation.

Rectourethral Fistula

This is the rectal anomaly most commonly seen in male patients. The fistula may be located at the bulbar level (see Figure 3-16B) or at the prostate (see Figure 3-16C). Infants with a *rectourethral fistula* require a colostomy in the newborn period before PSARP. This can be accomplished in the first few months of life.

A Foley catheter is inserted, the infant is then placed prone, and a midsagittal incision is performed from the lower portion of the sacrum down to and through the center of the sphincter. With rectoprostatic fistula, it may be possible to preserve the anterior limit of the sphincter. However, in those patients with rectobulbar fistulas, it is more convenient to continue the incision slightly beyond

the anterior limit of the sphincter (Figure 3-30A). The parasagittal fibers are separated, deepening the incision down to the levator and muscle complex. Once the muscle is incised, the rectum becomes evident, protruding through the defect in the levators. The rectum is then secured with fine silk sutures and is opened in the midline with a needle-tip electrocautery (Figure 3-30A). The fistula site in the lowest part of the rectum can now be identified. It is important to remember that rectum and urethra share a common wall immediately above the fistula site. The rectum is separated from the urethra by the use of rectal mucosal 6–0 silk traction sutures in order to avoid injury to the prostate, seminal vesicles, and vas deferens, which lie just below the anterior wall. Approximately 2 cm above the fistula, both structures are fully separate, and the dissection can be expedited (Figure 3-30B,C). The urethral fistula is then closed with interrupted 5–0 long-term absorbable sutures. A careful rectal dissection is carried out, using traction on the silk sutures to gain rectal length so that perineal reconstruction can be performed without tension (Figure 3-30D). If the rectum is ectatic and distended, tailoring is required to permit it to lie within the muscle structures (Figure 3-31A). The levator muscle must be constructed behind the rectum, with the distal bowel located within the confines of the muscle complex and external sphincter. The anterior extent of the muscle complex and external sphincter is reapproximated (Figure 3-31B). Sutures are placed in both levator muscle edges (Figure 3-31C), and the rectum is then passed anteriorly. The remainder of the levator muscle is sutured together. The posterior edge of the muscle complex is then reapproximated behind the rectum, with sutures that include the muscle complex and the rectal wall (Figure 3-31D). An anoplasty is performed, and the skin is closed with a subcuticular 5–0 Vicryl suture (Figure 3-31E). A urethral catheter is left in place for 7 days.

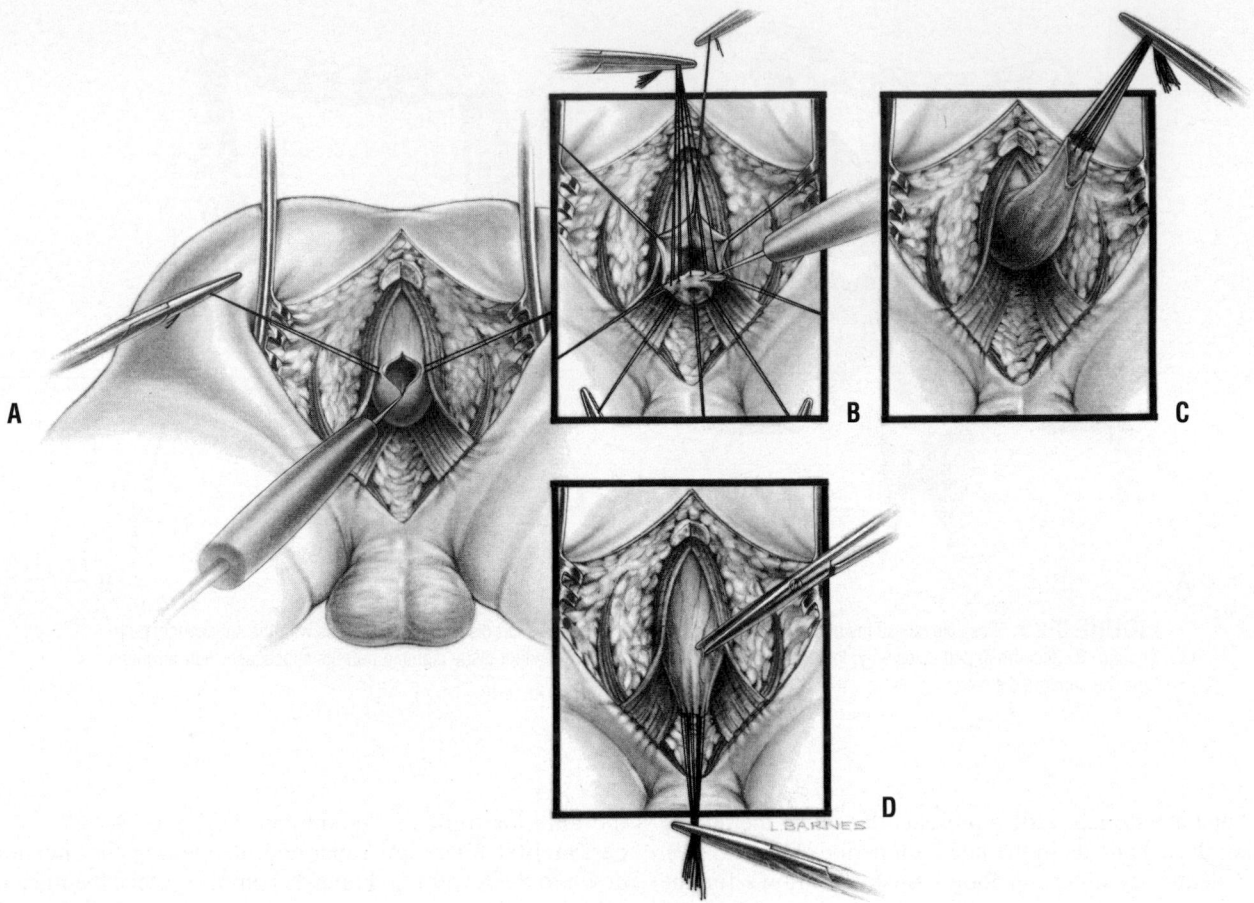

FIGURE 3-30. Repair of a rectourethral fistula. **A:** The incision extends beyond the limits of the external sphincter. The levator muscle is divided, and the rectum is opened. **B:** Separating the rectum from the urethra. **C:** The rectum separated from urethra. **D:** Dissection to gain rectal length.

Rectobladder Neck Fistula

These malformations represent the extreme in the spectrum of male anorectal defects. The rectum usually opens at the level of the bladder neck (see Figure 3-16D). The muscle complex and levator are frequently only rudimentary structures. Prognosis is not as good as that for the lower rectourethral fistulae. This malformation is often associated with varying degrees of sacral dysgenesis.

Because the rectum cannot be reached through a posterior sagittal approach, these children require a laparotomy or laparoscopy as well as a PSARP.[2,79,80] The entire body from axilla to feet is prepared preoperatively, and the abdomen is entered either through a midline laparotomy or with a laparoscopic approach. The retroperitoneal space at the presacral location is identified, and the rectum is dissected below the peritoneal reflection to the level of the bladder fistula. This is usually located approximately 2 cm below the reflection. Because it is a very high malformation, there is no problem with a common wall between rectum and bladder as is true for the lower malformations. The dissection, therefore, is rather straightforward, but the surgeon must be careful to avoid injury to the vas deferens, which frequently courses very near the area. The fistula site is closed with absorbable suture. The rectum is then mobilized so that it will reach the perineum. The rectum is tapered if needed, and then pulled to the perineum, bringing it through the presacral space. This area is opened via a small posterior sagittal incision with the legs lifted above the babies head. The operation is then completed with an anoplasty, and the abdomen is closed.

Imperforate Anus without Fistula

Surgical treatment for this defect in male and female patients is similar. The rectum is usually found 2 cm deep to the perineal skin. The technique is usually easier than that for patients with a fistula, but even in the absence of a communication between the rectum and vagina or urinary tract, one must be very cautious during the dissection of the anterior rectal wall in order to avoid injury to nearby structures.

Rectal Atresia or Stenosis

The repair of these malformations in the male patient is the same as that for the female. A presacral mass must be specifically sought through ultrasound and/or pelvic MRI.

Repair of Specific Defects in the Female
Rectoperineal Fistula

The most significant characteristic of this malformation is that the rectum and vagina are well separated without sharing a common wall. Therefore, the dissection between the two structures is relatively straightforward. Electrical stimulation will demonstrate that the fistula is not surrounded by muscle. Parasagittal fibers may be found on both sides of the fistula, but the anterior portion is usually devoid of muscle (see Figure 3-27).

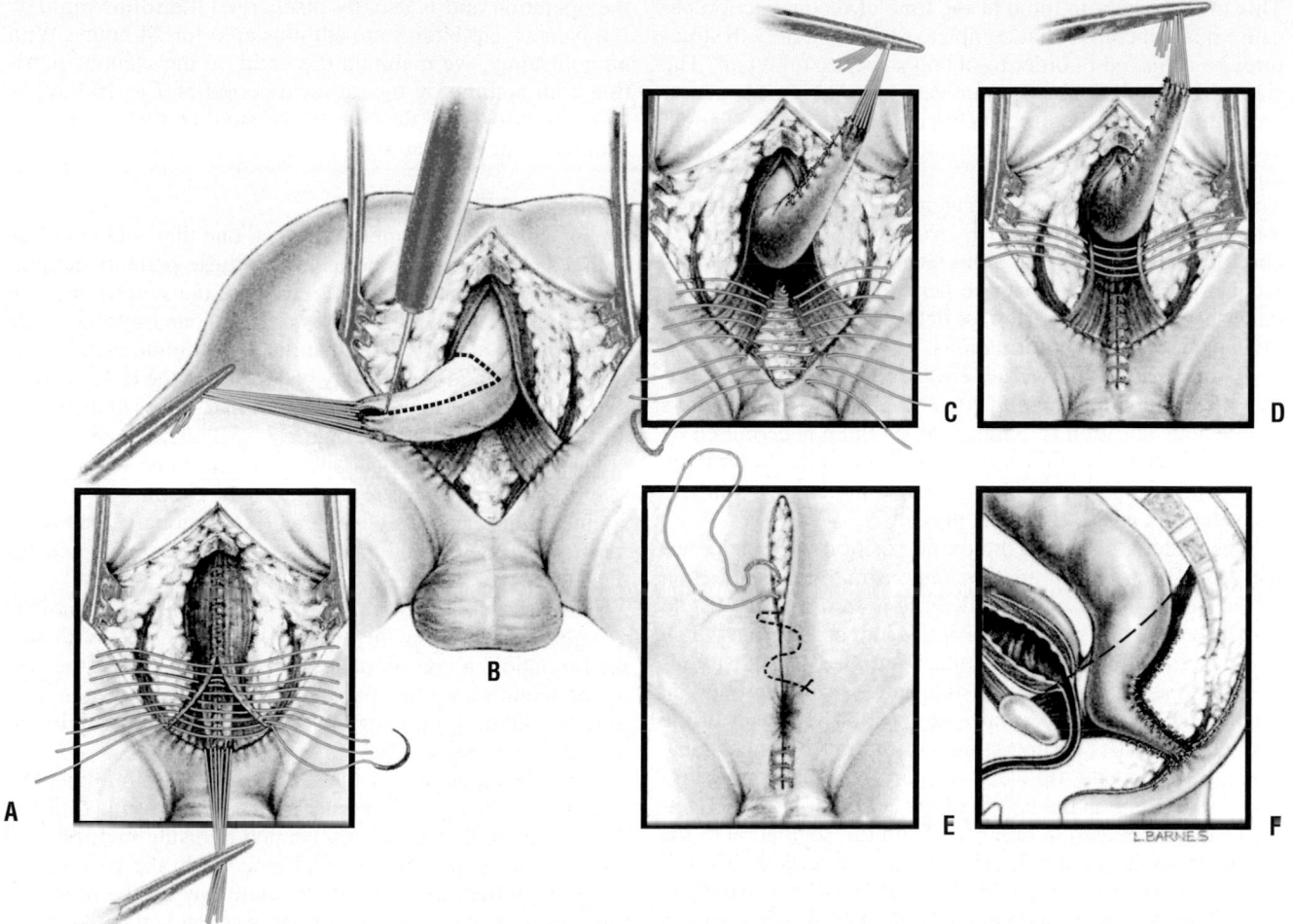

FIGURE 3-31. Repair of a rectourethral fistula. **A:** Tapering of the rectum. **B:** Repair of the perineal body. **C:** Sutures placed at the muscle complex and levator edge. **D:** Muscle complex sutures that will incorporate the rectal wall. **E:** Closure of the wound.

The operation is performed, ideally within the first few months of life. Sometimes the fistula is efficient in emptying the rectum, and the treatment can be delayed. This is especially important if the infant has additional anomalies. Another limiting factor may be the surgeon's experience, but if one is familiar with the fine structures of a newborn, the operation can be accomplished during the first few days of life.

The infant is placed in the prone position with the pelvis elevated to expose the perineal area. The incision encircles the fistula and extends posteriorly and midsagittally through the midportion of the sphincter mechanism (see Figure 3-27). Multiple 5–0 silk sutures are placed at the mucocutaneous junction of the fistula and are used for traction. A needle-tip electrocautery is advised for performing this dissection because special emphasis is placed on meticulous hemostasis. The dissection is undertaken as close as possible to the bowel wall in an attempt to preserve all the muscle lateral and posterior to the fistula. The dissection is also carried out as cephalad as is necessary in order to mobilize the rectum sufficiently so that it can be placed within the sphincter, without any tension on the suture line (see Figure 3-20).

After the mobilization has been completed, one is able to identify the vertical muscle fibers (i.e., muscle complex) that run parallel to the rectum and perpendicular to the parasagittal fibers (see Figure 3-20A). The vertical fibers and the parasagittal fibers cross at two places, creating two corners that mark the limits of the new anus. The dissection in this case does not reach deep enough to see the levator muscle. The rectum is then placed within the limits of the sphincter mechanism, and the perineal body is closed with 6–0 interrupted long-term absorbable sutures, bringing together the anterior limit of the muscle complex (see Figure 3-20A).

The posterior limit of the sphincter muscle is then sutured, incorporating part of the bowel wall to anchor the rectum and to prevent prolapse. An anoplasty is accomplished by suturing the rectum to the skin after trimming, but as much tissue as possible is preserved (see Figure 3-20B).

There is no need in the newborn for a bowel preparation, but prophylactic antibiotics are administered for 24 hours. The infant can eat after 5 to 7 days following surgery once it is clear that the perineal body is well healed. Recovery is usually uneventful, and rectal dilatation is instituted 2 weeks following the procedure.

Rectovestibular Fistula

The primary characteristic of this defect is that the rectum and vagina share a common wall distally (see Figure 3-21).

This must be kept in mind at the time of reconstruction because it is imperative that complete separation of both structures be achieved in order to obtain a successful repair. The size of the fistula orifice is quite variable. As a consequence, these infants may manifest different degrees of obstruction, although normal bowel movement patterns may be evident during the newborn period.

Traditionally, surgical management of this malformation required a diverting colostomy. However, if a surgeon feels comfortable with the meticulous technique necessary for this reconstruction, a repair can be performed without a stoma, either in the newborn period, or delayed, if the child has significant associated malformations.

At our institution, we adhere to a very strict preoperative bowel preparation, and for 7 to 10 postoperative days intravenous nutrition is maintained. Nothing is permitted by mouth. These precautions are employed in order to limit the likelihood of a perineal dehiscence and infection, complications that can adversely affect prognosis.

The child is placed in the prone position with the pelvis elevated. Electrical stimulation demonstrates the contraction of the sphincter muscle considerably posterior to the fistula site. The posterior sagittal incision is longer than that which was described for perineal fistula. Multiple 6–0 silk sutures are placed at the edge of the fistula and are used for traction. Because of the common wall, the most difficult part of the dissection consists in separating the rectum from the vagina. The use of a needle-tip electrocautery expedites the operation. Depending on the length of the common wall, the incision can be enlarged in order to obtain full separation of the rectum from the vagina. It must be made exactly in the midline so that the sphincter complex is divided into two equal parts. The sagittal incision extends into the muscle complex and sometimes into the inferior portion of the levator. This procedure is called a limited posterior (PSARP) because the dissection usually does not extend to the coccyx and levator muscles. With the application of an electrical stimulator, one can be certain that the dissection is in the midline. Mobilization of the rectum must be sufficiently adequate to permit relocation within the muscle complex and the sphincter complex without tension. One reaches an areolar plane that is the location of complete separation of the two walls. Tapering is usually not necessary with this malformation. The completed dissection reveals the intact vaginal wall, the anterior extent of the muscle complex, the perineal body with only subcutaneous fat, and the limits of the sphincter, marked by the crossing of the vertical and parasagittal fibers (see Figure 3-22A).

The anterior perineum is reconstructed with both anterior edges of the muscle complex approximated (see Figure 3-22B). The rectum is laid in position. The posterior limit of the muscle complex is also sutured together, along with a portion of the posterior rectal wall (see Figure 3-22C). This reduces the likelihood of a subsequent prolapse. An anoplasty is then created within the limits of the sphincter. The skin of the perineum is closed with interrupted 5–0 long-term absorbable sutures (see Figure 3-22D,E).

Postoperative. Postoperative care requires perineal cleansing and the use of antibiotic ointment daily for 1 week. Dilatations are begun 2 weeks following the procedure. If a colostomy is in place, the child can usually eat the day of the operation and is usually discharged the following day. Intravenous antibiotics are administered for 24 hours. With no colostomy, we maintain the child on intravenous nutrition with nothing by mouth for a period of 7 to 10 days in an attempt to avoid the passage of stool and to await good healing of the perineal body.

Rectovaginal Fistula

This is an extremely unusual defect, one that occurs in less than 1% of cases. The perineum in these patients demonstrates no obvious anal orifice. It is not unusual to find that the posterior rim of the hymen is missing, an important clue for detecting a low vaginal fistula. The communication between rectum and vagina may be located in the lower part of the vagina (most frequent; see Figure 3-23A) or in the upper portion (very unusual; see Figure 3-23B). The lower the fistula is located, the longer the common wall. The sacrum may demonstrate different degrees of dysplasia, and the sphincter muscles may be deficient. Occasionally, however, a patient with a vaginal fistula may have excellent sphincter muscles.

The operation can be performed in the first few months of age depending on the surgeon's experience. With this malformation, a considerable discrepancy between the size of the rectum and the space available between the levator muscle and the vagina may be found; this would require tapering (see Figure 3-23C).

Once the levator has been divided in the midline, the rectum must be opened in order to expose the fistula directly. The rectum and vagina are separated by using multiple 5–0 silk traction sutures in the rectal mucosa. In the presence of a very high malformation, the rectum may not be found by this approach; a laparotomy or laparoscopy is then required. When tapering is indicated, about 50% of the rectal wall is resected, depending on the magnitude of the discrepancy between the rectum and the available space. The bowel is then closed in two layers with interrupted 5–0 long-term absorbable sutures. The posterior wall of the vagina should be repaired. The rectum must then be relocated in front of the levator muscle and behind the vagina. It is then directed 90 degrees posteriorly, following the direction of the muscle complex (see Figure 3-23). The perineal body is reconstructed. The new anus is then created at the center of the sphincter, and the parasagittal fibers are reapproximated with interrupted 5–0 long-term absorbable sutures. The wound is closed with a subcuticular suture.

Perhaps because the operation is entirely accomplished through an incision in the midline raphe, it is relatively painless. A Foley catheter for urinary diversion is not used in any repair of perineal, vestibular, or vaginal fistulas.

Atresia and Stenosis of the Rectum

These children have the necessary anatomic structures for continence. The PSARP offers a unique opportunity for repairing this malformation because it permits excellent exposure to the anomaly. The operation usually requires a full PSARP, with or without a diverting colostomy, depending on the baby's circumstances and the surgeon's experience. A midline incision is carried down to the levator ani and to the atretic rectum following the principles mentioned in the previous descriptions. The narrowed or atretic section of rectum is incised posteriorly, and the circle becomes a hemicircle. The dentate line remains intact and becomes the anterior 180 degrees

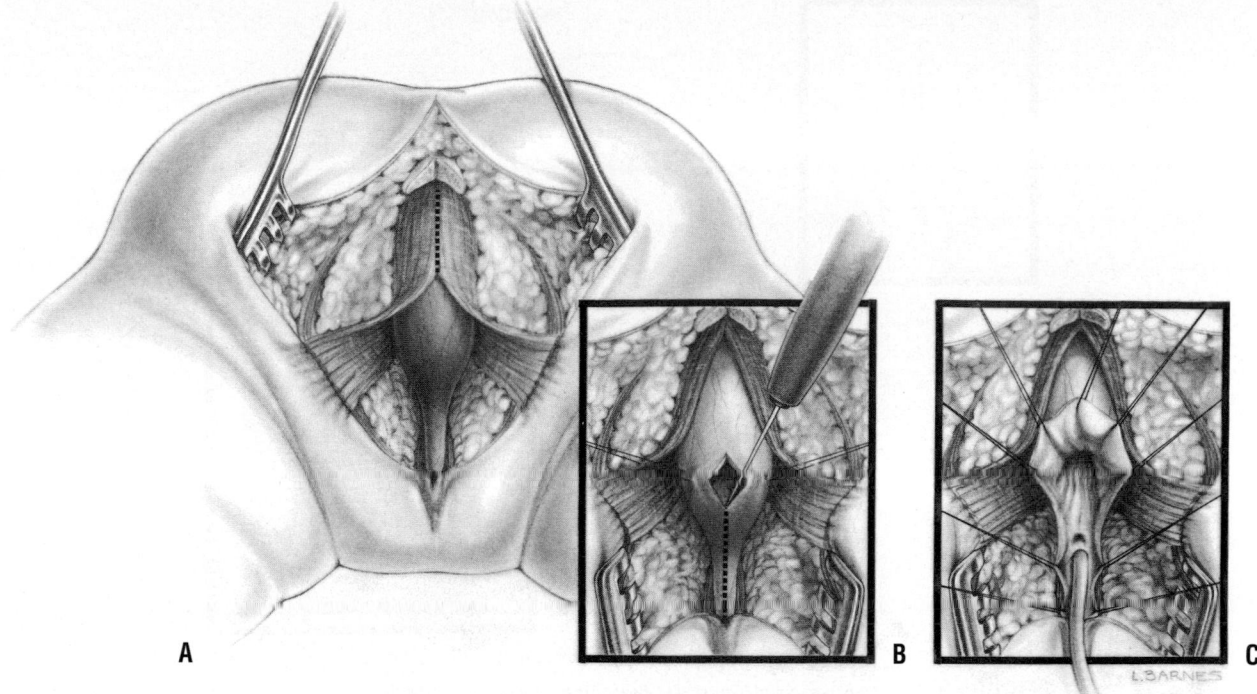

FIGURE 3-32. Repair of a persistent cloaca. **A:** The sphincter complex has been split in the midline. The levator is divided to expose the cloaca. **B:** Opening the rectum. **C:** The rectum and vagina are exposed; a catheter has been placed in the urethral orifice.

of the anastomosis. The proximal rectum is mobilized and becomes the posterior 180 degrees of the anoplasty. After this has been accomplished, the levator muscle, muscle complex, and parasagittal fibers are reapproximated. The skin is then closed. Even though the anus appears externally normal, an anastomotic stricture could develop. These children, therefore, require dilatation to be started at 1 month. Again, all such patients must be preoperatively screened for a presacral mass.

Persistent Cloaca

Management of the complex malformation of persistent cloaca requires a number of surgical maneuvers. The procedure is called a posterior sagittal anorectovaginourethroplasty.

The incision is shown in Figure 3-24, extending inferiorly from the lower portion of the sacrum. It passes through the center of the sphincter and ends at the single perineal opening. The parasagittal fibers, muscle complex, and levator are divided in the midline (Figure 3-32A). The rectum, including the common channel, is then opened exactly in the midline (Figure 3-32B). Once the entire visceral structure has been opened, one can identify the rectal, vaginal, and urethral orifices (Figure 3-32C). A Foley catheter is then inserted through the urinary opening. Attempts to pass the catheter before opening the cloaca are usually unsuccessful because one cannot be certain which opening was entered.

Because the rectum and vagina share a common wall, there is no natural plane of separation. By placing multiple 5–0 or 6–0 silk sutures into the rectal mucosa for traction, the maneuver is expedited. The submucosal dissection continues cephalad to the point where the vagina and the rectum separate. Then the maneuver becomes simplified because one is now dealing with the full thickness of the rectal wall. After the rectum has been successfully separated from the vagina, no attempt is made to separate the vagina from the

urinary tract. Rather, the entire urogenital sinus is dissected and mobilized (Figure 3-33). A total urogenital mobilization renders an excellent anatomic reconstruction.[82] Multiple fine silk sutures are placed at the edge of the vagina and the common channel. Another series of 6–0 silk sutures are then placed across the common channel (urogenital sinus) and between 5 and 10 mm dorsal to the clitoris. These sutures help to avoid tissue damage by distributing the tension on as many sutures as possible. The wall of the urogenital sinus is divided completely, ventral to the silk sutures. Anterior or ventral to the urogenital sinus, a well-defined space and plane separate this sinus from the pubis. The dissection must proceed lateral and ventral to the urogenital sinus in order to reach the retropubic space. Traction is exerted on the vaginal edges as the dissection continues in a circumferential manner, including vagina and urethra together as a single unit (Figure 3-34). The urethra and vagina are held in the pelvis by avascular supersensory fibrous ligaments attached to the pelvic rim. These ligaments must be divided to free the vagina, bladder, and urethra. The dissection continues circumferentially until enough length has been gained to connect the vaginal edges to the perineum. Thus, a urethral and vaginal opening of a near-normal appearance is created (Figure 3-35). The vaginal edges are then sutured to the skin or the labia of the perineum with interrupted 5–0 long-term absorbable sutures. The urethral opening will then be located 5 to 8 mm from the clitoris (Figure 3-36).

This maneuver allows the reconstruction of urethra and vagina in greater than 50% of the patients with cloacas, namely, those who have a common channel of less than 3 cm. Additional maneuvers are required for the vaginal reconstruction in cases of a longer common channel.

One must remember that persistent cloaca represents a spectrum of malformations. A relatively straightforward

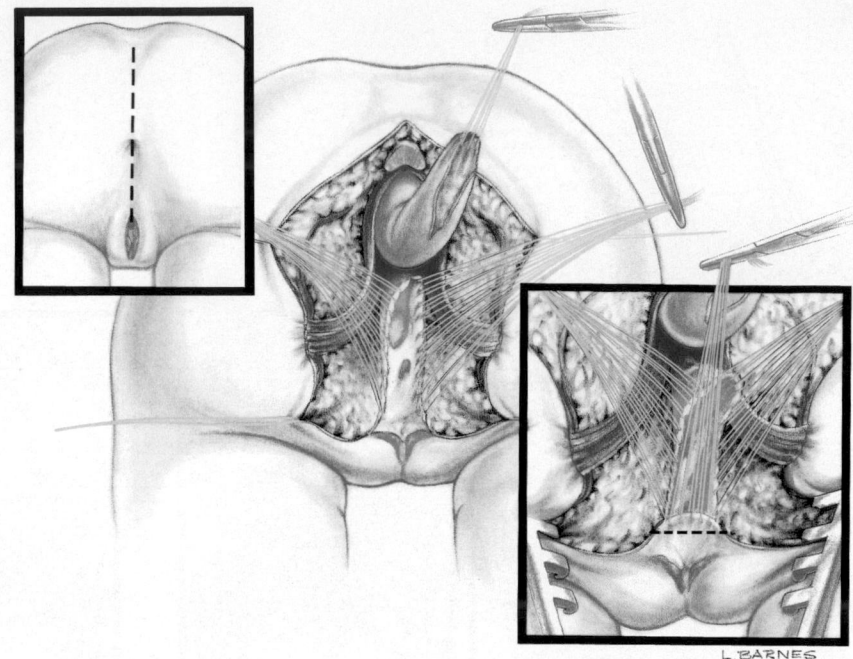

FIGURE 3-33. Management of a persistent cloaca. Total urogenital mobilization.

repair is that of a short common channel associated with a rather large vagina and a low rectum. Under these circumstances, rectum and vagina can be readily mobilized and reconstructed. At the other end of the spectrum, one may find a very high rectum that cannot even be seen during the posterior sagittal exploration. Under these circumstances, repair of this defect requires a laparotomy. Another difficult problem arises when one must deal with a long (e.g., 4 to 7 cm) common channel and a very small vagina that cannot be mobilized to the perineum. In this particular situation, several options are possible. For example, one can interpose a segment of small or large bowel between the lower vaginal

edge and the perineal skin.[61,89] If the surgeon is confronted with a rather large vagina but a short common channel, it may be feasible to create a flap of the dome for interposition between the vagina and the perineum.

Occasionally, patients have two very large hemivaginas (bilateral hydrocolpos) and a long common channel, indicating that both hemivaginas are located far away from the perineum. The distance from one hemicervix to the other (transverse diameter of both hemivaginas together) is longer than the vertical length of both structures (Figure 3-37). In this specific type of malformation, one can reconstruct the vagina with a maneuver called a vaginal switch (Figure 3-37).

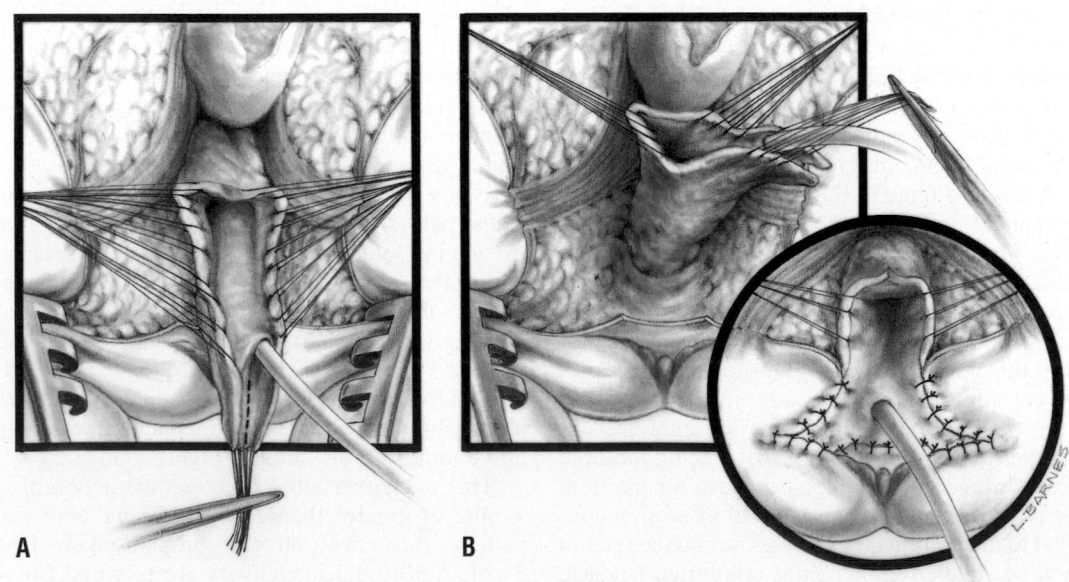

FIGURE 3-34. Management of a persistent cloaca. **A:** Mobilized urogenital sinus. **B:** Dissection of retropubic area. Reconstruction of the vulva (*inset*).

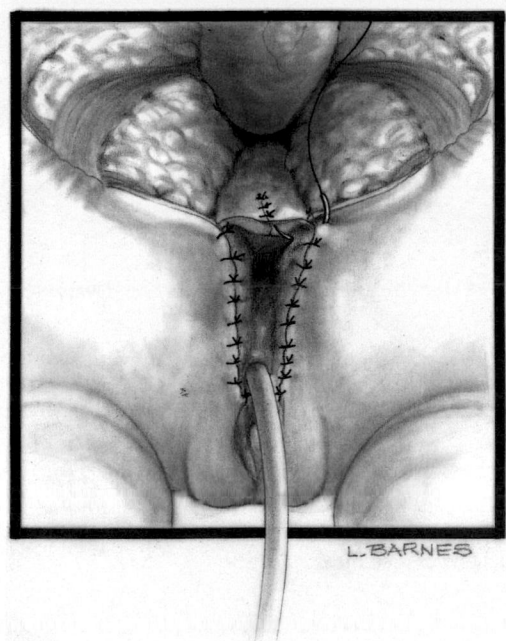

FIGURE 3-35. Management of a persistent cloaca. Total urogenital mobilization is completed.

With the aid of an electrical stimulator, the landmarks for the reconstruction, the center of the sphincter complex, and the anterior limit of the muscle complex are determined. Fine, long-term absorbable sutures are placed to reapproximate the anterior edge of the muscle complex and the anterior portion of the sphincter. The rectum now is located within the sphincter complex. The posterior limit of the muscle complex is then reapproximated behind the rectum with 5–0 long-term absorbable sutures, including a small bite of the bowel wall. An anoplasty is accomplished as described with the management of previous malformations, and the wound is closed in layers (Figure 3-36).

A urinary catheter is usually left in place for approximately 14 to 21 days. Anal dilatations are started 2 weeks following the operation as described for the postoperative management of other malformations.

Repair of these malformations represents the ultimate challenge in pediatric pelvic surgery and should be performed only by individuals who have considerable experience with these techniques.

Reoperations for the Treatment of Fecal Incontinence

Infants who were born with an anorectal malformation may suffer from fecal incontinence due to a persistent anatomic defect related to a mislocation of the rectal pull-through outside of the sphincter complex. The posterior sagittal approach can be used to relocate the rectum.[59]

The ideal candidate for this type of operation is a patient who has a favorable potential for continence: relatively normal sacrum and good quality muscles as evidenced by a good-looking perineum (e.g., midline raphe and anal dimple). The patient should have clinical evidence of an

One hemiuterus is resected, including the fallopian tube, with special care taken to preserve the ovary. The vaginal dome on that side is switched down to the perineum and will be reanastomosed to the introitus. After the urethra and vagina have been repaired, the rectum is reconstructed.

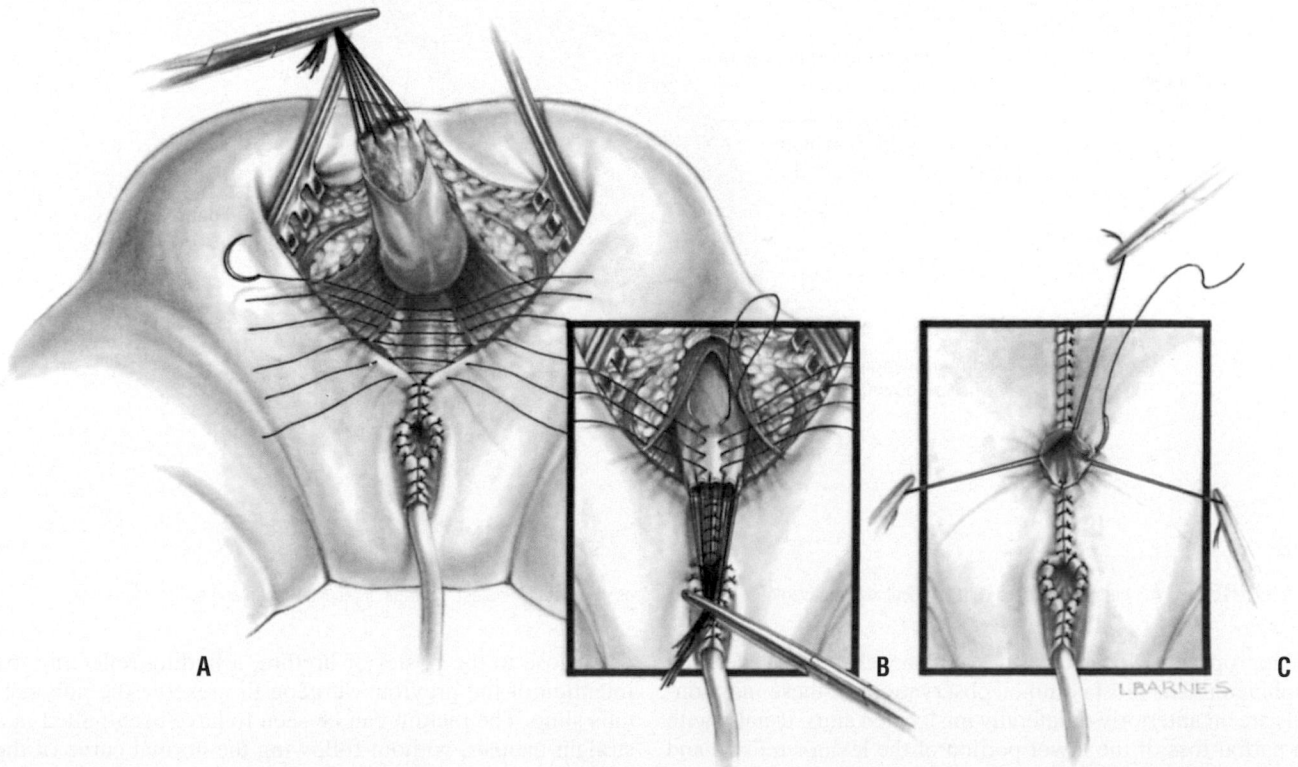

FIGURE 3-36. Repair of a persistent cloaca. **A:** The urethra and the vagina have been reconstructed. Sutures are placed in the perineum. The anterior edge of the muscle complex is approximated anterior to the rectum. **B:** The posterior edge of the muscle complex is approximated behind the rectum. The sutures include the rectum. **C:** Anoplasty.

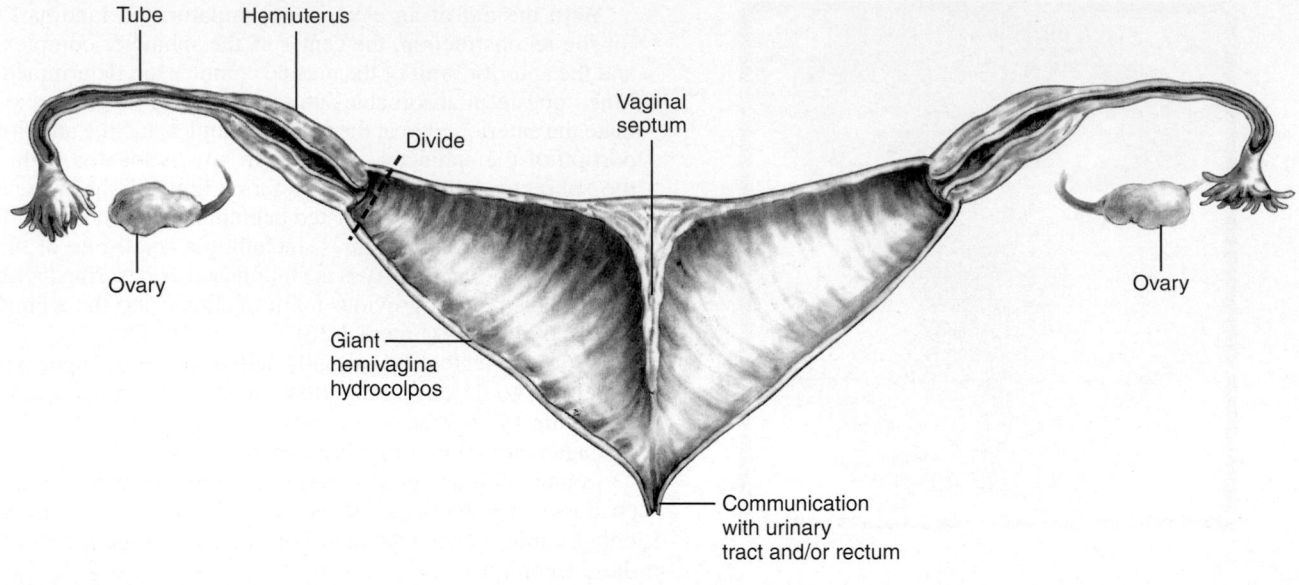

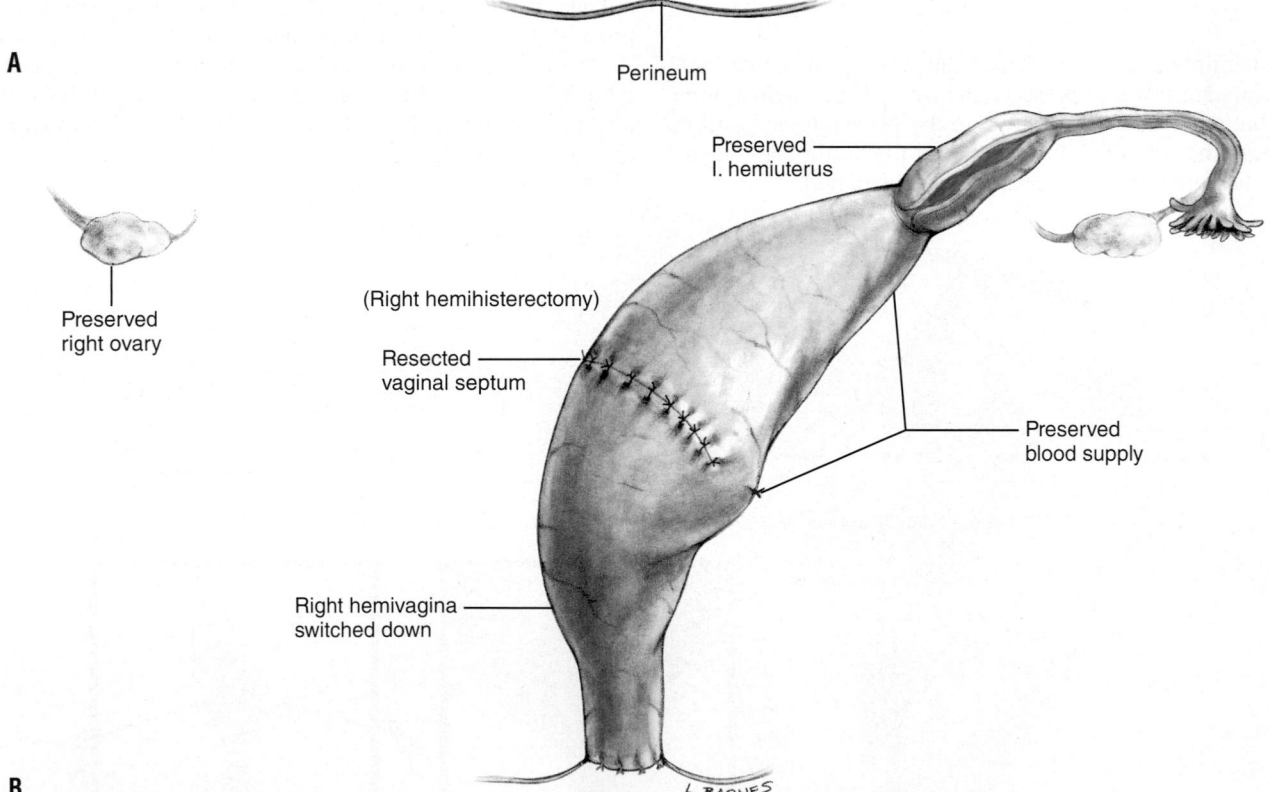

FIGURE 3-37. Persistent cloaca with hydrocolpos, hemivaginas, and hemiuterus. **A:** Anatomic defect. **B:** Vaginal reconstruction and switch maneuver.

inappropriately located rectum, with a well-preserved, intact sphincter. The most common observations in these individuals are an anteriorly or laterally mislocated anus, usually with a partial loss of the lower portion of the levator muscle and anterior aspect of the muscle complex (Figure 3-38). In those patients who had undergone an abdominoperineal procedure, considerable mesenteric fat may surround the rectum and interfere with muscle function. The rectum is usually identified

very close to the posterior urethra, a finding reflecting the intention of the previous surgeon to preserve the puborectalis sling. The rectum can be seen to have been pulled in a straight manner, without following the normal curve of the muscle complex (Figure 3-38).

The incision is carried out from the lower portion of the sacrum through the center of the sphincter and around the anus. Multiple 5–0 silk sutures are placed at the mucocutaneous

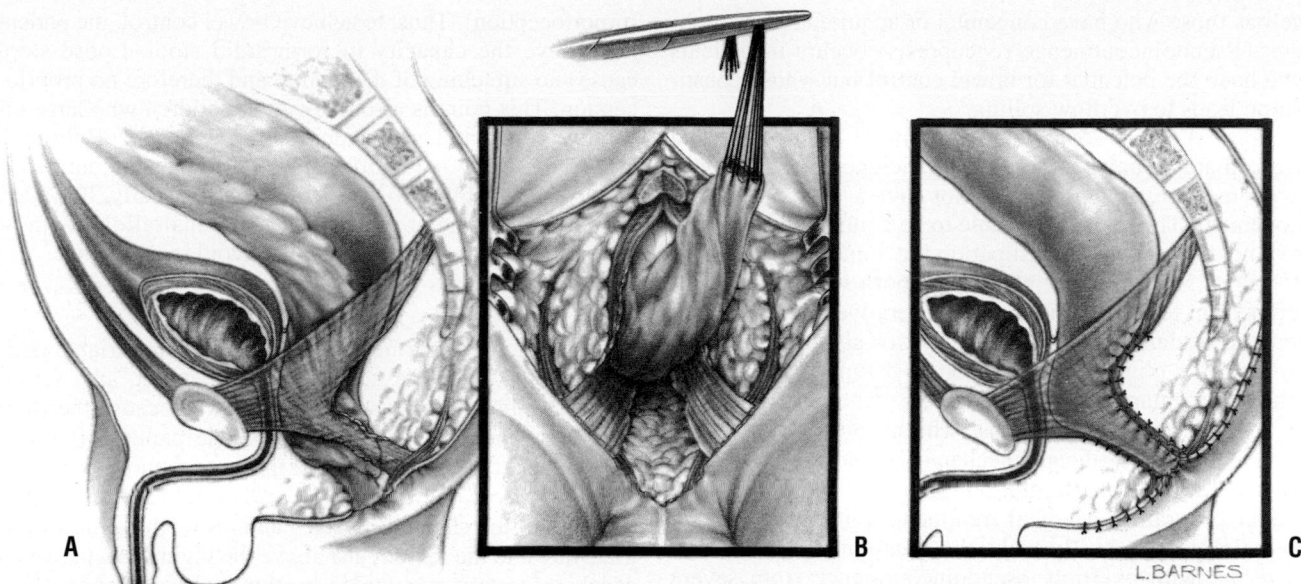

FIGURE 3-38. Secondary operation for the treatment of fecal incontinence. **A:** Preoperative findings. The levator and muscle complex are damaged. Mesenteric fat is surrounding the rectum. **B:** Rectum dissected. **C:** Operation completed. Mesenteric fat is removed, the rectum is relocated, and the muscle is reconstructed.

junction for traction. The incision is deepened, dividing the levator ani muscle and the muscle complex. Careful dissection is carried out as close as possible to the rectum, preserving all the striated muscle in the area. Figure 3-38B shows the rectum completely mobilized; the surrounding mesenteric fat can be easily appreciated. The repair consists of bringing together both anterior edges of the muscle complex and repairing the perineal body in a manner similar to that which has been previously described. The mesenteric fat is excised, with care taken to preserve adequate blood supply. Tapering of the rectum is rarely necessary, and the rectum is then relocated within the sphincter complex.

Because the urethra is not opened, a postoperative urinary catheter is not necessary. Anal dilatation is commenced 2 weeks following the operation.

Results of Treatment for Anorectal Malformations

Functional results vary even following a satisfactory repair because one is dealing with a spectrum of defects. For example, those individuals born with a poor sacrum or a spinal anomaly will have poor potential for fecal and urinary continence. Infants with a normal sacrum and good muscle structures usually attain fecal and urinary control. PSARP permits reconstruction of these defects by placing the rectum in the optimal position to achieve the best functional results. However, many patients continue to have bowel management problems, primarily because of sensory impairment, sphincter dysfunction, and motility disturbance. These can contribute to varying degrees of soiling and of constipation.

We have performed more than 1,600 primary reconstructive procedures for anorectal malformations.[88] Voluntary bowel movements were noted in 77% of those old enough to potty train and who are able to be evaluated. When separated by diagnosis, the percentages varied: 100% in patients with rectal atresia/stenosis and perineal fistulas, 92% in those with vestibular fistula, 82% with rectourethral-bulbar fistula, 71% with cloacas with common channels less than 3 cm, 44% in cloacas with 3 cm or greater common channels, 73% with

rectourethral-prostatic fistula, and 28% in individuals with bladder neck fistula. Of the entire series, 56% had voluntary bowel movements and never soiled their underwear. Constipation was a problem in 49% of all children and was more frequently noted in those with lower defects. Urinary incontinence was present in 7% of patients (excluding cloacal reconstructions) and really only seen when there was an associated spinal or sacral problem. In those with cloacas, urinary incontinence was found in 28% of girls having a common channel shorter than 3 cm and in 77% of those who had longer common channels.[61,89] This was well treated with intermittent catheterization because cloacas almost uniformly have a good bladder neck; thus, patients can be made dry. Sexual function and childbearing capacity is an emerging area of review in our series.[9]

Secondary operations for the treatment of fecal incontinence in patients with a normal sacrum revealed some improvement in approximately 80%. The same procedure, however, performed in individuals with an abnormal sacrum was found to achieve significant improvement in only 20%, and at least 50% failed to benefit in this last group.[59] We have learned to reserve this sort of reoperation for patients with good potential in whom improved anatomy may give them bowel control.

▶ PEDIATRIC FECAL INCONTINENCE

Fecal soiling is a common presenting problem that pediatric caregivers are asked to evaluate. It represents a devastating condition that may prevent a child from becoming socially accepted. Children affected include those born with surgical conditions such as anorectal malformations (ARMs) and Hirschsprung's disease (HD), as well as those who have spinal cord problems or injuries.

Patients can have true fecal incontinence or can suffer from overflow pseudoincontinence, both with completely different treatments. Those with true incontinence include a percentage of surgical patients (having ARMs and HD), as well as those who have congenital or acquired spinal problems. Pseudoincontinence (encopresis) occurs in patients who have the potential for bowel control but whose constipation leads to overflow soiling.

Approximately 25% of those operated on for anorectal malformations have enough of a deficiency in their continence mechanism that they cannot have a voluntary bowel movement. The rest may be able to be continent but require treatment, usually for constipation but sometimes for loose stool.[87] A small number of patients born with HD (<5%) suffer from fecal incontinence postoperatively,[4,57,114] usually because of damage to the anal canal or sphincters. Spinal problems or injuries can manifest as a limited capacity to achieve voluntary bowel movements.[53,121]

To treat these patients, those who have true fecal incontinence need an artificial (mechanical) mechanism to keep them clean and wearing normal underwear, and a tailored enema program.[86] Medical treatments with laxatives are not helpful and actually make the situation worse. Patients suffering with overflow pseudoincontinence from severe constipation, on the other hand, require adequate treatment of their constipation. This distinction is the key to determining correct management.

Physiologic Mechanisms of Fecal Continence

Fecal continence depends on voluntary sphincter muscles, anal canal sensation, and motility of the colon.[87]

Voluntary Sphincters

The voluntary sphincters include the levator ani, the muscle complex, and the external sphincter. These muscles are used only when stool in the rectum reaches the anorectal area, propelled there by the involuntary peristalsis of the rectosigmoid. A normal individual voluntarily holds the stool by contracting the sphincters and needs to do this only in the minutes prior to defecation. Otherwise, these muscles are used only occasionally the rest of the day and night. They also relax voluntarily at the appropriate time to allow the stool to exit the rectum.

The voluntary muscles in patients born with ARMs have varying degrees of hypodevelopment. Likewise, individuals who have spinal problems or injuries can have sphincter dysfunction.

Anal Canal

Voluntary sphincter muscles can be called upon only when the patient feels the need to use them, information that can only be derived from intact anal sensation. The anal canal provides this exquisite sensory output. Except for children born with rectal stenosis and atresia (those who have a normal anal canal), most patients who have ARMs are born without this distal anatomy, and for them sensation does not exist or is merely rudimentary. Patients who have HD are born with a normal anal canal, but this can be injured during the pull-through procedure if the canal is not carefully preserved.[57] Those who have spinal problems or pelvic trauma may have an injured, destroyed, denervated, or nonfunctional anal canal.

In order for the patient to perceive distention of the rectum, the rectum must be located precisely in the center of the sphincteric mechanism—a vital aspect of the pull-through procedure for imperforate anus. The stretching of the lumen by stool in the rectum is perceived by the patient (proprioception). Thus, to achieve bowel control, the patient must have the capacity to form solid stool. Loose stool causes no stretching of the rectum and therefore no proprioception. This point is also relevant in children who have ulcerative colitis and have undergone an ileoanal pull-through procedure. They may suffer from periods of incontinence due to their inability to form solid stool. Usually, however, the normal sphincter and intact anal canal allow them to overcome this hypermotility and to avoid incontinence.

Motility

The rectosigmoid normally remains quiet for variable periods (one to several days) and when quiescent, anal sensation and sphincteric muscles are inactive because the stool (if solid) remains inside the colon. The patient often can feel the peristaltic contraction of the rectosigmoid occurring prior to defecation. The normal individual can then voluntarily relax the skeletal muscles and allow the stool to migrate down to the rectum just above the highly sensitive anal canal. Information provided by the anal canal concerning the consistency and quality of the stool cues the patient to voluntarily push the rectal contents back up into the rectosigmoid and hold them there until the appropriate time for evacuation. The voluntary muscles then relax at the time of defecation.

The key factor that provokes emptying of the rectosigmoid is an involuntary peristaltic contraction helped along by a Valsalva maneuver. Patients born with an ARM may suffer from a disturbance of this mechanism. Those who have undergone a posterior sagittal anorectoplasty or any other type of sacroperineal approach in which the most distal part of the bowel has been preserved show evidence of an over-efficient reservoir, usually associated with a megarectum that manifests as constipation (particularly evident in patients born with lower type anorectal defects).[55,81]

The physiologic cause for this same scenario in patients not born with anatomic anomalies but who develop severe (idiopathic) constipation and encopresis remains unknown. It is clear that constipation that is not treated aggressively leads to more severe obstipation. A vicious cycle develops, with worsening constipation leading to more rectosigmoid dilation, leading to worse constipation and ultimately to soiling. We do not know why the enormously dilated rectosigmoid (possessing normal ganglion cells) is hypomotile initially and we do not know which comes first, constipation or loss of tone, leading to dilation.[87]

Patients born with ARMs who have had surgical procedures in which the most distal part of the colon was resected behave like patients who lack a rectal reservoir.[92] Depending on the amount of colon removed, the patient may have loose stools. In such cases, the child needs medical management. This consists of a constipating diet and medications to add bulk, such as pectin, and those that slow down colonic motility, such as loperamide. In children younger than 2 years of age, the use of loperamide must be monitored carefully because of the risk of central nervous system depression and rarely anaphylaxis. Resection of the distal aganglionic bowel is the basis of the operation performed on patients who have HD, but it is their normal anal canal and sphincters that allow the vast majority to remain continent despite the loss of the rectal reservoir. Interestingly, some patients afflicted with an injured anal canal and sphincters related to pelvic trauma can be continent if their motility is regular because the reliable contraction of the rectosigmoid can be translated into a successful voluntary bowel movement.

The clinician must distinguish between laxatives (which enhance motility by provoking peristalsis) and stool softeners and lubricants (which soften the stool and make it easier to pass). Many children who have slow moving colons, particularly those who have had surgery, need the provocative effect of laxatives and do not respond well to stool softeners. With stool softeners, the colon remains full of stool, albeit softer stool, but the stool still does not come out.

True Fecal Incontinence

The term *true fecal incontinence* refers to situations in which an underlying structural abnormality leads to fecal soiling, as opposed to pseudoincontinence, in which the soiling results from constipation and overflow of stool.

Patients with True Fecal Incontinence

Approximately 75% of children who have repaired ARMs have voluntary bowel movements after the age of 3 years.[88] About half of these patients soil their underwear on occasion, usually due to constipation; but when the constipation is treated properly, the soiling disappears. Thus, the majority of patients have voluntary bowel movements and no soiling and behave like normal children. Those who have bowel control may suffer from temporary episodes of fecal incontinence if they experience diarrhea.

About one-quarter of all children with ARMs suffer from true fecal incontinence. Some patients who have HD, as well as those afflicted with spinal problems, suffer from true fecal incontinence.[57] For these children, the clinician can apply similar principles of bowel management gleaned from the treatment of children who have ARMs.[86]

With knowledge of the specific type of ARM, the clinician can predict the functional prognosis. If the child's defect is one associated with a good prognosis (rectovestibular fistula, rectoperineal fistula, rectal atresia, rectourethral bulbar fistula, imperforate anus with no fistula or low cloaca), the child can be expected to have voluntary bowel movements by the age of 3 years. These children need careful supervision in order to avoid fecal impaction and constipation, which could lead to overflow pseudoincontinence.[55]

If the child has a type of defect that carries a poor prognosis (high cloaca with a common channel longer than 3 cm, rectobladder neck fistula), lacks normal sacral development, or has an associated spinal problem such as myelomeningocele, he or she most likely will need a bowel management program, with enemas in order to remain clean.[86] This regimen should be implemented when the child is 3 to 4 years old, before starting school.

Children born with an ARM and a rectoprostatic fistula have about a 50% chance of having voluntary bowel movements.[88] In these children, an attempt should be made to toilet train them by the age of 3 years. If unsuccessful, bowel management with enemas should be implemented. Each summer, after the school year, attempts can be made to reassess the child's ability to be trained.

In treating patients who have true fecal incontinence, the ideal approach is an enema program that involves teaching the patient and parents how to cleanse the colon mechanically once daily in order to stay completely clean between enemas. This result is achieved by choosing the correct enema and making certain that the colon remains quiescent between enemas. These children are not truly continent. They cannot have voluntary bowel movements, and it is for this reason that they require the artificial mechanism of a daily enema to empty their colons.

The program is implemented by trial and error during a period of 1 week, with the patient seen daily. Each day an abdominal radiograph is taken, so that he or she can be monitored for the amount and location of stool in the colon, as well as for any episodes of soiling. The daily radiographs are essential because they permit the clinician to make small adjustments in the regimen, such as modification of the type and volume of the enema, the doses of any medications, and the diet.[86] Enemas and laxatives are never combined because the enema will clean the colon but the laxative will provoke a bowel movement (and thus an incontinence episode) prior to the next enema washout.

Two well-defined groups of patients with fecal incontinence can be identified. The first and larger group includes those with a tendency toward constipation. The second group has a tendency toward loose stool. Those who manifest fecal incontinence after operations for ARM and HD and those who have spinal disorders usually fall into the constipated group, but some patients who have ARM and HD pass multiple loose stools and need treatment for hypermotility.[57]

Children with True Fecal Incontinence, Constipation, and a Slow Colon

In these children, colonic motility is slow. Because they are fecally incontinent and lack the ability to have voluntary bowel movements, the basis of their bowel management program is to cleanse the child's colon once a day with an enema. No specific diets or medications are necessary. Their constipation (hypomotility) helps them because the slow-moving colon remains quiescent between enemas. If the enema is adequate, no stool passes until the next enema 24 hours later. The challenge is to find the ideal enema capable of cleaning the rectosigmoid. Accidents or soiling episodes occur if the colon is not cleared by the enema, and stool subsequently passes. In such a case, a more potent enema is required. The enema itself may irritate the colon (phosphate enemas can do this) causing the patient to pass stool between enemas; yet, the radiograph is clean. In this case, a gentler enema is needed.

For those who have fecal incontinence and a firm stool, laxatives exacerbate soiling difficulties. These children require bowel management by means of a daily enema. Many children are categorized incorrectly and are treated with laxatives for many years, continuing to soil. Such children are easy to identify because typically they have an ARM as well as associated anomalies (abnormal sacrum, poor muscles) that carry a poor prognosis for continence.

Children with True Fecal Incontinence, Loose Stools, and a Rapid Transiting Bowel

In the years before the introduction of the posterior sagittal anorectoplasty for the repair of anorectal malformations, procedures frequently included resection of the rectosigmoid.[47,92] Such children have a tendency toward loose stool because of a hyperactive colon. They lack a rectal reservoir. Some patients who have HD behave as if they have hypermotility and can be managed similarly. Even when an enema cleanses the colon rather easily, new stool passes quickly through the colon. To prevent this effect, a constipating diet and agents such as loperamide and pectin to slow the colon and add bulk are needed. Foods that loosen bowel movements should be avoided. Diet is strictly enforced: banana, apple, baked bread, white pasta without sauce, and boiled meats. Fried and oily foods as well as dairy products must be avoided.

A successful bowel management program requires dedication and sensitivity from the medical team. The goals are to clean the colon once a day, to keep it quiescent, and to allow the child to remain soil-free for the 24 hours after the enema. The regimen is an ongoing process of trial and error that is individualized and usually is successful within 1 week.[86] During that time, the family, patient, physician, and nurse learn to tailor the enema routine.

Enema Program for Patients with True Fecal Incontinence

After a thorough history and examination are performed, the next step is to perform a contrast enema using water-soluble material—never barium because it can lead to impaction. The postevacuation radiograph is important and will show the type of colon: dilated (constipated) (Figure 3-39) or nondilated—(tendency toward loose stool) (Figure 3-40). The water-soluble contrast material also helps empty the colon. The enema type and volume can be estimated by the size of the colon on the study. We do not use manometry at our center because we have not found it helpful in evaluating or planning treatment nor does it provide information that we cannot already glean from the contrast study.

The results of the enema program are evaluated daily. Changes in the enema volume or content are made until we achieve the goal of a clean colon between enemas. A radiograph of the abdomen, taken every day, is vital in determining whether the colon is empty.

There are different types of enema solutions. We use 0.9% saline (from a pharmacy or home-made using the recipe of 1.5 teaspoons (7 cc) of salt added to 1,000 mL of water), usually in a volume somewhere between 350 and 750 cc. The saline enema can be combined with glycerine (10 to 30 cc) or castile soap (9 to 27 cc) to make a more potent solution.

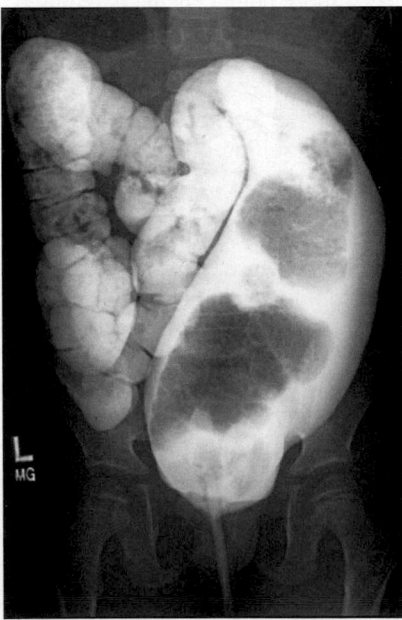

FIGURE 3-39. Contrast enema showing a megarectosigmoid. (Reprinted from Peña A, Levitt M. Colonic inertia disorders in pediatrics. In: Wells SA, ed. *Current Problems in Surgery.* Durham, NC: Mosby; 2002:681, with permission.)

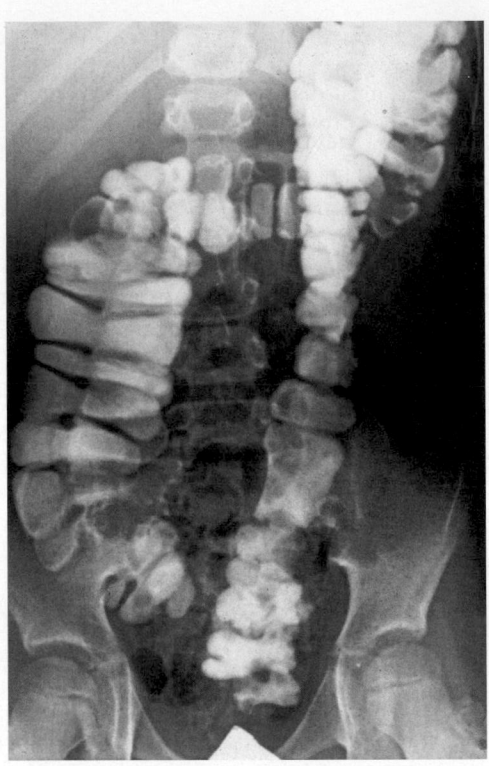

FIGURE 3-40. Contrast enema in a patient who has had the rectosigmoid resected. Note the absence of the sigmoid loop and the colonic haustra in the pelvis. (Reprinted from Levitt MA, Peña A. Treatment of chronic constipation and resection of the inert rectum. In: Holschneider AM, Hutson J, eds. *Anorectal Malformations in Children: Embryology, Diagnosis, Surgical Treatment, Follow-up.* Heidelberg, Germany: Springer; 2006:417, with permission.)

Phosphate enemas are convenient because they come in a prepared vial, but they sometimes irritate the colon and cannot be used in patients who have renal insufficiency.

The enema should result in a bowel movement within 30 to 45 minutes, followed by a period of 24 hours of complete cleanliness (Figure 3-41). If that enema does not clean the colon completely (as demonstrated by plain abdominal radiography, or if the child keeps soiling), the child requires a more aggressive treatment, and glycerine, castile soap, or phosphate is added to the saline solution. By learning from previous attempts and through a process of trial and error, the ideal enema can be determined, usually in 1 week's time.

For children with nondilated and hypermotile colons, parents learn which foods provoke loose stools and which help to constipate their children. The treatment starts with enemas (usually 250 cc to 400 cc of saline), a very strict diet, loperamide, and pectin. Most children respond to this management within 1 week. They stay on the diet until clean for 24 hours several days in a row and then are allowed to choose one new food every 2 to 3 days, observing the new food's effect on colonic motility. If the child soils after eating a newly introduced food, that food should be excluded from the diet. The most liberal diet possible is sought during several months, and the dose of the medications can gradually be reduced to the lowest effective amount required to keep the child clean for 24 hours.

Once the program is successful, parents often ask if the enemas will be needed for life. For children born with no potential for ultimate bowel control, the answer is yes. But because there is a wide spectrum of defects, many have some potential

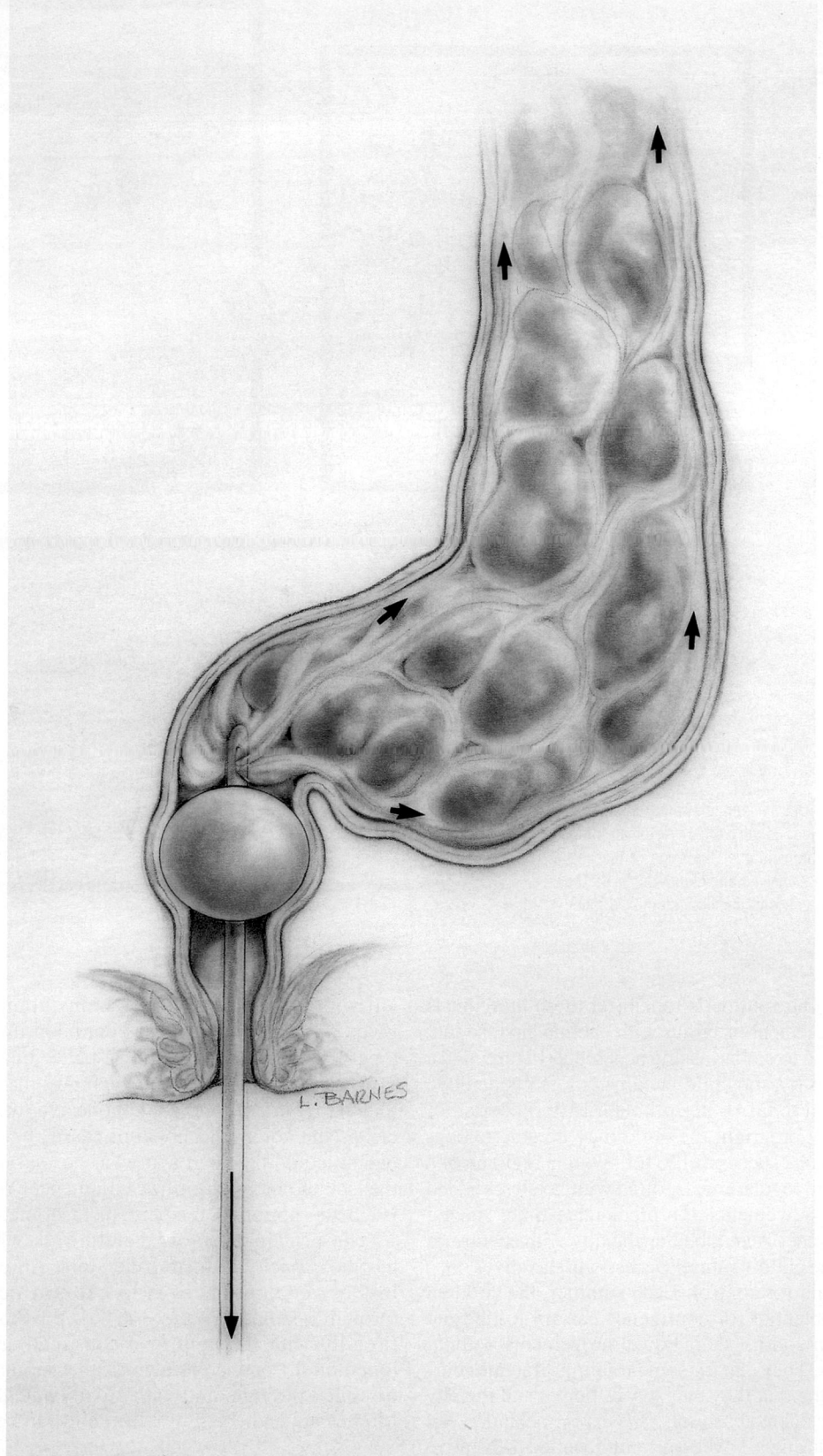

FIGURE 3-41. Enema given with Foley balloon. (Reprinted from Peña A, Guardino K, Tovilla JM, et al. Bowel management for fecal incontinence in patients with anorectal malformations. *J Pediatr Surg*. 1998;33(1):133–137, with permission.)

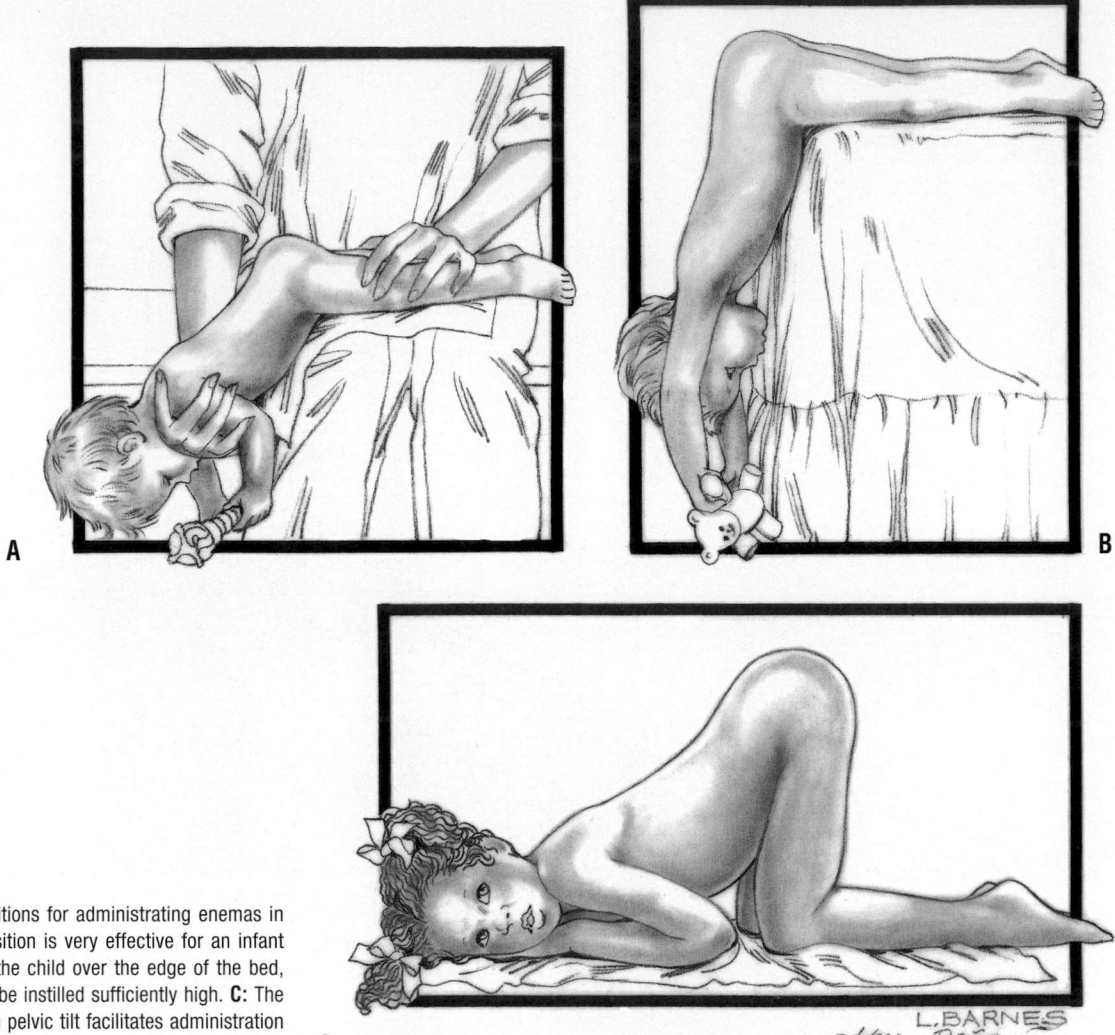

FIGURE 3-42. Positions for administrating enemas in children. **A:** The lap position is very effective for an infant or small child. **B:** With the child over the edge of the bed, the enema solution can be instilled sufficiently high. **C:** The knee-chest position with pelvic tilt facilitates administration and adequate evacuation.

for improvement. Our routine is to subject these individuals to the bowel management program with enemas first, so that they are not exposed to embarrassing accidents (Figure 3-42). Often, as time goes by, the child becomes more cooperative and more interested in his or her problem. After a period of a successful enema program, the child may be able to control bowel movements successfully, following a regimen of a disciplined diet with regular meals, often with laxatives added to provoke bowel movements at a predictable time. Having had time in clean underwear, albeit artificially with enemas, is advantageous to the child's future success with laxatives once he or she tries again for control. Each summer, the children who have some potential for continence can try to find out how well they can control their bowel movements without the help of enemas. They can try some training strategies during vacations, a time that they can stay at home, and thereby avoid having an accident at school. This experimentation can be accomplished during a 1-week program, called a "laxative trial," again with daily radiographs and tailoring of a laxative regimen with the goal of eliminating the enema.

Pull-Through versus Permanent Stoma

For children who have a colostomy and lack the potential for bowel control, the primary question is whether a pull-through operation should be performed or whether they should be left with a permanent stoma. Many clinicians believe that, given the lack of continence common in these individuals, a permanent stoma provides a better quality of life. However, given the success with the bowel management program (enema regimen), one could conceive that if a daily enema cleans the colon and no stool passes between enemas, the patient could be clean and wear normal underwear, despite the lack of potential for true continence. We believe that this is a better option than a permanent stoma.[56]

The principal factor, therefore, is whether the patient has the capacity to form solid stool. An option for children in these circumstances is to perform bowel management through a stoma (Figure 3-43). If the stoma remains quiet (usually with the help of a constipating diet, pectin, and loperamide) between enemas, that stoma could be closed or pulled through, and with a daily antegrade enema (via a Malone appendicostomy), the child can be kept clean.

Antegrade Enema

When children receiving enemas are young (below school age), they do not mind the enemas; but when they are older, many feel that their parents are intruding on their privacy, and it is difficult for them to administer an enema themselves. A reasonable surgical option exists for this specific group of children. A continent appendicostomy (Malone

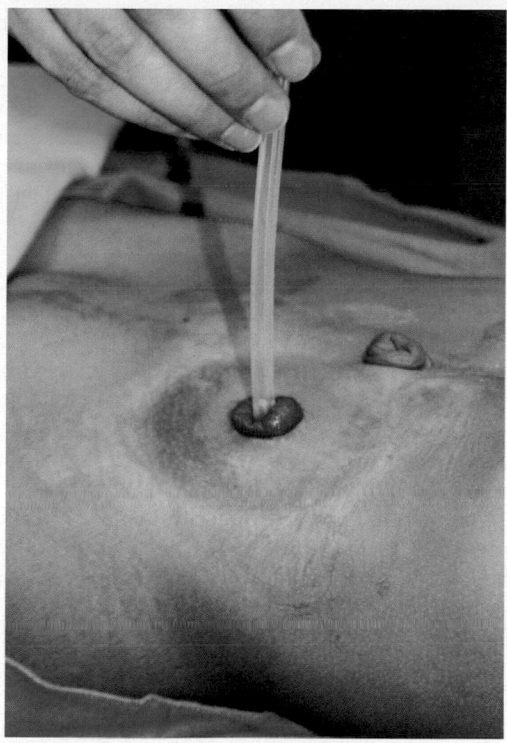

FIGURE 3-43. Bowel management administered through a colostomy. (From Bischoff A, Levitt MA, Bauer C, et al. Treatment of fecal incontinence with a comprehensive bowel management program. *J Pediatr Surg.* 2009;44(6):1278–1284, Elsevier, with permission.)

procedure—see below) can be performed whereby the appendix is connected to the umbilicus, through which an antegrade enema can be administered (Figure 3-44).[58,62,64] If the child has no appendix, a new one can be fashioned from a colonic flap. This opening is called a continent neo-appendicostomy (Figure 3-45). The Malone procedure only changes the route of enema administration; therefore, the child has to be perfectly clean with a bowel management regimen prior to the procedure. For those with spinal problems who are in a wheelchair, this is a particularly useful option.

Pseudoincontinence (Encopresis)

True fecal incontinence must be distinguished from overflow pseudoincontinence, which occurs when a patient behaves as if he or she is fecally incontinent, but really has severe constipation with overflow soiling (encopresis). Once the child is disimpacted and given sufficient laxatives to empty the colon on a daily basis, the soiling stops.

Normally, the rectosigmoid stores the stool. Then, every day or so, an active peristaltic wave occurs, which indicates that it is time to empty. A normal individual feels this sensation, tightens the muscles surrounding the anus, and then decides when to relax the sphincter mechanism. In many children, this process of relaxation is slow, leading over time to severe constipation.

If a child is fecally continent, constipation must be treated with laxatives, which are needed to provoke peristalsis and to overcome the hypomotility. Those who have undergone successful surgery for ARMs (associated with a good

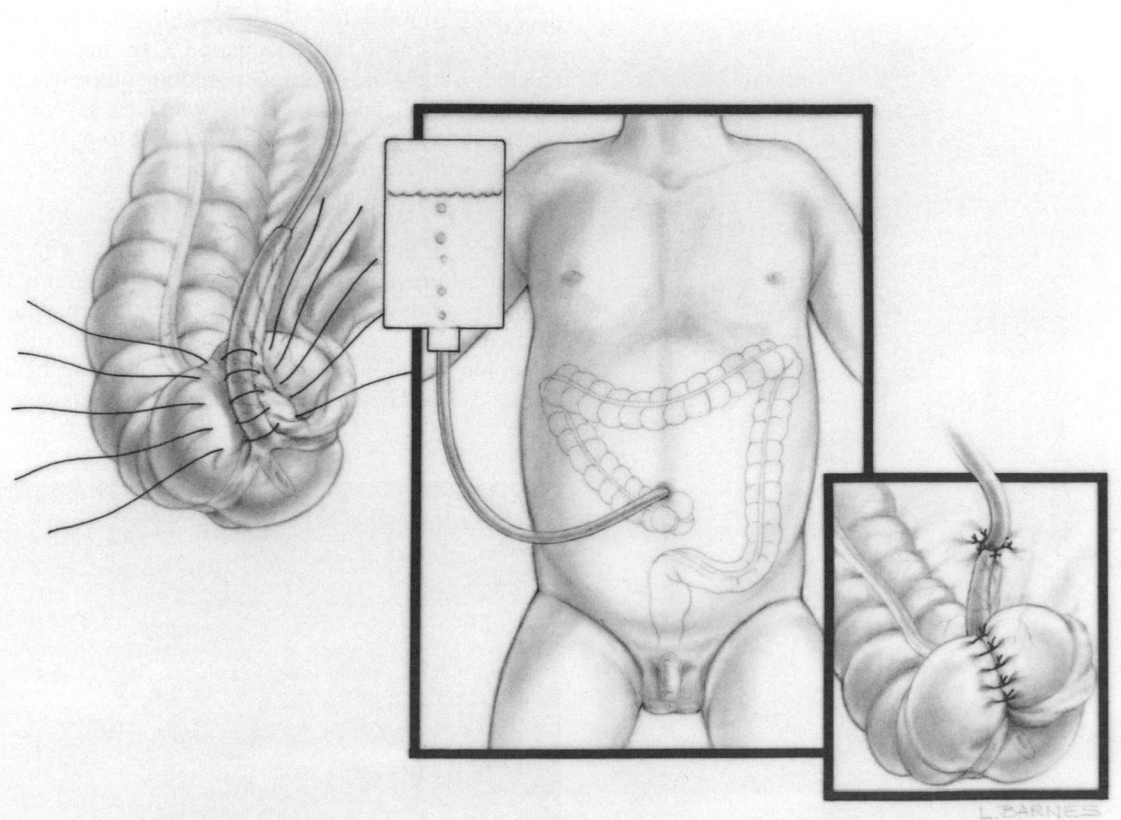

FIGURE 3-44. Malone appendicostomy. (From Levitt MA, Soffer SZ, Peña A. Continent appendicostomy in the bowel management of fecally incontinent children. *J Ped Surg.* 1997;32(11):1630–1633, Elsevier, with permission.)

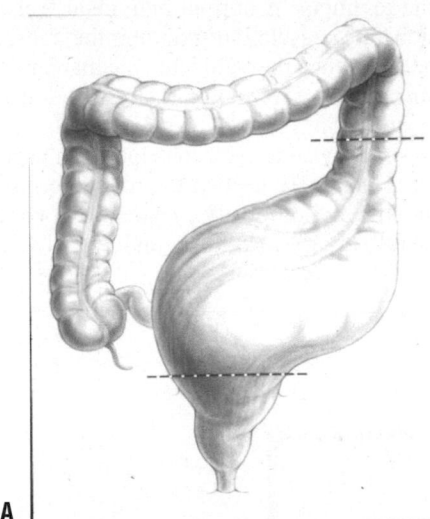

FIGURE 3-45. Neoappendicostomy. (Reprinted from Levitt MA, Peña A. Laparoscopy in the management of fecal incontinence and constipation. In: Holcomb GW III, Georgeson KE, Rothenberg SS, eds. *Atlas of Pediatric Laparoscopy and Thoracoscopy.* Philadelphia, PA: Saunders Elsevier; 2008:88, with permission.)

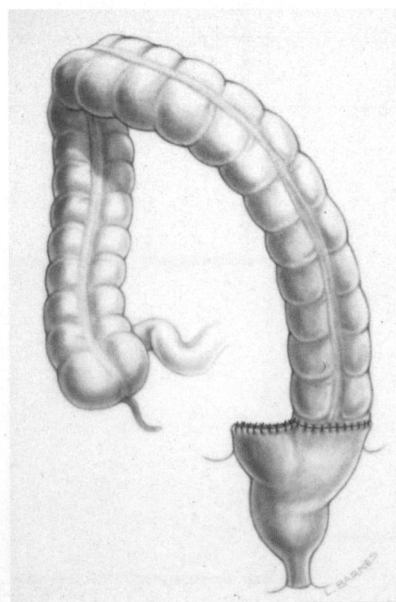

FIGURE 3-46. Diagram of a sigmoid resection. (From Peña A, El-Behery M. Megasigmoid: a source of pseudoincontinence in children with repaired anorectal malformations. *J Pediatr Surg.* 1993;28(2):199–203, Elsevier, with permission.)

prognosis type of anorectal defect and a normal spine), or HD, should be fecally continent. Patients who suffer from idiopathic constipation or encopresis also have an intact continence mechanism and should be capable of having voluntary bowel movements. These patients do not need enemas. We believe appendicostomies, described by some authors as indicated for this problem, are not needed.[12,48,65] These children need only the appropriate medical therapy with stimulant laxatives.

It is common to observe severe constipation in patients who have ARMs, especially in the more benign types[88]; in individuals following successful surgery for HD[57]; and in the large group of children considered to have idiopathic constipation. Untreated constipation can be extremely incapacitating for all of these patients.[55] In its most serious form, this can produce soiling, which really is overflow pseudoincontinence (encopresis).

The therapeutic value of dietary change is minimal in this group of patients. Passage of large, hard pieces of stool may provoke pain and make it appear as if these children are stool retainers. This can ultimately lead to soiling, which may have a pejorative psychological impact on the child.

Clinicians must determine the type of child they are dealing with. Those with a good prognosis for bowel control need an aggressive, proactive treatment of their constipation. If they do not have this capacity, laxatives will just cause them to have more soiling.

Usually these patients suffer from a megarectosigmoid (Figures 3-46 and 3-47), which results from a vicious cycle of hypomotility, constipation, inadequate colonic emptying, and colon dilatation.[33,84,88] This cycle is observed in children born with a good prognosis type of anorectal defect who underwent a technically correct operation but did not receive adequate treatment for constipation. Over time they develop fecal impaction and overflow pseudoincontinence. This outcome also can happen in children who have severe idiopathic constipation (encopresis) and who tend to have a similarly appearing dilated rectosigmoid. The resection can sometimes be accomplished transanally (Figure 3-48).

Diagnosis of Severe Idiopathic Constipation with Soiling

A contrast enema with a hydrosoluble material is the most valuable study. In the severely constipated patient, this study usually shows a megarectosigmoid with dilatation of the colon all the way down to the levator mechanism (see Figure 3-39). There is a dramatic size discrepancy between

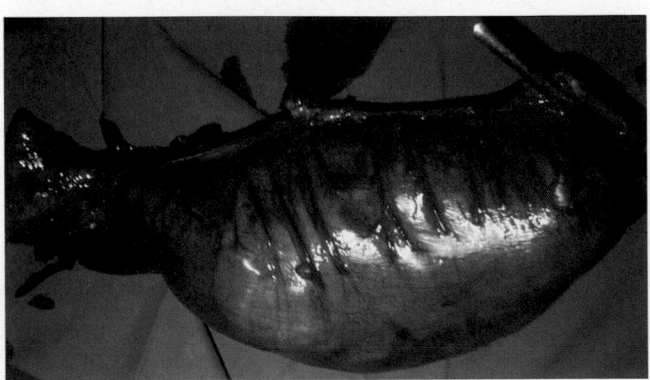

FIGURE 3-47. Specimen of sigmoid resection in a child with profoundly dilated sigmoid colon as a consequence of severe idiopathic constipation (encopresis).

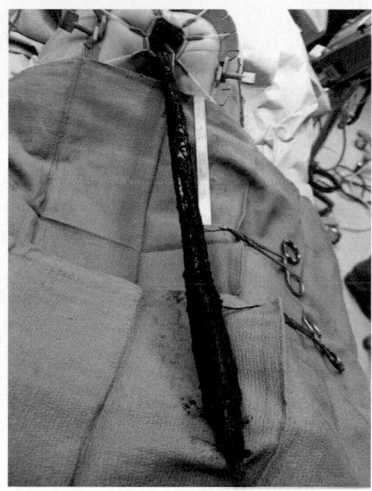

FIGURE 3-48. Transanal resection of a megarectosigmoid. (Reprinted from Levitt MA, Peña A. Laparoscopy in the management of fecal incontinence and constipation. In: Holcolm GW III, Georgeson KE, Rothenberg SS, eds. *Atlas of Pediatric Laparoscopy and Thoracoscopy.* Philadelphia, PA: Saunders Elsevier; 2008:83, with permission.)

a normal descending colon and a dilated megarectosigmoid. This is the exact opposite pattern from that seen in patients who have HD. The size of the colon guides the dosing of the laxatives.

Rectal and colonic manometry have been used in the evaluation of these patients.[19,22] However, we have not found these modalities helpful. Manometry, which places balloons at different levels of the colon and records the waves of contraction[22] or the electrical activity,[99] and scintigraphy, a nuclear medicine study, attempt to assess colonic motility objectively.[16] The key information the surgeon needs to know is if and when a colonic resection would benefit the patient who requires large doses of laxatives in order to evacuate. Unfortunately, these studies do not answer this question consistently. We are hopeful that more objective techniques will ultimately be developed.

When the histology of these colons is investigated, pathologists find hypertrophic smooth muscle in the area of the dilated colon and normal ganglion cells. More sophisticated histopathologic techniques would help understand what is the nature of the abnormality in these colons. These patients do not have HD but clearly have dysmotility. We find the concepts of "very low segment HD" or "internal sphincter achalasia"[19,67] confusing and are hopeful that further investigations will enhance our knowledge about colonic dysmotility and thus guide therapy.

Treatment of Severe Idiopathic Constipation with Soiling (Encopresis)

We treat patients based on an interpretation of the contrast study, inferring dysmotility in the dilated segment of the colon. The mandatory first step, which often is neglected, is to remove the child's fecal impaction. This is accomplished by enemas and sometimes by means of a bowel clean-out. Once the colon is empty, constipation is treated with large doses of stimulant laxatives, not stool softeners.

Stimulant laxatives provoke peristalsis; stool softeners merely soften the stool and do not ameliorate the motility problem. If the patient is not disimpacted first, laxatives cause cramping. In these cases, the laxatives we use often are the same as those that have been tried previously, but the protocol is more aggressive. The laxative dose is adapted to the patient's response, which is monitored daily with an abdominal radiograph. The laxative amount is adjusted until the amount that successfully empties the colon every day is reached. Almost always, the new dose is much greater than had been tried previously.

The colonic dysmotility seen in certain children who have HD, even after successful surgery that removed the aganglionic bowel, is not truly understood. These patients can behave like those who have ARMs and also benefit from early and proactive medical treatment of their constipation. Likewise, the cause of severe constipation and encopresis in many children cannot be determined. Proactive and aggressive laxative therapy helps these individuals. The dysmotility is incurable, but it is manageable. Treatments must be consistent with patients requiring close observation. Once treatments are tapered or interrupted, constipation will recur.

Some clinicians treat such "intractable" children with stomas or with antegrade enemas.[12,33,48,65,100] We feel that the preferred alternative is to employ stimulant laxatives. We reserve washouts for patients who have true fecal incontinence and who are incapable of having voluntary bowel movements.

If the child is incontinent, enemas as part of a bowel management regimen are appropriate. If continent, maintenance treatment of constipation with laxatives is the alternative of choice.

Determination of the Laxative Requirement

Once the colon is disimpacted, a dose of laxative is started empirically based on the contrast enema results. A senna derivative is ideal. The dose is given, and the patient is observed for the next 24 hours. If the child does not have a bowel movement in the first day after giving the laxative, the dose must have been inadequate and should be increased. An enema also should be given in order to remove the stool produced during the prior 24 hours. If the patient defecates multiple times and the radiograph is clean, the laxative dose can be decreased. The routine of choosing the laxative dose and giving an enema if needed is continued every night until the dose is found that provokes a voluntary bowel movement and empties the colon completely (as confirmed by abdominal radiograph). Sometimes the laxative empties the colon effectively, but the stool is too loose. In this circumstance, adding pectin provides bulk and causes the same laxative dose to be more efficacious.

Patients may have laxative requirements much greater than the manufacturer's recommendations. Usually, the dosage that the patient requires in order to empty the colon completely can be achieved. At that dose, the patient should stop soiling because he or she is emptying the colon effectively each day. Because the colon is empty, the patient remains clean until the next voluntary bowel movement. Occasionally, although during the process of increasing the amount of laxative, patients vomit before reaching an adequate effect or do not tolerate such a high dose because of side effects. Such children are candidates for surgical intervention.

Surgical Options: Rectosigmoid Resection

A sigmoid resection can be performed in selected patients who have a repaired anorectal malformation and who harbor severe constipation.[58,84] The very dilated megarectosigmoid is resected, and the descending colon is anastomosed to the rectum (see Figures 3-46 and 3-47). Because the rectum plays a vital reservoir function that allows the child to perceive rectal distention, it is preserved. The remaining rectum is abnormal, and without careful observation and treatment of constipation, the colon proximal to it can redilate.

In those who have intractable idiopathic constipation but who have normal sphincters and a normal anal canal, the rectosigmoid down to the pectinate line can be resected, in a similar manner used for patients who have HD. The nondilated colon (which is assumed to have normal motility) is anastomosed to the rectum above the pectinate line.[58] This procedure is a great alternative to traditional recommendations such as ileostomy, colostomy, or antegrade stomas for these most severely affected intractable patients.[12,13,33,58,65,100] Another option we have been employing is to perform both a resection and a Malone procedure for antegrade washouts. This combination of techniques is particularly effective for the most severe dysmotility cases.

The most dilated part of the colon is resected because it is considered empirically to be most seriously affected. The nondilated part of the colon is assumed to have a more normal motility, which we infer from the contrast enema. Perhaps emerging colonic motility diagnostic techniques will help with surgical planning. We have observed that the patients who have the most improvement are those who have a more localized form of megarectosigmoid. Those afflicted with a more generalized dilation of the colon do not respond as well and may require a more extensive resection. Perhaps in the future these observations can be corroborated, and results of resection predicted better by noninvasive modalities.

References

1. Aegineta P. On the imperforate anus. In: Adams F, trans. *The Seven Books, Book VI, Section LXXXI*. London, United Kingdom: Syndenham Society; 1844:405.
2. Albanese CT, Jennings RW, Lopoo JB, et al. One-stage correction of high imperforate anus in the male neonate. *J Pediatr Surg*. 1999;34(5):834–836.
3. Amussat JZ. Gustiure d'une operation d'anus artifical practiqué avec succàs par un nouveau procédé. *Gaz Med Paris*. 1835;3:735.
4. Bax KN. Duhamel lecture: the incurability of Hirschsprung's disease. *Eur J Pediatr Surg*. 2006;16(6):380–384.
5. Bealer JF, Natuzzi ES, Buscher C, et al. Nitric oxide synthase is deficient in the aganglionic colon of patients with Hirschsprung's disease. *Pediatrics*. 1994;93(4):647–651.
6. Belman AB, King LR. Urinary tract abnormalities associated with imperforate anus. *J Urol*. 1972;108(5):823–824.
7. Black CT, Sherman JO. The association of low imperforate anus and Down's syndrome. *J Pediatr Surg*. 1989;24(1):92–94.
8. Boley SJ. New modification of the surgical treatment of Hirschsprung's disease. *Surgery*. 1964;56:1015–1017.
9. Breech L. Gynecological concerns in patients with anorectal malformations. *Semin Pediatr Surg*. 2010;19(2):139–145.
10. Brenner EC. Congenital defects of the anus and rectum. *Surg Gynecol Obstet*. 1915;20:579–588.
11. Carcassonne M, Morisson LG, Letourneau JN. Primary corrective operation without decompression in infants less than three months of age with Hirschsprung's disease. *J Pediatr Surg*. 1982;17(3):241–243.
12. Cascio S, Flett ME, De la Hunt M, et al. MACE or caecostomy button for idiopathic constipation in children: a comparison of complications and outcomes. *Pediatr Surg Int*. 2004;20(7):484–487.
13. Cass DT. Neonatal one-stage repair of Hirschsprung's disease. *Pediatr Surg Int*. 1990;5:341–346.
14. Chassaignac M. Présentation de malades. *Bull Soc Chir*. 1856;20:410.
15. Cilley RE, Statter MB, Hirschl RB, et al. Definitive treatment of Hirschsprung's disease in the newborn with a one-stage procedure. *Surgery*. 1994;115(5):551–556.

16. Cook BJ, Lim E, Cook D, et al. Radionuclear transit to assess sites of delay in large bowel transit in children with chronic idiopathic constipation. *J Pediatr Surg*. 2005;40(3):478–483.
17. Curran TJ, Raffensperger JG. The feasibility of laparoscopic Swenson pull-through. *J Pediatr Surg*. 1994;29(9):1273–1275.
18. Davidson M. Alimentary canal. In: Code CF, Werner H, eds. *Handbook of Physiology*. 5th ed. Baltimore, MD: Williams & Wilkins; 1970:2783.
19. De Caluwé DD, Yoneda A, Akl U, et al. Internal anal sphincter achalasia: outcome after internal sphincter myectomy. *J Pediatr Surg*. 2001;36(5):736–738.
20. de la Torre-Mondragón L, Ortega-Salgado JA. Transanal endorectal pull-through for Hirschsprung's disease. *J Pediatr Surg*. 1998;33(8):1283–1286.
21. deVries PA, Peña A. Posterior sagittal anorectoplasty. *J Pediatr Surg*. 1982;17(5):638–643.
22. Di Lorenzo C, Flores A, Reddy S, et al. Use of colonic manometry to differentiate causes of intractable constipation in children. *J Pediatr*. 1992;120(5):690–695.
23. Dobbins WO III, Bill AH Jr. Diagnosis of Hirschsprung's disease excluded by rectal suction biopsy. *N Engl J Med*. 1965;272:990–993.
24. Docherty JG, Zaki A, Coutts JA, et al. Meconium ileus: a review 1972–1990. *Br J Surg*. 1992;79(6):571–573.
25. Duhamel B. Retrorectal and transanal pull-through procedure for the treatment of Hirschsprung's disease. *Dis Colon Rectum*. 1964;7:455–458.
26. Eek S, Knutrud O. Megacolon congenitum Hirschsprung. *J Oslo City Hosp*. 1962;12:245–270.
27. Ehrenpreis T. *Hirschsprung's Disease: Incidence*. Chicago, IL: Year Book; 1970.
28. Elema JD, deVries JA, Vos LJ. Intensity and proximal extension of acetylcholinesterase activity in the mucosa of the rectosigmoid in Hirschsprung's disease. *J Pediatr Surg*. 1973;8(3):361–368.
29. Fadda B, Pistor G, Meier-Ruge W, et al. Symptoms, diagnosis, and therapy of neuronal intestinal dysplasia masked by Hirschsprung's disease: report of 24 cases. *Pediatr Surg Int*. 1987;2:76–80.
30. Fewtrell MS, Tam PK, Thomson AH, et al. Hirschsprung's disease associated with a deletion of chromosome 10 (q11.2q21.2): a further link with the neurocristopathies? *J Med Genet*. 1994;31(4):325–327.
31. Georgeson KE, Cohen RD, Hebra A, et al. Primary laparoscopic-assisted endorectal colon pull-through for Hirschsprung's disease: a new gold standard. *Ann Surg*. 1999;229(5):678–682.
32. Georgeson KE, Fuenfer MM, Hardin WD. Primary laparoscopic pull-through for Hirschsprung's disease in infants and children. *J Pediatr Surg*. 1995;30(7):1017–1021.
33. Gladman MA, Scott SM, Lunniss PJ, et al. Systematic review of surgical options for idiopathic megarectum and megacolon. *Ann Surg*. 2005;241(4):562–574.
34. Goon HK. Repair of anorectal anomalies in the neonatal period. *Pediatr Surg Int*. 1990;5:246–249.
35. Graivier L, Sieber WK. Hirschsprung's disease and mongolism. *Surgery*. 1966;6(2):458–461.
36. Gross GW, Wolfson PJ, Peña A. Augmented-pressure colostogram in imperforate anus with fistula. *Pediatr Radiol*. 1991;21(8):560–562.
37. Hadra. *Berlin Klin Wochenschr*. 1886:7.
38. Hendren WH. Repair of cloacal anomalies: current techniques. *J Pediatr Surg*. 1986;21(12):1159–1176.
39. Hertzler DA II, DePowell JJ, Stevenson CB, et al. Tethered cord syndrome: a review of the literature from embryology to adult presentation. *Neurosurg Focus*. 2010;29(1):E1.
40. Hiatt RB. A further description of the pathologic physiology of congenital megacolon and the results of surgical treatment. *Pediatrics*. 1958;21(5):825–831.
41. Hirschsprung H. Stuhltrúgheit neugeboreher in Folge von dilatation und hypertrophie des colons. *Jahrb Kinderhkd*. 1888;27:1.
42. Holschneider AM, ed. *Hirschsprung's Disease*. Stuttgart, Germany: Hippokrates-Verlag; 1982.
43. Holschneider AM. Particular forms of Hirschsprung's disease. In: Holschneider AM, ed. *Hirschsprung's Disease*. Stuttgart, Germany: Hippokrates-Verlag; 1982:133.
44. Hong AR, Acuña MF, Peña A, et al. Urologic injuries associated with repair of anorectal malformations in male patients. *J Pediatr Surg*. 2002;37(3):339–344.
45. Howard ER. Hirschsprung's disease: a review of the morphology and physiology. *Postgrad Med J*. 1972;48(562):471–477.
46. Howard ER. Histochemistry in the diagnosis and investigation of congenital aganglionosis (Hirschsprung's disease). *Am Surg*. 1973;39(11):602–607.

47. Kiesewetter WB. Imperforate anus II. The rationale and technique of the sacroabdominoperineal operation. *J Pediatr Surg.* 1967;2:106–110.

48. King SK, Sutcliffe JR, Southwell BR, et al. The antegrade continence enema successfully treats idiopathic slow-transit constipation. *J Pediatr Surg.* 2005;40(12):1935–1940.

49. Ladd WE, Gross RE. Congenital malformations of anus and rectum: report of 162 cases. *Am J Surg.* 1934;23(1):167–183.

50. Langer JC, Durrant AC, de la Torre L, et al. One-stage transanal Soave pullthrough for Hirschsprung's disease: a multicenter experience with 141 children. *Ann Surg.* 2003;238(4):569–583.

51. Langer JC, Minkes RK, Mazziotti MV, et al. Transanal one-stage Soave procedure for infants with Hirschsprung's disease. *J Pediatr Surg.* 1999;34(1):148–151.

52. Leenders E, Sieber WK. Congenital megacolon observation by Frederick Ruysch—1691. *J Pediatr Surg.* 1970;5(1):1–3.

53. Lemelle JL, Guillemin F, Aubert D, et al. A multicentre study of the management of disorders of defecation in patients with spina bifida. *Neurogastroenterol Motil.* 2006;18(2):123–128.

54. Levitt MA, Dickie B, Peña A. Evaluation and treatment of the patient with Hirschsprung's disease patient who is not doing well after a pullthrough procedure. *Semin Pediatr Surg.* 2010;19(2):146–153.

55. Levitt MA, Kant A, Peña A. The morbidity of constipation in patients with anorectal malformations. *J Pediatr Surg.* 2010;45(6):1228–1233.

56. Levitt MA, Mak G, Falcone R, et al. Cloacal exstrophy—pull through or permanent stoma? A review of 53 patients. *J Pediatr Surg.* 2008;43(1):164–168.

57. Levitt MA, Martin C, Olesevich M, et al. Hirschsprung's disease and fecal incontinence: diagnostic and management strategies. *J Pediatr Surg.* 2009;44:271–277.

58. Levitt MA, Peña A. Laparoscopy in the management of fecal incontinence and constipation. In: Holcomb W, Georgeson K, Rothenberg S, eds. *Atlas of Pediatric Laparoscopy and Thoracoscopy.* Philadelphia, PA: Elsevier Saunders; 2008:81–90.

59. Levitt MA, Peña A. Reoperations in anorectal malformations In: Teich S, Caniano D, eds. *Reoperative Pediatric Surgery.* New York, NY: Humana Press; 2008:311 326.

60. Levitt MA, Peña A. Complications of surgery in anorectal malformations. In: Caty MG, ed. *Complications in Pediatric Surgery.* New York, NY: Informa Healthcare; 2009:301–315.

61. Levitt MA, Peña A. Cloacal malformations: lessons learned from 490 cases. *Semin Pediatr Surg.* 2010;19(2):128–138.

62. Levitt MA, Soffer SZ, Peña A. Continent appendicostomy in the bowel management of fecally incontinent children. *J Pediatr Surg.* 1997;32(11):1630–1633.

63. Luo Y, Ceccherini I, Pasini B, et al. Close linkage with the RET protooncogene and boundaries of deletion mutations in autosomal dominant Hirschsprung disease. *Hum Mol Genet.* 1993;2(11):1803–1808.

64. Malone PS, Ransley PG, Kiely EM. Preliminary report: the antegrade continence enema. *Lancet.* 1990;336(8725):1217–1218.

65. Marshall J, Hutson JM, Anticich N, et al. Antegrade continence enemas in the treatment of slow-transit constipation. *J Pediatr Surg.* 2001;36(8):1227–1230.

66. Martucciello G, Biocchi M, Dodero P, et al. Total colonic aganglionosis associated with interstitial deletion of the long arm of chromosome 10. *Pediatr Surg Int.* 1992;7(4):308–310.

67. Martucciello G, Pini Prato A, Puri P, et al. Controversies concerning diagnostic guidelines for anomalies of the enteric nervous system: a report from the fourth International Symposium on Hirschsprung's disease and related neurocristopathies. *J Pediatr Surg.* 2005;40(10):1527–1531.

68. Meier-Rouge W. Cause of colon disorder with symptoms of Hirschsprung's disease. *Verh Dtsch Ges Pathol.* 1971;55:506.

69. Meier-Rouge W. Hirschsprung's disease: its aetiology, pathogenesis and differential diagnosis. *Curr Top Pathol.* 1974;59:131–179.

70. Moore BG, Singaram C, Eckhoff DE, et al. Immunohistochemical evaluations of ultrashort-segment Hirschsprung's disease. Report of three cases. *Dis Colon Rectum.* 1996;39(7):817–822.

71. Moore TC. Advantages of performing the sagittal anoplasty operation for imperforate anus at birth. *J Pediatr Surg.* 1990;25(2):276–277.

72. Mundt E, Bates MD. Genetics of Hirschsprung disease and anorectal malformations. *Semin Pediatr Surg.* 2010;19(2):107–117.

73. Narasimharao KL, Prasad GR, Katariya S, et al. Prone cross-table lateral view: an alternative to the invertogram in imperforate anus. *AJR Am J Roentgenol.* 1983;140(2):227–229.

74. Noblett HR. A rectal suction biopsy tube for use in the diagnosis of Hirschsprung's disease. *J Pediatr Surg.* 1969;4(4):406–409.

75. Okamoto E, Ueda T. Embryogenesis of intramural ganglia of the gut and its relation to Hirschsprung's disease. *J Pediatr Surg.* 1967;2(5):437–443.

76. O'Kelly TJ, Davies JR, Tam PK, et al. Abnormalities of nitric-oxide-producing neurons in Hirschsprung's disease: morphology and implications. *J Pediatr Surg.* 1994;29(2):294–299.

77. Panuel M, Guys JM, Devred P, et al. Imagerie par résonance magnétique des malformations ano-rectales hautes. *Chir Pediatr.* 1988;29(5):243–246.

78. Peña A. Posterior sagittal anorectoplasty as a secondary operation for the treatment of fecal incontinence. *J Pediatr Surg.* 1983;18(6):762–773.

79. Peña A. *Posterior Sagittal Approach for the Correction of Anorectal Malformations.* Vol 19. Chicago, IL: Year Book; 1985.

80. Peña A. Surgical treatment of high imperforate anus. *World J Surg.* 1985;9(2):236–243.

81. Peña A. Anorectal malformations. *Semin Pediatr Surg.* 1995;4(1):35–47.

82. Peña A. Total urogenital mobilization: an easier way to repair cloacas. *J Pediatr Surg.* 1997;32(2):263–267.

83. Peña A, Devries PA. Posterior sagittal anorectoplasty: important technical considerations and new applications. *J Pediatr Surg.* 1982;17(6):796–811.

84. Peña A, El-Behery M. Megasigmoid: a source of pseudoincontinence in children with repaired anorectal malformations. *J Pediatr Surg.* 1993;28(2):199–203.

85. Peña A, Elicevik M, Levitt MA. Reoperations in Hirschsprung disease. *J Pediatr Surg.* 2007;42(6):1008–1013.

86. Peña A, Guardino K, Tovilla JM, et al. Bowel management for fecal incontinence in patients with anorectal malformations. *J Pediatr Surg.* 1998;33(1):133–137.

87. Peña A, Levitt MA. Colonic inertia disorders in pediatrics. *Curr Probl Surg.* 2002;39(7):666–730.

88. Peña A, Levitt MA. Imperforate anus and cloacal malformations. In: Ashcraft K, Holder T, Holcomb W, eds. *Pediatric Surgery.* 4th ed. Philadelphia, PA: WB Saunders; 2005:496–517.

89. Peña A, Levitt MA, Hong A, et al. Surgical management of cloacal malformations: a review of 339 patients. *J Pediatr Surg.* 2004;39(3):470–479.

90. Poenaru D, Borgstein E, Numanoglu A, et al. Caring for children with colorectal disease in the context of limited resources. *Semin Pediatr Surg.* 2010;19(2):118–127.

91. Pomeranz SJ, Altman N, Sheldon JJ, et al. Magnetic resonance of congenital anorectal malformations. *Magn Reson Imaging.* 1986;4(1):69–72.

92. Rehbein F. Imperforate anus: experiences with abdomino-perineal and abdomino-sacro-perineal pull-through procedures. *J Pediatr Surg.* 1967;2:99–105.

93. Rhoads JE, Piper RL, Randall JP. A simultaneous abdominal and perineal approach in operations for imperforate anus with atresia of the rectum and rectosigmoid. *Ann Surg.* 1948;127(3):552–556.

94. Robertson HE, Kernohan JW. The myenteric plexus in congenital megacolon. *Proc Staff Meet Mayo Clin.* 1938;13:123–125.

95. Sachs TM, Applebaum H, Touran T, et al. Use of MRI in evaluation of anorectal anomalies. *J Pediatr Surg.* 1990;25(7):817–821.

96. Sandgren K, Ekblad E, Larsson LT. Survival of neurons and interstitial cells of Cajal after autotransplantation of myenteric ganglia from small intestine in the lethal spotted mouse. *Pediatr Surg Int.* 2000;16(4):272–276.

97. Sane SM, Giardany BR. Total aganglionosis coli. Clinical and roentgenographic manifestations. *Radiology.* 1973;107(2):397–404.

98. Santulli TV. The treatment of imperforate anus and associated fistulas. *Surg Gynecol Obstet.* 1952;95(5):601–614.

99. Sarna SK, Bardakjian BL, Waterfall WE, et al. Human colonic electric control activity. *Gastroenterology.* 1980;78(6):1526–1536.

100. Scarpa M, Barollo M, Keighley MR. Ileostomy for constipation: long-term postoperative outcome. *Colorectal Dis.* 2005;7(3):224–227.

101. Sieber WK. Hirschsprung's disease. In: Welch KJ, Randolph JG, Ravitch MM, et al., eds. *Pediatric Surgery.* Vol 2. 4th ed. Chicago, IL: Year Book; 1986:995.

102. Smith BM, Steiner RB, Lobe TE. Laparoscopic Duhamel pullthrough procedure for Hirschsprung's disease in childhood. *J Laparoendosc Surg.* 1994;4(4):273–276.

103. So HB, Schwartz DL, Becker JM, et al. Endorectal "pull-through" without preliminary colostomy in neonates with Hirschsprung's disease. *J Pediatr Surg.* 1980;15(4):470–471.

104. Soave F. Hirschsprung's disease: a new surgical technique. *Arch Dis Child.* 1964;39:116–124.

105. Soper RT, Ortiz JM. Neonatal pneumoperitoneum and Hirschsprung's disease. *Surgery.* 1961;51:527–533.

106. Stephens FD. Imperforate rectum: a new surgical technique. *Med J Aust.* 1953;1(6):202–203.

107. Stephens FD, Smith ED. *Anorectal Malformations in Children*. Vol 4. Chicago, IL: Year Book; 1971.

108. Stephens FD, Smith ED. *Genito-urinary Anomalies and Their Complications*. Vol 4. Chicago, IL: Year Book; 1971.

109. Stephens FD, Smith ED. *Proposed International Classification*. Vol 4. Chicago, IL: Year Book; 1971.

110. Stephens FD, Smith ED. Classification, identification and assessment of surgical treatment of anorectal anomalies. *Pediatr Surg Int*. 1986;1:200.

111. Swenson O, Bill AH Jr. Resection of rectum and rectosigmoid with preservation of the sphincter for benign spastic lesions producing megacolon: an experimental study. *Surgery*. 1948;24(2):212–220.

112. Swenson O, Neuhauser EBD, Pickett LK. New concepts of the etiology, diagnosis and treatment of congenital megacolon (Hirschsprung's disease). *Pediatrics*. 1949;4(2):201–209.

113. Teitelbaum DH, Coran AG, Weitzman JJ, et al. Hirschsprung's disease and related neuromuscular disorders of the intestines. In: O'Neill JA Jr, Rowe MI, Grosfeld JL, et al., eds. *Pediatric Surgery*. St. Louis, MO: Mosby; 1998:1381–1424.

114. Teitelbaum DH, Drongowski RA, Chamberlain JN, et al. Long-term stooling patterns in infants undergoing primary endorectal pull-through for Hirschsprung's disease. *J Pediatr Surg*. 1997;32(7): 1049–1052.

115. Tiffin ME, Chandler LR, Faber HK. Localized absence of ganglion cells of the myenteric plexus in congenital megacolon. *Am J Dis Child*. 1940;59:1071–1082.

116. Tittle K. Uber eine angeborene Missbildung des Dickdarmes. *Wien Klin Wochenschr*. 1901;14:903–907.

117. Tobon F, Reid NC, Talbert JL, et al. Nonsurgical test for the diagnosis of Hirschsprung's disease. *N Engl J Med*. 1968;278(4): 188–193.

118. Tobon F, Schuster MM. Megacolon: special diagnostic and therapeutic features. *Johns Hopkins Med J*. 1974;135(2):91–105.

119. Torres R, Levitt MA, Tovilla JM, et al. Anorectal malformations and Down's syndrome. *J Pediatr Surg*. 1998;33(2):194–197.

120. Trusler GA, Wilkinson RH. Imperforate anus: a review of 147 cases. *Can J Surg*. 1962;5:269–277.

121. Vande Velde S, Van Biervliet S, Van Renterghem K, et al. Achieving fecal continence in patients with spina bifida: a descriptive cohort study. *J Urol*. 2007;178(6):2640–2644.

122. Wangensteen OH, Rice CO. Imperforate anus: a method of determining the surgical approach. *Ann Surg*. 1930;92(1):77–81.

123. Zuelzer WW, Wilson JL. Functional intestinal obstruction on congenital neurogenic basis in infancy. *Am J Dis Child*. 1948; 75(1):40–64.

4

Diet and Drugs in Colorectal Surgery

John L. Petrini, Jr.

A drug is a substance that, when injected into a rat, produces a scientific paper.

—ANONYMOUS

The role of diet in a healthy bowel has been a stimulating and controversial subject for two millennia. There are data to support numerous statements and recommendations, but controlled clinical trials defining the benefits of various foods and therapies are quite limited. In general, diets high in fiber and roughage help facilitate the normal passage of stool. In addition, they may be beneficial to the overall health of an individual by reducing cholesterol, maintaining blood sugar in the normal range, and decreasing the incidence of diverticulosis. Cruciferous plants also contain anticarcinogens that may reduce the incidence of colonic neoplasms. Furthermore, aspirin and other nonsteroidal anti-inflammatory drugs (NSAIDs) appear to reduce the incidence of colon cancer. Other claims—for example, that cow's milk and dairy products may be harmful for young children and most adults—have some validity. There are a host of other hypotheses, but the data in support of them are very weak.

Patients may solicit the opinion of a physician for concerns that do not necessarily require surgical intervention, or they may experience gastrointestinal symptoms that are consequences of an operation. For many, dietary manipulations and medical therapy may provide relief of the discomfort and disability. Initial therapy for most disorders of the colon and rectum often includes dietary adjustment. This approach is typically instituted by the patient himself or herself. The symptoms of certain conditions, such as irritable bowel syndrome (IBS), inflammatory bowel disease, diverticulitis, diarrhea, and constipation, can often be ameliorated by dietary manipulation, even though the cause of the disorder may not be related to a specific food. The addition of medication, either for symptomatic relief or to treat the specific disease state, may also contribute to the relief of a patient's symptoms. It is important, however, to understand the pathophysiology underlying the bowel symptoms in order to offer the appropriate treatment. Unfortunately, there is a paucity of information available for many disorders affecting the gastrointestinal tract that may aid the physician in appropriate therapeutic decision making. This chapter focuses on some of the more common symptoms and conditions for which patients seek the attention of physicians trained in gastrointestinal disease and gastrointestinal surgery.

▶ BOWEL MANAGEMENT PROBLEMS

Constipation

Constipation can be defined as either a decrease in the frequency of stools or an increase in the difficulty of passage of stool. Patients may also complain of hard bowel movements, small actions, inability to evacuate, or the sensation of incomplete evacuation. Some studies have demonstrated that 95% of healthy adults will have a minimum of three bowel movements per week.[24,33] Those with fewer than three stools a week are considered to have "constipation," but they may not be truly symptomatic or seek medical attention. Those who do request help usually complain of either decreased frequency or difficulty in passing stool. Therapy is therefore directed at either increasing the water content (i.e., softening the stool) or increasing the frequency of bowel movements.

History

In order to make a recommendation concerning therapy, a carefully obtained history is essential. This should include the duration of the complaints, dietary habits, the use of medications, and lifestyle. These often provide the information necessary to arrive at the source of the patient's complaints. It is not within the purview of this chapter to present a complete discussion of all the disease states, endocrine abnormalities, medications, neurologic disorders, and dietary issues that are associated with constipation. However, it is important to note the more common endocrine conditions that may affect the bowels and that should be considered: hypothyroidism, diabetes mellitus, and hyperparathyroidism. Other diseases that predispose to constipation include uremia, porphyria, amyloidosis, and short-segment Hirschsprung's disease.

As mentioned, medications are a frequent cause of constipation, so it is important to obtain a history of all medications used, including those available over the counter. Although the list is extensive, the more common ones to consider include the opiate/analgesics, antipsychotics (particularly the monoamine oxidase inhibitors and tricyclic antidepressants), anticholinergics, iron and other heavy metals, antacids, anticonvulsants, calcium channel blockers, and diuretics.

Evaluation

The perineum should be carefully inspected for obvious pathologic entities that may impede the passage of stool. Instrument examination, contrast studies, transit studies, gynecologic examination, ultrasonography, computed tomography, and physiologic studies may be required in selected patients. Certainly, gastrointestinal evaluation at some point must be accomplished to rule out the presence of a specific etiologic factor. These are discussed in the following chapters.

Treatment

The standard treatment of nonspecific constipation begins with dietary manipulation, usually through increasing dietary fiber and fluid intake. In addition, several classes of medication are available to increase stool water or stool frequency. These include bulk laxatives, stool softeners, osmotic or saline laxatives, cathartics, and motility-enhancing drugs (prokinetics).

Those who have constipation usually benefit from increasing the water content of the stool by increasing their intake of fiber and water. It is well known that individuals who live in so-called developing countries consume a large amount of unprocessed fiber. However, the diet in most developed countries contains inadequate roughage or unprocessed dietary fiber.[6,17] Dietary fiber consists of plant products that are not digested or absorbed by the small intestine. These include cellulose, lignin, gums, pectins, hemicelluloses, and polysaccharides. Increasing fluid intake without adding fiber to the diet is usually ineffective for correcting constipation. Fiber, however, will improve stool consistency irrespective of the water intake.[46] Interestingly, fiber with small amounts of water can be used to treat diarrhea. Some foods, particularly dairy products, actually decrease stool water content and contribute to constipation. Good sources of dietary fiber include fresh fruits and vegetables, whole grain cereals, and unprocessed carbohydrates such as bran, whole wheat, and brown rice (Table 4-1). Total daily fiber intake should be adjusted to approximately 30 g or more if tolerated by the patient.

Fiber Products

Those individuals whose diet remains inadequate in fiber can increase stool water-carrying capacity by adding a fiber-containing bulk laxative. Psyllium husk, either as powder or granules, is obtained from various species of plantain. Bran is a product of the milling of wheat. Flax seed and ground flax seeds are high sources of fiber as lignins. These products, when taken with adequate dietary water, will provide

TABLE 4-1 Fiber Content of Selected Dietary Items

FOOD GROUP	LOW FIBER	HIGH FIBER
Fruits	Apples (cooked) Oranges Pears Bananas Grapes Fruit juices	Prunes (stewed) Raspberries Apples (with peel) Dates (dried)
Vegetables	Cabbage Celery Lettuce Summer squash Vegetable juices Eggplant	Spinach Sweet potato Corn Broccoli Turnips Greens
Starches	Bagel White bread Flour, white Potato (mashed, chips) Pasta Popcorn	Lentils Bran Barley Kidney beans Peas Brown rice Granola Flour, whole wheat
Other	Meats, seafood Dairy products, eggs Nuts and seeds Oils	

additional bulk to the stool and increase the water content, trapping it in a mucin within the stool.

Other bulk laxatives use hydrophilic substances, such as polycarbophil and powdered karaya (sterculia) gum. The amount of bulking agents can be adjusted to what is required to alleviate the patient's constipation. This range is usually between 4 and 10 g/day, with the administration divided if a higher dose is required.

The major disadvantage of bulking agents is the bloating and gas commonly associated with the cellulose and lignin-based products. Fiber products with a base of hemicellulose or pectin seem to reduce these side effects, as does the use of the polycarbophil bulk agents. However, patients seem to require higher doses of the latter than of the cellulose-based products in order for similar results to be achieved. One of the side benefits of the use of bulk agents is the lowering of serum cholesterol. This is probably effected through the binding of bile salts and reducing their reabsorption, so that the bile salt pool is lowered. Problems associated with the use of bulking agents include intestinal obstruction and fecal impaction, particularly if there is an underlying pathologic entity. Additionally, allergic reactions have been reported.

Stool Softeners

Patients who are resistant to the bulking agents alone can increase the water content further with stool softeners or emollients. The principal agent is docusate (dioctyl sulfosuccinate), which is available as the sodium, calcium, or potassium salt. These products inhibit the normal water-absorptive capacity of the colon while producing only a minimal decrease in the transit of fecal contents. Once one of these products has been administered, it may take 1 to 3 days to see an effect. In essence, they act to soften the stool but do not promote defecation. The usual adult dose is from 50 to 250 mg/day. Docusate should not be given with mineral oil because absorption of the oil as well as other medications is enhanced.

Osmotic and Saline Laxatives

Should bulking agents and surfactants fail to enhance the passage of stool, the next preferred step would be to employ an osmotic or saline laxative. Magnesium phosphate, sodium sulfate, and potassium tartrate are poorly absorbed chemicals. Ingestion increases the stool water content through an osmotic effect. Surgeons are familiar with the use of saline laxatives for bowel preparations before operative or diagnostic procedures. In smaller doses, they can be used for their cathartic effect. Certain antacid products contain magnesium, and it is this agent that produces the side effect of diarrhea. There is, furthermore, some evidence that magnesium may actually increase motility of the small intestine through stimulation the release of cholecystokinin from the duodenum.[15] The phosphate-containing solutions may cause a high serum phosphate level and impair cardiac contractility. They should therefore be used with caution in individuals with renal, cardiac, or hepatic disease. Dehydration can also be a consequence of the use of saline laxatives. Patients should be cautioned to take adequate fluids when using these agents.

Modified doses of colonic purgatives used to clear the colon prior to surgery and gastrointestinal procedures are also available to treat constipation.[10] Miralax and Dulcolax Balance provide increased water to the colon by adding an osmotically neutral fluid to the gastrointestinal tract. The osmotically active agents, polyethylene glycol and a mixture of sodium and potassium sulfate, are not absorbed and remain in solution, carrying water to the colon. The usual dose is 17 g mixed with water; it can be given on a daily basis. There is minimal fluid or electrolyte shift, and side effects are rare.

Polysaccharides

Some carbohydrates are also poorly absorbed. This results in an osmotic effect that leads to enhanced water in the stool. These products include lactose, lactulose, and sorbitol. Lactulose has been particularly useful in the treatment of hepatic encephalopathy, but lower doses (30 to 60 mL/day) can be an effective laxative for patients with chronic constipation. Side effects include gas; bloating; cramps; flatulence; and, of course, fluid loss at high doses.

Lubricants

Mineral oil, a petroleum distillate, has been employed for the treatment of constipation. The mechanism of action appears to be penetration of the stool by the oil with resulting softening. However, because of the potential for complications, long-term use should be avoided. These include decreased absorption of fat-soluble vitamins and essential fatty acids. Furthermore, penetration of the mucosa can occur, and a foreign body reaction in the mesenteric lymph nodes, mucosa, and spleen has been reported. As previously mentioned, mineral oil should not be used with surfactants because there is the potential for increased absorption of the mineral oil.

Stimulant Laxatives

What rhubarb, senna or what purgative drug, would scour these English hence?
—WILLIAM SHAKESPEARE: *Macbeth* V, iii, 55

Cathartic laxatives are mucosally active agents that reduce net water and electrolyte absorption in addition to increasing bowel motility. The most frequently employed substances include phenolphthalein and the anthraquinone cathartics (senna, cascara sagrada, and danthron). These drugs act primarily to increase periodic mass movements within the colon and to decrease the segmental contractions that slow bowel activity. Generally, they become effective in 4 to 6 hours. The primary side effect, in addition to diarrhea, is that of cramping. Another drug, bisacodyl (Dulcolax), is a synthetic diphenylmethane that is similar to phenolphthalein. It is available not only for oral administration but also for rectal use. Because of the problem of gastric irritation, it is enteric coated. The standard adult dose is 10 to 15 mg.

Senna is an anthraquinone cathartic obtained from *Cassia acutifolia* or *Cassia angustifolia*. Preparations of the whole plant, leaflets, pods, and extracts are commercially available. Cascara sagrada is another anthraquinone; it is obtained from the bark of the buckthorn tree. Like all cathartics, these are variously effective depending on the dosage but can cause a problem with cramping. Furthermore, melanosis coli, a dark pigmentation of the colon mucosa, may be a consequence of long-term use of senna and cascara (see Figure 20-1).

Another cathartic, castor oil, is hydrolyzed in the small intestine to glycerol and ricinoleic acid. Ricinoleic acid acts in the small intestine by both decreasing net absorption of fluid and electrolytes and stimulating peristalsis. Because it is quite potent, it should be employed with special care. Long-term use should be avoided.

Motility Agents

Two agents are currently available that decrease transit time through acceleration of the muscular activity of the bowel. Gastrointestinal motility can be enhanced through the use of metoclopramide and erythromycin. Two other agents, cisapride and tegaserod, have been taken off the market in the United States. Metoclopramide and erythromycin have little or no effect on the colon and are not indicated for improving bowel function, but may be used for ameliorating gastric emptying.

Calcium Channel Stimulators

One medication approved for the treatment of constipation and constipation-predominate IBS is lubiprostone (Amitiza). Lubiprostone acts by stimulating intestinal chloride channels leading to fluid secretion. This increases intestinal motility. Lubiprostone is available in two doses, 8 μg and 24 μg, both given twice daily. The lower dose is approved for patients with IBS and pain that is associated with constipation, whereas the larger dose is indicated for chronic constipation.

Summary

Long-term use of intestinal stimulants and cathartics can lead to fluid and electrolyte disturbances, including dehydration, hypokalemia, hyponatremia, hypoalbuminemia, steatorrhea, protein-losing enteropathy, and secondary hyperaldosteronism. There is speculation that patients may become dependent on laxatives, and what is known as a "cathartic colon," or a chronically flaccid colon, may develop. However, there are no studies confirming that the presence or development of a so-called cathartic colon is a direct consequence of currently available laxatives or stimulants. A good general principle is that if laxatives are to be used, the lowest effective dose should be given. Long-term use should be discouraged. Most individuals will benefit from a program of increasing fiber and water content of the stool, with the addition of laxatives intermittently as needed to produce at least two or three bowel movements per week. The application of surgical intervention as a treatment for constipation should be offered only after an adequate trial of medical therapy and appropriate evaluation of the gastrointestinal tract (see Chapter 20).

Diarrhea

Diarrhea is a common complaint in numerous disorders, most of which are not attributable to colonic sources. A host of etiologic factors may produce an increase in stool water or stool frequency, including medications, infection, the consequences of radiation, hepatic or biliary disease, pancreatic insufficiency, intolerance to ingested food components, infiltration of the mucosa or submucosa with lymphocytes or eosinophils, neoplasm, inflammatory bowel disease, and IBS. It is beyond the scope of this chapter to offer a comprehensive discussion on the etiology and treatment of all the possible conditions that can lead to the symptom of diarrhea.

The most common presentation is that of increased stool water. This leads to loose stools, watery stools, and increased stool volume and/or frequency. The maximum number of bowel movements that is still considered within the normal range is three per day, assuming that this does not represent a change in the individual's normal bowel habits. By definition, diarrhea is classified as acute until symptoms have been present for more than 6 weeks. After this time, it is considered chronic.

Acute Diarrhea

Acute diarrhea is often caused by medication or an infectious process, including bacterial enteritis, toxin ingestion, and infestation by the common intestinal parasites (e.g., *Giardia*, *Cryptosporidium*, *Isospora*). A discussion of the infectious and noninfectious colitides can be found in Chapter 33. The use of broad-spectrum antibiotics, with resultant infection by *Clostridium difficile*, is a frequent source of acute diarrheal illness and represents one of the major hospital-acquired infections in the United States (see also Chapter 33).

Principles of Management

Treatment of acute diarrhea involves identification of the offending agent and initiation of whatever specific measures are necessary to eliminate the source or eradicate the organism. The use of medications that decrease gastrointestinal motility in acute, febrile diarrheal illnesses should be avoided because prolonged contact time can enhance the likelihood of transmucosal migration of the organism and systemic infection. A better alternative is the use of pectin or bismuth compounds, such as kaolin-pectin or bismuth subcitrate. These products bind shiga toxins and other cyclic guanosine monophosphate–stimulatory toxins associated with bacterial infection and decrease the net water and chloride secretion by the small bowel. If systemic signs and symptoms of infection are not present, the use of opiates to increase transit time and slow stool frequency offers symptomatic relief.

By prolonging contact time with the intestinal tract, fluid and electrolyte absorption will be enhanced.

Chronic Diarrhea

Chronic diarrheal illnesses may be caused by a wide variety of disorders that affect the hepatobiliary system, pancreas, and small or large bowel. Individuals with chronic diarrhea present a challenge in differential diagnosis. This inevitably may lead to an extensive and expensive workup. Assuming that such an evaluation fails to establish a specific cause for the patient's symptoms, the most likely disorder is the so-called IBS. Treatment for this complaint is to reduce the volume and frequency of bowel movements, so that the patient's lifestyle can be improved.

Treatment

The approach to the management of patients with chronic diarrhea without a definable cause begins with a carefully taken dietary history. An offending food or substance may be found in the patient's intake that increases the frequency of bowel action. For example, lactose-containing dairy products may induce symptoms of cramping or diarrhea in up to 65% of the adult population. Furthermore, caffeine-containing beverages may increase bowel activity and stool output. Additionally, sugarless candies, sodas, and fruits high in fructose or sorbitol may lead to symptoms of diarrhea. Therefore, removing the offending agent will usually improve symptoms.

Medical therapy encompasses a wide number of options. The following discussion focuses on those agents used specifically to treat diarrhea.

The fiber-containing bulk agents previously alluded to decrease stool water when they are given with less than the recommended volume of liquid. Any of the bulk agents taken under these circumstances decreases the absorption of water through the gastrointestinal tract. However, there are the side effects of bloating, gas, and cramping. Another means for binding stool water is through the use of bile salt–binding resins, such as cholestyramine (Questran). Bile salt–binding resins are the preferred drugs for the management of diarrhea associates with ileal resection.

Kaolin, a dehydrated aluminum silicate, and pectin, a carbohydrate (polygalacturonic acid), can also be used as adsorbents to treat diarrhea. Bismuth subcitrate may also be employed to bind stool water and ameliorate diarrheal symptoms, but these agents are less effective than are the opiates. The most efficacious use of these products may be to prevent or to treat traveler's diarrhea.

The opiates are the most effective form of therapy in the management of diarrheal illnesses. These are usually given in the form of diphenoxylate or loperamide, but they are available in many other substances, including codeine phosphate and tincture of opium (paregoric). Opiates are habit forming, but this risk is much less when they are taken orally. Still, loperamide, which fails to cross the blood–brain barrier, should be the initial choice. Studies have shown it to be comparable to diphenoxylate (Lomotil), which can cause euphoria in high doses. A patient whose diarrhea fails to resolve with the foregoing measures requires further evaluation.

Irritable Bowel Syndrome

IBS is defined as an abdominal pain with or without alterations in bowel habits and with no evidence of abnormality on diagnostic testing. Patients may present with a wide variety of complaints, but more than 90% will have two or more of the following: visible abdominal distension, increased frequency of bowel movements with the onset of pain, looser stools with the onset of pain, and relief of pain with defecation.[23] Most individuals typically complain of crampy, diffuse abdominal pains that are associated with alternating constipation and diarrhea. A consensus conference led to the publishing of the "Rome III" criteria for establishing the diagnosis of IBS.[22] These include recurrent abdominal pain or discomfort at least 3 days per month in the past 3 months associated with two or more of the following:

- Improvement with defecation
- Onset associated with a change in frequency of stools
- Onset associated with a change in stool form (appearance)

The criteria must be fulfilled for the last 3 months, with the onset of symptoms at least 6 months prior to diagnosis. One assumes, of course, that evaluation for other disorders is negative.

Etiology and Pathogenesis

The etiology of IBS is unknown. However, there is considerable evidence to implicate the roles of stress and psychiatric illness in the pathogenesis of this condition. Various psychiatric abnormalities can be seen in the majority of individuals with IBS. In 85% of these, psychiatric symptoms either preceded or occurred coincidentally with the onset of the abdominal complaints.[8,18,43] The condition is clearly associated with stress and emotional disturbances. Individuals frequently report exacerbation of their symptoms under these conditions. It has been shown that persons with IBS have a higher incidence of psychiatric illness when compared with those who do not or with those harboring other gastrointestinal disorders.[44] Finally, there is emerging evidence to suggest that a history of physical or sexual abuse may be associated with IBS.[11,42]

Numerous abnormalities have been implicated in the pathogenesis of IBS. Patients with this condition have been demonstrated to exhibit altered colonic motility in response to meals when compared with subjects without IBS. Balloon distension studies suggest that these individuals have an increased rectal sensitivity to pressure.[26] Further studies of the myoelectric activity of the bowel suggest that approximately 40% of patients have abnormalities or alterations. For example, a decrease is observed in the normal 6 cycles/minute of basic electrical rhythm to 3 cycles/minute. This decrease may persist despite treatment that effectively controls IBS symptoms.[37] Discomfort following distension of the ileum and the rectum is also increased in patients with IBS when compared with controls.[20,45] It is interesting that the perception of pain does not appear to be increased elsewhere in the body.

Treatment

The lack of a definable abnormality in patients with IBS contributes to our inability to correct the patients' symptoms in a uniformly effective manner. For the most part, IBS is a lifelong illness, with periods of health punctuated by episodes of symptoms. The approach to management begins with evaluation of the potential contributing factors, primarily emotional and dietary. If the patient's emotional or psychological history is probed in a careful and sensitive manner, the physician can often identify a source for the discomfort for which the patient has been unaware.

The use of psychiatric therapy in this condition has been the subject of numerous studies. Hypnotherapy, stress reduction psychotherapy, dynamic psychotherapy, and relaxation techniques have all been successfully employed. Unfortunately, when one reviews these approaches, there is a consensus that the trials are plagued with poor methodology. As a consequence, there is no general acceptance of any specific technique.[40] Still, these studies do suggest a place for psychotherapy in those individuals who are willing to consider this approach to treatment.

There is no doubt that dietary factors can play a role in IBS and lead to increased abdominal cramping or pain. Patients with diarrhea should be counseled with respect to foods that are likely to increase stool water and frequency. These include fiber, nonabsorbed carbohydrates, caffeine, and lactose. If constipation is the primary symptom, increased fiber and water intake may help reduce the difficulty in passing stools, but the consequences of bloating, cramps, and abdominal pain may make the use of this approach counterproductive.

For the majority of patients, crampy abdominal pain is the major reason for seeking medical care. The pain is often difficult to characterize but is usually diffuse, intermittent, and frequently localized to the left lower quadrant of the abdomen. The pain may be exacerbated by meals and relieved somewhat by defecation or the passage of flatus. Because the regulation of bowel movements may offer some relief from the discomfort, it should be part of the treatment for all patients with IBS. Although elimination of pain may not be successfully accomplished in everyone, a graduated approach provides the best chance of alleviating symptoms.

The current first line of medications is the anticholinergic class of drugs.[34] Anticholinergics can reduce the rate of spike activity, thereby decreasing tonic contractions in the colon. This may lead to decreased cramping and bloating. Anticholinergics may be administered alone or in combination with other sedative/hypnotic medications, such as atropine, scopolamine, hyoscyamine, and phenobarbital in combination (Donnatal) and a combination of clidinium and chlordiazepoxide (Librax). The addition of these drugs may also be useful for those patients in whom anxiety contributes to the symptoms. Short-acting anticholinergics can be administered sublingually or orally and can be used to suppress symptoms when they occur. Long-acting preparations may be helpful for the management of chronic symptoms.

Antidepressants have also been shown to provide relief from the pain of IBS, often at doses far lower than those used to achieve an antidepressant effect. Furthermore, this is seen at doses at which the anticholinergic effects are negligible. Imipramine, amitriptyline, or nortriptyline given at a starting dose of 10 mg at bedtime will often reduce or eliminate the abdominal pain associated with IBS. The dose can be increased, but at higher doses side effects are common. One side effect of the tricyclic class of antidepressants is constipation. Of course, this may help in those individuals who have diarrhea as a major component of their IBS, but it will certainly exacerbate symptoms for those whose primary complaint is constipation. In this latter group of patients, one may address this concern by switching to the selective serotonin reuptake inhibitors (SSRIs): fluoxetine (Prozac), paroxetine (Paxil), or sertraline (Zoloft), again at low doses. Although the SSRIs are less likely to be associated with constipation as a side effect, diarrhea may be aggravated. One must appreciate the importance of titration of the various medication choices in trying to identify the appropriate approach to the management of a given individual.

Various other medications have been used to treat the symptoms of IBS, but the data are preliminary, and the studies have been undertaken with only small groups of selected individuals.[21] Fedotozine, a gut κ receptor agonist, appears to decrease visceral sensitivity in animals. One study suggested improvement in the symptoms of bloating and abdominal pain when this drug was given during a 6-week trial.[9] Leuprolide, a gonadotropin-releasing hormone agonist, has been demonstrated to improve the symptoms of nausea, vomiting, bloating, abdominal pain, and early satiety in a group of women with functional gastrointestinal symptoms.[25] Octreotide has also been shown to improve the visceral perception of pain in patients with IBS without affecting the small intestinal muscle tone.[5,16] Cholecystokinin analogues have been demonstrated to offer some relief from the discomfort of IBS, but they are currently unavailable for use in the United States. Cromolyn sulfate has been shown in one study to improve the symptoms of IBS.[38] Patients were selected for diarrhea-predominant IBS, and the drug was compared with an elimination diet. Alosetron (Lotronex) is a selective serotonin 5-HT$_3$ receptor antagonist that has been approved for use in women with severe diarrhea predominate IBS. The drug was re-released by the Food and Drug Administration (FDA) with a black box warning for ischemic colitis, which was seen in 3/1,000 patients after more than 6 months of use. The drug is available in selected cases after patients have read an information brochure and signed a release. Initially released as 1 mg tablets, the drug is now given as 0.5 to 1 mg BID for patients who meet the criteria (diarrhea greater than 6 months without anatomic or pathologic abnormalities and who have failed conventional therapy).

A recent study suggests that poorly absorbed antibiotics with broad-spectrum activity against enteric bacteria may reduce the symptoms of IBS in some patients.[32] Using rifaximin, investigators were able to improve cramping, bloating, and diarrhea in some patients with IBS. Two identically designed, placebo-controlled trials assigned patients with abdominal pain and bloating without constipation-predominate IBS to either rifaximin 550 mg, three times daily, for 2 weeks or a placebo. In both studies, those taking rifaximin had significantly greater improvement in their symptoms when compared with those in the placebo arm. This advantage persisted during 10 weeks of follow-up (approximately 41% vs. 31%). Earlier studies from the same group suggested that some patients with symptoms of IBS following an episode of gastroenteritis had bacterial overgrowth in the small intestine that could be eliminated with antibiotics, with improvement in symptoms.[31] This data suggests that there may be a subset of IBS patients with abdominal pain and bloating due to bacterial overgrowth in the small intestine that may respond to poorly absorbed broad-spectrum antibiotics. Whether this data can be applied to the broader population of patients with IBS is questionable.

NSAIDs appear to have little role in the treatment of the pain of IBS, and there is absolutely no place for stronger pain medications such as opiates or narcotics. Obviously, it is essential to avoid potentially addictive psychotropic medications in those individuals whose disease state often has such a strong emotional component.

Short Bowel Syndrome

Patients who have undergone resection of the small intestine, particularly the distal ileum, may present with symptoms of urgency and diarrhea (especially after meals), weight loss, or dehydration. When an extensive portion of the small intestine has been resected, there may be insufficient surface area available for absorption of nutrients. It has been estimated that the minimal length of small intestine necessary to sustain adequate enteral nutrition is approximately 1 m, although the presence of the colon may reduce that requirement. Preservation of the proximal bowel (duodenum and jejunum) appears more likely to facilitate nutrient absorption than does the presence of ileum, with the exception of certain specific nutrients, such as vitamin B$_{12}$. Those individuals who are unable to achieve adequate enteral nutrition require parenteral hyperalimentation (see Chapter 30).

Studies have demonstrated that the colon actually is able to absorb a reasonable amount of calories, largely in the form of short-chain fatty acids.[28] In addition to providing nutrient value to the cells of the colonic mucosa itself, 500 kcal/day may actually be absorbed into the systemic circulation.

It has been demonstrated by using growth hormone and glutamine, with a diet of increased carbohydrates and decreased fat, that this combination is associated with an increase in the absorption of protein and a decrease in stool output.[7] In some individuals with small intestine too limited to provide adequate absorptive area, this regimen has been able to decrease or completely eliminate the need for parenteral hyperalimentation. The FDA has recently approved Zorbtive, a recombinant DNA human growth hormone produced in a mammalian cell line (mouse) for treatment of short bowel syndrome. Subcutaneous injection for 4 weeks, particularly when combined with a glutamine-enriched diet, has been associated with a decreased need for parenteral nutrition. The drug has not been approved for more than 4 weeks use, although studies have shown persistence of improvement up to 12 weeks following completion of therapy.

The proximal duodenum is the most efficient area for absorption of most nutrients, but jejunum and ileum can also adapt and increase absorption. This has been demonstrated following duodenal resection or bypass, provided there is adequate time for mixing of bile and pancreatic secretions with the ingested food. The distal ileum is the primary absorptive area for bile salts and for vitamin B$_{12}$, so that removal of this area can result in cholerrheic diarrhea and vitamin B$_{12}$ deficiency.

Those individuals who have undergone small bowel resection but still have adequate surface area for absorption may initially experience symptoms of rapid transit and diarrhea. In most cases, the remaining bowel can adapt to allow adequate nutrition, although a period of adjustment may be necessary. As previously suggested, patients with 100 cm of small bowel remaining should be able to subsist on an elemental diet, but the palatability of predigested food is very poor. Only very highly motivated individuals can tolerate oral elemental feedings, so usually a nasogastric tube, gastrostomy, or jejunostomy tube is required to achieve adequate caloric intake. With this regimen, patients often suffer an initial period of frequency, bloating, and loose stools. These symptoms gradually improve with time. Supplemental liquid nutrition given between meals may help maintain body weight. Additional therapy, including bile salt–binding resins and loperamide or diphenoxylate, will slow transit and should help improve absorption. The typical patient will initially suffer weight loss, but ultimately will achieve a new steady state at lower body mass. With this type of patient, oral intake is usually adequate to maintain metabolic balance. It is rare that parenteral nutrition will be required, and with appropriate management, individuals should be able to maintain a positive metabolic balance. However, those who have an inadequate small bowel surface area for absorption of nutrients will require some form of supplementation or parenteral nutrition.

Cholerrheic Diarrhea

Individuals who have undergone resection of the distal ileum, particularly if the ileocecal valve is removed, may exhibit symptoms of cramping, bloating, and diarrhea, often accompanying intake of food. The etiology of these complaints is not clear, but it appears to be related to deconjugation of nonabsorbed bile salts by the colonic bacteria. Deconjugated bile salts are toxic to the lining of the colon; they initiate fluid and electrolyte secretion and lead to symptoms of cramping and diarrhea (cholerrheic diarrhea). This theory is supported by the observation that bile salt–binding medications, such as cholestyramine, often ameliorate the symptoms associated with distal ileal resection and cholerrheic diarrhea. The dosage can be adjusted to achieve normal bowel movements without induction of constipation. Additional reduction in diarrhea can be afforded by the use of loperamide or diphenoxylate in those individuals whose diarrhea persists despite bile salt–binding medications.

Postoperative Ileus

Ileus is a common consequence of any abdominal operation and, obviously, of any operation on the intestinal tract. It may occur after minor surgical procedures, even those outside the abdomen, but it is clearly related to intra-abdominal surgery.[3] Why this occurs is not entirely clear, but it is thought to be due to the effects of the anesthetic, manipulation of the bowel, a generalized increase in sympathetic tone, or the opiates that may be used to control postoperative pain.[27] The effects of bowel manipulation are controversial, but it appears that less invasive surgical procedures are associated with less severe postoperative ileus. This, of course, is a contention of the advantage of minimally invasive surgery (see Chapter 19). The effects of the ileus appear most pronounced on the colon, with the small bowel and the stomach recovering function earlier.

Treatment

I do not presume to tell surgeons how to manage patients who have postoperative ileus. However, certain points are worth emphasizing, at least from the perspective of a gastroenterologist. Studies evaluating the efficacy of prokinetic agents (erythromycin, metoclopramide, and cisapride) have failed to generate consistent results that could suggest a reduced duration of postoperative ileus.[4,19,35,41] This lack of an effective medical approach mandates modification of oral intake following surgery. Traditionally, most surgeons have waited for evidence of bowel activity (the passage of flatus, the presence of bowel sounds, or a bowel movement) before resuming oral feedings. However, recent evidence suggests that one may, with caution, commence oral intake a lot sooner than had been previously recommended. This is based to some extent on the evidence gleaned from early alimentation following laparoscopic procedures.

There is no evidence that nasogastric tube suction in the absence of vomiting provides any benefit, but patients with distension and vomiting will have these symptoms ameliorated by gastric suction. With a nasogastric tube in place, the volume of aspirate can be ascertained, and this can be used as a guide for the initiation of oral feedings. Although there is a reasonable difference of opinion concerning when to remove the tube, the volume should be less than 50 mL/ hour before it is eliminated. Alternatively, clamping the tube for several hours or overnight and measuring the residual gastric fluid comprise a useful guide. If the residual is less than 100 mL after clamping for 4 hours, bowel activity may be presumed to have developed.

Clear liquids are usually offered initially, although the rationale for this concept remains murky. For example, there is no evidence to suggest that a regular diet should be initially avoided. This may be largely a consequence of the fact that it is easier to aspirate gastric retention if there is no residual solid material present. Diet is then advanced as tolerated, usually to a full liquid diet and then to a selected diet. However, certain clear liquids may produce untoward symptoms. For example, fruit juices that contain poorly absorbed carbohydrates, especially fructose, may lead to distension, bloating, and diarrhea. Apple juice, a staple in the clear liquid diet, is a particularly offending agent. Caffeine is a well-known gastric irritant. This may lead to substernal burning and to nausea. Full liquid diets may be high in dairy products and lactose. As mentioned, 65% of adults have varying degrees of intolerance to these substances.

A similar approach to avoiding items that may lead to dietary intolerance should be employed when enteral tube feedings are used. Tube feedings occasionally can cause diarrhea, possibly from the high osmolality of the feedings or to rapid feedings. However, the etiology of diarrhea is multifactorial and in the postoperative patient may include antibiotic use; the vehicles used to make medication soluble; the fact that it may be delivered by a tube, particularly sorbitol[13]; intra-abdominal infection; and the consequences of an anastomosis. Avoiding poorly tolerated carbohydrates, including fructose, lactose, lactulose, and sorbitol, can minimize the bowel discomfort often experienced by patients in the postoperative period.

Diverticular Disease

Diverticular disease is a frequently encountered condition in developed countries. The prevalence appears to be more than 30% in adults older than the age of 50 and rises with advancing age.[30] The presence of the mucosal herniations through the bowel wall is thought to be a consequence of decreased dietary fiber, a finding supported by epidemiologic data (see the discussion on diet in Chapter 27). In countries where the intake of dietary fiber is 5 to 10 times that of the United States, diverticular disease is a rare finding.[6,28] Patients with diverticulosis are usually asymptomatic, but abdominal pain has been attributed to spasm often seen in the presence of diverticula. Because IBS is found in approximately 12% of adults in the United States, it is not clear whether diverticulosis or IBS is responsible for the cramping abdominal pain in these individuals.[29] In one study, the poorly absorbed oral antibiotic, rifaximin, when given with fiber supplementation, reduced the discomfort of diverticular disease.[29]

Increasing dietary fiber is associated with an increase in the water content of stool and may ease its passage through the colon. If the theory that diverticula are more likely to occur in the setting of increased intraluminal pressure is correct, increased fiber should reduce the likelihood of new diverticula forming, but not eliminate the diverticula already present. Despite conventional wisdom, there is no evidence to suggest that seeds, nuts, popcorn husks, and other small, sharp, or firm food contents are responsible for acute attacks of diverticulitis. In fact one recent longitudinal study following a cohort of 47,228 men older than 18 years suggested that diet high in nuts, corn, and popcorn might actually reduce the incidence of attacks of diverticulitis.[38] Patients who ingested diet higher in nuts and popcorn (at least two servings a week) had an ordinate risk for developing diverticulitis or diverticular bleeding (0.80 and 0.72, respectively), compared to individuals who ingested fewer than one serving a month.[39]

When patients are experiencing the symptoms of diverticulitis, luminal narrowing is associated with distension, bloating, and alterations in bowel habits. With acute diverticulitis, reducing stool volume should decrease discomfort associated with the partial blockage of the bowel. Dietary therapy consists of clear liquid diet until normal fecal flow is established, followed by resumption of a high-fiber diet (if tolerated) once the inflammation has subsided. These measures are used to reduce bloating and distension, but the treatment of the acute episode remains broad-spectrum antibiotics.[12] Any one of a number of antibiotics is useful in this acute inflammatory condition, with surgery required for complications (see Chapter 27).

Chemoprophylaxis

Recent studies have renewed one's interest in probiotics, minerals, and NSAIDs in the prevention of gastrointestinal problems. Some of the more definitive therapies are discussed in the next sections.

Pouchitis

Patients who have undergone proctocolectomy with reservoir-anal procedures or continent pouches often present with inflammatory changes in the reservoir, a consequence of what has been attributed to bacterial overgrowth (see Chapter 29). Successful treatment usually consists of antibiotics such as metronidazole, 250 mg three times daily, or ciprofloxacin, 500 mg twice daily. However, some patients experience recurrent bouts of pouchitis that may be difficult to control. Studies using a probiotic, VSL-3, have suggested a prolonged remission from pouchitis.[14] The preparation contains multiple strains of bacteria that, theoretically, replenish the gut flora consortium that help to preserve a healthy colon mucosa. The medication is available online at http://www.questcor.com.

Colon Polyps and Cancer Prevention

Anecdotal reports and case-control studies suggest that patients taking aspirin, fiber, and vitamins and who consume vegetarian and low-fat diets have a reduced incidence of colon polyps. This has spurred interest in polyp chemoprevention. However, initial studies failed to demonstrate benefit with supplementary vitamins E, C, and β-carotene, as well as with fiber supplementation. A randomized, controlled trial found a reduction in new polyp formation through the use of calcium supplements.[1] Patients were given 1,200 mg of elemental calcium. Those treated had an adjusted risk ratio for the formation of new polyps of 0.85 compared with the placebo-treated population.

Reports that sulindac reduced the development of adenomatous polyps in familial adenomatous polyposis syndrome, as well as case-control studies in aspirin users, further stimulated interest in the use of NSAIDs to reduce new polyp formation. Prospective, randomized, controlled studies have suggested a reduction in the formation of new neoplastic polyps in patients with prior colorectal cancer or adenomas through the use of aspirin. Patients with previous colorectal cancer were placed on 325 mg of aspirin daily. They had an adjusted relative risk of forming new polyps of 0.65 compared with placebo-treated patients.[2] In the second study, two doses of aspirin, 325 mg or 81 mg, were compared with a placebo in preventing new polyps in patients with prior adenomas. Low-dose aspirin was associated with a modest risk reduction (0.81) compared with a placebo, but the regular aspirin tablet was no better than a placebo.[36] These studies suggest a modest effect of NSAIDs in reducing the formation of new polyps in patients prone to development of adenomas. However, the high rate of upper gastrointestinal complications associated with the use of NSAIDs, coupled with only a modest reduction in new polyp incidence, makes it difficult for one to advocate aspirin therapy at this time for this indication.

References

1. Baron JA, Beach M, Mandel JS, et al. Calcium supplements for the prevention of colorectal adenomas. Calcium Polyp Prevention Study Group. *N Engl J Med*. 1999;340(2):101–107.
2. Baron JA, Cole BF, Sandler RS, et al. A randomized trial of aspirin to prevent colorectal adenomas. *N Engl J Med*. 2003;348(10):891–899.
3. Benson MJ, Roberts JP, Wingate DL, et al. Small bowel motility following major intra-abdominal surgery: the effects of opiates and rectal cisapride. *Gastroenterology*. 1994;106(4):924–936.
4. Bonacini M, Quiason S, Reynolds M, et al. Effects of intravenous erythromycin on postoperative ileus. *Am J Gastroenterol*. 1993;88(2): 208–211.
5. Bradette M, Delvaux M, Staumont G, et al. Octreotide increases thresholds of colonic visceral perception in IBS patients without modifying muscle tone. *Dig Dis Sci*. 1994;39(6):1171–1178.
6. Burkitt DP, Walker AR, Painter NS. Effect of dietary fibre on stools and transit-times, and its role in the causation of disease. *Lancet*. 1972;2(7792):1408–1412.
7. Byrne TA, Persinger RL, Young LS, et al. A new treatment for patients with short-bowel syndrome. Growth hormone, glutamine, and a modified diet. *Ann Surg*. 1995;222(3):243–254.
8. Creed F, Guthrie E. Psychological factors in the irritable bowel syndrome. *Gut*. 1987;28(10):1307–1318.
9. Dapoigny M, Abitbol JL, Fraitag B. Efficacy of peripheral kappa agonist fedotozine versus placebo in treatment of irritable bowel syndrome. A multicenter dose-response study. *Dig Dis Sci*. 1995;40(10):2244–2249.
10. Di Palma JA, DeRidder PH, Orlando RC, et al. A randomized, placebo-controlled, multicenter study of the safety and efficacy of a new polyethylene glycol laxative. *Am J Gastroenterol*. 2000;95(2):446–450.
11. Drossman DA, Leserman J, Nachman G, et al. Sexual and physical abuse in women with functional or organic gastrointestinal disease. *Ann Intern Med*. 1990;113(11):828–833.
12. Duma RJ, Kellum JM. Colonic diverticulitis: microbiologic, diagnostic, and therapeutic considerations. *Curr Clin Topics Infect Dis*. 1991;11:218–247.
13. Edes TE, Walk BE, Austin JL. Diarrhea in tube-fed patients: feeding formula not necessarily the cause. *Am J Med*. 1990;88(2):91–93.
14. Gionchetti P, Rizzello F, Venturi A, et al. Oral bacteriotherapy as maintenance treatment in patients with chronic pouchitis: a double-blind, placebo-controlled trial. *Gastroenterology*. 2000;119(2):305–309.
15. Harvey RF, Read AE. Mode of action of the saline purgatives. *Am Heart J*. 1975;89(6):810–212.
16. Hasler WL, Soudah HC, Owyang C. Somatostatin analog inhibits afferent response to rectal distention in diarrhea-predominant irritable bowel patients. *J Pharmacol Exp Ther*. 1994;268(3):1206–1211.
17. Heller SN, Hackler LR. Changes in the crude fiber content of the American diet. *Am J Clin Nutr*. 1978;31(9):1510–1514.

18. Hislop IG. Psychological significance of the irritable colon syndrome. *Gut*. 1971;12(6):452–457.

19. Jepson S, Klaerke A, Nielsen PH, et al. Negative effect of Metoclopramide in postoperative adynamic ileus. A prospective, randomized, double blind study. *Br J Surg*. 1986;73(4):290–291.

20. Kellow JE, Phillips SF. Altered small bowel motility in irritable bowel syndrome is correlated with symptoms. *Gastroenterology*. 1987;92(6):1885–1893.

21. Longo WE, Vernava AM III. Prokinetic agents for lower gastrointestinal motility disorders. *Dis Colon Rectum*. 1993;36(7):696–708.

22. Longstreth GF, Thompson WG, Chey WD, et al. Functional bowel disorders. *Gastroenterol*. 2006;130(5):1480–1491.

23. Manning AP, Thompson WG, Heaton KW, et al. Towards positive diagnosis of the irritable bowel. *BMJ*. 1978;2(6138):653–654.

24. Martelli H, Devroede G, Arhan P, et al. Some parameters of large bowel motility in normal man. *Gastroenterology*. 1978;75(4):612–618.

25. Mathias JR, Clench MH, Reeves-Darby VG, et al. Effect of leuprolide acetate in patients with moderate to severe functional bowel disease. Double-blind, placebo-controlled study. *Dig Dis Sci*. 1994;39(6):1155–1162.

26. Munakata J, Naliboff B, Harraf F, et al. Repetitive sigmoid stimulation induces rectal hyperalgesia in patients with irritable bowel syndrome. *Gastroenterology*. 1997;112(1):55–63.

27. Ogilvy AJ, Smith G. The gastrointestinal tract after anesthesia. *Eur J Anaesthesiol Suppl*. 1995;10:35–42.

28. Painter NS, Burkitt DP. Diverticular disease of the colon: a deficiency disease of Western civilization. *BMJ*. 1971;2(5759):450–454.

29. Papi C, Ciaco A, Koch M, et al. Efficacy of rifaximin in the treatment of symptomatic diverticular disease of the colon. A multicentre double-blind placebo-controlled trial. *Aliment Pharmacol Ther*. 1995;9(1):33–39.

30. Parks TG. Natural history of diverticular disease of the colon. *Clin Gastroenterol*. 1975;4(1):53–69.

31. Pimentel M, Chow EJ, Lin HC. Normalization of lactulose breath testing correlates with symptom improvement in irritable bowel syndrome. A double-blind, randomized, placebo-controlled study. *Am J Gastroenterol*. 2003;98(2):412–419.

32. Pimentel M, Lembo A, Chey WD, et al. Rifaximin therapy for patients with irritable bowel syndrome without constipation. *N Engl J Med*. 2011;364(1):22–32.

33. Rendtdorff RC, Kashgarian M. Stool patterns of healthy adult males. *Dis Colon Rectum*. 1967;10(3):222–228.

34. Ritchie JA, Truelove SC. Treatment of irritable bowel syndrome with lorazepam, hyoscine butylbromide, and ispaghula husk. *BMJ*. 1979;1(6160):376–378.

35. Roberts JP, Benson MJ, Rogers J, et al. Effect of cisapride on distal colonic motility in the early postoperative period following left colonic anastamosis. *Dis Colon Rectum*. 1995;38(2):139–145.

36. Sandler RS, Halabi S, Baron JA, et al. A randomized trial of aspirin to prevent colorectal adenomas in patients with previous colorectal cancer. *N Engl J Med*. 2003;348(10):883–890.

37. Snape WJ Jr, Carlson GM, Cohen D. Colonic myoelectrical activity in the irritable bowel syndrome. *Gastroenterology*. 1976;70(3):326–330.

38. Stefanini GF, Saggioro A, Alvisi V, et al. Oral cromolyn sodium in comparison with elimination diet in the irritable bowel syndrome, diarrheic type. Multicenter study of 428 patients. *Scand J Gastroenterol*. 1995;30(6):535–541.

39. Strate LL, Liu YL, Syngal S, et al. Nut, corn, and popcorn consumption and the incidence of diverticular disease. *JAMA*. 2008;300(8):907–914.

40. Talley NJ, Owen BK, Boyce P, et al. Psychological treatments for irritable bowel syndrome: a critique of controlled treatment trials. *Am J Gastroenterol*. 1996;91(2):277–283.

41. Verlinden M, Michiels G, Boghaert A, et al. Treatment of postoperative gastrointestinal atony. *Br J Surg*. 1987;74(7):614–617.

42. Walker EA, Katon WJ, Roy-Byrne PP, et al. Histories of sexual victimization in patients with irritable bowel syndrome or inflammatory bowel disease. *Am J Psychiatry*. 1993;150(10):1502–1506.

43. Walker EA, Roy-Byrne PP, Katon WJ. Irritable bowel syndrome and psychiatric illness. *Am J Psychiatry*. 1990;147(5):565–572.

44. Walker EA, Roy-Byrne PP, Katon WJ, et al. Psychiatric illness and irritable bowel syndrome: a comparison with inflammatory bowel disease. *Am J Psychiatry*. 1990;147(12):1656–1661.

45. Whitehead WE, Holtkotter B, Enck P, et al. Tolerance for rectosigmoid distention in irritable bowel syndrome. *Gastroenterology*. 1990;98(5 pt 1):1187–1192.

46. Ziegenhagen DJ, Tewinkel G, Kruis W, et al. Adding more fluid to wheat bran has no significant effects on intestinal functions of healthy subjects. *J Clin Gastroenterol*. 1991;13(5):525–530.

5
Evaluation and Diagnostic Techniques

Paula I. Denoya and Marvin L. Corman

Come, come, and sit you down. You shall not budge!
You go not till I set you up a glass
Where you may see the inmost part of you.
—WILLIAM SHAKESPEARE: *Hamlet* III, iv, 18

This chapter addresses the evaluation of the symptoms frequently associated with diseases of the anus, rectum, and colon. In addition, the instrumentation, the studies, and the tests available for the diagnosis of these conditions are presented. Endoscopic options will be discussed separately. General principles of history taking and physical examination are introduced, but the reader is advised to consult the appropriate chapter for evaluation of a particular disease or condition.

▶ HISTORY

As in all fields of medicine, the patient's history is the single most important piece of information that the physician can obtain. A carefully obtained interview will in all probability either establish the diagnosis or at least suggest it. In consideration of the pathologic conditions affecting the anus, rectum, and colon, there are a limited number of issues and questions that are pertinent (Table 5-1).

Bleeding

Bleeding from the rectum has long been accepted as an important warning sign of bowel cancer, yet cancer is not the most likely cause of hematochezia. Blood may be pink, bright red, mahogany, black, or occult. It may be noticed on the toilet paper, in the toilet bowl, or both. None of these manifestations of blood loss is specifically diagnostic of the location or type of pathologic process; thus, it is important to keep an open mind. That stated, blood that appears solely on the toilet paper is suggestive of a distal cause (e.g., hemorrhoids, fissure). Altered (i.e., dark) blood suggests a more proximal lesion (e.g., carcinoma of the cecum). Blood found in the toilet bowl may or may not indicate a greater blood loss. One drop of blood will turn the water pink, and a few drops will turn it red. Blood that is not observed by the patient but is revealed through guaiac or orthotoluidine testing requires comprehensive gastrointestinal (GI) evaluation.

Rectal bleeding may not be an isolated symptom. When associated with a painful lump and unrelated to defecation, it is usually the result of a thrombosed hemorrhoid. When related to defecation and associated with pain, it is often the result of an anal fissure, the most common cause of bleeding in the infant. When bleeding accompanies diarrhea, inflammatory bowel disease must be considered.

The physician must have a reasonable index of suspicion, as well as competent clinical judgment, before embarking on additional studies to evaluate the cause of rectal bleeding. In exercising this judgment, it is proper to withhold radiologic studies and defer additional diagnostic procedures if the bleeding is from a readily apparent cause. However, bleeding is an important symptom not to have. If it is believed to be caused by hemorrhoids, appropriate treatment should be instituted to control the symptoms. If bleeding persists despite an attempt at treatment, it is the responsibility of the physician to order or to perform the studies necessary to establish a diagnosis or exclude within the limitations of the state of medical knowledge the presence of significant pathologic features.

TABLE 5-1 Differential Diagnosis of Anal Complaints

ACUTE PAIN	CHRONIC PAIN	BLEEDING	PRURITUS/DISCHARGE	LUMP/MASS
Anal fissure	Chronic fissure	Fissure	Fistula	Abscess
Abscess	Abscess or fistula	Anal or rectal neoplasm	Condylomata	Skin tag
Fistula	Anal stenosis	Inflammatory bowel disease	Anal incontinence or seepage	Anal or rectal neoplasm
Thrombosed hemorrhoid	Crohn's disease	Proctitis	Rectal prolapse	Rectal prolapse
	Thrombosed hemorrhoid	Internal hemorrhoids	Idiopathic pruritus	Crohn's disease
		Ruptured thrombosed external hemorrhoid	Hypertrophied anal papilla	Hypertrophied anal papilla
		Pruritus ani with fissuring	Prolapsed hemorrhoid	Thrombosed or prolapsed hemorrhoid
			Skin tag or external hemorrhoid	

Pain

Anorectal pain is a frequent complaint, one that can be most disabling to the patient. If it is continuous, unrelated to defecation, and associated with a lump, a thrombosed hemorrhoid is the probable diagnosis. An anorectal abscess is another possibility. If the pain is exacerbated during and following defecation, examination will usually reveal the presence of an anal fissure. If the pain is deep seated, intermittent, and unrelated to defecation, the patient is probably experiencing proctalgia fugax (i.e., levator spasm). If related to the coccyx and worsened by moving from a sitting to a standing position, coccygodynia is a possible cause. Anorectal pain is rarely associated with a tumor unless the lesion invades the anal canal or internal sphincter to produce tenesmus—a painful, ineffective desire to defecate.

Abdominal pain, if colicky in nature, may be caused by bowel obstruction but most commonly can be attributed to the irritable bowel syndrome. Physical examination and plain abdominal films readily distinguish the two entities. When abdominal pain is continuous, it may be a consequence of peritoneal irritation from any of a number of sources. Here again, physical examination and determination of the presence or absence of peritoneal signs will lead the physician to pursue the appropriate diagnostic and therapeutic course.

Anal and Perianal Masses

The differential diagnosis of an anal or perianal lump involves a spectrum of benign and malignant lesions as well as a host of dermatologic conditions. Probably the most common causes are a thrombosed hemorrhoid and a skin tag. Other frequently observed lumps include sebaceous cysts, lipomas, hypertrophied anal papillae, and condylomata. Protrusion or prolapse of hemorrhoids that reduces spontaneously or requires manual reduction may also be the cause of the mass. Uncommonly, rectal prolapse (i.e., procidentia) may present as a rectal mass. With lesions of uncertain nature, biopsy is mandatory.

Rectal Discharge

Mucous discharge and soiling of the underclothes are frequent complaints in the experience of most colon and rectal surgeons. The patient may have undergone prior anal surgery with resultant deformity and scarring or may have sustained sphincter injury from surgical, accidental, or obstetric trauma. Again, it is important to obtain an accurate history. Systemic disease (e.g., diabetes mellitus) or neurologic conditions may also be factors. Of course, when purulent discharge is accompanied by a painful swelling, the patient usually has an anal or perianal abscess.

Rectal discharge, however, is usually not related to the presence of a specific pathologic entity. Most individuals experience the difficulty because of dietary indiscretion or too vigorous attention to anal hygiene. Appropriate dietary and hygiene counseling may be all the treatment that is required. In patients with a lax anus, perineal strengthening exercises may be helpful.

Incontinence

Fecal incontinence is defined by most colon and rectal surgeons in accordance with the presenting complaint(s): incontinence of gas, soiling of the underclothes, incontinence for loose stool, incontinence for formed stool, and the requirement for the use of a pad. It is helpful to use a simple scoring system to quantify the incontinence at the time of the initial patient evaluation. Several validated scoring or quality-of-life surveys are available. The Cleveland Clinic

Florida Fecal Incontinence score is simple to use in the office setting while taking the patient's history.[13,62] Incontinence may be caused by anorectal disease, fecal impaction, laxative abuse, neurologic disease, and trauma (surgical, obstetric, blunt, and sharp). The complaint of fecal incontinence requires at least a minimal neurologic examination (e.g., sensory evaluation of the perianal area).[22] Repair or reconstruction is usually advocated for incontinence secondary to trauma or to congenital anomaly.

Change in Bowel Habits

The impression by the patient that the bowels have changed may have great significance. It is one of the symptoms suggestive of colonic neoplasm and almost always requires endoscopic or radiologic investigation for adequate assessment.

A change in bowel habits may be as obvious as diarrhea when the patient has had a long history of constipation or as subtle as the development of normal, easy bowel movements after many years of a difficult or irregular pattern. The presence of bleeding with a change in bowel habits increases exponentially the likelihood of the presence of a malignant neoplasm.

▶ PHYSICAL EXAMINATION

The evaluation of a colorectal complaint begins with the physical examination of the anus, rectum, and colon. The standard approach includes inspection, palpation, anoscopy, and proctosigmoidoscopy or flexible sigmoidoscopy. These findings then dictate any further radiologic evaluation. Generally, the term *proctosigmoidoscopy* is used interchangeably with the words *procto* and *sigmoidoscopy*. All three imply the use of the 25-cm rigid instrument.

Positioning the Patient for Rigid Sigmoidoscopy

The technique for rigid sigmoidoscopy is becoming a lost skill as flexible sigmoidoscopy has become available in the outpatient setting. However, there are certain advantages to the rigid examination. For example, ironing out the rectal valves can be more readily accomplished with a rigid instrument. Therefore, a better visualization of areas that are potentially awkward to view may be achieved. In addition, the rigid instrument permits accurate measurement of the level of a lesion. Very often, use of the flexible instrument results in a measurement that is falsely higher than is truly the case. The most commonly used patient positions for performing sigmoidoscopy are the prone jackknife position and the left lateral position (Figure 5-1).

The prone jackknife position requires a special table that tilts the patient's head down (Figure 5-2). The table is expensive, but it provides the easiest access and the best view for the examiner. It is the least comfortable position, however, for the patient.

The most comfortable position for an individual undergoing this examination is the left lateral (i.e., Sims') position. The patient lies on the left side on the examining table or bed with the buttocks protruding over the edge, hips flexed, knees slightly extended, and right shoulder rotated anteriorly. The examiner may sit or stand depending on the height of the table or bed. Although this position is the easiest of the three for the patient, it is not as convenient for the examiner as is the prone position. Some physicians believe that the sigmoidoscope can be inserted farther when an individual is in one position rather than another, but there is no evidence to suggest that position either interferes with or facilitates insertion of the instrument to its full length.

If one is to perform a satisfactory and reasonably comfortable examination and obtain all necessary information, it is essential to inform the patient continually what is to be expected and

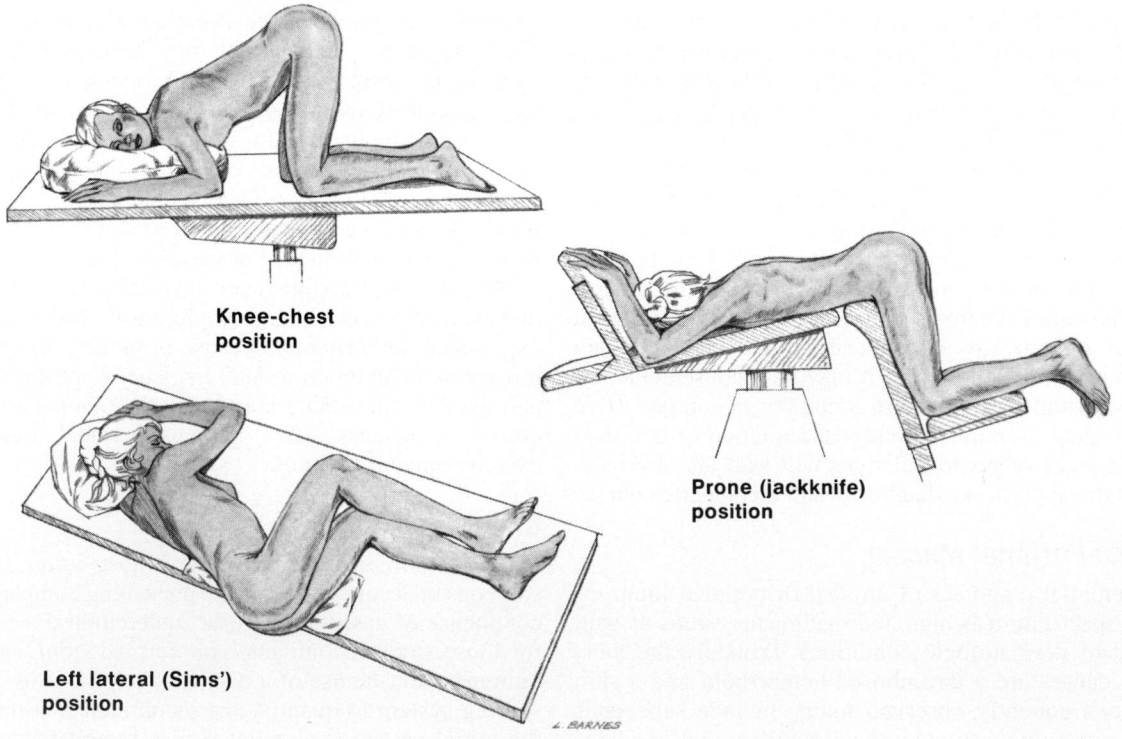

Knee-chest position

Prone (jackknife) position

Left lateral (Sims') position

L. BARNES

FIGURE 5-1. Positions used for performing sigmoidoscopy are the knee-chest, prone, and left lateral.

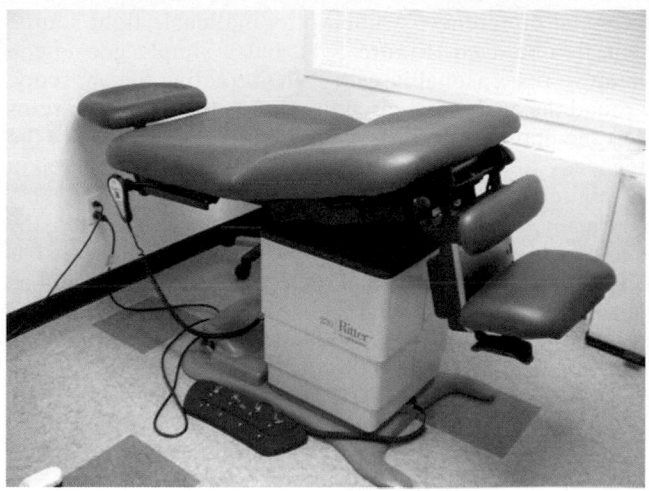

FIGURE 5-2. The Ritter table is used for examination in the prone jackknife position.

what is happening. Rectal examination may be a frustratingly unsuccessful experience for both the physician and the patient if proper concern is not demonstrated for the patient's understandable reluctance to submit to such an unpleasant intrusion of the intestinal tract. Warm hands and a reassuring demeanor are most helpful. Additionally, a relaxed and supportive attitude with due consideration for the patient's modesty is suggested, as is limiting the number of observers to no more than two.[31]

Inspection

Inspection of the anal area may reveal hemorrhoids, skin tags, a sentinel pile indicative of an underlying anal fissure, dermatologic problems including pruritic changes, an abscess, a fistula, a scar, or a deformity. Evaluation of the sacrococcygeal region may disclose a laminectomy scar, possibly suggesting a neurologic cause for any incontinence symptoms.[116] Pain on spreading the buttocks may indicate the presence of an anal fissure.

In addition to mere inspection of the perianal skin, evaluation of the resting state of the anal opening is possible. A patulous anal orifice may be seen. This may be due to a concomitant rectal prolapse, neurologic abnormality, or sphincter injury, or it may be a sign of an anoreceptive person.[129]

By asking the patient to strain, additional valuable information may be obtained. A rectal prolapse; hypertrophied anal papilla; or, most commonly, hemorrhoids may protrude. It should be remembered, however, that the prone jackknife position is least conducive to demonstrating conditions that tend to prolapse. If the physician suspects procidentia, then the examination should be conducted while the patient sits and attempts to strain while sitting on the toilet or commode.

Palpation

A water-soluble lubricant is applied to the gloved index finger. The patient is informed that a finger will be passed into the rectum and that this will make him or her feel as if the bowels will move. Again, it is imperative to inform, distract, and reassure the patient continually. The physician should examine the rectum and its surrounding structures in an organized approach. Assessment of sphincter tone and contractility is an important part of the rectal examination, and these should be noted routinely whenever a patient complains of problems with fecal control or discharge. Digital rectal examination may serve as a rudimentary gauge of anal sphincter weakness or defects. In a study comparing findings of digital examination, anal manometry, and anal ultrasound, the authors found that digital examination correlated well with manometric findings, and was accurately able to detect large sphincter defects.[24]

In the male patient, the prostate is felt anteriorly. It should be assessed for hypertrophy, nodularity, and firmness. In the female patient, the cervix can be palpated, unless it is surgically absent. The uterine body may be felt to be displaced posteriorly, and the presence of fibroid tumors may be noted. The uninitiated examiner may misinterpret the uterus or cervix as being an intrarectal tumor. Another common error of rectal palpation in women is to misjudge a vaginal tampon for a rectal wall lesion. With experience, however, there should be no confusion. A posteriorly displaced uterus may serve to warn the examiner that rigid proctosigmoidoscopy to the full length of the instrument may not be possible. Bidigital examination (i.e., one finger in the rectum and the other in the vagina) will readily distinguish any anatomic or pathologic variations.

The physician should then sweep the examining finger from anterior to posterior and back again, *consciously* thinking of a possible lesion that could be present. The conscious thought process is emphasized because all too often this phase of the examination is performed reflexively, with the assumption that any lesion will be identified by the instrument if it is not perceived by the examining finger. However, a submucosal rectal nodule may not be visible and would otherwise go undiagnosed if direct visualization alone were employed. It may even be possible to feel a tumor in the sigmoid colon or a diverticular mass. Asking the patient to strain down (i.e., Valsalva's maneuver—see Biography, Chapter 7) will sometimes reveal a lesion in the upper rectum or rectosigmoid that otherwise would not be palpable. Examination above the prostate in the male patient or in the cul-de-sac in the female patient may reveal Blumer's shelf,

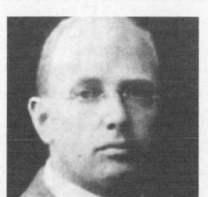

a hard mass on the anterior rectal wall caused by metastatic tumor, usually of gastric or pancreatic origin. Attention to the presacral area may reveal an extrinsic mass (e.g., cyst, tumor, or sacrococcygeal chordoma). Finally, as the finger is withdrawn, the presence of anal disease is noted (e.g., hypertrophied papilla, thrombosed hemorrhoid, stenosis, scarring).

Anoscopy

Anoscopy offers the best means to evaluate hemorrhoids, fissures, papillae, or other lesions of the anal canal. It is the requisite instrument if the physician is to perform an anal procedure or to treat a condition of the anal canal.

Numerous anoscopes and specula are available (Figure 5-3). The physician can purchase either reusable or disposable fiberoptic anoscopes; some have a light source that fits into the instrument. Although relatively expensive, lighted anoscopes are ideal for diagnostic purposes. However, they may be somewhat limiting when a procedure is attempted through the instrument. Still, the choice of instrument and light source are variables that are decided based on an individual's training, experience, and

personal preference. A fiberoptic, malleable light source can also be used (Figure 5-4), but a simple gooseneck lamp works reasonably well. When rotating the anoscope around the anal canal circumference, it is helpful to reinsert the obturator to turn the instrument. By doing so, the tendency to drag or pinch the anal canal or perianal skin is minimized.

Finally, when pathologic features are noted or treated, the site should be recorded as follows: right anterior, left lateral, and so forth. The use of o'clock descriptions should be abandoned because it requires a known patient position, and this may differ from one examination or examiner to another. Left posterior is left posterior even if the patient is hanging from a chandelier.

Rigid Proctosigmoidoscopy

The rigid sigmoidoscope is one of our most valuable diagnostic instruments available in the office setting. The examination is indicated to locate sources of bleeding, such as polyps and rectal cancer, and to evaluate proctitis. It may be used as part of the physical examination in asymptomatic

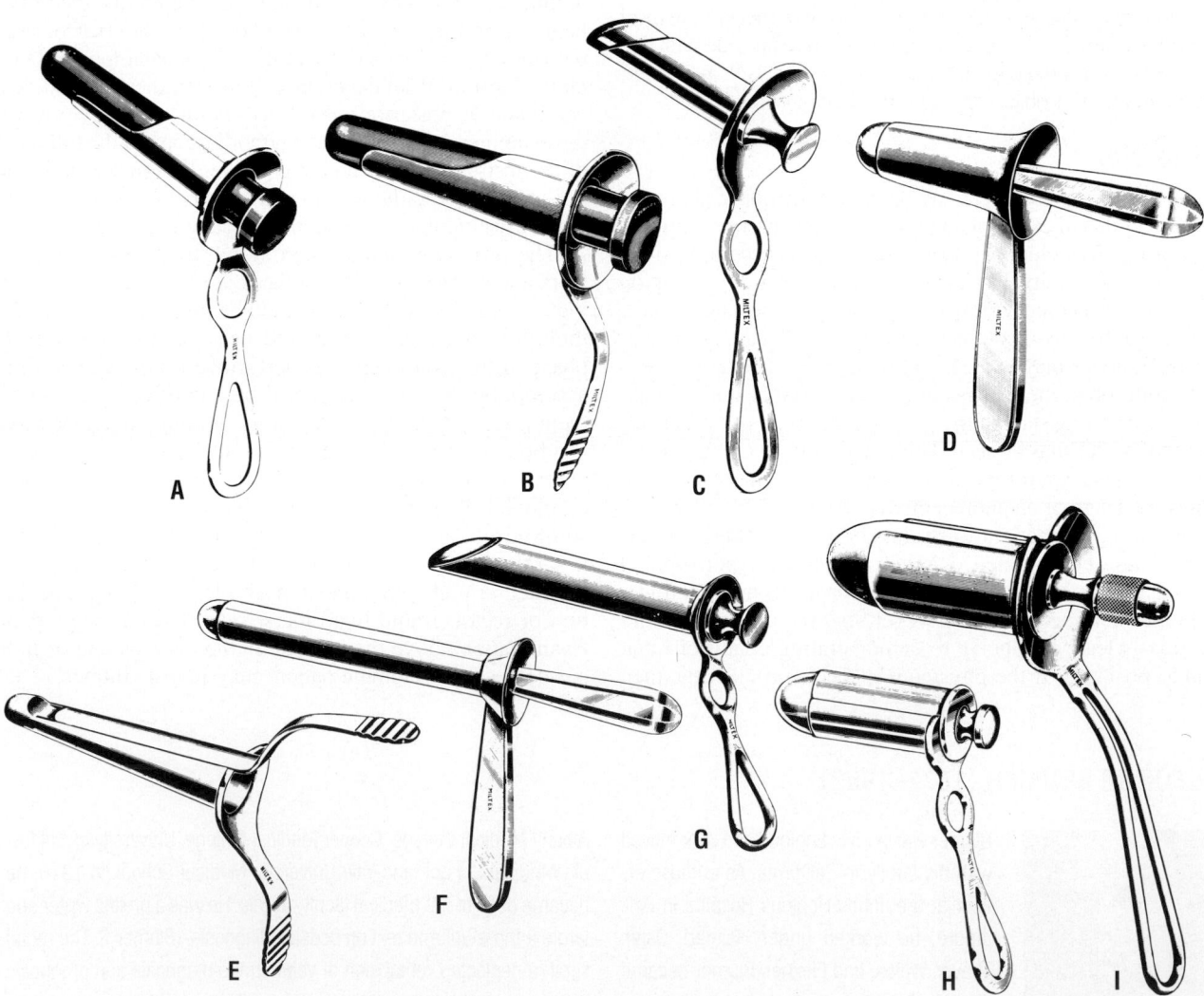

FIGURE 5-3. Anoscopes. **A:** Pennington. **B:** Fansler-Ives. **C:** Hirschman, available in three diameters: 7/8 in. (2.2 cm), 11/16 in. (1.75 cm), and 9/16 in. (1.43 cm). **D:** Kelly. **E:** Brinkerhoff. **F:** Kelly proctoscope. **G:** Hirschman proctoscope. **H:** Chelsea Eaton. **I:** Fansler operating speculum. (Courtesy of Miltex Instrument Co., Inc., York, PA.)

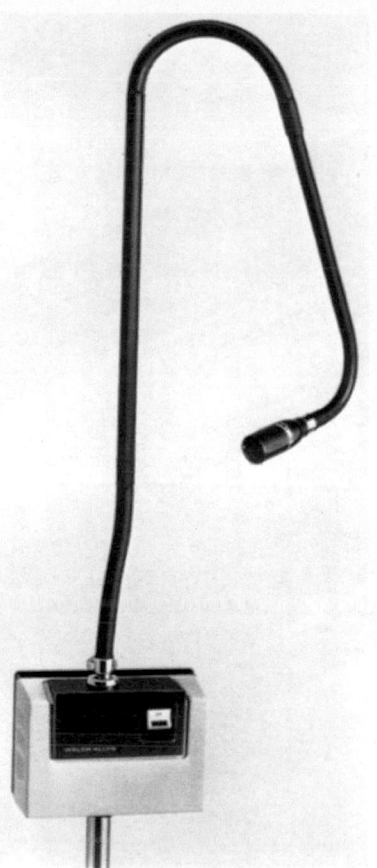

FIGURE 5-4. Fiberoptic malleable halogen examination light. (Courtesy of Welch Allyn, Inc., Skaneateles Falls, NY.)

patients as an initial screening tool.[108] Investigators have confirmed a relatively high yield of asymptomatic polyps when proctosigmoidoscopy is performed as part of a complete physical examination. Swinton reported an incidence of 5% in a series of 3,000 routine examinations.[134] Majarakis and Portes noted almost an 8% incidence in 50,000

asymptomatic patients.[87] In addition, it is often used intraoperatively to assess the location of lesions and the integrity of a colorectal or coloanal anastomosis. While leak testing for a colorectal anastomosis may be performed without direct visualization, it is beneficial to view the anastomosis. Direct visualization allows the surgeon to assess whether there is a patent, intact, and hemostatic anastomosis at a time when a decision to revise it or to perform a fecal diversion may be made without inconvenience.[81,112]

As previously mentioned, the rigid sigmoidoscope is the optimal instrument for evaluation of the rectum. Flexible sigmoidoscopy and colonoscopy are not as satisfactory as rigid sigmoidoscopy for evaluating ampullary lesions, unless a retroflexion maneuver is performed. Examination with the sigmoidoscope may reveal a mucosal excrescence, a polypoid lesion, cancer, inflammation, stricture, vascular malformation, or anatomic distortion from an extraluminal mass. It may also detect anal conditions, but it should not replace the anoscope for this purpose.

Equipment

Numerous reusable or disposable rigid sigmoidoscopes are available, with proximal or distal lighting, and with or without fiberoptics (Figures 5-5, 5-6, and 5-7). Reusable instruments require care and cleansing, with the need for sterilization equipment and with the burden of governmental regulations concerning ventilation and the use of hazardous materials (at least in the United States). Disposable ones are obviously discarded. If only a few examinations a day are performed, the reusable instrument may be more appropriate. If many examinations are undertaken every day, then the disposable instrument is usually preferred, unless the physician can afford the luxury of having a number of instruments and can justify the expense and inconvenience of cleansing them.

Reusable instruments are available in several diameters, ranging from 1.1 to 2.7 cm. The medium or 1.9-cm instrument is an excellent compromise that offers the physician the ability both to screen the patient and to perform procedures. The large-bore instrument is less useful for screening because of greater patient discomfort,

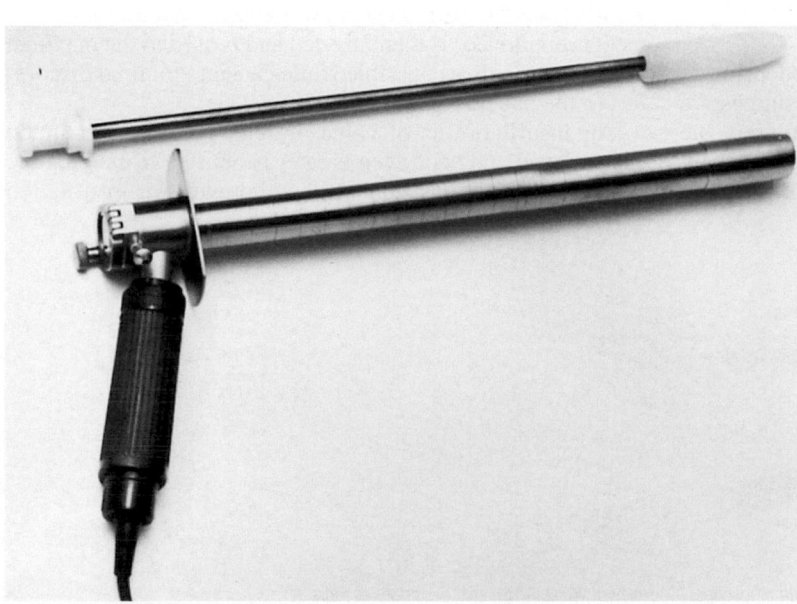

FIGURE 5-5. This reusable and autoclavable fiberoptic sigmoidoscope measures 1.9 cm in diameter and 25 cm in length. (Courtesy of Welch Allyn, Inc., Skaneateles Falls, NY.)

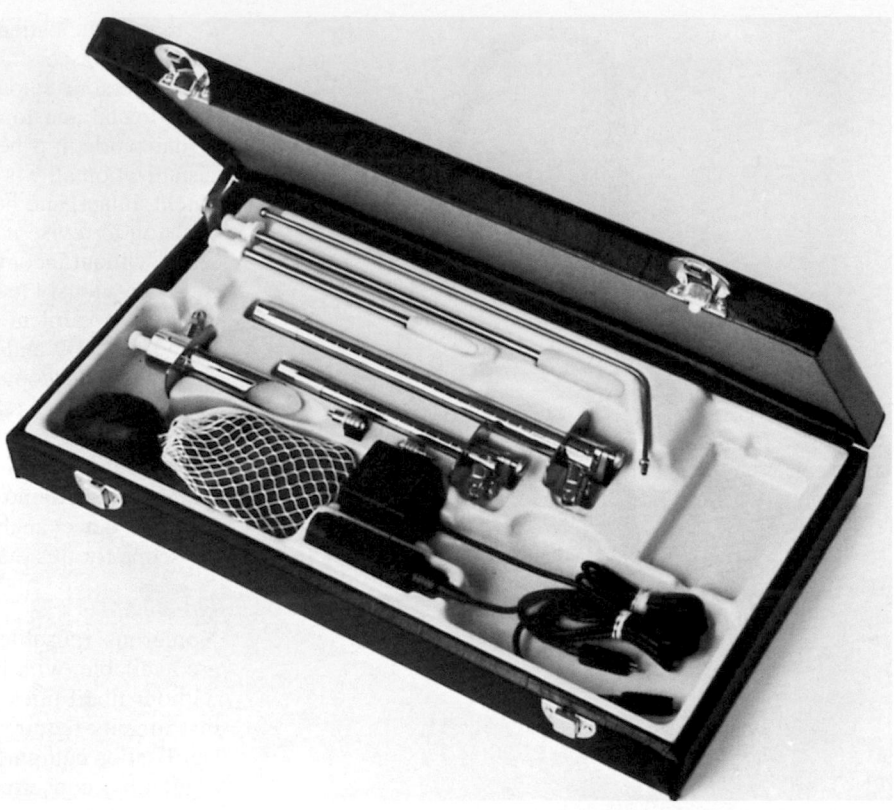

FIGURE 5-6. Fiberoptic endoscopic set including pediatric proctoscope. (Courtesy of Welch Allyn, Inc., Skaneateles Falls, NY.)

but may be invaluable for removing a large polyp. The narrow sigmoidoscope (1.1 cm) is a good screening tool and is particularly useful if an anal stricture precludes the use of the larger diameter instrument. It is very limiting, however, if one attempts to perform procedures with it. Disposable sigmoidoscopes are only available in one diameter (1.9 cm).

In addition to the speculum tube, the instrumentation includes a light source, a proximal magnifying lens, and an attachment for the insufflation of air. Another important detail is adequate provision for suction. This can be accomplished by attachment to a vacuum pump or a water tap. Long swabs (i.e., chimney sweeps) are also helpful (Figure 5-8).

Preparation

A small-volume enema (e.g., Fleet) is advised prior to the procedure unless the patient has a history suggestive of inflammatory bowel disease. Vigorous catharsis the day before the examination and dietary restrictions are unnecessary.

Technique

There are five principles that should be adhered to if the physician is to conduct a safe, competent sigmoidoscopic examination:

- Be expeditious.
- Insufflate minimal air.
- Always have a nurse or assistant available.
- Keep talking to the patient: explain, reassure, distract.
- Do no harm.

As mentioned earlier, a digital rectal examination should always precede instrumentation. In addition to providing valuable information, this procedure permits the sphincter to relax sufficiently to accept an instrument. The well-lubricated, warmed sigmoidoscope (if a reusable instrument is employed) is then inserted and passed to the maximal height as quickly as possible while causing minimal discomfort to the patient.

Air insufflation is of value in demonstrating the lumen of the bowel and is of even greater benefit in visualizing the mucosa when the instrument is withdrawn. Air insufflation

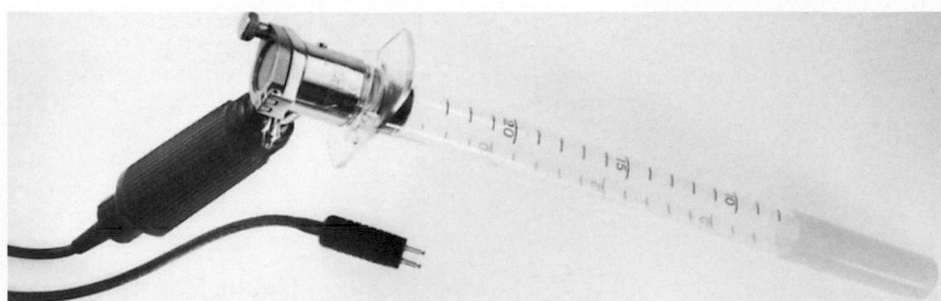

FIGURE 5-7. Disposable fiberoptic sigmoidoscope. (Courtesy of Welch Allyn, Inc., Skaneateles Falls, NY.)

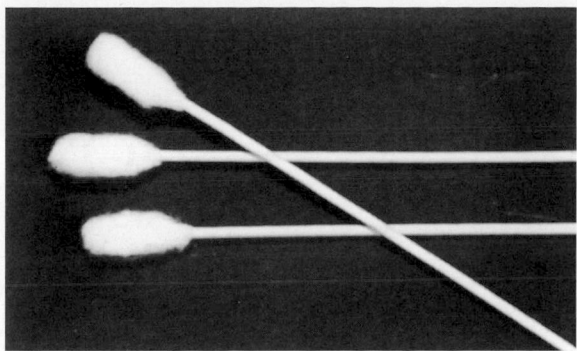

FIGURE 5-8. Chimney sweeps are long cotton-tip applicators useful for removing small amounts of stool.

should, however, be kept to a minimum because it tends to cause abdominal cramping that may persist for many hours. The novice should not pass the sigmoidoscope without clearly observing the lumen. However, as skill develops, the physician can determine the amount of gentle pressure that can be safely exerted as long as the mucosa is seen to be sliding past. When an obstacle is reached, the instrument is withdrawn slightly and redirected to view the lumen again; it is then readvanced.

The physician should withdraw in a rotating fashion, carefully viewing the entire circumference of the bowel wall and ironing out mucosal folds to be certain that no small lesion is missed. Several lateral folds are often encountered in the rectum, the so-called valves of Houston (see Biography, Chapter 1). Usually, three folds can be identified: the upper and lower are convex to the right, and the middle one is convex to the left (Figure 5-9). The valves can serve as useful sites for performing rectal biopsy when the mucosa is grossly normal because of technical ease as well as the limited risk for perforation. Particular care should be taken to view the posterior wall that sits in the hollow of the sacrum. This may necessitate the awkward placement of the examiner's head behind the patient's knees (if the prone jackknife position is employed).

Successful insertion of the sigmoidoscope requires familiarity with the anatomy of the rectum and sigmoid colon. Knowing where the lumen probably is located without actually visualizing it permits the experienced examiner considerable freedom in passing the instrument. When the sigmoidoscope is inserted, the low rectal and mid-rectal areas are midline structures. As the upper rectum is reached,

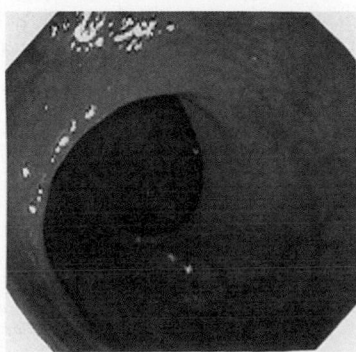

FIGURE 5-9. The middle and upper rectal valves of Houston.

the bowel bends slightly to the left. At the rectosigmoid junction, the tendency is for the instrument to turn to the right and ventrally. Therefore, if difficulty is encountered at the level of 15 or 16 cm, a maneuver to the left may reveal the proximal bowel. At a level of 18 or 19 cm, a more vigorous manipulation to the right and ventrally may permit the proximal colon to be entered.

In a report from the Mayo Clinic in Rochester, Minnesota, 25% of patients could not be examined beyond 20 cm.[119] Nivatvongs and Fryd reported the average depth of insertion to be 19.5 cm.[98] The two structures that may preclude complete examination (i.e., to 25 cm) are the uterus and the prostate gland. An enlarged prostate, a uterus containing fibroid tumors, or a uterus that is displaced posteriorly may make it impossible to pass the instrument beyond the 14- or 15-cm level. Persistence in attempting to achieve a higher penetration is usually unrewarding as well as potentially dangerous, and it is most uncomfortable for the patient. As mentioned previously, the potential for encountering this difficulty can often be predicted by careful digital examination.

Men are examined to the full length of the instrument much more often than women. Even when the uterus is surgically absent, fixation of the bowel in the pelvis may preclude further passage. A careful history will alert the examiner, thereby expediting the procedure and minimizing further discomfort.

Younger individuals are often more difficult to examine than older patients; because they usually have better sphincter tone, insertion of the instrument may cause more discomfort. The discomfort leads to apprehension and a tendency to bear down, making the examination more tedious. Also, pelvic organs are less lax in younger than in older women, causing it to be somewhat more difficult to displace the uterus and allow passage of the sigmoidoscope.

Complications
Perforation
The physician must take care when passing the instrument without visualizing the lumen. However, perforation from rigid sigmoidoscopy is extremely unusual. Gilbertsen reported five perforations in 103,000 examinations,[42] and Nelson and colleagues noted two in more than 16,000 proctosigmoidoscopies.[96] In a questionnaire of 277 British gastroenterologists, only five perforations were reported out of 328,815 rigid sigmoidoscopies with rectal biopsy.[114]

Perforation of the normal rectum or sigmoid colon is extremely rare from the instrument alone, but attempting to pass the rigid sigmoidoscope in a patient with inflammatory bowel disease, diverticulitis, radiation proctitis, or cancer can sometimes be a hazardous undertaking. Air insufflation can cause perforation of a diverticulum or of a walled-off abscess, and obviously such procedures as biopsy and electrocoagulation can result in perforation.

Bacteremia and Antibiotic Prophylaxis
Bacteremia can be associated with all endoscopic procedures.[2,23,67,75,78,115] Even rectal examination itself may predispose to such an occurrence, but there is considerable difference of opinion concerning the incidence (0% to approximately 25%) and significance of a transient nonfebrile episode.[56] Durack reported the following

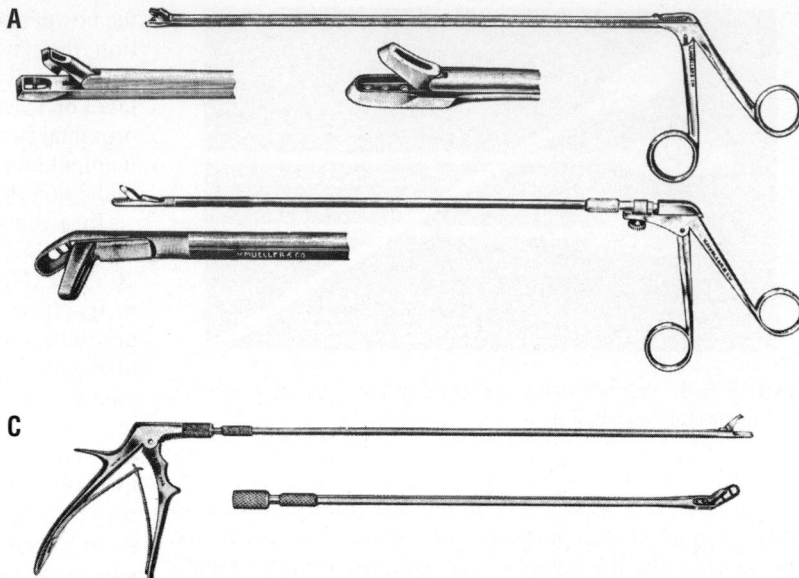

FIGURE 5-10. Rectal biopsy forceps. **A:** V. Mueller forceps (bite, 3.5 mm × 5.5 mm). **B:** Yeoman forceps (bite, 4 mm × 10 mm). **C:** Turell angulated specimen forceps. **D:** Biopsy forceps. The curved upper jaw has a 360-degree rotation feature. (Courtesy of V. Mueller, McGraw Park, IL.)

rates of bacteremia for a number of invasive colorectal procedures[26]:

Rates of Bacteremia

Procedure	*Incidence (Range), %*
Barium enema	10 (5–11)
Colonoscopy	5 (0–5)
Flexible sigmoidoscopy	0
Rigid sigmoidoscopy	5 (0–13)

Note, however, that in this study, brushing teeth had an incidence of 40% (range, 7% to 50%).[26]

In 1992, the Standards Task Force of the American Society of Colon and Rectal Surgeons published practice parameters for antibiotic prophylaxis during colon and rectal endoscopy.[6] These recommendations were updated in the year 2000[131] at which point, antibiotic prophylaxis had been recommended for endoscopic and anorectal procedures in high-risk cardiac patients. However, the more recently updated guidelines by the American Heart Association and the American Society for Gastrointestinal Endoscopy no longer advocate antibiotic prophylaxis solely for the purpose of preventing infectious endocarditis in gastrointestinal or genitourinary instrumentation.

A potential source of confusion and concern for some patients with cardiac lesions is that they have often been told that they must have antibiotic prophylaxis for all procedures. These individuals may be reassured that current recommendations are those of both the American Society for Gastrointestinal Endoscopy and the American Heart Association—that is, no antibiotic prophylaxis for routine endoscopic procedures (such as sigmoidoscopy and colonoscopy) even for high-risk patients. Parenthetically, the only *very* high-risk patients for infection are those with a prior history of endocarditis.[9,146] These changes were made due to the increased frequency of the development of antibiotic resistance and the low rates of bacteremia associated with these procedures when compared to bacteremia generated by daily activities such as teeth brushing.

Procedures Performed through the Sigmoidoscope

Three procedures are frequently performed through the rigid proctosigmoidoscope:

- Biopsy
- Electrocoagulation
- Snare excision

Gear and Dobbins have published a comprehensive review of the diagnostic usefulness of rectal biopsy, to which is appended an extensive bibliography.[39] It is interesting to note, however, the virtual absence of writings on rigid sigmoidoscopic procedures since the 1980s, owing to the fact that the technique has been essentially replaced by the flexible instruments. This is unfortunate because many diagnostic procedures are preferably performed through the rigid sigmoidoscope, not to mention measurement of the level of lesions that have been identified.

Instruments and Methods

Biopsy forceps are available with various biting tips (Figures 5-10 and 5-11). Some instruments are electrified

FIGURE 5-11. Buie rectal biopsy forceps. (Courtesy of V. Mueller, McGraw Park, IL.)

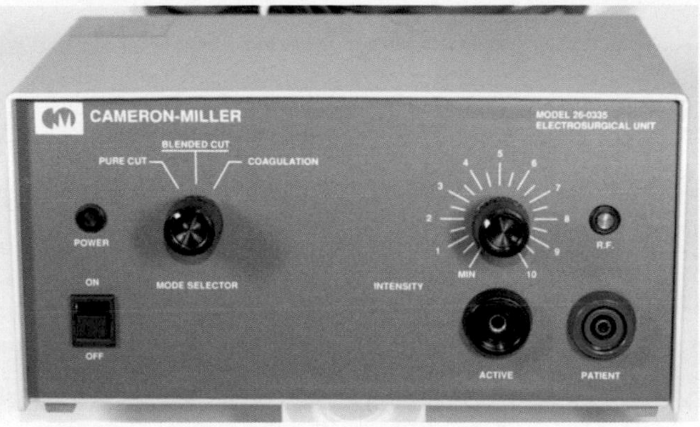

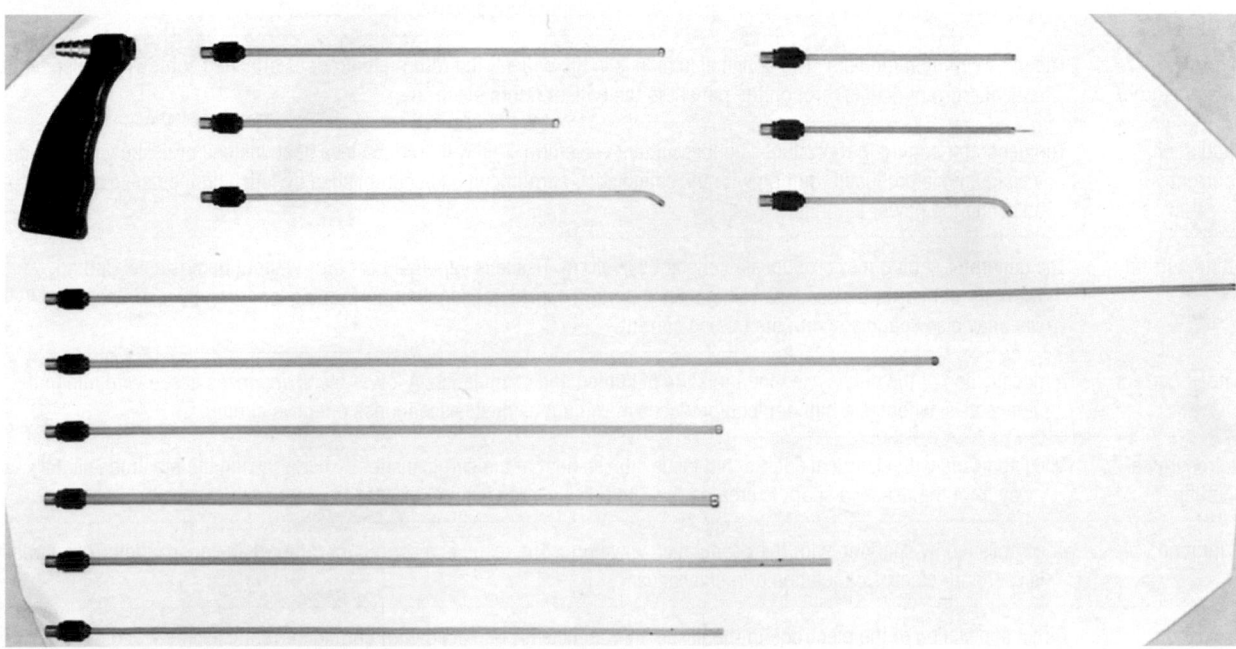

FIGURE 5-12. Cameron-Miller electrosurgery unit. (Courtesy of Cameron-Miller, Inc., Chicago, IL.)

for biopsy and coagulation, but this is usually not necessary as bleeding is rarely a problem when a biopsy is taken from an obvious lesion (see Complications of Procedures). Biopsy of the mucosa when a lesion is not present, such as is undertaken for amyloid, should always be performed on the posterior wall or on a valve of Houston. The valves are only mucosal structures, so perforation is virtually impossible. Conversely, biopsy of this area is not advisable if the physician wishes to obtain a sample of muscularis propria.

Electrocoagulation obviously requires familiarity with electrosurgical equipment (Figures 5-12 and 5-13). Most surgeons find the instrument setting that works well for the procedure performed, but the same maneuvers carried out in the hospital, with similar or different equipment, may produce inadequate or too vigorous electrocoagulation. The physician is advised to test any unfamiliar equipment on a bar of soap, adjusting the setting for the appropriate conditions. Although it is helpful to know that a small

lesion is a neoplasm (e.g., polypoid adenoma rather than a hyperplastic polyp), biopsy of every mucosal excrescence is meddlesome and unnecessary. The physician can feel content to fulgurate lesions smaller than 5 mm without biopsy. However, for larger tumors, it is preferable for one to obtain pathologic confirmation through either a biopsy or a snare excision.

Use of the *wire loop snare* (Figure 5-14) requires considerably more skill than fulguration alone. The technique usually permits complete excision with one application, although sometimes multiple snarings are required to remove larger growths. This is still can be an office procedure if the surgeon has the appropriate equipment.

The snare is passed around the polyp and the wire loop slowly closed; the instrument is jiggled as the wire tightens the base. This maneuver permits adjacent mucosa to escape and minimizes the risk of burning the bowel wall. Coagulation rather than cutting current is preferred for snare excision because greater control of the speed of cutting through tissue can be exerted. If a thick pedicle is present, the physician may take several minutes to excise the specimen. After the polyp is removed, it is helpful to have long alligator or biopsy forceps to retrieve it.

Principles of Electrosurgery

It is useful, especially for the resident who may not be familiar with electrosurgical equipment, to pen a few words about electrosurgical principles. The reader is encouraged to read a monograph on this subject that has been made available to members of the profession by Valleylab, a division of Covidien (Norwalk, CT). The following glossary (Table 5-2) of definitions and principles is useful.

Complications of Procedures
Bleeding

Bleeding is an unusual concern indeed if a biopsy is taken from a lesion, benign or malignant. The occasional incident

FIGURE 5-13. Suction coagulation electrodes. (Courtesy of Cameron-Miller, Inc., Chicago, IL.)

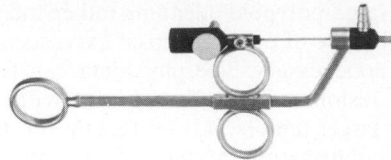

FIGURE 5-14. A wire loop snare and handle are used for polyp removal. (Courtesy of Cameron-Miller, Inc., Chicago, IL.)

TABLE 5-2 Glossary

TERMS	DEFINITIONS AND PRINCIPLES
Electrocautery	Direct current (electrons flow in one direction). Current does not enter the patient's body.
Electrosurgery	The patient is included in the circuit; current enters the patient's body.
Circuit	Pathway for the uninterrupted flow of electrons. The circuit is composed of the generator, active electrode, patient, and patient return electrode.
Ground	The position or portion of an electrical circuit that is at zero potential with respect to the earth; that is, a conducting connection to such a position. Pathways to ground may include the operating room table, surgeon, and equipment.
Voltage	Force pushing current through resistance, measured in volts.
Current	Flow of electrons during a period, measured in amperes.
Resistance	Obstacle to the flow of current, synonymous with impedance, measured in ohms. The patient's tissue provides the impedance. This produces heat as the electrons overcome this resistance.
Generator	A unit that converts 60 cycle current to more than 200,000 cycles/second. At this frequency, electrosurgical energy can pass through the patient with minimal neuromuscular electrostimulation and with no risk of electrocution.
Patient return electrode	Removes current from the patient safely. A burn occurs when the heat produced is not dissipated by its size or conductivity. Placing electrode over well-vascularized muscle mass is critical.
Bipolar electrosurgery	Both the active electrode and return electrode functions are performed at the site of the surgery; for example, two tines of a forceps in which only the tissue is grasped. No patient return electrode is necessary.
Monopolar electrosurgery	The most common modality. The active electrode is in the patient; the return electrode is attached somewhere else on the patient. Current flow is through the patient to the patient return electrode.
Coagulation current	The generator setting that produces an intermittent waveform. This will produce less heat. Instead of tissue vaporization, a coagulum is produced. Cutting with the coagulation current can be accomplished by touching the tissue and adjusting the power settings.
Cutting current	The generator setting that produces a constant waveform. Tissue is vaporized or "cut" without hemostasis. Cutting with the "cut current" uses less voltage, an important consideration when performing laparoscopy (see Chapter 19). One may also coagulate with the cutting current.
Blended current	A modification of the duty cycle, not a mixture of cutting and coagulation. A lower blend vaporizes tissue with minimal hemostasis, whereas a higher blend produces maximum hemostasis with less effective cutting.
Electrosurgical cutting	Dividing tissue with electrical sparks that focus intense heat at the surgical site. By withdrawing the electrode slightly away from the tissue, a spark is created that produces a large amount of heat to vaporize the tissue.
Fulguration	Accomplished by sparking with the coagulation waveform. The result is a coagulum rather than vaporization. This modality is useful for electrocoagulation of rectal cancer.
Desiccation	Direct application of the electrode to the tissue, more efficiently achieved with cutting current. Less heat is generated, and no cutting occurs.

of bleeding usually occurs when a specimen is obtained from a normal-appearing rectum, that is, when the physician is seeking a diagnosis of conditions such as Hirschsprung's disease or amyloidosis. Unless the bleeding is pulsatile, it is unnecessary to prolong the examination to await complete hemostasis. If persistent bleeding occurs, it may be treated by applying direct pressure with an epinephrine-soaked, cotton-tipped stick (i.e., a chimney sweep) or by saturation with the styptic, Monsel's solution, rather than by electrocoagulation. Electrocoagulating a bleeding area when a biopsy specimen has been taken from a grossly normal rectum may lead to perforation.[36]

If bleeding occurs from the pedicle of a snared polyp, it may be secured by fulguration, by application of pressure with an epinephrine-soaked chimney sweep, by the use of a long-armed (i.e., extended) rubber ring ligator, or by an endoscopic clip.

Explosion

In contrast to closed-system flexible endoscopy, electrocoagulation or snare excision with the open-ended sigmoidoscope does not require a full bowel preparation. Under these circumstances, an explosive gas mixture may be present. However, there are no adverse consequences because venting is sufficient to prevent proximal bowel injury. Although the "popping sound" or "firecracker-sounding explosion" may be quite disconcerting, no harm will ensue, at least to the patient.

Perforation

Bowel perforation from a biopsy, with or without electrocoagulation, or snare excision is a potential hazard that can lead to perforation. However, this is extremely uncommon for two reasons. First, the surgeon limits biopsy of grossly normal bowel to the area below the peritoneal reflection. Even a transmural injury at this location is generally harmless. Second, colonoscopy has supplanted polypectomy through the rigid sigmoidoscope. When a lesion is found within range of the short instrument, the patient is inevitably and appropriately submitted to complete colon evaluation.

As with colonoscopy perforation, the patient may develop signs and symptoms of bowel perforation within a few minutes of electrocoagulation, polyp excision, or biopsy,

or septic problems may develop as long as 10 days later. Anyone complaining of abdominal pain who has undergone such a procedure within that interval requires reevaluation and examination. The presence of free intra-abdominal or retroperitoneal gas establishes the diagnosis of a perforated viscus, but in the absence of obvious peritonitis, treatment may consist of in-hospital observation, restriction of oral intake, intravenous fluid replacement, and broad-spectrum antibiotics. Fever or leukocytosis is not necessarily an indication for surgical intervention. Each clinical situation must be addressed individually. In an equivocal circumstance, the physician may consider a water-soluble enema study (i.e., Gastrografin enema). However, no one should be critical of the surgeon who performs a negative exploratory laparotomy for an individual whose abdominal signs and symptoms are increasing in severity or who continues to manifest fever and leukocytosis. If patients are going to improve on conservative treatment, they almost always will do so within 24 hours. The principles of management are similar to those described for perforation following colonoscopy (see Chapter 6).

▶ RADIOLOGIC IMAGING OF THE SMALL BOWEL, COLON, AND RECTUM

Radiologic Evaluation of the Colon

Barium Enema

Walter D. Cannon is credited with the development of the contrast study of the GI tract through the use of bismuth. Until the advent of colonoscopy, the barium enema had been the standard procedure for evaluation of any mucosal abnormality.[15-17] Furthermore, with the development of computed tomography (CT), the barium enema study has been virtually replaced for extramucosal pathologic features as well. Barium enema is, in fact, an ideal study for demonstrating colonic anatomy (dolichocolon, redundancy, extrinsic compression, narrowing, intramural mass, incomplete rotation, etc.). At the very least, barium enema complements other investigations, facilitates the correct diagnosis, and thereby permits the implementation of proper treatment. It is a relatively simple examination to perform, it is time and cost efficient, and generally is well tolerated by patients.[43]

WALTER BRADFORD CANNON (1871–1945)

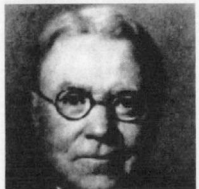

Born in Prairie du Chien, Wisconsin, Cannon was granted a scholarship to Harvard University, graduating summa cum laude in 1896. As a medical student at Harvard, he used the newly discovered roentgen ray to study the process of digestion in animals. His initial observations were made after administering mush mixed with bismuth to a goose. Following these studies, he focused his attention on gastrointestinal motility, tracing on toilet paper the fluoroscopic appearance of the gut. Cannon's ring was described as the tonic contraction often seen radiologically in the right transverse colon. He is credited with discovering sympathin E (i.e., the excitor factor) and sympathin I (i.e., the inhibitor), terms that have been replaced by epinephrine and norepinephrine. He discovered the chemical mediation of nerve impulses and coined the word *homeostasis*. Even though he established the principle of lining the fluoroscopy tube with lead to limit scattered radiation, he became a martyr to his work with x-rays, dying of complications of lymphoma. (Cannon WB. The movements of the intestines studied by means of the röentgen rays. *Am J Physiol.* 1901/1902;6:251.)

Indications

Historically, barium enema was one of the most effective means of identifying colon disorders (e.g., benign and malignant lesions, diverticular disease, inflammatory conditions, congenital anomalies, intrinsic and extrinsic abnormalities; Figure 5-15).[71,90] It has been employed in urgent or emergency circumstances to differentiate among small and large bowel obstruction, acute appendicitis, and periappendiceal abscess. It also had been used in the therapeutic setting to reduce volvulus and intussusception. However, in a recent review of the management of sigmoid volvulus, barium enema was found to have a recurrence rate of 11% and because the risk of barium peritonitis was felt to be too high, the technique was abandoned by the authors.[101]

Double-contrast, or air-contrast, barium enema (DCBE) is a technique that has some use in the screening of colorectal cancer. This technique employs air insufflated into the colon in order to serve as a contrast to the barium, which coats the colonic wall. It was adopted as part of the colorectal cancer screening guidelines in 1997 and is still one of the screening options used today.[147] DCBE has been found to have a sensitivity of 48% for adenomas ≥1 cm and 73% for adenomas >7 mm.[148] However, as other imaging modalities have become more popular, DCBE's use as a screening tool will continue to decline.[80]

Currently, contrast enema is used primarily as a preoperative "road map" to locate lesions found on colonoscopy, as an alternative when a colonoscopy is incomplete or cannot be performed; to evaluate for patency of a postoperative anastomosis; or to diagnose a colonic obstruction. However, because virtual colonoscopy is becoming more available, contrast enema's application for evaluating the colon after incomplete colonoscopy is diminishing.

Preparation

The procedure is essentially a meaningless exercise if the preparation has been inadequate. Without proper cleansing, it may be difficult to distinguish tumor from stool and impossible to exclude the presence of small neoplasms (Figure 5-16). Patients are usually required to follow a low residue diet for several days and a clear liquid diet on the day prior to the examination, along with taking a laxative solution. Sands was inspired to pen the following ode to the subject:

O for a colon that's pure and untrammeled,
O for a colon that's clean,
You may have a heart that's as pure as the snow,
And still have a bowel that's obscene.[120]

Technique of Examination Using a Single-Contrast Barium Enema

The colon is not the easiest organ to examine. To evaluate all of the twists, turns, and redundancies, it is inappropriate simply to instill a measured amount of barium and shoot a film with the patient lying supine on the table. Radiologists believe that 90% of the information from the study is gleaned during the fluoroscopic part of the examination. The final films are really a modus for creating a permanent record for future reference and comparison.

Cannon first instilled contrast material into the GI tract using bismuth subnitrate.[15] Shortly thereafter, barium began to be used because of its radiopacity, lack of absorption, ease of preparation, and low cost. Unfortunately, USP barium sulfate tends to settle and flocculate, and it is composed of varying-sized particles. Present preparations, however, are micronized with standard, small particles in a suspending

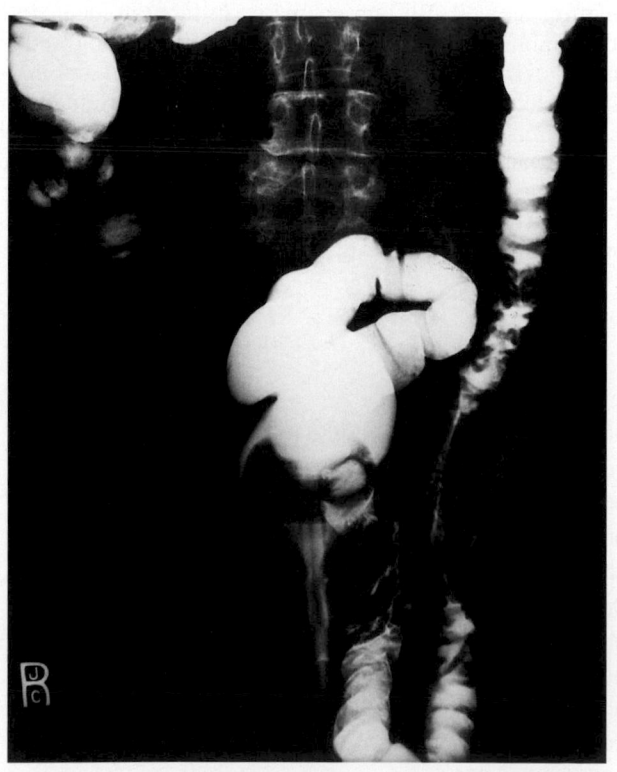

FIGURE 5-15. Barium enema demonstrates sigmoid colon in large scrotal hernia.

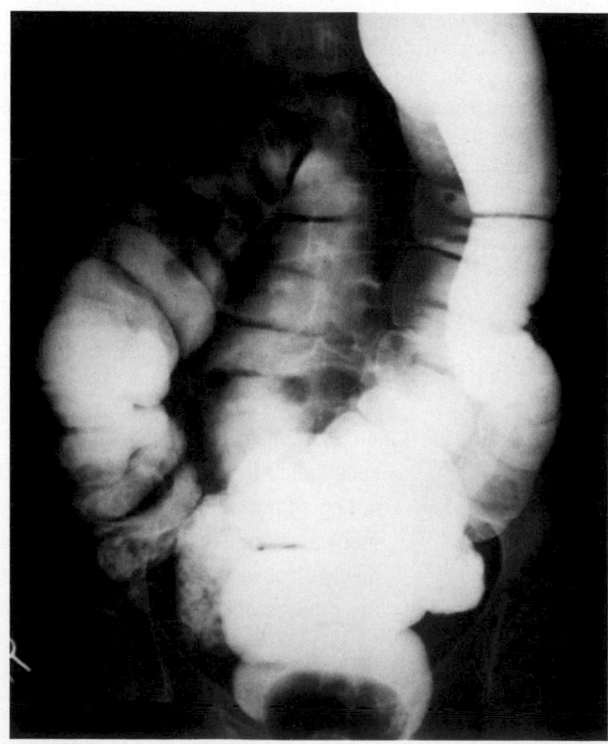

FIGURE 5-16. Barium enema with a large amount of retained stool makes diagnosis of an intraluminal lesion virtually impossible.

agent containing a measured amount of tannic acid. Barium is commercially available in a disposable bag, prepared for the addition of a specified amount of water. High voltage (approximately 100 kV) is used to ensure sufficient penetration of the barium column.

It is important to realize that administration of an opaque material within a hollow viscus does not fill the organ. What is seen is the contrast material against one wall of the colon with the nondependent wall not identified because it is not filled. That is why radiologists perform fluoroscopy with the patient in the supine position to evaluate the posterior wall of the bowel and make the overhead radiographs with the individual in the prone position to evaluate the anterior wall of the bowel. Questionable areas on the anterior wall then necessitate returning the patient to the x-ray table for fluoroscopy and respotting with the patient in the prone position.

Preliminary films of the abdomen are obtained to identify areas of calcification, the presence of air- or fluid-filled loops of intestine, residual fecal material, barium from prior contrast studies, and any soft tissue or bony abnormalities.

By means of an appropriate catheter, the barium–water mixture is inserted into the colon with the patient in the prone position until the column of barium reaches the splenic flexure. The tubing and tip must be of sufficient caliber to allow free flow of the contrast medium. A smooth enema tip with both end- and side-hole openings is preferred. For those individuals who have difficulty retaining an enema, it is helpful to use a tip with an inflatable cuff (Figure 5-17). It should be remembered, however, that an inflated balloon in the rectum will obscure the bowel wall. The barium enema is therefore inadequate for evaluation of the rectum or for identifying a lesion in this location. Endoscopic examination of the rectum should routinely be employed before this radiologic study.

As the barium flows, the radiologist looks for distensibility and interruption or deviation of the flow. Sometimes it is difficult to determine whether certain areas represent a fixed

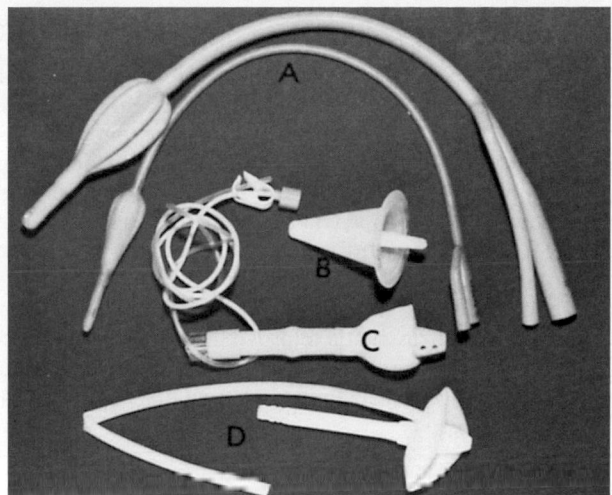

FIGURE 5-17. Barium enema catheter tips. **A:** Bardex retention balloon catheters (pediatric and adult). **B:** Colostotip for irrigating or performing contrast studies through a stoma. **C:** Catheter for air-contrast enema. **D:** Argyle retention cuff catheter.

or anatomic narrowing or whether the narrowing is physiologic (i.e., spasm). Many patients have been submitted to exploratory laparotomy for a suspected neoplasm because of this kind of misinterpretation (Figure 5-18). Anticholinergic agents have been employed to prevent spasm, but because of side effects they are no longer recommended and have been abandoned by most physicians. Glucagon (1 to 2 mg) given by the intramuscular or intravenous route has been shown to be an effective smooth muscle relaxant when administered parenterally.[91] It is as efficacious as anticholinergic drugs and has fewer side effects. Relaxation of the colon with reduction of discomfort allows the radiologist to perform a more satisfactory examination.

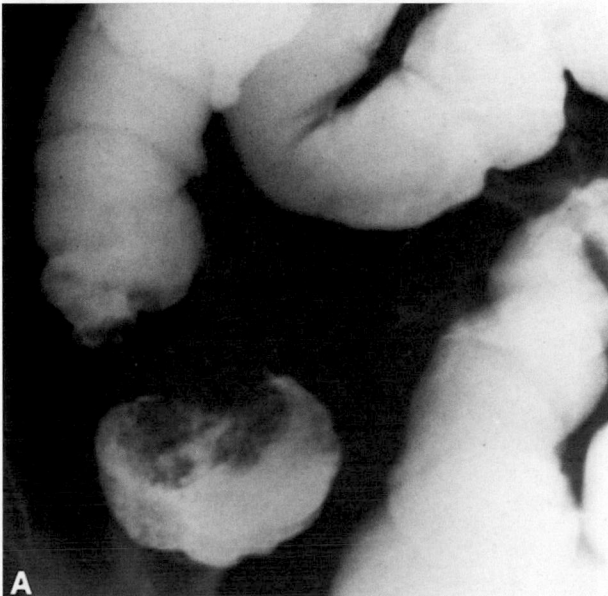

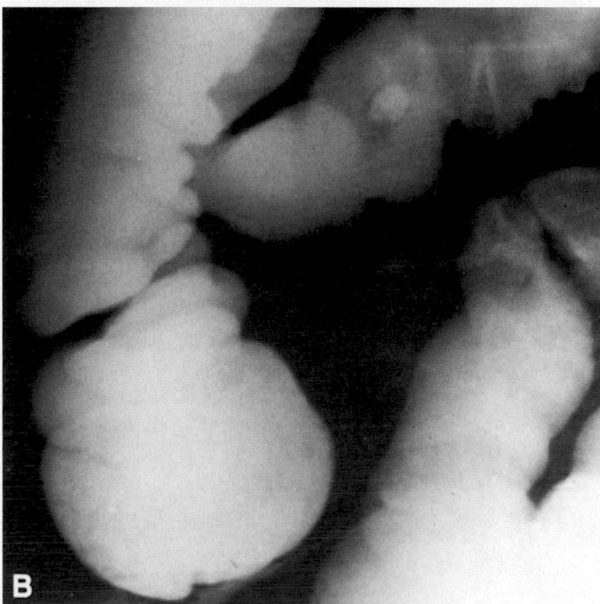

FIGURE 5-18. **A:** Barium enema study reveals an apparent mass in the cecum. **B:** A later film following administration of glucagon reveals no abnormality.

Spot films are usually taken of the rectosigmoid, hepatic flexure, splenic flexure, and cecum (Figure 5-19). Compression spot films are useful to identify small polyps (Figure 5-20). Angled views of the sigmoid colon (right anterior oblique in the prone position and left posterior oblique in the supine position) are most helpful in delineating this portion of the bowel for more thorough evaluation (Figure 5-21). The Chassard-Lapiné view (Figure 5-22) may be helpful in identifying sigmoid and rectosigmoid lesions, but it is hazardous in the reproductive years because of the increased radiation exposure.[27] Spot films of the cecum are made to prove that this area is indeed filled with barium, not necessarily because of difficulties with overlapping bowel. Peristalsis usually begins in the cecum, so that this area is frequently contracted or empty by the time the overhead films are taken.

How does the radiologist know that the cecum has been filled? Ideally, if the appendix fills or if reflux is seen in the terminal ileum, this would solve the issue, but the former is noted in only 30% of cases, and the latter no more than half the time. However, there are certain characteristics of the cecum to look for, such as the largest haustral marking and the ileocecal valve.

The rectum also requires special radiologic views. The radiologist is constantly endeavoring to move and massage the colon, to empty it and fill it. The rectum, however, is the only area of the bowel that the radiologist cannot manipulate by abdominal pressure. A lateral view must be obtained to visualize anterior and posterior wall lesions and to be certain

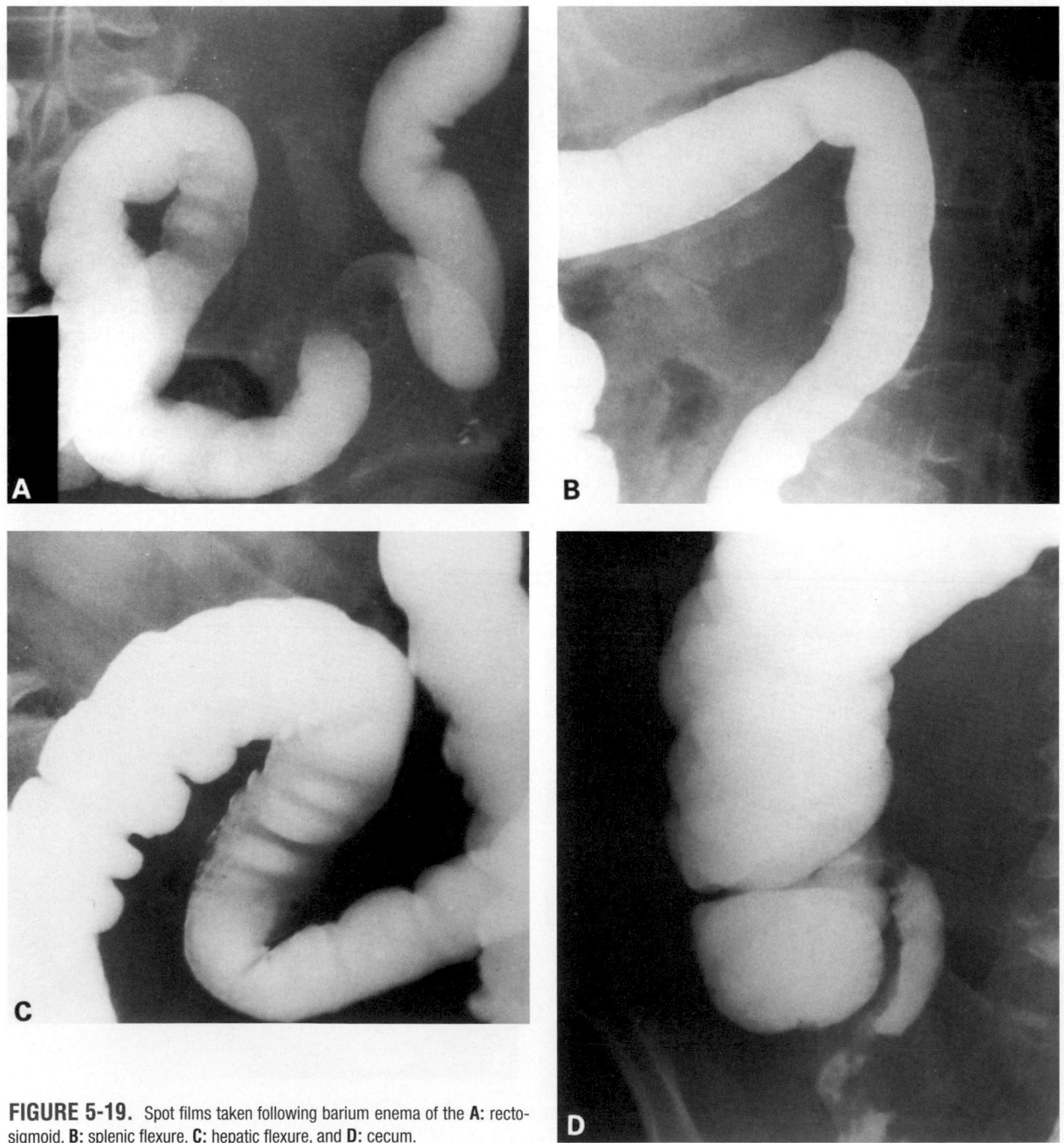

FIGURE 5-19. Spot films taken following barium enema of the **A:** rectosigmoid, **B:** splenic flexure, **C:** hepatic flexure, and **D:** cecum.

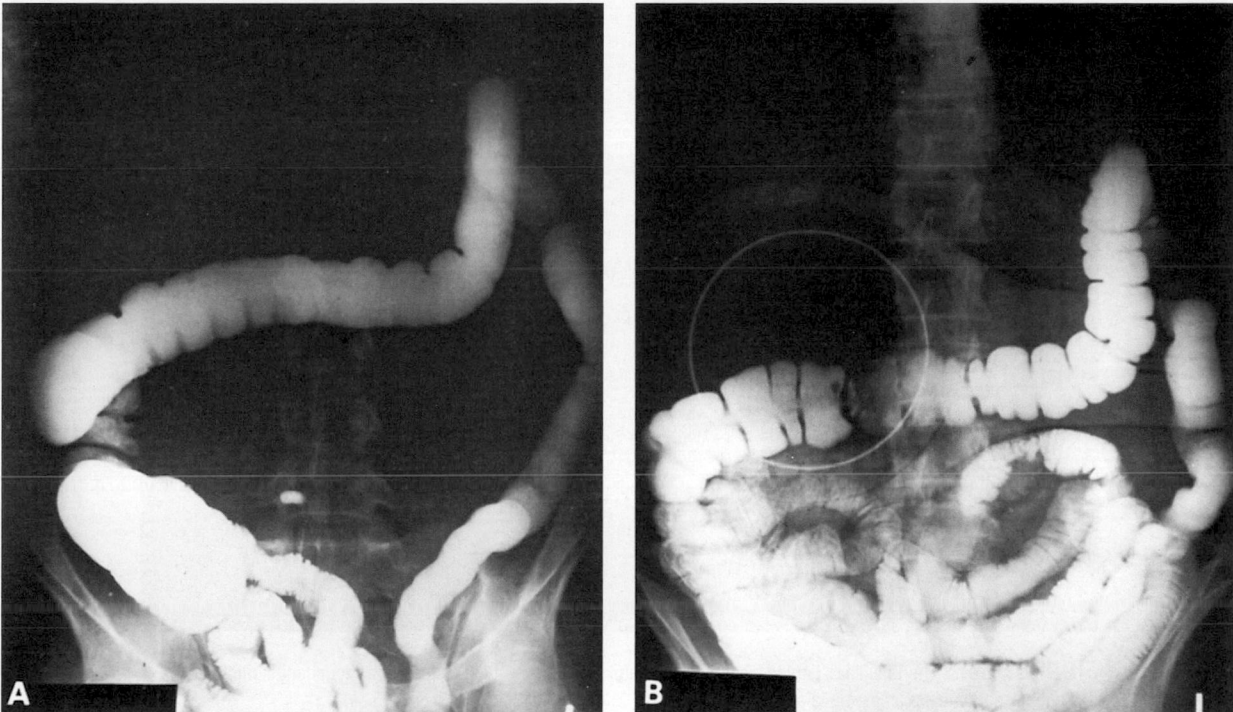

FIGURE 5-20. **A:** This transverse colon polyp is poorly seen after barium enema. **B:** A compression spot film demonstrates a small polyp.

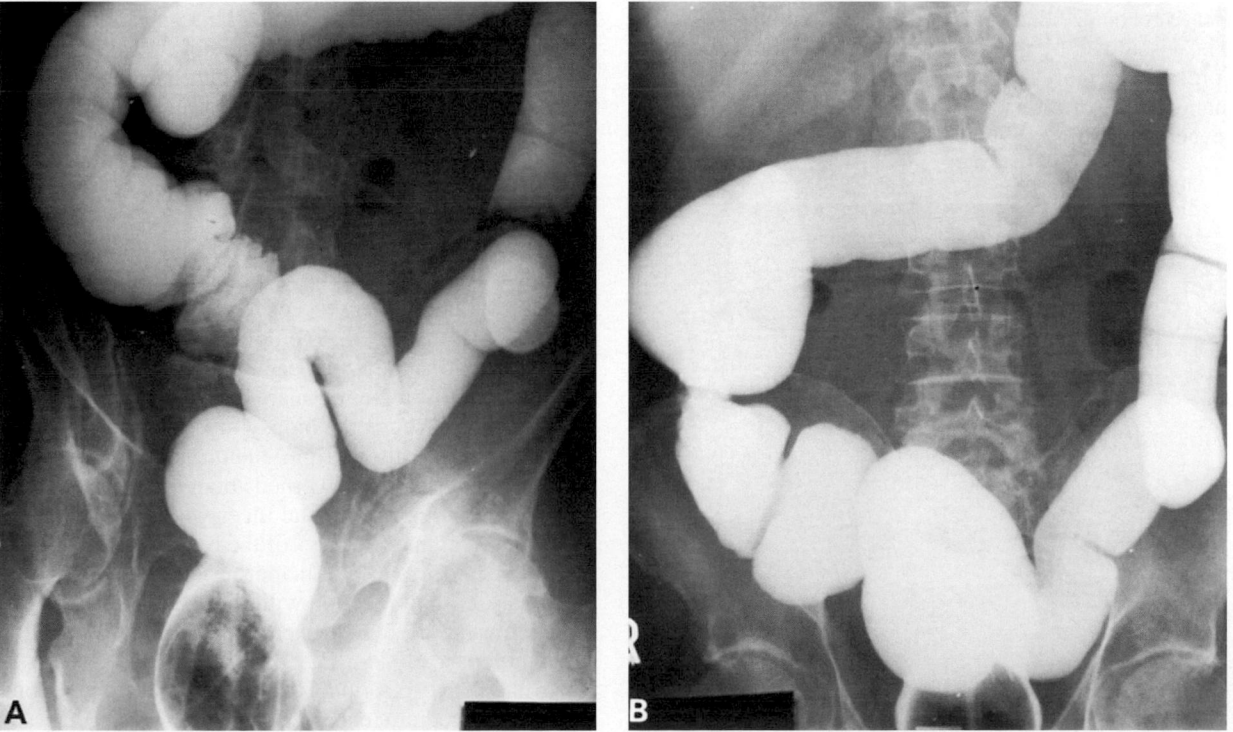

FIGURE 5-21. Barium enema. **A:** An oblique view of the sigmoid colon permits better evaluation. **B:** In the posteroanterior projection, the area would be obscured.

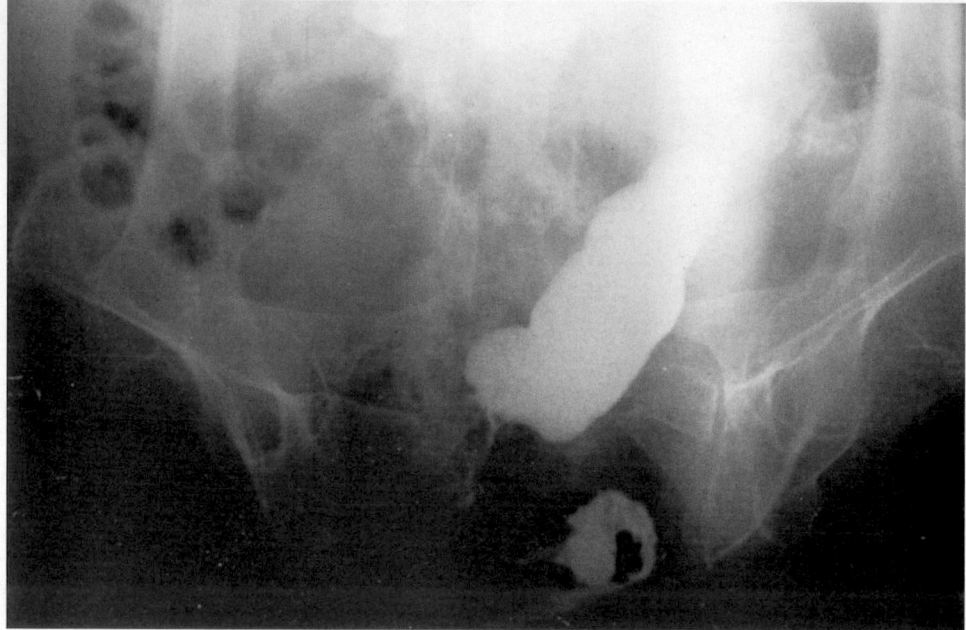

FIGURE 5-22. The Chassard-Lapiné view may be useful for demonstrating lesions in a redundant sigmoid colon. In this patient, an annular carcinoma is seen.

that the rectum lies well back in the hollow of the sacrum (Figure 5-23) and is not displaced forward by retrorectal inflammation or tumor (Figure 5-24).

Although the identification of intrinsic lesions of the colon is the primary purpose of the barium enema study, it is important to recognize that some organs, normal and abnormal, may be visualized by the defect produced through extrinsic compression (Figure 5-25). Probably the most important permanent film of the single-contrast barium enema is the postevacuation study (Figure 5-26). If there has been good

evacuation, it is the one time when all the walls of the colon are demonstrated. With a completely collapsed bowel, the physician can identify the mucosal pattern or lesions that disturb or destroy it.

To cover the colon satisfactorily, a small amount of tannic acid is added to the barium. This substance stimulates the bowel to empty more completely and effectively and causes the barium to contact the mucosa despite mucous secretion. Tannic acid is relatively contraindicated in patients with inflammatory bowel disease and in other ulcerative or inflammatory colon conditions because of the possibility of absorption and subsequent hepatic injury.

Alternatives to the Use of Barium

Barium is a substance that is potentially dangerous when used in a patient with a suspected bowel perforation. Barium peritonitis is often a lethal complication; that is why relative contraindications to barium enema include toxic megacolon, peritonitis, and biopsy or snare excision of a polyp within 24 hours. However, if the biopsy has been performed for an exophytic lesion, the barium enema need not be deferred. Some radiologists are concerned about the difficulty of interpreting the finding of a rectal ulcer when a barium study is performed within a few days of the biopsy, and that this may lead to the performance of inappropriate follow-up studies.[92] Obviously, communication with the radiologist is suggested if a contrast study is requested within a few days following a rectal biopsy.

An alternative to barium is one of the water-soluble solutions of diatrizoate sodium (e.g., Hypaque, Gastrografin). These solutions provide reasonable radiopacity, are nonirritating, and are relatively well tolerated if accidentally introduced into the peritoneal cavity. These solutions should be used whenever there is a possibility of intraperitoneal leak, such as in the postoperative evaluation of an anastomosis or possible fistula. Because they are hypertonic with respect to plasma, they can act as saline cathartics and may be of value for this reason in the diagnosis and management of acute, partial large bowel obstruction.[132] The result is

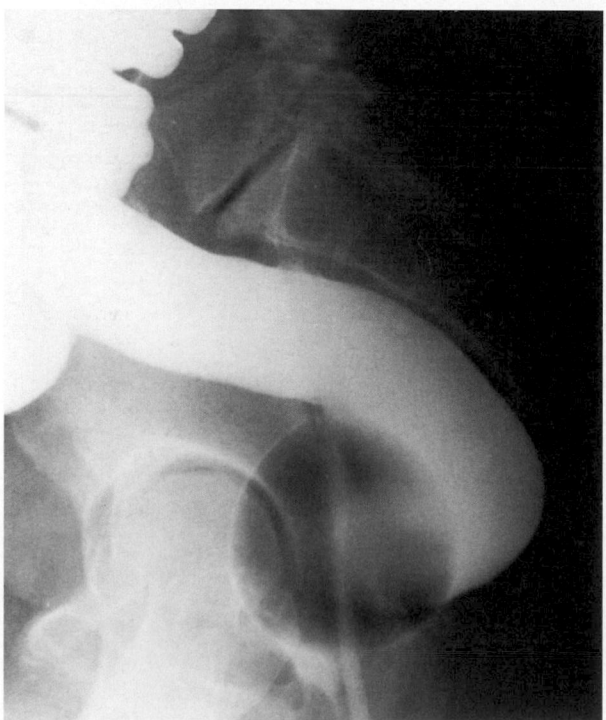

FIGURE 5-23. Normal lateral view of the rectum taken with a barium enema.

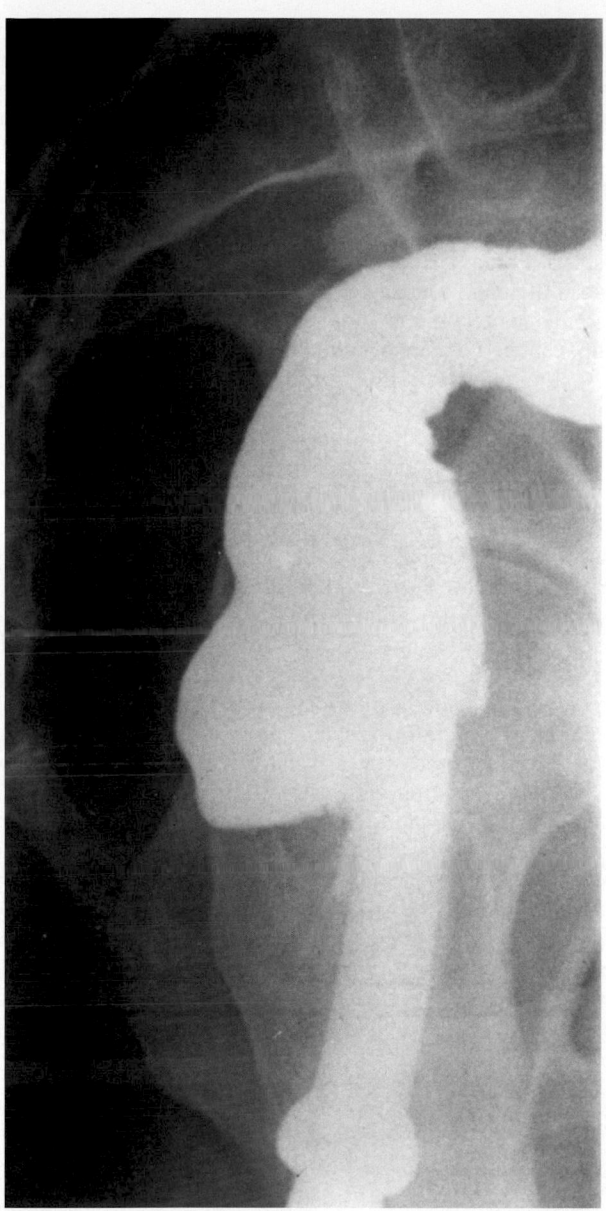

FIGURE 5-24. On lateral projection with barium enema, anterior displacement of the rectum from recurrent tumor is evident. Note the increased distance from the sacrum when compared with the normal position in Figure 5-23.

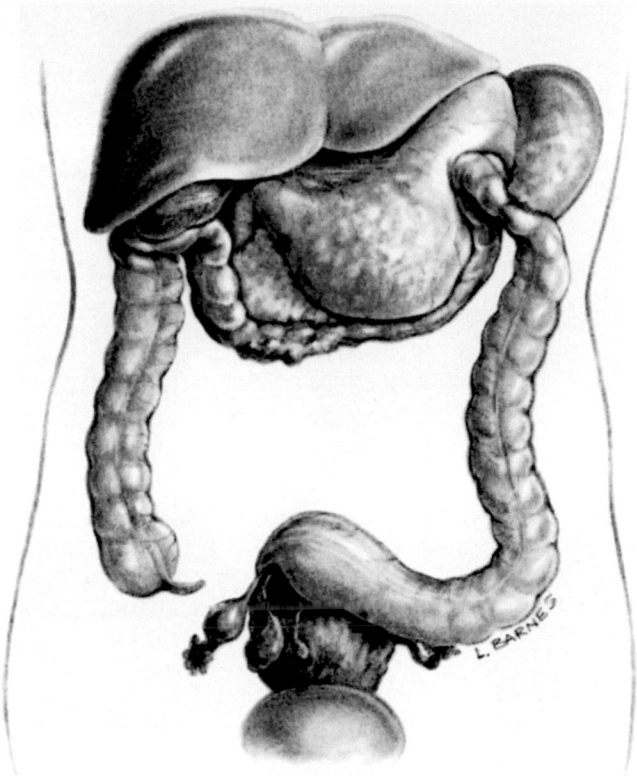

FIGURE 5-25. The colon and rectum can be deviated, distorted, compressed, or invaded as a consequence of problems in other organs, especially the spleen, pancreas, stomach, liver, gallbladder, uterus, ovaries, and prostate.

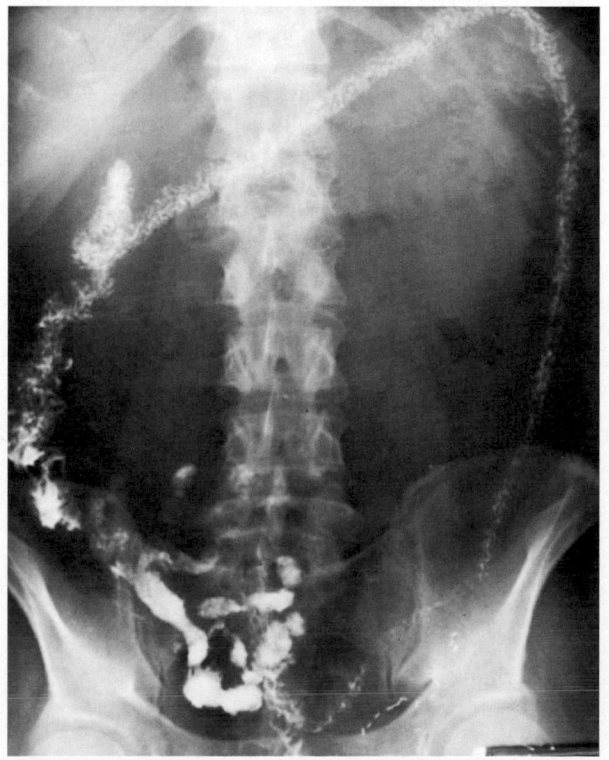

FIGURE 5-26. A postevacuation film following barium enema clearly demonstrates the normal mucosal pattern.

a rapid dilution of the opacity, but because of the cathartic effect they may be of benefit in the immediate preoperative situation.

There are, however, certain disadvantages of diatrizoate sodium. The major limitation is that because of reduced opacification, visualization is sometimes less than adequate. In essence, there is no postevacuation residual. Hypertonicity is a hazard in another respect; significant alteration in serum electrolytes can occur, especially in children and elderly patients. Individuals with cardiac or renal disease are also at increased risk when these agents are employed.

Double-Contrast or Air-Contrast Barium Enema

The double-contrast (i.e., air-contrast) barium enema study has been advocated as an improved means for evaluating the colon, identifying small mucosal lesions, and diagnosing inflammatory bowel disease.[76,77,143,144] Others suggest that either study may be optimal under a given circumstance.[41,88]

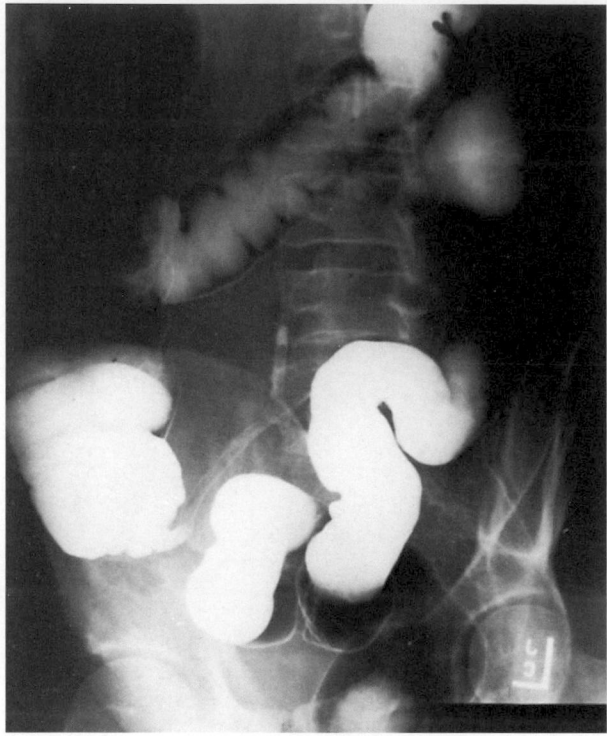

FIGURE 5-27. This double-contrast (air-contrast) barium enema study demonstrates a normal colon.

With the double-contrast examination, an attempt is made to coat the colon with a thin layer of contrast material and to distend the bowel with air so that the entire mucosal circumference is visualized (Figure 5-27). The barium used is a heavy-density, viscous material. To deliver this, a large-caliber enema tube is required. This has a soft tip and an inflatable cuff and uses a system that delivers air and barium separately (Figure 5-17C).

There are several disadvantages to the air-contrast enema. First, the study inevitably results in considerably more radiation exposure. An adequate examination necessitates 10 or 12 overhead films plus several spot films. Second, it requires a cooperative patient who is able to roll around, support his or her own weight, and comprehend instructions. A third relative disadvantage is that fluoroscopy has a lesser role in the course of the examination. The radiologist endeavors to move the viscous barium around the colon as expeditiously as possible and then depends largely on the permanent films for diagnosis. However, despite the foregoing concerns, with appropriate care, air-contrast enema can be accomplished in virtually all individuals.

Complications of Barium Enema Examination
Complications of barium enema examination are fortunately rare. However, when they occur, they can be of catastrophic consequence. Numerous complications have been reported, as listed here:

Rectal perforation from enema tip or excessive balloon inflation
Rectal tear or hemorrhage
Colonic perforation
Barium peritonitis
Barium submucosal granuloma
Toxic megacolon
Septicemia
Venous barium embolism
Retrograde GI filling with vomiting and aspiration in infants

In 1988, perforation of the colon or rectum during the course of barium enema study was estimated to occur in approximately 500 patients in the United States annually,[20] but certainly many fewer now may be anticipated with the decreased use of barium studies for colon evaluation. Rectal tearing or perforation is usually caused by trauma when the enema tip is inserted or by overinflation of a balloon catheter.[33,125] The tip or balloon can also lacerate the rectal wall and produce rectal bleeding. Use of a balloon for barium enema through a colostomy can produce colonic perforation at and below the stoma. This technique should never be employed; a Colostotip, catheter, or cone should be substituted (Figure 5-17B).

Colonic perforation with barium peritonitis has historically been associated with at least a 50% mortality rate (Figure 5-28; see also Figure 28-30), although there is a suggestion that the rate has fallen considerably because the availability of more effective antibiotics and early surgical intervention.[20,21,46,48] The mortality rate is influenced to a great extent by the volume of the extravasated barium. Although perforation at the site of tumor, diverticulitis, ischemic colitis, and nonspecific inflammatory bowel disease are the usual associated circumstances, perforation can occur in an otherwise normal bowel.[64,152] As implied, those who undergo barium contrast studies through stomas are at particular risk.

Idiopathic perforation has been reported to occur in 1 of 5,000 barium enema studies, usually in the right colon because of the lower bursting pressure in this area.[50] Between 1977 and 1996 at the Mayo Medical Center, 13,000 barium enema studies were performed.[48] Colorectal perforation occurred in five patients (incidence, 0.04%). Barloon and Shumway presented an interesting study on medical malpractice involving radiologic colon examinations.[11] The distribution of 18 cases of colon perforation in this group of litigious patients was as follows: cecum, one; transverse colon, one; extraperi-

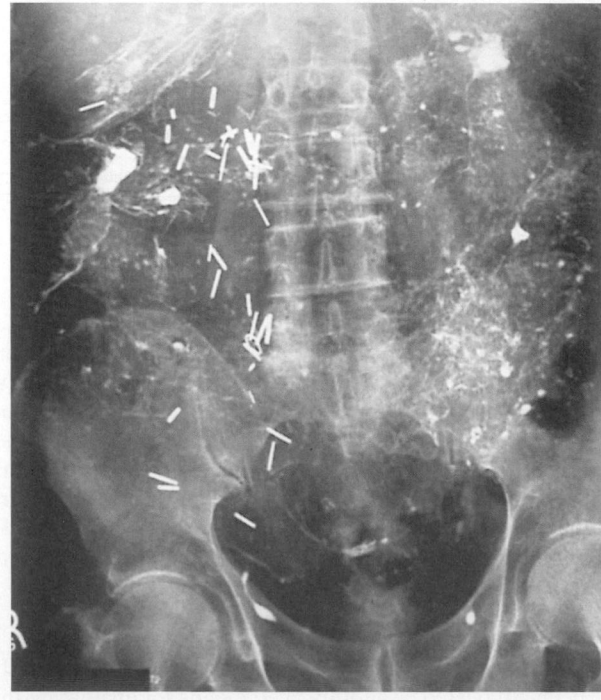

FIGURE 5-28. Barium peritonitis. Single view of the abdomen (kidneys, ureters, bladder) demonstrates extravasated barium. Note the dispersed appearance, with the barium outlining the inferior margin of the liver.

toneal rectum, seven; rectosigmoid, one; colostomy stoma, two; unspecified, six. In a recent review of colonic perforation during imaging studies, the rate of perforation during double-contrast barium enema was found to be 0.02% to 0.24%.[68]

It may be suspected that the term idiopathic is a euphemism for overfilling the colon or employing a high hydrostatic pressure. Fry and colleagues noted that 5 of 2,200 such studies were associated with perforation of the rectum or sigmoid colon, but only one bowel was considered normal.[37] The authors further observed the pressures created by a standard barium delivery set by using 1-m columns of water, 25% diatrizoate sodium (Hypaque), 20% barium, and 80% barium. The columns generated pressures of 70, 85, 95, and 120 mm Hg, respectively. They suggested the following options should be considered to reduce the incidence of perforation[37]:

Perform proctoscopy before barium enema study.
Avoid the use of a rectal balloon, especially with a known or suspected rectal lesion.
Avoid barium study in patients with active colitis.
Avoid generation of pressure greater than that created by a column of barium suspension of 1 m
Use a lower concentration of barium whenever possible.

As previously mentioned, the timing of a barium enema examination following biopsy of the rectum or colon has been the subject of considerable debate. Is there truly an increased risk for perforation? Many radiologists will not perform barium studies within 24 hours of such a procedure. Some insist on 48 hours and others on a delay of up to 1 week. On the basis of clinical studies and animal experiments, Harned and his associates suggest that a small biopsy with colonoscopic forceps requires no waiting period before a barium enema study is performed.[53]

Barium submucosal dissection with subsequent *granuloma formation* is very rarely seen today because of the decreased use of a barium enema study.[14,83] The resultant lesion may be attributed to healing of an ulcer or injury with entrapment of contrast material or to the performance of a barium enema right after biopsy. The barium poses no threat, but the differential diagnosis of a yellow, submucosal rectal nodule includes a carcinoid tumor. It is, therefore, important to limit the possibility of this complication, a circumstance that would otherwise necessitate a diagnostic biopsy or excision.

Management of Barium Enema Perforation

When free perforation is recognized, emergency surgical intervention is required. At laparotomy, it is necessary to remove as much of the contaminant as possible, an extremely tedious if not impossible task because of the paste-like consistency of the barium. Wiping the serosal surface with a moistened sponge or pad is a frustratingly unsuccessful exercise. Yamamura and colleagues describe the technique of irrigating the peritoneal cavity with a concentrated solution of urokinase (72,000 IU in 500 mL of normal saline solution).[149] With irrigation and mechanical wiping, this approach almost completely removed the barium from the surface of the peritoneum in their experience.

Barium and feces produce a severe exudative peritonitis. Large fluid and protein losses occur almost immediately. If the patient is fortunate enough to survive the initial hospitalization, there is a grave risk for the development of intestinal obstruction because of the dense adhesions that form.

Management of the patient with a rectal tear through which barium has extravasated poses a less clear-cut problem. Ultimately, a diversionary procedure may be required, but, depending on the extent of the injury, medical management

should be considered, at least initially. This should consist of vigorous intravenous fluid replacement, antibiotics, and dietary restriction. Three rectal perforations were managed conservatively in two individuals and by proximal diversion in one in the Mayo Clinic report.[48] All patients recovered. The authors opined that a localized, contained extraperitoneal rectal perforation can be managed conservatively in selected patients.

Perforation of the rectum or colon may also occur as a consequence of the double-contrast examination, with extravasation of air, but not necessarily of barium. Because clinical signs of peritonitis may not be evident, it has been suggested that asymptomatic patients with radiographic findings of perirectal, mediastinal, or cervical emphysema be managed in the hospital with close observation, rather than having to undergo immediate laparotomy.[37,103] The success achieved with this approach may be attributable to the fact that the patients generally have undergone a complete bowel cleansing. The risk for gross fecal contamination is therefore minimized. Parapharyngeal emphysema has been reported to cause a voice change, which may be the earliest recognizable symptom of the perforation.[107] Finally, approximately 12 cases of portal venous intravasation of contrast have been observed following barium enema study, a potentially devastating complication.[145] Virtually all these patients harbored a condition that disrupted mucosal integrity, such as inflammatory bowel disease or diverticulitis.

Computed Tomography

CT has become the radiologic "gold standard" for a host of conditions affecting the GI tract, both for diagnostic purposes and when performed with an interventional technique. Clearly, the diagnosis of diverticulitis is optimally made with CT. Metastatic cancer evaluation always includes CT. With the use of oral contrast, the site of a bowel obstruction may be identified, and the differential between partial and complete obstruction may be elucidated. Intravenous contrast CT allows for an accurate assessment of the urinary tract. CT scan with IV and oral contrast is the most commonly used initial evaluation of acute abdominal pain. In addition to the standard transverse views, coronal and sagittal reconstructions are useful to fully evaluate the images (Figure 5-29).

Important technical details in the performance of the examination include the following[7]:

- Fasting for 12 hours is preferred (although not always possible). Bowel cleansing limits interference due to fecal residue.
- Induction of intestinal hypomobility (0.1 mg of glucagon or 0.2 mg of scopolamine [Buscopan]) avoids peristaltic artifact and permits distension.
- Intravenous contrast enhancement is used.
- Adequate distension of the bowel with iodinated or hypodense (air, water, methylcellulose) contrast media introduced orally or rectally is ensured.

CT scan has a number of applications in the diagnosis and management of virtually every disease encountered by the colorectal surgeon, including malignancy, diverticulitis, bowel obstruction, inflammatory bowel disease, and hernias. In addition, CT scan is used to guide interventions, such as percutaneous drainage of intra-abdominal abscess. Each will be discussed in the relevant chapters in more detail.

Virtual Colonoscopy

Virtual colonoscopy (VC) or CT colonography (CTC) was first introduced by Vining and colleagues in 1994.[140,141]

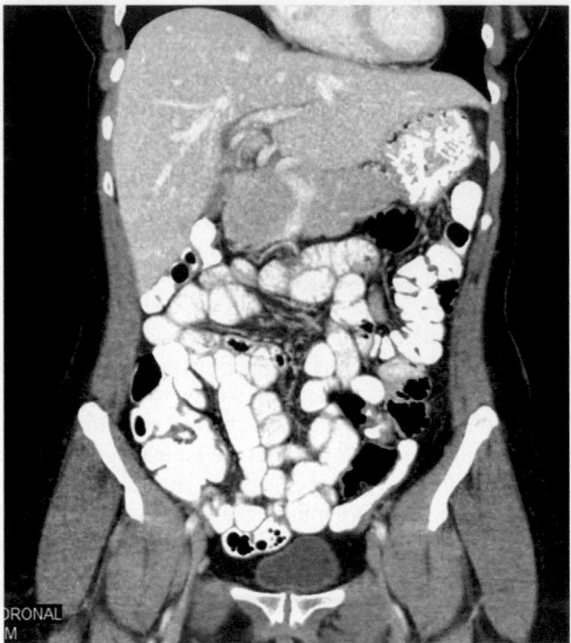

FIGURE 5-29. Normal CT scan with intravenous and oral contrast.

Because the x-ray tube is continuously rotating while the patient moves through the scanner, the beam describes a spiral pathway through the body, hence the term spiral CT.[49] Using a conventional workstation and a dynamic display of images, the radiologist can simulate an examination of the colon in much the same way as an endoscopist. The effect is to create images that are not dissimilar to those that are observed with optical colonoscopy (Figure 5-30). By the use of both two-dimensional and three-dimensional images, CTC has advantages over other imaging methods. It is able to examine the entire bowel wall as well as extracolonic organs. Furthermore, it can demonstrate tissue density, a singularly valuable asset in helping to characterize the nature of the lesion.

As with colonoscopy, the technique requires the patient to undergo a full bowel preparation. An intravenous smooth muscle relaxant may be administered, and the colon is insufflated with air until fully distended.[32] Intravenous contrast may also supplement the examination if indicated. If one is seeking a large or obvious lesion in a frail or elderly patient, the examination may be undertaken without a bowel cleansing.[49] There is also the potential for a limited bowel preparation with stool tagging to reduce patient discomfort.[105]

Published reports indicate that CTC affords great accuracy in the detection of colon polyps that exceed or are equal to 5 mm.[14,18,47,49,106,127,150] In a study of 2,531 patients who underwent CTC followed by optical colonoscopy, CTC identified 90% of lesions 10 mm or larger and 78% of those measuring 6 mm or more.[60] In another review of 3,120 patients who underwent CTC and 3,163 patients who underwent colonoscopy, the two modalities had similar rates of detection of advanced neoplasia, whereas CTC had a significantly lower perforation rate.[69] It is a relatively safe procedure without the risk of sedation or anesthesia and essentially without risk of perforation.[40] CTC has gained acceptance to evaluate the remaining colon after failed colonoscopy due to obstruction and as an alternative to optical colonoscopy for patients on anticoagulation (Figure 5-31).[84] At the time of this writing, in the United States CTC is not covered by most major insurance companies, including Medicare, for conventional colorectal cancer screening.

Radiologic Evaluation of the Anus and Rectum
Ultrasound
Ultrasound of the abdomen has been reported to be a helpful and a reasonably accurate diagnostic modality for a number of conditions affecting the bowel: Crohn's disease, cancer, diverticulitis, and intestinal obstruction.[113] Clearly, the technique is very much operator dependent. For practical purposes, however, despite the fact that it is noninvasive and well tolerated by patients, it is unlikely to replace or even to supplement barium enema, CT, or colonoscopy for any colonic condition. Ultrasound is still used occasionally for evaluation of abdominal pain in pregnant women or in settings where more advanced imaging technology is not available.

However, ultrasound is very widely used for evaluation of the rectum and anus. Ultrasound provides excellent imaging of the anal sphincter complex and the rectal wall, allowing for accurate delineation of sphincter defects, anal fistula tracts, and depth of penetration of rectal cancers.[93] Three-dimensional technology developed more recently is being used to provide improved representations of these entities, and work on dynamic pelvic floor studies is advancing. A group from the Netherlands evaluated 18 patients with fecal incontinence using both three-dimensional anal ultrasound and MRI.[19] Both technologies were equivalent for detecting external anal sphincter atrophy and defects.

Rectal ultrasound may be used for preoperative evaluation of rectal malignancy. When compared with surgical pathology reports, the accuracy of local staging has ranged from 62% to 91%.[122] In a study of 458 rectal cancer patients, an accuracy of 69% for T stage and 68% for N stage was identified. Moreover, it was found that T3 tumors were accurately staged most frequently (86%). Using a higher resolution machine improved results for the T1 tumors.[66]

Defecography
Defecography is a radiologic technique whereby the lower bowel is examined with the patient in the sitting or squatting position in the act of eliminating the barium. It has been recommended for the evaluation of individuals with irritable bowel syndrome, solitary rectal ulcer, rectal prolapse, proctalgia fugax, constipation, obstructed defecation (anismus), and internal procidentia (i.e., preprolapse).[12,30,74] It is for the last two conditions, however, that the technique is most usefully employed.

The procedure can be performed using a cineradiographic technique or simply by obtaining lateral spot films at different times during evacuation. Ekberg and colleagues reported 90 examinations performed on 83 patients with defecatory problems.[30] Whereas results of approximately one-third of the studies were normal, abnormalities such as intussusception, enterocele, proctocele, and fecal retention were clearly appreciated. This can be a valuable adjunctive study for assessing patients with defecation problems and should be included in the evaluation of these individuals before relegating them to the all-encompassing category of irritable bowel syndrome. However, confusion concerning interpretation and the significance of observed abnormalities still exists. In fact, there is a tendency to overinterpret every finding. This can lead to inappropriate treatment and unnecessary or unhelpful surgery. The technique and clinical applications of defecography are discussed in the appropriate chapters.

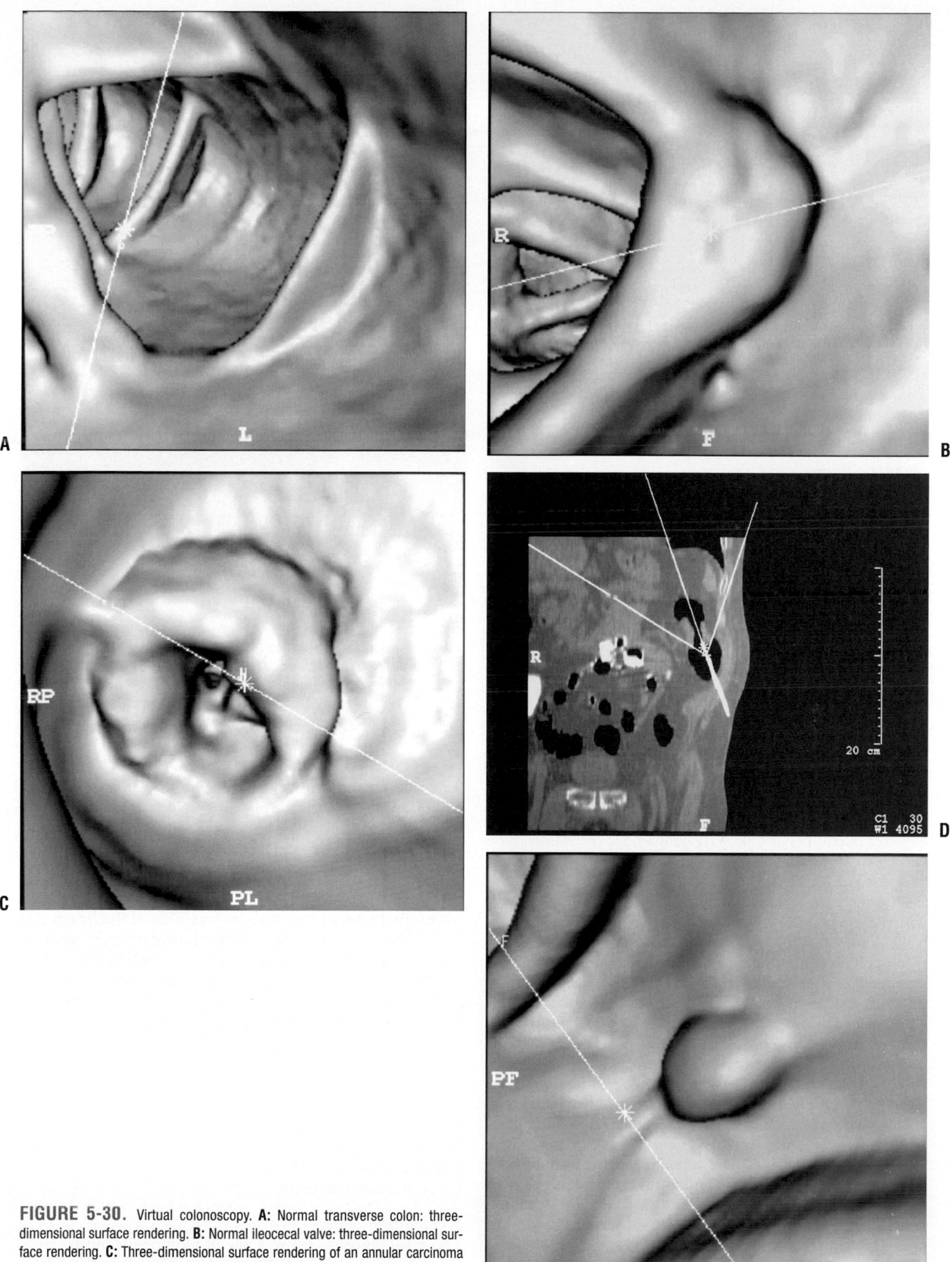

FIGURE 5-30. Virtual colonoscopy. **A:** Normal transverse colon: three-dimensional surface rendering. **B:** Normal ileocecal valve: three-dimensional surface rendering. **C:** Three-dimensional surface rendering of an annular carcinoma near the splenic flexure. **D:** Coronal view of annular carcinoma. **E:** Colonic polyp: three-dimensional surface rendering. (Courtesy of Victor J. Scarmato, MD.)

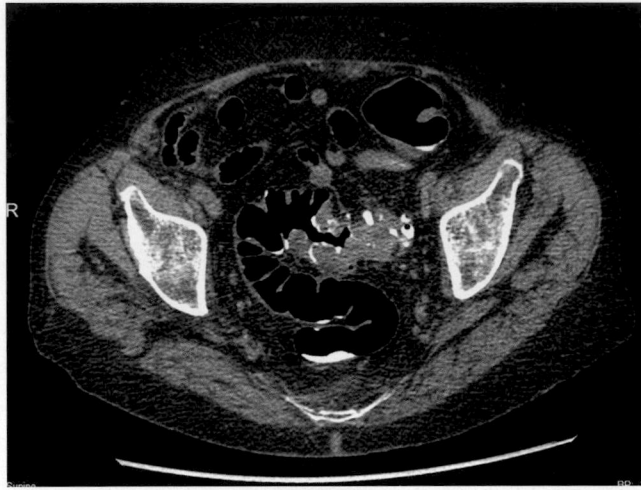

FIGURE 5-31. CT colonography (2D image) showing obstructing sigmoid colon mass. The patient could not undergo a complete colonoscopy because of this lesion.

Magnetic Resonance Imaging

Magnetic resonance imaging has become a very important diagnostic tool for colon and rectal conditions, especially for imaging the pelvis and for identifying normal and pathologic anorectal anatomy. As with endosonography, special application has been found for this modality in the evaluation of anorectal disease. Magnetic resonance imaging with endorectal coils can provide excellent imaging for anal and rectal cancer staging (including lymph nodes), fistula tracts, fluid collection and abscesses, and sphincteric defects (Figure 5-32).[133]

MRI is widely used for preoperative staging of rectal cancers. The technique uses gadolinium enhancement and is able to visualize the depth of penetration of the rectal cancer. It also reads lymph node metastases based on size criteria. Akasu and colleagues found an accuracy rate of 84% for transmural invasion, and 74% for mesorectal lymph node metastases by using high-resolution MRI and comparing the results with the pathologic diagnosis.[4] They also found an accuracy rate of 87% for lateral pelvic side wall lymph node metastasis. Kim and coworkers found that MRI provided an accuracy rate of 81% for T stage and 63% for N stage.[70] MRI was most accurate for more locally advanced disease. These results improve with the use of MRI with rectal coil, to 92% for T1–T2, 94% for T3, and 69% for N stage.[138] Addition of nodal enhancement with ultrasmall superparamagnetic iron oxide improved specificity of positive lymph nodes but did not change sensitivity when compared with standard MRI technique.[72]

In the last decade, magnetic resonance technology has been more widely used to evaluate the pelvic floor. MRI is being employed frequently for evaluation of anal sphincter defects and anal fistulas. In a study of 237 patients who underwent MRI and ultrasound evaluation for external anal sphincter defects followed by surgery, sensitivity and positive predictive values were 81% and 89%, respectively, for endoanal MRI and 90% and 85%, respectively, for endoanal ultrasound.[25] MR defecography is now able to be used to evaluate the pelvic floor during simulated defecation. Ultrasound gel is placed in the rectum to mimic stool. Images are then taken with the patient at rest and with feigned evacuation. An endoanal coil may be used during the same examination to obtain anatomic images of the pelvic floor.

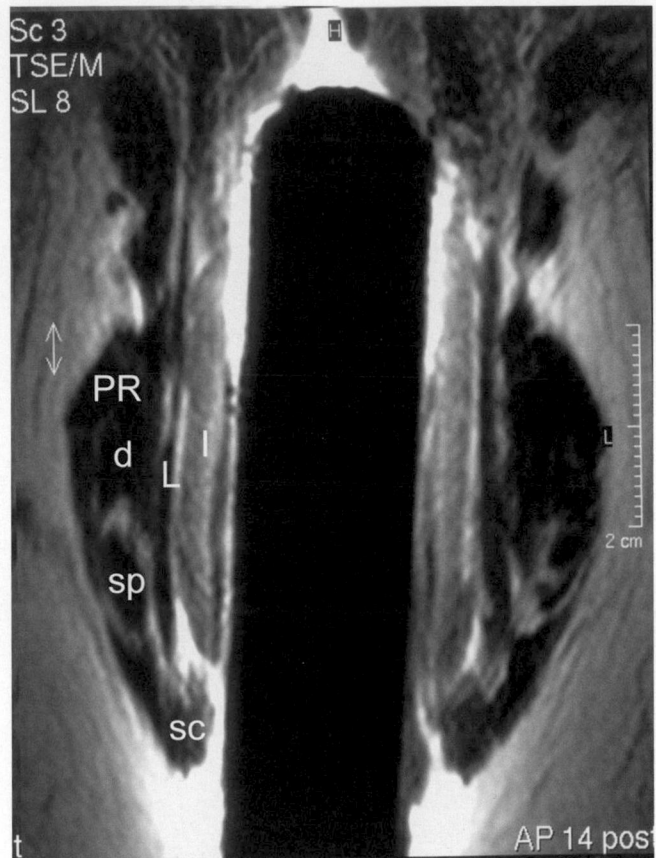

FIGURE 5-32. Endocoil magnetic resonance image of the anal canal in the coronal plane view. *I*, internal anal sphincter (moderate signal); *L*, longitudinal muscle (low signal); *PR*, puborectalis with *d*, deep part of the external anal sphincter; *sp*, superficial part; and *sc*, subcutaneous part. All the striated muscle is of low signal. The high signal on either side of the longitudinal muscle indicates a thin layer of fat. (Courtesy of Professor Clive Bartram, Harrow, United Kingdom.)

When compared with cinedefecography, MR defecography offers the advantage of being able to visualize pelvic floor muscle atrophy as well as other abnormalities, such as enterocele, cystocele, and uterine prolapse.[35,111]

Radiologic Evaluation of the Small Intestine

Although the small bowel represents 75% of the length and 90% of the mucosal surface of the alimentary tract, the incidence of small bowel disease is low.[86] For one to undertake a small bowel examination in every individual with complaints referable to the abdomen is generally a fruitless exercise. The following diseases often require imaging of the small intestine:

Crohn's disease
Polyposis
Unexplained iron-deficiency anemia
Unexplained GI bleeding
Diarrhea or steatorrhea
Unexplained abdominal pain
Fever of unknown origin

Small Bowel Series

The small bowel series was one of the first diagnostic techniques that became available to evaluate the small intestine. The small bowel is examined radiographically following

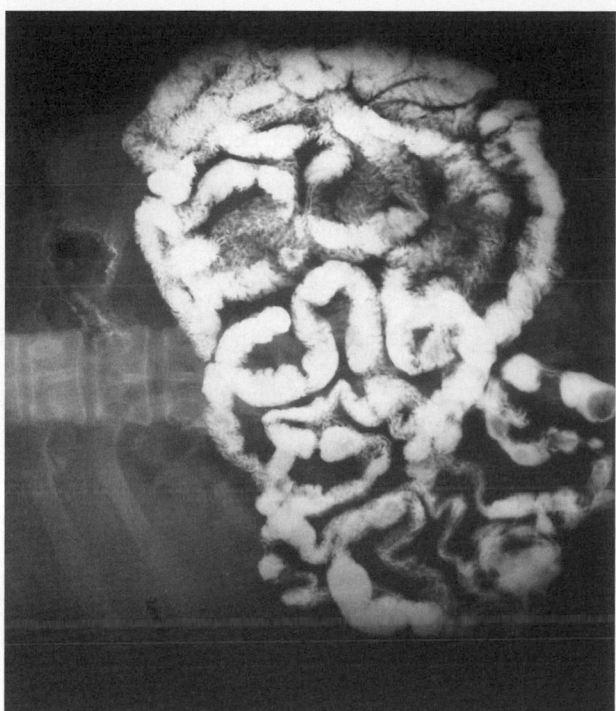

FIGURE 5-33. Small bowel series demonstrates normal mucosal pattern throughout. This is a study at 1.5 hours. The colon has not yet filled.

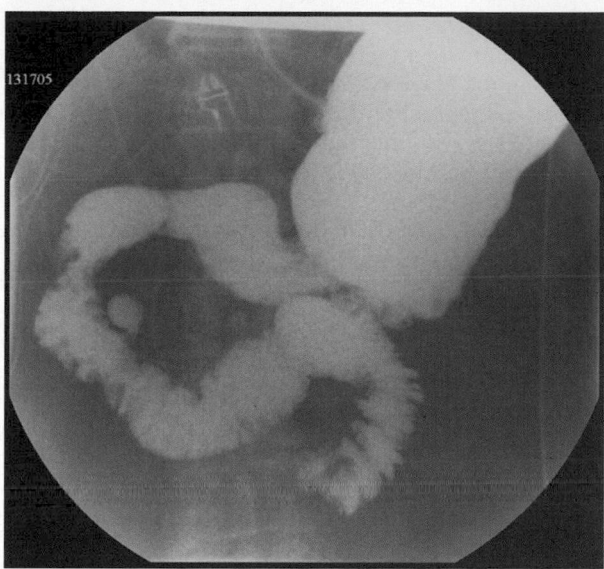

FIGURE 5-34. Small bowel series in postoperative patient demonstrating a small bowel obstruction in the proximal jejunum. Incidentally noted is a duodenal diverticulum.

administration of a mixture that is half barium sulfate and half water by mouth. A large volume of barium is especially helpful in interpretation of diffuse lesions of the small bowel. Compression studies are used whenever necessary for better delineation of a lesion, and they are routinely employed in demonstrating the terminal ileum.[89] Initially, the patient is examined fluoroscopically, and if the barium meal has progressed sufficiently, a film is taken. Further filming depends on the rate of passage of the barium and is usually performed once every 30 to 60 minutes until the material has reached the colon. In physiologically normal persons, the barium column may take from 2 hours to as long as 6 hours (Figure 5-33). The terminal ileum must always be compressed. This segment of bowel tends to be hidden by overlapping loops in the pelvis, and because it is the most frequent site of small bowel disease, special study is required. This is obviously particularly true in cases of Crohn's disease.

In cases of suspected perforation, fistula, or obstruction, the use of barium is contraindicated due to the risk of barium peritonitis. Under these circumstances, water-soluble contrast is administered. Although this contrast is not as sensitive for small mucosal abnormalities, because it becomes diluted by the time it reaches the distal bowel, it is very useful for identifying more obvious abnormalities, such as a fistula and obstruction (Figure 5-34).[59] It may be used to determine which patients with obstruction require urgent surgery or who will respond to nonoperative management.[63] It may even contribute to earlier resolution of partial small bowel obstructions, although the mechanism for this action is unclear.[1]

CT Enterography

CT enterography is becoming more frequently used in the place of small bowel series. It has the advantages of not only showing the abnormalities of the bowel lumen but also of

pathologic changes outside of the bowel. It is less operator dependent than small bowel series and permits better visualization of the distal ileum.[137] This is currently the recommended initial imaging study for the evaluation of newly diagnosed Crohn's disease according to the most recent American College of Radiology Appropriateness Criteria.[5]

The technique uses a multidetector CT scanner, intravenous contrast, and nonionic neutral oral contrast to distend the bowel wall. Patients must fast for 3 to 4 hours prior to the examination. In most protocols, they ingest approximately 1.5 L of neutral contrast over approximately 30 minutes in order to distend the small bowel and the stomach. Some protocols use water for at least part of this examination. Intravenous contrast is necessary in order to see mucosal enhancement. Intestinal wall thickening and mucosal enhancement are used to differentiate between acute and chronic inflammation, benign or neoplastic processes, edema, and ischemia, among other findings (Figure 5-35).[85]

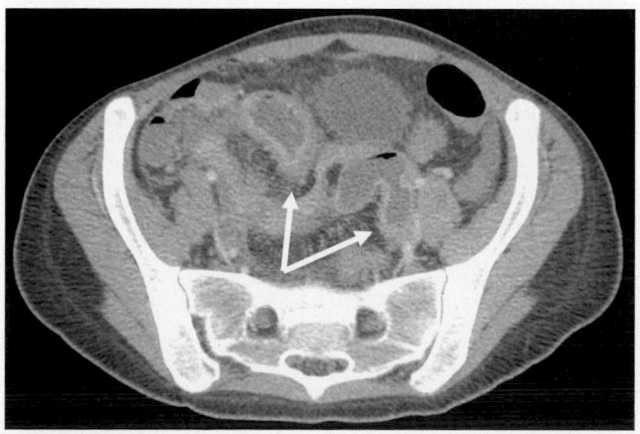

FIGURE 5-35. CT enterography showing active Crohn's disease of the ileum. Note the thickened bowel wall with mucosal enhancement with acute inflammation (*white arrows*).

MR Enterography

A new and emerging technique is MR enterography. In a study from the Mayo Clinic comparing the findings on CT and MR enterography in 30 Crohn's disease patients, the sensitivities of MR enterography and CT enterography for detecting active small bowel disease were similar (90.5% vs. 95.2%, respectively [$P = .32$]).[127] The image quality scores for MR enterography examinations were significantly lower than those for CT enterography ($P = .005$).

Enteroclysis

Enteroclysis is not used as frequently as it used to be but is included here for completeness. Enteroclysis involves the use of 250 mL of high-density barium. This is supplemented by methylcellulose, which acts to distend the small intestine. The material is inserted through a nasogastric tube with the tip of the small bowel ideally located at the ligament of Treitz. This permits a study equivalent to that of an air-contrast enema performed in the colon.

Enteroclysis has been the most accurate available technique for contrast examination of the small intestine. Its main advantage is that intubation beyond the pylorus bypasses its sphincteric restriction and makes possible the infusion of contrast material at a required rate.[54] There is the obvious disadvantage, however, of the need for intubation. The technique involves the infusion of a methylcellulose solution that follows the introduction of barium. The demonstration of small bowel detail is possible during single-contrast and double-contrast stages.[54] It should be remembered, however, that this technique is not the best method for evaluation of a problem related to the terminal ileal area.

CT and MR enteroclysis have been described. These techniques combine the enterography techniques described in the previous sections with duodenojejunal intubation for instillation of contrast. These procedures require sedation of the patient and are more invasive. They are, therefore, not recommended as first-line imaging techniques.[137]

Capsule Endoscopy

As implied, diseases affecting the small intestine are often difficult to diagnose because the traditional methods of radiology and endoscopy fail to provide a complete and accurate assessment of the entire organ. A newer and different concept has been developed to address this problem, that of capsule endoscopy. Introduced in 1998, the M2A Capsule Endoscopy Given Diagnostic System (Given Imaging, Ltd., Yoqneam, Israel; info@givenimaging.com) is a noninvasive diagnostic imaging device (Figure 5-36). An ingestible capsule device is equipped with a miniature video camera to visualize the small intestine (PillCam SB) and esophagus (PillCam ESO) for detection of damage or disease (Figure 5-37).

The capsule is swallowed and traverses the entire GI tract, transmitting color videos during its passage. The patient is fully ambulating and continues normal daily activities throughout the "endoscopic" examination. The smooth plastic capsule contains a miniature video camera and is equipped with a light source on one end, batteries, a radio transmitter, and antenna. After it is swallowed, the capsule transmits approximately

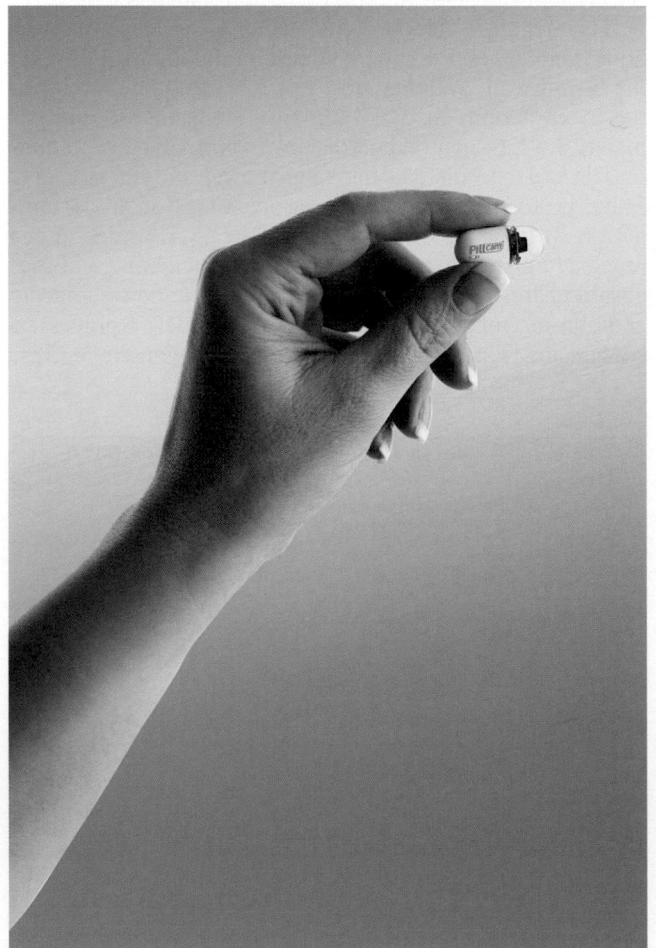

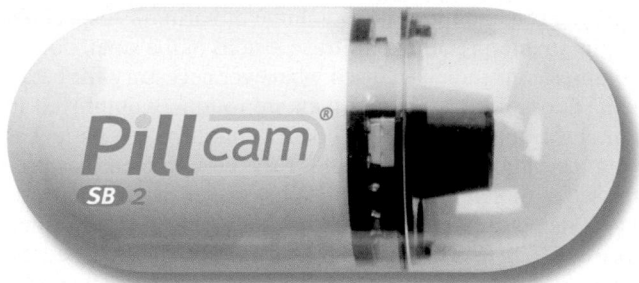

B

A

FIGURE 5-36. A: The PillCam SB video capsule measures 11 mm × 26 mm and weighs less than 4 g. **B:** PillCam SB 2 video capsule. (Courtesy of Given Imaging, Yoqneam, Israel.)

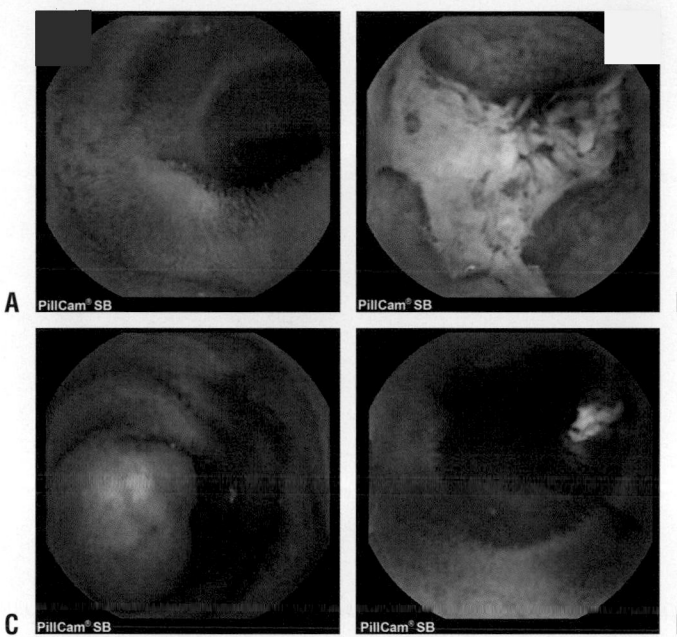

FIGURE 5-37. Capsule endoscopic appearance of small bowel lesions. **A:** Normal mucosa. **B:** Crohn's disease. **C:** Tumor. **D:** Hemorrhage. (Courtesy of Given Imaging, Yoqneam, Israel.)

50,000 images over the course of an 8-hour period (about two images per second) to a data recording device attached to a belt worn around the patient's waist. The small bowel images are then downloaded into a Given Workstation computer where a physician can review them in order to make a diagnosis. Once the patient swallows the capsule, he or she can continue with daily activities. The capsule is eliminated as a one-time use device. Numerous publications testify to the fact that capsule endoscopy is a valuable diagnostic tool for identifying Crohn's disease and bleeding lesions within the small bowel that could not be visualized by conventional imaging techniques.[29,34,55,82,121]

Positron Emission Tomography

The application of positron emission tomography (PET) for colorectal cancer was defined in 1982 and is based on the finding that the tracer 2-[^{18}F]fluoro-2-deoxy-D-glucose concentrates in malignant tissue as a consequence of increased glycolysis compared with the normal.[8,151] Whereas CT provides information on anatomy, PET specifically addresses metabolic or physiologic data. When used for the initial staging of colorectal cancer, PET alone is highly sensitive for detection of primary tumor and distant metastases but not for lymph node involvement.[65] However, when PET is combined with CT, the study affords an assessment of metabolic activity as well as spatial and anatomic relationships.

PET is a very expensive modality, with systems costing in the United States from $800,000 to $2.5 million and a cost per examination in the range of $2,000 (2001 figures).[8] The PET scan has its primary usefulness in the assessment of recurrent or metastatic colorectal cancer.[61]

Noninvasive Screening Methods for Colorectal Cancer

The commercially available guaiac-impregnated slide (Hemoccult II; Beckman Coulter, Inc., Fullerton, CA) has come to be used as the primary resource for this screening study. Guaiac is a chemical test for peroxidase activity that is present in both hemoglobin and certain foods.[117] Occult blood determination, however, is generally believed to be a suboptimal exercise unless strict dietary instructions are adhered to.[3] The real question is whether one wishes to substitute increased sensitivity for increased specificity. Interestingly, it has been shown that the method of stool collection affects the outcome of fecal occult blood testing. Stool obtained by digital rectal examination has a poorer positive predictive value for cancer and for polyps than stool obtained through routine screening.[94]

To increase the accuracy of the screening examination, the patient should be instructed to avoid rare meat, turnips, melons, horseradish, salmon, and sardines 48 hours prior to the collection of the first stool specimen in order to reduce the likelihood of false-positive determinations. A high-fiber diet is usually advised, but concern has been expressed that the increased fecal weight significantly lowers fecal hemoglobin concentration, with the implication of a false-negative result.[128] Medications such as aspirin and vitamin preparations, especially vitamin C (ascorbic acid) in excess of 250 mg/day, are excluded. Aspirin or other nonsteroidal anti-inflammatory drugs should be avoided for 7 days before and during the test period. The patient is then instructed to take stool samples from three consecutive bowel movements, smear some on the card, and then return the cards to the laboratory. If even one of the three cards is positive for occult blood, the physician then proceeds with more invasive studies, most commonly a colonoscopy. If the evaluation of the colon is negative, the upper gastrointestinal tract should be examined.[136]

Although Hemoccult is the most commonly used home screening test for occult blood, there are significant problems with compliance. Patients are reluctant to handle the stool or mail the cards. Delays in mailing the samples may lead to decreased sensitivity of the test as a consequence of false-negative results.[139] Problems with patient compliance and the high cost of false-positive results have stimulated the development of alternative screening approaches by other pharmaceutical companies. ColoCare (Helena Laboratories, Claremont, Ontario, Canada) and EZ Detect (Biomerica, Inc., Newport Beach, CA) are home detection products whose efficacy has not been clearly established. These generally involve placement of a specially prepared, chemically impregnated, biodegradable paper in the toilet bowl. The individual then observes the paper for a color change following defecation. An immunochemical test for occult stool human hemoglobin is also available (FlexSure OBT; Beckman Coulter, Inc.). Both this method and Hemoccult SENSA were compared in an endoscopic study by Rozen and colleagues to determine which to recommend for a population screening program.[117] Hemoccult SENSA had greater sensitivity, but FlexSure OBT had significantly greater specificity. A recent study from France found that the addition of the immunochemical test increased the sensitivity for neoplastic lesions in some anatomical locations more than others. The test was most useful for lesions in the rectum.[47]

Numerous reports of the beneficial results and cost-effectiveness of mass screening for colorectal cancer have been published.[38,44,45,51,52,73,95,99,104,118,130,135] Those patients found to harbor a malignant lesion usually have a much earlier stage tumor. Schnell and coworkers studied almost 30,000 individuals who returned their fecal blood test cards.[124] Eighty-two percent of all colorectal cancers that were detected by fecal occult blood testing were diagnosed at a favorable stage. However, the majority of known, advanced tumors (62%) escaped early detection by this method. The authors concluded that using this test alone may provide a false sense of security, especially in those individuals with advanced left-sided colorectal cancer.[124] Hardcastle and associates recruited approximately 75,000 individuals in a screening group and the same number as controls.[51] Of 893 cancers (20% stage Dukes' A) diagnosed in participants in the screening group, 26.4% were detected by fecal occult blood screening, 27.9% presented after a negative result on occult blood testing or investigation, and 44.8% presented in nonresponders. The incidence of cancer in the control group was 1.44 per 1,000 person-years. Three hundred sixty people died of colorectal cancer in the screening group, compared with 420 in the control group, a 15% reduction in cumulative colorectal cancer mortality by screening.[51] Leicester and colleagues studied 802 symptomatic patients with suspected colorectal disease.[79] There was good compliance (92.5%), and a high specificity for colorectal cancer was noted (85.4%). The false-positive rate was 8.6%, but the false-negative rate for rectal cancer was unacceptably high (45.4%). Of course, in these symptomatic patients, it is expected that at least a proctosigmoidoscopy would have been performed. Others have demonstrated that most known, advanced cases of colorectal cancer (62%) escape early detection with fecal occult testing.[124]

Given the poor sensitivity of this screening test, there is a need for new markers.[102] A variation on the theme of occult blood testing is the transferrin dipstick test, which was described by researchers in China.[126] They compared rates of positivity to immunochemical fecal occult blood testing and found significant differences in patients with advanced adenomas (72% vs. 44%, P < .05). Recently, work has also been done in detecting abnormal fecal DNA. Imperiale and colleagues compared results of Hemoccult II fecal test with a fecal DNA test, looking at abnormal DNA.[58] The fecal DNA panel detected 16 of 31 invasive cancers, whereas Hemoccult II identified 4 of 31 (51.6% vs. 12.9%, P = .003). When combining patients with invasive cancers and adenomas with high-grade dysplasia, the DNA panel detected 29 of 71 cases, whereas Hemoccult II identified 10 of 71 (40.8% vs. 14.1%, P < .001).[58]

A promising new marker is microRNA, which are small noncoding RNAs with posttranscriptional regulator functions.[123,142] Abnormal microRNAs are expressed in many types of cancers and may be involved in carcinogenesis.[123] These markers are actually found circulating in the blood and may eventually lead to a screening blood test, obviating the need for examining the stool at all.[57,97]

▶ FECES COLLECTION

Exfoliative Cytology

Exfoliative cytology has been recommended as a screening technique for the evaluation of iron-deficiency anemia, for early detection of colonic neoplasms, and to ascertain whether known lesions as determined by colonoscopy or roentgenography are benign or malignant.[109] The procedure involves a vigorous bowel cleansing.[10,28,100,109] Raskin and Pleticka advocate in-hospital evaluation to ensure such thoroughness.[110] Through a sigmoidoscope, a large diameter rubber catheter

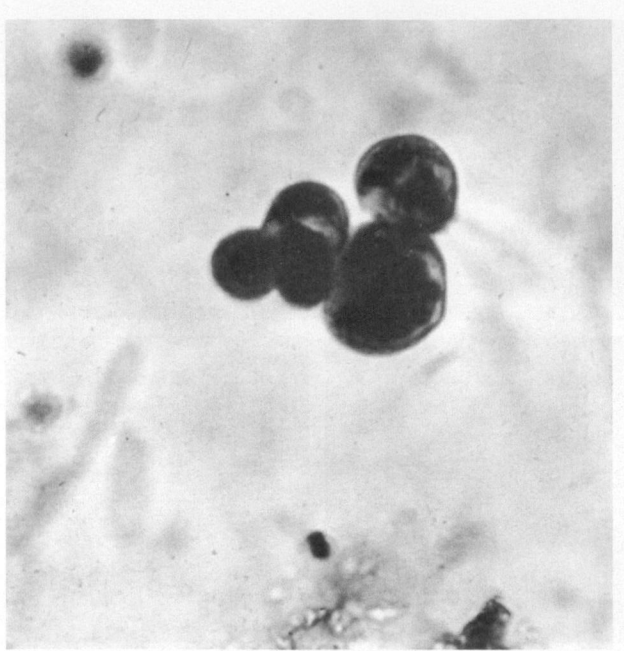

FIGURE 5-38. Exfoliative cytology demonstrates cancer cells in colonic washings (original magnification × 600). (Courtesy of Rudolf Garret, MD.)

is inserted and the instrument withdrawn. Irrigation is then carried out, usually by a trained technician, and slides are collected and reviewed by a pathologist (Figure 5-38).

Exfoliative cytology has never gained much acceptance, primarily because of the cumbersome methodology and the fact that colonoscopy is far superior for evaluation of the entire bowel. Outside of the veterinary population and for research, for all intents and purposes, this procedure has become obsolete.

Stool Culture (See also Chapter 33)

For stool culture, the stool should arrive in the laboratory within half an hour of having been taken unless it is placed in a transport medium. Refrigeration is contraindicated. Swabs should not be used for collection.

Stool cultures are made by placing a sterile swab into the specimen and streaking a portion of several agar plates containing various inhibitory and noninhibitory agents in order to allow the recovery of both intestinal flora and pathogenic organisms (e.g., *Salmonella*, *Shigella*, *Campylobacter*). The plates are examined at 24 hours, and suspect colonies are inoculated into identification media.

Certain organisms are somewhat unusual and difficult to identify in a stool specimen. A specific request is usually necessary for their culture because they require special techniques. These organisms include fungi (the test is generally limited to screening for *Candida*), *Mycobacterium*, pathogenic *Vibrio* (i.e., cholera), *Campylobacter*, and *Yersinia*. The discovery of certain organisms mandates reporting to the public health authority.

Stool Examination for Ova and Parasites (See also Chapter 33)

The specimen must be less than 1 hour old when received by the laboratory. Three specimens are recommended for screening over a 5-day period. Collection can be made by using a warm saline solution or Fleet enema. Bismuth, mineral oil, castor oil, psyllium, and magnesium compounds used as laxatives produce specimens that are unsatisfactory for evaluation. Also, stools should not be collected if a barium study has been performed within 1 week.

Stool specimens for parasites are examined macroscopically for color and appearance (e.g., formed or liquid, with mucus or blood). They are also checked for adult worms or tapeworm proglottids.

A wet-mount preparation of stool on a glass slide with a drop each of saline solution and iodine is cover slipped and examined microscopically for evidence of parasites (e.g., eggs, cysts, larvae) as well as for fecal leukocytes. A small portion of the specimen is also treated to concentrate the eggs and cysts and later examined microscopically with wet mounts. Finally, a slide is streaked, trichrome stained, and examined histologically with the oil immersion lens. For the diagnosis and treatment of a specific pathologic organism and disease, see the Index.

▶ FLEXIBLE SIGMOIDOSCOPY AND COLONOSCOPY

See Chapter 6.

▶ PHYSIOLOGIC STUDIES

See Chapter 7.

References

1. Abbas S, Bisset IP, Parry BR. Oral water soluble contrast for the management of adhesive small bowel obstruction. *Cochrane Database Syst Rev.* 2007;3:CD004651.
2. Adami B, Eckardt VF, Suermann RB, et al. Bacteremia after proctoscopy and hemorrhoidal injection sclerotherapy. *Dis Colon Rectum.* 1981;24(5):373–374.
3. Ahlquist DA, Wieand HS, Moertel CG, et al. Accuracy of fecal occult blood screening for colorectal neoplasia. A prospective study using Hemoccult and HemoQuant tests. *JAMA.* 1993;269(10):1262–1267.
4. Akasu T, Iinuma G, Takawa M, et al. Accuracy of high-resolution magnetic resonance imaging in preoperative staging of rectal cancer. *Ann Surg Oncol.* 2009;16(10):2787–2794.
5. American College of Radiology. ACR appropriateness criteria 2008. http://www.acr.org. Accessed.
6. American Society of Colon and Rectal Surgeons. Practice parameters for antibiotic prophylaxis to prevent infective endocarditis or infected prosthesis during colon and rectal endoscopy. The American Society of Colon and Rectal Surgeons. *Dis Colon Rectum.* 1992;35(3):277.
7. Angelelli G, Ianora AA, Scardapane A, et al. Role of computerized tomography in the staging of gastrointestinal neoplasms. *Semin Surg Oncol.* 2001;20(2):109–121.
8. Arulampalam TH, Costa DC, Loizidou M, et al. Positron emission tomography and colorectal cancer. *Br J Surg.* 2001;88(2):176–189.
9. ASGE Standards of Practice Committee, Banerjee S, Shen B, et al. Antibiotic prophylaxis for GI endoscopy. *Gastrointest Endosc.* 2008;67(6):791–798.
10. Bader GM, Papanicolaou GN. The application of cytology in the diagnosis of cancer of the rectum, sigmoid, and descending colon. *Cancer.* 1952;5(2):307–314.
11. Barloon TJ, Shumway J. Medical malpractice involving radiologic colon examinations: a review of 38 recent cases. *AJR Am J Roentgenol.* 1995;165(2):343–346.
12. Bartolo DC, Roe AM, Virjee J, et al. Evacuation proctography in obstructed defaecation and rectal intussusception. *Br J Surg.* 1985;72(suppl):S111–S116.
13. Baxter NN, Rothenberger DA, Lowry AC. Measuring fecal incontinence. *Dis Colon Rectum.* 2003;46(12):1591–1605.
14. Burnikel RH. Barium granuloma: an anorectal complication of barium enema x-ray studies. *Dis Colon Rectum.* 1962;5:224–227.
15. Cannon WB. The movements of the stomach studied by means of the Röntgen rays. *Am J Physiol.* 1898;1:360.
16. Cannon WB. The movements of the intestines studied by means of the Röntgen rays. *Am J Physiol.* 1901/1902;6:251–277.
17. Cannon WB, Moser A. The movements of the food in the esophagus. *Am J Physiol.* 1898;1:435–444.
18. Carrascosa P, Castiglioni R. Virtual colonoscopy: experience after 350 studies. *Dis Colon Rectum.* 2001;44:A5–A26.
19. Cazemier M, Terra MP, Stoker J, et al. Atrophy and defects detection of the external anal sphincter: comparison between three-dimensional anal endosonography and endoanal magnetic resonance imaging. *Dis Colon Rectum.* 2006;49(1):20–27.
20. Cordone RP, Brandeis SZ, Richman H. Rectal perforation during barium enema: report of a case. *Dis Colon Rectum.* 1988;31(7):563–569.
21. de Feiter PW, Soeters PB, Dejong CH. Rectal perforations after barium enema: a review. *Dis Colon Rectum.* 2006;49(2):261–271.
22. Dickinson VA. Maintenance of anal continence: a review of pelvic floor physiology. *Gut.* 1978;19(12):1163–1174.
23. Dickman MD, Farrell R, Higgs RH, et al. Colonoscopy associated bacteremia. *Surg Gynecol Obstet.* 1976;142(2):173–176.
24. Dobben AC, Terra MP, Deutekom M, et al. Anal inspection and digital rectal examination compared to anorectal physiology tests and endoanal ultrasonography in evaluating fecal incontinence. *Int J Colorectal Dis.* 2007;22(7):783–790.
25. Dobben AC, Terra MP, Slors JF, et al. External anal sphincter defects in patients with fecal incontinence: comparison of endoanal MR imaging and endoanal US. *Radiology.* 2007;242(2):463–471.
26. Durack DT. Prevention of infective endocarditis. *N Engl J Med.* 1995;332(1):38–44.
27. Dysart DN. Angled sigmoid view. In: Greenbaum EI, ed. *Radiographic Atlas of Colon Disease.* Chicago, IL: Year Book; 1980:31.
28. Ebeling WC, Little JW. The demonstration of malignant cells exfoliated from the proximal colon. *Ann Intern Med.* 1957;46(1):21–29.
29. Ellaklin R, Fischer D, Suissa A, et al. Wireless capsule video endoscopy is a superior diagnostic tool in comparison to barium follow-through and computerized tomography in patients with suspected Crohn's disease. *Eur J Gastroenterol Hepatol.* 2003;15(4):363–367.
30. Ekberg O, Nylander G, Fork FT. Defecography. *Radiology.* 1985;155(1):45–48.
31. Farmer KC, Church JM. Open sesame: tips for traversing the anal canal. *Dis Colon Rectum.* 1992;35(11):1092–1093.
32. Fenlon HM. Virtual colonoscopy. *Br J Surg.* 2002;89(1):1–3.
33. Fielding JF, Lumsden K. Large-bowel perforations in patients undergoing sigmoidoscopy and barium enema. *Br Med J.* 1973;1(5851):471–473.
34. Fireman Z, Mahajna E, Broide E, et al. Diagnosing small bowel Crohn's disease with wireless capsule endoscopy. *Gut.* 2003;52(3):390–392.
35. Fletcher JG, Busse RF, Riederer SJ, et al. Magnetic resonance imaging of anatomic and dynamic defects of the pelvic floor in defecatory disorders. *Am J Gastroenterol.* 2003;98(2):399–411.
36. Frühmorgen P, Bodem F, Reidenbach HD, et al. Endoscopic laser coagulation of bleeding gastrointestinal lesions with report of the first therapeutic application in man. *Gastrointest Endosc.* 1976;23(2):73–75.
37. Fry RD, Shemesh EI, Kodner IJ, et al. Perforation of the rectum and sigmoid colon during barium-enema examination. Management and prevention. *Dis Colon Rectum.* 1989;32(9):759–764.
38. Fujita M, Sugiyama R, Kumanishi Y, et al. Evaluation of effectiveness of mass screening for colorectal cancer. *World J Surg.* 1990;14(5):648–652.
39. Gear EV Jr, Dobbins WO 3d,+DOBBINS III: rectal biopsy. A review of its diagnostic usefulness. *Gastroenterology.* 1968;55(4):522–544.
40. Gelfand DW, Chen MY, Ott DJ. Preparing the colon for the barium enema examination. *Radiology.* 1991;178(3):609–613.
41. Gelfand DW, Ott DJ. Single- vs. double-contrast gastrointestinal studies: critical analysis of reported statistics. *AJR Am J Roentgenol.* 1981;137(3):523–528.
42. Gilbertsen VA. Proctosigmoidoscopy and polypectomy in reducing the incidence of rectal cancer. *Cancer.* 1974; 34(3 suppl):936–939.
43. Gourtsoyiannis N, Grammatikakis J, Prassopoulos P. Role of conventional radiology in the diagnosis and staging of gastrointestinal tract neoplasms. *Semin Surg Oncol.* 2001;20(2):91–108.
44. Greegor DH. Occult blood testing for detection of asymptomatic colon cancer. *Cancer.* 1971;28(1):131–134.
45. Greegor DH. A progress report. Detection of colorectal cancer using guaiac slides. *CA Cancer J Clin.* 1972;22(6):360–363.

46. Grobmyer AJ III, Kerlan RA, Peterson CM, et al. Barium peritonitis. *Am Surg*. 1984;50(2):116–120.

47. Guittet L, Bouvier V, Mariotte N, et al. Comparison of a guaiac and an immunochemical faecal occult blood test for the detection of colonic lesions according to lesion type and location. *Br J Cancer*. 2009;100(8):1230–1235.

48. Hakim NS, Sarr MG, Bender CE, et al. Management of barium enema-induced colorectal perforation. *Am Surg*. 1992;58(11):673–676.

49. Halligan S, Fenlon HM. Virtual colonoscopy. *BMJ*. 1999;319(7219): 1249–1252.

50. Han SY, Tishler JM. Perforation of the colon above the peritoneal reflection during the barium-enema examination. *Radiology*. 1982; 144(2):253–255.

51. Hardcastle JD, Chamberlain JO, Robinson MH, et al. Randomised controlled trial of faecal-occult-blood screening for colorectal cancer. *Lancet*. 1996;348(9040):1472–1477.

52. Hardcastle JD, Thomas WM, Chamberlain J, et al. Randomised, controlled trial of faecal occult blood screening for colorectal cancer. Results for first 107,349 subjects. *Lancet*. 1989;1(8648):1160–1164.

53. Harned RK, Consigny PM, Cooper NB, et al. Barium enema examination following biopsy of the rectum or colon. *Radiology*. 1982;145(1):11–16.

54. Herlinger H. Guide to imaging of the small bowel. *Gastroenterol Clin North Am*. 1995;24(2):309–329.

55. Herrerías JM, Caunedo A, Rodríguez-Téllez M, et al. Capsule endoscopy in patients with suspected Crohn's disease and negative endoscopy. *Endoscopy*. 2003;35(7):564–568.

56. Hoffman BI, Kobasa W, Kaye D. Bacteremia after rectal examination. *Ann Intern Med*. 1978;88(5):658–689.

57. Huang Z, Huang D, Ni S, et al. Plasma microRNAs are promising novel biomarkers for early detection of colorectal cancer. *Int J Cancer*. 2010;127(1):118–126.

58. Imperiale TF, Ransohoff DF, Itzkowitz SH, et al. Fecal DNA versus fecal occult blood for colorectal-cancer screening in an average-risk population. *N Engl J Med*. 2004;351(26):2704–2714.

59. Jobling C, Halligan S, Bartram C. The use of non-ionic water-soluble contrast agents for small bowel follow-through examination. *Eur Radiol*. 1999;9(4):706–710.

60. Johnson CD, Chen MH, Toledano AY, et al. Accuracy of CT colonography for detection of large adenomas and cancers. *N Eng J Med*. 2008; 359(12):1207–1217.

61. Johnson K, Bakhsh A, Young D, et al. Correlating computed tomography and positron emission tomography scan with operative findings in metastatic colorectal cancer. *Dis Colon Rectum*. 2001;44(3):354–357.

62. Jorge JM, Wexner SD. Etiology and management of fecal incontinence. *Dis Colon Rectum*. 1993;36(1):77–97.

63. Joyce WP, Delaney PV, Gorey TF, et al. The value of water-soluble contrast radiology in the management of acute small bowel obstruction. *Ann R Coll Surg Engl*. 1992;74(6):422–425.

64. Kahn SP, Lindenauer SM, Wojtalik RS. Perforation of the normal colon during barium contrast examination. *Am Surg*. 1976;42(10): 789–792.

65. Kantorová I, Lipská L, Bělohlávek O, et al. Routine (18)F-FDG PET preoperative staging of colorectal cancer: comparison with conventional staging and its impact on treatment decision making. *J Nucl Med*. 2003;44(11):1784–1788.

66. Kauer WK, Prantl L, Dittler HJ, et al. The value of endosonographic rectal carcinoma staging in routine diagnostics: a 10-year analysis. *Surg Endosc*. 2004;18(7):1075–1078.

67. Kelley CJ, Ingoldby CJ, Blenkharn JI, et al. Colonoscopy related endotoxemia. *Surg Gynecol Obstet*. 1985;161(4):332–334.

68. Khan JS, Moran BJ. Iatrogenic perforation at colonic imaging. *Colorectal Dis*. 2011;13(5):481–493.

69. Kim DH, Pickhardt PJ, Taylor AJ, et al. CT colonography versus colonoscopy for the detection of advanced neoplasia. *N Engl J Med*. 2007; 357(14):1403–1412.

70. Kim NK, Kim MJ, Park JK, et al. Preoperative staging of rectal cancer with MR: accuracy and clinical usefulness. *Ann Surg Oncol*. 2000;7(10):732–737.

71. Knutson CO, Williams HC, Max MH. Detection of intracolonic lesion by barium contrast enema. The importance of adequate colon preparation to diagnostic accuracy. *JAMA*. 1979;242(20):2206–2208.

72 Koh DM, George C, Temple L, et al. Diagnostic accuracy of nodal enhancement pattern of rectal cancer at MRI enhanced with ultrasmall superparamagnetic iron oxide: findings in pathologically matched mesorectal lymph nodes. *AJR Am J Roentgenol*. 2010;194(6):W505–W513.

73. Kronborg O, Fenger C, Olsen J, et al. Randomised study of screening for colorectal cancer with faecal-occult-blood test. *Lancet*. 1996;348(9040): 1467–1471.

74. Kuijpers HC, Bleijenberg G. The spastic pelvic floor syndrome. A cause of constipation. *Dis Colon Rectum*. 1985;28(9):669–672.

75. Kumar S, Abcarian H, Prasad ML, et al. Bacteremia associated with lower gastrointestinal endoscopy, fact of fiction? I. Colonoscopy. *Dis Colon Rectum*. 1982;25(2):131–134.

76. Laufer I. The radiologic demonstration of early changes in ulcerative colitis by double contrast technique. *J Can Assoc Radiol*. 1975;26(2):116–121.

77. Laufer I, Mullens JE, Hamilton J. Correlation of endoscopy and double-contrast radiography in the early stages of ulcerative and granulomatous colitis. *Radiology*. 1976;118(1):1–6.

78. LeFrock JL, Ellis CA, Turchik JB, et al. Transient bacteremia associated with sigmoidoscopy. *N Engl J Med*. 1973;289(9):467–469.

79. Leicester RJ, Lightfoot A, Millar J, et al. Accuracy and value of the Hemoccult test in symptomatic patients. *Br Med J(Clin Res Ed)*. 1983;286(6366):673–674.

80. Levin B, Lieberman DA, McFarland B, et al. Screening and surveillance for the early detection of colorectal cancer and adenomatous polyps, 2008: a joint guideline from the American Cancer Society, the US Multi-Society Task Force on Colorectal Cancer, and the American College of Radiology. *CA Cancer J Clin*. 2008;58(3):130–160.

81. Li VK, Wexner SD, Pulido N, et al. Use of routine intraoperative endoscopy in elective laparoscopic colorectal surgery: can it further avoid anastomotic failure? *Surg Endosc*. 2009;23(11):2459–2465.

82. Liangpunsakul S, Chadalawada V, Rex DK, et al. Wireless capsule endoscopy detects small bowel ulcers in patients with normal results from state of the art enteroclysis. *Am J Gastroenterol*. 2003;98(6): 1295–1298.

83. Lull GF Jr, Bryne JP, Sanowski RA. Barium sulfate granuloma of the rectum. A rare entity. *JAMA*. 1971;217(8):1102–1103.

84. Macari M, Berman P, Dicker M, et al. Usefulness of CT colonography in patients with incomplete colonoscopy. *AJR Am J Roentgenol*. 1999; 173(3):561–564.

85. Macari M, Megibow AJ, Balthazar EJ. A pattern approach to the abnormal small bowel: observations at MDCT and CT enterography. *AJR Am J Roentgenol*. 2007;188(5):1344–1355.

86. Maglinte DD, Kelvin FM, O'Connor K, et al. Current status of small bowel radiography. *Abdom Imaging*. 1996;21(3):247–257.

87. Majarakis JD, Portes C. Proctosigmoidoscopy-incidence of polyps in 50,000 examinations. *J Am Med Assoc*. 1957;163(6):411–413.

88. Margulis AR. Is double-contrast examination of the colon the only acceptable radiographic examination? *Radiology*. 1976;119(3):741–742.

89. Marshak RH, Lindner AE. *Radiology of Small Intestine*. Philadelphia, PA: WB Saunders; 1978:1–8.

90. Martel W, Robins JM. The barium enema: technique, value, and limitations. *Cancer*. 1971;28(1):137–143.

91. Miller RE, Chernish SM, Skucas J, et al. Hypotonic colon examination with glucagon. *Radiology*. 1974;113(3):555–562.

92. Millward SF, Chapman A, Somers S, et al. Rectal biopsy as a cause of rectal ulceration. *Radiology*. 1985;156(1):42.

93. Murad-Regadas SM, Regadas FS, Rodrigues LV, et al. The role of 3-dimensional anorectal ultrasonography in the assessment of anterior transsphincteric fistula. *Dis Colon Rectum*. 2010;53(7):1035–1040.

94. Nakama H, Zhang B, Fattah ASM, et al. Does stool collection method affect outcomes in immunochemical fecal occult blood testing? *Dis Colon Rectum*. 2001;44(6):871–875.

95. Nakama H, Zhang B, Zhang X, et al. Age-related cancer detection rate and costs for one cancer detected in one screening by immunochemical fecal occult blood test. *Dis Colon Rectum*. 2001;44(11):1696–1699.

96. Nelson RL, Abcarian H, Prasad ML. Iatrogenic perforation of the colon and rectum. *Dis Colon Rectum*. 1982;25(4):305–308.

97. Ng EK, Chong WW, Jin H, et al. Differential expression of microRNAs in plasma of patients with colorectal cancer: a potential marker for colorectal cancer screening. *Gut*. 2009;58(10):1375–1381.

98. Nivatvongs S, Fryd DS. How far does the proctosigmoidoscope reach? A prospective study of 1000 patients. *N Engl J Med*. 1980;303(7): 380–382.

99. Nivatvongs S, Gilbertsen VA, Goldberg SM, et al. Distribution of large-bowel cancers detected by occult blood test in asymptomatic patients. *Dis Colon Rectum*. 1982;25(5):420–421.

100. Oakland DJ. The diagnosis of carcinoma of the colon by exofoliative cytology. *Proc R Soc Med*. 1964;57:279–282.

101. Oren D, Atamanalp S, Aydinli B, et al. An algorithm for the management of sigmoid colon volvulus and the safety of primary resection: experience with 827 cases. *Dis Colon Rectum*. 2007;50(4):489–497.

102. Ottó S, Eckhardt S. Early detection for colorectal cancer: new aspects in fecal occult blood screening. *J Surg Oncol*. 2000;75(3):220–226.

103. Peterson N, Rohrmann CA Jr, Lennard ES. Diagnosis and treatment of retroperitoneal perforation complicating the double-contrast barium-enema examination. *Radiology.* 1982;144(2):249–252.

104. Petrelli NJ, Palmer M, Michalek A, et al. Massive screening for colorectal cancer. A single institution's public commitment. *Arch Surg.* 1990;125(8):1049–1051.

105. Pickhardt PJ, Choi JH. Electronic cleansing and stool tagging in CT colonography: advantages and pitfalls with primary three-dimensional evaluation. *AJR Am J Roentgenol.* 2003;181(3):799–805.

106. Pineau BC, Paskett ED, Chen GJ, et al. Virtual colonoscopy using oral contrast compared with colonoscopy for the detection of patients with colorectal polyps. *Gastroenterology.* 2003;125(2):304–310.

107. Rabin DN, Smith C, Witt TR, et al. Voice change after barium enema: a clinical sign of extraperitoneal colon perforation. *AJR Am J Roentgenol.* 1987;148(1):145–146.

108. Ransohoff DF, Lang CA. Screening for colorectal cancer. *N Engl J Med.* 1991;325(1):37–41.

109. Raskin HF, Palmer WL, Kirsner JB. Exfoliative cytology in diagnosis of cancer of the colon. *Dis Colon Rectum.* 1959;2(1):46–57.

110. Raskin HF, Pleticka S. Exfoliative cytology of the colon. Fifteen years of lost opportunity. *Cancer.* 1971;28(1):127–130.

111. Rentsch M, Paetzel C, Lenhart M, et al. Dynamic magnetic resonance imaging defecography: a diagnostic alternative in the assessment of pelvic floor disorders in proctology. *Dis Colon Rectum.* 2001;44(7):999–1007.

112. Ricciardi R, Roberts PL, Marcello PW, et al. Anastomotic leak testing after colorectal resection: what are the data? *Arch Surg.* 2009;144(5):407–411.

113. Richardson NG, Heriot AG, Kumar D, et al. Abdominal ultrasonography in the diagnosis of colonic cancer. *Br J Surg.* 1998;85(4):530–533.

114. Robinson RJ, Stone M, Mayberry JF. Sigmoidoscopy and rectal biopsy: a survey of current UK practice. *Eur J Gastroenterol Hepatol.* 1996;8(2):149–151.

115. Rodriguez W, Levine JS. Enterococcal endocarditis following flexible sigmoidoscopy. *West J Med.* 1984;140(6):951–953.

116. Rosen L. Physical examination of the anorectum: a systematic technique. *Dis Colon Rectum.* 1990;33(5):439–440.

117. Rozen P, Knaani J, Samuel Z. Comparative screening with a sensitive guaiac and specific immunochemical occult blood test in an endoscopic study. *Cancer.* 2000;89(1):46–52.

118. Saito H. Screening for colorectal cancer: current status in Japan. *Dis Colon Rectum.* 2000;43(10 suppl):S78–S84.

119. Salazar M, Jackman RJ. Reasons for incomplete proctoscopy. *Dis Colon Rectum.* 1969;12(1):19–21.

120. Sands J. Quoted by: Masel H, Masel JP, Casey KV. A survey of colon examination techniques in Australia and New Zealand, with a review of complications. *Australas Radiol.* 1971;15(2):140–147.

121. Scapa E, Jacob H, Lewkowicz S, et al. Initial experience of wireless-capsule endoscopy for evaluating occult gastrointestinal bleeding and suspected small bowel pathology. *Am J Gastroenterol.* 2002;97(11):2776–2779.

122. Schaffzin DM, Wong WD. Endorectal ultrasound in the preoperative evaluation of rectal cancer. *Clin Colorectal Cancer.* 2004;4(2):124–132.

123. Schepeler T, Reinert JT, Ostenfeld MS, et al. Diagnostic and prognostic microRNAs in stage II colon cancer. *Cancer Res.* 2008;68(15):6416–6424.

124. Schnell T, Aranha GV, Sontag SJ, et al. Fecal occult blood testing: a false sense of security? *Surgery.* 1994;116(4):798–802.

125. Seaman WB, Wells J. Complications of the barium enema. *Gastroenterology.* 1965;48:728–737.

126. Sheng JQ, Li SR, Wu ZT, et al. Transferrin dipstick as a potential novel test for colon cancer screening: a comparative study with immuno fecal occult blood test. *Cancer Epidemiol Biomarkers Prev.* 2009;18(8):2182–2185.

127. Siddiki HA, Fidler JL, Fletcher JG, et al. Prospective comparison of state-of-the-art MR enterography and CT enterography in small-bowel Crohn's disease. *AJR Am J Roentgenol.* 2009;193(1):113–121.

128. Slavin JL, Melcher EA, Sundeen M, et al. Effects of high-fiber diet on fecal blood content (HemoQuant assay) in healthy subjects. *Dig Dis Sci.* 1991;36(7):929–932.

129. Sohn N, Robilotti JG Jr. The gay bowel syndrome. A review of colonic and rectal conditions in 200 male homosexuals. *Am J Gastroenterol.* 1977;67(5):478–484.

130. Sontag SJ, Durczak C, Aranha GV, et al. Fecal occult blood screening for colorectal cancer in a Veterans Administration Hospital. *Am J Surg.* 1983;145(1):89–94.

131. Standards Task Force, American Society of Colon and Rectal Surgeons. Practice parameters for antibiotic prophylaxis to prevent infective endocarditis or infected prosthesis during colon and rectal endoscopy. The Standards Task Force. The American Society of Colon and Rectal Surgeons. *Dis Colon Rectum.* 2000;43(9):1193.

132. Stewart J, Finan PJ, Courtney DF, et al. Does a water soluble contrast enema assist in the management of acute large bowel obstruction: a prospective study of 117 cases. *Br J Surg.* 1984;71(10):799–801.

133. Stoker J, Rociu E, Wiersma TG, et al. Imaging of anorectal disease. *Br J Surg.* 2000;87(1):10–27.

134. Swinton NW. Polyps of rectum and colon. *J Am Med Assoc.* 1954;54(8):658–662.

135. Tate JJ, Northway J, Royle GT, et al. Faecal occult blood testing in symptomatic patients: comparison of three tests. *Br J Surg.* 1990;77(5):523–526.

136. Thomas WM, Hardcastle JD. Role of upper gastrointestinal investigations in a screening study for colorectal neoplasia. *Gut.* 1990;31(11):1294–1297.

137. Tochetto S, Yaghmai V. CT enterography: concept, technique, and interpretation. *Radiol Clin North Am.* 2009;47(1):117–132.

138. Torricelli P, Lo Russo S, Pecchi A, et al. Endorectal coil MRI in local staging of rectal cancer. *Radiol Med.* 2002;103(1–2):74–83.

139. van Rossum LG, van Rijn AF, van Oijen MG, et al. False negative fecal occult blood tests due to delayed sample return in colorectal cancer screening. *Int J Cancer.* 2009;125(4):746–750.

140. Vining D, Gelfand D. Noninvasive colonoscopy using helical CT scanning, 3D reconstruction and virtual reality. Paper presented at: The Meeting of the Society of Gastrointestinal Radiologists; February 13–18, 1994; Maui, HI.

141. Vining D, Gelfand D, Bechtold R. Technical feasibility of colon imaging with helical CT and virtual reality. *AJR Am J Roentgenol.* 1994; 162(suppl):104.

142. Wang YX, Zhang XY, Zhang BF, et al. Initial study of microRNA expression profiles of colonic cancer without lymph node metastasis. *J Dig Dis.* 2010;11:50–54.

143. Welin S. Results of the Malmö technique of colon examination. *JAMA.* 1967;199(6):369–371.

144. Welin S. Newer diagnostic techniques: the superiority of double-contrast roentgenology. *Dis Colon Rectum.* 1974;17(1):13–20.

145. Wheatley MJ, Eckhauser FE. Portal venous barium intravasation complicating barium enema examination. *Surgery.* 1991;109(6):788–791.

146. Wilson W, Taubert KA, Gewitz M, et al. Prevention of infective endocarditis: guidelines from the American Heart Association: a guideline from the American Heart Association Rheumatic Fever, Endocarditis and Kawasaki Disease Committee, Council on Cardiovascular Disease in the Young, and the Council on Clinical Cardiology, Council on Cardiovascular Surgery and Anesthesia, and the Quality of Care and Outcomes Research Interdisciplinary Working Group. *Circulation.* 2007;116(15):1736–1754.

147. Winawer SJ, Fletcher RH, Miller L, et al. Colorectal cancer screening: clinical guidelines and rationale. *Gastroenterology.* 1997;112(2):594–642.

148. Winawer SJ, Stewart ET, Zauber AG, et al. A comparison of colonoscopy and double-contrast barium enema for surveillance after polypectomy. National Polyp Study Work Group. *N Engl J Med.* 2000;342(24):1766–1772.

149. Yamamura M, Nishi M, Furubayashi H, et al. Barium peritonitis. Report of a case and review of the literature. *Dis Colon Rectum.* 1985;28(5):347–352.

150. Yee J, Akerkar GA, Hung RK, et al. Colorectal neoplasia: performance characteristics of CT colonography for detection in 300 patients. *Radiology.* 2001;219(3):685–692.

151. Yonekura Y, Benua RS, Brill AB, et al. Increased accumulation of 2-deoxy-2-[18F]Fluoro-D-glucose in liver metastases from colon carcinoma. *J Nucl Med.* 1982;23(12):1133–1137.

152. Yudis M, Cohen A, Pearce AE. Perforation of the transverse colon during barium enema and air-contrast studies. *Am Surg.* 1968;34(5): 334–336.

6

Flexible Sigmoidoscopy and Colonoscopy

Chris E. Lascarides

One look is worth a thousand listens.

—APHORISM

The ability to visualize the colon, rectum, and anus has essentially paralleled the precision with which the surgeon has been able to diagnose and treat individuals with diseases of this area of the digestive tract. In the mid-19th century, visualization was accomplished by means of a hollow tube illuminated by a candle and focused with a parabolic mirror. However, examination of the entire colon had not been possible prior to the introduction of x-rays (see Chapter 5). Although improved radiologic techniques facilitated the accuracy of colonic diagnoses, distal bowel visualization was limited to that which could be accomplished with the rigid proctosigmoidoscope. Illumination was provided by a lightbulb within the instrument or directed to the tip by means of straight fibers (see Chapter 5).

The origin of flexible endoscopy of the colon began with the introduction of semirigid and then flexible upper gastrointestinal instruments (esophagogastroscopy). Hopkins and Kapany are generally credited with describing the initial flexible fiberscope, in 1954.[84] Subsequently, a major improvement in the quality of light transmission was made with the establishment of a glass-coated fiber that permitted the transmission of illumination along nonlinear paths. When combined with a similar fiber bundle whose orientation was preserved, the illuminated image could be transmitted back to the observer. Initially, the technology was applied to the stomach, but this was quickly adapted to the colon. Short, flexible fiberoptic instrument examinations of the rectum and distal colon were performed, but soon longer instruments were developed, usually with the use of

gastroscopes applied to the bowel. It came to be appreciated, however, that successful colonic examination often required more forceful manipulation than was necessary for upper gastrointestinal endoscopy. Consequently, the later versions of the colonoscope that evolved were longer and more robust (see later).

A later advance in instrumentation has been the introduction of videoendoscopy. The image-transmitting fiberoptic bundle has been replaced by a charged coupled device that provides an electronic image of the field of view. The examiner no longer has to contend with broken fiber bundles and progressive degradation of the endoscopic picture. Furthermore, the endoscopist no longer needs to squint into the lens at the end of the instrument but can instead work directly from a high-resolution monitor. In addition, the digitized image can be handled like any electronic file: stored, printed, and annotated. This has proved to be a clearly superior method of record keeping and documentation.

▶ FLEXIBLE FIBEROPTIC SIGMOIDOSCOPY AND VIDEOENDOSCOPY

The term *endoscope* is derived from two Greek words: *endon*, meaning within, and *skopein*, to view. With the fiberoptic sigmoidoscope, the diameters of the individual glass fibers in the image-conveying aligned bundles are similar, ranging from 9 to 12 μm.[50] The individual fibers are bound together at their ends, whereas the rest of the fibers remain loose and flexible. The fiberoptic endoscope can be made as long as necessary because light loss is negligible over several meters.[50]

There is no doubt that flexible sigmoidoscopy (FS) inspects more bowel surface area than is possible with the rigid proctosigmoidoscope. Marks and associates reached 50 cm or more in approximately two-thirds of their patients.[107] The overall yield of pathology was more than three times greater with the flexible instrument. Wherry and Thomas recruited more than 4,000 asymptomatic patients in a screening program using FS.[171] Eleven carcinomas were detected, an overall rate of 3.2 per 1,000 subjects screened. Others also report considerable satisfaction in this regard,[14,21,59,134,174] but the length of bowel examined is often considerably less than it might appear. For example, Lehman and colleagues determined the anatomic extent of insertion by placing a clip on the bowel mucosa and subsequently identifying that point on a barium enema study.[101] A so-called 60-cm examination viewed the entire sigmoid in only 81% of patients. It is also important to recognize that if an individual were to undergo subsequent barium enema study, regardless of the endoscopic findings, there would be no appreciable difference between rigid proctosigmoidoscopy and FS in the incidence of detection of neoplasms.[152] This presupposes, of course, that the barium enema examination is of optimal quality (see Chapter 5).

FS is not a simple examination to master. The most difficult part of colonoscopy is negotiation of the sigmoid colon, and this problem pertains equally to FS; the only difference perhaps is that the physician does not usually employ various straightening maneuvers, although this can be accomplished if necessary (see Colonoscopy). The examination requires skill and patience, and there is no substitute for experience. To paraphrase Hedberg, "If only we could omit the first 100 endoscopies and begin with number 101, a more comprehensive examination would be obtained, and we would experience very few complications indeed" (S. E. Hedberg, personal communication,).

In addressing the assertion that the procedure is more comfortable than rigid proctosigmoidoscopy, this may be more a reflection of patient position than of the examination. As mentioned in Chapter 5, the lateral Sims' position is preferred for patient comfort, and this is the recommended approach for FS. The examination does, however, take longer; approximately one-half of the procedures took more than 5 minutes in a series by Marks and associates.[107] It has been shown, in fact, that women who have undergone hysterectomy have more difficult, painful, and more limited examinations.[4] Analgesia (i.e., conscious sedation) should perhaps be considered in this group of patients. With excessive air insufflation, gas cramping tends to persist for a much longer period following FS. The list here illustrates some real and theoretical disadvantages to this examination:

Cost
    Capital expense and repairs
    Personnel time for enema administration and/or bowel
      cleansing
    Duration
Communicable disease
Complications
    Perforation
    Hemorrhage with concomitant procedure
    Explosion with electrocautery
    Infection
    Compromise of adequate colon examination when colonoscopy is indicated

The first and most often quoted criticism of the technique is the cost of the equipment, which may exceed $15,000, including light source and accessories. In addition to the outlay for the capital expense and repairs, there are the costs of personnel (e.g., longer time for examination, need for cleansing the instrument, patient preparation). Of course, a critical consideration is the cost to the patient. In polling numerous medical centers and physicians, the fee for the examination ranged from a minimum of 25% more than for rigid proctosigmoidoscopy to as much as 200% more.

FS is an advance over rigid proctosigmoidoscopy as a screening tool, but it is not a substitute for colonic assessment. When a complete evaluation of the colon is indicated, such as when occult blood is present or when polyps have been documented, colonoscopy is the requisite procedure. There is, however, a place for rigid sigmoidoscopy. This technique is often preferred when a large biopsy is required, when a distal anastomosis needs to be visualized, when a culture needs to be obtained, or when an inflammatory disease is confined to the rectum.

FS is indicated in the following situations:

- As a substitute for rigid proctosigmoidoscopy in screening, in evaluation of gastrointestinal complaints, and in interim polyp and cancer surveillance between colonoscopic examinations for distal disease
- For evaluation of questionable radiologic findings in the sigmoid colon
- For confirmation of radiographic findings within range of the instrument
- For diagnostic and follow-up evaluation of a patient with inflammatory bowel disease, especially if the disease is confined to the left or distal colon
- For inspection of colon anastomosis when it is within range of the instrument

Therapeutically, FS may be employed to reduce sigmoid volvulus and in combination with the snare to remove a foreign body. Absolute contraindications to this examination include fulminant colitis, toxic megacolon, peritonitis, and acute diverticulitis. A poorly prepared bowel and an uncooperative patient are certainly limiting factors.

Instrumentation

The flexible fiberoptic sigmoidoscope is available in the United States through several companies (Olympus America [Melville, NY], Pentax [Orangeburg, NY], Fujinon [Wayne, NJ], and Vision Sciences [Natick, MA]). The specifications of the instruments vary somewhat among the manufacturers. Generally, the channel size ranges between 2.6 and 3.8 mm, the instrument diameter varies from 12.2 to 14.0 mm, and lengths range from 60 to 71 cm. Figure 6-1 illustrates a flexible fiberoptic sigmoidoscope, and a close-up view of the bending section is shown in Figure 6-2. Biopsy forceps, a cytology brush, or a snare and electrocautery may be passed through the working channel (Figure 6-3). The tip of the instrument is deflected by rotation of the larger dial in each direction (Figure 6-4). The smaller dial deflects the tip from side to side. If both dials are turned maximally, it produces a tight bend that causes the instrument to double back and impede further passage. When passing the instrument, it is advantageous to keep the dials in the neutral position as much as possible (see Colonoscopy).

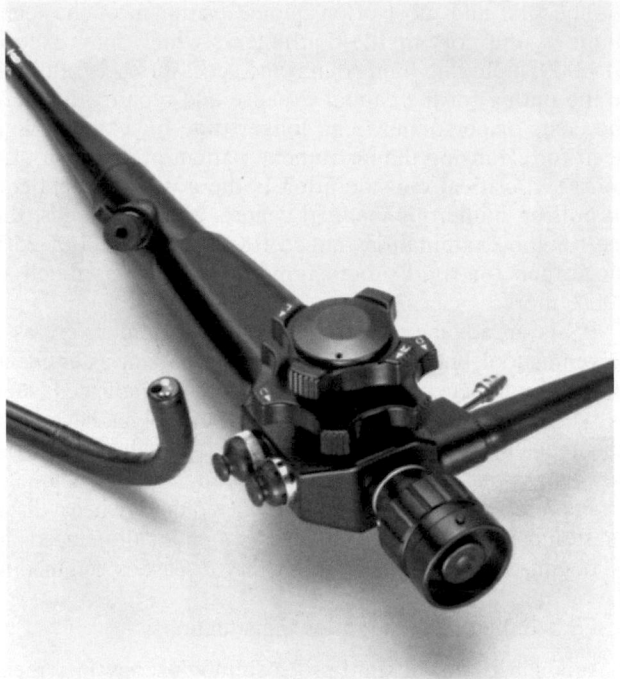

FIGURE 6-1. Pentax slim model (11.5-mm diameter) fiberoptic sigmoidoscope (model FS-34P2) with 70-cm working length. (Courtesy of Pentax Precision Instrument Corp., Orangeburg, NY.)

The 35-cm flexible instrument should be mentioned, especially regarding the relative merits of this shorter diagnostic endoscope. As a tool for screening, there seems to be little difference between the two fiberoptic instruments with respect to identification of neoplasms.[48,74] Furthermore, patients report that examination with the shorter instrument is, not surprisingly, more comfortable. I see, however, no

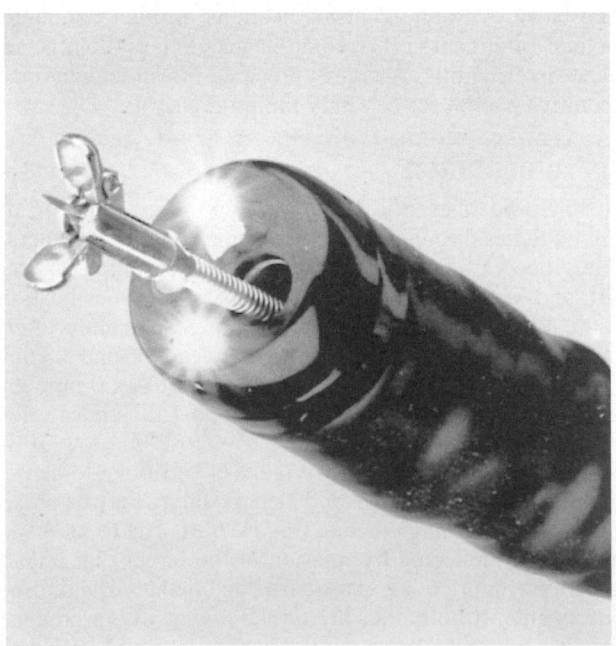

FIGURE 6-2. Close-up of the bending section with biopsy forceps of a fiberoptic sigmoidoscope (model CF-P20S). Channel size is 3.2 mm; diameter is 12.20 mm. (Courtesy of Olympus America, Melville, NY.)

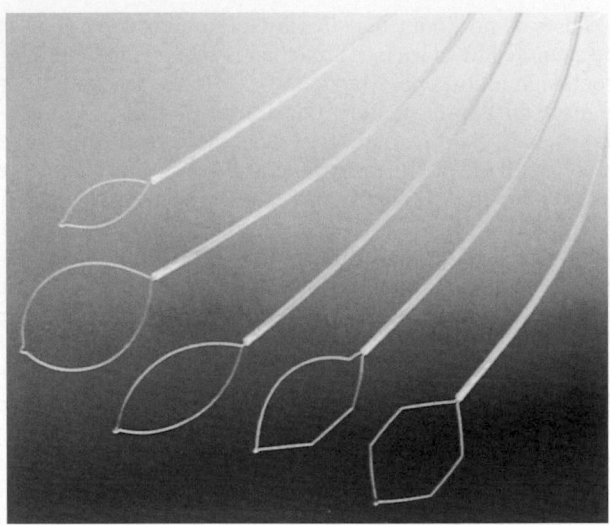

FIGURE 6-3. Variety of Captivator snares. (Courtesy of Microvasive, Boston Scientific Corp., Watertown, MA.)

great advantage in limiting the area of colon to be screened, and, in fact, with increased experience of the examiner, the length of time to perform the procedure should not be significantly different. The 35-cm flexible sigmoidoscope will in all probability be employed almost exclusively by the nonsurgeon and nonspecialist endoscopist.

Preparation

The use of FS requires only a limited bowel preparation. Two small enemas (e.g., Fleet) are given separately, the second approximately 10 minutes after the first has been eliminated. Dietary restrictions and oral laxatives are generally unnecessary. In some cases, oral preparations may be beneficial.

Technique

The patient is placed in the left lateral (Sims' position) on a relatively high-examining table. The patient's right leg is flexed more than the left, and the right shoulder is rotated anteriorly. It is usually easier for the physician to stand than to sit. Some physicians prefer a two-person team approach: one to handle the dials and the other to advance the instrument. Members of this school believe that in this way the procedure can be carried out much more expeditiously. This approach requires the use of a fiberoptic teaching attachment or videoendoscope (Figure 6-5). Conversely, most individuals believe that a single person should maneuver the dials with one hand and guide the instrument with the other, thereby permitting a more facile straightening maneuver. As a consequence, this may offer a more comfortable experience for the patient. The concept of discomfort has been addressed in a paper by Palakanis and colleagues on the effect of music therapy with individuals undergoing FS.[129] Not surprisingly, the authors discovered that those who listened to self-selected music tapes during the procedure had significantly decreased anxiety inventory measurements (State-Trait Anxiety Inventory). Furthermore, they had statistically significantly reduced heart rates and decreased arterial blood pressures in comparison with control subjects. The authors concluded that music

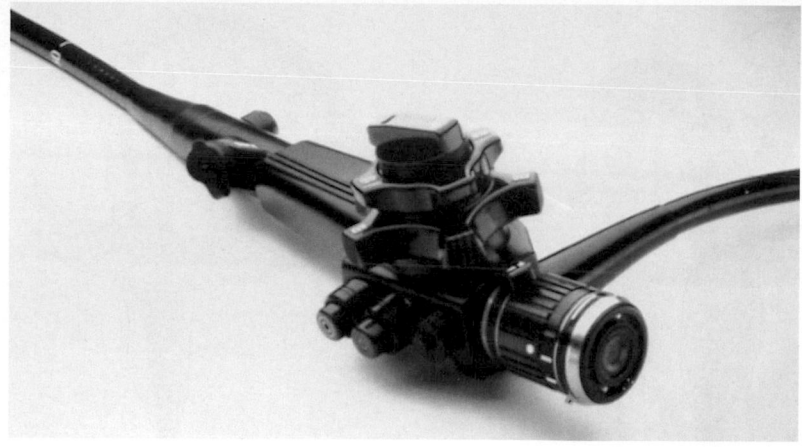

FIGURE 6-4. The control unit of the CF-P20S model fiberoptic sigmoidoscope has a maximum tip deflection of 180 degrees vertically, 160 degrees horizontally. (Courtesy of Olympus America, Melville, NY.)

is a very effective anxiolytic for the patient who undergoes FS.[129]

A well-lubricated finger is passed into the rectum, and then the instrument is inserted. Passing the blunt-ended endoscope through the anal canal without prior digital examination is difficult to accomplish and leads to considerable apprehension and discomfort for the patient.

What is usually encountered initially is a dull pink or orange haze, perhaps with some fecal debris or retained enema fluid. While insufflating air rather than redirecting the tip, the examiner passes the instrument to a depth of 10 or 12 cm. This will permit visualization of the rectal ampulla.

The instrument is passed with the lumen seen either under direct visualization or with the mucosa seen sliding past. Again, the endoscopist can judge how firmly to push while watching the mucosa rush by. This approach is quite similar to that applicable to rigid proctosigmoidoscopy, but this maneuver is not preferable to luminal visualization and must be undertaken with great caution.

If further passage is impeded, the instrument is withdrawn slightly, the lumen is searched out by dial manipulation and rotation, and the instrument is advanced again. Coller has described in detail various methods helpful in advancing the instrument. He calls them torquing, dithering, and dither-torquing (i.e., accordionization; see later).[32] By using the approach of dithering—the principle by which a person sitting on a chair with feet raised can move

it across the floor through abrupt, jerking motions of the body—staccato movements of the instrument forward and backward may permit the bowel virtually to intubate itself onto the instrument.[32]

Negotiation of the sigmoid colon is the most difficult part of the procedure. With an intended limited examination, straightening the sigmoid is, perhaps, of less importance than it is with colonoscopy. If all the physician accomplishes, however, is to stretch the colon through attempts at advancement, another maneuver must be tried. Counterclockwise rotation of the instrument produces the alpha loop (Figure 6-6). Clockwise rotation results in relative straightening of the sigmoid and the opportunity to advance the instrument into the descending colon. Sedation may be required to accomplish this, but this is usually not available for office examination. Another means of proceeding into the descending colon when the sigmoid loop has already been traversed is to withdraw the instrument while rotating it clockwise.

After the instrument has been passed to its full length or as far as is possible, it is carefully and slowly withdrawn. Suction, irrigation, and air insufflation are alternately employed as indicated to obtain clear visualization of the entire mucosa. Biopsy without electrocoagulation or brush cytology is obtained if appropriate, and the instrument is removed. It is important to remember that FS and colonoscopy are suboptimal tools for evaluation of ampullary or distal rectal disorders. Particular care is required for examination of this area, and retroflexion is strongly recommended as the ultimate maneuver (Figure 6-7).

Rectal Retroflexion

The importance of rectal retroflexion (RR) has been emphasized by Hanson and colleagues.[78] They compared 480 patients who had undergone FS without RR with a subsequent examination wherein RR was employed routinely. Discomfort precluded completion of this maneuver in 3.5%. There was a 1% increased yield of identifiable adenomas when RR was performed.[78]

The technique for accomplishing RR has been well described[78]:

- Advance the shaft approximately 10 cm above the mucocutaneous junction.
- Maximally deflect the shaft upward.
- Advance the instrument an additional 5 to 10 cm against the rectal fold.

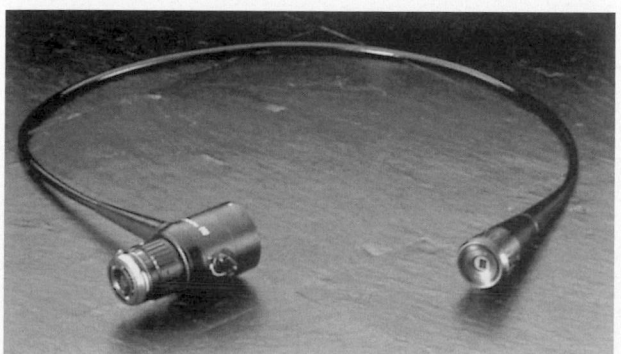

FIGURE 6-5. Fiberoptic teaching attachment, model LS-10. (Courtesy of Olympus America, Melville, NY.)

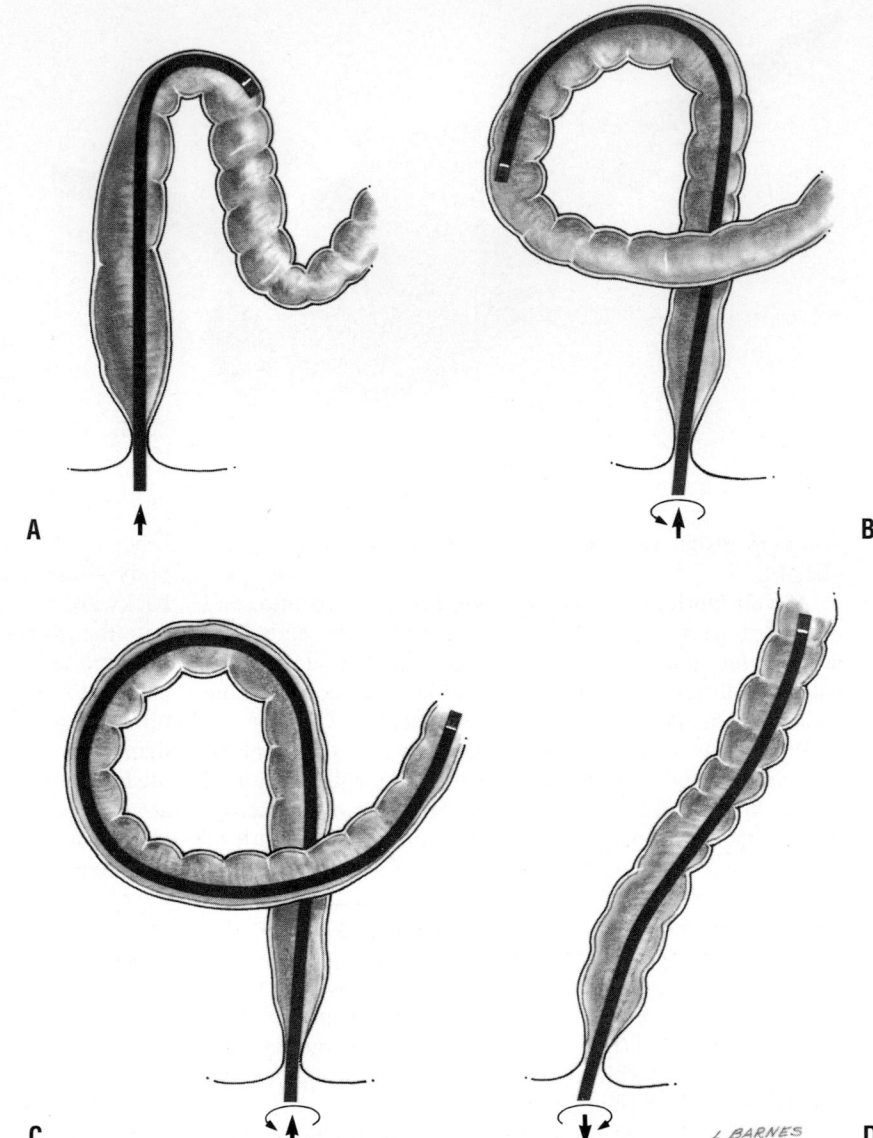

FIGURE 6-6. Alpha loop maneuver. **A:** The instrument is advanced into the sigmoid colon. **B:** Counterclockwise rotation during advancement results in the loop. **C:** The sigmoidoscope enters the descending colon. **D:** Clockwise torque during withdrawal permits straightening of the sigmoid colon.

- Rotate the retroflexed shaft to view the circumference of the anorectal junction.

Finally, the physician must not forget why the examination was being performed in the first instance. If bleeding were the indication, it is not sufficient to reassure the patient that FS was normal. Furthermore, the flexible sigmoidoscope is not the optimal tool for diagnosing pruritus ani, hemorrhoids, or fissure and obviously is not the ideal instrument for evaluating the anal canal (Figure 6-8). Anoscopy and additional studies may be required.

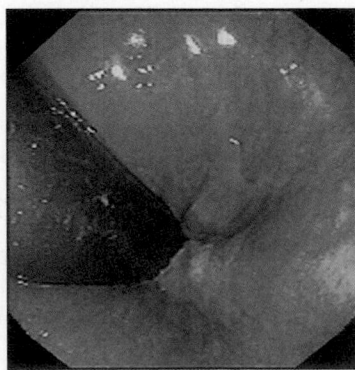

FIGURE 6-7. Retroflexion of the flexible sigmoidoscope.

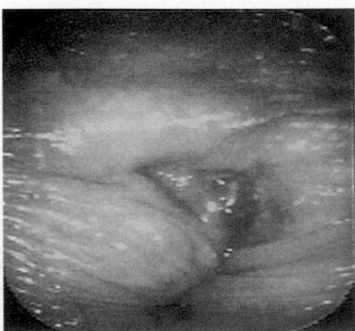

FIGURE 6-8. Anal fissure can be seen with the flexible sigmoidoscope. However, this is not the optimal way for making the diagnosis.

Gastroenterologists, however, because they do not generally perform anoscopy, seem quite comfortable with using FS and colonoscopy with RR as a diagnostic instrument for anal disorders. Although this is the standard of care for this specialty, anal lesions can be missed or misinterpreted if anoscopy is not performed when certain anal problems are suspected.

Videoendoscopy

In 1983, the Welch Allyn Corporation (Skaneateles Falls, NY) introduced a special feature for viewing the gastrointestinal tract, the videoendoscope. The endoscopic images are transmitted by a small electronic chip known as a charged coupled device.[142] Other companies have since entered the field, each producing video screen imagery with the ability to videotape examinations; to produce remote hard copy; and, of course, to serve as an excellent teaching modality (Figure 6-9). Information can be displayed on the monitor (i.e., patient's name, physician's name, pertinent history) to create a useful database for retrieval purposes.[148] Figure 6-10 shows the basic equipment. With the cost in excess of $75,000, this method is employed primarily in teaching centers and in endoscopy units, especially wherein there are numbers of patients sufficient to justify considerable capital investment. An attachment for converting the fiberoptic output to a video screen is also available (Figure 6-11). Their principles of passage are identical to those of FS with the fiberoptic instrument.

Complications of Flexible Sigmoidoscopy

Complications such as hemorrhage or perforation should not occur with any greater frequency with a flexible instrument than with the rigid, especially if the examiner does not force its passage—at least there are no randomized, clinical trials that demonstrate a difference. However, if an alpha or a straightening maneuver is undertaken, it is possible for the sigmoid colon to be torn and a perforation to occur. Attention to limiting patient discomfort is therefore an important concern. Furthermore, caution is obviously required whenever the procedure is undertaken in the presence of bowel disease. Depending on the acuteness of the process, especially with active inflammation, diverticulitis, or ischemia, FS may be

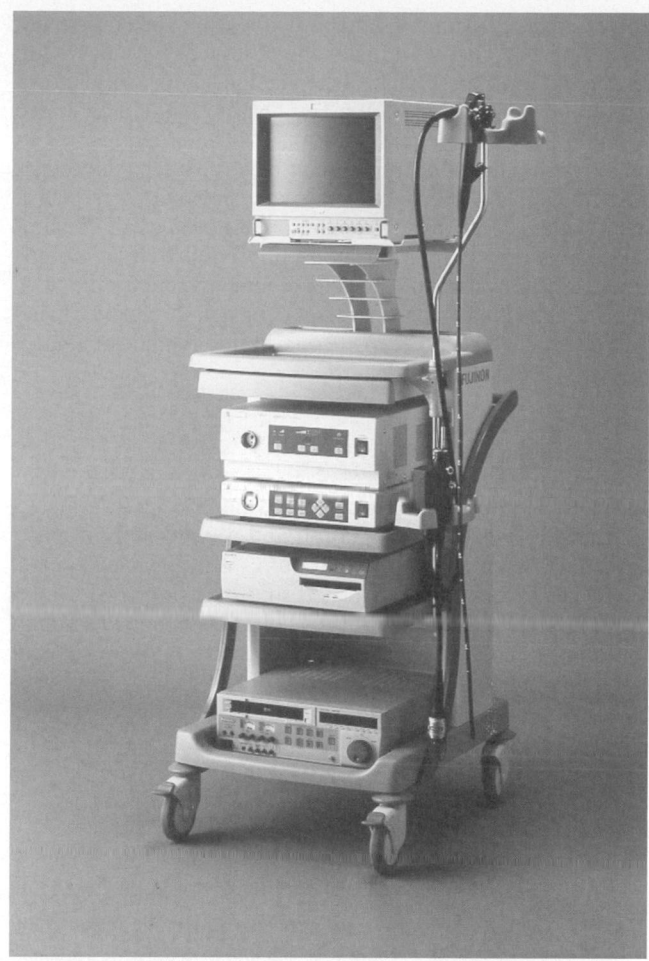

FIGURE 6-10. Videoendoscope system with colonoscope, light source, processor, and monitor. Remote switching gives the endoscopist the power to freeze images and to activate a number of hard copy devices. (Courtesy of Olympus America, Melville, NY.)

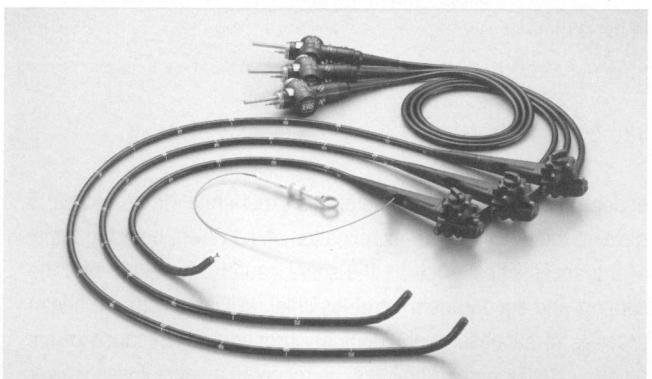

FIGURE 6-9. Videosigmoidoscope (73 cm [model CF-Q160S]) and videocolonoscopes (in two lengths: 133 cm [model CF-Q1601] and 168 cm [model CF-Q160L]). (Courtesy of Olympus America, Melville, NY.)

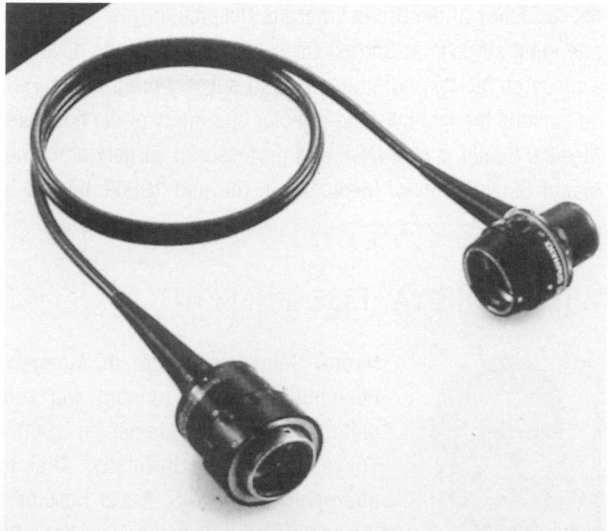

FIGURE 6-11. A direct video converter will convert standard endoscopic images for video–monitor viewing. (Courtesy of Olympus America, Melville, NY.)

contraindicated. Minimal air should be used when inflammation is present. Care should also be observed, especially with respect to insufflation of air, when an individual has a known inguinal hernia. Incarceration and obstruction of a herniated sigmoid colon from overdistension has been reported.[172] Explosions should not occur because electrocautery should not be employed for biopsy or snare excision with this instrument, unless a full bowel preparation has been used. The limited bowel preparation that is usually employed, combined with a closed system, presents a potential hazard for the presence of an explosive gas mixture. Biopsies should be carried out only with "cold" forceps. Brush cytology may, of course, be safely employed.

▶ COLONOSCOPY

In 1969, fiberoptic colonoscopy was introduced as a means of directly visualizing the colon and rectum and, in many instances, even the terminal ileum. Within a few years, Wolff and Shinya demonstrated that by using a wire loop snare and electrocautery, polyps could be removed through the instrument, thus virtually rendering colotomy and polypectomy obsolete.[175]

Instrumentation

As mentioned earlier, there are numerous suppliers of colonoscopes in the United States, most of which use similar optical or video structures. The instruments vary mainly in length, total diameter, and maneuverability and have a number of accessories. Working lengths vary from approximately 115 cm to almost 180 cm. They are forward viewing and may offer a field of view up to 160 degrees (Figure 6-12). Newer endoscopic systems additionally offer high-definition output for an even higher level of clarity on compatible monitors. Some individuals prefer a two-channel system in order to use two accessories for treatment, including that of polypectomy (Figure 6-13). As with FS, four-way angulation of the distal end is achieved from approximately 180 degrees up or down and 160 degrees right and left by manipulating the control knobs (Figure 6-4). Additional features include an air outlet, a forward water jet channel, and a suction/forceps channel. Air or carbon dioxide can be insufflated and liquid debris removed during the procedure. Accessories include a halogen light source (Figure 6-14) and an electrosurgical unit (Figure 6-15), as well as photographic equipment. Requisite items for procedures include biopsy forceps, a diathermy

WILLIAM IRWIN WOLFF (1916–2011)

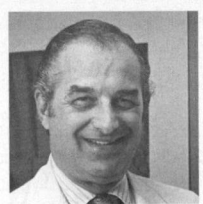

William Wolff was born in New York City and attended the University of Maryland School of Medicine, where he received the Prize Gold Medal. He then entered the Cornell and Columbia residency program at Bellevue Hospital in New York, with his training interrupted by World War II. While serving in a field hospital in Belgium after the Normandy invasion, he barely escaped capture during the Battle of the Bulge. After the war, he completed his residency at the Bronx Veterans Hospital in New York. As an attending surgeon at Cornell Division at Bellevue, he developed a research facility and an open-heart surgery program. In 1962, he became the first full-time director of surgery at the Beth Israel Medical Center in New York and professor of surgery at the new Mount Sinai School of Medicine. In the mid-1960s, he and his young associate, Hiromi Shinya, established an upper gastrointestinal fiberoptic endoscopic laboratory and clinical facility. Their work led to the development of the first flexible instruments for evaluating the entire colon. After a successful study, the era of colonoscopy and colonoscopic polypectomy was born. Their efforts resulted in what Francis Moore described as a "quantum advance in surgery." Their article was, in fact, selected by members of the American Society of Colon and Rectal Surgeons as among the top 11 literature contributions to 20th century colon and rectal surgery.[37] A founding member of the Society of American Gastrointestinal Endoscopic Surgeons, Wolff received the highest award given to an alumnus of his alma mater, the University of Maryland, for "outstanding contributions to medicine and distinguished service to mankind." He died at his home in Manhattan, August 20, 2011, in his 95th year.

HIROMI SHINYA (1935–PRESENT)

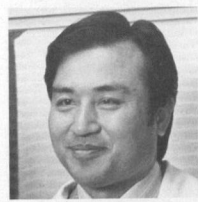

Hiromi Shinya was born in Yanagawa, Fukuoka prefecture, Japan, and completed his medical studies in 1960 at Tokyo's Juntendo University. After his internship at the U.S. Naval Hospital in Yokosuka, he arrived in New York City to begin his general surgical residency at the Beth Israel Medical Center. In 1967, while still in his residency, he became interested in the newly evolving instrumentation for upper gastrointestinal endoscopy. As a consequence of this experience, he moved on to develop the technique for examination of the colon, devising many of the accessories, such as the snare cautery. In 1969, with the support and encouragement of his chief, William Wolff, he began a series of successful polypectomy procedures. Because of his unique experience and abilities, he received a special visa waiver by order of the president of the United States to remain in the country and to continue his work. His colonoscopy experience to date exceeds 250,000 patients.

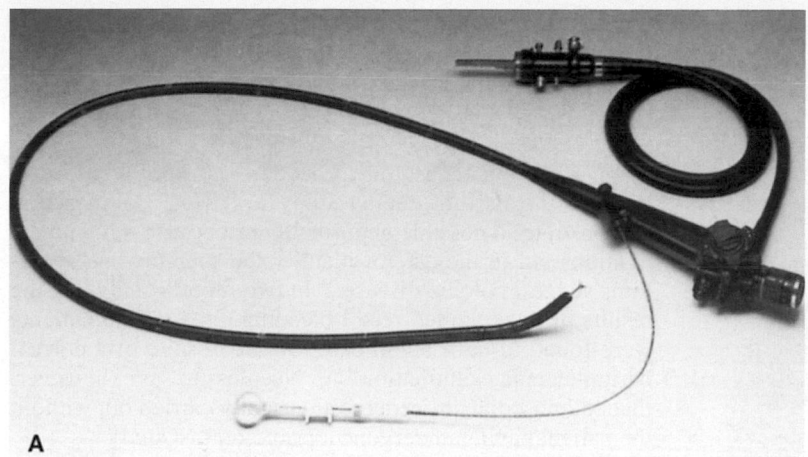

A

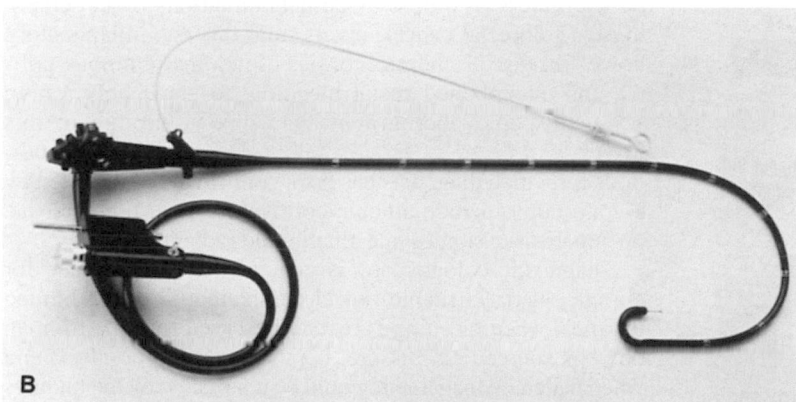

B

FIGURE 6-12. Colonoscopes. **A:** The fiberoptic colonoscope, model PCF-10 with biopsy instrument, is a 133-cm instrument. (Courtesy of Olympus America, Melville, NY.) **B:** Slim video colonoscope, model EC-3400. (Courtesy of Pentax Precision Instrument Corp., Orangeburg, NY.)

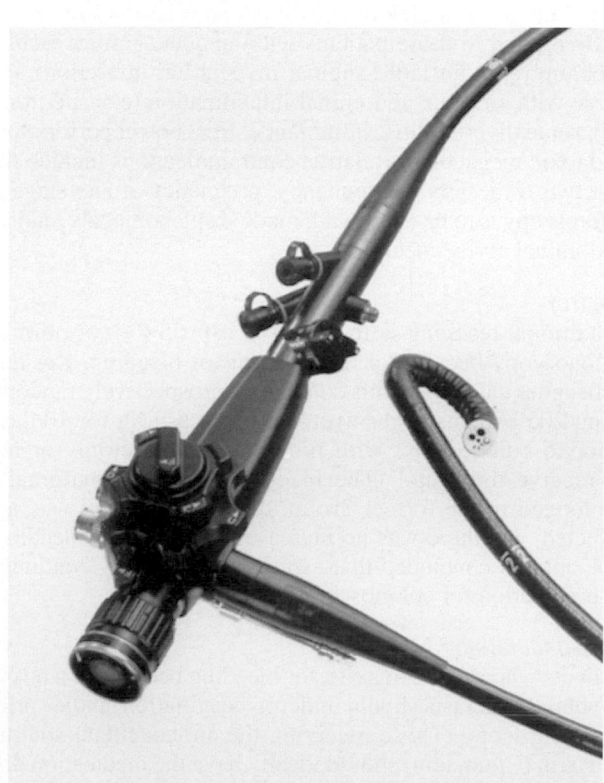

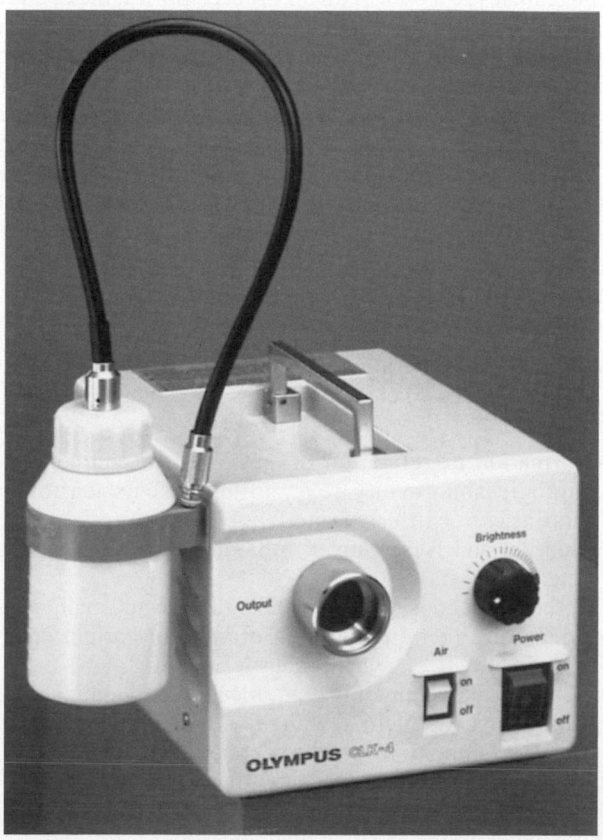

FIGURE 6-13. Two-channel therapeutic colonofiberscope (model FC-38TLH) features water jet. (Courtesy of Pentax Precision Instrument Corp., Orangeburg, NY.)

FIGURE 6-14. This simplified 150-W halogen light source includes an air pump and water container with pipe. (Courtesy of Olympus America, Melville, NY.)

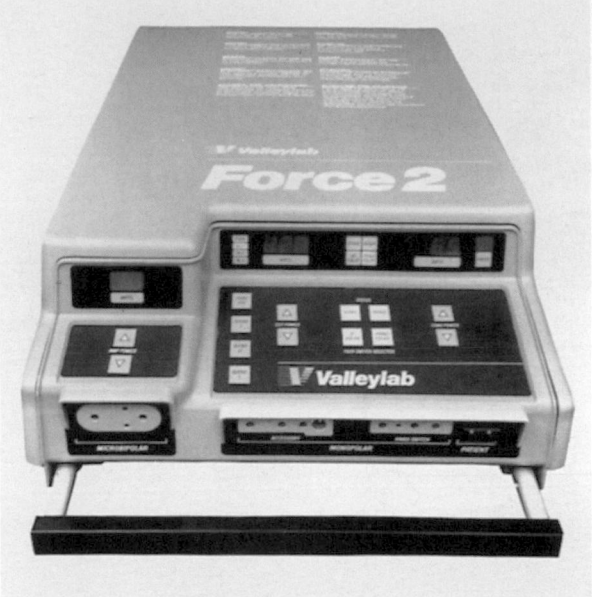

FIGURE 6-15. Electrosurgery generator. This unit has simultaneous independent coagulation ability, microbipolar mode, and handswitching and footswitching controls. (Courtesy of Tyco Valleylab, Inc., Boulder, CO.)

snare, and grasping forceps, in addition to an instrument for brush cytology.

Cost is also a major concern when contemplating the purchase of a colonoscope. The cost of a video colonoscope approximates $35,000. With all the accessories, the comprehensive unit could cost three times that amount. Repairs and the limited life expectancy of the instruments also must be considered in assessing the expense. However, there is universal agreement that, with the plethora of colon disorders in Western countries, especially neoplasms, colonoscopy and colonoscopy–polypectomy are among the most important advances for diagnosis and treatment to become available since the late 1960s.

Indications

It is generally agreed that colonoscopy has for the most part replaced the barium enema in the evaluation of colon disorders.[1] The list here summarizes the indications for this procedure:

Confirmation or refutation of suspected or equivocal radiologic abnormality (e.g., filling defects, narrowing [intrinsic vs. extrinsic lesion], polyps)
Evaluation and follow-up of inflammatory bowel disease (e.g., dysplasia)
Differential diagnosis of diverticular disease and malignancy
Presence of a rectal polyp with or without barium enema abnormality (e.g., synchronous lesions)
Gastrointestinal symptoms (e.g., bleeding, abdominal pain, iron-deficiency anemia) with or without radiologic investigation failing to reveal the source
Follow-up evaluation of patient with prior colon surgery
Colon and rectal cancer screening
Acute lower gastrointestinal bleeding
Clinically significant diarrhea of unexplained origin
Endoscopic polypectomy

Reduction of sigmoid volvulus
Decompression of dilated colon (e.g., Ogilvie's syndrome)
Intraoperative colonoscopy; confirmation of location of lesion at time of laparotomy or during laparoscopic procedures
Colonoscopic percutaneous colostomy

In some instances, the procedure is employed either because the barium enema study or virtual colonoscopy demonstrates a possible abnormality or because other investigations fail to indicate or identify the source when symptoms suggest colonic disease.[34] In two reports analyzing the results of unexplained rectal bleeding, 30% of the patients were found to have significant lesions in spite of a normal barium enema examination.[16,160] Needless to state, however, that colonoscopic procedures are usually carried out without the patient having undergone a prior contrast study.

Colonoscopy has been demonstrated to be of diagnostic usefulness in a host of clinical situations (e.g., screening for colorectal cancer, diverticular disease, inflammatory bowel disease, ischemic colitis, pseudomembranous colitis, and unexplained rectal bleeding, to name only a few; see endoscopic photographs that appear throughout this text).[13,16,17,41,43,58,61,67,76,83,97,104,113,118,149,156,159,160,164] Other conditions for which diagnosis has been confirmed or expedited by colonoscopy include amebic colitis, intestinal tuberculosis, pneumatosis cystoides intestinalis, and radiation colitis.[34,42,153]

Diagnostic colonoscopy is generally not appropriate for chronic, stable, irritable bowel complaints, in acute limited diarrhea, when bleeding is readily observed to come from an obvious source (e.g., fissure, hemorrhoids, peptic ulcer) and when patient management would be unaffected by the findings (e.g., metastatic carcinoma in the absence of bowel symptoms).

Contraindications and Concerns

Absolute contraindications to this examination are essentially limited to those patients with an acute cardiovascular problem (e.g., unstable angina, myocardial infarction) and those with an acute abdominal inflammation (e.g., peritonitis), acute diverticulitis, fulminant colitis, bowel perforation, and toxic megacolon. Relative contraindications include the last two trimesters of pregnancy, pregnancy at any stage if fluoroscopy is to be employed, marked splenomegaly, and an abdominal aortic aneurysm.[33]

Aspirin

Traditional teaching is to withhold aspirin 7 days prior to colonoscopy because of the concern for bleeding. Ker and colleagues challenged this concept by prospectively randomizing 205 patients to receive 650 mg of aspirin for 10 days prior to colonoscopy with biopsy or polypectomy or not to receive the drug.[94] The bleeding time was marginally prolonged in the former group, the platelet count was not affected, and there was no increased incidence of bleeding. The authors concluded that aspirin can be safely continued in preparation for colonoscopy.[94]

Anticoagulation

Patients who may be at a risk for bleeding because of a possible blood dyscrasia should undergo coagulation studies prior to colonoscopy. Those receiving the anticoagulant sodium warfarin (Coumadin) should ideally have the medication discontinued prior to the procedure.[33] Caliendo and coworkers performed a retrospective review of their patients with regard to anticoagulation.[19] They observed that colonoscopy without polypectomy may be performed safely without discontinuing therapy. However, resuming antiplatelet treatment immediately after colonoscopy–polypectomy was associated with a high risk of bleeding. There were no thromboembolic complications. Timothy and colleagues, also in a retrospective review involving 94 patients (109 examinations) on warfarin, noted that colonoscopy could be performed safely, but that there was a slightly increased incidence of hemorrhagic complications with biopsy or snare excision.[162] Their recommended approach to the patient on warfarin who can tolerate a "period" of "normal" coagulation is as follows[162]:

- Stop warfarin for 3 days.
- Obtain the prothrombin time/INR (international normalized ratio) prior to the procedure.
- If the INR is less than 2, proceed with colonoscopy and restart warfarin (using prior dosage) on the first postoperative day.
- If the INR is 2 or greater, postpone the procedure for 1 to 2 days or, alternatively, perform the diagnostic procedure and postpone restarting warfarin for 2 to 3 days if a therapeutic procedure is contemplated.
- If a diagnostic procedure is performed, restart warfarin at the prior dose on postprocedure day 1.

Privileging and Credentialing

Wexner, Eisen, and Simmang, in 2002, prepared a consensus document concerning endoscopic privileging and credentialing that has been endorsed by the Society of American Gastrointestinal and Endoscopic Surgeons, the American Society for Gastrointestinal Endoscopy, and the American Society of Colon and Rectal Surgeons.[170] They emphasized that the credentialing structure and process are the responsibility of the health care facility, and that uniform standards should be developed for performing specific endoscopic procedures regardless of the specialty in which an individual physician practices. Training may be accomplished through a formal surgery or gastroenterology residency program or through an equivalent "certification of experience by a skilled endoscopic practitioner." Determination of competence requires the following:

- Completion of a residency program with structured, documented experience in gastrointestinal endoscopy, or
- Demonstrated proficiency in technique and clinical judgment equivalent to that which is obtained in a residency program, and
- Confirmation in writing from the endoscopic director as to the applicant's training, experience, and observed level of competency

The consensus document also incorporates statements on training in new techniques, proctoring of applicants for privileges, criteria for competency, monitoring of performance, requirement for continuing medical education, and the renewal of privileges.[170]

Preparation of the Patient

As with barium enema examination, the importance of an adequately cleansed colon cannot be overemphasized.[157] There are two reasons for requiring a clean colon before proceeding with colonoscopic examination: safety and accuracy. The danger of causing injury when trying to intubate a feces-laden bowel is appreciable. The presence of formed stool may obscure the lumen and lead the endoscopist to apply forces in dangerous ways. Even a minor amount of stool can lead to confusion and misinterpretation. For example, a piece of stool that is firmly adherent to the lens may require removal of the instrument blindly and the necessity of starting all over again. When residual fecal matter is encountered, it is important to irrigate it free before passing on to other areas.

For most ambulatory patients, a vigorous cathartic followed by colonic irrigation or a small-volume enema (i.e., Fleet), along with appropriate dietary restriction, is generally satisfactory and can be commenced in the morning for an afternoon examination or in the evening prior to a morning endoscopy. However, sedentary or frail individuals may require several days to prepare the bowel adequately, especially if a less vigorous cleansing regimen is adopted. Care must be taken to maintain adequate fluid intake and to avoid electrolyte abnormalities because fluid loss may cause patients to lose as much as 7 lbs (3.2 kg).[10,171] This is of particular concern in individuals with cardiovascular or renal disease.

Davis and colleagues devised an electrolyte solution containing primarily sodium sulfate with polyethylene glycol (PEG) as an additional osmotic agent (i.e., Golytely).[40] Studies have been published that verify the safety and efficacy of this lavage method in preparation for colonoscopy and for barium enema examination, especially if bisacodyl (Dulcolax) is added to ensure evacuation of residual fluid.[45,51,70,71] It has become, at least for endoscopists, if not for patients, the most popular preparation in the United States for colonoscopy.

The preparation can be administered orally or by tube feedings. A dose of 4 L is usually sufficient to produce adequate cleansing. The most frequent complaint about this method of cleansing the bowel and the primary drawback are the discomfort and distaste associated with consumption of such a large quantity of fluid. "The preparation was worse than the procedure" is a frequently voiced statement. Another PEG preparation, Colyte, has been made available in various flavors to deal with the difficulties associated with poor patient compliance.[111]

It is because of patient complaints that some have used another colon-cleansing technique in these individuals. Fleet Phospho–Soda was a common component of colonoscopy preparations replacing PEG in most preparations. It was not applicable for those with renal failure, ascites, congestive heart failure, a diversionary stoma, a history of myocardial infarction within 6 months, or those taking a calcium channel blocker such as nifedipine (Procardia) or verapamil (Calan). In December 2008, this preparation was recalled from the market because there were several cases of renal toxicity in patients with no risk factors for renal insufficiency. Some of these patients had such pronounced renal insufficiency that they required hemodialysis and renal transplantation. It has been removed from general use in the preparation of patients undergoing colonoscopy and should not be prescribed.

Alternative Preparations

Magnesium citrate is an alternative preparation that was used as an intermediate volume preparation between the 1 gal PEG solutions and the 45-mL Fleet Phospho–Soda preps. This involves using two 10-oz bottles of magnesium citrate on the day prior to colonoscopy. It can be an effective preparation but carries some of the same electrolyte risks as the Fleet preparation and should not be used in patients with the previously detailed clinical conditions. Various other manufactures have come to market with alternative cleansing solutions, such as HalfLytely and MoviPrep (PEG + ascorbic acid).

They are all more or less based on PEG-type compounds, and one generally varies the volume used to cleanse the bowel. A common preparation in practice with gastroenterologists involves the use of Miralax, a tasteless laxative in powder form used in the treatment of constipation. It is often used in an off-label manor, with 238 g mixed with 64 oz of clear liquids, such as a sports drink or apple juice. This has supplanted Fleet Phospho–Soda as the preparation used in patients concerned about the taste of the preparation. Once again, use of this Miralax-based preparation is off of the FDA-approved label.

Timing of Preparations

It has been demonstrated that more important than the type of preparation used for bowel cleansing is the timing of administration. Traditionally, colonoscopy preparations have been administered as a single dose or in a divide dose on the evening prior to colonoscopy. Numerous recent studies have linked the quality of bowel cleansing, specifically of the right colon with "split-dose" regimens in which the second dose is given on the morning prior to the procedure.[108,130]

It has been deemed by many that the standard of care should include a colonic preparation when the second dose of laxative is begun 4 to 5 hours prior to the colonoscopy time and completed within 2 hours of the time of the procedure.

Sedation and Monitoring

Sedation with monitoring is usually employed whenever total colonoscopy is undertaken. The insufflation of air or carbon dioxide—the latter is more rapidly absorbed—and traction on the bowel from the instrument may cause considerable discomfort and anxiety. It is important for the examiner to be aware of any excessive discomfort that the patient is experiencing in order to avoid possible injury to the bowel wall, mesentery, or adjoining structures.

Certain combinations of medications have been advised to reduce discomfort, including meperidine hydrochloride (Demerol), fentanyl, diazepam (Valium), and midazolam (Versed).[34] Irrespective of the choice of medication, a heparin lock is recommended for intravenous access and is generally required by standardized conscious sedation regulations. Several publications have appeared cautioning one as to the risks of oversedation and the requirement for continuous monitoring, including electrocardiogram, blood pressure, pulse oximetry, nasal airflow by thermistor probe, and impedance pneumography.[79] Care should be taken to avoid respiratory depression and hypotension; elderly patients and those with respiratory and pulmonary difficulties are at particular risk. The most frequently employed monitoring device is the pulse oximeter, a method that provides continuous noninvasive measurement of arterial hemoglobin and oxygen saturation.

One of the real concerns about monitoring has been the cost. A manual sphygmomanometer is about $150; automatic pressure monitor, $3,000; electrocardiographic monitoring systems, $5,000 to $6,000; and pulse oximeters, $2,000 to $5,000.[56] Some recommendations concerning monitoring for conscious sedation have been offered by Fleischer.[56] However, there are no controlled studies that address the question of whether noninvasive monitoring decreases the incidence of complications. These guidelines have been fairly standardized and established at all hospitals and endoscopy centers. They generally include the following[56]:

- Monitoring should be part of the overall quality assurance program for the endoscopy unit.
- A competent assistant is the most important part of the monitoring process.
- The amount of monitoring should be proportional to the risk of the procedure for that individual.
- Minimal monitoring should include heart rate, blood pressure, and respiratory rate prior to, during, and immediately after the procedure and when the individual is about to leave the room.
- The requirement for sedation or analgesic medication must, perforce, be related to the technical facility of the examiner.

The American Society for Gastrointestinal Endoscopy has published a protocol for sedation and monitoring of patients undergoing endoscopic procedures. This is worth quoting:

> Every available means to ensure the safety of patients during endoscopic procedures is mandatory. This begins with a fully trained and knowledgeable endoscopist, thorough preparation of the unit to handle endoscopic procedures and potential adverse outcomes, appropriate patient preparation, skilled assistants, and monitoring of the patient's well-being before, during, and after the procedure.

The relative risks involved can be estimated from patient and procedural factors and should be determined for each examination. The level and type of monitoring during endoscopic procedures are dependent on a thorough understanding and assessment of the risk to the patient.

Monitoring of patients undergoing endoscopic procedures is mandatory and prudent. The ultimate responsibility for protecting the patient rests with the endoscopist and cannot be assigned to an assistant or to an electronic monitoring device. However, both may greatly improve the ability to detect patient distress at a time when intervention will prevent an otherwise adverse outcome.

Antibiotic Prophylaxis

The risk of infective endocarditis or other infectious complications from colonoscopy is quite low. Still, there is indeed a risk.[136] Recommendations for antibiotic prophylaxis are discussed in Chapter 5 and are equally applicable to colonoscopy and FS.

Technique of Examination: General Principles

If you don't know where you are going, all roads will get you there.

—Koran

Most colonoscopies require at least a modest amount of manipulation, and many are truly challenging. It is particularly important that the endoscopist has a thorough understanding of the interaction between a relatively unforgiving instrument and the variably compliant colon. Furthermore, a clear understanding of colonic anatomy is essential. For example, it is fixed at the rectum and is usually attached to the retroperitoneum at the descending, cecal, and ascending portions. Other areas, such as the hepatic and splenic flexures, although not fixed in the abdominal cavity, are intimately related to adjacent structures. Certain parts, notably the sigmoid and transverse colon, may have considerable mobility, being tethered only by the mesentery. Each portion of the colon has its own individual compliance. Successful intubation is in great part dependent on taking advantage of this compliance as well as overcoming the varied obstacles to passage.

There are certain properties of the colonoscope and maneuvers that must be employed in order to accomplish successful intubation. These include tip deflection, shaft torquing, and shaft dithering. These physical movements of the instrument are combined with air insufflation, deflation, patient positioning, and abdominal pressure.

Tip Deflection

The articulating deflection tip is the most critical element in the design of the colonoscope. The ability to move the viewing tip off center by more than 180 degrees in any direction enables the examiner to have active control of what happens at the far end of the instrument. Deflection permits the endoscopist to look around a bend or fold in order to see in just which direction one needs to proceed. Folds can be pressed against the wall so that small lesions, which would otherwise stay hidden, are exposed. This articulation is essential during therapeutic maneuvers in order to aim a snare or biopsy forceps in the proper direction. In selected instances, the deflection tip may be retroflexed in order to obtain a clearer view of an obscured area such as the top of the anal canal (Figure 6-7) or the cecal side of the ileocecal valve (see Figures 6-21 and 6-22 later).

The articulating deflection tip, as essential as it is to facilitating intubation, may at the same time be the single greatest impediment to successful passage, at least for the novice colonoscopist. As the tip is deflected from the straight position, a gentle curve forms along the distal 10 to 12 cm. With a relatively modest bend of 30 to 45 degrees, an advancement of the instrument shaft will not distort the contour of the colon. However, when one attempts to increase the deflection to more than 90 degrees, in an effort to see around a curve or angle of the bowel, the distribution of forces against the colon wall changes profoundly. In the latter situation, a greater proportion of the advancing force is distributed against the sidewall of the bowel rather than in the forward direction of the lumen. In addition, the application of extreme deflection to both knob controls further deviates force distribution and precludes all attempts at advancement. Longitudinal advancement of the scope no longer follows the tip of the instrument. Instead, the deflection bend now becomes the leading edge of the instrument, with forward force transmitted directly to the wall of the colon. As a consequence, blunt or tearing trauma can easily occur. This can take the form of splitting of the fibers of the muscle wall or frank perforation. The operator can avoid this complication by simply recognizing that extreme deflection is being employed, and that with attempted instrument advancement, the bowel under view seems to be getting further away rather than closer. Occasionally, extreme deflection is required in order to find the lumen. But once identified, the deflection should be eased, preferably to less than 90 degrees before attempting further advancement of the scope.

In summary, the least amount of deflection that is necessary in order to acquire the desired view is preferred. Limiting deflection to the use of the up–down dial only, while abjuring the simultaneous application of both controls, is helpful for minimizing inappropriate deflection.

Shaft Torquing

Torquing is an essential maneuver for effective intubation as well as for optimal surface visualization during extubation. Shaft torquing can produce three major effects. When left-handed or counterclockwise torque is applied, there is a tendency to produce a loop in the redundant sigmoid colon. Second, if clockwise torque is applied, the sigmoid colon tends to straighten. The third effect is produced at the tip of the scope. When the shaft is torqued in either direction in the presence of modest tip deflection, strong leverage is transmitted toward the entrance to the more proximal bowel. Using torque with modest tip deflection is generally more effective in locating an elusive proximal segment, as opposed to holding the shaft rigid while manipulating the deflection tip alone.

As more instrument is introduced, the response to torquing becomes more complex. If the scope is relatively straight, the torque will transmit nearly one to one to the viewing lens of the instrument. The field of view will simply be rotated; this facilitates identification of lesions or positioning of snares. However, if the scope shaft is within one or more loops, the results of torquing will have a much more profound effect on the bowel than on what is perceived through the viewing end of the instrument. If there is a so-called alpha loop present in the sigmoid colon, the effect of clockwise torquing (especially when combined with shaft withdrawal) is to reduce that loop by accordionizing the bowel onto the scope. This occurs without loss of intubation distance. However, once reduced, the sigmoid loop will have a tendency to form again, particularly if counterclockwise torque is applied during subsequent scope advancement. Therefore, in order to maintain reduction of a redundant sigmoid loop, one must advance the instrument while maintaining clockwise torque. The examiner can readily perceive this tendency to form the loop again by applying clockwise torque; the scope will appear to advance. Counterclockwise movement will reveal that the scope tends to lose ground.

Occasionally, an extremely redundant sigmoid colon will develop two complete loops during intubation. Nearly always, both are reducible. However, unlike the single-loop configuration, the first loop is removed by counterclockwise rotation and the second by clockwise rotation. Removing both loops is usually essential before proximal passage into the descending colon can be accomplished. After both loops have been straightened, the sigmoid colon is once again most likely to remain in this position only if clockwise torque is continued during further intubation.

Torque is also a very important maneuver in manipulations in the area of the hepatic flexure. If the transverse colon is held in the upper abdomen, the scope takes a straight line to the hepatic flexure. At this point, clockwise torque is usually beneficial as the gently deflected tip is directed down the ascending colon. Conversely, if the transverse colon is redundant, stretching down toward the pelvis, the hepatic flexure is then approached from below. When the ascending colon is viewed in this situation, there is a rather sharp deflection of the tip. Once again, gentle scope withdrawal along with clockwise torquing, as well as intermittent desufflation, all combine to broaden the hepatic flexure and to drop the instrument down into the ascending colon and cecum.

During extubation, torquing is an extremely important manipulation for efficient and thorough examination of the colon surface. As the instrument is withdrawn, the right hand is maintained on the shaft to apply torque. The left hand supports the scope head with the thumb free to move the up–down control. By combining back-and-forth torque with simultaneous small tip deflections, one can continuously examine the colon surface with minimal risk of overlooking lesions. This permits the colon that has been accordionized onto the scope to be dropped off, a bit at a time. If, rather than torquing, one simply withdraws while using both hands of the dial controls, the view behind prominent folds is likely to be inadequate. Furthermore, if the colon is redundant, the bowel will likely fly off the scope at an uncontrollable rate.

Advancement/Withdrawal ("Dithering")

Colonoscopic intubation would be a simple matter if the colon were a noncompliant tube without redundancy or irregularity. The procedure would be nothing more than an effortless advancement of the instrument. On occasion, especially after sigmoid colon resection, colonoscopic intubation may be no more demanding than this. However, under most circumstances, the in-and-out movements of the shaft are only effective when combined with appropriate tip deflection and torquing. There is a tendency for the inexperienced endoscopist to resist losing ground even though it is unclear in which direction the scope should be advanced. Almost always, when anatomy is unclear or visualization is difficult, it is best and certainly safest to withdraw rather than to continue blind manipulation or advancement.[169] The simple process of limited withdrawal is most likely to reveal the proper direction in which to proceed.

When progression of the instrument is not impeded by severe tip deflection, redundant colon can be encouraged to accordionize along its length. This is most likely to occur if the scope is repeatedly advanced and withdrawn, a process referred to as "dithering." When combined with torquing in the sigmoid/descending colon, short dithering strokes can often reduce sigmoid redundancy as the scope is advanced, thereby avoiding the creation of a full loop. In less tethered segments, such as with a redundant transverse colon, it is often advantageous to perform long (30- to 50-cm) dithering strokes in order to accordionize the excess bowel onto a limited segment of instrument.

Gas Insufflation

Insufflation of gas is essential for effective visualization during colonoscopy. However, insufflation should be used sparingly. Excess gas can lead to abdominal distension, which results in severe discomfort and a possible vasovagal reaction. Unfortunately, the design of the insufflation mechanism contributes to the possibility of inadvertent administration of unnecessary gas. This occurs because air is constantly being pumped to the insufflation trumpet valve on the control unit of the colonoscope. By simply covering the vent hole with a finger, one diverts a large volume of air into the colon. Depression of the trumpet valve diverts the air stream to the much smaller volume flow of the lens cleaning system. Consequently, if one develops the habit of resting the finger on part or all of the trumpet valve, colonic distension will inevitably result. If intubation of the distal ileum is performed, only a limited insufflation may lead to the accumulation of considerable small bowel gas.

Excessive intraluminal gas often works against the process of intubation, particularly at a flexure or when a redundant loop is being negotiated. Gas distension pushes the proximal end of the loop or flexure away from the end of the scope. As a consequence, the angle becomes more acute and therefore more difficult to pass. This is most evident at the hepatic flexure when the tip deflection is sharply angulated into the distal ascending colon. As air is introduced, the ileocecal valve is seen in the distance to move still further away. Conversely, when air is aspirated, the cecal area is observed to be almost sucked into the scope. This maneuver is facilitated by concomitant torquing.

Patient Position and Abdominal Pressure

Although there is no single position that is ideal, the construction of most endoscopes and the right-handedness of most physicians tend to favor the patients assuming the left lateral position. Patients with a colostomy or ileostomy may be more comfortable in either the lateral or supine position. In patients with poor abdominal wall muscle tone (e.g., paraplegia, large hernia, prior dehiscence), examination in the prone position may be helpful.

Changing positions during the examination when forward progress becomes stalled is often very beneficial. Rotating the patient 90 degrees to the left is analogous to torquing the scope 90 degrees to the right. Changing the patient position not only alters the relationship of the instrument to the colon, it also redistributes organ pressures within the abdominal cavity. Not infrequently, when one negotiates a difficult splenic flexure, the proximal bowel comes easily into view during the process of changing patient position. With the individual in the prone position, pressure in the abdominal cavity is increased. Once an excessively redundant sigmoid loop has been reduced, the broad pressure afforded by the prone position will discourage its reformation. To this one can add focal pressure by having an assistant push down on the abdomen in order to maintain straightening of the instrument.[168] Pressure from just to the right of the umbilicus and directed toward the left iliac fossa will discourage sigmoid looping. Similarly, central abdominal pressure will help keep the redundant transverse colon from dropping deeply into the pelvis.

If there is difficulty with entry into the ascending colon, the patient is rotated onto the right lateral decubitus position. This is an important and helpful maneuver when one must deal with a recalcitrant hepatic flexure. One presumes that pressure from the liver in this position flattens the flexure sufficiently to allow the scope to slip down the ascending colon.

Many endoscopists prefer to perform much of the examination with the patient in the supine position.[85,128,163] However, there are difficulties with this. If the scope is brought out between the patient's legs, there is minimal working room between the anus and the bed or gurney to allow adequate manipulation. If the instrument is brought out beneath the raised right leg, one must continually reposition the leg or use an assistant to attend to this.

General Preparations

Before actually starting the procedure, it is important to check that the instrument is in proper working order. This includes such basic maneuvers as switching on the suction and ensuring that the line is attached. Air insufflation and lens washing are tested. The deflection tip should be maximally flexed and examined for both the degree of deflection and integrity of the covering surface.

Some surgeons prefer to use a two-person approach to colonoscopy. One handles the dial-control housing while an assistant advances and torques the shaft. This team method is very difficult to coordinate because it is virtually impossible for each individual to have a sense of what the other is doing. Although it is helpful to have the assistant stabilize the shaft when positioning a snare onto a difficult polyp, it is strongly suggested that both shaft and dial controls be under the direction of a single mind.

The expert colonoscopist should be able to perform an expeditious and thorough examination by avoiding the formation of bowel loops that interfere with advancement. When loop formation is a problem, one should be able to widen the loop radius to facilitate intubation. The colonoscopist can detect the subtle clues that indicate a loop is starting to form the loss of the one-to-one correspondence of instrument insertion to image movement, a gradual increase in resistance to forward motion, and signs of patient discomfort. As mentioned previously, instrument withdrawal often facilitates subsequent passage. Advancement of the scope should nearly always be under direct vision. The "slide-by" technique, whereby the viewing tip is partially buried in the colon wall, should be avoided. Although it is often necessary to accept less than a totally clear view, insertion when one is blind to lumen orientation is strongly discouraged. One should be concerned about the possibility of causing injury if the colonic mucosa blanches or if the patient experiences pain.

There is always the desire not to lose ground, especially after spending considerable time reaching an area during a difficult colonoscopy. The endoscopist may be very reluctant to give up what has been accomplished even if there is no apparent outlet. This attitude will most likely impede passage rather than preserve it. By "periscoping" the deflection tip and stretching the colon, one inevitably embeds the instrument in a self-made recess, the consequence of an abrupt bend in the next segment. At the risk of redundancy, one cannot overemphasize the requirement for the endoscopist to withdraw shaft length whenever progress is arrested. Withdrawal is often the only means for visualizing the direction of the next segment of colon.

Fluoroscopy

Although not required for most examinations, the availability of fluoroscopy can be invaluable for difficult cases. When previous examinations have been inadequate or confusion as to the anatomy and lesion location exists, fluoroscopic guidance can be considered. In addition, fluoroscopy can be useful in training. How one perceives the configuration of the scope as compared with how it really exists in the bowel can be easily shown with fluoroscopic confirmation. A survey of members of the Society of American Gastrointestinal Endoscopic Surgeons and the American Society of Colon and Rectal Surgeons was undertaken to quantify the use of fluoroscopy and to elicit impressions regarding its capabilities, indications, and usefulness.[135] Seventy-five percent never used this modality, the most frequent reason being lack of need or inaccessibility of the equipment. Ninety-two percent of the frequent users reported that they would feel significantly impaired without having the capability of performing fluoroscopy.

Electronic Imaging

Real-time electromagnetic imaging has been applied as an aid for the performance of colonoscopy.[141] By this means, three sets of generator coils are placed beneath the endoscopy table, producing pulsed, low-strength electromagnetic fields outside of the patient. These fields are detected by a series of sensor coils positioned at 12-cm intervals along the length of a catheter that is inserted down the biopsy channel of the colonoscope. From the electrical signal produced in the sensor coil, the exact position and orientation of each can be calculated. In a controlled trial from the United Kingdom, Saunders and coworkers determined that there was no significant difference in intubation time and duration of loop formation. However, the number of attempts taken to straighten the colonoscope was less when the endoscopist was able to see the imager view.[141] Another study by Adam and colleagues in 2001 compared the amount of colon actually seen as assessed with this imaging technique with how far the endoscopists thought they had reached.[3] In 119 patients, clinical assessment was correct in only 92 (77%). When the endoscopist reported that cecal landmarks had been visualized, the instrument was found to be distal to the cecum in 8.2%. Without identification of cecal landmarks, the endoscopist was accurate in only 41%. The consequences of this report are particularly disturbing, especially in the circumstances when colonoscopy is being performed for occult blood positivity or for equivocal findings on radiologic study.

High-Magnification Chromoscopic Colonoscopy

The concept of trying to find small or flat cancers of the colon has led the Japanese to develop methods for early identification of cancer through magnification chromoscopy.[63] The technique involves the use of one of two stains, either indigo carmine (preferred) or crystal violet. The solution is flushed through a catheter placed within the biopsy channel of the colonoscope. Subtle endoscopic changes, such as pallor, erythema, unevenness, and superficial elevated lesions, may prompt the examiner to use a localized dye spraying or chromoscopy to aid in visualization.[87] Patterns of mucosal appearance suggestive of minute cancers or of an "invasive pit pattern" may lead one to consider a local treatment or a more radical one. The implication of detecting these lesions is potentially significant, but more study needs to be accomplished before the technique is applied routinely.

Sedation

Without sedation, colonoscopy of the entire colon may be an intolerably painful experience, thereby precluding a comprehensive evaluation. Although it has been demonstrated that some patients can undergo colonoscopy without sedation,[22] most colonoscopies are performed after administering intravenous doses of fentanyl and midazolam (Versed). This regimen may be supplemented, if necessary, depending on the patient's sensory and physiologic reactions. One should not strive to avoid medication but rather to provide a safe and reasonably comfortable examination for the patient (see previous discussion).

Performing the Examination

Rectal Examination

A digital rectal examination is a requisite initial step for every patient. As discussed in Chapter 5, it is not unusual to find important pathologic features, such as large hemorrhoids, an anal fissure, a prostatic nodule, or an anorectal mass. Furthermore, extrarectal lesions cannot be identified by the instrument alone. Digital examination also permits one to gauge anal sphincter tone. Knowing that an individual has poor tone will alert the examiner that it will be difficult for the patient to retain insufflated air. Alternatively, a tight or strictured anus may require gentle dilatation in order to accommodate the instrument. Finally, the examiner's finger prepares the patient for the subsequent insertion of the instrument.

Anorectal Intubation

Because the anus has been prelubricated with jelly during the digital examination, only a light coating needs to be placed along the shaft. Care should be taken to avoid the application of lubricant to the lens because it is not easily removed with the cleansing water jet. The scope should not be introduced end-on. Instead, the tip should be gently guided through the anal canal at an angle by using the index finger to support the flexible end. This will keep the tip from buckling during anal canal entry. Once inside the rectum, anatomic and technical factors may preclude clear visualization of the rectal ampulla during intubation. While the anal canal is oriented in the direction of the umbilicus, it joins the rectal ampulla, whose access is directed posteriorly toward the sacrum. The tip deflection mechanism responds poorly at this level because much of the deflection system still remains outside the anus. It is not until the deflecting section has completely traversed the sphincter that the examiner may begin to have control of tip deflection. Once the tip of the scope has been inserted approximately 10 cm above the anal verge, tip deflection will respond properly, and the middle and upper rectum can be readily visualized. The most frequent cause of poor visualization in the middle and upper rectum is not disease but rather the failure to provide adequate insufflation.

Sigmoid Intubation

Once the rectosigmoid has been reached, the stage is set for the technique of sigmoid intubation. With the instrument tip positioned in the rectosigmoid, one should take the control section with one's left hand while the right hand is positioned on the shaft. Throughout the remainder of the examination, this hand placement is the basic posture that will be employed. Both dial controls are maintained in the unlocked position. Tip deflection is managed virtually exclusively by rotation of the larger up–down control, using the thumb from beneath the control housing. This keeps the index or middle finger free to operate the suction or air insufflation.

Sigmoid-Descending Colon Intubation

As previously mentioned, proper and efficient negotiation of the sigmoid is often the most challenging aspect of colonoscopy, frequently determining the success of the entire procedure. Avoidance of bowel loop formation is not only more comfortable for the patient, but it also permits a more expeditious and more complete examination with a shorter length of instrument. While holding the control housing with the left hand, the right hand firmly grasps the shaft no more than 10 to 15 cm from the anus. A conscious effort is made to avoid bringing the right hand up to the dial controls. If one uses both hands simultaneously on the dial controls to periscope the deflection tip, although occasionally necessary, it usually results in overdeflection. Furthermore, this prevents one from using the very effective maneuver of simultaneous deflection and torquing. By keeping the hand on the shaft close to the anus, there is better control of the instrument and less tendency simply to push excess scope into the colon.

The three methods of traversing the sigmoid colon are intubation by elongation, by looping (alpha maneuver), and by accordionization (dither-torquing).[165] Although distinctly different techniques, they are not mutually exclusive solutions to the same problem. By using these principles, the operator can more deliberately and effectively control the process of intubation.

Intubation by Elongation

Intubation by elongation merely refers to the process by which the instrument is inserted until either there is no apparent place to go or there is no more scope left. Indeed, this is probably the most commonly used approach when one performs FS. No fancy maneuvers just advance the shaft and periscope the deflection tip to find the luminal direction. If the sigmoid is minimally redundant, there may be a reasonably straight shot through the sigmoid and descending colon to the level of the splenic flexure. Unfortunately, more often this technique merely stretches a redundant sigmoid until the sigmoid-descending colon junction is reached, if it is reached at all. At this point, entry into the descending colon is associated with an increased angle to 180 degrees. This angle at the deflection tip is too sharp to permit passage to progress. Additional shaft advancement therefore merely stretches the sigmoid further.

Intubation by Looping (Alpha Maneuver)

The relatively mobile sigmoid colon is fixed proximally at the descending colon junction and distally at the rectum. The best means to appreciate the varied configurations that can develop during sigmoid manipulation is to view the examination under fluoroscopic control (see earlier). In contrast to simple advancement, counterclockwise torque with gentle tip deflection stretches the midsigmoid, first in a ventral direction, and then toward the right lower quadrant of the abdomen (see Figure 6-6). As the scope is advanced using continuous counterclockwise torque, it courses back across the upper pelvis to the sigmoid-descending colon junction. Fluoroscopic examination will demonstrate a loop that resembles the Greek letter alpha (α). This intentionally created broad curve flattens the angle at the sigmoid-descending colon junction into a gentle curve. Once the tip of the scope has passed to the level of the mid-descending colon, reduction can be undertaken. In order to remove the loop, the instrument is simultaneously withdrawn while clockwise torque is applied (see Figure 6-6). It is evident that derotation is being accomplished when the endoscopist observes the advancement of the image in spite of the fact that the instrument is being withdrawn. Once the loop has been reduced, the scope can be readily advanced to the splenic flexure by maintaining clockwise torque during advancement of the shaft (see Figure 6-6). This is quite an efficient technique for negotiating a moderately redundant sigmoid colon if multiple tightly adherent loops are absent. However, if several adherent loops are present, this method cannot be successfully employed and only increases the level of discomfort for the patient. If the sigmoid loop is extremely large, it may not be able to be reduced by derotation until the proximal end of the instrument has been passed well into the transverse colon. The loop should be reduced either before the tip reaches the splenic flexure or after it has passed the distal transverse colon. Derotation with the deflection tip sharply angulated at the splenic flexure invites traction trauma to attachments that exist between the colon and the spleen (see Complications).

Intubation by Accordionization ("Dither-Torquing")

When the colon segment to be intubated is not a straight shot or when one is not able to create a large, gentle loop, it is often best to use a dither-torquing approach. This method

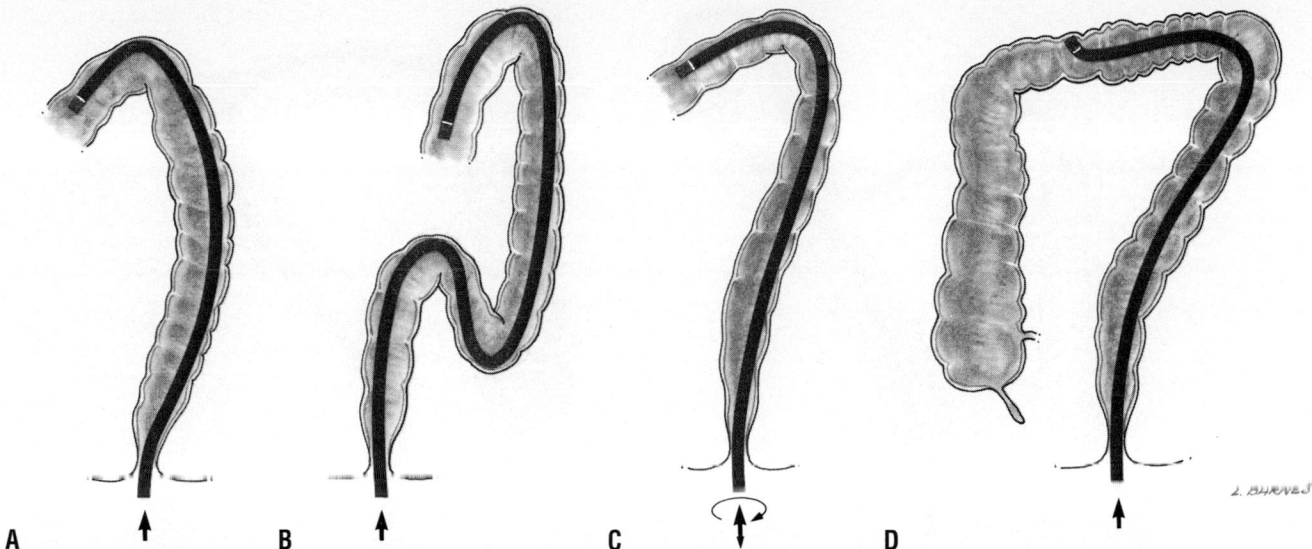

FIGURE 6-16. The colonoscope is maneuvered into the transverse colon by the following steps. **A:** "Hooking" the splenic flexure. **B:** Advancing the instrument. **C:** Withdrawing and straightening the tip while maintaining clockwise torque. **D:** Negotiating the transverse colon by hooking the bowel wall.

attempts to straighten a tightly nested colon as the scope is advanced. In this approach, one is trying to accordionize as much colon as possible onto a limited length of instrument.

The technique employs simultaneous application of both dithering and torquing. Dithering refers to the repeated in-and-out movement of the instrument shaft. While the shaft is being advanced proximally 6 to 10 cm, a small amount of counterclockwise torque of about 45 to 60 degrees is applied. The process is reversed by using clockwise torque during simultaneous withdrawal of the scope for the same length. This cycle is repeated in a rhythmic fashion at a rate of about 1 to 2 cycles/second, taking care to avoid net advancement of the shaft. The shaft is gripped with the right hand close to the anus in order to minimize premature advancement of the scope. Only after the lumen appears to be straight ahead with minimal tip deflection should one regrasp the shaft to a new position. If this precaution is not heeded, it is likely that the shaft will be inappropriately advanced, leading to the development of a large loop. Although the first few dither-torquing cycles may appear to accomplish little, by rhythmically continuing this motion, one will enable the bowel to accordionize onto the scope, straightening the colon as the examination proceeds. With experience, it becomes apparent that the cyclic rhythm, amount of torque, degree of tip deflection, and shaft advancement distance are all variables that can be altered to achieve the maximal effect. If successful, the descending colon as far as the splenic flexure may be intubated through the application of clockwise torque during shaft advancement with minimal deflection of the tip. In more proximal segments, such as in the transverse colon, the same dither-torquing maneuver may be used. Here, however, dithering can be extended by 50 to 60 cm at a time.

Splenic Flexure and Transverse Colon Intubation

If the sigmoid colon has been accordionized onto the scope and is straightened into a gentle, smooth curve, negotiation of the splenic flexure is usually not difficult. Even if the flexure is quite high and sharply angulated, the deflection tip

can be rotated into the distal transverse colon without much problem. It is at this point that one must remember the hazard of creating an excessive deflection bend. As soon as there is visual acquisition of the distal transverse colon lumen, the degree of the deflection should be eased in order to provide a gentle bend of less than 90 degrees. In order to achieve this less acute angle, one must course along the outside curve of the colon wall rather than view the center of the lumen. Although the lumen may be partially obscured by the outside wall, it should not be entirely lost. In fewer than 5% of patients, the splenic flexure must be intubated in essentially a reverse fashion, with the deflection tip stretching and coursing the flexure to the left and caudad, before proceeding into the transverse colon. Once the instrument has been passed to the level of the mid-transverse colon, this splenic flexure loop can generally be removed with a counterclockwise rotation (Figure 6-16).

Advancing the colonoscope through the transverse colon is usually uneventful. This part of the colon is distinguished by its well-defined triangular appearance (Figure 6-17). If the transverse colon is without redundancy, the intubation will proceed directly across the upper abdomen to the hepatic

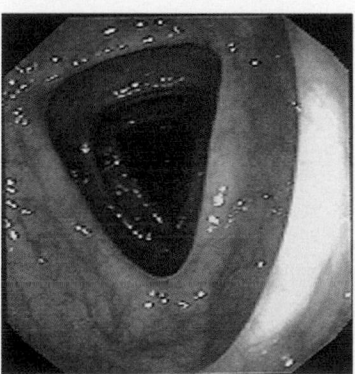

FIGURE 6-17. Normal transverse colon.

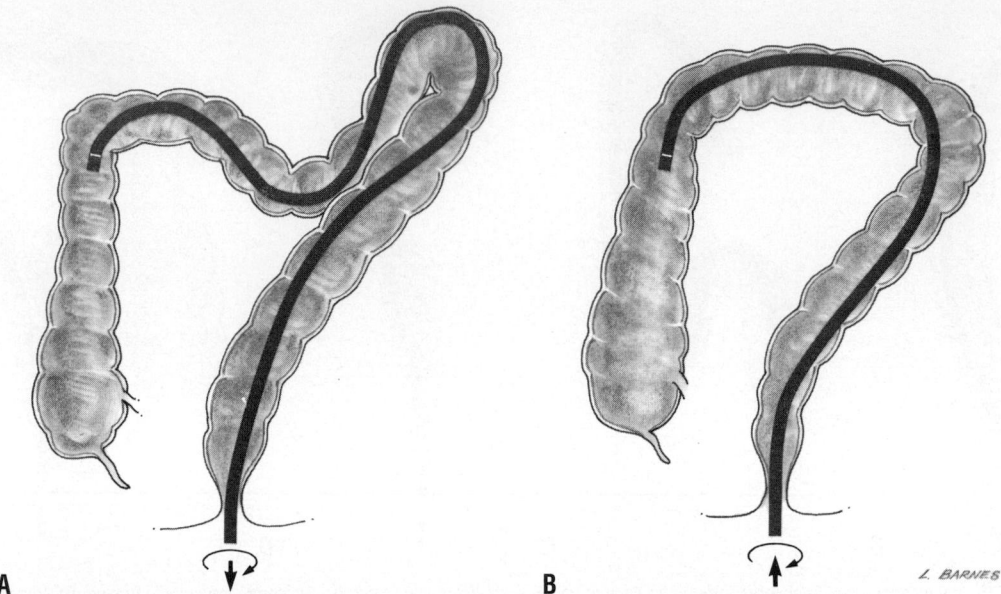

FIGURE 6-18. The colonoscope negotiates the ascending colon through the following steps. **A:** The tip is directed to visualize the ascending colon. **B:** Withdrawal produces advancement; this is expedited by the use of suction.

flexure (Figure 6-18). This redundancy can consume a considerable amount of scope length. When combined with a persistent sigmoid loop, there may be insufficient instrument left to complete the examination. Redundancy of the transverse colon may result in a loop that has the configuration of the Greek letter gamma (γ) when viewed by fluoroscopy. This loop is optimally removed by clockwise rotation of the shaft before attempting to proceed into the ascending colon. Once this has been accomplished, it will usually stay derotated. However, if it does tend to reform, external pressure at the umbilicus will often prevent this. If the transverse colon is redundant, one can also use the dither-torquing technique when progress is impeded. In this area, the dither-torquing maneuver is often best performed with longer, 30- to 60-cm strokes, rather than the short ones used in the sigmoid colon.

Hepatic Flexure and Ascending Colon Intubation

The hepatic flexure is often recognized by a bluish discoloration of the wall where the liver is in proximity (Figure 6-19). Not infrequently, however, the hepatic flexure is not immediately evident because of acute angulation. The deflection

tip may be sharply flexed with bowel lumen distorted by stretching. This often gives the endoscopist a false sense of accomplishment, leading him or her to believe that the cecum has been reached because there is apparently no colon left. If most of the colonoscope has been used and the specific cecal landmarks have not been identified, one is most likely at the hepatic flexure—not yet at the cecum. The true location is unlikely to be revealed until the shaft is withdrawn and torqued clockwise to bring the distal ascending colon into view.

If the transverse colon has been able to be negotiated straight across or straight down from a high splenic flexure, then intubation into the ascending colon is usually accomplished by clockwise torque, flattening of the deflection tip, and simultaneous gas aspiration. These three mechanisms combine to drop the scope into the cecum. If the transverse colon is excessively redundant, it may not be able to be maintained in the upper abdomen, even if abdominal pressure is applied. The instrument therefore approaches the hepatic flexure from below rather than from across. Inevitably, the deflection tip will require a 180-degree bend to negotiate this area. Once again, clockwise torque, flattening deflection, and gas aspiration, combined with what may be considerable shaft withdrawal, permit entry into the ascending colon. However, it is unlikely that the scope will drop into the ascending colon with a first attempt at torquing, flattening, and aspiration. Repeated efforts will usually be required to gather more colon progressively onto the instrument. Still, the maneuver that will finally drop the scope into the ascending colon and cecum will be the combination of clockwise torque, tip flattening, and gas aspiration (see Figure 6-18).

Finally, if negotiation of the hepatic flexure continues to be a problem, changing the position is often beneficial. Initially, the patient should be rotated to the prone position. If this is not helpful, the right lateral decubitus position should be attempted. The liver may have a flattening effect on the flexure in this position, thus permitting further passage.

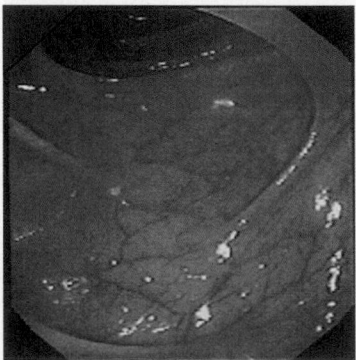

FIGURE 6-19. Hepatic flexure.

Cecum and Distal Ileum Intubation

The most reliable landmarks for visual confirmation of reaching the cecum are as follows:

- Appendiceal orifice (Figure 6-20)
- Ileocecal valve (Figures 6-21 and 6-22)
- Triangulation of the tinea (Figure 6-23)
- Intubation of the distal ileum (Figure 6-24)

Cirocco and Rusin believe that the ileocecal valve is the most reliable cecal landmark and is invariably visualized even when all other landmarks are obscure.[30] Palpation of the right lower quadrant with concomitant movement of the colon endoscopically and transillumination of the abdominal wall in the right iliac fossa are less dependable signs. When compressing the right lower quadrant, visual evidence of scope movement may be seen even if the viewing tip is at a considerable distance. Fluoroscopy as mentioned is helpful, but it must be kept in mind that the cecum is not always in the right iliac fossa. The same holds true if a plain abdominal film is completed at the end of the evaluation (Figure 6-25). Most newer equipment has a transillumination setting on the light source. However, the amount of interposing tissue can confuse interpretation, and difficulty with directing the light limits its applicability. Furthermore, a redundant transverse colon that extends into the right lower quadrant may mimic complete intubation if one were to rely on indirect criteria. Clearly, the least reliable indicator that the cecum has been reached is the impression that there is no remaining colon. If the usual landmarks of an ileocecal location are not present and there seems to be no remaining colon, the endoscopist has probably stretched a more proximal segment into a blind recess (e.g., the proximal transverse colon). Fleshner and colleagues suggest that there are mucosal spots or "freckles" that correlate microscopically with subepithelial and submucosal lymphoid follicles, an endoscopic feature of the cecum seen in approximately one-third of individuals.[57] Most experienced endoscopists can achieve the cecum more than 95% of the time.[167]

Sometimes it is important to intubate the distal ileum, especially for the evaluation of an individual with inflammatory bowel disease (see Figure 6-24). The success rate for accomplishing this maneuver increases with experience and is generally reported to be in the range of 80%.[15] Petrini visualized the ileum in 91% of the 97% in whom the cecum was reached (116 consecutive patients).[132] Muscular thickening of some ileocecal valves as well as the flutterlike configuration of others preclude a higher rate of intubation.

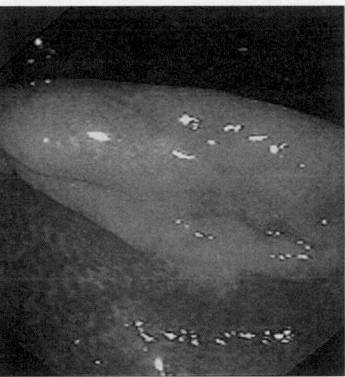

FIGURE 6-21. The ileocecal valve seen from a retroflexed instrument position.

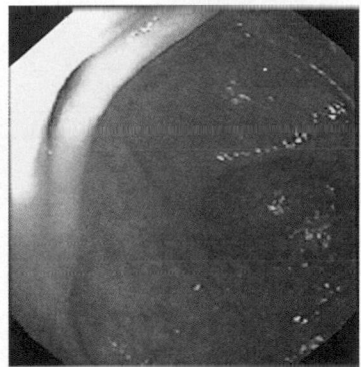

FIGURE 6-22. The ileocecal valve as is appears entering the cecum.

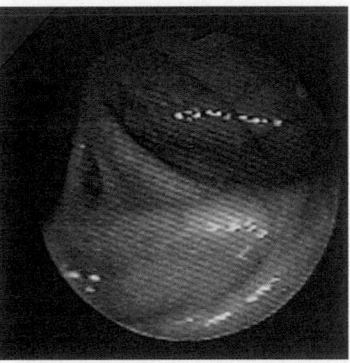

FIGURE 6-23. Normal cecal base with triangulation of the tinea.

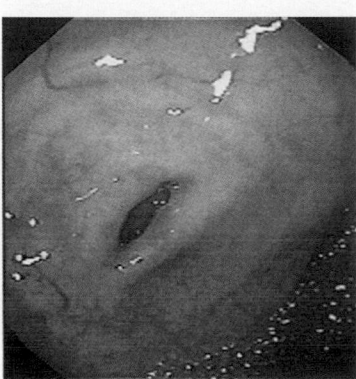

FIGURE 6-20. The appendiceal orifice.

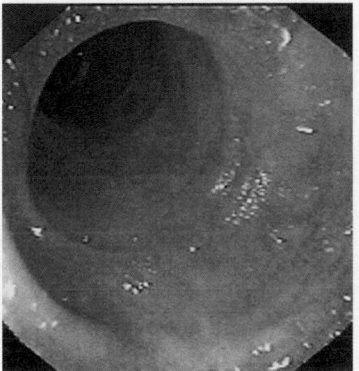

FIGURE 6-24. Normal terminal ileum.

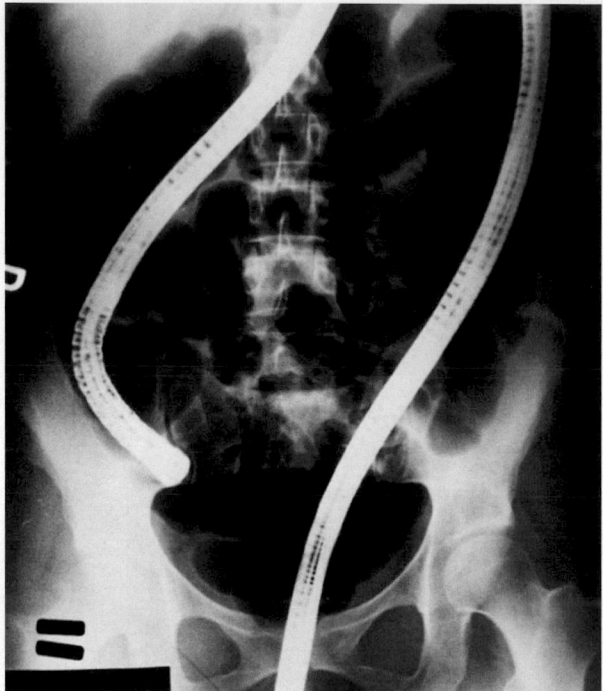

FIGURE 6-25. Plain abdominal film demonstrates a colonoscope that has reached the cecum.

Most endoscopists do not attempt ileocecal intubation on a routine basis unless clinically indicated. Furthermore, when one attempts to distend the valve, considerable air may be introduced into the ileum. The small bowel offers little resistance to the retrograde accumulation of air. Because it is not readily evacuated, it may lead to considerable postexamination discomfort.

When intubation of the distal ileum is indicated, one must recognize that the entrance is at an angle that is less than 90 degrees to the axis of the ascending colon. This angle is made even more acute because of the caudad displacement of the cecum produced by air insufflation when complete colon intubation has been accomplished. As viewed from the proximal ascending colon, only the prominent bilobar-shaped distal lip of the valve is in view (see Figure 6-21). The tip of the instrument must be positioned on the cecal side of the valve. The deflection tip is then angled toward the valve, prying the orifice open as the shaft is slightly withdrawn. A combination of torquing and suction will usually direct the scope into the terminal ileum. Others have developed their own methods for successful intubation.[23] The mucosal surface is recognized by its roughened, ground-glass appearance. This is in contrast to the smooth texture of the distended, adjacent cecum.

Withdrawal and Examination

Inspection of the colon should be a smooth and continuous process. If the instrument is simply withdrawn, the accordionized colon will fly off the end of the scope in an uncontrolled fashion at various points along the way. Hidden areas behind folds will go unexamined. In some instances, even long segments will evade adequate assessment. Expeditious withdrawal therefore usually results in poor evaluation of the colon.

Inspection of the mucosa for abnormalities will be facilitated if residual debris from the preparation has been removed during intubation. Conversely, if there is foreign material present, the endoscopist will have to aspirate frequently, collapsing the bowel lumen and interrupting the process of visual examination. Distension of the lumen will once again have to be established before inspection can proceed. When fluid must be removed, it is advantageous to position it at about 6 o'clock with respect to the viewing lens. This will permit removal without having to collapse the field from view completely. Sometimes muscular spasm or irritability of the colon interferes with optimal withdrawal visualization. This problem can sometimes be ameliorated by administering glucagon, 1 mg intravenously. However, this is not effective when the underlying impediment is due to a fibrotic stricture or bowel wall thickening associated with diverticulitis.

Examination of the colon during extubation is most efficiently performed by keeping the right hand on the shaft while controlling tip deflection with the left hand. The view of the lumen can be continuously readjusted while the shaft is being withdrawn. When there has been considerable redundancy and a substantial length of colon has been accordionized onto the scope, the instrument should be withdrawn by small amounts. A common practice is to withdraw 5 to 15 cm and then push the instrument back in. The excessive colon is released from the shaft, bit by bit. One must be particularly attentive at the flexures. The inner aspects of the proximal sides of both the hepatic and splenic flexures are areas that must be dropped from the scope very carefully in order to avoid missing what can be rather large lesions.

The ability to monitor quality during colonoscopy has been something that has been sought by those performing such procedures as a way to ensure a high standard of patient care. The concept of withdrawal time has been a fairly recent objective measure of said quality. It had been speculated that physicians who spent more time examining the colonic mucosa during removal of the colonoscope performed a more thorough evaluation of the colon than those who rushed through the procedure. Barclay and colleagues[10] demonstrated that those endoscopists who spent on average greater than 6 minutes during the withdrawal of the colonoscope from the cecum to the anus were more likely to detect colonic pathology. They demonstrated an increase in adenoma detection from 11.8% to 28.3% ($P < .001$) and a corresponding increase in advanced neoplasia detection from 2.6% to 6.4% ($P = .005$).

Cleansing the Instrument

The concern for transmitting disease may be exaggerated, but the fear of contracting hepatitis and AIDS has led to the marketing of numerous products for cleansing endoscopic equipment. Actually, the most common agents of infection transmitted by gastrointestinal endoscopy are *Salmonella* species and *Pseudomonas aeruginosa*.[151] In the United States, government regulations through the Centers for Disease Control and Prevention have produced numerous recommendations. Vigorous mechanical cleansing and the use of an enzymatic detergent immediately after the procedure, followed by a disinfectant and thorough rinsing, have been considered the most effective.[53,80,91,112,146] The channels should be likewise cleansed and air dried.

Gas sterilization is very effective but shortens the useful life of these very expensive instruments. Ultrasonic sterilizers, scope washers, and automatic computer-programmed disinfectors have been developed to reduce the possibility of toxic effects to the patient and to the personnel who handle the chemicals. Such products and companies are becoming numerous, and concepts are continuing to evolve in this area.

It is important to note that following disinfecting, the instruments should be thoroughly washed with plain water. A type of chemical colitis has been observed in some individuals, a complication believed to be due to contamination of the air–water channel with potentially toxic cleansing chemicals.[90]

Therapeutic Colonoscopy

Biopsy

Biopsy devices are available for sampling colonic mucosa and lesions. For reasons of reliability and the potential for contamination, these instruments are often disposable. Multiple specimens can be gathered within the cups of a large biopsy forceps, especially if a central spike is present to hold them (see Figure 6-2). This is particularly useful when gathering a large number of samples for dysplasia surveillance in chronic ulcerative and Crohn's colitis (see Chapter 29. Hot biopsy forceps are insulated and can be connected to a monopolar generator. This is particularly helpful for the management of small mucosal polyps. These lesions, which are usually not sufficiently defined to enable safe snare excision, can be grasped with forceps and removed during simultaneous electrocoagulation. With the polyp tented into the lumen, brief spurts of coagulation are applied until there is the first appearance of a whitish coagulum at the base of the forceps. Because the small surface area of contact results in a relatively high current density, electrocoagulation should be limited. Excessive or prolonged burning can result in full-thickness bowel injury. It is because of this concern that some endoscopists use a "cold biopsy" technique. The forceps will not sever the tissue in a scissorlike fashion; the instrument, therefore, must be abruptly pulled from the bowel wall. The specimen within the biopsy cut will be relatively unaffected by the coagulation current. Unlike a cold biopsy, the foregoing method will usually destroy any surrounding adenomatous tissue, thereby resulting in definitive treatment of small neoplastic polyps.

Blood vessel lesions, such as vascular ectasias (see Figure 28-6, are optimally treated by using a bipolar electrode. Complete destruction can be accomplished with minimal risk of bowel injury (see Chapter 28).

Snare Polypectomy

One of the most important advances in colon surgery during the past few decades has been the development of endoscopic polypectomy. The contrast between up to a 1-week hospitalization for an open colotomy–polypectomy and that of an outpatient colonoscopy–polypectomy performed in less than 1 hour is dramatic. The concept of following a polyp observed on barium enema examination in order to avoid a laparotomy, colotomy, and polypectomy has long been invalid (see Chapter 22). Using colonoscopy, most polyps can be removed or at least examined by biopsy. Patients who harbor a colon or rectal polyp require an aggressive approach to diagnosis and treatment.[35]

Equipment

As mentioned earlier, performance of polypectomy requires an electrical-generating power source that, for endoscopic use, is transmitted by means of a wire loop snare or coagulating electrode. Polypectomy is undertaken through the accessory channel of the instrument. Most commercially available high-frequency units permit tube or cutting current and a spark gap current, which produce coagulation or a blend of the two (see Figure 6-15 and Chapter 5).[62]

Gas insufflation during polypectomy is a matter of particular concern because of the potential hazard of an explosive mixtures being present.[9] The necessity for adequate bowel preparation has been discussed previously. The use of an inert gas—most commonly carbon dioxide—has been recommended by some experts but remains controversial. However, the requirements of tank storage and accessories have made this a rather impractical and, in the opinion of many, unnecessary alternative when other cathartic regimens are employed. Frühmorgen reported no instance of gas explosion using standard methods of bowel preparation in more than 2,700 colonoscopy–polypectomy procedures.[62] With respect to insufflation of air as a source of discomfort during colonoscopy, Church and Delaney performed a randomized trial with the use of air in one-half of patients and carbon dioxide in the other half.[29] There were 124 in the air group and 123 in the carbon dioxide group. There were no differences with respect to sedation/analgesia requirements during the procedure, but there was significantly less abdominal pain noted 10 minutes after conclusion of the examination when carbon dioxide was employed.

In addition to the previously mentioned equipment, many cold and hot biopsy forceps, snares, baskets, and hooks for retrieval are commercially available. Shapes include oval, eccentric, and hexagonal. Some prefer to use a hexagonal snare for most polyps. This configuration seems to hold its shape during difficult positioning or if multiple excisions are required. For polyps that are too large for hot biopsy excision, it is best to use a minisize snare. Milsom and Gottesman advise removing the snare wire and applying suction through the sheath for the removal of small polyps, especially from the right side of the colon.[117]

In 1976, Frühmorgen and others introduced the concept of applying the argon laser to the endoscopic treatment of a bleeding lesion.[64] The laser, an acronym for light amplification by stimulated emission of radiation, produces an intense monochromatic light, which can destroy tissue to varying depths of penetration. The argon laser is considered to be most useful for treating mucosal lesions because energy from this source penetrates only 1 mm of tissue; the neodymium:yttrium-aluminum-garnet laser is better for deeper and exophytic lesions because it penetrates 3 to 4 mm of tissue.[100] Optical fibers have been produced to fit through the open channel of most endoscopic instruments. Lasers have been used most effectively in the treatment of angiodysplastic lesions, but they have also been applied to benign and malignant tumors, as well as to a variety of anatomic abnormalities.[55,86,110]

Indications

The primary indications for the use of colonoscopy as a therapeutic tool are polypectomy and biopsy. Therapeutic colonoscopy is also indicated for treatment of bleeding lesions such as vascular anomalies, ulcerations, tumors, and those at the polypectomy site. Additional applications

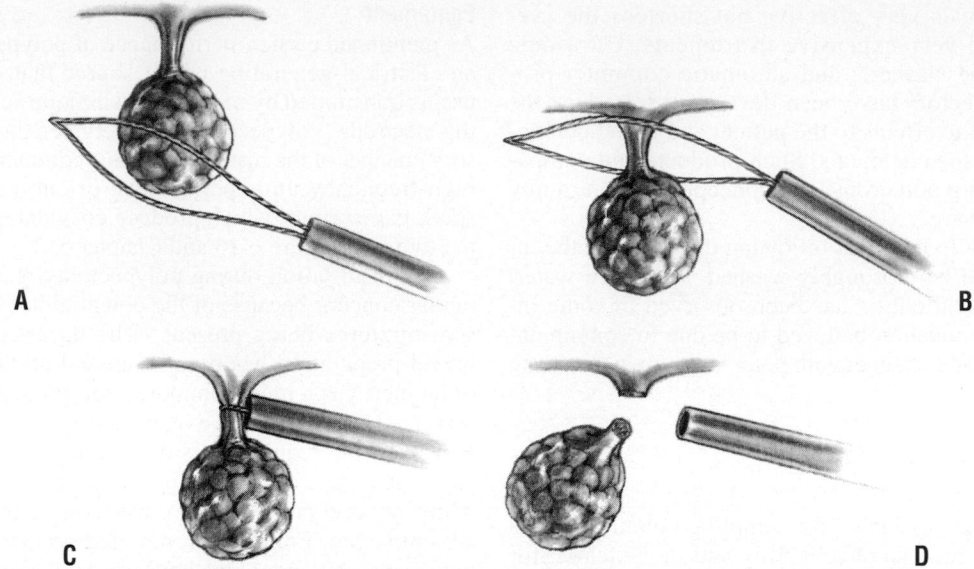

FIGURE 6-26. Techniques involved in polypectomy. **A,B:** The polyp is ensnared. **C:** Loop tightening results in coagulation and strangulation. **D:** The polyp is removed.

include decompression of cecal and sigmoid volvulus, colonic decompression in Ogilvie's syndrome, foreign body removal, balloon dilatation of stricture, and palliative treatment of stenosing or bleeding malignant lesions.

Technique

The technique for removal of a polyp is not dissimilar to that employed with the rigid sigmoidoscope, but maintaining adequate visualization and holding instrument position obviously pose more of a problem. The distal orifice for the snare exits the scope at the 5 o'clock position relative to the luminal view. If the polyp is on the opposite side (11 o'clock), the view will be lost when the snare is passed over the polyp. Consequently, whenever possible, it is best to rotate the scope so that the base of the polyp is located at the 5 o'clock position. This will ensure that the polyp remains in view while the snare loop is positioned.

The presence of an assistant is a requisite. Usually, the polyp is visualized 2 or 3 cm distal to the endoscope. By maneuvering the tip of the colonoscope and sometimes the patient, the wire loop is advanced and the head of the polyp encircled (Figure 6-26). Small lesions can be removed simply with the biopsy instrument (Figure 6-27). The loop is drawn

down to the pedicle until the latter is secured. The endoscope is then maneuvered to hold the polyp away from the bowel wall to avoid injury and possible perforation. The current is then applied and the polyp excised. It can then be removed using forceps, a hook or basket, or the suction device. When other polyps are present, they may be removed individually or collected by straining the stool following the procedure (Figure 6-28). Pathologic confirmation is, of course, required.

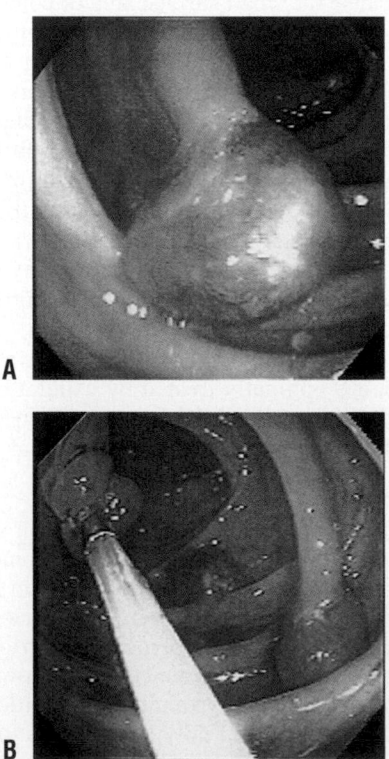

FIGURE 6-28. Technique of snare polypectomy. **A:** A polyp on a stalk is seen in the midsigmoid colon. **B:** The snare encompasses the head of the polyp; an adjacent pedunculated polyp can be seen.

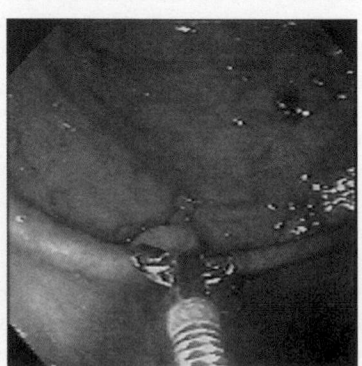

FIGURE 6-27. A small polyp is removed with biopsy forceps.

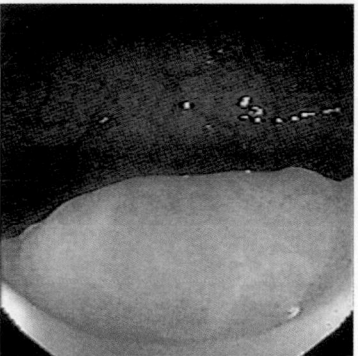

FIGURE 6-29. Sessile polypoid tumor of the rectosigmoid.

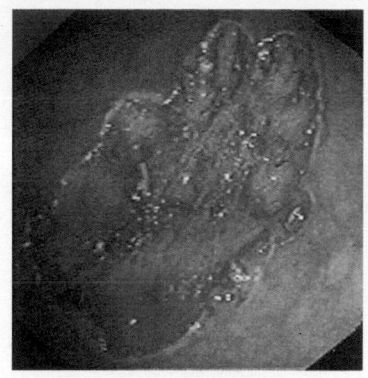

FIGURE 6-30. Removal of a tumor has been effected with snare cautery.

Large polyps (i.e., those greater than 2.5 cm) can be removed by the foregoing technique if adequate visualization of the pedicle is possible, and the head can be ensnared. Failing this, however, it can be removed piecemeal and the specimens collected as described. The expertise of the endoscopist determines the size and the nature of lesion one is willing to approach. Sessile and even submucosal lesions can be removed by endoscopy, but ulcerating tumors should not be.[25,26] Care must be taken to elevate the mucosa as the snare is tightened. Stripping the mucosa and submucosa is safe, but the physician must endeavor to leave intact the muscularis propria (Figures 6-29 through 6-31). Obviously, the risk of bowel perforation is increased when the physician attempts to remove such lesions.

A sessile polyp, however, may not permit adequate viewing of the entire lesion when the snare is applied. Under these circumstances, removal is accomplished in a piecemeal fashion so that each lobule that is excised can be clearly seen (Figure 6-32).

Several techniques may be used for removing larger sessile lesions. A two-channel scope permits the endoscopist to employ both a snare and a grasper to manipulate the polyp. The snare is passed through the one channel, and a grasper or large biopsy forceps is placed in the second. The latter is then passed out through the open loop of the snare. In this fashion, the polyp can be manipulated into the snare. Sometimes it is helpful to elevate a sessile polyp above the plane of the colon wall by injecting saline into the submucosa. This provides greater separation between the muscularis propria and the polyp base. In addition, the improved tissue hydration facilitates the electrocoagulation.

The proper application of electrocautery is essential for safe and effective polypectomy (see Chapter 5). There is no single combination of cutting and coagulation current or wattage that must be used or is preferred. A colonoscopist gradually develops confidence in his or her own electrosurgical method. What is remarkable is how varied these techniques may be. The general approach that many have employed uses short bursts of monopolar, blended, cutting current while one squeezes the snare. By using intermittent bursts, deep tissue cooling is permitted, thereby minimizing the likelihood of a full-thickness burn. Whenever possible, the polyp is suspended within the lumen to avoid adjacent tissue injury. If the polyp is too large to avoid touching the wall, then surface contact should intentionally be maximized in order to avoid pinpoint areas of high current density.

Although inpatient observation for 24 to 48 hours has been recommended in the past, this is no longer necessary, provided the patient is informed of the potential hazards and remains relatively close to the area for a day or so. At most institutions, virtually all patients are managed on an ambulatory basis.

Malignant polyps, even if technically removable at colonoscopy, may require a subsequent resection (see Chapter 22). Such lesions are unlikely to be palpable at the time of operation. Accurate localization is important, particularly if intraluminal landmarks are absent and fluoroscopic control is unavailable. Some have advised the performance of a localizing preoperative barium enema.[60] Another alternative is to place a clip on the lesion (e.g., HX-2U Clip-Fixing Device; Olympus America, Melville, NY) using a plain abdominal radiograph for localization.[155]

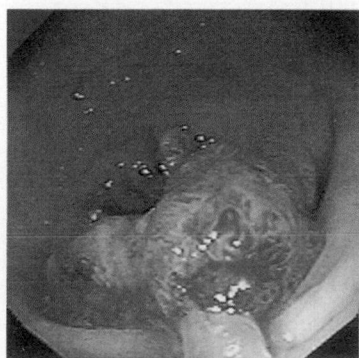

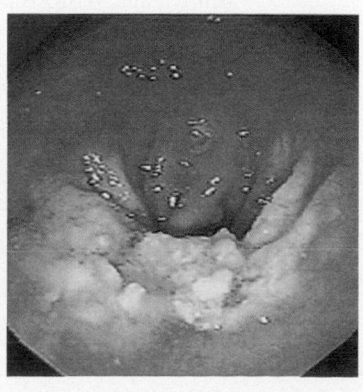

FIGURE 6-31. Snare excision of large polyp. **A:** Snare is passed around polypoid lesion. **B:** Coagulum appears at the site of polyp removal.

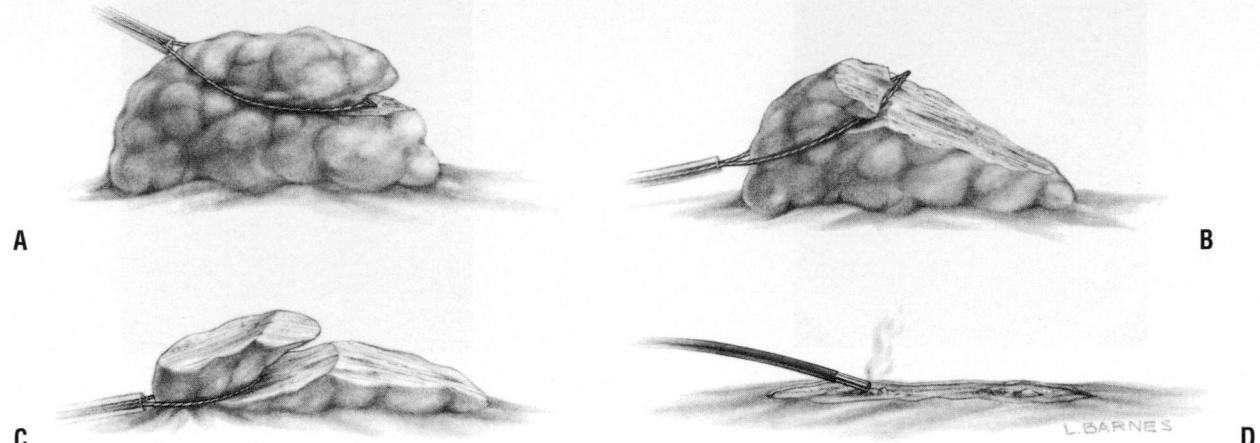

FIGURE 6-32. Technique for removal of a sessile polyp. **A:** The polyp is ensnared. **B:** The mucosa is elevated. **C:** Excision is done piecemeal. **D:** The residual polyp is removed and its base electrocoagulated.

An injection of particulate India ink applied submucosally with a sclerotherapy needle will persist indefinitely and allow identification of the dye on the serosal aspect at the time of laparotomy (Figure 6-33).[88,119,145] This technique is not without complications, however. Fat necrosis with inflammatory pseudotumor as well as colonic abscess and focal peritonitis have been reported secondary to India ink tattooing of the colon.[36,131] Tissue marking with submucosal injections of India ink or other similar marking agents has become the standard of care for lesions that are not located in the cecum or the rectum to ensure that the lesion is removed at the time of subsequent surgical excision.

Comment on Polypectomy

In the past, the decision of which large polyps should be removed endoscopically versus surgically was somewhat controversial and even arbitrary. Traditionally, gastroenterologists would remove the vast majority of polyps encountered during colonoscopy. The threshold for a gastroenterologist to refer a patient with a large adenoma for surgical resection has been based on several factors, including polyp size, percentage of luminal circumference occupied, number of folds involved and orientation, as well as the more subjective factor of endoscopist comfort level. It is generally thought that the surgeon may have a greater willingness to attempt removal because of his or her ability to deal with the potential complications. Depending on the experience of the gastroenterologist, the paradigm may have

changed somewhat. It is now common for many institutions to employ a therapeutic endoscopist. These physicians traditionally had been gastroenterologists who had additional training in endoscopic retrograde cholangiopancreatography (ERCP). More recently, training of these individuals has required an additional year of study, with this fourth year expanding to include such skills as endoscopic mucosal resection (EMR) and endoscopic submucosal dissection (ESD). These physicians have thus been trained to remove larger polyps endoscopically through more advanced techniques than traditional gastroenterologists and even most surgeons are qualified to employ. Thus, the management of complicated large/sessile polyps should involve a discussion between the gastroenterologist, his surgical colleague, and the patient. The input and the availability of specially trained advanced endoscopists should be considered in the decision-making process.

Results

Coller and colleagues reported colonoscopy on 146 patients with radiographically suspected polyps.[35] Of the 110 individuals found to have a neoplastic lesion, 62 were found to have an additional neoplasm (56%). It is because of this association that total colonoscopy is recommended for a patient found to harbor a colorectal neoplasm on imaging. Removing the lesion without such a complete evaluation is believed to be inadequate management because synchronous lesions can be missed.

Shinya and Wolff reported their experience of 7,000 polyps removed endoscopically.[147] There was no mortality. Most series, and the publications are indeed numerous, report approximately two-thirds of the lesions to be adenomatous polyps (i.e., tubular adenomas), a few as villous adenomas, and the remainder as malignant tumors, other benign neoplasms, and non-neoplastic conditions. The significance of polyps, their distribution, and the follow-up of patients are discussed in Chapter 22 .

Complications

The sheer volume of examinations that have been performed since the introduction of colonoscopy has resulted

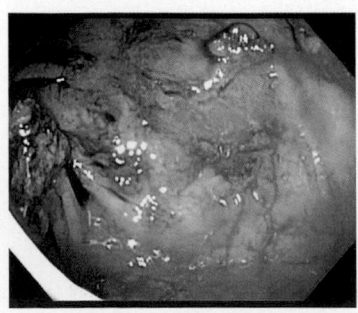

FIGURE 6-33. Endoscopic marking with India ink of a colorectal neoplasm.

in a broad spectrum of complications from both diagnostic as well as therapeutic endeavors. The frequency of complications, however, has remained fairly constant since the mid-1970s.

There are numerous complications that are associated with colonoscopy with and without polypectomy. Generally, they may be attributed to certain predisposing causes: bowel preparation and medication, equipment misuse or malfunction, patient factors (e.g., underlying comorbidities, such as cardiac, cerebral, pulmonary, and renal disease), and factors related to trauma coincident with the procedure.[73,106,137,139,144]

The following list enumerates the complications of colonoscopy with or without polypectomy:

Hemorrhage due to intraluminal or mesenteric injury, seromuscular tear, splenic trauma
Perforation
Retroperitoneal abscess
Retroperitoneal and mediastinal emphysema
Vertebral venous air embolism
Pneumoscrotum
Pneumothorax
Explosion
Postcolonoscopy distension
Postpolypectomy coagulation syndrome
Colonic obstruction
Loss of polyp
Volvulus
Internal hernia
Bacteremia
Infections
Medical problems (e.g., pulmonary, cardiovascular, renal)
Mechanical failure

In 1976, Smith polled members of the American Society of Colon and Rectal Surgeons.[150] He learned from the 162 respondents that more than 20,000 colonoscopies were performed. The overall complication rate was 0.4% for diagnostic colonoscopy and 1.8% for polypectomy. In like manner, Berci and colleagues questioned members of the Southern California Society for Gastrointestinal Endoscopy in 1974.[11] The incidence of perforation following colonoscopy and polypectomy (901 procedures) was 0.33%, whereas that following colonoscopy alone (3,850 procedures) was 0.25%. There was one death (0.02%). Bleeding occurred in 0.66% of polypectomized patients. Nivatvongs reported 19 complications following removal of 1,555 polyps, an incidence of 1.2%.[122] Bleeding was the most frequent problem. In these and in other studies, it becomes readily apparent that the incidence of complications decreases considerably as the examiner becomes more experienced. From the Ochsner Clinic group, in New Orleans, LA, over a 30-year period, more than 34,000 colonoscopies resulted in 31 perforations (0.09%).[8] It is probably axiomatic that therapeutic colonoscopy should not be performed until one achieves at least 50 diagnostic procedures.

Hemorrhage

Bleeding is the most common complication following polypectomy, representing 53% of all complications in the experience of Nivatvongs.[123] Hemorrhage can also be due to biopsy, laceration of the mucosa by the instrument, or tearing of the mesentery or the splenic capsule.[7,15,116,126] As previously suggested, those patients who are at an increased risk for bleeding must be identified and appropriate measures taken. Obtaining an adequate history before performing endoscopic procedures is therefore essential. Familiarity with the electrical equipment and use of coagulating current and the endoscopist's clinical experience reduce the risk of this complication (see Chapter 5). Inevitably, if the physician performs a sufficient number of examinations and procedures, bleeding will be encountered. Special caution should be employed when the endoscopist attempts removal of a polyp with a thick pedicle. Blended current is suggested by many experienced endoscopists under these circumstances. Intermittent application offers the best control and will most likely avoid precipitous transection.

The decision of how to manage the problem of bleeding depends on the magnitude of the hemorrhage. If bleeding is recognized at the time of polypectomy, the area should be re-snared (if the pedicle is still apparent) and strangulated for at least 5 minutes. Electrocautery should not be used, especially if no pedicle is present. If the area is within reach of the rigid proctosigmoidoscope, it may be controlled by one of the means suggested in Chapter 5. In-hospital observation is mandatory if control has not been established with reasonable certainty, and operative intervention may be necessary if bleeding persists. This is particularly true if bleeding is secondary to a mesenteric tear or to splenic injury, both of which may not be readily apparent for several hours. Symptoms include the usual signs of hemorrhage (i.e., weakness, syncope, pallor, hypotension, and tachycardia), but abdominal pain and distension as well as left shoulder pain may also be observed. A falling hematocrit is obviously ominous. Although computed tomography (CT) may be helpful, the greatest aid to an early diagnosis is the knowledge that this complication may indeed occur.[46,72] A splenic subcapsular hematoma may be observed by means of CT as long as 10 days after colonoscopy.[115,158]

Gibbs and colleagues reported the Ochsner Clinic experience with postpolypectomy colonic hemorrhage.[69] During a 5-year period, more than 12,000 colonoscopies were performed at that institution, of which approximately one-half required polypectomy or biopsy. The incidence of lower intestinal hemorrhage was 0.2% for individuals requiring hospitalization (13 patients). All episodes of bleeding occurred within 12 days following the procedure. Technetium-tagged red blood cell scintigraphy (see Chapter 28) was performed in all but one patient and was successful in localizing the bleeding in four (31%). In those with normal scintigrams, hemorrhage did not recur. Arteriography was performed in five individuals (38%), two of four with positive scintigrams; bleeding was controlled with selective vasopressin infusion. The fifth patient underwent vasopressin infusion without prior diagnostic study. In summary, of the 13 patients with hemorrhage, cessation occurred with rest and hydration in 9 (69%), selective vasopressin infusion in 3 (23%), and endoscopic cautery in 1 (8%). No individual required surgical intervention. The authors concluded that technetium-tagged red blood cell scintigraphy identifies those individuals who have ongoing bleeding and in whom additional invasive procedures, such as arteriography or repeat endoscopy, are warranted.[69]

Perforation

Perforation of the colon with pneumoperitoneum usually becomes manifest almost immediately or within a few hours following the procedure. The incidence of perforation has been reported to range from 0.03% to 0.65% for diagnostic colonoscopies and from 0.07% to 2.1% for therapeutic endoscopies.[39,89,120] Perforation may occur secondary to polypectomy, diseases of the colon itself (e.g., diverticulitis, colitis, or ischemia), or to vigorous manipulation, rotation, or angulation of the instrument. Overdistension with air or gas can also precipitate a perforation. The embarrassing observation of an epiploic appendage during colonoscopy establishes the diagnosis with certainty. Ileal perforation following colonoscopy has also been reported.[121] This has been attributed to the rigidity of the small intestine that may be produced by prior abdominal surgery or by adhesions.

The classic presentations of transmural burn are fever, localized abdominal pain, tenderness, focal peritoneal signs, distension, and leukocytosis.[123] Again, inpatient treatment is required. Occasionally the patient's symptoms may be minimal relative to the amount of gas that is apparent on abdominal roentgenogram. In selected cases in which the bowel has been well prepared, *cautious* continued observation may be considered.[2] This is particularly true if the patient presents many hours or a day or two after the procedure. Nonsurgical management may be considered reasonable under the following circumstances[8,20,27,77,82]:

- Stable condition
- Late diagnosis
- Good bowel preparation
- Pneumoperitoneum not expanding
- No evidence for peritonitis
- No distal obstruction
- Improvement with supportive care
- Absence of underlying pathologic features that would ultimately require resection

Frequent follow-up evaluation is, of course, required. Oral intake should be withheld, and intravenous fluid replacement with broad-spectrum antibiotics is advisable. A limited water-soluble (Gastrografin) enema may also be considered in the equivocal situation (see Chapter 5). The sigmoid colon is the most common site of perforation. This may be because it is the area of loop formation, and an expanding loop can longitudinally tear the sigmoid colon. Secondly, this is a frequent location for pathologic findings (e.g., polyp, diverticulitis).

Laparotomy should be undertaken if the patient exhibits signs and symptoms of peritonitis. Furthermore, surgery is most definitely indicated in the presence of a large perforation demonstrated either colonoscopically or radiographically and in the setting of generalized peritonitis or ongoing sepsis.[39] The presence of concomitant pathologic features at the time of the perforation, such as a large sessile polyp that may be malignant, intractable colitis, or a perforation proximal to a colonic lesion that will inevitably require surgery, generally mandates that the physician proceed to immediate operation.[39] Fever and leukocytosis alone or in combination are not necessarily absolute indications for surgical intervention, but the burden of responsibility falls on the surgeon for unwarranted delay. A perforation that has sealed or even a negative laparotomy should not evoke criticism.

When a perforation is recognized shortly following the endoscopy, the hole or tear usually can be closed primarily without the need for a diversionary procedure if the bowel has been well prepared. If a resection is considered advisable, it can be reasonably safely undertaken without the need for proximal colostomy or ileostomy unless sepsis or gross contamination is observed. Most surgeons and endoscopists agree that selective management of colonoscopic perforations is appropriate. It is recognized that perforations from therapeutic colonoscopy occur by a different mechanism than that from diagnostic colonoscopy and may be selectively managed without an operation.[8,92,105] Usually, perforations from diagnostic colonoscopy result in larger defects, and these are much more likely to require operative management.

As with prevention of hemorrhage, the risk of perforation is greatly reduced if intermittent bursts of current are applied. This reduces the likelihood of more extensive tissue injury, a consequence of transfer of heat into the deeper tissues or of contact of the polyp head with the bowel wall. When possible, an attempt should be made to suspend the polyp within the intestinal lumen during electrosurgical removal.[33]

Rectal perforation as a consequence of colonoscopy is extremely unusual.[127] One could expect that the frequency of this complication may be higher than that reported in the literature, especially with the recommendation to employ rectal retroflexion routinely.

Subcutaneous, retroperitoneal, and mediastinal emphysema after colonoscopy have been reported, as well as pneumoscrotum, pneumothorax, and vertebral venous air embolism.[5,24,54,103,143,177] These presentations do not necessarily constitute indications for surgical exploration because free perforation of the colon is not implied. It is therefore important to distinguish between retroperitoneal and intraperitoneal gas. In the former situation, nonsurgical treatment should be the initial approach (see Figure 29-37). In fact, as stated earlier, close observation with antibiotic administration may be considered reasonable even with a pneumoperitoneum.

Comment

Perforations occurring in the course of diagnostic colonoscopy are most frequently located in the sigmoid colon and appear to be a consequence of manipulation and intubation. Twisting and stretching a redundant, narrow, or diverticular-loaded sigmoid colon represent particular areas of relative difficulty. Consequently, when trauma ensues, it is more likely to be a broader injury. A large sigmoid colon loop in the colonoscope provides the potential for hidden injury, causing a longitudinal tear along the bowel wall, especially on the antimesenteric surface. Such defects, once created, are most likely to persist and require surgical intervention. A particularly jagged, broad defect usually requires resection. Conversely, perforation associated with polypectomy, hot biopsy excision, or laser therapy is usually a fairly discrete lesion that may seal rapidly. Under these circumstances, the perforation may be treated nonoperatively through bowel rest and antibiotics. In any case, the decision of whether to operate is based on clinical observation and a surgeon's judgment.

Explosion

Explosion should not occur in a well-prepared colon, although the use of mannitol as a bowel preparation has been implicated as a causative factor. The use of an inert gas, such as carbon dioxide, has been advocated by some, but is probably an unnecessary caution (see previous discussion).[12] It should be remembered, however, that with an essentially closed system such as is present when colonoscopy–polypectomy is performed, there is no means for gas to escape once ignited.

This is not true for the open-ended rigid proctosigmoidoscope. The examiner should be wary of using electric current if dissatisfied with the adequacy of the bowel preparation.

Postcolonoscopy Distension

A postcolonoscopy syndrome has been described, manifested by abdominal distension, discomfort, and dilated loops of bowel on the roentgenogram.[114,129] Patients do not exhibit signs of peritonitis. This is probably secondary to air insufflation, especially in a patient with an incompetent ileocecal valve. Treatment consists of observation, patient positioning (prone positioning), and medical management.

Postpolypectomy Coagulation Syndrome

Postpolypectomy coagulation syndrome was described by Waye in 1981.[166] The patient may develop localized signs of peritonitis—pain, fever, and leukocytosis—without evidence of perforation on radiologic examination. The condition is believed to be due to transmural thermal injury of the bowel at the site of the polypectomy.[31,166] Treatment may require inpatient observation, intravenous fluid therapy, and broad-spectrum antibiotics.

Obstruction and Incarcerated Hernia and Internal Hernia

Colonic obstruction can be precipitated by colonoscopy, usually at the site of underlying sigmoid disease. Volvulus has also been reported, possibly secondary to the alpha maneuver or to overinsufflation of air. Incarceration of the colonoscope in an inguinal hernia that does not permit reduction of the hernia nor removal of the instrument has been reported, along with the technique for extraction.[96,173] An acute small bowel obstruction has been described as a consequence of a rent in the mesentery caused by a diagnostic colonoscopy.[28]

Loss of Polyp

All removed polyps should be submitted to histologic examination. Those less than 8 mm in diameter may be suctioned through the accessory channel of the colonoscope with the aid of a mucus trap.[31] If the polyp cannot be removed by the standard methods of suctioning onto the tip of the instrument or snare recapture, an instrument such as a grasper or fabric basket can be used to capture the polyp. Polyps not retrieved with any of these techniques can sometimes be captured with the passage of fecal contents into a bedpan. Unfortunately, despite all reasonable efforts, a polyp is sometimes not recovered.

Bacteremia

Bacteremia has been reported to be associated with colonoscopy, but other studies have failed to confirm this observation.[38,44,98,124,125] Routine antibiotic prophylaxis, however, is no longer indicated for the high-risk patient (see Chapter 5).

Medical Problems

Hypotension, bradycardia, tachycardia, and myocardial infarction have all been observed during and after colonoscopy. Electrocardiogram monitoring with the addition of oxygen for patients at increased risk is worthy of consideration. Individuals with pacemakers may require a fixed rate if electrocoagulation is employed, even though there may be proper grounding and adequate shielding of the pacemaker. Herman and colleagues observed 233 consecutive patients who underwent colonoscopy for evidence of diaphoresis, bradycardia, or hypotension.[81] Of the 37 (16.5%) who demonstrated a vasovagal response, there was no difference with respect to the variables of examination difficulty, colon preparation, cardiopulmonary disease, or medications. However, there was a significantly greater dose of midazolam used in the vasovagal-response group. Furthermore, diverticulosis was more frequently observed in these patients.

Mechanical Failure

Numerous problems can develop from malfunction of the instruments and accessories (e.g., breakage of the colonoscope with entrapment of the instrument). Defective electrical equipment and inexperience with its use are two of the most common reasons for polypectomy hemorrhage and bowel wall necrosis. The snare wire can break or become fused with the polyp. Incomplete division of the pedicle can occur with the snare completely closed.

Conclusion

Despite the long list of complications, colonoscopy and colonoscopy with polypectomy can be undertaken with very low morbidity and very rare mortality—certainly lower mortality than may be anticipated after operative intervention.

Special Situations

Foreign Body Removal

The problems of removal of foreign bodies inserted into the rectum as well as ingested foreign bodies are addressed in Chapter 18. The colonoscope has been successfully employed for such extractions. For example, Frühmorgen removed a dental prosthesis as well as intestinal tubes by using this instrument (see Chapter 18).[63]

Volvulus

Colonoscopy has been successfully applied to the treatment of sigmoid volvulus.[68,140,154] Although rigid proctosigmoidoscopy is more readily available and easier to employ, there is the occasional situation when an attempt at reduction with a colonoscope may be indicated, especially when it involves more proximal bowel. The diagnosis and therapy of volvulus are discussed in Chapter 28.

Intraoperative Colonoscopy

Intraoperative colonoscopy may be considered in several situations:

When prior conventional colonoscopy has been unsuccessful

To evaluate the remainder of the colon when a partial resection is contemplated

To avoid contamination when an unsuspected polyp is found during a "clean" operation

To localize the site of a lesion or prior excision site, including with laparoscopic surgery

To complement arteriography in the diagnosis of the source of gastrointestinal hemorrhage[49,52,109,114,138]

The patient ideally is placed in the perineolithotomy position (see Figure 24-14) as if for combined abdominoperineal resection of the rectum. The abdominal surgeon guides the instrument through the bowel, thus expediting the procedure.

Comment

Although the application of this technique is limited, it may become of greater value in the diagnosis and treatment of lower gastrointestinal hemorrhage with improved methods for clearing liquid and clotted blood through the colonoscope.

Unfortunately, the requirement for intraoperative colonoscopy is often the result of failure to consider tattooing of the site of prior polyp removal (see Figure 6-33) or the willingness on the part of the surgeon to accept the information from the gastroenterologist as to the location of the lesion. The apothegm, "Don't let the enemy choose the territory!" when it comes to surgery for a small malignant tumor, the surgeon must be circumspect when informed as to the location of such a lesion. Too often, colon lesions are difficult to localize anatomically based on a colonoscopically reported distance of such lesions from the anus. One that is thought to be at 50 cm could be in the right or transverse colon, or even distal sigmoid. A straightforward operation then becomes an exercise in tedium and frustration, a situation that can usually be avoided. It would be imprudent and inappropriate indeed if a surgeon were to embark on a proposed low anterior resection without personally confirming the location of the lesion. With a more proximal tumor, however, the surgeon should at least feel reasonably confident that he or she knows exactly where that lesion is or, alternatively, expects to have no difficulty in finding it.

Pediatric Colonoscopy

Pediatric colonoscopy can be performed with a narrow-caliber endoscope or with the standard instrument, depending on the age of the patient. A general anesthetic is usually recommended for infants and young children. Preparation in infants usually consists of a clear liquid diet for 24 hours, but a laxative is usually advised for older children. Evaluation of rectal bleeding, suspicion of polyps, inflammatory bowel disease, and congenital anomalies are the most common indications for the procedure.[66,75,133,172] Colonoscopy is not useful in the evaluation of children with constipation and isolated recurrent abdominal pain.[93]

The technique for performing colonoscopy is somewhat modified when examination is undertaken in children, minimizing loop formation in order to provide greater comfort. Emphasis is made on intubating the terminal ileum as a standard part of pediatric colonoscopy because of its importance in the evaluation of Crohn's disease.[93] Obviously, children require close monitoring for respiratory depression, and resuscitation equipment with appropriate pediatric dosages should be readily available.

▶ BARIUM ENEMA AND VIRTUAL COLONOSCOPY VERSUS COLONOSCOPY

There is no disagreement that colonoscopy is more likely to detect small excrescences than will a barium enema examination, even with an optimal preparation and double-contrast technique.[44,47,95,161,176] It is fallacious to assume, however, that the radiologist can determine whether a polyp is benign or malignant. This is a distinction that must be made by histologic examination. CT colonography has a diagnostic sensitivity similar to that of standard colonoscopy for lesions at least 5 or 6 mm in diameter,[99] but as with barium enema, any polyp that is identified will require a repeat examination and procedure with the colonoscope (see Chapter 5).

Anderson and colleagues reviewed the radiographs and clinical records of 26 patients with colorectal cancer missed on barium enema study and subsequently detected by colonoscopy.[6] More than one-half were in the sigmoid colon and 8% in the rectum. In 76%, the cancer could be seen in retrospect. The most frequent error was caused by missing the lesion in a pool of barium, although the usual contributing factors, such as overlapping loops, were also observed. The authors advise double reporting of all barium enemas to improve detection rates.

For screening purposes, barium enema had once been considered the procedure of choice, but the new question is, which modality should be recommended for average risk colon cancer screening? Certainly, if it has been determined that the patient is in a higher risk group for the development of a neoplasm, periodic colonoscopy should be the diagnostic study employed (see Chapter 22). Furthermore, colonoscopy is recommended as the primary colonic evaluation for individuals with occult or obvious blood in the stool.[149]

The choice of screening method for the detection of colon polyps and cancers in an average-risk population is not a simple one. The possible diagnostic modalities include sigmoidoscopy, colonoscopy, barium enema, CT colonography, and stool-based tests (stool guaiac cards and DNA tests). Colonoscopy has become the screening method that generally has been chosen by many gastroenterologists and surgeons in the United States, but there is not sufficient physician capacity to screen the entire population of this country solely in this manor.

The multisociety task force has published guidelines for screening average-risk individuals for colon cancer.[102]

The task force suggests that all of the previously listed modalities may be used in the average-risk population. The intervals they recommend for screening are as follows: colonoscopy every 10 years, flexible sigmoidoscopy every 5 years, CT colonography every 5 years, double-contrast barium enema every 5 years, or annual fecal occult blood testing. The multitude of options afforded by the task force suggest that having multiple choices for screening is better than having only a single test. This allows the physician to tailor the screening recommendations on a patient-by-patient basis to allow for improved compliance. This philosophy stems from the idea that the best screening modality is the one that actually is performed. A more detailed discussion of colon cancer screening recommendation is beyond the scope of this chapter.

References

1. Abrams JS. A hard look at colonoscopy. *Am J Surg.* 1977;133(1):111–115.
2. Adair HM, Hishon S. The management of colonoscopic and sigmoidoscopic perforation of the large bowel. *Br J Surg.* 1981;68(6):415–416.
3. Adam IJ, Ali Z, Shorthouse AJ. Inadequacy of colonoscopy revealed by three-dimensional electromagnetic imaging. *Dis Colon Rectum.* 2001;44(7):978–983.
4. Adams C, Atkin W, Cook C, et al. Past hysterectomy reduces completion rate and polyp detection rate at flexible sigmoidoscopy. *Dis Colon Rectum.* 2002;45:A16.
5. Amshel AL, Shonberg IL, Gopal KA. Retroperitoneal and mediastinal emphysema as a complication of colonoscopy. *Dis Colon Rectum.* 1982;25(2):167–168.
6. Anderson N, Cook HB, Coates R. Colonoscopically detected colorectal cancer missed on barium enema. *Gastrointest Radiol.* 1991;16(2):123–127.
7. Anseline PF, Fazio VW. Management of massive postpolypectomy hemorrhage: report of a technique. *Dis Colon Rectum.* 1982;25(3):251–253.
8. Araghizadeh FY, Timmcke AE, Opelka FG, et al. Colonoscopic perforations. *Dis Colon Rectum.* 2001;44(5):713–716.
9. Avgerinos A, Kalantzis N, Rekoumis G, et al. Bowel preparation and the risk of explosion during colonoscopic polypectomy. *Gut.* 1984;25(4):361–364.

10. Barclay RL, Vicari JJ, Doughty AS, et al. Colonoscopic withdrawal times and adenoma detection during screening colonoscopy. *N Engl J Med*. 2006;355(24);2533–2541.

11. Berci G, Panish JF, Schapiro M, et al. Complications of colonoscopy and polypectomy. Report of the Southern California Society for Gastrointestinal Endoscopy. *Gastroenterology*. 1974;67(4):584–585.

12. Bigard MA, Gaucher P, Lassalle C. Fatal colonic explosion during colonoscopic polypectomy. *Gastroenterology*. 1979;77(6):1307–1310.

13. Blackstone MO, Riddell RH, Rogers BH, et al. Dysplasia-associated lesion or mass (DALM) detected by colonoscopy in long-standing ulcerative colitis: an indication for colectomy. *Gastroenterology*. 1981;80(2):366–374.

14. Bohlman TW, Katon RM, Lipshutz GR, et al. Fiberoptic pansigmoidoscopy. An evaluation and comparison with rigid sigmoidoscopy. *Gastroenterology*. 1977;72(4 pt 1):644–649.

15. Börsch G, Schmidt G. Endoscopy of the terminal ileum. Diagnostic yield in 400 consecutive examinations. *Dis Colon Rectum*. 1985;28(7):499–501.

16. Brand EJ, Sullivan BH Jr, Sivak MV Jr, et al. Colonoscopy in the diagnosis of unexplained rectal bleeding. *Ann Surg*. 1980;192(1):111–113.

17. Breiter JR, Hajjar JJ. Segmental tuberculosis of the colon diagnosed by colonoscopy. *Am J Gastroenterol*. 1981;76(4):369–373.

18. Burbige EJ, Bourke E, Tarder G. Effect of preparation for colonoscopy on fluid and electrolyte balance. *Gastrointest Endosc*. 1978;24(6):286–287.

19. Caliendo F, Eisenstat T, Oliver G, et al. Anticoagulants: do they need to be held in preparation for colonoscopy? *Dis Colon Rectum*. 2001;44:A5.

20. Carpio G, Albu E, Gumbs MA, et al. Management of colonic perforation after colonoscopy. Report of three cases. *Dis Colon Rectum*. 1989;32(7):624–626.

21. Carter HG. Short flexible fiberoptic colonoscopy in routine office examinations. *Dis Colon Rectum*. 1981;24(1):17–19.

22. Cataldo PA. Colonoscopy without sedation. *Dis Colon Rectum*. 1996;39(3):257–261.

23. Chen M, Khanduja KS. Intubation of the ileocecal valve made easy. *Dis Colon Rectum*. 1997;40(4):494–496.

24. Chorost MI, Wu JT, Webb H, et al. Vertebral venous air embolism: an unusual complication following colonoscopy: report of a case. *Dis Colon Rectum*. 2003;46(8):1138–1140.

25. Christie JP. Colonoscopic excision of sessile polyps. *Am J Gastroenterol*. 1976;66:23.

26. Christie JP. Colonoscopic excision of large sessile polyps. *Am J Gastroenterol*. 1977;67(5):430–438.

27. Christie JP, Marrazzo J III. "Mini-perforation" of the colon—not all postpolypectomy perforations require laparotomy. *Dis Colon Rectum*. 1991;34(2):132–135.

28. Chung H, Yuschak JV, Kukora JS. Internal hernia as a complication of colonoscopy: report of a case. *Dis Colon Rectum*. 2003;46(10):1416–1417.

29. Church J, Delaney C. Randomized, controlled trial of carbon dioxide insufflation during colonoscopy. *Dis Colon Rectum*. 2003;46(3):322–326.

30. Cirocco WC, Rusin LC. Confirmation of cecal intubation during colonoscopy. *Dis Colon Rectum*. 1995;38(4):402–406.

31. Cohen LB, Waye JD. Treatment of colonic polyps—practical considerations. *Clin Gastroenterol*. 1986;15(2):359–376.

32. Coller JA. Technique of flexible fiberoptic sigmoidoscopy. *Surg Clin North Am*. 1980;60(2):465–479.

33. Coller JA. Complications of endoscopy of the colon and rectum. In: Ferrari BT, Ray JE, Gathright JB, eds. *Complications of Colon and Rectal Surgery*. Philadelphia, PA: WB Saunders; 1985:69.

34. Coller JA, Corman ML, Veidenheimer MC. Diagnostic and therapeutic applications of fiberoptic colonoscopy. *Geriatrics*. 1974;29(10):67–73.

35. Coller JA, Corman ML, Veidenheimer MC. Colonic polypoid disease: need for total colonoscopy. *Am J Surg*. 1976;131(4):490–494.

36. Coman E, Brandt LJ, Brenner S, et al. Fat necrosis and inflammatory pseudotumor due to endoscopic tattooing of the colon with India ink. *Gastrointest Endosc*. 1991;37(1):65–68.

37. Corman ML. Landmark articles of the 20th century. *Sem Colon Rectal Surg*. 1999;10(4):247–252.

38. Coughlin GP, Butler RN, Alp MH, et al. Colonoscopy and bacteraemia. *Gut*. 1977;18(8):678–679.

39. Damore LJ II, Rantis PC, Vernava AM III, et al. Colonoscopic perforations. Etiology, diagnosis, and management. *Dis Colon Rectum*. 1996;39(11):1308–1314.

40. Davis GR, Santa Ana CA, Morawski SG, et al. Development of a lavage solution associated with minimal water and electrolyte absorption or secretion. *Gastroenterology*. 1980;78(5 pt 1):991–995.

41. Dean AC, Newell JP. Colonoscopy in the differential diagnosis of carcinoma from diverticulitis of the sigmoid colon. *Br J Surg*. 1973;60(8):633–635.

42. Desbaillets LG, Mangla JC. Pneumatosis cystoides intestinalis diagnosed by colonoscopy. *Gastrointest Endosc*. 1974;20(3):126–127.

43. Dickinson RJ, Dixon MF, Axon AT. Colonoscopy and the detection of dysplasia in patients with longstanding ulcerative colitis. *Lancet*. 1980;2(8195 pt 1):620–622.

44. Dickman MD, Farrell R, Higgs RH, et al. Colonoscopy associated bacteremia. *Surg Gynecol Obstet*. 1976;142(2):173–176.

45. DiPalma JA, Brady CE III, Stewart DL, et al. Comparison of colon cleansing methods in preparation for colonoscopy. *Gastroenterology*. 1984;86(5 pt 1):856.

46. Doctor NM, Monteleone F, Zarmakoupis C, et al. Splenic injury as a complication of colonoscopy and polypectomy. Report of a case and review of the literature. *Dis Colon Rectum*. 1987;30(12):967–968.

47. Dodds WJ, Stewart ET, Hogan WJ. Role of colonoscopy and roentgenology in the detection of polypoid colonic lesions. *Am J Dig Dis*. 1977;22(7):646–649.

48. Dubow RA, Katon RM, Benner KG, et al. Short (35-cm) vs. long (60-cm) flexible sigmoidoscopy: a comparison of findings and tolerance in asymptomatic patients screened for colorectal neoplasia. *Gastrointest Endosc*. 1985;31(5):305–308.

49. Eisenberg HW. Fiberoptic colonoscopy: intraoperative colonoscopy. *Dis Colon Rectum*. 1976;19(5):405–406.

50. Epstein M. Endoscopy: developments in optical instrumentation. *Science*. 1980;210(4467):280–285.

51. Ernstoff JJ, Howard DA, Marshall JB, et al. A randomized blinded clinical trial of a rapid colonic lavage solution (Golytely) compared with standard preparation for colonoscopy and barium enema. *Gastroenterology*. 1983;84(6):1512–1516.

52. Farinon AM, Vadora E. Endometriosis of the colon and rectum: an indication for peroperative coloscopy. *Endoscopy*. 1980;12(3):136–139.

53. Favero MS. Strategies for disinfection and sterilization of endoscopes: the gap between basic principles and actual practice. *Infect Control Hosp Epidemiol*. 1991;12(5):279–281.

54. Fishman EK, Goldman SM. Pneumoscrotum after colonoscopy. *Urology*. 1981;18(2):171–172.

55. Fleischer D. Lasers and colon polyps. Technology and pathology: the courtship continues. *Gastroenterology*. 1986;90(6):2024–2025.

56. Fleischer D. Monitoring the patient receiving conscious sedation for gastrointestinal endoscopy: issues and guidelines. *Gastrointest Endosc*. 1989;35(3):262–266.

57. Fleshner PR, Ackroyd FW, Shellito PC. The freckle sign—an endoscopic feature of the cecum. *Dis Colon Rectum*. 1990;33(10):836–839.

58. Forde KA, Lebwohl O, Wolff M, et al. The endoscopy corner: reversible ischemic colitis—correlation of colonoscopic and pathologic changes. *Am J Gastroenterol*. 1979;72(2):182–185.

59. Foster GE, Vellacott KD, Balfour TW, et al. Outpatient flexible fibreoptic sigmoidoscopy, diagnostic yield, and the value of glucagon. *Br J Surg*. 1981;68(7):463–464.

60. Frager DH, Frager JD, Wolf EL, et al. Problems in the colonoscopic localization of tumors: continued value of the barium enema. *Gastrointest Radiol*. 1987;12(4):343–346.

61. Franklin GO, Mohapatra M, Perrillo RP. Colonic tuberculosis diagnosed by colonoscopic biopsy. *Gastroenterology*. 1979;76(2):362–364.

62. Frühmorgen P. Therapeutic colonoscopy. In: Hunt RH, Waye JD, eds. *Colonoscopy: Techniques, Clinical Practice and Colour Atlas*. London, United Kingdom: Chapman and Hall; 1981:199.

63. Frühmorgen P. Therapeutic colonoscopy. In: Hunt RH, Waye JD, eds. *Colonoscopy: Techniques, Clinical Practice and Colour Atlas*. London, United Kingdom: Chapman and Hall; 1981:222.

64. Frühmorgen P, Bodem F, Reidenbach HD, et al. Endoscopic laser coagulation of bleeding gastrointestinal lesions with report of the first therapeutic application in man. *Gastrointest Endosc*. 1976;23(2):73–75.

65. Fujii T, Hasegawa RT, Saitoh Y, et al. Chromoscopy during colonoscopy. *Endoscopy*. 2001;33(12):1036–1041.

66. Gans SL. A new look at pediatric endoscopy. *Postgrad Med*. 1977;61(4):91–100.

67. Geboes K, Vantrappen G. The value of colonoscopy in the diagnosis of Crohn's disease. *Gastrointest Endosc*. 1975;22(1):18–23.

68. Ghazi A, Shinya H, Wolfe WI. Treatment of volvulus of the colon by colonoscopy. *Ann Surg*. 1976;183(3):263–265.

69. Gibbs DH, Opelka FG, Beck DE, et al. Postpolypectomy colonic hemorrhage. *Dis Colon Rectum*. 1996;39(7):806–810.

70. Girard CM, Rugh KS, DiPalma JA, et al. Comparison of Golytely lavage with standard diet/cathartic preparation for double-contrast barium enema. *AJR Am J Roentgenol*. 1984;142(6):1147–1149.

71. Goldman J, Reichelderfer M. Evaluation of rapid colonoscopy preparation using a new gut lavage solution. *Gastrointest Endosc*. 1982;28(1):9–11.

72. Gores PF, Simso LA. Splenic injury during colonoscopy. *Arch Surg.* 1989;124(11):1342.

73. Graham J, Eusebio EB. Complications of colonoscopy. *IMJ Ill Med J.* 1977;152(1):39–42.

74. Griffin JW Jr. Flexible fiberoptic sigmoidoscopy—longer may not be better for the "nonendoscopist". *Gastrointest Endosc.* 1985;31(5):347–348.

75. Habr-Gama A, Alves PR, Gama-Rodrigues JJ, et al. Pediatric colonoscopy. *Dis Colon Rectum.* 1979;22(8):530–535.

76. Hagihara PF, Ernst CB, Griffen WO Jr. Incidence of ischemic colitis following abdominal aortic reconstruction. *Surg Gynecol Obstet.* 1979;149(4):571–573.

77. Hall C, Dorricott NJ, Donovan IA, et al. Colon perforation during colonoscopy: surgical vs. conservative management. *Br J Surg.* 1991;78(5):542–544.

78. Hanson JM, Atkin WS, Cunliffe WJ, et al. Rectal retroflexion: an essential part of lower gastrointestinal endoscopic examination. *Dis Colon Rectum.* 2001;44(11):1706–1708.

79. Hartke RH Jr, Gonzalez-Rothi RJ, Abbey NC. Midazolam-associated alterations in cardiorespiratory function during colonoscopy. *Gastrointest Endosc.* 1989;35(3):232–238.

80. Hedrick E. Cleaning and disinfection of flexible fiberoptic endoscopes (FFE) used in gastrointestinal endoscopy. *APIC.* 1978;6(4):8–9.

81. Herman LL, Kurtz RC, McKee KJ, et al. Risk factors associated with vasovagal reactions during colonoscopy. *Gastrointest Endosc.* 1993;39(3):388–391.

82. Ho HC, Burchell S, Morris P, et al. Colon perforation, bilateral pneumothoraces, pneumopericardium, pneumomediastinum, and subcutaneous emphysema complicating endoscopic polypectomy: anatomic and management considerations. *Ann Surg.* 1996;62(9):770–774.

83. Hogan WJ, Hensley GT, Geenen JE. Endoscopic evaluation of inflammatory bowel disease. *Med Clin North Am.* 1980;64(6):1083–1102.

84. Hopkins HH, Kapany NS. A flexible fiberscope using static scanning. *Nature.* 1954;173:39.

85. Hunt RH, Waye JD, eds. *Colonoscopy: Techniques, Clinical Practice, and Colour Atlas.* London, United Kingdom: Chapman and Hall; 1981.

86. Hunter JG, Bowers JH, Burt RW, et al. Lasers in endoscopic gastrointestinal surgery. *Am J Surg.* 1984;148(6):736–741.

87. Hurlstone DP, Fujii T, Lobo AJ. Early detection of colorectal cancer using high-magnification chromoscopic colonoscopy. *Br J Surg.* 2002;89(3):272–282.

88. Hyman N, Waye JD. Endoscopic four quadrant tattoo for the identification of colonic lesions at surgery. *Gastrointest Endosc.* 1991;37(1):56–58.

89. Jentschura D, Raute M, Winter J, et al. Complications in endoscopy of the lower gastrointestinal tract. Therapy and prognosis. *Surg Endosc.* 1994;8(6):672–676.

90. Jonas G, Mahoney A, Murray J, et al. Chemical colitis due to endoscope cleaning solutions: a mimic of pseudomembranous colitis. *Gastroenterology.* 1988;95(5):1403–1408.

91. Kaczmarek RG, Moore RM Jr, McCrohan J, et al. Multi-state investigation of the actual disinfection/sterilization of endoscopes in health care facilities. *Am J Med.* 1992;92(3):257–261.

92. Kavin H, Sinicrope F, Esker AH. Management of perforation of the colon at colonoscopy. *Am J Gastroenterol.* 1992;87(2):161–167.

93. Kay M, Wylie R. Pediatric colonoscopy. *Practical Gastroenterol.* 1997;26:7.

94. Ker T, Run J, Beart R. Aspirin can be safely continued in preparation of colonoscopy. *Dis Colon Rectum.* 2002;45(12):A16–A19.

95. Kolts BE, Lyles WE, Achem SR, et al. A comparison of the effectiveness and patient tolerance of oral sodium phosphate, castor oil, and standard electrolyte lavage for colonoscopy or sigmoidoscopy preparation. *Am J Gastroenterol.* 1993;88(8):1218–1223.

96. Koltun WA, Coller JA. Incarceration of colonoscope in an inguinal hernia. "Pulley" technique of removal. *Dis Colon Rectum.* 1991;34(2):191–193.

97. Koo J, Ho J, Ong GB. The value of colonoscopy in the diagnosis of ileo-caecal tuberculosis. *Endoscopy.* 1982;14(2):48–50.

98. Kumar S, Abcarian H, Prasad ML, et al. Bacteremia associated with lower gastrointestinal endoscopy, fact or fiction? I. Colonoscopy. *Dis Colon Rectum.* 1982;25(2):131–134.

99. Laghi A, Iannaccone R, Carbone I, et al. Detection of colorectal lesions with virtual computed tomographic colonography. *Am J Surg.* 2002;183(2):124–131.

100. Lasers in medicine and surgery. Council on Scientific Affairs. *JAMA.* 1986;256(7):900–907.

101. Lehman GA, Buchner DM, Lappas JC. Anatomical extent of fiberoptic sigmoidoscopy. *Gastroenterology.* 1983;84(4):803–808.

102. Levin B, Lieberman DA, McFarland B, et al. Screening and surveillance for the early detection of colorectal cancer and adenomatous polyps, 2008: a joint guideline from the American Cancer Society, the US Multi-Society Task Force on Colorectal Cancer, and the American College of Radiology. *Gastroenterology.* 2008;134(5):1570–1595.

103. Lezak MB, Goldhamer M. Retroperitoneal emphysema after colonoscopy. *Gastroenterology.* 1974;66(1):118–120.

104. Lieberman DA, Weiss DG, Bond JH, et al. Use of colonoscopy to screen asymptomatic adults for colorectal cancer. Veterans Affairs Cooperative Study Group 380. *N Engl J Med.* 2000;343(3):162–168.

105. Lo AY, Beaton HL. Selective management of colonoscopic perforations. *J Am Coll Surg.* 1994;179(3):333–337.

106. Marino AWM. Complications of colonoscopy. *Dis Colon Rectum.* 1979;21:15.

107. Marks G, Boggs HW, Castro AF, et al. Sigmoidoscopic examinations with rigid and flexible fiberoptic sigmoidoscopes in the surgeon's office: a comparative prospective study of effectiveness in 1,012 cases. *Dis Colon Rectum.* 1979;22(3):162–168.

108. Marmo R, Rotondano G, Riccio G, et al. Effective bowel cleansing before colonoscopy: a randomized study of split-dosage vs. non-split dosage regimens of high-volume vs. low-volume polyethylene glycol solutions. *Gastrointest Endosc.* 2010;72(2):313–320.

109. Martin PJ, Forde KA. Intraoperative colonoscopy: preliminary report. *Dis Colon Rectum.* 1979;22(4):234–237.

110. Mathus-Vliegen EM, Tytgat GN. Nd:YAG laser photocoagulation in colorectal adenoma. Evaluation of its safety, usefulness, and efficacy. *Gastroenterology.* 1986;90(6):1865–1873.

111. Matter SE, Rice PS, Campbell DR. Colonic lavage solutions: plain vs. flavored. *Am J Gastroenterol.* 1993;88(1):49–52.

112. Matteucci DJ, Organ CH Jr, Dykstra M, et al. Efficacy of a simplified lower gastrointestinal flexible endoscope cleaning method. *Dis Colon Rectum.* 1985;28(9):653–657.

113. Max MH, Knutson CO. Colonoscopy in patients with inflammatory colonic strictures. *Surgery.* 1978;84(4):551–556.

114. Mendoza CB Jr, Watne AL. Value of intraoperative colonoscopy in vascular ectasia of the colon. *Am Surg.* 1982;48(4):153–156.

115. Merchant AA, Cheng EH. Delayed splenic rupture after colonoscopy. *Am J Gastroenterol.* 1990;85(7):906–907.

116. Millward SF, Chapman A, Somers S, et al. Rectal biopsy as a cause of rectal ulceration. *Radiology.* 1985;156(1):42.

117. Milsom JW, Gottesman L. A suction retriever to expedite recovery of colonic polyps. *Dis Colon Rectum.* 1987;30(8):644–646.

118. Myren J, Serck-Hanssen A, Solberg L. Routine and blind histological diagnoses on colonoscopic biopsies compared to clinical-colonoscopic observations in patients without and with colitis. *Scand J Gastroenterol.* 1976;11(2):135–140.

119. Naveau S, Bonhomme L, Preaux N, et al. A pure charcoal suspension for colonoscopic tattoo. *Gastrointest Endosc.* 1991;37(6):624–625.

120. Nelson RL, Abcarian H, Prasad ML. Iatrogenic perforation of the colon and rectum. *Dis Colon Rectum.* 1982;25(4):305–308.

121. Nemeh HW, Ranzinger MR, Dutro JA. Mid-ileal perforation secondary to colonoscopy. *Am Surg.* 1994;60(3):228–229.

122. Nivatvongs S. Complications in colonoscopic polypectomy. An experience with 1,555 polypectomies. *Dis Colon Rectum.* 1986;29(12):825–830.

123. Nivatvongs S. Complications in colonoscopic polypectomy: lessons to learn from an experience of 1576 polyps. *Am Surg.* 1988;54(2):61–63.

124. Norfleet RG, Mitchell PD, Mulholland DD, et al. Does bacteremia follow colonoscopy? II. Results with blood cultures obtained 5, 10, and 15 minutes after colonoscopy. *Gastrointest Endosc.* 1976;23(1):31–32.

125. Norfleet RG, Mulholland DD, Mitchell PD, et al. Does bacteremia follow colonoscopy? *Gastroenterology.* 1976;70(1):20–21.

126. Ong E, Böhmler U, Wurbs D. Splenic injury as a complication of endoscopy: two case reports and a literature review. *Endoscopy.* 1991;23(5):302–304.

127. Ostyn B, Bercoff E, Manchon ND, et al. Retroperitoneal abscess complicating colonoscopy polypectomy. *Dis Colon Rectum.* 1987;30(3):201–203.

128. Overholt BF. Colonoscopy. A review. *Gastroenterology.* 1975;68 (5 pt 1):1308–1320.

129. Palakanis KC, DeNobile JW, Sweeney WB, et al. Effect of music therapy on state anxiety in patients undergoing flexible sigmoidoscopy. *Dis Colon Rectum.* 1994;37(5):478–481.

130. Park JS, Sohn CI, Hwang SJ, et al. Quality and effect of single dose vs. split dose of polyethylene glycol bowel preparation for early-morning colonoscopy. *Endosopy.* 2007;39(7):616–619.

131. Park SI, Genta RS, Romeo DP, et al. Colonic abscess and focal peritonitis secondary to India ink tattooing of the colon. *Gastrointest Endosc.* 1991;37(1):68–71.

132. Petrini JL Jr. Terminal ileal intubation at colonoscopy. *Gastrointest Endosc.* 1989;35:182(abst 133).

133. Plucnar BJ. Colonoscopy in infancy and childhood with special regard to patient preparation and examination technique. *Endoscopy.* 1981;13(1):14–18.

134. Ransohoff DF, Lang CA. Sigmoidoscopic screening in the 1990s. *JAMA.* 1993;269(10):1278–1281.

135. Rauh SM, Coller JA, Schoetz DJ Jr. Fluoroscopy in colonoscopy. Who is using it and why? *Am Surg.* 1989;55(11):669–674.

136. Rodriguez W, Levine JS. Enterococcal endocarditis following flexible sigmoidoscopy. *West J Med.* 1984;140(6):951–953.

137. Rogers BH, Silvis SE, Nebel OT, et al. Complications of flexible fiberoptic colonoscopy and polypectomy. *Gastrointest Endosc.* 1975;22(2):73–77.

138. Saclarides TJ, Wolff BG, Pemberton JH, et al. Clean sweep of the colon. The use of intraoperative colonoscopy. *Dis Colon Rectum.* 1989;32(10):864–866.

139. Sands J. Quoted by Masel H, Masel JP, Casey KV. A survey of colon examination techniques in Australia and New Zealand, with a review of complications. *Australas Radiol.* 1971;15(2):140–147.

140. Sanner CJ, Saltzman DA. Detorsion of sigmoid volvulus by colonoscopy. *Gastrointest Endosc.* 1977;23(4):212–213.

141. Saunders BP, Bell GD, Williams CB, et al. First clinical results with a real time, electronic imager as an aid to colonoscopy. *Gut.* 1995;36(6):913–917.

142. Schapiro M. Electronic video endoscopy: a comprehensive review of the newest technology and techniques. *Practical Gastroenterol.* 1986;10:8.

143. Schmidt G, Börsch G, Wegener M. Subcutaneous emphysema and pneumothorax complicating diagnostic colonoscopy. *Dis Colon Rectum.* 1986;29(2):136–138.

144. Schwesinger WH, Levine BA, Ramos R. Complications in colonoscopy. *Surg Gynecol Obstet.* 1979;148(2):270–281.

145. Shatz BA, Thavorides V. Colonic tattoo for follow-up of endoscopic sessile polypectomy. *Gastrointest Endosc.* 1991;37(1):59–60.

146. Shields N. A survey of the costs of flexible endoscope cleaning and disinfection. *Gastroenterol Nurs.* 1993;16(2):53–60.

147. Shinya H, Wolff WI. Morphology, anatomic distribution and cancer potential of colonic polyps. *Ann Surg.* 1979;190(6):679–683.

148. Sivak MV. Video endoscopy. *Clin Gastroenterol.* 1986;15(2):205–234.

149. Smith GA, Oien KA, O'Dwyer PJ. Frequency of early colorectal cancer in patients undergoing colonoscopy. *Br J Surg.* 1999;86(10):1328–1231.

150. Smith LE. Fiberoptic colonoscopy: complications of colonoscopy and polypectomy. *Dis Colon Rectum.* 1976;19(5):407–412.

151. Spach DH, Silverstein FE, Stamm WE. Transmission of infection by gastrointestinal endoscopy and bronchoscopy. *Ann Intern Med.* 1993;118(2):117–128.

152. Spencer RJ, Wolff BG, Ready RL. Comparison of the rigid sigmoidoscope and the flexible sigmoidoscope in conjunction with colon x-ray for detection of lesions of the colon and rectum. *Dis Colon Rectum.* 1983;26(10):653–655.

153. Stevens AE. Colonoscopy in the irritable bowel syndrome. *Gut.* 1973;14(5):432.

154. Sugarbaker PH, Vineyard GC, Lewicki AM, et al. Colonoscopy in the management of diseases of the colon and rectum. *Surg Gynecol Obstet.* 1974;139(3):341–349.

155. Tabibian N, Michaletz PA, Schwartz JT, et al. Use of an endoscopically placed clip can avoid diagnostic errors in colonoscopy. *Gastrointest Endosc.* 1988;34(3):262–264.

156. Tawile NT, Priest RJ, Schuman BM. Colonoscopy in inflammatory bowel disease. *Gastrointest Endosc.* 1975;22(1):177–184.

157. Taylor EW, Bentley S, Youngs D, et al. Bowel preparation and the safety of colonoscopic polypectomy. *Gastroenterology.* 1981;81(1):1–4.

158. Taylor FC, Frankl HD, Riemer KD. Late presentation of splenic trauma after routine colonoscopy. *Am J Gastroenterol.* 1989;84(4):442–443.

159. Tedesco FJ. Antibiotic associated pseudomembranous colitis with negative proctosigmoidoscopy examination. *Gastroenterology.* 1979;77(2):295–297.

160. Tedesco FJ, Pickens CA, Griffin JW Jr, et al. Role of colonoscopy in patients with unexplained melena: analysis of 53 patients. *Gastrointest Endosc.* 1981;27(4):221–223.

161. Thoeni RF, Menuck L. Comparison of barium enema and colonoscopy in the detection of small colonic polyps. *Radiology.* 1977;124(3):631–635.

162. Timothy SK, Hicks TC, Opelka FG, et al. Colonoscopy in the patient requiring anticoagulation. *Dis Colon Rectum.* 2001;44(12):1845–1848.

163. Waye JD. Colonoscopy: a clinical view. *Mt Sinai J Med.* 1975;42(1):1–34.

164. Waye JD. Colitis, cancer, and colonoscopy. *Med Clin North Am.* 1978;62(1):211–224.

165. Waye JD. Colonoscopy intubation techniques without fluoroscopy. In: Hunt RH, Waye JD, eds. *Colonoscopy: Techniques, Clinical Practice and Colour Atlas.* London, United Kingdom: Chapman and Hall; 1981:170.

166. Waye JD. The postpolypectomy coagulation syndrome. *Gastrointest Endosc.* 1981;27:184.

167. Waye JD, Bashkoff E. Total colonoscopy: is it always possible? *Gastrointest Endosc.* 1991;37(2):152–154.

168. Waye JD, Yessayan SA, Lewis BS, et al. The technique of abdominal pressure in total colonoscopy. *Gastrointest Endosc.* 1991;37(2):147–151.

169. Webb WA. Colonoscoping the "difficult" colon. *Am Surg.* 1991;57(3):178–182.

170. Wexner SD, Eisen GM, Simmang C. Principles of privileging and credentialing for endoscopy and colonoscopy. *Dis Colon Rectum.* 2002;45(2):161–164.

171. Wherry DC, Thomas WM. The yield of flexible fiberoptic sigmoidoscopy in the detection of asymptomatic colorectal neoplasia. *Surg Endosc.* 1994;8(5):393–395.

172. Williams CB, Laage NJ, Campbell CA, et al. Total colonoscopy in children. *Arch Dis Child.* 1982;57(1):49–53.

173. Williard W, Satava R. Inguinal hernia complicating flexible sigmoidoscopy. *Am Surg.* 1990;56(12):800–801.

174. Winnan G, Berci G, Panish J, et al. Superiority of the flexible to the rigid sigmoidoscope in routine proctosigmoidoscopy. *N Engl J Med.* 1980;302(18):1011–1012.

175. Wolff WI, Shinya H. Polypectomy via the fiberoptic colonoscope. Removal of neoplasms beyond reach of the sigmoidoscope. *N Engl J Med.* 1973;288(7):329–332.

176. Wolff WI, Shinya H, Geffen A, et al. Comparison of colonoscopy and the contrast enema in five hundred patients with colorectal disease. *Am J Surg.* 1975;129(2):181–186.

177. Yassinger S, Midgley RC, Cantor DS, et al. Retroperitoneal emphysema after colonoscopic polypectomy. *West J Med.* 1978;128(4):347–350.

7

Setting Up a Colorectal Physiology Laboratory

Dana R. Sands and Steven D. Wexner

> *Pathology is the accomplished tragedy; physiology is the basis on which our treatment rests.*
>
> —SAMUEL BUTLER

The evaluation of patients with complex functional problems frequently requires multimodality testing for proper diagnosis. Beginning in the 1980s, physicians used the tools of the anorectal physiology laboratory to better understand the pathophysiology behind their patients' complaints. Over the ensuing decades, many clinicians have established their own physiology laboratories. An appreciation of the available testing modalities and their application to clinical practice is essential for the physician whose aim is the treatment of functional colorectal disorders. No longer is it suitable to rely solely on clinical examination. Sophisticated tools of the colorectal physiology laboratory will offer a greater depth of understanding of numerous disease states, including constipation, evacuatory dysfunction, fecal incontinence, and prolapse. Many of these conditions are underdiagnosed. As physicians become more aware of the prevalence of these conditions and also the incidence of concomitant anterior compartment pathology,[136] the use of the colorectal physiology laboratory will continue to increase. A team approach with urology and urogynecology counterparts facilitates accurate diagnosis with combined multimodality treatment regimens.

The components of a complete colorectal physiology laboratory include anal manometry, ultrasound of the anus and rectum, neurophysiologic assessment with pudendal nerve terminal motor latency, electromyographic evaluation, defecography, as well as transit studies of the small intestine and colon. No single test can adequately define the status of the anorectum, either in health or when diseased. Accurate diagnosis depends on the integration of a detailed history and clinical examination, along with the appropriate physiologic investigations. Thus, every laboratory must have the resources, space, and personnel to perform a wide array of physiologic studies. Setting up a new laboratory is an expensive venture, and administrative authorities may understandably require a cost-benefit analysis or business plan prior to considering whether this new cost center should be supported. Required data include anticipated case volumes and reimbursement expectations. Still, much of the capital outlay can be minimized if intradepartmental arrangements can be accommodated to share rooms, equipment, and ancillary personnel. For example, the computer hardware equipment, which can be used for both esophageal and anorectal manometry, can be purchased jointly by gastroenterology and colorectal divisions. Specific software packages and catheters can then be acquired. Similarly, an ultrasound scanner can be shared among gynecologists, urologists, and colorectal surgeons, with each using a specific probe. Defecography can be performed in a standard fluoroscopy suite, and electromyography (EMG) equipment can be shared with the neurology department.

Ideally, the various tests should be available in proximity, so that they can be performed in a relatively short time and with minimal inconvenience to the patient. The number of required personnel is dependent on the volume of tests undertaken each day. Many units have specifically trained nursing staff to perform these studies under appropriate supervision. The same nurses who undertake a given procedure for one department can also perform the analogous procedure for the department sharing the equipment.

▶ MANOMETRY

The first reports of anorectal manometry in the literature date back to 1972.[42] Since that time, there has been no standardization of the technique. The basic information provided, regardless of technique, should include an objective assessment of the anal muscular tone, rectal compliance, and anorectal sensation, as well as the determination of the integrity of the rectoanal inhibitory reflex. The lack of standardization creates some difficulty in comparing results from different institutions. In fact, institutions must determine a set of normal values for their patient population. There is often a difference noted between male and female subjects.[64]

Manometry has been useful in the diagnosis of patients suffering from fecal incontinence,[23] constipation,[135] Hirschsprung's disease,[127] and anal fissure.[57,152] It has been widely used in the investigation of individuals with fecal incontinence to identify the presence of sensory or muscular defects, as well as to define functional weakness of the internal and/or external anal sphincter. Those with fecal incontinence or proctitis may present with significant loss of the ability to sense rectal distension.[166] A maximal tolerable volume less than 100 mL may indicate visceral hypersensitivity, poor compliance, or rectal irritability.

Anorectal Manometry Systems

There are three basic types of systems used for performing manometric examinations: air- or water-filled balloon systems, water perfusion systems, and solid-state microtransducer systems.

Air- or Water-Filled Balloon Systems

In these systems, fluid- or air-filled balloons are placed within the anus and rectum and are connected to transducers via small catheters. One of the early designs was that of Schuster and colleagues.[149] This device consists of a hollow metal tube 4 in. in length surrounded by a latex balloon tied in such a way so as to create two separate compartments. Each balloon communicates with a pressure transducer via two plastic catheters. A further balloon can be placed into the rectum via the metal tube. The apparatus is placed in the rectum so that the internal balloon is surrounded by the internal sphincter, and the external balloon is encircled by the superficial fibers of the external anal sphincter (Figure 7-1).[148] The device is set by inflating the rectal balloon to elicit the rectoanal inhibitory reflex (RAIR), which automatically seats the catheter in position. Thereafter, mean resting and squeeze pressures, the presence of the RAIR, rectal sensitivity, and compliance can all be assessed.

Theoretically, this device should be able to assess pressures from the internal and external anal sphincter separately, but in practice the overlap of these two muscles is too great to allow differentiation.[149] Furthermore, because pressures within the anus are in part influenced by the distortion of the anal canal, a probe with a large balloon yields a greater pressure than does one with a smaller balloon in the same subject.[65,164] In addition, rapid distension of the balloon will generate a higher pressure.[65,164] One final area for confusion

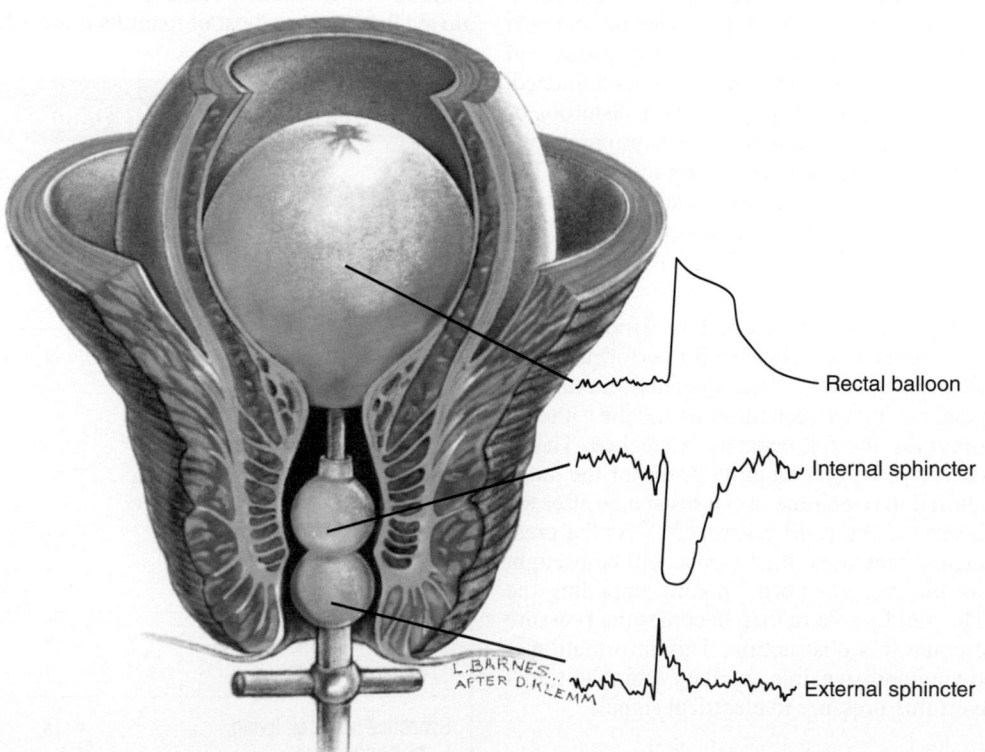

FIGURE 7-1. Anorectal manometric tracings indicate the pressure changes at each level after distension of the balloon in the ampulla. (Adapted from Rosen LS, Khubchandani IT, Sheets JA, et al. Management of anal incontinence. *J Am Fam Pract.* 1986;33:129, with permission.)

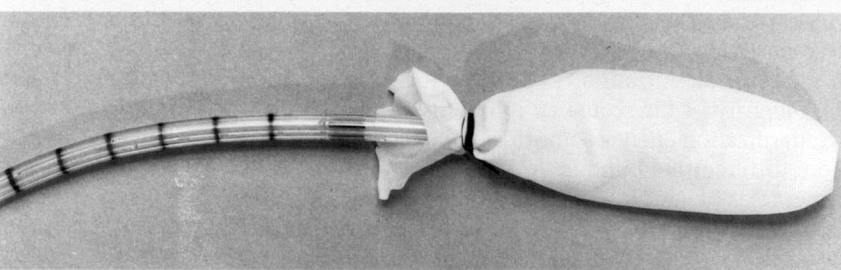

FIGURE 7-2. Water-perfused anorectal manometry catheters. **A:** Eight-channel radial catheter suitable for vector volume analysis. (Courtesy of Synectics Medical, Irving, TX.) **B:** Custom-built four-channel radial catheter with two intraballoon channels. (Courtesy of Arndorfer, Inc., Greendale, WI.)

with this method is that air is compressible, and the pressures recorded may be somewhat lower than the true values.

These disadvantages prompted the development of another balloon system that uses smaller, water-filled balloons (Marquat Company, Boissy-Saint-Léger Cedex, France).[65] However, although accurate assessments can be performed with these catheters, they permit measurement of only a limited area of the anal canal.[73]

Both of these systems are relatively simple, and once placed they do not require further movement. Investigations, therefore, can be performed by one operator. However, the information ascertainable from these systems is relatively limited because the pressure measured is the sum of all forces acting upon the balloon. Thus, only determinations of the global resting and squeeze pressures of the anal canal can be obtained. Indeed, because as implied, larger balloons produce more distortion of the anal canal, basal pressure measurements may be unreliable, with only the changes in pressure being reproducible.[65] The presence of the RAIR and information on rectal sensitivity and compliance can be obtained using either system.

Water-Perfused Systems

Water-perfused systems were developed by Arndorfer and colleagues and are the most widely used for performing manometry in the United States.[6] These systems function by creating an artificial cavity between the anus and the catheter. As perfusion continues, the full capacity is reached. Thereafter, fluid leaks into the rectal ampulla or out of the anus. The pressure required to overcome initial resistance after the space is filled is termed the *yield pressure*.[68,92] As the pressure in the anal canal increases, the mucosa will be brought into contact with the catheter ports, thereby impeding the flow of water. The yield pressure then becomes the pressure required to overcome this obstruction. This information is then transmitted via nondistensible capillary tubing to transducers that convert this pressure to electrical signals.

Equipment

Catheters. Catheters vary according to rigidity, diameter, and number and location of the ports. Rigid catheters tend to be easier to insert, but more flexible catheters cause less artifact

and are, therefore, often preferred. The external diameter should be 4 to 8 mm in order to minimize distortion of the anal canal.[56,113] The number of lumens and ports ranges from two to eight and may be arranged either radially or longitudinally in a spiral fashion at 5- to 8-mm intervals (Figure 7-2A). Additional ports for assessment of pressures inside rectal balloons can also be included (Figure 7-2B). Distal balloons may come preattached, but many investigators prefer to use either condoms or latex balloons made of a thinner and more compliant material. Radial catheters are used for assessment of the pressure profile of the anal canal, whereas spiral catheters are often preferred for elicitation of the RAIR. Many catheter varieties are available from a host of manufacturers (Table 7-1). These

TABLE 7-1 Manometry Catheters		
MANUFACTURER	**WATER PERFUSED**	**SOLID STATE**
Arndorfer, Inc., Greendale, WI 53129, USA	X	
Dantec Electronics, Bristol, UK	X	
Gaeltec Ltd., Isle of Skye, UK		X
Konigsberg Instruments, Pasadena, CA 91107, USA		X
Millar Instruments, Houston, TX 77023, USA		X
Mui Scientific, Mississauga, Ontario, Canada	X	
Synectics Medical, Irving, TX 75038, USA	X	
Synectics Medical AB, Stockholm, S-116 28, Sweden	X	

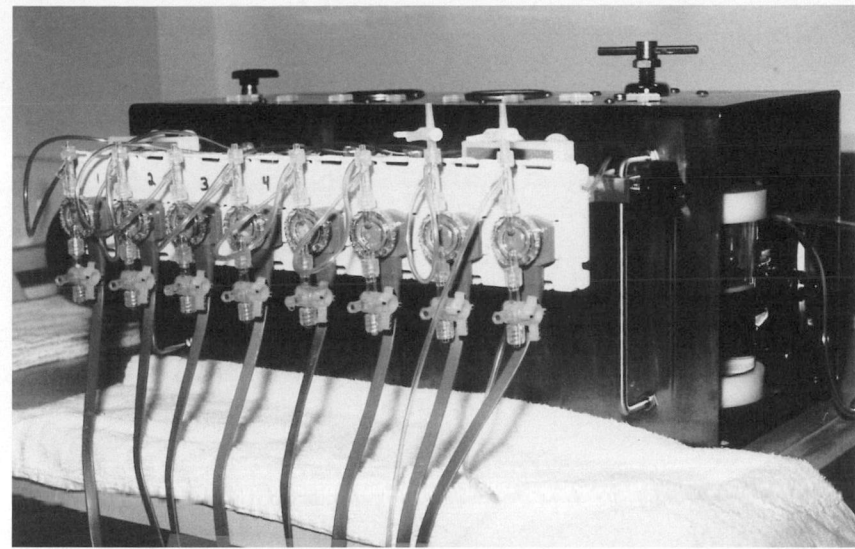

FIGURE 7-3. Eight-channel hydraulic capillary infusion system. (Courtesy of Arndorfer, Inc., Greendale, WI.)

are multiuse catheters with a life span of 1 to 2 years, depending on the number of evaluations performed. Satisfactory cleansing is therefore a priority. This can be accomplished by using activated dialdehyde solution (Cidex; Johnson & Johnson Medical, Inc., Arlington, TX). Proper facilities for the use of this chemical, especially adequate ventilation, are required.

Withdrawal Motor. Unlike balloon catheters, these devices are designed to measure pressures along the whole length of the anal canal. Some investigators prefer a manual pull-through technique that can be performed by a skilled technician. However, the rate of retraction is more easily standardized by using a withdrawal motor that can be controlled by computer software (Narco Bio-Systems, Austin, TX).

Perfusion Apparatus. Hydraulic capillary infusion systems use nitrogen gas or compressed air to force water from a reservoir through small capillary tubes, thereby allowing perfusion of each transducer and catheter channel separately (Figure 7-3).[6] The number of channels required is dependent on the type of catheter used. An apparatus with 4, 8, and 12 channels is available (Table 7-2). Other similar options are also manufactured (International Biomedical, Austin, TX) but are sold only in conjunction with complete motility and analysis systems (Narco Bio-Systems, Austin, TX). Figure 7-4 shows an integrated, computerized manometry biofeedback pudendal nerve terminal motor latency system.

Transducers. The number required depends on the number of channels within the catheter.

Recording Apparatus. Previously, most recordings were made on paper or smoked polygraph drums. Although real-time chart recording is available (MMS-200; Narco Bio-Systems, Austin, TX), computers have surpassed this method of data

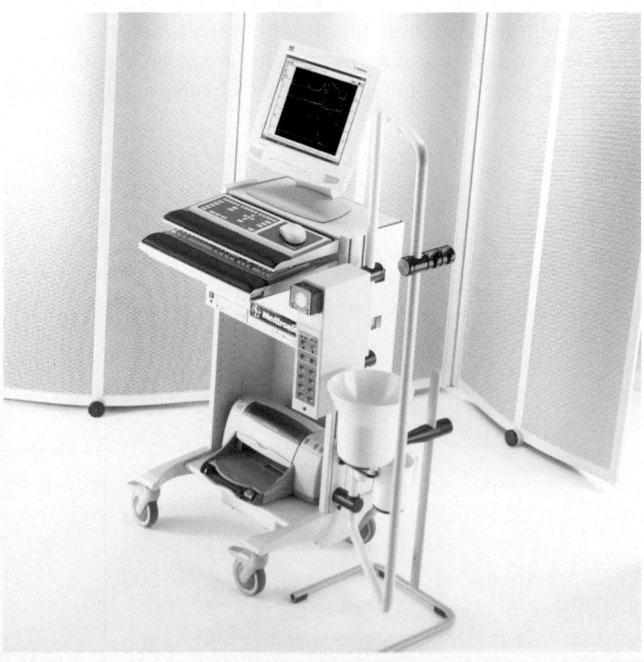

FIGURE 7-4. Duet Encompass System. Provides different configurations for specific uses, including cystometry, biofeedback applications, uroflowmetry, anorectal manometry, and neurodiagnostics with stimulation. (Courtesy of Medtronic, Inc., Minneapolis, MN.)

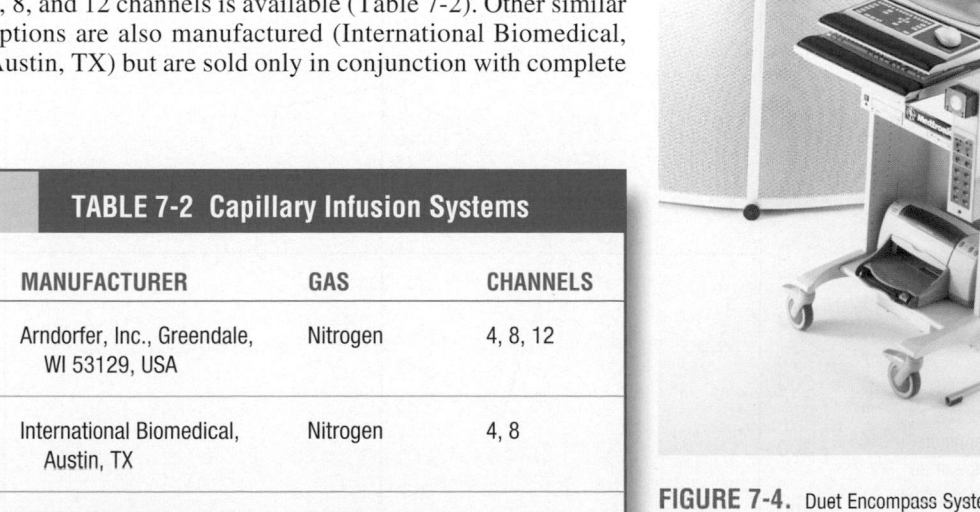

TABLE 7-2 Capillary Infusion Systems		
MANUFACTURER	GAS	CHANNELS
Arndorfer, Inc., Greendale, WI 53129, USA	Nitrogen	4, 8, 12
International Biomedical, Austin, TX	Nitrogen	4, 8
Mui Scientific, Mississauga, Ontario, Canada	Nitrogen/air compression	4, 6, 8, 12, 16

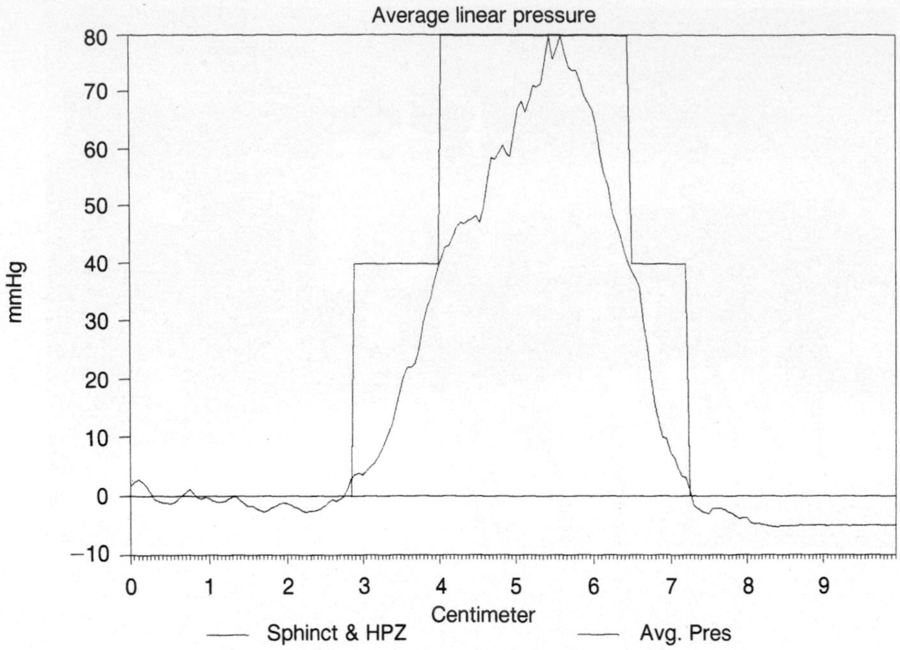

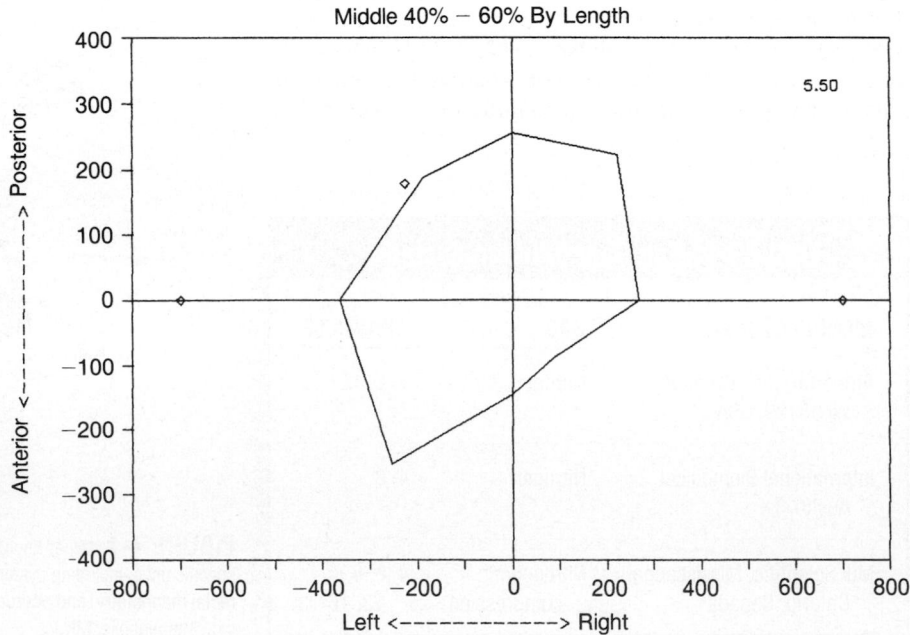

FIGURE 7-5. Normal longitudinal pressure profile of the anal sphincter provided by the Narco Bio-Systems MMS-200 physiologic recorder. The graph is made by pulling a radial catheter through the anal canal by computer control at the rate of 1 mm/second. Pressures are simultaneously acquired by eight radially positioned orifices; the average pressure is displayed in the graph. All pressures are referenced to a rectal pressure of zero so that atmospheric pressure will be a negative number. The maximum average resting pressure of the sphincter is approximately 80 mm Hg, and the sphincter length is 4.4 cm. (Courtesy of Narco Bio-Systems, Austin, TX, and John A. Coller, MD.)

collection for a number of reasons (Figure 7-5). For example, menu-driven software programs can be specially created that contain fixed protocols with instructions and prompts for performing various manometric investigations.[36,145,146] Software may also contain the mathematical algorithms for calculating pressure changes. Now, more complex programs are being created that automatically calculate many manometric parameters. Three-dimensional reconstruction of the pressure profile of the anal sphincter can demonstrate sphincter asymmetry and the presence of defects (Figures 7-6 through 7-8). Several systems now have the capability of integrating and displaying dynamic radiologic investigations with simultaneous motility studies. In addition, computers can also operate accessory equipment, such as probe withdrawal motors, and are excellent for storing data so that tests can be recalled and reviewed. Several manufacturers provide integrated hardware and software systems, some of which can also be used in combination with solid-state catheters (Table 7-3)

In summary, water perfusion systems provide a large amount of reproducible data about the status of the anal sphincters and rectum. The one limitation is that they require the patient to be in the lateral decubitus position, thereby precluding ambulatory study.

Solid-State Noninfusion Catheters. Noninfusion transducer catheters usually contain three or more pressure channels. Although not as versatile as infusion catheters, they eliminate concerns about positioning so that recordings can be made with patients sitting in the standard physiologic condition for evacuation.[11,139,181] Furthermore, these catheters can be used for ambulatory recordings. Several manufacturers produce suitable equipment (see Table 7-1).

FIGURE 7-6. Cross-sectional analysis of pressures in the midportion of an anal sphincter that has been damaged as a consequence of an obstetric injury. Note that anteriorly, especially in the right anterior position, pressures are considerably reduced when compared with those posteriorly. (Courtesy of John A. Coller, MD.)

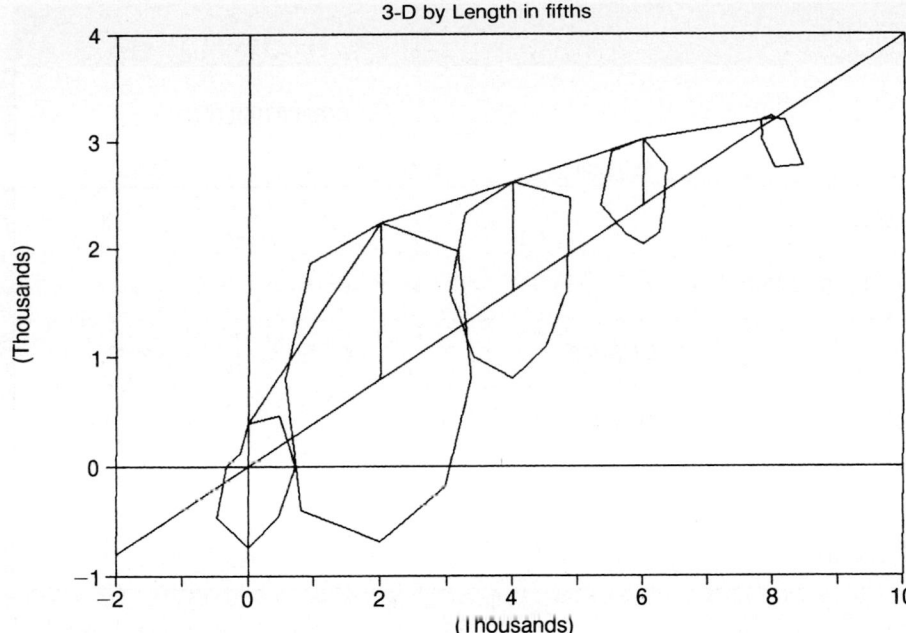

FIGURE 7-7. In this simple cross-sectional, computer-generated representation of the sphincter, there is a posterior predominance in the proximal portion of the anal canal and an anterior predominance in the distal portion (Courtesy of John A. Coller, MD.)

Technique of Manometric Evaluation

Our preference is to perform a station pull-through technique using a custom-built 4.8-mm diameter polypropylene flexible catheter with four radial ports located 8.5 cm from the tip (Arndorfer, Inc., Greendale, WI).[83,84] A further two ports are positioned 2 cm from the end of the catheter and are enclosed within a thin latex rubber balloon fashioned from the finger of an examination glove (Floor/exam latex glove no. 8857; Baxter Health Care Corporation, Valencia, CA). This balloon is secured at 3 cm from the tip of the catheter using a 2–0 silk ligature. An eight-channel hydraulic capillary infusion system (Arndorfer, Inc., Greendale, WI) is used with Medex transducers (M6677; Medex, Inc., Hilliard, OH).

Mechanical pressures are transmitted to a PC Polygraf HR (Synectics Medical, Inc., Irving, TX). The resulting electrical impulses are displayed on a computer using Polygram V6.4 software (Synectics Medical, Inc., Irving, TX).

With the patient in the left lateral decubitus position, the catheter is inserted to 6 cm; 20 to 30 seconds are allowed for the sphincter to recover from this insult and for the pressures to equilibrate. It is important to permit adequate time for the small cavity between the rectal wall and the catheter to fill with perfusate so that the yield pressure is reached.

Following this period of equilibration, various wave patterns may emerge that demonstrate the presence of intrinsic cyclic activity attributable primarily to the internal

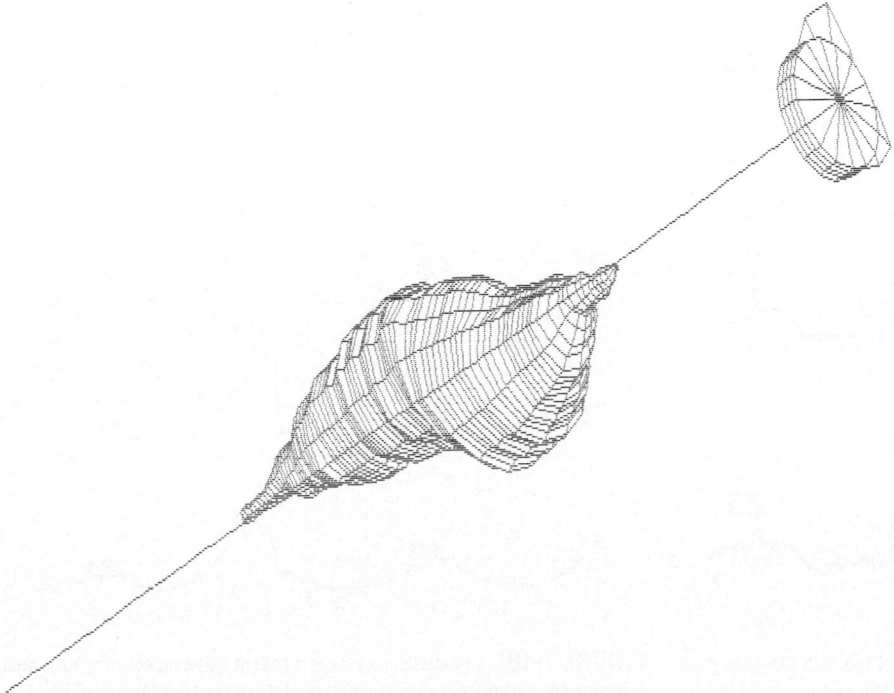

FIGURE 7-8. Three-dimensional reconstruction of same patient illustrated in Figure 7-7 using computer-aided design program. (Courtesy of John A. Coller, MD.)

TABLE 7-3 Manometry Systems

MANUFACTURER	SYSTEM	COMPATIBILITY	
		WATER PERFUSED	SOLID STATE
Medical Management Systems, Enschede, Holland			X
Medtronic Functional Diagnostics, Shoreview, MN 55126 USA	X	X	
Narco Bio-Systems, Austin, TX 78754, USA	MMS-200	X	X
Sandhill Scientific, Highlands Ranch, CO 80126, USA	BioLAB		X
Synectics Medical, Irving, TX 75038, USA	PC Polygraph	X	X
Synectics Medical AB, Stockholm, S-116 28, Sweden		X	X

sphincter.[175] Three basic patterns are observed. *Slow waves* are the most frequently encountered. These vary in frequency from 10 to 20 cycles/minute with an amplitude from just above physiologic baseline noise to 15 mm Hg (Figure 7-9).[146] They can most often be observed in the region between the proximal border of the sphincter and the area of the maximal average resting pressure.[36,130] The clinical significance of these waves is unknown.

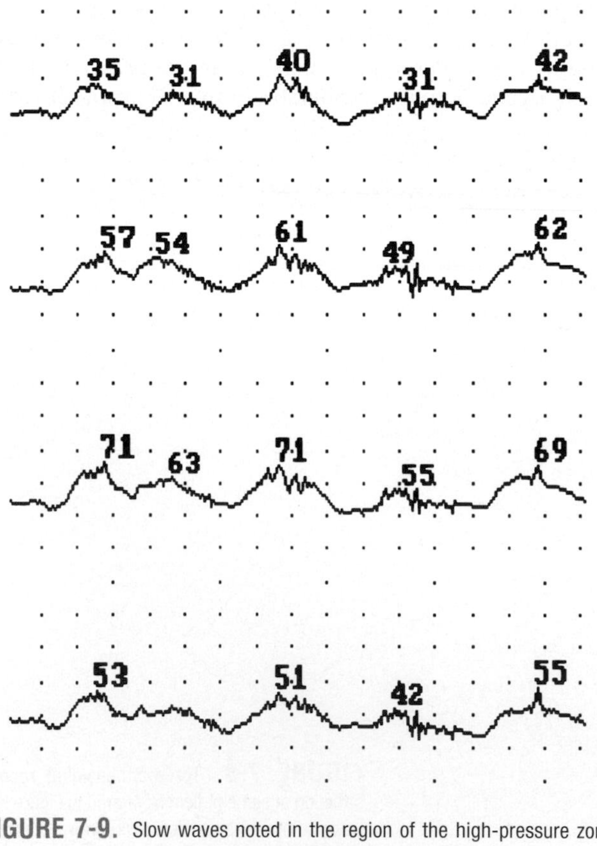

Ultraslow waves are the second most common waveforms recorded. They have a frequency of 0.5 to 1.5 cycles/minute and are of large amplitude (up to 100 mm Hg).[146] They are found more frequently in patients with high resting anal pressures,[69] such as in those individuals with an anal fissure,[66] hemorrhoids,[67] or primary anal sphincter hypertonia. They are seen most commonly in the region of maximal average resting pressure.

The *intermediate wave* is the least frequently observed type of oscillation (frequency, 4 to 8 cycles/minute). They are most often noted in patients with neurogenic fecal incontinence or following ileal pouch-anal anastomosis (Figure 7-10).[162] When present, they make interpretation of resting and squeeze pressures more difficult. *Resting pressure* should be assumed to be the mean of the peak and trough pressures at rest.

FIGURE 7-9. Slow waves noted in the region of the high-pressure zone. (Polygram software; courtesy of Synectics Medical, Irving, TX.)

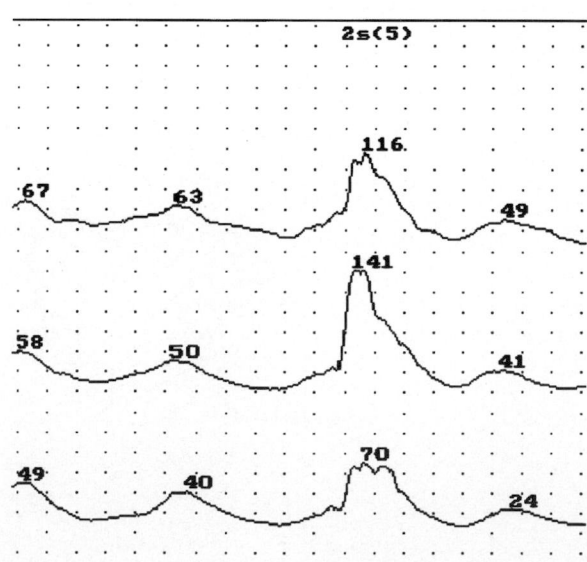

FIGURE 7-10. Intermediate waves in a patient following colonic pouch-anal anastomosis. (Polygram software; courtesy of Synectics Medical, Irving, TX.)

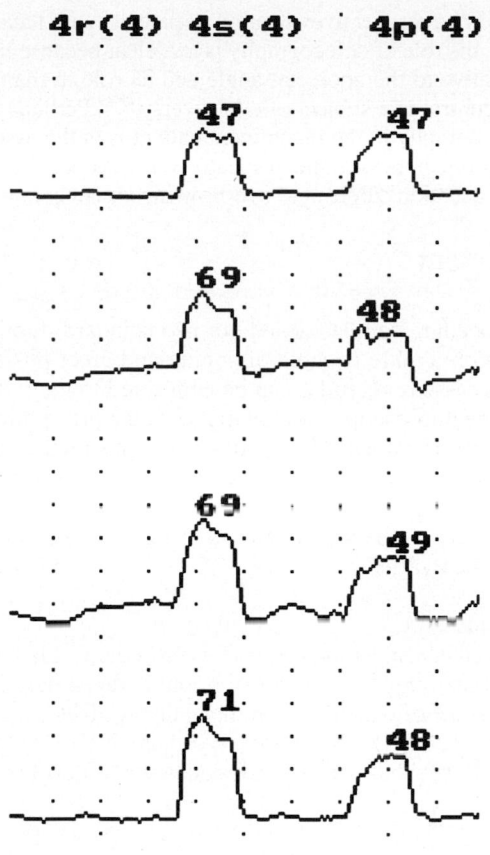

FIGURE 7-11. Rest, squeeze, and push phases of station pull-through manometry recorded at 4 cm from the anal verge. (Polygram software; courtesy of Synectics Medical, Irving, TX.)

Following equilibration of the pressures, the patient is asked to perform a single maximum squeeze effort followed by a period of rest, and then a maximal push effort (Figure 7-11). These measurements are repeated at a further five stations, separated by 1-cm intervals, as the catheter is progressively moved caudally. Thus, the rest and squeeze pressures over the entire length of the anal canal can be measured, and the mean resting and squeeze pressures over the *high-pressure zone* (HPZ) can be calculated. The HPZ is defined as that length of the anal canal through which pressures are greater than 50% of the average maximum pressure. This definition is similar to that used when a continuous pull-through technique is employed. Alternatively, the HPZ can be defined as that zone bounded caudally by a rise in pressure of 20 mm Hg and cephalad by a fall in pressure of 20 mm Hg in at least 50% of the channels. This latter definition may present a more accurate picture of the sphincters in incontinent patients because pressures are so low that there is no true HPZ. However, using the former definition, the HPZ will always be at least 1 cm, but this may be an inaccurate value in a patient with a patulous anus.

The catheter is then reinserted to a distance of 2 cm from the anal verge, and the latex balloon is insufflated with 40 mL of air over 2 to 3 seconds and kept inflated for 20 seconds in order to elicit the RAIR. In response to distension of the lower rectum and upper anal canal, external sphincter contraction is followed by internal sphincter relaxation

(Figure 7-12). If the reflex is not present, it is important to repeat the test with increased insufflation. Some patients, especially those with neurogenic fecal incontinence, decreased anal sensation, or megarectum, may respond only at a higher volume. The air is removed and the balloon reinflated with 50 or 60 mL until a reflex is observed. If the reflex is still undetectable, the catheter is inserted to 3 cm and repeat insufflations are performed. In our laboratory, we record only the presence or absence of the reflex. Some software programs contain the algorithms for calculating various reflex parameters, including duration, percentage of excitation, and excitation latency. Although some authors suggest that delayed, diminutive or absent excitation, or excitation only in response to large volumes may be used as a crude indicator of pudendal neuropathy, the clinical implications of these values are problematic.[145] Some prefer a spiral catheter to detect the presence of the RAIR over the entire length of the anal canal. However, the use of a radial catheter at the two stations where the reflex is most likely to be detected avoids this requirement for each investigation. In rare instances in which a reflex cannot be elicited and there is no evidence of megarectum, the spiral catheter may be useful. The most common reasons for absence of the RAIR are megarectum and a prior ileoanal or coloanal anastomosis.

The catheter is then inserted to a distance of 6 cm from the anal verge, positioning the balloon in the rectal ampulla. The balloon is then slowly filled with core temperature water at a

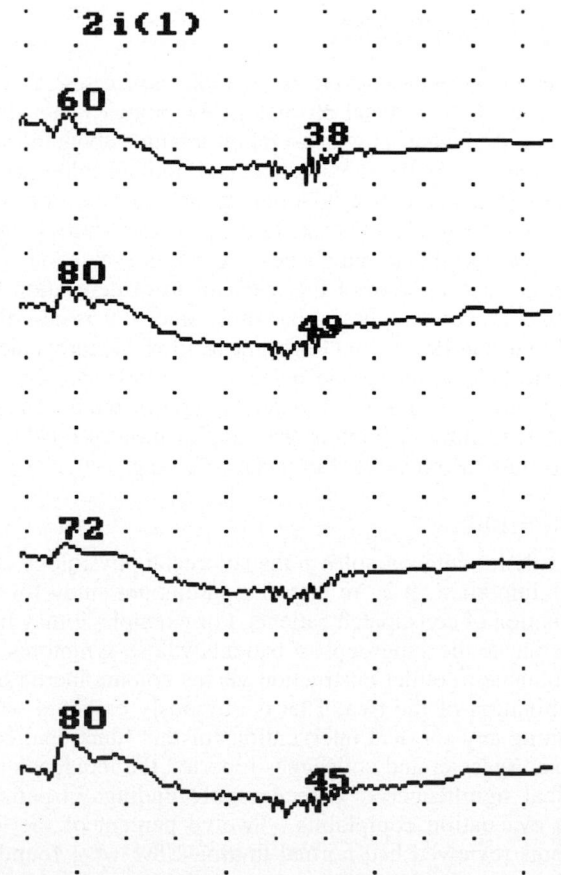

FIGURE 7-12. Rectoanal inhibitory reflex recorded at 2 cm from the anal verge in response to distension of the rectal balloon with 40 mL of air. (Polygram software; courtesy of Synectics Medical, Irving, TX.)

rate of approximately 1 mL/second. The first sensation perceived by the patient is noted as the minimal sensory volume, and the mean intraballoon pressure is noted. Thereafter, balloon filling is continued until the maximum tolerable volume is reached, and again the intraballoon pressure is noted. Using these values, rectal compliance can be calculated from the formula $\Delta V/\Delta P$.[84] Thus, with a large balloon volume and only a small increase in rectal pressure, the rectum is considered very compliant. In patients suffering from ulcerative colitis, Crohn's proctitis, or radiation proctitis, the rectum may be poorly compliant in that a small increase in volume will result in a large increase in pressure. When one uses this technique, it is important to know the compliance of the balloon at various stages of insufflation so that it can be subtracted from the pressure measured via the intraballoon ports. Latex balloons may deform along the longitudinal axis with increased infusion of water. This may give a false impression of high rectal compliance.[109] As a consequence, some clinicians prefer to use barostat equipment to calculate this parameter, using a noncompliant balloon that does not deform with increasing pressure.

The measurement of *compliance* is not a diagnostic test but supplements other investigations for evaluating the pathophysiology of anorectal disease. It is of particular value in patients with proctitis and incontinence through ascertaining whether the incontinence is due to lack of rectal reservoir function or diminished anal sphincter tone. Similarly, in some constipated patients, compliance may be abnormally high. This finding can reflect overaccommodation and, therefore, a sensory contribution to the outlet obstruction.

▶ DEFECOGRAPHY

Defecography or evacuation proctography is an essential component of the colorectal physiology laboratory. This study provides the physician with useful information about the anatomic interplay of the anus, rectum, and sigmoid colon as well as the vagina and pelvic floor during the defecatory process. Patients suffering from constipation, prolapse, solitary rectal ulcer, and rectal pain may benefit from this evaluation. This dynamic investigation of the mechanism of defecation has become an increasingly popular study since it was described by Wallden in 1952[174] and Burhenne in 1964.[26] Improvements in the technique, such as cinedefecography and videoproctography, have led to a better understanding of the evacuation process, thereby facilitating the identification of conditions that disturb the physiology of rectal emptying.

Indications

The role for defecography in the colorectal physiology center is important. It is, in fact, the paramount study for the evaluation of constipated patients. For example, it may help to delineate the subgroups of patients whose symptoms are attributable to outlet obstruction versus colonic inertia or a combination of the two. This is obviously essential when planning any surgical intervention for this functional condition. Agachan and colleagues reported the incidence and clinical significance of defecographic findings in patients with evacuation complaints.[2] Twelve percent of the 744 patients reviewed had normal findings, 8% were found to have rectal prolapse, 26% rectocele, 11% sigmoidocele, 13% intussusception, and 30% had a combination of findings.

The procedure may also be indicated for the investigation of individuals with solitary rectal ulcer syndrome[60,98,126] or rectal

pain.[144] With respect to evaluation of patients with fecal incontinence, the role of defecography is less clear because information relative to the anorectal angle and its role in maintaining bowel control is a subject of controversy.[48,49] Perhaps the role of defecography in the incontinent patient is in the assessment of the completeness to the evacuatory attempt because incomplete evacuation can lead to overflow incontinence.

Equipment

Imaging

The procedure can be carried out in a standard fluoroscopic suite, with a table capable of supine and erect positioning. A videocassette recorder can be connected to the video output of the fluoroscopic system to record the procedure. Static images are obtained at rest, squeezing, pushing, and postevacuation. Dynamic video imaging then captures the entire evacuation attempt. A standard examination will deliver 0.02 to 0.66 cGy to the skin of the right hip and 0.036 to 0.053 cGy to the ovaries.[12]

Commode

Almost all investigators perform this procedure with the patient in the seated position. A chair or commode is, therefore, required, some of which are commercially available, such as the Brunswick chair (E-Z-EM, Inc., Westbury, NY) and Portapotti (Figure 7-13), but several individuals have developed their

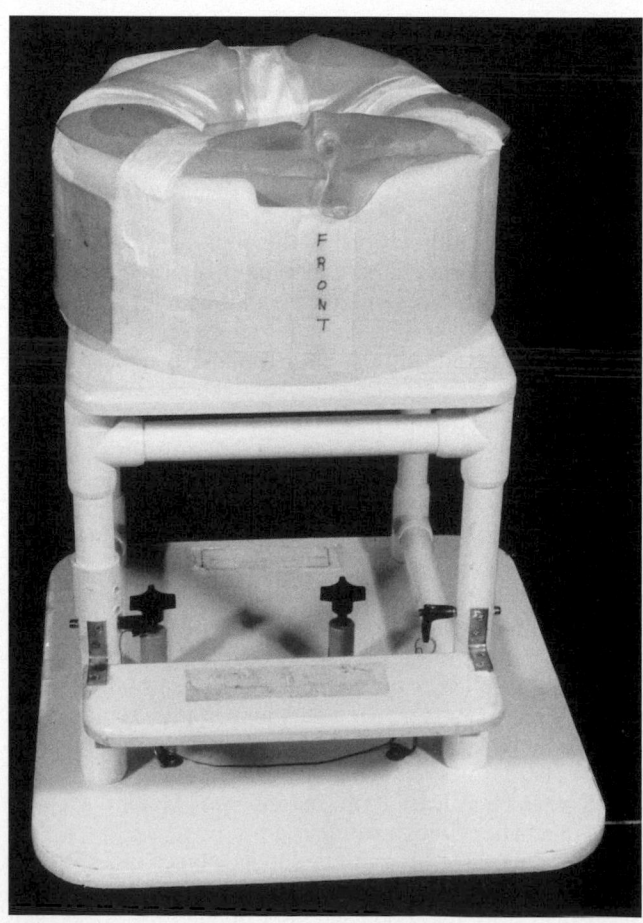

FIGURE 7-13. Defecography commode with modifications. The so-called blooming effect is diminished by the use of a water-filled rubber ring seat. (Courtesy of the Cleveland Clinic Florida, Weston, FL.)

own modifications. With the pelvis examined in profile, x-rays must pass through much tissue, thereby creating considerable absorption of the beam. Movement of the beam caudally, in order to examine anal movement during evacuation or to delineate rectoanal intussusception further, causes x-rays to pass through subcutaneous fat or air. This loss of tissue density and its resultant lack of absorption cause an excessive "flare" or "blooming," significantly detracting from the quality of the image. Various methods have been developed to address this problem, including the use of one or more water-filled rubber rings,[10] specifically designed Perspex water-filled commodes,[11] different thickness of leaded plexiglass,[134] and the use of carefully positioned copper or lead plates.[17]

Contrast Media

A varying amount of liquid barium of the type used for double-contrast enemas (58% weight/weight [wt/wt] barium sulfate suspension) can be administered using a standard enema-tipped catheter. In addition, many investigators use a high-density, high-viscosity barium paste to simulate stool. Others have prepared "home" recipes that involve thickening barium sulfate with methyl cellulose, porridge oats, potato starch, or Maizena.[11,101,110,139,150] The authors' preference is a combination of barium sulfate and oats to simulate stool consistency.

Author's Preferred Technique

Because most of our patients have several physiologic investigations performed on the same day, bowel preparation by means of a phosphate enema is usually performed before manometry. With the patient in the left lateral decubitus position, a digital rectal examination is performed to lubricate the anal canal, to ascertain the presence of any pathologic abnormality, and to ensure that the patient understands the instructions of how to squeeze and to push. Through an enema-tipped catheter, 50 mL of liquid barium (58% wt/wt barium sulfate suspension, Polybar) is introduced into the rectum followed by the insufflation of a small quantity of air to coat the mucosa of the sigmoid colon. Thickened barium paste is then introduced into the rectum until the patient experiences a feeling of fullness. A small quantity of paste is inserted into the anus in order to outline the anal canal, after which the vagina is opacified with Gastrografin. The patient is then turned to the right lateral side, and the table is slowly brought to the erect position. This enables one to slide down the table and to sit on the commode. The fluoroscopy tube is positioned so that the coccyx and the symphysis pubis are both visible on screening. Still pictures (*proctograms*) are taken at rest and at maximal squeeze prior to starting the video recording (Figure 7-14).

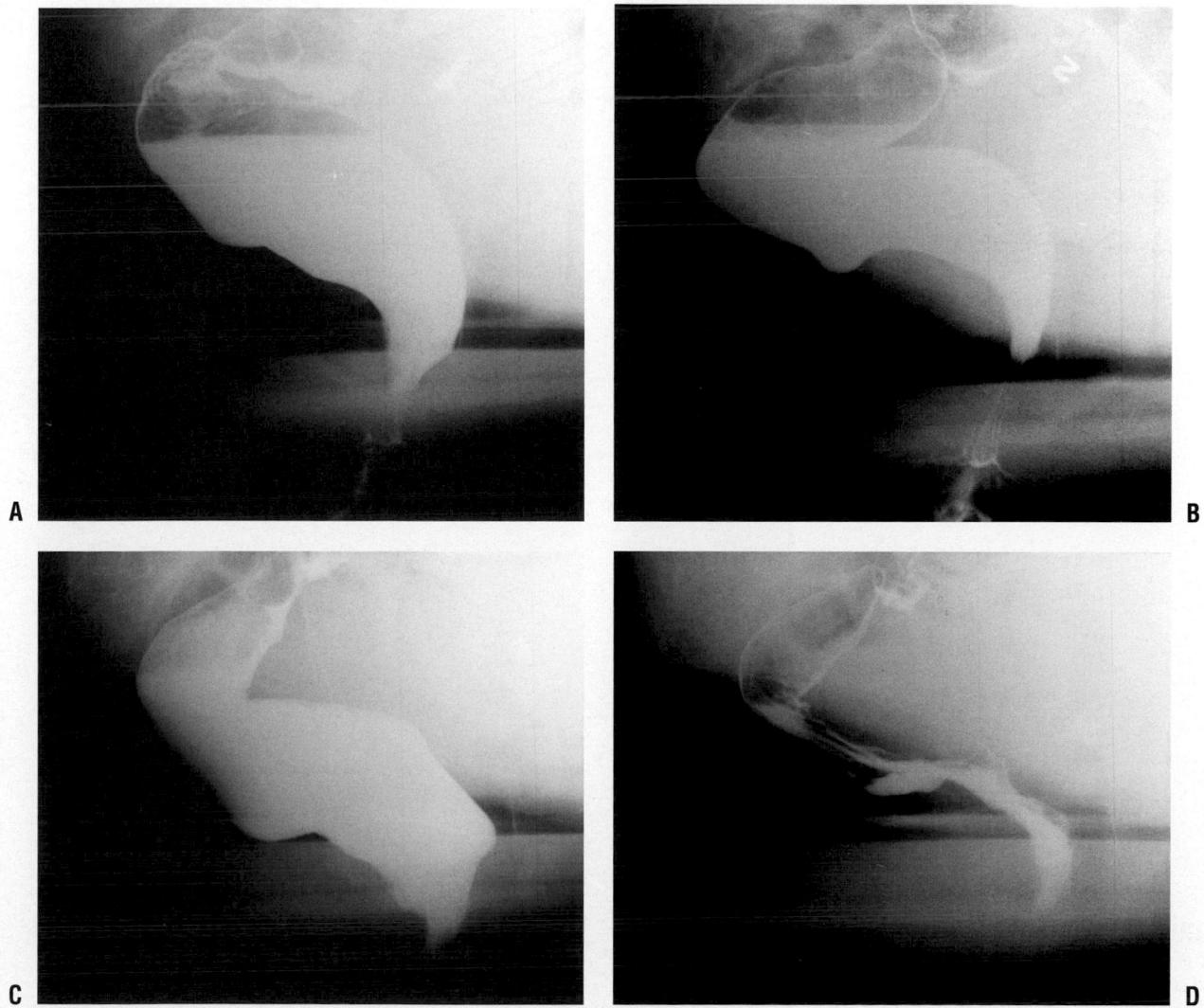

FIGURE 7-14. Proctogram series. **A:** Rest. **B:** Squeeze. **C:** Push. **D:** Postevacuation.

At the commencement of the video, the patients are asked to squeeze, to relax, and then to try to commence evacuation. As elimination starts, a further still picture is taken. Following evacuation, the recording is recommenced while the patient squeezes and pushes in order to check for the presence of an intussusception or nonemptying rectocele. A single still image of the evacuated rectum at rest is also obtained (Figure 7-15B).

With completion of the study, three lines of reference are drawn, so that the anorectal angle, puborectalis length, and extent of perineal descent can be assessed on the proctograms. First, a line is drawn between the tip of the coccyx and the anterosuperior surface of the symphysis pubis.

Lines are also drawn along the axis of the mid-anal canal and along the posterior rectal wall (Figure 7-15A).[86] Whereas some have proposed using the dynamic images alone,[156] the authors prefer to rely on the combination of the dynamic and still images. This has been shown to produce reliable and reproducible measurements.[35]

Anorectal Angle

Much attention has been directed to the *anorectal angle* since Parks (see Biography, Chapter 29) first proposed its role in maintaining fecal continence.[129] The anorectal angle

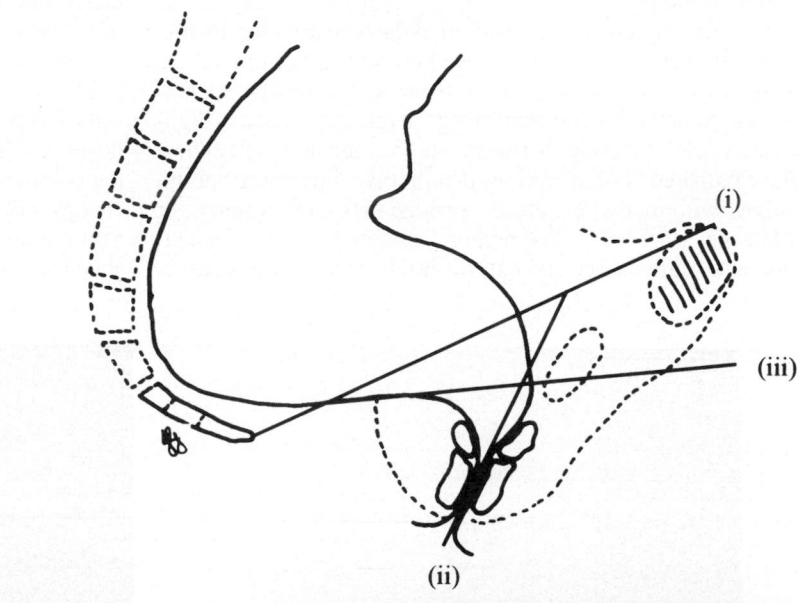

A

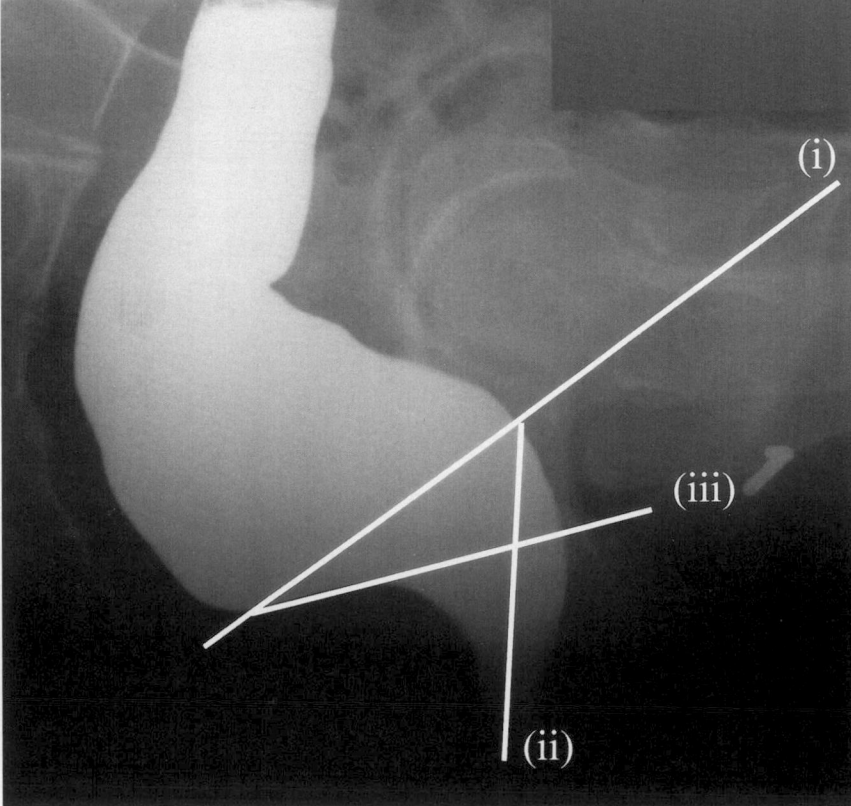

B

FIGURE 7-15. Lines of reference for analysis of proctograms. **A:** Diagrammatic representation of (*i*) pubococcygeal line, (*ii*) midanal line, and (*iii*) posterior rectal line. **B:** Resting proctogram with lines demonstrated.

is the angle formed by the axis of the posterior rectal wall and the axis formed by the anal canal; it is usually 70 to 140 degrees at rest.[59,110] This angle becomes more acute during the squeeze phase (75 to 90 degrees) and becomes more obtuse during evacuation (100 to 180 degrees at maximum strain).[86] Some investigators have reported greater anorectal angles in men,[153] but most clinicians believe that it is not affected by gender.[48] The wide variation in observed normal values is probably due to differences in interpretation.[49,59] It has even been suggested that a normal range is impossible to define.[153] Therefore, the change in angle seen during the squeeze and push phases is more important than the actual measurement.

Puborectalis Length and Perineal Descent

The *puborectalis length* is measured as the minimal distance between the anterosuperior aspect of the symphysis pubis and the puborectalis notch. This ranges between 14 and 16 cm in the rest position, shortens to between 12 and 15 cm during the squeezing phase, and is elongated to 15 to 18 cm during the push phase.[88] As with the anorectal angle determination, the change in these parameters is more important than their definitive value.

Perineal descent is assessed as the length of a perpendicular line drawn from the pubococcygeal line to the anorectal junction. Perineal descent of either more than 3 cm in the rest phase or a further increase of 3 cm in the push phase is considered abnormal.

Interpretation

As with all of the studies performed in the physiology laboratory, interpretation of the results of defecography should be combined with a thorough assessment of the patient's complaints through history and physical examination to ascertain the clinical significance of the findings. A normal defecogram should demonstrate relaxation of the puborectalis as indicated by (1) an increase in the anorectal angle, (2) lengthening of the puborectalis, and (3) a blunting of the puborectalis notch. These changes should be accompanied by symmetric opening of the anal canal to form a cone that is wider cephalad than it is caudad. This process takes ap-

proximately 4 to 5 seconds. Contrast material in the upper rectum should subsequently be passed into the lower rectum and out the anus by rectal contraction, a process that may be facilitated by Valsalva's maneuver, squeezing the rectum onto the levator plate.[108] Complete evacuation takes about 10 to 12 seconds when thickened contrast medium is used but is more rapid (8 to 9 seconds) when the mixture is more fluid.[97] Failure to relax the puborectalis is noted by the persistence of the puborectalis notch, failure of the anorectal angle to increase, and difficulty in emptying the rectum. Although these findings have been noted in normal individuals,[81] patients with complaints of difficult evacuation who have these radiologic findings should be treated for paradoxical puborectalis contraction.

In up to 50% of anatomically normal patients, some folding in of the mucosa on the posterior wall of the rectum is a common finding during evacuation (approximately 3 to 7 cm proximal to the anal canal).[151] If these folds become circumferential and form a ring pocket, then an intussusception is truly present. Obviously, if this intussusception is extruded outside the anal canal, then it is termed a rectal prolapse or procidentia. However, one should not need the radiologist to tell the clinician that a procidentia is present.

Bulging of the anterior or posterior wall of the rectum is a relatively common finding on defecography, particularly in women.[97] In female patients, an anterior *rectocele* 2 cm in size that empties on evacuation is considered within normal limits. The presence of a nonemptying rectocele may be considered pathologic, but this finding should be interpreted in accordance with the patient's symptoms. The presence of a *sigmoidocele* is assessed during the maximum straining phase. The presence of a first-degree sigmoidocele (a sigmoid loop that is present within the true pelvis but does not reach or cross the pubococcygeal line) is considered a normal finding. A second-degree sigmoidocele, one that extends to or below the pubococcygeal line, is considered abnormal. However, it may not be clinically significant. A sigmoid loop that extends below a line drawn between the coccyx and the ischial tuberosities is an uncommon finding and is termed a *third-degree sigmoidocele* (Figure 7-16).[87]

ANTONIO MARIA VALSALVA (1666–1723)

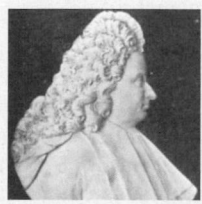

Antonio Maria Valsalva
Bas-relief in the library
of Imola, Italy

Valsalva was born in Imola, Italy on January 17, 1666, the son of a merchant and aristocrat. He was educated by the Jesuits and achieved his MD and PhD in 1687 from the University of Bologna. Upon graduation, he was appointed inspector of public health in Bologna. He was a pupil of Malpighi and teacher of Morgagni. Valsalva was a brilliant anatomist and became well recognized for his studies on the anatomy and physiology of the ear, a fact that culminated in the publication of his book, *De Aure Humana* (1704). His contributions to our understanding of a host of conditions were myriad. His name

is eponymously associated with the outpouching of the noncoronary sinus (aneurysm of the sinus of Valsalva), Valsalva's antrum, V's dysphagia, V's methods, V's muscle, V's ligaments, and of course, V's maneuver—the increase of intrapulmonic (and intraabdominal) pressure caused by forcible exhalation against the closed glottis—thereby facilitating pelvic floor descent and defecation. He wrote, "If the glottis be closed after a deep inspiration, and a strenuous and prolonged expiratory effort be then made, such pressure can be exerted upon the heart and intrathoracic vessels that the movement and flow of the blood are temporarily arrested." In 1705, Valsalva was appointed lecturer and demonstrator in anatomy at the university, a position he retained for the remainder of his life.

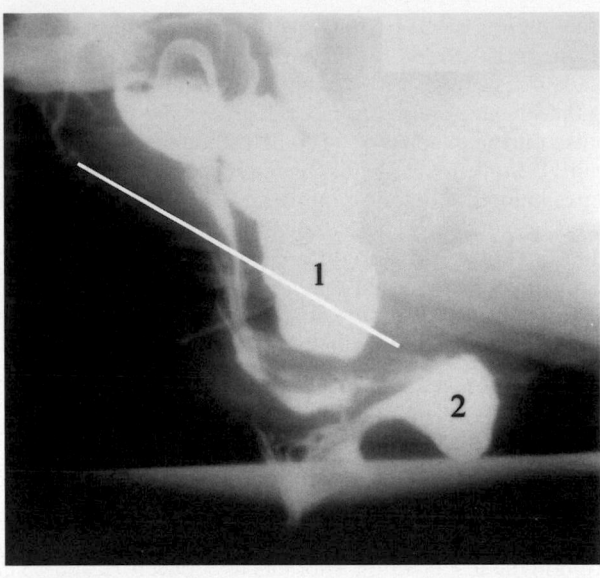

FIGURE 7-16. Lines of reference for classification of sigmoidoceles. **A:** Diagrammatic representation of (*i*) the pubosacral line, (*ii*) the pubococcygeal line, and (*iii*) the ischiococcygeal line. **B:** Evacuation proctogram demonstrating (*1*) a third-degree sigmoidocele with (*2*) a concomitant anterior rectocele. (From Jorge JM, Yang YK, Wexner SD. Incidence and clinical significance of sigmoidoceles as determined by a new classification system. *Dis Colon Rectum.* 1993;37(11):1112–1117, with permission.)

In summary, defecography is a useful test for the evaluation of patients suffering from constipation. It can provide important information as to the etiology of outlet obstructive symptoms.

MAGNETIC RESONANCE IMAGING

The use of MRI to diagnose pelvic floor abnormalities was first introduced in the early 1990s.[182] The overwhelming benefit when compared to standard defecography is the ability to visualize all of the pelvic organs and their interrelationships, thereby facilitating the diagnosis of concomitant pathology. In addition, there is the avoidance of ionizing radiation. Often, however, because of financial and logistical constraints, such as scheduling problems, the procedure may pose a challenge for one to obtain it.

There is also the concern for the positioning of the patient. If the study is undertaken in the supine position, there is the problem that pertinent pathologic entities could be missed or misinterpreted. With the patient in the nonphysiologic upright or sitting position, interpretation is subject to error.[18,171]

Several investigators have attempted to determine the normal values for this technique.[70,104,147] There has been, however, significant variability in the measurements and interpretation of the soft tissues of the pelvis with MRI.[105] Healy and coworkers proposed use of dynamic MRI in patients with obstructed defecation and in whom other physiologic studies were normal.[71] More recently, MRI has been shown to alter treatment plans in patients with obstructed defecation.[43]

MRI can be a useful adjunct to the colorectal physiology laboratory with complex patients suffering from a combination of anterior and posterior compartment pelvic pathology. Availability and financial constraints may again prevent this modality from becoming a first-line tool in the evaluation of the pelvic floor.

ULTRASOUND

Endoanal ultrasonography has become the cornerstone of the anorectal physiologic evaluation of fecal incontinence. It is an integral part of any anorectal physiology laboratory. Ultrasound gives the physician detailed information about the anatomy of the anal canal. It has been shown to be an accurate tool for the staging of rectal cancers (see Chapter 24),[94,103] as well as defining the anatomy of anal fistulas (see Chapter 14).[100,118] More recently, ultrasound has been used to evaluate the pelvic floor in patients with obstructed defecation.[25,112,117] Pulsed sound waves of a specific frequency are emitted from a transducer. As they traverse tissue planes, some of the sound waves are reflected back toward the transducer. The quantity reflected is dependent on the acoustic impedance of the different tissue densities. An image is generated by the digital sequential processing of these sound waves based on the time difference between sound transmission and reception of the echo. The study is well tolerated and avoids the use of ionizing radiation. It may not be feasible for patients who have a stenosis or other disease state that may be painful, such as an anal fissure.

Anal Ultrasound

The normal ultrasonographic anatomy of the anal canal is well described.[99,170] The efficacy of this technique was demonstrated by Sultan and colleagues who used cadaveric and surgical specimens to correlate ultrasonographic findings with anatomic dissection.[165] Their findings were further confirmed with histopathologic evaluation of the dissected specimens.

Examination takes place with the patient in the left lateral decubitus position, with the probe orientated so that the water spigot is in the upright position. Using this orientation, the anterior quadrant of the anal canal is seen in the superior aspect of the screen with the right quadrant seen on the left side of the screen. The different tissue densities and interfaces create a series of hyperechoic and hypoechoic images, corresponding to the different anatomic layers of the anal canal.[170] Using a 7-MHz probe, three distinct layers are seen. The mucosa/submucosa complex appears as a hyperechoic band surrounding the transducer. Outside this layer is a hypoechoic band that can be seen most clearly in the mid-anal canal; this represents the internal anal sphincter. The band has an average thickness of 2 to 4 mm. Parenthetically, it has been noted to increase with age.[27] The final layer is a thicker band of mixed echogenicity that represents the external anal sphincter. The junction between external sphincter and perirectal fat is not clearly defined, making it difficult to measure the thickness of the sphincter definitively (Figure 7-17).[164]

Localization of anal sphincter defects with ultrasound often forms the basis of the surgical management of fecal incontinence. Identification of the muscular layers throughout the levels of the anal canal can be accomplished with ease. The upper anal canal is identified by the U-shaped hy-

perechoic puborectalis muscle. It is important to recognize this level and to avoid confusing this normal anatomy with a sphincter defect. The mid-anal canal in normal patients is marked by the thickest portion of the hypoechoic internal anal sphincter and the circumferential mixed echogenic external anal sphincter. At the level of the distal anal canal, only the external sphincter is present. Also important in the evaluation of patients with fecal incontinence is the assessment of perineal body thickness (PBT). PBT less than 10 mm is considered abnormal, and those patients with PBT greater than 12 mm are considered unlikely to have a sphincter defect in the absence of prior reconstructive surgery.[123] The test is well tolerated and much less painful than the anal EMG. But the two have been shown to have excellent correlation.[45]

The use of ultrasound for the diagnosis of anal fistula and the delineation of the anatomy of the tract was first described by Law and associates.[100] It has subsequently been shown to

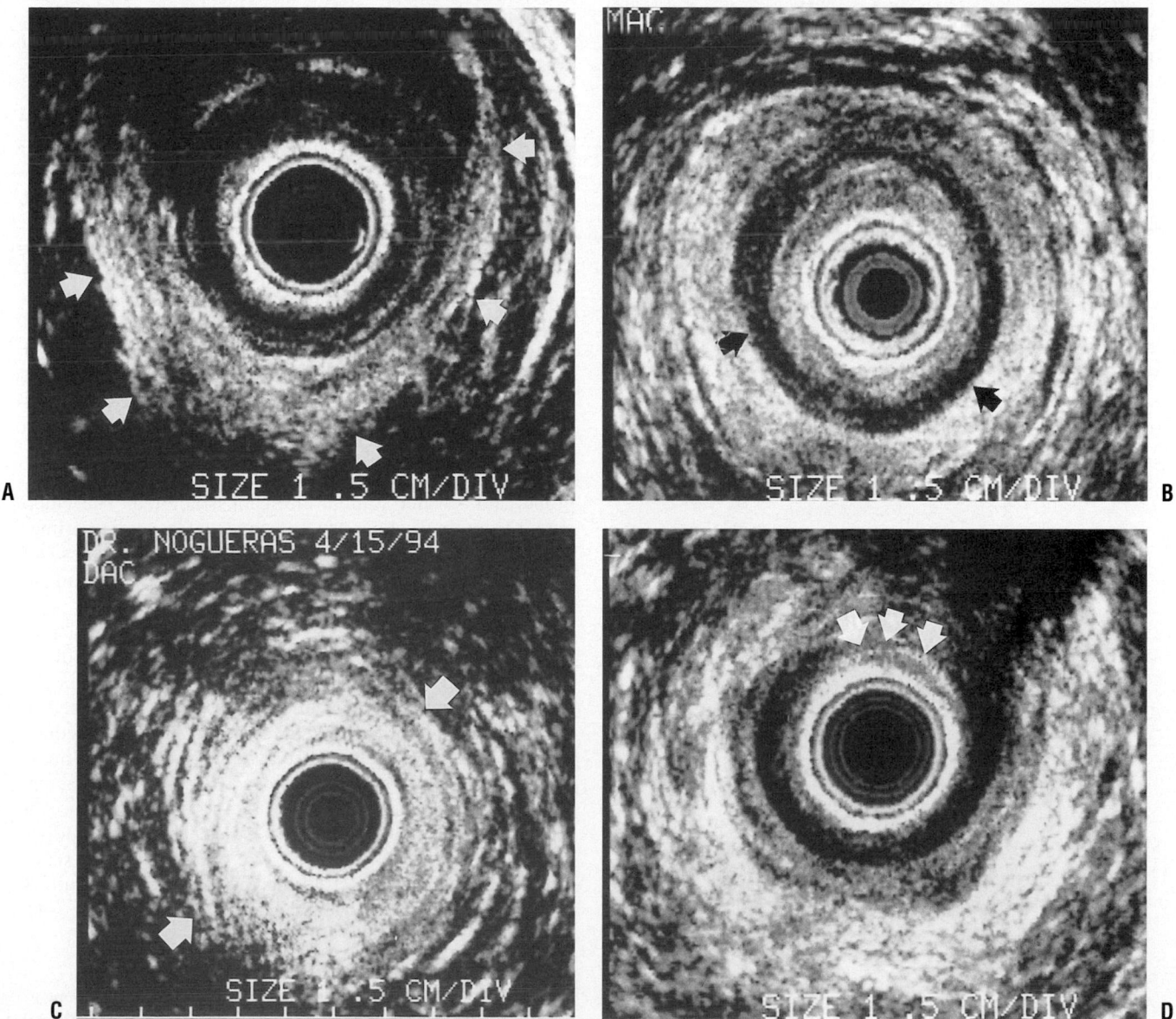

FIGURE 7-17. Endoanal ultrasound images. **A:** Upper anal canal: puborectalis sling posteriorly (*arrows*). **B:** Middle anal canal: the hypoechoic internal sphincter (*arrows*) is at its maximum thickness. **C:** Lower anal canal: the hypoechoic internal sphincter has disappeared and is replaced by hyperechoic external sphincter (*arrows*). **D:** Anterior sphincter defect in the midanal canal with absent external sphincter and scarring of the internal sphincter (*arrows*).

be helpful in determining the extent of the disease in those with Crohn's disease[157,169,172] and superior to MRI for the evaluation of complex fistulas.[125] Enhancement of the fistula tract with hydrogen peroxide has been shown to increase diagnostic accuracy for both standard and three-dimensional ultrasound.[163,177]

Dynamic Ultrasound

The concept of the use of dynamic ultrasound for the evaluation of the pelvic floor was first introduced in 2000.[9,90] The authors proposed that the ultrasound could be used to evaluate the anal sphincters as well as to diagnose patients with forms of outlet obstruction, including rectocele, intussusception, and enterocele. The technique of dynamic transperineal ultrasound was initially presented in 2002.[15] Transverse as well as sagittal images provided diagnostic accuracy similar to that of standard defecography, with the avoidance of ionizing radiation. Most recently, Murad-Regadas described the technique of echodefecography, noting that all of the pelvic floor structures were identifiable.[170] He concluded that this method was comparable to that of standard defecography. Further studies should help delineate the role of dynamic ultrasound in the physiology laboratory.

Ultrasound Equipment

Numerous ultrasound scanners and probes are available (Figures 7-18 and 7-19). Early versions did not have rotating transducer heads and could, therefore, only scan sectors of

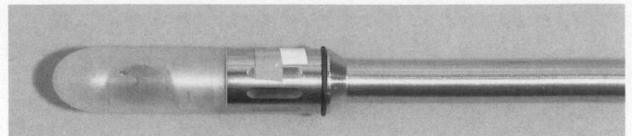

FIGURE 7-19. Transducer head of a 7-mHz rotating endoanal ultrasound probe (B & K 1850). (Courtesy of Brüel & Kjær Instruments, Inc., Billerica, MA.)

the anal canal ranging from 90 to 320 degrees. Even though accurate imaging was possible, it was difficult to ensure that pictures from different sectors were taken at the same level of the anus. Thus, it was problematic for the examiner to recreate the anatomy of the anal canal. This difficulty has been surmounted by the development of a 360-degree rotating transducer (Figure 7-18). Transducers of differing frequencies have also been used. Early models employed 4- and 5-MHz transducers,[32,61] but owing to focal length deficiencies these probes have been superseded by 7- and 10-MHz endoprobes. However, some controversy exists whether a 10-MHz transducer (focal length, 1 to 4 cm) gives a higher resolution of the anal sphincters than does the 7-MHz transducer (focal length, 2 to 5 cm). Based on ultrasonographic physics, higher frequency (number of cycles per second) improves resolution. Meanwhile, wave length (distance traveled by the ultrasonic wave per cycle) decreases as frequency increases, thus allowing better resolution but poorer tissue penetration.[141]

The transducer head is covered by a sonolucent hard cone, 1.7 cm in external diameter. This cone is carefully filled with water to ensure that all air bubbles are excluded because they will produce artifacts.

The newest three-dimensional ultrasound equipment houses the transducer within an outer casing. The transducer can move proximally and distally within the probe that lies still in the anal canal. This provides even greater comfort to the patient as there is less manipulation required.

A condom containing ultrasound gel is placed over the probe, and a water-soluble lubricant is applied. The video output from the scanner can be connected to a video printer so that still pictures can be taken. The dynamic images can be exported from the machine for further evaluation on a remote PC.

Ultrasonic probes are available in combination with various endoscopes to allow simultaneous observation of ultrasonic and endoscopic images. This technology is expensive, but because these endoscopes are widely used in gastroenterologic practice, shared equipment should reduce capital outlay. Two designs are available. A convex, longitudinal scanning system is preferred by some manufacturers because of improved reliability and the ease of use of accessory tools, such as biopsy needles. These endoscopes also provide color Doppler facility but only permit scanning through a sector of 100 degrees. Other manufacturers prefer a 360-degree mechanical radial scanner (Table 7-4).

Authors' Technique

Bowel preparation is not required for endoanal ultrasonography. After careful explanation of the procedure, a digital rectal examination is performed to lubricate the anal canal, to assess any anatomic defects, and to ensure that the probe can be introduced into the anal canal easily and without

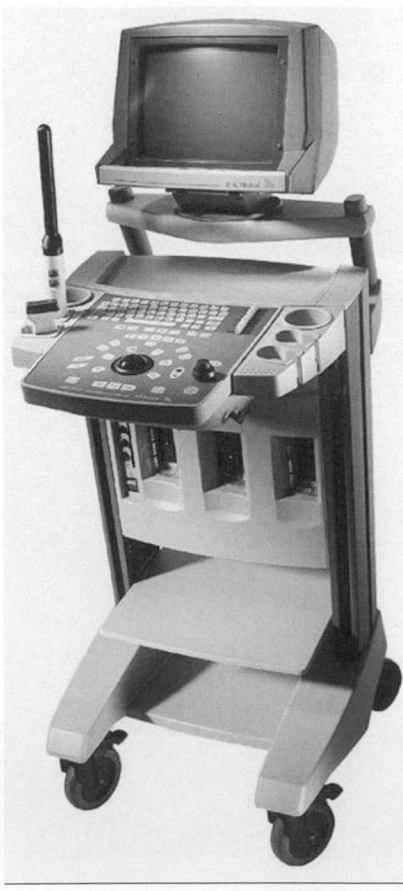

FIGURE 7-18. Falcon ultrasound scanner, probe, and monitor. (Courtesy of Brüel & Kjær Instruments, Inc., Billerica, MA.)

TABLE 7-4 Ultrasound Equipment Suppliers

MANUFACTURER	MODEL	TYPE	SCANNING SYSTEM	SCANNING ANGLE	FREQUENCY
Brüel & Kjær, North Billerica, MA 01862, USA	Probe 1850 Scanner 1846	Rigid	Mechanical, radial	360 degrees	7 or 10 MHz
Brüel & Kjær, Nærum, Denmark					
Olympus America Inc., Melville, NY 11747, USA	GF-UM20 gastroscope	Endoscopic	Mechanical, radial	360 degrees	7.5 or 12 MHz switchable
Olympus Keymed, Southport-on-Sea, SS2 5QH, UK	CF-UM20 colonoscope	Endoscopic	Mechanical, radial	360 degrees	7.5 or 12 MHz
Pentax Precision Instrument Corp., Orangeburg, NY 10962, USA	FG-32UA	Endoscopic	Convex, longitudinal	100 degrees	5 or 7.5 MHz switchable
Pentax UK Ltd., Slough, SL3 8PN, UK					

discomfort. The three-dimensional probe is inserted into the lower rectum and then is gradually withdrawn until the puborectalis sling can be most clearly identified. A three-dimensional scan of the anal canal commences from this level distally to the perineum. The anatomy of the anal musculature is assessed at the upper, middle, and distal anal canal levels. The perineal body is measured at the level of the mid-anal canal by gently inserting an examining finger into the vagina and resting it on the posterior wall. Still photos are generally taken at the three levels of the anal canal. If there is a sphincter defect evident, it is measured in degrees.

Conclusion

Ultrasound has a number of advantages when compared with other physiologic and anatomic investigations. First, it is usually painless and is, therefore, preferable to concentric needle EMG for mapping sphincter defects. Thus, patient compliance with respect to follow-up is generally not a problem. Second, ultrasound is less expensive than is other imaging modalities such as computed tomography or MRI. It is also quicker to perform than these two techniques, and the patient is not exposed to radiation. Finally, because the equipment is portable, it can be taken to the operating room or used in the clinician's examination room.

▶ NEUROPHYSIOLOGIC ASSESSMENT

Electromyography

EMG of the anal sphincter was first reported by Beck in 1930.[14] Anal EMG is a recording of the electrical activity from the muscle fibers of the external sphincter and puborectalis complex during rest, during maximum squeeze, during simulated defecation, and in response to various reflexes.

Electrical activity may be measured from individual fibers (fibrillation potentials). It is more common, however, to assess the summation of the electrical activity from a number of muscle fibers derived from a single motor unit. This activity forms a motor unit action potential. A motor unit is composed of an anterior horn cell, its axon and terminal branches, and the muscle fibers that it supplies. Depolarization of the motor end plate by the release of acetylcholine in response to a nerve impulse results in depolarization of the muscle fiber with resultant contraction. EMG records the change of electrical potential during muscle depolarization. Four techniques can be used to record this electrical activity: concentric needle EMG, monopolar wire electrode EMG, single-fiber EMG, and surface or anal plug electrode EMG. Anal EMG has been used for sphincter mapping in patients with fecal incontinence and is also of use in assessing the function of the pelvic floor in individuals with constipation. There have been recent reports of EMG correlating with success of treatment for fecal incontinence.[3]

Normal Anal Findings

The constant baseline EMG activity seen at rest is constantly changing.[52] During maximum voluntary contraction, the amplitude of the motor unit potential is, on average, 200 to 600 μV, with a maximum of 2 to 3 mV. However, amplitude depends on the number of fibers that discharge simultaneously. It also varies with the distance of the recording electrode from the motor unit. Amplitude values are, therefore, not useful for comparative purposes. Duration of the motor unit potential is more reproducible but has been noted to increase with age.[47] The mean duration of motor unit potentials of the adult anal sphincter during voluntary contraction is 5 to 7.5 milliseconds. Motor unit potentials are usually biphasic or triphasic. However, polyphasic potentials (with four or more phases) are observed in the normal external sphincter. Reported incidences vary between 7% and 25%.[46]

Abnormal Anal Findings

Damage to the anal sphincter often causes scarring resulting in a markedly decreased number of motor unit potentials at rest, during squeeze, and during reflex elicitation.[119] Damage to the nerve supply of a muscle will result in two different patterns of EMG activity, depending on the severity of the injury (Figure 7-20). In a severely injured sphincter, EMG activity is significantly decreased or even silenced. However, if the injury is incomplete, reinnervation will occur by either

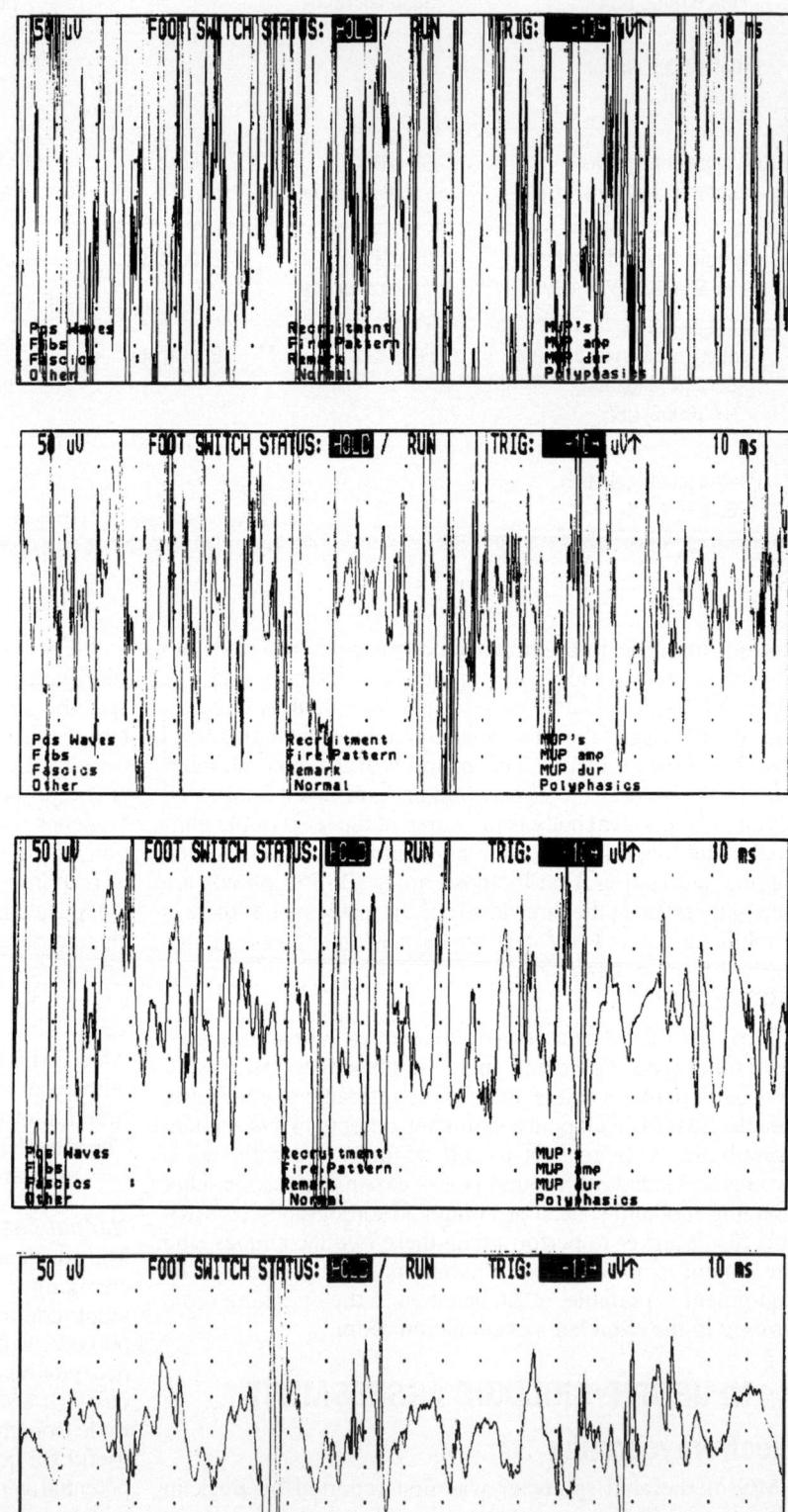

FIGURE 7-20. External anal sphincter electromyography during voluntary contraction. **Top to bottom:** Normal recruitment; mild decrease in recruitment; moderate decrease in recruitment; severe decrease in recruitment.

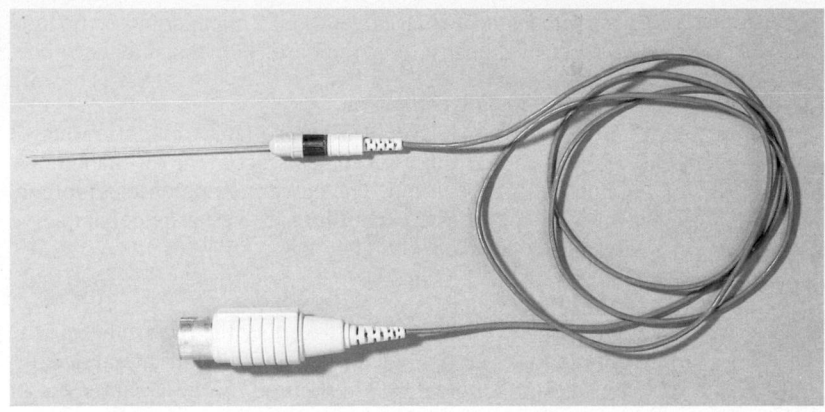

FIGURE 7-21. Bipolar concentric electromyographic needle (no. 53158). (Courtesy of Teca, Pleasantville, NY.)

regrowth of the damaged axons or sprouting of unaffected axons into different muscle fibers. Sprouting will alter the distribution of muscle fibers within motor units, a process known as fiber type grouping. This results in motor potentials of increased amplitude and prolonged duration and an increase in the number of polyphasic potentials.[45,50,120,154] These immature nerve fibers cannot conduct the nerve impulses quickly, which results in prolongation of the action potential.

During evacuation, EMG activity of the external sphincter and puborectalis should be almost silent. However, in patients with paradoxical contraction or nonrelaxation of the puborectalis, the EMG activity will increase or will remain unchanged during simulated defecation.[21,38,51,132,143] Fucini and colleagues evaluated patients with symptoms of obstructed defecation using EMG of the pelvic floor muscles.[54] They showed a lower frequency of pubococcygeal muscle inhibition in this specific study population.

Concentric Needle Electromyography

Adrian and Bronck designed the first concentric needle electrode in 1929.[1] This needle consisted of a bare-tipped steel wire, 0.1 mm in diameter, surrounded by a resin insulation (Figure 7-21). The needle can record electrical activity from a small area that includes a few motor units. Individual muscle fiber action potentials cannot be identified with this apparatus, however. The electrical activity is amplified and displayed using one of many recorders available from several commercial sources. Concentric needle EMG provides data on sphincter damage and reinnervation and is useful for sphincter mapping. However, it is painful, and patients will seldom be willing to undergo follow-up evaluation.

Single-Fiber Electromyography

A single-fiber EMG electrode consists of a needle slightly less than 0.1 mm in diameter that is filled with resin. A 25-μm diameter electrode projects through this needle. The cannula of the electrode acts as the reference electrode; a separate surface electrode to ground is also required. The single-fiber electrode measures electrical activity from a radius of 270 μm. An amplifier with a 500-Hz low-frequency filter setting and a trigger delay line are necessary, with the amplifier set at 2 to 5 milliseconds per division. Twenty different recordings are taken from each lateral hemisphere of the sphincter, and the fiber density is calculated as the mean number of single muscle fiber action potentials per position.[160] The normal fiber density is 1.5 ± 0.6.[120] The fiber density will increase during the period of reinnervation following nerve injury because more fibers are innervated by an individual axon.

The time interval between action potentials is called *neuromuscular jitter*. This parameter is an indication of variability in the speed of the transmission of impulses across the neuromuscular junction, but its clinical relevance is uncertain. This also can be assessed by using a single-fiber EMG electrode in such a manner that when the electrode is placed it records two fibers from the same motor unit.[41]

Surface Anal Plug Electromyography

Surface electrodes have been used to record the electrical activity of the sphincter apparatus, but they have since been replaced through the development of intra-anal plug EMG electrodes.[124] These plastic or sponge plugs have longitudinal or circular electrodes mounted on their surfaces and can be placed inside the anus with ease (Figure 7-22). Binnie and colleagues have demonstrated that longitudinal

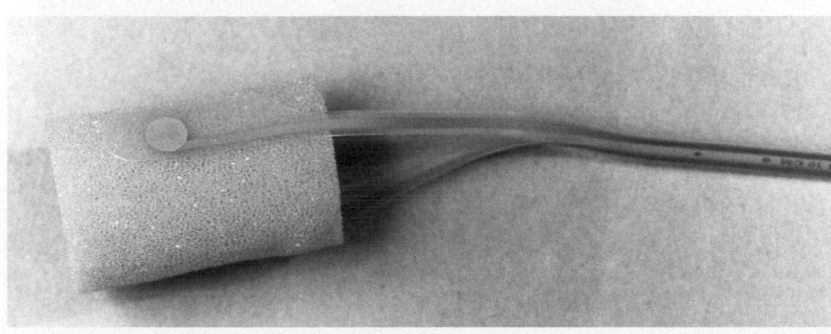

FIGURE 7-22. Intra-anal sponge plug electrode (model 13L81). (Courtesy of Dantec Medical, Inc., Allendale, NJ.)

electrodes are superior to the circular design because they correlate with fine-wire electrodes.[19] Furthermore, they are much better tolerated but only provide crude global information about the sphincter. As such, although they are useful in evaluating those with constipation, they cannot be applied for sphincter mapping in incontinent patients. A study by López and associates demonstrated a good correlation between surface electrodes and concentric needle electrodes in the diagnosis of paradoxical anal sphincter reaction.[106] EMG may also be an important adjunct to biofeedback in the management of patients with fecal incontinence and obstructed defecation.

Pudendal Nerve Terminal Motor Latency

Because the external anal sphincter is innervated by the pudendal nerve, the quantitative assessment of the speed of impulse transmission along this pathway can provide useful information in patients with incontinence, rectal prolapse, and constipation.[81,119] Based on the technique of electroejaculation, Kiff and Swash developed a fingerstall device containing stimulating and recording electrodes that could be used intrarectally to stimulate the pudendal nerve and to record the impulse distally.[24,93] The time taken for the impulse to be transmitted is known as the *pudendal nerve terminal motor latency* (PNTML). A disposable electrode based on this original design was developed by Rogers and colleagues.[140] In addition to bowel management concerns, the PNTML can be used to assess perineal nerve function indirectly in patients with urinary incontinence. There is a linear relationship between the terminal motor latencies of the perineal and pudendal nerves, the perineal nerve latencies being slightly longer. The clinical significance of pudendal neuropathy has been the subject of controversy in the management of patients with fecal incontinence.[7,53,80,128,138] Although this test may not alter surgical management, the authors believe that it is a useful adjunct for preoperative counseling of patients undergoing treatment for fecal incontinence.

Equipment
Electrode
The Dantec St. Mark's pudendal nerve stimulating device is used at most centers (Figure 7-23). This consists of a thin strip of paper with adhesive on the surface to be placed on the gloved finger. There are two stimulating electrodes, a larger anode and a smaller cathode, 1 cm apart at the tip, and two recording electrodes at the base, 4 cm distal to the anode.

Electromyographic Equipment
A unit that can deliver a 50-V square wave stimulus of 0.1 millisecond in duration and can record the resultant motor unit potential is required. The newer manometric equipment is outfitted with EMG capabilities as well as pudendal nerve assessment software.

Recommendations
A single Fleet enema is used to empty the rectum before the examination. The patient is placed in the left lateral decubitus position. An electrode is secured on the volar aspect of the examiner's gloved index finger. Following the application of electrode gel to the electrodes, the examiner's index finger is inserted into the rectum until the coccyx is palpated posteriorly. The finger is then moved laterally to the left, and the left ischial spine is palpated. The EMG equipment (Nicolet Viking IIe; Nicolet Biomedical, Inc., Madison, WI) is set to deliver 22- to 35-mA impulses controlled by a foot switch as the finger is moved across the pelvic side wall in order to determine the optimal site for assessing nerve latency. This point is recognized by a strong contraction of the external sphincter around the examiners finger and a coincident maximal amplitude motor unit potential of the recording apparatus (Figure 7-24). During recording, sensitivity is set at 50 μV, the low-frequency filter is set at 2 Hz, and the high-frequency filter is set at 5 kHz. The terminal motor latency is the time interval between the onset of the stimulus and the onset of the motor unit potential. Three values are taken from one nerve before rotating the finger and repeating the process on the contralateral nerve. The motor unit potential image will be inverted on this side. The normal value for PNTML in our laboratory is 2.0 ± 0.2 milliseconds.[93,155,179] Along with anal ultrasonography, these tests are the most important in the evaluation of fecal incontinence.

▶ TRANSIT STUDIES

Colon

The evaluation of colonic transit is important for patients suffering from constipation. Often, constipation is multifactorial, with contributory effects of poor diet, metabolic

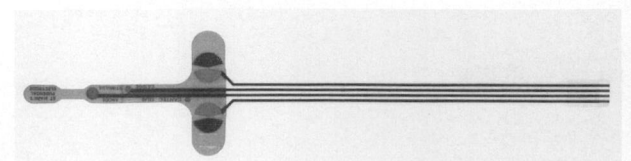
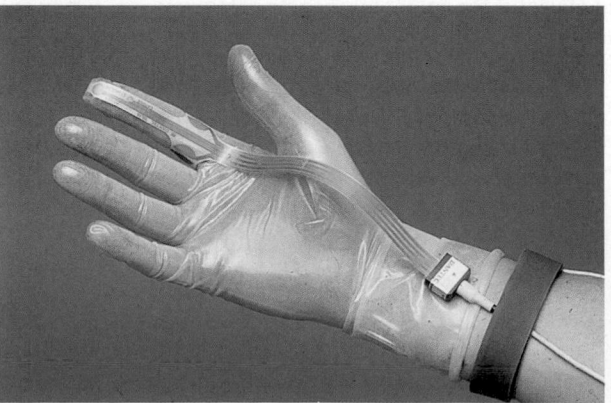

FIGURE 7-23. St. Mark's pudendal nerve stimulating device 13L40 showing arrangement of anode and cathode **(A)** and correct positioning for examination **(B)**. (Courtesy of Dantec Medical, Inc., Allendale, NJ.)

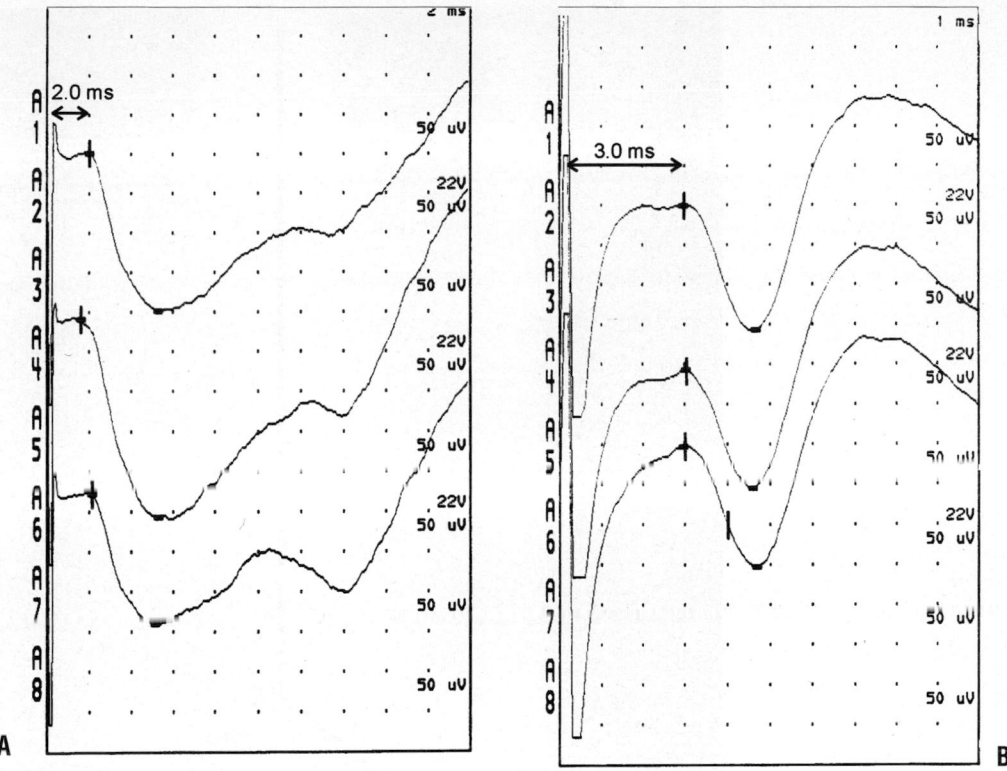

FIGURE 7-24. Pudendal nerve terminal motor latencies showing normal latency **(A)** and prolonged latency **(B)**.

causes, and outlet obstruction. Patients who have infrequent bowel movements and who are resistant to medical treatment with dietary manipulation and cathartics should be evaluated for colonic inertia. Historically, intestinal transit was assessed by the ingestion of nonabsorbable colored glass or plastic beads that were then collected following defecation.[4] This process was obviously aesthetically unpleasant for both patient and investigator. Similarly, other clinicians have used colored powders, such as indigo carmine and charcoal, or chemically detectable markers, such as chromium oxide and copper thiocyanate.[39,111,180] All of these methods have the same unaesthetic and cumbersome disadvantages and are no longer used. At the present time, assessment of colonic transit is most commonly accomplished through the use of radiopaque markers; colonic scintigraphy; or, most recently, wireless motility capsule.

Radiopaque Markers

In the initial use of this modality, radiopaque markers were ingested and their excretion in stool was monitored by serial radiographs of the feces.[75] Although this technique has the advantage of not exposing the individual to radiation, it is unpleasant for both the patient and the radiologist, and it gives no indication as to the anatomic distribution of markers over time. In 1981, Arhan and colleagues modified the procedure by taking serial x-ray studies of the abdomen every 24 hours for up to 7 days following ingestion of the markers.[5]

By using bony landmarks to divide the abdomen into three areas, some appreciation of segmental colonic transit can be obtained. For example, markers that are located to the right of the spinous processes of the vertebrae and above a line drawn from the fifth lumbar vertebra to the pelvic outlet are

in the right colon. Markers to the left of the vertebral spinous processes and above a line from the fifth lumbar vertebra to the iliac crest are in the left colon. Markers below the line of the pelvic brim on the right and the iliac crest on the left are said to be in the rectosigmoid and rectum (Figure 7-25). If a single bolus of 20 markers is given and serial x-ray studies are taken every 24 hours, Arhan's initial formula for the calculation of mean transit time (hours) per segment can be simplified to

$$\text{mean transit} = 1.2 \, (n_1 + n_2 + n_3 + \cdots + n_j)$$

where n equals the number of markers present on each film and j is the total number of films.

The problem with this approach, however, is that daily x-ray studies will expose the patient to more radiation than is necessary. This can be reduced without compromising the quality of the information by employing the technique described by Hinton and Lennard-Jones.[74] They suggested ingestion of a single capsule of 20 radiopaque rings followed by daily abdominal roentgenograms (see Figures 20-2 and 20-4). A normal study is one in which 16 or more of the markers have passed by the fifth postingestion day, and all have been evacuated by the seventh day. Metcalf and coworkers modified the test by suggesting the use of three boluses of 20 markers each, ingested at 24-hour intervals, and then taking two plain abdominal radiographs at 24 and 96 hours following the ingestion of the third bolus.[115] The same formula noted previously can be used to calculate segmental transit time.[114] Using modifications of these methods, transit through the right colon has been estimated to be from 6.9 to 13 hours, transit through the left colon from

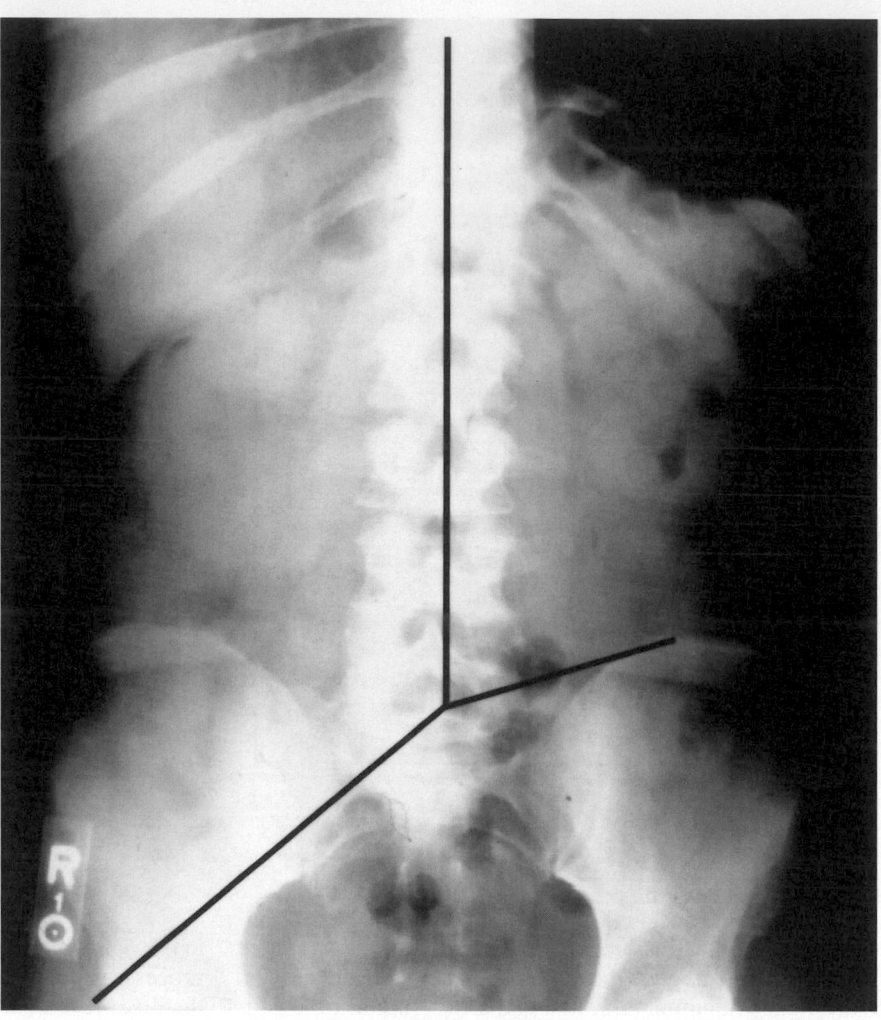

FIGURE 7-25. Plain abdominal x-ray study demonstrating lines of reference for segmental colonic transit marker studies.

9.1 to 15 hours, and transit through the rectosigmoid from 11 to 18.4 hours.[5,34,115] Because the radiopaque marker study is simple, inexpensive, and reproducible, it is the most widely performed colonic transit evaluation.

Although it is certainly intellectually gratifying and potentially useful to know the segmental transit, there is little to no clinical relevance.[107,131] Accordingly, the straightforward method on which we have settled is for the patient to ingest a single capsule containing 24 commercially available rings (see Figure 20-6, Sitzmarks, Konsyl Pharmaceuticals, Lafayette, TX). A single radiograph obtained 5 days after ingestion of the capsule can provide all of the necessary information. Specifically, retention of 20% or more of the markers can be interpreted as abnormal. There are three basic results to this single-capsule, single-radiograph study. First, if fewer than 20% of the markers are retained, this should be considered a "normal" study. Second, if 20% or more of the markers are retained in the rectosigmoid, a functional or anatomic pelvic outlet obstruction is thought to exist. Third, if 20% or more of the markers are retained and diffusely situated throughout the colon, this is suggestive of colonic inertia (see Chapter 20).

Colonic Scintigraphy

This procedure entails the tracking of a radionuclide-labeled bolus through the colon by using a gamma camera. It has been advocated as an accurate method of assessing colonic transit time but has the inconvenience of requiring that the radionuclide bolus be delivered to the cecum. This can be accomplished by direct installation into the cecum through either orocecal intubation or via colonoscopy.[89,96] Both of these methods are obviously invasive, and colonoscopic installation requires bowel preparation, which may confuse interpretation of colonic transit results. As an alternative, polystyrene pellets or resin particles labeled with ^{99m}Tc or indium (^{111}In) can be incorporated into a gelatin capsule coated with a methacrylate polymer.[133] Following ingestion, this capsule will remain intact through the acid pH of the stomach and duodenum but will dissolve in the distal small bowel where the pH is typically between 7.2 and 7.4.[46,176] Multiple images over 3 consecutive days can be obtained without increasing the radiation exposure.[79] However, this type of intensive study makes considerable time demands on gamma camera use and is inconvenient for the patient. These difficulties can be ameliorated by limiting data acquisition to three times: 28 hours, 52 hours, and 60 hours following ingestion.[122]

Sequential transit times can be calculated as the time difference between the initial detection of activity in one region of interest and initial detection of activity in the adjacent region of interest. This provides information about the rate of transit of the head of the meal and may differ from the transit time of the bulk of the meal. Furthermore, identification of the time when the meal enters a particular region is subject to further error, depending on the frequency with which images are obtained. To further confuse matters, image resolution is not ideal. This limitation leads to difficulty in interpreting the anatomic layout of the colon, loops of which may be superimposed or confused with small bowel.

Clearly, because of the complexity of this technique, it has limited clinical application. It does, however, remain as an investigational modality.

Recommendation

We prefer to use a modification of Hinton's and Lennard-Jones' original method.[74] No bowel preparation is carried out. The patient is given a single capsule containing 24 radiopaque markers. One is instructed to refrain from the use of laxatives or fiber products from the day before capsule ingestion until after completion of the study. Abdominal x-ray studies, which include the diaphragms and the pubis, are taken on days 3 and 5 following ingestion, and the total number of markers is counted on each film.[131] If most markers are delayed in the rectosigmoid area, outlet obstruction is probable.[178] The test is deemed to be normal if 80% of the markers have been evacuated by the fifth day.[5,75]

Motility Capsule

The use of capsule technology for the evaluation of gastrointestinal transit is a relatively new concept. The use of a wireless electronic radiotelemetry capsule to assess the GI tract dates back to the 1950s.[77,183] Initially, the technology was limited to the measurement of temperature, pressure, and pH. Recent advances and the development of video capabilities have led investigators to use capsule technology to assess motility.

The SmartPill (SmartPill Corp., Buffalo, NY) gives physicians the ability to assess whole gut transit time as well as segmental transit times. The study is performed in the ambulatory setting with the avoidance of any ionizing radiation. Once the capsule is activated and ingested, data regarding temperature, pH, and video images are transmitted to a receiver.

Transit time as well as mucosal abnormalities associated with dysmotility has been reported.[76] The technique was recently compared to the more standard radiopaque marker method of evaluating colonic motility and found to be comparable in a multicenter trial.[31] This technology is promising in the evaluation of GI transit but is not currently used in the authors' laboratory as a standard investigation.

Small Bowel

It has generally been believed that prolonged oroanal transit times reflect mainly colonic transit abnormality. However, many patients with delayed colonic transit times may have a generalized motility disturbance of the gastrointestinal tract. Thus, before submitting a patient to total colectomy, it may be advisable to obtain some measure of small bowel transit. Of course, an indication of small bowel transit time may be of benefit in the investigation of individuals with diarrhea, malabsorption, or increased stool frequency following colo-anal or ileal pouch-anal anastomosis.[22,95]

Breath Hydrogen Analysis

The investigation of small bowel transit time by the use of the breath hydrogen test was first described by Bond and

colleagues in 1975.[22] Strictly speaking, it is a measure of orocecal transit. Following an overnight fast, the subject ingests a nonabsorbable carbohydrate such as lactulose (1,4-β-galactofructose), which provides a value for liquid transit,[102] or consumes baked beans, which gives a figure for solid transit.[137] On entering the cecum, these substrates are metabolized by colonic bacteria to hydrogen and short-chain fatty acids. Hydrogen, which is highly diffusible and relatively insoluble in water, is rapidly absorbed into the blood, transported to the lungs, and exhaled.[102]

Although this is a relatively simple test, certain caveats may interfere with its interpretation. First, 5% to 20% of the population are so-called nonfermenters; they do not produce hydrogen.[20,21] In addition, oral bacteria may cause some breakdown of the substrate, but this can be easily overcome by the use of a mouthwash before the administration of the test meal.[168] Similarly, small intestinal bacterial overgrowth will result in early metabolism of the substrate.[37] This, unfortunately, is less easy to manage. Furthermore, antibiotics consumed within the prior 10 days may deplete the colonic flora and result in a falsely prolonged result. Smoking and vigorous exercise should also be avoided before the test because these factors may influence breath hydrogen. There may also be some difficulty in interpreting the first peak of breath hydrogen, thus making the results unreliable.[78]

Despite the limitations and the drawbacks, the breath hydrogen test has proven to be a simple, noninvasive technique to study small bowel transit time. Unfortunately, normal values often vary from center to center because of the different criteria used to identify the time of entry of the meal into the cecum. Certain investigators have used the first rise of breath hydrogen by 20 parts per million (ppm),[33] others 5 ppm,[142] still others 3 ppm,[8] or 2 ppm.[13] Some have calculated small bowel transit as the time from ingestion to maximal peak in breath hydrogen.[161]

Salicylazosulfapyridine

Another option for determining small bowel transit is this investigation. Following the oral administration of sulfasalazine (Azulfidine; Kabi Pharmacia, Piscataway, NJ), the azo bond is hydrolyzed by colonic bacteria, releasing mesalazine and sulfapyridine. Sulfapyridine is absorbed and can be detected within the patient's blood. This test of orocecal transit has the disadvantage of requiring multiple blood samples; up to 300 mL of blood may be removed. This test also may be adversely affected by small bowel bacterial overgrowth or by antibiotic ingestion. Because of its cost and more invasive nature, it is not frequently used.

Small Intestinal Scintigraphy

Gastric emptying and small bowel transit time can be assessed by the ingestion of polystyrene pellets labeled with either ^{99m}Tc or ^{111}In or by labeling a meal of mashed potatoes with ^{99m}Tc sulfur colloid or diethylenetriaminepentaacetic acid (DTPA).[30,137] Some physicians prefer ^{99m}Tc-HIDA. This tracer given intravenously is excreted in the bile and delivered into the duodenum, thereby avoiding any influence of gastric emptying rate on small bowel results.[63] Methods using polystyrene pellets measure the small bowel transit of nondigestible solids, whereas the mashed potato meal is probably a measurement of liquid transit. Small bowel transit time is calculated to be the time taken for a fixed quantity of the isotope (e.g., 10% or 50%) to empty from the stomach and enter the colon.[30,62] As with colonic scintigraphy, these radioisotope techniques are unaffected by bacterial overgrowth or antibiotics but do expose patients to low radiation doses. Interpretation may be made difficult if small bowel loops overly the cecum.[33] This can be clarified by allowing the test to continue so that accurate images of cecal filling can be obtained.

Recommendations

In our laboratory, small bowel transit is primarily used as an adjunct to colonic transit studies in order to identify individuals with generalized intestinal hypomotility.[16,173] We have found that measurements of orocecal transit using breath hydrogen are reliable, reproducible, and well tolerated.[85] After an overnight fast, patients are given 10 g/15 mL lactulose (UDL Laboratories, Inc., Rockford, IL) with 100 mL of water. This small dose produces values for orocecal transit that are more accurate; larger doses decrease transit times because of the osmotic effect.[22] Care is taken to ensure that the patient has refrained from antibiotics and bowel cleansing agents for the previous 7 days and from smoking on the morning of the test. End-expiratory breath samples (100 to 200 mL) are obtained every 15 minutes by having the patient exhale slowly into a 750-mL multipatient collection bag (QT 00841-P; Quintron, Milwaukee, WI). Samples are analyzed using a Microlyzer gas chromatograph analyzer (model 12i; Quintron, Milwaukee, WI) (Figure 7-26), which is calibrated using an air/hydrogen mixture (98.2 ppm hydrogen; Matheson Gas Products, Inc., Joliet, IL). Results are plotted as hydrogen (ppm) versus time (minutes), and sampling is continued for up to 3 hours or until the graph reaches a plateau, whichever is sooner.

In our laboratory, a rise of 3 ppm has been demonstrated to produce the lowest coefficient of variation between subjects and is, therefore, the value used to determine that the meal has reached the cecum.[85] Patients who fail to produce an appreciable rise (more than 2 ppm) or sustained rise (more than three consecutive measurements) in breath hydrogen within 3 hours of ingestion are assumed to be nonfermenters.[85]

▶ BIOFEEDBACK

There are no standardized treatment methods for biofeedback therapy. The process has been defined as

> A group of therapeutic procedures that utilizes electronic instrumentation to accurately measure, process, and feed back to persons and their therapists, meaningful physiological information with educational and reinforcing properties about their neuromuscular and autonomic activity, both normal and abnormal in the form of analog, binary, auditory and or visual feedback signals.[44]

The premise is that with a motivated patient and a skilled biofeedback therapist, the patient will develop heightened voluntary control over the physiologic process. There are numerous reports of utility in the treatment of migraines,[40] depression,[91] pain syndromes,[116] urinary incontinence, constipation,[58] and fecal incontinence. Biofeedback therapy for fecal incontinence requires several components. The patient must be capable of understanding the principles of the therapy and be highly motivated. There must be some baseline degree of rectal sensitivity and sphincter contraction.

The most common instrumentation used to deliver feedback to the patient is anal EMG with an intra-anal sensor to display electrical muscular activity or manometry with a display of sphincter pressures. These techniques are often coupled with rectal sensory training.[82] The use of ultrasound has also been described.[159] A program of home exercises is often used as well. One study paired an initial face-to-face treatment with ultrasound and manometry, followed by three telephone sessions and a final face-to-face assessment in an attempt to treat patients from geographically remote areas.[28] The ultimate goal is to improve the patient's ability to contract the external anal sphincter and puborectalis and to increase the ability to perceive rectal distension.

Biofeedback Results

Most recently, Byrne and colleagues reported their experience with biofeedback in 513 patients suffering from fecal

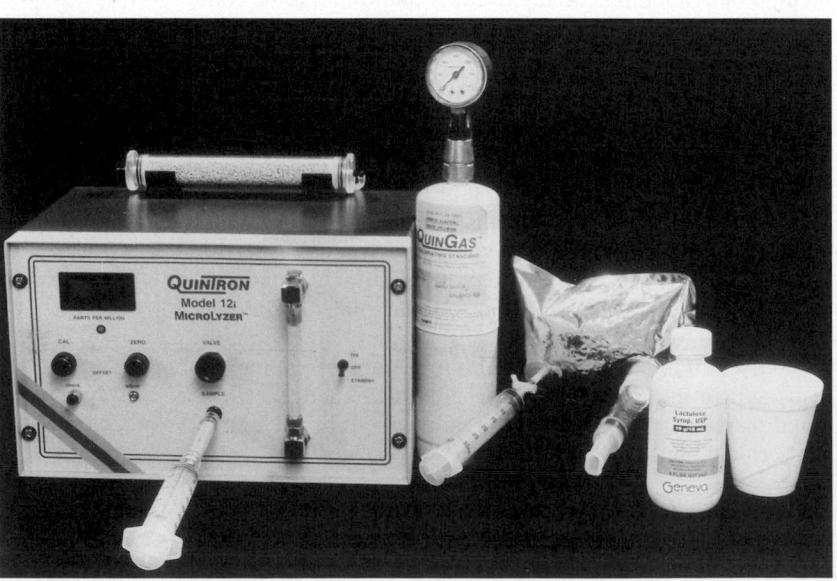

FIGURE 7-26. Microlyzer gas chromatograph analyzer (model 12). (Courtesy of Quintron, Milwaukee, WI.)

incontinence.[29] A manometry-based regimen of six monthly sessions along with a home exercise program was employed. Seventy-five percent (385) of patients completed the treatment. Success was determined by incontinence scores, nurse assessments, self-assessment scales, physiologic measures of sphincter function, and quality of life. Three-fourths reported improvement in quality of life and improved incontinence scores following treatment. Terra and coworkers used biofeedback to treat 281 patients suffering from fecal incontinence.[167] These individuals underwent nine weekly sessions of electrical stimulation, EMG guided biofeedback, and balloon sensory training. Subjective perception of improvement was reported by 60% (47% as slight and 13% as substantial). An increase in mean resting pressure was observed in 53%, and 56% had an increase in their mean squeeze pressures. Mean sensory thresholds and urge sensation increased in 45% and 54% of patients, respectively. Overall, there was a slight improvement in the majority of patients treated, with substantial improvement found in the minority of people.

Randomized Trials

Several randomized trials have attempted to define the utility of biofeedback for the treatment of fecal incontinence. Solomon and associates conducted a randomized trial of biofeedback with manometry, ultrasound, and digital examination alone.[158] One hundred twenty patients were enrolled to undergo monthly sessions for a total of 5 months. The treatment was completed by 85%. Improvement in symptom severity was noted by 70%, and 69% had improvement in quality-of-life assessments. There was no significant difference between the three groups with respect to quality-of-life improvements. There were some improvements noted in isotonic fatigue time and isometric fatigue contractions in the ultrasound group. However, this did not translate into betterment in symptom severity or quality-of-life improvement. Fynes and coworkers specifically evaluated patients with fecal incontinence after obstetric injury.[55] Forty patients underwent 12 weekly sessions of either sensory biofeedback using a perineometer in the vagina or augmented biofeedback with EMG and electrical stimulation with audiovisual feedback. There was improvement in continence scores in both groups. There was a greater improvement in the augmented group with associated increases in the manometric resting and squeeze pressures as well. Norton randomized 171 patients into four groups: advice, advice with instruction on sphincter exercises, hospital-based biofeedback, and hospital-based biofeedback with a home EMG biofeedback device.[121] The authors found no difference in the degree of improvement in incontinence scores, SF-36, disease-specific quality of life, and hospital anxiety and depression scale among the groups. There was improvement in all of the parameters with no differences between the four groups. They postulated that the beneficial results might have been more a result of the therapist–patient relationship rather than the specific type of therapy undertaken. This was also thought to confer an enhanced coping mechanism because the patients had a greater subjective satisfaction with treatment than actual decrease in the fecal incontinence scores.

Authors' Approach

At our institution, we prefer to use an intra-anal plug EMG to provide biofeedback (Figure 7-27). The intra-anal plug is

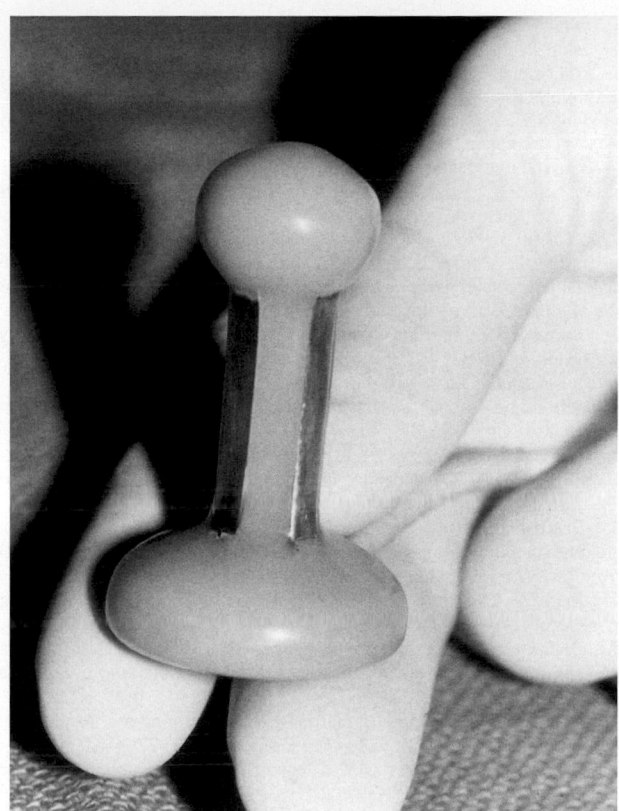

FIGURE 7-27. Perrymeter. (Courtesy of Synectics Medical, Irving, TX.)

equipped with longitudinal electrodes. Following insertion, the patient dresses. Biofeedback is carried out with the patient sitting on a chair. Sessions lasting 1 hour are scheduled regularly until the person has demonstrated control of the pelvic floor, and this has been accompanied by symptomatic improvement. We have not found the addition of balloon sensation training or home training to be helpful.[72]

▶ CONCLUSION

Not very long ago, anorectal physiology was considered a conglomeration of interesting but impractical investigations that provided novel but clinically irrelevant information. Currently, anorectal physiology is not only familiar to all who perform colorectal surgery but is also available to most practitioners. Viewed no longer as exclusively a research tool, anorectal physiology provides useful data for both clinical decision making and prognostic information. In this chapter, we outline some of the more widely available physiologic investigations. We endeavor to provide a comprehensive list of the tools necessary to complete these evaluations.

References

1. Adrian ED, Bronck DW. The discharge of impulses in motor nerve fibres: part II. The frequency of discharge in reflex and voluntary contractions. *J Physiol*. 1929;67(2):i3–i151.
2. Agachan F, Pfeifer J, Wexner SD. Defecography and proctography. Results of 744 patients. *Dis Colon Rectum*. 1996;39(8):899–905.
3. Altomare DF, Rinaldi M, Petrolino M, et al. Reliability of electrophysiologic anal tests in predicting the outcome of sacral nerve modulation for fecal incontinence. *Dis Colon Rectum*. 2004;47(6):853–857.
4. Alvarez WC, Freedlander BL. The rate of progress of food residues through the bowel. *JAMA*. 1924;83:576–580.

5. Arhan P, Devroede G, Jehannin B, et al. Segmental colonic transit time. *Dis Colon Rectum*. 1981;24(8):625–629.

6. Arndorfer RC, Stef JJ, Dodds WJ, et al. Improved infusion system for intraluminal esophageal manometry. *Gastroenterology*. 1977;73(1):23–27.

7. Baig MK, Wexner SD. Factors predictive of outcome after surgery for faecal incontinence. *Br J Surg*. 2000;87(10):1316–1330.

8. Barnett JL, Hasler WL, Camilleri M. American Gastroenterological Association medical position statement on anorectal testing techniques. American Gastroenterological Association. *Gastroenterology*. 1999;116(3):732–760.

9. Barthet M, Portier F, Heyries L, et al. Dynamic anal endosonography may challenge defecography for assessing dynamic anorectal disorders: results of a prospective pilot study. *Endoscopy*. 2000;32(4):300–305.

10. Bartolo DCC, Bartram CI, Ekberg O, et al. Symposium. Proctography. *Int J Colorectal Dis*. 1988;3(2):67–89.

11. Bartolo DC, Read NW, Jarratt JA, et al. Differences in anal sphincter function and clinical presentation in patients with pelvic floor descent. *Gastroenterology*. 1983;85(1):68–75.

12. Bartram CI, Turnbull GK, Lennard-Jones JE. Evacuation proctography: an investigation of rectal expulsion in 20 subjects without defecatory disturbance. *Gastrointest Radiol*. 1988;13(1):72–80.

13. Basilisco G, Bozzani A, Camboni G, et al. Effect of loperamide and naloxone on mouth-to-caecum transit time evaluated by lactulose hydrogen breath test. *Gut*. 1985;26(7):700–703.

14. Beck A. Electomyographische Untersuchungen am Sphinkter ani. *Arch Physiol*. 1930;224:278–292.

15. Beer-Gabel M, Teshler M, Barzilai N, et al. Dynamic transperineal ultrasound in the diagnosis of pelvic floor disorders: pilot study. *Dis Colon Rectum*. 2002;45(2):239–245.

16. Berman IR, Manning DH, Harris MS. Streamlining the management of defecation disorders. *Dis Colon Rectum*. 1990;33(9):778–785.

17. Bernier P, Stevenson GW, Shorvon P. Defecography commode. *Radiology*. 1988;166(3):891–892.

18. Bertschinger KM, Hetzer FH, Roos JE, et al. Dynamic MR imaging of the pelvic floor performed with patient sitting in an open-magnet unit versus with patient supine in a closed-magnet unit. *Radiology*. 2002;223(2):501–508.

19. Binnie NR, Kawimbe BM, Papachrysostomou M, et al. The importance of the orientation of the electrode plates in recording the external anal sphincter EMG by non-invasive anal plug electrodes. *Int J Colorectal Dis*. 1990;6(1):5–8.

20. Bjørneklett A, Jenssen E. Relationships between hydrogen (H2) and methane (CH4) production in man. *Scand J Gastroenterol*. 1982; 17(8):985–992.

21. Bleijenberg G, Kuijpers HC. Treatment of the spastic pelvic floor syndrome with biofeedback. *Dis Colon Rectum*. 1987;30(2):108–111.

22. Bond JH, Levitt MD, Prentiss R. Investigation of small bowel transit time in man utilizing pulmonary hydrogen (H2) measurements. *J Lab Clin Med*. 1975;85(4):546–555.

23. Bordeianou L, Lee KY, Rockwood T, et al. Anal resting pressures at manometry correlate with the Fecal Incontinence Severity Index and with presence of sphincter defects on ultrasound. *Dis Colon Rectum*. 2008;51(7):1010–1014.

24. Brindley GS. Electroejaculation: its technique, neurological implications and uses. *J Neurol Neurosurg Psychiatry*. 1981;44(1):9–18.

25. Brusciano L, Limongelli P, Pescatori M, et al. Ultrasonographic patterns in patients with obstructed defaecation. *Int J Colorectal Dis*. 2007;22(8):969–977.

26. Burhenne HJ. Intestinal evacuation study: a new roentgenologic technique. *Radiol Clin*. 1964;33:79–84.

27. Burnett SJ, Bartram CI. Endosonographic variations in the normal internal anal sphincter. *Int J Colorectal Dis*. 1991;6(1):2–4.

28. Byrne CM, Solomon MJ, Rex J, et al. Telephone vs. face-to-face biofeedback for fecal incontinence: comparison of two techniques in 239 patients. *Dis Col Rectum*. 2005;48(12):2281–2288.

29. Byrne CM, Solomon MJ, Young JM, et al. Biofeedback for fecal incontinence: short-term outcomes of 513 consecutive patients and predictors of successful treatment. *Dis Col Rectum*. 2007;50(4):417–427.

30. Camilleri M, Colemont LJ, Phillips SF, et al. Human gastric emptying and colonic filling of solids characterized by a new method. *Am J Physiol*. 1989;257(2 pt 1):G284–G290.

31. Camilleri M, Thorne NK, Ringel Y, et al. Wireless pH-motility capsule for colonic transit: prospective comparison with radiopaque markers in chronic constipation. *Neurogastroenterol Motil*. 2010;22(8):874–882.

32. Cammarota T, Discalzo L, Corno F, et al. First experiences with trans-rectal echotomography in perianal abscess pathology. *Radiol Med*. 1986;72(11):837–840.

33. Caride VJ, Prokop EK, Troncale FJ, et al. Scintigraphic determination of small intestinal transit time: comparison with the hydrogen breath technique. *Gastroenterology*. 1984;86(4):714–720.

34. Chaussade S, Roche H, Khyari A, et al. Mesure du temps de transit colique (TTC): Description et validation d'une nouvelle technique [Measurement of colonic transit time: description and validation of a new method]. *Gastroenterol Clin Biol*. 1986;10(5):385–389.

35. Choi JS, Wexner SD, Nam YS, et al. Intraobserver and interobserver measurements of the anorectal angle and perineal descent in defecography. *Dis Colon Rectum*. 2000;43(8):1121–1126.

36. Coller JA, Sangwan YP. Computerized anal sphincter manometry performance and analysis. In: Smith LE, ed. *Practical Guide to Anorectal Testing*. 2nd ed. New York, NY: Igaku-Shoin; 1995:51–100.

37. Corazza GR, Menozzi MG, Strocchi A, et al. The diagnosis of small bowel bacterial overgrowth: reliability of jejunal culture and inadequacy of breath hydrogen testing. *Gastroenterology*. 1990;98(2):302–309.

38. Dahl J, Lindquist BL, Tysk C, et al. Behavioral medicine treatment in chronic constipation with paradoxical anal sphincter contraction. *Dis Colon Rectum*. 1991;34(9):769–776.

39. Dick M. Use of cuprous thiocyanate as a short-term continuous marker for faeces. *Gut*. 1969;10(5):408–412.

40. Dodick DW, Silberstein SD. Migraine prevention. *Pract Neurol*. 2007;7(6):383–393.

41. Ekstedt J. Human single muscle fibre action potentials. Extracellular recording during voluntary and chemical activation. With some comments on end-plate physiology and on the fiber arrangement of the motor unit. *Acta Physiol Scand Suppl*. 1964;suppl 226:1.

42. el-Shafie M, Suzuki H, Schnaufer L, et al. A simplified method of anorectal manometry for wider clinical application. *J Pediatr Surg*. 1972;7(2):230–235.

43. Elshazly WG, El Nekady Ael A, Hassan H. Role of dynamic magnetic resonance imaging in management of obstructed defecation case series. *Int J Surg*. 2010;8(4):274–282.

44. Enck P. Biofeedback training in disordered defecation. A critical review. *Dig Dis Sci*. 1993;38(11):1953–1960.

45. Enck P, von Giesen HJ, Schäfer A, et al. Comparison of anal sonography with conventional needle electromyography in the evaluation of anal sphincter defects. *Am J Gastroenterol*. 1996;91(12):2539–2543.

46. Evans DF, Pye G, Bramley R, et al. Measurement of gastrointestinal pH profiles in normal ambulant human subjects. *Gut*. 1988; 29(8):1035–1041.

47. Farouk R. Electromyographic techniques. In: Smith LE, ed. *Practical Guide to Anorectal Testing*. 2nd ed. New York, NY: Igaku-Shoin; 1995:195–206.

48. Felt-Bersma RJ, Luth WJ, Janssen JJ, et al. Defecography in patients with anorectal disorders. Which findings are clinically relevant? *Dis Colon Rectum*. 1990;33(4):277–284.

49. Ferrante SL, Perry RE, Schreiman JS, et al. The reproducibility of measuring the anorectal angle in defecography. *Dis Colon Rectum*. 1991;34(1):51–55.

50. Ferrara A, Lujan JH, Cebrian J, et al. Clinical, manometric, and EMG characteristics of patients with fecal incontinence. *Tech Coloproctol*. 2001;5(1):13–18.

51. Fleshman JW, Dreznik Z, Meyer K, et al. Outpatient protocol for biofeedback therapy of pelvic floor outlet obstruction. *Dis Colon Rectum*. 1992;35(1):1–7.

52. Fletcher JG, Busse RF, Riederer SJ, et al. Magnetic resonance imaging of anatomic and dynamic defects of the pelvic floor in defecatory disorders. *Am J Gastroenterol*. 2003;98(2):399–411.

53. Fowler AL, Mills A, Durdey P, et al. Single-fiber electromyography correlates more closely with incontinence scores than pudendal nerve terminal motor latency. *Dis Colon Rectum*. 2005;48(12):2309–2312.

54. Fucini C, Ronchi O, Elbeltti C. Electromyography of the pelvic floor musculature in the assessment of obstructed defection symptoms. *Dis Colon Rectum*. 2001;44(8):1168–1175.

55. Fynes MM, Marshall K, Cassidy M, et al. A prospective, randomized study comparing the effect of augmented biofeedback with sensory biofeedback alone on fecal incontinence after obstetric trauma. *Dis Col Rectum*. 1999;42(6):753–758.

56. Gibbons CP, Read NW. Anal hypertonia in fissures: cause or effect? *Br J Surg*. 1986;73(6):443–445.

57. Gil J, Luján J, Hernández Q, et al. Screening for the effectiveness of conservative treatment in chronic anal fissure patients using anorectal manometry. *Int J Colorectal Dis*. 2010;25(5):649–654.

58. Gilliland R, Heymen S, Altomare DF, et al. Outcome and predictors of success of biofeedback for constipation. *British J Surg*. 1997; 84(8):1123–1126.

59. Goei R. Anorectal function in patients with defecation disorders and asymptomatic subjects: evaluation with defecography. *Radiology.* 1990;174(1):121–123.

60. Goei R, Baeten C, Arends JW. Solitary rectal ulcer syndrome: findings at barium enema study and defecography. *Radiology.* 1988;168(2):303–306.

61. Goldman S, Glimelius B, Norming U, et al. Transanorectal ultrasonography in anal canal carcinoma. A prospective study of 21 patients. *Acta Radiol.* 1988;29(3):337–341.

62. Greydanus MP, Camilleri M, Colemont LJ, et al. Ileocolonic transfer of solid chyme in small intestinal neuropathies and myopathies. *Gastroenterology.* 1990;99(1):158–164.

63. Grybäck P, Jacobsson H, Blomquist L, et al. Scintigraphy of the small intestine: a simplified standard for study of transit with reference to normal values. *Eur J Nucl Med Mol Imaging.* 2002;29(1):39–45.

64. Gundling F, Seidl H, Scalercio N, et al. Influence of gender and age on anorectal function: normal values from anorectal manometry in a large caucasian population. *Digestion.* 2010;81(4):207–213

65. Hallböök O, Sjödahl R. Techniques of rectal compliance measurement. *Semin Colon Rect Surg.* 1992;3:88–91.

66. Hancock BD. The internal sphincter and anal fissure. *Br J Surg.* 1977;64(2):92–95.

67. Hancock BD. Internal sphincter and the nature of haemorrhoids. *Gut.* 1977;18(8):651–655.

68. Harris LD, Winans CS, Pope CE II. Determination of yield pressures: a method for measuring anal sphincter competence. *Gastroenterology.* 1966;50(6):754–760.

69. Haynes WG, Read NW. Ano-rectal activity in man during rectal infusion of saline: a dynamic assessment of the anal continence mechanism. *J Physiol.* 1982;330:45–56.

70. Healy JC, Halligan S, Reznek RH, et al. Dynamic MR imaging compared with evacuation proctography when evaluating anorectal configuration and pelvic floor movement. *AJR Am J Roentgenol.* 1997;169(3):775–779.

71. Healy JC, Halligan S, Reznek RH, et al. Magnetic resonance imaging of the pelvic floor in patients with obstructed defaecation. *Br J Surg.* 1997;84(11):1555–1558.

72. Heymen S, Vickers D, Weiss EG, et al. A prospective randomized trial comparing four biofeedback techniques for patients with constipation. *Gastroenterology.* 1996;110:A678.

73. Hill JR, Kelley ML Jr, Schlegel JF, et al. Pressure profile of the rectum and anus of healthy persons. *Dis Colon Rectum.* 1960;3:203–209.

74. Hinton JM, Lennard-Jones JE. Constipation: definition and classification. *Postgrad Med J.* 1968;44(515):720–733.

75. Hinton JM, Lennard-Jones JE, Young AC. A new method for studying gut transit times using radioopaque markers. *Gut.* 1969;10(10):842–847.

76. Hoog CM, Lindberg G, Sjoqvist U. Findings in patients with chronic intestinal dysmotility investigated by capsule endoscopy. *BMC Gastroenterol.* 2007;7:29.

77. Hopkins HH, Kapany NS. A flexible fibrescope, using Static Scanning. *Nature.* 1954;173:39–41.

78. Howard PJ, Lazarus C, Maisey MN, et al. Interpretation of postprandial breath hydrogen excretion in relation to small bowel transit and ileocecal flow patterns of a radiolabeled solid meal in man. *J Gastrointest Motil.* 1990;2(3):194–201.

79. Hutchinson R, Kumar D. Colonic and small bowel transit studies. In: Wexner SD, Bartolo DCC, eds. *Constipation: Etiology, Evaluation and Management.* Oxford, United Kingdom: Butterworth-Heinemann; 1995:52–62.

80. Johnson E, Carlsen E, Steen TB, et al. Short- and long-term results of secondary anterior sphincteroplasty in 33 patients with obstetric injury. *Acta Obstet Gynecol Scand.* 2010;89(11):1466–1472.

81. Jones PN, Lubowski DZ, Swash M, et al. Is paradoxical contraction of the puborectalis muscle of functional importance? *Dis Colon Rectum.* 1987;30(9):667–670.

82. Jorge JJ, Habr-Gama A, Wexner SD. Biofeedback therapy in colon and rectal practice. *Appl Psychophysiol Biofeedback.* 2003;28(1):47–61.

83. Jorge JM, Wexner SD. Anorectal manometry: techniques and clinical applications. *South Med J.* 1993;86(8):924–931.

84. Jorge JM, Wexner SD. A practical guide to basic anorectal physiology investigations. *Contemp Surg.* 1993;43(4):214–224.

85. Jorge JM, Wexner SD, Ehrenpreis ED. The lactulose hydrogen breath test as a measure of orocaecal transit time. *Eur J Surg.* 1994;160(8):409–416.

86. Jorge JM, Wexner SD, Marchetti F, et al. How reliable are currently available methods of measuring the anorectal angle? *Dis Colon Rectum.* 1992;35(4):332–338.

87. Jorge JM, Yang YK, Wexner SD. Incidence and clinical significance of sigmoidoceles as determined by a new classification system. *Dis Colon Rectum.* 1994;37(11):1112–1117.

88. Jorge MJ, Ger GC, Gonzalez L, et al. Patient position during cinedefecography. Influence on perineal descent and other measurements. *Dis Col Rectum.* 1994;37(9):927–931.

89. Kamm MA, Lennard-Jones JE, Thompson DG, et al. Dynamic scanning defines a colonic defect in severe idiopathic constipation. *Gut.* 1988;29(8):1085–1092.

90. Karaus M, Neuhaus P, Wiedenmann TB. Diagnosis of enteroceles by dynamic anorectal endosonography. *Dis Colon Rectum.* 2000;43(12):1683–1688.

91. Karavidas MK, Lehrer PM, Vaschillo E, et al. Preliminary results of an open label study of heart rate variability biofeedback for the treatment of major depression. *Appl Psychophysiol Biofeedback.* 2007;32(1):19–30.

92. Katz LA, Kaufman HJ, Spiro HM. Anal sphincter pressure characteristics. *Gastroenterology.* 1967;52(3):513–518.

93. Kiff ES, Swash M. Slowed conduction in the pudendal nerves in idiopathic (neurogenic) faecal incontinence. *Br J Surg.* 1984;71(8):614–616.

94. Kim NK, Kim MJ, Yun SH, et al. Comparative study of transrectal ultrasonography, pelvic computerized tomography, and magnetic resonance imaging in preoperative staging of rectal cancer. *Dis Colon Rectum.* 1992;42(6):770–775.

95. Kmiot WA, O'Brien JD, Awad R, et al. Estimation of small bowel transit time following colectomy and ileal reservoir construction. *Br J Surg.* 1992;79(7):697–700.

96. Krevsky B, Malmud LS, D'Ercole F, et al. Colonic transit scintigraphy: a physiologic approach to the quantitative measurement of colonic transit in humans. *Gastroenterology.* 1986;91(5):1102–1112.

97. Kuijpers HC. Defaecography. In: Wexner SD, Bartolo DCC, eds. *Constipation: Etiology, Evaluation and Management.* Oxford, United Kingdom: Butterworth-Heinemann; 1995:77–85.

98. Kuijpers HC, Schreve RH, ten Cate Hoedemakers H. Diagnosis of functional disorders of defecation causing the solitary rectal ulcer syndrome. *Dis Colon Rectum.* 1986;29(2):126–129.

99. Law PJ, Bartram CI. Anal endosonography: technique and normal anatomy. *Gastrointest Radiol.* 1989;14(4):349–353.

100. Law PJ, Talbot RW, Bartram CI, et al. Anal endosonography in the evaluation of perianal sepsis and fistula in ano. *Br J Surg.* 1989;76(7):752–755.

101. Lesaffer LPA. Digital subtraction defecography. In: Smith LE, ed. *Practical Guide to Anorectal Testing.* 2nd ed. New York, NY: Igaku-Shoin; 1995:161–184.

102. Levitt MD. Production and excretion of hydrogen gas in man. *N Engl J Med.* 1969;281(3):122–127.

103. Li JC, Liu SY, Lo AW, et al. The learning curve for endorectal ultrasonography in rectal cancer staging. *Surg Endosc.* 2010;24(12):3054–3059.

104. Lienemann A, Sprenger D, Janssen U, et al. Functional MRI of the pelvic floor. The methods and reference values. *Radiologe.* 2000;40(5):458–464.

105. Lockhart ME, Fielding JR, Richter HE, et al. Reproducibility of dynamic MR imaging pelvic measurements: a multi-institutional study. *Radiology.* 2008;249(2):534–540.

106. López A, Nilsson BY, Mellgren A, et al. Electromyography of the external anal sphincter: comparison between needle and surface electrodes. *Dis Colon Rectum.* 1999;42(4):482–485.

107. Lundin E, Karlbom U, Påhlman L, et al. Outcome of segmental colonic resection for slow-transit constipation. *Br J Surg.* 2002;89(10):1270–1274.

108. MacDonald A, Paterson PJ, Baxter JN, et al. Relationship between intra-abdominal and intrarectal pressure in the proctometrogram. *Br J Surg.* 1993;80(8):1070–1071.

109. Madoff RD, Orrom WJ, Rothenberger DA, et al. Rectal compliance: a critical reappraisal. *Int J Colorectal Dis.* 1990;5(1):37–40.

110. Mahieu P, Pringot J, Bodart P. Defecography: I. Description of a new procedure and results in normal patients. *Gastrointest Radiol.* 1984;9(3):247–251.

111. Manousos ON, Truelove SC, Lumsden K. Transit times of food in patients with diverticulosis or irritable colon syndrome and normal subjects. *Br Med J.* 1967;3(5568):760–762.

112. Martellucci J, Naldini G. Clinical relevance of transperineal ultrasound compared with evacuation proctography for the evaluation of patients with obstructed defaecation. *Colorectal Dis.* 2011;13(10):1167–1172. doi:10.1111/j.1463-1318.2010.02427.x

113. McHugh SM, Diamant NE. Effect of age, gender, and parity on anal canal pressures. Contribution of impaired anal sphincter function to fecal incontinence. *Dig Dis Sci.* 1987;32(7):726–736.

114. Metcalf AM. Transit time. In: Smith LE, ed. *Practical Guide to Anorectal Testing.* 2nd ed. New York, NY: Igaku-Shoin; 1995:17–21.

115. Metcalf AM, Phillips SF, Zinsmeister AR, et al. Simplified assessment of segmental colonic transit. *Gastroenterology*. 1987;92(1):40–47.

116. Morone NE, Greco CM. Mind-body interventions for chronic pain in older adults: a structured review. *Pain Med*. 2007;8(4):359–375.

117. Murad-Regadas SM, Regadas FS, Rodrigues LV, et al. A novel three-dimensional dynamic anorectal ultrasonography technique (echodefecography) to assess obstructed defecation, a comparison with defecography. *Surg Endosc*. 2008;22(4):974–979.

118. Murad-Regadas SM, Regadas FS, Rodrigues LV, et al. The role of 3-dimensional anorectal ultrasonography in the assessment of anterior trans-sphincteric fistula. *Dis Colon Rectum*. 2010;53(7):1035–1040.

119. Neill ME, Parks AG, Swash M. Physiological studies of the anal sphincter musculature in faecal incontinence and rectal prolapse. *Br J Surg*. 1981;68(8):531–536.

120. Neill ME, Swash M. Increased motor unit fibre density in the external anal sphincter muscle in ano–rectal incontinence: a single fibre EMG study. *J Neurol Neurosurg Psychiatry*. 1980;43(4):343–347.

121. Norton C, Chelvanayagam S, Wilson-Barnett J, et al. Randomized controlled trial of biofeedback for fecal incontinence. *Gastroenterology*. 2003;125(5):1320–1329.

122. Notghi A, Hutchinson R, Kumar D, et al. Simplified method for the measurement of segmental colonic transit time. *Gut*. 1994; 35(7):976–981.

123. Oberwalder M, Thaler K, Baig MK, et al. Anal ultrasound and endosonographic measurement of perineal body thickness: a new evaluation for fecal incontinence in females. *Surg Endosc*. 2004; 18(4):650–654.

124. O'Donnell P, Beck C, Doyle R, et al. Surface electrodes in perineal electromyography. *Urology*. 1988;32(4):375–379.

125. Orsoni P, Barthet M, Portier F, et al. Prospective comparison of endosonography, magnetic resonance imaging and surgical findings in anorectal fistula and abscess complicating Crohn's disease. *Br J Surg*. 1999;86(3):360–364.

126. Ortega AE, Klipfel N, Kelso R, et al. Changing concepts in the pathogenesis, evaluation, and management of solitary rectal ulcer syndrome. *Am Surg*. 2008;74(10):967–972.

127. Osatakul S, Patrapinyokul S, Osatakul N. The diagnostic value of anorectal manometry as a screening test for Hirschsprung's disease. *J Med Assoc Thai*. 1999;82(11):1100–1105.

128. Osterberg A, Graf W, Edebol Eeg-Olofsson K, et al. Results of neurophysiologic evaluation in fecal incontinence. *Dis Colon Rectum*. 2000;43(9):1256–1261.

129. Parks AG. Royal Society of Medicine, Section of Proctology; Meeting 27 November 1974. President's Address. Anorectal incontinence. *Proc R Soc Med*. 1975;68(11):681–690.

130. Penninckx F, Debruyne C, Lestar B, et al. Observer variation in the radiological measurement of the anorectal angle. *Int J Colorectal Dis*. 1990;5(2):94–97.

131. Picirillo MF, Reissman P, Wexner SD. Colectomy as treatment for constipation in selected patients. *Br J Surg*. 1995;82(7):898–901.

132. Preston DM, Lennard-Jones JE. Anismus in chronic constipation. *Dig Dis Sci*. 1985;30(5):413–418.

133. Proano M, Camilleri M, Phillips SF, et al. Unprepared human colon does not discriminate between solids and liquids. *Am J Physiol*. 1991; 260(1 pt 1):G13–G16.

134. Rafert JA, Lappas JC, Wilkins W. Defecography: techniques for improved image quality. *Radiol Technol*. 1990;61(5):368–373.

135. Rao SS, Singh S. Clinical utility of colonic and anorectal manometry in chronic constipation. *J Clin Gastroenterol*. 2010;44(9):597–609.

136. Raza-Khan F, Cunkelman J, Lowenstein L, et al. Prevalence of bowel symptoms in women with pelvic floor disorders. *Int Urogynecol J*. 2010;21(8):933–938.

137. Read NW, Miles CA, Fisher D, et al. Transit of a meal through the stomach, small intestine, and colon in normal subjects and its role in the pathogenesis of diarrhea. *Gastroenterology*. 1980;79(6):1276–1282.

138. Ricciardi R, Mellgren AF, Madoff RD, et al. The utility of pudendal nerve terminal motor latencies in idiopathic incontinence. *Dis Colon Rectum*. 2006;49(6):852–857.

139. Roberts JP, Womack NR, Hallan RI, et al. Evidence from dynamic integrated proctography to redefine anismus. *Br J Surg*. 1992; 79(11):1213–1215.

140. Rogers J, Henry MM, Misiewicz JJ. Disposable pudendal nerve stimulator: evaluation of the standard instrument and new device. *Gut*. 1988;29(8):1131–1133.

141. Rozycki GS. Ultrasonography: surgical applications. In: American College of Surgeons, ed. *Principle and Practice*. American College of Surgeons; 2003:1–15.

142. Rubinoff MJ, Piccione PR, Holt PR. Clonidine prolongs human small intestine transit time: use of the lactulose-breath hydrogen test. *Am J Gastroenterol*. 1989;84(4):372–374.

143. Rutter KR. Electromyographic changes in certain pelvic floor abnormalities. *Proc R Soc Med*. 1974;67(1):53–56.

144. Salzano A, Carbone M, Rossi E, et al. Defecography and treatment of essential anal pain. *Radiol Med*. 1999;98(1–2):48–52.

145. Sangwan YS, Coller JA, Barrett RC, et al. Distal rectoanal excitatory reflex: a reliable index of pudendal neuropathy? *Dis Colon Rectum*. 1995;38(9):916–920.

146. Sangwan YP, Coller JA, Schoetz DJ Jr, et al. Relationship between manometric anal waves and fecal incontinence. *Dis Colon Rectum*. 1995;38(4):370–374.

147. Schoenenberger AW, Debatin JF, Guldenschuh I, et al. Dynamic MR defecography with a superconducting, open-configuration MR system. *Radiology*. 1998;206(3):641–646.

148. Schuster MM. Colon motility and anosphincteric manometric recordings by air-filled balloon technique. In: Smith LE, ed. *Practical Guide to Anorectal Testing*. 2nd ed. New York, NY: Igaku-Shoin; 1995:37–50.

149. Schuster MM, Hookman P, Hendrix TR, et al. Simultaneous manometric recording of the internal and external anal sphincter reflexes. *Bull Johns Hopkins Hosp*. 1965;116: 79–88.

150. Sentovich SM, Rivela LJ, Thorson AG, et al. Simultaneous dynamic proctography and peritoneography for pelvic floor disorders. *Dis Colon Rectum*. 1995;38(9):912–915.

151. Shorvon PJ, McHugh S, Diamant NE, et al. Defecography in normal volunteers: results and implications. *Gut*. 1989;30(12):1737–1749.

152. Simkovic D, Smejkal K, Siroký M, et al. Importance of the anorectal manometry in chronic anal fissure. *Acta Medica (Hradec Kralove)*. 2001;44(3):105–107.

153. Skomorowska E, Hegedüs V. Sex differences in anorectal angle and perineal descent. *Gastrointest Radiol*. 1987;12(4):353–355.

154. Snooks SJ, Barnes PR, Swash M, et al. Damage to the innervation of the pelvic floor musculature in chronic constipation. *Gastroenterology*. 1985;89(5):977–981.

155. Snooks SJ, Swash M. Nerve stimulation techniques. In: Henry MM, Swash M, eds. *Coloproctology and the Pelvic Floor: Pathophysiology and Management*. London, United Kingdom: Butterworths; 1985:112–128.

156. Sobrado CW, Pires CE, Araújo SE, et al. Computerized videodefecography versus defecography: do we need radiographs? *Sao Paulo Med J*. 2005;123(3):105–107.

157. Solomon MJ. Fistulae and abscesses in symptomatic perianal Crohn's disease. *Int J Colorectal Dis*. 1996;11(5):222–226.

158. Solomon MJ, Pager CK, Rex J, et al. Randomized, controlled trial of biofeedback with anal manometry, transanal ultrasound, or pelvic floor retraining with digital guidance alone in the treatment of mild to moderate fecal incontinence. *Dis Col Rectum*. 2003;46(6):703–710.

159. Solomon MJ, Rex J, Eyers AA, et al. Biofeedback for fecal incontinence using transanal ultrasonography: novel approach. *Dis colon Rectum*. 2000;43(6):788–792.

160. Stålberg E, Thiele B. Motor unit fibre density in the extensor digitorum communis muscle: single fibre electromyographic study in normal subjects at different ages. *J Neurol Neurosurg Psychiatry*. 1975; 38(9):874–880.

161. Staniforth DH, Rose D. Statistical analysis of the lactulose/breath hydrogen test in the measurement of orocaecal transit: its variability and predictive value in assessing drug action. *Gut*. 1989;30(2):171–175.

162. Stein BL, Roberts PL. Manometry and the rectoanal inhibitory reflex. In: Wexner SD, Bartolo DCC, eds. *Constipation: Etiology, Evaluation and Management*. Oxford, United Kingdom: Butterworth-Heinemann; 1995:63–76.

163. Sudol-Szopin;aaska I, Jakubowski W, Szczepkowski M, et al. Usefulness of hydrogen peroxide enhancement in diagnosis of anal and anovaginal fistulas. *Eur Radiol*. 2003;13(5):1080–1084.

164. Sultan AH, Kamm MA, Talbot IC, et al. Anal endosonography for identifying external sphincter defects confirmed histologically. *Br J Surg*. 1994;81(3):463–465.

165. Sultan AH, Nicholls RJ, Kamm MA, et al. Anal endosonography and correlation with in vitro and in vivo anatomy. *Br J Surg*. 1993;80(4):508–511.

166. Sun WM, Read NW, Prior A, et al. Sensory and motor responses to rectal distention vary according to rate and pattern of balloon inflation. *Gastroenterology*. 1990;99(4):1008–1015.

167. Terra MP, Dobben AC, Berghmans B, et al. Electrical stimulation and pelvic floor muscle training with biofeedback in patients with fecal incontinence: a cohort study of 281 patients. *Dis Col Rectum*. 2006;49(8):1149–1159.

168. Thompson DG, Binfield P, De Belder A, et al. Extra intestinal influences on exhaled breath hydrogen measurements during the investigation of gastrointestinal disease. *Gut.* 1985;26(12):1349–1352.

169. Tio TL, Mulder CJ, Wijers OB, et al. Endosonography of peri-anal and peri-colorectal fistula and/or abscess in Crohn's disease. *Gastrointest Endosc.* 1990;36(4):331–336.

170. Tjandra JJ, Milsom JW, Stolfi VM, et al. Endoluminal ultrasound defines anatomy of the anal canal and pelvic floor. *Dis Colon Rectum.* 1992;35(5):465–470.

171. Vanbeckevoort D, Van Hoe L, Oyen R, et al. Pelvic floor descent in females: comparative study of colpocystodefecography and dynamic fast MR imaging. *J Magn Reson Imaging.* 1999;9(3):373–377.

172. Van Outryve MJ, Pelckmans PA, Michielsen PP, et al. Value of transrectal ultrasonography in Crohn's disease. *Gastroenterology.* 1991;101(5):1171–1177.

173. Vasilevsky CA, Nemer FD, Balcos EG, et al. Is subtotal colectomy a viable option in the management of chronic constipation? *Dis Colon Rectum.* 1988;31(9):679–681.

174. Wallden L. Defecation block in cases of deep rectogenital pouch. *Acta Chir Scand.* 1952;103(3):236–238.

175. Wankling WJ, Brown BH, Collins CD, et al. Basal electrical activity in the anal canal in man. *Gut.* 1968;9(4):457–460.

176. Watson BW, Meldrum SJ, Riddle HC. pH profile of gut as measured by radiotelemetry capsule. *Br Med J.* 1972;2(5805):104–106.

177. West RL, Zimmerman DD, Dwarkasing S, et al. Prospective comparison of hydrogen peroxide-enhanced three-dimensional endoanal ultrasonography and endoanal magnetic resonance imaging of perianal fistulas. *Dis Colon Rectum.* 2003;46(10):1407–1415.

178. Wexner SD, Cheape JD, Jorge JM, et al. Prospective assessment of biofeedback for the treatment of paradoxical puborectalis contraction. *Dis Colon Rectum.* 1992;35(2):145–150.

179. Wexner SD, Marchetti F, Salanga VD, et al. Neurophysiologic assessment of the anal sphincters. *Dis Colon Rectum.* 1991;34(7):606–612.

180. Whitby LG, Lang D. Experience with the chromic oxide method of fecal marking in metabolic balance investigations on humans. *J Clin Invest.* 1960;39:854–863.

181. Womack NR, Williams NS, Holmfield JH, et al. New method for the dynamic assessment of anorectal function in constipation. *Br J Surg.* 1985;72(12):994–998.

182. Yang A, Mostwin JL, Rosenshein NB, et al. Pelvic floor descent in women: dynamic evaluation with fast MR imaging and cinematic display. *Radiology.* 1991;179(1):25–33.

183. Zworkin VK. "A radio pill." *Nature.* 1957;179:898.

8

Analgesia in Colon and Rectal Surgery

Theodore J. Saclarides

The art of life is the art of avoiding pain.
—THOMAS JEFFERSON (1743–1826)
Letter to Maria Cosway, October 12, 1786

With the exception of pudendal nerve block and local infiltration of the anal and perianal areas, there is no specific anesthetic situation that is unique to the field of colon and rectal surgery.[22,48,54] The principles and techniques of anesthetic induction and maintenance during major surgery should be of interest to any surgeon. However, such a discussion is not within the purview of this text. Still, the management of pain is a situation that every surgeon must confront and for which he or she must provide direction and care. The surgeon should be familiar with what options are available as well as their potential complications as they relate to patient outcome.

The severity of postoperative pain encountered is often not adequately appreciated, and as a consequence, is often inadequately treated.[11] One method for analyzing the efficacy of pain control has been the development of the visual analog pain score. If one assumes that a score of 3 for pain with movement is unacceptably high,[31] a multi-institutional study demonstrated that more than 80% of individuals experienced more pain than was considered appropriate both with the use of epidural and with patient-controlled analgesia (PCA).[40]

The management of postoperative pain is often difficult not only because of variation in analgesic requirements, but also because of the variability of pathophysiologic interactions with different therapies and, of course, the individual's subjective pain experiences. Recent concepts in the management of postoperative pain use the assessment of pain in three situations: when moving (e.g., during physical therapy), when in bed, and the worst pain during a day.

There are numerous approaches to controlling pain depending on the individual circumstances, each with varying degrees of effectiveness. For example, it has been demonstrated that epidural analgesia provides more effective pain relief than does either PCA or intramuscular drug administration.[60] It is not simply the route of administration that one must consider, however. Epidural catheter placement is accompanied by potential complications not seen with PCA, such as infection, paralysis, and bleeding. It has been established that pain control with this method may actually not be required with advances in surgical technique such as laparoscopic colectomy. Opiate tolerance effects, as manifested by comorbid preoperative use of these medications, certainly affect postoperative consumption.[58] Furthermore, preoperative pain and opiate use generally are associated with a greater degree of postoperative pain.[9]

▶ OPIATES

Opiates affect neuronal activity at the pain control apparatus (substantia gelatinosa, spinal trigeminal nucleus, periaqueductal gray, medullary raphe nucleus, and hypothalamus). Receptors are present in the limbic system, thalamus, striatum, hypothalamus, midbrain, and spinal cord. These receptors have been given various Greek letter identifications based on their location. For example, the *mu receptor* is found in the pain control apparatus of the central nervous system (CNS) and spinal cord. The *kappa receptor* is found in the deep layers of the cerebral cortex. The *delta receptor* is localized to the limbic system. The *sigma receptor* is involved in the dysphoric (excessive pain, anguish, agitation) and dyschronic-stimulating effects of opiates. Agonist activity at the mu and kappa receptors produce analgesia, miosis, and increased body temperature. It is the mu receptor activity that is responsible for opiate dependency. Respiratory depression is, in all probability, mediated through the mu and kappa activity.

Actions and Effects

Opiates have profound and varied effects on the CNS. For example, large doses may induce *excitation* or *seizures*. Normeperidine, the principal metabolite of meperidine (Demerol), is well known to induce "pseudoseizures" particularly in individuals who have renal insufficiency. This is because the metabolite is long-lived in these circumstances, accumulates, and is cleared slowly. Opiates also *suppress the cough reflex* by direct activity on the medulla. Furthermore, through a direct effect on the brain stem (pons, medulla), opiates *alter respiratory rhythm* and voluntary control as well as decrease responsiveness to carbon dioxide tension. Normally, as arteriole carbon dioxide tension rises, cerebrovascular dilatation occurs, with the resultant increase in cerebral blood flow and cerebrospinal fluid (CSF) pressure. This response is diminished with the use of opiates, an effect that is much more likely with intravenous administration.

Another effect is *nausea*, which develops as a consequence of orthostatic hypotension or by direct stimulation of a chemotactic trigger zone in the medulla oblongata. *Orthostasis* may occur as a result of vasodilatation from histamine release or from the suppression of sympathetic outflow from the vasomotor medullary center. The medullary nuclei may also be stimulated to cause *bradycardia*. The one exception to this phenomenon is the opiate, meperidine, which is usually associated with tachycardia. Finally, there is increased vestibular activity observed with opiates as well.

As can be readily appreciated, there are numerous and profound effects produced by the administration of opiates. In addition to the foregoing, opiates *increase smooth muscle tone* throughout the gastrointestinal tract, including the gastric antrum, duodenum, large bowel, and the various gastrointestinal and biliary sphincters. When measured, the amplitude of nonpropulsive contractions is increased, but the intensity of propulsive contractions is decreased. The exception is meperidine. Whereas it does have some sympathomimetic (anticholinergic-like, atropine-like) effects, it may produce less smooth muscle spasm. Therefore, this drug should be considered the preferred opiate to use after bowel surgery because it is least likely to affect return of intestinal function. The effects are not always uniform with opiates, however. For example, biliary spasm does not always occur. Some individuals have no change in ductal diameter or pressure. Increased smooth muscle tone, resulting in reduce motility of the affected part, is variable according to the drug, being greatest for morphine, followed in order by methadone, meperidine, and codeine.

Another effect of opiates is increased tone of the bladder sphincter, *impeding urination*. There is also increased tone and contraction in the lower one-third of the ureter. Furthermore, tone of the detrusor muscle is increased, which may result in urinary urgency. Finally, opiates may increase secretion of vasopressin, a consequence of which may be oliguria.

Opiates can also have a profound effect on the endocrine system. Inhibition of the release of thyrotropin from the adenohypophysis leads to a decrease in thyroid hormone. Opiates may also produce *hyperglycemia* by stimulating receptors near the foramen of Monro or by releasing epinephrine. This may be associated with a decrease in the metabolic rates by about 10% to 20%.

The relative potency of the various opiates is summarized in Table 8-1.

Metabolism

Opiates are primarily metabolized by the microsomes in the endoplasmic reticulum of the liver. Additionally, metabolism also occurs in the CNS, kidneys, lungs, and placenta. This is accomplished by hydrolysis, oxidation, and conjugation with glucuronide.

Mechanism of Action

All opiate receptors appear to function primarily by exerting inhibitory modulation of transmission of synapses in the spinal cord, the myenteric plexus, and the CNS. When located at a presynaptic terminal, these receptors act to reduce neurotransmitter release and, therefore, to decrease conductance. All appear to be linked to guanine nucleotide-binding regulator proteins (G proteins). Opioids regulate the so-called transmembrane signaling system—adenylate cyclase activity, ion channel activity, and the activity of phospholysasis or phosphoinositol. So-called kappa agonistic activity inhibits N-type voltage-dependent calcium channels, specifically in the myenteric plexus and the dorsal root ganglia. Stimulation of mu receptors in the locus coeruleus produces membrane hyperpolarization by an inward potassium rectifying current. The opioid receptors on terminals of afferent nerves in the CNS and in the spinal cord mediate inhibition of the release of neurotransmitters, including

TABLE 8-1 Potency of Opiates			
	EQUIVALENT	**CONVERSION**	
Analgesic	**Potency IM**	**Oral (mg)**	**IV (mg)**
Morphine	10	40–60	10
Codeine	130	200	—
Heroin	5	60	5
Hydromorphone	1.5	7.5	1.0
Levorphanol	2	4	1.5
Meperidine	75	400	75
Methadone	10	20	10
Oxycodone	15	30	—
Fentanyl	—	500 μg	100 μg

substance P. Enhanced activity in descending aminergic bulbospinal pathways then exerts inhibitory effects on the processing of nociceptive information. Specifically, mu opioids in the ventral tegmentum activate certain dopaminergic and γ-aminobutyric acidergic neurons that project to the nucleus accumbens. This is the site that is postulated to be the central point producing opiate euphoria and the self-reinforcing effects well known to individuals familiar with addiction.[34]

Within the *intestinal tract*, enterocytes themselves possess opioid receptors. As a consequence, opiates inhibit transfer of fluid and electrolytes into the intestinal lumen through their actions on the intestinal mucosa. Through effects on the submucosal plexus, there is a decrease in enterocyte basal secretion. Additionally, there is an inhibition of stimulatory effects of acetylcholine, prostaglandin E_2, and vasoactive intestinal peptides. The pressure of opiates at the periaqueductal gray or in the spinal cord will also inhibit gastrointestinal activity as long as the extrinsic innervation to the bowel is intact. This may explain why agents with poor penetration of the CNS (e.g., paregoric) can produce constipation at subanalgesic dosages.

Postoperative ileus is the temporary cessation of coordinated bowel motility, and its presence may prevent transit of bowel contents or tolerance of oral intake. Ileus is an expected occurrence after abdominal surgery; it usually lasts 3 to 4 days. It may be more prolonged if there is a complication such as an anastomotic leak. Endogenous opioids (endorphins, enkephalins, dynorphins) and prescribed opioids activate the mu receptor within the bowel and affect motility, secretion, and transport of fluids and electrolytes. The total dose of exogenous opioid administered correlates significantly with the return of bowel function as measured by the presence of bowel sounds, time to passage of first flatus, and time to first bowel movement. Return of bowel function also correlates with hospital length of stay.[5,10,45]

Patient-Controlled Analgesia

Intravenous (IV) PCA, a technique that allows patients to medicate themselves, dates back to the mid-1960s. The development of electronic devices or pumps that deliver small amounts of medicine on demand has been an essential ingredient for the success of this pain management system. Improvements in device design have increased security and data output capacity, introduced error reduction programs, and offered a choice of electrical or battery power. Based on a literature review, Dolin and coworkers concluded that IV PCA provided better pain relief than intermittent IM opioid analgesia.[18] Three meta-analyses have confirmed these results, although the magnitude of the differences was small.[2,30,59] Certainly, conventional forms of opioid administration, that is, given by nursing staff, can be as effective as IV PCA, but this requires patient care settings where the nurse-to-patient ratio is high. Typically, such a unit is an intensive care area, which is neither a cost-effective organization for all levels of patient care nor an acceptable use of nursing services.

In the postoperative setting, a PCA device is used primarily for the administration of opiates to alleviate pain. Usually, morphine, hydromorphone (Dilaudid), fentanyl, or meperidine is used. A PCA device can also be programmed for use with epidural infusions, patient-controlled epidural

analgesia. The goal of the PCA is to administer more timely drug doses and thereby to enhance patient satisfaction. White suggested it may decrease the amount of drug administered because it is more closely matched to the painful activity or stimulus encountered.[61] Others have shown that opioid consumption may be higher with IV PCA when compared with conventional opioid analgesia, but there does not appear to be a difference in the incidence of opioid-related side effects.[2,30] If morphine is used, the dosage range is from 1 to 3 mg/hour following abdominal surgery. Self-reporting scales that have been assessed with this drug note effective analgesia.[61]

The choice of agent is often a determination made by the surgeon based on his or her comfort level. Because of its roughly eightfold higher potency, faster onset, and greater lipid solubility (hence greater CNS penetration), hydromorphone (Dilaudid) is usually selected for more severe pain. Certainly, for those who require more close matching of drug delivery, time of onset, and proximity to painful stimulus, hydromorphone is a sound alternative. Owing to the accumulation of a normeperidine metabolite, meperidine (Demerol) at the usual clinical doses is recommended by many individuals familiar with pain control only when the specific advantages (sympathomimetic anticholinergic properties, known anaphylaxis to alternative opiates, etc.) outweigh this disadvantage. The use of fentanyl in PCA should be approached with caution. Although its potency, speed of onset, and density of analgesic action are perhaps desirable, the likelihood of respiratory suppression, accumulation of drug-inhibiting gastrointestinal function, and sedation limit this opiate to management by only those specially qualified.

In initially programming a PCA device, a target hourly "safe" dose should be selected. Then, the "demand" and "interval time" can be set according to the half-life alpha distribution times and times to peak analgesia. Morphine is typically set at 1 mg every 8 minutes. This results in a maximum dose of 7 mg/hour. The peak effect of morphine occurs in about 10 minutes after intravenous administration. Less than 0.1% of intravenously administered morphine enters the CNS at the time of peak plasma concentrations.[42] Therefore, the demand interval is set slightly less than that. The peak effect of hydromorphone is approximately 5.5 minutes; its interval is set at about 3 to 4 minutes. The total analgesic administered per hour is dependent on the volume of distribution, acid–base status, plasma protein–binding capacity, ventilatory mechanics, cerebral blood flow patterns, and presence of metabolic abnormalities (e.g., hypothyroidism), as well as a number of other subtle factors.

One should certainly consider the use of basal infusions when using PCA. In monitored areas such as intensive care units or operating suites, overdosing can be quickly recognized and treated. Because basal (continuous) infusions are not patient regulated, sedation and other side effects may accumulate rapidly; therefore, this method should be used with caution in less monitored patient care areas. Although one may achieve more "stable" pharmacologic plasma levels by the use of basal infusions, annoying pruritus, nausea, and prolonged ileus may result.

The choice of opiate depends on the volume and the route of administration, the side effects and toxicities, and the physiologic factors of the individual that affect drug excretion. For example, fentanyl has a membrane-stabilizing influence that may potentiate the activity of local anesthetics.

Alternatively, with respect to its anesthetic effectiveness, morphine may be more desirable when a greater spread involving more dermatomes is necessary. This is because of morphine's hydrophilicity and lack of segmental spinal cord binding (lipophilic binding). Ultimately, the surgeon uses whichever agent he or she feels most familiar with and most comfortable.

Complications relating to the use of PCA can be operator related, patient related, equipment related, and those secondary to the agent chosen. The most common operator-related complications are (in decreasing frequency) improper opioid dose or quantity, unauthorized drug, omission error, and prescribing error (wrong drug, inappropriate use of concurrent medications).[57] Approximately 30% of all PCA errors may result from incorrect programming of PCA pumps, which is twice as likely to cause injury or death than mishaps involving general-purpose infusion pumps.[21] Innovations applied to avoid this include systems that use internal software to check the doses prescribed against preset limits. The programmer is then alerted. Patient-related errors may be offset by proper initial education and by limiting access to the drug reservoir and microprocessor program with the use of a key or access code. This may reduce tampering by family members.

Opioid side effects include respiratory depression, nausea and vomiting, and pruritus. Risk factors for respiratory depression include the use of continuous (background) infusions, concurrent administration of sedatives, advanced patient age, and hypovolemia. The addition of antiemetics directly to the PCA solution is controversial; perhaps separate administration is preferable and allows more accurate dosing.

▶ KETOROLAC

Ketorolac (Toradol) is a nonsteroidal anti-inflammatory drug that is available for oral or intravenous use. It possesses no sedative or anxiolytic properties and has its peak analgesic effect within 2 to 3 hours following administration. It is principally metabolized in the liver and excreted in the urine. In several prospective, randomized studies comparing it with morphine and meperidine, ketorolac has been shown to have a longer duration of efficacy. Furthermore, when given in combination with opioids, this drug significantly reduces the requirement for narcotics. Another benefit is blunting of the inflammatory response leading to a reduction in the influx of macrophages and mast cells into the area of surgical trauma as well as a reduction in nitric oxide, prostaglandin, and proinflammatory cytokines. All of which side effects potentiate postoperative ileus. Ketorolac does not reduce colonic contractions, and it has become an invaluable addition to postoperative analgesia protocols. The primary concern with the use of this agent, however, is an increased risk for gastrointestinal bleeding, presumably because of its effect on platelet aggregation, especially in the elderly. Therefore, ketorolac is contraindicated in individuals with a history of gastrointestinal bleeding and those with peptic ulcer disease. The combined duration for its use must not exceed 5 days.

Place and colleagues evaluated ketorolac in a prospective, randomized study in patients undergoing anorectal surgery.[44] They found that the addition of this drug (60 mg), either given intravenously or injected in combination with a local anesthetic, decreased the risk of urinary retention as well as that of analgesic requirements.

▶ EPIDURAL ANALGESIS

Continuous epidural infusions of local anesthetics at dilute concentrations, in combination with epidural opioids, are effective means for treating pain.[14] All epidural opiates will achieve some plasma systemic levels. The use of epidural analgesia has particular value in that it appears to be associated with faster resolution of postoperative ileus[37,51] and it decreases the inflammatory sequelae in the perioperative period.[27] In a landmark study to assess the basis for using intensive postoperative analgesia, Mangano and colleagues evaluated patients who had undergone coronary artery bypass grafts and found intensive prolonged analgesia reduced the number and severity of postoperative ischemic episodes.[41]

Epidural analgesics reduce not only postoperative morbidity from all causes but also length of hospitalization.[17,62] Epidural analgesia appears to have the greatest potential to improve perioperative outcome and morbidity when high-risk patients undergo major operations. This has been demonstrated for perioperative cardiovascular morbidity, pulmonary complications, and infection.[17,55,62]

Several randomized controlled trials comparing epidural anesthetics/analgesics with systemic opioids have shown a benefit in favor of the former.[28] There is a demonstrable reduction in time to passage of first flatus, first stool, or both. Epidural infusions containing local anesthetic or dilute local anesthetic plus opioid are associated with more rapid return of bowel function and earlier hospital discharge than either epidural opioids alone or intravenous PCA.[38] As mentioned, with the increasing use of minimally invasive surgery, however, epidural infusions may become unnecessary for many patients.

Epidural Opiates

Epidural opiates act both by venous absorption, thereby producing systemic plasma levels, and by dispersion into the CSF. Approximately 10% to 15% of epidural morphine reaches the CSF. Activity may result from direct binding at the mu receptor complex in the substantia gelatinosa, direct binding onto nerve roots, or spread and assimilation of morphine through the CSF to the periaqueductal gray of the CNS. Despite their acknowledged efficacy, opiates alone are inadequate for complete intraoperative and postoperative pain relief. Local anesthetics are the agents responsible for affording anesthesia. However, by means of synergistic activity with opiates, the concentrations can be reduced, thereby minimizing motor blockade or total sensory blockade.

Epidural local anesthetic infusions in combination with opiates may inhibit efferent sympathetic pathways and neural reflex arcs.[6] Through this action, the incidence of perioperative increase in coagulation tendency can be reduced, with concomitant decrease in venous and arterial thrombosis.[53,55]

Cousins and colleagues studied selective spinal analgesia and demonstrated the difference between analgesia obtained with nonselective axonal conduction block by a local anesthetic and that of spinal opiates.[12] They observed that selective block of nociception through the use of opiates at the spinal cord does not cause sympathetic block or orthostasis. Furthermore, this selectivity permits ambulation without motor blockade. Additionally, it is not associated with seizures or hypotension. Spinal opiates, however, do cause both early and late respiratory depression. This is usually slow in onset and is augmented by parenteral sedative, hypnotic agents. Unique to spinal opiates is the fact that they cause pruritus and are more likely to be associated with nausea and vomiting. Still, they have about the same incidence of urinary retention as is associated with the use of local anesthetics.

Onset of epidural opiate analgesia is directly related to the lipid partition coefficient. The higher the lipid solubility, the more rapid is the onset of analgesia. The duration of analgesia is inversely related to lipid solubility, but it is also influenced by the rate of dissociation from receptors and perhaps by the deposition in the lipid of the epidural space.

It has been demonstrated that if similar dosages of opiates are given intramuscularly and epidurally, blood concentrations are similar. However, analgesia is significantly greater for epidural opiates when compared with the intramuscular route.[24] This points to a central or spinal effect. It has also been shown that analgesia is longer lasting and denser when equivalent doses of fentanyl have been given epidurally rather than intramuscularly.[39] Others have demonstrated in a study of 14,000 patients given epidural morphine at a dose of 4 mg that delayed respiratory depression occurred at a rate of 1 in 1,000.[47] This compares with a rate for the intrathecal use of morphine (0.2 to 0.8 mg) of 1 in 275. Those patients who had never been exposed to opiates, and presumably having no tolerance, were found to have rare respiratory depression as long as no other opiates had been administered by other routes.[25] One must weigh the potential benefit of the superior analgesia obtained with epidural opiates against the greater invasiveness and the possible complications of respiratory depression, pruritus, nausea, and urinary retention. Alternatively, as discussed previously, infusions of opioids may provide similar analgesia, albeit not as satisfactory in some respects, but they do so less invasively and with a lower rate of complications.[50]

Complications

Clearly, as with all invasive techniques, complications can arise from their use. With respect to epidural analgesia, these include toxicity and seizures, urinary retention, epidural abscess, hematoma, inadvertent dural puncture, backache, and nerve root injury. Two of these complications are discussed.

Epidural Abscess

Epidural abscess is a rare complication of epidural analgesia. Baker and colleagues reviewed a series of 39 abscesses and found that 38 were associated with simultaneous systemic infections.[1] The diagnosis was made based on the patient complaining of severe back pain, local tenderness, and fever. Leukocytosis was also present. Subsequent myelography demonstrated obstruction to flow.

Epidural Hematoma

Epidural hematoma as a consequence of epidural anesthesia and analgesia is most probably the result of needle or catheter trauma to the epidural veins. Generally, in a patient free of bleeding tendencies, bleeding is minimal and ceases rapidly. There has only been one reported case of hematoma formation with the potential for neurologic compromise when the coagulation profile had been determined to be normal.[36] However, when anticoagulant therapy is administered (e.g., aspirin, heparin), an epidural hematoma may develop from catheter insertion or simply by the placement of a needle.[15,36] Still, there may be some confusion as to the cause because there have been more than 100 instances of hematoma

formation spontaneously produced in this area and not associated with epidural management in patients who are on anticoagulants.[23] Interestingly, the risk of epidural hematoma or related neurologic injury is not increased by preoperative oral anticoagulation with warfarin (Coumadin).[26,43] This is also true for intraoperative anticoagulation with heparin in patients undergoing regional blockade for major vascular surgery.[46] However, both these studies recommend against the use of regional anesthesia if thrombocytopenia is present, if antiplatelet agents are given, or if there is a qualitative defect in platelets (e.g., an abnormal bleeding time). If anticoagulation is continued in the postoperative period, the potential movement of the epidural catheter as a consequence of ambulation poses a risk for venous trauma and hematoma formation. Consequently, anesthesiologists are opposed to the use of continuous catheter techniques under such circumstances.

Low-dose heparin therapy for deep venous thrombosis prophylaxis represents a controversial area for the use of epidural analgesia. Obviously, the risks and benefits of epidural blockade need to be weighed against the risks and benefits of deep venous thrombosis prophylaxis with heparin or enoxaparin. One should not consider epidural block if therapeutic intravenous heparin administration has been previously given. Because there is a small chance of trauma and bleeding with an indwelling catheter, even with the patient receiving low-dose or mini-dose heparin, the anesthesiologist may well be advised to decline placement and/or continuation of this technique.

Venous thromboembolism (VTE) is a significant concern in the postoperative patient. Nearly every hospitalized patient has at least one risk factor; approximately 40% have several risk factors and are therefore candidates for thromboprophylaxis. The use of regional anesthetics and epidural catheters poses a challenge in the face of VTE prevention because of concerns about bleeding. A review of the literature in this regard is beyond the scope of this chapter. However, the following conclusions can be found in the American Society of Regional Anesthesia (Third Edition) 2010 guidelines[29]:

1) There is no contraindication to VTE prophylaxis with unfractionated heparin, 5,000 U twice a day, simultaneous with epidural or spinal blockade.
2) The patient's medical record should be reviewed daily to rule out concurrent medications that may interfere with the clotting cascade.
3) Doses of unfractionated heparin more than 10,000 U daily or administration more than twice daily should be used cautiously. There may be an increased incidence of surgical site bleeding, but it is unclear if the incidence of spinal hematoma is increased.
4) Patients who have been receiving IV heparin for several days should be screened for heparin-induced thrombocytopenia before regional block is instituted and before catheter removal.
5) Catheter insertion before the injection of subcutaneous unfractionated heparin may be preferable, but there is little data to suggest the reverse order is harmful.
6) The use of epidural analgesia is probably safe in patients receiving low-molecular-weight heparin once a day unless the patient is receiving additional anticoagulation medication. Guidelines have consistently advised against the use of epidurals in patients receiving twice a day dosing.
7) Epidural catheters should be removed prior to starting low-molecular-weight heparin VTE prophylaxis.

8) If blood is seen during needle or catheter placement, low-molecular-weight heparin should be withheld for 24 hours.
9) Catheter placement should be withheld until 10 to 12 hours after the previous low-molecular-weight dose.
10) For patients who have been taking warfarin, catheter insertion should be withheld for 4 to 5 days. International normalized ratio (INR) should be checked and verified to be normal.

Duration of Catheter Placement

The duration for epidural catheter use is variable. A fibrous tissue reaction occurs at about 72 hours.[20] A distinct advantage of an epidural catheter, however, is that it does not break the protective barrier of the dura, thereby limiting the likelihood of an infection developing in the CSF. Furthermore, use of epidural catheters avoids the headache associated with puncture of the dura when intrathecal catheters are placed.

One study evaluated the use of percutaneous catheters on a long-term basis (72 days).[63] Complications included catheter dislodgement, obstruction, and localized site infection. There were two instances of nonfatal meningitis in a total of 139 patients. In a study of 105 individuals in whom a total of 215 catheters were placed, no infectious complications were observed.[13] A Silastic catheter can be tunneled and left in place for more than 1 year, particularly if a silver–silver chloride cuff (Vitacuff) is used at the exit site.[19] In most instances, however, an epidural catheter is left in place for about 7 days before a change of sites is recommended.

A very rare occurrence is the migration of the catheter into the intravascular, subdural, or subarachnoid space.[12] Vertebral column movement, ligamentum flavum movement, and respiratory-induced space pressure variations make epidural catheters mobile, but catheter tip design and integrity of dural arachnoid membrane generally prevent this from occurring.

Factors Affecting Epidural Blockade

With respect to adult body weight, there appears to be no correlation between this variable and the spread of the analgesia. As may be expected, blockade is most intense and has the most rapid onset close to the site of injection. Studies by Bromage have demonstrated the mass of drug itself determines the spread of analgesia.[7] If one increases the dose or mass of the pharmacologic agent, the amount of sensory blockade and its duration are increased. In addition, by increasing the concentration of the drug, the onset time is reduced, and greater motor block is achieved. Furthermore, the intensity of sensory and motor blockade increases with subsequent injections. This intensification and deepening of blockade is important with the use of dilute local anesthetic solutions that are applied for differential postoperative blockade (sensory vs. motor).

An example of spread is as follows. The four-segment spread for 2% lidocaine is 15 ± 5 minutes. This can be compared to 18 ± 10 minutes for 0.5% bupivacaine. The two-segment repression time is 100 ± 40 minutes, compared with 200 ± 80 minutes (the "wear-off" time of the block).[8] The duration of the blockade is related to the commencement of the regression of the block. The onset time (four-segment spread) indicates that all blocks take time to establish. It requires the patience of all individuals involved while the local anesthetic "takes."

In summary, then, the use of epidural analgesics introduces risks that must be balanced against the benefits. That said, epidural analgesia has proven to be an extremely safe and effective technique.[17,49,52]

▶ BALANCED ANALGESIA

Henrik Kehlet and his colleagues at Copenhagen University Hospital have been singularly important contributors to the concept of expediting the recovery process through what they have termed *balanced analgesia*.[3,4,28,32,33] This is defined as the achievement of optimal pain relief and return of normal function through a combination of different analgesics and methods of administration. It is well known that limiting factors for early discharge from the hospital (in addition to pain) include ileus, organ dysfunction, and fatigue.[33] Through a multimodality program, including intraoperative spinal-epidural anesthesia, postoperative epidural analgesia for 48 hours, and immediate oral nutrition and mobilization, Kehlet and Mogensen were able to discharge their patients following open sigmoid colectomy at a median of 2 days.[33] In another study involving patients who underwent restoration of continuity following Hartmann's operation, postoperative stay was reduced to 3 days through continuous epidural analgesia with local anesthetic, enforced oral nutrition and mobilization, a laxative, and a "planned 2-day hospital stay."[4] The same protocol with similar results was applied to abdominal rectopexy for prolapse.[3] In a prospective, randomized, controlled trial, Delaney and colleagues evaluated 64 patients who underwent intestinal or rectal resection.[16] The authors found through the application of a postoperative care pathway using controlled rehabilitation with early ambulation and diet (CREAD), *without epidural analgesia*, that patients had a shorter hospital stay with no adverse consequences. With increasing focus on cost containment and with limitation on hospital resources, it seems prudent for one to encourage surgeons to increase their collaboration with anesthesiologists and to minimize pain while preventing ileus, thus improving patient outcomes.[16,28,32]

▶ NONPHARMACOLOGIC THERAPY

The use of adjuvant nonpharmacologic analgesic techniques may diminish the cumulative dose of analgesic drugs used and are essentially free of side effects. These techniques have not gained wide acceptance in Western medicine, yet they are an integral component of complementary/alternative medicine. Acupuncture, acupressure, and moxibustion are rooted in ancient Eastern Asian medicine practices, whereas transcutaneous electrical nerve stimulation (TENS) and percutaneous electrical nerve stimulation (PENS) have undergone their development in the West. The unifying theme with these therapies involves the use of subnoxious to noxious stimuli at discrete locations to produce counterirritation and a state of heightened analgesia.

Acupuncture is based on the philosophy that the flow of energy in the universe is in a state of constant balance between the forces of yin and yang. Energy flow, or qi, travels through the human body along 14 traditional pathways known as *meridians*. If these meridians are obstructed, the qi will no longer flow, and disease will then occur. Acupuncture points (approximately 360 in number) connect the meridians, and stimulation of these points, with periodic twirling or flicking of needles, produces afferent stimuli that redirect the flow of qi.

Clinical research has suggested that acupuncture releases endogenous opioids. Naloxone, an opioid-specific antagonist, can negate the beneficial effects of acupuncture. Trials investigating the use of acupuncture for postoperative pain control have shown that acupuncture may not change verbal or visual pain intensity scores. However, researchers have noted significant improvements in analgesic consumption, time to first pain medication request, and duration of the pain-free period.[35,56]

References

1. Baker AS, Ojemann RG, Swartz MN, et al. Spinal epidural abscess. *N Engl J Med.* 1975;293(10):463–468.
2. Ballantyne JC, Carr DB, Chalmers TC, et al. Postoperative patient-controlled analgesia: meta-analyses of initial randomized control trials. *J Clin Anesth.* 1993;5(3):182–193.
3. Basse L, Billesbølle P, Kehlet H. Early recovery after abdominal rectopexy with multimodal rehabilitation. *Dis Colon Rectum.* 2002;45(2):195–199.
4. Basse L, Jacobsen DH, Billesbølle P, et al. Colostomy closure after Hartmann's procedure with fast-track rehabilitation. *Dis Colon Rectum.* 2002;45(12):1661–1664.
5. Bauer AJ, Boeckxstaens GE. Mechanisms of postoperative ileus. *Neurogastroenterol Motil.* 2004;16(suppl 2):54–60.
6. Blomberg SG, Emanuelsson H, Kvist H, et al. Effects of thoracic epidural anesthesia on coronary arteries and arterioles in patients with coronary artery disease. *Anesthesiology.* 1990;73(5):840–847.
7. Bromage PR. Mechanism of action of extradural analgesia. *Br J Anaesth.* 1975;47(suppl):199–211.
8. Bromage PR. *Epidural Analgesia.* Philadelphia, PA: WB Saunders; 1978.
9. Burns JW, Hodsman NB, McLintock TC, et al. The influence of patient characteristics on the requirements of postoperative analgesia. A reassessment using patient-controlled analgesia. *Anaesthesia.* 1989;44(1):2–6.
10. Cali RL, Meade PG, Swanson MS, et al. Effect of Morphine and incision length on bowel function after colectomy. *Dis Colon Rectum.* 2000;43(2):163–168.
11. Cousins M. Acute and postoperative pain. In: Wall PD, Melzack R, eds. *Textbook of Pain.* New York, NY: Churchill Livingstone; 1994:357.
12. Cousins MJ, Glynn CJ, Wilson PR, et al. Epidural morphine. *Anaesth Intensive Care.* 1980(2);8:217–219.
13. Crawford ME, Andersen HB, Augustenborg G, et al. Pain treatment on outpatient basis utilizing extradural opiates: a Danish multicenter study comprising 105 patients. *Pain.* 1983;16(1):41–47.
14. Dahl JB, Rosenberg J, Hansen B, et al. Differential analgesic effects of low-dose epidural morphine and morphine-bupivacaine at rest and during mobilization after major abdominal surgery. *Anesth Analg.* 1992;74(3):362–365.
15. DeAngelis J. Hazards of subdural and epidural anesthesia during anticoagulant therapy: a case report and review. *Anesth Analg.* 1972;51(5):676–679.
16. Delaney CP, Zutshi M, Senagore AJ, et al. Prospective, randomized, controlled trial between a pathway of controlled rehabilitation with early ambulation and diet and traditional postoperative care after laparotomy and intestinal resection. *Dis Colon Rectum.* 2003;46(7):851–859.
17. de Leon-Casasola OA, Parker B, Lema MJ, et al. Postoperative epidural bupivacaine-morphine therapy. Experience with 4,227 surgical cancer patients. *Anesthesiology.* 1994;81(2):368–375.
18. Dolin SJ, Cashman JN, Bland JM. Effectiveness of acute postoperative pain management: I. Evidence from published data. *Br J Anaesth.* 2002;89(3):409–423.
19. Dupen SL. Silastic long term epidural catheters. *Anesthesiology.* 1986;65:195.
20. Durant PA, Yaksh TL. Epidural injections of bupivacaine, morphine, fentanyl, lofentanil and DADL in chronically implanted rats: a pharmacologic and pathologic study. *Anesthesiology.* 1986;64(1):43–53.
21. Emergency Care Research Institute. Patient-controlled analgesic infusion pumps. *Health Devices.* 2006;35(1):5–35.
22. Gabrielli F, Chiarelli M, Cioffi U, et al. Day surgery for mucosal-hemorrhoidal prolapse using circular stapler and modified regional anesthesia. *Dis Colon Rectum.* 2001;44(6):842–844.
23. Gingrich TF. Spinal epidural hematoma following continuous epidural anesthesia. *Anesthesiology.* 1968;29(1):162–163.
24. Gustafsson LL, Johannisson J, Garle M. Extradural and parenteral pethidine as analgesia after total hip replacement: effect and kinetics. A controlled clinical study. *Eur J Clin Pharmacol.* 1986;29(5):529–534.
25. Gustafsson LL, Schildt B, Jacobsen K. Adverse effects of extradural and intrathecal opiates: report of a nationwide survey in Sweden. *Br J Anaesth.* 1982;54(5):479–486.
26. Harik SI, Raichle ME, Reis DJ. Spontaneously remitting spinal epidural hematoma in a patient on anticoagulants. *N Engl J Med.* 1971;284(24):1355–1357.
27. Hendolin H, Lahtinen J, Länsimies E, et al. The effect of thoracic epidural analgesia on postoperative stress and morbidity. *Ann Chir Gynaecol.* 1987;76(4):234–240.
28. Holte K, Kehlet H. Postoperative ileus: a preventable event. *Br J Surg.* 2000;87(11):1480–1493.
29. Horlocker TT, Wedel DJ, Rowlingson JC, et al. Regional anesthesia in the patient receiving antithrombotic or thrombolytic therapy: American Society of Regional Anesthesia and Pain Medicine Evidence-Based Guidelines (Third Edition). *Reg Anesth Pain Med.* 2010;35(1):64–101.
30. Hudcova J, McNicol E, Quah C, et al. Patient controlled intravenous opioid analgesia versus conventional opioid analgesia for postoperative pain control: a quantitative systematic review. *Acute Pain.* 2005;7:115–132.
31. Kehlet H. Postoperative pain relief—what is the issue? *Br J Anaesth.* 1994;72(4):375–378.
32. Kehlet H. Balanced analgesia: a prerequisite for optimal recovery. *Br J Surg.* 1998;85(1):3–4.
33. Kehlet H, Mogensen T. Hospital stay of 2 days after open sigmoidectomy with a multimodal rehabilitation programme. *Br J Surg.* 1999;86(2):227–230.
34. Koob GF, Bloom FE. Cellular and molecular mechanisms of drug dependence. *Science.* 1988;242(4879):715–723.
35. Lao L, Bergman S, Hamilton GR, et al. Evaluation of acupuncture for pain control after oral surgery: a placebo-controlled trial. *Arch Otolaryngol Head Neck Surg.* 1999;125(5):567–572.
36. Lerner SM, Gutterman P, Jenkins F. Epidural hematoma and paraplegia after numerous lumbar punctures. *Anesthesiology.* 1973;39(5):550–551.
37. Liu SS, Carpenter RL, Mackey DC, et al. Effects of perioperative analgesic technique on rate of recovery after colon surgery. *Anesthesiology.* 1995;83(4):757–765.
38. Liu S, Carpenter RL, Neal JM. Epidural anesthesia and analgesia. Their role in postoperative outcome. *Anesthesiology.* 1995;82(6): 1474–1506.
39. Lomessey A, Magnin C, Viale JP, et al. Clinical advantages of fentanyl given epidurally for postoperative analgesia. *Anesthesiology.* 1984;61(4):466–469.
40. Lynch EP, Lazor MA, Gellis JE, et al. Patient experience of pain after elective noncardiac surgery. *Anesth Analg.* 1997;85(1):117–123.
41. Mangano DT, Silicano D, Hollenberg M, et al. Postoperative myocardial ischemia. Therapeutic trials using intensive analgesia following surgery. The Study Perioperative Ischemia (SPI) Research Group. *Anesthesiology.* 1992;76(3):342–353.
42. Mule SJ. Physiological dispositions of narcotic agonists and antagonists. In: DH Clouet, ed. *Narcotic Drugs: Biochemical Pharmacology.* New York, NY: Plenum Press; 1971.
43. Odoom JA, Sih IL. Epidural analgesia and anticoagulant therapy. Experience with one thousand cases of continuous epidurals. *Anaesthesia.* 1983;38(3):254–259.
44. Place RJ, Coloma M, White PF, et al. Ketorolac improves recovery after outpatient anorectal surgery. *Dis Colon Rectum.* 2000;43(6):804–808.
45. Prasad M, Matthews JB. Deflating postoperative ileus. *Gastroenterology.* 1999;117(2):489–492.
46. Rao TL, El-Etr AA. Anticoagulation following placement of epidural and subarachnoid catheters: an evaluation of neurological sequelae. *Anesthesiology.* 1981;55(6):618–620.
47. Rawal N, Arnér S, Gustafsson LL, et al. Present state of extradural and intrathecal opioid analgesia in Sweden. A nationwide follow-up survey. *Br J Anaesth.* 1987;59(6):791–799.
48. Read TE, Henry SE, Hovis RM, et al. Prospective evaluation of anesthetic technique for anorectal surgery. *Dis Colon Rectum.* 2002;45(11):1553–1558.
49. Ready LB, Loper KA, Nessly M, et al. Postoperative epidural morphine is safe on surgical wards. *Anesthesiology.* 1991;75(3):452–456.
50. Rosenberg PH, Heino A, Scheinin B. Comparison of intramuscular analgesia, intercostal block, epidural morphine and on-demand-i.v.-fentanyl in the control of pain after abdominal surgery. *Acta Anaesthesiol Scand.* 1984;28(6):603–607.
51. Scheinin B, Asantila R, Orko R. The effect of bupivacaine and morphine on pain and bowel function after colonic surgery. *Acta Anaesthesiol Scand.* 1987;31(2):161–164.

52. Senagore AJ, Delaney CP, Mekhail N, et al. Randomized clinical trial comparing epidural anaesthesia and patient-controlled analgesia after laparoscopic segmental colectomy. *Br J Surg.* 2003;90(10): 1195–1199.

53. Sharrock NE, Ranawat CS, Urquhart B, et al. Factors influencing deep vein thrombosis following total hip arthroplasty under epidural anesthesia. *Anesth Analg.* 1993;76(4):756–771.

54. Tan PY, Vukasin P, Chin ID, et al. The WAND local anesthetic delivery system: a more pleasant experience for anal anesthesia. *Dis Colon Rectum.* 2001;44(5):686–689.

55. Tuman KJ, McCarthy RJ, March RJ, et al. Effects of epidural anesthesia and analgesia on coagulation and outcome after major vascular surgery. *Anesth Analg.* 1991;73(6):696–704.

56. Usichenko TI, Lysenyuk VP, Groth MH, et al. Detection of ear acupuncture points by measuring the electrical skin resistance in patients before, during, and after orthopedic surgery performed under general anesthesia. *Acupunct Electrother Res.* 2003;28(3–4): 167–173.

57. US Pharmacopeia Quality Review. Patient-controlled analgesia pumps. US Pharmacopeia Web Site. http:/www.usp.org/patientsafety/newsletters/qualityreview/qr812004-09-01.html. Accessed.

58. Voulgari A, Lykouras L, Papanikolaou M, et al. Influence of psychological and clinical factors on postoperative pain and narcotic consumption. *Psychother Psychosom.* 1991;55(2–4):191–196.

59. Walder B, Schafer M, Henzi I, et al. Efficacy and safety of patient-controlled opioid analgesia for acute postoperative pain. A quantitative systematic review. *Acta Anaesthesiol Scand.* 2001;45(7):795–804.

60. Weller R, Rosenblum M, Conard P, et al. Comparison of epidural and patient-controlled intravenous morphine following joint replacement surgery. *Can J Anaesth.* 1991;38(5)582–586.

61. White PF. Patient controlled analgesia: a new approach to the management of postoperative pain. *Semin Anesth.* 1985;4:255.

62. Yeager MP, Glass DD, Neff RK, et al. Epidural anesthesia and analgesia in high-risk surgical patients. *Anesthesiology.* 1987;66(6): 729–736.

63. Zenz M, Piepenbrock S, Tryba M. Epidural opiates: long-term experiences in cancer pain. *Klin Wochenschr.* 1985;63(5):225–229.

9
Cutaneous Conditions

Julia Zakhaleva and Marvin L. Corman

What's the matter, you dissentious rogues
That, rubbing the poor itch of your opinion,
Make yourselves scabs?
—WILLIAM SHAKESPEARE: *Coriolanus* I, i, 168

Dermatologic anal problems are often trivialized by the surgeon, who may categorize them as complaints attributable to a psychoneurotic or anal-obsessive personality. The patient may be referred directly to a dermatologist or may be given any one of a number of proprietary creams or the ubiquitous topical steroid, without the benefit of a physical examination. Dermatologists are understandably more adept at establishing the diagnosis of skin problems and usually perform a biopsy for confirmation in questionable cases, but the dermatologist is loath to perform a rectal examination and rarely has endoscopic equipment available. In our opinion, therefore, patients with anal complaints, including perianal dermatologic problems, should be seen by a physician or surgeon who has the knowledge and the instruments necessary to perform a complete rectal evaluation. If the condition appears to be limited to the skin and of uncertain diagnosis, consultation with a dermatologist is certainly appropriate.

The purpose of this chapter is to describe the skin conditions that affect the perianal area, emphasizing the differential diagnosis, indications for biopsy, and treatment of the relevant diseases. Those conditions that may be found in the anal area that are only incidental to a systemic cutaneous process are mentioned en passant if recognition of the disease in the area is believed to be unique or of particular interest. However, this chapter is not meant to be a précis of a textbook of dermatology.

▶ CLASSIFICATION

Dermatologic diseases may be categorized in a number of ways: based on the type of lesion (e.g., flat, elevated, depressed), according to whether they are primary or secondary, histopathologically, or by the commonly employed classifications of inflammation, infection, and neoplasm. A modification using this last method is illustrated as follows:

Dermatologic Anal Conditions
Inflammatory Diseases
Pruritus ani
Psoriasis
Lichen planus
Lichen sclerosus et atrophicus
Atrophoderma
Contact (i.e., allergic) dermatitis
Seborrheic dermatitis
Atopic dermatitis
Radiodermatitis
Behçet's syndrome
Lupus erythematosus
Dermatomyositis
Scleroderma
Erythema multiforme
Familial benign chronic pemphigus (i.e., Hailey-Hailey)
Pemphigus vulgaris
Cicatricial pemphigoidpa

Infectious Diseases
Nonvenereal
    Pilonidal sinus
    Suppurative hidradenitis
    Anorectal abscess and anal fistula
    Crohn's disease
    Tuberculosis
    Actinomycosis
    Fournier's gangrene

Ecthyma gangrenosum
Herpes zoster
Vaccinia
Tinea cruris
Majocchi's granuloma
Candidiasis (i.e., moniliasis)
"Deep" mycoses
Amebiasis cutis
Trichomoniasis
Schistosomiasis cutis
Bilharziasis
Oxyuriasis (e.g., pinworm, enterobiasis)
Creeping eruption (i.e., larva migrans)
Larva currens
Cimicosis (i.e., bedbug bites)
Pediculosis
Scabies
Venereal
Gonorrhea
Syphilis
Chancroid
Granuloma inguinale
Lymphogranuloma venereum (*Chlamydia* infection)
Molluscum contagiosum
Herpes genitalis
Condylomata acuminata

Premalignant and Malignant Diseases

Acanthosis nigricans
Leukoplakia
Mycosis fungoides
Leukemia cutis
Basal cell carcinoma
Squamous cell carcinoma
Malignant melanoma
Bowen's disease
Extramammary Paget's disease

In addition, a glossary of dermatologic terms (provided at the end of this chapter) may aid the reader in interpreting the description of the lesions.[120,155]

▶ INFLAMMATORY CONDITIONS

Pruritus Ani

Itching in the perianal area, pruritus ani, is a frequently voiced complaint. In fact, it is a symptom that was well recognized in antiquity. In the earliest manuscript exclusively devoted to anorectal disorders, the Chester Beatty Medical Papyrus, 10 of its 41 remedies were devoted to the management of anal itching and irritation.[29] By far the most common anorectal symptom presenting to the dermatologist is pruritus ani.[11] The rich nerve supply to the perianal area is thought to be the primary reason for the sensitivity to potential irritants.[270]

Symptoms

Itching is usually noted in the anal or occasionally the genital areas, but the condition is not generalized. Although the anus is frequently the site for autoeroticism, most individuals do not appear to fall into this category. The condition tends to be worse at night, awakening the patient from sleep. This leads to scratching, which exacerbates the complaint even further. Pruritus ani is more common in men.

Differential Diagnosis

Although the symptoms may be associated with a specific condition (e.g., hemorrhoids,[286] anal fissure, scarring from prior anal surgery, or with constipation or diarrhea), most patients are not found to have significant anorectal pathology except for the obvious skin changes. Besides anorectal disease, allergic dermatitis (i.e., contact), mycoses, seborrhea, diabetes, and oxyuriasis (pinworm) have all been implicated as causative factors. Other dermatologic problems, such as psoriasis (see later), should be considered. In addition, the possibility of harboring a systemic disease, such as diabetes, may necessitate further studies. Anal neurodermatitis may cause violent itching, which may lead to tearing of the perianal area (Figure 9-1). With chronicity, the skin can become atrophic or hypertrophic, with nodularity and scarring (Figure 9-2).

Special Studies

Physiologic studies have demonstrated that in patients with idiopathic pruritus ani, the anal sphincter relaxes in response to rectal distension more readily than in those with no anal disease.[148] Allan and colleagues showed that individuals harboring pruritic symptoms without coexisting anal pathologic features had a significantly greater fall of anal pressure when a rectal balloon was inflated (57%) than did a control population (40%).[13] Others have observed that patients with idiopathic pruritus ani have an abnormal rectoanal inhibitory reflex and a lower threshold for internal sphincter relaxation during such studies as the saline continence test.[150] It is therefore postulated that pruritus and soiling in some patients may occur as a result of a defect in anal sphincter function.

Evaluation

Physical examination should include anoscopy and proctosigmoidoscopy to look for a local cause of the symptoms. Daniel and colleagues reviewed 109 individuals with pruritus ani as the only presenting symptom and concluded that those with complaints of long duration should undergo evaluation

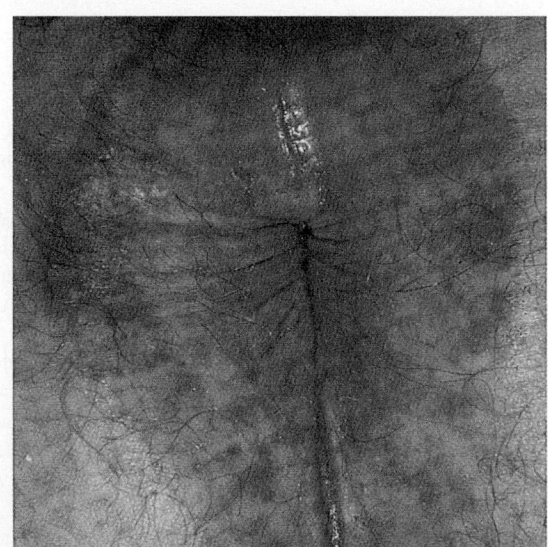

FIGURE 9-1. Perianal neurodermatitis is manifested with severe erythema and fissuring.

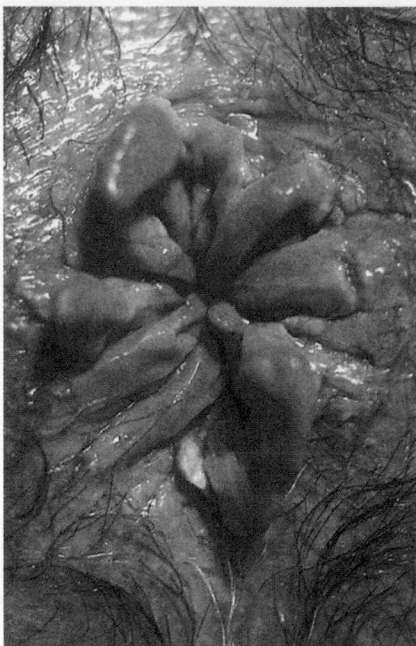

FIGURE 9-2. Marked edema with papillomatosis and nodularity resulting from chronic abrading is characteristic of pruritus ani. (Courtesy of William G. Robertson, MD.)

for proximal colon and anorectal neoplasms.[109] Usually, however, the procedures are unrewarding. Examination with a magnifying lens may be helpful.[107] Evaluation with Wood's lamp may reveal fluorescence,[356] but this equipment is usually not readily available in the office practice of most physicians and surgeons. If suspicion warrants, skin scrapings of the perianal area may be examined using a potassium hydroxide slide preparation and should be cultured on Sabouraud's medium for yeast and fungi (see Fungal Infections). However, because there is no good evidence to suggest that abnormal fecal flora contributes to the symptoms, neither qualitative nor quantitative assessment of the stool is considered appropriate.[351]

Treatment

Pruritus ani has traditionally been considered a condition that eludes all attempts at cure. Numerous potions, nostrums, and lotions have been employed with varying degrees of success, as well as more aggressive treatment, such as injection of local anesthetics, phenol, and alcohol.[366,367] Excision and skin grafting have also been suggested. Eusebio and colleagues reported "long-term cure" with the use of up to 30 mL of 0.5% methylene blue (i.e., methylthionine chloride) injected intradermally and subcutaneously in 23 individuals with intractable pruritus ani.[147]

Psychological factors have been thought to play a role in contributing to symptoms. However, there has never been objective evidence to demonstrate a statistically significant deviation from a normal personality.[14] It is reasonable to assume that severe perianal itching, 24 hours a day, every day, is likely to make an individual rather irascible.

In recent years, attention has been drawn to the role of diet in the cause of the condition; therefore, an accurately obtained history will often dictate the appropriate treatment. Items that have been implicated include the following:

- Coffee (caffeine)
- Tea (caffeine)
- Carbonated beverages, especially caffeinated colas
- Milk products
- Alcohol, particularly wine and beer
- Tomatoes and tomato products, such as ketchup
- Cheese
- Chocolate
- Citrus fruits, grapes, prunes, figs[349]
- Nuts[163,373]

Cigarette smoking is another factor. It is postulated that all these products induce mucous discharge, probably through a systemic route, or possibly in some instances by changing the pH of the stool.

Because most individuals indulge in one or more of the foregoing substances, it is probable that the physician will receive at least one affirmative response when inquiring about the dietary history. By recognizing the association of one of these agents with pruritus ani, a patient will become an ally of the surgeon. It is therefore important to solicit an individual's understanding and cooperation.[29] A patient may have been previously told that the problem is psychoneurotic, so that the physician's reassurance and sympathy are beneficial factors that contribute to a satisfactory resolution. Removing or changing the dietary factor may cause the symptoms to disappear. Gradual reintroduction of the potentially causative dietary substance is then used to calculate the acceptable daily level.[349] Additionally, promoting complete evacuation with increased fluids and bulking agents (e.g., bran, psyllium) may help avoid the irritation.[42] Rectal irrigation and a bowel management program also may be necessary for those individuals who experience incontinence or leakage of stool (see Chapter 16).

Despite the validity of the previous suggestions, the most important advice that can be given is usually directed toward the management of anal hygiene. Many individuals perceive their problem to be one of lack of cleanliness; the opposite is more likely. Vigorous scrubbing of the area with soap and water will cause the skin to be defatted, and contact dermatitis may supervene. Rarely have I identified a patient with pruritus who was not scrupulous with respect to anal cleanliness (one rather stoic individual even used steel wool); the difficulty is to convince the person that the anal area need not be sterilized.

One should advise the patient to remove the soap from the area! The perineum should be cleansed with plain water, particularly when bathing or showering, and ideally even following defecation. Irrigating the rectum with warm water through a bulb syringe is often ameliorating. Some individuals may actually be allergic to toilet paper, so that in stubborn cases a moist cloth should be used for cleansing. Even in a public toilet, a moistened paper towel is preferable to the irritative effects of continued rubbing with toilet paper. For those with copious discharge, a cotton ball placed at the anal verge, changed as necessary, may be helpful.

Heat and sweat tend to exacerbate pruritus. Although there is no evidence concerning the causative effect of clothes, patients should wear garments and underwear that allow air circulation and dryness. Residue remaining on the clothes after the use of detergents based on biologic enzymes may result in itching, and these should be avoided.[349]

A wealth of topical creams and ointments, obtained over the counter and by prescription, is available for the pruritus ani sufferer. The use of anesthetic ointments and creams (e.g., dibucaine [Nupercainal], pramoxine [Tronolane], benzocaine [Americaine], lidocaine [ELA-Max 5]) is not advised except on a highly limited basis. Symptoms are only temporarily masked, the underlying problem is not addressed, and allergic dermatitis can develop. Soothing creams and lotions are generally preferred to ointments; many are quite satisfactory (e.g., mineral oil and lanolin [Balneol], witch hazel and glycerin [Tucks], pramoxine [Prax]). For more severe skin cracking, bath treatment with Aveeno colloidal oatmeal may be quite helpful.

The brief, severe, burning sensation produced by topical capsaicin results in an inhibitory feedback, which may eliminate the need to scratch. A randomized crossover study showed topical 0.006% capsaicin cream applied three times a day to be effective in those who had pruritus ani for greater than 3 months.[261]

When the proprietary preparation fails, one must consider using a topical steroid; this almost inevitably will bring immediate relief. My own preference is to use Proctocort (1% hydrocortisone cream) or 2.5% Analpram-HC (hydrocortisone and pramoxine) because they are nicely packaged with a plastic applicator. The medication is applied at bedtime and once or twice more during the day, if necessary. It should be discontinued, however, as soon as symptoms resolve, in order to avoid skin atrophy (see Atrophoderma). Prolonged use of topical steroids can also result in the rebound itch after cessation requiring further use; this has often been described as an addiction.[230] Dasan and colleagues opine that patients with unresolved, long-standing pruritus ani and with no other symptoms to suggest colorectal disease should be referred to a dermatologist for assessment and patch testing (see Allergic Dermatitis).[111]

Systemic antihistamines may reduce nocturnal scratching,[43] thus aiding sleep rather than addressing local inhibition. However, there have been no randomized trials evaluating the usefulness of antihistamines in the management of pruritus ani.

Anal tattooing, or intradermal injection of methylene blue, may be considered in those who have failed other treatment measures, have become steroid dependent, or in whom symptoms severely impact quality of life. The postulated mechanism of action is destruction of nerve endings. However, the adverse effects include skin ulceration and necrosis.[269] In the intractable case, sedatives and tranquilizers may be considered. In addition, biofeedback and self-hypnosis have been of demonstrable benefit with some patients. Consultation with a professional familiar with these techniques may be advisable.

Psoriasis

Psoriasis is a common, immune-mediated, chronic inflammatory disease of the skin, characterized by rounded, circumscribed, erythematous, dry, scaling patches covered by grayish white or silvery white scales.[291] The lesions have a predilection for the scalp, nails, extensor surfaces of the limbs, elbows, knees, and the sacral region.[112] When the condition occurs in the anal area, it may cause severe pruritic symptoms. Perianal psoriasis is usually sharply marginated, with a characteristic butterfly distribution extending over the coccyx and sacrum (Figure 9-3). Psoriatic lesions are often present at other sites on the body. Smoking is associated with an increased risk of psoriasis and also with increased severity.[160,190,288] Psoriasis is an independent risk factor for myocardial infarction, coronary artery disease,

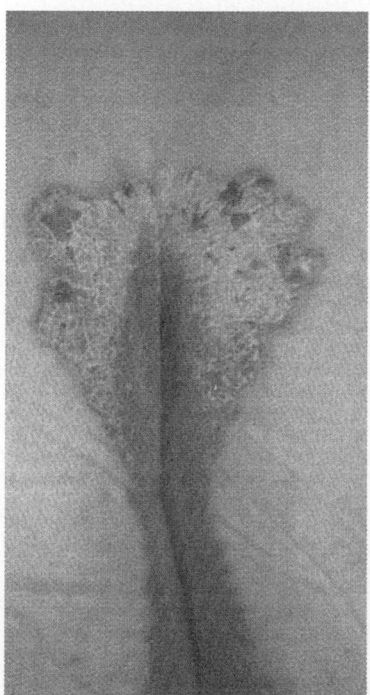

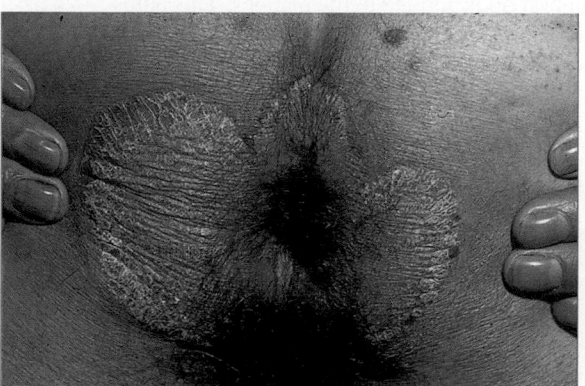

FIGURE 9-3. Well-marginated erythematosquamous plaque with characteristic silvery scales indicates psoriasis. **A:** (Courtesy of Arnold Medved, MD.) Characteristic butterfly appearance of psoriasis in this area, with extension over the coccyx and sacrum. Note absence of changes in the patient's nails. Perianal psoriasis presents prior to systemic skin and nail manifestations in approximately 10% of cases **(B)**.

and atherosclerotic disease in noncardiac sites.[169,316] A recent large observational study suggests the association of psoriasis with malignancy unrelated to the treatment with immunosuppressants.[56] Histologically, characteristic features include epidermal thickening (i.e., acanthosis), regular elongation of the rete ridges with broadening of the deeper aspect, and elongation with edema of the dermal papillae (Figure 9-4). There may be increased mitotic activity in the epidermis. Cells of the stratum corneum usually have retained nuclei (i.e., parakeratosis). Focal collections of neutrophils in the subcorneum are known as Munro's microabscesses.

Treatment may simply consist of moisturizers (emollients) and agents containing salicylic acid. Topical agents include corticosteroids, coal tar products, anthralin, retinoid (tazarotene), a vitamin D_3 derivative (calcipotriene), or a combination of these. In addition, the application of sunlight (not terribly practical for perianal disease) and the use of ultraviolet light B (UVB) have been found to be beneficial. More recently, the so-called PUVA treatment has been advocated. This consists of a combined systemic-external therapy, using a potent photoactive agent (i.e., psoralen) followed by administration of a special light system emitting long-wave UVA. Cancer chemotherapeutic drugs, such as methotrexate and cyclosporine, have also been advocated.

One may understandably be reluctant to treat psoriasis without dermatologic consultation unless the condition is localized to the perianal area and then only for a limited course.

Lichen Planus

Lichen planus is a skin condition that consists of an eruption of small, flat-topped papules with a distinct violaceous color and polypoid configuration. The cutaneous manifestations begin on the volar aspects of the wrists and forearms. The lesion is characteristically found on the flexor surfaces, mucous membranes, genitalia (25%), and occasionally in the perianal area. Wickham striae are intersecting gray lines that can be seen if mineral oil is applied to the plaques. This helps to establish the diagnosis.[269] There have been rare reports of squamous cell carcinoma developing within lichen planus in

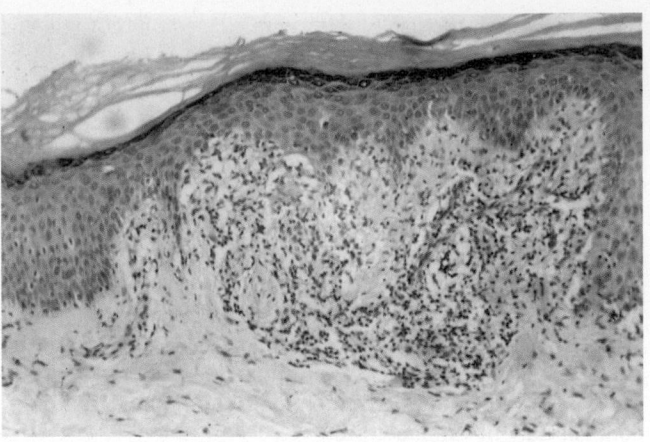

FIGURE 9-5. Characteristics of lichen planus include moderate hyperkeratosis, thickening of the stratum granulosum, sawtooth configuration of the rete ridges, and lymphocytic infiltration of the dermis and basal cell layer. Note the sharp demarcation of the lymphocytic infiltrate. (Original magnification × 120; courtesy of Rudolf Garret, MD.)

the anal area.[164] This condition may be seen in patients with disease processes characterized by altered cell-mediated immune responses.[269]

Histologically, the papule shows focal thickening of the granular layer, degeneration of the basement membrane and basal cells, and a bandlike lymphocytic infiltrate in the upper dermis (Figure 9-5). Biopsy of the skin establishes the diagnosis.

Treatment often has less than satisfactory results, with corticosteroids appearing to be the most helpful for this condition. Topical preparations with occlusive dressings are quite useful, and systemic administration and intralesional injections have also been employed. In mild cases, antipruritic lotions and antihistamines are suggested. Rest is also helpful.

Lichen Sclerosus et Atrophicus

Lichen sclerosus et atrophicus is an unusual condition of unknown cause. It occurs much more frequently in women than in men. The genital area appears to be the most commonly involved site.

Physical examination may reveal the characteristic "inverted keyhole" distribution. In this situation, the disease extends beyond the mucocutaneous border to involve the skin of the vulva, perineum, and perianal area. In the vulva, the condition affects the labia, vestibule, and introitus (Figure 9-6). Discomfort, pruritus, dysuria, and dyspareunia are common complaints.

The characteristic histologic changes in lichen sclerosus et atrophicus are edema and homogenization of the collagen below the epidermis (Figure 9-7). The epidermis also shows variable hyperkeratosis and follicular plugging. Lichen sclerosus et atrophicus may be associated with squamous cell carcinoma of the vulva. An association between the condition and squamous cell carcinoma of the perianal region has also been noted.[354]

Because of the small risk of malignancy, all nonresponders or those with recurrent sclerosis should have a skin biopsy.[349]

Treatment is primarily directed to the relief of the pruritic complaints in the hope of lessening the risk for leukoplakia

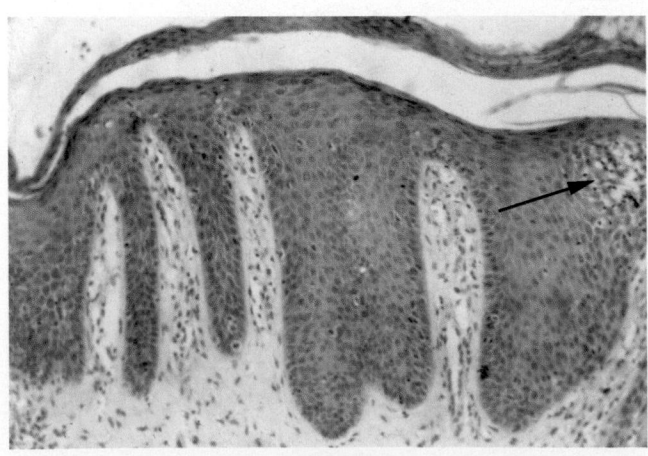

FIGURE 9-4. Psoriasis. Elongation of the rete ridges and edema of the dermal papillae are characteristic features of psoriasis. Note parakeratosis, Munro abscess (*arrow*), and the absence of a granular cell layer. (Original magnification × 180; courtesy of Rudolf Garret, MD.)

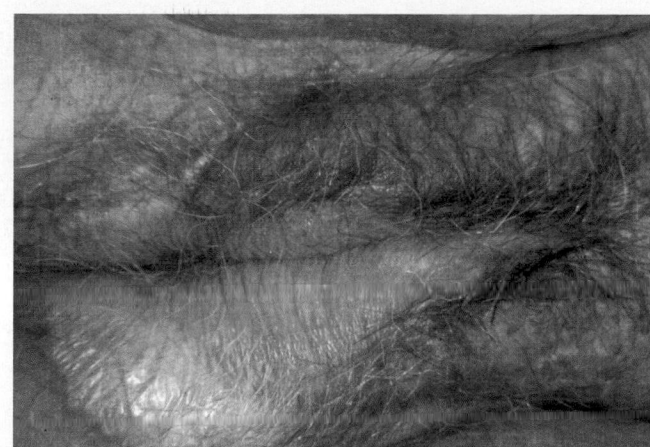
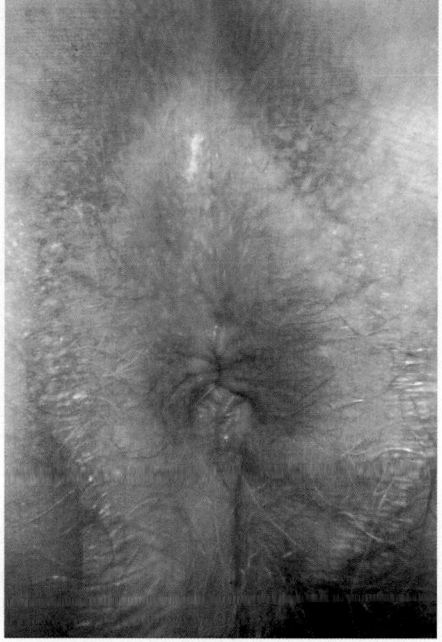

A

B

FIGURE 9-6. Characteristic of lichen sclerosus et atrophicus is a sharply defined dermatosis in the **(A)** vulvar area and **(B)** perianum with hypopigmentation centrally and hyperpigmentation peripherally. Note the lichenoid papules about the periphery. (Courtesy of John A. Clark, MD.)

and carcinoma. A mild topical steroid sufficient to control the symptoms is advocated. Retinoids and testosterone creams have also been described.[275,345] Secondary infection should be treated with appropriate antibiotics.

Atrophoderma or Atrophy of the Skin

Atrophy of the skin is a reaction to the repeated and prolonged application of topical corticosteroids; it may also follow local injection of these products.[173] Telangiectasia occurs, indicating loss of dermal collagen, and the patient who initially complained of pruritus subsequently reports discomfort and burning.[357] The friction of walking rubs the already atrophic and thinned epidermis.

Patients usually report a history of self-application of topical corticosteroids for many years. Attempting to remove the medication is frequently unsuccessful. Biopsy may

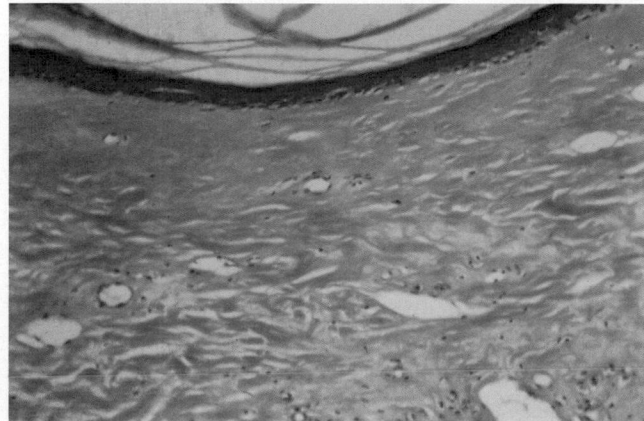

FIGURE 9-7. Atrophy of the epidermis and hyalinization of the dermis in lichen sclerosis et atrophicus. (Original magnification × 120; courtesy of Rudolf Garret, MD.)

reveal atrophy and hyperkeratosis. Because of the risk for development of this condition, it is important to discontinue the use of cortisone treatment as soon as possible.

Irritant and Contact or Allergic Dermatitis

Two types of dermatitis are caused by substances coming into contact with the skin:

- Irritant dermatitis (caused by a nonallergic reaction following exposure to an irritating substance)
- Allergic (contact) dermatitis caused by allergic sensitization to a number of agents[122]

Irritants include alkalis, acids, metal salts, dusts, gases, and hydrocarbons. Allergic contact dermatitis results from hypersensitivity of the delayed type, also known as *cell-mediated hypersensitivity or immunity*.[122] A person may be exposed to an allergen for many years before hypersensitivity develops. The allergens are numerous and varied, as follows:

- Dyes
- Oils
- Resins
- Chemicals used for fabrics, cosmetics, and insecticides
- Products or the substances of bacteria, fungi, and parasites[122]

The most common causes of contact dermatitis are as follows, in order of frequency:

1. Poison ivy, oak, and sumac
2. Paraphenylenediamine
3. Nickel
4. Common rubber compounds
5. Neomycin
6. Dichromates[154]

The patch test is used to detect hypersensitivity to a substance that is in contact with the skin (see Pruritus Ani). A nonirritating concentration of agents suspected to be the cause of the contact dermatitis is applied. The patches remain in place for 48 hours, less if burning or itching occurs. A positive reaction will produce severe pruritus and erythema or vesicles. It is wise to defer this test, however, until the rash has cleared to limit the likelihood of a severe exacerbation.

Therapy obviously is directed toward removing the underlying cause of the skin problem or the allergen. Iodine and adhesive tape are common dermatitis-inducing products in patients who undergo anal surgery. Soothing compresses such as Aveeno colloidal oatmeal, in addition to corticosteroids and possibly antipruritics, may be advisable.

Seborrheic Dermatitis

Seborrheic dermatitis is a chronic, superficial, inflammatory disease of the skin, with a predilection for the scalp, eyebrows, nasolabial crease, ears, axillae, submammary folds, umbilicus, groin, and natal cleft. The disease is characterized by dry, moist, or greasy scales and by crusted, pink-yellow patches of diverse size and shape.[124] The condition is believed to be caused by hypersecretion of sebum and is apparently exacerbated by increased perspiration and emotional stress. A high fat intake is frequently noted.

Histologically, the picture is not dissimilar to that of psoriasis, but Munro's abscesses are not seen. According to one school of thought, the two conditions are so similar that there is some justification for thinking their origin may be the same. However, more recent evidence favors a role for yeast organisms in the etiology of the condition, with therapy being directed accordingly. Still, application of corticosteroids is the primary therapy.

Atopic Dermatitis or Atopic Eczema

The term *atopy* is derived from the Greek word meaning "out of place" or "strange." It is defined as the tendency for allergies to manifest themselves by systemic symptoms, such as asthma, hay fever, and eczema.[121] The condition is believed to be either a form of immunologic deficiency or possibly a blockade of β-adrenergic receptors in the skin.

Atopic dermatitis can occur as localized, erythematous, scaly, papular, or vesicular patches or in the form of pruritic, lichenified lesions.[124] The condition is often paroxysmal, with an emotional upset initiating some attacks. Other factors exacerbating the problem may be clothing, certain foods, and dryness of the skin. Superimposed infections such as intertrigo and dermatophytosis may produce further recurrences. The most common secondary skin infections in atopic dermatitis are caused by herpes simplex virus (HSV) and *Staphylococcus aureus*.[303] In the absence of clinical signs of infection, most atopic dermatitis patients are also colonized with *S. aureus* on their skin lesions. This pathogen produces proinflammatory factors that trigger the cutaneous immune system.[340] The severity of dermatitis correlates with the density of *S. aureus* colonization of skin lesions.[406] Anti-*S. aureus* antibiotics have been shown to improve the severity of atopic dermatitis.[59] Histologically, hyperkeratosis and parakeratosis with acanthosis are noted (Figure 9-8). When lichenification is present, the acanthosis is increased, and there is papillomatosis, with long papillary bodies reaching to the stratum corneum. These changes may somewhat resemble those seen in psoriasis.

Treatment consists of avoiding emotional stress, if possible; avoiding extremes of cold and heat; limiting the use

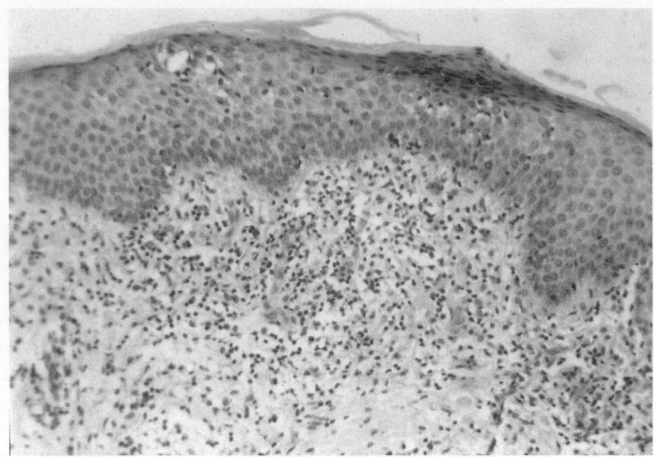

FIGURE 9-8. Histologic characteristics of atopic dermatitis include mild acanthosis, spongiosis, focal parakeratosis, and dermal mononuclear cell infiltrate. (Original magnification × 180; courtesy of Rudolf Garret, MD.)

of stimulant beverages; and using oral antihistamines and topical corticosteroids. Prednisone, 30 to 40 mg orally for 4 to 6 weeks or possibly longer, is usually recommended. Alternatively, a parenteral preparation may be substituted.

Radiodermatitis

Radiodermatitis is a particular problem in the anal area because current therapy for carcinoma of the rectum, anus, and prostate often involves ionizing radiation. In some individuals, unfortunately, the side effects of the cancer treatment may actually lead to worse symptoms than the original disease (see Chapters 24 and 25).

Many changes are found in the cell as the result of radiation therapy. Mitoses are temporarily arrested, chromosomal abnormalities occur, and there is at least a temporary halt in the normal cell cycle. The amount of skin change resulting from radiotherapy depends on the dose. These alterations may be manifested as erythema, edema, and ulceration, and symptoms may include burning, itching, or severe pain. After a period, telangiectasia, atrophy, and freckling may appear. The skin becomes dry, thin, smooth, and shiny (Figure 9-9). Radiation injury may result in the subsequent development of malignancy, in most cases following a rather prolonged latent period. The manifestations of this complication increase with the passage of time.

Results of treatment are often less than satisfactory. However, symptomatic improvement has been reported with a regimen consisting of oral vitamin A, 8,000 IU, given twice daily.[251] Hyperbaric oxygen treatment has also been recommended. Cleansing the area with mild soap and water, in addition to the use of an emollient, a corticosteroid preparation, or both, may be of help. Biopsy specimens should be taken from any suspected lesions.

Behçet's Syndrome

Behçet's syndrome is characterized by four main symptoms: recurrent aphthous ulcers in the mouth, skin lesions, eye lesions, and genital ulcerations.[197] Genital ulcerations may be found in persons of both sexes on the genitocrural fold, on the anus, on the perineum, or in the rectum. Scrotal scarring secondary to ulcers is rarely found in conditions other

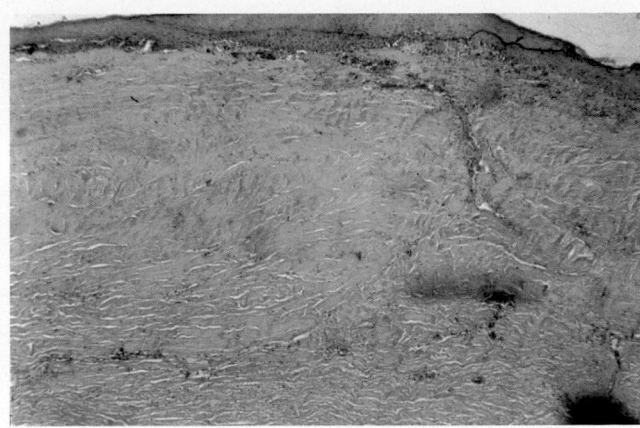

A

B

FIGURE 9-9. Radiodermatitis. **A:** Erythematous, smooth, and shiny buttocks skin with associated linear necrotic ulceration that developed during the course of neoadjuvant radiation therapy for rectal cancer. **B:** Histologic findings of radiodermatitis include fibrosis of the dermis with sclerosis, atrophy of the epidermis, and the absence of skin appendages. (Original magnification × 120; courtesy of Rudolf Garret, MD.)

than Behçet's syndrome. Although the cause of the condition is unknown, there is some evidence to suggest that it is of viral origin or possibly represents an autoimmune disease. Behçet's is one of the few forms of vasculitis in which there is a known genetic predisposition. Histologically, the lesions usually show vasculitis involving vessels of all sizes—small, medium, and large—on both the arterial and venous sides of the circulation.

The anal condition may be misdiagnosed as hemorrhoids, fissure, Crohn's disease, condylomata, or STI.[197] Surgery is contraindicated, and corticosteroid treatment, systemically or topically, is the preferred treatment (see also Chapter 28).

Lupus Erythematosus

Lupus erythematosus, like other connective tissue diseases, only rarely occurs in the anal area and still more rarely develops as an isolated finding in this location. The cutaneous manifestation is called *discoid lupus erythematosus* (DLE). It may begin with single or multiple lesions involving entire regions of the body, especially the head and neck, sternum, vulva, and perineum. The typical plaque is approximately 1 cm or more in diameter, with characteristic scales. Removal of the scales reveals patulous follicular orifices with dry, horny, keratinous plugs.[123] Occasionally, basal cell or squamous cell carcinoma may develop in long-standing DLE lesions.

In laboratory investigation, the LE cell test usually yields a negative result in DLE. Results of the direct immunofluorescence test are usually positive, however, as are antinuclear antibody test results.

Treatment consists of avoidance of strong sunlight, extremes in temperature, and localized trauma. Smoking cessation is recommended because smokers tend to have more active disease.[159,170] Corticosteroid creams and ointments are particularly beneficial, with intralesional steroid therapy often helpful. Systemic therapy with antimalarials and immunosuppressive agents also has been advised.

Dermatomyositis

Dermatomyositis (polymyositis) is an inflammatory condition that produces angiopathy in the skin, subcutaneous tissue, and muscles. Women are twice as likely to be affected as men. Many clinical and serologic features of the disease vary widely among affected individuals, depending on the patient's immunogenetic profile and a host of potential environmental triggers.[344,300] The disease usually starts on the face and eyelids as a heliotrope rash and may spread to other areas forming a "shawl sign" of diffuse, flat, erythematous lesions over the chest and shoulders and affecting the metacarpophalangeal and interphalangeal joints in a symmetric fashion (so-called Gottron's sign). It is associated with a number of other disturbances, including Raynaud's phenomenon, alopecia, urticaria, and erythema multiforme. Of particular interest to the surgeon is that in patients older than 40 years of age, visceral cancer is frequently associated with the condition. The spectrum of malignancies usually parallels the distribution in the general population with a few exceptions. Dermatomyositis carries an increased risk of cancer mortality compared with the general population.[63,350,417] Additional risk factors for malignancy include evidence of capillary damage on muscle biopsy,[390] cutaneous necrosis of the trunk,[34] cutaneous leukocytoclastic vasculitis,[195] and older age (older than 65) at the diagnosis of dermatomyositis.[267] Histologic changes are similar to those of lupus erythematosus. Treatment consists of rest, salicylates, steroids, methotrexate, and azathioprine.

Scleroderma or Progressive Systemic Sclerosis

Scleroderma is characterized by the appearance of areas that are immobile and give the skin the appearance of being "hidebound."[123] The skin becomes smooth, yellowish, and firm, and it shrinks so that the underlying structures are bound down. Although the condition frequently involves the face and hands, leading to an expressionless appearance on the former and a clawlike appearance of the latter, it can progress to involve most of the internal organs. Involvement of the small intestine may cause constipation, diarrhea, and abdominal distension. Although the colon is only rarely affected, it can produce the signs and symptoms of Ogilvie's syndrome (see Chapter 20). Systemic sclerosis appears to be associated with a modest increase in the overall risk of malignant disease.[114] The most significant association appears to be with lung cancer.[46,76] There is also an association with skin cancer, hepatoma, and hematopoietic malignancies,[314] and there is a marked increase in the risk of esophageal carcinoma and oropharyngeal carcinoma.[334] Treatment consists of supportive measures, baths, a high-protein diet, corticosteroids, and a number of other medications, including immunosuppressives.

Erythema Multiforme

Erythema multiforme is a clinically and histologically distinctive skin disease that is precipitated by the following conditions, among others:

- Viral infections
- Bacterial infections
- Radiotherapy
- Carcinomatosis
- Pregnancy
- Connective tissue diseases
- Drug reactions

The mechanism for this particular reaction is unknown. The lesions present as flat, dull red maculopapules that may be rather small or may increase to 1 or 2 cm in 48 hours. The periphery may remain red, whereas the center is purpuric. The lesions look almost like targets. They commonly appear in the oral mucous membrane, but genital lesions are also frequent.

Histologically, the abnormality is confined to the upper dermis and lower epidermis. In more severe cases, there is necrosis of the whole epidermis. Bullae usually are subepidermal.

Treatment consists of symptomatic relief in mild cases, but in severe instances the use of corticosteroids has been suggested. Antibiotics are advised if secondary infection develops.

Familial Benign Chronic Pemphigus or Hailey-Hailey

Familial benign chronic pemphigus is a hereditary disease characterized by a recurrent bullous and vesicular dermatitis of the neck, axillae, flexors, and surfaces that appose. The condition has been found localized to the perianal area and may pose confusion in differential diagnosis (Figure 9-10).[404] The disease is transmitted as an autosomal dominant trait. It generally presents between the second and the fourth decade. Usually, the disease persists throughout life and is triggered by UV light, friction, sweating, and bacterial infections.

The condition is caused by a defect in keratinocyte adhesion based on the mutation of the ATP2C1 gene

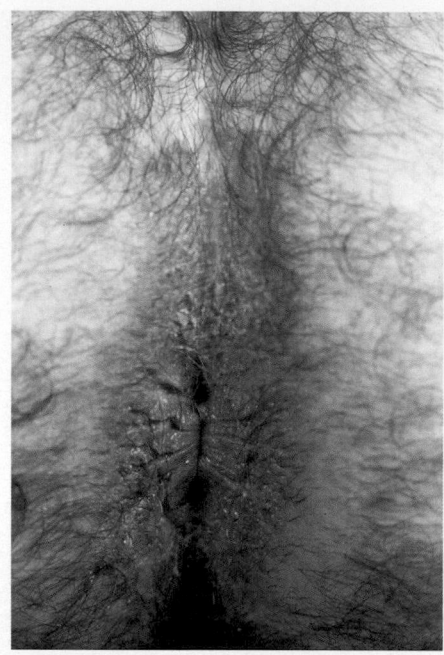

FIGURE 9-10. Hailey-Hailey. A macerated erythematous patch has well-defined borders. (Courtesy of Samuel L. Moschella, MD.)

on chromosome 3q21-q24.[67] The histologic pattern is unique, with prominent intraepidermal vesicles and bullae (Figure 9-11).

Treatment consists of local or systemic antibiotics and the use of topical corticosteroids. Additionally, low-dose radiation treatment has been recommended. Localized areas have been treated by excision and skin grafting.

Pemphigus Vulgaris

Pemphigus vulgaris is characterized by bullae appearing on apparently normal skin and mucous membranes.[127] The lesions usually begin first in the mouth and next

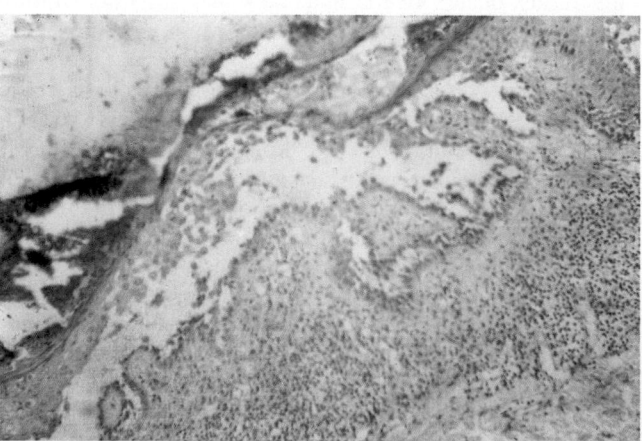

FIGURE 9-11. Benign familial chronic pemphigus (Hailey-Hailey) is characterized by suprabasal bullae, such as the one shown here, containing detached prickle cells and good preservation of acantholytic cells. Note the moderate inflammatory reaction in the underlying dermis. (Original magnification × 180; courtesy of Rudolf Garret, MD.)

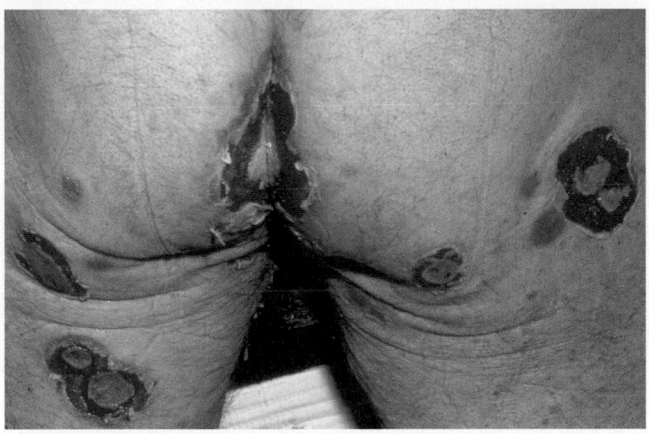

FIGURE 9-12. Pemphigus vulgaris. Bullae affect the perineum and buttocks with characteristic lesions.

in the groin, scalp, face, neck, axillae, and genitals (Figure 9-12). It appears that an autoimmune mechanism is the cause. The condition occurs equally in both sexes, usually in adults in their fifth and sixth decades. Circulating intercellular antibodies directed against desmoglein, an adhesion molecule, may be demonstrated in these individuals.[18,364]

The pathologic changes are acantholysis, cleft and blister formation in the intraepidermal areas just above the basal cell layer, and the formation of acantholytic cells (Figure 9-13).[127] Characteristic of the separation of keratinocytes is the presence of Tzanck's cell lining the bulla, as well as lying free in the cavity.

Because of the pain associated with advanced cases, prolonged daily baths with permanganate solution may be advised. Silver sulfadiazine (Silvadene) cream, which is effective in the treatment of burns, is also useful in this condition. High-dose corticosteroids (160 mg of prednisone daily) remain the primary therapy. Immunosuppressive agents, such as azathioprine, cyclophosphamide, cyclosporine, and methotrexate, are part of the

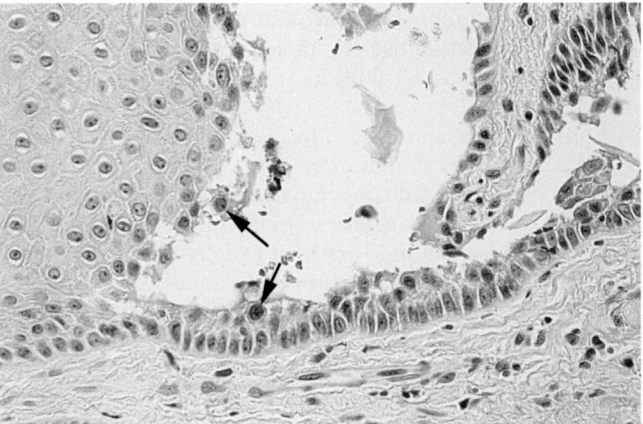

FIGURE 9-13. Intraepithelial vesicles such as this one are characteristic of pemphigus vulgaris. The *arrows* indicate cells with large hyperchromatic nuclei (Tzanck's cells). There is an absence of inflammatory reaction in the dermis. (Original magnification × 600.)

multimodality approach, which may include antibiotics, antimalarials, gold, and plasmapheresis. Treatment with rituximab with or without intravenous immunoglobulin appears to be an effective therapy in patients with refractory disease.[7,189,196]

Cicatricial Pemphigoid or Benign Mucosal Pemphigoid

Cicatricial pemphigoid is characterized by the presence of transient vesicles that heal by scarring of mucous membranes. The condition most commonly occurs in the mouth and conjunctivae. Other areas of involvement include the pharynx, esophagus, genitalia, and anus. In rare cases, the lesion has been confined to the genital and anal areas.[393] Direct immunofluorescence of the lesion reveals the presence of antibodies at the basement membrane. Individuals with autoantibodies directed at epiligrin (laminin 5) appear to have a high risk for adenocarcinoma.[139] The absence of acantholysis differentiates the condition from pemphigus vulgaris.

There is no effective medication for cicatricial pemphigoid. Obstructing areas in the larynx and esophagus may require tracheostomy or gastrostomy.

▶ INFECTIOUS CONDITIONS

For the purposes of discussion, we have taken the liberty of classifying the infectious processes as those that are nonvenereal and those that are usually attributable to venereal causes.

Nonvenereal Infections
Pilonidal Sinus

Pilonidal sinus is a common infective process occurring in the natal cleft and sacrococcygeal region. It primarily affects young adults and teenagers. There is a 3:1 male predominance. In the military in particular, it has been a considerable source of concern regarding personnel and economics. For example, more than 77,000 soldiers were admitted to army hospitals for symptoms from pilonidal sinus disease from 1942 through 1945, and they remained for an average of 44 days.[332] In 1973, more than 70,000 patients were admitted to nongovernmental hospitals in the United States with the primary diagnosis of a pilonidal sinus.[264] As recently as 1980, more than 40,000 patients with pilonidal disease were hospitalized in the United States, averaging more than 5 days of in-hospital care.[31] Of course, this was before government and insurance company restrictions were applied in the United States concerning permissible days in the hospital for a given illness.

The condition was originally described by Anderson in a letter to the editor of the *Boston Medical Surgical Journal* of 1847 and was subsequently named "pilonidal sinus" by Hodges in 1880.[19,192] The term literally means "nest of hair"; this is because the epithelium-lined sinus usually is found to contain hair.

When the sinus becomes infected, commonly after puberty, it drains from an opening or openings overlying the coccyx and sacrum (Figure 9-14). The infected abscess may extend to the perianal area in a presentation that may be

ABRAHAM WENDELL ANDERSON (1804–1876)

Anderson was born in Windham, Maine, the son of the first settlers in the town. He attended Gorham Academy and in 1829 graduated from Bowdoin Medical School. He established his practice in the town of Gray Corner, where he remained all his life. In 1868, he participated in the founding of the Cumberland County Medical Society and was elected its first president. In his letter, Anderson reports a 21-year-old man with what was thought to be a scrofulous sore on his back.[19] The author found "a fistula opening near the os coccygis," which he drained. Three weeks later, he drew out of the cavity "a hair, very finely matted, and about two inches in length." The discharge stopped, and the wound healed rapidly.

RICHARD MANNING HODGES (1827–1896)

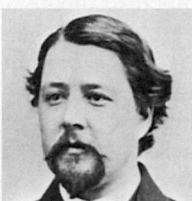

Hodges was born in Bridgewater, Massachusetts. He graduated from Harvard College in the class of 1847 and subsequently received his MA and MD at Harvard Medical School. He then joined the faculty there in the department of anatomy as a demonstrator, a position he held until 1861. He was befriended by the renowned Boston surgeon, Henry Bigelow, who helped launch him toward a successful career in surgery. Hodges served on the Board of Overseers of Harvard College and as a visiting surgeon at the Massachusetts General Hospital. He was a member of the American Academy of Arts and Sciences. Although many of his writings were on orthopedics and trauma, it is because of his article, read before the Boston Society for Medical Improvement, in which he names the condition "pilonidal sinus" that he is recognized today.

mistaken for an anal fistula. The disease can also be confused with suppurative hidradenitis (see later). Although the condition is by no means life threatening, it does cause considerable disability for many individuals. Time lost from school or work can amount to months.

Etiology

The etiology of the condition has been the subject of some controversy and discussion. One possible theory that has been espoused is the failure of fusion in the embryo, with resultant entrapment of hair follicles in the sacrococcygeal region. Proponents of this theory are quick to point out the frequent incidence of eyebrow hair that meets in the midline in such patients. Another theory attributes the problem to the result of trauma, with the introduction of hair shafts into the subdermal area. Mechanical forces, such as suction, assist the hairs in penetrating deeper in the subcutaneous tissue. As a person sits or bends, this draws the skin of the natal cleft more taut, lifting it away from the underlying sacrococcygeal fascia. This creates negative pressure in the subcutaneous tissue, which draws hair deeper into the space. It has long been observed that the natal cleft is often deeper in patients with a pilonidal sinus, one of the variables that one may consider in determining the choice of surgical management, especially with those that flatten the cleft.[8] Doll and colleagues observed that a family history of pilonidal sinus predisposes to an earlier onset of the condition and is associated with as much as a 50% long-term recurrence rate.[119]

Lord observed a number of interesting features of the condition.[259] He believed that there was a constant relationship between the lateral sinus openings and the midline pits; the openings were always cephalad to the pits. Lord further observed the presence of 23 hairs of exactly the same length, diameter, color, and orientation in a patient. He postulated that it would be impossible for this number of hairs to follow each other into a pilonidal sinus and be identical in every respect. Lord applied this observation by proposing that the treatment of pilonidal sinus could therefore be made quite simple. He suggested that all that is required is the removal of the offending hair follicle and the hairs that have been shed. These observations were subsequently confirmed by Bascom, a concept that led to his proposed surgical approach (see later).[31]

FIGURE 9-14. Pilonidal sinus. Note the multiple openings overlying the sacrum and buttocks.

Symptoms and Findings

The patient usually presents with pain, swelling, and purulent drainage at and around the site of the pilonidal opening. A solitary midline opening or pit may be observed, or there may be numerous openings, with pus draining and hair protruding. The typical appearance of an abscess that can be found anywhere in the skin and subcutaneous tissue may be evident. Fever and leukocytosis may also accompany the symptoms.

Most individuals may merely observe periodic discharge or intermittent swelling and discomfort. The process may resolve spontaneously or progress to more obvious drainage, an abscess, and severe pain. Long-standing disease may be associated with the development of squamous cell carcinoma (see later). A critical symptom, *bleeding* in a sinus that has been present for many years, warrants special attention and surgical intervention.[408] An association with condylomata and HIV has also been described with squamous cell cancer.[51] Other reported complications of the condition are sacral osteomyelitis, necrotizing fasciitis, toxic shock syndrome, and meningitis.[394,408]

Treatment

As with other septic processes in the perianal area, antibiotics have little place in the therapy, except possibly as an adjunct to the surgical procedure in a septic or immunocompromised patient. For acute pilonidal abscess, incision and drainage should relieve the patient's symptoms. Regardless of the size of the septic process, this can usually be accomplished in a physician's office or in an ambulatory care facility. Whenever possible, it is advisable to drain the abscess and curette or excise the infected sinus simultaneously. The Standards Task Force of the American Society of Colon and Rectal Surgeons has established certain practice parameters for the performance of ambulatory surgery.[363] The following represents their complete statement:

> Localized pilonidal abscesses, either primary or recurrent, can usually be incised and drained under local anesthesia in an outpatient setting. For uncomplicated pilonidal sinuses, definitive surgical treatment, including but not limited to excision, curettage, and unroofing, can be accomplished as an outpatient procedure.

More complicated surgical procedures, including but not limited to wide excision, creation of skin flaps, and grafting, may require inpatient stay for concern over skin viability or bleeding. Extensive cellulitis in association with pilonidal disease may require inpatient intravenous antibiotic therapy.[363]

Definitive elective treatment of pilonidal disease includes excision and primary closure, excision and grafting, excision leaving the wound open to close secondarily, incision and curettage, follicle excision, and cryosurgical destruction.

Drainage with or without Excision. Incision or excision with drainage is rather simple to accomplish, requires minimal hospital stay, and in fact usually can be accomplished with a local anesthetic in the office. A probe is passed from opening to opening, and the sinus is unroofed (Figure 9-15A). Alternatively, the multiple openings can be excised en bloc, with further extensions or side tracts curetted out (Figure 9-15B). If the procedure is undertaken on an ambulatory basis, the patient is instructed to remove the packing the following morning, usually while taking a bath.

Shpitz and colleagues perform what they term a "controlled excision" by means of loop diathermy.[346] The procedure consists of incision and drainage of any pus, followed by excision of diseased tissue and lateral sinuses. With this approach, an expeditious surgical procedure and a shortened or eliminated hospital stay are, in essence, exchanged for a prolonged postoperative convalescence, especially if one is dealing with extensive or deep tissue involvement. All too often, these difficult wounds require frequent treatments, necessitating cauterization, shaving, cleansing, and packing,[27,313] although there is a real question whether prophylactic hair epilation reduces the likelihood of recurrence. An approach to dealing with this problem has been suggested by Rosenberg.[333] He advocates taping the buttocks apart to flatten the intergluteal cleft during the healing process. However, there is little existing evidence to support the use of antimicrobial agents for chronic wound healing.[301]

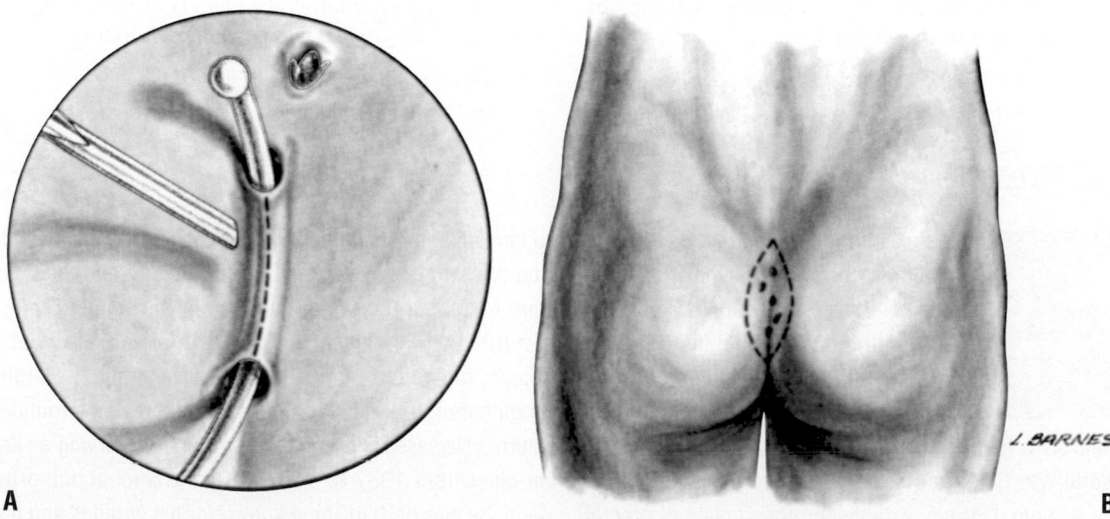

A   **B**

FIGURE 9-15. Excision and packing for the treatment of pilonidal sinus can be accomplished by **(A)** unroofing of the individual tract or by **(B)** an all-encompassing excision.

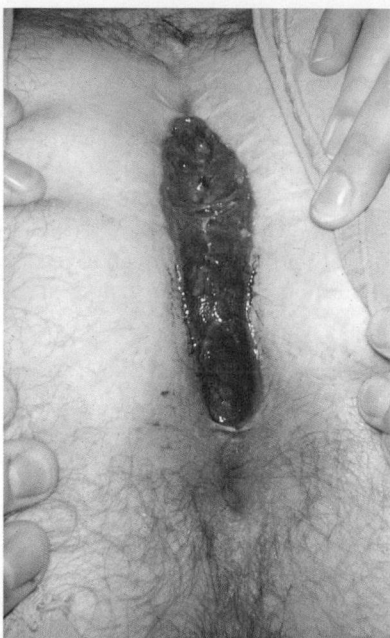

FIGURE 9-16. Indolent, granulating, nonhealing wound of a recurrent (persistent) pilonidal sinus.

It is not uncommon for pilonidal sinus wounds that extend toward the anal verge to take 6 months or longer to heal (Figure 9-16). Delayed healing may persist to the point where re-excision is advised; multiple operative procedures are frequent sequelae under these circumstances. It is for this reason that one may be reluctant to advise this particular approach except for relatively small sinuses.

A more recent option for the postoperative management of a complex or large pilonidal sinus is *vacuum-assisted closure.*[274] This technique employs a subatmospheric pressure dressing that consists of a foam pad cut to the internal shape of the wound and inserted with a plastic fenestrated tube applied to the center.[274] In theory, the vacuum device assists wound contraction by exerting a centripetal force and increases blood flow while reducing edema and tissue bacterial counts.[274] Disadvantages include the initial hospital charges, the relative immobility of the patient, and the cost associated with the use of the pump.

Marsupialization. Excision with marsupialization is a compromise between a completely open wound and a completely closed one. This approach was initially described by Buie in 1937 and amplified later in his article on "jeep disease."[65] This operation permits a somewhat smaller opening than does the technique in which the wound is left totally open (Figure 9-17). If the catgut or long-term absorbable suture succeeds in holding the edges together, more rapid healing should occur. Unfortunately, the sutures frequently pull out, and the individual is left with as wide a wound as would have resulted had excision and packing been employed. Even without this complication, the wound still requires careful attention, including packing, perhaps shaving, cauterization and cleansing.

Oncel and coworkers undertook a prospective, randomized study in which 40 consecutive patients with "limited, chronic pilonidal disease" were operated on with either excision or marsupialization.[302] Operation time, hospital stay, and time lost from work were all shorter in the former group. Furthermore, patient satisfaction was significantly greater in this group, primarily because the procedure was undertaken on an outpatient basis.

Excision with Primary Closure. Excision with primary closure can be performed in an ambulatory surgical facility if the sinus is relatively small. However, for more extensive lesions, inpatient therapy is recommended. This approach has the disadvantage of a relatively prolonged hospital stay, but it provides the potential benefit of a healed wound within perhaps 10 to 14 days. For large, complex pilonidal sinus problems, particularly when multiple procedures have been previously performed (see Figure 9-16), the excision and primary closure technique may be very effective.

The pilonidal sinus is excised to the gluteal fascia (Figure 9-18A). The fascia is incised, and a periosteal elevator is used to lift the fascia off the sacrum (Figure 9-18B). This maneuver permits the placement of heavy retention sutures through all layers. These are laid into position, and the fascia is reapproximated with absorbable suture material (Figure 9-19A). The wound is copiously irrigated, and the skin is closed (Figure 9-19B). The retention sutures are secured over a stent dressing, and the dressing is left in place for approximately 10 days (Figure 9-19C). When the pilonidal sinus extends near the anal opening, it is better to

LOUIS A. BUIE (1890–1975)

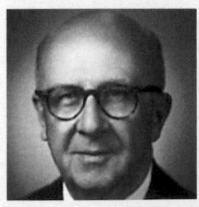

Buie was born in Kingstree, South Carolina and received his bachelor's degree from the University of South Carolina in 1911. He graduated from the University of Maryland Medical School, and after internship in Maryland, he entered the Mayo Clinic as a fellow in surgery. Following service in Italy during World War I, he returned to the Mayo Clinic and, at the request of William J. Mayo, established the section of proctology. A founder of the American Board of Proctology and twice president of the American Proctologic Society, he played a leading role in the development of proctology and, later, of colon and rectal surgery as a specialty in the United States. Other contributions included designs of a sigmoidoscope, proctoscopic table, and biopsy forceps. In addition, he authored or coauthored three texts on proctology and was a founder of the journal *Diseases of the Colon and Rectum*, serving as its editor-in-chief from 1957 to 1967. An international authority in the field, he was perhaps best known for his writings and treatment of pilonidal sinus.

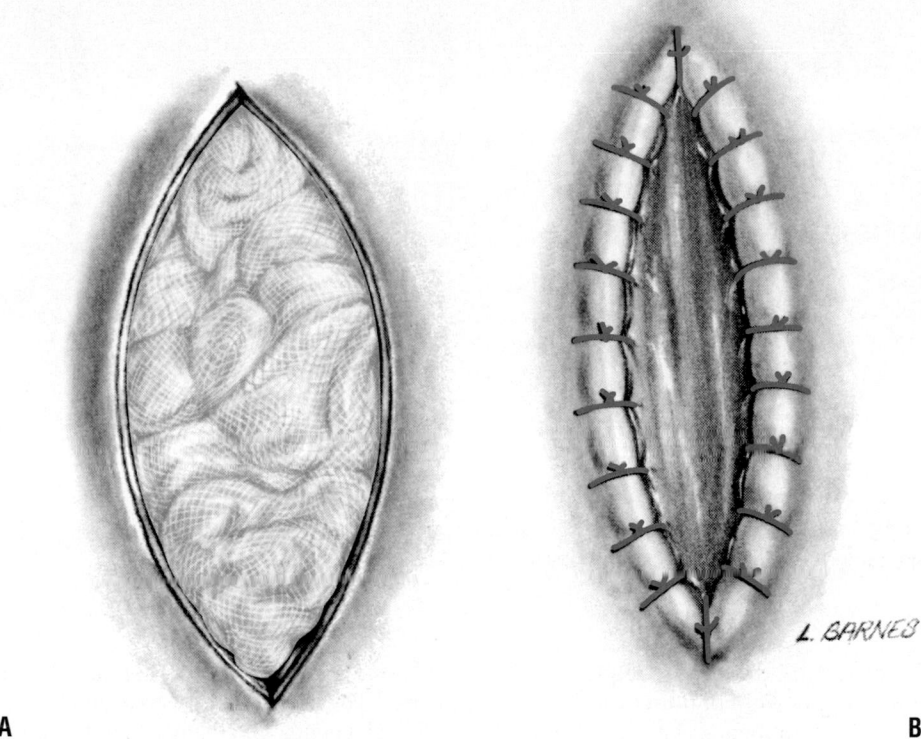

FIGURE 9-17. Appearance of the pilonidal sinus after two different surgical approaches: **(A)** open and packed, usually with iodoform gauze and **(B)** marsupialized, suturing the full thickness of the skin to the underlying epithelialized tract or fascia.

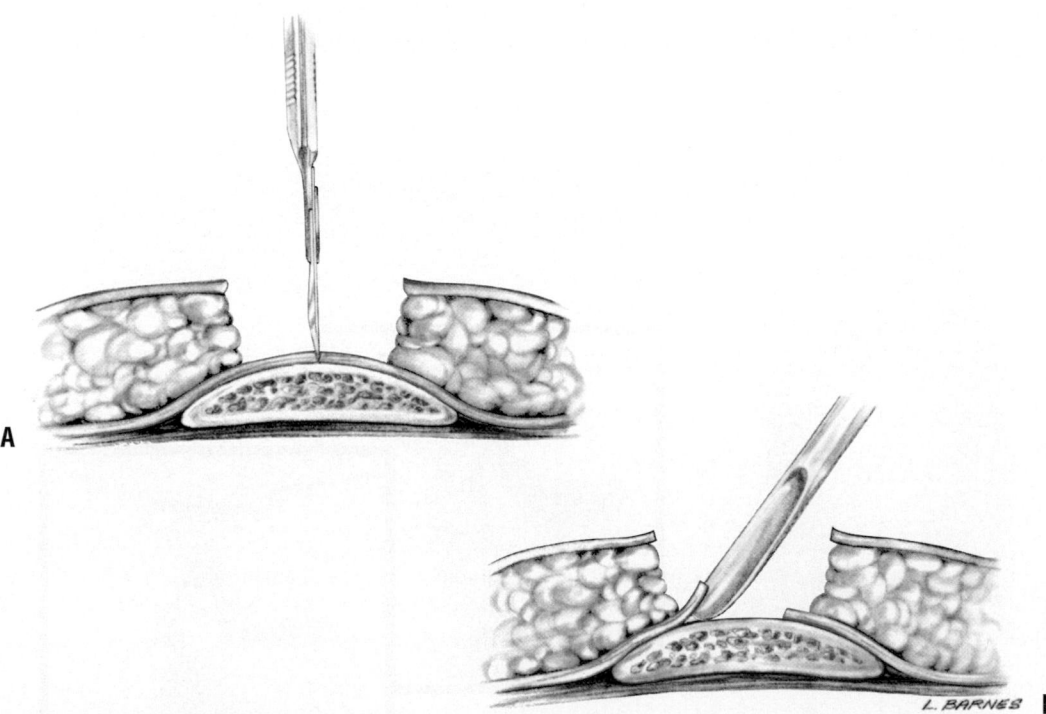

FIGURE 9-18. The first two steps in the primary closure technique for the treatment of pilonidal sinus infection. **A:** The fascia is incised. **B:** The fascia is elevated.

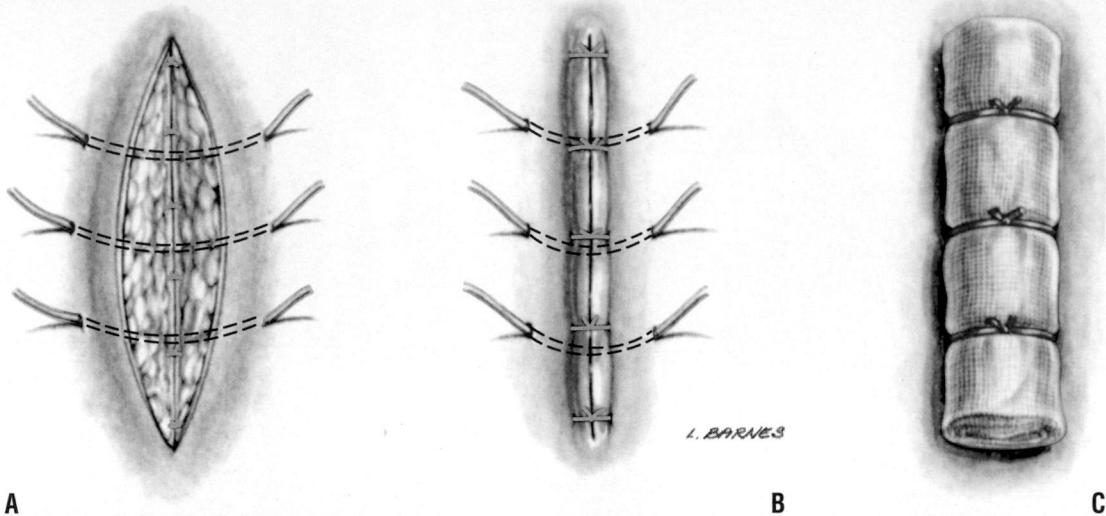

A   **B**   **C**

FIGURE 9-19. The last three steps in the primary closure technique for treating pilonidal sinus infection. **A:** With retention sutures in place, the fascia is closed. **B:** The skin is closed. **C:** A stent dressing is secured.

confine the bowels for several days. This requires a clear liquid diet and the use of a bowel-confining regimen—deodorized tincture of opium, diphenoxylate hydrochloride, and codeine.

Excision with Grafting. With considerable skin loss, as may occur following multiple operations, or as a primary procedure, it is sometimes useful to rotate skin flaps to cover the resultant wound defect.[181] This can be performed using the principles described in Chapter 11; advancement or rotation flaps (see Anoplasty for Severe Stenosis); or even, as has been

suggested, by means of a gluteus maximus myocutaneous flap.[311] To eliminate the deep natal cleft and the conventional vertical wound, which tends to pull apart, some surgeons recommend a Z-plasty.[52,225,264,273,281–283,382] Others suggest excision in a rhomboid fashion, with coverage effected by means of a so-called Limberg buttock flap (Figure 9-20).[17,381,391] Another modification of the rhomboid flap design is the so-called Dufourmentel technique.[265] In the Z-plasty, the depth of the intergluteal fold with the associated pilonidal sinus disease is excised; skin flaps are then mobilized, rotated, and interdigitated (Figure 9-21).

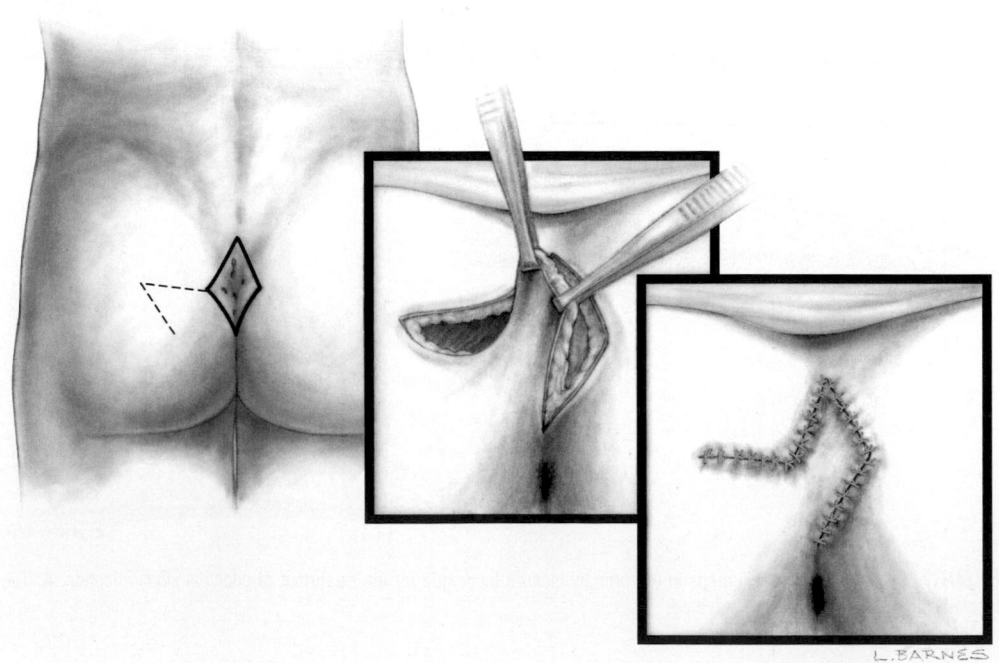

FIGURE 9-20. Pilonidal sinus treated by excision with a rhomboid design and a Limberg flap.

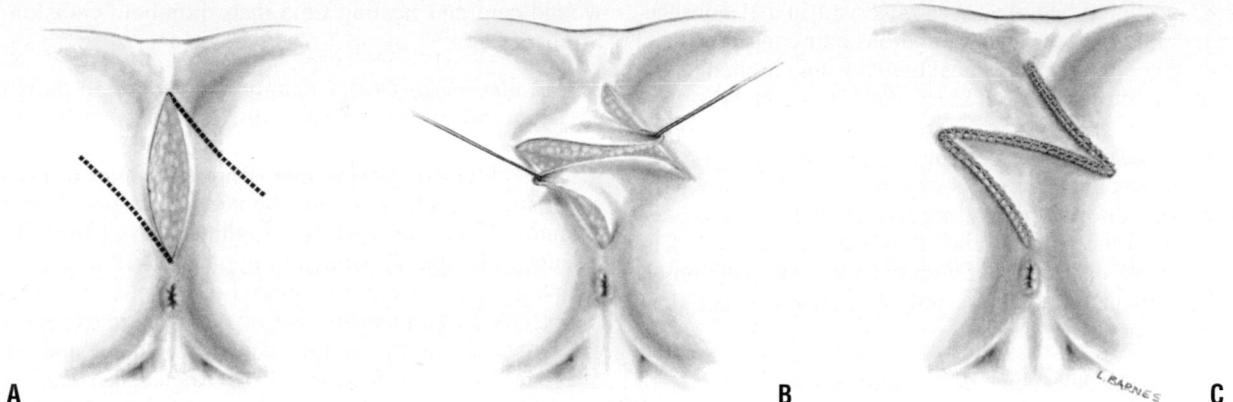

FIGURE 9-21. Treatment of pilonidal sinus by Z-plasty. **A:** Incisions outlined. **B:** Skin flaps rotated. **C:** Primary closure obliterates the natal cleft defect.

Karydakis described a technique for limiting the likelihood of recurrence following excision of pilonidal sinus by means of a variation of excision with primary closure and grafting in more than 6,000 patients.[220] By this technique, each sinus is completely excised through a vertical, eccentric, elliptical incision. A thick flap is created by undermining the medial edge and advancing it across the midline so that the whole suture line is lateralized in order to reduce the risk for recurrence.[228]

Sinus Extraction. The importance of avoiding the creation of a midline incision has been emphasized by Lord and Bascom.[31,32,259] This approach consists of lateral drainage of the abscess, removal of the hair, and excision of the hair follicle (if present). Minimal excision of a sinus tract may be performed. The cavity is cleansed through incisions adjacent to but not inside the pilonidal sinus. The cavity walls are not excised but are permitted to collapse. The procedure may be carried out in the office or at an ambulatory surgical facility. An alternative approach is to drain the acute abscess and allow the infection to subside before follicle removal is attempted.[32] According to Bascom, the enlarged follicles should be excised individually, leaving only small midline wounds, 2 to 4 mm in diameter (Figure 9-22).[32] Alternatively, these may be closed primarily to reduce healing time.

This technique may be analogous to that of the management of a "horseshoe" fistula, in which one endeavors merely to remove the crypt-bearing area and establish adequate drainage. Certainly, if one can accomplish this satisfactorily, healing will result with minimal deformity. The same "less is more" approach appears equally valid for selected instances of pilonidal sinus.

Sclerosing Injection. Hegge and colleagues suggest a "conservative" approach to the treatment of pilonidal disease, injection of phenol (80%) into the sinus tract.[186] The procedure was carried out on 48 patients after they had undergone minimal drainage and hair removal. They were considered cured if there was no evidence of recurrent disease within 1 year of treatment. The authors reported a low recurrence rate—only 6.3%.

Cryosurgery. The use of cryosurgical destruction has also been advocated in the surgical management of pilonidal sinus.[168,297] The technique consists of surgery (opening of the tracts and side branches), curettage, and electrocoagulation of bleeding points. The open wound is then sprayed with liquid nitrogen for approximately 5 minutes

We have had no experience with this technique, but O'Connor has stated that there is less deformity and scarring than with a wider excision.[297] However, because it has been generally recognized that a wide excision is not a necessary part of the treatment, the comparison may be inappropriate.

Nonoperative Management. As previously mentioned, the military has been quite concerned about the lost time associated with the surgical management of pilonidal sinus and its adverse consequences. Armstrong and Barcia examined the role of conservative, nonoperative treatment of pilonidal sinus disease at an army community hospital.[26] Complete healing

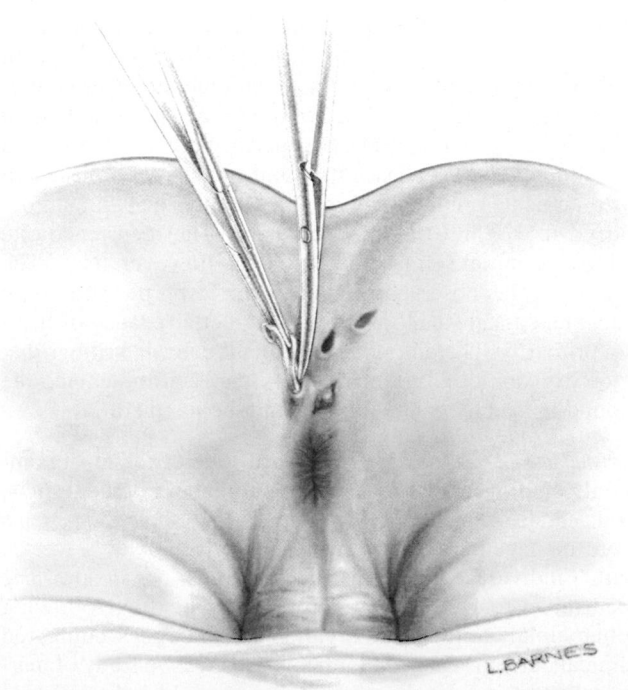

FIGURE 9-22. Pilonidal sinus excision by extraction technique (Bascom's). Each individual sinus opening is excised. The midline wounds are closed whenever possible, leaving the lateral wounds open to drain.

over 83 occupied bed days was observed in 101 consecutive cases managed through meticulous hair control by natal cleft shaving, improved perineal hygiene, and limited lateral incision and drainage for abscess. This was compared with 4,760 occupied bed days in 229 patients who had undergone 240 operative procedures during the previous 2 years. The prolonged hospitalization was explained by the army basic trainee population, who, by regulation, could not be discharged from the hospital until they were fit for duty. The authors further observed that with the application of conservative treatment over 17 years, only 23 excisional operations were performed.

Results of the Various Methods of Management

It is interesting to note that almost irrespective of the method of treatment applied, very few patients are troubled with symptoms of persistent pilonidal sinus disease beyond the age of 40 years. Perhaps one simply outgrows the condition. It is therefore important to understand that ultimate cure is an almost inevitable result when one compares the value of the various surgical alternatives. Another problem with analyzing the data is that there are very few so-called prospective, randomized, controlled studies that can survive critical review. One such report by Füzün and colleagues randomly compared primary closure with excision in 110 consecutive patients.[165] Although primary closure was associated with hospital stays significantly longer than those in the open-treatment group, the patients returned to work earlier. The primary closure group also had an increased risk for infection and a higher recurrence rate (4.1% vs. 0%). The authors concluded that both treatments have their place. Therefore, the recommendation should be based on individual preference, especially employment status. Others concur in uncontrolled studies that the primary advantage of the closed techniques over open drainage is more rapid recovery, but this must be balanced against the risk of infection.[304,362]

Incision or Excision and Drainage. Hanley has been an advocate of emergency surgery for acute pilonidal abscess by excision and open treatment.[183] With this technique, he reported uniform healing with no evidence of recurrence in a small group of patients. Jensen and Harling performed simple incision and drainage of 73 consecutive individuals who presented with an acute pilonidal abscess.[208] Healing per primam occurred in 42 (58%) within 10 weeks. The recurrence rate following initial primary healing was, however, 21%. The authors further observed that those with fewer pits and lateral tracts had a statistically significantly better chance of healing primarily. There is agreement in all current writings that wide excision of all tissue down to the sacrum, leaving the wound to heal by granulation, cannot be justified.[15]

Excision and Marsupialization. This is still one of the most commonly employed options for the treatment of pilonidal sinus. Solla and Rothenberger reported that 125 of their 150 patients were managed.[361] The average healing time was 4 weeks, with 3 individuals requiring up to 20 weeks for closure. The recurrence rate was 6%, all ultimately healing following remarsupialization. Karakayali and colleagues compared clinical outcomes in a randomized, prospective study of marsupialization versus rhomboid excision and Limberg flap in 140 consecutive patients. They concluded that the former approach provides more clinical benefits with respect to convenience but is associated with more inconvenience as to

wound care and healing time than rhomboid excision and Limberg flap.[219]

Excision with Primary Closure. Zimmerman reported outpatient excision and primary closure in 32 patients.[418] Follow-up was for a mean of 24 months. In all cases, primary healing was obtained, a result that is not dissimilar to my own experience. In addition, Obeid noted primary healing in all 27 individuals managed by a modification of the primary closure technique illustrated in Figures 19-18 and 19-19.[296] Kronborg and colleagues reported the results of a randomized trial of treatment by one of three methods: excision, excision with suture, and excision with suture and antibiotic coverage with clindamycin.[239] Recurrence rates were, respectively, 13%, 25%, and 19%. As expected, healing was much quicker after primary suture than after excisional therapy alone (median, 14 days vs. 64 days). Tritapepe and Di Padova reported 243 consecutive patients who underwent excision and primary closure with the use of a closed-suction drain for 24 hours, followed by wound irrigation with an antiseptic solution.[386] With a follow-up of 5 to 15 years, there were no wound breakdowns and no recurrences.

Petersen and colleagues undertook a meta-analysis of data published over a period of 35 years with various primary closure techniques.[312] Seventy-four publications included a total of 10,090 patients. These investigators concluded that there appears to be a significant benefit with respect to healing when the asymmetric-oblique closure or the full-thickness flap technique is employed when compared with midline closure.[312]

Excision and Grafting. Reports of the success of excision and grafting are somewhat difficult to interpret in light of the lack of a control in these studies.[181,264] In the report from the Cleveland Clinic in Ohio, 58 patients were reviewed who underwent extensive or recurrent pilonidal disease surgery with primary skin grafting.[181] More than 72% had recurrent disease when initially seen. The average hospital stay was 10 days, and the time lost from work averaged 28 days. The recurrence rate was 1.7%, and the failure rate was 3.4%. Using the Z-plasty technique, Mansoory and Dickson treated 120 patients.[264] There were two recurrences, a very favorable experience. Alver and colleagues reported 35 selected individuals with "small and moderate extent disease" treated by the fasciocutaneous Limberg flap method.[17] The rate of wound infection or dehiscence was 17%, with all individuals ultimately healing. Urhan and coworkers initially reported 110 Limberg flap procedures with five recurrences (4.9%),[391] with no further failures when 90 later patients were added.[381] Manterola and colleagues used the similar Dufourmentel technique in 25 patients and noted two instances of infection or dehiscence.[265] Kitchen reported 141 patients treated by the Karydakis operation and noted a recurrence rate of 4%.[228]

When skin is lost as a consequence of pilonidal sinus disease, particularly in the recurrent situation, mobilizing skin to cover the defect will more reliably lead to a satisfactory result. Bascom reported 30 patients with open midline wounds from recurrence.[33] All healed by closure of the natal cleft through the raising of skin flaps.

During the past decade, the literature is replete with techniques on the treatment of pilonidal sinus, almost exclusively using either one of the primary closure methods, with or without skin mobilization, or some modification of a Bascom-like minimal procedure. Almost all are nonrandomized publications of an individual surgeon's experience or that of his or her group. A few references are cited here for the convenience of the reader.[4,20,44,118,146,237,258,263,285,378]

Sinus Extraction (Lord-Bascom Procedure). Bascom and Edwards reported their experiences with the Lord treatment: removal only of the follicles and hairs.[31,135] In an earlier report, 50 patients were treated in the office, and local anesthesia was used. Acute abscesses were treated by excision of the enlarged follicles from the midline skin. One to 10 follicles were removed, individually if possible. Because incisions were kept smaller than 7 mm, the specimens weighed less than 1 g per patient. Follow-up averaged 24 months. The mean disability was 1 day, and the mean wound healing time was 3 weeks. Recurrences appeared in four patients (8%); all were healed 3 weeks following reoperation. There was no incident of a second recurrence. A later publication by Bascom of 161 patients treated revealed comparable results.[32]

Edwards reported 102 patients treated by this technique.[135] The median number of days lost from work was 10, and the median number of days requiring healing was 39. Eighty-nine percent of these patients were free of recurrent disease provided they attended the follow-up clinic. Because some patients failed to attend, it is difficult to interpret the results of this study. It appears, however, that the author was not as successful as Bascom.

Senepati and associates performed 218 Bascom's operations as day cases.[343] Ten percent developed recurrences requiring reoperation. Theodoropoulos and colleagues opine, based on their experience with this operation in a military hospital, that this operation is safe, with minimal morbidity, and can be reliably used as a second-line alternative for recurrent disease.[379]

Gips and colleagues reported the use of a trephine technique to accomplish a limited procedure in 1,358 patients. Each crypt opening was cored out with the use of Keyes trephines of various diameters. The recurrence rate was 6.5% at 1 year and 11.5% after 4 years.[172]

Meta-analysis of Results. Brasel and coworkers undertook a meta-analysis comparing healing by primary closure techniques with that of open healing in randomized controlled trials.[55] Eighteen trials were included. They concluded that wounds heal more quickly after primary closure than after open healing but at the expense of increased risk of recurrence. They recommend that off-midline closure should become the standard management for pilonidal disease when closure is desired.[55]

Comment. It is now generally agreed that minimal surgery should be applied to the treatment of pilonidal disease whenever possible. The concept of Lord and of Bascom in removing the hair follicles and the hairs themselves without extensive excision and debridement is an excellent one. Every attempt should be made to keep the patient out of the hospital and to limit the morbidity of the procedure. However, there are some individuals who will benefit from a more generous excision, particularly those who have undergone multiple procedures or have extensive disease. Under these circumstances, inpatient hospital treatment with excision and primary closure, with or without grafting, may offer a lower morbidity, shortened convalescence, and more rapid healing.

Pilonidal Sinus and Squamous Cell Carcinoma

Squamous cell carcinoma has been reported to arise in pilonidal sinus tracts, almost all inevitably involving long-standing active inflammation. Fasching and colleagues reviewed 36 cases that they identified in the literature.[151] As of 1996, there were 44 reported.[112] Treatment consisted of wide excision and grafting. This is similar to the management of squamous cell carcinoma of the skin anywhere in the body that can lend itself to this approach. More recently, it has been suggested that because of the high recurrence rate of the malignancy, consideration should be given to adjuvant chemotherapy and radiation.[112,241]

Suppurative Hidradenitis (Hidradenitis Suppurativa)

Suppurative hidradenitis is an uncommon, chronic, recurrent, indolent infection involving the skin and subcutaneous tissue arising in the apocrine glands (i.e., axillary, inguinal, genital, perineal, and mammary). The most frequent area of involvement is the axilla. The condition was originally described in 1839 by Velpeau.[395] The overall incidence is higher in women, with most cases occurring between the ages of 16

ALFRED-ARMAND-LOUIS-MARIE VELPEAU (1795–1867)

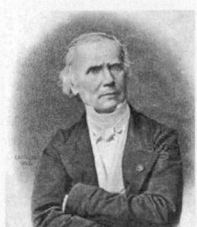

A native of Brèches, Indre-et-Loire, Velpeau was a student and assistant to Pierre Bretonneau. During his early medical career, he was a surgeon in several hospitals in Paris. In 1833, he succeeded Alexis de Boyer as chair of clinical surgery at the University of Paris, a position he maintained until his death in 1867. He was a skilled surgeon and renowned for his knowledge of surgical anatomy. He published more than 340 titles on surgery, embryology, anatomy, obstetrics, and other subjects, and in 1830, he wrote an important book on obstetrics, entitled *Traité elementaire de l'art des accouchements.* In 1827, he is credited for providing the first accurate description of leukemia. The eponymous "Velpeau bandage" that is used for arm support is named after him. There are several other medical terms named after him; however, these are now primarily used for historical purposes, including *Velpeau hernia* for the femoral hernia, *Velpeau's disease* for hidradenitis suppurativa, *Velpeau's canal* for the inguinal canal, and *Velpeau's fossa,* which is the ischiorectal fossa. Despite being one of the top surgeons in his time, Velpeau believed that pain-free surgery was a fantasy, and that surgery and pain were inseparable. With the advent of the anesthetics ether and chloroform in the 1840s, Velpeau was amazed, saying *"On the subject of ether, that it is a wonderful and terrible agen[t]; I will say of chloroform, that it is still more wonderful and more terrible."*

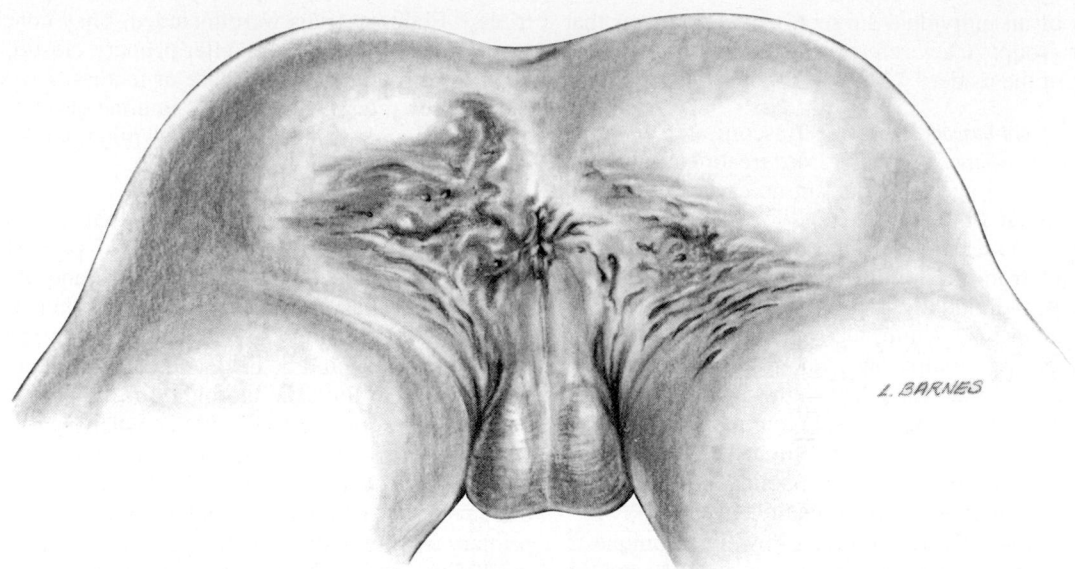

FIGURE 9-23. Artist's concept of suppurative hidradenitis with extensive involvement of perianal area and buttocks.

and 40 years, but most studies of operated cases affecting the perineum indicate a larger number of men.

Etiology

Suppurative hidradenitis does not occur before puberty because it is believed that the effect of sex hormones on the apocrine glands is the inciting factor. An androgen-based endocrine disorder has also been postulated. Harrison and colleagues demonstrated an androgen excess and a progesterone decrease through detailed hormonal profiles in 36 women and 14 controls.[184] The proposed mechanism for the possible role of androgens being associated with suppurative hidradenitis lies in end organ sensitivity, rather than in absolute plasma levels. Although the etiology is unknown, acne appears to be a predisposing factor, with stress, poor skin hygiene, obesity, excessive heat, hyperhidrosis, and chemical depilatories possibly playing a role.[94] There has been no documentation of an increased association with diabetes mellitus, but impaired glucose tolerance has been observed. There may be a genetic predisposition based on an increased familial incidence. Some observe an increased frequency in those with Crohn's disease, irritable bowel syndrome, herpes simplex, certain kinds of arthritis, and a number of other conditions. Squamous cell carcinoma arising in long-standing suppurative hidradenitis has been reported in at least 16 cases,[21,62,128,277,416] with one-half of these patients dying of metastatic disease.

Pathophysiology

Suppurative hidradenitis commences with obstruction of the hair follicle rather than the apocrine gland duct. This is due to a defect in terminal differentiation that impedes follicular epithelial shedding.[415] After follicular keratinocyte multiplication occurs, folliculitis proceeds to occlude the apocrine gland duct with resultant inspissated secretions. The gland may then rupture, which can lead to extension of the process into the dermis, with consequent secondary involvement of other glands and ducts. In rare instances, the process can extend through the fascia into the underlying muscle.

Differential Diagnosis

The condition may be confused with anal fistula, Crohn's disease, tuberculosis, pilonidal sinus, infected sebaceous cyst, furunculosis, granuloma inguinale, lymphogranuloma venereum, and other infections in the anal area.

Physical Examination

Examination reveals painful, tender, erythematous, purulent lesions (Figure 9-23). These may be associated with adenopathy and systemic signs (i.e., fever, malaise, leukocytosis). The condition frequently produces burrowing sinuses that can extend for many inches around the anus, into the scrotum, buttocks, labia, medial thighs, and sacrum (Figures 9-24 and 9-25).

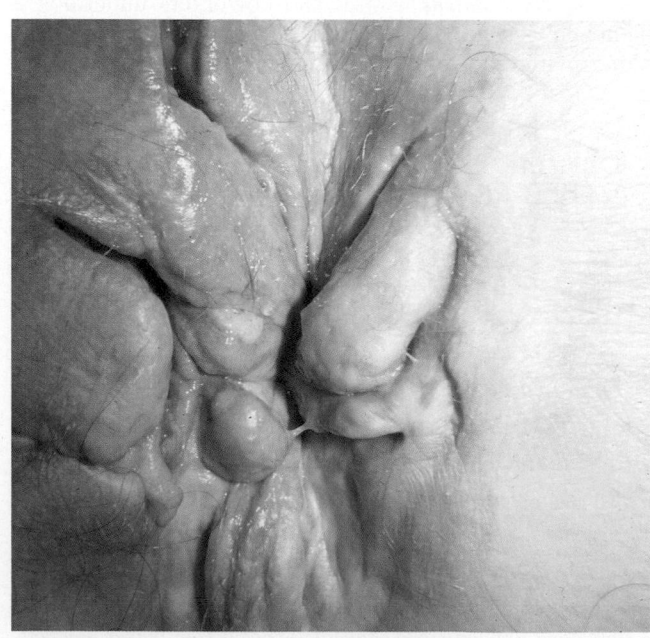

FIGURE 9-24. Suppurative hidradenitis with extensive perianal sinuses may be confused with horseshoe fistula or Crohn's disease.

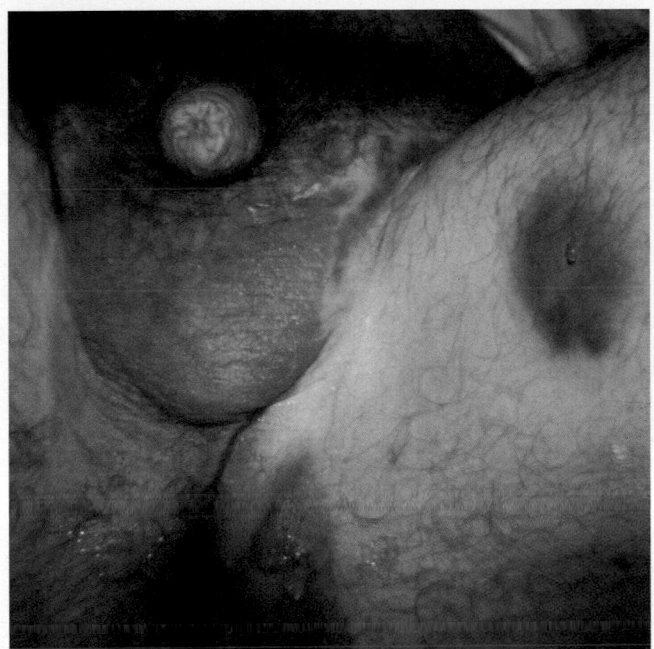

FIGURE 9-25. Suppurative hidradenitis affecting the groin, scrotum, perineum, and thigh.

Although the tracts are usually relatively superficial, they can actually invade deeply and extend to involve the area around the femoral vessels. Urethral and rectal fistulas have been noted, but these are more likely caused by aggressive surgery rather than aggressive disease.

Histopathology

Microscopically, the earliest inflammatory changes are seen within and around the apocrine glands, the ducts of which may be distended with leukocytes (Figure 9-26). In the chronic stage, multiple abscesses, intercommunicating sinus tracts, and irregular hypertrophied scars form.[81] The scars, ulceration, and infection extend within the subcutaneous tissue to the fascia (Figure 9-27). Sebaceous gland involvement is not a component of suppurative hidradenitis, either by histologic examination or by measuring the sebum secretion rate.[205,206]

Treatment

There is no cure for suppurative hidradenitis. However, various medical and surgical strategies can help to eliminate existing lesions and prevent development of new ones. Such general care measures as avoiding heat and humidity, limiting friction from tight synthetic clothing, and addressing perspiration help to alleviate the symptoms. Regular use of antiperspirants is acceptable, but these agents, along with shaving and depilation, may cause additional irritation in affected areas.

It is generally believed that antibiotic therapy early in the course of the disease is of considerable value. Numerous bacteria have been isolated, including staphylococci, streptococci, *Escherichia coli*, and *Proteus* species. It is interesting to note, however, that in one study, a sample of the drained pus sent for culture and antibiotic sensitivity revealed no growth in approximately one-half of the patients.[380] Still, local and systemic broad-spectrum antibiotics are advisable. These include penicillin, erythromycin, clindamycin, and tetracycline in those cases when acne is noted in other areas. The antibiotics should be used until resolution of the process is complete. Some patients require treatment for months or even years. Isotretinoin (Accutane) has been shown to benefit some patients. Antiandrogen therapy has been investigated in multiple trials and occasionally found to be more effective than oral antibiotics.[236] Systemic steroids are not typically used for treatment of suppurative hidradenitis. However, intralesional injection of glucocorticoids appears to be effective for individuals with a few isolated tender and early lesions,[290] but it is not appropriate for patients with extensive disease.[411]

TNF-α inhibitors provide rapid control of the inflammatory component of the disease, and the response to them can be dramatic.[12] In many patients, they are effectively used as a short-term course to limit disease activity prior to surgical intervention. This provides easier definition of the disease and improves the healing process.[199] Unfortunately, there is a group of individuals who do not respond to any medical regimen, and disability is such that surgical intervention is required to treat the extensive sinus tracts and abscesses.

Operative Approaches

With minimal involvement and inadequate palliation by medical means, incision and drainage of an abscess may

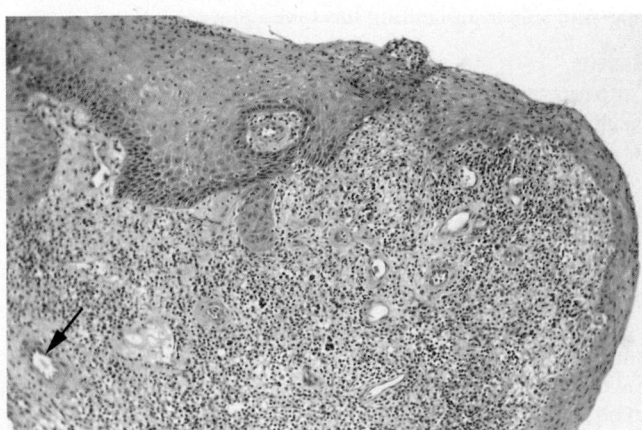

FIGURE 9-26. Suppurative hidradenitis. An apocrine gland *(arrow)* has surrounding inflammation. (Original magnification × 120.)

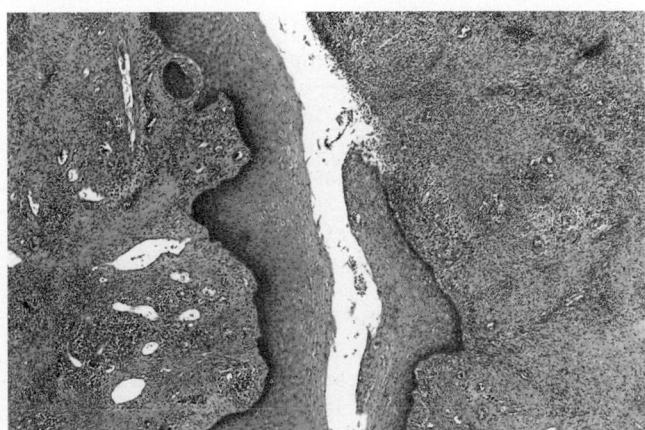

FIGURE 9-27. Suppurative hidradenitis. The sinus tract is lined by squamous epithelium with surrounding acute and chronic inflammation. (Original magnification × 120.)

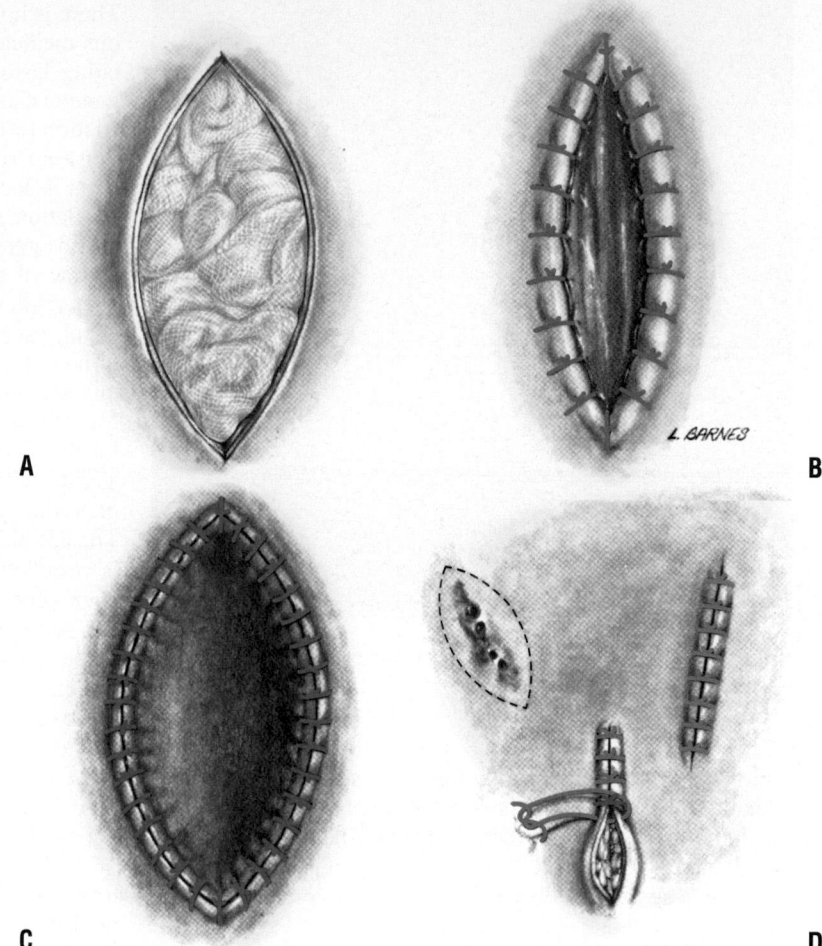

FIGURE 9-28. Four methods of treatment for suppurative hidradenitis. **A:** Excision with packing. **B:** Excision with marsupialization. **C:** Excision with grafting. **D:** Excision and primary closure.

result in cure. When the condition progresses to extensive sinus formation, excision is the only means by which the condition can be effectively ameliorated.

The four methods of surgical treatment are as follows (Figure 9-28):

1. Excision with primary closure
2. Excision with grafting
3. Excision with marsupialization
4. Excision with packing

All four methods can be applied usefully, even in the same patient. Primary closure usually requires a relatively narrow wound, but often by elevating the full thickness of skin on either side of the excision site, the wound may be approximated without tension. Wide excision, leaving the wound open to heal by second intention, is probably the most common method of surgical treatment. This has the obvious disadvantage of a prolonged healing time (Figure 9-29).

Methods for closing the wound include the application of a split-thickness graft or some form of plastic procedure similar to that previously described for pilonidal sinus (e.g., Z-plasty or Limberg flap).[326] It is certainly preferable to close the wound by some means if this is possible. Occasionally, it is necessary to perform a diverting colostomy if extensive surgery and grafting are required in the perianal area (Figure 9-30). Fortunately, the anal canal itself is usually spared. Involvement of the sphincter muscle is so unusual that this observation should encourage the surgeon to consider another diagnosis for the problem. Rarely does the disease progress to the point where there is such significant deformity of the anal canal that a permanent colostomy becomes necessary. For those who harbor bilateral, circumferential, or anterior and posterior disease in the perineal area, it may be wise from the perspective of patient discomfort and disability to perform surgery on one side only and to treat the opposite side after healing has taken place.

Results

Culp reported the Mayo Clinic (Rochester, Minnesota) experience with 132 patients observed with anogenital hidradenitis suppurativa during a 6-year period.[105] Of the 30 individuals whose disease was limited to the anal canal and adjacent areas, two-thirds were men. Most had undergone previous multiple attempts at surgical drainage or excision. The author commented that although excision with grafting had been used extensively in the past, such a program had not been necessary in recent years. Extensive excision was the method employed in 17 of the 30 patients; the wounds healed within 8 weeks in all cases. A diverting colostomy was not believed to be necessary. There was no recurrence in more than 1 year of follow-up.

Thornton and Abcarian reviewed 104 patients who underwent surgery for the condition at the Cook County

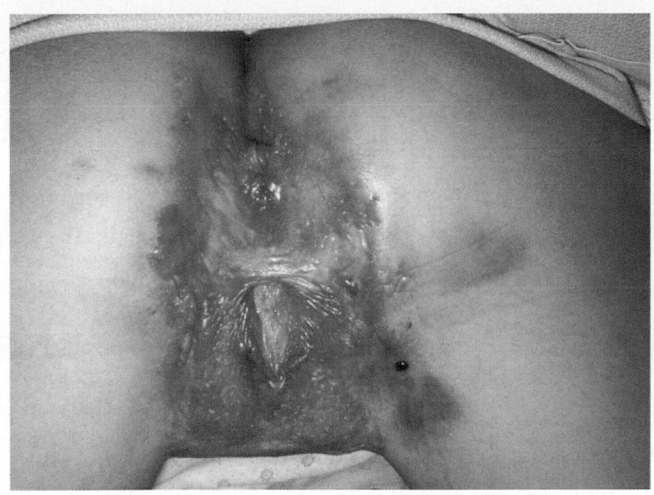 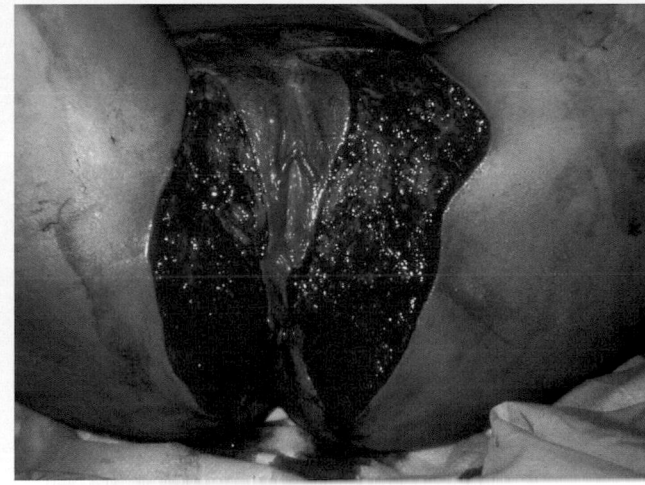

A

B

FIGURE 9-29. Suppurative hidradenitis. **A:** Extensive perineal disease. **B:** Treatment by wide excision.

Hospital in Chicago.[380] Approximately two-thirds were men. The operative procedure for all patients consisted of wide excision down to normal fat or fascia using electrocautery. The wounds were then packed with iodoform gauze, and the patients were followed on a biweekly basis. The average hospital stay was approximately 1 week. However, those more than 40 years old had an average hospital stay of approximately 19 days. Healing times ranged from approximately 1 month for relatively small wounds to 2 months for larger ones. In four individuals, a recurrence developed.

Broadwater and colleagues reviewed their experience of 23 patients treated between 1967 and 1981.[60] Sixty-one percent were male, the average age was 30 years, and the mean duration of symptoms was in excess of 5 years. The authors' primary treatment included wide and deep excision with selective (i.e., individualized) closure. Although it is difficult to evaluate the reasons for selection of the procedure, the overall recurrence rate in those undergoing

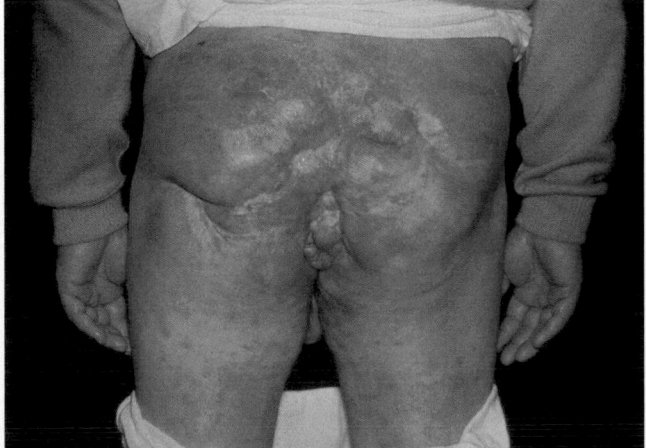

FIGURE 9-30. Suppurative hidradenitis. Healed wounds with extensive scarring and deformity involving the buttocks and perineum. Patient did not require fecal diversion because the anus and perianal skin were spared.

primary closure was 30%. Those who underwent excision with application of a split-thickness graft had a 13% incidence of recurrence. In one-half of the patients treated by excision, with the wound left open to heal by secondary intention, recurrence developed. However, only four individuals were treated.

Wiltz and colleagues reviewed the Lahey Clinic (Boston) experience involving 43 individuals.[409] Recurrence developed in two-thirds after either wide excision with healing allowed by secondary intention or incision and drainage with or without limited local excision. Jemec reported a very limited cure rate with excision—only 21%.[204] However, patient satisfaction was quite high, implying that even temporary relief through surgical excision is preferable to the chronic draining illness. Others believe that wide excision is the preferred treatment and the one most likely to effect cure.[49]

Banerjee reviewed a number of publications reporting the results of surgical treatment of suppurative hidradenitis and concluded that no method satisfies all requirements for the ideal treatment.[28] Furthermore, good reports of the relative cure rates of the different surgical options are scarce, with controlled trials nonexistent. He considered that the preferred option in most instances is wide local excision, with healing taking place by secondary intention.[28]

Comment

Suppurative hidradenitis is a complicated condition to treat, and the approach to each case must be individualized. Whenever possible, one should adequately excise the involved tissue and to perform primary closure if possible. For large lesions, it is probably preferable to excise widely and to marsupialize or to leave the area to granulate. In some situations with extensive involvement, one may consider the application of a split-thickness graft 4 or 5 days after initial excision or a grafting maneuver to expedite the healing process. Repeated operations may also be required for extension of the disease process that was inapparent at the time of the initial procedure.

Anorectal Abscess and Anal Fistula

Anorectal abscess and fistula (Figure 9-31) are perianal infective processes that may be confused with pilonidal sinus

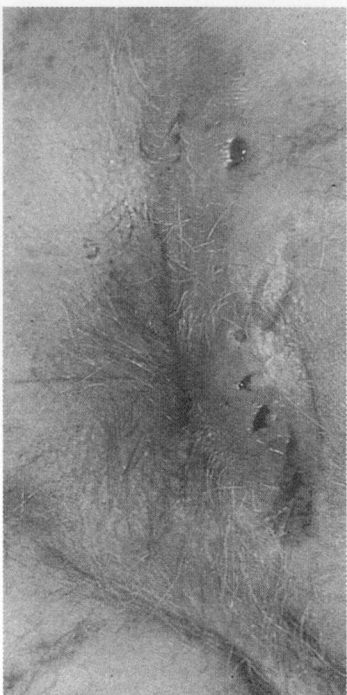

FIGURE 9-31. Multiple external openings are present in this patient with fistula-in-ano.

and suppurative hidradenitis. Chapters 13 and 14 are dedicated to the diagnosis and management of these conditions.

Crohn's Disease

Anal and perianal Crohn's disease present difficult management problems. This condition is discussed in Chapter 14, and the diagnosis and management of Crohn's disease are presented in Chapter 30.

Tuberculosis

Tuberculosis distal to the ileocecal valve is uncommon, and it is seldom even considered in the differential diagnosis when the disease process is located in the large intestine.[179] When it affects the perianal area, it can be confused with Crohn's disease, actinomycosis, anal fistula, colloid carcinoma, sarcoidosis, and other skin conditions. Anal fistula is the most frequent presentation of anorectal tuberculosis (80% to 90%), but there are no obvious distinguishing characteristics from that of cryptoglandular fistula.[375] Most reported cases occur in developing countries. The disease is seen most commonly in men, usually associated with pulmonary tuberculosis, but there have been case reports of the process occurring in the absence of pulmonary infection.[235,403] Primary inoculation of the mycobacteria may result from trauma to the skin or mucosa. Other postulated mechanisms by which tubercle bacilli reach the perianal region include hematogenous spread from a primary lung focus with later reactivation, ingestion of bacilli in sputum from an active pulmonary focus, ingestion of contaminated cow's milk, direct spread from adjacent organs, and through lymph channels from infected lymph nodes.[180]

The lesion may appear as a brownish red papule that can progress into an ulcerating plaque; this is known as a tuberculous chancre. The ulcers are usually painful and indolent, with blue, irregular edges. Regional lymphadenopathy

is common. A high index of suspicion is necessary if one is to establish the diagnosis early and to initiate appropriate therapy. It has been suggested that an anal fissure in an unusual location that is slow to heal should be pathologically confirmed with appropriate staining and cultures to rule out the presence of the bacterium.[249]

The diagnosis can be established by the determination of acid-fast bacilli in the biopsy specimen (Ziehl-Nielsen stain), by positive guinea pig culture, and by the presence of caseating granulomas in the histologic examination of skin lesions. Because culture results take about 4 weeks, newer approaches may be more useful, such as the detection of the bacterial DNA by means of genomic amplification by polymerase chain reaction, a 48-hour test.[375] Chaudhary and Gupta and Gupta and colleagues suggest that the biopsy be performed using an anesthetic because considerable effort is required to obtain representative tissue from the depths of any fibrotic or strictured area.[77,179] Demonstration of active disease in the lungs and a positive tuberculin skin test result are helpful in confirming the true nature of the lesion (see Chapter 33).

In developed countries, tuberculosis is not likely to be considered in the differential diagnosis of a perianal ulcer.[6,211] In the absence of a pulmonary lesion, it would be very difficult for one *not* to work up and treat the patient, initially at least, for Crohn's disease. One should certainly consider performing a tuberculin skin test and obtaining cultures in individuals who harbor wounds that fail to heal, especially if the person comes from a developing country.

Obviously, antituberculous drugs are the treatment of choice. Therapy with isoniazid, rifampin, and ethambutol will usually resolve the anal condition in a matter of 2 or 3 weeks. However, treatment should be continued for many months following resolution of the local or systemic manifestations.

Actinomycosis

Actinomycosis is a chronic infectious disease involving the cervicofacial area, thorax, or abdomen. It is caused by an anaerobic, gram-positive bacterium, *Actinomyces israelii*. It produces a suppurative, fibrosing inflammation that forms sinus tracts, discharging granules (Figure 9-32). In the abdominal

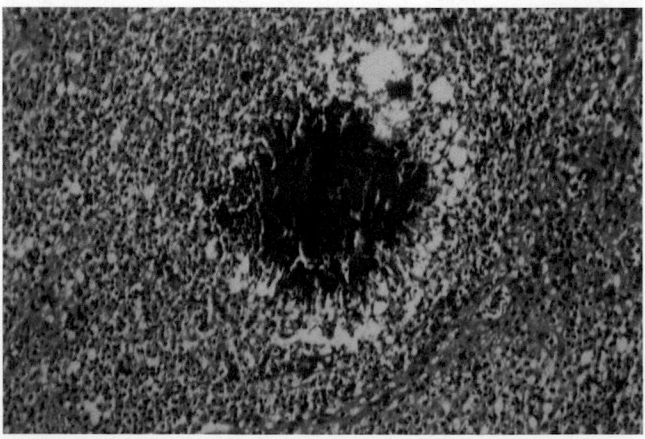

FIGURE 9-32. The basophilic "sulfur granule" of *Actinomyces* in actinomycosis. Note the homogeneous center and the club-shaped filaments at the periphery. (Original magnification × 120; courtesy of Rudolf Garret, MD.)

form, a mass is usually present, and a psoas abscess occasionally occurs (see Chapter 33). Perianal actinomycosis has a predilection for men, with a male to female ratio of 9.5:1; other predispositions for developing this condition include diabetes mellitus and inflammatory or neoplastic processes.[97] The disease develops almost exclusively by direct invasion and rarely by hematogenous spread, having a tendency to disregard anatomical barriers.[40]

The diagnosis is established by identification of the microorganism in cultures of tissue or the exudate of the lesion; it is almost invariably isolated as a part of the polymicrobial flora.[202] The finding of sulfur granules leaves no doubt as to the diagnosis. In the anal area, sinus tracts and fistulas may resemble Crohn's disease, anal fistula, suppurative hidradenitis, and tuberculosis.[16] The presence of the disease elsewhere, particularly in the abdomen, is helpful in alerting the surgeon to the nature of the problem. The possibility of perianal actinomycosis should be entertained in any individual who has extensive fistula tracts and in whom recurrence develops after what are considered adequate attempts at surgical treatment.

Management consists of surgical excision and drainage of the abscess, as well as antibiotics, usually penicillin. A 4-week period of treatment is recommended.

Viral Infections

Virtually any viral infection that affects the skin can involve the perianal area. This may occur as part of a generalized cutaneous process or by autoinoculation from another site. When lesions are seen in an intertriginous zone, they may not resemble the typical appearance seen elsewhere. This may cause the physician to misdiagnose the condition as secondary syphilis.[222] Two common viral infections that are presumed to be nonvenereal in origin are mentioned briefly.

Herpes Zoster

Herpes zoster, caused by reactivation of varicella, may involve the anal area. The condition, also known as shingles, affects both sexes equally and may be particularly troublesome in patients who have been immunosuppressed by treatment for malignancy. Age is the most important factor for the development of zoster. A dramatic increase in rates begins to occur after 50 years.[193,305,323] The lesion is characterized by groups of vesicles on an erythematous base along the distribution of a spinal nerve leading to a posterior ganglion. Itching, tenderness, and pain are characteristically located along the region supplied by the nerve. Jellinek and Tulloch described seven patients with retention, loss of sensation, or incontinence.[203]

Diagnosis can be established by means of tissue culture and by demonstration of antibodies in the serum by immunofluorescent techniques. Histologically, vesicles are seen to be intraepidermal; within these vesicles are found large, swollen cells called "balloon cells" (Figure 9-33).

Treatment consists of medical measures, including rest and the application of heat. Analgesics are advisable for acute neuralgia. Acyclovir (Zovirax), 800 mg orally four to five times per day for 7 to 10 days, is extremely helpful if initiated early in the course of the disease. For older patients with severe pain, systemic corticosteroid therapy may be considered.

Vaccinia

Vaccinia virus is an attenuated cowpox virus that has been propagated in laboratories for immunization against smallpox.

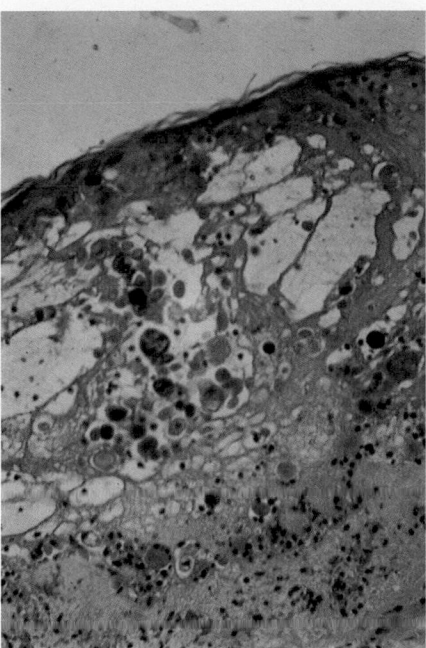

FIGURE 9-33. Ballooning degeneration of prickle cells with the formation of multilocular vesicles in herpes zoster. Note the cells with large inclusion bodies. (Original magnification × 240; courtesy of Rudolf Garret, MD.)

Perianal vaccinia is a rare complication of vaccination and usually occurs in young children.[99] It has also been reported as a complication of diarrhea, with probable transmission to the excoriated area by the fingers.[102] In adults, the condition may be confused with syphilis or with herpes simplex infection. The history is helpful if the patient has undergone a recent vaccination or was exposed to someone who had done so. There are reports of vaccinia being sexually transmitted from a partner who had recently received smallpox vaccine.[73,138]

Treatment is generally supportive because complete recovery usually occurs spontaneously. However, vaccinia immune globulin has been recommended in severe cases or to expedite resolution of the process.

Bacterial Infections

Infective processes associated with bacterial organisms, such as pilonidal sinus and suppurative hidradenitis, have already been discussed. There is however a unique infective condition in the perianal area that is worthy of discussion, Fournier's gangrene.

Fournier's Gangrene or Necrotizing Perineal Infection

In 1883, Fournier described a necrotizing soft tissue infection of the perineum, groin, and genitalia that almost invariably ended fatally. Because of the prevalence of two or more species of bacteria in the infection, the term *synergistic gangrene* has been employed. *Necrotizing fasciitis* is another expression that has been used to describe the condition. It is important to distinguish this entity from clostridial myonecrosis because the treatment is obviously different.[48]

Why such a fulminant septic process develops in some patients with seemingly trivial septic problems in the rectum, perianal area, or urinary tract is not known. The basic pathologic mechanism of the disease process is believed to be an obliterative end arteritis caused by the

JEAN-ALFRED FOURNIER (1832–1914)

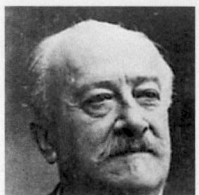

Fournier was born in Paris. He became a pupil of Ricord, who exerted considerable influence over him and was responsible for stimulating Fournier to pursue investigations on STDs. In 1860, he graduated from the University of Paris Medical School, his thesis dealing with syphilitic contagion. Fournier is recognized as one of the pioneers in the diagnosis and management of STIs. In 1863, he became physician to the hospitals of Paris and Professeur Agrégé in the faculty of medicine. In 1868, he was appointed chief of service at the Lourcine Hospital, and in 1876, he was advanced to the Hôpital St. Louis, where he remained until retirement in 1902. The Academy of Medicine admitted Fournier to its ranks in 1879. His activities in writing and teaching brought him worldwide recognition and probably the largest clientele in the history of syphilology. Among the honors he received were the presidency of the French Society of Dermatology and Syphilology, commander of the Legion of Honor, and the Order of Leopold of Belgium. In later years, his particular interest was the Society of Sanitary and Moral Prophylaxis, of which he was the founder and first president.

spread of the pathogens aided by distal arterial disease (e.g., diabetes mellitus) and by being immunocompromised.[140,187,212,320,324] Delay in making the correct diagnosis and in initiating appropriate treatment of minor infections probably is the major contributing factor. The high mortality rate associated with these infections may in part be attributable to its occurrence in patients with debilitating illnesses, including diabetes.[30,232,246] Urinary tract infection, instrumentation, and surgery have all been implicated as contributing factors. Patients who undergo chemotherapy and those with AIDS are also more susceptible, implying that immunosuppression may play a role (see later and Chapters 10 and 33).[321] Some patients have a history of prior anorectal surgery or pelvic surgery for an infective process (e.g., perforated diverticulitis), but sometimes, especially when an anorectal procedure is performed, an underlying infection may not be recognized. Rubber ring ligation of hemorrhoids has been reported to be the precipitating event in a number of cases (see Chapter 11). Virtually all patients in published series have a demonstrable port of entry for the organism; specifically, perianal infection has become the most common cause.[115] Interestingly, the well-recognized entity in children of perianal cellulitis, caused by hemolytic streptococci, does not seem to predispose to the development of this complication.[328]

Stephens and colleagues reviewed the English language literature to determine whether there have been changes in demography, etiology, and outcome, compared with cases dating back to 1763.[365] They noted that in the decade 1970s to 1980s, 449 cases were reported. The average age was 50 years, with 14% of cases occurring in females. The most common etiologic factors were colorectal (33%), idiopathic (26%), and genitourinary (21%).[365] The authors noted that the mortality associated with the disease as a consequence of colorectal disease was highest (1 of 3 died). The overall mortality in the series was 22%.

Symptoms and Findings

The usual presenting complaints are perineal pain and swelling. Frank suppuration or even gangrene of the overlying skin may be apparent in advanced cases (Figure 9-34). Fever and leukocytosis are invariably present.

Bacteriology

There has been considerable disagreement about the specific bacteria involved in the infection. Numerous organisms have been identified, both aerobic and anaerobic, including *Clostridium welchii*.[191] More commonly, the gangrene is caused by such mixed bacterial flora as microaerophilic *Streptococcus*, *Staphylococcus aureus* and *Staphylococcus albus*, *Bacteroides*, *Klebsiella*, *E. coli*, *Enterococcus*, *Proteus*, and *Citrobacter*.[224] The highest rates of isolation in diabetic patients have been reported to be *Streptococcus* spp., *Staphylococcus* spp., and mixed anaerobic flora.[247,294] Gram stain and aerobic and anaerobic cultures should be obtained from the margins where infection is advancing.[224]

Treatment

Broad-spectrum antibiotic therapy is of course recommended. Because most anaerobic isolates are reported to be sensitive to clindamycin and metronidazole, these have been suggested to be the first-line antibiotics of choice.[315] However, vigorous surgical excision and debridement of all nonviable tissue are imperative (Figure 9-35).[30,115,143,224,234,317] Treatment with hyperbaric oxygen is controversial and may be contraindicated unless the infection is caused by *C. welchii*.[115,143,224] A colostomy may be advisable to reduce fecal contamination of the area but is mandatory if anorectal or colonic disease is the cause of the perineal sepsis. Debridement must be radical and should be continued until the skin and subcutaneous tissue cannot be readily separated from the fascia.[143] Histologic examination of the margins of excised tissue may be useful in determining the

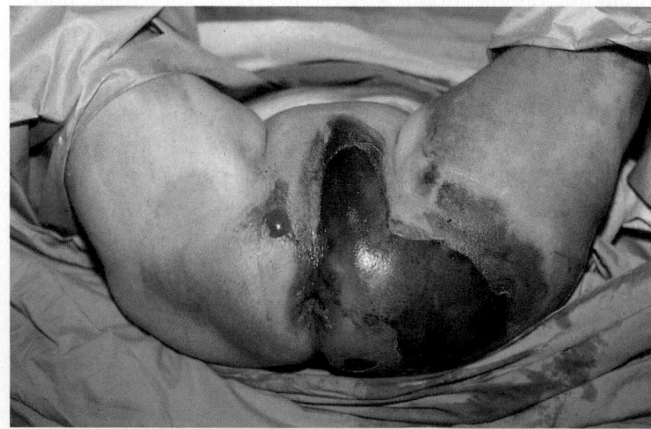

FIGURE 9-34. Fournier's gangrene. Note the necrotic areas of perianal skin, bullae, and introital edema. (Courtesy of Paul J. Kovalcik, MD.)

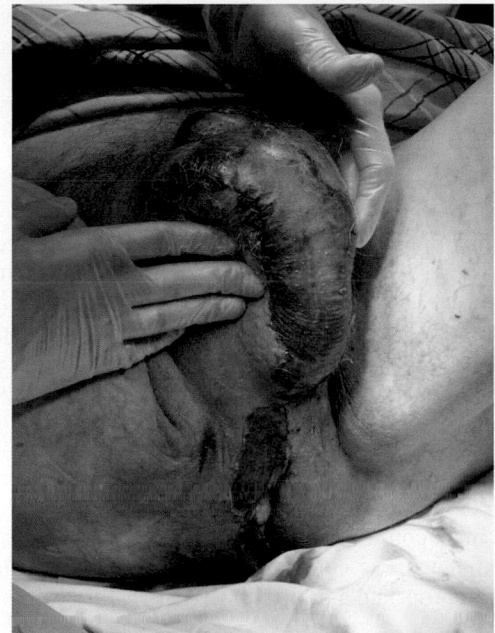

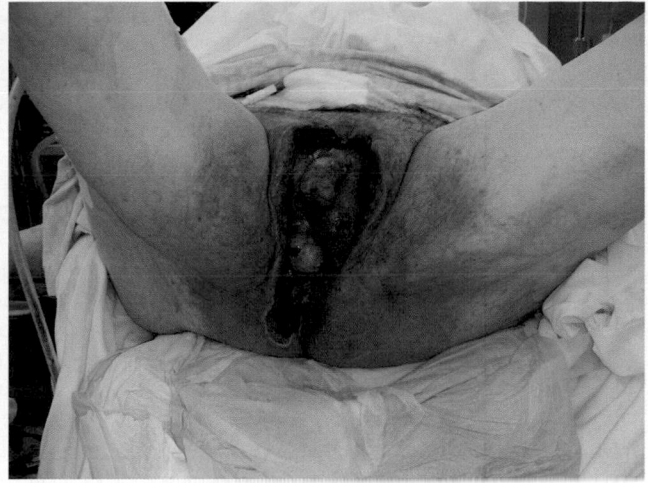

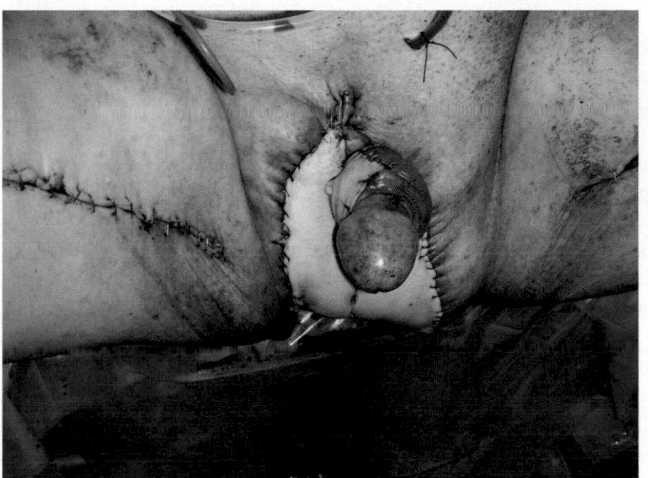

FIGURE 9-35. **A:** Fournier's gangrene of scrotum and perineum. **B:** Debridement of scrotum with testicular sparing. **C:** Grafting of scrotal defect with partial closure of other debrided sites. (Courtesy of Jason Ganz, MD and Paula Denoya, MD.)

adequacy of debridement.[317] Because of the life-threatening nature of the illness, one should not be concerned about the need for subsequent skin coverage or reconstruction.[115,143] One exception to this dictum is the need to protect exposed testes from desiccation. Because the scrotal skin has considerable elastic properties, this can often be used.[317] If this is not possible, the testicles can be implanted in thigh pouches.[325] Urinary diversion (in the form of suprapubic cystostomy) is advocated by some authors, whereas others recommend that this should be reserved only for those with extensive urethral or penile pathology.[233,412] The wounds are left open and packed, and the patient is returned to the operating room if further debridement is deemed advisable. Vigorous irrigation with antiseptic solution (e.g., peroxide, sodium hypochlorite [Dakin solution]) is recommended. Delayed primary closure, skin grafting, and other reconstructive procedures are often ultimately required.

HENRY DRYSDALE DAKIN (1880–1952)

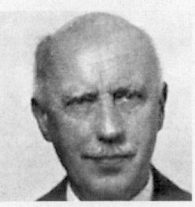

Dakin was born in London, the son of a Leeds iron and steel merchant. In 1898, he entered Yorkshire College, now the University of Leeds, to study under the famous organic chemist, Julius Cohen. Because of Dakin's particular interest in enzyme chemistry, Cohen gave him the nickname "Zyme," which became his mode of address by friends for the rest of his life. Indeed, he became one of the founding leaders in the emerging field of biochemistry. In 1902, Dakin was awarded a scholarship to study in other laboratories—the Jenner Institute in London and with Kossel in Heidelberg. While there, he shared in the discovery of arginase.

When World War I broke out, he offered his services and was asked to cooperate with Alexis Carrel in a research effort in the treatment of injuries suffered by the French wounded at Compiègne. It was there that he developed the buffered hypochlorite solution that bears his name. Later, in the Dardenelles, the ship *Aquitania* was fitted with a special tank for the electrolysis of seawater, through which an unlimited supply of hypochlorite disinfectant solution was made available. On this converted hospital ship, an immediate reduction in the incidence of infection was noted. Among his other notable achievements were the synthesis of epinephrine, the discovery of glyoxalase, and the oxidation of fatty acids. The French government made him a Chevalier of the Legion of Honor.

An interesting approach to the management of Fournier's gangrene was proposed by Efem from the University Department of Surgery in Calabar, Nigeria.[136] He postulated that the organisms commonly associated with the condition are sensitive to the antimicrobial activity of unprocessed honey. In 20 consecutive cases, the author applied the honey topically along with systemic antibiotics. Using historic controls, he observed that the response to treatment and the reduction of morbidity were better in the honey-treated group. It is theorized that its effectiveness is based on a combination of wound debridement, topical antibacterial activity, and local generation of oxygen.

Results

Generally, the results of treatment for this condition, applying the principles outlined earlier, have improved considerably.[223] Eke identified 1,726 patients with Fournier's gangrene in the literature since the 1950s.[140] Enriquez and colleagues described 28 patients with necrotizing genital and perianal infections and noted an overall mortality of 25%.[143] Anorectal infections were more severe and carried a higher mortality than those from primary urologic causes. Di Falco and colleagues reported 5 patients with one death.[115] Full-thickness skin grafts were required in 3 individuals. Barkel and Villalba reported eight cases, six of which were anorectal in origin.[30] One died following treatment by means of an abdominoperineal resection, and another expired of an unrelated cause. The interval from the onset of clinical symptoms to initial surgical intervention is the most important factor that contributes to a successful outcome.[232]

Clayton and colleagues identified 57 men in whom necrotizing fasciitis of the male genitalia developed.[87] Forty-seven (82%) survived. Survival was associated with a younger age, a serum blood urea nitrogen level of less than 50 mg/dL at presentation, and fewer major complications after initial debridement. Interestingly, the authors found that the survival of those with a localized process was no better than that of individuals in whom extension into the abdominal wall or thigh developed. In the experience of Stephens and coworkers, the highest mortality was associated with a colorectal cause (33%).[365] Female mortality (49%) was not significantly greater than male mortality (17%) when obstetric origin was excluded. The overall mortality for the 11 reported cases was 22%.[365]

A Fournier's gangrene severity index score (FGSI) has been proposed to predict the outcome. A score greater than 9 is suggested to have a 75% probability of death, and an index score of 9 or less is associated with a 78% likelihood of survival, but the accuracy of this index remains controversial.[95,215,389,413] The importance of combined aggressive surgical and medical management, using a team comprising an infectious disease specialist, a surgeon, and, if necessary, a urologist, cannot be overestimated.

Ecthyma Gangrenosum

Ecthyma gangrenosum is a skin condition found most commonly in immunocompromised children, such as those with leukemia.[161] It is usually caused by infection with the organism *Pseudomonas aeruginosa*. Most of the lesions are located in the anogenital area, axillae, and extremities. They begin as a small area of edema and quickly evolve into painless nodular lesions with central hemorrhage, ulceration, and necrosis. This disease results from perivascular bacterial invasion of the media and adventitia of arteries and veins with secondary ischemic necrosis. Ecthyma lesions typically progress rapidly and can be single or multiple. A report of the need for perineal reconstruction as a consequence of tissue destruction from this condition has been described.[161]

Perianal Streptococcal Dermatitis

This infectious dermatitis predominantly affects younger children and is caused primarily by group A β-hemolytic streptococci. Most children are diagnosed by pediatricians, but occasionally a colon and rectal surgeon is called on to evaluate the condition. The clinical picture is that of a sharply demarcated perianal erythema. Jongen and colleagues reported a case series of 124 children.[214] Symptoms include itching, anal discomfort, bleeding, constipation, and pain during defecation. The condition is usually characterized by perianal erythema with a mostly well-defined margin. PSD was the most common infectious disease in their practice.[214]

The diagnosis is confirmed by swab culture with treatment by appropriate antibiotics.

Fungal Infections

The primary site of involvement of recognized superficial fungal infections is the skin. This is presumably because fungi digest and live on keratin. These superficial fungi are called dermatophytes; they include *Microsporum*, *Trichophyton*, and *Epidermophyton*.[125]

Tinea Cruris (Jock Itch, Crotch Itch)

Tinea cruris, also known as ringworm of the groin, is caused by a species of *Trichophyton*. The condition occurs most commonly in the intertriginous areas and is exacerbated by heat and humidity (Figure 9-36). The differential diagnosis includes candidiasis, erythrasma, seborrheic dermatitis, psoriasis, and vegetative pemphigus. Demonstration of the fungus by potassium hydroxide microscopic examination and culture confirms the diagnosis (Figure 9-37).

Treatment consists of reduction of perspiration and enhancement of evaporation from the crural area. Daily application of talcum or other desiccant powders to keep the area dry helps prevent recurrence. Loose-fitting clothes are suggested. Griseofulvin has been considered the most

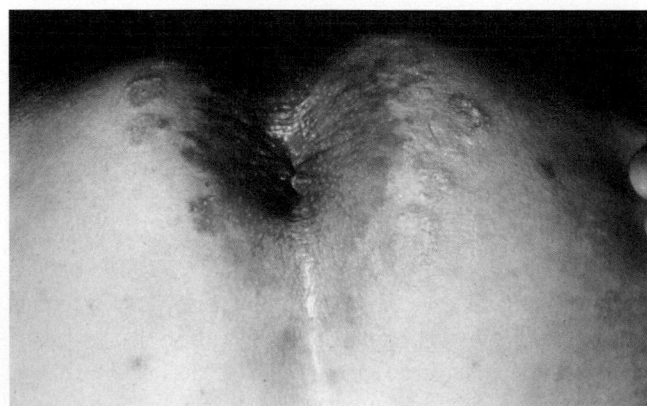

FIGURE 9-36. Dermatophytosis (tinea cruris), a superficial fungal infection. Note that patches have annular borders with scaling and a tendency toward central clearing. (Courtesy of Samuel L. Moschella, MD.)

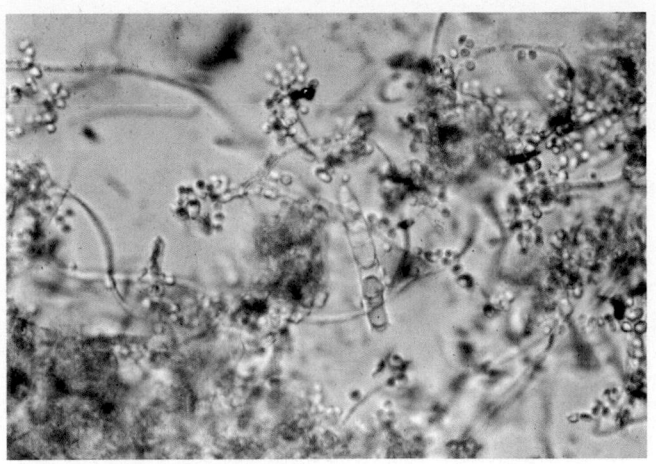

FIGURE 9-37. *Trichophyton mentagrophytes,* as seen in a potassium hydroxide preparation, a species of *Trichophyton* that can cause tinea cruris (ringworm) of the groin. (Original magnification × 600; courtesy of Rudolf Garret, MD.)

effective drug in the treatment of all dermatophytes, but it is rarely needed.[400] Its action is believed to modify keratin so that the fungus will not invade. Treatment for 3 to 4 weeks is advised if topical fungicides such as tolnaftate, clotrimazole, miconazole, econazole, and ciclopirox are not helpful.[400]

Majocchi's Granuloma

Majocchi's granuloma is a rare type of tinea corporis in which the dermatophyte invades the dermis and subcutaneous tissue, instead of being limited to the epidermis. *Trichophyton rubrum* is the most frequent organism.[355] The condition is precipitated by trauma to the skin or occlusion of hair follicles, leading to the disruption of hair follicles and passage of the dermatophyte into the dermis.[82,171] The clinical findings are characterized by a localized area of erythematous, perifollicular papules or small nodules. Pustules may also be present. Rarely systemic disease may occur.[295,355]

A presumptive diagnosis is confirmed with a skin biopsy exhibiting fungal forms in the dermis.[355] Tissue culture can identify the causative organism, but a KOH preparation may remain negative.[152,201,227,355] Topical treatment of superficial fungal infections with glucocorticoids can lead to local immunosuppression and promote the development of Majocchi's granuloma.[82,141] Topical antifungals are unlikely to penetrate deeply enough for effective treatment of this condition. Treatment with an oral antifungal is recommended. Terbinafine taken for 2 to 4 weeks has been successfully used for treatment of this condition.[178,396]

Candidiasis or Moniliasis

Candidiasis is caused by the yeastlike fungus, *Candida albicans.* The fungus is a frequent commensal in humans and is present in the alimentary tract and vagina of many healthy people.[400] Intertriginous areas are commonly affected, including the perianal and inguinal folds and the axillae.

The organism is usually found outside the epidermis and behaves primarily as an opportunistic infection, especially in patients who have impaired resistance (e.g., AIDS). The condition may be somewhat difficult to recognize. Pustules without surrounding inflammation may leave a "collarette" of scale, and satellite lesions can be often seen in adjacent

skin (Figure 9-38). Some eruptions in the inguinal area may resemble tinea cruris, but usually there is less scaling and a greater tendency to fissure.[125] When the condition occurs in children, it is called diaper or napkin (nappy) dermatitis.

The diagnosis of candidiasis is made by demonstrating the yeast, spores, or pseudomycelium under the microscope with potassium hydroxide (see Figure 33-23). Culture on Sabouraud's glucose agar shows a growth of creamy, grayish, moist colonies in about 4 days.[125]

Treatment consists of topical nystatin, clotrimazole, or miconazole. For very severe cases, usually in those patients with an immunologic deficiency, oral ketoconazole Nizoral), 200 mg, or intravenous amphotericin B can be administered.

Sporotrichosis, Coccidioidomycosis, Histoplasmosis, North American Blastomycosis, Chromomycosis, Cryptococcosis, Nocardiosis, and Mycetoma

These fungal infections are generally known as the "deep" mycoses. They usually come from inhalation of dust contaminated with the fungus, from droppings of animals infected by it, or from contamination from other sources.[125] All have associated skin lesions, which have a good prognosis in the case of primary cutaneous infections. However, when skin involvement is the result of dissemination from a visceral focus, the prognosis is usually much worse. Generally, skin biopsy will reveal the presence of the fungi.

Treatment varies with the type of fungus and with the extent of disease, either localized or systemic. The reader is referred to a textbook of medicine for the clinical features, diagnosis, and management of these conditions.

Parasitic Diseases

Numerous parasitic diseases exhibit cutaneous manifestations and many of these also affect the alimentary tract. Included are infections caused by protozoa (i.e., single-cell organisms), nematodes (i.e., roundworms), arthropods, trematodes (i.e., flukes), cestodes (i.e., flatworms), annelids (i.e., leeches), and chordates. Some of these conditions are addressed in Chapter 33. The discussion that follows is limited to those cutaneous manifestations that may be of interest to the surgeon.

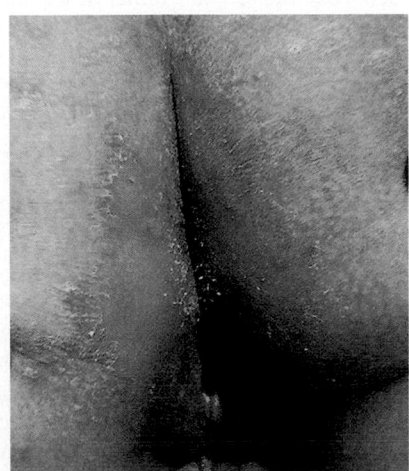

FIGURE 9-38. Perianal candidiasis and vulvovaginitis. Superficial infections of skin and mucosal membranes may cause local inflammation and commonly discomfort.

Amebiasis Cutis

Entamoeba histolytica is an organism that causes disease that is most common in the tropics. Cutaneous amebiasis occurs less frequently than the intestinal condition, except for cutaneous manifestations in the genitalia and perianal area. It is believed that the reason for its presentation in this location is direct extension from the involved bowel. Lesions begin as deep abscesses that rupture and form exquisitely tender distinct ulcerations; there is usually an erythematous halo around the ulcer. Perianal lesions can extend to involve the genitalia and may be mistaken for condylomata lata or squamous cell carcinoma. Characteristically, skin lesions spread rapidly and may terminate fatally.

Histologically, there are areas of necrotic ulceration, with many lymphocytes, neutrophils, plasma cells, and eosinophils. The organism is frequently demonstrated in the fresh material from the base (see Chapter 33). Serologic tests are usually negative in early cases and in the absence of hepatic or invasive intestinal involvement.

Although abscesses may require surgical drainage, the cutaneous manifestation will usually respond to either metronidazole or emetine.

Trichomoniasis

Trichomonas vulvovaginitis causes vaginal pruritus, burning, and leukorrhea. The condition is caused by the protozoan *T. vaginalis*. Because of the discharge and pruritic symptoms, the anal area may be secondarily involved by the irritation. Eliciting a history of the vaginal discharge will alert the physician to the source of the problem. Treatment is metronidazole (Flagyl), 250 mg for 10 days.

Schistosomal Dermatitis (Schistosomiasis Cutis, Swimmer's Itch)

Schistosomal dermatitis is a severe pruritic, papular dermatitis caused by cercarial species of *Schistosoma*, a genus of trematodes. Exposure to the cercariae (see Figure 33-41) occurs by swimming or wading in freshwater containing them. They attach by burrowing into the skin. Clinically, there is severe itching at the time of the exposure secondary to an urticarial reaction. The resultant papular, pruritic lesion spontaneously regresses after a few days, disappearing by 2 weeks. Antipruritic measures are used for treatment.

Visceral schistosomiasis (i.e., bilharziasis) may produce cutaneous manifestations as a result of deposition of eggs in the dermis. Fistulous tracts may develop in the perineum and buttocks, associated with hard masses, sinus tracts, and seropurulent discharge with a characteristic foul odor. In the severe vegetating form, malignant change in the granulomas has been noted. Treatment consists of trivalent antimony compounds (e.g., tartar emetic, stibophen, trivalent sodium antimonyl gluconate [Triostam], astiban).

Nematode Infections

Oxyuriasis (Pinworm, Threadworm, Enterobiasis)

Enterobius (Oxyuris) vermicularis is the helminth that most commonly infects humans. Children are more frequently affected than adults, and the condition is more common in temperate climates than in the tropics. The worm lives in the proximal colon and is often found in the appendix (Figure 9-39), but the disease is not truly related to the bowel itself. The worms migrate to the rectum at night and emerge on the perianal skin to deposit thousands of ova

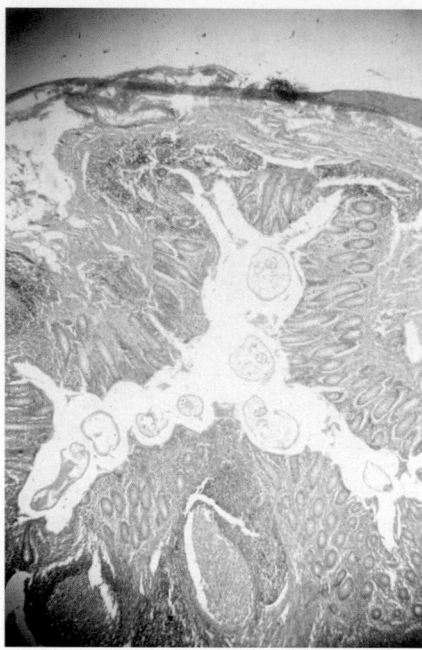

FIGURE 9-39. *Enterobius vermicularis* infection. In a cross-sectional view, pinworms are seen in the appendix. (Original magnification × 80; courtesy of Rudolf Garret, MD.)

(Figures 9-40 and 9-41). The ova are returned to the mouth by the patient through scratching. The larvae then hatch in the duodenum and migrate to the small and large intestine. Fertilization occurs in the cecum, completing the life cycle.

The primary complaint is usually itching, especially interfering with the patient's sleep. Friction and maceration by tight-fitting clothes may lead to superficial or deep folliculitis of the buttocks and perineum.[157] Anal abscess complicating

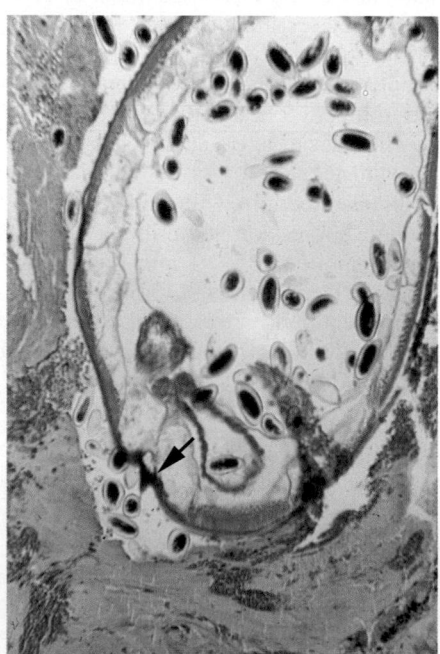

FIGURE 9-40. Adult pinworm (*Enterobius vermicularis*). Note the prominent lateral alae (*arrow*). Numerous ova are seen. (Original magnification × 170; courtesy of Rudolf Garret, MD.)

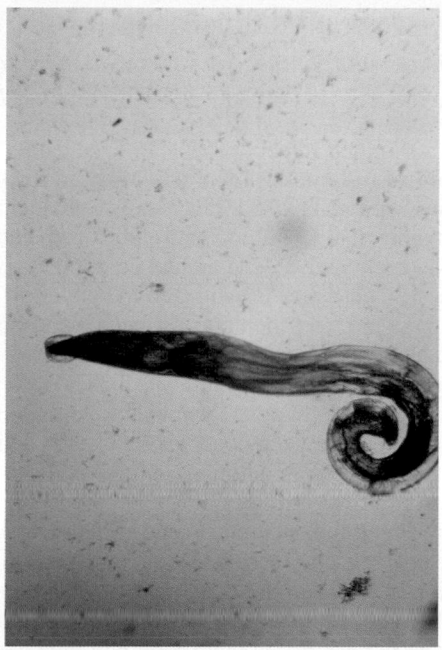

FIGURE 9-41. *Enterobius vermicularis*, the adult pinworm (female). (Courtesy of Rudolf Garret, MD.)

the condition has also been reported,[284] as has a perineal, subcutaneous nodule.[242] Other symptoms include restlessness and insomnia.[210] Secondary bacterial infections can result if the excoriation is severe.

The diagnosis is usually established by demonstration of the ova in smears taken from the anal area early in the morning. Applying cellophane tape against the perianal region, adding a drop of iodine, and examining the tape under a microscope slide may facilitate detection of the ova. Demonstration of the pinworm in the stool is rarely successful, but occasionally the adult worms may be seen on the perianal skin. Because of the high likelihood of communication, it is appropriate to study members of the patient's family.

Current management of pinworm infestation is mebendazole (Vermox), 100 mg, as a chewable tablet, taken once. Other effective medications for the treatment of the condition are piperazine (Antepar) and pyrvinium pamoate (Povan). The former is given in single daily doses of 65 mg/kg (not to exceed 2,500 mg) taken 1 hour before breakfast for 8 consecutive days, and the latter is given in a single dose of 5 mg/kg; a second dose may be given 1 week after the first treatment.[126] Undergarments, towels, sheets, pajamas, and other clothing should be thoroughly laundered separately from those of other members of the family.

Creeping Eruption or Larva Migrans
Larva migrans is a cutaneous eruption caused by larvae of several nematodes, most commonly the cat or dog hookworm, *Ancylostoma braziliense* or *A. caninum*. The ova of these hookworms are deposited in the soil and hatch into infectious larvae that penetrate the skin. People who go barefoot at the beach, children playing in sandboxes, carpenters and plumbers working under homes, and gardeners are the most common victims.[126] The feet, buttocks, hands, and genitals are most frequently involved by the process. Raised, pruritic, thin, linear, tunnel-like lesions that contain serous

fluid are noted. Rare pulmonary involvement occurs due to larval hematogenous dissemination to the lungs.

The disease is usually self-limited, but freezing of the larvae with ethyl chloride or liquid nitrogen is effective. An alternative internal treatment is thiabendazole (Mintezol). Systemic treatment with ivermectin or albendazole is also acceptable.[9]

Larva Currens
Larva currens is a form of cutaneous larva migrans caused by *Strongyloides stercoralis*. The condition is so called because of the speed of larval migration. It is caused in essence by an autoinfection, penetration of the perianal skin by larvae excreted in the feces. The eruption is usually associated with intestinal strongyloidiasis, beginning in the skin around the anus, and may involve the buttocks, thighs, and back. The itching is quite severe. As the larvae leave the skin to enter the bloodstream and settle in the intestinal mucosa, the rash disappears. The skin demonstrates a papular eruption with edema and urticaria. Treatment consists of thiabendazole, 25 to 50 mg/kg for 2 to 4 days.

Insect Diseases
Cimicosis or Bedbug Bites
The bedbug (i.e., *Cimex lectularius*) hides in crevices during the daytime and feeds on human blood at night.[175] The bedbug usually produces a linear series of bites on the ankles and buttocks. Because the bites are painless, the patient may not be aware of what has happened until finding the bedclothes stained with blood. Some individuals may react with severe urticaria and pain. Treatment consists of soothing antipruritic lotions. The pests are eliminated by means of fumigation (e.g., with malathion).

Pediculosis Pubis (Phthiriasis)
Several varieties of *Pediculus* affect humans, but the one that concerns us for the purpose of this discussion is *Phthirus pubis* (*P. pubis*), the pubic or crab louse. The condition is usually transmitted by sexual intercourse or acquired from contaminated bedding. Teenagers and young adults are most commonly affected. The lice are found on the hair or skin and appear as yellowish brown or gray, glistening specks.[126] The so-called nits are attached to the hair shaft and are best seen under Wood's light. Symptoms include intense pruritus and the secondary effects of persistent excoriation. Inguinal lymphadenopathy is present in some patients. The condition frequently coexists with other sexually transmitted diseases. A thorough sexual history and screening for other sexually transmitted diseases is warranted in patients with pediculosis pubis. Treatment consists of 1% γ-benzene hexachloride cream or lotion to the pubic area, lindane (Kwell), or crotamiton (Eurax). Bed linen and clothing essentially require sterilization.

Arachnid Infection
Scabies
Scabies is a skin condition resulting from infestation by the mite *Sarcoptes scabiei*. Transmission is usually from person to person by direct contact or through clothing. The female burrows into the stratum corneum and there deposits her eggs. Patients complain primarily of itching that is worse at night. The itching is the result of a delayed type IV

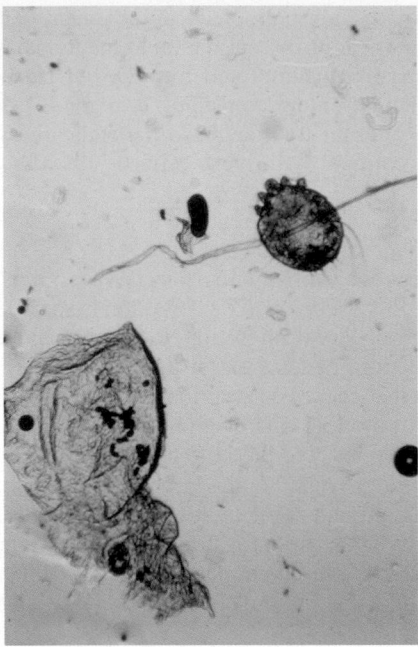

FIGURE 9-42. Scrapings from a scabies lesion showing the female mite. (Original magnification × 240; courtesy of Rudolf Garret, MD.)

hypersensitivity reaction to the mite, mite feces, and mite eggs.[106] Areas commonly involved include the interdigital folds; flexor aspects of the wrist, nipples, navel, genitals, buttocks; and outer aspects of the feet. The lesion appears as a whitish burrow that is rather tortuous and threadlike. Papules and pustules are frequently seen. The condition is usually contracted by close contact with a person harboring the mite. The diagnosis is made by microscopic examination of scrapings or shave excision of suspected skin for eggs, larvae, adult mites, or feces (Figures 9-42 and 9-43).[156] Treatment consists of permethrin (Elimite) cream, 10% crotamiton cream (Eurax), oral ivermectin, or thiabendazole, as well as decontamination of clothing. Any complicating pyoderma should be treated with appropriate systemic antibiotics.

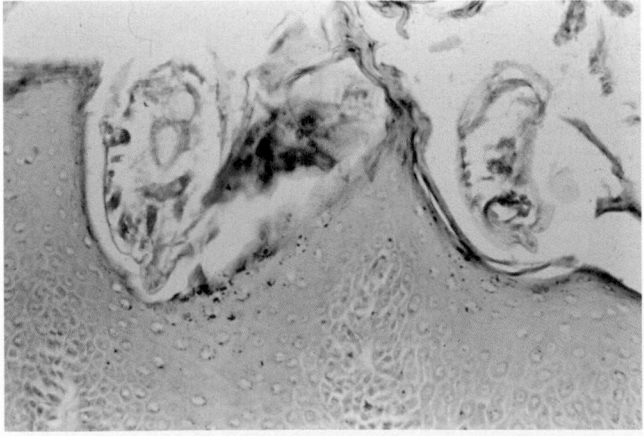

FIGURE 9-43. A biopsy specimen showing the female mite burrowing into the epidermis. (Original magnification × 280; courtesy of Rudolf Garret, MD.)

Sexually Transmitted Diseases

Two minutes with Venus, two years with mercury.
—J. EARLE MOORE: *Aphorism*

Sexually transmitted infections (STIs), once called STD, are among the most common infectious diseases in the United States today. More than 20 STIs have now been identified, and they affect more than 13 million men and women in the United States alone each year.[299] The annual comprehensive cost of STIs in the United States is estimated to be well in excess of $10 billion. STIs affect men and women of all backgrounds and economic levels but are most prevalent among teenagers and young adults. Nearly two-thirds of all STIs occur in people younger than 25 years of age. The incidence of STIs continues to rise, in part because young people are sexually active earlier yet are marrying later. In addition, divorce is more common. The net result is that sexually active people today are more likely to have multiple sex partners during their lives. Sohn and Robilotti coined the phrase "gay bowel syndrome" to indicate a constellation of diseases and conditions to which male homosexuals fall victim.[360] Receptive anal intercourse is a particular risk factor because of the greater fragility of the rectal mucosa in comparison with the squamous mucosa of the vagina.[306]

Most of the time, STIs cause no symptoms, particularly in women. When and if symptoms develop, they may be confused with those of other diseases not transmitted through sexual contact. Health problems caused by STIs tend to be more severe and more frequent for women than for men, in part because the frequency of asymptomatic infection means that many women do not seek care until serious problems have developed. Some STIs can spread into the uterus and fallopian tubes to cause pelvic inflammatory disease, which, in turn, is a major cause of both infertility and ectopic pregnancy. STIs in women also may be associated with cervical cancer. One STI, human papillomavirus (HPV) infection, causes genital warts and cervical and other genital cancers. The following is a list of STIs and the organisms responsible:

Disease	*Organism*
AIDS HIV	
Bacterial vaginosis	*Bacteroides, Gardnerella vaginalis, Mobiluncus* sp., *Mycoplasma hominis, Ureaplasma urealyticum*
Chancroid	*Haemophilus ducreyi*
Chlamydial infections	*Chlamydia trachomatis*
Cytomegalovirus infections	Cytomegalovirus
Genital herpes	Herpes simplex virus
Genital (venereal) warts	HPV
Gonorrhea	*Neisseria gonorrhoeae*
Granuloma inguinale (donovanosis)	*Calymmatobacterium granulomatis*
Leukemia-lymphoma	Human T-cell lymphotrophic virus I and II
Lymphogranuloma venereum	*Chlamydia trachomatis*
Molluscum contagiosum	Molluscum contagiosum virus
Pubic lice	*Pediculus pubis*
Scabies	*Sarcoptes scabiei*
Syphilis	*Treponema pallidum*
Trichomoniasis	*Trichomonas vaginalis*
Vaginal yeast infections	*Candida albicans*

The epidemic venereal conditions today are condylomata acuminata, anogenital herpes, and HIV/AIDS (see Chapter 10). With the changes in mores and attitudes toward sexual matters, it is incumbent on the surgeon to be knowledgeable about the manifestations, differential diagnosis, and treatment of STIs.

Gonorrhea

Gonorrhea is a bacterial infection caused by *Neisseria gonorrhoeae*, a gram-negative diplococcus. Humans are the only known reservoir. The disease affects mucous membranes of the urethra, cervix, rectum, and oropharynx. During the 1980s, the incidence of the disease declined markedly, but still the condition is diagnosed at least 10 times more often than syphilis. The 2003 summary of reported cases by the U.S. Centers for Disease Control and Prevention (CDC) reached an all-time low of 116.2 cases per 100,000 population.[72] More than 300,000 cases of gonorrhea are reported to the CDC each year. Gonorrhea appears to facilitate both the transmission and acquisition of HIV.[89,244] The incidence in the black population has been reported to be almost 40 times that of whites.

The most common symptoms of gonorrhea are a discharge from the vagina or penis and painful or difficult urination. Gonococcal dermatitis is a rare infection that may develop in a wound that has come in contact with the bacterium, including wounds of the genital area. The most common and serious complications occur in women and, as with chlamydial infection, these complications include pelvic inflammatory disease, ectopic pregnancy, and infertility. The complication of gonorrheal proctitis is of particular interest to the surgeon. This is usually seen in the homosexual population as a result of infection from anal intercourse (see Chapter 10). In women, the condition is frequently caused by spread to the rectum from the genital tract. The vast majority of anorectal gonorrheal infections in women are asymptomatic. When symptoms occur, they include anal itching, rectal discharge, rectal fullness, and painful defecation.[229] In one study of 228 women with gonorrhea, culture of the anal canal using a blind swab technique was as reliable as rectal swab samples collected under direct visualization.[231] Historically, penicillin has been used to treat gonorrhea, but since the mid-1990s, antibiotic resistance has emerged. New antibiotics or combinations of drugs must be used to treat these resistant strains. Due to the increasing prevalence of quinolone-resistant *N. gonorrhoeae*, the CDC has issued recommendations for the use of third-generation cephalosporins as first-line therapy.[74] The reader is referred to Chapter 33 for a discussion of gonococcal proctitis and its treatment.

Syphilis (Lues)

*Know syphilis in all its manifestations
and relations, and all things clinical
will be added unto you.*

—WILLIAM OSLER: *Aequanimitas*

According to the U.S. Public Health Service, the incidence of primary and secondary syphilis in the United States is about 130,000 cases annually, with 3 cases in men reported for every 1 in a woman.[156] The disease is caused by the spirochete *Treponema pallidum*.

The organism enters the skin or mucous membrane, producing a chancre approximately 3 weeks following the infection. This is the primary stage of the disease. The lesion is usually single and is most commonly found as an open sore on the penis or vagina, but it can also be seen on the lips, tongue, tonsillar area, and in the anus. In women,

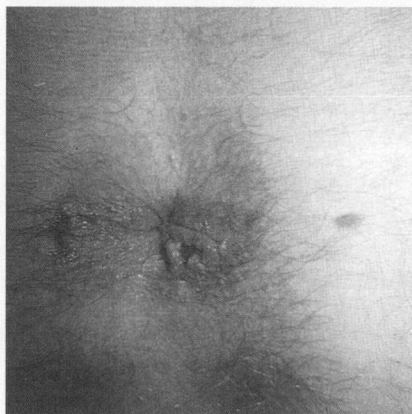

FIGURE 9-44. A noninflamed, punched out–appearing ulcerated chancre that was dark field positive for *Treponema pallidum*.

it may be inapparent because of its location within the vagina or cervix. In the homosexual population, the chancre is usually situated at the anal margin or in the anal canal (Figure 9-44). The lesion is usually painless, but near the anal opening there may be severe discomfort, tenesmus, difficulty with defecation, and discharge. Unless there is a high index of suspicion, the condition may be confused with an anal fissure, but the presence of inguinal adenopathy should alert the examiner to this possibility. The aberrant location of the fissure (e.g., lateral) may create some suspicion, but this also could be a finding consistent with anal Crohn's disease.

Most writings on the subject state that the diagnosis can be established based on identification of the organism by means of dark-field examination (Figure 9-45).

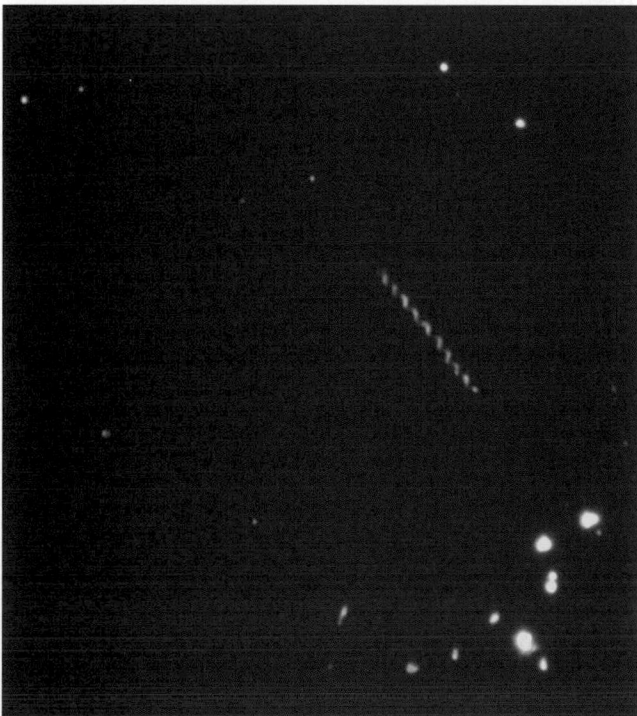

FIGURE 9-45. *Treponema pallidum*, the causative agent of syphilis, appears as a corkscrew-shaped organism on dark-field examination. (Original magnification × 600; courtesy of Rudolf Garret, MD.)

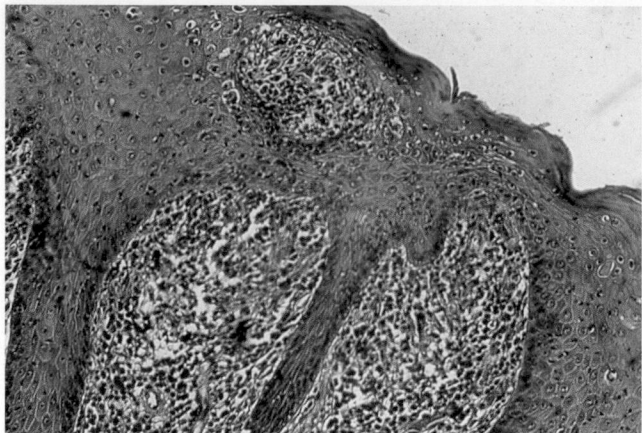

FIGURE 9-46. Syphilitic chancre demonstrating pseudoepitheliomatous hyperplasia and plasma cell infiltration of the dermis with dilated lymphatics. (Original magnification × 250; courtesy of Rudolf Garret, MD.)

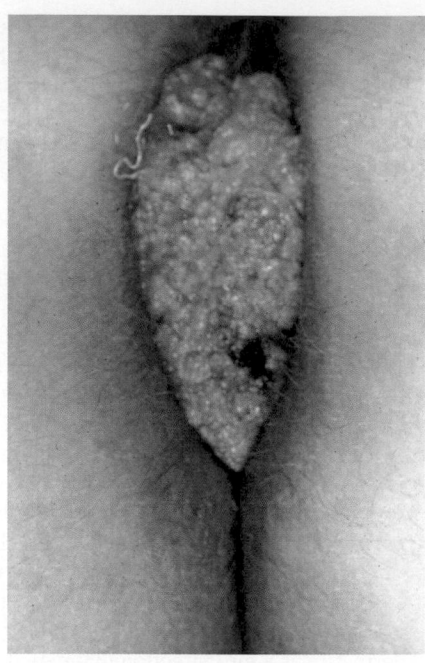

FIGURE 9-47. Condylomata lata. This large, perianal, mucoid, warty mass is composed of smooth-surfaced lobules. (Courtesy of Rudolf Garret, MD.)

Because the absence of a positive test result does not exclude the diagnosis, it is probably preferable to treat patients with suspected clinical lesions and await the results of serologic evaluation. It is important to remember, however, that serologic tests for syphilis do not yield positive results until the primary chancre has been present for several weeks.

Although excision of the lesion is not recommended, there are characteristic histopathologic changes (Figure 9-46).[131] There is dense infiltration by round cells, plasma cells, and fibroblasts. Proliferation of endothelial cells results in progressive arteritis.

Treatment
Benzathine penicillin is the treatment of choice in nonallergic patients, 2.4 million U intramuscularly, repeated 7 days later. For those who are allergic to penicillin, tetracycline, 500 mg orally four times daily for 15 days, is recommended.[131] Other tetracyclines can be used as well as erythromycin, 500 mg orally four times daily for 15 days (see Chapter 10).

Condylomata Lata
The other cutaneous manifestation of lues is the secondary stage of syphilis, condylomata lata. The signs and symptoms of secondary syphilis may develop 2 to 6 months after infection and usually 6 to 8 weeks after the appearance of the primary chancre. Both lesions may exist synchronously. A maculopapular rash develops, which gives rise to a proliferating, weeping mass containing the spirochetes. The lesions may appear rather flat, scaling, red, and indurated. In the anal area particularly, they may become papillomatous and vegetative with an associated foul odor (Figure 9-47). Although most literature suggests that the lesions are nonpruritic, some believe that this may be the primary complaint.[90]

The diagnosis may be established by demonstrating the organism using dark-field microscopic examination, but results of serologic tests are virtually always positive. The histopathology of secondary syphilis varies depending on the clinical presentation. The lesions of condylomata lata show acanthosis and edema in the epidermis with broadening of the rete ridges (Figure 9-48). Some lesions may demonstrate a nonspecific chronic inflammatory reaction with a large number of plasma cells (Figure 9-49).

Treatment with penicillin, erythromycin, or tetracycline is effective. An important part of the management of the patient includes the tracing of all sexual contacts, which, in the case of secondary syphilis, necessitates a 1-year retrospective review.

Chancroid
Chancroid is a rare sexually transmitted disease, but recent years have seen an increase in the incidence in the United States, presumably based on individuals emigrating from the Caribbean, Mexico, and Southeast Asia.[156] The condition is most common in tropical and subtropical areas and in the poorer populations. The disease is caused by the gram-negative bacillus, *Haemophilus ducreyi*.

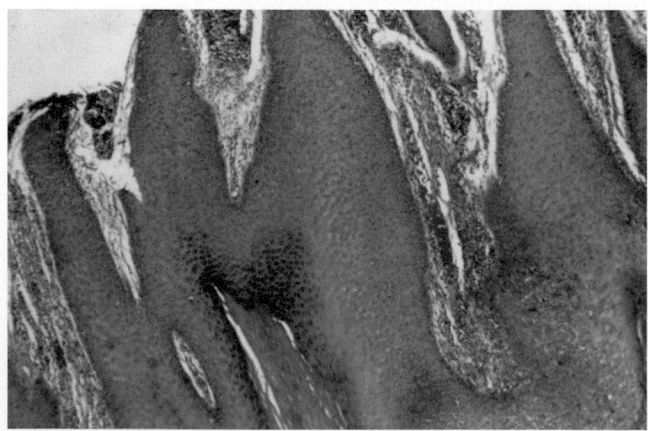

FIGURE 9-48. Condylomata lata demonstrating dilated lymphatics, proliferation of the prickle cell layer (acanthosis), and an inflammatory exudate. (Original magnification × 250; courtesy of Rudolf Garret, MD.)

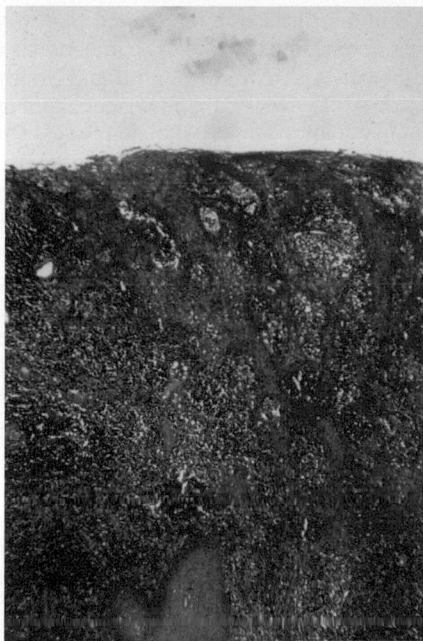

FIGURE 9-49. Condylomata lata showing pseudoepitheliomatous hyperplasia of the squamous epithelium. A heavy plasma cell infiltrate is evident in the dermis, with dilated lymphatics. (Original magnification × 250; courtesy of Rudolf Garret, MD.)

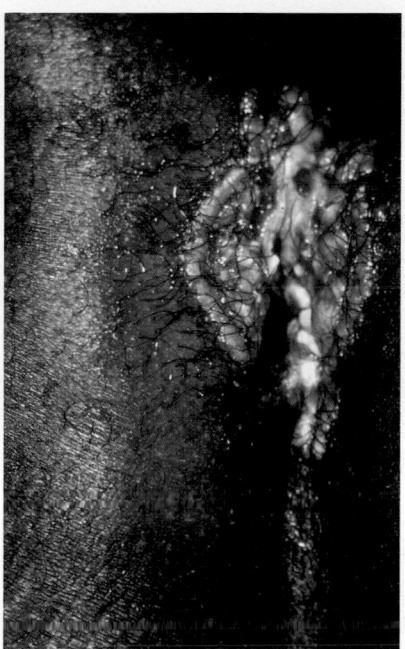

FIGURE 9-50. Cicatricial granulomatous nodule with a surrounding erythematous border, characteristic of granuloma inguinale. (Courtesy of Rudolf Garret, MD.)

Chancroid begins on the genitals as an inflammatory macule or pustule; the latter ruptures, forming a punched-out ulcer with irregular edges. Within a few days to 2 weeks, inguinal adenitis frequently develops, which may lead to perforation of the lymphatics. The inguinal node is called a *bubo*. Characteristic of chancroid is its tendency to auto-inoculation. In addition to involvement of the anal area, extragenital lesions may be noted on the hands, eyelids, and elsewhere. The diagnosis is established by demonstrating the bacterium in smears from the ulcer grown on enhanced chocolate agar vancomycin[156] or on an enriched medium containing hemin.[385] When examined on Gram stain, organisms from culture often clump in long parallel strands, producing a so-called school of fish appearance. Because many cases are resistant to tetracycline, treatment usually consists of sulfonamides (i.e., double-strength trimethoprim-sulfamethoxazole), one tablet orally every 12 hours for 14 days. Third-generation cephalosporins are also effective. Patients with suspected chancroid also should be empirically treated for syphilis because of frequent coinfection.[75] Data from the era before effective antimicrobial therapy suggested that failure to aspirate fluctuant buboes results in the development of draining fistulas or secondary ulcers at the site of spontaneous rupture.[374] A recent study found that there is no difference in the clinical outcomes between needle aspiration and incision and drainage of fluctuant lymphadenitis associated with chancroid. However, those who have undergone needle aspiration often require repeated aspirations.[144]

Granuloma Inguinale (Granuloma Venereum, Donovanosis)
Granuloma inguinale is a chronic, granulomatous, ulcerative skin disease caused by *Calymmatobacterium granulomatis*, formerly known as *Donovania granulomatis*. In the United States, fewer than 100 cases are reported annually, almost exclusively in homosexual, African American men.[156]

There is some question whether it may be transmitted non-venereally as well as venereally. The lesions appear as cauliflower-like proliferations from which develop pustules and papules (Figure 9-50). Sinuses and scars are characteristic, with healed areas often devoid of pigment (Figure 9-51). The lesions may be quite uncomfortable. Adenopathy is not necessarily present, but secondary infection with abscess of

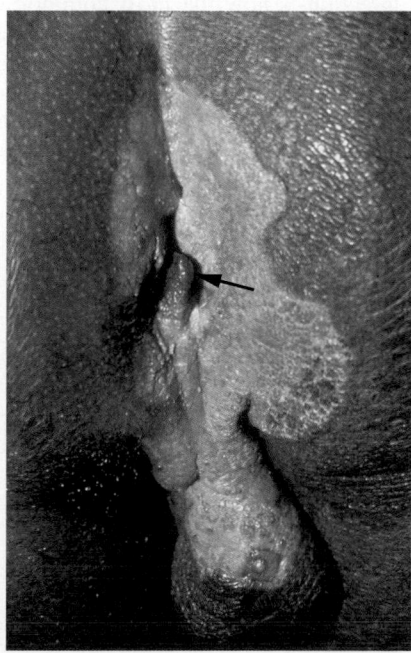

FIGURE 9-51. Granuloma inguinale. This is a chronic, irregularly shaped, enlarging ulceration of the perianal area (*arrow*). Note the hypertrophic scarring devoid of pigment. (Courtesy of Samuel L. Moschella, MD.)

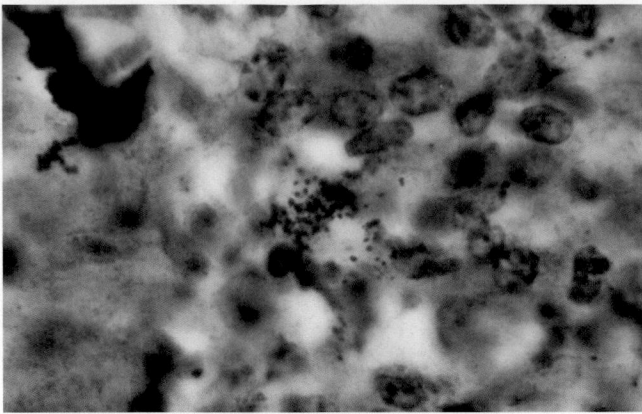

FIGURE 9-52. Granuloma inguinale. Donovan bodies in macrophages are demonstrated by Leishman's stain. (Original magnification × 600; courtesy of Rudolf Garret, MD.)

inguinal nodes can occur. Squamous cell carcinoma may develop in long-standing, untreated lesions.

The diagnosis is usually established by the appearance, by the history, and by the staining of a punch biopsy specimen. Donovan bodies appear as deeply staining, bipolar, safety pin–shaped rods in the cytoplasm of macrophages (Figure 9-52). Biopsy usually reveals a massive, predominantly polymorphonuclear inflammatory reaction, thickening of the epidermis at the periphery, and pale-staining macrophages, usually in the upper parts of the granuloma (Figure 9-53).

Many antibiotics have been successful in the treatment; the recommended alternative is azithromycin, 1 g weekly until complete healing is achieved.[298] If irreversible tissue destruction develops, resective surgery may be necessary.

Chlamydia Infection, Lymphogranuloma Venereum (Lymphogranuloma Inguinale, Lymphopathia Venereum)

Chlamydia infection is now the most common of all bacterial STIs in the United States, with an estimated 4 to 8 million new cases occurring each year. It is most frequently seen in the homosexual population, with a particularly high incidence among African Americans. Lymphogranuloma venereum is a suppurative STI caused by *C. trachomatis*. It has

been an uncommon disease in the United States, with fewer than 400 cases noted annually.[156,260] The infection is more common in Southeast Asia, Africa, Central and South America, and the Caribbean. However, the incidence is increasing as a complication in patients with AIDS patients (see Chapter 10).

Lymphogranuloma venereum is predominantly a disease of lymphatic tissue. It induces a lymphoproliferative reaction through direct extension from the primary infection site to the draining lymph node basins. The nodes are filled with areas of necrosis, followed by abscess formation.[262] The microorganism appears to bind to epithelial cells via heparin sulfate receptors.[79] Early symptoms are referable to the genitourinary tract, although 25% of men and 50% of women experience no initial symptoms. In both men and women, chlamydial infection may cause an abnormal genital discharge and burning with urination. Late untreated or undertreated disease is characterized by fibrosis and strictures. In women, untreated chlamydial infection may lead to pelvic inflammatory disease, one of the most common causes of ectopic pregnancy and infertility. A case of the disease presenting as a rectovaginal fistula has been described.[260]

The lesion initially appears as a herpetiform vesicle on the genitalia or anal area. Complaints, when they occur, include dysuria, pyuria, and mucopurulent discharge. Lower abdominal pain may also be noted, especially in women. The diagnosis can be established by noting the clinical pattern of the genital lesion, followed 1 to 4 weeks later by marked unilateral lymphadenopathy and systemic symptoms. The nodes enlarge, form a large mass, become fluctuant, and drain.

Lymphogranuloma venereum may also start in the rectum as a proctitis. Clinical symptoms under these circumstances are rectal discharge, bleeding, and tenesmus. An associated anal fissure is not uncommon. Perianal and rectovaginal fistulas may develop, and in late cases, progression to severe rectal stricture can occur. Approximately 2 weeks following the appearance of the primary lesion, inguinal lymphadenopathy is evident. Characteristically, in men the nodes fuse together in a large mass. If the primary lesion appears on the cervix or in the rectum, the perirectal and deep iliac nodes will enlarge.[156] Intestinal obstruction and elephantiasis of the genitals are late sequelae.

Histologically, the changes consist of an infectious granuloma with the formation of stellate abscesses (Figure 9-54).

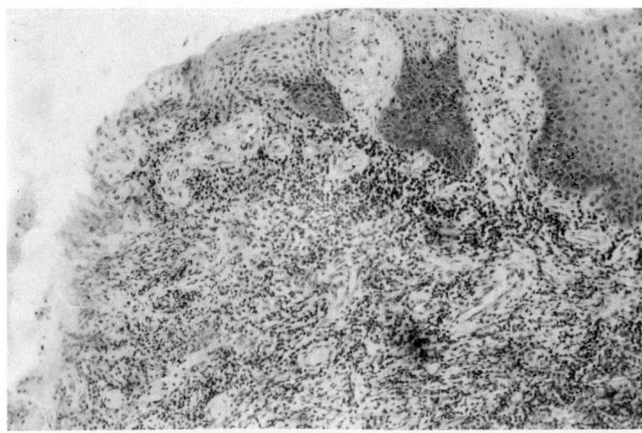

FIGURE 9-53. Granuloma inguinale. Mononuclear cell infiltrate in the dermis with an ulcer on the left is seen. (Original magnification × 120; courtesy of Rudolf Garret, MD.)

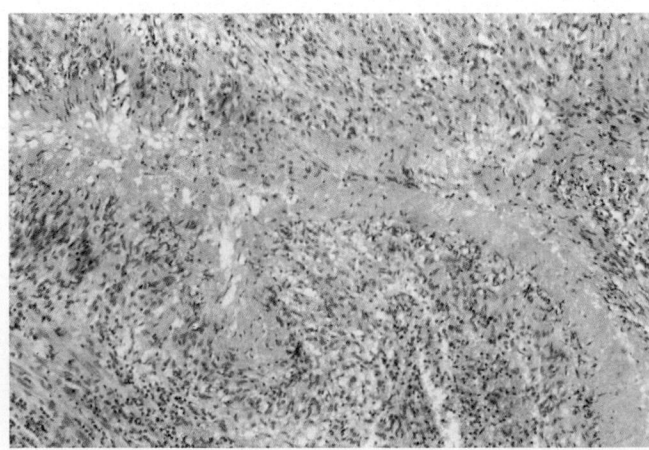

FIGURE 9-54. Lymphogranuloma venereum. Stellate granuloma in a lymph node is evident. (Original magnification × 280; courtesy of Rudolf Garret, MD.)

Laboratory studies reveal characteristic abnormalities, such as the frequently observed inversion of the albumin-globulin ratio. The so-called Frei test had been employed to establish the diagnosis of lymphogranuloma venereum; this is an intradermal test similar to the tuberculin test. However, the procedure has fallen into disrepute and generally is not available. The lymphogranuloma venereum complement fixation test is considered positive at 1:80 or higher, but the microimmunofluorescent test is regarded as being more sensitive.[156] Elevated titers are noted approximately 1 month after the onset of the illness. A positive serologic test for IgG antibodies, in the presence of a compatible clinical syndrome, is considered adequate for a presumptive diagnosis. Most authorities recommend a titer of greater than 1:256 in order to establish the diagnosis, whereas a titer of less than 1:32 rules it out.[262] Nucleic acid amplification testing (NAAT) of rectal specimens is not currently approved by the U.S. Food and Drug Administration (FDA). However, the current literature suggests that sensitivity and specificity of NAAT is greater than 95% when compared with culture.[35,78,182,254,339,392] Recommended treatments include the following: tetracycline, 500 mg orally four times daily for 21 days; erythromycin, 500 mg orally four times daily for 21 days; and double-strength trimethoprim-sulfamethoxazole, every 12 hours for 21 days.[108,156] Needle aspiration or incision and drainage of buboes may be required to prevent their rupture and sinus tract formation. Patients with a clinical syndrome consistent with lymphogranuloma venereum proctocolitis are treated with empiric therapy of doxycycline, 100 mg, orally twice a day for 7 days and ceftriaxone, 125 mg, once intramuscularly, pending results of laboratory tests.[75] Rectal stenosis may require a resective procedure or fecal diversion (Figure 9-55).[98]

Molluscum Contagiosum

Molluscum contagiosum is a communicable skin disease caused by a poxvirus. It is seen principally in preschool and elementary school children. In adults, it is most closely associated with underlying cellular immunodeficiency, such as HIV, and also in the setting of chemotherapy or corticosteroid administration. The condition can involve the skin of the

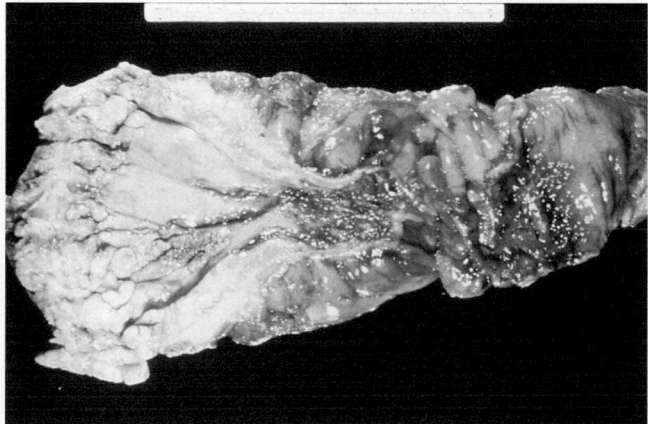

FIGURE 9-55. Severe rectal stricture caused by lymphogranuloma venereum necessitated proctectomy. If resection is necessary, reestablishment of intestinal continuity should be attempted if possible. (From Corman ML, Veidenheimer MC, Swinton NW. *Diseases of the Anus, Rectum and Colon. Part I: Neoplasms.* New York, NY: Medcom; 1972, with permission.)

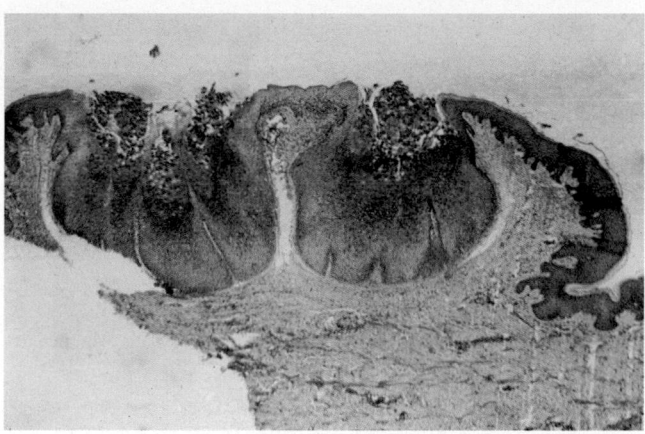

FIGURE 9-56. Proliferation of squamous cells with formation of pear-shaped lobules and molluscum bodies in the central, craterlike area, characteristic of molluscum contagiosum. (Original magnification × 120; courtesy of Rudolf Garret, MD.)

abdomen, thighs, groin, genitalia, buttocks, and, in homosexual men, the perianal area. The lesions begin as papules, often develop central umbilication, and may be widely disseminated. They are often asymptomatic but may be pruritic.

Molluscum contagiosum has a characteristic histopathology. There is a downward proliferation of the rete ridges and envelopment by the connective tissue to form a deep crater. So-called molluscum bodies are found in the cytoplasm of the cells of the stratum malpighii (Figure 9-56).

Treatment may not be required because the lesions usually heal without scarring unless secondarily infected. Curettage can be employed using ethyl chloride spray for freezing. Liquid nitrogen, electrocoagulation, 20% podophyllin, trichloroacetic acid, carbon dioxide laser, and pulsed dye laser have also been effective.[414]

Herpes Genitalis, Genital Herpes, Herpes Simplex Infection, Herpes

Herpes simplex is a ubiquitous infection caused by a virus that has been associated with a number of acute, limited, vesicular eruptions near mucocutaneous junctions. Synonyms include fever blister, cold sore, herpes febrilis, herpes labialis, and genital herpes. According to the CDC, approximately 500,000 new cases occur annually, with 60 million Americans believed to be harboring the virus.[156]

Classically, herpes simplex virus type 1 (HSV-1) commonly appeared above the waistline and was not usually sexually acquired, whereas with the type 2 form (HSV-2), the opposite was often the case.[156] With the increased frequency of oral-genital sex, however, both types may be found in each location. The likelihood of reactivation of herpes simplex infection differs between HSV-1 and HSV-2 infections; the frequency of clinical recurrence with the genital form is six times that of the oral-labial type.[243]

The major symptoms of herpes infection are painful blisters or open sores in the genital area (Figure 9-57). These may be preceded by a tingling or burning sensation in the legs, buttocks, or genital region. The herpes sores usually disappear within 2 to 3 weeks, but the virus remains in the body for life, and the lesions may recur from time to time. Cutaneous lesions associated with herpes simplex infections are usually characteristic vesicles in small groups. However, patients are often not seen until the vesicles have ulcerated.

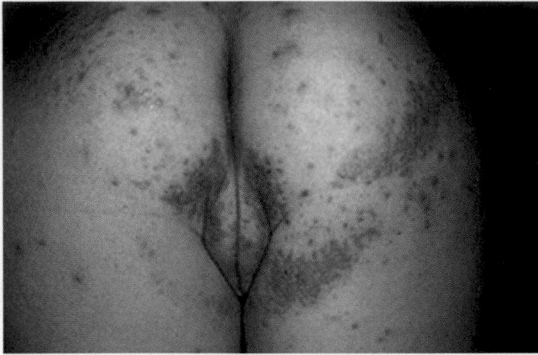

FIGURE 9-57. Genital herpes. Extensive herpetic rash involving buttocks, vulvar area, and perineum.

In the genital area, painful lesions may appear on the prepuce, glans, shaft of the penis, labia, vulva, clitoris, and cervix. The inguinal nodes may be firm and tender. Healing is usually complete by 10 days.

The anal area and medial buttocks are also commonly involved, especially in homosexual men. Jacobs reported 16 patients with herpes simplex infection of the perianal skin and anal canal over a 2-year period.[200] There were 14 men and 2 women; all were either homosexual or bisexual. Chronic perianal herpes is also more frequently seen in immunocompromised patients (see Chapter 10).[216]

Following infection, the virus travels by an afferent nerve to the associated ganglion (e.g., HSV-2 goes to the sacral ganglion) and remains in the body in a latent state. At this stage, there are no clinical manifestations, but reactivation of the virus may occur usually two or three times a year, sometimes after a fever, emotional upset, trauma, or perhaps menstruation. Prodromal symptoms of exacerbation include itching, tingling, and radiating pain to the pelvis and legs. Recurrent episodes tend to be of shorter duration and intensity. Once infected, the patient is condemned to have herpes for life.

Concerns about herpes infections relate not only to the primary cutaneous process, but also to adverse psychological effects and to the risk for transmission from pregnant mothers to newborns. There may also be an increased frequency of cervical cancer. Untreated neonatal herpes is associated with a 50% mortality rate, but this risk can be reduced by cesarean delivery.

To determine the risk for sexual transmission of herpes simplex virus, Mertz and colleagues prospectively studied heterosexual couples in which one partner had symptomatic recurrent disease.[278] They concluded that transmission appeared to result from sexual contact during periods of asymptomatic viral shedding in 70% of individuals. Furthermore, they noted that the risk for acquisition of HSV was higher in women than in men.

Diagnosis

A direct fluorescent antibody technique using the fluid from a vesicle is a rapid means for confirmation. Tzanck's preparation, in which scrapings are placed on a slide and stained, will reveal intranuclear inclusion bodies and giant cells. The most definitive method for the diagnosis of HSV infection is viral culture, but this is a cumbersome, expensive study. The clinical picture of grouped vesicles on an erythematous base anywhere in the body suggests herpes infection, so that laboratory studies serve primarily for confirmation.

Treatment

Current therapy for the condition is the use of an antiviral preparation, acyclovir (Zovirax), but it does not cure the disease.[129,177,279,293,329,369] Acyclovir is a synthetic acyclic purine nucleoside analog that exhibits in vitro inhibitory activity against the virus. Treatment is directed to three areas: management of the initial episode, management of the recurrence, and maintenance between attacks. Primary herpes of less than 7 days' duration is treated by oral acyclovir, 200 mg, five times daily for 10 days. Intermittent therapy, given at the first sign of recurrence, consists of 200 mg five times daily for 5 days. Long-term suppressive therapy for recurrent disease is 400 mg, two times daily for up to 12 months. Patients who present after 1 week but who still have early vesicular lesions or constitutional symptoms may also benefit from therapy. However, acyclovir is not recommended for the management of crusted lesions and for patients who are asymptomatic.[177] Recurrent episodes must be treated within 48 hours if beneficial results are to be expected, but some clinicians believe that acyclovir has no measurable effect on the natural history of the disease.[177] Suppressive therapy is probably most effective in those patients who are subject to frequent exacerbations, but asymptomatic shedding of the virus implies that the individual is still infectious. Continuous or episodic oral acyclovir therapy has been demonstrated to be safe and reasonably effective, with annual rates of recurrence substantially reduced.[218,280] Some recommend interrupting any prolonged treatment to assess further need.[368]

Topical care should include frequent gentle cleansing of the area with alcohol. A cortisone-antibiotic ointment may be employed when the lesions are crusted but not vesicular. Acyclovir ointment applied to the affected area may also be of value during an attack.

Condylomata Acuminata (Venereal Warts)

Condylomata acuminata represent the most common STI in the practice of most surgeons. The condition is also among the most troublesome to eliminate. Health officials estimate that genital or anal warts develop in 1 million Americans annually, and two-thirds of their sexual partners acquire the condition. The disease is caused by HPV, a double-stranded DNA virus that is a member of the papovavirus group.[47] Evidence suggests that the virus is antigenically, biochemically, and immunologically distinct from the virus of the common wart, verruca vulgaris.[47] Its incubation period after exposure ranges from 3 weeks to 8 months. Most infections are transient and cleared within 2 years.[68] Although the condition may occur in heterosexual men and women, it is most commonly seen in male homosexuals. It may be found in association with other diseases, such as gonorrhea, lymphogranuloma venereum, and syphilis, especially in those who have had homosexual contact.[268] A retrospective review of 677 patients who tested positive for HIV revealed that 119 (19%) had anal condylomata.[39] The condition has also been reported in a child with HIV infection.[248] Because there is such a strong association, all patients who are observed to have anal condylomata should undergo appropriate blood testing for HIV (see Chapter 10).

Condylomata acuminata can also occur in infants and children. The increased incidence of anogenital warts in children is rising, with sexual abuse having been implicated as a potential cause.[64] It is therefore important to be aware of this relationship and to report suspected cases of sexual abuse to the appropriate authorities, including child protection services.

Symptoms

Patients usually complain of a lump or lumps and often think that the problem is caused by hemorrhoids. Other symptoms include discharge, pruritus, difficulty with defecation, anal pain, tenesmus, foul odor, and rectal bleeding.

A characteristic scenario is one in which the patient reports having received some form of topical external therapy over many weeks or months. The fact that the treatment has failed precipitates the second opinion or referral. Clearly, treatment of the external component should not be undertaken unless the patient has undergone an adequate anoscopic examination. External application of various medicaments and even the various ablative therapies are doomed to failure if disease is present in the anal canal. It therefore should be self-evident that no clinician, irrespective of medical specialty, should treat perianal condylomata without having performed an internal anal assessment. However, one is probably preaching to the choir because the initial treatment is often rendered by a nonsurgeon.

Examination

The appearance of the warts usually makes the diagnosis quite obvious. However, topical application of 5% acetic acid facilitates identification by making the lesions white, but this is not specific for condylomata. The warts are usually small, discrete, elevated, pink to gray, vegetative excrescences in the anal canal, perianal skin, and urogenital region (Figure 9-58). They may be single or multiple or may coalesce to form polypoid masses. Lesions in the anal canal rarely extend into the rectum but are confined to the squamous epithelium and transitional zones. The wart itself is histologically a hyperplastic epithelial growth with irregular acanthosis and marked hyperkeratosis (Figure 9-59).

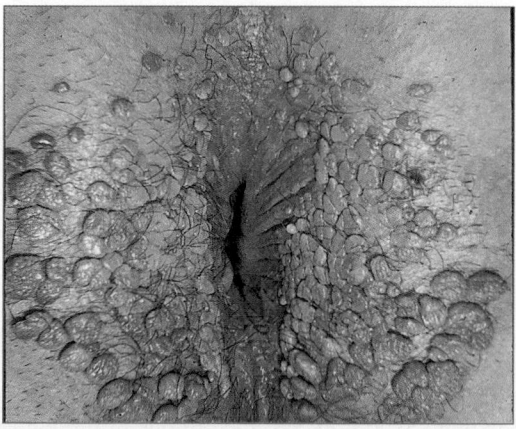

FIGURE 9-58. Condylomata acuminata. Multiple, closely grouped papillomas create a cauliflower-like appearance. (From Corman ML, Veidenheimer MC, Swinton NW. *Diseases of the Anus, Rectum and Colon. Part I: Neoplasms.* New York, NY: Medcom; 1972, with permission.)

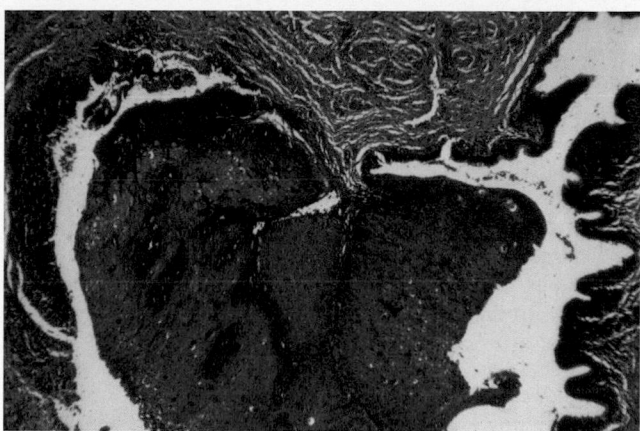

FIGURE 9-59. Condylomata acuminata in an anal duct. Note the proliferation of squamous cells, vacuolated squamous cells, and hyperchromatic nuclei, and the absence of a cornified layer. Note also the columnar epithelium lining the anal duct. (Original magnification × 120; courtesy of Rudolf Garret, MD.)

Treatment

The Standards Task Force of the American Society of Colon and Rectal Surgeons has recommended certain practice parameters for ambulatory surgery of anal condylomata.[363] The statement reads as follows:

> When condylomata are limited to the perianal skin, treatment with topical medications, local destruction, or harvesting and immunotherapy can be administered in an outpatient setting. Patients with extensive perianal or anal canal condylomata or those patients with associated genital condylomata may require inpatient care.

Numerous methods of treating anal condylomata have been proposed, including the following:

- Podophyllin
- Bichloracetic acid
- Trichloroacetic acid
- Immunotherapy
- Immunomodulation
- Chemotherapy
- Sublesional injection of interferon alfa
- Antimicrobials
- Cryotherapy
- Laser therapy
- Electrocoagulation
- Ultrasonic-driven Harmonic scalpel
- Surgical excision

Podophyllin. Podophyllin is a chemical agent that is cytotoxic for the warts, but it has the disadvantage of being quite irritating to the skin. It is therefore important to apply the liquid with care, and then only to the warts. Podophyllum resin, derived from the plants *Podophyllum emodi* and *P. peltatum*, contains many biologically active lignin compounds, including podofilox, the most thoroughly characterized and the most active against genital warts.[45] The technique has the advantage of being simple and inexpensive, but its application is limited to external warts. The drug is teratogenic and must not be used in pregnancy or suspected pregnancy. Adverse effects range from mild skin irritation to ulceration and pain, depending on the concentration and the length of time over which it is applied to the skin. As with all topical methods, no specimen is available for pathologic determination;

this also is a theoretical disadvantage. Dysplasia has been reported with prolonged use, but whether this is from the warts or from the chemical itself has been a matter of some conjecture. Multiple treatments are often required.

Simmons performed a randomly allocated double-blind study of 10% and 25% podophyllin in 140 men with anogenital warts.[352] There was no significant difference in the effect of the two preparations; only 22% of the patients were free of warts following 3 months of therapy. Beutner and colleagues used a technique whereby patients applied the chemical to themselves without systemic adverse reactions and with satisfactory results.[45]

Bichloracetic Acid or Dichloroacetic Acid. Bichloracetic acid, an extremely powerful keratolytic and cauterant, has also been successfully employed in the management of condylomata. The chemical rapidly penetrates and cauterizes the skin, keratin, and other tissues. Like podophyllin, it is simple to apply and is inexpensive. Additionally, it has the advantage of being applicable to the anal canal. Multiple office visits are usually required, however, and there is the concern for skin irritation and discomfort.[402]

Swerdlow and Salvati treated 34 patients by bichloracetic acid only in an uncontrolled study comparing patients who had undergone other forms of therapy.[376] The authors concluded that the recurrence rate was lower and discomfort was less.

Trichloroacetic Acid. Trichloroacetic acid (80% to 90% concentration) physically destroys the wart tissue by protein coagulation. Clearance rates and adverse effects are similar to podophyllin, but trichloroacetic acid may be successfully used for internal lesions[271] and during pregnancy, when some consider it to be first-line therapy. Repeated application is required. The solution is very caustic and should not be applied to skin surrounding the lesion. A barrier of petroleum jelly may help to protect unaffected areas.

Immunotherapy. Abcarian and Sharon stimulated considerable interest in 1982 by employing another approach to the management of anal condylomata, that of immunotherapy.[2] A vaccine is created by excising and washing the condyloma tissue, and a 10% suspension is prepared in Medium 199 supplemented with antibiotics. Following homogenization and freezing, it is then centrifuged, and the supernatant is heated. The inactivated material is then centrifuged again, and the supernatant is collected and tested for bacterial sterility. The patient is vaccinated with six consecutive weekly injections of 0.5 mL, subcutaneously administered in the deltoid area, with the vaccine frozen between injections.[1-3]

Two hundred consecutive patients were studied during an 8-year period.[3] Excellent results were seen in 84%, and fair results in 11%; no improvement was noted in 5%. There were no adverse reactions or complications. The authors concluded that immunotherapy should be the recommended method of treatment for extensive, recurrent, or persistent anal condylomata.

Eftaiha and colleagues reported their own experience with immunotherapy and compared it with other more conventional forms of treatment.[137] Condylomata were successfully eradicated in approximately 94% of patients by this means. It was the authors' opinion, however, that this treatment modality should be reserved for recurrent and giant anal condylomata. Wiltz and coworkers compared surgical excision followed by vaccination using an autogenous condylomata acuminata vaccine for primary and recurrent

perianal warts with other modalities.[410] They found this approach far superior to excision alone, bichloracetic acid, podophyllin, and interferon alfa. The recurrence rate with a mean follow-up of 13 months was only 4.6%.

Although the results of immunotherapy are really quite good, the application of this modality has become a moot issue because convincing a laboratory to prepare it is virtually impossible. Because of the potential liability hazards and the considerable financial investment needed to perform the clinical and laboratory trials required by the U.S. FDA, no laboratory has been willing to assume the responsibility. However, if the physician is able to convince the appropriate personnel to become involved, the technique used for vaccine preparation is well within the capacity of a standard hospital laboratory.

Immunomodulators

IMIDAZOQUINOLINES. The imidazoquinolines are a new class of immune response modifiers (immunomodulators) that have been introduced for the treatment of *external* genital and perianal warts. Imiquimod (Aldara) cream 5% (3M Pharmaceuticals) does not possess direct antiviral activity nor does it cause direct, nonspecific cytolysis.[388] Although its mechanism of action is unknown, it is thought to play a role in the cytokine-induced activation of the immune system.

The product is self-applied three times per week at bedtime. The primary side effect is that of local skin reaction, especially erythema. Treatment is continued until the warts are eradicated or until 16 weeks have elapsed. Results of clinical studies have demonstrated early promise in the treatment of those affected with external condylomata.

CIDOFOVIR (HPMPC). Another immunomodulator has been reported from Belgium, cidofovir (Vistide Pharmacia, Brussels, Belgium).[96] This antiviral topical agent has been demonstrated to be effective in HPV infections. Coremans and colleagues found that this drug compared favorably with electrocoagulation in a noncontrolled study, but its primary value was to supplement conventional electrosurgery when recurrence developed.[96]

COMMENT. Further publications are awaited concerning the merits of both of these immunomodulators, but the fact that they are applicable only to the external component causes one to be quite circumspect as to the relative value for the practice of colon and rectal surgeons.

Topical Cytostatics. Various chemotherapeutic agents have been advocated in the treatment of this condition, including 5-fluorouracil,[289] thiotepa,[80] and bleomycin.[153,318] Figueroa and Gennaro injected bleomycin intralesionally in 10 patients at intervals of every 2 to 3 weeks.[153] An overall success rate of 70% was achieved. Three individuals experienced total resolution of the condylomata after the first treatment, but 3 patients failed to respond after several sessions. With the exception of discomfort, there were no systemic effects following the treatment.

5-Fluorouracil. Fluorouracil is a pyrimidine antimetabolite that interferes with DNA synthesis. A gel consisting of 5-fluorouracil and epinephrine can be injected intralesionally. One study evaluated the safety and efficacy of this treatment in 401 patients randomly assigned to one of three groups.[377] Each lesion was injected with fluorouracil and epinephrine gel, fluorouracil gel, or placebo once a week for 6 weeks. The complete response rate was higher in individuals treated with fluorouracil and epinephrine gel when compared with fluorouracil and placebo groups (61% vs. 43% and 5%, respectively). The recurrence rate in patients with complete response to drug therapy was 50% to 60% at 3 months.

Interferon. Human leukocyte interferon (Alferon N), because of its antiproliferative and antiviral properties, has been demonstrably effective in the treatment of condylomata acuminata.[145,162,194] Interferons are produced and secreted in response to viral infections and to a variety of other synthetic and biologic inducers. Alferon N is manufactured from pooled units of human leukocytes that have been induced by incomplete infection with an avian virus to produce interferon alfa-n3.

Eron and colleagues performed a randomized, controlled study involving 257 patients and injected the substance intralesionally into each wart.[145] There was a statistically significant reduction in wart area in the treated group. A later report revealed complete clearance of warts in 62% of patients.[162] Fleshner and Freilich performed a prospective, randomized controlled study in which one group of patients underwent surgical excision and fulguration immediately followed by an injection of 500,000 IU (0.1 mL) of interferon alfa-n3 into each quadrant of the anal canal.[159] The other group underwent surgical excision and fulguration but then received four injections of saline solution into each quadrant. After a mean follow-up of 3.8 months, condylomata recurred in 23%, but only 12% were noted to have recurrence in the interferon-treated group. A 39% recurrence rate was observed in the controls. The difference was statistically significant.

Individual warts may be readily treated by this technique, but patient intolerance would probably preclude its application for larger lesions. Under these circumstances, the recommendation of excision combined with interferon treatment has been demonstrated to have merit.[93]

The most commonly observed adverse effects are mild, transient, flulike symptoms. Cyclic therapy with low-dose interferon has also been believed to be very effective.[176] In asymptomatic individuals affected with HIV, the therapeutic response to intralesional treatment with interferon is considerably reduced.[130] The management of condylomata by this technique is also very expensive (see Chapter 10).

Current recommendation is to inject each wart with 0.05 mL (250,000 IU), twice weekly for up to 8 weeks. The maximum dose per session should not exceed 0.5 mL (2.5 million IU).

Antimicrobials. A new approach involves topical application of antimicrobials, such as cidofovir and bacillus Calmette–Guérin (BCG). Cidofovir undergoes cellular phosphorylation, after which it completely inhibits viral DNA synthesis. A double-blind, randomized trial compared topical 1% cidofovir gel to a placebo in 30 patients with condylomata acuminata.[358] Patients treated with cidofovir were more likely than placebo recipients to have a complete or partial response (47% vs. 0% and 37% vs. 18%, respectively). In one series, 10 patients were treated with topical BCG with a response in six and a partial response in one (mean, 9-month follow-up).[50] Both therapies require further investigations.

Cryotherapy. Cryotherapy is an approach that is also advocated for the treatment of this condition.[287,338] Savin reported one failure in six patients.[338] It is certainly one of the most frequently used techniques by dermatologists for removal of conventional warts on the fingers and hands. Topical application of liquid nitrogen is simple to accomplish and requires the use of very little special equipment. This can be performed with a spray or with the use of a cotton-tipped applicator and can be applied with limited success within the anal canal. As with the foregoing methods, no pathologic specimen is obtained. Some patients report sufficient discomfort that either a local or regional anesthetic may be required.

Laser Therapy. Some have recommended laser therapy in the treatment of condylomata, with early success noted in the range of 88% to 95%.[117,347] Contact lasers have been said to produce more predictable, sharply defined areas of thermal necrosis than electrosurgery, although noncontact neodymium:yttrium-aluminum-garnet and carbon dioxide lasers have been successfully employed.[347] One of the concerns that has been expressed is the possibility of vaporizing the viral particles, with consequent risk to the surgeon and to the operating room team. Special mask precautions have therefore been recommended by some, but evidence for this requirement is more theoretical than scientific. Other disadvantages are the absence of a pathologic specimen and the expensive equipment that is required.

Billingham and Lewis reported a controlled study of 38 patients.[47] Surgical therapy was performed on the left half of the anus (i.e., electrocoagulation), whereas the right half was treated with the carbon dioxide laser. The authors concluded that the laser was associated with at least as much pain as electrocoagulation. Furthermore, recurrences were seen more often on the laser side. These factors, along with the high cost of the equipment, implied no advantage to this form of treatment.

Another randomized trial also compared carbon dioxide laser therapy with conventional electrocoagulation.[133] There was no difference between the two groups with respect to number of recurrences, postoperative pain, healing time, and rate of scar formation. The authors believed that treatment of recalcitrant condylomata acuminata with the laser did not offer any advantages over traditional surgery.

A randomized, prospective trial was reported from Greece in which the argon plasma coagulator combined with imiquimod cream was compared with the argon plasma coagulator alone in the treatment of intra-anal condylomata.[397] The former approach resulted in earlier clearance of the warts but did not affect the frequency of recurrence.

Electrocoagulation and Surgical Excision. Electrocoagulation with excision of a portion of the specimen to submit for pathologic examination is the "gold standard" for the management of *anal canal* condylomata. The procedure can be undertaken in the office if there are only a few warts present. A local anesthetic injection is generally required because of the anticipated pain, however. For more extensive warts, a general anesthetic, field block, or spinal or epidural anesthetic is recommended.

The technique of electrocoagulation requires the creation of a first- or at most a second-degree burn. When the needle-tip electrode is used, the wart is virtually exploded, and the residual tissue is wiped away with a dry sponge (Figure 9-60). It is helpful to remove a sampling of the warts to submit for pathologic examination, especially if there are any suspicious areas. This can be accomplished by simple scissors dissection. If the "burn" is not undertaken too deeply, pain is not very severe; it can usually be controlled with a nonnarcotic prescription. Creating a burn deep into the dermis or fat implies an incorrect technique. Patients will likely complain bitterly of pain, and there is a risk for the subsequent development of an anal stricture if a large area is to be treated. The patient is advised to take sitz baths and is seen every 2 weeks for evaluation and further treatment if necessary.

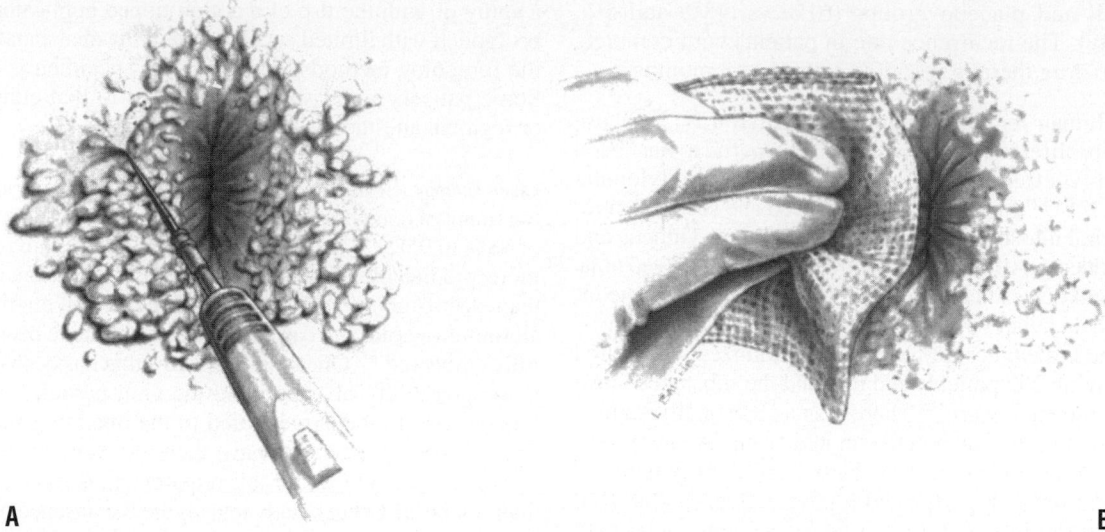

A **B**

FIGURE 9-60. Technique of diathermy excision of anal condylomata. **A:** With a needle-tip electrode, warts are individually electrocoagulated. **B:** Wiping the debris with a dry sponge should leave behind intact skin, with evidence only of a first- or second-degree burn.

Results

Close follow-up examination is required to treat recurrent lesions as soon as they are evident, without, it is hoped, the need to return the patient to the operating room. Unfortunately, fewer than one-half of our patients have resolution of the process after only one treatment. It is important, therefore, for one to understand that therapy may be rather prolonged. However, once the warts have been removed and the wounds have healed, the condition usually does not recur.

Preoperative immune status has been shown to affect the likelihood of recurrence following surgical excision. de la Fuente and coworkers performed a retrospective review on 63 consecutive patients with anal condylomata who underwent excision.[113] Forty-five were immunocompromised (HIV-positive patients, patients with leukemia, transplant recipients), and 18 were immunocompetent. Recurrence developed with a statistically significantly increased frequency and within a shorter period in the immunocompromised group.

Khawaja prospectively compared podophyllin versus scissor excision in the treatment of condylomata acuminata.[226] With the former method, initial complete clearance was noted in 89% versus 79% with podophyllin. However, only one-third were free of recurrence at 42 weeks with podophyllin, compared with 72% in the scissor excision group. A similar trial from another institution revealed comparable results.[207]

Harmonic Scalpel. Any method that will destroy tissue should, in principle, have some value in the expiration of anal condylomata. For example, Colombo-Benkmann and colleagues undertook a prospective evaluation of the ultrasound-driven Harmonic scalpel in 11 patients with preliminarily satisfactory results.[91]

Opinion

External condylomata without evidence of internal warts can usually be effectively treated by chemical means (e.g., podophyllin, trichloroacetic acid, imiquimod). If the response is unsatisfactory, physical destruction by electrocoagulation is the preferred approach. If there are only a few warts, the use of a local anesthetic will permit adequate office treatment. For more extensive lesions, a general anesthetic administered

on an outpatient basis is recommended. Obtaining tissue for pathologic confirmation, especially with respect to premalignant or malignant change, is a prudent philosophy.

Anal Intraepithelial Neoplasia in Condylomata

Anal intraepithelial neoplasia (AIN) is a lesion that is thought to be a precursor of anal squamous cell carcinoma (see Chapter 25) and has been observed in those with HIV and AIDS (see Chapter 10). The incidence of subclinical AIN in patients with anal condylomata has been studied by the Cleveland Clinic Florida group.[92] Thirty-one percent of 97 specimens were found to harbor unsuspected AIN. The incidence was higher in the HIV-positive group (51%) as compared with the HIV-negative patients (17%). The authors stress the importance of obtaining pathologic material.

Giant Condyloma Acuminatum or Buschke-Löwenstein Tumor and Malignant Degeneration

The Buschke-Löwenstein tumor, also known as giant condyloma acuminatum, is a variant of anal condylomata that tends to behave in a locally malignant fashion, burrowing deeply into adjacent structures (Figure 9-61).[10,142] According to Trombetta and Place, 52 cases were reported in the English literature from 1958 to 2000.[387]

A number of articles have described the development of squamous cell carcinoma in these rare "giant" cases.[104,250,257,315] Creasman and colleagues hypothesize that this entity represents an intermediate lesion in a pathologic continuum from condyloma acuminatum to squamous cell carcinoma.[100] Chu and coworkers analyzed 42 cases in the English literature and reviewed the behavior and management of the lesion.[84] They observed the hallmark of the disease to be the high rate of recurrence (66%) and the high incidence of malignant transformation (56%). Recurrences developed in 50% of those who were initially treated with radical surgery.

Wide local excision, however, is the recommended initial surgical approach. If the margins are free of tumor, no further treatment is warranted. Occasionally, however, the lesion may be so extensive that it is deemed unresectable. Butler and colleagues reported a case successfully managed by intravenous 5-fluorouracil, mitomycin C, and extended-field

ABRAHAM BUSCHKE (1868–1943)

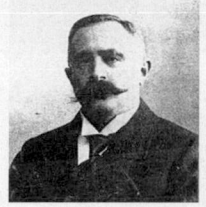

Abraham Buschke was a German Jewish dermatologist and native of Prussia, from the Province of Posen, now part of Poland. He was educated in Berlin where he received his doctorate in 1891. He worked in Greifswald, a town in northeastern Germany, as a surgical assistant. After his brief time in Greifswald, he joined the Dermatological University Clinic in Breslau under the mentorship of Albert Neisser (known for discovering the pathogen for gonorrhea). This is where his interest in bacteriologic research in infectious diseases developed. Later, he was called to the University of Berlin where he worked with Edmund Lesser, an authority in the field of syphilis. By 1902, Buschke was part of the German Society for the Prevention of Venereal Diseases. In 1906, he became head of the Department of Dermatology at Rudolf Virchow Hospital in Berlin. At the time, this was the largest hospital in the world; the department of dermatology alone had a 600-bed capacity. Based on his training, Buschke focused his research efforts mostly on venereal diseases. In 1926, he published a treatise on syphilis with the help of Martin Grumpert, an American physician and writer. Buschke was a prolific writer who had written more than 250 titles of books and articles. Additionally, he is credited with describing several dermatologic disorders, including the Buschke-Löwenstein tumor. Other disorders include Buschke's scleroderma, the Buschke-Ollendorff syndrome (disseminated lenticular dermatofibrosis), and Busse-Buschke disease, an infection caused by *Cryptococcus neoformans*. In 1943, at the age of 73, Abraham Buschke died in a Nazi concentration camp at Theresienstadt, Bohemia. (Attributions: Casper WA. Abraham Buschke—Centennial of his birth. *Arch Derm*. 1968;98:12. Abraham Buschke. Wikipedia. http://en.wikipedia.org/wiki/Abraham_Buschke; with appreciation to Michael S. Halbreiner, MD.)

radiation.[69] Adjuvant chemoradiation therapy has been found to be associated with an improved cure rate in comparison with surgery alone.[84] Others have report successful regression with radiation therapy.[359] Adjuvant therapy with lesions of this type should be considered in accordance with the protocol described in Chapter 25. In addition, malignant transformation in a virally caused illness, especially a condition that is common in the immunocompromised population, should alert the physician to the possibility of AIDS (see Chapter 10).

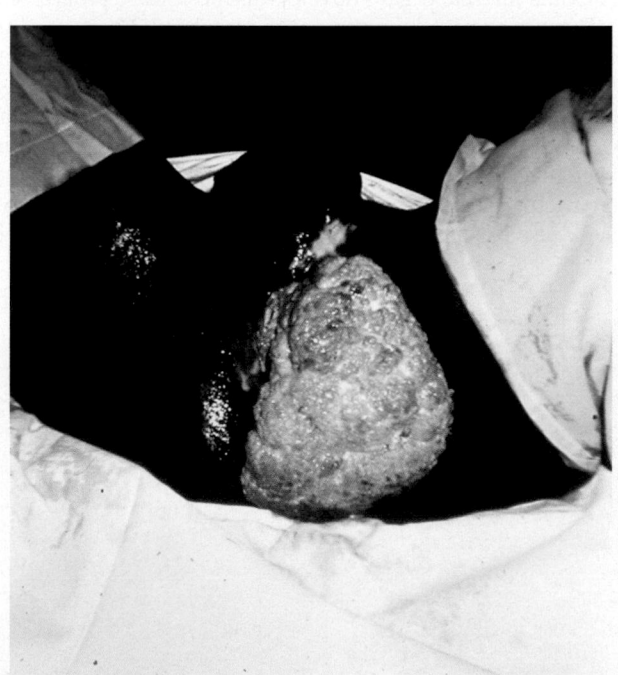

FIGURE 9-61. Verrucous squamous carcinoma or tumor of Buschke-Löwenstein. (From Corman ML, Veidenheimer MC, Swinton NW. *Diseases of the Anus, Rectum and Colon. Part I: Neoplasms*. New York, NY: Medcom; 1972, with permission.)

HIV Infection and AIDS

AIDS was first reported in the United States in 1981. It is caused by the HIV. In August 2008, the CDC published the first national HIV incidence (new infections) estimates using new technology and methodology that more directly measure the number of new HIV infections in the United States. The first analyses, published in the August 6, 2008 issue of the *Journal of the American Medical Association* (*JAMA*), showed that in 2006, an estimated 56,300 new HIV infections occurred—a number that is substantially higher than the previous estimate of 40,000 annual new infections. It should be noted that the new incidence estimate does not represent an actual increase in the numbers of HIV infections but reflects a more accurate way of measuring new infections. An estimated 900,000 people in the United States are currently infected. Transmission of the virus primarily occurs during sexual activity and by sharing needles used to inject intravenous drugs. The colorectal manifestations are discussed in Chapter 10.

▶ PREMALIGNANT AND MALIGNANT DERMATOSES

Malignant neoplasms of the anal margin and perianal skin include basal cell carcinoma, extramammary Paget's disease, Bowen's disease, malignant melanoma, and epidermoid carcinoma. The last two conditions are discussed in Chapter 25. Leukemic and lymphomatous infiltration also may involve the anal area. In addition to these, two other cutaneous lesions may be premalignant or associated with cancer elsewhere: acanthosis nigricans and leukoplakia.

Acanthosis Nigricans

Acanthosis nigricans is known chiefly to surgeons for its ominous association with abdominal cancer in adults.[57] Regions affected include the face, neck, axillae, external genitalia, groin, inner thighs, umbilicus, and anus (Figure 9-62). The condition appears usually as a grayish, velvety thickening or roughening of the skin. The pathologic changes are epidermal,

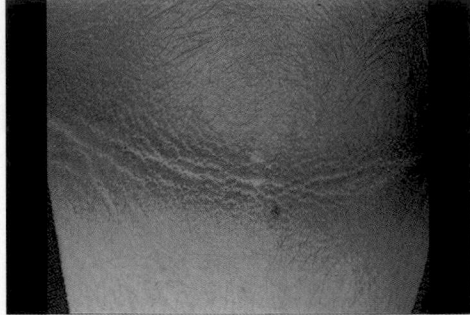

FIGURE 9-62. Acanthosis nigricans. Thickened velvety patches, especially in the folds of skin in the axilla (armpit—as in this photo), groin, and back of the neck. (From Weinberg S, Prose NS, Kristal L. *Color Atlas of Pediatric Dermatology.* 3rd ed. New York, NY: McGraw-Hill; 2007. Copyright 2008, 1998, 1990, 1975, by the McGraw-Hill Companies, Inc.)

with papillomatosis, hyperkeratosis, and hyperpigmentation (Figure 9-63). Pruritus is the most frequent symptom.

The malignant form of acanthosis nigricans may antedate, accompany, or follow the onset of the internal cancer. Most abdominal malignancies are adenocarcinomas, usually of gastric origin (60%). The tumor itself is usually advanced at the time of discovery and has a rapid progression. Treatment is directed to the primary malignant condition.

Leukoplakia

Leukoplakia is a whitish thickening of the mucous membrane epithelium occurring in patches of diverse size and shape. In the anal canal, it is seen mostly in men and is occasionally associated with delayed wound healing (e.g., following excision of a fissure, hemorrhoids, and condylomata; Figure 9-64). Although the anal condition itself does *not* represent a malignancy, when it occurs in the gingival and buccal mucosa, there is a high risk for the development of epidermoid carcinoma. Bleeding, discharge, and pruritic symptoms are the most common complaints.

Microscopically, hyperkeratosis and squamous metaplasia are seen (Figure 9-65). Excision of the lesion has been unsuccessful in my experience; the condition simply recurs. However, the likelihood of recurrence may be reduced if an anoplasty is performed, covering the defect with new, full-thickness skin (see Chapter 10). Because of

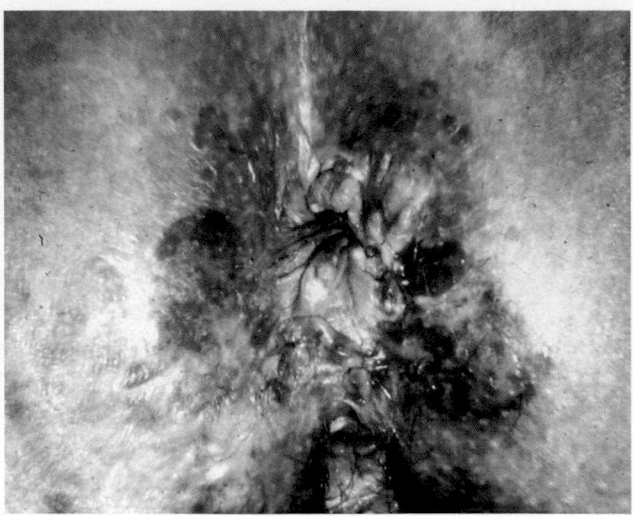

FIGURE 9-64. Leukoplakia. Thickening of the mucosa and perianal skin occurring in whitish patches. This patient underwent fissure excision and partial hemorrhoidectomy.

the theoretical potential for malignancy, annual proctosigmoidoscopy (anoscopy) with biopsy of any suspected area is advised.

Mycosis Fungoides

Mycosis fungoides is a pruritic, usually fatal cutaneous malignant neoplasm of the lymphoreticular system, specifically the thymus-derived lymphocytes (T cells). It is the most common form of cutaneous T-cell lymphomas.[54,103,405] Typically, the lymphocytes display the immunophenotype of mature memory T cells.[384] Subsequent involvement of lymph nodes and internal organs develops as the disease progresses.

The cutaneous lesion can occur anywhere. The overlying skin may have only telangiectasia or be violaceous, often of varied vivid color (Figure 9-66). As the tumor advances, ulcerations occur (Figure 9-67), and pain is a predominant symptom. Microscopic changes include epidermal invasion of small groups of abnormal-appearing lymphocytes and perivascular accumulation of lymphocytic cells. Clinically, the disease has an indolent and chronic course characterized

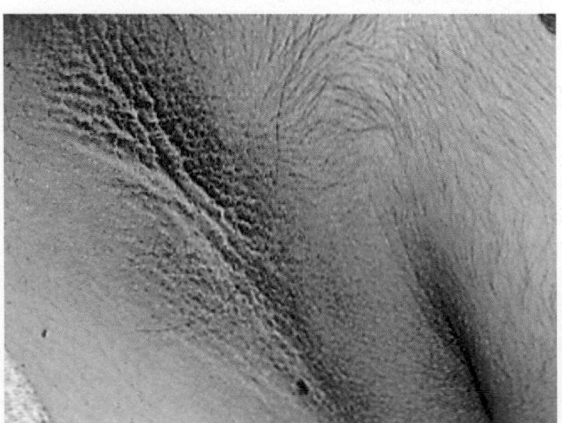

FIGURE 9-63. Acanthosis nigricans, hyper pigmented area around the neck. The dark color is readily evident.

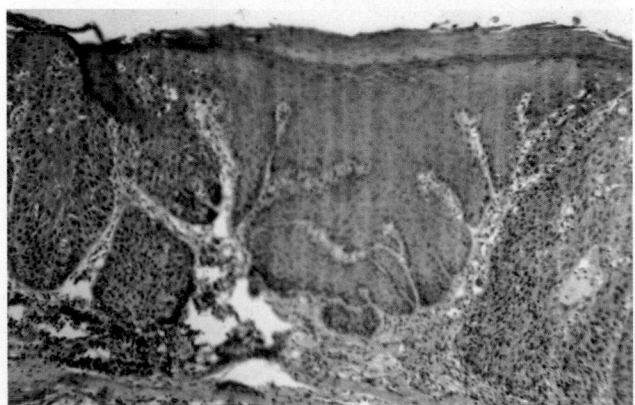

FIGURE 9-65. Leukoplakia. Parakeratosis with atrophy of the epidermis and fibrosis of the dermis is seen. Note the few cells with hyperchromatic nuclei close to the basal cell layer. (Original magnification × 240; courtesy of Rudolf Garret, MD.)

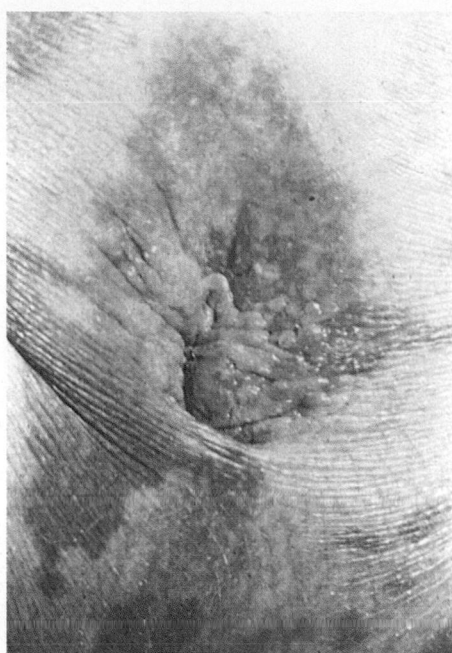

FIGURE 9-66. A violaceous tumor with adjacent reddish brown, irregularly shaped plaques is indicative of mycosis fungoides. (From Corman ML, Veidenheimer MC, Swinton NW. *Diseases of the Anus, Rectum and Colon. Part I: Neoplasms.* New York, NY: Medcom; 1972, with permission.)

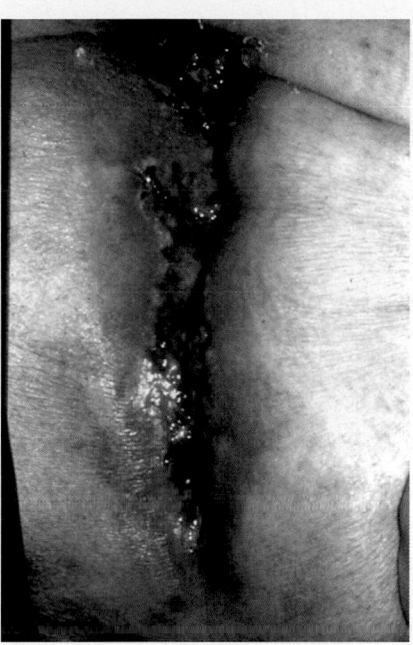

FIGURE 9-67. Perianal ulceration, nodules, and skin infiltration by biopsy-proven lymphomatous infiltrate. (Courtesy of Daniel Rosenthal, MD.)

by episodes of treatment-associated remissions and subsequent relapses. Progression to extracutaneous involvement is estimated to occur in approximately 30% of patients and is associated with a poor prognosis.[5]

As the disease progresses, increased numbers of abnormal, malignant cells are demonstrated (Figure 9-68). Skin-directed therapy is accepted as treatment of choice for patients with early disease stages,[221] whereas careful observation without active treatment is also considered a valid option. Interestingly, mycosis fungoides, together with other types of cutaneous T-cell lymphomas, is the only malignant disease treated with ultraviolet radiation.[384] Systemic and more aggressive treatments should be reserved for high-disease stages, progression, or lack of appropriate response.

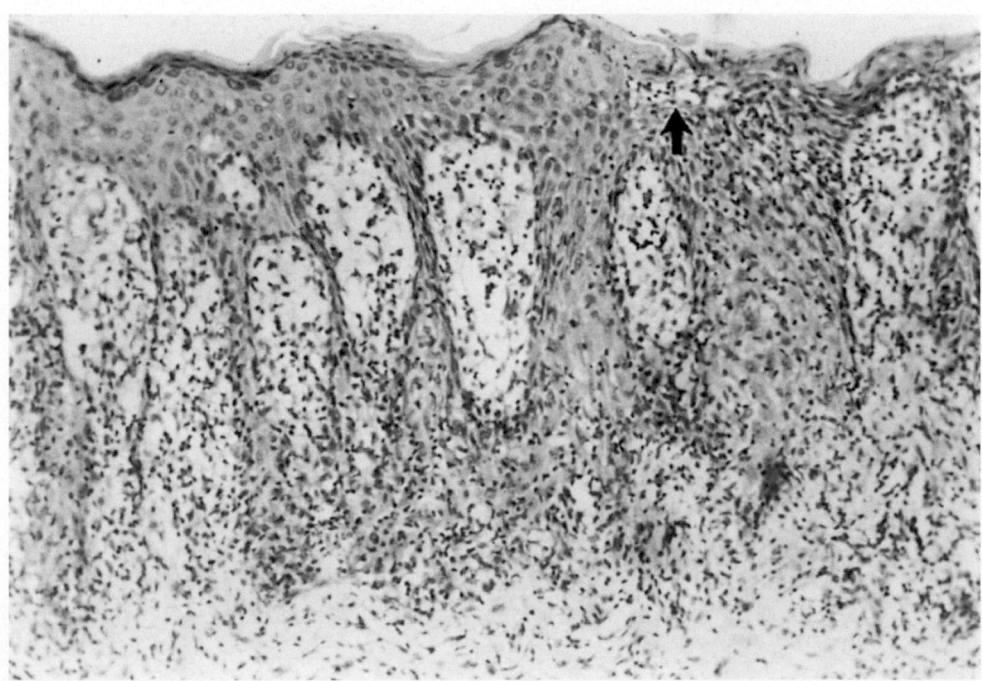

FIGURE 9-68. Mycosis fungoides, pleomorphic infiltrate of the dermis with characteristic Pautrier's abscess (*arrow*) within the epidermis. (Original magnification × 280; courtesy of Rudolf Garret, MD.)

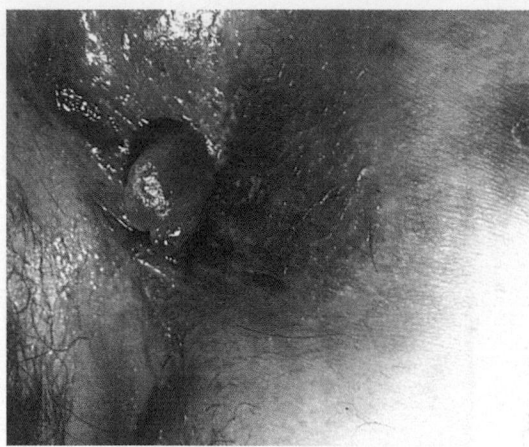

FIGURE 9-69. An ulcerating, violaceous nodule demonstrated leukemic cells on biopsy, indicating leukemia cutis. (From Corman ML, Veidenheimer MC, Swinton NW. *Diseases of the Anus, Rectum and Colon. Part I: Neoplasms.* New York, NY: Medcom; 1972, with permission.)

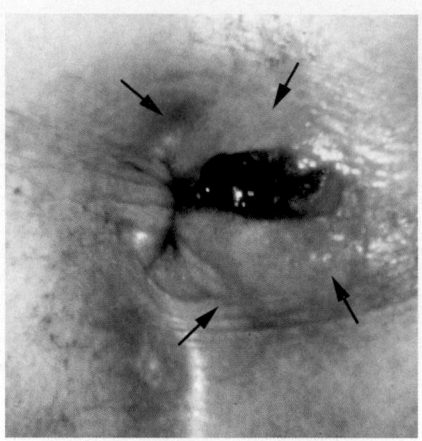

FIGURE 9-70. Leukemia cutis (lymphocytic leukemia). Diffuse swelling and infiltration (*arrows*) with ulceration are noted. (Courtesy of Daniel Rosenthal, MD.)

Leukemia Cutis

Infiltration of the perianal area by leukemic cells is quite uncommon.[101,104,132,353,399] Occasionally, this may be the first manifestation of the malignancy. Leukemia of the skin may consist of a diffuse infiltration, erythema, and ulceration (Figure 9-69). Lymphocytic leukemia characteristically may have a discrete nodular appearance (Figure 9-70). It may present as a fistula, an abscess, or a tender, erythematous area. Cellulitis may be quite marked.

Histologically, masses of cells may be seen in the upper dermis or as nodules in the dermis (Figure 9-71). The type of cells and immature forms are those of the systemic process. Mitoses are infrequently seen in the skin lesions.

Infections in the perianal area are relatively common in patients with myeloproliferative disorders. The incidence in those with acute leukemia is approximately 8% to 9%, with mortality rates as high as 55%.[70] Because the initial symptoms may be confined to the anal area, biopsy and appropriate hematologic studies as well as immunophenotyping may be the only means for establishing an early diagnosis because leukemia cutis alone is nonspecific.[71,83] In acute leukemia, the course of the neutrophil count is an important prognostic factor as to the appropriateness of operative intervention.[70]

The reader is referred to Chapter 13 for a discussion of the management of perianal complications of leukemia. Leukemia cutis is a local manifestation of an underlying

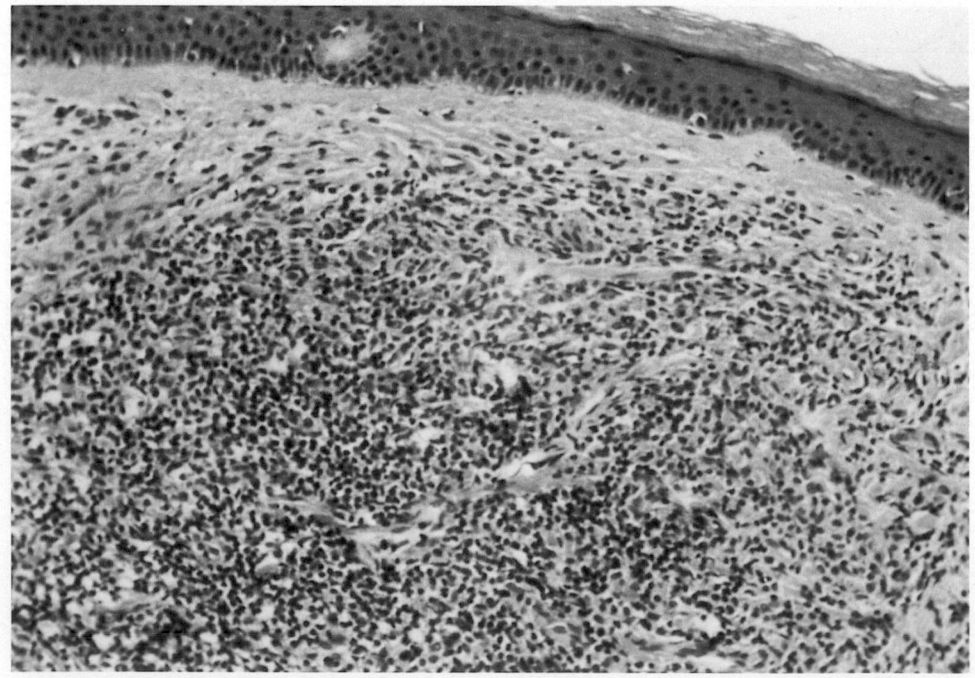

FIGURE 9-71. Leukemia cutis. Infiltration of the dermis by leukemic cells. Note the collagen bundle separating the mass of tumor cells from the underlying epidermis. (Original magnification × 240; courtesy of Rudolf Garret, MD.)

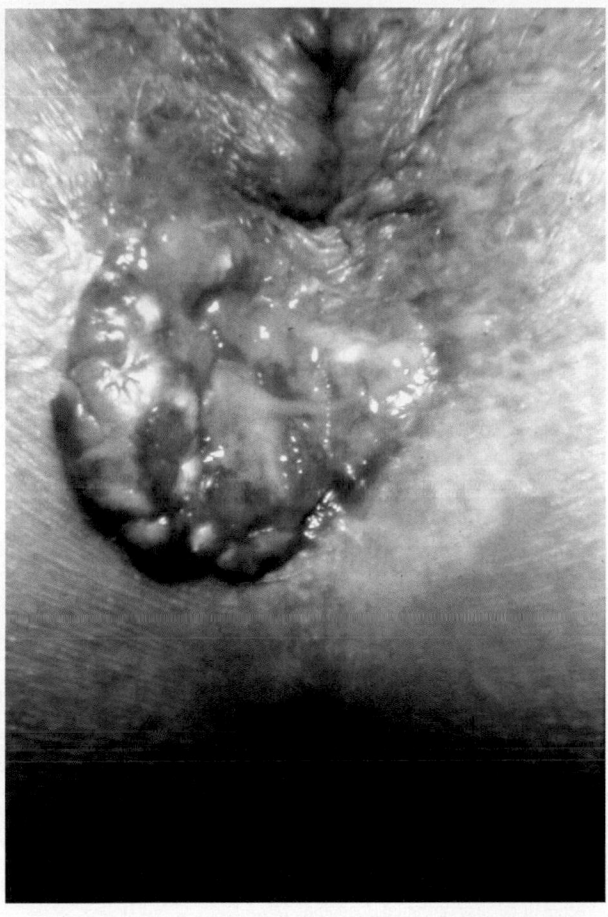

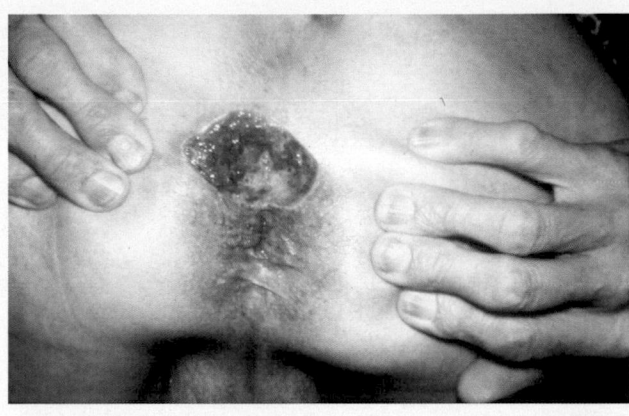

FIGURE 9-72. Basal cell carcinoma. **A:** With characteristic pearly borders and **B:** a typical rodent ulcer. (Courtesy of Daniel Rosenthal, MD.)

systemic disease; therefore, the treatment should be aimed at eradicating the systemic condition by using appropriate chemotherapy, as well as local therapy. In general, the development of leukemia cutis portends a poor prognosis.[139,371]

Basal Cell Carcinoma

Basal cell carcinoma is the most common cutaneous malignancy, but in the anal area it is an extremely rare tumor. Only one case was reported in Gabriel's experience of 1,700 malignant tumors of the anus and rectum.[166] Most published reports involve one or two patients.[24,66,238,335] Nielsen and Jensen published the largest single series; 34 patients were treated over a 30-year period.[292] There was no gender predominance. Tumors were usually between 1 and 2 cm in size and localized to the anal margin. Symptoms include the sensation of a lump or of an ulcer in two-thirds of patients. Bleeding, pain, pruritus, and discharge were other observed complaints. Paterson and colleagues reported their experience with 21 patients, 17 of whom were treated by local excision, 1 by electrocautery, and 1 by Mohs' surgery.[310] No tumor recurred. One-third of the individuals were found to have basal cell cancers at other sites, leading the reviewers to recommend careful assessment of the total skin surface rather than limiting oneself to the perhaps obvious primary complaint.

The characteristic appearance of the lesion is that of a chronic, indurated growth with rolled edges (i.e., pearly border) and a central depression or ulceration (Figure 9-72A,B). Histologically, the tumor arises from the basal cells of the malpighian layer of the skin (Figure 9-73). Sheets of basophilic-staining cells are seen to contain large, blue-staining nuclei with minimal cytoplasm.

Local excision with adequate margins is the preferred treatment. Abdominoperineal resection is performed for

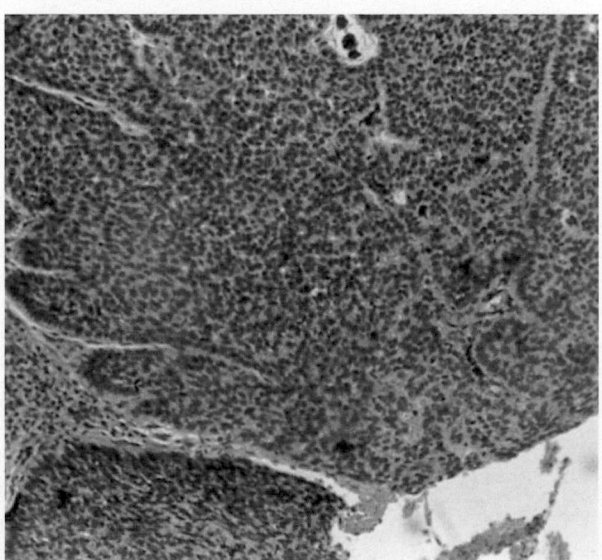

FIGURE 9-73. Basal cell carcinoma. Proliferating basal cells infiltrate the dermis. Note the peripheral palisading. (Original magnification × 240; courtesy of Rudolf Garret, MD.)

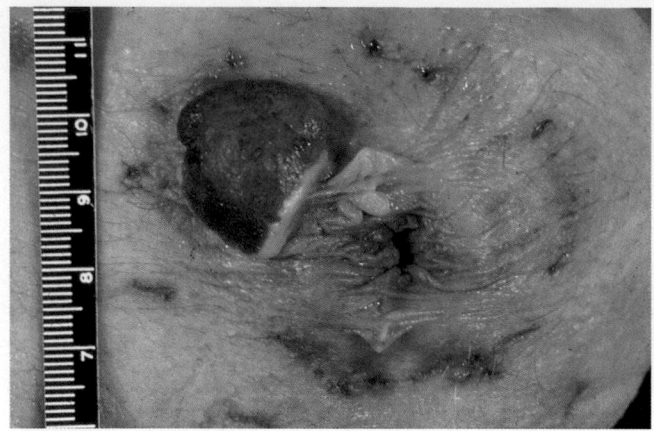

FIGURE 9-74. Squamous cell carcinoma. An ulcerating, friable tumor is noted. (Courtesy of Rudolf Garret, MD.)

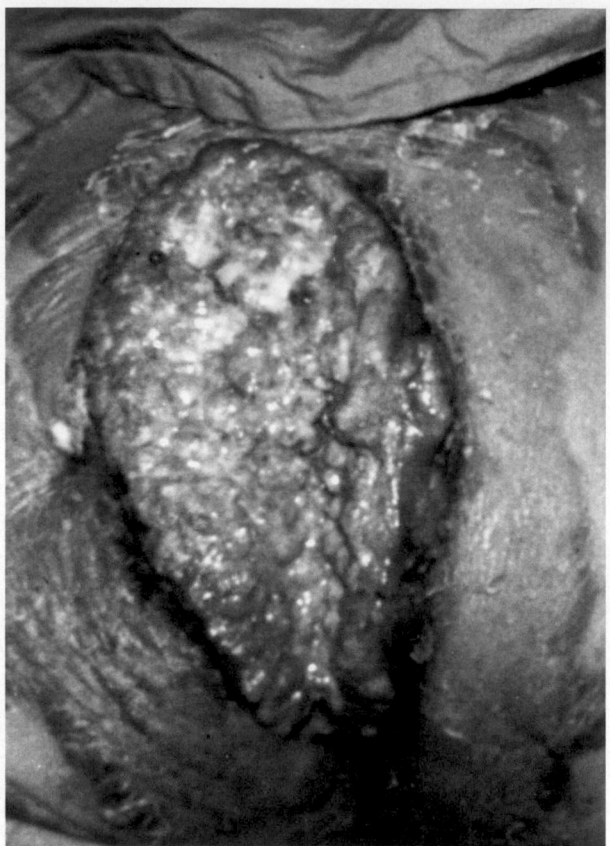

FIGURE 9-75. Squamous cell carcinoma. A fungating, cauliflower-like mass is present. (Courtesy of Daniel Rosenthal, MD.)

neglected, extensive, or infiltrating tumors. There were no deaths caused by basal cell carcinoma in the series of Nielsen and Jensen.[292] Those tumors in other series that were reported to have metastasized were probably basaloid (i.e., cloacogenic) carcinomas with both squamous and basal cell histologic features (see Chapter 25).

Squamous Cell or Epidermoid Carcinoma

Squamous cell carcinoma of the perianal skin is manifested in the same way as lesions occurring in the skin elsewhere on the body. The tumor may appear superficial, discrete, and hard. With progression, it may ulcerate (Figure 9-74) or become papillomatous or cauliflower-like (Figure 9-75). Although this tumor is relatively slow growing, metastases to regional lymph nodes can occur. Wide local excision is the treatment of choice for most lesions (Figure 9-76).[116,319] If the anal canal or anal margin is involved, treatment in accordance with the protocol described in Chapter 25 is suggested.

Malignant Melanoma

Malignant melanoma is described in Chapter 25.

Bowen's Disease

Bowen's disease is an intraepidermal squamous cell carcinoma that tends to spread intraepidermally, but it may also invade. As with AIN, it is a precursor to squamous cell carcinoma of the anus, and it, too, is associated with HPV infection.[37,88,401] Additional risk factors in men include a history of rectal discharge, a history of genital warts,[309] intravenous drug use, and cigarette smoking.[308] Additional risk factors in women include a history of cervical cancer,[276] vulvar cancer,[341] and iatrogenic immunosuppression, such as in solid organ transplantation.[341,383] The condition is eponymously recognized through the author of the 1912 article.[53] It is more commonly seen on the trunk, but more than 100 cases involving the anus have been reported.[319] Graham and Helwig noted a relationship of this condition to malignant tumors elsewhere (e.g., thymoma, bronchogenic carcinoma,

JOHN TEMPLETON BOWEN (1857–1940)

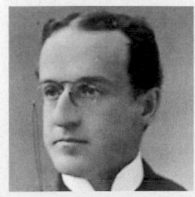

Bowen was born in Boston, Massachusetts, the son of a prominent family. He attended Boston Latin School and graduated from Harvard College in 1879 and from Harvard Medical School in 1884. For most of the ensuing 3 years, he studied in Berlin, Munich, and Vienna. He must have developed an interest in dermatologic problems during this time because in 1889 he was appointed assistant physician to outpatients with diseases of the skin at the Massachusetts General Hospital. In 1907, he became the first Wigglesworth Professor of Dermatology at Harvard Medical School, before which he was elected president of the American Dermatological Association. Bowen is best remembered for his description of precancerous dermatoses. A man who loved quiet and solitude, he is recognized as one of the preeminent figures in the field of dermatology.

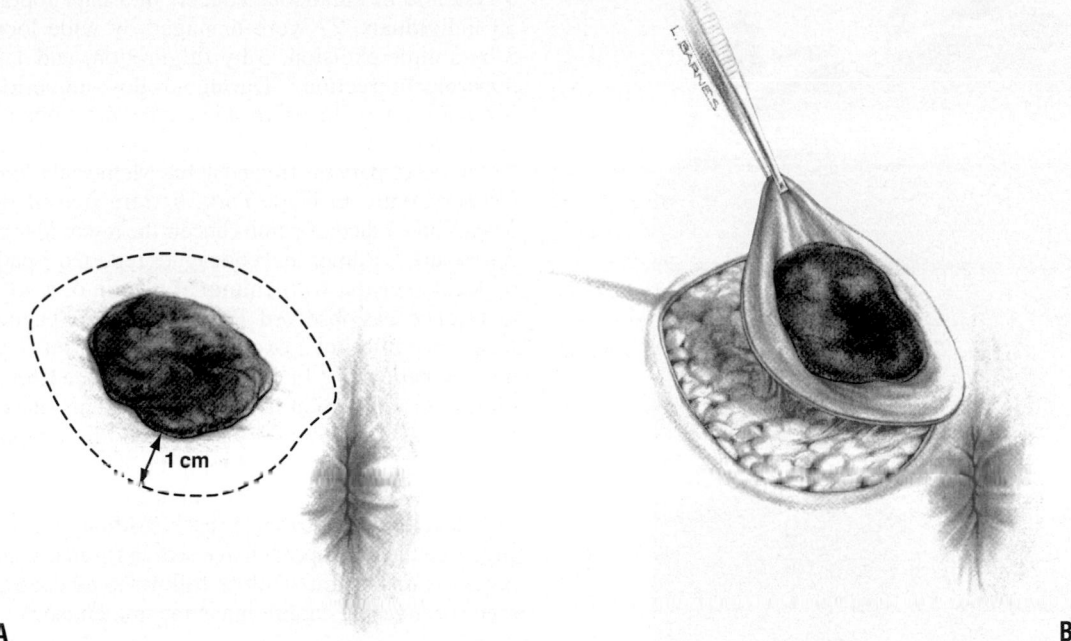

A   **B**

FIGURE 9-76. Technique for wide local excision of perianal skin cancer. **A:** At least a 1-cm margin of normal skin should be excised with the lesion. **B:** Full thickness of skin completes the excision. Margins should be checked by means of frozen section to ensure adequacy of removal. Depending on the size of the defect, various skin-grafting approaches may be used.

hypernephroma, gastrointestinal cancer).[174,175] Neoplasms developed in one-third of their patients within 10 years of the original diagnosis. They suggested that Bowen's disease could represent a cutaneous manifestation of a predisposition to the development of cancer. However, Reymann and colleagues, in a retrospective statistical study of 581 patients with Bowen's disease, failed to support the view that the condition is a marker for internal malignancy.[330] Others have also come to adopt this opinion, so the current consensus is that there is no such relationship.[58,85,86] Parenthetically, a case of Bowen's disease in association with Crohn's colitis has been described.[38]

Symptoms

The disease usually presents with itching and burning, although pain and bleeding may be noted.[342] Strauss and Fazio, in their report from the Cleveland Clinic of 12 patients, noted that the diagnosis was usually made as an incidental finding after anorectal surgery.[370] In a later publication from the same institution involving 33 patients with perianal Bowen's disease, 20 (61%) presented with symptoms, whereas 13 individuals (39%) were noted to harbor the condition on pathologic evaluation of hemorrhoidectomy specimens.

Clinical Appearance and Histology

The lesion appears as an erythematous, slightly crusted, plaquelike area with well-defined margins (Figure 9-77). The condition may be confused with psoriasis and with Paget's disease. Topical staining with toluidine blue has been successfully applied as a screening technique for intraepithelial carcinoma of the cervix and vulva.[61] This approach may prove to have value in the diagnosis of Bowen's disease.

Microscopically, the epidermis is thickened by hyperkeratosis, and there may be parakeratosis and acanthosis (Figure 9-78). In contrast to what is noted in Paget's disease, a bowenoid cell does not pick up aldehyde fuchsin stain (Figure 9-79).[319] Anal Bowen's disease and high-grade squamous intraepithelial lesions are histologically and immunochemically indistinguishable.[401]

Treatment

Treatment requires wide local excision with frozen-section examination to ensure adequate margins, although radical

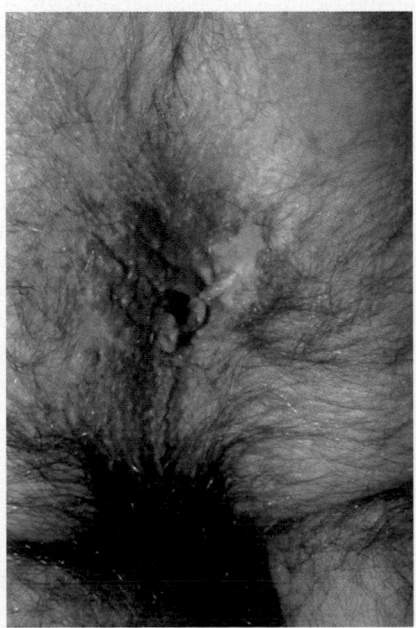

FIGURE 9-77. Bowen's disease. An indurated erythematosquamous patch involves the perianal area (*arrows*).

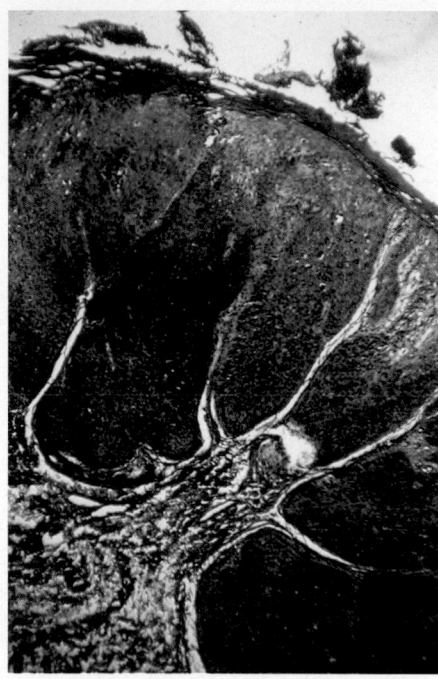

FIGURE 9-78. Bowen's disease. Disturbance of architecture of the squamous epithelium is noted. (Original magnification × 250; courtesy of Rudolf Garret, MD.)

surgical extirpation has been used when this procedure fails.[134] The condition has also been reported to respond to topical dinitrochlorobenzene and 5-fluorouracil.[322] Photodynamic therapy has been described for the management of residual disease.[337]

Results

In the 12 individuals reviewed by the Cleveland Clinic group, there was no recurrence or metastasis when adequate excision with or without grafting was employed.[370] Seven of the patients previously had or subsequently developed a systemic or cutaneous cancer. In a later report involving 33 individuals, 27 were managed by wide local excision, 3 by simple excision, 3 by fulguration, and 1 by abdominoperineal resection.[37] During a follow-up period averaging 3.7 years, a new invasive skin cancer developed in 1 person, and a second was found to have recurrent Bowen's disease.

Of the 11 patients treated at the Memorial Sloan-Kettering Cancer Center in New York, 5 were free of disease after 5 years and 1 died of colon cancer; the remainder had a limited follow-up.[319] Ramos and colleagues reported 7 patients treated by local excision with "minimal margin of resection."[327] No recurrence was observed. Reynolds and colleagues noted one recurrence after total excision of the anal mucosa and grafting in 6 patients.[331] In the experience of the Cleveland Clinic Florida group, which involved 25 patients, no concomitant carcinomas were found by computed tomography and colonoscopy.[149] There were no recurrences in the 15 individuals without HPV or HIV infection, but 5 (50%) with this association developed recurrent disease. Although newer evidence suggests that a comprehensive search for malignancy in other organs is unwarranted, close follow-up evaluation for recurrence or invasive carcinoma is recommended.[266]

Bowenoid Papulosis

Bowenoid papulosis was described in 1979 by Wade and colleagues as a dermatosis affecting the genitalia, a condition that is quite similar to Bowen's disease.[398] The condition is often associated with anal condylomata or genital herpes. HPV is believed to be the causative agent. Immunocompromised individuals, especially those with AIDS, may be at a higher risk for development of cancer based on bowenoid papulosis.[336]

The lesions are described as multiple reddish brown or violaceous papules. Most individuals are asymptomatic or have pruritic complaints. Because the microscopic picture is essentially identical to that of Bowen's disease, the differential diagnosis between the two conditions is made based on age (i.e., patients with bowenoid papulosis tend to be younger) and the fact that bowenoid lesions are small, papular, and multiple.[250] Local excision is the treatment of choice, but the prognosis following removal is unclear.

Extramammary Paget's Disease

In 1874, Sir James Paget described a cutaneous lesion of the breast that histologically demonstrated the presence of large, round, clear-staining cells with large nuclei.[307] Darier and Couillaud subsequently described the condition in the perineal area, the lesions of extramammary Paget's disease being not unlike those seen in the breast.[110] This is a relatively rare condition, with only about 125 cases reported in the literature.[213] It is more common in women.[213] The mean age of onset has been reported to be from 59 to 65 years.[41,188]

Presentation and Histopathology

Most patients complain of ulceration, discharge, pruritus, and occasionally bleeding and pain in the areas harboring apocrine sweat glands. They may be asymptomatic or have a florid type of eczema.[41] The centrifugal growth pattern leads to formation of a polygonal border, which may provide a diagnostic clue.

Helwig and Graham reviewed material from the Armed Forces Institute of Pathology; 40 patients were identified

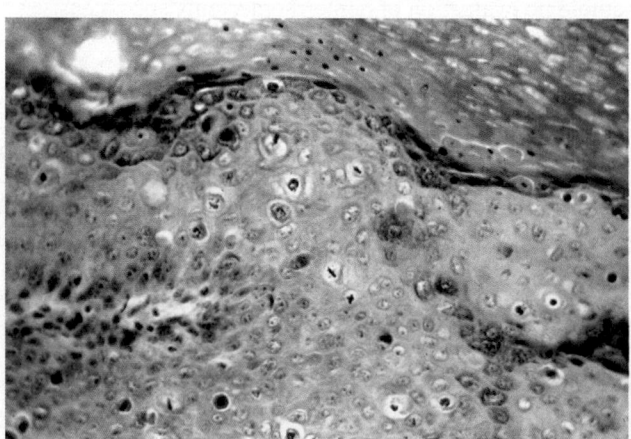

FIGURE 9-79. Bowen's disease. Note the cells with hyperchromatic nuclei (bowenoid cells) scattered throughout the epithelium. Many mitotic figures are seen. (Original magnification × 600; from Corman ML, Veidenheimer MC, Swinton NW. *Diseases of the Anus, Rectum and Colon. Part I: Neoplasms.* New York, NY: Medcom; 1972, with permission.)

JAMES PAGET (1814–1899)

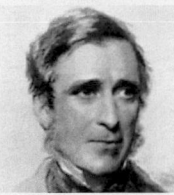

Paget was born one of 17 children. He studied at St. Bartholomew's Hospital in London, where he made his first observation. Small, hard specks were often seen in muscle at that time, and he became quite curious as to their nature. Because St. Bartholomew's did not have a microscope, Paget traveled to the British Museum and discovered *Trichinella spiralis*. In 1842, he began to assist in the cataloging of the College of Surgeons' Museum. In the next year, he was given the lectureship in physiology at St. Bartholomew's and was appointed warden of the new residential college for medical students at that hospital. The professorship of anatomy and surgery of the College of Surgeons came next. In 1849, the *Pathological Catalogue of the College of Surgeons Museum*, of which he was the greatest contributor, was completed; this volume formed an exact description of more than 3,500 specimens. Paget established himself as one of the most notable pathologists of all time, with 30 learned bodies conferring distinction on him. Although he did not describe the disease as it affects the anus, only the breast condition, Darier and Couillaud credit him with the identification of the peculiar cells that may be found in these locations. (From Graham H. *Surgeons All*. New York, NY: Philosophical Library; 1957:370; and Power D. *British Masters of Medicine*. Baltimore, MD: W. Wood; 1936:131.)

with lesions in this area.[188] These investigators found that the dermatosis usually appeared erythematous to whitish gray, elevated, crusty, scaly, eczematoid, and occasionally papillary (Figure 9-80). The pattern of metastasis in primary extramammary Paget's disease is characterized by continuous lymphogenous, or less often, hematogenous spread.[185] The secondary form of the disease is defined as an expression of continuous intraepithelial metastasis.

Microscopically, hyperkeratosis, parakeratosis, acanthosis, and pale vacuolated cells are seen (pagetoid cells) within the epidermis (Figure 9-81). Sialomucin may be identified by periodic acid–Schiff stain (Figure 9-82). Conversely, Bowen's disease does not show this positive staining.

Association with Malignancy

Carcinoma in adjacent areas is found in a high percentage of patients, especially in the anal canal and rectum (Figure 9-83). The frequency of cancer related to extramammary Paget's disease varies by affected site. The risk is higher for perianal Paget's than for vulvar disease, but generally only about 25% of patients have an associated neoplasm identified.[217,255,419] Thirteen of the 40 patients in the series of Helwig and Graham had an immediate underlying cutaneous carcinoma.[188] Another 7 had primary internal or extracutaneous cancer. Lock and associates reported 4 patients, in 3 of whom carcinoma developed.[256] Others note a similar association—for example, with cloacogenic carcinoma and with villous adenoma of the rectum.[23,198,319,372,407] In addition, a familial occurrence has been described.[240] A special staining technique has been employed to assist in the distinction between Paget's disease and so-called pagetoid spread as a consequence of an anorectal malignancy,[25] but further studies are awaited.

Treatment

Treatment depends on the presence or absence of an underlying invasive carcinoma. The use of a retinoid, etretinate,

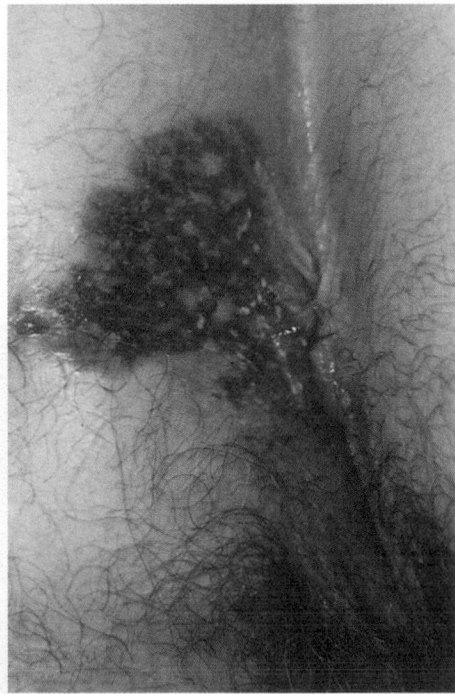

FIGURE 9-80. Extramammary Paget's disease has caused an irregular but well-marginated erythematous erosive patch with slightly indurated edges in this patient. (Courtesy of Arnold Medved, MD.)

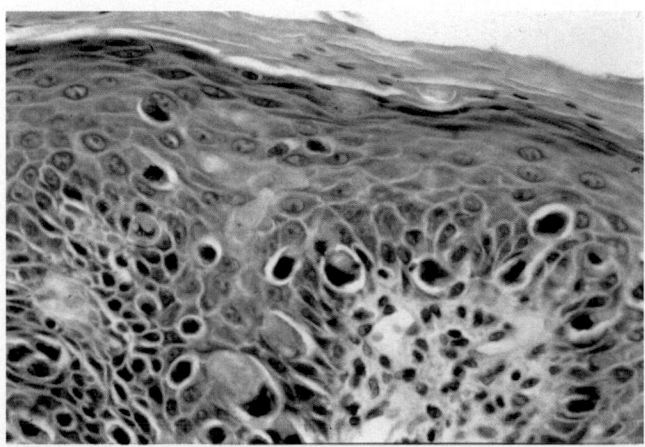

FIGURE 9-81. Extramammary Paget's disease. Note the large, pagetoid cells within the epithelium. These were mucicarmine positive (Figure 9-82), thus ruling out Bowen's disease. (Original magnification × 240; courtesy of Rudolf Garret, MD.)

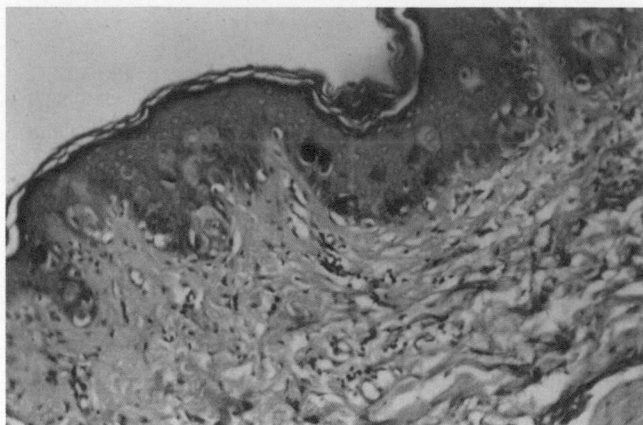

FIGURE 9-82. Extramammary Paget's disease. Mucicarmine-positive cells are present within the epithelium. (Original magnification × 240; courtesy of Rudolf Garret, MD.)

taken orally may be beneficial in the treatment of the chronic or recurrent form when there is no concomitant invasive carcinoma.[253] It should be self-evident that all these individuals require a careful proctosigmoidoscopy and anoscopy. Linder and Myers suggest that a distinction be made between a carcinoma in situ and an infiltrating growth.[252] In the latter situation, abdominoperineal resection may be required, or consideration may be given to neoadjuvant therapy (see Chapter 25). Wide local excision with or without grafting should be adequate for noninvasive disease, however (Figure 9-84).[22,167,245,272] Usually, mapping biopsies with frozen section are used. Some have suggested that one can determine the extent of the disease by means of photodynamic diagnosis.[22] This is a noninvasive tool that uses a 20% 5-aminolevulinic acid (ALA) ointment applied around the lesion, which is then protected from light.[22] When pagetoid or cancer cells are exposed to ALA, they accumulate intrinsic protoporphyrin IX, which emits red fluorescence with ultraviolet light.[22]

Shutze and Gleysteen suggest a management classification based on the depth of invasion, a modification of which follows[348]:

Stage I. Localized perianal disease without carcinoma: wide local excision

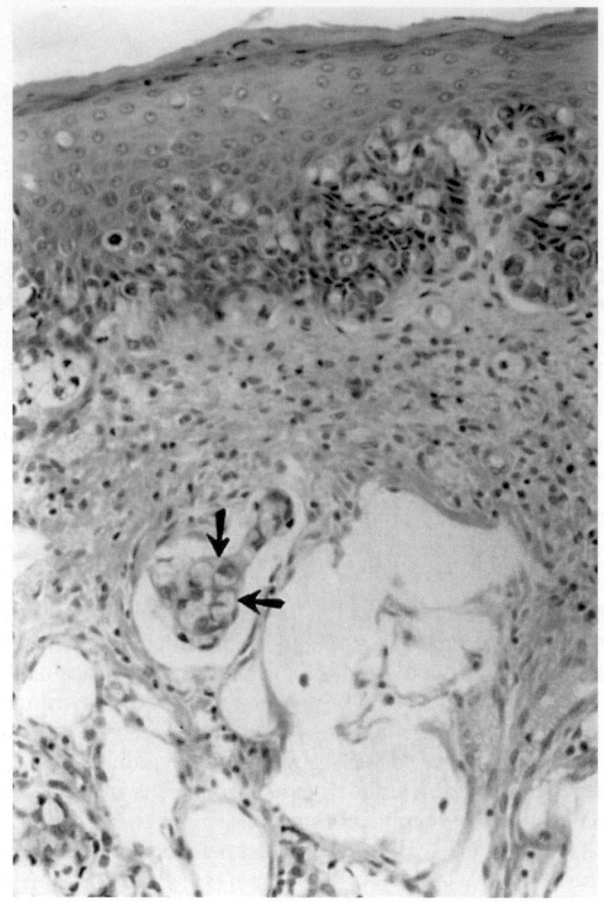

FIGURE 9-83. Perianal skin shows infiltration of lower portion of epidermis by Paget's cells. These are characterized by clear cytoplasm and nuclear pleomorphism. In the underlying dermis, a nest of mucin-secreting carcinoma is seen. The cells show a typical signet-ring appearance (*arrows*). The spaces represent pools of mucin. On resection, the tumor was proved to arise from anal glands. (Original magnification × 240.)

Stage IIA. Localized disease with underlying malignancy: wide local excision

Stage IIB. Localized disease with associated anorectal carcinoma: abdominoperineal resection

Stage III. Associated carcinomatous spread to regional lymph nodes: abdominoperineal resection plus chemo-

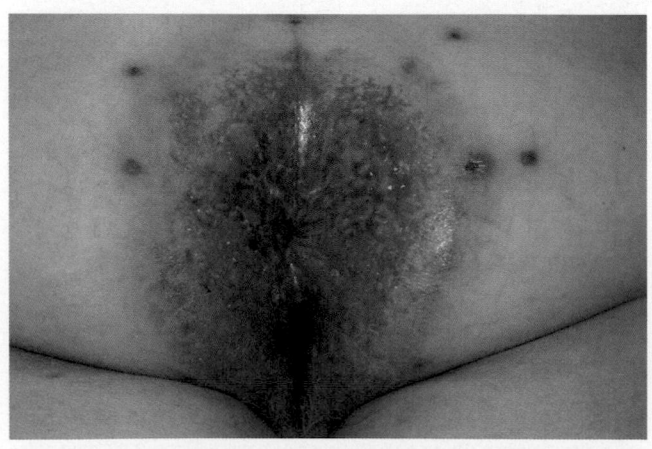

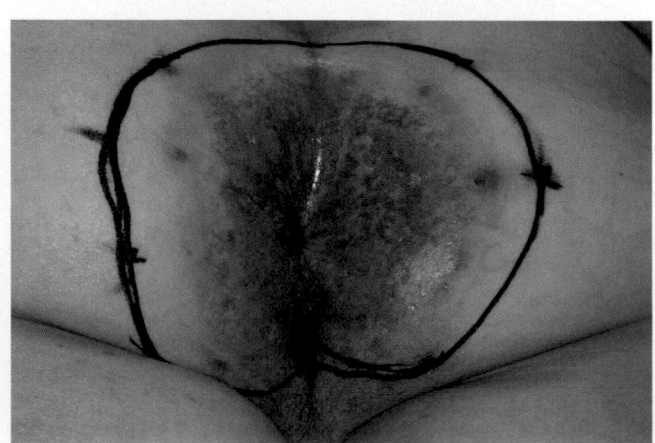

FIGURE 9-84. **A:** Technique of wide excision of perianal Paget's disease. **B:** Outline of the incision. *(continued)*

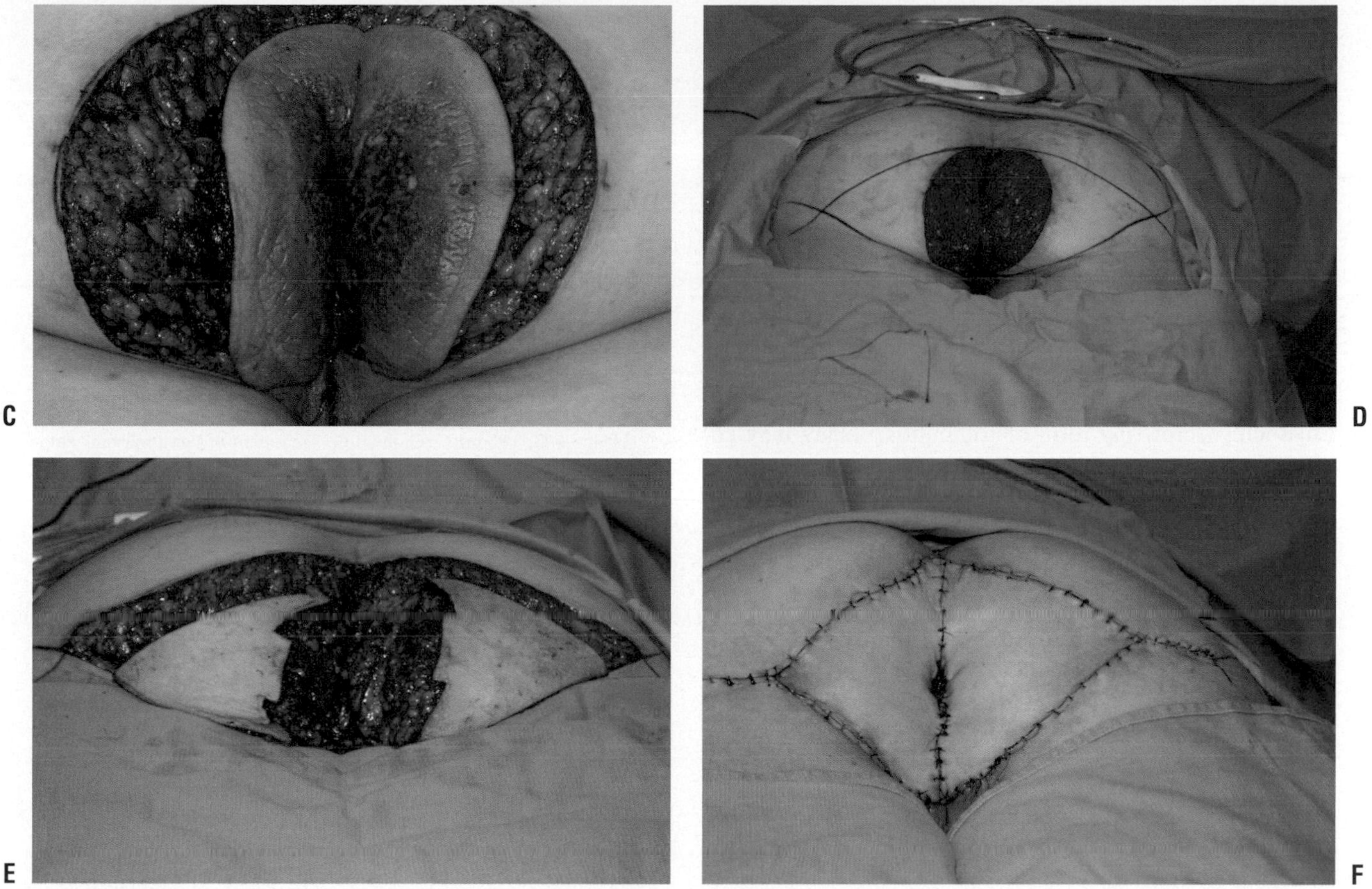

C

D

E

F

FIGURE 9-84. *(continued)* **C:** Excision of the lesion with adequate margin. **D:** Outlining incisions for coverage of the defect. **E:** Full-thickness buttock skin is mobilized bilaterally. **F:** Completed closure with anal canal reconstructed.

radiation therapy; possible radical inguinal node dissection

Stage IV. Distant metastases: standard palliative cancer management

Results

In the experience of the Cleveland Clinic group (10 patients), most were free of disease when wide, local excision and skin grafting were performed.[36] The 3 patients in whom metastatic disease developed all presented with invasive carcinoma.

Jensen and colleagues evaluated 22 patients with Paget's disease of the anal margin.[209] Approximately three-fourths suffered from persistent pruritus ani, and about one-third had a malignancy. The 5- and 10-year crude survival rates of 54% and 45%, respectively, were significantly lower than that which would be anticipated in the normal population. The Memorial Sloan-Kettering Cancer Center experience was reported in 2003 and involved 27 patients who were identified between 1950 and 2000.[272] The median age was 63 years. Three-fourths were treated with wide local excision, and the overall recurrence rate was 37%. Forty-four percent had an invasive component. The overall and disease-free survivals at 5 years were 59% and 64%, respectively, decreasing to 33% and 39%, respectively, at 10 years.[272]

Careful follow-up is considered essential, with recurrence probably dictating a wider excision, provided, of course, that there is no evidence of malignancy (Figure 9-85). Photodynamic therapy for recurrent disease has also been advocated.[337] Those managed by local excision should undergo frequent biopsy of any pruritic areas or skin lesions.[209]

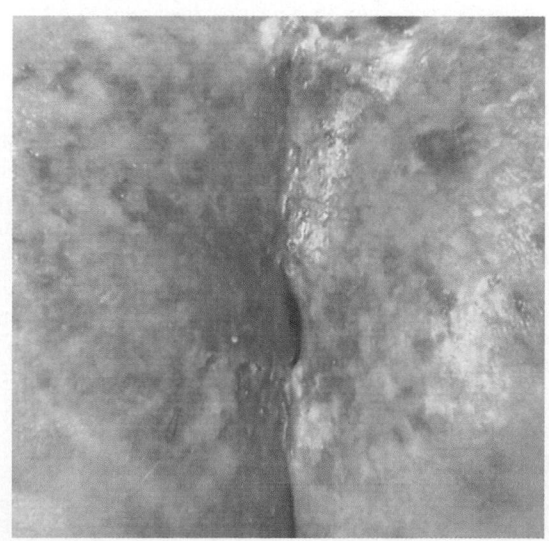

FIGURE 9-85. Extramammary Paget's disease that recurred after excision and skin grafting. (Courtesy of William G. Robertson, MD.)

▶ GLOSSARY OF DERMATOLOGIC TERMS

Elevated Lesions

Abscess localized collection of pus

Bulla (bullae) bleb; blisters containing serous or seropurulent fluid

Crusts dried masses of serum, pus, or blood, with epithelial and bacterial debris

Cyst sac containing liquid or semisolid material

Desquamation scales; results from abnormal keratinization and exfoliation of cornified epithelial cells

Exfoliation scales; laminated masses of keratin; desquamated epidermis

Exudate crusts; dried blood or pus

Furuncle necrotizing form of folliculitis; many may coalesce to form a carbuncle

Hyperkeratosis increased thickening of the stratum corneum

Keratosis (keratotic) horny growth

Lichenification (lichenoid) thickened, leathery; exaggerated skin markings resembling a mosaic

Nodule (nodular) larger papule

Papule (papular, papilloma, papillomatosis) circumscribed solid elevations with no fluid

Plaque minimal height, relatively large surface area

Pustule "pimple"; elevation of the skin containing pus

Urticaria wheals

Vegetation (vegetative) luxuriant, funguslike growth

Vesicle blister; circumscribed epidermal elevation

Wheal evanescent, edematous, variably sized flat elevation

Flat Lesions

Macule (macular) circumscribed change in skin color

Sclerosis (sclerotic) induration or hardening

Telangiectasia condition caused by dilatation of capillary vessels and minute arteries

Depressed Lesions

Atrophy (atrophic) thin, almost transparent epidermis

Excoriation mechanical abrasion

Gangrene death and decay of body tissue characterized by both liquefactive and coagulative necrosis

Scar cicatrix secondary to injury or disease

Sinus tract from a suppurative cavity to skin surface

Ulcer excavation of variable depth involving loss of dermis as well as epidermis

From Domonkos AN, Arnold HL Jr, Odom RB. Cutaneous symptoms, signs and diagnosis. In: Domonkos AN, Arnold HL, eds. *Andrew's Diseases of the Skin*. 7th ed. Philadelphia, PA: WB Saunders; 1982:15; Fitzpatrick TB. Fundamentals of dermatologic diagnosis. In: Fitzpatrick TB, Eisen AZ, Wolff K, et al, eds. *Dermatology in General Medicine*. 2nd ed. St. Louis, MO: McGraw-Hill; 1979:10; and Rook A, Wilkinson DS. The principles of diagnosis. In: Rook A, Wilkinson DS, Ebling FJG, eds. *Textbook of Dermatology*. 3rd ed. Oxford, United Kingdom: Blackwell Scientific; 1979:57.

References

1. Abcarian H, Sharon N. The effectiveness of immunotherapy in the treatment of anal condyloma acuminatum. *J Surg Res*. 1977;22(3):231–236.
2. Abcarian H, Sharon N. Long-term effectiveness of immunotherapy of anal condyloma acuminatum. *Dis Colon Rectum*. 1982;25(7):648–651.
3. Abcarian H, Smith D, Sharon N. The immunotherapy of anal condyloma acuminatum. *Dis Colon Rectum*. 1976;19(3):237–244.
4. Abdelrazeq AS, Rahman M, Botterill ID, et al. Short-term and long-term outcomes of the cleft lift procedure in the management of nonacute pilonidal disorders. *Dis Colon Rectum*. 2008;51(7):1100–1106.
5. Agar NS, Wedgeworth E, Crichton S, et al. Survival outcomes and prognostic factors in mycosis fungoides/Sézary syndrome: validation of the revised International Society for Cutaneous Lymphomas/European Organisation for Research and Treatment of Cancer staging proposal. *J Clin Oncol*. 2010;28(31):4730–4739.
6. Ahlberg J, Bergstrand O, Holmström B, et al. Anal tuberculosis. A report of two cases. *Acta Chir Scand*. 1980;500:45–47.
7. Ahmed AR, Spigelman Z, Cavacini LA, et al. Treatment of pemphigus vulgaris with rituximab and intravenous globulin. *N Engl J Med*. 2006;355:1772–1779.
8. Akinci OF, Kurt M, Terzi A, et al. Natal cleft deeper in patients with pilonidal sinus: implications for choice of surgical procedure. *Dis Colon Rectum*. 2009;52(5):1000–1002.
9. Albanese G, Venturi C, Galbiati G. Treatment of larva migrans cutanea (creeping eruption): a comparison between albendazole and traditional therapy. *Int J Dermatol*. 2001;40(1):67–71.
10. Alexander RM, Kaminsky DB. Giant condyloma acuminatum (Buschke-Lowenstein tumor) of the anus: case report and review of the literature. *Dis Colon Rectum*. 1979;22(8):561–565.
11. Alexander S. Dermatological aspects of anorectal disease. *Clin Gastroenterol*. 1975;4(3):651–657.
12. Alexis AF, Strober BE. Off-label dermatologic use of anti-TNF-a therapies. *J Cutan Med Surg*. 2005;9(6):296–302.
13. Allan A, Ambrose NS, Silverman S, et al. Physiological study of pruritus ani. *Br J Surg*. 1987;74(7):576–579.
14. Allan A, Keighley MRB. Treatment for pruritus ani. *Surg Rounds*. 1988;7:69.
15. Allen-Mersh TG. Pilonidal sinus: finding the right track for treatment. *Br J Surg*. 1990;77:123–132.
16. Alvarado-Cerna R, Bracho-Riquelme R. Perianal actinomycosis—a complication of a fistula-in-ano. Report of a case. *Dis Colon Rectum*. 1994;37:378–380.
17. Alver O, Kayabasi B, Ozcan M, et al. The complete rhombic excision of pilonidal sinus with primary closure by the use of fasciocutaneous Limberg flap. *Contemp Surg*. 1988;33:54–56.
18. Amagai M, Klaus-Kovtun V, Stanley JR. Autoantibodies against a novel epithelial cadherin in pemphigus vulgaris, a disease of cell adhesion. *Cell*. 1991;67:869–877.
19. Anderson AW. Hair extracted from an ulcer. *Boston Med Surg J*. 1847;36:74.
20. Anderson JH, Yip CO, Nagabhushan JS, et al. Day-case Karydakis flap for pilonidal sinus. *Dis Colon Rectum*. 2008;51:134–138.
21. Anstey AV, Wilkinson JD, Lord P. Squamous cell carcinoma complicating hidradenitis suppurativa. *Br J Dermatol*. 1990;123:527–531.
22. Araki Y, Noake T, Hata H, et al. Perianal Paget's disease treated with a wide excision and gluteal fold flap reconstruction guided by photodynamic diagnosis: report of a case. *Dis Colon Rectum*. 2003;46:1563–1565.
23. Arminski TC, Pollard RJ. Paget's disease of the anus secondary to a malignant papillary adenoma of the rectum. *Dis Colon Rectum*. 1973;16:46–55.
24. Armitage G, Smith I. Rodent ulcer of the anus. *Br J Surg*. 1955;42:395–398.
25. Armitage NC, Jass JR, Richman PI, et al. Paget's disease of the anus: a clinicopathological study. *Br J Surg*. 1989;76:60–63.
26. Armstrong JH, Barcia PJ. Pilonidal sinus disease. The conservative approach. *Arch Surg*. 1994;129:914–917.
27. Aygen E, Arslan K, Dogru O, et al. Crystallized phenol in nonoperative treatment of previously operated, recurrent pilonidal disease. *Dis Colon Rectum*. 2010;53:932–935.
28. Banerjee AK. Surgical treatment of hidradenitis suppurativa. *Br J Surg*. 1992;79(9):863–866.
29. Banov L Jr. Pruritus ani and anal hygiene. *J S C Med Assoc*. 1985;81(10):557–558.
30. Barkel DC, Villalba MR. A reappraisal of surgical management in necrotizing perineal infections. *Am Surg*. 1986;52(7):395–397.
31. Bascom J. Pilonidal disease: origin from follicles of hairs and results of follicle removal as treatment. *Surgery*. 1980;87(5):567–572.
32. Bascom J. Pilonidal disease: long-term results of follicle removal. *Dis Colon Rectum*. 1983;26(12):800–807.
33. Bascom JU. Repeat pilonidal operations. *Am J Surg*. 1987;154(1):118–122.

34. Basset-Seguin N, Roujeau JC, Gherardi R, et al. Prognostic factors and predictive signs of malignancy in adult dermatomyositis. A study of 32 cases. *Arch Dermatol.* 1990;126(5):633–637.

35. Bauwens JE, Orlander H, Gomez MP, et al. Epidemic Lymphogranuloma venereum during epidemics of crack cocaine use and HIV infection in the Bahamas. *Sex Transm Dis.* 2002;29(5):253–259.

36. Beck DE, Fazio VW. Perianal Paget's disease. *Dis Colon Rectum.* 1987;30(4):263–266.

37. Beck DE, Fazio VW, Jagelman DG, et al. Perianal Bowen's disease. *Dis Colon Rectum.* 1988;31(6):419–422.

38. Beck DE, Harford FJ, Roettger RH. Perianal Bowen's disease associated with Crohn's colitis. Report of a case. *Dis Colon Rectum.* 1989;32(3):252–255.

39. Beck DE, Jaso RG, Zajac RA. Surgical management of anal condylomata in the HIV-positive patient. *Dis Colon Rectum.* 1990;33(3):180–183.

40. Belmont MJ, Behar PM, Wax MK. Atypical presentations of actinomycosis. *Head Neck.* 1999;21(3):262–268.

41. Berardi RS, Lee S, Chen HP. Perianal extramammary Paget's disease. *Surg Gynecol Obstet.* 1988;167(4):359–366.

42. Berman IR. Mechanisms, diagnosis, and management of anal irritation and itching. In: Schrock TR, ed. *Perspectives in Colon and Rectal Surgery.* Vol 3. St. Louis, MO: Quality Medical; 1990:83.

43. Bernhard, JD. *Itch: Mechanisms and Management of Pruritis.* New York, NY: McGraw-Hill; 1994.

44. Bessa SS. Results of the lateral advancing flap operation (modified Karydakis procedure) for the management of pilonidal sinus disease. *Dis Colon Rectum.* 2007;50(11):1935–1940.

45. Beutner KR, Conant MA, Friedman-Kien AE, et al. Patient-applied podofilox for treatment of genital warts. *Lancet.* 1989;1(8642):831–834.

46. Bielefeld P, Meyer P, Caillot D, et al. [Systemic scleroderma and cancers: 21 cases and review of the literature]. *Rev Med Interne.* 1996;17(10):810–813.

47. Billingham RP, Lewis FG. Laser versus electrical cautery in the treatment of condylomata acuminata of the anus. *Surg Gynecol Obstet.* 1982;155(6):865–867.

48. Blanchard RJ. Fulminating nonclostridial gas-forming infection: a case of necrotizing fasciitis. *Can J Surg.* 1975;18(4):339, 341, 344.

49. Bocchini SF, Habr-Gama A, Kiss DR, et al. Gluteal and perianal hidradenitis suppurativa: surgical treatment by wide excision. *Dis Colon Rectum.* 2003;46(7):944–949.

50. Bohle A, Büttner H, Jocham D. Primary treatment of condylomata acuminata with viable bacillus Calmette-Guerin. *J Urol.* 2001;165(3):834–836.

51. Borges VF, Keating JT, Nasser IA, et al. Clinicopathologic characterization of squamous-cell carcinoma arising from pilonidal disease in association with condylomata acuminatum in HIV-infected patients: report of two cases. *Dis Colon Rectum.* 2001;44(12):1873–1877.

52. Bose B, Candy J. Radical cure of pilonidal sinus by Z-plasty. *Am J Surg.* 1970;120(6):783–786.

53. Bowen JT. Precancerous dermatoses: a study of two cases of chronic atypical epithelial proliferation. *J Cutan Dis.* 1912;30:241–255.

54. Bradford PT, Devesa SS, Anderson WF, et al. Cutaneous lymphoma incidence patterns in the United States: a population-based study of 3884 cases. *Blood.* 2009;113(21):5064–5073.

55. Brasel KJ, Gottesman L, Vasilevsky CA, et al. Meta-analysis comparing healing by primary closure and open healing after surgery for pilonidal sinus. *J Am Coll Surg.* 2010;211(3):431–444.

56. Brauchli YB, Jick SS, Miret M, et al. Psoriasis and risk of incident cancer: an inception cohort study with a nested case-control analysis. *J Invest Dermatol.* 2009;129(11):2604–2012.

57. Braverman IM. *Skin Tags of Systemic Disease.* Philadelphia, PA: WB Saunders; 1981:669.

58. Braverman IM. Bowen's disease and internal cancer. *JAMA.* 1991;266(6):842–843.

59. Breuer K, Häussler S, Kapp A, et al. *Staphylococcus aureus:* colonizing features and influence of an antibacterial treatment in adults with atopic dermatitis. *Br J Dermatol.* 2002;147(1):55–61.

60. Broadwater JR, Bryant RL, Petrino RA, et al. Advanced hidradenitis suppurativa. Review of surgical treatment in 23 patients. *Am J Surg.* 1982;144(6):668–670.

61. Broen EM, Ostergard DR. Toluidine blue and colposcopy for screening and delineating vulvar neoplasia. *Obstet Gynecol.* 1971;38(5):775–778.

62. Brown SC, Kazzazi N, Lord PH. Surgical treatment of perineal hidradenitis suppurativa with special reference to recognition of the perianal form. *Br J Surg.* 1986;73(12):978–980.

63. Buchbinder R, Forbes A, Hall S, et al. Incidence of malignant disease in biopsy-proven inflammatory myopathy. A population-based cohort study. *Ann Intern Med.* 2001;134(12):1087–1095.

64. Budayr M, Ankney RN, Moore RA. Condyloma acuminata in infants and children. A survey of colon and rectal surgeons. *Dis Colon Rectum.* 1996;39(10):1112–1115.

65. Buie LA. Jeep disease (pilonidal disease of mechanized warfare). *South Med J.* 1944;37:103.

66. Bunstock WH. Basal cell carcinoma of the anus. *Am J Surg.* 1958;95(5):822–825.

67. Burge SM. Hailey-Hailey disease: the clinical features, response to treatment and prognosis. *Br J Dermatol.* 1992;126(3):275–282.

68. Burk RD, Kelly P, Feldman J, et al. Declining prevalence of cervicovaginal human papillomavirus infection with age is independent of other risk factors. *Sex Transm Dis.* 1996;23(4):333–341.

69. Butler TW, Gefter J, Kletto D, et al. Squamous-cell carcinoma of the anus in condyloma acuminatum. Successful treatment with preoperative chemotherapy and radiation. *Dis Colon Rectum.* 1987;30(4):293–295.

70. Büyükaşik Y, Ozcebe OI, Sayinalp N, et al. Perianal infections in patients with leukemia: importance of the course of neutrophil count. *Dis Colon Rectum.* 1998;41(1):81–85.

71. Carle G. Anorectal involvement in leukaemia. *J R Coll Surg Edinb.* 1982;27(2):118.

72. Centers for Disease Control and Prevention. *Sexually Transmitted Disease Surveillance, 2003.* Atlanta, GA: U.S. Department of Health and Human Services, Centers for Disease Control and Prevention; 2004.

73. Centers for Disease Control and Prevention. Vulvar vaccinia after sexual contact with a military smallpox vaccinee—Alaska, 2006. *MMWR Morb Mortal Wkly Rep.* 2007;56(17):417–419.

74. Centers for Disease Control and Prevention. *Sexually Transmitted Diseases Surveillance, 2008.* Atlanta, GA: U.S. Department of Health and Human Services, Centers for Disease Control and Prevention; 2009.

75. Centers for Disease Control and Prevention, Workowski KA, Berman SM. Sexually transmitted diseases treatment guidelines, 2006. *MMWR Recomm Rep.* 2006;55(RR11):1–94.

76. Chatterjee S, Dombi GW, Severson RK, et al. Risk of malignancy in scleroderma: a population-based cohort study. *Arthritis Rheum.* 2005;52(8):2415–2424.

77. Chaudhary A, Gupta NM. Colorectal tuberculosis. *Dis Colon Rectum.* 1986;29(11):738–741.

78. Chen CY, Chi KH, Alexander S, et al. A real-time quadriplex PCR assay for the diagnosis of rectal lymphogranuloma venereum and non-lymphogranuloma venereum *Chlamydia trachomatis* infections. *Sex Transm Infect.* 2008;84(4):273–276.

79. Chen JC, Stephens RS. Trachoma and LGV biovars of *Chlamydia trachomatis* share the same glycosaminoglycan-dependent mechanism for infection of eukaryotic cells. *Mol Microbiol.* 1994;11(3):501–507.

80. Cheng SF, Veenema RJ. Topical application of thio-tepa to penile and urethral tumors. *J Urol.* 1965;94(30):259–262.

81. Ching CC, Stahlgren LH. Clinical review of hidradenitis suppurativa: management of cases with severe perianal involvement. *Dis Colon Rectum.* 1965;8(5):349–352.

82. Cho HR, Lee MH, Haw CR. Majocchi's granuloma of the scrotum. *Mycoses.* 2007;50(6):520–522.

83. Cho-Vega JH, Medeiros LJ, Prieto VG, et al. Leukemia cutis. *Am J Clin Pathol.* 2008;129(1):130–142.

84. Chu QD, Vezeridis MP, Libbey NP, et al. Giant condyloma acuminatum (Buschke-Löwenstein tumor) of the anorectal and perianal regions. Analysis of 42 cases. *Dis Colon Rectum.* 1994;37:950–957.

85. Chuang TY, Reizner GT. Bowen's disease and internal malignancy. A matched case-control study. *J Am Acad Dermatol.* 1988;19 (1 pt 1):47–51.

86. Chute CG, Chuang TY, Bergstralh EJ, et al. The subsequent risk of internal cancer with Bowen's disease. A population-based study. *JAMA.* 1991;266(6):816–819.

87. Clayton MD, Fowler JE Jr, Sharifi R, et al. Causes, presentation and survival of fifty-seven patients with necrotizing fasciitis of the male genitalia. *Surg Gynecol Obstet.* 1990; 170(1):49–55.

88. Cleary RK, Schaldenbrand JD, Fowler JJ, et al. Perianal Bowen's disease and anal intraepithelial neoplasia: review of the literature. *Dis Colon Rectum.* 1999;42(7):945–951.

89. Cohen MS, Hoffman IF, Royce RA, et al. Reduction of concentration of HIV-1 in semen after treatment of urethritis: implications for prevention of sexual transmission of HIV-1. AIDSCAP Malawi Research Group. *Lancet.* 1997;349(9069):1868–1873.

90. Cole GW, Amon RB, Russell PS. Secondary syphilis presenting as a pruritic dermatosis. *Arch Dermatol.* 1977;113(4):489–490.

91. Colombo-Benkmann M, Tübergen D, Buchweitz O, et al. Ultrasonic technology: a new treatment option for anal condylomata acuminata. *Dis Colon Rectum.* 2008;51(11):1681–1685.

92. Colquhoun P, Efron J, Eze G, et al. The incidence of subclinical anal intraepithelial neoplasia (AIN) in patients with anal condylomata. *Dis Colon Rectum*. 2001;44:A5.

93. Congilosi SM, Madoff RD. Current therapy for recurrent and extensive anal warts. *Dis Colon Rectum*. 1995;38(10):1101–1107.

94. Conway H, Stark RB, Climo S, et al. The surgical treatment of chronic hidradenitis suppurativa. *Surg Gynecol Obstet*. 1952;95(4):455–464.

95. Corcoran AT, Smaldone MC, Gibbons EP, et al. Validation of the Fournier's gangrene severity index in a large contemporary series. *J Urol*. 2008;180(3):944–948.

96. Coremans G, Margaritis V, Snoeck R, et al. Topical cidofovir (HPMPC) is an effective adjuvant to surgical treatment of anogenital condylomata acuminate. *Dis Colon Rectum*. 2003;46(8):1103–1108.

97. Coremans G, Margaritis V, Van Poppel HP, et al. Actinomycosis, a rare and unsuspected cause of anal fistulous abscess: report of three cases and review of the literature. *Dis Colon Rectum*. 2005;48(3):575–581.

98. Corman ML, Veidenheimer MC, Swinton NW. *Diseases of the Anus, Rectum, and Colon. Part I: Neoplasms*. New York, NY: Medcom; 1972:64.

99. Crapp AR, Macbeth WAAG. Perianal vaccinia: a case report. *Aust NZ J Surg*. 1976;46:83.

100. Creasman C, Haas PA, Fox TA Jr, et al. Malignant transformation of anorectal giant condyloma acuminatum (Buschke-Löwenstein tumor). *Dis Colon Rectum*. 1989;32:481–487.

101. Cresson DH, Siegal GP. Chronic lymphocytic leukemia presenting as an anal mass. *J Clin Gastroenterol*. 1985;7(1):83–87.

102. Crighton JL. Diarrhoea and perianal vaccinia. *Br Med J*. 1976;2(6038):732–733.

103. Criscione VD, Weinstock MA. Incidence of cutaneous T-cell lymphoma in the United States, 1973–2002. *Arch Dermatol*. 2007;143(7):854–859.

104. Croxson T, Chabon AB, Rorat E, et al. Intraepithelial carcinoma of the anus in homosexual men. *Dis Colon Rectum*. 1984;27(5):325–330.

105. Culp CE. Chronic hidradenitis suppurativa of the anal canal. A surgical skin disease. *Dis Colon Rectum*. 1983;26(10):669–676.

106. Currie BJ, McCarthy JS. Permethrin and ivermectin for scabies. *N Engl J Med*. 2010;362(8):717–725.

107. Dailey TH. Pruritus ani. *Pract Gastroenterol*. 1980;4:30.

108. Dan M, Rotmensch HH, Eylan E, et al. A case of lymphogranuloma venereum of 20 years' duration. Isolation of *Chlamydia trachomatis* from perianal lesions. *Br J Vener Dis*. 1980;56(5):344–346.

109. Daniel GL, Longo WE, Vernava AM III. Pruritus ani. Causes and concerns. *Dis Colon Rectum*. 1994;37(7):670–674.

110. Darier J, Couillaud P. Sur un cas de maladie de Paget de la région périnéo-anale et scrotale. *Soc Fr Dermatol Syphilogr*. 1893;4:25.

111. Dasan S, Neill SM, Donaldson DR, et al. Treatment of persistent pruritus ani in a combined colorectal and dermatological clinic. *Br J Surg*. 1999;86(10):1337–1340.

112. Davis KA, Mock CN, Versaci A, et al. Malignant degeneration of pilonidal cysts. *Am Surg*. 1994;60(3):200–204.

113. de la Fuente SG, Ludwig KA, Mantyh CR. Preoperative immune status determines anal condyloma recurrence after surgical excision. *Dis Colon Rectum*. 2003;46(3):367–373.

114. Derk CT, Rasheed M, Artlett CM, et al. A cohort study of cancer incidence in systemic sclerosis. *J Rheumatol*. 2006;33(6):1113–1116.

115. Di Falco G, Guccione C, D'Annibale A, et al. Fournier's gangrene following a perianal abscess. *Dis Colon Rectum*. 1986;29(9):582–585.

116. Dillard BM, Spratt JS Jr, Ackerman LV, et al. Epidermoid cancer of anal margin and canal. Review of 79 cases. *Arch Surg*. 1963;86:772–777.

117. Dixon JA, Gilbertson JJ. Cutaneous laser therapy. *West J Med*. 1985;143(6):758–763.

118. Doll D, Krueger CM, Schrank S, et al. Timeline of recurrence after primary and secondary pilonidal sinus surgery. *Dis Colon Rectum*. 2007;50(11):1928–1934.

119. Doll D, Matevossian E, Wietelmann K, et al. Family history of pilonidal sinus predisposes to earlier onset of disease and a 50% long-term recurrence rate. *Dis Colon Rectum*. 2009;52(9):1610–1615.

120. Domonkos AN, Arnold HL Jr, Odom RB. Cutaneous symptoms, signs and diagnosis. In: Domonkos AN, Arnold HL, eds. *Andrew's Diseases of the Skin*. 7th ed. Philadelphia, PA: WB Saunders; 1982:15.

121. Domonkos AN, Arnold HL Jr, Odom RB. Cutaneous symptoms, signs, and diagnosis. In: Domonkos AN, Arnold HL, eds. *Andrew's Diseases of the Skin*. 7th ed. Philadelphia, PA: WB Saunders; 1982:75.

122. Domonkos AN, Arnold HL Jr, Odom RB. Cutaneous symptoms, signs, and diagnosis. In: Domonkos AN, Arnold HL, eds. *Andrew's Diseases of the Skin*. 7th ed. Philadelphia, PA: WB Saunders; 1982:97.

123. Domonkos AN, Arnold HL Jr, Odom RB. Cutaneous symptoms, signs, and diagnosis. In: Domonkos AN, Arnold HL, eds. *Andrew's Diseases of the Skin*. 7th ed. Philadelphia, PA: WB Saunders; 1982:175.

124. Domonkos AN, Arnold HL Jr, Odom RB. Cutaneous symptoms, signs, and diagnosis. In: Domonkos AN, Arnold HL, eds. *Andrew's Diseases of the Skin*. 7th ed. Philadelphia, PA: WB Saunders; 1982:228.

125. Domonkos AN, Arnold HL Jr, Odom RB. Cutaneous symptoms, signs, and diagnosis. In: Domonkos AN, Arnold HL, eds. *Andrew's Diseases of the Skin*. 7th ed. Philadelphia, PA: WB Saunders; 1982:341.

126. Domonkos AN, Arnold HL Jr, Odom RB. Cutaneous symptoms, signs, and diagnosis. In: Domonkos AN, Arnold HL, eds. *Andrew's Diseases of the Skin*. 7th ed. Philadelphia, PA: WB Saunders; 1982:526.

127. Domonkos AN, Arnold HL Jr, Odom RB. Cutaneous symptoms, signs, and diagnosis. In: Domonkos AN, Arnold HL, eds. *Andrew's Diseases of the Skin*. 7th ed. Philadelphia, PA: WB Saunders; 1982:581.

128. Donsky HJ, Mendelson CG. Squamous cell carcinoma as a complication of hidradenitis suppurativa. *Arch Dermatol*. 1964;90(5):488–491.

129. Douglas JM, Critchlow C, Benedetti J, et al. A double-blind study of oral acyclovir for suppression of recurrences of genital herpes simplex virus infections. *N Engl J Med*. 1984;310(24):1551–1556.

130. Douglas JM Jr, Rogers M, Judson FN. The effect of asymptomatic infection with HTLV-III on the response of anogenital warts to intralesional treatment with recombinant alpha 2 interferon. *J Infect Dis*. 1986;154(2):331–334.

131. Drusin LM, Homan WP, Dineen P. The role of surgery in primary syphilis of the anus. *Ann Surg*. 1976;184(1):65–67.

132. Dubois JD, Dilly SA, Gazet JC. Leukaemic infiltration of the anus. *Eur J Surg Oncol*. 1985;11(4):365–367.

133. Duus BR, Philipsen T, Christensen JD, et al. Refractory condylomata acuminata: a controlled clinical trial of carbon dioxide laser versus conventional surgical treatment. *Genitourin Med*. 1985;61(1):59–61.

134. Edwards M. Bowen's disease: a case report. *Dis Colon Rectum*. 1965;8:297–299.

135. Edwards MH. Pilonidal sinus: a 5-year appraisal of the Millar-Lord treatment. *Br J Surg*. 1977;64(12):867–868.

136. Efem SE. Recent advances in the management of Fournier's gangrene: preliminary observations. *Surgery*. 1993;113(2):200–204.

137. Eftaiha MS, Amshel AL, Shonberg IL, et al. Giant and recurrent condyloma acuminatum: appraisal of immunotherapy. *Dis Colon Rectum*. 1982;25(2):136–138.

138. Egan C, Kelly CD, Rush-Wilson K, et al. Laboratory-confirmed transmission of vaccinia virus infection through sexual contact with a military vaccinee. *J Clin Microbiol*. 2004;42(11):5409–5411.

139. Egan CA, Lazarova Z, Darling TN, et al. Anti-epiligrin cicatricial pemphigoid: clinical findings, immunopathogenesis, and significant associations. *Medicine (Baltimore)*. 2003;82(3):177–186.

140. Eke N. Fournier's gangrene: a review of 1726 cases. *Br J Surg*. 2000;87(6):718–728.

141. Elgart ML. Tinea incognito: an update on Majocchi granuloma. *Dermatol Clin*. 1996;14(1):51–55.

142. Elliot MS, Werner ID, Immelman EJ, et al. Giant condyloma (Buschke-Loewenstein tumor) of the anorectum. *Dis Colon Rectum*. 1979;22(7):497–500.

143. Enriquez JM, Moreno S, Devesa M, et al. Fournier's syndrome of urogenital and anorectal origin: a retrospective, comparative study. *Dis Colon Rectum*. 1987;30(1):33–37.

144. Ernst AA, Marvez-Valls E, Martin DH. Incision and drainage versus aspiration of fluctuant buboes in the emergency department during an epidemic of chancroid. *Sex Transm Dis*. 1995;22(4):217–220.

145. Eron LJ, Judson F, Tucker S, et al. Interferon therapy for condylomata acuminata. *N Engl J Med*. 1986;315(17):1059–1064.

146. Eryilmaz R, Okan I, Coskun A, et al. Surgical treatment of complicated pilonidal sinus with a fasciocutaneous V-Y advancement flap. *Dis Colon Rectum*. 2009;52(12):2036–2040.

147. Eusebio EB, Graham J, Mody N. Treatment of intractable pruritus ani. *Dis Colon Rectum*. 1990;33(9):770–772.

148. Eyers AA, Thomson JP. Pruritus ani: is anal sphincter dysfunction important in aetiology? *Br Med J*. 1979;2(6204):1549–1551.

149. Eze G, Park T, Efron J, et al. Perianal Bowen's disease: result of wide local excision and association with other carcinomas. *Dis Colon Rectum*. 2001;44:A27–A59.

150. Farouk R, Duthie GS, Pryde A, et al. Abnormal transient internal sphincter relaxation in idiopathic pruritus ani: physiological evidence from ambulatory monitoring. *Br J Surg*. 1994;81(4):603–606.

151. Fasching MC, Meland NB, Woods JE, et al. Recurrent squamous-cell carcinoma arising in pilonidal sinus tract—multiple flap reconstructions. Report of a case. *Dis Colon Rectum*. 1989;32(2):153–158.

152. Feng WW, Chen HC, Chen HC. Majocchi's granuloma in a 3-year-old boy. *J Pediatr Infect Dis.* 2006;25(7):658–659.

153. Figueroa S, Gennaro AR. Intralesional bleomycin injection in treatment of condyloma acuminatum. *Dis Colon Rectum.* 1980;23(8): 550–551.

154. Fisher AA. New advances in contact dermatitis. *Int J Dermatol.* 1977;16(7):552–568.

155. Fitzpatrick TB. Fundamentals of dermatologic diagnosis. In: Fitzpatrick TB, Eisen AZ, Wolff K, et al, eds. *Dermatology in General Medicine.* 2nd ed. St. Louis, MO: McGraw-Hill; 1979:10.

156. Fiumara NJ. *Pictorial Guide to Sexually Transmitted Diseases.* Secaucus, NJ: Hospital Publications; 1987.

157. Fiumara NJ, Tang S. Folliculitis of the buttocks and pinworms. A case report. *Sex Transm Dis.* 1986;13(1):45–46.

158. Fleshner PR, Freilich MI. Adjuvant interferon for anal condyloma. A prospective, randomized trial. *Dis Colon Rectum.* 1994;37(12): 1255–1259.

159. Formica MK, Palmer JR, Rosenberg L, et al. Smoking, alcohol consumption, and risk of systemic lupus erythematosus in the Black Women's Health Study. *J Rheumatol.* 2003;30(6):1222–1226.

160. Fortes C, Mastroeni S, Leffondre K, et al. Relationship between smoking and the clinical severity of psoriasis. *Arch Dermatol.* 2005;141(12):1580–1584.

161. Freud E, Farkash U, Prieto F, et al. Perineal reconstruction for severe sequela of ecthyma gangrenosum: report of a case. *Dis Colon Rectum.* 1999;42(7):961–963.

162. Friedman-Kien AE, Eron LJ, Conant M, et al. Natural interferon alfa for treatment of condylomata acuminata. *JAMA.* 1988;259(4):533–538.

163. Friend WG. The cause and treatment of idiopathic pruritus ani. *Dis Colon Rectum.* 1977;20(1):40–42.

164. Fundarò S, Spallanzani A, Ricchi E, et al. Squamous-cell carcinoma developing within anal lichen planus: report of a case. *Dis Colon Rectum.* 1998;41(1):111–114.

165. Füzün M, Bakir H, Soylu M, et al. Which technique for treatment of pilonidal sinus—open or closed? *Dis Colon Rectum.* 1994;37(11):1148–1150.

166. Gabriel WB. *The Principles and Practice of Rectal Surgery.* 4th ed. London, United Kingdom: HK Lewis; 1948:469.

167. Gaertner WB, Hagerman GF, Goldberg SM, et al. Perianal Paget's disease treated with wide excision and gluteal skin flap reconstruction: report of a case and review of the literature. *Dis Colon Rectum.* 2008;51(12): 1842–1845.

168. Gage AA, Dutta P. Cryosurgery for pilonidal disease. *Am J Surg.* 1977;133(2):249–254.

169. Gelfand JM, Neimann AL, Shin DB, et al. Risk of myocardial infarction in patients with psoriasis. *JAMA.* 2006;296(14):1735–1741.

170. Ghaussy NO, Sibbitt W Jr, Bankhurst AD, et al. Cigarette smoking and disease activity in systemic lupus erythematosus. *J Rheumatol.* 2003;30(6):1215–1221.

171. Gill M, Sachdeva B, Gill PS, et al. Majocchi's granuloma of the face in an immunocompetent patient. *J Dermatol.* 2007;34(10):702–704.

172. Gips M, Melki Y, Salem L, et al. Minimal surgery for pilonidal disease using trephines: description of a new technique and long-term outcomes in 1,358 patients. *Dis Colon Rectum.* 2008;51(11):1656–1662.

173. Goldman L, Kitzmiller KW. Perianal atrophoderma from topical corticosteroids. *Arch Dermatol.* 1973;107(4):611–612.

174. Graham JH, Helwig EB. Bowen's disease and its relationship to systemic cancer. *Arch Dermatol.* 1959;80(2):133–159.

175. Graham JH, Helwig EB. Bowen's disease and its relationship to systemic cancer. *Arch Dermatol.* 1961;83:738–758.

176. Gross G. Interferon and genital warts. *JAMA.* 1988;260(14):2066.

177. Guinan ME. Oral acyclovir for treatment and suppression of genital herpes simplex virus infection. A review. *JAMA.* 1986;255(13):1747–1749.

178. Gupta AK, Prussick R, Sibbald RG, et al. Terbinafine in the treatment of Majocchi's granuloma. *Int J Dermatol.* 1995;34(7):489.

179. Gupta AS, Sharma VP, Rathi GL. Ano-rectal tuberculosis simulating carcinoma. *Am J Proctol.* 1976;27(1):33–38.

180. Gupta PJ. Ano-perianal tuberculosis—solving a clinical dilemma. *Afr Health Sci.* 2005;5(4):345–347.

181. Guyuron B, Dinner MI, Dowden RV. Excision and grafting in treatment of recurrent pilonidal sinus disease. *Surg Gynecol Obstet.* 1983;156(2):201–204.

182. Hampton T. Lymphogranuloma venereum targeted: those at risk identified; diagnostic test developed. *JAMA.* 2006;295(22):2592.

183. Hanley PH. Acute pilonidal abscess. *Surg Gynecol Obstet.* 1980;150(1):9–11.

184. Harrison BJ, Read GF, Hughes LE. Endocrine basis for the clinical presentation of hidradenitis suppurativa. *Br J Surg.* 1988;75(10):972–975.

185. Hatta N, Yamada M, Hirano T, et al. Extramammary Paget's disease: treatment, prognostic factors and outcome in 76 patients. *Br J Dermatol.* 2008;158(2):313–318.

186. Hegge HG, Vos GA, Patka P, et al. Treatment of complicated or infected pilonidal sinus disease by local application of phenol. *Surgery.* 1987;102(1): 52–54.

187. Hejase MJ, Simonin JE, Bihrle R. Genital Fournier's gangrene: experience with 38 patients. *Urology.* 1996;47(5):734–739.

188. Helwig EB, Graham JH. Anogenital (extramammary) Paget's disease. A clinicopathological study. *Cancer.* 1963;16(3):387–403.

189. Herrmann G, Hunzelmann N, Engert A. Treatment of pemphigus vulgaris with anti-CD20 monoclonal antibody (rituximab). *Br J Dermatol.* 2003;148(3):602–603.

190. Herron MD, Hinckley M, Hoffman MS, et al. Impact of obesity and smoking on psoriasis presentation and management. *Arch Dermatol.* 2005;141(12):1527–1534.

191. Himal H, McLean AP, Duff JH. Gas gangrene of scrotum and perineum. *Surg Gynecol Obstet.* 1974;139(2):176–178.

192. Hodges RM. Pilo-nidal sinus. *Boston Med Surg J.* 1880;103:485–486.

193. Hope-Simpson RE. Postherpetic neuralgia. *J R Coll Gen Pract.* 1975;25(157):571–575.

194. Horowitz BJ. Interferon therapy for condylomatous vulvitis. *Obstet Gynecol.* 1989;73(3 pt 1):446–448.

195. Hunger RE, Dürr C, Brand CU. Cutaneous leukocytoclastic vasculitis in dermatomyositis suggests malignancy. *Dermatology.* 2001;202(2):123–126.

196. Ishii N, Hashimoto T, Zillikens D, et al. High dose intravenous immunoglobulin (IVIG) therapy in autoimmune skin blistering diseases. *Clin Rev Allergy Immunol.* 2010;38(2–3):186–195.

197. Iwama T, Utzunomiya J. Anal complication in Behçet's syndrome. *Jpn J Surg.* 1977;7(3):114–117.

198. Jackson BR. Extramammary Paget's disease and anaplastic basaloid small-cell carcinoma of the anus: report of a case. *Dis Colon Rectum.* 1975;18(4):339–345.

199. Jacob AF, Kerdel SA. Biologics for hidradenitis suppurativa (Verneuil's disease in the Era of biologics). In: Jemec GBE, Revuz J, Leyden J, eds. *Hidradenitis Suppurativa.* Berlin, Germany: Springer; 2006.145.

200. Jacobs E. Anal infections caused by herpes simplex virus. *Dis Colon Rectum.* 1976;19(2):151–157.

201. Jacobs PH. Majocchi's granuloma (due to therapy with steroid and occlusion). *Cutis.* 1986;38(1):23.

202. Jacobs RF, Schutze GE. Actinomycosis. In: Behrman ER, ed. *Nelson Textbook of Pediatrics.* 16th ed. Philadelphia, PA: WB Saunders; 2000.

203. Jellinek EH, Tulloch WS. Herpes zoster with dysfunction of bladder and anus. *Lancet.* 1976;308(7997):1219–1222.

204. Jemec GB. Effect of localized surgical excisions in hidradenitis suppurativa. *J Am Acad Dermatol.* 1988;18(5 pt 1):1103–1107.

205. Jemec GB, Gniadecka M. Sebum excretion in hidradenitis suppurativa. *Dermatology.* 1997;194(4):325–328.

206. Jemec GB, Hansen U. Histology of hidradenitis suppurativa. *J Am Acad Dermatol.* 1996;34(6):994–999.

207. Jensen SL. Comparison of podophyllin application with simple surgical excision in clearance and recurrence of perianal condylomata accuminata. *Lancet.* 1985;326(8465):1146–1148.

208. Jensen SL, Harling H. Prognosis after simple incision and drainage for a first-episode acute pilonidal abscess. *Br J Surg.* 1988;75(1):60–61.

209. Jensen SL, Sjolin KE, Shokouh-Amiri MH, et al. Paget's disease of the anal margin. *Br J Surg.* 1988;75(11):1089–1092.

210. Jones JE. Pinworms. *Am Fam Physician.* 1988;38(3):159–164.

211. Jones LM. Rectal tuberculosis. *Contemp Surg.* 1985;26:41–43.

212. Jones RB, Hirschmann JV, Brown GS, et al. Fournier's syndrome: necrotizing subcutaneous infection of the male genitalia. *J Urol.* 1979;122(3):279–282.

213. Jones RE Jr, Austin C, Ackerman AB. Extramammary Paget's disease. A critical reexamination. *Am J Dermatopathol.* 1979;1(2):101–132.

214. Jongen J, Eberstein A, Peleikis HG, et al. Perianal streptococcal dermatitis: an important differential diagnosis in pediatric patients. *Dis Colon Rectum.* 2008;51(5):584–587.

215. Kabay S, Yucel M, Yaylak F, et al. The clinical features of Fournier's gangrene and the predictivity of the Fournier's Gangrene Severity Index on the outcome. *Int Urol Nephrol.* 2008;40(4):997–1004.

216. Kalb RE, Grossman ME. Chronic perianal herpes simplex in immunocompromised hosts. *Am J Med.* 1986;80(3):486–490.

217. Kanitakis J. Mammary and extramammary Paget's disease. *J Eur Acad Dermatol Venereol.* 2007;21(5):581–590.

218. Kaplowitz LG, Baker D, Gelb L, et al. Prolonged continuous acyclovir treatment of normal adults with frequently recurring genital herpes simplex virus infection. The Acyclovir Study Group. *JAMA.* 1991;265(6):747–751.

219. Karakayali F, Karagulle E, Karabulut Z, et al. Unroofing and marsupialization vs. rhomboid excision and Limberg flap in pilonidal disease: a prospective, randomized, clinical trial. *Dis Colon Rectum*. 2009;52(3):496–502.

220. Karydakis GE. Easy and successful treatment of pilonidal sinus after explanation of its causative processes. *Aust N Z J Surg*. 1992;62(5):385–389.

221. Kaye FJ, Bunn PA Jr, Steinberg SM, et al. A randomized trial comparing combination electron-beam radiation and chemotherapy with topical therapy in the initial treatment of mycosis fungoides. *N Engl J Med*. 1989; 321(26):1784–1790.

222. Kennedy CTC, Lyell A. Perianal orf. *J Am Acad Dermatol*. 1984; 11(1):72–74.

223. Kent RB, Richards JJ. Fournier's perianal gangrene. *Surg Rounds*. 1989;8:33.

224. Khan SA, Smith NL, Gonder M, et al. Gangrene of male external genitalia in a patient with colorectal disease. Anatomic pathways of spread. *Dis Colon Rectum*. 1985;28(7):519–522.

225. Khatri VP, Espinosa MH, Amin AK. Management of recurrent pilonidal sinus by simple V-Y fasciocutaneous flap. *Dis Colon Rectum*. 1994;37(12):1232–1235.

226. Khawaja HT. Podophyllin versus scissor excision in the treatment of perianal condylomata acuminata: a prospective study. *Br J Surg*. 1989;76(10):1067–1068.

227. Kim ST, Baek JW, Kim TK, et al. Majocchi's granuloma in a woman with iatrogenic Cushing's syndrome. *J Dermatol*. 2008;35(12):789–791.

228. Kitchen PR. Pilonidal sinus: experience with the Karydakis flap. *Br J Surg*. 1996;83(10):1452–1455.

229. Klein EJ, Fisher LS, Chow AW, et al. Anorectal gonococcal infection. *Ann Intern Med*. 1977;86(3):340–346.

230. Kligman AM, Frosch PJ. Steroid addiction. *Int J Dermatol*. 1979;18(1):23–31.

231. Kolator B, Rodin P. Comparison of anal and rectal swabs in the diagnosis of anorectal gonorrhea in women. *Br J Vener Dis*. 1979;55(3):186–187.

232. Korkut M, İçöz G, Dayangaç M, et al. Outcome analysis in patients with Fournier's gangrene: report of 45 cases. *Dis Colon Rectum*. 2003;46(5):649–652.

233. Koukouras D, Kallidonis P, Panagopoulos C. Fournier's gangrene, a urologic and surgical emergency: presentation of a multi-institutional experience with 45 cases. *Urol Int*. 2011;86(2):167–172.

234. Kovalcik PJ, Jones J. Necrotizing perineal infections. *Am Surg*. 1983;49(3):163–166.

235. Kraemer M, Gill SS, Seow-Cheon F. Tuberculous anal sepsis: report of clinical features in 20 cases. *Dis Colon Rectum*. 2000;43(11):1589–1591.

236. Kraft JN, Searle GE. Hidradenitis suppurativa in 64 female patients: retrospective study comparing oral antibiotics and antiandrogen therapy. *J Cutan Med Surg*. 2007;11(4):125–131.

237. Krand O, Yalt T, Berber I, et al. Management of pilonidal sinus disease with oblique excision and bilateral gluteus maximus fascia advancing flap: result of 278 patients. *Dis Colon Rectum*. 2009;52(6):1172–1177.

238. Kraus EW. Perianal basal cell carcinoma. *Arch Dermatol*. 1978;114(3):460–461.

239. Kronborg O, Christensen K, Zimmermann-Nielsen C. Chronic pilonidal disease: a randomized trial with a complete 3-year follow-up. *Br J Surg*. 1985;72:303–304.

240. Kuehn PG, Tennant R, Brenneman AR. Familial occurrence of extramammary Paget's disease. *Cancer*. 1973;31(1):145–148.

241. Kulaylat MN, Gong M, Doerr RJ. Multimodality treatment of squamous cell carcinoma complicating pilonidal disease. *Am Surg*. 1996;62(11):922–929.

242. Kumar N, Sharma P, Sachdeva R, et al. Perineal nodule due to enterobiasis: an aspiration cytologic diagnosis. *Diagn Cytopathol*. 2003;28(1):58–60.

243. Lafferty WE, Coombs RW, Benedetti J, et al. Recurrences after oral and genital herpes simplex virus infection. *N Engl J Med*. 1987;316(23):1444–1449.

244. Laga M, Manoka A, Kivuvu M, et al. Non-ulcerative sexually transmitted diseases as risk factors for HIV-1 transmission in women: results from a cohort study. *AIDS*. 1993;7(1):95–102.

245. Lam DT, Batista O, Weiss EG, et al. Staged excision and split-thickness skin graft for circumferential perianal Paget's disease. *Dis Colon Rectum*. 2001;44(6):868–870.

246. Lamerton AJ. Fournier's gangrene: non-clostridial gas gangrene of the perineum and diabetes mellitus. *J R Soc Med*. 1986;79(4):212–215.

247. Laor E, Palmer JE, Tolia BM, et al. Outcome prediction in patients with Fournier's gangrene. *J Urol*. 1995;154(1):89–92.

248. Laraque D. Severe anogenital warts in a child with HIV infection. *N Engl J Med*. 1989;320(18):1220–1221.

249. LaVoo JW. Bowenoid papulosis. *Dis Colon Rectum*. 1987;30(1):62–64.

250. Lee SH, McGregor DH, Kuziez MN. Malignant transformation of perianal condyloma acuminatum: a case report with review of the literature. *Dis Colon Rectum*. 1981;24(6):462–467.

251. Levitsky J, Hong JJ, Jani AB, et al. Oral vitamin A therapy for a patient with a severely symptomatic postradiation anal ulceration: report of a case. *Dis Colon Rectum*. 2003;46(5):679–682.

252. Linder JH, Myers RT. Perianal Paget's disease. *Am Surg*. 1970;36(6):342–345.

253. Lingam MK, O'Dwyer PJ. Clinicopathological study of perineal Paget's disease. *Br J Surg*. 1997;84(2):231–232.

254. Lister NA, Tabrizi SN, Fairley CK. Validation of Roche COBAS Amlicor assay for detection of Chlamydia trachomatis in rectal and pharyngeal specimens by an omp1 PCR assay. *J Clin Microbiol*. 2004;42(1):239–241.

255. Lloyd J, Flanagan AM. Mammary and extramammary Paget's disease. *J Clin Pathol*. 2000;53(10):742–749.

256. Lock MR, Katz DR, Parks A, et al. Perianal Paget's disease. *Postgrad Med J*. 1977;53:768–772.

257. Longo WE, Ballantyne GH, Gerald WL, et al. Squamous cell carcinoma in situ in condyloma acuminatum. *Dis Colon Rectum*. 1986;29(8):503–506.

258. Lorant T, Ribbe I, Mahteme H, et al. Sinus excision and primary closure versus laying open in pilonidal disease: a prospective randomized trial. *Dis Colon Rectum*. 2011;54(3):300–305.

259. Lord PH. Anorectal problems: etiology of pilonidal sinus. *Dis Colon Rectum*. 1975;18(8):661–664.

260. Lynch CM, Felder TL, Schwandt RA, et al. Lymphogranuloma venereum presenting as a rectovaginal fistula. *Infect Dis Obstet Gynecol*. 1999;7(4):199–201.

261. Lysy J, Sistiery-Ittah M, Israelit Y, et al. Topical capsaicin—a novel and effective treatment for idiopathic intractable pruritus ani: a randomized, placebo controlled, crossover study. *Gut*. 2003;52(9):1323–1326.

262. Mabey D, Peeling RW. Lymphogranuloma venereum. *Sex Transm Infect*. 2002;78(2):90–92.

263. Mahdy T. Surgical treatment of the pilonidal disease: primary closure or flap reconstruction after excision. *Dis Colon Rectum*. 2008;51(12):1816–1822.

264. Mansoory A, Dickson D. Z-plasty for treatment of disease of the pilonidal sinus. *Surg Gynecol Obstet*. 1982;155(3):409–411.

265. Manterola C, Barroso M, Araya JC, et al. Pilonidal disease: 25 cases treated by the Dufourmentel technique. *Dis Colon Rectum*. 1991;34(8):649–652.

266. Marfing TE, Abel ME, Gallagher DM. Perianal Bowen's disease and associated malignancies. Results of a survey. *Dis Colon Rectum*. 1987;30(10):782–785.

267. Marie I, Hatron PY, Levesque H, et al. Influence of age on characteristics of polymyositis and dermatomyositis in adults. *Medicine (Baltimore)*. 1999;78(3):139–147.

268. Marino AW Jr. Proctologic lesions observed in male homosexuals. *Dis Colon Rectum*. 1964;7:121–128.

269. Markell KW, Billingham RP. Pruritus ani: etiology and management. *Surg Clin North Am*. 2010;90(1):125–135.

270. Marks MM. The influence of the intestinal pH on anal pruritus. *South Med J*. 1968;61:1005–1006.

271. Maw RD. Treatment of anogenital warts. *Dermatol Clin*. 1998;16(4):829–834.

272. McCarter MD, Quan SH, Busam K, et al. Long-term outcome of perianal Paget's disease. *Dis Colon Rectum*. 2003;46(5):612–616.

273. McDermott FT. Pilonidal sinus treated by Z-plasty. *Aust N Z J Surg*. 1967;37(1):64–69.

274. McGuinness JG, Winter DC, O'Connell PR. Vacuum-assisted closure of a complex pilonidal sinus. *Dis Colon Rectum*. 2003;46(2):274–276.

275. Meffert J. Lichen sclerosis et atrophicus. Emedicine Web site. http://emedicine.mescape.com/article/1123316-overview. Updated January 29, 2009.

276. Melbye M, Sprøgel P. Aetiological parallel between anal cancer and cervical cancer. *Lancet*. 1991;338(8768):657–659.

277. Mendonça H, Rebelo C, Fernandes A, et al. Squamous cell carcinoma arising in hidradenitis suppurativa. *J Dermatol Surg Oncol*. 1991;17(10):830–832.

278. Mertz GJ, Benedetti J, Ashley R, et al. Risk factors for the sexual transmission of genital herpes. *Ann Intern Med*. 1992;116(3):197–202.

279. Mertz GJ, Critchlow CW, Benedetti J, et al. Double-blind placebo-controlled trial of oral acyclovir in first-episode genital herpes simplex virus infection. *JAMA*. 1984;252(9):1147–1151.

280. Mertz GJ, Jones CC, Mills J, et al. Long-term acyclovir suppression of frequently recurring genital herpes simplex virus infection. A multicenter double-blind trial. *JAMA*. 1988;260(2):201–206.

281. Middleton MD. Treatment of pilonidal sinus by Z-plasty. *Br J Surg.* 1968;55(7):516–518.

282. Monro RS. A consideration of some factors in the causation of pilonidal sinus and its treatment by Z-plasty. *Am J Proctol.* 1967;18(3): 215–225.

283. Monro RS, McDermott FT. The elimination of causal factors in pilonidal sinus treated by Z-plasty. *Br J Surg.* 1965;52:177–181.

284. Mortensen NJ, Thomson JP. Perianal abscess due to *Enterobius vermicularis.* Report of a case. *Dis Colon Rectum.* 1984;27(10):677–678.

285. Müller K, Marti L, Tarantino I, et al. Prospective analysis of cosmesis, morbidity, and patient satisfaction following Limberg flap for the treatment of sacrococcygeal pilonidal sinus. *Dis Colon Rectum.* 2011;54(4):487–494.

286. Murie JA, Sim AJ, Mackenzie I. The importance of pain, pruritus and soiling as symptoms of haemorrhoids and their response to haemorrhoidectomy or rubber band ligation. *Br J Surg.* 1981;68(4):247–249.

287. Nahra KS, Moschella SL, Swinton NW Sr. Condyloma acuminatum treated with liquid nitrogen: report of five cases. *Dis Colon Rectum.* 1969;12(2):125–128.

288. Naldi L, Chatenoud L, Linder D, et al. Cigarette smoking, body mass index, and stressful life events as risk factors for psoriasis: results from an Italian case-control study. *J Invest Dermatol.* 2005;125(1):61–67.

289. Nel WS, Fourie ED. Immunotherapy and 5 percent topical 5-fluorouracil ointment in the treatment of condylomata acuminata. *S Afr Med J.* 1973;47(2):45–49.

290. Newell GB. Treatment of hidradenitis suppurativa. *JAMA.* 1973;223: 556–557.

291. Nickoloff BJ, Nestle FO. Recent insights into the immunopathogenesis of psoriasis provide new therapeutic opportunities. *J Clin Invest.* 2004;113(12):1664–1775.

292. Nielsen OV, Jensen SL. Basal cell carcinoma of the anus—a clinical study of 34 cases. *Br J Surg.* 1981;68(12):856–857.

293. Nilsen AE, Aasen T, Halsos AM, et al. Efficacy of oral acyclovir in the treatment of initial and recurrent genital herpes. *Lancet.* 1982;2(8298): 571–573.

294. Nisbet AA, Thompson IM. Impact of diabetes mellitus on the presentation and outcomes of Fournier's gangrene. *Urology.* 2002;60(5):775–779.

295. Novick NL, Tapia L, Bottone EJ. Invasive trichophyton rubrum infection in an immunocompromised host. Case report and review of the literature. *Am J Med.* 1987;82(2):321–325.

296. Obeid SA. A new technique for treatment of pilonidal sinus. *Dis Colon Rectum.* 1988;31(11):879–885.

297. O'Connor JJ. Surgery plus freezing as a technique for treating pilonidal disease. *Dis Colon Rectum.* 1979;22(5):306–307.

298. O'Farrell N, Moi H. European guideline for the management of donovanosis, 2010. *Int J STD AIDS.* 2010;21(9):609–610.

299. Office of Communications and Public Liaison, National Institute of Allergy and Infectious Diseases. Bethesda, MD: National Institutes of Health; 1999.

300. O'Hanlon TP, Carrick DM, Targoff IN, et al. Immunogenetic risk and protective factors for the idiopathic inflammatory myopathies: distict HLA-A, -B, -Cw, -DRB1, and -DQA1 allelic profiles distinguish European American patients with different myositis autoantibodies. *Medicine (Baltimore).* 2006;85(2):111–127.

301. O'Meara SM, Cullum NA, Majid M, et al. Systematic review of antimicrobial agents used for chronic wounds. *Br J Surg.* 2001;88(1):4–21.

302. Oncel M, Kurt N, Kement M, et al. Excision and marsupialization versus sinus excision for the treatment of limited chronic pilonidal disease: a prospective, randomized trial. *Tech Coloproctol.* 2002;6(3):165–169.

303. Ong PY, Leung DY. The infectious aspects of atopic dermatitis. *Immunol Allergy Clin North Am.* 2010;30(3):309–321.

304. Orland PJ, Rhei E, Brolin RE, et al. Comparison of open versus closed excision of chronic pilonidal sinus. *Contemp Surg.* 1992;41:13.

305. Oxman MN. Immunization to reduce the frequency and severity of herpes zoster and its complications. *Neurology.* 1995;45(12 suppl 8): S41–S46.

306. Owen RL. Role of biopsy in diagnosis of rectal infections. *Gastroenterology.* 1986;91(3):770–772.

307. Paget J. On disease of the mammary areola preceding cancer of the mammary gland. *St Barth Hosp Rep.* 1874;10(5):87–89.

307. Palefsky JM, Holly EA, Ralston MI, et al. Anal cytological abnormalities and anal HPV infection in men with Centers for Disease Control Group IV HIV disease. *Genitourin Med.* 1997;73(3):174–180.

309. Palefsky JM, Holly EA, Ralston MI, et al. Anal squamous intraepithelial lesions in HIV-positive and HIV-negative homosexual and bisexual men: prevalence and risk factors. *J Acquir Immune Defic Syndr Hum Retrovirol.* 1998;17(4):320–326.

310. Paterson CA, Young-Fadok TM, Dozois RR. Basal cell carcinoma of the perianal region: 20-year experience. *Dis Colon Rectum.* 1999;42(9): 1200–1202.

311. Perez-Gurri JA, Temple WJ, Ketcham AS. Gluteus maximus myocutaneous flap for the treatment of recalcitrant pilonidal disease. *Dis Colon Rectum.* 1984;27(4):262–264.

312. Petersen S, Koch R, Stelzner S, et al. Primary closure techniques in chronic pilonidal sinus: a survey of the results of different surgical approaches. *Dis Colon Rectum.* 2002;45(11):1458–1467.

313. Petersen S, Wietelmann K, Evers T, et al. Long-term effects of postoperative razor epilation in pilonidal sinus disease. *Dis Colon Rectum.* 2009;52(1):131–134.

314. Pontifex EK, Hill CL, Roberts-Thomson P, et al. Risk factors for lung cancer in patients with scleroderma: a nested case-control study. *Arthritis Rheum.* 2007;66(4):551–553.

315. Prasad ML, Abcarian H. Malignant potential of perianal condyloma acuminatum. *Dis Colon Rectum.* 1980;23(3):191–197.

316. Prodanovich S, Kirsner RS, Kravetz JD, et al. Association of psoriasis with coronary artery, cerebrovascular, and peripheral vascular diseases and mortality. *Arch Dermatol.* 2009;145(6):700–703.

317. Pruitt BA Jr. Invited commentary to Diettrich NA, Mason JH. Fournier's gangrene: a general surgery problem. *World J Surg.* 1983;7(2): 288–294.

318. Pyrhönen SO. Treatment of condyloma acuminatum and other warts. *Infect Surg.* 1988;7:674.

319. Quan SH. Anal and para anal tumors. *Surg Clin North Am.* 1978;58(3): 591–603.

320. Quie PG, Cates KL. Clinical conditions associated with defective polymorphonuclear leukocyte chemotaxis. *Am J Pathol.* 1977;88(3):711–726.

321. Quinn TC. Gastrointestinal manifestations of AIDS. *Pract Gastroenterol.* 1985;9:23–24.

322. Raaf JH, Krown SE, Pinsky CM, et al. Treatment of Bowen's disease with topical dinitrochlorobenzene and 5-fluorouracil. *Cancer.* 1976;37(4): 1633–1642.

323. Ragozzino MW, Melton LJ III, Kurland LT, et al. Population-based study of herpes zoster and its sequelae. *Medicine (Baltimore).* 1982;61. 310–316.

324. Rajbhandari SM, Wilson RM. Unusual infections in diabetes. *Diabetes Res Clin Pract.* 1998;39(2):123–128.

325. Ramanujam PS, Taylor LG, DeLaPava D, et al. Fournier's gangrene: importance of aggressive management. *Contemp Surg.* 1989;35:21.

326. Ramasastry SS, Conklin WT, Granick MS, et al. Surgical management of massive perianal hidradenitis suppurativa. *Ann Plast Surg.* 1985;15(3): 218–223.

327. Ramos R, Salinas H, Tucker L. Conservative approach to the treatment of Bowen's disease of the anus. *Dis Colon Rectum.* 1983;26(11):712–715.

328. Rehder PA, Eliezer ET, Lane AT. Perianal cellulitis. Cutaneous group A streptococcal disease. *Arch Dermatol.* 1988;124(5):702–704.

329. Reichman RC, Badger GJ, Mertz GJ, et al. Treatment of recurrent genital herpes simplex infections with oral acyclovir: a controlled trial. *JAMA.* 1984;251(16):2103–2107.

330. Reymann F, Ravnborg L, Schou G, et al. Bowen's disease and internal malignant disease. A study of 581 patients. *Arch Dermatol.* 1988;124(5): 677–679.

331. Reynolds VH, Madden JJ, Franklin JD, et al. Preservation of anal function after total excision of the anal mucosa for Bowen's disease. *Ann Surg.* 1984;199(5):563–568.

332. Rook A, Wilkinson DS. The principles of diagnosis. In: Rook A, Wilkinson DS, Ebling FJG, eds. *Textbook of Dermatology.* 3rd ed. Oxford, United Kingdom: Blackwell Scientific; 1979:57.

333. Rosenberg I. The dilemma of pilonidal disease: reverse bandaging for cure of the reluctant pilonidal wound. *Dis Colon Rectum.* 1977;20(4): 290–291.

334. Rosenthal AK, McLaughlin JK, Linet MS, et al. Incidence of cancer among patients with systemic sclerosis. *Cancer.* 1995;76(5):910–914.

335. Rosenthal D. Basal cell carcinoma of the anus: report of two cases. *Dis Colon Rectum.* 1967;10(5):397–400.

336. Rüdlinger R, Buchmann P. HPV 16-positive bowenoid papulosis and squamous-cell carcinoma of the anus in an HIV-positive man. *Dis Colon Rectum.* 1989;32(12):1042–1045.

337. Runfola MA, Weber TK, Rodriguez-Bigas MA, et al. Photodynamic therapy for residual neoplasms of the perianal skin. *Dis Colon Rectum.* 2000;43(4):499–502.

338. Savin S. The role of cryosurgery in management of anorectal disease: preliminary report on results. *Dis Colon Rectum.* 1975;18(4):292–297.

339. Schachter J, Moncada J, Liska S, et al. Nucleic acid amplification tests in the diagnosis of chlamydial and gonococcal infections of the

oropharynx and rectum in men who have sex with men. *Sex Transm Dis.* 2008;35(7):637–642.

340. Schlievert PM, Strandberg KL, Lin YC, et al. Secreted virulence factor comparison between methicillin-resistant and methicillin-sensitive *Staphylococcus aureus*, and its relevance to atopic dermatitis. *J Allergy Clin Immunol.* 2010;125(1):39–49.

341. Scholefield JH, Sonnex C, Talbot IC, et al. Anal and cervical intraepithelial neoplasia: possible parallel. *Lancet.* 1989;2(8666):765–769.

342. Scoma JA, Levy EI. Bowen's disease of the anus: report of two cases. *Dis Colon Rectum.* 1975;18(2):137–140.

343. Senepati A, Cripps NP, Thompson MR. Bascom's operation in the day-surgical management of symptomatic pilonidal sinus. *Br J Surg.* 2000;87(8):1067–1070.

344. Shamim EA, Rider LG, Pandey JP, et al. Differences in idiopathic inflammatory myopathy phenotypes and genotypes between Mesoamerican Mestizos and North Ameracan Caucasians: ethnogeographic influences in the genetics and clinical expression of myosis. *Arthritis Rheum.* 2002;46(7):1885–1893.

345. Sheth S, Schechtman AD. Itchy perianal erythema. *J Fam Pract.* 2007;56(12):1025–1027.

346. Shpitz B, Kaufman Z, Kantarovsky A, et al. Definitive management of acute pilonidal abscess by loop diathermy excision. *Dis Colon Rectum.* 1990;33(5):441–442.

347. Shumaker BP. Treatment of condylomata acuminata with the contact laser system. In: *Clinical Procedures Review.* Vol 9. San Antonio, TX: Surgical Laser Technologies; 1991.

348. Shutze WP, Gleysteen JJ. Perianal Paget's disease. Classification and review of management: report of two cases. *Dis Colon Rectum.* 1990;33(6):502–507.

349. Siddiqi S, Vijay V, Ward M, et al. Pruritus ani. *Ann R Coll Surg Engl.* 2008;90(6):457–463.

350. Sigurgeirsson B, Lindelöf B, Edhag O, et al. Risk of cancer in patients with dermatomyositis or polymyositis. A population-based study. *N Engl J Med.* 1992;326:363–367.

351. Silverman SH, Youngs DJ, Allan A, et al. The fecal microflora in pruritus ani. *Dis Colon Rectum.* 1989;32(6):466–468.

352. Simmons PD. Podophyllin 10% and 25% in the treatment of ano-genital warts. A comparative double-blind study. *Br J Vener Dis.* 1981;57(3):208–209.

353. Slater DN. Perianal abscess: "Have I excluded leukaemia?" *Br Med J.* 1984;289(6459):1682.

354. Sloan PJ, Goepel J. Lichen sclerosus et atrophicus and perianal carcinoma: a case report. *Clin Exp Dermatol.* 1981;6(4):399–402.

355. Smith KJ, Neafie RC, Skelton HG III, et al. Majocchi's granuloma. *J Cutan Pathol.* 1991;18(1):28–35.

356. Smith LE, Henrichs D, McCullah RD. Prospective studies on the etiology and treatment of pruritus ani. *Dis Colon Rectum.* 1982;25:358–363.

357. Sneddon IB. Atrophy of the skin. The clinical problems. *Br J Dermatol.* 1976;94(suppl 12):121–123.

358. Snoeck R, Bossens M, Parent D, et al. Phase II double-blind, placebo-controlled study of the safety and efficacy of cidofovir topical gel for the treatment of patients with human papillomavirus infection. *Clin Infect Dis.* 2001;33(5):597–602.

359. Sobrado CW, Mester M, Nadalin W, et al. Radiation-induced total regression of a highly recurrent giant perianal condyloma: report of case. *Dis Colon Rectum.* 2000;43(2):257–260.

360. Sohn N, Robilotti JG Jr. The gay bowel syndrome. A review of colonic and rectal conditions in 200 male homosexuals. *Am J Gastroenterol.* 1977;67(5):478–484.

361. Solla JA, Rothenberger DA. Chronic pilonidal disease. An assessment of 150 cases. *Dis Colon Rectum.* 1990;33(9):758–761.

362. Spivak H, Brooks VL, Nussbaum M, et al. Treatment of chronic pilonidal disease. *Dis Colon Rectum.* 1996;39(10):1136–1139.

363. Standards Task Force of the American Society of Colon and Rectal Surgeons. Practice parameters for ambulatory anorectal surgery. *Dis Colon Rectum.* 1991;34:285.

364. Stanley JR, Amagai M. Pemphigus, bullous impetigo, and the staphylococcal scalded-skin syndrome. *N Engl J Med.* 2006;355(17):1800–1810.

365. Stephens BJ, Lathrop JC, Rice WT, et al. Fournier's gangrene: historic (1764–1978) versus contemporary (1979–1988) differences in etiology and clinical importance. *Am Surg.* 1993;59(3):149–154.

366. Stone HB. A treatment for pruritus ani. *Johns Hopkins Hosp Bull.* 1916;27:242.

367. Stone HB. Pruritus ani: treatment by alcohol injection. *Surg Gynecol Obstet.* 1926;42:565.

368. Straus SE, Croen KD, Sawyer MH, et al. Acyclovir suppression of frequently recurring genital herpes. Efficacy and diminishing need during successive years of treatment. *JAMA.* 1988;260:2227–2230.

369. Straus SE, Takiff HE, Seidlin M, et al. Suppression of frequently recurring genital herpes. A placebo-controlled double-blind trial of oral acyclovir. *N Engl J Med.* 1984;310:1545–1550.

370. Strauss RJ, Fazio VW. Bowen's disease of the anal and perianal area. A report and analysis of twelve cases. *Am J Surg.* 1979;137(2):231–234.

371. Su WP. Clinical, histopathologic, and immunohistochemical correlations in leukemia cutis. *Semin Dermatol.* 1994;13(3):223–230.

372. Subbuswamy SG, Ribeiro BF. Perianal Paget's disease associated with cloacogenic carcinoma: report of a case. *Dis Colon Rectum.* 1981;24(7):535–538.

373. Sullivan ES, Garnjobst WM. Symposium on colon and anorectal surgery. Pruritus ani: a practical approach. *Surg Clin North Am.* 1978;58(3):505–512.

374. Sullivan M. Chancroid. *Am J Syphilis Gonorrhea Venereal Dis.* 1940;24:480–521.

375. Sultan S, Azria F, Bauer P, et al. Anoperineal tuberculosis: diagnostic and management considerations in seven cases. *Dis Colon Rectum.* 2002;45(3):407–410.

376. Swerdlow DB, Salvati EP. Condyloma acuminatum. *Dis Colon Rectum.* 1971;14(3):226–231.

377. Swinehart JM, Sperling M, Phillips S, et al. Intralesional fluorouracil/epinephrine injectable gel for treatment of condylomata acuminata. A phase 3 clinical study. *Arch Dermatol.* 1997;133(1):67–73.

378. Tezel E, Bostanci H, Anadol AZ, et al. Cleft lift procedure for sacrococcygeal pilonidal disease. *Dis Colon Rectum.* 2009;52(1):135–139.

379. Theodoropoulos GE, Vlahos K, Lazaris AC, et al. Modified Bascom's asymmetric midgluteal cleft closure technique for recurrent pilonidal disease: early experience in a military hospital. *Dis Colon Rectum.* 2003;46(9):1286–1291.

380. Thornton JP, Abcarian H. Surgical treatment of perianal and perineal hidradenitis suppurativa. *Dis Colon Rectum.* 1978;21(8):573–577.

381. Topgül K, Ozdemir E, Kiliç K, et al. Long-term results of limberg flap procedure for treatment of pilonidal sinus: a report of 200 cases. *Dis Colon Rectum.* 2003;46(11):1545–1548.

382. Toubanakis G. Treatment of pilonidal sinus disease with the Z-plasty procedure (modified). *Am Surg.* 1986;52(11):611–612.

383. Tramujas da Costa e Silva I, de Lima Ferreira LC, Santos Gimenez F, et al. High-resolution anoscopy in the diagnosis of anal cancer precursor lesions in renal graft recipients. *Ann Surg Oncol.* 2008;15(5):1470–1475.

384. Trautinger F. Phototherapy of mycosis fungoides. *Photodermatol Photoimmunol Photomed.* 2011;27(2):68–74.

385. Trees DL, Morse SA. Chancroid and *Haemophilus ducreyi*: an update. *Clin Microbiol Rev.* 1995;8:357–375.

386. Tritapepe R, Di Padova C. Excision and primary closure of pilonidal sinus using a drain for antiseptic wound flushing. *Am J Surg.* 2002;183(2):209–211.

387. Trombetta LJ, Place RJ. Giant condyloma acuminatum of the anorectum: trends in epidemiology and management: report of a case and review of the literature. *Dis Colon Rectum.* 2001;44(12):1878–1886.

388. Tyring SK. Immune-response modifiers: a new paradigm in the treatment of human papillomavirus. *Curr Ther Res Clin Exp.* 2000;61(9):584–596.

389. Unalp HR, Kamer E, Derici H, et al. Fournier's gangrene: evaluation of 68 patients and analysis of prognostic variables. *J Postgrad Med.* 2008;54(2):102–105.

390. Urbano-Márquez A, Casademont J, Grau JM. Polymyositis/dermatomyositis: the current position. *Ann Rheum Dis.* 1991;50(3):191–195.

391. Urhan MK, Kücükel F, Topgül K, et al. Rhomboid excision and Limberg flap for managing pilonidal sinus: results of 102 cases. *Dis Colon Rectum.* 2002;45(5):656–659.

392. Van der Bij AK, Spaargaren J, Morré SA, et al. Diagnostic and clinical implications of anorectal lymphogranuloma venereum in men who have sex with men: a retrospective case-control study. *Clin Infect Dis.* 2006;42(2):186–194.

393. van Joost T, Faber WR, Manuel HR. Drug-induced anogenital cicatricial pemphigoid. *Br J Dermatol.* 1980;102(6):715–718.

394. Velitchkov N, Djedjev M, Kirov G, et al. Toxic shock syndrome and necrotizing fasciitis complicating neglected sacrococcygeal pilonidal sinus disease: report of a case. *Dis Colon Rectum.* 1997;40(11):1386–1390.

395. Velpeau A. *Dictionnaire en 30 Volumes.* Articles: Aiselle, II, 91; Anus, III, 304; Mamelles, XIX, 1839; Clinique chirurg, II, 133. Quoted by Conway H, Stark RB, Climo S, et al. The surgical treatment of chronic hidradenitis suppurativa. *Surg Gynecol Obstet.* 1952;95:455–464.

396. Verma GK, Sharma NL, Shanker V, et al. Amoebiasis cutis: clinical suspicion is the key to early diagnosis. *Australas J Dermatol.* 2010;51(1):52–55.

397. Viazis N, Vlachogiannakos J, Vasiliadis K, et al. Earlier eradication of intra-anal warts with argon plasma coagulator combined with imiquimod cream compared with argon plasma coagulator alone: a prospective, randomized trial. *Dis Colon Rectum*. 2007;50(12):2173–2179.

398. Wade TR, Kopf AW, Ackerman AB. Bowenoid papulosis of the genitalia. *Arch Dermatol*. 1979;115(3):306–308.

399. Walsh G, Stickley CS. Acute leukemia with primary symptoms in the rectum: a rapid increase in the white cells and fatal outcome. *South Med J*. 1934;96:684–689.

400. Warin RP. Antifungal agents. *Practitioner*. 1974;213(1276 spec no):494–507.

401. Welton M, Amerhauser A, Litle V, et al. Anal Bowen's disease and high-grade squamous intraepithelial lesions are histologically and immunohistochemically indistinguishable. *Dis Colon Rectum*. 2001;44:A27.

402. Wexner SD. Managing common anorectal sexually transmitted diseases. *Infect Surg*. 1990;9:9.

403. Whalen TV Jr, Kovalcik PJ, Old WL Jr. Tuberculous anal ulcer. *Dis Colon Rectum*. 1980;23(1):54–55.

404. Wilkin JK. Chronic benign familial pemphigus. Minimal involvement mimicking chronic perianal candidiasis. *Arch Dermatol*. 1978;114(1):136.

405. Willemze R, Jaffe ES, Burg G, et al. WHO-EORTC classification for cutaneous lymphomas. *Blood*. 2005;105(10):3768–3785.

406. Williams RE, Gibson AG, Aitchison TC, et al. Assessment of a contact-plate sampling technique and subsequent quantitative bacterial studies in atopic dermatitis. *Br J Dermatol*. 1990;123(4):493–501.

407. Williams SL, Rogers LW, Quan SH. Perianal Paget's disease: report of seven cases. *Dis Colon Rectum*. 1976;19(1):30–40.

408. Williamson JD, Silverman JF, Tafra L. Fine-needle aspiration cytology of metastatic squamous-cell carcinoma arising in a pilonidal sinus, with literature review. *Diagn Cytopathol*. 1999;20(6):367–370.

409. Wiltz O, Schoetz DJ Jr, Murray JJ, et al. Perianal hidradenitis suppurativa. The Lahey Clinic experience. *Dis Colon Rectum*. 1990;33(9):731–734.

410. Wiltz OH, Torregrosa M, Wiltz O. Autogenous vaccine: the best therapy for perianal condyloma acuminata? *Dis Colon Rectum*. 1995;38(8):838–841.

411. Wiseman MC. Hidradenitis suppurativa: a review. *Dermatol Ther*. 2004;17(1):50–54.

412. Wolach MD, MacDermott JP, Stone AR, et al. Treatment and complications of Fournier's gangrene. *Br J Urol*. 1989;64(3):310–314.

413. Yeniyol CO, Suelozgen T, Arslan M, et al. Fournier's gangrene: experience with 25 patients and use of Fournier's gangrene severity index score. *J Urol*. 2004;64(2):218–222.

414. Yoshinaga IG, Conrado LA, Schainberg SC, et al. Recalcitrant molluscum contagiosum in a patient with AIDS: combined treatment with CO_2 laser, trichloroacetic acid, and pulsed dye laser. *Lasers Surg Med*. 2000;27(4):291–294.

415. Yu CC, Cook MG. Hidradenitis suppurativa: a disease of follicular epithelium, rather than apocrine glands. *Br J Dermatol*. 1990;122(6):763–769.

416. Zachary LS, Robson MC, Rachmaninoff N. Squamous cell carcinoma occurring in hidradenitis suppurativa. *Ann Plast Surg*. 1987;18(1):71–73.

417. Zantos D, Zhang Y, Felson D. The overall and temporal association of cancer with polymyositis and dermatomyositis. *J Rheumatol*. 1994;21(10):1855–1859.

418. Zimmerman CE. Outpatient excision and primary closure of pilonidal cysts and sinuses. *Am J Surg*. 1978;136(5):640–642.

419. Zollo JD, Zeitouni NC. The Roswell Park Cancer Center Institute experience with extramammary Paget's disease. *Br J Dermatol*. 2000;142(1):59–65.

10

Colorectal Manifestations of Acquired Immunodeficiency Syndrome (HIV Infection)

Pranat Kumar and Lester Gottesman

In human affairs the best stimulus for running is to have something we must run from.
—ERIC HOFFER: *The Ordeal of Change* (1964)

► ACQUIRED IMMUNODEFICIENCY SYNDROME

Acquired immunodeficiency syndrome (AIDS) is caused by human immunodeficiency virus (HIV), a *Lentivirus*, from the family of retroviruses, with an RNA genome. The disease was first recognized in the United States in 1981. HIV has since become the sixth leading cause of death worldwide, with an estimated 40 million men, women, and children infected according to 2004 figures.[290] In the United States, the number of new cases appears to be increasing.[39] There were 41,113 new cases diagnosed in 2000.[38] In 2006, that number jumped to 56,300 new cases.[113] Improved medical therapy, with the development of highly active antiretroviral therapy (HAART) in the mid-1990s, decreased the number of AIDS-related deaths, thus resulting in increased numbers of persons living with AIDS. In 2000, this number was estimated to be

337,731 in the United States.[38] Whereas AIDS was initially confined to the homosexual population, intravenous drug users, and recipients of contaminated blood, there has been a noticeable increase in the incidence among the heterosexual population.

Mechanism of Viral Replication

HIV infects immune cells, thereby enabling replication of the virus. The HIV glycoprotein, gp120, interacts with the cell surface CD4 molecule and either the CXCR4 chemokine receptor (expressed in CD4$^+$ T cells) or the CCR5 chemokine receptor (expressed in macrophages and primary T cells) to permit cellular entry of HIV. The viral RNA is reverse-transcribed into complementary DNA (cDNA) by the enzyme reverse transcriptase (RT). The cDNA is then transported to the host cell nucleus and is integrated into the host cell DNA by the enzyme integrase, thereby permitting replication of the viral RNA and the synthesis of viral proteins. The enzyme, protease, sections the viral proteins into shorter pieces, which then encapsulate, allowing release of new virions.

HIV infection results in immune dysfunction, which, if untreated, leads to a progressive, profound immunocompromised state, with decreased cellular and humoral immunity, opportunistic infections, rare malignant tumors, and, ultimately, death.

Symptoms and Associated Conditions

HIV often causes a brief, flulike illness at the time of infection, but the virus may be harbored for many years without producing clinical manifestations. Because the acute infection generally produces mild, nonspecific symptoms, HIV infection is usually not diagnosed until several years after infection. Immunoglobulin M (IgM) antibodies to various HIV proteins are detectable within 2 weeks of infection by enzyme-linked immunoabsorbent assay and Western blot.[156] IgG antibody is generally detected by 6 weeks after the onset of acute infection, although Imagawa and colleagues demonstrated that HIV infection may actually occur 35 months before detection of antibodies.[126] However, this observation is generally thought to be the exception.

Acute HIV infection may manifest itself through fever, lymphadenopathy, pharyngitis, rash, weight loss, and fatigue.[50] Gastrointestinal symptoms such as abdominal pain, diarrhea, nausea, and anorexia have also been reported during the acute illness.[219,231] Immunologically, there is a precipitous drop in peripheral T-cell populations during the acute phase.[55] This is transient and is followed by a lymphocytosis 3 to 4 weeks later, although there is a decrease in CD4$^+$ cells relative to CD8$^+$ cells.[294]

Progression of HIV results in a gradual decline of CD4$^+$ cells and an increase in the number of virions ("viral load"). CD4$^+$ lymphocyte counts are used as an indicator of disease progression. Individuals with CD4$^+$ cell counts lower than 200 are considered to have advanced immunodeficiency, and, by definition, AIDS, and those with CD4$^+$ cell counts lower than 50 have end-stage disease. HIV continually destroys resident T cells at a fairly constant rate and, after initial infection, stabilizes the rate of viral replication (called the *set point*) in each individual. This continues until the capacity of the immune system to restore itself is exhausted. Because T4 cells are constantly being replenished and destroyed, measurement of plasma HIV-1 RNA now appears to be a better prognostic indicator of disease activity than the CD4 count.[85] Disease progression leads to increased opportunistic infections, AIDS-related malignancies, and, ultimately, death.

Colonic and anorectal problems in individuals who are HIV positive are mainly infectious in origin, as can be predicted from the immunodeficient status of the patients. Certain enteric infections have a high prevalence among homosexual men with and without AIDS, but especially if the latter condition supervenes. These include gonorrhea, syphilis, shigellosis, condylomata acuminata, campylobacteriosis, amebiasis, giardiasis, cryptosporidiosis, cytomegalovirus infection, isosporiasis, candidiasis, and infection with *Chlamydia trachomatis*, *Salmonella typhimurium*, and *Mycobacterium avium*.[197] Gastrointestinal tract hemorrhage is an uncommon manifestation.[36] Miles and colleagues noted that the most frequent reason for surgical referral was anorectal disease (5.9% of all HIV-positive patients), and warts comprised the single most common indication.[170]

Certain malignant tumors are seen more frequently in patients with AIDS. The most common are Kaposi's sarcoma and non-Hodgkin's lymphoma (NHL), both of which may have colonic involvement. The incidence of anal squamous carcinoma is also increased in patients with AIDS.[229]

Intestinal and Anorectal Immunology and HIV

The mucosal layer on the surface of the gut provides a barrier to the large number of bacteria within the intestinal tract. Nonspecific mucosal defenses are extrinsic to the mucosa and form a protective barrier. These include the mucous coat; resident microflora, which prevent overgrowth of pathogenic organisms; proteolytic secretions; and glycocalyx. Secretory IgA, the primary immunoglobulin in external secretions, is the main immunologic defense in the gastrointestinal tract, and it acts as a non–complement-binding antibody that captures pathogens before they can invade the mucosal surface. An antigen that succeeds in penetrating this defense is processed by specialized epithelial cells on the mucosal surface, microvillus (M) cells, and is presented to immunologically competent cells in the lamina propria. Gut-associated lymphoid tissue is found in Peyer's patches, solitary lymphoid follicles, and local, activated T cells within the lamina propria. Intraluminally, these lymphoid aggregates are covered with follicle-associated epithelium that contains M cells. M cells function to transport antigen to dendritic cells and tissue macrophages within the lymphoid aggregates, which, in turn, present antigen to CD4$^+$ T cells and B cells.[190] Once activated, resident T cells initiate cellular immunity by release of cytokines and modulation of other cellular immune elements, and B cells produce antigen-specific antibody.

HIV can gain access to lymphoid tissue within the lamina propria either through a break in the mucosa or by M cell–mediated transport. Within the lamina propria and epithelium of the intestinal tract, HIV infects resident T-cell and macrophage populations in the lymphoid aggregates and diffuses activated memory T cells. As described earlier, this is mediated through the cell surface coreceptors CXCR4 and CCR5. Gut-associated lymphoid tissue contains more than 50% of total lymphocytes in the body and as such represents an important HIV reservoir. It is unique in the proportion of activated memory T cells it contains, which is higher than in peripheral blood and lymph nodes. It has been postulated to be an early site of HIV infection and replication because the virus replicates more efficiently in activated memory T cells.[224,262,295] In a primate model using simian immunodeficiency virus (SIV), activated memory CD4 T cells were found to be rapidly depleted within days of SIV infection. The early, selective, rapid infection and depletion of intestinal lymphoid tissue led the authors to hypothesize that acute HIV and SIV infection is primarily a disease of the mucosal/intestinal immune system.[262] The early infection and apoptosis of intestinal mucosal CD4 T cells may explain the abdominal complaints common in early HIV infection described earlier. The depletion of CD4 T cells adversely affects immunoglobulin production and mucosal integrity, thereby promoting translocation of bacteria and subsequent bacterial invasion.[96] A similar phenomenon has been more recently described for vaginal mucosal CD4 T cells, which likewise serves as an early site of entry and replication of HIV.[263]

The squamous epithelium of the anal canal and anal verge also has immunologic function. Both CD4 and CD8 T lymphocytes and dendritic cells, which function as antigen-presenting cells, are present in the anal mucosa.[30,97] Dendritic cells, also known as *Langerhans cells* after migration to the epithelium, act as antigen-presenting cells to activate a cellular immune response.[254] In their capacity as antigen-presenting cells, epithelial and subepithelial dendritic cells of the anal canal may act to facilitate access of HIV to the mucosal lymphoid system. The capacity to migrate from initial points of entry, together with their capacity to activate the cellular immune response by recruiting and activating large numbers of T cells, led some researchers to propose that these cells play an integral role in sexual transmission of HIV.[144]

The interaction of HIV, anal canal dendritic cells, and mucosal T cells may explain the effect of HIV on other viral infections of the anal canal in HIV-positive patients, including human papillomavirus (HPV). Persistent HPV infection in HIV-positive patients may be secondary to local immune dysfunction rather than to generalized immunosuppression.[61] Sobhani and coworkers have shown a decrease in the number of dendritic cells in the anal mucosa of HIV-positive patients with HPV infection compared with HIV-negative controls,[243] a finding that may explain the more aggressive nature of HPV infection in HIV-positive patients.

New antiviral therapies and mucosal vaccines are being investigated that would block the transmission of HIV to T cells by dendritic cells via the membrane protein, DC-SIGN, which binds the HIV-1 envelope.[198]

Antiretroviral Therapy

HAART has profoundly affected the progression of HIV disease. HAART reduces plasma viral load, increases CD4 T-cell counts, and reduces the incidence of opportunistic infections in HIV-infected patients.[83,189] HAART is a combination of three or more antiretroviral drugs from two or, sometimes, three different classes of drugs. Class-sparing regimens have been advocated to allow for second-line therapy in case of resistance.[1] The three classes of drugs used in HAART are the nucleoside RT inhibitors (NRTIs), the nonnucleoside RT inhibitors (NNRTIs), and the protease inhibitors (PIs). More recently, a fourth class, the fusion inhibitors, has been introduced and approved by the U.S. Food and Drug Administration (FDA). The NRTIs were the first class of antiretroviral drugs, introduced with zidovudine (formerly known as azidothymidine or AZT).[114] The NRTIs are dideoxynucleoside analogues that, once phosphorylated, can be incorporated into the cDNA, causing early chain termination and preventing HIV replication. The NNRTIs, like the NRTIs, prevent the transcription of the HIV RNA into cDNA. However, unlike the NRTIs, the NNRTIs do not act as substrates for the enzyme but rather bind to the active site of the enzyme, preventing viral DNA synthesis. PIs, introduced in 1995, inhibit the enzyme HIV protease, blocking the final cleavage of HIV proteins and preventing the assembly of new virions.[69] Combination antiviral therapy with a PI is more effective in reducing plasma HIV-1 RNA compared with regimens without a PI.[111] In March 2003, the FDA approved enfuvirtide (Fuzeon), the first fusion inhibitor to be approved for use in combination with other antiretroviral drugs. The fusion inhibitors, a novel class of drug, differ from previous HIV medications in that they do not disrupt the replication and release of HIV but rather prevent the entry of HIV into the target cell.[130] Unlike other antiretrovirals, enfuvirtide lacks oral availability and is administered by subcutaneous injection twice daily. However, this class of drugs has had limited clinical use because of rapid induction of resistance.[118]

The impact of HAART on the intestinal mucosal immune system has not been shown to be as effective as it is in the peripheral immune system.[256] As mentioned earlier, the gut-associated lymphoid tissue represents a large reservoir for HIV infection and is affected by HIV early in the course of infection with a dramatic loss of lymphoid cells and, by extension, decrease in the immune function of the intestinal mucosa. Talal and coworkers examined the effects of HAART on gut-associated lymphoid tissue in a small, prospective study with eight patients. In all individuals, levels of HIV-1 RNA fell to less than detectable levels after 6 months of therapy in both gut-associated lymphoid tissue and plasma. Immune reconstitution, however, was less dramatic in intestinal lymphoid tissue compared with peripheral blood.[253] Other authors have documented a similar decrease in HIV-1 RNA but with a significant increase in CD4 T-cell counts in rectal biopsies.[149]

Although HAART has not yet been definitively shown to result in immune reconstitution of gut-associated lymphoid tissue, combination antiviral therapy has had a tremendous impact on intestinal manifestations of HIV. The incidence of AIDS-associated intestinal malignancies and opportunistic infections has decreased since the advent of HAART. The prevalence of opportunistic pathogens in endoscopic biopsy specimens in HIV-infected patients decreased from 69% to 13% following the introduction of HAART.[173] Similarly, the incidence of opportunistic infections causing chronic diarrhea in patients with AIDS decreased from 53% to 13% following the introduction of HAART.[30] However, the overall incidence of diarrhea remains high, a concern that may be secondary to PIs. Diarrhea is a common side effect of these inhibitors and is noted in up to 70% of patients. Treatment for opportunistic pathogens in HIV-infected patients with chronic diarrhea is more successful in patients receiving HAART. In a study of 282 individuals, those receiving PIs had a significantly higher response rate to the treatment for pathogen-identified diarrhea.[18] Immune reconstitution of gut-associated lymphoid tissue with an increase in CD4 T cells and recovery from cryptosporidiosis in an HIV-infected patient following initiation of HAART have been described.[221]

Surgery and Surgical Outcome

Surgical consultation is often sought in patients with HIV infection or AIDS for complaints of abdominal pain. Many of the opportunistic gastrointestinal diseases that are seen in patients with AIDS may present with severe abdominal pain that can mimic standard surgical conditions. The majority of these can safely be managed nonoperatively. Generally, the goal in management of the acute abdomen in a patient with HIV is to *try to avoid surgery*.[84,228] Evaluating by means of computed tomography and endoscopy, understanding the natural history of the colonic manifestations, and knowing the expected responses from pharmacologic intervention will usually allow the surgeon to avoid an unnecessary and unhelpful laparotomy. However, intestinal perforation, gastrointestinal bleeding, and obstruction as a consequence of infection or malignancy may be seen in HIV-positive patients, and these manifestations often necessitate surgical intervention.

Numerous articles have been published on the results of surgery in individuals who harbor the AIDS virus and in those who have the full-blown picture of AIDS or AIDS-related complex.[66,107,225,282] Wolkomir and colleagues reported

474 patients who underwent abdominal and anorectal surgery with these conditions.[288] None required surgery for complications secondary to cytomegalovirus, visceral lymphoma, or visceral Kaposi's sarcoma. Although no deaths occurred within 30 days, the morbidity rate was 72%. The rate of wound healing was inversely related to the white blood cell count. Deneve and coworkers reported their single institution experience in 77 patients with a preoperative diagnosis of HIV or AIDS.[70] They found that a lower CD4 count was associated with a higher likelihood of urgent operation, increased overall complication rate, and higher mortality. Wilson and colleagues submitted their experience of 36 major abdominal operations performed on 35 patients with AIDS.[287] Cytomegalovirus was the most common pathogen. Mycobacterial infections presented as retroperitoneal adenopathy or splenic abscess, and NHL was the most common malignancy identified.[112] Elective mortality was 9% at 30 days and 46% when an emergency operation was necessary. In a study by Chambers and Lord, the outcome of laparotomy in patients with AIDS who were found to have AIDS-related pathology was compared with those with non–AIDS-related pathology.[41] Those in the former group were found at the time of laparotomy to have lower mean body weights, serum albumin levels, and CD4 T-cell counts. The most frequent postoperative AIDS-related pathology was B-cell NHL. The 30-day mortality rate was 17%, and the complication rate was 70%, with no significant difference between patients with AIDS or with AIDS-related pathology and those with non–AIDS-related pathology. More than 50% of postoperative complications were infectious in origin (pulmonary, wound, and systemic sepsis). This is in contrast to an earlier study in which a slightly higher mortality rate in patients with AIDS-related pathology at laparotomy was observed (47%) compared with patients with non–AIDS-related pathology.[20] Postoperative complications have been noted to occur with a higher frequency (61% vs. 7%) in patients with AIDS than in asymptomatic HIV-infected patients. Again, most complications were infectious in origin.[290]

With the addition of highly active antiretroviral therapies, there has been a significant reduction in abdominal complications associated with opportunistic infections.[204] Monkemuller and associates reported a decrease in opportunistic infections from 69% in the pre-HAART era to 13% currently.[173] Antiretroviral therapy has also been associated with a reduction in operative mortality when compared to outcomes in the pre-HAART era. Mortality rates ranged from 57% to 86% in HIV/AIDS patients before the advent of HAART.[210,216,281] Recent studies have shown that operative mortality is as low as 11% to 19% for emergency abdominal surgery in patients on HAART.[66,257,291]

In contrast to intra-abdominal surgical procedures, perianal surgical procedures do not appear to carry a higher morbidity and mortality in HIV-infected patients.[34] Barrett and coworkers reported a 2% complication rate in 485 anorectal procedures, and there were no deaths.[10] This is consistent with our own experience.

However, surgeons must not forget that illnesses common in non-HIV patients may also occur in the immunocompromised HIV patient. In fact, conditions such as appendicitis, diverticulitis, cholecystitis, pancreatitis, hepatitis, peptic ulcer disease, ischemic bowel disease, and symptomatic abdominal aortic aneurysm have been reported to occur with the same frequency in HIV and in non-HIV patient groups.[210,239,293]

Postoperative Complications and Wound Healing

Early reports about poor wound healing and fear of becoming infected through inadvertent exposure have contributed to the reluctance of many surgeons to operate on HIV-positive patients. Analysis of data suggests an inverse relationship between CD4 T-cell count and wound healing—that is, poor wound healing is associated with low CD4 T-cell counts in lesions not expected to heal, such as malignancies and ulcers.[53] More recently, a greater incidence of wound complications in HIV-positive patients has been reported.[68] CD4 T-cell counts do appear to be a prognostic factor in surgical outcome in patients with AIDS. Albaran and coworkers found that patients with CD4 T-cell counts lower than 200 cells/mm^3 had increased morbidity and mortality rates following surgery.[7] An increased incidence of surgical infection, regardless of the type of operative procedure, has been noted in HIV-positive patients with CD4 T-cell counts lower than 200 cells/mm^3.[81] In experimental studies, abdominal wounds in thymectomized rats with depletion of CD4 lymphocytes have been found to have a significant decrease in strength, resilience, and toughness.[67] The effect of viral load on postoperative outcomes has also been studied. In their retrospective study, Horberg and colleagues found that a viral load equal to or greater than 30,000 copies per milliliter was associated with increased postsurgical complications.[124]

Similar results of lower CD4 T-cell counts on wound healing and outcome following anorectal surgery have been reported. Viral load has also been studied as a prognostic indicator following surgery in HIV-positive patients,[281] although as noted earlier, more recent studies found no increased incidence of complications following anorectal surgery. Studies have demonstrated that viral load is the best single predictor of clinical outcome, followed by CD4 T-cell counts.[19,165] Unfortunately, no studies have examined the prognostic value of the extent of viremia on postoperative outcome.

Given the evidence available, increased wound and other infective complications should be expected following abdominal and, possibly, anorectal surgery.[128] The prognostic values of CD4 T-cell counts and viral load indicates that optimization of the patient with immune reconstitution through HAART should be beneficial before semielective and elective procedures. Obviously, this is not possible in the emergency situation.

▶ COLONIC MANIFESTATIONS OF HIV INFECTION

Gastrointestinal disease is seen frequently in HIV-infected patients. Specifically, a variety of disease processes may affect the colon in an individual who harbors HIV. These may present in a number of ways. Diarrhea has been reported to affect up to 50% of patients with AIDS in North America and is a significant cause of morbidity and mortality among such persons.[241] Chronic diarrhea is seen more frequently in male homosexual HIV-infected patients and in those with severely depleted CD4 T-cell counts.[135,206] Gastrointestinal bleeding and perforation are most commonly seen in enteroinvasive infections, such as those caused by cytomegalovirus and *Clostridium difficile*, but they may be secondary to gastrointestinal involvement by HIV-associated malignancies. Obstruction may be seen with malignant disease, primarily Kaposi's sarcoma and NHLs. Finally, lymphadenopathy itself may cause severe abdominal pain and compression of viscera, primarily through a *M. avium* complex (MAC) infection.

Diarrheal Conditions

Diarrhea is seen in approximately 50% of patients with AIDS.[241] Chronic diarrhea results in a decreased quality of life and contributes to the morbidity of HIV infection. The etiology is multifactorial. Certainly, the ability to identify an organism depends on how vigorously the cause is pursued.[23] Infection with HIV is thought to cause minor alterations in architecture of the villi, which may lead to mild malabsorption of carbohydrates;[136] this can cause diarrhea also. Furthermore, increased permeability resulting from cytokine activation by foreign antigens, as well as bacterial overgrowth in the small bowel, may also contribute to pathogen-negative diarrhea.[13] HIV has amino acid sequences similar to those of vasoactive intestinal peptide (VIP) and may induce diarrhea by upregulation of VIP receptors.[264] HIV infection of the intestinal tract may also affect the barrier function of the intestinal epithelium. Stockmann and coworkers have proposed a leak-flux mechanism for diarrhea in HIV-infected individuals, secondary to intestinal mucosal cytokine release with resultant disruption of the epithelial barrier.[250]

Patients who present with diarrhea and abdominal pain should be assessed with a detailed history and physical examination, routine laboratory studies, and stool studies. The patient's immune status should be assessed by CD4 T-cell count and viral load. Recent exposure history can be obtained by careful attention to sexual history, travel, diet (to rule out food intolerance), and medications (specifically, PIs and antibiotic use). The characteristics of the diarrhea should be assessed, including duration, severity, associated abdominal pain, hematochezia, weight loss, and fever. Frequent, small movements with associated tenesmus are more indicative of an anorectal cause, whereas bloody movements and fever suggest an enteroinvasive, colonic pathogen. Physical examination should include a careful abdominal examination with attention to organomegaly, tenderness, and distension; an anorectal examination to assess for perianal lesions that may highlight an infectious source (e.g., herpes simplex); and a general physical evaluation to determine temperature, the presence or absence of cachexia, and lymphadenopathy.[175]

The American Gastroenterological Society created guidelines for the evaluation and management of chronic diarrhea in HIV-infected patients.[285] Recommendations include stool samples for bacteria and parasites, as well as for *C. difficile* if there is a risk for antibiotic-associated diarrhea. In the febrile patient, blood cultures should be drawn for bacteria and, in severely immunocompromised patients with CD4 T-cell counts lower than 100 cells/mm³, for mycobacteria. For those in whom stool studies fail to identify an infectious cause, endoscopy and mucosal biopsy are recommended, particularly in patients whose symptoms indicate a rectal or colonic cause. Flexible sigmoidoscopy with mucosal biopsies for microscopic examination and for bacterial and mycobacterial culture should be performed. Total colonoscopy may be necessary in certain patients, particularly when cytomegalovirus infection is suspected, given the high incidence of isolated proximal colonic involvement. Finally, esophagogastroduodenoscopy should be performed with duodenal biopsies

when other investigations have failed to reveal a source. This may aid in identifying *Giardia*, MAC, microsporidia, or *Isospora*. With a comprehensive investigation, an etiologic agent can be found in 90% of patients.[23] Among identified causes of diarrhea in patients with AIDS and chronic diarrhea, the most common opportunistic pathogens are cytomegalovirus, MAC, and the protozoans *Cryptosporidia* and *Microsporidia*.[285] Treatment of pathogen-negative diarrhea consists of rehydration and somatostatin analogues.[237]

Cytomegalovirus Infection

Cytomegalovirus is a double-stranded DNA virus from the herpesvirus family. It was first isolated in 1956 and has been found in urine, feces, semen, saliva, breast milk, blood, and cervical and vaginal secretions.[207] Although ubiquitous in humans, cytomegalovirus does not produce symptoms; it becomes an opportunistic infection as immune function deteriorates. Infection with cytomegalovirus is extremely common in patients with AIDS.[176] Disseminated cytomegalovirus has been identified in 90% of patients with AIDS at autopsy, with 94% of homosexual men testing positive at some venereal disease clinics.[282] Colonic cytomegalovirus is a common cause of diarrhea and abdominal pain in patients with AIDS, with resultant morbidity and mortality.[285]

Gastrointestinal manifestations of cytomegalovirus infection include ulcers, which may occur anywhere along the gastrointestinal tract, enteritis, colitis, ileocecal obstruction, perforation, and gastrointestinal hemorrhage. The colon is the main target in the gastrointestinal tract, and ileocolitis is the major colorectal manifestation.[75,205,277] In a study examining the colonoscopic findings of cytomegalovirus infection in patients with AIDS, ulcerations, colitis, and subendothelial hemorrhage were the most common findings. Disease limited to the right colon was seen in 13% of patients, again emphasizing the need for complete colonoscopy in those with suspected cytomegalovirus.[284] The diagnosis of cytomegalovirus colitis should always be considered in patients with AIDS who develop an acute abdomen, especially if a free perforation is diagnosed on radiographic study (see later).

Symptoms and Findings

The most common manifestation of colonic cytomegalovirus infection is watery diarrhea.[72,73,167] Bloody stools are common and may be seen in the absence of diarrhea. Abdominal pain may be severe, mimicking an acute surgical abdomen.[284] Up to 30% of patients may complain of fever and weight loss *without* diarrhea.[72] As the virally induced vasculitis progresses, thrombosis, occlusion, and ischemia of the affected area may occur. Toxic megacolon, hemorrhage, and perforation have been reported; this is of obvious interest to the surgeon.[101,271,282] Cytomegalovirus enterocolitis was the single most common reason for abdominal surgery in the AIDS population in the experience of Wilson and colleagues and is the most frequent life-threatening condition requiring emergency celiotomy in these individuals.[151,287] However, effective antiviral therapy has reduced the incidence of these severe complications.[271]

Diagnosis

The accurate diagnosis of cytomegalovirus colitis is sometimes quite difficult. Endoscopically, the mucosa in cytomegalovirus colitis is diffusely erythematous and friable with ulcerations. The ulcers themselves range from shallow, punctate lesions to deeply coalescing ulcers, the appearance of which may be difficult to distinguish from that of other colitides. Submucosal hemorrhage, secondary to cytomegalovirus-induced vasculitis, may be seen. Colonic involvement is patchy or limited to one region. As mentioned, patchy colitis localized to the right colon may be seen in 13% to 40% of patients, necessitating full colonoscopy rather than sigmoidoscopy.[72,151,284] However, in 25% of those with cytomegalovirus colitis, the mucosa appears endoscopically normal. For diagnosis, biopsy samples are taken randomly from the cecum, ascending colon, transverse colon, descending colon, and sigmoid colon. Cytomegalovirus may be demonstrated on histologic examination of grossly normal mucosa; therefore, samples of both inflamed and noninflamed areas should be taken.

Pathology

Biopsy usually reveals an inflammatory infiltrate, including lymphocytes and plasma cells with, in some areas, polymorphonuclear leukocytes and histiocytes.[74,209] Cellular changes seen under light microscopy are colonic mucosal cell enlargement with basophilic intranuclear inclusions, surrounded by a clear halo that gives the characteristic "owl's eye" appearance (Figure 10-1).[121] The retrieval of cytomegalovirus inclusions appears to depend on the number of biopsy specimens, the skill of the pathologist, and whether the material was taken from an endoscopically abnormal colon.[103,167] Cultures for cytomegalovirus have been inconsistent in predicting the presence of active infection. In situ hybridization staining and polymerase chain reaction may increase the sensitivity of histologic analysis.[59,227] Polymerase chain reaction amplification of cytomegalovirus DNA offers the best method for both diagnosis and monitoring of the efficacy of therapy.[58]

Radiologic investigation, specifically computed tomography, usually reveals the nonspecific changes of colitis, with colonic thickening and diffuse ulcerations.

Management

Medical management includes the antiviral agents ganciclovir, valganciclovir, and foscarnet. Ganciclovir is given intravenously at a dose of 5 mg/kg twice a day, and valganciclovir is given as a single 900-mg dose orally. Ganciclovir is the treatment of choice for induction of gastrointestinal disease, and recent reports show that valganciclovir may be as effective for mild disease. However, valganciclovir is not recommended in severe disease where absorption may be compromised.[9] Ganciclovir usually improves both the histologic and macroscopic appearance within 3 weeks. If there is no improvement, foscarnet, at a dose of 60 to 90 mg/kg intravenously three times daily, should be used. Complete response to ganciclovir and/or foscarnet therapy can be expected in approximately 90%. However, because relapse is very common (50%), maintenance therapy should always be considered.[19,63] Patients receiving such treatment and those taking PIs have been demonstrated to have the lowest recurrence rates and an improved survival.[19]

Surgical intervention is reserved for perforation, massive bleeding, and toxic megacolon. However, a patient with mild peritoneal signs, without free air, and with the presumptive diagnosis of cytomegalovirus colitis may be treated with both ganciclovir and appropriate antibiotics for aerobic and anaerobic organisms while he or she is observed carefully. Most individuals will respond without the need for surgical intervention. However, when emergency surgery is required, resection of the involved segment of colon is necessary. No anastomosis should be performed under these circumstances.

Results of Surgery

Approximately two-thirds of patients with AIDS who underwent emergency bowel resection by Wexner and colleagues had cytomegalovirus ileocolitis.[282] The postoperative mortality was 28% at 1 day, 71% at 1 month, and 86% at 6 months. Death often is a consequence of sepsis and pneumonia caused by *Pneumocystis jiroveci*.[151] Elective resection of eight patients reported by Söderlund and coworkers resulted in one death.[245] Recurrent or persistent symptoms of cytomegalovirus enterocolitis occurred in four patients after a mean of 7 months.

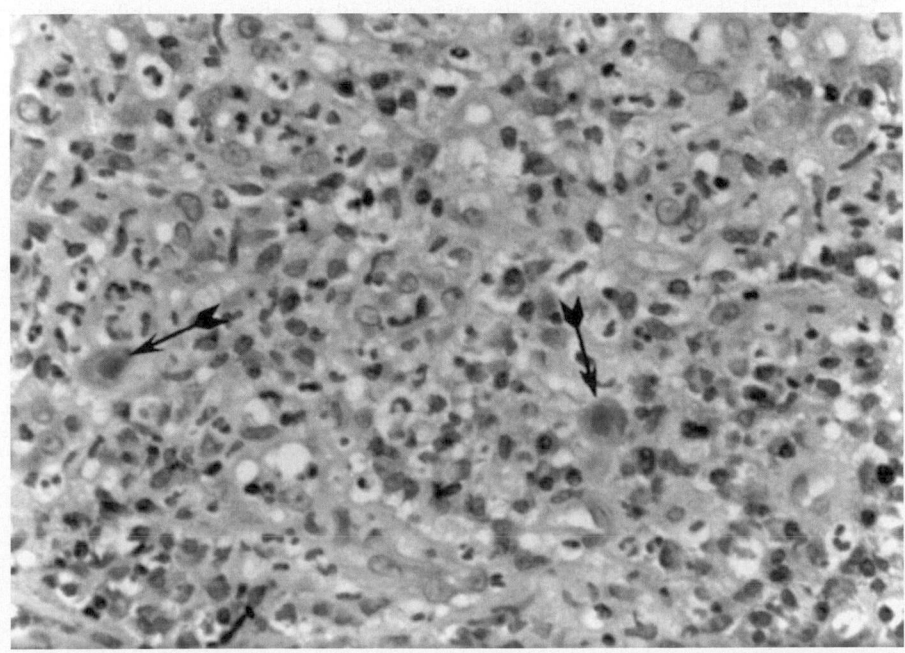

FIGURE 10-1. Cytomegalovirus enterocolitis. Acutely inflamed granulation tissue with cells positive for cytomegalovirus demonstrating intranuclear inclusions (*arrows*). (Original magnification × 400.)

Mycobacterium Avium Complex Infection

MAC affects about 5% of severely immunocompromised HIV patients and is diagnosed in 50% of those with AIDS.[76] This is an environmental bacterium that enters through both the gastrointestinal and respiratory tracts.[16] Typically, patients with gastrointestinal MAC infection have low CD4 T-cell counts. In addition to severe diarrhea, patients may report abdominal pain, anorexia, and weight loss. Anemia may be identified upon laboratory evaluation. Abdominal pain may be secondary to intra-abdominal lymphadenopathy. This is readily diagnosed by computed tomography and needle aspiration.[5] Colonic infection may result in obstruction, fistula formation, and perforation, although these are uncommon, and surgery is rarely indicated in the management of gastrointestinal MAC.[111]

Diagnosis is made on biopsy of either affected small intestine or colon. The endoscopic appearance of MAC is quite distinctive, with granular, small (4-mm) white nodules with surrounding erythema. Colonic mucosa may be edematous and, uncommonly, ulcerated. Biopsy cultures are used to confirm the diagnosis and permit sensitivity typing. Because MAC is a systemic disease, blood cultures may be taken to confirm the diagnosis and have been reported to be more helpful than either stool or respiratory specimens for establishing the diagnosis with certainty.[46]

Medical treatment of gastrointestinal MAC is with a combination of antituberculous drugs. Ethambutol (15 to 25 mg/kg daily), ciprofloxacin (500 to 750 mg twice daily), rifampin (600 mg daily), rifabutin (450 to 600 mg daily), amikacin (10 to 15 mg/kg daily), clofazimine (50 to 200 mg daily), and azithromycin (500 mg daily) may be used in three or four drug regimens for a 12-week treatment period.[14,32] Response to quadruple therapy is good, with more than one-half of patients demonstrating complete response and resolution of symptoms.[138]

Protozoal Infections

Microsporidia Infection

Microsporidia, of which *Enterocytozoon bieneusi* accounts for the majority of cases in patients with AIDS, are obligate intracellular, spore-forming protozoa. Microsporidia have been identified in up to 60% of patients with AIDS with chronic diarrhea.[172,244] Microsporidiosis is usually seen in those with advanced AIDS with CD4 T-cell counts lower than 100 cells/mm^3. Patients present with frequent, watery bowel movements (nonbloody), abdominal pain, and nausea.

Diagnosis. Microsporidiosis most frequently affects the proximal jejunum. Upper endoscopy with a pediatric colonoscope is necessary to obtain biopsies. Histologically, characteristic small, round/oval plasmodia and spores within the infected enterocyte cytoplasm, typically supranuclear in the apical cytoplasm, are demonstrated.[181] Atrophy of intestinal villi and crypt hyperplasia are seen microscopically, and the resultant changes in absorption contribute to the diarrhea.[195]

Colonoscopy with terminal ileal biopsies may permit visualization of the organisms and should be performed when microsporidiosis is suspected. Although examination of biopsy specimens is the most sensitive method for detection, microscopic examination of stool samples, both with trichrome staining and indirect immunofluorescence, using polyclonal and monoclonal antibodies, may diagnose the condition.[273,296]

Treatment. Treatment of microsporidiosis is difficult and generally does not result in eradication of the infection. The destruction of the resident T cells in the lamina propria of the gut is probably responsible for the persistence of these protozoal infections.[158] Albendazole, 400 mg twice daily, is the recommended drug. Clinically, a partial response of more than 50% reduction in bowel movements was noted in one study, although repeat endoscopy revealed persistence of infection in all regardless of clinical response.[71] More recently, thalidomide has been investigated as a drug to treat the condition. Thalidomide, 100 mg daily for 30 days, was found to result in a complete clinical response in 7 of 28 patients.[232] Immune reconstitution with HAART has been noted to result in a complete clinical response in patients with microsporidiosis and cryptosporidiosis.[33]

Cryptosporidium Infection

Cryptosporidium is a protozoan parasite that primarily affects the small intestine and causes a profuse, watery diarrhea (see Chapter 33). *Cryptosporidium* oocysts are spread by person-to-person contact and by contaminated water transmission. It is a common source of diarrhea in immunocompetent individuals worldwide but is usually self-limiting in the nonimmunocompromised host. In HIV-positive patients, cryptosporidiosis is self-limited in up to one-third of patients with CD4 T-cell counts higher than 200/μL. However, in patients with AIDS with lower CD4 T-cell counts, *Cryptosporidium* may result in a serious, chronic disease with abdominal pain, nausea, vomiting, and anorexia, in addition to diarrhea.[87] Infection can be fatal, with severe dehydration and electrolyte imbalances, and wasting.

Diagnosis. *Cryptosporidium* affects primarily the jejunum and ileum, resulting in villous atrophy, malabsorption, and altered permeability.[104] *Cryptosporidium* may produce an enterotoxin that results in hypersecretion of fluid into the bowel and the large-volume diarrhea seen clinically.[110] Diagnosis is made by stool examination with modified acid-fast stain and light microscopy to detect oocysts (see Figure 33-31). Alternatively, immunofluorescence antibody may be used with increased sensitivity.[95] Endoscopic biopsy demonstrates the intracellular protozoa, villous atrophy, and inflammation of the lamina propria.

Treatment. Treatment of cryptosporidiosis is difficult, and there still remains no ideal regimen. As noted earlier, immune reconstitution with HAART may result in resolution of symptoms. A more recent study demonstrated that a combination of azithromycin and paromomycin may be promising, with almost complete eradication of oocyst excretion at 12 weeks.[240] Preventive measures include avoiding drinking water directly from lakes and waters, careful hand washing after contact with human and animal feces, and avoidance of oral-anal sexual practices.

Clostridium Difficile Infection (See also Chapter 33)

C. difficile colitis is the most common cause of bacterial diarrhea in HIV patients.[217] It is common among AIDS victims because many who are infected with HIV receive a variety of antimicrobial agents, either for prophylaxis or for treatment of bacterial illnesses. In addition, repeat hospital admissions predispose the patient to colonization with the organism.

The observed frequency of *C. difficile*–associated diarrhea among patients with AIDS has actually decreased in the era of HAART. It has been postulated that this is secondary to the reduced number of hospital visits in patients with restored immunity on antiretroviral therapy.[217]

The typical presentation includes mucoid diarrhea, abdominal pain, and fever (see Chapter 33). The condition may progress to that of acute megacolon as well as to life-threatening diarrhea.[137]

Diagnosis is made by testing stool for toxin A or toxin B, both of which are produced by *C. difficile*. Endoscopy is usually not indicated and, in fact, should be discouraged in patients with severe disease without suspicion of necrosis. Endoscopically, the colonic mucosa appears inflamed. Ulcerations and pseudomembranes may be present. However, in the patient with AIDS, the colitis may lack characteristic pseudomembranes and may also involve a secondary pathogen, such as cytomegalovirus.[35]

Treatment is with either oral vancomycin (125 mg, four times daily) or metronidazole (250 mg, four times daily). In severe disease, a combination of intravenous metronidazole (Flagyl) and oral vancomycin is recommended. With profuse diarrhea, oral cholestyramine may be used to bind toxin and to reduce stool frequency. Fidaxomicin, a potential new agent in the treatment of *C. difficile*, is a macrolide antibiotic that has recently been shown in a clinical trial to be as effective as vancomycin in treating infection with this organism and may be superior for preventing recurrence.[160] Current investigations of fecal transplant to reconstitute the flora of the colon are also underway. The reader is referred to Chapter 33 for a comprehensive discussion of antibiotic-associated colitis.

Histoplasmosis

Histoplasma capsulatum is a fungus that usually causes subclinical infection when its airborne spore is inhaled.[108] The risk of developing histoplasmosis and the severity of disease are dependent on the immune status of HIV-infected individuals. Disseminated histoplasmosis is usually seen in patients with CD4 T-cell counts lower than 200 cells/mm^3.[283] Gastrointestinal involvement is common in disseminated histoplasmosis, although symptomatic gastrointestinal disease is only seen in a small percentage of patients.

Symptoms of gastrointestinal histoplasmosis are nonspecific and include abdominal pain, diarrhea, nausea, anorexia, and weight loss. Gastrointestinal histoplasmosis may also present with gastrointestinal bleeding, obstruction, or perforation.[89,119,139,248] Dissemination of the fungus may cause focal lesions affecting any segment of the gastrointestinal tract. However, the terminal ileum and ascending colon are the most frequently involved sites, probably because of the presence of considerable lymphoid tissue.[11] The lesions may appear as polyps or may coalesce to form inflammatory masses that may mimic carcinoma.[8] An additional discussion concerning this fungal infection is found in Chapter 33.

Non-Hodgkin's Lymphoma

NHL is an AIDS-defining malignancy. HIV infection increases the risk of systemic NHL by 200-fold, with the greatest increase in high-grade NHL.[57] Extranodal NHL occurs in approximately 10% of HIV-infected individuals, and it had become the most common malignant disease associated with

AIDS in certain areas until the mid-1990s.[109] However, after a steady increase in the number of NHL cases up until 1995, there has since been a decline.[65] Unlike Kaposi's sarcoma (see later), there is little variation in the incidence of NHL between different HIV exposure groups. It tends to occur in advanced disease in those individuals with a CD4 cell count of less than 50/mm^3.[202]

Pathogenesis

The biology and presentation of NHL in HIV-positive individuals are different from those of the general population in that high-grade lymphomas are more frequent with HIV infection. The biology of these lymphomas varies in relationship to morphologic type, anatomic site, and overall state of immunodeficiency.[145] Large cell immunoblastic lymphomas are the most common (see Figure 26-28).[15] Many AIDS-associated large cell lymphomas represent polyclonal proliferation suggestive of lymphokine induced expansion of a B-cell population.[226] In addition, most patients with HIV infection and NHL present with advanced disease; 90% have extranodal disease at presentation, and more than 50% present with stage IV disease.[133,143] Age older than 35 years, advanced stage at diagnosis, and a CD4 count of less than 100 cells/mm^3 are adverse prognostic factors. HAART is associated with a decreased incidence of NHL and an improved prognosis.[162] The gastrointestinal tract is the most common site of extranodal NHL, and in approximately 25% of the time, the gastrointestinal tract is the only site of disease.[127] More than 90% of these lymphomas are B-cell lymphomas, and Epstein–Barr virus expression is seen in the majority.[147,234]

It has been postulated that HIV infection results in immune dysfunction and altered cytokine release that, when combined with chronic antigenic exposure to other viral pathogens, namely, the Epstein–Barr virus or human herpesvirus-8, result in proliferation of B-cell clones that subsequently undergo malignant transformation secondary to genetic instability.[146] More recently, it has been hypothesized that integration of the HIV genome into the genome of infected macrophages results in overexpression of stimulatory cytokines that enhances B-cell proliferation and potentiates malignant transformation.[163]

Diagnosis

NHL may present as a rectal or colonic mass causing abdominal pain, bleeding, or obstruction.[31] Radiographically, a nodule or nodules that may be ulcerated can be seen on a computed tomography scan. These may be quite large and show evidence of central necrosis. Endoscopically, submucosal masses may be noted, and these should undergo biopsy for tissue diagnosis. If tumors cannot be safely accessed or sampled for biopsy by means of endoscopy, percutaneous biopsy or surgery may be necessary in order to obtain a tissue diagnosis.

Treatment and Results

Chemotherapy is generally an effective treatment, with surgery reserved for bleeding, perforation, or obstruction (see Chapter 26).[129] One of the complications of chemotherapy, however, is perforation; fortunately, this is quite rare. Resection should be reserved for localized disease, and then only after an extensive search has been made for a disseminated process. A primary anastomosis may be safely performed in the absence of concomitant severe colitis.

In the past, survival was quite limited once the diagnosis of NHL was made, but with improvement in the treatment of HIV, especially with the introduction of HAART, as well as improvement in life expectancy in those with AIDS, patients with NHL are being treated more aggressively.[247,260] Results of the survival benefits of these regimens is awaited.

Kaposi's Sarcoma

Kaposi's sarcoma is usually an indolent cutaneous disorder in older men of central European origin, but the neoplasm is more aggressive in immunocompromised patients and resembles the more aggressive "endemic" form of Kaposi's sarcoma seen in sub-Saharan Africa.[52] The increased incidence of Kaposi's sarcoma early in the AIDS epidemic resulted in its becoming a specific diagnostic criterion for this condition in HIV-positive individuals. The recognition of an increased incidence of Kaposi's sarcoma in the homosexual population was made in the early 1980s.[93] This was identified as a much more aggressive form, with frequent metastatic spread to lymph nodes and the gastrointestinal tract.

Epidemiology, Etiology, and Pathogenesis

The incidence of Kaposi's sarcoma peaked at approximately 32 per 100,000 white men in the early 1990s, but since the advent of HAART, much like NHL, it has steadily declined to approximately 2.8 per 100,000 white men in 1998.[79] In fact, it has been noted that triple-antiretroviral therapy may decrease the incidence of Kaposi's sarcoma by 50% in HIV-infected homosexual men.[131] Kaposi's sarcoma is predominantly a disease of homosexual men with AIDS and is not commonly seen among other HIV exposure groups. This prompted the search for an infective cofactor as the etiologic agent. Initially, cytomegalovirus was implicated but could not be consistently identified by in situ hybridization probes.[4,75] Eventually, a herpes-like virus was identified as the cause of Kaposi's sarcoma,[43] and it has since been named Kaposi's sarcoma–associated herpesvirus or human herpesvirus-8. The mode of transmission of human herpesvirus-8 is still not clear. However, a sexual mode of transmission has been hypothesized because the incidence of Kaposi's sarcoma is related to the number of sexual partners in men who have sex with men.[22,179] Interestingly, heterosexual transmission is not common; in the endemic form of the disease in Africa, transmission via saliva is hypothesized.[201]

It is postulated that Kaposi's sarcoma lesions are fed by the massive cytokine levels that circulate in the HIV-infected patient.[80] Kaposi's sarcoma is more common in HIV-1 infection than in HIV-2 infection in patients with similar herpesvirus-8 infection rates, a finding raising the possibility that HIV-1 may have an etiologic role in Kaposi's sarcoma.[6] In an experimental animal model, Vogel and coworkers have demonstrated a role for HIV tat, which is an angiogenesis factor and induces secretion of inflammatory cytokines, in the development of Kaposi's sarcoma–like lesions in mice.[266] In addition, it appears that female sex hormones are inhibitory for Kaposi's sarcoma and may be used in treatment.[116]

Clinical Presentation

Kaposi's sarcoma lesions vary in their clinical presentations. The lesions range in color from light pink to purple and may appear as papules, plaques, and nodules. Although skin lesions are the most common, up to 50% of patients with AIDS

and with cutaneous lesions also have oral and gastrointestinal manifestations.[203,215] The gastrointestinal tract appears to be uniquely susceptible to dissemination by this tumor, and occasionally gastrointestinal lesions antedate skin changes.[272] The stomach, duodenum, small bowel, and colon may be affected simultaneously, or the tumor may be localized to one site.[119] Rectal involvement is quite common.[82]

Symptoms

Symptoms may include diarrhea, mucous discharge, bleeding, rectal pain, and incontinence, but patients are more often troubled with systemic problems related to opportunistic infections. The presence of characteristic raised, purple, nontender skin lesions, especially on the feet, should alert the physician to the diagnosis.

In view of the increased incidence in AIDS, a diagnosis of Kaposi's sarcoma should be considered in homosexual men presenting with persistent diarrhea for which no infectious cause can be ascertained.[272] Advanced gastrointestinal disease may present with both upper and lower gastrointestinal bleeding. Large lesions may result in acute obstruction, either directly or through intussusception of the affected bowel. Rectal lesions may be mistaken for thrombosed external hemorrhoids, given their purple, nodular appearance.

Endoscopy

The lesions appear submucosal, purple, spongy, and irregularly shaped.[246] When viewed endoscopically, they may vary in size from a few millimeters up to 2 cm.[52] There may be a resemblance to angiodysplasia, characterized by maculopapular tumors with a stellate vascular pattern (Figure 10-2).[278] In larger lesions, a central umbilication may develop in the ulcerated area.[177] Biopsy specimens can be taken if clinical management may be altered by the results. A deep biopsy is usually needed because of the location of the lesions. Because of the tendency to hemorrhage following rectal biopsy, Sohn recommends performing a rubber band ligation of the site and then sampling the more superficial portion.[246] However, attempts at biopsy confirmation may be frustrating because of the submucosal nature of the lesions and the sometimes firm consistency.[52,78] False-negative biopsy

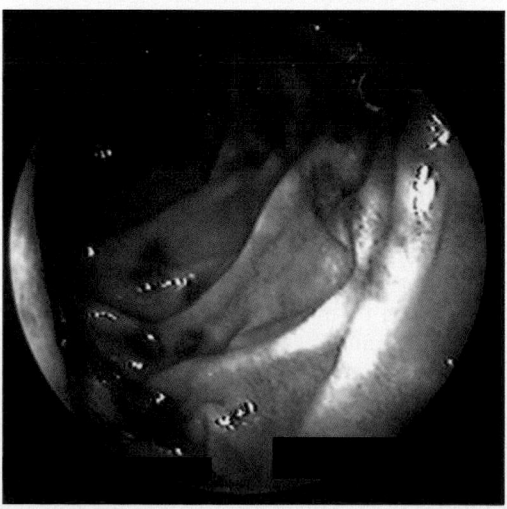

FIGURE 10-2. Kaposi's sarcoma. Colonoscopy reveals characteristic maculopapular lesions resembling angiodysplasia. (From Buckley RM, Gluckman SJ. *HIV Infection in Primary Care.* Philadelphia, PA: WB Saunders; 2002.)

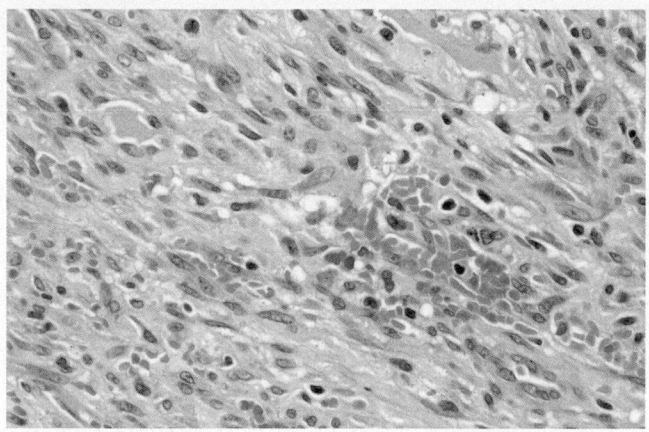

FIGURE 10-3. Kaposi's sarcoma. Spindle cell proliferation with slitlike vascular spaces. There are a few inflammatory cells. Endothelial cellular atypia is noted and some extravasated red cells are seen. (Original magnification × 400.)

results are common, and rates of up to 77% have been reported.[92] Oral cavity and skin lesions are more accessible and are therefore preferred for biopsy.

Histopathology

When the biopsy is successful in obtaining histologic material, spindle-like cells with hemorrhage are frequently demonstrated (Figure 10-3).[177] Kaposi's sarcoma cells are thought to arise from the mesenchymal cells and are characterized by intense neovascularization with spindle cells.[171,276] Three features make up the histologic appearance of Kaposi's sarcoma: proliferation of vascular spaces, a background of spindle cells, and extravasation of red cells. Cytochemical and phenotypic marker studies have demonstrated Kaposi's sarcoma cells to have features of vascular channel and endothelial cell lineage.

Radiologic Studies

Contrast study may reveal changes in the stomach and duodenum suggestive of diffuse nodularity, multiple polypoid lesions, or the presence of an infiltrative mass. In the small bowel, thickening and irregularity of the folds may be noted. In the limited number of articles published to date, barium enema investigation sometimes reveals any one or more of the changes seen in the upper gastrointestinal tract.[91,269]

Computed tomography of the rectum reveals a high incidence of rectal and perirectal abnormalities, but the changes are nonspecific because many of these patients harbor other inflammatory conditions of the rectum.[3] Identification of the site of massive bleeding by means of angiography has been demonstrated in a patient with ileal Kaposi's sarcoma.[177]

Treatment

"Aggressive" attempts at surgical management are not indicated except for the rare case of bleeding or obstruction.[157,159] Medically, antiretroviral therapy in the HAART era with immune reconstitution is essential to the management of Kaposi's sarcoma. Immune reconstitution may not only decrease active human herpesvirus-8 infection but may also decrease HIV viral load. Controlling HIV replication would decrease levels of the HIV tat protein and decrease the cytokine-driven proliferation of the sarcoma. In addition, certain PIs have direct antineoplastic effects in Kaposi's sarcoma.[194,230]

Local therapies include intralesional injection with vinblastine or 3% sodium tetradecyl sulfate, interferon alfa, and cryotherapy.[208,274] Cutaneous lesions have been irradiated successfully.[52] Gastrointestinal lesions, if symptomatic, necessitate systemic therapy. Chemotherapy includes recombinant human interferon alfa, the vinca alkaloids, etoposide, and doxorubicin.[52,134,155,272] Interferon alfa as a single agent has been found to have a 20% response rate.[267] High-dose interferon alfa (8 million units daily, subcutaneously) plus the antiretroviral, zidovudine, resulted in a 31% response rate.[152] Systemic chemotherapy may be used for symptomatic gastrointestinal disease and rapidly progressive disease. It may have an indolent course or progress aggressively with significant mortality and morbidity. The single agents approved for use in Kaposi's sarcoma by the FDA are liposomal doxorubicin, liposomal daunorubicin, and paclitaxel.[268]

▶ ANORECTAL DISEASE IN THE HIV-INFECTED PATIENT

A host of coexisting factors can make evaluation of the anorectum in the HIV-infected patient perplexing. The anorectum in the practicing homosexual is infected by a variety of pathogens, some living comfortably and clandestinely and some wreaking havoc. To this must be added the effects of HIV infection on the integrity of the mucosal cells (making them extremely friable), of anoreceptive intercourse on sphincter function, and of intermittent, indolent infections (herpes simplex) and routine anorectal diseases (fissures, fistulas). It is hoped that the following contribution will help the clinician to understand these varied, unusual processes.

Examination and Diagnosis: General Principles

Despite increased reliance on expensive laboratory evaluation, much can be ascertained by clinical examination in the HIV-positive patient. Visual inspection of the perineum may reveal condylomata, the blisters of herpes simplex, the linear lesions of a sacral root herpes zoster, the erythema of an ischiorectal abscess, or the excoriated anus of a patient with intractable diarrhea and a lax sphincter. Before performing a digital examination, it is important to manipulate the perianal tissue and to look for the discharge of pus or air bubbles that would suggest a deep infection. Spreading the buttocks gently can identify an anal fissure. Palpation of the anus and low rectum may demonstrate a mass or an ulcer. Careful attention should be paid to the prostate because a patient with a prostatic abscess may present with vague, deep-seated rectal pain and fever, and the condition can be mistaken for an ischiorectal abscess. Rigid sigmoidoscopy will assess the rectal mucosa for evidence of proctitis. In any patient in whom evaluation is too painful, it is wise to proceed to an examination under anesthesia.

An examination under anesthesia should be performed before any definitive therapy is entertained, including sphincterotomy. A few caveats are helpful as well as cost effective. Any exudate associated with a fistula or ulcer should be sent for acid-fast stain and culture. Rarely is useful information obtained from routine aerobic and anaerobic culture. Furthermore, *any exudate found in the anus or distal rectum without a demonstrable fistula should be cultured and stained for Neisseria gonorrhoeae, Chlamydia, amoebae, acid-fast bacilli,* and *herpes simplex virus (HSV).*

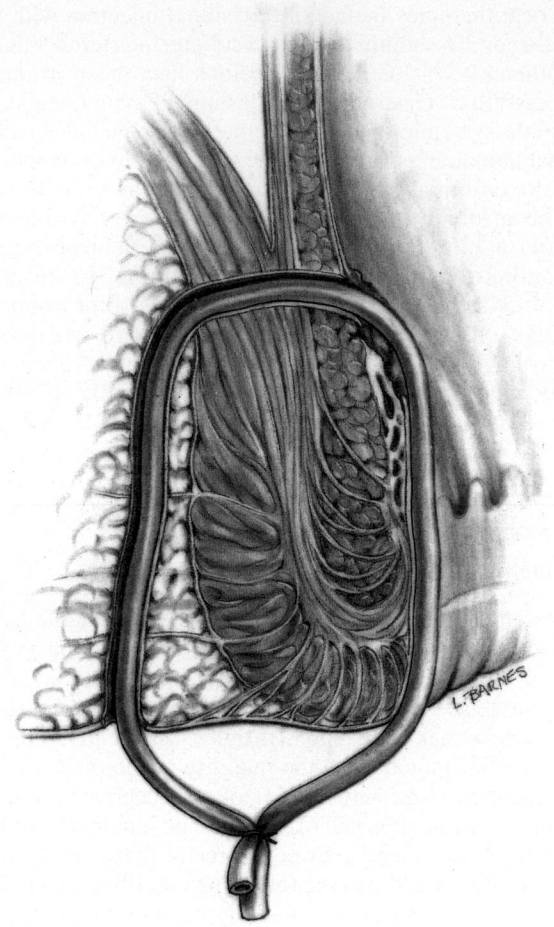

FIGURE 10-4. Noncutting seton placed for a high anal fistula in HIV-positive patients.

For inflammation extending proximal to 15 cm from the anal verge, cultures for all enteric pathogens, ova and parasites, and *C. difficile* should be requested and colonoscopy performed if preliminary results are nondiagnostic. Tissue from all ulcerative lesions that are shallow and not suggestive of an idiopathic AIDS-related ulcer should be sent for cytomegalovirus and HSV culture as well as for histopathology. A noncutting seton should be placed in all identified fistula tracts (Figure 10-4). Biopsy should be performed on any mass. Frozen-section examination generally does not alter immediate therapy and should therefore be used judiciously. One should not risk complications such as bleeding by obtaining large biopsy specimens for tissue typing in patients with NHL. It is safer to oversew biopsy sites in a patient with a friable mucosa with 2–0 long-term absorbable sutures. Thinner material may cut through with resultant bleeding. This adds to everyone's concerns because postoperative hemorrhage poses a hazard for both patient and health care providers.

Nonsexually Transmitted Anal Disease

The anus of the HIV-infected patient may be affected by a number of conditions not necessarily related to HIV. This is important to note because in addition to the reluctance of many physicians to treat HIV-positive patients, there is the natural tendency to ascribe all diseases in this population to specifically HIV-related problems.

Anal Fissure

The differentiation of an anal fissure from an idiopathic AIDS-related ulcer is critical to proper management. This is discussed later and also in Chapter 12. Anal fissures present with pain and bleeding, the same as in the general population. Chronic diarrhea and anoreceptive intercourse may contribute to the development of anal fissures and may delay their healing. Benign anal fissure should be initially managed conservatively with sitz baths and fiber supplements. Sources of chronic diarrhea are sought and appropriately treated. If conservative management fails, topical therapy with 0.2% nitroglycerin cream, 2% diltiazem, or botulinum toxin injection (10 to 20 U) may be tried before surgical therapy (see Chapter 12).

Uncontrolled diarrhea is a relative contraindication to a definitive procedure, such as lateral internal anal sphincterotomy. Generally, the results of internal anal sphincterotomy are satisfactory.[213] However, if there is heightened concern about the possibility of impairment for bowel control, anorectal manometry can be performed to assess the anal canal pressure preoperatively and to determine whether the procedure can be undertaken with minimal morbidity.

Perianal Suppuration

Perianal abscess in the HIV-positive patient is analogous to the problem observed in an individual with Crohn's disease. One must distinguish between the standard cryptoglandular infection and that caused by erosion from ulcer or malignancy. Studies have shown that incision and drainage of abscesses can be successful, with salutary results.[275] Therefore, there is no place for nonoperative management in the presence of perianal suppuration.

A generous incision should be made, but the wound should not be packed. If a fistula is found, a noncutting seton should be placed (Figure 10-4). Any purulent material should be sent for acid-fast stain and for culture. Untreated perianal sepsis may progress to necrotizing gangrene (see Chapter 9) or can lead to disseminated abscesses.[54]

Fistula-in-Ano

Generally, any anal fistula should be treated conservatively, without performing a definitive operation. As previously mentioned, diarrhea can lead to disabling incontinence in many of the patients with attenuated sphincters. A fistulotomy may be considered only when the tract is superficial. High fistulas can be managed with seton drainage, changed or removed if necessary (see also Chapter 14). Spontaneous healing can occur, but this is unpredictable and may be related to the response to treatment of an underlying specific infection (Figure 10-5).

Hemorrhoids

The frequency of hemorrhoidal symptoms does not appear to be increased in HIV-infected patients. In fact, the physician needs to be aware that many so-called exacerbations of hemorrhoidal disease are in reality acute HSV infections.

External thrombosed hemorrhoids may be safely excised, with similar indications for surgery as in the HIV-negative patient. Rubber band ligation of symptomatic hemorrhoids has been reported to result in a higher complication rate.[222] However, we have not found this to be true in our practice and offer it to appropriate patients as a therapeutic option. Although hemorrhoidectomy has been reported to

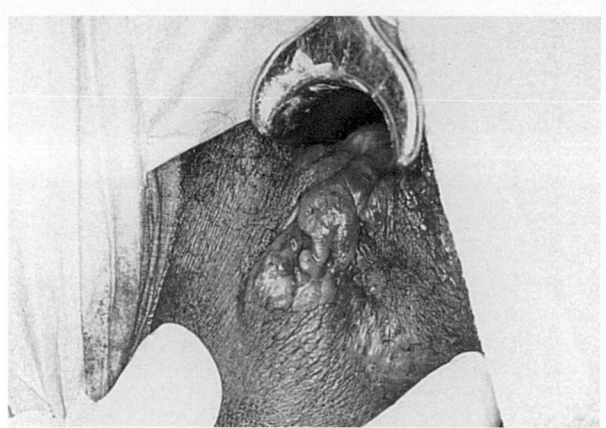

FIGURE 10-5. Fistula caused by *Mycobacterium avium* complex that spontaneously healed.

be safe in HIV-positive individuals,[120] only one-third actually underwent a full hemorrhoidectomy. It is our practice to offer surgical hemorrhoidectomy to the patient with symptomatic grade III hemorrhoids if the HIV disease is early in its course. However, it is extremely difficult to treat grades III and IV hemorrhoids in advanced AIDS. The accompanying diarrhea aggravates hemorrhoidal prolapse and is a significant source of morbidity. In such cases, injection sclerotherapy has been shown to be an effective treatment option.[218]

Pruritus Ani

Severe pruritus occurs secondary to leakage of pus, fecal incontinence, and fungal overgrowth. This is readily treated by antifungal powders and the avoidance of sensitizing over-the-counter preparations (see Chapter 9). If possible, the source of the excessive moisture should be eliminated. Persistence of pruritus despite therapy should lead one to consider biopsy to rule out Bowen's disease and other specific perianal conditions (see Chapter 9).

Sexually Transmitted Disease in the HIV-Infected Population

Gonorrhea

Gonorrhea is caused by *Neisseria gonorrhoeae* and is considered to be the most common sexually transmitted disease in homosexual men. Historically, carrier rates have been reported in up to 55% of homosexual men.[132] Although the incidence of gonorrhea initially declined with the advent of safe-sex practices, more recently the incidence has been reported to be increasing (see also Chapters 9 and 33).[233,261] The gonorrheal organism is thought to be a cofactor in the transmission of HIV.[60]

Presentation and Diagnosis

The classic clinical presentation of rectal gonorrhea is that of a thick, yellow mucopurulent discharge, with or without proctitis, occurring 5 days after inoculation. In addition to mucoid rectal discharge, patients may present with tenesmus, pruritus, or rectal bleeding. Evaluation of the anorectum reveals friable, erythematous rectal mucosa with mucopurulent exudates. Mucopurulent discharge may be noted from the anal crypts or may be elicited by gentle external pressure. Diagnosis is confirmed by the presence of gram-negative

intracellular diplococci on culture of rectal swabs on Thayer-Martin medium (see Figure 33-20). At the time of diagnosis, patients should also be screened for syphilis.

Treatment

Rectal gonorrhea has been reported to be more resistant to therapy because of the antibiotic inactivation attributed to the microflora of the rectum.[88] Empiric treatment is initiated with a single dose of ceftriaxone, 125 mg intramuscularly, while awaiting culture results. Alternative regimens are ciprofloxacin, 500 mg orally, or levofloxacin, 500 mg orally, in a single dose. Because of the high coinfection rate with *C. trachomatis*, current recommendations are to treat with a regimen effective against uncomplicated chlamydial infection.[289]

If left untreated, gonorrhea may progress to disseminated gonococcal infection. Disseminated infection results in petechial skin lesions, septic arthritis, and tenosynovitis. Less commonly, it may manifest as fulminant perihepatitis, meningitis, or endocarditis. Hospitalization with intravenous antibiotics is recommended for disseminated gonococcal infection. Endocarditis requires 4 weeks of therapy. The reader is referred to Chapters 9 and 33 for a more comprehensive discussion of this infection.

Chlamydia Infection and Lymphogranuloma Venereum

C. trachomatis is the most common sexually transmitted infectious pathogen in the United States. Anal chlamydial infection is transmitted by anal receptive intercourse and oral-anal intercourse. After a 10-day incubation period, symptomatic chlamydial infection may occur, although the large number of asymptomatic infections explains the high prevalence among sexually active individuals. Depending on the serotype, the infection may present as mild proctitis or may progress to lymphogranuloma venereum. Ten days after inoculation, nonlymphogranuloma venereum proctitis presents with pain, tenesmus, fever, and nonulcerative proctitis, with a bloody or mucoid discharge. Upon proctoscopy, the rectal mucosa appears erythematous, friable, and granular. When lymphogranuloma venereum develops, ulceration, abscesses, and strictures mimicking Crohn's disease occur. However, whereas lymphadenopathy is present in lymphogranuloma venereum, it is absent with Crohn's disease. Once a stricture develops, fecal diversion is the preferred option.

Diagnosis is most reliably made with culture of a rectal biopsy. Unfortunately, the biopsy needs to be transported on ice for tissue culture, thus making it expensive and time consuming. Antichlamydial antibodies can be assayed with a complement fixation test. A titer of 1:80 or greater is confirmatory of chlamydial infection. Elevated titers are not seen, however, less than 1 month after infection. A newly developed urinary polymerase chain reaction test for chlamydia may allow for more rapid confirmation.[161]

Chlamydial infection is treated with a single dose of azithromycin, 1 g orally, or doxycycline, 100 mg orally, twice a day for 21 days. As mentioned in the section on gonorrhea, treatment for concurrent gonorrhea infection is recommended. Further details concerning epidemiology, symptoms, and treatment of this condition are found in Chapter 9.

Syphilis

Anal syphilis, caused by *Treponema pallidum*, is a condition that develops 2 to 6 weeks following inoculation. The primary lesion of syphilis is the chancre, a rounded ulcer with well-defined margins that may be mistaken for an anal fissure. Although typically painless at other sites, anal chancres may result in severe anal pain. The ulcerative lesions may be single (most common) or multiple. When multiple and situated opposite one another, the pathognomonic "kissing" ulcers may be observed. Additionally, one may find mild proctitis. Even without treatment, the primary chancre of syphilis heals within 3 to 6 weeks.

The disease progresses in approximately one-third of patients, and in one-third it remains latent. When it progresses, the second stage usually is recognized 2 months following resolution of the chancre. The presentation at this time is that of verrucous, flat lesions (condylomata lata) that are associated with pruritus and discharge, a maculopapular rash on the soles of the feet and the palms of the hand, fever, and malaise.

Diagnosis is made by dark-field immunofluorescent microscopy and nontreponemal serology testing, that is, the Venereal Disease Research Laboratory (VDRL) assay. Although the classic treatment consists of intramuscular benzathine penicillin, complicating factors in the HIV-positive population include the high incidence of neurosyphilis and the lack of a predictable serologic response to treatment.[27,292] This translates into either doing a spinal tap at the time of diagnosis or empirically treating all patients for neurosyphilis. Following treatment, patients should undergo quantitative serologic testing at 3-month intervals for 1 year in order to document falling titers and to aid in identifying treatment failures. The reader is referred to Chapter 9 for an additional discussion.

Herpes Simplex

HSV is a large DNA virus transmitted by anal intercourse (HSV type 2, accounting for 90% of anal herpes) and oral-anal contact (HSV type 1, accounting for 10% of anal herpes).[56,280] HSV infection is important not only because of its high incidence, but also because the associated break in the epithelial integrity of the skin probably facilitates the transmission of HIV.[105,235] The incubation period for HSV type 2 infections is 4 to 21 days. Initially, small vesicles with associated perivesicular erythema develop that may then coalesce to form larger ulcers within the anal canal and distal rectum and on the perianal skin. The disease is usually self-limiting, and ulcers heal after 2 weeks. In severely immunocompromised individuals, the disease may persist. Persistence of herpetic vesicles and ulcers beyond 1 month is an AIDS-defining condition (Figure 10-6). Recent studies have even shown that HSV may be spread when there are no visible lesions or symptoms. Given that genital HSV-2 increases the infectiousness of persons with HIV, suppressive therapy aimed at controlling HSV should be undertaken to limit the transmissibility of HIV.[37]

Clinically, patients typically complain of exquisite anorectal pain, which is exacerbated by defecation and ano-receptive intercourse, pruritus, and tenesmus. The initial infection may be accompanied by systemic signs, including fever, general malaise, and inguinal lymphadenopathy.[100] Following resolution of the initial infection, the virus remains latent in the sacral root ganglia with frequent reactivations. Upon reactivation, in addition to anorectal ulcerations, it can cause root symptoms along the affected dermatomes, leading to urinary dysfunction, paresthesias, constipation, and impotence.

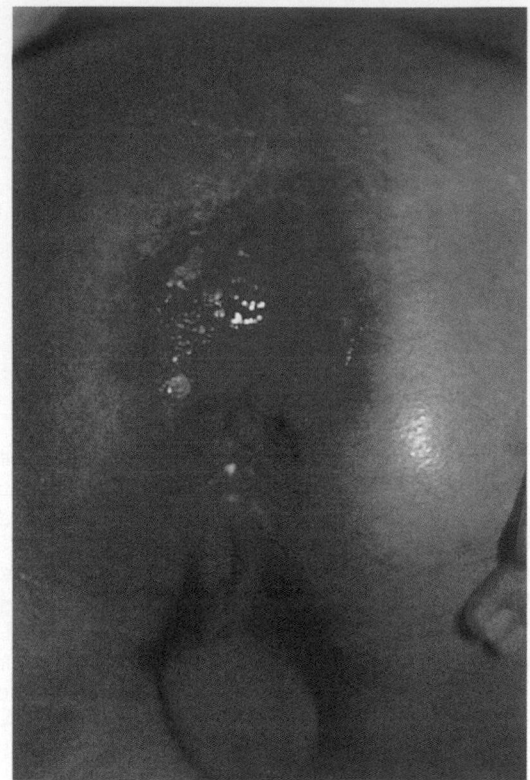

FIGURE 10-6. Severe erosive perianal herpes simplex.

Both tissue culture and biopsy specimens for histopathology are recommended, rather than the use of simple swabs. Biopsies of ulcer beds reveal the typical multinucleated giant cells or intranuclear inclusion bodies as seen in Figure 10-7. Tissue should be sent for cell culture to isolate HSV. However, sensitivity declines after healing of lesions starts. Therefore, empiric treatment with antiviral therapy should be undertaken before results of biopsy are obtained. Acyclovir promotes healing of lesions and decreases the duration of anorectal pain.[212] The dosage of acyclovir used for herpetic proctitis (400 to 800 mg, five times per day for 7 days) is higher than the recommended regimen for genital herpes. However, no studies have documented a clear advantage to the higher dosage. Alternative drugs for the acute treatment

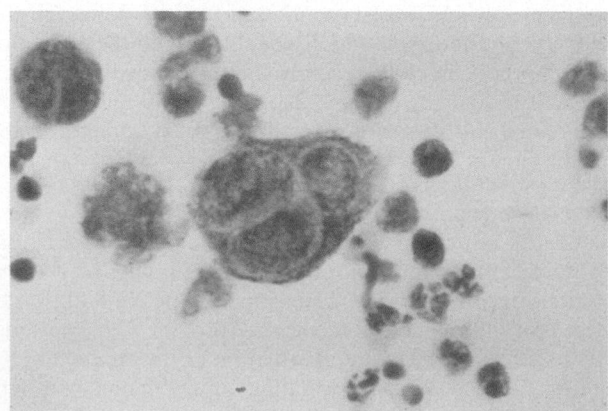

FIGURE 10-7. Characteristic multinucleated giant cell of herpes simplex virus infection.

of herpes are valacyclovir (1,000 mg, twice/day) and famciclovir (500 mg, twice/day). Both have been shown to have comparable efficacy to acyclovir in the treatment of anogenital herpes in HIV-infected patients.[51,211] The twice-daily dosing regimens of valacyclovir and famciclovir offer the added advantage of a reduced medication burden. Supportive care, including sitz baths and topical anesthetic agents, help to minimize pain during the active infection. Those who are acyclovir resistant (thymidine kinase–deficient HSV-2 mutants) usually respond well to foscarnet (Foscavir).[7,214] Suppressive therapy with antivirals reduces the frequency of herpetic recurrences with no cumulative toxicity. They should be considered in patients with frequent recurrence or in severely immunocompromised patients because the severity and frequency of recurrences vary inversely with the CD4 count.[7,44,168] The daily suppressive dose of acyclovir is 400 mg twice daily. Topical acyclovir, however, has little utility in the HIV-positive patient. Valacyclovir, at a dose of 500 mg, twice a day, has been shown to have comparable efficacy to that of acyclovir as suppressive therapy in patients with CD4 T-cell counts greater than 200 cells/mm³.[51] Patients with severe disease or with evidence of disseminated disease (i.e., pneumonitis, meningitis, or hepatitis) should be hospitalized and treated with intravenous acyclovir therapy at a dose of 5 to 10 mg/kg body weight, every 8 hours, until clinical improvement is noted.[289]

Herpes genitalis is also discussed in Chapter 9, and herpes simplex proctitis is discussed in Chapter 33.

Cytomegalovirus Infection

Cytomegalovirus has been implicated in causing anorectal ulceration.[125] Because cytomegalovirus is ubiquitous in the AIDS population, it may actually be a nonpathogenic bystander or secondary pathogen rather than a primary cause of disease. In addition, it has a predilection for endothelial cells found in the granulation tissue of many inflammatory anal conditions.

It has been suggested that a diagnosis of cytomegalovirus infection can be made by an "erosive or ulcerative process in the wall of the gut in which the presence of cytomegalovirus is shown by routine histologic examination, culture, or antigen or DNA staining, and in a person in whom other explanations for the lesion(s) have been excluded."[102]

Opinion

Our skepticism in implicating cytomegalovirus in anal disease arises from the lack of ability to retrieve cytomegalovirus from anal lesions and the lack of predictable response to therapy from lesions in which cytomegalovirus has been identified. It is our opinion that cytomegalovirus plays very little role in anal disease in HIV-infected patients.

Anal Condylomata Acuminata
Etiology and Pathogenesis

Condylomata are caused by HPV, a sexually transmitted virus. HPV is a double-stranded DNA virus. More than 80 subtypes have been identified, with subtypes 6 and 11 responsible for most anal condylomata acuminata.[252] Certain subtypes, notably 16, 18, and perhaps 31, 33, 45, and 46, have a greater oncogenic potential. HPV typically causes infection by direct inoculation, infecting basal keratinocytes, but anoreceptive intercourse is not required for anal infection. Viral replication occurs in basal keratinocytes, and the viral genome is carried to upper layers of the epithelium. As the virus propagates upward through the layers of the epithelium, the characteristic lesions are seen.

Anogenital HPV infection is more common in HIV-infected patients. The prevalence of anal HPV ranges from 72% to 90% in HIV-positive homosexual men, whereas the prevalence of anal HPV in homosexual men who are HIV negative has been found to be in the range of 57% to 61%.[47,188] Among HIV-positive men, HPV infection is more common in the homosexual population.[27,142] In one study, the prevalence of anal HPV infection in HIV-positive homosexual men was found to be 85%, compared with 46% in HIV-positive heterosexual men with no history of anal receptive sex.[199] The prevalence of this virus is probably a confounding factor in a variety of pathologic conditions affecting the anorectum in the HIV-positive patient.[17] Shedding of HPV, extent of disease, and recurrence of anal condylomata all increase as CD4 T-cell counts decrease.[49,184]

Malignant transformation is believed to be secondary to integration of the HPV DNA into the host genome. The integration of the viral DNA results in loss of the regulatory viral genes *E1* and *E2* and leads to overexpression of the *E6* and *E7* viral genes. The *E6* gene binds to the tumor suppressor protein p53, resulting in its degradation. *E7* binds to pRB, a cellular protein that normally inhibits transcriptional activity. Together, the result is increased DNA synthesis and decreased DNA repair of the host cell producing a malignant transformation.[77,220,255,280] HIV may be a cofactor in *E6* and *E7* gene expression.[29]

Presentation

Clinically, patients with anal warts may present with only a complaint of perianal lesions, or they may complain of perianal discomfort, itching, bleeding, or discharge. On examination, anal warts are easily identified by their white or pigmented, exophytic, hyperkeratotic appearance (see Chapter 9). Acetic acid may be used to help illuminate the warts in order to aid in their identification, particularly small warts or the less common flat warts. Microscopic changes show characteristic orderly papillomatosis, poikilocytosis, and hyperkeratosis (Figure 10-8).

Anal Intraepithelial Neoplasia

As previously noted, HPV infection is more common in HIV-infected individuals. Infection with multiple subtypes of HPV and more extensive disease are seen in HIV-positive

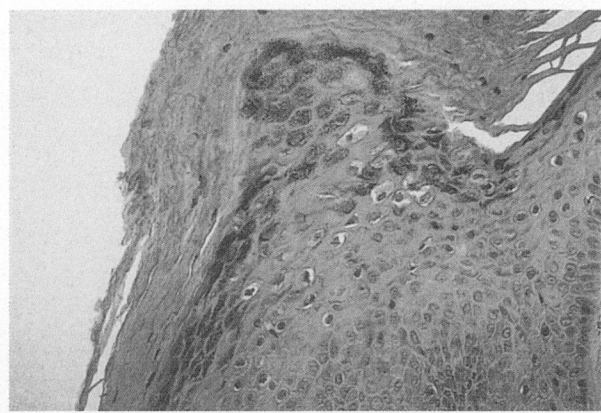

FIGURE 10-8. Histopathology of anal condyloma acuminatum, showing orderly papillomatosis, poikilocytosis, and hyperkeratinization.

patients. The incidence of anal cancer is higher in HIV-infected individuals, with a relative risk of 6.8 in women and 37.9 in men.[94] Sobhani and coworkers examined the prevalence of anal dysplasia and anal cancer with respect to HIV status, CD4 T-cell counts, and HPV. They found HIV positivity, HIV viral loads (but not CD4 counts), and condyloma relapse to be risk factors for high-grade dysplasia and invasive carcinoma. Of note, the same study found decreased local immunity, as measured by Langerhans cells in the anal mucosa, and increased prevalence of oncogenic HPV subtypes in HIV-positive patients.[97,242] A prospective study examining HPV as a risk factor for anal and perianal skin cancer found an increased risk in patients seropositive for IgG antibodies to HPV-16 and HPV-18.[21] It should be noted that anal HPV infection and anal intraepithelial neoplasia (AIN) can be observed in HIV-positive patients in the absence of prior anal intercourse.[199]

The association among HPV infection, HIV-positivity, AIN, and the possible progression of these dysplastic lesions to invasive anal carcinoma have stimulated a great deal of debate on screening and management in the HIV-positive patient. Initially, a similarity was found between AIN and cervical intraepithelial neoplasia, a precursor to cervical cancer (Figure 10-9).[12] The finding of AIN in routine scrapings from the anus of HIV-positive male patients, in addition to an increase in both prevalence and progression of cytologic changes, engendered fear of a potential epidemic of anal cancer.[183,186] It appears that in HIV-infected men, HPV infection may occur with clinically normal but histologically abnormal epithelium.[251] Progression to AIN appears to be directly related to the level of immunosuppression rather than to the specific subtype of HPV retrieved. However, recent reports indicate that the introduction of HAART has not yielded a benefit in reducing the incidence of high-grade AIN or in the regression of existing high-grade lesions.[45,62,169,270] In a study examining the natural history of AIN following initiation of HAART in 200 patients, rates of progression or regression of AIN remained unchanged in the first 6 months after HAART use was started, even though there was an increase in the CD4 T-cell counts of treated patients.[188] Because the benefits of HAART do not appear to extend to AIN and do not affect progression of low-grade lesions to high-grade lesions, the question of screening and treatment of subclinical lesions in the HIV-infected patient has been raised. Presumably, as life expectancy of these patients is improved,

rates of progression to invasive squamous carcinoma will increase. Adding further to the confusion is the observation of infection with multiple concurrent subtypes, variability of retrieval of HPV by different methods used, and overall higher retrieval rate of oncogenic HPV subtypes in the immunosuppressed patient.[28,236,238]

Palefsky and coworkers have proposed an AIN-screening protocol in which anal cytologic examination is performed in a fashion similar to the Papanicolaou's smear for cervical cytology with a water-moistened Dacron swab of the anal canal. Anal cytology is categorized similar to cervical cytology in the Bethesda system: normal, atypical squamous cells of undetermined significance (ASC-US), low-grade squamous intraepithelial lesion (LSIL), high-grade squamous intraepithelial lesion (HSIL), atypical squamous cells, and cannot rule out HSIL (ASC-H). Anal histology is graded based on severity where mild abnormalities are graded as AIN I, moderate abnormalities are graded as AIN II, and severe abnormalities are graded as AIN III or HGAIN (high-grade anal intraepithelial neoplasia). In their protocol, all patients with abnormal cytology are then referred for high-resolution anoscopy (HRA), which may be aided by acetic acid illumination of abnormal tissue and biopsy of all visualized lesions. According to their protocol, any patient with HGAIN on biopsy should then be treated.[187,192] However, there are currently no randomized controlled trials of AIN treatment from which to make management recommendations. Additionally, no studies have clearly documented progression to anal invasive squamous cell carcinoma, and, in fact, two small reports failed to demonstrate progression of AIN to squamous cell cancer. Despite the lack of conclusive evidence, ablative therapy for treatment of AIN has been proposed.[48,86,90,178] Chin-Hong and Palefsky recommend treating lesions smaller than 1 cm² with local topical therapy and treating larger lesions with surgery, although for very large and/or circumferential disease, they recommend no treatment because of the high morbidity of the extensive surgical procedure involved.[48] Given that progression rates to invasive cancer remain unknown as well as the high rates of persistent or recurrent AIN following surgical treatment (23 of 29 patients in one study), one may be legitimately concerned that vigorous screening for subclinical lesions will lead to unnecessarily debilitating surgery.[42]

Principles of Management

Anal warts should be destroyed, with follow-up every 2 months. Topical treatments that are available include podophyllin, bichloroacetic acid, and imiquimod. Podophyllin is cytotoxic to warts provided it is applied directly to the external component. However, its use is limited by its local toxicity. The success rate with podophyllin is problematic. In a study comparing surgical therapy versus podophyllin, the recurrence rate at 42 weeks was 68% for podophyllin versus 28% in the surgery group.[140] Bichloroacetic acid, a caustic agent, is similarly limited in its utility because of the poor response and high recurrence rate. Imiquimod is a newer agent that was approved for use in 1997. Application of imiquimod results in a local release of cytokines, including interferon.[258] Although it does have efficacy against anal warts, it does not appear to be effective as monotherapy in our experience.[106] However, in our practice, we have found imiquimod effective as adjunctive therapy in select patients following cytodestruction. This is used in patients who have shown a high recurrence rate after conventional therapy and

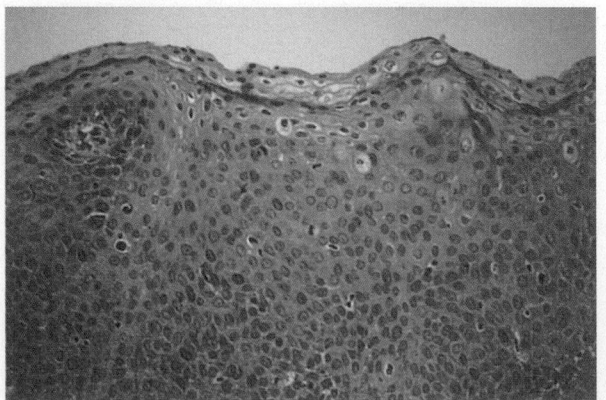

FIGURE 10-9. Histopathology of a flat lesion showing anal intraepithelial neoplasia (AIN III) with severe dysplasia.

not after the first treatment. Imiquimod 5% cream should be administered topically three times per week for a duration of at least 8 weeks for external anal warts. It can be used off label to insert into the anal canal after treatment of internal anal condyloma. Because of the poor response and high recurrence rates following topical therapy, our preferred alternative is cytodestruction (electrocautery) after acetic acid staining (Figure 10-10). This technique combines the antiproliferative and antiviral properties of imiquimod with cytodestruction to maximize eradication of both clinical and subclinical disease. It is our belief that aggressive treatment of clinical lesions should be performed in all patients with good performance status. Larger flat lesions should be excised. Noninvasive flat lesions that are determined to be carcinoma in situ with negative margins do not require additional therapy.[174] *HPV subtyping* should be reserved for research protocols only because it is expensive and really does not affect treatment and many patients have multiple subtype infection and determination of one subtype does not affect prognosis. We also believe that *anal cytology* is a tool for the primary care physician as it will allow referral to an appropriate colorectal consultant who then can assess the perianal and intra-anal regions. Furthermore, ablative prophylactic therapy for AIN is not indicated. These patients should be observed at 3-month intervals. Biopsy specimens can safely be taken from any suspected lesions, which can be treated as they become apparent.

Although various methods have been described for treating anal condyloma acuminata, high recurrence rates remain a problem. However, decreased relapse rates in HIV-positive patients with improved management of their underlying HIV infection with HAART have been reported.[182]

Research has focused on the development of both prophylactic and therapeutic HPV vaccines. Prophylactic vaccines are based on the viral capsid protein L1.[150] In a multicenter, randomized controlled trial of more than 4,000 healthy men, the quadrivalent HPV vaccine (active against HPV types 6, 11, 16, and 18) was found to reduce the incidence of condyloma acuminatum over a 3-year period.[98]

This study showed a 60% efficacy for the vaccine in preventing external genital lesions. The vaccine was also found to have 47% efficacy against persistent HPV infection. Whether the prevention of HPV infection reduces the incidence of anal cancer will have to be determined in future studies.[98]

Therapeutic vaccines to eradicate infected cells are being investigated as potential treatments for HPV intraepithelial neoplasia and invasive cancer. The HPV proteins, E6 and E7, are overexpressed in cells undergoing malignant transformation. Therefore, therapeutic vaccines have largely been based on these oncoproteins and the establishment of a cytotoxic T-cell response to cells expressing the E6 and E7 proteins. A vaccine developed from fusing the HPV-16 E7 protein to the bacille Calmette–Guérin heat-shock protein 65 was tested in patients with persistent high-grade squamous intraepithelial lesions in an open-label trial. Goldstone and coworkers reported complete resolution of warts in 3 of 14 patients at baseline, at week 24 following vaccination, and a 70% to 95% reduction in warts in 10 of the 14 patients.[99] At 15 months, 95% of men with high-grade anal dysplasia showed at least a reduction in pathologic staging to low-grade anal dysplasia, and 44% demonstrated a complete pathologic response.[185] Other therapeutic vaccines, including a HPV-6 L2/E7 fusion protein, initially showed promise, but after phase II trials, it was not found to be effective in reducing recurrence of disease nor in primary clearance of lesions.[153,154] In time, the development of prophylactic and therapeutic vaccines will, we hope, allow for the gradual eradication of anogenital warts (see also Chapter 9).

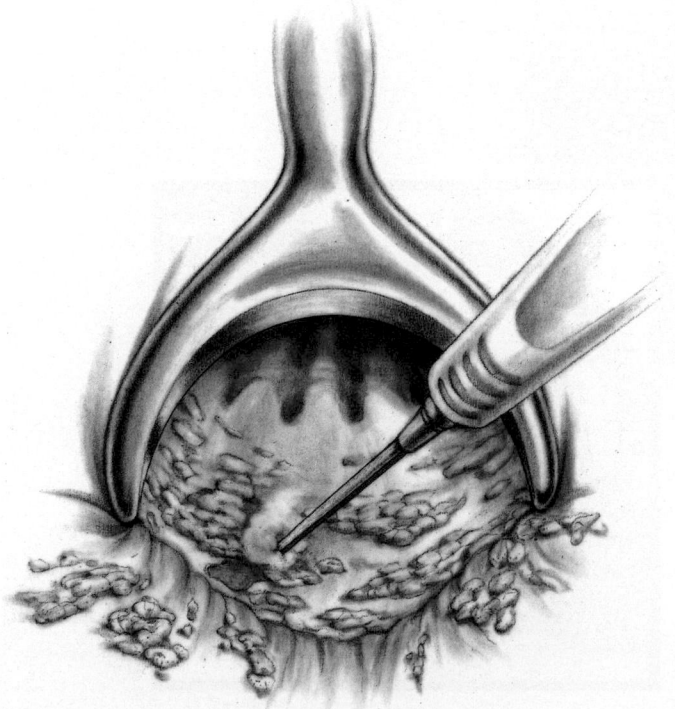
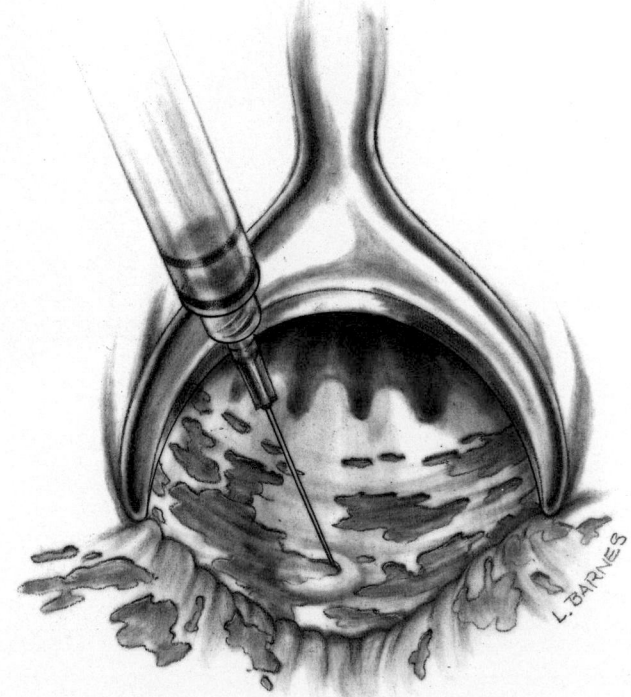

A

B

FIGURE 10-10. Fulguration **(A)** after acetic acid staining of anal condyloma acuminatum **(B)**.

AIDS-Specific Disease

The most debilitating lesions seen in the anorectum of patients with AIDS are idiopathic AIDS-related ulcers. These occur in advanced disease, usually when the CD4 T-cell counts fall to less than 200 cells/μL. Although no study has examined the effect of immune reconstitution on the natural history of idiopathic AIDS-related ulcers, the incidence of these anal ulcers in the era of HAART has predictably decreased. Their characteristic appearance is one of an extremely erosive and ulcerative process that occurs more proximally than do benign anal fissures, undermines what appears to be normal mucosa, and traverses normal tissue planes (Figures 10-11 through 10-14).[265] Whereas benign fissures are associated with hypertonia, idiopathic HIV-associated anal ulcers typically are associated with hypotonia of the anal sphincter. Symptoms include a sensation of pressure caused by pocketing of stool, pus, and vegetable matter and severe pain that is worse on defecation.

An aggressive workup for the cause of idiopathic AIDS-related ulcers is usually a fruitless exercise, except, of course, for an underlying malignancy.[159,223] Neither HSV nor cytomegalovirus is considered a causative agent, so therapy against retrieved pathogens is futile. In our experience, one-half of these patients harbor oncogenic HPV in adjacent mucosa.[191] This may be purely coincidental or may suggest HPV-induced initiation of a cytodestructive cytokine cascade.[166]

Treatment consists of operative debridement to eliminate the pocketing effect and injection of a depot steroid preparation into the base and sides of the ulcers (Figures 10-15 and 10-16). As we have reported, this protocol has produced uniformly satisfying results.[265] It is thought that the steroids may downregulate cytokine reduction in aphthous ulceration in the same way as a model seen in the esophagus.[148] Another agent, thalidomide, has been used anecdotally in both anal and oral aphthous ulceration.[193] Its presumed mechanism of action is also downregulation of cytokine production. Some authors have advocated operative debridement and a rectal mucosal advancement flap and have reported favorable results.[53] In patients with severe pain in whom anal procedures have failed, fecal diversion may be considered. Laparoscopic stoma creation has been reported to have the benefit of improved postoperative recovery and decreased compromise of immune function when compared with laparotomy.[180]

Anorectal Malignancy

As stated previously, the anorectum may be the initiating site for NHL (Figure 10-17). It may present as either a mass or a fissure; biopsy is diagnostic. Because chemotherapy is so effective, a diverting stoma is now rarely used in the management of NHL. With respect to Kaposi's sarcoma, this is usually an incidental finding and rarely causes significant anorectal symptoms.[159]

The greatest controversy in the AIDS-infected individual concerns the management of squamous cell carcinoma (Figure 10-18). The incidence of this tumor in the homosexual population has been rising, and with the onset of HIV, incidence rates have further increased.[164,286] Combined-modality therapy replaced abdominoperineal resection in the

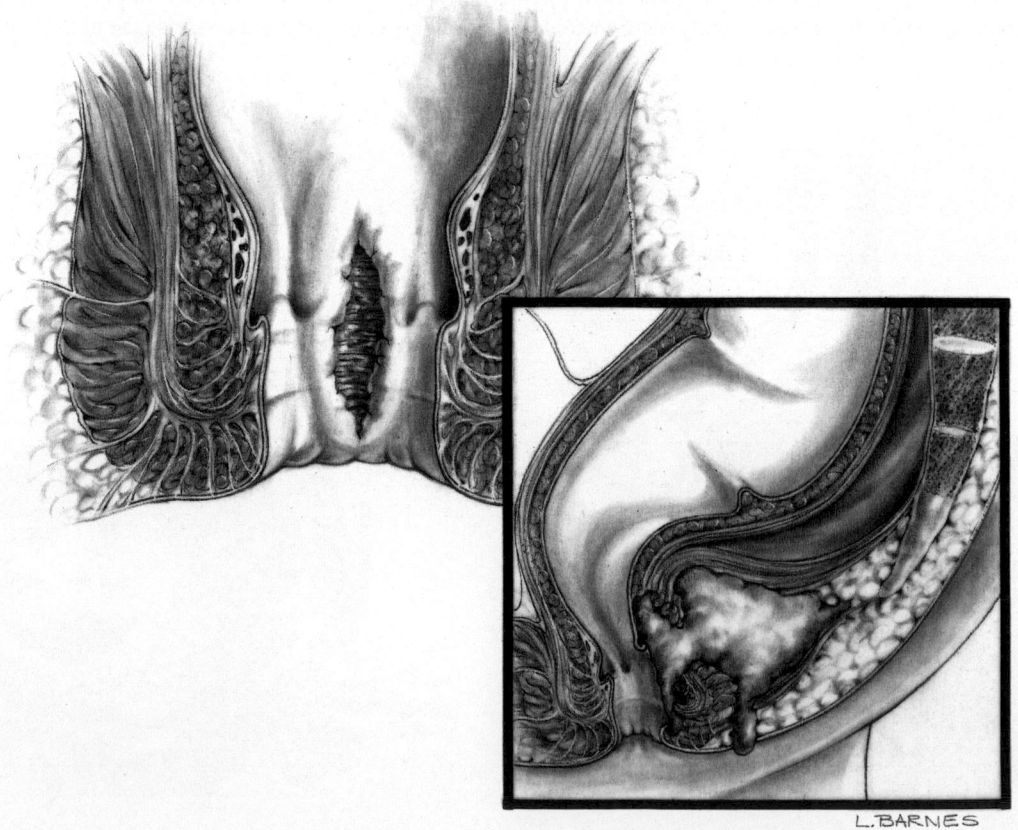

FIGURE 10-11. AIDS-related ulcer showing erosion in submucosal planes with destruction of the intersphincteric plane and formation of a deep postanal space collection (*inset*). The "bottleneck" causes a sensation of pressure.

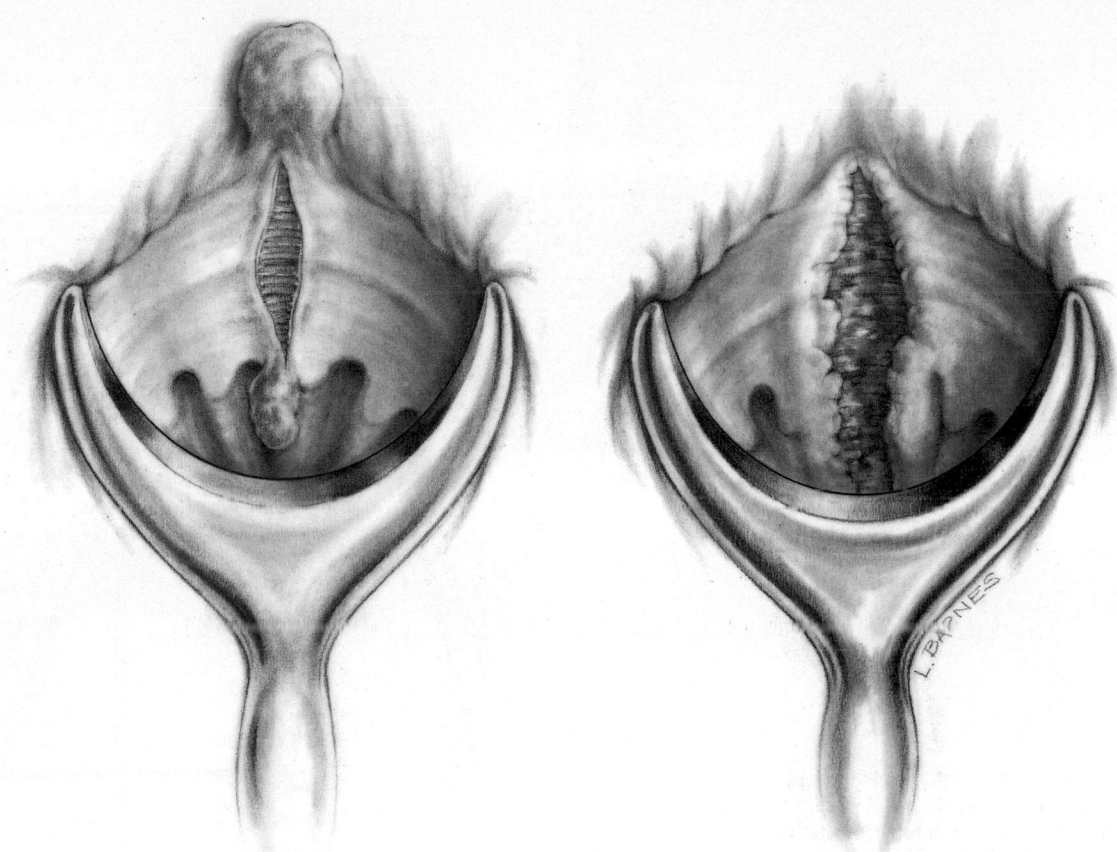

A   B

FIGURE 10-12. Anal ulcers. Artist's conception of the clinical appearances differentiating between a so-called benign lesion **(A)** and an idiopathic AIDS-related ulcer **(B)**.

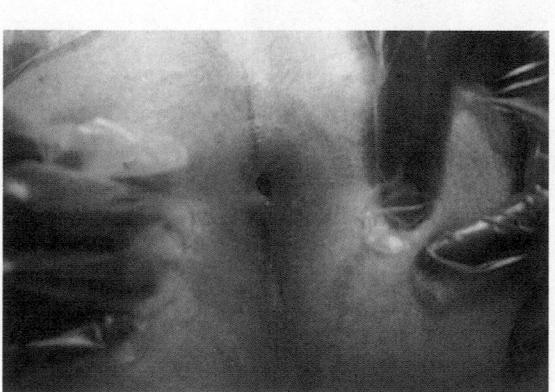

FIGURE 10-13. Erosion of an idiopathic AIDS-related ulcer into the deep postanal space, exiting into the perianal skin.

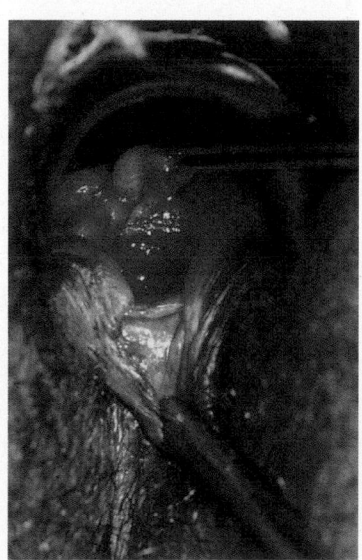

FIGURE 10-14. Idiopathic AIDS-related ulcer showing dissection in the submucosal and intersphincteric plane.

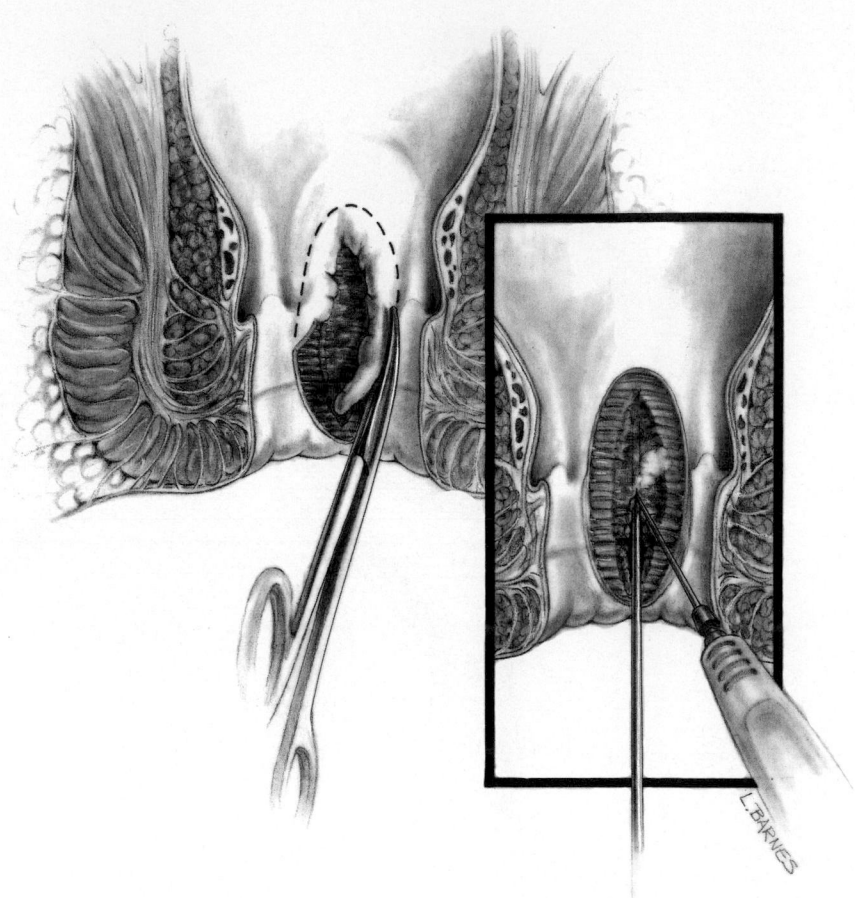

FIGURE 10-15. Treatment of an AIDS-related ulcer by debridement of the mucosal overhanging edges and incision of the internal anal sphincter to allow better drainage (*inset*).

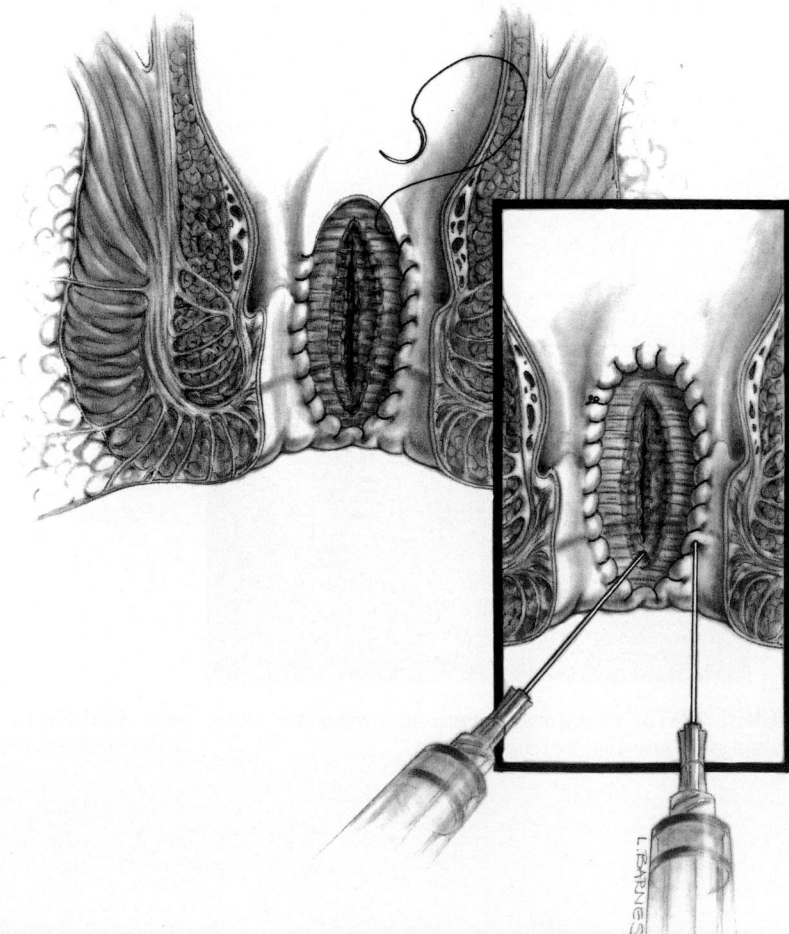

FIGURE 10-16. Treatment of an AIDS-related ulcer by marsupialization of the mucosal edges with heavy absorbable suture and injection of methylprednisolone (Depo Medrol) into the submucosal and deep tissues (*inset*).

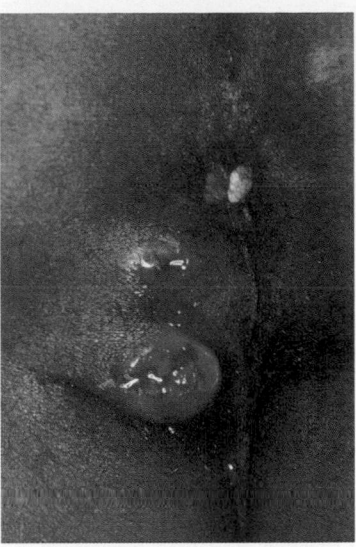

FIGURE 10-17. Large non-Hodgkin's rectal lymphoma eroding through the perianal skin.

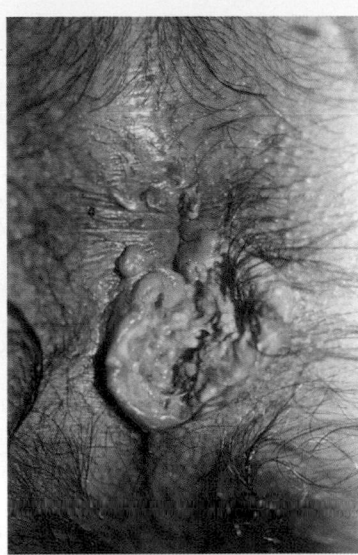

FIGURE 10-18. Squamous cell carcinoma of the anus in a patient with AIDS.

1980s and remains the standard of care (see Chapter 25).[64] Prior to the introduction of HAART, combined-modality therapy was often difficult for the patient and was associated with a high morbidity. Adverse effects of radiation therapy included desquamation of the perineal region, diarrhea, and severe anal pain. Anal stenosis and ulcers were late manifestations of radiation toxicity. Toxic effects of chemotherapy included exacerbation of chronic diarrhea, weight loss (in an already nutritionally challenged patient), and bone marrow suppression. Several small series, including our unpublished experience, have documented the inability of patients with advanced HIV disease or coincidental diarrhea to complete the protocol without intolerable consequences.[26,40,117,123] Hoffman and coworkers found that in patients with a CD4 count lower than 250 undergoing combined-modality therapy, 50% of patients required a colostomy for control of symptoms.[122] In another study of patients who underwent combined-modality therapy prior to HAART, higher rates of acute toxicity were found in HIV-positive patients when compared with HIV-negative patients (80% vs. 30%). Late toxic effects of combined-modality therapy were likewise increased (38% vs. 15%).[141] In an attempt to limit the toxicity of therapy, the dose of radiation therapy was lowered to 30 Gy in one small study, with no impact on local control. However, this was a small study limited to patients with stage II disease and no prior opportunistic infections.[196]

In recent years, the impact of HAART on the toxicity profile of combined-modality therapy has been studied. Blazy and colleagues found that in HIV-positive patients on HAART who underwent concomitant chemoradiation therapy, acute toxicity occurred at a similar rate as observed in non–HIV-infected patients.[24] In their retrospective review of those undergoing combined-modality therapy for SCC of the anal canal, Hammad and coworkers found the incidence of grade 3 and grade 4 toxicities was similar in HIV-infected patients on HAART when compared with noninfected patients. The only difference in toxicity was seen with radiation dermatitis, which actually occurred more frequently in the noninfected group. In their study, HIV-infected patients

received similar doses of radiation when compared with the noninfected group at a lower dose of chemotherapy. These dose reductions were planned and were not due to observed toxicity. The authors assert that lower dose chemotherapy may be required in HIV-positive patients with SCC, but in the era of HAART this can help achieve adequate local control with acceptable toxicity.[115] In patients with advanced HIV disease, however, studies have shown that there is an increased risk for hematologic toxicity. Because toxicity may lead to treatment breaks, decreased local control in HIV-positive patients is likely to result.[279]

The outcome of combined-modality therapy in anal squamous cell cancers in HIV-positive patients on HAART has also been examined. In a retrospective study, poor local control and persistent disease were noted in more than 50% of patients with invasive cancer prior to the HAART era.[200] Kim and coworkers found that only 62% of HIV-positive patients in the pre-HAART era had a complete response to combined-modality therapy as compared with 85% of HIV-negative patients.[141] However, since the initiation of HAART, response rates and local failure rates have improved. In a retrospective review of individuals with invasive SCC who underwent combined-modality therapy, Stadler and coworkers found that the 24-month survival was 17% in HIV-infected patients who were not on HAART and 67% for those on HAART. The survival rate for the HAART group is favorable to rates reported for the non-HIV population (between 73% and 86%).[249] Particularly in cases where the diagnosis is made early, local failure rates are similar. In a retrospective review of 32 HIV-positive patients treated with combined-modality therapy for anal squamous cell cancer, Wexler and associates found a 16% local failure rate. This is similar to local failure rates in HIV-negative patients. The authors attributed some of the success of treatment to the early diagnosis made by experienced primary providers. Further studies, including randomized multicenter trials, will be needed to optimize the chemoradiation regimen while reducing morbidity in the treatment of invasive anal squamous cell carcinoma in patients with advanced AIDS.

▶ PROTECTION OF THE SURGEON

Seroconversion to an HIV-positive state following percutaneous exposure with a hypodermic needle (0.3%) and mucous membrane exposure (0.09%) has been documented. However, there have been no reported seroconversions after being stuck with a suture needle.[259] This is thought to be a consequence of the fact that the needle is solid. Furthermore, there have been no seroconversions following exposure when the skin is intact. The quantification of viral load in assessing risk of transmission of HIV following occupational exposure has not been established. Although universal precautions should be routinely instituted, certain special efforts should be made when operating on an identified or suspected HIV-infected individual. The following recommendations should be enforced:

- Safety glasses should be worn, in addition to water-resistant foot covering.
- Double gloves with a disposable sleeve insert should be used to prevent blood from reaching the wrists of the surgeon.
- Scalpels should be disposed of once skin incisions have been made.
- A choreographed procedure is dictated by the senior surgeon when suturing is being performed.[271]
- Triple therapy is recommended if a serious exposure occurs.

▶ CONCLUSIONS

The introduction of HAART has radically changed the clinical course of HIV infection and AIDS. Although not curative, HAART does lead to significant and sustained elevations in CD4 T-cell counts and immune function as well as decreased serum viral levels to almost undetectable levels. This has resulted in a reduction in the number of opportunistic infections and malignancies associated with AIDS and an improved survival and life expectancy.

In this chapter, we attempt to discuss the major colonic and anorectal problems encountered in the HIV-positive patient. Controversies remain in the management of several disorders, including AIN and invasive squamous cell carcinoma of the anal canal. The roles of therapeutic vaccines in HPV are yet to be elucidated. However, there is promising evidence that prophylactic vaccines will reduce the morbidity of HPV and its associated diseases. Lest we be lulled into a false sense of security, it should be remembered that the incidence of HIV is once again rising, and the compliance of HIV-positive patients, particularly younger people with HAART regimens, is dropping. Sadly, although HAART improves life expectancy through inhibition of viral replication and immune reconstitution, 90% of the world's HIV-infected individuals do not have access to these drugs.

References

1. AIDSinfo Web site. http://Aidsinfo.nih.gov. Accessed August 2003.
2. Albaran RG, Webber J, Steffes CP. CD4 cell counts as prognostic factor of major abdominal surgery in patients infected with the human immunodeficiency virus. *Arch Surg.* 1998;133(6):626–631.
3. Albin J, Lewis E, Eftekhari F, et al. Computed tomography of rectal and perirectal disease in AIDS patients. *Gastrointest Radiol.* 1987;12(1):67–70.
4. Andersen CB, Karkov J, Bjerregaard B, et al. Cytomegalovirus infection in classic endemic and epidemic Kaposi's sarcoma analyzed by in situ hybridization. *APMIS.* 1991;99(10):893–897.
5. Angelici A, Palumbo P, Piermattei A, et al. Exploratory laparotomy for diagnosis of abdominal painful syndromes in HIV-positive patients. *Int Conf AIDS.* 1993;9:447.

6. Ariyoshi K, Schim van der Loeff M, Cook P, et al. Kaposi's sarcoma in the Gambia, West Africa is less frequent in human immunodeficiency virus type 2 than in human immunodeficiency type 1 infection despite a high prevalence of human herpesvirus 8. *J Hum Virol.* 1998;1(3):193–199.
7. Bagdades EK, Pillay D, Squire SB, et al. Relationship between herpes simplex virus ulceration and CD4$^+$ cell counts in patients with HIV infection. *AIDS.* 1992;6(11):1317–1320.
8. Balthazar EJ, Megibow AJ, Barry M, et al. Histoplasmosis of the colon in patients with AIDS: imaging findings in four cases. *AJR Am J Roentgenol.* 1993;161(3):585–587.
9. Baroco AL, Oldfield EC. Gastrointestinal cytomegalovirus disease in the immunocompromised patient. *Curr Gastroenterol Rep.* 2008;10(4):409–416.
10. Barrett WL, Callahan TD, Orkin BA. Perianal manifestations of human immunodeficiency virus infection: experience with 260 patients. *Dis Colon Rectum.* 1998;41(5):606–612.
11. Becherer PR, Sokol-Anderson M, Joist JH, et al. Gastrointestinal histoplasmosis presenting as hematochezia in human immunodeficiency virus–infected hemophiliac patients. *Am J Hematol.* 1994;47(3):229–231.
12. Beck DE, Jaso RG, Zajac RA. Surgical management of anal condylomata in the HIV-positive patient. *Dis Colon Rectum.* 1990;33(3):180–183.
13. Belitsos PC, Greenson JK, Yardley JH, et al. Association of gastric hypoacidity with opportunistic enteric infections in patients with AIDS. *J Infect Dis.* 1992;166(2):277–284.
14. Benson CA. Treatment of disseminated disease due to the *Mycobacterium avium* complex in patients with AIDS. *Clin Infect Dis.* 1994;18(suppl 3):S237–S242.
15. Beral V, Peterman T, Berkelman R, et al. AIDS-associated non-Hodgkin lymphoma. *Lancet.* 1991;337(8745):805–809.
16. Bermudez LE. Immunobiology of *Mycobacterium avium* infection. *Eur J Clin Microbiol Infect Dis.* 1994;13(11):1000–1006.
17. Bernard C, Mougin C, Madoz L, et al. Viral co-infections in human papillomavirus-associated anogenital lesions according to the serostatus for the human immunodeficiency virus. *Int J Cancer.* 1992;52(5):731–737.
18. Bini EJ, Cohen J. Impact of protease inhibitors on the outcome of human immunodeficiency virus-infected patients with chronic diarrhea. *Am J Gastroenterol.* 1999;94(12):3553–3559.
19. Bini EJ, Gorelick SM, Weinshel EH. Outcome of AIDS-associated cytomegalovirus colitis in the era of potent antiretroviral therapy. *J Clin Gastroenterol.* 2000;30(4):414–419.
20. Bizer LS, Pettorino R, Ashikari A. Emergency abdominal operations in the patient with acquired immunodeficiency syndrome. *J Am Coll Surg.* 1995;180(2):205–209.
21. Bjørge T, Engeland A, Luostarinen T, et al. Human papillomavirus as a risk factor for anal and perianal skin cancer in a prospective study. *Br J Cancer.* 2002;87(1):61–64.
22. Blackbourn DJ, Osmond D, Levy JA, et al. Increased human herpesvirus 8 seroprevalence in young homosexual men who have multiple sex contacts with different partners. *J Infect Dis.* 1999;179(1):237–239.
23. Blanshard C, Gazzard BG. Natural history and prognosis of diarrhoea of unknown cause in patients with acquired immunodeficiency syndrome (AIDS). *Gut.* 1995;36(2):283–286.
24. Blazy A, Hennequin C, Gornet J, et al. Anal carcinomas in HIV-positive patients: high dose chemoradiotherapy is feasible in the era of highly active antiretroviral therapy. *Dis Colon Rectum.* 2005;48(6):1176–1181.
25. Bordón J, Martínez-Vásquez C, Alvarez M, et al. Neurosyphilis in HIV–infected patients. *Eur J Clin Microbiol Infect Dis.* 1995;14(10):864–869.
26. Bottomley D, Gershuny A, Govindaraju S, et al. Epidermoid anal cancer in HIV infected patients. *Br J Cancer.* 1994;70(suppl 22):17.
27. Breese PL, Judson FN, Penley KA, et al. Anal human papillomavirus infection among homosexual and bisexual men: prevalence of type-specific infection and association with human immunodeficiency virus. *Sex Transm Dis.* 1995;22(1):7–14.
28. Brown DR, Bryan JT, Cramer H, et al. Detection of multiple human papillomavirus types in condylomata acuminata from immunosuppressed patients. *J Infect Dis.* 1994;170(4):759–765.
29. Buonaguro FM, Tornesello ML, Buonaguro L, et al. Role of HIV as cofactor in HPV oncogenesis: in vitro evidence of virus interactions. *Antibiot Chemother.* 1994;46:102–109.
30. Call SA, Heudebert G, Saag M, et al. The changing etiology of chronic diarrhea in HIV-infected patients with CD4 cell counts less than 200 cells/mm^3. *Am J Gastroenterol.* 2000;95(11):3142–3146.
31. Cappell MS, Botros N. Predominantly gastrointestinal symptoms and signs in 11 consecutive AIDS patients with gastrointestinal lymphoma: a multicenter, multiyear study including 763 HIV-seropositive patients. *Am J Gastroenterol.* 1994;89(4):545–549.

32. Cappell MS, Mandell W, Grimes MM, et al. Gastrointestinal histoplasmosis. *Dig Dis Sci.* 1988;33(3):353–360.

33. Carr A, Marriott D, Field A, et al. Treatment of HIV-1-associated microsporidiosis and cryptosporidiosis with combination antiretroviral therapy. *Lancet.* 1998;351(9098):256–261.

34. Carr ND, Mercey D, Slack WW. Non-condylomatous, perianal disease in homosexual men. *Br J Surg.* 1989;76(10):1064–1066.

35. Case records of the Massachusetts General Hospital. Weekly clinicopathological exercises. Case 17-1996. A 48-year-old man with the acquired immunodeficiency syndrome, abdominal pain, and bloody diarrhea. *N Engl J Med.* 1996;334(22):1461–1467.

36. Cello JP, Wilcox CM. Evaluation and treatment of gastrointestinal tract hemorrhage in patients with AIDS. *Gastroenterol Clin North Am.* 1988;17(3):639–648.

37. Celum C, Wald A, Lingappa JR, et al. Acyclovir and transmission of HIV-1 from persons infected with HIV-1 and HSV-2. *N Eng J Med.* 2010;362(5):427–439.

38. Centers for Disease Control and Prevention. Diagnosis and reporting of HIV and AIDS in states with HIV/AIDS surveillance—United States, 1994–2000. *MMWR Morb Mortal Wkly Rep.* 2002;51(27):595–598.

39. Centers for Disease Control and Prevention. Advancing HIV prevention: new strategies for a changing epidemic—United States, 2003. *MMWR Morb Mortal Wkly Rep.* 2003;52(15):329–332.

40. Chadha M, Rosenblatt EA, Malamud S, et al. Squamous cell carcinoma of the anus in HIV-positive patients. *Dis Colon Rectum.* 1994;37(9): 861–865.

41. Chambers AJ, Lord RS. Incidence of acquired immune deficiency syndrome (AIDS)-related disorders at laparotomy in patients with AIDS. *Br J Surg.* 2001;88(2):294–297.

42. Chang G, Berry J, Jay N, et al. Surgical treatment of high-grade anal squamous intraepithelial lesions: a prospective study. *Dis Colon Rectum.* 2002;45(4):453–458.

43. Chang Y, Cesarman E, Pessin MS, et al. Identification of herpesvirus–like DNA sequences in AIDS-associated Kaposi's sarcoma. *Science.* 1994;266(5192):1865–1869.

44. Change E, Absar N, Beall G. Prevention of recurrent herpes simplex virus (HSV) infections in HIV-infected persons. *AIDS Patient Care.* 1995;9(5):252–255.

45. Chaturvedi AK, Madeleine MM, Biggar RJ, et al. Risk of human papillomavirus-associated cancers among persons with AIDS. *J Natl Cancer Inst.* 2009;101(16):1120–1130.

46. Chin DP, Hopewell PC, Yajko DM, et al. *Mycobacterium avium* complex in the respiratory or gastrointestinal tract and the risk of *M. avium* bacteremia in patients with the human immunodeficiency virus. *J Infect Dis.* 1994;169(2):289–295.

47. Chin-Hong PV, Berry JM, Cheng SC, et al. Comparison of patient- and clinician-collected anal cytology samples to screen for human papillomavirus-associated anal intraepithelial neoplasia in men who have sex with men. *Ann Intern Med.* 2008;149(5):300–306.

48. Chin-Hong PV, Palefsky JM. Natural history and clinical management of anal human papillomavirus disease in men and women infected with human immunodeficiency virus. *Clin Infect Dis.* 2002;35(9): 1127–1134.

49. Chopra KF, Tyring SK. The impact of the human immunodeficiency virus on the human papillomavirus epidemic. *Arch Dermatol.* 1997;133(5):629–633.

50. Clark SJ, Saag MS, Decker WD, et al. High titers of cytopathic virus in plasma of patients with symptomatic primary HIV-1 infection. *N Engl J Med.* 1991;324(14):954–960.

51. Conant MA, Schacker TW, Murphy RL, et al. Valaciclovir versus aciclovir for herpes simplex virus infection in HIV-infected individuals: two randomized trials. *Int J STD AIDS.* 2002;13(1):12–21.

52. Cone LA, Woodard DR, Potts BE, et al. An update on the acquired immunodeficiency syndrome (AIDS). Associated disorders of the alimentary tract. *Dis Colon Rectum.* 1986;29(1):60–64.

53. Consten EC, Slors FJ, Noten HJ, et al. Anorectal surgery in human immunodeficiency virus-infected patients. Clinical outcome in relation to immune status. *Dis Colon Rectum.* 1995;38(11):1169–1175.

54. Consten EC, Slors JF, Danner SA, et al. Severe complications of perianal sepsis in patients with human immunodeficiency virus. *Br J Surg.* 1996;83(6):778–780.

55. Cooper DA, Tindall B, Wilson EJ, et al. Characterization of T lymphocyte responses during primary infection with human immunodeficiency virus. *J Infect Dis.* 1988;157(5):889–896.

56. Corey L, Nahmias AJ, Guinan ME, et al. A trial of topical acyclovir in genital herpes simplex virus infections. *N Engl J Med.* 1982;306(22): 1313–1319.

57. Coté TR, Biggar RJ, Rosenberg PS, et al. Non-Hodgkin's lymphoma among people with AIDS: incidence, presentation and public health burden. AIDS/Cancer Study Group. *Int J Cancer.* 1997;73(5):645–650.

58. Cotte L, Drouet E, Bailly F, et al. Cytomegalovirus DNA level on biopsy specimens during treatment of cytomegalovirus gastrointestinal disease. *Gastroenterology.* 1996;111(2):439–444.

59. Cotte L, Drouet E, Bissuel F, et al. Diagnostic value of cytomegalovirus-DNA amplification from gastrointestinal biopsies in HIV-infected patients [abstract]. *Int Conf AIDS.* 1993;9(1):346.

60. Craib KJ, Meddings DR, Strathdee SA, et al. Rectal gonorrhoea as an independent risk factor for HIV infection in a cohort of homosexual men. *Genitourin Med.* 1995;71(3):150–154.

61. Critchlow CW, Hawes SE, Kuypers JM, et al. Effect of HIV infection on the natural history of anal human papillomavirus infection. *AIDS.* 1998;12(10):1177–1184.

62. Critchlow CW, Surawicz CM, Holmes KK, et al. Prospective study of high grade anal squamous intraepithelial neoplasia in a cohort of homosexual men: influence of HIV infection, immunosuppression and human papillomavirus infection. *AIDS.* 1995;9(11):1255–1262.

63. Crumpacker CS. Ganciclovir. *N Engl J Med.* 1996;335(10):721–729.

64. Cummings BJ. Concomitant radiotherapy and chemotherapy for anal cancer. *Semin Oncol.* 1992;19(4 suppl 11):102–108.

65. Dal Maso L, Franceschi S. Epidemiology of non-Hodgkin lymphomas and other haemolymphopoietic neoplasms in people with AIDS. *Lancet Oncol.* 2003;4(2):110–119.

66. Davidson T, Allen Morah TG, Miloo AJ, et al. Emergency laparotomy in patients with AIDS. *Br J Surg.* 1991;78(8):924–926.

67. Davis PA, Corless DJ, Aspinall R, et al. Effect of CD4(+) and CD8(+) cell depletion on wound healing. *Br J Surg.* 2001;88(2):298–304.

68. Davis PA, Corless DJ, Gazzard BG, et al. Increased risk of wound complications and poor healing following laparotomy in HIV-seropositive and AIDS patients. *Dig Surg.* 1999;16(1):60–67.

69. Deeks SG, Volberding PA. HIV-1 protease inhibitors. *AIDS Clin Rev.* 1997–1998:145–185.

70. Deneve JL, Shantha JG, Page AJ, et al. CD4 count is predictive of outcome in HIV-positive patients undergoing abdominal operations. *Am J Surg.* 2010;200(6):694–699.

71. Dieterich DT, Lew EA, Kotler DP, et al. Treatment with albendazole for intestinal disease due to *Enterocytozoon bieneusi* in patients with AIDS. *J Infect Dis.* 1994;169(1):178–183.

72. Dieterich DT, Rahmin M. Cytomegalovirus colitis in AIDS: presentation in 44 patients and a review of the literature. *J Acquir Immune Defic Syndr.* 1991;4(suppl 1):S29–S35.

73. Drew WL. Cytomegalovirus infection in patients with AIDS. *J Infect Dis.* 1988;158(2):449–456.

74. Drew WL, Buhles W, Erlich KS. Herpesvirus infections (cytomegalovirus, herpes simplex virus, varicella-zoster virus). How to use ganciclovir (DHPG) and acyclovir. *Infect Dis Clin North Am.* 1988;2(2):495–509.

75. Drew WL, Mills J, Hauer LB, et al. Declining prevalence of Kaposi's sarcoma in homosexual AIDS patients paralleled by fall in cytomegalovirus transmission. *Lancet.* 1988;1(8575–8576):66.

76. Dryden MS, Shanson DC. The microbial causes of diarrhoea in patients infected with the human immunodeficiency virus. *J Infect.* 1988;17(2):107–114.

77. Dyson N, Howley PM, Münger K, et al. The human papilloma virus-16 E7 oncoprotein is able to bind to the retinoblastoma gene product. *Science.* 1989;243(4893):934–937.

78. Ell CH, Matek W, Gramatzki M, et al. Endoscopic findings in a case of Kaposi's sarcoma with involvement of the large and small bowel. *Endoscopy.* 1985;17(4):161–164.

79. Eltom MA, Jemal A, Mbulaiteye SM, et al. Trends in Kaposi's sarcoma and non-Hodgkin's lymphoma incidence in the United States from 1973 through 1998. *J Natl Cancer Inst.* 2002;94(16):1204–1210.

80. Emmanoulides C, Miles SA, Mitsuyasu RT. Pathogenesis of AIDS—related Kaposi's sarcoma. *Oncology.* 1996;10(3):335–341.

81. Emparan C, Iturburu IM, Ortiz J, et al. Infective complications after abdominal surgery in patients infected with human immunodeficiency virus: role of CD4+ lymphocytes in prognosis. *World J Surg.* 1998;22(8):778–782.

82. Endean ED, Ross CW, Strodel WE. Kaposi's sarcoma appearing as a rectal ulcer. *Surgery.* 1987;101(6):767–769.

83. Eron JJ, Benoit SL, Jemesk J, et al. Treatment with lamivudine, zidovudine, or both in HIV-positive patients with 200 to 500 CD4+ cells per cubic millimeter. North American HIV Working Party. *N Engl J Med.* 1995;333(25):1662–1669.

84. Fauci AS. AIDS in 1996. Much accomplished, much to do. *JAMA.* 1996;276(2):155–156.

85. Feinberg MB. Changing the natural history of HIV disease. *Lancet.* 1996;348(9022):239–246.

86. Fenger C, Nielsen VT. Precancerous changes in the anal canal epithelium in resection specimens. *Acta Pathol Microbiol Immunol Scand A*. 1986;94(1):63–69.

87. Flanigan T, Whalen C, Turner J, et al. *Cryptosporidium* infection and CD4 counts. *Ann Intern Med*. 1992;116(10):840–842.

88. Fluker JL, Deherogoda P, Platt DJ, et al. Rectal gonorrhoea in male homosexuals. Presentation and therapy. *Br J Vener Dis*. 1980;56(6):397–399.

89. Forsmark CE, Wilcox CM, Darragh TM, et al. Disseminated histoplasmosis in AIDS: an unusual case of esophageal involvement and gastrointestinal bleeding. *Gastrointest Endosc*. 1990;36(6):604–605.

90. Foust RL, Dean PJ, Stoler MH, et al. Intraepithelial neoplasia of the anal canal in hemorrhoidal tissue: a study of 19 cases. *Hum Pathol*. 1991;22(6):528–534.

91. Frager DH, Frager JD, Brandt LJ, et al. Gastrointestinal complications of AIDS: radiologic features. *Radiology*. 1986;158(3):597–603.

92. Friedman SL, Wright TL, Altman DF. Gastrointestinal Kaposi's sarcoma in patients with acquired immunodeficiency syndrome. Endoscopic and autopsy findings. *Gastroenterology*. 1985;89(1):102–108.

93. Friedman-Kien A, Laubenstein L, Marmor M, et al. Kaposi's sarcoma and *Pneumocystis* pneumonia among homosexual men—New York City and California. *MMWR Morb Mortal Wkly Rep*. 1981;30(25):305–308.

94. Frisch M, Biggar RJ, Engels EA, et al. Association of cancer with AIDS-related immunosuppression in adults. *JAMA*. 2001;285(13):1736–1745.

95. Garcia LS, Brewer TC, Bruckner DA. Fluorescence detection of *Cryptosporidium* oocysts in human fecal specimens by using monoclonal antibodies. *J Clin Microbiol*. 1987;25(1):119–121.

96. Gautreaux MD, Gelder FB, Deitch EA, et al. Adoptive transfer of T lymphocytes to T-cell-depleted mice inhibits *Escherichia coli* translocation from the gastrointestinal tract. *Infect Immun*. 1995;63(10):3827–3834.

97. Gervaz E, Dauge-Geffroy MD, Sobhani I, et al. Quantitative analysis of the immune cells in the anal mucosa. *Pathol Res Pract*. 1995;191(11):1067–1071.

98. Giuliano AR, Palefsky JM, Goldstone S, et al. Efficacy of quadrivalent HPV vaccine against HPV infection and disease in males. *N Engl J Med*. 2011;364(5):401–411.

99. Goldstone SE, Palefsky JM, Winnett MT. Activity of HspE7, a novel immunotherapy, in patients with anogenital warts. *Dis Colon Rectum*. 2002;45(4):502–507.

100. Goodell SE, Quinn TC, Mkrtichian E, et al. Herpes simplex virus proctitis in homosexual men. Clinical, sigmoidoscopic, and histopathological features. *N Engl J Med*. 1983;308(15):868–871.

101. Goodgame MD, Porter DD. Cytomegalovirus vasculitis with fatal colonic hemorrhage. *Arch Pathol*. 1973;96(4):281–284.

102. Goodgame RW. Gastrointestinal cytomegalovirus disease. *Ann Intern Med*. 1993;119(9):924–935.

103. Goodgame RW, Genta RM, Estrada R, et al. Frequency of positive tests for cytomegalovirus in AIDS patients: endoscopic lesions compared with normal mucosa. *Am J Gastroenterol*. 1993;88(3):338–343.

104. Goodgame RW, Kimball K, Ou CN, et al. Intestinal function and injury in acquired immunodeficiency syndrome-related cryptosporidiosis. *Gastroenterology*. 1995;108(4):1075–1082.

105. Gottesman L. Ulcerative disease of the anorectum in AIDS. *Int J STD AIDS*. 1995;6(1):4–6.

106. Gottesman L. Adjuvant operative bed alfa-interferon 2b in the treatment of persistent and recalcitrant anal condylomata acuminata [abstract]. American Society of Colon and Rectal Surgery, Seattle; 1996.

107. Gottesman LG, Miles AJ, Milsom JW, et al. The management of anorectal disease in HIV-positive patients. *Int J Colorectal Dis*. 1990;5(2):61–72.

108. Graybill JR. Histoplasmosis and AIDS. *J Infect Dis*. 1988;158(3):623–626.

109. Grulich AE, Li Y, McDonald AM, et al. Decreasing rates of Kaposi's sarcoma and non-Hodgkin's lymphoma in the era of potent combination anti-retroviral therapy. *AIDS*. 2001;15(5):629–633.

110. Guarino A, Canani R, Pozio E, et al. Enterotoxic effect of stool supernatant of Cryptosporidium-infected calves on human jejunum. *Gastroenterology*. 1994;106(1):28–34.

111. Gulick RM, Mellors JW, Havlir D, et al. Treatment with indinavir, zidovudine, and lamivudine in adults with human immunodeficiency virus infection and prior antiretroviral therapy. *N Engl J Med*. 1997;337(11):734–739.

112. Haddad FS, Ghossain A, Sawaya E, et al. Abdominal tuberculosis. *Dis Colon Rectum*. 1987;30(9):724–735.

113. Hall HI, Song R, Rhodes P, et al. Estimation of HIV incidence in the United States. *JAMA*. 2008;300(5):520–529.

114. Hamilton JD, Hartigan PM, Simberkoff MS, et al. A controlled trial of early versus late treatment with zidovudine in symptomatic human immunodeficiency virus infection. Results of the Veterans Affairs Cooperative Study. *N Engl J Med*. 1992;326(7):437–443.

115. Hammad N, Heilbrun LK, Gupta S, et al. Squamous cell cancer of the anal canal in HIV-infected patients receiving highly active antiretroviral therapy: a single institution experience. *A J Clin Oncol*. 2011;34(2):135–139.

116. Harris PJ. Treatment of Kaposi's sarcoma and other manifestations of AIDS with human chorionic gonadotropin. *Lancet*. 1995;346:118–119.

117. Harrison M, Tomlinson D, Stewart S. Squamous cell carcinoma of the anus in patients with AIDS. *Clin Oncol*. 1995;7(1):50–51.

118. He Y, Cheng J, Lu H, et al. Potent HIV fusion inhibitors against Enfuvirtide-resistant HIV-1 strains. *Proc Natl Acad Sci USA*. 2008;105(42):16332–16337.

119. Heneghan SJ, Li J, Petrossian E, et al. Intestinal perforation from gastrointestinal histoplasmosis in acquired immunodeficiency syndrome. Case report and review of the literature. *Arch Surg*. 1993;128(4):464–466.

120. Hewitt WR, Sokol TP, Fleshner PR. Should HIV status alter indications for hemorrhoidectomy? *Dis Colon Rectum*. 1996;39(6):615–618.

121. Hinant KL, Rotterdam HZ, Bell ET, et al. Cytomegalovirus infection of the alimentary tract: a clinicopathological correlation. *Am J Gastroenterol*. 1986;81(10):944–950.

122. Hoffman R, Welton ML, Klencke B, et al. The significance of pretreatment CD4 count on the outcome and treatment tolerance of HIV-positive patients with anal cancer. *Int J Radiat Oncol Biol Phys*. 1999;44(1):127–131.

123. Holland JM, Swift PS. Tolerance of patients with human immunodeficiency virus and anal carcinoma to treatment with combined chemotherapy and radiation therapy. *Radiology*. 1994;193(1):251–254.

124. Horberg MA, Hurley LB, Klein DB, et al. Surgical outcomes in human immunodeficiency virus-infected patients in the era of highly active antiretroviral therapy. *Arch Surg*. 2006;141(12):1238–1245.

125. Horn TD, Hood AF. Cytomegalovirus is predictably present in perineal ulcers from immunosuppressed patients. *Arch Dermatol*. 1990;126(5):642–644.

126. Imagawa DT, Lee MH, Wolinsky SM, et al. Human immunodeficiency virus type 1 infection in homosexual men who remain seronegative for prolonged periods. *N Engl J Med*. 1989;320(22):1458–1462.

127. Imrie K, Sawka CA, Kutas G, et al. HIV-associated lymphoma of the gastrointestinal tract [abstract]. *Proc Ann Meeting Am Soc Clin Oncol*. 1993;12:A1.

128. Irizarry E, Gottesman L. Rectal sexual trauma including foreign bodies. *Int J STD AIDS*. 1996;7(3):166–169.

129. Jarrin G, Kemeny M, Lee M. Abdominal surgery in patients with AIDS-related lymphomas: bacteremia in patients with human immunodeficiency virus infection [abstract]. *J Infect Dis*. 1994;169:289; *Proc Ann Meeting Am Soc Clin Oncol*. 1992;11:A17.

130. Jiang S, Zhao Q, Debnath AK. Peptide and non-peptide HIV fusion inhibitors. *Curr Pharm Des*. 2002;8(8):563–580.

131. Jones JL, Hanson DL, Dworkin MS, et al. Incidence and trends in Kaposi's sarcoma in the era of effective antiretroviral therapy. *J Acquir Immune Defic Syndr*. 2000;24(3):270–274.

132. Judson FN, Penley KA, Robinson ME, et al. Comparative prevalence rates of sexually transmitted diseases in heterosexual and homosexual men. *Am J Epidemiol*. 1980;112(6):836–843.

133. Kaplan LD, Abrams DI, Feigal E, et al. AIDS-associated non-Hodgkin's lymphoma in San Francisco. *JAMA*. 1989;261(5):719–724.

134. Kaplan LD, Wofsy CB, Volberding PA. Treatment of patients with acquired immunodeficiency syndrome and associated manifestations. *JAMA*. 1987;257(10):1367–1374.

135. Kaslow RA, Phair JP, Friedman HB, et al. Infection with the human immunodeficiency virus: clinical manifestations and their relationship to immunodeficiency. A report from the Multicenter AIDS Cohort Study. *Ann Intern Med*. 1987;107(4):474–480.

136. Keating J, Bjarnason I, Somasundaram S, et al. Intestinal absorptive capacity, intestinal permeability and jejunal histology in HIV and their relation to diarrhoea. *Gut*. 1995;37(5):623–629.

137. Kelly CP, Pothoulakis C, LaMont JT. *Clostridium difficile* colitis. *N Engl J Med*. 1994;330(4):257–262.

138. Kemper CA, Meng TC, Nussbaum J, et al. Treatment of *Mycobacterium avium* complex bacteremia in AIDS with a four-drug oral regimen. Rifampin, ethambutol, clofazimine, and ciprofloxacin. The California Collaborative Treatment Group. *Ann Intern Med*. 1992;116(6):466–472.

139. Kerr A, Dix J, Quinnonez C. A case of fatal hemorrhage caused by intestinal histoplasmosis. *Am J Gastroenterol*. 1991;86(7):910–912.

140. Khawaja HT. Podophyllin versus scissor excision in the treatment of perianal condylomata acuminata: a prospective study. *Br J Surg*. 1989;76(10):1067–1068.

141. Kim JH, Sarani B, Orkin BA, et al. HIV-positive patients with anal carcinoma have poorer treatment tolerance and outcome than HIV-negative patients. *Dis Colon Rectum.* 2001;44(10):1496–1502.

142. Kiviat N, Rompalo A, Bowden R, et al. Anal human papillomavirus among human immunodeficiency virus-seropositive and -seronegative men. *J Infect Dis.* 1990;162(2):358–361.

143. Klencke B, Kaplan L. Advances and future challenges in non-Hodgkin's lymphoma. *Curr Opin Oncol.* 1998;10(5):422–427.

144. Knight SC, Patterson S. Bone marrow-derived dendritic cells, infection with human immunodeficiency virus, and immunopathology. *Annu Rev Immunol.* 1997;15(15):593–615.

145. Knowles DM. Biologic aspects of AIDS-associated non-Hodgkin's lymphoma. *Curr Opin Oncol.* 1993;5(5):845–851.

146. Knowles DM. Etiology and pathogenesis of AIDS-related non-Hodgkin's lymphoma. *Hematol Oncol Clin North Am.* 1996;17(3):785–820.

147. Knowles DM, Chadburn A. AIDS-associated lymphoid proliferations. In: Knowles DM, ed. *Neoplastic Hematopathology.* Baltimore, MD: Williams & Wilkins; 1992.

148. Kotler DP, Reka S, Orenstein JM, et al. Chronic idiopathic esophageal ulceration in the acquired immunodeficiency syndrome. Characterization and treatment with corticosteroids. *J Clin Gastroenterol.* 1992;15(4):284–290.

149. Kotler DP, Shimda T, Snow G, et al. Effect of combination antiretroviral therapy upon rectal mucosal HIV RNA burden and mononuclear cell apoptosis. *AIDS.* 1998;12(6):597–604.

150. Koutsky LA, Ault KA, Wheeler CM, et al. A controlled trial of a human papillomavirus type 16 vaccine. *N Engl J Med.* 2002;347(21):1645–1651.

151. Kram HB, Shoemaker WC. Intestinal perforation due to cytomegalovirus infection in patients with AIDS. *Dis Colon Rectum.* 1990;33(12):1037–1040.

152. Krown SE, Gold JW, Niedzwiecki D, et al. Interferon-alpha with zidovudine: safety, tolerance, and clinical and virologic effects in patients with Kaposi sarcoma associated with the acquired immunodeficiency syndrome (AIDS). *Ann Intern Med.* 1990;112(11):812–821.

153. Lacey CJ. Therapy for genital human papillomavirus-related disease. *J Clin Virol.* 2005;32(suppl 1):S82–S90.

154. Lacey CJ, Thompson IIS, Monteiro EF, et al. Phase IIa safety and immunogenicity of a therapeutic vaccine, TA-GW, in persons with genital warts. *J Infect Dis.* 1999;179(3):612–618.

155. Laine L, Amerian J, Rarick M, et al. The response of symptomatic gastrointestinal Kaposi's sarcoma to chemotherapy: a prospective evaluation using an endoscopic method of disease quantification. *Am J Gastroenterol.* 1990;85(8):959–961.

156. Lange JM, Parry JV, de Wolf F, et al. Diagnostic value of specific IgM antibodies in primary HIV infection. *AIDS.* 1988;2(1):31–35.

157. Lew EA, Dieterich DT. Severe hemorrhage caused by gastrointestinal Kaposi's syndrome in patients with the acquired immunodeficiency syndrome: treatment with endoscopic injection sclerotherapy. *Am J Gastroenterol.* 1992;87(10):1471–1474.

158. Lim SG, Condez A, Lee CA, et al. Loss of mucosal CD4 lymphocytes is an early feature of HIV infection. *Clin Exp Immunol.* 1993;92(3):448–454.

159. Lorenz HP, Wilson W, Leigh B, et al. Kaposi's sarcoma of the rectum in patients with the acquired immunodeficiency syndrome. *Am J Surg.* 1990;160(6):681–682.

160. Louie TJ, Miller MA, Mullane KM, et al. Fidaxomicin versus vancomycin for Clostridium difficile infection. *N Engl J Med.* 2011;364(5):422–431.

161. Marrazzo JM, Whittington WL, Celum CL, et al. Urine-based screening for *Chlamydia trachomatis* in men attending sexually transmitted disease clinics. *Sex Transm Dis.* 2001;28(4):219–225.

162. Matthews GV, Bower M, Mandalia S, et al. Changes in acquired immunodeficiency syndrome-related lymphoma since the introduction of highly active antiretroviral therapy. *Blood.* 2000;96(8):2730–2734.

163. McGrath MS, Shiramizu B, Herndier BG. Clonal HIV in the pathogenesis of AIDS-related lymphoma: sequential pathogenesis. In: Goedert JJ, ed. *Infectious Causes of Cancer: Targets for Intervention.* Totowa, NJ: Humana Press; 2000:231–244.

164. Melbye M, Coté TR, Kessler L, et al. High incidence of anal cancer among AIDS patients. The AIDS/Cancer Working Group. *Lancet.* 1994;343(8898):636–639.

165. Mellors JW, Rinaldo CR Jr, Gupta P, et al. Prognosis in HIV-1 infection predicted by the quantity of virus in plasma. *Science.* 1996;272(5265):1167–1170.

166. Memar OM, Arany I, Tyring SK. Skin-associated lymphoid tissue in human immunodeficiency virus-1, human papillomavirus, and herpes simplex virus infections. *J Invest Dermatol.* 1995;105(1 suppl):99S–104S.

167. Mentec H, Leport C, Leport J, et al. Cytomegalovirus colitis in HIV-1-infected patients: a prospective research in 55 patients. *AIDS.* 1994;8(4):461–467.

168. Mertz GJ, Jones CC, Mills J, et al. Long-term acyclovir suppression of frequently recurring genital herpes simplex virus infection. A multicenter double-blind trial. *JAMA.* 1988;260(2):201–206.

169. Metcalf AM, Dean T. Risk of dysplasia in anal condyloma. *Surgery.* 1995;118(4):724–726.

170. Miles AJ, Mellor CH, Gazzard B, et al. Surgical management of anorectal disease in HIV-positive homosexuals. *Br J Surg.* 1990;77(8):869–871.

171. Mitsuyasu RT. Kaposi's sarcoma in the acquired immunodeficiency syndrome. *Infect Dis Clin North Am.* 1988;2(2):511–523.

172. Molina JM, Sarfati C, Beauvais B, et al. Intestinal microsporidiosis in human immunodeficiency virus-infected patients with chronic unexplained diarrhea: prevalence and clinical and biological features. *J Infect Dis.* 1993;167(1):217–221.

173. Mönkemüller KE, Call SA, Lazenby AJ, et al. Declining prevalence of opportunistic gastrointestinal disease in the era of combination antiretroviral therapy. *Am J Gastroenterol.* 2000;95(2):457–462.

174. Morgan AR, Miles AJ, Wastell C. Anal warts and squamous carcinoma-in-situ of the anal canal. *J R Soc Med.* 1994;87(1):15.

175. Mortensen NJ, Thomson JP. Perianal abscess due to *Enterobius vermicularis.* Report of a case. *Dis Colon Rectum.* 1984;27(10):677–678.

176. Murray JG, Evans SJ, Jeffrey PB, et al. Cytomegalovirus colitis in AIDS: CT features. *AJR Am J Roentgenol.* 1995;165(1):67–71.

177. Neff R, Kremer S, Voutsinas L, et al. Primary Kaposi's sarcoma of the ileum presenting as massive rectal bleeding. *Am J Gastroenterol.* 1987;82(3):276–277.

178. Northfelt DW. Anal neoplasia in persons with HIV infection. *AIDS Clin Care.* 1996;8(8):63–66.

179. O'Brien TR, Kedes D, Ganem D, et al. Evidence for concurrent epidemics of human herpesvirus 8 and human immunodeficiency virus type 1 in US homosexual men: rates, risk factors, and relationship to Kaposi's sarcoma. *J Infect Dis.* 1999;180(4):1010–1017.

180. Oliveira L, Wexner SD. Laparoscopically assisted sigmoid colectomy in human immunodeficiency virus (HIV) patients: a good indication for laparoscopic surgery. *Surg Laparosc Endosc.* 1996;6(5):414–416.

181. Orenstein JM, Tenner M, Kotler DP. Localization of infection by the microsporidian *Enterocytozoon bieneusi* in the gastrointestinal tract of AIDS patients with diarrhea. *AIDS.* 1992;6(2):195–197.

182. Orlando G, Fasolo MM, Signori R, et al. Impact of highly active antiretroviral therapy on clinical evolution of genital warts in HIV-infected patients. *AIDS.* 1999;13(2):291–293.

183. Palefsky JM, Gonzales J, Greenblatt R, et al. Anal intraepithelial neoplasia and anal papillomavirus infection among homosexual males with group IV HIV disease. *JAMA.* 1990;263(21):2911–2916.

184. Palefsky JM. Cutaneous and genital HPV-associated lesions in HIV-infected patients. *Clin Dermatol.* 1997;15(3):439–447.

185. Palefsky JM, Goldstone SE, Winnett M, et al. HspE7 treatment of anal dysplasia: results of an open label trial of HspE7 and comparison with a prior controlled trial of low dose HspE7 [abstract]. Paper presented at: 41st Interscience Conference on Antimicrobial Agents and Chemotherapy; 2001; Chicago, IL.

186. Palefsky JM, Holly EA, Gonzales J, et al. Natural history of anal cytologic abnormalities and papillomavirus infection among homosexual men with group IV HIV disease. *J Acquir Immune Defic Syndr.* 1992;5(12):1258–1265.

187. Palefsky JM, Holly EA, Hogeboom CJ, et al. Anal cytology as a screening tool for anal squamous intraepithelial lesions. *J Acquir Immune Defic Syndr Hum Retrovirol.* 1997;14(5):415–422.

188. Palefsky JM, Holly EA, Ralston ML, et al. Effect of highly active antiretroviral therapy on the natural history of anal squamous intraepithelial lesions and human papillomavirus infection. *J Acquir Immune Defic Syndr.* 2001;28(5):422–428.

189. Palella FJ Jr, Delaney KM, Moorman AC, et al. Declining morbidity and mortality among patients with advanced human immunodeficiency virus infection. HIV Outpatient Study Investigators. *N Engl J Med.* 1998;338(13):853–860.

190. Panja A, Mayer L. Diversity and function of antigen-presenting cells in mucosal tissue. In: Ogra PL, Lamm ME, McGhee JR, eds. *Handbook of Mucosal Immunology.* San Diego, CA: Academic Press; 1994:177.

191. Pare A, Gottesman L. Oncogenic human papillomavirus in idiopathic AIDS ulcers: cause or bystander? *Presentation, NY Soc Colon Rect Surg.* 1995.

192. Park IU, Palefsky JM. Evaluation and management of anal intraepithelial neoplasia in HIV-negative and HIV-positive men who have sex with men. *Curr Infect Dis Rep.* 2010;12(2):126–133.

193. Paterson DL, Georghiou PR, Allworth AM, et al. Thalidomide as treatment of refractory aphthous ulceration related to human immunodeficiency virus infection. *Clin Infect Dis.* 1995;20(2):250–254.

194.   Pati S, Pelser CB, Dufraine J, et al. Antitumorigenic effects of HIV protease inhibitor ritonavir: inhibition of Kaposi sarcoma. *Blood.* 2002;99(10):3771–3779.

195.   Peacock CS, Blanshard C, Tovey DG, et al. Histological diagnosis of intestinal microsporidiosis in patients with AIDS. *J Clin Pathol.* 1991;44(7):558–563.

196.   Peddada AV, Smith DE, Rao AR, et al. Chemotherapy and low-dose radiotherapy in the treatment of HIV-infected patients with carcinoma of the anal canal. *Int J Radiat Oncol Biol Phys.* 1997;37(5):1101–1105.

197.   Peppercorn MA. Enteric infections in homosexual men with and without AIDS. *Contemp Gastroenterol.* 1989;2:23–32.

198.   Piguet V, Blauvelt A. Essential roles for dendritic cells in the pathogenesis and potential treatment of HIV disease. *J Invest Dermatol.* 2002;119(2):365–369.

199.   Piketty C, Darragh TM, Da Costa M, et al. High prevalence of anal human papillomavirus infection and anal cancer precursors among HIV-infected persons in the absence of anal intercourse. *Ann Intern Med.* 2003;138(6):453–459.

200.   Place RJ, Gregorcyk SG, Huber PJ, et al. Outcome analysis of HIV-positive patients with anal squamous cell carcinoma. *Dis Colon Rectum.* 2001;44(4):506–512.

201.   Plancoulaine S, Abel L, van Beveren M, et al. Human herpesvirus 8 transmission from mother to child and between siblings in an endemic population. *Lancet.* 2000;356(9235):1062–1065.

202.   Pluda JM, Venson DJ, Tosato G, et al. Parameters affecting the development of non-Hodgkin's lymphoma in patients with severe human immunodeficiency virus infection receiving antiretroviral therapy. *J Clin Oncol.* 1993;11(6):1099–1107.

203.   Port JH, Traube J, Winans CS. The visceral manifestations of Kaposi's sarcoma. *Gastrointest Endosc.* 1982;28(3):179–181.

204.   Powderly WG, Landay A, Lederman MM. Recovery of the immune system with antiretroviral therapy: the end of opportunism? *JAMA.* 1998;280(1):72–77.

205.   Puy-Montbrun T, Ganansia R, Lemarchand N, et al. Anal ulcerations due to cytomegalovirus in patients with AIDS. Report of six cases. *Dis Colon Rectum.* 1990;33(12):1041–1043.

206.   Rabeneck L, Crane MM, Risser JM, et al. Effect of HIV transmission category and CD4 count on the occurrence of diarrhea in HIV-infected patients. *Am J Gastroenterol.* 1993;88(10):1720–1723.

207.   Rabinowitz M, Bassan I, Robinson MJ. Sexually transmitted cytomegalovirus proctitis in a woman. *Am J Gastroenterol.* 1988;83(8):885–887.

208.   Ramírez-Amador V, Esquivel-Pedraza L, Lozada-Nur F, et al. Intralesional vinblastine vs. 3% sodium tetradecyl sulfate for the treatment of oral Kaposi's sarcoma. A double blind, randomized clinical trial. *Oral Oncol.* 2002;38(5):460–467.

209.   Rene E, Marche C, Chevalier T, et al. Cytomegalovirus colitis in patients with acquired immunodeficiency syndrome. *Dig Dis Sci.* 1988;33(6):741–750.

210.   Robinson G, Wilson SE, Williams RA. Surgery in patients with acquired immunodeficiency syndrome. *Arch Surg.* 1987;122(2):170–175.

211.   Romanowski B, Aoki FY, Martel AY, et al. Efficacy and safety of famciclovir for treating mucocutaneous herpes simplex infection in HIV-infected individuals. Collaborative Famciclovir HIV Study Group. *AIDS.* 2000;14(9):1211–1217.

212.   Rompalo AM, Mertz GJ, Davis LG, et al. Oral acyclovir for treatment of first-episode herpes simplex virus proctitis. *JAMA.* 1988;259(19): 2879–2881.

213.   Safavi A, Gottesman L, Dailey TH. Anorectal surgery in the HIV+ patient: update. *Dis Colon Rectum.* 1991;34(4):299–304.

214.   Safrin S. Treatment of acyclovir-resistant herpes simplex virus infections in patients with AIDS. *J Acquir Immune Defic Syndr.* 1992;5(suppl 1):S29–S32.

215.   Saltz RK, Kurtz RC, Lightdale CJ, et al. Kaposi's sarcoma. Gastrointestinal involvement correlation with skin findings and immunologic function. *Dig Dis Sci.* 1984;29(9):817–823.

216.   Saltzman DJ, Williams RA, Gelfand DV, et al. The surgeon and AIDS: twenty years later. *Arch Surg.* 2005;140(10):961–967.

217.   Sanchez TH, Brooks JT, Sullivan PS, et al. Bacterial diarrhea in persons with HIV infection, United States, 1992–2002. *Clin Infect Dis.* 2005;41(11):1621–1627.

218.   Scaglia M, Delani GG, Destefano I, et al. Injection treatment of hemorrhoids in patients with acquired immunodeficiency syndrome. *Dis Colon Rectum.* 2001;44(3):401–404.

219.   Schacker T, Collier AC, Hughes J, et al. Clinical and epidemiologic features of primary HIV infection. *Ann Intern Med.* 1996;125(4):257–264.

220.   Scheffner M, Whitaker NJ. Human papillomavirus-induced carcinogenesis and the ubiquitin-proteasome system. *Semin Cancer Biol.* 2003;13(1):59–67.

221.   Schmidt W, Wahnschaffe U, Schäfer M, et al. Rapid increase in mucosal CD4 T cells followed by clearance of intestinal cryptosporidiosis in an AIDS patient receiving highly active antiretroviral therapy. *Gastroenterology.* 2001;120(4):984–987.

222.   Schmitt SL, Wexner SD. Treatment of anorectal manifestations of AIDS: past and present. *Int J STD AIDS.* 1994;5(1):8–10.

223.   Schmitt SL, Wexner SD, Nogueras JJ, et al. Is aggressive treatment of perianal ulcers in homosexual HIV-seropositive men justified? *Dis Colon Rectum.* 1993;36(3):240–246.

224.   Schnittman SM, Lane HC, Greenhouse J, et al. Preferential infection of CD4⁺ memory T cells by human immunodeficiency virus type 1: evidence for a role in the selective T-cell functional defects observed in infected individuals. *Proc Natl Acad Sci USA.* 1990;87(16):6058–6062.

225.   Scholefield JH, Northover JM, Carr ND. Male homosexuality, HIV infection and colorectal surgery. *Br J Surg.* 1990;77(5):493–496.

226.   Schulz TF, Boshoff CH, Weiss RA. HIV infection and neoplasia. *Lancet.* 1996;348(9027):587–591.

227.   Schwartz DA, Wilcox CM. Atypical cytomegalovirus inclusions in gastrointestinal biopsy specimens from patients with the acquired immunodeficiency syndrome: diagnostic role of in situ nucleic acid hybridization. *Hum Pathol.* 1992;23(9):1019–1026.

228.   Science and Technology. Hope. *Economist.* 1996:82–84.

229.   Selik RM, Rabkin CS. Cancer death rates associated with human immunodeficiency virus infection in the United States. *J Natl Cancer Inst.* 1998;90(17):1300–1302.

230.   Sgadari C, Barillari G, Toschi E, et al. HIV protease inhibitors are potent anti-angiogenic molecules and promote regression of Kaposi sarcoma. *Nat Med.* 2002;8(3):225–232.

231.   Sharpstone D, Gazzard B. Gastrointestinal manifestations of HIV infection. *Lancet.* 1996;348(9024):379–383.

232.   Sharpstone D, Rowbottom A, Francis N, et al. Thalidomide: a novel therapy for microsporidiosis. *Gastroenterology.* 1997;112(6):1823–1829.

233.   Sherrard J, Forsyth JR. Homosexually acquired gonorrhoea in Victoria, 1983–1991. *Med J Aust.* 1993;158(7):450–453.

234.   Shiramizu BS, Herndier BG, McGrath MS. Identification of a common clonal human immunodeficiency virus integration site in human immunodeficiency virus-associated lymphomas. *Cancer Res.* 1994;54(8):2069–2072.

235.   Siegel FP, Lopez C, Hammer GS, et al. Severe acquired immunodeficiency in male homosexuals, manifested by chronic perianal ulcerative herpes simplex lesions. *N Engl J Med.* 1981;305(24):1439–1444.

236.   Sillman FH, Sedlis A. Anogenital papillomavirus infection and neoplasia in immunodeficient women. *Obstet Gynecol Clin North Am.* 1987;14(2):537–558.

237.   Simon DM, Cello JP, Valenzuela J, et al. Multicenter trial of octreotide in patients with refractory acquired immunodeficiency syndrome-associated diarrhea. *Gastroenterology.* 1995;108(6):1753–1760.

238.   Skyldberg B, Hagmar B, Johansson B, et al. HPV detection in cytological cases with condylomatous or dysplastic changes: a study with PCR and in situ hybridization on cytological material. *Diagn Cytopathol.* 1995;13(1):8–14.

239.   Slaven EM, Lopez F, Weintraub SL, et al. The AIDS patient with abdominal pain: a new challenge for the emergency physician. *Emerg Med Clin North Am.* 2003;21(4):987–1015.

240.   Smith NH, Cron S, Valdez LM, et al. Combination drug therapy for cryptosporidiosis in AIDS. *J Infect Dis.* 1998;178(3):900–903.

241.   Smith PD, Quinn TC, Strober W, et al. NIH conference. Gastrointestinal infections in AIDS. *Ann Intern Med.* 1992;116(1):63–77.

242.   Sobhani I, Vuagnat A, Walker F, et al. Prevalence of high-grade dysplasia and cancer in the anal canal in human papillomavirus-infected individuals. *Gastroenterology.* 2001;120(4):857–866.

243.   Sobhani I, Walker F, Aparicio T, et al. Effect of anal epidermoid cancer-related viruses on the dendritic (Langerhans') cells of the human anal mucosa. *Clin Cancer Res.* 2002;8(9):2862–2869.

244.   Sobottka I, Schwartz DA, Schottelius J, et al. Prevalence and clinical significance of intestinal microsporidiosis in human immunodeficiency virus-infected patients with and without diarrhea in Germany: a prospective coprodiagnostic study. *Clin Infect Dis.* 1998;26(2):475–480.

245.   Söderlund C, Bratt GA, Engström L, et al. Surgical treatment of cytomegalovirus enterocolitis in severe human immunodeficiency virus infection. Report of eight cases. *Dis Colon Rectum.* 1994;37(1):63–72.

246.   Sohn N. Surgical conditions of the anus and rectum in male homosexuals. *Pract Gastroenterol.* 1985;9:46.

247.   Sparano JA. Clinical aspects and management of AIDS-related lymphoma. *Eur J Cancer.* 2001;37(10):1296–1305.

248.   Spivak H, Schlasinger MH, Tabanda-Lichauco R, et al. Small bowel obstruction from gastrointestinal histoplasmosis in acquired immune deficiency syndrome. *Am Surg.* 1996;62(5):369–372.

249. Stadler RF, Gregorcyk SG, Euhus DM, et al. Outcome of HIV-infected patients with invasive squamous-cell carcinoma of the anal canal in the era of highly active antiretroviral therapy. *Dis Colon Rectum.* 2004;47(8):1305–1309.

250. Stockmann M, Schmitz H, Fromm M, et al. Mechanisms of epithelial barrier impairment in HIV infection. *Ann N Y Acad Sci.* 2000;915:293–303.

251. Surawicz CM, Critchlow C, Sayer J, et al. High grade anal dysplasia in visually normal mucosa in homosexual men: seven cases. *Am J Gastroenterol.* 1995;90(10):1776–1778.

252. Sykes NL Jr. Condyloma acuminatum. *Int J Dermatol.* 1995;34(5):297–302.

253. Talal AH, Monard S, Vesanen M, et al. Virologic and immunologic effect of antiretroviral therapy on HIV-1 in gut-associated lymphoid tissue. *J Acquir Immune Defic Syndr.* 2001;26(1):1–7.

254. Teunissen MB. Dynamic nature and function of epidermal Langerhans cells in vivo and in vitro: a review, with emphasis on human Langerhans cells. *Histochem J.* 1992;24(10):697–716.

255. Thomas M, Massimi P, Jenkins J, et al. HPV-18 E6 mediated inhibition of p53 DNA binding activity is independent of E6 induced degradation. *Oncogene.* 1995;10(2):261–268.

256. Tincati C, Biasin M, Bandera A, et al. Early initiation of highly active antiretroviral therapy fails to reverse immunovirological abnormalities in gut-associated lymphoid tissue induced by acute HIV infection. *Antivir Ther.* 2009;14(3):321–330.

257. Tran HS, Moncure M, Tarnoff M, et al. Predictors of operative outcome in patients with human immunodeficiency virus infection and acquired immunodeficiency syndrome. *Am J Surg.* 2000;180(3):228–233.

258. Tyring S. Imiquimod applied topically: a novel immune response modifier. *Skin Therapy Lett.* 2001;6(6):1–4.

259. United States Public Health Service. Updated U.S. Public Health Service Guidelines for the management of occupational exposures to HBV, HCV, and HIV and recommendations for postexposure prophylaxis. *MMWR Recommen Rep.* 2001;50(RR-11):1–52.

260. Vaccher E, Spina M, Tirelli U. Clinical aspects and management of Hodgkin's disease and other tumours in HIV-infected individuals. *Eur J Cancer.* 2001;37(10):1306–1315.

261. van den Hoek JA, van Griensven GJ, Coutinho RA. Increase in unsafe homosexual behaviour. *Lancet.* 1990;336(8708):179–180.

262. Veazey RS, DeMaria M, Chalifoux LV, et al. Gastrointestinal tract as a major site of $CD4^+$ T cell depletion and viral replication in SIV infection. *Science.* 1998;280(5362):427–431.

263. Veazey RS, Marx PA, Lackner AA. Vaginal $CD4^+$ T cells express high levels of CCR5 and are rapidly depleted in simian immunodeficiency virus infection. *J Infect Dis.* 2003;187(5):769–776.

264. Veljkovic V, Metlas R, Raspopovic J, et al. Spectral and sequence similarity between vasoactive intestinal peptide and the second conserved region of human immunodeficiency virus type 1 envelope glycoprotein (gp120): possible consequences on prevention and therapy of AIDS. *Biochem Biophys Res Commun.* 1992;189(2):705–710.

265. Viamonte M, Dailey TH, Gottesman L. Ulcerative disease of the anorectum in the HIV^+ patient. *Dis Colon Rectum.* 1993;6(9):801–805.

266. Vogel J, Hinrichs SH, Reynolds RK, et al. The HIV tat gene induces dermal lesions resembling Kaposi's sarcoma in transgenic mice. *Nature.* 1998;335(6191):606–611.

267. Volberding PA, Mitsuyasu RT, Golando JP, et al. Treatment of Kaposi's sarcoma with interferon alpha-2b (Intron A). *Cancer.* 1987;59(suppl 3):620–625.

268. Von Roenn JH. Clinical presentations and standard therapy of AIDS-associated Kaposi's sarcoma. *Hematol Oncol Clin North Am.* 2003;17(3):747–762.

269. Wall SD, Friedman SL, Margulis AR. Gastrointestinal Kaposi's sarcoma in AIDS: radiographic manifestations. *J Clin Gastroenterol.* 1984;6(2):165–171.

270. Wallace M, Bower M, Allen-Mersh T. The severity of anal intraepithelial neoplasia is not affected by antiretroviral therapy in HIV positive men. *Dis Colon Rectum.* 2002;45:A30.

271. Wastell C, Corless D, Keeling N. Surgery and human immunodeficiency virus-1 infection. *Am J Surg.* 1996;172(1):89–92.

272. Weber JN, Carmichael DJ, Boylston A, et al. Kaposi's sarcoma of the bowel—presenting as apparent ulcerative colitis. *Gut.* 1985;26(3):295–300.

273. Weber R, Bryan RT, Owen RL, et al. Improved light-microscopical detection of microsporidia spores in stool and duodenal aspirates. The Enteric Opportunistic Infections Working Group. *N Engl J Med.* 1992;326(3):161–166.

274. Webster GF. Local therapy for mucocutaneous Kaposi's sarcoma in patient's with acquired immunodeficiency syndrome. *Dermatol Surg.* 1995;21(3):205–208.

275. Weiss EG, Wexner SD. Surgery for anal lesions in the HIV-infected patients. *Ann Med.* 1995;27(4):467–475.

276. Welch HA, Salahuddin SZ, Gill P, et al. AIDS-associated Kaposi's sarcoma-derived cells in long-term culture express and synthesize smooth muscle alpha-actin. *Am J Pathol.* 1991;139(6):1251–1258.

277. Weller IV. The gay bowel. *Gut.* 1985;26(9):869–875.

278. Weprin L, Zollinger R, Clausen K, et al. Kaposi's sarcoma: endoscopic observations of gastric and colon involvement. *J Clin Gastroenterol.* 1982;4(4):357–360.

279. Wexler A, Berson AM, Goldstone SE, et al. Invasive anal squamous-cell carcinoma in the HIV-positive patient: outcome in the era of highly active antiretroviral therapy. *Dis Colon Rectum.* 2008;51(1):73–81.

280. Wexner SD. Sexually transmitted diseases of the colon, rectum, and anus. The challenge of the nineties. *Dis Colon Rectum.* 1990;33(12):1048–1062.

281. Wexner SD, Smithy WB, Milsom JW, et al. The surgical management of anorectal diseases in AIDS and pre-AIDS patients. *Dis Colon Rectum.* 1986;29(11):719–723.

282. Wexner SD, Smithy WB, Trillo C, et al. Emergency colectomy for cytomegalovirus ileocolitis in patients with the acquired immune deficiency syndrome. *Dis Colon Rectum.* 1988;31(10):755–761.

283. Wheat J. Endemic mycoses in AIDS: a clinical review. *Clin Microbiol Rev.* 1995;8(1):146–159.

284. Wilcox CM, Chalasani N, Lazenby A, et al. Cytomegalovirus colitis in acquired immunodeficiency syndrome: a clinical and endoscopic study. *Gastrointest Endosc.* 1998;48(1):39–43.

285. Wilcox CM, Rabeneck L, Friedman S. AGA technical review: malnutrition and cachexia, chronic diarrhea, and hepatobiliary disease in patients with human immunodeficiency virus infection. *Gastroenterology.* 1996;111(6):1724–1752.

286. Williams GR, Talbott IC. Anal carcinoma—a histological review. *Histopathology.* 1994;25(6):507–516.

287. Wilson SE, Robinson G, Williams RA, et al. Acquired immune deficiency syndrome (AIDS). Indications for abdominal surgery, pathology, and outcome. *Ann Surg.* 1989;210(4):428–434.

288. Wolkomir AF, Barone JE, Hardy HW III, et al. Abdominal and anorectal surgery and the acquired immune deficiency syndrome in heterosexual intravenous drug users. *Dis Colon Rectum.* 1990;33(4):267–270.

289. Workowski KA, Levine WC. Selected topics from the Centers for Disease Control and Prevention sexually transmitted diseases treatment guidelines 2002. *HIV Clin Trials.* 2002;3(5):421–433.

290. World Health Organization. The top 10 causes of death. http://www.who.int/mediacentre/factsheets/fs310/en/index.html. Updated June 2011. Accessed June 12, 2011.

291. Yii MK, Saunder A, Scott DF. Abdominal surgery in HIV/AIDS patients: indications, operative management, pathology and outcome. *Aust N Z J Surg.* 1995;65(5):320–326.

292. Yinnon AM, Coury-Donger P, Polito R, et al. Serologic response to treatment of syphilis in patients with HIV infection. *Arch Intern Med.* 1996;156(3):321–325.

293. Yoshida D, Caruso JM. Abdominal pain in the HIV infected patient. *J Emerg Med.* 2002;23(2):111–116.

294. Zaunders J, Carr A, McNally L, et al. Effects of primary HIV-1 infection on subsets of $CD4^+$ and $CD8^+$ T lymphocytes. *AIDS.* 1995;9(6):561–566.

295. Zeitz M, Greene WC, Peffer NJ, et al. Lymphocytes isolated from the intestinal lamina propria of normal nonhuman primates have increased expression of genes associated with T-cell activation. *Gastroenterology.* 1988;94(3):647–655.

296. Zierdt CH, Gill VJ, Zierdt WS. Detection of microsporidian spores in clinical samples by indirect fluorescent-antibody assay using whole-cell antisera to *Encephalitozoon cuniculi* and *Encephalitozoon hellem. J Clin Microbiol.* 1993;31(11):3071–3074.

11

Hemorrhoids

Marvin L. Corman

And the men that died not were smitten with the emerods; and the cry of the city went up to heaven.
—1 Samuel 5:12*

*It is always stimulating to receive comments from readers of prior editions, especially those that are not merely flattering but from which I may learn of mistakes and omissions. The following communication was received from Professor Samuel Argov in Haifa, Israel.

MLC

I read the Bible in its original Hebrew, and, being a colorectal surgeon, I have investigated the story of the Holy Ark, the Philistines, and the Israelites, as narrated in Samuel 1, Chapters 5, 6. It would appear that the Philistines were struck by an epidemic which is almost certainly bubonic plague, caused by *Yersinia pestis*. As is well-known, the disease is transmitted by mice and rats through their fleas. The epidemic swept quickly through the population (Samuel 1, Chapters 5, 11, 12). It is difficult to conceive of an epidemic of hemorrhoids. The fact that the Philistines gave an offering of five golden mice implies that they knew the pathogenesis of the plague (Samuel 1, Chapter 6, verse 4). This confusion of interpretation arises from an early incorrect translation of the Hebrew word *Tchorim* by the vulgata and later copiers to mean hemorrhoids. In actuality, the original Hebrew word *Tchorim* meant a ball or bubo. The mistake was carried forward into modern Hebrew. Even today in Israel, everyone uses the biblical term for the wrong disease.

Hemorrhoid disease affects more than 1 million Americans per year.[37] It has been estimated that over a period of 3 years, approximately 4.4% of the US population will have symptoms attributed to hemorrhoids.[142] Although the condition is rarely life threatening, the complications of therapy can be. This fact led to the beatification of St. Fiachre, the patron saint of gardeners and hemorrhoid sufferers.[239,269] From the patient's perspective, the complaint of "hemorrhoids" simply represents the diagnosis for a host of anal problems, including itching, a lump, pain, swelling, bleeding, and protrusion. In most physicians' office practices, it is as likely that an individual's symptoms will be attributable to another cause as they are to hemorrhoids.

Hemorrhoid complaints are one of the most common afflictions of Western civilization. The problem can occur at any age and can affect both sexes. It has been estimated that at least 50% of individuals older than the age of 50 years have at some time experienced symptoms related to hemorrhoids. Johanson and Sonnenberg analyzed data from governmental sources and concluded that the prevalence rate in the United States is 4.4%.[142] In their study, Whites were affected more frequently than African Americans, and there was an increased frequency in those of higher socioeconomic status. It is also more common in rural than in urban areas. Some reports have commented on the relative rarity of the condition in rural Africa.[43]

The following have been suggested as factors that contribute to the development of hemorrhoids:

• Heredity
• Anatomic features
• Nutrition

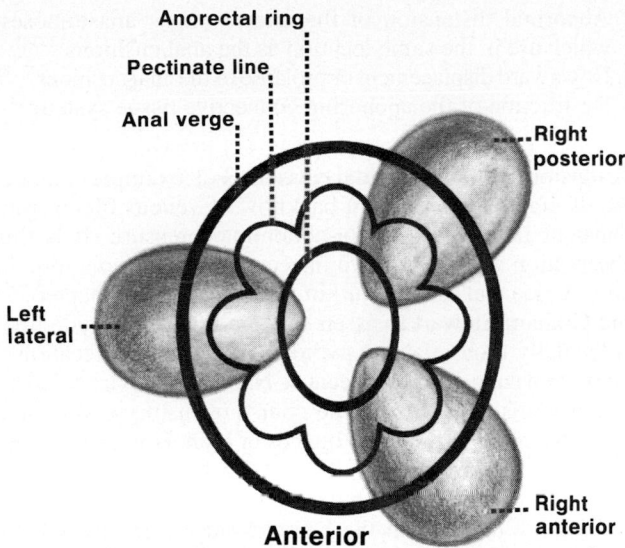

FIGURE 11-1. The three primary hemorrhoidal groups.

- Occupation
- Climate
- Psychological problems
- Senility
- Endocrine changes
- Food and drugs
- Infection
- Pregnancy
- Exercise
- Coughing
- Straining
- Vomiting
- Constrictive clothing
- Constipation[19,79]

Burkitt and Graham-Stewart refute most of these concepts and provide their own theories of pathogenesis (see the following section).[43] This report and those of others have clarified the anatomy and attempted to establish the etiology on a more scientific footing.

▶ ETIOLOGY AND ANATOMY

In 1975, Thomson published his master's thesis based on anatomic and radiologic studies and introduced the term *vascular cushions*.[290] According to this theory, the submucosa does not form a continuous ring of thickened tissue in the anal canal, but rather a discontinuous series of cushions; the three main cushions are found in the left lateral, right anterior, and right posterior positions (Figure 11-1). The submucosal layer of each of these thicker regions is rich with blood vessels and muscle fibers, the latter known as the *muscularis submucosa* (Figure 11-2).[225,312] These fibers, arising from the internal sphincter and from the conjoined longitudinal muscle, are important in maintaining adherence of mucosal and submucosal tissues to the underlying internal sphincter and in supporting the blood vessels of the submucosa. It is postulated that the cushions, by filling with blood during the act of defecation, protect the anal canal from injury. The muscularis submucosa and its connective tissue fibers return the anal canal lining to its initial position after the temporary downward displacement that occurs during defecation.

The anal cushions receive their blood supply primarily from the terminal branches of the superior hemorrhoidal artery (i.e., superior rectal artery) and, to a lesser extent, from branches of the middle hemorrhoidal arteries.[32,225] These branches communicate with one another and with branches of the inferior hemorrhoidal arteries, which supply the lower portion of the anal canal. The superior, middle, and inferior hemorrhoidal veins, which drain blood from the

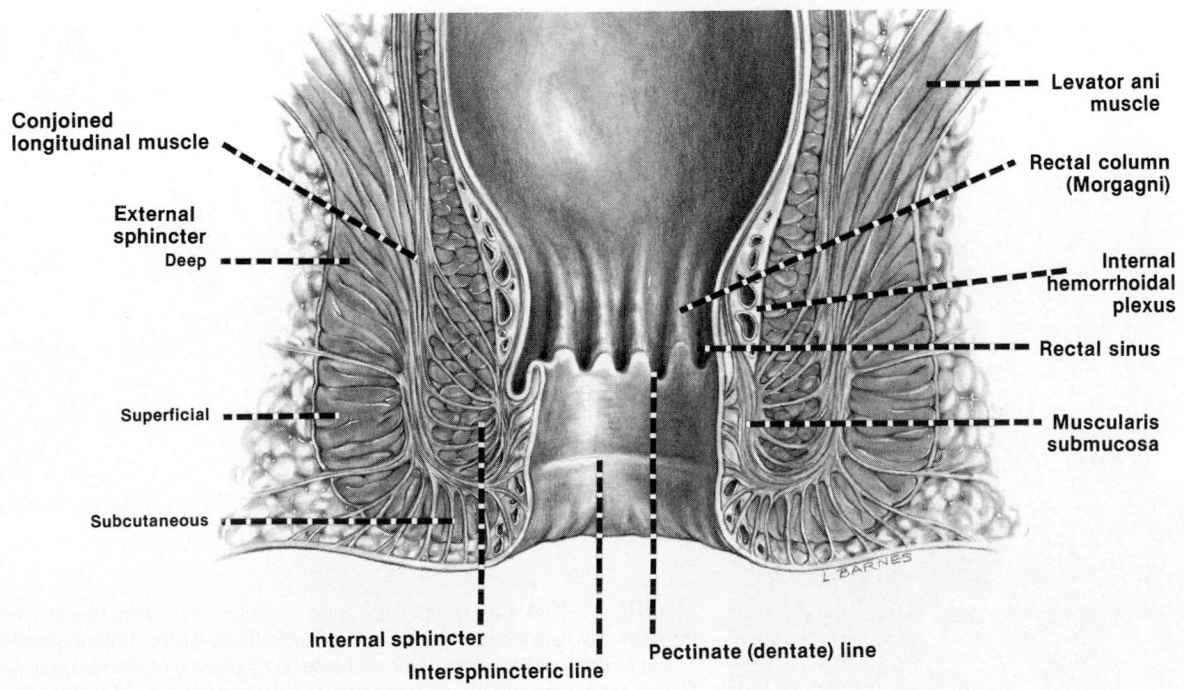

FIGURE 11-2. Anatomy of the anal region.

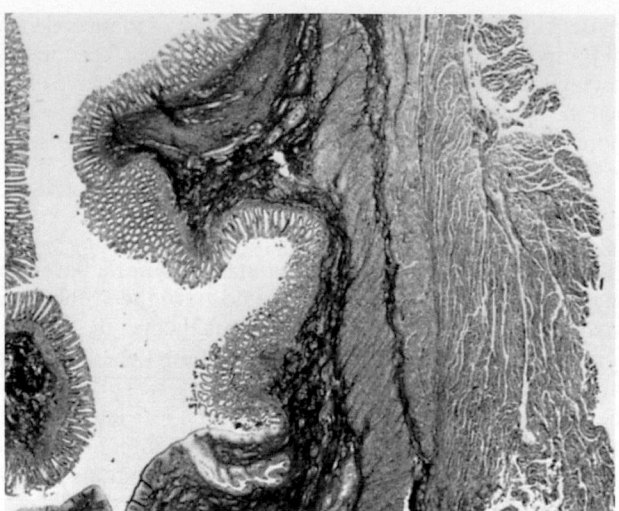

FIGURE 11-3. Longitudinal section through the anal canal of a newborn. Note the well-organized, firm connective tissue fibers that support the vessels within the hemorrhoidal pad and anchor them to the internal sphincter and conjoined longitudinal muscle. (Original magnification × 16; courtesy of Peter A. Haas, MD.)

tissues of the anal canal, correspond to each of the hemorrhoidal arteries.[32,126,225]

Anatomic studies by Haas and colleagues reveal that anchoring and supporting tissue deteriorates with aging, and that this phenomenon becomes apparent in the third decade of life (Figure 11-3).[124] This ultimately produces venous distension, erosion, bleeding, and thrombosis (Figure 11-4).

The following are the four major theories regarding the causes of hemorrhoids.

1. Abnormal dilatation of the veins of the internal hemorrhoidal venous plexus, a network of the tributaries of the superior and middle hemorrhoidal veins[43,223]

2. Abnormal distension of the arteriovenous anastomoses, which are in the same location as the anal cushions[126,127]
3. Downward displacement or prolapse of the anal cushions[77,289]
4. Destruction of the anchoring connective tissue system[124]

Other theories have been proposed to explain abnormal distension of hemorrhoidal vessels. For example, hemorrhoids may be caused by a backflow of venous blood from transient increases in intra-abdominal pressure. It is this observation and the relative infrequency of the condition in rural Africa that caused Burkitt (see Biography, Chapter 27) and Graham-Stewart to assert the importance of crude fiber in the daily food intake to avoid straining with defecation.[43] They even suggested that because Napoleon was troubled by hemorrhoids at Waterloo, the course of history could have been changed but for a few ounces of bran. However, others have called the presumption of causality between straining or constipation and hemorrhoids into question.[142]

Pressure exerted on the hemorrhoidal veins by a fetus explains the exacerbation of the condition in pregnant women.[176,226] Engorgement of vessels may result from a defect in venous drainage, which, in turn, may be caused by failure of the internal sphincter to relax as it should during defecation. Vascular distension may be attributed to augmented arterial flow; this would account for why some with hemorrhoids feel additional discomfort after a heavy meal. More blood is delivered to the digestive system through the mesenteric artery, of which the superior hemorrhoidal artery is a branch.[281] Hemorrhoids, however, are not varicose veins. They are structures that are normally present but do not produce symptoms until the fibromuscular supporting tissue above the cushions deteriorates.[34] This permits the cushions to slide, engorge, prolapse, and bleed.

Hemorrhoids may be caused by more than one factor. Although some evidence suggests that hemorrhoids are familial, it is not known whether this is caused by hereditary influences (e.g., weak-walled veins, atrophied or weakened

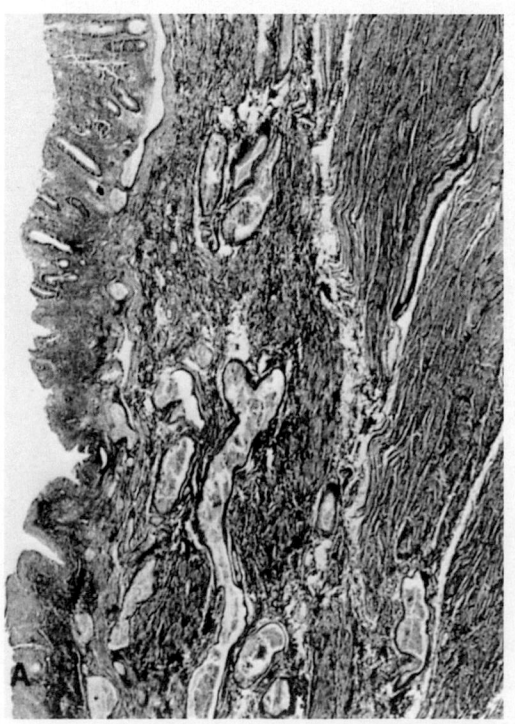

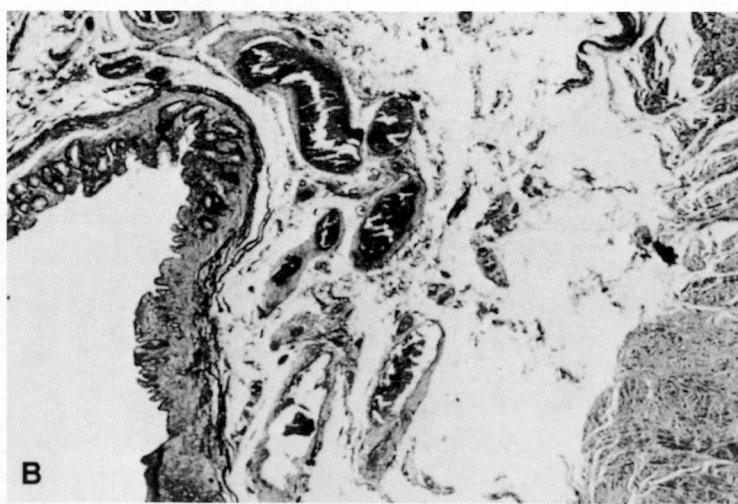

FIGURE 11-4. **A:** Early disintegration of the connective tissue fibers. Venous sinuses in the submucosa have lost their support and are moderately distended. (Original magnification × 16.) **B:** Complete breakdown of the anchoring and supporting connective tissue system. Mucosa and perianal skin are separated from the internal sphincter. (Original magnification × 20; courtesy of Peter A. Haas, MD.)

fibrocollagenous supporting tissue) or environmental factors (e.g., family members may have similar dietary or bowel habits).

Despite a vast literature on the subject of hemorrhoids, the pathogenesis and even the function of this tissue remain controversial. Furthermore, there still exists a difference of opinion as to the definition of hemorrhoidal disease. The high prevalence of anoscopic evidence of this pathologic entity and its problematic relationship to symptoms suggests that perhaps these findings may be more a consequence of the aging process than truly a disease entity.[172]

Wexner and Baig opine, however, that hemorrhoidal tissue performs three main functions besides that of the veins providing drainage of blood from the area.[306] These functions theoretically include the following:

- Maintenance of continence through the filling of the vascular cushions (15% to 20% of resting anal pressures)
- "Protection" of the sphincter mechanism by providing a cushion
- Augmentation of the anal closure mechanism[306]

Portal Hypertension and Rectal Varices

What is the relationship of hemorrhoids to portal hypertension? The most common manifestation of hemorrhage in patients with liver disease is upper gastrointestinal bleeding, not lower gastrointestinal bleeding. Numerous studies have failed to demonstrate an increased incidence of hemorrhoids in this population. However, rectal varices may be seen as enlarged portal-systemic collateral veins in patients with portal hypertension.[304] This collateral circulation from the portal vein passes into the systemic circulation through the middle and inferior hemorrhoidal veins. In other words, hemorrhoids and rectal varices must be recognized as two separate entities. Hosking and colleagues evaluated 100 consecutive patients with cirrhosis and noted that 44% had anorectal varices.[134] Goenka and associates performed a prospective study to evaluate the prevalence of this finding in 75 individuals with known portal hypertension.[115] Sixty-seven (89.3%) were demonstrated to have lower gastrointestinal varices, the rectum being the most common site. There was no correlation, however, between the presence of these varices and the severity of esophagogastric mucosal changes of portal hypertension.

It is essential to differentiate anorectal varices from bleeding hemorrhoids because the treatment is so obviously different. Endoscopic ultrasonography and magnetic resonance imaging are noninvasive modalities for diagnosis and control after treatment.[91]

Bleeding from varices may be treated by transanal suture technique, by transhepatic inferior mesenteric venography and embolization, or by any one of the methods of portal-systemic shunting and decompression.[91,135,205,304]

PHYSIOLOGY

The anal sphincters of many patients with hemorrhoids demonstrate an abnormal rhythm of contraction and exert a greater force of contraction than those of asymptomatic control subjects. Whether this sphincter abnormality is a cause or an effect of hemorrhoids is not known, but it may relate to any of the hypotheses outlined. An overactive sphincter could contribute to venous congestion, expose the anal cushions to greater shearing forces, or do both by constricting the anal canal.[12,125] Objective anorectal manometric studies reveal increased anal canal pressure in patients with symptomatic hemorrhoids when they are compared with control subjects.[88,129,284] Sun and colleagues performed a combined manometric and ultrasonographic study of the internal anal sphincter in 20 individuals with hemorrhoids and in 20 age-matched normal controls.[283] As expected, mean basal anal pressures were significantly higher in the patients with hemorrhoids than in the control patients. The mean maximal residual pressure was significantly higher in these individuals. Furthermore, direct pressure measurement in the anal canal cushions of the patients with hemorrhoids demonstrated abnormally high median pressure in comparison with that in controls. However, ultrasonographic study of the anal canal revealed a clear image of the internal sphincter that could easily be measured and was essentially no different from that of controls. The authors conclude that the absence of any significant differences in internal sphincter thickness between subjects without hemorrhoids and patients with hemorrhoids suggests that the high anal pressure observed in those with hemorrhoids is of a vascular origin.[283] This elevated pressure usually returns to normal levels following hemorrhoidectomy.

The hypothesis that this condition results from chronic constipation was investigated by Gibbons and colleagues, who studied bowel habits, anal pressure profiles, and anal compliance.[110] Hemorrhoids were associated with significantly longer anal high-pressure zones and significantly greater maximal resting pressures at all levels of anal distension. However, constipated women had normal pressure profiles and pressures. The study affirmed that patients with hemorrhoids are not necessarily constipated, and that chronically constipated individuals do not necessarily have hemorrhoids.

Other physiologic studies have been performed on patients with enlarged, symptomatic hemorrhoids. Various abnormalities have been reported, including increased electromyographic activity, increased external sphincter fiber density, prolonged pudendal nerve terminal motor latencies, reduced anal electrosensitivity, reduced temperature sensation, and reduced rectal compliance.[306]

CLASSIFICATION

Hemorrhoids are classified by location (i.e., external, internal, or mixed) or by degree (i.e., first, second, third, and fourth).[101] External hemorrhoids arise from the inferior hemorrhoidal plexus and are covered by modified squamous epithelium. They occur below the pectinate line and may become thrombotic and ulcerate. Internal hemorrhoids occur above the pectinate line. They may prolapse, ulcerate, bleed, and/or thrombose. They may be reducible or irreducible. Internal hemorrhoids arise from the superior hemorrhoidal plexus and are covered by mucosa. Mixed hemorrhoids (i.e., external-internal) may be prolapsed, irreducible, thrombosed, or ulcerated. They arise from the inferior and superior hemorrhoidal plexus and their anastomotic connections.

A grading system has been established for hemorrhoids, but this classification applies only to the internal variety. In first-degree hemorrhoids, the veins of the anal canal are increased in number and size, and they may bleed at the time of defecation. They do not prolapse but merely project into the lumen. Second-degree hemorrhoids present to the outside of the anal canal during defecation but return spontaneously to within the anal canal where they remain the rest of the time. Third-degree hemorrhoids protrude outside the anal canal and require manual reduction. Fourth-degree hemorrhoids are irreducible and constantly remain in the prolapsed state.

External Hemorrhoids

Two types of hemorrhoids are found at the external anal orifice. One occurs predominantly in the form of dilatation and engorgement of the veins beneath the skin, and the other is manifested as a thrombosis of these veins. When the clot forms, the patient becomes aware of its presence. The degree of pain depends on the size of the clot and the relationship it bears to the anal sphincters. A large clot will cause pain, but even if a clot is small, it can be quite uncomfortable if it lies within the anal musculature. Small, thrombosed hemorrhoids rarely ulcerate and bleed.

When the process spreads into external and internal tissue surrounding hemorrhoidal veins, considerable external swelling develops as edematous fluid fills the subcutaneous area at the anal margin. This may result in acute external and internal hemorrhoidal venous thrombosis and prolapse.

External Tags or Skin Tabs

External tags or skin tabs are deformities of the skin of the external anal margin and occur as redundant folds (Figure 11-5). These may be the residual of prior thrombosed hemorrhoids that have become organized into fibrous appendages. More than likely the patient will have no antecedent history that would suggest the origin of the tags. Women, however, will often state that the tags arose during pregnancy, especially during the third trimester, persisting following delivery.[18]

The practice of removing hemorrhoids in three primary groups usually leaves bridges of tissue between the sites of the hemorrhoidal masses. When hemorrhoid disease is extensive, some of the diseased veins remain beneath these bridges of skin; these, too, may become fibrous skin tags after the wounds have healed (discussed later in this chapter).

Internal Hemorrhoids

The usual internal hemorrhoid is not evident on visual inspection of the anal area, especially if the patient is not bearing down. When an individual strains, a bulging mass may

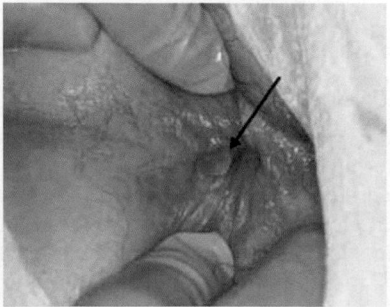

FIGURE 11-5. Anal tag (*arrow*). (From Pfenninger JL, Zainea GG. Common anorectal conditions: part II. Lesions. *Am Fam Physician.* 2001;64(1):77–88.)

appear that involves all or part of the anal canal. The full extent of pressure is exerted on the anorectal outlet only during defecation or straining. Therefore, a truly reliable examination cannot be made with the patient in either the recumbent or the inverted jackknife position. Optimally, to assess the full extent of the process, examination with the patient seated on a commode is preferred.

Thrombosed Hemorrhoids

Thrombosed hemorrhoids (i.e., clotted hemorrhoids) are seen most often in patients who strain while defecating or when lifting heavy objects; those who have frequent bowel actions, such as occurs with inflammatory bowel disease or malabsorption; and those who sit for long periods (e.g., long-distance truck drivers, motorcycle policemen, airline pilots, operators of heavy construction equipment). Theoretically, direct trauma to the area creates an inflammatory response, which leads to thrombosis. Additionally, the Valsalva action during straining can lead to protrusion, which, if irreducible, can precipitate this complication. Stasis of the blood flow during straining is another possible explanation.

One of the most common etiologic associations of thrombosed hemorrhoids is the maintenance of a "library" in the toilet. Virtually every patient who experiences recurrent thromboses will harbor such a home resource. Death from Fournier's gangrene has been reported in a nonoperated patient with thrombosed hemorrhoids,[30] but this must be a unique occurrence and calls into question the issue of the person being immunocompromised.

▶ DIFFERENTIAL DIAGNOSIS

Polyp, Adenoma, and Carcinoma

Sessile, polypoid masses (e.g., adenomas), and carcinomas, which are easily palpated or seen, should be readily differentiated from hemorrhoidal tissue. Internal hemorrhoids uncomplicated by thrombosis, edema, prolapse, or other factors are usually simple to diagnose. However, biopsy and microscopic study of any suspicious lesion are essential to establish the diagnosis with certainty. The old adage, "when in doubt, biopsy," is worth remembering.

Hypertrophied Anal Papilla

A firm mass that seems to arise from an attached pedicle in the region of the dentate line is most likely to represent a hypertrophied anal papilla (Figures 11-6 and 11-7; see Figure 12-3). Anoscopy will clarify any confusion by revealing that the pedicle arises from the dentate margin and that the entire lesion is invested by skin.

Rectal Prolapse

Rectal prolapse may be either partial, involving only the mucosal layer of the rectal wall, or complete, involving the full thickness. Partial prolapse may affect either part or all of the circumference of the anal outlet. Differentiating prolapsed internal hemorrhoids from partial or mucosal prolapse may be somewhat confusing at times, but internal hemorrhoids are separated by sulci that radiate peripherally from the center of the anal outlet, whereas mucosal prolapse usually exhibits a more uniformly concentric protrusion.

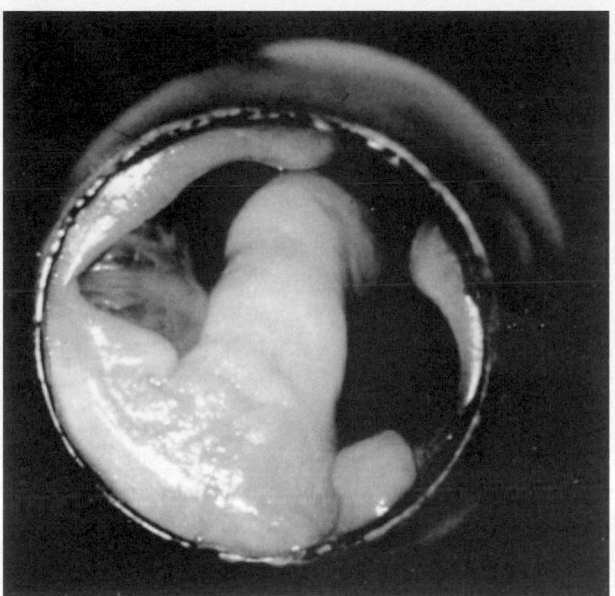

FIGURE 11-6. Anoscopic view of hypertrophied anal papilla. (Courtesy of Elliot D. Prager, MD.)

Often there is some element of mucosal prolapse when a circumferential rosette of hemorrhoids becomes irreducible and thrombosed (Figure 11-8). Complete rectal prolapse, however, should be readily distinguished by its concentrically arranged mucosal folds, which are strikingly different from the radiating sulci separating prolapsed internal hemorrhoids.

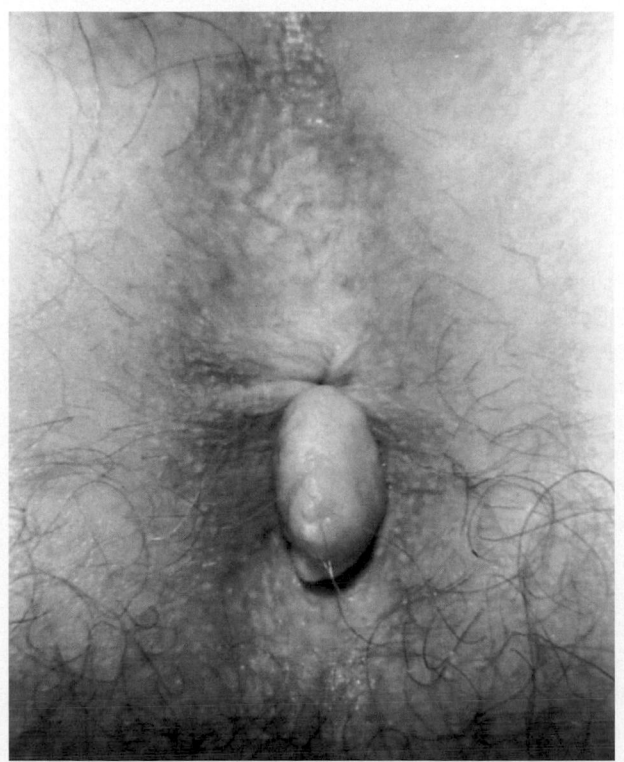

FIGURE 11-7. Prolapsed hypertrophied anal papilla. The fact that the lesion is covered by skin should eliminate confusion regarding the diagnosis.

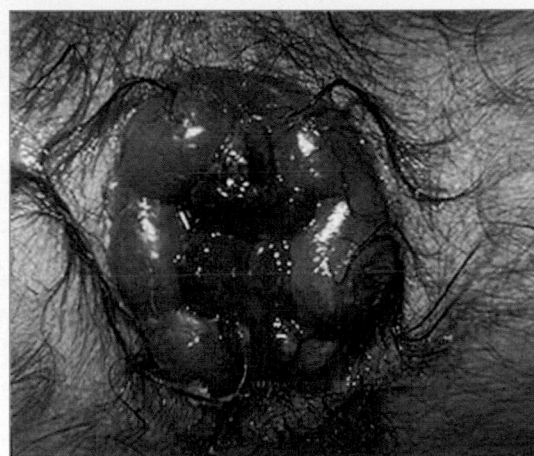

FIGURE 11-8. Prolapsed, thrombosed hemorrhoids. These are irreducible and have an element of mucosal prolapse.

► SIGNS AND SYMPTOMS

The most common presenting complaint of patients with hemorrhoids is bleeding. This usually occurs during or after defecation and is exacerbated by straining and by frequent bowel actions. Blood can be evident on the paper, in the toilet bowl, or both. Occasionally, blood loss may be severe enough to produce profound anemia. Pain is usually not caused by hemorrhoids, unless the hemorrhoidal vein is thrombosed, ulcerated, or gangrenous. The most common cause of anal pain is fissure. Prolapse, either with spontaneous return or requiring manual reduction, is a common presentation of hemorrhoids. The hemorrhoids may also be irreducible. Pruritus ani is often attributed to hemorrhoids, but frequently the examination fails to reveal significant hemorrhoidal disease. That is why, unfortunately, many patients who undergo operative hemorrhoidectomy for this indication discover that the pruritic symptoms persist. Pruritus ani is a condition whose treatment includes diet, bowel management, anal hygiene, and perhaps medication (see Chapter 9).

Constipation is not a symptom of hemorrhoids, but defecation may be difficult when thrombosis or gangrene produces pain. Patients tend to avoid the toilet if hemorrhoidal symptoms are exacerbated by defecation; this can lead to refusal of the urge to pass stool and can result in constipation or even obstipation.

► EXAMINATION

Physical examination should include proctosigmoidoscopy and anoscopy. Colonoscopy or a barium enema study must be performed in all patients who have rectal bleeding when the source is not readily apparent from these examinations. In patients older than 50 years of age, an evaluation of the colon should be performed at some time, even if hemorrhoids are the apparent cause of the patient's symptoms. This may be deferred if an individual's symptoms or inconvenience preclude carrying out such studies at the time of the examination.

Kluiber and Wolff at the Mayo Clinic in Rochester, Minnesota reviewed in a retrospective fashion the incidence of hemorrhoidal bleeding that produced anemia.[158] The incidence of bleeding attributed to hemorrhoids that caused anemia was found to be 0.5/100,000 population per year in Olmsted County, Minnesota from 1976 to 1990. The authors found that recovery from anemia after definitive treatment by means of hemorrhoidectomy was quite rapid. From a mean hemoglobin concentration before treatment of 9.4 g/dL, it was found that the hemoglobin concentration increased to 12.3 g/dL after 2 months. By 6 months, the mean hemoglobin concentration was 14.1 g/dL. The authors concluded that failure to recover hemoglobin concentration should prompt further or repeated evaluation for other causes of the anemia.[158]

▶ GENERAL PRINCIPLES OF TREATMENT

Bleeding

Bleeding, if occasional and related to straining or to diarrhea, can often be managed without specific treatment of the hemorrhoids; in other words, treatment should be directed to the cause of the bleeding. Constipation may be controlled by appropriate dietary measures, a bowel management program, stool softeners, laxatives, or a combination of these. Moesgaard and colleagues, in a prospective double-blind trial of a bulk agent (i.e., psyllium) versus a placebo in patients with bleeding and pain at defecation, noted a statistically significant difference in improvement of symptoms during a 6-week period ($P < .025$).[192] They recommended the use of a high-fiber diet as the initial approach to the treatment of patients with symptomatic hemorrhoids. Diarrhea or frequent defecation may be managed with antidiarrheal medications and diet. Attention should also be given to improvement of anal hygiene. No less a sage than Moses Maimonides wrote in the 12th century of the importance of the nonoperative management of hemorrhoids.

The use of commercial topical creams, lotions, and suppositories is worthy of comment. These preparations include Tucks pads and cream, Anusol cream and suppositories, Balneol lotion, Prax, ProctoFoam, Calmol 4, micronized purified flavonoid fractions, and the most ubiquitous self-medication employed by the average American for "symptomatic hemorrhoids," Preparation H. Preparation H has been alleged in the past to contain shark liver oil as well as a "skin respiratory factor" of unknown formulation that is supposed to improve wound healing. Its active ingredient today is phenylephrine hydrochloride (0.25%), a vasoconstrictor that may lead to temporary relief of burning and itching. Subramanyam and colleagues created rectal ulcers by performing rectal biopsy on volunteer subjects, determined the speed of healing with use of this product in suppository form, and compared it with a placebo.[282] Although healing was quicker and more complete in the Preparation H group, the number of patients in the study was too small to achieve statistical significance. In my personal opinion, Preparation H acts essentially to soothe skin irritation and is as effective for this purpose as virtually any topical cream, lotion, or ointment. Symptoms of pruritus ani may be ameliorated, but there is no evidence that Preparation H causes hemorrhoids to shrink. There are also commercially available mechanical devices and products that are used to facilitate cleansing of the anus, such as mini-bidets, the Shower Mini, and the Water-pic.

MOSES MAIMONIDES (1138–1204)

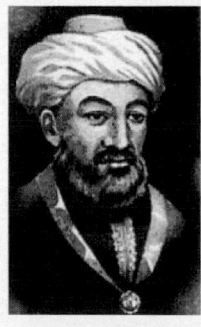

Maimonides' full Arabic name was Abū ʿImrān Mūsā bin Maimūn bin ʿUbaidallāh al-Qurṭubī, or Mūsā ibn Maymūn in short. His full Hebrew name was Rabbi Moshe ben Maimon whose acronym forms "Rambam," his nickname. In Latin, the Hebrew "ben" (son of) becomes the Greek-style suffix "-ides" to form "Moses Maimonides." He was born in Cordova, Spain in 1138. His family was forced into exile in 1148, finally settling in Fez, Morocco after traveling for 10 years. Little is known of Maimonides' formal education, but it is thought that he was essentially self-educated, evincing knowledge of Greek and Muslim writers. Hippocrates, Galen, Aristotle, Al Rhazes, and Ibn Zuhr were quoted frequently in his works. Maimonides moved again in 1165 to Fustat (now part of Old Cairo). He was later appointed court physician to the Regent of Egypt while the sultan was fighting in the crusades, and later became physician to the sultan's son. He was also known for declining an offer from Richard the Lionhearted to be his personal physician. Maimonides was well recognized as a spiritual leader of the Jewish community in Egypt. He was one of history's most famous rabbis. He wrote numerous books, the most famous of which was the *Mishneh Torah* ("Repetition of the Torah"). Compiled between 1170 and 1180, this code of Jewish religious law (*Halakha*) in 14 books is regarded as Maimonides' *magnum opus*. He also wrote 10 medical works. His fourth such effort was a *Treatise on Hemorrhoids*, written for a nobleman who was thought to be a member of the sultan's family. The paper provides an early insight into the etiology and management of hemorrhoids. Maimonides believed that surgery should be reserved for severe hemorrhoids or "closed" type (strangulated hemorrhoids). He describes the importance of changes to one's lifestyle, diet alteration to soften stool, topical treatments, and fumigation. Maimonides died on December 12, 1204. He was buried in Tiberias, in what is now a city on the western shore of the Sea of Galilee, Israel. (Magrill D, Sekaran P. Maimonides: an early but accurate view on the treatment of haemorrhoids. *Postgrad Med J.* 2007;83(979):352–354; Rosner F. *The Medical Legacy of Moses Maimonides*. Hoboken, NJ: KTAV Publishing House; 1998; Davidson HA. *Moses Maimonides, The Man and His Works*. New York, NY: Oxford University Press; 2005; Picture. htpp://www.pneuro. com/publications/oaths/ [Courtesy of Hussna Wakily, MD.])

Suppositories have been employed since the civilization of ancient Egypt for three basic reasons:

- To promote defecation
- To introduce medications into the body
- To treat anorectal disease[19]

It is difficult to assess the actual efficacy of suppositories regarding this last condition. Because the anorectal disease is often self-limited, resolution may occur irrespective of this treatment. Furthermore, the physician cannot gainsay the psychological benefit that vigorous promotional effort of such products produces for the patient. Finally, the bullet-shaped suppository often used in the treatment of anal conditions cannot exert its primary benefit within the anal canal because it must advance at least as far as the rectum. To be truly useful, Banov suggested that the suppository be hourglass or collar button shaped to maintain effective contact with the anal mucosa.[22] Such a modification has yet to be produced.

If bleeding persists despite the foregoing approaches, some form of interventional treatment should be offered. If the patient believes that bleeding is caused by hemorrhoids and does not seek medical attention, or if the surgeon accepts this diagnosis without attempting to address the bleeding, a neoplasm may develop and go unrecognized. Such a situation could jeopardize the opportunity for early diagnosis and treatment.

Prolapse

Prolapsed hemorrhoids that return spontaneously or are manually reducible can usually be treated by a number of the office procedures discussed later. Attempting reduction is important because persistent prolapse predisposes the patient to thrombosis and possibly even necrosis. If the prolapse is irreducible or if an external component is present, an excisional approach may be indicated.

Pain

If pain is caused by gangrenous, ulcerated, or thrombosed hemorrhoids, a surgical procedure is the best means of treatment. If symptomatic or extensive hemorrhoids are associated with an anal fissure, hemorrhoidectomy should be considered and the fissure treated by internal anal sphincterotomy (discussed later in this chapter; see also Chapter 12). A thrombosed external hemorrhoid that produces pain is ideally managed by local excision.

The physician should consider the value of warm sitz baths in the treatment of any anal problem. Subjectively, there is little question that pain is ameliorated by the application of heat. Studies suggest there may be an explanation for how heat contributes to this response. Dodi and colleagues performed anorectal manometry on volunteers and on patients with anorectal problems (e.g., hemorrhoids, anal fissure) and determined pressure changes after immersion in warm (40° C) and cold (5° C and 23° C) water.[84] In all subjects, a statistically significant decrease in resting pressure was observed after immersion in the warm water. No change was seen when patients were exposed to the colder temperatures. Because individuals with certain anal conditions often have elevated pressures, the lowering of resting anal canal pressure probably produces the observed symptomatic improvement.

▶ AMBULATORY TREATMENT

In 1993, practice parameters for ambulatory anorectal surgery were established by the Standards Task Force of the American Society of Colon and Rectal Surgeons (ASCRS) and were subsequently revised in 2003.[59,279] A disclaimer was incorporated recognizing that the guidelines were not inclusive of all proper methods and did not exclude other reasonable options. Their purpose is to provide information on which decisions can be made rather than dictate a specific form of treatment.[59] Cataldo and coworkers authored another set of parameters in 2005 for the management of hemorrhoids on behalf of the ASCRS.[46] Fundamentally, they concluded that the ultimate judgment regarding the propriety of any specific procedure falls within the purview of the treating physician. The subject of *parameters* and *guidelines* is discussed in other chapters where such management issues are addressed.

Gastroenterologists, internists, and family practitioners have all invaded the hitherto sacrosanct domain of the surgeon through the invasive treatment of hemorrhoids. This contemporary change seems reasonable when specialized training that nonsurgeons may receive in the management of other invasive techniques is considered.[265] In fact, some of the tools that are advocated for the outpatient treatment of hemorrhoids are directly marketed to nonsurgeons by mail and at meetings and conventions. I believe that it is fitting and proper for any physician to perform many of the following discussed procedures, with the proviso that they are held to the same standards of care that are demanded of surgeons. Likewise, surgeons must be held to the very same criteria for competence as are gastroenterologists when they perform colonoscopy or colonoscopy-polypectomy.

Sclerotherapy: Injection Treatment of Hemorrhoids

The first attempt to obliterate hemorrhoids by means of injection was reported in 1869 by John Morgan. Morgan used iron persulfate to treat external hemorrhoids, varicose veins, and vascular lesions. In 1871, this unique form of therapy, using phenol and other chemical agents, was introduced in the United States. It was advertised as a "painless cure for piles without surgery (probably from the Latin, *pila* "a ball" presumably because of the shape)."[10] Because specula were not available at that time, only prolapsed hemorrhoids were selected for treatment, with a single massive injection given to slough off the hemorrhoid. In 1879, Edmund Andrews, president of the Chicago Medical Society, presented a report of 3,295 patients, collected through correspondence, who had undergone injection therapy.[10] Many of the patients had been treated by itinerant charlatans and inadequately trained physicians. Numerous complications, including severe pain, sloughing, and even death (nine cases), were reported. Despite these problems, Andrews believed that cautious application of the procedure was appropriate if the following criteria were met: internal hemorrhoids were treated, the patient was kept at bed rest for at least 8 hours after the procedure, and carbolic acid in oil or glycerine was employed. At about this time, Kelsey in the United States and Edwards in England recognized that the injection method was beneficial and substituted a

JOHN MORGAN (1820–1891)

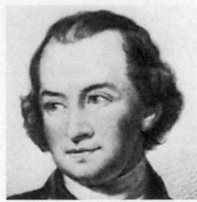

Morgan was born in Bath, England, the son of a physician. After the death of his father, he moved to London and entered King's College. As was the custom of the day, he became apprenticed to a surgeon and attended lectures, especially at St. George's Hospital. He established himself as a surgeon in London in 1845 in the neighborhood of Hyde Park, the area being the "resort of the wealthy and successful." Little is known about how Morgan came to employ the technique of injection, but he did achieve a significant reputation in the medical community as an anatomist and surgeon. (Morgan J. Varicose state of saphenous haemorrhoids treated successfully by the injection of tincture of persulphate of iron. *Med Press Circular*. 1869:29.)

EDMUND ANDREWS (1824–1904)

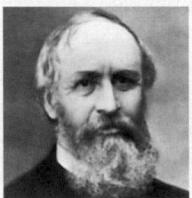

Andrews was born in Putney, Vermont. At the age of 16, he moved to Detroit and completed his literary studies at the University of Michigan, graduating in 1849. He received his medical degree 3 years later from the same university. After several years on the faculty in the department of anatomy at the university, he joined the Department of Surgery at the Rush Medical College. In 1854, Andrews founded the Chicago Academy of Sciences. During the Civil War, he served as chief of surgery at one of the camp hospitals and directed mobile surgical units in Tennessee and Mississippi, with the responsibility for maintaining the records of surgery during the war. As professor of surgery at Rush, he ultimately became dissatisfied and severed his connections there. With several other well-recognized physicians in Chicago, Andrews established the Lind University Medical School, which eventually became the Medical School of Northwestern University; for 46 years he was professor of surgery. An innovative surgeon, Andrews developed many instruments, including braces for correction of spinal curvature, an appliance for trephining, and an early endoscope that paved the way for modern cystoscopy. Following a trip to England in 1867, he was the first surgeon in the West to use and promote Lister's antiseptic methods.

CHARLES BOYD KELSEY (1850–1917)

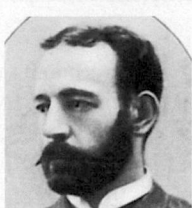

Kelsey was born in Farmington, Connecticut, the son of a Protestant minister. He received his medical degree from the College of Physicians in New York in 1873 and became a house surgeon at St. Luke's Hospital in New York. There followed a period of 5 years in the department of anatomy at his alma mater as a demonstrator, during which time he developed a commitment to the treatment of anorectal diseases. In 1880, he was instrumental in the establishment of a hospital in New York that was "founded on the same general plan as St. Mark's Hospital in London." St. Paul's Infirmary for Hemorrhoids, Fistula, and Other Diseases of the Rectum survived for only a few years, but Kelsey became recognized as one of the leading authorities on rectal surgery in the United States. His books, *Surgery of the Rectum and Pelvis* and *Diseases of the Rectum and Anus: Their Pathology, Diagnosis and Treatment*, were considered the most authoritative texts in the United States at the time on the subject of rectal disease. Kelsey became professor in the Department of Diseases of the Rectum at the University of Vermont in 1889 and 2 years later occupied the same chair at the New York Postgraduate School. (Kelsey CB. *Surgery of the Rectum and Pelvis*. New York, NY: W. Wood; 1902; Kelsey CB. *Diseases of the Rectum and Anus: Their Pathology, Diagnosis and Treatment*. New York, NY: W. Wood; 1890; Banov L Jr. St. Paul's infirmary for haemorrhoids, fistula, and other diseases of the rectum. *South Med J*. 1978;71(12):1559–1561.)

weaker solution of 5% to 7.5% carbolic acid in glycerine and water; this resulted in less sloughing.[86,150] Phenol (5%) in almond or vegetable oil is still the primary sclerosing agent used in Great Britain today; 3 mL is usually injected into each hemorrhoid site.

The combination of quinine and urea hydrochloride, widely used as a local anesthetic agent before the introduction of procaine, was associated with the development of fibrous tissue proliferation and sometimes sloughing at the site of injection.[287] In 1913, Terrell first used this substance in the injection treatment of internal hemorrhoids, with dramatic results. He concluded that a 5% solution was satisfactory from the standpoint of effectiveness and the patient's safety.[287] The historical implications of the development of the injection method are well described by Anderson in his 1924 review.[8] Sclerosants include sodium morrhuate and sodium tetradecyl sulfate (i.e., Sotradecol), but the safest continues to be phenol (5%) in vegetable oil. A new sclerosing agent has been recently described and advocated from a group in Japan, that of aluminum potassium sulfate/tannic acid.[291] In essence, all the ambulatory, nonexcisional treatments of hemorrhoids produce fibrosis of the submucosa, thereby obliterating the redundant tissue.

Indications and Contraindications

The nonprolapsing internal hemorrhoid is most amenable to injection treatment. Sometimes, a large, slightly protruding hemorrhoid can be successfully treated in this manner. Injection usually affords only temporary relief of symptoms when hemorrhoids are voluminous, contain a great deal of fibrous tissue, or require digital replacement after defecation. External hemorrhoids should never be treated by injection. Internal hemorrhoids that are infected or contain thrombi likewise should not be injected. Hemorrhoids with evidence of inflammation, such as ulceration and gangrene, are also unsuitable for injection treatment. Tags, fistulas, tumors, and anal fissures are complicating conditions that contraindicate use of the injection method.

Technique

With the patient in the semi-inverted jackknife or left lateral (i.e., Sims') position, an anoscope is inserted and the anal canal observed (Figure 11-9). The entire region is inspected so that, ideally, a diagram of the position of the hemorrhoids can be drawn on the patient's chart (see Figure 11-1). This is especially useful when long intervals elapse between injections. The point at which each injection is made, the amount of solution used, and the date of the injection should be recorded on the chart, or at least clearly documented in the notes. The term *o'clock* should not be used to describe the location of the treatment or the location of the hemorrhoids. Left lateral is left lateral whether the patient is in the prone jackknife position, in the lithotomy position, or hanging from the chandelier. The use of the word *o'clock* mandates that the position of the patient be described, and this is inevitably absent in most office notes and communications.

Figure 11-10 shows the syringe and long, angled needle used for sclerotherapy. Although this type of needle is very well known to head and neck surgeons, its value for the colon and rectal surgeons is not generally appreciated. More to the point, however, is the fact that standard, straight, disposable needles are a requisite for every physician's office. Still, the longer the needle that is used (e.g., a spinal needle), the better the visualization is of the pile site.

The needle is introduced through the mucous membrane into the center of the mass of veins (Figure 11-11). No antiseptic is necessary. Care must be taken to avoid bringing the point of the needle into contact with the sensitive margin

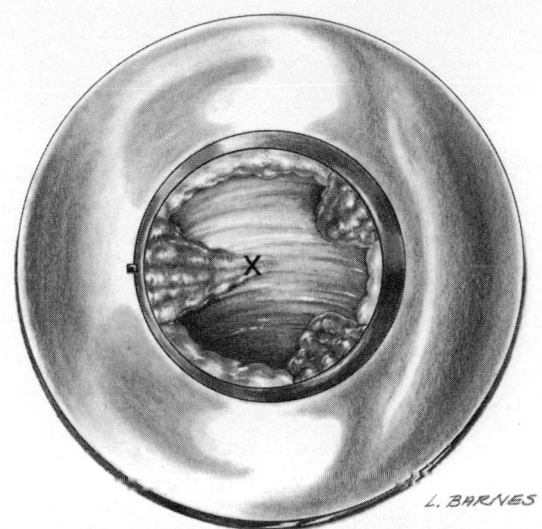

FIGURE 11-9. Hemorrhoids in commonly seen locations in the anal canal as viewed through the anoscope. The *X* indicates the planned site for injection of the left lateral pile, in an insensitive area of the anal canal.

of the pectinate line. Because of the extremely remote possibility that the needle could enter the lumen of a vein and that the solution could be injected into the circulation, some surgeons withdraw the plunger of the syringe to see whether blood appears. Unlike sclerotherapy for varicose veins, this technique requires that intraluminal injection be avoided, but in actuality it is virtually impossible to perform an intravenous injection.

After the needle is in position, 0.5 mL of sodium morrhuate, quinine, and urea hydrochloride, or Sotradecol is slowly injected submucosally into each pile site. Alternatively, the physician may employ a 5% solution of phenol in almond, vegetable, or arachis oil. A wheal should form, indicating that the injection was given in the proper plane. No more than 3 mL should be used in total if a commercial sclerosant is being used. Conversely, with the phenol in oil solution, 3 mL may be injected into each pile site. All hemorrhoids should be injected at the first treatment session.

A modification has been adopted by some gastroenterologists, that is, injection via a catheter passed through the channel of a colonoscope. Because gastroenterologists generally do not use anoscopy, they look at the anal canal (as best they can) through a retroflexed, long instrument. This technique is mentioned only to condemn it. However, having never attempted it, I can only imagine what a cumbersome exercise it must be to endeavor to perform sclerotherapy by this technique.

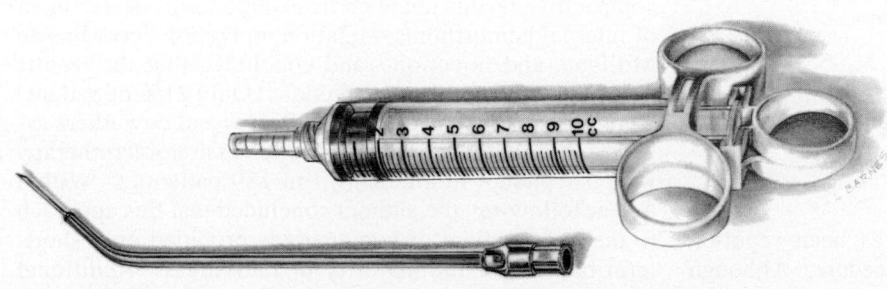

FIGURE 11-10. Syringe and angled hemorrhoid needle used for sclerotherapy. An angled needle permits better visualization than does a straight one. Alternatively, a fine-bore hypodermic needle can be employed.

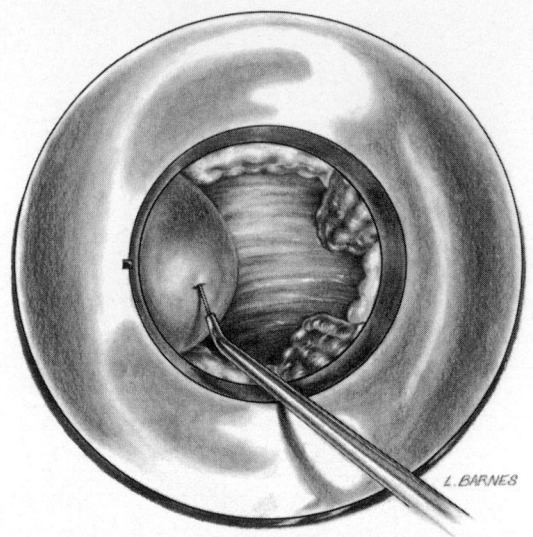

FIGURE 11-11. Sclerotherapy. If a wheal is not produced, the injection is too deep, and the needle should be withdrawn. An injection that is too superficial can cause necrosis of the lining of the anal canal.

Complications
Sloughing

If sloughing follows the injection of a sclerosant, one or more of three errors are usually responsible:

- The injection was too superficial.
- Too much solution was injected into one area.
- A second injection was made into a hemorrhoid too soon after the first.

Expectant management usually results in resolution without long-term sequelae. However, anal stricture can be a consequence of extensive tissue destruction.[251]

Thrombosis and Necrosis (Sloughing)

Thrombosed hemorrhoids, whether internal, external, or both, are uncommon consequences of properly performed sclerotherapy. However, necrosis of anal mucosa or perianal skin is usually the result of too superficial an injection, the injection of too much sclerosant, or the injection of overlapping areas. Generally, treatment is conservative and consists of sitz baths, analgesics, and topical anal creams. If scarring or stricture supervenes, an anoplasty should be considered (see later).

Burning

Burning in the anal canal is a late consequence of repeated sclerotherapy. The discomfort can in some patients be quite disabling, unremitting, and unresponsive to the usual local measures. Systemic pain medication may be the only effective therapy. I do not recommend repeated injections primarily because of my fear of this complication.

Local Abscess and Paraffinoma

Submucous abscess and paraffinoma (i.e., oleogranuloma) have been reported, the latter after the use of oil-based sclerosing agents (see Chapter 26).[82,199]

Bacteremia and Sepsis

Bacteremia following sclerotherapy has been reported in 8% of patients who undergo this procedure.[2] Although septicemia did not develop in any of the patients, antibiotic prophylaxis had for a long time been recommended for those individuals at an increased risk (e.g., valvular heart disease). However, recent evidence suggests that most people with heart conditions are actually at substantially lower risk for endocarditis than previously believed, and therefore do not need endocarditis prophylaxis. Accordingly, the American Heart Association made a major revision in their guidelines on endocarditis prophylaxis in 2007, so that prophylaxis is now recommended for many fewer patients, and for fewer procedures, than previously. Endocarditis prophylaxis is now recommended only for people who are at the highest risk for endocarditis. These include

- patients with artificial heart valves,
- patients who have had heart repairs using prosthetic material (note: this does not include coronary artery *stents*),
- patients with a prior history of endocarditis,
- patients with certain unrepaired or incompletely repaired *congenital heart disease*, and
- patients who have transplanted hearts who now have developed heart valve problems.

It is worth noting that the current guidelines do not recommend endocarditis prophylaxis for most patients with aortic or mitral valve disease (including those with *mitral valve prolapse*), or for patients with hypertrophic cardiomyopathy. The new guidelines recommend prophylaxis only for

- dental procedures involving manipulation of the gums or the roots of the teeth,
- procedures of the respiratory tract, and
- procedures involving infected tissues.

Prophylaxis is no longer recommended for procedures of the gastrointestinal or genitourinary systems.

Other extremely rare reported complications include urologic sepsis, prostatic abscess, epididymitis, seminal vesicle abscess, urinary-perineal fistula, retroperitoneal sepsis, perineal and scrotal necrotizing fasciitis, septic shock, and rectal perforation with retroperitoneal abscess.[123,245] In the era of HIV and the immunocompromised patient, one must be sensitive to the potential for an increased risk of septic complications in these individuals.

Results

Few reports of sclerotherapy have been published in contemporary English language publications. Khoury and colleagues conducted a randomized trial that compared single versus multiple phenol injections in the treatment of hemorrhoids.[152] Results were assessed up to 1 year later. Most patients fell into the category of mild-to-moderate hemorrhoid disease. The authors demonstrated that a single session of injection treatment using "adequate doses of sclerosant" (i.e., 3 to 5 mL) was as effective as multiple treatments. Dencker and colleagues reported on the comparative results obtained from three forms of treatment of internal hemorrhoids—ligation, operation according to Milligan, and injection—and concluded that the results obtained with injection were poor.[78] Only 21% of patients were well at the time of review. Santos and coworkers assessed the outcome following single-session sclerotherapy with 5% phenol in almond oil in 189 patients.[261] With a 4-year follow-up, the authors concluded that this approach to the management of hemorrhoids provided only short-term benefit for the majority of individuals. Additional

EDWARD THOMAS CAMPBELL MILLIGAN (1886–1972)

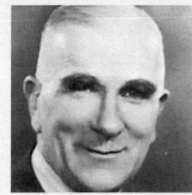

Milligan was born at Waterloo, near Ballarat, Victoria, Australia, the son of a gold miner. He attended Ballarat College and received his medical training at Melbourne University, graduating with honors in 1910. In 1914, he went to France with the Australian Expeditionary Force and distinguished himself by the application of the radical exploration and debridement of wounds. At the conclusion of the war, he received the Order of the British Empire and settled in London to become a consultant to a number of hospitals, including St. Mark's. He developed an interest in anal diseases and became extremely adept in performing a combined abdominoperineal resection. It was said that he was a "master of surgical planes and deft atraumatic dissection, and even after the most major procedures his patients looked undisturbed." One of his outstanding achievements was the work that he and his junior colleagues prepared on the detailed anatomy of the pelvis, the sphincter mechanism, and the treatment of hemorrhoids. (Milligan ETC, Morgan CN, Jones LE, et al. Surgical anatomy of the anal canal, and the operative treatment of haemorrhoids. *Lancet.* 1937;233:1119–1124.)

studies demonstrate sclerosant therapy to be less effective than a number of other options.[7,105,168,272] Because other methods afforded Dencker and colleagues better results, they did not think that injection treatment should be used routinely for internal hemorrhoids.

Alexander-Williams and Crapp, in a report on conservative management of hemorrhoids, stated that they had used sclerotherapy extensively in the past and as part of clinical comparative trials. They found that it gave satisfactory short-term results, particularly in the treatment of patients with first-degree hemorrhoids.[4]

Opinion

I believe injection treatment is a reasonable option for the management of a limited number of individuals who have symptomatic hemorrhoids, especially bleeding, and in whom rubber band ligation cannot be tolerated (see next section). Because of my concern for the complication of intractable burning and discomfort from multiple injections, only one treatment of all pile sites is advisable. If symptoms persist, an alternative approach should be offered.

Rubber Ring Ligation

Ligation of hemorrhoids was first described by Hippocrates in 460 BC, writing about using thread to tie off the hemorrhoids. Tissue necrosis and fixation can also be produced by rubber ring ligation.[80,81] In 1954, Blaisdell described an instrument for ligation of internal hemorrhoids as an outpatient procedure.[36] In 1962, Barron modified this instrument and presented two series reporting excellent results (Figure 11-12).[24,25] The results of the ligation technique have been so gratifying that this approach has replaced surgical hemorrhoidectomy for approximately 80% of my patients and is the primary office procedure for hemorrhoid management by surgeons in the United States.[69]

Any individual who has hemorrhoids manifested by bleeding, prolapse, or both is a candidate for this procedure. No anesthetic is required, but the rubber rings must be placed on an insensitive area, usually at or just above the dentate line. Skin tags or hypertrophied anal papillae cannot be treated by ligation because the patient would experience too much discomfort.

After a small cleansing enema has been given, proctosigmoidoscopy and anoscopy are performed. If the patient's history is suggestive of colonic disease, colonoscopy or barium enema examination is completed before any treatment of the hemorrhoids is considered. Several treatments, spaced over 3- to 4-week intervals, may be required, depending on how many pile sites must be eliminated to alleviate the symptoms. Generally, I do not recommend multiple bandings in the first treatment session. I make exceptions to this policy based on patient insistence or convenience, lack of discomfort with a prior treatment, or the necessity of the patient to travel a considerable distance for subsequent therapy. However, multiple bandings are offered or routinely employed by some physicians.

Technique

Figure 11-13 shows the McGivney ligator; I prefer this instrument to the Barron ligator. It has a much more secure shaft, which may be rotated in a 360-degree arc to facilitate placement. All nonsuction instruments have the relative disadvantage of requiring two people to perform the procedure: one to maintain the anoscope or retractor in position and the other to hold the ligator and grasping forceps. Alternatively, the physician may use a suction hemorrhoidal ligator such as the Lurz-Goltner (Figure 11-14) or the McGown ligator (Figure 11-15). These instruments draw the hemorrhoid into the cup through suction and therefore do not require a grasping forceps. Because the Lurz-Goltner ligator is a side-application device, maneuvering the ligator onto the pile is quite easy. An end-suction instrument, such as the McGown ligator, is also very simple to use, but it requires slightly more manipulation to fit onto the hemorrhoid. Conversely, the disadvantage of the side-suction ligator is that mechanical problems occasionally prevent the instrument from working optimally. Treatment with a suction ligator seems to be associated with less patient discomfort, but this is perhaps

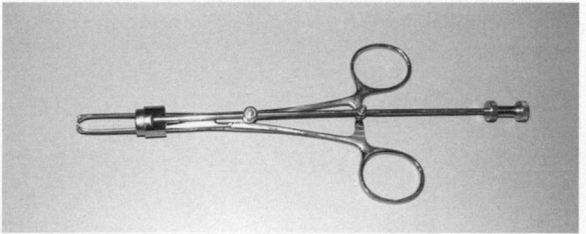

FIGURE 11-12. Original Barron hemorrhoid ligator. (Courtesy of Theodore E. Eisenstat, MD.)

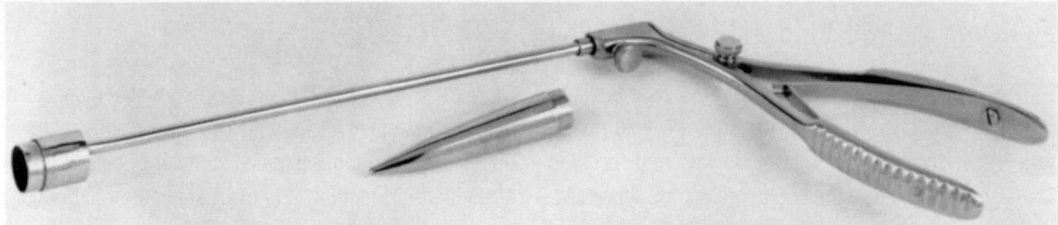

FIGURE 11-13. McGivney hemorrhoid ligator. This improved model has an offset handle for better vision; working length is 7 in. There are two thumb screws: one to assemble and secure the handle on the shaft and the other to permit rotation of the shaft in a 360-degree arc to facilitate placement on to the pile. (Courtesy of Miltex Instrument Co., Lake Success, NY.)

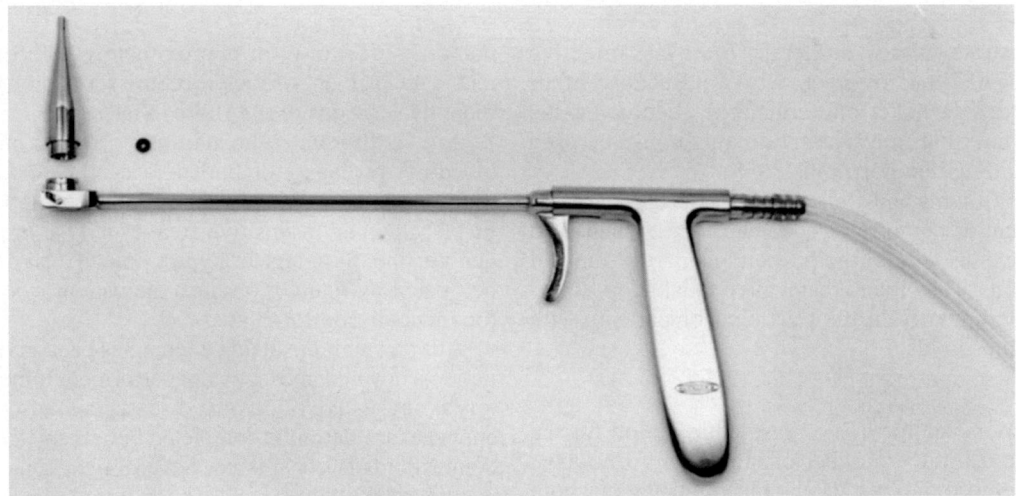

FIGURE 11-14. Lurz-Goltner suction hemorrhoidal ligator. (Courtesy of Scanlan International, St. Paul, MN.)

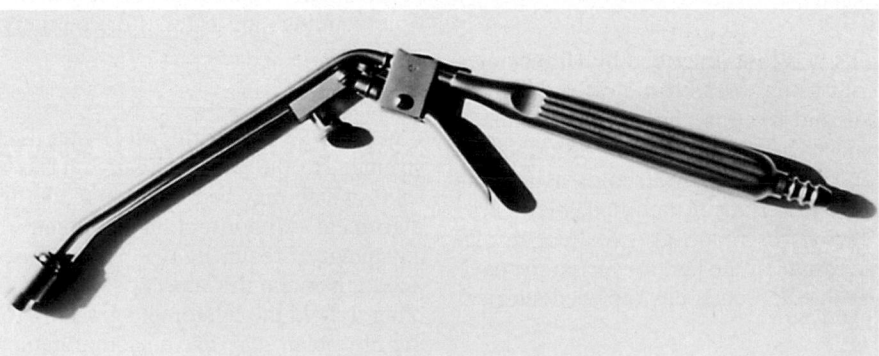

FIGURE 11-15. McGown one-hand hemorrhoidal ligator. This instrument has two interchangeable heads and a thumb suction activator. (Courtesy of George P. McGown, MD.)

because the drum incorporates a smaller volume of tissue. This factor, of course, is a potential disadvantage because the open-barrel device can permit incorporation of very large hemorrhoids and even redundant rectal mucosa.

Figure 11-16 shows an anal canal in which the ligator and alligator forceps have been inserted. I personally prefer to use the long alligator forceps because they securely grab the tissue, but more importantly they facilitate clear visualization of the site to be treated. However, most surgeons are familiar with and use Allis forceps. This short instrument is less than ideal because one's hand is often in the way, but the angled Allis forceps help somewhat in ameliorating this difficulty.

The most prominent hemorrhoid is treated first. It is grasped with the forceps as illustrated in Figure 11-17A and pulled up through the drum of the ligator (Figure 11-17B). If the patient experiences pain, a slightly more proximal point is selected, and this step is repeated. If the patient is still very uncomfortable, the wise course is to abandon this method of treatment and consider one of the alternatives. The tissue is drawn into the drum until it is taut, and the trigger is released, expelling two rubber rings (Figure 11-17C). Two

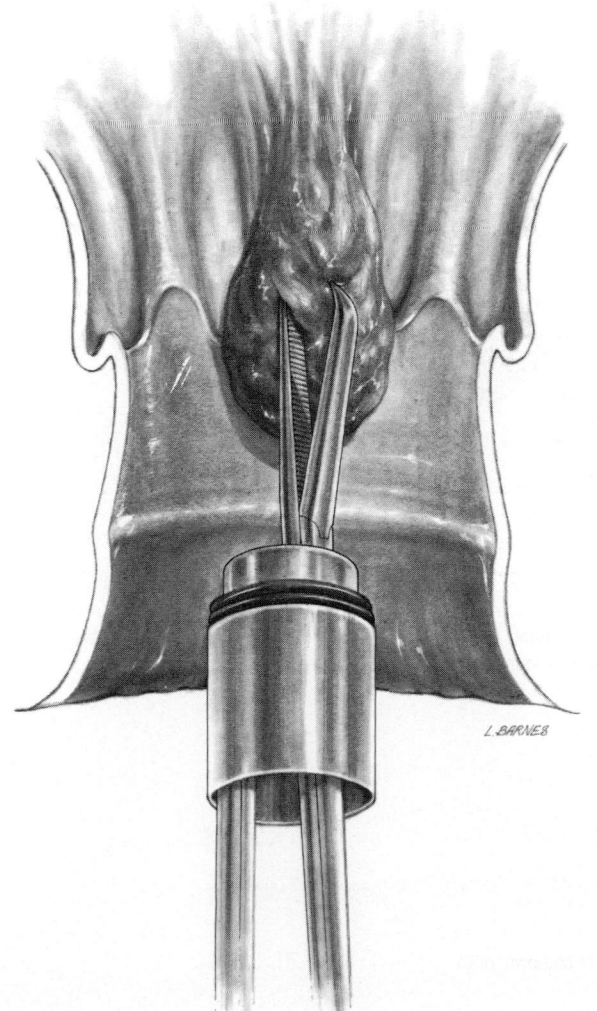

FIGURE 11-16. Rubber ring ligation. Alligator forceps are used to grasp the hemorrhoid. The forceps pass through the drum of the ligator.

rings are advised in case one breaks; there is considerable variation in the form and force of the rubber rings available on the market.[147] When the rings are in place, the anoscope is withdrawn (Figure 11-17D). As previously mentioned, if the physician uses the suction ligator, no grasping instrument is required.

The patient rarely experiences pain so severe that removal of the rings is necessary, but if required, this can be done by interposing the end of a conventional disposable suture-removal scissors or the application of a crochet hook. George McGown (Pembroke Pines, FL) has designed a cutting hook for this sole purpose (Figure 11-18). Other methods for removing the rings, such as cutting with a scalpel, tend to precipitate bleeding. Removal of the rubber rings can be accomplished with minimal trauma within a few minutes after application. However, if the patient returns at a later time because of pain, the associated edema precludes the possibility of safe removal. Adequate analgesic medication, therefore, is the preferred option. This presupposes that sepsis is not the cause (see Complications).

A more recent modification of a rubber band ligator has been developed, that of a disposable instrument, the O'Regan System (Figures 11-19 and 11-20). This device is a self-contained syringe-like instrument that eliminates the need for wall suction and tubing. As with the reusable instrument, it requires only one person, but clearly the primary advantage is that of disposability. In an era of concern for reprocessing costs, occupational health issues, and the risks of cross-contamination, this alternative has real merit. The technique is illustrated in Figure 11-21.

Armstrong has developed a modified anoscope with lateral apertures at the left lateral, right anterior, and right posterior quadrants in order to enable synchronous exposure and concomitant multiple hemorrhoidal ligations (Figures 11-22 and 11-23).[14] Another innovation that facilitates the performance of multiple ligations in one sitting is a multiple-banding instrument, the ShortShot Saeed Hemorrhoidal Multi-Band Ligator (Figure 11-24—Cook Medical, Bloomington, IN). This is a fully disposable suction ligating device that permits up to four bandings with the one instrument. A similar product called Haemoband is also available preloaded with four rubber bands and a multiaction handle that fires and reloads the bands (Haemoband Surgical, Belfast, Northern Ireland). And speaking of loading the bands, this may be an exercise in frustration as the rings fly across the room when one uses the conventional applicator to set the ring onto the barrel. A simple attachment, the "magic loading cone," (George Percy McGown, Brooklyn, NY) has been developed to address this concern (Figure 11-25).

Care Following Treatment

Bowel actions should be maintained without the patient straining. Appropriate dietary instructions, bulk agents, or a stool softener should be considered. The individual should be forewarned that some bleeding may be noted initially and again when the rubber rings are dislodged.

One of the major advantages of rubber ring ligation is its convenience. The patient need not return at fixed intervals for further ligation. Nothing is lost if one chooses to return 3 months, 6 months, or even years later. Other areas subsequently can be treated equally well despite such delays. However, the patient should realize that if symptoms are

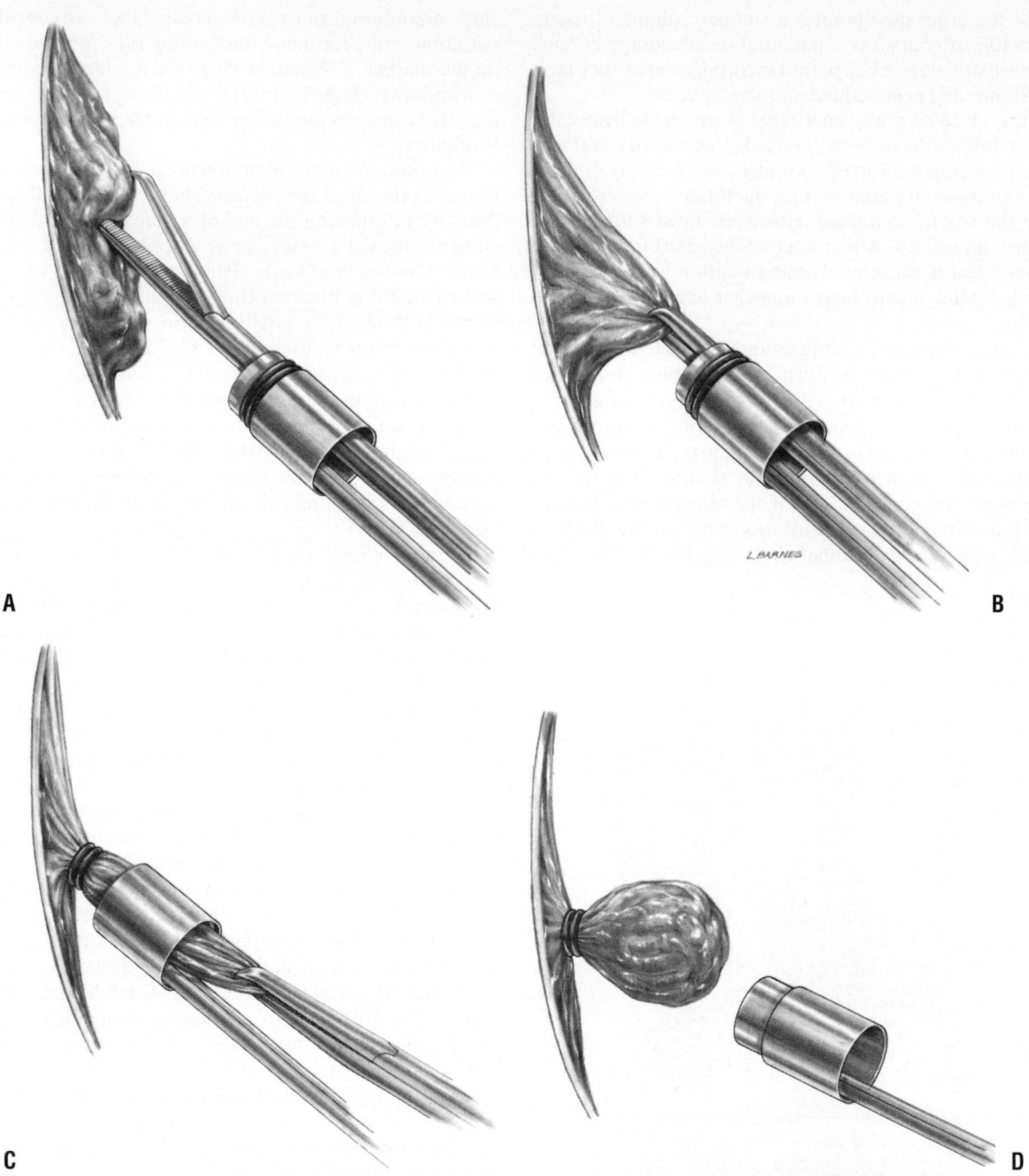

A

B

C

D

FIGURE 11-17. Rubber ring ligation. **A,B:** The hemorrhoid is grasped and firmly tethered. **C:** The tissue is drawn into the drum. If the patient tolerates the maneuver, ligation can be performed with minimal or no discomfort. **D:** The two rubber rings are released.

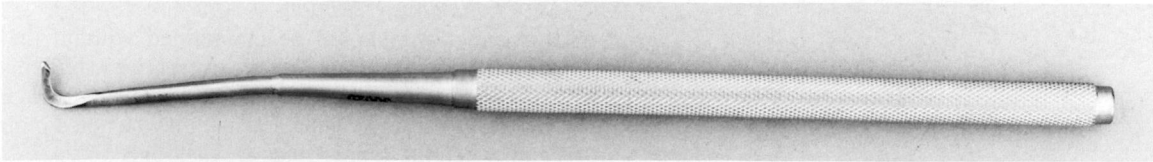

FIGURE 11-18. Rubber band cutter (model 30020). (Courtesy of George P. McGown, MD.)

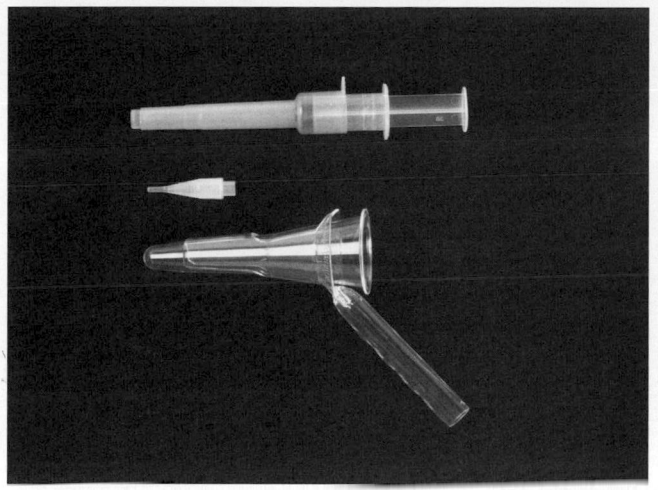

FIGURE 11-19. O'Regan Disposable Banding System. This includes (from **top**): suction-ligating syringe with band pusher, rubber band applicator, and slotted anoscope with obturator. (Courtesy of CRH Medical Corporation Vancouver, British Columbia, Canada.)

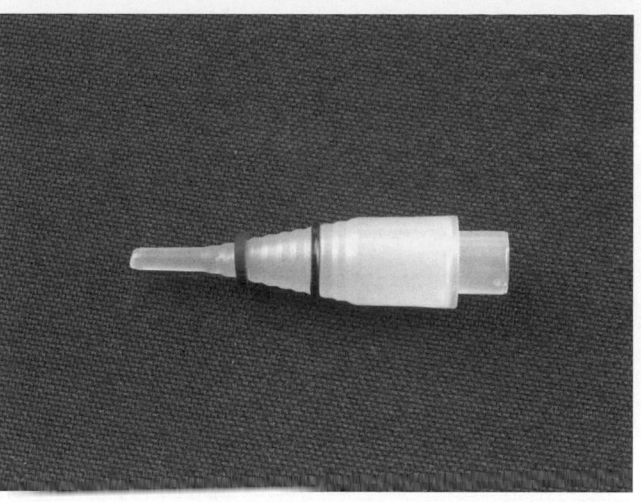

FIGURE 11-20. O'Regan Disposable Banding System. Rubber band applicator with rings. (Courtesy of Medsurge Medical Products Corp., North Vancouver, Canada.)

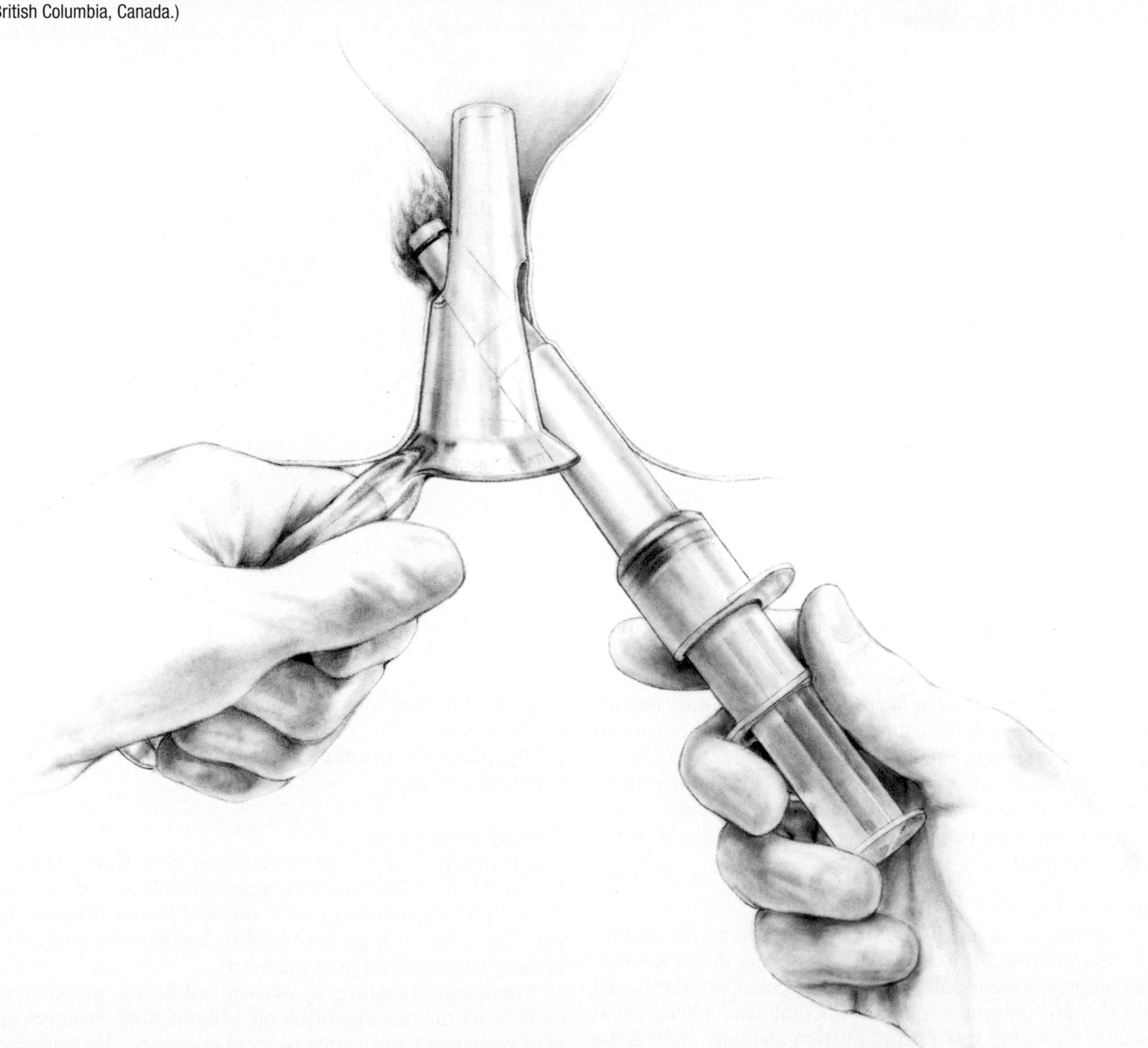

A

FIGURE 11-21. Technique of ligation using the O'Regan Ligating System. Ligator positioned through lateral slot of anoscope **(A)**. Plunger withdrawn and locked in first position to effect initial suction *(continued)*

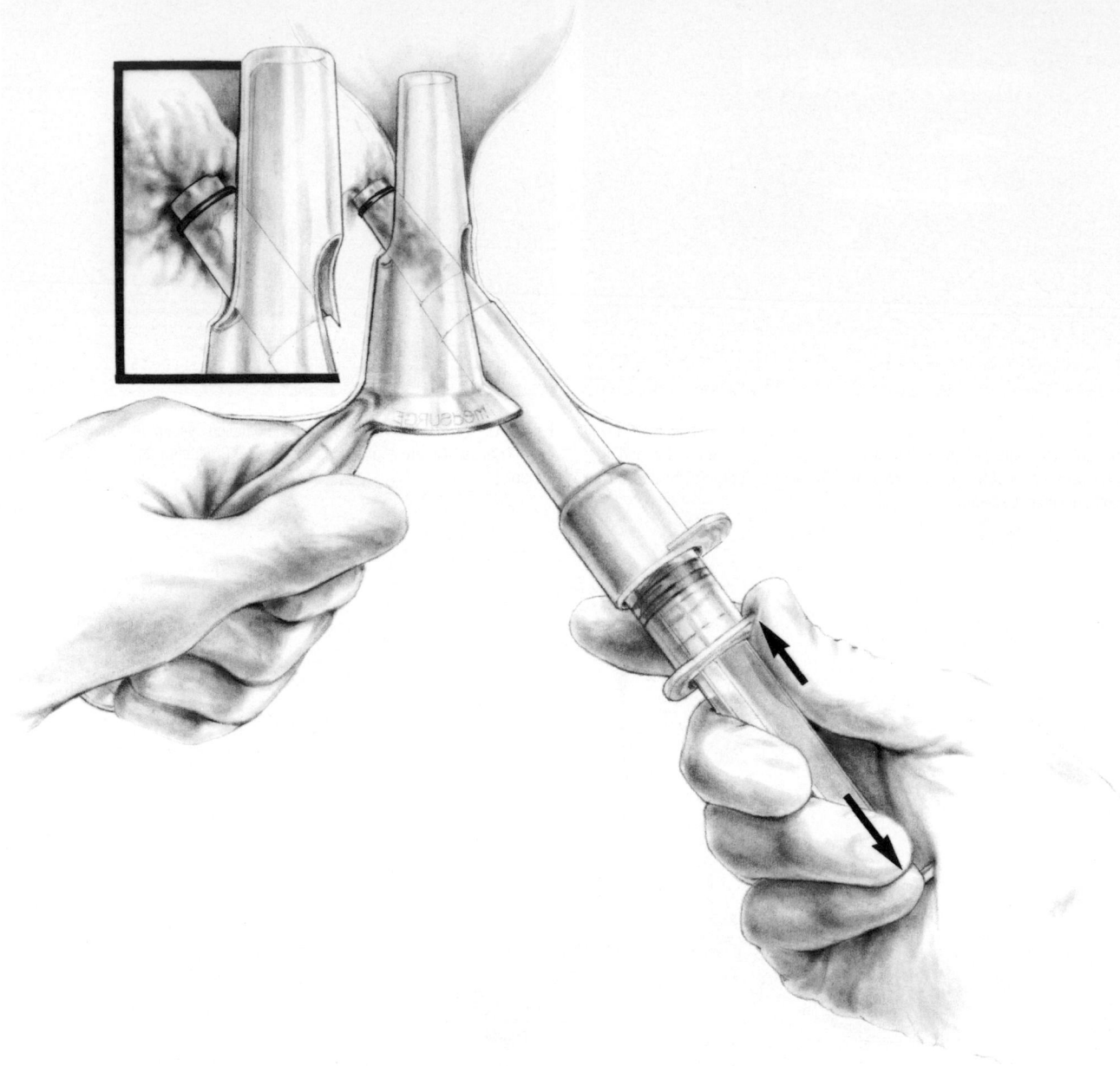

B

FIGURE 11-21. *(continued)* **(B)**; plunger withdrawn to second position to create maximum suction *(continued)*

not completely relieved, it is probably because other hemorrhoidal areas need to be addressed, assuming of course that there is no other explanation for the bleeding. Conversely, if the individual experiences complete relief after the initial ligation, there is no need to continue therapy. Under these circumstances, the patient is advised to return if and when symptoms recur.

Complications

A moderate sense of discomfort or fullness in the rectum can be anticipated for a few days following the procedure, but complaints are usually minimal and can often be relieved by sitz baths and mild analgesics. Complications are occasionally seen after rubber ring ligation and may include the following:

- Delayed hemorrhage
- Severe pain
- External hemorrhoidal thrombosis
- Ulceration
- Slippage of the ligature
- Fulminant sepsis

Delayed Hemorrhage

Late hemorrhage (i.e., 1 to 2 weeks after treatment) following rubber ring ligation occurs in approximately 1% of patients. As with late hemorrhage after surgical hemorrhoidectomy (see later), this may be attributed to sepsis in the pedicle or to early cutting through of the tissue.

Significant bleeding, as determined by the presence of clots or by the passage of blood without stool, requires urgent assessment, even emergency management. Patients may be evaluated in the emergency department or, if convenient, in the surgeon's office. Anoscopic examination is mandatory. If the patient is unstable, hypotensive, or tachycardic,

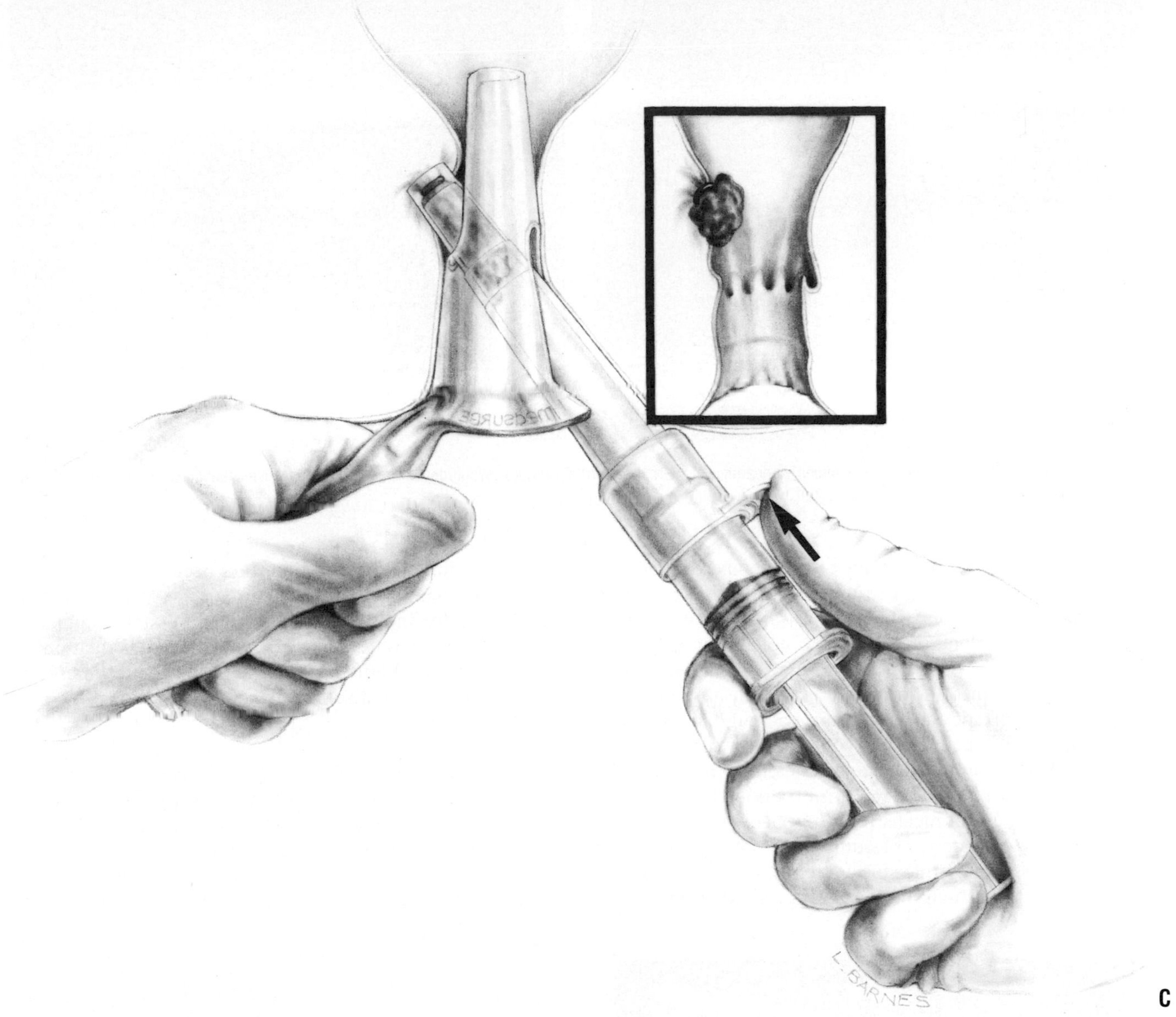

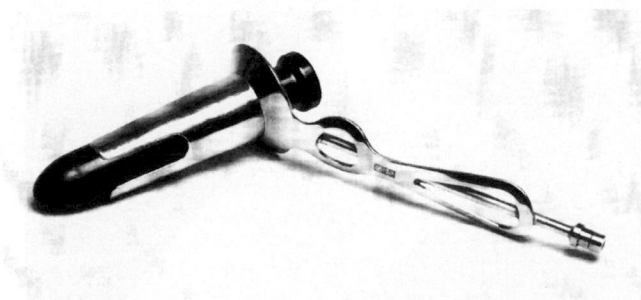

FIGURE 11-21. *(continued)* **(C)**; the pusher is advanced to release rings. The *inset* shows a ligated hemorrhoid pedicle.

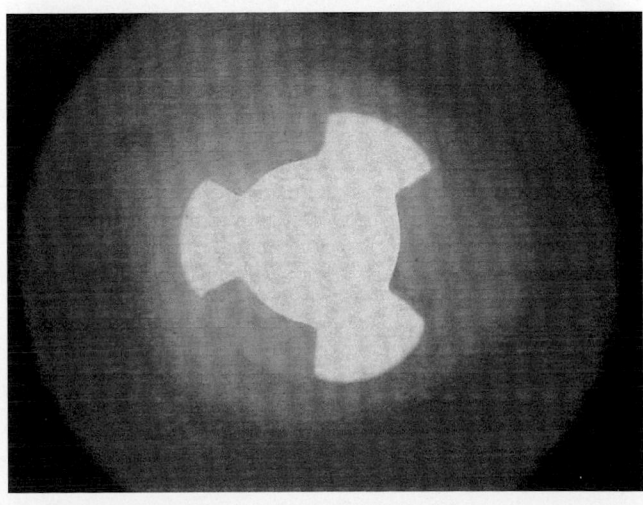

FIGURE 11-22. Armstrong anoscope for synchronous hemorrhoidal ligation. (Courtesy of David N. Armstrong, MD.) **A:** With obturator in place. **B:** End view without obturator. Note the lateral apertures.

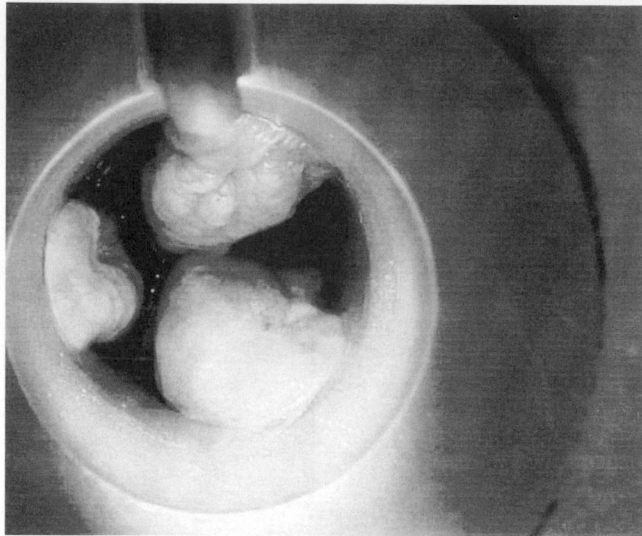

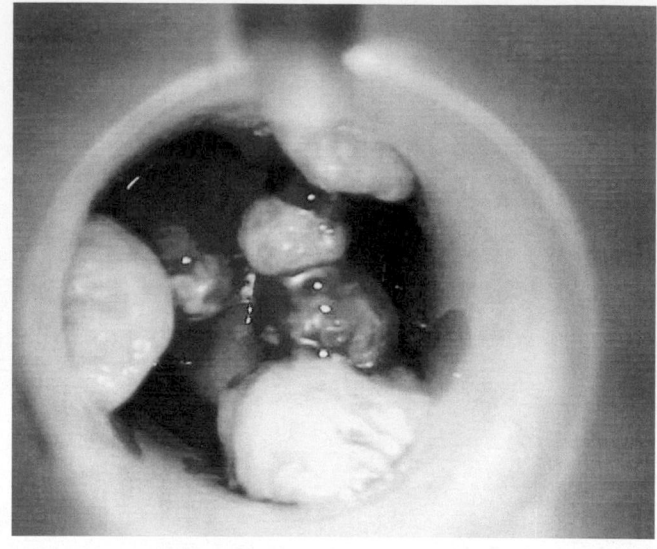

FIGURE 11-23. Multiple hemorrhoid ligations. Appearance of internal hemorrhoids prior to synchronous ligation **(A)** and following ligations **(B)**. (Courtesy of David N. Armstrong, MD.)

hospitalization is required. It must be remembered that individuals who have undergone rubber ring ligation can bleed massively. Transfusion may be necessary. Usually a local anesthetic, field block (see later), or general or spinal anesthetic is required. If the bleeding site is identified, suture ligation is performed. If the facilities are unsatisfactory for adequate visualization and suturing, packing the anus with gauze and with a hemostatic agent such as Surgicel, Gelfoam, or Avitene may be effective on a temporary basis. The use of a Foley catheter with a 30-mL balloon has also been suggested as a useful means for tamponading the bleeding. Often, however, no active bleeding site is appreciated at the time of assessment. Under these circumstances, the use of a hemostatic agent may be reassuring, in addition to hospital admission and observation. It is because of the risk of late hemorrhage that rubber ring ligation is absolutely contraindicated for individuals who are taking anticoagulants. An excisional option, sclerotherapy, infrared coagulation, or one of the other alternatives may be considered, unless the anticoagulant can be discontinued.

Pain

Pain requiring removal of the rings and measures to alleviate discomfort have been mentioned previously. Tchirkow and colleagues recommend injection of a local anesthetic solution into the hemorrhoid bundle.[286] In my experience, however, in most patients who complain of pain, this symptom develops after the anesthetic effect would have dissipated.

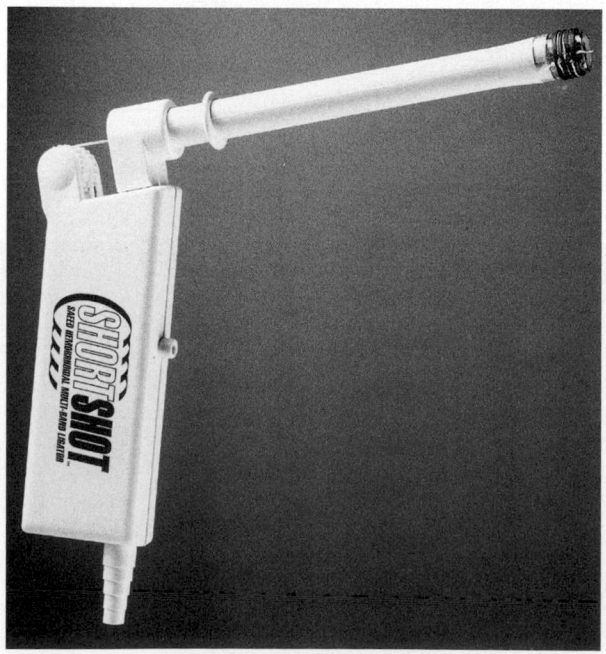

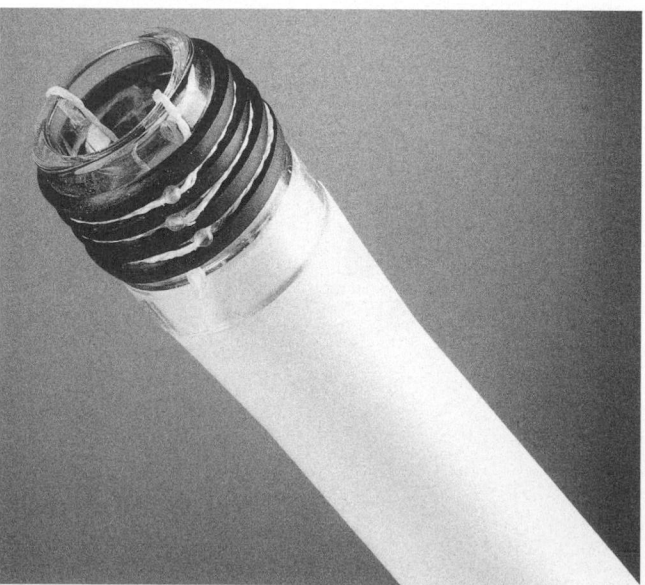

FIGURE 11-24. ShortShot Saeed Hemorrhoidal Multi-Band Ligator. **A:** Suction instrument. **B:** Close-up view of the instrument head shows the four rubber bands in place. (Courtesy of Cook Medical, Bloomington, IN.)

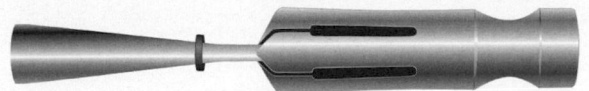

FIGURE 11-25. Magic Loading Cone. (Courtesy George Percy McGown, Brooklyn, NY.)

However, a local anesthetic at the time of treatment may be a valuable adjunct if the patient is particularly apprehensive.

In my opinion, pain is much more likely to be a source of concern if multiple bandings are attempted. Although this statement is not supported by controlled studies, it seems reasonable to conclude that the simultaneous ligation of three or more pile sites will inevitably lead to an exponential risk of discomfort. Pain that seems to worsen a few days following treatment merits reevaluation of the patient, especially if fever supervenes or if a problem with micturition develops. Anal and perineal sepsis can lead to gangrene and result in death (see Sepsis).

In the usual scenario, however, sitz baths and an over-the-counter or nonnarcotic prescription pain medication should be sufficient to relieve discomfort associated with rubber ring ligation. If the patient returns within a few hours of banding with exquisite pain, attempt at removal of the rubber rings is generally a bloody, unhappy exercise for both patient and surgeon. It is better to offer a stronger, even a narcotic prescription, rather than to struggle trying to remove the rings. Removal, if advisable, should only be performed, in my opinion, soon after banding (see Technique). With respect to subsequent management, it seems reasonable to conclude that if the patient tolerated the initial ligation poorly, an alternative approach should be considered if additional treatment be required.

Thrombosis
With ligation of internal hemorrhoids, the risk for subsequent thrombosis of corresponding external hemorrhoids is 2% to 3%. If thrombosis occurs, sitz baths and stool softeners are recommended. Occasionally, excision of the thrombosed hemorrhoid is required (see later).

Ulceration
Anal ulceration is a normal consequence of ligation. The rubber rings cause tissue necrosis, and they generally fall off in 2 to 5 days, leaving an ulcerated area. On rare occasions, a large ulcer, sometimes associated with a fissure, may be a troublesome complication. Treatment consists of sitz baths and perhaps a topical cortisone preparation, but if the fissure persists, internal anal sphincterotomy should be considered (see Chapter 12).

Slippage
The rubber rings can slip or break at any time, but this usually happens after the initial bowel movement. Breakage may be caused by a defective rubber ring, hence, the reason I prefer to use two. A more likely explanation is that it is a consequence of tension produced by a large bulk of tissue that has been ligated. The use of a mild laxative, bulking agent, or stool softener can help prevent the passage of a hard stool and, it is hoped, avoid precipitous dislodgement of the rings. If necessary, a repeat ligation of the same pile site can be reasonably performed 3 to 4 weeks after the initial procedure.

Sepsis
Aside from the normal sloughing that occurs from necrosis of tissue, sepsis following rubber ring ligation had been unknown for more than 20 years since rubber ring ligation had been generally available. A case of tetanus was reported as a possible consequence of treatment in 1978,[199] but the first reported incident of a profound infection was reported by O'Hara in 1980, that of a patient who developed fatal clostridial sepsis following rubber ring ligation.[215] Since this observation, others have described the same or a similar complication.[62,237,253,264,275,303] There seems to be a characteristic scenario of events. Young male patients appear to be at the greatest risk. A complaint of increasing anorectal pain, perineal pain, scrotal swelling, and difficulty urinating mandates emergency evaluation. So horrendous is this complication that I specifically inform all young male patients to be aware of the warning signs.

The origin of this potentially devastating complication is unclear, but some have suggested that many of these individuals may actually be in an immunocompromised state. For example, the initial reports of this complication originated from the San Francisco Bay area before the recognition of HIV, in a community with a large gay population. Still, Moore and Fleshner report that rubber band ligation can be safely performed in selected HIV-positive patients.[194] Another possible explanation is that the physician failed to recognize a septic process as the cause of the patient's so-called hemorrhoid complaints. Obviously, the physician should vigorously seek alternative causes of anorectal complaints, especially pain, before embarking on rubber ring ligation.[272] Still, there are highly experienced colon and rectal surgeons who have had the rare patient develop this complication and for whom there has been no satisfactory explanation. For example, Eugene Salvati, a former president of the ASCRS reported in a podium presentation at the society's annual meeting that he had performed in excess of 25,000 rubber band ligations and encountered only one individual who developed a septic complication.

Findings on physical examination may include fever, perineal edema, scrotal edema, perineal ulceration, cellulitis, or frank gangrene. Rectal examination usually demonstrates a boggy, edematous anal canal that is exquisitely tender. Computed tomography and magnetic resonance imaging of the pelvis are useful, especially to identify thickening of the rectal wall, gas within the wall of the bowel or within the pelvis, a pelvic fluid collection, or any other extrarectal disorder.[264]

Treatment requires massive antibiotic therapy, vigorous debridement, and possibly hyperbaric oxygen treatment. A colostomy may be necessary. Survival is problematic in the advanced case; those who recovered were inevitably recognized early and treated aggressively. Suggestions for prevention have included using prebanding enemas, prophylactic antibiotics, and even meticulous sterile technique (whatever that may be).[148] I believe that such measures are neither appropriate nor helpful. However, I routinely administer a small-volume Fleet enema before all anorectal procedures, primarily for aesthetic purposes (I simply do not enjoy the presence of stool in the field) and the fact that usually the patient need not be concerned about defecating for the remainder of the day.

Error in Diagnosis
A theoretical disadvantage of rubber ring ligation and all the nonexcisional methods for treating hemorrhoids is that no

EUGENE PHILIP SALVATI (1923–PRESENT)

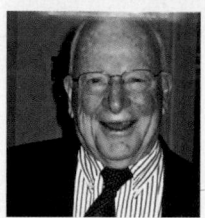

Eugene Salvati was born in Purslove, West Virginia, on September 7, 1923, the son and grandson of Italian immigrants. He attended college at West Virginia University, graduating from the University of Maryland Medical School in 1947. After beginning his postgraduate training at the Muhlenberg Hospital in New Jersey, he ultimately completed his general surgery residency in Indiana at the St. Vincent's Hospital in Indianapolis. During the Korean War, he served with the United States Medical Corps, receiving the Bronze Star and the Combat Medical Badge. He returned to complete his fellowship in colon and rectal surgery in Allentown, Pennsylvania, and began his practice in that specialty in Plainfield, New Jersey. In 1969, he established the first residency program in the specialty in the greater New York metropolitan area. In 1982, he was appointed professor of surgery at the University of Medicine and Dentistry of New Jersey—Rutgers University Medical School. During his career, Salvati championed many innovative and important contributions to the field, including local treatment of rectal cancer, the management of acute diverticulitis, the use of local anesthesia in anal surgery, and the value of hemorrhoid ligation. Salvati served as president of the American Society of Colon and Rectal Surgeons, the American Board of Colon and Rectal Surgery, as well as the New York, Pennsylvania, and New Jersey Societies. The Salvati Colon and Rectal Residency Program has trained more than 100 surgeons as of 2010, "not bad for a West Virginia country boy," as he has been fond of saying. (With appreciation to Theodore E. Eisenstat, MD.)

pathologic specimen is obtained. Invasive epidermoid carcinoma or other tumor occasionally has been reported in an excised hemorrhoid specimen (perhaps in less than 1% of cases). In the rare instance of its occurrence, such a lesion will obviously be missed. However, the physician should not condemn the procedure and limit its application because of an apparently reasonable, albeit truly unwarranted, concern. One must be mindful of the fact that the standard of care no longer requires submission of a pathologic specimen even when a surgical hemorrhoidectomy is performed. Cataldo and MacKeigan reviewed more than 20,000 hemorrhoid operations over a 20-year period.[47] Only one example of an unsuspected carcinoma of the anus was diagnosed solely by microscopic analysis. The authors conclude that selective rather than routine pathologic evaluation of hemorrhoidectomy specimens should be the policy. I concur. As stated previously, however, if there is any doubt or concern about the presence of a lesion or the possibility of an underlying malignancy, biopsy should be performed.

Results

In 1977, Bartizal and Slosberg published a retrospective review of the records of 670 patients who underwent 3,208 rubber ring ligations for internal hemorrhoids.[26] The degree of discomfort after banding and the presence and amount of rectal bleeding were assessed. All were followed for a minimum of 1 month after the completion of banding.

Complications were confined to pain and bleeding. Only 21 patients (4%) had any pain. Mild pain was defined as that which did not require treatment; moderate pain required analgesics, and severe pain caused limitation of activities. No bleeding at all was reported by 642 (96%). Bleeding to a slight degree was noted by 19 (3%) but required no specific treatment. Bleeding to a significant degree occurred in 9 patients (1%). Most were treated successfully with bed rest, but two required hospitalization. When those patients who had moderate and severe pain were combined with those who had severe bleeding, only 13 (2% of all patients treated) had complications severe enough to interfere with daily activity.

Bat and coworkers performed a prospective study involving in excess of 500 patients who underwent rubber band ligation.[28] The hospitalization rate was 2.5%, with approximately half of these admissions based on delayed massive rectal bleeding. There was no incident of overwhelming sepsis. An additional 4.6% suffered minor complications, including thrombosed hemorrhoids, mild bleeding, and urinary retention.

Steinberg and colleagues, by means of a questionnaire answered by 125 of 147 patients, conducted a long-term assessment (mean, 4.8 years) of the value of rubber ring ligation as a treatment for hemorrhoids.[280] Most (89%) considered themselves cured or greatly improved; however, only 44% were completely free of symptoms. Intermittent mild discomfort, occasional spotting of blood, and an awareness of lumps at the anus were the principal residual symptoms. Nevertheless, many were reportedly happier with this condition than with their state before treatment. Patients who suffered persistent or severe recurrent symptoms after rubber ring ligation were treated by further conservative measures. Fifteen patients (12%) had another rubber ring ligation, anal dilatation, or lateral sphincterotomy.

My colleagues and I reported our long-term results with rubber ring ligation (mean, 60 months).[318] Of 352 patients who were sent a questionnaire, 266 (76%) responded. Although many continued to have some symptoms, the condition of 80% of the respondents was improved by the procedure. The best results were obtained in patients who had grade I hemorrhoids. Patients with grade IV hemorrhoids were less likely to have had a good result ($P < .02$). The effectiveness of treatment did not depend on the number of hemorrhoids ligated. Those who had a single pile site treated were as likely to have had a good result as those in whom two or more bands were applied. Perhaps the most meaningful conclusion of our study is that a single treatment can achieve satisfactory results.[318] If more than three sessions are required to control symptoms, the procedure should probably be abandoned and hemorrhoidectomy performed.

The Cleveland Clinic group reported that 77% of their patients were asymptomatic following treatment.[107] Their technique differed in that approximately 90% of patients were treated by multiple ligations in a single session. Although the long-term results indicated fewer symptoms, pain after treatment was more frequently observed and was more severe.

Lau and colleagues performed rubber ring ligation on all three primary hemorrhoids at each single outpatient session.[164] Good to excellent results were noted in 91%, but moderate to severe pain was reported by 58 patients (29%). Although the authors strongly endorsed this approach, their rate of complications (i.e., hemorrhage, urinary retention, anal stenosis) was 3.5%. Khubchandani conducted a controlled study of single, double, and triple bandings.[153] There was no significant difference in the incidence of complaints of bleeding or pain following any of these three approaches; however, some patients had to have the rubber bands removed because of discomfort. Poon and colleagues compared single versus multiple ligations in a prospective, randomized trial.[235] Both methods were effective, and the incidence of complications and complaints was similar. The authors recommend multiple ligations—the patients are less inconvenienced, and they anticipated there should be some cost savings. The Mayo Clinic experience also reflects an acceptably low rate of complications.[165]

Other studies have demonstrated that rubber ring ligation is far superior to sclerosing agents.[105,272] Better long-term results, significantly more effective management of symptoms of protrusion, and greater likelihood of control of bleeding symptoms can be anticipated with this method of treatment. Chew and colleagues, however, recommend combining sclerotherapy with rubber band ligation.[53]

In order to compare this modality with surgical hemorrhoidectomy, Murie and colleagues randomly allocated 80 patients to ligation or to surgery.[198] Follow-up results at varying intervals for up to 3 years revealed no significant difference in the frequency of amelioration of symptoms, although it was not clear to me whether patients with more severe hemorrhoidal manifestations were excluded.

Comment

Rubber ring ligation is an excellent alternative to surgical hemorrhoidectomy for most patients. However, one must understand that the results may not equal those that can be achieved by surgery. Nevertheless, because of the limited morbidity, adequate long-term effectiveness, convenience, and patient acceptability, I recommend this procedure as the primary outpatient therapy for bleeding and for reducible hemorrhoid prolapse. However, in the presence of an external component, hypertrophied anal papilla, associated fissure, or large (grade IV) hemorrhoids, surgical treatment is unquestionably more effective.

Cryosurgery

Cryosurgery is based on the concept of cellular destruction through rapid freezing followed by rapid thawing. The treatment of hemorrhoids by this technique had been advocated by Lewis and colleagues and by others as painless, effective, and especially recommended for those patients who are medically unable to undergo general anesthesia.[64,111,171,307,309] The principle of cryosurgery is well described in these cited articles.

Technique

The following protocol has been recommended by most authors:

- The procedure is explained, and the patient is advised of the probability of profuse drainage and considerable swelling. If necessary, an intravenous injection of a sedative is administered, and a local anesthetic is usually recommended.

- The patient is placed in either the left lateral or prone jackknife position. The surgeon's fingers, a plastic vaginal speculum, or a modified plastic proctoscope are used to isolate one primary hemorrhoidal plexus at a time. A metal instrument is not employed because it would conduct cold, and a water-soluble jelly is used to achieve good contact between the cryoprobe and the hemorrhoid.

- The cryoprobe is applied. The tissue freezes around the tip. Thus, the distance between the tip and the outer border of the ice ball equals the depth of the ice ball. This allows the surgeon to determine visually how much tissue is being destroyed. Only that tissue encompassed within the ice ball allegedly will undergo irreversible cellular destruction. Changes at the boundary between the ice ball and normal tissue are reversible, and theoretically, no true cellular destruction occurs.

Theoretically, both internal and external hemorrhoids can be treated in one operation. The tip of the cryoprobe is placed in the center of either the internal or external hemorrhoidal plexus and remains there until the tissue to be destroyed is enveloped by the ice ball (Figure 11-26). The period of freezing varies according to the cooling power of the probe. With a liquid nitrogen probe at $-196°$ C or a liquid nitrous oxide probe at $-89°$ C, the application time is about 2 minutes per hemorrhoid area. The greater the vascularity of the hemorrhoid, the greater is the cooling power required to freeze it. Therefore, the liquid nitrogen probe is more effective for large hemorrhoids than is the nitrous oxide probe. When an adequate amount of tissue has been frozen, the probe is switched off, rewarmed, and detached from the hemorrhoid; each plexus in turn is treated the same way.

Care Following Treatment

Considerable swelling and edema occur within 24 hours of the procedure, but generally these effects do not interfere with normal bowel function and elimination. Drainage usu-

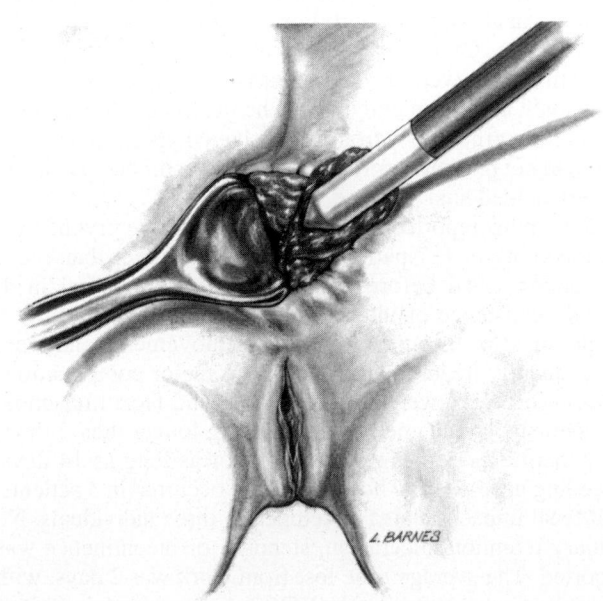

FIGURE 11-26. Cryosurgical destruction. The cryoprobe is applied to a combined internal-external hemorrhoid.

ally starts several hours later; it is fairly heavy for the first 3 to 4 days but decreases during the following 2 to 3 weeks. Patients are instructed to use some form of sterile pad and to change the pad several times a day during the first 3 to 4 days.

Two to 3 hours after freezing, the tissue becomes swollen and erythematous. Within 72 hours, pale spots appear on the surface, and these coalesce to form irregular patches by the fourth day. By the fifth or sixth day, the whole hemorrhoidal area is pale; black, gangrenous areas may then appear. Necrosis is usually complete between postoperative days 7 and 9. Thereafter, the hemorrhoid begins to disintegrate and should come away completely by the 18th postoperative day, leaving, it is hoped, a normal-appearing anus.

Results

It should be noted that many of the following references are older. Wilson and Schofield reported 100 consecutive cases of hemorrhoids treated by cryosurgery.[310] All were managed on an ambulatory basis, usually without an anesthetic. A nitrous oxide cryoprobe was used. Watery discharge has been said to occur in all patients, but in this study many did not notice a discharge at all, and only one complained that the discharge was a nuisance. Four patients experienced immediate pain during the freezing process; three required a general anesthetic. An additional six patients underwent elective general anesthesia. Only one complained of pain during the first 5 days after treatment, and many returned to work the following day. No major hemorrhages were encountered, although the watery discharge was sanguineous in some. The patients were assessed at 6 weeks and 3 months, with satisfactory results obtained in 94%.

Savin reported 444 operations performed with a nitrous oxide probe.[263] Excellent results were obtained, according to the author, in that all hemorrhoidal tissue and symptoms were eliminated in 431 of 434 patients. Ten patients were lost to follow-up study, and 3 patients had some residual hemorrhoidal tissue. Additionally, cryosurgery was successful in removing 97% of the concomitant pathologic conditions treated, such as anal fissure, anal fistula, hypertrophied anal papilla, condyloma acuminatum, and mucosal prolapse. Of 155 patients evaluated 1 to 2 years after operation, 151 were graded as having excellent results; 3 had small, asymptomatic internal hemorrhoids; 1 had an external hemorrhoid; 3 were found to have hypertrophied anal papillae not present before; and 2 patients still had persistent hypertrophied anal papillae.

O'Connor reported results of nitrous oxide cryohemorrhoidectomy in 117 patients.[209] Skin tags larger than those the patients had before the procedure were found in 4; 5 had persistence of internal hemorrhoids. Three of the 5 complained of bleeding with bowel movements and were subsequently treated by ligation. The major complications after cryosurgery were pain, bleeding, and fecal impaction. Six patients complained of pain lasting longer than 2 days, 2 of them experiencing discomfort for as long as 14 days. Bleeding necessitating hospitalization occurred in 3 patients, and fecal impaction also developed in three individuals. No urinary retention, ulceration, stenosis, or incontinence was reported. The average time lost from work was 2 days, with a range of none to 14 days. O'Connor concluded that internal hemorrhoids were easily treated by cryosurgery, and that thrombosed and edematous hemorrhoids should be managed

by methods other than cryosurgery. He further advised that thick skin tags and large prolapsing hemorrhoids should be treated by excisional surgery. It would appear from the author's subsequent report, however, that he had abandoned this method for the indications outlined in favor of infrared coagulation (see Infrared Coagulation).

Oh initially reviewed 100 patients who had undergone cryohemorrhoidectomy, and he subsequently reported on 1,000 of these individuals.[212,213] In his original report, two-thirds experienced pain, 2 suffered massive hemorrhage, and 5 encountered urinary difficulties. Effectiveness of cryotherapy was 90%, similar to that for rubber ring ligation, but the discomfort, prolonged drainage, and prolonged recovery were believed to be distinct disadvantages when cryohemorrhoidectomy was compared with ligation. MacLeod, in his report on 528 patients treated by cryotherapy, recommended that this modality be used only on internal hemorrhoids and that the treatments be staged.[177]

Traynor and Carter reported a prospective study on the treatment of second- and third-degree hemorrhoids by cryotherapy.[292] Approximately half of the 125 patients analyzed were hospitalized for less than 24 hours. Profuse serous discharge was reported by two-thirds; more than 90% returned to work within 3 weeks. The principal long-term disadvantage appeared to be the failure to eliminate skin tags.

Smith and colleagues reported a study in which closed hemorrhoidectomy and cryotherapy were performed on 26 patients.[277] One side of the anus was designated at random for surgery and the other for cryotherapy. Although pain was initially less after cryosurgery (only 1 patient noted severe pain on the cryotherapy side), 12 had pain for more than 2 weeks on the cryotherapy side, compared with only 3 patients who experienced pain after 2 weeks on the surgical side. Interestingly, patients could determine which side had been surgically treated and which side had been "frozen." Of 24 patients examined 1 year after treatment, 13 had residual hemorrhoids, 12 of which were at the cryosurgical site. Six of these 13 patients requested further treatment. When patient opinion was ascertained, 65% said they preferred operative hemorrhoidectomy and 35% said they preferred cryosurgery.

Comment

When cryosurgical hemorrhoidectomy was first introduced, it was claimed to be painless, did not require an anesthetic, and was effective for external tags and hypertrophied papillae. Since that time, reports have confirmed that it is not painless—local or general anesthetic has been suggested by almost all observers—and that it is less effective, and in many ways ineffective, for the treatment of hypertrophied anal papillae and skin tags. For internal hemorrhoids, rubber ring ligation is demonstrably superior to cryosurgery. It is quicker and cheaper and requires no anesthetic. For the external component or hypertrophied papilla, excision after local infiltration rapidly removes the offending tissue. Complete healing takes place in 7 to 10 days. Cryosurgical destruction requires the use of relatively expensive equipment and is time consuming to perform—some authors recommend hospitalization or an outpatient setting. In addition, it results in profuse drainage and sometimes delayed healing. True, the initial postanesthetic pain may be somewhat less than with surgical hemorrhoidectomy, but this pain usually can be controlled with a mild analgesic (see later).

In my opinion, cryosurgery adds nothing to the treatment of hemorrhoids that is not available by other means at lower cost, at greater efficiency, with fewer complications, and with as good if not better results. Others must agree, because I have not been able to identify more recent references in peer-reviewed publications with this technique since the second edition of this text (1989). In fact, in a poll of members of the ASCRS at a national meeting in the year 2000, no individual was performing cryosurgical destruction of hemorrhoids at that time. Moreover, the genuine fear of causing severe tissue injury, scarring, deformity, and incontinence, as well as the plethora of lawsuits, have destroyed all semblance of enthusiasm within the profession.

Infrared Coagulation

In 1979, Neiger described a method for the treatment of hemorrhoids using infrared coagulation.[200] Leicester and associates reported a prospective, randomized trial using this technique and found that it compared favorably with injection sclerotherapy and rubber ring ligation, except perhaps for the management of prolapse.[169,160]

The apparatus produces infrared radiation and is focused by a photoconductor (Figure 11-27). It was developed as an offshoot of laser technology, but it is not a laser (see Laser Surgery). Infrared light penetrates the tissue to a predetermined level at the speed of light and is converted to heat.[210] The amount of tissue destruction can be regulated by direct visualization and by adjusting the pulse setting on the instrument.

Technique

The procedure is relatively simple and easy to learn. A sterile, disposable sheath is placed over the light guide. An anoscope is inserted, and the light guide is placed in direct contact with the mucosa at the base of the hemorrhoid (Figure 11-28). A 1- or 1.5-second pulse is usually used in the treatment of hemorrhoids, with the probe applied at the same site where the physician would normally inject. The radiation causes protein coagulation 3 mm wide and 3 mm deep. The manufacturer recommends the application

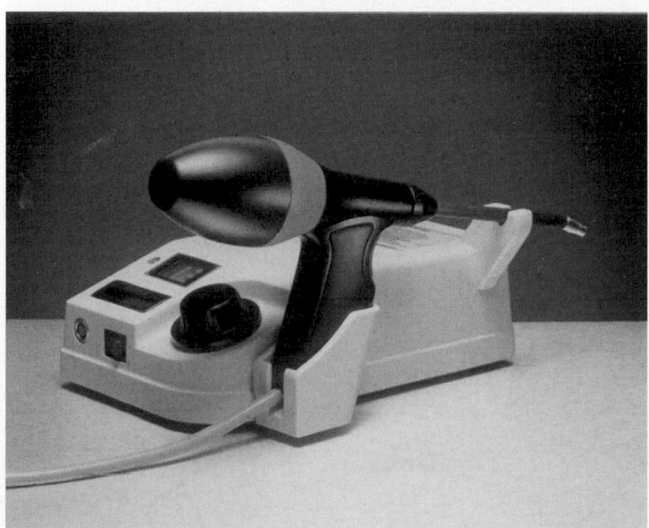

FIGURE 11-27. Infrared coagulator: power supply unit and applicator. (Courtesy of Redfield Corporation, Montvale, NJ.)

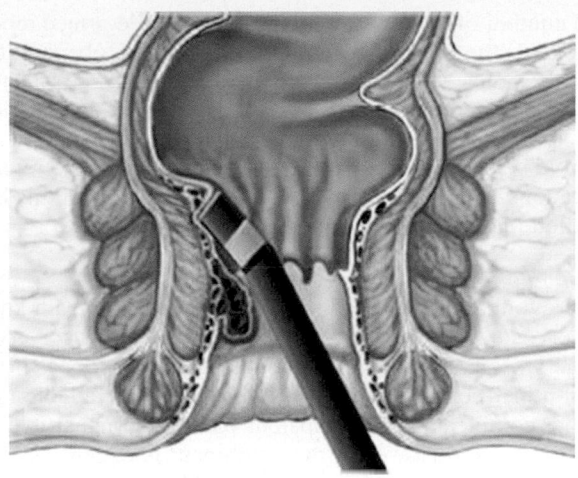

FIGURE 11-28. Application of the infrared coagulator probe to the hemorrhoid. (Courtesy of Digestive Disorders Associates, Annapolis, MD.)

of three to five pulses.[219] Following coagulation, the tissue appears as a whitish, circular eschar. Over the following week, a dark eschar forms, ultimately leaving a slightly puckered, pink to red scar.[210] The physician may elect to treat one area at a time or to ablate all evident hemorrhoids. Additional treatments may be repeated every 2 or 3 weeks if necessary. Although some authors can perform the procedure without a local anesthetic, particularly if the coagulator is applied above the dentate line, infiltrating the area with 0.5% bupivacaine (Marcaine) is often recommended. Of course, if an external tag is to be treated, a local anesthetic is required.

Results

Infrared coagulation of hemorrhoids has an excellent record of safety with minor bleeding and some discomfort occasionally observed. There have been no reported incidents of sepsis or stricture. Ambrose and colleagues compared photocoagulation and rubber ring ligation in the treatment of hemorrhoids by means of a randomized controlled study of 268 patients.[6] There was no difference in the symptomatic outcome between these two groups up to 1 year following the procedure. A higher incidence of bleeding and pain was noted following banding that was statistically significant, but additional outpatient procedures were more frequently encountered with photocoagulation. Another study from the same surgical unit compared photocoagulation with injection sclerotherapy.[7] The results were considered comparable, although the injection group required fewer additional treatments. Weinstein and colleagues noted a different result in their prospective, randomized trial of rubber ring ligation and infrared coagulation.[305] A significantly better result at 1 month and at 6 months was achieved by the former method. There was no difference with respect to pain, although banding was associated with two complications: thrombosed hemorrhoids and delayed bleeding. In the manufacturer's rebuttal to this article, Osur noted that the infrared coagulator was not designed to achieve optimal results in a single treatment session.[219] In their survey, only 3.7% of users employed just one session.

Comparison studies of the use of infrared coagulation and of bipolar diathermy (BICAP; see Bipolar Diathermy) revealed no significant difference in rate of complications and number of treatments required.[82] In a three-armed report involving the infrared technique, the heater probe, and the Ultroid device (Microvasive, Watertown, MA; see later), it was concluded that all three methods are effective modalities for first- and second-degree hemorrhoids, but that the Ultroid was associated with less discomfort and fewer complications.[321] Furthermore, the authors believed that this last method may be more applicable for larger piles.

Comment

I believe that infrared coagulation has rung the death knell for cryosurgery; the most outspoken enthusiasts for cryosurgery seem now to prefer photocoagulation. It is as if the option of freezing hemorrhoids is no longer available (see earlier comments), if the apparent void in journal articles is any indication. However, the equipment is expensive, and rubber rings are not. Moreover, even the manufacturer concurs that the technique is not recommended for the management of prolapsing hemorrhoids.

My own approach is to use infrared coagulation as the preferred alternative to injection therapy. Symptomatic hemorrhoids that are too small to band are optimally treated by this technique. I also occasionally offer it to patients for treatment of the external component (with a local anesthetic) when I do not wish to employ excisional therapy.

Ultroid

The Ultroid device is another tool for the ambulatory treatment of hemorrhoids. It is a monopolar, low-voltage instrument that includes a generator unit, an attachable handle, single-use sterile probes, a grounding pad, and a nonconductive anoscope (Figure 11-29). Some have commented that it is confusing to have two electrodes, yet the instrument is not bipolar.[81] The Ultroid Hemorrhoid Management System delivers, according to the manufacturer, Ultroid Technologies (Tampa, FL), a very low direct current to the hemorrhoid, causing a reaction in the structure. Although some people experience immediate relief, the hemorrhoid shrinks over the next 7 to 10 days. There is no need for bowel preparation, anesthesia, or surgery. And there is allegedly no healing time because there is no cutting or tissue destruction: one apparently leaves the physician's office and resumes normal activities. The company contends that the mode of action of this device is not thermal but rather is a consequence of the production of sodium hydroxide at the negative electrode. It strains credulity for me that this is the mechanism, but as I am not a biophysicist, I can merely offer healthy skepticism. The fact is that I have no experience with this device.

Technique

By means of the nonconductive anoscope (Figure 11-30), the probe tip is placed at the apex of the hemorrhoid, above the dentate line. The amperage is slowly increased to the level of patient tolerance as the probe is inserted into the hemorrhoid. The usual treatment range is 6 to 16 mA. The probe is left in position for approximately 10 minutes, or until the "popping" sounds cease. Once the treatment has been completed, the current is gradually decreased to zero. Failure to do this will result in pain on removal of the probe. One site is usually treated per session, usually because of time constraints

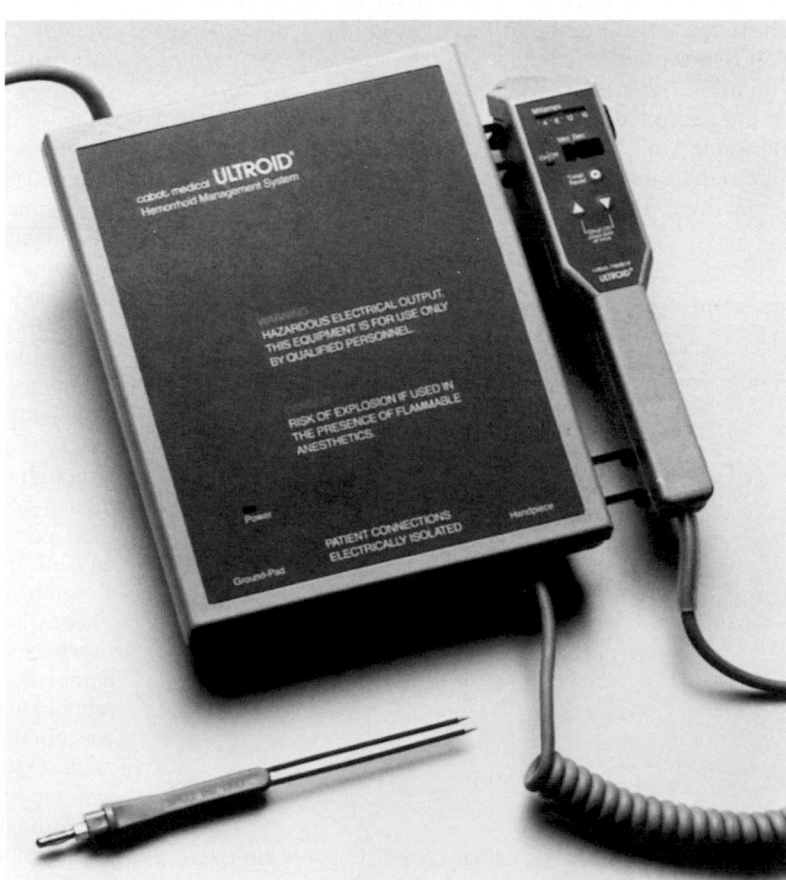

FIGURE 11-29. This Ultroid device with a generator source and handle uses disposable probes. (Courtesy of Ultroid Technologies, Inc., Tampa, FL.)

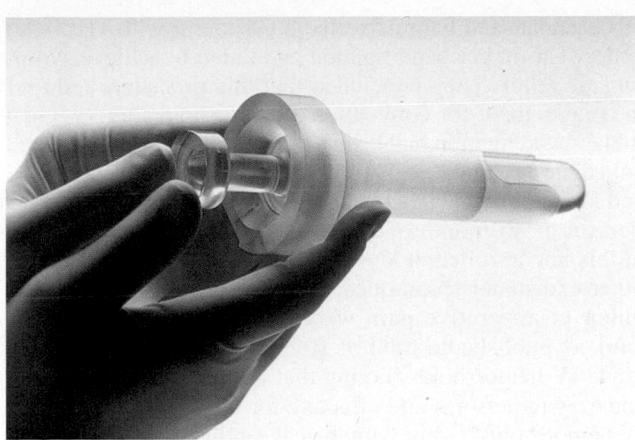

FIGURE 11-30. Nonconductive anoscope. (Courtesy of Ultroid Technologies, Inc., Tampa, Fl.)

and the fact that the patient does not usually appreciate a prolonged anoscopy.

Results

Norman and colleagues reported the application of this technique in 120 patients.[206] Ablation of the hemorrhoids was directly correlated with the amount of current employed and the duration of the treatment. The procedure was completely successful, according to the authors in every patient (i.e., all became asymptomatic), and there were no complications. Most hemorrhoid disease (78%) was successfully treated with one application of direct current. The group included 46 individuals with grade III hemorrhoids and 37 with grade IV, a most remarkable accomplishment indeed.

Dennison and colleagues comment that they achieved results comparable with those of other techniques in their 25 patients, but the time required for treatment was a particular disadvantage.[81] In addition, the operator is required to hold the probe quite still for a period of time.[80] Zinberg and colleagues noted good results in 85% of those with grade III hemorrhoids, but none of four persons with grade IV disease could be classified as having good results.[321] As previously stated, Zinberg and colleagues affirmed that Ultroid therapy was associated with less discomfort and fewer complications than either infrared coagulation or heater probe coagulation therapy. Hinton and Morris observed that the technique was effective in 26 patients, including those with large, prolapsing piles.[130] Wright and coworkers reported a prospective study from the Division of Gastroenterology at the University of Louisville, Kentucky, comparing direct current electrotherapy with standard medical therapy for symptomatic hemorrhoidal disease.[317] Those who did not respond to initial treatment were crossed over at 8 weeks, receiving alternate therapy twice. The authors concluded that no difference could be found between the standard medical therapy and that of direct current electrotherapy. The obvious extension of this conclusion is that because direct current electrotherapy is no better than standard medical treatment, it cannot be recommended for the management of symptomatic hemorrhoid disease.[317]

Comment

There is a paucity of articles in the surgical literature on the Ultroid device, perhaps because the device is also marketed to family practitioners and gastroenterologists. Personally, I am skeptical that this approach will be high on the list of options for surgeons in the ambulatory management of hemorrhoids. Most surgeons have neither the time nor the patience to stand around holding the probe for up to 10 minutes. Given the choice, it is unlikely that patients themselves will elect to have a "poker" in their anus for any more time than is necessary to get the job done.

Bipolar Diathermy

Like photocoagulation, BICAP is a method of treating hemorrhoids that is designed to produce tissue destruction, ulceration, and fibrosis by the local application of heat.[81] The diathermy system was originally developed for the treatment of bleeding peptic ulcers and was later employed to palliate esophageal and rectal carcinomas,[80] The disposable Circon ACMI BICAP hemorrhoid probe uses bipolar RF current to coagulate the blood vessels (Figure 11-31). The principle of action is the passage of current through tissue as it travels between adjacent electrodes located at the tip of the probe. The espoused, perhaps theoretical, advantage of this technique over other methods such as monopolar coagulation, laser coagulation, or photocoagulation is that the BICAP device maintains a short current path, thereby producing a limited depth of penetration even after multiple applications.

Technique

With the use of a disposable, nonconductive anoscope, the side of the probe tip is applied directly and firmly to the hemorrhoid above the dentate line.[80] The generator is used on the infinity setting and is activated by a foot switch. A white coagulum approximately 3 mm deep is produced. All hemorrhoids are treated in one session, and no local anesthetic is usually required.

Results

Numerous controlled trials have been published comparing BICAP with other ambulatory methods in the management of hemorrhoids. Hinton and Morris randomly allocated patients with third-degree hemorrhoids to either this technique or to the Ultroid.[130] Both were believed to be effective, essentially equally so. There were no particular complications in either group, but the time advantage, and therefore better patient

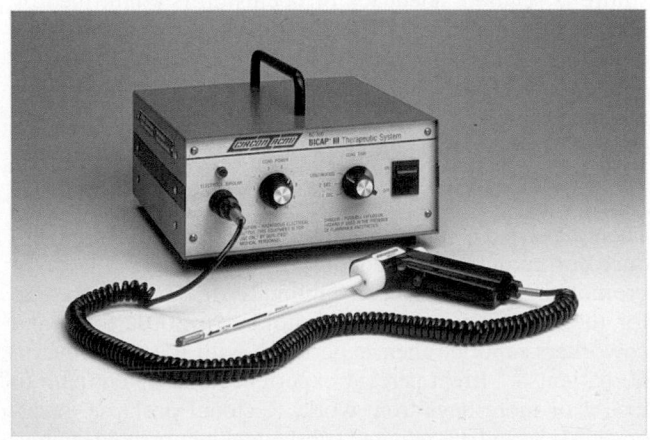

FIGURE 11-31. Bipolar diathermy (BICAP) hemorrhoid probe and generator. (Courtesy of Circon ACMI, Santa Barbara, CA.)

acceptability, was enjoyed by BICAP. Dennison and colleagues compared BICAP with infrared photocoagulation.[82] The authors opined that BICAP permits multiple applications to the same site without producing excessive tissue penetration, whereas infrared photocoagulation produces further penetration under these circumstances. Overheating and breakdown were problems more frequently encountered with the infrared coagulator. Griffith and colleagues randomized 110 patients to receive either BICAP or rubber ring ligation.[121] There were no substantive differences in the results when the two methods were compared.

Randall and coworkers compared direct current (Ultroid) and bipolar electrocoagulation (BICAP).[242] There were no statistically significant differences with respect to the two modalities, but because of the speed of the latter technique, the authors recommended it. Yang and others concurred with the issue of pain in their randomly assigned study with direct current versus bipolar electrocoagulation.[319] In addition, however, there was a statistically significantly increased incidence of pain with the Ultroid device.

Ultrasonic Doppler-Guided Transanal Hemorrhoidal Ligation (Dearterialization—THD)

In 1995, a Japanese surgeon, Kazumasa Morinaga and his colleagues, conceived of a novel way to treat hemorrhoids. He identified the hemorrhoidal arteries by means of a Doppler (ultrasound) transducer.[196] This specially designed instrument contained a Doppler transducer and a window, which permitted the surgeon to identify and ligate the hemorrhoidal arteries by placing a suture around them.

Technique

A progressive anal dilation is performed, and a modified anoscope with built-in ultrasound transducer, light, and special window Echo sounder is inserted, with reduction of any prolapsing tissue and anoderm, and rotated to locate the artery to be ligated (Figure 11-32). The arterial sound is clearly audible when the Doppler transducer is directly over the hemorrhoidal artery. The vessel is then suture ligated. At each location (the typical procedure requires treatment of six to eight locations), the hemorrhoidal arterial branch is identified and ligated through the aperture in the anoscope with a figure-of-eight or purse-string suture. Each time a suture is secured, adequacy of occlusion is confirmed by loss of Doppler signal. The completeness of suture hemorrhoidopexy is also confirmed circumferentially and, if needed, additional plication sutures are placed to achieve the desired results. A local anesthetic may be injected to control postoperative pain.

Results

There has been a number of published reports of this procedure during the past decade, especially because it is being promoted as an alternative, minimally invasive procedure for the management of hemorrhoids. In 2001, Sohn and coworkers reported their experience with the technique in 60 patients.[278] Eight percent experienced sufficient pain to lose 2 or more days from work. Residual prolapse developed in 7%, and 3% required subsequent hemorrhoidectomy. They concluded that the procedure is an effective alternative to hemorrhoidectomy.

Conaghan and Farouk treated 203 patients with THD who underwent rubber band ligation and failed to achieve symptomatic relief. They concluded that this procedure reduced the requirement for conventional hemorrhoid surgery when rubber band ligation had been unsuccessful.[63] Dal Monte and colleagues performed THD in 330 patients with grade III and IV hemorrhoids, two-thirds of whom were followed for a mean of 46 months.[75] The efficacy and recurrence rates in this uncontrolled study were felt to be similar to that of other excisional techniques. A low complication rate and minor postoperative pain were noted. Faucheron and coworkers published a total of 100 consecutive patients with grade IV hemorrhoids, noting that the procedure was "safe and easy to perform and effective for the treatment of grade IV hemorrhoids"—but with the caveat that there was lack of a long-term follow-up as well as the absence of a controlled comparison with other surgical options.[92] However, Bursics and associates found comparable results with a 1-year follow-up comparing conventional hemorrhoidectomy with THD.[44] Others note satisfactory results in the treatment of grade III and grade IV hemorrhoids.[288]

Opinion

There is confusion in the literature whether this procedure is truly applicable to grade IV hemorrhoidal disease. Still, the primary advantage of this technique is that there is no cutting; hence, there is less discomfort. Historically, however, the concept of hemorrhoid ligation without excision was associated with a high rate of persistent symptoms, and, as a consequence, the procedure fell into disrepute. However, perhaps the ability to clearly identify and ligate the arteries will permit long-term benefit. Longer follow-up is required before one can adequately assess the merits of this new approach, as well as meaningful prospective randomized controlled clinical trials.[98,114,243]

Lord's Dilatation

In addition to the nonexcisional methods of treatment for hemorrhoids that have been discussed, another procedure, that of anal dilatation, should be included in this category. In 1968, Lord reported a method he had devised for the treatment of hemorrhoids.[174] He based his approach on the hypothesis that increased anal canal pressure contributes to the hemorrhoid problem, and that dilatation reduces this pressure, thereby ameliorating the condition. Although this method requires a general or spinal anesthetic, hospitalization can often be limited to a 1-day stay, or the patient can be discharged from an ambulatory care facility or similar surgical center.

Technique

Lord stated, "The procedure takes a little less time to perform than to describe."[175] The instruments are not sterile. The patient is placed on the left side and given an intravenous anesthetic. A constriction to the outlet, which Lord believes is present in all patients with third-degree hemorrhoids, is identified.

Two fingers of one hand are pulled upward, and the index finger of the other hand presses downward to feel the constriction. The aim is to dilate the lower part of the rectum and anal canal gently and firmly until no constrictions remain. It is an "ironing out" process that is carried out by a circular movement through all four quadrants. Tearing should be avoided. During the procedure, eight fingers are inserted as

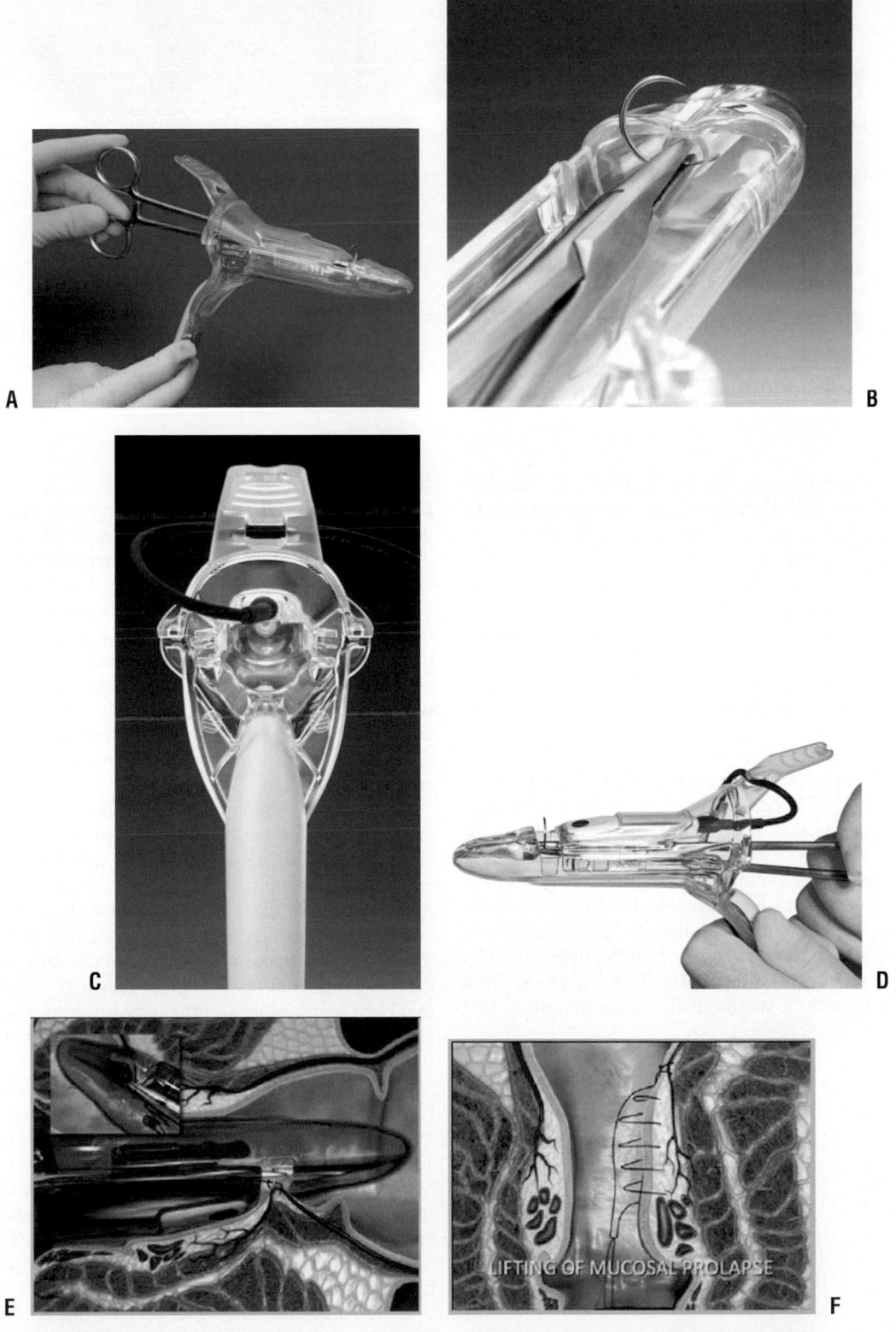

FIGURE 11-32. Ultrasonic Doppler-guided transanal hemorrhoidal dearterialization (THD). **A:** Side view with needle holder inserted into the pivot. **B:** Cutaway detailed view of needle holder inserted into the pivot. **C:** Rear view showing unencumbered direct visualization. **D:** Side view fully assembled. Note precise needle location and rotation. **E:** Dearterialization: Doppler detection and ligation (anchor stitch). **F:** Running mucopexy stitch. *(continued)*

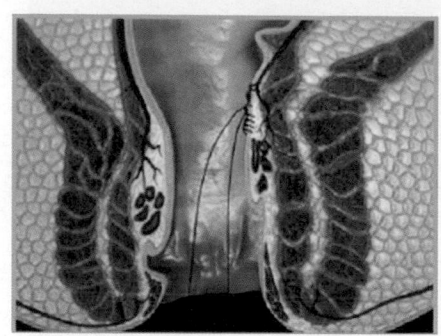
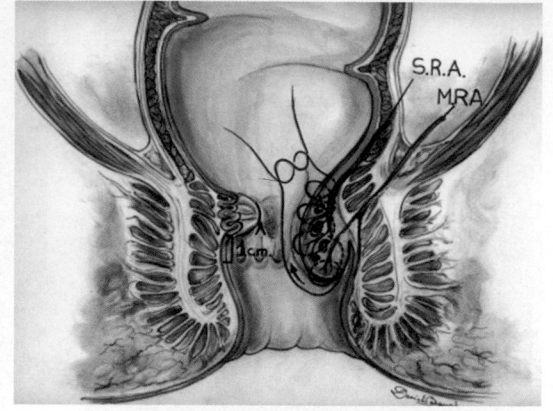

G

H

FIGURE 11-32. *(continued)* **G:** Tissue lifted using figure of 8 stitch tied to original anchor stitch. **H:** Different view, not completed mucopexy at left. (Courtesy of THD America.)

high as they will reach, actually dilating not only the anal canal, but also the rectal ampulla. Not all patients can be dilated safely to this extent, and Lord cautions that it is much better to do too little than too much.

As dilatation is achieved, an assistant inserts a sponge, usually by means of ring forceps. The sponge presses on the walls of the lower part of the rectum and anal canal and is apparently used to reduce the risk for postoperative hematoma formation. The sponge is left in place for 1 hour, and the patient is discharged when alert.

Postoperative Care

The patient is instructed on the insertion of a dilating cone (Figure 11-33), which can be used as required for anal symptoms, but even Lord wondered whether it is vital to the success of the method. Vellacott and Hardcastle randomly allocated one group of patients to a bulk laxative and the other to a dilator.[297] Because there was no difference in results, they concluded that an anal dilator was not necessary. However, Greca and colleagues reported the opposite to be true.[120] The patient is advised to take 2 or 3 days off from work and be seen after 2 weeks. If free of symptoms at that time, the patient is discharged.

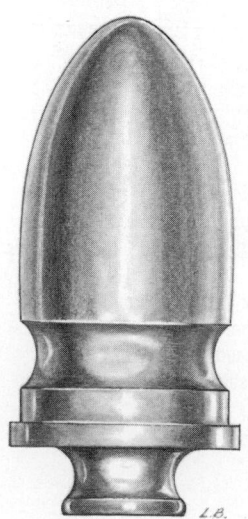

FIGURE 11-33. Lord's dilator.

Results

Lord claimed that less pain and postoperative morbidity occur after dilatation than after hemorrhoidectomy. He states that his method does not cause urinary retention, deep vein thrombosis, postoperative bleeding, or fecal impaction. The patients are free of pain during defecation, operating room time is saved, and the hospital stay is greatly shortened. Still, in Lord's opinion, rubber ring ligation is the treatment of choice for most hemorrhoid problems, and dilatation should be used as an alternative to surgical hemorrhoidectomy. However, he suggested that hemorrhoidectomy should be considered when hypertrophied papillae and external tags are present.

Creve and Hubens noted the effect of the procedure on anal pressure.[73] They found a significant lowering of pressure following dilatation compared with that occurring after conventional hemorrhoidectomy. Keighley and colleagues, in a prospective trial, compared dilatation, sphincterotomy, and a high-fiber diet in patients classified into two groups: those with low maximal resting anal pressure and those with elevated maximal resting anal pressure.[149] They concluded that Lord's procedure significantly lowered resting anal pressure, but it should be the treatment of choice in those patients with a preoperative elevation in pressure.

A 5-year follow-up study of 100 patients who underwent Lord's dilatation for hemorrhoids was reported by Walls and Ruckley.[299] Hemorrhoids were first-degree lesions in 15 patients, second-degree in 48, and third-degree in 37. Seventy-five patients were free of symptoms or greatly improved following dilatation, but the treatment was unsuccessful in 22. All except 1 of these patients reported failure within 3 months, and 19 were subsequently treated by hemorrhoidectomy.

A prospective study was carried out by McCaffrey on 50 patients with hemorrhoids treated by the Lord method and followed for at least 4 years.[183] Of 36 individuals who were free of symptoms, 19 still had evidence of anal congestion but no distinct hemorrhoids, and 4 subsequently underwent a standard hemorrhoid operation for persistent prolapse and bleeding.

Jones compared three different methods of treatment (i.e., surgical hemorrhoidectomy, rubber ring ligation, and maximal anal dilatation) used successively, with 100 patients in each group.[144] Follow-up was obtained at 4 weeks and at

6 months. The author believed that a reasonable effort should be made to avoid excisional surgery except when one of the other methods fails to relieve symptoms. Older patients who underwent anal dilatation occasionally reported control problems, so Jones recommends that Lord's procedure be limited to those younger than 55 years of age. Twenty (40%) of McCaffrey's patients had mild incontinence from 4 to 26 days after operation.[183] The problem was primarily limited to flatus and mucus, with minimal impairment of control of feces.

Lewis and colleagues randomly allocated 112 patients with prolapsing hemorrhoids to maximal anal dilatation, rubber ring ligation, cryosurgery, and hemorrhoidectomy.[170] Five weeks after treatment, anal dilatation was found to be as effective as surgical removal in control of symptoms, but residual hemorrhoids were more evident after Lord's procedure. The other methods were less successful. Follow-up as long as 5 years revealed that surgical hemorrhoidectomy offered the best results for this group of patients.

In the most recent published paper (2000), Konsten and Baeten followed patients for a median of 17 years in a prospective, randomized trial of hemorrhoidectomy versus Lord's method.[139] Recurrent hemorrhoids were noted in 26% of patients who underwent hemorrhoidectomy but in 46% with the operative dilation (with the postoperative dilation program). Interestingly, those who were not dilating postoperatively did better (39% recurrence). Fifty-two percent of those who underwent Lord's procedure experienced incontinence symptoms. The authors concluded that the procedure should be abandoned.

Opinion

When one performs this maneuver, it has been facetiously remarked that the surgeon (or more likely the patient) will chant, "Lord, Lord!" I do not recommend Lord's dilatation for the treatment of hemorrhoids. Failure to deal with tags and papillae, as well as the risk of incontinence, especially in patients older than 60 years of age, should preclude the application of this technique. The physician must recognize that sphincter stretch inevitably must attenuate the external sphincter as well as the internal. With the plethora of innovations for the treatment of hemorrhoids, excisional and nonexcisional, I expect that the procedure inevitably will be referred to as a historical curiosity.

Internal Anal Sphincterotomy

Using the principle that many patients who harbor hemorrhoids have elevated anal canal pressure, Schouten and van Vroonhoven selected those with such elevations for sphincterotomy as the primary treatment of symptomatic hemorrhoids.[266] For a discussion of the techniques and indications for internal anal sphincterotomy, see Chapter 12. Individuals with normal or low anal pressures were treated by rubber ring ligation or hemorrhoidectomy. About 75% of patients who were managed by sphincterotomy alone were considered successfully treated. The authors suggest that this procedure is a good alternative in selected patients.

Opinion

Seventy-five percent is usually considered a passing grade in an examination, not for a surgical procedure. There is a real morbidity associated with internal anal sphincterotomy (see Chapter 12). Sphincterotomy alone for the primary treatment of hemorrhoids should not be done—full stop.

▶ TREATMENT OF THROMBOSED HEMORRHOIDS

External Hemorrhoids

The patient with thrombosed external hemorrhoids usually presents with a painful, tender, bluish mass (Figure 11-34) and may report that the lump appeared following a bout of constipation or diarrhea. If one or the other is a frequent occurrence, appropriate counseling needs to be implemented. An important predisposing factor for the development of recurrent thrombosed hemorrhoids is spending too much time on the toilet. Counseling should also include the suggestion of removing the library from the bathroom as a prophylactic measure.

If the problem has been present for more than 2 or 3 days, the discomfort usually has begun to subside. Under these circumstances, medical management should be offered. This consists of appropriate counseling in the use of sitz baths and stool softeners. A mild analgesic may be recommended. Topical nifedipine (0.3% nifedipine and 1.5% lidocaine ointment, every 12 hours), a calcium channel antagonist, has also been demonstrated to afford excellent pain relief in a prospective, randomized clinical trial.[229] The control group received only the lidocaine.

The mass will usually resolve in 7 to 10 days, especially if the patient makes a vigorous effort to apply heat to the area. If the area involved corresponds to the location where the patient reports a tendency for prolapse, rubber ring ligation should be considered following resolution of symptoms. If

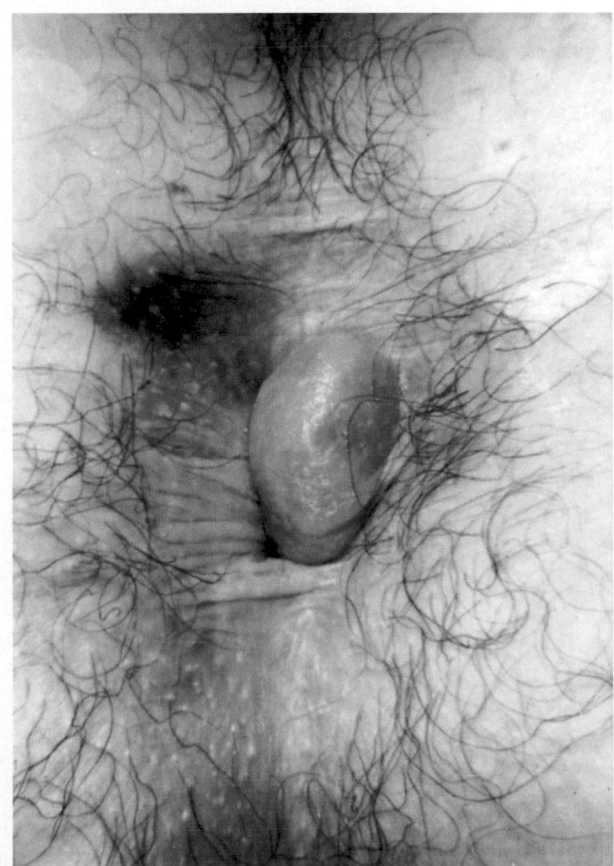

FIGURE 11-34. A thrombosed external hemorrhoid.

ulceration or rupture has occurred, or if the patient is seen within 48 hours, it is usually advisable to excise the lesion. Certainly, if the pain is severe, excision is preferred.

Technique

The hemorrhoid should be excised, not incised. Making a small incision and shelling the clot out like a pea from a pod often results in recurrent hemorrhage into the subcutaneous tissue and clot reaccumulation. Simple incision often produces more swelling and pain with recurrent bleeding than did the original thrombosis. This necessitates a visit to the emergency facility with the inevitable consequence of an angry patient.

Figure 11-35 demonstrates the proper technique for performing the excision, albeit with a bit of artistic license

and exaggeration of the size of the defect to make a point. The principle is to leave the wound open a bit to permit drainage. The area is infiltrated with a local anesthetic of choice (e.g., a solution of 0.5% bupivacaine [Marcaine] in 1:200,000 epinephrine). The bupivacaine solution as commercially prepared is quite acidic and is often associated with extreme burning pain upon injection[67]; however, pH adjustment through increased alkalinization ameliorates this problem considerably.[185,186,195,216,224] The alkalinization of bupivacaine has been said to be difficult because precipitation occurs rapidly, thus limiting the increase in pH.[40] Because epinephrine is unstable in alkaline solution, it is important that administration take place within 6 hours after alkalinization. It is therefore recommended that 1 mL of 8.4% sodium

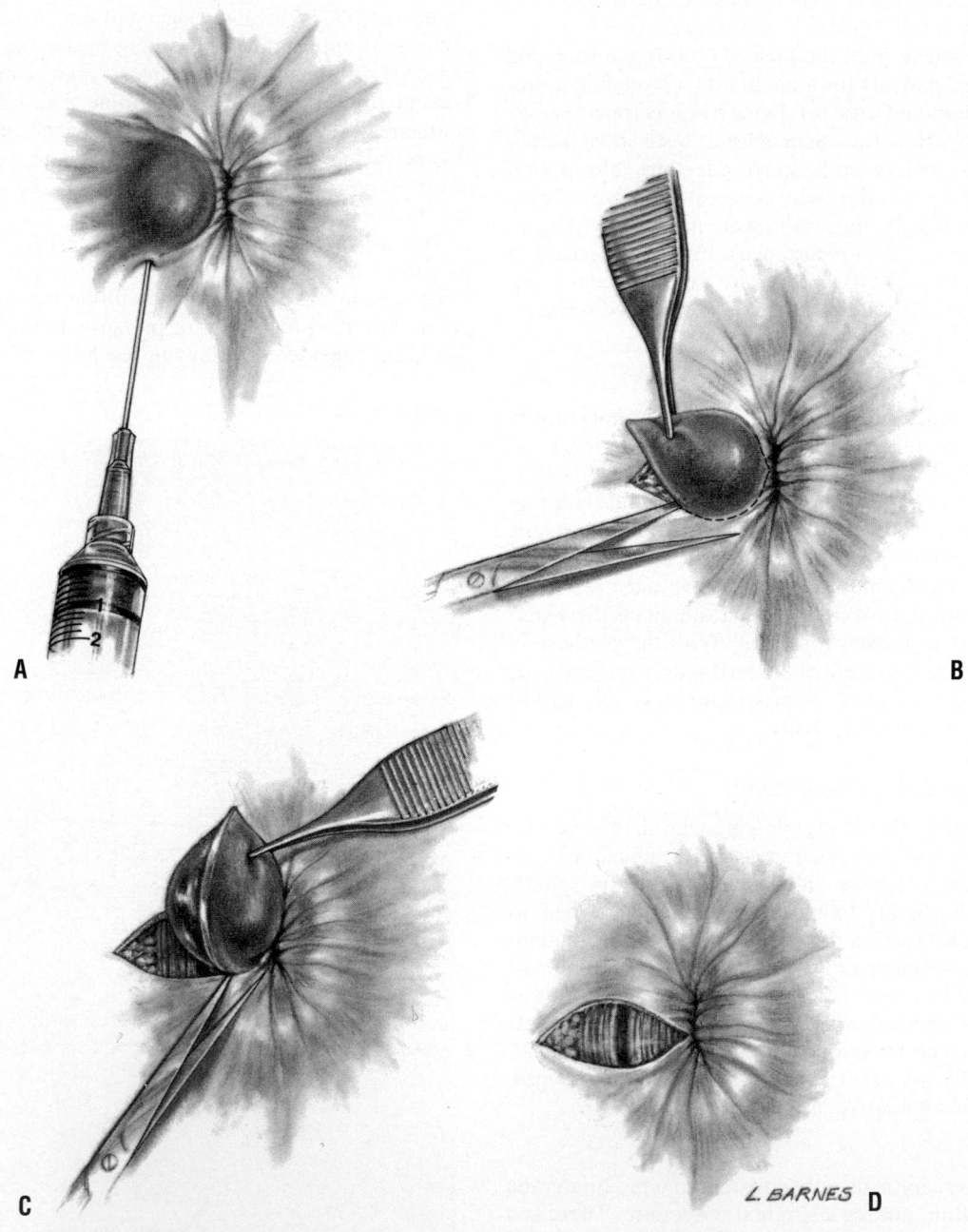

FIGURE 11-35. Excision of a thrombosed hemorrhoid. **A:** The area is infiltrated with 0.5% bupivacaine in 1:200, epinephrine. **B,C:** The thrombosis is excised with the underlying vein and with a wedge of skin. **D:** Skin edges are sufficiently separate to permit adequate drainage, thereby preventing reaccumulation of a clot.

bicarbonate solution, USP, be added to 9 mL of bupivacaine with epinephrine. This markedly improves the discomfort associated with the injection. We have also had a favorable experience with the WAND local anesthetic delivery system (Milestone Scientific, Inc., Livingston, NJ).[285] This foot pedal-controlled, computer-automated apparatus allows precise delivery of anesthesia at a constant flow rate. As such it is quite effective in providing a more comfortable experience for the patient.

The underlying hemorrhoid is excised, as is a wedge of skin (Figure 11-35). Bleeding is controlled with pressure, topically applied epinephrine, or electrocautery.[145] Another option is Monsel's solution, a chemical styptic agent (ferric subsulfate).[141] A pressure dressing is used.

Postoperative Care

The patient is instructed to maintain the pressure dressing in place for a few hours. By this time there is usually some discomfort, and the dressing is then removed. Sitz baths are then commenced. If bleeding occurs, it can usually be controlled by the application of direct pressure on the wound with a cloth or compress. A small dressing or pad can be used to avoid soiling clothing. Twice-daily sitz baths are recommended until the wound heals (i.e., 7 to 10 days). A mild analgesic and a topical anesthetic cream are usually salutary.

Internal Hemorrhoids

In addition to the previously mentioned factors that may cause thrombosis of external hemorrhoids, prolapse with inadequate reduction may cause thrombosis of internal hemorrhoids. As a result, stasis develops within the vein and thrombosis occurs.

The treatment of thrombosed internal hemorrhoids is not as straightforward as that for external hemorrhoids. Fortunately, however, pain is not as frequent a complaint. Excision of a thrombosed internal hemorrhoid, however, requires instrumentation and a more extensive local infiltration or field block. Suturing within the anal canal is always necessary to maintain hemostasis, simply because the application of adequate direct pressure is virtually impossible.

Because operative intervention for the acute problem is rarely indicated, sitz baths are recommended, as well as a mild systemic analgesic and a topical anesthetic cream or suppository. A stool softener is also advisable. If the patient has concurrent extensive hemorrhoids, tags, hypertrophied papillae, or associated anal fissure, a surgical approach may ultimately be advocated.

► GANGRENOUS, PROLAPSED, EDEMATOUS HEMORRHOIDS

The patient who presents with severely disabling, irreducibly prolapsed, gangrenous hemorrhoids requires urgent medical measures and, ideally, some form of surgical intervention. A carefully conceived hemorrhoidectomy within 24 hours is the preferred approach if convenient for the patient, but there are other options. Pain, swelling, bleeding, foul-smelling discharge, and difficulty defecating are common presenting complaints. Of prior hemorrhoidal difficulties, prolapse is the most frequent. Proctosigmoidoscopic and anoscopic examination reveal edematous, thrombosed, irreducible hemorrhoids (Figures 11-8 and 11-36).

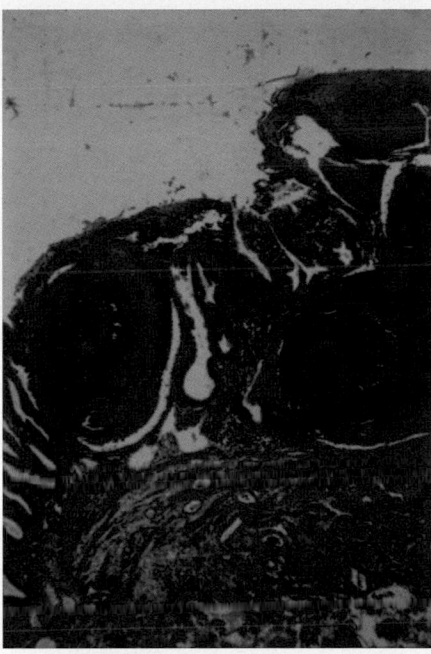

FIGURE 11-36. Hemorrhoidal tissue with hemorrhage is seen in a patient who underwent urgent hemorrhoidectomy. Note the dilated veins close to the surface containing recent blood clots. (Original magnification × 180.)

Nonoperative alternatives consist of warm sitz baths, analgesics, stool softeners, creams, lotions, and suppositories. Ice packs and bed rest with the legs elevated have also been recommended, but confining a patient under such circumstances suggests to me 19th-century medicine rather than 21st, especially because the end point may not be reached for 2 or 3 weeks. Other options include reduction of the mass by means of a field block (see later) followed by the application of pressure, the injection of hyaluronidase to dissipate the edema, and the evacuation of the clots, with or without concomitant rubber band ligations.

Technique of Creating a Field Block

A perianal field block is established by using a local anesthetic solution. My own preference is to employ an alkalinized solution of 0.5% bupivacaine (Marcaine) with 1:200,000 epinephrine, and ideally adding to this two 1 mm ampules of hyaluronidase (300 NF units of hyaluronidase [Wydase]). Unfortunately, the use of hyaluronidase in the United States has been called into question because of the potential for allergic reaction as well as its interaction with certain commonly used prescription medications. A subcutaneous circumanal wheal is infiltrated into the edematous hemorrhoidal tissue (Figure 11-37). Four deep injections are made in the intersphincteric groove in each quadrant to effect paralysis of the sphincter mechanism and to create total perianal anesthesia. A finger may be inserted into the rectum during introduction of the needle to avoid penetrating the lumen of the bowel, but this is unlikely to occur. Care should also be taken to avoid entering the vagina, prostate, or urethra anteriorly. After a few minutes, in order to allow the medication to take effect, direct massaging pressure is applied with a sterile pad to reduce the hemorrhoidal mass. A pressure dressing is used, and the buttocks are taped if no further intervention is planned at

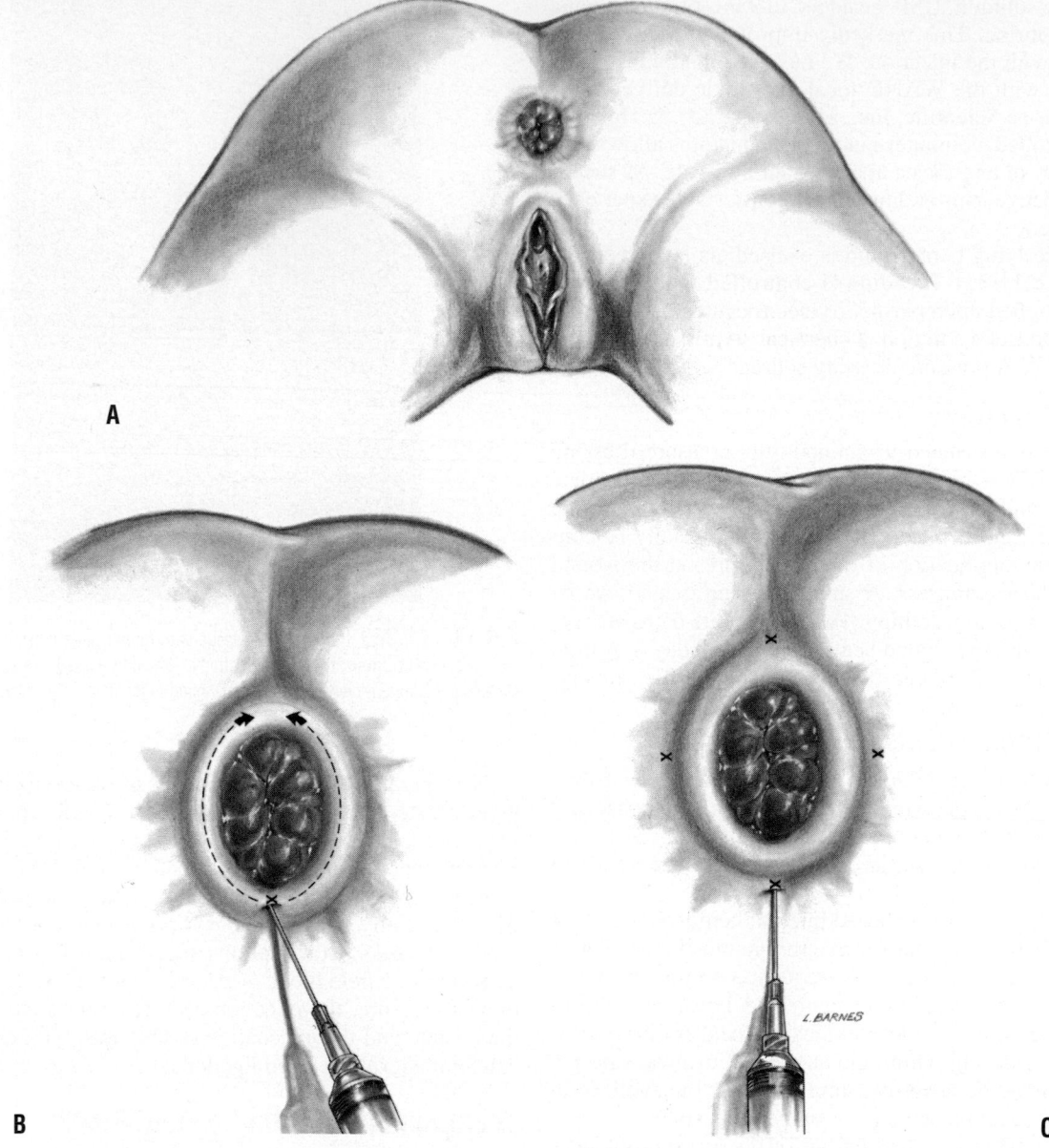

FIGURE 11-37. Method of establishing perianal field block. **A:** The patient is placed in the prone (i.e., jackknife) position. **B:** A subcutaneous perianal wheal is raised. **C:** Deep injections are made at four sites to effect further anesthesia and paralysis of sphincter muscles.

the time. Alternatively, one may elect to evacuate the clots and even to perform multiple rubber band ligations, as has been advocated by some surgeons.

My personal approach is, ideally, to admit the patient to the hospital on an emergency basis, and a hemorrhoidectomy is performed the same day or the following. With reduction maintained, the patient is usually reasonably comfortable, and an adequate, safe operation can be performed with less edema than would be present without reduction (see Surgical Hemorrhoidectomy).

Results of Emergency Surgery

Historically, the concept of surgical hemorrhoidectomy in the presence of thrombosed, ulcerated, gangrenous hemorrhoids was considered unwise because of the risks for pyelophlebitis, perianal sepsis, hemorrhage, and the sub-

sequent development of anal stricture. However, with the application of proper surgical technique, the complication rate should be minimal. Ackland reported 25 patients with prolapsed and strangulated hemorrhoids who underwent emergency operations.[1] The results were compared with those in a similar group who had elective surgery for chronic hemorrhoids. According to this study, operation for prolapsed and strangulated hemorrhoids in the acute stage was safe and effective, comparable to that of elective operation for chronic hemorrhoidal complaints. Postoperative pain was not significantly different. Anal stenosis, however, developed in one individual. Shieh and Gennaro reported 23 patients who underwent "semiemergency" hemorrhoidectomy 12 to 24 hours after manual reduction by a method similar to that described previously.[273] Early hemorrhage developed in one person, and an episode of late bleeding in another, but there were no other complications, save urinary retention, that could be directly attributed to the procedure. Others have also reported success with this management.[89,128] Eisenstat and colleagues used the aforementioned field block and then performed multiple rubber ring ligations, incising any thromboses, rather than performing a surgical hemorrhoidectomy.[87] They reported gratifying results without significant complication.

Comment

As suggested, because conservative treatment of strangulated hemorrhoids (i.e., sitz baths, analgesics, and stool softeners) entails the prolongation of disability and perhaps financial hardship, urgent operation is advised for all such individuals. It must be remembered, however, that the patient may harbor colonic pathology (e.g., inflammatory bowel disease or neoplasm) that may be the predisposing factor for the hemorrhoid problem. At minimum, a proctosigmoidoscopic examination should be performed prior to hemorrhoidectomy. The decision whether to embark on a more extensive evaluation before or after the operation should rest on the surgeon's judgment in the individual case.

▶ OPERATIVE APPROACHES TO THE TREATMENT OF HEMORRHOIDS

Surgical hemorrhoidectomy should be considered when the anorectal architecture has been severely compromised (e.g., with an external component, ulceration, gangrene, extensive thrombosis, hypertrophied papillae, or associated fissure). In 1993, the previously mentioned Standards Task Force of the American Society of Colon and Rectal Surgeons stipulated that excision of a "solitary external hemorrhoid can be performed as an outpatient procedure. For the satisfactory surgical treatment of internal hemorrhoids, with or without external hemorrhoids, ambulatory or inpatient stay is determined by the operating surgeon based on the preoperative clinical findings or the pathologic findings at surgery."[279] In 2003, "Practice Parameters for Ambulatory Anorectal Surgery" were published by the Standards Task Force.[234] The following were some of the conclusions:

- Anorectal surgery may be safely and cost-effectively performed in an ambulatory surgery center.
- Approximately 90% of anorectal cases may be suitable for ambulatory surgery.
- Patients with American Society of Anesthesiologists classifications I and II are generally considered suitable; selected category III patients may also be appropriate candidates.
- The choice of preoperative investigations should be determined by the history and physical examination.
- Most anorectal surgery may be safely and cost-effectively performed with a local anesthetic; regional and general anesthesia can be used depending on physician and patient preference.

One should add, however, that in the United States, the decisions on the facility for undertaking the procedure (hospital, ambulatory surgery facility, or office) and whether hospitalization is optimal for the patient are always determined by a third-party payer. The likelihood that the patient will be permitted hospitalization beyond what is termed "a 23-hour stay" is virtually nonexistent.

Preoperative, Intraoperative, and Postoperative General Principles

The most useful preoperative measure, in my opinion, is a small-volume enema (e.g., Fleet) the morning of operation. Vigorous mechanical cleansing by means of laxatives is counterproductive. The patient should be able to defecate as soon as possible after the operation and yet be empty of stool that could be a nuisance to the surgeon during the procedure.

No antibiotics are indicated, absent those conditions that require prophylaxis (see Chapter 5). Minimal intravenous fluids should be administered before and during the anesthesia, and the patient should be encouraged to void following the procedure. However, I do not increase fluid intake in the recovery room in order to stimulate urinating and have no aversion about overruling some hospital's policy that mandates voiding before discharge (see Complications, Urinary Retention). Patients do better in the peacefulness of their own familiar environment when compared with the public performance that is sometimes demanded in the recovery area. A small area may be shaved in the operating room if the situation warrants.

Conventional Surgical Approaches

Ideally, the goal of conventional hemorrhoidectomy is to excise completely all the hemorrhoidal tissue without postoperative complication. Unfortunately, this is sometimes an unrealized objective. Part of the failure may be attributable to the low priority that operations in the anal area command in most general surgery residency training programs, at least in the United States. As a consequence, the performance of surgical hemorrhoidectomy too frequently involves instruction of the surgical resident by an inexperienced surgeon. No less an authority than the late John Goligher stated, "Anal surgery is usually a matter of the novice being taught by the incompetent."

Hemorrhoidectomy should be planned at the operating table and should proceed according to the dictates of the individual case. Inserting a dry sponge into the rectum and withdrawing it is an excellent way to demonstrate hemorrhoidal tissue, tags, papillae, and the extent of redundant mucosa. Not every patient will have hemorrhoids in the classical three-quadrant distribution previously mentioned. The surgeon should, therefore, be prepared to excise any and all hemorrhoidal disease and redundant mucosa, irrespective of the location within and outside the anal canal. However, a bridge of intact skin and mucosa should be left between excised hemorrhoidal sites to avoid subsequent stricture formation (see Complications). This is particularly important when operating for acute, edematous, or gangrenous hemorrhoids.

Numerous approaches have been used for the surgical removal of hemorrhoids. Some eponymous operations include those of Buie, Fansler, Ferguson, Milligan-Morgan, Parks, Salmon, and Whitehead and their colleagues.[42,90,96,189,223,258,308] The procedure that I favor is a modification of Ferguson or closed hemorrhoidectomy.

Closed (Ferguson) Hemorrhoidectomy
Anesthesia and Patient Position
The patient is placed in the prone jackknife position with the buttocks taped apart (Figure 11-38). Having the patient in the lithotomy position is awkward for the assistant because a moderate amount of suturing is required when the primary closure technique is used. However, many surgeons in the

CLIFFORD NAUNTON MORGAN (1901–1986)

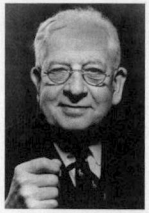

Naunton Morgan was born in Penygraig, Glamorgan, Wales on December 20, 1901. He was educated at the Royal Masonic School, Bushey, and at University College Cardiff, Wales, before entering St. Bartholomew's Hospital Medical College. Having received his fellowship in the Royal College of Surgeons in 1927, he subsequently became an anatomy demonstrator at St. Bartholomew's. Following several years, initially as assistant surgeon and then as chief assistant to Charles Gordon-Watson, he ultimately was appointed surgeon to St. Mark's Hospital as well as assistant director of the Professorial Surgical Unit at St. Bartholomew's Hospital. Following the outbreak of World War II, Naunton Morgan joined the Royal Army Medical Corps and was appointed officer-in-charge of a surgical division with the rank of lieutenant colonel, ultimately achieving the rank of brigadier to the East African Command. He remained a consultant surgeon to the navy, army, and air force until his retirement. Naunton Morgan contributed numerous articles and chapters in colon and rectal surgery, receiving many awards and recognitions, including honorary fellow of the American College of Surgeons, president of the Association of Surgeons of Great Britain and Ireland, and president of the section of proctology of the Royal Society of Medicine. He died February 24, 1986 at the age of 84. (Photograph, Courtesy of St. Mark's Hospital, Harrow, United Kingdom.)

WALTER WHITEHEAD (1840–1913)

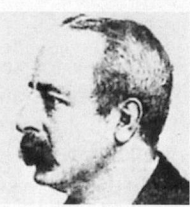

Whitehead was born at Haslem Hey, Bury, England, where his father's family had resided for more than 200 years. At the age of 19, he decided to study medicine and practiced initially in Mansfield, where he organized a small cottage hospital. In 1867, he was appointed to the St. Mary's Hospital for Women and Children in Manchester. He became involved in a number of charitable organizations and was instrumental in the introduction of a bill before the House of Commons on the protection of infant life. In 1885, he was elected president of the Manchester Medical Society, and at his inaugural address he attracted much attention for initially recognizing the increased incidence of cancer. Whitehead's operative technique seemed to be characterized by originality as well as by a certain simplified approach. Two operations bear his name: his method of excising the tongue and his method of hemorrhoidectomy. This latter operation was severely criticized even in his own day because of the "deformity," perhaps in some cases the result of misapplication of "drawing down the divided surface of mucous membrane and attaching [it] by several fine silk sutures to the denuded border at the verge of the anus." (Whitehead W. The surgical treatment of haemorrhoids. *Br Med J*. 1882;1(1101):148–150.)

JAMES A. FERGUSON (1915–2005)

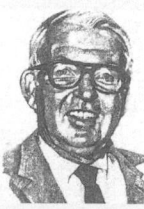

James Ferguson was born in Grand Rapids, Michigan and attended Grand Rapids Junior College, completing his undergraduate work and medical degree at the University of Michigan in Ann Arbor. His surgical residency was undertaken in Lexington, Kentucky, and after completion he returned to Grand Rapids, Michigan in July 1941. "Dr. Jim," as he was fondly called, was made the first new partner of Ferguson-Droste-Ferguson Clinic, a medical center established by his father and uncle. However, his tenure was interrupted by induction into the medical battalion of the Army Air Force in 1942. Returning to Grand Rapids from World War II overseas duty in 1945, Ferguson renewed and expanded his certifications in proctology (later colon and rectal surgery). In 1952, he established his place as president of the Ferguson-Droste-Ferguson Clinic, later changed to the Ferguson Clinic. His career was dominated by special awards, certifications, and innovations in the field of colon and rectal surgery, including presidency of the American Society of Colon and Rectal Surgeons. To this day, his papers and teachings are standards in the field. Under the influence of leading Midwestern proctologists, he established this specialty at the Ferguson-Droste-Ferguson Clinic. Ferguson was highly influential as an educator, establishing one of the first residency programs through the American Board of Proctology. He was a master at building team spirit and loyalty among the staff and residents. He provided free housing and an apartment in the hospital for on-call residents, long before the concept became routine for teaching hospitals. Ferguson suggested that it was possible to close the wounds after hemorrhoidectomy without risking infection. By this technique, a procedure he performed more than 10,000 times, he felt that there was more rapid healing, better hemostasis, reduced likelihood of stricture, less pain, and a more cosmetic result. "Dr. Jim" retired from the Ferguson Clinic in 1978 and maintained a residence in Fort Myers, Florida until a move in 1995 to Austell, Georgia. He died at his home on February 6, 2005. (Courtesy of John M. MacKeigan, MD.)

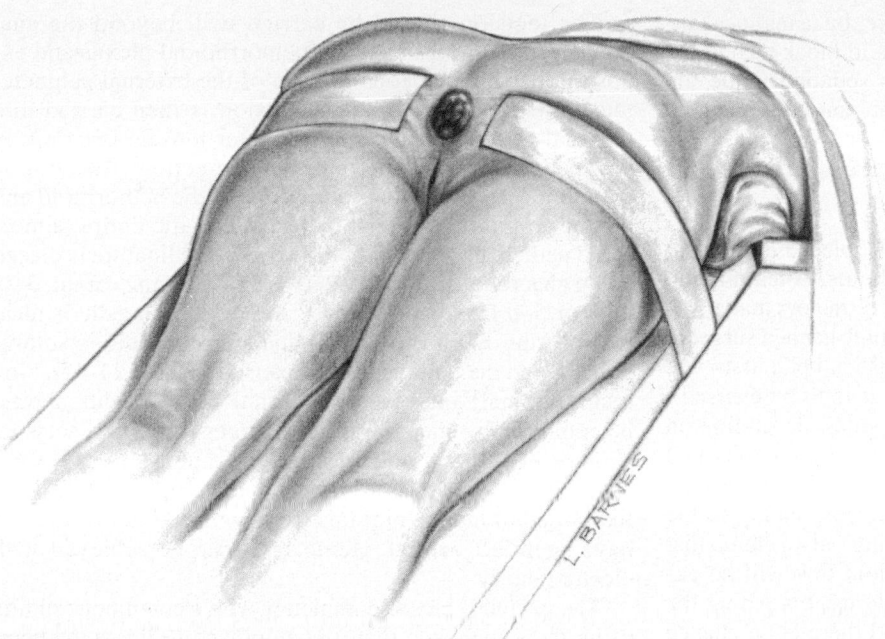

FIGURE 11-38. Position of the patient for hemorrhoidectomy. Local anesthesia with intravenous sedation is ideal. However, spinal, caudal, or general endotracheal anesthesia is frequently employed.

United Kingdom prefer lithotomy, although this is changing. Often the choice of position is dictated by demands made by the anesthesiologist, especially if the patient is obese or has breathing problems. Given the opportunity, most anesthesiologists would never elect to place the patient in the prone jackknife position because of airway concerns, but with reasoned communication between congenial colleagues the optimal solution can usually be achieved, even though our compatriots at the head of the table always manage to contain their enthusiasm. Having had considerable experience with both approaches, in Britain as a senior registrar and in the United States, I think there is no comparison between the two. Admittedly, however, if one leaves the wounds open, the differing advantages in patient position is less evident. The lateral decubitus position has been recommended for many years by the Ferguson Clinic Group and their disciples, a compromise between the other two alternatives. In my opinion, this position is also very inconvenient for the assistant.

Read and colleagues prospectively analyzed anesthetic technique for anorectal surgery on 413 consecutive patients.[244] Most underwent their procedures in the prone position (389 patients). Two-thirds of these patients received intravenous sedation with local anesthesia (260 patients). All but one of the others received a caudal or epidural anesthetic. Although patients were obviously not randomized to one or the other position, and the study does imply a certain selectivity bias, two conclusions could be reached. First, only two patients (0.8%) of the 260 patients required turning to the supine position before completion of the surgery, and second, discharge from recovery was much sooner when compared with those undergoing regional anesthesia.

The anus is infiltrated with a solution of approximately 20 mL of 0.5% bupivacaine in 1:200,000 epinephrine (Figure 11-39). This low dose usually does not affect the heart rate or the blood pressure. The infiltration technique minimizes bleeding, and the anatomic plane between the hemorrhoidal masses and the underlying internal sphincter

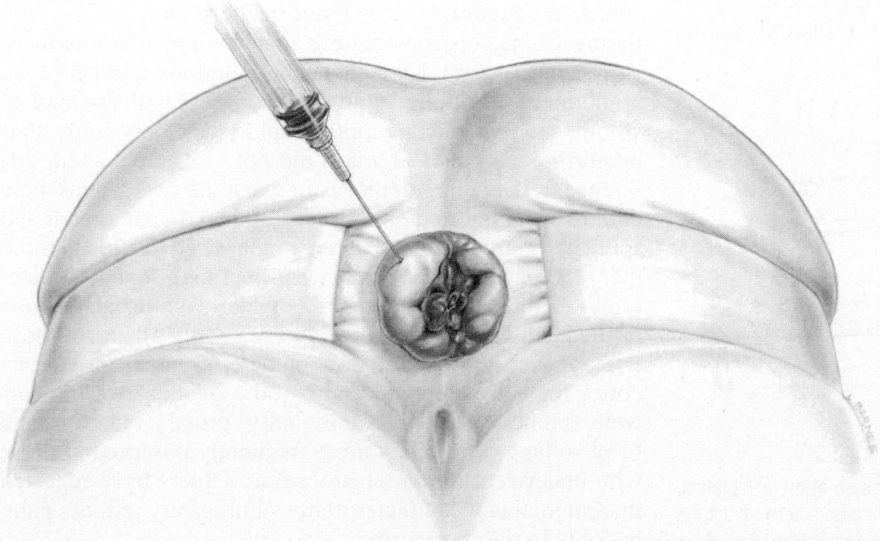

FIGURE 11-39. In preparation for hemorrhoidectomy, the anus is infiltrated with a local anesthetic of bupivacaine in epinephrine.

muscle is clearly delineated. Furthermore, by using local anesthesia and the previously discussed field block technique, often with supplementary intravenous sedation while the medication is administered, no additional anesthesia is necessary. As mentioned, a general, caudal, or spinal anesthetic may be used.

Technique

A Hill-Ferguson retractor (Figure 11-40) placed in the anal canal reveals the extent of the hemorrhoids. Alternatively, there are many other rectal specula and retractors that a surgeon may prefer (Figure 11-41). For a right-handed surgeon, it is usually best to deal with the more difficult pile first—the one in the right posterior quadrant (if it is to be excised). Alternatively, one may elect to switch sides, depending on the hemorrhoid side one is treating, and the comfort and handedness of the surgeon. Some surgeons like to place an anchoring suture in the distal rectum corresponding to the site of the hemorrhoid, but I prefer placing only a clamp that incorporates the skin tag and hemorrhoid that will be excised (Figure 11-42). The reason for doing this is that the suture tends to limit the dissection, and there is no chance of cutting a stitch out that has *not* been placed. Excision can be performed with a knife, scissors, electrocautery, laser, or with the Harmonic scalpel.[15,109] There has not been good evidence to indicate an advantage of one cutting method over another. However, in a prospective, randomized trial comparing the Harmonic scalpel, bipolar scissors, and ordinary scissors in hemorrhoidectomy, Chung and colleagues found the Harmonic scalpel to be superior because less pain was associated with it.[57] The observed benefits were small and did not affect time off from work and other activities. Others compared the Harmonic scalpel with bipolar electrocautery in a randomized, controlled trial of hemorrhoidectomy. They, too, noted reduced postoperative pain in the former group and attributed this is avoidance of excessive lateral thermal injury. Whether this postulate is factual is problematic because patients often complain bitterly of pain following hemorrhoidectomy, even when "cold scissors" or a "cold scalpel" is employed for the dissection, with suturing for hemostasis.

A more recent approach to hemorrhoid excision is the use of the *LigaSure* device (Figure 11-43—Valleylab, Boulder, CO). Having been designed primarily for abdominal surgery, it can seal vessels up to 7 mm in diameter; it has also found some acceptance for the treatment of hemorrhoids.[58,99,188,220] Historically, this is not dissimilar to that of the old "clamp and cautery" method (see later discussion).

The incision should be carried well beyond the anal verge, removing the external hemorrhoidal plexus and exposing the subcutaneous portion of the external sphincter muscle (Figure 11-44). The incision is then carried into the anal canal; the internal sphincter muscle is carefully dropped away from the plane of dissection. Bleeding is avoided when the dissection is outside the hemorrhoid and medial to the internal sphincter. When the entire hemorrhoid pedicle has been mobilized, a suture ligature is placed using absorbable material (2–0 or 3–0 chromic catgut, 3–0, 4–0, or 5–0 Dexon or Vicryl). A 5/8 circle needle is ideal for suturing within the anal canal. The pedicle is suture-ligated, and the hemorrhoid is excised (Figure 11-45). Any residual small internal or external hemorrhoids should be removed by means of Allis forceps and fine scissors (Figure 11-46). By undermining the mucosa or skin for a short distance and removing the veins, one can limit the likelihood of later symptoms from hemorrhoidal veins that have been left behind. Hemostasis can be achieved with electrocautery.

The wound is closed completely with a continuous suture, using the same stitch that was employed to ligate the hemorrhoid pedicle (Figure 11-47). When the mucocutaneous junction is reached, the skin is closed in either a subcuticular fashion or by a continuous simple suture. In like manner, the remaining pile sites are excised, ligated, and primarily closed (Figure 11-48). Aside from the cosmetic appearance of the wounds, the fact that the physician is able to close all incisions and maintain the retractor in place as is illustrated implies that the anal canal opening is adequate. The physician need not be concerned about the subsequent development of a stricture under these circumstances.

The wounds are cleansed, and povidone-iodine (Betadine) ointment and a small dressing are applied. A bulky pressure dressing is avoided; no packing is necessary. Packing or anything else placed within the anal canal is uncomfortable. If the surgeon is concerned about hemostasis, he or she should take a few extra moments to ensure that it has been established.

Hemorrhoidectomy and Sphincterotomy

If a fissure is present, usually in the posterior position, an internal anal sphincterotomy is undertaken in the lateral pile site by dividing the lower one-third of the internal anal sphincter (Figure 11-49). Even in the absence of an anal fissure, some surgeons believe that this procedure reduces complaints of pain. Khubchandani undertook a prospective, randomized, controlled study involving 42 patients, half of whom underwent concomitant sphincterotomy with their hemorrhoidectomies and half did not.[155] There was no difference in the perception of pain when the two groups were compared. Asfar and colleagues compared anal stretch and sphincterotomy in a prospective randomized fashion in more than 250 patients who underwent operative hemorrhoidectomy.[17] The sphincterotomy was undertaken usually at one of the lateral hemorrhoidectomy sites. Only 18.4% of those who underwent concomitant sphincterotomy required narcotics for pain, compared with 100% of those who underwent sphincter stretch. Additionally, urinary retention and fecal soilage were much more frequently observed in those who underwent the latter procedure. Others have reported that internal anal sphincterotomy significantly reduces pain, but only in the short term.[83]

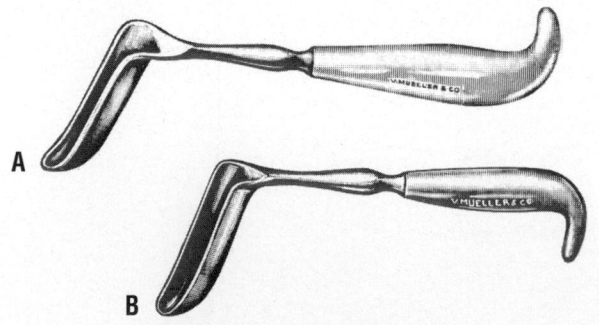

FIGURE 11-40. Anorectal retractors. **A:** The Ferguson-Moon rectal retractor is available in two depths and widths. **B:** The Hill-Ferguson rectal retractor is available in three depths and widths. (Courtesy of V. Mueller, McGraw Park, IL.)

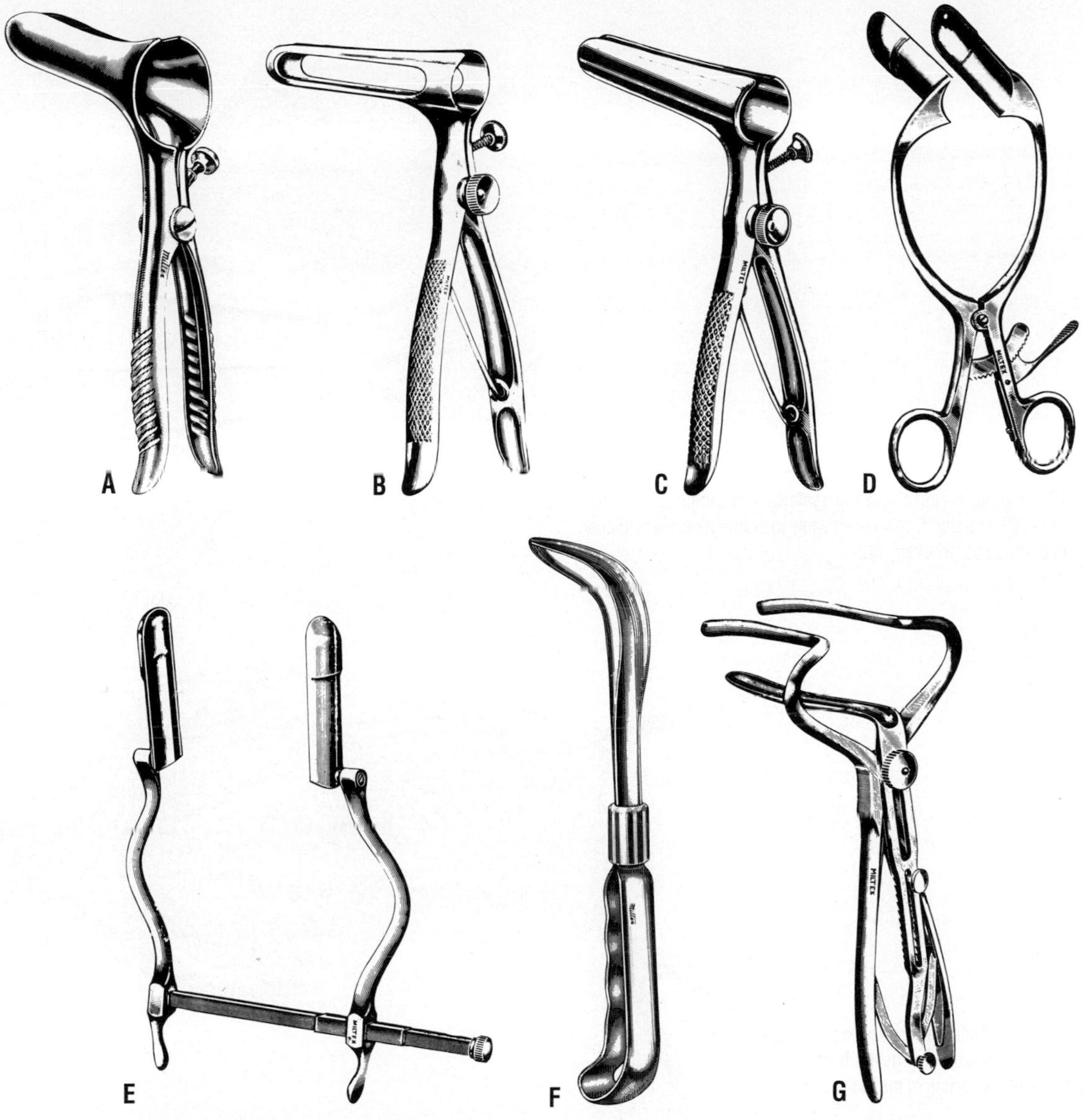

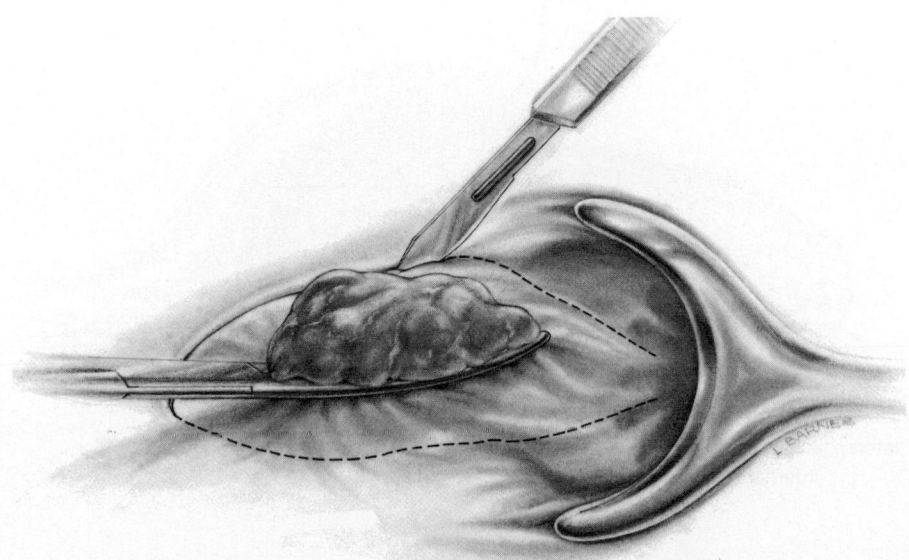

FIGURE 11-41. Rectal retractors. **A:** Pratt. **B:** Sims. **C:** Bodenhammer. **D:** Barr. **E:** Smith (or Buie). **F:** Sawyer. **G:** Cook. (Courtesy of Miltex Instrument Co., Lake Success, NY.)

FIGURE 11-42. The hemorrhoid is identified and grasped with a clamp. The area for excision is outlined by a broken line.

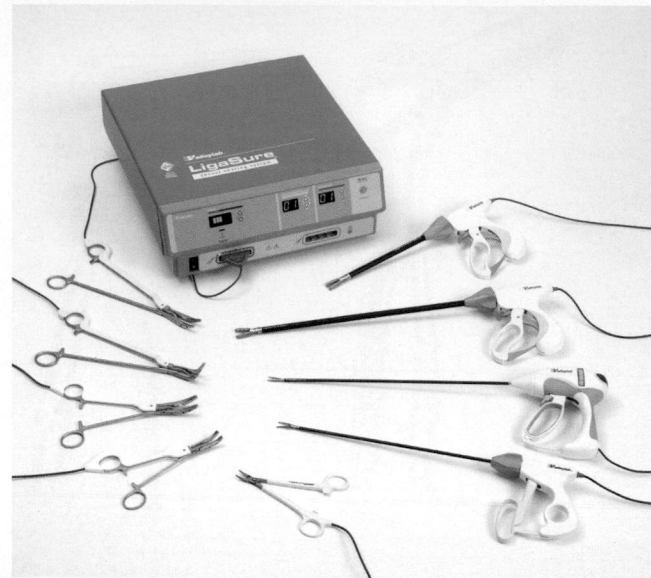

FIGURE 11-43. LigaSure vessel-sealing system. The LigaSure system's technology is a hemostatic tool that fuses vessel walls to create a permanent seal. (Courtesy of Valleylab Products, Boulder, CO.)

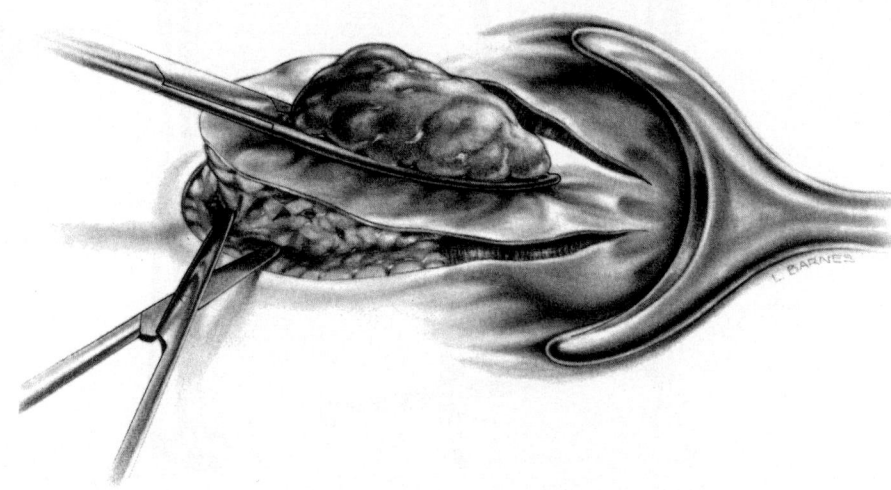

FIGURE 11-44. After the area for excision is outlined, the hemorrhoidal plexus is removed from the underlying subcutaneous portion of the external and internal sphincters.

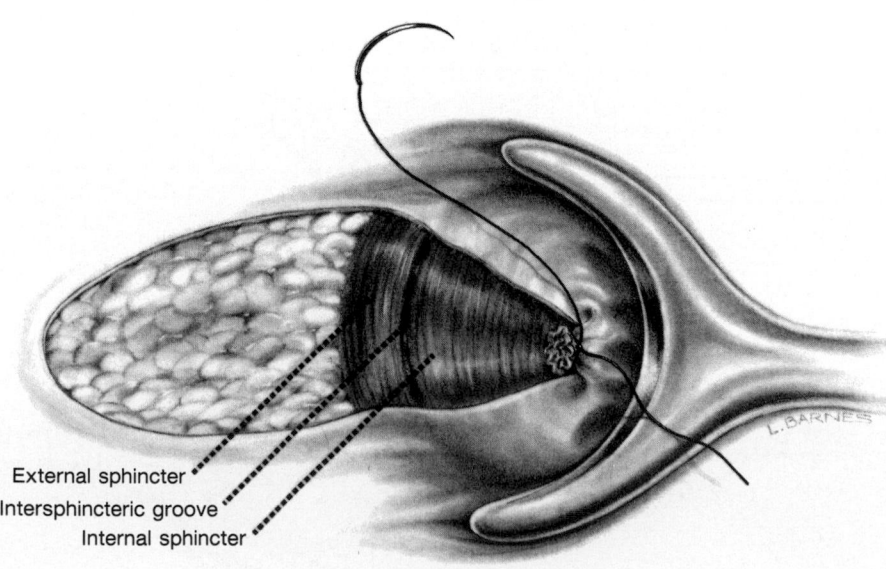

External sphincter
Intersphincteric groove
Internal sphincter

FIGURE 11-45. Open wound after excision of the hemorrhoid. No external or internal veins remain.

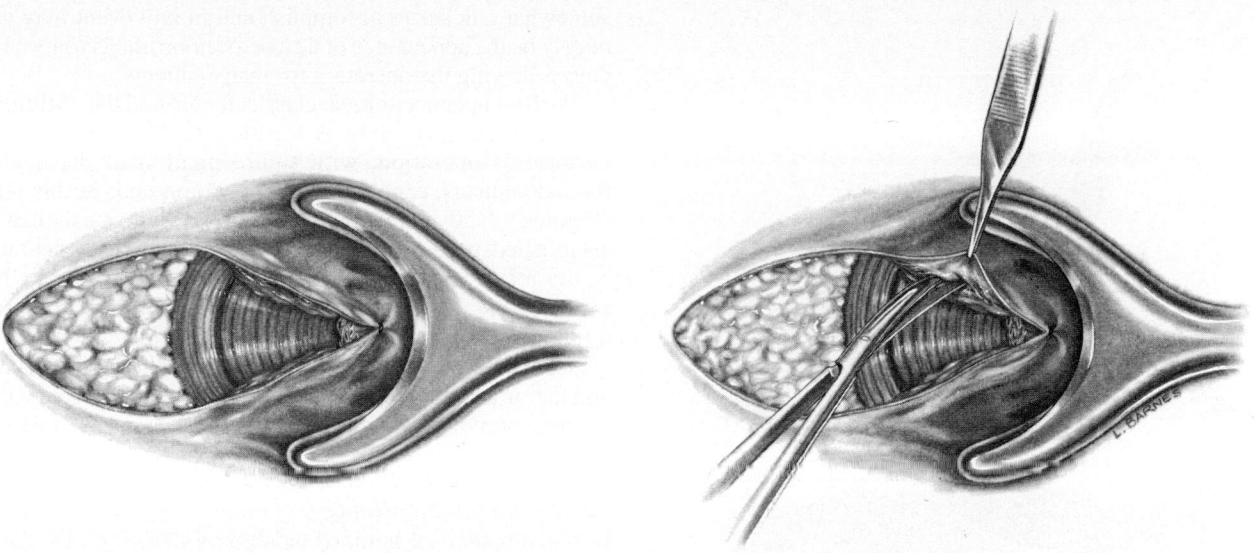

FIGURE 11-46. Residual hemorrhoids are removed by undermining the mucosa.

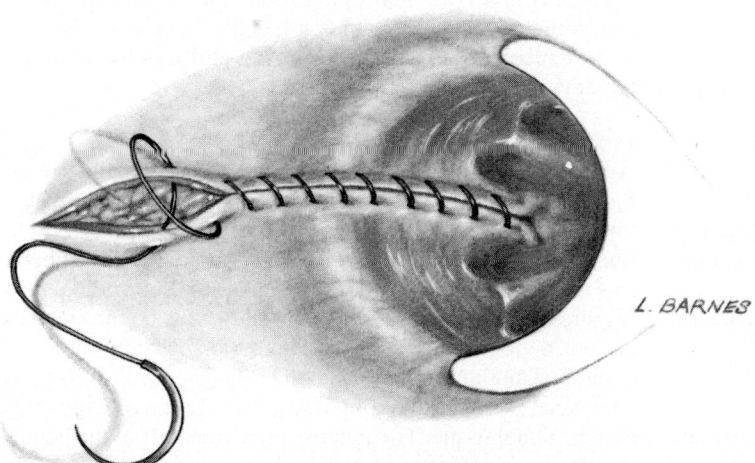

FIGURE 11-47. The wound is primarily closed.

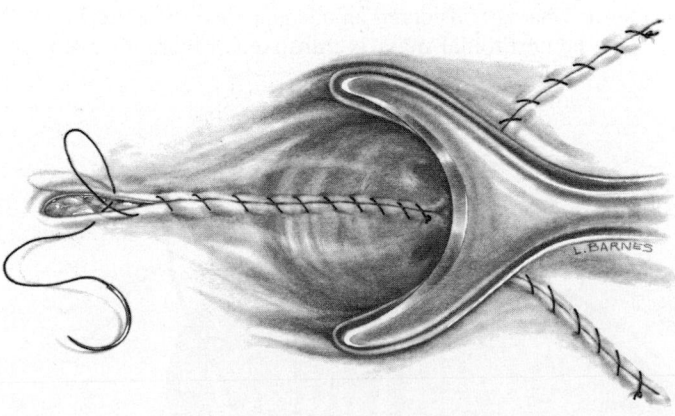

FIGURE 11-48. Completed closed (i.e., Ferguson) hemorrhoidectomy. With a Hill-Ferguson retractor in place, there can be no anal canal narrowing.

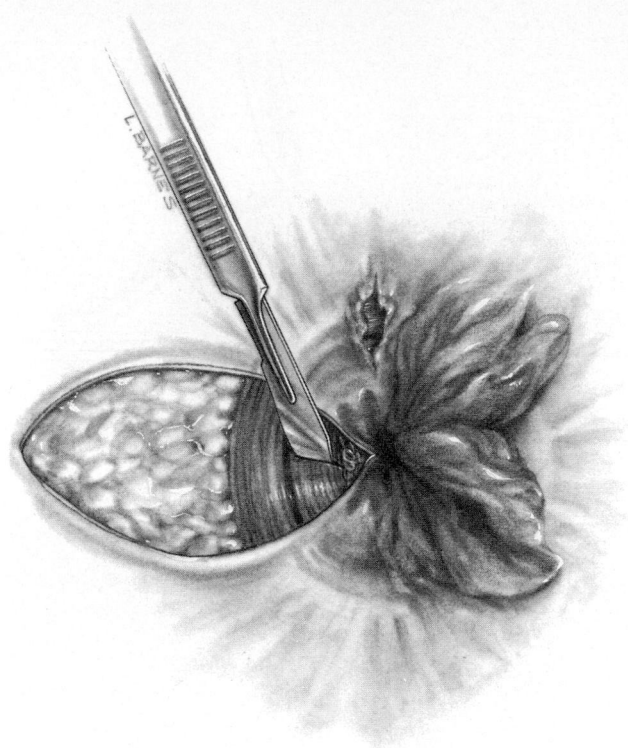

FIGURE 11-49. An internal anal sphincterotomy is performed at the site of excision of a left lateral pile in a patient with anal fissure.

Opinion

I do not employ sphincterotomy in the absence of a fissure. It is meddlesome, does not ameliorate the pain of hemorrhoidectomy in my experience, and may result in morbidity—infection, fistula, and some degree of impairment for bowel control (see Chapter 12).

Open Hemorrhoidectomy

Modifications of a closed or open hemorrhoidectomy are myriad. In the previous procedure, the wounds are completely closed. When hemorrhoids are gangrenous or circumferential, or when closure of wounds cannot be carried out with even a narrow retractor in place (generally a technical judgmental error), an open approach at one, two, or all of the pile sites may be indicated. Certainly, the open hemorrhoidectomy is somewhat quicker to accomplish and in any event may ultimately be the appearance of a closed hemorrhoidectomy a few days following the operation for many patients.

With an open technique, classically termed the "Milligan-Morgan," the procedure is identical to that described for Ferguson's operation, with suture ligation of the hemorrhoidal pedicles, except that the operation ends at this point (Figures 11-50 and 11-51). Additional hemostasis can be established with electrocautery. The aesthetic appearance of the result is reflected by the aphorism, "If it looks like a clover, the operation is over; if it looks like a dahlia, it's a failure." Alternatively, one or two sites may be left open, closed, or partially closed, depending on the circumstances and the surgeon's preference. Good results are possible with a combination of open and closed approaches to each pile site.

Submucosal Hemorrhoidectomy or Parks' Hemorrhoidectomy

In the submucosal hemorrhoidectomy described by Parks, the mucosa of the anal canal and rectum is incised, and the hemorrhoidal tissue beneath is removed.[222] The mucosa is then reapproximated. The goal of this method is to excise all the hemorrhoidal tissue without injuring the overlying squamous and columnar epithelium. The advantage of this procedure is that the wounds allegedly heal more quickly, with reduced induration and scarring and less likelihood of the development of a stricture.

Technique

A self-retaining anal (i.e., Parks) retractor is usually recommended, primarily by United Kingdom surgeons; however, virtually any conventional anal retractor may be used. A solution of 0.5% bupivacaine or lidocaine in 1:200,000 epinephrine is injected into the submucosa and the hemorrhoidal mass (Figure 11-52A). The skin incision starts outside the anus and is carried around the forceps holding the anal skin, removing a minimal amount of anal canal mucosa (Figure 11-52B). The anal canal is undermined by scissor dissection to expose the hemorrhoidal tissue. The mucosa is elevated off of the hemorrhoidal vessels (Figure 11-52C). The upper limit of the dissection should be about 4 cm above the mucocutaneous junction. The external and internal sphincters are identified as the hemorrhoidal mass is elevated and stripped off the internal sphincter to what is considered an adequate level (Figure 11-52D). The hemorrhoidal mass is transfixed (Figure 11-52E), and

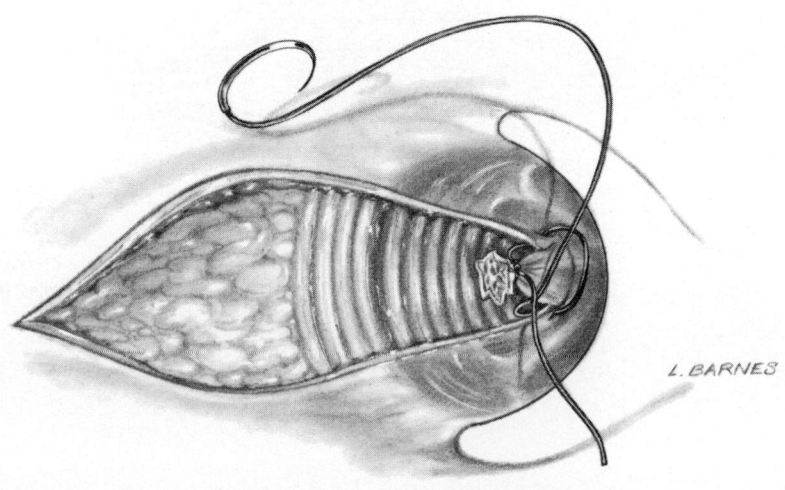

FIGURE 11-50. Open hemorrhoidectomy: technique of burying the hemorrhoidal pedicle.

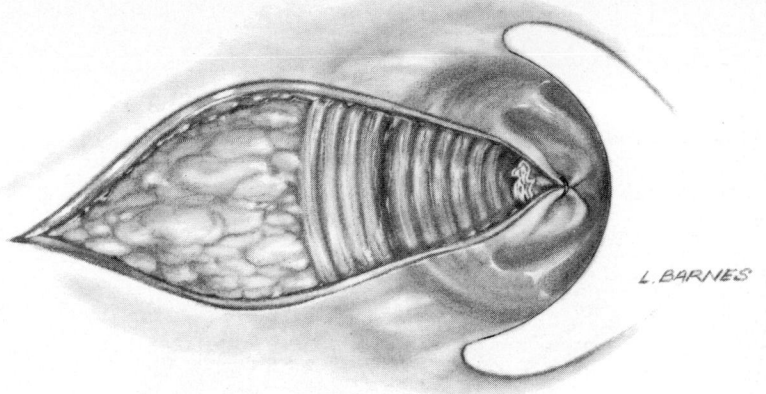

FIGURE 11-51. Completed open hemorrhoidectomy. Partial closure to the mucocutaneous junction is another option.

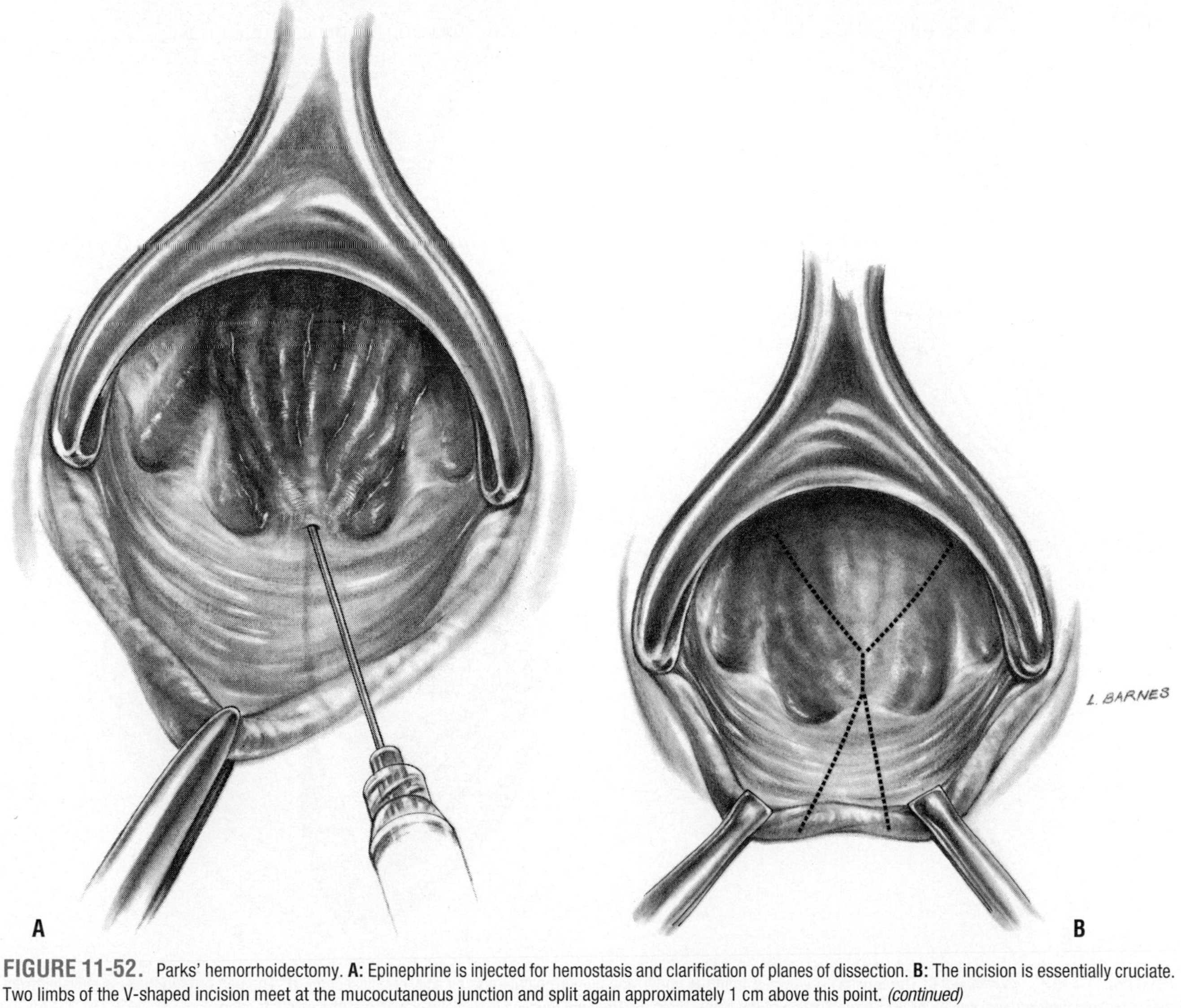

A

B

FIGURE 11-52. Parks' hemorrhoidectomy. **A:** Epinephrine is injected for hemostasis and clarification of planes of dissection. **B:** The incision is essentially cruciate. Two limbs of the V-shaped incision meet at the mucocutaneous junction and split again approximately 1 cm above this point. *(continued)*

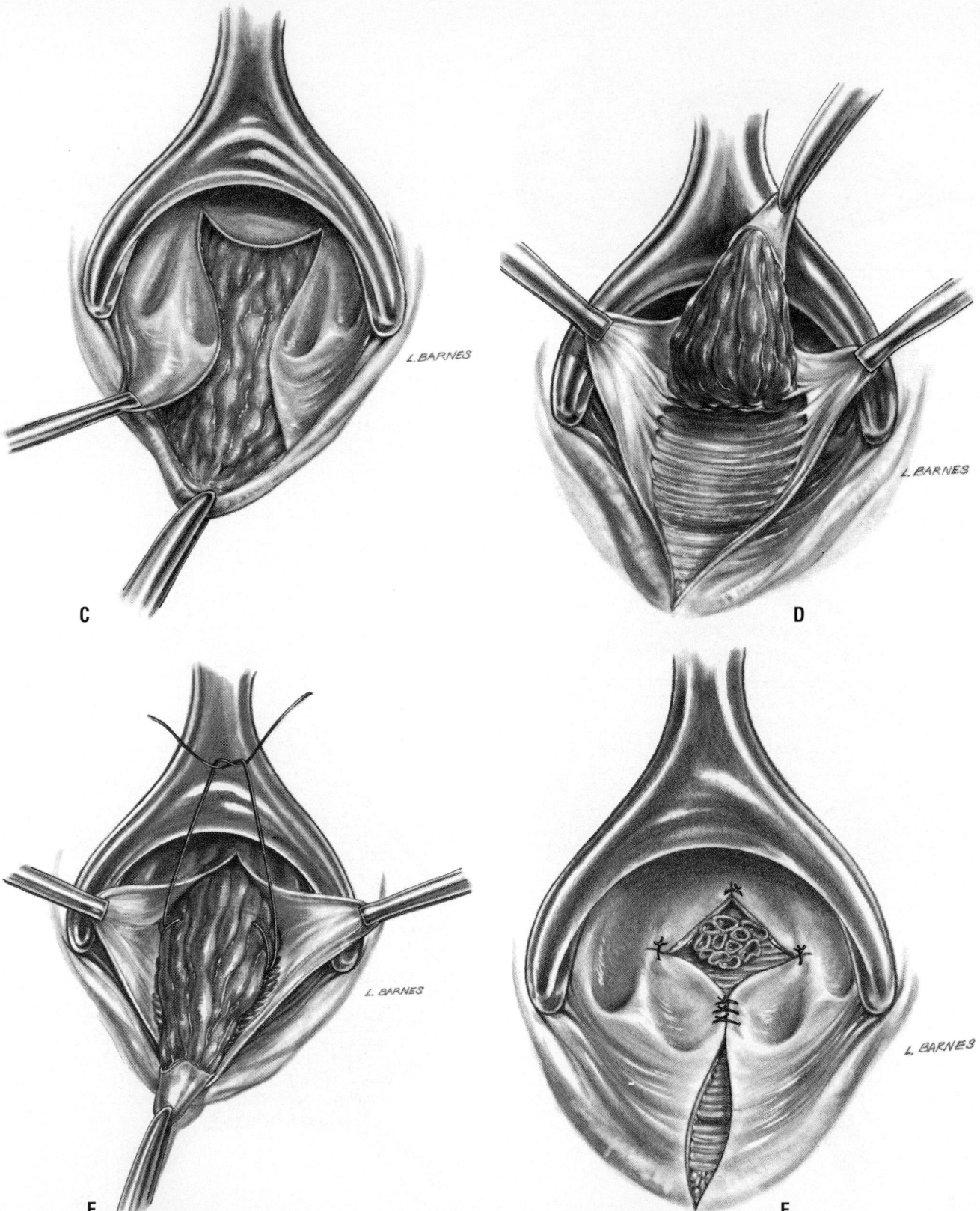

FIGURE 11-52. *(continued)* **C:** The mucosa is elevated from the underlying hemorrhoidal mass by scissors dissection. **D:** The hemorrhoid mass is elevated from the underlying internal anal sphincter. **E:** Suture ligation of the hemorrhoid. **F:** The anal mucosa is partially closed and the skin left open.

the hemorrhoid is excised. The flaps of the mobilized anal canal mucosa are reapproximated, and the underlying internal sphincter is incorporated with the sutures to prevent dislodgement (Figure 11-52F). The skin may be left open or closed.

A modification of the Parks operation has been offered by Selvaggi and colleagues.[268] They describe a technique that allegedly permits excision of circumferential hemorrhoids and grafting via an open technique (Figure 11-53).

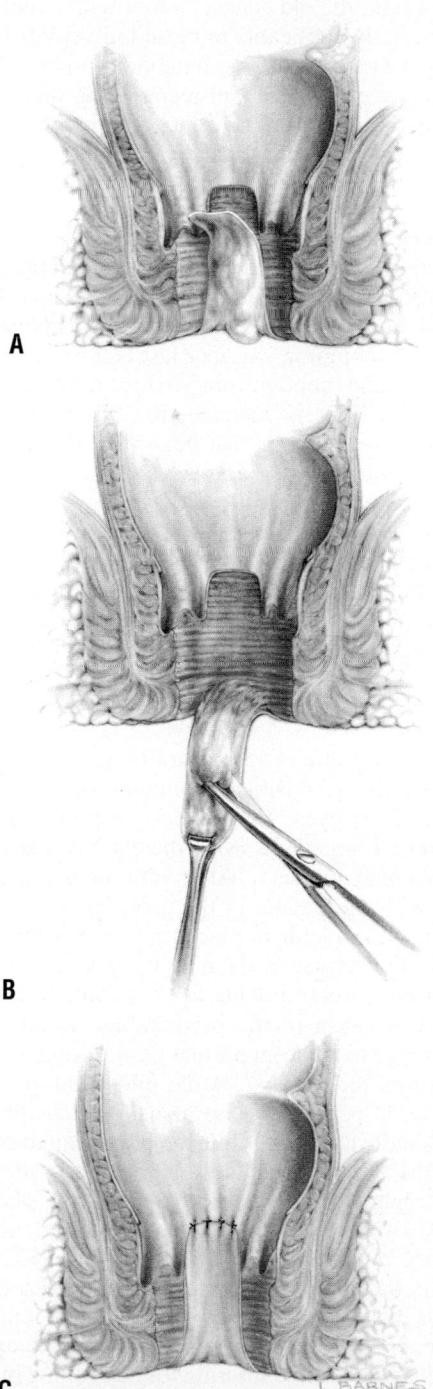

FIGURE 11-53. Submucosal hemorrhoidectomy as advocated by Selvaggi and colleagues. **A:** If large residual hemorrhoids are identified, a transverse incision is made above the apex. **B:** Allis forceps are used to apply tension to the anodermal flap, and the submucosal plexus is removed. **C:** Absorbable sutures are used to reanchor the flap to the cut edge of the rectum and the underlying internal sphincter.

Opinion

The Parks hemorrhoidectomy is an elegant approach that minimizes tissue loss, but, as described, does not deal with the external component, hypertrophied anal papillae, or redundant mucosa. The development of a stricture is virtually impossible unless the overlying mucosa has been devascularized. However, I do not feel that the effort required for one to accomplish the procedure is justified. In my opinion, it should be relegated to that of historic interest except to emphasize and to illustrate the value of submucosal dissection in removing residual hemorrhoidal veins.

Whitehead's Hemorrhoidectomy

As previously suggested, Whitehead's hemorrhoidectomy is very rarely employed by surgeons today because of the complications of stricture and ectropion, but the procedure that frequently results in these complications is not truly the one that was described by the author.[308] As originally recommended by Whitehead, the mucosa was sutured to the anal canal above the level of the pectinate line, but later surgeons misinterpreted this description and anchored the mucosa to the skin at the anal verge (Figure 11-54). All too often, the suture line dehisced, and the wound was left to granulate and heal by secondary intention. More commonly, a mucosal ectropion, the so-called wet anus or Whitehead deformity, was the consequence (Figure 11-55). Poor Dr. Whitehead was tarred with this same brush, achieving eponymous immortality for a complication for which he was not truly responsible.

Results

Although favorable results have been reported with a modified Whitehead procedure, it is my impression that the authors are merely performing a variation of an open hemorrhoidectomy.[39,314] In other words, whether the physician simply anchors the cut edge of the rectum to the underlying

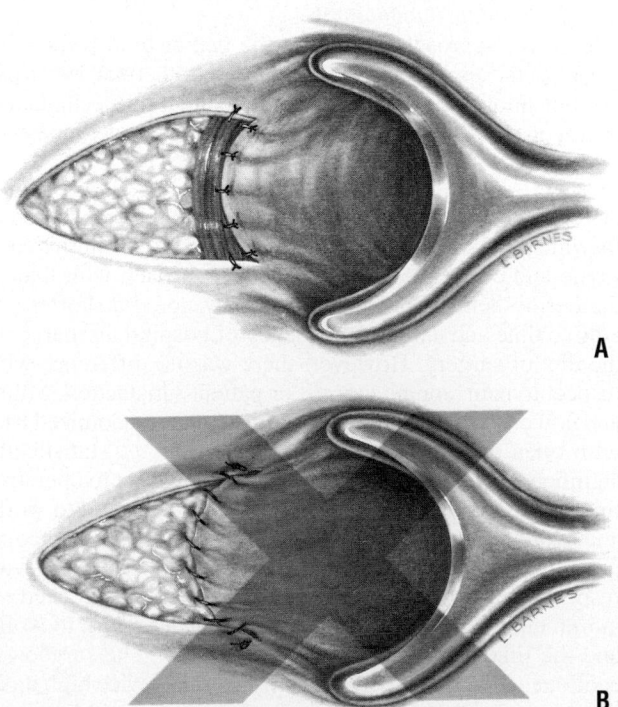

FIGURE 11-54. Whitehead's hemorrhoidectomy. **A:** Proper mucosal anchoring to the underlying internal sphincter. **B:** Improper anchoring may lead to an ectropian.

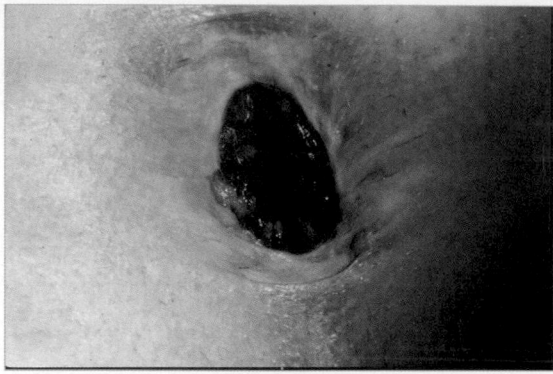

FIGURE 11-55. Whitehead's deformity. Note the mucosal ectropion that developed after excision of all of the anal canal, the characteristic "wet anus."

internal sphincter or combines an amputative hemorrhoidectomy with advancement of the perianal skin into the anal canal, the results should be quite satisfactory. Clearly, the mucosa should never be anchored to the skin outside the anus.

Barrios and Khubchandani related their experience with a modified Whitehead operation.[23] Their modification involved removal of the entire anoderm, but the perianal skin was preserved and the edges of the anal mucosa were sutured to the subcutaneous tissue, not to the skin. Although reporting satisfactory results in 41 patients, they noted a 32% incidence of urinary retention, a 5% incidence of hemorrhage, and a 10% incidence of late complications (i.e., stenosis, ectropion, and incontinence). A later report from one of the authors on the results of Whitehead's operation on 84 patients revealed late complications in 13%.[156] Among these were varying problems with continence in 3 patients and the development of anal strictures in 3. There was no instance of ectropion.

LigaSure Hemorrhoidectomy

The newer approach of sealing the hemorrhoid pedicle by means of the application of a bipolar electrothermal device has been mentioned previously. I suggested that this technique is analogous to that of the outmoded clamp and cautery method.

Results

Several prospective, randomized trials have been published in which LigaSure was compared with other alternatives. Jayne and colleagues compared this approach with that of diathermy hemorrhoidectomy.[139] They noted a shorter operative time and a higher frequency of hospital discharge on the day of surgery. However, there was no difference with respect to pain, complications, or patient satisfaction. Milito and coworkers compared this approach in a randomized trial with open diathermy hemorrhoidectomy.[188] A statistically significant advantage was observed with respect to operative time, pain medication requirements, time to return to work, and wound healing. Others report advantages when compared with conventional hemorrhoidectomy, especially with respect to operative time, postoperative pain, the reduced requirement for analgesic medications, earlier return to work, and the time for wound healing.[5,35,204,220,255] The surgeon is cautioned, however, to avoid applying this device high up in the rectum because of the risk of pelvic infection. Moreover, because there is a 2-mm thermal spread into adjacent tissue, it is critical not to be aggressive with tissue removal.

Opinion

The LigaSure method of performing a hemorrhoidectomy is qualitatively and quantitatively different from that of conventional hemorrhoidectomy. For example, the amount of tissue actually removed should be less than with the former approach, unless excessively applied. Furthermore, it is not clear what (if anything) is being done with the external component. The length of follow-up in publications is short—a few months (if it is mentioned at all). There are inherent risks in the use of all surgical equipment, including scissors and scalpel. However, the old adage, "a fool with a tool is still a fool," is especially applicable to those individuals who substitute alleged avant-garde instruments in order to advance their personal agendas, without recognizing their own and the instruments' limitations. For me, before considering the possibility of adopting this alternative, I would require a randomized trial that compares it with rubber band ligation.

Laser Surgery

As discussed in Chapter 6, the laser has been applied to the treatment of polyps and other lesions. It has also been advocated in the management of hemorrhoids (Figure 11-56). The three most common surgical lasers are the carbon dioxide, argon, and neodymium:yttrium-aluminum-garnet (Nd:YAG). The different wavelengths of their light produce characteristic tissue effects that determine their usefulness in surgery. The carbon dioxide laser primarily cuts and is awkward to use endoscopically. Conversely, the argon laser coagulates surface vessels quite well, whereas the noncontact Nd:YAG can be used with deep vessels. Both, however, are limited by their unsatisfactory cutting qualities. A distinct advantage is the fact that Nd:YAG light will pass through optical fibers and can therefore be used through the operating channel of most endoscopy equipment.

Technique

Use of the laser requires special training and precautions. Because the light is invisible, the operator must wear goggles to protect the eyes. Yu and Eddy reported the results of treatment of 134 patients using the Nd:YAG laser to perform hemorrhoidectomies.[320] After administration of a local anesthetic, with the patient in the prone position and with a Hill-Ferguson retractor in place, the laser beam is aimed directly onto the surface of the pile. Iwagaki and colleagues believe that the carbon dioxide laser is suitable for hemorrhoidectomy because of the predictable biologic effects, minimal damage to adjacent normal tissue, good hemostasis, and precision of technique.[138] A red pilot light, provided by low-power laser, permits precise focusing of the therapeutic beam. The handle is moved while the laser beam destroys the tissue until the area is covered by a white membrane. Internal and external hemorrhoids are treated similarly. The authors required 30 to 45 minutes for each operation, and the patients were discharged the same day but were followed daily in the office for the first week. Sankar and Joffe suggest that large hemorrhoids may be treated by a submucosal technique.[260] It is, therefore, essentially a Parks' hemorrhoidectomy, except that the laser augments the suturing for controlling blood loss.

Results

Narcotic pain medication is necessary for the first few days according to Yu and Eddy, and usually, healing was accomplished in about 1 month.[320] The early and late complication rates were not significantly different from those of conventional

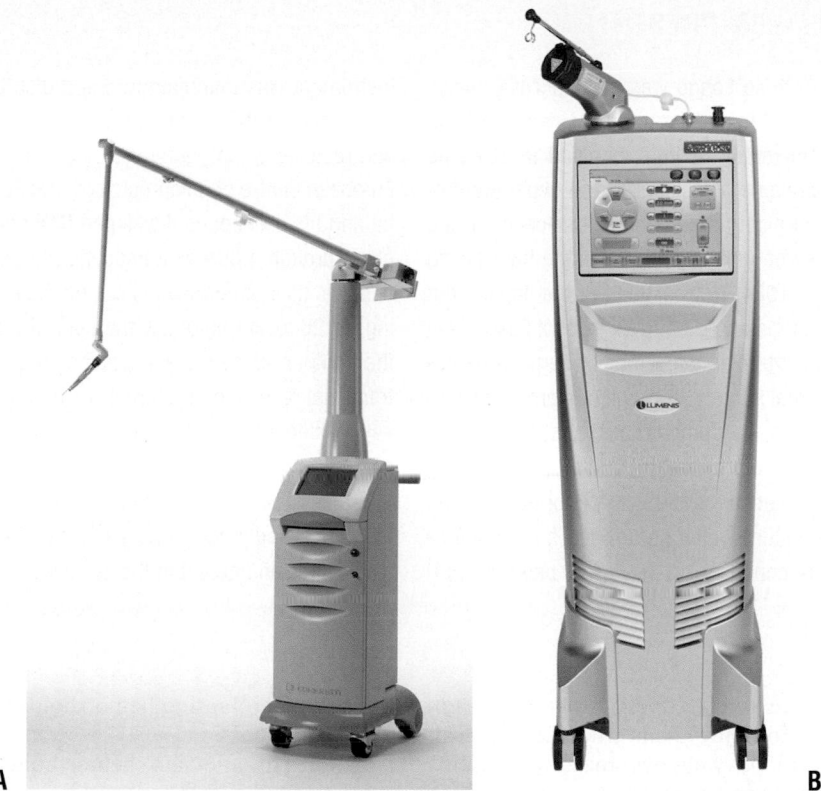

FIGURE 11-56. Carbon dioxide lasers like the UltraPulse Encore (**A**) and AcuPulse Wave-Guide FiberLase (**B**) can be used to cut, ablate, and coagulate tissue and are especially useful for hemorrhoidectomy. (Courtesy of Lumenis, Inc., Santa Clara, CA.)

surgical hemorrhoidectomy, although an anal stenosis developed in three patients. Other physicians have also reported a favorable experience with laser hemorrhoidectomy.[138]

Wang and colleagues performed a randomized trial of hemorrhoidectomy either by means of Nd:YAG laser phototherapy or Ferguson's technique in 88 patients.[300] There was a statistically significant difference in the need for narcotic medication (laser, 11%; Ferguson, 56%); additionally, postoperative urinary retention was much less frequent when the laser was used (7% vs. 39%). Postoperative stay was also much shorter with the laser hemorrhoidectomy. Conversely, Nicholson and colleagues noted no advantage in using the sapphire-tip Nd:YAG laser in treating grade III or IV hemorrhoids.[202] When they compared this approach with closed hemorrhoidectomy in a randomized, controlled way, they observed no differences in the duration of hospitalization, requirement for catheterization, operative time, blood loss, or narcotic use. Wound healing was also similar in both methods.

Chia and coworkers randomized 28 patients to either receive carbon dioxide laser hemorrhoidectomy or the conventional surgical approach.[54] The laser group required less postoperative pain medication. They were also able to demonstrate that the carbon dioxide laser did not cause any alteration in anorectal physiology. Others have concluded that laser hemorrhoidectomy compares favorably.[132]

Leff performed a prospective study that compared hemorrhoidectomy by means of a carbon dioxide laser (170 patients) with conventional, closed hemorrhoidectomy (56 patients).[166] The author observed no differences with respect to pain, wound healing, or complication rate.

Similarly, Senagore and colleagues performed a prospective, randomized trial comparing sharp dissection using a scalpel with that of the contact Nd:YAG laser.[270] Both techniques involved the standard, Ferguson-closed hemorrhoidectomy in a total of 86 patients. There were no significant differences between the groups, except that there was actually more inflammation and a greater incidence of dehiscence with the laser procedure. Because of the increased cost for the laser group, there was a significant price differential also. The authors concluded that the therapeutic efficacy and cost-benefit ratio with the application of lasers to the treatment of hemorrhoids could not be supported.

Comment

Proponents of this approach usually claim that hemorrhoid laser surgery is associated with earlier healing, less pain, and reduced scarring or deformity. In my opinion, there is no advantage of hemorrhoid laser surgery over that of scalpel surgery. Even properly performed, laser surgery is associated with the same operative and postoperative risks and results. It assuredly requires specialized, expensive equipment that mandates a period of education and is not without unique concerns. In some of the earlier writing on the application of lasers, those who have had the most experience with laser hemorrhoidectomy seem to be the same surgeons who previously had been the enthusiastic advocates of cryosurgery. I do not mean to imply criticism, merely skepticism. As with all laser applications, safety is an important concern. In light of the dearth of recent publications on this subject, I am not motivated to abandon the technique that has served me, most

ANTONIO LONGO (1953–PRESENT)

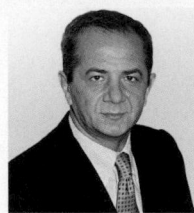

Antonio Longo was born in Tusa, Sicily. He obtained his medical degree at the University of Palermo, and in 1979 he became a resident in the department of surgical and anatomical sciences at the same university, completing his training in 1984. He remained in the department of surgery as assistant, ultimately rising to the post of head of the department. His primary interests were that of surgical pathophysiology and experimental surgery. Through numerous clinical-defecographic observations, he demonstrated that prolapse of hemorrhoids is associated with an internal rectal prolapse and a cause of obstructed defecation. In 1993, he performed the first hemorrhoidopexy, a procedure which he devised for the operative management of this condition. In 1998, his patented PPH instrument was manufactured and distributed. In 1999, he proposed the STARR technique to correct internal rectal prolapse and rectocele. That same year, he moved to Vienna to head the European Centre of Coloproctology and Pelvic Diseases. In Vienna, he and his colleagues developed RMI and RX Dynamic Pelvigraphy. Through 4,000 examinations, he demonstrated that a host of pelvic floor abnormalities can be the result of excessive straining. In 2000, he patented the curved stapler, manufactured as the Contour 40 for rectal resections and the Contour Transtar for transanal resection of internal rectal prolapse. Longo has served as president of the Italian Society of Coloproctology. An extraordinarily innovative and creative surgeon, he holds, as of this writing, 18 patents. He is active in colorectal surgery education, with his theoretical and practical workshops in Vienna, a destination for all who evince an interest in the specialty.

other surgeons, and patients so effectively—that is, conventional excisional (scissors or knife) hemorrhoidectomy—although stapled hemorrhoidopexy has become quite tempting for selected patients (see the following).

Stapled Hemorrhoidopexy

There has truly been a renascent interest in surgical hemorrhoidectomy since the introduction of the circular stapling device for the treatment of hemorrhoid prolapse by Longo in 1998.[173] A plethora of publications have appeared in the past few years on this approach, primarily from Europe and Asia, but more recently also in the United States.[16,29,38,49,71,93,103,131,151,180,187,217,218,228,231,238,252,276,301]

In accordance with recommendations proposed in the 1993 by the Standards Task Force of the ASCRS on the treatment of hemorrhoids,[279] as well as the reported complications,[52,61,123,181,182,193,247] it was thought prudent to examine this new modality in light of the publicity, both within the profession and in the lay press. An international working party was convened in July 2001. This consisted of 11 individuals with experience in the performance of the hemorrhoid operation by means of the circular stapler (Figure 11-57), the so-called stapled hemorrhoidectomy. The conference resulted in the development of a consensus paper to establish the criteria for performing this procedure.[68] The following were the recommendations:

Name of Procedure
- Stapled hemorrhoidopexy

The panel believed that the operation is *not* a hemorrhoidectomy. Neither anal mucosa nor hemorrhoidal tissue is removed if the procedure is performed properly. Therefore, the term, "stapled hemorrhoidectomy," should not be applied.

Indications
- Prolapsing hemorrhoids requiring manual reduction (grade III)
- Uncomplicated hemorrhoids, irreducible by the patient but reducible at surgery (grade IV)
- Irreducible hemorrhoids at surgery but by a modified surgical technique (see later)

- Selected prolapsing hemorrhoids with spontaneous reduction (grade II)
- Failure to alleviate hemorrhoidal symptoms by other methods (e.g., rubber band ligation)

Issues and Concerns (Different from Those of Conventional Hemorrhoidectomy)
- Anal intercourse (male or female)
- Anal fissure (see Chapter 12)
- Anal fistula (see Chapter 14)
- Skin tags
- Hypertrophied anal papillae
- Thrombosis
- Preexisting sphincter injury or loss
- Excessive rectal mucosal prolapse

Anal intercourse is a unique concern. Although the staples generally slough out or ultimately become completely

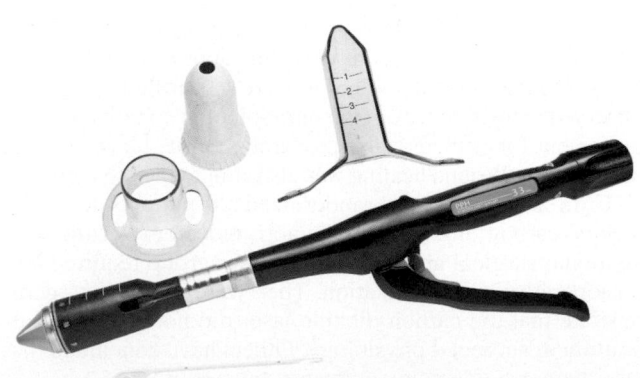

FIGURE 11-57. Proximate HCS procedure for prolapse and hemorrhoids (PPH) set with hemorrhoid circular stapler (HCS33), circular anal dilator (CAD33), purse-string suture anoscope, and suture threader (ST100). (Courtesy Ethicon Endo-Surgery, Inc.)

buried within the mucosa and submucosa, there still remains a small risk of penile injury with anal intercourse during the first several months following operation. *Anal fissure* is traditionally managed at the time of conventional hemorrhoidectomy by sphincterotomy at one of the pile sites. Because no wound is created within the anal canal by stapled hemorrhoidopexy, a concomitant or independent procedure would be necessary (if indicated). As with anal fissure, concomitant *anal fistula* requires a procedure that could not be performed at the site of hemorrhoid removal. The surgeon is advised to use his or her good judgment as to the appropriateness of concomitant stapled hemorrhoidopexy when this condition is present. *Skin tags* and *hypertrophied papillae* need to be managed individually (if indicated).

The presence of *acute thrombosis* is a very real concern if a stapled hemorrhoidopexy is to be performed. It is strongly recommended that the thrombotic area be incised and removed if this procedure is to be undertaken.

Preexisting sphincter injury or loss and *anal incontinence* were considered by the panel to be very real concerns if stapled hemorrhoidopexy is to be performed. The reason is that the operation requires the insertion of a relatively large circular anal dilator (CAD [33 mm]). The stretching associated with the placement of this instrument can lead to further impairment of bowel control. Finally, *excessive mucosal prolapse* is considered a concern because of the inability of the instrument to adequately encompass all of the redundant tissue (see later).

Contraindications
- Abscess
- Gangrene
- Anal stenosis
- Full-thickness rectal prolapse

Performance of stapled hemorrhoidopexy in the presence of *gangrenous* or *infected tissue* is absolutely contraindicated because the operation fails to remove the source of sepsis. Furthermore, opening additional tissue planes may expose the patient to pelvic sepsis and to the possibility of Fournier's gangrene (see later). The presence of *anal stenosis* is a contraindication because of one's inability to insert the CAD. *Full-thickness rectal prolapse* is not appropriately treated by this operation. There is no evidence, even anecdotal, that the operation can ameliorate true procidentia.

Informed Consent (Unique to the Procedure)
- Urgency and rectal irritation
- Pain and swelling (thrombosis of residual hemorrhoids)
- Anastomotic stenosis
- Anal intercourse

Because the procedure is undertaken within the rectum, itself, and in effect is associated with a staple line that is somewhat analogous to that of a distal rectal anastomosis, patients may experience *urgency* to defecate and may have transient problems with *discharge* and *irritation*. With respect to *pain* and *swelling*, especially as a consequence of thrombosed hemorrhoids that develop during the postoperative period, this must be considered a complication of the procedure. Because the dissection is not undertaken within the anal canal and hemorrhoidal veins are *not* removed, stapled hemorrhoidopexy can lead to this complication in the occasional patient. *Anastomotic stenosis* has been reported but should be quite unusual with the PPH instrument, given

its relatively large diameter. The major precaution is that the surgeon must create the staple line *above the anal canal* (see later).

Patient Position (Surgeon's Preference)
Surgeons should choose the position with which they are most comfortable as if conventional hemorrhoidectomy were to be performed.

Anesthesia (Surgeon's Preference)
- Local (conscious sedation is required)
- Regional
- General

If local anesthesia is elected, conscious sedation is strongly recommended. Placement of the purse-string suture into the rectal mucosa can be associated with discomfort that would not necessarily be adequately controlled by means of a local anesthetic alone.

Technique
The hemorrhoids are assessed, and the CAD is inserted and anchored to the skin by means of a heavy suture on a cutting needle; the procedure is aborted if stenosis precludes passage (Figure 11-58). Countertraction is applied to the skin to facilitate insertion. It is important to reduce the external component as much as possible manually. The purse-string suture anoscope is introduced through the CAD. Its rotation allows the placement of a circumferential purse string at the correct height (3 to 4 cm above the dentate line) and depth (only mucosa and submucosa). Small bites placed close together are advised. A 2–0 monofilament suture on a 25- to 30-mm curved needle is used (Figure 11-59). One must confirm the completeness of the purse string to ensure that there

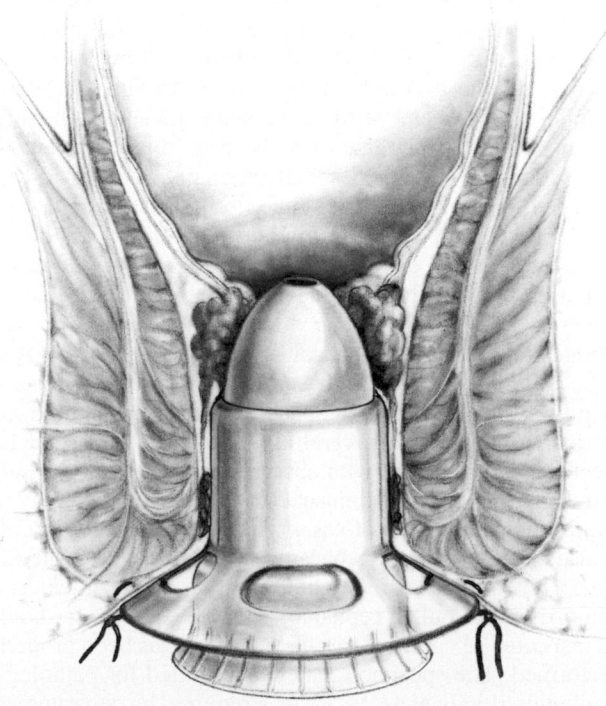

FIGURE 11-58. The circular anal dilator (CAD33) is inserted, and the obturator is removed. The prolapse is reduced and the dentate line identified. The device should remain in position throughout the procedure and may be secured to the skin with sutures.

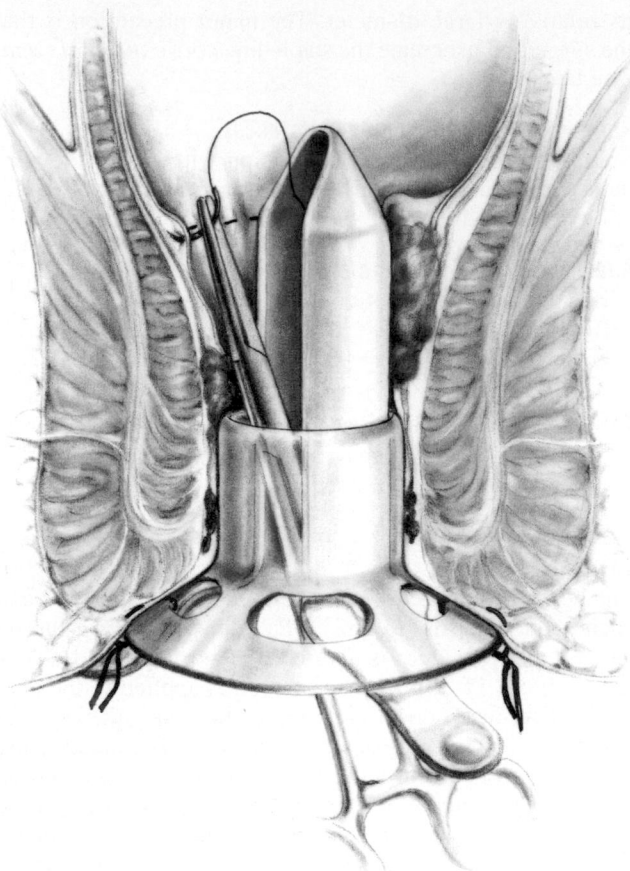

FIGURE 11-59. Placement of the purse-string suture 3 to 4 cm above the dentate line.

(see previous discussion). An internal anal sphincterotomy would, of necessity, require either an open or closed procedure in accordance with the surgeon's personal preference.

Credentialing

Since the 1970s, numerous innovations have been developed in the field of colon and rectal surgery alone. Examples are colonoscopy and colonoscopy/polypectomy, stapled anastomotic techniques, intestinal reservoirs, and laparoscopic colectomy. There is ample precedent for determining the means for proper introduction of new technology. The following represents the consensus of the Working Party as minimal requirements. These are not meant to be standards but recommended guidelines.

- Experience with anorectal surgery and an understanding of anorectal anatomy should be a requisite.
- Experience with circular stapling devices is essential.
- The surgeon should attend a formal course—including lectures, videos, the application of the instrument in models, and observation of the operation performed by a surgeon recognized by his or her peers—leading ultimately to undertaking the procedure while being observed by an experienced surgeon. Following satisfactory completion of the foregoing, independent responsibility should be determined by each individual's surgical department.

are no gaps or "dog ears" present. The fully opened stapler head is then inserted through the purse string (Figure 11-60). The purse string is then tied with just one throw knot. One then draws the two tails of the suture through the lateral channels in the head of the anvil with the suture threader (Figure 11-60). The purse string is secured under direct visualization. The tails are knotted externally or clamped with forceps (Figure 11-61). The stapler is aligned along the axis of the anal canal and closed while maintaining moderate downward tension on the purse string (Figure 11-62). At the end of the closure, the 4-cm mark should be at the level of the anal verge. If the patient is a woman, it is advisable to pass a finger into the vagina, checking the posterior vaginal wall to be certain that it has not been incorporated. The stapler is then fired. The head is then opened and the stapler removed. At this point, one should carefully inspect the staple line for bleeding and reinforce with absorbable sutures if necessary (Figure 11-63). It is not unusual that a suture or two may be required (at least 50% of cases). Electrocoagulation should be used only with caution because of the presence of the staples. The anal mucosa with both internal and even external hemorrhoids is pulled cephalad. The mucosal sleeve should be inspected to confirm that the technique has been properly performed. The specimen may be submitted for pathologic evaluation if judged necessary or if required by departmental or hospital policy.

Because no procedure is performed within the anal canal with the stapled hemorrhoidopexy, concomitant excision may be indicated for skin tags, papillae, or thromboses

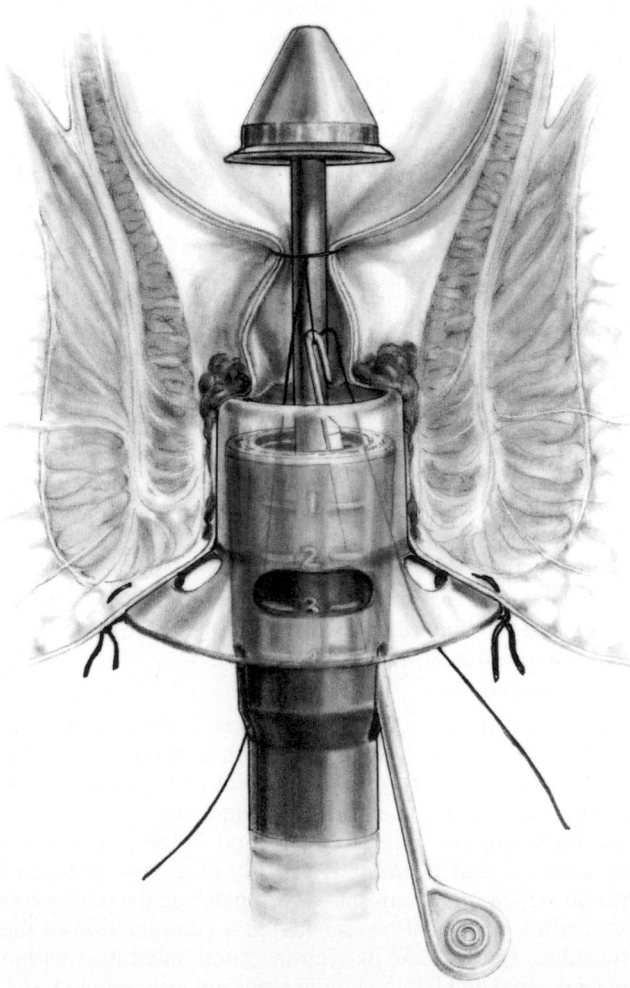

FIGURE 11-60. The hemorrhoid circular stapler (HCS33) is fully opened prior to insertion. One throw knot secures the purse-string suture. By using the suture threader, the tails are drawn through the lateral channels.

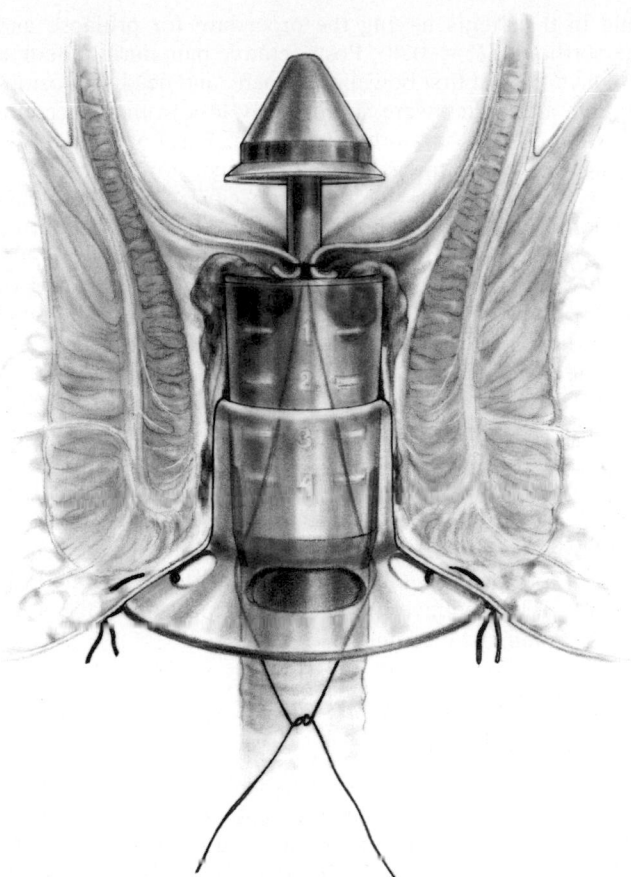

FIGURE 11-61. External knotting or clamping of suture tails.

Complications

There have been some disconcerting complications that are unique to the procedure of stapled hemorrhoidopexy as well as a suggestion of an increased risk of septic complications. These include retropneumoperitoneum, pneumomediastinum,[247] pelvic sepsis,[182,193] persistent severe pain and fecal urgency,[52] rectal perforation,[104,316] rectal stricture,[232] rectal obstruction,[61] rectovaginal fistula, and obstructed defecation (anismus).[85] Sepsis has been recognized, albeit rarely, as a complication of conventional hemorrhoidectomy, however. An increased incidence of inconsequential bacteremia has been reported in a prospective, randomized trial.[181] Some have recommended the routine application of prophylactic antibiotics, but there is no evidence to suggest that this is appropriate or likely to be helpful. As mentioned previously, one must be circumspect when considering this procedure in those who practice anal sex. A penile laceration from an exposed staple, when the partner has a sexually acquired disease, may have serious consequences.[191] It has become abundantly clear that this operation should be performed only by surgeons experienced with the technique and who are truly mindful of the potential complications.

Results

There have been many published studies, often prospectively randomized, that are worthy of mentioning. In every study comparing this approach with hemorrhoidectomy by any method, there is a highly significant reduction in postoperative pain.[16,38,49,71,103,131,146,151,180,187,217,218,252] This also translates to earlier return to normal activity and to greater patient

satisfaction.[252,276] This is not surprising in light of the fact that there is no "cutting" within the anal canal or in perianal skin. What is being excised is a circumferential column of mucosa and submucosa above the anal canal. There may, however, be an increased risk of postoperative bleeding according to some investigators.[311] Others opine that there should be no such concern.[131,252] There is also some reports of fecal urgency, late-onset pain, and the possibility of having to undergo a secondary procedure at a later date, especially because of a symptomatic external component[51] or recurrent prolapse.[218] Short and intermediate follow-up studies (up to 1 year) are favorable,[29,103,228] but long-term results are truly needed.

Bona and colleagues reported the outcome of their 400 patients who underwent this procedure after at least a 6-month follow-up.[38] Early postoperative bleeding was noted in 3.5%, half of whom required return to the operating room. With a median follow-up of 6.1 years, 4 patients required reoperation for recurrent symptoms. There was a statistically significant improvement in obstructed defecation scores. Ceci and coworkers noted an 18.2% recurrence rate in their 291 patients with grade III and grade IV hemorrhoids following PPH.[49] Reoperation for persistent complaints was required for 7.2%. Ommer and associates analyzed 257 patients with a mean follow-up of 6.3 years.[217] Of these, 87.1% were satisfied. Reoperation was required in 3.6%.

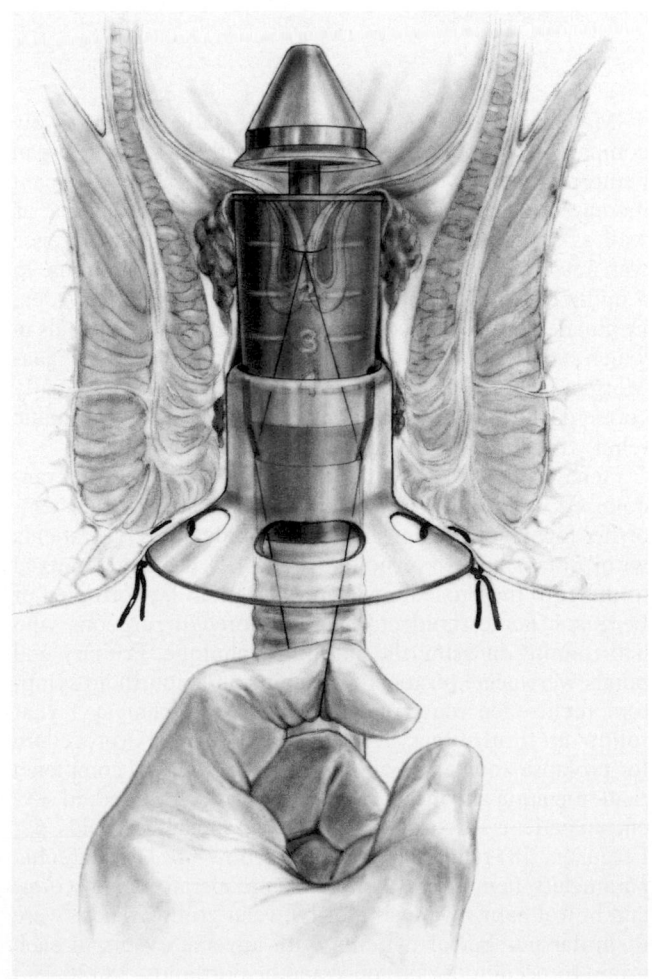

FIGURE 11-62. The instrument is closed and fired with continued downward traction on the purse-string suture. This draws the mucosa into the head of the stapler.

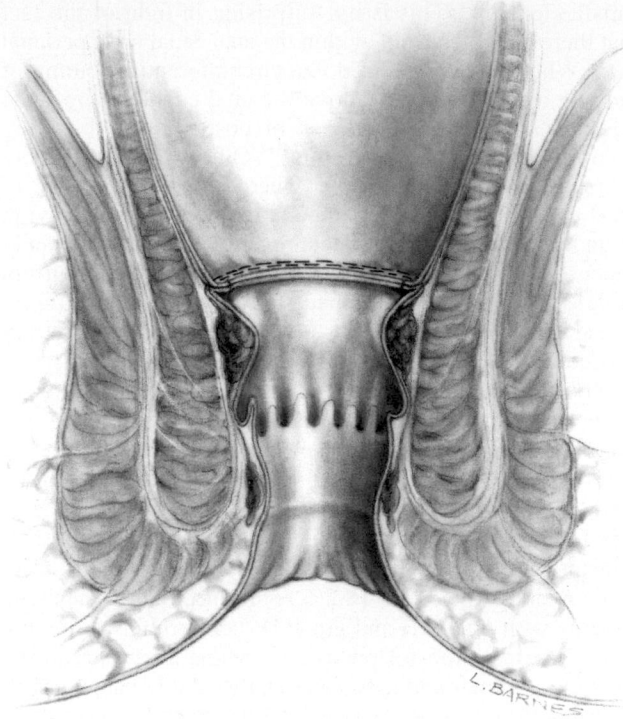

FIGURE 11-63. A strip of mucosa above the hemorrhoids has been removed with resultant "anal lifting." The circular staple line, ideally at least 2 cm proximal to the dentate line, is evident.

Mattana and his group from Rome, Italy, retrospectively compared stapled hemorrhoidopexy with Milligan-Morgan hemorrhoidectomy.[180] There was a statistically significant increased incidence of bleeding with the PPH technique as well as an increased incidence of tenesmus. No difference was noted in patient satisfaction or recurrent symptoms. In a multicenter, prospective, randomized trial from Sweden, Denmark, and the United Kingdom involving 18 hospitals in which stapled hemorrhoidopexy was compared with Milligan-Morgan hemorrhoidectomy, at 1 year prolapse was equally corrected, but hemorrhoidectomy offered better symptomatic relief with the downside of being more painful.[208]

Senagore and coworkers undertook a prospective, randomized, controlled multicenter trial comparing stapled hemorrhoidopexy and Ferguson hemorrhoidectomy.[271] Patients with prolapsing hemorrhoids (grade III) were randomized to undergo the procedure for prolapse and hemorrhoids or Ferguson hemorrhoidectomy by colorectal surgeons who had training in using the stapling technique. Primary end points were acute postoperative pain and hemorrhoid symptom recurrence requiring additional treatment at 1-year follow-up from surgery. A total of 156 patients (procedure for prolapse and hemorrhoids, 77; Ferguson, 79) completed randomization and the surgical procedure. One hundred seventeen patients (procedure for prolapse and hemorrhoids, 59; Ferguson, 58) returned for 1-year follow-up. Demographic parameters, hemorrhoid symptoms, preoperative pain scores, and bowel habits were similar between groups. There were a similar number of patients with adverse events in each group (procedure for prolapse and hemorrhoids, 28 [36.4%] vs. Ferguson, 38 [48.1%]; P = .138). Reoperation for an adverse effect was required in 6 (7.6%) Ferguson patients

and in 0 patients having the procedure for prolapse and hemorrhoids (P = .028). Postoperative pain during the first 14 days, pain at first bowel movement, and need for postoperative analgesics were significantly less in the procedure for prolapse and hemorrhoids group. Control of hemorrhoid symptoms was similar between groups; however, significantly fewer patients having the procedure for prolapse and hemorrhoids required additional anorectal procedures during 1-year follow-up (procedure for prolapse and hemorrhoids, 2 [2.6%], vs. Ferguson, 11 [13.9%]; P = .01). Only 4 of the Ferguson patients (five interventions) required additional procedures more than 30 days after surgery.

These data demonstrate that stapled hemorrhoidopexy offers the benefits of less postoperative pain, less requirement for analgesics, and less pain at first bowel movement, while providing similar control of symptoms and need for additional hemorrhoid treatment at 1-year follow-up from surgery.

Arroyo and his colleagues evaluated the long-term benefits of a newer version of the PPH 33-01 stapler, the PPH 33-03.[16] They believe this latest development reduces the risks of pain and bleeding.

Care Following Hemorrhoidectomy (Personal Opinion)

Each surgeon has his or her personal preference as to the follow-up management after any surgical procedure. Hemorrhoid operations are no exceptions. Rather than express the whole range of options, I will simply provide my personal preferences. The reader should understand, however, that surgeons who are otherwise quite objective, sensitive, and reasonable and who are worthy of great respect become quite exorcised over this issue. They will vigorously defend their personal approaches to postoperative management, virtually unto death. Nevertheless, I shall charge on.

Anal dressings are indeed painful. I try to avoid them and simply use a pad or panty liner for the expected discharge. Any dressing, however, should ideally be removed the evening of the operation, and 20-minute warm sitz baths can be commenced. A warm water bath, three or four times a day, is probably the most salutary experience possible for an individual who has undergone anal surgery. A topical cream or lotion, such as Tucks, Balneol, Proctodan, Anusol, Analpram, or Prax (among others) may be applied. I avoid local anesthetic creams unless the patient is obstreperous, but ointments should not be used. They are too difficult and painful to remove. The cream should be left at the bedside, used liberally, and applied frequently. A small dressing such as a Tucks pad, also kept at the bedside, helps to prevent soiling of sheets and garments. Tape should be avoided. Medications include a prescription analgesic (ideally a nonconstipating agent), a bulking agent (I prefer Konsyl), a stool softener, or a stimulant laxative if necessary.

The patient is not seen until 3 or 4 weeks after discharge, at which time the wounds are usually healed. By delaying a follow-up visit until this time, one is protected from much complaining. It is much more pleasant to talk with a grateful patient who has hopefully suppressed the memory of any suffering. To undertake a digital examination at an earlier time in order to evaluate the possibility of a stricture, or worse, to dilate the anus, is cruel and inhuman punishment. A properly performed operation is not likely to result in stricture formation; thus, weekly digital examinations are not necessary and merely serve to cause a mass exodus from one's waiting area.

Complications of Surgical Hemorrhoidectomy

To avoid the pitfalls of hemorrhoid surgery, conscientious effort is required—not only with respect to meticulous surgical technique, but also with regard to a compulsive approach to postoperative management. The following is a partial list of the potential problems of surgical hemorrhoidectomy:

- Pain
- Urinary retention
- Urinary tract infection
- Constipation
- Fecal impaction
- Hemorrhage
- Infection and sepsis
- Anal tags
- Mucosal prolapse
- Mucosal ectropion
- Rectal stricture
- Anal stenosis
- Anal fissure
- Pseudopolyps
- Epidermal cysts
- Anal fistula
- Pruritus ani
- Fecal incontinence
- Recurrent hemorrhoids

Pain

Although pain is not actually a complication of surgery but is an anticipated consequence, it is nonetheless the single most important reason that patients avoid hemorrhoidectomy. I am certain that it is because of this fear that so few surgeons elect the operation for themselves, often despite having a severe hemorrhoid problem. It has been mentioned previously that internal anal sphincterotomy or sphincter stretch concomitant with hemorrhoidectomy had been thought by some to ameliorate this concern, but I believe that this has been disproved to most surgeons' satisfaction. Sphincter stretch, particularly in the older patient, may be associated with the complications of soilage and incontinence, and no prospective, randomized trial supports that this maneuver ameliorates pain. Internal anal sphincterotomy likewise can cause similar problems (see Chapter 12). Mortensen and colleagues performed a randomized study comparing surgical hemorrhoidectomy with and without anal dilatation.[197] They concluded that the combination did not improve cure rates compared with hemorrhoidectomy alone, but the addition of a sphincter stretch increased the risk for continence disturbances.[197] As mentioned previously, in the absence of a fissure or some other pathologic condition, I do not advocate either of these additional procedures.

A great deal of emphasis has been given to the management of pain in the posthemorrhoidectomy patient, not only because of the pain itself, but also because of the role it plays in causing urinary complications (see the following section). Recent literature abounds with newer alternatives in the management of discomfort. Epidural morphine has been employed for analgesia after hemorrhoidectomy at some

centers,[162] but with the requirement for early discharge, this approach has become a moot issue except for the individual who remains in the hospital. An ambulatory alternative that has been promoted is the STA Cath attachable infusion catheter. This consists of a special catheter that is sutured into the rectum above the dentate line. A topical anesthetic medication is delivered to the affected area by means of an infusion pump (Advanced Infusion, Inc., Snellville, GA). A volume of 2 to 4 mL/hour is perfused into the rectum, an amount which is believed to provide adequate flow of the topical anesthetic in order to minimize pain. Injection of a long-acting local anesthetic (ropivacaine) has also been proved effective in at least one prospective, randomized, double-blind study.[298]

Goldstein and colleagues have employed a subcutaneous morphine pump in postoperative pain management.[116] Although this was not a controlled study in the true sense, the authors concluded that the combination of *outpatient hemorrhoidectomy* and the pump was cost effective when compared with the inpatient stay.

Chiu and coworkers performed a prospective, randomized trial using transcutaneous electrical nerve stimulation in one arm of the study.[55] They found a statistically significant improvement in pain relief and in the frequency of urinary retention when compared with individuals receiving a more conventional pain management alternative. Others have found that pudendal nerve block with bupivacaine following successful pudendal nerve stimulation provided excellent analgesia, reducing the requirement for opioids in a randomized, double-blind study.[137] The efficacy was up to 24 hours.

Ketorolac tromethamine (Toradol) has also been advocated following anal surgery.[211,246] Many surgeons believe this is the most effective medication alternative for the posthemorrhoidectomy patient. One option is to inject 60 mg (2 mL) directly into the anal sphincter musculature at the time of its operative exposure. Studies suggest that there is a much reduced incidence not only of pain, but also of urinary retention.[211,246] Ketorolac is also quite effective following discharge when administered orally for pain control. Likewise, ibuprofen injection (Caldolor), 800 mg, through intravenous infusion over 5 to 7 minutes, has been shown to be a safe and effective opioid-sparing approach when compared with placebo.

Another pain management option is the application of transdermal fentanyl (Duragesic).[157] Fentanyl has been recommended as an effective analgesic alternative that essentially improves the transition to outpatient management with a nonnarcotic pain medication. In a letter to the editor, however, criticism was expressed for encouraging the use of a "contraindicated" medication.[33] It was believed that there is an unacceptably high incidence of hypoventilation with possible respiratory depression. In fact, recommendations against this use have been included with the package insert by the manufacturer.

Metronidazole (Flagyl) has been recommended as an effective medication for pain following hemorrhoidectomy, but in one randomized, double-blind trial this conclusion could not be supported.[21] However, in another randomized, placebo-controlled study following hemorrhoidectomy, there was a statistically significant reduction in postoperative pain in the treated group.[3] Nitroglycerin ointment (0.2%) and Nitroderm TTS band application have been demonstrated in prospective, randomized trials to reduce pain after hemorrhoidectomy.[72,301] Headache, however, is a potential problem. Davies and colleagues undertook a double-blind study of 50 consecutive patients who underwent Milligan-Morgan hemorrhoidectomy and assigned an internal sphincter injection of 0.4 mL of a solution containing either botulinum toxin (20 U; Botox) or normal saline.[76] Those who received the toxin injection had a significant pain reduction.

Topical nifedipine with lidocaine ointment was compared with lidocaine ointment alone in a prospective, randomized, double-blind study after hemorrhoidectomy.[230] Although some benefit was achieved at times, the results were, at best, mixed. And finally, topical sucralfate cream has been found to decrease pain following hemorrhoidectomy at days 7 and 14 while promoting faster wound healing when compared with that of a placebo.[122] It was subsequently pointed out by others that in the United States, smaller pharmacies do not have the capability to compound this 7% chemical in a petrolatum base.[50] However, although the larger chains could do so, the cost was not prohibitive—varying from $34 to $50 for a 4-week supply.

Opinion

It is my opinion that a simple and reasonably effective pain management approach is either ketorolac (Toradol) or an oral narcotic analgesic medication, administered in adequate doses and given frequently, such as oxycodone (Percocet) or hydrocodone (Vicodin). I fully recognize that the latter medications are quite constipating. Therefore, it is very important to provide a concomitant laxative to deal with this expected consequence.

Urinary Retention

Urinary retention is the most common complication following hemorrhoidectomy. Bleday and coworkers reported a 20% incidence of postoperative urinary complications.[37] Factors often held responsible include the following:

- Fluid overload
- Spinal anesthesia
- Rectal pain and spasm
- High ligation of the hemorrhoidal pedicle
- Rough handling of tissue
- Heavy suture material
- Numerous sutures
- Rectal packing
- Tight, bulky dressings
- Anticholinergics
- Narcotics[74,160,201,259]

Bailey and Ferguson demonstrated the effectiveness of fluid restriction in a carefully controlled, prospective randomized study of 500 patients.[20] One group was given free access to oral fluids after the operation. The other was permitted neither coffee nor tea, and oral fluids were limited to 250 mL until voiding was spontaneous or until a catheter was inserted. Both groups were treated identically in all respects except for the postoperative fluid intake. Each patient was instructed to empty the bladder before going to the operating room. Anesthesiologists were asked to limit intravenous fluids to the amount they considered a safe minimum. Patients were not routinely catheterized; this was carried out only in the case of bladder distension diagnosed by a physician.

Only 3.5% of the patients in the group having limited fluids required catheterization, versus 14.9% with unlimited fluids. No recognized postoperative complication was attributable to fluid restriction. The authors concluded that the postoperative catheterization rate was dramatically reduced by restricting fluids and delaying catheterization until the bladder was distended.

Scoma reported a similar study in an effort to eliminate this common postoperative complication.[267] The charts of 100 patients who underwent hemorrhoidectomy before the trial were reviewed. A second group consisted of 100 consecutive patients undergoing hemorrhoidectomy procedures performed by the author using local anesthesia (i.e., bupivacaine hydrochloride with epinephrine and hyaluronidase). None received atropine or scopolamine. The anesthesiologist was asked to give diazepam (Valium) intravenously with small doses of thiopental sodium (Pentothal), if necessary, at the beginning of the local infiltration. Amounts of intraoperative fluids were limited to 200 mL, and the infusion was terminated as the dressings were being applied.

Postoperatively, 100 mg of meperidine hydrochloride (Demerol) was given intramuscularly 4 hours after hemorrhoidectomy was completed and every 2 hours thereafter as needed. Patients were told to take only sips of water until they voided. Nurses catheterized the patient only after approval by the physician and were instructed not to urge the patient to void. The morning after operation, the patient sat in a bath of hot water and was encouraged to void. Those who did not urinate immediately in the bath stood under a hot shower to encourage voiding.

In the first group, 52% of the patients were catheterized, and in the second group, no one was catheterized. Of those in the second group, 86% voided before they took the hot bath, and the remaining voided in the bath or shower.

The incidence of urinary retention is not generally believed to be altered by the prophylactic administration of bethanechol chloride (Urecholine).[41] However, Gottesman and colleagues found that this drug, given in a dose of 10 mg subcutaneously, significantly lowered the incidence of postoperative urinary retention after anorectal surgery.[118] Prophylactic α-adrenergic blockade has failed to prevent this complication, as has the administration of anxiolytic agents.[48,118]

It is important to recognize that all reports indicate that with the promotion of ambulatory anorectal surgery, the incidence of urinary retention is significantly lower than that of the historical in-hospital rate. It has also been observed that the use of local anesthesia is associated with a significantly lower incidence of urinary retention when compared with spinal anesthesia.[97] Hoff and colleagues noted that only one of their 190 patients required catheterization following ambulatory surgical hemorrhoidectomy.[133]

Comment

Pain and fluid overload are the primary factors that cause urinary retention. If pain medication is inadequate, the patient cannot relax the sphincter mechanism sufficiently to urinate—it simply hurts too much. Clearly, one must limit fluid intake. This requires education of the anesthesiologists, the nurses, and the house officers. Threatening the patient with a catheter or leaving standing orders for catheterization is a self-fulfilling prophecy for its subsequent insertion. The minimal intravenous infusion necessary is given during the operation, and the infusion is terminated in the recovery room. If hospital regulations require that an intravenous line must be maintained, a heparin lock will suffice. Oral fluids are restricted until the following morning. Finally, patients are not routinely catheterized; this is undertaken only when the bladder is distended or if the patient complains, and then only after examination by a physician.

The policy in many ambulatory surgical facilities is that the patient must void before discharge. I overrule any such dictum and mandate that the nurses not even ask about urinating, much less insist upon it. Later that day or evening, or the following morning, with the commencement of sitz baths or hot showers, virtually every patient will void. Once the nursing service and the patient have been educated, the incidence of retention and the associated complication of urinary tract infection will be virtually eliminated. However, if urinary retention does develop, the inconvenience, discomfort, and anxiety are, for the patient, not inconsiderable.

If catheterization becomes necessary (in the hospital, in the emergency room, at the patient's home, or in the physician's office), it should be performed with a balloon catheter. If the residual urine is determined to be greater than 500 mL, the catheter should be left in place for 24 hours because it is unlikely that the patient will be able to void subsequently. Conversely, with a residual of less than 500 mL, the catheter can be removed with the reasonable expectation that spontaneous urination will occur.

Urinary Tract Infection

Urinary tract infection is usually a direct consequence of catheterization for urinary retention. The most common offending organisms are coliform bacteria. Appropriate antibiotics and catheter removal usually result in rapid resolution, but chronic infection, cystitis, and pyelonephritis can be late sequelae. Here again, the value of avoiding urinary retention cannot be overestimated.

Constipation

Patients who undergo hemorrhoidectomy await their postoperative bowel evacuation less than enthusiastically and always view the possibility of an enema intended to facilitate this function with apprehension. Constipation after anorectal surgery must be either relieved effectively or prevented because if it is untreated, it may lead to fecal impaction—a matter of special concern in this group of patients. Despite awareness of this possibility, as long as 72 hours may elapse before one considers the value of administering a laxative agent.[201,294] Factors that contribute to this delay include the effects of analgesic medications given before or after the operation; the consequences of the anesthetic, itself; and local physiologic dysfunction resulting from surgical manipulation, as well as the tendency for the patient not to ambulate and the fear of painful defecation. A history of irregular bowel function and colonic hypomotility may complicate the problem further.

Johnson and colleagues prospectively randomized 30 hemorrhoidectomy patients into two groups: one received wheat fiber and the other a laxative regimen of sterculia, magnesium sulfate, and mineral oil.[143] Those who received the fiber had a significantly shorter hospital stay, less painful bowel actions, and less discharge and soiling.

I evaluated the efficacy of senna (Senokot S) tablets in a prospective fashion on 50 patients who underwent anal operations in an in hospital setting.[65] Patients took two tablets with a full glass of water on the evening of the first day after operation. If no bowel movement occurred by the evening of the second day, the dose was changed to two tablets at bedtime and two tablets the following morning. If no stool was passed by the evening of the third day of treatment, the dose at bedtime was increased to three tablets. Enemas or other suitable forms of treatment were administered if function of the bowel was not restored by the evening of the fourth day. One of the options was to increase the dose of the test medication to a maximum of four tablets. No other laxatives or stool modifiers were taken during the trial period. The test preparation was administered for a maximum of 4 days. All patients achieved bowel movements during the study, and none required enemas. None passed hard stools on the day of release from the hospital.

Comment

As with the management of urinary retention, the patient can no longer be permitted the luxury of remaining in the hospital to await the first bowel action. Discharge instructions should include a bowel management program conducive to satisfactory bowel evacuation (e.g., a bulk laxative and a stimulant laxative). I believe that a stimulant laxative should be given on the evening of the operation and continued in increasing doses until defecation occurs, as described earlier. By the third postoperative day with no bowel action, a vigorous laxative (e.g., magnesium citrate, Dulcolax, Miralax) should be considered. If no bowel movement occurs by the fourth day, a gentle enema may be administered. If this fails to be rewarding, the patient will require reevaluation for the possibility of fecal impaction.

Hemorrhage

Massive hemorrhage that occurs in the recovery room is always the result of a technical error and can usually be attributed to improper or inadequate ligation of the hemorrhoid pedicle. This most commonly occurs if the pedicle is simply hand-tied rather than suture-ligated (Figure 11-64). Such a complication requires emergency surgical intervention. This should be quite unusual when Ferguson's hemorrhoidectomy is performed because care is taken in closing the wounds. Although management of active bleeding soon after hemorrhoidectomy may include submucosal injection with 1 to 2 mL of 1:100,000 epinephrine, direct pressure with a finger or gauze, and the use of topical epinephrine, returning the patient promptly to the operating room for direct visualization of the operative site with suture ligation is the most effective, most reassuring, and safest alternative.[207]

Delayed hemorrhage (i.e., 3 to 14 days postoperatively) is probably the result of sepsis in the pedicle or erosion of

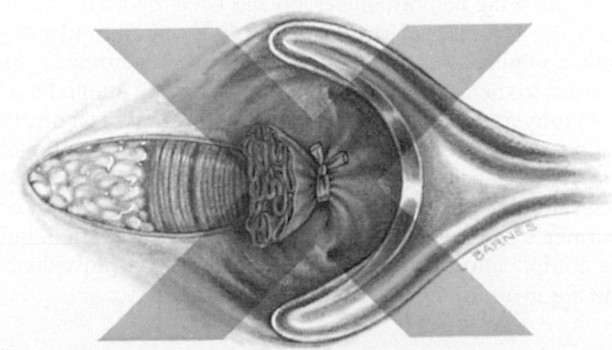

FIGURE 11-64. Incorrect mass ligation technique of the hemorrhoid pedicle. The pedicle must be suture ligated to limit the risk for early postoperative hemorrhage.

the suture. This occurs in approximately 1% to 2% of hemorrhoidectomies.[37] Patients may experience renewed slight bleeding, the passage of clots, or massive hemorrhage. Bleeding 1 week or longer following surgery, when the patient has previously ceased bleeding, warrants examination. Treatment varies from expectant management to in-hospital observation, transfusion, and resuture. Rosen and colleagues identified 27 patients with the complication of delayed hemorrhage over an 8-year period (1983 to 1990), an incidence of 0.8%.[250] The mean interval from the operation to hemorrhage was 6 days. Three-fourths of the patients were treated by bedside anal packing, 18% by observation alone, and two individuals required suture ligation. Although initial packing was successful in all those treated, 15% required repeated operation because of rebleeding. The packing material employed was a rolled, slightly moistened, absorbable gelatin sponge (Gelfoam). Basso and Pescatori observed an incidence of delayed bleeding of approximately 2%, with a mean interval from the operation to hemorrhage of 4 days.[27] They employed a Foley catheter technique for tamponading of the bleeding point, with complete success in all five individuals treated. In my opinion, delayed hemorrhage usually is not a preventable complication.

Local Infection and Overwhelming Sepsis

It seems surprising that, because hemorrhoidectomy is carried out in a field with numerous and varied bacterial organisms present, there is not a higher incidence of septic complications following the operation. As Lal and Levitan have pointed out, hemorrhoidectomy may be followed by transient bacteremia and low-grade fever as a result of the relatively constant release of bacteria into the bloodstream from a feeding focus.[163] For example, an 8.5% rate of bacteremia has been reported following proctoscopic examination of patients with no evidence of lower intestinal disease.[167] However, despite the presence of potentially virulent organisms (e.g., clostridia, anaerobic streptococci, bacteroides, *Escherichia coli*), local infection and more generalized septic problems are indeed extremely rare.

It has been hypothesized that the major venous drainage of the rectum, by passing through the superior hemorrhoidal veins into the portal system, is cleared of organisms by the reticuloendothelial system of the liver.[167] This hepatic clearance, by effectively removing the bacteria released into the circulation, may be important in minimizing the impact of rectal colonic flora in the systemic circulation and may be the reason that infection is so uncommon, although liver abscess following hemorrhoidectomy has been reported.[221] Guy and Seow-Choen performed a MEDLINE search to identify septic complications after surgical hemorrhoidectomy.[123] As opposed to the case reports of sepsis following stapled mucosectomy and rubber band ligation, there simply is a dearth of reported cases of overwhelming sepsis with conventional hemorrhoidectomy despite the well-recognized transient bacteremia. There have been, however, isolated reports of Fournier's gangrene as a consequence of this operation, but this complication appears to be associated with individuals who are in an immunocompromised state.[60]

Comment

Because sitz baths are a routine part of the postoperative management, most skin problems (e.g., cellulitis, abscess) theoretically might be treated in an essentially prophylactic manner.

In an experience of more than 2,000 hemorrhoidectomies, I cannot recall ever seeing even cellulitis, much less draining an abscess. However, one must be circumspect if surgery on the anus is contemplated in an individual with AIDS or with leukemia, or in someone with agranulocytosis, receiving chemotherapy, or is otherwise immunocompromised.

Anal Tag

Anal tags, which can interfere with proper cleansing of the anus and thus lead to skin irritation, can usually be avoided by excising redundant skin at the time of operation. I suspect, however, that tags more often than not are the result of the manner in which the wounds heal, perhaps analogous to keloid formation in other incision sites. Bothersome tags can be excised as an office procedure if symptoms warrant.

Mucosal Prolapse

Inadequate removal of redundant or mobile rectal mucosa at the time of hemorrhoidectomy may result in mucosal prolapse. Patients may complain of a lump that requires manual reduction. Problems with mucous discharge and pruritic symptoms are common.

Treatment usually consists of rubber ring ligation of the prolapsed mucosa. If there seems to be extensive or circumferential involvement, the surgeon should conduct the examination while the patient strains on the toilet in order to look for procidentia.

Prevention of this complication requires that the surgeon remove any redundant mucosa at the time of hemorrhoidectomy. It will be interesting to note whether there is an increased incidence of recurrent prolapse following stapled hemorrhoidopexy.

Ectropion

Because the mucosa is more mobile than the perianal skin, the tendency for mucosal descent is greater than the likelihood of the skin ascending to reline the denuded anal canal (see Figure 11-55). If redundant mucosa above the site of the excised hemorrhoid tissue is not properly anchored to the underlying internal sphincter, the mucosa can heal outside the anal verge (see Figure 11-54). If the entire anal canal is removed, and the cut edge of the rectum is sutured to the perianal skin, a characteristic Whitehead deformity may be produced. If the surgeon anchors the mucosa to the skin in one or more quadrants, a partial ectropion may result. Interestingly, Khubchandani has reported treatment of anal stenosis by doing just what has been condemned—advancing the mucosa, albeit not beyond the anal verge.[154] Ectropion can lead to mucous discharge, skin irritation, and pruritus ani.[25,119] Prevention requires excising the redundant mucosa and anchoring the cut edge as described.

Treatment of an ectropion that is evident in only one quadrant is shown in Figure 11-65. As long as no stricture is present, a simple excision and transverse suture of the rectum to the underlying internal anal sphincter will suffice. The open wound should heal without the mucosal extrusion. An alternative approach is to perform an anoplasty (discussed later).

Anal Stricture

A considerable area of mucosa and anoderm may be denuded when the physician attempts to remove extensive, encircling hemorrhoids. If hemorrhoids are present in many areas, only minimal sections of intact, elastic anal tissue may be left

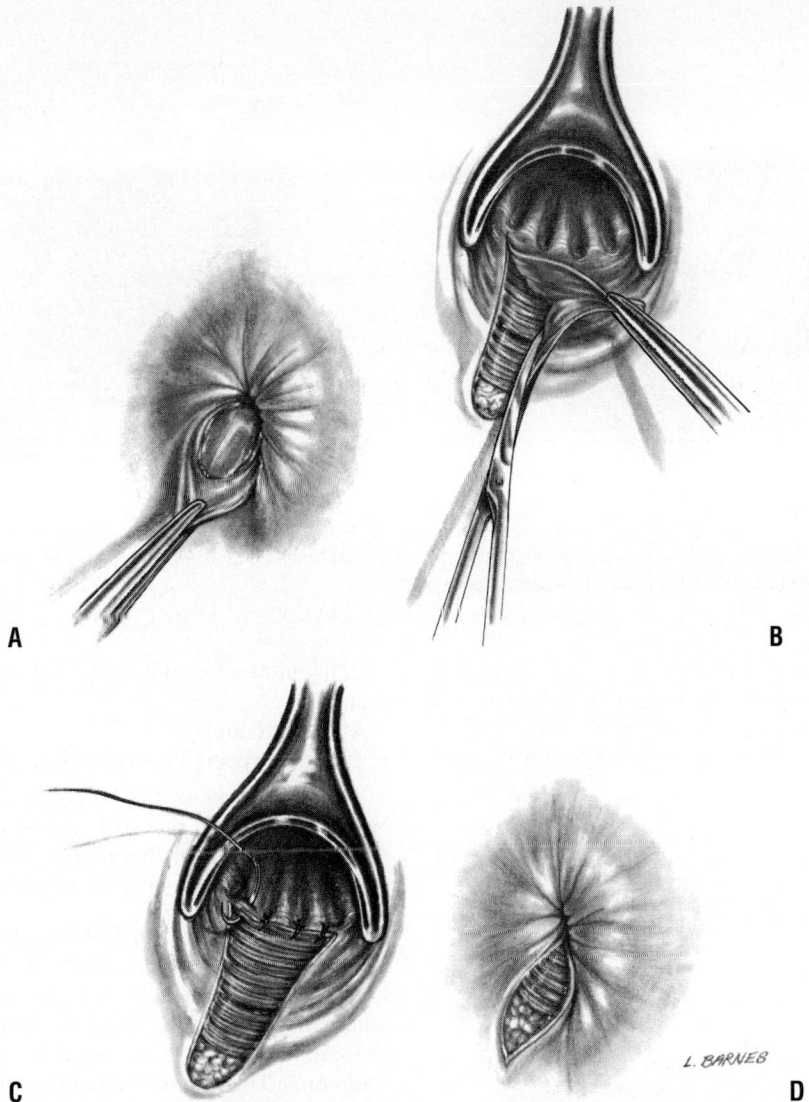

FIGURE 11-65. Treatment of mucosal ectropion. **A:** The mucosa projects in one quadrant. **B:** The mucosa is excised. **C:** The edge of the rectum is sutured to the underlying internal sphincter. **D:** The wound is left open to granulate.

following excision. With progressive healing, fibrous scar tissue may proliferate and contract the anorectal outlet.[302] When healing is complete, a narrow, foreshortened stenotic orifice may remain.

As with ectropion, anal stenosis is a preventable complication. If adequate skin bridges are preserved, the risk for reducing the circumference of the anal canal is minimized. However, in the presence of gangrenous hemorrhoids, distortion of the anal canal, fibrosis, chronic fissure, external tags, and hypertrophied anal papillae, extensive removal of the anal canal is often necessary to accomplish an adequate hemorrhoidectomy. Under these circumstances, the surgeon has two options: either compromise on the amount of tissue removed and accept the consequences of patient complaints of residual disease, or consider the possibility of performing an anoplasty at the time of hemorrhoidectomy.

The surgeon must attempt to preserve skin bridges; even one bridge is better than none (Figure 11-66). If because of sepsis, sloughing, or radical surgery, the potential for stricture formation becomes evident, digital examination of the rectum is advisable. This is an exception to my approach of not performing rectal examinations on posthemorrhoidectomy patients. It is probably worthwhile to advise insertion of a dilator two or three times daily in patients at risk for stricture (Figure 11-67). Weekly office visits are also suggested. Prevention of anal stricture when there is legitimate justification for concern is, in my opinion, the only indication for frequent digital examinations and the use of a dilator. If the wound heals without a stricture, digital examination and the use of a dilator can be discontinued, usually within 6 to 8 weeks. However, if a healed, fixed stricture develops, I prefer to perform an anoplasty rather than to have the patient use a dilator indefinitely.

Anoplasty

Anoplasty is a procedure whereby perianal skin is moved to cover a defect in the anal canal. This defect is usually the result of an operative procedure, such as excision of a portion or all of the anal canal, hemorrhoidectomy, excision of an anal fissure, or excision of a lesion of the anal canal.

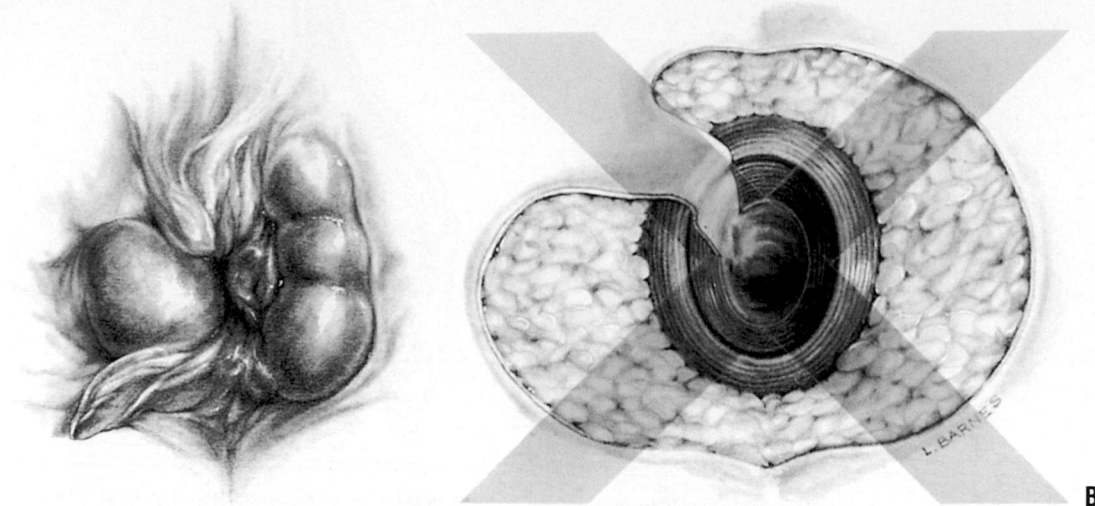

A   **B**

FIGURE 11-66. **A:** Artist's conception of extensive circumferential hemorrhoids. **B:** Virtual complete removal of the hemorrhoids with an inadequate attempt to preserve a mucocutaneous bridge.

Anoplasty may be performed to correct an anal stenosis or coincidentally with repair of a rectovaginal fistula or with sphincteroplasty for sphincteric injury.[66,70,95,136,179,203,214,241,262] The following list summarizes the indications for this procedure.

Indications
    Anal stricture
    Congenital
    Inflammatory (e.g., fistula, abscess)
    Trauma
        Operative (e.g., hemorrhoidectomy, fissurectomy, pull-through procedure, excisional procedures)
        Accidental
    Disuse caused by laxatives, enemas, chronic diarrhea
    Coincident with excision of anal lesions
    Ulcer
Concomitant with reconstructive anorectal operations
    Rectovaginal fistula repair
    Anterior fistula in women
    Sphincter repair
    Congenital anomaly (e.g., imperforate anus, ectopic anus)
    Tumor excision

Anal stricture can be one of the most disabling complications of anal surgery or of anal disease. Stenosis can occur as a consequence of numerous conditions:

- Benign and malignant tumors
- Inflammations, especially Crohn's disease
- Congenital anomalies (e.g., ectopic anus and imperforate anus)
- Abuse of laxatives
- Trauma, especially surgical trauma

However, overzealous hemorrhoidectomy continues to be one of the reasons that patients require an anoplasty. In the experience of Milsom and Mazier, 88% of 212 patients treated for anal stenosis had a history of prior hemorrhoidectomy.[190]

Symptoms, Findings, and Differential Diagnosis

The most troublesome complaint of individuals with anal stenosis is difficulty with defecation. Constipation, obstipation, painful bowel movements, narrow caliber of the stool, abdominal cramping, and bleeding are frequently associated symptoms. The fear of fecal impaction or pain usually causes the patient to rely on daily laxatives or enemas.

Physical examination readily reveals the problem. It may be impossible to perform a digital examination, or only the small finger may be tolerated. Proctosigmoidoscopy and anoscopy require narrow-caliber instruments. If there is any question concerning the etiology of the stenosis or the possibility of a proximal lesion, a barium enema or colonoscopy should be performed, if such examinations are technically possible. Sometimes, it is difficult to distinguish true stenosis with tissue loss from the sphincter spasm associated with an anal fissure. Administration of a local anesthetic may be helpful, but on occasion a general anesthetic may be required. The anesthetic abolishes the spasm associated with an acute fissure but will not produce an increased luminal diameter in a patient with true stenosis.[295]

It is important to ascertain the cause of the stricture in order to determine proper therapy. Anal Crohn's disease is an absolute contraindication to anoplasty in my opinion, and obviously a malignant process must be treated by excision or resection. Perhaps the most useful diagnostic tool is an accurate history. If the patient associates the onset of the problem with prior hemorrhoidectomy or with electrocoagulation of anal condylomata, for example, the condition may be appropriately treated by an anoplasty. Conversely, with no such history, such as in someone with long-term laxative use, correction of the stricture may produce anal incontinence. This

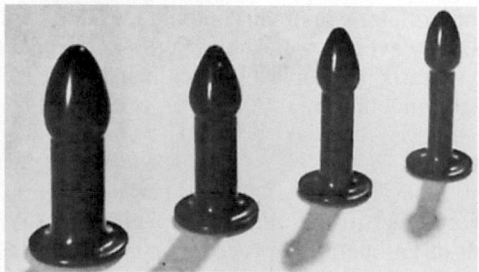

FIGURE 11-67. Young's Bakelite rectal dilators in a set of four adult sizes.

problem occurs when sphincter muscle wasting accompanies an anal stricture, a consequence of passing small, narrow bowel actions over many years. Mineral oil is notorious for leading to stenosis, probably because the lubricated stool fails to dilate the anal canal.

Symptoms present from birth imply a congenital origin. Most common is an anteriorly situated ectopic anus, usually at the introitus in female patients.[31] A hooded anus (see Figure 3-17) and anorectal atresia are also congenital lesions that may be associated with stenosis despite treatment early in life.

Medical Treatment

As mentioned, the conservative management of anal stenosis includes laxatives, suppositories, dilatation, and enemas. These approaches may effect defecation, but they do not specifically treat the cause of the problem, a narrow diameter of the anal canal. A dilator may tear the canal. In fact, a complication from its use may itself precipitate the need for surgical intervention.[293]

Surgical Treatment

Excision of Eschar and Sphincterotomy. The classic surgical treatment of an anal stricture is lysis of the stricture and excision of the eschar, ideally transverse suturing of the rectal mucosa to the underlying internal sphincter, and sphincterotomy—the same procedure described for the treatment by excision of chronic anal fissure (see Figure 12-23). Although the results have been reported as excellent (i.e., several hundred patients of Pope, more than 200 patients of Turell and Gelernt, 17 patients of Shropshear, and 224 patients of Malgieri),[179,236,274,296] it is difficult to interpret whether the patients had significant narrowing or merely spasm associated with an anal fissure. Furthermore, the term *anoplasty* should be limited, in my opinion, to those procedures that actually replace the anal canal with new tissue.

TECHNIQUE An artist's conception of a deformed, narrowed anal orifice that does not admit the index finger is shown

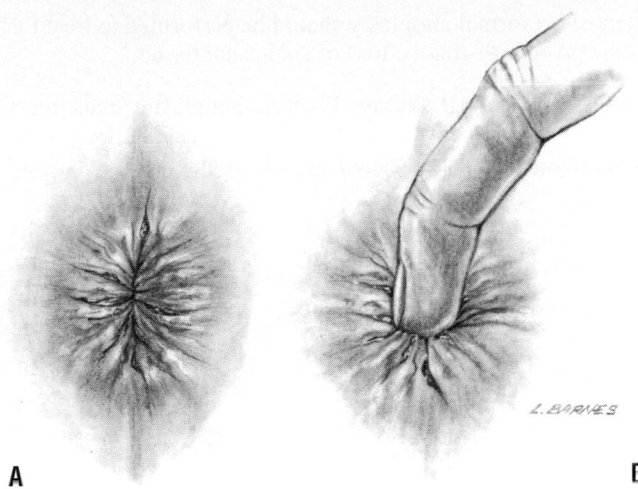

FIGURE 11-68. **A:** Anal deformity with stricture. **B:** This stricture does not permit digital examination.

in Figure 11-68. When the stricture is excised or lysed, a 29-mm (medium-size) Hill-Ferguson retractor is inserted. The cut edge of the rectum can be sutured to the underlying internal anal sphincter in a transverse fashion, thereby widening the anal canal (Figure 11-69A,B). If the lumen is still inadequate, the same maneuver can be performed on the opposite side (Figure 11-69C).

This is a perfectly acceptable technique that will yield satisfactory results if sufficient skin bridges remain. However, if this is not the case, frequent digital examinations must be performed or dilators employed to prevent restricture. As with sphincterotomy or sphincter stretch (see Chapter 12), this operation does not create a new anal canal lining with sensory-bearing mucosa. However, this procedure, or even sphincterotomy alone, may be quite adequate for a patient with a mild degree of narrowing. For more profound

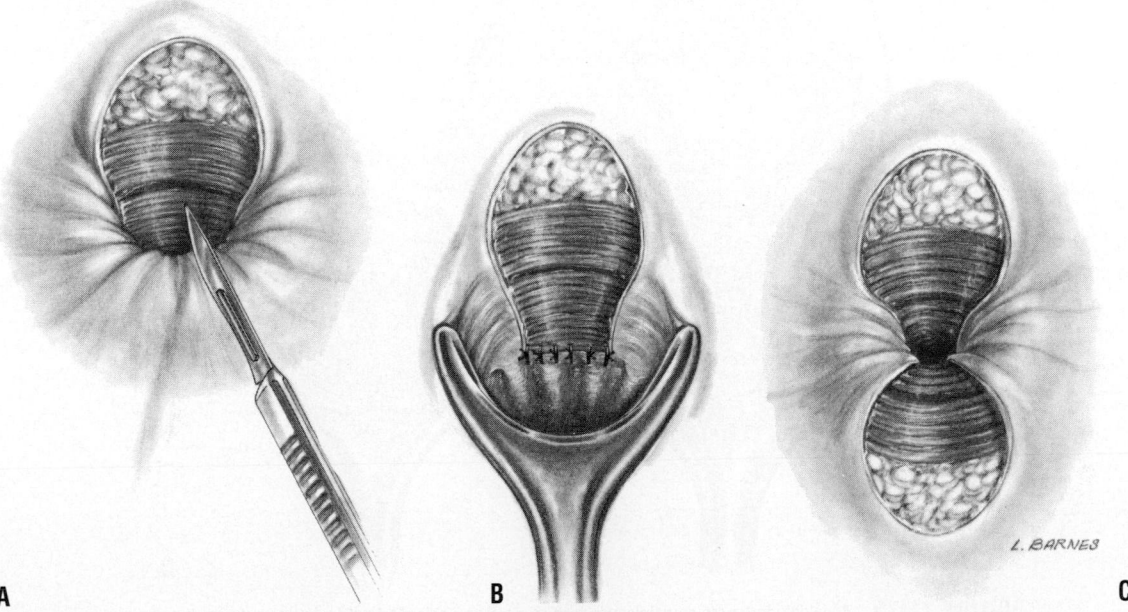

FIGURE 11-69. **A:** Lysis of the anal stricture permits insertion of a 29-mm Hill-Ferguson retractor. **B:** The rectum is sutured to the underlying internal anal sphincter. **C:** When further widening is required, this can be done on the opposite side.

stenosis, a formal anoplasty should be performed to treat the basic problem—that is, loss of anal canal tissue.

Anoplasty for Minimal Stenosis. Esoteric anoplastic maneuvers should be reserved for loss of anal canal tissue, but even mild anal stenosis can be treated by skin replacement. A small advancement flap (Y-V) may be useful for stenosis accompanying chronic posterior anal fissure.

PREOPERATIVE MANAGEMENT How aggressive should a bowel preparation be when the physician performs an anoplastic procedure? Probably all that is necessary is a small-volume enema,

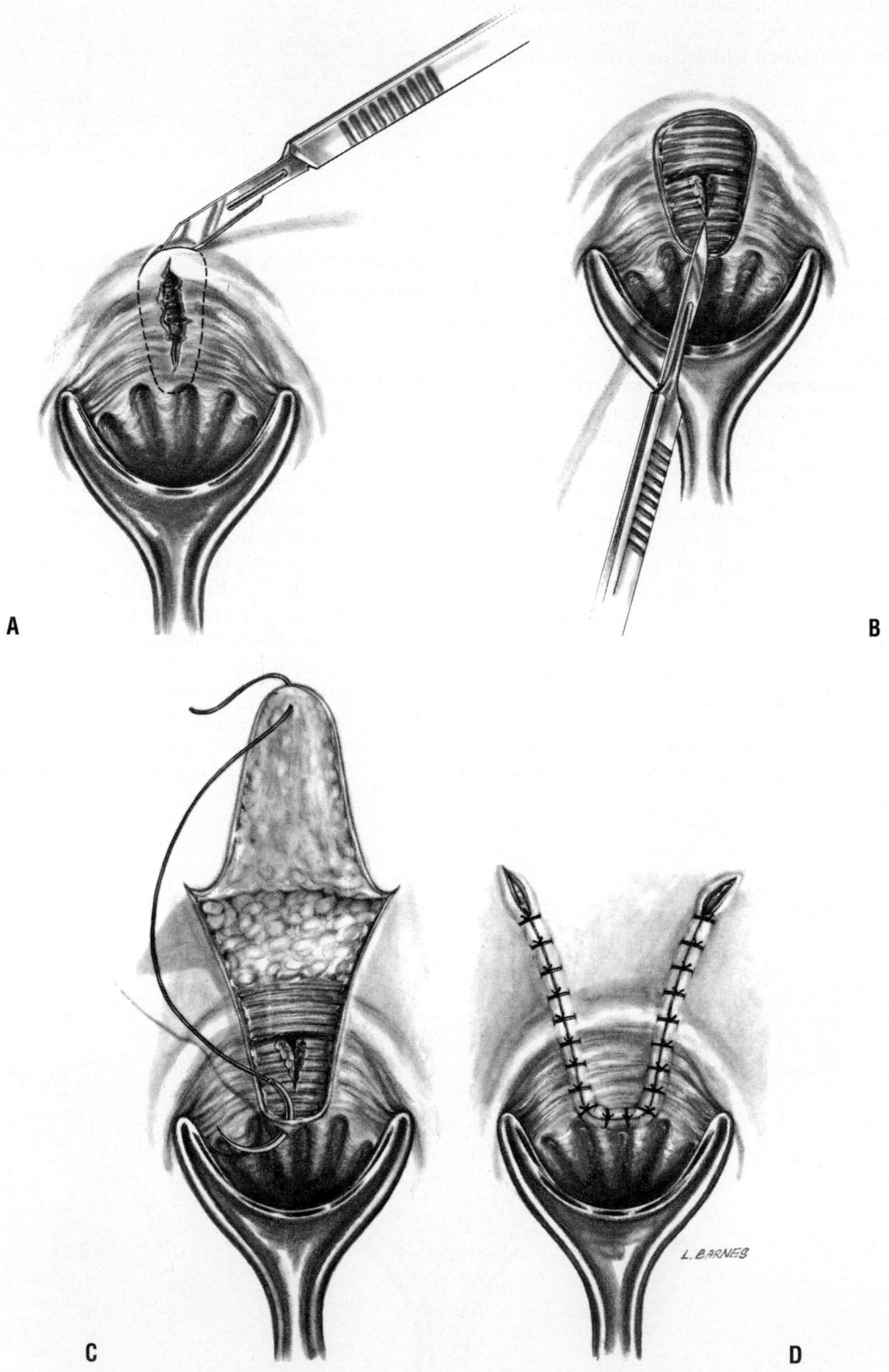

FIGURE 11-70. Anoplasty for chronic anal fissure with minimal stenosis. **A:** The *dashed line* shows the planned incision. **B:** An internal anal sphincterotomy is performed. **C:** The skin flap is elevated. **D:** The flap is advanced and sutured to the rectum.

but some advocate a full mechanical bowel preparation. Broad-spectrum, perioperative, systemic antibiotics have also been suggested. The more extensive the skin mobilization, the more concerned I am about the possibility of infection. A cleansing enema before surgery is probably the most important. One does not wish to deal with stool in the field if performing skin grafting.

OPERATIVE TECHNIQUE The patient is placed in the prone jackknife position with the buttocks taped apart. Spinal, caudal, general endotracheal, or local anesthesia may be employed. The stricture is incised (Figure 11-70A), and an internal anal sphincterotomy may be performed, if indicated (Figure 11-70B). A full-thickness flap of skin is elevated in the posterior midline (Figure 11-70C). A 29-mm Hill-Ferguson retractor is kept in place for the entire operation to maintain the adequacy of the lumen. If the canal can be reconstructed with the retractor in place, the anal opening will inevitably be adequate.

Incisions are carried proximally for 5 to 8 cm. Care must be taken to avoid creating a narrow pedicle that could compromise the blood supply to the apex of the flap. Mobilization over the sacrum is unnecessary for this degree of anal canal defect. The full thickness of the skin is sutured to the rectal mucosa and to the underlying internal anal sphincter with interrupted long-term absorbable sutures. The completed repair is shown in Figure 11-70D. The external aspect may be left open if tension is produced by closure, or the entire wound may be closed primarily. The final, healed wounds can be seen in Figure 11-71 in a patient who underwent the operation for mild anal stenosis.

This technique is simple and quite useful for stricture associated with an anal fissure. However, if more than 25% of the circumference of the anal canal needs to be covered, another anoplastic approach is indicated.

A so-called V-Y or island flap anoplasty is another option for the management of mild anal stenosis or the treatment of a limited mucosal ectropion.[45,248] The full thickness of perianal skin is mobilized and advanced into the anal canal to create a new lining (Figure 11-72). Care must be taken to preserve the blood supply to the graft. A similar modification has been termed the house advancement flap.[56] Its theoretical advantages are that (1) it provides a broad skin flap for the

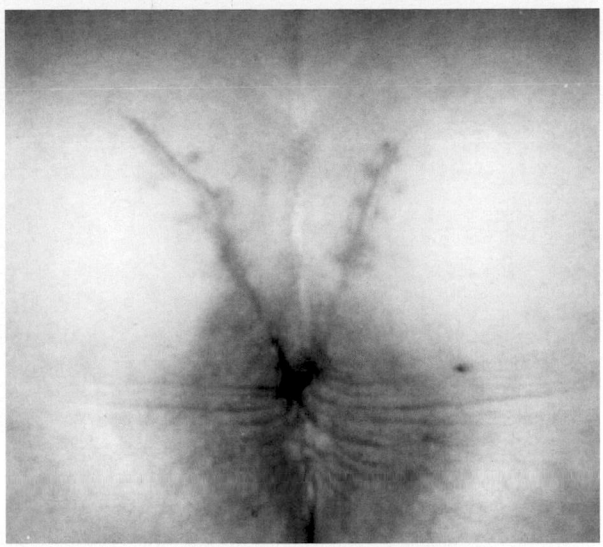

FIGURE 11-71. Postoperative appearance of **Y-V** anoplasty at 8 weeks.

entire length of the entire anal canal and (2) it allows for primary closure of the donor site. The word *house* denotes the schematic representation of a house in terms of the way the flap is created. The technique is illustrated in Figure 11-73.

POSTOPERATIVE MANAGEMENT The postoperative care of any patient who undergoes some type of anorectal reconstruction—that is, using skin or muscle—is the subject of much debate. There are no prospective, randomized trials with bowel-confining regimens or with antibiotics (neither type nor duration). Therefore, one must resort to discussing *art*, not *science*. In all operations involving an anoplasty, an antibiotic, usually a cephalosporin, is given perioperatively. Whether it is continued postoperatively, orally or parenterally, for 1, 2, or more days, depends on the extent of the reconstruction and the surgeon's personal preference. Again, the decision of whether to prevent bowel action postoperatively is also the surgeon's choice. Generally, however, because only a small graft is created in an anoplasty for mild stenosis, confining the bowels is unnecessary. Furthermore, the more

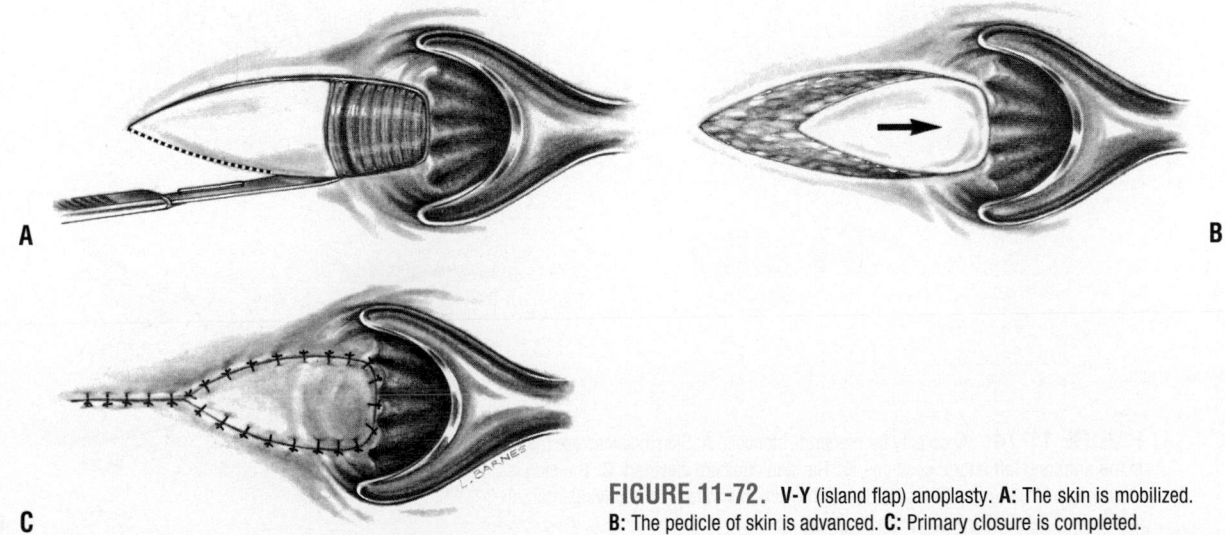

FIGURE 11-72. **V-Y** (island flap) anoplasty. **A:** The skin is mobilized. **B:** The pedicle of skin is advanced. **C:** Primary closure is completed.

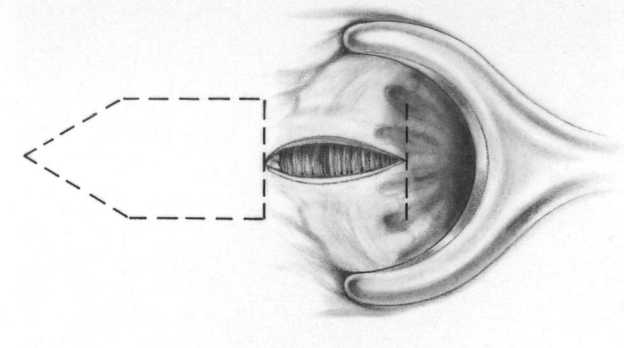
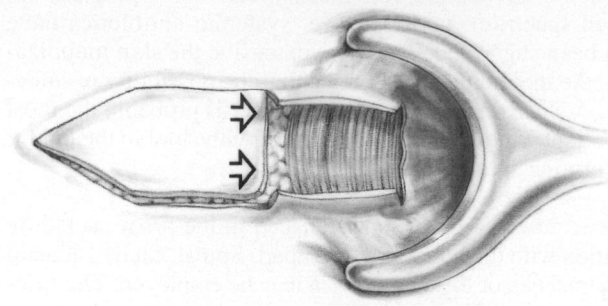
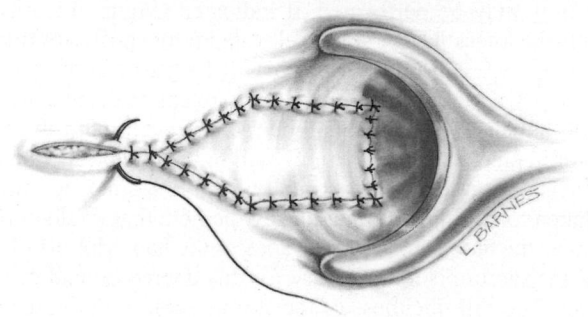

FIGURE 11-73. House advancement flap for anal stenosis. **A:** A longitudinal incision is made laterally for the length of the anal canal. **B:** After the wound edges are undermined, the incision assumes a rectangular shape. **C:** The completed house flap is advanced, lining the entire length of the anal canal, and sutured into place. (After Christensen MA, Pitsch RM Jr, Cali RL, et al. "House" advancement pedicle flap for anal stenosis. *Dis Colon Rectum.* 1992;35(2):201–203.)

vigorous the postoperative regimen, the longer one tends to stay in the hospital. Without a bowel-confining regimen, the patient is permitted a regular diet supplemented by a bulk laxative containing psyllium or a stool softener. Showers are permitted, but sitz baths are not recommended. Simple cleansing of the wound is all that is required. Rarely is it necessary to probe under the skin flap to evacuate a hematoma or purulent collection, but even under these circumstances the viability of the graft is usually not compromised. The patient is discharged when a bowel movement occurs (insurance company permitting) and is then seen weekly or every 2 weeks until the wounds heal, usually in 5 to 6 weeks.

Anoplasty for Moderate Stenosis. When a greater area needs to be covered than can be accomplished with a single advancement flap, sufficient skin can often be obtained by performing bilateral advancements in the right lateral and left lateral positions. This will permit resurfacing of up to 50% of the anal canal circumference.

OPERATIVE TECHNIQUE The patient is placed in the prone jackknife position with the buttocks taped apart. A local anesthetic is not advised because of the extensive infiltration required and its associated discomfort. Figure 11-74 illustrates the technique. The full thickness of the skin is sutured to the cut edge of the rectum

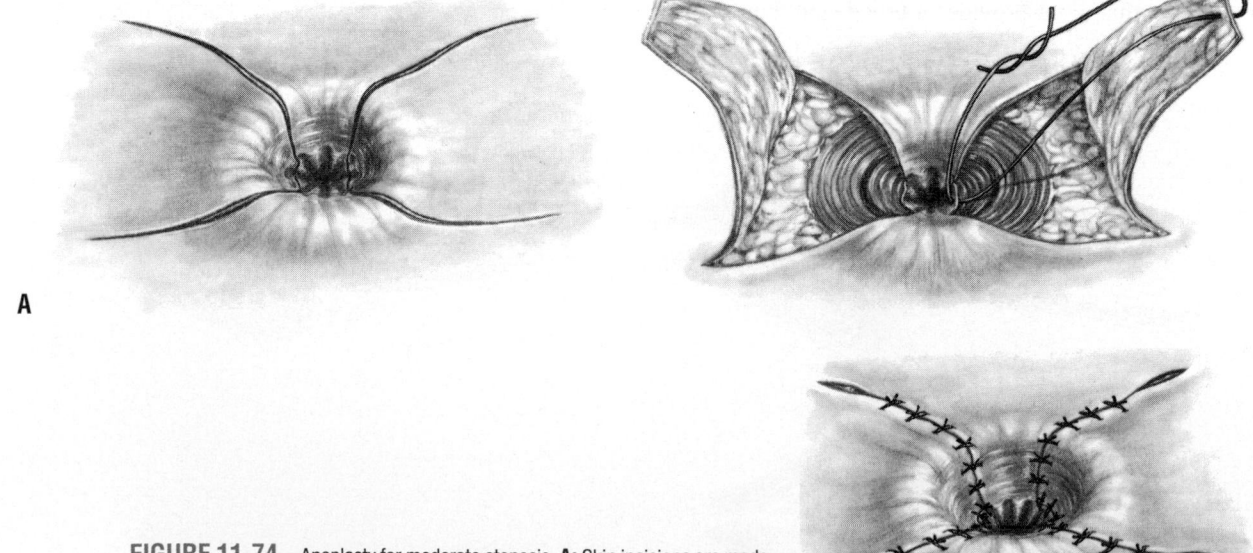

FIGURE 11-74. Anoplasty for moderate stenosis. **A:** Skin incisions are made in the right and left lateral positions. **B:** The skin flaps are elevated. **C:** The skin is advanced and sutured to the cut edge of the rectum and to the underlying internal sphincter. The Hill-Ferguson retractor is not shown.

and the underlying internal sphincter with long-term absorbable sutures. This effectively increases the diameter of the anal canal.

POSTOPERATIVE MANAGEMENT It may be advisable to confine the bowels after this procedure because of the extent of the skin coverage attempted, but here again it becomes a matter of surgeon preference and one's ability to prolong the patient's hospitalization. This is accomplished with diphenoxylate hydrochloride (Lomotil), up to eight tablets a day; codeine, up to 240 mg daily; and deodorized tincture of opium, up to 80 drops a day. As with all skin grafts, sitz baths are withheld. The wounds are cleansed with an antiseptic such as hydrogen peroxide or povidone-iodine four times daily.

My own, frequently changing preference is to discontinue the medications after 3 days. A regular diet is instituted, supplemented with a bulk laxative and a stool softener. Some small separation of the wound may occur, but satisfactory healing with an adequate anal opening may be anticipated. The patient is ideally discharged when bowel function has returned or at the insistence of the low dull normal insurance mafia who determine how one should practice medicine. The patient is seen usually every 10 to 14 days until complete healing has taken place.

Anoplasty for Severe Stenosis or for Major Coverage of the Anal Canal. The plastic maneuvers previously described are useful for minimal or moderate problems of skin coverage. However, if 50% or more of the anal canal needs to be reconstructed, a rotation flap of skin should be considered. The reason for using this type of graft is that rotation flaps can cover a greater surface area without tension and with less concern for viability than can advancement flaps. Conditions that may necessitate this maneuver include stricture secondary to radical hemorrhoidectomy, concomitant tissue loss with excision of an anal

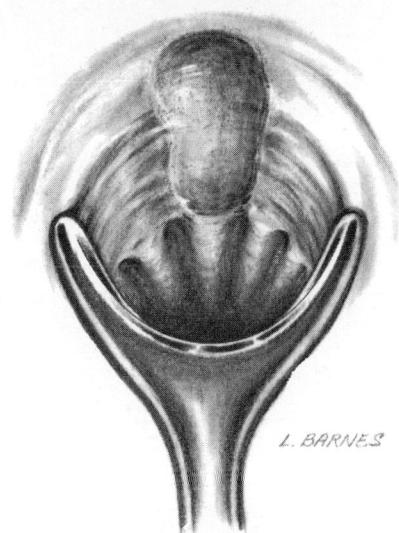

FIGURE 11-76. Artist's conception of a keyhole deformity, a consequence of excision of an anal fissure in the posterior midline.

canal lesion, and mucosal ectropion. This last problem may be seen not only following the so-called Whitehead hemorrhoidectomy (see Figure 11-55), but also after an abdominal-anal pull-through procedure or after any operation for imperforate anus. Another indication for this operation is to correct the "keyhole" deformity that may be a consequence of excision of an anal fissure or excision of an anal fistula.

OPERATIVE TECHNIQUE The patient is placed in the prone jackknife position, and the buttocks are taped apart. In most instances, a single rotation flap will provide adequate skin coverage (Figure 11-75). Figure 11-76 illustrates a keyhole deformity in the posterior midline, a consequence of excisional fissure surgery. After excision of the scar, an outline of the incision is made, the flap is elevated and rotated medially, and the wound is closed, primarily with interrupted, long-term absorbable sutures (Figure 11-77).

In the correction of Whitehead's deformity or when the entire anal canal must be replaced, a bilateral rotation flap (S-plasty) should be performed. Spinal, caudal, or general endotracheal anesthesia is employed; a locally administered anesthetic is not advised. The anal canal is incised posteriorly, and the lower portion of the internal sphincter is divided. The anal canal is incised farther to permit insertion of a Hill-Ferguson retractor.

A full-thickness flap of skin is elevated, and the incision is begun in the midline and carried laterally in a curvilinear fashion for approximately 8 to 10 cm. A longer length can be obtained by incising farther laterally and, eventually, somewhat medially. Care should be taken to avoid necrosis; a thick flap that includes subcutaneous tissue is preferred. As mentioned, more than one flap is rarely required because a new anal canal along one-half of the circumference is more than adequate. However, if the entire anal canal needs to be reconstructed, as has been mentioned with Whitehead's deformity or ectropion associated with surgery for imperforate anus (in which all the mucosa must be excised completely, thereby denuding the anal canal), a similar incision is performed on the opposite side. Hemostasis is effected with electrocautery. The wound is irrigated with saline solution,

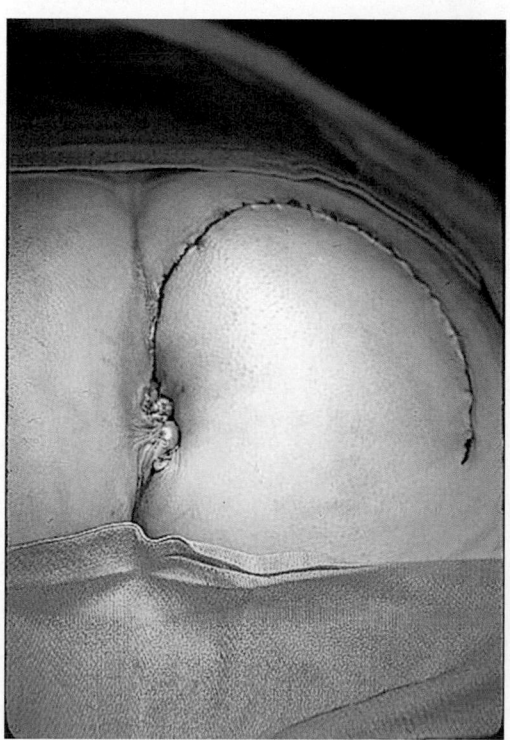

FIGURE 11-75. Immediate postoperative appearance of rotation skin flap repair for severe anal stenosis.

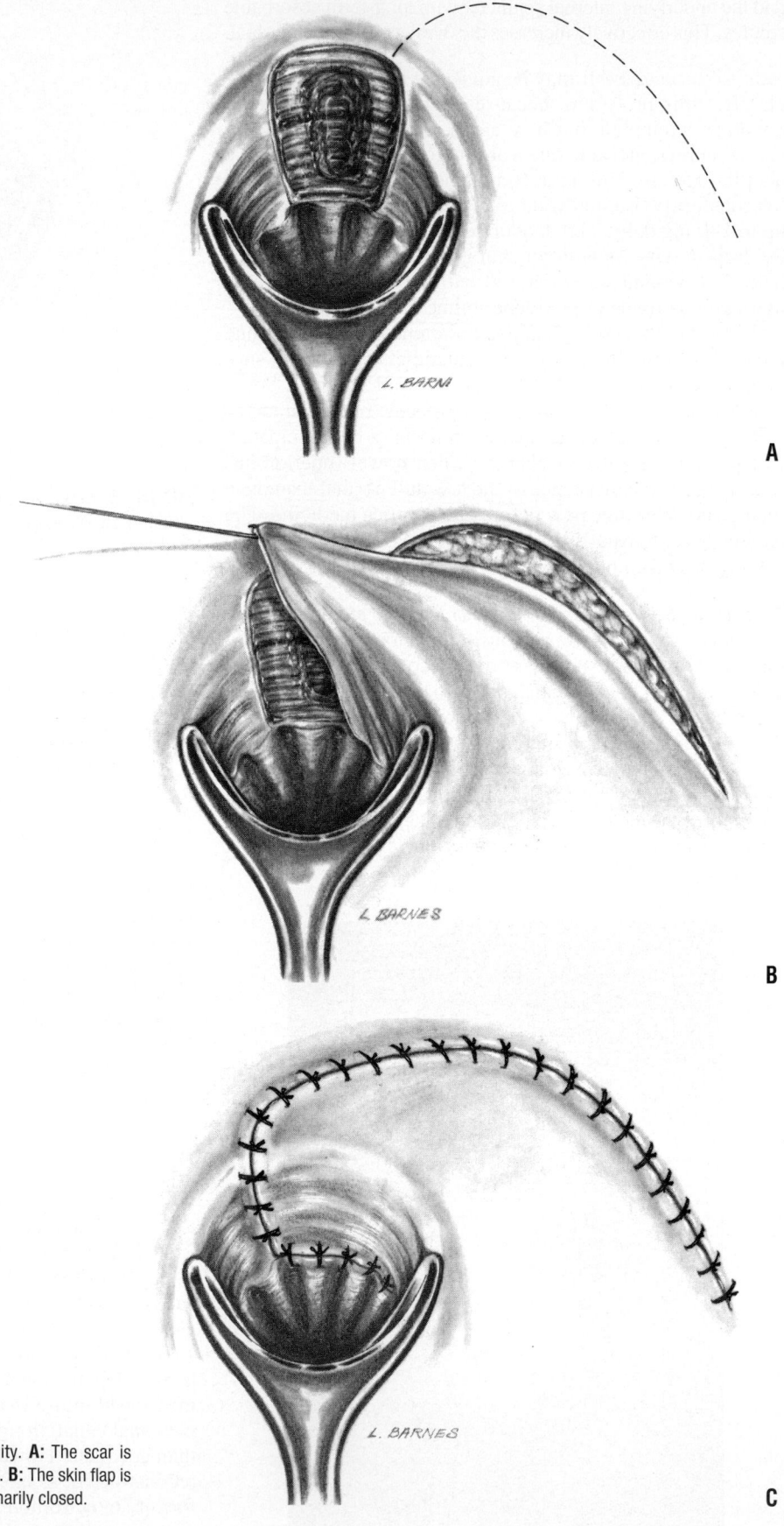

FIGURE 11-77. Correction of keyhole deformity. **A:** The scar is excised; note the outline of the skin flap (*dashed line*). **B:** The skin flap is mobilized and rotated medially. **C:** The wound is primarily closed.

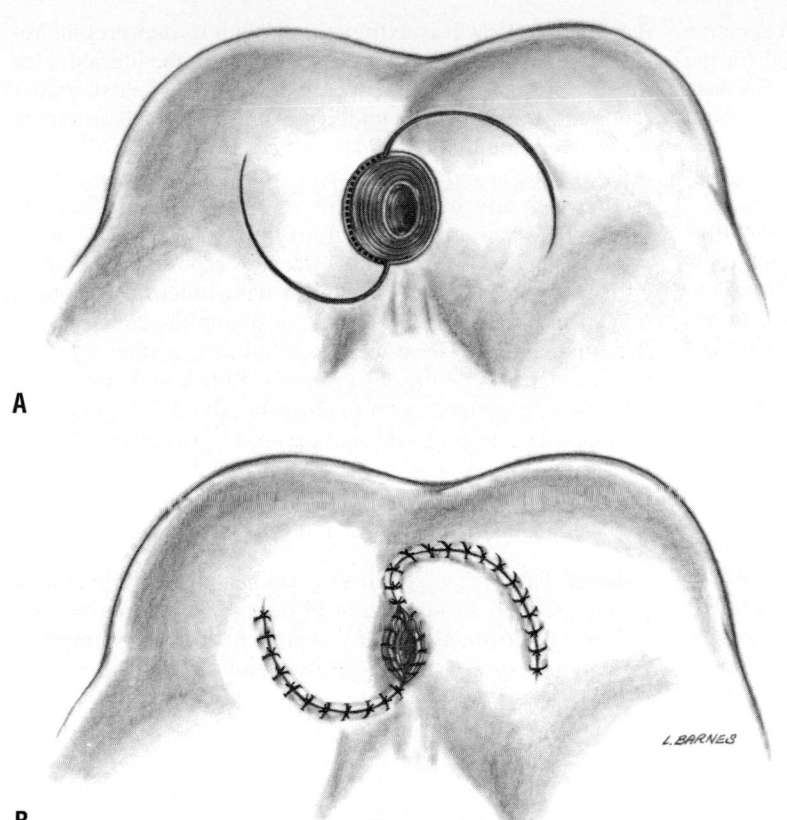

A

B

FIGURE 11-78. Anoplasty is used for severe anal stenosis or for significant loss of anal canal tissue. **A:** The skin flaps are outlined; the eschar has been excised. **B:** The flaps are rotated and sutured to the rectum and underlying internal sphincter. The Hill-Ferguson retractor is not shown.

and the skin is rotated medially and sutured to the rectum and to the underlying internal sphincter with long-term absorbable sutures (Figure 11-78). Because there is a greater tendency for the mucosa to be mobile and to protrude quite readily, it is important to excise any redundant rectal mucosa. After the new mucocutaneous junction has been completed, continuous subcuticular 3–0 long-term absorbable or interrupted simple sutures of similar material are used, and the wounds are closed completely by mobilizing a full-thickness flap of skin cephalad and laterally (Figure 11-79). If there still is too much tension, the easiest alternative is to leave the lateral aspect open to granulate. If there is a very large defect, one may apply a split-thickness skin graft from the thigh, but this is rarely indicated.

POSTOPERATIVE MANAGEMENT The bowel-confining regimen that has been described previously may be carried out for 3 days.

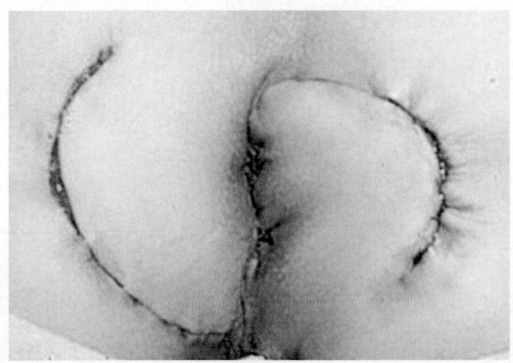

FIGURE 11-79. S-plasty with bilateral rotation flaps is shown immediately after correction of a Whitehead deformity.

Systemic antibiotic coverage is continued during this time. Rarely, a hematoma or an abscess will develop underneath one of the flaps. By insertion of a hemostat between the sutures, evacuation of the collection usually can be achieved without compromising the graft.

An anal stenosis of long duration or Whitehead's deformity usually results in an attenuated sphincter mechanism. With a widely patent anal orifice, discharge of mucus and incontinence for flatus or even for feces may occur during the initial few weeks after operation. It is therefore advisable to start a regimen of perineal strengthening exercises (see Chapter 16) to be performed 10 to 15 times a day. Significant improvement in control may take many weeks, but relatively normal continence should be achievable except in the patient who has an anal stenosis with an atrophied sphincter. These individuals should be carefully selected before an anoplastic operation is considered. If surgery is believed to be advisable, a less than generous opening should be created. The patient needs to be forewarned that incontinence is a possibility.

Lateral Mucosal Advancement Anoplasty. Another approach to the treatment of anal stricture that has been recommended is to advance the rectal mucosa downward, but only to the level of the intersphincteric groove (see Figure 11-54A).[240] As previously discussed, this risks the possibility of creating a mucosal ectropion, but if performed carefully (with limited mucosal mobilization and excision of any mucosal redundancy) there may be value in the selective application of this alternative.

Internal Pudendal Flap Anoplasty. Another option for reconstructing the anal canal is the internal pudendal flap anoplasty.[256] This solitary case report was applied when extensive coverage was required concomitant with excision of Paget's disease of the anus. This flap is based on the terminal branches of the internal pudendal vessels. Because in my opinion one is most likely to require the services of a plastic surgeon, I have not included illustrations for this approach.

Foreskin Anoplasty. An interesting operation has been described by Freeman for the treatment of mucosal ectropion—the foreskin anoplasty.[100] The procedure, which obviously implies that a prepuce be present and suitable, uses the foreskin to provide a full-thickness skin graft to the anal canal. The technique is shown in Figure 11-80. Freeman reported his experience with six children in 1984,[100] but no further publications have been noted since this initial report.

Anoplasty with Sphincteroplasty for Ectopic Anus, Perineal Body Reconstruction, and Management of Rectovaginal Fistulas and Obstetric Injury. In restorative procedures of the anal sphincter mechanism as described in Chapter 16, the skin often must be mobilized concomitantly to effect an adequate repair. The anoplasty described in that chapter is most useful in women with an ectopic anus, rectovaginal fistula, or sphincter injury.

Results of Anoplasty. It is extremely difficult to interpret the results of the various anoplastic maneuvers in the literature for the obvious reason that prospective trials do not exist. Sarner reported 21 patients who underwent one to four advancement flaps for symptomatic anal stenosis.[262] He stated, "Adequate relief was achieved in all cases."[262] Others have noted satisfaction with advancement flaps.[113,179,190,241,249] Ferguson and others have had an equally gratifying experience by using rotation flaps.[95,214] Pearl and colleagues reported 20 patients with benign anal strictures and 5 with mucosal ectropion treated by means of either a U- or diamond-shaped island flap anoplasty.[237] There were two failures, neither attributable to lack of viability of the flaps. Pidala and coworkers reviewed 28 patients who underwent island flap anoplasty for mucosal ectropion and anal stenosis.[233] In those individuals available for follow-up, 91% judged their symptoms to be improved. In reality, every publication reflects contentment and success on the part of all authors.[11,117]

Comment. There are no controlled studies on the comparative advantages and disadvantages of the various anoplastic procedures; however, almost any approach will at least improve the patient's symptoms. Certainly, in my experience of more

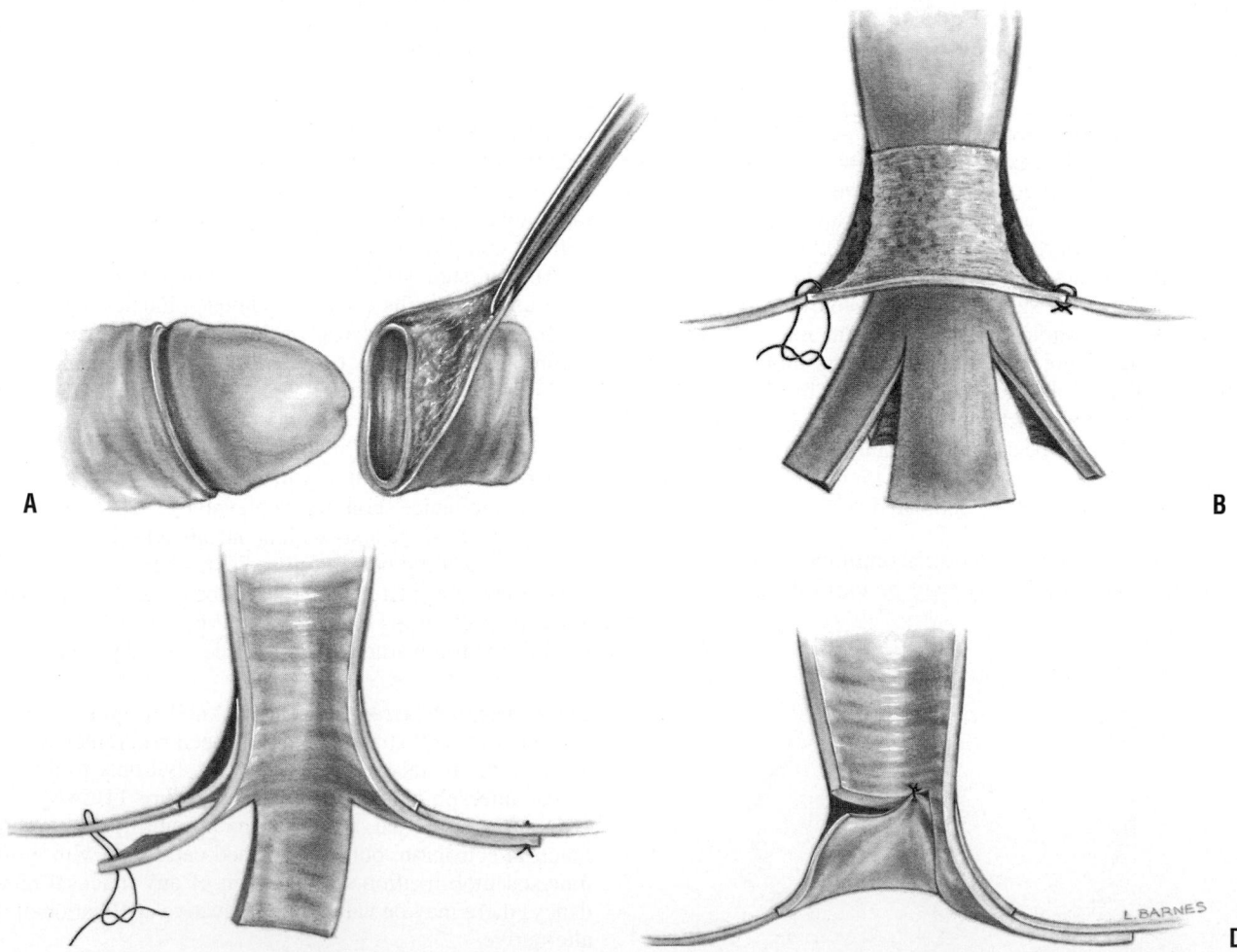

FIGURE 11-80. Foreskin anoplasty. **A:** Circumcision is performed, and the two layers of foreskin are unfolded into a cylinder, with the raw surface exposed externally. **B:** The caudal end of the cylinder is sutured at the anal verge. The rest of the graft lies against the rectum; the latter is split into quadrants. **C:** The split bowel compresses the graft into its new position. **D:** Redundant bowel is freed by removing stay sutures, cutting off the rectum deep within the anal canal, and suturing the proximal end to the foreskin. (Adapted from Freeman NV. The foreskin anoplasty. *Dis Colon Rectum.* 1984;27(5):309–313, with permission.)

than 300 anoplasties, no patient failed to have the condition ameliorated. Interestingly, stenosis following hemorrhoidectomy has become a rare indication for anoplasty. This is either a tribute to improvement in surgical technique or, more likely, to the much reduced application of conventional surgical hemorrhoidectomy (at least in the United States).

The methods described for plastic reconstruction of the anal canal and perianal skin should be employed only in selected individuals. Routine application for the uncomplicated hemorrhoidectomy, fissure operation, or fistula repair is inappropriate. However, with anal stenosis, mucosal ectropion, sphincter injury, rectovaginal fistula, obstetric injury, or tissue loss from any reason, one of these procedures should be extremely effective in ensuring a successful result.

Rectal Stricture

Stricture of the rectum is a rare complication of hemorrhoidectomy and usually is misdiagnosed as an anal stricture. The complication is caused by vigorous high ligation of the hemorrhoid pedicles that may strip the rectal mucosa in several areas or even circumferentially (Figure 11-81). This is most likely to occur if the patient has an element of prolapse or a laxity of the rectal mucosa. As with virtually all complications, prevention is the best approach. Care must be taken to avoid gathering a mass of rectal lining into the ligatures.

Management of this complication may require dilatation, either with Young's dilators (see Figure 11-67) if the stricture is distal, or a Hegar dilator (see Figure 24-89) if the stricture is higher. Operative lysis may be necessary, possibly including either advancement of the rectal mucosa or proctoplasty (see Figure 24-91).

Fissure or Ulcer

An anal fissure may develop in a patient who has a contracted anorectal outlet after hemorrhoidectomy. Usually, the fissure is situated posteriorly. Repeated trauma from defecation results in laceration of the eschar, which may become a chronic, painful anal ulcer. Such postoperative fissures may respond to conservative management (e.g., laxatives, enemas, suppositories, topical creams such as cortisone)

and dilatation. However, often an additional procedure is required, most commonly an internal anal sphincterotomy (see Chapter 12). Excision of the ulcer concomitant with the sphincterotomy may be of benefit, but some form of anoplasty may ultimately be required to increase anal canal circumference.

Pseudopolyps

Hemorrhoidectomy usually requires ligation of the stump of the hemorrhoid. Tissue strangulation will take place at the site of ligation, resulting in sloughing of the stump. This leaves a defect that heals by granulation, the end result of which may be a pseudopolyp. Another possible contributing factor is a foreign body granuloma, which may be a consequence of the prolonged presence of suture material.[106,112] This may be manifested by an edematous, polypoid, or sessile tumor at the site of the suture. Pseudopolyps can be excised with a local anesthetic or be electrocoagulated.

Epidermal Cyst

In rare instances, some months after hemorrhoidectomy, asymptomatic inclusion cysts may appear in the anal canal or in the immediate perianal region. Their origin has been attributed to retention of keratin elements, hair particles, or exfoliated squamous epithelial cells in the wound.[177] If these cysts are bothersome, they can be removed by local excision.

Anal Fistula

Anal fistula is an unusual complication of hemorrhoidectomy, occurring in approximately 1% of patients. It is allegedly more common after the closed operation than the open, but the incidence is so low that this observation is probably more theoretical than factual. The fistula is inevitably low and subcutaneous, not transsphincteric or even intersphincteric unless the finding is coincidental. Fistulotomy is the appropriate treatment and can often be accomplished in the office.

Pruritus Ani

Most causes of pruritus ani are related to diet or are caused by overaggressive attention to anal hygiene (see Chapter 9). However, pruritic symptoms following hemorrhoidectomy are not unusual and may actually have an anatomic basis. A mucosal ectropion or Whitehead's deformity, for example, can produce mucous discharge, which can contribute to the pruritus. With a specific anatomic abnormality, anoplasty may be advisable. The medical management of pruritus ani is discussed in Chapter 9.

Fecal Incontinence

Fecal soilage or incontinence following hemorrhoidectomy, although infrequent, is not as rare as the physician would expect. A possible explanation is the loss of anal canal sensation resulting from removal of sensory-bearing tissue and its replacement by scar. I do not subscribe to such a theory, however.

A high percentage of patients who develop impairment for fecal control following hemorrhoidectomy are elderly. If the physician takes a careful history, it will probably be discovered that many of these individuals have experienced some soilage before the operation, although the procedure may have exacerbated the problem. This is often the case when the patient has some degree of mucosal or rectal prolapse, and it is a particular concern in women. Special care

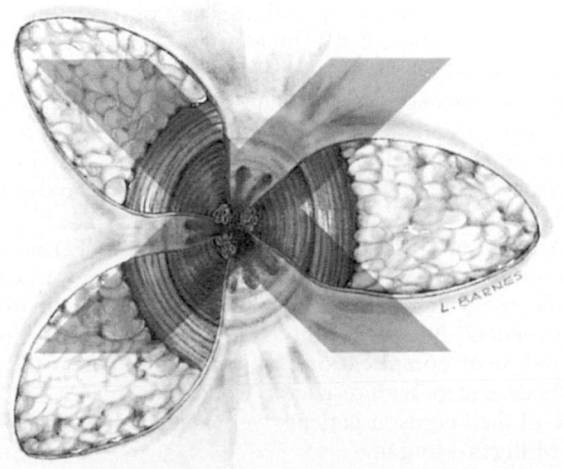

FIGURE 11-81. High ligation of rectal mucosa in an effort to remove mucosal redundancy or prolapse can result in stricture of the rectum.

should be taken when performing this operation in the older age group; it is important to avoid unnecessary sphincter stretch or sphincterotomy. As previously mentioned, many surgeons are fond of sphincterotomy because they believe it ameliorates the postoperative pain problem. When it is performed at the posterior pile site, a keyhole deformity can result. It is a potentially hazardous maneuver in an individual without a concomitant fissure and should be avoided, especially in someone older than 60 years of age.

Recurrence

Most patients who complain of recurrent hemorrhoids usually are describing skin tags or have pruritic symptoms. However, in some cases true hemorrhoidal veins have developed that have become symptomatic after an assumed complete hemorrhoidectomy. "Doctor, I had the operation 10 years ago, and now the hemorrhoids are back," is usually the expressed observation. However, piles that have been removed cannot recur. The "recurrence" consists of veins that, either because of their normal appearance at the time of hemorrhoidectomy or in an effort to preserve adequate mucosal bridges, were left undisturbed. With increased engorgement, collateral circulation, or cushion laxity developing over the years, symptomatic hemorrhoids result.

Because of this potential problem, ideally all hemorrhoidal veins should be removed at the time of the surgical procedure. Tunneling out small vessels from the underlying mucosa and debriding all veins over the external sphincter are important prophylactic maneuvers (see Figure 11-46). When recurrent piles become symptomatic, treatment can usually be accomplished by one of the office procedures, especially rubber ring ligation or office excision.

Retroperitoneal Air

A solitary case of retroperitoneal air following hemorrhoidectomy was reported by Kriss and colleagues.[161] The patient had been receiving steroids for rheumatoid arthritis, so this medication may have played some part in its occurrence. The authors suggest that air was introduced either during the dissection or subsequently, when the patient coughed or strained. A third explanation, not offered by the authors, is the possibility that this complication was unrelated to the operation. The patient responded well to nonoperative management.

Results of Surgical Hemorrhoidectomy

Few contemporary studies evaluate the results of hemorrhoidectomy, and those published reports that attempt to address the issue with long-term follow-up are subject to a number of criticisms. There are very few prospective studies, and retrospective interpretations tend to be rather self-serving. Simply stated, every surgeon who has made the effort to submit the results for publication is satisfied with the procedure. In 1971, Ganchrow and colleagues published the results of a retrospective study of 2,038 consecutive hemorrhoidectomies employing the Ferguson technique, together with 5-year follow-up results.[102] Eighty-two patients (4%) had postoperative complications, 40 patients (2%) had minimal bleeding, 27 patients (1.3%) needed subsequent suture ligation, and two postoperative deaths occurred (0.1%). One patient died at home 10 days after the operation following an uneventful course; postmortem examination was not performed. The other patient died of gram-negative sepsis secondary to a urinary tract infection 37 days after operation.

Between the fifth and seventh postoperative days, 700 patients (34.3%) were discharged from the hospital, 524 (26%) were discharged on the eighth postoperative day, and 770 were discharged after the eighth day. Fortunately or unfortunately, we shall never see reports of postoperative in-hospital recoveries of that duration again.

Questionnaires were returned by 1,018 persons (50%). Of the responses, 970 patients (95%) answered that they had relief of symptoms, 892 patients (88%) answered that they had satisfactory bowel movements since the operation, 732 (72%) had no rectal complaints whatsoever during the 5 years, and 293 (28%) had some complaints, of which pruritus was the most common.

McConnell and Khubchandani evaluated by questionnaire and by examination 441 patients who had undergone closed hemorrhoidectomy up to 7 years previously.[184] One patient required another hemorrhoidectomy. Residual hemorrhoid problems required treatment in 34 individuals (7.7%). Interestingly, of those responding to the questionnaire, 7.3% were dissatisfied with the results, and an additional 4.7% would not recommend the procedure. The authors state that the dissatisfaction was the result of failure to treat the preoperative complaints adequately. The implication, however, is that the indications for surgery may not have been sufficiently restrictive.

Wolfe and colleagues sent a questionnaire to members of the ASCRS in 1979.[313] There was no statistically significant difference among the various techniques employed with respect to pain, complications, and length of hospital stay. However, the open technique was believed to have a slightly more rapid healing time and was associated with a lower incidence of stenosis in this flawed study.

Andrews and coworkers randomly allocated 20 consecutive patients to either diathermy hemorrhoidectomy or scissors dissection using the open technique (Milligan-Morgan).[9] There was no statistically significant difference between the two groups with respect to pain, length of hospitalization, or frequency of bowel movement. Others, in a prospective, pundomized study combining open and closed techniques opine that despite the longer healing time, pain is less when the operation is performed open.[108]

Eu and associates compared emergency and elective hemorrhoidectomy in a total of 704 patients.[89] Five hundred underwent an elective operation. They observed after the elective operation a 5.4% incidence of secondary hemorrhage, a very high incidence. After emergency surgery, secondary hemorrhage developed in 4.9%, also very high. There was also no statistically significant difference with respect to the other variables: incontinence (5.2% vs. 4.4%), anal stenosis (5.9% vs. 3.0%), and recurrent hemorrhoids (7.6% vs. 6.9%).

Arbman and associates compared closed (Ferguson's) hemorrhoidectomy with open (Milligan-Morgan) hemorrhoidectomy in a prospective, randomized trial involving 77 patients.[13] No statistically significant differences in the incidence of complications were found between the two methods, except with respect to wound healing. At 3 weeks, 86% of the Ferguson patients were healed but only 18% of the Milligan-Morgan.

Peng and coworkers randomized 55 patients with grade III and "small" grade IV hemorrhoids to either rubber band ligation or stapled hemorrhoidopexy.[227] Statistically significantly increased pain was noted with an increased analgesia requirement in the latter group. The complication rate was also significantly increased.

Felt-Bersma and colleagues revealed unsuspected sphincteric defects following anorectal surgery by means of anal endosonography.[94] This observation is not unusual after fistula operations, but it is certainly a potential source of concern in the occasional patient following hemorrhoidectomy.

MacRae and McLeod performed a meta-analysis involving a total of 18 trials to assess whether any method of hemorrhoid treatment has been demonstrably superior.[178] The following were their conclusions:

- Hemorrhoidectomy was found to be significantly more effective than manual dilation, with less need for further therapy.
- No significant difference was observed in the incidence of complications.
- Hemorrhoidectomy was found to be associated with significantly more pain.
- Patients undergoing hemorrhoidectomy had a better response to treatment than those treated with rubber band ligation.
- Hemorrhoidectomy was associated with more complications than rubber band ligation.
- Rubber band ligation was better than sclerotherapy in the treatment of all grades of hemorrhoids.

Comment

Although I have not reviewed my experience with Ferguson's hemorrhoidectomy, I have been very pleased with the technical aspects and the results of this operation. I, therefore, have used this technique almost exclusively in all individuals who have been candidates for the surgical removal of hemorrhoids. Usually, the patient's only regret is inappropriate procrastination before permitting operative intervention. With respect to stapled hemorrhoidopexy, I must confess that I initially was extremely skeptical about its value and its efficacy. Now that I have had a moderate experience, I have been converted. This is truly an exciting concept. No, it is not a hemorrhoidectomy, but it may prove to be the preferable way of addressing the physiologic and anatomic problems that result in hemorrhoidal complaints, especially in those individuals whose primary complaint is prolapse. The fact is that it works, patients usually have little discomfort, it is technically relatively straightforward, and it is associated with minimal morbidity. However, the reported (albeit rare) complications may be so devastating (rectovaginal fistula, overwhelming sepsis), that one still must be wary of becoming too much the enthusiast. And equally important, long-term follow-up as well as prospective trials with other methods of hemorrhoidectomy are in progress.

▶ HEMORRHOIDS IN INFLAMMATORY BOWEL DISEASE

Exacerbation of hemorrhoidal complaints is not at all uncommon in patients with inflammatory bowel disease, or for that matter, with any of the infectious or noninfectious colitides. Jeffery and associates reported a retrospective review of 42 patients with ulcerative colitis and 20 with Crohn's disease who were treated for hemorrhoids and inflammatory bowel disease between 1935 and 1975.[140] Both surgical and conservative treatment of hemorrhoids in those with ulcerative colitis had low complication rates (i.e., four complications after 50 courses of treatment). In Crohn's disease, the complication rate was high, 11 complications after 26 courses of treatment. One of the 42 patients with ulcerative colitis and 6 of the 20 with Crohn's disease required rectal excision for complications apparently dating from the treatment of hemorrhoids. Wolkomir and Luchtefeld performed surgical hemorrhoidectomy on 17 patients with known Crohn's disease.[315] All but two healed without complication. Although no individual had acutely active disease, four had inflammatory changes in the rectum.

Comment

Despite the foregoing observation, in my opinion any procedure performed on the anus or perianal skin in patients with inflammatory bowel disease should be limited to the minimal maneuvers that will effectively treat the patient's complaint. Definitive or extensive surgical treatment of any anorectal problem in such individuals could result in delayed healing or nonhealing, with greater disability to the patient than before the operation (see Chapters 14 and 30; see Figure 14-52). Occasionally, when disease is quiescent and sepsis, fistula formation, and scarring are not present, bleeding or protrusion of hemorrhoids may reasonably be treated by rubber ring ligation.

▶ HEMORRHOIDECTOMY IN THE HIV-POSITIVE PATIENT

One of the most remarkable characteristics of the anus and rectum is the extraordinary resistance to infection in that area. This feature permits a successful outcome following a plethora of surgical procedures.[254] Safavi and colleagues presented a series of 75 consecutive surgical procedures on 40 HIV-positive individuals and 22 patients with AIDS.[254] Only those with the hemorrhoid manifestation of thrombosis were surgically treated, however. This represented 4 patients, 3 of whom healed; 1 obtained no relief.

Although not clearly documented by statistics in the literature, definitive surgical hemorrhoidectomy in HIV-positive patients is probably contraindicated (see also Chapter 10).

▶ HEMORRHOIDECTOMY DURING PREGNANCY

As mentioned earlier in this chapter, women are often troubled by hemorrhoidal complaints during the latter part of pregnancy. Most such problems can be treated adequately by bowel management (e.g., laxatives, stool softeners) and by sitz baths. A thrombosed hemorrhoid can be excised in the usual way. There is no clear-cut answer to the question of what should be done when a woman has a sufficiently profound complication that surgical hemorrhoidectomy appears to be the best recourse.

Saleeby and colleagues performed operative hemorrhoidectomies on 25 of 12,455 pregnant women (0.2%) who delivered in their institution.[257] All but three were in their third trimester. The operations were of the closed type and were accomplished with a local anesthetic. Other than one instance of postoperative hemorrhage, there were no other maternal or fetal complications.

References

1. Ackland TH. The treatment of prolapsed gangrenous haemorrhoids. *Aust N Z J Surg.* 1961;30(3):201–203.

2. Adami B, Eckardt VF, Suermann RB, et al. Bacteremia after proctoscopy and hemorrhoidal injection sclerotherapy. *Dis Colon Rectum.* 1981;24(5):373–374.

3. Ala S, Saeedi M, Eshghi F, et al. Topical metronidazole can reduce pain after surgery and pain on defecation in postoperative hemorrhoidectomy. *Dis Colon Rectum.* 2008;51(2):235–238.

4. Alexander-Williams J, Crapp AR. Conservative management of haemorrhoids. Part I: injection, freezing and ligation. *Clin Gastroenterol.* 1975;4(3):595–618.

5. Altomare DF, Milito G, Andreoli R, et al. Ligasure Precise vs. conventional diathermy for Milligan-Morgan hemorrhoidectomy: a prospective, randomized, multicenter trial. *Dis Colon Rectum.* 2008;51(5):514–519.

6. Ambrose NS, Hares MM, Alexander-Williams J, et al. Prospective randomised comparison of photocoagulation and rubber band ligation in treatment of haemorrhoids. *Br Med J.* 1983;286(6375):1389–1391.

7. Ambrose NS, Morris D, Alexander-Williams J, et al. A randomized trial of photocoagulation or injection sclerotherapy for the treatment of first- and second-degree hemorrhoids. *Dis Colon Rectum.* 1985;28(4):238–240.

8. Anderson HG. The "injection" method for the treatment of haemorrhoids. *Practitioner.* 1924;113:399–409.

9. Andrews BT, Layer GT, Jackson BT, et al. Randomized trial comparing diathermy hemorrhoidectomy with the scissor dissection Milligan-Morgan operation. *Dis Colon Rectum.* 1993;36(6):580–583.

10. Andrews E. The treatment of hemorrhoids by injection. *Med Rec.* 1879;15:451.

11. Angelchik PD, Harms BA, Starling JR. Repair of anal stricture and mucosal ectropion with Y-V or pedicle flap anoplasty. *Am J Surg.* 1993;166(1):55–59.

12. Arabi Y, Alexander-Williams J, Keighley MR. Anal pressures in hemorrhoids and anal fissure. *Am J Surg.* 1977;134(5):608–610.

13. Arbman G, Krook H, Haapaniemi S. Closed vs. open hemorrhoidectomy—is there any difference? *Dis Colon Rectum.* 2000;43(1):31–34.

14. Armstrong DN. Multiple hemorrhoidal ligation: a prospective, randomized trial evaluating a new technique. *Dis Colon Rectum.* 2003;46(2):179–186.

15. Armstrong DN, Frankum C, Schertzer ME, et al. Harmonic scalpel hemorrhoidectomy: five hundred consecutive cases. *Dis Colon Rectum.* 2002;45(3):354–359.

16. Arroyo A, Pérez-Legaz J, Miranda E, et al. Long-term clinical results of double-pursestring stapled hemorrhoidopexy in a selected group of patients for the treatment of chronic hemorrhoids. *Dis Colon Rectum.* 2011;54(5):609–614.

17. Asfar SK, Juma TH, Ala-Edeen T. Hemorrhoidectomy and sphincterotomy: a prospective study comparing the effectiveness of anal stretch and sphincterotomy in reducing pain after hemorrhoidectomy. *Dis Colon Rectum.* 1988;31(3):181–185.

18. Avsar AF, Keskin HL. Haemorrhoids during pregnancy. *J Obstet Gynaecol.* 2010;30(3):231–237.

19. Bacon HE. *Anus, Rectum and Sigmoid Colon.* 3rd ed. Vol 1. Philadelphia, PA: JB Lippincott; 1949:453.

20. Bailey HR, Ferguson JA. Prevention of urinary retention by fluid restriction following anorectal operations. *Dis Colon Rectum.* 1976;19(3):250–252.

21. Balfour L, Stojkovic SG, Botterill ID, et al. A randomized, double-blind trial of the effect of metronidazole on pain after closed hemorrhoidectomy. *Dis Colon Rectum.* 2002;45(9):1186–1190.

22. Banov L Jr. Suppositories: are they effective? *J S C Med Assoc.* 1985;81(7):407.

23. Barrios G, Khubchandani M. Whitehead operation revisited. *Dis Colon Rectum.* 1979;22(5):330–332.

24. Barron J. Office ligation of internal hemorrhoids. *Am J Surg.* 1963;105:563–570.

25. Barron J. Office ligation treatment of hemorrhoids. *Dis Colon Rectum.* 1963;6:109–113.

26. Bartizal J, Slosberg PA. An alternative to hemorrhoidectomy. *Arch Surg.* 1977;112(4):534–536.

27. Basso L, Pescatori M. Outcome of delayed hemorrhage following surgical hemorrhoidectomy [letter]. *Dis Colon Rectum.* 1994;37(3):288–289.

28. Bat L, Melzer E, Koler M, et al. Complications of rubber band ligation of symptomatic internal hemorrhoids. *Dis Colon Rectum.* 1993;36(3):287–290.

29. Beattie GC, Loudon MA. Follow-up confirms sustained benefit of circumferential stapled anoplasty in the management of prolapsing haemorrhoids. *Br J Surg.* 2001;88(6):850–852.

30. Becker de Moura H, Ribeiro-Silva A. Death resulting from fournier gangrene secondary to thrombosis of very large hemorrhoids: report of a case. *Dis Colon Rectum.* 2007;50(10):1715–1718.

31. Bentley JFR. Developmental anomalies and other diseases in children. In: Morson BC, ed. *Diseases of the Colon, Rectum and Anus.* New York, NY: Appleton-Century-Crofts; 1969:64.

32. Bernard A, Parnaud E, Guntz M, et al. Radioanatomie normale du réseau vasculaire hémorrhoidal. (Note préalable à propos d'une étude portant sur 15 cas). *Ann Radiol (Paris).* 1977;20(5):483–489.

33. Bernstein KZ, Klausner MA. Potential dangers related to transdermal fentanyl (Duragesic) when used for postoperative pain [letter]. *Dis Colon Rectum.* 1994;37(12):1339–1340.

34. Bernstein WC. What are hemorrhoids and what is their relationship to the portal venous system [editorial]? *Dis Colon Rectum.* 1983;26(12):829–834.

35. Bessa SS. Ligasure™ vs. conventional diathermy in excisional hemorrhoidectomy: a prospective, randomized study. *Dis Colon Rectum.* 2008;51(6):940–944.

36. Blaisdell PC. Prevention of massive hemorrhage secondary to hemorrhoidectomy. *Surg Gynecol Obstet.* 1958;106(4):485–488.

37. Bleday R, Pena JP, Rothenberger DA, et al. Symptomatic hemorrhoids: current incidence and complications of operative therapy. *Dis Colon Rectum.* 1992;35(5):477–481.

38. Bona S, Battafarano F, Fumagalli Romario U, et al. Stapled anopexy: postoperative course and functional outcome in 400 patients. *Dis Colon Rectum.* 2008;51(6):950–955.

39. Bonello JC. Who's afraid of the dentate line? The Whitehead hemorrhoidectomy. *Am J Surg.* 1988;156(3 pt 1):182–186.

40. Bonhomme L, Benhamou D, Martre H, et al. Chemical stability of bupivacaine and epinephrine in pH-adjusted solutions [abstract]. *Anesthesiology.* 1987;37:279.

41. Bowers FJ, Hartmann R, Khanduja KS, et al. Urecholine prophylaxis for urinary retention in anorectal surgery. *Dis Colon Rectum.* 1987;30(1):41–42.

42. Buie LA. *Practical Proctology.* Philadelphia, PA: WB Saunders; 1937.

43. Burkitt DP, Graham-Stewart CW. Haemorrhoids—postulated pathogenesis and proposed prevention. *Postgrad Med J.* 1975;51(599):631–636.

44. Bursics A, Morvay K, Kupcsulik P, et al. Comparison of early and 1-year follow-up results of conventional hemorrhoidectomy and hemorrhoid artery ligation: a randomized study. *Int J Colorectal Dis.* 2004;19(2):176–180.

45. Caplin DA, Kodner IJ. Repair of anal stricture and mucosal ectropion by simple flap procedures. *Dis Colon Rectum.* 1986;29(2):92–94.

46. Cataldo PA, Ellis CN, Gregorcyk S, et al. Standards Practice Task Force of the American Society of Colon and Rectal Surgeons. Practice parameters for the management of hemorrhoids (revised). *Dis Colon Rectum.* 2005;48(2):189–194.

47. Cataldo PA, MacKeigan JM. The necessity of routine pathologic evaluation of hemorrhoidectomy specimens. *Surg Gynecol Obstet.* 1992;174(4):302–304.

48. Cataldo PA, Senagore AJ. Does alpha sympathetic blockade prevent urinary retention following anorectal surgery? *Dis Colon Rectum.* 1991;34(12):1113–1116.

49. Ceci F, Picchio M, Palimento D, et al. Long-term outcome of stapled hemorrhoidopexy for Grade III and Grade IV hemorrhoids. *Dis Colon Rectum.* 2008;51(7):1107–1112.

50. Chaudhary ND, Rivadeneira DE, Ranire-Maguire M, et al. Topical sucralfate post-hemorrhoidectomy: an affordable and feasible treatment option. *Dis Colon Rectum.* 2008;51(12):1857.

51. Cheetham MJ, Cohen CR, Kamm MA, et al. A randomized, controlled trial of diathermy hemorrhoidectomy vs. stapled hemorrhoidectomy in an intended day-care setting with longer-term follow-up. *Dis Colon Rectum.* 2003;46(4):491–497.

52. Cheetham MJ, Mortensen NJ, Nystrom PO, et al. Persistent pain and faecal urgency after stapled haemorrhoidectomy. *Lancet.* 2000;356(9231):730–733.

53. Chew SS, Marshall L, Kalish L, et al. Short-term and long-term results of combined sclerotherapy and rubber band ligation of hemorrhoids and mucosal prolapse. *Dis Colon Rectum.* 2003;46(9):1232–1237.

54. Chia YW, Darzi A, Speakman CT, et al. CO$_2$ laser haemorrhoidectomy: does it alter anorectal function or decrease pain compared to conventional haemorrhoidectomy? *Int J Colorectal Dis.* 1995;10(1):22–24.

55. Chiu JH, Chen WS, Chen CH, et al. Effect of transcutaneous electrical nerve stimulation for pain relief on patients undergoing hemorrhoidectomy: prospective, randomized, controlled trial. *Dis Colon Rectum.* 1999;42(2):180–185.

56. Christensen MA, Pitsch RM Jr, Cali RL, et al. "House" advancement pedicle flap for anal stenosis. *Dis Colon Rectum.* 1992;35(2):201–203.

57. Chung CC, Ha JP, Tai YP, et al. Double-blind, randomized trial comparing Harmonic scalpel hemorrhoidectomy, bipolar scissors hemorrhoidectomy, and scissors excision: ligation technique. *Dis Colon Rectum.* 2002;45(6):789–794.

58. Chung YC, Wu HJ. Clinical experience of sutureless closed hemorrhoidectomy with LigaSure. *Dis Colon Rectum.* 2003;46(1):87–92.

59. Church J, Simmang C; Standards Task Force, American Society of Colon and Rectal Surgeons. Practice parameters for the treatment of patients with dominantly inherited colorectal cancer (familial adenomatous polyposis and hereditary nonpolyposis colorectal cancer). *Dis Colon Rectum.* 2003;46(8):1001–1012.

60. Cihan A, Mentes BB, Sucak G, et al. Fournier's gangrene after hemorrhoidectomy: association with drug-induced agranulocytosis: report of a case. *Dis Colon Rectum.* 1999;42(12):1644–1648.

61. Cipriani S, Pescatori M. Acute rectal obstruction after PPH stapled hemorrhoidectomy. *Colorectal Dis.* 2002;4(5):367–370.

62. Clay LD III, White JJ Jr, Davidson JT, et al. Early recognition and successful management of pelvic cellulitis following hemorrhoidal banding. *Dis Colon Rectum.* 1986;29(9):579–581.

63. Conaghan P, Farouk R. Doppler-guided hemorrhoid artery ligation reduces the need for conventional hemorrhoid surgery in patients who fail rubber band ligation treatment. *Dis Colon Rectum.* 2009;52(1):127–130.

64. Cooper IS, Lee AS. Cryostatic congelation: a system for producing a limited, controlled region of cooling or freezing of biologic tissues. *J Nerv Ment Dis.* 1961;133:259–263.

65. Corman ML. Management of postoperative constipation in anorectal surgery. *Dis Colon Rectum.* 1979;22(3):149–151.

66. Corman ML. Anoplasty. In: Maingot R, ed. *Abdominal Operations.* 7th ed. New York, NY: Appleton-Century-Crofts; 1980:2367.

67. Corman ML. pH of local anesthetic solutions. *Dis Colon Rectum.* 1990;33(2):166–167.

68. Corman ML, Gravié JF, Hager T, et al. Stapled haemorrhoidopexy: a consensus position paper by an international working party—indications, contra-indications and technique. *Colorectal Dis.* 2003;5(4):304–310.

69. Corman ML, Veidenheimer MC. The new hemorrhoidectomy. *Surg Clin North Am.* 1973;53(2):417–422.

70. Corman ML, Veidenheimer MC, Coller JA. Anoplasty for anal stricture. *Surg Clin North Am.* 1976;56(3):727–731.

71. Correa-Rovelo JM, Tellez O, Obregón L, et al. Stapled rectal mucosectomy vs. closed hemorrhoidectomy: a randomized, clinical trial. *Dis Colon Rectum.* 2002;45(10):1367–1374.

72. Coskun A, Duzgun SA, Uzunkoy A, et al. Nitroderm TTS band application for pain after hemorrhoidectomy. *Dis Colon Rectum.* 2001;44(5):680–685.

73. Creve U, Hubens A. The effect of Lord's procedure on anal pressure. *Dis Colon Rectum.* 1979;22(7):483–485.

74. Crystal RF, Hopping RA. Early postoperative complications of anorectal surgery. *Dis Colon Rectum.* 1974;17(3):336–341.

75. Dal Monte PP, Tagariello C, Sarago P, et al. Transanal haemorrhoidal dearterialisation: nonexcisional surgery for the treatment of haemorrhoidal disease. *Tech Coloproctol.* 2007;11(4):333–338.

76. Davies J, Duffy D, Boyt N, et al. Botulinum toxin (botox) reduces pain after hemorrhoidectomy: results of a double-blind, randomized study. *Dis Colon Rectum.* 2003;46(8):1097–1102.

77. Davy A, Duval C. Modifications macroscopiques et microscopiques du réseau vasculaire hémorrhoidal dans la maladie hémorrhoidaire. *Arch Fr Mal App Dig.* 1976;65(7):515–521.

78. Dencker H, Hjorth N, Norryd C, et al. Comparison of results obtained with different methods of treatment of internal haemorrhoids. *Acta Chir Scand.* 1973;139(8):742–745.

79. Denis J. Étude numérique de quelques facteurs étiopathogéniques des troubles hémorrhoidaires de l'adulte. *Arch Fr Mal App Dig.* 1976;65(7):529–536.

80. Dennison AR, Wherry DC, Morris DL. Hemorrhoids: nonoperative management. *Surg Clin North Am.* 1988;68(6):1401–1409.

81. Dennison AR, Whiston RJ, Rooney S, et al. The management of hemorrhoids. *Am J Gastroenterol.* 1989;84(5):475–481.

82. Dennison AR, Whiston RJ, Rooney S, et al. A randomized comparison of infrared photocoagulation with bipolar diathermy for the outpatient treatment of hemorrhoids. *Dis Colon Rectum.* 1990;33(1):32–34.

83. Diana G, Guercio G, Cudia B, et al. Internal sphincterotomy reduces postoperative pain after Milligan Morgan haemorrhoidectomy. *BMC Surg.* 2009;9:16.

84. Dodi G, Bogoni F, Infantino A, et al. Hot or cold in anal pain? A study of the changes in internal anal sphincter pressure profiles. *Dis Colon Rectum.* 1986;29(4):248–251.

85. Dowden JE, Stanley JD, Moore RA. Obstructed defecation after stapled hemorrhoidopexy: a report of four cases. *Am Surg.* 2010;76(6):622–625.

86. Edwards FS. The treatment of piles by injection. *Br Med J.* 1888;2(1450):815–816.

87. Eisenstat T, Salvati EP, Rubin RJ. The outpatient management of acute hemorrhoidal disease. *Dis Colon Rectum.* 1979;22(5):315–317.

88. El-Gendi MA, Abdel-Baky N. Anorectal pressure in patients with symptomatic hemorrhoids. *Dis Colon Rectum.* 1986;29(6):388–391.

89. Eu KW, Seow-Choen F, Goh HS. Comparison of emergency and elective haemorrhoidectomy. *Br J Surg.* 1994;81(2):308–310.

90. Fansler WA, Anderson JK. A plastic operation for certain types of hemorrhoids. *JAMA.* 1933;101(14):1064–1066.

91. Fantin AC, Zala G, Risti B, et al. Bleeding anorectal varices: successful treatment with transjugular intrahepatic portosystemic shunting (TIPS). *Gut.* 1996;38(6):932–935.

92. Faucheron JL, Poncet G, Voirin D, et al. Doppler-guided hemorrhoidal artery ligation and rectoanal repair (HAL-RAR) for the treatment of grade IV hemorrhoids: long-term results in 100 consecutive patients. *Dis Colon Rectum.* 2011;54(2):226–231.

93. Fazio VW. Early promise of stapling technique for haemorrhoidectomy. *Lancet.* 2000;355(9206):768–769.

94. Felt-Bersma RJF, van Baren R, Koorevaar M, et al. Unsuspected sphincter defects shown by anal endosonography after anorectal surgery: a prospective study. *Dis Colon Rectum.* 1995;38(3):249–253.

95. Ferguson JA. Repair of Whitehead deformity of the anus. *Surg Gynecol Obstet.* 1959;108(1):115–116.

96. Ferguson JA, Heaton JR. Closed hemorrhoidectomy. *Dis Colon Rectum.* 1959;2(2):176–179.

97. Fleischer M, Marini CP, Statman R, et al. Local anesthesia is superior to spinal anesthesia for anorectal surgical procedures. *Am Surg.* 1994;60(11):812–815.

98. Forrest NP, Mullerat J, Evans C, et al. Doppler-guided haemorrhoidal artery ligation with recto anal repair: a new technique for the treatment of symptomatic haemorrhoids. *Int J Colorectal Dis.* 2010;25(10):1251–1256.

99. Franklin EJ, Seetharam S, Lowney J, et al. Randomized, clinical trial of Ligasure vs conventional diathermy in hemorrhoidectomy. *Dis Colon Rectum.* 2003;46(10):1380–1383.

100. Freeman NV. The foreskin anoplasty. *Dis Colon Rectum.* 1984;27(5):309–313.

101. Gabriel WB. *The Principles and Practice of Rectal Surgery.* 4th ed. London, United Kingdom: HK Lewis; 1948.

102. Ganchrow MI, Mazier WP, Friend WG, et al. Hemorrhoidectomy revisited: a computer analysis of 2,038 cases. *Dis Colon Rectum.* 1971;14(2):128–133.

103. Ganio E, Altomare DF, Gabrielli F, et al. Prospective randomized multicentre trial comparing stapled with open haemorrhoidectomy. *Br J Surg.* 2001;88(5):669–674.

104. Gao XH, Wang HT, Chen JG, et al. Rectal perforation after procedure for prolapse and hemorrhoids: possible causes. *Dis Colon Rectum.* 2010;53(10):1439–1445.

105. Gartell PC, Sheridan RJ, McGinn FP. Out-patient treatment of haemorrhoids: a randomized clinical trial to compare rubber band ligation with phenol injection. *Br J Surg.* 1985;72(6):478–479.

106. Gaskin ER, Childers MD Jr. Increased granuloma formation from absorbable sutures. *JAMA.* 1963;185:212–214.

107. Gehamy RA, Weakley FL. Internal hemorrhoidectomy by elastic ligation. *Dis Colon Rectum.* 1974;17(3):347–353.

108. Gençosamoğlu R, Sad O, Koç D, et al. Hemorrhoidectomy: open or closed technique? A prospective, randomized clinical trial. *Dis Colon Rectum.* 2002;45(1):70–75.

109. Giamundo P, Salfi R, Geraci M, et al. The hemorrhoid laser procedure technique vs rubber band ligation: a randomized trial comparing 2 mini-invasive treatments for second- and third-degree hemorrhoids. *Dis Colon Rectum.* 2011;54(6):693–698.

110. Gibbons CP, Bannister JJ, Read NW. Role of constipation and anal hypertonia in the pathogenesis of haemorrhoids. *Br J Surg.* 1988;75(7):656–660.

111. Gill W, Fraser J, Da Costa J, et al. The cryosurgical lesion. *Am Surg.* 1970;36(7):437–445.

112. Gillman T, Penn J, Bronks D, et al. Reactions of healing wounds and granulation tissue in man to auto-Thiersch, autodermal, and homodermal grafts: with an analysis of the implications of the phenomena encountered for an understanding of the behaviour of grafted tissue and the genesis of scars, keloids, skin carcinomata, and other cutaneous lesions. *Br J Plast Surg.* 1953;6(3):153–223.

113. Gingold BS, Arvanitis M. Y-V anoplasty for treatment of anal stricture. *Surg Gynecol Obstet.* 1986;162(3):241–242.

114. Giordano P, Overton J, Madeddu F, et al. Transanal hemorrhoidal dearterialization: a systematic review. *Dis Colon Rectum.* 2009;52(9): 1665–1671.

115. Goenka M, Kochhar R, Nagi B, et al. Rectosigmoid varices and other mucosal changes in patients with portal hypertension. *Am J Gastroenterol.* 1991;86(9):1185–1189.

116. Goldstein ET, Williamson PR, Larach SW. Subcutaneous morphine pump for postoperative hemorrhoidectomy pain management. *Dis Colon Rectum.* 1993;36(5):439–446.

117. González AR, de Oliveira O Jr, Verzaro R, et al. Anoplasty for stenosis and other anorectal defects. *Am Surg.* 1995;61(6):526–529.

118. Gottesman L, Milsom JW, Mazier WP. The use of anxiolytic and parasympathomimetic agents in the treatment of postoperative urinary retention following anorectal surgery: a prospective, randomized, double-blind study. *Dis Colon Rectum.* 1989;32(10):867–870.

119. Granet E. Hemorrhoidectomy failures: causes, prevention and management. *Dis Colon Rectum.* 1968;11(1):45–48.

120. Greca F, Hares M, Keighley MRB. Anal dilatation [letter]. *Br J Surg.* 1981;68(2):141.

121. Griffith CDM, Morris DL, Wherry DC, et al. Outpatient treatment of haemorrhoids: a randomised trial comparing contact bipolar diathermy with rubber ring ligation. *Coloproctology.* 1987;9:332–334.

122. Gupta PJ, Heda PS, Kalaskar S, et al. Topical sucralfate decreases pain after hemorrhoidectomy and improves healing: a randomized, blinded, controlled study. *Dis Colon Rectum.* 2008;51(2):231–234.

123. Guy RJ, Seow-Choen F. Septic complications after treatment of haemorrhoids. *Br J Surg.* 2003;90(2):147–156.

124. Haas PA, Fox TA Jr, Haas GP. The pathogenesis of hemorrhoids. *Dis Colon Rectum.* 1984;27(7):442–450.

125. Hancock BD. Internal sphincter and the nature of haemorrhoids. *Gut.* 1977;18(8):651–655.

126. Hansen HH. Neue Aspekte zur Pathogeneses und Therapie des Hämorrhoidalleidens. *Dtsch Med Wochenschr.* 1977;102(35):1244–1248.

127. Hansen HH. Pathomorphologie und Therapie des Hämorrhoidalleidens. *Hautarzt.* 1977;28(7):364–367.

128. Heald RJ, Gudgeon AM. Limited haemorrhoidectomy in the treatment of acute strangulated haemorrhoids. *Br J Surg.* 1986;73(12):1002.

129. Hiltunen KM, Matikainen M. Anal manometric findings in symptomatic hemorrhoids. *Dis Colon Rectum.* 1985;28(11):807–809.

130. Hinton CP, Morris DL. A randomized trial comparing direct current therapy and bipolar diathermy in the outpatient treatment of third-degree hemorrhoids. *Dis Colon Rectum.* 1990;33(11):931–932.

131. Ho YH, Cheong WK, Tsang C, et al. Stapled hemorrhoidectomy—cost and effectiveness. Randomized, controlled trial including incontinence scoring, anorectal manometry, and endoanal ultrasound assessments at up to three months. *Dis Colon Rectum.* 2000;43(12):1666–1675.

132. Hodgson WJ, Morgan J. Ambulatory hemorrhoidectomy with CO_2 laser. *Dis Colon Rectum.* 1995;38(12):1265–1269.

133. Hoff SD, Bailey HR, Butts DR, et al. Ambulatory surgical hemorrhoidectomy—a solution to postoperative urinary retention? *Dis Colon Rectum.* 1994;37(12):1242–1244.

134. Hosking SW, Smart HL, Johnson AG, et al. Anorectal varices, haemorrhoids, and portal hypertension. *Lancet.* 1989;1(8634):349–352.

135. Hsieh JS, Huang CJ, Huang YS, et al. Demonstration of rectal varices by transhepatic inferior mesenteric venography. *Dis Colon Rectum.* 1986;29(7):459–461.

136. Hudson AT. S-plasty repair of Whitehead deformity of the anus. *Dis Colon Rectum.* 1967;10(1):57–60.

137. Imbelloni LE, Vieira EM, Gouveia MA, et al. Pudendal block with bupivacaine for postoperative pain relief. *Dis Colon Rectum.* 2007;50(10):1656–1661.

138. Iwagaki H, Higuchi Y, Fuchimoto S, et al. The laser treatment of hemorrhoids: results of a study on 1816 patients. *Jpn J Surg.* 1989;19(6):658–661.

139. Jayne DG, Botterill I, Ambrose NS, et al. Randomized clinical trial of Ligasure versus conventional diathermy for day-case haemorrhoidectomy. *Br J Surg.* 2002;89(4):428–432.

140. Jeffery PJ, Ritchie JK, Parks AG. Treatment of haemorrhoids in patients with inflammatory bowel disease. *Lancet.* 1977;1(8021):1084–1085.

141. Jetmore AB, Heryer JW, Conner WE. Monsel's solution: a kinder, gentler hemostatic. *Dis Colon Rectum.* 1993;36(9):866–867.

142. Johanson JF, Sonnenberg A. The prevalence of hemorrhoids and chronic constipation. An epidemiologic study. *Gastroenterology.* 1990;98(2):380–386.

143. Johnson CD, Budd J, Ward AJ. Laxatives after hemorrhoidectomy. *Dis Colon Rectum.* 1987;30(10):780–781.

144. Jones CB. A comparative study of the methods of treatment for haemorrhoids. *Proc R Soc Med.* 1974;67(1):51–53.

145. Jongen J, Bach S, Stübinger SH, et al. Excision of thrombosed external hemorrhoid under local anesthesia: a retrospective evaluation of 340 patients. *Dis Colon Rectum.* 2003;46(9):1226–1231.

146. Kairaluoma M, Nuorva K, Kellokumpu I. Day-case stapled (circular) vs. diathermy hemorrhoidectomy: a randomized, controlled trial evaluating surgical and functional outcome. *Dis Colon Rectum.* 2003;46(1):93–99.

147. Katchian A. Hemorrhoids. Measuring the constrictive force of rubber bands. *Dis Colon Rectum.* 1984;27(7):471–474.

148. Katchian A. Rubber band ligation [letter]. *Dis Colon Rectum.* 1985;28(10):759.

149. Keighley MRB, Buchmann P, Minervini S, et al. Prospective trials of minor surgical procedures and high-fibre diet for haemorrhoids. *Br Med J.* 1979;2(6196):967–969.

150. Kelsey CB. How to treat haemorrhoids by injections of carbolic acid. *N Y Med J.* 1885;42:546.

151. Khalil KH, O'Bichere A, Sellu D. Randomized clinical trial of sutured versus stapled closed haemorrhoidectomy. *Br J Surg.* 2000;87(10): 1352–1355.

152. Khoury GA, Lake SP, Lewis MC, et al. A randomized trial to compare single with multiple phenol injection treatment for haemorrhoids. *Br J Surg.* 1985;72(9):741–742.

153. Khubchandani IT. A randomized comparison of single and multiple rubber band ligations. *Dis Colon Rectum.* 1983;26(11):705–708.

154. Khubchandani IT. Mucosal advancement anoplasty. *Dis Colon Rectum.* 1985;28(3):194–196.

155. Khubchandani IT. Internal sphincterotomy with hemorrhoidectomy does not relieve pain: a prospective, randomized study. *Dis Colon Rectum.* 2002;45(11):1452–1457.

156. Khubchandani M. Results of Whitehead operation. *Dis Colon Rectum.* 1984;27(11):730–732.

157. Kilbride M, Morse M, Senagore A. Transdermal fentanyl improves management of postoperative hemorrhoidectomy pain. *Dis Colon Rectum.* 1994;37(11):1070–1072.

158. Kluiber RM, Wolff BG. Evaluation of anemia caused by hemorrhoidal bleeding. *Dis Colon Rectum.* 1994;37(10):1006–1007.

159. Konsten J, Baeten CG. Hemorrhoidectomy vs. Lord's method: 17-year follow-up of a prospective, randomized trial. *Dis Colon Rectum.* 2000;43(4):503–506.

160. Kratzer GL. Improved local anesthesia in anorectal surgery. *Dis Colon Rectum.* 1974;40(10):609–612.

161. Kriss BD, Porter JA, Slezak FA. Retroperitoneal air after routine hemorrhoidectomy: report of a case. *Dis Colon Rectum.* 1990;33(11): 971–973.

162. Kuo RJ. Epidural morphine for post-hemorrhoidectomy analgesia. *Dis Colon Rectum.* 1984;27(8):529–530.

163. Lal D, Levitan R. Bacteremia following proctoscopic biopsy of a rectal polyp. *Arch Intern Med.* 1972;130(1):127–128.

164. Lau WY, Chow HP, Poon GP, et al. Rubber band ligation of three primary hemorrhoids in a single session. A safe and effective procedure. *Dis Colon Rectum.* 1982;25(4):336–339.

165. Lee HH, Spencer RJ, Beart RW Jr. Multiple hemorrhoidal bandings in a single session. *Dis Colon Rectum.* 1994;37(1):37–41.

166. Leff EI. Hemorrhoidectomy—laser versus nonlaser: outpatient surgical experience. *Dis Colon Rectum.* 1992;35(8):743–746.

167. LeFrock JL, Ellis CA, Turchik JB, et al. Transient bacteremia associated with sigmoidoscopy. *N Engl J Med.* 1973;289(9):467–469.

168. Leicester RJ, Nicholls RJ, Mann CV. Comparison of infrared coagulation with conventional methods and the treatment of hemorrhoids. *Coloproctology.* 1981;5:313–315.

169. Leicester RJ, Nicholls RJ, Mann CV. Infrared coagulation: a new treatment for hemorrhoids. *Dis Colon Rectum.* 1981;24(8):602–605.

170. Lewis AA, Rogers HS, Leighton M. Trial of maximal anal dilatation, cryotherapy and elastic band ligation as alternatives to haemorrhoidectomy in the treatment of large prolapsing haemorrhoids. *Br J Surg.* 1983;70(1):54–56.

171. Lewis MI. Cryosurgical hemorrhoidectomy: a follow-up report. *Dis Colon Rectum.* 1972;15(2):128–134.

172. Loder PB, Kamm MA, Nicholls RJ, et al. Haemorrhoids: pathology, pathophysiology and aetiology. *Br J Surg.* 1994;81(7):946–954.

173. Longo A. Treatment of hemorrhoid disease by reduction of mucosa and hemorrhoid prolapse with a circular-suturing device: a new procedure. In: Proceedings of the Sixth World Congress of Endoscopic Surgery; 1998; Rome, Italy. 777–784.

174. Lord PH. A new regime for the treatment of haemorrhoids. *Proc R Soc Med.* 1968;61(9):935–936.

175. Lord PH. Diverse methods of managing hemorrhoids: dilatation. *Dis Colon Rectum*. 1973;16(3):180–183.

176. Lurz KH, Göltner E. Hämorrhoiden in Schwanger-schaft und Wochenbett. *Munch Med Wochenschr*. 1977;119(48):1551–1552.

177. MacLeod JH. In defense of cryotherapy for hemorrhoids: a modified method. *Dis Colon Rectum*. 1982;25(4):332–335.

178. MacRae HM, McLeod RS. Comparison of hemorrhoidal treatment modalities: a meta-analysis. *Dis Colon Rectum*. 1995;38(7):687–694.

179. Malgieri JA. Anoplasty to correct anal stricture. *Dis Colon Rectum*. 1961;4:289–291.

180. Mattana C, Coco C, Manno A, et al. Stapled hemorrhoidopexy and Milligan Morgan hemorrhoidectomy in the cure of fourth-degree hemorrhoids: long-term evaluation and clinical results. *Dis Colon Rectum*. 2007;50(11):1770–1775.

181. Maw A, Concepcion R, Eu KW, et al. Prospective randomized study of bacteraemia in diathermy and stapled haemorrhoidectomy. *Br J Surg*. 2003;90(2):222–226.

182. Maw A, Eu KW, Seow-Choen F. Retroperitoneal sepsis complicating stapled hemorrhoidectomy: report of a case and review of the literature. *Dis Colon Rectum*. 2002;45(6):826–828.

183. McCaffrey J. Lord treatment of haemorrhoids. Four year follow-up of fifty patients. *Lancet*. 1975;1(7899):133–134.

184. McConnell JC, Khubchandani IT. Long-term follow-up of closed hemorrhoidectomy. *Dis Colon Rectum*. 1983;26(12):797–799.

185. McKay W, Morris R, Mushlin P. Sodium bicarbonate attenuates pain on skin infiltration with lidocaine, with or without epinephrine. *Anesth Analg*. 1987;66(6):572–574.

186. McLeskey CH. pH of local anesthetic solutions. *Anesth Analg*. 1980;59(11):892–893.

187. Mehigan BJ, Monson JR, Hartley JE. Stapling procedures for haemorrhoids versus Milligan-Morgan haemorrhoidectomy: randomized controlled trial. *Lancet*. 2000;355(9206):782–785.

188. Milito G, Gargiani M, Cortese F. Randomised trial comparing LigaSure haemorrhoidectomy with the diathermy dissection operation. *Tech Coloproctol*. 2002;6(3):171–175.

189. Milligan ETC, Morgan CN, Jones LE, et al. Surgical anatomy of the anal canal, and the operative treatment of haemorrhoids. *Lancet*. 1937;2:119–124.

190. Milsom JW, Mazier WP. Classification and management of postsurgical anal stenosis. *Surg Gynecol Obstet*. 1986;163(1):60–64.

191. Mlakar B. Should we avoid stapled hemorrhoidopexy in males and females who practice receptive anal sex? *Dis Colon Rectum*. 2007;50(10):1727.

192. Moesgaard F, Nielsen ML, Hansen JB, et al. High-fiber diet reduces bleeding and pain in patients with hemorrhoids: a double-blind trial of Vi-Siblin. *Dis Colon Rectum*. 1982;25(5):454–456.

193. Molloy RG, Kingsmore D. Life threatening pelvic sepsis after stapled haemorrhoidectomy. *Lancet*. 2000;355(9206):810.

194. Moore BA, Fleshner PR. Rubber band ligation for hemorrhoidal disease can be safely performed in select HIV-positive patients. *Dis Colon Rectum*. 2001;44(8):1079–1082.

195. Moore DC. The pH of local anesthetic solutions. *Anesth Analg*. 1981;60(11):833–834.

196. Morinaga K, Hasuda K, Ikeda T. A novel therapy for internal hemorrhoids: ligation of the hemorrhoidal artery with a newly devised instrument (Moricorn) in conjunction with a Doppler flowmeter. *Am J Gastroenterol*. 1995;90(4):610–613.

197. Mortensen PE, Olsen J, Pedersen IK, et al. A randomized study on hemorrhoidectomy combined with anal dilatation. *Dis Colon Rectum*. 1987;30(10):755–757.

198. Murie JA, Sim AJ, Mackenzie I. Rubber band ligation versus haemorrhoidectomy for prolapsing haemorrhoids: a long term prospective clinical trial. *Br J Surg*. 1982;69(9):536–538.

199. Murphy KJ. Tetanus after rubber-band ligation of haemorrhoids. *Br Med J*. 1978;1(6127):1590–1591.

200. Neiger A. Hemorrhoids in everyday practice. *Proctology*. 1979;2:22–28.

201. Nesselrod JP. *Clinical Proctology*. 3rd ed. Philadelphia, PA: WB Saunders; 1964.

202. Nicholson JD, Halleran DR, Trivisonno DP, et al. The efficacy of the contact sapphire tip Nd:YAG laser hemorrhoidectomy. Poster presentation at: 89th Annual Meeting of the American Society of Colon and Rectal Surgeons; April 29 to May 4, 1990; St. Louis, MO.

203. Nickell WB, Woodward ER. Advancement flaps for treatment of anal stricture. *Arch Surg*. 1972;104(2):223–224.

204. Nienhuijs SW, deHingh IH. Pain after conventional versus Ligasure haemorrhoidectomy. A meta-analysis. *Int J Surg*. 2010;8(4):269–273.

205. Nivatvongs S. Suture of massive hemorrhoidal bleeding in portal hypertension. *Dis Colon Rectum*. 1985;28(11):878–879.

206. Norman DA, Newton R, Nicholas GV. Direct current electrotherapy of internal hemorrhoids: an effective, safe, and painless outpatient approach. *Am J Gastroenterol*. 1989;84(5):482–487.

207. Nyam DC, Seow-Choen F, Ho YH. Submucosal adrenaline injection for posthemorrhoidectomy hemorrhage. *Dis Colon Rectum*. 1995;38(7):776–777.

208. Nyström PO, Qvist N, Raahave D, et al. Randomized clinical trial of symptom control after stapled anopexy or diathermy excision for haemorrhoid prolapse. *Br J Surg*. 2010;97(2):167–176.

209. O'Connor JJ. Cryohemorrhoidectomy: indications and complications. *Dis Colon Rectum*. 1976;19(1):41–43.

210. O'Connor JJ. Infrared coagulation of hemorrhoids. *Pract Gastroenterol*. 1986;10:8–14.

211. O'Donovan S, Ferrara A, Larach S, et al. Intraoperative use of Toradol facilitates outpatient hemorrhoidectomy. *Dis Colon Rectum*. 1994;37(8):793–799.

212. Oh C. The role of cryosurgery in management of anorectal disease: cryohemorrhoidectomy evaluated. *Dis Colon Rectum*. 1975;18(4):289–291.

213. Oh C. One thousand cryohemorrhoidectomies: an overview. *Dis Colon Rectum*. 1981;24(8):613–617.

214. Oh C, Zinberg J. Anoplasty for anal stricture. *Dis Colon Rectum*. 1982;25(8):809–810.

215. O'Hara VS. Fatal clostridial infection following hemorrhoidal banding. *Dis Colon Rectum*. 1980;23(8):570–571.

216. Okamura RK, Reisner LS, Kalichman MW. Effects of pH-adjusted lidocaine solutions on the compound action potential in intact rat sciatic nerves [abstract]. *Anesthesiology*. 1987;37:281.

217. Ommer A, Hinrichs J, Möllenberg H, et al. Long-term results after stapled hemorrhoidopexy: a prospective study with a 6-year follow-up. *Dis Colon Rectum*. 2011;54(5):601–608.

218. Ortiz H, Marzo J, Armendariz P. Randomized clinical trial of stapled haemorrhoidopexy versus conventional diathermy haemorrhoidectomy. *Br J Surg*. 2002;89(11):1376–1381.

219. Osur D. [letter]. *Surg Gynecol Obstet*. 1988;167:148.

220. Palazzo FF, Francis DL, Clifton MA. Randomized clinical trial of Ligasure versus open haemorrhoidectomy. *Br J Surg*. 2002;89(2):154–157.

221. Parikh SR, Molinelli B, Dailey TH. Liver abscess after hemorrhoidectomy. Report of two cases. *Dis Colon Rectum*. 1994;37(2):185–189.

222. Parks AG. The surgical treatment of haemorrhoids. *Br J Surg*. 1956;43(180):337–351.

223. Parks AG. Hemorrhoidectomy. *Adv Surg*. 1971;5:1–50.

224. Parnass SM, Baughman VL, Miletich DJ, et al. The effects of pH on the oxidation rate of epinephrine [abstract]. *Anesthesiology*. 1987;67:A280.

225. Parnaud E, Guntz M, Bernard A, et al. Anatomie normale macroscopique et microscopique du réseau vasculaire hémorrhoidal. *Arch Fr Mal App Dig*. 1976;65(7):501–514.

226. Parturier-Albot M, Rouzotte P, Elizalde N. Hémorrhoides et vue génitale de la femme. *Arch Fr Mal App Dig*. 1976;65(7):537–540.

227. Peng BC, Jayne DG, Ho YH. Randomized trial of rubber band ligation vs. stapled hemorrhoidectomy for prolapsed piles. *Dis Colon Rectum*. 2003;46(3):291–297.

228. Pernice LM, Bartalucci B, Bencini L, et al. Early and late (ten years) experience with circular stapler hemorrhoidectomy. *Dis Colon Rectum*. 2001;44(6):836–841.

229. Perrotti P, Antropoli C, Molino D, et al. Conservative treatment of acute thrombosed external hemorrhoids with topical nifedipine. *Dis Colon Rectum*. 2001;44(3):405–409.

230. Perrotti P, Dominici P, Grossi E, et al. Topical nifedipine with lidocaine ointment versus active control for pain after hemorrhoidectomy: results of a multicentre, prospective, randomized, double-blind study. *Can J Surg*. 2010;53(1):17–24.

231. Pescatori M. Stapled rectal prolapsectomy [letter]. *Dis Colon Rectum*. 2000;43(6):876–878.

232. Pescatori M. Management of post-anopexy rectal stricture. *Tech Coloproctol*. 2002;6(2):125–126.

233. Pidala MJ, Slezak FA, Porter JA. Island flap anoplasty for anal canal stenosis and mucosal ectropion. *Am Surg*. 1994;60(3):194–196.

234. Place R, Hyman N, Simmang C, et al; Standards Task Force of the American Society of Colon and Rectal Surgeons. Practice parameters for ambulatory anorectal surgery. *Dis Colon Rectum*. 2003;46(5):573–576.

235. Poon GP, Chu KW, Lau WY, et al. Conventional vs triple rubber band ligation for hemorrhoids. A prospective, randomized trial. *Dis Colon Rectum*. 1986;29(12):836–838.

236. Pope CE. An anorectal plastic operation for fissure and stenosis and its surgical principles. *Surg Gynecol Obstet*. 1959;108(2):249–252.

237. Quevedo-Bonilla G, Farkas AM, Abcarian H, et al. Septic complications of hemorrhoidal banding. *Arch Surg*. 1988;123(5):650–651.

238. Raahave D, Jepsen LV, Pedersen IK. Primary and repeated stapled hemorrhoidopexy for prolapsing hemorrhoids: follow-up to five years. *Dis Colon Rectum*. 2008;51(3):334–341.

239. Racouchot JE, Pétouraud C, Rivoire J. Saint Fiacre. The healer of haemorrhoids and patron saint of protology. *Am J Proctol*. 1971;22(2):175–179.

240. Rakhmanine M, Rosen L, Khubchandani I, et al. Lateral mucosal advancement anoplasty for anal stricture. *Br J Surg*. 2002;89(11):1423–1424.

241. Rand AA. The sliding skin-flap graft operation for hemorrhoids: a modification of the Whitehead procedure. *Dis Colon Rectum*. 1969;12(4):265–276.

242. Randall GM, Jensen DM, Machicado GA, et al. Prospective randomized comparative study of bipolar versus direct current electrocoagulation for treatment of bleeding internal hemorrhoids. *Gastrointest Endosc*. 1994;40(4):403–410.

243. Ratto C, Donisi L, Parello A, et al. Evaluation of transanal hemorrhoidal dearterialization as a minimally invasive therapeutic approach to hemorrhoids. *Dis Colon Rectum*. 2010;53(5):803–811.

244. Read TE, Henry SE, Hovis RM, et al. Prospective evaluation of anesthetic technique for anorectal surgery. *Dis Colon Rectum*. 2002;45(11):1553–1558.

245. Ribbans WJ, Radcliffe AG. Retroperitoneal abscess following sclerotherapy for hemorrhoids. *Dis Colon Rectum*. 1985;28(3):188–189.

246. Richman IM. Use of Toradol in anorectal surgery. *Dis Colon Rectum*. 1993;36(3):295–296.

247. Ripetti V, Caricato M, Arullani A. Rectal perforation, retropneumoperitoneum, and pneumomediastinum after stapling procedure for prolapsed hemorrhoids: report of a case and subsequent considerations. *Dis Colon Rectum*. 2002;45(2):268–270.

248. Rosen L. V-Y advancement for anal ectropion. *Dis Colon Rectum*. 1986;29(9):596–598.

249. Rosen L. Anoplasty. *Surg Clin North Am*. 1988;68(6):1441–1446.

250. Rosen L, Sipe P, Stasik JJ, et al. Outcome of delayed hemorrhage following surgical hemorrhoidectomy. *Dis Colon Rectum*. 1993;36(8):743–746.

251. Rosser C. Chemical rectal stricture. *JAMA*. 1931;96(21):1762–1763.

252. Rowsell M, Bello M, Hemingway DM. Circumferential mucosectomy (stapled haemorrhoidectomy) versus conventional haemorrhoidectomy: randomised controlled trial. *Lancet*. 2000;355(9206):779–781.

253. Russell TR, Donohue JH. Hemorrhoidal banding: a warning. *Dis Colon Rectum*. 1985;28(5):291–293.

254. Safavi A, Gottesman L, Dailey TH. Anorectal surgery in the HIV⁺ patient: update. *Dis Colon Rectum*. 1991;34(4):299–304.

255. Sakr MF, Moussa MM. LigaSure hemorrhoidectomy versus stapled hemorrhoidopexy: a prospective, randomized clinical trial. *Dis Colon Rectum*. 2010;53(8):1161–1167.

256. Saldana E, Paletta C, Gupta N, et al. Internal pudendal flap anoplasty for severe anal stenosis: report of a case. *Dis Colon Rectum*. 1996;39(3):350–352.

257. Saleeby RG Jr, Rosen L, Stasik JJ, et al. Hemorrhoidectomy during pregnancy: risk or relief? *Dis Colon Rectum*. 1991;34(3):260–261.

258. Salmon F. *A Practical Essay on Stricture of the Rectum Illustrated by Cases, Showing the Connexion of that Disease with Affections of the Urinary Organs and the Uterus, with Piles and Various Constitutional Complaints*. 3rd ed. London, United Kingdom: Whitaker, Treacher & Arnot; 1829:208.

259. Salvati EP, Kleckner MS. Urinary retention in anorectal and colonic surgery. *Am J Surg*. 1957;94(1):114–117.

260. Sankar MY, Joffe SN. Technique of contact laser hemorrhoidectomy: an ambulatory surgical procedure. *Contemp Surg*. 1987;30:9–11.

261. Santos G, Novell JR, Khoury G, et al. Long-term results of large-dose, single-session phenol injection sclerotherapy for hemorrhoids. *Dis Colon Rectum*. 1993;36(10):958–961.

262. Sarner JB. Plastic relief of anal stenosis. *Dis Colon Rectum*. 1969;12(4):277–280.

263. Savin S. Hemorrhoidectomy: how I do it? Results of 444 cryorectal surgical operations. *Dis Colon Rectum*. 1977;20(3):189–196.

264. Scarpa FJ, Hillis W, Sabetta JR. Pelvic cellulitis: a life-threatening complication of hemorrhoidal banding. *Surgery*. 1988;103(3):383–385.

265. Schapiro M. The gastroenterologist and the treatment of hemorrhoids: is it about time? *Am J Gastroenterol*. 1989;84(5):493–495.

266. Schouten WR, van Vroonhoven TJ. Lateral internal sphincterotomy in the treatment of hemorrhoids: a clinical and manometric study. *Dis Colon Rectum*. 1986;29(12):869–872.

267. Scoma JA. Hemorrhoidectomy without urinary retention and catheterization. *Conn Med*. 1976;40(11):751–752.

268. Selvaggi F, Scotto di Carlo E, Silvestri A, et al. Surgical treatment of circumferential hemorrhoids. *Dis Colon Rectum*. 1990;33(10):903–904.

269. Senagore AJ. Surgical management of hemorrhoids. *J Gastrointest Surg*. 2002;6(3):295–298.

270. Senagore AJ, Mazier WP, Luchtefeld MA, et al. Treatment of advanced hemorrhoidal disease: a prospective, randomized comparison of cold scalpel vs. contact Nd:YAG laser. *Dis Colon Rectum*. 1993;36(11):1042–1049.

271. Senagore AJ, Singer M, Abcarian H, et al. A prospective, randomized, controlled multicenter trial comparing stapled hemorrhoidopexy and Ferguson hemorrhoidectomy: perioperative and one-year results. *Dis Colon Rectum*. 2004;47(11):1824–1836.

272. Shemesh EI, Kodner IJ, Fry RD, et al. Severe complication of rubber band ligation of internal hemorrhoids. *Dis Colon Rectum*. 1987;30(3):199–200.

273. Shieh CJ, Gennaro AR. Treatment of acute prolapsed hemorrhoids: manual reduction followed by semi-emergent hemorrhoidectomy. *Am J Proctol Gastroenterol Colon Rectal Surg*. 1985;36:12.

274. Shropshear G. Posterior and anterior anal proctotomy: a simplified technic for postoperative anal stenosis. *Dis Colon Rectum*. 1971;14(1):62–66.

275. Sim AJ, Murie JA, Mackenzie I. Three year follow-up study on the treatment of first and second degree hemorrhoids by sclerosant injection or rubber band ligation. *Surg Gynecol Obstet*. 1983;157(6):534–536.

276. Singer MA, Cintron JR, Fleshman JW, et al. Early experience with stapled hemorrhoidectomy in the United States. *Dis Colon Rectum*. 2002;45(3):360–367.

277. Smith LE, Goodreau JJ, Fouty WJ. Management of hemorrhoids: operative hemorrhoidectomy versus cryosurgery. *Dis Colon Rectum*. 1979;22(1):10–16.

278. Sohn N, Aronoff JS, Cohen FS, et al. Transanal hemorrhoidal dearterialization is an alternative to operative hemorrhoidectomy. *Am J Surg*. 2001;182(5):515–519.

279. Standards Task Force, American Society of Colon and Rectal Surgeons. Practice parameters for the treatment of hemorrhoids. *Dis Colon Rectum*. 1993;36(12):1118–1120.

280. Steinberg DM, Liegois H, Alexander-Williams J. Long term review of the results of rubber band ligation of haemorrhoids. *Br J Surg*. 1975;62(2):144–146.

281. Stelzner F, Staubesand J, Machleidt H. The corpus cavernosum recti: basis of internal hemorrhoids. *Langenbecks Arch Klin Chir Ver Dtsch Z Chir*. 1962;299:302–312.

282. Subramanyam K, Patterson M, Gourley WK. Effects of preparation-H on wound healing in the rectum of man. *Dig Dis Sci*. 1984;29(9):829–832.

283. Sun WM, Peck RJ, Shorthouse AJ, et al. Haemorrhoids are associated not with hypertrophy of the internal anal sphincter, but with hypertension of the anal cushions. *Br J Surg*. 1992;79(6):592–594.

284. Sun WM, Read NW, Shorthouse AJ. Hypertensive anal cushions as a cause of the high anal canal pressures in patients with haemorrhoids. *Br J Surg*. 1990;77(4):458–462.

285. Tan PY, Vukasin P, Chin ID, et al. The WAND local anesthetic delivery system: a more pleasant experience for anal anesthesia. *Dis Colon Rectum*. 2001;44(5):686–689.

286. Tchirkow G, Haas PA, Fox TA Jr. Injection of a local anesthetic solution into hemorrhoidal bundles following rubber band ligation. *Dis Colon Rectum*. 1982;25(1):62–63.

287. Terrell EH. The treatment of hemorrhoids by a new method. *Trans Am Proctol Soc*. 1916:65.

288. Testa A, Torino G, Gioia A. DG-RAR (Doppler-guided recto-anal repair): a new mini invasive technique in the treatment of prolapsed hemorrhoids (grade III–IV): preliminary report. *Int Surg*. 2010;95(3):265–269.

289. Thomson H. A new look at hemorrhoids. *Med Times*. 1976;104(11):116–123.

290. Thomson WH. The nature of haemorrhoids. *Br J Surg*. 1975;62(7):542–552.

291. Tokunaga Y, Sasaki H, Saito T. Evaluation of sclerotherapy with a new sclerosing agent and stapled hemorrhoidopexy for prolapsing internal hemorrhoids: retrospective comparison with hemorrhoidectomy. *Dig Surg*. 2010;27(6):469–472.

292. Traynor OJ, Carter AE. Cryotherapy for advanced haemorrhoids: a prospective evaluation with 2-year follow-up. *Br J Surg*. 1984;71(4):287–289.

293. Turell R. Postoperative anal stenosis. *Surg Gynecol Obstet*. 1950;90(2):231–233.

294. Turell R. Preoperative and postoperative management in anorectal surgery. In: Turell R, ed. *Diseases of the Colon and Anorectum*. 2nd ed. Vol 2. Philadelphia, PA: WB Saunders; 1969:883.

295. Turell R, Gelernt IM. Anal stenosis. In: Turell R, ed. *Diseases of the Colon and Anorectum*. 2nd ed. Vol 2. Philadelphia, PA: WB Saunders; 1969:1046.

296. Turell R, Gelernt IM. Anal stenosis. In: Turell R, ed. *Diseases of the Colon and Anorectum*. 2nd ed. Vol 2. Philadelphia, PA: WB Saunders; 1969:1051.

297. Vellacott KD, Hardcastle JD. Is continued anal dilatation necessary after a Lord's procedure for haemorrhoids? *Br J Surg*. 1980;67(9):658–659.

298. Vinson-Bonnet B, Coltat JC, Fingerhut A, et al. Local infiltration with ropivacaine improves immediate postoperative pain control after hemorrhoidal surgery. *Dis Colon Rectum*. 2002;45(1):104–108.

299. Walls AD, Ruckley CV. A five-year follow-up of Lord's dilatation for haemorrhoids. *Lancet*. 1976;1(7971):1212–1213.

300. Wang JY, Chang-Chien CR, Chen JS, et al. The role of lasers in hemorrhoidectomy. *Dis Colon Rectum*. 1991;34(1):78–82.

301. Wasvary HJ, Hain J, Mosed-Vogel M, et al. Randomized, prospective, double-blind, placebo-controlled trial of effect of nitroglycerin ointment on pain after hemorrhoidectomy. *Dis Colon Rectum*. 2001;44(8):1069–1073.

302. Watts JM, Bennett RC, Duthie HL, et al. Healing and pain after hemorrhoidectomy. *Br J Surg*. 1964;51:808–817.

303. Wechter DG, Luna GK. An unusual complication of rubber band ligation of hemorrhoids. *Dis Colon Rectum*. 1987;30(2):137–140.

304. Weinshel E, Chen W, Falkenstein DB, et al. Hemorrhoids or rectal varices: defining the cause of massive rectal hemorrhage in patients with portal hypertension. *Gastroenterology*. 1986;90(3):744–747.

305. Weinstein SJ, Rypins EB, Houck J, et al. Single session treatment for bleeding hemorrhoids. *Surg Gynecol Obstet*. 1987;165(6):479–482.

306. Wexner SD, Baig K. The evaluation and physiologic assessment of hemorrhoidal disease: a review. *Tech Coloproctol*. 2001;5(3):165–168.

307. White AC. Liquid air: its application in medicine and surgery. *Med Rec*. 1899;56:109–112.

308. Whitehead W. The surgical treatment of haemorrhoids. *Br Med J*. 1882;1(1101):148–150.

309. Williams KL, Haq IU, Elem B. Cryodestruction of haemorrhoids. *Br Med J*. 1973;1(5854):666–668.

310. Wilson MC, Schofield P. Cryosurgical haemorrhoidectomy. *Br J Surg*. 1976;63(6):497–498.

311. Wilson MS, Pope V, Doran HE, et al. Objective comparison of stapled anopexy and open hemorrhoidectomy: a randomized, controlled trial. *Dis Colon Rectum*. 2002;45(11):1437–1444.

312. Wilson PM. Anorectal closing mechanisms. *S Afr Med J*. 1977;51(22):802–808.

313. Wolfe JS, Munoz JJ, Rosin JD. Survey of hemorrhoidectomy practices: open versus closed techniques. *Dis Colon Rectum*. 1979;22(8):536–538.

314. Wolff BG, Culp CE. The Whitehead hemorrhoidectomy: an unjustly maligned procedure. *Dis Colon Rectum*. 1988;31(8):587–590.

315. Wolkomir AF, Luchtefeld MA. Surgery for symptomatic hemorrhoids and anal fissures in Crohn's disease. *Dis Colon Rectum*. 1993;36(6):545–547.

316. Wong LY, Jiang JK, Chang SC, et al. Rectal perforation: a life-threatening complication of stapled hemorrhoidectomy: report of a case. *Dis Colon Rectum*. 2003;46(1):116–117.

317. Wright RA, Kranz KR, Kirby SL. A prospective crossover trial of direct current electrotherapy in symptomatic hemorrhoidal disease. *Gastrointest Endosc*. 1991;37(6):621–623.

318. Wrobleski DE, Corman ML, Veidenheimer MC, et al. Long-term evaluation of rubber ring ligation in hemorrhoidal disease. *Dis Colon Rectum*. 1980;23(7):478–482.

319. Yang R, Migikovsky B, Peicher J, et al. Randomized, prospective trial of direct current versus bipolar electrocoagulation for bleeding internal hemorrhoids. *Gastrointest Endosc*. 1993;39(6):766–769.

320. Yu JC, Eddy HJ Jr. Laser, a new modality for hemorrhoidectomy. *Am J Proctol Gastroenterol Colon Rectal Surg*. 1985;36:9–13.

321. Zinberg SS, Stern DH, Furman DS, et al. A personal experience in comparing three nonoperative techniques for treating internal hemorrhoids. *Am J Gastroenterol*. 1989;84(5):488–492.

12
Anal Fissure

Sanjay P. Jobanputra

Wisdom is nothing more than healed pain.
—ROBERT E. LEE

Anal fissure (fissure-in-ano) is a common anorectal condition, which is also one of the most painful. It can be very troubling because, if acute, the severity of patient discomfort and extent of disability far exceed that which would be expected from a seemingly trivial lesion.

An anal fissure is a cut or crack in the anal canal or anal verge that may extend from the mucocutaneous junction to the dentate line. It can be acute or chronic. It may occur at any age (it is the most common cause of rectal bleeding in infants) but is usually a condition of young adults, with both sexes being affected equally. Anal fissures are most commonly found in the posterior midline. However, in 10% of women it will be seen in the anterior midline.[37] This compares with only 1% incidence in men in this location.[37] Abramowitz and colleagues prospectively studied 165 consecutive women during their last 3 months of pregnancy and following delivery and noted that one-third develop thrombosed external hemorrhoids or anal fissures.[3] They attributed the most important predisposing factor to that of dyschezia (difficult or painful evacuation).

▶ ETIOLOGY AND PATHOGENESIS

Anal fissure has been attributed to constipation or to straining at stool; theoretically, the passage of a hard fecal bolus through a relatively tight anal sphincter is thought to crack the anal canal. Patients will often remember the exact time the fissure developed based on the symptoms. Classically, this will almost always be associated with an episode of constipation. To identify risk factors for the development of an anal fissure, Jensen studied 174 patients with chronic anal fissure and compared them with controls with respect to diet, beverage consumption, occupational exposures, and medical/surgical history.[47] A decreased risk was associated with increased consumption of raw fruits, vegetables, and whole grain bread. A significantly increased risk was noted with frequent consumption of white bread, sauces thickened with a roux, bacon, and sausage. Risk was not related to consumption of coffee, tea, or alcohol.

Even though usually associated with constipation, anal fissure can also be a consequence of frequent defecation and diarrhea. It may be noted with nonspecific inflammatory bowel disease and must be considered in the differential diagnosis of certain specific inflammatory conditions (e.g., syphilis, tuberculosis, gonorrhea, chlamydial infection, herpes, acquired immunodeficiency syndrome [AIDS], carcinoma, and others). If there is cause for concern as to the true nature of the ulcer or fissure, biopsy, stool culture, serology, and gastrointestinal evaluation may be indicated. When anal fissure occurs in an unusual location, especially laterally, the physician must entertain the possibility that the patient harbors nonspecific inflammatory bowel disease, likely Crohn's disease.

Why the fissure is most commonly located in the posterior anal canal is a subject of some controversy. Lockhart-Mummery believed that the explanation can be found in the structure of the external sphincter.[63] The lower portion of this muscle is not truly circular but rather consists of a band of muscle fibers that pass from posterior to anterior and split around the anus. He postulated that the anal mucosa is, therefore, best supported laterally and is weakest posteriorly. The decreased anterior support in women is believed to account for the greater occurrence in this location than in men. Additional evidence reinforcing the Lockhart-Mummery concept may be apparent when the physician inserts an anal retractor too vigorously at the time of hemorrhoid surgery. The split

JOHN PERCY LOCKHART-MUMMERY (1875–1957)

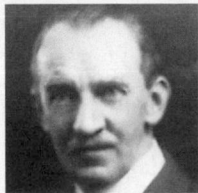

Lockhart-Mummery was born at Islip Manor, Northolt, England, the eldest son of a distinguished dental surgeon. He was educated at Leys School and Caius College, Cambridge. He was an outstanding student and in 1897 was appointed an assistant demonstrator in anatomy at his alma mater. In 1900, he became a fellow of the Royal College of Surgeons and subsequently received several hospital appointments. In 1903, having developed a special interest in proctology, he was appointed assistant surgeon at St. Mark's Hospital. In 1904, he was Hunterian professor at the Royal College of Surgeons, and in 1909, he was Jacksonian prizewinner at the college. He contributed extensively to the literature throughout his career. Among his writings were six books on colorectal surgery, in addition to two collections of essays on nonmedical subjects. He was a very energetic man, even "hopping up the steps to the hospital"—a rather relevant observation; while a student at Cambridge, he had undergone a leg amputation for sarcoma by Lord Lister himself. He was the first secretary of the British Proctological Society and was instrumental in establishing it as an independent section of the Royal Society of Medicine. In 1937, he was elected as a fellow of the American College of Surgeons. In 1940, after 37 years at St. Mark's Hospital, Lockhart-Mummery was made an honorary consulting surgeon. (Lockhart-Mummery P. Fissure-in-ano. In: *Diseases of the Rectum and Anus: A Practical Handbook.* New York, NY: William Wood; 1944:169.)

that may occur is almost invariably located posteriorly. Likewise, if the sphincter is stretched in the cadaver, tearing almost always occurs posteriorly.[64]

Another theory that has been suggested is related to the blood supply to the area. Klosterhalfen and associates visualized the inferior rectal artery by means of postmortem angiography, by manual preparations, and by histologic study following vascular injection.[56] They determined that in 85% of specimens, the posterior commissure is less well perfused than other areas of the anal canal. Hence, ischemia may be an important etiologic factor in causing anal fissure, especially in the posterior location. The authors further suggest that the blood supply, which is already tenuous, may be further compromised by compression and contusion as the branch of the inferior rectal artery passes through the internal anal sphincter. Others have confirmed in cadaveric studies that there is a significant trend to an increasing number of arterioles from posterior to anterior in the subanodermal space at all levels.[67]

Schouten and colleagues assessed microvascular perfusion of the anoderm by means of Doppler flowmetry in 27 patients.[104] Anodermal blood flow at the fissure site was significantly lower at the posterior commissure of the controls. Reduction of anal pressure by sphincterotomy improved anodermal blood flow, resulting in healing of the fissure. These observations lend further support to the concept that ischemia is the etiologic factor that contributes to the development of fissure disease. A later study by the same authors, this time involving 178 subjects, confirmed that anodermal blood flow was less in the posterior midline than in other segments of the anal canal.[105]

Why some fissures heal spontaneously and others become chronic is an unresolved question. Ischemia, infection, or lymphatic obstruction secondary to persistent inflammation may be responsible. A characteristic skin tag (i.e., a sentinel pile) may develop distally, whereas proximally, a hypertrophied anal papilla may be seen (Figures 12-1 through 12-3). If one wishes to attempt an anthropomorphic explanation for

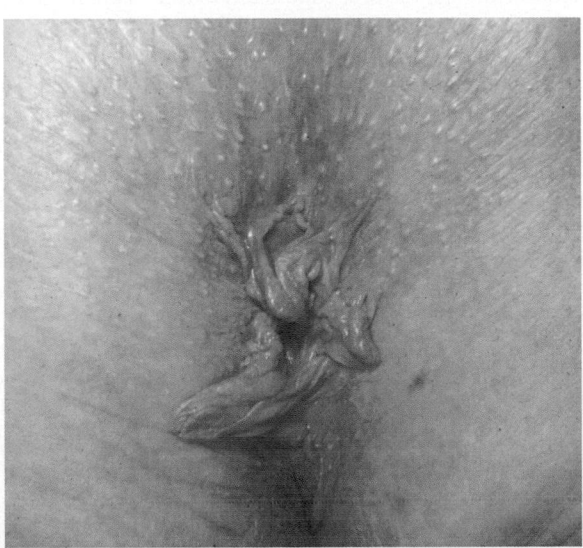

FIGURE 12-1. Posterior anal fissure and associated skin tags are clearly seen upon inspection.

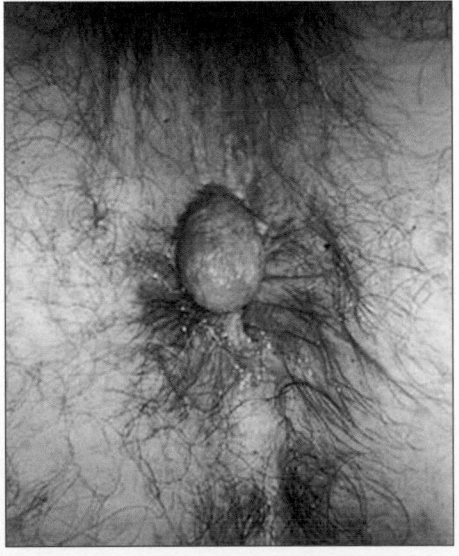

FIGURE 12-2. Prolapsed, hypertrophied anal papilla associated with anal fissure. This condition must be distinguished from an external hemorrhoid in order to provide the appropriate treatment.

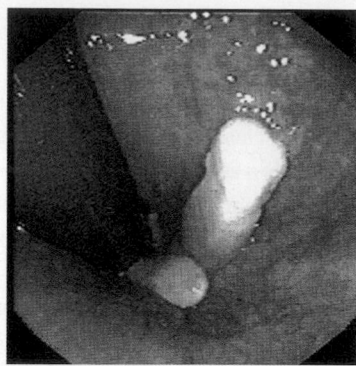

FIGURE 12-3. Hypertrophied anal papillae are seen through a retroflexed video endoscope in a patient with chronic anal fissure.

the occurrence of skin tags and papillae, it is as if healing cannot take place across the defect produced by the fissure, so the body attempts to heal it through overgrowth on the proximal and distal ends of the defect. One often observes that the internal anal sphincter muscle fibers can be seen at the base of the open wound (Figures 12-1 and 12-4).

▶ PHYSIOLOGIC STUDIES

Anal manometric pressure studies in patients with anal fissure have interested investigators for some time. Duthie and Bennett in 1964 were among the earliest who measured anal

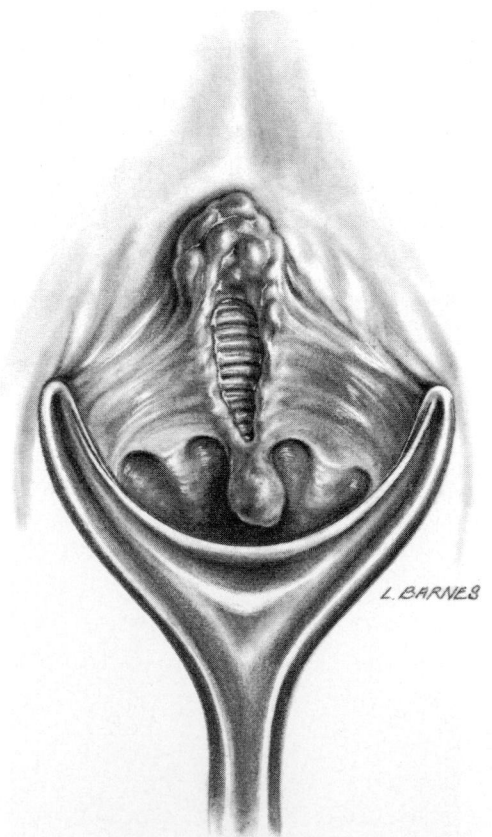

L. BARNES

FIGURE 12-4. Artist's concept of chronic posterior anal fissure with skin tag and hypertrophied anal papilla. Note fibers of the internal anal sphincter at the base of the wound.

canal pressures. They used an open-ended tube connected to a recording device by a strain gauge.[21] Although all patients had demonstrable spasm of the sphincter based on digital examination, no increase in the resting pressure was found when they were compared with control subjects. When sphincter stretch was performed, a moderate fall in pressure was noted, but it returned virtually to normal by the eighth postoperative day. It appeared to the authors that the therapeutic effect of sphincter stretch was not related so much to reduction in anal pressure as to prevention of the spasm.[21] Others have observed a similar pattern in which the pressure falls after internal anal sphincterotomy.[5,14,41,105]

However, Gibbons and Read employed perfusion probes of varying diameters in patients with chronic anal fissure.[34] Resting pressures were *elevated* in all subjects when compared with controls, irrespective of probe size. They, therefore, postulated that resting pressures are indeed elevated in individuals with an anal fissure and that this observed phenomenon is not caused by spasm. They postulated that ischemia of the anal canal mucosa may be the cause of pain and the failure of fissures to heal.

Nothmann and Schuster performed balloon rectosphincteric manometry on patients with anal fissure.[84] Resting pressures were twice as high as those measured in control subjects. Technique is important, however. One must recognize that resting pressures measured with an open-tipped tube in patients with anal fissure may be normal, whereas those measured by balloon catheter are usually elevated.[106] Following distension of the rectum by the balloon, there is the expected internal sphincter relaxation, but this is followed by a *marked and prolonged contraction above the initial baseline*, termed the "overshoot" phenomenon.[84] Nothmann and Schuster concluded that this reflexively stimulated sphincter spasm is involved in the etiology of the condition.[84]

Keck and colleagues examined manometric findings in patients with anal fissure by the use of a computer-assisted system.[53] They concluded that the primary abnormality in fissure is persistent hypertonia affecting the entire internal sphincter.

One can add another possibility to the theories and observations of the ameliorative effect of sphincterotomy. Abcarian and associates, by their manometric evaluation of patients with anal fissure, concluded that the benefit is really the consequence of an anatomic widening of the anal canal that occurs during sphincterotomy.[2]

Roe and coworkers have described a technique for quantifying anal canal sensation by means of two platinum electrodes placed 1 cm apart and connected to copper wires passed to a constant current generator.[99] Patients with acute anal fissure exhibited a lower threshold of sensation at the site of the fissure. The authors propose that the findings may reflect stimulation of exposed nerve endings at the base of the fissure rather than actual heightened sensory awareness in this group of patients. The value of this experimental modality in the diagnosis and therapy of patients with anorectal disorders, particularly incontinence, has yet to be determined.

Another potentially useful investigative study is that of anal canal ultrasonography. Reissman believes that this investigation may be important in identifying unrecognized obstetrically related sphincteric injuries before performance of internal anal sphincterotomy.[95] Although it is recognized that anal ultrasound may be rather difficult to perform in the presence of an acute, painful fissure, one could consider the advisability of identifying such at-risk individuals. Ultrasound may also be considered in patients who have had previous internal sphincterotomy and present with recurrent fissure.

▶ HISTOPATHOLOGY

Nothing in particular is histologically diagnostic of an anal fissure (Figure 12-5). If the lesion is excised and submitted for pathologic examination, usually typical nonspecific inflammatory changes are observed. Brown and colleagues prospectively studied 18 consecutive patients who underwent internal anal sphincterotomy for chronic anal fissure and took a biopsy specimen from the base and also from the muscle before division.[13] Histologic evaluation confirmed the presence of fibrosis throughout the internal sphincter, but no such finding was identified in controls.

▶ SYMPTOMS

The diagnosis of an anal fissure can usually be made based on the history alone. The characteristic complaints of a patient with an acute anal fissure are pain and bleeding. The pain usually occurs with and immediately after defecation. One usually describes the pain as severe and sharp, often stating he or she feels as if glass is cutting the person during the act of defecation. Often, the pain ceases in a few minutes, but occasionally it may persist for hours. The patient often relates that constipation is the antecedent event, but once pain develops, the fear of the act of defecation and refusal of the call to stool can exacerbate this problem. This anxiety leads to fecal impaction, particularly in children and in the elderly. Bleeding is usually minimal and frequently occurs only on the toilet paper, but sometimes blood will be seen in the toilet bowl. It is not uncommon for patients to report no evidence of bleeding.

The pain of anal fissure can be differentiated from that of proctalgia fugax (see Chapter 20) in that the latter condition produces discomfort, which is usually not related to bowel action. In addition, the patient with a fissure feels the discomfort in the anal area; the pain of proctalgia fugax is higher and more deep-seated. The other anal condition that commonly produces pain is a thrombosed hemorrhoid (see Chapter 11), but with this complaint, the patient also reports feeling a lump. This will not be present if an acute anal fissure is the cause of the pain.

Those individuals with a long-standing (i.e., chronic) anal fissure will present with a different symptom complex. They may complain of a lump representing the sentinel tag, drainage or discharge from the open wound, pruritus, or a combination of several symptoms. Bleeding may or may not be present, and pain is usually mild and frequently absent. Problems with micturition (e.g., retention, urgency, frequency) and dyspareunia occasionally accompany the symptoms of both acute and chronic fissure.

▶ EXAMINATION

Acute Fissure

As suggested, the patient's history is usually so characteristic that the diagnosis can be easily established. By mere inspection or gentle retraction of the perianal skin, the open wound often can be seen (Figure 12-6). If the physician is unable to pry the buttocks apart to view the area, the presence of an acute anal fissure is a virtual certainty. However, other pathologic entities such as abscess should be entertained. Under such circumstances, to attempt digital examination or to insert an instrument is usually unnecessary, counterproductive, and an inhumane exercise. Careful visual inspection of the area will often reveal the fissure, especially in the classic posterior midline. Appropriate treatment may be initiated without more specific confirmatory evidence. It is, however, important that follow-up by means of a more thorough anorectal examination when symptoms improve should be accomplished to rule out other pathologic entities, including distal anorectal carcinoma.

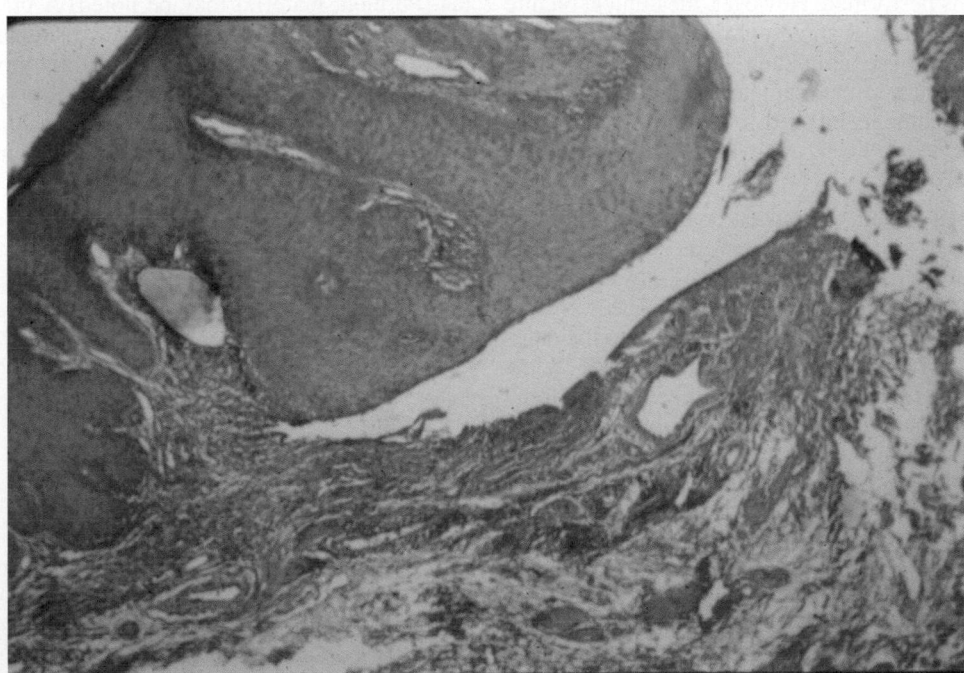

FIGURE 12-5. This anal fissure is an elongated defect surrounded by granulation tissue on one side and acanthotic squamous epithelium on the other. (Original magnification × 180.)

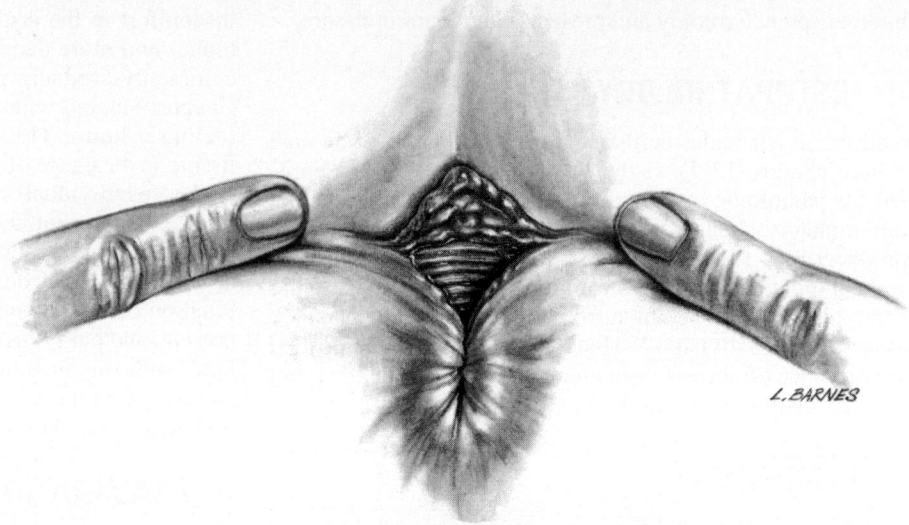

L. BARNES

FIGURE 12-6. Artist's concept of a "sentinel pile," or skin tab, at the lower edge of an anal fissure. These can easily be recognized without instrumentation.

Examination may still be possible if the examiner is so committed and the patient is forbearing. A topical anesthetic jelly may be usefully employed. Palpation will usually demonstrate a spastic anal sphincter or a tight anal canal, and, of course, the examination will exacerbate the patient's discomfort. The open wound is often not appreciated by the examining finger in an individual with an acute anal fissure. Because the cut is relatively superficial, there is usually no fibrosis.

Anoscopic examination, if possible, confirms the location of the fissure. The ability to perform this examination, however, may reflect the chronicity of the problem. As previously mentioned, ideally, proctosigmoidoscopic examination should be carried out prior to performing any surgical procedure to establish that the rectum, at least, is not involved by inflammatory bowel disease or any other pathologic entity. This should be a self-evident policy when an examination under anesthesia is performed. However, the clinical picture is usually so characteristic that most physicians appropriately tend to omit or defer this examination. However, if anoscopy and sigmoidoscopy are to be attempted, it is suggested that narrow-caliber instruments be used.

Chronic Fissure

There is no real agreement as to what constitutes a chronic anal fissure.[90] One definition is that a fissure is chronic when it has become a clearly recognized, well-circumscribed ulcer.[83] Others suggest that it is a fissure that has been present for at least 2 months. Many physicians subscribe to the rationale that is perhaps analogous to the comment made by the U.S. Supreme Court justice, Potter Stewart, when he offered his opinion with respect to a ruling on pornography. It is as follows: ". . . [in certain cases one is] faced with the task of trying to define what may be indefinable. . . . But I know it when I see it." As with Justice Potter, surgeons seem to know it (chronic anal fissure) when they see it.

Examination of the patient with a chronic anal fissure often reveals the characteristic sentinel pile. This can at times become rather large (i.e., 3 to 4 cm). Digital examination characteristically permits palpation of the fissure, open wound, induration, and fibrosis. A hypertrophied anal papilla often can be felt at the apex of the ulcer; sometimes it may be mistaken for a tumor (Figures 12-2 through 12-4).

Because pain and tenderness are generally minimal or absent, anoscopy frequently can be accomplished without difficulty. However, scarring may result in some degree of narrowing of the anal canal, and it may be necessary to use a narrow-diameter anoscope. Characteristically, the internal anal sphincter fibers are clearly seen at the base of a chronic anal fissure. Proctosigmoidoscopy or flexible sigmoidoscopy should be performed to rule out the possibility of a concurrent tumor or distal inflammatory bowel disease.

Occasionally, the base of the fissure may become infected and form an abscess that may discharge as a fistula (Figure 12-7; see Chapter 14). When it occurs, the fistula is inevitably superficial—in fact, truly subcutaneous. Examination may reveal an external opening, virtually always in the midline, usually no more than 1 or 2 cm distal to the skin tag. Purulent material may be noted. A probe passed from the external opening emerges at the distal end of the fissure; usually, the internal anal sphincter is not traversed.

As suggested, chronic anal fissure may sometimes be associated with anal stenosis, particularly if the fissure is the result of prior anal surgery (e.g., hemorrhoidectomy

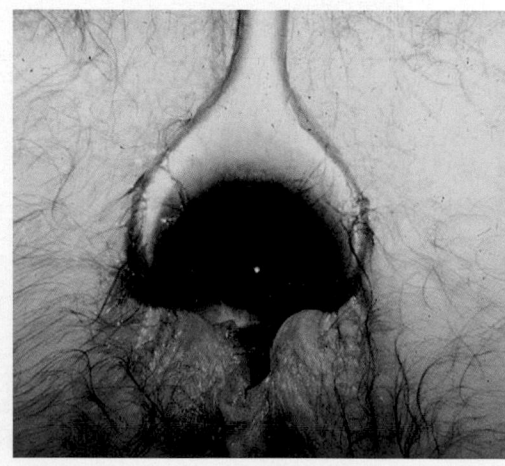

FIGURE 12-7. Anal fissure with associated fistula-in-ano. (Courtesy of Daniel Rosenthal, MD.)

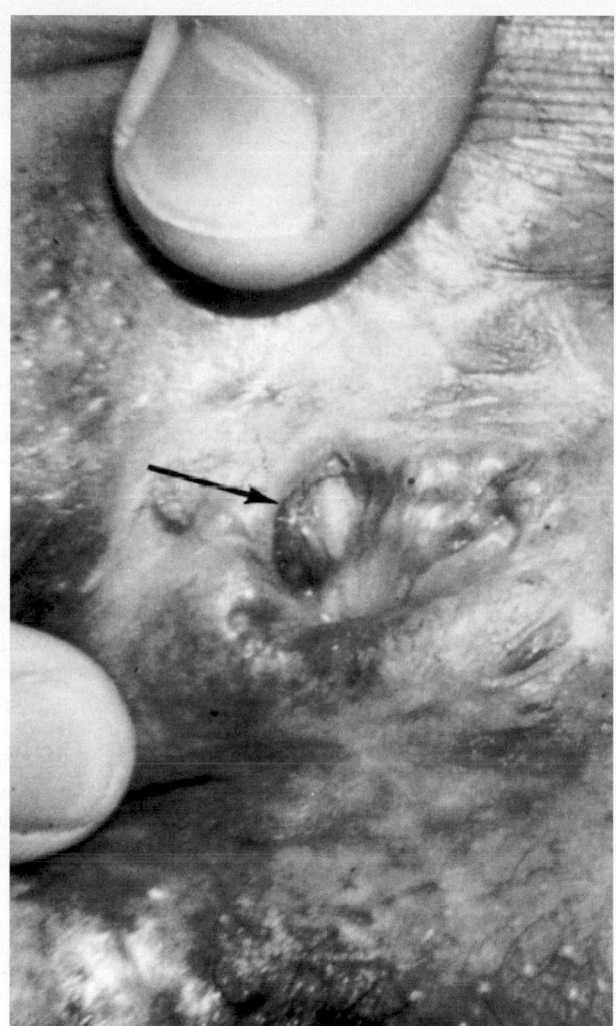

FIGURE 12-8. An anal fissure (*arrow*) resulting from stenosis following hemorrhoidectomy. (Courtesy of Daniel Rosenthal, MD.)

[Figure 12-8]). Under this circumstance, treatment may require an anoplasty (see Chapter 11).

▶ TREATMENT

Medical Management

In 2010, the Standards Practice Task Force of the American Society of Colon and Rectal Surgeons published guidelines for the management of anal fissure.[89] The statement cautioned, however, that "ultimate judgment regarding the propriety of any specific procedure must be made by the physician in light of all the circumstances presented by the individual patient." Those with a history suggestive of anal fissure of relatively recent onset are usually successfully treated by conservative measures, such as stool softeners (e.g., docusate sodium), bulking agents (e.g., psyllium), a high-fiber diet, increased water intake, and sitz baths. Preparations containing mineral oil are not advised because of difficulty in cleansing the area following defecation. Suppositories also are not recommended because they do not act effectively within the anal canal. Inserting any one of several proprietary creams (i.e., hydrocortisone-based creams and ointments in the area, with or without a local anesthetic)

may offer some transient relief. To prevent recurrence, the patient should be encouraged to continue with the diet and bulk laxative agent, even after symptoms have resolved.

Topical anesthetic preparations (i.e., lidocaine 5% cream or ointment) that are applied just before defecation and/or afterward may offer transient relief of pain. Injection of a long-acting local anesthetic may also afford temporary relief and may permit examination, but its use on an ambulatory basis is impractical. Anal dilators should not be employed (see later), and the application of silver nitrate without a local anesthetic will usually succeed in clearing the physician's waiting room, so dramatic is the patient's response. The task force concludes that nonoperative treatment continues to be safe, has few side effects, and should usually be the first step in therapy.

Sclerotherapy

Periodic reports have surfaced in the literature concerning the use of sclerotherapy with that of a local anesthetic. In a nonrandomized, noncontrolled study, Antebi and colleagues treated acute anal fissure by injection of Sotradecol (i.e., sodium tetradecyl sulfate) directly into the fissure.[4] In 96 patients with a 1-year follow-up, 80% were free of symptoms and had no evidence of fissure. These investigators recommended the technique for those individuals who fail to respond to conservative management. However, this approach seems to have faded in both clinical practice and in the literature.

Solcoderm

Chen and coworkers reported the topical use of Solcoderm (Solco, Basel, Switzerland) in the treatment of anal fissure.[15] The product has been employed for the management of a variety of skin diseases. In a controlled study involving 25 patients in each group, a statistically significantly better healing rate was shown with the drug at 1 month (84% vs. 28%) and at 1 year (84% vs. 44%).

Comment

This is another treatment method that has never gained much popularity in clinical practice and has virtually disappeared from current literature.

Hyperbaric Oxygen

On the theory that hypoxia is an important factor leading to the development of an anal fissure, Cundall and colleagues treated eight patients in whom conservative treatment, including glyceryl trinitrate (GTN) ointment (see later), had failed.[20] Each patient received 15 hyperbaric treatments over 3 weeks. This consisted of 90 minutes of breathing 100% oxygen at 2.3 atmospheres. At the end of 3 months, five had healed. There were no side effects.

Comment

This approach to the medical management of a fissure has likewise disappeared from the literature, probably as a consequence of its considerable cost as well as compliance issues. Fundamentally, this treatment and others have been supplanted by the availability of other treatment options.

Glyceryl Trinitrate Ointment

The concept of a "chemical sphincterotomy" through the use of a nitric acid donor, topical nitroglycerine (GTN), has been the subject of numerous articles and considerable debate in both the medical literature and the lay press in recent years.[39,46,65,66,68,71,89,114] Nitric oxide is a neurotransmitter that leads to relaxation of the internal sphincter. When applied topically to the anal canal, GTN diffuses across the mucosa causing a reduction in internal anal sphincter pressure.[71] This leads to improvement of anal blood flow with the consequence of increased likelihood for healing of the fissure.

McLeod and Evans, in an article published in 2002, identified a total of nine randomized, controlled trials in which the efficacy of GTN was studied.[71] Lund and Scholefield randomized 80 consecutive patients to receive treatments with topical 0.2% GTN ointment or a placebo.[68] After 8 weeks, healing was observed in 26 of 38 patients treated with GTN (68%) but in only 3 of 39 treated with the placebo (8%). These differences were highly significant. The authors concluded that topical GTN provides rapid, sustained relief of pain in individuals with anal fissure. A multi-institutional investigation was conducted in 17 centers with the aim of determining the optimal dosage and dosing interval for the use of GTN.[6] There were no significant differences observed in fissure healing among any of the treatment groups, but those who received 0.4% (1.5 mg) GTN ointment had a statistically significant decrease in pain intensity. The primary side effect was headache. Pitt and colleagues treated 1,998 patients with 0.2% GTN ointment.[91] They found that the presence of a sentinel pile adversely affected the outcome. To put it another way, the longer the fissure is present, the less likely GTN will be helpful. In a systematic review by Poh et al., healing rates for GTN range from 40.4% to 68%, with the most common concentration used being 0.2%.[92] Reported recurrence rates were 7.9% to 50%, with the most common complication being headaches. The frequency of this complication ranged from 5.9% to 56.4%. As would be expected, incontinence was not a significant issue in the reviewed studies.

Emami and coworkers applied a 0.2% GTN *suppository* for the management/healing of chronic anal fissure.[25] However, the long-term results were not statistically different.

Karanlik and associates used GTN following hemorrhoidectomy in a prospective, randomized, double-blind, placebo-controlled trial.[52] They observed that GTN ointment significantly decreased postoperative pain following this procedure as well as reducing analgesic requirements in the immediate postoperative period. The use of the ointment also appeared to achieve more rapid wound healing. The aforementioned Standards Practice Task Force opined that anal fissures may be treated with topical nitrates, although nitrates are (only) marginally superior to placebo with respect to healing.

Calcium Channel Blockers

Calcium ions are important for smooth muscle contraction. It has, therefore, been suggested that calcium channel blockers may be an effective treatment for anal fissure. This represents a second method for relaxing the internal anal sphincter.

Nifedipine and *diltiazem* have been shown to be effective calcium channel antagonists. Cook and coworkers undertook a study with oral nifedipine in healthy volunteers and in 15 patients with chronic anal fissure.[18] A highly significant decrease in maximum resting pressure was observed along with a reduction in pain scores. Nine patients experienced complete healing after 8 weeks. Side effects included flushing and mild headache. Perotti and colleagues employed topical nifedipine (0.3%) with lidocaine ointment (1.5%) every 12 hours for 6 weeks in a prospective, randomized, double-blind study.[88] The control group received topical lidocaine ointment (1.5%) with hydrocortisone acetate (1%). They found a 94.5% incidence of healing in the nifedipine group

but only 16.4% of the controls had healed. A total of 110 patients with chronic anal fissure were entered into the trial.[88]

Diltiazem (DTZ) is another calcium channel blocker that has been proffered as an alternative for the treatment of chronic anal fissure. In a prospective assessment of 71 such patients, Knight and coworkers found a rate of healing of 75%.[57] They concluded that topical 2% DTZ has a high success rate. Jonas and colleagues employed DTZ in patients in whom GTN had failed.[49] Thirty-nine individuals were treated, with 49% healing within 8 weeks. Side effects included headache, drowsiness, mood swings, and perianal itching. The same group compared oral versus topical DTZ and noted that the topical application is more effective and is associated with fewer side effects.[48] Kocher and associates performed a randomized trial in which the side effects of GTN were compared with those of DTZ.[58] These investigators found no difference in healing rates, but because of much fewer side effects associated with DTZ (especially headache), they opined that DTZ "may be the preferred first-line treatment for chronic anal fissure."[58]

Despite the similar rates of healing between GTN and calcium channel blockers, Jonas and associates found 2% diltiazem ointment to be an effective treatment in patients who failed GTN treatment.[49] They found 44% healing in this group. The Standards Practice Task Force felt that anal fissures may be treated with topical calcium channel blockers, with (the expectation of) a lower incidence of adverse effects than topical nitrates. However, there are insufficient data to conclude whether they are superior to placebo in healing anal fissures.[89]

Botulinum Toxin

In 1993, Jost and Schimrigk, in a letter to the editor, originally reported the injection of botulinum toxin (BNT) into the anal sphincter as a new mode of treatment for anal fissure.[50] In a subsequent report involving 12 patients, two doses (each consisting of 0.1 mL of diluted toxin corresponding to 2.5 E BoTox; BoTox Allergan, Irvine, CA) were injected into the external anal sphincter on both sides lateral to the fissure.[51] Maria and coworkers conducted a double-blind, placebo-controlled study in 30 patients, with the use of saline injections for the control group.[69] They used 20 U of botulinum A for the treatment group. After 2 months, 11 individuals in the treated group had healed, whereas only 2 in the control group were healed ($P = .003$).

BNT is a powerful poison that inhibits neuromuscular transmission. While acting through a different mechanism than GTN, its beneficial effect should be to increase blood flow to the area. Some have warned that this drug needs greater regulation, with a careful review of the risks and benefits.[12] Although not common, side effects of its various applications have included increased urinary residual volume, heart block, skin and allergic reactions, muscle weakness, postural hypotension, and changes in heart rate and blood pressure.[12] A case of Fournier's gangrene has been reported after an injection of BNT.[117] Transient incontinence for flatus is not unusual.

Lindsey and colleagues employed BNT in a high-concentration, low-volume solution in the treatment of patients in whom GTN therapy had failed.[62] Two milliliters of 0.9% saline were injected into a 100-U vial of BNT, and a 0.4-mL aliquot was drawn into a 1-mL syringe. With the use of a 27-gauge needle, a solution of 0.2 mL was injected into the internal sphincter on either side but at some distance from the fissure.[62] With this "second-line therapy," approximately one-half of the fissures healed. The authors concluded as follows: "A policy of first line GTN and second line BNT . . . avoids surgical sphincterotomy and its risks *in the short term* [italics mine] in almost 90 percent of cases."[62] Others have concluded that although GTN and BNT have negligible side effects, the success rates are no better than 80% initially, dropping to 55% with longer term follow-up.[3] Samim et al. performed a double-blind, randomized, controlled trial in which BNT had a higher healing rate than that of topical diltiazem in the short term.[103] However, at 3 months, both groups were found to have equal rates of healing, and there were also no significant differences in pain reduction in either group. They concluded that there was not a significant advantage of one treatment over the other. In the systematic review by Poh et al., the healing rates with BNT in the literature range from 27% to 96%, with most studies reporting dosing between 20 and 25 U.[92] A systematic review by Yiannakopoulou concluded that BNT should be considered a treatment option for anal fissure.[117] However, he further stated that "well designed randomized trials are needed for the valid estimation of the efficacy and safety of botulinum toxin in this therapeutic indication."[117]

The Standards Practice Task Force comments that botulinum toxin injection has been associated with healing rates superior to that of a placebo.[89] However, they note that there is inadequate consensus on dosage, precise site of administration, number of injections, or efficacy.

Gonyautoxin is another agent that has been studied with promising results. Garrido and coworkers demonstrated 98% healing at 28 days, with only one recurrence at 14 months.[33] However, there is the absence of published experience from other centers.

Comment

The true efficacy of chemical sphincterotomy, whether topical or by injection, remains to be seen. There is no doubt that many patients benefit, at least in the short term. However, until better evidence from further clinical trials become available, chemical sphincterotomy will remain a reasonable alternative for the surgeon who evinces an interest in the management of anal fissure. But the surgical alternative should be considered, even initially, especially in those with severe pain.

The statement published by Helton in 2002, reflecting a consensus statement on behalf of a panel representing three organizations: the Society for Surgery of the Alimentary Tract, the American Gastroenterological Association, and the American Society for Gastrointestinal Endoscopy, has as much validity today.[43] The last version of this position statement reads in part, "Pharmacologic treatment should balance efficacy, short- and long-term side effects, convenience, and expense."[89] It further states that "surgery is consistently superior to medical therapy and may be offered without a pharmacological treatment failure."[89]

Surgical Management

The previously mentioned set of practice parameters devoted to the management of anal fissures was published by the Standards Practice Task Force of the American Society of Colon and Rectal Surgeons in 2010 (3rd revision).[89] This committee concluded that lateral internal sphincterotomy is the surgical treatment of choice for refractory anal fissures. Still, reasonable surgeons believe that there are preferred alternatives to this operation for reasons that will be discussed next.

The choice of operative approach to the treatment of anal fissure depends on the duration of symptoms and on the physical findings. For an acute anal fissure without a tag, hypertrophied papilla, or significant hemorrhoids, the two procedures that have historically been advocated are sphincter stretch and internal anal sphincterotomy. For chronic anal fissure with an external component, or when the condition is associated with symptomatic large hemorrhoids, at least partial excisional therapy with sphincterotomy is the preferred option.

Sphincter Stretch

Sphincter stretch was originally described by Récamier in 1838 for the treatment of proctalgia fugax and for anal fissure. The procedure can be carried out with a local infiltration, but a brief general anesthetic is preferable. An ambulatory surgical facility is ideal. The patient is placed in the lithotomy position; sterile draping is unnecessary. There are incorrect (Figure 12-9) and correct methods (Figure 12-10) for performing sphincter stretch. The index finger of one hand is inserted into the rectum, followed by the index finger of the opposite hand. Gentle lateral retraction with each finger

---

JEAN-CLAUDE-ANTHELME RÉCAMIER (1774–1852)

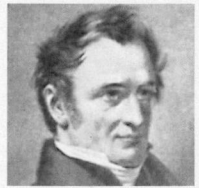

Récamier was born at Rochefort-en-Bugey to a well-educated, important local family. He studied medicine at the Belley Hospital and then at Bourg, where he was called for military service. In 1797, he went to Paris, and in 1806, at the age of 33, he became chief physician at the Hôtel-Dieu. He became interested in diseases of women and is considered a pioneer in gynecologic surgery, inventing the cylindric vaginal speculum and the bivalve speculum. His interest in uterine cancer led him to perform the first colpohysterectomy in 1829. He introduced the curette in the treatment of endometritis and incised pelvic abscesses through the posterior cul-de-sac. He is also recognized as the first person to apply forcible dilatation in the treatment of anal fissure. Récamier was named as one of the original members of the L'Académie Nationale de Médecine when it was founded in 1820. He was later appointed professor in the faculty of medicine, and in 1826, he succeeded Laennec to the chair of the College of France. He died of apoplexy. (Récamier JCA. Extension, massage et percussion cadencée dans le traitement des contractures musculaires. *Rev Med Fr.* 1838;1:74. Originally published in English in: *Dis Colon Rectum.* 1980;23(5):362–367.)

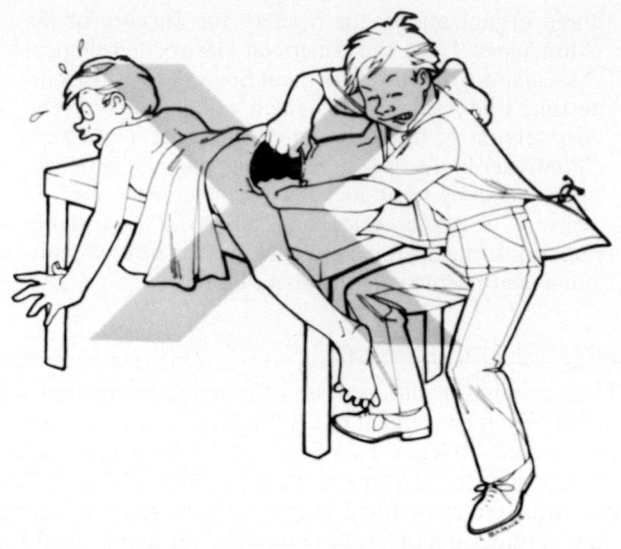

FIGURE 12-9. Incorrect technique for performing a sphincter stretch. A meticulous routine is required, not merely avulsion or distraction of the anal outlet.

commences for approximately 30 seconds. The long finger is inserted and then the other long finger. With four fingers in place, the anal canal is stretched (massaged) cautiously for 4 minutes. In men, it is easier to stretch the sphincter in the anteroposterior plane because of the narrowness of the pelvic outlet. Sphincter stretch in women, however, should always be performed in the transverse plane (if undertaken at all). Narrowness is not a concern, but disruption of anterior sphincteric support is a real possibility.

Results

Watts and associates performed sphincter stretch for anal fissure in 99 patients.[115] All were followed for at least 5 months. Three-fourths of the patients achieved symptomatic relief within 48 hours; pain was resolved within 2 weeks in 20%. Six patients continued to have a fissure, although two were free of pain, and in five others recurrent discomfort developed without evidence of fissure. The most troublesome complication in this series was related to control, usually for flatus alone but occasionally for feces. Some swelling was also reported. Twenty-eight percent were noted to have at least one of these complaints.

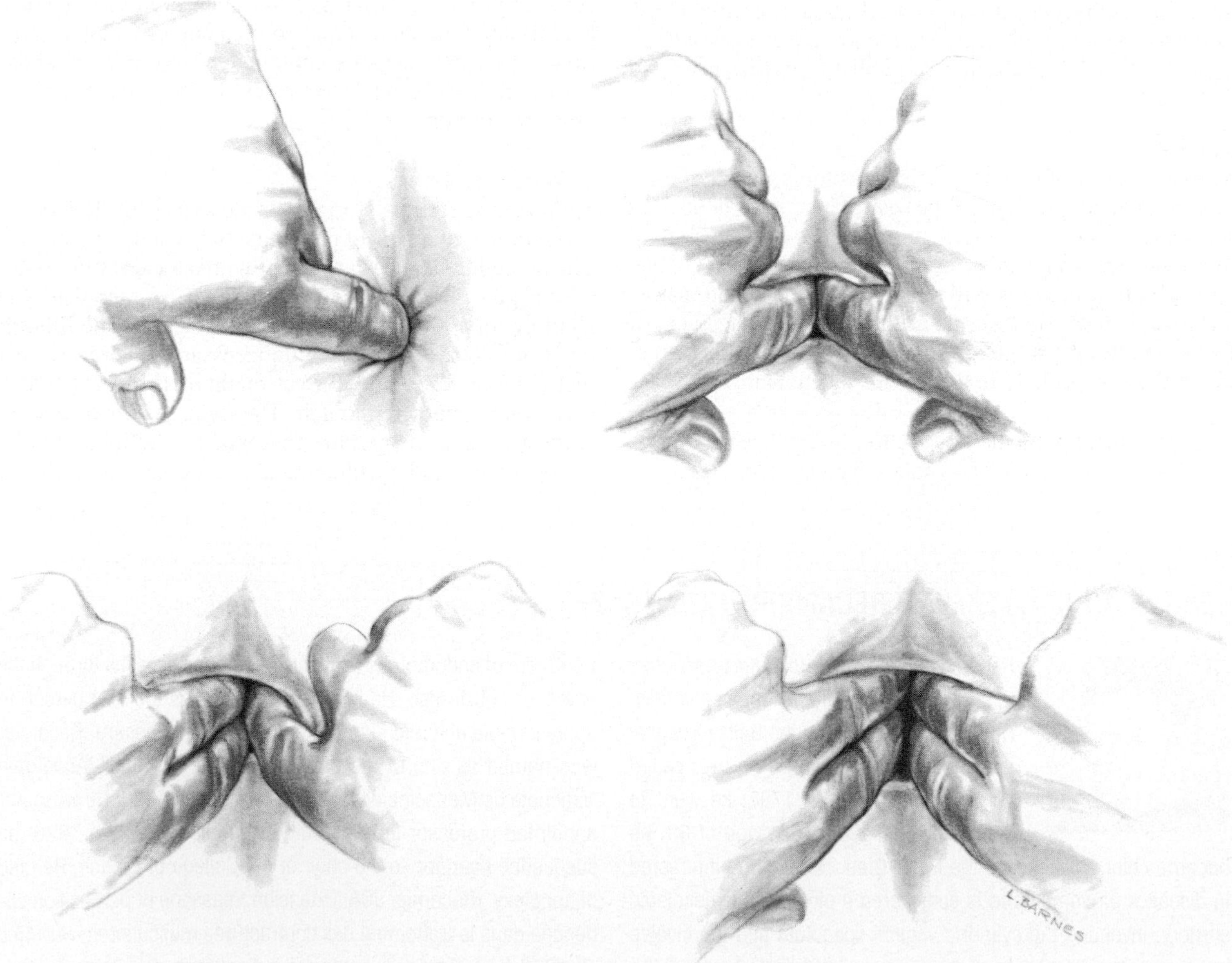

FIGURE 12-10. Proper approach to performing a sphincter stretch. Male patients may require an anteroposterior stretch because of the limitations of a narrow outlet and close approximation of the ischial spines. Female patients should always undergo a lateral stretch.

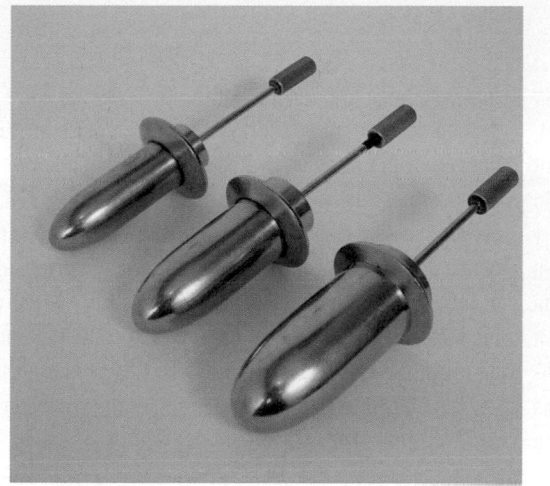 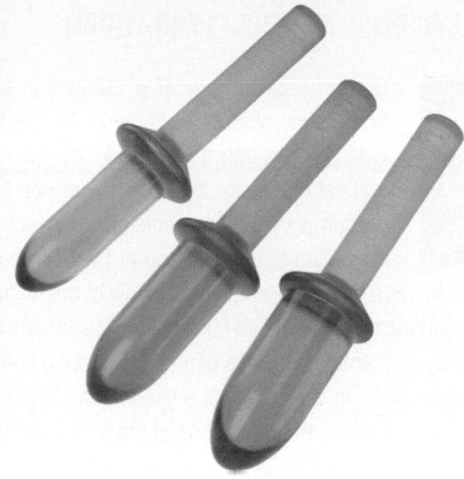

FIGURE 12-11. Sohn's dilators. **A:** Original stainless steel instruments in three sizes: 30 mm, 35 mm, and 40 mm. **B:** The amber-colored instruments are made of a lightweight autoclavable plastic called "polysulfone." (Courtesy of Arnold R. Leiboff, MD.)

Sohn and colleagues precisely performed anorectal sphincter dilatation with a Parks retractor opened to 4.8 cm or with a 40-mm balloon.[107] The dilatations were sustained for exactly 5 minutes. The cure rates were 93% and 94%, respectively. There was no incident of incontinence in the latter group (66 patients). Two of 105 with the Parks dilatation noted incontinence.

It seemed, at least from the literature, that interest in sphincter stretch had been waning, but in recent years, there has been a recrudescent interest in "controlled dilatation" as a means of avoiding incontinence and leakage problems. Sohn's dilators have been developed for this purpose (Figure 12-11—Tools for Surgery, Stony Brook, NY). Others have described and recommended endoscopic anal dilatation, with results comparable with that of lateral sphincterotomy while limiting the risk of incontinence.[86,118] Balloon dilatation has also been advocated as a simple and safe procedure.[96,97,112]

Sphincter injury after anal dilatation has been assessed by anal endosonography.[79,109] In those individuals complaining of fecal incontinence, fragmentation or disruption of the internal sphincter is usually observed, in addition to defects in the external sphincter (Figure 12-12).[109] Sphincteric defects were found in 11 of 18 incontinent patients in a University of Copenhagen study.[79] However, as implied from the previous discussion, manometric evaluation following balloon dilatation is not associated with the degree of sphincteric damage that manual sphincter stretch often produces.[96]

As discussed in Chapter 6, antibiotic prophylaxis should be considered with any patient who cannot afford an infection. Goldman and colleagues evaluated 100 patients who underwent anal dilatation for fissure and noted positive blood cultures in 8%.[36] There appeared to be some correlation with the extent of trauma as determined by the levels of elevation of serum muscle enzymes.

Internal Anal Sphincterotomy

In 1839, Brodie was the first person to perform an anal sphincterotomy. He advocated the operation for "preternatural contraction of the anal sphincter." In 1863, Hilton also suggested that the treatment for anal ulcer should be sphincterotomy. However, Miles (see Biography, Chapter 24) is usually credited as the surgeon who gave the operation real

credence, although Miles believed that he was dividing what he called "the pecten band."[38,75] In 1951, Eisenhammer was the first person to advocate internal anal sphincterotomy for anal fissure and to truly understand which muscle he was dividing.[22]

The internal anal sphincter is the continuation of the distal portion of the circular muscle of the rectum (see Figure 11-2). Its length is essentially equal to that of the anal canal. Distally, it can usually be felt medial to the intersphincteric groove outside the anal verge. The subcutaneous portion of the external sphincter is lateral to the groove.

The internal sphincter maintains the anal canal in the closed position; action is involuntary. The external sphincter is a striated muscle. The external sphincter and the levator ani are the muscles involved in voluntary control. Complete division of the internal anal sphincter is possible without

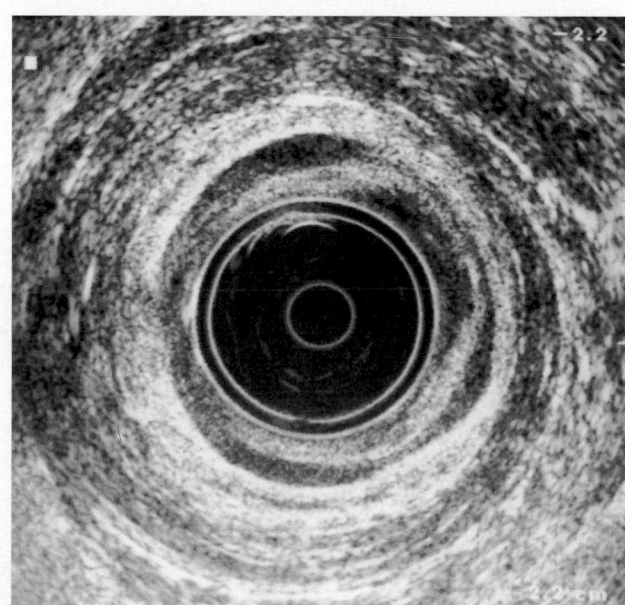

FIGURE 12-12. A fragmented internal anal sphincter can be appreciated in this endorectal ultrasonogram. (Courtesy of C. I. Bartram, MD, Department of Radiology, St. Mark's Hospital, Harrow, United Kingdom.)

BENJAMIN COLLINS BRODIE (1783–1862)

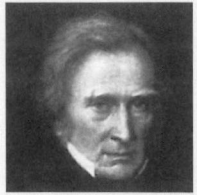

Brodie was the son of a clergyman in Winterslow, Wiltshire, England. In 1798, when he was only 15 years old, he fought against Napoleon. In 1801, he decided to pursue a career in medicine, eventually becoming house surgeon at St. George's Hospital in 1822. In 1810, he was elected as a fellow of the Royal Society after presenting a paper entitled "Dissection of a Fetus." It was because of this presentation that he began to achieve a considerable reputation, not only as a surgical anatomist but also as a writer and speaker. In 1813, Brodie described the joint disease that was later to bear his name. So universal were his writings that he seemed as comfortable discussing the subject of the influence of the nervous system on the production of animal heat as describing the pathology of anal fissure. In 1828, he became surgeon to King George IV. He held many prestigious positions, including president of the Medico-Chirurgical Society and president of the General Medical Council. He was the first surgeon to hold the position of president of the Royal Society. He died of a malignant disease, probably sarcoma, that originated in his shoulder. (Brodie BC. Preternatural contraction of the sphincter ani. *London Med Gazette*. 1835;16:26.)

JOHN HILTON (1805–1878)

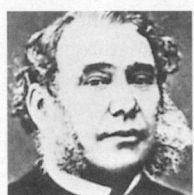

Hilton was born in the village of Sible Hedingham in Essex, England. He was accepted at Guy's Hospital, and after completing his studies, he was appointed as a demonstrator in anatomy. During this period, he recognized that an inflamed joint not only referred pain to the skin over it but also caused muscle spasms that immobilized and protected the joint from further injury; this phenomenon became known as Hilton's law. In 1844, Hilton was appointed assistant surgeon at Guy's Hospital and was promoted to full surgeon in 1849. He was one of the first surgeons to advocate a lumbar colostomy, and in 1846, he performed one of the first recorded operations for the relief of strangulated hernia. In 1860, Hilton was appointed professor of Anatomy and Surgery at the Royal College of Surgeons. In 1863, he presented 18 lectures, including one on the treatment of anal ulcer in which he mentions that the internal sphincter can be transected safely using the whitish area over the groove between the internal and external sphincters as a landmark (i.e., the white line of Hilton). Unfortunately, this incorrectly became synonymous with the mucocutaneous junction. (Hilton J. *On the Influence of Mechanical and Physiological Rest in the Treatment of Accidents and Surgical Diseases, and the Diagnostic Value of Pain*. London, United Kingdom: *Bell & Daldy*; 1863:279. Reprinted in part by Bonello JC. Classic articles in colonic and rectal surgery. John Hilton 1805-1878. On the influence of mechanical and physiological rest in the treatment of accidents and surgical diseases, and the diagnostic value of pain. *Dis Colon Rectum*. 1987;30(4):304–313.)

STEPHEN EISENHAMMER (1906–1995)

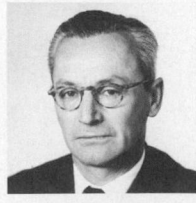

Eisenhammer was born in Middleburg, Cape Province, South Africa, of parents of Viennese descent and grew up on a farm in what was then Southern Rhodesia. He began his medical studies at the University of Cape Town before moving to the University of Edinburgh, Scotland, from which he graduated in 1930. After various surgical appointments, he became house surgeon and resident surgical officer at St. Mark's Hospital. At the outbreak of World War II, he joined the London Emergency Medical War Services before returning to South Africa, where in 1942 he joined the South African Medical Corps, seeing service in Madagascar. In 1944, he started private practice in Johannesburg with the decision to specialize in proctology. In spite of not having a teaching appointment at any hospital or medical school, he proved to be a prolific researcher and writer in his chosen field. Beginning in the 1950s, he began to make notable contributions to a better understanding of hemorrhoids, anal fistula, anal abscess, and the application of internal anal sphincterotomy for fissure. In 1962, he was elected an honorary member of the Section of Proctology of the Royal Society of Medicine. He continued researching and publishing into the mid-1980s, by which time he was well into his 70s. (Photograph and biographic information courtesy of John Eisenhammer and with special appreciation to Gary R. Gecelter, MD.)

creating significant impairment of fecal continence.[23] The reader is referred to Chapters 1, 2, and 16 for further discussion on the anatomy and physiology of the sphincter mechanism.

Technique

The procedure of internal anal sphincterotomy has classically been performed in the posterior midline. Although this approach usually cures the condition, it is associated with the complication of the so-called keyhole deformity (see Complications section). Bennett and Goligher reported a high incidence of impairment for flatus with posterior internal anal sphincterotomy (34%) and a 15% incidence of difficulty controlling feces.[9] After a time, however, further improvement was evident, with a cure rate of 93%, but an appreciable morbidity remained.

Eisenhammer advocated the lateral position for sphincterotomy, dividing one-half of the muscle in an open fashion.[23] In 1969, Notaras reported a technique using a narrow-bladed scalpel to perform an internal anal sphincterotomy in a closed fashion in the lateral position.[80] In 66 patients treated, he reported a 6% incidence of fecal soiling. Notaras subsequently described his procedure in detail by a technique in which he employed a scalpel used for cataract surgery.[81,82] His method involved submucosal insertion of a knife, followed by an outward incision to the intersphincteric groove. This has the advantage of minimizing the risk of mucosal injury, but it has at least the theoretical disadvantage of one not knowing how deep to cut, risking injury to the external sphincter.

The procedure can be performed in the office using a local anesthetic (e.g., 0.5% bupivacaine [Marcaine] in 1:200,000 epinephrine) or in an ambulatory surgical facility, using a short-acting general anesthetic, spinal anesthetic, or local with conscious sedation. If the former method is used, the patient may be placed in stirrups, in the left lateral position, or in the prone jackknife position, depending on the surgeon's preference and the availability of the appropriate table. Women are obviously more accustomed to the lithotomy stirrups and are more tolerant of assuming that position. Men, however, are usually quite self-conscious, if not downright obstreperous, in the lithotomy position. If there is any concern that the patient may not tolerate the procedure in the office, it should be scheduled with the support of anesthesia.

In the office the fissure is infiltrated, as well as the site for insertion of the knife—either the right lateral or left lateral position. A narrow anal retractor (e.g., Hill-Ferguson) is employed. The intersphincteric groove is usually easily felt (Figure 12-13), and the knife blade is inserted into the left lateral aspect (Figure 12-14A). Some surgeons use a No. 11 blade, scissors (by the open technique; see later), or a hooked knife, but a Beaver (catalog no. 375220, Becton Dickinson and Company, Franklin Lakes, NJ) cataract blade (size 25.5 × 2.2 mm) is preferable. The knife is used as a stiletto and creates a very small wound. For a left-handed surgeon, operating on the right lateral aspect is easier. There is a theoretical advantage in cutting on the right side because the hemorrhoid sites are usually in the anterior and posterior positions, but it requires a right-handed surgeon to operate backhanded, depending on the patient's position, of course. Therefore, I perform the sphincterotomy on the patient's left and accept the increased risk for a hematoma if the left lateral pile is lacerated. The foregoing admonitions refer to a patient placed in the lithotomy position.

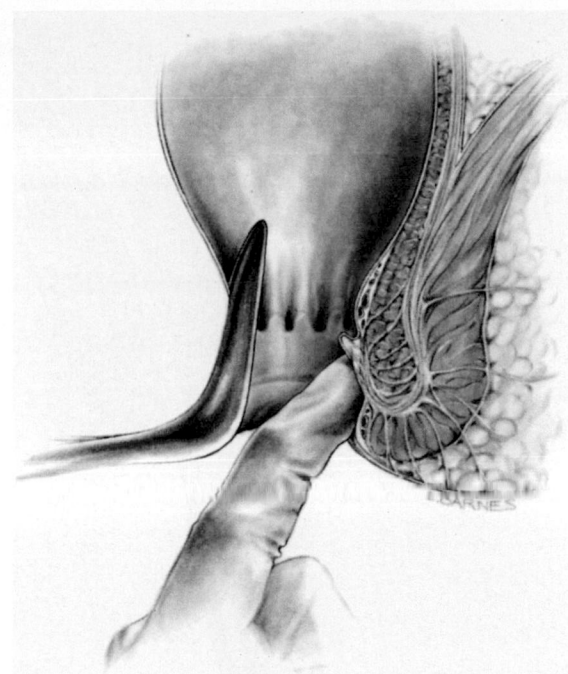

FIGURE 12-13. Digital examination to identify the intersphincteric groove. The novice should practice palpating the groove on numerous asymptomatic patients before embarking on closed sphincterotomy. The location of the groove can be quite variable. The finger may be used to protect the external sphincter as the knife blade is inserted.

The tip of the blade is angled medially (Figure 12-14B), pointing just above the dentate line, and the lower one-third to one-half of the internal anal sphincter is divided. When the knife is seen beneath the intact anal mucosa, it is withdrawn. The side of the finger is then used to break any residual sphincter fibers (Figure 12-14C). If the physician pushes with the fingertip, there is a tendency to tear the mucosa, which may then lead to bleeding and possibly the subsequent development of a fistula. If bleeding occurs at the wound puncture site, it can be readily controlled by a few moments of direct pressure. If a tag or papilla is present, it can be removed by excision with scissors or electrocautery. No dressings are required, and the patient is discharged when alert.

An alternative approach is to undertake the operation without a retractor in place. The index finger senses the knife blade beneath the anal mucosa, and the residual internal anal sphincter fibers are broken by the side of the finger (Figure 12-15).

Another variation of the lateral sphincterotomy is the open technique. This, too, can be performed either in the office or in the hospital. The disadvantages are that it takes longer to perform and usually requires suturing. Many surgeons prefer this approach in order to visualize the internal and the external sphincter directly for security of anatomy.

A small, radial incision is made laterally, at the lower border of the internal sphincter and continued into the intersphincteric groove (Figure 12-16). Alternatively, a curvilinear incision outside the anal verge can be used. Because of the open wound and the possibility of bleeding, it is helpful to infiltrate the area with a local anesthetic containing epinephrine solution. The distal internal sphincter is grasped with forceps and bluntly freed. The lower one-third to one-half is divided with scissors. The wound is closed with absorbable suture material, and a small dressing is applied.

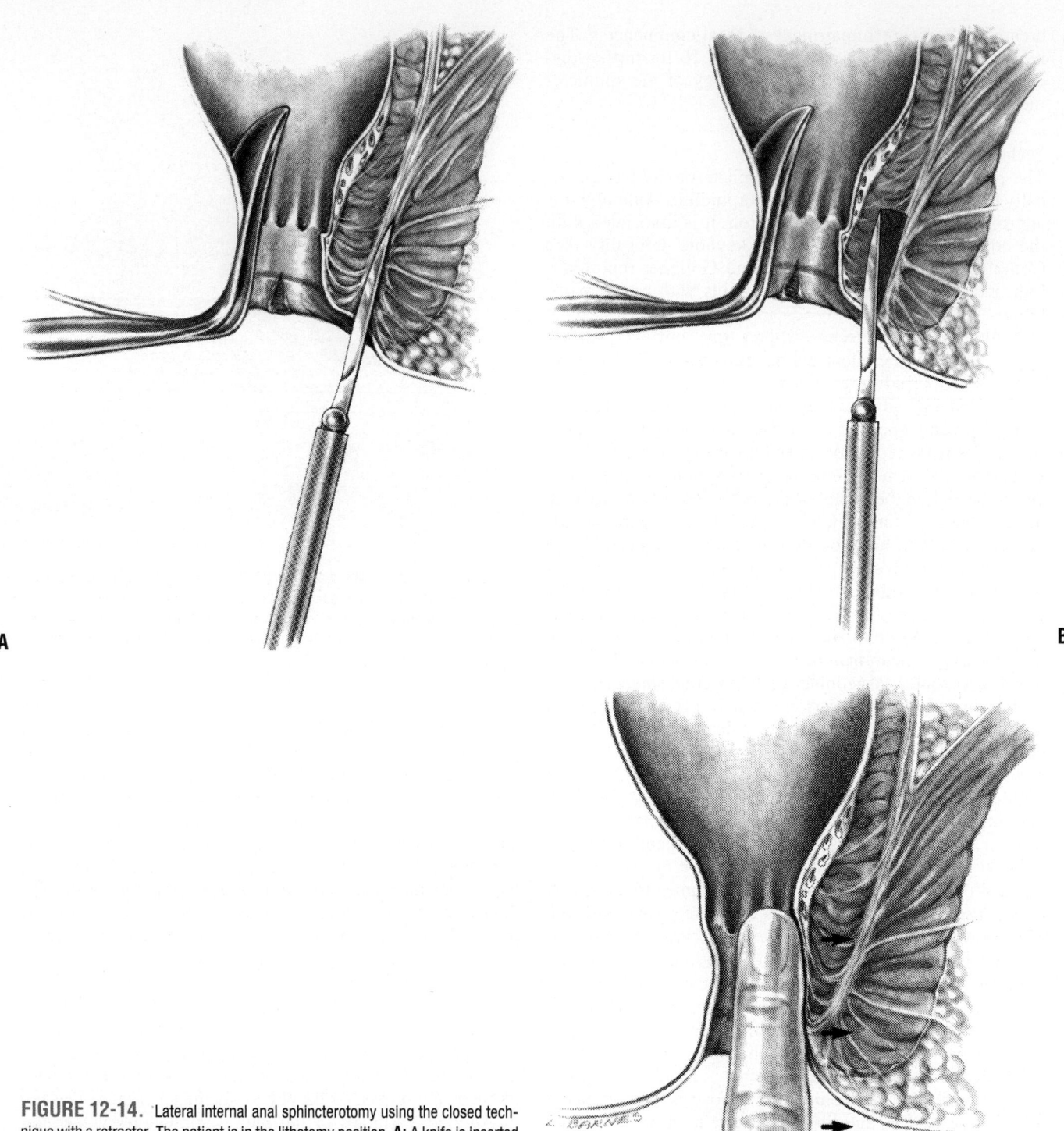

A

B

C

FIGURE 12-14. Lateral internal anal sphincterotomy using the closed technique with a retractor. The patient is in the lithotomy position. **A:** A knife is inserted into the intersphincteric groove. **B:** The lower one-third to one-half of the internal sphincter is divided. **C:** The residual fibers are broken with the finger.

Postoperative Care
Warm (sitz) baths and a mild analgesic are the only postoperative measures advised. Pain is often less than that experienced preoperatively, and most patients resume their normal activities within 48 to 72 hours.

Complications
Surgery for anal fissure is associated with numerous complications, most of which are preventable by the application of judicious surgical technique and, of course, by familiarity with anorectal anatomy.

Ecchymosis is frequently noted around the entrance wound if the closed technique is used, but this is of no concern. A *hematoma* is rare and usually the result of failure to apply adequate pressure to the site. Likewise, *hemorrhage* is extremely unusual by either the closed or open method, but is much more likely to occur with the open procedure. Suture ligation may be required.

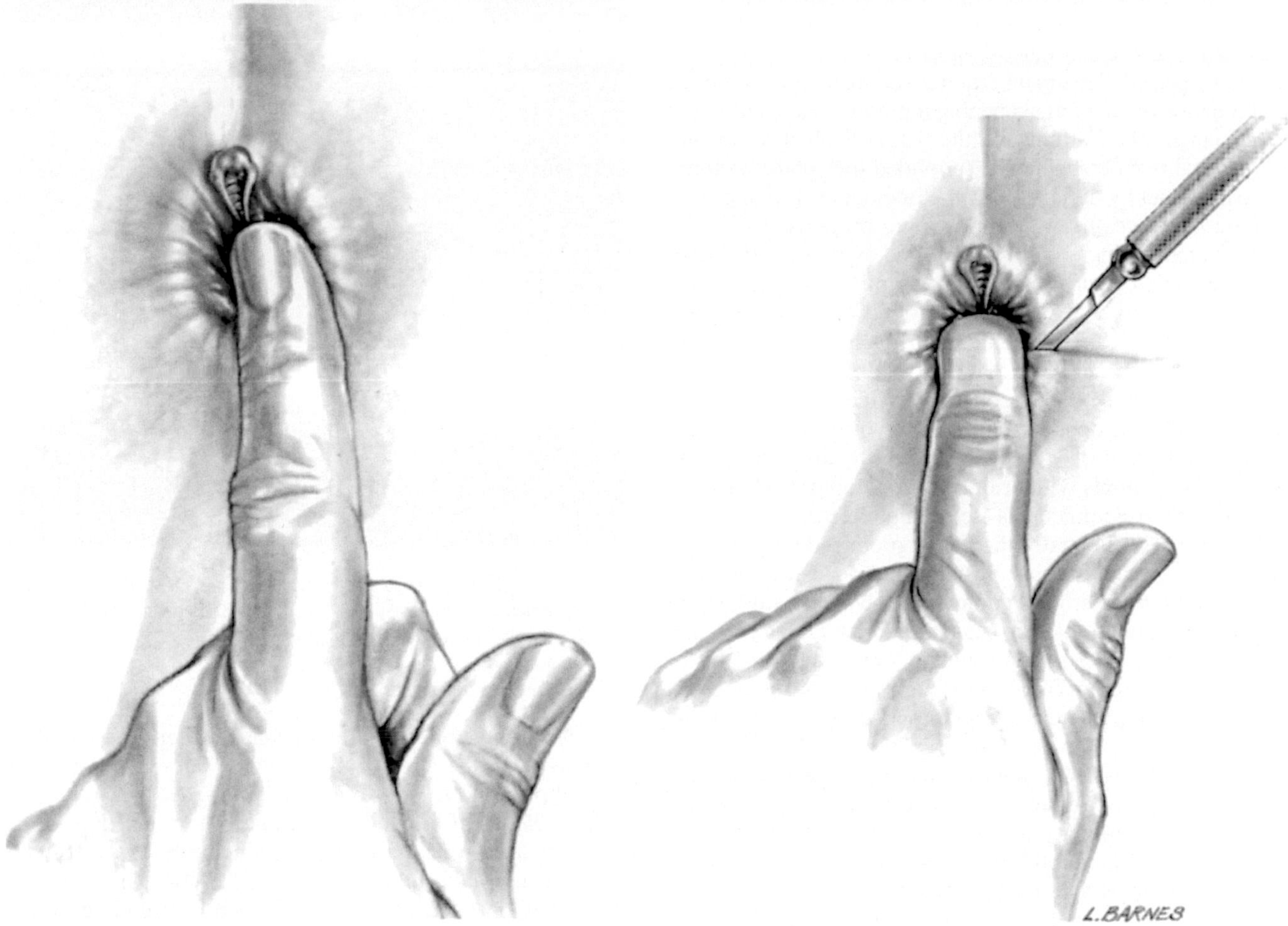

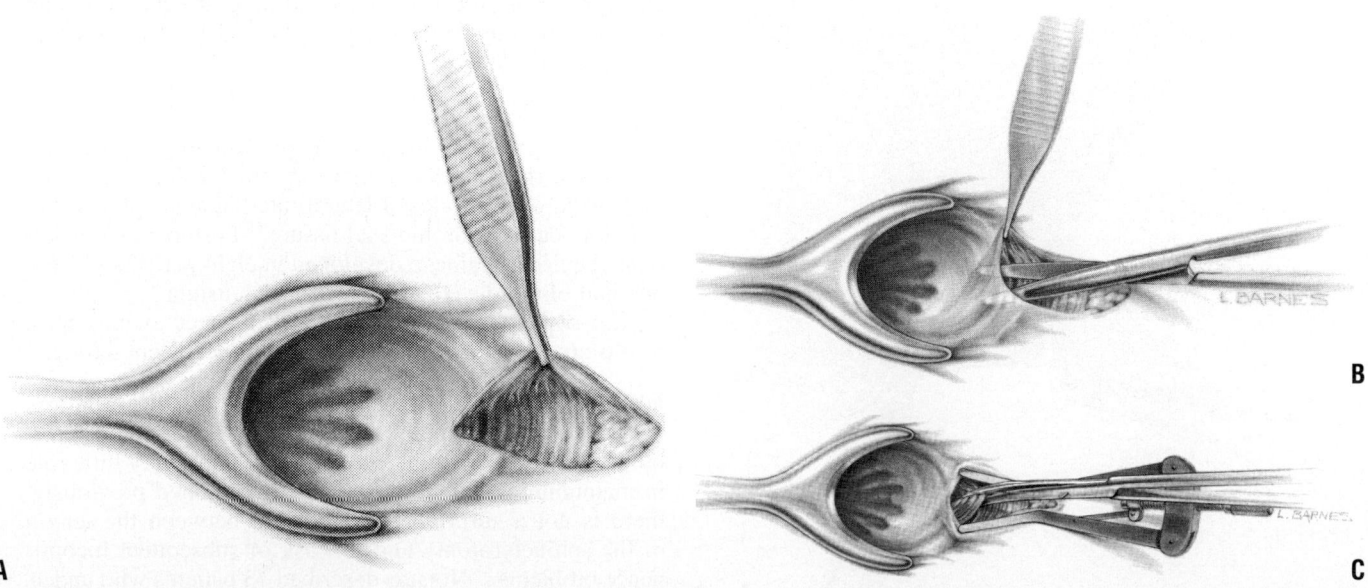

FIGURE 12-15.   Lateral internal anal sphincterotomy using the closed technique, no retractor, and a local anesthetic. **A:** A finger is inserted into the anal canal after anesthesia is established. **B:** The sphincterotomy is performed with the finger in place.

FIGURE 12-16.   Lateral internal anal sphincterotomy using the open technique with the patient placed in the lateral or the prone (i.e., jackknife) position. **A:** A radial incision is made across the intersphincteric groove. A narrow Hill-Ferguson retractor is in place. **B:** The internal sphincter is separated from the anoderm by blunt dissection. **C:** The internal sphincter is divided. The wound may be closed or left open.

Perianal *abscess* occurs after 1% of closed internal anal sphincterotomies. It is virtually always associated with an anal fistula. This presumably is the result of penetration of the mucosa of the anal canal by the knife blade (Figure 12-17). It is surprising that this complication is not seen more frequently because the anal canal mucosa must be breached more often than is suspected. Treatment requires drainage of the abscess, identification of an internal opening if present, and fistulotomy (see Chapter 14). Fortunately, the fistula is always low and submucosal or intersphincteric, provided the sphincterotomy was carried out by dividing only the internal anal sphincter.

True *fecal incontinence* following a properly performed internal anal sphincterotomy should be extraordinarily rare. However, as is discussed later, it is not that unusual for a patient to experience *soiling* of underclothes and *incontinence for flatus*. This is a particular problem in some women. Sultan and colleagues note that the performance of an internal anal sphincterotomy frequently divides more sphincter in women than it does in men.[110] They attribute this to the shorter anal canal of women. Particular caution should be exercised in patients with prior obstetric trauma and in those women with an ectopic anus (see Chapter 16).

Figure 12-18 illustrates the defect produced by lateral internal anal sphincterotomy through the means of endoanal ultrasonography. García-Aguilar and coworkers studied the anatomic and functional consequences of lateral internal anal sphincterotomy in 13 patients with incontinence and 13 who had no such symptoms.[31] The only significant difference was that incontinent patients had undergone longer sphincterotomies. The fact that the external sphincter was also thinner in the incontinent patients suggests that a preoperative abnormality predisposed some to an increased risk of fecal incontinence, a problem that became unmasked by the addition of internal anal sphincterotomy. Menteş and coworkers undertook a study by using an anal calibrator up to a diameter of 30 mm in a randomized, prospective fashion to "control" the

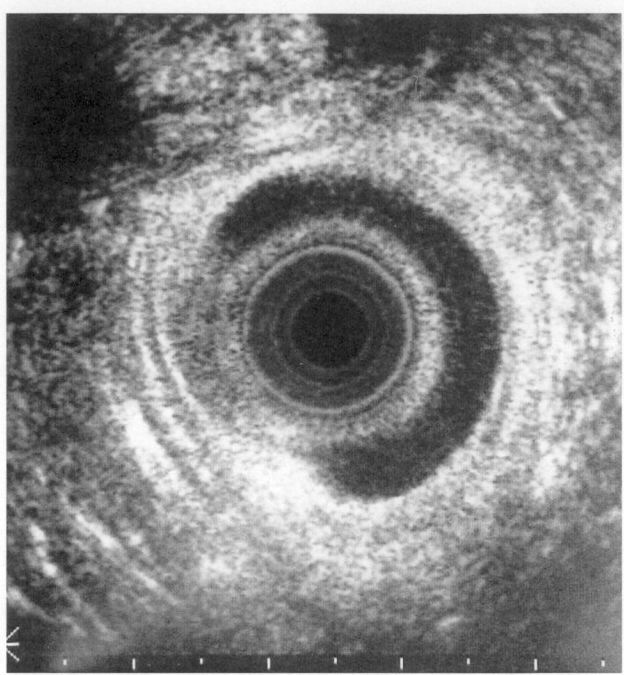

FIGURE 12-18. Ultrasonography demonstrates internal sphincter defect following sphincterotomy. (Courtesy of C. I. Bartram, MD, Department of Radiology, St. Mark's Hospital, Harrow, United Kingdom.)

sphincterotomy for a specific distance rather than carrying the incision to the apex of the fissure.[73] They noted a faster relief of pain and a lower rate of incontinence.

A *keyhole deformity* is a troublesome consequence of fissure excision or internal anal sphincterotomy performed in the posterior midline (see Figure 11-76). The resultant defect may produce symptoms of mucous discharge, pruritus, and soiling of undergarments. Excision of an uncomplicated acute fissure with a posterior midline sphincterotomy should be avoided; a lateral internal anal sphincterotomy is preferred (Figure 12-19). With persistent symptoms despite an appropriate bowel management program and cleansing methods, the deformity may be treated by an anoplasty (see Chapter 11).

Results

Infection. The primary initial concern following sphincterotomy is the risk of infection. We reported 350 patients who underwent open or closed lateral internal anal sphincterotomy for acute or chronic anal fissure.[61] Postoperative infections requiring drainage developed in eight patients (2.3%); one-half of these were associated with a fistula.

The two concerning issues with respect to long-term results are incontinence and recurrent or persistent fissure.

Incontinence. Complete fecal incontinence (i.e., the total loss of bowel control) should not occur following sphincterotomy because the internal anal sphincter plays very little role in maintaining anal continence. As mentioned previously, there is not a surprising relationship between the length of the sphincterotomy and the risk of subsequent incontinence problems.[31] Notaras described 73 patients who underwent this procedure and found 4 who experienced soiling of the underclothes, 2 who had imperfect control of flatus, and 1 who had occasional fecal soilage.[81] This last patient

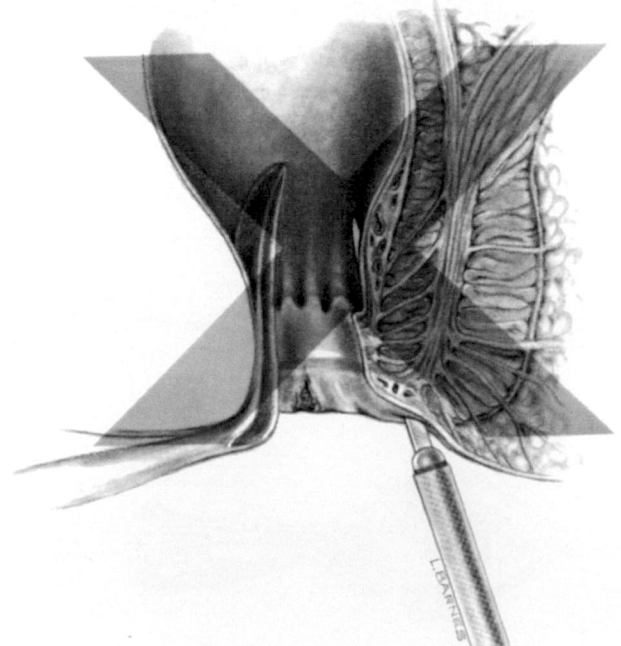

FIGURE 12-17. Sphincterotomy that penetrates through the anal mucosa may result in anal abscess and fistula.

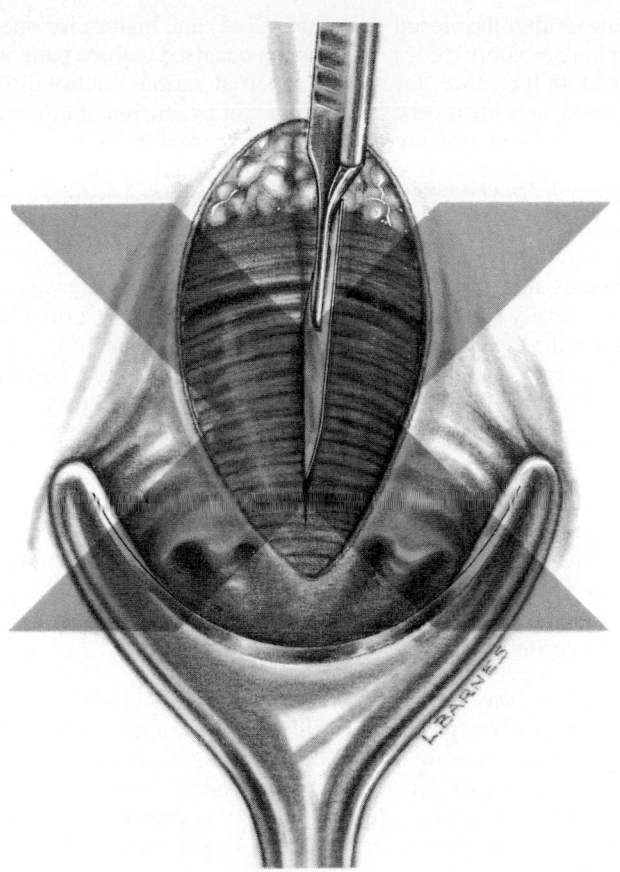

FIGURE 12-19. Excision of a fissure with posterior internal anal sphincterotomy is not a recommended technique.

was thought to have been a poor candidate for the procedure. Millar reported either a mucous discharge or flatus-control problems in 3 of 99 patients treated.[76] Hoffmann and Goligher noted that 12 of 99 patients had some minor deficiency of anal control.[44] Pernikoff and colleagues reviewed 500 patients who underwent internal anal sphincterotomy and identified fecal incontinence in 8%.[87] In our experience, 60 individuals (17%) complained of incontinence for flatus or for stool, but for two-thirds this was transient.[61]

It is probably wise to record the patient's preoperative bowel control status, especially if there is some degree of impairment reported during the preoperative interview. However, if significant incontinence does supervene, it is most likely the result of inadvertent or inappropriate division of a portion of the external sphincter. This may occur with the closed technique (Figure 12-20) or with the open method (Figure 12-21). If symptoms warrant, apposition or overlapping of the divided muscle will usually ameliorate the problem (see Chapter 16).

Recurrence. The incidence of delayed healing or recurrence is the standard of measurement for the success or failure of the operation. Millar reported that 88% of patients were healed at 2 weeks, and 100% healed eventually.[76] Hoffman and Goligher noted that 2% were unhealed at 9 months.[44] Notaras and Ray and colleagues had an astounding rate of healing of 100%.[81,94] Marya and colleagues reported a 2% incidence of nonhealing, and Gingold noted a rate of approximately 4%.[35,70] Rudd evaluated 200 patients and found only one unhealed; Crohn's disease subsequently developed in that person.[101] In the experience of Pernikoff and coworkers, 1% failed to heal.[87]

If the fissure persists despite conservative therapy (e.g., sitz baths, stool softeners), repeat sphincterotomy, during which a more generous portion of the internal sphincter is divided,

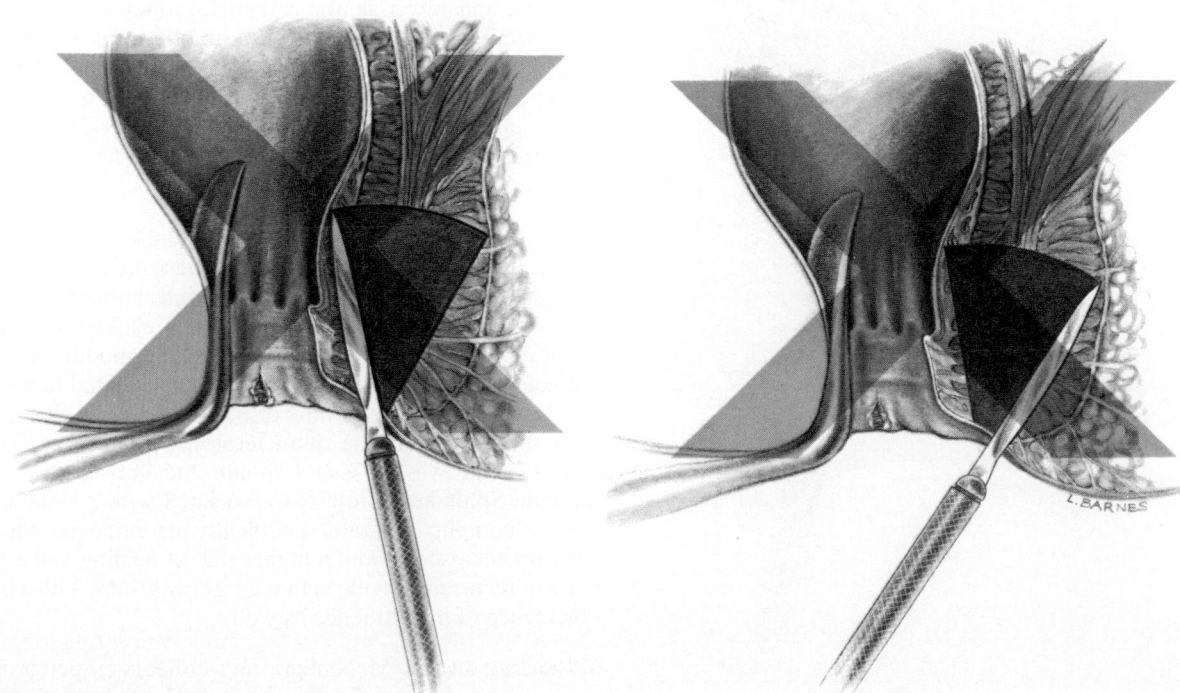

FIGURE 12-20. Incorrect closed internal anal sphincterotomy. **A:** The external sphincter can be divided inadvertently if the incision is made toward the anal canal. **B:** The risk for injury is even greater with a lateral incision.

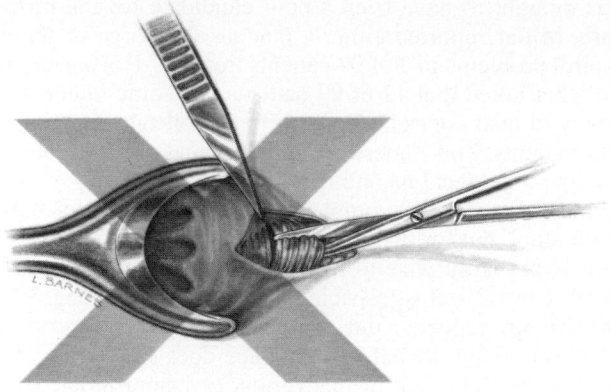

FIGURE 12-21. Improper open "external" anal sphincterotomy. Simply opening the area to visualize the site for sphincterotomy does not guarantee the absence of complications. Knowledge of the anatomy is still a requisite.

is the appropriate treatment (Figure 12-22). If healing still does not take place, the patient should undergo gastrointestinal investigation to seek for the possibility of concurrent inflammatory bowel disease, assuming that this had not been accomplished previously (see Anal Fissure and Crohn's Disease section).

Open versus Closed. Walker and colleagues reviewed their experience with lateral internal anal sphincterotomy for anal fissure and stenosis in more than 300 patients.[113] Sphincterotomy was performed by several techniques (open, closed, multiple) and under diverse circumstances, so it is difficult to interpret the results. It is apparent, however, that complications were

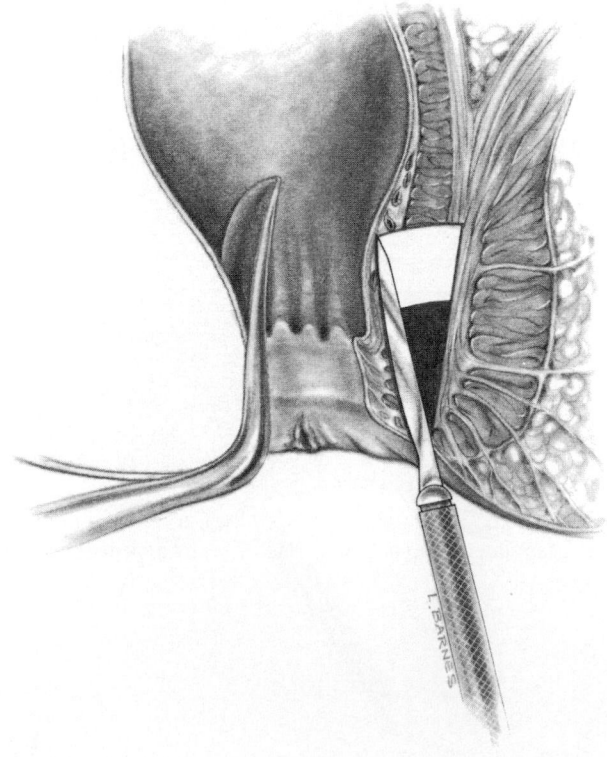

FIGURE 12-22. An anal fissure that fails to heal within a reasonable time may be treated by a more generous internal anal sphincterotomy.

lowest after the closed procedure (20%) and highest for open sphincterotomy (55%). Anal fistula occurred in three patients (1%). In the entire series, 15% reported various control difficulties, and when very strict criteria for evaluation of morbidity were used, minor complications occurred in 36%.

In our reported experience mentioned earlier, 21 of 350 patients (6%) failed to heal or had a recurrence during the follow-up period (mean = 14 months).[61] Five subsequently were found to have Crohn's disease. Excluding these individuals, the incidence of nonhealing was 4.6%. There was no statistically significant difference in healing rate or morbidity when the open was compared with the closed method.

Nelson undertook an analysis of 19 publications encompassing 3,083 patients to determine whether a preferred technique could be identified.[78] He concluded as follows:

- Anal stretch is associated with a higher risk of persistent fissure.
- Anal stretch has a higher risk for minor incontinence.
- There is no difference in complication rate between open and closed sphincterotomy.
- Open and closed sphincterotomies are equally efficacious in curing anal fissure.

Anesthetic Type. Keighley and associates compared lateral sphincterotomy performed with a local anesthetic versus lateral sphincterotomy undertaken with a general anesthetic.[54] They found a 50% incidence of delayed healing with a local and a 3% incidence after a general anesthetic. They concluded that the operation should not be performed with local infiltration.

Sphincterotomy versus Nitroglycerin. A randomized, controlled trial was undertaken by the Canadian Colorectal Surgical Trials Group.[98] This involved 82 patients who were assessed at 6 weeks and 6 months. The study concluded that internal anal sphincterotomy is superior to topical nitroglycerin paste (NG) (0.25%), with a high rate of healing, few side effects, and low risk for early incontinence.[98] In another prospective trial from Australia involving 65 patients, the results and the recommendations were similar.[26] Although NG paste healed the majority of anal fissures, many patients experienced little improvement or developed side effects that required subsequent sphincterotomy. Some fissures recurred after initially healing with NG.

Sphincterotomy versus Botulinum Toxin. Mentes and colleagues undertook a prospective, randomized trial in which internal anal sphincterotomy was compared with BNT.[74] In the BNT group (n = 61), a single injection resulted in complete healing in 74% of patients at the second month. A second injection, in those willing to undergo it, resulted in an overall healing rate at 6 months of 87%. At 1 year, the success rate fell to 75%. In the sphincterotomy group (n = 50), the success rate was 82% at 1 month and 98% at the second month. Sphincterotomy was associated with a significantly higher complication rate, specifically incontinence. Nasr and coworkers also showed a higher rate of healing and a lower rate of recurrence in the sphincterotomy group, with a higher incidence of incontinence as well.[77]

Physiologic Studies. McNamara and colleagues performed a prospective, anorectal, manometric evaluation on 13 patients before and after closed internal anal sphincterotomy.[72] As expected, the resting pressure fell to normal levels following successful operation, which suggests that it is the internal anal sphincter that is responsible for the preoperative resting pressure elevation. Many investigators have concluded that healing of the anal fissure is a consequence of reduced anal pressure.[105]

García-Granero and associates used anal endosonography to evaluate the extent of internal anal sphincter division following closed sphincterotomy to determine its role with respect to recurrence and incontinence.[32] They found that significant symptomatic recurrence was associated with an incomplete sphincterotomy.

Children. Cohen and Dehn performed lateral subcutaneous sphincterotomy on 23 *children* (between the ages of 8 and 168 months).[17] All were healed by 8 weeks.

▶ CHRONIC ANAL FISSURE

Chronic anal fissure usually produces symptoms of pain and bleeding, but the pain is not as severe as that with an acute fissure. Frequently, the patient's symptoms are attributable to secondary changes, such as the presence of a lump. Other common complaints include mucous discharge, soiling of the underclothes, and pruritus. If the patient is concerned primarily with the pruritic symptoms, cleansing the area with warm water following defecation is usually helpful. Many patients believe that itching is caused by a lack of cleanliness, and they vigorously scrub the area with soap and water; this only serves to exacerbate the problem. The patient should be cautioned not to use soap in the perianal area; this is not an area that requires sterilization. Avoiding coffee, alcoholic beverages, smoking, and spicy foods should also have an ameliorative effect (see Chapter 9). If discharge is a problem and surgery is not considered appropriate, or if the patient refuses surgery, a ball of cotton can be placed at the anal opening and changed as necessary to avoid soiling underclothes and exacerbating pruritic symptoms.

Surgical Treatment

The classic operative approach for chronic anal fissure is excision and internal anal sphincterotomy in the posterior position. This removes the eschar, skin tag, and papilla, but it may produce the complication of the previously mentioned keyhole deformity. Excision of the tag and papilla is helpful, but the sphincterotomy should still be accomplished in the lateral position. Unless the edges of the fissure are very fibrotic, removal of the tag and papilla by snipping with scissors should suffice. However, a more formal excision can be accomplished if the surgeon prefers (Figure 12-23). The underlying internal anal sphincter should not be incised. As mentioned, the sphincterotomy can then be performed at a lateral site by one of the methods described previously.

Results

There is confusion in the literature with respect to interpretation of the results of surgery for chronic anal fissure. It is often not clear whether patients truly fulfill the criteria, such as a sentinel tag, hypertrophied anal papilla, and thickened, fibrotic appearance. That stated, reports of the treatment of chronic anal fissure by lateral internal anal sphincterotomy have been quite enthusiastic.[59] Bell noted one failure in 56 patients.[8] Ravikumar and colleagues reported all fissures healed by 5 weeks, and all but two within 3 weeks.[93] Kortbeek and

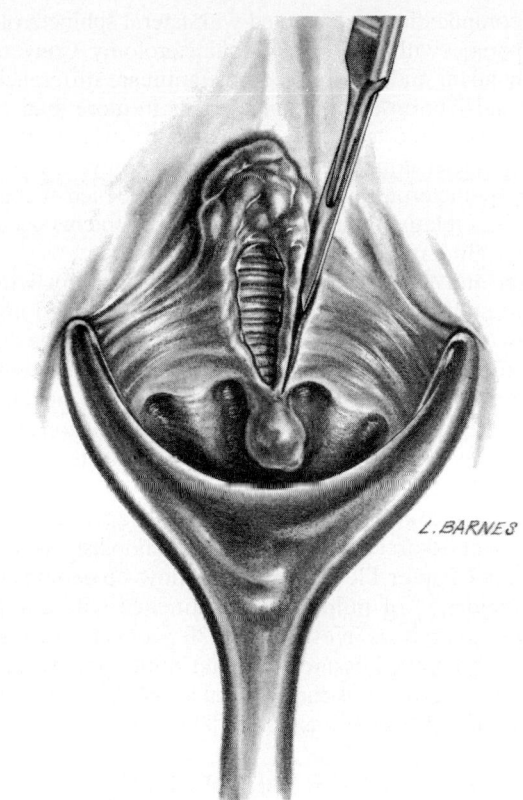

FIGURE 12-23. Chronic anal fissure is treated by excision of the fibrous tissue skin tag and hypertrophied anal papilla. Sphincterotomy should not be performed at this site.

associates, in a controlled study, found that healing was similar for the subcutaneous (96.6%) and open (94.4%) groups.[59] Anal canal pressure studies have repeatedly demonstrated that pressure reduction occurs and is maintained in patients who undergo open or closed lateral internal anal sphincterotomy for chronic anal fissure.[11,16,100]

Abcarian retrospectively analyzed 300 patients, one-half of whom underwent lateral internal anal sphincterotomy, and the other half underwent fissurectomy and midline sphincterotomy.[1] Although both groups had the same incidence of delayed healing (two patients), no one experienced fecal soilage in the former group. Five percent noted this problem after the latter operation. Bode and colleagues performed fissurectomy with "superficial" midline sphincterotomy in 121 individuals.[10] No patient was found to have a keyhole deformity during a mean follow-up of more than 8 years. The recurrence rate was approximately 5%. García-Aguilar and coworkers, in a retrospective analysis, found that closed sphincterotomy was preferable to open because it was associated with a similar rate of cure and fewer control complaints.[30]

Hawley reported a prospective study of three methods of treatment of chronic anal fissure: sphincter stretch, posterior sphincterotomy, and lateral sphincterotomy.[42] He found that lateral internal anal sphincterotomy was the preferred operation because it resulted in earlier wound healing, less postoperative discomfort, and fewer problems with soiling. Hsu and MacKeigan reported the treatment of more than 1,700 patients with chronic anal fissure by five different methods.[45]

Fewer complications were noted with lateral sphincterotomy in comparison with excision and sphincterotomy. Conversely, Khubchandani and Reed noted no significant differences in patient satisfaction or functional results in more than 1,000 patients, irrespective of the method of treatment, whether lateral sphincterotomy, bilateral sphincterotomy, or posterior midline sphincterotomy.[55] However, the incidence of complications was relatively high: flatus control problems occurred in 35%, soiling in 22%, and "accidents" in 5%.

Engel and associates performed fissurectomy without sphincterotomy in 17 consecutive patients who did not respond to conservative measures using the nitric oxide donor, isosorbide dinitrate cream postoperatively.[25] All wounds healed within 10 weeks, with no recurrence at a median follow-up of 29 months. The authors concluded that one should consider this approach as a sphincter-sparing technique to minimize the risk of impairment for bowel control.

Hancke and colleagues used dermal flap coverage for chronic anal fissure, similar to that of an anoplasty as recommended in Chapter 11.[40] Long-term follow-up demonstrated a low incidence of mild anal incontinence with complete healing of the fissure in every case (30 patients). Baraza and associates employed fissurectomy and botulinum toxin injection for the treatment of chronic anal fissure in women, but a high rate of recurrence was noted (50%).[7]

Chronic Anal Fissure with Stenosis

Difficulty with defecation secondary to narrowing of the anal canal from chronic fissure can occasionally occur. The problem is more commonly seen, however, when excess anal canal mucosa is removed at the time of hemorrhoidectomy. Stenosis and fissure may supervene. Conservative medical management with stool softeners and a dilator is often advised, but an anoplasty is recommended (see Chapter 11).[19,27]

Even in the absence of stenosis, concomitant anoplasty has been recommended. Leong and Seow-Choen randomized 40 patients with chronic anal fissure to lateral sphincterotomy or to anal advancement flap.[60] However, all healed with the former operation, and 15% failed to heal with the flap. Nyam and colleagues advise an island advancement flap as an alternative when resting or squeeze pressures are reduced or when there is increased risk through the performance of a "sphincter-weakening procedure."[85]

Anal Fissure and Hemorrhoids

When a patient harbors an anal fissure as well as a hemorrhoid problem sufficient to warrant surgical treatment, a hemorrhoidectomy with sphincterotomy should be performed concurrently (see Figure 12-1 and Chapter 11). The sphincterotomy should be carried out laterally, usually at the site of the left lateral pile (see Figure 11-49).

Anal Fissure and Crohn's Disease

If the fissure is ectopic, extends proximal to the dentate line, is particularly broad based, or is especially purulent, the association with underlying inflammatory bowel disease must be considered (see Chapters 14 and 30). A history of diarrhea or abdominal pain is highly suggestive. Fielding reported in a prospective study of 153 patients with Crohn's disease that more than one-half had anal fissures, most of which were asymptomatic.[28] When doubt exists about the cause of the condition, intestinal evaluation, including small bowel series and colonoscopy, should be performed before a definitive surgical procedure is undertaken. It may be worthwhile to perform a small biopsy of the anal area, possibly to demonstrate a characteristic granuloma of Crohn's disease. Other conditions may produce an anal fissure or ulcer, but the differential diagnosis usually poses little problem. Anal canal carcinoma, carcinoma of the anal margin, and tuberculosis all exhibit more extensive changes than a solitary anal fissure. Conservative (i.e., medical) treatment is the prudent course. If a surgical procedure is undertaken, the resultant wound often tends to be indolent and leads to more symptoms than did the original condition. Furthermore, the patient's wound may be so debilitating that the need for a diversionary procedure may be precipitated. Still, some published studies have testified to a high rate of healing when internal anal sphincterotomy is performed, even in the presence of active Crohn's disease.[29,108,116] Certainly, the physician should consider the possibility of underlying inflammatory bowel disease in any patient whose fissure fails to heal following surgery.

Anal Fissure in the Anoreceptive Individual

Anal fissures are common among patients, both male and female, who practice anal receptive intercourse, presumably as a consequence of trauma or stretching.[102] However, numerous anal and perianal ulcers occur in these individuals that may pose a problem in differential diagnosis. Certainly, a primary syphilitic chancre may be confused with anal fissure (see Figure 9-44). Because a high index of suspicion is necessary for the diagnosis of these conditions, any fissure or perianal ulcer should be cultured and a biopsy performed in this group of patients.[102] Besides syphilis, the causes of such lesions have been reported to include *Chlamydia*, *Haemophilus ducreyi*, cytomegalovirus, herpes simplex virus, human immunodeficiency virus (HIV) (see Chapters 9, 10, and 33), and neoplasms (e.g., squamous cell carcinoma, non-Hodgkin's lymphoma, and Kaposi's sarcoma; see Chapters 25 and 26).[102] Those HIV-positive individuals with no identifiable associated cause may be helped with aggressive debridement or intralesional steroid therapy.[111] Sphincterotomy for uncomplicated fissure can be performed with the expectation of healing if symptoms warrant and if medical management has been unsuccessful.[102]

References

1. Abcarian H. Surgical correction of chronic anal fissure: results of lateral internal sphincterotomy vs. fissurectomy—midline sphincterotomy. *Dis Colon Rectum*. 1980;23(1):31–36.
2. Abcarian H, Lakshmanan S, Read DR, et al. The role of internal sphincter in chronic anal fissures. *Dis Colon Rectum*. 1982;25(6):525–528.
3. Abramowitz L, Sobhani I, Benifla JL, et al. Anal fissure and thrombosed external hemorrhoids before and after delivery. *Dis Colon Rectum*. 2002;45(5):650–655.
4. Antebi E, Schwartz P, Gilon E. Sclerotherapy for the treatment of fissure in ano. *Surg Gynecol Obstet*. 1985;160(3):204–206.
5. Arabi Y, Alexander-Williams J, Keighley MR. Anal pressures in hemorrhoids and anal fissure. *Am J Surg*. 1977;134(5):608–610.
6. Bailey HR, Beck DE, Billingham RP, et al. A study to determine the nitroglycerine ointment dose and dosing interval that best promote the healing of chronic anal fissures. *Dis Colon Rectum*. 2002;45(9):1192–1199.
7. Baraza W, Boereboom C, Shorthouse A, et al. The long-term efficacy of fissurectomy and botulinum toxin injection for chronic anal fissure in females. *Dis Colon Rectum*. 2008;51(2):239–243.
8. Bell GA. Lateral internal sphincterotomy in chronic anal fissure—a surgical technique. *Am Surg*. 1980;46(10):572–575.
9. Bennett RC, Goligher JC. Results of internal sphincterotomy for anal fissure. *Br Med J*. 1962;2(5318):1500–1503.

10. Bode WE, Culp CE, Spencer RJ, et al. Fissurectomy with superficial midline sphincterotomy: a viable alternative for the surgical correction of chronic fissure/ulcer-in-ano. *Dis Colon Rectum*. 1984;27(2):93–95.

11. Boulos PB, Araujo JG. Adequate internal sphincterotomy for chronic anal fissure: subcutaneous or open technique? *Br J Surg*. 1984;71(5):360–362.

12. Brisinda D, Maria G, Fenici R, et al. Safety of botulinum neurotoxin treatment in patients with chronic anal fissure. *Dis Colon Rectum*. 2003;46(3):419–420.

13. Brown AC, Sumfest JM, Rozwadowski JV. Histopathology of the internal anal sphincter in chronic anal fissure. *Dis Colon Rectum*. 1989;32(8):680–683.

14. Cerdán FJ, Ruiz de León A, Azpiroz F, et al. Anal sphincteric pressure in fissure-in-ano before and after lateral internal sphincterotomy. *Dis Colon Rectum*. 1982;25(3):198–201.

15. Chen J, Michowitz M, Bawnik JB. Solcoderm as alternative conservative treatment for acute anal fissure: a controlled clinical study. *Am Surg*. 1992;58(11):705–709.

16. Chowcat NL, Araujo JG, Boulos PB. Internal sphincterotomy for chronic anal fissure: long-term effects on anal pressure. *Br J Surg*. 1986;73(11):915–916.

17. Cohen A, Dehn TC. Lateral subcutaneous sphincterotomy for treatment of anal fissure in children. *Br J Surg*. 1995;82(10):1341–1342.

18. Cook TA, Humphreys MM, McC Mortensen NJ. Oral nifedipine reduces resting anal pressure and heals chronic anal fissure. *Br J Surg*. 1999;86(10):1269–1273.

19. Crapp AR, Alexander-Williams J. Fissure-in-ano and anal stenosis. Part I: conservative management. *Clin Gastroenterol*. 1975;4(3):619–628.

20. Cundall JD, Gardiner A, Laden G, et al. Use of hyperbaric oxygen to treat chronic anal fissure. *Br J Surg*. 2003;90(4):452–453.

21. Duthie HL, Bennett RC. Anal sphincteric pressure in fissure in ano. *Surg Gynecol Obstet*. 1964;119:19–21.

22. Eisenhammer S. The surgical correction of chronic internal anal (sphincteric) contracture. *S Afr Med J*. 1951;25(28):486–489.

23. Eisenhammer S. The evaluation of the internal anal sphincterotomy operation with special reference to anal fissure. *Surg Gynecol Obstet*. 1959; 109:583–590.

24. Emami MH, Sayedyahossein S, Aslani A. Safety and efficacy of new glyceryl trinitrate suppository formula: first double blind placebo-controlled clinical trial. *Dis Colon Rectum*. 2008;51(7):1079–1083.

25. Engel AF, Eijsbouts QA, Balk AG. Fissurectomy and isosorbide dinitrate for chronic fissure in ano not responding to conservative treatment. *Br J Surg*. 2002;89(1):79–83.

26. Evans J, Luck A, Hewett P. Glyceryl trinitrate vs. lateral sphincterotomy for chronic anal fissure: prospective, randomized trial. *Dis Colon Rectum*. 2001;44(1):93–97.

27. Ferguson JA. Fissure-in-ano and anal stenosis. Part II: radical surgical management. *Clin Gastroenterol*. 1975;4(3):629–634.

28. Fielding JF. *An Enquiry into Certain Aspects of Regional Enteritis* [MD thesis]. Dublin, Ireland: National University of Ireland; 1967.

29. Fleshner PR, Schoetz DJ Jr, Roberts PL, et al. Anal fissure in Crohn's disease: a plea for aggressive management. *Dis Colon Rectum*. 1995;38(11):1137–1143.

30. García-Aguilar J, Belmonte C, Wong WD, et al. Open vs. closed sphincterotomy for chronic anal fissure: long-term results. *Dis Colon Rectum*. 1996;39(4):440–443.

31. García-Aguilar J, Belmonte Montes C, Perez JJ, et al. Incontinence after lateral internal sphincterotomy: anatomic and functional evaluation. *Dis Colon Rectum*. 1998;41(4):423–427.

32. García-Granero E, Sanahuja A, García-Armengol J, et al. Anal endosonographic evaluation after closed lateral subcutaneous sphincterotomy. *Dis Colon Rectum*. 1998;41(5):598–601.

33. Garrido R, Lagos N, Lagos M, et al. Treatment of chronic anal fissure by gonyautoxin. *Colorectal Dis*. 2007;9(7):619–624.

34. Gibbons CP, Read NW. Anal hypertonia in fissures: cause or effect? *Br J Surg*. 1986;73(6):443–445.

35. Gingold BS. Simple in-office sphincterotomy with partial fissurectomy for chronic anal fissure. *Surg Gynecol Obstet*. 1987;165(1):46–48.

36. Goldman G, Zilberman M, Werbin N. Bacteremia in anal dilatation. *Dis Colon Rectum*. 1986;29(5):304–305.

37. Goligher JC. *Surgery of the Anus, Rectum and Colon*. 4th ed. New York, NY: Macmillan; 1980:136.

38. Goligher JC. *Surgery of the Anus, Rectum and Colon*. 4th ed. New York, NY: Macmillan; 1980:147.

39. Gorfine SR. Treatment of benign anal disease with topical nitroglycerin. *Dis Colon Rectum*. 1995;38(5):453–456.

40. Hancke E, Rikas E, Suchan K, et al. Dermal flap coverage for chronic anal fissure: lower incidence of anal incontinence compared to lateral internal sphincterotomy after long-term follow-up. *Dis Colon Rectum*. 2010;53(11):1563–1568.

41. Hancock BD. The internal sphincter and anal fissure. *Br J Surg*. 1977;64(2):92–95.

42. Hawley PR. The treatment of chronic fissure-in-ano. A trial of methods. *Br J Surg*. 1969;56(12):915–918.

43. Helton WS; SSAT, AGA, ASGE Consensus Panel. 2001 consensus statement on benign anorectal disease. *J Gastrointest Surg*. 2002;6(3): 302–303.

44. Hoffmann DC, Goligher JC. Lateral subcutaneous internal sphincterotomy in treatment of anal fissure. *Br Med J*. 1970;3(5724):673–675.

45. Hsu TC, MacKeigan JM. Surgical treatment of chronic anal fissure. A retrospective study of 1753 cases. *Dis Colon Rectum*. 1984;27(7):475–478.

46. Hyman NH, Cataldo PA. Nitroglycerin ointment for anal fissures: effective treatment or just a headache? *Dis Colon Rectum*. 1999;42(3): 383–385.

47. Jensen SL. Diet and other risk factors for fissure-in-ano. Prospective case control study. *Dis Colon Rectum*. 1988;31(10):770–773.

48. Jonas M, Neal KR, Abercrombie JF, et al. A randomized trial of oral vs. topical diltiazem for chronic anal fissures. *Dis Colon Rectum*. 2001;44(8):1074–1078.

49. Jonas M, Speake W, Scholefield JH. Diltiazem heals glyceryl trinitrate-resistant chronic anal fissures: a prospective study. *Dis Colon Rectum*. 2002;45(8):1091–1095.

50. Jost WH, Schimrigk K. Use of botulinum toxin in anal fissure [letter]. *Dis Colon Rectum*. 1993;36(10):974.

51. Jost WH, Schimrigk K. Therapy of anal fissure using botulin toxin. *Dis Colon Rectum*. 1994;37(12):1321–1324.

52. Karanlik H, Akturk R, Camlica H, et al. The effect of glyceryl trinitrate ointment on posthemorrhoidectomy pain and wound healing: results of a randomized, double-blind, placebo-controlled study. *Dis Colon Rectum*. 2009;52(2):280–285.

53. Keck JO, Staniunas RJ, Coller JA, et al. Computer-generated profiles of the anal canal in patients with anal fissure. *Dis Colon Rectum*. 1995;38(1):72–79.

54. Keighley MR, Greca F, Nevah E, et al. Treatment of anal fissure by lateral subcutaneous sphincterotomy should be under general anesthesia. *Br J Surg*. 1981;68(6):400–401.

55. Khubchandani IT, Reed JF. Sequelae of internal sphincterotomy for chronic fissure in ano. *Br J Surg*. 1989;76(5):431–434.

56. Klosterhalfen B, Vogel P, Rixen H, et al. Topography of the inferior rectal artery: a possible cause of chronic, primary anal fissure. *Dis Colon Rectum*. 1989;32(1):43–52.

57. Knight JS, Birks M, Farouk R. Topical diltiazem ointment in the treatment of chronic anal fissure. *Br J Surg*. 2001;88(4):553–556.

58. Kocher HM, Steward M, Leather AJ, et al. Randomized clinical trial assessing the side-effects of glyceryl trinitrate and diltiazem hydrochloride in the treatment of chronic anal fissure. *Br J Surg*. 2002;89(4):413–417.

59. Kortbeek JB, Langevin JM, Khoo RE, et al. Chronic fissure-in-ano: a randomized study comparing open and subcutaneous lateral internal sphincterotomy. *Dis Colon Rectum*. 1992;35(9):835–837.

60. Leong AF, Seow-Choen F. Lateral sphincterotomy compared with anal advancement flap for chronic anal fissure. *Dis Colon Rectum*. 1995;38(1):69–71.

61. Lewis TH, Corman ML, Prager ED, et al. Long-term results of open and closed sphincterotomy for anal fissure. *Dis Colon Rectum*. 1988;31(5):368–371.

62. Lindsey I, Jones OM, Cunningham C, et al. Botulinum toxin as second-line therapy for chronic anal fissure failing 0.2 percent glyceryl trinitrate. *Dis Colon Rectum*. 2003;46(3):361–366.

63. Lockhart-Mummery P. *Diseases of the Rectum and Anus*. New York, NY: William Wood; 1914:169.

64. Lockhart-Mummery P. *Diseases of the Rectum and Anus*. New York, NY: William Wood; 1914:171.

65. Loder PB, Kamm MA, Nicholls RJ, et al. 'Reversible chemical sphincterotomy' by local application of glyceryl trinitrate. *Br J Surg*. 1994;81(9):1386–1389.

66. Lund JN, Armitage NC, Scholefield JH. Use of glyceryl trinitrate ointment in the treatment of anal fissure. *Br J Surg*. 1996;83(6):776–777.

67. Lund JN, Binch C, McGrath J, et al. Topographical distribution of blood supply to the anal canal. *Br J Surg*. 1999;86(4):496–498.

68. Lund JN, Scholefield JH. A randomised, prospective, double-blind, placebo-controlled trial of glyceryl trinitrate ointment in treatment of anal fissure. *Lancet*. 1997;349(9044):11–14.

69. Maria G, Cassetta E, Gui D, et al. A comparison of botulinum toxin and saline for the treatment of chronic anal fissure. *N Engl J Med*. 1998;338(4):217–220.

70. Marya SK, Mittal SS, Singla S. Lateral subcutaneous internal sphincterotomy for acute fissure in ano. *Br J Surg*. 1980;67(4):299.

71. McLeod RS, Evans J. Symptomatic care and nitroglycerin in the management of anal fissure. *J Gastrointest Surg*. 2002;6(3):278–280.

72. McNamara MJ, Percy JP, Fielding IR. A manometric study of anal fissure treated by subcutaneous lateral internal sphincterotomy. *Ann Surg*. 1990;211(2):235–238.

73. Menteş BB, Güner MK, Leventoglu S, et al. Fine-tuning of the extent of lateral internal sphincterotomy: spasm-controlled vs. up to the fissure apex. *Dis Colon Rectum*. 2008;51(1):128–133.

74. Menteş BB, Irkörücü O, Akin M, et al. Comparison of botulinum toxin injection and lateral internal sphincterotomy for the treatment of chronic anal fissure. *Dis Colon Rectum*. 2003;46(2):232–237.

75. Miles WE. *Rectal Surgery*. London, United Kingdom: Cassell & Co; 1939.

76. Millar DM. Subcutaneous lateral internal anal sphincterotomy for anal fissure. *Br J Surg*. 1971;58(10):737–739.

77. Nasr M, Ezzat H, Elsebae M. Botulinum toxin injection versus lateral internal sphincterotomy in the treatment of chronic anal fissure: a randomized controlled trial. *World J Surg*. 2010;34(11):2730–2734.

78. Nelson RL. A review of operative procedures for anal fissure. *J Gastrointest Surg*. 2002;6(3):284–289.

79. Nielsen MB, Rasmussen OO, Pedersen JF, et al. Risk of sphincter damage and anal incontinence after anal dilatation for fissure-in-ano. An endosonographic study. *Dis Colon Rectum*. 1993;36(7):677–680.

80. Notaras MJ. Lateral subcutaneous sphincterotomy for anal fissure—a new technique. *Proc R Soc Med*. 1969;62(7):713.

81. Notaras MJ. The treatment of anal fissure by lateral subcutaneous internal sphincterotomy—a technique and results. *Br J Surg*. 1971;58(2):96–100.

82. Notaras MJ. Fissure-in-ano: lateral subcutaneous internal anal sphincterotomy. In: Todd IP, ed. *Operative Surgery: Colon, Rectum, and Anus*. 3rd ed. London, United Kingdom: Butterworth; 1977:354.

83. Notaras MJ. Anal fissure and stenosis. *Surg Clin North Am*. 1988;68(6):1427–1440.

84. Nothmann BJ, Schuster MM. Internal anal sphincter derangement with anal fissures. *Gastroenterology*. 1974;67(2):216–220.

85. Nyam DC, Wilson RG, Stewart KJ, et al. Island advancement flaps in the management of anal fissures. *Br J Surg*. 1995;82(3):326–328.

86. Pérez-Miranda M, Robledo P, Alcalde M, et al. Endoscopic anal dilatation for fissure-in-ano: a new outpatient treatment modality. *Rev Esp Enferm Dig*. 1996;88(4):265–272.

87. Pernikoff BJ, Eisenstat TE, Rubin RJ, et al. Reappraisal of partial lateral internal sphincterotomy. *Dis Colon Rectum*. 1994;37(12):1291–1295.

88. Perrotti P, Bove A, Antropoli C, et al. Topical nifedipine with lidocaine ointment vs. active control for treatment of chronic anal fissure: results of a prospective, randomized, double-blind study. *Dis Colon Rectum*. 2002;45(11):1468–1475.

89. Perry WB, Dykes SL, Buie WD, et al; Standards Practice Task Force of the American Society of Colon and Rectal Surgeons. Practice parameters for the management of anal fissures (3rd revision). *Dis Colon Rectum*. 2010;53(8):1110–1115.

90. Phillips R. Pharmacologic treatment of anal fissure with botoxin, diltiazem, or bethanechol. *J Gastrointest Surg*. 2002;6(3):281–283.

91. Pitt J, Williams S, Dawson PM. Reasons for failure of glyceryl trinitrate treatment of chronic fissure-in-ano: a multivariate analysis. *Dis Colon Rectum*. 2001;44(6):864–867.

92. Poh A, Tan KY, Seow-Choen F. Innovations in chronic anal fissure treatment: a systematic review. *World J Gastrointest Surg*. 2010;2(7):231–241.

93. Ravikumar TS, Sridhar S, Rao RN. Subcutaneous lateral internal sphincterotomy for chronic fissure-in-ano. *Dis Colon Rectum*. 1982;25(8):798–801.

94. Ray JE, Penfold JC, Gathright JB Jr, et al. Lateral subcutaneous internal anal sphincterotomy for anal fissure. *Dis Colon Rectum*. 1974;17(2):139–144.

95. Reissman P. Significance of anal canal ultrasound before sphincterotomy in multiparous women with anal fissure [letter]. *Dis Colon Rectum*. 1996;39(9):1060.

96. Renzi A, Brusciano L, Pescatori M, et al. Pneumatic balloon dilatation for chronic anal fissure: a prospective, clinical, endosonographic, and manometric study. *Dis Colon Rectum*. 2005;48(1):121–126.

97. Renzi A, Izzo D, Di Sarno G, et al. Clinical, manometric, and ultrasonographic results of pneumatic balloon dilatation vs. lateral internal sphincterotomy for chronic anal fissure: a prospective, randomized, controlled trial. *Dis Colon Rectum*. 2008;51(1):121–127.

98. Richard CS, Gregoire R, Plewes EA, et al. Internal sphincterotomy is superior to topical nitroglycerin in the treatment of chronic anal fissure: results of a randomized, controlled trial by the Canadian Colorectal Surgical Trials Group. *Dis Colon Rectum*. 2000;43(8):1048–1057.

99. Roe AM, Bartolo DC, Mortensen NJ. New method for assessment of anal sensation in various anorectal disorders. *Br J Surg*. 1986;73(4):310–312.

100. Romano G, Rotondano G, Santangelo M, et al. A critical appraisal of pathogenesis and morbidity of surgical treatment of chronic anal fissure. *J Am Coll Surg*. 1994;178(6):600–604.

101. Rudd WW. Lateral subcutaneous internal sphincterotomy for chronic anal fissure, an outpatient procedure. *Dis Colon Rectum*. 1975;18(4):319–323.

102. Safavi A, Gottesman L, Dailey TH. Anorectal surgery in the HIV⁺ patient: update. *Dis Colon Rectum*. 1991;34(4):299–304.

103. Samim M, Twigt B, Stoker L, et al. Topical diltiazem cream versus botulinum toxin A for the treatment of chronic anal fissure: a double-blind randomized clinical trial [published online ahead of print June 16, 2011]. *Ann Surg*.

104. Schouten WR, Briel JW, Auwerda JJ. Relationship between anal pressure and anodermal blood flow: the vascular pathogenesis of anal fissures. *Dis Colon Rectum*. 1994;37(7):664–669.

105. Schouten WR, Briel JW, Auwerda JJ, et al. Ischaemic nature of anal fissure. *Br J Surg*. 1996;83(1):63–65.

106. Schuster MM. The riddle of the sphincters. *Gastroenterology*. 1975;69(1):249–262.

107. Sohn N, Eisenberg MM, Weinstein MA, et al. Precise anorectal sphincter dilatation—its role in the therapy of anal fissures. *Dis Colon Rectum*. 1992;35(4):322–327.

108. Sohn N, Korelitz BI. Local operative treatment of anorectal Crohn's disease. *J Clin Gastroenterol*. 1982;4(4):395–399.

109. Speakman CT, Burnett SJ, Kamm MA, et al. Sphincter injury after anal dilatation demonstrated by anal endosonography. *Br J Surg*. 1991;78(12):1429–1430.

110. Sultan AH, Kamm MA, Nicholls RJ, et al. Prospective study of the extent of internal anal sphincter division during lateral sphincterotomy. *Dis Colon Rectum*. 1994;37(10):1031–1033.

111. Viamonte M, Dailey TH, Gottesman L. Ulcerative disease of the anorectum in the HIV⁺ patient. *Dis Colon Rectum*. 1993;36(9):801–805.

112. Walfisch S, Silberstein E. Balloon anal dilatation for anal fissure. *Tech Coloproctol*. 1998;2:73–75.

113. Walker WA, Rothenberger DA, Goldberg SM. Morbidity of internal sphincterotomy for anal fissure and stenosis. *Dis Colon Rectum*. 1985;28(11):832–835.

114. Watson SJ, Kamm MA, Nicholls RJ, et al. Topical glyceryl trinitrate in the treatment of chronic anal fissure. *Br J Surg*. 1996;83(6):771–775.

115. Watts JM, Bennett RC, Goligher JC. Stretching of anal sphincters in treatment of fissure-in-ano. *Br Med J*. 1964;2(5405):342–343.

116. Wolkomir AF, Luchtefeld MA. Surgery for symptomatic hemorrhoids and anal fissures in Crohn's disease. *Dis Colon Rectum*. 1993;36(6):545–547.

117. Yiannakopoulou E. Botulinum toxin and anal fissure: efficacy and safety systematic review [published online ahead of print August 6, 2011]. *Int J Colorectal Dis*. doi:10.1007/s00384-011-1286-5.

118. Yucel T, Gonullu D, Oncu M, et al. Comparison of controlled-intermittent anal dilatation and lateral internal sphincterotomy in the treatment of chronic anal fissures: a prospective, randomized study. *Int J Surg*. 2009;7(3):228–231.

13

Anorectal Abscess

Brett E. Ruffo

Staphylococcus Aureus
By Gram and Koch he swore
He would invade new regions
Unconquered heretofore—
By Gram and Koch he swore it,
To take a patient's life,
And called the Cocci, young and old,
From all his colonies of gold
To aid him in the strife
　　　　St. Bartholomew's Hospital Journal 1909;17:13
　　　　　　　—"THE BATTLE OF FURUNCULUS"

▶ ETIOLOGY AND PATHOGENESIS

Anorectal abscess is an acute inflammatory process that often is the initial manifestation of an underlying anal fistula. An abscess in this area may also be a consequence of other causes and associations. These include the following:

- Foreign body intrusion
- Trauma
- Malignancy
- Radiation
- Immunocompromised state (e.g., leukemia, AIDS)
- Infectious dermatitides (e.g., suppurative hidradenitis)
- Tuberculosis
- Actinomycosis
- Crohn's disease
- Anal fissure[4,42]

Additionally, anorectal abscess may develop as a complication of anal operations, such as hemorrhoidectomy (rarely—see Chapter 11) and internal anal sphincterotomy (see Chapter 12).

The cause of nonspecific anorectal abscess and fistula is believed to be plugging of the anal ducts; this is known as the *cryptoglandular theory*. Credit for introducing the concept of gland infection in the pathogenesis of anal fistula is generally attributed to Chiari (1878)[17] and to Herrmann and Desfosses (1880).[38] Klosterhalfen and colleagues examined 62 autopsy specimens by means of conventional and special immunohistologic staining methods and confirmed that anal intramuscular glands should be the anatomic correlate of anal fistulas.[46] Between 6 and 10 of these glands and ducts are located around the anal canal and enter at the base of the crypts (see Figure 11-2). Parks (see Biography, Chapter 29) demonstrated by meticulous histologic review that one-half of all crypts are not entered by glands, that the ducts usually end blindly, and that the most common direction of spread is downward into the submucosa.[63] Of particular interest is his observation that in two-thirds of the specimens, one or more branches enter the sphincter, and in one-half, the branches cross the internal sphincter completely to end in the longitudinal layer (Figure 13-1). In his study, however, no branches crossed into the external sphincter. The implication is that plugging or infection of the duct can result in an abscess that can spread in several directions. This may ultimately lead to the development of an anal fistula. In theory, therefore, an intersphincteric fistula may develop when the duct traverses the internal sphincter, and a transsphincteric fistula may be a consequence of the duct traversing the external sphincter.

Shafer and colleagues performed surgery for anal fistula in 52 infants and noted a markedly irregular, thickened dentate line.[78] They attributed the condition to a defect in the dorsal portion of the cloacal membrane, which fuses with the hindgut during week 7 of gestation. In essence, then, contemporary theory implies that fistula-in-ano is the result of a congenital anomaly or a predisposition.[20]

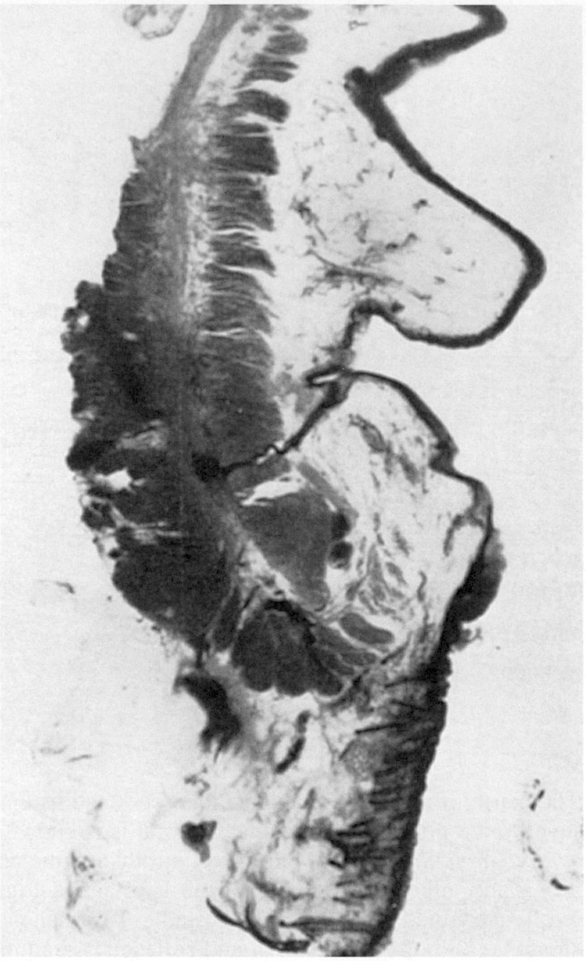

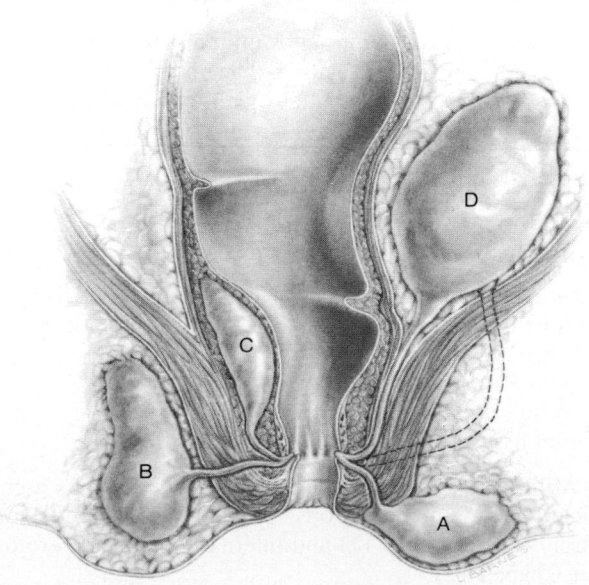

FIGURE 13-1. This thick section through the anal canal shows an anal gland penetrating the internal sphincter, terminating in the longitudinal layer. (From Parks AG. Fistula-in-ano. In: Morson BC, ed. *Diseases of the Colon, Rectum and Anus*. New York, NY: Appleton-Century-Crofts; 1969:277, with permission.)

be a seasonal occurrence for the condition, with the highest incidence in the spring and summer. Despite the opinions of some, there does not appear to be a correlation between the development of anal abscess and personal hygiene or bowel habits, such as diarrhea.[89]

Hill reported a personal experience of 626 patients[40]; the youngest was 2 months of age, and the oldest was 79 years. The number of male patients was almost twice the number of females. In his experience, most developed symptoms in the fourth, fifth, and sixth decades.

Infants younger than 2 years of age represent a different spectrum of the disease when compared with older children and adults. There is an overwhelming male predominance with abscess and with concomitant anal fistula, that is, in excess of 85%.[1,46,67] However, the distribution in older children tends to resemble that seen in adults.

▶ TYPES OF ABSCESS

Four presentations of anorectal abscess have been described:

- Perianal
- Ischiorectal
- Intersphincteric (also known as *submucosal*)
- Supralevator

These types are illustrated in Figure 13-2. It is important to distinguish among these presentations because the etiology, therapy, and implications for the presence or subsequent development of anal fistula are different for each.

Perianal Abscess

Perianal (or perirectal) abscess is identified as a superficial, tender mass outside the anal verge (Figure 13-3). It is arguably the most common type of anorectal abscess, occurring in perhaps 40% to as much as 60% of cases, but the relatively high incidence may be a reflection of the nature of one's practice. The patient can present with a short history of

Further support for the proposition of a congenital origin, albeit by different mechanisms, has been offered by several authors. One theory holds that an excess of androgens may lead to the formation of abnormal glands in utero and that these abnormal glands are predisposed to infection.[27] Pople and Ralphs postulated that the "inappropriate" presence of columnar and transitional epithelium along the length of the excised fistula tracts of four infants is further evidence of a congenital abnormality presenting in the first few months of life.[68] They suggest that migratory cells from the urogenital sinus of the primitive hindgut become locally displaced and entrapped. Because fusion in females is less extensive, this could explain, according to the authors, the higher incidence of fistula in males.

▶ AGE, SEX, AND EPIDEMIOLOGY

Abscess and fistula occur more commonly in men than in women. McElwain and colleagues reported a ratio of three men to one woman, whereas two large series from Cook County Hospital in Chicago were noted to have a two-to-one ratio.[58,70,71] At the time of presentation, two-thirds of patients are in the third or fourth decade of life.[58,70] There seems to

FIGURE 13-2. Infection of the anal duct can present as an abscess in a number of locations. **A:** Perianal. **B:** Ischiorectal. **C:** Intersphincteric. **D:** Supralevator.

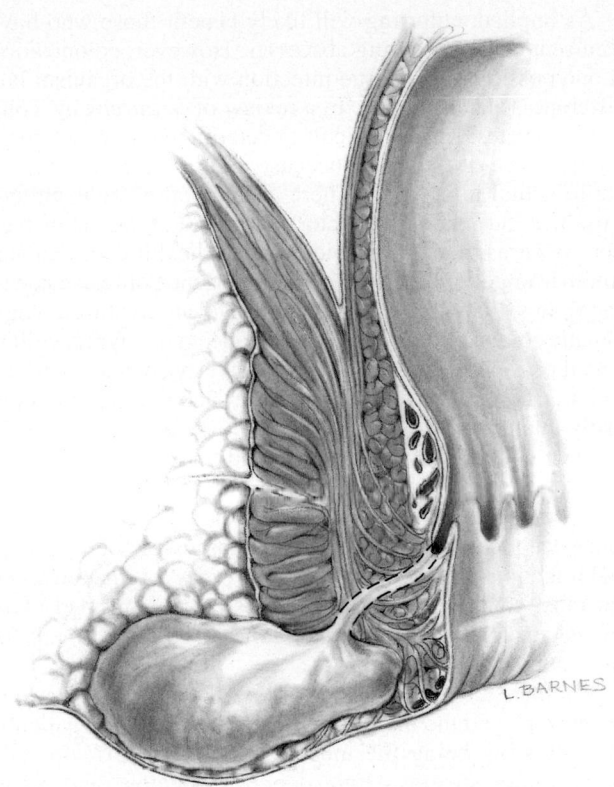

FIGURE 13-3. Perianal abscess. Only a few of these lesions are associated with an underlying fistula. The *dashed lines* illustrate the possible course of a fistula tract if it is present.

painful swelling that may be exacerbated by defecation and by sitting. Not uncommonly, however, one may complain of a recurrent lump that resolves or drains spontaneously. A history of having undergone a prior incision and drainage is not unusual. Fever and leukocytosis are rare.

Physical examination reveals an area of erythema, induration, or possibly fluctuance. Proctosigmoidoscopic examination may be difficult to perform because of pain, but even when it can be accomplished, it is usually unrewarding. Occasionally, however, anoscopic examination demonstrates pus exuding from the base of a crypt or at the site of a chronic anal fissure.

Treatment

As mentioned in other chapters, the American Society of Colon and Rectal Surgeons (ASCRS) has established guidelines for the treatment of numerous conditions. These include the parameters for the management of abscess and anal fistula.[81]

Acute Suppuration (Abscess)
Presentation and Management

An abscess should be drained in a timely manner; lack of fluctuance is not a reason for delay in treatment. If the abscess is superficial, it may be drained in the office setting using a local anesthetic. If the patient is too tender to permit examination and drainage, then these measures should be undertaken in the operating room. Antibiotics may have a role as adjunctive therapy in special circumstances, including certain heart valve conditions, immunosuppression, extensive cellulitis, and diabetes. Laboratory tests are usually not required unless the patient harbors systemic symptoms. Further evaluation by means of endoanal ultrasound, computed tomography (CT), or magnetic resonance imaging (MRI) is unnecessary except perhaps when the etiology of the patient's symptoms is in question. Location of the abscess should be documented. If possible, anoscopy should be performed to reveal the primary site of infection. Patients should notify the physician if pain recurs after abscess drainage.

It is important to distinguish an anal abscess from other pathologic entities, such as hidradenitis, skin furuncles, herpes, HIV, tuberculosis, syphilis, and actinomycosis.[19] One must always be cognizant of the fact that thickened skin tags, multiple fissures, eccentric location of a fissure, or concomitant fistula may suggest Crohn's disease. Any suspicion requires a more comprehensive workup than might otherwise be indicated (see later). When only erythema is present with no apparent mass, the surgeon may be misled into believing that incision and drainage will not be beneficial. Under such circumstances, the patient may be instructed to take sitz baths or may be given a broad-spectrum antibiotic and advised to return in 24 to 48 hours. Despite the absence of fluctuance or significant induration, an abscess is usually present. A patient who is dismissed without undergoing drainage may return a few hours or days later, distressed that spontaneous discharge has taken place, even though the discomfort may have been ameliorated. There is no place for antibiotics alone in the management of anorectal abscess. As I. J. Kodner has stated in numerous panel discussions on the subject, "The presence of pain suggests the need to drain."

The procedure is usually readily performed in the office with a local anesthetic. Alternatively, an emergency department setting or ambulatory surgical facility may be preferred. A large-bore hypodermic needle inserted into the region of induration is a simple diagnostic test, but establishing adequate drainage is critical to success. If purulence is present, a small incision is made using a local anesthetic. The pus is drained; a small gauze wick, gauze, or drain may be inserted, depending on the surgeon's personal preference; and a dressing is applied. Aggressive manipulation and breaking of loculations is not only unnecessary but may also risk sphincter injury. The patient is instructed to remove the dressing and the drain in 24 hours while taking a warm bath. Baths three times daily are advised, and the patient is reexamined in 7 to 10 days. Replacing the wick, drain, or packing (if it had been placed previously) is not necessary. At this time, proctosigmoidoscopic and anoscopic examinations are performed. If an external opening persists and a fistula tract is identified, a definitive procedure is indicated (see Chapter 14, "Anal Fistula").

Postoperative Antibiotics

The value of postoperative antibiotics for someone who has undergone incision and drainage is open to question. However, those at an increased risk based on the criteria outlined in Chapter 5 should be treated.

Antibiotics given after drainage of a perianal abscess have been an issue of debate for some time. Sözener and colleagues undertook a randomized, placebo-controlled, double-blind, multicenter study in order to determine whether antibiotics are important in preventing the subsequent development of an anal fistula after initial drainage of an anal abscess.[80] A total of 151 patients were analyzed; 76 received antibiotics and 75 did not. Those with prior anorectal surgery, inflammatory bowel disease (IBD), recent antimicrobial use, recurrent abscess, pregnant, or who were immunocompromised were excluded. No preoperative antibiotic was given. Augmentin 875 mg was given twice daily for 10 days, and the controls were given similar pills without content. Blinding was applicable to both staff surgeon and research assistants. A follow-up at 1 year revealed that a fistula developed in almost 30% (45 of 151). Fistula development was found in 22.4% of those treated with the placebo and in 37.3% in the antibiotic-treated group. Their conclusion was that antibiotics had no protective or effective means of decreasing the rate of fistula formation and may actually increase the incidence after first-time drainage of an anal abscess.[80]

Drainage has been shown to be the most important aspect in the treatment regimen for anal abscess. Although antibiotics may be beneficial for those with more severe illnesses such as IBD, HIV, and those with an associated cellulitis, for the straightforward anal abscess, incision and drainage is considered appropriate as the sole treatment.

Microbiology

The purpose of culturing the pus following drainage of a perianal or ischiorectal abscess is also a subject of some interest. Usually, the physician performs a culture to determine the appropriate antibiotic for treatment. As previously mentioned, however, antibiotics are usually unnecessary, but culture does have some benefit in determining the likelihood for the subsequent development of a fistula. If the culture demonstrates no bowel-derived organisms (i.e., skin bacteria), the chance of a subsequent fistula is virtually nil.[31,37] Conversely, if enteric organisms are identified, the probability of the presence of a fistula is increased. Lunniss and Phillips, in a prospective trial involving 22 patients, found culture of gut organisms to be quite sensitive for detecting an underlying fistula, but not particularly specific (80%).[53] Conversely, when an infection was present in the anorectal space, culture was 100% sensitive and 100% specific for the detection of an underlying fistula. Certainly, in this group of patients, surgical assessment is a better predictor of the subsequent development or presence of a fistula than is culture.

The increased incidence of methicillin-resistant *Staphylococcus aureus* (MRSA), especially in hospital populations, may lead to an increased frequency of the surgeon obtaining wound cultures. The question, however, is whether such colonization mandates antibiotics against MRSA simply because the organism is present in the culture. Conversely, should the presence of systemic signs and symptoms dictate antibiotic management? The answer today: surgeon's judgment.

The study of the bacteriology of perirectal abscess in *children*, as in adults, has demonstrated that anaerobic organisms are the predominant isolates, although *S. aureus* is frequently found.[11,48] Although no studies have been performed in children concerning the implication of the different culture results, it is reasonable to assume that the principle is identical.

A recent study by Liu and coworkers reviewed the microbiology of 183 patients, both diabetic and nondiabetic.[52] The purpose was to identify the most common organism involved in perianal abscess. In nondiabetics, most commonly identified was *Escherichia coli*, whereas *Klebsiella pneumoniae* was found to be the dominant organism. The authors also noted that first-generation cephalosporins will eradicate *Klebsiella* in 90% of cases.[52]

As implied, culturing will likely benefit those who have recurrent or nonresolving abscesses. However, colonization is one possible factor; true infection with the organism is a different issue altogether. In a review of *S. aureus* by Tong and associates, it was difficult to determine the most appropriate course of treatment because multiple factors contribute to actual infection.[86] There are numerous concomitant variables, such as host factors, immune status, skin barrier concerns, age, comorbidities, and health care contact. Another important concern is the emergence of resistance to antibiotics; there is, therefore, a downside to treating asymptomatic colonization. Albright and colleagues suggest culturing all perianal abscesses with extensive erythema, cellulitis, and lack of purulent material because such findings are more likely related to MRSA.[2]

Stelzmueller and coworkers found, in a retrospective review of perianal infections, that group milleri streptococci (GMS), a heterogeneous group of bacteria, was involved in more deep, complex, and recurrent abscesses.[82] Polymicrobial infections with *E. coli* and *Bacteroides fragilis* remained the most common pathogens. These patients needed more intensive surgical therapy and an increased requirement for antibiotics in their experience.[82]

Another study by Ulug and associates found that *aerobic bacteria* played the major role in the etiology in 81 patients, the following being the most common: *Escherichia coli*, *Bacteroides* species, *Enterococcus* species, and skin-derived organisms, such as coagulase-negative staphylococci, *S. aureus*, and *Peptostreptococcus*.[87] They supported the concept that antibiotics should be used only in selected cases with drainage but did recommend routine wound culture because of increasing emergence of antibiotic-resistant bacteria and their varying virulent factors.[87]

Practice parameters by the ASCRS advise those with bacterial endocarditis, prosthetic heart valves, congenital heart disease, or a heart transplant should all receive preoperative antibiotics prior to drainage. There is no longer evidence to support preoperative antibiotics in patients with mitral valve prolapse.[10]

Recurrence

The incidence of recurrence of perianal abscess or fistula development after initial drainage is approximately 35%. Determining the risk factors that predispose to these consequences has been somewhat controversial.

Hamadani and coworkers looked at recurrence of an abscess or development of a fistula following treatment for first-time perianal abscess in a retrospective study of 148 patients.[33] Age younger than 40 years was the single most important factor related to an increased recurrence risk in a 38-month follow-up. The peak incidence of developing an abscess was age older than 40, however, but recurrence was twofold higher in patients younger than 40. Those with HIV, IBD, recurrent abscesses or fistulas, and inadequate follow-up were excluded. Smoking, gender, and antibiotics did not seem to be a relevant issue. It was noted that diabetes may actually be "protective" against subsequent fistula development. In this study, gender, although not relevant to development of a fistula or abscess recurrence, revealed a 71% predominance in males.

Yano and associates attempted to determine the factors that may lead to recurrence of an anal abscess following drainage in 205 first-time patients followed during 5 years, excluding those with prior abscess, fistula, anorectal surgery, and IBD.[95] Parameters included gender, age, body mass index (BMI), type of anesthesia, location of abscess, anatomic classifications, drain usage, presence of diabetes, and time to drainage after symptoms developed (early was within 7 days and late was after 8 days). A total of 74 patients developed a recurrence. The only significant factor associated with recurrence was the timing from the development of symptoms to subsequent abscess drainage. Those with early drainage had a lower rate of recurrence.

It has been shown that men are two to four times more likely to develop a fistula after an abscess. In a recent study in San Diego at the Veterans Administration health care system, it was proposed that a history of recent smoking is a risk factor in developing an anal fistula after drainage of an anal abscess.[19] A case-controlled study was initiated using a tobacco questionnaire. Three disease processes were excluded: diabetes, IBD, and HIV. Recent smokers were defined as currently smoking or those who quit within the previous year. These were compared with nonsmokers and former smokers. Seventy-four abscess/fistula cases were identified along with 816 controls. There were 22 nonsmokers, 24 current smokers, and 28 previous smokers (12 quit within a year, 27 within 5 years, and 28 within 10 years). Those who smoke or who quit within a year had the highest incidence of developing an anal fistula. Almost a twofold higher risk was noted, an increased association with smoking lasting up to 5 years of quitting. The 5-year mark appears important because after that date, the risk appear to be that of nonsmokers. Limitations to the study are selection bias, definitions of smoking, recall bias, and a nonstandardized questionnaire used to obtain the data. But this publication does demonstrate a strong correlation between smoking and the subsequent development of recurrent abscess and anal fistula. This conclusion should inspire additional research.[19] In an editorial by Zimmerman regarding this study, educating patients on the importance of cessation of smoking was felt to be an obvious health care benefit that may offer this additional advantage.[96]

Synchronous Fistulotomy

A fistula with an internal opening may be seen at the time that the abscess is drained. The incidence as reported from numerous centers is somewhat variable. This may be attributed to the differences in aggressiveness of examiners in attempting to identify a fistula and perhaps also to demographic factors. Vasilevsky and Gordon reported recurrent abscess or the development of an anal fistula in 48% of patients who underwent drainage of a perianal or ischiorectal abscess.[89] Table 13-1 illustrates the results from the Cook County Hospital with the various types of fistulas.

If the internal opening is low lying, the surgeon may elect to perform fistulotomy at the same time the abscess is drained in order to avoid the need for a second procedure. However, the literature is rather contradictory on this point because it is not always clear from the article what type of fistula or abscess the author is treating. A recurrence rate of a mere 3.4% was reported by McElwain and colleagues following initial drainage and fistulotomy, but this is old data.[57] Their subsequent report demonstrated the rate of recurrence of abscess, fistula, or both to be 3.6%, which compared quite favorably with their own recurrence rate of 6% when an established fistula was excised.[58] Waggener also recommends primary fistulotomy.[90]

Scoma and coworkers reported a retrospective review of 232 patients with anal abscess who underwent initial office drainage only.[76] A fistula subsequently developed in two-thirds. Unfortunately, the authors failed to breakdown the incidence of fistula according to the type of abscess. They recommended that fistulotomy be delayed until the fistula becomes manifest. Others concur, although it is not always clear whether a vigorous attempt was made to identify a fistula at the initial procedure.[34] Tang and associates compared incision and drainage alone with concurrent fistulotomy for perianal abscess with a demonstrated internal opening in a prospective, randomized study involving 45 patients.[85] They concluded that incision with drainage alone was not associated with a statistically significantly higher incidence of recurrence of anal fistula when compared with concomitant fistulotomy. Therefore, a simple drainage procedure was essentially as good as a definitive fistula operation.

With respect to *incontinence*, Stremitzer and colleagues reviewed 173 patients over a 121-month follow-up period.[83] If synchronous fistulotomy were performed, severe incontinence developed in 4% and mild in 9%, with a higher rate of incontinence noted in those with multiple procedures.

TABLE 13-1 Incidence of Fistula in Various Types of Anorectal Abscess

TYPE OF ABSCESS	NUMBER OF ABSCESSES	NUMBER WITH FISTULAS	PERCENTAGE (%)
Perianal	437	151	34.5
Ischiorectal	233	59	25.3
Intersphincteric	219	104	47.4
Supralevator	75	32	42.6
Submucous of intermuscular	59	9	15.2

From Ramanujam PS, Prasad ML, Abcarian H, et al. Perianal abscesses and fistulas. A study of 1,023 patients. *Dis Colon Rectum*. 1984;27(9):593–597, with permission.

In a review by Holzheimer and Siebeck of 63 studies from 1964 to 2004, there were no data that effectively compared the different available treatment options.[41] Many flaws were found in the randomization of, especially that of definitions, abscess type and management approach. Their conclusion was that neither primary nor secondary fistulotomy could be recommended based on the reviewed data. One must rely on the experience of the surgeon to adequately evaluate each individual situation in order to determine the appropriate management strategy.[41]

This subject was also studied by Malik and colleagues in a Cochrane database review in which data from six randomized trials were analyzed from 1997 to 2008.[55] The concern was that synchronous fistulotomy may either lead to increased incontinence or subject the patient to unnecessary surgery because some abscesses will probably resolve spontaneously. Of the 479 patients included, there was no statistically significant increased incidence of incontinence reported within 1-year follow-up of drainage and synchronous fistulotomy. There was, however, a slight increase in incontinence with transsphincteric, high, and complex fistulas. This review concluded that the data is "weak," concerning any increased incontinence risk with fistula surgery at the time of initial abscess drainage. Emphasized again is the need for sound surgical judgment in order to help ensure appropriate selection of those who will benefit from this approach and those who need another alternative. Their conclusion is that a concomitant fistulotomy should be considered, but only in carefully selected patients.[55]

If the sphincter anatomy is unclear, loose seton drainage is always safe with essentially no risk of incontinence unless aggressive manipulation of loculations is performed. Stremitzer and associates recommend referral to a surgeon who has experience in managing these potentially complicated entities in order to minimize recurrence, ongoing sepsis, and to limit incontinence.[83] They also emphasize the importance of supervising and educating residents because they are often the initial contacts for the patient.[83]

Opinion

In my own experience, an anal fistula is usually not recognized at the time of drainage of a perianal abscess. However, if a low-lying fistula is encountered, I recommend incision of the tract if it can be easily accomplished at that time. In accordance with my own preference, the patient usually undergoes drainage as an office procedure. Therefore, discomfort often precludes a more thorough evaluation, the identification of a fistula tract (if present), and the ability to perform definitive fistulotomy. Certainly, if an individual is to undergo a regional or general anesthetic, concomitant fistulotomy is a reasonable plan, recognizing that the use of setons is prudent if there is any uncertainty as to sphincteric anatomy.

Ischiorectal Abscess

Ischiorectal abscess may present as a large, erythematous, indurated, tender mass of the buttock or may be virtually inapparent, the patient complaining only of severe pain (Figure 13-4). This type of abscess is seen in 20% to 25% of patients. Pus is almost always present. Waiting for the abscess to "mature" causes the patient to suffer needlessly. As with other suspected abscesses, needle aspiration will usually resolve the issue. Proctosigmoidoscopy and anoscopy are usually deferred because of the patient's discomfort, although the physician should

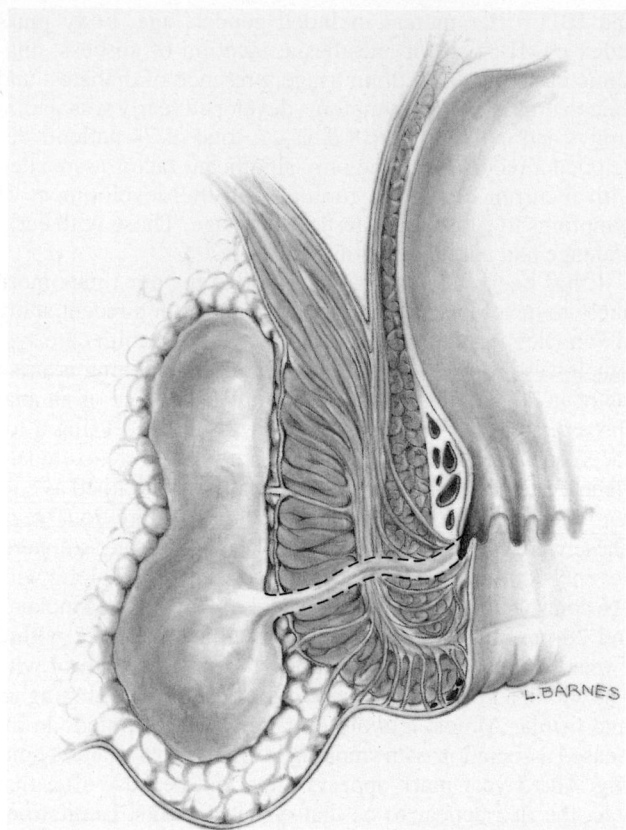

FIGURE 13-4. Ischiorectal abscess. This type of presentation often is inapparent on physical examination. One must maintain a high index of suspicion. The *dashed lines* illustrate the possible course of a fistula tract if it is present.

keep in mind the possibility of rectal or anal cancer or other colorectal condition producing this manifestation.[2] Therefore, a thorough rectal evaluation at some point is mandatory.

Techniques of Drainage

Drainage of an ischiorectal abscess requires some planning because the condition may well be associated with the subsequent development of a transsphincteric fistula (see Chapter 14). In fact, most patients with this type of abscess will require a subsequent fistula procedure. It is important, therefore, to drain the abscess by creating an external opening as close to the anal verge as is possible (Figure 13-5). If this is not considered, the subsequent fistulotomy may result in a large wound that requires a long time to heal (Figure 13-6). The abscess cavity can be readily entered and adequate drainage established without "attacking" the point of presentation or the most indurated or fluctuant area.

The technique for drainage of a large ischiorectal abscess is little different from that of a small perianal abscess. Neither necessarily requires a general anesthetic nor vigorous operative manipulation. After administration of a local anesthetic, a small incision is made and the pus is evacuated. The cavity is irrigated, and a small gauze wick or drain is inserted (not vigorously packed in). The concept of creating a large, cruciate incision and breaking up loculations is unnecessary and extremely uncomfortable. All one needs to accomplish is to establish adequate external drainage. Any residual pus will quickly drain if a small skin opening is maintained with gauze or some form of drain. A dressing is applied, and the

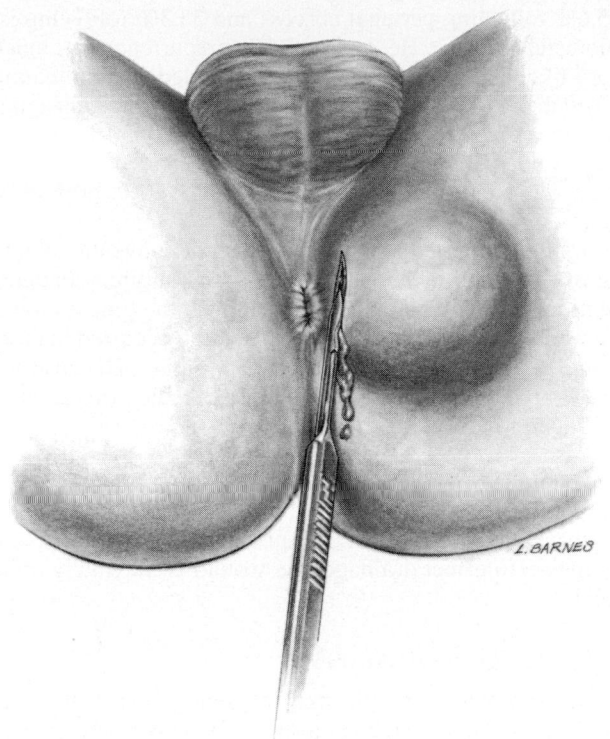

FIGURE 13-5. Proper drainage of an ischiorectal abscess requires that the incision be made as medially as possible, not necessarily at the point of maximal fluctuance. This enables the surgeon to avoid a subsequent long fistulotomy incision.

patient is instructed to take warm baths. The patient removes the drain in 48 to 72 hours and is seen again in 1 week, at which time probing of the external opening, proctosigmoidoscopy, and anoscopic examinations are performed. MRI, ultrasound, and sinography/fistulography at this time may be helpful in selected patients if there is a suspicion of a fistula and to identify possible tracts.

In-Hospital Drainage

Several factors may contraindicate drainage of an ischiorectal abscess in the office. First, a general, spinal, or caudal anesthetic may be required because of patient insistence or

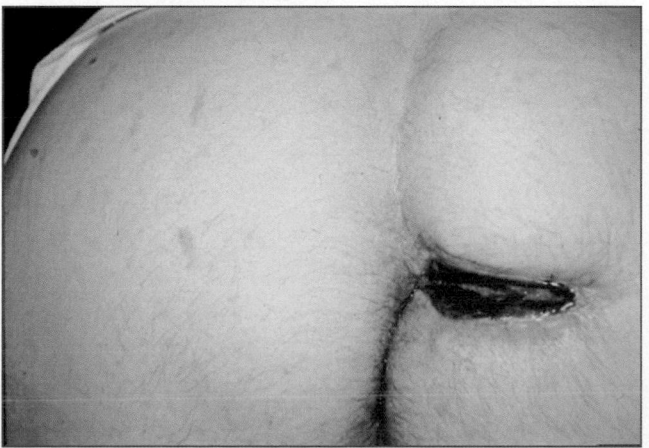

FIGURE 13-6. Drainage of a buttock abscess too far laterally results in a long fistula wound that requires a prolonged healing time.

because the patient is unable to tolerate the manipulation associated with a local procedure. Second, the surgeon may not have ideal space or office facilities. Contamination of the floor, walls, countertops, and instruments will certainly limit the use of the examining room for a time. Third, an ischiorectal abscess should not be drained in the office when the patient is septic, except as a preamble to hospitalization. Others who are at particular risk for ambulatory treatment are those with insulin-dependent diabetes and those who are immunocompromised. Systemic antibiotics and more vigorous irrigations than are possible with an office procedure may be advisable.

In-hospital drainage follows essentially the same procedure advocated for office treatment. The incision should be minimal and medial. Irrigation with saline or an antiseptic solution is followed by insertion of a small drain or wick. Administration of an anesthetic also permits proctosigmoidoscopy and anoscopy, which may help to identify a specific cause for the abscess and localize an internal opening.

A simple method for determining whether an internal opening is present is to pass an anoscope while compressing the mass before drainage. Pus may be seen to exude from a crypt. If an opening is identified, its presence is noted for subsequent definitive treatment, usually after 2 weeks. I do not advocate fistulotomy of a transsphincteric fistula synchronously with drainage of an ischiorectal abscess if for no other reason than providing adequate *informed consent* (see Chapter 14).

Once started, antibiotics are usually continued for 48 hours. Longer treatment may be appropriate in those individuals with signs and symptoms of sepsis, who are immunocompromised, and who harbor other comorbidities. As previously implied, although a culture of the pus may be taken in the operating room, it is rarely of use in treatment, except in predicting the possibility of a fistula. Ischiorectal abscesses are known to have a higher incidence of subsequent fistula development. Drainage is the definitive therapy, and the patient almost invariably becomes afebrile within a short time following the procedure.

Endoanal Ultrasonography

The use of intraoperative ultrasonography for the evaluation of anorectal abscess and fistula has been a subject of some interest in the last few years. Cataldo and colleagues published their experience in 24 individuals with suspected perianal abscess and fistula.[16] All 19 patients subsequently were proved to harbor an abscess that was correctly identified preoperatively by this evaluation. Furthermore, the technique helped to determine the relationship between the abscess and the sphincter muscles in approximately two-thirds of the cases. However, whereas internal openings of fistula tracts were surgically found in 14 of 19 individuals, in only 28% were they identified by endoanal ultrasonography (EAU). The authors concluded that EAU may be of value in certain clinical situations, but most patients with abscesses can be managed without this modality.

EAU is normally used for preoperative evaluation for an anal fistula but can be applicable for complicated anal abscess in order to facilitate the operative approach and to minimize risk of incontinence by clearly identifying the underlying anatomy. Limitations accurately identifying the ischiorectal space and its relationship to both abscess and possible fistula. Other limitations include locating the internal opening, differentiating between high transsphincteric from suprasphincteric, low transsphincteric from intersphincteric fistula, and scar from fistula. With three-dimensional imaging, accuracy can be increased to 98% for primary fistula and 96% for the internal opening. Some believe that hydrogen peroxide injection of the tract concomitant with EAU facilitates identification, but others are more circumspect.[44]

With a new computer postprocessing technique called volume-rendered mode, three-dimensional EAU can demonstrate an improved accuracy by means of digital enhancement. Anal abscesses were correctly identified in 19 of 20 patients, but more importantly, there was improved imaging of the sphincter muscle.[84] This may help enhance the ability to assess muscle damage since atrophy was clearly identified. This may have some benefit in potentially reducing postoperative incontinence concerns. It may also lead to more accurate evaluation of deep ischiorectal abscess. Sudoł-Szopi ska and coworkers have commented that research is ongoing, with further benefit expected along with optimizing imaging through the use of hydrogen peroxide.[84]

CT Scan Efficacy

Although the evaluation for suspected perianal abscess should be primarily clinical, there are many CT scans being performed having been ordered by the initial physician who assesses these patients (i.e., emergency room doctors). One must remember, however, that fluctuance is an advanced sign. If the physician waits for this finding to develop, he or she is denying the patient-needed surgical treatment and may be exposing that individual to an unacceptable risk. Caliste and colleagues retrospectively analyzed CT for its value in patients with anal abscess who present with "subtle" or "atypical" signs and symptoms, such as when the area of so-called fluctuance is not readily apparent.[14] In an analysis of 113 patients, the authors concluded that CT lacked sensitivity and missed approximately 25% of surgically proven abscesses. Moreover, some drained spontaneously 24 to 48 hours following a negative CT. The authors concluded that a negative CT does not necessarily negate the need for surgical drainage because the sensitivity was determined to be only 77%.

MRI has become the preferred modality if one is to consider radiologic investigation. Li and coworkers demonstrated high accuracy in the diagnosis of anal abscess in a variety of locations in 51 patients.[50] The anatomy of abscess and anal canal is generally clearly visualized.[50]

Opinion

Although an unusual presentation or a complicated history may reasonably justify the use of CT and/or MRI, the high cost associated with these investigations strongly favors EAU and surgical drainage.

Primary Closure

Ellis advocated incision, curettage, and primary suture with antibiotic coverage in the treatment of anorectal abscess.[24,25] Although he reported excellent results in which primary healing took place in the vast majority of cases, one wonders about the likelihood of subsequent fistula development. Wilson reported on 100 of 120 patients treated and followed for an average of more than 2 years.[93] Approximately two-thirds initially had a perianal abscess; the remainder had an ischiorectal abscess. The overall recurrence rate was 22%

(15.6% following perianal abscess and 33.3% following ischiorectal abscess). He, too, noted that recurrence was much more likely if the culture initially revealed predominantly *E. coli* than if it yielded *S. aureus*. Mortensen and colleagues enrolled 107 patients in a study of primary suture with intraoperative parenteral antibiotics.[61] The incidence of recurrence was about the same, approximately 20%, in the two groups.

Goligher reported a prospective trial of conventional laying open versus incision, curettage, and suture.[29] Patients identified as having an internal opening at the time of drainage were excluded from the study. Healing occurred in more than 90% of those treated by primary suture. Because the follow-up period was less than 1 year, the rate of recurrence is difficult to judge.

Opinion

I have had no experience with this technique. Still, I can see no advantage in adopting it. Because I advocate minimal manipulation to effect drainage, the wound is inevitably quite small.

Deep Postanal Abscess

A transsphincteric fistula may present as an abscess in the deep postanal space (Figure 13-7). This space is deep (posterior) to the external sphincter and inferior to the levator ani muscle. The patient will usually complain of severe rectal discomfort, often with radiation to the sacrum, coccyx, or buttock, or it will display a sciatic distribution. It may be exacerbated by sitting, defecation may be impaired, and a fecal impaction may be present. Symptoms may mimic proctalgia fugax, coccygodynia, or lumbosacral strain. A helpful finding that implies the true nature of the problem is that the patient is frequently febrile. Someone with posterior rectal pain and rectal tenderness of relatively short duration (i.e., less than 48 hours), with pain that is continuous rather than intermittent and not affected by position, must be suspected of harboring an infection in the deep postanal space.

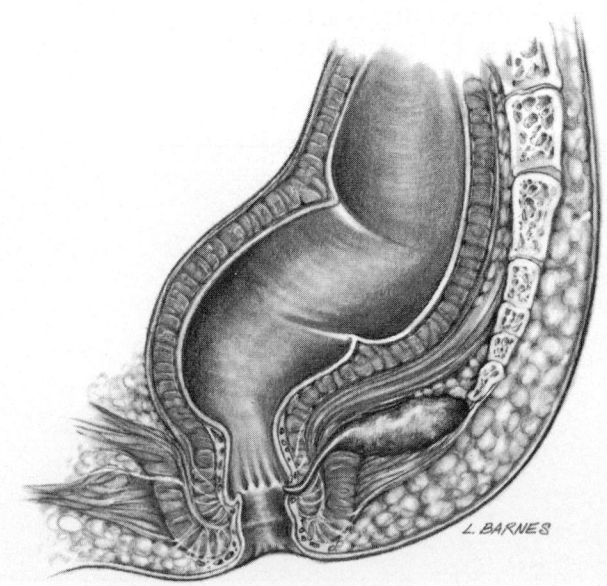

FIGURE 13-7. Deep postanal abscess originating from a posterior crypt. Drainage is effected through an incision from the internal opening to the coccyx.

Examination

Physical examination may be unrevealing except for exquisite posterior rectal tenderness. Very often the diagnosis is missed, and the patient is sent home with instructions concerning warm baths and perineal exercises and is told to take an analgesic medication. Eventually, the abscess will usually present at the skin or drain spontaneously through the rectum. There is, however, the risk of sepsis and even Fournier's gangrene (see Chapter 9) if the condition is unrecognized and treatment is delayed. A high degree of suspicion, therefore, may be required if appropriate management is to be initiated. An attempt at aspiration between the rectum and coccyx in the midline will prove diagnostic. If an extrarectal mass is felt, the differential diagnosis includes presacral cyst, presacral lipoma, teratoma, chordoma, and a host of unusual retrorectal conditions, but these are all rarely tender. The physician must also be aware of the fact that postanal infections often communicate with the ischiorectal fossae on either side. The presentation may therefore be that of bilateral ischiorectal abscesses, also known as a *horseshoe abscess.*

Treatment

Management requires drainage of the deep postanal space, a procedure that cannot be accomplished adequately in the office with only a local anesthetic. Almost inevitably an internal opening in the posterior midline is identified at the time of drainage.

The best access to the deep postanal space to effect drainage was initially described by Hanley (see Biography, Chapter 14).[36] He advocated placing a probe in the primary opening in the posterior midline and making an incision over the probe toward the tip of the coccyx. This incision divides the internal sphincter and the superficial and subcutaneous portions of the external sphincter in order to enter and to decompress the cavity. Counterincisions may be made to drain the ischiorectal fossae if necessary (e.g., horseshoe abscess). Packing is advised and should be left in place for 24 to 48 hours (see Figure 14-27). By today's standards, there is no other appropriate method for establishing drainage with this condition.[1,35]

Rosen and colleagues performed a retrospective review of horseshoe abscess and fistula during the 11 years from 1990 to 2001.[72] This manifestation represented 15% of all patients with anorectal sepsis at Cleveland Clinic Florida (31 patients). A higher incidence was noted in those individuals who were found to have Crohn's disease. The authors recommend unroofing and counter-drainage of the ischiorectal spaces. Another option would be to use a cutting seton once the initial perirectal sepsis has been drained and controlled.

This group also used imaging techniques, such as EAU and MRI. Despite the cost, with the availability of an experienced radiologist, MRI is becoming more reliable for interpreting the anatomy and the nature of the pathology.

Intersphincteric Abscess

Intersphincteric abscess was initially described by Eisenhammer (see Biography, Chapter 12) and subsequently subdivided by him into a high type and a low type.[21,22] The condition arises from an infected crypt in the anal canal, but in this situation, the infection usually burrows cephalad to present as a mass within the lower part of the rectum. It dissects in the intersphincteric plane, not under the mucosa, although it is frequently mistakenly called a "submucous"

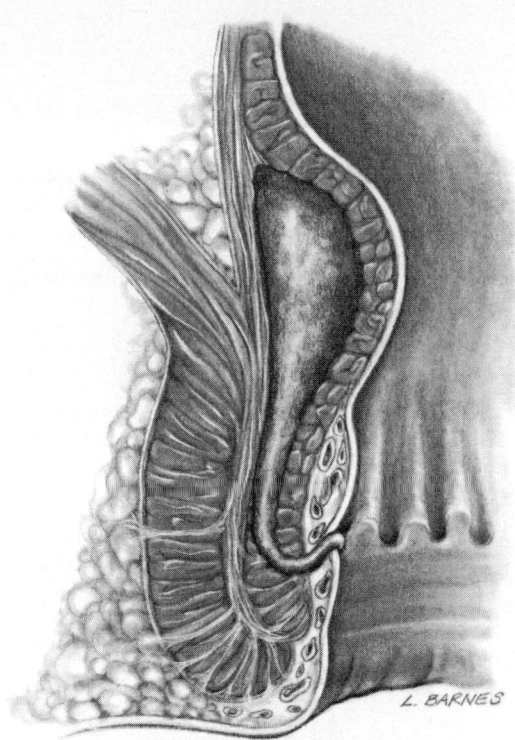

FIGURE 13-8. Intersphincteric abscess. The internal opening is at the level of the crypt with extension cephalad in the intermuscular plane.

abscess (Figure 13-8). Intersphincteric abscess is also sometimes classified as a submucous fistula, but this is an improper term because the condition does not fulfill the criterion for the definition of a fistula: a tract between two epithelial surfaces. Intersphincteric abscess represents between 2% and 5% of perirectal abscesses.

The patient usually complains of rectal or anal discomfort, which may be exacerbated by defecation. A sense of fullness in the rectum is often felt. Pus or mucous discharge may be noted. The individual may or may not be febrile.

Rectal examination may reveal a tender submucosal mass, which may not be readily apparent by anoscopy or proctosigmoidoscopy. The condition can be confused through palpation alone with a thrombosed internal hemorrhoid, but visual examination should distinguish the deep purple hemorrhoid from an abscess. The surface is edematous and indurated. An anal fissure is associated with the abscess in about 25% of patients.[65] Pus from the associated crypt should leave no doubt as to the nature of the lesion (Figure 13-9).

Treatment

Treatment usually requires a general, caudal, or spinal anesthetic, but a field block with conscious sedation may be attempted. However, this should *not* be considered an office procedure. A Hill-Ferguson retractor or other appropriate anal retractor is inserted. The abscess is *excised* through the internal sphincter, removing the associated crypt-bearing area (Figure 13-10). Finally, the cut edge of the rectum and the underlying internal sphincter can be sutured for hemostasis, leaving the wound open for drainage (Figure 13-11). No packing is required. The patient is discharged and advised to take a stool softener and warm baths. Healing usually takes place within 3 to 4 weeks; no further procedure is required.

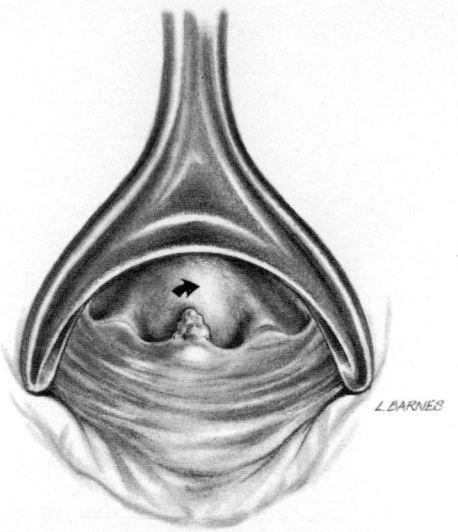

FIGURE 13-9. Opening of an intersphincteric abscess at the level of the crypt. Induration (*arrow*) is usually present proximal to this point.

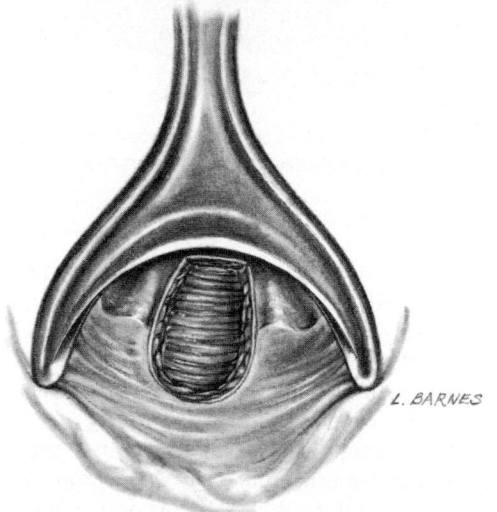

FIGURE 13-10. Intersphincteric abscess. The mucosa and the underlying internal sphincter are excised.

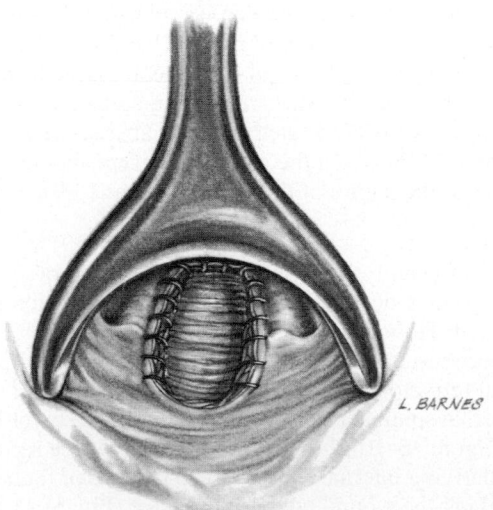

FIGURE 13-11. Intersphincteric abscess. The cut mucosal edge with the internal anal sphincter is sutured for hemostasis.

Supralevator Abscess

A high intersphincteric abscess can extend into the supralevator space to produce what is termed a *supralevator abscess*. This presentation is relatively rare, comprising fewer than 2.5% of abscesses as published in most series (Figure 13-12).[7,12,30,45] However, Goldenberg and Prasad and colleagues reviewed the Cook County Hospital experience and found the incidence to be higher, 7.5% and 9.1%, respectively.[28,69] It is difficult to explain this variation in incidence; however, these reporters attribute their large experience to the low socioeconomic status of the patients, although I do not fully understand why this should be a factor. Obesity and diabetes mellitus were considered important contributing factors; one or the other was observed in 23% of their patients. Other rare causes are diverticulitis, gynecologic infections, appendicitis, Crohn's disease, and systemic infectious sources.

Perianal and buttock pain are the most common presenting complaints. Most patients are febrile and demonstrate a leukocytosis.

Urgent management by means of surgical drainage has often led to spreading infection and the development of problems with delayed healing and nonhealing, as well as a

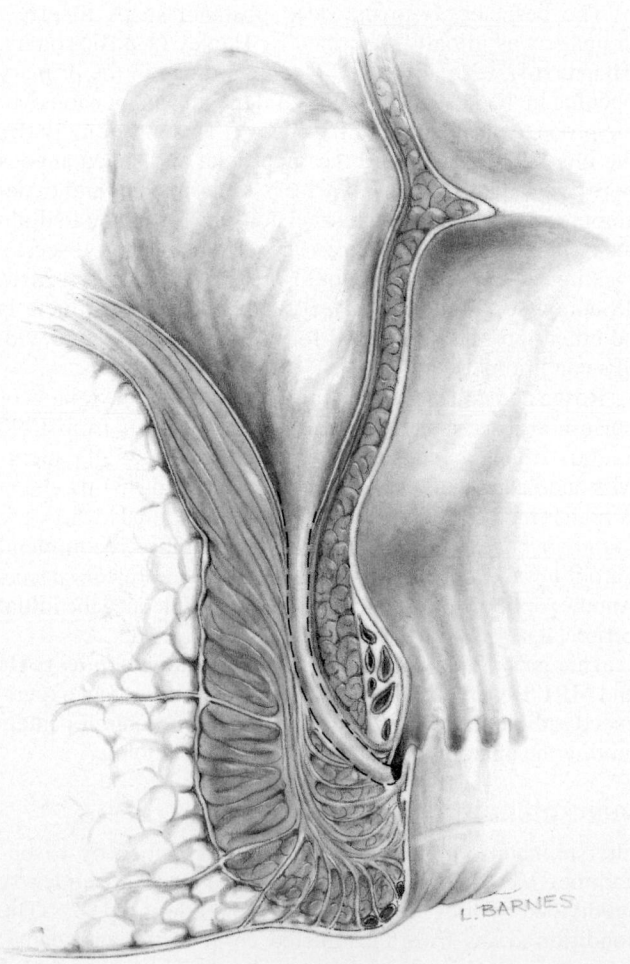

FIGURE 13-12. Supralevator abscess. As implied and as illustrated, the abscess is located in the space above the levatores and adjacent to the rectum. The *dashed lines* illustrate the possible course of a fistula tract if it is present.

high incidence of recurrence. In a study by Millan and colleagues, in which 9 of 21 abscesses were of the high type, it was found that preoperative imaging with EAU and/or MRI (if available) should be accomplished prior to undertaking any procedure.[60] Once appropriately evaluated, catheter drainage is advised. This should include division of the internal sphincter and unroofing of the abscess cavity if possible. This will result in a reduced risk of muscle injury and minimize the likelihood of recurrence. Endoanal ultrasound needle aspiration has also been attempted with some success by Epstein and Giordano.[26] Patients were followed for 12 to 18 months without any complication or recurrence, but the sample size was small. Despite the above concerns, establishing open drainage remains the standard.

Comment

In my experience, most individuals who present with a supralevator abscess have a characteristic history—namely, an underlying pelvic inflammatory process, prior recent abdominal surgery, or Crohn's disease. Parks and Gordon reported a number of cases of perineal fistula that developed secondary to an intra-abdominal process.[64] Supralevator abscess may also occur as an in-continuity cephalad extension of a transsphincteric or rarely an intersphincteric abscess (see Figure 13-2).

Principles of Treatment of Anal/Perianal Abscess

The cause of the abscess determines the therapy: transrectal or transvaginal drainage for abscess caused by pelvic sepsis and external drainage for abscess secondary to transsphincteric fistula. To perform transrectal drainage when an internal opening is present at the level of the crypt is an invitation to disaster. Similarly, to drain an abscess to the perineum when a communication is present above the levators may result in a high extrasphincteric fistula. Management of this unfortunate consequence is notably highly complicated (see Chapter 14).

Effective treatment, therefore, mandates an understanding of the etiology of the septic process. To accomplish this, an appreciation of the history is very helpful (e.g., knowledge that the patient has Crohn's disease or has recently undergone abdominal surgery). More important, however, is to evaluate the situation by using an anesthetic and by attempting to identify an internal opening at the level of the crypt. If such an opening is found, the drainage procedure should be external; if absent, drainage probably should be internal (Figure 13-13).

Internal Drainage

For *internal drainage*, the patient is optimally placed in the prone position if the abscess is located anteriorly or in the lithotomy position if the abscess is situated posteriorly. However, because the drainage procedure can be performed relatively quickly and anesthesiologists are rather disinclined to place patients face down, the lithotomy position is generally favored.

Following aspiration, an incision is made into the cavity, either sharply with a knife or bluntly with a curved clamp (Figure 13-14). A de Pezzer (i.e., mushroom), Malecot, or Foley catheter may be inserted into the cavity and delivered

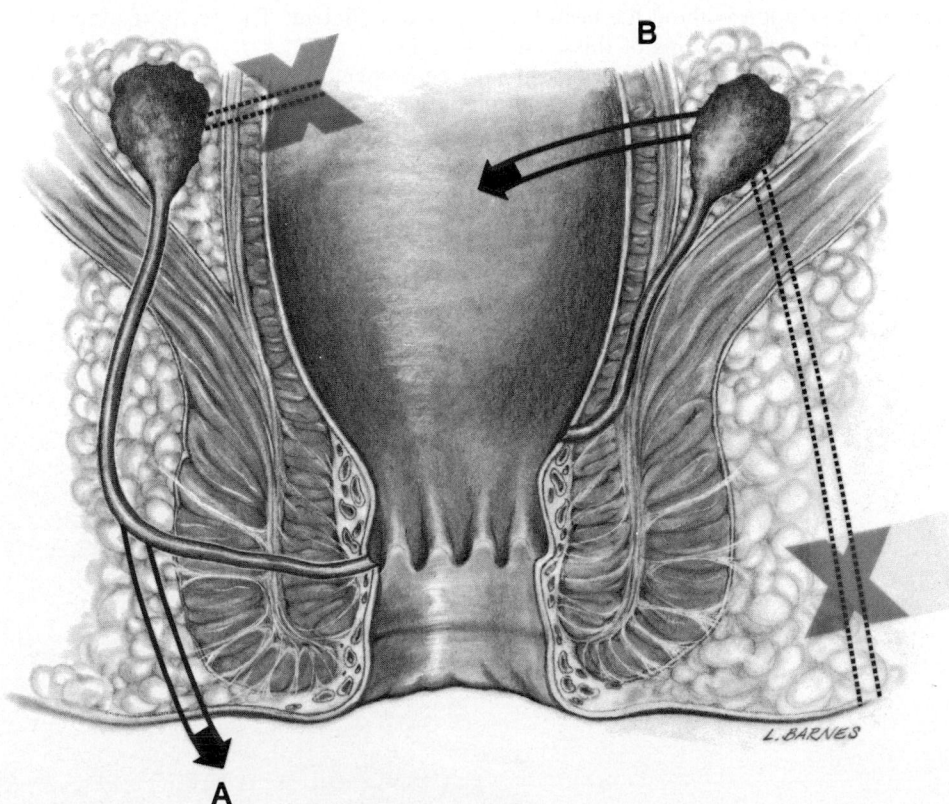

FIGURE 13-13. Methods of drainage for supralevator abscess. **A:** Perineal drainage secondary to transsphincteric fistula. **B:** Transrectal drainage from pelvic sepsis. Unfortunately, the clearly defined possible scenarios illustrated do not necessarily facilitate decision making in individual cases.

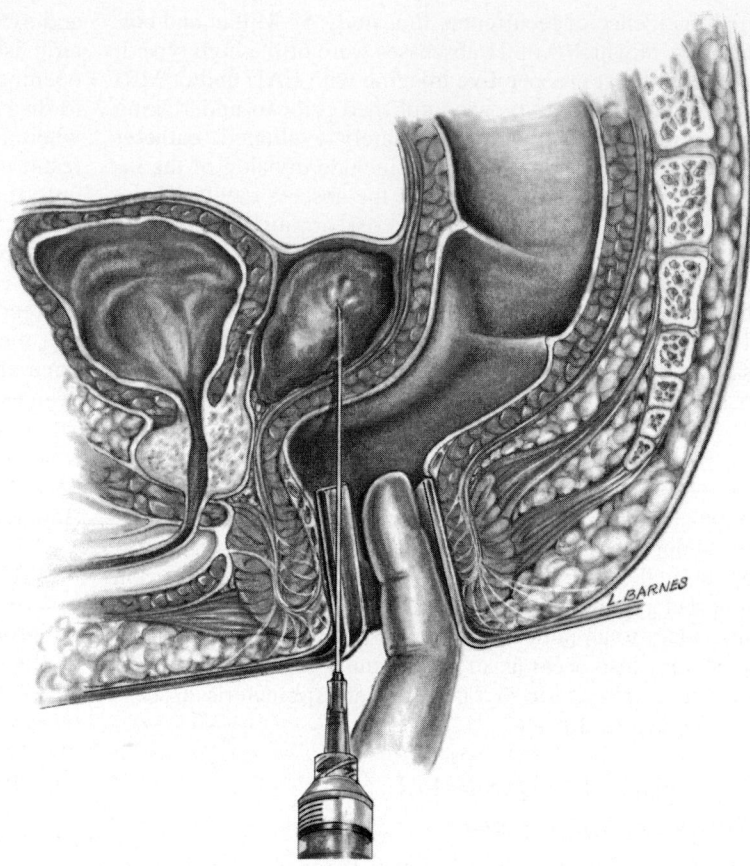

FIGURE 13-14. Aspiration of a supralevator abscess confirms the location for drainage and may be performed with a retractor in position or by manual assessment.

through the anal verge. The opening is made small enough for the catheter to remain in position without the need for suturing (Figure 13-15). Other modifications of this technique include placing a cut piece of rubber catheter through the tip of another to hold it in place or using a T tube. However, many surgeons believe that placement of a drain is not required; evacuation of the purulent material is considered sufficient. The drain, if used, is removed in 24 to 48 hours.

In women, whenever possible, an anterior abscess should be drained transvaginally through the posterior cul-de-sac (Figure 13-16). Drainage is technically easier to perform,

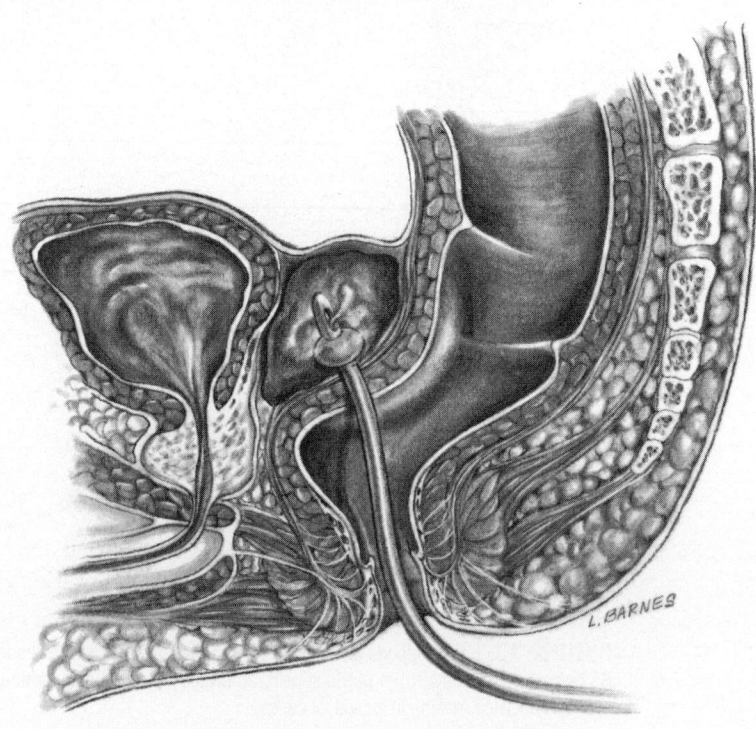

FIGURE 13-15. A catheter is inserted into the supralevator abscess cavity to maintain adequate drainage.

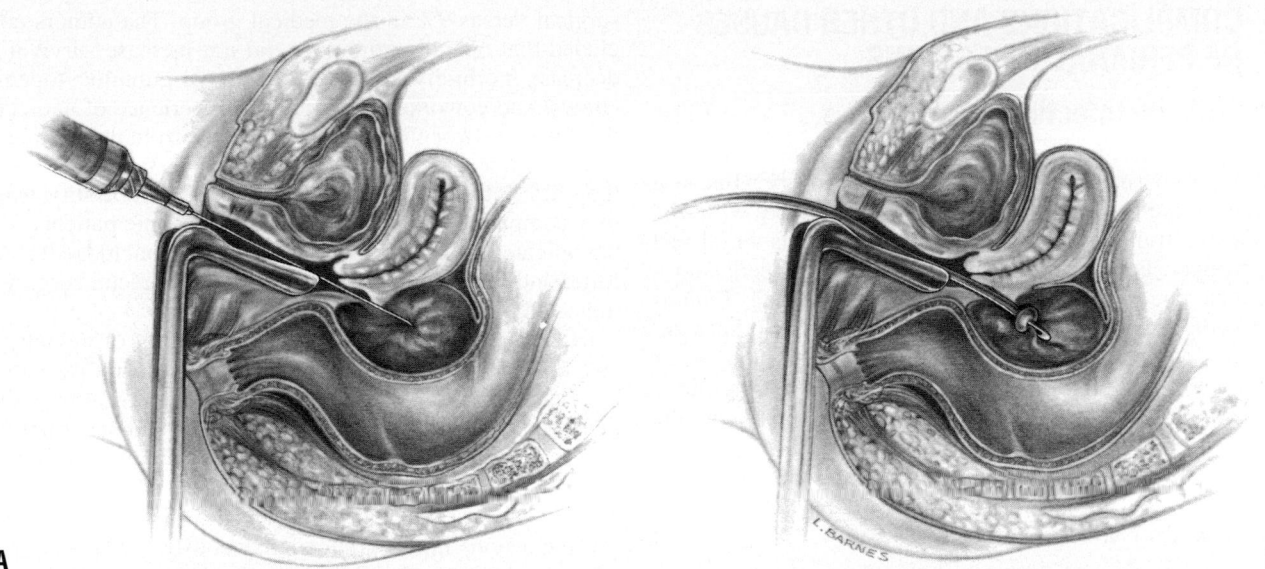

FIGURE 13-16. Drainage of pelvic abscess is performed transvaginally. **A:** Needle aspiration. **B:** Insertion of a catheter into the cavity

and the patient is more comfortable if the intact anal sphincter is avoided should a drain be inserted.

External Drainage

If *external drainage* is deemed appropriate, the patient is placed in the prone jackknife position. A larger external wound is required than for other abscesses because it is imperative to drain the supralevator collection adequately. Again, the location of the incision should be as medial as possible. The supralevator space may be packed, or a Foley, de Pezzer (i.e., mushroom), or Malecot catheter can be placed in the cavity and left for 24 to 48 hours (Figure 13-17). Irrigation through the catheter may also be considered.

Results

It is essentially impossible to find any meaningful data in the literature on the results of surgery following drainage of supralevator abscesses. In the series of Prasad and associates, primary fistulotomy was performed in two-thirds of patients who were found to have concurrent fistulas.[69] In my opinion, however, definitive fistula surgery probably should be undertaken during a subsequent hospitalization following the initial drainage.

Commentary on Drains and Drainage Procedures

CT-guided drainage is an alternative whenever there is material to drain and whenever there is a portal as well as the availability of a skilled invasive radiologist. Surgeons should feel comfortable getting their hands dirty, but radiologists rarely feel so inclined. Sometimes it is easier to ask another specialist to take care of the problem, especially if it is in the middle of the night. Unfortunately for the patient, CT-guided drainage involves a procedure, which most individuals consider uncomfortable at best, that is associated with some morbidity, with sometimes inadequate drainage, with the placement of a catheter for 10 days or more (always a very uncomfortable experience), and with the need for additional radiologic studies, as well as its rather uncomfortable removal. The fact is that the physician may credibly

argue that drains are probably unnecessary. Once the abscess has been effectively evacuated, the cavity usually collapses and heals rather quickly. In any event, with the exception of the radiologist's manipulations, most drains fall out within a short time.

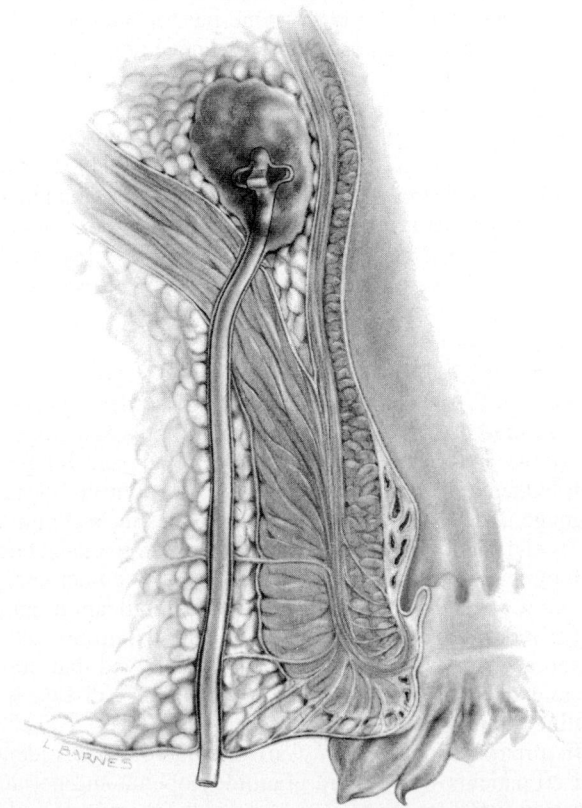

FIGURE 13-17. External drainage of a supralevator abscess with insertion of a catheter. This rather unusual approach is often undertaken in individuals whose complication is secondary to Crohn's disease. Long-term drainage is often necessary.

► COMPLICATIONS AND OTHER CAUSES OF PERIANAL INFECTIONS

Necrotizing Infection

Necrotizing infection (i.e., Fournier's gangrene; see Chapter 9) can be a consequence of anorectal abscess.[7,10,56] Because diabetes mellitus is so frequently associated with the disease, it truly merits etiologic status.[23] This is why I feel so strongly about diabetic patients who develop perianal infections require treatment within a hospital setting. *Tetanus* following drainage of anorectal abscess has also been reported.[51,62] Delay in diagnosis and treatment—a week or more in most cases—as well as associated conditions (diabetes, obesity, malignancy, AIDS, tuberculosis, and the immunocompromised state) are contributing factors (see also Chapter 10).[3,59,91,94] Treatment requires antibiotics, nutritional support, wide debridement, adequate drainage, and usually proximal diversion.

Hematologic Disease

Abscess, fistula, and perirectal infections are commonly seen in patients with hematologic abnormalities (e.g., leukemia, granulocytopenia, lymphoma; see Chapter 9). These problems represent 3% to 8% of hematology admissions.[8,11,12,15,32,39,47,48,75,77,88] In the experience from one center in Turkey, the incidence of perianal infections was found to be 7.3% in 259 patients with acute leukemia, but only 1% in those with chronic leukemia.[13] In another study of more than 200 individuals with acute leukemia, perianal infections developed in 7.9%.[6] The incidence in granulocytopenia, defined as a polymorphonuclear neutrophil count of less than 500/mm³, has been reported to be 11%.[88] One-half of the patients die within 1 month of diagnosis, most of septic complications.

Symptoms and Findings

Patients usually present with anal pain, but fever, septicemia, and shock may also be evident. Often, neither fluctuation nor pus is present. Urinary retention, peritoneal signs, and infection of the genitalia are common.[6] Of interest is the fact that cultured organisms may be quite different from those usually identified with uncomplicated perirectal septic processes.[39]

Treatment and Results

The prognosis is closely correlated with the response to management of the underlying hematologic disorder. Conservative treatment (e.g., antibiotics, warm baths, granulocyte infusions) and perhaps radiotherapy are advised for those with leukemia if the disease is under poor control. Surgical drainage under such circumstances may result in fulminant sepsis and death. Shaked and colleagues showed that patients with agranulocytosis who underwent operative intervention had slow wound healing, prolonged hospitalization, and a higher mortality rate when compared with the group that received antibiotics alone.[79] The authors believed that drainage may be performed, however, if the patient's disease is in relative remission.

In a retrospective review, Carlson and colleagues identified 20 patients with severe granulocytopenia and perianal infection.[15] Eleven were managed medically, and 9 underwent operative drainage. With the exception of a higher frequency of positive blood cultures in those who had surgery, the two groups were similar. Mortality was 44.4% in the

surgical versus 9% in the medical group. The authors concluded that operative drainage did not increase survival or decrease morbidity in those with severe granulocytopenia. Grewal and coworkers reported the experience of anorectal disease in neutropenic leukemia patients from the Memorial Sloan-Kettering Cancer Center in New York.[32] Because they did not observe excess morbidity or mortality when they compared operated neutropenic leukemic patients with nonoperated patients (20% vs. 18%), they concluded that selected individuals should not be denied anorectal surgery if indicated.

Hiatt and colleagues support the concept of an aggressive approach, stating that hemodynamic instability should be regarded as an indication for surgical intervention rather than a contraindication.[39] In addition to broad-spectrum antibiotic coverage, they advise wide debridement and end-sigmoid colostomy with closure of the distal rectum. Some recommend a drainage procedure if there is persistent fever and the lesions fail to drain spontaneously.[6] Others suggest baths, suppositories, antibiotics, and judicious surgical drainage.[9] Even abdominoperineal resection has been performed in a patient with extensive perirectal sepsis.[66] Although it is obvious that controversy exists concerning management options in these patients, a nonoperative approach is generally recommended, especially for the neutropenic individual. In others words, treatment should be directed to restoring the granulocyte count in these situations. The neutrophil count and its course during the infection are the most significant variables with respect to the evolution of perianal lesions and the ultimate prognosis.[13] However, with appropriate support, and with an adequate neutrophil count, perianal septic problems can reasonably be treated surgically.

Anorectal Abscess in the Cancer Patient

As previously implied, mortality rates approach 50% in immunocompromised patients if an anal abscess develops and is felt to require surgery. Perianal sepsis was and still leads to a high-associated morbidity as well as a potentially lethal consequence for those receiving chemotherapy. Treatment is distinctly different from that of noncancer patients. Cancer patients are affected by a variety of factors, including chemotherapy, steroid use, immunosuppression, other medications, prior radiation, and even ethical issues.

Badgwell and associates evaluated the presentation and treatment of anorectal infection in 100 cancer patients.[5] Forty-two were managed nonoperatively, and 58 underwent surgery, the most common being incision and drainage (79%). Others underwent seton insertion (9%), fistulotomy (3%), and wide debridement (2 patients for a necrotizing infection process). The 90-day mortality was 1%. Thrombocytopenia (platelet count <50,000) is a poor prognostic sign that mandates a nonoperative approach because mortality rates have been found to exceed 59% with surgical intervention. Another factor is severe neutropenia, wherein the operative mortality approaches 44% as compared with a 9% mortality with nonoperative management. Lehrnbecher and associates satisfactorily treated 52 of 82 patients with antibiotics alone, reserving surgery for progressive infections and for abscesses with "concerning clinical features."[49] They also suggest the possibility of needle aspiration and close follow-up in sicker patients with a more developed abscess. Others opine that without progressive infection, withholding surgery is probably preferred in this patient population. Neutropenia remains an area of "debate and controversy," but when an immunocompromised patient in need of chemotherapy presents with an abscess, he or she should undergo incision and drainage with seton insertion when possible until such time as the immune system recovers.[5,49]

Bone Marrow Transplantation

Perianal infection is a rare complication of bone marrow transplantation. Cohen and colleagues performed a retrospective review over a 10-year period that involved almost 1,000 patients at the City of Hope National Medical Center near Los Angeles.[18] Twenty-four were diagnosed with perianal infections following transplants (2.5%). The authors concluded that the management of this complication is essentially the same as that described for patients with hematologic diseases. In general, perianal wound healing is not prolonged in those undergoing surgical drainage for infection following bone marrow transplantation.[18]

AIDS

Patients with AIDS are extremely susceptible to opportunistic infections in the anorectal area. Wexner and colleagues reported their experience with 340 such individuals from the St. Luke's–Roosevelt Hospital in New York City.[92] The incidence of anorectal disease, most commonly abscess and fistula, was 34%.

Due to the variety of etiologic factors that may contribute to perianal sepsis in these patients, consultation by surgeons experienced with these disease processes is pivotal. The reader is referred to a discussion of the colorectal manifestations of AIDS in Chapter 10.

Anal Abscess in Crohn's Disease

For acute perianal suppuration, management with drainage, antibiotics, and seton placement remains the primary strategy. This is discussed further in Chapter 14.

Jones and Finlayson looked at the surgical trends in patients with Crohn's disease since the emergence of Remicade (infliximab) as an effective medication for this condition.[43] It has been shown in many studies that infliximab may lead to closure of perianal fistulas, but in this study, it was demonstrated that this drug may actually increase the incidence of perianal abscesses.

Limited incision and drainage is appropriate for a localized abscess. However, in those individuals receiving this medication for anal fistula, close monitoring is important because the requirement for surgery in the perianal region does appear to increase. This may be due to closing of the external (secondary) opening while the internal opening remains patent. This is in contrast to the publication by Sands and coworkers (2004) in which they recommend infliximab maintenance therapy for fistulizing Crohn's disease.[73] EAU and MRI may be useful for identifying potential recurrent sources of infection.[43,73]

Surgical Specialization

There is data to support that individuals trained in colorectal surgery have better outcomes and different management strategies than other specialists for the treatment of perianal abscess and fistula. A retrospective study by Malik and associates reviewed 147 cases of anal abscesses (28%,

recurrent), many with concomitant anal fistula.[54] Fistulas were identified in 30 patients, with more than half identified by specialist consultants ($P = .00001$). Consultants performed fistulotomy and seton insertion in 50% and 17% of patients, respectively, whereas registrars (surgical residents) performed these procedures in only 4% and 8% of patients ($P < .00001$). The authors concluded that although surgical management of perianal abscess is one of the most common emergency procedures performed by the surgical trainee, input from a senior clinician improves the identification and definitive management of an underlying fistula.

Tuberculous Anal Sepsis
See Chapter 9.

Perianal Actinomycosis
See Chapter 9.

▶ SUMMARY POINTS

1. Clinical examination will usually identify the abscess. Waiting for fluctuance to develop is inappropriate and delays needed treatment. If in doubt, needle aspiration to confirm the presence of an abscess can be performed, and then drain appropriately.
2. MRI has emerged as the most accurate investigation, but it costs more, and equipment with a skilled interpreter may be unavailable. Imaging studies such as CT, EAU, and MRI are not usually necessary except with complicated fistulas, such as suprasphincteric, extrasphincteric, high intersphincteric, and recurrence.
3. Drainage *not* antibiotics is the required treatment, with antibiotics reserved for specific conditions, such as Crohn's disease, the immunocompromised state, cellulitis, and sepsis. The use of setons, when possible, permits resolution of severe inflammation in complicated cases. Most cancer and immunocompromised patients can be managed conservatively unless acute suppuration is noted.
4. Office drainage is appropriate for most perianal abscesses but operative drainage for complex abscesses and septic or immunocompromised patients is needed.
5. Drain close to the anus.
6. There is generally no reason to repack drainage sites following initial removal.
7. Avoid aggressive manipulation and disruption of loculations.
8. Primary closure is not appropriate.
9. Do not hesitate to return to the operating room for re-exploration and drainage if fever, cellulitis, or signs of sepsis develop.
10. Use caution with drainage of a supralevator abscess whether intersphincteric or ischioanal in origin to avoid the creation of inappropriate fistula.
11. Limit synchronous fistulotomy to that of involvement of only superficial muscle.
12. When in doubt, seek consultation or input from someone with more experience.
13. Although a rare source of concern, recurrent abscesses and fistulas requiring multiple treatments and nonhealing wounds should be biopsied to ensure that the process is benign. Perineal mucinous adenocarcinoma was found in both abscesses and fistulas.[74]

14. The importance of a discussion with the patient in both preprocedure and postprocedure follow-up cannot be overestimated.
15. One must be aware of the possibility that multiple procedures may be required to resolve the condition.
16. A discussion of incontinence risk is beneficial in formulating the best management strategy.

References

1. Abcarian H. Surgical management of recurrent anorectal abscesses. *Contemp Surg.* 1982;21:85.
2. Albright JB, Pidala MJ, Cali JR, et al. MRSA-related perianal abscesses: an under recognized disease entity. *Dis Colon Rectum.* 2007;50(7): 996–1003.
3. Allen-Mersh TG. Symposium: the management of anorectal disease in HIV-positive patients. *Int J Colorectal Dis.* 1990;5:61.
4. Avill R. The management of carcinoma of the rectum presenting as an ischiorectal abscess. *Br J Surg.* 1984;71(9):665.
5. Badgwell BD, Chang GJ, Rodriguez-Bigas MA, et al. Management and outcomes of anorectal infection in the cancer patient. *Ann Surg Oncol.* 2009;16(10):2752–2758.
6. Barnes SG, Sattler FR, Ballard JO. Perirectal infections in acute leukemia. Improved survival after incision and debridement. *Ann Intern Med.* 1984;100(4):515–518.
7. Bevans DW Jr, Westbrook KC, Thompson BW, et al. Perirectal abscess: a potentially fatal illness. *Am J Surg.* 1973;126(6):765–768.
8. Blank WA. Anorectal complications in leukemia. *Am J Surg.* 1955; 90(5):738–741.
9. Boddie AW Jr, Bines SD. Management of acute rectal problems in leukemic patients. *J Surg Oncol.* 1986;33(1):53–56.
10. Bode WE, Ramos R, Page CP. Invasive necrotizing infection secondary to anorectal abscess. *Dis Colon Rectum.* 1982;25(5):416–419.
11. Brook I, Martin WJ. Aerobic and anaerobic bacteriology of perirectal abscess in children. *Pediatrics.* 1980;66(2):282–284.
12. Buchan R, Grace RH. Anorectal suppuration: the results of treatment and the factors influencing the recurrence rate. *Br J Surg.* 1973;60(7):537–540.
13. Büyükaşik Y, Ozcebe OI, Sayinalp N, et al. Perianal infections in patients with leukemia: importance of the course of neutrophil count. *Dis Colon Rectum.* 1998;41(1):81–85.
14. Caliste X, Nazir S, Goode T, et al. Sensitivity of computed tomography in detection of perirectal abscess. *Am Surg.* 2011;77(2):166–168.
15. Carlson GW, Ferguson CM, Amerson JR. Perianal infections in acute leukemia. Second place winner: Conrad Jobst Award. *Am Surg.* 1988; 54(12):693–695.
16. Cataldo PA, Senagore A, Luchtefeld MA. Intrarectal ultrasound in the evaluation of perirectal abscesses. *Dis Colon Rectum.* 1993;36(6): 554–558.
17. Chiari H. Ueber die analen Divertikel der Rectumsschleimhaut und ihre Beziehung zu den Analfisteln. *Med Jahr.* 1878;8:419–427.
18. Cohen JS, Paz IB, O'Donnell MR, et al. Treatment of perianal infection following bone marrow transplantation. *Dis Colon Rectum.* 1996;39(9):981–985.
19. Devaraj B, Khabassi S, Cosman BC. Recent smoking is a risk factor for anal abscess and fistula. *Dis Colon Rectum.* 2011;54(6):681–685.
20. Duhamel J. Anal fistulae in childhood. *Am J Proctol.* 1975;26(6): 40–43.
21. Eisenhammer S. The internal anal sphincter; its surgical importance. *S Afr Med J.* 1953;27(13):266–270.
22. Eisenhammer S. The internal anal sphincter and the anorectal abscess. *Surg Gynecol Obstet.* 1956;103(4):501–506.
23. Eke N. Fournier's gangrene: a review of 1726 cases. *Br J Surg.* 2000;87(6):718–728.
24. Ellis M. The use of penicillin and sulphonamides in the treatment of suppuration. *Lancet.* 1951;1(6658):774–775.
25. Ellis M. Recurrence of infection following treatment of anorectal abscesses by primary suture. *Proc R Soc Med.* 1962;55:757.
26. Epstein J, Giordano P. Endoanal ultrasound-guided needle drainage of intersphincteric abscess. *Tech Coloproctol.* 2005;9(1):67–69.
27. Fitzgerald RJ, Harding B, Ryan W. Fistula-in-ano in childhood: a congenital etiology. *J Pediatr Surg.* 1985;20(1):80–81.
28. Goldenberg HS. Supralevator abscess diagnosis and treatment. *Surgery.* 1982;91(2):164–167.
29. Goligher JC. Fistula-in-ano: management of perianal suppuration. *Dis Colon Rectum.* 1976;19(6):516–517.
30. Goligher JC. *Surgery of the Anus, Rectum and Colon.* 4th ed. New York, NY: Macmillan; 1980:156.
31. Grace RH, Harper IA, Thompson RG. Anorectal sepsis: microbiology in relation to fistula-in-ano. *Br J Surg.* 1982;69(7):401–403.
32. Grewal H, Guillem JG, Quan SH, et al. Anorectal disease in neutropenic leukemic patients: operative vs. nonoperative management. *Dis Colon Rectum.* 1994;37(11):1095–1099.
33. Hamadani A, Haigh PI, Liu IL, et al. Who is at risk for developing chronic anal fistula or recurrent anal sepsis after initial perianal abscess? *Dis Colon Rectum.* 2009;52(2):217–221.
34. Hämäläinen KP, Sainio AP. Incidence of fistulas after drainage of acute anorectal abscesses. *Dis Colon Rectum.* 1998;41(11):1357–1361.
35. Hamilton CH. Anorectal problems: the deep postanal space—surgical significance in horseshoe fistula and abscess. *Dis Colon Rectum.* 1975;18(8):642–645.
36. Hanley PH. Conservative surgical correction of horseshoe abscess and fistula. *Dis Colon Rectum.* 1965;8(5):364–368.
37. Henrichsen S, Christiansen J. Incidence of fistula-in-ano complicating anorectal sepsis: a prospective study. *Br J Surg.* 1986;73(5):371–372.
38. Herrmann G, Desfosses L. Sur la muqueuse de la région cloacale du rectum. *C R Acad Sci (Paris).* 1880;90:1301–1304.
39. Hiatt JR, Kuchenbecker SL, Winston DJ. Perineal gangrene in the patient with granulocytopenia: the importance of early diverting colostomy. *Surgery.* 1986;100(5):912–915.
40. Hill JR. Fistulas and fistulous abscesses in the anorectal region: personal experience in management. *Dis Colon Rectum.* 1967;10(6): 421–434.
41. Holzheimer RG, Siebeck M. Treatment procedures for anal fistulous cryptoglandular abscess—how to get the best results. *Eur J Med Res.* 2006;11(12):501–515.
42. Jackman RJ, Buie LA. Tuberculosis and anal fistula. *J Am Med Assoc.* 1946;130:630–632.
43. Jones DW, Finlayson SR. Trends in surgery for Crohn's disease in the era of infliximab. *Ann Surg.* 2010;252(2):307–312.
44. Kim Y, Park YJ. Three-dimensional endoanal ultrasonographic assessment of an anal fistula with and without H_2O_2 enhancement. *World J Gastroenterol.* 2009;15(38):4810–4815.
45. Kline RJ, Spencer RJ, Harrison EG Jr. Carcinoma associated with fistula-in-ano. *Arch Surg.* 1964;89:989–994.
46. Klosterhalfen B, Offner F, Vogel P, et al. Anatomic nature and surgical significance of anal sinus and anal intramuscular glands. *Dis Colon Rectum.* 1991;34(2):156–160.
47. Kott I, Urca I. Perianal abscess as a presenting sign of leukemia. *Dis Colon Rectum.* 1969;12(5):338–339.
48. Krieger RW, Chusid MJ. Perirectal abscess in childhood. *Am J Dis Child.* 1979;133(4):411–412.
49. Lehrnbecher T, Marshall D, Gao C, et al. A second look at anorectal infections in cancer patients in a large cancer institute: the success of early intervention with antibiotics and surgery. *Infection.* 2002;30(5):272–276.
50. Li X, Qiang JW, He C, et al. Magnetic resonance imaging study of perianal abscess. *Zhonghua Wei Chang Wai Ke Za Zhi.* 2011;14(11): 868–870.
51. Lichtenstein D, Stavorovsky M, Irge D. Fournier's gangrene complicating perianal abscess: report of two cases. *Dis Colon Rectum.* 1978;21(5):377–379.
52. Liu CK, Liu CP, Leung CH, et al. Clinical and microbiological analysis of adult perianal abscess. *J Microbiol Immunol Infect.* 2011;44(3):204–208.
53. Lunniss PJ, Phillips RKS. Surgical assessment of acute anorectal sepsis is a better predictor of fistula than microbiological analysis. *Br J Surg.* 1994;81(3):368–369.
54. Malik A, Hall D, Devaney R, et al. The impact of specialist experience in the surgical management of perianal abscesses. *Int J Surg.* 2011;9(6):475–477.
55. Malik AI, Nelson RL, Tou S. Incision and drainage of perianal abscess with or without treatment of anal fistula. *Cochrane Database Syst Rev.* 2010;7(7):CD006827.
56. Marks G, Chase WV, Mervine TB. The fatal potential of fistula-in-ano with abscess: analysis of 11 deaths. *Dis Colon Rectum.* 1973;16(3):224–230.
57. McElwain JW, Alexander RM, MacLean MD. Primary fistulectomy for anorectal abscesses: clinical study of 500 cases. *Dis Colon Rectum.* 1966;9(3):181–185.
58. McElwain JW, MacLean MD, Alexander RM, et al. Anorectal problems: experience with primary fistulectomy for anorectal abscess, a report of 1,000 cases. *Dis Colon Rectum.* 1975;18(8):646–649.
59. Miles AJ, Mellor CH, Gazzard B, et al. Surgical management of anorectal disease in HIV-positive homosexuals. *Br J Surg.* 1990;77(8): 869–871.

60. Millan M, García-Granero E, Esclápez P, et al. Management of intersphincteric abscesses. *Colorectal Dis.* 2006;8(9):777–780.

61. Mortensen J, Kraglund K, Klaerke M, et al. Primary suture of anorectal abscess: a randomized study comparing treatment with clindamycin versus clindamycin and Gentacoll. *Dis Colon Rectum.* 1995;38(4):398–401.

62. Myers KJ, Heppell J, Bode WE, et al. Tetanus after anorectal abscess. *Mayo Clin Proc.* 1984;59(6):429–430.

63. Parks AG. Pathogenesis and treatment of fistula-in-ano. *Br Med J.* 1961;1(5224):463–469.

64. Parks AG, Gordon PH. Perineal fistula of intra-abdominal or intrapelvic origin simulating fistula-in-ano: report of seven cases. *Dis Colon Rectum.* 1976;19(6):500–506.

65. Parks AG, Thomson JP. Intersphincteric abscess. *BMJ.* 1973;2(5865):537–539.

66. Paterson FW, Wonke B, Piper JV. Abdominoperineal resection in acute myeloblastic leukemia. *Br Med J.* 1976;1(6018):1124.

67. Piazza DJ, Radhakrishnan J. Perianal abscess and fistula-in-ano in children. *Dis Colon Rectum.* 1990;33(12):1014–1016.

68. Pople IK, Ralphs DN. An aetiology for fistula in ano. *Br J Surg.* 1988;75(9):904–905.

69. Prasad ML, Read TR, Abcarian H. Supralevator abscess: diagnosis and treatment. *Dis Colon Rectum.* 1981;24(6):456–461.

70. Ramanujam PS, Prasad ML, Abcarian H, et al. Perianal abscesses and fistulas: a study of 1023 patients. *Dis Colon Rectum.* 1984;27(9):593–597.

71. Read DR, Abcarian H. A prospective survey of 474 patients with anorectal abscess. *Dis Colon Rectum.* 1979;22(8):566–568.

72. Rosen SA, Colquhoun P, Efron J, et al. Horseshoe abscesses and fistulas: how are we doing? *Surg Innov.* 2006;13(1):17–21.

73. Sands BE, Anderson FH, Bernstein CN, et al. Infliximab maintenance therapy for fistulizing Crohn's disease. *N Engl J Med.* 2004;350(9):876–885.

74. Schaffzin DM, Stahl TJ, Smith LE. Perianal mucinous adenocarcinoma: unusual case presentations and review of the literature. *Am Surg.* 2003;69(2):166–169.

75. Schimpff SC, Wiernik PH, Block JB. Rectal abscesses in cancer patients. *Lancet.* 1972;2(7782):844–847.

76. Scoma JA, Salvati EP, Rubin RJ. Incidence of fistulas subsequent to anal abscesses. *Dis Colon Rectum.* 1974;17(3):357–359.

77. Sehdev MK, Dowling MD, Seal SH, et al. Perianal and anorectal complications in leukemia. *Cancer.* 1973;31(1):149–152.

78. Shafer AD, McGlone TP, Flanagan RA. Abnormal crypts of Morgagni: the cause of perianal abscess and fistula-in-ano. *J Pediatr Surg.* 1987;22(3):203–204.

79. Shaked AA, Shinar E, Freund H. Managing the granulocytopenic patient with acute perianal inflammatory disease. *Am J Surg.* 1986;152(5):510–512.

80. Sözener U, Gedik E, Kessaf Aslar A, et al. Does adjuvant antibiotic treatment after drainage of anorectal abscess prevent development of anal fistulas? A randomized, placebo-controlled, double-blind, multicenter study. *Dis Colon Rectum.* 2011;54(8):923–929.

81. Standards Task Force, American Society of Colon and Rectal Surgeons. Practice parameters for treatment of fistula-in-ano. The American Society of Colon and Rectal Surgeons. *Dis Colon Rectum.* 1996;39(12):1361–1372.

82. Stelzmueller I, Aigner F, Albright J, et al. Group Milleri Streptococci in perianal infections. *Colorectal Dis.* 2010;12(7 online):e121–e127.

83. Stremitzer S, Strobl S, Kure V, et al. Treatment of perianal sepsis and long-term outcome of recurrence and continence. *Colorectal Disease.* 2001;13(6):703–707.

84. Sudoł-Szopińska I, Kołodziejczak M, Szopiński TR. The accuracy of a post-processing technique—volume render mode—in three-dimensional endoanal ultrasonography of anal abscesses and fistulas. *Dis Colon Rectum.* 2011;54(2):238–244.

85. Tang CL, Chew SP, Seow-Choen F. Prospective randomized trial of drainage alone vs. drainage and fistulotomy for acute perianal abscesses with proven internal opening. *Dis Colon Rectum.* 1996;39(12):1415–1417.

86. Tong SY, Chen LF, Fowler VG Jr. Colonization, pathogenicity, host susceptibility, and therapeutics for *Staphylococcus aureus*: what is the clinical relevance [published online ahead of print December 11, 2011]? *Semin Immunopathol.* 2012;34(2):185–200.

87. Ulug M, Gedik E, Girgin S, et al. The evaluation of bacteriology in perianal abscesses of 81 adult patients. *Braz J Infect Dis.* 2010;14(3):225–229.

88. Vanheuverzwyn R, Delannoy A, Michaux JL, et al. Anal lesions in hematologic diseases. *Dis Colon Rectum.* 1980;23(5):310–312.

89. Vasilevsky CA, Gordon PH. The incidence of recurrent abscesses or fistula-in-ano following anorectal suppuration. *Dis Colon Rectum.* 1984;27(2):126–130.

90. Waggener HU. Immediate fistulotomy in the treatment of perianal abscess. *Surg Clin North Am.* 1969;49(6):1227–1233.

91. Wexner SD. Managing common anorectal sexually transmitted diseases. *Infect Surg.* 1990;9:9.

92. Wexner SD, Smithy WB, Milsom JW, et al. The surgical management of anorectal diseases in AIDS and pre-AIDS patients. *Dis Colon Rectum.* 1986;29(11):719–723.

93. Wilson DH. The late results of anorectal abscess treated by incision, curettage, and primary suture under antibiotic cover. *Br J Surg.* 1964;51:828–831.

94. Wolkomir AF, Barone JE, Hardy HW III, et al. Abdominal and anorectal surgery and the acquired immune deficiency syndrome in heterosexual intravenous drug users. *Dis Colon Rectum.* 1990;33(4):267–270.

95. Yano T, Asano M, Matsuda Y, et al. Prognostic factors for recurrence following the initial drainage of an anorectal abscess. *Int J Colorectal Dis.* 2010;25(12):1495–1498.

96. Zimmerman DD. The impact of smoking on perianal disease. *Dis Colon Rectum.* 2011;54(6):658–659.

14

Anal Fistula

Alex Jenny Ky and Emily Steinhagen

Bertram: What is it, my good lord, the King languishes of?
Lafew: A fistula, my lord.

—WILLIAM SHAKESPEARE:
All's Well That Ends Well, I.1.37

A fascinating narrative of Shakespeare and the literary history of anal fistula has been written by Cosman.[44]

▶ HISTORY

Anal fistula is a condition that has been described virtually from the beginning of medical history. Hippocrates, in about 430 BCE, suggested that the disease was caused by "contusions and tubercles occasioned by rowing or riding on horseback."[4] He was the first person to advocate the use of a seton in treatment (from the Latin *seta*, a bristle) "taking a very slender thread of raw lint, uniting it into five folds of the length of a span, and wrapping them round with a horse hair."[4] Numerous commentaries have been written on the historical implications associated with anal fistula (see Abu Marwan bio). For example, it has been known that the Sun King, Louis XIV, developed an abscess on February 18, 1685, and by May 2 a fistula had appeared. His doctors tried to treat him, unsuccessfully, with enemas and poultices. Eventually, Charles-François Felix was sent for. Felix recommended an operation, and Louis agreed to it. Felix, however, requested 6 months to prepare himself. He had never done such an operation before, and he needed to practice. He performed the procedure on 75 peasants, men who didn't actually need the operation. Not all of them lived. On November 18, 1686, at 7 o'clock in the morning, Felix operated on the king. The king was calm, but the surgeon was terrified. The operation was performed without anesthetic. Felix had devised a special curved scalpel and unique retractor. The operation was

a success. King Louis was able to sit up in bed within a month, and in another 3 months he was able to ride again. Word of his great courage during the operation spread throughout the court, and some of the nobles took to wearing bandages on their buttocks in the king's honor. The procedure became known as "the Royal," and at least 30 nobles asked Felix to perform the same operation on them. They were greatly disappointed when he told them that they didn't need it. In gratitude for his services, Felix was given a large sum of money, a title, and an estate. The status of surgeons was greatly improved by the event, and in 1731 Louis XV, Louis XIV's grandson, would establish the Royal Academy of Surgeons. As for Charles-François Felix, he was apparently greatly shaken by his experience. He never touched a scalpel again.

The fascination with anal fistula for more than 2,000 years is manifested by the numerous papers and books on the subject. In fact, Salmon established a hospital in London devoted to the treatment of anal fistula and other rectal conditions—St. Mark's. Allingham also established his reputation through operations for anal fistula. His book on rectal surgery was published through numerous editions.

It has been said that more surgeons' reputations have been impugned because of the consequences of fistula operations than from any other operative procedure. Complications of fistula surgery are myriad and include fecal soilage, mucous discharge, varying degrees of incontinence (gas and/or stool), recurrent abscess, and recurrent fistula. In the United States, impairment for bowel control from even a properly performed operation for anal fistula is one of the most frequent reasons in the field of colon and rectal surgery for a patient to pay a visit to an attorney. It is for this reason that the prescient surgeon will make a special effort to explain in detail the attendant risks of the procedure. Moreover, it is critically important to

ABU MARWAN ABD AL-MALIK IBN ABI AL-ALA ZUHR (1091–1161)

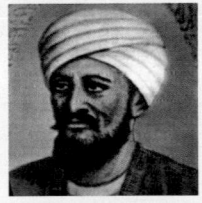

Also known as Ibn Zuhr or Avenzoar was born in Seville, Spain. He was considered the most renowned physician of Muslim Spain. His most famous book is *Al-Taisir* in which he introduced the experimental method into surgery, one example being the tracheostomy he performed first on a goat. He was also the first to perform postmortem autopsies and dissections and also contributed to developing feeding tubes and parenteral nutrition. He established surgery as an independent field of medicine by introducing a training course for future surgeons. He was also known for his contributions to the field of pharmacology, neurology, and parasitology. He was one of the first physicians to use anesthesia for surgical procedures. He belonged to a family of physicians who served the Almohad ruler, but due to political turmoil he fell out of favor with the Almoravid ruler. He fled Seville but was imprisoned in Marrakesh. It was during that time when he wrote *"Verrucae That Occur in the Stomach"* in which he gives the first detailed description of a prisoner suffering from advanced colon cancer. He describes symptoms of diarrhea, bloody stools, palpation of an apple-sized tumor in the lower abdomen, change in stool caliber, cyclical fevers, and cachexia. He attributed his tumor to the diet of his community, which consisted of cured camel meat. In 1147 when the Almohad dynasty conquered Seville, he returned and continued to practice medicine and teaching. He died in 1161 in Seville. (References: Glick TF, Livesey SJ, Wallis F, eds. *Medieval Science, Technology, and Medicine: An Encyclopedia.* New York, NY: Psychology Press; 2005; Azar H. *The Sage of Seville: Ibn Zuhr, His Time and His Medical Legacy.* New York, NY: The American University in Cairo Press; 2008; Azar HA, McVaugh MR, Shatzmiller J. Ibn Zuhr (Avenzoar)'s description of a verrucous malignancy of the colon (with an English translation from Arabic and notes on its Hebrew and Latin versions). *Can Bull Med Hist.* 2002;19(2):431–440; Picture from http://www.nndb.com/people/643/000097352/.) (With appreciation to Hussna Wakily, MD.)

FREDERICK SALMON (1796–1868)

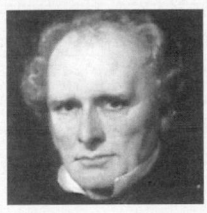

Salmon was born in Bath, England. He received his medical education at St. Bartholomew's Hospital and became a member of the Royal College of Surgeons in 1818. After several years in the General Dispensary, Aldersgate Street, Salmon resigned his position, and in 1835 he opened an institution that was named "The Infirmary for the Relief of the Poor, Afflicted With Fistula and Other Diseases of the Rectum." After relocation two additional times, it was reopened on April 25, 1854 (St. Mark's Day)—hence, the adoption of the name St. Mark's Hospital. Salmon seemed to have more than his share of critics; the following is a quote from an obituary statement that appeared in the *British Medical Journal*: "How far the course which he took was prompted by difficulties in pursuing an useful and honourable career in a general hospital, where his labours would have been more useful and more instructive, it is now difficult to say. It was, we fully believe, contrary to the best interests both of the profession and of the public; and the success of St. Mark's Hospital was of unfortunate omen and has since borne bad fruit in encouraging similar enterprises."

document the state of that individual's continence prior to embarking on any procedure. The fact is that no one goes whole to the grave with perfect anal control following surgery if an anal fistula traverses a significant portion of the external sphincter. Clearly, the surgeon who is fortunate enough to have the opportunity to treat the patient initially is the one most likely to effect a cure, to limit morbidity, and to minimize disability.

▶ SYMPTOMS

The most frequent presenting complaints of patients with an anal fistula are swelling, pain, and discharge. The former two symptoms usually are associated with an abscess when the external or secondary opening has closed or has failed to develop. Discharge may be from the external opening or may be reported by the patient as mucus or pus mixed with the stool. Most patients with an overt fistula have an antecedent history of abscess that drained spontaneously or for which surgical drainage had been performed.

Anal fistula may be confused with suppurative hidradenitis and pilonidal sinus (see Chapter 9). However, they may also occur secondary to inflammatory bowel disease (IBD) (see later and Chapter 30), anal or rectal carcinoma, tuberculosis, actinomycosis, lymphogranuloma venereum, radiation, trauma, or iatrogenic injury.

▶ CLASSIFICATION

The most commonly referred classification was suggested by Parks and colleagues.[137]

Intersphincteric
  Simple low tract
  High blind tract
  High tract with opening into rectum
  High fistula without a perineal opening
  High fistula with extrarectal or pelvic extension
  Fistula from pelvic disease

WILLIAM ALLINGHAM (1829–1908)

William Allingham was educated for the profession of architecture at University College, where he gained numerous prizes. He even practiced as an architect, exhibited studies at the exhibitions of the Royal Academy, and obtained honorable mention for a design of a building to house the Great Exhibition of 1851. In this year, however, he decided to abandon architecture for medicine. Entering as a student at St. Thomas's Hospital, he carried off prize after prize—the Descriptive Anatomy Prize, the Anatomy Prize (1854), the Medicine Prize, the Clinical Medicine President's Prize, and the Clinical Medicine Treasurer's Prize (1855). After qualifying in 1855, he volunteered as surgeon in the Crimean War. He was in time to be present at the siege of Sebastopol and to see a vast amount of practical surgery in the most arduous circumstances at the hospitals at Scutari. During a large part of his war services, he was attached to the French Army, which was extremely poorly provided with surgical aid, and there is no doubt that under the strenuous nature of the duties which devolved upon him, Allingham gained the courage and sense of responsibility, which marked him out as a successful operating surgeon from the beginning of his career. After his return home, he was surgical tutor, demonstrator of anatomy, and then surgical registrar at St. Thomas's Hospital. He set up in practice in 1863 as a consultant at 36 Finsbury Square, EC, but removed to Grosvenor Street, where he soon became a well-known authority on diseases of the rectum and enjoyed a large practice. In 1871, he published his classical book on *Diseases of the Rectum*.[7] It was accepted at once as an authoritative and inclusive work, although some surgeons differed from the author on points of technique. William Allingham was not attached to the staff of any of the great London hospitals possessing a medical school, but was for many years surgeon to the Great Northern Central Hospital and to St. Mark's Hospital for Fistula and Diseases of the Rectum. He was also consulting surgeon to the Farringdon General Dispensary and to the Surgical Aid Society, of which, together with some of his relatives and others, he was one of the founders in 1862. He was a member of the Council of the Royal College of Surgeons from 1884 to 1886 and retired from practice in 1894. Allingham was one of the first surgeons in England to specialize in the treatment of diseases of the rectum, out of which he made a considerable fortune. After his retirement, he lived for some time at St. Leonards, and then at Worthing, where he died on February 4, 1908. (Courtesy of Muath Bishawi, MD.)

Transsphincteric
    Uncomplicated
    High blind tract
Suprasphincteric
    Uncomplicated
    High blind tract
Extrasphincteric
    Secondary to transsphincteric fistula
    Secondary to trauma
    Secondary to anorectal disease (e.g., Crohn's)
    Secondary to pelvic inflammation
Combined
Horseshoe
    Intersphincteric
    Transsphincteric

Although not included in this classic schema, "complex fistula" is defined as other than an intersphincteric or low extrasphincteric fistula. The implication is that they are more difficult to treat than conventional fistulas and, in addition, are associated with increased risk of recurrence as well as a greater likelihood for impairment of control. These fistulas have also been labeled "problematic" by some.[1,167] Frenkel proposed a classification based on the level of the fistula: low, mid, and high/complex.[57] However, five types of fistulas are generally described by most authors. They are as follows:

- Submucous
- Intersphincteric (Figure 14-1)
- Transsphincteric (Figure 14-2)
- Suprasphincteric (Figure 14-3)
- Extrasphincteric (Figure 14-4)

The *submucous fistula* is a misnomer. See the discussion in Chapter 13.

As its name suggests, an *intersphincteric fistula* passes through the internal sphincter to the skin. Occasionally, an extension may be observed to proceed cephalad in the intersphincteric plain (i.e., high blind tract), but this has no consequence in one's therapeutic decision making. It has also been

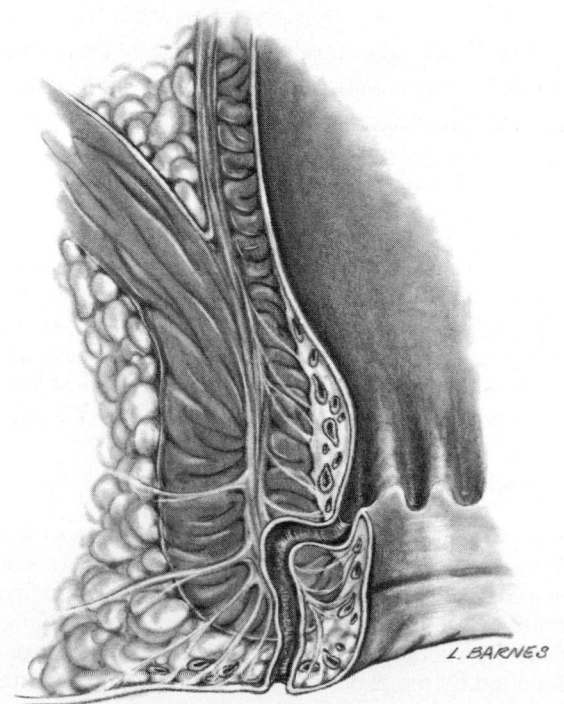

FIGURE 14-1. Intersphincteric fistula. The tract passes through the internal sphincter and in the intersphincteric plane.

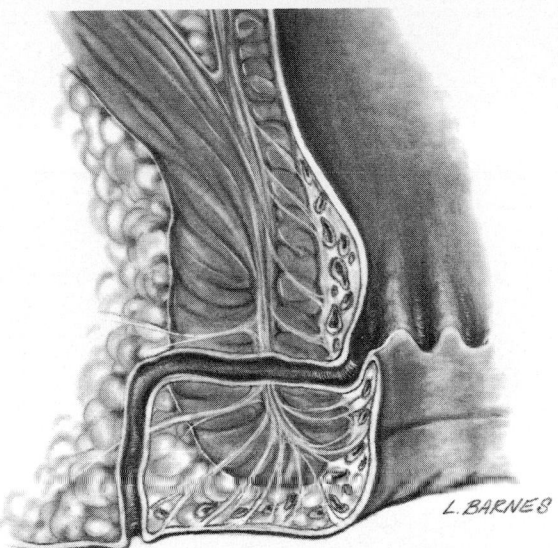

FIGURE 14-2. Transsphincteric fistula. The tract passes through both the internal and external sphincters, into the ischiorectal fossa, and to the skin.

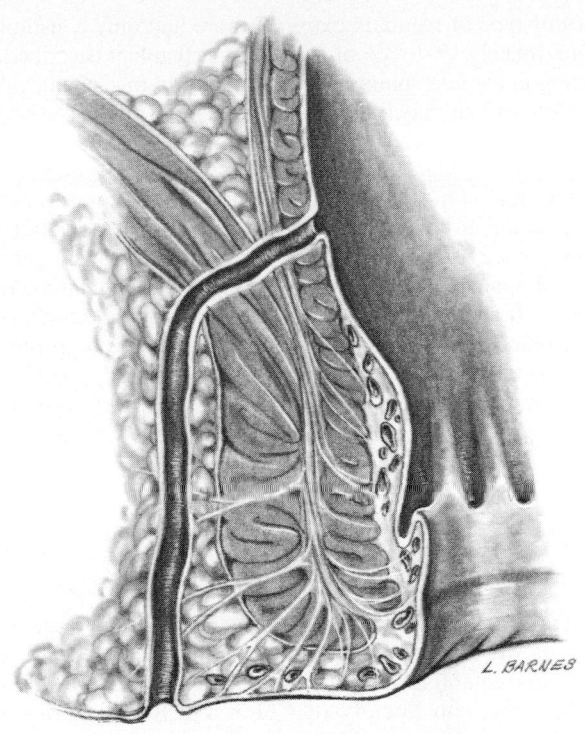

FIGURE 14-4. Extrasphincteric fistula. The internal opening is above the level of the levator ani muscle, and the tract passes to the skin deep to the external sphincter in the ischiorectal space.

reported to extend cephalad and present with another opening in the rectum.[137] Only the most superficial or subcutaneous portions of the external sphincter may be divided when a fistulotomy is undertaken. Intersphincteric fistulas are the most common type of fistula, with an incidence of 55% to 70%.

A *transsphincteric fistula* passes through both the internal and external sphincters before exiting to the skin. It usually results from an ischiorectal abscess. The level of the tract determines how much sphincter will need to be divided and the risk of impairment for bowel control if a fistulotomy is performed. This type of fistula is observed in 20% to 25% of most series. Occasionally, a supralevator extension of a transsphincteric fistula is identified (Figure 14-5). Treatment

requires recognition of this condition, curettage, irrigation, and packing of the supralevator extension. Under no circumstances should the extension be drained into the rectum.

A *suprasphincteric fistula* was noted by Parks and colleagues to comprise 20% of their series.[137] Other series have reported

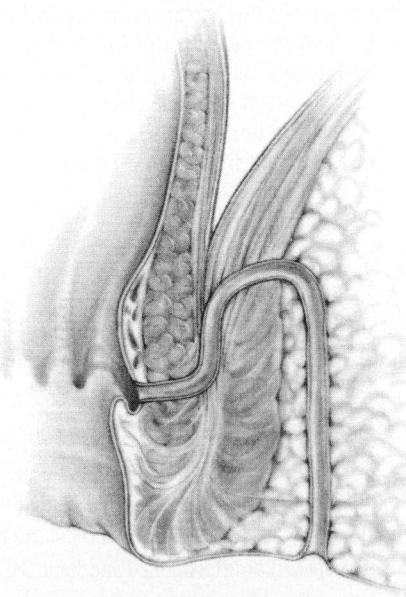

FIGURE 14-3. Suprasphincteric fistula. The tract courses above the puborectalis muscle after initially passing cephalad as an intersphincteric fistula. It then traverses downward through the ischiorectal fossa to the skin.

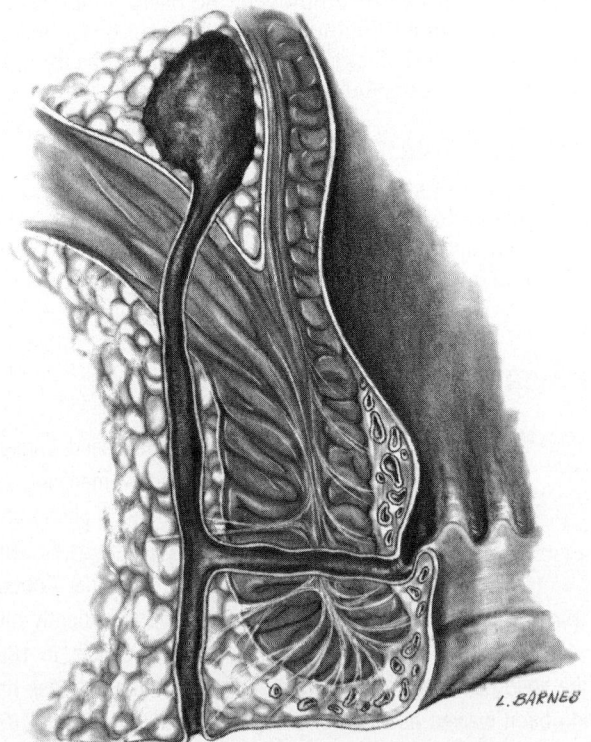

FIGURE 14-5. Transsphincteric fistula with supralevator extension. Drainage of the extension into the rectum is contraindicated.

that this type of fistula is extremely rare and only constitutes approximately 1% to 3% of fistulas.[4] The fistula is described as starting in the intersphincteric plane, passing to a supralevator location, and ultimately tracking between the puborectalis and the levator ani muscles to end in the ischiorectal fossa.

The *extrasphincteric fistula* involves a supralevator internal opening with a tract that passes through the entire sphincter mechanism torward its exit at the skin. It is usually a consequence of trauma (e.g., foreign body, surgical manipulation, impalement), Crohn's disease, or pelvic inflammatory disease. It can also develop when a supralevator abscess or transsphincteric fistula with supralevator extension ruptures spontaneously into the rectum. This type of fistula represents approximately 2% to 3% of fistulas, but if the physician's practice encompasses many individuals with inflammatory bowel disease, the incidence could be higher.

▶ PRACTICE PARAMETERS FOR TREATMENT

As has been mentioned in prior chapters, practice parameters for the treatment of a number of colorectal conditions have been established by the Standards Practice Task Force of the American Society of Colon and Rectal Surgeons. These recommendations have also been established for the evaluation and treatment of fistula-in-ano.[178] The reader is advised to review the society's guidelines with respect to the latest revisions concerning evaluation and treatment of this condition.

▶ IDENTIFICATION OF THE FISTULA TRACT

How does the physician identify the type of fistula, the course of the tract, and the location of the internal opening? Numerous methods can be employed, the basic principles and procedures of which include the application of Goodsall's rule,[67] careful physical examination, probing of the tract, and a variety of injection and radiologic techniques.

Goodsall's Rule

When the external opening lies anterior to the transverse plane, the internal opening tends to be located radially. Conversely, when the external opening lies posterior to the plane, the internal opening is usually (but not always) located in the

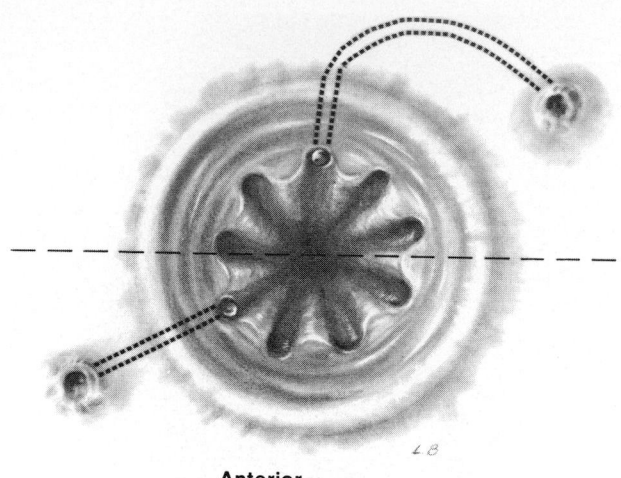

Anterior

FIGURE 14-6. Typical courses of fistula tracts according to Goodsall's rule.

posterior midline (Figure 14-6). One must remember that this is a "rule," not a "law." There *are* exceptions to "rules."

There is some controversy over the reasons for the disparate manifestations. However, the reason for this eventuality probably lies with the fact that the posterior course is the result of a defect in fusion of the longitudinal muscle and the external sphincter in the posterior midline. A transsphincteric fistula is, therefore, more likely to occur in this position; the tract can then dissect into one or both ischiorectal fossae.

Cirocco and Reilly analyzed the predictive accuracy of this rule by reviewing 216 patients who underwent fistula surgery.[41] Only 49% of those who harbored an external opening anterior to the transverse plane had radially directed fistulas, but the accuracy rate of Goodsall's rule regarding posterior secondary openings was much greater.

Essentially, the rule should merely be used as a guide to help the surgeon find the tract when it may not be apparent. It is not a substitute for meticulous technique, clear identification of the direction of the tract, and location of the internal opening.

Usually, there is only one external or secondary opening. Most commonly, fistulas pass in the intersphincteric plane, but with transsphincteric fistulas, multiple openings can develop from communication with the deep postanal space and from the ischiorectal fossae; this is the origin of the so-called transsphincteric horseshoe fistula (see later).

DAVID HENRY GOODSALL (1843–1906)

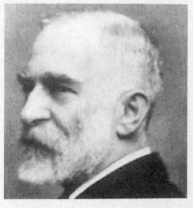

Goodsall was born in Gravesend, England. His father had decided on medicine as a career. While performing a postmortem examination as a student at St. Bartholomew's Hospital, the elder Goodsall injured his hand and subsequently died, presumably because of sepsis. In 1865, the young Goodsall entered that same institution, his fees having been waived because of his father's tragic death. In 1870, he was appointed house surgeon to St. Mark's Hospital, and he became full surgeon in 1888. It was there that he developed his

lifelong interest in rectal surgery. He contributed many articles to the surgical literature, including reports on foreign bodies of the rectum, pilonidal sinus, colostomy, and anal fissure. However, his best-remembered work was accomplished in concert with W. Ernest Miles, a book entitled *Diseases of the Anus and Rectum*. In Goodsall's chapter on anal fistula, the rule is espoused that has become eponymously associated with Goodsall. He is thought to have died of a myocardial infarction. (Goodsall DH. Anorectal fistula. In: Goodsall DH, Miles WE, eds. *Diseases of the Anus and Rectum*. London, United Kingdom: Longmans, Green & Co; 1900:92.)

Physical Examination and Endoscopy

Careful palpation may reveal the thickened tract proceeding into the anal canal if the fistula assumes a relatively superficial position. This finding is most characteristic of an intersphincteric fistula. Bidigital examination, placing the thumb on the outside and the index finger within the anal canal, may also help to reveal the course of the tract. Failure to identify the tract by palpation implies that it is deep and, therefore, more likely to be a transsphincteric fistula. Anoscopic examination may demonstrate an internal opening or purulent material exuding from the base of the crypt. By gentle probing with a crypt hook or malleable probe (Figure 14-7), the presence of the tract may

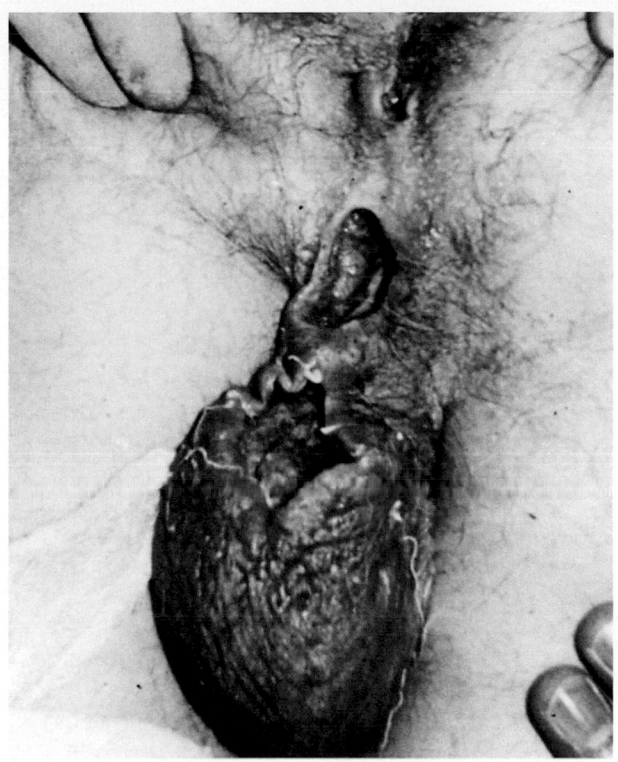

FIGURE 14-8. Scrotal fistula. The multiple openings are due to extensive subcutaneous tracking. Although on cursory examination the fistula may appear to be difficult to treat, the tract is usually quite superficial.

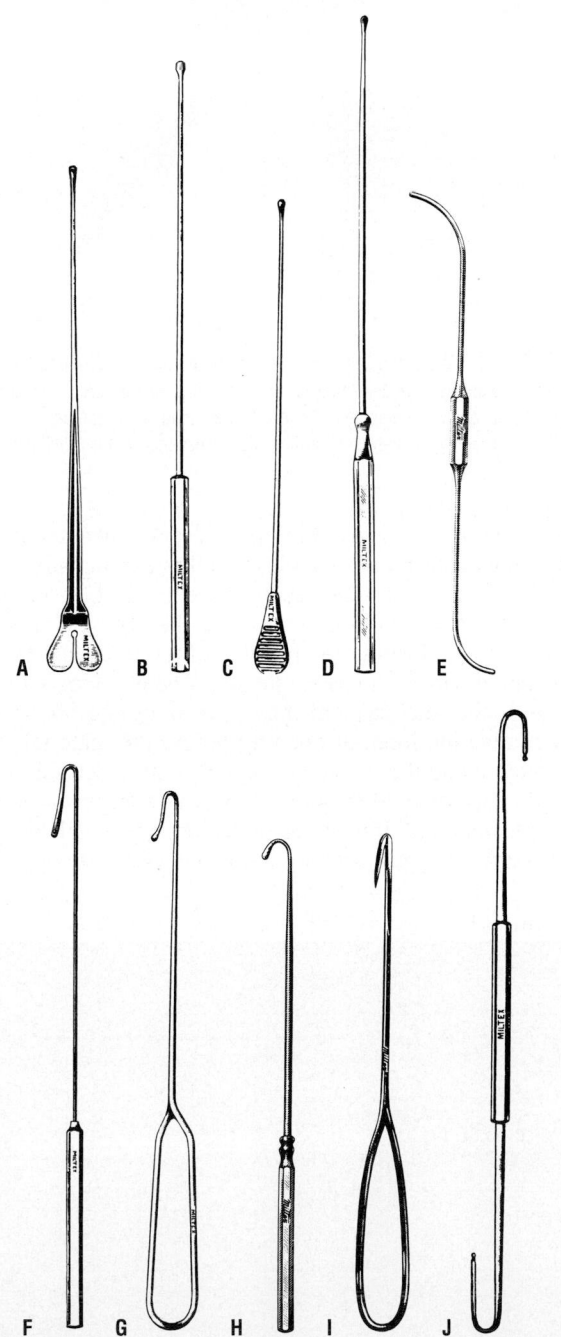

FIGURE 14-7. Anorectal probes. **A:** Larry. **B:** Barr. **C:** Buie. **D:** Pratt. **E:** Barr double-ended. **F:** Pratt crypt hook. **G:** Stewart crypt hook. **H:** Rosser crypt hook. **I:** Blanchard cryptotome. **J:** Barr crypt hook.

be confirmed. This maneuver is easier to accomplish for a radially located fistula than for one that opens in the posterior midline. Occasionally, the tract will pass subcutaneously for a considerable distance and end in the perineum, scrotum, labia, or thigh (Figure 14-8). Failure to identify the internal opening does not mean that it has closed, however. Angulation or narrowing of the tract may preclude the possibility of adequate evaluation by probing, and excessive manipulation will certainly lead to considerable discomfort for the patient. Under these circumstances, examination under an anesthetic may be required to adequately delineate the course of the tract unless one wishes to perform special studies.

At the time of bidigital examination, baseline sphincter tone, bulk, and squeeze should be assessed because this may affect the risk of incontinence with a surgical procedure.

Passing a Probe

As implied, passage of a probe can be attempted from both the external and the internal openings. Sometimes it is easier to identify the tract from the internal opening, but probing through the external one will usually reveal the course more readily. Simultaneous passage of two probes, from the internal and the external openings, may confirm the tract's location if the tips of the probes touch. A stenotic or sharply angulated area within the tract may preclude complete passage from either end. The probe should never be forced, merely gently maneuvered in order to avoid creating another tract or sinus (Figure 14-9).

Traction on the Tract

Theoretically, if the physician mobilizes a small portion of the tract from the secondary (i.e., external) opening and

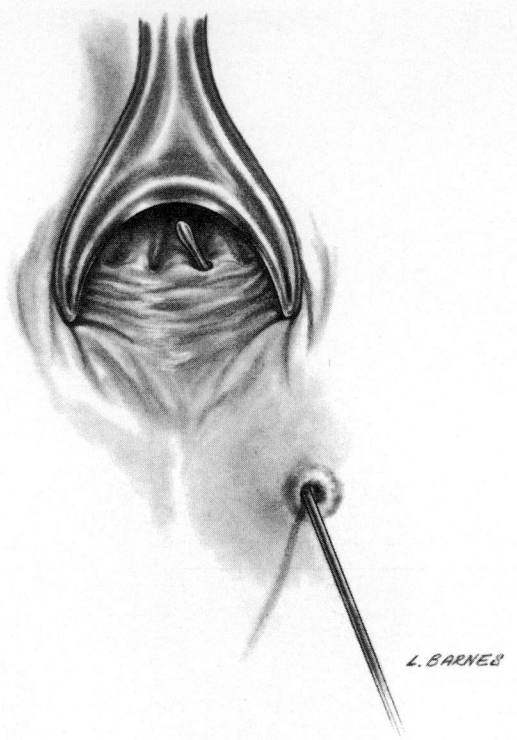

FIGURE 14-9. A malleable probe is passed from the external to the internal openings to confirm the course of the tract.

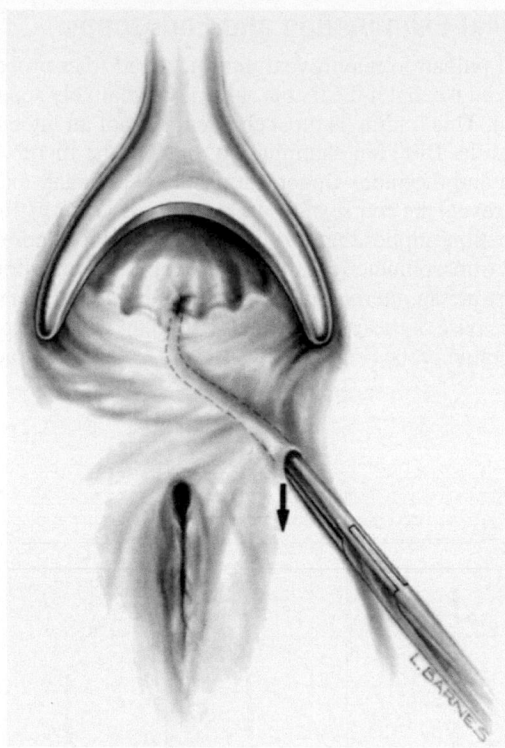

FIGURE 14-10. Attempt at identification of the primary (i.e., internal) opening by pulling on the epithelialized tract with a clamp. This may create a "dimpling" at the internal opening because of tethering, indicating where the opening should be. This approach is unlikely to be successful unless the tract is radially located.

applies traction, an indentation or dimpling will be evident at the level of the crypt—the site of the internal opening (Figure 14-10). With the exception of the most simple, radially directed tracts, we have not found this particular maneuver to be helpful especially when the tract is friable and with little substance to pull on. The variable and often curvilinear course of more complex fistulas lessens the potential benefit of this method for tract identification.

Injection Techniques
Dye
A DeBakey olive-end needle may be used to inject material through the opening and into the tract while an anoscope is in position in the rectum (Figure 14-11). We like to cut a 20-gauge angiocatheter at an angle to facilitate cannulation of the fistula tract. If a substance such as methylene blue or indigo carmine is injected through the tract, the dye may appear in the rectum, confirming the patency of the tract and its communication with an internal opening. The problem with such agents is that the surgeon may have only one opportunity to visualize the internal opening before the material stains the mucosa and the whole anal canal. It has been said that it would be as sensible to pour ink on a newspaper in order to facilitate reading.[51] If the surgeon has no other available agent except dye, I suggest diluting it down to one part per 20.

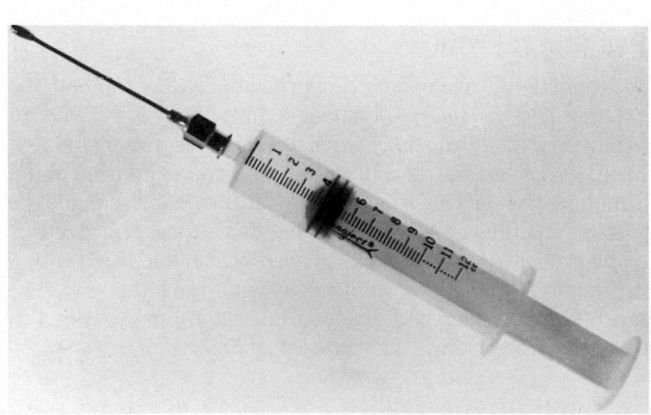

A

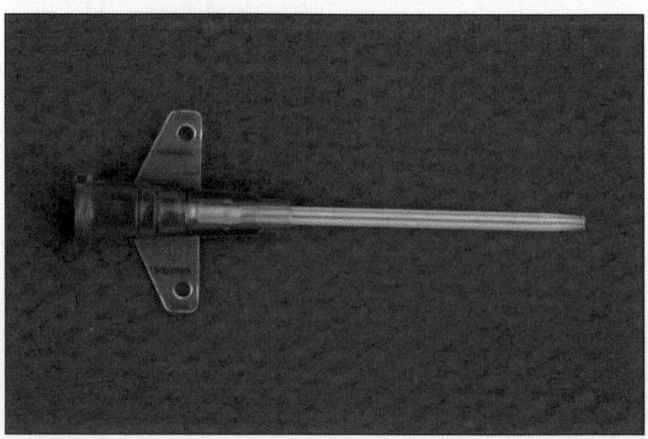

B

FIGURE 14-11. A DeBakey olive-end needle has a bulbous tip that permits insertion into the external opening without penetrating the wall of the tract **(A)**. Alternatively, an Angiocath may be used **(B)**.

Milk

Milk can also be used to identify the tract and the internal opening; sterility is not required. The milk can be wiped away without staining the tissue, permitting repeated attempts to inspect the internal opening. Failure to demonstrate communication with the internal opening implies stenosis of the tract, but if the milk is seen in the submucosa of the anal canal, even without escaping into the lumen, the associated crypt-bearing area should be excised with the presumption that the internal opening has closed.

Hydrogen Peroxide

Hydrogen peroxide injection is an ideal means for identifying the internal opening. The liberated oxygen may be seen to bubble through the internal opening. The pressure created by the gas may be sufficient to penetrate even a stenotic tract and pass into the anal canal. Additionally, staining of the tissue does not occur.

Imaging

Fistulography

Fistulography, the radiologic delineation of a fistula tract with a water-soluble contrast agent, is thought generally to be of limited value, having essentially been completely replaced by endoluminal sonography and magnetic resonance imaging (MRI).[181] However, the technique is quite simple to perform. The patient is placed on the x-ray table, usually in the left lateral position, and a small-bore catheter is inserted into the external opening. A few milliliters of water soluble contrast material are injected, and films are taken in several projections (Figures 14-12 and 14-13).

This technique does not directly image the sphincters. Thus, the relationship between the fistula and sphincter muscle cannot be determined with certainty. Additionally, the specific location of the internal opening within the anal canal is often impossible to determine. Furthermore, extensions

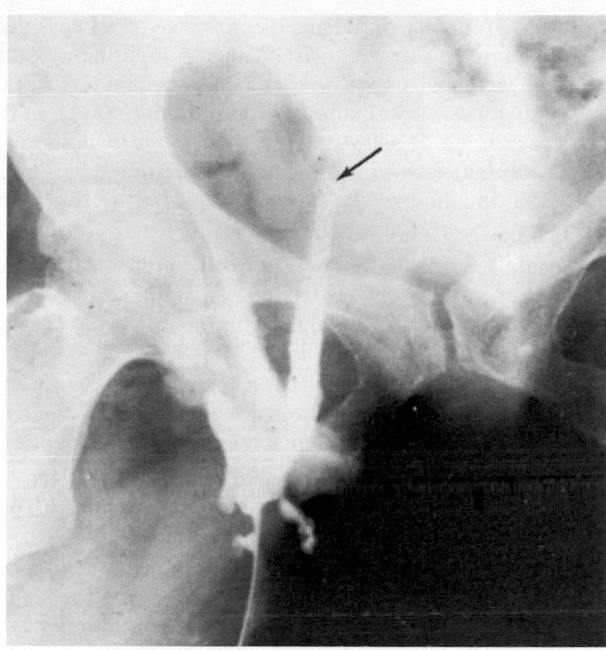

FIGURE 14-13. Fistulogram of an extrasphincteric fistula. The tract enters the rectum at the level of the *arrow*.

from the primary tract may not fill, and, therefore, will not be visualized.[72]

Several small studies have come to conflicting results about the usefulness of this technique. In one retrospective review of fistulography compared with subsequent surgical findings in 25 cases, fistulograms were accurate in only 16%, and false-positive results were identified in 10%.[100] However, another retrospective review of 27 patients who underwent anal fistulography noted that 48% harbored unexpected pathologic features that led to an alternative surgical treatment.[9] One prospective study involving 50 patients came to the conclusion that fistulography provided "helpful information."[197]

The limitations of fistulography have led most specialists in colon and rectal surgery to abandon it because more precise imaging modalities are now available.

Endoanal Ultrasound

Endoanal ultrasound (EUS) may be used to image the anal canal and surrounding pelvic structures. The technique is simple to perform, although it is operator-dependant. It is noninvasive, inexpensive, and generally well tolerated. Most studies examining the accuracy of endoanal ultrasound report excellent correlation with surgical findings, particularly in visualizing the primary tract.[36,46,105,187] One report noted that the surgical procedure was influenced by ultrasonographic findings in up to 38% of cases.[110] In one study that compared digital examination with ultrasound, the two were equally able to identify intersphincteric and transsphincteric tracts, but ultrasound was unable to assess superficial, suprasphincteric, extrasphincteric, and supralevator or infralevator tracts. Digital examination was, therefore, considered more reliable.[36]

The inability to identify all extensions of complex fistulas or even primary tracts when they are beyond the reach of the instrument is a limitation of this technique. Furthermore,

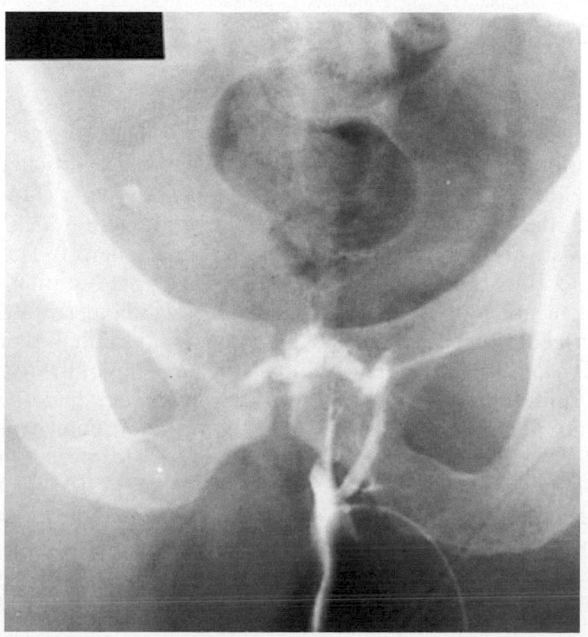

FIGURE 14-12. Fistulogram with water-soluble contrast material demonstrates the course of a transsphincteric fistula with an internal opening at the level of the anorectal ring.

scar or inflammatory tissue and the presence of abscess may limit the ability to distinguish the anatomic structures that otherwise are usually seen on endoanal ultrasound. Abscess, in particular, can appear similar to adipose tissue seen in the ischiorectal fossa. It has also typically been difficult to identify the internal opening of a fistula in the mucosa. To aid in the identification of the internal opening, the following criteria have been suggested by Cho[35]:

- Criterion I. Rootlike budding formed by the intersphincteric tract, which contacts the internal sphincter.
- Criterion II. Rootlike budding within the internal sphincter defect.
- Criterion III. Subepithelial breach connecting to the intersphincteric tract through an internal sphincter defect. Using these criteria, the internal opening may be identified in approximately 76% of cases.

However, it is unclear how many were able to be identified based on physical examination alone.

The addition of hydrogen peroxide appears to improve the accuracy of endoanal ultrasound, particularly for identifying the internal opening and secondary extensions of the fistula tract (Figure 14-14).[106,144,148] The hydrogen peroxide

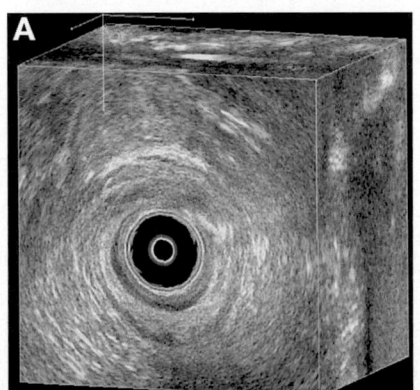
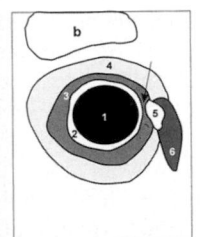
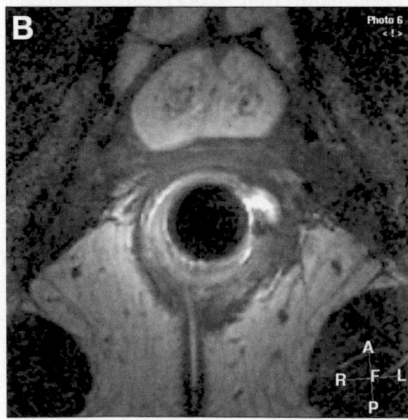
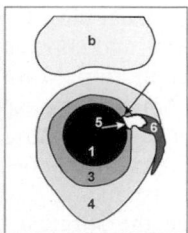

FIGURE 14-14. Transsphincteric fistula and the internal opening. Axial hydrogen peroxide–enhanced three-dimensional endoanal ultrasonography image **(A)** and axial endoanal magnetic resonance imaging (T2-weighted, gradient echo) image **(B)** showing the endoprobe *(1)* and anal coil *(1)*, submucosa *(2)*, the internal anal sphincter *(3)*, the external anal sphincter *(4)*, the fistula and the internal opening *(5; black arrow)*, fibrosis *(6)*, and the bulbocavernous muscle *(b)*. *A*, anterior; *R*, right; *F*, feet; *L*, left; and *P*, posterior. (From West RL, et al. Prospective comparison of hydrogen peroxide-enhanced three-dimensional endoanal ultrasonography and endoanal magnetic resonance imaging of perianal fistulas. *Dis Colon Rectum.* 2003;46(10):1407–1415, with permission.)

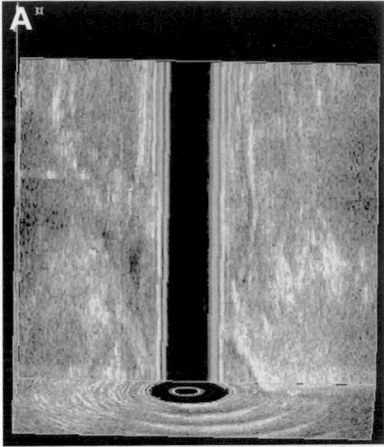
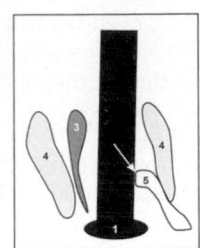
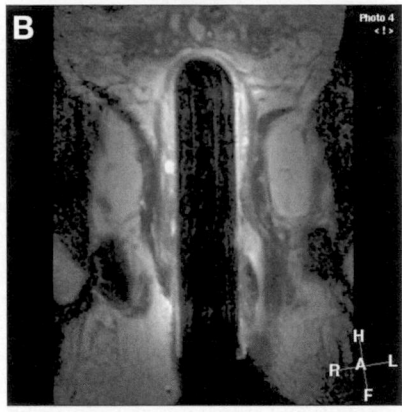
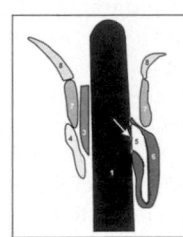

FIGURE 14-15. Coronal image of a transsphincteric fistula. Hydrogen peroxide–enhanced three-dimensional endoanal ultrasonography image **(A)** and endoanal magnetic resonance (T2-weighted, fast spin echo) image **(B)** showing the endoprobe *(1)* and anal coil *(1)*, the internal anal sphincter *(3)*, the external anal sphincter *(4)*, the fistula and the internal opening *(5; arrow)*, fibrosis *(6)*, puborectal muscle *(7)*, and levator ani muscle *(8)*. *H*, head; *A*, anterior; *L*, left; *R*, right; and *F*, feet. (From West RL, et al. Prospective comparison of hydrogen peroxide-enhanced three-dimensional endoanal ultrasonography and endoanal magnetic resonance imaging of perianal fistulas. *Dis Colon Rectum.* 2003;46(10):1407–1415, with permission.)

forms hyperechoic gas bubbles that can enhance visualization of the tract (Figure 14-15). This has been particularly helpful for recurrent or complex disease in some studies, but other authors note that the improved imaging does not necessarily translate to changes in management.[27] Three-dimensional ultrasound has also been suggested to improve the accuracy of endoanal ultrasound. It can be used to create reconstructed images of the coronal and sagittal planes; this can be helpful in clarifying the relationship of the fistula to surrounding structures. The two techniques have been combined, but some have reported no additional benefit over three-dimensional imaging alone.[95,99] Postprocessing, volume-rendered imaging has also been suggested for the enhancement of the image created by traditional ultrasound. This approach may improve contrast between structures so that primary tracts can be classified more accurately and potentially detect an abscess. However, it has not been found to affect treatment planning.[20]

Endoanal ultrasound may be particularly helpful in the evaluation of Crohn's fistulas. Accuracy has been reported to be up to 91%.[134,162] When a patient is treated with infliximab, the superficial opening of the fistula may appear to have healed. However, a persistent fistula may be demonstrated on ultrasound.[11] Anal ultrasound is typically not used for the characterization of straightforward fistulas. It may, however, be helpful in specific situations, such as the inability to demonstrate an internal opening, recurrent or persistent fistula following surgery, Crohn's disease, or complicated cases.

Magnetic Resonance Imaging

MRI produces detailed images of the perianal region and of fistula tracts via magnetic fields and radiofrequency energy. A variety of sequences and techniques, some using endoluminal anal coils, have been used. It is useful for demonstrating the relationship between the sphincters, soft tissues, and fistulas in all planes. An advantage over that of EUS is the ability to image the entire pelvic region and to, at least theoretically, see all extensions of a fistula. MRI appears to have the greatest concordance with clinical and surgical findings when compared with EUS or CT, with reported accuracy rates of 85% or greater.[28,84,113] In one study, when discordance was noted between tracts on MRI not identified during surgery, there was a 52% recurrence rate following surgery.[127] Subsequent findings confirmed the MRI in all cases. In contrast, the failure rate was 13% when there was concordance between surgical and MRI findings. However, in this study, surgeons acted on the MRI in 21% of cases, which biased the results. The same authors note in another small series that even though MRI can alter plan of surgery, in many instances the disagreement between imaging and examination findings did not affect the treatment plan because the classification differences were not clinically significant.[30]

Dynamic contrast-enhanced MRI has been compared with physical examination and surgical exploration.[16] It appears to have a high sensitivity and specificity and is able to identify more secondary tracts. Moreover, it is felt to be more accurate in identifying complex fistulas than either digital rectal examination alone or surgical exploration.

Because of the ability to visualize extensions or areas of abscess in the pelvis not accessible by physical examination, one small study suggested that MRI may be superior to EUS at predicting outcomes of surgery.[177] Spencer and colleagues

reported positive and negative predictive values of 73% and 87%, respectively, for MRI and 57% and 56% for EUS.[177] Others have noted that MRI may provide helpful additional information beyond what is found at EUS. In one study, MRI was particularly useful in Crohn's disease and in classifying recurrent fistulas, thus providing helpful additional information in 40% and 24% of these situations, respectively.[17] However, in two studies evaluating the use of EUS and MRI for Crohn's fistulas, EUS was superior.[162] Importantly, when any two methods were combined in one of the studies, the accuracy was reportedly to be 100%.[134] This suggests that a multimodality approach may be beneficial. As with EUS, MRI can be used to evaluate the response of Crohn's fistulas to infliximab, often showing the persistence of a fistula in the presence of superficial healing.

It is important that an MRI used to delineate fistula anatomy be read by a radiologist with experience in pelvic anatomy because there is a learning curve associated with its interpretation.[161] The cost and accessibility of the machine must also be taken into account, as should medical contraindications, such as pacemakers or the inability of the patient to tolerate the contrast material. In all studies comparing imaging to either physical examination or surgical findings, the "true" or correct classification of the fistula is not known with certainty. In difficult cases, it may be impossible to truly delineate the course of the fistula. Therefore, critical review of such reports is required.

Additional Gastrointestinal Studies

Gastrointestinal evaluation, in addition to rigid or flexible sigmoidoscopy, is generally unnecessary for patients with conventional anal fistula. However, in the presence of known or suspected inflammatory bowel disease, colonoscopic examination and a small bowel series are strongly encouraged.

▶ PRINCIPLES OF SURGICAL TREATMENT

Although the history of the treatment of anal fistula by means of a seton can be traced to ancient Greece (see earlier discussion), al-Zahrawi (Albucasis) is recognized as the first to use cauterization for this condition (10th century). The

ABUL QASIM KHALAF IBN AL-ABBAS AL-ZAHRAWI, ALSO KNOWN AS AL-ZAHRAWI OR ALBUCASIS (936–1013)

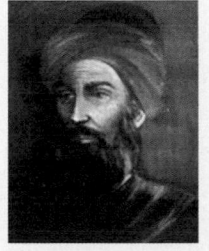

Al-Zahrawi was born in El-Zahra, northwest of Córdoba, Spain. He is known as one of the fathers of modern surgery for his contributions to advancing the field. He dedicated his life to medical ethics and to encouraging the knowledge of anatomy. He had great respect for the surgical theories and the works of the Greeks but introduced new surgical techniques and instruments. He is most famously known for his publication, the *Al-Tasrif*, a comprehensive and illustrated textbook of surgery. This monumental text is composed of 30 volumes, the last part of which deals with surgery, which in itself is divided into three books. The first deals with cauterization;

the second discusses general surgery, trauma, obstetrics, gynecology, and urology; and the last covers orthopedics. He was the first to describe the use of cauterization in the treatment of anal fistula and hemorrhoids but recommended it only if the surgeon could avoid damage to the sphincter. Alternatively, he recommended the initial use of a cutting seton, which he describes in detail to treat anal fistulas. He has also been credited for performing the first thyroidectomy, being among the initial proponents of the use of anesthesia, using absorbable catgut sutures, ligation to control bleeding, and much more. The *Al-Tasrif* has illustrations of 200 surgical instruments, many of which are still in use today. He died in Córdoba in 1013 but his books continued to be used as resources for centuries in Europe. (Courtesy of Hussna Wakily, MD.)

management of anal fistula by division or "laying open" the tract was initially described by John of Arderne in the 14th century.[10] With minor variations, this is the same method that is most commonly employed today. Percivall Pott suggested that there are essentially three means for cure: caustic, ligature, and incision.

The surgeon who initially treats the patient has the best opportunity to identify the tract, find the internal opening, and effect a cure. When this is not accomplished in the first instance, further surgery may be more complex, and the patient will be subjected to an increased risk of complications.

Failure to cure the patient is usually the result of either *timorousness* or *temerity*. If the surgeon traces the tract from the external opening to the level of the crypt but cannot pass the probe into the anal canal and subsequently desists from excising the crypt-bearing area, one is being too timid. In this situation, it is reasonable to assume that the crypt opening has sealed and that it is, indeed, the source of the fistula (Figure 14-16A). Likewise, if the surgeon identifies the internal opening of a "virgin fistula" but is reluctant to lay it open because of fear that the opening is too high, that decision may jeopardize the opportunity of curing the pa-

tient. The fistula will inevitably persist, and the subsequent procedure will be performed without the security of knowing that the observed internal opening occurred as a natural consequence. With few exceptions (e.g., Crohn's disease, a history of trauma), the surgeon should be able to open the tract at the time of the initial operation without fear of causing significant impairment for bowel control. If there is concern about the safety of dividing at the level of the internal opening, a seton can be temporarily employed (see later).

Conversely, if the tract is identified only partially (i.e., not to the level of the crypt), and the surgeon elects to guess or to assume where the opening should be, thereby creating an "artificial" internal opening, one is being too aggressive (Figure 14-16B). The actual opening and the tract have not been appreciated. When the surgeon is subsequently confronted with a persistent fistula after such an ill-conceived maneuver, both the natural and the artificial internal openings must be considered.

The previously mentioned injection techniques may confirm the presence of the fistula and the internal opening. They do not, however, identify the course of the tract. If a probe can be passed, it is only necessary to incise down onto it.

JOHN ARDERNE (1307–1380?)

Arderne, or de Arderne, claimed descent from Saxon times. His family was one of the first to assume a surname in imitation of the Normans. He stated that he was 70 in the first year of the reign of Richard II (i.e., 1377), hence our ability to deduce the year of his birth. He was a surgeon of the pre-Renaissance period and quite well educated, but little is known about him except for information that was gleaned from autobiographic details in some of his manuscripts. Scholars surmise that he was educated at Montpellier and served on the English side in France during the early period of the One Hundred Years War.

He treated patients in Newark, Nottinghamshire, from 1349 to 1370 and then came to London. In 1376, Arderne issued his *Treatise on Fistula-in-ano*. A prolific writer in colloquial Latin, it was soon translated into English. Although he was apparently a brilliant surgeon, he still adhered to and promulgated astrology, keeping his medicaments and plasters secret. In fact, his fame as a pharmacist was said to have long outlasted his reputation as a surgeon. (Arderne J. *Treatises of Fistula-in-Ano, Hemorrhoids and Clysters*. Power D, trans. London, United Kingdom: Kegan Paul, Trench, Trubner; 1910.)

PERCIVALL POTT (1714–1788)

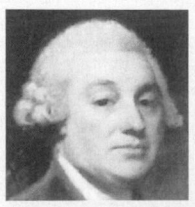

Pott was born in London, the son of a scrivener, in a house on Threadneedle Street at which location now sits the Bank of England. With the assistance of a relation, the Bishop of Rochester, Pott was able to attend a private school in Kent. At the age of 16, he demonstrated an interest in surgery and was apprenticed to Edward Nourse, an assistant surgeon at St. Bartholomew's Hospital. It was Pott's responsibility to prepare anatomic subjects for Nourse's lectures. In 1736, Pott received his diploma and was admitted to the Company of Barber-Surgeons. Following dissolution of the company in 1745, Pott allied himself with the surgeons, having been appointed assistant surgeon at St. Bartholomew's. In his *Treatise on Fistula*, Pott stressed the

advisability of minimal dissection, that is, the performance of limited fistulotomy. In 1756, Pott was thrown from his horse and suffered a compound fracture of the ankle. Despite having been advised to undergo amputation, he successfully managed to preserve the limb. The term Pott's fracture is still used to describe this particular injury. In 1786, the Royal College of Surgeons at Edinburgh elected Pott an honorary fellow, the first gentleman of the faculty to whom this honor was given. He served St. Bartholomew's Hospital for one-half century, and when he died, the place in the Court of Assistants of the Surgeon's Company was filled by his eminent pupil, John Hunter. (Pott P. *The Chirurgical Works*. Vols 1–3. London, United Kingdom: J Johnson; 1808; adapted from Parks AG, Gordon PH, Hardcastle JD. A classification of fistula-in-ano. *Br J Surg*. 1976;63(1):1–12.)

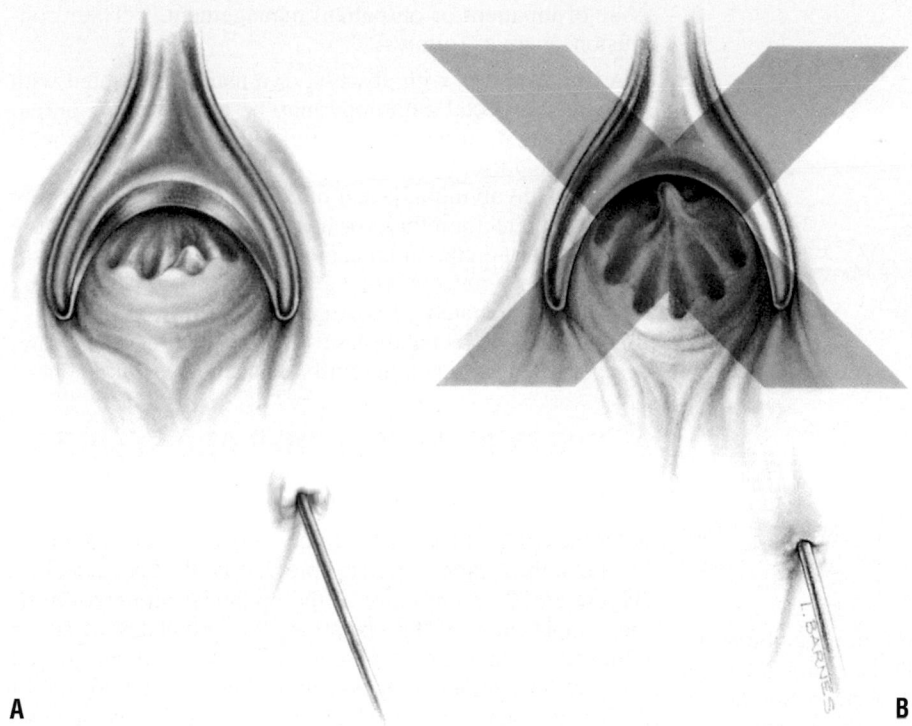

A **B**

FIGURE 14-16. Probing the tract may reveal that the internal opening has sealed. **A:** If the tip of the probe can be appreciated at the level of the crypt, a fistulotomy may be undertaken with safety. **B:** However, creating an "artificial" internal opening is contraindicated at a higher level.

However, if this cannot be accomplished and should a fistulotomy be elected, the dissection must be carried out slowly and meticulously, following the epithelialized tract until it communicates with the anal canal (Figure 14-17).

A fistula operation should always be performed with electrocautery. Identification of the tract requires a dry operative field. In such a vascular area, this is the best means for maintaining hemostasis.

Fistulotomy versus Fistulectomy

Whether to perform fistulectomy or fistulotomy has been a source of controversy. Kronborg randomly allocated patients with anal fistula to either an incisional or an excisional approach.[98] Times to healing were significantly shorter when the fistula was laid open in comparison with excision, but recurrence rates were comparable. Fistulotomy is preferable because of the prolonged healing time associated with excisional techniques (Figures 14-18 and 14-19). However, a small portion of the tract may be removed for pathologic examination, especially if there is a concern about the possibility of Crohn's disease or malignancy (see later).

Office Fistulotomy

Office fistulotomy may be undertaken synchronously with drainage of an abscess if the internal opening is low or if it is an intersphincteric fistula. It may also be performed in the office as an interval procedure following abscess drainage. Local anesthesia or a field block is usually adequate for analgesia (see Chapters 8 and 11). For the majority of patients, however, definitive fistula surgery should be performed in the operating room with a general, spinal, or caudal anesthetic under optimal conditions. A local anesthetic with conscious sedation may also be used in selected individuals. With the exception of certain complex fistulas or those in whom concomitant sphincter repair is undertaken,

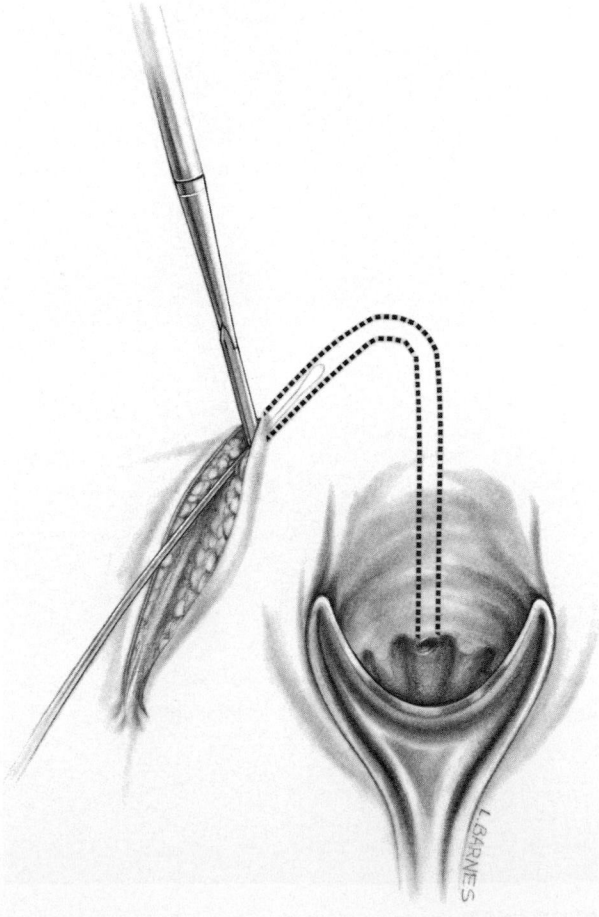

FIGURE 14-17. Progressive unroofing of a fistula with electrocautery, following the tract with the aid of a probe.

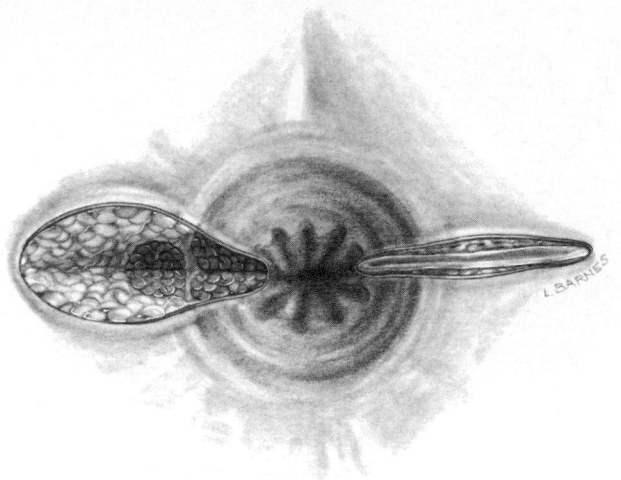

FIGURE 14-18. Fistulectomy versus fistulotomy, matters of prolonged wound healing, scarring, and deformity.

the operation can usually be performed on an ambulatory basis. This is also in accordance with the recommendations of the Standards Task Force of the American Society of Colon and Rectal Surgeons.[179] However, the most current set of recommendations does not specifically address the

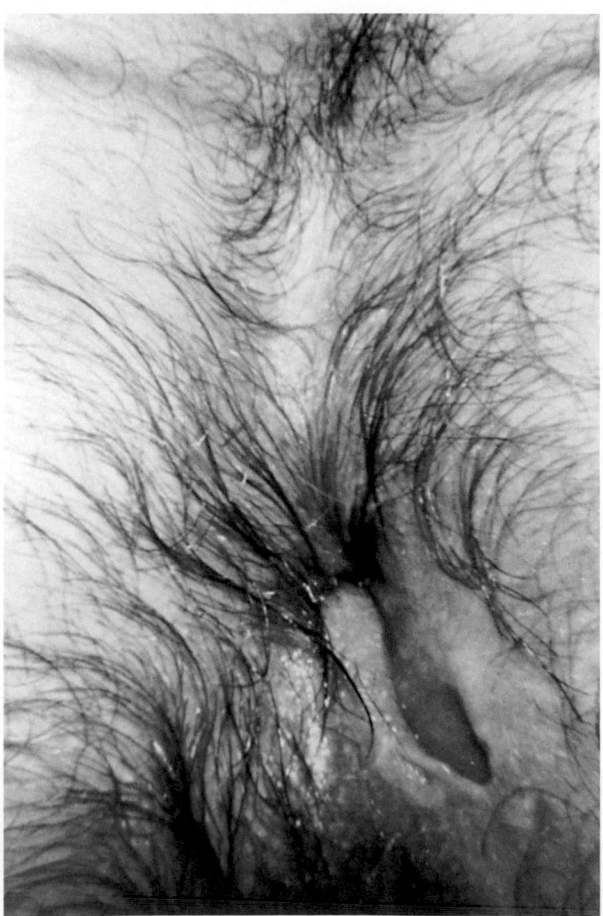

FIGURE 14-19. Anal fistulectomy may require prolonged healing time. This wound is still open 6 weeks after the operation.

issue of inpatient or outpatient management.[180] Their conclusions were as follows:

- A fistula, fistula with abscess, or a fistula associated with limited anorectal pathology may be treated on an outpatient basis if, in the judgment of the operating surgeon, it is safe to do so.
- Fistulas involving adjacent organs or structures (i.e., rectovaginal, rectourethral, or horseshoe) often require more extensive surgery, and inpatient postoperative care is usually needed.
- Fistulas associated with extensive cellulitis or abscess or additional anorectal disease may require inpatient care, especially if intravenous antibiotics are necessary.[179]

▶ SURGICAL APPROACHES AND RESULTS

Treatment of Conventional Fistula

After the external and internal openings have been identified by one of the means mentioned previously, the tract is incised (Figure 14-20). Continuity of the epithelial lining confirms the completeness of the operation, and granulation tissue is removed by curettage. A portion of the tract may be excised and sent for pathologic examination. The external portion of the incision may be widened relative to the size of the opening in the anal canal because skin tends to heal more rapidly than anal mucosa. If this is not done, delayed healing within the anal canal may result. The cut edges of the anal mucosa and the underlying internal anal sphincter can be oversewn with absorbable suture for hemostasis (Figure 14-21). The wound is otherwise left open and gently packed. Petroleum jelly gauze is preferred by some surgeons because subsequent removal is less likely to induce bleeding. Others endorse the use of iodoform

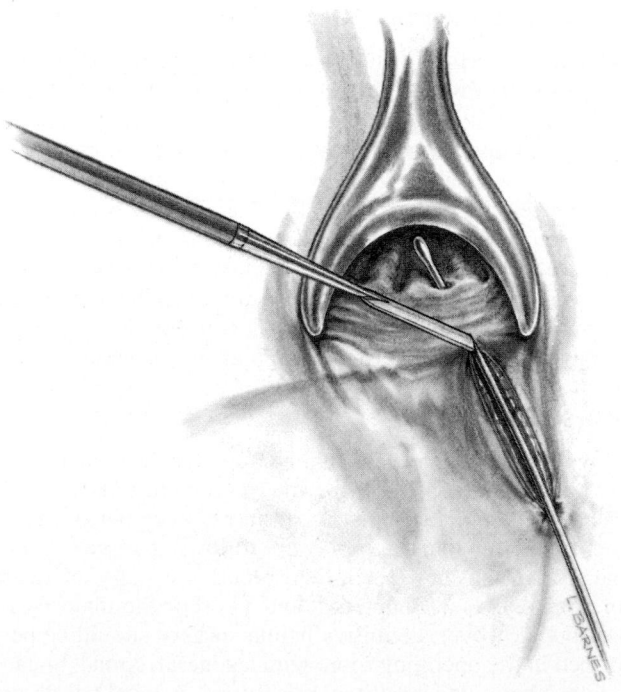

FIGURE 14-20. Conventional fistulotomy. With the use of electrocautery, the tract is laid open between the internal and external openings.

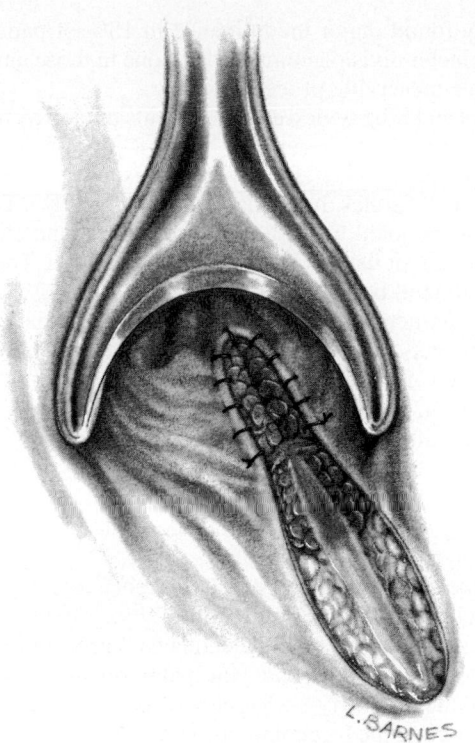

FIGURE 14-21. Conventional fistulotomy. The anal opening with the underlying internal sphincter is sutured for hemostasis.

gauze, Surgicel, Telfa, or simply a gauze sponge. Tight packing should be avoided because it can lead to cellulitis and abscess.

To reiterate, the principles of operative treatment are as follows:

- Identify the tract.
- Incise the tract.
- Excise a portion for biopsy material (if considered potentially useful).
- Widen the external wound.
- Suture the cut edge of the anal canal.
- Gently pack the wound.

The dressing is removed the evening of surgery or the next day, and sitz baths should be performed. Vigorous mechanical cleansing of the wound is encouraged with either a washcloth or a gauze pad. The use of a Water-Pic device or comparable irrigating equipment has merit in postoperative wound management. One should be as vigorous as possible, maintaining the wound in a well-debrided and clean state. An office visit is recommended 10 days later to assess healing, and usually every 1 to 2 weeks thereafter until healing is complete. Less frequent appointments may be appropriate for individuals with straightforward fistulas if the patient understands the need for and is committed to vigorous cleansing.

If a large portion of the external sphincter must be divided, consideration should be given to primary sphincter repair or possibly to seton division (see later discussion). An anterior fistula in a woman should always be considered for either reconstruction or another alternative to limit sphincter damage (Figure 14-22). When a fistula occurs anteriorly in a

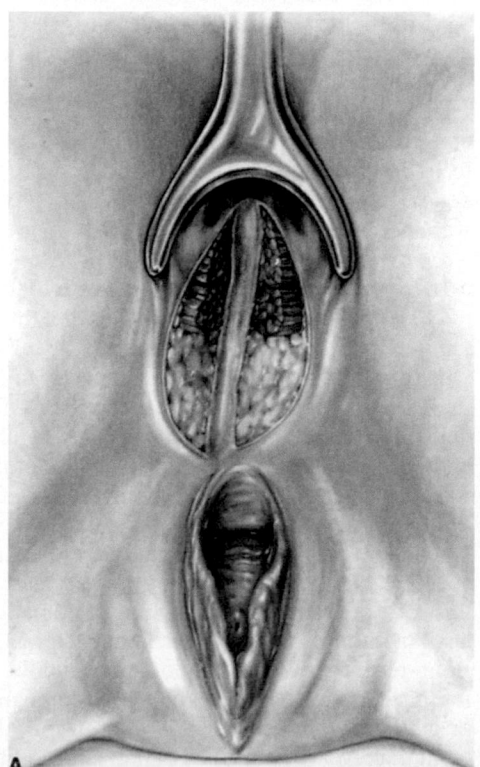
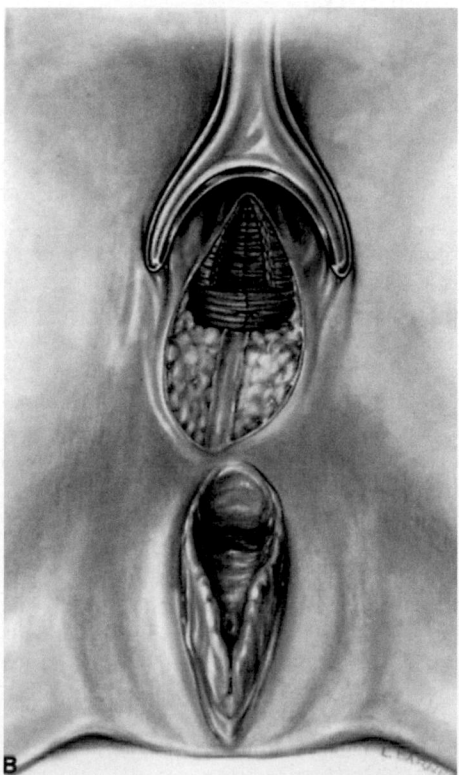

FIGURE 14-22. Anterior fistula in a female patient may be treated by repair of the external sphincter. **A:** Fistulotomy dividing a portion of the external sphincter. **B:** Repair of the sphincter is effected, and the wound is left open.

woman, surgical treatment inevitably will create some degree of impaired control. To minimize the disability, sphincter reconstruction should be attempted at the time of fistulotomy. Another alternative for managing such a problem is to use a seton or to perform a closure of the internal opening with a sliding endorectal flap, such as that which may be recommended for rectovaginal fistula repair and high transsphincteric anal fistulas.

Results

It is difficult to interpret the results of treatment for anal fistula for a number of reasons. One attempts to analyze variables that include an individual surgeon's personal operative preferences and technique, the type of fistula encountered, and the cause of the problem. Not only are the variables poorly defined in the numerous published papers, but also the clinical material often consists of a melange of fistula manifestations. Most important, there is a dearth of prospective, randomized trials.

The three primary criteria for determining success or failure of fistula surgery are the following:

- Recurrence
- Delayed healing
- Incontinence

A few generalizations can be made in attempting to interpret the published results:

- The more "complex" the fistula is, the higher the internal opening will be.
- The more sphincter that is divided, the longer it takes to heal, the greater the likelihood of recurrence, and the higher risk of fecal soiling.
- The most likely cause of recurrence is the failure to identify and adequately treat the internal opening.

As mentioned, the results of surgery for anal fistula are extremely difficult to interpret from the published articles. Virtually all of the studies are retrospective and reflect the individual author's personal preference for management. Despite the fact that many of these series incorporate hundreds of patients, there is no consensus that can be derived. Generally, recurrence rates vary from 4% to 10%, with missed internal openings at the initial surgery accounting for the vast majority of such recurrences.[159] Certainly, those individuals with high openings, posterior openings, or fistula extensions are at increased risk for developing recurrence.[192] In the experience of the University of Minnesota group, factors associated with recurrence included complex type of fistula, horseshoe extension, lack of identification or lateral location of the internal fistulous opening, prior fistula surgery, and even the variable of the surgeon.[63]

Besides the issue of recurrence, the other major concern is incontinence. This is reported to be noted in 10% to 50%. Again, from the Minnesota group, greater than 50% complained of some degree of postoperative incontinence.[63] Articles have been published concerning manometric evaluation and anorectal function following fistula surgery.[18,155,157] The self-evident conclusion is that the more one divides or fails to preserve the sphincter, the lower the resting and squeeze pressures of the anal canal. Anorectal physiology and continence were assessed prospectively before and after surgery in 50 individuals with anal infection at St. Bartholomew's and St. Mark's Hospitals in London.[114] Functional deficit occurred in 8 of 15 patients. Bokhari and Lindsey reported on 128 patients treated with sphincter division and noted higher healing rates compared with sphincter-conserving treatment, but they found major incontinence in 13% of patients who had sphincter division compared to none in those undergoing sphincter-preserving procedures.[23]

Parks and Stitz reviewed 158 patients treated by the senior author over a 15-year period.[138] Follow-up of at least 1 year was available in 142. There were 12 instances of recurrence (9%) and 10 fistulas that remained unhealed (7%). The recurrences were noted with all types of fistulas, and all but two of the recurrent fistulas healed with reoperation. The authors also evaluated bowel control and found that 17% who had an intersphincteric fistula had difficulty with flatus control or occasional soiling. One-third of those with transsphincteric fistulas reported one complaint or the other. It is worth recognizing, however, that, depending on the definition, no patient in either group became truly incontinent.

Hidaka and coworkers performed fistula operations on 2,242 patients, almost one-half of whom underwent "sphincter-preserving surgery."[80] They concluded that failure rates were similar and low (less than 5%).

Kuypers reported an overall recurrence rate of 4%, and a 10% incidence of some control difficulty.[103] Bennett noted in 114 patients that 12% had inadequate control for feces, 16% had poor flatus control, and 24% had frequent soiling of their underclothes.[19] Thirty-six percent of patients complained of one or more of the foregoing problems. Adams and Kovalcik reported an overall recurrence rate of 4% in 133 individuals.[3] Hill followed 476 patients for up to 20 years.[81] Delayed wound healing occurred in only 7; 4 experienced recurrence, and 19 had varying degrees of control difficulties. Results of treatment of fistula-in-ano were analyzed in 260 consecutive patients by Vasilevsky and Gordon.[194] Continence problems were observed in 6% and recurrence in 6.3%. Sainio and Husa reported minor defects in bowel control in 34% of their patients.[156] Of interest is their opinion that the amount of divided muscle did not influence the incidence of incontinence. Toyonaga and coworkers examined factors affecting continence after fistulotomy and found low preoperative contraction pressure and multiple previous surgeries to be independently associated with postoperative incontinence.[186] However, location and level of the internal opening were not associated.

A review of the experience at St. Mark's Hospital over a 10-year period found that fistulotomy led to closure rates of 96% to 98%, depending on the height of the opening. Only two patients in their series of 180 had a recurrence. Operation-induced incontinence, mostly to flatus, was noted in 30% to 44% of cases.[13] In a large study from the Netherlands, the 3-year recurrence rate after fistulotomy was 7%, and some soiling was noted in up to 40% of patients.[191] There were no clear predictors of increased risk for either failure or impaired control.

Outcomes after fistula surgery were examined on a prospective, multicenter basis by Hyman and colleagues.[87] In this series, 25 surgeons contributed 245 patients. The overall healing rate was 19.5% after 1 month and 63.2% at 3 months. Long-term follow-up was not yet available. However, fistulotomy had the highest healing rates compared with draining or cutting setons, anal fistula plug, fibrin glue, or advancement flap. Nearly one-third of patients required an additional procedure during the study period, and nearly one-third were being treated for recurrent fistulas. Those treated for recurrent fistulas were less likely to heal. As noted in other studies, seton drainage did not improve success rates.

Horseshoe Fistula

Horseshoe fistula may be intersphincteric but is much more frequently transsphincteric. It is so called because it is composed of multiple external openings joined by a subcutaneous communication in a U or horseshoe shape (Figure 14-23). The arms of the U are almost always directed anteriorly, and the internal opening is in the posterior midline. Rarely, a horseshoe fistula may present with the opposite configuration; that is, the internal opening is in the anterior midline, and the arms of the U are directed posteriorly.

Treatment of this condition has evolved to be much less radical than originally described. The classic procedure required identification of the tracts and internal opening and unroofing or excision of each of them (Figure 14-24). This inevitably resulted in a huge, gaping wound, which required a prolonged healing time (Figure 14-25). Disability after this operation can last for many months.

In 1965, Hanley described a rather conservative approach to the management of horseshoe fistula that limits the number and extent of the incisions.[75] The most important aspects of the operation are to eliminate the internal opening and to establish adequate external drainage.[58,75] Because all of the tracts and external openings communicate, if the internal opening has been removed, the external openings will close. Most surgeons have successfully adopted this approach to the treatment of horseshoe anal fistula.

If the fistula is transsphincteric, the deep postanal space must be entered, curetted, and irrigated (Figure 14-26). This involves incision of both the internal sphincter and a portion of the external sphincter. It is then necessary only to unroof the external openings, curette the tracts, and drain the wounds (Figure 14-27). The cut edges of the anal canal and underlying internal sphincter are sutured for hemostasis. The deep postanal space is packed loosely, usually with iodoform gauze, and a dressing is applied.

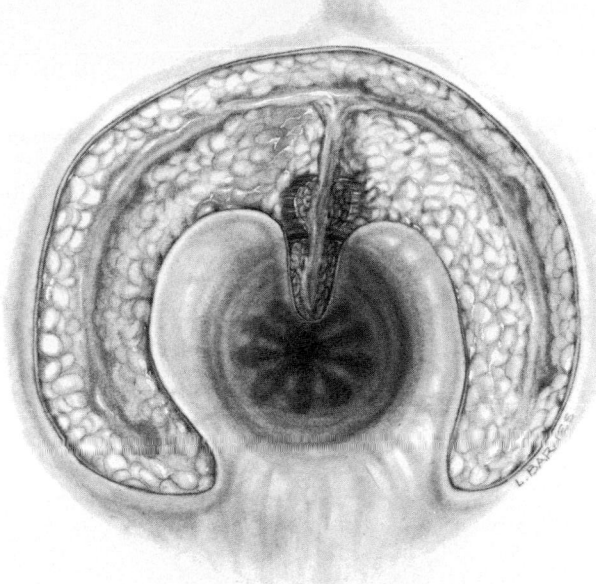

FIGURE 14-24. Classic treatment of horseshoe fistula with excision of all openings.

When the fistula is approached in this way, healing is generally rapid, and the risk of functional impairment to the anus from scarring and deformity is decreased. Duration of disability is also markedly reduced.

Postoperatively, the packing is removed in 24 to 48 hours, and the patient may begin sitz baths. Weekly office visits are recommended until the wounds have healed.

Results

Hanley and colleagues reported their results in 41 patients with horseshoe fistula.[76] There was no problem with healing, recurrence, or incontinence using the technique previously described. Hamilton, using the same approach, reported

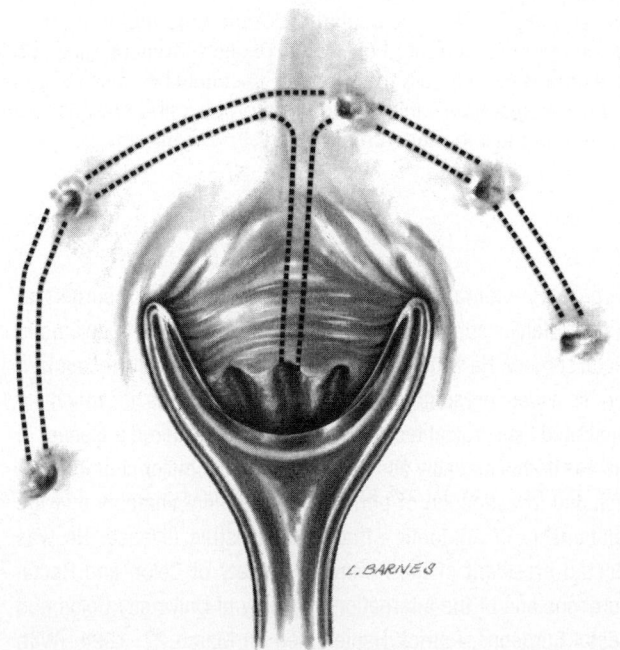

FIGURE 14-23. Representation of a horseshoe anal fistula. The internal opening is in the posterior midline.

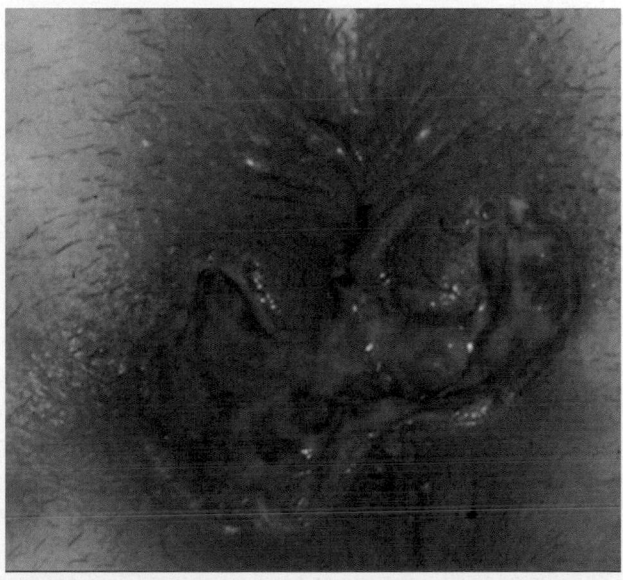

FIGURE 14-25. Treatment of an anterior horseshoe fistula by the classic technique leaves a large, gaping wound that requires prolonged healing time.

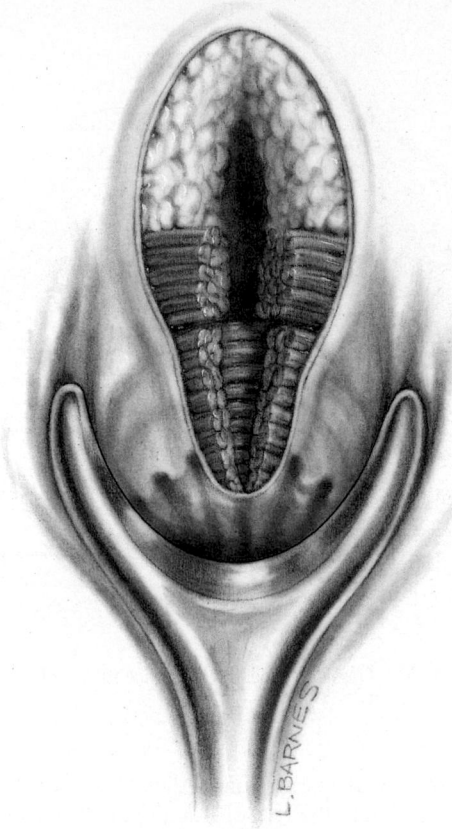

FIGURE 14-26. Successful management of a typical posterior horseshoe fistula requires entrance to the deep postanal space even though a portion of the internal and external sphincter must be divided.

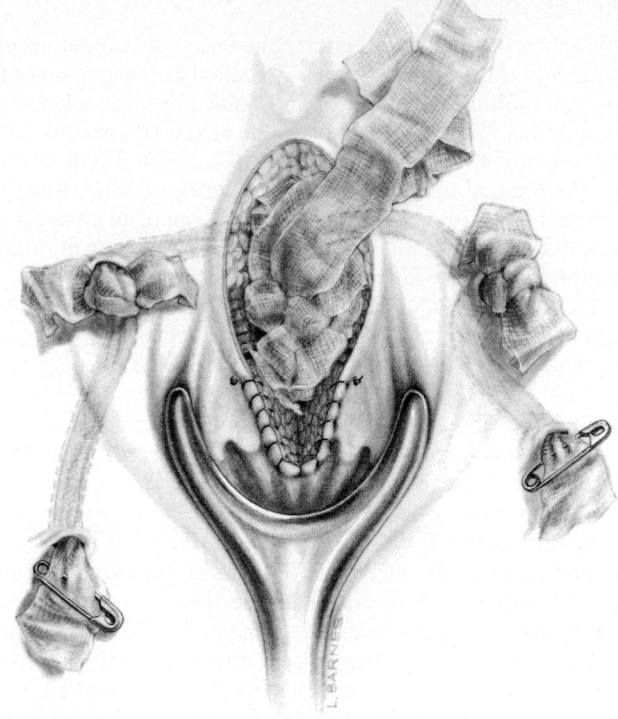

FIGURE 14-27. Treatment of horseshoe fistula-in-ano requires unroofing in the posterior midline to drain the deep postanal space adequately. The external openings are individually drained, with curettage only of the underlying tracts. Packing is placed through each opening and in the deep postanal space.

Treatment of Suprasphincteric Fistula

The management of suprasphincteric fistula is comparable to that of other complex fistulas. Options include endorectal advancement flap, primary closure and drainage, and seton division. In general, once the fistula has been recognized as such, fistulotomy can be accomplished distal to the internal opening by dividing the lower portion of the internal and external sphincters (Figure 14-28). The cephalad component, including the internal opening, is treated by means of seton division (see later). It is important to assess the length of the canal because men tend to have longer anal canals, whereas women tend to have shorter. Sufficient muscle must remain to preserve continence.

four recurrences in 57 patients.[74] Held and coworkers noted a recurrence rate of 18% and advised more frequent use of a seton to promote drainage and to avoid premature closure.[77] Others have adopted a similar philosophy and used seton division with drainage in the management of this condition.[188] In 11 patients so treated, 2 developed recurrences (18.1%). Pezim also emphasized the importance of unroofing the deep postanal space and achieved healing in 92% of his 24 patients.[142]

PATRICK H. HANLEY (1909–1994)

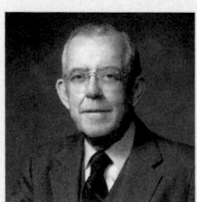

Courtesy Ochsner Clinic Foundation, New Orleans, Louisiana

Patrick Hanley was born February 2, 1909, in Lockport, Louisiana. He graduated from Southwestern Louisiana Institute in 1929 and received his medical degree from Tulane University School of Medicine in 1933. He completed his surgical residency at Charity Hospital in New Orleans under the guidance of Alton Ochsner. During World War II, he served as a lieutenant commander in Bahia, Brazil, where he devoted himself to communicable disease prevention and to health education. After the war, he returned to New Orleans and to the Ochsner Clinic, at which institution he developed a training program in colon and rectal surgery. He ultimately was promoted to professor of surgery at Tulane. Hanley supervised the training of 40 fellows in colon and rectal surgery. He wrote extensively and was especially recognized for his video presentations at national meetings in which he illustrated his surgical techniques. He was considered a pioneer in the use of this modality as a teaching tool. His major contributions included investigation of perineal and perianal anatomy and the relationship of anatomic structures to fistula disease. He was elected president of the American Society of Colon and Rectal Surgeons and of the International Society of University Colon and Rectal Surgeons. Patrick Hanley died on March 27, 1994. (With appreciation to David E. Beck, MD, chairman, Department of Colon and Rectal Surgery, Ochsner Clinic Foundation, New Orleans, LA.)

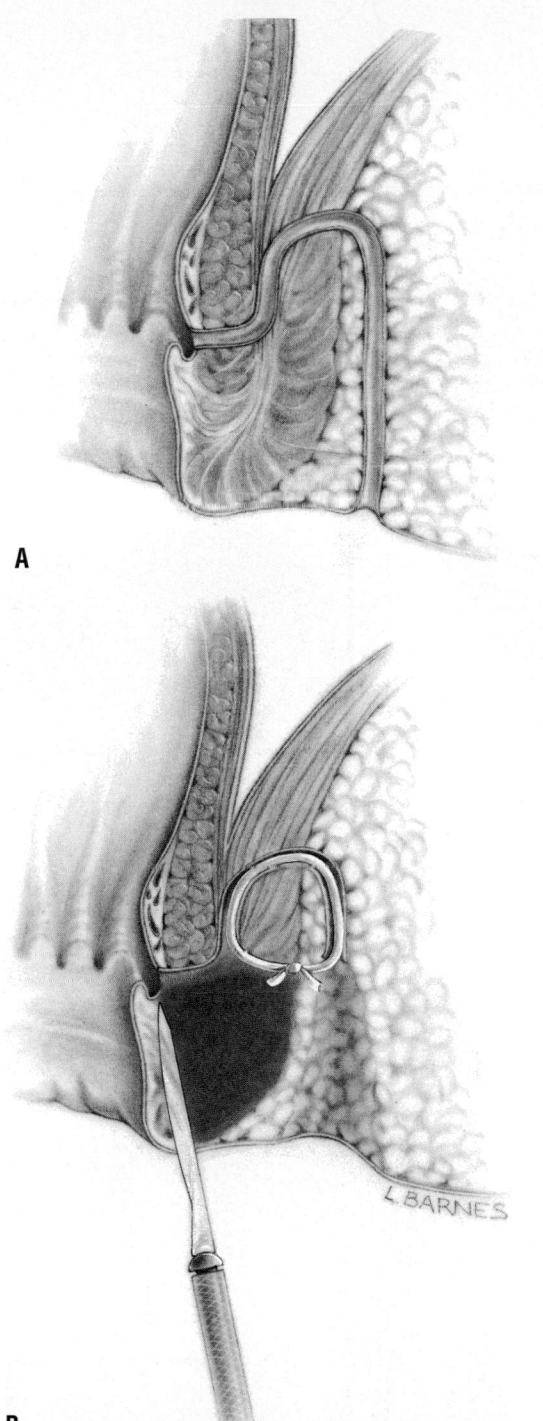

A

B

FIGURE 14-28. Suprasphincteric fistula. **A:** The tract courses above the levators, passing through to the skin in the ischiorectal fossa. **B:** The internal and external sphincters have been incised, but the high opening is treated by seton division to minimize the risk of fecal incontinence.

Treatment of Extrasphincteric Fistula

When the internal opening is thought to lie above the levators, division of the tract may result in fecal incontinence. If the puborectalis sling is completely divided, anal incontinence will ensue. When doubt exists as to the level of the internal opening, a seton can be employed as a diagnostic tool. This involves placing a vessel loop through the tract and out the anal canal. This can be facilitated by passing the vessel loop

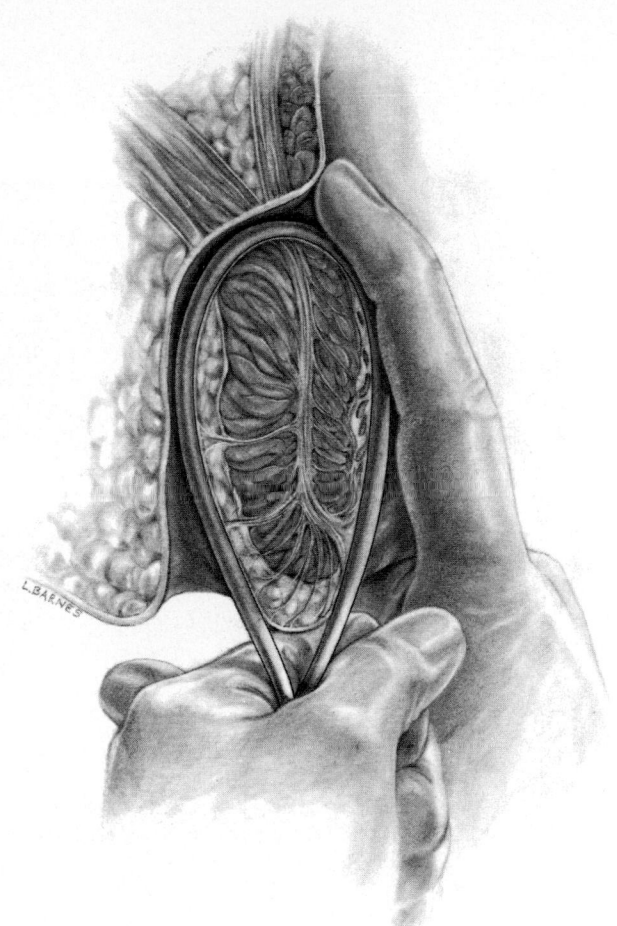

FIGURE 14-29. A seton is used to evaluate the level of the internal opening.

through the eye of a probe. The seton is loosely tied, and no further procedure is undertaken at that time.

When the patient is alert, rectal examination is performed. While he or she alternately tightens and relaxes the sphincter, the seton can be felt to lie above or below the levators (Figure 14-29). If it is below, a fistulotomy can be performed safely. Conversely, if the internal opening is above the level of the levators, an alternative procedure must be undertaken. Several possible operative approaches exist for the treatment of extrasphincteric fistula (see later).

Results

It is virtually impossible to analyze the results of treatment for extrasphincteric fistula because (absent Crohn's disease or a specific cause) the condition is extremely rare. Furthermore, those who do report some experience generally comingle the results or even confuse the condition with that of a high transsphincteric fistula. In the series of Parks and Stitz, only 2 of 13 patients who harbored extrasphincteric fistulas were incontinent. However, the method of treatment was not clearly stated.[138]

Cavanaugh and colleagues suggested that a more accurate interpretation of the functional results for fistula surgery (specifically fecal incontinence) could be achieved through the use of the Fecal Incontinence Severity Index (FISI, see Chapter 16).[33] The median score was 6, with 36% having a score of 0. As could be anticipated, direct correlation was identified with the amount of sphincter divided. Furthermore, there was an adverse effect on quality-of-life issues

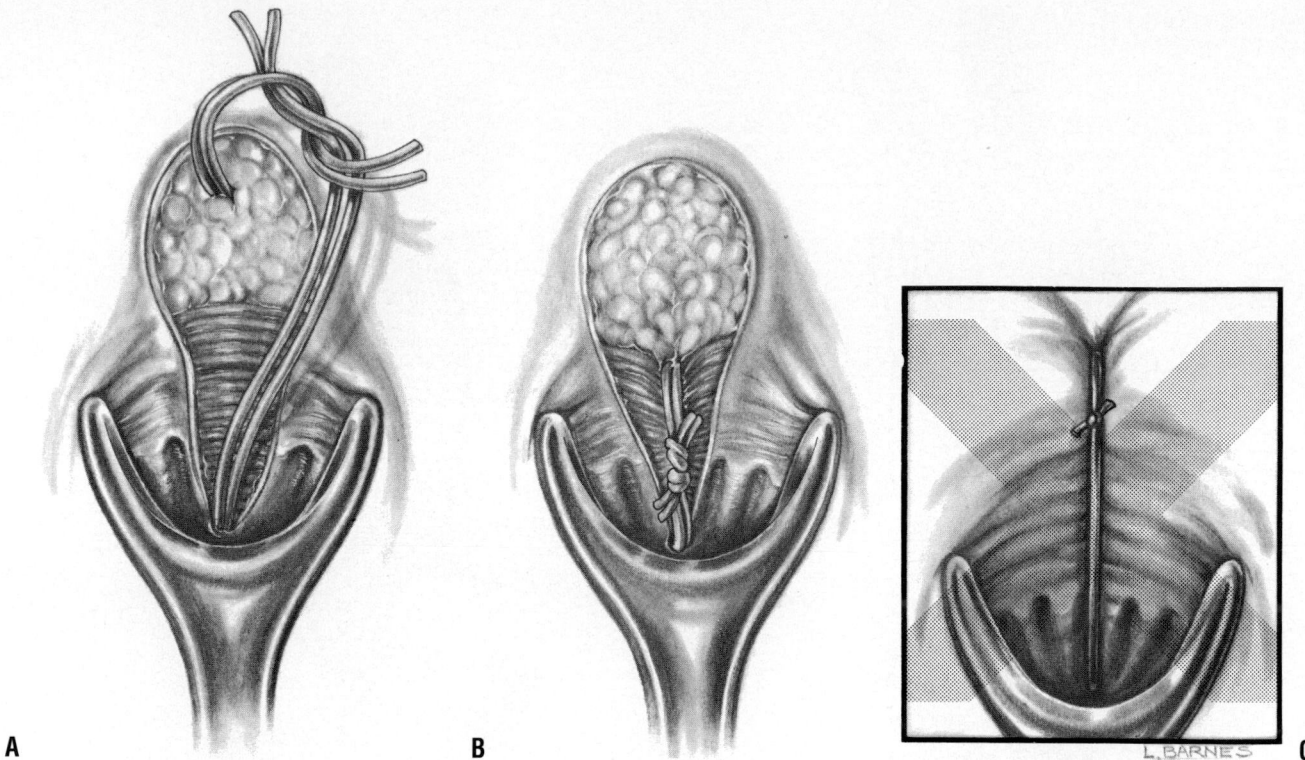

FIGURE 14-30. Application of a seton in the treatment of extrasphincteric fistula. **A:** Doubled heavy sutures (silk is preferred with this technique) are passed through the external and internal openings. **B:** The sutures are firmly secured. **C:** The skin must be divided.

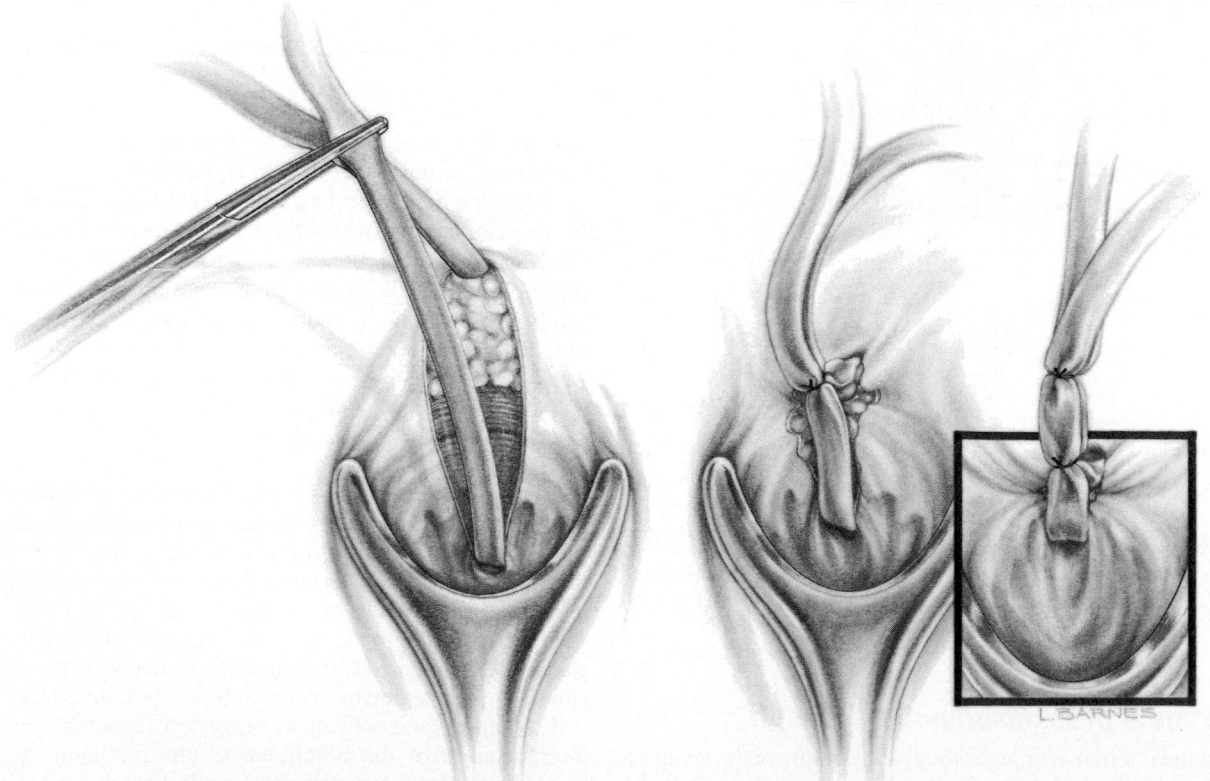

FIGURE 14-31. A 1/4-in. Penrose drain is used to effect seton division. The *inset* demonstrates subsequent ligation of the drain at a higher level. (Adapted from Culp CE. Use of Penrose drains to treat certain anal fistulas: a primary operative seton. *Mayo Clin Proc.* 1984;59(9):613–617, with permission.)

(depression, embarrassment) that was directly proportional to a FISI score in excess of 30.[33]

Seton Division

Seton division was described by Hippocrates in the 5th century BC in his medical works known as the *Hippocratic Collection*.[4] His concepts are still applicable today for the management of difficult fistula problems. It is certainly the simplest of the methods available for the treatment of extrasphincteric fistula and probably produces results comparable to other approaches, at least with respect to cure rate.[37,102,147] Bowel control, however, may be less satisfactory when compared with other options.

The principle involved in the use of the seton as a therapeutic tool is analogous to that of a wire cutting through a block of ice. The ice is still adherent after division by the wire. Theoretically, by tightening the suture and permitting it to cut through over a number of days or weeks, the resultant inflammatory response keeps the sphincter muscle from retracting and separating. A caveat, however, is not to use this technique if the patient is suspected of harboring Crohn's disease. The seton will often slice through the inflamed tissue rapidly, increasing the risk of incontinence.

Technique

The skin and anal canal mucosa between the openings must be initially incised. Then the suture is passed (Figure 14-30A). Some surgeons prefer doubled no. 2 silk, but other alternatives include elastic bands (e.g., vessel loops) or a 1/4-in. Penrose drain (Figure 14-31).[45] The seton is securely tied, usually with moderate tension (Figure 14-30B). The use of a rubber ring ligator has been suggested to subsequently tighten the ligature (Figure 14-32).[42] Another method of securing and tightening the seton involves the use of a so-called hangman's knot (Figure 14-33).[111] Still another alternative is to insert multiple setons initially, securing only one.[65] As each cuts through, another one is tied. If an elastic band, vessel loop, or Penrose drain is used, one may secure the drain to itself with a ligature, thereby creating some compression of the tissue (Figure 14-34).

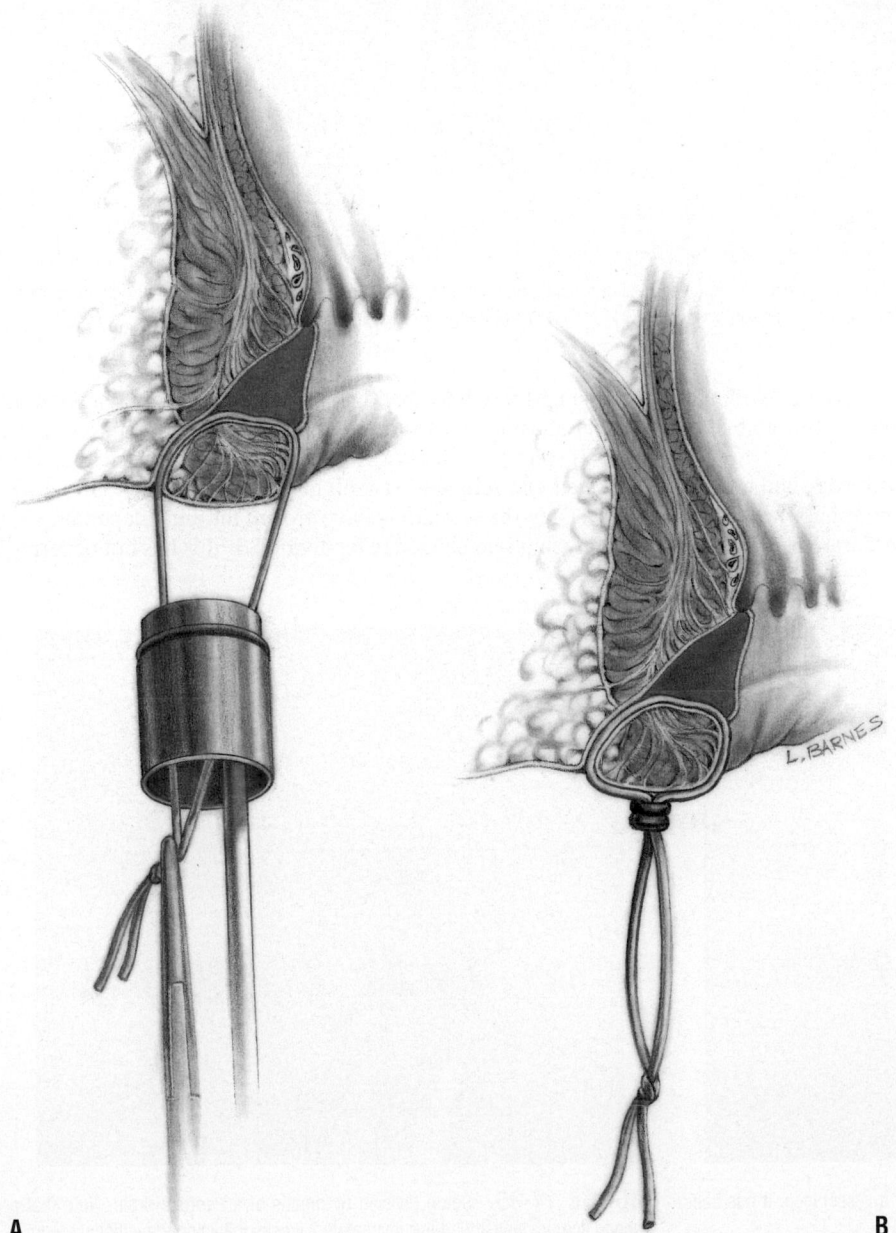

A

B

FIGURE 14-32. Seton fistulotomy using elastic bands applied by rubber ring ligator as suggested by Cirocco and Rusin.[42] **A:** A rubber band ligator is introduced. **B:** Rubber bands are secured.

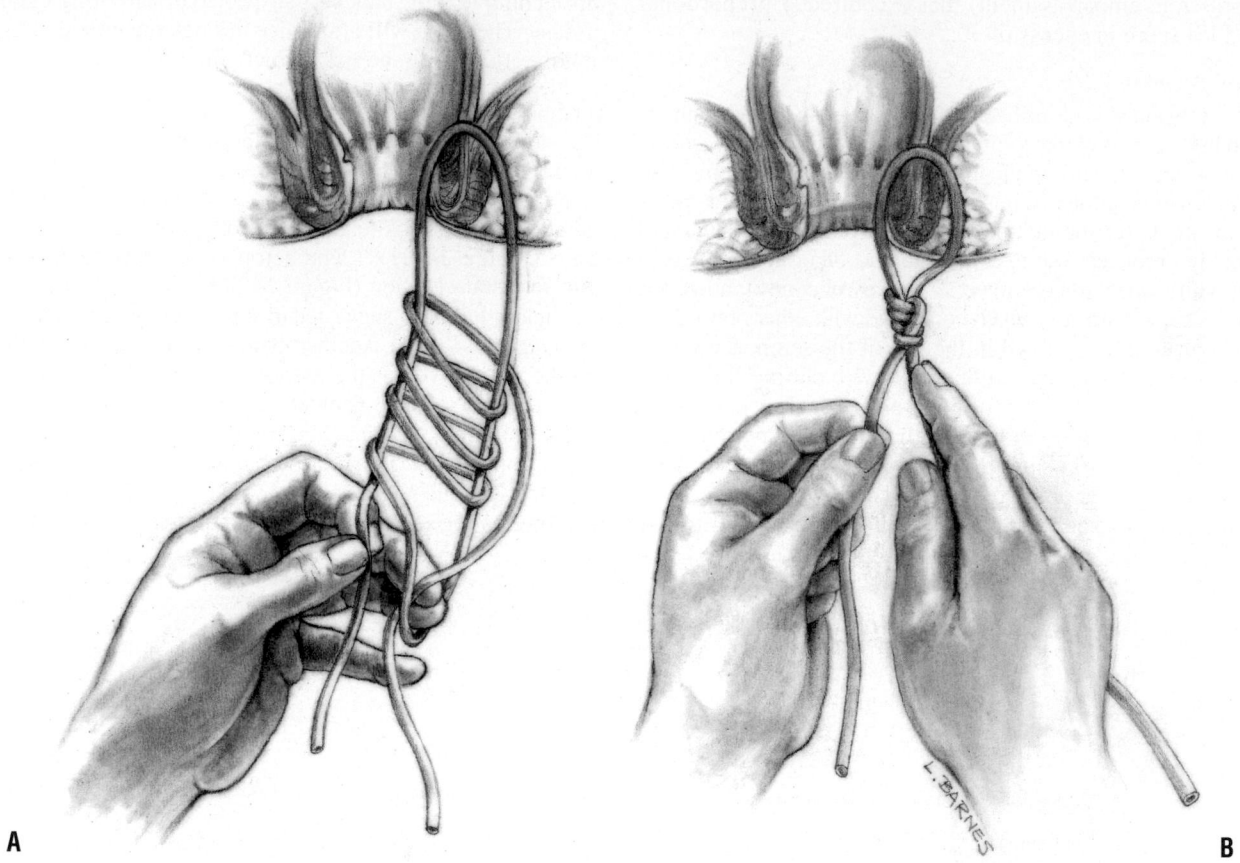

A   **B**

FIGURE 14-33. Securing the seton in such a matter that it permits tightening using a hangman's tie. (Adapted from Loberman Z, Har-Shai Y, Schein M, et al. Hangman's tie simplifies seton management of anal fistulas. *Surg Gynecol Obstet.* 1993;177(4):413–414, with permission.)

The approach we prefer is to use a vessel loop, tied with silk such that it is a continuous loop. This is more comfortable for the patient because it avoids sitting on a knot.

The patient is usually discharged the same day and is reexamined 1 week later. By this time, the suture has either loosened or, if minimal tissue has been incorporated, passed by necrosing through the residual muscle. Following injection of a local anesthetic into the sphincter, a second suture can be used. If some type of elastic band has been employed, it can be stretched and religated at a higher level (Figure 14-35). Two weeks later, the seton may have eroded through, depending on how much tissue needed to be divided. If this has not occurred

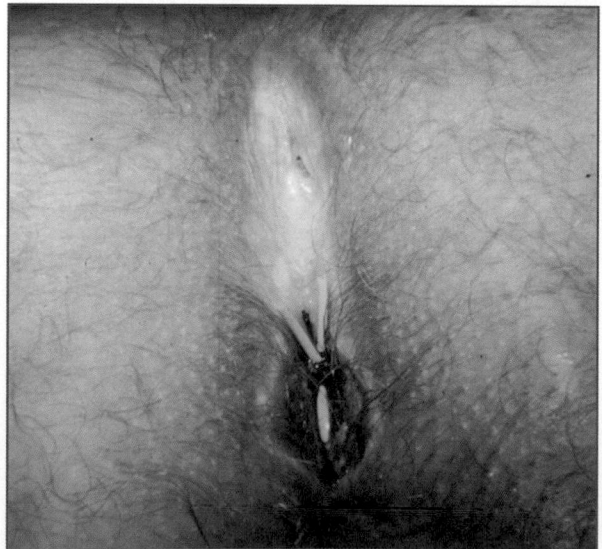

FIGURE 14-34. Seton fistulotomy by means of a vessel loop. It has been secured with a ligature.

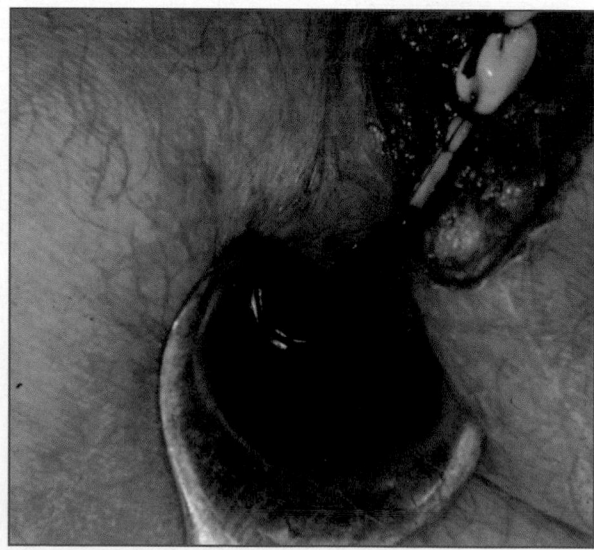

FIGURE 14-35. Seton division by means of a Penrose drain. Note that a second ligature was added approximately 2 weeks following the initial procedure.

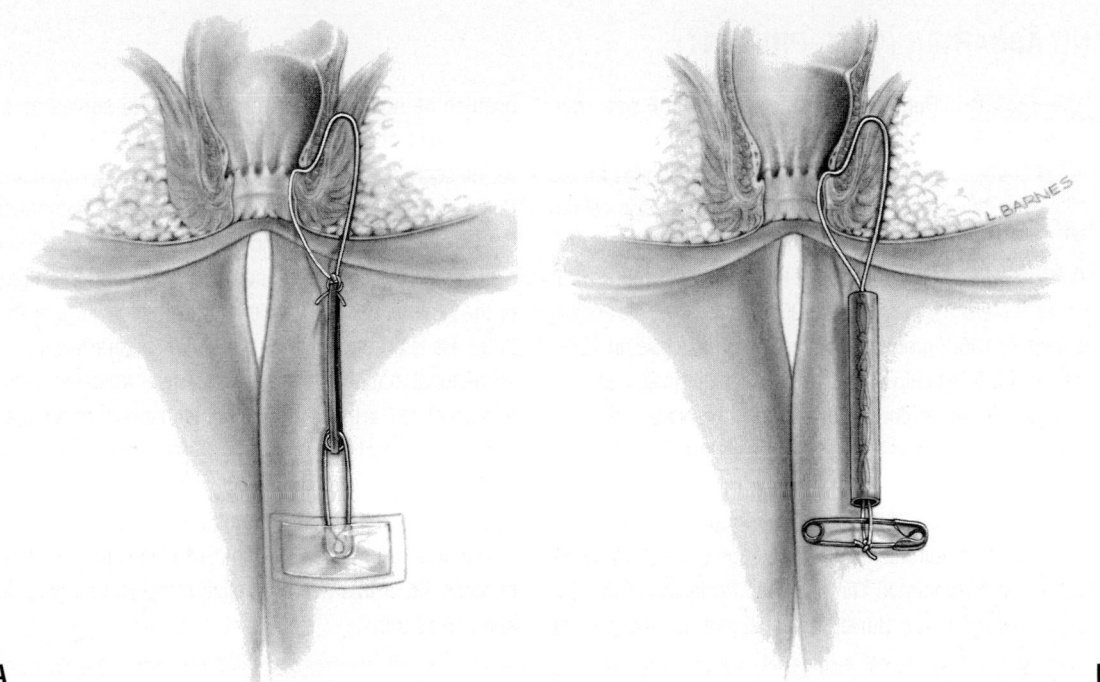

A   **B**

FIGURE 14-36. Adjustable seton in the management of a suprasphincteric anal fistula. **A:** Variable tension is produced by the elastic secured to the thigh. **B:** An adjustable tourniquet accomplishes the same ends. (Adapted from Thompson JE Jr, Bennion RS, Hilliard G. Adjustable seton in the management of complex anal fistula. *Surg Gynecol Obstet.* 1989;169(6):551–552, with permission.)

and there is minimal residual tissue, the fistulotomy can be completed in the office. However, if the surgeon prefers, a third tightening or even more can be performed, if indicated.

Thompson and colleagues suggest the use of a seton technique that can apply varying amounts of tension to accomplish sphincter division.[183] A no. 1 nylon or polypropylene suture or vessel loop is threaded around the sphincter in the usual way and tied loosely. A heavy elastic band is secured to the suture, and a safety pin is attached. The pin is then taped to the thigh with a small amount of tension, and the patient is instructed to adjust the amount that will produce minimal discomfort until the seton has cut through (Figure 14-36A). The authors offer another method of accomplishing patient-controlled seton division—tightening the noose by means of an adjustable tourniquet (Figure 14-36B).[183] This approach has two theoretical advantages. First, pain, a consequence of tissue ischemia and necrosis, is a well-recognized problem with seton division. Using a system that permits the patients to adjust the tension for minimal discomfort would certainly appear to be reasonable, provided, of course, that it was effective. Second, this seton technique is, in essence, a one-stage procedure.

Results

Kuypers reported his experience with the use of the seton in the treatment of extrasphincteric fistula.[102] No recurrences were observed in his 10 patients; 6 experienced slight soiling, and 1 was incontinent. A more recent report from the same unit in the Netherlands included 34 patients.[193] Of the 29 available for follow-up, 12 had normal bowel control, 5 had no control for flatus, 11 were incontinent for liquid stool, and 1 had continued fecal leakage. The authors concluded that this technique is *not* recommended for fistulas with high openings.

Williams and colleagues reviewed their experience with 74 patients who underwent seton division of "high" anal fistulas by four techniques: staged fistulotomy, cutting seton, short-term

drainage, and long-term drainage for Crohn's disease.[200] None who was treated with a cutting seton (13 patients) developed a recurrence. Minor instances of incontinence developed in 54% of those treated by two-stage fistulotomy or by cutting seton.

Much of the work on the place of setons in contemporary anal surgery and their innovative applications is based on the huge experience of Abcarian and his colleagues. Pearl and co-workers, reporting from the Cook County Hospital in Chicago, accomplished seton fistulotomy in 116 patients.[139] Major fecal incontinence requiring the use of a pad occurred in 5%, with recurrent fistulas identified in 3%. The authors concluded that seton fistulotomy is a safe and effective method for treating high or complicated anorectal fistulas. García-Aguilar and associates retrospectively reviewed patients who were treated by seton fistulotomy or by placement of the seton to "stimulate fibrosis" and subsequent one-stage fistulotomy.[64] No difference was noted with respect to recurrence rates, incontinence, and incontinence scores. Other studies confirm the safety and efficacy of seton fistulotomy, although gas incontinence is a concern in up to 10%.[83,89,94,122] A meta-analysis of 37 different studies that examined the incidence of incontinence following cutting seton use reported a rate of 12%, increasing proportionally with the height of the internal opening.[150] The authors note heterogeneity in the type of seton, tightening technique, definitions of incontinence, and an overall poor quality of evidence. This highlights the difficulty in making any generalizations about this strategy and others in the absence of common definitions and end points.

Long-term Seton Drainage

The concept of seton drainage without definitive fistulotomy has been applied to the management of extrasphincteric fistulas, especially those associated with Crohn's disease (see later).[154,168] However, some surgeons have used this concept for the "therapeutic" management of low

HERAND ABCARIAN (1941–PRESENT)

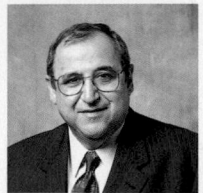

Herand Abcarian was born in Ahvaz, Iran, in January 1941, the third child of Joseph and Stella. The family lived in Shiraz for the following 6 years, but he grew up in Tehran and completed his primary and high school education there. He entered the Tehran University Faculty of Medicine in the fall of 1958 and received his doctorate in medicine in 1965, graduating at the top of his class. In 1966, Abcarian started his internship at Cook County Hospital in Chicago and went on to complete his residencies in general surgery and colon and rectal surgery, becoming certified in both specialties in 1972. That same year, he was appointed as chief of the Division of Colon and Rectal Surgery and director of the Residency Program, remaining in these positions until his retirement from Cook County Hospital in 1995.

In 1989, he was appointed Turi Josefsen Professor in the Department of Surgery at the University of Illinois at Chicago, the position he holds at the present time. He served as head of the Department of Surgery from 1989 to 2006. Abcarian has served as the secretary and later the president of the American Society of Colon and Rectal Surgeons and its research foundation and was the associate editor of the journal *Diseases of the Colon and Rectum*. He served as the executive director and secretary/treasurer of the American Board of Colon and Rectal Surgery from 1986 to 2008. He is on the editorial boards of six journals; is a member of 18 regional, national, and international surgical societies; and has published 117 articles and 20 book chapters on a variety of topics in colon and rectal surgery. As a warm and generous person, as an extraordinary raconteur, and as an accomplished lecturer, it is rare indeed to fail to see his name on a prominent international or national program in the field of colon and rectal surgery. He remains, as of this writing, active in clinical surgery, in teaching, and in research.

transsphincteric and intersphincteric anal fistulas.[107] In the experience of Lentner and Wienert, the suture eventually either cut through the anal and perianal skin on its own, or the authors elected to perform fistulotomy at a subsequent operation.[107] The mean duration of the presence of the seton was in excess of 1 year. The recurrence rate was only 3.7%, and fewer than 1% experienced problems with bowel control. As long as the seton is in the proper position, it will prevent an abscess from occurring.

A drainage seton can either be used long-term to control sepsis or as the first stage prior to a definitive procedure. This approach, however, may not increase the success of the secondary

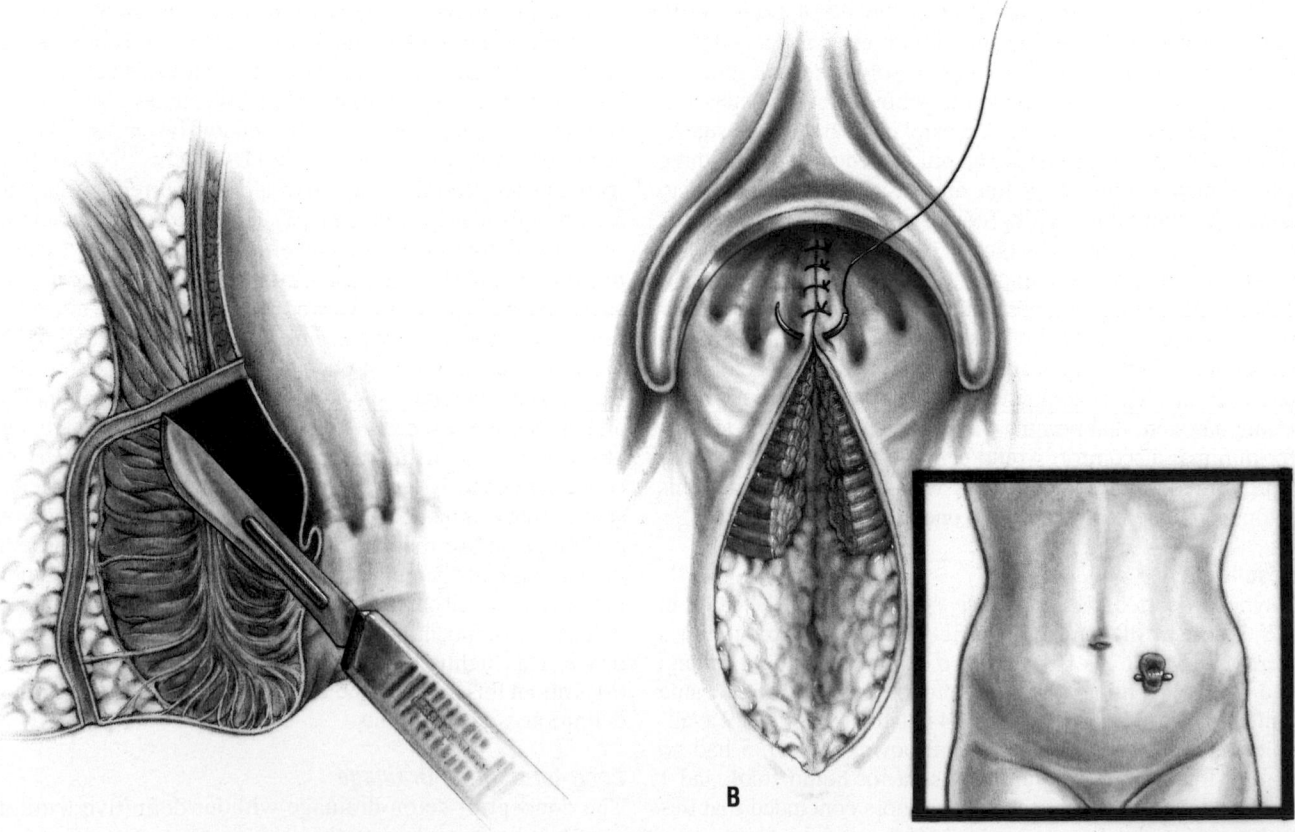

FIGURE 14-37. **A:** Primary fistulotomy for extrasphincteric fistula. **B:** Reconstruction is undertaken after excision of the tract. **C:** A diverting colostomy or ileostomy is recommended for this approach.

procedure. For example, Mitalas and colleagues examined this technique for advancement flaps and found no difference in success rates based on preoperative seton drainage.[125]

Fistulotomy with Sphincter Repair

Complete division of an extrasphincteric fistula is a hazardous undertaking. Although direct repair can be performed immediately, breakdown is common. It should still be considered, however, to be an alternative technique for the treatment of high-level fistulas and, as has been mentioned previously, in the management of transsphincteric anterior fistulas in women.

Technique

The entire tract is divided. The epithelial lining is excised and the wound irrigated. A layered closure is performed using long-term absorbable sutures (e.g., 0 or 2–0 Vicryl), closing the rectal wall, and reconstructing the sphincter muscles. The ischiorectal fossa is widely drained externally. A protective colostomy or ileostomy is strongly suggested if fistulotomy with sphincter repair is contemplated for an extrasphincteric fistula (Figure 14-37).

Closure of the Internal Opening and Drainage of the Extrasphincteric Tract

Closure of the internal opening and drainage of the extrasphincteric tract are less destructive of tissue than fistulotomy with sphincter repair, but the operation has a prohibitively high failure rate. The procedure involves debridement and closure of the internal opening through a transanal operation. Adequate external drainage is established, and the supralevator area is vigorously curetted, irrigated, and packed (Figure 14-38). A concomitant colostomy or ileostomy should certainly be considered to enhance the possibility of a successful outcome.

Another option for conservation of the sphincter mechanism in high anal fistula is to perform the same operation with primary closure through the intersphincteric plane. This has been described from the St. Mark's Hospital group (Figure 14-39).[121] In their operation, the entire tract is excised

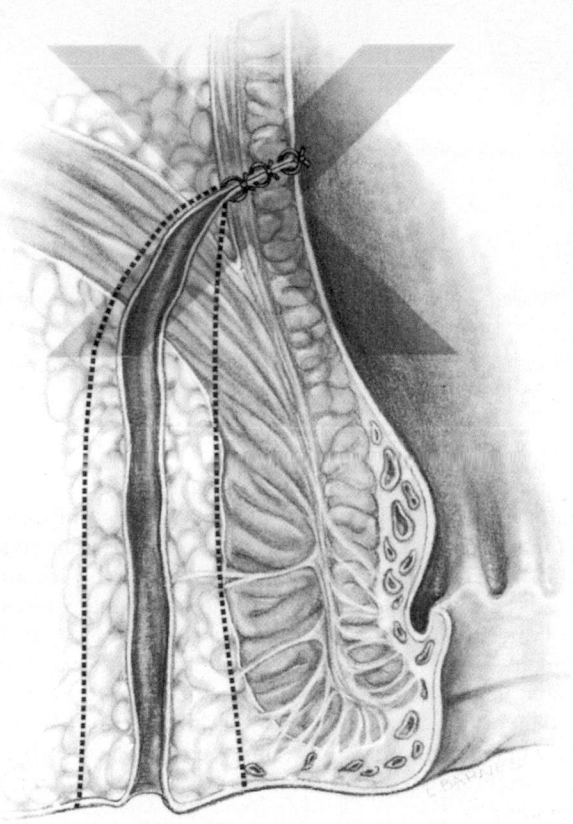

FIGURE 14-38. Treatment of extrasphincteric fistula by closure of the internal opening and wide drainage of the supralevator space and ischiorectal fossa (*broken line*). The *X* indicates one's concerns about the usefulness of this approach.

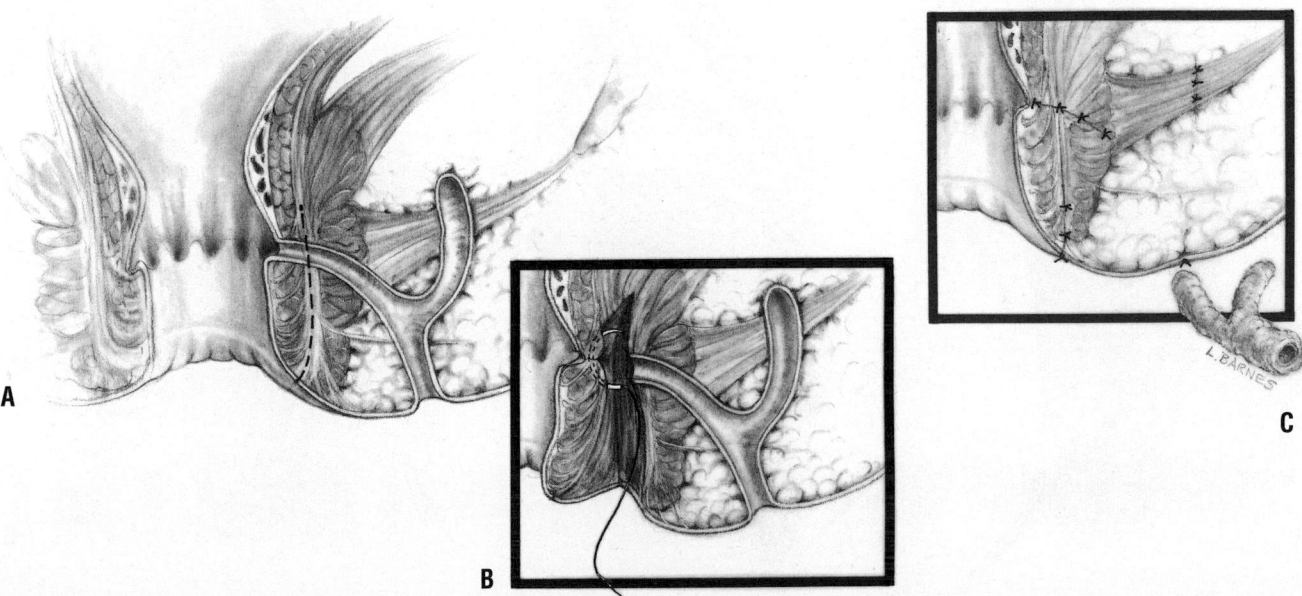

FIGURE 14-39. Total sphincter conservation in a high anal fistula. **A:** A curvilinear incision is made over the intersphincteric groove between the external opening and the anus, deepening the incision in the intersphincteric space to divide the tract just deep to the internal opening. **B:** The opening in the internal sphincter is oversewn with long-term absorbable sutures from within the intersphincteric space. **C:** The tract outside the external sphincter is excised, and the defects in the muscle are repaired prior to primary wound closure. (Adapted from Matos D, Lunniss PJ, Phillips RK. Total sphincter conservation in high fistula in ano: results of a new approach. *Br J Surg.* 1993;80(6):802–804, with permission.)

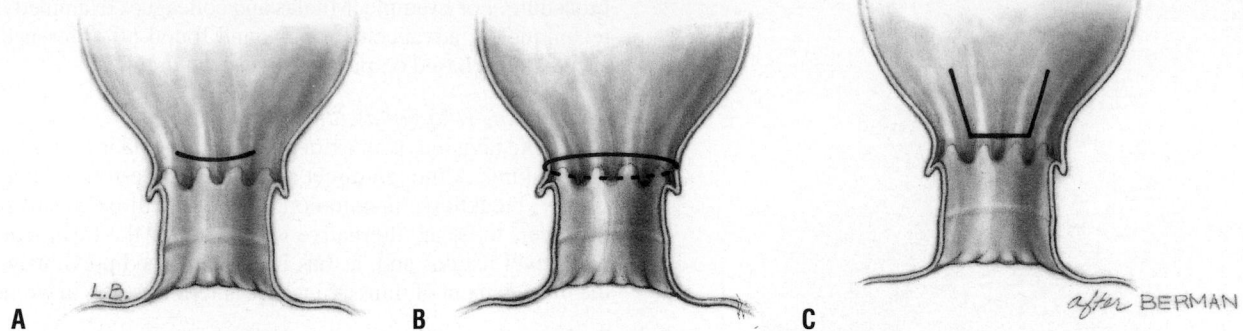

FIGURE 14-40. Endorectal mucosal advancement. **A:** Semilunar flap. **B:** Tubal or sleeve flap. **C:** Vertical or tongue flap. (After Berman IR. Sleeve advancement anorectoplasty for complicated anorectal/vaginal fistula. *Dis Colon Rectum.* 1991;34(11):1032–1037, with permission.)

through this approach, and the defects in the sphincter muscle that are produced as a consequence of tract removal are primarily closed. Although the authors report a failure rate of approximately 30%, they conclude that, if successful, continence is better than after other approaches. Sometimes, it may not be easy to excise the tract as described when it is not sufficiently fibrosed to be removed as a whole.

Results

Gustafsson and Graf reported their experience with the discredited operation of simple closure of the internal opening in 42 patients.[70] Core excision of the primary tract was performed with closure of the internal opening by suturing the internal sphincter and then mucosal layers. However, after eight cases, the authors switched to the advancement flap and combined the results.

Endorectal Advancement Flap

Aguilar and colleagues have advocated preservation of the sphincter muscle by extrasphincteric fistulectomy, closure of the sphincteric defect, and endorectal mucosal advancement.[5] Their approach is a modification of the techniques described by Noble[131] and by Elting.[54] Berman stated that the concept of endoanal or endorectal mucosal advancement has evolved into three principal methods: vertical tongue flaps, semilunar lip flaps, and circumferential tubal or sleeve flaps (Figure 14-40).[20] The concept of mucosal advancement may also be employed for the treatment of rectourethral fistula and selected rectovaginal fistulas (see Chapter 15).

Figure 14-41 describes the principles of the procedure. The incision begins *distal* to the internal opening, and the flap is mobilized, excising the scar. The method of flap construction

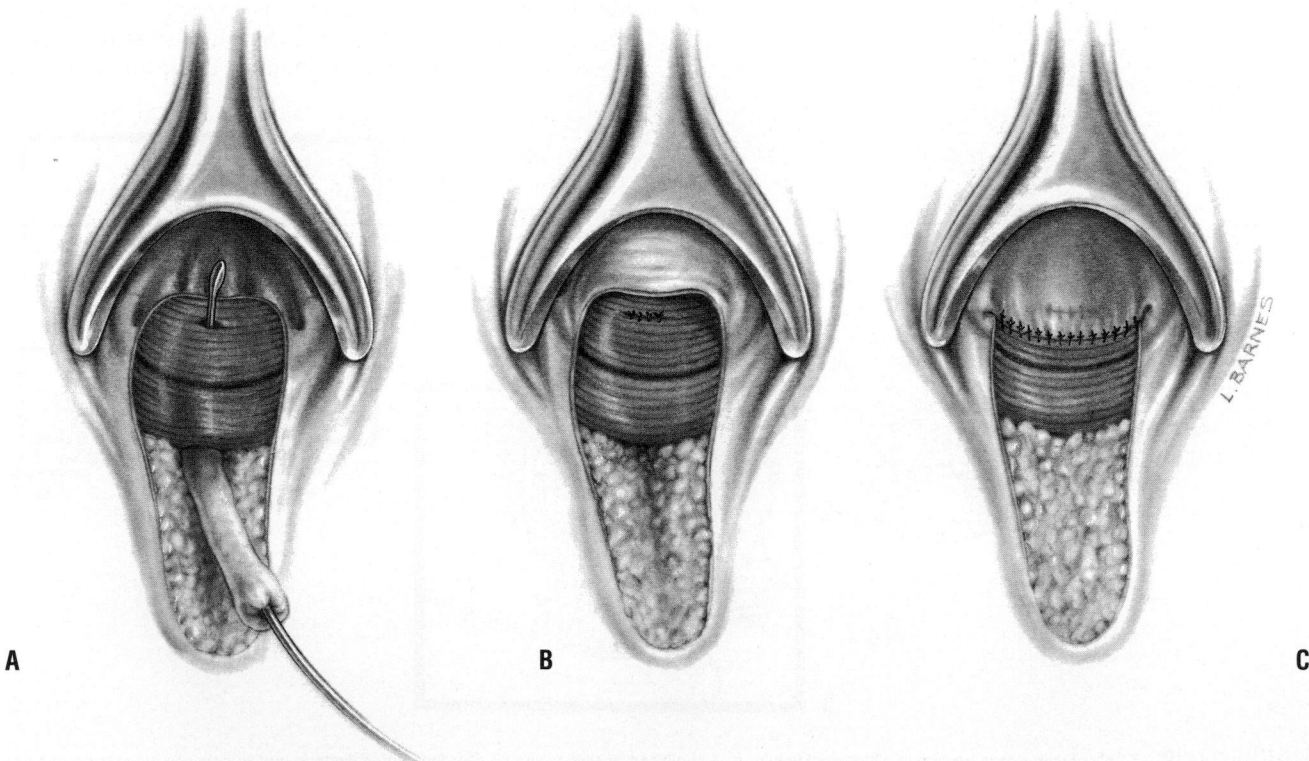

FIGURE 14-41. Mucosal advancement is performed by the following steps. **A:** Excision of skin and mucosa with probe through fistula tract. **B:** Repair of defect in sphincter. **C:** Mucosa advanced and sutured over closed internal opening. (Adapted from Aguilar PS, Plasencia G, Hardy TG Jr, et al. Mucosal advancement in the treatment of anal fistula. *Dis Colon Rectum.* 1985;28(7):496–498, with permission.)

is a matter of opinion. Some suggest an oblique incision, but this risks ischemic necrosis at the apex. Others prefer mobilization in a circumferential fashion, incorporating as much as 50% of the rectum. The dissection can be facilitated by means of infiltration with a dilute epinephrine solution. The *optimal depth* of the flap is another subject of dispute. It is the general contention that incorporating the mucosa alone is not adequate, and that part of the muscularis propria is also required. Others believe that the flap should contain the full thickness of the rectal wall in order to limit the likelihood of dehiscence.[109] Using mucosa alone results in a higher failure rate. Incorporation of at least some muscle appears to improve success of this procedure. It is also important to ensure that the base is sufficiently broad in order to prevent necrosis of the tip. The internal opening is closed separately, perhaps in two layers and tested so that a probe can no longer pass through.

Tun and Choi emphasize the important components of the procedure.[92] They are as follows:

- Excision of the internal opening
- Excision or curettage of the tract
- Closure of the internal opening by an anal, anorectal, rectal, or anocutaneous flap
- External drainage

Realistically, the pathologic process that is illustrated in Figure 14-41 is more consistent with that of a high trans-sphincteric fistula than an extrasphincteric fistula. However, the principles outlined earlier are still relevant. The technique for accomplishing such a repair by means of endorectal advancement is shown also in Figure 14-42, using the muscularis propria.

Management of the external portion of the tract is a matter of some controversy regarding "coring out" versus simple debridement. However, the external opening needs to be large enough so that it does not close prematurely. Berman also has suggested application of a sleeve advancement for individuals who have even more extensive fistula problems.[20] For example, a patient who has combined rectovaginal and cryptogenic fistulas may be managed by this approach. This is illustrated in Figure 14-43.

Results

One of the more popular methods for managing high anal and rectal (i.e., extrasphincteric) fistulas is the advancement flap.[47] Here again, however, the literature is confusing. Articles are published that mix extrasphincteric with transsphincteric fistulas. The advancement technique of Aguilar and colleagues was initially limited to transsphincteric horseshoe fistula, but subsequently was advocated for all fistulas when considerable sphincter muscle would otherwise be divided.[5] They noted three recurrences in 189 patients, but it is a potpourri of lesions. Wedell and coworkers employed a similar technique in 30 patients; no recurrence was observed, but one individual

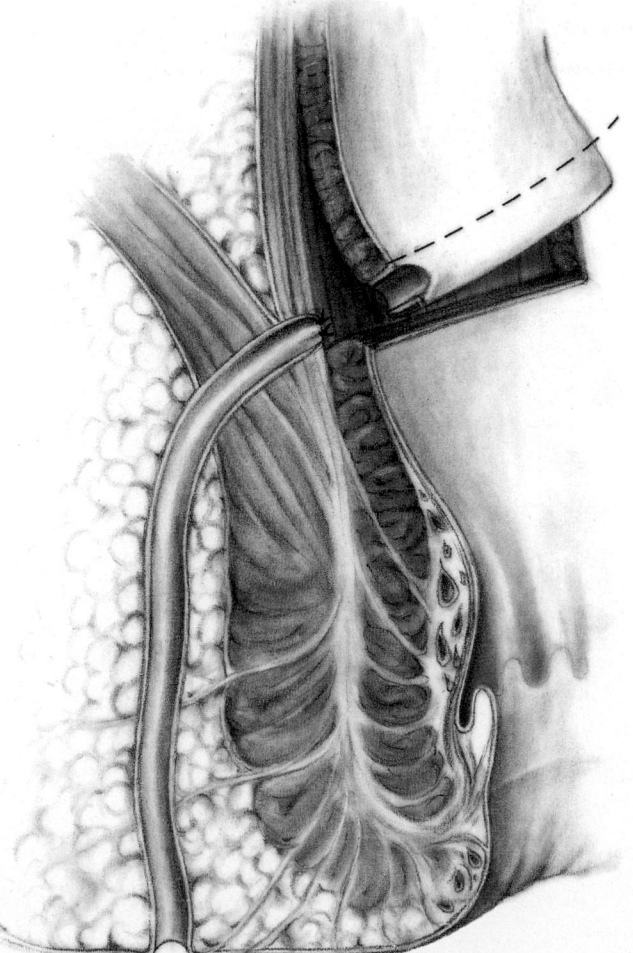
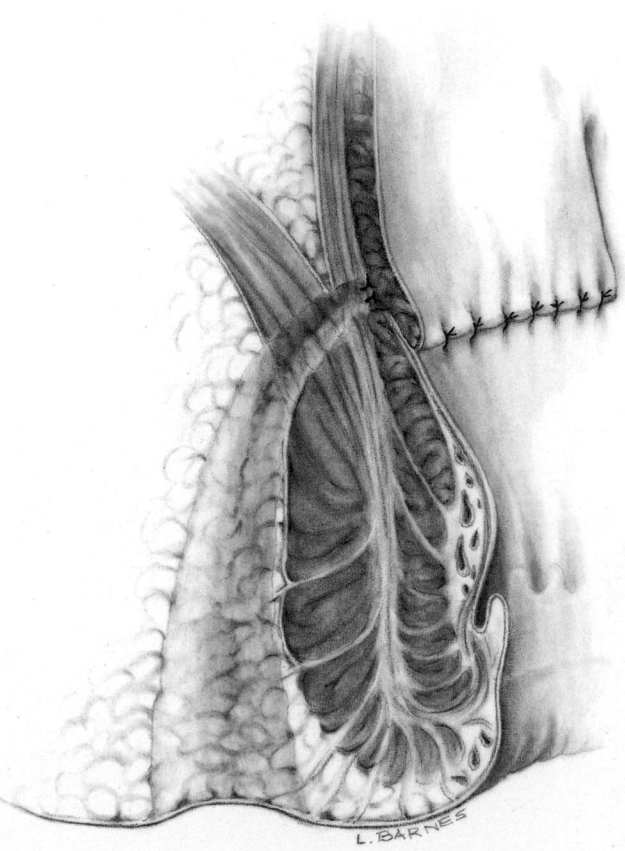

FIGURE 14-42. Extrasphincteric fistulectomy with endorectal flap advancement. A "mucosal" flap (including muscularis) is elevated, beginning distal to the opening. **A:** The internal opening may be closed. **B:** The "mucosa" is advanced and sutured distally. The external wound is then widely and adequately drained.

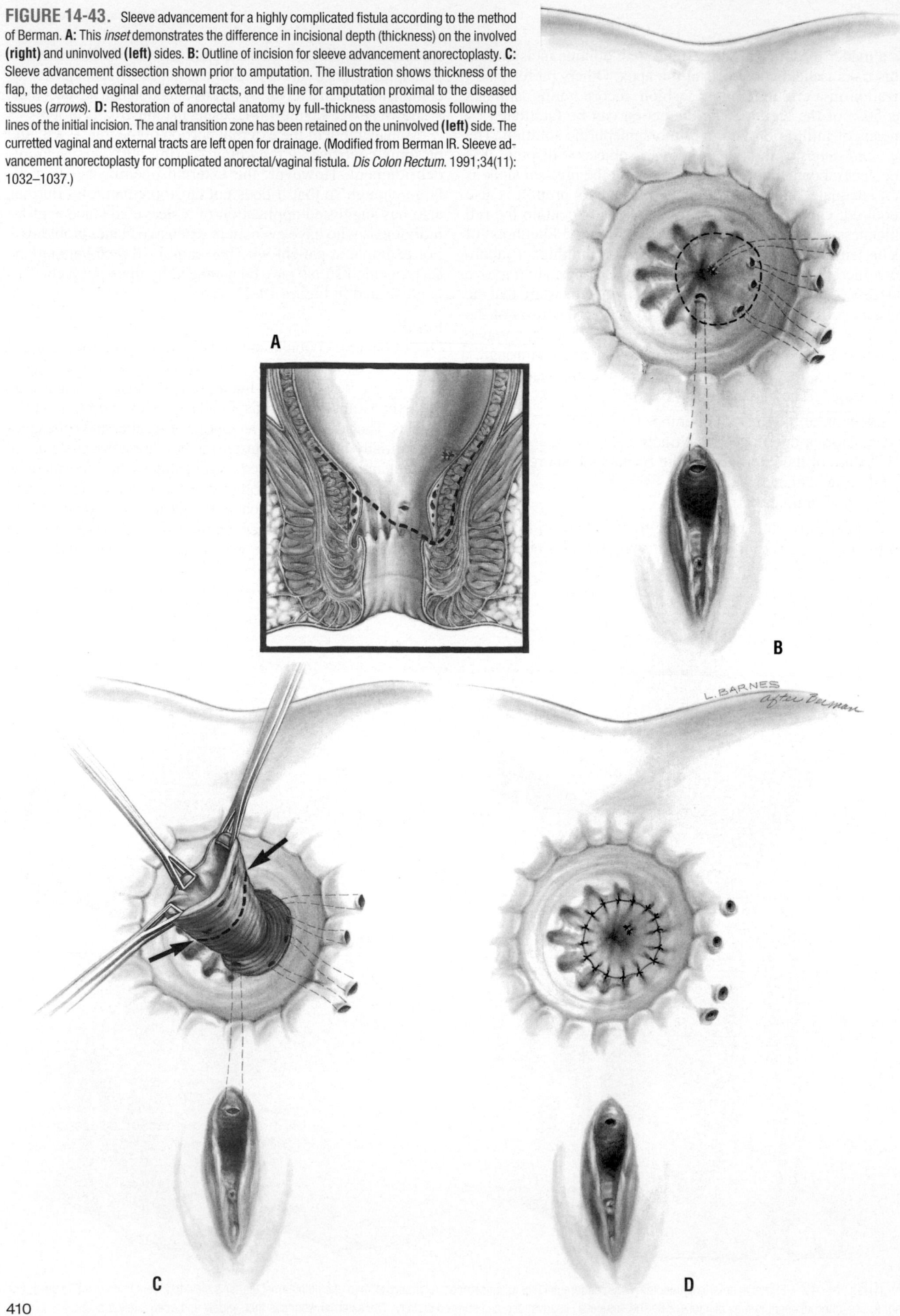

FIGURE 14-43. Sleeve advancement for a highly complicated fistula according to the method of Berman. **A:** This *inset* demonstrates the difference in incisional depth (thickness) on the involved **(right)** and uninvolved **(left)** sides. **B:** Outline of incision for sleeve advancement anorectoplasty. **C:** Sleeve advancement dissection shown prior to amputation. The illustration shows thickness of the flap, the detached vaginal and external tracts, and the line for amputation proximal to the diseased tissues (*arrows*). **D:** Restoration of anorectal anatomy by full-thickness anastomosis following the lines of the initial incision. The anal transition zone has been retained on the uninvolved **(left)** side. The curretted vaginal and external tracts are left open for drainage. (Modified from Berman IR. Sleeve advancement anorectoplasty for complicated anorectal/vaginal fistula. *Dis Colon Rectum.* 1991;34(11): 1032–1037.)

A

B

L. BARNES
after Berman

C

D

developed necrosis of the flap.[196] Reznick and Bailey reported seven individuals treated by this method with one recurrence (14%).[149] Oh noted that 2 of his 15 (13%) patients required reoperation for recurrence.[132] Lewis and Bartolo applied this principle to eight people (six with Crohn's disease), all of whom had not been cured by prior fistula procedures.[109] One of the two patients without Crohn's disease experienced a recurrence as did one individual with the condition.

In a meta-analysis specifically addressing advancement flap in cryptoglandular Crohn's fistulas, the weighted success rate was 81%.[174] The specific problem of fistulas in Crohn's disease is discussed later, but from these results advancement flap seems to be a good option for these patients. The authors offer reasonable opinions—that healing seems more rapid than with the other methods, there is less tissue destruction, and postoperative discomfort is minimal. Certainly, bowel control should be optimal when compared with the other methods, and if recurrence develops, it is still possible to redo the repair without necessarily expecting deterioration of function.

The Cleveland Clinic group reported their experience with transanal advancement flap in the management of rectovaginal fistula and other complicated fistulas involving the anorectum.[136] There were 52 individuals with a rectovaginal fistula, 46 with anal/perineal fistulas, and 3 with rectourethral fistulas. Overall recurrence was seen in 29% (total, 101 patients). The fact that a large percentage of these patients had Crohn's disease did not statistically affect the recurrence rates in this report.[136] Another study from the Cleveland Clinic group was published nearly 15 years later, consisting of patients from a distinct period.[90] Again, they included a significant proportion with IBD. At mean follow-up of 7 years, primary healing occurred in 72% of patients; 28% had a second flap procedure and 57% of those healed. Four of six patients who underwent a third procedure also healed. The overall healing rate in this series was 93%, although it was significantly lower in patients with Crohn's disease.

Zimmerman and coworkers analyzed a consecutive series of 105 patients with respect to numerous variables that could affect the outcome.[206] These included age, sex, number of prior repair attempts, preoperative seton drainage, fistula type, presence of horseshoe extensions, location of the internal opening, postoperative drainage, body mass index, and the number of cigarettes smoked per day. Although those with Crohn's disease were excluded from the study, the investigators found that only smoking affected the outcome of this operation.

Advancement flap repair for anal fistula is today a very popular choice despite the fact that published results vary from the sublime to the woeful. The extraordinary success reported by some is especially curious because this approach is very often applied to the most complex fistula problems. For example, Jun and Choi treated 40 individuals with high transsphincteric or suprasphincteric fistulas, with only one failure.[92] Ortíz and Marzo reported a 98% success rate in 96 patients.[135] Amin and colleagues noted an 83% rate of success in their 18 patients.[8]

Sonoda and coworkers, in 2001, expressed a cautionary tone with the following statement: "[While] mucosal advancement flap is effective for the treatment of fistula, . . . success may not be as optimistic as previously reported."[175] It turns out that their recurrence rate, as noted in a subsequent article, was 36%.[176] Kreis and associates were initially successful in curing 20 of 24 patients, but ultimately five more recurred, for an overall failure rate of 37.5%.[97] In all fairness to these investigators, some of the patients had Crohn's disease. Still, Zimmerman and associates reported success in only 12 of 26 patients (46%), all with high transsphincteric fistulas.[205] The Cleveland Clinic Florida group (total, 94 patients) noted a failure rate of 57% with fistulas in Crohn's disease and 33% without underlying disease, clearly a different experience from that of their Cleveland Clinic Ohio colleagues.[126]

In a randomized trial that compared advancement flap to fistulotomy with sphincter reconstruction, no differences were noted between Wexner scores or manometric measurements.[140] Recurrence rates were also similar. Of note, recurrence rates may be lower with advancement flap than with other nonsphincter cutting modalities. Data is somewhat conflicting in this regard. One randomized trial of advancement flap versus fistula plug was terminated early because the recurrence rates were significantly higher in the plug group compared to the flap group.[18] In a multicenter, double-blinded study of 60 patients, the recurrence rates were 52% with advancement flap compared with 71% with the plug. The authors concluded that although both were disappointing, there were no significant differences in recurrence rates, function, or quality of life between the two.[190]

As with other nonsphincter cutting procedures, if the advancement flap fails, other options are available. Therefore, this approach may be favored in some situations.

Transposition of the Fistula Tract
A unique concept in the management of extrasphincteric fistula has been proffered by Mann and Clifton. They advise rerouting the extrasphincteric portion of the tract into an intersphincteric position (Figure 14-44A).[118] The external sphincter is immediately repaired, and the newly positioned intersphincteric fistula is treated by a delayed procedure (Figure 14-44B). The intersphincteric tract may be further transposed at a later time into the submucous plane by division and immediate repair of the internal sphincter (Figure 14-44C). A third operation may be performed if it is elected to lay open the now submucosal fistula (Figure 14-44D). The authors reported five cases with complete healing and good functional results. No further publications exist regarding this technique since the initial 1985 paper.

Fibrin Glue
The use of fibrin glue to seal wounds began in the 1940s. It gained attention in the United States in the late 1990s when it was approved for treatment.[195] Initially, the product was formulated from the patient's own tissue and then activated by mixing with thrombin.[207] However, commercial preparations such as Tisseel VH Fibrin Sealant are now available that mix fibrinogen with thrombin and calcium in a double syringe (Figure 14-45). This mimics the clotting cascade, while an added inhibitor prevents fibrinolysis. In some instances, antibiotics are also added.[172,208] The presence of a fibrin clot then promotes tissue healing and collagen production while gradually dissolving via fibrinolysis. Any infection issues should be completely resolved at the time when the "glue" is instilled.

Technique
Numerous modifications for preparing the tract have been proposed. The principles (which are subject to individual variation) are as follows:

- Identify the internal and external openings of the fistula.
- Cleanse and debride the tract using a curette, gauze strip, or pipe cleaner.

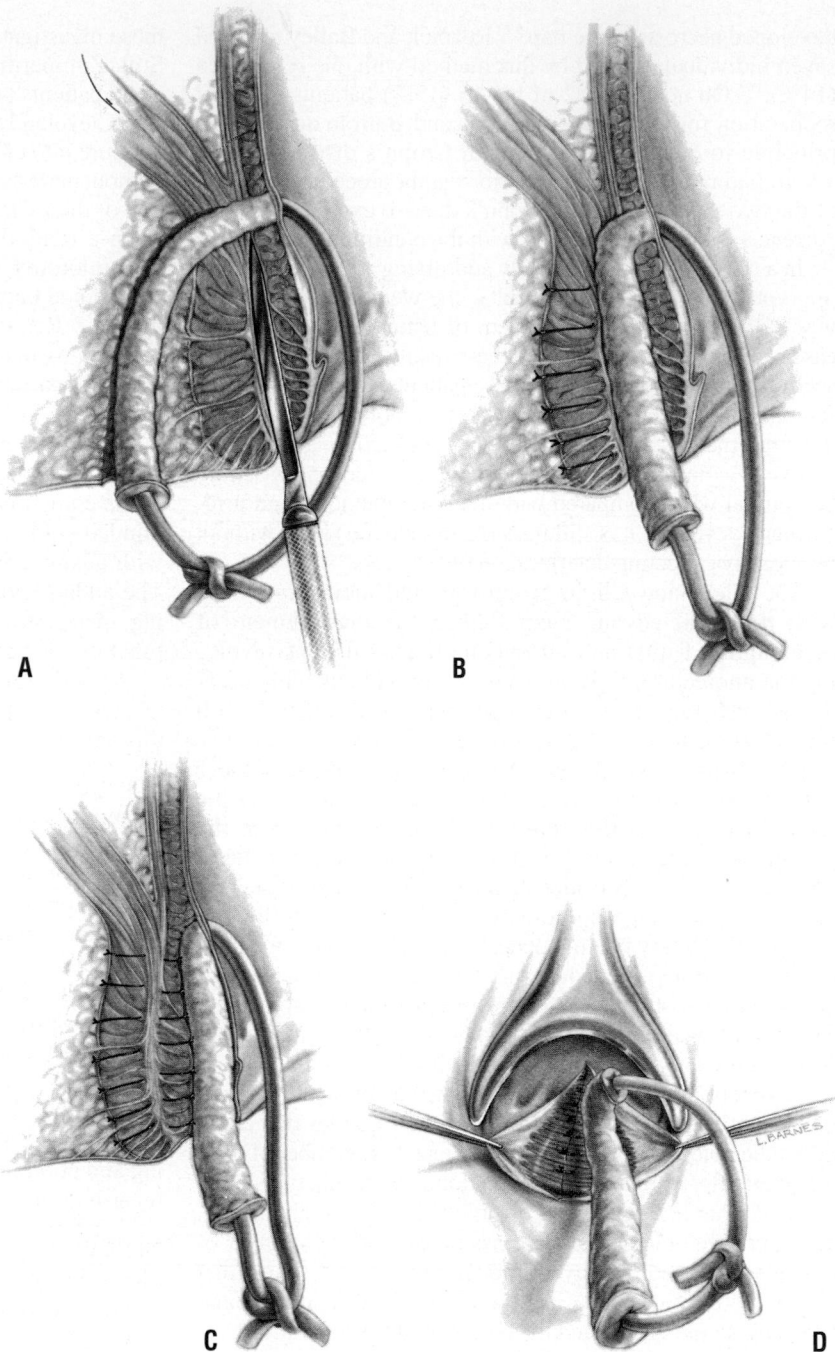

FIGURE 14-44. Transposition of the fistula tract. **A:** Placement of a seton and division of the external sphincter. **B:** Repair of the external sphincter with the tract now in the intersphincteric position. **C:** The intersphincteric tract may be transposed by division and repair. **D:** Completed fistula operation. (Adapted from Mann CV, Clifton MA. Re-routing of the track for the treatment of high anal and anorectal fistulae. *Br J Surg.* 1985;72(2):134–137, with permission.)

- Inject the fibrin glue until it is seen to be exuding from the internal opening.

Performing the procedure in the presence of local sepsis or active inflammation is not recommended. A vessel loop, placed as a seton for 6 to 8 weeks prior to the fibrin glue treatment, is strongly advised.[166]

Results

Initial studies of the use of fibrin glue were promising, but later evaluations failed to achieve comparable results. Healing rates have been in the range of 14% to 80%.[2,26,39,82,112,165,195,207] Interestingly, when some authors extended their initially promising series to include more patients and longer follow-up, failure rates seemed to increase.[39,40,165,166]

When compared with other techniques that do not cut the sphincters, fibrin glue was better only than seton drainage alone. The healing rate with glue was 39.1%, whereas the fistula plug, advancement flap, and seton drainage had healing rates of 59.3%, 60.4%, and 32.6% at 12 weeks of follow-up, respectively.[38] Compared with the "conventional treatments" of fistulotomy or advancement flap, fibrin glue led to successful healing in 50% of "simple" cases, whereas 100% healed following fistulotomy in one study.[110] Conversely, for complex fistulas, fibrin glue healed 69% of fistulas, whereas conventional treatment led to healing in 13%.[110]

The wide variation in the results in the literature may be partially attributable to differences in technical factors, inclusion criteria, definitions of healing, and length of follow-up.

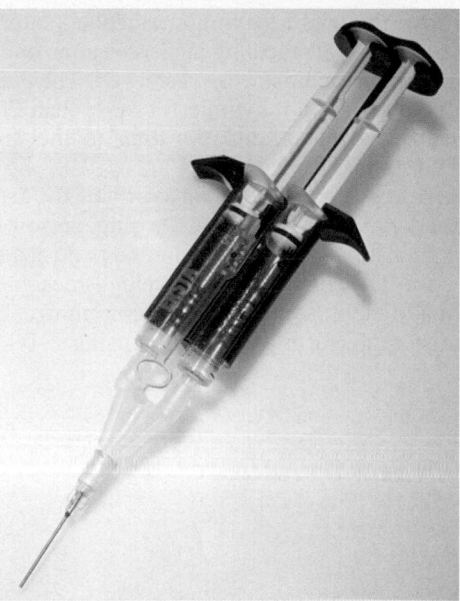

FIGURE 14-45. Tisseel Duploject System. This consists of a clip for two identical disposable syringes and a common plunger that ensures equal volumes of the two components are fed through a common joining piece before mixing in the application needle and being ejected. (Courtesy of Baxter Healthcare Corporation, One Baxter Way, Glendale, CA.)

Different authors describe various methods of preparing the tract, including hydrogen peroxide, curettage, or debridement with gauze or a pipe cleaner. In some series, antibiotics are mixed with the fibrin as noted earlier. The use of preoperative bowel preparation and postoperative bowel regimens vary. Some studies include all fistulas, whereas others include only complex fistulas; and the inclusion of Crohn's disease patients varies. Subgroup analysis in one study suggested that intersphincteric fistulas were more likely to heal with fibrin glue (82% vs. 40%).[40] However, this group is at the lowest risk for incontinence with conventional approaches; employing a technique with inferior results may, therefore, not be useful. Moreover, success may be defined as the absence of drainage from the fistula, a normal appearance on physical examination, or complete resolution demonstrated on imaging. Imaging appears to be the most stringent criterion for success or failure. Buchanon and colleagues, in a prospective trial, determined that at a median of 14 months, only 14% of patients were healed on MRI.[26] Of note, at first follow-up, almost 75% of these patients appeared to have healed on physical examination.[26]

Many studies are limited by their length of follow-up. Zmora and coworkers as well as Haim and associates, in well-controlled, prospective studies, were able to assess 72% of the subjects by phone and found that for those who were healed at 6 months, 74% remained were disease free.[110,208] Four of the six patients who experienced recurrence underwent an additional surgical treatment and the other two were treated with antibiotics alone. Late recurrence was noted at an average of 4.1 years but was found at 6 years in only one patient. Based on these results, it appears that if a fistula heals initially with fibrin glue application, the results are likely to be durable.

Because early failure occurs when the fibrin plug formed by the glue is extruded prior to healing, a method of closing the internal opening has been suggested. The combination of advancement flap and fibrin glue has also been explored. One retrospective review found that this led to decreased recurrence compared with fibrin glue alone (although the rate of healing was not lower than that for advancement flap alone at the same institution).[207] A prospective randomized study compared advancement flap with or without fibrin glue for transsphincteric fistulas.[71] Patients treated with advancement flap alone had a lower recurrence rate compared with those who underwent advancement flap with fibrin glue (20% vs. 46.4%), thus suggesting rather than the advancement flap improving the results of closure with fibrin glue, the fibrin glue was preventing healing in those fistulas treated with advancement flap repair.[71,207]

According to a study by Ellis and Clark for patients with well-controlled Crohn's disease, fibrin glue (with extra aprotinin to increase the sealing properties) led to clinical remission in 38% of fistulas at 16 weeks of follow-up, compared with 16% of those who had observation alone.[53] The benefit seemed to be greater in those with simple Crohn's fistulas. These were defined as having a single tract, no ulceration at the internal opening, and no vaginal involvement.[53] In other studies, fistulas related to Crohn's disease are often grouped into the "complex" category and not analyzed separately.

The advantages of fibrin glue for anal fistula include easy application, no risk of damage to the sphincter complex, minimal patient discomfort, and the ability to repeat applications for treatment failures.[71] Despite the overall low healing rates, its use does not preclude performing other procedures if initially unsuccessful. Therefore, it is a reasonable method to use, especially if there is concern about complications related to other techniques. However, both the surgeon and the patient should be aware of the limited expectations for success when attempting fistula closure with fibrin glue.

Anal Fistula Plug

The fistula plug also holds promise as a successful alternative for the treatment of anal fistula. Cook Medical's Surgisis Fistula Plug was approved by the U.S. Food and Drug Administration (FDA) in 2005 and became the first commercially available anal plug in the United States designed to treat fistulas. Since then, W.L. Gore and Associates entered the fistula plug field, developing their BIO-A Fistula Plug, which was in turn approved by the FDA in 2009. Both have been studied with variable results. As with other fistula repair techniques, the variability of fistula anatomy, differences in inclusion criteria, and differing end points have made it difficult to determine the efficacy of the plug. Therefore, there is no consensus among case series about the success rates of this technique. Closure of all external openings, along with absence of drainage and perineal abscess, are generally regarded as determinants of success.[69]

Cook Surgisis Biodesign Fistula Plug

Developed from lyophilized porcine intestinal submucosa, this device has an inherent resistance to infection, does not initiate an immune response, and becomes repopulated with host cell tissue during a period of 3 months.[31] Healing rates range between 13.9% and 87%.[69] A common cause of failure is that of plug dislodgment and migration out of the fistula tract.[69] Extrusion occurs mostly with shorter, more superficial tracts and can possibly be attributed to an inadequate amount of supporting tissue associated with the fistula.[69]

Technique

The following technique and illustrations are supplied by the Cook Medical (Bloomington, IN) and are the corporate recommendations for undertaking this procedure (Figure 14-46):

A. Place a seton if any signs of sepsis or infection are present. Allow the tract to mature and stabilize for 6 to 8 weeks before placing the plug.

B. Irrigate the tract with hydrogen peroxide.

C. Use the Cook Fistula Brush to clean and gently debride the fistula tract, removing nonvascularized tissue. A small amount of blood at the tract and on the brush bristles indicates adequate debridement.

D. Remove the brush leaving an attached suture within the tract. Hydrate the plug in sterile saline until desired handling characteristics are achieved. The plug should not be allowed to rehydrate for more than 2 minutes. After hydration, secure the plug to the previously placed suture.

E. Use hydrogen peroxide again to irrigate the fistula tract.

F. (Superficial placement) Pull the plug, narrow end first, into the fistula tract until the button is flush against the mucosa. The Biodesign fistula plug is designed with a button to facilitate fixation and to minimize the risk of extrusion. Perform plug fixation using 2–0 long-term

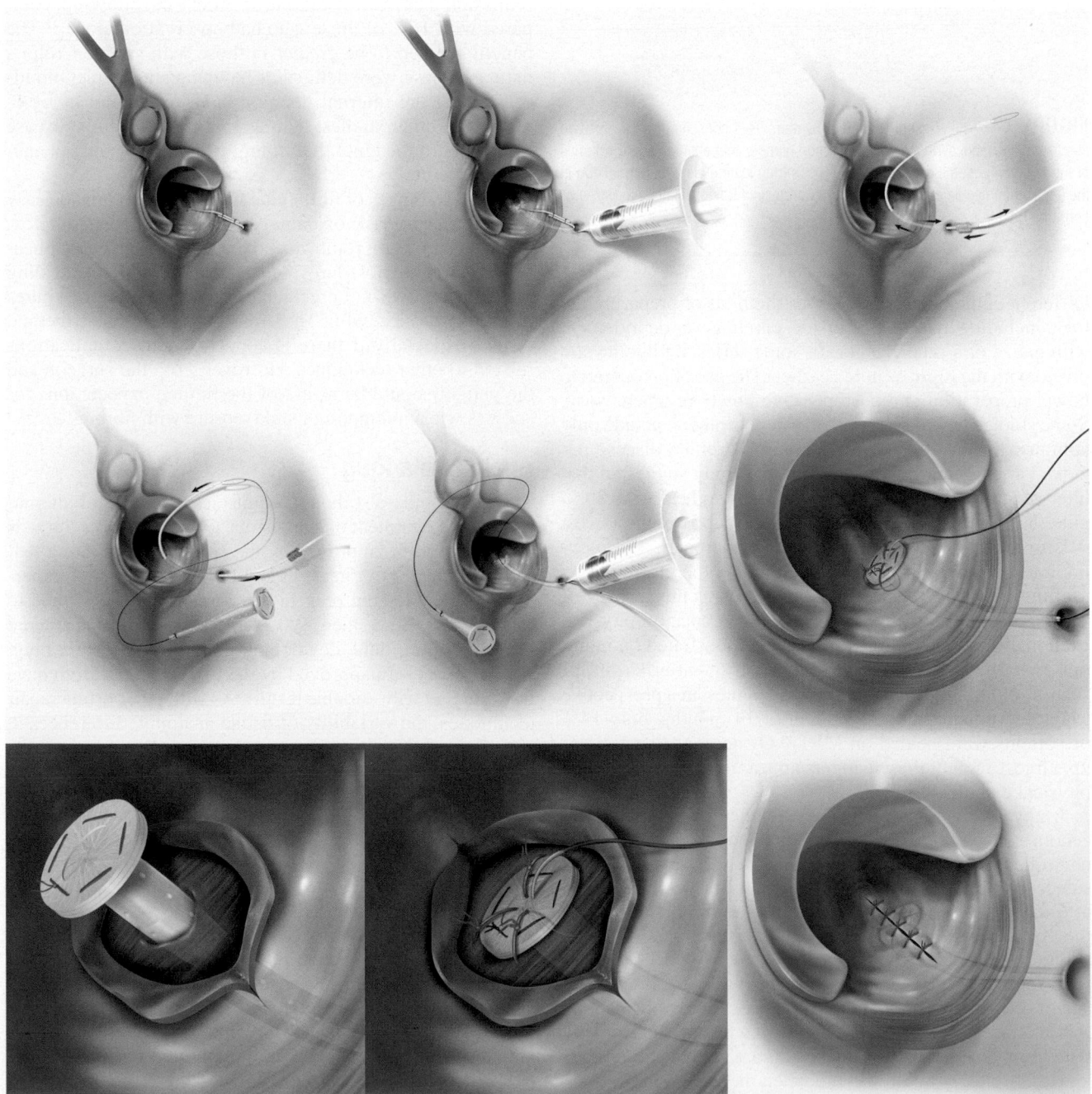

FIGURE 14-46. Technique for insertion of Cook Surgisis Biodesign Fistula Plug. (©2010, Lisa Clark, courtesy of Cook Medical Inc.)

On May 19, 2007, a Consensus Conference was held in Chicago, Illinois for the purpose of developing uniformity of opinion from individuals who have had considerable experience with this technique in the management of fistula-in-ano. They formed the Surgisis (AFP) Consensus Committee. The following is their report.

PURPOSE OF THE CONFERENCE

Of the 15 surgeons in attendance, 5 had performed 50 or more anal fistula plug procedures. Success rates with this approach have been reported to be as high as 85%.[1] However, other often anecdotal communications have been less sanguine. Plug extrusion and inadequacy of long-term follow-up have been expressed concerns. It was thought prudent to hold this gathering because despite a number of publications attesting to the safety and efficacy of the procedure, to date, there has not been uniformity of opinion with respect to indications and to technique nor has there been level 1 evidence of the actual benefit.

PLUG MATERIAL, MECHANISM, AND APPLICATIONS

Small intestinal submucosa (SIS) is a natural biomaterial harvested from porcine small intestine and fabricated into a biomedical product of various shapes and thicknesses.[3] As such, it has been applied for a host of potential indications. These include reinforcement of soft tissue for incisional and inguinal herniorrhaphy, urethral sling placement in urogynecology, staple line reinforcement, paraesophageal hernia repair, and in the treatment of anal fistula.[4,5,6,8–10,15,16,18,19,179] The fact that it has been demonstrably useful as a bioprosthetic material in infected fields makes the application in fistula surgery quite reasonable. The Surgisis AFP anal fistula plug ("the plug") has a rolled configuration suitable for fistula disease. When SIS is implanted, host tissue cells and blood vessels colonize the "graft." In essence, SIS provides a scaffold or matrix for the patient's connective tissue growth and differentiation. The material is supplied in a sterile, peel-open package and is intended for one-time use.

RECOMMENDATIONS

All of the following recommendations and opinions of the consensus panel were unanimous unless indicated otherwise:

Inclusion/Exclusion Criteria

Indications for the use of the plug include the following:

Transsphincteric Fistula. This is considered to be the ideal indication for the use of the plug.

Anovaginal Fistula. Although it is recognized that the shorter the tract the less likely the procedure will be successful, the plug was felt to be a reasonable alternative to the other operations. In other words, outside of the financial cost of failure, there appeared to be no downside in attempting its use.

Intersphincteric Fistula. The consensus panel opined that the use of the plug for this indication is valid if conventional fistulotomy poses a significant risk for incontinence. This would include those patients who have inflammatory bowel disease and those who had previously undergone *radiation therapy*.

Extrasphincteric Fistula. Although this is recognized as an uncommon indication for fistula surgery, this manifestation clearly is an indication for the use of the plug. Whether the plug can actually be sutured based on the level of the internal opening, and the likelihood of its success, is considered problematic.

The plug is *not recommended* for conventional, uncomplicated intersphincteric fistula because success approaches 100% with minimal morbidity with standard fistulotomy. Thus, the cost/failure rate with the use of the plug cannot be justified. In addition, the following conditions were felt to be inappropriate uses of the plug because of the extremely low probability of success:

- Pouch-vaginal fistula
- Rectovaginal fistula (because of the short length of the tract)
- Fistula with a persistent cavity

Contraindications to plug insertion include fistulas with any suggestion of infection. Examples are those with associated anorectal abscess, persistent cavity (as above), and a fistula with induration or purulent drainage. *Allergy* to porcine products would obviously preclude implantation, and one's inability to identify both the external and internal openings is an absolute contraindication for undertaking this procedure.

Preoperative Preparation

Some surgeons who are experienced with the plug have prepared the bowel as if for a major colon resection, including laxatives and antibiotics. The consensus panel queried its purpose—should there be an attempt to delay defecation? Is liquid stool preferable to solid for prevention of extrusion of the plug? Even with respect to a preoperative small-volume enema, there was no consensus—1/2 used it and 1/2 did not. These concerns could not be addressed with any evidence. Therefore, in the absence of data, the panel concluded that a bowel preparation and/or the use of a small-volume enema should be left to the individual surgeon's personal preference. However, oral antibiotics were *not recommended*. The panel did recommend that a single preoperative dose of systemic antibiotics be given.

Intraoperative Management

Anesthetic. Patient/surgeon preference.

Positioning the Patient. In essence, this, too, is a matter of the surgeon's personal preference. The critical element, however, is to ensure adequate visualization of the internal opening in order to place the suture correctly.

Identifying the Internal and External Openings. The plug cannot be inserted unless there is clear delineation of the primary and secondary openings. Irrigation of the tract with saline or peroxide is recommended.

Passing a Probe. Gentle passage of a probe is essential in order to confirm the position of the tract and to facilitate insertion of the plug. The panel unanimously affirmed that debridement, curettage, or brushing of the tract should *not* be performed. Such maneuvers will enlarge the fistula tract.

Using a Seton. There was uniformity of opinion that a seton should always be employed temporarily until there is no evidence of acute inflammation, purulence, or excessive drainage. This often takes 6 to 12 weeks. However, the use of a seton prior to implantation is unnecessary if there is no acute inflammatory process.

Preparing the Plug. The AFP plug should be completely immersed in sterile saline for 2 minutes. Allowing immersion for more than 5 minutes risks fragmentation of the plug. Conversely, implantation of a nonhydrated plug is extremely painful.

Managing the Recessed Internal Opening. If there is epithelialization of the internal opening (dimpled or recessed), one should consider limited mobilization of the mucosal edges and debridement prior to suture placement.

Passing the Plug. Use a suture or ligature to pull the narrow end of the plug from the internal opening through the external opening until the plug is snug. Clearly, this is a subjective determination.

Trimming the Plug. Excess plug should be trimmed at the level of the internal opening (the wide end) and sutured with 2–0 long-term, braided, absorbable material (e.g., Vicryl), incorporating the underlying internal anal sphincter. Monofilament material should not be used. There was no consensus, however, whether one needs to bury the plug under the mucosa. The excess external plug should be trimmed flush with the skin *without* fixation. The external opening may be enlarged if necessary to facilitate drainage.

Postoperative Care. The panel had a stimulating discussion as to a host of postoperative management alternatives. However, in the absence of meaningful data, opinions revolved around what seemed reasonable and appropriate and had less to do with "science" and more with the "art" of medicine. Still, there were several unanimous conclusions.

- Diet. No dietary restrictions.
- Activity. No strenuous activity, exercise, or heavy lifting for 2 weeks. Abstinence from sexual intercourse for 2 weeks.
- External dressing. For patient comfort only.
- Topical antibiotics are not indicated.
- Cleansing. Showers with gentle cleaning.
- Bowel management. Medications as necessary to prevent constipation or diarrhea.
- Follow-up visits. Surgeon's preference. The tract should *not* be probed during these visits.

Defining Failure. Early extrusion of the plug is either a technical error (the tract being too large, the plug pulled too tightly, or by faulty fixation [i.e., to the mucosa rather than to the internal sphincter]) or the presence of infection. The panel unanimously determined that the overwhelming majority of patients who heal do so within 3 months. However, some will take longer. The decision whether the operation should be considered a failure rests with the individual surgeon, but it should not be considered as such for a minimum of 3 months.

CONCLUSIONS

Implantation of the anal fistula plug is felt to be a reasonable alternative for the surgical management of anal fistula disease. The panel members were polled as to what was felt to be a reasonable success rate. They concluded that a rate of 50% to 60% should be considered acceptable. In order to achieve the highest probability of success, the panel concluded that patient selection, avoidance of local infection, and meticulous technique are required. Still, outside of the cost, the patient should be affected no more adversely than prior to plug implantation, and all other options of management are still available. However, even with observed healing, the recurrence rate is unknown. Ideally, a prospective, randomized trial comparing the anal fistula plug with that of seton fistulotomy will be forthcoming.

Finally, although it should be intuitively obvious, it is important to state that the procedure should be undertaken only by individuals familiar with anorectal anatomy and who are experienced with conventional anal fistula surgery and the management of its complications.

absorbable suture on a UR6 or comparable needle. Four sutures should be placed through the center of the plug, deep to the internal sphincter.

G. (Submucosal placement) Create small mucosal flaps or undermine the mucosa circumferentially to create a small pocket to accommodate the button portion of the fistula plug.

H. (Submucosal placement) Pull the plug, narrow end first, into the fistula tract until the button is flush against the surface of the internal sphincter. Perform plug fixation using 2–0 long-term absorbable suture on a UR6 or comparable needle. Four sutures should be placed through the center of the plug, deep to the internal sphincter.

I. (Submucosal placement) Reapproximate the mucosal edges, completely covering the button portion of the plug. Trim any external portion of the plug flush with the skin. Slightly enlarge the external opening to facilitate drainage. Drainage is to be expected for a minimum of 2 weeks and can continue up to 12 weeks.

Buchberg and colleagues conducted a study over a 28-month period, comparing the Cook Biodesign (Surgisis) and Gore BIO-A products.[69] The median time to success for the BIO-A plug was 47 days compared with 45 days for the Surgisis plug; but the overall success rate was 12.5%, compared with 54.5% for the Surgisis plug. Four patients initially treated with the BIO-A plug who experienced failure had a Surgisis plug placed, which subsequently healed. Another prospective study, published 2 years after the Surgisis plug was made commercially available, resulted in a success rate of 41%.[34] Dislodgement was claimed as a particularly common reason for failure. However, there have been good results as well.

Champagne and coworkers published a study of 46 patients, all of whom underwent placement of the Surgisis plug.[31] At follow-up (median, 12 months), 83% had successful closure, with only 15% of all fistulas persisting. Furthermore, out of the eight failures, seven were within 30 days of the initial surgery, and one was 9 months after surgery. They also demonstrated no statistically significant difference between closure rates and the use of a preoperatively placed seton.

O'Riordan and associates identified 76 articles or abstracts relevant to the anal fistula plug for those with and without Crohn's-related fistula-in-ano (see later discussion concerning Crohn's-associated fistula).[133] Twenty studies involving 530 patients were ultimately included. The authors determined that the study was limited by the variability of operative technique. Healing was achieved by the anal fistula plug in approximately 54% of patients without Crohn's disease, but they could reach no definitive conclusion in those with the condition.

Gore BIO-A Fistula Plug

In 2009, the FDA approved the BIO-A plug. This is a porous, fibrous polymer composed of 67% polyglycolide and 33% trimethylene carbonate (Figure 14-47). Biocompatible and nonantigenic, it differs from the Surgisis in that it has a 16-mm diameter disk attached to six tubes, 9 cm each in length. The disk sits internally and is sutured into the muscle while the tubes (however, many are necessary to fill the fistula's diameter) are pulled through the tract to the external surface. The tubes are trimmed at the level of the external opening.[48] Cells migrate into the scaffold, and tissue is generated as the body gradually absorbs the material, leaving no permanent synthetic material.[79] The internally seated and secured disk has proven to be advantageous in limiting plug migration, which is a frequent problem with the Surgisis plug.

Similar to the Surgisis model, the BIO-A product has had successful healing rates—ranging from 14% to 88%.[69,79] In one prospective study with 25 patients, at final follow-up 44% had complete healing, whereas 40% still had a remaining fistula requiring fistulotomy, and 8% had persistent transsphincteric fistulas.[123] Other studies report less successful outcomes, including one which noted only 3 of 19 patients had complete healing (15.8%).[123] The authors note, however, that there may have been serious limitations to the study, including the small number of patients, many of which had high transsphincteric, complex fistulas. Moreover, the surgeons' learning curve and the absence of a preoperatively placed seton may have diminished the success rate. In

another case study, however, that considered 20 fistulas in 12 patients, the success rate was 75%.[34]

Ligation of Intersphincteric Fistula Tract

There has been increasing interest in the treatment of *intersphincteric* fistula by means of ligation of the fistula tract (LIFT). In 1993, Matos and colleagues described a technique of excision of intersphincteric anal gland infection through an intersphincteric approach.[121] They reported a technique of excising the entire fistula tract, in addition to primary repair, by means of an intersphincteric approach to the fistula excision and by suturing the internal anal sphincter defect. However, their success with 20 patients was only 45%. These poor results were attributed to blood supply issues that resulted in wound breakdown.

In 2007, Rojanasakul and coworkers at Chulalongkorn University in Bangkok, Thailand, noted a success rate of 94%.[152] Their technique is based on a secure closure of the internal opening and removal of the infected cryptoglandular tissue through the intersphincteric plane. The principles are as follows[151]:

- Identify the internal opening
- Incision at the intersphincteric groove
- Dissection of the intersphincteric gland
- Identify the intersphincteric fistula tract (Figure 14-48)
- Ligation of the intersphincteric tract (Figure 14-49)
- Excision of the tract
- Open and curette the external opening
- Close the sphincter defect
- Close the wound

There are also variations to the conventional LIFT procedure. Neal Ellis describes the use of a bioprosthetic graft to reinforce the ligation, calling it the BioLIFT procedure (Figure 14-50).[128] In order for this procedure to be effective, a well-formed and epithelialized tract is advised. Therefore, a seton should be placed until the inflammation has resolved (see Figure 14-46A). If the tract is inflamed or in the presence of granulation tissue, there may not be adequate tissue strength to permit ligation.

Results

The early results of the LIFT have been promising. As mentioned, Rojanasakul reported a 94% success rate.[152] Ellis' BioLIFT also noted a 94% success rate with his modified technique.[128] Several small observational studies on the LIFT have been reported. An Italian study of 18 "complex" fistula cases was found to have a healing rate of 83% and with no impairment for continence.[171] Three patients required additional surgical intervention. When 33 patients with transsphincteric fistulas and 12 with complex fistulas were followed, including 5 with recurrent fistulas, 82% healed at a median of 7 weeks.[170] There was no significant morbidity. Bleier and colleagues reported 39 patients, 74% of whom had failed previous attempts at repair.[22] Their overall closure rate was 57%. The low success rate reported in this study may be tempered by the consideration that many of these patients had previously undergone multiple procedures. A group from Singapore reported 93 patients with 78% success.[182]

Special Situations

Tubercular Fistulas

Anorectal fistula on rare occasions may be a consequence of tubercular disease (see Chapter 9). Index of suspicion should be heightened in endemic countries and in patients with a history of a draining fistula for many years, the presence of multiple openings, the failure of a fistula wound

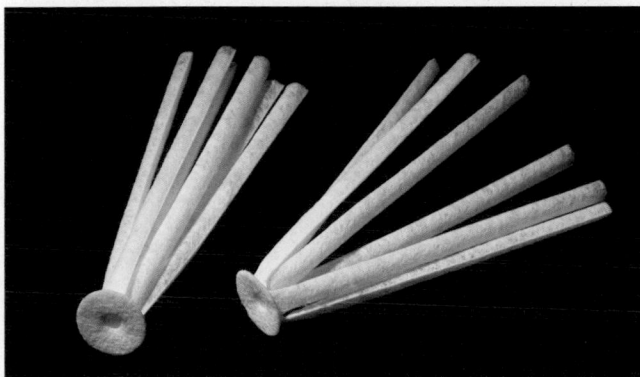

FIGURE 14-47. GORE BIO-A Fistula Plug. (Courtesy of W. L. Gore & Associates, Inc., Flagstaff, AZ.)

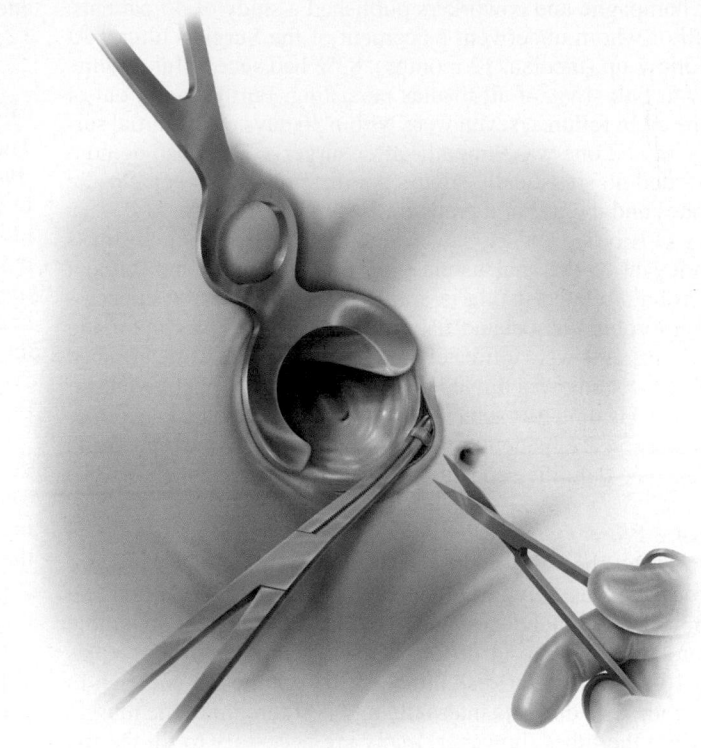

FIGURE 14-48. LIFT procedure. Create a 3-cm incision along the intersphincteric groove. Dissection should be carried out 1 to 2 cm proximal and lateral to fistula tract. Once identified, isolate the tract with forceps and excise the tract within the intersphincteric plane. (©2010, Lisa Clark, courtesy of Cook Medical Inc.)

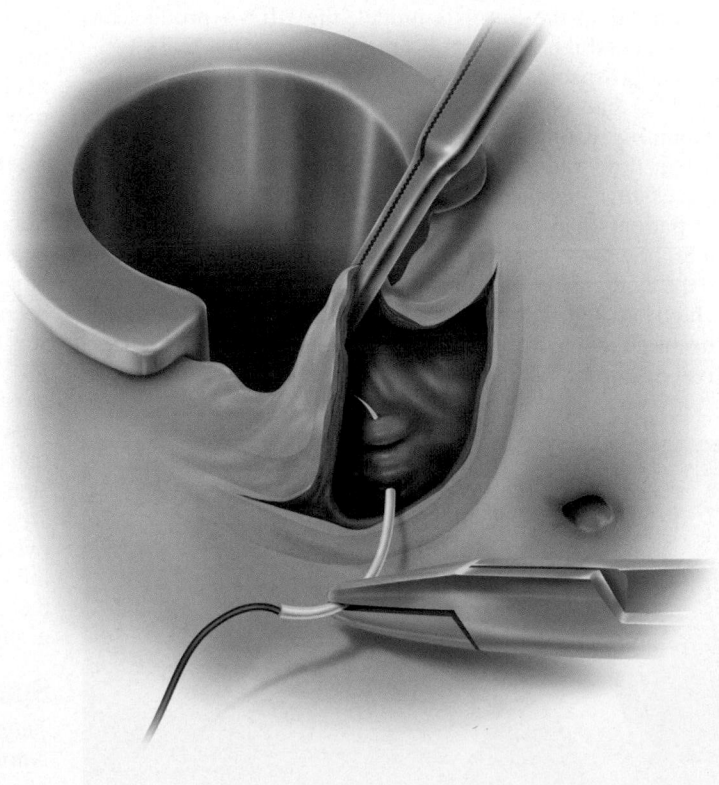

FIGURE 14-49. LIFT procedure. Suture the primary opening of the fistula tract closed from within the intersphincteric plane using absorbable suture. The secondary tract should be left open to drain. (©2010, Lisa Clark, courtesy of Cook Medical Inc.)

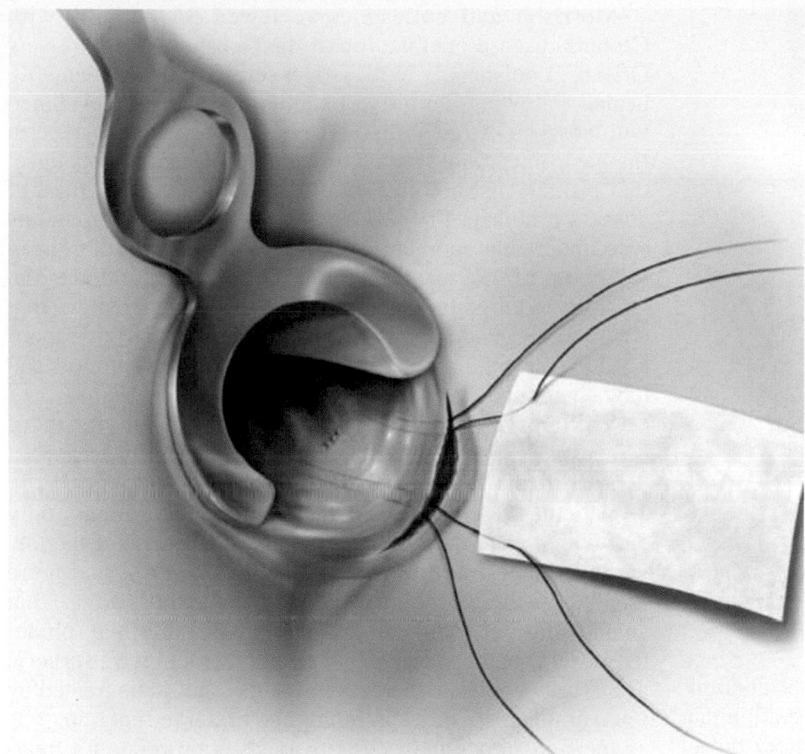

FIGURE 14-50. LIFT procedure with graft. Parachute the Biodesign graft into place within the intersphincteric plane using anchoring sutures through the external sphincter muscle. To ensure adequate coverage of the repaired fistula tract, a minimum 1 to 2 cm of overlap should be achieved proximal, distal, and lateral to the repaired fistula opening. (©2010, Lisa Clark, courtesy of Cook Medical Inc.)

to heal after 6 months following surgery, the presence of inguinal adenopathy, and the presence of caseation on histologic specimen. The diagnosis is usually established by microscopic evaluation using Ziehl-Neelsen stain and mycobacterial culture.[169]

Anal Fistula and Crohn's Disease

Fistula and abscess are among the most difficult manifestations of Crohn's disease to manage (see Chapter 30). In the experience of Williams and colleagues, anal fissures, fistulas, and abscesses occurred as complications in 22% of 1,098 patients. This was more common with colonic inflammation (52%) than with small bowel involvement (14%).[199] The incidences in most other series are comparable.[32,78,100,120,202]

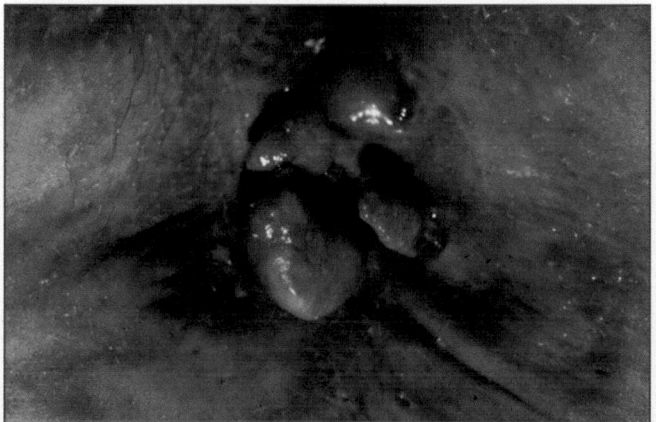

FIGURE 14-51. Anal Crohn's disease. Note the thickened, edematous tags with furrowing and fissuring of the skin. (From Corman ML, Veidenheimer MC, Nugent FW, et al. *Diseases of the Anus, Rectum and Colon. Part II: Non-specific Inflammatory Bowel Disease.* New York, NY: Medcom; 1976.)

Clinical Features

Lesions in these patients tend to be chronic, indurated, and cyanotic, but they are often painless unless an abscess is present.[43] The typical perineum of an individual with anal Crohn's disease is shown in Figure 14-51. Alexander-Williams found that one-half of his patients with anal fistula and Crohn's disease had no symptoms.[6] Skin irritation is frequently noted but may be due to diarrhea rather than to intrinsic disease of the anus. The fistula may be low lying, with an internal opening at the level of the crypt. More commonly, however, the fistula is associated with a deep ulcer, and the internal opening may either be inapparent or found in a supralevator location. In women, vaginal communication is not unusual (see Figure 15-3).

Treatment

The presence or absence of symptoms is the criterion upon which to determine therapy. Particularly in those with Crohn's disease, the goal of therapy is to ameliorate fistula-related symptoms, rather than necessarily to accomplish complete healing. Many individuals with fistulas are relatively asymptomatic; approximately 25% of patients in one series did not even require specific treatment.[189] At the Mayo Clinic, 86 individuals were followed for a minimum of 10 years to determine the course of the disease.[203] The overall cumulative probability of avoiding proctectomy was 91.6% at 10 years and 82.5% at 20 years. Resection of all proximal Crohn's disease did not improve the anorectal condition, except in those with all proximal disease removed previously *and* who had no recurrence.[203]

It is important to distinguish between anal Crohn's disease with fistula and Crohn's disease of the intestinal tract and a coincidental fistula-in-ano. This distinction is critical because a definitive fistula procedure can be performed with relative safety in a patient with Crohn's disease in whom

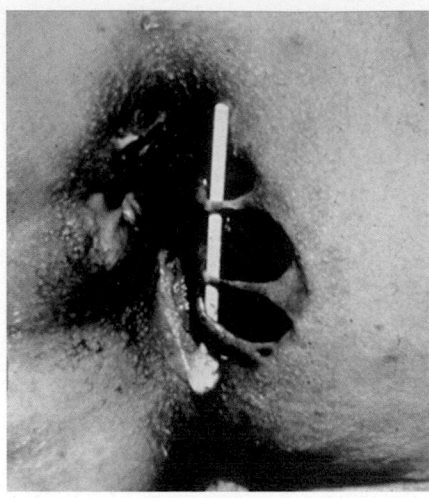

FIGURE 14-52. This indolent, ulcerating wound resulted from an ill-conceived fistulectomy in a patient with Crohn's disease. (Corman ML, Veidenheimer MC, Nugent FW, et al. *Diseases of the Anus, Rectum and Colon. Part II: Non-specific Inflammatory Bowel Disease.* New York, NY: Medcom; 1976.)

the disease does not involve the anus, provided the abdominal condition is quiescent. A definitive fistula operation that is undertaken in the presence of active inflammatory bowel disease, however, is hazardous. The resulting wound may be a greater management problem than was the original condition (Figure 14-52). Alexander-Williams stated that "incontinence in Crohn's disease is due to aggressive surgeons and not to progressive disease." Another important precaution is to evaluate the entire gastrointestinal tract before embarking on surgery for suspected anal Crohn's disease.

In the presence of known anal Crohn's disease, it may be possible to ameliorate the patient's condition and to relieve the discomfort associated with anal abscess and fistula without resorting to definitive fistulotomy. Long-term seton placement can be extremely effective in relieving symptoms.[184] However, superficial fistulas of a cryptoglandular nature can be successfully treated by fistulotomy.[173]

Morrison and colleagues reviewed 35 patients with Crohn's disease operated on at the Ochsner Clinic in New Orleans, Louisiana.[127] With proper selection, more than 90% healed following definitive fistulotomy. Success correlated with absence of rectal disease and quiescence elsewhere in the gastrointestinal tract. The authors particularly counsel that primary fistulotomy should be avoided at the time of abscess drainage. Fry and associates evaluated 73 patients who underwent anorectal surgical procedures, with a mean follow-up of 4.6 years.[60] Nine healed after fecal diversion, and nine required proctectomy. They and others believe that anal and perianal suppurative disease can usually be managed by careful drainage with the expectation that most can have their sphincters preserved.[60,146]

Williams and coworkers reviewed the University of Minnesota experience with "aggressive" surgical treatment of anal fistula in Crohn's disease.[201] Forty-one fistulas in 33 patients were treated by conventional fistulotomy, only 5 of which were transsphincteric, and these were of the low variety. Three-fourths were healed at 3 months, and more than 90% were healed by 6 months. The authors advise that anal fistulas in Crohn's disease that involve minimal sphincter muscle can be successfully treated by definitive surgery. They further suggest that higher fistulas should be treated by seton drainage to limit symptoms and preserve function.[200,201]

Incision and drainage are obviously appropriate for treating perianal and ischiorectal abscesses. Makowiec and associates found that of 126 patients with Crohn's disease who were seen regularly at an outpatient clinic, almost one-half developed at least one abscess during the mean follow-up period of 32 months.[117] As with abscess in the absence of Crohn's disease, the incision should be as medial as possible (see Management of Abscess in Chapter 13). Long-term, continuous drainage can be facilitated by insertion of a Pessar (i.e., mushroom) or Malecot catheter or by the application of seton drainage (Figures 14-53 through 14-55). Another method of treating patients with Crohn's disease is to establish adequate drainage of the internal opening. This is best accomplished by excising the internal opening and the underlying internal anal sphincter in the same manner described for the treatment

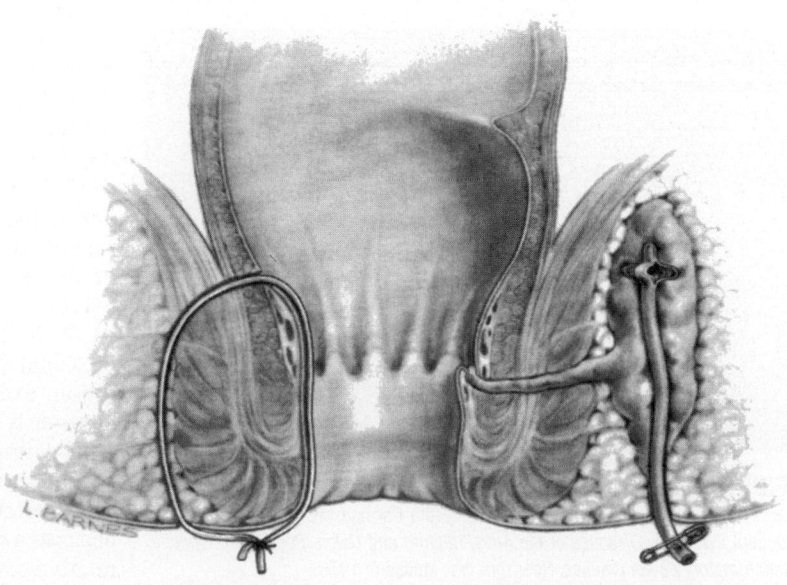

FIGURE 14-53. Sagittal view shows the seton drain in place on the **left**, with catheter drainage of the ischiorectal fossa on the **right**.

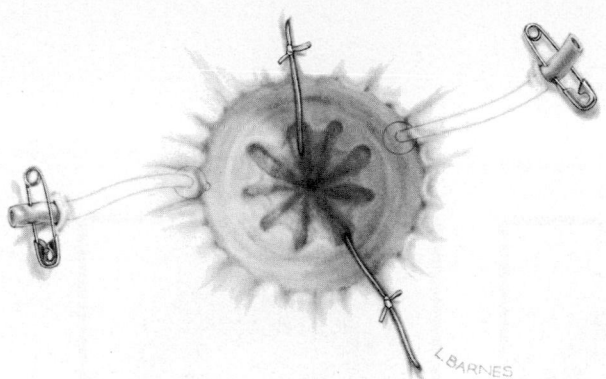

FIGURE 14-54. Seton drainage in combination with catheter drainage is an effective way to manage perineal septic problems in the patient with Crohn's disease.

of intersphincteric abscess. The external opening can then be unroofed, and drainage can be established between the external sphincter and the external opening (Figure 14-56). This is not a conventional fistulotomy but is a complete drainage of the fistula on either side of the external sphincter. However, because this lesion frequently heralds the onset of intestinal manifestations, the most prudent course of action is to incise and drain the abscess when it becomes symptomatic.

A third alternative is to use a rectal mucosal advancement flap.[104] Fry and Kodner recommend placing a mushroom catheter through the external opening to permit adequate drainage (Figure 14-57).[59] If the physician wishes to attempt a definitive repair, this is the safest method for treating anterior fistulas in women, extrasphincteric fistulas, and high anal canal fistulas, especially in Crohn's disease.

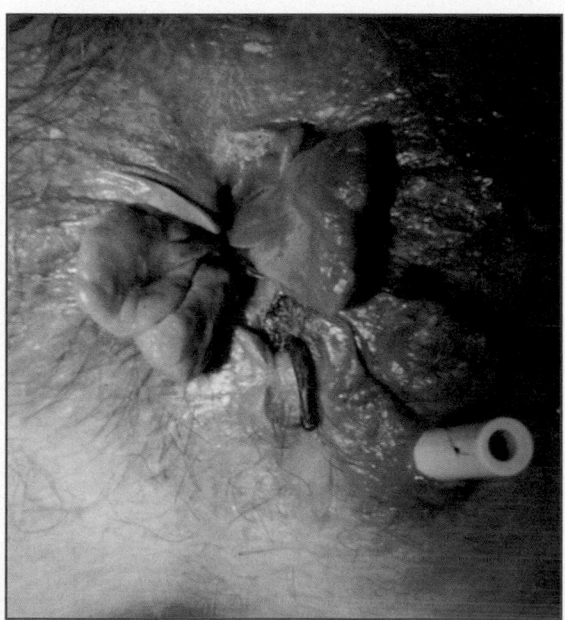

FIGURE 14-55. Perineum of a patient with Crohn's disease and multiple fistulas. Note the presence of two setons as well as a mushroom catheter to establish adequate drainage. This, one hopes, will maintain the patient in relative comfort and will obviate the need for more extensive surgical intervention.

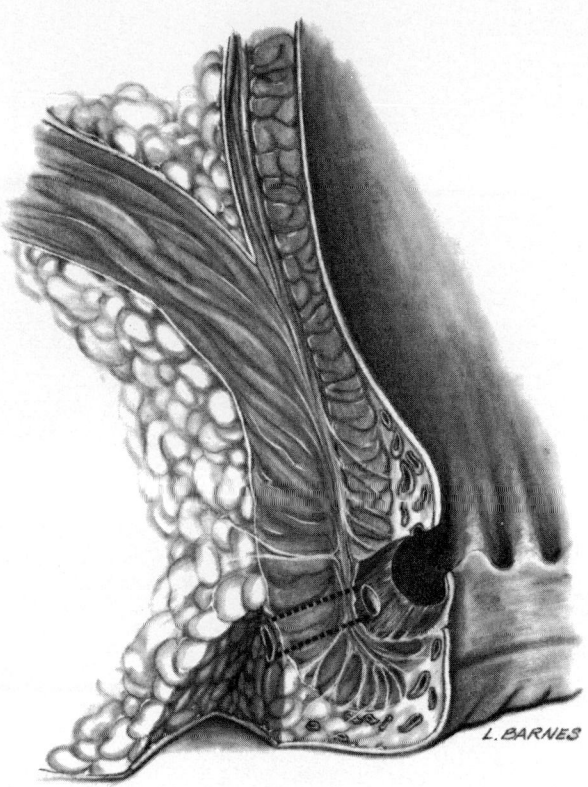

FIGURE 14-56. Treatment of a fistula in the presence of anal Crohn's disease. The internal opening and a portion of the internal sphincter are excised. The external opening has been adequately drained. A fistula tract through the external sphincter is indicated (*dotted lines*); this is not incised.

Results

Makowiec and colleagues reported their experience in 32 patients.[116] Of the 36 repairs, 4 failed initially. In addition, 11 developed a recurrence after a median of 7 months, and a new fistula developed in six patients. Other reports have noted approximately a 50% "success rate."[119] A review of the Cleveland Clinic experience reveals a healing rate of 89%, with a mean follow-up of 7 years in individuals treated with loose seton drainage followed by advancement flap, although some patients required a second procedure.[90] An analysis of 35 studies by Soltani and Kaiser demonstrated that 64% of Crohn's-related fistulas were treated successfully, with 9.4% developing incontinence following the procedure.[174]

Fibrin glue and the anal fistula plug have also been used in Crohn's-associated fistulas with the expectation that these procedures would not pose any risk of incontinence and do not preclude additional procedures if necessary (see Fibrin Glue and Anal Fistula Plug sections). It appears that these procedures may lead to short-term improvement of symptoms, but ultimately do not have high rates of long-term success.

Medical Treatment

Medical therapy can play an important role in the treatment of Crohn's fistulas. It has been suggested that metronidazole may produce symptomatic improvement in some patients with perianal disease, but there is no irrefutable proof that fistulas are likely to close with continued therapy (see Chapter 30).[21,24] Furthermore, antitumor necrosis factor-alpha medications, such as infliximab, have altered the treat-

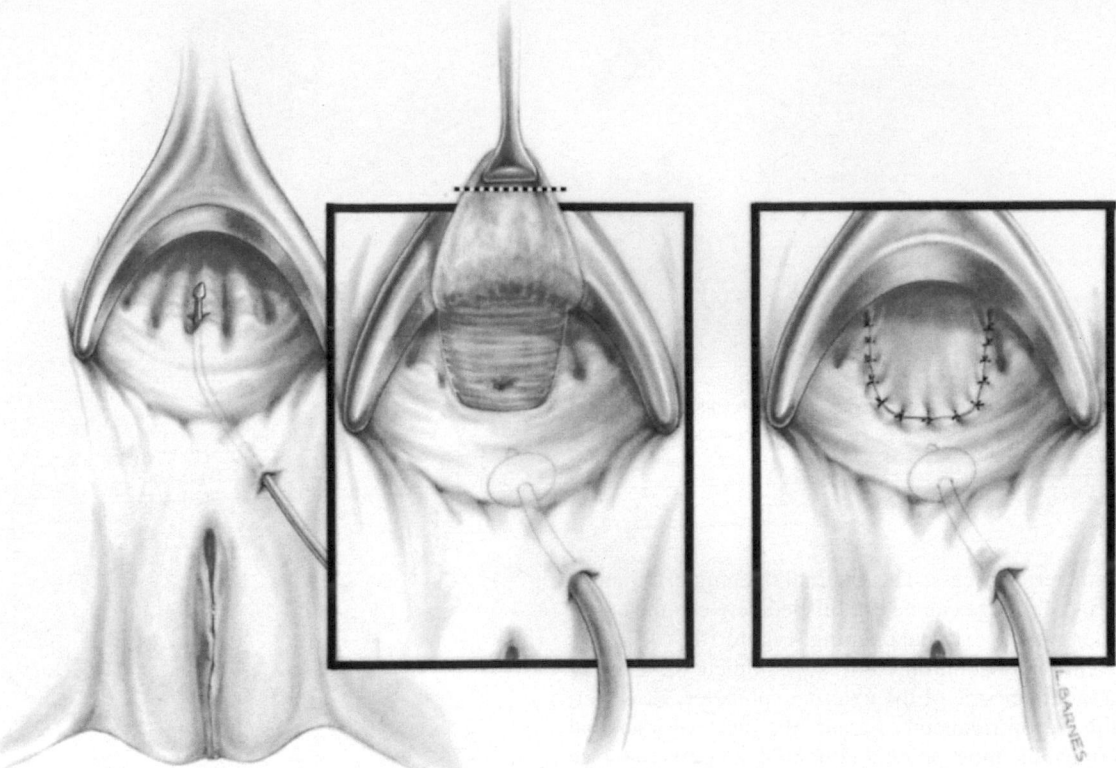

FIGURE 14-57. Advancement flap for anal fistula. This has been successfully used for fistulas in patients with Crohn's disease, with the addition of a mushroom catheter drain. The technique is otherwise comparable to the other advancement techniques. Amputation of the internal opening site is indicated (*dotted line*).

ment paradigm for perianal Crohn's disease. Whereas some have demonstrated a decreased need for surgical intervention with infliximab, others have shown no difference in subsequent fistula surgery rates since the introduction of these agents in population-based studies.[91] However, the ACCENT II trial demonstrated that infliximab must be continued as maintenance therapy to increase the change of any sustained response.[158] In cases refractory to infliximab, adalimumab can be used. Long-term response rates of approximately 41% without surgical intervention have been reported.[52,56] The combination of surgery and infliximab appears to decrease the time for fistula healing.[163] Other studies have demonstrated that combined approaches achieve response rates of 18% to 90%.[61,85,185] However, when 79 patients who underwent surgery combined with infliximab were compared with 147 who had surgery alone, there was no significant difference in healing rates.[61] This is perhaps a more significant end point than the time to healing. Direct injection of these agents has also been suggested, but no large studies have been undertaken. In a pilot project, only 4 of 11 patients achieved long-term remission with infliximab injections.[12]

Medical treatment or a minimal surgical procedure may be preferred for complex fistulas, for high transsphincteric fistulas, or for extensive or active inflammatory bowel disease in order to maintain sphincter integrity.[198] Conversely, most are willing to adopt the position that in carefully selected patients, definitive fistulotomy is a relatively safe procedure.[15,73,108,141,160,164] However, in refractory cases, fecal diversion or proctectomy may ultimately be required. Although fecal diversion does not necessarily lead to healing, it can ameliorate symptoms and may improve patient's quality of life.[93]

Comment

In analyzing the results of treatment for anal fistulas associated with Crohn's disease, the physician is confronted with the same difficulties of interpretation that one experiences when attempting to review the literature of anal fistula in

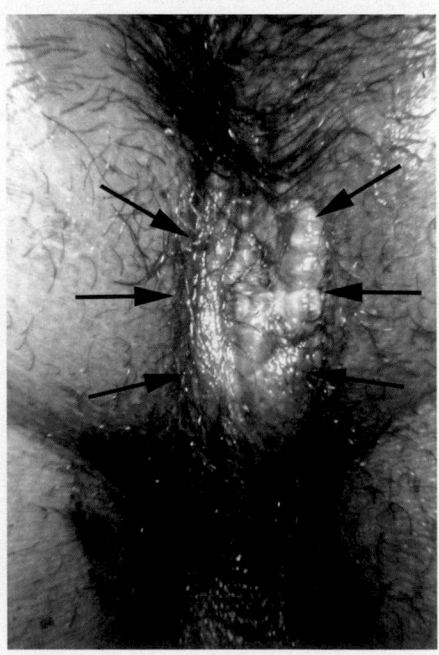

FIGURE 14-58. Adenocarcinoma (*arrows*) is seen arising in an anal fistula. (Courtesy of Daniel Rosenthal, MD.)

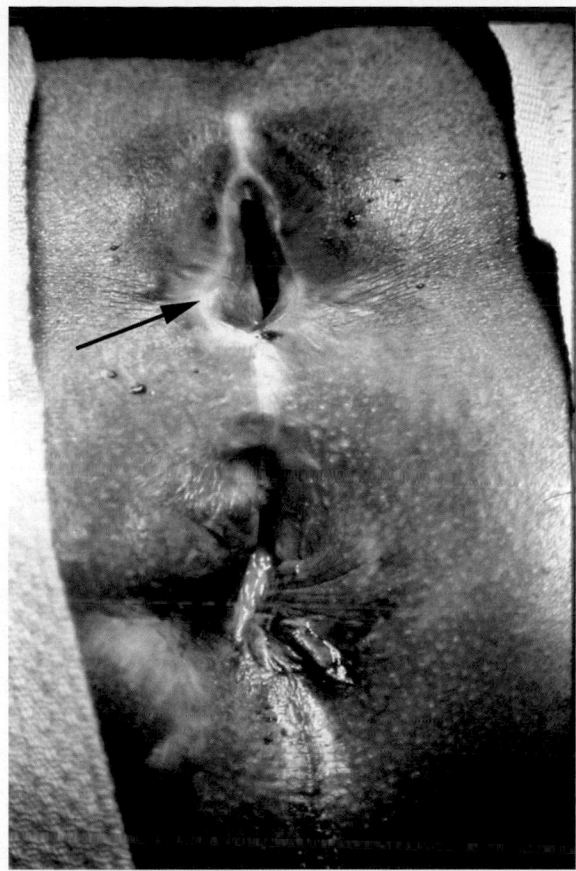

FIGURE 14-59. Squamous cell carcinoma (*arrow*) developed in a patient with a fistula that had been present for 4 years. (Courtesy of Daniel Rosenthal, MD.)

the absence of Crohn's disease. This, as well as the plethora of approaches employed and the varied presentations of the condition, may lead to confusion in the decision-making process. The following offers a reasonable starting point for developing some principles of management:

- Absence of symptoms: no treatment
- Active Crohn's disease: systemic treatment and surgical

drainage or long-term drainage only
- Quiescent Crohn's disease with anal and rectal sparing, and with superficial, intersphincteric, and low transsphincteric fistulas: definitive fistulotomy
- High transsphincteric or complex fistulas: long-term seton drainage with consideration given to advancement flap, fistula plug, or fibrin glue
- Low threshold for creating a "temporary" stoma concomitant with any definitive repair, especially an advancement flap

Anal Fistula and Carcinoma

Rarely, carcinoma can develop in a chronic anal fistula (Figures 14-58 through 14-60). A nationwide pathology database in the Netherlands identified only four cases of malignant transformation of a fistula, and all occurred in individuals with Crohn's disease.[14] As noted, both adenocarcinomas and squamous cell carcinomas have been reported. Getz and associates and others reported two cases and observed that there were fewer than 150 cases reported in the literature.[50,66,145] Ky and coworkers related 7 patients with carcinoma arising in anorectal fistulas associated with Crohn's disease and identified 33 more in the literature.[104] A later report included a total of 65 patients.[88] They observed that most had a long history of perianal fistula as well as mucinous histologic features. Millar described three cases of villous tumors arising in anal fistulas.[124] Long-standing, chronic inflammation in the region of the anal glands is believed by some to lead to malignant degeneration. However, immunohistochemical staining has revealed that the origin of these cancers may be from the rectal mucosa rather than the anal glands in one small series.[130] The presence of a tumor mass, bloody discharge, and mucin secretion are suggestive of the presence of an underlying tumor.[101] Delay in diagnosis, unfortunately, is not unusual. Therefore, long-standing anorectal disease should raise the suspicion for fistula-associated anal carcinoma.[62]

Differential diagnosis includes anal canal carcinoma (e.g., epidermoid, cloacogenic) with fistula, carcinoma of the rectum with fistula, suppurative hidradenitis with malignant degeneration, and carcinoma arising in an anal duct.[55,66,129] Carcinoma of the colon has also been reported to seed into a preexisting fistula.[86,153] Recurrent colon carcinoma has also

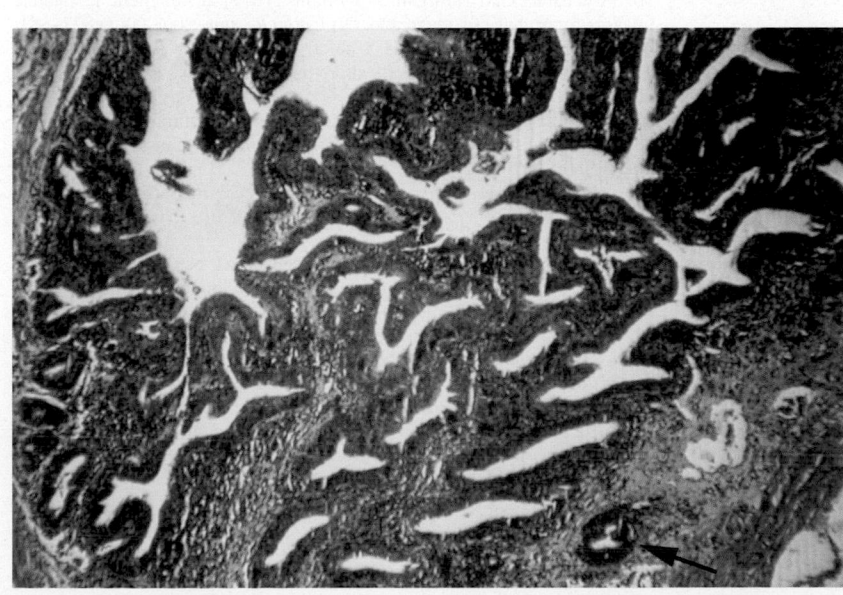

FIGURE 14-60. Adenocarcinoma arising in an anal fistula. Tortuous glandular structures are lined by proliferating epithelial cells. Note the infiltration of the wall of the fistula (*arrow*). (Original magnification × 260; courtesy of Rudolf Garret, MD.)

been found in a previously benign fistula.[68] This is believed to occur via exfoliation of tumor cells into the lumen that then settles into the inflamed tissue of the tract. These observations corroborate the opinion that the entire colon should be evaluated when a perianal malignancy is identified. Biopsy, especially of long-standing fistulas, is highly recommended. The importance of histologic examination of all tissues recovered from an anal fistula in an individual who is suspected of harboring a tumor is obviously extremely important. Endorectal ultrasound and pelvic MRI may be very helpful in evaluating fistula-associated carcinoma by delineating the extent of local involvement.

Potentially curative treatment depends on the etiology of the carcinoma. Adenocarcinoma usually requires abdominoperineal resection, perhaps with preoperative chemoradiation therapy. Good results have been reported with aggressive treatment.[62] Sphincter-sparing approaches have also been reported in highly selected cases.[204]

Anal Fistula in Infants and Children

The anomaly of a congenital anal fistula without an imperforate anus is rare, representing fewer than 1% of anorectal malformations.[25] There is an overwhelming male predominance in infants with abscess and concomitant anal fistula.[143] However, only 20% of abscesses are associated with the presence of a fistula.[115] The embryologic basis for this congenital malformation in a normally placed anus remains speculative and may not be the same for the two sexes.[25] In the experience of Duhamel, the onset of the condition in 70% was in the first 10 months of life, most arising in the first month (22%).[49] Presenting symptoms and signs include diarrhea, inguinal adenopathy, and proctitis. The fistula is usually simple, with a tract running directly between a crypt and the external opening.[49] In children, fistulas are almost always superficial and intersphincteric. Again, in the experience of Duhamel, multiple fistulas are fairly common, but these consist of separate tracts; he noted six double fistulas and four triple fistulas.[49]

Treatment consists of identification of the tract by one of the means described earlier and standard fistulotomy.[25,49,96] Recurrence or lack of healing after definitive fistulotomy should alert the physician to consider the possibility of Crohn's disease.[115]

References

1. Abcarian H, Dodi G, Gironi J, et al. Fistula-in-ano. *Int J Colorectal Dis*. 1987;2(2):51–71.
2. Abel ME, Chiu YS, Russell TR, et al. Autologous fibrin glue in the treatment of rectovaginal and complex fistulas. *Dis Colon Rectum*. 1993; 36(5):447–449.
3. Adams D, Kovalcik PJ. Fistula in ano. *Surg Gynecol Obstet*. 1981; 153(5):731–732.
4. Adams F. On fistulae. In: *The Genuine Works of Hippocrates: Translated from the Greek with a Preliminary Discourse and Annotation*. New York, NY: William Wood; 1849.
5. Aguilar PS, Plasencia G, Hardy TG Jr, et al. Mucosal advancement in the treatment of anal fistula. *Dis Colon Rectum*. 1985;28(7):496–498.
6. Alexander-Williams J. Fistula-in-ano: management of Crohn's fistula. *Dis Colon Rectum*. 1976;19(6):518–519.
7. Allingham W. *Fistula, Haemmorrhoids, Painful Ulcer, Stricture, Prolapsus, and Other Diseases of the Rectum: Their Diagnosis and Treatment*. 4th ed. New York, NY: Birmingham; 1882:9–252.
8. Amin SN, Tierney GM, Lund JN, et al. V-Y advancement flap for treatment of fistula in-ano. *Dis Colon Rectum*. 2003;46(4):540–543.
9. Ani AN, Lagundoye SB. Radiological evaluation of anal fistulae: a prospective study of fistulograms. *Clin Radiol*. 1979;30(1):21–24.
10. Arderne J. *Treatises of Fistula-in-Ano, Hemorrhoids and Clysters*. Power D, trans. London, United Kingdom: Kegan Paul, Trench, Trubner; 1910.
11. Ardizzone S, Maconi G, Colombo E, et al. Perianal fistulae following infliximab treatment: clinical and endosonographic outcome. *Inflamm Bowel Dis*. 2004;10(2):91–96.
12. Asteria CR, Ficari F, Bagnoli S, et al. Treatment of perianal fistulas in Crohn's disease by local injection of antibody to TNF-alpha accounts for a favourable clinical response in selected cases: a pilot study. *Scand J Gastroenterol*. 2006;41(9):1064–1072.
13. Atkin GK, Martins J, Tozer P, et al. For many high anal fistulas, lay open is still a good option. *Tech Coloproctol*. 2011;15(2):143–150.
14. Baars JE, Kuipers EJ, Dijkstra G, et al. Malignant transformation of perianal and enterocutaneous fistulas is rare: results of 17 years of follow-up from The Netherlands. *Scand J Gastroenterol*. 2011;46(3):319–325.
15. Bayer I, Gordon PH. Selected operative management of fistula-in-ano in Crohn's disease. *Dis Colon Rectum*. 1994;37(8):760–765.
16. Beckingham IJ, Spencer JA, Ward J, et al. Prospective evaluation of dynamic contrast enhanced magnetic resonance imaging in the evaluation of fistula in ano. *Br J Surg*. 1996;83(10):1396–1398.
17. Beets-Tan RG, Beets GL, van der Hoop AG, et al. Preoperative MR imaging of anal fistulas: does it really help the surgeon? *Radiology*. 2001;218(1):75–84.
18. Belliveau P, Thomson JP, Parks AG. Fistula-in-ano. A manometric study. *Dis Colon Rectum*. 1983;26(3):152–154.
19. Bennett RC. A review of the results of orthodox treatment for anal fistulae. *Proc R Soc Med*. 1962;55:756–757.
20. Berman IR. Sleeve advancement anorectoplasty for complicated anorectal/vaginal fistula. *Dis Colon Rectum*. 1991;34(11):1032–1037.
21. Bernstein LH, Frank MS, Brandt LJ, et al. Healing of perineal Crohn's disease with metronidazole. *Gastroenterology*. 1980;79(2):357–365.
22. Bleier JI, Moloo H, Goldberg SM. Ligation of the intersphincteric fistula tract: an effective new technique for complex fistulas. *Dis Colon Rectum*. 2010;53(1):43–46.
23. Bokhari S, Lindsey I. Incontinence following sphincter division for treatment of anal fistula. *Colorectal Dis*. 2010;12(7 online):e135–e139.
24. Brandt LJ, Bernstein LH, Boley SJ, et al. Metronidazole therapy for perineal Crohn's disease: a follow-up study. *Gastroenterology*. 1982;83(2):383–387.
25. Brem H, Guttman FM, LaBerge JM, et al. Congenital anal fistula with normal anus. *J Pediatr Surg*. 1989;24(2):183–185.
26. Buchanan GN, Bartram CI, Phillips RK, et al. Efficacy of fibrin sealant in the management of complex anal fistula: a prospective trial. *Dis Colon Rectum*. 2003;46(9):1167–1174.
27. Buchanan GN, Bartram CI, Williams AB, et al. Value of hydrogen peroxide enhancement of three-dimensional endoanal ultrasound in fistula-in-ano. *Dis Colon Rectum*. 2005;48(1):141–147.
28. Buchanan GN, Halligan S, Bartram CI, et al. Clinical examination, endosonography, and MR imaging in preoperative assessment of fistula in ano: comparison with outcome-based reference standard. *Radiology*. 2004;233(3):674–681.
29. Buchanan GN, Halligan S, Williams AB, et al. Effect of MRI on clinical outcome of recurrent fistula-in-ano. *Lancet*. 2002;360(9346):1661–1662.
30. Buchanan GN, Halligan S, Williams AB, et al. Magnetic resonance imaging for primary fistula in ano. *Dis Colon Rectum*. 2003;90(7):877–881.
31. Buchberg B, Masoomi H, Choi J, et al. A tale of two (anal fistula) plugs: is there a difference in short-term outcomes? *Am Surg*. 2010; 76(10):1150–1153.
32. Buchmann P, Keighley MR, Allan RN, et al. Natural history of perianal Crohn's disease. Ten year follow-up: a plea for conservatism. *Am J Surg*. 1980;140(5):642–644.
33. Cavanaugh M, Hyman N, Osler T. Fecal incontinence severity index after fistulotomy: a predictor of quality of life. *Dis Colon Rectum*. 2002;45(3):349–353.
34. Champagne BJ, O'Connor LM, Ferguson M, et al. Efficacy of anal fistula plug in closure of cryptoglandular fistulas: long-term follow-up. *Dis Colon Rectum*. 2006;49(12):1817–1821.
35. Cho DY. Endosonographic criteria for an internal opening of fistula-in-ano. *Dis Colon Rectum*. 1999;42(4):515–518.
36. Choen S, Burnett S, Bartram CI, et al. Comparison between anal endosonography and digital examination in the evaluation of anal fistulae. *Br J Surg*. 1991;78(4):445–447.
37. Christensen A, Nilas L, Christiansen J. Treatment of transsphincteric anal fistulas by the seton technique. *Dis Colon Rectum*. 1986;29(7): 454–455.
38. Chung W, Kazemi P, Ko D, et al. Anal fistula plug and fibrin glue versus conventional treatment in repair of complex anal fistulas. *Am J Surg*. 2009;197(5):604–608.

39. Cintron JR, Park JJ, Orsay CP, et al. Repair of fistulas-in-ano using autologous fibrin tissue adhesive. *Dis Colon Rectum.* 1999;42(5):607–613.

40. Cintron JR, Park JJ, Orsay CP, et al. Repair of fistulas-in-ano using fibrin adhesive: long-term follow-up. *Dis Colon Rectum.* 2000;43(7):944–950.

41. Cirocco WC, Reilly JC. Challenging the predictive accuracy of Goodsall's rule for anal fistulae. *Dis Colon Rectum.* 1992;35(6):537–542.

42. Cirocco WC, Rusin LC. Simplified Seton management for complex anal fistulas: a novel use for the rubber band ligator. *Dis Colon Rectum.* 1991;34(12):1135–1137.

43. Cohen Z, McLeod RS. Perianal Crohn's disease. *Gastroenterol Clin North Am.* 1987;16(1):175–189.

44. Cosman BC. All's well that ends well: Shakespeare's treatment of anal fistula. *Dis Colon Rectum.* 1998;41(7):914–924.

45. Culp CE. Use of Penrose drains to treat certain anal fistulas: a primary operative seton. *Mayo Clin Proc.* 1984;59(9):613–617.

46. Deen KI, Williams JG, Hutchinson R, et al. Fistulas in ano: endoanal ultrasonographic assessment assists decision making for surgery. *Gut.* 1994;35(3):391–394.

47. Del Pino A, Nelson RL, Pearl RK, et al. Island flap anoplasty for treatment of transsphincteric fistula in ano. *Dis Colon Rectum.* 1996;39(2):224–226.

48. de la Portilla F, Rada R, Jiménez-Rodriguez R, et al. Evaluation of a new synthetic plug in the treatment of anal fistulas: results of a pilot study. *Dis Colon Rectum.* 2011;54(11):1419–1422.

49. Duhamel J. Anal fistulae in childhood. *Am J Proctol.* 1975;26(6):40–43.

50. Dukes CE, Galvin C. Colloid carcinoma arising within fistulae in the anorectal region. *Ann R Coll Surg Engl.* 1956;18(4):246–261.

51. Dunphy JE, Pikula J. Fact and fancy about fistula-in-ano. *Surg Clin North Am.* 1955;35:1469–1477.

52. Echarri A, Castro J, Barreiro M, et al. Evaluation of adalimumab therapy in multidisciplinary strategy for perianal Crohn's disease patients with infliximab failure. *J Crohns Colitis.* 2010;4(6):654–660.

53. Ellis CN, Clark S. Fibrin glue as an adjunct to flap repair of anal fistulas: a randomized, controlled study. *Dis Colon Rectum.* 2006;49(11):1736–1740.

54. Elting AW. X. The treatment of fistula in ano: with especial reference to the Whitehead Operation. *Ann Surg.* 1912;56(5):744–752.

55. Fincato M, Corsi C, Perrone A, et al. Perianal fistulous abscesses and cloacogenic cancer. *Proctology.* 1980;2:105.

56. Fortea-Ormaechea JI, González-Lama Y, Casis B, et al. Adalimumab is effective in long-term real life clinical practice in both luminal and perianal Crohn's disease. The Madrid experience. *Gastroenterol Hepatol.* 2011;34(7):443–448.

57. Frenkel I. Fistula-in-ano: a new classification system for perirectal fistulas. *Dis Colon Rectum.* 2002;45:A25–A28.

58. Friend WG. Anorectal problems: surgical incisions for complicated anal fistulas. *Dis Colon Rectum.* 1975;18(8):652–656.

59. Fry RD, Kodner IJ. Management of anal and perineal Crohn's disease. *Infect Surg.* 1989:209.

60. Fry RD, Shemesh EI, Kodner IJ, et al. Techniques and results in the management of anal and perianal Crohn's disease. *Surg Gynecol Obstet.* 1989;168(1):42–48.

61. Gaertner WB, Decanini A, Mellgren A, et al. Does infliximab infusion impact results of operative treatment for Crohn's perianal fistulas? *Dis Colon Rectum.* 2007;50(11):1754–1760.

62. Gaertner WB, Hagerman GF, Finne CO, et al. Fistula-associated anal adenocarcinoma: good results with aggressive therapy. *Dis Colon Rectum.* 2008;51(7):1061–1067.

63. García-Aguilar J, Belmonte C, Wong DW, et al. Anal fistula surgery. Factors associated with recurrence and incontinence. *Dis Colon Rectum.* 1996;39(7):723–729.

64. García-Aguilar J, Belmonte C, Wong DW, et al. Cutting seton versus two-stage seton fistulotomy in the surgical management of high anal fistula. *Br J Surg.* 1998;85(2):243–245.

65. García Olmo D, Vázquez Aragón P, López Fando J. Multiple setons in the treatment of high perianal fistula. *Br J Surg.* 1994;81(1):136–137.

66. Getz SB Jr, Ough YD, Patterson RB, et al. Mucinous adenocarcinoma developing in chronic anal fistula: report of two cases and review of the literature. *Dis Colon Rectum.* 1981;24(7):562–566.

67. Goodsall DH. Anorectal fistula. In: Goodsall DH, Miles WE, eds. *Diseases of the Anus and Rectum, Part I.* London, United Kingdom: Longmans, Green & Co; 1900:92.

68. Gravante G, Delogu D, Venditti D. Colosigmoid adenocarcinoma anastomotic recurrence seeding into a transsphincteric fistula-in-ano: a clinical report and literature review. *Surg Laparosc Endosc Percutan Tech.* 2008;18(4):407–408.

69. Grimaud JC, Munoz-Bongrand N, Siproudhis L, et al. Fibrin glue is effective healing perianal fistulas in patients with Crohn's disease. *Gastroenterology.* 2010;138(7):2275–2281, 2281.e1.

70. Gustafsson UM, Graf W. Excision of anal fistula with closure of the internal opening: functional and manometric results. *Dis Colon Rectum.* 2002;45(12):1672–1678.

71. Haim N, Neufeld D, Ziv Y, et al. Long-term results of fibrin glue treatment for cryptogenic perianal fistulas: a multicenter study. *Dis Colon Rectum.* 2011;54(10):1279–1283.

72. Halligan S, Stoker J. Imaging of fistula in ano. *Radiology.* 2006;239(1):18–33.

73. Halme L, Sainio AP. Factors related to frequency, type, and outcome of anal fistulas in Crohn's Disease. *Dis Colon Rectum.* 1995;38(1):55–59.

74. Hamilton CH. Anorectal problems: the deep postanal space—surgical significance in horseshoe fistula abscess. *Dis Colon Rectum.* 1975;18(8):642–645.

75. Hanley PH. Conservative surgical correction of horseshoe abscess and fistula. *Dis Colon Rectum.* 1965;8(5):364–368.

76. Hanley PH, Ray JE, Pennington EE, et al. Fistula-in-ano: a ten-year follow-up study of horseshoe-abscess fistula-in-ano. *Dis Colon Rectum.* 1976;19(6):507–515.

77. Held D, Khubchandani I, Sheets J, et al. Management of anorectal horseshoe abscess and fistula. *Dis Colon Rectum.* 1986;29(12):793–797.

78. Hellers G, Bergstrand O, Ewerth S, et al. Occurrence and outcome after primary treatment of anal fistulae in Crohn's disease. *Gut.* 1980;21(6):525–527.

79. Heydari A, Attina G, Merolla E, et al. Treatment of anal fistulas with GORE BIO-A fistula plug. Poster session presented at: 6th Scientific & Annual Meeting of the European Society of Coloproctology; September 21–24, 2011; Copenhagen, Denmark.

80. Hidaka H, Kuroki M, Hirokuni T, et al. Follow-up studies of sphincter-preserving operations for anal fistulas. *Dis Colon Rectum.* 1997;40(10 suppl):S107–S111.

81. Hill JR. Fistulas and fistulous abscesses in the anorectal region: personal experience in management. *Dis Colon Rectum.* 1967;10(6):421–434.

82. Hjortrup A, Moesgaard F, Kjaergård J. Fibrin adhesive in the treatment of perineal fistulas. *Dis Colon Rectum.* 1991;34(9):752–754.

83. Ho KS, Tsang C, Seow-Choen F, et al. Prospective randomised trial comparing ayurvedic cutting seton and fistulotomy for low fistula-in-ano. *Tech Coloproctol.* 2001;5(3):137–141.

84. Hussain SM, Stoker J, Schouten WR, et al. Fistula in ano: endoanal sonography versus endoanal MR imaging in classification. *Radiology.* 1996;200(2):475–481.

85. Hyder SA, Travis SP, Jewell DP, et al. Fistulating anal Crohn's disease: results of combined surgical and infliximab treatment. *Dis Colon Rectum.* 2006;49(12):1837–1841.

86. Hyman N, Kida M. Adenocarcinoma of the sigmoid colon seeding a chronic anal fistula: report of a case. *Dis Colon Rectum.* 2003;46(6):835–836.

87. Hyman N, O'Brien S, Osler T. Outcomes after fistulotomy: results of a prospective, multicenter regional study. *Dis Colon Rectum.* 2009;52(12):2022–2027.

88. Iesalnieks I, Gaertner WB, Glass H, et al. Fistula-associated anal adenocarcinoma in Crohn's disease. *Inflamm Bowel Dis.* 2010;16(10):1643–1648.

89. Isbister WH, Al Sanea N. The cutting seton: an experience at King Faisal Specialist Hospital. *Dis Colon Rectum.* 2001;44(5):722–727.

90. Jarrar A, Church J. Advancement flap repair: a good option for complex anorectal fistulas. *Dis Colon Rectum.* 2011;54(12):1537–1541.

91. Jones DW, Finlayson SR. Trends in surgery for Crohn's disease in the era of infliximab. *Ann Surg.* 2010;252(2):307–312.

92. Jun SH, Choi GS. Anocutaneous advancement flap closure of high anal fistulas. *Br J Surg.* 1999;86(4):490–492.

93. Kasparek MS, Glatzle J, Temeltcheva T, et al. Long-term quality of life in patients with Crohn's disease and perianal fistulas: influence of fecal diversion. *Dis Colon Rectum.* 2007;50(12):2067–2074.

94. Kennedy M, Perera D, Sydney D. Fistula-in-ano: cutting seton in the management of fistula-in-ano. *Dis Colon Rectum.* 2002;45:A25–A28.

95. Kim Y, Park YJ. Three-dimensional endoanal ultrasonographic assessment of an anal fistula with and without H_2O_2 enhancement. *World J Gastroenterol.* 2009;15(38):4810–4815.

96. Klingbeil JK, Toyama WM. Fistula-in-ano in infants and children. *Contemp Surg.* 1995;46:133.

97. Kreis ME, Jehle EC, Ohlemann M, et al. Functional results after transanal rectal advancement flap repair of trans-sphincteric fistula. *Br J Surg.* 1998;85(2):240–242.

98. Kronborg O. To lay open or excise a fistula-in-ano: a randomized trial. *Br J Surg.* 1985;72(12):970.

99. Kruskal JB, Kane RA, Morrin MM. Peroxide-enhanced anal endosonography: technique, image interpretation, and clinical applications. *Radiographics.* 2001;21 spec no:S173–S189.

100.   Kuijpers HC, Schulpen T. Fistulography for fistula-in-ano. Is it useful? *Dis Colon Rectum.* 1985;28(2):103–104.

101.   Kulaylat MN, Doerr RJ, Karamanoukian H, et al. Basal cell carcinoma arising in a fistula-in-ano. *Am Surg.* 1996;62(12):1000–1002.

102.   Kuypers HC. Use of the seton in the treatment of extrasphincteric anal fistula. *Dis Colon Rectum.* 1984;27(2):109–110.

103.   Kuypers JH. Diagnosis and treatment of fistula-in-ano. *Neth J Surg.* 1982;34(4):147–152.

104.   Ky A, Sohn N, Weinstein MA, et al. Carcinoma arising in anorectal fistulas of Crohn's disease. *Dis Colon Rectum.* 1998;41(8):992–996.

105.   Law PJ, Talbot RW, Bartram CI, et al. Anal endosonography in the evaluation of perianal sepsis and fistula in ano. *Br J Surg.* 1989;76(7):752–755.

106.   Lengyel AJ, Hurst NG, Williams JG. Pre-operative assessment of anal fistulas using endoanal ultrasound. *Colorectal Dis.* 2002;4(6):436–440.

107.   Lentner A, Wienert V. Long-term, indwelling setons for low transsphincteric and intersphincteric anal fistulas. Experience with 108 cases. *Dis Colon Rectum.* 1996;39(10):1097–1101.

108.   Levien DH, Surrell J, Mazier WP. Surgical treatment of anorectal fistula in patients with Crohn's disease. *Surg Gynecol Obstet.* 1989;169(2):133–136.

109.   Lewis P, Bartolo DC. Treatment of trans-sphincteric fistulae by full thickness anorectal advancement flaps. *Br J Surg.* 1990;77(10):1187–1189.

110.   Lindsey I, Smilgin-Humphreys MM, Cunningham C, et al. A randomized, controlled trial of fibrin glue vs. conventional treatment for anal fistula. *Dis Colon Rectum.* 2002;45(12):1608–1615.

111.   Loberman Z, Har-Shai Y, Schein M, et al. Hangman's tie simplifies seton management of anal fistulas. *Surg Gynecol Obstet.* 1993;177(4):413–414.

112.   Loungnarath R, Dietz DW, Mutch MG, et al. Fibrin glue treatment of complex anal fistulas has low success rate. *Dis Colon Rectum.* 2004;47(4):432–436.

113.   Lunniss PJ, Barker PG, Sultan AH, et al. Magnetic resonance imaging of fistula-in-ano. *Dis Colon Rectum.* 1994;37(7):708–718.

114.   Lunniss PJ, Kamm MA, Phillips RK. Factors affecting continence after surgery for anal fistula. *Br J Surg.* 1994;81(9):1382–1385.

115.   Macdonald A, Wilson-Storey D, Munro F. Treatment of perianal abscess and fistula-in-ano in children. *Br J Surg.* 2003;90(2):220–221.

116.   Makowiec F, Jehle EC, Becker HD, et al. Clinical course after transanal advancement flap repair of perianal fistula in patients with Crohn's disease. *Br J Surg.* 1995;82(5):603–606.

117.   Makowiec F, Jehle EC, Becker HD, et al. Perianal abscess in Crohn's disease. *Dis Colon Rectum.* 1997;40(4):443–450.

118.   Mann CV, Clifton MA. Re-routing of the track for the treatment of high anal and anorectal fistulae. *Br J Surg.* 1985;72(2):134–137.

119.   Marchesa P, Hull TL, Fazio VW. Advancement sleeve flaps for treatment of severe perianal Crohn's disease. *Br J Surg.* 1998;85(12):1695–1698.

120.   Marks CG, Ritchie JK, Lockhart-Mummery HE. Anal fistulas in Crohn's disease. *Br J Surg.* 1981;68(8):525–527.

121.   Matos D, Lunniss PJ, Phillips RK. Total sphincter conservation in high fistula in ano: results of a new approach. *Br J Surg.* 1993;80(6):802–804.

122.   McCourtney JS, Finlay IG. Cutting seton without preliminary internal sphincterotomy in management of complex high fistula-in-ano. *Dis Colon Rectum.* 1996;39(1):55–58.

123.   Meshkat B, Pakravan F, Helms C. Results of the bioabsorbable fistula plug for management of anal fistulas. Poster session presented at: 6th Scientific & Annual Meeting of the European Society of Coloproctology; September 21–24, 2011; Copenhagen, Denmark.

124.   Millar DM. Villous neoplasms in anorectal fistulas. *Proctology.* 1979;2:50.

125.   Mitalas LE, van Wijk JJ, Gosselink MP, et al. Seton drainage prior to transanal advancement flap repair: useful or not? *Int J Colorectal Dis.* 2010;25(12):1499–1502.

126.   Mizrahi N, Wexner SD, Zmora O, et al. Endorectal advancement flap: are there predictors of failure? *Dis Colon Rectum.* 2002;45(12):1616–1621.

127.   Morrison JG, Gathright JB Jr, Ray JE, et al. Surgical management of anorectal fistulas in Crohn's disease. *Dis Colon Rectum.* 1989;32(6):492–496.

128.   Neal Ellis C. Outcomes with the use of bioprosthetic grafts to reinforce the ligation of the intersphincteric fistula tract (BioLIFT procedure) for the management of complex anal fistulas. *Dis Colon Rectum.* 2010;53(10):1361–1364.

129.   Nelson RL, Prasad ML, Abcarian H. Anal carcinoma presenting as a perirectal abscess or fistula. *Arch Surg.* 1985;120(5):632–635.

130.   Nishigami T, Kataoka TR, Ikeuchi H, et al. Adenocarcinomas associated with perianal fistulae in Crohn's disease have a rectal, not an anal, immunophenotype. *Pathology.* 2011;43(1):36–39.

131.   Noble GH. A new operation for complete laceration of the perineum designed for the purpose of eliminating danger of infection from the rectum. *Trans Am Gynecol Soc.* 1902;27:357.

132.   Oh C. Management of high recurrent anal fistula. *Surgery.* 1983;93(2):330–332.

133.   O'Riordan JM, Datta I, Johnston C, et al. A systematic review of the anal fistula plug for patients with Crohn's and non-Crohn's related fistula-in-ano. *Dis Colon Rectum.* 2012;55:351.

134.   Orsoni P, Barthet M, Portier F, et al. Prospective comparison of endosonography, magnetic resonance imaging and surgical findings in anorectal fistula and abscess complicating Crohn's disease. *Br J Surg.* 1999;86(3):360–364.

135.   Ortíz H, Marzo J. Endorectal flap advancement repair and fistulectomy for high trans-sphincteric and suprasphincteric fistulas. *Br J Surg.* 2000;87(12):1680–1683.

136.   Ozuner G, Hull TL, Cartmill J, et al. Long-term analysis of the use of transanal rectal advancement flaps for complicated anorectal/vaginal fistulas. *Dis Colon Rectum.* 1996;39(1):10–14.

137.   Parks AG, Gordon PH, Hardcastle JD. A classification of fistula-in-ano. *Br J Surg.* 1976;63(1):1–12.

138.   Parks AG, Stitz RW. The treatment of high fistula-in-ano. *Dis Colon Rectum.* 1976;19(6):487–499.

139.   Pearl RK, Andrews JR, Orsay CP, et al. Role of the seton in the management of anorectal fistulas. *Dis Colon Rectum.* 1993;36(6):573–577.

140.   Perez F, Arroyo A, Serrano P, et al. Randomized clinical and manometric study of advancement flap versus fistulotomy with sphincter reconstruction in the management of complex fistula-in-ano. *Am J Surg.* 2006;192(1):34–40.

141.   Pescatori M, Interisano A, Basso L, et al. Management of perianal Crohn's disease. Results of a multicenter study in Italy. *Dis Colon Rectum.* 1995;38(2):121–124.

142.   Pezim ME. Successful treatment of horseshoe fistula requires deroofing of deep postanal space. *Am J Surg.* 1994;167(5):513–515.

143.   Piazza DJ, Radhakrishnan J. Perianal abscess and fistula-in-ano in children. *Dis Colon Rectum.* 1990;33(12):1014–1016.

144.   Poen AC, Felt-Bersma RJ, Eijsbouts QA, et al. Hydrogen peroxide-enhanced transanal ultrasound in the assessment of fistula-in-ano. *Dis Colon Rectum.* 1998;41(9):1147–1152.

145.   Prioleau PG, Allen MS Jr, Roberts T. Perianal mucinous adenocarcinoma. *Cancer.* 1977;39(3):1295–1299.

146.   Pritchard TJ, Schoetz DJ Jr, Roberts PL, et al. Perirectal abscess in Crohn's disease. Drainage and outcome. *Dis Colon Rectum.* 1990;33(11):933–937.

147.   Ramanujam PS, Prasad ML, Abcarian H. The role of seton in fistulotomy of the anus. *Surg Gynecol Obstet.* 1983;157(5):419–422.

148.   Ratto C, Gentile E, Merico M, et al. How can the assessment of fistula-inano be improved? *Dis Colon Rectum.* 2000;43(10):1375–1382.

149.   Reznick RK, Bailey HR. Closure of the internal opening for treatment of complex fistula-in-ano. *Dis Colon Rectum.* 1988;31(2):116–118.

150.   Ritchie RD, Sackier JM, Hodde JP. Incontinence rates after cutting seton treatment for anal fistula. *Colorectal Dis.* 2009;11(6):564–571.

151.   Rojanasakul A. LIFT procedure: a simplified technique for fistula-in-ano. *Tech Coloproctol.* 2009;13(3):237–240.

152.   Rojanasakul A, Pattanaarun J, Sahakitrungruang C, et al. Total anal sphincter saving technique for fistula-in-ano; the ligation of intersphincteric fistula tract. *J Med Assoc Thai.* 2007;90(3):581–586.

153.   Rollinson PD, Dundas SA. Adenocarcinoma of sigmoid colon seeding into pre-existing fistula in ano. *Br J Surg.* 1984;71(9):664–665.

154.   Safavi A, Gottesman L, Dailey TH. Anorectal surgery in the HIV+ patient: update. *Dis Colon Rectum.* 1991;34(4):299–304.

155.   Sainio P. A manometric study of anorectal function after surgery for anal fistula, with special reference to incontinence. *Acta Chir Scand.* 1985;151(8):695–700.

156.   Sainio P, Husa A. Fistula-in-ano. Clinical features and long-term results of surgery in 199 adults. *Acta Chir Scand.* 1985;151(2):169–176.

157.   Sainio P, Husa A. A prospective manometric study of the effect of anal fistula surgery on anorectal function. *Acta Chir Scand.* 1985;151(3):279–288.

158.   Sands BE, Anderson FH, Bernstein CN, et al. Infliximab maintenance therapy for fistulizing Crohn's disease. *N Engl J Med.* 2004;350(9):876–885.

159.   Sangwan YP, Rosen L, Riether RD, et al. Is simple fistula-in-ano simple? *Dis Colon Rectum.* 1994;37(9):885–889.

160.   Sangwan YP, Schoetz DJ Jr, Murray JJ, et al. Perianal Crohn's disease. Results of local surgical treatment. *Dis Colon Rectum.* 1996;39(5):529–535.

161.   Scholefield JH, Berry DP, Armitage NC, et al. Magnetic resonance imaging in the management of fistula in ano. *Int J Colorectal Dis.* 1997;12(5):276–279.

162. Schwartz DA, Wiersema MJ, Dudiak KM, et al. A comparison of endoscopic ultrasound, magnetic resonance imaging, and exam under anesthesia for evaluation of Crohn's perianal fistulas. *Gastroenterology*. 2001;121(5):1064–1072.

163. Sciaudone G, Di Stazio C, Limongelli P, et al. Treatment of complex perianal fistulas in Crohn disease: infliximab, surgery or combined approach. *Can J Surg*. 2010;53(5):299–304.

164. Scott HJ, Northover JM. Evaluation of surgery for perianal Crohn's fistulas. *Dis Colon Rectum*. 1996;39(9):1039–1043.

165. Sentovich SM. Fibrin glue for all anal fistulas. *J Gastrointest Surg*. 2001;5(2):158–161.

166. Sentovich SM. Fibrin glue for anal fistulas: long-term results. *Dis Colon Rectum*. 2003;46(4):498–502.

167. Seow-Choen, Phillips RK. Insights gained from the management of problematical anal fistulae at St. Mark's Hospital, 1984–88. *Br J Surg*. 1991;78(5):539–541.

168. Shah N, Remzi F, Massmann A, et al. Fistula-in-ano: management and treatment outcome of pouch-vaginal fistulas following restorative proctocolectomy. *Dis Colon Rectum*. 2002;45:A25–A28.

169. Shan YS, Yan JJ, Sy ED, et al. Nested polymerase chain reaction in the diagnosis of negative Ziehl-Neelsen stained *Mycobacterium tuberculosis* fistula-in-ano: report of four cases. *Dis Colon Rectum*. 2002;45(12):1685–1688.

170. Shanwani A, Nor AM, Amri N. Ligation of the intersphincteric fistula tract (LIFT): a sphincter-saving technique for fistula-in-ano. *Dis Colon Rectum*. 2010;53(1):39–42.

171. Sileri P, Franceschilli L, Angelucci GP, et al. Ligation of the intersphincteric fistula tract (LIFT) to treat anal fistula: early results from a prospective observational study. *Tech Coloproctol*. 2011;15(4):413–416.

172. Singer M, Cintron J, Nelson R, et al. Treatment of fistulas-in-ano with fibrin sealant in combination with intra-adhesive antibiotics and/or surgical closure of the internal fistula opening. *Dis Colon Rectum*. 2005;48(4):799–808.

173. Sohn N, Korelitz BI, Weinstein MA. Anorectal Crohn's disease: definitive surgery for fistulas and recurrent abscesses. *Am J Surg*. 1980;139(3):394–397.

174. Soltani A, Kaiser AM. Endorectal advancement flap for cryptoglandular or Crohn's fistula-in-ano. *Dis Colon Rectum*. 2010;53(4):486–495.

175. Sonoda T, Hull T, Piedmonte M. Factors affecting successful repair of anal fistulas using mucosal advancement flap (MAF). *Dis Colon Rectum*. 2001;44:A27–A59.

176. Sonoda T, Hull T, Piedmonte MR, et al. Outcomes of primary repair of anorectal and rectovaginal fistulas using the endorectal advancement flap. *Dis Colon Rectum*. 2002;45(12):1622–1628.

177. Spencer JA, Chapple K, Wilson D, et al. Outcome after surgery for perianal fistula: predictive value of MR imaging. *AJR Am J Roentgenol*. 1998;171(2):403–406.

178. Standards Practice Task Force, American Society of Colon and Rectal Surgeons. Practice parameters for treatment of fistula-in-ano. *Dis Colon Rectum*. 1996;39(12):1361–1362.

179. Standards Task Force, American Society of Colon and Rectal Surgeons. Practice parameters for ambulatory anorectal surgery. *Dis Colon Rectum*. 1991;34:285.

180. Steele SR, Kumar R, Feingold DL, et al. Practice parameters for the management of perianal abscess and fistula-in-ano. *Dis Colon Rectum*. 2011;54(12):1465–1474.

181. Stoker J, Rociu E, Wiersma TG, et al. Imaging of anorectal disease. *Br J Surg*. 2000;87(1):10–27.

182. Tan KK, Tan IJ, Lim FS, et al. The anatomy of failures following the ligation of intersphincteric tract technique for anal fistula: a review of 93 patients over 4 years. *Dis Colon Rectum*. 2011;54(11):1368–1372.

183. Thompson JE Jr, Bennion RS, Hilliard G. Adjustable seton in the management of complex anal fistula. *Surg Gynecol Obstet*. 1989;169(6):551–552.

184. Thornton M, Solomon MJ. Long-term indwelling seton for complex anal fistulas in Crohn's disease. *Dis Colon Rectum*. 2005;48(3):459–463.

185. Topstad DR, Panaccione R, Heine JA, et al. Combined seton placement, infliximab infusion, and maintenance immunosuppressives improve healing rate in fistulizing anorectal Crohn's disease: a single center experience. *Dis Colon Rectum*. 2003;46(5):577–583.

186. Toyonaga T, Matsushima M, Kiriu T, et al. Factors affecting continence after fistulotomy for intersphincteric fistula-in-ano. *Int J Colorectal Dis*. 2007;22(9):1071–1075.

187. Toyonaga T, Tanaka Y, Song JF, et al. Comparison of accuracy of physical examination and endoanal ultrasonography for preoperative assessment in patients with acute and chronic anal fistula. *Tech Coloproctol*. 2008;12(3):217–223.

188. Ustynoski K, Rosen L, Stasik J, et al. Horseshoe abscess fistula. Seton treatment. *Dis Colon Rectum*. 1990;33(7):602–605.

189. van Dongen LM, Lubbers EJ. Perianal fistulas in patients with Crohn's disease. *Arch Surg*. 1986;121(10):1187–1190.

190. van Koperen PJ, Bemelman WA, Gerhards MF, et al. The anal fistula plug treatment compared with the mucosal advancement flap for cryptoglandular high transsphincteric perianal fistula: a double-blinded multicenter randomized trial. *Dis Colon Rectum*. 2011;54(4):387–393.

191. van Koperen PJ, Wind J, Bemelman WA, et al. Long-term functional outcome and risk factors for recurrence after surgical treatment for low and high perianal fistulas of cryptoglandular origin. *Dis Colon Rectum*. 2008;51(10):1475–1481.

192. van Tets WF, Kuijpers HC. Continence disorders after anal fistulotomy. *Dis Colon Rectum*. 1994;37(12):1194–1197.

193. van Tets WF, Kuijpers JH. Seton treatment of perianal fistula with high anal or rectal opening. *Br J Surg*. 1995;82(7):895–897.

194. Vasilevsky CA, Gordon PH. The incidence of recurrent abscesses or fistula-in-ano following anorectal suppuration. *Dis Colon Rectum*. 1984;27(2):126–130.

195. Venkatesh KS, Ramanujam P. Fibrin glue application in the treatment of recurrent anorectal fistulas. *Dis Colon Rectum*. 1999;42(9):1136–1139.

196. Wedell J, Meier zu Eissen P, Banzhaf G, et al. Sliding flap advancement for the treatment of high level fistulae. *Br J Surg*. 1987;74(5):390–391.

197. Weisman RI, Orsay CP, Pearl RK, et al. The role of fistulography in fistula-in-ano. Report of five cases. *Dis Colon Rectum*. 1991;34(2):181–184.

198. White RA, Eisenstat TE, Rubin RJ, et al. Seton management of complex anorectal fistulas in patients with Crohn's disease. *Dis Colon Rectum*. 1990;33(7):587–589.

199. Williams DR, Coller JA, Corman ML, et al. Anal complications in Crohn's disease. *Dis Colon Rectum*. 1981;24(1):22–24.

200. Williams JG, MacLeod CA, Rothenberger DA, et al. Seton treatment of high anal fistulae. *Br J Surg*. 1991;78(10):1159–1161.

201. Williams JG, Rothenberger DA, Nemer FD, et al. Fistula-in-ano in Crohn's disease. Results of aggressive surgical treatment. *Dis Colon Rectum*. 1991;34(5):378–384.

202. Williams NS, MacFie J, Celestin LR. Anorectal Crohn's disease. *Br J Surg*. 1979;66(10):743–748.

203. Wolff BG, Culp CE, Beart RW Jr, et al. Anorectal Crohn's disease. A long-term perspective. *Dis Colon Rectum*. 1985;28(10):709–711.

204. Yamaguchi T, Kagawa R, Sakata S, et al. Successful sphincter-sparing local excision for mucinous adenocarcinoma associated with chronic fistula in ano using preoperative MRI evaluation. *Int Surg*. 2008;93(4):220–225.

205. Zimmerman DD, Briel JW, Gosselink MP, et al. Anocutaneous advancement flap repair of transsphincteric fistulas. *Dis Colon Rectum*. 2001;44(10):1474–1480.

206. Zimmerman DD, Delemarre JB, Gosselink MP, et al. Smoking affects the outcome of transanal mucosal advancement flap repair of transsphincteric fistulas. *Br J Surg*. 2003;90(3):351–354.

207. Zmora O, Mizrahi N, Rotholtz N, et al. Fibrin glue sealing in the treatment of perineal fistulas. *Dis Colon Rectum*. 2003;46(5):584–589.

208. Zmora O, Neufeld D, Ziv Y, et al. Prospective, multicenter evaluation of highly concentrated fibrin glue in the treatment of complex cryptogenic perianal fistulas. *Dis Colon Rectum*. 2005;48(12):2167–2172.

15

Rectovaginal and Rectourethral Fistula

Paula I. Denoya and Marvin L. Corman

Mothers love their children more than fathers, because parenthood costs the mothers more trouble.
—ARISTOTLE: *Nicomachean Ethics* IX, vii

▶ RECTOVAGINAL FISTULA

Anovaginal or rectovaginal fistula is not usually a manifestation of anal fistula because it is rarely a consequence of cryptoglandular infection. The condition most commonly occurs following trauma, especially obstetric injury. Venkatesh and colleagues studied the incidence of complications following vaginal delivery in 20,500 women.[80] Five percent of all normal deliveries resulted in episiotomy-associated third- and fourth-degree lacerations (Figure 15-1). Of the fourth-degree lacerations, 10% disrupted after primary repair (Figure 15-2).

In addition to obstetrically related causes, other etiologic factors related to the development of rectovaginal fistula include the following:

- Inflammatory bowel disease—the second most frequent cause (Figure 15-3)
- Carcinoma
- Radiation
- Diverticulitis
- Foreign body
- Penetrating trauma
- Infectious processes
- Congenital anomalies
- Pelvic, perineal, and rectal surgery, especially vaginal hysterectomy and low anterior resection
- Anorectal eroticism
- Ergotamine induced[54]

Symptoms and Classification

Patients usually complain of passage of flatus, feces, or pus from the vagina. Depending on the etiology, location, extent, and associated injury, the woman may also have difficulty with the control of flatus and feces per rectum.

Although there is no official classification scheme for rectovaginal fistulae, a commonly used approach is to base categorization on the location of the rectal opening: anal, low rectal, and high rectal. The equivalent gynecologic classification is low vaginal, midvaginal, and high vaginal. The location of the fistula is important because it will determine the operative approach.

A low fistula is usually readily apparent on inspection or upon anoscopy. One usually has little difficulty in identifying the tract and passing a probe, but careful assessment of the tone and contractility of the muscle above the fistula should be made. A midrectal (midvaginal) fistula is also relatively easy to visualize, particularly when one attempts to pass a probe from vagina to rectum. A high fistula may be quite difficult to diagnose, especially if the opening is small. This type is usually a complication of diverticulitis or of hysterectomy. It may also develop as a consequence of an anastomotic leak or staple injury following low anterior resection (Figure 15-4). This type of fistula may originate from the colon, rather than the rectum.

Evaluation

Physical examination should include both rectal and vaginal evaluations. Proctosigmoidoscopic examination and gastrointestinal contrast studies may be indicated, especially if there is doubt concerning the origin of the fistula. With

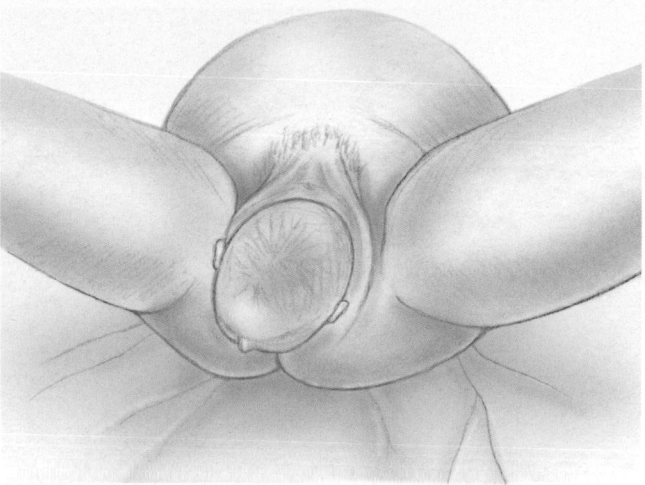

FIGURE 15-1. Infant's head presenting during vaginal delivery. Although vaginal delivery may be a normal physiologic phenomenon, the consequences both short term and long term may be anatomically and functionally problematic.

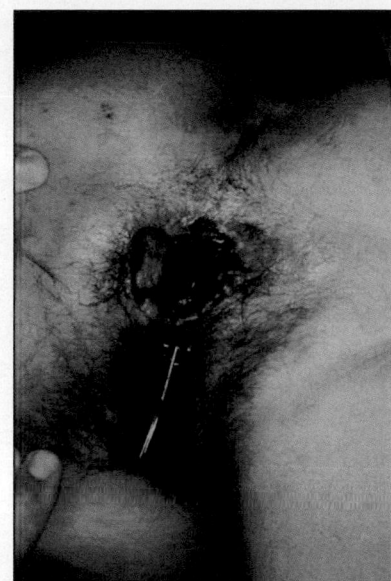

FIGURE 15-3. Rectovaginal fistula secondary to Crohn's disease. Note the marked disruption of the anal architecture.

high fistulas, proctosigmoidoscopic examination seldom will demonstrate the opening, but gentle probing at the apex of the vagina will often identify the defect. Barium enema examination may show opacification of the vagina (Figure 15-5). A biopsy should be performed if the fistula is secondary to radiation injury in order to determine the presence or absence of tumor.

If the patient's symptoms are characteristic, but the surgeon is unable to confirm a fistula by one of the foregoing means, there are two other approaches worth attempting. One procedure is to place the patient in the lithotomy position and insert a proctoscope in the rectum. With the woman in a slight Trendelenburg position, the vagina is filled with warm water. Air is then insufflated through the proctoscope; if bubbles are seen in the vagina, the diagnosis is confirmed. Another alternative is to give the patient a methylene blue small retention enema and leave a tampon in the vagina. The tampon is removed after 1 hour to see whether the blue color appears on it.

Depending on the origin of the fistula, it may be appropriate to evaluate the proximal colon before definitive repair. This is usually readily accomplished by means of either colonoscopy or barium enema examination. Occasionally, however, it may be difficult to advance the endoscope above the fistula site, and contrast may preferentially pass completely out of the vagina. Under these circumstances, a combination of guidewire passage of the instrument and placement of a Foley catheter above the communication will facilitate proximal evaluation.[70]

Yee and coworkers reviewed their experience with endoanal ultrasound in patients with rectovaginal fistulas in order to define what role this modality has in preoperative assessment.[84] Although the authors believed that noncontrast ultrasound was not helpful for evaluation, they recommended its

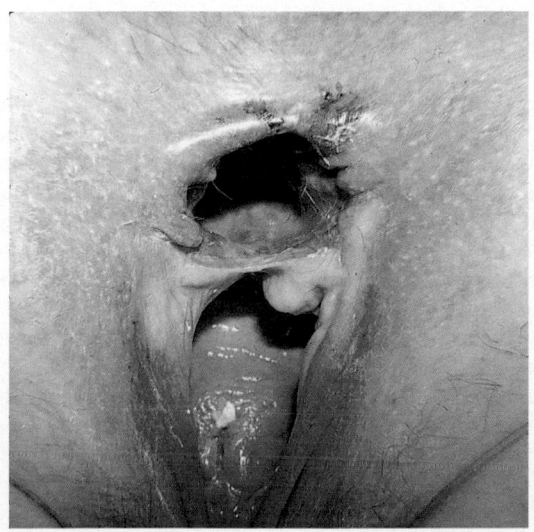

FIGURE 15-2. Cloacal-like defect, a consequence of vaginal delivery of a large infant, a third-degree laceration, and breakdown of the repair.

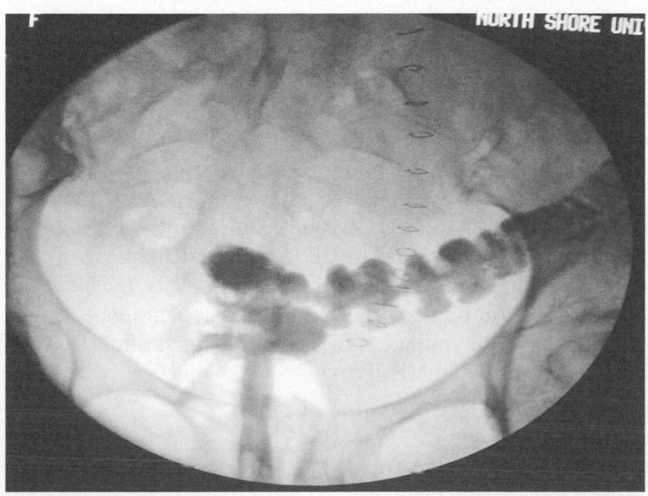

FIGURE 15-4. Barium enema reveals contrast material in the vagina as a consequence of the stapling device incorporating a portion of the posterior vaginal wall.

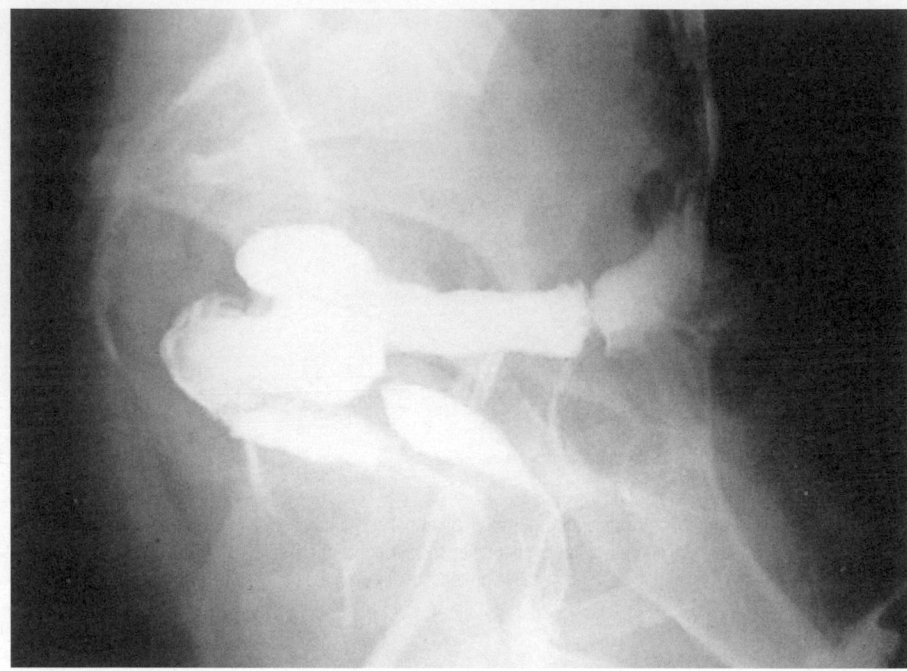

FIGURE 15-5. Rectovaginal fistula following hysterectomy. A barium enema demonstrates contrast material in the vagina.

use in order to identify occult sphincter defects. The primary purpose, therefore, is to alert the surgeon to consider performing a sphincter reconstruction, which greatly improves successful repair in patients with sphincter defects.[76]

Magnetic resonance imaging (MRI) may also be used to identify the presence of an occult fistula and to assess the integrity of the anal sphincter muscles. In a retrospective study, MRI was able to detect 100% of anal canal internal openings and 95% of vaginal openings. MRI was also able to identify secondary fistula tracts, abscesses, and sphincter defects.[17]

Treatment

As suggested, the treatment of rectovaginal fistula depends on the location and the cause. High rectovaginal fistulas are generally approached transabdominally and involve a bowel resection if colon or rectal disease precipitated the communication. If the fistula occurred secondary to hysterectomy, it may suffice to separate the bowel from the vagina; close the opening; and interpose omentum, a peritoneal flap, or fascia. For midvaginal and low rectovaginal fistulas, numerous operative approaches have been advocated, including transvaginal, perineal, transanal, and transsphincteric. One operation that should rarely be considered, however, even for anovaginal or introital fistulas, is simple fistulotomy. Dividing the perineum, even for a relatively superficial fistula, will inevitably cause some degree of incontinence (see Chapter 16) unless a concomitant sphincteroplasty is accomplished to repair any divided sphincter.[60] The following summarizes the various operative alternatives:

Operations for Rectovaginal Fistula
Perineal
    Fistulotomy alone (placed here for completeness—see previous comment)
    Fistulotomy with muscle repair
        Anoplasty
    Interposition (e.g., bulbocavernosus-labial flap [Martius])

Transanal
    Repair in layers
    Repair in layers with sliding flap
        Anterior rectal wall
        Internal sphincter
Transsphincteric (Mason)
    Repair in layers
        With sliding vaginal flap (Warren)
        With interposition
Abdominal
    Simple closure
        With interposition
    Resection (low anterior, pull-through, abdominosacral, coloanal)
        With interposition
    Colostomy

The following discussion is confined to low-level and midlevel fistulas. Operations that require an abdominal approach are similar to those performed for other conditions; these are discussed in Chapters 23 and 24.

Most surgeons prefer to place the patient on a mechanical bowel preparation as if for colon resection. This includes a vigorous laxative 1 day before and a tap water enema the morning of surgery until the returns are clear. Others suggest that no cleanout is required, but even if there is no demonstrable increase in septic complications or breakdown of the repair, few enjoy wallowing in stool. Broad-spectrum intravenous antibiotics are also suggested within one-half hour prior to incision time. A Foley catheter should be inserted before surgery and kept in place as long as is reasonable or convenient. Standard vaginal antiseptic preparation should also be performed at the time of surgery.

Techniques for Repair of Anovaginal and Low Rectovaginal Fistulas
Any attempt at repair must primarily address the anal or rectal opening, even though the fistula may have arisen from a vaginal source (e.g., obstetric trauma). Many surgeons and

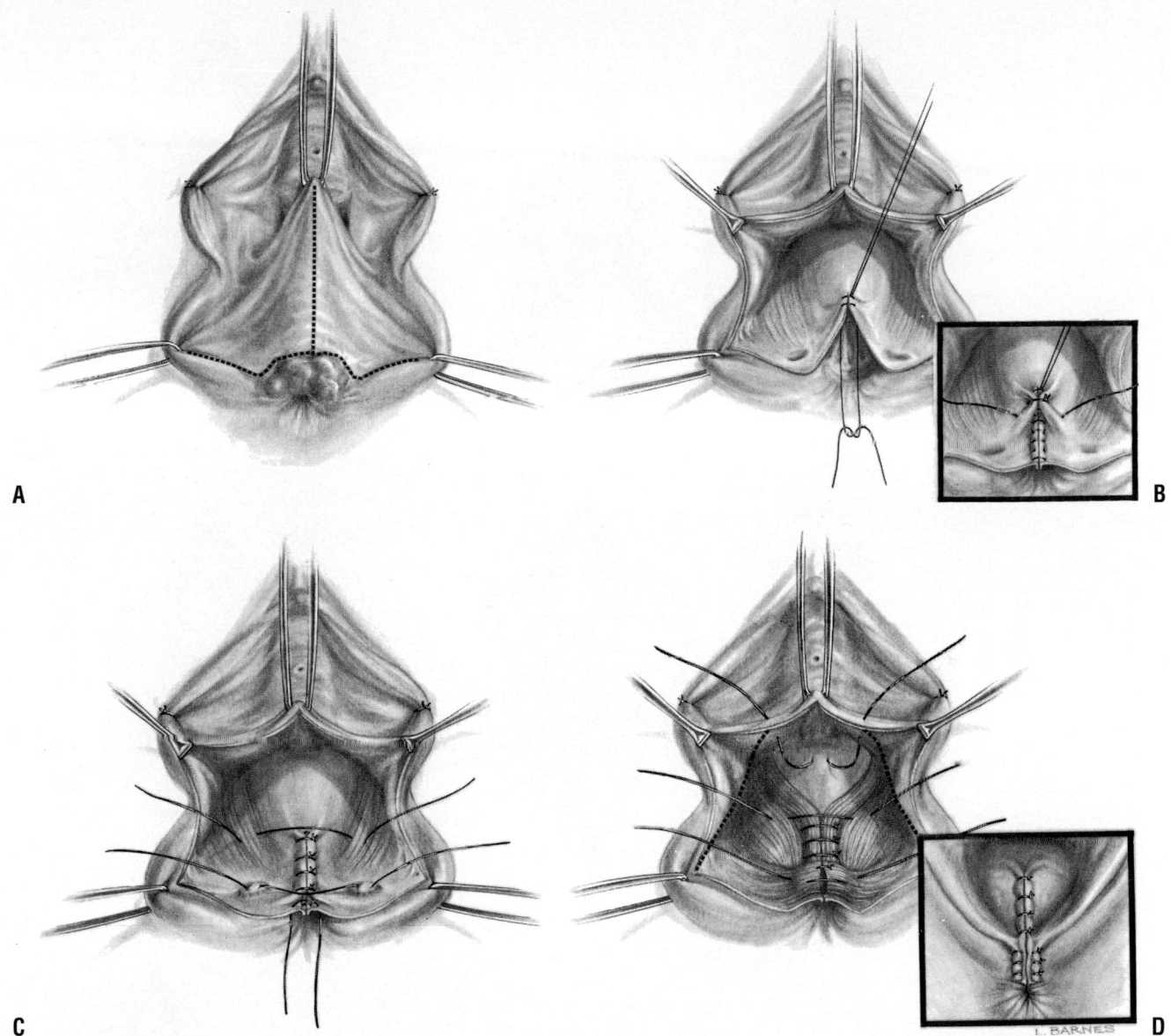

FIGURE 15-6. Repair of complete perineal body disruption with or without rectovaginal fistula. **A:** Incisions in the posterior vaginal wall and perineum are indicated (*dotted lines*). **B:** Repair of the anterior rectal wall. A second layer is placed through the muscularis (*inset*). **C,D:** The external sphincter and levator ani are sutured together. The wound is primarily closed (*inset*). (Adapted from Howkins J, Hudson CN. *Shaw's Textbook of Operative Gynaecology.* 4th ed. Edinburgh, NY: Churchill Livingstone; 1977.)

all gynecologists prefer to repair a rectovaginal fistula using the transvaginal approach.[73] This is not recommended because the high-pressure zone is in the rectum. If the repair of the rectal opening is satisfactorily accomplished, it is not even necessary to deal with the vagina. Conversely, no matter how meticulous the technique is when performed through the vagina, if the rectal closure does not remain secure, failure will result.

With an anal canal or low-rectal fistula occurring as a consequence of an obstetric injury, the ideal choice is to perform a perineal operation with a concomitant anoplasty and sphincteroplasty (see Chapter 16). The condition is usually the result of anterior displacement of the rectum (i.e., the anal opening is abnormally close to the vagina; see Figures 16-50 through 16-60). Most of these patients will have a concomitant anterior sphincter defect. Many will have significant impairment for the control of feces even if they

do not actually have a rectovaginal fistula. To effect a satisfactory repair, the surgeon should reconstruct the perineal body, and to accomplish this, an anoplasty is preferred.[15,63] The operative technique for this procedure is discussed in Chapter 16.

Numerous other approaches to the management of this type of fistula have been described.[5,6,7,24,27,29,37,59,63] In general, gynecologists prefer a transvaginal repair—excising or dividing the fistula tract, closing the defects in the rectal and vaginal walls, and repairing the perineum. Three methods of transvaginal repair are illustrated in Figures 15-6 through 15-8.

In recent years, surgeons have begun selectively to employ the *endorectal advancement flap* technique to repair anal and low-rectal fistulas.[36,71] This is the same principle described in Chapter 14 for fistula-in-ano. In brief, a mucosal flap is raised, which starts distal to the internal opening. The base should be twice as wide as the apex of the flap and should

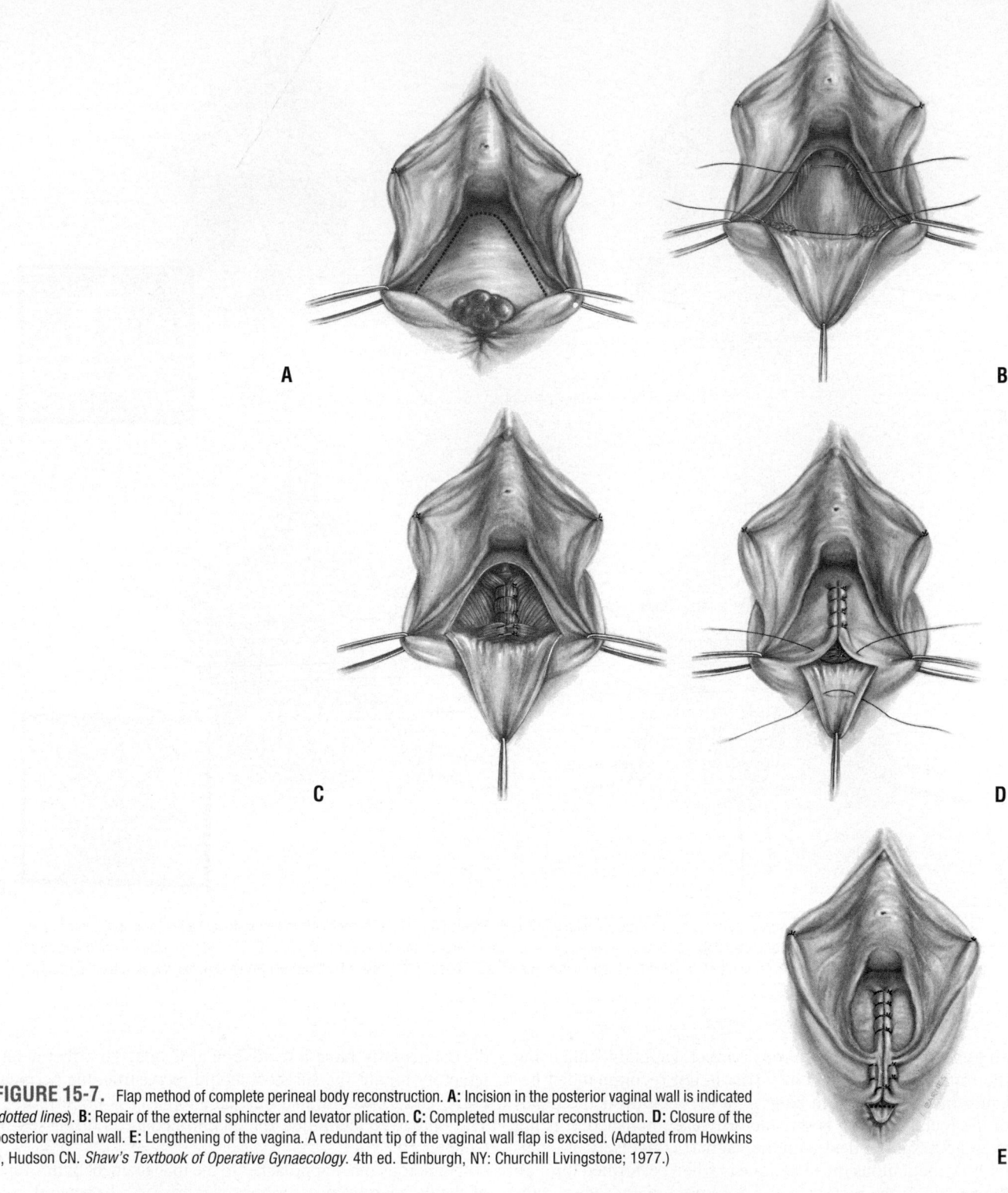

FIGURE 15-7. Flap method of complete perineal body reconstruction. **A:** Incision in the posterior vaginal wall is indicated (*dotted lines*). **B:** Repair of the external sphincter and levator plication. **C:** Completed muscular reconstruction. **D:** Closure of the posterior vaginal wall. **E:** Lengthening of the vagina. A redundant tip of the vaginal wall flap is excised. (Adapted from Howkins J, Hudson CN. *Shaw's Textbook of Operative Gynaecology.* 4th ed. Edinburgh, NY: Churchill Livingstone; 1977.)

extend at least 4 cm proximal to the internal opening in order to allow a tension-free and well-vascularized repair. The flap is mobilized distally to cover the fistula opening and the excess, including the internal opening, is trimmed off. Repair is accomplished using absorbable sutures. The vaginal opening should remain open to allow for drainage. This operation is more likely to be successful for low rectovaginal fistulas than for anovaginal fistulas, however. Berman advocates a

sleeve advancement technique for complicated anorectal and rectovaginal fistulas (see Figure 14-43).[6] This approach is believed to be particularly useful for individuals in whom the fistulas encompass an extensive portion of the anal or rectal wall or in those with multiple internal openings. The transanal approach with endorectal advancement flap has become the most popular method for treating this complication today.[30,33,36,51,59,68] Kodner and colleagues reported their

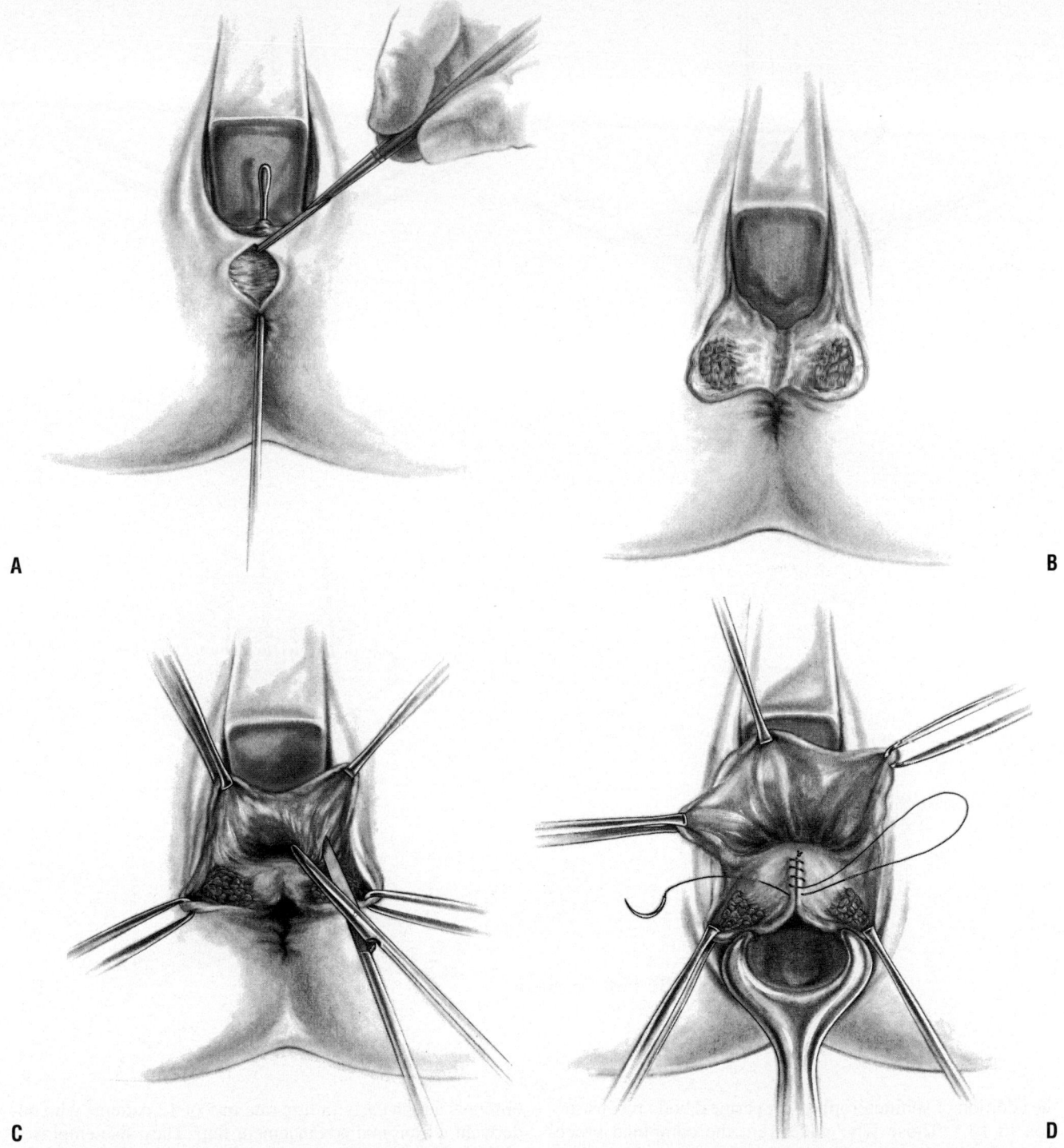

A

B

C

D

FIGURE 15-8. Transsphincteric rectovaginal fistula repair. **A,B:** The fistula is divided. **C:** Separation of the vagina from the rectum. **D:** The rectal mucosa is closed. **E:** Levator plication. **F:** The external sphincter is repaired. **G:** The perineal body is reconstructed by a layered closure. (Adapted courtesy of James A. Breen, MD, and Caterina A. Gregori, MD.)

experience on 107 individuals who underwent this technique for rectovaginal and other complicated anorectal fistulas.[36] Their experience is summarized in Table 15-1.

Persistence of the fistula or recurrence developed in 17 patients (16%). Ultimately, the overall success rate in excess of 90% for this complicated group of patients, with the avoidance of fecal diversion, even on a temporary basis, is excellent.

The University of Minnesota group initially reported 91% success with 35 patients.[59] However, a later publication involving 81 patients noted that this was reduced to 83%.[40] The Cleveland Clinic group observed a 77% success rate for this procedure.[33] The primary factor as noted in another publication from the same institution that adversely affected results was Crohn's disease.[71] Wise and colleagues performed endorectal advancement flaps in 40 women, with

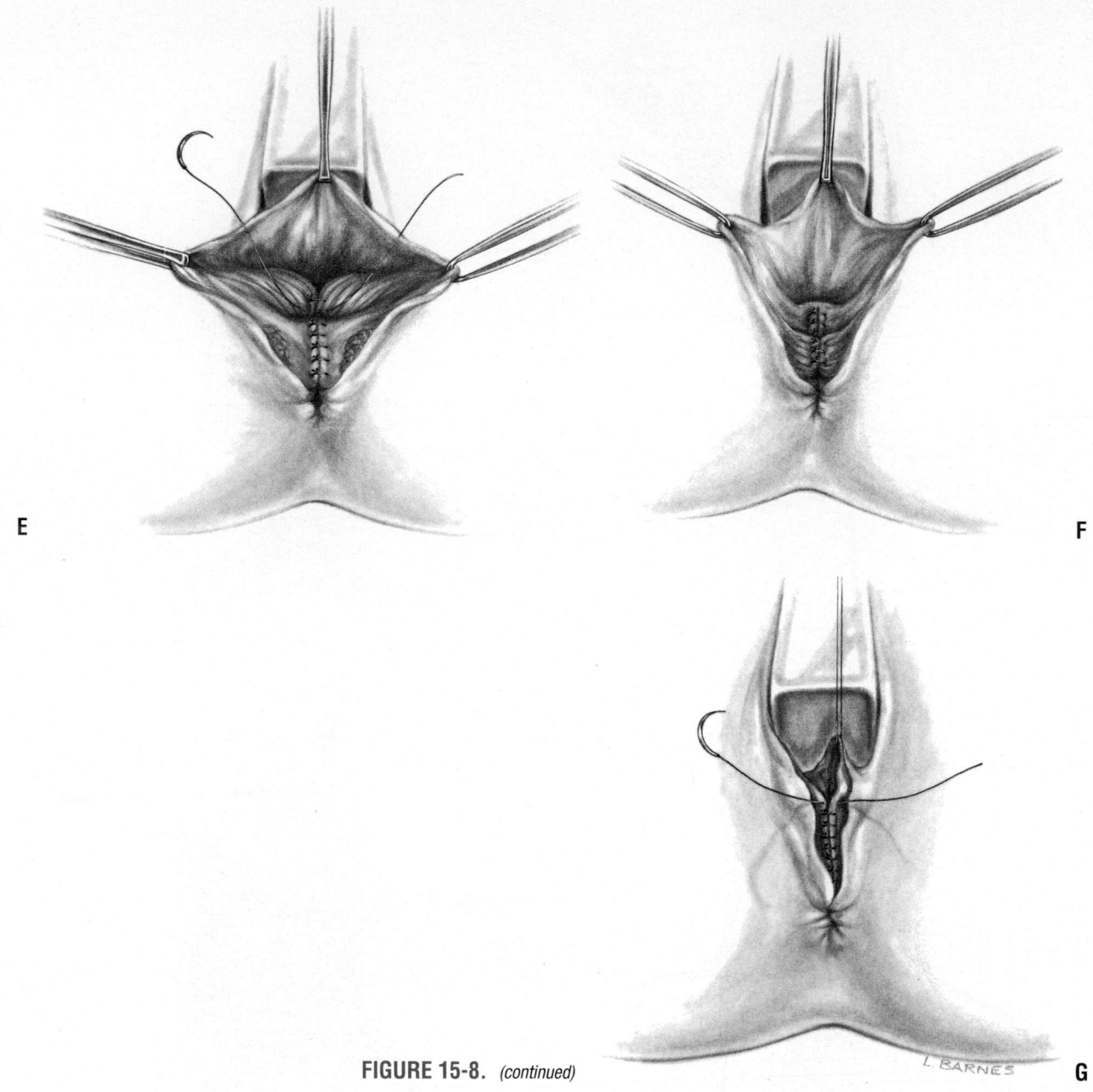

E

F

G

L. BARNES

FIGURE 15-8. *(continued)*

the addition of sphincteroplasty or perineal body reconstruction in 15.[83] Those who underwent the combined procedures were continent, whereas seven of those who had not undergone either sphincteroplasty or perineal body reconstruction, in addition to the endorectal advancement flaps, reported impairment for control. It appears, therefore, that the importance of perineal body reconstitution is justified (see Chapter 16). MacRae and coworkers, reporting from Toronto, caution that persistence of a rectovaginal fistula after failed repair should not be managed by advancement flap.[41] In essence, they recommend that the patient has one shot at this approach. If it does indeed fail, another option should be selected. Watson and Phillips, reporting from St. Mark's Hospital in the United Kingdom, experienced overall success in all but 3 of their 26 patients with rectovaginal fistula.[82] However, the authors cautioned that this result

obscures a high early failure rate in 5 of 12 patients who underwent a transanal advancement flap. They also employed a temporary stoma in 11 individuals.

Techniques for Repair of Midrectal Fistula

A midrectal (i.e., midvaginal) fistula is the most difficult type of gynecologic/intestinal fistula to repair satisfactorily. Fistula in this location is often a consequence of concomitant Crohn's disease, of tumor, of radiation injury, and of trauma (including obstetric and surgical). A theoretically simple approach would be to convert the fistula to that of a "fourth-degree laceration." However, this would of necessity require division of the entire sphincter mechanism. Although this can certainly be accomplished, and it will provide excellent exposure indeed, the risk of breakdown and fecal incontinence should stay the surgeon's hand. In patients who

TABLE 15-1 Results of Endorectal Advancement Flap Repair of Fistulas According to Cause

CAUSE	HEALED PRIMARILY (%)	HEALED INCLUDING FURTHER TREATMENT (%)
Obstetric injury	42/48 (88)	45/48
Cryptoglandular	27/31 (87)	30/31
Crohn's disease	17/24 (71)	22/24
Trauma (two after sphincterotomy)	4/4 (100)	4/4
Total	90/107	101/107

From Kodner IJ, Mazor A, Shemesh EI, et al. Endorectal advancement flap repair of rectovaginal and other complicated anorectal fistulas. *Surgery.* 1993;114(4):682–689, with permission.

already have impaired continence due to sphincter injury, performing a perineoproctotomy may be considered to allow adequate access to both the fistula tract and the sphincter defect. Given reported 32 operative repairs for rectovaginal fistula that were undertaken by 16 surgeons.[24] In 10 cases, the entire perineal body was incised, converting the fistula into a complete laceration; this laceration was then repaired in layers. Primary healing took place in all patients. Other procedures were less successful, but the reasons may have had more to do with the level of the fistula and with the underlying pathology than with the method employed. In a retrospective study of 87 patients, Hull and coworkers reported similar success in obtaining healing of the fistula by rectal advancement flap or perineoproctotomy (62% vs. 78%, $P = .1$), but improved outcomes relating to fecal continence ($P < .001$) and sexual function ($P = .04$).[31]

Transvaginal Approaches

Vaginal advancement flap is favored by most gynecologists and has some advantages and disadvantages. The procedure is performed in the lithotomy position. Vaginal mucosa is mobilized as an advancement flap to cover the vaginal opening. After mobilizing the mucosal flap, the muscular wall is approximated to cover the fistula tract prior to closing the mucosa. The rectal opening is usually left open. This approach is generally viewed as inferior by most colorectal surgeons due to the fact that the rectum is at a higher pressure than that of the vagina. By not closing the rectal opening, it is believed that the fistula will more likely recur. However, there are some advantages to this approach. Specifically, in circumstances where the rectal mucosa may be abnormal, such as in Crohn's disease, there may be more success if the flap is made of healthy tissue such as the vaginal mucosa. When combined with a diverting ostomy, this approach has been reported to be more successful. A group from the Mount Sinai Hospital in New York described their experience with 14 patients with Crohn's disease and rectovaginal fistulas. All were treated by vaginal advancement flap and a diverting ileostomy—13 healed successfully.[4,69] A systematic review by Ruffolo and associates found a healing rate of 69.4% (range, 0% to 92.9%) following vaginal advancement flap repair of rectovaginal fistula due to any etiology.[62]

Lawson described a transvaginal approach to high rectovaginal fistulas that developed following obstetric injury.[37] This procedure involved incising the vagina, sometimes dividing the cervix, and opening the pouch of Douglas. As previously mentioned, it would seem that such a fistula could be more easily treated by an abdominal approach.

Simple Closure or Advancement Flap

This operation can readily be performed transvaginally, but a transanal or transcoccygeal approach is preferred (see earlier).[71] The principles of excision, layered closure, and endorectal advancement flaps are illustrated in Chapter 14 and in Figure 15-9.

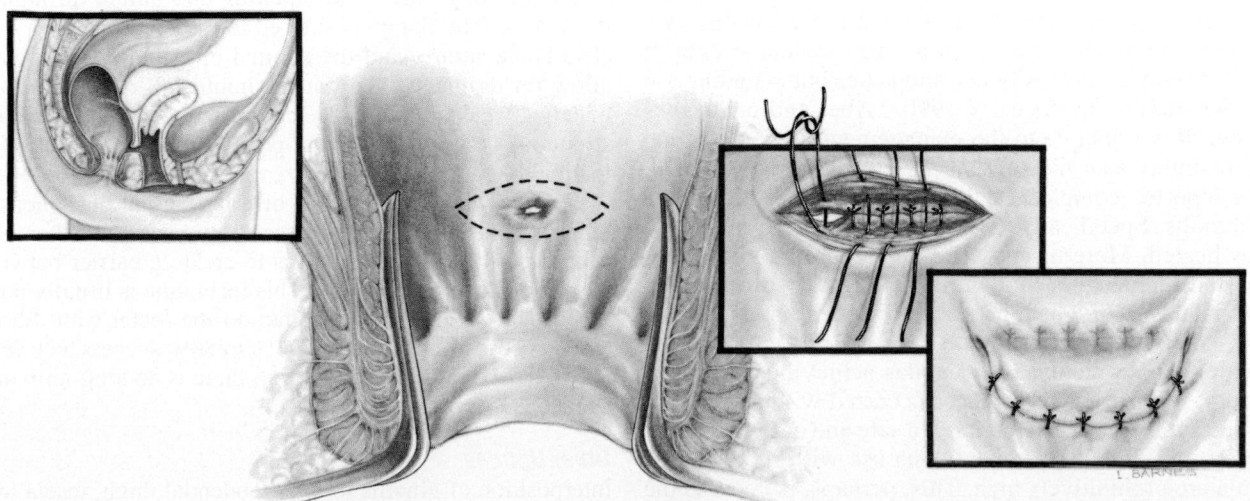

FIGURE 15-9. Transanal repair of a low to midrectovaginal fistula. The importance of the location is that it permits a layered closure with mucosal advancement. If the high-pressure zone in the rectum is successfully repaired, a vaginal approach or vaginal closure is unnecessary.

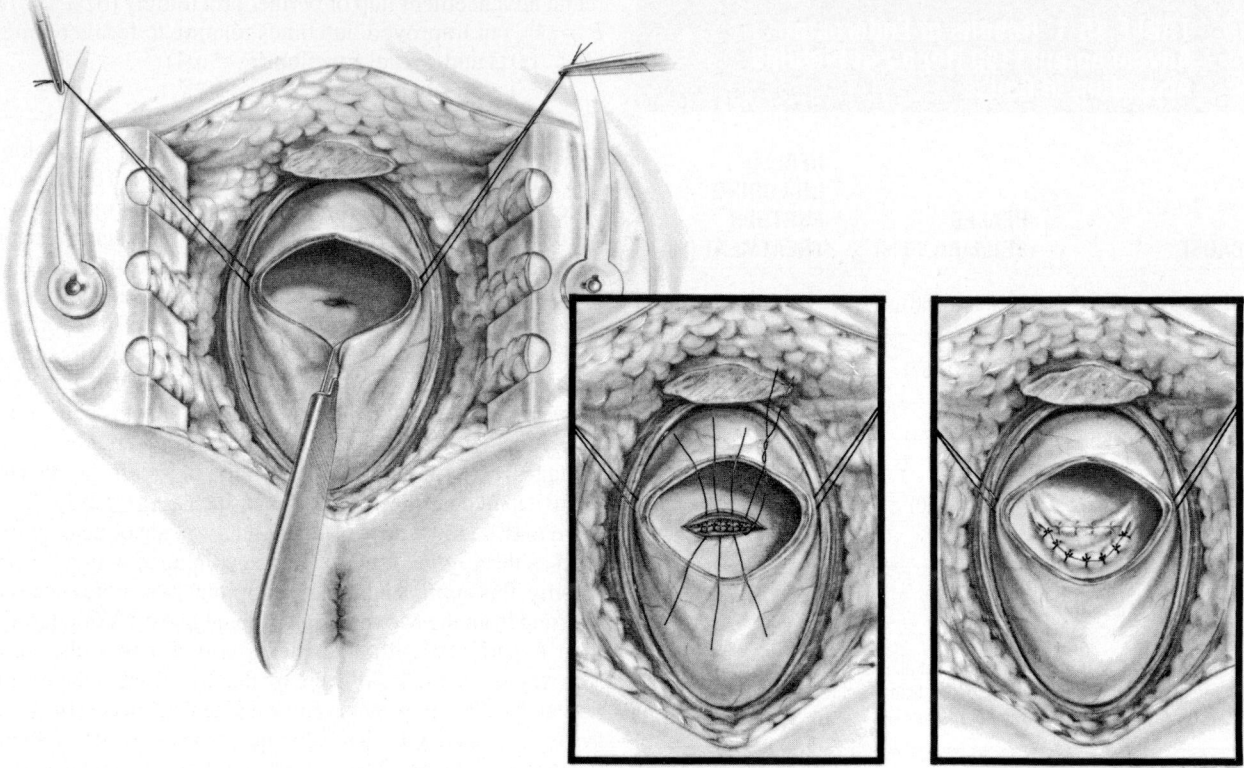

FIGURE 15-10. Transcoccygeal repair of rectovaginal or rectourethral fistula. The so-called Kraske operation permits excellent exposure for low or midrectal fistulas. Through a posterior proctotomy, the fistula site is identified and repaired by suture closure and mucosal advancement.

Transcoccygeal Repair

A transcoccygeal (or transsacral) alternative is shown in Figure 15-10. This approach is essentially the same as that described in Chapter 24 for the management of certain types of rectal tumors. It can also be a very helpful exposure for closure of a rectourethral fistula (see later).

Use of Fibrin Glue

The use of fibrin to seal surgical openings has been applied for almost a century (see Chapter 14). With the development of microsurgical techniques, there has come into application, particularly in Europe, but more recently also in the United States, the use of a fibrin sealant system. It has been applied primarily in orthopedics but is finding use in other fields.[1] In the early 1990s, Abel and colleagues applied this principle to the management of rectovaginal and complex anal fistulas.[1] In the 10 individuals treated, 60% reported complete healing with a follow-up of 3 to 12 months. Specifically, four of the five rectovaginal fistulas healed. More recently, Loungnarath and colleagues reported their experience with 42 patients with complex anal fistulas, 3 of whom had a rectovaginal fistula.[39] They reported an overall healing rate of only 31%, with 1 of the 3 patients with rectovaginal fistulas achieving successful closure. Most of the recurrences occurred within 3 months of glue application. Although it is a safe and easy procedure to perform, the failure rates for its use with rectovaginal fistula are prohibitively high. This, perhaps, is because the tract is too short to be filled by the sealant. In any event, its application for this fistula complication has been all but abandoned for that reason.

Use of Bioprosthetics

Recently, bioprosthetics such as porcine intestinal submucosa meshes and plugs have been introduced for a variety of uses. The Surgisis Biodesign Fistula Plug (Cook Medical Inc., Bloomington, IN), which was initially introduced for anal fistula, now has been adapted for use in rectovaginal fistula repair. The plug has a small plastic flange on the rectal end, which helps to secure it in place, because the rectovaginal fistula tends to be too short to adequately maintain the plug in position (Figure 15-11). The plug is inserted through the rectal opening and pulled through to the vagina. The flange is sutured to the rectal mucosa with absorbable suture, and the vaginal opening is left open to allow for drainage. The flange should fall out in approximately 4 weeks. Patients are counseled to abstain from any strenuous activity or vaginal penetration for 6 weeks following the repair.

Repairs with transperineal or transvaginal placement of bioprosthetic mesh into the rectovaginal septum has also been described. The purpose is to create a barrier between the vaginal and rectal walls. This technique is usually combined with an advancement flap on the rectal wall. Short-term success has been good (71% to 80% success at 1 year) in two small studies[18,65]; however, there is no long-term data available as of this writing.

Other Options

Interposition of gracilis muscle, pudendal thigh, fascia lata, and fat has been advocated by various authors in order to minimize the likelihood of breakdown and recurrence.[12,41] These techniques are more invasive and are often reserved

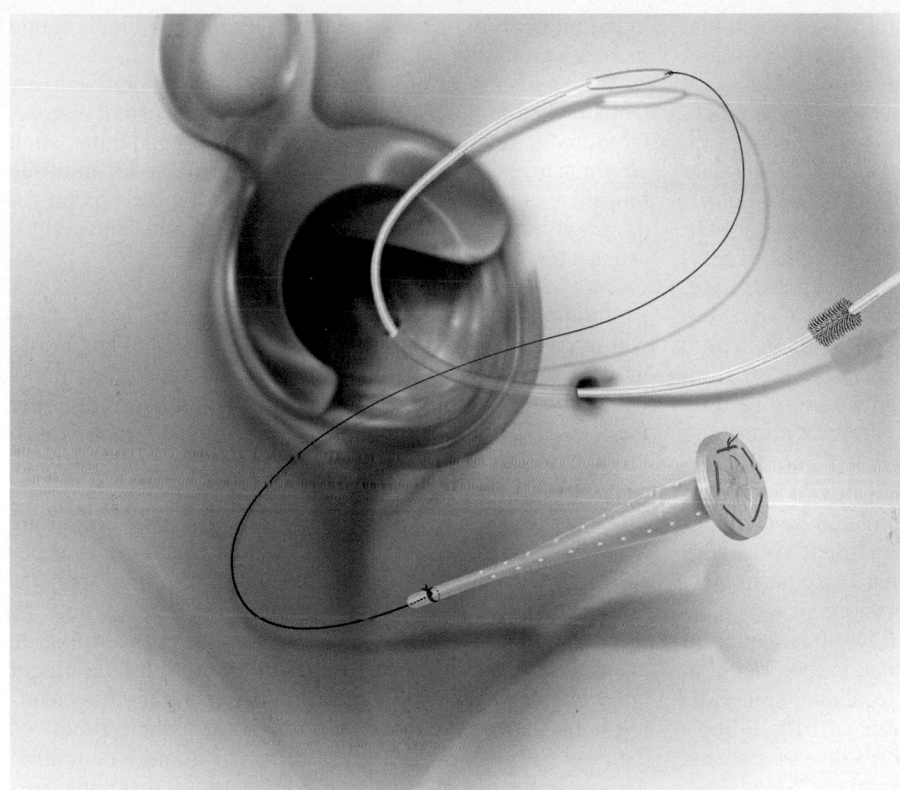

FIGURE 15-11. The Biodesign® Fistula Plug is available with or without an end button for facilitating placement and suturing. The end button modification is used for recto-vaginal fistulas. (©2010, Lisa Clark courtesy of Cook Medical Inc.)

for after simpler approaches have failed and for patients with radiated tissue. The advantage of a muscle interposition technique is that it allows introduction of healthy, well-vascularized tissue into the field. The flap is harvested as described in Chapter 16. The technique is simpler than that used for reconstruction in anal trauma and incontinence because the muscle does not need to be wrapped around the anus for this repair. A transverse perineal incision is made and the rectovaginal septum, which is usually very thin, is dissected to create a space. The flap is then tunneled into the rectovaginal septum to physically separate the rectum from the vagina. It is placed in such a manner as to completely cover the fistula tract and then sutured loosely into place with absorbable sutures. The perineal incision is then closed, leaving the center open to allow for drainage. Use of a drain may be preferred by some surgeons.

Rectovaginal Fistula in Crohn's Disease

One of the most challenging problems in patients with Crohn's disease is the management of rectovaginal fistula (see Figure 15-3 and also Chapter 14).[2] At St. Mark's Hospital, 1 in 10 women with the disease developed a rectovaginal fistula, a higher percentage than that usually reported by others.[58] The authors attributed this elevated rate to the theory that more patients attending St. Mark's have colorectal involvement. Certainly, rectovaginal fistula is more frequently associated with granulomatous colitis than with small bowel disease. This complication may ultimately require a diversionary procedure or a proctectomy; diversion alone, however, is unlikely to cure the condition. The endorectal advancement flap is probably the only definitive surgical option that the physician should consider if repair of the fistula is to be attempted. Besides the obvious, the

major advantages of this approach are that no sphincter is divided, continence is not impaired, there is no perineal wound with which to contend, and rarely is the underlying condition exacerbated.

Technical considerations that should be implemented in the endorectal advancement flap advancement procedure include the following:

- Use the prone jackknife position.
- Ensure precise anatomic definition of the fistula.
- Infiltrate with epinephrine to facilitate dissection and minimize bleeding.
- Make the advancement flap quite thick; this may necessitate taking a portion of the internal sphincter for anovaginal fistulas.
- Mobilize without creating tension.
- Perform excision, curettage, and watertight closure, with closure of the defect in the muscularis.
- Strongly consider temporary fecal diversion.

Results

Several factors adversely influence the outcome of the advancement flap procedure:

- An internal opening higher than 2 cm from the dentate line
- Active Crohn's disease elsewhere
- Severe proctitis
- Persistent or undrained sepsis in the rectovaginal septum (long-term drainage should be performed initially).
- With proper patient selection, successful results are possible.[5,14,20,46,78]

Many patients with this complication are managed nonoperatively, whereas those who do come to the operating room are often submitted to proctectomy. More than one-half of the patients with rectovaginal fistula from St. Mark's Hospital underwent rectal excision.[58] Scott and colleagues noted that only 13 of 38 women with perianal Crohn's disease without vaginal fistula required a stoma or proctectomy, whereas 18 of 29 with vaginal fistulization underwent one of these procedures.[67] These differences were statistically significant.

It should be kept in mind that rectovaginal fistula can, on occasion, be seen in individuals with *ulcerative colitis*. Froines and Palmer reported 3 patients who underwent ileo-anal pouch procedures for this complication, with successful results.[22] However, for patients with Crohn's disease, the preferred method of repair is the endorectal advancement flap.[19,58] With this technique, the Cleveland Clinic group noted a rate of success of 60%.[33] A later report from the same institution revealed the recurrence rate to be only 29%.[49] They concluded that the failure rate was influenced only by the prior number of repairs. As noted from the earlier table, Kodner and coworkers experienced a 71% healing rate in individuals with Crohn's disease treated by endorectal advancement flap.[36] Bauer and Sher and their colleagues reported 14 patients from the Mount Sinai Hospital in New York who underwent a transvaginal operation, all with a diverting ostomy.[4,69] All but one healed. Follow-up ranged from 9 to 68 months. The authors emphasize that, in their opinion, success depends on the use of temporary fecal diversion. Ruffolo et al. reported an overall healing rate of 81% following rectovaginal fistula repair in 52 Crohn's disease patients treated with rectal or vaginal advancement flaps.[61] However, many patients required more than one attempt at repair. The primary healing rate was 56%, and secondary healing was achieved in 57% of the patients. Forty-four percent received perioperative anti-TNF therapy. There was no significant effect on healing due to the anti-TNF therapy. Thirty-five percent of the patients had a covering ostomy created.

For persistent fistulas, interposing a muscle flap into the rectovaginal septum may be considered. Pitel and associates found a 60% success rate using a Martius flap for low rectovaginal fistula repair.[55] The majority of their patients had Crohn's disease. They found a 50% success rate in this group, with a 35-month follow-up period.

It is important to keep in mind that the presence of active abdominal Crohn's disease may influence the success of healing perianal and rectovaginal fistulas. Also, the role of anti-TNF medication has not been determined yet. Twenty-five (18%) of the patients included in the ACCENT II study harbored rectovaginal fistulas[64]; 60.7% (17 of 28) and 44.8% (13 of 29) of them closed at weeks 10 and 14, respectively, following infusions of infliximab. The duration of rectovaginal fistula closure was longer in the infliximab 5 mg/kg maintenance group (median, 46 weeks) than in the placebo group (33 weeks). These patients did not undergo concomitant surgical repairs.

Rectovaginal Fistula After Radiotherapy

Rectovaginal fistula after radiation therapy presents a particularly difficult problem in management (see Chapter 28). However, there are some patients for whom repair may produce quite satisfactory results.

Individuals with this condition often give a history of having undergone radiotherapy many years previously, usually for carcinoma of the cervix. In more recent years, such a complication may be the result of radiation treatment for cancer of the anal canal, rectum, or bladder. Most of these patients present with a fistula above the sphincters, usually in the midrectum or upper rectum. Often the fistula is found in a background of radiation proctitis.

With a history of prior malignancy, it is imperative to establish whether the patient has evidence of recurrent disease. Obviously, reconstruction is contraindicated under such circumstances. Complete evaluation by means of multiple biopsies; radiologic investigation, including computed tomography; and hematologic studies is required. The genitourinary tract should also be investigated.

Techniques and Results

Numerous operative approaches to the repair of radiation-induced rectovaginal fistula have been described.[10,11,26,42,52,74] Optimally, normal, nonradiated tissue should be brought to the area. This would involve a resection, such as the pull-through operation, coloanal anastomosis, bowel interposition, or the abdominosacral resection (see Chapter 24).[10,42,43,52,72,74]

Layered closure has also been used successfully, along with the sartorius muscle and the gracilis muscle interpositions.[11,26] The endorectal advancement flap is probably a poor choice because radiated bowel inevitably would be used. There is genuine risk of the patient's developing an even more difficult management problem, that is, a bigger hole. Boronow reported his experience using a bulbocavernosus fat flap with transvaginal repair for radiation-induced fistulas.[9] Successful closure was effected in more than 80%. Although this is a relatively simple operation that could justifiably be applied as first-line therapy,[9] our own preference is to perform a colostomy at the time of the repair if a nonresection operation is carried out. Of course, if the patient is not a candidate for reconstruction, a diversionary procedure is indicated.

▶ RECTOVAGINAL CYST

Benign cysts of the vagina, especially inclusion cysts, are quite common. These are usually located near the introitus or in episiotomy scars. Most of these lesions are simple inclusion cysts, but one-third of the reported cases in one series were of müllerian origin.[16] Other cystic lesions that may appear in the area are Gartner's duct cysts, Bartholin's duct cysts, endometriosis, adenosis, and vaginitis emphysematosa.[66] The lesion is often asymptomatic, but it may be associated with constipation; mucus discharge; and, if ulcerated, rectal bleeding. In the experience of Pradhan and Tobon with 41 patients, most complained of a swelling or mass in the vagina accompanied by stress incontinence in some, dyspareunia, dysfunctional uterine bleeding, or a history of episiotomy or vaginal lacerations.[56]

Physical examination usually reveals a mass in the rectovaginal septum, but endoscopy will fail to identify a mucosal abnormality. The size of the cyst may be quite variable (up to 7 cm in diameter), but most are smaller than 2 cm.[56]

Most of these lesions can be excised transvaginally, but if the cyst seems to be extending into the submucosa of the rectum, transanal excision as described in Figure 15-12 is warranted.

▶ RECTOURETHRAL FISTULA

Rectourethral fistula is, fortunately, a rare condition. It is seen as a complication of prostatectomy, especially when performed through the perineal route (see Figure 24-82).

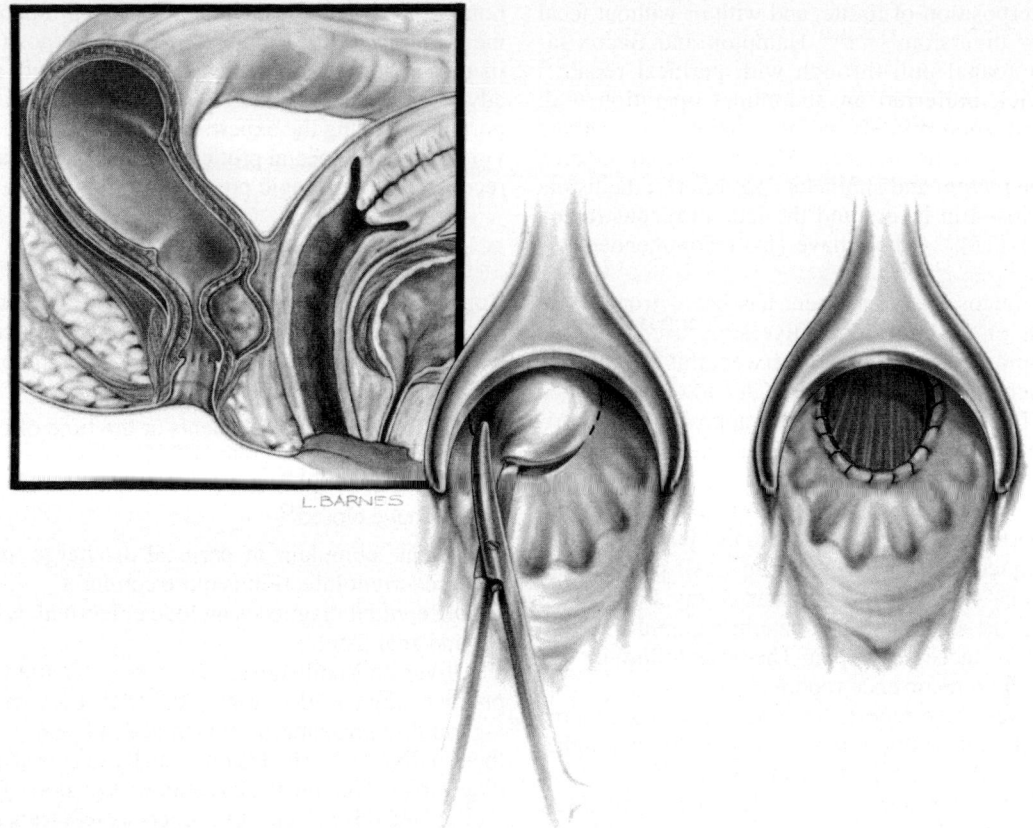

FIGURE 15-12. Transanal excision of a rectovaginal cyst. For a posterior presentation, the lesion is excised with care to avoid entering the vagina. The open wound is sutured for hemostasis but is left open to drain. Healing usually takes place within a few weeks.

It may be seen as a consequence of radiation therapy for carcinoma of the bladder or prostate. Specifically, brachytherapy for prostatic cancer is probably the most common cause today. Trauma, infection, and Crohn's disease are more unusual causes. Even in the adult, a congenital anomaly may be the cause.[28]

Looser and colleagues reported the experience of colorectal–urinary tract fistulas at the Memorial Hospital in New York and found only two cases of rectourethral communication during a 17-year period.[38] One followed a low anterior rectal resection and the other a radical perineal prostatectomy. Thompson and colleagues reported the Mayo Clinic (Rochester, MN) experience over a 30-year period.[75] There were 36 rectourethral fistulas. Fourteen followed prostatectomy, 6 occurred after trauma, 3 were associated with Crohn's disease, and 4 resulted from other causes. Nine patients had malignant fistulas. Although the authors did not distinguish between the symptoms of rectovesical and rectourethral fistulas, 90% had urinary tract infections, and 83% reported urine issuing from the rectum. More than one-half of the patients noted pneumaturia and fecaluria. Bleeding through the rectum implied a malignant process. Cystoscopy established the diagnosis in 84%, and proctoscopy was of value in 70%.

Garofalo and colleagues reported the Cleveland Clinic (Ohio) experience with 23 men.[23] The cause was iatrogenic from prostatic or rectal surgery in 10 patients, Crohn's disease in 9, and radiation in 3. One patient developed a fistula

following an automobile accident. The high incidence of fistula secondary to Crohn's disease is undoubtedly a reflection of the unique referral situation at that institution. Symptoms were multiple in 43%, urine per rectum in 39%, and pneumaturia in 9%, and one patient (5%) presented with fecaluria. Diagnosis was confirmed most frequently by cystoscopy, followed by proctoscopy, cystography, and rectal contrast. The most sensitive test today, however, is computed tomography with rectal contrast.

Kheterpal and associates reviewed their experience with 4,400 men who underwent robotic prostatectomy for prostate cancer.[35] They reported 10 (0.2%) intraoperative rectal injuries that were suture repaired in layers. Of these, 1 patient progressed to develop a rectourethral fistula that required secondary repair.

Netsch and coworkers reported eight (2.2%) rectourethral fistulas in 363 consecutive cases of prostate cancer treated with high-intensity focused ultrasound (HIFU).[47] These developed after one or two sessions of HIFU, and generally presented 3 weeks after the session. The risk of fistula formation increased with more HIFU sessions. All eight fistulas required surgical repair to close.

Treatment and Results

Many approaches have been used to treat rectourethral fistula—transanal, transperineal, transcoccygeal (Figure 15-12), transabdominal (including pouch-anal anastomosis), with or without interposition of tissue, and with or without fecal and/or urinary diversion.[13,25,48,81] Hampton and Bacon favored abdominoanal pull-through with perineal repair.[28] Turner-Warwick preferred an abdominal operation with interposition of appropriately tailored omentum.[77] Others have interposed gracilis muscle.[85] Mason exposed the area by dividing the rectum and sphincters posteriorly; the fistula can then be closed in layers and the rectum reconstructed (see Figure 24-115).[44] Others have also recommended this technique.[57]

Transanal mucosal advancement has been strongly advocated, with or without fecal diversion.[21,32,33,53] In the Cleveland Clinic report, 12 men underwent this operation.[23] All seven patients whose fistulas were due to trauma healed successfully. The authors advocate this approach for all primary operations as well as repeat surgical procedures if this can be accomplished technically. They further advise that all patients undergo concomitant fecal diversion. Joshi and associates reported their experience with five patients treated by transanal mucosal advancement flap.[34] All patients had iatrogenic fistulas resulting from prostatectomy. Four (80%) were closed in one stage, and one patient required a second flap procedure for successful repair. The mean follow-up was 11 months, with no recurrence reported.

Recently, a few case reports have been published on the use of transanal endoscopic microsurgery to allow a higher fistula to be treated by rectal advancement flap.[3,8]

Zmora and coworkers reported the Cleveland Clinic (Florida) experience with the transperineal operation and gracilis muscle interposition.[85] Six patients had prior radiotherapy, and five others had failed repairs. Nine patients healed following this procedure. The authors emphasize the importance of obtaining pathologic material when there is a history of prior malignancy. In contrast to their northern colleagues, they consider this operation to be the procedure of choice. They also recommend fecal diversion. Likewise, the Mayo Clinic group concludes that patients with rectourethral fistula following prostatectomy or radiotherapy should undergo fecal (and urinary) diversion with muscle transposition.[48]

A recent retrospective review from the Lahey Clinic reported 74 patients with rectourethral fistulas who underwent repair with an anterior perineal approach and muscle interposition flap (68 gracilis muscle interposition flaps, 6 other muscle interposition flaps).[79] A buccal mucosal graft urethral patch onlay was used selectively. At a mean follow-up of 20 months, 100% of nonradiated rectourethral fistulas and 84% of radiated rectourethral fistulas were closed in a single stage. Most of the patient had also undergone fecal diversion.

In those individuals with nonresectable malignant disease, a diversionary procedure is the treatment of choice. If the tumor is resectable, pelvic exenteration is the optimal course. When radiation injury is the causative factor or associated concern, hyperbaric oxygen treatment prior to reconstruction may have some value.[50] For benign conditions, successful repair generally requires long-term catheter or suprapubic drainage of the urinary tract.

Opinion

This is a rare condition for one to treat. That is perhaps why it is difficult to be convinced that one technique is preferable. Alternatives that are generally quite satisfactory for the nonirradiated patient include a transanal mucosal advancement, a transperineal approach with interposition of gracilis muscle, or a transcoccygeal operation with sliding rectal advancement flap. We strongly believe, however, in the importance of using the expertise of a urologist, ideally an individual who has special proficiency and interest in performing reconstructive urologic procedures.

► ANTERIOR PERINEAL SINUS OR CYST

Congenital cysts of the genitoperineal raphe are extremely rare. Their initial description has been attributed to Mermet, who reported the condition in 1895.[45] Two theories concerning their etiologies have been proposed:

- Infolding of dermal elements at the time of closure of the genital folds
- Outgrowth of epithelial cells in the raphe after the genital folds have closed[49]

Patients complain of perineal discharge, irritation, and pain; recurrent infection is quite common.

Differential diagnoses include epidermal cyst, hidradenitis, and anal fistula.

Oliver and colleagues identified 31 patients from their practice during a 20-year period.[49] Male predominance (87%) and midlife presentation (mean age, 44 years) characterized these individuals. The lesions usually occurred along the median raphe. Treatment consisted of excision of any nodules with laying open of the sinus tracts. A recurrence rate of 15% was reported.

References

1. Abel ME, Chiu YS, Russell TR, et al. Autologous fibrin glue in the treatment of rectovaginal and complex fistulas. *Dis Colon Rectum.* 1993;36(5):447–449.
2. Alexander-Williams J, Buchmann P. Perianal Crohn's disease. *World J Surg.* 1980;4(2):203–208.
3. Andrews EJ, Royce P, Farmer KC. Transanal endoscopic microsurgery repair of rectourethral fistula after high-intensity focused ultrasound ablation of prostate cancer. *Colorectal Dis.* 2011;13(3):342–343.
4. Bauer JJ, Sher ME, Jaffin H, et al. Transvaginal approach for repair of rectovaginal fistulae complicating Crohn's disease. *Ann Surg.* 1991;213(2):151–158.
5. Beecham CT. Recurring rectovaginal fistula. *Obstet Gynecol.* 1972;40(3):323–326.
6. Berman IR. Sleeve advancement anorectoplasty for complicated anorectal/vaginal fistula. *Dis Colon Rectum.* 1991;34(11):1032–1037.
7. Block IR, Rodriguez S, Olivares AL. The Warren operation for anal incontinence caused by disruption of the anterior segment of the anal sphincter, perineal body, and rectovaginal septum: report of five cases. *Dis Colon Rectum.* 1975;18(1):28–34.
8. Bochove-Overgaauw DM, Beerlage HP, Bosscha K, et al. Transanal endoscopic microsurgery for correction of rectourethral fistulae. *J Endourol.* 2006;20(12):1087–1090.
9. Boronow RC. Repair of the radiation-induced vaginal fistula utilizing the Martius technique. *World J Surg.* 1986;10(2):237–248.
10. Bricker EM, Johnston WD. Repair of postirradiation rectovaginal fistula and stricture. *Surg Gynecol Obstet.* 1979;148(4):499–506.
11. Byron RL Jr, Ostergard DR. Sartorius muscle interposition for the treatment of the radiation-induced vaginal fistula. *Am J Obstet Gynecol.* 1969;104(1):104–107.
12. Cardon A, Pattyn P, Monstrey S, et al. Use of a unilateral pudendal thigh flap in the treatment of complex rectovaginal fistula. *Br J Surg.* 1999;86(5):645–646.
13. Celebrezze JP Jr, Medich DS. Rectal ulceration as a result of prostatic brachytherapy: a new clinical problem: report of three cases. *Dis Colon Rectum.* 2003;46(9):1277–1279.
14. Cohen JL, Stricker JW, Schoetz DJ Jr, et al. Rectovaginal fistula in Crohn's disease. *Dis Colon Rectum.* 1989;32(10):825–828.
15. Corman ML. Anal incontinence following obstetrical injury. *Dis Colon Rectum.* 1985;28(2):86–89.

16. Deppisch LM. Cysts of the vagina: classification and clinical correlations. *Am J Obstet Gynecol.* 1975;45(6):632–637.

17. Dwarkasing S, Hussain SM, Hop WC, et al. Anovaginal fistulas: evaluation with endoanal MR imaging. *Radiology.* 2004;231(1):123–128.

18. Ellis CN. Outcomes after repair of rectovaginal fistulas using bioprosthetics. *Dis Colon Rectum.* 2008;51(7):1084–1088.

19. Farkas AM, Gingold BS. Repair of rectovaginal fistula in Crohn's disease by rectal mucosal advancement flap. *Mt Sinai J Med.* 1983;50(5): 420–423.

20. Faulconer HT, Muldoon JP. Rectovaginal fistula in patients with colitis: review and report of a case. *Dis Colon Rectum.* 1975;18(5):413–415.

21. Fazio VW, Jones IT, Jagelman DG, et al. Rectourethral fistulas in Crohn's disease. *Surg Gynecol Obstet.* 1987;164(2):148–150.

22. Froines EJ, Palmer DL. Surgical therapy for rectovaginal fistulas in ulcerative colitis. *Dis Colon Rectum.* 1991;34(10):925–930.

23. Garofalo TE, Delaney CP, Jones SM, et al. Rectal advancement flap repair of rectourethral fistula: a 20-year experience. *Dis Colon Rectum.* 2003;46(6):762–769.

24. Given FT Jr. Rectovaginal fistula. A review of 20 years' experience in a community hospital. *Am J Obstet Gynecol.* 1970;108(1):41–46

25. Goligher JC. *Surgery of the Anus, Rectum and Colon.* 4th ed. New York, NY: Macmillan; 1980:193.

26. Graham JB. Vaginal fistulas following radiotherapy. *Surg Gynecol Obstet.* 1965;120:1019–1030.

27. Greenwald JC, Hoexter B. Repair of rectovaginal fistulas. *Surg Gynecol Obstet.* 1978;146(3):443–445.

28. Hampton JM, Bacon HE. Diagnosis and surgical management of rectourethral fistulas. *Dis Colon Rectum.* 1961;4:177.

29. Hibbard LT. Surgical management of rectovaginal fistulas and complete perineal tears. *Am J Obstet Gynecol.* 1978;130(2):139–141.

30. Hilsabeck JR. Transanal advancement of the anterior rectal wall for vaginal fistulas involving the lower rectum. *Dis Colon Rectum.* 1980;23(4):236–241.

31. Hull TL, El-Gazzaz G, Gurland B, et al. Surgeons should not hesitate to perform episioproctotomy for rectovaginal fistula secondary to cryptoglandular or obstetrical origin. *Dis Colon Rectum.* 2011;54(1):54–59.

32. Johnson WR, Druitt DM, Masterson JP. Anterior rectal advancement flap in the repair of benign rectoprostatic fistula. *Aust N Z J Surg.* 1981;51(4):383–385.

33. Jones IT, Fazio VW, Jagelman DG. The use of transanal rectal advancement flaps in the management of fistulas involving the anorectum. *Dis Colon Rectum.* 1987;30(12):919–923.

34. Joshi HM, Vimalachandran D, Heath RM, et al. Management of iatrogenic recto-urethral fistula by transanal rectal flap advancement. *Colorectal Dis.* 2011;13(8):918–920.

35. Kheterpal E, Bhandari A, Siddiqui S, et al. Management of rectal injury during robotic radical prostatectomy. *Urology.* 2011;77(4):976–979.

36. Kodner IJ, Mazor A, Shemesh EI, et al. Endorectal advancement flap repair of rectovaginal and other complicated anorectal fistulas. *Surgery.* 1993;114(4):682–689.

37. Lawson J. Rectovaginal fistulae following difficult labour. *Proc R Soc Med.* 1972;65(3):283–286.

38. Looser KG, Quan SH, Clark DG. Colo-urinary-tract fistula in the cancer patient. *Dis Colon Rectum.* 1979;22(3):143–148.

39. Loungnarath R, Dietz DW, Mutch MG, et al. Fibrin glue treatment of complex anal fistulas has low success rate. *Dis Colon Rectum.* 2004;47(4):432–436.

40. Lowry AC, Thorson AG, Rothenberger DA, et al. Repair of simple rectovaginal fistulas. Influence of previous repairs. *Dis Colon Rectum.* 1988;31(9):676–678.

41. MacRae HM, McLeod RS, Cohen Z, et al. Treatment of rectovaginal fistulas that have failed previous repair attempts. *Dis Colon Rectum.* 1995;38(9):921–925.

42. Marks G. Combined abdominotranssacral reconstruction of the radiation-injured rectum. *Am J Surg.* 1976;131(1):54–59.

43. Marks G, Mohiudden M. The surgical management of the radiation-injured intestine. *Surg Clin North Am.* 1983;63(1):81–96.

44. Mason AY. The place of local resection in the treatment of rectal carcinoma. *Proc R Soc Med.* 1970;63(12):1259–1262.

45. Mermet P. Congenital cysts of the genitoperineal raphe. *Rev Chir.* 1895;15:382.

46. Morrison JG, Gathright JB Jr, Ray JE, et al. Results of operation for rectovaginal fistula in Crohn's disease. *Dis Colon Rectum.* 1989;32(6): 497–499.

47. Netsch C, Bach T, Gross E, et al. Rectourethral fistula after high-intensity focused ultrasound therapy for prostate cancer and its surgical management. *Urology.* 2011;77(4):999–1004.

48. Nyam DC, Pemberton JH. Management of iatrogenic rectourethral fistula. *Dis Colon Rectum.* 1999;42(8):994–997.

49. Oliver GC, Rubin RJ, Salvati EP, et al. Anterior perineal sinus. *Dis Colon Rectum.* 1991;34(9):777–779.

50. O'Reilly KJ, Hampson NB, Corman JM. Hyperbaric oxygen in urology. *AUA Update Series.* 2001:21.

51. Ozuner G, Hull TL, Cartmill J, et al. Long-term analysis of the use of rectal advancement flaps for complicated anorectal/vaginal fistulas. *Dis Colon Rectum.* 1996;39(1):10–14.

52. Parks AG, Allen CL, Frank JD, et al. A method of treating post-irradiation rectovaginal fistulas. *Br J Surg.* 1978;65(6):417–421.

53. Parks AG, Motson RW. Perianal repair of rectoprostatic fistula. *Br J Surg.* 1983;70(12):725–726.

54. Pfeifer J, Reissman P, Wexner SD. Ergotamine-induced complex rectovaginal fistula. A report of a case. *Dis Colon Rectum.* 1995;38(11): 1224–1226.

55. Pitel S, Lefevre JH, Parc Y, et al. Martius advancement flap for low rectovaginal fistula: short- and long-term results. *Colorectal Dis.* 2011;13(6):e112–e115.

56. Pradhan S, Tobon H. Vaginal cysts: a clinicopathological study of 41 cases. *Int J Gynecol Pathol.* 1986;5(1):35–46.

57. Prasad ML, Nelson R, Hambrick E, et al. York Mason procedure for repair of postoperative rectoprostatic urethral fistula. *Dis Colon Rectum.* 1983;26(11):716–720.

58. Radcliffe AG, Ritchie JK, Hawley PR, et al. Anovaginal and rectovaginal fistulas in Crohn's disease. *Dis Colon Rectum.* 1988;31(2): 94–99.

59. Rothenberger DA, Christenson CE, Balcos EG, et al. Endorectal advancement flap for treatment of simple rectovaginal fistula. *Dis Colon Rectum.* 1982;25(4):297–300.

60. Rothenberger DA, Goldberg SM. The management of rectovaginal fistulae. *Surg Clin North Am.* 1983;63(1):61–79.

61. Ruffolo C, Penninckx F, Van Assche G, et al. Outcome of surgery for rectovaginal fistula due to Crohn's disease. *Br J Surg.* 2009;96(10): 1190–1195.

62. Ruffolo C, Scarpa M, Bassi N, et al. A systematic review on advancement flaps for rectovaginal fistula in Crohn's disease: transrectal vs transvaginal approach. *Colorectal Dis.* 2010;12(12):1183–1191.

63. Russell TR, Gallagher DM. Low rectovaginal fistulas. Approach and treatment. *Am J Surg.* 1977;134(1):13–18.

64. Sands BE, Blank MA, Patel K, et al. Long-term treatment of rectovaginal fistulas in Crohn's disease: response to infliximab in the ACCENT II Study. *Clin Gastroenterol Hepatol.* 2004;2(10):912–920.

65. Schwandner O, Fuerst A, Kunstreich K, et al. Innovative technique for the closure of rectovaginal fistula using Surgisis mesh. *Tech Coloproctol.* 2009;13(2):135–140.

66. Scott JR, DiSaia PJ, Hammond CB, et al, eds. *Danforth's Obstetrics and Gynecology.* 6th ed. Philadelphia, PA: JB Lippincott; 1990:967.

67. Scott NA, Nair A, Hughes LE. Anovaginal and rectovaginal fistula in patients with Crohn's disease. *Br J Surg.* 1992;79(12):1379–1380.

68. Shemesh EI, Kodner IJ, Fry RD, et al. Endorectal sliding flap repair of complicated anterior anoperineal fistulas. *Dis Colon Rectum.* 1988; 31(1):22–24.

69. Sher ME, Bauer JJ, Gelernt I. Surgical repair of rectovaginal fistulas in patients with Crohn's disease: transvaginal approach. *Dis Colon Rectum.* 1991;34(8):641–648.

70. Silverman WB, Marmolya G. Endoscopic placement of a Foley catheter across a stricture and rectovaginal fistula to perform a barium enema. *Am J Gastroenterol.* 1991;86(1):99–101.

71. Sonoda T, Hull T, Piedemonte MR, et al. Outcomes of primary repair of anorectal and rectovaginal fistulas using the endorectal advancement flap. *Dis Colon Rectum.* 2002;45(12):1622–1628.

72. Steichen FM, Barber HK, Loubeau JM, et al. Bricker-Johnston sigmoid colon graft for repair of postradiation rectovaginal fistula and stricture performed with mechanical sutures. *Dis Colon Rectum.* 1992;35(6): 599–603.

73. Tancer ML, Lasser D, Rosenblum N. Rectovaginal fistula or perineal and anal sphincter disruption, or both, after vaginal delivery. *Surg Gynecol Obstet.* 1990;171(1):43–46.

74. Thomford NR, Smith DE, Wilson WH. Pull-through operation for radiation-induced rectovaginal fistula: report of a case. *Dis Colon Rectum.* 1970;13(6):451–453.

75. Thompson JS, Engen DE, Beart RW Jr, et al. The management of acquired rectourinary fistula. *Dis Colon Rectum.* 1982;25(7):689–692.

76. Tsang CB, Madoff RD, Wong WD, et al. Anal sphincter integrity and function influences outcome in rectovaginal fistula repair. *Dis Colon Rectum.* 1998;41(9):1141–1146.

77.   Turner-Warwick R. The use of pedicle grafts in the repair of urinary tract fistulae. *Br J Urol*. 1972;44(6):644–656.

78.   Tuxen PA, Castro AF. Rectovaginal fistula in Crohn's disease. *Dis Colon Rectum*. 1979;22(1):58–62.

79.   Vanni AJ, Buckley JC, Zinman LN. Management of surgical and radiation induced rectourethral fistulas with an interposition muscle flap and selective buccal mucosal onlay graft. *J Urol*. 2010;184(6): 2400–2404.

80.   Venkatesh KS, Ramanujam PS, Larson DM, et al. Anorectal complications of vaginal delivery. *Dis Colon Rectum*. 1989;32(12):1039–1041.

81.   Visser BC, McAninch JW, Welton ML. Rectourethral fistulae: the perineal approach. *J Am Coll Surg*. 2002;195(1):138–143.

82.   Watson SJ, Phillips RK. Non-inflammatory rectovaginal fistula. *Br J Surg*. 1995;82(12):1641–1643.

83.   Wise WE Jr, Aguilar PS, Padmanabhan A, et al. Surgical treatment of low rectovaginal fistulas. *Dis Colon Rectum*. 1991;34(3):271–274.

84.   Yee LF, Birnbaum EH, Read TE, et al. Use of endoanal ultrasound in patients with rectovaginal fistulas. *Dis Colon Rectum*. 1999;42(8):1057–1064.

85.   Zmora O, Potenti FM, Wexner SD, et al. Gracilis muscle transposition for iatrogenic rectourethral fistula. *Ann Surg*. 2003;237(4):483–487.

Fecal Incontinence

R. John Nicholls

My wind exploded like a thunder-clap
Iaso blushed a rosy red
And Panacea turned her head
Holding her nose:
My wind's not frankincense.

—ARISTOPHANES: *Plutus*

Fecal incontinence is common, especially in the elderly, and can cause considerable morbidity and diminution of quality of life. It may not be life threatening, but it is traumatizing and often disabling. Many patients feel too embarrassed to discuss the symptom with a physician. Incontinence can result from intestinal disease causing irritability and urgency of defecation due to inflammation or loss of capacity of the rectum or neorectum, or from a defective anal sphincter mechanism. Both factors can be present in the same patient. The management of incontinence associated with intestinal diseases is part of the treatment of those conditions. Most patients suffering from incontinence will, however, fall into the category of having an incompetent sphincter mechanism. This chapter will deal predominantly with these.

There have been several advances in the understanding and management of fecal incontinence in the past 10 years. Previously, the condition had been regarded more as a mechanical disorder, but it has become increasingly apparent that there is a large functional component. Behavioral therapies have been developed, and their value is now established. Importantly, surgical correction is reserved for patients who have a mechanical disruption of the sphincter mechanism. Its use has, therefore, declined having been largely replaced by neuromodulation in many centers, which includes stimulation of the sacral nerve (SNS or SNM) and more recently of the posterior tibial or pudendal nerves or the dorsal nerve of the clitoris. Artificial sphincters either biologic in the form of gracioplasty (stimulated or nonstimulated) or prosthetic in that of the artificial bowel sphincter (ABS [Acticon, AMS]) have been found to be less effective than was originally hoped. Anal procedures including the injection of bulking agents into the anal canal lining and so-called radio frequency energy delivery (SECCA) to promote scarring of the anal canal have been developed, particularly for patients with passive incontinence due to failure of the internal sphincter.

Clinical assessment combined with anal ultrasound to establish the anatomy of the sphincter and physiologic testing by manometry will result in reasonable decision making in most circumstances. Anal ultrasound is now routinely applied for the assessment of continence. The axial view of a normal anal canal shown in Figure 16-1 demonstrates the concentric layers of the submucosa, internal sphincter, longitudinal muscle, and external anal sphincter. Some of the physiologic parameters thought to be important in the past, such as electromyography and others (see Chapter 7), are regarded by many to be no longer useful in clinical practice.

The outcome for the patient is now expressed as much by quality of life as by the frequency of incontinent episodes. The important symptom of urgency, which may be the only manifestation of a continence disturbance, can now be quantified, thus enabling improved assessment. The development of continence scoring systems has also improved our ability to assess the effectiveness of treatment.

As with other areas in colorectal surgery, there has been a general tendency toward specialization. The treatment

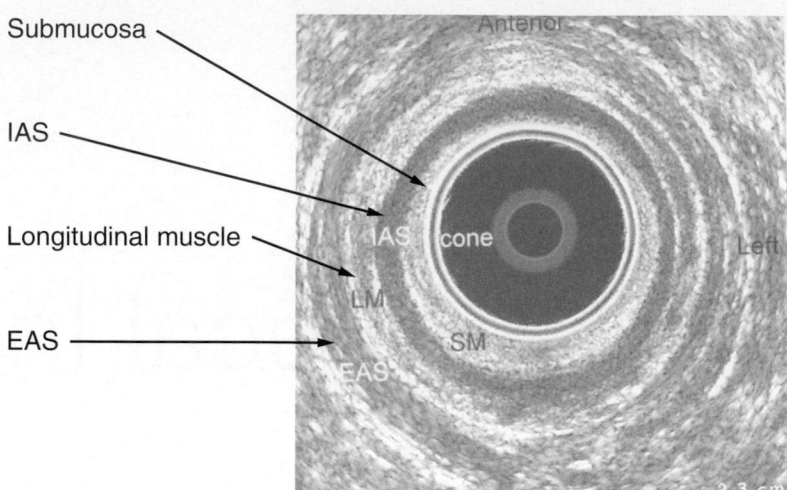

FIGURE 16-1. Normal axial image. Orientation and five-layer pattern.

options for incontinence are now such that the patient is best served in a unit with the capacity to investigate and maintain continuity of care. Thus, a patient suitable for neuromodulation, for example, should be managed in a formally constituted physiology unit.[60]

The techniques used for the evaluation of incontinence overlap with those used for other functional disturbances, including difficulty in defecation and prolapsing disorders. Furthermore, some patients with incontinence may, in reality, have another associated condition—for example, an evacuation disorder such as constipation. It is therefore essential for the physician to be aware of such a possibility.

▶ SCORING SYSTEMS

The development of scoring systems has been an important feature of practice. Their use is now widespread in the reporting of results. Parks introduced a simple system based on the degree of leakage with **A**, being normal; **B**, incontinent to flatus; **C**, incontinent to liquid stool; and **D**, incontinent to solid stool.[350] Pescatori and colleagues[358] identified 13 classifications suggested by various authors, including one by Corman. It took into account both the degree and frequency of symptoms in which **A**, **B**, and **C** reflect increasing problems with incontinence for stool and the number system indicates the frequency of the problem (occasional, weekly, and daily).

In 1993, Jorge and Wexner proposed a continence grading scale, which is now termed the Cleveland Clinic Incontinence Score (Table 16-1) and has now come to be used by many investigators.[216]

The score is determined by adding points from this table, which includes the type and frequency of incontinence and the extent to which it alters the patient's life. This was one of the first attempts by a scoring system to assess quality of

TABLE 16-1 The Jorge–Wexner Incontinence Scoring System

Type of Incontinence	FREQUENCY				
	Never	Rarely	Sometimes	Usually	Always
Solid	0	1	2	3	4
Liquid	0	1	2	3	4
Gas	0	1	2	3	4
Wears pad	0	1	2	3	4
Lifestyle alteration	0	1	2	3	4

0 = Perfect
20 = Complete incontinence
Never = 0 (never)
Rarely = <1/month
Sometimes = <1/week, >1/month
Usually = <1/day, >1/week
Always = >1/day

life. Being a benign condition, this is the most important end point for a patient with fecal incontinence, a determination that has been emphasized by several investigators.[54,388]

Although these scoring systems were useful in comparing the severity of continence before and after treatment, an attempt at standardization was made by a consensus group consisting of representation from five well-recognized academic divisions of colon and rectal surgery in the United States. This resulted in the publication in 1999 of the *Fecal Incontinence Severity Index (FICI)*.[216] Four incontinence events were used to determine the FICI score, all calculated based on the frequency of incontinence of flatus, mucus, liquid stool, and solid stool. Each included five frequencies: one to three times per month, once per week, twice per week, once per day, and twice per day. The same group also turned its attention to the development of a health-related quality of life (HRQoL) scale.[378] This self-completing questionnaire addressed four domains including lifestyle, coping/behavior, depression/self-perception, and embarrassment.

More recently, a scoring system was developed at St. Mark's Hospital,[465] which combined the Pescatori and Wexner scales along with a system developed for the assessment of artificial bowel sphincter by American Medical Systems (AMS). It added further points, including the need for antidiarrheal medication, and improved the assessment of urgency by classifying this symptom to be more or less than 15 minutes. Used in 33 patients, the score that ranged from 0 to 24 (completely incontinent) more accurately coincided with the clinician's assessment than did the other scoring systems. In a further study of 390 patients, the score agreed moderately well with the patients' opinions.[277]

Scoring systems have considerable value, particularly when comparing symptoms before and after treatment. They may also allow some comparison between different units. Being a numerical scale, however, they have the weakness that an idea is being replaced by a figure, and it can be easy to forget what the scale really means in practice. For example, a fall from a score of 14 to 9 sounds impressive, but the patient is still left with troublesome symptoms. A more meaningful statement would include the number of incontinent episodes per unit time—for example, a week or the interval between the arrival of the stimulus and the actual time the patient has in minutes to get to the bathroom. These are also quantifiable in digit integer form and are immediately understandable to patient and physician alike.

▶ PREVALENCE AND ETIOLOGIC FACTORS

Available studies indicate the prevalence of incontinence in the general population to be around 2%, with an increased incidence in the elderly and those in psychiatric, geriatric, and community-based accommodations as high as 50%. It is the second most common cause of institutionalization in the elderly, and in 1993, it accounted for one-half billion dollars per year in the United States for the cost of adult diapers.[216] Significant positive associations for fecal incontinence in the nursing home population include urinary incontinence, tube feeding, loss of activity, diarrhea, pressure ulcers, dementia, impaired vision, fecal impaction, constipation, male gender, age, and increased body mass index (BMI).[323]

In an earlier article, Nelson and colleagues attempted to determine the prevalence and characteristics of anal incontinence in the general community.[324] A total of 2,570 households comprising almost 7,000 individuals were surveyed. The overall incidence of anal incontinence was 2.2%. Thirty percent of those affected were older than 65 years, and approximately two-thirds were women. Of those with anal incontinence, 36% were incontinent for formed stool, 54% for liquid stool, and 60% for gas. This figure is similar to that reported by Varma and coworkers who studied a randomly selected group of women (average age, 56 years) from the Reproductive Risks of Incontinence Study at the Kaiser Permanente facility. Although self-reported incontinent episodes in the prior year were recorded by 24% of patients, in only 2.1% was this weekly or more.[474]

Goode and colleagues studied 1,000 individuals aged 65 to 106 years who were recipients of State Medicare benefits.[160] The prevalence of fecal incontinence was 12.0% (12.4% males; 11.6% females). In a subsequent study from the same group, Markland and associates found the incidence of fecal incontinence over a 4-year period in three rural and two urban districts of Alabama to be 17%, with 6% experiencing episodes at least monthly.[286]

Although age and sex are regarded to be risk factors, definitions are important. This may have accounted for the results of a telephone interview study of 1,153 households in Winnipeg (population, 650,000) in which the overall incidence of an incontinent episode in the previous 12 months was 3.7% (2.0% when physician-diagnosed disease was removed from the analysis) and was not related to age or sex. The average age of the respondents was 47 years; the lower age limit for inclusion in the study was 18 years.[203]

In a study of 271 identical twin pairs, Abramov and colleagues analyzed the returns of the Colorectal Anal Distress Inventory.[5] They found the following variables to be associated with fecal incontinence: age older than 40 years, menopause, parity >2, and urinary stress incontinence. Obesity was very significantly related to incontinence ($P < .007$). Cesarean delivery was not significantly related to a lower incidence, but no patient having delivery by this means experienced fecal incontinence.

Male Patients

There is a difference in the type of lesion responsible for incontinence between men and women. The published data from 1990 to 2007 were reviewed by Shamliyan and associates.[413] They extracted information from 21 observational studies and 4 randomized, controlled trials among community-dwelling elderly men. The pooled prevalence of fecal incontinence was 5%. This was primarily related to age in men older than 85 years, but also to the prevalence of kidney disease.

In a prospective study of 59 males with incontinence, there were 36 with fecal incontinence and 23 with leakage. Overall there were only 5 patients with a sphincter defect (4/36 and 1/23, respectively), 4 of whom had had previous anal surgery. Anal pressures were normal in patients with leakage but were reduced in those with incontinence (resting pressure, 58 vs. 85 [normal]; squeeze, 167 vs. 248 [normal]).[453] In another prospective study of 85 consecutive males presenting over 1 year (408 females in the same period), the etiology was determined in 72%. The most important causes were prior anal surgery (23), treatment for cancer of the prostate (9), and spinal injury (9). Eight patients had soiling of unknown origin. A sphincter defect was present in 35%, compared with 70% in female patients. Treatment resulted in complete resolution of symptoms in 17%, and a further 48% were improved.[78]

Comorbidity

It is clear that incontinence is not only common in society, especially in the elderly and in those who are institutionalized, but it is also related to comorbid and social factors. In a recent systematic review, Hägglund and colleagues[172] evaluated 48 publications on the assessment, management, and prevention of dementia with respect to urinary and fecal incontinence. The prevalence of fecal incontinence among the elderly population aged 75 to 90 years was 17%,[429] whereas among demented patients it was 32%[47] and 34.8%[181] in two studies, a prevalence higher than the available data for the normal elderly population.

In a randomly selected group of women, aged 56 years, gleaned from the Reproductive Risks of Incontinence Study, not surprisingly fecal incontinence reduced the quality of life and increased the "bother." It was also related to obesity (odds ratio [OR] = 1.2), pulmonary obstructive airways disease (OR = 1.9), irritable bowel syndrome (OR = 2.4), urinary incontinence (OR = 2.1), and colectomy (OR = .9).[474] Incontinence was related to chronic diarrhea (OR = 4.55), urinary incontinence (OR = 2.65), hysterectomy (OR = 1.93), poor self-perceived health status (OR = 1.88), geriatric depression score >5 (OR = 2.83), living alone (OR = 2.38), transient ischemic attacks (OR = 3.11), and prostatic symptoms (OR = 2.29).[160] In females, risk factors included white race, depression, chronic diarrhea, and urinary incontinence. In males, only urinary incontinence was associated.[286] Other risk factors include kidney disease (OR = 1.9) and prostatic surgery or radiotherapy.[272] Impaired cognition is also related to incontinence.[413]

Obesity

There is an extensive literature linking fecal incontinence to obesity. Erekson and colleagues[127] measured BMI in 519 new patients attending a clinic for pelvic floor disorders and found a significant correlation with the presence of fecal incontinence (OR = 1.25 [95% CI, 1.09–1.44]) while the relationship with a defecatory disorder was not significant. Looked at from the other perspective, of the 256 women (BMI mean, 49.3 ± kg/m^2) attending a bariatric surgery seminar, 61% were found on questionnaire to have experienced incontinence, with a median Wexner score of 7 (1–20) and a score of 10 or more in 34%. Multivariate analysis showed that obstetric injury (OR = 2.4) and urinary infection (OR = 1.2) were significantly related to incontinence, but age, BMI, parity, diabetes, and hypertension were not.[485] There is a link between obesity, urinary incontinence, and fecal incontinence. Among 336 women aged 53 ± 10 years with more than 10 or more episodes of urinary incontinence over 7 days, 55 (16%) had fecal incontinence. This was related to low-fiber intake, a high depressive index, and urinary tract infection.[287]

The connection between urinary and fecal incontinence with obesity was further amplified in a report of the outcome of bariatric surgery in 404 patients whose symptoms were determined by questionnaire. Of the females, 78% had experienced urinary incontinence prior to the operation, of whom 39% felt that they had improved postoperatively. Only 21% of men experienced urinary incontinence preoperatively. The prevalence of fecal incontinence to liquid stool before bariatric surgery was 42% and 48% when comparison is made between the sexes—21% and 30% for solid stool, respectively. The operation resulted in worsening incontinence in 55% of women and in 31% of men. This was attributed to postoperative diarrhea.[377] In an age of increasing obesity surgery, this is an important consideration when advising patients and obtaining consent, as is discussed in a Bharucha's editorial article.[30]

In summary, fecal incontinence is related to generalized morbidities, including renal, pulmonary, cardiovascular disease, and obesity. It is related to intestinal symptoms, such as diarrhea and the irritable bowel syndrome, and to dementia. Social factors and psychiatric status are also important. The causes associated conditions differ between the sexes.

► MECHANISMS OF INCONTINENCE

Normal Continence

Continence is a balance between the ability of the anal sphincter mechanism to withstand the propulsive efforts of the distal intestine, which depends on motility patterns and adequate rectal capacitance. The anal sphincter and pelvic floor form a complex mechanism with motor and sensory nerve components.

Take your hands if you will and cup them.
Put in them a mixture of gas, liquid and solid,
And try to let only the gas escape—your will fail!
The anal sphincter mechanism can do this.
Furthermore, the sphincter mechanism can tell
Whether you are with friends or alone,
Whether you are sitting or standing, or whether you
have your pants on or off.
There is no muscle that is so prepared to preserve the
dignity of mankind
Yet so ready to come to one's relief.
—ROBERT W. BEART, JR, MD

The anal sphincter mechanism includes the anal sphincter itself and the levator ani (see Chapter 1). The latter forms the pelvic floor. It is composed of three parts, including the ischiococcygeus, the pubococcygeus, and the puborectalis (see Figures 1-11 and 1-12). The first two form a muscular sheet across the pelvic outlet with attachments to the back of the pubis, the obturator fascia, and the coccyx. This is penetrated in the midline by the urethra, vagina, and gut tube in female and by the urethra and gut tube in male. The puborectalis arises on each side from the back of the pubis and passes posteriorly to form a sling around the gut tube. This and the levator ani are in a constant state of tonic activity mediated by muscle spindles located in the levator ani. As a result, the puborectalis draws the gut tube forward to create an angle between the rectum and anal canal. Under normal resting conditions, the long axes of each form an angle, the anorectal angle, which is about 90 to 100 degrees. The puborectalis sling marks the functional junction between the anal canal and the rectum and is easily palpable on digital examination (Figure 16-2).

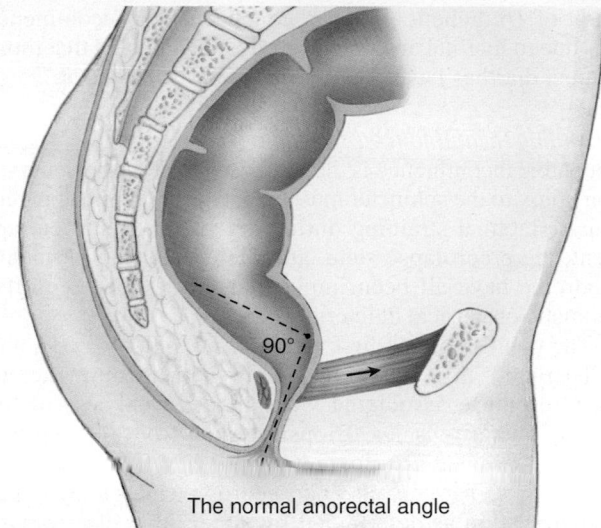

FIGURE 16-2. Normal anorectal angle.

The anal canal comprises the internal and external sphincters and its epithelial lining, which is richly supplied by sensory nerves. The internal sphincter is responsible for 70% of the resting tone.[27] It is maximally contracted at rest and shows reflex relaxation in response to distension of the rectum. This is referred to as the rectoanal inhibitory reflex (RAIR), which is under autonomic control and requires an intact submucous nervous plexus for it to function.[267] The pelvic floor musculature relaxes during defecation. Sensory factors include the sampling reflex that is disordered in incontinence.[178] It has been estimated that about 15% of anal resting tone is due to the hemorrhoidal complexes.[261] The longitudinal length of the anal sphincter complex in female is less than that of male.[493]

Causes of Incontinence

A classification of the causes of incontinence is shown in Table 16-2.

Increased Intestinal Propulsion

Fecal incontinence can be due to uncontrollable defecation as a result of inflammatory or functional disease of the rectum and more proximal bowel. Diarrheal disorders associated with urgency include any form of proctitis, but in clinical practice ulcerative colitis or Crohn's disease are the most important. Infective proctocolitides, dysentery, is usually self-limiting or responds to treatment, but it is necessary to consider this in the differential diagnosis of incontinence, particularly because the incidence of infective proctocolitis is increasing in Western society, especially in institutions (see Chapter 33). Organisms responsible include among others *Shigella*, *Clostridium difficile*, and *Campylobacter*. *C. difficile* and ulcerative colitis can present in an identical manner. There has been an "alarming" increase in *C. difficile*–associated disease (CDAD) in the United States. This has been dramatic in patients with inflammatory bowel disease (IBD). Rodemann and colleagues reported that between 1998 and 2004 in the United States, CDAD in ulcerative colitis patients rose from 18.4 to 57.6 (more than threefold) per 1,000 admissions.[379] In endemic areas, *Entamoeba histolytica* should be borne in mind.

Urgency may be the predominant feature in some patients with irritable bowel syndrome. It is important to recognize this because surgery has no role to play in the treatment, although neuromodulation may have a place.

Urgency incontinence may also occur as a result of inadequate capacitance of the rectum or "neorectum" in patients who have undergone restorative surgery or radiotherapy. In colorectal practice where many patients will have had a low anterior resection, for example, this form of incontinence is fairly common. Functional symptoms after anterior resection are referred to as the *anterior resection syndrome* and include the frequent passage of small-volume stool with passive and sometimes urgency incontinence. Those with this disorder may also have a weak sphincter (see next section).

Intrinsic Sphincter Incompetence

The anal sphincter mechanism may be unable to retain stool and flatus if it suffers damage to its nerve supply or as a consequence of direct trauma. Myopathic degeneration can also occur. There is a gradual physiologic weakening with age that can be identified by physiologic testing.[205]

Age

Attempts have been made to compare functional estimations of anal sphincter capacity in the elderly population with younger individuals. Bannister and coworkers measured anorectal function in 37 elderly patients and compared the results with 48 young, physiologically normal subjects.[18] The former had lower anal pressures, required lower rectal volumes to inhibit anal sphincter tone, and had increased rectal pressures as measured by balloon distension, implying lower compliance. Some suggest that internal anal sphincter dysfunction may be the important factor.[21] Others believe that, especially in women, the pudendal and somatic pelvic nerves are injured when there is perineal descent on straining such as occurs with aging or during childbirth.[244] Many geriatricians believe that fecal incontinence is more likely to be due to a remediable cause, such as fecal

TABLE 16-2 Causes of Incontinence

Increased intestinal propulsion
    Inflammatory bowel disease
    Functional bowel disease
Incompetent sphincter mechanism
    Age
    Neurologic disease
    Myopathy
Anorectal disease
Congenital anomaly
Extrarectal fistula
Trauma
    Obstetric injury
    Anorectal surgery
    Accidental trauma
Reduced rectal capacity
    Anterior resection
    Radiotherapy
Activation of the anorectal inhibitory reflex in fecal impaction

impaction, rather than to dementia, the postmenopausal state, or to old age.[283]

Neurologic Disease

Any neurologic disease may affect bowel control. Upper and lower motor neuron lesions seen in general neurologic diseases, injury to the spinal cord or cauda equina, spina bifida, and neuropathies can all be responsible. In diabetes mellitus,[484] there may be the dual factors of diarrhea from autonomic neuropathy and diffuse sphincter weakness due to the neuropathy.

General neurologic diseases including multiple sclerosis[206] and Parkinson's disease can be associated with incontinence. It is clearly necessary to be aware of the possibility of these when assessing the patient. Dementia due to cerebral degeneration in the elderly has already been mentioned. It and presenile dementia are among the most common causes of incontinence. Other conditions leading to cerebral damage include cardiovascular accident, trauma, and tumor.

Spinal cord injury results in weakness of the pelvic floor muscles, but it can also lead to failure of rectal evacuation, impaction, and soiling. Reflex defecation precipitated by sensory cutaneous stimulation above the level of the lesion may be maintained.

Trauma to the cauda equina, with damage to sacral 4 and 5 segments, causes lower motor paralysis of the pelvic floor and sphincter muscles. Voluntary contraction of the levator ani and external sphincter is reduced or absent depending on the severity of the lesion. Internal sphincter tone is preserved, however, because this is mediated by autonomic activity. There is sensory loss of the perineal skin and of the anorectum and patulousness after digital examination (Figure 16-3).

Spina bifida occurs in association with meningocele or myelomeningocele. Involvement of sensory or motor nerves may produce urinary and fecal incontinence and, with time, rectal prolapse, which will further exacerbate the incontinence. This condition is described in Chapter 21.

Rectal impaction causes internal sphincter relaxation through activation of the RAIR, owing to distension of the rectum by stool. This is a temporary effect that will resolve once the impaction is treated. Schiller and colleagues, in their

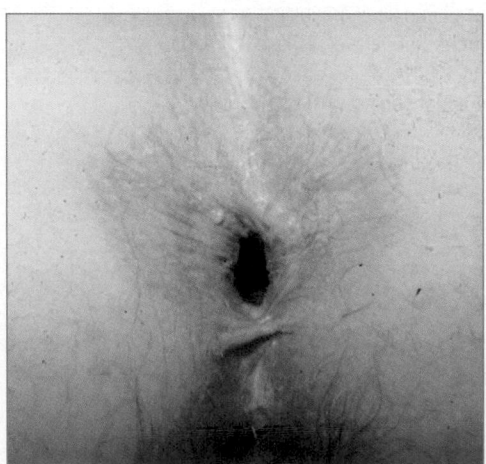

FIGURE 16-3. Patulous appearance of the anus immediately following rectal examination. Patient's incontinence was a consequence of spinal nerve injury.

study of 16 diabetic patients, concluded that incontinence was due to internal anal sphincter dysfunction and that those without diarrhea have no impairment of fecal control.[400]

Idiopathic Incontinence (Pudendal Neuropathy)

Idiopathic incontinence is the term used to describe denervation injury to the sphincter muscle that occurs for no apparent cause. Habitual straining during defecation, nerve entrapment, the preprolapse state, and the descending perineum syndrome have all been implicated. It may be seen after traumatic obstetrical delivery.

The condition was first formally defined by Parks and colleagues[352] in a group of patients with incontinence or rectal prolapse associated with diffuse weakness of the anal sphincter muscles. Biopsies taken from the external sphincter showed histologic evidence of atrophy of type I fibers. These patients also had neurophysiologic evidence of denervation as determined by single-fiber electromyographic (EMG) studies. This technique enables an estimate of the ratio of nerve to muscle fibers in the motor neuron unit. When denervation occurs, there is reinnervation by branching of intact nerve axons in an attempt to reach denervated muscle fibers. Consequently, the ratio of nerve to muscle fibers increases, and this can be detected neurophysiologically by direct recording of a needle electrode introduced through the skin into a nerve ending.[320] In addition, measurement of the speed of conduction in the pudendal nerve showed the latency to be increased.[227] Further studies in patients with idiopathic incontinence identified that most also have degenerative changes in the internal sphincter.[245,266] It was postulated that the neuropathic changes might be due to damage to the pudendal nerve through stretching, thereby causing a degree of apraxia as might occur with excessive descent of the pelvic floor, such as in the descending perineum syndrome or during childbirth. It is unlikely that stretching occurs at the level of the ischial spine because at this level the pudendal nerve has not yet branched to supply the sphincter, perineum, and clitoris. Computer modeling has hypothesized that potential stretch during delivery is more likely to damage the inferior rectal nerve.[263]

Objective evidence of a sensory deficit can be found in patients with idiopathic neuropathic incontinence, as would be expected in the presence of nerve damage. Others have supported the hypothesis that sensory function may be an independent factor contributing to continence.[22,31]

The normal anal canal is extremely sensitive to temperature. Moreover, there appears to be a temperature gradient between the rectum and the anal canal.[308,309] Ambulatory pressure monitoring has shown that the sphincter relaxes several times an hour, allowing equalization of rectal and anal pressures, which permits entry of small amounts of rectal contents into the anal canal.[307] This so-called sampling reflex may be lost with neuropathic change. Patients with idiopathic incontinence have reduced thermal sensation at all levels within the anal canal when compared with normal individuals.[306] Another report from the same unit involving patients with hemorrhoids and others with incontinence showed reduced sensation in incontinence but also in those with hemorrhoids, albeit to a lesser degree.[308] Others have challenged the importance of thermal sensitivity on the basis that the maximum temperature difference was merely 0.13° and was in the region of the anorectal junction.[381] Such a difference was considered too small in their view to have a meaningful role in sampling.

Myopathic Disease
Physiologic
Estrogen and progesterone receptors have been found in the internal sphincter, derived from tissue obtained from hemorrhoidectomy specimens in premenopausal and postmenopausal women. Although none of the differences was considered to be statistically significant, the numbers (17 in each group) were small—a type II error. In premenopausal patients, estrogen receptors were present in 23.5% compared with 11.8% in postmenopausal women. The respective proportions of progesterone receptors were 41.2% and 11.8%.[348]

Internal Sphincter Degeneration
Internal sphincter degeneration was described by Vaizey and colleagues in 1997.[466] They reported a series of 45 patients (35 females) who presented with passive incontinence associated with reduced resting anal and normal squeeze pressures. The pudendal nerve terminal motor latencies (PNTMLs) were normal. The internal sphincter on ultrasound was thinned and showed hypoechoic changes (Figure 16-4). The increased thickening seen with normal aging is not seen. Such patients may be suitable for neuromodulation (see later).

Scleroderma
Scleroderma is a chronic multisystem disorder characterized by excess deposition of connective tissue in skin and internal organs, associated with microvascular changes and immunologic abnormalities leading to nerve and muscle degeneration. This results in motility disturbances of the gastrointestinal tract. Thus, gastric emptying is delayed in up to 75% of patients, with small bowel involvement occurring in 17% to 57% of patients. The migrating motor complexes are reduced or absent, predisposing to bacterial overgrowth. Barium enema examination demonstrates pancolonic involvement in 10% to 50% of patients associated with

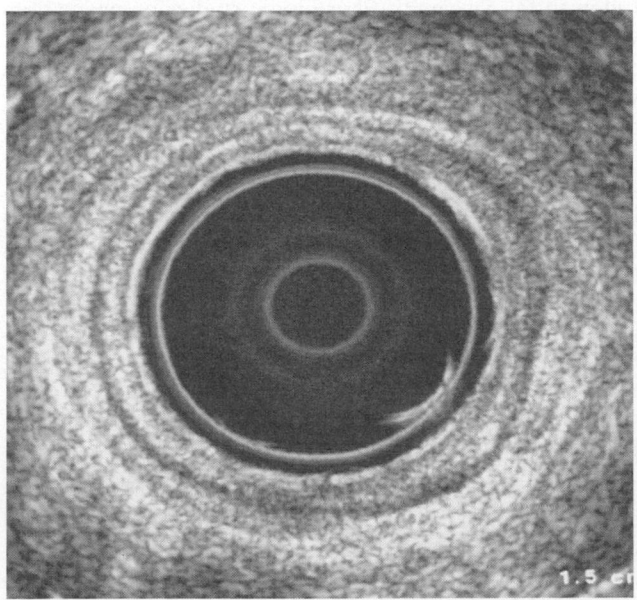

FIGURE 16-4. Anal ultrasound demonstrates internal sphincter degeneration.

wide-mouthed diverticula. Pseudoobstruction may occur. Complications include pneumatosis cystoides intestinalis, stercoral ulceration, and perforation.

Systemic sclerosis may produce incontinence on either a neurologic or a myopathic basis.[66,257] The condition affects the internal sphincter, which shows morphologic changes compatible with both neuropathy and myopathy, with atrophy and fibrosis. Resting tone is reduced, and the RAIR may be absent.[114]

Anal manometry may demonstrate a reduction or loss of the RAIR. Treatment includes biofeedback, sacral nerve stimulation, and surgery.[114,232]

Anorectal Disease
Soiling may occur in anorectal disease from such conditions as hemorrhoids, fissure, and anal fistula, even without surgical intervention. Prolapse of rectal mucosa or hemorrhoids and true procidentia may interfere with closure of the anal canal. With time, the protruding mass stretches the sphincter and may lead to further weakening. In addition, the rectal prolapse is likely to be associated with internal sphincter atrophy and pudendal neuropathy, both of which are factors responsible for its occurrence in the first place. The incontinence is often ameliorated with definitive treatment of the prolapse (see Chapter 21).[395]

Congenital Anomaly (See also Chapter 3)
Failure of embryologic development of the hindgut, pelvic floor, and related structures results in varying degrees of anatomical and functional deformity. The condition occurs in approximately 1 in 5,000 births. There are several classifications that mostly divide patients into those with a low, intermediate, or high anomaly. A high anomaly is often associated with a degree of sacral agenesis and in addition to anatomical loss of the lower gut tube; there is also sensory and functional loss of that part of the rectum that is present. The anal sphincter mechanism is not developed and may be too weak to maintain continence even after surgical procedures, such as pull-through operations and posterior sagittal anorectoplasty (PSARP). A megarectum may be present.

The adult colorectal surgeon may encounter patients with a congenital anomaly after leaving pediatric care. Many will have undergone surgery in infancy, either in the form of a pull-through procedure or a PSARP.[62,355,356]

Those with a low anomaly may have been satisfactorily managed by surgical recanalization when the lumen is absent by dilatation of the stenosed anal segment. The functional results may be disappointing. The condition is described in greater detail in Chapter 3.

Extrarectal Fistula
In this condition, there is an abnormal communication between the intestine above the level of the anal sphincter and the outside, usually the perianal skin. Etiologies and associated conditions include neoplasms, inflammatory conditions (Crohn's disease, diverticular disease), and anastomotic leakage. A fistula from an intra-abdominal organ to the perineum or vagina will result in fecal incontinence. A pouch-vaginal fistula is one of the most common conditions encountered in colorectal surgical practice.[185,412] Management is directed to the cause of the fistulization. This can be located in the intestine, the female genital tract, or to the urologic system. Figure 16-5 demonstrates a fistula to

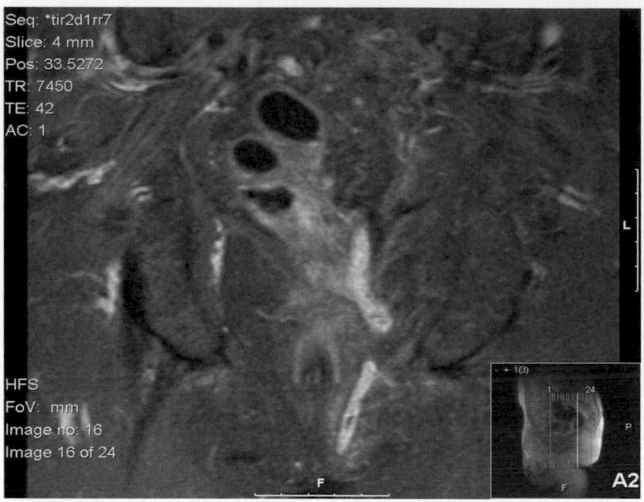

FIGURE 16-5. Magnetic resonance imaging of a fistula from the sigmoid colon to the perineum as a complication of diverticular disease.

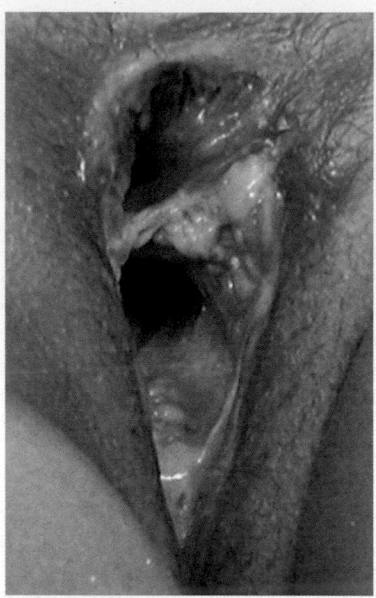

FIGURE 16-6. Cloacal defect following obstetrical injury. There is only a limited separation between the rectum and vagina.

the perineum from a segment of diverticular disease of the sigmoid colon. The diagnosis and management of extrarectal fistula will be dealt with in Chapter 14.

Trauma

The anal sphincter mechanism can be damaged by direct injury in the form of surgery, itself, or by civilian or military trauma. It can also be damaged during childbirth. In the practice of colon and rectal surgery, childbirth injury is now the most common cause of traumatic incontinence.

Obstetrical Injury

Direct Sphincter Trauma and Nerve Damage

During delivery, the pelvic floor is at risk from trauma due to stretching by the fetal head on the perineum. This may cause a tear in the anterior part of the sphincter. Such an injury may involve only the sphincter ring or it may result in a cloacal deformity if a complete rupture of the anal canal opens into the introitus (Figure 16-6). In recent years, more emphasis has been placed on this form of damage than on denervation injury. Both are, however, important and often occur simultaneously. Subclinical nerve damage during delivery may be a cause of incontinence years later as the natural process of neuromuscular degeneration leads to a situation where the sphincter is no longer competent. This may account for somewhat disappointing results following surgical repair.

Evidence of pudendal nerve damage from childbirth was first reported by Snooks and colleagues in 1984 who measured fiber density and PNTMLs in 79 women 2 months following delivery. Compared with controls, fiber density (1.37 vs. 1.67) and PNTML (1.9 vs. 2.1) were both abnormal in multiparous women, with recovery being evident in those who were primiparous.[418,419] Rieger and colleagues[375] found a fall in resting and squeeze pressures at 6 weeks after delivery among 53 primiparous women. Although a sphincter defect was found in 41%, this was not associated with lowered anal canal pressures. In a series of 259 women assessed at 6 weeks prior to and 8 weeks following delivery, a sphincter defect occurred in 16.7% and only in those undergoing a vaginal delivery. Multivariate analysis showed forceps delivery (OR = 12), perineal tear (OR = 16), episiotomy (OR = 6.6), and parity (OR = 8.8) to be risk factors for

incontinence. Overall, 9% had symptoms of incontinence, but of these only 45% were found to have a defect.

It has become clear that incontinence after childbirth can occur without a sphincter defect.[6] When pudendal nerve function was measured in 128 unselected women before and at 6 to 8 weeks after delivery, there was a significant increase in PNTML determinations in both primipara and multiparous women but not in 7 patients who underwent elective cesarean delivery, although not in those having a section after a trial of labor. Twelve women with increased PNTML at 6 weeks were reexamined at 6 months; 8 had returned to normal values.[435] In incontinent patients, the PNTML was increased and related to perineal descent, indicating the presence of neurologic damage to the whole pelvic floor in some patients.[245] Persistent evidence of pudendal neuropathy was evident among 14 multiparous women who were followed for 5 years.[422] Physiologic studies on postpartum women have shown that multiparity, forceps delivery, increased duration of the second stage of labor, and high birth weight may lead to pudendal nerve damage and to sphincter atrophy.[421]

Anal ultrasound has demonstrated a high incidence of subclinical sphincter damage following delivery (Figure 16-7). In many cases, the presence of a defect on ultrasound has been interpreted as an indication for surgical repair. Many of these instances, however, are not associated with disruption of the sphincter ring, and repair offers, therefore, no benefit in this circumstance. Poor case selection may be another factor to explain some of the unsatisfactory results following repair.

Incidence

The use of ultrasound (Figure 16-8) has enabled the incidence of sphincter injury during childbirth to be studied objectively. In a group of 202 women who had an anal ultrasound prior to delivery, a repeat examination was undertaken in 150 at 6 weeks and in 32 at 6 months after delivery. Symptoms of anal incontinence were present in 10/79 (13%)

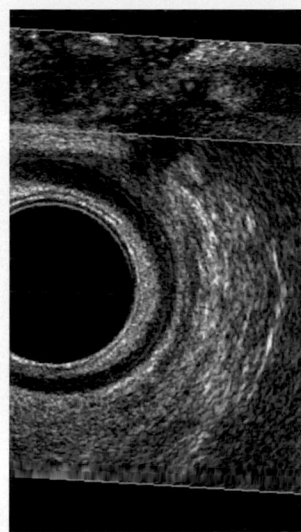

FIGURE 16-7. Three-dimensional ultrasound image of an occult tear of the external anal sphincter in the left anterior position. Note that the internal anal sphincter is intact.

of primiparous individuals and in 11/48 (23%) of those who were multiparous. A sphincter defect was found in 28/79 (35%) and 19/48 (40%) at 6 weeks and in 22/79 (28%) of primiparae at 6 months. None of the 23 patients who had a cesarean delivery were found to have a defect. Eight of 10 patients who had forceps assistance developed a defect compared with none who had vacuum extraction. There was a correlation between a sphincter defect and symptoms of incontinence, including urgency as well as soiling.[436]

A similar finding was reported by Pollack and colleagues from a questionnaire survey of 349 nulliparous women who then became pregnant.[366] Of these, 242 returned the questionnaire at 5 and 9 months and 5 years after delivery. At 5 years, incontinent symptoms were reported in 53% of women who had a sphincter tear and in 32% of those who did not. Age, sphincter tear, and subsequent childbirth were all risk factors for incontinent symptoms at 5 years. It is important to point out that in most of these patients "incontinence" was no more than occasional loss of flatus and that fecal incontinence was rare. de Leeuw and colleagues found that 12 (35%) of their 34 patients who suffered a sphincter injury at the time of delivery experienced difficulty with bowel control.[98] Sphincter defects were demonstrated in the majority. The protective effect of cesarean delivery was demonstrated in a study of 1,200 women, half of whom underwent assessment after delivery.[503] In those who had a vaginal delivery, there was a fall in anal canal resting pressure, although this did not occur after cesarean delivery. The first vaginal delivery appeared to cause a permanent lowering of resting anal pressure. Frudinger and colleagues found that anal continence deteriorated in 27.6% of women following delivery, 43.2% of whom had sonographic evidence of sphincter trauma.[144] Others have shown a high prevalence of anal sphincter defects on ultrasound (up to 62%) in incontinent, parous women without a prior history of anal surgery.[91,318]

In a study of 3,002 primiparous women who delivered between 1983 and 1986 recorded on the U.K. National Health Service database, 62% responded to a questionnaire sent two decades later. Of the 985 with adequate data, 54% recorded some form of pelvic floor symptom. About 5% had

severe impairment of continence to solid stool. Cesarean delivery was protective for both urinary (OR = 0.47) and fecal (OR = 0.32) incontinence, but of 76 who had only a cesarean delivery, 9 (12%) had experienced some degree of fecal continence disturbance.[107]

In most patients, fecal incontinence when present resolves spontaneously within the first year. Thus, in a series of 86 primiparous women having vaginal delivery, 19 (25%) had flatus incontinence at 5 months, but this had fallen threefold by 12 months.[319] In some patients symptoms persist, with the rate estimated to be approximately 3%.[111] Macarthur and colleagues followed 4,214 women by mail questionnaire for 6 years.[270] The prevalence of fecal incontinence at 6 years was 3.6%. Interestingly, only 10% of patients had any symptom after the first delivery. Cesarean delivery was not related to the development of symptoms (OR = 1.04), but forceps-assisted delivery at any time was (OR = 1.48). Other risk factors included high maternal age, multiparity, and Asian ethnicity. There is other evidence indicating that African Americans have a lower incidence of pelvic floor trauma than other racial groups.[14,200] In their study of 128 unselected women, Sultan and associates found that a heavy baby and a prolonged second stage of labor were associated with abnormal pudendal function following delivery.[435]

Patients who have persisting symptoms of postpartum incontinence, or present with late onset fecal incontinence, have a high prevalence of sphincter injury. Thus, the presence of a sphincter defect among 335 patients with fecal incontinence was 65%, rising to 88% in those who had had a vaginal delivery and proctologic surgery. This compared with 43% of patients without symptoms of incontinence and with 22% in asymptomatic volunteers, the latter suggesting that the criteria for determining a sphincter defect may have been too liberal.[220] Not all reports have indicated obstetrical

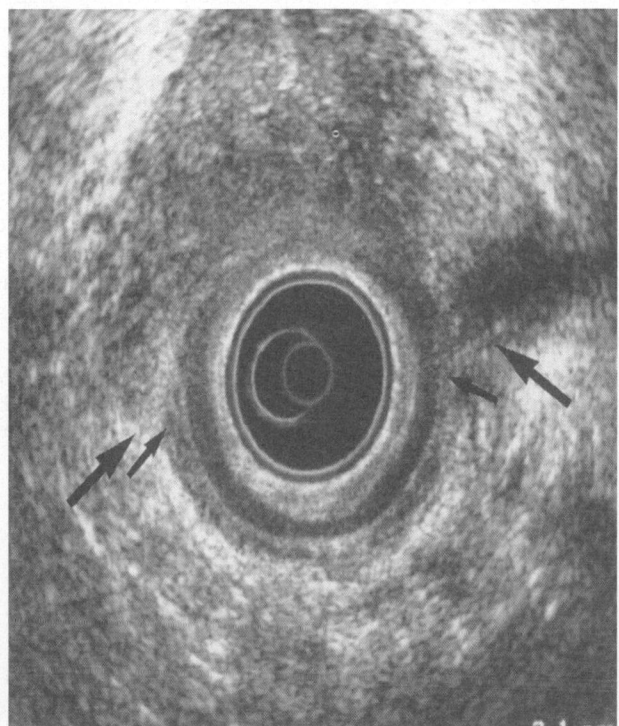

FIGURE 16-8. Anal ultrasound demonstrates external sphincter anterior defect (*large arrows*) with associated internal sphincter defect (*small arrows*).

injury is associated with incontinence. In another questionnaire survey, Fritel and coworkers received a response from 85% of 3,114 women aged 50 to 61 years.[141] Fecal incontinence within the prior 12 months was experienced by 250 (9.5%) and was related to depression (OR = 2.1), obesity (OR = 1.5), previous surgery for urinary incontinence (OR = 3.5), and anal surgery (OR = 1.7), but not to any obstetrical variable, such as parity, mode of delivery, birth weight, episiotomy, or third-degree perineal tear.

The symptoms and prognosis of incontinence may be related to the severity of the obstetrical injury. In a series of 52 women having a third- or fourth-degree tear treated by repair, 31 (61%) had persisting symptoms. The prevalence of a defect in each group was 39 (75%) and 10 (20%).[362] A mail survey by questionnaire was carried out in 180 women out of 5,123 who experienced a vaginal delivery in one Norwegian county between 1999 and 2000. Of these, 156 (87%) responded. At a median of 25 months, 88 (59%) experienced incontinence symptoms that were restricted to flatus in 53 (35%). Fourteen (9%) patients had urgency as the only symptom. It is noteworthy that only 3 of 29 women who regarded themselves to be severely disabled had sought medical help.[331] Others, however, have not found a correlation with the severity of the tear and symptoms. In a study of 330 patients with fecal incontinence, Voyvodic and colleagues found no correlation between the ultrasonic severity of external and internal sphincter defects and symptoms.[483] Resting tone was not related to whether or not there was a defect of the internal sphincter, although patients with a fragmented sphincter did have a low resting pressure. In contrast, however, Nichols and colleagues carried out a prospective study of 56 women who sustained a third- or fourth-degree tear of whom 39 were enrolled.[328] Those with a fourth-degree tear were more likely to have bowel symptoms (59% vs. 28%) and a persistent defect (48% vs. 8%).

In another study of 55 women having their first baby, ultrasound evidence of trauma was found in 13 (29%), but clinical significance was confined to the 5 patients with evidence of external sphincter damage.[490]

Encopresis

Encopresis, or psychogenic soiling, is defined as the passage of formed or semiformed stool in a child's underclothes (or other inappropriate places) that occurs regularly after the age of 4 years. It is essentially an involuntary evacuation of the bowel not caused by organic factors. Encopresis is at least four times more common in boys than in girls and is analogous to enuresis as it pertains to urinary incontinence.

The condition was first described by Weissenberg who recognized that this form of fecal incontinence was associated with emotional disturbance. Behavioral factors that may contribute to the problem include the following:

- Excessive parental attention to toilet habits
- Laxative use
- Harsh or lax toilet training methods
- Fear of the toilet or the loss of feces
- Desire for attention
- Family or personal stress

In time, the increasing retention of feces leads to attenuation of the rectal wall, lax sphincter contractility, progressive constipation, obstipation, and fecal impaction. Anal fissure and hemorrhoidal difficulties may develop. Loening-Baucke observed a common clinical history with children exhibiting chronic constipation and soiling, often many years of infrequent and abnormal stools, a dilated rectal ampulla, and the presence of an abdominal fecal mass.

Treatment is usually directed toward bowel management, stress reduction, and child and family psychological counseling. Laxatives, enemas, and dietary regimens are recommended, as well as encouraging the child to sit on the toilet for 10 minutes twice daily at the same time each day. The goal is to establish a practical time for defecation and, ultimately, a spontaneous bowel evacuation habit. Uridine-5-triphosphate has been suggested to have some limited success. Although the mechanism of action of this drug has not been ascertained, it is believed to stimulate the cortical substance of the brain to make the child more aware of the need to defecate.

Loening-Baucke used anorectal manometry to evaluate 20 healthy children, 12 with constipation, and 20 with chronic constipation and encopresis. Mean values for anal resting tone and anal pull-through pressure were lower in the constipated and the encopretic children than in the controls. The study was repeated up to 4 years after treatment for the condition; abnormal anorectal function was still apparent even years after cessation of treatment and apparent recovery. In a later study of 97 children, also by Loening-Baucke, the author reported that 57% had not recovered. Using a host of training techniques, Loening-Baucke noted that there was no difference in recovery rates for boys and girls, and that the likelihood of success or failure could not be predicted a priori.

Summary

The incidence of fecal incontinence after delivery is about 3%. Certainly, disturbance of control of flatus is common. The incidence of a sphincter defect ranges from 10% to 40% depending on the study and the woman's parity. There is evidence of pudendal nerve damage in a high proportion of primiparous women as well as multiparous, but resolution of abnormal latency occurs in at least two-thirds of cases. However, it may be permanent in a few cases. Obstetric factors, which have been related to continence after delivery, include sphincter tear, perineal tear, episiotomy, forceps assistance, long second stage, epidural anesthesia, and birth weight of more than 4 kg. Damage to the external sphincter is more clinically significant than that of the internal sphincter.

Prevention

Prevention of sphincter injury during childbirth is dependent on numerous factors. First is the recognition of risk. Patients at greater risk include multiparous individuals; those with prior history of obstetrical trauma, especially if an episiotomy or repair of a tear had been required; and those with general risk factors for incontinence, such as obesity and advanced maternal age. Second known obstetrical risk factors should be avoided as far as they are possible to avoid. Some of these can be recognized before labor commences. A large baby should be identified in advance although prenatal estimation of birth weight. However, such estimates are prone to inaccuracy. Clinical assessment seems to be as accurate as ultrasound estimation.[113,175,182,438] An estimated weight of more than 4 kg should prompt one to perform a cesarean delivery. A history of obstetrical difficulty or of large bowel surgery, such as a restorative proctocolectomy, should lead the obstetrician to advise a cesarean delivery.

Once labor has started, delay in the second stage should be recognized early and thought given to performing a cesarean delivery if the time is significantly prolonged.[108] This might reduce the need for episiotomy or instrumental assistance. In the United States, an episiotomy was performed in 25% of deliveries in 2003 with a range of 13% to 95%.[167,236] This approach leads to a higher incidence of sphincter injury, with a greater risk associated with midline than with mediolateral episiotomy.[79,415] Forceps assistance is needed in approximately 4% of deliveries.[313] This method is indicated based on the duration of the second stage of labor.[64] The reality is that every type of instrumentation can cause damage to the sphincter,[113] with new symptoms of fecal incontinence reported to occur in as many as 59% of women requiring forceps assistance.[138] Despite some evidence to the contrary, ventouse extraction (vacuum assisted) appears to be no less traumatic when compared with forceps assistance.[148,458]

Cesarean delivery is protective against sphincter damage unless it is carried out late in the second stage.[145] Its incidence is increasing, and recent reports indicate that in the United States 29% of all deliveries are by this means[316]; the figure in the United Kingdom is approximately 23%.[475]

Diagnosis

Third- and fourth-degree injuries are diagnosed immediately in about 1.5% to 9% of deliveries. Occult injury can be difficult to identify in the acute phase, owing to the presence of blood and edema.[92] It is clear that the incidence varies with experience in that in one study the incidence was estimated in turn by midwives, junior doctors, specialist trainees, and consultants as 87%, 28%, 14%, and 1% of cases, respectively.[13]

As indicated previously in patients with a chronic sphincter injury, ultrasound is more sensitive than is clinical examination,[437,439,442] but the clinician should be aware of overdiagnosis. Evidence of a scar on ultrasound may be called a "defect," when in reality it does not represent a true disruption of the anal ring. Therefore, a repair in this circumstance is not indicated because it cannot improve the mechanical integrity of the anal sphincter. It is helpful for the clinician to be familiar with the Starck scoring system for ultrasonic defects.[428]

Treatment

Obstetrical injury causing a tear should be treated by immediate repair if recognized. When it is not accomplished or if after repair a defect persists, then the question may be asked whether a surgical repair or some other treatment should be offered. This is discussed next.

Anal Surgery

Fistula-in-Ano. The adverse effect of fistula surgery on continence has been recognized for many years (Figure 16-9).[34,36] Varying degrees of impairment for control are seen even after what is considered to be a limited division of the sphincter muscle. Complete incontinence (for formed stool) that follows anorectal surgery is usually the result of inappropriate division of the anorectal ring. This is most likely to occur when a high fistula is laid open or an artificial internal opening is created (see Chapter 14).

Internal Anal Sphincterotomy. Internal anal sphincterotomy (Figure 16-10) has been the preferred surgical treatment for anal fissure for many years (see Chapter 12). It is still the most effective approach to the management of this condition when

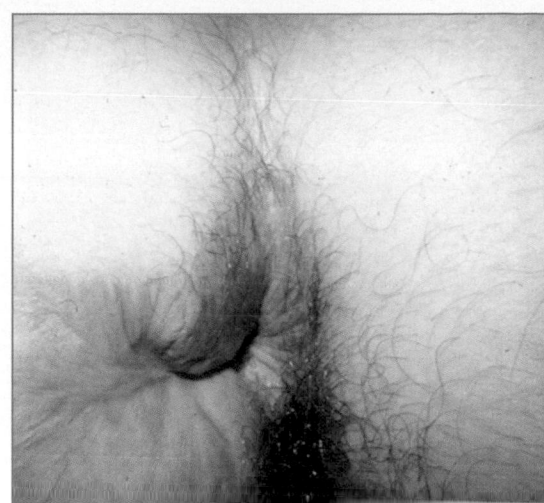

FIGURE 16-9. Scarring, deformity, and partial sphincter loss as a consequence of anal fistulectomy.

conservative treatment fails. Unfortunately, there is a small incidence of incontinence associated with this operation. The literature, however, confuses minor with major incontinence, and in many of the reports, preoperative continence has not been recorded. The results of medical and surgical treatment have been summarized by Nelson in two excellent Cochrane reviews,[321,322] with a commentary in an editorial by this author.[326] The incidence is probably well below 5% and the type of soiling is minor, with mostly small amounts of mucous discharge or flatus. It may be that a form of "tailored" sphincterotomy will avoid this possibility.[119,190] There is a more detailed discussion of this topic in Chapter 12.

Anal Dilatation. Sphincter stretch for anal fissure or manual dilatation as a treatment for hemorrhoids (Lord's procedure) is also associated with fecal incontinence. This was first reported by Snooks and colleagues before anal ultrasound was available.[417] In a series of 10 patients who had undergone a Lord's anal dilatation, they demonstrated impairment of both the external and internal sphincters. Subsequent reports of the ultrasonographic changes showed disintegration of both sphincters.[330,424] Damage caused in this manner results in a

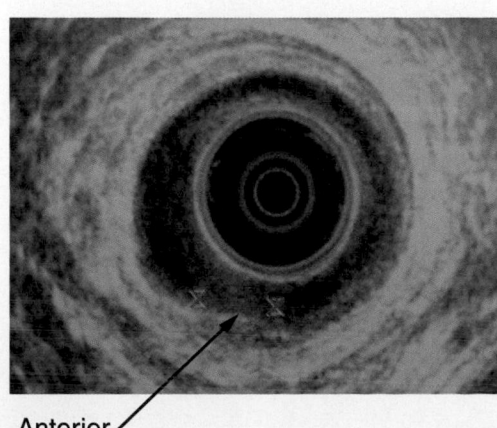

Anterior

FIGURE 16-10. Anal ultrasound showing internal anal sphincter defect (*arrow*) following sphincterotomy.

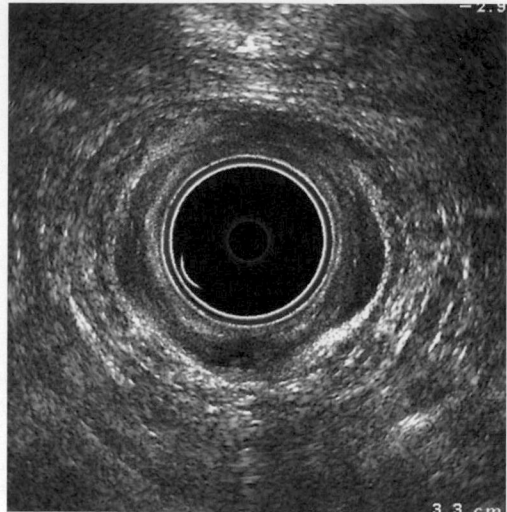

FIGURE 16-11. Anal ultrasound demonstrates fragmented sphincter following anal dilatation.

destruction of the normal sphincter anatomy and is untreatable by conventional repair (Figure 16-11). For this and other reasons, hemorrhoids are no longer treated by manual dilatation.

Other Anal Operations. Partial incontinence may follow hemorrhoidectomy. This may further impair closure of the canal and allow continuous discharge of mucus (see Chapter 11).[168]

Accidental Trauma

Trauma to the perineum can injure the sphincter mechanism (Figure 16-12). Impalement on a spike or pole as well as social injuries (e.g., fist fornication) may result in rupture of the sphincter and contamination of the extrarectal spaces.[53,89,265,343,494] Sepsis can supervene and lead to excessive scar formation with a resultant patulous anal canal and an incompetent sphincter (see also Chapters 17 and 18).

Reduced Rectal Capacity
Anterior Resection

In low anterior resection, there are several factors that can impair continence. These include the loss of the rectal reservoir, damage to the anal sphincter mechanism, reduced sensation, and the effect of radiotherapy. This last factor may cause direct radiation damage to the sphincter if this is in the field of irradiation. If radiation is given postoperatively, it will reduce neorectal compliance (see later). Bowel resection designed to preserve the anal sphincter (e.g., low anterior resection, various pull-through procedures, coloanal anastomosis, abdominosacral resection) frequently results in discharge of mucus or incontinence for flatus and stool by the effect of anterior resection on the rectal capacitance, sphincter function, and neural regulation. Injury to the levator ani and external sphincter or to their innervation, and the decreased capacity of the neorectum, are contributing factors.[192,295,327]

Some degree of sphincter stretch occurs when a low coloanal or ileoanal anastomosis is carried out, either by transanal stapling or manually.[197] Even after a stapled ileoanal anastomosis, resting tone falls in 50% of patients.[68] This gradually improves with time (up to 2 years) but never fully recovers. In a prospective, randomized study of transanal-stapled anastomosis compared with the use of biofragmentable ring, 5 of 18 patients in the former group had ultrasound evidence of fragmentation of the internal sphincter that was associated with symptoms.[193]

Clinically, the patient will suffer from frequent small-volume evacuations, often without warning and often associated with incontinence usually of the soiling type.[345,497]

Pelvic Radiotherapy

Radiotherapy will cause direct injury to the anal sphincter if this is in the field of irradiation as is the case of patients having treatment for anal carcinoma.[425,473] Damage to the rectum can also occur following radiotherapy for prostatic carcinoma.[272,365,445] When used for the treatment of rectal cancer, radiotherapy doubles the risk of poor function because

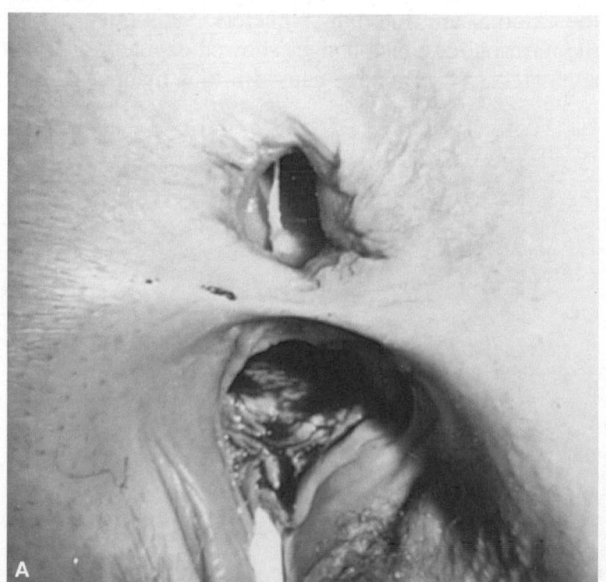
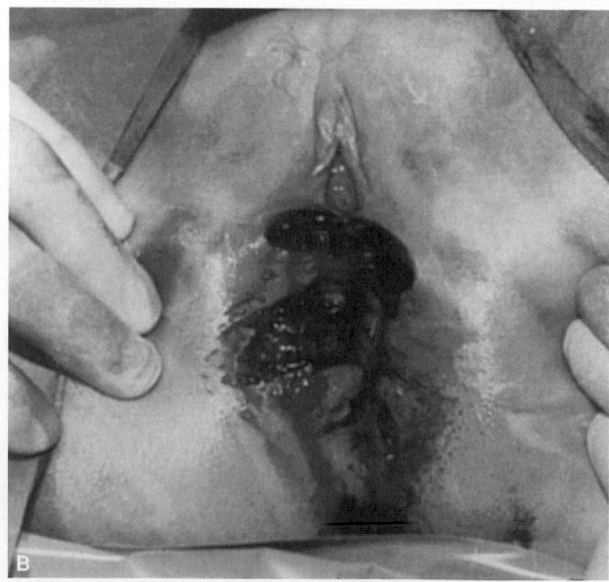

FIGURE 16-12. Perineal injuries as a consequence of accidental trauma. **A:** Patulous anus with avulsed sphincter from impalement on a picket fence. **B:** Severe perineal trauma from impalement on a bedpost as a consequence of jumping in bed.

it is superimposed on the anterior resection.[122] This is particularly true when given postoperatively.[269] The long-term effects of adjuvant radiotherapy that was employed in the Swedish trials, especially those involving five 25 Gy fractions, have been reviewed by Birgisson and colleagues.[33] Surgical options are limited, with every operative approach having a high complication and failure rate (see Chapter 24). Most patients are, therefore, usually managed conservatively by antidiarrheal agents and a bowel management program or by fecal diversion.[179] Sacroneuromodulation has been used in four patients after anterior resection with chemoradiotherapy, of whom three appeared to benefit from permanent implantation.[372]

Activation of the Anorectal Inhibitory Reflex
Patients with fecal impaction often are incontinent owing to the reflex development of internal sphincter relaxation. This results in passive leakage of stool associated with a physiologically patulous sphincter.

▶ ASSESSMENT

Symptoms
The history is the key for a proper assessment of the patient. It should not be hurried and should not be obtained by a tick box method performed by the patient alone or a nonmedical person. A pro forma history is useful, however, because it results in full capture of all aspects of the background of the incontinence. However, it should be filled in by the physician seeing the patient. The first aim of the history is to determine the nature of the symptoms, their severity, and the degree to which they are affecting the patient's life (now called "quality of life"). The frequency of incontinent episodes and the volume of stool lost on each occasion should be established. This last can range from a normal fecal bolus to a stain on the underwear. It is useful to ask the patient whether the stool lost is three or two dimensional. Frequency should be expressed as episodes per unit time such as 24 hours (not "day"), week, or month. The ability to hold flatus should be noted. The consistency of the stool will often have a bearing on incontinence. A gradation from watery to thin porridge to thick porridge to sausages (normal) to golf balls or rocks is a useful means of recording consistency.

It is essential to determine the presence of urgency and to quantify it. It is not sufficient to state that urgency is "mild, moderate, or severe" because this form of assessment can vary according to the patient's interpretation. Urgency should be recorded objectively in minutes as stated by the patient when asked the question, "When you want to go to the bathroom, how many minutes do you have?" The answer—for example, "less than 1," "5," or "15"—can be used quantitatively in the assessment of any improvement after treatment. This was employed with useful effect in the assessment of patients entered in the multicenter prospective undertaking, the 301 study of sacral nerve stimulation (Figure 16-13).[291] Urgency may be the patient's most troublesome symptom.

The history should also record whether the patient uses pads and if so how many per 24 hours. It should determine the social incapacity experienced by the patient—for example, the degree to which normal activity such as shopping or social occasions is limited.

Other Factors in the History
The second aim of the history is to determine the cause of the incontinence. It must, therefore, include details of previous obstetrical deliveries, anal operations, and symptoms that may possibly indicate neurologic, intestinal, or anal disease. The occurrence of rectal prolapse should be inquired about. Previous treatment such as rectal surgery or radiotherapy for cervical or prostatic cancer should be determined.[272] The obstetrical history should include details of the type and number of deliveries, whether vaginal or cesarean, the duration of labor, any forceps or ventouse assistance, any tears whether episiotomy or inadvertent, and the birth weight of the infant.

The overall health of the patient, including an assessment of comorbidities such as pulmonary, renal, and cardiovascular disease, should be ascertained. A drug history is essential. A past or present history of psychiatric disease or dementia must be obtained and the social circumstances of the patient established.

Conclusion
Patients with loss of sphincter function through injury, whether surgical, obstetrical, or accidental, are the most amenable to reconstructive surgery, whereas those with incontinence due to disease or a locally diffuse weakness of the pelvic muscles are generally poor candidates for an attempt at repair. For these individuals, conservative treatment in the form of dietary advice, antidiarrheal medication, and behavioral therapy such as biofeedback should be the initial approach along with treatment of any underlying disease. Some of these patients will be candidates for neuromodulation if conservative management is not successful (see later).

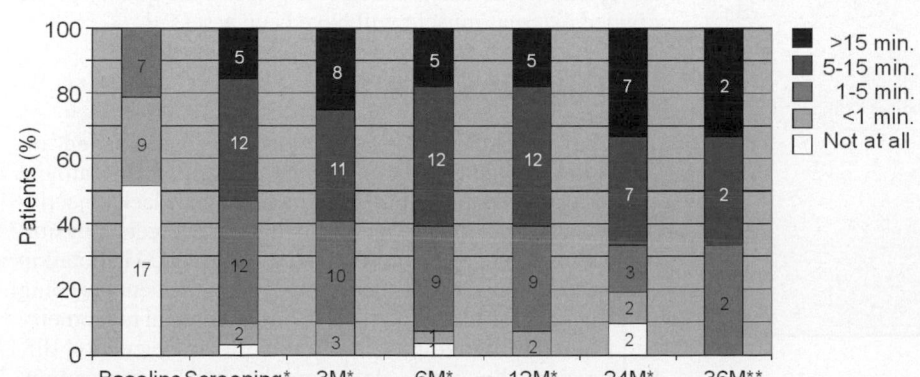

FIGURE 16-13. Quantitative change in urgency after sacral neuromodulation: The 310 Study. (From Matzel KE, Kamm MA, Stösser M, et al. Sacral spinal nerve stimulation for fecal incontinence: multicentre study. *Lancet.* 2004;363(9417):1270–1276.)

Having obtained the history, the physician will know the nature of incontinence, its severity, the likely cause, and the degree to which the patient's life is being affected.

Physical Examination

A general medical evaluation should include an assessment of the skin, oral cavity, lymph nodes, and a brief neurologic examination. This involves patient orientation and cognitive ability and motor and sensory defects in the perineum and lower limbs. A rectoscopy will identify proctitis if present. Anorectal examination by inspection and palpation should reveal the information that will dictate treatment.

Inspection

Fecal soiling around the anus may be noted. On spreading the patient's buttocks, it will be possible to determine whether the anus is patulous, implying a weak internal sphincter from neuromuscular impairment. Inspection will determine whether the anal sphincter ring is intact or whether it is ruptured. This is one of the most important signs that will determine whether a sphincter repair is likely to help the patient. The presence of a scar alone does not indicate disruption if, for example, it represents the site of a previous repair or an episiotomy and when the sphincter ring is intact. A scar with a disrupted ring, however, may be a sign that a repair may be necessary or appropriate. The most obvious example of this abnormality is the presence of a cloacal deformity. This is usually caused by complete disruption of the anterior sphincter into the posterior vaginal wall (see Figure 16-6). A deliberate attempt to identify a mucosal ectropion (Figure 16-14) or a rectal prolapse (Figure 16-15) must be made because this will involve a different management plan from other causes of incontinence. If a prolapse is suspected from the history but is not initially evident during the examination, the patient should be asked to strain while sitting on the toilet (see Chapter 21). The presence of perineal descent during staining should be noted. Spontaneous opening of the anal canal or sphincteric relaxation is said to be indicative of anoreceptive sexual intercourse or it may suggest neurologic impairment.

Palpation

Palpation allows the resting tone of the anal canal to be assessed. Most of the effects are due to contraction of the internal sphincter. The patient is then asked to "tighten up," and the degree of contraction or the "squeeze pressure" is

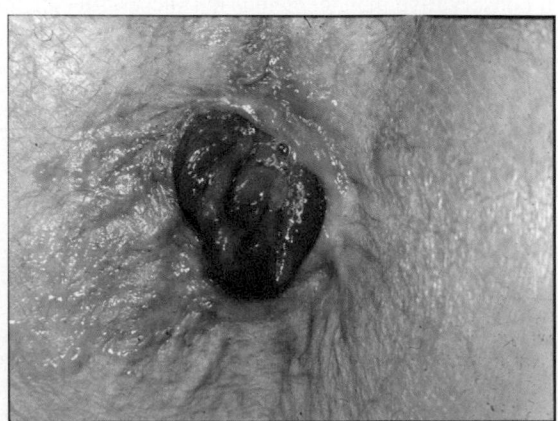

FIGURE 16-14. Mucosal ectropion.

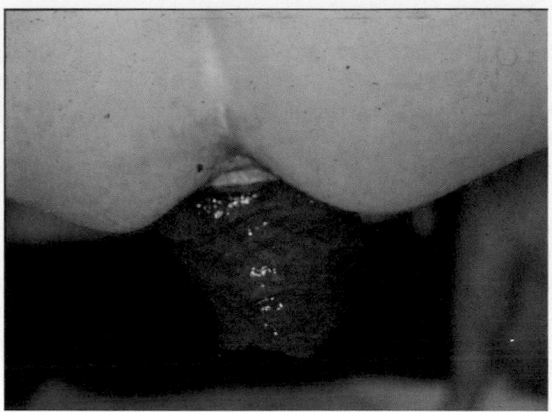

FIGURE 16-15. Full-thickness rectal prolapsed.

evaluated. The examiner will be able to judge whether the contraction is normal or reduced. In extreme cases, it may be absent. The key question is whether any weakness felt is diffuse or localized. Diffuse weakness is a feature of pudendal neuropathy as occurs in idiopathic incontinence (see previous discussion). A localized weakness may be the site of a sphincter injury. In patients with disruption of the anal ring, an assessment of the quality or contractility of the divided external sphincter can only be obtained by palpation. With the finger in contact with the muscle, it is possible to gauge the power of its contraction. This is not possible by the physiologic tests currently available because pressure recording in a disrupted anal canal will not reflect the activity of either sphincter.

In neurologic conditions, including lesions of the spinal cord and cauda equina, the tone may initially seem to be normal. However, when gentle traction is applied to the anorectal ring, the anal orifice is seen to gape (see Figure 16-3).[177] Thus, Hill and colleagues performed a prospective study on 237 patients with idiopathic fecal incontinence and were able to demonstrate that an informed history and digital examination can predict the manometric findings and specialized anorectal physiologic studies with a high degree of accuracy.[188] Others have reported the same conclusions.[173,221] Sensory testing of the perineal skin is essential in patients with neurologic disease. Spinal and cauda equina lesions result in reduced sensation of sacral segments, S4 and S5, which will be apparent by soliciting numbness of the perineum and buttocks.

At the end of the examination, it should be possible to state whether the anal ring is intact, whether the anal muscle is diffusely weak, and whether the muscle is normal but interrupted by a defect. If a defect is present, the quality of the divided external muscle will have been assessed.

▶ INVESTIGATION

The clinical history and examination will give sufficient information to enable one to make the most suitable treatment choice for most patients but, unfortunately, they lack objectivity. Such information is obtained by tests of anorectal physiology and imaging. Physiologic testing is described in detail in Chapter 7. In current practice, almost all patients undergoing investigation for incontinence will have anorectal manometry and anal endosonography. In those with an evacuation difficulty, cineradiography, defecography, balloon evacuation, and estimation of intestinal transit may also be performed—the first two particularly for patients with suspected rectal external or internal prolapse and the last for those with defecatory disorders (e.g., constipation, fecal impaction).[46,106] If incontinence is believed to be due to a neurologic disorder, the opinion of a neurologist should be solicited.

Physiologic Studies

Physiologic evaluation of the gastrointestinal tract is now routinely performed in any specialized unit treating incontinence.[134] This is useful not only for research but also for assisting in the management of the patient. The reader is referred to Chapter 7 for information on setting up such a laboratory. A working party comprising some prominent investigators who had contributed extensively to the literature on anorectal physiology was established in 1988 to determine indices of anorectal physiology.[223] Their recommendations were useful at the time, but during the subsequent 20 plus years, there have since been changes in the value placed upon various aspects of these studies. This applies particularly to EMG and pudendal nerve latency, both of which have declined in importance in the evaluation of incontinence in the opinion of many investigators.

EMG was first studied by Beck in the 1930s for the investigation of the sphincter (see Chapter 7).[24] The working party felt at the time that it was still a useful test. Since then, however, it has been less frequently employed owing to the pain caused by insertion of the needle electrode as well as the introduction of anal ultrasonography. This latter study is now the first-line investigation for assessing the state of the musculature.[459] The recommendations also supported the value of pudendal nerve latency as an indication of the degree of denervation of the pelvic floor musculature.[189,444] Since then, however, it has been felt by many in the field that the poor reproducibly and the unreliability of action potential recording have reduced its value. It is now more of research than of clinical interest in my opinion. Further details of this technique are given in Chapter 7.

Anal Manometry

Manometry involves measurement of the resting tone. This is mostly due to the contraction of the internal sphincter (resting pressure), the functional length of the anal canal, the increase in anal canal pressure due to the voluntary contraction of the external sphincter (squeeze pressure), and the RAIR.[27] Computerized vector manometry was developed because conventional manometry is not able to determine whether a lowered anal canal pressure is due to a diffuse or to a focal sphincter lesion.[40,357] As a research tool, this technique has been able to construct a three-dimensional anal pressure vectorgram from the data obtained by manometry and has allowed the anus to be viewed from all angles (see Figures 7-5 through 7-8). It was hoped that it would reveal occult anal sphincter injury to improve the selection of patients for sphincter repair, but despite its promise the technique has not become part of routine investigation.

Technique

Anal manometry can be undertaken using various techniques, such as open-tipped or closed-tipped catheters, perfused catheters, macroballoons, and microballoons (see Chapter 7). Most units today use an open-tipped perfused catheter

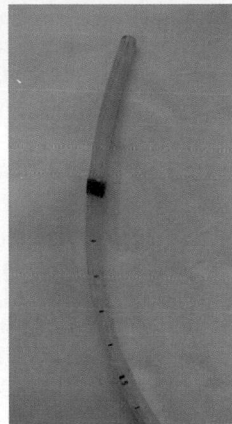

FIGURE 16-16. Open-tipped manometric catheter.

(Figure 16-16). Variations in recording instrument diameter consistently affect measurements of resting anal canal pressure and the maximum squeeze pressure (MSP).[296] Interpretation of physiologic studies is made difficult by incomplete knowledge of the physiology of defecation.[80] Ambulant manometry is technically difficult to accomplish and remains a research tool.[15]

Normal Values

Pedersen and Christiansen studied 78 healthy volunteers to determine the range of normal physiologic variations with anal manometry.[354] They found that the maximum intraindividual variations in the length of the anal high-pressure zone, the resting pressure, and the squeeze pressure were 10, 26, and 68 mm Hg, respectively. The median length of the pressure zone was 4 mm (14 mm Hg resting and 48 mm Hg squeeze). No gender difference was found in the length of the high-pressure zone, whereas resting pressures and squeeze pressures were higher in men than in women. One study has shown that male patients with so-called idiopathic fecal seepage may have a long anal sphincter with an abnormally high resting tone.[347] Standard tests of anorectal sensorimotor function have been reproducible by different investigators, suggesting that comparison of data from different institutions is probably valid, provided the methods employed are clearly defined.[382]

The working party agreed that maximum resting anal pressure (MRP) should be used to denote the highest recorded pressure at any site in the anal canal at rest, and the MSP should be defined as the highest recorded pressure at any site in the anal canal during maximum voluntary (squeeze) contraction.[223] Despite their recommendation to report pressure in kilopascals (100 cm of water = 9.8 kPa), most continue to use centimeters of water or millimeters of mercury.

Applications

Anorectal manometry is a useful objective measure to assess the power of the internal sphincter in patients with an intact sphincter ring and of the external sphincter during voluntary contraction. In patients with a disrupted ring, the pressure in the anal canal at rest or during maximal squeeze will not be a reflection of the intrinsic function of either sphincter.

Generally, patients suffering from problems with bowel control have lower anal canal pressures at rest and during maximum voluntary contraction than normal. There is also overlap of the value of squeeze pressures between asymptomatic patients and those with impairment for bowel control. Many factors contribute to the mechanism for continence, and impairment of one may be compensated by the combined function of others.[238]

Pudendal Nerve Terminal Motor Latency

The PNTML used to be regarded as one of the most useful of physiologic parameters for the evaluation of incontinence, for determining prognosis, and for ascertaining response to treatment. The prevalence of increased latency (defined as a PNTML greater than 2.2 m/second) in 96 patients with fecal incontinence was 70% overall (75% female; 50% male) and was greater in patients with perineal descent or in those having had a difficult labor or excessive straining during defecation.[383] Others have compared measurement of the PNTML with anal manometry in individuals with anal incontinence. In a study of 38 females and 14 males with fecal incontinence, the prevalence of an increased PNTML was 52%, being greater in females, but there was no relationship between increased PNTML and anal resting or voluntary squeeze pressures. PNTML might have been related to a shorter sphincter length, however.[477] Manometry alone is, therefore, not helpful in identifying neuropathy, although Sangwan and coworkers found a good correlation between PNTML, single-fiber density estimation, and the RAIR. They felt that the RAIR was a good indication of the presence of neuropathy.[398] Despite some slight discrepancy, the investigators believed that RAIR compared favorably with PNTML in diagnosing pudendal neuropathy.

PNTML requires training to reduce inaccuracy. Yip and colleagues compared the measurement of PNTML by students and teacher in 50 patients (41 females, 34 with fecal incontinence) and found a false-positive rate of about 20% among the students. The difference reduced, however, with experience and was abolished after 40 or more examinations.[506] Despite this observation, no correlation between the PNTML and sphincter defect was found in a study of 124 females with late onset fecal incontinence, of whom 88 (71%) had a defect on ultrasound.[340] Pudendal neuropathy was less common in those with (15% to 20%) than in those without (30% to 35%) a defect. The value of PNTML in the assessment of patients can be questioned further from the results of a study of 1,404 patients with fecal incontinence attending a pelvic floor outpatient clinic, of whom 83 were found to have an intact sphincter on anal ultrasound. Of these, only 28% had a raised PNTML (threshold >2.2 milliseconds), and although there was a correlation between PNTML and resting tone and fecal incontinence score, there was none with voluntary contraction pressure. This might have been expected if PNTML is an indication of pudendal neuropathy.[373]

In practice, PNTML is used less now than it had been 10 years ago for both diagnosis and assessment. It is susceptible to observer variation and may not correlate with the outcome after treatment. Anal ultrasound is a far more useful diagnostic modality because it gives an accurate picture of the anatomy of the anal sphincters as well as the possible occurrence of sphincter damage.

Sensation

Anal sensation is measured in the anal canal and the lower rectum by determining the current in milliamperes required to be felt by the patient on electrical stimulation—the higher the threshold, the greater the sensory deficit.[380] The normal values of anal and rectal sensation are 2.0 to 9.4 mA and 7.0 to 36 mA, respectively. Anal sensation is reduced in neurologic diseases and in patients with injury to the spinal nerves supplying the perineum. Those with idiopathic incontinence associated with pudendal neuropathy have reduced sensation.

Rectal Sensation
Volumetry
Being a capacitance organ, the rectum is distensible. It can detect different degrees of distension from the first perception of the presence of a balloon introduced into the rectum to a sense of urgency with greater distension, and to a final point of maximal tolerable volume. The volumes at which these sensations occur will be a reflection of the capacitance of the rectum and also a reflection of its nerve supply.

The patient lies in the left lateral position. A balloon mounted on a catheter with a three-way tap is inserted into the rectum (Figure 16-17). The balloon is gently inflated with air or water from a 60-mL bladder syringe. The patient is asked to state when the balloon is first felt, and this volume is recorded. Inflation continues until the patient senses urgency and finally with further inflation, the patient is no longer able to tolerate the degree of distension. There is a large range of the threshold, urge, and maximal tolerable volumes as follows: 10 to 30 mL, 30 to 70 mL, and 120 to 250 mL. The volumes will be reduced where there is chronic inflammation of the rectal wall that leads to rigidity and loss of compliance, such as occurs in IBD and radiation proctitis. The volumes will also be reduced if the rectum has been replaced by colon or ileum in reconstructive surgery unless a reservoir has been constructed. They will also be increased with a megarectum and in neurologic disorders where denervation has occurred.

The Rectoanal Inhibitory Reflex
The patient lies in the left lateral position. A rectal balloon is inserted, and an anal balloon or open-tipped catheter is placed in the anal canal and fixed to the perianal skin in order to maintain its position. The anal pressure is continuously recorded. After a steady state has been achieved, 50 mL of air or water is introduced into the rectal balloon. This will induce a reflex fall of anal pressure. This maneuver is repeated, and the tracing is kept as a record of the investigation.

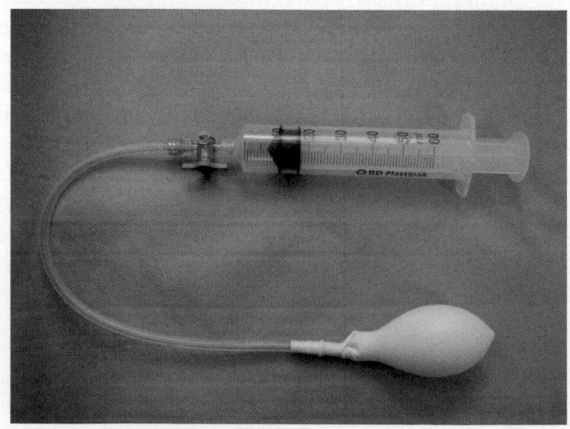

FIGURE 16-17. Balloon for estimation of rectal volume.

The reflex is absent in Hirschsprung's disease; this is the most sensitive test in the diagnosis of this disorder. Sun and coworkers were able to demonstrate a close association between rectal distension and external sphincter contraction.[443] Fecal incontinence occurred in some patients in their study as a result of delayed or absent external anal sphincter contraction when the internal sphincter relaxed. Bannister and colleagues analyzed the responses to rectal distension in 18 women with idiopathic fecal incontinence.[19]

Imaging

Anal Endosonography

This technique was developed and introduced into clinical practice by Bartram who modified the probe used for endorectal ultrasound, replacing the balloon with a sheath of adequate diameter to permit acoustic contact with the anal canal lining (Figure 16-18).[249] The space between the sheath and the sensor on the probe, itself, was filled with degassed water. This technique has revolutionized the diagnosis of many anal and pelvic floor disorders, and in the case of incontinence, it allows identification of both internal and external sphincters. It can demonstrate the thickness of the former and the integrity of the sphincter ring. A normal anal sonograph is shown in Figure 16-1. Defects appear as amorphous areas of varying echogenicity that interrupt the normal striated pattern (see Figure 16-8).[248]

The technique was compared with electromyography in 15 women who had sustained an obstetrical injury, and the results demonstrated for the first time that an objective picture of the sphincter could be obtained, including the presence of a defect.[247] The examination was well tolerated, much more so than electromyography, and a subsequent study revealed significant abnormalities in most of 44 patients with incontinence.[248] Its ability to detect defects was confirmed in a second publication.[52] Voyvodic and coworkers demonstrated a correlation between the size of the tear and anal pressures.[483] Endoanal ultrasound has been used extensively for the identification and detection of defects in the anal sphincter as described previously.[90,99,116,120,128,133,376,436] Sultan and colleagues have also used vaginal endosonography to image the anal sphincters.[440] Anterior internal and external sphincteric defects can be clearly identified with both techniques, but obviously vaginal endosonography is limited to the anterior sphincter.

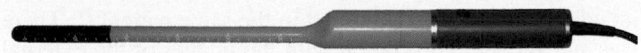

FIGURE 16-19. Brüel & Kjær Medical 2050 probe for three-dimensional endosonography. (Courtesy Brüel & Kjær, Wilmington, MA.)

Three-dimensional Endoanal Sonography

BK Medical Systems (Brüel & Kjær, Wilmington, MA) introduced the 2050 Transducer with built-in, three-dimensional imaging capability (Figure 16-19). The scanning head is moved along a 60-mm distance inside a fully encapsulated probe by using two control buttons on the handle of the transducer.[169] Thus, the technique differs from conventional two-dimensional ultrasound in that multiple images are acquired during automatic withdrawal of the probe in short steps. Interpretation is not made in real time as it is with two-dimensional ultrasound. The images of three-dimensional ultrasound can be obtained by a technician and interpreted by the radiologist or clinician at a convenient time later.

Gold and coworkers at St. Mark's Hospital used this multiplanar imaging technique to reveal the length and radial extent of a sphincter tear (Figure 16-20).[159] Twenty controls and 24 patients with fecal incontinence were studied. They were also able to clearly demonstrate the sex differences in sphincter configuration. Bollard and colleagues attempted to quantify the nature, characteristics, and frequency of variations in female anal sphincter anatomy.[38] They observed that nulliparous women have a variable natural "defect" occurring along the anterior length of the sphincter, a factor that may contribute to overinterpretation of the existence of defects. Three-dimensional ultrasound imaging may ultimately prove to be the most useful diagnostic tool in the assessment of an individual with anal incontinence.

Magnetic Resonance Imaging

The application of high-resolution imaging of the anal sphincter mechanism has been achieved by means of an endoanal coil.[100] The St. Mark's Hospital group affirmed that an external sphincter injury can be readily assessed by means of endosonography.[492] Williams who also compared this technique with that of three-dimensional endosonography analyzed the anal anatomy at similar levels by a graphic. Williams and colleagues used an overlay technique, whereby the images of three-dimensional ultrasound and magnetic resonance

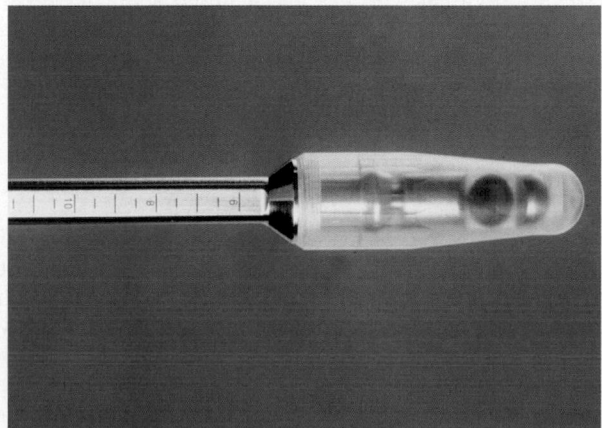

FIGURE 16-18. Two-dimensional endosound probe (7.5 MHz). (Courtesy Brüel & Kjær, Wilmington, MA.)

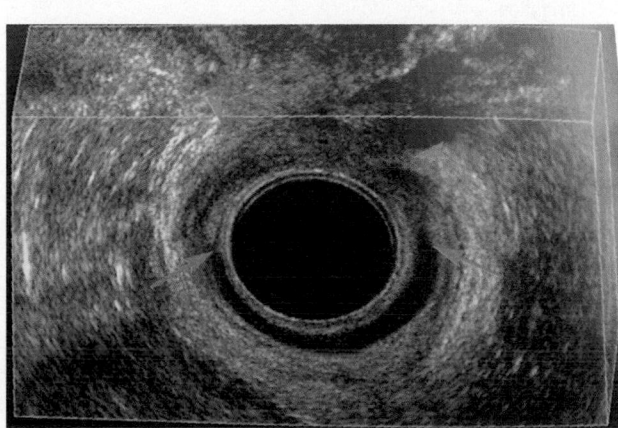

FIGURE 16-20. Three-dimensional ultrasound image of sphincter tear (*arrows*, internal sphincter; *arrowheads*, external sphincter).

imaging (MRI) were combined in the same patient.[491] There was an excellent correlation with the images of the external and internal sphincters but not with the longitudinal muscle.

Magnetic imaging is expensive and given the accuracy and easy availability of ultrasound, it has remained primarily a research tool. It may, however, be a method of quantifying atrophy of the external sphincter. Briel and colleagues were the first to use MRI to assess this.[44] They studied 20 female patients aged 50 years (range, 28 to 75) and found atrophy in 8 (40%). Its presence was related to the clinical outcome. They subsequently studied 25 women with fecal incontinence who had a sphincter repair following obstetrical injury. Biopsies of the external sphincter were taken at operation. The MRI showed atrophy in 9 (36%), which was confirmed histologically in 8.[45] Williams and colleagues studied 25 female patients, none of whom had a normal resting pressure and 16 had a low squeeze pressure. The respective cross-sectional area of the external sphincter was 240, and the mean fat content was 23%.[492]

► MANAGEMENT STRATEGY

Result of the Assessment

The clinical examination and investigations will allow the following to be determined:

- *Severity of incontinence* from the history
- *Intact or ruptured anal ring* by inspection and confirmed by anal ultrasound
- *Diffuse or localized sphincter weakness* by palpation and anal ultrasound
- *Presence or absence of sensory loss* by clinical sensation testing, electrical sensitivity, and balloon volumetry

---

TABLE 16-3 Fecal Incontinence: Treatment Options

Noninvasive

Conservative treatment
 General measures
 Drugs
 Biofeedback
 Irrigation
 Anal plug

Invasive

Injectables
SECCA
Neuromodulation
 Sacral nerve
 Pudendal nerve
 Posterior tibial nerve
 Dorsal nerve of penis/clitoris
Surgical repair
Artificial sphincter
Gracioplasty
Artificial bowel sphincter (ABS)
Stoma

TABLE 16-4 Algorithm for the Management of Fecal Incontinence

Sphincter intact	Medical treatment Failure → SNS Failure → ? Artificial sphincter Failure → Colostomy
Sphincter defect	Repair if large, SNS if small Failure → Repeat repair or SNS Failure repeat repair → SNS Failure SNS → ? Artificial sphincter/colostomy

SNS, sacral nerve stimulation.

This will permit the surgeon to make a recommendation as to the management plan. The options available are shown in Table 16-3.

Algorithm for the Management of Anal Incontinence

An algorithm for the management of fecal incontinence based on current evidence is shown in Table 16-4.

The key to decision making depends on whether the sphincter ring is intact or not. This is determined on clinical examination by inspection and by anal ultrasound. Failure of all reasonable attempts to relieve incontinence will then require fecal diversion as the optimal surgical alternative.

A patient with a *complete sphincter ring* will not respond to repair because surgery cannot improve on the anatomical situation. Conservative treatment should be attempted. If this fails, operations include neuromodulation, anal canal injection, SECCA, or irrigation.

A patient with a *disrupted sphincter ring* will be helped by surgical repair if the displacement is large, such as may be present with a cloacal deformity. Where sphincter disruption is of a lesser degree, the patient may be suitable for a sphincter repair or for neuromodulation (sacroneuromodulation being the only approach that has been tried thus far). An individual who has had a failed sphincter repair, and in whom the muscle is still of good contractility, may benefit from a second attempt at repair. Irrigation is also an option in this group of patients when the aforementioned treatments fail.

► GENERAL APPROACH

The first question to answer is whether the patient should be treated conservatively in the first instance. The answer to this will depend on two factors, including the severity of the incontinence and the capability of other methods to improve the situation. In general, conservative treatment should be attempted unless it is obvious that some form of invasive treatment is inevitable. A cloacal deformity with severe incontinence is an example of a condition when repair is indicated. In most patients, however, conservative treatment should at least be tried.

When should conservative measures be abandoned in favor of invasive treatment? The answer to this question is the same for all functional conditions; it is when the patient feels, with full knowledge of the options, including their disadvantages, that another treatment should be tried. When this position has been arrived at, treatment options divide according to whether the sphincter ring is intact or not, such as is described previously.

▶ NONINVASIVE TREATMENT
Conservative Management

Unless the patient has a lesion that obviously requires surgery, such as occurs with acute perineal trauma, or a chronic traumatic lesion with wide displacement, conservative measures should be tried. This will comprise most patients. Conservative treatment includes a set of measures such as education, promotion of healthy living, dietary advice, and drug treatment. The patient may also feel improvement simply by receiving the attention of a therapist, having perhaps previously had little support, sympathy, and information.

General Measures

The measures to be taken will depend to a considerable extent on the type of incontinence and the age and social circumstances of the patient. General principles include education of the patient as to the anatomy and function of the pelvic floor as well as the mechanism of defecation. Weight reduction in the obese and daily exercise for everyone should be advised.[23,402] Smoking may reduce intestinal transit time, a habit that may aggravate a tendency to urgency.[406] If individuals are living in community-based accommodations, particularly when they require help from a caregiver, it is essential that a routine be established. This includes regular visits to the bathroom and the maintenance of a clean and well-ordered environment. Unfortunately, this is not always the case when it comes to many institutions. Therefore, education of the management personnel and caregivers is an important part of the program for improving the patient's life. Such a regimen should emphasize the importance of avoiding constipation; clearly, if impaction develops, incontinence will ensue. It is also important to avoid urgency incontinence by anticipating the individual's need for nearby bathroom access. In selected individuals, rectal irrigation may have a place (see later).[69]

Drugs that the patient is taking should be reviewed. This will include any nonstandard medications such as herbal treatments. Laxatives and products which thin the consistency of the stool should be identified. It should be recognized that patients with incontinence often manipulate their diets.[176] This may involve avoiding meals or reducing the volume of food ingested. It is important to bear the possibility of nutritional deficiencies in mind and to check the blood count for anemia. In general, any dietary advice should be personalized with inquiry made as to foods that in the patient's experience may tend to induce loose stools. There is some evidence that increasing dietary fiber may be beneficial,[35] but in another study it was not found to be helpful.[246]

Drug treatment for incontinence includes antidiarrheal agents as well as those used to treat constipation. Loperamide is generally considered the drug of choice for diarrhea. It has no irreversible side effects, although it can be associated with bloating and abdominal cramps in some patients. In those with passive incontinence, phenylephrine theoretically might be beneficial through its direct effect on the smooth muscle of the internal sphincter. There is precious little information on this, however.

Perineal Exercises

In 1950, Kegel suggested an exercise regimen that appeared to be beneficial in both fecal and urinary incontinence.[222] Since that time, numerous articles have been published attesting to the validity of this approach. Although it probably is not possible to increase internal anal sphincter tone by perineal strengthening exercises, muscle bulk and voluntary contractility of the external anal sphincter, puborectalis sling, and levatores may be improved by such a regimen.

Biofeedback

This is a difficult area because of the numerous subjective influences to which behavioral treatments in general are liable

ARNOLD HENRY KEGEL (1894–1981)

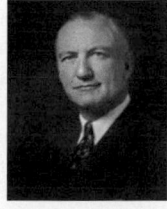

Kegel was a California gynecologist who invented the Kegel perineometer (used for measuring vaginal air pressure) and Kegel exercises (squeezing of the muscles of the pelvic floor) as a nonsurgical treatment for genital relaxation, urinary incontinence, and fecal incontinence. The following is a quote from his paper:

Experience with muscle education and resistive exercises of the pubococcygeus has proved gratifying whenever these procedures have been applied to conditions due to, or connected with, impaired function of the pelvic musculature. On the basis of therapeutic results achieved, it seems possible that other ill-defined complaints referable to the genital tract in women might profitably be studied from the standpoint of muscular dysfunction. For instance, it has been found that dysfunction of the pubococcygeus exists in many women complaining of lack of vaginal feeling during coitus and that in these cases sexual appreciation can be increased by restoring function of the pubococcygeus. The field of physiologic therapy of the pelvic muscles is thus much wider than at first suspected.

Today, pelvic floor exercises are widely held as first-line treatment for urinary stress incontinence and female genital prolapse, with evidence supporting its use from systematic reviews of randomized trials in the Cochrane Library among others. Kegel first presented his ideas in 1948. He was assistant professor of gynecology at the University of Southern California School of Medicine. (Photo courtesy of Gladser Studios; biographic sketch through Wikipedia.)

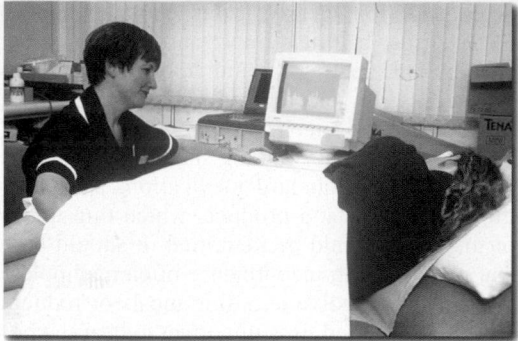

FIGURE 16-21. Patient in biofeedback treatment room with therapist and monitor.

and, in addition, to the particular effect the therapist is likely to have on the patient. Biofeedback involves the combination of monitoring of anal pressure, which the patient can relate to his or her own attempts at contraction of the pelvic floor and the attention of a therapist (Figure 16-21). An interesting observation on the value of exercise was made by Engel and colleagues in a report of six patients who had severe fecal incontinence from diverse causes.[125] They inserted a 50-mL balloon into the rectum and recorded the response to sphincter contraction on a polygraph. By verbal reinforcement, each patient was able to sense the rectal distension and associated this stimulus with attempts to tighten the sphincter. This technique became known as biofeedback and has become one of the mainstays of conservative treatment. It is emphasized, however, that it is one part of a routine consisting of many features as outlined previously.

There are useful reviews on biofeedback, one of the first being that of Heymen and colleagues.[186] Norton and associates reviewed the published trials of biofeedback and found 70 noncontrolled and 11 controlled studies.[334,336] All reported that biofeedback resulted in improvement, but the dropout rate was approximately 20%. The treatment groups often contained patients with various conditions, and few papers revealed long-term results. Most of the studies contained small numbers, and all were from single centers. In the 11 controlled studies, there were 592 patients; improvement occurred in 70%.

In a recent randomized, controlled trial aimed at determining whether the availability of biofeedback added value to pelvic floor exercises, there were 108 patients (83 females) with incontinence of at least 1 teaspoon of feces per week.[187] They were randomized to pelvic exercises alone and pelvic exercises plus biofeedback. The patients entered a 4-week period of education and medical treatment. Those who experienced success were then excluded from the trial. The remainder went on to exercises (63) and exercises plus biofeedback (45). They each had six 1-hour training visits once in 2 weeks for 3 months. The patients were then evaluated (53 vs. 40) at 3 months. Those who had a successful result were then assessed at 1 year. The biofeedback included display of rectal and anal canal pressures to the patient, with the end points of perception of a 10-mL rectal balloon and a squeeze of 125 mm Hg maintained for 10 seconds. At 3-month assessment on an intention to treat basis, 20 (44%) of 48 biofeedback and 13 (23%) of 63 exercises only patients were free of incontinence. The frequency of days per week with fecal incontinence was 0.83 ± 1.5 and

1.6 ± 2.0 days per week ($P = .083$). At 12 months, 24 of the 45 biofeedback patients had "adequate relief" compared with 22 of the 63 exercises only patients.[187]

Electrical Stimulation

Electrical stimulation in incontinence has also been the subject of a Cochrane review.[199] These authors found four eligible trials containing a total of 260 patients. The results were contradictory, although symptoms improved in the stimulation group in each report. The authors concluded, however, that it was not possible to determine that stimulation was the factor responsible.

Electrical stimulation with biofeedback was compared with biofeedback alone in a multicenter (six center) randomized trial. One hundred fifty-eight patients with incontinence for any reason (sphincter damage, rectocele, fistula surgery, previous hysterectomy, etc.) were randomized to receive amplitude-modulated, medium-frequency stimulation with EMG-biofeedback ("triple treatment") or EMG-biofeedback alone twice daily for 9 months. At randomization, there were 79 patients in each group, but this had fallen to 52 and 62 at 6 months and to 19 and 43 at 9 months. Patients were lost to follow-up largely because they were satisfied with the results, because they had become discouraged, or did not have the time. The Cleveland Clinic scores at baseline were 10.9 ± 4.2 and 11 ± 4.8 in the EMG-biofeedback alone and the triple treatment groups, and these were 7.8 ± 5.1 versus 6.0 ± 5.3 at 6 months and 7.3 ± 5.2 versus 4.8 ± 5.7 at 9 months.[403] In an invited editorial, Norton comments on the high attrition rate of the study.[333] In addition, the patients had various causes for their incontinence, and the variance of the continence scores was quite considerable. Thus, the conclusions from the study that stimulation adds to biofeedback were not secure.

Anal Plug

In 1984, Prager described a device for control of feces from an end colostomy.[368] Although this fell from use owing to the occurrence of local pressure necrosis in some cases, the balloon used was adapted for anal use. Mortensen and Humphreys investigated three different designs of an anal continence plug made of polyurethane sponge coated with a water-soluble surface in 10 patients (Figure 16-22).[310] Patients were able to tolerate them for a median of 12 hours, indicating their potential usefulness in selected patients with anal incontinence.

Deutekom and Dobben reviewed the literature and found four trials of the anal plug.[101] Two compared plug to no plug,[472] one compared two plugs of the same brand,[335] and one compared two plugs of different brands. There was no report of the outcome related to the severity of symptoms. Moreover, there were methodologic defects, including incompleteness of follow-up, failure to blind (three studies), and failure to assess on an intention to treat basis (three studies). Of 20 individuals tested, 14 were not able to tolerate the plug because of discomfort.[335] There is a suggestion that plugs made of polyurethane function are better than those of polyvinyl alcohol.[101]

Colonic Irrigation
Antegrade

In 1990, Malone and colleagues described an antegrade colonic irrigation technique for the management of anal incontinence through the creation of a tube appendicostomy.[280]

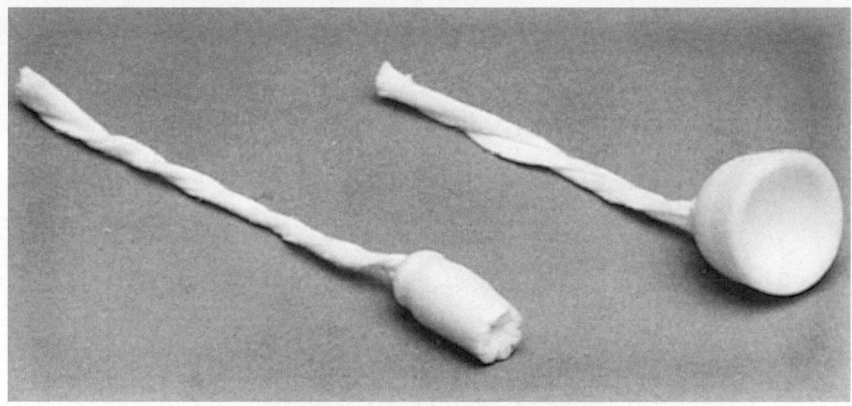

FIGURE 16-22. Prototype conceal anal continence plug. The plug is wrapped in a water-soluble coat **(left)** and is inserted like a suppository with the gauze tape outside the anal canal. The expanded plug sits in the upper portion of the anal canal to facilitate bowel control **(right)**. (Courtesy of Neil Mortensen, MD, John Radcliffe Hospital, Oxford, United Kingdom.)

This has been applied to the treatment of defecatory disorders in children with intractable constipation and for fecal incontinence. Levitt and colleagues developed a modification of this approach and reported their experience in 20 children with anal incontinence, for whom bowel management with conventional enemas was unsuccessful (Figures 16-23 and 16-24).[262] Krogh and Laurberg reported 16 adults who underwent this approach, 10 of whom had fecal incontinence.[237]

Marked improvement was noted in 8, with all experiencing improvement in quality of life. Poirier and colleagues reported the results of the Malone operation in 18 patients with a defecation disorder followed for a mean of 18.5 months (range, 3 to 67).[364] Five had incontinence, 4 of whom reported a satisfactory result.

Hughes and Williams described a colonic conduit that incorporated an intussuscepting valve to manage fecal

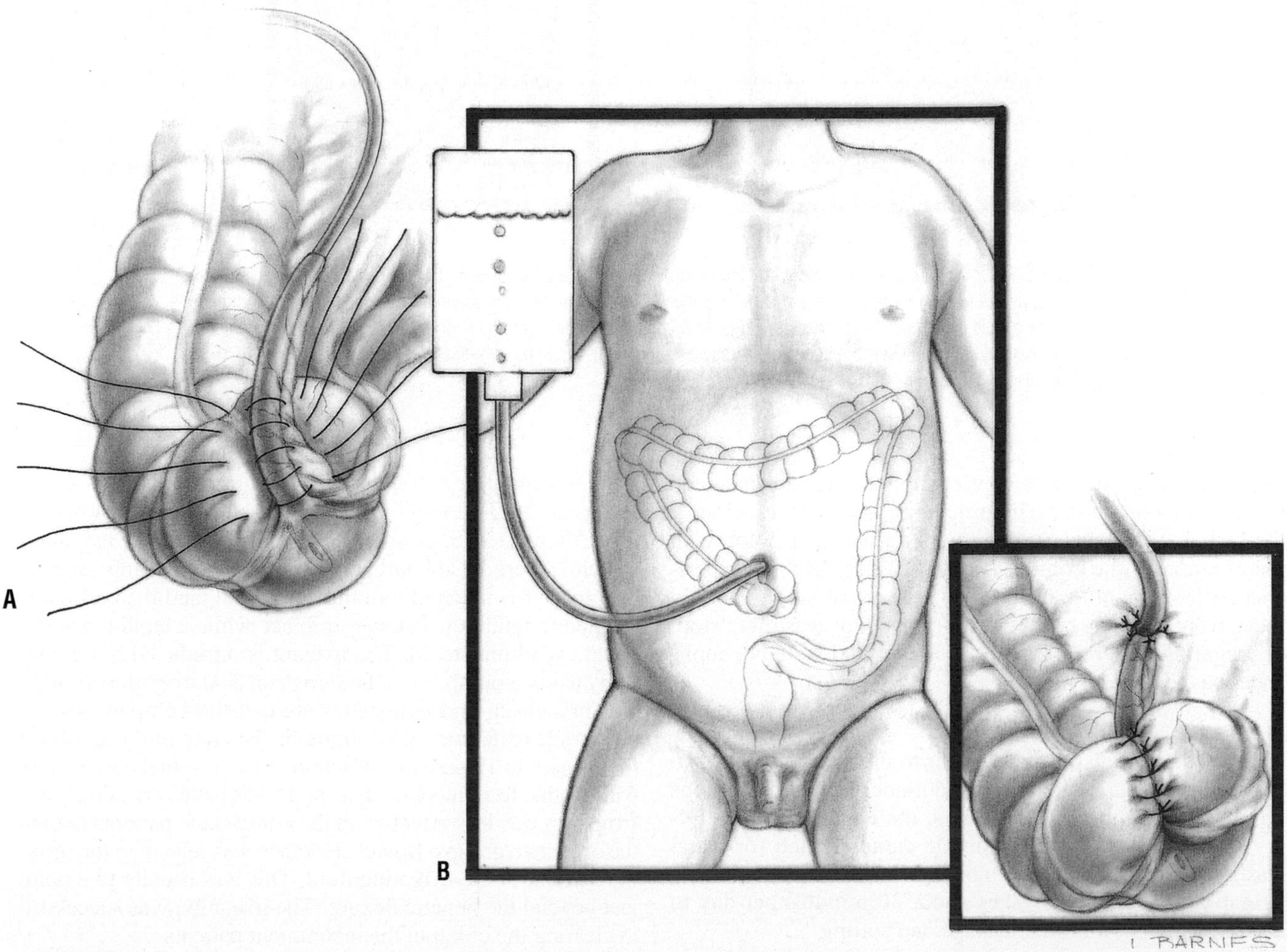

FIGURE 16-23. Appendicostomy. Cecal plication around the native appendix. **A:** Appendix overlying cecum. **B:** Administration of an enema through the umbilicus. **C:** Completed plication. (From Levitt MA, Soffer SZ, Peña A. Continent appendicostomy in the bowel management of fecally incontinent children. *J Pediatr Surg.* 1997;32(11):1630–1633, with permission.)

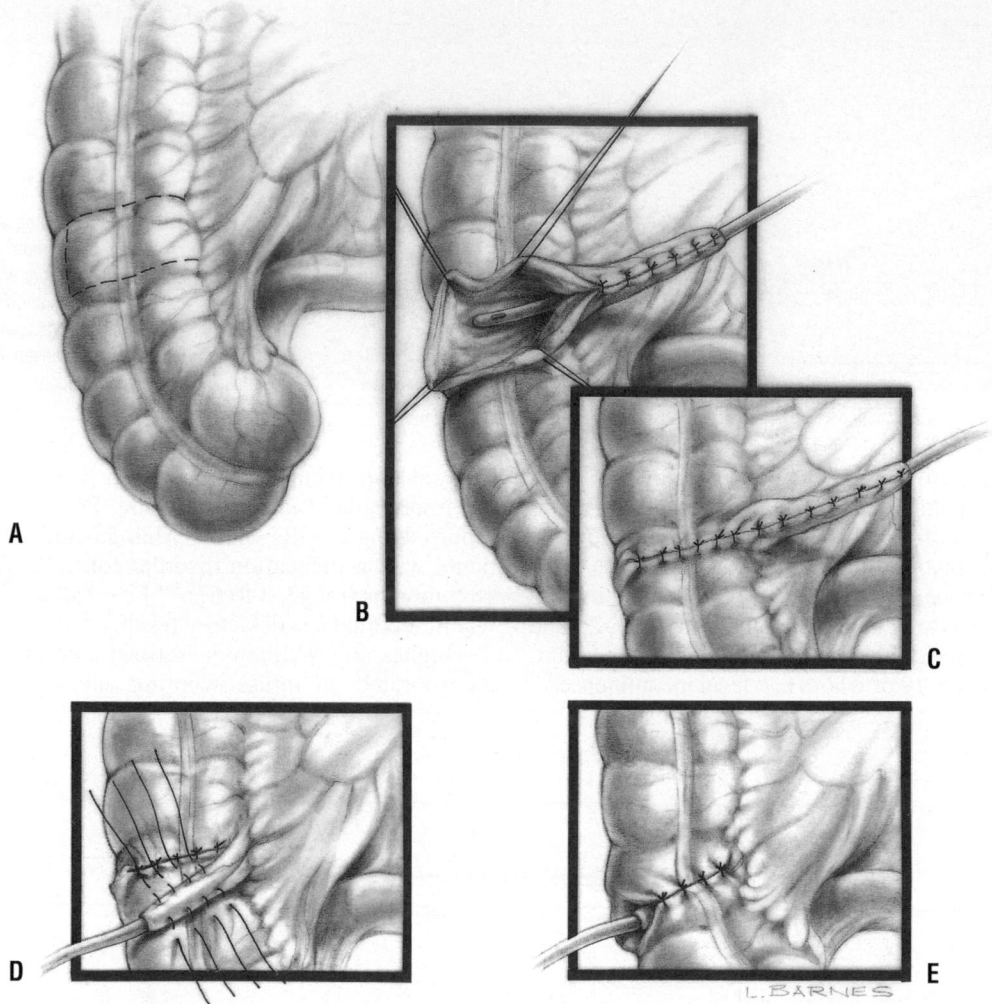

A

B

C

D

E

L. BARNES

FIGURE 16-24. Neoappendicostomy. **A:** Flap of cecum with mesenteric vessels at its base. **B:** Tubularization of the cecal flap over a feeding tube. **C:** Completed neoappendix. **D:** Plication of cecum around the neoappendix (neoappendix suture line should not appose the cecal suture line). **E:** Completed plication. (From Levitt MA, Soffer SZ, Peña A. Continent appendicostomy in the bowel management of fecally incontinent children. *J Pediatr Surg.* 1997;32(11):1630–1633, with permission.)

incontinence and disordered evacuation through an antegrade irrigation technique.[201] The procedure involves division of the bowel at the level of the proximal transverse colon with the creation of the conduit (Figure 16-25). In their experience, after 1 month there was no leakage of solid or liquid feces from the anus between irrigations, nor was there stool or irrigating fluid refluxing to the abdominal wall. No appliance was required.

Retrograde

Retrograde administration is easier to undertake because no surgical procedure is required and associated complications are avoided. In the last few years, the apparatus for delivery has improved from the simple catheter used for rectal washout. Closed systems are now available, which will allow irrigation that normally takes about 30 minutes per day to accomplish with minimal leakage and soiling.

Technique

The commercial systems available for transanal irrigation use either a rectal balloon catheter (Peristeen anal irrigation

system; Coloplast A/S, Kokkedal, Denmark or Mallinckrodt, St. Louis, MO—Figure 16-26) or a cone-shaped colostomy tip (Coloplast A/S, Humlebæk, Denmark; Qufora irrigation system; Allerød, Denmark; or Biotrol irrimatic pump; Braun). The former is inserted into the anal canal, and the balloon is inflated to retain the catheter in place while a tepid tap water enema is administered. The irrigant is introduced by gravity or by using a pump, as in the Peristeen anal irrigation system.

Christensen and colleagues studied the completeness of retrograde irrigation by scintigraphic labeling of the stool and the irrigant in 19 patients, of whom 5 had a spinal cord lesion, 6 idiopathic fecal incontinence, and 8 idiopathic constipation.[72] Irrigation was less effective in the constipated patients than in the other two groups. Bowel clearance was related to the proximal extent of the irrigating fluid. This was usually to a point just beyond the hepatic flexure. The irrigation was successful in clearing the colon in the incontinent patients.

Results

Briel and colleagues applied the system used for colostomy irrigation to 32 patients with soiling (16) or frank fecal

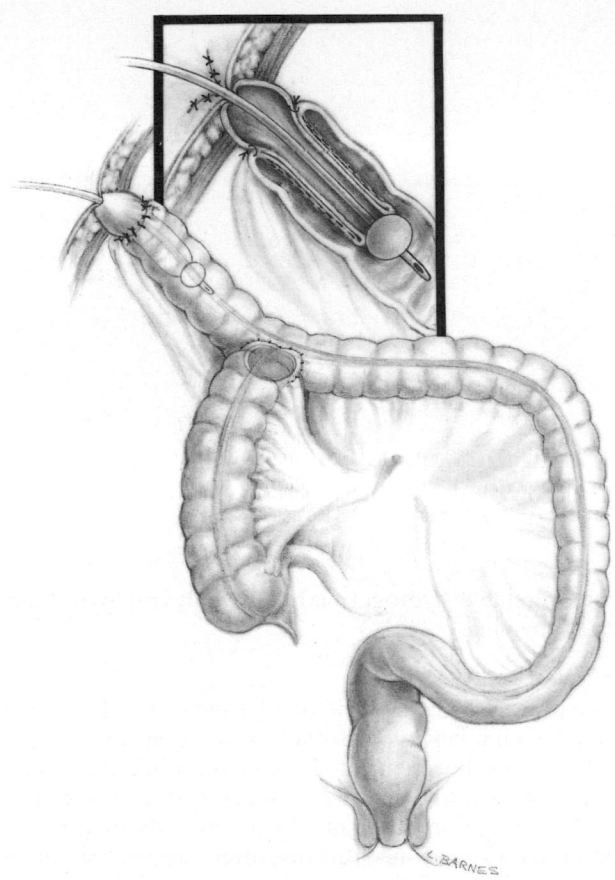

FIGURE 16-25. The colon is divided, and the proximal transverse colon is used to construct the conduit. An intussuscepting valve is created and fixed with sutures and staples. The conduit is exteriorized with skin flaps. (After Hughes SF, Williams NS. Continent colonic conduit for the treatment of faecal incontinence associated with disordered evacuation. *Br J Surg.* 1995;82(10):1318–1320.)

incontinence (16).[43] Ten were unable to tolerate the treatment and stopped within 1 month. The remaining 22 continued irrigation, and over a median follow-up period of 18 months, "success" was experienced by 92% with soiling and 60% with frank incontinence.

In a retrospective study of 92 patients having irrigation for incontinence or constipation assessed by questionnaire, there were 48 (52%) responses.[88] Of these, 44 were still irrigating at the time, of whom 20 were irrigating twice (2) daily or daily (18). There were 33 patients with incontinence, of whom 16 (48%) recorded success using a visual analogue scale. No difference in the quality of life or physiologic assessments between patients who had a successful or nonsuccessful result was observed, however.

In 267 patients treated by retrograde rectal irrigation between 1989 and 2001 for incontinence or defecation disorders, 239 were available for follow-up.[163] These individuals received a questionnaire from whom 190 (79%) responded. Of these, 21 (11%) never started irrigation. This left 169 patients for analysis. Of these, 332 had soiling and 71 had fecal incontinence. Irrigation was effective in 47% and 41% of the two groups, although 10 and 5 patients in each had stopped irrigating despite the benefit it offered.

Cazemier and colleagues reported the results of 201 adults and children with constipation or incontinence treated from 1980 to 2005.[58] Of 28 adults with fecal incontinence, 63% were still irrigating at a mean of 8.5 years. Of these, 88% were satisfied. Similar results were obtained in the children. In a prospective study of retrograde irrigation for fecal incontinence and constipation, Koch and coworkers found that 17 of 28 patients with fecal incontinence were continent at 3 months and had low incontinence scores at 12 months.[230] Christensen and associates reported 348 patients having anal irrigations for defecation disorders and incontinence.[71] In the whole series, perforation not requiring surgery occurred in 2 of 110,000 irrigations.

Spinal Cord Injury

Patients with spinal cord injury pose a special problem in that their treatment options are limited. Christensen and colleagues conducted a multicenter (five centers), randomized trial comparing conservative bowel management with conservative bowel management plus retrograde irrigation over 10 weeks in 87 patients with this condition.[69] At the end of this period, the St. Mark's continence scores in the two groups were 7.3 (4.0) and 5.0 (4.6), being significantly in favor of the irrigation group. The American Society of Colon and Rectal Surgeons (ASCRS) fecal incontinence scores for depression and embarrassment also favored the irrigation group.

Anterior Resection Syndrome

Koch and colleagues studied the application of irrigation in 30 patients with incontinence following anterior resection.[231] Data were available on 26, of whom 21 still used irrigation at the time of assessment. Of these, 5 had stopped; but of the remaining 21, 12 (57%) had complete continence, 3 (14%) had incontinence for flatus, and 6 (29%) had incontinence for liquid stool. The authors concluded that irrigation was a successful treatment option for these individuals.

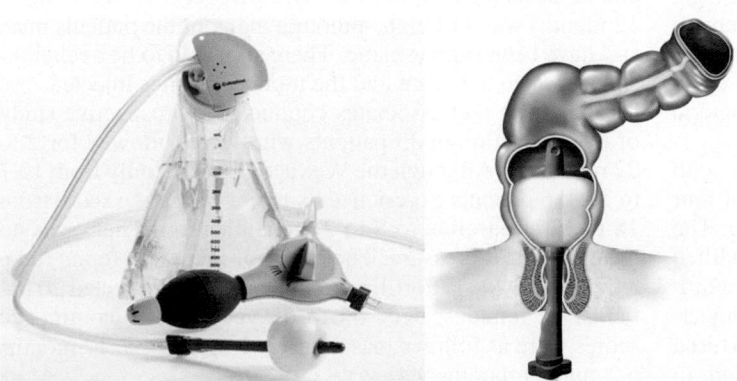

FIGURE 16-26. Equipment for performing retrograde irrigation.

Overall Assessment. In a review, Tod and colleagues concluded that at the time, 2005, there was only limited evidence to support rectal irrigation for fecal incontinence and they indicated the need for further research.[460] They summarized their position by demonstrating in the studies reviewed a continuation rate of irrigation of 40% to 69% over periods ranging from 6 weeks to 56 months. The most common reason for discontinuance was lack of effectiveness of the regimen, followed by perceived benefit but no need to continue, and third by technical difficulty.

In another review, 17 articles on irrigation in adults were analyzed.[70] These included 1,229 patients, of whom 648 (53%) were said to have had "success." Only one of these studies was randomized.[69] In the incontinent patients, success was recorded in 47%. None of the studies addressed long-term outcome. The most recent review analyzed 25 eligible studies and reaffirmed that rectal irrigation improved symptoms in patients with spinal cord injury.[121] It also indicated that it was particularly helpful in children with spina bifida.

Comment. Retrograde irrigation is easy to perform and has a very low morbidity. The available evidence strongly indicates that it can be usefully applied to various forms of incontinence, including anterior resection syndrome, idiopathic incontinence, and neurogenic incontinence. One may anticipate a success rate of at least 50%. It may be sufficiently beneficial that one may be able to avoid a colostomy when all other treatment methods have been tried and failed. In current practice, this option is probably underused.

▶ INVASIVE TREATMENT

Bulking Agent Injection

Patients with passive seepage due to weakness of the internal sphincter have been treated by injection of bulking agents into the submucous and intersphincteric plane in the upper anal canal. Shafik was the first to report this approach using Teflon (polytetrafluoroethylene) paste (DuPont, Texas).[409] He then tried autologous fat injection in 14 patients in whom complete continence was achieved at a follow-up of 18 months in all patients following up to three injections.[410]

Technique

The procedure can be carried out in the office or in a day center. The bowel is prepared with a Fleet enema (CB Fleet Co., Inc., Lynchburg, VA). The procedure is covered by a single dose of antibiotic such as a second-generation cephalosporin with metronidazole. With the patient in the left lateral position under mild sedation and after infiltration of a local anesthetic, a finger is inserted in the anus. An 18-gauge, 2.5-in. needle attached to a ratchet gun or other convenient syringe, depending on the viscosity of the material, is placed through the skin just to the side of the anus. It is advanced under digital control into the submucosa or intersphincteric space and also into any obvious defect (Figure 16-27).

Durasphere is delivered using a prepacked syringe with an 18-gauge, 4-cm long needle. Injections are made at four evenly spaced positions using about 2 mL at each site. The technique of injection through a proctoscope was modified by Tjandra and colleagues by the use of ultrasound guidance.[457] This improves the accuracy of placement of injectable silicone PTQ implants (Bioplastique), with textured polydimethylsiloxane elastomer particles suspended in

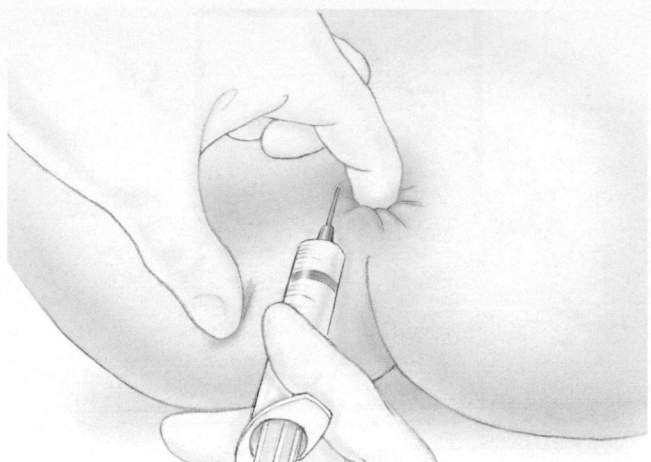

FIGURE 16-27. Injection of bulking agent.

a bioexcretable hydrogel carrier of polyvinylpyrrolidone (PVP, povidone).

Results

Bernardi and colleagues reported a case of a 34-year-old woman with a keyhole deformity who became fully continent after two injections of autologous fat into the defect.[28] Kumar and coworkers used anal glutaraldehyde cross-linked (GAX) collagen injection in 17 patients with idiopathic incontinence (9) and incontinence after various anal procedures (8).[239] The injections were given submucosally, using a Gabriel syringe, after an intradermal injection to exclude allergy, with particular attention to a defect if present. At a mean follow-up of 8 months (range, 4 to 12), 11 patients had marked improvement without any leakage of liquid stool or soiling. Malouf and coworkers injected a silicone-based product, Bioplastique (Uroplasty, Ltd., Reading, United Kingdom), in 10 patients with fecal incontinence.[282] Although the procedure was clinically effective over the short term, the benefit was maintained in only a few individuals.

Davis and colleagues used biocompatible carbon-coated beads suspended in a water-based carrier gel containing beta glucan, Durasphere (Advanced UroScience, St. Paul, MN).[94] The beads are three times the migration threshold of 80 μm and cannot be absorbed by the body. Eighteen patients of average age 60 years with fecal soiling or leakage were treated and followed for a mean of 28.5 months. There was no change from baseline for 6 months, but at 12 months there were improvements in continence scores from 11.9 $\pm$ 5.1 to 8.1 $\pm$ 3.7, patient satisfaction, depression, coping, and embarrassment. It is noteworthy, however, that the score at 12 months was still high, although many of the patients must still have been symptomatic. There appeared to be a relationship between the score and the number of sites injected.

Soerensen and associates conducted a prospective study of PTQ injection in 33 patients who were followed for 2 to 22 months.[423] Although the Wexner score fell only from 12.7 to 10.4, 6 patients experienced a major fall in the score from 18 to 13 at baseline to 8 to 2 after injection. There was no change in anal pressure. The effect of PTQ was found to be temporary by de la Portilla and colleagues who treated 20 patients, 12 females, aged 55 to 65 years.[96] The continence scores were as follows: baseline 13, 1 month 4.5, 12 months 6.2, and 24 months 9.4.

Randomized Controlled Trials

Maeda and colleagues have carried out a Cochrane review[273] and indentified four published randomized, controlled trials.[278,416,455,457] In the trial by Tjandra and colleagues, 82 patients were randomized to intersphincteric silicone injections with (42) or without (40) endosound guidance.[457] Of the 82, 71 had an intact internal sphincter, and 60% of the patients had an increase in the PNTML. At a mean of 6 months (range, 1 to 12), the respective proportions of patients who had more than 50% improvement in the Wexner score were 69% and 40%, a statistically significant difference. A high proportion of patients in each group (93% and 92%) had an increase in the quality-of-life score of more than 50%. The authors concluded that ultrasound guidance improved the results.[457]

In the trial by Maeda and colleagues, 10 patients underwent injection with Bulkamid (hydrogel cross-linked with polyacrylamide) or Permacol (porcine dermal collagen). The St. Mark's continence score fell from 15 to 12.5 at 6 weeks but was 14 at 12 months. The authors concluded that neither agent offered benefit in the intermediate term.

The trial carried out by Siproudhis and coworkers randomized 44 women to injection, with polydimethylsiloxane (PDMS) elastomer implant (22) and normal saline (22). There was no difference in the percentage of patients improved at 3 months (23% and 27%), and the continence scores were 11.7 and 11.4. There was, thus, no evidence that PDMS was effective.[416]

In the last randomized, controlled trial that compared the safety and efficacy of injectable silicone biomaterial, PTQ (Uroplasty, Ltd., Geleen, The Netherlands) with Durasphere, Tjandra and colleagues randomized 40 patients to each type of injection.[455] Age (59 years), gender (9/1, F/M), and resting tone (22 and 25 mm Hg) were well matched. The injections were placed in the intersphincteric space under ultrasound control. Both resulted in an improvement in continence; this was maintained at 12 months. There were no complications after PTQ injection, but pain (1), erosion of the material (2), and hypersensitivity reaction (1) occurred after Durasphere injection. From a baseline Wexner score of 11.45 in each group, the score at 12 months was 3.8 and 7.0 in favor of PTQ. There was no difference in resting tone between the two groups, although there was a 50% rise at 12 months compared with baseline.

Summary

Anal injection of bulking agents improves passive incontinence in the short term in more than 50% of patients, but the improvement is often short-lived and may reduce the continence score only slightly, thus still leaving the patient with significant symptoms. Repeated injections may be necessary. It is not known whether intersphincteric or submucosal injection is more effective. PTQ may be preferable to Durasphere injection. The procedure can be carried out in the office or day center. More trials of this treatment approach are needed.

Radiofrequency Energy Delivery for the Treatment of Fecal Incontinence (SECCA Procedure)

Radiofrequency (RF) energy has been used for electrosurgery techniques (cutting and coagulation) since the 1920s. When delivered to tissue in the frequency range of 200 kHz to 3.3 MHz, RF energy results in vibration of water molecules and subsequent frictional heating. The Secca System (Mederi Therapeutics, Inc., Greenwich, CT) was designed to deliver temperature-controlled RF energy to the muscle of the anal canal to induce fibrosis in the hope that this would improve anal canal closure.

The RF energy handpiece is composed of a clear anoscopic barrel with four nickel-titanium curved needle electrodes (22 gauge, 6 mm in length; Figure 16-28). The needle electrodes are deployed through the mucosa of the anal canal and into the internal sphincter muscle. When this occurs, there is a reduction in electrical impedance, indicating penetration of the electrode below the mucosal surface. Temperature is monitored automatically and a temperature-control mechanism adjusts the RF output to achieve a target temperature of 85° C at the tip of the needle electrode (Figure 16-29). Anoderm temperature is continuously monitored, and energy delivery automatically ceases if the temperature exceeds a preset limit of 42°.

Indications and Technique

SECCA has been used mainly for patients with passive incontinence associated, therefore, with internal sphincter weakness. It is a day case outpatient procedure undertaken in

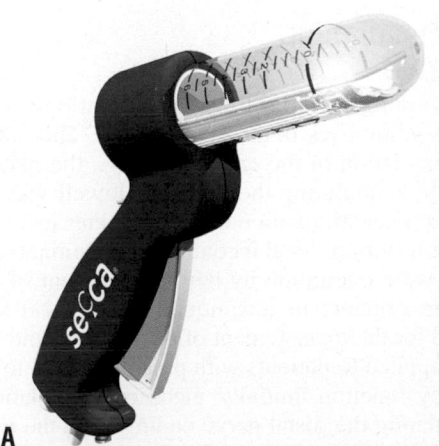
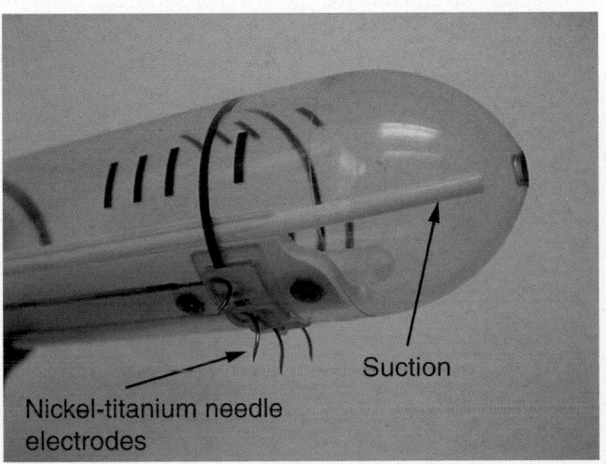

Suction

Nickel-titanium needle electrodes

A

B

FIGURE 16-28. Secca handpiece. **A:** Unit with handle/anoscope, light attachment, radiofrequency delivery connector, suction, and irrigation. **B:** Close-up view with needles deployed. (Courtesy of Mederi Therapeutics, Inc., Greenwich, CT.)

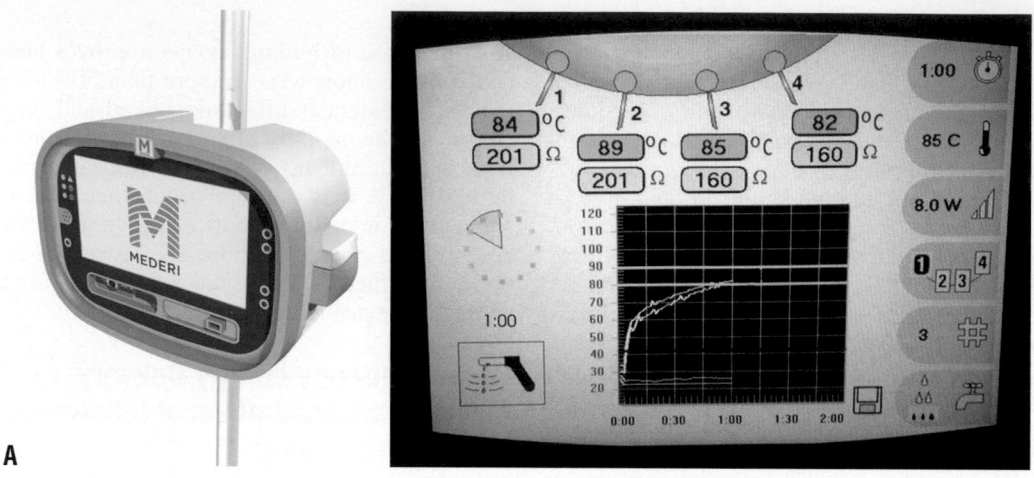

A   B

FIGURE 16-29. Pole-mounted monitor screen **(A)**. Monitor with schematically shown four electrodes and corresponding temperatures (84° C to 86° C) with impedances. Note that the temperature range over time is in the therapeutic range. Also note the flat two lines at the bottom of the graph showing cool surface temperatures **(B)**. (Courtesy of Mederi Therapeutics, Inc., Greenwich, CT.)

an ambulatory surgical or endoscopy unit, under local anesthesia with sedation. With the patient in the prone jackknife position, the handpiece is introduced into the anal canal so that the needles, when inserted, will enter the tissues below the dentate line. Once appropriate tissue penetration by the needles is achieved, energy is then delivered to all four electrodes for 1 minute to achieve a target temperature of 85° C (Figure 16-30). Care must be taken to avoid damage to the vagina. The procedure takes approximately 30 minutes.

Results

Efron and colleagues reported the results in 50 patients treated in five centers who had not responded to conservative measures.[117] At 6 months, the Wexner score had changed from 14.8 to 11.1, with corresponding improvements in the different domains of the SF-36 assessment. Whether this change was clinically significant is another question. In a study of 10 patients, there was an improvement at 2 years with a reduction of the incontinence score from 13.8 to 7.3.[446] In another small study of 11 patients, 6 had improved at 12 months. The Vaizey continence score fell from 18.9 to 11.5. There was no change in anal pressure measurements.[135] In still another small series of 15 patients, the Wexner score at

12 months after treatment had fallen from 14.07 to 12.33, which has to be regarded as not clinically significant. Again, there was no change in the ultrasound appearances or physiologic measurements. Lefebure and colleagues reported another small series of 15 patients whose Wexner score fell from 14.07 to 12.33 without any change in the ultrasound or physiologic parameters.[250] In another report of SECCA of 8 patients, none was improved.[228] A recent publication of 24 patients of whom 16 were evaluable at 12 months showed a reduction of the incontinence score from 15.6 to 12.9 at 1 year.[389]

Comment

The numbers of patients in these studies are small, and the reductions in the incontinence scores have been very limited. The results of the planned prospective, randomized, sham-controlled study have never been produced nor published, perhaps because at a time the original company (Curon Medical) entered bankruptcy proceedings. The present company who bought the assets (Mederi Therapeutics, Inc.) has been resurrecting the product, but for the present one must consider that the role of SECCA in the treatment of anal incontinence appears to be marginal.

Neuromodulation

Introduction

There is a long history of nerve stimulation for functional disorders going back to the 19th century. This was either by direct stimulation of the end organ (e.g., the bladder) or indirectly by stimulating the nerve. Caldwell was the first to apply electrical stimulation to the sphincter in a patient with a 30-year history of fecal incontinence.[55] Initial technical difficulties were overcome by the development of equipment and improvements in technique.[196] Electrical stimulation was used for the management of pain (1965) and was subsequently applied to patients with paraplegia and to those with urinary dysfunction. Initially, electrical stimulation focused on stimulating the distal nerve endings and the pelvic floor, but as of the 1990s, interest developed in applying electrical stimulation directly to the peripheral nerves responsible for continence. The concept of recruiting the unused residual

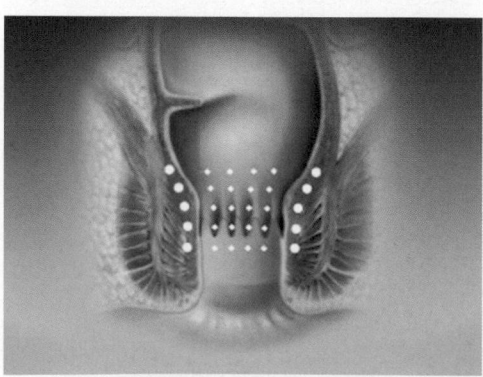

FIGURE 16-30. Schematic illustration of electrode deployment sites. Four quadrants are treated in a similar manner. (Courtesy of Mederi Therapeutics, Inc., Greenwich, CT.)

function of an inadequate urinary continence organ by electrostimulation of its peripheral nerve supply through the sacral nerves had been implemented in urology by Tanagho and colleagues during the 1980s.[449,450] They treated patients with urinary urgency by sacral nerve stimulation and reported that 90% of such individuals were suitable for this approach. Of these, 70% were improved. This concept was used experimentally in the management of fecal incontinence by application of direct stimulation of the dorsal nerve of the penis,[32,401] but this did not take hold for several more years. Matzel and coworkers were the first to stimulate the sacral nerve roots for fecal incontinence.[294] They noted encouraging results in three patients. Since then, the technique has been prospectively assessed, with sacral nerve stimulation or modulation being used for the treatment of fecal incontinence and more recently for that of constipation. The term "modulation" is now preferred because it gives recognition to the sensory as well as the motor effect of the electrical impulse.

There is now an extensive literature on sacral nerve modulation. More recently, other peripheral nerves including the posterior tibial nerve, pudendal nerve, and the dorsal nerve of the clitoris or penis have been used.

Mechanism of Action

Although the mode of action is not known, the available information is reviewed by Gourcerol and colleagues.[164] There are, however, three hypotheses: influence by neuromodulation on the somato-visceral reflex, modulation of perception of afferent information, and increase on external sphincter activity. Somato-visceral reflex activity involves peripheral stimulation, which then inhibits colonic activity and increases internal sphincter activity via the autonomic nervous system. It is known that stimulation of myelinated afferent fibers leads to inhibition of neuronal activity to the bladder.[87]

Animal experiments have shown a similar effect in the colon.[480] This also occurs when the somatic afferent branches of the sciatic nerve are stimulated, supporting the action of posterior tibial nerve stimulation. The situation is less clear in humans in whom sacral nerve stimulation may reduce propulsive activity in the colon and reduce postprandial rectal motility. This probably occurs by inhibiting the increase in rectal tone without affecting its phasal motor activity. The picture is confusing, however, because there is evidence that sacral nerve stimulation can increase colonic activity and facilitate defecation, as demonstrated clinically by its effect on some patients with slow-transit constipation. Also, there is evidence in humans that sacral nerve stimulation increases rectal blood flow, an effect that is contrary to that demonstrated in animals.

Modulation of perception by activation of somatic large afferent fibers reduces the activity of C fibers in the dorsal horn. This would block input from the rectum to the pontine center and thus inhibit defecation. There is immunochemical evidence that substance P, which is expressed by C fibers, is more elevated in patients with fecal incontinence than in controls. It returns to the level of control patients after sacral nerve stimulation.[161] This might be associated with its effect on reducing rectal hypersensitivity, thus explaining the fall of urgency in patients with irritable bowel syndrome. Sacral nerve stimulation also influences blood flow to the brain. There is an observed decreased flow in the midbrain and basal ganglia, which might be related to a decreased sensation of urgency and fullness of the bladder. These observations do not explain, however, why no associated physiologically measureable changes in rectal compliance or capacitance can be found.

Third, it is possible that sacral nerve stimulation may cause activation of somatic large afferent fibers, which reflexly enhance external sphincter activity. Such an action may be through cerebral cortical centers concerned with anal function that alter the excitability of the external sphincter. The difficulty here again is that objective changes of the external sphincter function during sacral nerve stimulation are not consistent, but in any event this effect is probably of minor importance.

Sacral Nerve Modulation

Indications

There is general agreement that patients who might be eligible for sacroneuromodulation should undergo an initial course of biofeedback. Thus, this approach is reserved for those who have failed conservative treatment. Still, there is currently some debate whether it should be the first treatment modality in patients with a chronic sphincter defect. Most surgeons are of the view that a patient with a cloacal injury or a defect in the sphincter ring of more than 90 degrees is better treated by an initial surgical repair. If this is unsuccessful, then sacroneuromodulation is still available as a secondary treatment. Others would recommend SNM in the first instance owing to the less than favorable long-term outcome of repair.

SNS was first attempted in patients who had evidence of pelvic floor muscle dysfunction without any evidence of structural sphincter injury.[224,294,317,458,468] With less rigid inclusion criteria, SNS was found to be of benefit in patients with fecal incontinence secondary to idiopathic weakness of the pelvic floor.[385] Leroi and colleagues published a position statement derived from the responses to a questionnaire sent to French units involved in the use of SNM for fecal incontinence.[258] There was general agreement that SNM should be offered to patients in whom any defect of the external sphincter was less than 30% (100 degrees) of the circumference of the anal ring. Other indications agreed by the respondents included scleroderma and neurologic lesions, provided that they were incomplete. Flatus incontinence and incontinence associated with intestinal disease were regarded as contraindications. Other indications now include iatrogenic injury to the internal sphincter,[212] neurologic causes including incomplete spinal cord lesions,[29,208,385] scleroderma,[225] rectal prolapse,[210] anal fissure,[504] and fecal incontinence secondary to low anterior resection.[209] SNS has also been used as a treatment for anal pain.[129,194,505] Moreover, SNS has been applied for the management of slow-transit constipation,[218,315] although others have not found it to be of great benefit.[26] There appears to be a high incidence of loss of efficacy in the experience of some authors.[274,275]

Sacral nerve stimulation is unlikely to be beneficial in patients with a complete spinal cord injury. When a complete lower motor lesion with interruption of the reflex arc occurs, there is risk for autonomic dysreflexia. For the same anatomical reasons, patients with congenital spinal abnormalities, such as spina bifida and complete sacral agenesis, are not suitable. In the case of partial congenital sacral agenesis, a preoperative x-ray is essential to assess the patency and accessibility of the vertebral foramina. Additional absolute contraindications include pregnancy, untreated pilonidal disease, and patients with severe immune deficiency. There is a real risk of implant infection.

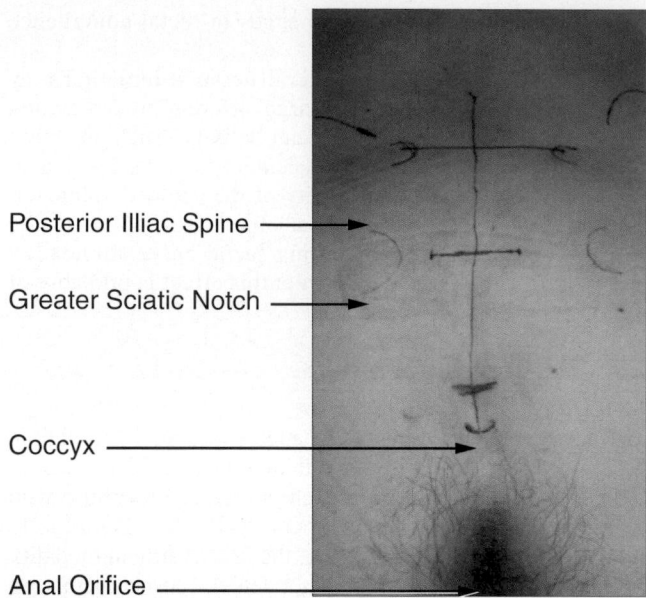

Posterior Illiac Spine

Greater Sciatic Notch

Coccyx

Anal Orifice

FIGURE 16-31. Peripheral nerve evaluation. Anatomical landmarks.

Technique

Any form of neuromodulation has the advantage of a trial period of peripheral nerve evaluation (PNE). This approach will demonstrate whether the patient will benefit and, therefore, be a candidate for a permanent electrode implant. There is almost no other treatment that will allow this strategy. General considerations include caution in the presence of a cardiac pacemaker and cessation of anticoagulants. Antibiotic coverage including immersion of the device in antibiotic solution just prior to implantation is recommended. In the case of local anesthesia being used for the PNE stage, occasionally, the sacral nerve root may become anesthetized and result in a false-negative response. In the case of general anesthesia, with the patient prone, intubation will be necessary. Long-acting neuromuscular relaxants are contraindicated, but if considered essential, a short-acting opioid may be given. Care should be taken with the use of electrocautery not to damage the lead electrode; for hemostasis, bipolar low amplitude coagulation should be employed.

Peripheral Nerve Evaluation

This part of the procedure is carried out under a local or general anesthetic. If the latter is used, then no neuromuscular blocking agents should be given. The patient is placed in the prone jackknife position, and the buttocks are gently strapped apart and draped, leaving the area over the sacrum and the perineum exposed. This allows direct visualization of the anus. The legs are extended with the feet and great toe exposed beyond the drapes.

Sacral Foramina

The sacral foramina lie about one fingerbreadth lateral to the midline. The S3 foramina are level with a transverse line joining the upper margin of the greater sciatic notch on each side (Figure 16-31). This is the same level as the most prominent part of the sacrum as demonstrated by the point at which a pen balances evenly on the skin when viewed laterally, as shown in Figure 16-32. The foramina lie about one fingerbreadth lateral to the midline at this level. The S3 site is preferred because this usually gives the best response, but if not successful S2 or S4 can be tried. The third sacral nerve root is a major component of the pudendal nerve and contains mixed autonomic and somatic motor fibers and sensory fibers.

If a local anesthetic is used, correct positioning is judged by the patient feeling a sensation in the perineum in the region of the anus and introitus. This is somewhat unreliable, however. For general anesthesia, correct placement of the electrode is judged by a motor response of the pelvic floor, external sphincter, and foot. Stimulation of S2, S3, and S4 all produce a bellows contraction in which the perineum is seen to rise during the application of current. Stimulation of S3 usually produces flexion of the great toe, but if the whole foot or the lower leg moves, stimulation at S2 is likely. S4 stimulation does not cause flexion of the great toe.

Needle Electrode Insertion

Many units have used the Medtronic Model 3886 electrode (Medtronic, Inc., Minneapolis, MN), which is cheap and expendable. In 2002, Medtronic introduced a lead fitted with barbs or "tines" (Medtronic InterStim A Model 3889/3093), which prevented or at least reduced lead migration. This is increasingly being employed even for the PNE stage because the majority of patients will be likely to be eligible for insertion of a permanent electrode. Although initial studies have suggested that the PNE phase has a 100% positive predictive value,[458] this has not been found by others.[311]

The needle electrode is inserted through the skin and advanced with a slight lateral inclination (Figure 16-33). If successful, it will be felt to pass through the posterior sacral foramen to a depth of several centimeters. It is then connected to an extracorporeal pulse generator using the attachment (Figure 16-34), and the current is switched on. Several

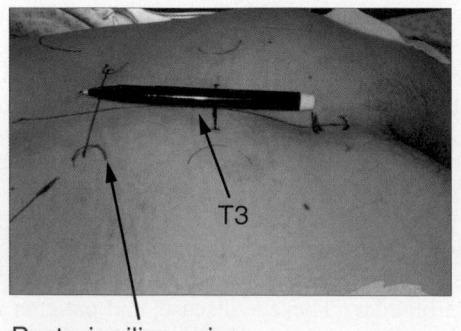

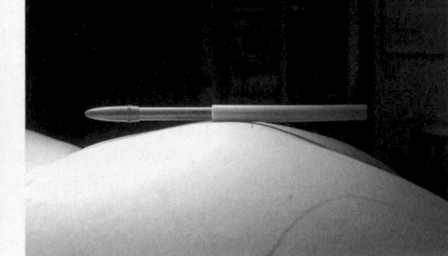

T3

FIGURE 16-32. Peripheral nerve evaluation. Lateral view of landmarks.

Posterior iliac spine

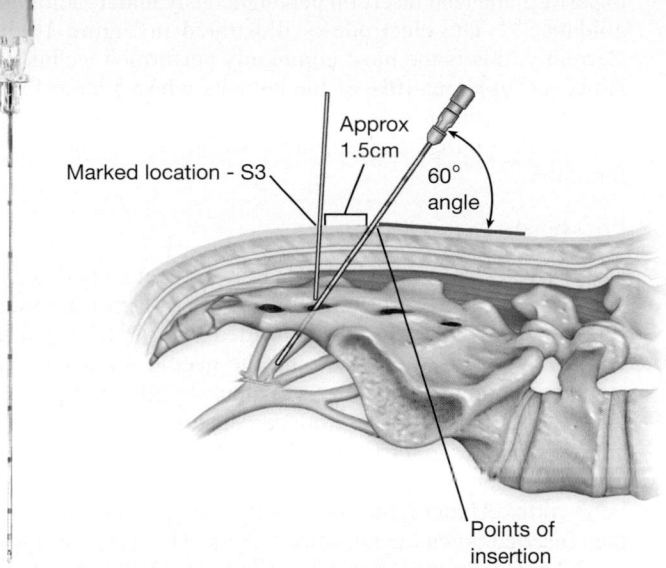

Marked location - S3

Approx 1.5cm

60° angle

Points of insertion

FIGURE 16-33. Peripheral nerve evaluation. Insertion of the electrode. (From Wexner SD, Fleshman J. *Colon and Rectal Surgery: Anorectal Operations (Master Techniques in General Surgery)*. Philadelphia, PA: Lippincott Williams & Wilkins; 2012.)

passes of the needle electrode may be required to enter the foramina of S2–4 on each side in order to determine the best response at the lowest voltage possible. When the optimal response has been ascertained, a wire electrode is passed down the needle that is then withdrawn to leave the wire in situ, but ensuring that a motor response is still preserved. The electrode is secured to the skin by an adhesive dressing, and the lead is connected to an extracorporeal pulse generator, having placed an earth pad to the skin by an adhesive to complete the electrical circuit. Stimulation is set at a pulse-width of 210 μs and a frequency of 14 Hz at the lowest voltage that produces a response.

Diary Recording
The patient then records function, entering details into a diary over the following 2 to 3 weeks, having done so for a week prior to stimulation. If a satisfactory reduction in incontinent episodes and urgency is demonstrated, the patient is eligible for a permanent implant. This is usually established as more than a 50% reduction in the frequency of incontinent episodes.

PNE is reversible and has a low morbidity and complication rate.[211,260,291,467] The responses gained with temporary stimulation tend to be clear cut, making the decision on whether to proceed to permanent implantation straightforward in most cases. When there is uncertainty, the bowel

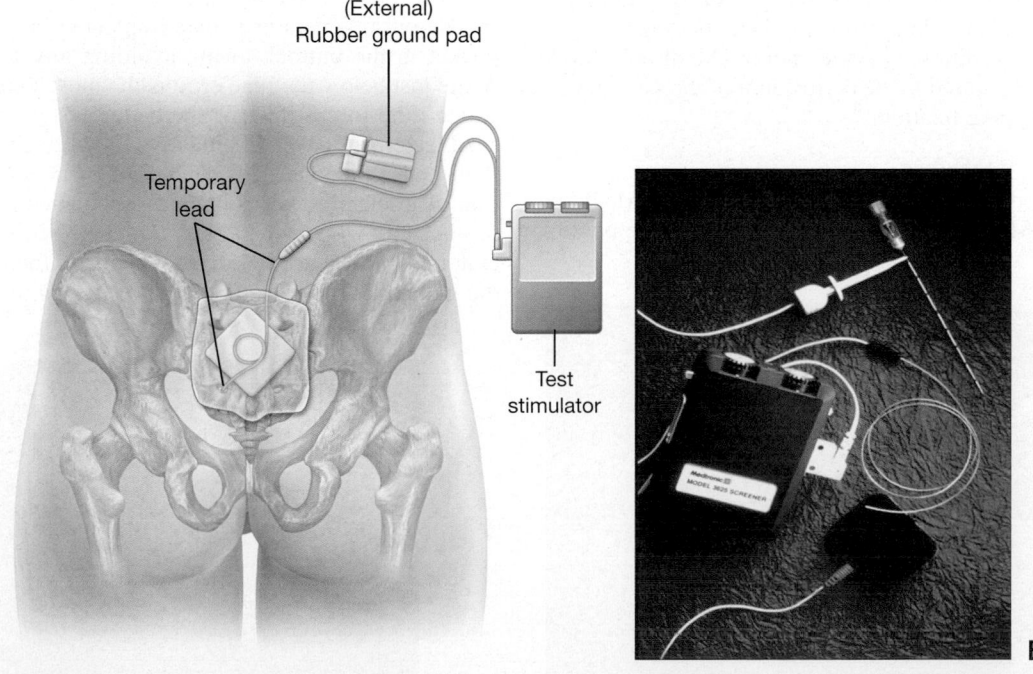

(External) Rubber ground pad

Temporary lead

Test stimulator

A   B

FIGURE 16-34. Peripheral nerve evaluation. **A:** Artistic representation of the setup for stimulation. **B:** PNE stimulation kit. (From Wexner SD, Fleshman J. *Colon and Rectal Surgery: Anorectal Operations (Master Techniques in General Surgery)*. Philadelphia, PA: Lippincott Williams & Wilkins; 2012.)

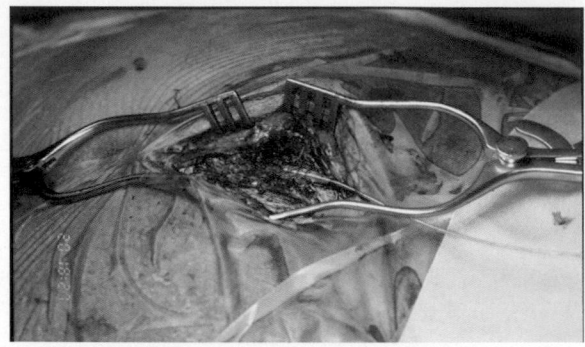

FIGURE 16-35. Open placement of the permanent electrolyte (historical technique).

diary in conjunction with a discussion with the patient will enable one to make the ultimate decision.

Permanent Lead Insertion

Two permanent implants are available: InterStim I (Medtronic Model 3023) and InterStim II (Medtronic Model 3058). The latter is smaller and does not require a lead extension. It is slightly less expensive but has a shorter battery life. This device should, therefore, be used in thin patients and for whom the larger InterStim I may be uncomfortable.

Open Technique

Prior to 2002, the permanent lead was implanted using an open surgical approach. A vertical incision was made over the sacrum and the temporary lead identified as it passes through the posterior sacral foramen. This was then replaced under direct vision by a permanent lead electrode, which was sewn in place by sutures passed around it and fixed to the periosteum (Figure 16-35).[414] This had the disadvantages of an open procedure, with its associated wound and also a certain incidence of lead migration. The early lead models had no mechanism to hold them in place, but the next generation had an additional plastic anchor (Medtronic Model 3080) that was sutured to the periosteum of the sacrum in an attempt to improve fixation.[110]

Percutaneous Technique

With the introduction of the "tined" (barbed) lead (Medtronic InterStim A Model 3889/3093) in 2002, it became possible to perform the lead insertion percutaneously under radiologic guidance.[426] The electrode is illustrated in Figure 16-36. Currently, this is the most commonly performed technique. However, in about 10% of the patients who undergo PNE, electrode placement using the percutaneous technique proves impossible owing to anatomical variations of the sacral foramina.[212]

Electrode Insertion

The wire electrode of the PNE is removed, and a permanent electrode is placed under radiologic control into the same foramen. A needle electrode is inserted as for PNE. A guidewire is then passed down it and the needle removed. The skin at the point of puncture is opened slightly by a pointed (no. 11) scalpel, and an introducer sheath (Figure 16-37) is passed over the guidewire and advanced under radiologic control so that its tip comes to the level of the anterior sacral bone cortex. Under radiologic control, the permanent lead is then inserted down the introducer again. There are two types available (Medtronic Model 3889 and Model 3093); either is suitable. Both have four electrodes placed at short intervals from the tip. The electrode should be inserted to a depth at which a motor response is obtained by stimulation of each electrode at as low an amplitude as possible. Some adjustment may be necessary to achieve this. Satisfactory insertion is inferred if the two distal electrodes project anteriorly to the sacral cortex with the third at the level of the cortex, and the most proximal still within the sacral foramen.

The next step is to remove the sheath. This will deploy the tines (barbs) after which further adjustment of the position of the electrode is not possible. Removal of the sheath is therefore a crucial part of the procedure. There are two markings on the sheath that indicate the point of exposure of the electrodes and the point at which the electrodes begin to be deployed. During withdrawal of the sheath, frequent stimulation of the electrode is performed to check that a motor response is maintained.

The pulse generator is then implanted in a subcutaneous pocket in the buttock away, avoiding any pressure point. A site just below the iliac crest is the most suitable. In a thin patient, the InterStim II is the better system because of its small size. An incision is made in the buttock, and a pocket in the subcutaneous fat is developed by gentle blunt dissection. The electrode is tunneled subcutaneously to emerge through the wound. It is then connected to the pulse generator as shown in Figure 16-38. This is then inserted into the wound with the lead deep to its casing to minimize the

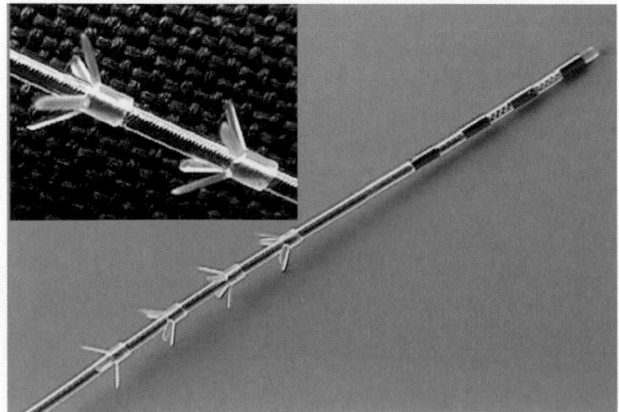

FIGURE 16-36. The "tined" (barbed) electrolyte.

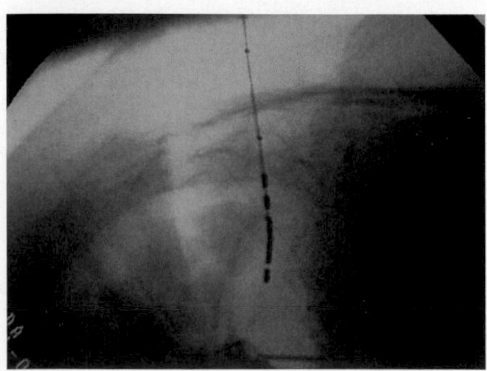

FIGURE 16-37. Radiologic screening and positioning of the electrode.

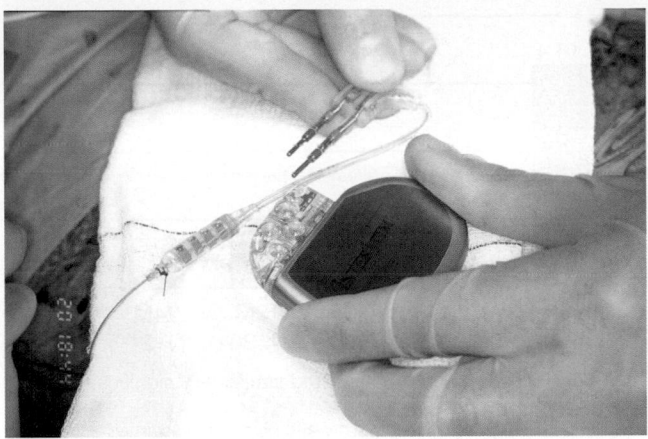

FIGURE 16-38. Connecting the electrode to the pulse generator.

chance of lead damage if future surgery should be needed. The skin wound is closed with sutures.

The operation can be performed as a day case procedure. A few weeks later, the patient should be evaluated for the wound to be checked and the settings verified or adjusted if necessary. There should be a degree of open access to the unit in the event that the patient is having postoperative difficulty. The settings can be controlled using the patient programmer (Figure 16-39).

Other Techniques of Electrode Insertion
Laparoscopic
A laparoscopic approach for placement of the stimulating electrode was described using sheep in which a fine endoscope was introduced into the perirectal space. Successful stimulation was achieved in all animals.[162] Possover has described the laparoscopic implantation of a neuroprosthesis in humans (the LION procedure), and in eight patients with paralysis after spinal cord injury, successful placement was achieved in six. In the remaining two, the sacral nerve roots were shown to have irretrievable destruction.[367] The advantage of this approach is that implantation of the stimulating electrode is accomplished under direct visualization.[367]

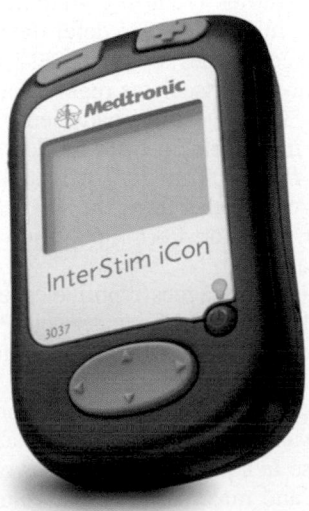

FIGURE 16-39. Patient programmer for sacroneuromodulation.

Transcutaneous
Transcutaneous electrical nerve stimulation (TENS) of S3 has also been used. In a study of 17 patients followed for a mean of 19.7 months, 69% were improved after 3 months of stimulation.[65] Although larger multicenter studies are required to confirm its efficacy, this nontraumatic approach to SNS may hold some promise.

Adverse Events
The NICE (National Institute for Health and Clinical Excellence, United Kingdom) guidelines summarized adverse events recorded from six studies for both the PNE and chronic stimulation phases (Table 16-5).[140]

Importantly, all the infections were from studies that did not adhere to the original protocol of implantation.[291,468] The original percutaneous temporary test electrode (Medtronic 041830-004) was a simple nonhelical, nonflexible wire with no retaining mechanism. This became dislodged before the end of the PNE period in one-third of patients. With the development of the new helical temporary electrode, lead displacement is much less likely. No infections have been reported since the new wire has been introduced. In addition, the new barbed ("tined") permanent quadripolar electrode lead (Medtronic 3093) can now be placed percutaneously, thus minimizing the risk of infection associated with open procedures.[464] The original protocol suggested that the pulse generator should be implanted in the anterior abdominal wall. Due to pain from the cable running over the iliac crest, the site of implantation was changed to the upper buttock. No reported case of pain from the lead has been documented with this new location.

Wexner and colleagues[487] reported 120 patients enrolled from 16 units in the United States and Australia who

TABLE 16-5 The Results of Peripheral Nerve Evaluation (PNE) in 266 Patients Assessed for Sacral Neuromodulation	
PNE No. of Patients	**266**
No improvement	58
Insufficient improvement	44
Lead dislodgement	9
Successful PNE but refused permanent implantation	5
Successful PNE but awaiting IPG at time of study	1
Superficial skin infection	1
Permanent Electrode No. of Patients	**149**
Lead migration	8
Pain from leads	3
Pain at IPG site	1
Pain (unspecified)	2
Infection	3
Interruption of electrode	1
Superficial wound dehiscence	1

IPG, implantable pulse generator.
From National Institute for Health and Clinical Excellence (NICE) guidelines on sacral nerve stimulation 2004.[140]

underwent implantation.[140] Of these, 12 developed infections, 6 of which resolved, but 6 required removal. Late infection (>1 year) occurred in 4 patients.

Faucheron and coworkers reported the reasons for surgical revision in 87 patients undergoing SNM.[132] There were 34 such cases. These included infection (4), electrode displacement (2), breakage (2), increased impedance to stimulation (4), pain (7), battery depletion (8), and loss of effectiveness (7). Repositioning of the electrode was possible in 12 patients. Michelsen and colleagues reported a removal rate of 15 (12%) of 126 patients, with infection being the reason in two.[303]

Maeda and associates reported 592 adverse events at a median of 11 months in 150 of 176 patients having a permanent implant out of 245 patients initially assessed.[276] Most of these (397 [66.9%]) were issues of reprogramming of the stimulation parameters, but there were 40 events (6.8% of all adverse events) of lead removal and replacement. Most of the remainder (212 [35.8%] of all events) were due to loss of efficacy experienced (87 patients at a median of 19 [IQR 11–36] months). Pain and discomfort were reported in 21.3% of all events by 67 patients at 11 months. In summary, of the 245 patients, 176 had a permanent device implanted, and of these 103 had a favorable outcome and 35 an acceptable outcome. These amounted to about 42% on an intention to treat basis.

Clinical Results

Early reports include the original article by Matzel and colleagues.[294] Their 3 patients had fecal incontinence for 18 to 36 months. All showed a clinical and physiologic response to PNE, which was reversed on removal of the stimulus. At 6 months following implantation of a permanent electrode, 2 patients were fully continent and the third was greatly improved. This was followed by a publication by Vaizey and colleagues of 12 patients with fecal incontinence for solid or liquid stool of at least 6 years duration who underwent PNE.[468] All had a structurally intact anal sphincter on ultrasound. Full anorectal physiology studies including 24-hour ambulatory manometry were performed both at baseline and 1 and 7 days after electrode placement. A 1-week, bowel diary card was filled in at baseline prior to stimulation and repeated during the 7-day screening process. Temporary stimulation was performed using a percutaneous wire in 10 patients and by operative placement of a permanent electrode in 2 others. Two patients experienced displacement of the lead within the first 24 hours, and a further 2 showed displacement before the evaluation was completed. A total of 9 patients had an evaluable result, of which 7 were fully continent on temporary stimulation. One patient had marked reduction in incontinent episodes, and another had no response. Resting anal pressure did not improve on stimulation, but there was a change in the MSPs in some patients.

There are now many large published studies on the outcome of permanent sacral nerve modulation. An international, multicenter, prospective, nonrandomized trial involving eight institutions reported on 37 patients with fecal incontinence resistant to conventional treatment.[291] Eight had a history of previous sphincter repair, whereas 29 had not undergone prior surgery. All patients had an intact sphincter for at least 50% of its longitudinal length on ultrasound. Of 34 patients (92%) progressing to permanent implantation, continence improved from a median of 16.4 incontinent

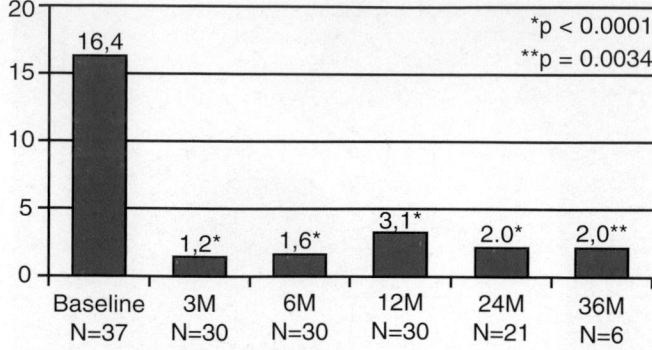

FIGURE 16-40. Incontinent episodes after permanent sacral neuromodulation.

episodes per week at baseline to a median of two incontinent episodes per week at 24 months following SNM ($P < .0001$); see Figure 16-40. Thirty-seven percent of patients were reported to be fully continent, 83% had a 50% or greater improvement in the number of incontinent episodes a week, and 71% showed a 50% or greater improvement in the total number of days of incontinence per week. Patients were found to have less passive incontinence and increased ability to defer defecation with a corresponding improvement of continence and quality-of-life scores. Social functioning as investigated by the SF-36 evaluation improved significantly ($P = .0002$). The effect on urgency was particularly noteworthy.

Numerous studies have shown good short- and medium-term follow-up results in patients who underwent sacral nerve stimulation.[11,148,212,224,259,371,385,462] A systematic review by Jarrett and coworkers summarized the available data.[149,211,212,259,290,385,461] They analyzed the data on 266 patients who underwent temporary screening. Of these, 149 (57%) progressed to permanent implantation. Follow-up ranged from 1 to 99 months. Complete continence was achieved in 41% to 75% of patients, whereas an improvement in the number of incontinent episodes per unit time of more than 50% occurred in 75% to 100%. In some studies, 96% of patients had improved symptoms, whereas 48% were reported "cured."[212,260,385] The reported reduction in episodes of fecal incontinence varied from 67% to 98%, with the larger studies recording statistical significance. An improvement in the ability to defer defecation was also noted. Leroi and colleagues reported a 52% reduction in urgency, and Ganio and associates reported a 52% reduction in pad usage.[149,260] Three authors had used a scoring system, and all showed improvement from 57% to 71% ($P < .01$, $P < .0001$, and $P = .003$).[149,212,291] All studies that reported quality of life through either using the ASCRS quality-of-life assessment[378] or the Short Form-36[214] showed an improvement in all domains.

Melenhorst and colleagues reported a series of 134 patients (age 56, 117 females) who underwent PNE.[297] Of these, 100 (74.6%) went on to a permanent implant. They were followed for 25.5 months (range, 2.5 to 63.2). The number of incontinent episodes per 3 weeks fell from 31.3 to 4.8 at 3 years. There was no change in resting anal pressure, but a marginal increase in squeeze pressure was observed. Rectal sensation, urge, and maximal tolerable volumes decreased. Failure, defined as loss of efficacy to less than 50% of the baseline value, occurred in 21 patients. There was no case of lead migration. In another large study of 177 patients (160 females; age 59.5 years) who underwent PNE, 142 showed a greater than 50% reduction in incontinent episodes.

In a still large series, Michelsen and colleagues reported the results in 177 patients (160 females; age 59.5 years) treated between 2001 and 2007 mostly for idiopathic or obstetric-related incontinence.[303] Of these, 121 were PNE positive. After taking into account the 21 patients who were positive on a second PNE assessment, there were 143 candidates for SNM, of whom 126 underwent implantation. These were followed for 24 months (range, 3 to 72). Removal of the device was carried out in 15 (12%). The incontinence score fell in successful patients from 16 to 10. The results were sustained at 6 years in 10 patients followed for this length of time.

The North American and Australian experience has recently been reported by Wexner and colleagues.[487] In an institutional review board–approved multicenter prospective trial of SNM in 16 United States and Australian units between 2002 and 2007, 133 patients underwent PNE. Of these, 120 (110 women [90%]) had a permanent implant. At 24 months (76 patients), therapeutic success was reported in 85% of patients, with a decrease of incontinent episodes from 9.4 per week at baseline to 2.9. There were 13 infections, which included five device removals and two having reimplantations.

Efficacy against Controls

Double-Blind Crossover and Randomized Controlled Trials

Vaizey and colleagues published a double-blind crossover study of two patients who had already undergone chronic stimulation for 9 months.[467] Stimulating at a subsensory threshold, the implantable pulse generator was switched randomly by an independent operator either on or off for 2 weeks and then off or on for 2 weeks. Both patient and main investigator were blinded to the status of the stimulation. Both patients had a good clinical response to chronic stimulation below the sensory threshold with deterioration of continence when the stimulator was switched off. Although the sample size was small, these results suggest that the improvement of symptoms with stimulation is not due to a placebo effect.

A larger double-blind crossover study was subsequently undertaken by Leroi and colleagues.[260] Twenty-seven patients were randomized to having stimulation on or off for 1 month. They then had another month with the on or off positions reversed. At the end of the second month, the patients were asked to choose which setting they preferred. They then had a further 3-month period exclusively according to their choice. Twenty-four patients completed the 2-month period, of whom 19 chose the on and 5 the off position. During the 3-month period, episodes of incontinence per week were significantly reduced during the 19 with an "on" setting (3.5 to 0.5, $P = .005$). Urgent episodes per week fell (2.3 to 1, $P = .01$), and symptom severity scores also fell, although by not much (16 to 13, $P = .0004$). In the five patients with an "off" setting, fecal incontinent episodes per week deteriorated.

Tjandra and colleagues conducted a prospective trial in which 120 patients with fecal incontinence were randomized to SNM (60) or to best supporting treatment (60).[454] The latter included pelvic floor exercises, bulking agents, and dietary adjustment. All domains of quality of life improved with SNM in contrast to supportive treatment where there was no change. These studies demonstrate that SNM results in an objective improvement in incontinence.

Using matched patients who underwent artificial bowel sphincter implantation (15) as the control and 15 having permanent SNM implantation, Meurette and colleagues found that the mean postoperative continence score was higher (9.4 vs. 5.7 [$P < .01$]), but constipation was more common after artificial sphincter insertion.[302] This comparison was made with ABS patients who had succeeded in the sense that they still had a functioning anus (see later) and may not, therefore, be entirely equivalent.

Risk Factors for Failure

Sacral neuromodulation is costly. Therefore, it is important for one to determine in those with a borderline PNE whether permanent implantation will be successful. There are now some indicators that may be helpful in this regard. In a study of 81 patients who had PNE over a 10-year period, the outcome was not affected by gender, age, BMI, or the severity or duration of symptoms. Factors indicative of failure included multiple attempts at PNE and evidence of previous sphincter injury. A low threshold to obtain a motor response was associated with an improved outcome.[109] Govaert and colleagues, in a series of 245 patients (226 females, age 56.6 years) who underwent PNE, identified three factors that were related to a successful result.[165] These included older age, the presence of a sphincter defect, and repeated procedures. When the 173 patients underwent the permanent implant, no factors influencing the result in these individuals could be found.

Giani and colleagues measured the latency of cerebral-evoked potentials following an electrical stimulus administered to the perineum in a group of 23 female patients with fecal incontinence.[156] Those with an increased latency were more likely to have a successful clinical result at 6 months of SNM. This had the effect of bringing this parameter to within the normal range. There is evidence that the clinical result is related to the degree of response during the PNE stage.[276]

Long-term Outcome

Long-term results are only just being reported. One of the first was from Matzel and colleagues who reported 12 patients operated on from 1994 to 1999.[292] Of these, 9 had been assessed over a minimum of 7 years. At the time of evaluation, 3 had had the device removed, and of the 6, remaining incontinent episodes at baseline of 9 per week had reduced to 0 per week. Quality-of-life assessment was improved in every domain. Of the 9 patients, the pulse generator had required a battery change at approximately 7.4 years in eight cases. Uludağ and coworkers reported the results at a median of 7.1 years (range, 5.6 to 8.7) in 50 patients operated on from 2000.[463] Eight had experienced deterioration of function, of whom 3 required a colostomy and 3 needed irrigation. The device had been removed in 7. There had been 9 reoperations for electrode dislocation (7) and fracture (2). In those patients still retaining the device, the frequency of incontinent episodes per week had fallen from approximately eight at baseline to one at 4 years. There was also a significant fall in the number of incontinence days per week. Hollingshead and associates reported 118 patients seen over a 10-year period, of whom 91 (77%) were eligible for a permanent implant based on a positive PNE.[195] Of these, 86 underwent implantation. Seventy were followed for 1 year, with success in 63 (90%); 18 were followed for 5 years. There was loss of efficacy over time, with life table analysis showing 83% with a good result just after implantation to 47% at 5 years. This is reminiscent of the outcome noted following anal sphincter repair.

To summarize the results among the 245 patients reported by Maeda and colleagues, 176 had a permanent device implanted.[276] Of these, 103 had a favorable outcome and 35 an acceptable outcome. These amounted to about 42% on an intention to treat basis when followed over a period of a median of 33 months (IQR 20–52). Results at a median follow-up period of 33 months were disappointing in 45 patients reported by Vallet and colleagues who underwent PNE.[470] Of these, 32 (71%) had a permanent implant. When analyzed at 33 months, only 25 patients still had a functioning device. Of these, 12 had good function, and in 5 it was satisfactory. In 6 it was poor. Gallas and coworkers, in a large French study of 200 patients, found that the results of permanent implantation were not influenced by age, gender, duration of symptoms, cause of fecal incontinence, physiologic, or ultrasound findings.[147] Only the consistency of the stool and low intensity of stimulation were related to a good outcome. They concluded that preoperative assessment was a poor predictor of success or failure. In another study reporting 52 patients having a permanent implant available for long-term follow-up of 5 years or more, out of 94 patients who were initially assessed, Altomare and colleagues reported a fall in the Wexner score from 15 (baseline) to 5, with a 50% improvement in continence in 74% of patients.[9] Quality of life was improved in all domains, with an overall improvement in SF-36 scores of 40%. These authors did not give an overall satisfaction rate nor did they comment on the low number of patients with a good result compared with the initial 94 patients.

SNM in the Presence of a Sphincter Defect

The majority of studies of sacral nerve stimulation have been reported on patients with a functionally weak but structurally intact anal sphincter. Anal manometry in these studies has been conflicting whether anal squeeze pressure is increased or unaltered by stimulation.[11,148,213,291,371,385,462] If the mechanism of action of SNM does not involve an improvement of external sphincter function, then patients with a sphincter defect may benefit from SNM without the need for a preceding repair.

Leroi and coworkers were the first to report the use of sacral nerve stimulation as a first-line surgical treatment in four patients with an external sphincter defect.[259] In three, the defect was limited to less than or equal to 30 degrees of the circumference of the muscle as measured by two-dimensional endoanal ultrasonography, whereas in the third this was 60 degrees. Chronic stimulation showed an improvement in continence and reduction in urgency in all four patients. Jarrett and associates found temporary sacral nerve stimulation to be beneficial in eight patients with a combined external and internal anal sphincter defect.[213] All benefited from temporary stimulation, with reduction in incontinent episodes and improvement of continence score.

Maslekar and colleagues reported 20 women, median age 42 years, with external and internal anal sphincter disruption who had undergone sacral nerve modulation as the primary treatment for fecal incontinence.[288] Of 19 permanently implanted, there was a reduction in symptoms of incontinence as measured by the Cleveland Clinic Continence Score from a median of 16 before treatment to a median of 3 at a follow-up of 48 months. The ability to defer defecation was

improved from less than 5 before to more than 5 minutes after the implant in all but 1 patient at 48 months. The use of constipating medication during follow-up was, however, not reported. Conaghan and Farouk reported that benefit was maintained with sacral nerve modulation in 3 patients who had obstetrically caused sphincter disruption affecting between one-quarter and one-third of the circumference of the sphincter ring at 18 to 24 months of follow-up.[81] Two were fully continent, and the third was continent for solid stool.

Given the results of sacral nerve modulation in patients with a failed sphincter repair as well as when used as the first procedure in those individuals presenting with sphincter disruption, combined with the uncertain long-term results of sphincter repair, a randomized controlled trial is needed to compare repair with direct SNM.

Summary

Sacral nerve modulation for fecal incontinence is simple and well tolerated. It can be carried out as a day case procedure. The availability of PNE identifies patients suitable for a permanent implant, thus avoiding unnecessary treatment. In patients with a diffusely weak sphincter or those who have failed sphincter repair, SNM has about a 70% chance of resulting in satisfactory continence provided there is neuromuscular integrity. It may be suitable for patients with a sphincter defect without the requirement for a failed repair. This chapter has devoted a great deal of space to discussion of this exciting alternative, but further data clearly are needed before one can state that this modality should be considered for all individuals in whom a procedure is contemplated.

Posterior Tibial Nerve Modulation

In 1983, Nakamura and colleagues reported that transcutaneous stimulation of the posterior tibial nerve reduced urinary urgency and irritable bladder.[314] This approach was an extension of the development of TENS, as described by Melzack and Wall.[299] Its effects on the parameters of urinary function have been described by others.[12] van Balken and colleagues had tried to use it for pelvic pain,[471] and in the same year, Shafik and coworkers reported its value in the treatment of incontinence.[411] They studied 32 patients who had not responded to other treatments, of whom 26 appeared to have rectal urgency. The posterior tibial nerve was stimulated for 20 minutes every other day for 4 weeks via a needle electrode inserted through the skin at 0.5 to 10 mA and a frequency of 20 Hz by using a Stoller afferent nerve stimulator (UroSurge, Coralville, IA). Seventeen patients had a good result, with a score of 1.7 out of a possible value of 20. Five did not respond. Mentes and colleagues described 2 patients treated, both of whom responded with improvement in the Wexner score of 30%.[300]

Technique

Posterior tibial nerve modulation can be effected by direct stimulation by an electrode in contact with the nerve inserted through the skin (percutaneous) or indirectly through the skin by an electrode fixed over the nerve by an adhesive plaster (transcutaneous).

Percutaneous Stimulation

The Urgent PC neuromodulation system (Uroplasty, Ltd., Berkshire, United Kingdom) uses a 34-gauge inert stainless steel needle (Urgent 1 PC catalogue #250-12). With the patient

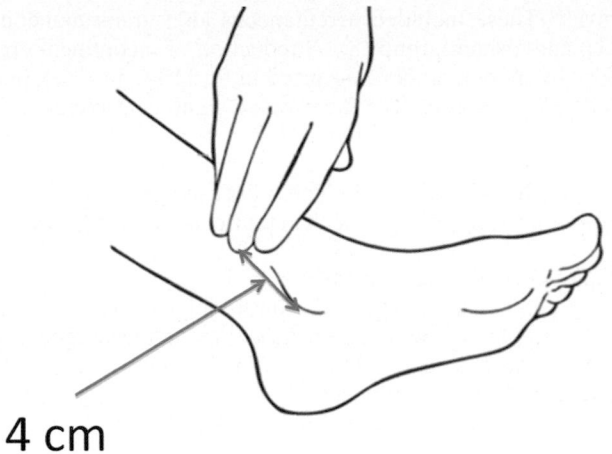

4 cm

FIGURE 16-41. Posterior tibial nerve modulation. Surface marking of the nerve.

supine, the soles of the feet are placed together and the knees abducted. After cleansing of the skin, a fine (34-gauge) needle electrode is inserted through the skin one fingerbreadth posterior and three fingerbreadths (4 cm) superior to the medial malleolus (between the posterior margin of the tibia and soleus muscle—Figure 16-41). A neutral surface adhesive electrode is placed on the same leg near the arch of the foot. The needle and electrode are connected to an external pulse generator (Urgent PC stimulator; Uroplasty, Inc., Minnetonka, MN) with an adjustable pulse intensity of 0 to 9 mA, a fixed pulse-width of 200 μs, and a frequency of 20 Hz (Figure 16-42).

The amplitude of stimulation is gradually increased until the great toe begins to flex and the patient experiences a tingling sensation radiating to the toes. If these responses do not occur, the position of the needle is adjusted, and stimulation is tried again. The stimulation then continues for 30 minutes before the needle electrode is removed, and gentle pressure is applied to the skin if any bleeding occurs.

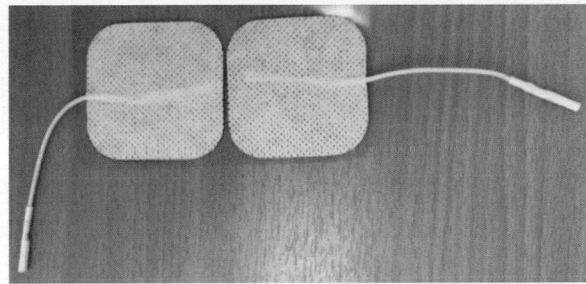

FIGURE 16-43. Surface electrodes.

Transcutaneous Stimulation

Transcutaneous stimulation is applied via two 50 mm × 50 mm self-adhesive surface electrodes (Figure 16-43) using a NeuroTrac continence neurostimulator (NeuroTrac continence; Premier Medical Products, Bedford, United Kingdom) connected to two 50 mm × 50 mm self-adhesive surface electrodes (Model VS.5050; Premier Medical Products, Bedford, United Kingdom—Figure 16-44). The negative electrode is placed behind the medial malleolus, and the positive electrode 10 cm above it. Generally, a higher amplitude of stimulation is required in order to obtain the sensory and motor responses as the electrode is further away from the nerve than with percutaneous stimulation. The stimulation settings include a pulse-width of 200 milliseconds and a frequency of 10 or 20 Hz. Stimulation at 20 Hz may cause its effect through two mechanisms, namely conversion of fast-twitch to slow-twitch fibers[229] and a reflex inhibition.[301] Stimulation is maintained for 30 minutes after which the electrodes are removed.

Results

Further studies were carried out by percutaneous and others by transcutaneous stimulation. Using a surface electrode, Queralto and colleagues applied stimulation daily for

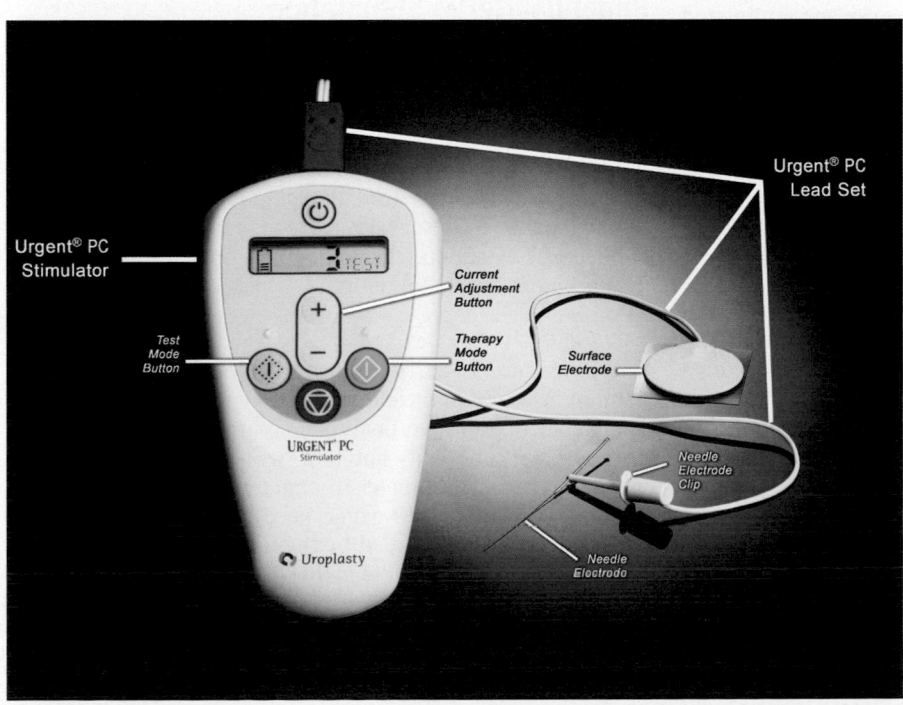

Urgent® PC Stimulator

Urgent® PC Lead Set

Current Adjustment Button

Test Mode Button

Therapy Mode Button

Surface Electrode

URGENT PC Stimulator

Uroplasty

Needle Electrode Clip

Needle Electrode

FIGURE 16-42. Urgent uroplasty stimulator.

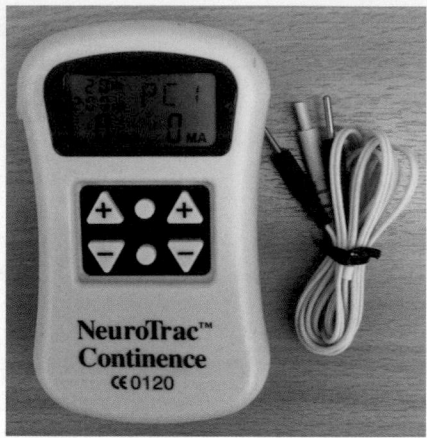

FIGURE 16-44. NeuroTrac continence neurostimulator.

20 minutes for 4 weeks (10 to 35 mA, pulse-width of 200 μs, 10 Hz) in 8 of 10 women (two had withdrawn voluntarily).[370] There was a 66% fall in the Wexner score (4–15 vs. 0–10). In those showing benefit, the effect lasted at least 12 weeks. Percutaneous posterior tibial stimulation resulted in an initial improvement in 10 of 16 patients with a mean incontinence score of 13.3 ± 4.1 before treatment to 9 ± 5.2. Five patients were free of incontinence at 6 months, having not had more than two initial treatments.[97] There was an improvement in quality of life, coping, depression, and embarrassment. In a larger prospective study over 14 months of 31 patients with urgency fecal incontinence, 21 (68%) showed improvement at a median follow-up of 9 (3 to 14) months and remained satisfied.[39] The median number of incontinent episodes fell from 4 (0–30) to 0 (0–27) per week, and the incontinence score improved from 13 (5–20) to 7 (0–20). Percutaneous stimulation was also employed in a multicenter study of 22 patients, using the Urgent PC neuromodulation system (Uroplasty, Inc., Geleen, The Netherlands).[166] A 34-gauge needle electrode was inserted into the nerve and stimulated by a 9-V battery at up to 9 mA, with a fixed pulse-width of 200 μs and a fixed frequency of 20 Hz. Fourteen patients had a reduction in the frequency of incontinent episodes per 3 weeks from 19.6 ± 21.0 to 9.9 ± 15.5, and this fell further to 3.6 ± 4.8 at 1 year. The urgency time rose from about 1 minute to 5 at 6 weeks and 10 at 1 year.

In another recent article involving 24 patients who underwent transcutaneous stimulation daily for 3 months, 13 (54%) were improved.[482] It is noteworthy, however, that the Wexner score fell from 14 to 12 only. At 15 months, the authors reported that 11 of the 13 still showed improvement. Eléouet and colleagues reported the results in 32 patients with a Wexner score of 14.5 ± 28.[118]

They experienced subjective improvement after treatment for 20 minutes per day for 3 months, with 32% experiencing an improvement of more than 25%.

Findlay and Maxwell-Armstrong reviewed the literature.[137] They, themselves, had treated 13 female patients with incontinence of varying causes. At the end of treatment at 12 weeks, episodes of flatus and liquid and solid stool incontinence had fallen to 0, but 1 month later this was not sustained for fecal continence. George and colleagues carried out a prospective trial in which patients were randomized to three treatment arms.[154] These included percutaneous (11), transcutaneous (11), and a sham group (8). A reduction of incontinent episodes by more than 50% occurred in 9 (82%), 5 (45%), and 1 (12.5%), respectively. There was a significant increase of urgency time of <1 to 7 minutes, 2 to 5 minutes, and <1 to 2.5 minutes. There were small falls in the continence scores (19–12, 18–14, and 16–14). These data suggest that percutaneous may be more effective than transcutaneous stimulation.

Inflammatory Bowel Disease

One group has applied percutaneous tibial nerve (PTN) stimulation to patients with incontinence, including urgency, in IBD.[481] Transcutaneous stimulation for 3 months was given to 12 patients with incontinence associated with IBD (Crohn's disease, 7; indeterminate colitis, 2; and ulcerative colitis, 3). Although only one individual showed an improvement in the continence score at 3 months, five experienced a significantly better quality of life. Further information is required before any useful comment on this indication can be made.

Summary

Posterior tibial nerve stimulation demonstrates short-term improvement in continence score and frequency of incontinence episodes from 30% to more than 70%. It appears that percutaneous stimulation is more effective than transcutaneous. The question, of course, is whether improvement as quantified by a scoring scale is clinically important. For example, is a fall from 14 to 12 useful to the patient? To some extent, this question is answered by the evident improvement in the quality of life when this had been assessed. Nevertheless, the positive results reported have been made by enthusiasts, and only by long-term assessment will the true value of this treatment be known. Furthermore, there is some difference in the rate at which an initially successful result is maintained (from less than a month to up to 12 months). The advantages include easy administration, low cost, and the ability to repeat the treatment at the patient's convenience. The prime disadvantage is its variable effectiveness.

Pudendal Nerve Stimulation

Patients who fail sacral nerve stimulation may have a more distal neurologic lesion or may simply not have responded to PNE. In these individuals, stimulation of the pudendal nerve may offer the possibility of clinical success. Direct stimulation of the pudendal nerve has been described by Spinelli and colleagues.[427] This is a difficult technique, however. A modification has been described in a cadaveric study, and when applied to 12 patients, there was only one case of electrode displacement over 12 months.[154]

Technique

The procedure is carried out under local anesthesia. The point of insertion of the electrode shown in Figure 16-45 is at the intersection of a vertical line passing through the middle of the ischial tuberosity and a horizontal line level with the upper aspect of the greater trochanter. With a finger in the rectum, an insulated 20-gauge needle is introduced via the perineum and its tip guided by the finger to the ischial spine (Figure 16-46). The needle is then directed medially toward the ischial fossa to Alcock's canal. A custom-made cable is used to connect the Keypoint equipment (Medtronic, Inc., Minneapolis, MN) to the auxiliary screener cable. The wire (Medtronic, Inc. 041831) is connected to the negative pole,

Line through middle of ischial tuberosity

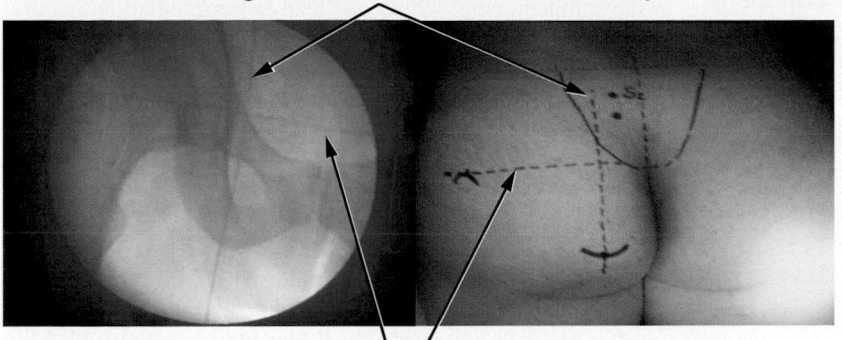

Line level with upper aspect of greater trochanter

FIGURE 16-45. Pudendal nerve stimulation. Surface marking of insertion of the electrode.

whereas the positive pole is connected to a ground pad. Electrical stimulation is applied, and external sphincter activity is recorded. On increasing the stimulation current, the responses obtained are viewed, and the position of the needle is adjusted until the trace is reproducible. Once the needle is in the correct position (Figure 16-47), it is possible to place a temporary stimulation lead or a definitive quadripolar tined lead along the pudendal nerve in Alcock's canal.

Results

In 15 patients with neurogenic urinary incontinence (nontraumatic [8], vascular myelopathy [3], myelitis [3], syringomyella [1], cerebellum neoplasia [1], traumatic [7], incomplete lesion at the cervical level at level D12–L1 [3], complete dorsal lesion [2]), the daily average number of incontinent episodes fell from 7 ± 3.3 to 2.6 ± 3.3 per 24 hours. Eight of the 25 became continent.[427] Bock and colleagues claim to have been the first to have applied this technique for fecal incontinence.[37] They describe two patients, one with Parkinson's disease and the other with incontinence associated with previous aneurysm surgery. Both experienced a cessation of incontinent episodes in the short term. George and coworkers conducted a study of pudendal nerve stimulation in 20 patients (18 females): 13 secondary to a complete cauda equina lesion and 7 with fecal incontinence who had failed sacral nerve stimulation.[154] Twelve responded in the temporary phase and underwent a permanent implant. Two who initially failed went on to have a reinsertion and then to a permanent implant. Six (3 cauda equina, 3 failed SNS) failed and did not have an implant. Over a median follow-up of 10 (range, 2 to 14) months, all the patients experienced benefit. There was one failure at 4 months (lead detachment), and one lead became infected.

Stimulation of the Dorsal Nerve of the Clitoris or Penis

The dorsal nerve of the clitoris or penis offers another peripheral nerve for access to the central nervous system. The use of the pudendo-anal reflex was first described by Binnie and colleagues.[32] Frizelle and coworkers reported the results in 67 patients who received pudendal nerve stimulation using a device manufactured by the Department of Medical Physics and Bioengineering, Christchurch, New Zealand, of whom 42 had sufficient evaluable data.[142] A square pulse of 0.1 millisecond duration was delivered at a frequency of 10 Hz for 5 minutes three times daily for 8 weeks placed at the base of the penis or clitoris. The pulse voltage of 30 to 90 mV was self-titrated to result in a perceived stimulus by the patient. Of the 42 evaluable patients, 39 (92%) were female. The pretreatment score of 9.3 fell to 6 afterwards. The need for pads fell from 74% to 14%.

Position of the ischial spine

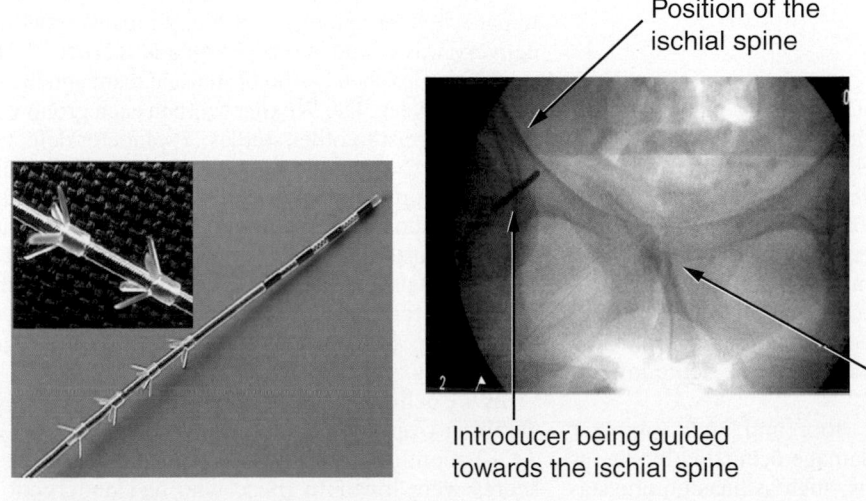

Introducer being guided towards the ischial spine

Finger *per anum* guiding the introducer towards the ischial spine

FIGURE 16-46. Pudendal nerve stimulation. Introduction of electrode guided by finger in the rectum.

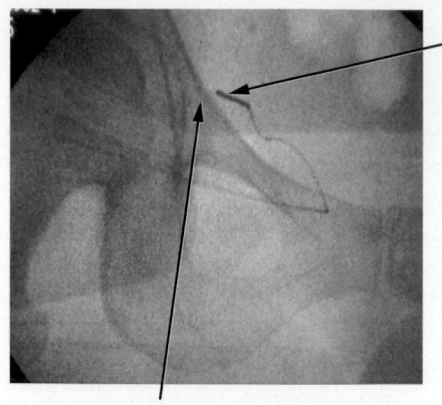

Permanent
stimulating
electrode in
position

Position of the ischial spine

FIGURE 16-47. Final position of the pudendal nerve electrode.

More recently, Worsøe and colleagues reported similar results in a pilot study of dorsal genital nerve stimulation in fecal incontinence.[501]

Surgical Repair

Before the 1990s, the mainstay of treatment of fecal incontinence was sphincter repair. This was applied in two forms of sphincter dysfunction. These included (1) diffuse weakness of the pelvic floor musculature and (2) localized sphincter trauma. Postanal repair for the former had a long-term satisfactory outcome in 30% of patients. Local trauma with sphincter disruption was treated by direct repair to correct the anatomical displacement. In the case of acute obstetrical injury recognized at the time of delivery, repair was carried out by the obstetrician usually by an end-to-end technique. It is now known that there is a high incidence of early attenuation of the repair. Many of the patients who continued to experience incontinence would come under the care of a colorectal surgeon usually months to years later.

In the 1980s and 1990s, there were many publications that demonstrated improvement in continence after delayed sphincter repair in up to 80% of patients,[20,123,219,387] but the report of Malouf and associates as well as others subsequently showed that in many cases an initially good result was followed by deterioration with time, although it is noteworthy that 50% of the patients regarded the operation as a success.[281]

Sphincter Repair

Acute Perineal Injury

Patients can present with an acute injury caused by direct laceration or blunt trauma that may be associated with other injuries (see also Chapter 17). There may be fecal contamination of the injured field. Management will involve a decision whether or not to perform a defunctioning stoma along with debridement of the wound, removing nonviable tissue and foreign material. After recovery of the patient, any pelvic floor damage can be repaired electively. It is recommended that reconstruction should not be performed for at least 3 months to allow the acute inflammation to settle.

Acute trauma to the pelvic floor and anal sphincter mechanism may also be due to damage occurring by the introduction of surgical instruments, such as anastomotic stapling devices, a large foreign body, or a fist during sexual activity.[193] Here the injury is more the result of dilatation of the sphincter ring, which can lead to fragmentation and disruption of the muscles. Management will depend on whether there is contamination and the degree of incontinence. Fecal diversion may be necessary. Where it is not, a localized rupture should be repaired. If the sphincter has been diffusely damaged, long-term management may be necessary, although the prognosis for patients with a severely fragmented sphincter is poor.

Acute Obstetrical Trauma

A third- or fourth-degree tear is detected in approximately 1.5% to 9% of deliveries.[7,111] It may not be recognized at the time, however, and it is important for the obstetrician to have a high degree of suspicion.[143,170,436] Antenatal factors such as nulliparity, large baby (>4,000 g), persistent occipito-posterior position, and induction of labor and intrapartum factors such as epidural anesthesia, a long second stage (>1 hour), instrumental delivery, and midline episiotomy are indications that a tear may have occurred.[2] Immediate repair of an injury of the perineum or the sphincter muscle has the best chance to obtain an optimal functional result, although there is a high incidence of ultrasound evidence of the development of a subsequent defect occurring over the following months (see later).

There is a debate whether the technique should involve overlapping of the sphincter or whether an end-to-end repair is as good.[430,441] In the short term, there is no evidence in favor of one technique over the other. In a randomized trial, Garcia and colleagues randomized 41 women who had had a third- or fourth-degree tear to end-to-end (23) and overlapping (18) repair.[150] Only 26 were followed, but at 4 months there was no difference in the two groups clinically or on ultrasound. The repair was felt to be intact in approximately 90%. The incidence of anorectal symptoms was the same in each group (42%). Over a longer period, however, there seems to be an advantage to an overlapping repair. Tjandra and associates conducted a small randomized, controlled trial of overlapping (11) and end-to-end repair (12).[456] Two in the former group experienced impaction. At a median follow-up of 18 months, there was no difference in the continence scores (17 to 3 and 17 to 3), although there may have been a greater difficulty in evacuation in the overlapping group.

A randomized controlled trial of 119 patients (60 end-to-end; 59 overlapping) of primary repair immediately after delivery was conducted by Rygh and Körner.[393] The repairs were accomplished by the obstetrical team and the results assessed at 1 year. The Wexner score in each group was 2.4 and 2.2. In contrast to other studies, a sphincter defect was present in only 2 of 46 and none of 42 patients after end-to-end and overlapping repair, respectively. In marked contrast, another randomized controlled trial of 149 primiparae with a third- or fourth-degree tear were randomized to primary end-to-end (75) or overlapping (74) repair. At 6 months, the results in the former group were better with flatus incontinence in 35% and 61% and fecal incontinence in 8% and 15%, respectively.[130]

In a Cochrane review, three studies of 279 women undergoing overlapping or end-to-end repair were analyzed. At 12 months, urgency was less and fecal incontinence scores were lower in those who had undergone an overlapping repair.[136] Residual defects may persist in 29% to

36% of women who have had a primary sphincter repair, but the relevance of this in the context of an asymptomatic patient is unclear.[2] Samarasekera and colleagues analyzed the long-term status of 54 patients who had a primarily repaired third-degree tear between 1981 and 1983 and compared them with 71 matched normal vaginal deliveries and 54 cesarean deliveries, with a mean follow-up in each group of 14.8, 14.2, and 14.2 years.[397] The respective prevalence of fecal incontinence in each group was 28 (53%), 13 (19%), and 6 (11%).

There is evidence that a primary repair should be carried out when possible because the long-term quality of life appears to be better than in patients who have a delayed repair. Tan and coworkers reviewed studies reporting the results of 103 primary and 777 delayed sphincter repairs from 1976 to 2006.[447] At 10 years, there were respective gains in QUALYs of 5.72 and 3.73, making primary repair about twice as cost effective.

Delayed Sphincter Repair

In many women who develop a tear during delivery, there is an obvious defect of the anal ring with disruption of the sphincter muscles. These are treated at the time by a repair. In others, however, the sphincter damage goes undetected and such patients may present months or years later. These individuals often undergo a delayed repair, usually by a colorectal surgeon.

For many years, this operation was carried out in fairly large numbers, and many series were reported in the literature. It became apparent on publication of the results that an initially satisfactory delayed repair often deteriorated with time.[281] This assessment coincided with the expanded use of ultrasound. With the advent of sacroneuromodulation, the number of repair operations has decreased, at least in Europe. There are nevertheless patients with severe defects of the anal sphincter and perineum for whom reconstruction is indicated. Those with a cloacal deformity in which the anterior anal canal and posterior vaginal wall have become one structure will require restoration of the anatomy.

The three standard methods for repairing the injured sphincter include apposition, overlapping, and plication or reefing. Each has its advocates, but none can be consistently employed with success. In principle, the surgeon usually attempts to repair the displaced muscle. In the case of a pure sphincter repair, the internal sphincter is taken with the external sphincter as one structure. Repair of each individually is not necessary although there is no evidence base for this statement.

Technique

Principles. The aim of sphincter repair is to reconstruct normal anatomy. The incision should be centered on the scar. This will allow identification of the normal anatomy, which is the first step to reconstruction. Too much mobilization of the sphincter muscle will increase the risk of denervation. The surgeon should remember when electrocoagulating a blood vessel that a nerve is close by. Sutures placed through the muscle will cause necrosis if tied too tightly. It is logical to place them through the scar tissue when possible. The material used should be absorbable but of sufficient duration to allow adequate healing before being hydrolyzed.[7] Nonabsorbable sutures may lead to abscess formation and persistent sinus formation.[268]

In the postoperative period, impaction must be avoided. Pelvic floor exercises should not begin until the wound has fully healed (several weeks to months). Early exercises are analogous to instructing a patient to lift heavy weights after an inguinal hernia repair.

Preoperative Preparation. It is advantageous to have an empty rectum at the time of operation, and a preoperative enema is considered good practice.[235] The orally administered antibiotic regimen of erythromycin base and neomycin, as popularized by Nichols and colleagues, is not felt to be helpful.[329] Antibiotic use in sphincter repair has been the subject of a Cochrane review.[51] Of 37 studies, only one was selected as being of a sufficiently satisfactory design to allow a meaningful conclusion. This involved 147 patients randomized to a second-generation cephalosporin against a placebo. Wound disruption or purulent discharge occurred in 8% and 24%, respectively.[112]

▶ THE OPERATION

Simple Sphincter Repair

An indwelling urinary catheter is inserted and the patient placed in the prone jackknife position. A curvilinear circumferential incision centered around the scar outside the anal verge will usually provide an adequate exposure of the underlying muscle (Figure 16-48A). However, if additional skin coverage is needed to close a defect, a concomitant anoplasty may be necessary, although leaving the wound open does not greatly affect the healing time.

The skin is mobilized laterally. This will reveal the superficial part of the external sphincter on each side. The skin on the anal side of the incision is then dissected from the subcutaneous tissues up into the lower anal canal to identify the scar tissue of the defect. The plane between the vagina and the scar tissue is dissected to a level above the sphincter. The maneuver in which the vagina is steadied by two fingers in the vagina to separate it from the anal canal is useful when performing this dissection because it minimizes damage to the vagina and the anorectum. Once the dissection has freed the scar in continuity with the sphincter on each side, it is divided to produce two limbs (Figure 16-48B). Each is then dissected laterally for a distance sufficient to produce a limb of sufficient mobility to allow an overlapping repair. The repair is then carried out using an end-to-end technique (Figure 16-48C) or an overlapping reconstruction as shown in Figure 16-48D. Some surgeons add a plication of the levator ani and puborectalis, but care should be taken to avoid narrowing the anal orifice. A finger or retractor placed into the anal canal during the tying of the sutures minimizes this risk (Figure 16-49).

The skin is then closed as far as is possible without tension. This may leave a small raw area in the middle to close by secondary intention. Hemostasis is important, and it may be helpful to insert a pack in the vagina to exert gentle pressure on the wound. Imbrication rather than an overlapping repair of an attenuated anterior sphincter has been reported, but there are insufficient data to determine whether it has a place.[341]

Rectovaginal Fistula and Cloacal Deformity

In patients who have a rectovaginal fistula associated with a divided anterior sphincter, reconstruction will depend on

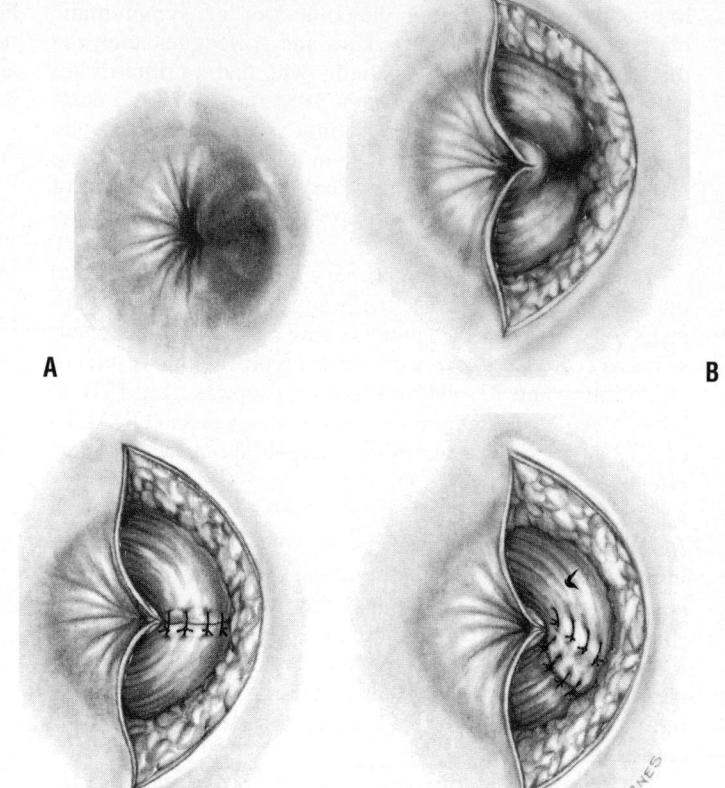

A

B

C

D

FIGURE 16-48. Technique of direct sphincter repair. **A:** A defect on the right side as a consequence of tissue loss. **B:** The ends of the divided sphincter are identified. Eschar is not debrided. **C:** Technique of apposition. **D:** Technique of overlapping.

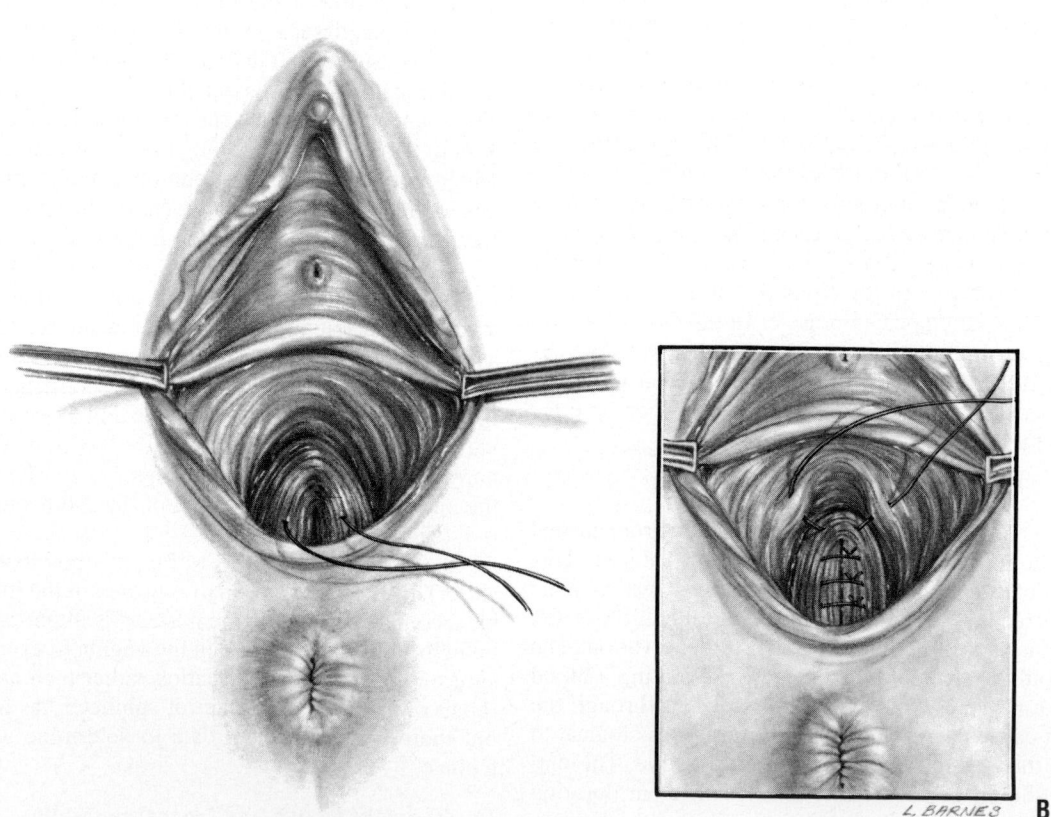

A

B

FIGURE 16-49. The reefing procedure as performed anteriorly in women. **A:** The vaginal mucosa has been elevated and the sphincter identified. **B:** The sphincter is reefed, and the perivaginal fascia is used to complete the repair.

the level of the fistula (see Chapter 15). For a fistula between the vagina and the anal canal, the easiest solution is to close the vagina and the gut tube in layers with a repair of the sphincter. This technique is the same as that for a cloacal deformity. Although there are a number of ways of accomplishing reconstruction, the method described by Corman in prior editions of this text is a reasonable alternative for providing skin coverage and for reconstruction of the posterior vaginal and anterior rectal walls.

Technique of Repair

The patient is placed in the prone jackknife position. If the perineal body must be reconstituted, and/or it becomes necessary to find tissue to reconstruct the posterior vaginal wall and distal rectum, it may be useful to perform bilateral advancement flaps. If one elects this approach, a cruciate incision is made across the perineal body, and full-thickness flaps of skin are developed as illustrated (Figure 16-50). However, if the perineal body is thought to be adequate, most surgeons prefer a curvilinear incision between the anus and the vagina (Figure 16-51). A retractor is kept in the anal canal for the entire operation in order to maintain adequacy of the lumen while the muscle repair is completed. The rectovaginal septum is infiltrated with 0.5% bupivacaine (Marcaine) with 1:200,000 epinephrine (Figure 16-52). This aids in hemostasis and facilitates the dissection. The rectum is separated from the vagina, and any concomitant fistula tract, if present, is identified (Figure 16-53). The cephalad limit is reached, and plication of the levator ani muscle may be carried out anterior to the rectum (see earlier admonition—Figure 16-54). This usually requires three or four long-term absorbable sutures.

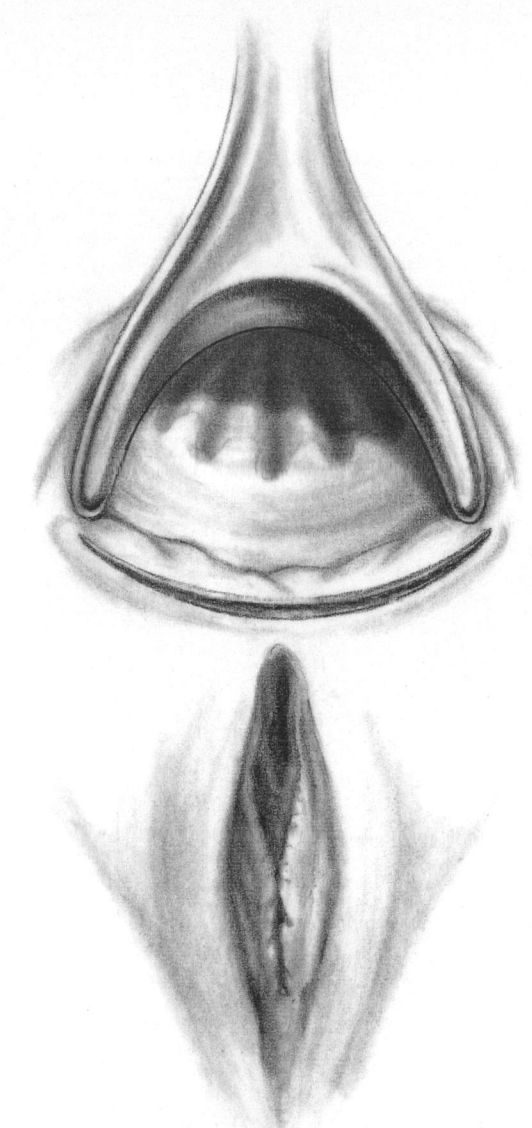

FIGURE 16-51. Standard transverse, curvilinear incision across the perineal body.

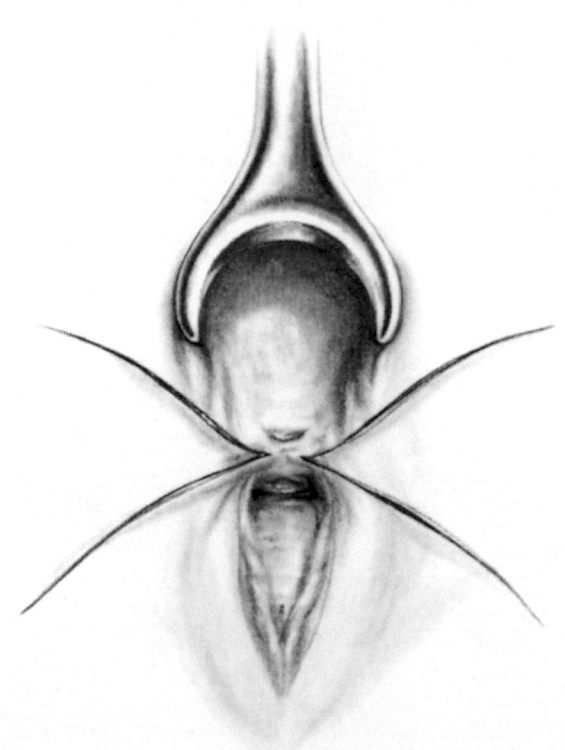

FIGURE 16-50. In anovaginal reconstruction, a cruciate incision is made across the perineal body. Note the close proximity between the anal verge and the introitus.

Often, rectovaginal fistula repair requires a concomitant sphincter reconstruction (see Chapter 15). How the approach is effected depends on the location of the openings and the origin of the problem. For a fistula between the vagina and the anal canal, one may effect the repair through a transperineal approach, with a concomitant anoplasty. For a higher level fistula, the option of mucosal advancement should be considered (see Chapter 14), although it may be possible to approach the fistula through the perineum. For still higher fistulas, either a mucosal advancement or an abdominal operation (low anterior resection, pull-through, or coloanal anastomosis) is suggested. Most women with rectovaginal fistula as a consequence of an obstetrical injury have an ectopic anus (Figure 16-55). To achieve the best functional results, reconstruction of the perineal body should also be undertaken in this group of patients.

The redundant mucosa, including any fistula, is excised from the vagina and the rectum (Figure 16-56). The external

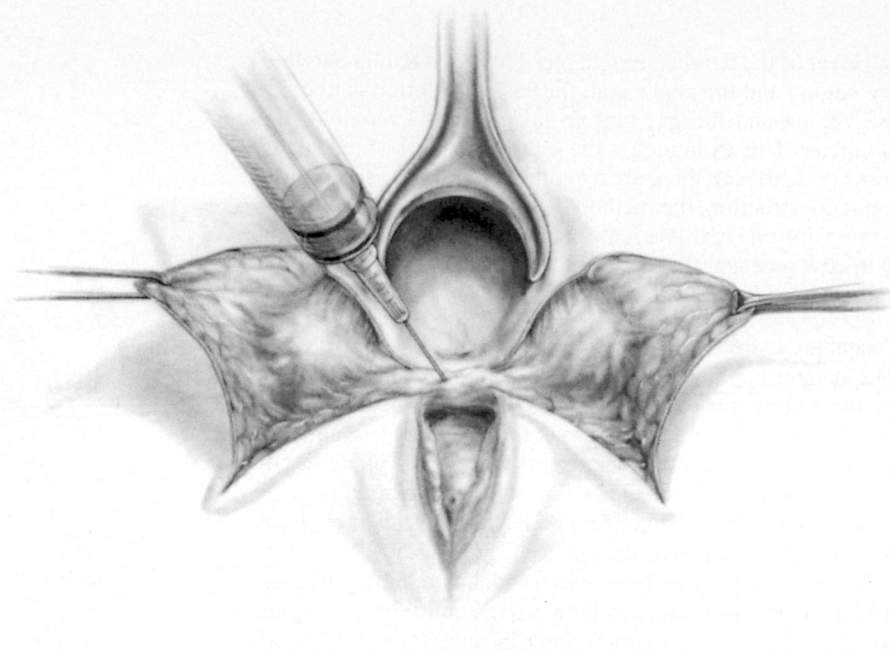

FIGURE 16-52. Anovaginal reconstruction: skin flaps are elevated, and a dilute epinephrine solution is injected into the rectovaginal septum to facilitate the dissection.

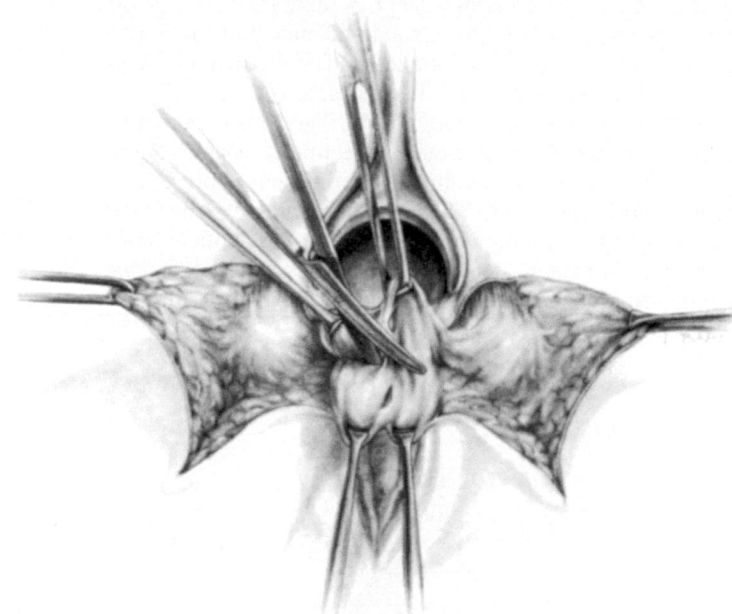

FIGURE 16-53. Anovaginal reconstruction: the rectum is separated from the vagina by careful sharp dissection.

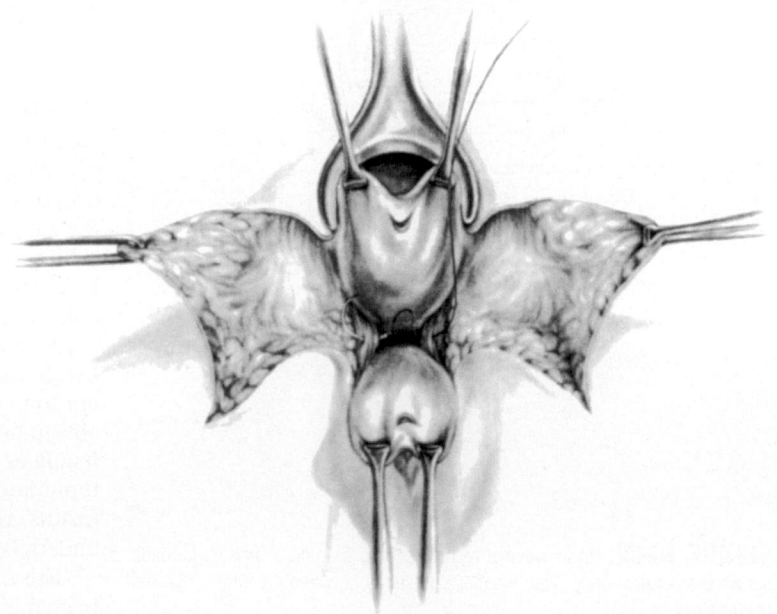

FIGURE 16-54. Anovaginal reconstruction: mobilization has been completed, and the levatores may be reefed. Three sutures of heavy, long-term absorbable material are recommended. Maintaining the retractor in place prevents the rectal lumen from being narrowed.

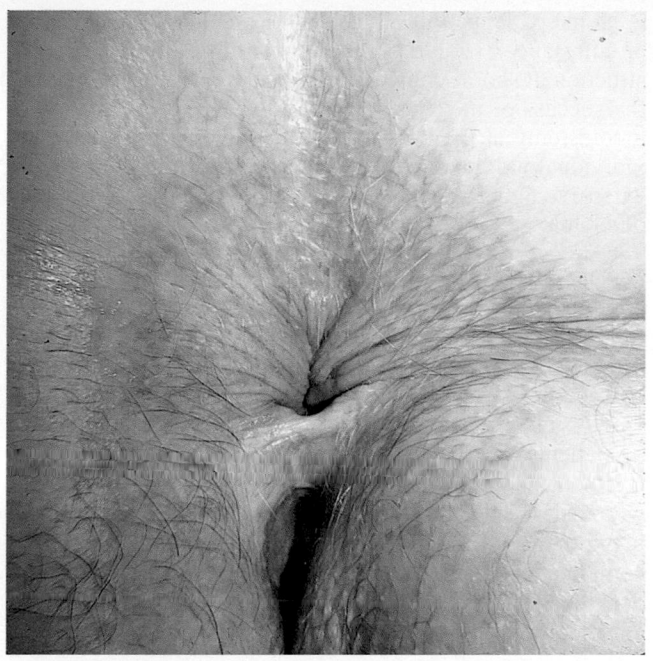

FIGURE 16-55. Ectopic anus. Anal opening is seen in close proximity to the vagina, a situation observed in 10% of women. This woman was completely asymptomatic.

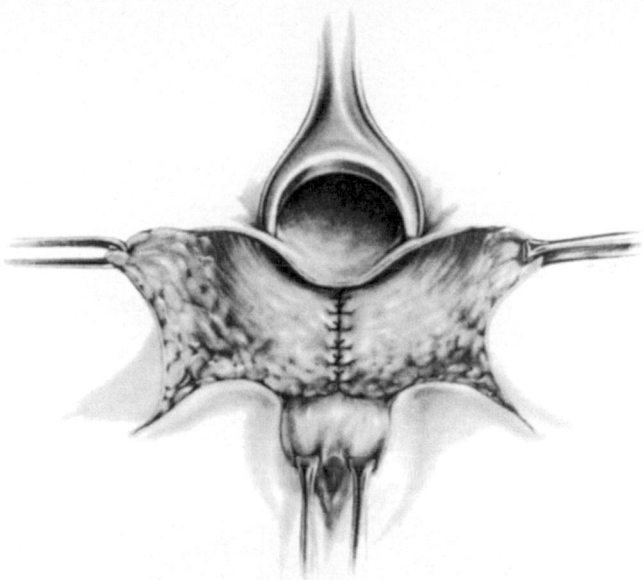

FIGURE 16-57. Anovaginal reconstruction: external sphincter repair has been completed in one or two layers.

sphincter muscle is reapproximated in one or two layers, using the same suture material (Figure 16-57). The final step in the operation is to advance and interdigitate the two triangular flaps of skin (Figure 16-58). With adequate mobilization of the skin, the suture line will partly lie within the anal canal and vagina.

Robertson suggests a different method of covering the skin defect, that of advancing bilateral, full-thickness islands of skin (Figure 16-59).

A flat Silastic drain may be placed under the skin flaps and brought out through a stab wound in the buttock; it is then attached to continuous suction. The drain is removed in 48 to 72 hours. A firm pressure dressing is applied. When a transverse incision is initially employed, the ultimate skin closure actually becomes longitudinal (Figure 16-60). This is a consequence of the muscle repair, bringing much more tissue into the midline to build up the perineal body. However, the midportion of the incision usually is left open because of tension. Figures 16-61 and 16-62 show women who sustained obstetrical trauma and who underwent reconstruction with skin advancement.

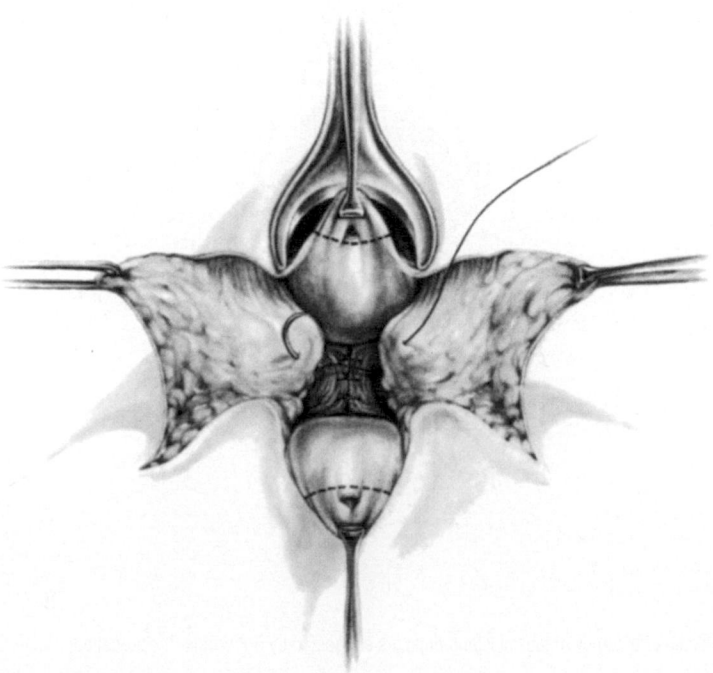

FIGURE 16-56. Anovaginal reconstruction: the fistula openings and redundant mucosa in both the rectum and vagina, if present, are excised (*dashed lines*). The external sphincter repair is then begun.

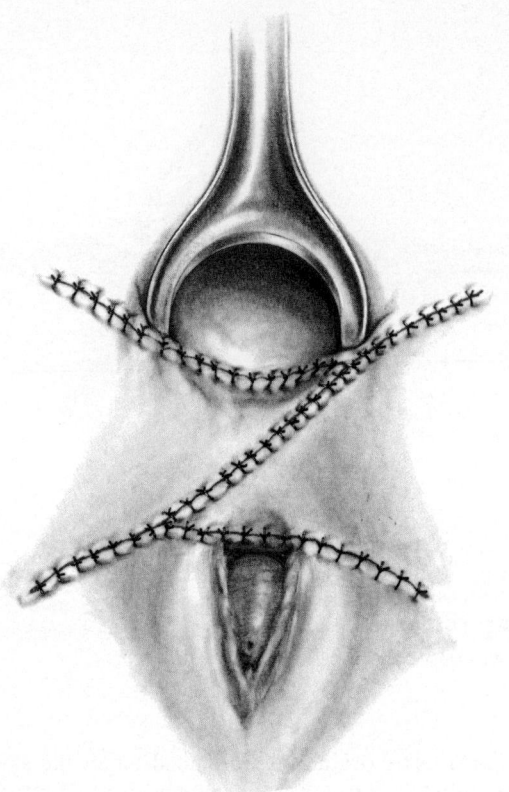

FIGURE 16-58. Anovaginal reconstruction: the skin flaps are advanced and interdigitated, thereby permitting the widened perineal body to be closed completely.

Some patients will already have a colostomy. Under no circumstances should this be closed at the time of reconstruction. It should remain until the wounds are healed when the success of the repair can be judged. The indication of a colostomy at the time of repair, however, is a matter of individual judgment. In line with common sense, the more extensive the reconstruction, the more one should consider diversion.

Postoperative Care

Although there was no difference in a randomized controlled trial of bowel confinement compared with no confinement, impaction requiring intervention to clear is very likely to damage the repair, possibly irretrievably.[279] Nessim and co-workers conducted a prospective, randomized trial involving 54 patients, one-half of whom received a bowel-confining regimen and the other a regular diet.[325] In the 32 individuals who underwent a sphincter repair, there were no differences between the two groups in the incidence of septic or urologic complications, and there were cost savings due to reduced hospital stay. Impaction is a particular concern, however. When mechanical disimpaction is required, the repair is at risk.

Results

There are now many reports of sphincter repair in the literature (Table 16-6). Many of these do not distinguish between its application to obstetrical injury and injury from other causes such as anal surgery or general trauma. The lack of prospective randomized trials makes it difficult to assess the results not only between different techniques of repair but also between repair and nonsurgical treatment. If there is little or no residual sphincter, an attempt at resuture is unlikely to be successful. With respect to the value of preoperative physiology, Buie and colleagues demonstrated that clinical

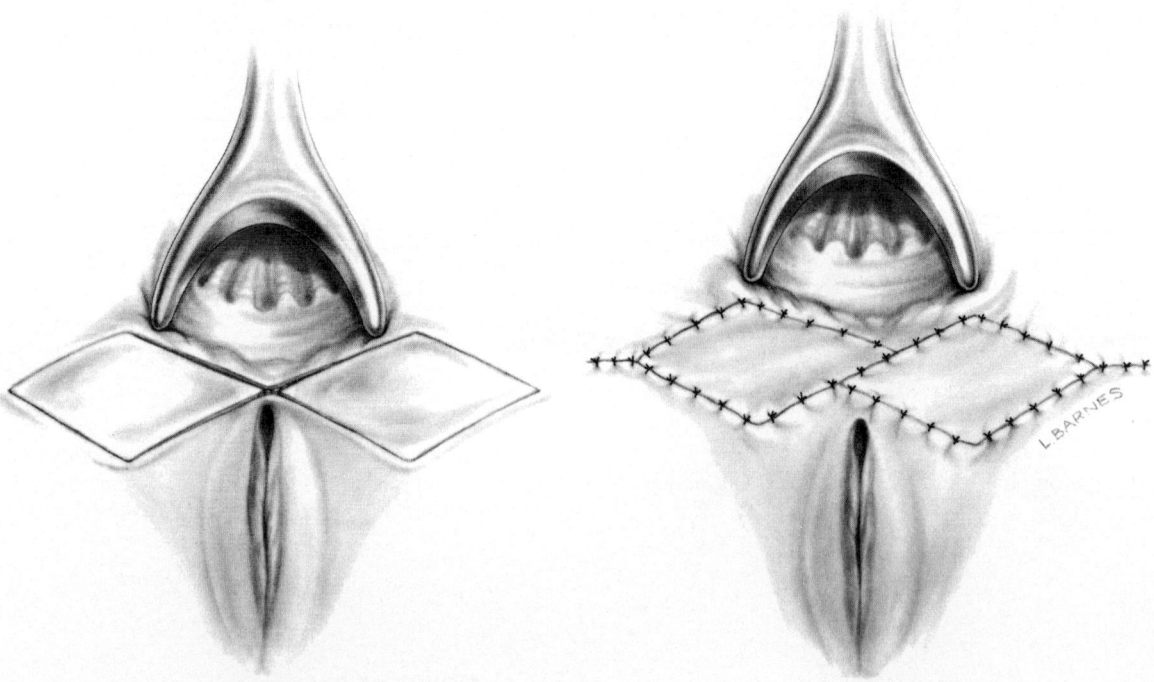

A   B

FIGURE 16-59. Anovaginal reconstruction: skin closure can also be effected by means of island flaps, as suggested by Robertson, the so-called Texas double diamond.

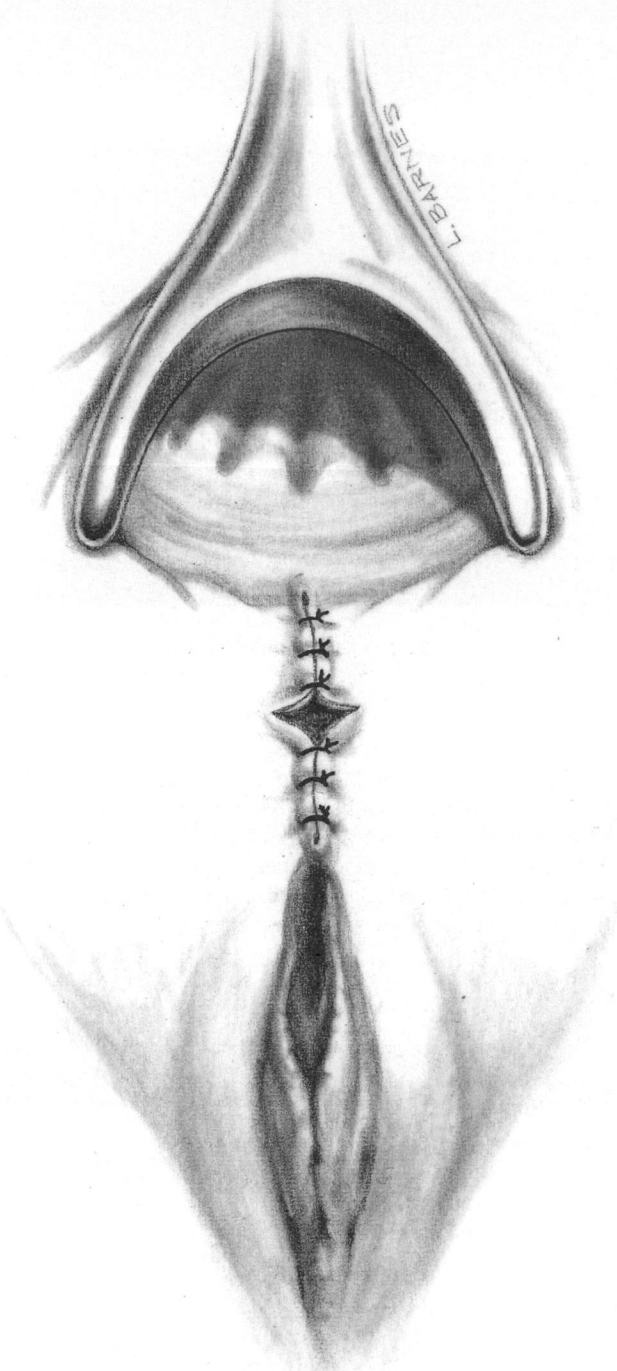

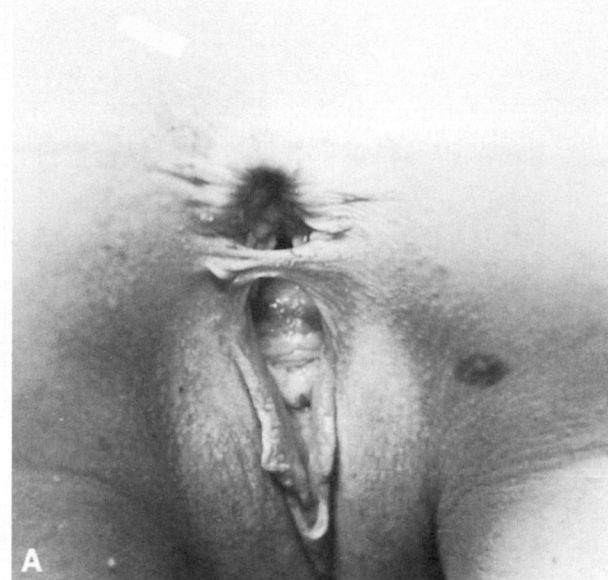

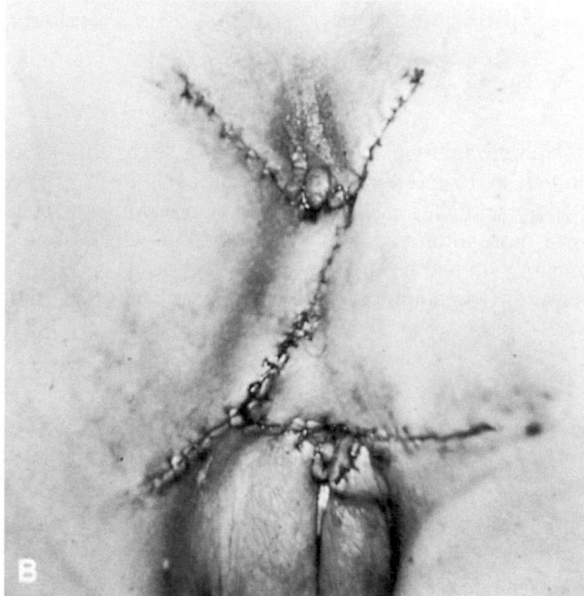

FIGURE 16-61. Rectovaginal fistula secondary to obstetrical injury. **A:** Note the ectopic (anterior) displacement of the anorectum. **B:** Reconstruction completed by advancement of skin flaps. The distance between the anus and the vagina is essentially normal.

FIGURE 16-60. Following repair, the original transverse incision becomes longitudinal, further separating the anal verge from the introitus. Usually one cannot close the midportion of the wound.

rather than manometric assessment predicts continence after sphincter repair.[50]

Sphincter repair is followed by deterioration of an initially good result in many patients. Fleshman and coworkers performed overlapping sphincteroplasty in 55 women whose incontinence was primarily the result of obstetrical injury.[139] Although most patients were satisfied, complete continence was restored in only about one-half of the patients. In a later article from the same group, they noted that the only factor that correlated with the return to normal sphincter function

following overlapping sphincteroplasty was an increase in squeeze pressure.[171] Physiologic improvement was related to clinical improvement by Oliveira and colleagues who reported the results in 55 female patients followed for 29 months.[342] Of these, 39 had a successful result. The functional length of the anal canal increased from 1.0 cm to 2.2 cm, and the Wexner score fell from 15.3 to 5.8. This fall was independent of age, with patients older than 60 years having a similar result.

Since the publication by Malouf and colleagues,[281] there have been many reports demonstrating a decline in function over time after an initially successful repair.[20,41,174,281] Malouf and coworkers[281] were able to study 55 patients longitudinally who were previously reported at a median interval of 15 months following the repair.[123] These were then reassessed at 77 months (range, 60 to 96) by postal questionnaire and

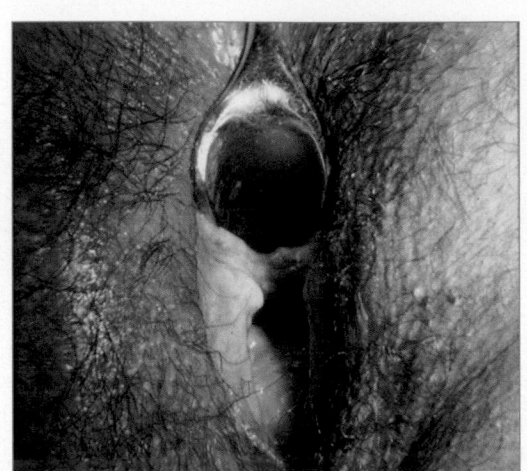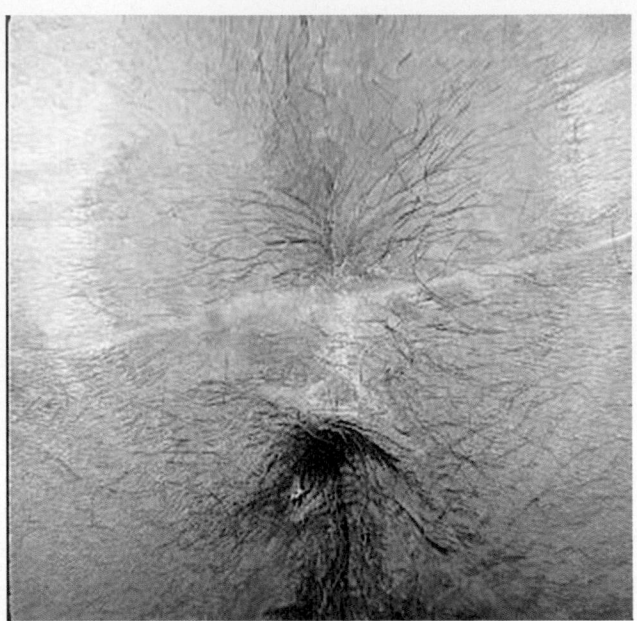

FIGURE 16-62. Anal incontinence secondary to obstetrical injury. **A:** Preoperative appearance. **B:** Appearance 8 weeks following surgery.

by telephone interview. At the original assessment, 42 were continent at 15 months. Of the 55 patients, 46 (86%) were contactable. Of these, 23 (50%) rated their bowel control to be 50% or more improved. However, only four were completely continent. Six had no urgency, and 8 had no passive soiling. Twenty of 38 patients in whom this detail was ascertained needed to wear a pad, and 25 had a lifetime restriction. It is noteworthy, however, that half of the patients felt that the result was "successful." For a benign condition such as incontinence, this is the most important end point. Bravo Gutierrez and colleagues reported a large series of 191 patients who had undergone a repair. After excluding death and the occurrence

TABLE 16-6 Results of Delayed Sphincter Repair

AUTHOR	YEAR	PATIENTS	FU MO	PARKS I/II %	PARKS III/IV %
Fleshman	1991	55	12	72	28
Rothbarth	2000	39	12	62	38
Engel	1994	55	15	76	24
Pinta	2003	39	22	59	41
Karoui	2000	86	40	51	49
Buie	2001	158	43	62	38
Halverson	2002	49	69	46	54
Malouf	2000	38	77	11	89
Barisic	2006	65	80	48	52
Bravo Guttierrez	2004	130	120	22	78

of dementia, there were 182 eligible for assessment. Of these, 130 (71%) returned a questionnaire. At a follow-up of 10 years, 6% had no fecal incontinence, 16% had incontinence of flatus only, and 19% had soiling. In contrast, 57% had incontinence of solid stool. These symptoms worsened between 3 and 10 years. Preoperative physiology was not predictive of the clinical outcome.[41] There is some evidence that the results of sphincter repair may be improved by biofeedback, although there may be a question of statistical significance.[95,215]

Factors Relating to Failure

It is possible that the repair itself causes damage to the muscle directly or to its nerve supply.[281] Age may be a factor, bearing in mind that the actual test of competence of the muscle can only be judged after the repair, which for the first time in years in some instances may have been put to the test.[202]

Several studies have reported the early development of a further defect following repair. Whether this is related to poor technique or the result of infection or natural parting of the integrity of the repair due to tension on the suture line is not known. Reports of a continuing defect after repair may truly reflect a disruption of the repair or the "defect" may simply be due to the fact that any repair will, by definition, leave evidence of scarring even when there is no loss of integrity of the anal ring. Some of the patients said to have a defect in this circumstance may be the subject of a radiologic misinterpretation. Thus, rates of a defect of up to 90% may be an overestimate because none of the reports stated whether the anal ring was intact or not.[332,301,362]

Norderval and colleagues reported much better results following repair in 74 women having had a vaginal delivery who underwent primary repair of a tear.[332] At a follow-up of 27 months (range, 14 to 39), anal endosound was performed in 62. Of these, 22 had "incontinence," but on closer reading this was for stool in only 5 (8%) and for flatus in 17 (27%). The authors state, furthermore, that the symptoms were mild in 11 women, and in only 6 did they occur more than once per month. Only 3 (4%) had urgency alone, and here it occurred less than once per week. None of 17 women with normal ultrasonography results was incontinent compared with 20 of 45 with an ultrasonographic defect ($P = .001$). The mean sphincter length, squeeze pressure, and resting pressure were significantly higher in women with Wexner scores of 0 to 2 compared with women with a score of more than 2. Sphincter length was inversely related to the degree of incontinence ($P < .001$). These authors used the ultrasound criteria of sphincter defect as defined by Williams and colleagues.[490] The article, however, does not give any measure of a defect and furthermore does not define the criteria for disruption of the anal ring in any objective form.

Pudendal neuropathy may also be a factor which if progressive would explain a continuing deterioration in function. In some reports, patients with pudendal neuropathy have been found to have worse results than those without, whereas others have not found this to be the case.[41,50,61,151,157,387,510] Atrophy may be due to factors other than neuropathy, but whatever its cause it may be associated with failure.[44,45,492] Briel and colleagues, in applying MRI to 20 patients with incontinence and with an anterior sphincter defect after obstetrical injury, found atrophy in 8 (40%).[44] Clinical success in those with and without atrophy was 2 (25%) of 8 and 11 (92%) of 12 patients.

As might be expected, therefore, success after a sphincter repair following obstetrical injury is related to the quality of the sphincter muscle as judged by denervation and atrophy. It is possible that the degenerative disorder may be progressive.

Summary

The conclusion from these studies is that evidence of a sphincter defect after repair is common. The definition of a defect is unclear, however. Of course, scarring at the site of a repair is an inevitable consequence of the repair itself. The degree of angular extent is usually not given. In addition, as the article by Norderval and colleagues demonstrates, the state of "incontinence" has many degrees of severity.[332] Thus, of the 22 patients in their study who were said to have incontinence, it would appear to be mild both in volume and frequency in all cases. Assessment by questionnaire encourages overreporting. It is vital, therefore, that clinicians understand the sources of error in the reporting of the results of treatment for incontinence. In the case of sphincter repair, it would be a great disservice to the patient if this treatment fell into disuse without a more detailed and objective assessment of the results. The degree of patient satisfaction is the most important end point, more so than the number of incontinent episodes.

Cloacal Defect

This is an extreme form of sphincter injury in which the anterior defect extends into the vagina and for a limited distance into the lower rectum. In patients with healthy muscle, continence may be satisfactory despite the complete disruption of the sphincter ring. Nevertheless, repair as described previously is advisable because function may deteriorate with time.

Corman reported 28 women such patients.[85] All had varying degrees of incontinence for flatus or feces, and most wore a pad. Twenty (71%) had undergone a midline episiotomy. Approximately one-half of the patients had a prior attempt at repair. This type of anovaginal reconstruction has since been applied to 135 patients. Eight percent noted some degree of impairment of incontinence for gas. Four experienced no improvement compared with the preoperative status. All of these individuals had pudendal neuropathy. Ninety-two percent reported complete continence for loose stool. Abcarian and coworkers reported excellent results in 43 patients who sustained a cloacal defect.[3] Others noted generally satisfactory results with conventional sphincter repair for a host of anorectal complications associated with vaginal delivery, including sphincter disruption, rectovaginal fistula, cloacal defect, and fistula-in-ano.[139,433,476] Khanduja and colleagues performed repair of obstetrical injuries associated with a vaginal repair on 52 patients.[226] At a mean of 16 months, continence was observed in 64%, including 56% of those with a rectovaginal fistula.

Repeat Repair

Some patients who experience failure after a sphincter repair may be salvaged by a repeat operation. Pinedo and colleagues reported the results in 26 women who had had a failed initial repair following obstetrical injury.[360] All were judged to have good contraction of the disrupted external sphincter muscle when the patient was asked to tighten the perineum. The period of urgency rose from less than 5 minutes to more than 15 minutes in one-half the patients. This benefit was maintained at 5 years on follow-up.[469] Others have reported a similar experience.[50,158]

Crohn's Disease

Sphincter repair has been applied to selected patients with Crohn's disease. Scott and colleagues carried out a repair in patients for whom the alternative would have been a proctocolectomy.[404] All but one underwent successful repair, and only one had a permanent stoma.

Postanal Repair (Parks)

Parks (see Biography, Chapter 29) emphasized the importance of restoration of the anorectal angle by what he called a "postanal repair."[350] He believed that one of the major contributing factors for maintaining continence is the valve effect caused by the anorectal angle that is created by the tonic contraction of the puborectalis muscle. At the time, the operation was advocated for patients with incontinence associated with pudendal neuropathy and also for rectal prolapse and the descending perineum syndrome. For 10 to 15 years, it was used frequently owing to its apparent early effectiveness and the limited treatment options available at the time. It has now almost died out, although there is a small population of patients who have benefited in the long term.

Technique

The operation was originally described with the patient in the lithotomy position but it is much easier in the prone jackknife position as the illustrations show. A V-shaped incision is made approximately 6 cm posterior to the anal verge (Figure 16-63A). The skin is then dissected anteriorly to re-

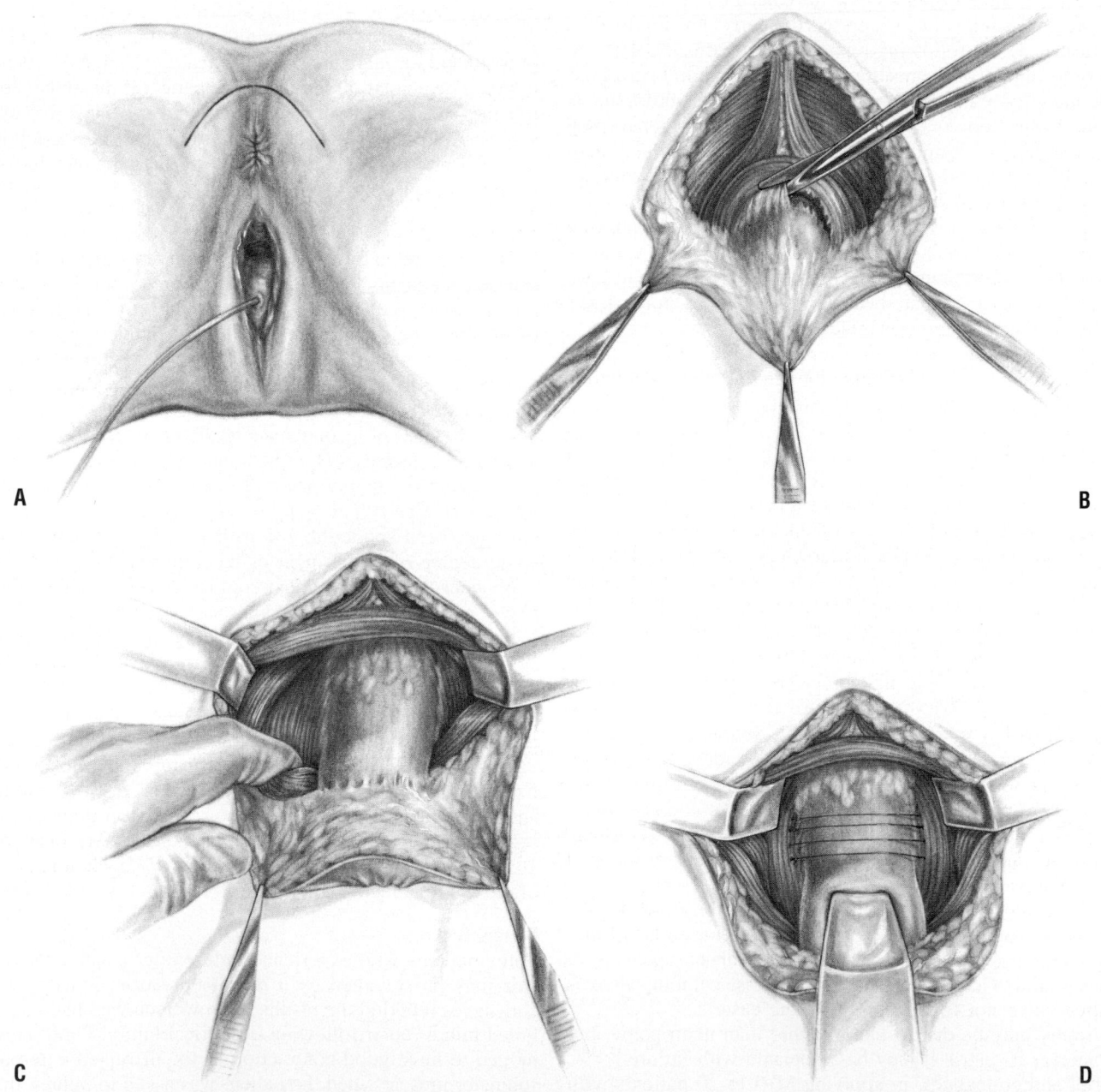

FIGURE 16-63. Parks' postanal pelvic floor repair. **A:** V-shaped incision is made ~6 cm posterior to the anal verge. **B:** The internal sphincter is separated from the external sphincter through one-half of its circumference. **C:** The rectum is lifted off the upper portion of the external sphincter reaching the puborectalis muscle. **D:** Sutures of polypropylene are placed across the two limbs of the iliococcygeus muscle. Approximately three layers are placed at this topmost level and are tied loosely, without tension, to form a lattice across the pelvis. *(continued)*

veal the subcutaneous border of the external sphincter. The interspincteric plane is identified, and the dissection is continued proximally between the two sphincters (Figure 16-63B). This is a bloodless plane through which dissection should not cause bleeding or nerve injury. Dissection is then carried out in the intersphincteric plane, displacing the posterior portion of the external sphincter through one-half of its circumference. The dissection is continued above the puborectalis (Figure 16-63C) to the level of the coccyx taking care to remain anterior to the fascia covering the levator ani muscles. In this manner, the perineal branch of S4 that supplies the levator plate is avoided because it lies deep to the fascia.

The dissection proceeds cephalad by lifting the rectum off the upper part of the external sphincter. The internal

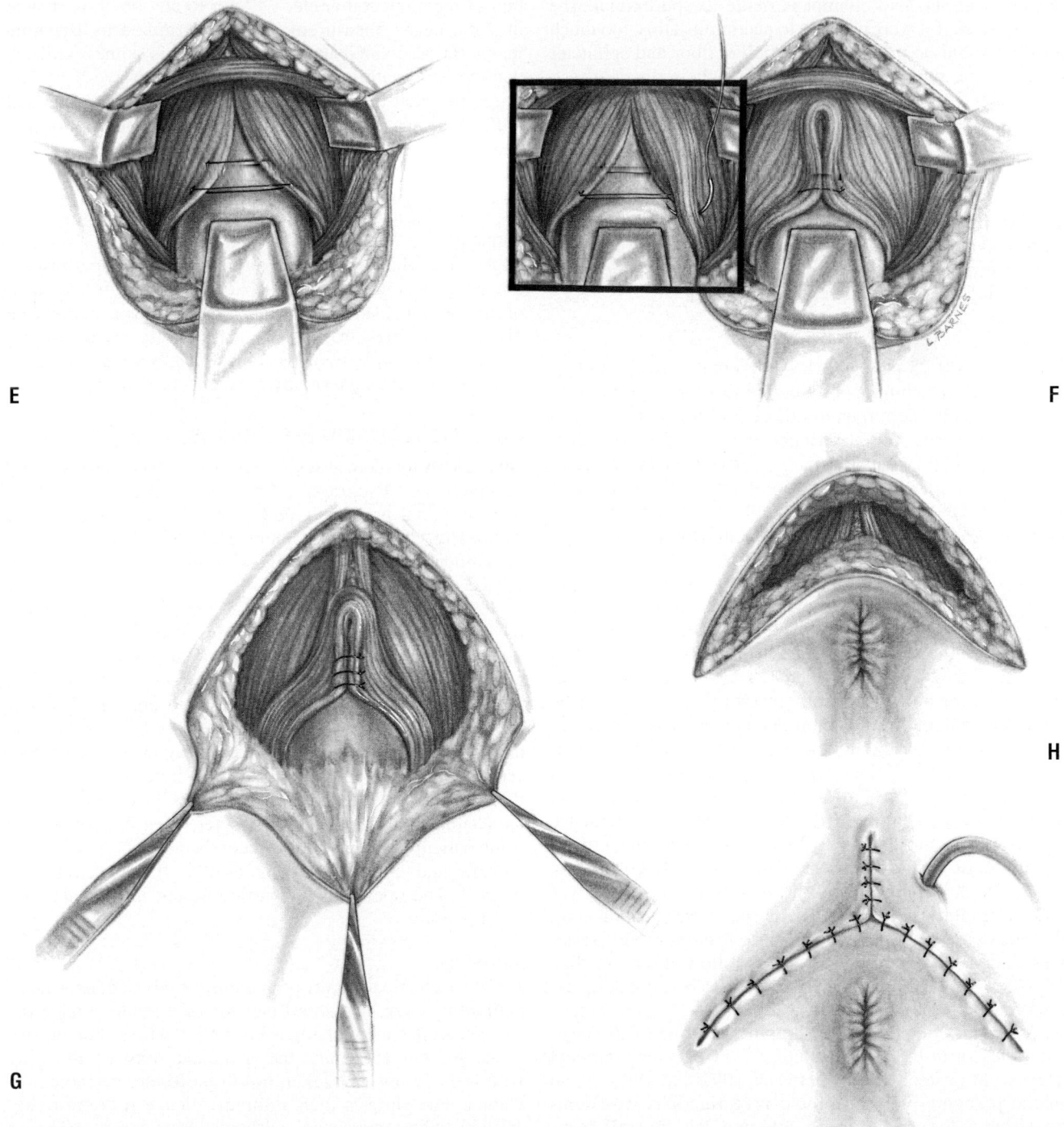

FIGURE 16-63. *(continued)* **E:** The next layer is placed in the upper part of the pubococcygeus muscle as a lattice. The lower part, closer to the midline, can be approximated. **F:** The puborectalis is now plicated. This is the strongest and thickest part and the muscle that is most easily visualized. **G:** The external sphincter is sutured. **H:** Repair results in the drawing forward of the anterior skin flap; simple reconstitution would be under tension. **I:** Skin closure is Y shaped. (Adapted from Parks AG, Percy J. Postanal pelvic floor repair for anorectal incontinence. In: Todd IP, Fielding LP, eds. *Operative Surgery*. London, United Kingdom: Butterworths; 1983:433, with permission.)

sphincter becomes contiguous with the circular muscle of the rectum at about the level of the puborectalis muscle. Above the puborectalis, the fascia of Waldeyer is encountered, and the mesorectal fat and posterior rectal wall are exposed.

The highest and most lateral point of the levatores is identified close to the spines of the ischium (i.e., the iliococcygeus muscle). With exposure of the levator ani, a lattice darn of monofilament or floss nylon in two or three layers is constructed, either by continuous or interrupted sutures (Figure 16-63D). No attempt is made to approximate the muscle; even if it were possible to accomplish this, too much tension would be produced. The pelvic floor and sphincter muscles are approximated, displacing them anteriorly to increase the anorectal angle (Figure 16-63E–G). Drainage of the subcutaneous tissue is recommended and the skin is closed (Figure 16-63 H,I).[351]

Postoperative Care

The bowels can either be confined or the patient given laxatives to avoid impaction. In females, the bladder is catheterized. Antibiotics are given for 2 to 3 days. The importance of avoiding straining should be emphasized.

Results

Parks reported 75 patients who underwent postanal repair, approximately two-thirds of whom had a rectal prolapse.[350] The best results were found in those without prolapse, with an overall success of 83%. Henry and Simson reported the results of all postanal repairs performed by the surgical staff at St. Mark's Hospital during the period 1978 through 1983.[183] There were 242 patients, with an overall complication rate of 20%, mostly due to wound infections. A satisfactory result was achieved in almost 60%.

Yoshioka and Keighley reported the results in 124 patients.[509] There was improvement in incontinence in 81%, but 76% still leaked stool, and 52% required pads. The quality of continence after the operation was generally poor. A report from the Lahey Clinic of 14 patients showed that 9 had initial improvement with two subsequent failures.[433] Similarly, there was a fall in the initial improvement in 36 patients evaluated at 6 months, and in only 50% of those improved was this maintained.[207] A long-term assessment (median of 6.2 [5 to 8] years) in 30 of 54 women operated on between 1984 and 1986 showed, however, that 9 had either no incontinence or incontinence to flatus only, and only 4 were incontinent to solid stool. Of the 54 patients, only 1 needed a colostomy, and of the 30 patients, only 2 were housebound. There was a deterioration of the PNTMS and fiber density, indicating that the denervation process was progressive.[408] This result was similar to a report of 19 patients followed for a median of 8 (2 to 10) years, of whom 7 had a successful result, and 4 more were significantly improved.[374]

A similar conclusion was drawn from one of the largest series from the United States.[289] Twenty-one patients underwent postanal repair between 1992 and 1998. None of the preoperative physiologic investigations was demonstrated to be predictive of outcome. The overall "success rate" was 35%. The authors concluded that in spite of the low success rate, the absence of mortality and the low morbidity should at least permit its application in selected instances. Engel and colleagues also showed reasonable results at 43 (15 to 126) months in 38 patients, 19 of whom were satisfied with the operation. These individuals tended to have a higher resting pressure than those who were not satisfied.[124] Further reports indicate that about 30% to 50% of patients had an adequate result at intervals of 2 to 3 years postoperatively.[42] A report of 47 patients out of a series of 66 operated on between 1994 and 2001 showed that at a follow-up of 3 (2 to 9) years, 4 patients were continent, and 30 were significantly improved.[1] Fourteen were no better nor worse.

The reasons for improvement are not related to accentuation of the anorectal angle,[344,498] nor to any obvious change in static pelvic measurements as determined by dynamic magnetic resonance imaging.[180] There is some evidence that the neuropathic changes may be progressive.[408,420] The suggestion that the result is related to improvement in anal pressures[344] was not borne out by others.[509] No relationship between clinical outcome and the preoperative physiologic assessment has been found despite the finding that anal canal pressures may rise after the operation.[399,405]

Summary

At the time when postanal repair was commonly performed, the general conclusion was that the operation produced disappointing results, but when looked at from a distance of 20 years, these results are surprisingly good. This is especially true in light of those obtained by sphincter repair and even in the long term after sacroneuromodulation.

Anal Encirclement Procedures

Anal encircling procedures were originally described by Thiersch (see Biography, Chapter 21) for the management of rectal prolapse (see Chapter 21), but Gabriel (see Biography, Chapter 24) recommended its application to fecal incontinence.[146] He reported good results in 11 patients with the use of silver wire.

This approach offers a simple alternative to the transposition of the gracilis or gluteus muscle for supplementing the sphincter mechanism. Various materials for ameliorating fecal incontinence have been used, including fascia lata, Teflon, Marlex, catgut, Mersilene, and Dacron-impregnated Silastic sheet, as a prosthesis encircling the anus (Figure 16-64). Labow and colleagues originally described the use of this material as an alternative to wire in the treatment of rectal prolapse.[242] Others have found it to be an adequate substitute anal sphincter when implanted into some patients who have fecal incontinence.[84,85,198,241,243,264,433] Devesa and colleagues have used a flat Jackson-Pratt drain.[102] The operation is contraindicated in patients with constipation.

Technique

A full mechanical bowel preparation is advised, and under antibiotic cover, two small incisions are made outside the anal verge. A curved clamp is inserted into the subcutaneous tissue and passed around the anal canal drawing the sling with it. Care must be taken not to perforate the rectum or vagina. The sling is then sutured to leave it comfortably applied to the anal canal without undue tension (Figure 16-65). Figure 16-66 illustrates the preoperative and later postoperative results in an older woman with presumed pudendal nerve injury as the cause of her incontinence. Most recently, Cook Biotech developed their Biodesign (Surgisis) implantable device for use as a sling to narrow the anus (Figure 16-67).

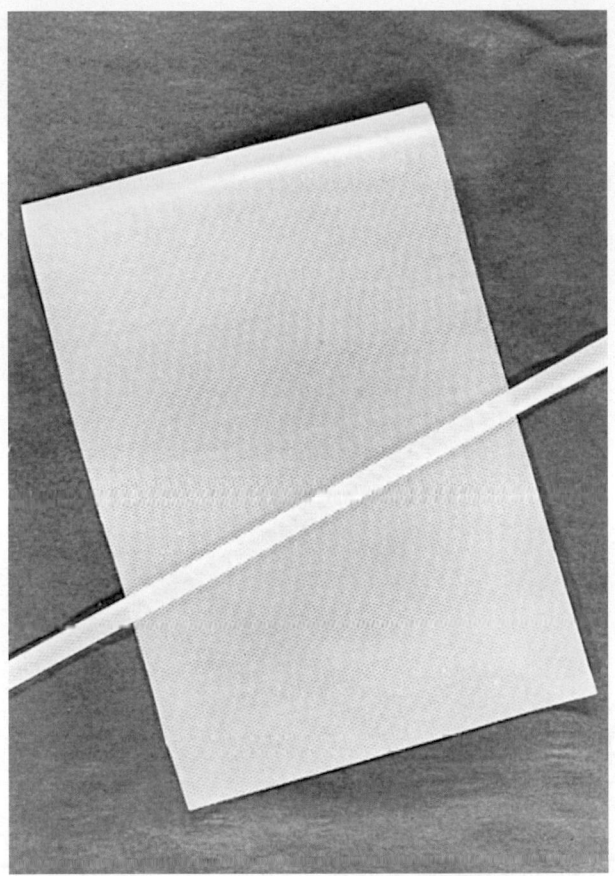

FIGURE 16-64. The elasticity of the 1.5-cm wide strip can be readily appreciated (Dow Corning, Midland, MI). Care must be taken to trim the sheet along the proper axis.

Results

Corman reported an overall failure rate of approximately 40%, but the Lahey Clinic group reported good to excellent results in about 75% of patients.[198] They emphasized that the sling should be positioned at least 2 cm from the anal verge to limit the likelihood of erosion and pain.[433] Sainio and colleagues performed anal encirclement with polypropylene mesh for rectal prolapse as well as for anal incontinence.[394] All three patients operated on for the latter indication improved.

There has been little in the literature since the 1990s, but Devesa and colleagues have recently reported the results of insertion of a flat band silicone sling in 33 patients (20 females) followed for a mean of 37 months over a range of 2 to 60 months.[102] The indication was incontinence due to a host of factors, including iatrogenic (5), obstetrical (5), idiopathic (5), restorative proctocolectomy (5), rectal prolapse (4), congenital (4), neuropathic (3), and other trauma (1). The sling had to be removed in 13 patients of whom 10 were able to be reimplanted. Early infection occurred in two and late skin erosion in another two patients. Quality of life improved in all domains, and the Wexner score fell from 15 ± 5 to 7 ± 4.

Complications include infection, stricture, fecal impaction, persistent incontinence, and pain. It is primarily because of this last problem that removal of the sling becomes necessary. Migration and erosion are not uncommon, and

Labow and colleagues have suggested fixing Dacron felt to the sheeting to prevent this from occurring.[241]

Removal of the sling is usually simple to undertake because of encapsulation. This can be accomplished under local anesthetic as an office procedure. Interestingly, many patients experience improvement of symptoms when the mesh is removed. Perhaps the scarring and capsule formation around the implant narrow the anal canal sufficiently to produce a comparable effect.

Comment

It is difficult to assess this treatment against other sling procedures such as a graciloplasty or artificial bowel sphincter. It is, however, a much simpler and less traumatic procedure. A prospective, randomized trial with another form of treatment would be useful.

Artificial Sphincter

Artificial sphincters, including dynamic graciloplasty (Medtronic, Inc., Minneapolis, MN) and the artificial bowel sphincter (ABS; American Medical Systems, Minnetonka, MN), were tested in the 1990s and the early part of the 2000s during which period sacral nerve modulation was just coming into use. Dynamic graciloplasty has often been followed by complications and technical difficulties with the stimulator.[152] ABS was less prone to early complications, but infection and extrusion occurred as a late complication. Function, however, was usually satisfactory when the device remained in place. The overall complications and functional results of each form of artificial sphincter were similar in a comparative review.[500]

Standards for anal sphincter replacement were considered by an international group of surgeons who recommended that the artificial bowel sphincter and electrically stimulated muscle neosphincter were suitable procedures for end-stage fecal incontinence. Indications, function and quality of life, choice of therapy, and diffusion of the technique were all considered.[271] The group recommended that the ASCRS incontinence-specific quality-of-life scale be used for evaluation and analysis and that dissemination of the technique should be carried out in a controlled manner. In summary, it was agreed that the artificial bowel sphincter could be offered where there was no other option to the status quo than a stoma.

Artificial Muscle Plastic Procedures

Procedures to create an autologous neosphincter using the gracilis or the gluteus maximus muscles have been developed over the last 60 years.[73,105] Initially, the gracilis muscle was used,[359] but in the 1990s the operation was modified by the inclusion of a stimulator working at a frequency that converted the muscle fiber type from fast twitch (type II) to slow action (type I).[73,105] The idea was to simulate the constant tonic activity of the pelvic floor.[16,17,496] There is now a large literature on these procedures, and the clinical results, including complications and function, have been extensively reported. Although improved in some cases, improvement in continence is often disappointing. With the decline of reconstructive surgery and the rise of behavioral treatments and neuromodulation, gracilis and gluteus maximus sphincter replacements have been little used in the last 10 years.

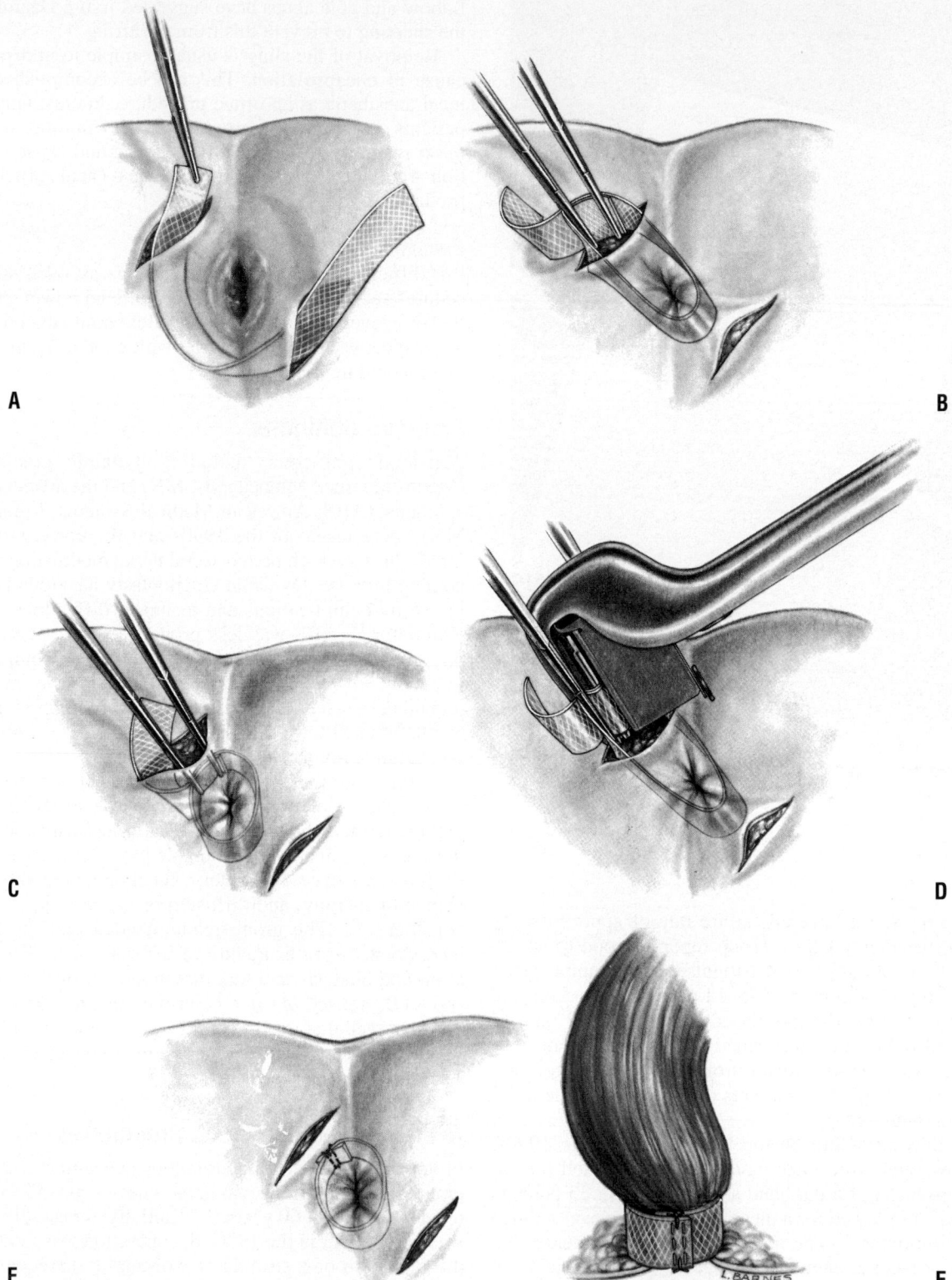

FIGURE 16-65. FIGURE 16-65. Silastic-Dacron implant. **A:** Appropriately tailored sheet is passed circumferentially in the ischiorectal fossa. **B:** Mesh is secured with paired straight clamps. **C:** Implant is replaced and adequacy of the lumen determined by the index finger. **D:** The ends are secured by stapling. **E,F:** Final position of the implant.

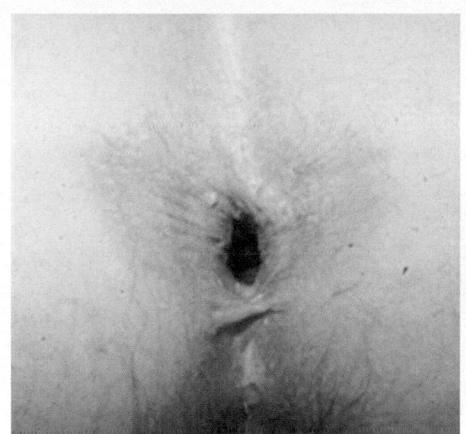
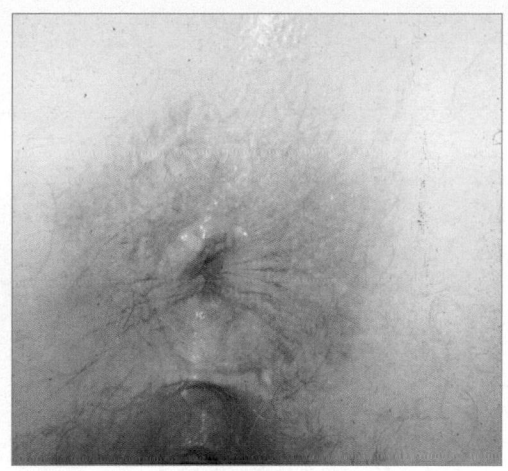

FIGURE 16-66. Incontinence of uncertain origin in an elderly woman presumably based on pudendal nerve injury. **A:** Patulous anus is evident on mere spreading of the buttocks. **B:** Postoperative appearance 2 months following insertion of an elastic fabric sling.

Gracioplasty (Gracilis Muscle Transposition)

Nonstimulated

In 1952, Pickrell and colleagues developed a procedure using the gracilis muscle as a substitute anal sphincter.[359] Corman found this to be a very effective operation for selected patients when a supplementary sphincter was required or when multiple attempts at direct repair had been unsuccessful.[82-84]

Indications

Gracilis muscle transposition (GMT) is a complex and technically difficult procedure with a high failure rate. The primary indication has been when fecal incontinence could not be controlled by nonoperative means or where sphincteroplasty had failed. Gracioplasty has also been used for reconstruction of the anus after abdominoperineal resection and in the management of postirradiation necrosis.[337,495]

In modern practice, there are few indications but there is no question that potential candidates should be treated in a center familiar with the procedure. Contraindications include irritable bowel, diarrhea or constipation, patients with anal disease, an irradiated perineum, radiation proctitis, and older age. It has myriad technical pitfalls and intraoperative and postoperative complications.

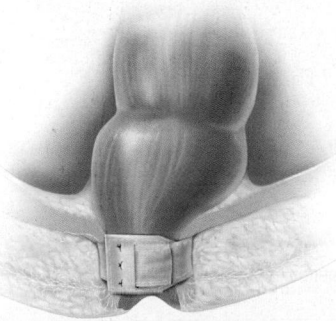

FIGURE 16-67. Cook Biodesign (Surgisis) Sling follows the same principles of implantation described in Figure 16-63. Note the closing mechanism. However, anchoring sutures are still required. (©2009, Lisa Clark courtesy of Cook Medical Inc.)

Technique

The patient is placed in the lithotomy position giving access to the leg and the perineum. Although not demonstrated to reduce morbidity, some surgeons prefer always to create a colostomy. A mechanical bowel preparation is given and the operation is carried out under antibiotic coverage.

The primary blood supply of the gracilis muscle is almost always proximal, and, therefore, dividing it at its insertion into the tibia usually does not compromise viability. Occasionally, however, distal mobilization may result in ischemia, and care should be taken to recognize this. The muscle can be mobilized using three incisions or by dissection through a laparoscope introduced through a single wound. Distally, the gracilis tendon lies deep to the sartorius and can be difficult to isolate.

The muscle is mobilized to the neurovascular bundle (Figures 16-68 and 16-69) and delivered through the wound at the top of the thigh (Figure 16-70). It is important to conserve as much length as possible for the anal neosphincter. Any distal wound is closed.

A curvilinear incision is then made approximately 1.5 cm from the anal verge anteriorly and posteriorly. In a modification of this, a bridge of skin is left that minimizes breakdown of the wounds (one of the most frequent causes of failure) while allowing access to the rectovaginal plane and ischiorectal fossae for circumferential passage of the muscle and tendon.[217]

A tunnel is developed between the proximal thigh incision and the anterior perianal incision and is enlarged to accommodate the muscle belly without constriction. The muscle is then pulled through the anterior perianal wound (Figure 16-71).

A circumferential tunnel is developed around the anus by blunt dissection in the ischiorectal fossa on either side of the anal canal and in the deep postanal space. The rectovaginal plane should be developed as cephalad as possible. It is easier and safer to perform this maneuver in the male patient. The tendon is passed clockwise if the right or counterclockwise if the left gracilis muscle is being transposed. The tendon is passed around the anal canal and fixed to the contralateral ischial tuberosity either

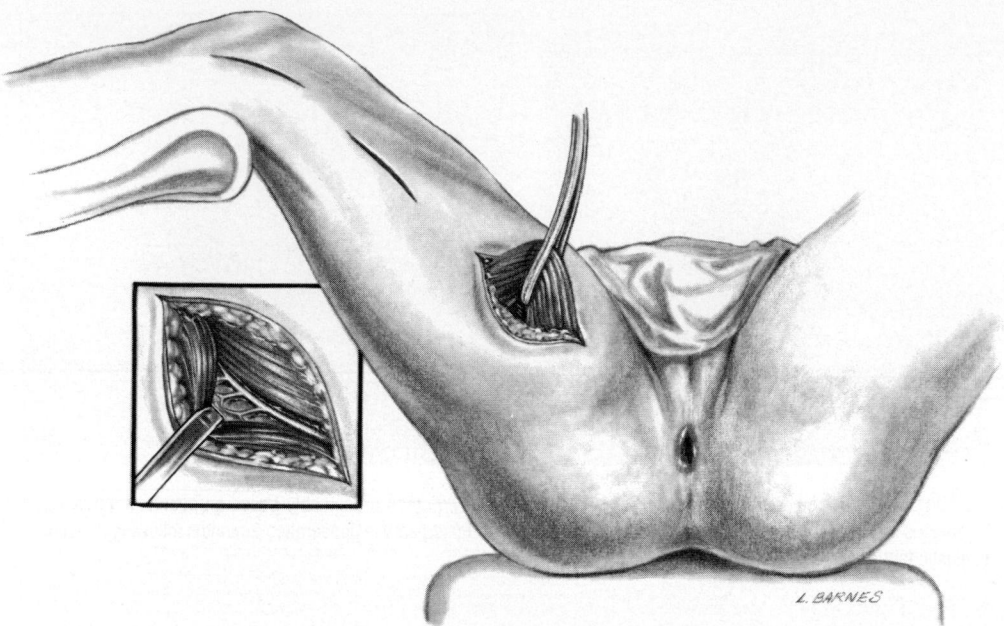

FIGURE 16-68. Gracilis muscle transposition: two incisions are made in the thigh and one across the knee joint for mobilizing the gracilis muscle. A Penrose drain is placed around the muscle proximally; this tethers the muscle and facilitates identification of the neurovascular bundle (*inset*).

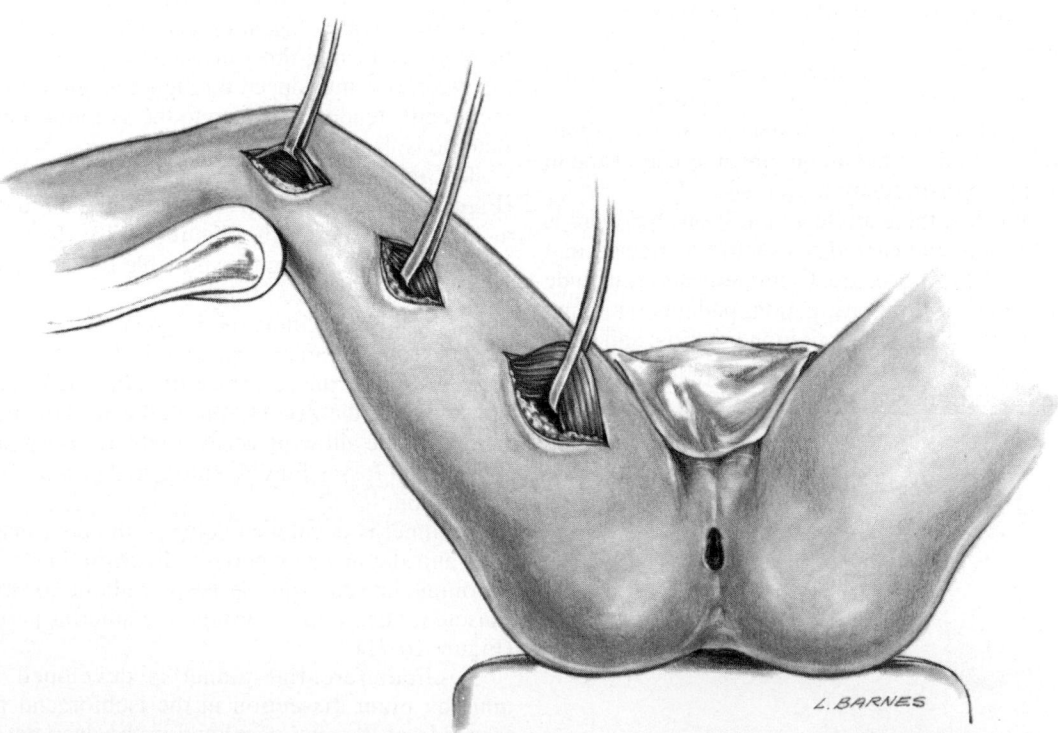

FIGURE 16-69. Gracilis muscle transposition: complete mobilization of muscle and tendon.

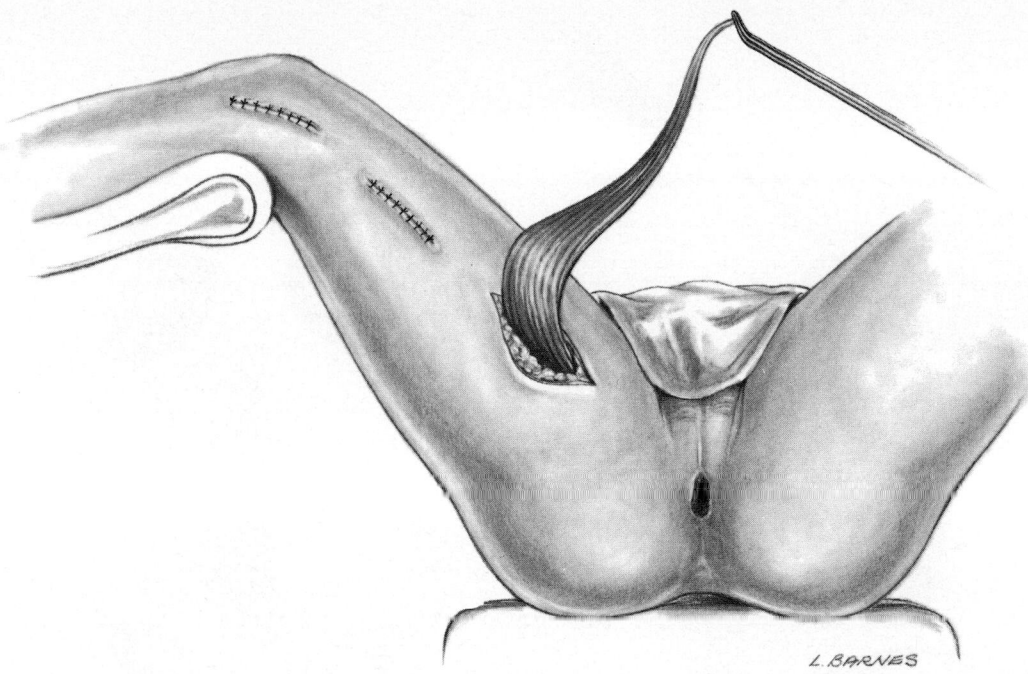

FIGURE 16-70. Gracilis muscle transposition: the muscle is delivered through the proximal incision.

by nonabsorbable (Prolene) sutures or staples introduced through a small separate incision (Figures 16-72 through 16-76). The donor leg is removed from the stirrup and adducted to release tension on the muscle. If the tendon were to be anchored without adduction, the neosphincter would be too loose. With the leg in maximal adduction, the tendon is pulled taut to render the anal canal to be snugly closed judged by a finger inserted into the rectum (Figure 16-77). If it is too tight, the anal orifice may be enlarged by gentle dilatation. All incisions are closed without drainage (Figure 16-78). The final position is illustrated in Figure 16-79.

Figure 16-80 illustrates the appearance before and after GMT in a young man who sustained severe perineal trauma from a motorcycle accident, rendering him completely incontinent. A concomitant anoplasty was required to create a new anal canal. Five years later, the patient experienced no difficulty with bowel control.

Postoperative Care

Postoperatively, the bowels should be confined for 3 to 5 days and the patient kept on bed rest for 72 hours after which progressive ambulation is permitted. Lack of success may be due to inadequate attention in the postoperative

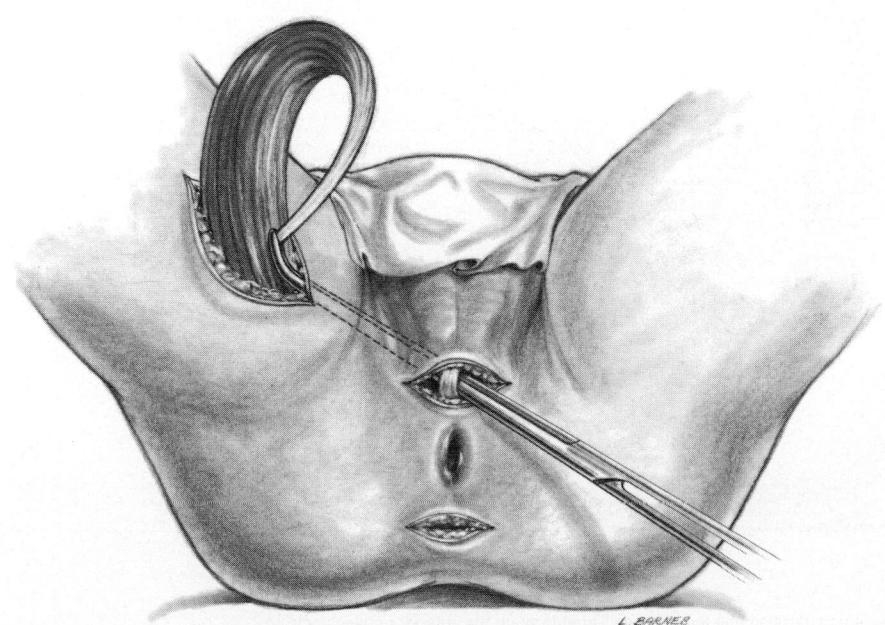

FIGURE 16-71. Gracilis muscle transposition: incisions are made anteriorly and posteriorly outside the anus, preserving the raphes. The placental forceps serve to deliver the tendon through the thigh tunnel.

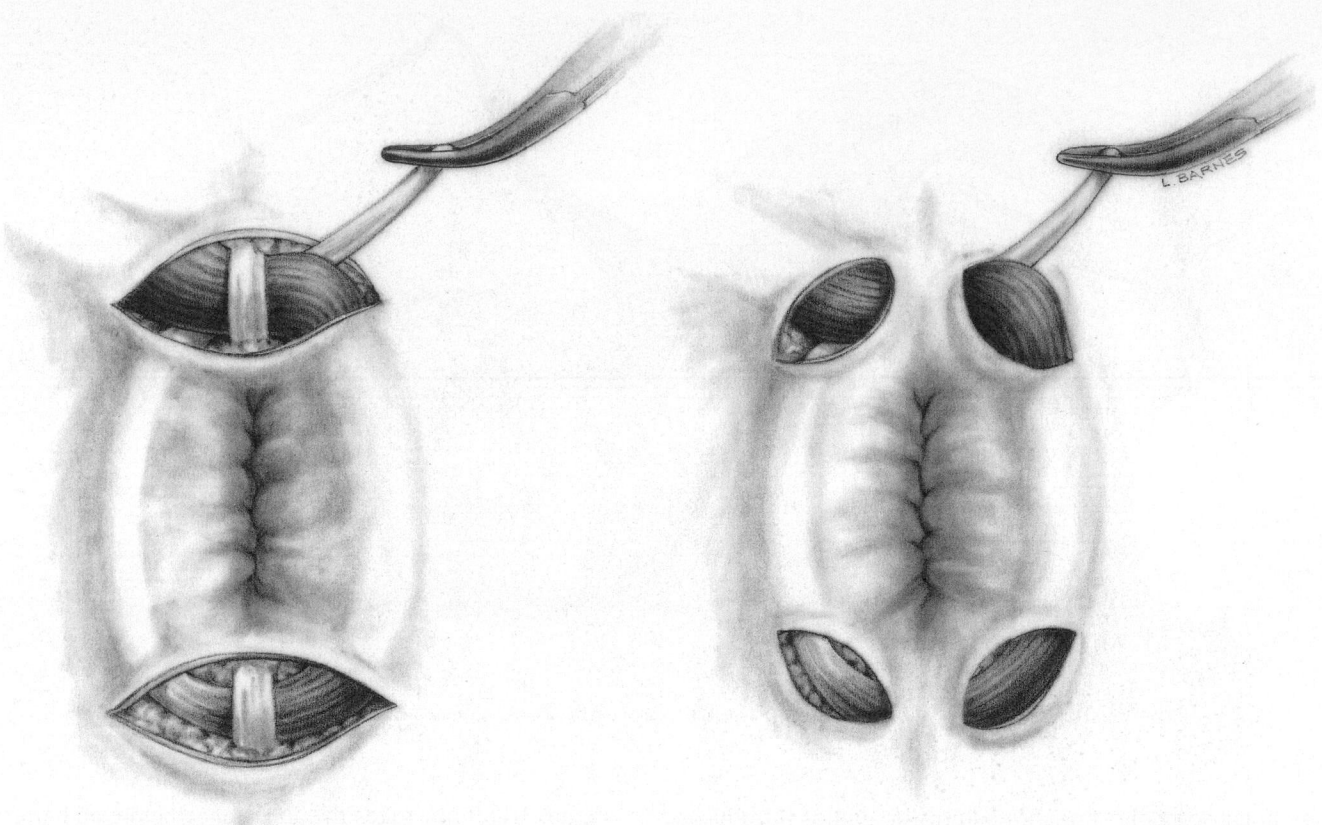

FIGURE 16-72. Gracilis muscle transposition. **Left:** Conventional anterior and posterior incisions. Both raphes are preserved. **Right:** Suggested perianal approach. Two anterior and posterior incisions are made, but the skin bridge in the middle is preserved. The raphes (if present) are therefore reinforced by the intact skin coverage. (From Kaiser AM, Corman ML. Modified perianal incisions in graciloplasty for fecal incontinence. *Dis Colon Rectum.* 2002;45(5):703–704, with permission.)

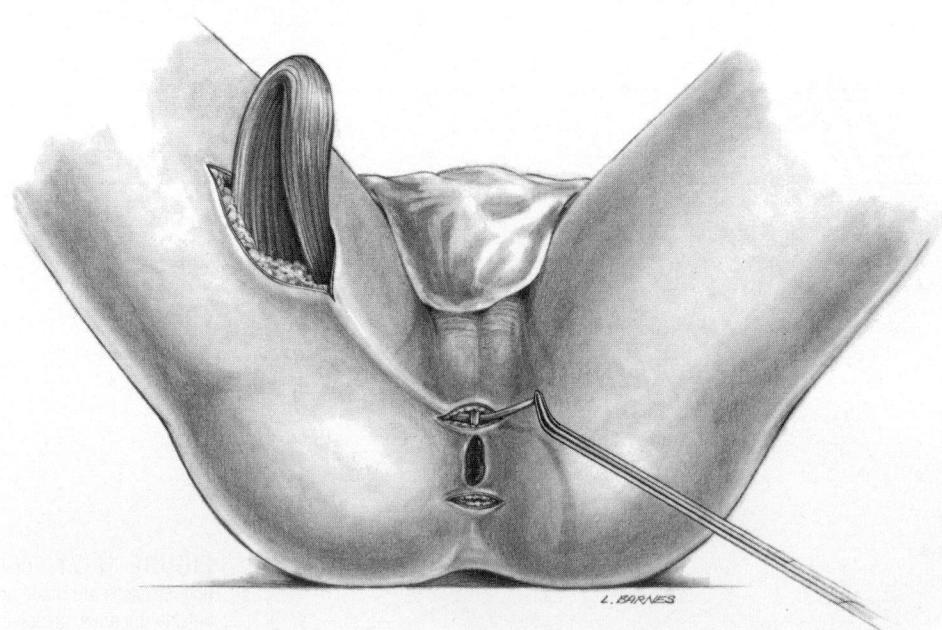

FIGURE 16-73. Gracilis muscle transposition: the tendon is delivered through the anterior perianal incision.

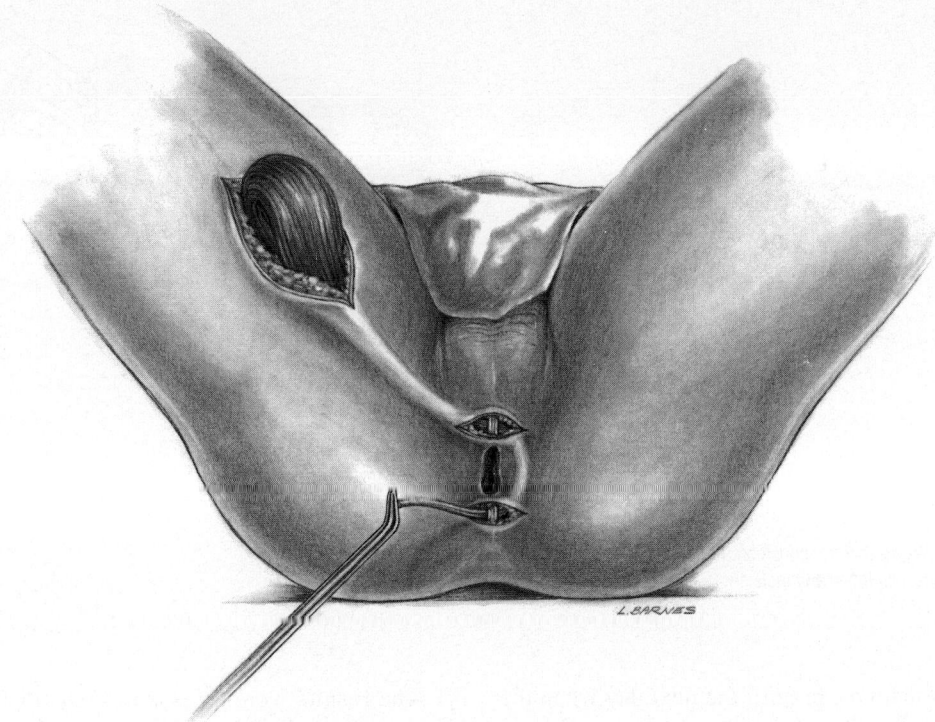

FIGURE 16-74. Gracilis muscle transposition: the tendon is brought out through the posterior incision.

period. The repair is analogous to the Thiersch operation in that the anal orifice is narrowed, but unlike the Thiersch sling, it is theoretically expandable and dynamic. Some surgeons believe that the patient can learn to adjust to the new circumstance but this is an illusion. Rather, a successful GMT works by the simple expedient of producing a corklike effect. It can open when the patient squats, the position of maximal relaxation, and is maximally tight with the person in the upright posture, an ideal arrangement most of the time.

The aim should be to establish a regular time for defecation. For most people, this is in the morning. Ideally, evacuation is achieved by a suppository, such as bisacodyl, inserted immediately after breakfast. With luck, the patient

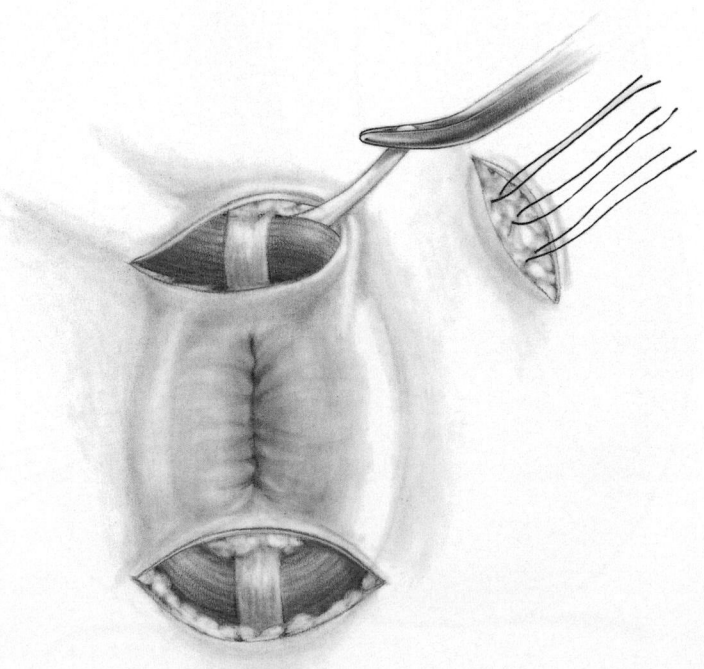

FIGURE 16-75. Gracilis muscle transposition: the tendon has encircled the anus. An incision is made over the contralateral ischial tuberosity, and sutures are placed in the gluteal fascia.

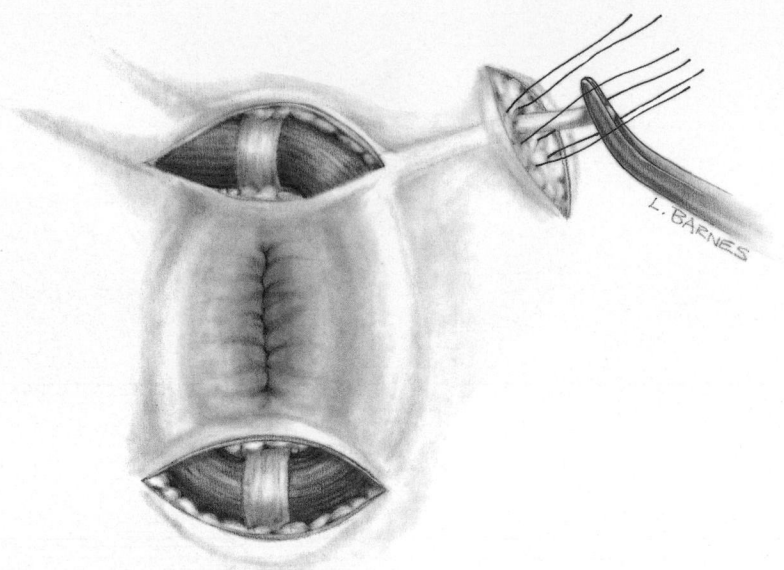

FIGURE 16-76. Gracilis muscle transposition: the tendon is brought out through the ischial tuberosity incision.

will defecate and remain clean until the next day when the procedure is repeated. Ultimately, it may be possible to establish a pattern that avoids the need for a suppository.

Results

Corman reported the long-term results in 14 patients followed for 5 or more years out of a total experience of 22. He emphasized that only patients in whom a sphincter reconstruction was not possible were selected for the procedure. The indication in the 14 included congenital anomaly (3), trauma (4), and previous anal or gynecologic surgery (4). The results were assessed as excellent (7), good, fair (4), and poor (3).[86] Leguit and coworkers suggested that GMT is the procedure of choice for the management of total incontinence in individuals who have no functional anal sphincter.[251] Patients with incontinence due to obstetrical injury are better treated by sphincter reconstruction or neuromodulation.

Yoshioka and Keighley reported their experience with six GMTs, all with poor results.[508] No objective improvement was seen, and every patient required a colostomy. It should be noted, however, that severe postoperative

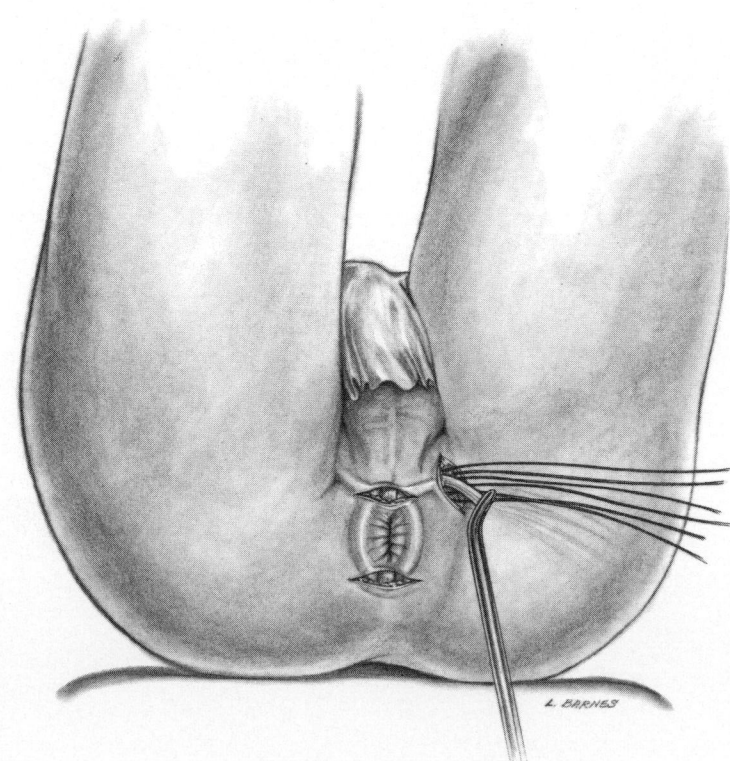

FIGURE 16-77. Gracilis muscle transposition: adduction of the thigh before the tendon is secured is an extremely important maneuver.

gracilis, can be converted to a fatigue-resistant slow-twitch muscle by means of low-frequency electrical stimulation.[396] In 1988, Baeten and colleagues reported a patient with a suboptimal GMT who improved after implantation of electrodes connected to a pulse generator (Itrel Model 7420; Medtronic, Inc., Minneapolis, MN).[17] Later, the same group demonstrated histologic changes in the transposed muscle whereby the percentage of type I slow-twitch, fatigue-resistant fibers in the transposed gracilis muscle increased from 46% before to 64% following electrical stimulation.[233] The external sphincters in cadavers were found to have a predominance of type I fibers (80%). Others have shown the same phenomenon.[155] In a series of 11 patients with fecal incontinence and 8 who had had a total rectal excision, George and coworkers found a significant increase in type I fibers and reduced axon diameter at 80 (49 to 137) days after low-frequency electrical stimulation. Compared with the prestimulation state, with a shift in the frequency response curve and a prolongation of the time course of individual muscle twitches, this suggested transformation to a slow-twitch, fatigue-resistant muscle type.

Technique

The technique of preparation of the gracilis muscle is the same as described previously. It is modified, however, by the placement of an electrode on or near the nerve to the gracilis muscle. The electrode is connected to a pulse generator that is implanted subcutaneously into the anterior abdominal wall.[234] Intramuscular stimulation of the nerve was compared with direct nerve stimulation carried out in Maastricht by Baeten and colleagues (intramuscular, 200) and in London by Williams and associates (direct, 81). Clinical success (74% vs. 57%) and the incidence of electrode failure (2.7% vs. 26%) showed the former technique to be superior. This is now the accepted method.

After mobilization of the gracilis muscle, a platinum/iridium electrode (Model 4300; Medtronic, Inc., Minneapolis, MN) is then inserted. The cathode is passed through the belly of the gracilis muscle close to the entry of the nerve and the anode connected about 4 cm distally into the epimysium (the fibrous sheath). Both are fixed in place with a suture. The electrodes are then connected to wires, which are led to the subcutaneous of the anterior abdominal wall, where they are connected to a pulse generator (IPG InterStim Model 3023 or more recently InterStim II Model 3058; Medtronic, Inc., Minneapolis, MN—Figure 16-82). This is then placed to lie well away from any bony prominence and to be accessible to the patient when applying the control switch.

Stimulation is begun about 1 month postoperatively after the surgical wounds have healed. This can either be continuous with a gradually increasing frequency, starting from 2 Hz to 15 Hz after 6 to 8 weeks. Alternatively, it can be phasic, with stimulation at 15 Hz oscillating between on and off over a few seconds, gradually increasing the on-periods until it has attained 100% by 8 weeks. The voltage setting is the minimum to achieve adequate muscle contraction, with a pulse-width of 200 milliseconds.

The patient can switch the pulse generator on and off, and the amplitude, frequency, pulse-width, and polarity can be adjusted.

Results

In a patient with anal atresia, Baeten was the first to add electrical stimulation to graciloplasty.[17] He and Williams subsequently developed the technique independently.[496] Williams and colleagues reported 20 patients with incontinence and 12 having perineal anorectal reconstruction. They introduced the staged technique of vascular delay. This was carried out during a first operation in which the distal arterial vessels to the muscle are divided in order to promote collateral vessel formation and to reduce the chances of ischemia following the graciloplasty, itself.

In 1995, Baeten and colleagues published the largest initial series, 52 patients who had undergone preoperative and postoperative assessment of function and quality of life. At a median of 2.1 (0.2 to 7.4) years, 38 (73%) were continent. The device had to be removed for infection in 7 patients. The frequency of defecation fell from 5 to 2 per 24 hours,

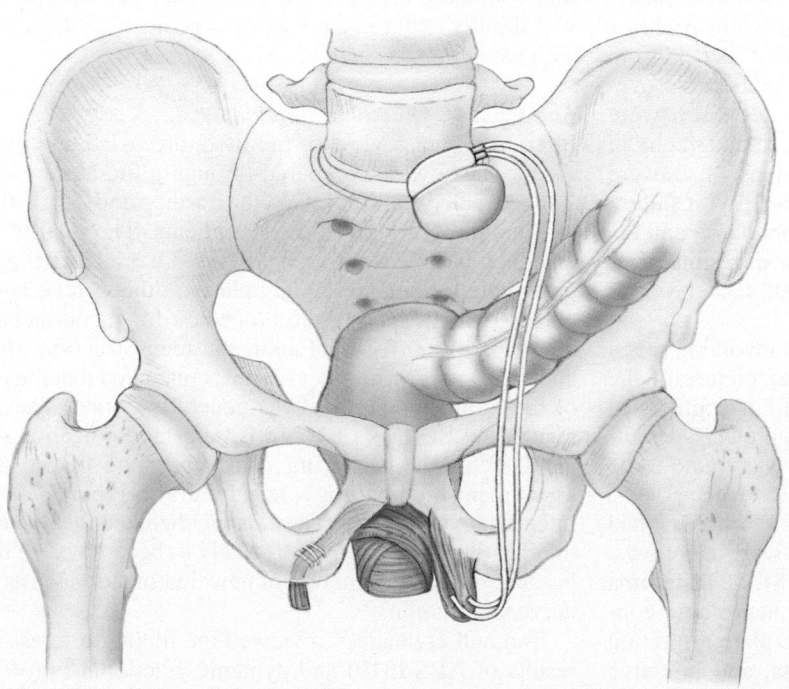

FIGURE 16-82. Stimulated graciloplasty.

and the ability to defer rose from 9 seconds to 19 minutes. In 30 patients assessed for quality of life, anxiety, social coping, personal relationships, and sexual function, all improved.[16] In a later report involving 67 patients, 53 complications were identified in 36.[152] Failures were attributable to poor muscle contraction, perforation of the anal canal during stimulation, infection at the stimulator or lead site, and poor function. In a subsequent publication from Maastricht of 200 patients followed for 261 (145 to 200) weeks, Rongen and colleagues reported normal continence or leakage to flatus in 145 (71%). This was lower in the 28 individuals for whom the indication was congenital anomaly (52%) and highest in those with trauma (82%), neurologic disease (80%), and pudendal neuropathy (82%). There were 138 complications, which included a high incidence of infections in the first 100 patients, but this fell to 6% in the second 100. Of the 46 failures, 32 were due to persisting fecal incontinence and 14 to technical problems. The median survival of the implanted pulse generator until battery expiration was 405 weeks.[384]

Wexner and coworkers,[488] similar to Williams and colleagues,[496] used a distal vascular delay technique. Despite a very high morbidity, 13 of the 15 eligible patients had the stoma reversed. Based on questionnaires, 60% reported improvement in continence and quality of life. However, one-third used daily enemas to assist evacuation. The incidence of complications was reported in greater depth by the Dynamic Graciloplasty Therapy Study Group.[293] There were 211 complications in 93 patients. Of these, 89 (46%) in 61 patients were severe, with major infection (19) being the most important cause.

Chapman and colleagues undertook a systematic review of the literature up to November 1999.[59] There was no high level evidence for the effectiveness of the procedure, and there were no comparative studies. Nevertheless, the published results indicated that 42% to 85% of patients were continent, but there was a significant risk of complications. Of 383 identified patients, there were 105 infections (28%) and 59 stimulator and lead faults (15%), including erosion, breakage, and displacement. In a publication of pooled data from 129 patients with end-stage fecal incontinence operated on between 1996 and 1999 in units in North America and Europe, 115 fulfilled the entry criteria. Of these, 88 were without a colostomy. Using the criterion of >50% improvement in the number of incontinent episodes, 62% were considered to be a success.[486] In a study of defecography in 38 patients who underwent dynamic graciloplasty for severe fecal incontinence, the results correlated well with failure and success among the 24 who achieved continence and the 14 who did not.[478] Significant improvement in resting pressures, pressure volume, and anal canal length have been reported as well.[293,392,507]

Perhaps the prospective multicenter trial involving seven specialist centers worldwide gives the best picture of the outcome of the operation, although it should be appreciated that all but eight of the implants used plate electrodes directly attached to the nerve. This method was found to be less effective than fixation to the muscle close to the nerve.[234] Mander and colleagues recruited 64 patients of whom 60 had a colostomy.[285] The causes of incontinence were as follows: obstetrical injury (22), iatrogenic injury (8), other trauma (8), pudendal neuropathy (10), and other neurologic conditions (6). Technical problems, including plate migration and lead fracture, occurred in 16 patients, and infective

complications occurred in 22. Of the 64, 9 never had the colostomy closed. This left 55 for analysis. At 1 month, a poor result had been obtained in 11 patients, leaving 44 who were said to have had a good result. The 44 patients were assessed at a median follow-up of 10 (1 to 35) months. Of these, 29 were found to have a good result—there having been failures due to evacuation difficulty (5), technical failure (5), and others (lost to follow-up [3], died [1], awaiting reimplantation [1]). The authors concluded that a good result at just less than 1 year was obtained in 29 patients, 53% of 55 patients or 45% of the original number of 64.

A prospective study was carried out by Tillin and colleagues of 49 patients undergoing dynamic graciloplasty between 1997 and 2002.[452] The indications were for obstetrical trauma (24), other trauma (17), cancer (1), and congenital anomaly (6). They were compared with two groups of patients with similar bowel disorders, including those refusing surgery (38) and patients not offered surgery (40). The groups were not completely matched because the severity of the incontinence at baseline was considerably worse in the dynamic graciloplasty than in the refused surgery group. Fifteen individuals experienced failure over a 3-year period. At 2 years after surgery, nearly two-thirds (23 of 37) of patients who underwent dynamic graciloplasty (DGP) were never or rarely incontinent to solid and liquid stool. Although the actual Wexner scores were not given, 11 of 17 patients had a greater than 20% improvement at the 2-year assessment. One-third experienced disordered bowel evacuation. The authors concluded that despite a high morbidity, the operation deserves to be considered in patients with refractory incontinence in whom conventional treatments have failed. Similar results were reported by Thornton and colleagues in 33 of 38 evaluable patients operated on over a 10-year period and followed for a median of 60 months.[451] Leg pain, swelling, or paresthesias occurred in 72%, and 27% had sexual difficulties. A colostomy was required in 16% for incontinence and 11% for obstructed defecation. Of the patients with a functioning graciloplasty, 50% had a degree of obstructed defecation, and 64% stated that their bowel function had a negative impact on their life. Quality of life was slightly better in patients with a colostomy than in those with a continence score of >12.

ABS versus Dynamic Graciloplasty

In an excellent review of the literature, ABS and dynamic graciloplasty were compared through a literature search.[392] This revealed 23 studies of the former and 52 of the latter, including a total of 1,510 patients. The quality of the evidence base was never below 3b. Overall, ABS appears preferable to dynamic graciloplasty, although the latter includes patients having the procedure for incontinence and others having it for total anorectal reconstruction. Belyaev and colleagues, in another review, concluded that the quality of the published studies was generally poor.[25] They commented on the lack of controls, nonstandardization of surgical technique, differing continence and quality-of-life assessment methodology, and failure to report data on an intention to treat basis. They also recognized that the indication for these treatments was likely to become more limited because of the introduction of new treatments, such as sacral nerve stimulation.

Tan and colleagues reviewed the literature to assess the results of ABS (319) and dynamic graciloplasty (301) and

TABLE 16-7 ABS and Dynamic Graciloplasty Comparing 75 Studies Including 1,510 Patients

	ABS 23 ARTICLES	DG 52 ARTICLES
Infection	95/437 (22%)	303/865 (35%)
Revision	164/437 (37%)	352/856 (35%)
Removal	131/437 (30%)	128/701 (18%)
Score (Wexner)	8 articles	9 articles
Before vs. after	17.9 vs. 4.7	17.6 vs. 7.5
Pressure resting mm Hg	Increased 50% (15 studies)	Increased 49% (20 studies)
Pressure voluntary contraction mm Hg	Increased 30% (7 studies)	Increased 50% (13 studies)
Cost	€10,000	€30,000

ABS, artificial bowel sphincter; DG, dynamic graciloplasty.
From Tan EK, Vaizey CJ, Cornish J, et al. Surgical strategies for faecal incontinence—a decision analysis between dynamic graciloplasty, artificial bowel sphincter and end stoma. *Colorectal Dis.* 2008;10(6): 577–586.

compared them with end stoma (ES) regarding relative cost—Table 16-7.[448] Over 5 years, ES gave a QALY (quality-adjusted life year) gain of 3.45 for £16,280, giving an incremental cost-effectiveness ratio (ICER) of £4,719/QALY. ABS produced a gain of 4.38 QALYs for £23,569 (ICER £5,387/QALY), and dynamic graciloplasty produced a gain of 4.00 QALYs for £25,035 (ICER £6,257/QALY). With the willingness-to-pay threshold set at £30,000/QALY, ES was the most cost-effective initial intervention, with ABS being the most cost effective after 10 years.

Summary

The results show that dynamic graciloplasty is associated with considerable morbidity, including infective complications and technical problems. The functional results are difficult to gauge because they often do not supply the frequency of incontinent episodes. It is clear, however, that evacuation difficulty occurs in a quarter to more than one-third of patients. Given the availability of neuromodulation and improved conservative management for incontinence, it is not surprising that dynamic graciloplasty is little used for treatment today.

Gracilis Muscle Transposition Following Rectal Excision

Cavina and colleagues, having developed a double-wrap nonstimulated graciloplasty to act as a neosphincter after total rectal excision, reported the functional results in 26 out of series of 31 (24 electrically stimulated).[57] Of these,

22 (85%) were continent to liquid and solid stool. In another publication, the results were reviewed in 81 patients in whom a complication occurred in 30 (37%).[56] Among 37 survivors, 90% had continence for stool.

Mander and colleagues employed dynamic graciloplasty following abdominoperineal resection.[284] Over a four and a half year period, 12 patients were treated (10 rectal cancer, 1 malignant melanoma, 1 sweat gland tumor), and 8 had the colostomy closed. All had evacuation difficulties and episodes of incontinence to solid stool; all wore a pad. However, the authors stated that no patient wanted to return to a colostomy. Seccia and coworkers reported an experience of 75 patients who underwent electrostimulated graciloplasty following removal of the rectum for cancer.[407] Of these, 42 were available for assessment. When simulation was intermittent, 29 (71%) were incontinent, but when it was made constant, all became continent. Rullier and coworkers performed a double dynamic graciloplasty in 15 individuals.[391] Early and late morbidity occurred in 11, mostly due to stenosis of the neosphincter. Of 12 evaluable patients, 7 had satisfactory continence. The results of others are summarized in Table 16-8.[10,153,191,386,479]

Summary

These are certainly remarkable results for such an extensive nonphysiologic operation. Clearly, patients should be carefully selected not only based on their desire to have such a major reconstruction, but also on the prognosis of the tumor. It is noteworthy that this type of surgery has been undertaken by only a handful of colon and rectal surgeons.

Gluteus Maximus Transposition

In 1926, Stone reported the use of fascia as a purse-string suture about the anus.[431] Although this did not permit voluntary control, it narrowed the anal outlet so that the patient had

TABLE 16-8 The Results of Dynamic Graciloplasty in Patients Having Total Anorectal Reconstruction after Rectal Excision

AUTHOR	YEAR	NUMBER	SUCCESS	%	LOOP
Rullier	2000	15	7	45	Double
Seccia	1994	42	42	100	Double
Mander	1996	12	8	67	Single
Geerdes	1997	15	8	64	Double
Altomare	1998	4	2	50	Single
Rosen	1998	18	10	56	Single
Violi	2004	16	12	75	Double
Ho	2005	17	10	58	Single

HARVEY BRINTON STONE (1882–1977)

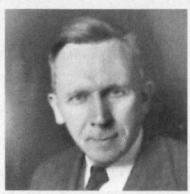

Harvey Stone was born in Baltimore, Maryland, and graduated from Johns Hopkins University in 1902 and from its medical school in 1906. He completed his internship and residency also at Johns Hopkins. He then joined the faculty of the University of Virginia in Charlottesville, returning to Baltimore as associate professor of surgery in 1908. In 1916, he published an article on the treatment of pruritus ani by alcohol injection, a method that was adopted by many proctologists for some years. Stone served in France during World War I, ultimately becoming the hospital base commander. He published approximately 100 articles, often on experimental surgery, and did some of the original work on endocrine gland transplantation. Stone was president of the Southern Surgical Association and the American Surgical Association. (Photograph courtesy of the Alan Mason Chesney Medical Archives of the Johns Hopkins Medical Institutions, Baltimore, MD.)

some degree of continence. The operation was subsequently extended and revised to encircle the fascia around the anus and to anchor the free ends to the gluteus maximus muscle on each side, a method popularized by Wreden.[502] The anal canal was, thus, enclosed in a fascial ring, which could theoretically be tightened by contraction of the gluteal muscle. Satisfactory results were reported in 30 patients, but no one seems to have reported this technique since 1941.[432] The use of the gluteus, however, as a substitute anal muscle has been reported by many authors.[48,49, 67,126,184,204,353]

Technique

The blood supply of the gluteus maximus comes from the superior and inferior gluteal arteries, supplemented by branches of the medial and lateral femoral circumflex arteries.[353] Motor innervation is from the inferior gluteal nerve (L5, S1, S2). Several techniques for harvesting the muscle, tunneling, and suturing have been described.

The patient is placed in the prone jackknife position. An incision is made lateral to the anal verge on each side. Another pair of incisions is made parallel to the caudal border of the gluteus maximus muscle, exposing its medial portion (Figure 16-83). A part of the muscle is then mobilized, taking care to safeguard the neurovascular bundle. A similar mobilization is undertaken on the other side (Figure 16-84). The muscle flaps are then brought through tunnels between the incisions and secured to their opposite member anteriorly and posteriorly (Figure 16-85). Devesa and colleagues emphasized the importance of the use of a nerve stimulator to monitor contractility, as well as of the placement of a tape around the neurovascular pedicle to keep it protected.[105] They also advised that an end colostomy should be performed and that only one side should be used. A bowel-confining regimen is recommended in the early postoperative period.

Results

The obvious advantage of the gluteus muscle is that contraction will more effectively result in closure of the anal orifice.[184] Whether this is effective is doubtful, however. As with graciloplasty, stenosis of the anal orifice may also be a factor contributing to improved function. This is consistent with the observation that nighttime control is more likely to be impaired.[369]

There are few data concerning long-term function and morbidity of this procedure because the literature, such as it is, essentially consists of articles noting one or two cases. However, a few groups have a larger experience. Chen and Zhang performed the operation on 6 patients, with "success" in 4.[63] Prochiantz and Gross point to the difficulty in obtaining sufficient length to encircle the rectum.[369] In their series, this could not be accomplished in 4 patients, and in 11 in whom an adequate repair was effected, four failures occurred (overall failure rate, 36%). Pearl and colleagues carried out the procedure in 7 patients with one failure.[353] Devesa and coworkers initially preferred to use only one side but subsequently reported bilateral transpositions.[103,105] Abou-Zeid and Marzouk noted improvement in all but 2 of their 10 patients (one infection and one "bad selection").[4] Christiansen and colleagues performed this operation on seven individuals for varying indications, with three improved and no change in four.[73] They concluded that gluteus maximus transposition is no better than nonstimulated graciloplasty.

ROMAN R. WREDEN (1867–1934)

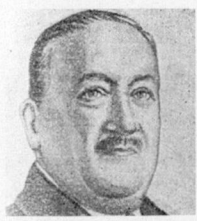

Roman Wreden was a Russian surgeon who is known as the founder of Russian operative orthopedics. He graduated from the Military Medical Academy in 1890, completing his surgical training under Professor V. A. Ratimov. Wreden was awarded a PhD in 1893 for his dissertation on cystitis. From 1893 to 1896 he was an attending surgeon in the Kiev Military Hospital. In 1896, Wreden became an assistant professor at the Military Medical Academy and professor in 1900. Wreden organized and became head of the first Russian Orthopedic Institute in 1906, which he directed until his death. He published 80 scientific works, including a number of books. (Photograph courtesy of the Bakulev AN, ed. *Medical Encyclopedia*. Moscow, Russia: Government Medical Publishing; 1958.)

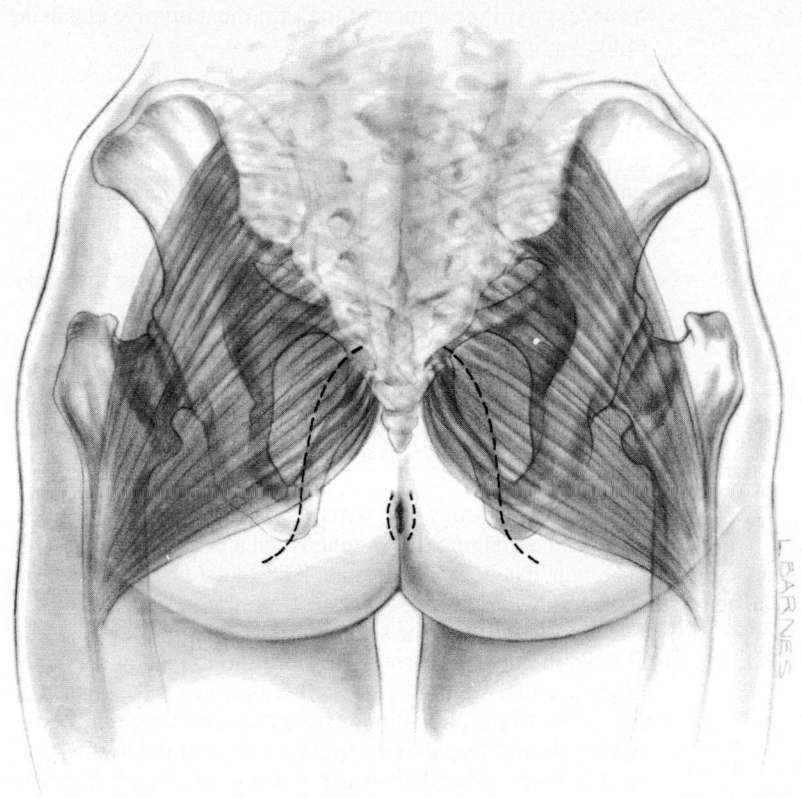

FIGURE 16-83. Gluteus maximus muscle transposition: a pair of lateral circumanal incisions is made to permit mobilization and suturing of the bifurcated ends of the transposed muscle. (Adapted from Hentz VR. Construction of a rectal sphincter using the origin of the gluteus maximus muscle. *Plast Reconstruct Surg.* 1982;70(1):82–85; Pearl RK, Prasad ML, Nelson RL, et al. Bilateral gluteus maximus transposition for anal incontinence. *Dis Colon Rectum.* 1991;34(6):478–481, with permission.)

Conclusion

Gluteus maximus transposition is rarely applied today, and in light of the more recent alternatives is probably more of historical interest.

The Artificial Bowel Sphincter (Acticon [AMS] Device)

The artificial urinary sphincter has been successfully employed for the treatment of urinary incontinence for many years, but its application to fecal incontinence was first reported in 1987 by Christiansen and Lorentzen.[74] They used the AMS 800 artificial urinary sphincter (American Medical Systems, Minnetonka, MN) for this indication. A subsequent report involved five patients with presumed neuromuscular anal incontinence, with no occurrence of late erosion.[75,77] It was concluded that the operation was a reasonable alternative to a permanent colostomy. The urinary device has since been modified for use in the treatment of fecal incontinence.

The system consists of a cuff, which is placed surgically around the upper anal canal. This is connected by tubing to a pump, which is inserted into the labia or scrotum in order

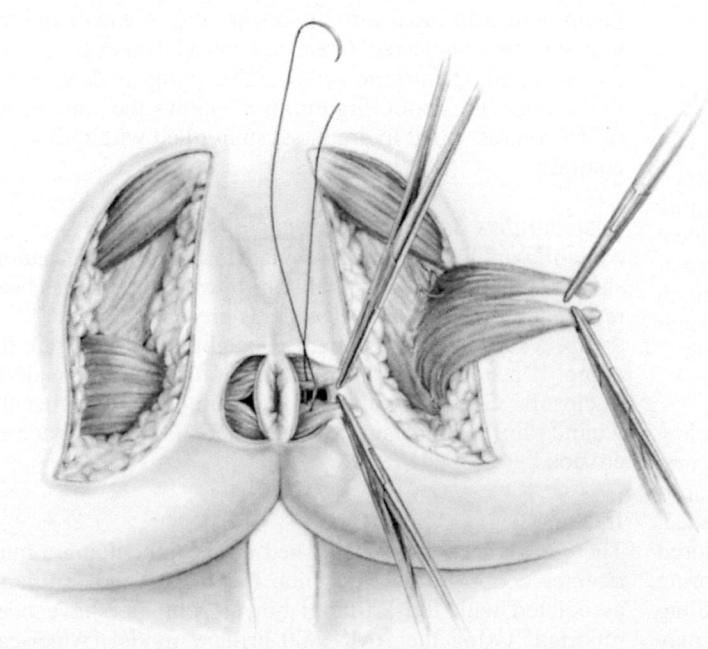

FIGURE 16-84. Gluteus maximus muscle transposition: a tunnel is created around the rectum. The freed muscle on each side is split to make two tails. Each side is passed anteriorly and posteriorly. (Adapted from Hentz VR. Construction of a rectal sphincter using the origin of the gluteus maximus muscle. *Plast Reconstruct Surg.* 1982;70(1):82–85; Pearl RK, Prasad ML, Nelson RL, et al. Bilateral gluteus maximus transposition for anal incontinence. *Dis Colon Rectum.* 1991;34(6):478–481, with permission.)

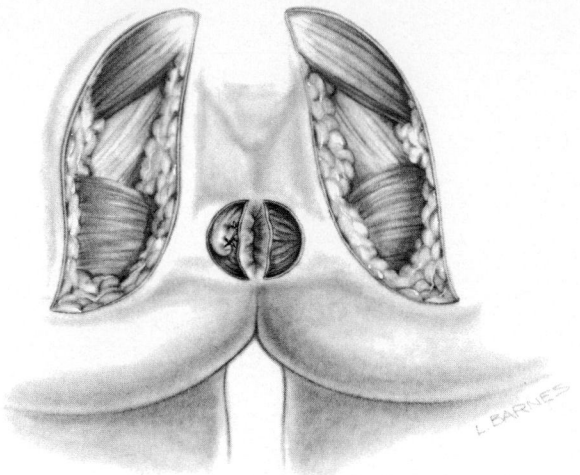

FIGURE 16-85. Gluteus maximus muscle transposition: the muscle tails from each side are secured to each other and to itself. All wounds are closed primarily. (Adapted from Hentz VR. Construction of a rectal sphincter using the origin of the gluteus maximus muscle. *Plast Reconstruct Surg.* 1982;70(1):82–85; Pearl RK, Prasad ML, Nelson RL, et al. Bilateral gluteus maximus transposition for anal incontinence. *Dis Colon Rectum.* 1991;34(6):478–481, with permission.)

to be accessible to the patient. The pump is connected to a reservoir or pressure regulating balloon of about 40 mL capacity, implanted in the abdominal wall. The whole system is filled with radiopaque hydraulic fluid, which can be moved by the pump to control the flow to and from the anal cuff. In the neutral position the cuff is full, thus occluding the anal canal. When the patient wishes to defecate, she or he squeezes the pump. This causes the fluid to flow from the anal cuff to the balloon, thereby allowing defecation to occur. On completing evacuation, the pump is released, and the fluid then flows back into the cuff spontaneously over the next few minutes, occluding the anal canal once again.

The cuff is available in different lengths and widths, and there are several pressure balloons available to deliver pressures from 60 to 90 mm of water. In practice, the smallest cuff size diameter is the most suitable for general use.

Indications and Contraindications

With the current availability of neuromodulation and the high incidence of erosion of the implant through the skin (see later), the indications for the artificial bowel sphincter have diminished in the last 10 years. It still has a place, however, because there are many examples of long-term success. Relative or absolute contraindications include impaired healing potential, such as following irradiation; the presence of local sepsis (e.g., anal fistula, Crohn's disease); severe diarrhea or irritable bowel disease; intractable constipation; evacuation disorder; and reduced manual dexterity, such as might occur in rheumatoid arthritis or after a cerebrovascular accident.

Preparation of the Patient

It is essential to observe strict sterile precautions including preoperative baths with antiseptic solution as well as mechanical bowel preparation. Prophylactic intravenous antibiotics are mandatory. A covering colostomy is not needed, but if there is one already in place, it should not be closed until it is clear that the operation has been a success. During the operation itself, great care should be taken when handling the device, and frequent changes of the surgeon's gloves may

be necessary. Preparation of the skin must involve cleansing of the vagina.

Technique

The operation can be undertaken by an abdominal and a perineal surgeon working synchronously, with the former implanting the reservoir, connecting the pump, and priming the tubing and connections, whereas the latter inserts the anal cuff. Thus, the patient should be placed in the lithotomy position in order to allow simultaneous access to the abdomen and the perineum.

Placement of the anal cuff can be made through two lateral incisions, with blunt finger dissection to encircle the gut tube separating the upper anal canal from the vagina. Alternatively, an anterior incision is made and the anovaginal septum formally dissected to a sufficient level. Then one proceeds with blunt dissection to encircle the anal canal laterally and posteriorly. This technique is safer, with less chance of damaging the vagina, when a prior anterior sphincter repair has been performed. The incision is deepened to separate the anterior rectal wall from the vagina for at least 5 cm. This will permit sufficient space to implant the cuff at a depth adequate enough to limit the risk of cuff erosion (Figure 16-86). The ischiorectal fossae are then entered on each side using blunt finger dissection to create a circular tunnel around the anus in order to accommodate the cuff. A cuff sizer (provided in the Acticon package) is passed around the anal canal to determine the diameter of cuff to be implanted. This should be about 1 cm greater than the measurement on the sizer. In almost all cases, a 12-cm cuff is used. The longitudinal length of the cuff is available in several sizes. In practice, the 1.5 cm cuff is almost always selected.

The abdominal operation is undertaken through a low transverse incision. The choice of side is opposite to the handedness of the patient. The anterior rectus sheath is opened, and a balloon calibrated to generate a pressure of between 80 and 90 cm of water is chosen. The tubing from the cuff is attached to a metal tunneler and brought into the groin incision. A tunnel is also developed between the incision and the labium or scrotum using Hegar dilators. The pump is then inserted into the pocket thus created, and the tubing is then connected. Great care must be taken to prevent air from getting into the system. The pump is deactivated in the operating room. Figure 16-87 shows the appearance of the contrast-filled hydraulic system filled with radiologic contrast.

Postoperative Care and Subsequent Management

Systemic antibiotics are continued for 5 days. The patient should be kept in the hospital until bowel function has been restored, unless of course a stoma is present.

Six weeks later, the patient is taught how to operate the pump. If a stoma is present, a decision should be made as to closure. Criteria should be based simply on whether the wounds are healed and whether there is no evidence of erosion.

Results

There have been many published articles, including a multicenter cohort study, in which the merits and problems associated with the artificial bowel sphincter have been reported. Using the AMS 800 urinary model (American

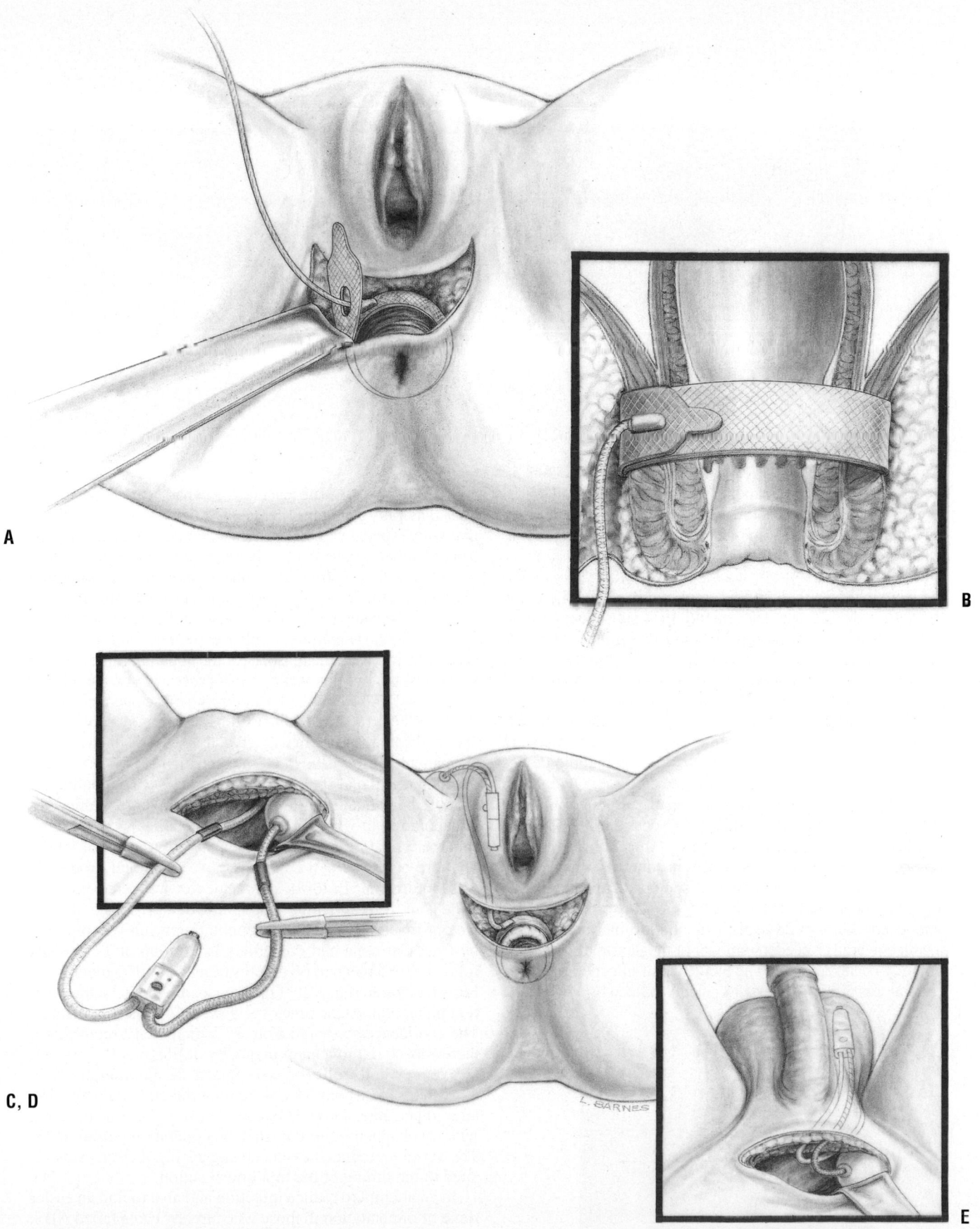

FIGURE 16-86. Artificial anal sphincter implantation. **A:** The cuff is wrapped around the anorectum. **B:** The cuff is secured by means of a knob and tab locking mechanism. The connecting tubing should be placed on either the right or left side, depending on which side of the groin will be dissected. All connections are completed. **C:** The tubing to the cuff and the tubing to the balloon are each clamped with an atraumatic Silastic-shod mosquito clamp. The excess tubing is trimmed to the appropriate length so that the pump sits properly in the labium **(D)** or scrotum **(E).** *(continued)*

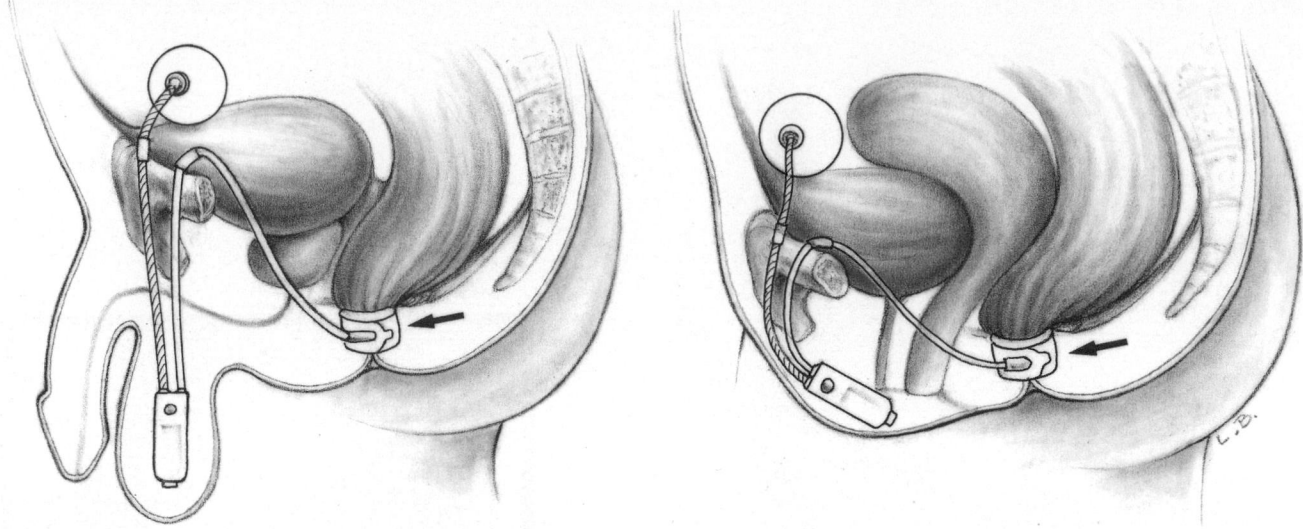

F   G

FIGURE 16-86. *(continued)* Schematic final position in the male **(F)** and in the female **(G)** patient.

Medical Systems, Minneapolis, MN), Lehur and colleagues (Nantes, France) reported their initial results in 13 patients.[254] Three required removal, and 9 of the remaining 10 were continent to stool at a median interval of 20 (4 to 60) months. Four patients had mild difficulty in evacuation. There was one technical failure due to a ruptured cuff. Reimplantation of another device was successful. In a subsequent report of 13 patients, presumably the same individuals as in the previous study, now followed for 30 (5 to 76) months, 11 had a functioning device after reimplantation in 2 of them.[252] Quality of life assessed in 16 individuals improved in each domain assessed, and, not surprisingly, correlated with the clinical result.[256] In a three-center series, 24 patients were followed for 20 (10 to 35) months.[255] Seven had the device removed, but it had been reimplanted in three. Overall, 18 (75%) were found to have a good result, although mild (7) and severe (2) evacuation difficulties occurred in 9 patients.

It had been clear from the outset that infection and erosion were common complications. This is in contrast with the experience of using the artificial urinary sphincter. Apparently, the deep placement away from the skin is probably protective. Erosion occurred in 4 of 28 patients in a multicenter Italian study in which overall, 7 needed removal of the device.[8] Evacuation difficulty occurred in 12. The incidence of infection requiring removal was 50% in the first 12 patients treated by Michot and

colleagues, but in the subsequent 25, 23 had no early complications, and only 5 required removal.[304] This served to indicate that with experience complications can be reduced. They attributed this improvement to better patient selection, excluding those with a scarred or irradiated perineum or those with diarrhea. Of the 20 with a functioning device, continence was normal in 16, although evacuation difficulties were seen in 7.

These authors maintained that experience and improved case selection were the reasons for the apparent improvement in the results, but this was not the experience of Parker and colleagues.[349] They divided patients into those operated on between 1989 to 1992 and 1997 to 2001. The removal rates were 4/10 and 14/35, and there was a high rate of revisional surgery (13 patients; 21 revisions). Of the 35 patients, 17 (49%) had a functional artificial sphincter in whom the fecal incontinence score fell and quality of life improved. In a large multicenter collaboration in which a common protocol was followed by each participating unit, 112 patients were treated, of whom 55 were reviewed at 12 months.[500] A revisional procedure was required in 51 (46%), and the device was removed in 41 (37%). Of the 53% with a functioning device, 85% had satisfactory function. A similar disappointing result was reported by Ruiz Carmona and coworkers in a group of 17 patients followed for a mean of 68 months (range, 3 to 133 months).[390] Eleven required removal of the device, of whom 7 underwent reimplantation. At the time of review, only 9 were assessable. The continence score fell from 17.5 to 10 at 12 months, but there was no improvement in quality of life.

Wexner and colleagues reported 52 implantations in 47 patients, of whom 54% were undertaken for dysfunction after imperforate anus.[489] Overall, 23 (41%) became infected, with this happening in the early postoperative period in 18. The authors produced evidence suggesting that this was related to the timing of the first bowel action.

In an attempt to reduce infection and also to find an easier route of implantation in those who already had a failed ABS, Michot and colleagues carried out transvaginal implantation in 32 individuals, 9 (28%) of whom had had a previous failed ABS.[305] Nine (28%) required removal as a consequence of sepsis in seven. Of the 23 (72%) who retained the device,

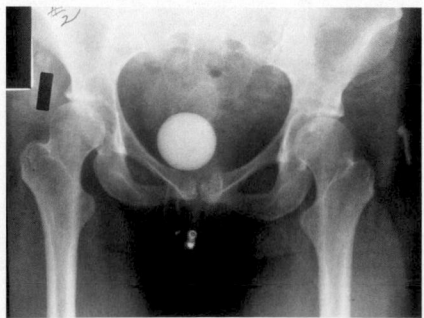

FIGURE 16-87. Artificial bowel sphincter. The artificial bowel sphincter in place filled with radiopaque contrast, showing the cuff, pump, and balloon.

the incontinence score fell from 18.4 to 6.8. Most published reports present a short-term experience of up to 3 or 4 years. Over this duration, failure is in the range of 25% to 50%.[104,339] Ortiz and colleagues inserted 24 artificial anal sphincter devices in 22 patients and found the cumulative probability of device removal to be 44% at 48 months.[346] In the series of Christiansen and associates, of 17 patients followed for up to 16 years, 2 died of unrelated causes, 3 had removal for infection, and 4 were removed for malfunction, leaving 8 (47%) with a satisfactory long-term result. Melenhorst and colleagues, in 33 patients, reported 7 who required removal of the device.[298] The complication of constipation was studied by Gallas and coworkers in 44 patients, of whom 57% had some degree of constipation or evacuation difficulty. Despite these issues, the artificial bowel sphincter was felt to offer a better quality of life in those in whom it continued to function as opposed to those who were being managed conservatively. O'Brien and colleagues carried out a randomized trial comparing the artificial bowel sphincter with best supportive care.[338] Complications after ABS (3/7) were more common than with conservative treatment (0/7), but continence scores (4.8 vs. 14.3), change in continence (6/6 vs. 1/7), and quality of life (82.7 vs. 54.7) favored ABS.

In a review of the literature in which all articles even those containing the lowest level of evidence were included, Mundy and associates found 14 publications (Table 16-9).[312] In none was the results analyzed on an intention to treat basis, and no data were given for the outcome of patients whose device was removed. They concluded that the procedure was of uncertain benefit.

In another review, 5,390 articles were identified, of which 38 fulfilled the criteria for inclusion.[25] These dealt with dynamic graciloplasty and the artificial bowel sphincter. There was one randomized controlled trial[338] and two comparisons between graciloplasty and ABS.[93,346] The 15 studies included 444 patients. Of these, the results were as follows: success (189 [42.6%]), complications (302 [68%]), removal (146 [32%]), and revision (202 [45.5%]).

TABLE 16-9 Results of the Artificial Bowel Sphincter

AUTHOR/YEAR	PATIENTS	FOLLOW-UP MO	DEFINITIVE REMOVAL	WEXNER SCORE BEFORE	WEXNER SCORE AFTER
Lehur, 2002	16	25	4/16		
Lehur, 2000	24	20	4/24		
Lehur, 1998	13	30	2/13	13 17.0 (1.8)	11 4.5 (3.4)
Altomare, 2001	28	19	5/28	28 14.9 (11–20)	21 2.6 (0–6)
Christiansen, 1999	17	60	7/17		
Devesa, 2002	53	26	10/53	53 17 (3)	43 4 (3)
Dodi, 2000	8	10	2/8		
Michot, 2003	25	34	5/25		
O'Brien, 2000	13	NA	3/13	13 18.7 (14–20)	10 2.1 (2–6)
Ortiz, 2002	22	28	7/22	22 18 (14–20)	15 4 (0–14)
Vaizey, 1998	6	10	1/6	6 19.5 (0–8)	6 4.5 (4–9)
Wong, 1996	12	58	3/12		
Wong, 2002	112	12	34/112		
Gelet, 1997	1	24	0/1		

From Mundy L, Merlin TL, Maddern GL, et al. Systematic review of safety and effectiveness of an artificial bowel sphincter for faecal incontinence. *Br J Surg.* 2004;91(6):665–672.

Erosion or Infection

When this serious complication occurs, removal of the device is mandatory if infection supervenes or if erosion of the cuff occurs. There is no place for antibiotics in an attempt to save the implant. Conversely, it may be possible to preserve the pump and reservoir if the problem is limited to the cuff, but this is rarely successful. Mechanical problems, however, may be individually addressed with replacement and reconnection of the affected part. It is also possible to repressurize the system without removing all of the components.

Summary

The artificial bowel sphincter has been used in a relatively small number of patients. There is a high complication rate due mostly to infection and erosion. The rates of failure requiring removal of the device range from 20% to 40% over periods of follow-up of no more than 5 years. Reoperation is common. In those with a functioning sphincter, function is good in approximately 80% of patients, although evacuation difficulty occurs in 10% to 30%.

The Magnetic Anal Sphincter

A magnetic prosthesis, the magnetic anal sphincter (MAS), has been developed.[253] It consists of a ring of magnetic titanium beads sealed within a casing. The technique of insertion is similar to the cuff phase of the ABS. In a preliminary report, Wong and colleagues describe 10 female patients aged 64.5 years with incontinence for 1 to 40 years. At an interval of 8 (6 to 13) months, the incontinence score fell from 17 (baseline) to 6.[499]

► FECAL DIVERSION

The performance of a colostomy or ileostomy in a patient with fecal incontinence is thought generally to be an admission of failure, but it should not be regarded as such. Many individuals should not be submitted to the rigors of an esoteric sphincter-saving operation. For example, the likelihood of success in those who have severe neurologic deficit, who are retarded or senile, or who have profound bowel function problems is extremely limited. Fecal diversion is virtually always the optimal choice for a patient confined to a nursing home or to a convalescent facility. Irrespective of the method of treatment, perhaps more frequently than any other condition discussed in this text, patients with fecal incontinence need to be willing partners in the decision-making process.

When to close a colostomy that had been placed prior to reconstruction of the anal sphincter is often a difficult decision. The surgeon may consider physiologic studies such as those discussed previously. Other options include encouraging the patient to hold an enema or the use of a more formed substance that simulates feces (e.g., psyllium). This latter method has been advocated by Pittman and colleagues.[363] A mixture of psyllium and water is instilled through the distal limb of a loop stoma or through the mucous fistula.

References

1. Abbas SM, Bissett IP, Neill ME, et al. Long-term outcome of postanal repair in the treatment of faecal incontinence. *ANZ J Surg*. 2005;75(9):783–786.
2. Abbott D, Atere-Roberts N, Williams A, et al. Obstetric anal sphincter injury. *BMJ*. 2010;341:C3414.
3. Abcarian H, Orsay CP, Pearl RK, et al. Traumatic cloaca. *Dis Colon Rectum*. 1989;32(9):783–787.
4. Abou-Zeid AA, Marzouk DM. Gluteus maximus neosphincter is a viable option for patients with end-stage fecal incontinence. *Dis Colon Rectum*. 2000;43(11):1635–1636.
5. Abramov Y, Sand PK, Botros SM, et al. Risk factors for female anal incontinence: new insight through the Evanston-Northwestern twin sisters study. *Obstet Gynecol*. 2005;106(4):726–732.
6. Abramowitz L, Sobhani I, Ganansia R, et al. Are sphincter defects the cause of anal incontinence after vaginal delivery? Results of a prospective study. *Dis Colon Rectum*. 2000;43(5):590–596.
7. Adams E, Fernando RJ. *Management of Third- and Fourth-Degree Perineal Tears Following Vaginal Delivery. Guideline No. 29*. London, United Kingdom: RCOG Press; 2001.
8. Altomare DF, Dodi G, La Torre F, et al. Multicentre retrospective analysis of the outcome of artificial anal sphincter implantation for severe faecal incontinence. *Br J Surg*. 2001;88(11):1481–1486.
9. Altomare DF, Rinaldi M, Lobascio P, et al. Factors affecting the outcome of temporary sacral nerve stimulation for faecal incontinence. The value of the new tined lead electrode. *Colorectal Dis*. 2011;13(2):198–202.
10. Altomare DF, Rinaldi M, Pannarale OC, et al. Electrostimulated gracilis neosphincter for faecal incontinence and in total anorectal reconstruction: still an experimental procedure? *Int J Colorectal Dis*. 1997;12(5):308–312.
11. Altomare DF, Rinaldi M, Petrolino M, et al. Permanent sacral nerve modulation for fecal incontinence and associated urinary disturbances. *Int J Colorectal Dis*. 2004;19(3):203–209.
12. Amarenco G, Ismael SS, Even-Schneider A, et al. Urodynamic effect of acute transcutaneous posterior tibial nerve stimulation in overactive bladder. *J Urol*. 2003;169(6):2210–2215.
13. Andrews V, Sultan AH, Thakar R, et al. Occult anal sphincter injuries—myth or reality? *BJOG*. 2006;113(2):195–200.
14. Angioli R, Gómez-Marín O, Cantuaria G, et al. Severe perineal lacerations during vaginal delivery: the University of Miami experience. *Am J Obstet Gynecol*. 2000;182(5):1083–1085.
15. Auwerda JJ, Schouten WR. New device for adequate fixation of recording instruments in ambulant anorectal manometry. *Dis Colon Rectum*. 1994;37(4):383–385.
16. Baeten C, Geerdes BP, Adang EM, et al. Anal dynamic graciloplasty in the treatment of intractable fecal incontinence. *N Engl J Med*. 1995;332(24):1600–1605.
17. Baeten C, Spaans F, Fluks A. An implanted neuromuscular stimulator for fecal continence following previously implanted gracilis muscle. Report of a case. *Dis Colon Rectum*. 1988;31(2):134–137.
18. Bannister JJ, Abouzekry L, Read NW. Effect of aging on anorectal function. *Gut*. 1987;28(3):353–357.
19. Bannister JJ, Read NW, Donnelly TC, et al. External and internal anal sphincter responses to rectal distension in normal subjects and in patients with idiopathic faecal incontinence. *Br J Surg*. 1989;76(6):617–621.
20. Barisic GI, Krivokapic ZV, Markovic VA, et al. Outcome of overlapping anal sphincter repair after 3 months and after a mean of 80 months. *Int J Colorectal Dis*. 2006;21(1):52–56.
21. Barrett JJ, Brocklehurst JC, Kiff ES, et al. Anal function in geriatric patients with faecal incontinence. *Gut*. 1989;30(9):1244–1251.
22. Bartolo DC, Jarratt JA, Read NW. The cutaneo-anal reflex: a useful index of neuropathy? *Br J Surg*. 1983;70(11):660–663.
23. Bates-Jensen BM, Alessi CA, Al-Samarrai NR, et al. The effects of an exercise and incontinence intervention on skin health outcomes in nursing home residents. *J Am Geriatr Soc*. 2003;51(3):348–355.
24. Beck A. Electromyographische Untersuchungen am Sphincter ani. *Pflugers Arch Ges Physiol*. 1930;224:278–292.
25. Belyaev O, Müller C, Uhl W. Neosphincter surgery for fecal incontinence: a critical and unbiased review of the relevant literature. *Surg Today*. 2006;36(4):295–303.
26. Benini L, Gabbrielli A, Agugiaro F, et al. Sacral nerve stimulation for intractable constipation: was it really an intractable constipation? *Gut*. 2010;59(8):1156–1157.
27. Bennett RC, Duthie HL. The functional importance of the internal anal sphincter. *Br J Surg*. 1964;51:355–357.
28. Bernardi C, Favetta U, Pescatori M. Autologous fat injection for treatment of fecal incontinence: manometric and echographic assessment. *Plast Reconstr Surg*. 1998;102(5):1626–1628.
29. Bernstein AJ, Peters KM. Expanding indications for neuromodulation. *Urol Clin North Am*. 2005;32(1):59–63.
30. Bharucha A. Incontinence: an underappreciated problem in obesity and bariatric surgery. *Dig Dis Sci*. 2010;55(9):2428–2430.

31. Bielefeldt K, Enck P, Erckenbrecht JF. Sensory and motor function in the maintenance of anal continence. *Dis Colon Rectum.* 1990;33(8):674–678.

32. Binnie NR, Kawimbe BM, Papachrysostomou M, et al. Use of the pudendo-anal reflex in the treatment of neurogenic faecal incontinence. *Gut.* 1990;31(9):1051–1055.

33. Birgisson H, Påhlman L, Gunnarsson U, et al. Late adverse effects of radiation therapy for rectal cancer—a systematic overview. *Acta Oncol.* 2007;46(4):504–516.

34. Blaisdell P. Repair of the incontinent sphincter ani. *Surg Gynecol Obstet.* 1940;70:692.

35. Bliss DZ, Jung HJ, Savik K, et al. Supplementation with dietary fiber improves fecal incontinence. *Nurs Res.* 2001;50(4):203–213.

36. Block IR. Repair of the incontinent sphincter ani following operative injury. *Surg Gynecol Obstet.* 1959;109(1):111–116.

37. Bock S, Folie P, Wolff K, et al. First experiences with pudendal nerve stimulation in fecal incontinence: a technical report. *Tech Coloproctol.* 2010;14(1):41–44.

38. Bollard RC, Gardiner A, Lindow S, et al. Normal female anal sphincter: difficulties in interpretation explained. *Dis Colon Rectum.* 2002;45(2):171–175.

39. Boyle DJ, Prosser K, Allison ME, et al. Percutaneous tibial nerve stimulation for the treatment of urge fecal incontinence. *Dis Colon Rectum.* 2010;53(4):432–437.

40. Braun JC, Treutner KH, Dreuw B, et al. Vectormanometry for differential diagnosis of fecal incontinence. *Dis Colon Rectum.* 1994;37(10):989–996.

41. Bravo Gutierrez A, Madoff RD, Lowry AC, et al. Long-term results of anterior sphincteroplasty. *Dis Colon Rectum.* 2004;47(5):727–731.

42. Briel JW, Schouten WR. Disappointing results of postanal repair in the treatment of fecal incontinence. *Ned Tijdschr Geneeskd.* 1995;139(1):23–26.

43. Briel JW, Schouten WR, Vlot EA, et al. Clinical value of colonic irrigation in patients with continence disturbances. *Dis Colon Rectum.* 1997;40(7):802–805.

44. Briel JW, Stoker J, Rociu E, et al. External anal sphincter atrophy on endoanal magnetic resonance imaging adversely affects continence after sphincteroplasty. *Br J Surg.* 1999;86(10):1322–1327.

45. Briel JW, Zimmerman DD, Stoker J, et al. Relationship between sphincter morphology on endoanal MRI and histopathological aspects of the external anal sphincter. *Int J Colorectal Dis.* 2000;15(2):87–90.

46. Brocklehurst JC. Management of anal incontinence. *Clin Gastroenterol.* 1975;4(3):479–487.

47. Brocklehurst JC, Dickinson E, Windsor J. Laxatives and faecal incontinence in long-term care. *Elder Care.* 1998;10(4):22–25.

48. Bruining H, Bos KE, Colthoff EG, et al. Creation of an anal sphincter mechanism by bilateral proximally based gluteal muscle transposition. *Plast Reconstr Surg.* 1981;67(1):70–73.

49. Brummelkamp W, Leguit P Jr, van Baal JG. Pedicle muscle grafts for rectal incontinence: a review. *Surg Rounds.* 1986;9:66.

50. Buie WD, Lowry AC, Rothenberger DA, et al. Clinical rather than laboratory assessment predicts continence after anterior sphincteroplasty. *Dis Colon Rectum.* 2001;44(9):1255–1260.

51. Buppasiri P, Lumbiganon P, Thinkhamrop J, et al. Antibiotic prophylaxis for fourth-degree perineal tear during vaginal birth. *Cochrane Database Syst Rev.* 2005;4:CD005125.

52. Burnett SJ, Speakman CT, Kamm MA, et al. Confirmation of endosonographic detection of external anal sphincter defects by simultaneous electromyographic mapping. *Br J Surg.* 1991;78(4):448–450.

53. Busch DB, Starling JR. Rectal foreign bodies: case reports and a comprehensive review of the world's literature. *Surgery.* 1986;100(3):512–519.

54. Byrne CM, Pager CK, Rex J, et al. Assessment of quality of life in the treatment of patients with neuropathic fecal incontinence. *Dis Colon Rectum.* 2002;45(11):1431–1436.

55. Caldwell KP. The electrical control of sphincter incompetence. *Lancet.* 1963;2(7300):174–175.

56. Cavina E. Outcome of restorative perineal graciloplasty with simultaneous excision of the anus and rectum for cancer. A ten-year experience with 81 patients. *Dis Colon Rectum.* 1996;39(2):182–190.

57. Cavina E, Seccia M, Banti P, et al. Anorectal reconstruction after abdominoperineal resection. Experience with double-wrap graciloplasty supported by low-frequency electrostimulation. *Dis Colon Rectum.* 1998;41(8):1010–1016.

58. Cazemier M, Felt-Bersma RJ, Mulder CJ. Anal plugs and retrograde colonic irrigation are helpful in fecal incontinence or constipation. *World J Gastroenterol.* 2007;13:3101–3105.

59. Chapman A, Geerdes B, Hewett P, et al. Systematic review of dynamic graciloplasty in the treatment of faecal incontinence. *Br J Surg.* 2002;89:138–153.

60. Chatoor D, Soligo M, Emmanuel A. Organising a clinical service for patients with pelvic floor disorders. *Best Pract Res Clin Gastroenterol.* 2009;23(4):11–20.

61. Chen AS, Luchtefeld MA, Senagore AJ, et al. Pudendal nerve latency. Does it predict outcome of anal sphincter repair? *Dis Colon Rectum.* 1998;41(8):1005–1009.

62. Chen CJ. The treatment of imperforate anus: experience with 108 patients. *J Pediatr Surg.* 1999;34(11):1728–1732.

63. Chen YL, Zhang XH. Reconstruction of rectal sphincter by transposition of gluteus muscle for fecal incontinence. *J Pediatr Surg.* 1987;22(1):62–64.

64. Cheng YW, Hopkins LM, Caughey AB. How long is too long: does a prolonged second stage of labor in nulliparous women affect maternal and neonatal outcomes? *Am J Obstet Gynecol.* 2004;191(3):933–938.

65. Chew SS, Sundaraj R, Adams W. Sacral transcutaneous electrical nerve stimulation in the treatment of idiopathic faecal incontinence. *Colorectal Dis.* 2010;13(5):567–571.

66. Chiou AW, Lin JK, Wang FM. Anorectal abnormalities in progressive systemic sclerosis. *Dis Colon Rectum.* 1989;32(5):417–421.

67. Chittenden A. Sphincter muscle and reconstruction. *Ann Surg.* 1930;92:152–154.

68. Choen S, Tsunoda A, Nicholls RJ. Prospective randomized trial comparing anal function after hand sewn ileoanal anastomosis with mucosectomy versus stapled ileoanal anastomosis without mucosectomy in restorative proctocolectomy. *Br J Surg.* 1991;78(4):430–434.

69. Christensen P, Bazzocchi G, Coggrave M, et al. A randomized, controlled trial of transanal irrigation versus conservative bowel management in spinal cord-injured patients. *Gastroenterology.* 2006;131(3):738–747.

70. Christensen P, Krogh K. Transanal irrigation for disordered defecation: a systematic review. *Scand J Gastroenterol.* 2010;45(5):517–527.

71. Christensen P, Krogh K, Buntzen S, et al. Long-term outcome and safety of transanal irrigation for constipation and fecal incontinence. *Dis Colon Rectum.* 2009;52(2):286–292.

72. Christensen P, Olsen N, Krogh K, et al. Scintigraphic assessment of retrograde colonic washout in fecal incontinence and constipation. *Dis Colon Rectum.* 2003;46(1):68–76.

73. Christiansen J, Hansen CR, Rasmussen O. Bilateral gluteus maximus transposition for anal incontinence. *Br J Surg.* 1995;82(7):903–905.

74. Christiansen J, Lorentzen M. Implantation of artificial sphincter for anal incontinence. *Lancet.* 1987;2(8553):244–245.

75. Christiansen J, Lorentzen M. Implantation of artificial sphincter for anal incontinence. Report of five cases. *Dis Colon Rectum.* 1989;32(5):432–436.

76. Christiansen J, Sørensen M, Rasmussen OO. Gracilis muscle transposition for faecal incontinence. *Br J Surg.* 1990;77(9):1039–1040.

77. Christiansen J, Sparro B. Treatment of anal incontinence by an implantable prosthetic anal sphincter. *Ann Surg.* 1992;215(4):383–386.

78. Christoforidis D, Bordeianou L, Rockwood TH, et al. Fecal incontinence in men. *Colorectal Dis.* 2011;13(8):906–913.

79. Coats PM, Chan KK, Wilkins M, et al. A comparison between midline and mediolateral episiotomies. *Br J Obstet Gynaecol.* 1980;87(5):408–412.

80. Coller JA. Clinical application of anorectal manometry. *Gastroenterol Clin North Am.* 1987;16(1):17–33.

81. Conaghan P, Farouk R. Sacral nerve stimulation can be successful in patients with ultrasound evidence of external anal sphincter disruption. *Dis Colon Rectum.* 2005;48(8):1610–1614.

82. Corman M. Gracilis muscle transposition. *Contemp Surg.* 1978;13:9.

83. Corman ML. Follow-up evaluation of gracilis muscle transposition for fecal incontinence. *Dis Colon Rectum.* 1980;23(8):552–555.

84. Corman ML. The management of anal incontinence. *Surg Clin North Am.* 1983;63(1):177–192.

85. Corman ML. Anal incontinence following obstetrical injury. *Dis Colon Rectum.* 1985;28(2):86–89.

86. Corman ML. Gracilis muscle transposition for anal incontinence: late results. *Br J Surg.* 1985;72(suppl):S21–S22.

87. Craggs M, McFarlane J. Neuromodulation of the lower urinary tract. *Exp Physiol.* 1999;84(1):149–160.

88. Crawshaw AP, Pigott L, Potter MA, et al. A retrospective evaluation of rectal irrigation in the treatment of disorders of faecal continence. *Colorectal Dis.* 2004;6(3):185–190.

89. Critchlow JF, Houlihan MJ, Landolt CC, et al. Primary sphincter repair in anorectal trauma. *Dis Colon Rectum.* 1985;28(12):945–947.

90. Cuesta MA, Meijer S, Derksen EJ, et al. Anal sphincter imaging in fecal incontinence using endosonography. *Dis Colon Rectum.* 1992;35(1):59–63.

91. Damon H, Henry L, Barth X, et al. Fecal incontinence in females with a past history of vaginal delivery: significance of anal sphincter defects detected by ultrasound. *Dis Colon Rectum.* 2002;45(11):1445–1450.

92. Damon H, Henry L, Bretones S, et al. Postdelivery anal function in primiparous females: ultrasound and manometric study. *Dis Colon Rectum.* 2000;43(4):472–477.

93. da Silva GM, Jorge JM, Belin B, et al. New surgical options for fecal incontinence in patients with imperforate anus. *Dis Colon Rectum.* 2004;47(2):204–209.

94. Davis K, Kumar D, Poloniecki J. Preliminary evaluation of an injectable anal sphincter bulking agent (Durasphere) in the management of faecal incontinence. *Aliment Pharmacol Ther.* 2003;18(2):237–243.

95. Davis KJ, Kumar D, Poloniecki J. Adjuvant biofeedback following anal sphincter repair: a randomized study. *Aliment Pharmacol Ther.* 2004;20(5):539–549.

96. de la Portilla F, Fernandez A, Leon E, et al. Evaluation of the use of PTQ implants for the treatment of incontinent patients due to internal anal sphincter dysfunction. *Colorectal Dis.* 2008;10(1):89–94.

97. de la Portilla F, Rada R, Vega J, et al. Evaluation of the use of posterior tibial nerve stimulation for the treatment of fecal incontinence: preliminary results of a prospective study. *Dis Colon Rectum.* 2009;52(8):1427–1433.

98. de Leeuw JW, Vierhout ME, Struijk PC, et al. Anal sphincter damage after vaginal delivery: relationship of anal endosonography and manometry to anorectal complaints. *Dis Colon Rectum.* 2002;45(8):1004–1010.

99. Deen K, Kumar D, Williams JG, et al. Anal sphincter defects. Correlation between endoanal ultrasound and surgery. *Ann Surg.* 1993;218(2):201–205.

100. deSouza NM, Hall AS, Puni R, et al. High resolution magnetic resonance imaging of the anal sphincter using a dedicated endoanal coil. Comparison of magnetic resonance imaging with surgical findings. *Dis Colon Rectum.* 1996;39(8):926–934.

101. Deutekom M, Dobben A. Plugs for containing faecal incontinence. *Cochrane Database Syst Rev.* 2005;20(3):CD005086.

102. Devesa JM, Hervás PL, Vicente R, et al. Anal encirclement with a simple prosthetic sling for faecal incontinence. *Tech Coloproctol.* 2011;15(1):17–22. doi:10.1007/s10151-010-0673-1.

103. Devesa JM, Madrid JM, Gallego BR, et al. Bilateral gluteoplasty for fecal incontinence. *Dis Colon Rectum.* 1997;40(8):883–888.

104. Devesa JM, Rey A, Hervas PL, et al. Artificial anal sphincter: complications and functional results of a large personal series. *Dis Colon Rectum.* 2002;45(9):1154–1163.

105. Devesa JM, Vicente E, Enríquez JM, et al. Total fecal incontinence—a new method of gluteus maximus transposition: preliminary results and report of previous experience with similar procedures. *Dis Colon Rectum.* 1992;35(4):339–349.

106. Dickinson VA. Maintenance of anal continence: a review of pelvic floor physiology. *Gut.* 1978;19(12):1163–1174.

107. Dolan LM, Hilton P. Obstetric risk factors and pelvic floor dysfunction 20 years after first delivery. *Int Urogynecol J.* 2010;21(5):535–544.

108. Donnelly V, Fynes M, Campbell D, et al. Obstetric events leading to anal sphincter damage. *Obstet Gynecol.* 1998;92(6):955–961.

109. Dudding TC, Parés D, Vaizey CJ, et al. Predictive factors for successful sacral nerve stimulation in the treatment of faecal incontinence: a 10-year cohort analysis. *Colorectal Dis.* 2008;10(3):249–256.

110. Dudding TC, Parés D, Vaizey CJ, et al. Comparison of clinical outcome between open and percutaneous lead insertion for permanent sacral nerve neurostimulation for the treatment of fecal incontinence. *Dis Colon Rectum.* 2009;52(3):463–468. 410.1007/DCR.1000b1013e318197e318131f.

111. Dudding TC, Vaizey CJ, Kamm MA. Obstetric anal sphincter injury: incidence, risk factors, and management. *Ann Surg.* 2008;247(2):224–237.

112. Duggal N, Mercado C, Daniels K, et al. Antibiotic prophylaxis for prevention of postpartum perineal wound complications: a randomized controlled trial. *Obstet Gynecol.* 2008;111(6):1268–1273.

113. Dupuis O, Madelenat P, Rudigoz RC. Fecal and urinary incontinence after delivery: risk factors and prevention. *Gynecol Obstet Fertil.* 2004;32(6):540–548.

114. Ebert EC. Gastric and enteric involvement in progressive systemic sclerosis. *J Clin Gastroenterol.* 2008;42(1):5–12.

115. Eccersley AJ, Lunniss PJ, Williams NS. Unstimulated graciloplasty in traumatic faecal incontinence. *Br J Surg.* 1999;86(8):1071–1072.

116. Eckardt VF, Jung B, Fischer B, et al. Anal endosonography in healthy subjects and patients with idiopathic fecal incontinence. *Dis Colon Rectum.* 1994;37(3):235–242.

117. Efron J, Corman ML, Fleshman J, et al. Safety and effectiveness of temperature-controlled radio-frequency energy delivery to the anal canal (Secca procedure) for the treatment of fecal incontinence. *Dis Colon Rectum.* 2003;46(12):1606–1616.

118. Eléouet M, Siproudhis L, Guillou N, et al. Chronic posterior tibial nerve transcutaneous electrical nerve stimulation (TENS) to treat fecal incontinence (FI). *Int J Colorectal Dis.* 2011;25(9):1127–1132.

119. Elsebae MM. A study of fecal incontinence in patients with chronic anal fissure: prospective, randomized, controlled trial of the extent of internal anal sphincter division during lateral sphincterotomy. *World J Surg.* 2007;31(10):2052–2057.

120. Emblem R, Dhaenens G, Stien R, et al. The importance of anal endosonography in the evaluation of idiopathic fecal incontinence. *Dis Colon Rectum.* 1994;37(1):42–48.

121. Emmanuel A. Review of the efficacy and safety of transanal irrigation for neurogenic bowel dysfunction. *Spinal Cord.* 2010;48(9):664–673.

122. Emmertsen KJ, Laurberg S. Bowel dysfunction after treatment for rectal cancer. *Acta Oncol.* 2008;47(6):994–1003.

123. Engel AF, Kamm MA, Sultan AH, et al. Anterior anal sphincter repair in patients with obstetric trauma. *Br J Surg.* 1994;81(8):1231–1234.

124. Engel AF, van Baal SJ, Brummelkamp WH. Late results of postanal repair for idiopathic faecal incontinence. *Eur J Surg.* 1994;160(11):637–640.

125. Engel BT, Nikoomanesh P, Schuster MM. Operant conditioning of rectosphincteric responses in the treatment of fecal incontinence. *N Engl J Med.* 1974;290(12):646–649.

126. Enriquez-Navascues J, Devesa-Mugica M. Traumatic anal incontinence. Role of unilateral gluteus maximus transposition supplementing and supporting direct anal sphincteroplasty. *Dis Colon Rectum.* 1994;37(8):766–769.

127. Erekson EA, Sung VW, Myers DL. Effect of body mass index on the risk of anal incontinence and defecatory dysfunction in women. *Am J Obstet Gynecol.* 2008;198(5):596.e1–596.e4.

128. Falk PM, Blatchford GJ, Cali RL, et al. Transanal ultrasound and manometry in the evaluation of fecal incontinence. *Dis Colon Rectum.* 1994;37(5):468–472.

129. Falletto E, Masin A, Lolli P, et al. Is sacral nerve stimulation an effective treatment for chronic idiopathic anal pain? *Dis Colon Rectum.* 2009;52(3):456–462.

130. Farrell S, Gilmour D, Turnbull GK, et al. Overlapping compared with end-to-end repair of third- and fourth-degree obstetric anal sphincter tears: a randomized controlled trial. *Obstet Gynecol.* 2010;116(1):16–24.

131. Faucheron JL, Hannoun L, Thome C, et al. Is fecal continence improved by nonstimulated gracilis muscle transposition? *Dis Colon Rectum.* 1994;37(10):979–983.

132. Faucheron JL, Voirin D, Badic B. Sacral nerve stimulation for fecal incontinence: causes of surgical revision from a series of 87 consecutive patients operated on in a single institution. *Dis Colon Rectum.* 2010;53(11):1501–1507.

133. Felt-Bersma RJ, Cuesta MA, Koorevaar M, et al. Anal endosonography: relationship with anal manometry and neurophysiologic tests. *Dis Colon Rectum.* 1992;35(10):944–949.

134. Felt-Bersma RJ, Klinkenberg-Knol EC, Meuwissen SG. Anorectal function investigations in incontinent and continent patients. Differences and discriminatory value. *Dis Colon Rectum.* 1990;33(6):479–485.

135. Felt-Bersma RJ, Szojda MM, Mulder CJ. Temperature-controlled radiofrequency energy (SECCA) to the anal canal for the treatment of faecal incontinence offers moderate improvement. *Eur J Gastroenterol Hepatol.* 2007;19(7):575–580.

136. Fernando R, Sultan AH, Kettle C, et al. Methods of repair for obstetric anal sphincter injury. *Cochrane Database Syst Rev.* 2006;3:CD002866.

137. Findlay J, Maxwell-Armstrong C. Posterior tibial nerve stimulation and faecal incontinence: a review. *Int J Colorectal Dis.* 2011;26(3):265–273. doi:10.1007/s00384-010-1085-4.

138. Fitzpatrick M, Behan M, O'Connell PR, et al. Randomised clinical trial to assess anal sphincter function following forceps or vacuum assisted vaginal delivery. *BJOG.* 2003;110(4):424–429.

139. Fleshman J, Peters WR, Shemesh EI. Anal sphincter reconstruction: anterior overlapping muscle repair. *Dis Colon Rectum.* 1991;34(9):739–743.

140. Fraser C, Glazener C, Grant A, et al. *Systemic Review of the Efficacy and Safety of Sacral Nerve Stimulation for Faecal Incontinence.* Aberdeen, United Kingdom: University of Aberdeen, Health Services Research Unit; 2004.

141. Fritel X, Ringa V, Varnoux N, et al. Mode of delivery and fecal incontinence at midlife: a study of 2,640 women in the Gazel cohort. *Obstet Gynecol.* 2007;110(1):31–38.

142. Frizelle F, Gearry RB, Johnston M, et al. Penile and clitoral stimulation for faecal incontinence: external application of a bipolar electrode for patients with faecal incontinence. *Colorectal Dis.* 2004;6(1):54–57.

143. Frudinger A, Bartram CI, Spencer JA, et al. Perineal examination as a predictor of underlying external anal sphincter damage. *Br J Obstet Gynaecol.* 1997;104(9):1009–1013.

144.   Frudinger A, Halligan S, Bartram CI, et al. Assessment of the predictive value of a bowel symptom questionnaire in identifying perianal and anal sphincter trauma after vaginal delivery. *Dis Colon Rectum.* 2003;46(6):742–747.

145.   Fynes M, Donnelly VS, O'Connell PR, et al. Cesarean delivery and anal sphincter injury. *Obstet Gynecol.* 1998;92(4 pt 1):496–500.

146.   Gabriel W. *The Principles and Practice of Rectal Surgery.* 5th ed. London, United Kingdom: HK Lewis; 1963.

147.   Gallas S, Michot F, Faucheron JL, et al. Predictive factors for successful sacral nerve stimulation in the treatment of faecal incontinence: results of trial stimulation in 200 patients. *Colorectal Dis.* 2011;13(6):689–696.

148.   Ganio E, Ratto C, Masin A, et al. Neuromodulation for fecal incontinence: outcome in 16 patients with definitive implant. The initial Italian Sacral Neurostimulation Group (GINS) experience. *Dis Colon Rectum.* 2001;44(7):965–970.

149.   Ganio E, Realis LA, Ratto C, et al. Sacral nerve modulation for fecal incontinence: functional results and assessment of quality of life. Colorep Web site. http://www.colorep.it. Accessed 2002.

150.   Garcia V, Rogers RG, Kim SS, et al. Primary repair of obstetric anal sphincter laceration: a randomized trial of two surgical techniques. *Am J Obstet Gynecol.* 2005;192(5):1697–1701.

151.   Gearhart S, Hull T, Floruta C, et al. Anal manometric parameters: predictors of outcome following anal sphincter repair? *J Gastrointest Surg.* 2005;9(1):115–120.

152.   Geerdes BP, Heineman E, Konsten J, et al. Dynamic graciloplasty. Complications and management. *Dis Colon Rectum.* 1996;39(8):912–917.

153.   Geerdes BP, Zoetmulder FA, Heineman E, et al. Total anorectal reconstruction with a double dynamic graciloplasty after abdominoperineal reconstruction for low rectal cancer. *Dis Colon Rectum.* 1997;40(6):698–705.

154.   George AT, Dudding TC, Nicholls RJ, et al. A new minimally invasive technique for pudendal nerve stimulation. *Colorectal Dis.* 2012;14(1):98–103. doi:10.1111/j.1463-1318.2010.02485.x.

155.   George BD, Williams NS, Patel J, et al. Physiological and histochemical adaptation of the electrically stimulated gracilis muscle to neoanal sphincter function. *Br J Surg.* 1993;80(10):1342–1346.

156.   Giani I, Novelli E, Martina S, et al. The effect of sacral nerve modulation on cerebral evoked potential latency in fecal incontinence and constipation. *Ann Surg.* 2011;254(1):90–96.

157.   Gilliland R, Altomare DF, Moreira H Jr, et al. Pudendal neuropathy is predictive of failure following anterior overlapping sphincteroplasty. *Dis Colon Rectum.* 1998;41(12):1516–1522.

158.   Giordano P, Renzi A, Efron J, et al. Previous sphincter repair does not affect the outcome of repeat repair. *Dis Colon Rectum.* 2002;45(5):635–640.

159.   Gold DM, Bartram CI, Halligan S, et al. Three-dimensional endoanal sonography in assessing anal canal injury. *Br J Surg.* 1999;86(3):365–370.

160.   Goode PS, Burgio KL, Halli AD, et al. Prevalence and correlates of fecal incontinence in community-dwelling older adults. *J Am Geriatr Soc.* 2005;53(4):629–635.

161.   Gooneratne M, Facer P, Knowles CH, et al. Normalization of substance P levels in rectal mucosa of patients with faecal incontinence treated successfully by sacral nerve stimulation. *Br J Surg.* 2008;95(4):477–483.

162.   Goos M, Haberstroh J, Baumann T, et al. New selective endoscopic sacral nerve root stimulation—an advance in the treatment of fecal incontinence. *Neurogastroenterol Motil.* 2011;23(2):e104–e109.

163.   Gosselink MP, Darby M, Zimmerman DD, et al. Long-term follow-up of retrograde colonic irrigation for defaecation disturbances. *Colorectal Dis.* 2004;7(1):65–69.

164.   Gourcerol G, Vitton V, Leroi AM, et al. How sacral nerve stimulation works in patients with faecal incontinence. *Colorectal Dis.* 2011;13(8):e203–e211.

165.   Govaert B, Melenhorst J, Nieman FH, et al. Factors associated with percutaneous nerve evaluation and permanent sacral nerve modulation outcome in patients with fecal incontinence. *Dis Colon Rectum.* 2009;52(10):1688–1694.

166.   Govaert B, Pares D, Delgado-Aros S, et al. A prospective multicentre study to investigate percutaneous tibial nerve stimulation for the treatment of faecal incontinence. *Colorectal Dis.* 2010;12(12):1236–1241.

167.   Graham ID, Carroli G, Davies C, et al. Episiotomy rates around the world: an update. *Birth.* 2005;32(3):219–223.

168.   Granet E. Hemorrhoidectomy failures: causes, prevention and management. *Dis Colon Rectum.* 1968;11(1):45–48.

169.   Gravante G, Giordano P. The role of three-dimensional endoluminal ultrasound imaging in the evaluation of anorectal diseases: a review. *Surg Endosc.* 2008;22(7):1570–1578.

170.   Groom KM, Paterson-Brown S. Can we improve on the diagnosis of third degree tears? *Eur J Obstet Gynecol Reprod Biol.* 2002;101(1):19–21.

171.   Ha HT, Fleshman JW, Smith M, et al. Manometric squeeze pressure difference parallels functional outcome after overlapping sphincter reconstruction. *Dis Colon Rectum.* 2001;44(5):655–660.

172.   Hägglund D. A systematic literature review of incontinence care for persons with dementia: the research evidence. *J Clin Nurs.* 2010;19(3–4):303–312.

173.   Hallan RI, Marzouk DE, Waldron DJ, et al. Comparison of digital and manometric assessment of anal sphincter function. *Br J Surg.* 1989;76(9):973–975.

174.   Halverson AL, Hull TL. Long-term outcome of overlapping anal sphincter repair. *Dis Colon Rectum.* 2002;45(3):345–348.

175.   Handa VL, Danielsen BH, Gilbert WM. Obstetric anal sphincter lacerations. *Obstet Gynecol.* 2001;98(2):225–230.

176.   Hansen JL, Bliss DZ, Penden-McAlpine C. Dietary strategies used by women managing fecal incontinence. *J Wound Ostomy Continence Nurs.* 2006;33(1):52–62.

177.   Hardcastle J, Porter NH. Anal continence. In: Morson BC, ed. *Diseases of the Colon, Rectum, and Anus.* New York, NY: Appleton-Century-Crofts; 1969:251.

178.   Hautmann RE, Egghart G, Frohneberg D, et al. The ileal neobladder. *J Urol.* 1988;139(1):39–42.

179.   Hayne D, Vaizey CJ, Boulos PB. Anorectal injury following pelvic radiotherapy. *Br J Surg.* 2001;88(8):1037–1048.

180.   Healy JC, Halligan S, Bartram CI, et al. Dynamic magnetic resonance imaging evaluation of the structural and functional results of postanal repair for neuropathic fecal incontinence. *Dis Colon Rectum.* 2002;45(12):1629–1634.

181.   Hellström L, Ekelund P, Milsom I, et al. The influence of dementia on the prevalence of urinary and faecal incontinence in 85-year-old men and women. *Arch Gerontol Geriatr.* 1994;19(1):11–20.

182.   Hendrix NW, Grady CS, Chauhan SP. Clinical vs. sonographic estimate of birth weight in term parturients. A randomized clinical trial. *J Reprod Med.* 2000;45(4):317–322.

183.   Henry MM, Simson JN. Results of postanal repair: a retrospective study. *Br J Surg.* 1985;72(suppl):S17–S19.

184.   Hentz V. Construction of a rectal sphincter using the origin of the gluteus maximus muscle. *Plast Reconstr Surg.* 1982;70(1):82–85.

185.   Heriot AG, Tekkis PP, Smith JJ, et al. Management and outcome of pouch-vaginal fistulas following restorative proctocolectomy. *Dis Colon Rectum.* 2005;48(3):451–458.

186.   Heymen S, Jones KR, Ringel Y, et al. Biofeedback treatment of fecal incontinence: a critical review. *Dis Colon Rectum.* 2001;44(5):728–736.

187.   Heymen S, Scarlett Y, Jones K, et al. Randomized controlled trial shows biofeedback to be superior to pelvic floor exercises for fecal incontinence. *Dis Colon Rectum.* 2009;52(10):1730–1737.

188.   Hill J, Corson RJ, Brandon H, et al. History and examination in the assessment of patients with idiopathic fecal incontinence. *Dis Colon Rectum.* 1994;37(5):473–477.

189.   Hill J, Hosker G, Kiff ES. Pudendal nerve terminal motor latency measurements: what they do and do not tell us. *Br J Surg.* 2002;89(10):1268–1269.

190.   Ho K, Ho YH. Randomized clinical trial comparing oral nifedipine with lateral anal sphincterotomy and tailored sphincterotomy in the treatment of chronic anal fissure. *Br J Surg.* 2005;92(4):403–408.

191.   Ho KS, Seow-Choen F. Dynamic graciloplasty for total anorectal reconstruction after abdominoperineal resection for rectal tumour. *Int J Colorectal.* 2005;20(1):38–41.

192.   Ho YH, Brown S, Heah SM, et al. Comparison of J-pouch and coloplasty pouch for low rectal cancers: a randomized, controlled trial investigating functional results and comparative anastomotic leak rates. *Ann Surg.* 2002;236(1):49–55.

193.   Ho YH, Tsang C, Tang CL, et al. Anal sphincter injuries from stapling instruments introduced transanally: randomized, controlled study with endoanal ultrasound and anorectal manometry. *Dis Colon Rectum.* 2000;43(2):169–173.

194.   Hollingshead J, Dudding TC, George AC, et al. Sacral nerve stimulation (SNS) for the treatment of chronic functional anal pain. *Colorectal Dis.* 2010;12:34.

195.   Hollingshead JR, Dudding TC, Vaizey CJ. Sacral nerve stimulation for faecal incontinence: results from a single centre over a 10-year period. *Colorectal Dis.* 2011;13(9):1030–1034. doi:10.1111/j.1463-1318.2010.02383.x.

196.   Hopkinson BR, Lightwood R. Electrical treatment of anal incontinence. *Lancet.* 1966;1(7432):297–298.

197.   Horgan PG, O'Connell PR, Shinkwin CA, et al. Effect of anterior resection on anal sphincter function. *Br J Surg.* 1989;76(8):783–786.

198. Horn HR, Schoetz DJ Jr, Coller JA, et al. Sphincter repair with a Silastic sling for anal incontinence and rectal procidentia. *Dis Colon Rectum.* 1985;28(11):868–872.

199. Hosker G, Cody JD, Norton CC. Electrical stimulation for faecal incontinence in adults. *Cochrane Database Syst Rev.* 2007;18(3):CD001310.

200. Howard D, Davies PS, DeLancey JO, et al. Differences in perineal lacerations in black and white primiparas. *Obstet Gynecol.* 2000;96(4): 622–624.

201. Hughes SF, Williams NS. Continent colonic conduit for the treatment of faecal incontinence associated with disordered evacuation. *Br J Surg.* 1995;82(10):1318–1320.

202. Hull TL. Invited editorial. *Dis Colon Rectum.* 2004;47(5):731–732.

203. Ilnyckyj A. Prevalence of idiopathic fecal incontinence in a community-based sample. *Can J Gastroenterol.* 2010;24(4):251–254.

204. Iwai N, Kaneda H, Tsuto T, et al. Objective assessment of anorectal function after sphincter reconstruction using the gluteus maximus muscle. Report of a case. *Dis Colon Rectum.* 1985;28(12):973–977.

205. Jameson JS, Chia YW, Kamm MA, et al. Effect of age, sex, and parity on anorectal function. *Br J Surg.* 1994;81(11):1689–1692.

206. Jameson JS, Rogers J, Chia YW, et al. Pelvic floor function in multiple sclerosis. *Gut.* 1994;35(3):388–390.

207. Jameson JS, Speakman CT, Darzi A, et al. Audit of postanal repair in the treatment of fecal incontinence. *Dis Colon Rectum.* 1994;37(4):369–372.

208. Jarrett ME, Matzel KE, Christiansen J, et al. Sacral nerve stimulation for faecal incontinence in patients with previous partial spinal injury including disc prolapse. *Br J Surg.* 2005;92(6):734–739.

209. Jarrett ME, Matzel KE, Stösser M, et al. Sacral nerve stimulation for faecal incontinence following a rectosigmoid resection for colorectal cancer. *Int J Colorectal Dis.* 2005;20(5):446–451.

210. Jarrett ME, Matzel KE, Stösser M, et al. Sacral nerve stimulation for fecal incontinence following surgery for rectal prolapse repair: a multicenter study. *Dis Colon Rectum.* 2005;48(6):1243–1248.

211. Jarrett ME, Mowatt G, Glazener CM, et al. Systematic review of sacral nerve stimulation for faecal incontinence and constipation. *Br J Surg.* 2004;91(12):1559–1569.

212. Jarrett ME, Varma JS, Duthie GS, et al. Sacral nerve stimulation for faecal incontinence in the UK. *Br J Surg.* 2004;91(6):755–761.

213. Jarrett ME, Vaizey CJ, Cohen R, et al. Sacral nerve stimulation for faecal incontinence secondary to obstetric damage: superior to sphincter repair. *Colorectal Dis.* 2004;6(suppl 1):67.

214. Jenkinson C, Coulter A, Wright L. Short form 36 (SF36) health survey questionnaire: normative data for adults of working age. *BMJ.* 1993;306(6890):1437–1440.

215. Jensen L, Lowry AC. Biofeedback improves functional outcome after sphincteroplasty. *Dis Colon Rectum.* 1997;40(2):197–200.

216. Jorge JM, Wexner SD. Etiology and management of fecal incontinence. *Dis Colon Rectum.* 1993;36(1):77–97.

217. Kaiser AM, Corman ML. Modified perianal incisions in graciloplasty for fecal incontinence. *Dis Colon Rectum.* 2002;45(5):703–704.

218. Kamm MA, Dudding TC, Melenhorst J, et al. Sacral nerve stimulation for intractable constipation. *Gut.* 2010;59(3):333–340.

219. Karoui S, Leroi AM, Koning E, et al. Results of sphincteroplasty in 86 patients with anal incontinence. *Dis Colon Rectum.* 2000;43(6):813–820.

220. Karoui S, Savoye-Collet C, Koning E, et al. Prevalence of anal sphincter defects revealed by sonography in 335 incontinent patients and 115 continent patients. *AJR Am J Roentgenol.* 1999;173(2):389–392.

221. Kaushal JN, Goldner F. Validation of the digital rectal examination as an estimate of anal sphincter squeeze pressure. *Am J Gastroenterol.* 1991;86(7):886–887.

222. Kegel A. Active exercise of the pubococcygeus muscle. In: Meigs JV, Strugis SH, eds. *Progress in Gynecology: Vol. 2.* New York, NY: Grune & Stratton; 1950.

223. Keighley MR, Henry MM, Bartolo DC, et al. Anorectal physiology measurement: report of a working party. *Br J Surg.* 1989;76(4):356–357.

224. Kenefick NJ, Vaizey CJ, Cohen CR, et al. Medium-term results of permanent sacral nerve stimulation for faecal incontinence. *Br J Surg.* 2002;89(7):896–901.

225. Kenefick NJ, Vaizey CJ, Nicholls RJ, et al. Sacral nerve stimulation for faecal incontinence due to systemic sclerosis. *Gut.* 2002;51(6):881–883.

226. Khanduja KS, Yamashita HJ, Wise WE Jr, et al. Delayed repair of obstetric injuries of the anorectum and vagina. A stratified surgical approach. *Dis Colon Rectum.* 1994;37(4):344–349.

227. Kiff ES, Swash M. Slowed conduction in the pudendal nerves in idiopathic (neurogenic) faecal incontinence. *Br J Surg.* 1984;71(8):614–616.

228. Kim DW, Yoon HM, Park JS, et al. Radiofrequency energy delivery to the anal canal: is it a promising new approach to the treatment of fecal incontinence? *Am J Surg.* 2009;197(1):14–18.

229. Klingler HC, Pycha A, Schmidbauer J, et al. Use of peripheral neuromodulation of the S3 region for treatment of detrusor overactivity: a urodynamic-based study. *Urology.* 2000;56(5):766–771.

230. Koch SM, Melenhorst J, van Gemert WG, et al. Prospective study of colonic irrigation for the treatment of defaecation disorders. *Br J Surg.* 2008;95(10):1273–1279.

231. Koch SM, Rietveld MP, Govaert B, et al. Retrograde colonic irrigation for faecal incontinence after low anterior resection. *Int J Colorectal Dis.* 2009;24(9):1019–1022.

232. Koh CE, Young CJ, Wright CM, et al. The internal anal sphincter in systemic sclerosis. *Dis Colon Rectum.* 2009;52(2):315–318.

233. Konsten J, Baeten CG, Havenith MG, et al. Morphology of dynamic graciloplasty compared with the anal sphincter. *Dis Colon Rectum.* 1993;36(6):559–563.

234. Konsten J, Rongen MJ, Ogunbiyi OA, et al. Comparison of epineural or intramuscular nerve electrodes for stimulated graciloplasty. *Dis Colon Rectum.* 2001;44(4):581–586.

235. Kovavisarach E, Sringamvong W. Enema versus no-enema in pregnant women on admission in labor: a randomized controlled trial. *J Med Assoc Thai.* 2005;88(12):1763–1767.

236. Kozak LJ, Lees KA, DeFrances CJ. National Hospital Discharge Survey: 2003 annual summary with detailed diagnosis and procedure data. *Vital Health Stat 13.* 2006;160:1–206.

237. Krogh K, Laurberg S. Malone antegrade continence enema for faecal incontinence and constipation in adults. *Br J Surg.* 1998;85(7):974–977.

238. Kuijpers HC, Scheuer M. Disorders of impaired fecal control. A clinical and manometric study. *Dis Colon Rectum.* 1990;33(3):207–211.

239. Kumar D, Benson MJ, Bland JE. Glutaraldehyde cross-linked collagen in the treatment of faecal incontinence. *Br J Surg.* 1998;85(7):978–979.

240. Kumar D, Hutchinson R, Grant E. Bilateral gracilis neosphincter construction for treatment of faecal incontinence. *Br J Surg.* 1995;82(12): 1645–1647.

241. Labow SB, Hoexter B, Moseson MD, et al. Modification of Silastic sling repair for rectal procidentia and anal incontinence. *Dis Colon Rectum.* 1985;28(9):684–685.

242. Labow S, Rubin RJ, Hoexter B, et al. Perineal repair of rectal procidentia with an elastic fabric sling. *Dis Colon Rectum.* 1980;23(7):467–469.

243. Larach SW, Vazquez B. Modified Thiersch procedure with silastic mesh implant: a simple solution for fecal incontinence and severe prolapse. *South Med J.* 1986;79(3):307–309.

244. Laurberg S, Swash M. Effects of aging on the anorectal sphincters and their innervation. *Dis Colon Rectum.* 1989;32(9):737–742.

245. Laurberg S, Swash M, Snooks SJ, et al. Neurologic cause of idiopathic incontinence. *Arch Neurol.* 1988;45(11):1250–1253.

246. Lauti M, Scott D, Thompson-Fawcett MW. Fibre supplementation in addition to loperamide for faecal incontinence in adults: a randomized trial. *Colorectal Dis.* 2008;10(6):553–562.

247. Law PJ, Kamm MA, Bartram CI. A comparison between electromyography and anal endosonography in mapping external anal sphincter defects. *Dis Colon Rectum.* 1990;33(5):370–373.

248. Law PJ, Kamm MA, Bartram CI. Anal endosonography in the investigation of faecal incontinence. *Br J Surg.* 1991;78(3):312–314.

249. Law PJ, Talbot RW, Bartram CI, et al. Anal endosonography in the evaluation of perianal sepsis and fistula in ano. *Br J Surg.* 1989;76(7): 752–755.

250. Lefebure B, Tuech JJ, Bridoux V, et al. Temperature-controlled radio frequency energy delivery (Secca procedure) for the treatment of fecal incontinence: results of a prospective study. *Int J Colorectal Dis.* 2008;23(10):993–997.

251. Leguit P Jr, van Baal JG, Brummelkamp WH. Gracilis muscle transposition in the treatment of fecal incontinence. Long-term follow-up and evaluation of anal pressure recordings. *Dis Colon Rectum.* 1985;28(1):1–4.

252. Lehur PA, Glemain P, Bruley des Varannes S, et al. Outcome of patients with an implanted artificial anal sphincter for severe faecal incontinence. A single institution report. *Int J Colorectal Dis.* 1998;13:88.

253. Lehur PA, McNevin S, Buntzen S, et al. Magnetic anal sphincter augmentation for the treatment of fecal incontinence: a preliminary report from a feasibility study. *Dis Colon Rectum.* 2010;53(12):1604–1610.

254. Lehur PA, Michot F, Denis P, et al. Results of artificial sphincter in severe anal incontinence. Report of 14 consecutive implantations. *Dis Colon Rectum.* 1996;39(12):1352–1355.

255. Lehur PA, Roig JV, Duinslaeger M. Artificial anal sphincter: prospective clinical and manometric evaluation. *Dis Colon Rectum.* 2000;43(8):1100–1106.

256. Lehur PA, Zerbib F, Neunlist M, et al. Comparison of quality of life and anorectal function after artificial sphincter implantation. *Dis Colon Rectum.* 2002;45(4):508–513.

257. Leighton JA, Valdovinos MA, Pemberton JH, et al. Anorectal dysfunction and rectal prolapse in progressive systemic sclerosis. *Dis Colon Rectum*. 1993;36(2):182–185.

258. Leroi AM, Damon H, Faucheron JL, et al. Sacral nerve stimulation in faecal incontinence: position statement based on a collective experience. *Colorectal Dis*. 2009;11(6):572–583.

259. Leroi AM, Michot F, Grise P, et al. Effect of sacral nerve stimulation in patients with fecal and urinary incontinence. *Dis Colon Rectum*. 2001;44(6):779–789.

260. Leroi AM, Parc Y, Lehur PA, et al. Efficacy of sacral nerve stimulation for fecal incontinence: results of a multicenter double-blind crossover study. *Ann Surg*. 2005;242(5):662–669.

261. Lestar B, Penninckx F, Kerremans R. The composition of anal basal pressure. An in vivo and in vitro study in man. *Int J Colorectal Dis*. 1989;4(2):118–122.

262. Levitt MA, Soffer SZ, Peña A. Continent appendicostomy in the bowel management of fecally incontinent children. *J Pediatr Surg*. 1997;32(11):1630–1633.

263. Lien KC, Morgan DM, Delancey JO, et al. Pudendal nerve stretch during vaginal birth: a 3D computer simulation. *Am J Obstet Gynecol*. 2005;197(5):1669–1676.

264. Lomas MI, Cooperman H. Correction of rectal procidentia by polypropylene mesh (Marlex). *Dis Colon Rectum*. 1972;15(6):416–419.

265. Lou MA, Johnson AP, Atik M, et al. Exteriorized repair in the management of colon injuries. *Arch Surg*. 1981;116(7):926–929.

266. Lubowski DZ, Nicholls RJ, Burleigh DE, et al. Internal anal sphincter in neurogenic fecal incontinence. *Gastroenterology*. 1988;95(4):997–1002.

267. Lubowski DZ, Nicholls RJ, Swash M, et al. Neural control of internal anal sphincter function. *Br J Surg*. 1987;74(8):668–670.

268. Luck AM, Galvin SL, Theofrastous JP. Suture erosion and wound dehiscence with permanent versus absorbable suture in reconstructive posterior vaginal surgery. *Am J Obstet Gynecol*. 2005;192(5):1626–1629.

269. Lundby L, Krogh K, Jensen VJ, et al. Long-term anorectal dysfunction after postoperative radiotherapy for rectal cancer. *Dis Colon Rectum*. 2005;48(7):1343–1349.

270. Macarthur C, Glazener C, Lancashire R, et al. Faecal incontinence and mode of first and subsequent delivery: a six-year longitudinal study. *BJOG*. 2005;112(8):1075–1082.

271. Madoff RD, Baeten CG, Christiansen J, et al. Standards for anal sphincter replacement. *Dis Colon Rectum*. 2000;43(2):135–141.

272. Maeda Y, Høyer M, Lundby L, et al. Faecal incontinence following radiotherapy for prostate cancer: a systematic review. *Radiother Oncol*. 2011;98(2):145–153. doi:10.1016/j.radonc.2010.12.004.

273. Maeda Y, Laurberg S, Norton C. Perianal injectable bulking agents as treatment for faecal incontinence in adults. *Cochrane Database Syst Rev*. 2010;5:CD007959. doi:10.1002/14651858.CD007959.pub2.

274. Maeda Y, Lundby L, Buntzen S, et al. Sacral nerve stimulation for constipation: loss of efficacy and reoperations. *Colorectal Dis*. 2009;11:6.

275. Maeda Y, Lundby L, Buntzen S, et al. Sacral nerve stimulation for constipation: suboptimal outcome and adverse events. *Dis Colon Rectum*. 2010;53(7):995–999.

276. Maeda Y, Lundby L, Buntzen S, et al. Suboptimal outcome following sacral nerve stimulation for faecal incontinence. *Br J Surg*. 2011;98(1):140–147.

277. Maeda Y, Parés D, Norton C, et al. Does the St. Mark's incontinence score reflect patients' perceptions? A review of 390 patients. *Dis Colon Rectum*. 2008;51(4):436–442.

278. Maeda Y, Vaizey CJ, Kamm MA. Pilot study of two new injectable bulking agents for the treatment of faecal incontinence. *Colorectal Dis*. 2008;10(3):268–272.

279. Mahony R, Behan M, O'Herlihy C, et al. Randomized, clinical trial of bowel confinement vs. laxative use after primary repair of a third-degree obstetric anal sphincter tear. *Dis Colon Rectum*. 2004;47(1):12–17.

280. Malone PS, Ransley PG, Kiely EM. Preliminary report: the antegrade continence enema. *Lancet*. 1990;336(8725):1217–1218.

281. Malouf AJ, Norton CS, Engel AF, et al. Long-term results of overlapping anterior anal-sphincter repair for obstetric trauma. *Lancet*. 2000;355(9200):260–265.

282. Malouf AJ, Vaizey CJ, Norton CS, et al. Internal anal sphincter augmentation for fecal incontinence using injectable silicone biomaterial. *Dis Colon Rectum*. 2001;44(4):595–600.

283. Mandelstam D. Faecal incontinence: social and economic factors. In: Henry MM, Swash M, eds. *Coloproctology and the Pelvic Floor*. London, United Kingdom: Butterworth; 1985:217.

284. Mander BJ, Abercrombie JF, George BD, et al. The electrically stimulated gracilis neosphincter incorporated as part of total anorectal reconstruction after abdominoperineal excision of the rectum. *Ann Surg*. 1996;224(6):702–709.

285. Mander BJ, Wexner SD, Williams NS, et al. Preliminary results of a multicentre trial of the electrically stimulated gracilis neoanal sphincter. *Br J Surg*. 1999;86(12):1543–1548.

286. Markland AD, Goode PS, Burgio KL, et al. Incidence and risk factors for fecal incontinence in black and white older adults: a population-based study. *J Am Geriatr Soc*. 2010;58(7):1341–1346.

287. Markland AD, Richter HE, Burgio KL, et al. Fecal incontinence in obese women with urinary incontinence: prevalence and role of dietary fiber intake. *Am J Obstet Gynecol*. 2009;2009(5):566.e561–566.e566.

288. Maslekar SK, Gardiner AB, Duthie GS. Sacral nerve neuromodulation as primary treatment for faecal incontinence with disrupted anal sphincters: medium and long-term results. Paper presented at: Digestive Disease Week, 2006; Los Angeles, CA.

289. Matsuoka H, Mavrantonis C, Wexner SD, et al. Postanal repair for fecal incontinence—is it worthwhile? *Dis Colon Rectum*. 2000;43(11):1561–1567.

290. Matzel KE, Bittorf B, Stadelmaier U, et al. Sacral nerve stimulation in the treatment of faecal incontinence. *Chirurg*. 2003;74(1):26–32.

291. Matzel KE, Kamm MA, Stösser M, et al. Sacral spinal nerve stimulation for fecal incontinence: multicentre study. *Lancet*. 2004;363(9417):1270–1276.

292. Matzel KE, Lux P, Heuer S, et al. Sacral nerve stimulation for faecal incontinence: long-term outcome. *Colorectal Dis*. 2009;11(6):636–641.

293. Matzel KE, Madoff RD, LaFontaine LJ, et al. Complications of dynamic graciloplasty: incidence, management, and impact on outcome. *Dis Colon Rectum*. 2001;44(10):1427–1435.

294. Matzel KE, Stadelmaier U, Hohenfellner M, et al. Electrical stimulation of sacral spinal nerves for treatment of faecal incontinence. *Lancet*. 1995;346(8983):1124–1127.

295. Matzel KE, Stadelmaier U, Muehldorfer S, et al. Continence after colorectal reconstruction following resection: impact of level of anastomosis. *Int J Colorectal Dis*. 1997;12(2):82–87.

296. McHugh SM, Diamant NE. Effect of age, gender, and parity on anal canal pressures. Contribution of impaired anal sphincter function to fecal incontinence. *Dig Dis Sci*. 1987;32(7):726–736.

297. Melenhorst J, Koch SM, Uludag O, et al. Sacral neuromodulation in patients with faecal incontinence: results of the first 100 permanent implantations. *Colorectal Dis*. 2007;9(8):725–730.

298. Melenhorst J, Koch SM, van Gemert WG, et al. The artificial bowel sphincter for faecal incontinence: a single centre study. *Int J Colorectal Dis*. 2008;23(1):107–111.

299. Melzack R, Wall PD. Pain mechanisms: a new theory. *Science*. 1965;150(3699):971–979.

300. Mentes BB, Yüksel O, Aydin A, et al. Posterior tibial nerve stimulation for faecal incontinence after partial spinal injury: preliminary report. *Tech Coloproctol*. 2007;11(2):115–119.

301. Messelink EJ. The overactive bladder and the role of the pelvic floor muscles. *BJU Int*. 1999;83(suppl 2):31–35.

302. Meurette G, La Torre M, Regenet M, et al. Value of sacral nerve stimulation in the treatment of severe faecal incontinence: a comparison to the artificial bowel sphincter. *Colorectal Dis*. 2009;11(6):631–635.

303. Michelsen HB, Thompson-Fawcett M, Lundby L, et al. Six years of experience with sacral nerve stimulation for fecal incontinence. *Dis Colon Rectum*. 2010;53(4):414–421.

304. Michot F, Costaglioli B, Leroi AM, et al. Artificial anal sphincter in severe fecal incontinence: outcome of prospective experience with 37 patients in one institution. *Ann Surg*. 2003;237(1):52–56.

305. Michot F, Lefebure B, Bridoux V, et al. Artificial anal sphincter for severe fecal incontinence implanted by a transvaginal approach: experience with 32 patients treated at one institution. *Dis Colon Rectum*. 2010;53(8):1155–1160.

306. Miller R, Bartolo DC, Cervero F, et al. Anorectal temperature sensation: a comparison of normal and incontinent patients. *Br J Surg*. 1987;74(6):511–515.

307. Miller R, Bartolo DC, Cervero F, et al. Anorectal sampling: a comparison of normal and incontinent patients. *Br J Surg*. 1988;75(1):44–47.

308. Miller R, Bartolo DC, Roe A, et al. Anal sensation and the continence mechanism. *Dis Colon Rectum*. 1988;31(6):433–438.

309. Miller R, Lewis GT, Bartolo DC, et al. Sensory discrimination and dynamic activity in the anorectum: evidence using a new ambulatory technique. *Br J Surg*. 1988;75(10):1003–1007.

310. Mortensen N, Humphreys MS. The anal continence plug: a disposable device for patients with anorectal incontinence. *Lancet*. 1991;338(8672):295–297.

311. Mowatt G, Glazener C, Jarrett M. Sacral nerve stimulation for fecal incontinence and constipation in adults: a short version Cochrane review. *Neurour Urodyn.* 2008;27(3):155–161.

312. Mundy L, Merlin TL, Maddern GJ, et al. Systematic review of safety and effectiveness of an artificial bowel sphincter for faecal incontinence. *Br J Surg.* 2004;91(6):665–672.

313. Murphy DJ, Liebling RE, Verity L, et al. Early maternal and neonatal morbidity associated with operative delivery in second stage of labour: a cohort study. *Lancet.* 2001;358(9289):1203–1207.

314. Nakamura M, Sakurai T, Tsujimoto Y, et al. Transcutaneous electrical stimulation for the control of frequency and urge incontinence. *Hinyokika Kiyo.* 1983;29(9):1053–1059.

315. Naldini G, Martellucci J, Moraldi L, et al. Treatment of slow-transit constipation with sacral nerve modulation. *Colorectal Dis.* 2010;12(11):1149–1152.

316. National Center for Health Statistics. Centers for Disease Control and Prevention Web site. http://www.cdc.gov/nchs. Accessed 2006.

317. National Institute for Health and Clinical Excellence. *Sacral Nerve Stimulation for Faecal Incontinence.* London, United Kingdom; National Institute for Health and Clinical Excellence; 2004.

318. Nazir M, Carlsen E, Jacobsen AF, et al. Is there any correlation between objective anal testing, rupture grade, and bowel symptoms after primary repair of obstetric anal sphincter rupture? An observational cohort study. *Dis Colon Rectum.* 2002;45(10):1325–1331.

319. Nazir M, Carlsen E, Nesheim BI. Do occult anal sphincter injuries, vector volume manometry and delivery variables have any predictive value for bowel symptoms after first time vaginal delivery without third and fourth degree rupture? A prospective study. *Acta Obstet Gynecol Scand.* 2002;81(8):720–726.

320. Neill ME, Swash M. Increased motor unit fibre density in the external anal sphincter muscle in anorectal incontinence: a single fibre EMG study. *J Neurol Neurosurg Psychiatry.* 1980;43(4):343–347.

321. Nelson R. Non surgical therapy for anal fissure (Review). *Cochrane Database Syst Rev.* 2006;4:CD003431. doi:10.1002/14651858.CD003431.pub2.

322. Nelson R. Operative procedures for fissure in ano. *Cochrane Database Syst Rev.* 2009;18(2):CD002199. doi:10.1002/14651858.CD002199.pub2.

323. Nelson R, Furner S, Jesudason V. Fecal incontinence in Wisconsin nursing homes: prevalence and associations. *Dis Colon Rectum.* 1998;41(10):1226–1229.

324. Nelson R, Norton N, Cautley E, et al. Community-based prevalence of anal incontinence. *JAMA.* 1995;274(7):559–561.

325. Nessim A, Wexner SD, Agachan F, et al. Is bowel confinement necessary after anorectal reconstructive surgery? A prospective, randomized, surgeon-blinded trial. *Dis Colon Rectum.* 1999;42(1):16–23.

326. Nicholls J. Anal fissure: surgery is the most effective treatment. *Colorectal Dis.* 2008;10(6):529–530.

327. Nicholls RJ, Lubowski DZ, Donaldson DR. Comparison of colonic reservoir and straight colo-anal reconstruction after rectal excision. *Br J Surg.* 1988;75(4):318–320.

328. Nichols CM, Lamb EH, Ramakrishnan V. Differences in outcomes after third-versus fourth-degree perineal laceration repair: a prospective study. *Am J Obstet Gynecol.* 2005;193(2):530–534.

329. Nichols RL, Broido P, Condon RE, et al. Effect of preoperative neomycin-erythromycin intestinal preparation on the incidence of infectious complications following colon surgery. *Ann Surg.* 1973;178(4):453–462.

330. Nielsen MB, Rasmussen OO, Pedersen JF, et al. Risk of sphincter damage and anal incontinence after anal dilatation for fissure-in-ano. An endosonographic study. *Dis Colon Rectum.* 1993;36(7):677–680.

331. Norderval S, Nsubuga D, Bjelke C, et al. Anal incontinence after obstetric sphincter tears: incidence in a Norwegian county. *Acta Obstet Gynecol Scand.* 2004;83(10):989–994.

332. Norderval S, Oian P, Revhaug A, et al. Anal incontinence after obstetric sphincter tears: outcome of anatomic primary repairs. *Dis Colon Rectum.* 2005;48(5):1055–1061.

333. Norton C. Triple target treatment versus biofeedback. *Dis Colon Rectum.* 2010;53(7):971–972.

334. Norton C, Cody JD, Hosker G. Biofeedback and/or sphincter exercises for the treatment of faecal incontinence in adults. *Cochrane Database Syst Rev.* 2006;3:CD002111.

335. Norton C, Kamm MA. Anal plug for faecal incontinence. *Colorectal Dis.* 2001;3(5):323–327.

336. Norton C, Whitehead WE, Bliss DZ, et al. Management of fecal incontinence in adults. *Neurourol Urodyn.* 2010;29(1):199–206.

337. Nowacki MP, Towpik E. Reconstruction of the anus, rectovaginal septum, and distal part of the vagina after postirradiation necrosis. Report of a unique case. *Dis Colon Rectum.* 1989;31(8):632–634.

338. O'Brien PE, Dixon JB, Skinner S, et al. A prospective, randomized, controlled clinical trial of placement of the artificial bowel sphincter (Acticon Neosphincter) for the control of fecal incontinence. *Dis Colon Rectum.* 2004;47(11):1852–1860.

339. O'Brien PE, Skinner S. Restoring control: the Acticon Neosphincter artificial bowel sphincter in the treatment of anal incontinence. *Dis Colon Rectum.* 2000;43(9):1213–1216.

340. Oberwalder M, Dinnewitzer A, Baig MK, et al. The association between late-onset fecal incontinence and obstetric anal sphincter defects. *Arch Surg.* 2004;139(4):429–432.

341. Oberwalder M, Dinnewitzer A, Nogueras JJ, et al. Imbrication of the external anal sphincter may yield similar functional results as overlapping repair in selected patients. *Colorectal Dis.* 2008;10(8):800–804.

342. Oliveira L, Pfeifer J, Wexner SD. Physiological and clinical outcome of anterior sphincteroplasty. *Br J Surg.* 1996;83(4):502–505.

343. Oreskovich M, Carrico CJ, Baker LW. Complications of penetrating colon injury. *Infect Surg.* 1983;2:101.

344. Orrom WJ, Miller R, Cornes H, et al. Comparison of anterior sphincteroplasty and postanal repair in the treatment of idiopathic fecal incontinence. *Dis Colon Rectum.* 1991;34(4):305–310.

345. Ortiz H, Armendariz P. Anterior resection: do the patients perceive any clinical benefit? *Int J Colorectal Dis.* 1996;11(4):191–195.

346. Ortiz H, Armendariz P, DeMiguel M, et al. Prospective study of artificial anal sphincter and dynamic graciloplasty for severe anal incontinence. *Int J Colorectal Dis.* 2003;18(4):349–354.

347. Parellada CM, Miller AS, Williamson ME, et al. Paradoxical high anal resting pressures in men with idiopathic fecal seepage. *Dis Colon Rectum.* 1998;41(5):593–597.

348. Parés D, Iglesias M, Pera M, et al. Expression of estrogen and progesterone receptors in the anal canal of women according to age and menopause. *Dis Colon Rectum.* 2010;53(12):1687–1691.

349. Parker SC, Spencer MP, Madoff RD, et al. Artificial bowel sphincter: long-term experience at a single institution. *Dis Colon Rectum.* 2003;46(6):722–729.

350. Parks A. Anorectal incontinence. *Proc R Soc Med.* 1975;68:681–690.

351. Parks A, Percy J. *Postanal Pelvic Floor Repair for Anorectal Incontinence.* London, United Kingdom: Butterworth; 1983.

352. Parks AG, Swash M, Urich H. Sphincter denervation in anorectal incontinence and rectal prolapse. *Gut.* 1977;18(8):656–665.

353. Pearl RK, Prasad ML, Nelson RL, et al. Bilateral gluteus maximus transposition for anal incontinence. *Dis Colon Rectum.* 1991;34(6):478–481.

354. Pedersen IK, Christiansen J. A study of the physiological variation in anal manometry. *Br J Surg.* 1989;76(1):69–70.

355. Peña A. Posterior sagittal anorectoplasty: results in the management of 332 cases of anorectal, malformations. *Pediatr Surg Int.* 1988;3(2–3):94–104.

356. Peña A, Amroch D, Baeza C, et al. The effects of the posterior sagittal approach on rectal function (experimental study). *J Pediatr Surg.* 1993;28(6):773–778.

357. Perry RE, Blatchford GJ, Christensen MA, et al. Manometric diagnosis of anal sphincter injuries. *Am J Surg.* 1990;159(1):112–116.

358. Pescatori M, Anastasio G, Bottini C, et al. New grading and scoring for anal incontinence. Evaluation of 335 patients. *Dis Colon Rectum.* 1992;35(5):482–487.

359. Pickrell KL, Broadbent TR, Masters FW, et al. Construction of a rectal sphincter and restoration of anal continence by transplanting gracilis muscle: report of four cases in children. *Ann Surg.* 1952;135(6):853–862.

360. Pinedo G, Vaizey CJ, Nicholls RJ, et al. Results of repeat anal sphincter repair. *Br J Surg.* 1999;86(1):66–69.

361. Pinta T, Kylänpää-Bäck ML, Salmi T, et al. Delayed sphincter repair for obstetric ruptures: analysis of failure. *Colorectal Dis.* 2003;5(1):73–78.

362. Pinta T, Kylänpää ML, Salmi TK, et al. Primary sphincter repair: are the results of the operation good enough? *Dis Colon Rectum.* 2004;47(1):18–23.

363. Pittman RD, Medwell SJ, Friend WG. A method for determining fecal continence prior to closure of colostomy. *Surg Gynecol Obstet.* 1985;161(4):388–389.

364. Poirier M, Abcarian H, Nelson R. Malone antegrade continent enema: an alternative to resection in severe defecation disorders. *Dis Colon Rectum.* 2006;50(1):22–28.

365. Pollack J, Holm T, Cedermark B, et al. Long-term effect of preoperative radiation therapy on anorectal function. *Dis Colon Rectum.* 2006;49(3):345–352.

366. Pollack J, Nordenstam J, Brismar S, et al. Anal incontinence after vaginal delivery: a five-year prospective cohort study. *Obstet Gynecol.* 2004;104(6):1397–1402.

367. Possover M. The laparoscopic implantation of neuroprosthesis to the sacral plexus for therapy of neurogenic bladder dysfunctions after failure of percutaneous sacral nerve stimulation. *Neuromodulation.* 2010;13(2):141–144.

368. Prager E. The continent colostomy. *Dis Colon Rectum.* 1984;27(4):235–237.

369. Prochiantz A, Gross P. Gluteal myoplasty for sphincter replacement: principles, results and prospects. *J Pediatr Surg.* 1982;17(1):25–30.

370. Queralto M, Portier G, Cabarrot PH, et al. Preliminary results of peripheral transcutaneous neuromodulation in the treatment of idiopathic fecal incontinence. *Int J Colorectal Dis.* 2006;21(7):670–672.

371. Rasmussen OO, Buntzen S, Sørensen M, et al. Sacral nerve stimulation in fecal incontinence. *Dis Colon Rectum.* 2004;47(7):1158–1162; discussion 1162–1163.

372. Ratto C, Grillo E, Parello A, et al. Sacral neuromodulation in treatment of fecal incontinence following anterior resection and chemoradiation for rectal cancer. *Dis Colon Rectum.* 2005;48(5):1027–1036.

373. Ricciardi R, Mellgren AF, Madoff RD, et al. The utility of pudendal nerve terminal motor latencies in idiopathic incontinence. *Dis Colon Rectum.* 2006;49(6):852–857.

374. Rieger NA, Sarre RG, Saccone GT, et al. Postanal repair for faecal incontinence: long-term follow-up. *Aust N Z J Surg.* 1997;67(8):566–570.

375. Rieger N, Schloithe A, Saccone G, et al. A prospective study of anal sphincter injury due to childbirth. *Scand J Gastroenterol.* 1998;33(9):950–955.

376. Rieger N, Tjandra J, Solomon M, Endoanal and endorectal ultrasound: applications in colorectal surgery. *ANZ J Surg.* 2004;74(8):671–675.

377. Roberson EN, Gould JC, Wald A. Urinary and fecal incontinence after bariatric surgery. *Dig Dis Sci.* 2010;55(9):2606–2613.

378. Rockwood TH, Church JM, Fleshman JW, et al. Fecal Incontinence Quality of Life Scale: quality of life instrument for patients with fecal incontinence. *Dis Colon Rectum.* 2000;43(1):9–16.

379. Rodemann JF, Dubberke ER, Kimberly A, et al. Incidence of *Clostridium difficile* infection in inflammatory bowel disease. *Clin Gastroenterol Hepatol.* 2007;5(3):339–344.

380. Roe AM, Bartolo DC, Mortensen NJ. New method for assessment of anal sensation in various anorectal disorders. *Br J Surg.* 1986;73(4):310–312.

381. Rogers J, Hayward MP, Henry MM, et al. Temperature gradient between the rectum and the anal canal: evidence against the role of temperature sensation as a sensory modality in the anal canal of normal subjects. *Br J Surg.* 1988;75(11):1083–1085.

382. Rogers J, Laurberg S, Misiewicz JJ, et al. Anorectal physiology validated: a repeatability study of the motor and sensory tests of anorectal function. *Br J Surg.* 1989;76(6):607–609.

383. Roig JV, Villoslada C, Lledó S, et al. Prevalence of pudendal neuropathy in fecal incontinence. Results of a prospective study. *Dis Colon Rectum.* 1995;38(9):952–958.

384. Rongen MJ, Uludag O, El Naggar K, et al. Long-term follow-up of dynamic graciloplasty for fecal incontinence. *Dis Colon Rectum.* 2003;46(60):716–721.

385. Rosen HR, Urbarz C, Holzer B, et al. Sacral nerve stimulation as a treatment for fecal incontinence. *Gastroenterology.* 2001;121(3):536–541.

386. Rosen HR, Urbarz C, Novi G, et al. Long-term results of modified graciloplasty for sphincter replacement after rectal excision. *Colorectal Dis.* 2001;4(4):266–269.

387. Rothbarth J, Bemelman WA, Meijerink WJ, et al. Long-term results of anterior anal sphincter repair for fecal incontinence due to obstetric injury/with invited commentaries. *Dig Surg.* 2000;17(4):390–393; discussion 394.

388. Rothbarth J, Bemelman WA, Meijerink WJ, et al. What is the impact of fecal incontinence on quality of life? *Dis Colon Rectum.* 2001;44(1):67–71.

389. Ruiz D, Pinto RA, Hull TL, et al. Does the radiofrequency procedure for fecal incontinence improve quality of life and incontinence at 1-year follow-up? *Dis Colon Rectum.* 2010;53(7):1041–1046.

390. Ruiz Carmona MD, Alós Company R, Roig Vila JV, et al. Long-term results of artificial bowel sphincter for the treatment of severe faecal incontinence. Are they what we hoped for? *Colorectal Dis.* 2009;11(8):831–837.

391. Rullier E, Zerbib F, Laurent C, et al. Morbidity and functional outcome after double dynamic graciloplasty for anorectal reconstruction. *Br J Surg.* 2000;87(7):909–913.

392. Ruthmann O, Fischer A, Hopt UT, et al. Dynamic graciloplasty vs artificial bowel sphincter in the management of severe fecal incontinence. *Chirurg.* 2006;77(10):926–938.

393. Rygh AB, Körner H. The overlap technique versus end-to-end approximation technique for primary repair of obstetric anal sphincter rupture: a randomized controlled study. *Acta Obstet Gynecol Scand.* 2010;89(10):1256–1262.

394. Sainio AP, Halme LE, Husa AI. Anal encirclement with polypropylene mesh for rectal prolapse and incontinence. *Dis Colon Rectum.* 1991;34(10):905–908.

395. Sainio AP, Voutilainen PE, Husa AI. Recovery of anal sphincter function following transabdominal repair of rectal prolapse: cause of improved continence? *Dis Colon Rectum.* 1991;34(9):816–821.

396. Salmons S, Henriksson J. The adaptive response of skeletal muscle to increased use. *Muscle Nerve.* 1981;4(2):94–105.

397. Samarasekera DN, Bekhit MT, Wright Y, et al. Long-term anal continence and quality of life following postpartum anal sphincter injury. *Colorectal Dis.* 2008;10(8):793–799.

398. Sangwan YP, Coller JA, Barrett RC, et al. Unilateral pudendal neuropathy. Impact on outcome of anal sphincter repair. *Dis Colon Rectum.* 1996;39(6):686–689.

399. Scheuer M, Kuijpers HC, Jacobs PP. Postanal repair restores anatomy rather than function. *Dis Colon Rectum.* 1989;32(11):960–963.

400. Schiller LR, Santa Ana CA, Schumulen AC, et al. Pathogenesis of fecal incontinence in diabetes mellitus: evidence for internal-anal-sphincter dysfunction. *N Engl J Med.* 1982;307(27):1666–1671.

401. Schmidt RA, Kogan BA, Tanagho EA. Neuroprostheses in the management of incontinence in myelomeningocele patients. *J Urol.* 1990;143(4):779–782.

402. Schnelle JF, Alessi CA, Simmons SF, et al. Translating clinical research into practice: a randomized controlled trial of exercise and incontinence care with nursing home residents. *J Am Geriatr Soc.* 2002;50(9):1476–1483.

403. Schwandner T, König IR, Heimerl T, et al. Triple target treatment (3T) is more effective than biofeedback alone for anal incontinence: the 3T-AI Study. *Dis Colon Rectum.* 2010;53(7):1007–1016.

404. Scott A, Hawley PR, Phillips RK. Results of external sphincter repair in Crohn's disease. *Br J Surg.* 1989;76(9):959–960.

405. Scott AD, Henry MM, Phillips RK. Clinical assessment and anorectal manometry before postanal repair: failure to predict outcome. *Br J Surg.* 1990;77(6):628–629.

406. Scott AM, Kellow JE, Eckersley GM, et al. Cigarette smoking and nicotine delay postprandial mouth-cecum transit time. *Dig Dis Sci.* 1992;37(10):1544–1547.

407. Seccia M, Menconi C, Balestri R, et al. Study protocols and functional results in 86 electrostimulated graciloplasties. *Dis Colon Rectum.* 1994;37(9):897–904.

408. Setti Carraro P, Kamm MA, Nicholls RJ. Long-term results of postanal repair for neurogenic faecal incontinence. *Br J Surg.* 1994;81(1):140–144.

409. Shafik A. Polytetrafluoroethylene injection for the treatment of partial fecal incontinence. *Int Surg.* 1993;78(2):159–161.

410. Shafik A. Perianal injection of autologous fat for treatment of sphincteric incontinence. *Dis Colon Rectum.* 1995;38(6):583–587.

411. Shafik A, Ahmed I, El-Sibai O, et al. Percutaneous peripheral neuromodulation in the treatment of fecal incontinence. *Eur Surg Res.* 2003;35(2):103–107.

412. Shah NS, Remzi F, Massmann A, et al. Management and treatment outcome of pouch–vaginal fistulas following restorative proctocolectomy. *Dis Colon Rectum.* 2003;46(7):911–917.

413. Shamliyan TA, Bliss DZ, Du J, et al. Prevalence and risk factors of fecal incontinence in community-dwelling men. *Rev Gastroenterol Disord.* 2009;9(4):E97–E110.

414. Siegel SW. Management of voiding dysfunction with an implantable neuroprosthesis. *Urol Clin North Am.* 1992;19(1):163–170.

415. Signorello LB, Harlow BL, Chekos AK, et al. Midline episiotomy and anal incontinence: retrospective cohort study. *BMJ.* 2000;320(7227):86–90.

416. Siproudhis L, Morcet J, Lainé F. Elastomer implants in faecal incontinence: a blind, randomized placebo-controlled study. *Aliment Pharmacol Ther.* 2007;25(9):1125–1132.

417. Snooks S, Henry MM, Swash M. Faecal incontinence after anal dilatation. *Br J Surg.* 1984;71(8):617–618.

418. Snooks SJ, Henry MM, Swash M. Faecal incontinence due to external anal sphincter division in childbirth is associated with damage to the innervation of the pelvic floor musculature: a double pathology. *Br J Obstet Gynaecol.* 1985;92(8):824–828.

419. Snooks SJ, Setchell M, Swash M, et al. Injury to innervation of pelvic floor sphincter musculature in childbirth. *Lancet.* 1984;2(8402):546–550.

420. Snooks SJ, Swash M, Henry M. Electrophysiologic and manometric assessment of failed postanal repair for anorectal incontinence. *Dis Colon Rectum.* 1984;27(11):733–736.

421. Snooks SJ, Swash M, Henry MM, et al. Risk factors in childbirth causing damage to the pelvic floor innervation. *Br J Surg.* 1985;72(suppl):S15–S17.

422. Snooks SJ, Swash M, Mathers SE, et al. Effect of vaginal delivery on the pelvic floor: a 5-year follow-up. *Br J Surg*. 1990;77(12):1358–1360.

423. Soerensen MM, Lundby L, Buntzen S, et al. Intersphincteric injected silicone biomaterial implants: a treatment for faecal incontinence. *Colorectal Dis*. 2009;11(1):73–76.

424. Speakman CT, Burnett SJ, Kamm MA, et al. Sphincter injury after anal dilatation demonstrated by anal endosonography. *Br J Surg*. 1991;78(12):1429–1430.

425. Speakman CT, Hoyle CH, Kamm MA, et al. Abnormal internal anal sphincter fibrosis and elasticity in fecal incontinence. *Dis Colon Rectum*. 1995;38(4):407–410.

426. Spinelli M, Giardiello G, Arduini A, et al. New percutaneous technique of sacral nerve stimulation has high initial success rate: preliminary results. *Eur Urol*. 2003;43(1):70–74.

427. Spinelli M, Malaguti S, Giardiello G, et al. A new minimally invasive procedure for pudendal nerve stimulation to treat neurogenic bladder: description of the method and preliminary data. *Neurourol Urodyn*. 2005;24(4):305–309.

428. Starck M, Bohe M, Valentin L. Results of endosonographic imaging of the anal sphincter 2–7 days after primary repair of third- or fourth-degree obstetric sphincter tears. *Ultrasound Obstet Gynecol*. 2003;22(6):609–615.

429. Stenzelius K, Mattiasson A, Hallberg IR, et al. Symptoms of urinary and faecal incontinence among men and women 75+ in relation to health complaints and quality of life. *Neurourol Urodyn*. 2004;23(3):211–222.

430. Stepp KJ, Siddiqui NY, Emery SP, et al. Textbook recommendations for preventing and treating perineal injury at vaginal delivery. *Obstet Gynecol*. 2006;107(2 pt 1):361–366.

431. Stone HB. Plastic operation for anal incontinence. *Tr South Surg Assoc*. 1926;41:235.

432. Stone HB, McLanahan S. Results with the fascia plastic operation for anal incontinence. *Ann Surg*. 1941;114(1):73–77.

433. Stricker JW, Schoetz DJ Jr, Coller JA, et al. Surgical correction of anal incontinence. *Dis Colon Rectum*. 1988;31(7):533–540.

434. Sultan AH, Johanson RB, Carter JE. Occult anal sphincter trauma following randomized forceps and vacuum delivery. *Int J Gynaecol Obstet*. 1998;61(2):113–119.

435. Sultan AH, Kamm MA, Hudson CN. Pudendal nerve damage during labour: prospective study before and after childbirth. *Br J Obstet Gynaecol*. 1994;101(1):22–28.

436. Sultan AH, Kamm MA, Hudson CN, et al. Anal-sphincter disruption during vaginal delivery. *N Engl J Med*. 1993;329(26):1905–1911.

437. Sultan AH, Kamm MA, Hudson CN, et al. Endosonography of the anal sphincters: normal anatomy and comparison with manometry. *Clin Radiol*. 1994;49(6):368–374.

438. Sultan AH, Kamm MA, Hudson CN, et al. Third degree obstetric anal sphincter tears: risk factors and outcome of primary repair. *BMJ*. 1994;308(6933):887–891.

439. Sultan AH, Kamm MA, Talbot IC, et al. Anal endosonography for identifying external sphincter defects confirmed histologically. *Br J Surg*. 1994;81(3):463–465.

440. Sultan AH, Loder PB, Bartram CI, et al. Vaginal endosonography. New approach to image the undisturbed anal sphincter. *Dis Colon Rectum*. 1994;37(12):1296–1299.

441. Sultan AH, Monga AK, Kumar D, et al. Primary repair of obstetric anal sphincter rupture using the overlap technique. *Br J Obstet Gynaecol*. 1999;106(4):318–323.

442. Sultan AH, Nicholls RJ, Kamm MA, et al. Anal endosonography and correlation with in vitro and in vivo anatomy. *Br J Surg*. 1993;80(4):508–511.

443. Sun WM, Read NW, Miner PB. Relation between rectal sensation and anal function in normal subjects and patients with faecal incontinence. *Gut*. 1990;31(9):1056–1061.

444. Swash M. Anorectal incontinence: electrophysiological tests. *Br J Surg*. 1984;72(suppl):S14–S15.

445. Syndikus I, Morgan RC, Sydes MR, et al. Late gastrointestinal toxicity after dose-escalated conformal radiotherapy for early prostate cancer: results from the UK Medical Research Council RT01 trial (ISRCTN47772397). *Int J Radiat Oncol Biol Phys*. 2009;77(3):773–783.

446. Takahashi T, Garcia-Osogobio S, Valdovinos MA, et al. Extended two-year results of radio-frequency energy delivery for the treatment of fecal incontinence (the Secca procedure). *Dis Colon Rectum*. 2003;46(6):711–715.

447. Tan EK, Jacovides M, Khullar V, et al. A cost-effectiveness analysis of delayed sphincteroplasty for anal sphincter injury. *Colorectal Dis*. 2008;10(7):653–662.

448. Tan EK, Vaizey C, Cornish J, et al. Surgical strategies for faecal incontinence—a decision analysis between dynamic gracioplasty, artificial bowel sphincter and end stoma. *Colorectal Dis*. 2007;10(6):577–586.

449. Tanagho EA, Schmidt RA. Bladder pacemaker: scientific basis and clinical future. *Urology*. 1982;20(6):614–619.

450. Tanagho EA, Schmidt RA, Orvis BR. Neural stimulation for control of voiding dysfunction: a preliminary report in 22 patients with serious neuropathic voiding disorders. *J Urol*. 1989;142(2 pt 1):340–345.

451. Thornton MJ, Kennedy ML, Lubowski DZ, et al. Long-term follow-up of dynamic gracioplasty for faecal incontinence. *Colorectal Dis*. 2004;6(6):470–476.

452. Tillin T, Gannon K, Feldman RA, et al. Third-party prospective evaluation of patient outcomes after dynamic gracioplasty. *Br J Surg*. 2006;93(11):1402–1410.

453. Titi M, Jenkins JT, Urie A, et al. Prospective study of the diagnostic evaluation of faecal incontinence and leakage in male patients. *Colorectal Dis*. 2007;9(7):647–652.

454. Tjandra JJ, Chan MK, Yeh CH, et al. Sacral nerve stimulation is more effective than optimal medical therapy for severe fecal incontinence: a randomized, controlled study. *Dis Colon Rectum*. 2008;51(5):494–502.

455. Tjandra JJ, Chan MK, Yeh HC. Injectable silicone biomaterial (PTQ) is more effective than carbon-coated beads (Durasphere) in treating passive faecal incontinence—a randomized trial. *Colorectal Dis*. 2009;11(4):382–389.

456. Tjandra JJ, Han WR, Goh J, et al. Direct repair vs. overlapping sphincter repair: a randomized, controlled trial. *Dis Colon Rectum*. 2003;46(7):937–942; discussion 942–943.

457. Tjandra JJ, Lim JF, Hiscock R, et al. Injectable silicone biomaterial for fecal incontinence caused by internal anal sphincter dysfunction is effective. *Dis Colon Rectum*. 2004;47(12):2138–2146.

458. Tjandra JJ, Lim JF, Matzel K. Sacral nerve stimulation: an emerging treatment for faecal incontinence. *ANZ J Surg*. 2004;74(12):1098–1106.

459. Tjandra JJ, Milsom JW, Schroeder T, et al. Endoluminal ultrasound is preferable to electromyography in mapping anal sphincteric defects. *Dis Colon Rectum*. 1993;36(7):689–692.

460. Tod AM, Stringer E, Levery C, et al. Rectal irrigation in the management of functional bowel disorders: a review. *Br J Nurs*. 2007;16(14):858–864.

461. Uludağ O, Darby M, Dejong CH, et al. [Sacral neuromodulation is effective in the treatment of fecal incontinence with intact sphincter muscles; a prospective study]. *Ned Tijdschr Geneeskd*. 2002;146(21):989–993.

462. Uludağ O, Koch SM, van Gemert WG, et al. Sacral neuromodulation in patients with fecal incontinence: a single-center study. *Dis Colon Rectum*. 2004;47(8):1350–1357.

463. Uludağ O, Melenhorst J, Koch SMP, et al. Sacral neuromodulation: long term outcome and quality of life in patients with faecal incontinence. *Colorectal Dis*. 2011;13(10):1162–1166. doi:10.1111/j.1463-1318.2010.02447.x.

464. Vaizey CJ. Invited editorial. *Dis Colon Rectum*. 2004;47:1162–1163.

465. Vaizey CJ, Carapeti E, Cahill JA, et al. Prospective comparison of faecal incontinence grading systems. *Gut*. 1999;44(1):77–80.

466. Vaizey CJ, Kamm MA, Bartram CI. Primary degeneration of the internal anal sphincter as a cause of passive faecal incontinence. *Lancet*. 1997;349(9052):612–615.

467. Vaizey CJ, Kamm MA, Roy AJ, et al. Double-blind crossover study of sacral nerve stimulation for fecal incontinence. *Dis Colon Rectum*. 2000;43(3):298–302.

468. Vaizey CJ, Kamm MA, Turner IC, et al. Effects of short term sacral nerve stimulation on anal and rectal function in patients with anal incontinence. *Gut*. 1999;44(3):407–412.

469. Vaizey C, Norton C, Thornton MJ, et al. Long-term outcome of repeat sphincter repair. *Dis Colon Rectum*. 2004;47(6):858–863.

470. Vallet C, Parc Y, Lupinacci R, et al. Sacral nerve stimulation for faecal incontinence: response rate, satisfaction and the value of preoperative investigation in patient selection. *Colorectal Dis*. 2010;12(3):247–253.

471. van Balken MR, Vandoninck V, Messelink BJ, et al. Percutaneous tibial nerve stimulation as neuromodulative treatment of chronic pelvic pain. *Eur Urol*. 2003;43(2):158–163.

472. Van Winckel M, Van Biervliet S, Van Laecke E, et al. Is an anal plug useful in the treatment of fecal incontinence in children with spina bifida or anal atresia? *J Urol*. 2006;176(1):342–344.

473. Varma JS, Smith AN, Busuttil A. Function of the anal sphincters after chronic radiation injury. *Gut*. 1986;27(5):528–533.

474. Varma MG, Brown JS, Creasman JM, et al. Fecal incontinence in females older than aged 40 years: who is at risk? *Dis Colon Rectum*. 2006;49(6):841–851.

475. VEGA Group. *Galileo System Simulation Facility*. Darmstadt, Germany: VEGA Informations-Technologien GmbH; 2005.

476. Venkatesh KS, Ramanujam PS, Larson DM, et al. Anorectal complications of vaginal delivery. *Dis Colon Rectum*. 1989;32(12):1039–1041.

477. Vernava AM III, Longo WE, Daniel GL. Pudendal neuropathy and the importance of EMG evaluation of fecal incontinence. *Dis Colon Rectum.* 1993;36(1):23–27.

478. Versluis PJ, Konsten J, Geerdes B, et al. Defecographic evaluation of dynamic gracioplasty for fecal incontinence. *Dis Colon Rectum.* 1995;38(5):468–473.

479. Violi V, Boselli AS, De Bernardinis M, et al. Surgical results and functional outcome after total anorectal reconstruction by double gracioplasty supported by external-source electrostimulation and/or implantable pulse generators: an 8-year experience. *Int J Colorectal Dis.* 2004;19(3):219–227.

480. Vitton V, Abysique A, Gaige S, et al. Colosphincteric electromyographic responses to sacral root stimulation: evidence for a somatosympathetic reflex. *Neurogastroenterol Motil.* 2008;20(4):407–416.

481. Vitton V, Damon H, Roman S, et al. Transcutaneous posterior tibial nerve stimulation for fecal incontinence in inflammatory bowel disease patients: a therapeutic option? *Inflamm Bowel Dis.* 2009;15(3):402–405.

482. Vitton V, Damon H, Roman S, et al. Transcutaneous electrical posterior tibial nerve stimulation for faecal incontinence: effects on symptoms and quality of life. *Int J Colorectal Dis.* 2010;25(8):1017–1020.

483. Voyvodic F, Rieger NA, Skinner S, et al. Endosonographic imaging of anal sphincter injury: does the size of the tear correlate with the degree of dysfunction? *Dis Colon Rectum.* 2003;46(6):735–741.

484. Wald A, Tununguntla AK. Anorectal sensorimotor dysfunction in fecal incontinence and diabetes mellitus. Modification with biofeedback therapy. *N Engl J Med.* 1984;310(20):1282–1287.

485. Wasserberg N, Haney M, Petrone P, et al. Fecal incontinence among morbid obese women seeking for weight loss surgery: an underappreciated association with adverse impact on quality of life. *Int J Colorectal Dis.* 2008;23(5):493–497.

486. Wexner SD, Baeten C, Bailey R, et al. Long-term efficacy of dynamic gracioplasty for fecal incontinence. *Dis Colon Rectum.* 2002;45(6):809–818.

487. Wexner SD, Coller JA, Devroede G, et al. Sacral nerve stimulation for fecal incontinence: results of a 120-patient prospective multicenter study. *Ann Surg.* 2010;251(3):441–449.

488. Wexner SD, Gonzalez-Padron A, Rius J, et al. Stimulated gracilis neosphincter operation. Initial experience, pitfalls, and complications. *Dis Colon Rectum.* 1996;39(9):957–964.

489. Wexner SD, Jin HY, Weiss EG, et al. Factors associated with failure of the artificial bowel sphincter: a study of over 50 cases from Cleveland Clinic Florida. *Dis Colon Rectum.* 2009;52(9):1550–1557.

490. Williams AB, Bartram CI, Halligan S, et al. Anal sphincter damage after vaginal delivery using three-dimensional endosonography. *Obstet Gynecol.* 2001;97(5 pt 1):770–775.

491. Williams AB, Bartram CI, Halligan S, et al. Endosonographic anatomy of the normal anal canal compared with endocoil magnetic resonance imaging. *Dis Colon Rectum.* 2002;45(2):176–183.

492. Williams AB, Bartram CI, Modhwadia D, et al. Endocoil magnetic resonance imaging quantification of external anal sphincter atrophy. *Br J Surg.* 2001;88(6):853–859.

493. Williams AB, Cheetham MJ, Bartram CI, et al. Gender differences in the longitudinal pressure profile of the anal canal related to anatomical structure as demonstrated on three-dimensional anal endosonography. *Br J Surg.* 2000;87(12):1674–1679.

494. Williams L, Lewis E. Identification of small rectal perforations. *Surg Gynecol Obstet.* 1987;164(5):475.

495. Williams NS, Hallan RI, Koeze TH, et al. Restoration of gastrointestinal continuity and continence after abdominoperineal excision of the rectum using an electrically stimulated neoanal sphincter. *Dis Colon Rectum.* 1990;33(7):561–565.

496. Williams NS, Patel J, George BD, et al. Development of an electrically stimulated neoanal sphincter. *Lancet.* 1991;338(8776):1166–1169.

497. Williamson ME, Lewis W, Finan P, et al. Recovery of physiologic and clinical function after low anterior resection of the rectum for carcinoma: myth or reality? *Dis Colon Rectum.* 1995;38(4):411–418.

498. Womack NR, Morrison JF, Williams NS. Prospective study of the effects of postanal repair in neurogenic faecal incontinence. *Br J Surg.* 1988;75(1):48–52.

499. Wong MT, Meurette G, Stangherlin P, et al. The magnetic anal sphincter versus the artificial bowel sphincter: a comparison of 2 treatments for fecal incontinence. *Dis Colon Rectum.* 2011;54(7):773–779.

500. Wong WD, Congliosi SM, Spencer MP, et al. The safety and efficacy of the artificial bowel sphincter for fecal incontinence: results from a multicenter cohort study. *Dis Colon Rectum.* 2002;45(9):1139–1153.

501. Worsøe J, Fynne L, Laurberg S, et al. Electrical stimulation of the dorsal genital nerve reduces incontinence episodes in idiopathic fecal incontinent patients: a pilot study. *Colorectal Dis.* 2012;14(3):349–355.

502. Wreden R. A method of reconstructing a voluntary sphincter ani. *Arch Surg.* 1929;18:841–844.

503. Wynne JM, Myles JL, Jones I, et al. Disturbed anal sphincter function following vaginal delivery. *Gut.* 1996;39(1):120–124.

504. Yakovlev A, Karasev SA. Successful treatment of chronic anal fissure utilizing sacral nerve stimulation. *Dis Colon Rectum* 2010;54:324–327.

505. Yang KS, Kim YH, Park HJ, et al. Sacral nerve stimulation for treatment of chronic intractable anorectal pain—a case report. *Korean J Pain.* 2010;23(1):60–64.

506. Yip B, Barrett RC, Coller JA, et al. Pudendal nerve terminal motor latency testing: assessing the educational learning curve: can we teach our own? *Dis Colon Rectum.* 2002;45(2):184–187.

507. Yip B, Barrett RC, Coller JA, et al. Linear pressure profiles and symmetric findings in the stimulated gracilis muscle. *Dis Colon Rectum.* 2003;46(1):77–80.

508. Yoshioka K, Keighley MR. Clinical and manometric assessment of gracilis muscle transplant for fecal incontinence. *Dis Colon Rectum.* 1988;31(10):767–769.

509. Yoshioka K, Keighley MR. Critical assessment of the quality of continence after postanal repair for faecal incontinence. *Br J Surg.* 1989;76(10):1054–1057.

510. Young CJ, Mathur MN, Eyers AA, et al. Successful overlapping anal sphincter repair: relationship to patient age, neuropathy, and colostomy formation. *Dis Colon Rectum.* 1998;41(3):344–349.

17

Colorectal Trauma

Robert W. Beart, Jr. and George C. Velmahos

The profession of medicine and surgery must always rank as the most noble that men can adopt. The spectacle of a doctor in action among soldiers, in equal danger and with equal courage, saving life where all others are taking it, allaying pain where all others are causing it, is one which must always seem glorious, whether to God or man. It is impossible to imagine any situation from which a human being might better leave this world and embark on the hazards of the unknown.

—WINSTON S. CHURCHILL:
The Story of the Malakand Field Force

Hippocrates regarded abdominal wounds as deadly while Celsus advised that their cure be left to nature.[30] The injury may be caused by blunt or penetrating trauma of the abdomen or perineum. It may result in damage to the intraperitoneal or retroperitoneal bowel, or it may interrupt its blood supply. If the trauma is to the rectum or perineum, the sphincter mechanism may be injured, as may adjacent organs (e.g., bladder, urethra, and vagina).

The colon is involved in 25% of gunshot wounds, 5% of stab wounds, and 2% of blunt abdominal injuries.[104] It is expected that this will continue to be a pervasive problem in our society because of the frequency of motor vehicle accidents and the ready availability of firearms, especially in the United States. There still remains considerable controversy concerning the appropriate management of colorectal injuries. Many of the issues, such as the method of repair for simple colon injuries, have been resolved. Other concerns, such as the role of colostomy in extraperitoneal rectal injuries, have not reached consensus. This chapter will describe the options for the diagnosis and treatment of colorectal injuries.

▶ HISTORY

The first recorded injury to the colon was described in the Old Testament in the book of Judges. For centuries, such injuries were untreatable and virtually always resulted in the victim's demise. The first instance of a successful repair of a musket ball injury to the colon was performed in 1831 by Lucien Baudens, a French military surgeon in Algeria.[5] Baudens digitally explored the wound and felt a loop of intestine seemingly hardened by the marked contraction of its muscle coat. Upon pulling his finger out, Baudens noticed that it was covered with feces. He enlarged the abdominal wound and asked the patient to cough. This resulted in a large expulsion of gas from within the peritoneal cavity and caused the injured segment of colon to protrude. The large intestine was noted to have a large, tangential laceration that he repaired with the use of Lembert sutures. The colon was replaced in the abdomen, the abdomen was closed, and the patient recovered.

During the American Civil War, penetrating abdominal injuries were treated nonoperatively and were thus associated with a 90% mortality rate. The decision about nonoperative intervention was made simply because such injuries were virtually always fatal, regardless of the method of treatment. Furthermore, such a noninterventionist approach was probably based on the fact that surgeons at that time had no good idea of what to do when confronted with such a problem. One of the earliest operations for a gunshot wound of the abdomen in the United States was performed by William Bull.

Encouraged by the success of elective surgery following the introduction of anesthesia and of aseptic surgical technique, World War I surgeons began to operate on casualties suffering from abdominal wounds. The standard at that time was primary repair, a considerable improvement over nonoperative management, but the mortality rate was 60%.

WILLIAM TILLINGHAST BULL (1849–1909)

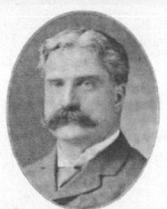

William Bull was born in Newport, Rhode Island, a direct descendent of Henry Bull, one of the nine original settlers of Aquidneck and twice governor of the colony. He graduated with honors from Harvard College in 1869 and attended the College of Physicians and Surgeons in New York where he received the degree of doctor of medicine in 1872. After completing an internship at Bellevue Hospital, Dr. Bull travelled to Europe where he spent 2 years. He studied surgical pathology in Germany and learned operative technique in France. On his return in 1875, Bull became house surgeon to the New York Dispensary, and in 1876 he was appointed surgeon-in-chief to the Chambers Street Hospital (House of Relief, Department of New York Hospital), a position which he held for 11 years. There he performed one of the earliest laparotomies for abdominal gunshot wound. Prior to his intervention such injuries had been almost uniformly fatal, and his surgery greatly reduced the mortality. In 1880 to 1883, Dr. Bull became assistant demonstrator of anatomy and adjunct professor of surgery. In 1888, he was appointed professor of the practice of surgery and clinical surgery at the College of Physicians and Surgeons. He was also visiting surgeon to the St. Luke's Hospital and attending surgeon to the New York Hospital. He later served as an attending surgeon at Roosevelt Hospital, the New York Cancer Hospital, and many others. William Bull died in his 60th year of cancer of the neck. (Leonardo RA. *Lives of Master Surgeons.* New York, NY: Froben Press; 1948; with appreciation to Julia Zakhaleva, MD.)

With the advent of World War II came weapons with a much greater potential for creating massive intestinal injury. Primary repair resulted in a prohibitively high rate of sepsis and death. As a consequence, Major General W. Heneage Ogilvie (see Biography, Chapter 20), senior surgical consultant for the British forces in the North African theater, mandated in 1942 that all colonic injuries should be exteriorized or treated with concomitant colostomies.[87] In 1943, the surgeon general of the American forces in North Africa adopted the same policy.[86] This succeeded in lowering the mortality rate from colonic injury to 35%.

During the Korean conflict and the war in Vietnam, the mortality rate for colonic injuries was reduced still further to 15% and 10%, respectively. This was largely attributed to the institution of a rapid evacuation system through the use of helicopters, the immediate availability of antibiotics and blood products, and the improvement in methods of resuscitation. There was concern, however, about excessive reliance on modern medical technology in that it appeared to lead to some reports of disastrous results. This led to the call for a return to a more "conservative" approach in the management of intestinal war injuries.

Following World War II, the combat-trained surgeon returned to civilian life and began to apply the principles of management that had been used for colon injuries experienced in warfare (Figure 17-1). Exteriorization of the injured segment, as well as the use of colostomy, became the standard treatment for all colorectal injuries. However, some began to consider that for civilian injuries, typically produced by low-velocity missiles, primary repair could be an appropriate alternative. Numerous studies since the mid-1970s have demonstrated repeatedly that this form of treatment in selective instances is safe.

Today in the United States, a victim of penetrating abdominal trauma is frequently transported to the hospital within a few minutes following injury. Sophisticated radiographic equipment is readily available, as well as intravenous fluids, blood, blood products, and antibiotics. Evaluation by trauma teams and transfer to the operating room is rapid. Under these conditions, it is little wonder that the mortality rate for civilian colorectal injuries is now less than 5%.

A singular advance in the management of individuals with colonic injuries was made by Stone and Fabian in their 1979 publication in which they conducted a randomized trial of patients meeting so-called good-risk criteria.[112] Patients with colonic injuries who were believed to be good risks were randomly allocated to either undergo a primary repair or a colostomy. Fewer septic complications were observed in the former group. This study succeeded in inspiring others to implement primary repair more frequently. Numerous articles have since been published demonstrating the efficacy of primary repair, especially as applied to civilian trauma centers in the United States.[1,4,11,20,22,28,31,38,40,42–44,47,54,55,56,61,62,69,73,81,83,98,103,105,113,115,127,132]

This trend continued in the 1990s, with numerous contributors advocating primary repair as the objective of management for both civilian and wartime colon injuries.[10,12,13,24,26,64,82,96,102] Furthermore, anastomotic failure rates have been quite low, reinforcing the fact that primary repair, at least today, is the ideal approach for the treatment of colonic injury.

▶ ETIOLOGY AND EVALUATION

Penetrating Trauma

Most colon injuries result from penetrating wounds to the abdomen. Twenty percent of all such wounds are associated with injury to the large bowel. Septic morbidity is a real danger because of the combination of fecal spillage, soft tissue injury, and bleeding, all of which predispose to subsequent infection. Furthermore, gunshot wounds of the colon are typically associated with more tissue destruction and result in an increased number of associated injuries in comparison with stab wounds (Figures 17-2 through 17-7).

With respect to etiology, it is generally self-evident as to the nature of the causative agent when one is confronted with a penetrating injury to the abdomen. However, how one proceeds with evaluation and treatment is subject to some controversy. Stab wounds of the abdomen, which more than 20 years ago were frequently managed by routine laparotomy, are now subjected to selective nonoperative management. Only patients with diffuse abdominal tenderness or hemodynamic

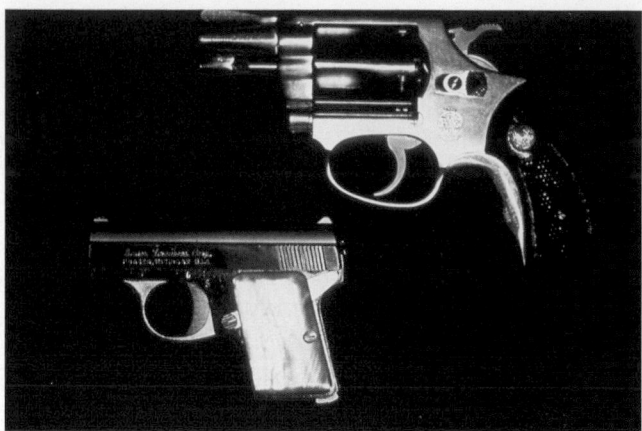
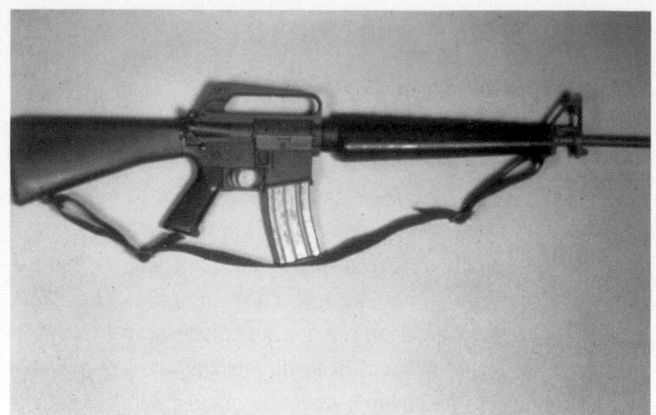
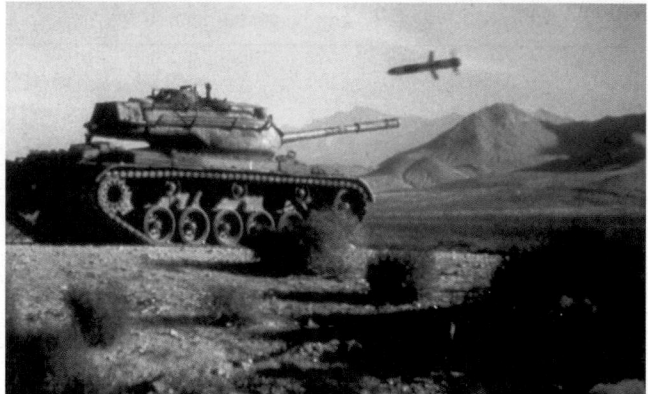

FIGURE 17-1. Progressively more destructive penetrating wounds depend on the velocity and the mass of the projectile. **A:** Bad. **B:** Worse. **C:** Worst. (Courtesy of Daniel Rosenthal, MD.)

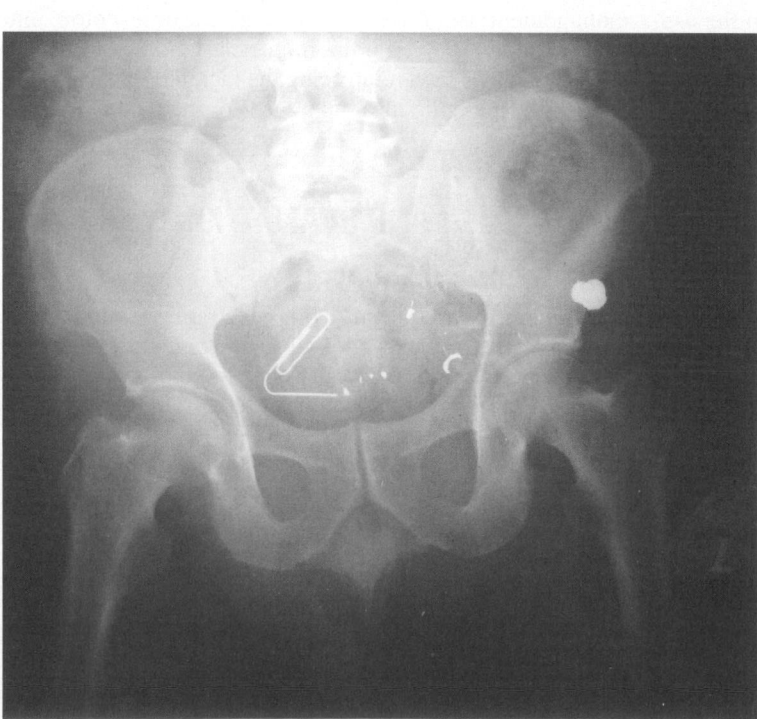
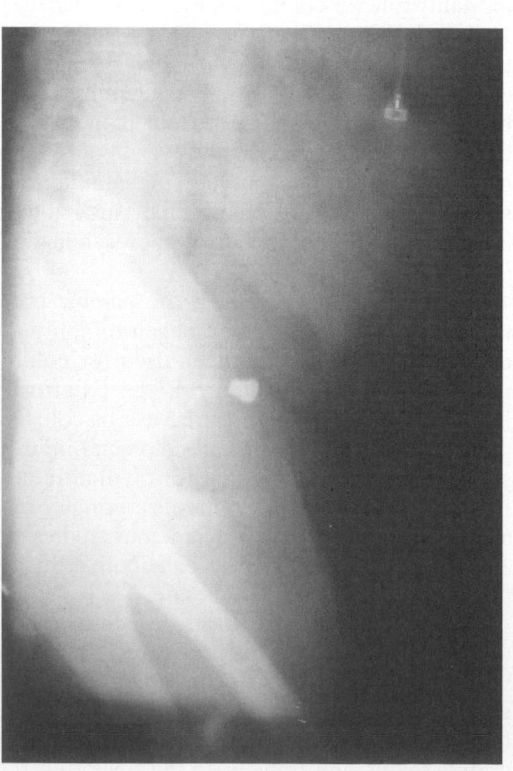

FIGURE 17-2. Bullet wound of the pelvis. **A:** High-caliber bullet overlying the left ilium. Metallic fragments are consistent with striking bone. The tip of the paper clip indicates the entrance wound. The bullet traversed the sigmoid colon. **B:** Lateral view in the same patient.

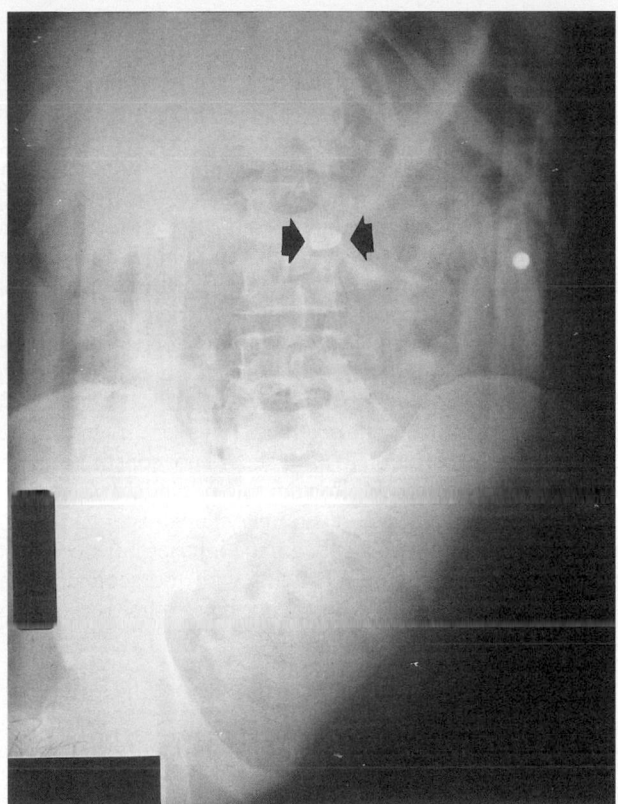

FIGURE 17-3. Bullet wound of the abdomen. The missile can be seen overlying the vertebra (*arrows*). The missile traversed the transverse colon and the aorta. The patient survived this injury.

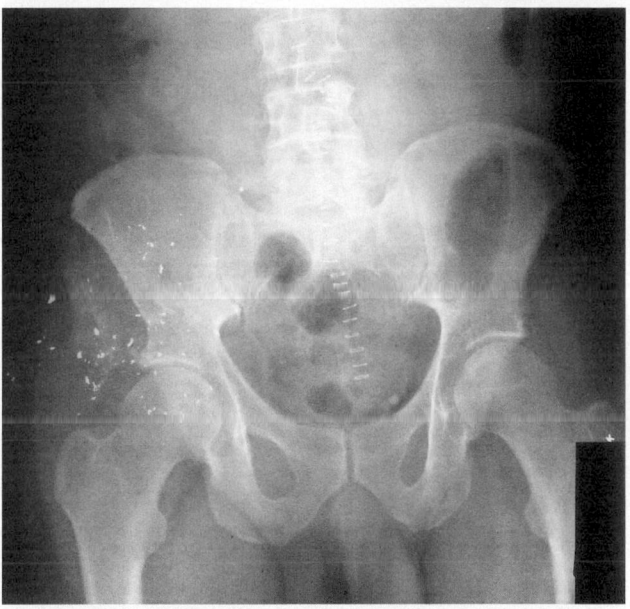

FIGURE 17-4. Metallic fragments overlying the right ilium imply that the missile struck bone. The distal small bowel and right colon were virtually vaporized.

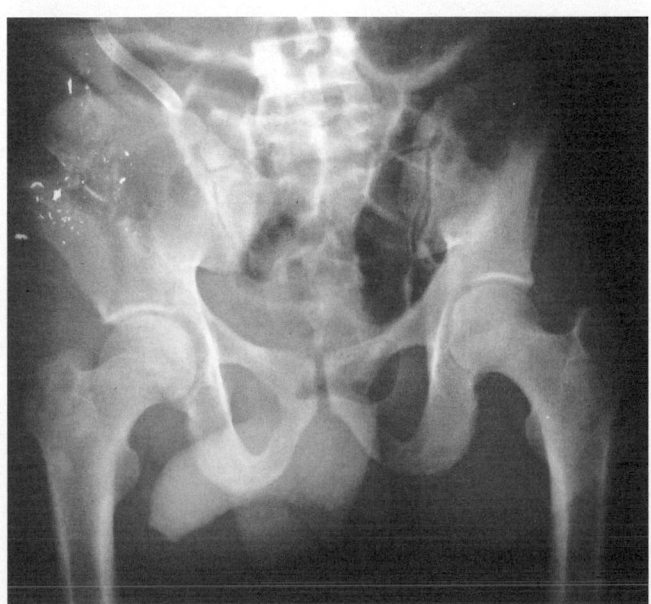

FIGURE 17-5. A similar injury was created from this bullet wound to that noted in Figure 17-3. However, note that the ilium was shattered. The patient also suffered major vessel injury to the right leg.

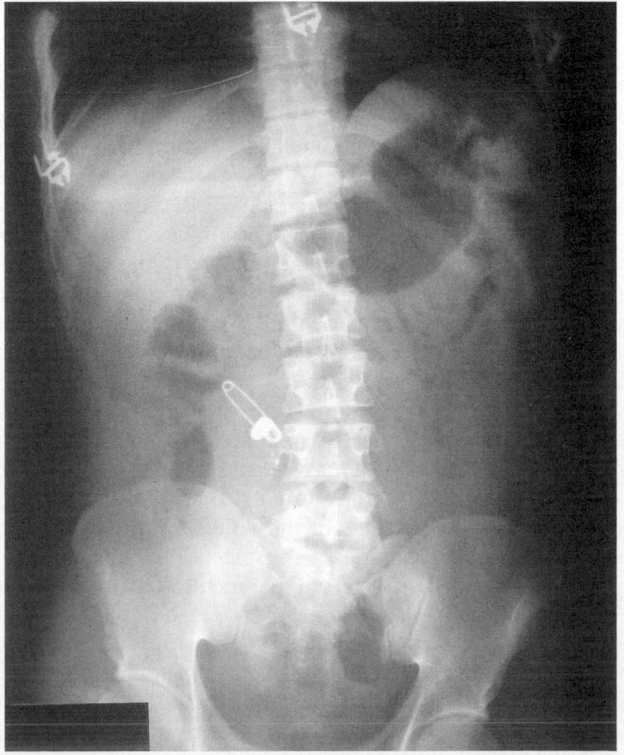

FIGURE 17-6. This bullet traversed the small bowel, the transverse colon, and the vena cava. The entrance wound is marked by a safety pin.

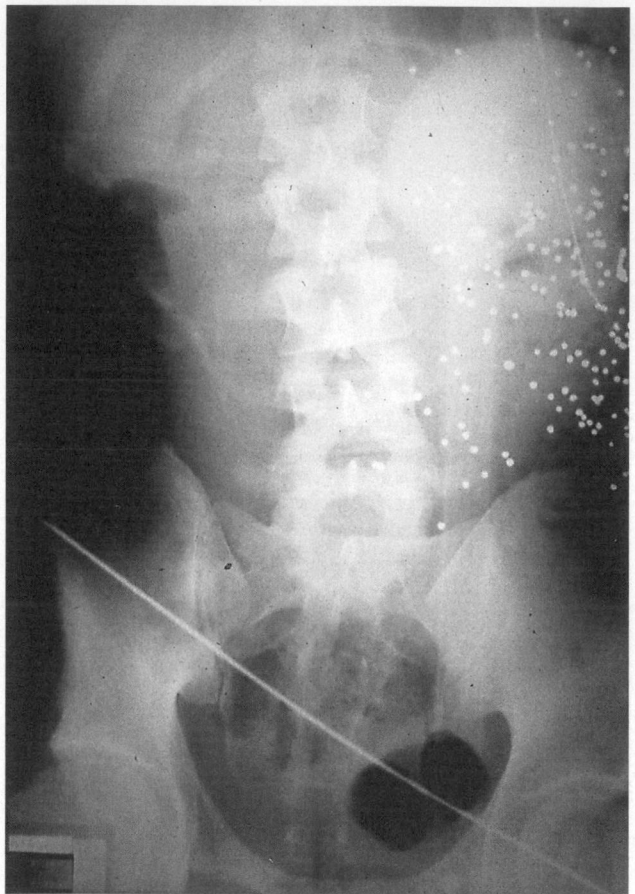

FIGURE 17-7. Shotgun wound to the left upper quadrant resulted in destruction of the splenic flexure, spleen, tail of pancreas, and kidney. Such low-velocity wounds can create devastating injury at close range.

instability are rushed to the operating room. All other patients who can be reliably evaluated should be monitored closely and observed for the development of abdominal signs. For abdominal gunshot wounds, the tendency to treat by means of laparotomy is much more frequent. Based on reports of a high incidence of intraperitoneal organ injury after a gunshot wound to the abdomen and on the relatively "benign" consequences of a negative laparotomy, many surgeons operated routinely with this presentation. However, the frequency of significant abdominal injuries has been found to be approximately 70%, and the incidence of complications following a negative exploration ranges from 20% to 40%.[29,119,121,122,124,125] Therefore, a policy of selective nonoperative management for abdominal gunshot wound may be as prudent as it is for stab wounds. In the largest study to date, that of 1,856 abdominal gunshot wounds, 34% of the anterior and 68% of the posterior abdominal injuries were selected for nonoperative management.[125] The rate of nontherapeutic laparotomy was 9%. Of complications related to nonoperative management (0.3%, five cases), all were treated successfully. The concept of selective nonoperative management was applied to different populations and found to be equally valid.[122–124]

Laparoscopy

The use of laparoscopy has also been suggested for the evaluation of patients with penetrating abdominal trauma.[33,36,53,63,99,106,108,109,136] In stable individuals, laparoscopy is a highly sensitive test for determining peritoneal penetration. It can be particularly helpful for thoracoabdominal wounds when local exploration may not be possible or may actually be contraindicated. Laparoscopy is sensitive for detecting a diaphragmatic injury, a situation in which observation, diagnostic peritoneal lavage, or focused sonography may be unhelpful.[76] Although laparoscopy is sensitive for determining peritoneal penetration, it should be noted that this technique is not nearly as reliable for identifying intra-abdominal injury. Retroperitoneal or hollow viscus injuries can be missed with laparoscopic exploration. Furthermore, the benefit of repeated clinical examinations to detect evolving tenderness is lost for an individual postlaparoscopy. Most investigators have cautioned against using laparoscopy for purposes other than determining peritoneal penetration. However, given the fact that peritoneal penetration in itself should not constitute an absolute criterion for laparotomy, the role of diagnostic laparoscopy is still indeterminate. In summary, laparoscopy is useful in determining whether diaphragmatic injuries have occurred in hemodynamically stable patients with thoracoabdominal penetrating injuries and who do not have other reasons for surgical exploration.

Computed Tomography and Focused Abdominal Sonographic Assessment

Focused abdominal sonographic assessment for trauma (FAST) and high-resolution computed tomography (CT) have both been employed as adjunctive techniques to that of clinical assessment of the abdomen following penetrating trauma. These procedures may be useful in the decision-making process with respect to the advisability of operative versus nonoperative intervention in stable patients with penetrating wounds.[16,118] Although CT is frequently used in patients who do not require immediate exploration, there is still debate about its sensitivity and specificity.[119] FAST appears more useful in blunt trauma. Because penetrating injury may occur without an associated large volume of free fluid within the abdominal cavity, the sensitivity of FAST is low in this circumstance.[70]

Blunt Trauma

Blunt trauma to the abdomen causes colonic injury in fewer than 5% of these cases. Mobile segments of the colon (e.g., cecum, transverse colon, and sigmoid colon) are more susceptible to injury, although other areas of the bowel can be affected. Most perforations are found in the sigmoid colon, an observation that can be explained by its redundancy, its tendency to form a closed loop, and/or to be subjected to acceleration/deceleration forces. The right side of the colon, however, is the most common site for devascularizing injuries.[21] These patients are usually victims of motor vehicle accidents and therefore commonly have multisystem and multiorgan injuries (Figures 17-8 and 17-9).[14,21] The use of seat belts seems to be a predisposing factor.[2,7,48,92] Appleby and Nagy caution that a high degree of suspicion should be maintained in individuals who are found to have bruising of the abdominal wall as a consequence of the use of seat belts.[2] These individuals have a high incidence of gastrointestinal injuries and, in addition, associated lumbar spinal injuries.

Bubenik and colleagues describe three patients who sustained blunt colonic injury.[9] In their experience, a characteristic scenario was observed. Perforation was discovered 7 to 10 days following the incident, indicated by findings suggestive

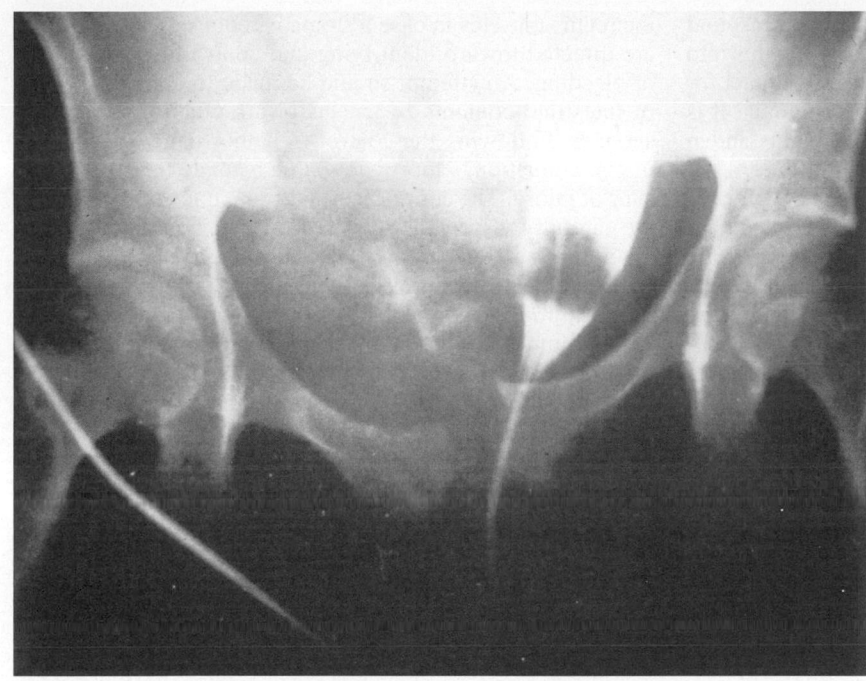

FIGURE 17-8. Motor vehicle accident causing severe blunt trauma resulted in a displaced pelvic fracture. The patient sustained bladder injury as well as major trauma to the sigmoid colon.

of sepsis. A particularly prominent sign of occult infection was the syndrome of posttraumatic pulmonary insufficiency.

Wisner and coworkers identified 56 individuals who sustained blunt intestinal injury, but only 6 of these were colonic.[133] Most injuries occurred in the proximal and distal small bowel at points of fixation, with devascularization most frequently seen in the ileum and in the sigmoid colon. The same principles of treatment as those discussed with respect to penetrating injuries apply here, but the authors caution that delay in diagnosis is one of the major concerns. They note that CT was not especially helpful in the preoperative assessment, but this may have improved with advancements in CT technology.

Howell and colleagues identified 19 patients who sustained blunt trauma to the colon.[49] They advise that careful inspection of pericolic, subserosal, and mesenteric hematomas at the time of laparotomy is essential for the detection and management of such injuries. Unfortunately, some individuals present many days following the initial injury and are found on exploratory laparotomy to have considerable

contamination and sepsis. Under these circumstances, resection and a diversionary procedure are indicated. As with other types of colonic trauma, infections are the major source of morbidity, but the nature of associated injuries is the principal determinant of survival.[49]

Diagnosis

Fortunately, blunt trauma to the abdomen rarely produces injury to the colon. However, when it occurs, the consequences can be devastating. Alterations in the patient's level of consciousness, as well as the presence of associated injuries, present problems in diagnosis and therapeutic priorities. Peritoneal lavage, CT of the abdomen, and abdominal ultrasonography have been described as adjunctive measures for evaluating patients with such injuries. Peritoneal lavage may be useful if the returns are grossly positive with stool, but frankly this is an antiquated approach. The risk of oversensitivity by which a lavage is deemed positive even with a minimal amount of free blood has been the main reason for abandoning this technique. In most modern trauma centers, CT has almost exclusively replaced peritoneal lavage. It is readily available, and it avoids the risk associated with intervention-related complications.

The results of CT may be difficult to interpret. Certainly, the presence of free fluid without evident liver or spleen injury is worrisome, as is the presence of mesenteric inflammatory change, edema, or hematoma. Free air is a pathognomonic sign of hollow visceral injuries.

FAST will not detect an injury to the colon unless sufficient fluid or blood is present. Still, McElveen and Collin found an overall sensitivity of 88% and a 98% specificity when comparing this test with others in individuals with blunt abdominal trauma.[67] FAST is quite helpful when it is positive; the reported specificity rate is high for detecting hemoperitoneum (in the range of 95% to 100%).[77,91] When the ultrasound scan is negative, the results are not as beneficial; the reported specificity rates range from 42% to 87%. The wide discrepancy in sensitivity and specificity serves to

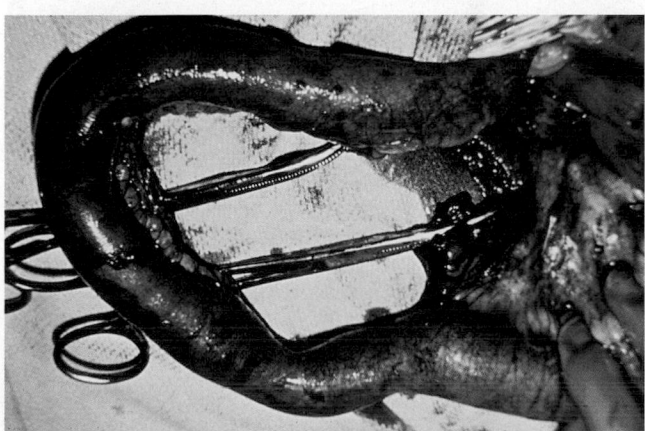

FIGURE 17-9. Mesenteric rent in the small bowel from blunt trauma as a consequence of a motor vehicle accident.

emphasize another potential weakness of the ultrasound examination—that is, operator dependency. Taking this into consideration, the FAST examination is a useful adjunct for abdominal assessment during resuscitation for trauma. It is most helpful in patients with hemodynamic instability and in those who cannot readily be moved to the CT scanner.

A large volume of literature supports the use of CT for patient assessment following abdominal trauma.[68] CT scan has been shown to be highly sensitive and specific. However, the Achilles heel of CT scanning has been the presence of a mesenteric tear or an early hollow viscus injury. Still, the newer generation of CT scanners is more sensitive than prior technology, but such injuries can still be missed. A high degree of suspicion with appropriate clinical correlation improves the overall accuracy. Additional signs of colon or small bowel injury include mesenteric hematoma; edema; bowel wall thickening; and, as mentioned, the presence of free fluid without evident solid organ injury. Nolan and colleagues opine that physicians should entertain the possibility of mesenteric injury in all patients presenting with blunt abdominal trauma, even if few clinical findings are initially present and/or CT fails to demonstrate a definitive abnormality or injury.[85]

▶ SURGICAL MANAGEMENT

General Principles

Once the decision has been made to perform an exploratory laparotomy, the abdomen is entered through a midline incision. It is important to preserve the area overlying the rectus muscles in case a stoma is required. Initial efforts are directed toward identifying and controlling any source of bleeding. An attempt should be made to contain spillage of intestinal contents by means of atraumatic clamps and sponges. Following the control of hemorrhage and sources of contamination, a thorough search is made for all possible sites of injury. The entire gastrointestinal tract and mesentery are carefully inspected. Special attention should be given to the number and location of all wounds. Usually, there is an even number of openings in the bowel, compatible with a typical through-and-through injury pattern. However, when an odd number of wounds is identified, the surgeon should make a great effort to look for the "missing hole." The bowel should be carefully reinspected, especially the region adjacent to the mesentery, where breaches of the bowel wall may be hidden. It is suggested that the entire gastrointestinal tract be inspected twice, even when all wounds appear to be accounted for. Obviously, a missed visceral injury can have catastrophic consequences.

Once the injuries have been identified, the surgeon then proceeds with the repair. When primary repair is attempted, care must be taken to avoid narrowing the lumen; therefore, this is often accomplished in a transverse fashion (Figure 17-10). Whether a two-layer or a single-layer technique is employed is a matter of each individual surgeon's personal preference. When the colon is destroyed or its blood supply is compromised, resection is mandatory (Figure 17-11). If diversion of the fecal stream is required, either the injured segment is brought out to the abdominal wall or a proximal portion of bowel is selected as a

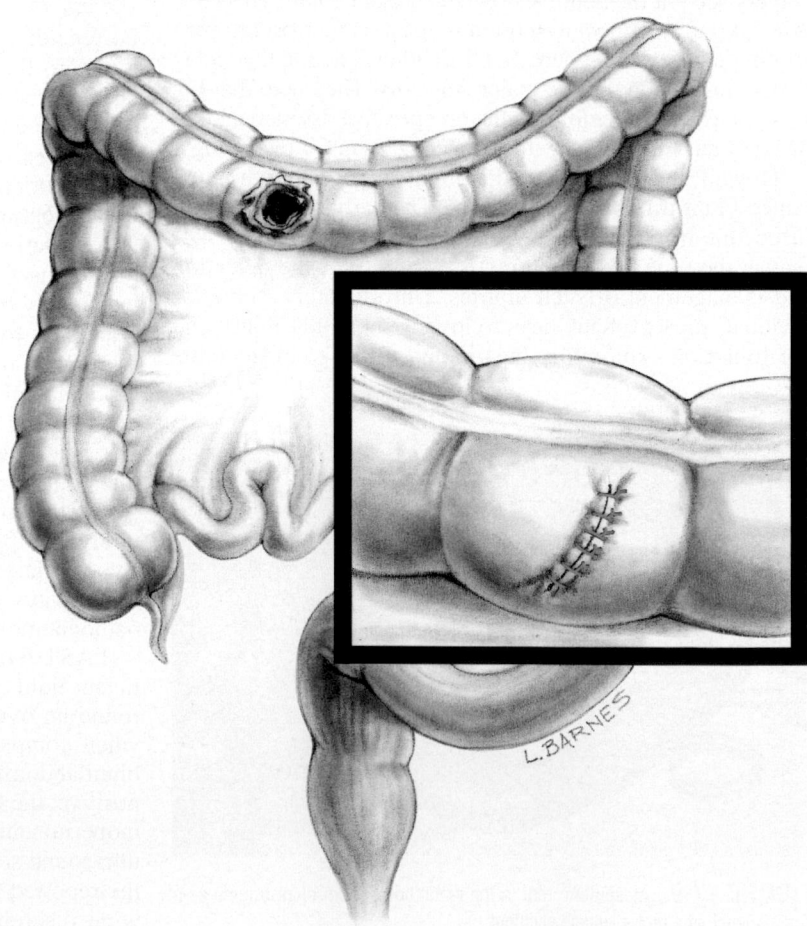

FIGURE 17-10. Artist's concept of a penetrating wound of the transverse colon that is treated by primary closure in a transverse fashion (*inset*).

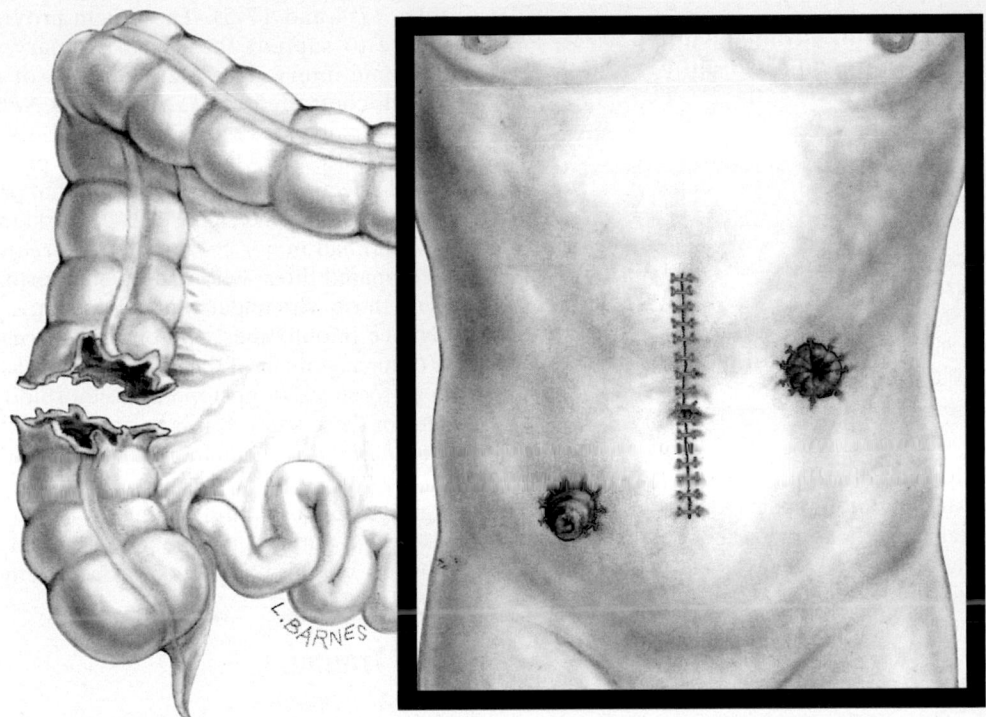

FIGURE 17-11. Artist's representation of a massive injury to the right colon requiring resection. This illustration demonstrates creation of an ileostomy with a mucous fistula.

colostomy or ileostomy. Meticulous attention should be given to creating a satisfactory stoma; some reports have suggested that complication rates for stomal construction in conditions of trauma are higher than those reported for elective surgery.[90,107,135] This may be attributed to the fact that sufficient attention is not paid to the creation of a satisfactory stoma when the surgeon is dealing with an emergency problem in a critically ill patient. It is often suggested that the skin wound be left open or sutures placed for delayed primary repair, although this remains a subject of controversy. Wound infections range from a relatively minor problem to a serious event, leading to a fascial dehiscence, to a potentially life-threatening complication, and to necrotizing soft tissue infections.[128] The presence of concomitant shock, soft tissue injury, and fecal contamination creates an environment unlike that of elective colon surgery, one that may encourage the development of overwhelming sepsis.

Operative Alternatives for Treating Penetrating Colonic Injury

Many different operative techniques are available for managing the injured colon (Table 17-1). However, they can all be classified into one of three primary approaches: fecal diversion, primary repair, or exteriorization repair. The last one is mostly of historic interest and as such it will be described next.

Exteriorization Repair

Exteriorization repair was initially suggested by Mason in 1945.[66] It is a hybrid of primary repair and fecal diversion in which the colon wound is repaired and brought out to the abdominal wall. Subsequently, if the enterotomy closure

breaks down, it is then matured into a standard ostomy. However, if it heals, it is then replaced into the peritoneal cavity. Theoretically, exteriorization repair takes advantage of the benefits of the two approaches. It avoids a colostomy for those individuals whose repairs heal, while preventing contamination that could result in an anastomotic leak. Although some investigators have recommended this type of approach, conversion rates to an ostomy range between 21% and 50%.[75,116] This is considerably higher than the incidence of clinically significant leaks associated with a primary repair.

Another concern is that the technique requires special postoperative management to prevent defecation. This problem can lead to breakdown of the wound. Additionally, exteriorization repair does not preclude the possibility of intra-abdominal sepsis. Breakdown with abscess and/or fecal fistula is still possible once the bowel is returned to the abdomen.[62,79]

TABLE 17-1 Operative Alternatives for Treating Penetrating Colonic Injury

The choices of operations are summarized as follows:

Simple closure
Resection with primary anastomosis
Resection with primary anastomosis and proximal diversion
Resection with end colostomy and Hartmann's pouch
Exteriorization with repair (not used anymore)
Exteriorization of injury site (not used anymore)

TABLE 17-2 Factors Predisposing to Increased Morbidity and Mortality

Increased age
Associated organ injury
Multiple blood transfusions
Left colon injury
Preoperative shock
Gross fecal contamination
Delay in initiating therapy
Extensive colonic injury
Questionable viability of the bowel

In summary, although this approach has certain theoretical advantages, exteriorization repair requires more postoperative attention than the other options and is associated with a higher complication rate. Most investigators have abandoned this approach. For the purposes of this discussion, it is not recommended.[64]

Fecal Diversion versus Primary Repair

Fecal diversion had been the mainstay of the management of civilian colonic injuries until relatively recently. Mandatory colostomy, even today, is conceptually attractive because it eliminates or at least minimizes the complications associated with the creation of an anastomosis. In many patients, the colostomy will not be subsequently closed. If closure is attempted, there is a significant morbidity and mortality associated with this, the second operation.[6] In 1951, Woodhall and Ochsner suggested that primary repair could be appropriately applied to civilian practice.[134] Since that time, a vigorous debate has surrounded the management of colonic injuries. Variables that affect these decisions are summarized in Table 17-2.

Table 17-3 illustrates five prospective, randomized trials that compare the two approaches.[15,35,46,100,112] In addition to these randomized studies, numerous large series have been reported that also compare these alternatives

(Tables 17-4 and 17-5). These data provide very strong evidence to support the use of primary repair following colonic injury. In a meta-analysis of published randomized, controlled trials, Singer and Nelson found that primary repair was favored over fecal diversion for penetrating injuries.[105] All concluded that primary repair was safe and effective. Recently, in a seminal prospective multicenter study, Demetriades and coworkers evaluated patients who had major colonic injuries requiring resection and compared those who underwent a primary anastomosis with those who underwent a colostomy.[27] There was no difference in outcomes, and on multivariate analysis, the type of management of the colon injury was not associated with differences in postoperative morbidity. As a consequence of these studies, it is believed that the great majority of colon injuries can be repaired primarily. Colostomy seems to offer no benefits in terms of time spent in the operating room or complications. It is reserved only for a few selected patients in whom anatomical or physiologic conditions would make a colonic anastomosis extremely vulnerable.

Rectal Trauma

Clinical Examination

Physical examination should include digital rectal examination and careful palpation of the perineal area. In female patients, a vaginal examination should be performed. Asking the patient to "tighten up" will help evaluate the efficacy of the sphincteric mechanism and whether it is intact.

Diagnostic Studies

The most important diagnostic technique is sigmoidoscopy. This can be done at the bedside or, if a decision for operation is already made, at the operating room table after the patient is intubated and before an abdominal incision is made. Gentle lavage may help visualization. However, it is important to realize that the diagnosis of rectal injury is made by the mere presence of blood in the rectum. Precise inspection of the site of penetration is desirable but not necessary.

A barium enema examination is contraindicated if rectal injury is suspected; a water-soluble technique should be

TABLE 17-3 Randomized Prospective Trials: Primary Repair versus Colostomy

ARTICLE (REF.)	PRIMARY REPAIRS	RESECTIONS AND ANASTOMOSES	PRIMARY REPAIR LEAKS	RESECTIONS AND ANASTOMOTIC LEAKS	COLOSTOMY/ EXTERIORIZATION
Stone and Fabian[112]	67	0	1	—	72
Chappuis et al.[15]	17	11	0	0	28
Falcone et al.[35]	0	11	—	0	11
Sasaki et al.[101]	31	12	0	0	28
Gonzalez et al.[46]	51	5	0	1	53
Total	166	39	1 (0.6%)	1 (2.6%)	192

TABLE 17-4 Colon Trauma: Prospectively Obtained Data

ARTICLE (REF.)	PRIMARY REPAIRS	RESECTIONS AND ANASTOMOSES	PRIMARY REPAIR LEAKS	RESECTIONS AND ANASTOMOTIC LEAKS	COLOSTOMY/ EXTERIORIZATION
George et al.[44]	83	12	0	1	7
Baker et al.[4]	172	0	1	—	217
Demetriades et al.[26]	76	0	2	—	24
Ivatury et al.[52]	159	26	0	2	67
Total	490	38	3 (0.6%)	3 (7.9%)	315

employed. Obviously, the presence of intraperitoneal gas implies a perforated viscus. Still, simple contrast evaluation is rarely done now, having been replaced by CT. The CT scan can map the bullet trajectory and provide additional information about the pelvic tissues. The introduction of contrast into the rectum may increase the diagnostic sensitivity of CT.

Intraoperative Management

Weil reported 66 patients who sustained retroperitoneal trauma to the colon and rectum.[130] These injuries usually affected both the intraperitoneal anterior and retroperitoneal posterior walls. The authors emphasize that the retroperitoneum must be inspected when an intraperitoneal hole is found or whenever the wound is in the flank or the back. The retroperitoneal rectum has been dreaded as a source of pelvic sepsis in case a suture line leaked. Because of the lack of serosa and the difficult approach to it, especially in the male pelvis, suture lines are thought to be at a high risk. Therefore, a proximal diverting colostomy has been recommended as part of the treatment. The old concept of distal bowel washout and presacral drainage has been generally abandoned because it has not been shown to yield any significant improvement in outcomes.[45] Thus, the choices for management of retroperitoneal rectal injuries have been narrowed to three: primary repair, proximal colostomy, or primary repair and proximal colostomy. In one comparative study, it has been shown that a colostomy alone is adequate and avoids the problems associated with opening the retroperitoneum and potentially contaminating the peritoneal cavity.[126] For injuries close to the anus produced by low-velocity bullets, transanal repair or even nonoperative management may be acceptable.

Whether to perform a direct sphincter repair as part of the initial management is a matter of some debate because no meaningful statistics are available. Of course, every effort must initially be directed to saving the patient's life; therefore, it is not surprising that most articles place little or no emphasis on sphincter reconstruction. An important principle to remember, however, is that the surgeon should endeavor to preserve sphincter muscle if vigorous debridement of the perineum is required. Identification of the cut muscle can be subsequently facilitated by marking the ends with nonabsorbable sutures. Direct repair should also be performed at the time if prolonging the surgery does not compromise the patient's safety and if the surgeon is satisfied with the viability of the tissue. The sphincters should be approximated with mattress sutures of absorbable material and the wound left open. Delayed reconstruction should be considered in accordance with the principles outlined in Chapter 16. Finally, the likelihood of septic complications is reduced if perineal skin wounds are left open to heal by second intention or closed in accordance with a delayed primary repair technique.[51]

Timing of Closure of Colostomy

Most surgeons recommend closure of the stoma when the patient has completely recovered, usually in 3 to 4 months. However, Renz and colleagues prospectively studied the safety of same-admission colostomy closure in individuals who suffered rectal wounds.[94] In principle, all patients underwent a contrast enema on the 10th day following creation of the colostomy. Those who demonstrated no radiologic leakage, no infection, and no problem with bowel control underwent colostomy closure. Sixty percent with such injuries were considered candidates, 53% of whom were discharged with their colostomies closed. There were no rectal injury–related complications following colostomy closure. The same findings were corroborated in the only prospective, randomized study that exists on the issue.[120] Same-admission colostomy closure was safe in appropriate patients who were not particularly ill at the time of closure.

Strategies to Prevent Infection

As previously implied, the combination of soft tissue injury, hypotension, and fecal contamination provide all the elements necessary for infection (a nutritive medium, a susceptible host, and the presence of bacteria). This triad is invariably present when the injury is caused by high-velocity missile or close-range shotgun wounds. Debridement of devitalized tissue is necessary. For major soft tissue injury, debridement should be succeeded by pressurized, pulsatile irrigation. Such an approach is very effective for removing bacteria and microparticulate debris.

TABLE 17-5 Colon Trauma: Retrospective Data Collection

ARTICLE (REF.)	PRIMARY REPAIRS	RESECTIONS AND ANASTOMOSES	PRIMARY REPAIR LEAKS	RESECTIONS AND ANASTOMOTIC LEAKS	COLOSTOMY/ EXTERIORIZATION
Thigpen et al.[115]	35	0	U	—	37
Wiener et al.[132]	85	0	U	—	57
Dang et al.[20]	24	0	0	—	58
Karanfilian et al.[55]	17	9	0	3	106
Adkins et al.[1]	36	0	0	—	20
Cook et al.[18]	27	0	U	U	180
Nallathambi et al.[80]	43	16	0	0	77
Shannon and Moore[103]	80	30	1	0	118
Dawes et al.[22]	21	13	0	1	103
Miller et al.[69]	0	16	—	0	12
George et al.[43]	73	0	0	—	41
Frame et al.[40]	30	0	U	—	35
Nelken and Lewis[83]	34	3	1	0	39
Ridgeway et al.[95]	30	U	0	—	35
Orsay et al.[89]	1	2	U	U	230
Levison et al.[62]	98	8	1	0	133
Burch et al.[12]	564	50	9	4	344
Morgado et al.[74]	60	32	1	2	9
Schultz et al.[102]	40	17	0	0	43
Taheri et al.[114]	43	12	0	0	91
Sasaki et al.[101]	50	52	0	0	52
Bostick et al.[8]	59	U	2[a]	U	155
Stewart et al.[110]	0	43	—	6	7
Total	1,450	303	15 (1.0%)	16 (5.0%)	1,982

[a]Combined primary repair and resection and anastomosis without stating numbers of each.
U, unstated in article.
Modified from Timothy Fabian, MD, with permission.

Antibiotics

It should be self-evident that antibiotics are considered an important part in the postoperative management of individuals with colonic trauma. No prospective, randomized clinical trial has compared the use of prophylactic antibiotics with that of a placebo following colonic injury. However, there are certainly data to support the use of such drugs in this circumstance.[41] Based simply on the principles of effective use of antibiotics in other clinical settings and the diverse colonic flora, a nontoxic drug directed at gram-negative aerobes and anaerobes should be administered as soon as possible after the injury. The tissue level should be high at the time the skin incision is made to ensure maximum effectiveness. One trial concluded that aztreonam with clindamycin is superior to gentamicin and clindamycin in the prevention of infections following penetrating abdominal trauma.[34] Most surgeons treating trauma patients use either a broad-spectrum, second-generation cephalosporin (cefoxitin, cefotetan) or a broad-spectrum beta-lactam plus beta-lactamase inhibitor (ticarcillin-clavulanate, ampicillin-sulbactam, piperacillin-tazobactam). The use of second-generation cephalosporins has been associated with an increased incidence of enterococci as pathogens identified in superficial wound infections. However, no difference has been observed in deep infection rates.[129] Probably, numerous antibiotic regimens and combinations are safe and effective for the management of patients who sustain colonic injury.

Generally, it is unnecessary to continue the antibiotics after 24 hours. Prospective, double-blind, randomized trials have demonstrated that 5 days of antibiotic therapy is not superior to 24 hours of therapy.[32] If intraoperative bleeding is a problem or the operation is longer than two drug half-lives, the antibiotics should be readministered intraoperatively. Prolonged use of antibiotics may be associated with superinfection, resistant organisms, and pseudomembranous colitis. In another prospective, randomized study of patients with severe abdominal trauma and colon injuries, Cornwell and associates also showed that one day of a single, broad-spectrum antibiotic is as effective as more prolonged regimens.[19]

Nichols and colleagues demonstrated by logical regression analysis of 145 patients that a statistically significantly increased risk for infection was associated with increased age, injury to the left colon, the administration of a greater number of units of blood or blood products, and associated organ injury.[84] Others have confirmed the prognostic importance of these risk factors and advise colostomy as a minimal treatment if these are present.[22] Some antibiotic regimens have been employed that seem to be equally efficacious, but the single most important factor contributing to a low rate of infection is prompt surgical intervention.[23,84,97]

Hypothermia

Another factor that may be associated with an increased risk for the development of infection is hypothermia.[59] Therefore, avoidance of this complication should be added to adequate resuscitation in order to prevent infection during the intraoperative period.

Foreign Body

Another issue that has stimulated some interest is the presence of a retained foreign body—specifically the missile. Poret and colleagues reviewed a series of wounds, comparing patients who harbored missiles with those who did not.[93] They discovered that after the bullet passed through the colon, a retained foreign body was frequently the source of postoperative abscess. Others have not been able to demonstrate an increased rate of infection that is related to a retained bullet.[25,39] Currently, the general consensus is that a missile should be removed if it is easy to do or can be accomplished without extensive dissection. Missiles that are lodged away from the operative field and may require extensive surgical maneuvers to localize are best left alone. An abscess around a bullet or a more serious complication are rather rare events.

Nutrition

The value of nutritional support is undoubted. Two randomized trials have reported the use of jejunostomy followed by immediate enteral feeding.[57,71] Fewer abscesses and pulmonary infections have been noted in the enteral feeding groups. Another trial compared a standard elemental formula to one enhanced with arginine, omega-3 fatty acids, and glutamine (immune-enhancing diet).[72] The immune-enhancing regimen was associated with a statistically significantly reduced incidence of infections when compared with the standard regimen. The use of early enteral feeding is strongly recommended except in those individuals with severe hypotension or prolonged ileus. The placement of a small-bore feeding jejunostomy has itself been associated with a low complication rate.[78]

Right versus Left Colon Injuries

There is a controversy about whether penetrating injuries of the right colon should be treated differently from those of the left. Thompson and colleagues compared their experience in patients who sustained injury to the right colon with those who had left colon injury.[117] Both groups were similar with respect to the mechanism of injury, presence of shock at admission, degree of fecal contamination, severity of trauma, and frequency of associated intra-abdominal problems. The number of patients managed by primary repair, resection, resection with exteriorization, and colostomy was comparable for right and left injuries, but it must be remembered that these were historical controls. The management of right colon injuries resulted in a morbidity rate of 32% and a mortality rate of 2%; left-sided injuries were found to have a 33% morbidity rate and a 4% mortality rate. Because of the comparable results, the authors concluded that penetrating trauma to the right and left colon should be managed similarly for the same degree of injury, contamination, and so forth. Stewart and colleagues also found no difference in leak or abscess rates in a group of severely injured patients with destructive colon wounds.[110] Similarly, Demetriades and coworkers stated that the clinical significance of the different anatomy, physiology, and bacteriology of the right and the left colon has been overemphasized.[28] They wrote that in most cases primary repair can be safely performed irrespective of the location of the injury unless gross fecal contamination, extensive tissue destruction, or a considerable amount of retained feces is present. However, these and other studies have the drawback of being retrospective.[81] Another approach that may be useful in selective circumstances is a primary repair followed by a proximal, protective loop

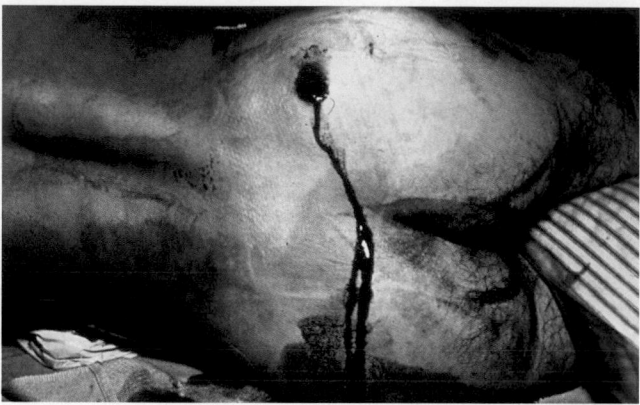

FIGURE 17-12. Entrance wound to the right buttock from a bullet fired from an M16 rifle. Understanding the course of the projectile is critical in surgical decision making. (Courtesy of Daniel Rosenthal, MD.)

ileostomy, which can be easily closed at a second stage through a local incision.

Gunshot Wounds to the Buttocks

Gunshot wounds to the gluteal region warrant special consideration because this type of injury often poses a challenging diagnostic and therapeutic dilemma (Figure 17-12). The question is whether it represents pure soft tissue injury—that is, injury unrelated to the colorectal area—or whether there is concern for associated bowel problems. Velmahos and colleagues identified 59 consecutive patients with wounds of the buttocks during a 1-year period at Los Angeles County, University of Southern California Medical Center.[127] The buttocks were defined as the body area confined between the posterior superior iliac spines superiorly, the gluteal folds inferiorly, and the projection of the midaxillary lines laterally. Superficial wounds and those tracking away from the retroperitoneum were excluded. The postulate in the study was the opinion of the investigators that clinical examination is a safe and reliable tool for triage in individuals with these types of injuries. In other words, it was believed that patients could be managed selectively based on clinical findings alone. Based on these observations, approximately one-third (19 patients) underwent surgery, with all but 2 individuals found to have significant intra-abdominal injuries. The remaining 40 patients (two-thirds) were successfully observed. There were no missed injuries or delays in diagnosis. The authors concluded that clinical examination is a safe method for selecting patients with gunshot wounds to the buttocks for nonoperative treatment.[127]

A particular caveat should be introduced, however, concerning the role of *sigmoidoscopy* in this situation. Ferraro and coworkers reviewed sigmoidoscopy in patients who sustained gunshot wounds to the buttocks.[37] Sixteen individuals underwent this examination, and a rectal injury was demonstrated in 7. There were no missed injuries and no morbidity in the remaining patients managed without sigmoidoscopy (an additional 52 patients). The authors concluded that sigmoidoscopy can be performed *selectively* in individuals who have sustained a

gunshot wound to the buttocks when the possibility of involvement of the rectum is in doubt.[37] An abdominal/pelvic CT scan may also help to determine the missile tract in these patients.

Damage Control Procedures

The principles of management of severely injured patients have evolved considerably since the mid-1990s, but still the main determinant of survival is the extent of the initial injury. The triad of coagulopathy, acidosis, and hypothermia is a well-recognized harbinger of poor outcome. Strategies to control hemorrhage, minimize contamination, and reduce operative time are essential if one is to improve the prognosis. In a damage control approach, the goals are to minimize operative time while attempting to restore normal physiology.[60] To meet these goals, the celiotomy must be abbreviated. Operative bleeding is controlled as rapidly as possible with the most expedient technique that is consistent with this objective. Visceral contamination is limited through the use of clamps followed by either an *expeditious* primary repair or resection with a stapling device. Alternatively, in the absence of special equipment, the bowel can be ligated with the use of an umbilical tape or equivalent and divided. No reconstruction is attempted during the initial stage of the damage control procedure. Once operative bleeding and visceral contamination are controlled, nonsurgically induced bleeding is controlled with packing. When possible, a nonadherent or hemostatic interface between the packing and the bleeding surface should be used in order to control hemorrhage better and to prevent rebleeding upon removal of the pack. The abdomen is then closed using a technique that does not injure the fascia. This usually entails either rapidly closing the skin or implanting a plastic prosthesis attached to the skin. Another popular technique involves placing a cover over the bowel and using a large self-adhesive drape over the abdominal wall, with closed-suction drains placed underneath the drape to control drainage (vacuum-assisted drainage). Commercially available systems minimize the time of assembling the multiple elements and provide optimal suction effect. Resuscitation to restore normal physiology is continued, with special attention to maintaining adequate oxygen delivery, correcting any coagulopathy, and addressing hypothermia.

Following establishment of normal physiologic parameters, the patient is returned to the operating room where the abdomen is reexplored. The packs are removed, hemostasis is secured, and hollow viscus reconstruction or an ostomy is performed. For colon injuries, a primary repair is preferable, as mentioned previously, although a colostomy may be necessary in cases of extensive edema, loss of bowel, mesocolic retraction, or other anatomical burdens. If a colostomy is selected, care should be taken to allow sufficient distance between the stoma and the wound in order to avoid interference with subsequent reconstruction of the abdominal wall. At the second operation, appropriate drains and enteral tubes are placed. These may include closed-suction drains for liver, pancreatic or genitourinary injuries, and gastrostomy or jejunostomy tubes. If the abdomen cannot be closed primarily, numerous options are available.[88] In general, we prefer to use a biologic mesh with closure of the skin over it after undermining the subcutaneous tissue, in addition to generous mobilization of dermocutaneous flaps toward the midline.

Colon Injury in Military Conflict

A military physician close to a battlefield or a civilian surgeon far from a specialized trauma center could be faced with a mass casualty situation and have to treat colon injuries under less than optimal conditions. The following are principles of management under these circumstances.

When exploring the abdomen, colon wounds should be temporarily closed with clamps and the area of injury covered with gauze packs to minimize contamination. War wounds of the colon are typically extensive and may require colostomy more frequently than civilian injuries. Additionally, patients operated in battlefield hospitals are often moved along different echelons of care. They therefore cannot be monitored adequately for anastomotic leaks or the development of sepsis. Injuries are typically multiple with resuscitation not always optimal. Debridement and sterility may be inadequate. Under these conditions, a colostomy may constitute a safer option, although this has not been tested under protocol. Although the approach of creating colostomies for military colon injuries has been supported through extensive experience during World War II, in Korea, and in Vietnam, the studies are old and do not reflect current standards of care.[3,17,50,65,86,87,131] Even in the precarious situation of war surgery, the technique of primary repair merits consideration.[73] For several reasons, many who work in developing countries may favor this approach when they are faced with gunshot wounds of the abdomen. First, follow-up is practically impossible in many cases, and therefore leaving a patient with a stoma may not be an option. Second, stoma appliances are a luxury that may not be obtainable. Third, mortality and morbidity conferences are seldom held in the developing world during periods of conflict, neither in the countryside nor in urban areas.

Complex Perineal Injuries

Complex wounds to the perineum with or without pelvic fracture present a considerable challenge to the surgeon.[58]

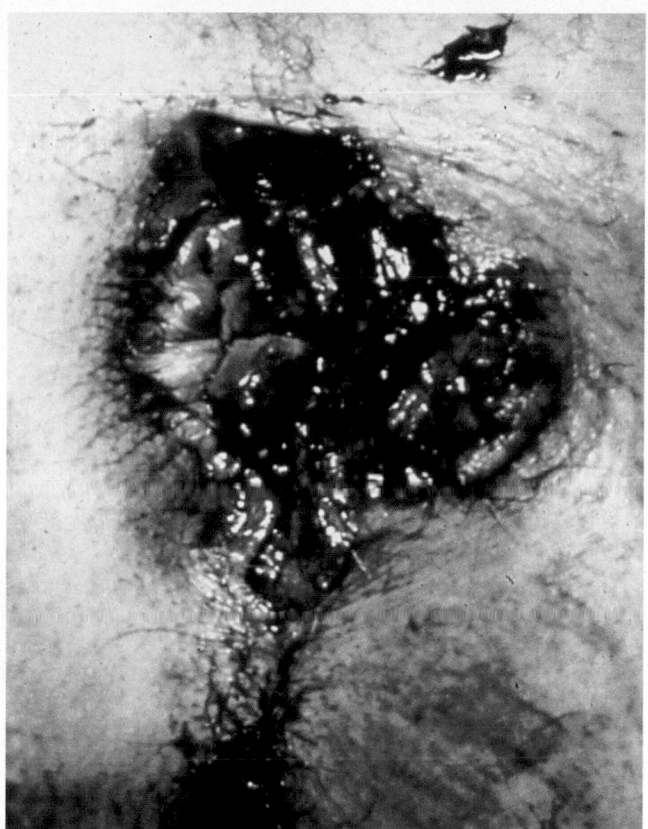

FIGURE 17-14. Anorectal impalement injury. The anus is displaced to the right side.

Such injuries are usually the result of high-speed motor vehicle or motorcycle accidents and historically have been associated with a very high mortality rate (Figures 17-13 and 17-14). Early death is usually a consequence of bleeding and pelvic sepsis, whereas pulmonary embolism and multiple organ failure are the causes of late demise in these individuals. There is often associated extensive soft tissue injury. An organized approach is essential to prevent complications following these devastating wounds. The principles are summarized in Table 17-6.[111]

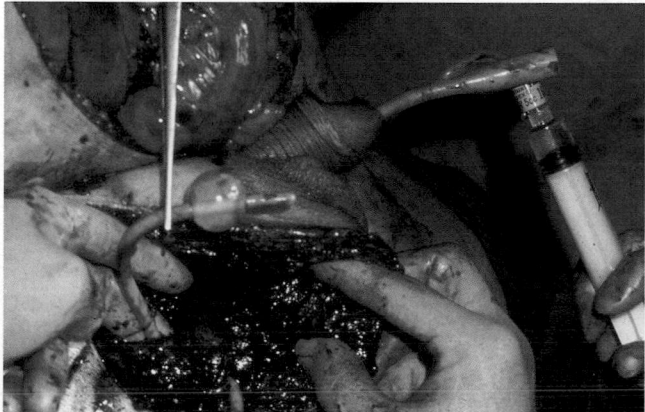

FIGURE 17-13. Perineal trauma. Severe avulsion injury from a motorcycle accident with laceration of the urethra and rectum. Note the Foley catheter emerging from the defect in the urethra.

TABLE 17-6 Complex Perineal Wounds Management Guidelines

- Resuscitation with hemorrhage control
- Identification and treatment of associated injuries
- Fecal diversion (consider feeding jejunostomy at same time)
- Urinary diversion for complex urologic injuries
- Aggressive initial debridement with pressurized pulsatile irrigation
- Immediate fracture fixation
- Early enteral nutrition
- Daily intraoperative debridement
- Wound coverage with skin graft as soon as feasible
- Deep venous thrombosis prophylaxis

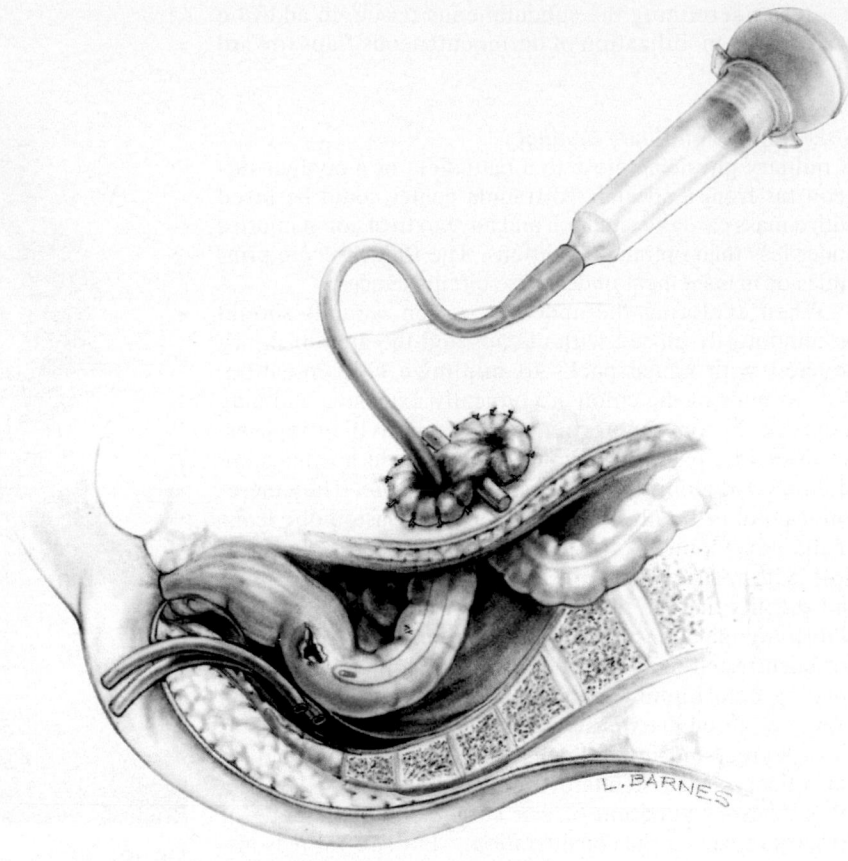

FIGURE 17-15. Management of an extra-peritoneal rectal injury. A colostomy is created; irrigation and presacral drainage may be effected although these are not frequently used.

Colostomy with distal irrigation is probably important, as is aggressive soft tissue debridement, often by means of frequent examinations under anesthesia (Figure 17-15). This approach greatly reduces the incidence of pelvic sepsis. Although it is imperative to remove all nonviable tissue, every effort should be made to preserve the anal sphincter mechanism. Debridement of the muscle should be conservative. As stated earlier, repair should be delayed under these circumstances. One is advised to pay particular attention to the prevention of deep venous thrombosis because pulmonary embolism is a frequent cause of morbidity and mortality, especially following pelvic injury with fracture.

▶ CONCLUSIONS AND RECOMMENDATIONS

The history of colorectal wound injuries and their management is fascinating, but it has often been surrounded by controversy. However, prospective, randomized, controlled trials have helped to clarify what should be the appropriate management for most patients. It is certainly clear that a reasonably consistent approach may be established for the treatment of nondestructive colon wounds. Unfortunately, the data are less conclusive for more extensive wounds and for rectal injuries.

In summary, all uncomplicated colon wounds (which represent 80% to 90% of all colon injuries) may be safely managed by means of primary repair. Destructive or devitalized colonic injuries require resection and, perforce, have a higher complication rate if an anastomosis is attempted. However, it appears that this complication rate is no worse than the rate associated with colostomy. Most such patients can still be managed by primary repair but selected individuals may require diversion.

Extraperitoneal rectal injuries are managed preferentially by fecal diversion, although this issue is still debated. The addition of primary repair or the use of primary repair without diversion are considered acceptable alternatives in appropriate patients.

References

1. Adkins RB Jr, Zirkle PK, Waterhouse G. Penetrating colon trauma. *J Trauma.* 1984;24(6):491–499.
2. Appleby JP, Nagy AG. Abdominal injuries associated with the use of seatbelts. *Am J Surg.* 1989;157(5):457–458.
3. Artz CP. Battle casualties in Korea: studies of the surgical research team. In: *Battle Wounds: Clinical Experiences.* Vol 3. Washington, DC: Medical Service Graduate School; 1955.
4. Baker LW, Thomson SR, Chadwick SJ. Colon wound management and prograde colonic lavage in large bowel trauma. *Br J Surg.* 1990;77(8): 872–876.
5. Baudens L. Clinique des plaies d'armes à feu (1836). Reported in: *Medical and Surgical History of the War of Rebellion.* Part 2. Vol 2. Washington, DC: United States Government Printing Office; 1876:124.
6. Berne JD, Velmahos GC, Chan LS, et al. The high morbidity of colostomy closure after trauma: further support for the primary repair of colon injuries. *Surgery.* 1998;123(2):157–164.
7. Blumenberg RM. The seat belt syndrome: sigmoid colon perforation. *Ann Surg.* 1967;165(4):637–639.
8. Bostick PJ, Heard JS, Islas JT, et al. Management of penetrating colon injuries. *J Natl Med Assoc.* 1994;86(5):378–382.

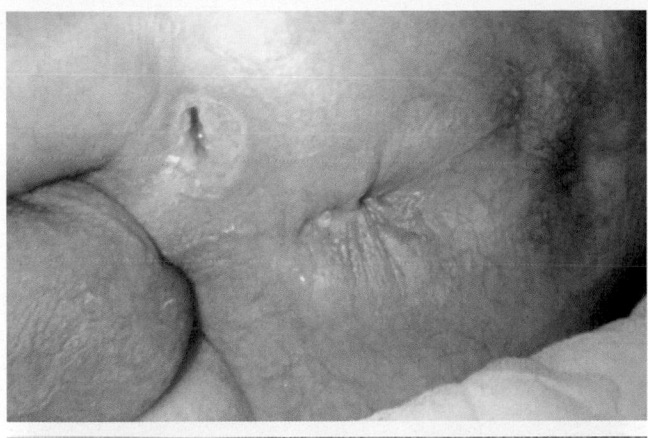

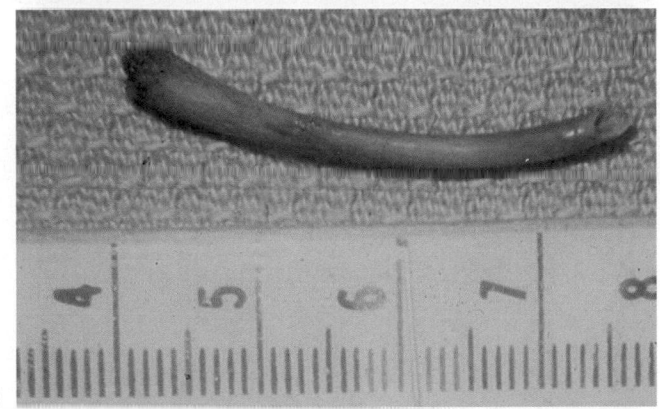

FIGURE 18-1. **A:** Perforation of the rectum from an ingested foreign body that produced an ischiorectal abscess. **B:** A chicken bone was the cause of the perforation. (Courtesy of Daniel Rosenthal, MD.)

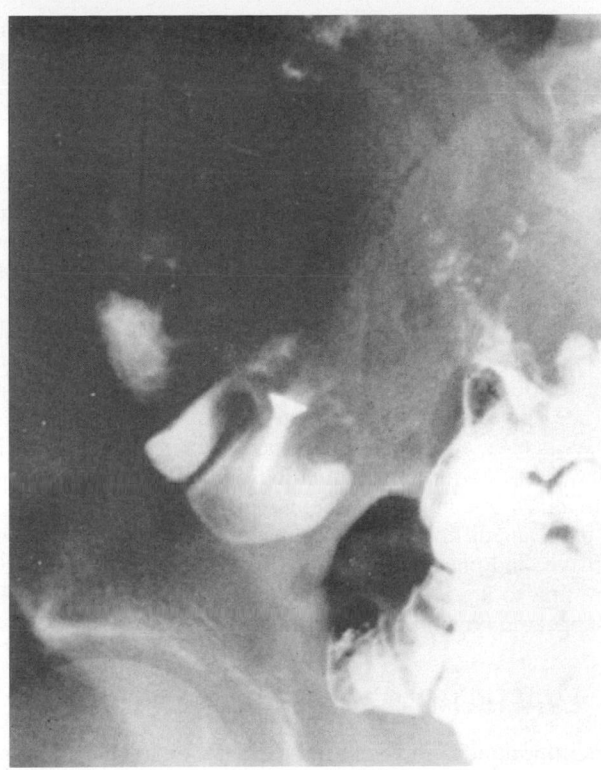

FIGURE 18-2. An accidentally swallowed wood screw is lodged in the cecum. Because of peritoneal signs, a laparotomy was undertaken. (Courtesy of Albert Medwid, MD.)

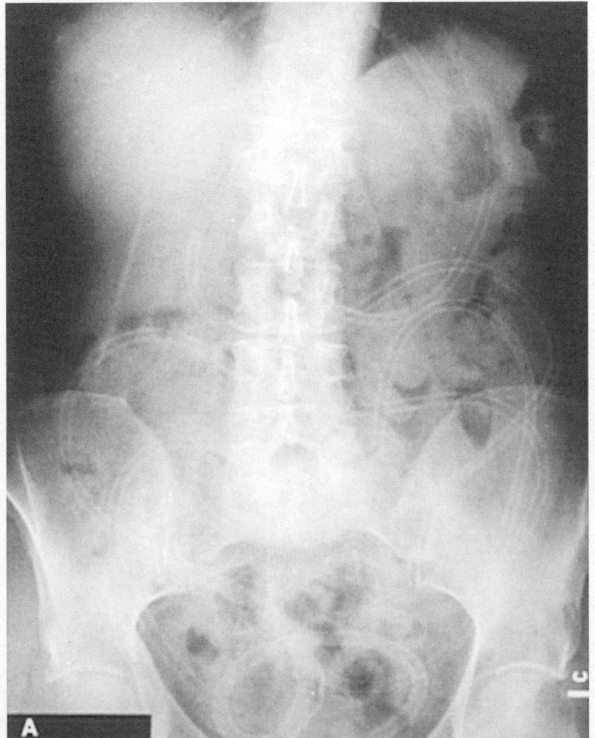

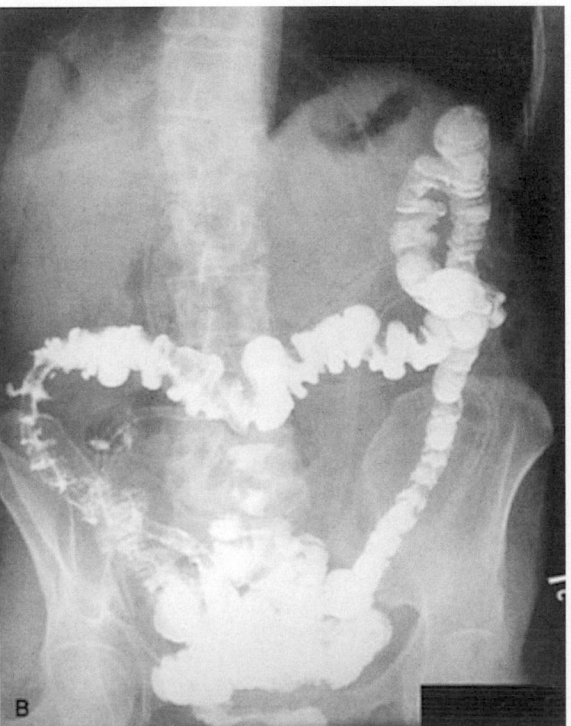

FIGURE 18-3. Miller–Abbott tube lodged in the intestine several years after it had been divided in the oropharynx with the expectation that it would pass **(A)**. Barium enema examination reveals that the distal end reaches the mid-transverse colon **(B)**. Despite attempted removal via colonoscopy, a laparotomy was necessary.

and reduce exposure to ionizing radiation. Obviously, any individual with peritoneal signs needs radiologic investigation and/or exploratory laparotomy.

▶ FOREIGN BODIES OF THE RECTUM

The list of objects that have been removed from the rectum is virtually endless (e.g., lightbulbs, catheters, pens and pencils, glass tubes, candles, vibrators, dildos, bottles and jars; Figures 18-4 through 18-10). The story of the discovery of a deceased gerbil in the rectum is probably of questionable authenticity. Busch and Starling identified 182 cases from the world's literature and noted the recovery of objects from A (i.e., apple) to Z (i.e., zucchini).[5]

As can be appreciated, the variety of foreign bodies is limited only by one's imagination. Individuals may present with a host of complaints, including rectal bleeding, anorectal pain, and difficulty with micturition. Embarrassed, apprehensive, and uncomfortable, many deny the incident, often claiming to have fallen on the object, which miraculously disappeared beyond his or her reach.

▶ EVALUATION

It is important to evaluate the patient's abdomen for signs and symptoms suggestive of peritoneal irritation. An indwelling catheter may be necessary if there is any concern about urinary retention. Inspection and palpation of the anal canal and rectum may reveal the foreign body. Note should be made of sphincter tone and contractility, especially if

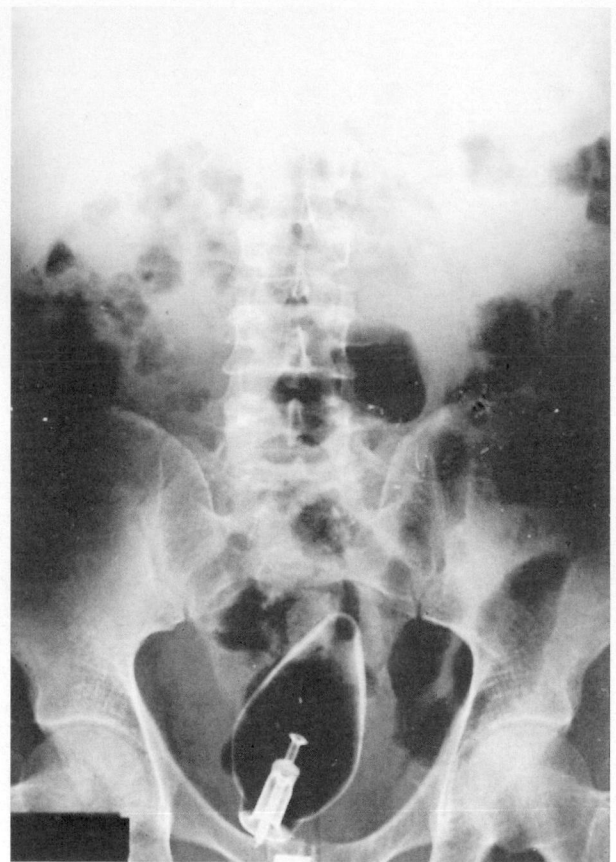

FIGURE 18-5. Foreign body: lightbulb in the rectum.

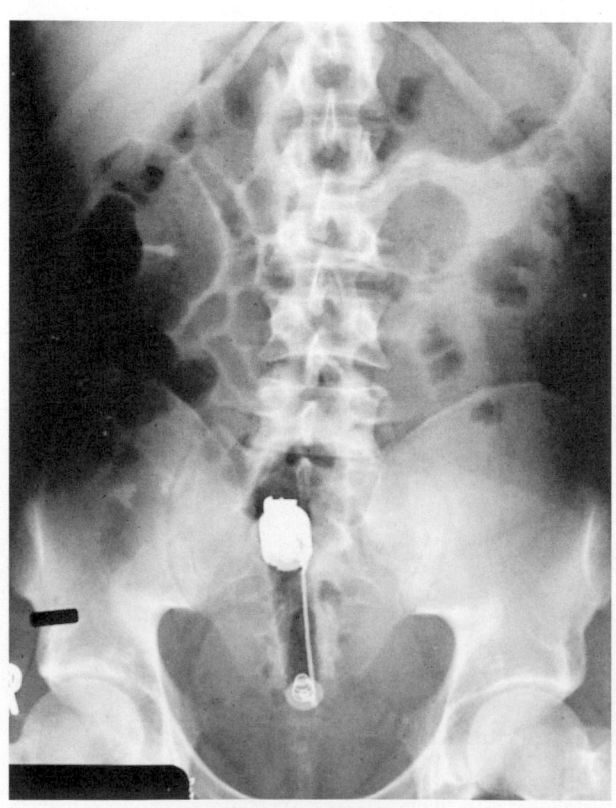

FIGURE 18-4. Foreign body: vibrator in the rectum.

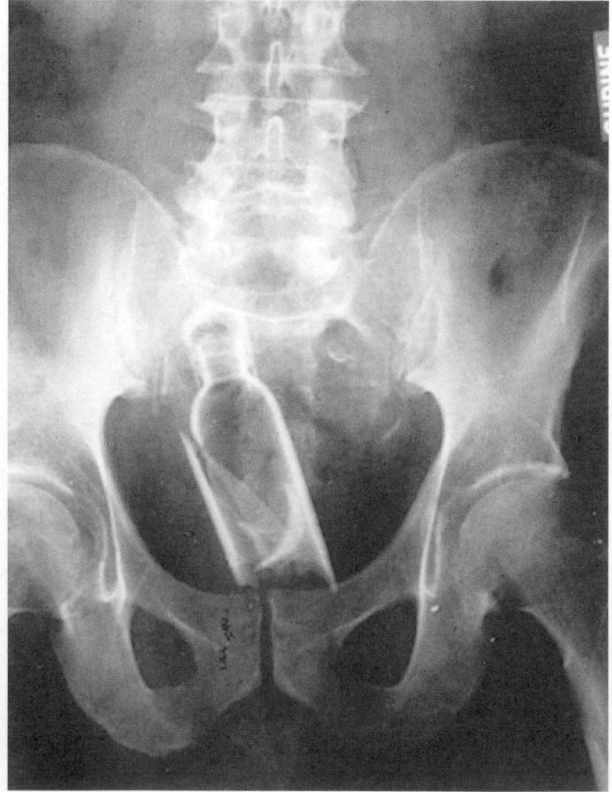

FIGURE 18-6. Foreign body. Extraction of broken bottle in the rectum presents a particularly challenging problem.

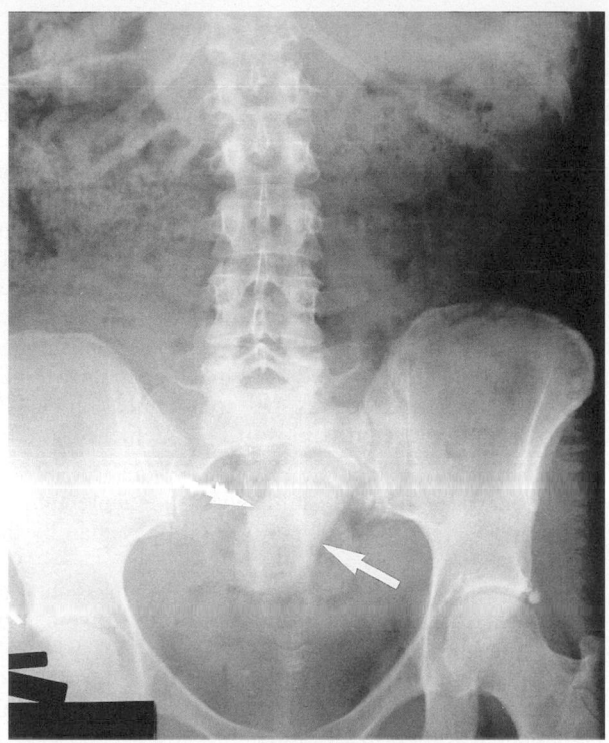

FIGURE 18-7. Foreign body: dildo in the rectum (*arrows*).

signs of anoreceptivity are evident. Such a situation may actually facilitate evaluation of the patient and extraction of the foreign body. An x-ray film of the pelvis will demonstrate the contours of any radiopaque foreign material. One should also seek to identify any unsuspected second foreign body.

One may attempt extraction of colonic foreign bodies by means of the colonoscope, but if symptoms of peritoneal irritation develop, removal will require laparotomy and colotomy.[21] Removal by appendicostomy has also been suggested if the object is small.[15] Rocklin and Apelgren, in a literature review, found 29 instances of colonoscopic removal of a variety of objects reported in 14 publications.[18] Biopsy forceps, polypectomy snares, and stone-extracting baskets have all been successfully employed. Removal techniques must be individualized to deal with the specific object. For example, in one instance the surgeon attached a lightbulb socket on the end of a stick, screwed the socket into the bulb, and ultimately pulled out the bulb.[3]

The following protocol has been recommended for management of colon objects[18]:

- Plain abdominal radiograph for nature and location
- Immediate attempt at colonoscopic extraction if the foreign body is associated with bleeding or obstruction
- Barium enema or water-soluble contrast enema for difficult-to-localize, suspected, or known radiolucent foreign body

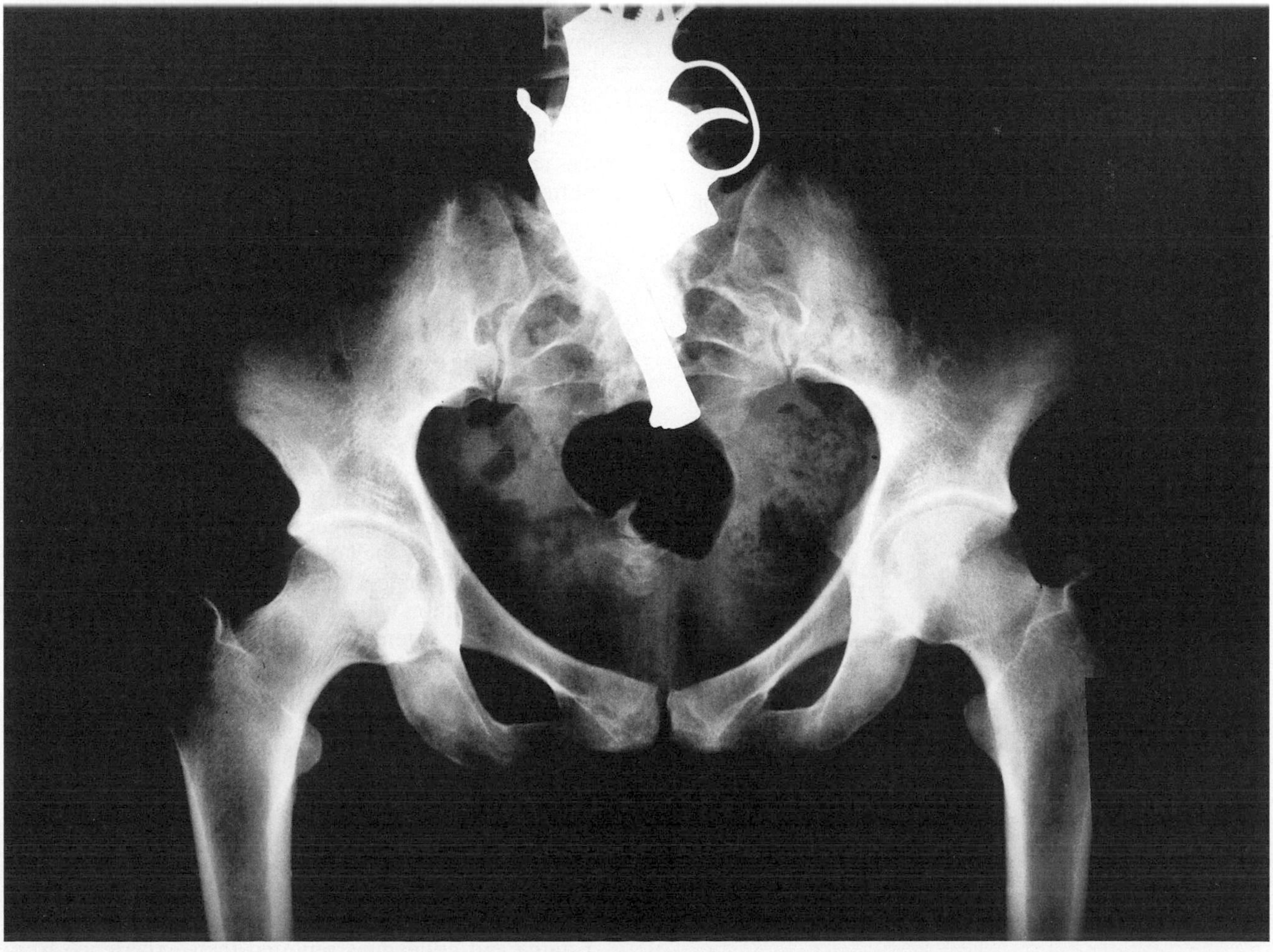

FIGURE 18-8. Foreign body. A pistol in the rectosigmoid gives a special meaning to the expression "a shot in the dark." (Courtesy of Daniel Rosenthal, MD.)

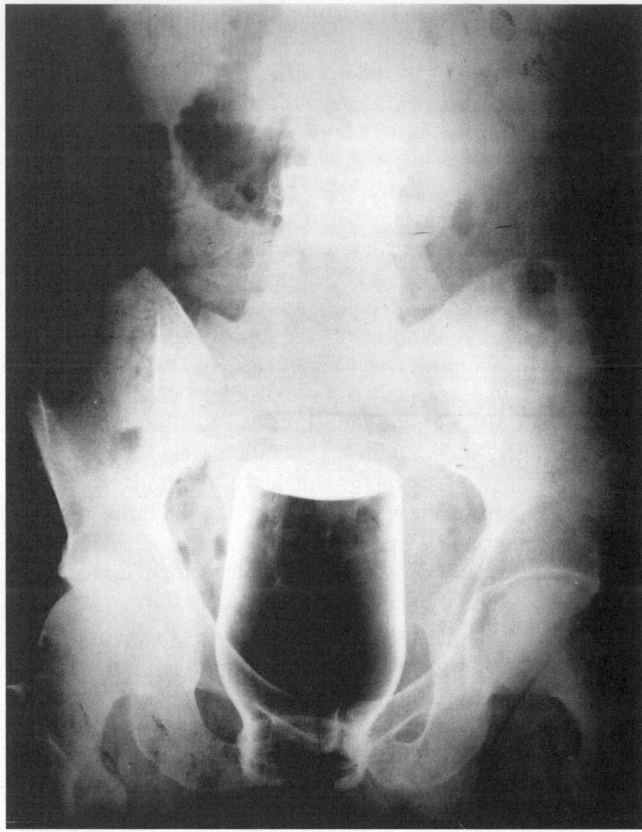

FIGURE 18-9. Foreign body: bottle in the rectum.

- High-fiber diet, bulk laxative, mineral oil (no cathartics)
- Serial radiographs to follow progression
- Enemas before the procedure to enhance visualization
- Broad-spectrum antibiotics before the procedure
- Colonoscopic extraction if the object fails to progress on serial radiographs during 48 hours
- Observation for 24 hours after removal

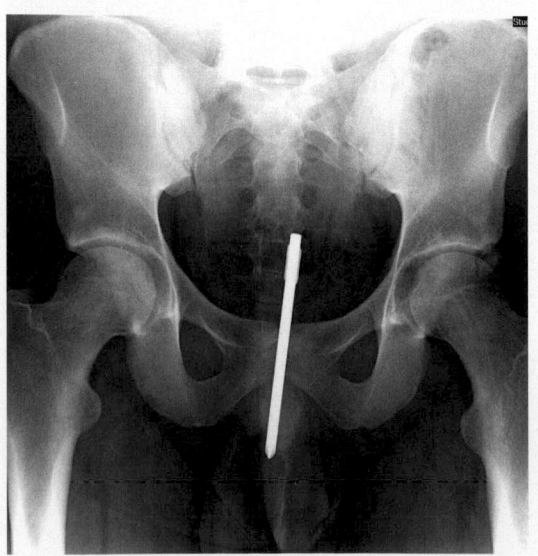

FIGURE 18-10. Foreign body: end of Phillips screwdriver in the rectum.

► PRINCIPLES OF MANAGEMENT OF RECTAL FOREIGN BODIES

The requirement for extracting foreign bodies from the rectum has become virtually epidemic. The presence of these objects in the rectum often poses unique difficulty in management, especially when dealing with the risk of breaking glass. The administration of glucagon, spinal anesthesia, or general anesthesia assists in relaxation of the sphincter, greatly facilitating removal of the object.[19] In general, foreign bodies located within the rectum can be extracted as an outpatient procedure or in the emergency department. Those positioned above the rectum should be removed in the operating room.

Stewart (Stewart RM, personal communication, 1997) outlines the following principles of management of rectal foreign bodies:

- More damage is generally inflicted on the anorectum by a forceful attempt to remove a foreign body than by the original insertion.
- Never attempt to remove a foreign body unless the patient's anal sphincter is fully relaxed by local, spinal, or general anesthesia.
- Never attempt to extract a foreign body using instruments in an uncooperative patient because a sudden move can precipitate tearing or perforation.
- Large foreign bodies are preferentially removed in the operating room under a spinal or general anesthetic.
- Following retrieval of the object, meticulous endoscopic examination should be undertaken and repair effected for any associated lacerations.
- Rectal perforation, whether intraperitoneal or extraperitoneal, requires a diverting stoma.

Senile patients with a patulous anus can usually have foreign bodies removed without an anesthetic. Thermometers are the most frequently encountered foreign objects in this age group.

► SPECIAL TECHNIQUES

Numerous techniques have been suggested to remove objects from the rectum, including the use of blunt hooks or sponge holders, bimanual manipulation, and the use of a nasogastric tube as a lasso.[10] A Foley catheter is particularly useful for a hollow body, such as a jar.[9,12] Drilling a hole in the bottom of a bottle or jar and inserting a Foley catheter is another means for removing such an item if the open end is directed cephalad. Garber and colleagues suggest using the more rigid endotracheal tube for such objects.[11] Foley catheters may be inserted above an object into the proximal bowel lumen. Gentle distal traction while inserting air above the object to break the vacuum often will result in successful extraction.[17] Aquino and Turner advise the use of three lubricated Tauber vaginal spatulas to break the suction and rock the object out.[1] Rubber-shod clamps may be employed to remove broken glass. Under these circumstances, with careful follow-up by means of computed tomography, looking for retroperitoneal air, an exploratory laparotomy may not be needed. Berci and Morgenstern describe the use of an operating proctoscope and tenaculum for extraction of foreign bodies.[4] Johnson and Hartranft recommend the use of an obstetric vacuum extractor to remove glass foreign bodies.[13]

Eftaiha and colleagues reported their experience from the Cook County Hospital in Chicago with the removal of

31 objects from the rectum.[8] They employed the principles of biplane abdominal roentgenograms to identify the location, type, and number of foreign materials, and they emphasize the necessity of an anesthetic. It is crucial that once the presence of the foreign body has been determined, it must be removed while the patient is under adequate anesthesia to avoid the possibility of further injury. This is of particular concern if the object is glass. Whenever possible, transanal extraction should be used and laparotomy undertaken only as a last resort. Proctosigmoidoscopic examination should be performed after removal of the foreign body to be certain that no injury to the bowel has been sustained. It is also advisable to keep the patient in the hospital until a bowel movement has been achieved and the surgeon is convinced that sepsis or perforation is unlikely. A later report of 55 patients from the same institution confirms the wisdom of the policies stated earlier.[23] Conversely, in the experience of Barone and coworkers, of 112 patients who sustained trauma of the rectum or sigmoid from foreign bodies, most were able to have the foreign bodies removed on an outpatient basis.[2] These investigators do not believe that admission after removal is mandatory. Only one patient required a laparotomy, and this was performed because of signs and symptoms of peritonitis.

If a laparotomy is required, an attempt should be made to "milk" the foreign body down into the field of vision of the perineal operator; hence, the perineolithotomy position should be used. If injury to the rectum has occurred, the previously discussed principles apply. If the object cannot be removed transanally, a colotomy should be undertaken. In the controlled situation, without fecal contamination, no colostomy is performed.

References

1. Aquino MM, Turner JW. A simple technique for removing an impacted aerosol-can cap from the rectum. *Dis Colon Rectum*. 1986;29(10):675.
2. Barone JE, Yee J, Nealon TF Jr. Management of foreign bodies and trauma of the rectum. *Surg Gynecol Obstet*. 1983;156(4):453–457.
3. Benjamin HB, Klamecki B, Haft JS. Removal of exotic foreign objects from the abdominal orifices. *Am J Proctol*. 1969;20(6):413–417.
4. Berci G, Morgenstern L. An operative proctoscope for foreign-body extraction. *Dis Colon Rectum*. 1983;26(3):193–194.
5. Busch DB, Starling JR. Rectal foreign bodies: case reports and a comprehensive review of the world's literature. *Surgery*. 1986;100(3):512–519.
6. Caes F, Vierendeels T, Welch W, et al. Aortocolic fistula caused by an ingested chicken bone. *Surgery*. 1988;103(4):481–483.
7. Dinnick T. The origins and evolution of colostomy. *Br J Surg*. 1934;22(85):142–154.
8. Eftaiha M, Hambrick E, Abcarian H. Principles of management of colorectal foreign bodies. *Dis Colon Rectum*. 1977;112(6):691–695.
9. Floyd WF, Walls EW. Electromyography of the sphincter ani externus in man. *J Physiol*. 1953;122(3):599–609.
10. French GW, Sherlock DJ, Holl-Allen RT. Problems with rectal foreign bodies. *Br J Surg*. 1985;72(3):243–244.
11. Garber HI, Rubin RJ, Eisenstat TE. Removal of a glass foreign body from the rectum. *Dis Colon Rectum*. 1981;24(4):323.
12. Hughes JP. Foreign body of the rectum removal. *Am J Proctol Gastroenterol Colon Rectal Surg*. 1983;34:16.
13. Johnson SO, Hartrantt TH. Nonsurgical removal of a rectal foreign body using a vacuum extractor. Report of a case. *Dis Colon Rectum*. 1996;39(8):935–937.
14. McDowell GC II, Henry M, Ellison EC. Ingestion of sharpened pencils. *Surg Rounds*. 1988;11:77–80.
15. Mizrahi S, Eyal I, Shtamler B. Foreign body removal through an appendicostomy. *Dis Colon Rectum*. 1990;33(10):902.
16. Mortensen NJ, Irvin TT. Disembowelment per rectum: a fatal rectal injury. *Br J Surg*. 1984;71(4):289.
17. Nehme Kingsley AN, Abcarian H. Colorectal foreign bodies. Management update. *Dis Colon Rectum*. 1985;28(12):941–944.
18. Rocklin MS, Apelgren KN. Colonoscopic extraction of foreign bodies from above the rectum. *Am Surg*. 1989;55(2):119–123.
19. Shillingstad RB, Marks JM, Ponsky JL. Endoscopic management of gastrointestinal foreign bodies. *Contemp Surg*. 1997;50:87.
20. Silverberg D, Menes T, Kim U. Surgery for "body packers"—a 15-year experience. *World J Surg*. 2006;30(4):541–546.
21. Sorenson RM, Bond JH Jr. Colonoscopic removal of a foreign body from the cecum. *Gastrointest Endosc*. 1975;21(3):134–135.
22. White SW. Remarkable case of the swallowing of a silver spoon and the excision of it from the intestinal canal with the recovery of the patient. *Med Repository*. 1807;4:367.
23. Whitehead WE, Burgio KL, Engel BT. Biofeedback treatment of fecal incontinence in geriatric patients. *J Am Geriatr Soc*. 1985;33(5):320–324.

19

Laparoscopic Colon and Rectal Surgery

Roberto C. M. Bergamaschi, Sergio W. Larach, Alessio Pigazzi, Slawomir Marecik, Elsa B. Valsdottir, and Salim Amrani

A little learning is a dangerous thing.
—ALEXANDER POPE (1688–1744),
Essay on Criticism, Part ii

*A learning curve is not a valid justification for
patient injury.*
—State of New York Department of Health
Memorandum—Series 92-20, June 12, 1992

▶ HISTORY

Laparoscopic colorectal surgery has evolved considerably, especially over the past 20 years. In 1991, Schlinkert[193] described the surgical technique of laparoscopic-assisted right hemicolectomy for cancer in a single case report. A lateral-to-medial dissection was performed with intracorporeal vessel ligation through the use of five ports. A horizontal laparotomy with division of the right rectus muscle was carried out to resect, anastomose, and retrieve the specimen. In 1991, Fowler and White[75] described the surgical technique of laparoscopic-assisted sigmoid resection with intracorporeal vessel ligation, also in a case report. A muscle-splitting laparotomy was carried out in the left lower abdominal quadrant in order to resect the bowel and to fashion a purse-string suture around the circular stapler's anvil. The suture was placed in the proximal end of the descending colon. Also in 1991, Jacobs and colleagues[101] reported a case series of 20 patients who underwent laparoscopic-assisted right hemicolectomy or sigmoid resection for benign and malignant diseases.

Following these reports, colorectal surgeons in Germany and the United States undertook laboratory investigations. Kockerling and associates[80,116] performed an experimental surgery using intracorporeal anastomotic techniques in large animals and developed a reusable laparoscopic purse-string suture instrument (Figure 19-1). Cohen and coworkers[49] presented the initial experimental results in pigs with intracorporeal anastomoses and with mesenteric closure with the use of staples. Böhm and colleagues[34] performed an oncologic right colectomy with intracorporeal ileocolic anastomosis in a canine model.

In 1992, Phillips and associates[166] published a series of 51 patients who underwent a variety of colorectal resections with a laparoscopic, intracorporeal, hand-sewn purse-string suture and transanal natural orifice specimen extraction (NOSE). In 1993, Bleday and coworkers[33] described a similar intracorporeal technique using a colonoscopic snare for transanal NOSE (Figure 19-2). In 1995, Mentges and associates described a technique that involved a proctotomy in the anterior rectal wall in order to insert the anvil of a circular stapler into the peritoneal cavity and to perform a NOSE by means of transanal endoscopic microsurgery (TEM) (Figure 19-3).[142] Also in 1994, Darzi and colleagues described a left colon resection with transanal NOSE followed by a triple-stapled intracorporeal colorectal anastomosis (Figure19-4).[55] In 2000, the use of a 33-mm port (Figure 19-5), which allowed the insertion of the anvil of a circular stapler into the abdominal cavity, was described to circumvent the requirement to use transanal NOSE for this purpose (Figure 19-6).[20]

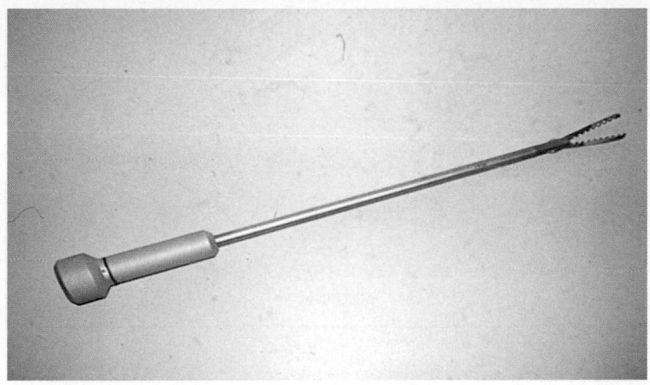

FIGURE 19-1. Reusable laparoscopic purse-string suture device. (Courtesy of Professor Ferdinand Kockerling.)

Most of the aforementioned intracorporeal techniques have not stood the test of time. In fact, nonrandomized and randomized data have established similar outcomes following intracorporeal and laparoscopic-assisted sigmoid colectomy.[28,29] However, attention has been drawn to the specimen extraction site. The traditional lower abdominal quadrant muscle-splitting incision for performing left colectomy was being challenged. For example, a Pfannenstiel incision affords direct visualization of the colorectal anastomosis fashioned at the level of the sacral promontory, thus obviating the requirement for reestablishing a pneumoperitoneum prior to performing the anastomosis (Figure 19-7).[17] In 2005, Chang

and coworkers popularized hand-assisted laparoscopic sigmoid colectomy using this incision.[41]

At first glance, one might interpret that the earlier literature seemed to be focused on technical feasibility. However, as early as 1992, Wexner and colleagues reported no immediately recognizable benefits for patients undergoing laparoscopic total colectomy, shifting the focus to that of clinical outcomes.[221] That same year, Pezet and coworkers warned about seeding the abdominal wall during laparoscopic cholecystectomy for gallbladder cancer.[165] In 1993, their report was echoed by a number of case reports of incisional recurrences after laparoscopic surgery for colon cancer.[5,77,160,219] Although the 1994 American Society of Colon and Rectal Surgeons registry data published an incisional recurrence rate of 0.4% after laparoscopic surgery for colon cancer,[174] the aforementioned anecdotal reports generated widespread concern. Colorectal surgeons in Europe and in the United States went back to the laboratory generating at least 72 articles on animal studies, the validity of which has been questioned.[15] In Norway, the consensus was not to attempt laparoscopic surgery for cure of colon cancer prior to level 1 evidence becoming available.[25] Eventually, the results of three adequately powered, randomized controlled trials reported no significant differences in oncologic outcomes at 3- and 5-year follow-up.[88,154,217] Although all three randomized controlled trials did not include transverse colon cancer, the Medical Research Council conventional versus laparoscopic-assisted surgery in colorectal cancer (CLASICC) trial did incorporate patients with rectal cancer and concluded that routine use of laparoscopic surgery for rectal cancer is *not* justified.[88,103] As of this

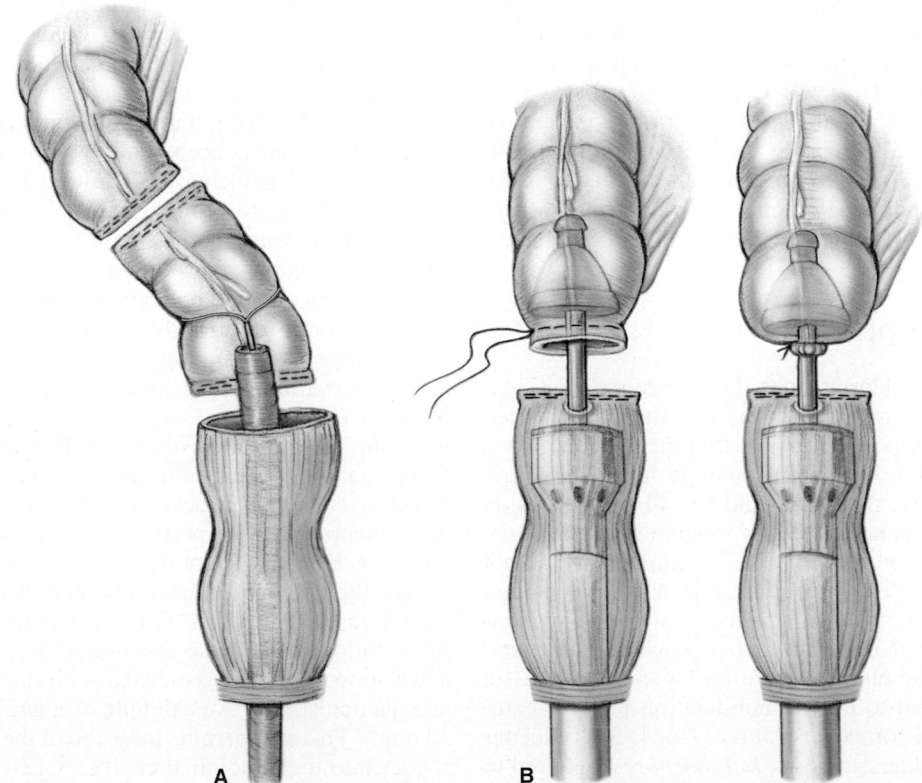

FIGURE 19-2. **A:** Colonoscopic snare transanal retrieval of specimen. **B:** Laparoscopic double-stapled colorectal anastomosis.

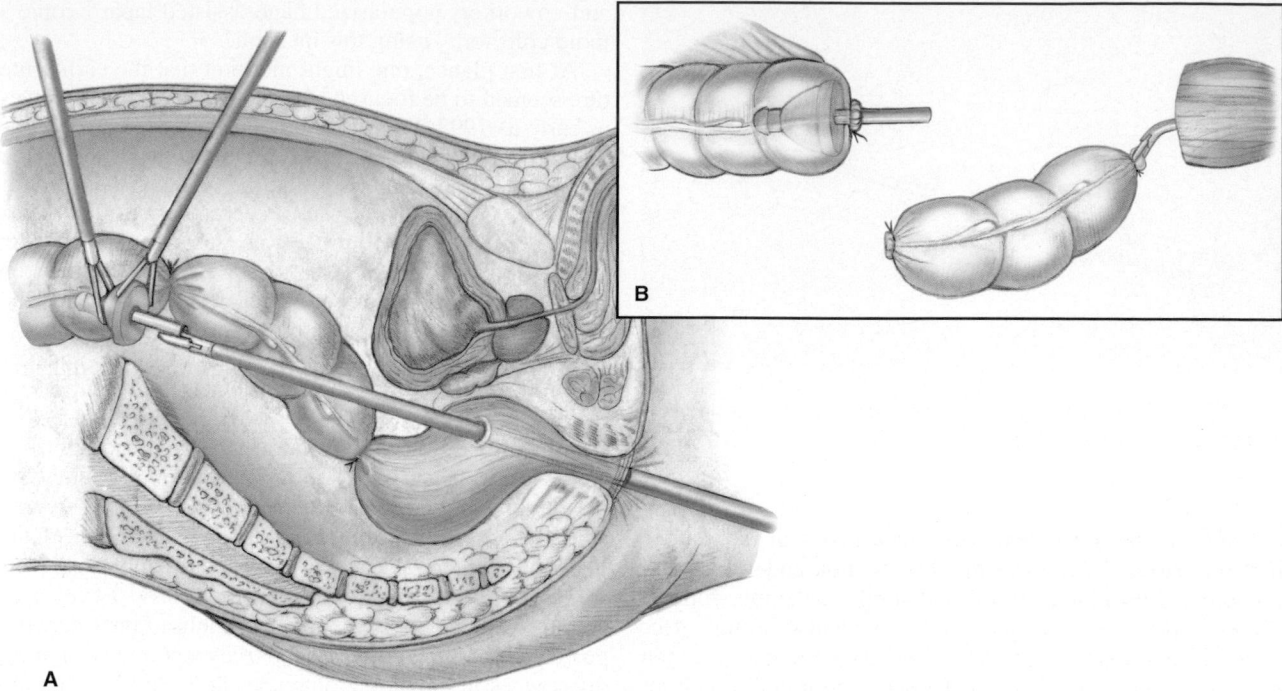

FIGURE 19-3. A: Proctotomy performed in order to insert the anvil into the peritoneal cavity and proximal colon. **B:** Retrieval of specimen by means of transanal endoscopic microsurgery (TEM) rigid scope. (Redrawn after Mentges B, Buess G, Schäfer D, et al. Transanal endoscopic microsurgery and combined operations. In: Moreno-González E, Escartín P, Lygidakis NJ, eds. *Joint Meeting of Surgery, Gastroenterology and Endoscopy.* Madrid, Spain: Jarpyo; 1995:339–345.)

writing, at least two randomized controlled trials are evaluating laparoscopic surgery for rectal cancer.[23]

The 20th century saw the development of an organized approach to performing laparoscopic colorectal surgery. For example, Senagore pioneered standardization of surgical technique, introducing sequential operative steps for accomplishing sigmoid colectomy.[197] Evolution of laparoscopic right colectomy resulted initially in performing 5 operative steps,[231] then 8,[196] and ultimately 10.[27] "Hindered" or facilitated, gasless or with gas, extracorporeal or intracorporeal, multiple- or single-port laparoscopic colon and rectal surgery is still evolving, with many more authors and players entering the fray.

▶ INTRODUCTION

Twenty years have elapsed since the first reports on laparoscopic colectomy appeared in the literature.[75,101,193] Yet, readers might be surprised to know that there has not been a consistent use of a defined terminology in the literature. When in its infancy, there was understandable confusion regarding the nomenclature, mostly reflecting its evolution. The term *laparoscopic facilitated*,[180] although it did not gain popularity, described exteriorizing the colon through a limited laparotomy following lateral-to-medial mobilization. The term *laparoscopic-assisted*, however, appeared frequently in the literature, indicating laparoscopic vessel ligation with medial-to-lateral mobilization prior to exteriorizing the bowel for *extracorporeal* (for lack of a better term) resection and anastomosis. *Intracorporeal* referred to the adoption of laparoscopic bowel transection and laparoscopic anastomosis with specimen retrieval in a plastic bag. Even the term *minimally invasive* (which could function as

an umbrella term, encompassing all such concepts) has been challenged by the supporters of the phrase *minimal access surgery*. It is now recognized that defined terminology is a prerequisite for allowing a meaningful flow of information for any nascent field to develop and grow. For example, NOTES is an acronym for natural orifice transluminal endoscopic surgery, which is actually endoscopic surgery, an established concept that does not include skin incisions.[2] Curiously, the one concept that seems intuitive, and one that would not need an elaborate definition, has generated a publication dedicated to define surgery performed through a single port (laparoendoscopic single site [LESS]).[83] Currently, LESS colectomy is considered a "boutique procedure," a niche, or specialized application (from French for "shop," via Latin from Greek ἀποθήκη [apothēkē], "storehouse").[134] On the subject of etymology, the definition of a trocar (variant: *trochar*; from French: alteration of *trois-carré* from *trois* [three] + *carré* [square]—i.e., "three-edged," triangular) and its evolution is an interesting one. The term initially identified a cannula several millimeters in diameter. Later, it was broadened to include trocars several centimeters in diameter. Needlescopic surgery performed using instruments with a diameter of 2 mm did not represent an option for conducting minimally invasive colorectal surgery because of technical limitations of the optics. Other concerns include improper illumination, inadequate resolution, and lack of clarity, in addition to problems associated with instrument sturdiness and manipulability. An example of a larger port is that of a 33 mm.[20] This size permits insertion of the anvil of a circular stapler into the abdominal cavity. A 12-cm port allows insertion of the surgeon's hand. Interestingly, these two large ports reflect opposite visions. The former is the intracorporeal vision with the unresolved issue of specimen extraction.

Colorectal anastomosis following laparoscopic left colon resection differs from its right-sided counterpart because the rectum cannot be exteriorized. Following proximal colon transection, a purse-string suture of the proximal colon end may be hand-sewn extracorporeally. The laparoscopic, intracorporeal, hand-sewn purse-string suture, although feasible, has not become popular among colorectal surgeons, mainly because of lack of training in laparoscopic suturing. The advent of robotic technology will most likely have an impact on implementation of intracorporeal suturing with its requisite intracorporeal knot-tying. In fact, the robot has given back to surgeons the two degrees of freedom lost by the use of laparoscopic, nonwristed instrumentation. Nevertheless, the fact remains that safe specimen extraction still requires at least the enlargement of a port site incision unless transvaginal NOSE is considered in female patients.[162] As mentioned, the port allowing insertion of the surgeon's hand reflects a different vision for accomplishing laparoscopic surgery. However, hand-assisted laparoscopic surgery (HALS) does provide reasonable solutions to some legitimate concerns. For example, HALS allows manual palpation of a rectal tumor for providing adequate distal transection of the rectum as well as decreased operating time for laparoscopic total colectomy by expediting transverse colon mobilization and safe vessel ligation.[130]

This chapter represents current opinion on the impact of laparoscopic colon and rectal surgery performed with

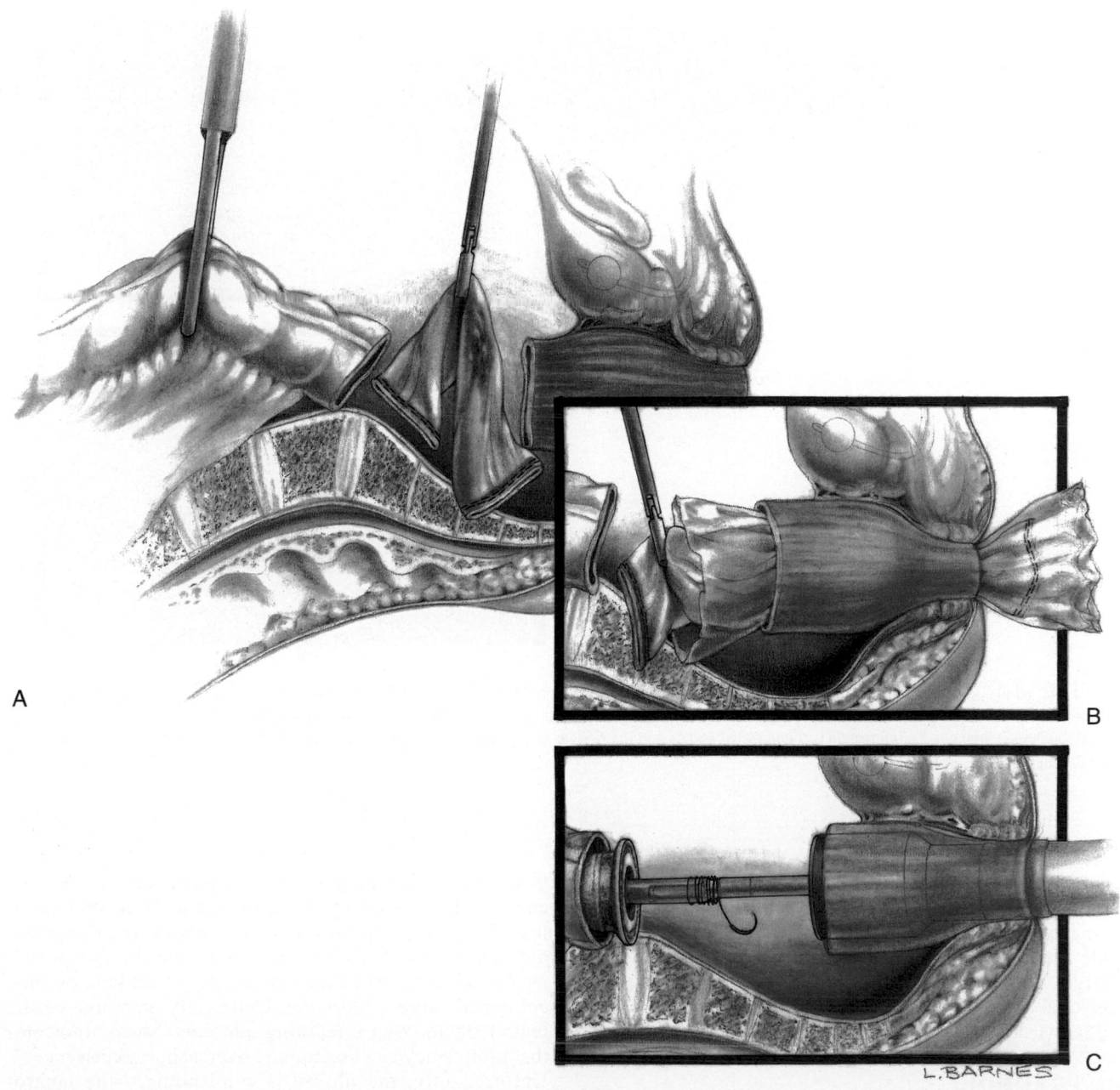

FIGURE 19-4. Intracorporeal anastomotic technique. **A:** The proximal bowel is occluded, and the specimen stapled at both resection margins. **B:** A plastic bag is introduced through the rectum. It is then opened to receive the specimen, which is then withdrawn. **C:** The circular stapler is inserted into the rectum. A suture is secured to the anvil. *(continued)*

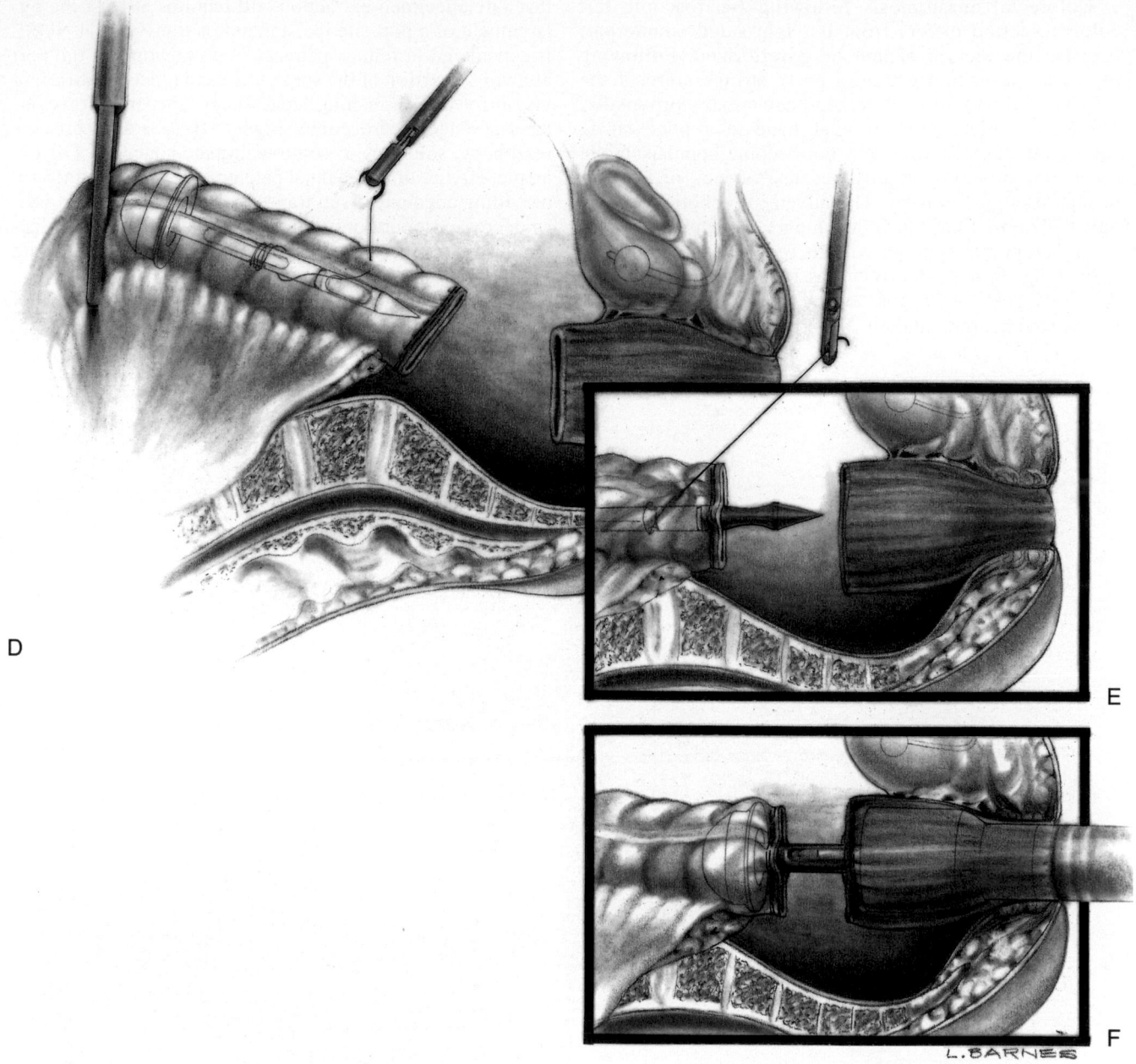

FIGURE 19-4. *(continued)* **D:** The anvil is placed into the proximal colon, and the circular stapler is withdrawn from the anus. The suture is passed from within the bowel lumen to provide a "handle." The proximal bowel is stapled. **E:** The anvil is controlled by means of the suture and brought through the staple line. The staple line is then cut. **F:** The rectum is then stapled across and the circular stapler inserted in accordance with the standard, "double-stapling" technique (see Chapter 24).

pneumoperitoneum through multiple ports on several diseases of the colon and rectum. Herein, however, no attempt is made to provide a systematic review of the evidence available in the literature because the objective is to present an insight into laparoscopic surgical techniques, the authors' personal opinions, and an overview of the literature dealing with this subject.

▶ LEARNING

The subject of learning the technique for performing any surgery, especially that of laparoscopic colorectal surgery,

is of paramount concern and importance. A *learning curve* is defined as a graphical description of the rate of learning.[181] Initially introduced in educational psychology, these two words have acquired considerable prominence and have been used extensively in the laparoscopic colorectal surgery literature. Classically, it is noteworthy that characterizing a learning curve as "steep" indicates that proficiency can be attained over a short experience.[175] Unfortunately, the phrase is a misnomer—the laparoscopic colorectal surgery literature refers to a steep learning curve as indicative of the opposite—that is, a rather long time for acquiring the skill.

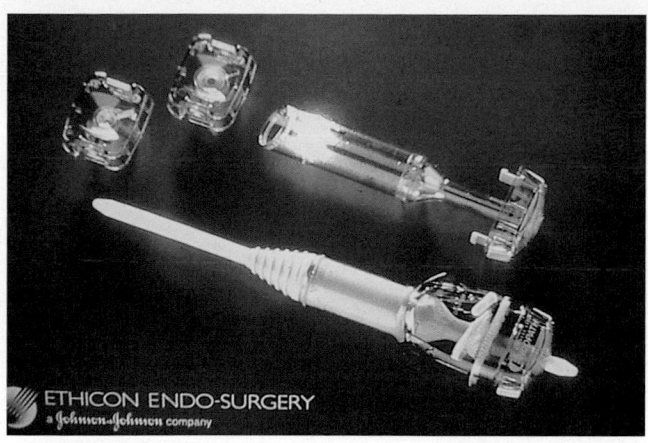

FIGURE 19-5. A 33-mm port with obturator. (Courtesy of Ethicon Endo-Surgery.)

Goodness of Fit Metrics

The goodness of fit of a given model describes how the model fits a set of data.[194] The term, *goodness of fit*, is used here as an analogy to characterize the complexity of evaluating the learning curve in laparoscopic colorectal surgery. The metrics used in the literature to appraise the learning curve include operating time, conversion rates, and complication rates. However, readmission rates should probably be added. A study involving chronologic groups reported a decrease in operating time from 250 to 156 minutes over the first 75 cases, following which operating time remained stagnant.[227] Another study observed that surgeons were getting faster despite the increasing complexities of caseloads, suggesting improved skills.[1] Dinçler and associates suggested shifting the focus from solely decreased operating time to a multidimensional analysis, which would take into account the conversion and complication rates as well.[60] Chen and colleagues came to the conclusion that operating time seemed to be a poor surrogate for evaluating the learning curve.[43] Thus, the question becomes, *Do we need to get faster?*[227]

Conversion to open surgery has also been viewed as a metric for evaluating the learning curve. There are, however, a number of other factors impacting on conversion rates, such as a patient's American Society of Anesthesiologist (ASA) and body mass index (BMI) scores, the type of resection; operative findings, such as the presence of an internal fistula and/or an intra-abdominal abscess; and more.[206] The complication rate is probably the single most important metric. Bennet and coworkers reported a significant decrease in postoperative complication rates after one performs 40 operations.[16] Reissman and colleagues showed that complication rates were significantly higher after total colectomy (42%) as compared with segmental colectomy (19%) and nonresectional procedures (12%).[176]

So what is the magic number? Several studies have been published in an attempt to identify that figure. Although Simons and associates suggested 11 to 15 procedures in

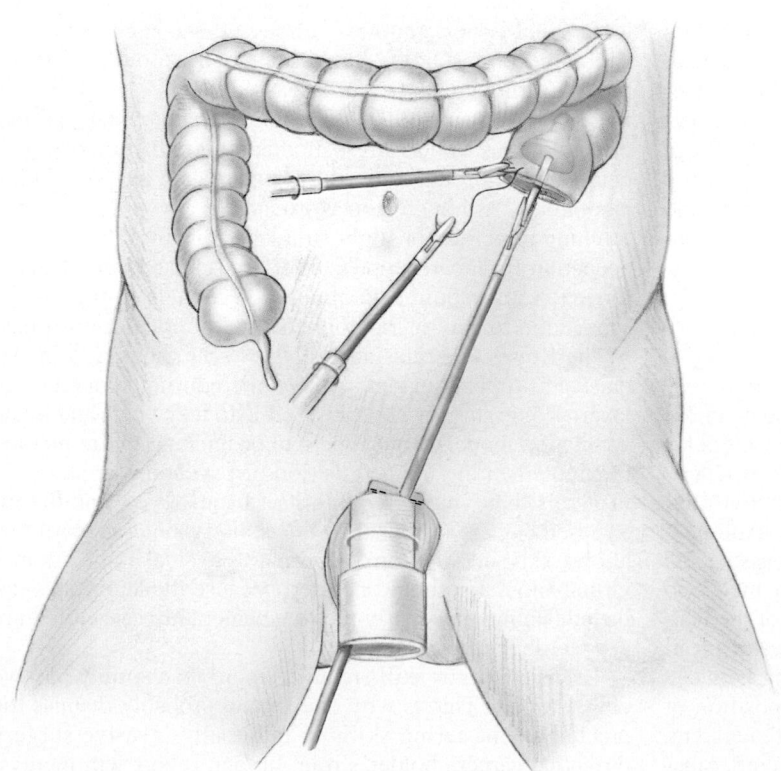

FIGURE 19-6. Insertion of anvil through 33-mm suprapubic port and intracorporeal hand-sewn purse-string suture.

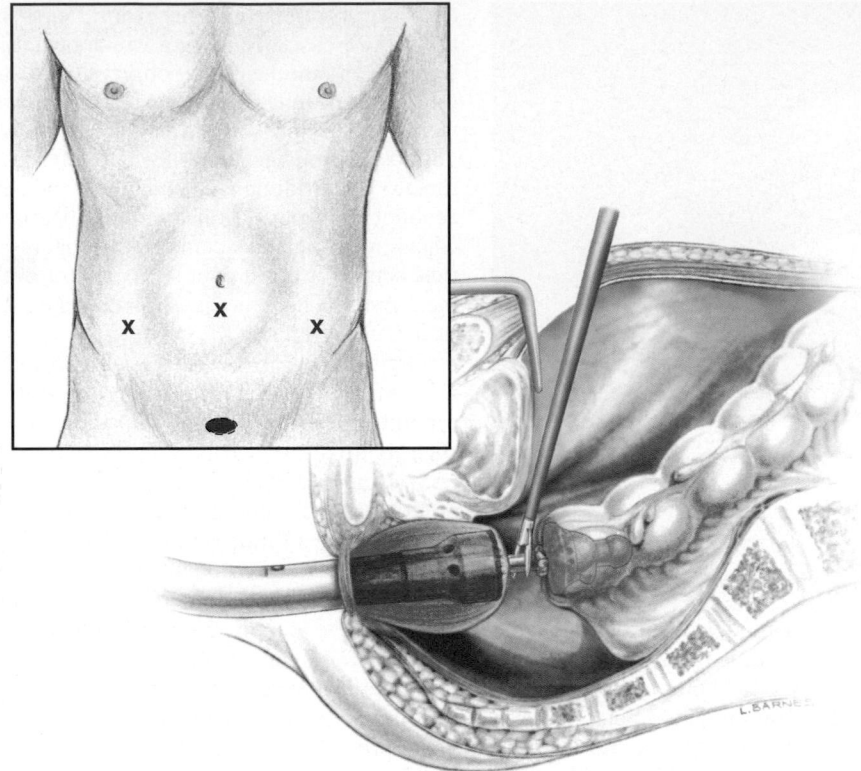

FIGURE 19-7. Conventional colorectal anastomosis through a suprapubic incision without reestablishing a pneumo-peritoneum.

1995,[201] that same year Wishner and colleagues increased that number to 35 to 50.[227] A decade later, Tekkis and coworkers estimated 55 right colectomies and 62 left colectomies to be the "right numbers."[207] Interestingly, both COST (Clinical Outcomes of Surgical Therapy) and COLOR (Colon Cancer Laparoscopic or Open Resection) trials required participating surgeons to perform 20 laparoscopic colectomies before entering patients in the trials. In conclusion, there is truly a "poorness of fit" in comparing learning models to the literature data with respect to the learning curve in laparoscopic colorectal surgery.

Simulation

Psychomotor Skills

Surgical training remains to a great extent, even today, mired in William Halsted's century-old apprenticeship model.[90] Although in the past the Halstedian method has produced generations of fine technical surgeons, its adequacy for training future laparoscopic surgeons is questionable. Among a number of possible factors, such as the problems associated with the fulcrum effect, the loss of tactile sensation, increased complexity of the techniques, less independence of the residents, shorter work hours, the most important factor probably is the disruption of the constrained coupling between the surgeon's hands and eyes through the interposition of a video camera, moving independently. Thus, although cut, sew, and tie remain the staples of one's surgical craft, laparoscopic surgery requires the development of a new skill set. Several factors including random educational opportunities,

concern for the patient, time constraints, surreptitious dissection by the attending surgeon or faculty, distractions, interpersonal issues, and cost, among others, suggest that the operating room (OR) is a suboptimal classroom to obtain a proper learning experience, at least initially.

Training outside of the OR offers a structured educational opportunity as well as stress modulation (reduction of a resident's stress through procedures undertaken in a simulation laboratory). Although isoperformance is a well-documented teaching principle for flight simulation, its introduction into education for laparoscopic surgery raises the issue of transferring skills acquired in simulation models to the OR. A systematic review of randomized and nonrandomized data by the Royal Australasian College of Surgeons was inconclusive as to what extent skills learned during simulation in laparoscopic surgery are transferable to the OR.[204] Inanimate simulation models would seem to be an appropriate method for implementing the acquisition of psychomotor skills. In fact, it is the dynamic coupling of hands, eyes, and the interposed camera (rather than the static graphic display) that allows skill acquisition. Inanimate physical rather than a virtual simulator should be used because the latter does not include an independently moving camera nor does it feature any tactile feedback.[104]

Learning motor skills requires more than simply passive observation.[21] That is why one should probably dismiss the practice of mastering skills in minimally invasive surgery through a camera holder's role. In fact, robots will increasingly hold the telescope and allow the surgeon to steer an otherwise independently moving camera.[212]

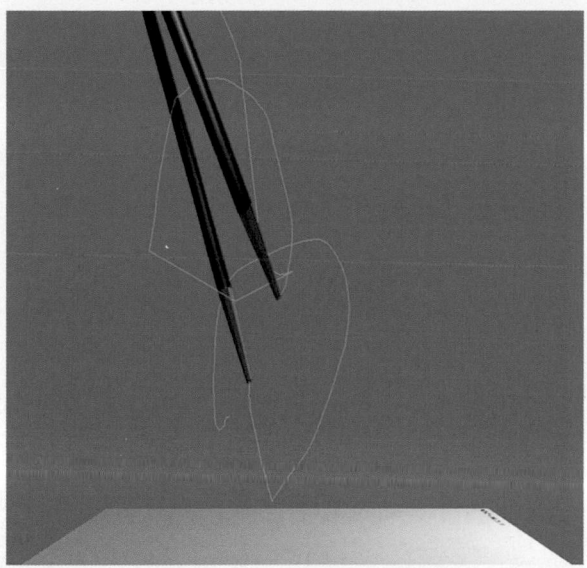
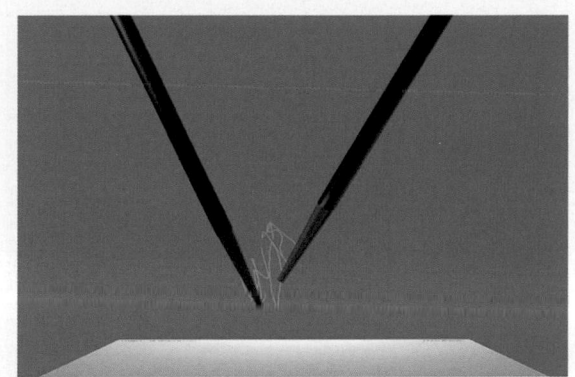

FIGURE 19-8. **A:** Path length, the measurement in millimeters of the movement of the laparoscopic instrument tips during simulation, as used by a novice; **(B)** as used by an expert.

The process of acquisition of motor skills may be broken down into three phases.[108] Both stand-up and CD-ROM tutorials are adequate for task understanding (phase 1). The interaction between task practicing (phase 2) and feedback is essential to skill acquisition. (For phase 3, see Procedural Skills.) Novices compare their own performance to that of CD-ROM to minimize the difference (internal feedback). Experts (external feedback) provide learners with information about the procedure's effectiveness and quality of the operative end product. The former can be evaluated by objective assessment of a number of outcome measures (goal- and nongoal-directed actions, forces and torques, and operating time), and the latter can be assessed by end product analysis (accuracy error, tissue damage, water tightness, etc.). The reported poor correlation between the two may indicate that a range of pattern of movements may result in a similar quality of end product. A number of advantages (construct validity, time and cost efficiency, resident autonomy in performance, and reduced examiner bias) suggest that product analysis is suited for skill assessment despite its low reliability. There is no consensus on which dexterity drills should be incorporated into simulation models for the acquisition of motor skills.[18] Reliability and validity (content, construct, criterion, concurrent, and predictive) of current simulation models have been evaluated only to a limited extent.[54]

Metrics

A fundamental issue for training with simulators has been the need for metrics.[52] Examples of previously validated content-valid metrics include accuracy error, knot slippage, leakage, operating time, and tissue damage.[213] Hybrid simulators (combination of real instruments and box trainer with computer monitoring) offer software-generated metrics not available in the operating room, such as path length (Figure 19-8) and smoothness of laparoscopic instrument movement. However, studies have shown no correlation between simulator-generated metrics and content-valid metrics except for operating time.[40] Most simulation studies compare metrics at baseline testing with metrics at unmentored final testing. This is the definition of responsiveness, which is a change in performance over time.[95,207] Nonetheless, additional challenges to the validity of any simulation metrics derive from the so-called ceiling effect, learning the drill without acquiring the skill.

Procedural Skills

A stepwise draft for learning outside of the OR involves the acquisition of procedural skills without distinct cognitive awareness (phase 3). Learning the setup and exposure for a surgical procedure requires simulation models, such as anatomical. Ethical issues, limited availability, and high costs have limited the use of live animal or fresh human cadaver models. An alternative bench model consists of en bloc resected fresh animal organs placed in a simulator and artificially perfused. Whether this model has the potential for transferring skills to the OR remains to be proven, particularly in the specific case of colorectal surgery. Currently, hybrid simulators specially designed for laparoscopic colorectal surgery feature an anal opening (Figure 19-9) and include a disposable abdominal tray (Figure 19-10). Unfortunately, the human anatomy associated with such trays is questionably accurate and valid and is costly. Nevertheless, simulation studies with laparoscopic sigmoidectomy have reported good responsiveness among surgery residents, with significantly decreased operating time and lower anastomotic leak rates.[70]

Recently, task analysis of skills involved in laparoscopic colorectal surgery has been performed according to the Likert scale* and the Delphi process†.[188] When responding to a Likert questionnaire item, individuals specify their level of agreement or disagreement on a symmetric agree–disagree

---

*A Likert scale is commonly used in research. It employs questionnaires such as survey research.
†The Delphi process is a structured communication technique for a panel of experts.

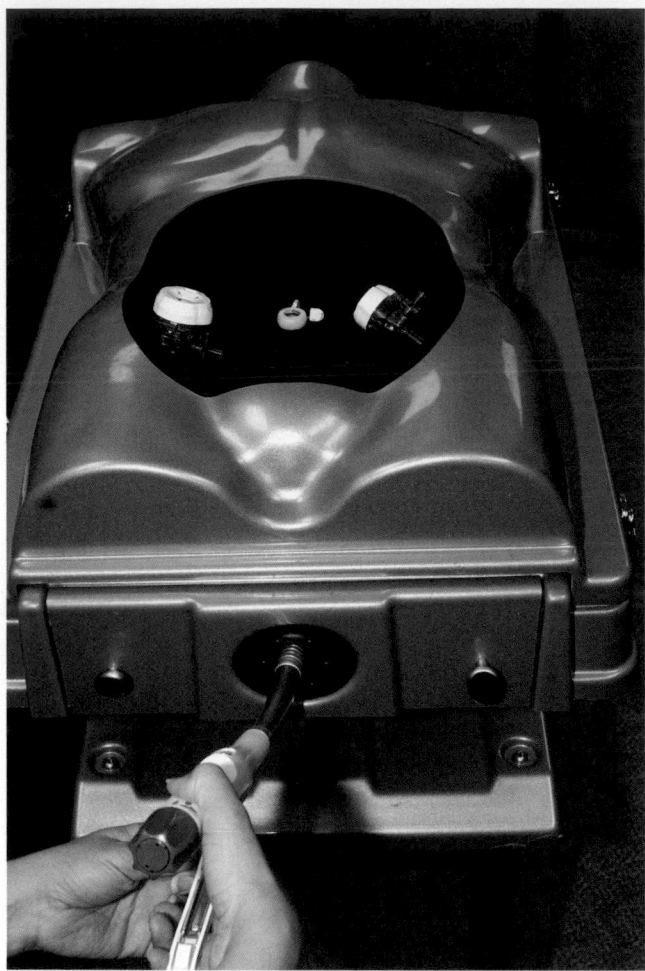

FIGURE 19-9. Hybrid simulator allowing transanal anastomosis.

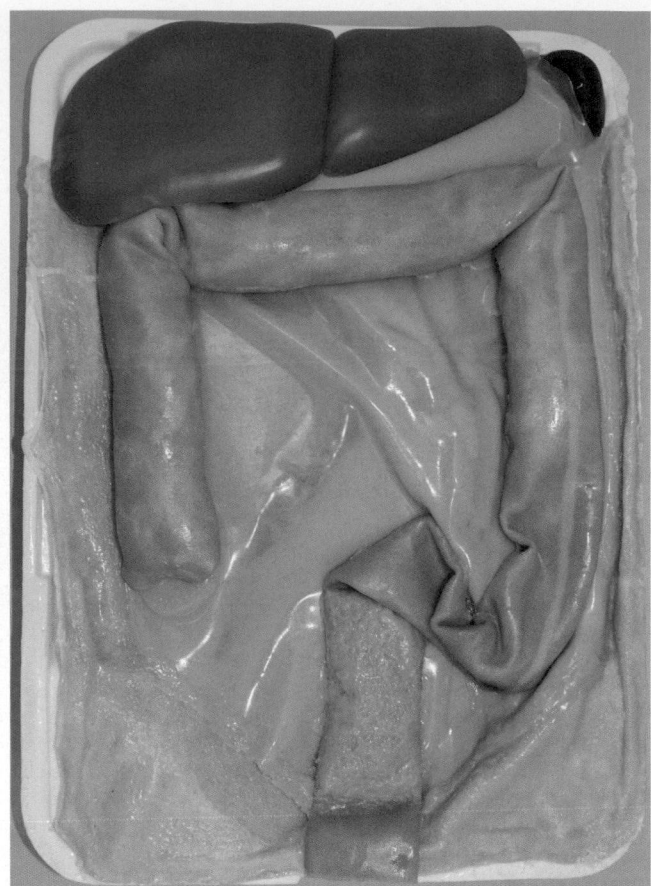

FIGURE 19-10. Abdominal tray.

scale for a series of statements. Delphi is based on the principle that decisions from a structured group of individuals are more accurate than those from unstructured groups. The experts answer questionnaires in two or more rounds. After each round, a facilitator provides an anonymous summary of the experts' decisions from the previous round as well as the reasons they provided for their judgments. Thus, experts are encouraged to revise their earlier answers in light of the replies of other members of their panel. Simulation research is an educational challenge that requires a change of attitude in the surgical community in addition to funding.[178] The primary end point of educational research studies should be to provide evidence that proper instruction has an impact on the quality of patient care.

▶ OPERATING ROOM

The First Port

Safe access to the abdominal cavity is the initial critical step during surgery. Although surgeons may have a personal preference for the open or the blind (Veress) technique, the fact remains that many of the access-related complications are due to the first trocar insertion. The Hasson technique was initially described as an alternative for accessing the abdominal cavity in previously operated

patients (Figure 19-11).[93] By choosing a cutdown approach, the surgeon can introduce a blunt tip trocar into the abdominal cavity under direct visualization, as opposed to a blind entry with the Veress needle. In fact, most surgeons favor a cutdown technique for reoperative surgery.

When dealing with a reoperation, it is advisable to avoid scars because the risk of inadvertent injury to intra-abdominal organs is increased. Assuming that the patient will undergo a midline laparotomy, the most frequently encountered scenario, the initial trocar should be placed

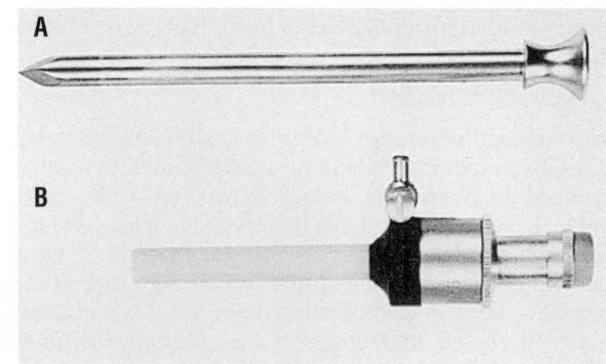

FIGURE 19-11. Reusable Hasson port. **A:** Sharp obturator. **B:** Cannula with a 12 mm in diameter.

lateral to the rectus muscle sheath in the midpoint between the lower edge of the rib cage and the anterior superior iliac spine along the anterior axillary line. The surgeon must also be careful not to place the trocar too far laterally because of the risk of injuring the descending colon. Detailed awareness of the patient's prior abdominal operations will, of course, assist in determining which side of the abdomen the first trocar should be placed. For example, if the patient is to undergo a left colectomy, the first trocar should be inserted on the right side of the abdomen. The opposite concept is true for surgeries performed on the right side of the patient. Optical access trocar systems have been developed, which allow the surgeon to visualize the abdominal wall layers as the trocar enters the peritoneal cavity. These ports are made with the intention of minimizing organ injury while gaining laparoscopic access. There are currently two optical view trocars: one of them uses a blade and the other uses a rotating, sharp, plastic, clear tip, both under direct laparoscopic view. Regardless of what type of trocar the surgeon chooses, the insertion technique should involve minimal force and *consistent direct visualization.*

Vascular Injuries

Although the Hasson technique will not completely eliminate the risk for major vascular injuries, there is evidence that suggests this risk is decreased. Although vascular injuries are rare, they must be recognized and repaired by means of an immediate laparotomy. Prior to converting, the surgeon may attempt to control the bleeding vessel with a laparoscopic Satinsky clamp. Much of the evidence related to vascular injuries secondary to laparoscopic trocar insertion comes from case reports. In a review of 629 trocar incident reports, 408 cases were associated with major vascular injuries, resulting in 26 deaths. The vessels most commonly injured were the aorta (23%) and the vena cava (15%).[32] Optical view ports had been used, which indicates that such accessories cannot completely prevent trocar insertion-related injuries.

Bowel Injuries

Unfortunately, neither the rate of bowel injuries nor related death rates have been reduced by the Hasson technique. It is worth repeating that the Hasson approach should be employed at a site away from preexisting scars. In fact, 40% of bowel injuries have been reported to be due to insertion of additional trocars. Therefore, insertion of ports must be performed under direct vision with sufficient intraperitoneal space. This entails adequate relaxation of the abdominal wall musculature by the anesthesiologist.

Pneumoperitoneum

There is no question about the need for adequate pneumoperitoneum. Surgeons should have a thought process that evaluates all possible causes of insufficient pneumoperitoneum. Once all common causes are ruled out, the surgeon should communicate with the anesthesiologist to ensure that proper paralysis of the anterior abdominal wall has been provided. It is beneficial for patients to be operated on with the lowest possible intra-abdominal pressure. In fact, there is very little difference in the exposure provided with 10 versus 15 mm Hg.[157] If the operation is performed mostly in the pelvis, it may be sufficient to operate with an intra-abdominal pressure of less than 10 mm Hg because the pelvis is a bony structure.

The surgeon must also take into account the patient's body habitus when inducing and maintaining pneumoperitoneum. An abdominal wall thickness of 10 cm or more will require a 15-cm long port, rather than the ordinary 10-cm length. If the trocar is too short for the abdominal wall thickness, insufflation of CO_2 will lead to subcutaneous emphysema with subsequent increase in tidal volume. Certain medical comorbidities such as chronic obstructive pulmonary disease, other respiratory diseases, and congestive heart failure are considered contraindications to prolonged pneumoperitoneum. In fact, as the intra-abdominal pressure increases, the splanchnic flow, cardiac output, and renal cortical blood flow all decrease.[97] An alternative for these patients may include the use of nitrous oxide or helium. However, one must consider that the former is combustible and the latter not soluble.

Laparoscope

There is usually no role for a 0-degree laparoscope for such complex procedures as colorectal surgery. The surgeon will often need to look around adhesions rather than straight forward. The minimal degree of angulation required is 30 degrees, but sometimes 45 degrees may prove to be useful. An alternative is the deflectable tip laparoscope (Figure 19-12). The camera holder should be familiar with the device. The authors' preference is to use a video laparoscope, as opposed to an optical system with an interphase between the instrument and the camera. In fact, the latter may be associated with fogging and sterility hazards when the hose is positioned. Furthermore, the surgeon should be aware that camera chips are located on the tip of the video laparoscope, as opposed to the classical system where the camera chip is outside the patient's abdomen.

Camera Holder

In laparoscopic surgery, the disruption of the constrained coupling between the surgeon's hands and eyes by the interposition of a camera, moving independently of the surgeon, is a drawback that is not encountered in conventional surgery. The camera is usually held by a junior resident or a medical student, and individual who may be unfamiliar

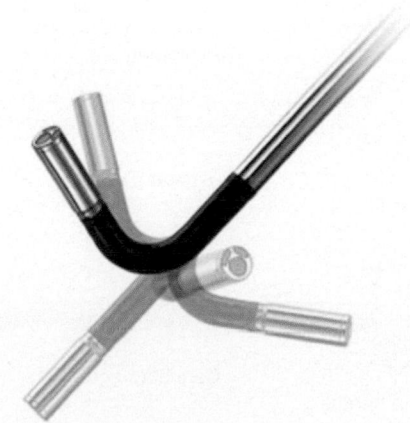

FIGURE 19-12. Deflectable tip laparoscope.

with the surgical procedure, who may be standing in an uncomfortable position, or who may be easily distracted. As a result, the camera may rotate away from the horizon and/or drift away from the surgical field, with the potential for increased risk of causing technical errors.[78] In fact, errors that lead to injury mostly stem from misperception rather than lack of knowledge or poor judgment.[220] Mechanical camera holders (passive or voice-controlled) may provide a more stable image and enable surgeons to control their own view direction.[102] Several reports have suggested that voice-controlled camera holders may offer advantages when compared with a human camera holder.[118,120,144,168,212]

Ports

A laparoscopic port represents, in itself, a limitation of laparoscopic surgery; this is known as the fulcrum effect. A port consists of a trocar and a cannula (Figure 19-13). In general, cannula sleeves should be transparent and threaded with no metallic parts in order to allow visual control, stability within the abdominal wall, and minimal electrical risk. Bladed trocars require a retractable shield to minimize the risk of injury to intra-abdominal organs. The insertion of additional trocars does not require an open access but should be performed under direct visualization. The geometry of multiple port placements on the anterior abdominal wall should be triangular whenever possible in order to avoid injuries to the inferior epigastric vessels. Following insertion of the first port, space in the abdominal cavity may be very limited if dense adhesions are present. In such a case, bladeless trocars are not recommended because they require significant force during insertion. This may result in inward tenting of the abdominal wall. Bladed trocars or ultrasonic-guided ports (Figure 19-14) are safer for reoperative surgery because excessive force is not required during insertion.

Instruments

Laparoscopic instruments offer only four degrees of freedom of movement (Figure 19-15), as opposed to that of the human hand. This is obviously because of the loss of the ability to move one's wrist (Figure 19-16). Surgeons have been traditionally using instruments with a finger loop handle, with in-line configuration to perform conventional surgery.

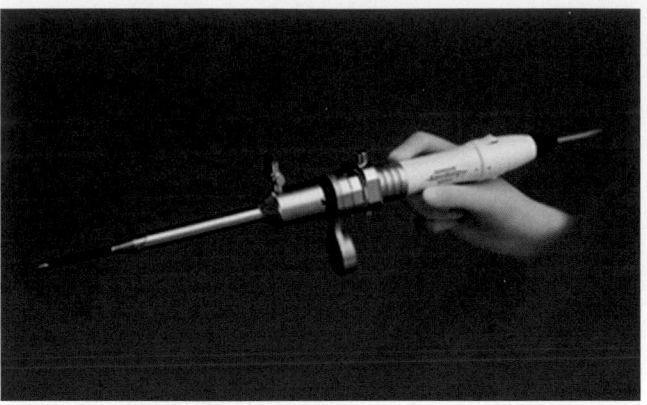

FIGURE 19-14. Ultrasonic-guided laparoscopic port.

In the early 1990s, disposable laparoscopic instruments became available, mostly with a pistol grip–shaped handle. Simulation evaluations as well as surveys report concern whether pistol grip handles meet standard ergonomic requirements.[137,216] However, studies measuring surgeon forearm workload by electromyogram have been inconclusive.[31,69,211] Eventually, reusable laparoscopic instruments became available, featuring various types of in-line handles.

Laparoscopic colorectal surgery may be reasonably safely accomplished with the aid of the following instruments: fenestrated bowel grasper with in-line handle (Figure 19-17) and without finger loops (Figure 19-18), right-angle clamp (Figure 19-19), curved scissors (Figure 19-20) with in-line ring handle (Figure 19-21), curved-tip needle driver (Figure 19-22) with in-line ring handle (Figure 19-23), and

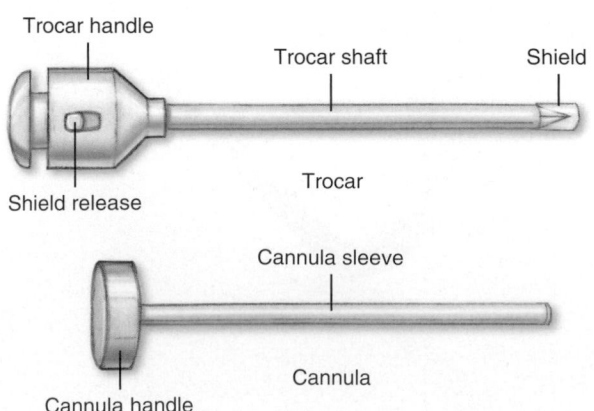

FIGURE 19-13. Laparoscopic port.

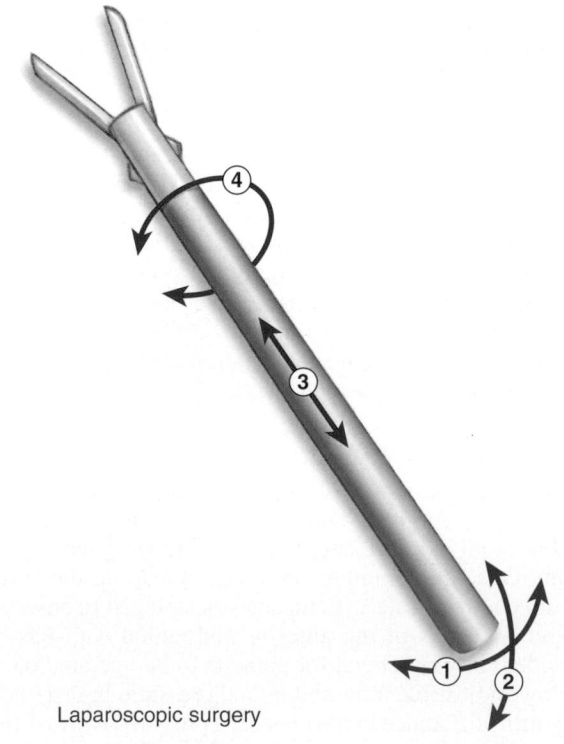

Laparoscopic surgery

FIGURE 19-15. Laparoscopic instrument with four degrees of freedom.

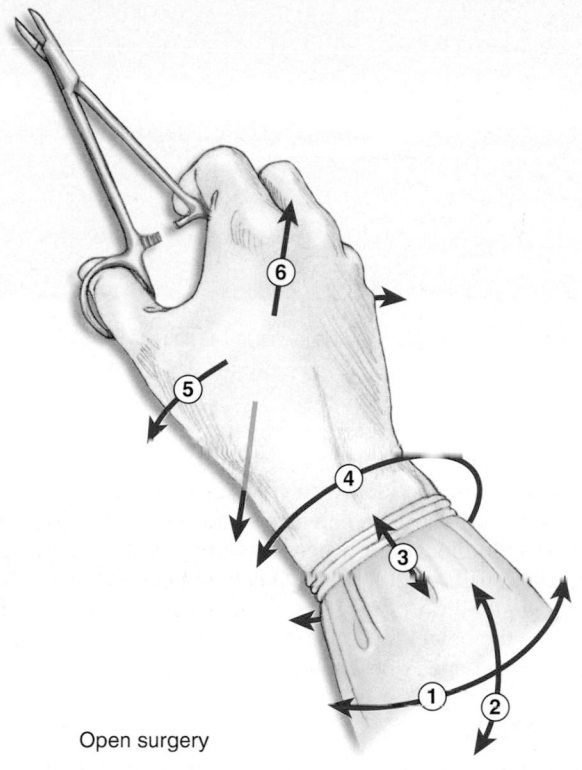

Open surgery

FIGURE 19-16. Human hand with six degrees of freedom.

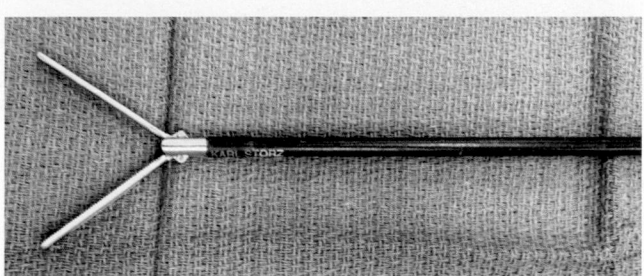

FIGURE 19-17. Laparoscopic fenestrated bowel grasper tip.

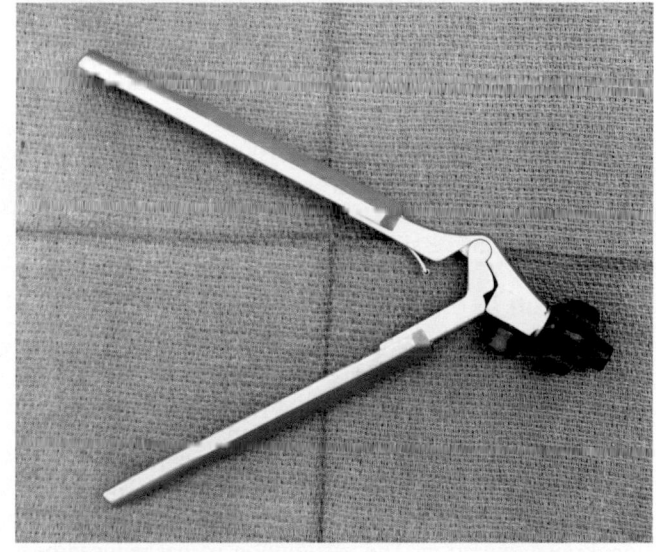

FIGURE 19-18. Bowel grasper in-line handle without finger loops.

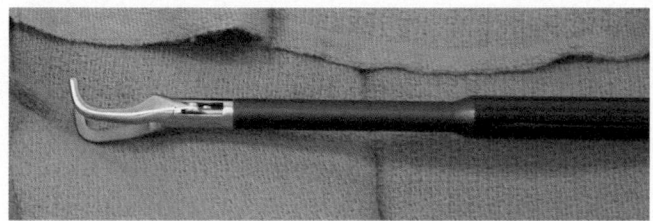

FIGURE 19-19. Right-angle clamp tip.

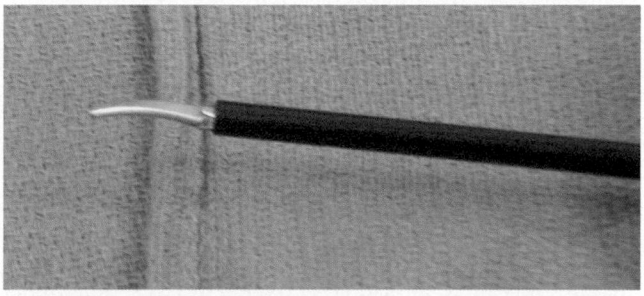

FIGURE 19-20. Curved scissors tip.

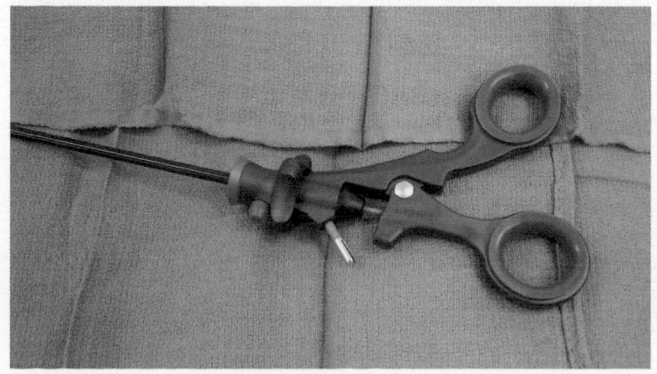

FIGURE 19-21. Curved scissors with in-line ring handle.

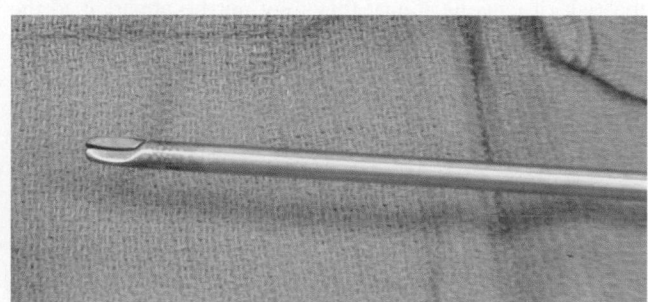

FIGURE 19-22. Needle driver with curved tip.

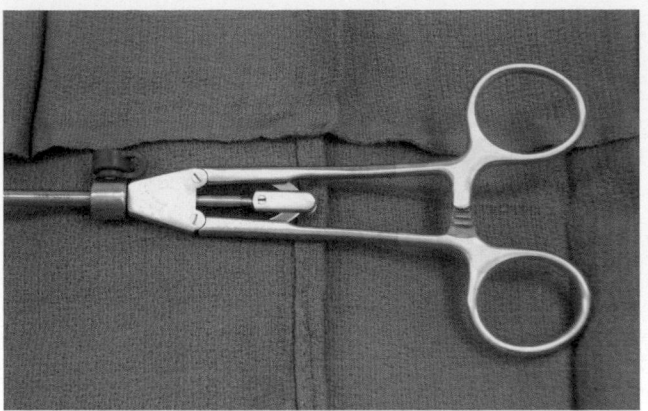

FIGURE 19-23. Needle driver with in-line ring handle.

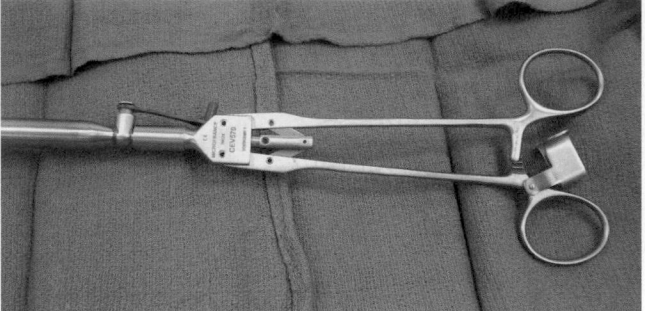

FIGURE 19-25. Satinsky vascular clamp in-line ring handle.

Satinsky vascular clamp (Figure 19-24) with in-line ring handle (Figure 19-25). Laparoscopic instruments are currently available in short (more than 30 cm) and long (more than 40 cm) shaft versions.

Dissection

Sharp dissection with cold instruments is undoubtedly the standard. Blunt dissection should be considered in laparoscopic surgery only after an areolar plane has been accessed by gentle traction applied with a laparoscopic "peanut" dissector. In the case of fused planes in between organs, surgeons should not be tempted to apply force with laparoscopic instruments and should convert to HALS or conventional open operation. The assumption is that reduced heat production may minimize thermal tissue damage.[30] The use of monopolar coagulation devices should be discouraged for dissection purposes because of the high risk of thermal tissue damage. Multifunctionality and reduced heat production are among the appealing features that made ultrasonic-activated devices attractive for use in laparoscopic surgery. These allow coagulation and cutting, thereby minimizing the need for frequent instrument changes and may contribute to reducing operating time. It has been confirmed in animal models that heat production by ultrasonic-activated devices is decreased when compared with the heat generated by monopolar coagulation. The assumption is that reduced heat production may minimize thermal tissue damage.[30] There are currently three ultrasonic-activated devices: AutoSonix (Tyco, Pembroke, Bermuda), SonoSurg (Olympus, Tokyo, Japan), and UltraCision (Johnson & Johnson, Cincinnati, OH)—see Table 19-1. The use of ultrasonic-activated devices near hollow organs must be discouraged because of the risk of causing injury that may not be apparent to the surgeon, such as to the small bowel and ureter. Adhesions

between the anterior abdominal wall and intra-abdominal organs should be divided with cold scissors. In cases of extremely dense adhesions between small bowel loops and the anterior abdominal wall, where it is not possible to create a safe plane of dissection, it may become necessary to excise en bloc a small portion of the parietal peritoneum in order to release the bowel loop. This, of course, may be necessary even when an open operation is performed.

Hemostasis

In conventional surgery, vessels are secured with either ties or suture ligation prior to being severed. Suturing and knotting techniques in laparoscopic surgery, however, have not been embraced by the majority of surgeons. The adoption of laparoscopic clips has gained considerable popularity, but clips can limit one's application of staplers. The inherent tedium of mastering intracorporeal knot-tying techniques probably accounts for greater interest in energy-based alternatives.

In the early 1990s, laparoscopic vessel-sealing devices became available as a safe option to divide arteries up to 7 mm in diameter (Figure 19-26). Burst pressure testing in animal models has demonstrated that 3 to 7 mm arteries managed with ties, clips, or vessel-sealing devices can withstand a maximum pressure of 900 mm Hg.[110] Interestingly, the same experiment reported that 3 to 7 mm arteries managed with ultrasonic-activated devices could burst at pressures less than 100 mm Hg. Nevertheless, there are no data regarding safety of laparoscopic vessel-sealing devices when applied to large, calcified arteries.

Hemostasis can be a challenge in laparoscopic surgery. Excessive bleeding may be due to preexisting comorbidities, intraoperative findings, and such is not uncommon during reoperations. Adhesions can alter the anatomy that may complicate dissection. Medications such as cortisone, thrombocyte aggregation inhibitors, and anticoagulants can decrease tissue consistency and increase the risk of oozing that can impede the view. Bleeding due to intraoperative findings tends to occur with inadequate exposure or inability to appropriately manipulate the tissue or to equipment failure. Prevention of bleeding begins with correctly understanding the anatomy and choice of the appropriate instruments. The following materials for management of hemostasis should be available in the operating room, especially for reoperative cases: clips, collagen fleece, coagulation (bipolar and monopolar), endoloops, fibrin adhesive, sutures, and a vessel-sealing device.

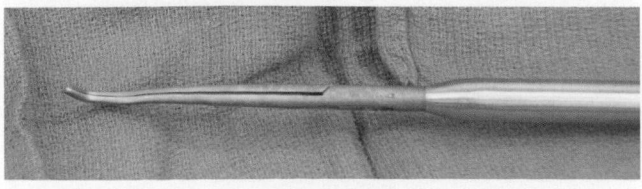

FIGURE 19-24. Satinsky vascular clamp tip.

TABLE 19-1 Comparison of Characteristics and Settings of Three Ultrasonic-Activated Devices

	AUTOSONIX	SONOSURG	ULTRACISION
Active blade			
Length (mm)	13	15.5	15
Type	Blunt	Blunt	Blunt
Cutting mechanism	Increase power	Increase power	Increase power
Handle ergonomics	Pistol grip	Pistol grip	Pistol grip
Vibration setting			
Amplitude (mm)	70	100	80
Frequency (kHz)	55.5	23.5	55.5
Use	Disposable	Reusable	Disposable
Working shaft			
Axial rotation	Available	Available	Unavailable
Diameter (mm)	5	11	10
Length (mm)	29	33	34

From Bergamaschi R, Yavuz Y, Marvik R. Laparoscopic bowel resection: a comparison of three ultrasonically activated devices. *JSLS*. 2003;7(1):19–22.

It should be axiomatic that every member of the operating room staff, before assisting, should attend an in-service session or sessions for all devices. The operating room team including the scrub and circulating nurses should discuss preoperatively the algorithms established to handle acute bleeding events and especially to familiarize themselves with the nomenclature of the devices. For example, in the case of a spurting vessel, the camera holder should immediately retract the telescope into the port to avoid obstruction of view. The surgeon should apply compression with his or her nondominant hand to temporarily control the bleeding. For venous bleeding, compression can be achieved with a small sponge introduced into the abdomen via a 10-mm trocar. Bleeding from arteries with a diameter of 7 mm or less can be controlled by using endoloops, clips, suture ligation with intracorporeal knot-tying, or vessel-sealing devices. Before final hemostasis is ensured, it is necessary to ascertain that the bleeding vessel is "expendable." If the vessel is not expendable, a laparoscopic Satinsky vascular clamp should be applied temporarily to achieve vascular control while a laparotomy is performed in preparation for vascular reconstruction. Oozing from the liver, pancreas, spleen, mesentery, or retroperitoneum can be treated effectively by compression and definitive hemostasis with collagen fleece and a fibrin adhesive. Before a hemostyptic is applied, compression should be

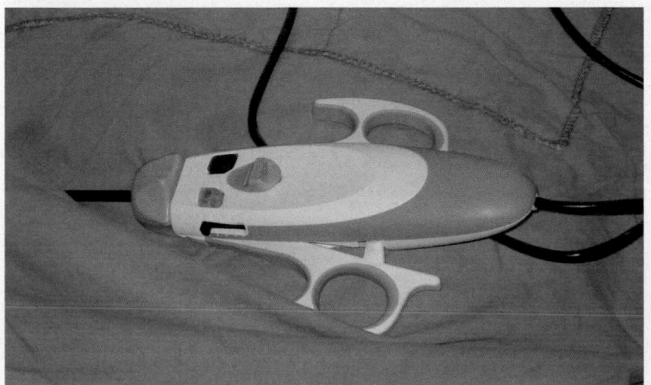
FIGURE 19-26. Laparoscopic vessel-sealing device with an in-line handle, with finger loops, and 5-mm shaft.

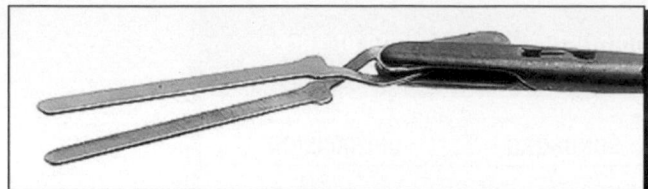

FIGURE 19-27. Laparoscopic bulldog clamp.

carried out patiently for a sufficient period. In complicated reoperative procedures, use of a drain can be considered. A drain with active suction is effective, but it should not be placed directly near the source of the previously controlled bleeding site.

Intraoperative Endoscopy

Intraoperative endoscopy is a tool that may be helpful in reoperative surgery and should preferably be made available prior to the beginning of the operation. Intraoperative gastroscopy and enteroscopy are unlikely to be indicated during reoperative surgery for colon and rectal diseases. The benefit of an intraoperative gastroscopy should always be weighed against the likely increase in small bowel distention that inevitably follows. Options for minimizing small bowel distention include applying a laparoscopic bulldog clamp (Figure 19-27) on the proximal jejunum just distal to the Treitz ligament and/or using CO_2 for insufflation during endoscopy. Intraoperative enteroscopy, if indicated, should preferably be performed as push enteroscopy, given the relative ease of use and the fact that low capital investment and maintenance are involved. On the other hand, double-balloon enteroscopy requires specialized training, significant capital investment, and is time consuming. Spiral enteroscopy is still under evaluation. One advantage of positioning the patient in the lithotomy position is to make intraoperative colonoscopy easily feasible. Intraoperative colonoscopy may become necessary for the assessment of ischemia, perforation, neoplasia, anastomoses, and other indications. Again, insufflation with CO_2 is to be preferred in order to prevent prolonged distention of the large bowel. Rigid proctoscopy is also a requirement in

emergency colorectal cases because it is the ideal instrument for evaluating the rectum.

Closure

Following a successful performance of a laparoscopic-performed operation, the technique for closure of the ports should not be trivialized because complications may occur. Port site hernias may include an asymptomatic fascial defect or, more threatening, an incarcerated or strangulated hernia. Surgeons should always make an attempt to close all ports. Fascial defects of 10 mm or greater in diameter should always be sutured even in the case of oblique trocar insertion. Fascia closure may preferentially be performed with an open technique using a robust needle (UR-6) in order to minimize the chances of needle fracture within the abdominal wall. Open suture closure of a 5-mm port site is often not possible unless the patient has a low BMI. In most cases, it is, therefore, preferable to close a 5-mm defect laparoscopically using a suture passer. Should the patient have a preexisting large incisional hernia requiring a mesh, the repair may have to be postponed. This is particularly true if an enterotomy or bowel resection is included in the surgery.

Room Setup

Sir Charles Bell stated, "If it be a great operation, and especially if the assistants and nurses are not habituated, be careful to appoint them their places and their duties; for nothing tends more to the right performance of an operation of magnitude, than that composure and quietness which result from arrangement." (*The Principles of Surgery*, London, T. Cadell & EW Davis, 1826–1828.)

The foregoing comment was made in 1821, yet it is still extremely important to the contemporary operating room scene (Figure 19-28). There is no doubt that laparoscopic colorectal procedures are "operations of magnitude." With so many distractions of equipment—individuals, often in unfamiliar circumstances—it is essential to consider all that is required to ensure quietness and composure.

A nostalgic view of the bittersweet world of conventional surgery (Figure 19-29) is succeeded by a humorous

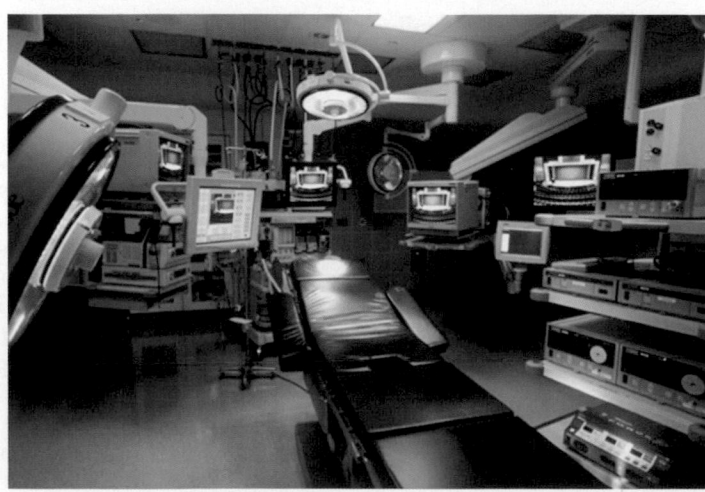

FIGURE 19-28. The author's fully integrated operating suite.

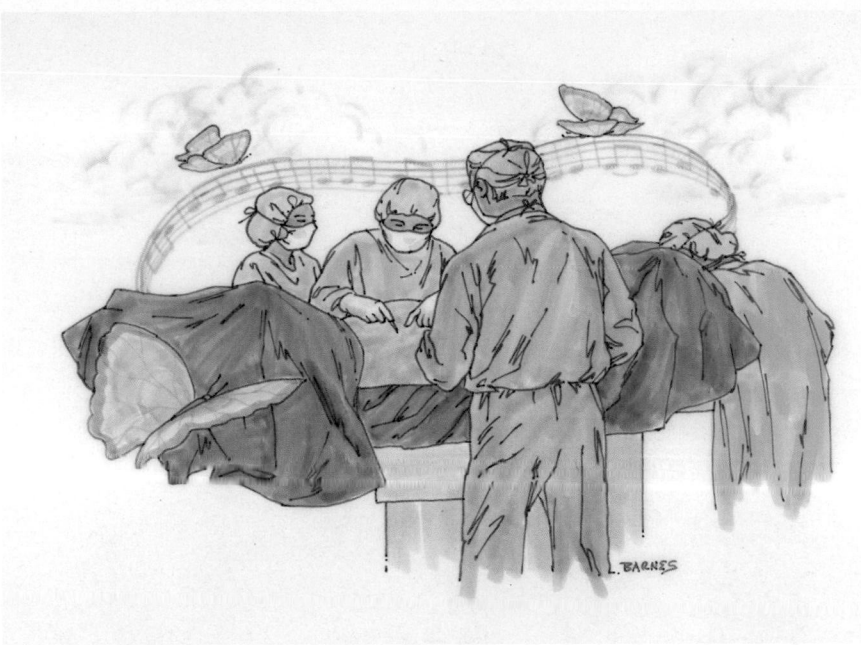

FIGURE 19-29. A nostalgic view of the world of conventional surgery. (Courtesy of Marvin L. Corman, MD.)

depiction of the perceived chaos and associated stress that accompanies the hard-won, successful transition to laparoscopic surgery (Figure 19-30). The perplexities or entanglements experienced by many surgeons when HALS becomes paramount are shown in Figure 19-31. Figure 19-32 reveals an entertainingly common, albeit unenlightened view of the field of robotics, a new technology that requires further exploration.

► SURGICAL PROCEDURES

Laparoscopic-Assisted Colonoscopic Polypectomy for Difficult Right Colon Polyps

Introduction

Not all right colon polyps discovered at colonoscopy are amenable to safe colonoscopic snare polypectomy. Large polyps or those positioned in a difficult location are often too risky to remove or are not completely resectable by standard snare polypectomy. As such, standard practice has been to biopsy such lesions in order to obtain a histologic diagnosis and to exclude cancer, marking the site through using a tattoo agent, and then referring the patient for right colectomy. Laparoscopic-assisted colonoscopic polypectomy (LACP) has been reported and practiced at selected centers for the management of large polyps without histologic evidence of cancer.[232] This is a procedure performed in the operating room in which the surgeon and gastroenterologist work together to remove the polyp without removing the colon. Colonoscopy is accomplished using CO_2 rather than air in order to allow faster desufflation of colon.[152] Although LACP has been recognized as an acceptable form of treatment for the past 5 to 10 years, it has not been compared with laparoscopic right colectomy in randomized, controlled trials. Currently, throughout the United States, right colectomy for large polyps is more commonly practiced than LACP.

Indications

Patients found to have a right colon polyp at colonoscopy in which the polyp is deemed unresectable by the gastroenterologist can be offered LACP based on the following criteria: polyp spanning two or more colonic folds, polyp >20 mm, polyp spanning greater than 50% of the colonic circumference, positive "lift sign" following submucosal injection of saline beneath the polyp, and difficult location or position of the polyp, thus limiting one's ability to determine that removal can be adequately and completely accomplished.

Patients with the following criteria should not be offered LACP: polyps with histologic evidence of adenocarcinoma, patients with known inflammatory bowel disease, patients with known familial adenomatous polyposis, polyps without known histology, and polyps with large ulcerations or those that demonstrate a "nonlift sign" during submucosal injection at the time of colonoscopy.

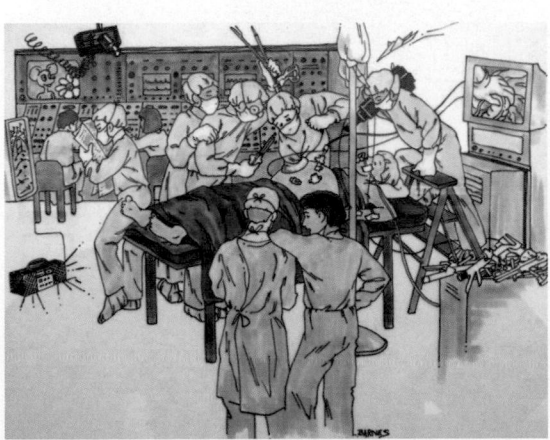

FIGURE 19-30. A hyperbolic view of the hard fought transition to laparoscopic surgery. (Courtesy of Marvin L. Corman, MD.)

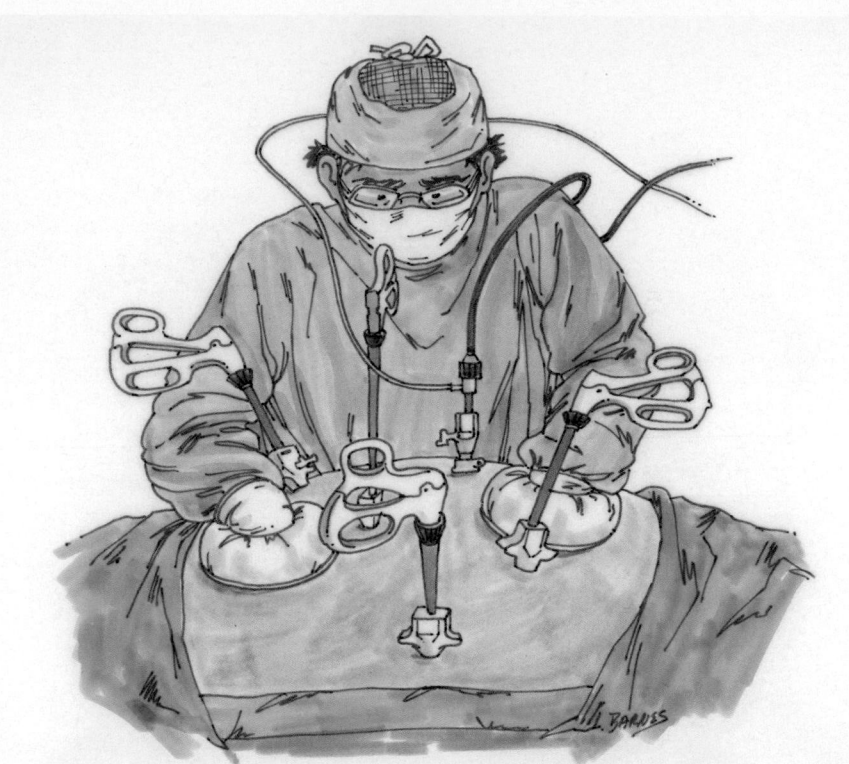

FIGURE 19-31. A humorous view of hand-assisted laparoscopic surgery (HALS). (Courtesy of Marvin L. Corman, MD.)

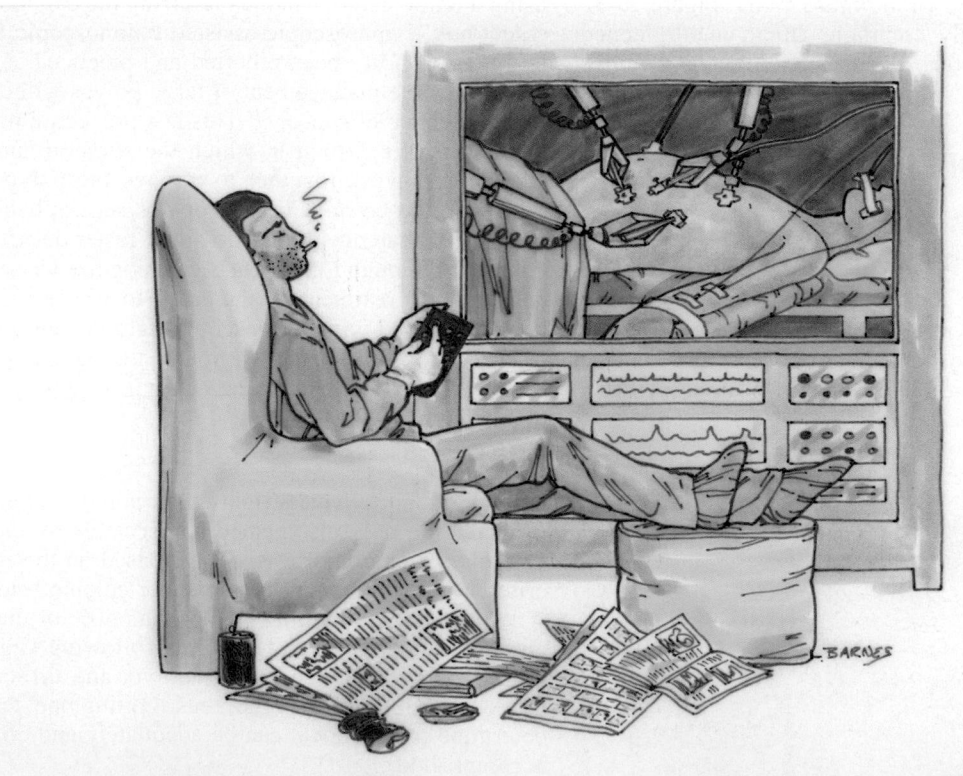

FIGURE 19-32. An entertaining view of the world of robotics. (Courtesy of Marvin L. Corman, MD.)

Preoperative Workup

The preoperative workup includes colonoscopy and marking the polyp site with a tattooing agent. A mechanical bowel preparation is achieved by using polyethylene glycol ingested orally the day before surgery.

Operating Room

The operating room includes a third area for colonoscopy in addition to the classical surgery and anesthesia areas. Patients in lithotomy position receive general anesthesia with endotracheal intubation and undergo placement of adequate intravenous access, nasogastric tube, and urinary catheter. Intravenous antibiotics are given. Sequential compression devices are applied to the legs. The patient with both arms tucked is securely strapped to the table at the chest and thighs because tilting the table will be necessary. The abdomen is prepped and sterilely draped. The surgeon, assistant, and scrub nurse stand on the patient's left side. The laparoscopy monitor is located at the patient's right side. Colonoscopy is performed using CO_2. The gastroenterologist stands in between the patient's legs.

Surgical Technique

Pneumoperitoneum is established with carbon dioxide insufflated to a pressure of 12 mm Hg and by placement of a reusable Hasson trocar of 10 mm in diameter in the infraumbilical skin using a cutdown technique. Two reusable, threaded 5-mm ports are inserted under direct visual control in the left upper and lower quadrants lateral to the rectus muscle sheath. The table is turned into a left lateral tilt as well as into the Trendelenburg position. Laparoscopic instruments include bowel graspers, needle holders, and a laparoscopic bulldog clamp (Figure 19-27). After identification of the tattoo, a laparoscopic bulldog clamp is placed on the terminal ileum to prevent distention of the small bowel by the CO_2 insufflated via the colonoscope. The laparoscopic shaft is then disconnected from the bulldog clamp, thereby allowing the surgeon to use two ports. The remainder of the operation consists of providing laparoscopic assistance to the gastroenterologist in order to accomplish a complete polypectomy. Should a full-thickness colon burn or perforation occur, the surgeon performs laparoscopic suturing with intracorporeal knot-tying. However, in selected cases, laparoscopic cecal wall excision may be an option. A leak test using CO_2 insufflation through the colonoscope and immersion of the bowel segment under saline is performed. The specimen is retrieved with an endoscopic net, extracted transanally and sent to pathology.

Laparoscopic Ileocolic Resection with Intracorporeal Mesentery Division for Crohn's Disease

Introduction

The thickened and foreshortened mesentery of the terminal ileum in patients with Crohn's disease has been safely divided by conventional surgery for decades. The introduction of a laparoscopic-facilitated ileocolic resection entails the exteriorization of the mobilized bowel and mesentery with extracorporeal division of the mesentery. However, extracorporeal ligation of a foreshortened mesentery exteriorized through a short laparotomy can be technically difficult to accomplish.[150] Still, laparoscopic intracorporeal

division of the mesentery for Crohn's disease has been successfully reported.[23]

Indications

Patients presenting with refractory Crohn's disease confined to terminal ileum and cecum with or without internal fistula, localized abscess, or chronic obstruction can be managed by laparoscopic ileocolic resection unless the patient presents with massive small bowel distention (Figure 19-33). Patients are not eligible for this approach if any one of the following findings is present: frozen abdomen due to large fixed mass, recurrent Crohn's disease following prior resection, or perforated disease requiring emergency surgery.

Preoperative Workup

A thorough history and physical exam and a preoperative consultation with a gastroenterologist specializing in inflammatory bowel disease are essential. The preoperative workup includes esophagogastroduodenoscopy, proctoscopy, colonoscopy, and CT enterography. A mechanical bowel preparation is achieved by using 2 L of polyethylene glycol ingested orally the day before surgery.

Operating Room

Patients receive general anesthesia with endotracheal intubation and undergo placement of a nasogastric tube and urinary catheter. A right ureteral stent may be placed by a urologist if considered prudent. Adequate intravenous access must be ensured. Broad-spectrum intravenous antibiotics are given. Sequential compression devices are applied to the legs. Patients are placed in the supine position with both arms tucked. Individuals should be securely strapped to the table at the chest and thighs because tilting the table will be necessary. The abdomen is prepped and sterilely draped. The surgeon and the scrub nurse stand on the patient's left side, and the assistant stands on the patient's right. One assistant is needed to control the camera unless a robotic camera holder is available. The television monitor is located at the patient's right foot (Figure 19-34).

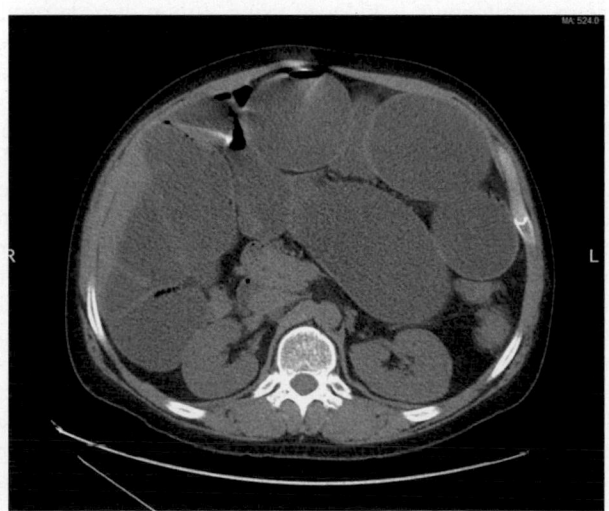

FIGURE 19-33. Profound small bowel distention in a patient with an ileal stricture.

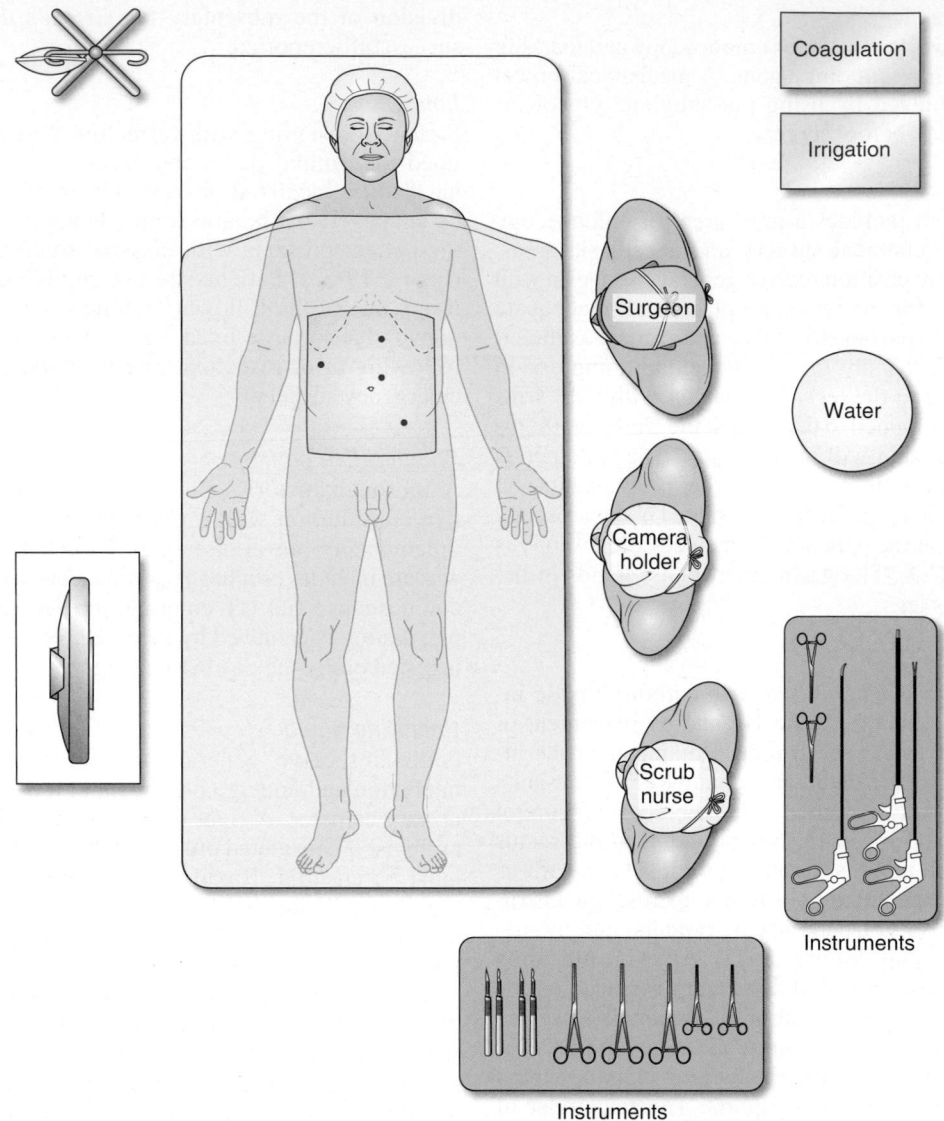

FIGURE 19-34. Operating room setup for laparoscopic ileocolic resection for Crohn's disease.

Surgical Technique

Pneumoperitoneum is induced using carbon dioxide insufflated to a pressure of 12 mm Hg by placement of a reusable Hasson trocar 10 mm in diameter in the supraumbilical skin by using a cutdown technique. A 30-degree telescope is inserted. A reusable, threaded 5-mm port is placed in the right upper quadrant lateral to the rectus muscle sheath. A disposable, threaded 12-mm port is placed in the left lower quadrant lateral to the rectus muscle sheath and caudal to the umbilicus. A reusable, threaded 5-mm port is placed on the midline above the umbilicus (Figure 19-35). The table is turned into a moderate left tilt and into a Trendelenburg position. Reusable instruments include long laparoscopic instruments (more than 40-cm long shaft), bowel graspers, scissors, right-angle forceps, needle holders, and Satinsky vascular clamp. The disposable instruments include laparoscopic stapler, bipolar vessel-sealing device, and specimen bag. Laparoscopic ileocolic resection involves a lateral-to-medial approach encompassing at least nine sequential steps:

1. The ligament of Treitz is identified and the small bowel inspected to the ileocecal valve. Care is taken not to grasp the intestine directly, and atraumatic bowel graspers are applied to the mesentery.

2. The terminal ileum is carefully inspected to rule out internal fistulas. Ileosigmoid, ileoileal, or ileovesical fistulas are repaired prior to embarking on the ileocolic resection. The site of transaction on the terminal ileum is chosen to achieve macroscopically uninvolved resection margins. The terminal ileum is transected with a laparoscopic stapler after having scored the mesentery in a window beneath it.

3. A lateral-to-medial mobilization of the terminal ileum and cecum off of the retroperitoneum is performed. A combination of sharp and blunt dissection is used.

4. The right ureter is identified by inspection and by gentle palpation with a blunt instrument if necessary.

5. The mesentery of the terminal ileum is transected with a bipolar vessel-sealing device or stapler near the bowel wall in a proximal to distal direction. Each staple line is meticulously inspected for evidence of bleeding prior to proceeding to the next stapler application. In case of oozing, compression is attempted first followed by oversewing with intracorporeal knot-tying if this becomes necessary.

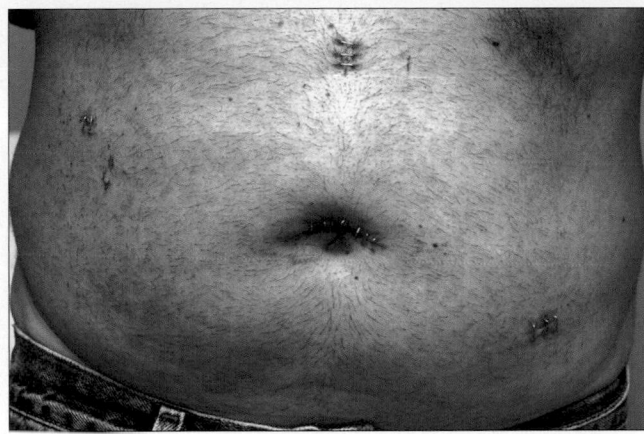

FIGURE 19-35. Port placements for laparoscopic ileocolic resection for Crohn's disease.

Uncontrolled bleeding is addressed with prompt application of a Satinsky vascular clamp followed by oversewing. Care is taken to avoid dividing the ileocolic vessels in order to preserve blood supply to the ascending colon.

6. The cecum is transected with the laparoscopic stapler.
7. The ileum and the ascending colon are aligned side-to-side by a stay suture placed at their antimesenteric sides; the suture is tied intracorporeally and held by the assistant. An enterotomy and a colotomy are made at the antimesenteric sites of the staple ends of the ileum and ascending colon, respectively. A side-to-side anastomosis is fashioned with a laparoscopic stapler using one 60-mm long cartridge. Following stapler extraction, stay sutures are placed on the remaining enterotomy; this, in turn, is closed in two layers of interrupted sutures.
8. The mesenteric defect is left open.
9. The specimen is delivered via a bag through the umbilical port site. The fascia is enlarged along the midline, whereas the skin is enlarged in a curved fashion.

Postoperative Care

The nasogastric or orogastric tube can be removed in the operating room at the end of the procedure. On postoperative day 1, the patient is allowed to drink clear fluids, encouraged to ambulate, and the urinary catheter is removed. If liquids are tolerated, intravenous fluid volume is decreased, a low-fiber diet is initiated, and mobilization of the patient is increased on postoperative day 2. The patient may be advanced to a regular diet on postoperative day 3 if passing flatus and comfortable. Analgesic medication is switched from epidural to oral. On postoperative day 4, intravenous fluids are discontinued, and the patient may be discharged if comfortable and is tolerating the diet.

Opinion

An outsider to the field of surgery would probably take it for granted that surgeons have a highly developed rationale for choosing a laparoscopic approach for the management of Crohn's disease.[19] However, this is not quite true. The most likely preservation of the abdominal wall, body image,[64] and small bowel obstruction rates represent all the rationalities for undertaking a laparoscopic approach.[9,26] Incisions for specimen extraction and port placement should be planned in advance, keeping in mind that temporary defunctioning stomas

may become necessary when severe perianal disease is present or in selected patients with refractory Crohn's colitis. In fact, 30% of patients with colorectal Crohn's disease may require a permanent ileostomy. Furthermore, right colectomy should be avoided because it deprives patients of useful water-absorbing colonic mucosa. Unfortunately, laparoscopic ileocolic resection does not decrease disease recurrence rates.[26]

Laparoscopic Right Colectomy with Intracorporeal Anastomosis for Cancer

Introduction

Although laparoscopic-assisted right colectomy was first reported in 1991,[193] descriptions of a standardized surgical technique became available in recent years. The first consisted of a five-step lateral-to-medial approach with extracorporeal vascular ligation and ileocolic anastomosis.[233] The second included eight steps with a medial-to-lateral approach in which vascular ligation was performed intracorporeally, whereas the anastomosis was fashioned extracorporeally.[197] Laparoscopic intracorporeal right colectomy entails 10 steps with intracorporeal anastomosis followed by specimen removal in a bag.[27]

Indications

Resection of malignant tumors (adenocarcinomas, carcinoid tumors, neoplastic polyps) localized to the distal ileum, ileocecal valve, appendix, cecum, ascending colon, or hepatic flexure can be managed by right hemicolectomy. This procedure entails complete mobilization of the terminal ileum and right colon to the level of the midportion of the transverse colon. This technique is contraindicated for T4 right colon cancer invading the right kidney, duodenum, or abdominal wall. However, it can be used in the cases of T4 tumors invading the greater omentum.

Preoperative Evaluation

Undertaking a thorough history and performing a complete physical exam are essential. Chest x-ray and electrocardiogram (EKG) should be performed in patients older than the age of 50. Preoperative workup includes a complete blood count, blood chemistry determination, and a coagulation profile. Colonoscopy, CT scan of the abdomen and pelvis with intravenous and oral contrast, or positron emission tomography (PET) scan can establish the exact location of the malignancy and the tumor TNM grading (tumor size, lymph nodes, and systemic metastasis).

Operating Room

Patients receive general anesthesia with endotracheal intubation and undergo placement of a nasogastric tube and urinary catheter. If the individuals cannot tolerate general anesthesia, the procedure can be done with a spinal or epidural, with the addition of a transverse block. A mechanical bowel preparation is achieved by using 2 L of polyethylene glycol ingested orally during the day before surgery. Adequate intravenous access should be ensured. Broad-spectrum intravenous antibiotics are given. Sequential compression devices are applied to the legs. Patients are supine in a beanbag with the right arm abducted and the left arm tucked. The patient should be securely strapped to the table at the chest because tilting the table is necessary. The abdomen is prepped and draped sterile. The surgeon, the camera holder, and the scrub nurse stand on the patient's left side

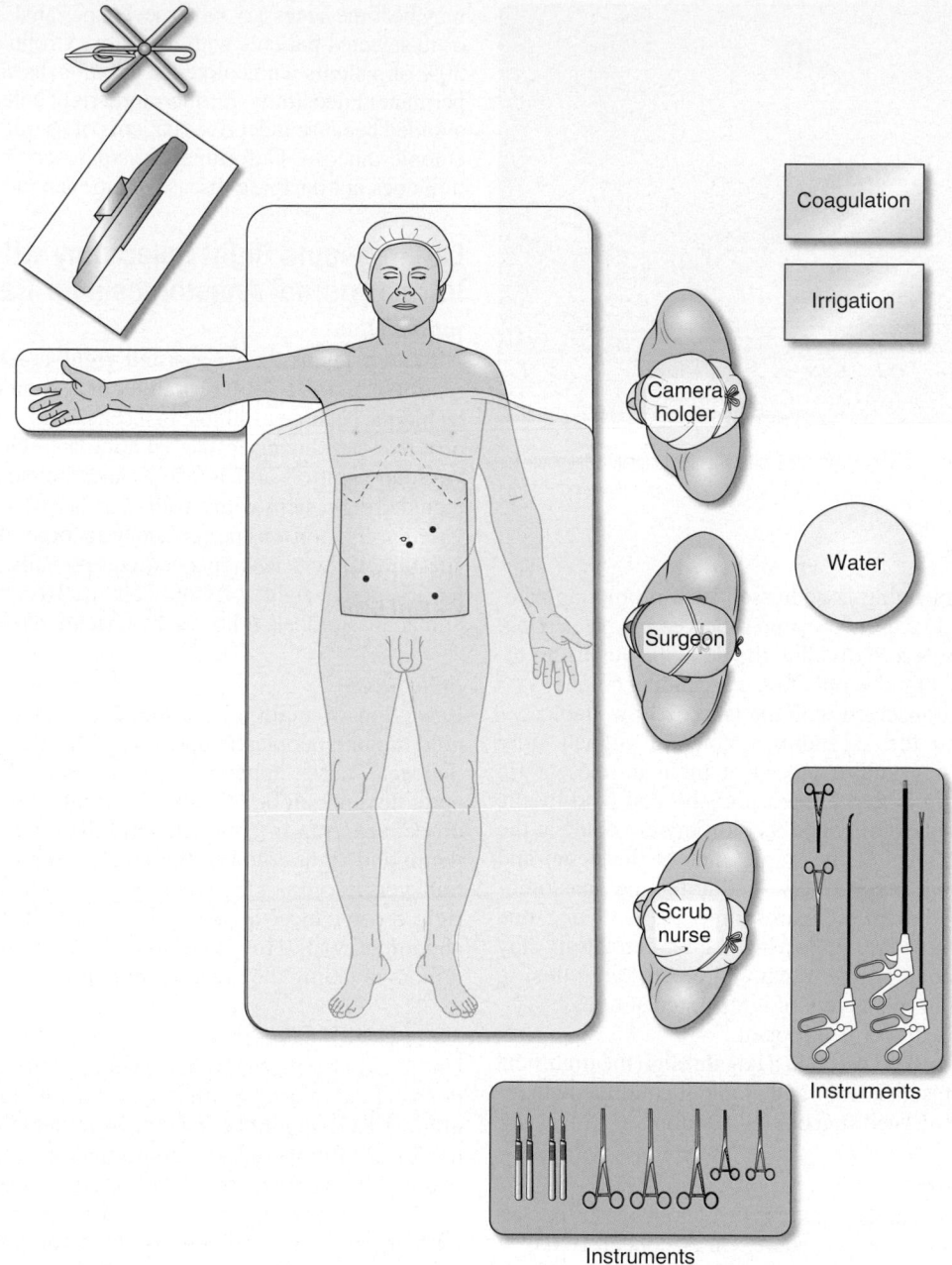

FIGURE 19-36. Operating room setup for laparoscopic right colectomy.

(Figure 19-36). One assistant is needed to control the camera unless a robotic camera holder is available.

Surgical Technique

Pneumoperitoneum is induced using carbon dioxide insufflated to a pressure of 12 mm Hg by placement of a reusable Hasson trocar of 10 mm in diameter in the infraumbilical skin using a cutdown technique. A 30-degree telescope is introduced for peritoneal inspection. A reusable, threaded 5-mm port is placed 3 cm medial to the right anterior superior iliac spine. A disposable, threaded 12-mm port is placed in the left upper quadrant lateral to the rectus muscle sheath and above the umbilicus. A reusable, threaded 5-mm port is placed 3 cm proximal to the pubic tubercle just left to the midline. The table is turned into a moderate left tilt as well as

into a Trendelenburg position. Reusable devices include long instruments (43 cm shaft): bowel graspers, scissors, right-angle forceps, and needle holders. The disposables include an ultrasonic-activated device and staplers. Laparoscopic intracorporeal right colectomy involves a medial-to-lateral approach, encompassing the following 10 sequential steps:

1. The ileocolic vessels are identified by gentle traction applied by the assistant to the cecum; the superior mesenteric vein (SMV) is located; a window beneath the ileocolic vessels is opened, incising the peritoneum close to the SMV and gently lifting the ileocolic vessels with a closed grasper; the ileocolic artery crossing to the SMV is assessed as anterior or posterior, and the ileocolic vessels were divided after the duodenum had been identified (Figure 19-37).

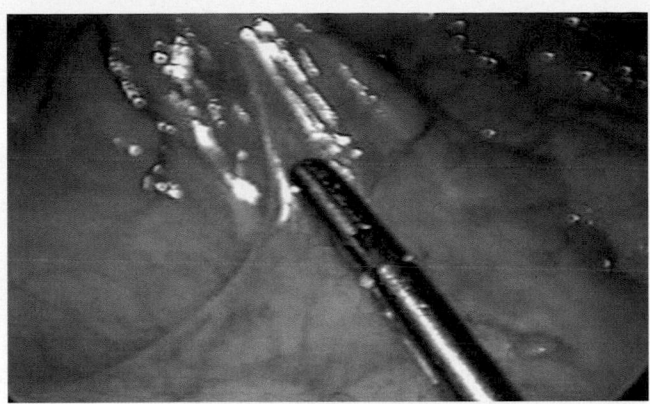

FIGURE 19-37. Ileocolic vessels. (From Bergamaschi R, Schochet E, Haughn C, et al. Standardized laparoscopic intracorporeal right colectomy for cancer: short-term outcome in 111 unselected patients. *Dis Colon Rectum*. 2008;51(9):1350–1355.)

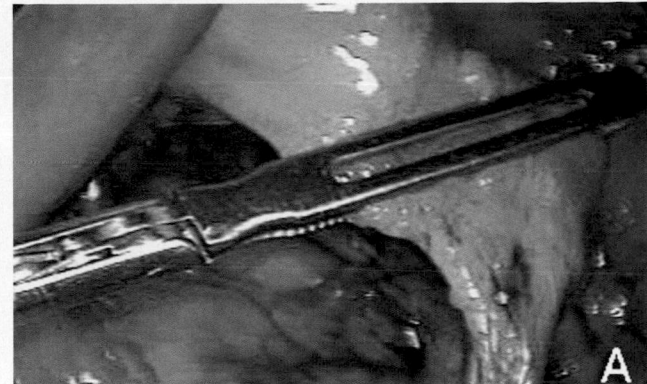

FIGURE 19-39. Identification of right ureter. (From Bergamaschi R, Schochet E, Haughn C, et al. Standardized laparoscopic intracorporeal right colectomy for cancer: short-term outcome in 111 unselected patients. *Dis Colon Rectum*. 2008;51(9):1350–1355.)

2. The right ureter is identified by inspection and, if necessary, by gentle palpation with a blunt instrument (Figure 19-38) while the assistant gently elevates the stump of the ileocolic vessels (specimen side) off the retroperitoneum (Figure 19-39).

3. The dissection starts at the origin of the ileocolic vessels proceeded along the SMV in a cephalad direction; if present, the right colic vessels are divided after having assessed whether the right colic artery crosses anteriorly or posteriorly to the SMV; the dissection ends at the origin of Henle's gastrocolic trunk from the SMV; the mesentery of the proximal transverse colon is gently elevated off the duodenum (Figure 19-40).

4. The table is leveled from the Trendelenburg position but kept in a moderate left tilt; the omentum is divided and the lesser sac entered; the division of the omentum is performed in a medial-to-lateral direction, caudal to the right gastroepiploic vessels by using an ultrasonic-activated device (Figure 19-41).

5. The middle colic vessels are identified by gentle elevation of the transverse colon off of the duodenum and retroperitoneum; the right branch of the middle colic vessel is divided while the proximal transverse colon is gently elevated by the assistant (Figure 19-42).

6. The proximal transverse colon is transected with a laparoscopic stapler (Figure 19-43).

7. The hepatic flexure is mobilized in a medial-to-lateral direction using an ultrasonic-activated device; if present, the superior right colic vein is divided; the mesentery of the ascending colon is mobilized off the retroperitoneum, and the lateral peritoneal reflection of the ascending colon is divided along the white line of Toldt in a caudal to cephalad direction using an ultrasonic-activated device (Figure 9-44).

8. The terminal ileum is transected with a laparoscopic stapler and held by the assistant to prevent rotation of its mesentery (Figure 19-45).

9. The table is leveled from the left tilt; the antimesenteric side of the stapled ends of the transverse colon and terminal ileum are approximated by a stay suture tied intracorporeally and then held by the assistant; an antimesenteric enterotomy and an antimesenteric colotomy are made 10 cm distal to the stapled ends of the transverse colon and terminal ileum, respectively; a side-to-side anastomosis is fashioned with a laparoscopic stapler (Figure 19-46); the enterotomy after stapler extraction is closed by two layers of silk sutures tied intracorporeally (Figure 19-47); the mesenteric defect is left open.

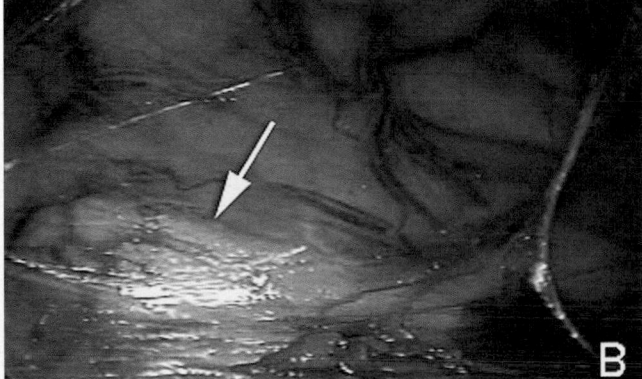

FIGURE 19-38. Lifting transected ileocolic vessel stump. (From Bergamaschi R, Schochet E, Haughn C, et al. Standardized laparoscopic intracorporeal right colectomy for cancer: short-term outcome in 111 unselected patients. *Dis Colon Rectum*. 2008;51(9):1350–1355.)

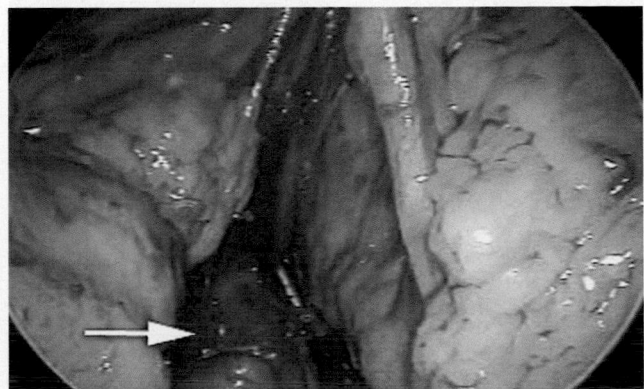

FIGURE 19-40. Identification of duodenum. (From Bergamaschi R, Schochet E, Haughn C, et al. Standardized laparoscopic intracorporeal right colectomy for cancer: short-term outcome in 111 unselected patients. *Dis Colon Rectum*. 2008;51(9):1350–1355.)

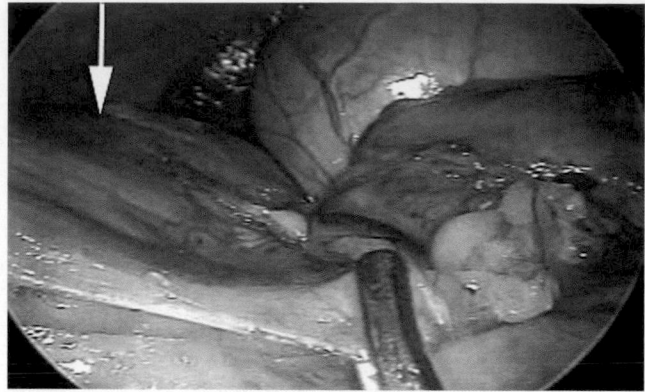

FIGURE 19-41. Accessing the lesser sac. (From Bergamaschi R, Schochet E, Haughn C, et al. Standardized laparoscopic intracorporeal right colectomy for cancer: short-term outcome in 111 unselected patients. *Dis Colon Rectum.* 2008;51(9):1350–1355.)

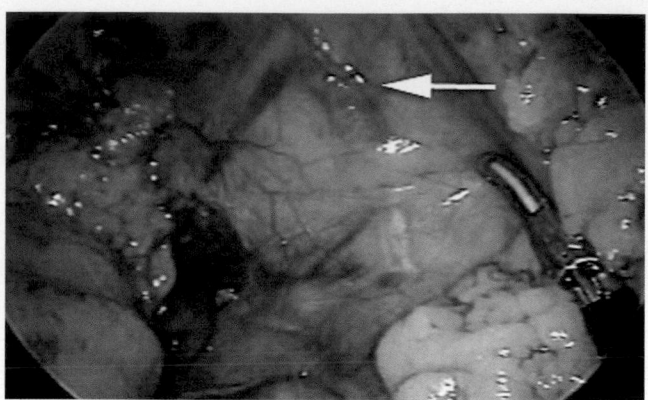

FIGURE 19-42. Identification of the right branch of the middle colic vessel. (From Bergamaschi R, Schochet E, Haughn C, et al. Standardized laparoscopic intracorporeal right colectomy for cancer: short-term outcome in 111 unselected patients. *Dis Colon Rectum.* 2008;51(9):1350–1355.)

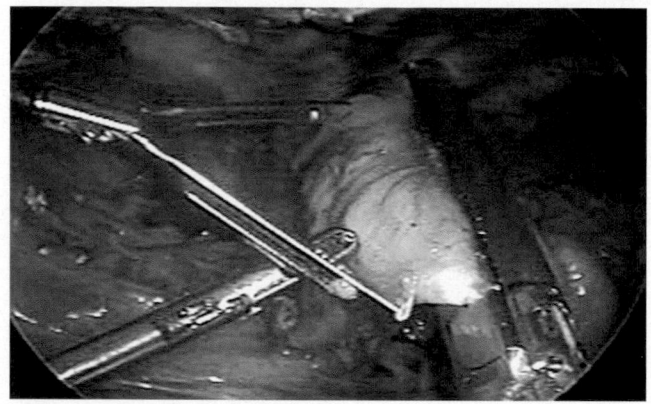

FIGURE 19-43. Transecting transverse colon. (From Bergamaschi R, Schochet E, Haughn C, et al. Standardized laparoscopic intracorporeal right colectomy for cancer: short-term outcome in 111 unselected patients. *Dis Colon Rectum.* 2008;51(9):1350–1355.)

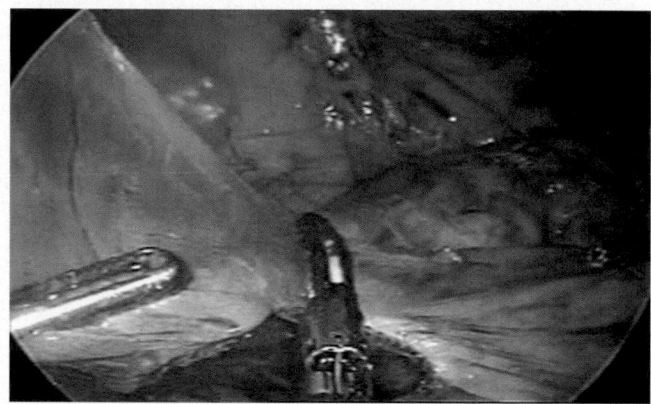

FIGURE 19-44. Mobilization of right colon along the line of Toldt. (From Bergamaschi R, Schochet E, Haughn C, et al. Standardized laparoscopic intracorporeal right colectomy for cancer: short-term outcome in 111 unselected patients. *Dis Colon Rectum.* 2008;51(9):1350–1355.)

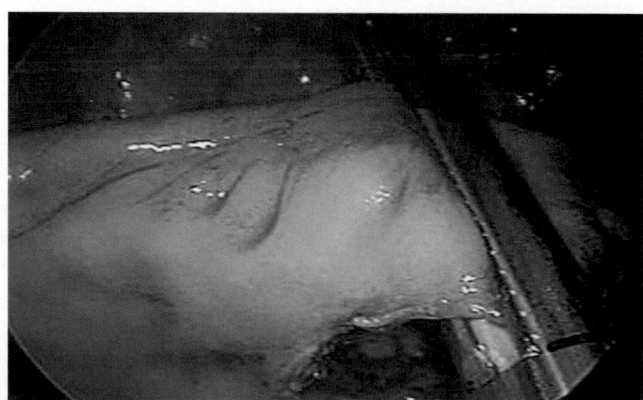

FIGURE 19-45. Transecting the terminal ileum. (From Bergamaschi R, Schochet E, Haughn C, et al. Standardized laparoscopic intracorporeal right colectomy for cancer: short-term outcome in 111 unselected patients. *Dis Colon Rectum.* 2008;51(9):1350–1355.)

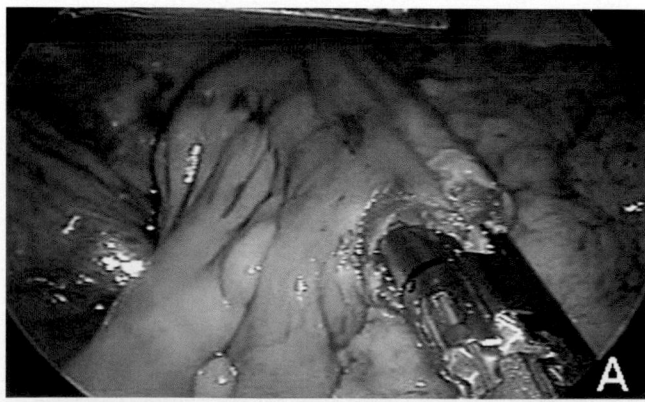

FIGURE 19-46. Stapled side-to-side ileocolic anastomosis. (From Bergamaschi R, Schochet E, Haughn C, et al. Standardized laparoscopic intracorporeal right colectomy for cancer: short-term outcome in 111 unselected patients. *Dis Colon Rectum.* 2008;51(9):1350–1355.)

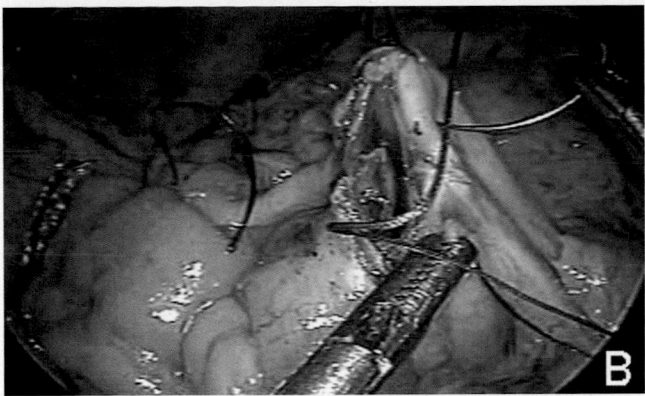

FIGURE 19-47. Hand-sewing enterotomy laparoscopically. (From Bergamaschi R, Schochet E, Haughn C, et al. Standardized laparoscopic intracorporeal right colectomy for cancer: short-term outcome in 111 unselected patients. *Dis Colon Rectum*. 2008;51(9):1350–1355.)

10. The specimen is delivered in a bag through an enlarged umbilical or suprapubic port site. Fascial defects are closed with 0-polyglycolic acid sutures. Skin incisions are closed with running subcuticular 4–0 polyglycolic acid sutures.

Postoperative Care

The nasogastric or orogastric tube can be removed in the operating room at the end of the procedure. On postoperative day 1, the patient is allowed clear fluids, encouraged to ambulate, and the urinary catheter is removed. If liquids are tolerated, a low-fiber diet is commenced on postoperative day 2, intravenous fluid replacement is discontinued, analgesic medication is prescribed orally, and mobilization of the patient increased. On postoperative day 3, the patient may be discharged if comfortable, tolerating the diet, and passing gas. If patients do not tolerate a solid diet, they are not pushed to start eating, but intravenous fluid and analgesic administration are withdrawn because both of them prolong ileus.

Opinion

Potential advantages of intracorporeal ileocolic anastomosis include (1) anastomosing at some distance from the abdominal wall—this may reduce surgical site infection rates; (2) no manipulation of the abdominal cavity by the surgeon's hands can reduce the risk of creating adhesions and perforce the rate of adhesive small bowel obstruction; (3) a 50% reduction in the abdominal wall incision length for specimen extraction could lead to clinically relevant benefits; (4) laparoscopic visualization during the creation of the anastomosis should minimize the risk of unrecognized twisting of the terminal ileal mesentery; and (5) no requirement for mobilization of the transverse colon. Intracorporeal ileocolic anastomosis following laparoscopic right colectomy may be fashioned either partially stapled, hand-sewn, or totally stapled.

Potential disadvantages of totally stapled intracorporeal ileocolic anastomosis (Figure 19-48) are as follows: (1) leads to an everted anastomosis with the potential for increased risk of complications as opposed to its hand-sewn inverted counterpart; (2) requires usage of 60-mm long cartridge for side-to-side ileocolic stapling; it inevitably excises tissue and thereby potentially reduces the size of the anastomosis; (3) most likely requires an additional port if performed on the transverse colon; (4) does not obviate the need for intracorporeal suturing because stay stitches are required to ensure safe stapler application on the enterocolotomy; (5) may require multiple firings, depending on the size of the enterocolotomy or whether the previous staple line is being excised; and (6) leads to higher costs due to additional cartridges. The author's preferred option is to hand-sew the enterotomy (Figure 19-49).

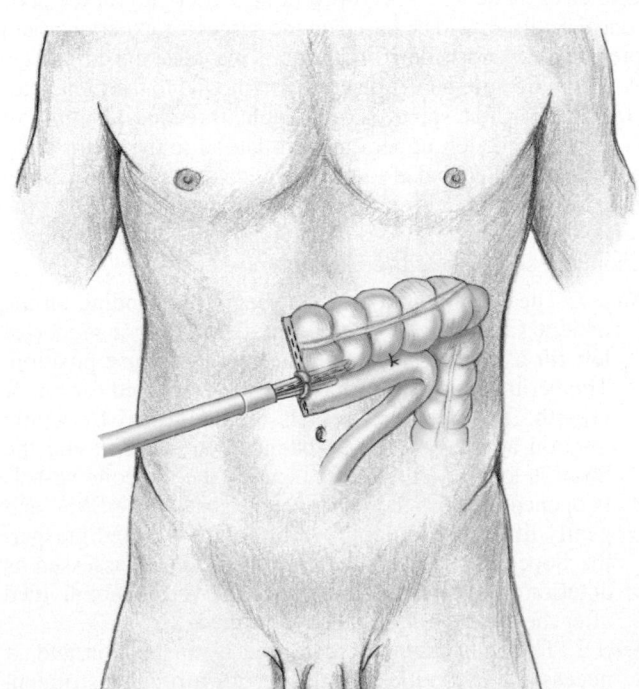

FIGURE 19-48. Totally stapled intracorporeal ileocolic anastomosis.

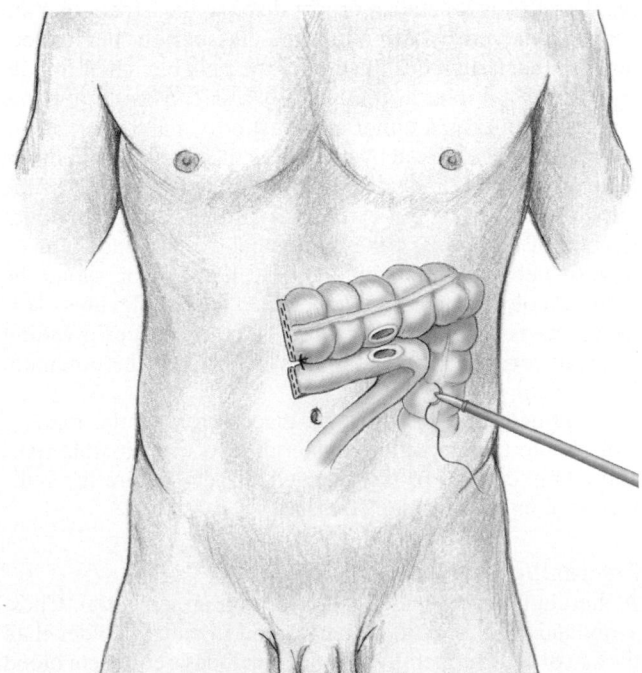

FIGURE 19-49. Stapling anastomosis prior to hand-sewing the enterotomy.

Laparoscopic-Extended Right Hemicolectomy for Transverse Colon Cancer

Introduction

Tumors in the transverse colon pose several challenges for the surgeon. The tumors can receive blood supply from the right colic, middle colic, as well as the left colic artery, and, hence, the lymph-bearing area can be wide and variable. A segmental resection of the transverse colon can result in tension on the anastomosis secondary to the fixity of the ascending and descending colon to the retroperitoneal structures. In addition, there is an increased risk of anastomotic leak when performing colon-to-colon anastomosis as compared with ileocolic anastomosis. To avoid this and to ensure that all the lymph-bearing areas of the tumor have been removed, it is common practice to perform either an extended right or left hemicolectomy rather than a segmental resection of the transverse colon. An extended right hemicolectomy requires division of the middle colic artery, which can be challenging laparoscopically and requires advanced laparoscopic skills.

Due to these complexities, tumors of the transverse colon have been omitted from the large, randomized controlled trials that compare laparoscopic colon resection for cancer to open resection, such as COST, COLOR, and CLASICC. The results of these trials are, therefore, not directly applicable to transverse colon tumors; doubt remains regarding the optimal approach for the management of lesions in this location. Because cancer of the transverse colon is rare (10% of all colon cancer cases), unfortunately it is unlikely that separate trials will be conducted to settle this issue. However, in the literature, there are a few single-institution, nonrandomized cohort studies and quantitative comparisons that strongly suggest that laparoscopic surgery for transverse colon cancer is as safe and feasible as other laparoscopic surgeries for colon cancer.[114,122,192]

Indications

A tumor that is located at or just distal to the hepatic flexure can be removed by extending the classic right hemicolectomy so that it includes ligation of the right branch of middle colic artery, as long as that permits a safe, 5-cm tumor-free margin. Similarly, a tumor at or just proximal to the splenic flexure can be removed by extending the classic left hemicolectomy so that it includes ligation of the left branch of the middle colic artery. An extended right hemicolectomy with ligation of the trunk of the middle colic artery and an anastomosis between the ileum and descending colon should be used for colon cancer arising between the two flexures. This technique is contraindicated for T4 colon cancer invading adjacent organs, except for cases where only the omentum is involved.

Treatment options must be discussed with the patient. One should understand the material facts and possible risks and complications of the planned surgery before the individual signs an informed consent.

Preoperative Workup

A thorough history and physical exam are essential. Chest x-ray and EKG should be performed in patients older than the age of 50. Preoperative workup includes a complete blood count, chemistries, coagulation profile, and a carcinoembryonic antigen (CEA) level. Preoperative localization of colon cancer is always important, but for transverse colon cancers, it is imperative. Colonoscopy alone is not adequate for this determination. CT scan of chest, abdomen, and pelvis with intravenous and oral contrast and PET scan can establish the exact location of the tumor and the TNM stage, respectively. To further confirm the exact localization of the tumor, India ink injection can be performed at the time of colonoscopy. The bowel should be prepared orally with laxatives and antibiotics in accordance with each institution's protocol, unless there is a narrow stricture. In such cases, no oral bowel preparation should be used.

Operating Room

The patient should be identified with an appropriate time out prior to the induction of general anesthesia with endotracheal intubation. Intravenous antibiotics should be administered perioperatively. A Foley catheter and nasogastric or orogastric tube should be inserted. The patient is supine on the operating table with the lower limbs either in stirrups or spread apart. Sequential compression devices are applied to the legs. Both arms should be tucked. The patient should be securely strapped to the table at the chest because tilting the table will be necessary. All equipment including monitors should be placed on the patient's right side in clear view of the surgeon, who stands on the patient's left side. One assistant is needed to control the camera unless a robotic camera holder is available. The abdomen and perineum should be prepped and draped in a sterile manner.

Surgical Technique

The procedure for extended right hemicolectomy begins exactly like a standard right hemicolectomy. The instruments used are long bowel graspers, scissors, right-angle forceps, and a needle holder. The dissecting energy source can be either an ultrasonic-activated device or an electrosurgical vessel-sealing device. If an ultrasonic machine is employed, a vascular stapler should be used for the vascular pedicles. Choice of mode of access (open or laparoscopic) for the peritoneal cavity should be based on the surgeon's experience and preference. A reusable 10-mm port is placed at the umbilicus. A reusable 5-mm port is placed 3 cm medial to the right anterior superior iliac spine. A disposable, threaded 12-mm port is placed in the left upper quadrant lateral to the rectus muscle sheath and cephalad to the umbilicus. A reusable 12-mm port is placed 3 cm proximal to the pubic tubercle just to the left of the midline. A 30-degree videoscope (5 or 10 mm in diameter) should be placed at the umbilicus.

Step 1: The surgeon and assistant begin by standing on the patient's left side. The table is turned into a moderate left tilt as well as into a slight Trendelenburg position. The peritoneal surfaces and liver are inspected for tumor growth. The ileocolic vessels are identified by gentle traction applied by the assistant to the cecum, and the SMV is located. A window beneath the ileocolic vessels is opened incising the peritoneum close to the SMV and gently lifting the ileocolic vessels with a closed grasper; the ileocolic artery crossing to the SMV is assessed as anterior or posterior, and the ileocolic vessels are divided after the duodenum has been identified.

Step 2: The right ureter is identified by inspection and, if necessary, by gentle palpation with a blunt instrument while the assistant gently elevates the stump of the ileocolic vessels (specimen side) off of the retroperitoneum.

Step 3: The dissection starts at the origin of the ileocolic vessels and proceeds along the SMV in a cephalad direction; if present, the right colic vessels are divided after one has assessed whether the right colic artery crosses anteriorly or posteriorly to the SMV. At this point, the dissection ends at the origin of the Henle's gastrocolic trunk from the SMV. The mesentery of the proximal transverse colon is gently elevated off the duodenum.

Step 4: The table is leveled from the Trendelenburg position but kept in a moderate left tilt; the omentum is divided and the lesser sac entered; the division of the omentum is performed in a medial-to-lateral direction caudal to the right gastroepiploic vessels using a dissecting device.

Step 5: The hepatic flexure is mobilized in a medial-to-lateral direction, the lateral peritoneal reflection of the ascending colon is divided along the white line of Toldt in a caudal to cephalad direction, and the mesentery of the ascending colon is mobilized off the retroperitoneum.

Step 6: The terminal ileum is transected with a laparoscopic stapler, and the pole of the cecum is mobilized.

Step 7: The surgeon and assistant now move to the patient's right side. The surgeon uses the right-sided and suprapubic ports. The table is tilted to the right and in reversed Trendelenburg position, and the transverse colon is gently elevated off the duodenum to identify the middle colic vessels. It is important to recognize the anatomic location of the SMV as well as the gastrocolic trunk of Henle.[99] These vessels are short, and excessive traction can lead to profuse bleeding at the inferior border of the pancreas. The middle colic vessels are divided while the transverse mesentery is held up.

Step 8: Division of the greater omentum is continued toward the patient's left by grasping the gastrocolic ligament, thus fully opening the lesser sac and always avoiding traction on the spleen. The splenic flexure is mobilized laterally by retracting the colon gently medially, dividing the lateral attachments, and lifting the colon off of the retroperitoneum, carefully avoiding the tail of the pancreas. To fully mobilize the flexure, the retroperitoneum is incised 1 cm below the pancreas, and the colon is peeled off of Gerota's fascia.

Step 9: The descending colon is transected with a laparoscopic stapler, coming in from the right-sided port.

Step 10: The table is leveled from the right tilt; the antimesenteric side of the stapled ends of the descending colon and terminal ileum are approximated by a stay suture tied intracorporeally and then held by the assistant. An antimesenteric enterotomy and an antimesenteric colotomy are made 10 cm distal to the stapled ends of the transverse colon and terminal ileum, respectively, and a side-to-side anastomosis is fashioned with a laparoscopic stapler, placed at the suprapubic port. The enterotomy after stapler extraction is closed by two layers of silk sutures tied intracorporeally. The mesenteric defect is left open.

Step 11: The specimen is delivered in a bag, or using a wound protector, through an enlarged umbilical or suprapubic port site. Fascial defects larger than 5 mm are closed with 0-polyglycolic acid sutures. Skin incisions are closed with running subcuticular 4–0 polyglycolic acid sutures.

Postoperative Care

If a nasogastric or orogastric tube is used intraoperatively, this should be removed at the end of the procedure. The patient is encouraged to ambulate on the day of the procedure because early mobilization is imperative for helping to prevent complications, such as atelectasis, pneumonia, or vein thrombosis. A liquid diet should be started on postoperative day 1 if there are no clinical signs of ileus. Usually, oral pain medications are tolerated on postoperative day 1. The Foley catheter should also be removed on postoperative day 1 unless there are clinical signs of hypovolemia. Most patients are ready for discharge from the hospital on postoperative days 3 to 4. Follow-up should be at 2 and 6 weeks and after that according to each institution's protocol for colon cancer.

Laparoscopic-Assisted Left Colon Resection for Recurrent Diverticulitis

Introduction

The natural history of diverticulitis was described in the first half of the last century. Parks observed in 1969,[161] in his review of more than 500 patients, that 10% to 25% of those with diverticular disease will develop symptoms at some time in their lives. Furthermore, nearly one-fourth of those successfully treated medically after a first episode of acute diverticulitis were readmitted with a second episode. Parks also found that the disease behaved more aggressively in younger patients. Subsequent studies confirm this as well as suggesting that recurrent episodes of uncomplicated diverticulitis are a risk factor for developing complicated diverticulitis. This has led to guidelines that were followed during the second half of the last century, in which elective surgery was recommended following two episodes of acute diverticulitis and after one episode in patients younger than 40 years of age. More recent studies have challenged this approach. Simply stated it appears that the era of recommending elective surgery based on the strict criteria of the number of prior episodes and the patient's age appears to have passed. We have now begun an era of individualized treatment.

Guidelines from major surgical societies (European Association for Endoscopic Surgery [EAES],[117] American Society of Colon and Rectal Surgeons [ASCRS], and the Society for Surgery of the Alimentary Tract [SSAT]) agree that for elective resection for recurrent, uncomplicated diverticulitis, one must consider the risks of death using the colorectal POSSUM score and to what extent the frequency and severity of the episode(s) and/or persisting symptoms following the acute episode impact one's quality of life. Because the sigmoid colon is most frequently the site of disease, a complete sigmoid resection is recommended. It is important that the level of the distal resection is accomplished in the upper rectum and not the distal sigmoid colon in order to reduce the risk of recurrence.[208] There is no need to extend the resection proximally, even if there are diverticula present in the proximal colon, as long as they are not inflamed.[228] There is general consensus that laparoscopic surgery for diverticular disease is safe and even advantageous; this has been confirmed in a recent randomized, controlled trial.[115]

Indications

The decision whether resection is indicated for recurrent uncomplicated diverticular disease needs to be made on a case-by-case basis, that is, the severity of the disease and the patients' preoperative risk. The former may be quantified by means of a careful history, whereas the POSSUM score may be useful to measure the latter. Surgical access to the abdomen, be it conventional or laparoscopic, should have no bearing on whether a patient undergoes an operation. It is important to preoperatively attempt to distinguish recurrent, uncomplicated diverticulitis from other conditions likely to cause pain in the lower abdomen, such as the irritable bowel syndrome or endometriosis.

The authors of this chapter suggest that the indications for laparoscopic resection for recurrent uncomplicated diverticulitis may include frequent episodes of left lower quadrant abdominal pain with signs of inflammation (fever, chills, change in bowel habits, etc.), leading to absence from work or affecting quality of life; severe frequent attacks leading to hospitalization; persistent symptoms between acute episodes, such as spasms and bowel irregularity not relieved by antispasmotics and bulking agents and that do not fulfill the Rome criteria for irritable bowel syndrome; and patients who require chronic immunosuppression. The finding of stricture in the sigmoid colon places the case in the category of complicated diverticulitis and constitutes an indication for resection because of one's inability to rule out colonic carcinoma.

Treatment options must, of course, be discussed with the patient. The patient should understand the material facts and possible risks and complications of the planned surgery before signing the informed consent form.

Preoperative Workup
As with any recommended surgery, whether open or laparoscopic, a thorough history and physical examination are essential, detailing number, frequency, and severity of episodes. The time from the last episode is important because it is optimal to perform surgery at least 6 to 8 weeks later. In patients with more frequent episodes, however, this may not be possible. Additional assessment should include a colonoscopy as well as an imaging study, usually computed tomographic (CT) scan, to provide information on location of the disease process, extent of disease, and coexisting intra-abdominal abnormalities. Blood work should include typing and screen. Chest x-ray and EKG should be routinely performed for those at the age of 50. The bowel should be prepared orally with laxatives and intravenous antibiotics in accordance with each institution's protocol. However, if narrowing of the bowel is evident, no laxative preparation should be administered, but an enema should be given the night before surgery and the morning of the procedure.

Operating Room
The patient should be identified with an appropriate time-out prior to the induction of the anesthetic. A Foley catheter, a left ureteral stent, and an orogastric tube should be inserted. The patient is placed supine on the operating table with the lower limbs either in stirrups or abducted. Sequential compression devices are applied to the legs. Both arms should be tucked. The patient should be securely strapped to the table at the chest because tilting the table will inevitably be necessary. All equipment, including monitors, should be placed on the patient's left side. The surgeon stands on the patient's right side (Figure 19-50). One assistant is needed to control the camera unless a robotic camera holder is available. The abdomen and perineum should be prepped and sterilely draped.

Surgical Technique
A 30-degree laparoscope (5 or 10 mm in diameter) should be placed in the midline slightly above the umbilicus. Two additional 10 to 12 mm trocars are placed in the right side of the abdomen: one lateral to the rectus muscle sheath proximal to the umbilicus and the other in the right lower quadrant at the level of the anterior superior iliac spine. If there is a need for additional retraction or suction, 5-mm ports can be placed in the left side lateral to the rectus sheath, as well as suprapubically in the midline. The surgeon uses an atraumatic bowel grasper in the left hand and alternates the use of scissors, right-angle clamp, ultrasonic or bipolar vessel-sealing devices, and staplers in the right hand.

To ensure a tension-free anastomosis, the splenic flexure should be mobilized. This is accomplished initially with the camera at the umbilical port and the table tilted to the right and in reverse Trendelenburg. The gastrocolic ligament is grasped, the lesser sac opened and the mobilization continued in an antegrade fashion toward the spleen. The descending colon is then mobilized in a retrograde fashion by placing gentle retraction on the appendices epiploicae of the colon in order to expose the white line of Toldt; this is incised sharply. The transverse colon is peeled off Gerota's fascia by incising the retroperitoneum 1 cm below the pancreas and by using blunt dissection to lift the colon.

Once the splenic flexure has been adequately mobilized, the table is positioned in steep Trendelenburg. The omentum and small bowel are placed in the right upper quadrant. A lateral-to-medial approach is then used to mobilize the sigmoid colon. First, the left ureter and the left iliac vein are identified. The retroperitoneum is then incised from the right side at the sacral promontory with the colon retracted anteriorly, and the avascular plane underneath the colonic mesentery visualized. The following branches of the inferior mesenteric artery are identified: left colic, sigmoidal, and superior hemorrhoidal. The left colic and sigmoidal branches are divided using a bipolar vessel-sealing device. The superior hemorrhoidal artery should be spared in order to preserve the proximal blood supply to the rectal stump. It is not necessary to divide the inferior mesenteric vein for this dissection, unless there is a problem with the length of the remaining colon ensuring a tension-free anastomosis. It can be helpful to divide the mesentery of the colon at the point where the proximal resection is planned in order to facilitate extraction of the specimen.

Once the colon is completely mobilized, the dissection is carried on to the proximal rectum because it is imperative that the division of the colon be undertaken below the rectosigmoid junction. Care is taken to stay in the avascular plane around the mesorectum to avoid injury to the left ureter and the hypogastric nerves. The rectum is then divided using a linear stapler with staples that are 3.5 mm (blue cartridge). Ideally, one is able to obtain a single staple line perpendicular to the rectum, but often more than one firing of the stapler is required to accomplish the task. The stapled end of the colon is grasped with a locking grasper, and an incision is made to extract the specimen. This can be performed by making a 4- to 6-cm long suprapubic (Pfannenstiel) incision. The wound edges are protected with a wound protector, and the stapled end of the colon delivered through the incision. Once the sigmoid colon is resected, the proximal end is prepared for a circular anastomosis, either in an end-to-end fashion or by a side-to-end approach if there are extensive diverticula present proximally. The colon with the anvil secured is placed back in the abdominal cavity and the abdomen re-insufflated. The anastomosis is then carried out in

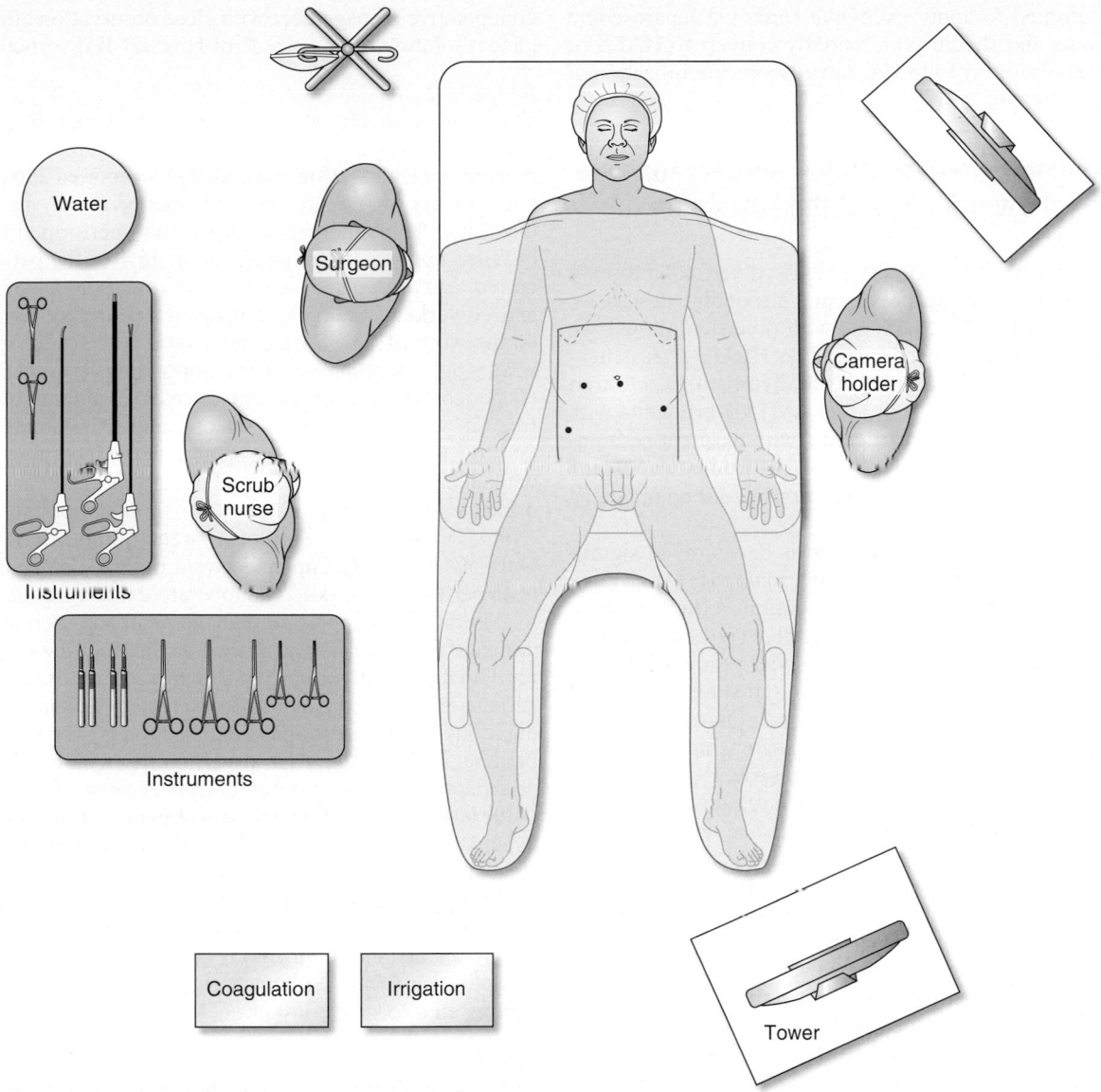

FIGURE 19-50. Operating room setup for left colon resection for recurrent diverticulitis.

the usual fashion, using the circular stapler. The integrity of the anastomosis should be checked with an air-water test. Drains should not be used routinely. The final steps are to check for hemostasis, to suction all fluid from the pelvis, and to ascertain that there are no loops of small bowel herniated underneath the descending colon. The fascia at the extraction site is closed with a running, nonabsorbable suture. If any 10- to 12-mm ports are used, the fascia should be closed. The skin can be closed with staples.

Postoperative Care
If a nasogastric or orogastric tube is used intraoperatively, this should be removed at the end of the procedure. A liquid diet should be started on postoperative day 1 if there are no clinical signs of ileus. Also, usually oral pain medications are tolerated on postoperative day 1. The Foley catheter should also be removed on that day unless there are clinical signs of hypovolemia. Early mobilization with chest physical therapy is imperative to prevent complications like atelectasis, pneumonia, and vein thrombosis. Most patients are ready

for discharge from the hospital on postoperative days 3 to 4. Follow-up should be at 2 and 6 weeks. Flexible sigmoidoscopy is generally undertaken by 6 months. If there are no recurrent symptoms at 12 months, the patient can return to routine colonoscopic screening appropriate for age and risk factors for colon cancer.

Opinion
Laparoscopic sigmoid colectomy is currently performed by most surgeons through the use of a laparoscopic-assisted method with a suprapubic horizontal or infraumbilical midline incision. In fact, nonrandomized and randomized data reported similar clinical outcomes following intracorporeal sigmoid colectomy as compared to its laparoscopic-assisted counterpart. Laparoscopic intracorporeal hand-sewn purse-string suture at the proximal colon end is not popular due to a combination of lack of training in laparoscopic suturing and ergonomic difficulties. The advent of robotic technology may impact intracorporeal suturing in the future. In the case of woody diverticulitis or complex phlegmon, surgeons should

not be tempted to apply excessive force via laparoscopic instruments and should preferentially convert to HALS or conventional surgery following laparoscopic mobilization of the splenic flexure.

Laparoscopic Nonresectional Surgery for Hinchey II Diverticulitis of the Left Colon

Introduction

Besides the acute inflammatory process, diverticular disease can be complicated by pelvic and mesocolic abscesses. In fact, 20% to 30% of patients with diverticulitis will be classified as having an abscess. The Hinchey classification (see Chapter 27) stratifies acute diverticulitis into four classes: diverticulitis without abscess (I), diverticulitis with abscess (II), perforated diverticulitis with purulent peritonitis (III), and perforated diverticulitis with fecal peritonitis (IV). Hinchey class II or higher is considered complicated diverticulitis.

Management of acute diverticulitis has evolved significantly and is based on severity of the acute disease process, prior diverticulitis history, and patient comorbidities. Historically, recommendation for elective sigmoid resection was made after resolution of two episodes of uncomplicated or Hinchey I diverticulitis, or following just one episode of Hinchey II diverticulitis. The reason for this recommendation was based on the possibility of increasing severity of complications with each subsequent episode. However, there are now data to suggest that more than one-half of patients presenting with perforated diverticulitis had not had a prior episode of diverticulitis.[42] In other words, individuals do not necessarily have an increased risk of perforation with each subsequent episode. The treatment for diverticulitis with a Hinchey II abscess has evolved as percutaneous CT-guided drainage techniques have improved. Currently, the preferred approach for these patients is to place them on bowel rest with intravenous antibiotics and percutaneously drain the abscess if it is larger than 3 cm. These individuals are then offered elective sigmoid colon resection after the acute episode has resolved and a colonoscopy has been accomplished. However, the natural history after percutaneous drainage has not been very well defined. There is little data on the recurrence rates of diverticulitis after resolution of one acute episode of Hinchey II diverticulitis. This is because all available data is retrospective and includes a mixed patient population with different severity of disease. In addition, surgical resection does not always resolve the symptoms, with some studies reporting as high as a 20% incidence of persistent complaints after adequate resection.[67] Surgical resection exposes patients to the operative risks, including anastomotic leak, the need for an ostomy, cardiac and pulmonary complications, surgical site infections, thromboembolic events, and mortality.

There are some authors who advocate not considering diverticulitis with a mesocolic abscess as an indication for surgery.[6] Understanding the risks of surgery, many patients and doctors fear recurrent diverticulitis less than they fear surgery. Moreover, patients undergoing elective sigmoid resection may experience up to a 38.5% postoperative complication rate, whereas those undergoing nonoperative management (with percutaneous drainage) have only a 5% complication rate.[202] There is no level 1 evidence in the literature that defines the role of elective surgery versus nonoperative management with close observation after complete resolution of an episode of Hinchey II diverticulitis.

Indications

The goal of nonoperative management is clearly to avoid emergency surgery. The optimal way to achieve this goal remains unclear. Nelson and colleagues reported 256 patients with abscess or free air managed nonoperatively in 39% of the cases.[156] No emergency surgery was performed because of failed nonoperative management; 46% of the patients recurred, and 20% underwent elective resection. Dharmarajan and coworkers[58] suggested using a grading system based on the work of Siewert and associates[200] to stratify patients who would be candidates for nonoperative management: (1) pericolonic free air without abscess, (2) amount of distant free air <2 cm or abscess <4 cm, and (3) amount of distant free air >2 cm or abscess >4 cm.[58] Except for patients with an abscess >4 cm who had undergone CT scan–guided drainage, all other patients were treated nonoperatively (NPO, IV antibiotics, and total parenteral nutrition [TPN]). Only 5% of 136 patients underwent urgent surgery that had been performed for failed nonoperative management.[58]

Although nonoperative management with percutaneous drainage of a diverticular abscess is the first line of therapy for Hinchey II diverticulitis, laparoscopic nonresectional surgery may be considered for selected patients. The indications for laparoscopic nonresectional surgery include patients with Hinchey IIb diverticulitis where CT-guided percutaneous drainage is not feasible because of the location of the abscess, or in situations where interventional radiology expertise is not available, and the patient is deteriorating despite appropriate medical treatment. Treatment options must be discussed with the patient. Advantages and disadvantages of such alternatives should be explained in lay terms. One should understand the material facts and possible risks and complications of the planned surgery prior to the patient signing an informed consent.

Preoperative Workup

A thorough history and physical exam are, of course, essential. A peripheral intravenous line should be placed on arrival in the hospital. A CT scan of the abdomen and pelvis with intravenous contrast helps establish the Hinchey class. Intravenous antibiotics should be started as soon as the diagnosis of complicated diverticulitis is confirmed. Blood work should include typing and screening. A chest x-ray and EKG should be performed in those older than the age of 50. No bowel preparation should be used.

Operating Room

The patient should be identified with an appropriate time-out prior to the induction of general anesthesia with endotracheal intubation. If the patient cannot tolerate a general anesthetic, the procedure can be accomplished with a spinal or epidural, with the addition of a transverse block. Adequate intravenous access should be ensured. If the patient is hemodynamically unstable, an arterial line and/or a central venous catheter should be considered, and a Foley catheter and nasogastric or orogastric tube inserted. The patient is placed supine on the operating table with the lower limbs either in stirrups or abducted. Sequential compression devices are applied to the legs. Both arms should be tucked. The patient should be securely strapped to the table at the chest because tilting the table will be necessary. All equipment including monitors should be placed on the patient's left side in clear view of the surgeon, who stands on the patient's right side. One assistant is needed to control the camera. The abdomen should be prepped and draped sterile. Because most diverticular abscesses are located in the sigmoid colon, the preparation and draping should be the same as that for a laparoscopic sigmoid resection. Intraoperative endoscopy should be available. The surgeon should consider having ureteral stents placed, in case the operative plan changes to resectional surgery.

Surgical Technique

There is great variation in the literature on how nonresectional surgery should be performed. This ranges from drainage of an abscess with irrigation of the abdominal cavity to creation of a diverting loop ileostomy. The following are general guidelines that need to be modified as deemed necessary for each case. Choice of access to the peritoneal cavity should be based on the surgeon's experience. However, if the abdomen is distended, an open method of entry is safer than the use of a Veress needle. A 30-degree laparoscope (5 or 10 mm in diameter) should be placed slightly above the umbilicus. Placement of additional trocars depends on the location of the perforation. Most commonly, 5-mm ports are placed in the right abdominal quadrants lateral to the rectus muscle sheath. Intraoperative rigid or flexible endoscopy should be considered early in the procedure to rule out bowel perforation. If, after thorough inspection of the abdomen, the abscess site is found and the intent of surgery is to perform lavage only, irrigation is carried out in all four quadrants with copious amounts of warmed saline solution until the abdomen has been cleansed. A high-pressure laparoscopic irrigation system is necessary to accomplish this. The use of antibiotic solution or dilute Betadine solution has been described. Either can be used at the surgeon's discretion. If a more definitive approach becomes necessary, lysis of adhesions and blunt lateral-to-medial mobilization are performed in order to separate the inflamed segment of colon from adjacent structures. Purulent fluid should be aspirated and cultured. If an obvious bowel perforation is found at intraoperative endoscopy, the operative plan is changed to that of resectional surgery. The decision to add a diverting stoma depends on whether the source of contamination has been adequately controlled. An air-leak test with a proctoscope can be helpful to determine the status. Irrigation is then carried out in the same manner as described earlier. The placement of drains in the pelvis is advisable.

Postoperative Care

The nasogastric or orogastric tube can be removed at the end of the procedure. A liquid diet should be started on postoperative day 1 if there are no clinical signs of ileus. Drains should be removed within 5 days. Antibiotics should be continued intravenously until the patient is afebrile, blood work is normalizing, and the patient is able to take medication by mouth. However, the total duration of antibiotics should be at least 10 days. After the initial course of the acute illness has passed, a full evaluation of the colon needs to be carried out by means of a colonoscopy to rule out malignant disease. Ultimately, the need for resectional surgery needs to be addressed at a later time for the diverticular disease. This decision needs careful risk–benefit assessment, wherein the risks of subsequent attacks are compared with the risks of elective surgery.

Laparoscopic Hartmann's Procedure for Perforated Diverticulitis with Peritonitis

Introduction

Free perforation with peritonitis is a life-threatening complication of diverticulitis. Although uncommon, the prevalence of perforated diverticulitis has increased in developed countries with the sigmoid colon affected in 98%. A recent retrospective review of a large database indicates a trend toward decreased use of the Hartmann procedure (HP) in emergency surgery for diverticulitis (from 61% in 2002 to 54% in 2007).[136] According to the same database, the use of resection with primary anastomosis (PRA) in emergency surgery for diverticulitis has increased by 7%.[136] A few retrospective studies have suggested that PRA may be a safe alternative to the HP for perforated diverticulitis with peritonitis.[195,235] Moreover, a still recent review reported that adverse event rates following PRA and HP might be similar.[210]

The Standard Task Force of the ASCRS states that the role and safety of PRA in perforated diverticulitis with peritonitis remains unsettled.[171] The literature offers also interesting data from nonrandomized studies. A systematic review of 98 studies published between 1957 and 2003 reported that adverse event rates following PRA and HP for perforated diverticulitis with peritonitis did not differ significantly (see also Chapter 27). There were 569 PRA patients from 50 studies and 1,051 HP patients from 54 studies. Mortality rates were 9.9% and 18.6%, respectively.[186] Another systematic review of 15 studies noted that mortality rates were similar following PRA and HP for perforated diverticulitis with peritonitis provided that the patients were matched for severity of peritonitis. There were 547 PRA patients and 416 HP patients. Mortality rates were 14.1% and 14.4%, respectively.[51]

The evolution of surgical technique for perforated diverticulitis consists of a transition from three-stage surgery to two-stage surgery. According to a retrospective review of a large database from 2002 to 2007, a diverting loop ileostomy was rarely added in the context of PRA for perforated diverticulitis with peritonitis (1%).[158] The literature suggests that anastomotic leakage rate after PRA is approximately 10%.[186] Unfortunately, two-stage surgery entails a second operation in order to close the stoma. It is known that HPs are not restored in a troublingly high proportion. In fact, a study of 11,582 hospital admissions for diverticulitis reported that 35% of 1,176 HP patients had not undergone closure at a 4-year follow-up.[132] Moreover, a review of 6,619 patients undergoing emergency surgery for perforated diverticulitis with peritonitis reported a reversal rate of 73%.[50] Although HP was originally described for rectal cancer and thereby involved low rectal transection,[91] the term HP has been extended to include any left colon resection with end colostomy. There are only a few reports of laparoscopic HP for perforated diverticulitis with fecal peritonitis in the literature.[46]

Indications

When surgery is indicated for perforated diverticulitis of the sigmoid colon with peritonitis, the choice of the type of surgery should be based on the extent of the disease and the patient's preoperative risk. The former may be quantified using the Mannheim Peritonitis Index, whereas APACHE or POSSUM scores may be useful to measure the latter. Resection remains the standard of care for perforated diverticulitis with peritonitis because of the reported lower postoperative death rates (low evidence level). HP should be performed in case of fecal peritonitis, whereas those with purulent peritonitis should undergo PRA with loop ileostomy.

Operating Room

The patient is placed supine on the operating table with the lower limbs either in stirrups or abducted. Sequential compression devices are applied to the legs. Both arms should be tucked. The patient should be securely strapped to the table at the chest because tilting the table will be necessary. All equipment including monitors should be placed on the patient's left side in clear view of the surgeon, and the surgeon stands on the patient's right side. One assistant is needed to operate the camera. The abdomen is prepped and draped in a sterile manner.

Surgical Technique

A 10-mm Hasson port is inserted infraumbilically using an open technique. Pneumoperitoneum is established, and the camera is introduced in order to perform a diagnostic laparoscopy. Three additional ports are inserted in the right upper and lower quadrants (5 mm and 12 mm in diameter) and in the left lower quadrant at the site of the projected end colostomy (12 mm in diameter).

After establishing the diagnosis of diverticulitis with fecal peritonitis, the first step of the procedure is to withdraw a peritoneal fluid sample for culture. Positive pressure peritoneal irrigation is then performed using warm 0.9% saline. The inferior mesenteric artery is ligated following identification of the left ureter in a medial-to-lateral fashion. The diseased left colon is mobilized in a lateral-to-medial direction. The right and left leaflets of the peritoneum at the level of the sacral promontory are incised beyond the macroscopically inflamed colon but medial to the ureters. Mobilization is limited to thickened inflamed colon and always includes the rectosigmoid junction. The upper rectum is transected with a stapler. The splenic flexure of the colon is not mobilized. The skin is then incised around the 12-mm trocar at the site of the projected end colostomy, and a core of tissue is excised all the way down to the fascia, which is incised in a cross fashion to fit two fingerbreadths. The rectus muscle is spread along its fibers, and the posterior rectus muscle sheath is opened in a cruciate manner. The specimen may be exteriorized through a suprapubic horizontal incision or through the projected end colostomy site. In both cases, an abdominal wound protector is mandatory. Following bowel transection, the macroscopically normal colonic stump is matured as an end colostomy. Reinsufflation is then accomplished, and additional positive-pressure peritoneal lavage is performed to verify hemostasis. One drain is placed in the pelvis.

Opinion

An increasing number of case reports on laparoscopic nonresectional surgery for perforated diverticulitis with peritonitis have been published since 1996.[4] Surgery consists of irrigation with or without drainage, ignoring or addressing the perforation with biologic glue or sutures and/or omental patch, and with or without the addition of a stoma. Interestingly, intraoperative endoscopy is not included in the aforementioned literature, and there is an inconsistent policy whether elective resection should follow laparoscopic nonresectional surgery. It is unclear what happened to close the circle as Mayo and colleagues described irrigation with drainage and diverting ostomy in 1907.[138]

TABLE 19-2 A Method for Grading Recommendations According to Scientific Evidence[a]

GRADE OF RECOMMENDATION	LEVEL OF EVIDENCE	STUDY DESIGNS
A	1a	Systematic review of RCTs
	1b	Individual RCT
	1c	All or none case series
B	2a	Systematic review of cohort studies
	2b	Individual cohort study
	2c	Outcomes research
	3a	Systematic review of case-control studies
	3b	Individual case-control study
C	4	Case series
D	5	Expert opinion

RCT, randomized controlled trial.
[a]Data from Sackett DL, Straus SE, Richardson WS, et al. *Evidence-Based Medicine: How to Practice and Teach EBM.* 2nd ed. London, United Kingdom: Churchill Livingstone; 2000.

There are at least three categories for discussion. Editorial responsibility is one; in fact, too few editors have expressed their views such as those that appear in Arregui's "friendly disclaimer."[8] [‡] Another is how innovation in surgery should be implemented. There are currently no federal regulations governing new surgical procedures in the United States. Moreover, implementation of the American College of Surgeon's Committee on Emerging Surgical Technology and Education (CESTE) statement may be inadequate due to its voluntary nature.[7] As much as there is a need for innovation in surgery, it is necessary that this takes place in accordance with the rules of evidence.[141,177]

A third category for discussion is to what extent clinical guidelines are likely to increase compliance or impact patient outcomes.[140] In fact, both the EAES[189] and the Association of Coloproctology of Great Britain and Ireland (ACPGBI) guidelines[76] sound glorified when they ambiguously refer to "some patients" having been given a grade of recommendation C for laparoscopic nonresectional surgery (Table 19-2).

In conclusion, patients with perforated diverticulitis should undergo resection or nonresectional surgery regardless of whether the access to the abdomen is conventional or laparoscopic. And there is no gainsaying the fact that a surgeon should perform the same operation laparoscopically as he or she would accomplish by the open technique.[187]

[‡]Maurice E. Arregui is coeditor of a laparoscopic surgery journal. He decried the publications of papers describing unethical surgical procedures.

Laparoscopic Left Colectomy for Cancer

Introduction

What defines the left colon resection? Unfortunately, the answer is not as clear as it is with a right colon resection. That is because the left colon resection can involve resection of the colonic segment anywhere between the left transverse colon and the upper rectum, with the anastomosis located somewhere in that part of the colon. There does, however, appear to be one common denominator in patients requiring a left colon resection, and that is the need to mobilize the left portion of the colon.

It is important for surgeons who undertake a laparoscopic left colon resection to become familiar with all options available for mobilizing the left colon. Therefore, they must understand that one's preferred technique may not work in all cases. Thus, the surgeon should be prepared to use an alternative method depending on the specific situation. It is the author's preferred technique to use a medial-to-lateral approach with initial vascular control. In certain circumstances, the lateral-to-medial approach should be initially considered, such as in cases where there is an inability to retract the small bowel effectively or in those with an obese body habitus. Of course, even with the medial-to-lateral approach, there is not just one method available for accomplishing this maneuver. If the inferior mesenteric artery (IMA) cannot be easily identified and the inferior mesenteric vein (IMV) is visible, then dissection can be started with the IMV. Likewise, if a purely laparoscopic technique seems either impossible or dangerous because of unclear anatomy, then the surgeon should be familiar with the hand-assisted technique and the use of a Pfannenstiel incision. This approach can often avoid conversion to a laparotomy.

The goal of this chapter is to demonstrate that the approach to laparoscopic colon resection can and should be flexible. Because our work involves physicians in training, it is our responsibility to provide this in a way that can be structured, yet easy to remember. Herein, we describe a technique in which the majority of the dissection is performed by the qualified assistant (physician in training), whereas the primary surgeon remains in control of the overall procedure by holding the camera, retracting, and exposing the operating field. It is important at the outset to stress the value of adequate basic laparoscopic training for *both* surgeons, as well as the need for surgeons to be proficient in operating with both hands.

Indications

Indications for laparoscopic left colon resection include the presence of cancer or benign disease (diverticulitis, stricture, and Crohn's disease). Contraindications are a completely obstructing lesion, tumor invasion into other organs (small bowel, stomach, tail of pancreas, spleen, or kidney), and bulky lymphadenopathy at the root of the IMA.[36] Abdominal wall or omental invasion is not an absolute contraindication. Under such circumstances, modification of the laparoscopic approach by use of the hand-assisted technique through a Pfannenstiel incision is a very reasonable alternative.[145]

The spectrum of indications consists of a heterogeneous group of conditions and patients, with the common denominator being the requirement for full mobilization of the left colon. By this maneuver, the surgeon can perform an adequate resection with a secure, tension-free anastomosis. Full mobilization includes that of the left transverse colon, splenic flexure, descending colon, sigmoid colon, and upper rectum. In the majority of cancer cases, oncologic resection requires IMA lymphadenectomy, whereas in those involving diverticulitis, resection of the distal sigmoid is necessary. In both situations, a colorectal anastomosis is required. Rarely, a colo-colonic anastomosis is performed, such as may be appropriate with an early malignancy at the splenic flexure. Under these circumstances, only the left colic arterial branch is sacrificed. Principles of colonic resection for cancer are also discussed in Chapter 23.

Preoperative Workup

Patients must be medically cleared prior to undergoing this major abdominal procedure. Most have already undergone CT scan as part of their preoperative assessment. Important information pertaining to the planned surgical dissection can also be obtained from a detailed analysis of the CT scan. Generally, a colonoscopy has also been performed with India ink marking having already been accomplished.

Operating Room

After undergoing general and often epidural anesthesia, the patient is placed on a beanbag in a modified lithotomy position (Figure 19-51). Gel pads are used to protect all bony prominences, as well as potential sites of nerve compression, in order to avoid peripheral neuropathy. The beanbag is molded around the patient's body with special attention paid to the right side because the patient will spend most of the time tilted to that side. The beanbag is further supported with shoulder pads and brackets to prevent the patient from

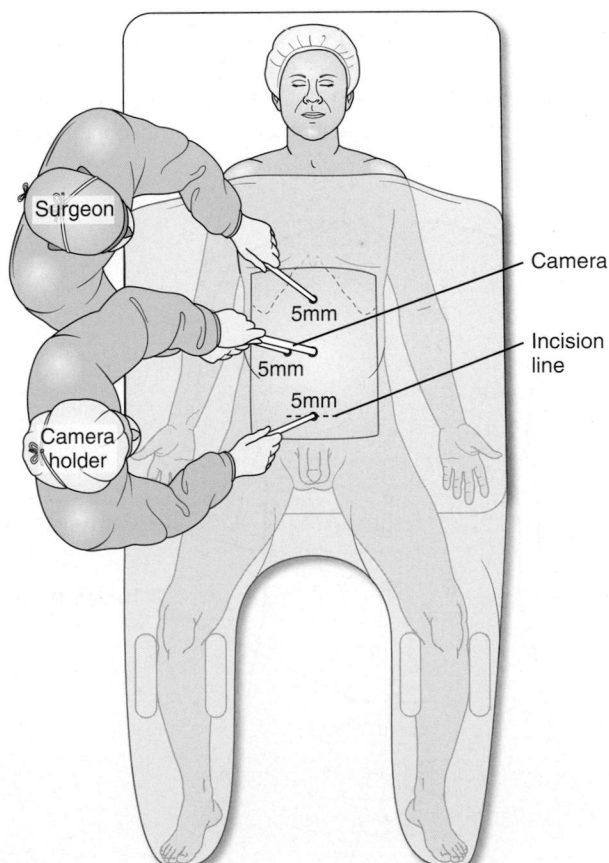

FIGURE 19-51. Operating room setup for laparoscopic left colectomy.

sliding while in the Trendelenburg position. The chest is also taped to the bed to prevent any sideways sliding.

An orogastric tube (removed at the end of operation) and Foley catheter are inserted. In cases where the circular stapler is used to create the anastomosis, it is our preference to insert a rectal irrigation system. This is made up of a large Foley catheter, water bag, and collection bag. These are all joined by a three-way connector. Once this has been accomplished, the patient is draped in the standard fashion. It is helpful to use the Ioban (3M US) foil to prevent the draping towels from sliding down and exposing the unsterile field. As with any laparoscopic operation, side pockets are also useful.

The operation is performed by two surgeons using a four-hand technique. The surgeon stands by the patient's right hip while the assistant (often the physician-in-training) stands on the left side of the surgeon. The scrub nurse is situated either in between the patient's legs or by the left leg of the patient. The active monitor is placed on the left side of the patient.

Surgical Technique

The goal of the procedure described next is to perform complete laparoscopic mobilization of the left colon. Resection of the requisite colonic segment and subsequent reconstruction can be performed in an extracorporeal fashion through the small incision (most often the Pfannenstiel). If one chooses to limit the amount of extracorporeal work to be performed, then the small incision can be used to extract the specimen, and in most cases to insert the anvil for the circular end-to-end colorectal anastomosis.

We prefer to use the Veress needle to establish the pneumoperitoneum when we believe it is safe to do so, such as when there is no scar around the umbilicus. In other cases, the Hasson technique can be employed. The pneumoperitoneum pressure should be set at 15 mm Hg. The entire procedure can be performed using four 5-mm ports with a high resolution 5-mm camera scope (Figure 19-52). If a good quality 5-mm camera is not available, then a 10-mm scope through a 12-mm umbilical port is suggested. This will prevent frequent fogging of the lens. This technique allows for major vascular control, with a 5-mm energy device and complete mobilization of the left colon. In the majority of cases, we use a 0-degree camera, although a 30-degree downward lens is useful for a difficult splenic flexure.

The instruments necessary for our preferred technique include two atraumatic bowel graspers, one cautery hook (ideally hand-controlled), and a 5-mm energy device that is able to seal and divide a 7-mm vascular pedicle (our preferred instrument is Enseal by Ethicon). The first port is placed in the umbilical area and will accommodate the scope. The next two 5-mm ports are placed in the midline in the epigastrium and suprapubic areas. Finally, the third 5-mm port is placed approximately 6 to 7 cm lateral to the umbilicus (as measured on the insufflated abdomen). Next, one mobilizes the left colon using the medial-to-lateral approach; this initially involves division of the vascular pedicles.

The patient is placed in the Trendelenburg position with a steep tilt to the right. The primary surgeon, situated at the patient's right hip, holds the camera in the left hand and the atraumatic bowel grasper in the right (introduced through the suprapubic port). The assistant stands on the left side of the primary surgeon and holds another atraumatic grasper in his left hand (epigastric port) and a cautery hook in his right hand (lateral port).

The first step is to clear the base of the left mesocolon by retracting the small bowel and pushing it into the right upper quadrant. It is helpful to identify the important landmarks so that both the primary surgeon and the assistant have the same reference points. These landmarks include the sacral promontory, IMA pedicle, and IMV pedicle (Figure 19-53). In addition, we determine how much sigmoid colon is located in the pelvis and what attachment points are involved.

The second step requires exposing and retracting the mesocolon of the rectosigmoid at the level of the sacral promontory. The primary surgeon pulls up on the rectosigmoid ventrally in order to create tension on the peritoneum at its base. A line is then marked with a cautery between the origin of the IMA pedicle and the sacral promontory. The arc of the superior hemorrhoidal artery (SHA) and the pedicle of the IMA are visualized. Dissection is performed below the artery arc. The undersurface of the artery is exposed with preservation of the autonomic nerve plexus. For better orientation, the top of the presacral space can be visualized, and

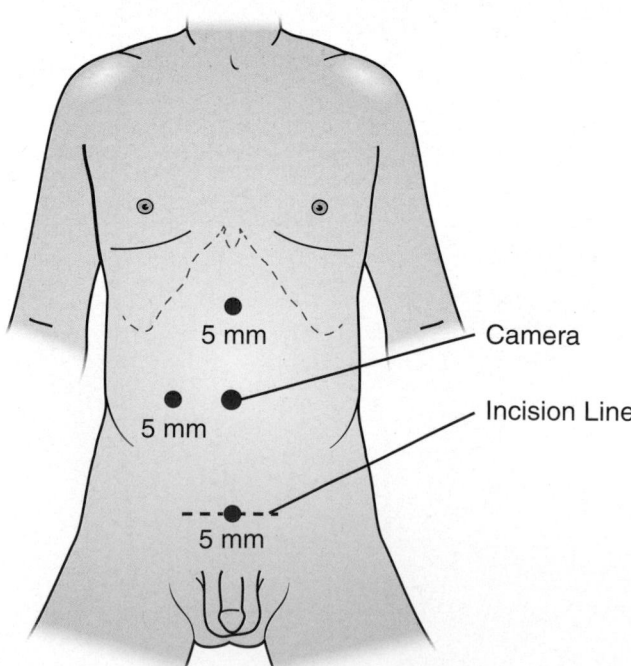

FIGURE 19-52. Port placement for laparoscopic left colectomy.

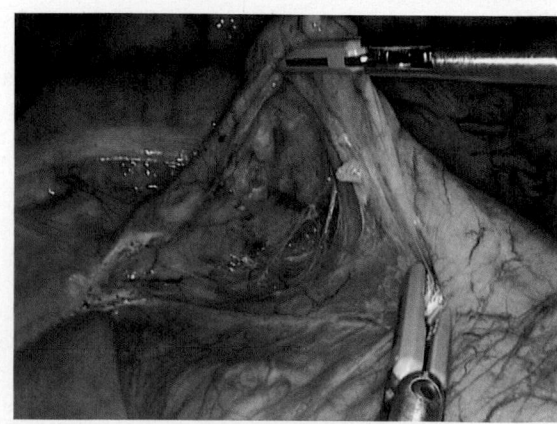

FIGURE 19-53. Identifying inferior mesenteric vein (IMV).

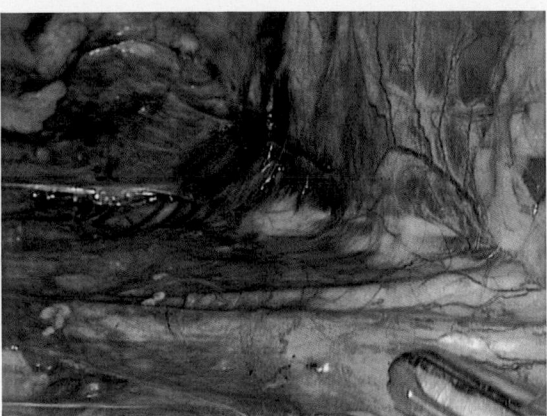

FIGURE 19-54. Left ureter is identified.

dissection can continue toward the left ureter. The left iliac artery can be seen or felt. It is important to leave a layer of areolar tissue covering the iliac arteries in order to ensure that the dissection is not performed too deeply or in the wrong tissue plane. The left ureter can then be seen (Figure 19-54).

It is potentially hazardous when performing the dissection to expose the ureter, leaving the periureteric vessels on the mesenteric side of dissection. If this occurs, it is often necessary to incise the fascial reflection in order to reach the correct, more superficial layer and to leave the vessels on the retroperitoneal (down) side of dissection. Once the arc of the SHA is released and sufficient retroperitoneal dissection is performed, the next step is to isolate the IMA pedicle (Figure 19-55). Because more of an upward retraction can now be provided to the pedicle, it is easy to isolate it. The base of the mesentery cephalad from the IMA is incised. Some of the retroperitoneum is separated from the mesocolon in a similar manner that was accomplished earlier. Both planes of dissection are joined behind the IMA. Fibrosis underneath the origin of the IMA pedicle is frequently seen and involves lymphatic vessels, as well as the autonomic nerve fibers, which are located on the surface of the aorta. Dissection in this area should be performed meticulously. The authors do so using the cautery hook, although cautery scissors are a good option as well. As long as the dissection is kept directly underneath the pedicle, the autonomic nerves should be able to be preserved.

Division of the IMA pedicle is frequently performed beneath the takeoff of the left colic artery (LCA). The SHA and the LCA branches can be taken separately if the pedicle is very thick or if calcifications are suspected. Prior to division of the pedicle, it is important to ensure that the left ureter is at a safe distance. We routinely use the 5-mm sealing/cutting device to control the pedicle (any of three working ports can be used in these circumstances). The alternative is to use a laparoscopic vascular stapler; however, this device requires a 12-mm laparoscopic port. In our experience, we very rarely encounter cases in which the standard clipping and cutting technique can be used easily.

Because the strongest attachments of the left mesocolon have previously been released, it is straightforward to detach the rest of the mesocolon from the aorta. This is accomplished up to the level of the IMV origin. Occasionally, some of the duodenal/small bowel attachments need to be taken down in order to visualize the IMV pedicle. Initial dissection is then performed in the proper retroperitoneal plane. Subsequently, a window is created in a thin avascular area of the mesentery just above the takeoff of the left colic vein (the branch supplying the splenic flexure). The main pedicle is then divided using the energy device (Figure 19-56). The epigastric port can often be used to provide a good angle for vascular division.

Once the base of the mesentery is completely released, the next step is to divide the mesentery from the retroperitoneum. This, of course, should be performed in the proper plane. The primary goal for performing the dissection is to leave no remaining layers of the tortuous, small vessels on the mesenteric undersurface. The dissection should be accomplished along the inferior border of the pancreas, toward the left upper quadrant in the direction of splenic hilum. This part of the dissection is easier to accomplish than beneath the SHA arc. If a special effort is required to separate the layers, it means that the dissection is being performed too deeply. In such a circumstance, gradual separation should be performed in a caudal direction. The lateral limit of dissection is marked by exposure of the colonic wall. In the left lower quadrant, the ureter and the gonadal vessels, as well as the psoas muscle, are encountered, but all of these structures are to be left behind the distinct layer of an intact Gerota's fascia.

Retroperitoneal dissection is then performed in a blunt fashion, as long as it is carried out in the proper plane. Typically, the primary surgeon lifts up the edge of the mesentery

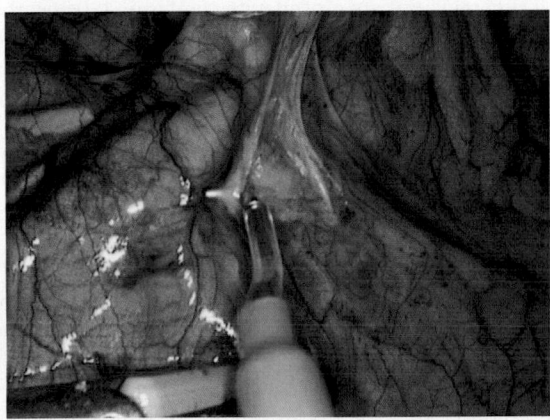

FIGURE 19-55. Dissection of inferior mesenteric artery (IMA).

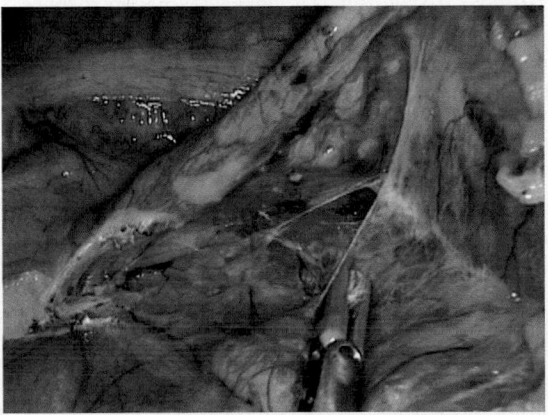

FIGURE 19-56. Dividing inferior mesenteric vein (IMV).

with his or her right hand, using the grasper introduced through the suprapubic port (macroretraction). The assistant then provides the upward microretraction in the working niche underneath the mesentery using his left hand. The right hand is used to hold the blunt instrument (e.g., energy device) to perform downward movement while dissecting the planes.

Once the retroperitoneum is separated from the mesentery, the dissection can be moved from beneath the mesentery to the lateral aspect of the proximal sigmoid. In a standard fashion (the same as in the open technique), the lateral attachments are divided, joining the space already created under the bowel. It is then relatively easy to continue incision of Toldt's fascia in the cephalad direction in order to detach the descending colon up to the highest level (in the area of the splenic flexure). At this point in the dissection, it is our preference to come back to the area of the sigmoid colon. The released bowel is then brought medially, exposing the sigmoid colon attachments in the pelvis. These are separated carefully, using a cautery hook held in the assistant's left hand, and again identifying the psoas muscle, gonadal vessels, and left ureter. If dissection is continued toward the pelvic brim, it is important to stay close to the pericolic/perirectal fat in order to avoid injury to the hypogastric nerves.

At this point, the dissection is directed to the splenic flexure. If easily accessible, omental attachments to the spleen can be divided. Otherwise, one moves to the distal transverse colon. The assistant grasps the omentum with the left hand, and the primary surgeon grasps the bowel wall with his or her right hand. The assistant separates the bowel from the omentum using a cautery hook held in the right hand. Initially, the superficial leaf of the omentum is detached. In most cases, it is necessary to separate the second, deeper leaf from the transverse mesocolon in order to gain access to the lesser sac. In the area of the splenic flexure, we prefer to use cautery rather than other energy devices. It provides precision of dissection and minimizes the risk of thermal bowel injury. If the use of a sealing device is elected in order to separate the omentum from the splenic flexure, special care is required not to inadvertently seal the marginal branch of the colon in the area of the lienocolic ligament. Because the IMV had been taken down at its origin, the amount of tethering adhesions should be minimal once the splenic flexure is mobilized.

This completes mobilization of the left colon. Although the order in which it is accomplished can vary, we prefer to take down the IMV prior to the IMA. Subsequent retroperitoneal dissection is then easier because there is no fibrosis beneath its origin. There are also no lymphatics in this region, meaning a more rapid identification of the proper tissue plane.

There are some instances when access to the base of the mesentery is very difficult, limiting the medial-to-lateral approach or making it impossible to safely accomplish. This can be seen with an obese individual, a small patient with little intra-abdominal domain, and with distended small bowel. In these circumstances, the lateral-to-medial approach is a reasonable alternative.

When the left colon is successfully mobilized, the segment for resection is identified. In the majority of instances, one transects the bowel in the upper rectum. That is dictated by oncologic principles and the blood supply (for cancer of the descending, sigmoid, and rectosigmoid colon), obtaining a

disease-free segment, a low-pressure anastomosis distally (for diverticular disease), and the practicality of using the circular stapler to create the anastomosis. In our experience, we rarely perform a stapled side-to-side anastomosis on the left colon because emptying problems can lead to stercoral ulceration and a greater risk of incorporating diverticula in the anastomosis. For a splenic flexure tumor, when the main IMA pedicle does not have to be sacrificed and some of the sigmoid colon can be preserved, we prefer an end-to-end or end-to-side, hand-sewn colo-colonic anastomosis.

There are several options for completing the resection and constructing the anastomosis. The simplest way is to create a small Pfannenstiel incision, exteriorize the specimen, transect the bowel and the mesentery, and create an end-to-end colorectal anastomosis. This is the standard, very familiar technique used by most surgeons. It also allows for creation of a single-stapled, double purse-string anastomosis (the authors' preferred technique). The second option is to divide the mesentery proximally and distally by means of laparoscopy through the use of an energy-sealing device. The distal bowel transection (upper rectum level) can be accomplished using a laparoscopic stapler introduced through a 12-mm port. The camera port can be used for this purpose when the lens is switched to a 5-mm size and introduced through the side port. A small incision can then be created (again a Pfannenstiel incision is preferred) through which the required segment of the bowel is exteriorized and transected at the skin level. The anvil is inserted into the proximal colon and secured with a purse-string suture. The bowel is then placed into the abdominal cavity, the wound closed, and pneumoperitoneum reestablished. The circular stapler is introduced through the anus into the rectal stump, and a colorectal double-stapled anastomosis is performed under laparoscopic guidance.

In rare cases, when the IMA trunk is preserved and only the left colic branch is sacrificed, it is our preference to transect the mesentery laparoscopically. Once this is done, the next step is to exteriorize the bowel, usually through the supraumbilical midline minilaparotomy incision. The bowel is then transected at the skin level where the hand-sewn, colo-colonic end-to-end or side-to-end anastomosis is created.

The specimen is always delivered through a wound protector. Every upper rectal anastomosis is tested by flexible sigmoidoscopy. Not only is the air-water test performed, but also the anastomosis itself is evaluated for integrity. Drains are used rarely and very selectively and introduced through the 5-mm port (umbilical port included).

All skin incisions are closed with staples or 4–0 absorbable sutures. The fascial layer of any 12-mm port site, if present, is closed with a #0 figure-of-eight, long-term absorbable suture. The fascial layer of the minilaparotomy incision is closed with a loop #1 long-term absorbable suture. In our experience, the Pfannenstiel incision results in a minimal hernia rate as compared with midline mini-incisions.[57]

Postoperative Care

The orogastric tube is removed at the conclusion of the procedure. The Foley catheter is removed on the first postoperative day. No additional antibiotics are given, and a clear liquid diet is started on the day following surgery and advanced once the patient's bowel function returns. In most cases, epidural analgesia is sufficient for controlling pain if placed preoperatively.

Laparoscopic Approach for Rectal Prolapse

Introduction

More than 150 years have elapsed since the first report on full-thickness rectal prolapse (FTRP) surgery appeared in the literature.[130] There are a number of abdominal procedures available for the treatment of this condition, which differ whether rectopexy and/or sigmoid resection are added to mobilization of the rectum (see Chapter 21). A meta-analysis of randomized controlled trials by the Cochrane Library concluded in 2008 that there is not enough evidence to support one abdominal surgical procedure over another regarding recurrence rates.[209]

Indications

Rectopexy versus Mobilization Only

Controversies have not yet been resolved on which step of the abdominal surgery for FTRP contributes the most to minimizing recurrence rates. The addition of rectopexy may have certain disadvantages, such as added operating time, problems associated with implantation of foreign material, bleeding from sacral veins, and nerve injury to the presacral plexus. On the other hand, the literature on rectal mobilization only (without rectopexy) is very limited (data on resection not taken into account). In fact, in a series of 13 patients who underwent rectal mobilization only, 15% had a recurrence rate at a median follow-up of 1 year (range, 0.39–1.88).[155]

Another potential issue is that published recurrence rates are often unreliable. In a recent meta-analysis on individual patient data, published recurrence rates differed by as much as 47% from recurrence rates reestimated by actuarial analysis.[59] A recent randomized controlled trial reported that adding pexy to mobilization of the rectum significantly decreased 5-year recurrence rates.[107]

Suture Rectopexy

Suture rectopexy was first described by Cutait[53] in 1959 (see Biography, Chapter 24). The rationale for using sutures has been to maintain the rectum in its new position in order to allow its eventual fixation to the sacrum by scar tissue.[112] There are a few technical details about the surgical technique of suture rectopexy that deserve attention. Most authors suture the fascia propria of the posterior mesorectum to the presacral fascia.[86,96,112] Some also include a partial thickness of the posterior rectum.[112] Another option is to suture the right and left peritoneal flaps to the presacral fascia. The sutures are placed onto the sacral promontory.[96] The exact location on the promontory should be lateral to the hypogastric nerves and medial to the ureters on both sides of the rectum (Figure 19-57). Alternative sites on the sacrum below the promontory have been suggested (Figure 19-58). Most surgeons agree that two sutures are adequate, but some prefer more.[96,112]

Mesh Rectopexy

The literature suggests that rectopexy is as effective with sutures as with mesh.[66,173,209] A multicenter pooled analysis of 643 patients demonstrated no difference in recurrence rates between suture rectopexy and mesh rectopexy (Figure 19-59).[173] This leads to the question whether a mesh should be used at all because it may increase the incidence of postoperative constipation and also carry the potential risk of infection.[190]

Sigmoid Resection

Sigmoid resection is suggested only in cases of well-documented constipation and should be avoided in incontinent patients. Adding resection to rectopexy does not seem to decrease recurrence rates as compared with rectopexy alone.[209] In addition to a history of intractable constipation, clustering of radiopaque rings in the sigmoid should be documented by means of colonic transit time. If resection is indicated at the time of the rectal prolapse procedure, the amount of colon removed should be limited to the redundant portion of sigmoid. The superior rectal artery should be spared because preserving the blood supply to a long rectal stump will minimize the risk of an anastomotic leak.[24] Moreover, avoiding dissection of the inferior mesenteric artery is particularly relevant in the rare male patient undergoing resection for rectal prolapse because of potential damage to sympathetic nerves. Alternative, perineal approaches should be discussed with such an individual.

Preoperative Evaluation

Risk Assessment

The following discussion of principles is equally applicable to that of open surgery. Patients with FTRP are a heterogeneous group with a variety of additional symptoms. Hence, a single treatment approach will not be adequate,[59] and alternative treatment options should be evaluated. The first step of the algorithm is to assess the potential for mortality for someone undergoing a major operation. This evaluation should be based on the colorectal POSSUM score rather than on the ASA score.[173] Actually, the colorectal POSSUM score can be quickly evaluated online by entering four physiologic and four operative data points.[209] If the patient is unfit for abdominal surgery with a general anesthetic and with endotracheal intubation, a perineal procedure with a spinal or epidural anesthetic may be offered. All who are fit for a general anesthesia should be considered as candidates for an abdominal operation regardless of chronologic age. One exception is the occasional male patient with true FTRP. The risk of iatrogenic impotence following abdominal surgery should be thoroughly explained and the advantages and disadvantages of perineal procedures considered.

There are four risk areas for autonomic nerve injury during rectal dissection.[5] Damage to the sympathetic nerves may occur when dissecting the inferior mesenteric artery and during posterior rectal mobilization at the promontory close to the hypogastric nerves. Injury to the parasympathetic nerves may occur during dissection of the lateral stalks of the rectum as well as anterior rectal mobilization between the seminal vesicles and prostate gland.

Surgical Technique

Laparoscopic Suture Rectopexy

If the rectum is prolapsed, it should be reduced prior to starting the procedure. It is this author's preference to achieve pneumoperitoneum through an open technique as opposed to using the Veress needle. A 10-mm incision is made just below the umbilicus, and the umbilical stalk is dissected and then grasped with a Kocher clamp and pulled in a cephalad direction. The fascia is incised with a knife along the midline under direct visual control. A bladeless Hasson trocar is then inserted into the peritoneal cavity. The trocar is secured into position by two sutures placed on each side of the incision. It is not usually necessary to exceed an intra-abdominal

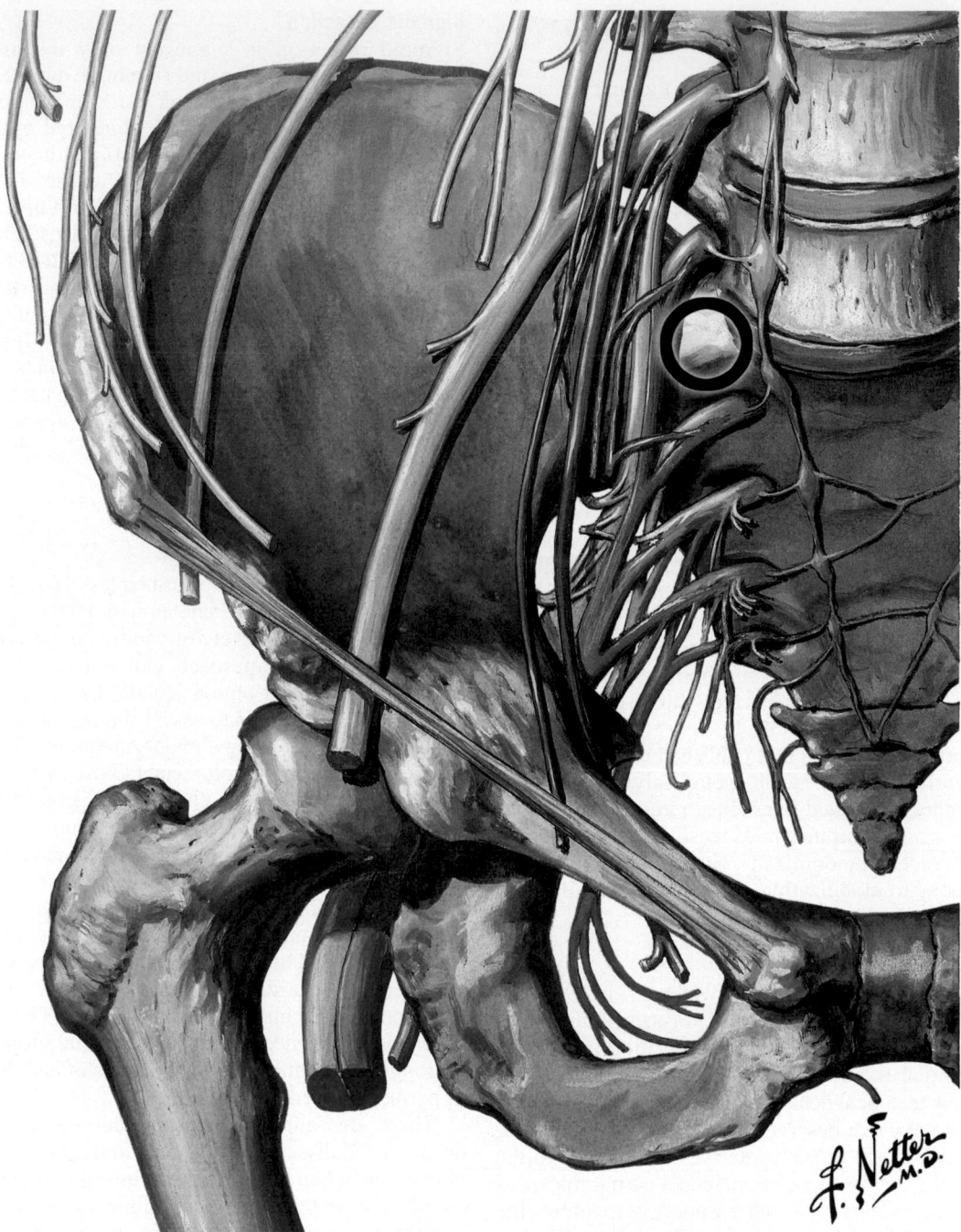

FIGURE 19-57. Suture rectopexy on sacral promontory. (From the Netter Collection of Medical Illustrations; a Novartis Publication)

pressure of 10 mm Hg because the procedure will be accomplished primarily within the bony pelvis. Two ports (10 and 5 mm) are placed in the right lower quadrant in a triangulating fashion with the umbilical site. The 10-mm port allows the surgeon to insert the curved suture needle into the abdominal cavity to accomplish the rectopexy. A final 5-mm port is placed in the left lower quadrant for use of the assistant's instruments.

The patient is placed in the Trendelenburg position. This facilitates the freeing of the small bowel and omentum out of the pelvis into the upper abdominal cavity. The assistant proceeds to lift the rectosigmoid colon. However, the sigmoid colon should not require mobilization. The second step includes identification of the left ureter. This can be facilitated by prior insertion of lighted ureteral stents. Visualization of the iliac bifurcation as well as the gonadal vessels can also help with identification. The pelvic peritoneum should be incised toward the pouch of Douglas. This will define the extent of the lateral dissection. The dissection is begun above the level of the sacral promontory. The peritoneum is divided at least 2 cm from the rectum in order to create peritoneal "wings" to be used for pexy. The peritoneum of the sigmoid mesentery is opened and connected with the lateral dissection just posterior to the inferior mesenteric pedicle. This last structure is elevated as the rectosigmoid colon is maintained on tension. One then extends the medial peritoneal dissection

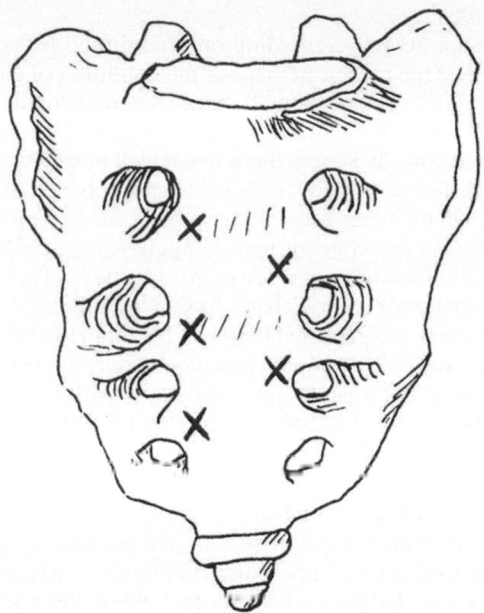

FIGURE 19-58. Alternative sites for rectopexy. (From Graf W, Stefánsson T, Arvidsson D, et al. Laparoscopic suture rectopexy. *Dis Colon Rectum.* 1995;38(2): 211–212.)

over the sacral promontory along the sulcus toward the pouch of Douglas to mirror the lateral dissection. At the level of the sacral promontory, the hypogastric nerves are amenable to injury. In order to avoid this complication, one should keep the dissection close to the fascia propria of the rectum. Then the surgeon should continue to lift and provide appropriate tension to the rectosigmoid colon. This dissection is often facilitated by the frequently observed lack of fixation of the rectum to the sacrum, a part of the pathophysiology of prolapse. The presacral fascia and hypogastric nerves should remain out of the field of dissection.

One should be mindful of the presacral vessels as the dissection approaches the pelvic floor. When the levator ani muscles become apparent, the rectum will have become parallel to the pelvic floor. The angle of dissection should then be adjusted to avoid injury to the presacral vessels. Vigorous bleeding may occur if these vessels are inadvertently injured. The posterior dissection is completed to the level of the coccyx. The lateral dissection should spare the lateral stalks (ligaments). The rectum is lifted by the assistant, and a point is selected for the rectopexy. The rectum should not be placed on tension, but the prolapse should still be reduced. Silk sutures are secured to the right and left sacral promontory. The sites of sutures on the promontory should be placed lateral to the hypogastric nerves and medial to the ureter on both sides of the rectum. Attention to the position of the hypogastric nerves and the presacral vessels will guide suture placement. The assistant should maintain the anatomic position of the rectum while the surgeon secures the two previously placed sutures to the peritoneal "wings." Once the mobilization and rectopexy are complete, hemostasis should be reaffirmed. The pelvis is irrigated with saline. No drain is required. The Foley catheter should be left in place, but the oral-gastric tube may be discontinued.

Laparoscopic Sigmoid Resection Sparing Superior Rectal Artery

The previously mentioned technical steps remain the same for resection, yet there are some important points worth amplifying upon. While performing the circumferential rectal mobilization, the posterior mesorectum is dissected off the posterior wall of the rectum at approximately 14 cm from the anal verge. This distance can be verified by an intraoperative rigid sigmoidoscopy. The sigmoid colon is then divided by a laparoscopic linear stapler that is positioned perpendicular to the axis of the sigmoid colon. The mesentery of the sigmoid colon is divided close to the bowel, and the mesorectum is not divided, thereby sparing the superior rectal artery (Figure 19-60). The specimen is retrieved through a Pfannenstiel incision. One then proceeds to perform a double-stapled colorectal anastomosis without the need for reestablishment of a pneumoperitoneum.

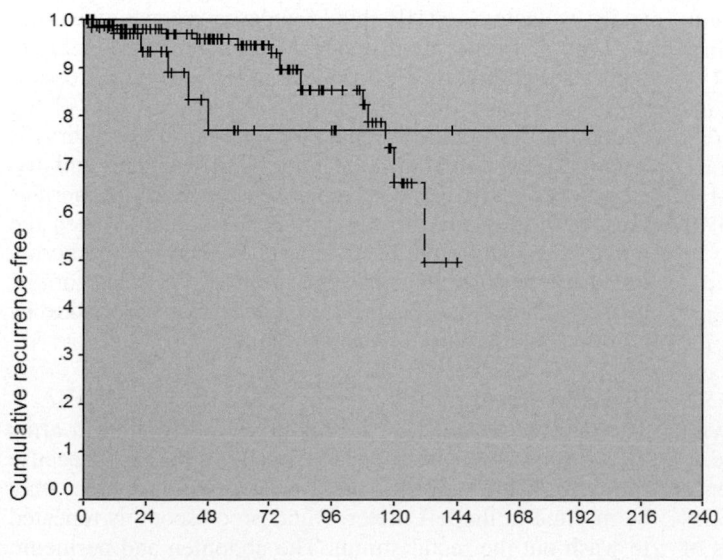

FIGURE 19-59. No difference is shown in recurrence rates between suture and mesh rectopexy in 643 patients. (From Raftopoulos Y, Senagore AJ, Di Giuro G, et al; Rectal Prolapse Recurrence Study Group. Recurrence rates after abdominal surgery for complete rectal prolapse: a multicenter pooled analysis of 643 individual patient data. *Dis Colon Rectum.* 2005;48(6):1200–1206.)

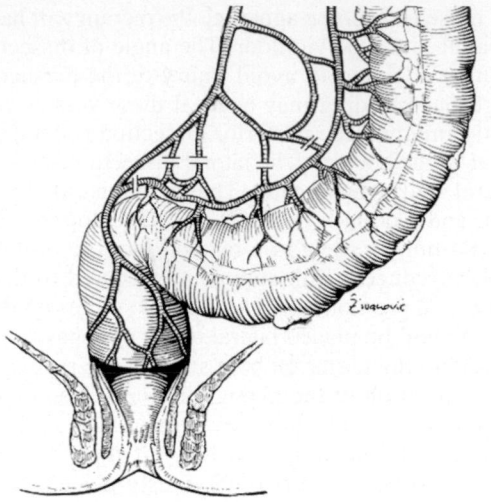

FIGURE 19-60. Sparing the superior rectal artery during laparoscopic sigmoid resection for rectal prolapse. (From Bergamaschi R, Lovvik K, Marvik R. Preserving the superior rectal artery in laparoscopic sigmoid resection for complete rectal prolapse. *Surg Laparosc Endosc Percutan Tech.* 2003;13(6):374–376.)

Postoperative Care

The Foley catheter can be removed on the first postoperative day. Pain is initially controlled with an epidural catheter with local anesthetic. Diet is advanced with return of bowel function, and the pain medication is transitioned to oral formulations. Upon discharge, the patient is instructed to avoid heavy lifting. Bowel management should be discussed. In my opinion, the patient should be seen in the office within 2 weeks of discharge. Continued follow-up will assist the surgeon in his or her evaluation of the success of the repair.

Laparoscopic Hartmann's Reversal

Introduction

Comparison has been made of the laparoscopic approach to Hartmann's reversal (LHR) to that of open Hartmann's reversal (OHR) with respect to such issues as postoperative morbidity and mortality rates.[11] In fact, patients undergoing LHR have been found to have decreased complication and reoperation rates at 6-month follow-up when compared with their OHR counterparts.[94] This is not surprising because in OHR patients most complications and reoperations at 6-month follow-up are abdominal wall–related. In fact, the avoidance of a long midline laparotomy is the primary factor impacting the rates of complications and reoperations. However, the frequency of readmission to the hospital at 6 months following surgery may be similar in both OHR and LHR patients.[94]

Complications at 30 days generally include surgical site infection (SSI), such as wound infection and intra-abdominal abscess, anastomotic leak, and postoperative ileus.[11] A 1.7% 30-day mortality rate after OHR was reported by Aydin and colleagues.[11] This may be a reflection of a preoperative ASA grade of 3 to 5 in these patients (58.9%). No deaths with LHR were reported in a recent review of the literature.[183] However, selection bias most likely accounts for the absence of mortality because most studies reviewed were case series and included up to 22 patients. Still in a similar series of 27 patients, there were no postoperative deaths.[111]

Indications

There is controversy regarding optimal timing for performing an HR. One reason perhaps is the definition of early and late reversal. This has varied between 4 and 8 months.[11,109,182] In the 1990s, proponents of early reversal favored patients' preference. Simply stated, there was a lack of data to demonstrate a difference in adverse event rates between early and late HR. On the other hand, the argument supporting late HR was based on the concept that delaying reversal allows for edema, inflammation, and sepsis to subside.[164] This subject still is a matter of some debate. In fact, in a recent review, a wide lag time was reported between HP and HR (less than 3 to 13.5 months).[214] A population-based study also noted that the timing of HR was directly associated with the risk for a second stoma being created during this second operation.[185] The rate of a second stoma creation was 5% when the lag time was less than 6 months as opposed to 12.5% when the lag time exceeded 12 months.

Patients with higher ASA classes are more likely to experience adverse events. Comorbidities such as cardiovascular disease, diabetes, chronic obstructive pulmonary disease (COPD), hypertension, and renal disease have also been evaluated as predictors of postoperative adverse events. The presence of chronic renal failure requiring dialysis is the only independent predictor of adverse event rates at multilogistic regression.[159] Those with renal disease are 21 times more likely to experience adverse events. Because HR remains an operation with a reported morbidity ranging up to 50% and a mortality up to 5%, patients with chronic renal failure requiring dialysis are not candidates for HR.[214]

Preoperative Evaluation
Risk Assessment

Patients with comorbidities such as cardiovascular disease, diabetes, COPD, hypertension, and renal disease should be informed of the likelihood of postoperative adverse events. All should be informed at the time of consenting that the feasibility of performing an HR is not 100% and that another, hopefully temporary, stoma may become necessary.

Workup

Regardless whether the emergency left colectomy with end colostomy was performed in another institution, patients under evaluation for HR should undergo preoperative colonoscopy and rigid proctoscopy. A review of the operative report and pathology report of the index emergency operation is necessary. Meticulous physical examination of the abdominal wall (supplemented by CT scan if necessary) is helpful to rule out an incisional hernia. Advantages and disadvantages of simultaneous repair of large incisional hernias must be discussed with the patient, particularly when the repair may require the use of mesh. Postponing the hernia repair is a reasonable alternative in those scheduled for HR given the high risk of SSI related to the colostomy and to its closure (Figure 19-61—see also Chapter 31).

Operating Room

The patient is placed in the lithotomy position with arms tucked and securely strapped to the table at the chest because tilting the table will ultimately be necessary. A stent may be inserted in the left ureter. Rigid proctoscopy is repeated to wash out the rectal stump. The abdomen and perineum are prepped and draped in a sterile fashion. The colostomy

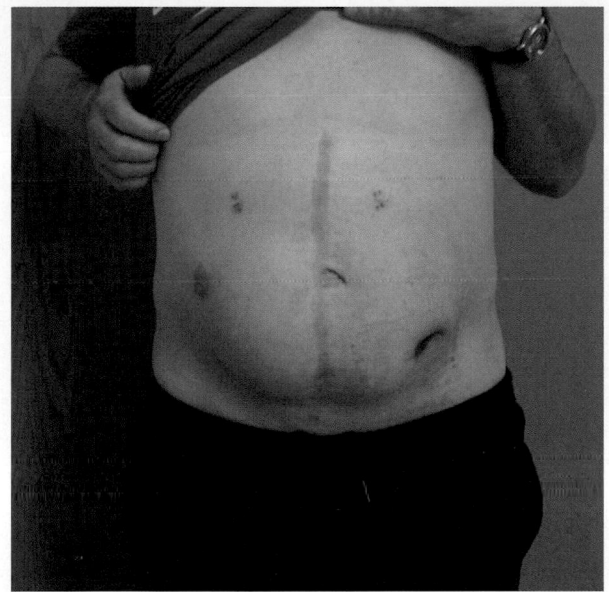

FIGURE 19-61. Postoperative view of a patient who underwent Hartmann reversal with untreated preexisting incisional hernia.

site is covered with disposable adhesive sterile drape. All equipment including two monitors should be placed on the patient's left side in clear view of the surgeon. The surgeon stands on the patient's right side (Figure 19-62).

Surgical Technique
The first incision is made lateral to the right rectus muscle sheath along the anterior axillary line. A Hasson port is inserted and a pneumoperitoneum established. An evaluation of the complexity of the intra-abdominal adhesions is carried out and the feasibility and safety of proceeding laparoscopically reassessed. Second and third ports are inserted under direct visual control in the right upper and lower quadrants, avoiding excessive tenting of the abdominal wall. During the lysis of adhesions, creation of an enterotomy is a real concern, especially if it is actually missed during the operation. A missed enterotomy can occur with laparotomy as well; however, the risk with laparoscopy is higher. The risk of enterotomy can be minimized by following sound surgical techniques.

Fenestrated bowel graspers with nonlocking handles should be used to gently run the bowel. Exposure can be achieved by pushing with closed tools rather than by grasping the bowel with instruments. The small bowel should be inspected in a retrograde fashion commencing at the cecum or with decompressed bowel, and any point of transition identified. Cold scissors should be used to divide matted adhesions or an adhesive band. Energy-based devices should be avoided when dividing adhesions. The following statement should always be one's guiding principle: *a low threshold should be maintained for conversion to conventional, open surgery.* Conversion is not a sign of failure; instead, it represents good clinical judgment. The goals of lysing of adhesions include identification of the rectal stump and mobilization of the small bowel out of the left lower quadrant. The former is a mandatory step prior to proceeding to the takedown of the colostomy. The latter step is essential for the avoidance of tension at the intended colorectal anastomosis. The rectal stump is then fully freed from the retroperitoneum and additional resection performed as required.

Temporary exsufflation of the pneumoperitoneum is then accomplished. The stoma site is fully mobilized extracorporeally. The anvil of the circular stapler is introduced into the colon and secured with a hand-sewn purse-string suture using nonabsorbable monofilament 3–0 suture. The colon is reinserted into the abdomen, the fascia at the stoma site is closed with interrupted nonabsorbable monofilament #1 sutures, and the pneumoperitoneum recreated. The splenic flexure is mobilized. A single- or double-stapled anastomosis is performed with a circular stapler inserted transanally. An air-leak test is accomplished. No drains are used. All three port sites are closed layer by layer. The skin at the stoma site is left open and the wound packed wet to dry.

Postoperative Care
The urinary catheter can be removed on the first postoperative day. Pain is initially controlled with local anesthetic through an epidural catheter and as soon as possible transitioned to oral medication. Diet is advanced with passage of flatus. Upon discharge from hospital, dietary goals should be addressed. The patient is seen in the office within 2 weeks of discharge during which time daily dressing changes of the open wound at the prior ostomy site are necessary.

Laparoscopic Resection of Rectum for Cancer
Introduction
Laparoscopic resection of the rectum for cancer is not a simple operation, and indeed claims of its clinical benefits still remain to be proven. The purpose of laparoscopic rectal cancer resection is neither for feasibility nor for theoretical benefits, such as a magnified view of the pelvis.[146] Meaningful examples of potential clinical advantages are the achievement of negative radial margins, spared autonomic nerves, and the avoidance of ureteral injury. A 12% rate of radial margin positivity after laparoscopic surgery was reported in the CLASICC trial (Medical Research Council trial of laparoscopically assisted vs. open surgery for colorectal cancer). This compared with a 6% rate in the conventional study arm.[88] Nonrandomized data revealed a 47% rate of impotence or retrograde ejaculation after laparoscopic surgery in sexually active men as opposed to 4.5% rate following conventional surgery.[169] Unfortunately, such data do not correlate with the impressive photographs that have been published, which clearly demonstrate laparoscopic autonomic nerve identification.[92] By implication, one can only hope that the more judicious use of energy-based instruments will lead to a decreased incidence of autonomic nerve injury.

A Cochrane review (2006) identified more than 4,000 patients in 48 publications.[37] Three of these studies were randomized controlled trials; they accounted for more than 600 patients. However, these trials did not comply with the CONSORT statement (**CON**solidated **S**tandards **o**f **R**eporting Trials) on allocation concealment[149] and, therefore, may not have been truly randomized. Because two of these three randomized, controlled trials provided no data on tumor distance from the anal verge[125,126] it is quite possible that such studies included patients with sigmoid cancer rather than rectal cancer. In light of the suboptimal quality of the data generated by such randomized controlled trials, there is hardly any point in performing meta-analyses to conclude that laparoscopic surgery is associated with longer operating time and fewer complications.[79] Early recovery, as suggested in another meta-analysis,[12] is an example of a surrogate end

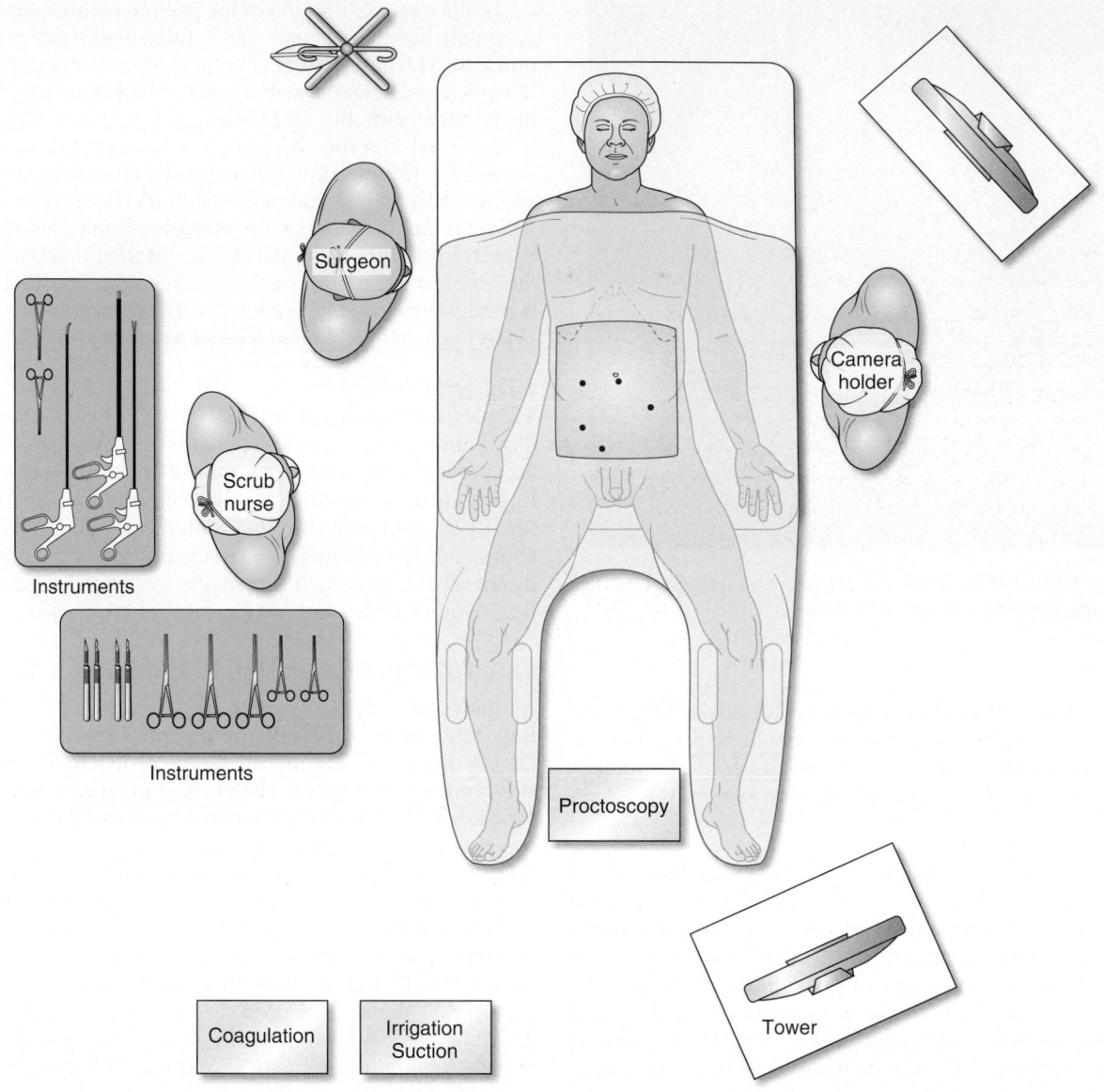

FIGURE 19-62. Operating room setup for laparoscopic Hartmann reversal.

point, particularly when studies are conducted in socialized health care systems or derived from administrative databases.[71] While the COLOR II (Randomized clinical trial comparing laparoscopic and open surgery for rectal cancer) and ACOSOG (American College of Surgeons Oncology Group) randomized controlled trials are still under way, the CLASICC trial provides the only source of truly randomized data. It is important to note, however, that there was a 57% conversion rate.[88] Such a high figure reflects the nonselection of the patients and the surgeons "good" judgment. However, it also suggests that the surgeons' learning curve in laparoscopic resection of the rectum for cancer was included in the randomized controlled trials.

In fact, it is questionable whether the randomized study design is the most appropriate for evaluating the impact of surgical technique on clinical outcomes. The random operation design is biased in favor of prerandomized controlled trial routine operations and technically more straightforward, perhaps easier, procedures.[215] Alternative study designs such as process of care should be considered to minimize the

inclusion of the learning curve into randomized controlled trials.[179] The best example of process of care studies in rectal surgery is the Norwegian Rectal Cancer Project.[223,224] A 34% local recurrence rate prompted the retraining of colorectal surgeons and the implementation of a standardized total mesorectal excision technique. This resulted in lowering the recurrence rate to 6%. In my opinion, laparoscopic resection of the rectum for cancer will be a short-lived phenomenon unless further research is conducted, focusing on clinical outcome measures rather than surrogate end points.[22]

Indications

Patients presenting with resectable, histologically proven adenocarcinoma of the rectum without documented involvement of the external sphincter are candidates for laparoscopic resection of the rectum with anastomosis. Those with cancer of the upper third of the rectum should be considered for low anterior resection (LAR) with partial mesorectal excision as long as an adequate distal resection margin is achieved. Patients with cancer of the mid-third of the rectum should be considered for LAR with total mesorectal excision (TME) and at least a 1 cm distal resection margin. Individuals with cancer of the lower third of the rectum involving the internal anal sphincter may be considered for intersphincteric resection (ISR) with TME and hand-sewn coloanal anastomosis. Patients with cancer of the lower third of the rectum involving the external anal sphincter should undergo an abdominoperineal resection (APR). Those with a resectable T4 rectal cancer should be evaluated for the possibility of undergoing a pelvic exenteration, provided that there is no evidence of distant metastases.

Surgical Technique

The patient is placed in the lithotomy position with arms tucked and the chest strapped to the table because tilting the table will be necessary. A stent may be inserted in the left ureter. Rigid proctoscopy is repeated to wash out the rectal stump. The abdomen and perineum are prepped and draped in a sterile manner. All equipment, including two monitors, should be placed in clear view. The surgeon stands on the patient's right side.

Pneumoperitoneum is established through an open technique at the umbilicus. Four ports can be used, in addition to the umbilical site where a 10-mm, 30-degree laparoscope is inserted. One 12-mm port placed in the right lower quadrant lateral to the rectus muscle sheath allows the use of a stapling device. Three 5-mm ports are inserted under direct vision in the right upper quadrant, suprapubic midline, and in the left lower quadrant. The left port is used by the assistant. The table is airplaned to the right. The IMA is divided with a stapler after identification of the left ureter. Such identification may be facilitated by the insertion of a lighted stent. Division of the IMA with a stapler is preferred to that of using laparoscopic vessel-sealing devices because of the concern for arterial calcification. Identification and ligation of the IMV follows. Medial-to-lateral mobilization of the left mesocolon is the next step.

Mobilization of Splenic Flexure

Prior to tilting the table into the Trendelenburg position, the splenic flexure must be completely mobilized. The rationale for performing this maneuver is to ensure adequate length of the proximal colon for a tension-free anastomosis, as well as a tension-free mesentery that will not compromise the blood supply. The following situations warrant special precautions: a history of aortic surgery (this can interrupt or reverse the normal circulation in the marginal artery), prior radical left nephrectomy (this can compromise certain intraperitoneal vessels), and previous colonic surgery with concern on arterial flow in the marginal artery. An antegrade mobilization is preferred to that of retrograde. Technical steps include division of the gastrocolic omental attachments, mobilization of the left colonic mesentery, and division of the root of the mesentery of the transverse colon.

Preservation of Autonomic Nerves

Blunt dissection of the rectum as well as excessive use of energy-based devices must be avoided. As previously discussed, there are four key zones where autonomic nerve injuries are most likely to occur during resection of the rectum for cancer: the superior hypogastric plexus during dissection of the IMA, the hypogastric nerves during posterior mobilization of the rectum, the pelvic plexus during lateral rectal mobilization, and the anterior cavernous nerves during anterior dissection.[129]

Distal Rectal Transection

There are technical limitations to performing safe laparoscopic distal rectal transection. One such factor is the fulcrum effect of operating a stapler through a port that is placed in the abdominal wall. Another limitation is the degree of angulation of the currently available staplers. A virtual simulation study has shown that present-day staplers will actually have to go through the iliac bone to achieve a 90-degree angle of rectal transection at the level of the levator ani muscle (Figure 19-63).[35] A third limitation is the number of cartridges required for stapled distal rectal transection. Ideally, distal rectal transection should be accomplished with a single firing. Nonrandomized data indicate that multiple firings lead to increased anastomotic leak rates when compared with a single firing.[100] However, this cannot be performed by using laparoscopic staplers with a 45-degree angulation. Tilting the mobilized rectum to the left has been suggested in order to achieve a 90-degree angle of transection with such staplers, but this is not always feasible.[121] Battery-powered laparoscopic staplers with a 90-degree angulation may have a positive impact on the angle of transection (Figure 19-64). Double-stapling following oblique transection of the rectum may result in an anastomotic stricture because of the potential for suboptimal blood supply in the acute angle of transection (Figure 19-65). In order to avoid multiple firings, a conventional surgery stapler may be inserted through a suprapubic incision. This is subsequently oversewn around the stapler shaft.[87] The fulcrum effect, however, will remain unresolved, and the pneumoperitoneum may become unstable. An alternative method is to insert a conventional stapler through a gel port. However, this is, of course, associated with an increased cost. There are three advantages to the last option: the fulcrum effect is ameliorated by the consistency of the gel, pneumoperitoneum is stabilized by the seal of the

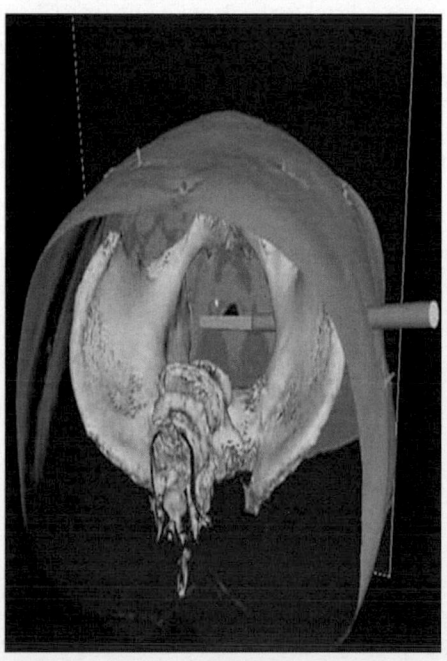

FIGURE 19-63. Simulation of a stapler passing through the iliac bone to achieve a 90-degree low rectal transection. (From Brannigan AE, De Buck S, Suetens P, et al. Intracorporeal rectal stapling following laparoscopic total mesorectal excision: overcoming a challenge. *Surg Endosc.* 2006;20(6):952–955.)

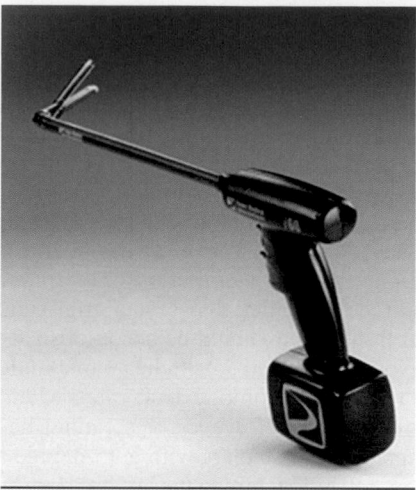

FIGURE 19-64. Battery-powered stapler with a 90-degree angulation. (Copyright ©2012 Covidien. All rights reserved. Used with permission of Covidien.)

hand port, and the port permits the reassurance of one palpating the tumor and the distal margin prior to rectal transection.

The double-stapled colorectal anastomosis is carried out in accordance with the same principles described in conventional surgery. The air-leak test is performed under endoscopic view using a rigid proctoscope, with the bowel clamped proximal to the anastomosis.

Intersphincteric Resection

ISR was first described by Schiessel in 1994.[191] When ISR is indicated, patients must undergo a preoperative evaluation of the external anal sphincters by means of manometry, ultrasound, and defecogram to ensure adequate preoperative sphincter function. ISR entails transanal circumferential incision of the anal mucosa at the intersphincteric groove, which is located distal to the dentate line (see Chapter 24).[184] The dissection between the internal sphincter and the external sphincter starts posteriorly, extends laterally, and is completed anteriorly. ISR leads to en bloc resection of the rectum and internal sphincter; these are extracted transanally. Coloanal anastomosis is performed transanally with

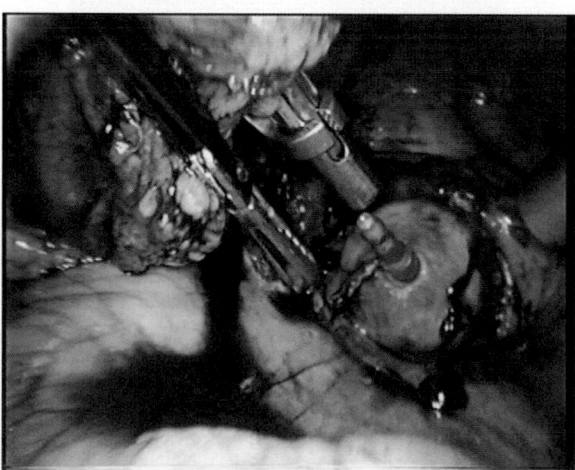

FIGURE 19-65. Laparoscopically transected rectum on an angle less than 90 degrees.

interrupted absorbable sutures. ISR should be reserved for selected patients with tumors not amenable to LAR. Such individuals must be informed preoperatively of the possible functional outcomes of ISR with hand-sewn coloanal anastomosis.

Loop Ileostomy

Fecal diversion in the form of a defunctioning loop ileostomy may be considered. Some believe that by diverting the fecal stream and maintaining the anastomosis free of contamination, leakage will be less likely. Although defunctioning stomas are widely practiced and supported in principle by the literature, there is ample evidence to suggest that the notion that fecal diversion has any influence on anastomotic leak rates is erroneous.[85] The clinical significance of a leak, however, is obviously quite different. Karanjia and colleagues initially recommended fecal stream diversion in all low anastomosis,[106] but they later found that the leak rates were similar whether or not the stool was diverted.[105] A prospective study in 2005 concluded that a defunctioning ileostomy has no influence over whether a low rectal anastomosis leaks after surgery. Rather, the authors concluded that a loop ileostomy minimizes the consequences of a leak but has significant morbidity and should, therefore, be used judiciously.[229]

Opinion

There is evidence to suggest that training, volume of surgery, and an individual's skill may have an impact on the quality of care in rectal cancer surgery (Tables 19-3 and 19-4).[98]

TABLE 19-3 Selected Studies Comparing Outcome of Rectal Surgery Performed by Colorectal Surgeons and General Surgeons

ARTICLE	PTS #	MORTALITY %		LRR %		SURVIVAL %	
		CRS	GS	CRS	GS	CRS	GS
Porter et al.	683	0.9	2.3	13.4	37.4	67.3	49.0[a]
		P = NS		*P* < .001		*P* < .001	
Rosen et al.	2,805	1.4	7.3				
		P < .001					
Wibe et al.[b]	3,319			6	12.9	73	60
						P = .03	
Smedh et al.	277	1	8				
		P = .002					
Read et al.	384			7	16	77	68
				P < .005		*P* < .005	

[a]Months
[b]CRS with TME training and CRS without TME training course
Empty boxes, data not reported; CRS, colorectal surgeons; GS, general surgeons; pts, patients; LRR, local recurrence rates; NS, not significant.
From Ignjatovic D, Bergamaschi R. Rectal cancer: from outcomes of care to process of care. *Scand J Gastroenterol.* 2006;41(6):636–639. Table 1.

TABLE 19-4 Selected Studies Comparing Outcome of Rectal Surgery Performed by High-Volume Surgeons and Low-Volume Surgeons

ARTICLE	PATIENTS #	MORTALITY % HVS	LVS	LRR % HVS	LVS	SURVIVAL % HVS	LVS
Porter et al.	683			26.0	42.2	53.5	38.8
				P < .001		*P* = .001	
Parry et al.	927	10	15				
		P > .05					
Schrag et al.	384	4.3	1.7			66	76
		P < .20				*P* = .001	
Dowdall et al.	82	4		6.1		67	
Martling et al.	652	11	18	4	10		
		P = .007		*P* = .02			
Hodgson et al.	9,843	1.6	4.8			76.6	83.7
		P < .001				*P* < .001	
Holm et al.	1,399	3.4	4.4	20	26	47	53
		P = NS		*P* = .06			

LRR, local recurrence rates; HVS, high-volume surgeons; LVS, low-volume surgeons; Empty boxes = data not reported.
From Ignjatovic D, Bergamaschi R. Rectal cancer: from outcomes of care to process of care. *Scand J Gastroenterol.* 2006;41(6):636–639. Table 2.

uninvolved circumferential resection margins (CRMs) remains the most relevant determination with respect to the technical approach, whether open or laparoscopic. As a corollary to this critical issue, because a standard, combined (two-person) APR may involve considerable rectal dissection through the perineum (as opposed to the abdomen), the variable also with the laparoscopic approach is how much dissection should be performed abdominally and how much perineally (see also Chapter 24). Certainly, in the one-stage APR, less emphasis is placed on the perineal phase as one attempts to maximize dissection from within the abdomen. Laparoscopy may have further prompted this trend.

Studies on laparoscopic APR infrequently report CRM involvement rates. Among 17 studies published from 1994 to date on oncologic outcomes of laparoscopic APR, only six included data on CRM involvement. In 1999, Fleshman and colleagues reported a 12% CRM involvement in 33 laparoscopic APRs.[73] In another study, a 20.7% CRM involvement rate was reported for 53 patients undergoing laparoscopic APR,[199] In still another study, 74 consecutive patients who underwent a laparoscopic APR were found to have a 16.2% CRM involvement rate.[172] The same study indicated that tumor size (35 vs. 16 cm^3) and stage (T4 vs. T3) may impact CRM involvement rates. This finding was confirmed by the Dutch TME trial, which reported a similar association between high tumor staging and CRM involvement.[56] Studies on conventional APR have demonstrated an even higher rate of CRM involvement. According to a multicenter trial of 434 patients who underwent conventional APR, the rate of CRM involvement was 30%.[56]

Performing an APR laparoscopically does not decrease the rate of CRM involvement. Therefore, attention should be focused on the technical aspects of the plane of dissection rather than the issue of how much access to the abdomen may be preferred.

Although outcomes of care with respect to rectal cancer surgery contain data on many thousands of patients, their quality is not sufficient to draw definitive conclusions on whether surgeons are a variable in these outcomes. The data acquired from selected reports seem to point in the direction of identifying critical steps in the process of care. This may be why process of care studies might in the future render outcome of care research relatively unimportant. The fact is that we should measure outcomes, modify processes, and measure outcomes again, and then repeat the continuous cycle in order to achieve the optimal quality of care.

Laparoscopic Abdominoperineal Resection

Introduction
Despite surgical options to spare the anal sphincter, APR is still required in 18% of patients with rectal cancer.[158] Performing APR laparoscopically offers the benefits of avoiding a minilaparotomy for specimen removal because the specimen is extracted perineally, and the left port site is adapted for an end colostomy. Obtaining a specimen with

Operating Room
The patient is placed in the lithotomy position with arms tucked and securely strapped to the table at the chest because tilting the table will be necessary. A stent may be inserted in the left ureter. All equipment including two monitors should be placed on the patient's left side in clear view of the surgeon. The surgeon stands on the patient's right side.

Surgical Technique
Standard Abdominoperineal Resection
Abdominal Procedure. The pneumoperitoneum is established through an open technique at the umbilicus. Four ports can be used. Additionally, one at the umbilical site is used for a 10-mm, 30-degree laparoscope (Figure 19-66). One 12-mm port placed in the right lower quadrant lateral to the rectus muscle sheath allows the use of a stapling device. Three 5-mm ports are inserted under direct vision in the right upper quadrant, suprapubic midline, and in the left lower quadrant. The left port is inserted at a premarked ostomy site and used by the assistant. The table is tilted head down and airplaned to the right.

Prior to dividing the inferior mesenteric vessels, the left ureter is identified. The bowel can be divided at the junction of the sigmoid colon with the descending colon by

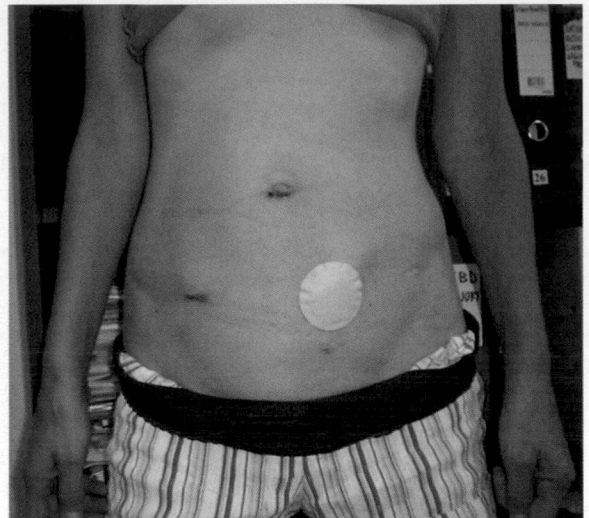

FIGURE 19-66. Postoperative appearance showing scars from port placement for laparoscopic abdominoperineal resection with colostomy patch.

using a stapler. The posterior rectal dissection starts with the identification of the hypogastric plexus and proceeds along the avascular plane. However, Waldeyer's fascia should be divided and entered approximately at the level of S4. In other words, the posterior rectal dissection should not continue as low as possible following the tapering of the mesorectum until the anorectal junction is achieved (Figure 19-67).[170] One must take care during the lateral rectal dissection not to injure the pelvic plexus (Figure 19-68).[48]

At the conclusion of the abdominal dissection, a drain is left in the pelvis and brought out through the anterior abdominal wall. All incisions are closed and dressed before the colostomy is matured.

Perineal Procedure. The bottom end dissection is the same as that described in detail in Chapter 24. With the patient in the lithotomy position, an elliptical skin incision is made in the perineum around the anus outside of the sphincter muscles, including a generous margin of perianal skin. During the perineal dissection, care is taken not to perforate the rectum. The inferior hemorrhoidal vessels are encountered lying anteriorly and posteriorly on either side in the ischiorectal fat. Once the ischiorectal fossa has been entered, a self-retaining retractor facilitates the exposure. The presacral space is entered by dividing the rectococcygeus muscle, commencing at the level of the tip of the coccyx. The coccyx is not excised. The proximal end of the intended specimen is delivered out of the pelvis posteriorly. In male patients, the remaining attachments of the rectourethralis muscle and fascia in the region of the urethra are sharply divided. If one dissects along an imaginary line to the promontory of the sacrum, the transverse perineal and rectourethralis muscles are divided anteriorly, and the posterior aspect of the prostate gland is identified. The peritoneal cavity is entered. In female patients, unless the tumor is quite small and exophytic or localized only to the posterior wall of the rectum, an en bloc posterior vaginectomy is performed (see also Chapter 24). After the specimen is removed, the perineal wound is copiously irrigated with saline solution. The perineal incision is closed in layers with interrupted absorbable sutures. The perineal skin is sutured until the forchette has been reconstituted.

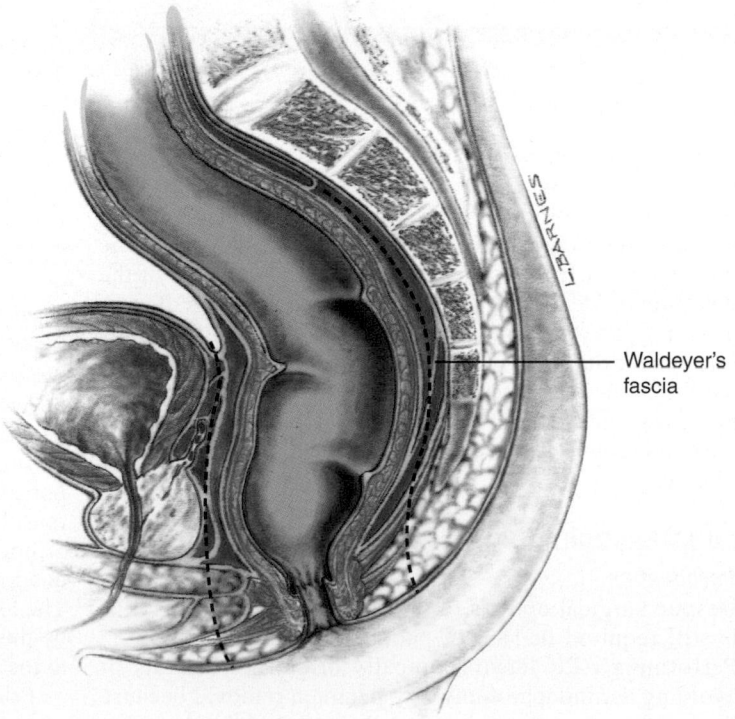

FIGURE 19-67. Posterior plane of dissection dividing Waldeyer's fascia.

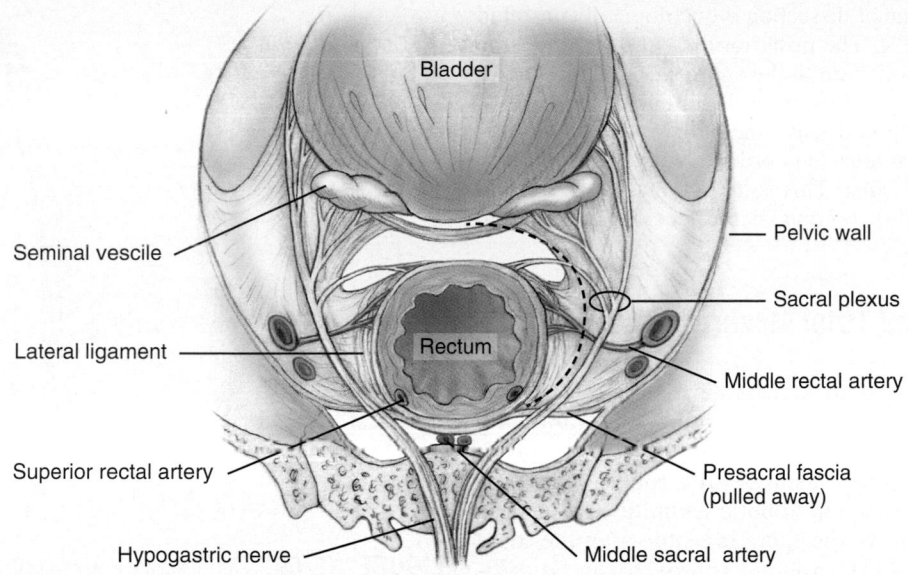

FIGURE 19-68. Avoiding pelvic plexus injury during lateral dissection.

The posterior vaginal defect is left open, but the cut edges are sutured with an absorbable material for hemostasis. A drain is brought out through the defect in the vaginal wall rather than through the perineum.

Extralevator Abdominoperineal Resection

Abdominal Procedure. The patient is placed in the supine position for the abdominal procedure but prone for the perineal procedure. The abdominal procedure for extralevator APR is identical to the abdominal procedure described earlier for standard APR with one exception. Rectal dissection concludes higher in the extralevator APR than in the standard APR. In the extralevator APR, the dissection stops at the origin of the levator ani muscle. A vertical rectus abdominis myocutaneous (VRAM) flap may be created, if necessary, prior to closure of the abdomen. The stoma is created, and the patient is rotated from supine to prone position.

VRAM Flap. VRAM flap harvest technique is identical to that which has been reported in the literature.[39] The skin paddle is placed cephalically overlying the rectus abdominis muscle and centered over the musculocutaneous perforators. The anterior rectus sheath is incised and included with the skin paddle, subcutaneous fat, and rectus abdominis muscle. The posterior rectus sheath is left intact, thereby allowing for closure of the abdominal wall. This technique affords a large amount of well-vascularized tissue with a large arc of rotation, as well as a predictable vascular pedicle. This makes it ideal for pelvic and perineal reconstruction. By this approach, one obliterates the large pelvic/perineal dead space created after some APRs as well as providing well-vascularized soft tissue to counteract the effects of possible radiation. The VRAM is harvested at the end of the abdominal portion of the operation. The flap is mobilized and placed in the pelvis directly behind the mobilized rectum. The colostomy is brought out on the left side of the abdomen, and the abdominal wall is then closed. The patient is moved into the prone position to complete the perineal portion of the APR. Once the specimen is resected, the VRAM flap is brought out of the pelvis and positioned in such a manner as to close the perineal incision.

Perineal Procedure. The patient is placed in the prone position. The perineal dissection is commenced with an elliptical incision made outside of the sphincter muscle, including a generous margin of perianal skin. As previously described, the inferior hemorrhoidal vessels are encountered lying anteriorly and posteriorly on either side in the ischiorectal fat. Once the ischiorectal fossas have been entered, a self-retaining retractor facilitates the exposure. The presacral space is entered by dividing the rectococcygeus muscle, commencing at the level of the tip of the coccyx. The levator ani muscle is divided near the pelvic wall attachments. This involves removal of the entire sphincter complex, following the inferior surface of the levators up to a lateral point where they originate on the pelvic sidewall. This point should be just inferior to the level where the abdominal procedure was terminated and where the abdominal and perineal procedures meet. The coccyx may be removed in continuity with the rectum in order to improve direct visualization during the dissection. In a woman, if the tumor is located anteriorly, a portion of the vaginal wall may also be removed. The pedicle VRAM flap can be used to close the perineal wound if the defect is of sufficient magnitude.

Opinion
There are, unfortunately, a number of misconceptions surrounding the planes of dissection for cancer of the lower third of the rectum. The most common is the confusion

between the plane of dissection for LAR and the plane for APR. The TME plane of dissection is oncologically unsound when applied to APR. The posterior dissection follows the tapering of the mesorectum to the anorectal junction, rather than entering Waldeyer's fascia at S4 aiming at the coccyx. Lateral dissection should leave the TME plane at the origin of the levator ani muscle in order to achieve a specimen without a so-called waist. This is the rationale for rejecting the practice of "trial dissection" before deciding whether to perform LAR or APR.

Robotic-Assisted Total Mesorectal Excision

Introduction

Robotic-assisted total mesorectal excision (RTME) is increasingly being recognized as a promising minimally invasive alternative procedure for rectal resection.[167] RTME can be performed using a fully robotic approach or as a hybrid laparoscopic/robotic technique.[13] Because of the inability to move the operating table after the robot has been docked, a fully robotic approach can be difficult and time consuming, especially when splenic flexure mobilization is required. Our preferred approach is to perform a hybrid procedure with laparoscopic mobilization of the splenic flexure followed by robotic proctectomy, unless a full splenic flexure release can be avoided. Because it has been described elsewhere in this chapter, I will not discuss the technique of laparoscopic splenic flexure mobilization and will limit myself to the robotic steps of the procedure.

Surgeon Selection

The experience of many centers across the world seems to indicate that RTME has a shorter learning curve compared with laparoscopic TME (see earlier discussion on the meaning of the phrase *learning curve*). Nevertheless, it must be stressed that this is a complex procedure and is best suited for high-volume rectal surgeons who have had broad experience with conventional laparoscopic colorectal operations and who have gone through extensive training in robotics. The presence of an experienced proctor in the operating room during the first few cases performed by a novice robotic rectal surgeon can be very beneficial and is highly recommended.

Patient Selection

I use robotic TME for all patients presenting with primary, localized rectal cancer. Ideal cases at the beginning of one's experience are thin individuals with relatively high tumors. The robotic approach to the female pelvis is usually easier regardless of tumor location. The use of neoadjuvant chemoradiotherapy does not preclude a robotic approach.

Patient Positioning

My preference is to place a large foam mat under the patient in order to prevent sliding. The upper chest is secured with a strap attached to the operating bedside rails. After induction of general anesthesia, the patient is moved to a modified lithotomy position. The perineum is prepped sterile only if a transanal extraction and hand-sewn coloanal anastomosis are anticipated. The routine use of ureteral stents is not considered necessary.

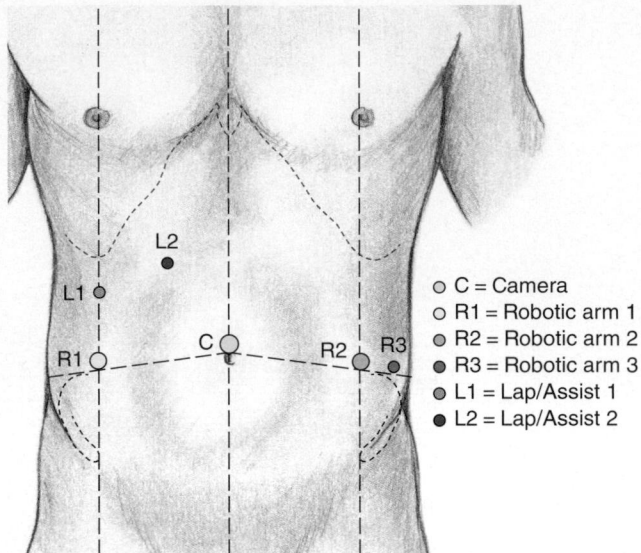

FIGURE 19-69. Port placement for robotic transanal mesorectal excision (TME).

○ C = Camera
○ R1 = Robotic arm 1
◑ R2 = Robotic arm 2
● R3 = Robotic arm 3
◔ L1 = Lap/Assist 1
● L2 = Lap/Assist 2

Port Placement

Pneumoperitoneum can be established with the Veress needle or via a Hasson approach in the midline where the scope will be inserted. This trocar is placed halfway between the pubis and the xiphoid, usually at or a few centimeters above the umbilicus (Figure 19-69, port C). The minimum distance between trocars is typically four fingerbreadths. A 12-mm trocar (Figure 19-69, R1) is then inserted approximately halfway between C and the right anterior superior iliac spine (ASIS) at approximately the midclavicular line (MCL). R1 will be the main stapling port and can also be used as the site of a protective loop ileostomy. A robotic 8 mm trocar (Figure 19-69, R2) will be inserted in the same position on the left side. The third robotic port (Figure 19-69, R3) will be about 8 to 10 cm more lateral to R2, usually just above the left ASIS. Two laparoscopic-assistant ports are inserted: one is placed about 10 cm above R1 in the MCL (Figure 19-69, L1), and the other is placed halfway between the MCL and the midline (Figure 19-69, L2). Robotic trocars can be also used during the laparoscopic portion of the procedure. Some variations in this port setup will be required from case to case. Experience has taught us that the narrower the pelvic inlet, the more medial the robotic ports will need to be.

Laparoscopic Mobilization of Splenic Flexure and Left Colon

Both surgeon and assistant stand on the patient's right side. I normally begin my medial-to-lateral dissection under the inferior mesenteric vein (IMV—Figure 19-70) and free the left mesocolon from its attachment to the retroperitoneum. The IMV is divided close to the pancreas with a vessel-sealing device or with a vascular stapler. The splenic flexure is mobilized according to the individual surgeon's preference and the descending and sigmoid colon are medialized. Port R2 can be used as well to reach a high flexure from the left side of the abdomen. The inferior mesenteric

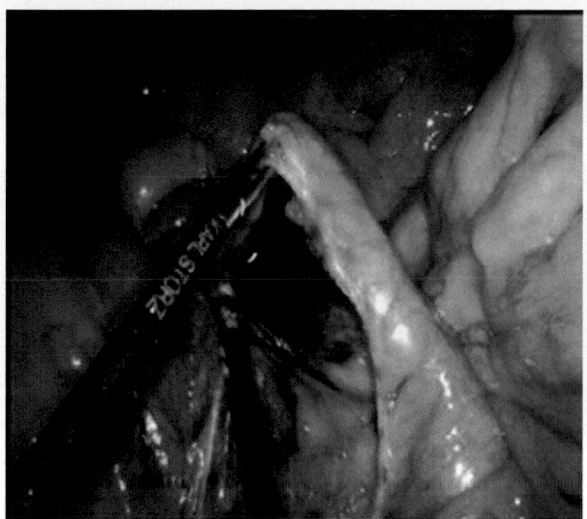

FIGURE 19-70. Laparoscopic dissection of the inferior mesorectal vein (IMV).

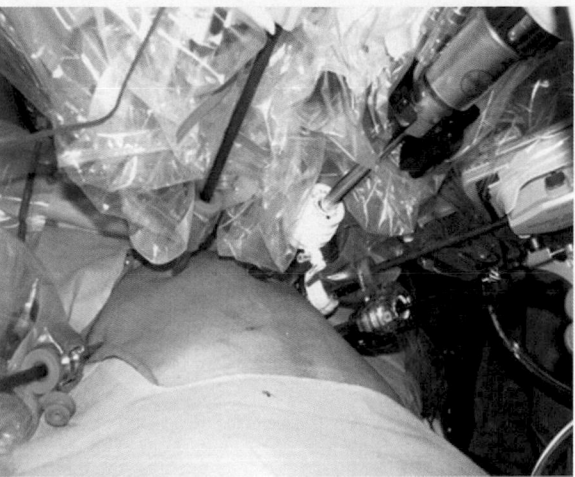

FIGURE 19-72. Robotic arms.

artery (IMA) can be divided laparoscopically or robotically as described next.

Robotic Vascular Control and Pelvic Dissection

After completing the colonic mobilization, the robotic part of the procedure can begin. The patient is maintained in sufficient Trendelenburg position to permit retraction of the small intestine out of the pelvis. A four-arm da Vinci S or Si is the robotic system of choice. I prefer to dock the system from the left hip instead of in between the legs (Figure 19-71). This is because this setup allows for ready access to the anus for performing intraoperative digital or endoscopic examinations as well as an eventual transanal extraction with the system in place.

A 0-degree scope at port C is ideal for the robotic part of the procedure, especially for the pelvic dissection. Robotic arm 1 will slide into the 12-mm R1 port, whereas arms 2 and 3 will be docked to trocars R2 and R3, respectively

(Figure 19-72). The robotic instrumentation is optimized with a hook cautery or scissors in arm 1, a bipolar grasper in 2, and a "prograsp" instrument in 3. A competent assistant on the right side of the patient is very helpful, and he or she will use ports L1 and L2 mostly for suctioning and retraction.

The dissection starts at the sacral promontory, where the parietal peritoneum medial to the right common iliac artery is incised. The plane is developed out under the superior hemorrhoidal artery following the areolar tissue. The left ureter is identified and preserved. The dissection proceeds toward the left, defining the IMA origin from the aorta. This can be skeletonized precisely using the robotic scissors or hook and subsequently divided with a stapler or between clips. In order to gain length and facilitate a tension-free anastomosis, I also routinely divide the left colic branch at its origin from the IMA.

The total mesorectal excision begins at the promontory. Whereas the assistant retracts the sigmoid colon anteriorly and superiorly, the robotic surgeon follows the areolar plane under the superior hemorrhoidal artery along the presacral fascia (Figure 19-73). Laterally, the hypogastric nerves are identified and preserved (Figure 19-74). Scissors is an ideal instrument for the TME in that it allows a

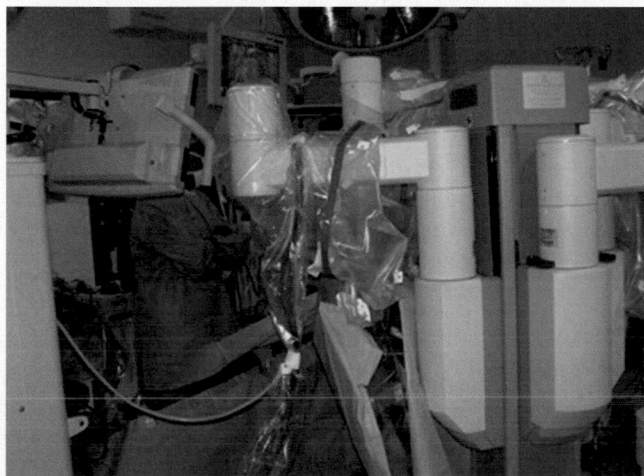

FIGURE 19-71. Docking the robot.

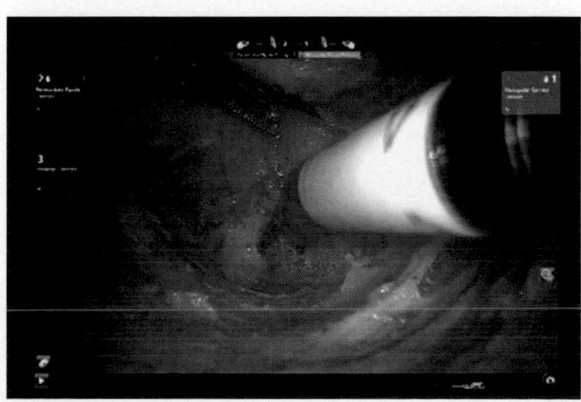

FIGURE 19-73. Robotic posterior dissection of the rectum.

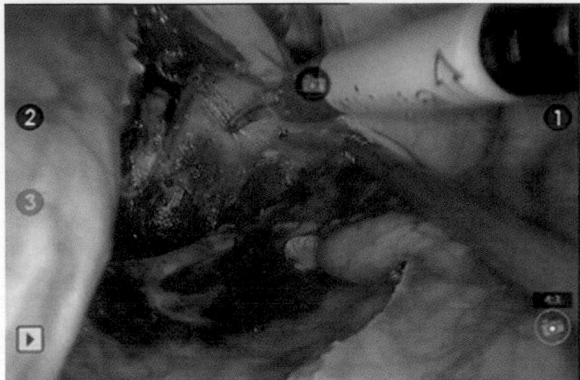

FIGURE 19-74. Robotic identification of the hypogastric nerves.

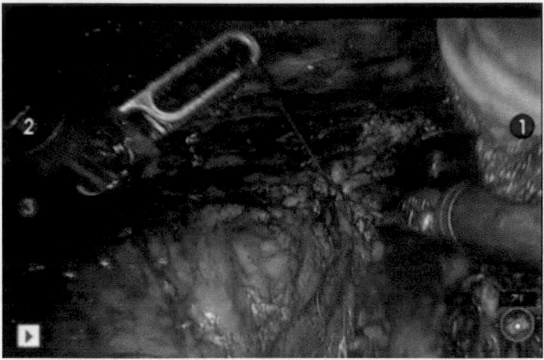

FIGURE 19-76. Robotic purse-string suture distal to rectal tumor.

rapid development of the plane while minimizing the use of electrical energy. The TME proceeds first posteriorly, then laterally, and finally anteriorly. It is important to point out that the left hand of the robotic surgeon (arm 2) should not grasp the mesorectum during the dissection because the robotic instruments are particularly powerful and can lacerate the mesorectal fascia and cause bleeding. With this arm configuration, arm 3 is used chiefly as an anterior retractor to keep the bladder, uterus, vagina, or prostate out of the field of dissection (Figure 19-75). On the side walls, autonomic nerve preservation is performed, and the middle hemorrhoidal vessels can be controlled with bipolar cautery. The dissection proceeds down to the pelvic floor where the levators can be easily identified under robotic visualization.

The "canonical principles" of the open TME are followed during RTME, emphasizing minimal manipulation of the rectum, identification of the embryologic planes, and tumor clearance with negative circumferential and distal margins. Large anterior tumors close to the vagina or prostate and seminal vesicles are clearly more challenging, especially given the lack of haptic (the sense of touch) feedback from the robotic arms. This can render the identification of the proper planes difficult.

To ascertain the appropriate level for rectal division, frequent digital rectal examinations under robotic vision are performed in order to obtain adequate distal resection

margins. For tumors that are at least 2 to 3 cm from the anorectal ring, a double-stapled colorectal anastomosis can be used. The articulating robotic arms allow for easy placement of a purse-string suture distal to the tumor. This will occlude the rectal lumen and supply a convenient handle to retract the rectum (Figure 19-76). For rectal division, my preference is to insert the articulating linear stapler through port R1 with the robotic arm removed, or alternatively to add another 12-mm port just lateral and superior to R1. A 45-mm green stapler load or the purple Tristaple cartridge is recommended, especially if preoperative radiation has been given. This is a delicate part of the procedure, and care must be taken to apply the stapler sequentially without crossing the previous transection line. An average of 2.5 firings is needed.

For tumors that are closer than 2 to 3 cm above the anorectal ring, a double-stapled anastomosis may be difficult to accomplish under robotic or laparoscopic control without compromising the distal resection margin. In properly selected patients, an intersphincteric resection with transanal extraction and hand-sewn coloanal anastomosis may be used for an ultra-low tumor that does not invade the external sphincter or levators.

Anastomosis
The robot is undocked after transecting the rectum. I recommend removing the specimen via a Pfannenstiel minilaparotomy covered with a wound protector. The proximal bowel and mesentery are divided and an anvil secured with a purse-string suture. After pushing the colon back into the abdomen, a circular anastomosis can be created laparoscopically (Figure 19-77). The decision whether to perform a fecal diversion by means of a loop ileostomy will depend on the individual case and the surgeon's preference, but is generally recommended to protect a very low anastomosis.

Transanal Minimally Invasive Surgery
Introduction
Transanal excision of both benign and malignant lesions of the rectum can be a challenging procedure for even a well-experienced surgeon. This is primarily because exposure and visualization can be difficult, resulting in compromised specimen quality. For this reason, other techniques have

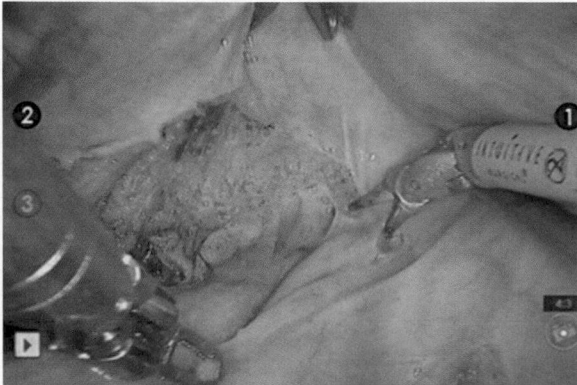

FIGURE 19-75. Robotic anterior dissection of the rectum.

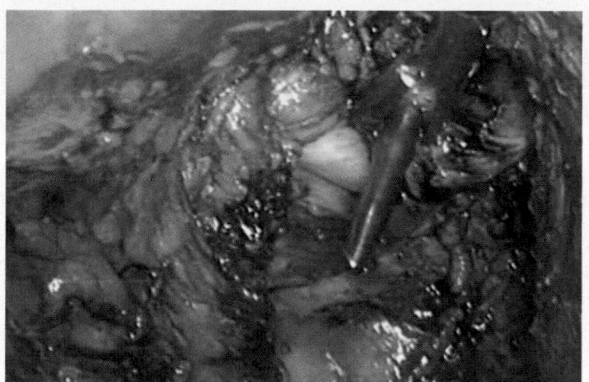

FIGURE 19-77. Robotic colorectal anastomosis.

been explored, most notably transanal endoscopic microsurgery (TEM—see Chapters 22 and 23).[38]

It has been well demonstrated that TEM provides superior quality of resection, with decreased local recurrence and improved survival when compared with standard peranal methods.[47,61,87,128,139,151,153,161,222,226] This is primarily because TEM allows for a better field of view, thereby improving the rate of negative resection margins and even permitting one to remove lesions at higher levels within the rectum, levels which cannot be obtained with the standard peranal approach. Despite these attractive advantages, TEM has failed to achieved widespread usage among colorectal surgeons because of its steep learning curve, its more complicated operative setup, and the sometimes prohibitive cost of the specialized instrumentation.[135]

Transanal minimally invasive surgery (TAMIS) is a newly developed method for peranal resection of rectal lesions. TAMIS has the same advantages as TEM, without some of the shortcomings. It was first developed in 2009[10] and has since become the preferred approach for transanal resection of benign rectal neoplasms and well-selected early stage rectal cancers. TAMIS offers the same quality of visualization as TEM, but unlike standard TEM, expensive, specialized instrumentation is not required. Furthermore, surgeons are not required to complete supplementary training because this approach uses the same familiar instruments that are used in laparoscopy. Knowledge and experience with single-port laparoscopy is, however, strongly recommended.

TAMIS incorporates the laparoscopic advancement of a single-port technique so that the confined rectal lumen can be easily accessed and visualized. Ultimately, this allows for full-thickness resection of lesions with the ability to harvest mesorectal tissue en bloc. With TAMIS, even complete rectal mobilization is possible. Furthermore, TAMIS, like TEM, permits resection of lesions at a greater distance from the anal verge than can normally be accessed with the standard peranal approach. For these reasons, TAMIS shows promise for gaining widespread acceptance in the future.

Indications

Patients suitable for TAMIS resection should have histologically favorable, mobile neoplasms amenable to transanal excision. Typically, those who meet TEM criteria also meet TAMIS resection criteria. TAMIS should not be considered as an alternative to standard oncologic resection. Although TAMIS has been successfully performed in the lower, mid-, and upper rectum, it is perhaps best suited for mid- and lower rectal lesions, providing a less morbid alternative to anterior resection or APR in highly selected patients.

Preoperative Workup

All patients who have been selected to undergo TAMIS resection should have had a colonoscopy to assess the possibility of the presence of synchronous lesions and to obtain a biopsy of the rectal lesion. For malignant, early stage tumors of the rectum, endorectal ultrasound or pelvic MRI is performed to determine preoperative T and N stage. Currently, only patients with uTis or uT1 and uN0 cancer are considered candidates for TAMIS. More advanced lesions require adjuvant or neoadjuvant chemoradiation therapy. The local approach has not been validated with prospective, randomized clinical trials. CT scan of the chest, abdomen, and pelvis are also performed to assess for tumor metastasis. Patients with stage IV disease are not candidates for TAMIS unless the intent is palliation.

Operating Room

Preparation includes full mechanical bowel cleansing and the administration of parenteral antibiotics less than 30 minutes preoperatively. Patients are placed in the lithotomy position regardless of the location of the lesion on the rectal wall. The prone jackknife position is another alternative. The operating room should be fitted with standard laparoscopic equipment, including light source, video monitor, and CO_2 insufflator. General anesthesia with muscle paralysis is required in order to avoid collapse of the rectal wall with spontaneous respiration.

Surgical Technique

A single-incision laparoscopic surgery port (SILS port; Covidien, Mansfield, MA) is deployed into the anal canal with lubricant and gentle maneuvering. Although this is an off-label use of the Covidien SILS port, it provides a naturally conforming fit. Once in place, three 5-mm ports allow access to the rectum so that TAMIS can be performed. Using a standard laparoscopic tower, pneumorectum with CO_2 is established to 16 mm Hg through the insufflation-dedicated cannula. The current Covidien SILS port is designed to allow an exchange of a 5 mm access to 12 mm. Once the SILS trocars are placed, standard laparoscopic instruments including graspers, thermal energy devices, and needle drivers can be used to perform the procedure. A 5-mm, 30-degree or 45-degree angled camera is inserted with triangulation of the instrument facilitating the surgical dissection (Figure 19-78). Resection using TAMIS is typically performed by demarcating the perimeter of the lesion, thereby providing an appropriate margin. This is accomplished by using electrocautery (Figure 19-79). I find that simple, short bursts of suction, and the use of a laparoscopic suction-irrigator device, maintains image clarity quite well. The specimen may be tented gently by using a grasper, and electrocautery on a spatula-tip or needle-tip allows for full-thickness excision. Interestingly, CO_2 insufflation provides a natural "pneumo-dissection," thereby augmenting the ease and clarity of TAMIS. By using this approach, TAMIS permits an R0 resection, with complete

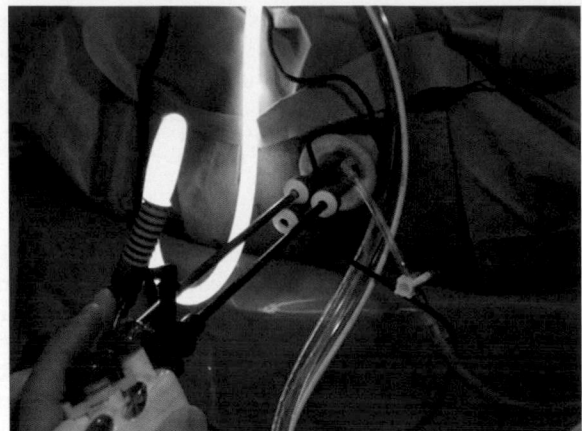

FIGURE 19-78. Operating room setup for transanal minimally invasive surgery (TAMIS).

en bloc removal in the majority of instances. Once the specimen has been excised, it can be retrieved by removing the single-incision port. The specimen is then sent to the pathology laboratory so that clear margins can be confirmed. Next, the SILS port is quickly reintroduced. Suturing of the rectal wall defect is facilitated by bending of the swaged needle and by securing knots with the help of a standard knot pusher. Alternatively, the Endo Stitch (Covidien) can be used to perform endoluminal suturing. Also, V-Loc 180 (Covidien) can be used because the suture can be secured without knots. Generally, it is preferred to close the rectal wall defect transversely in order to prevent luminal narrowing. Once surgical closure is achieved, an endoscopic examination should be performed in order to ensure that the luminal diameter has not been compromised.

Postoperative Care

One advantage to transanal resection using TAMIS is that postoperative pain is minimal. Patients are typically admitted for observation and are discharged on the first postoperative day. Perioperative intravenous antibiotics are administered, and patients are transitioned to oral antibiotics with anaerobic and gram-negative coverage for a period of 7 days. There are

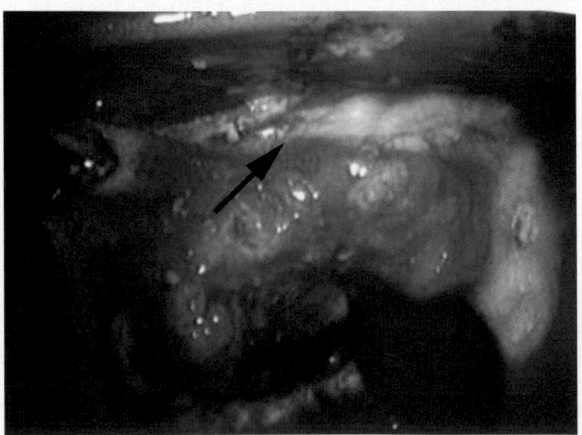

FIGURE 19-79. Marking resection margin with electrocautery during transanal minimally invasive surgery (TAMIS).

no dietary restrictions. Follow-up is recommended to be at 2 and 6 weeks. Rigid proctoscopy is performed at those visits to assess healing. Patient follow-up conforms to the National Comprehensive Cancer Network guidelines, depending on the final pathology results.

Laparoscopic Loop Ileostomy and Colostomy

Introduction

The first laparoscopic loop colostomy was described by Lange and coworkers in 1991.[124] This was performed on a 48-year-old patient with severe fecal incontinence. Laparoscopic loop ileostomy was first described by Khoo and associates in 1993 for a 45-year-old female with a rectovaginal fistula.[113] Although I believe these techniques have since gained wide acceptance along with the development of laparoscopic colon surgery, the frequency of use remains unknown, and only a few series have been published. To this date, there is no randomized controlled study comparing laparoscopic loop stoma creation to that of the open technique. Despite this limitation, the potential advantages are believed to be the following: avoidance of a large incision, the ability to perform a diagnostic laparoscopy, obtaining biopsies if needed at the time of the stoma creation, reduced pain and ileus, shorter hospitalization, and better cosmetic appearance. As with any laparoscopic surgical procedure, if the operation cannot be accomplished with reasonable safety, it should not be performed by this means.

Indications

The indications for laparoscopic loop ostomy are identical to those for conventional loop ostomy (see Chapter 31). It is a valid approach if one wishes to obtain a temporary or even a permanent diversion of the fecal stream, such as in an individual with severe perianal Crohn's disease, fecal incontinence, rectovaginal fistula, perianal sepsis, perineal burn, anorectal trauma, a near-obstructing rectal cancer prior to initiating chemoradiation therapy, advanced rectal cancer or other advanced pelvic tumors, colonic inertia, and paraplegia. The choice between ileostomy and colostomy will depend on the indication and the surgeon's preference.

Preoperative Workup

Preoperatively and ideally, a wound/ostomy, continence (WOC) nurse should be involved in educating the patient and in marking the proposed stoma site(s) (see Chapter 32). This will minimize the risk of complications related to the ostomy as well as avoiding a prolonged hospital stay for stoma teaching. Mechanical bowel preparation is left to the surgeon's preference because its value has been challenged in recent years. It is important to take into consideration that for a patient with a nearly obstructing tumor, a mechanical bowel preparation may not be tolerated well. This could result in profound bowel distention, thereby rendering the laparoscopic approach more difficult to accomplish. Perioperative antibiotic prophylaxis should be part of the routine.

Operating Room

The patient is placed under a general anesthesia in the supine position with arms tucked. For laparoscopic loop ileostomy, the surgeon and the assistant are located on the left side of the patient. The monitor should be positioned in the right side toward the feet. The surgeon then will move to the right side after the loop is ready to be matured. For laparoscopic loop colostomy, the patient could be in the same position or in a modified lithotomy position. The surgeon and assistant will be located on the right side of the patient, or the surgeon could be in between the patient legs if the lithotomy position is elected. One monitor should be positioned toward the patient's left shoulder and another monitor toward the left foot. The surgeon will move to the patient's left in order to mature the colostomy.

Operative Technique
Laparoscopic Loop Ileostomy

A 5-mm port is placed in the supraumbilical area, and a 5-mm, 30-degree laparoscope is inserted. A 12-mm port is preferred in the right lower abdominal quadrant at the in tended ileostomy location. An additional 5-mm trocar may be placed in the suprapubic area or the left lower quadrant if technically necessary. After a diagnostic laparoscopy has been completed, the terminal ileum is identified and the distal loop is grasped with a laparoscopic ratcheted nontraumatic bowel grasper. Care must be taken to identify the afferent and efferent limbs, and no tension should be encountered when elevating the loop toward the anterior abdominal wall. The skin is then incised around the 12-mm trocar, and a core of tissue is excised all the way down to the fascia. This is then incised in a cruciate fashion to accommodate two finger-breadths. The rectus muscle is split, and the posterior rectus sheet is incised transversely. At this time, the pneumoperitoneum is lost. The 12-mm trocar is removed en bloc with the laparoscopic grasper. The loop of ileum is then grasped with a Babcock clamp. The pneumoperitoneum is then restored. The loop of bowel can be visualized and identified as to the afferent and efferent limbs in order to confirm that there is no twisting. The pneumoperitoneum is then released, and the loop ileostomy is then matured in the usual fashion. My preference is to create an opening in the mesentery, and a rod or rubber catheter is placed to form a supporting bridge. The distal limb is opened transversely about 5 mm above the skin level, and the proximal cut edge is everted and sutured to the skin, tacking seromuscular bites similar to that of a Brooke ileostomy. Conversion to an open procedure should be carried out if one is unable to proceed laparoscopically or if complications ensue.

Laparoscopic Loop Colostomy

With this procedure, a 5-mm port is used in the umbilical area and a 5-mm, 30-degree laparoscope is employed. A 12-mm trocar is placed in the proposed colostomy site. Another 5-mm trocar is placed in the right lower quadrant. The patient should be secured to the operating table as with a laparoscopic colon resection and should be tilted right-side down in steep Trendelenburg. The sigmoid colon or descending colon is retracted medially, and using endoshears, the lateral attachments are taken down so that a mobile sigmoid or descending colon is obtained. The loop of desired colon should easily reach the abdominal wall without tension. It is then grasped with a locking laparoscopic Babcock through the 12-mm port. The skin is then excised around the 12-mm trocar. A core of tissue is excised to the level of the fascia. This is incised in a cruciate fashion with the rectus muscle fibers spread apart and the posterior sheet opened. The

opening needs to be sufficiently capacious to accommodate the loop of colon. The trocar and the laparoscopic Babcock holding the colon are removed en bloc. The colon is grasped with the Babcock clamp and matured in a similar fashion to that of the open technique.

Laparoscopic Management of Adhesive Small Bowel Obstruction
Introduction

Adhesions were of little clinical significance prior to the development of anesthesia and when antisepsis permitted widespread use of laparotomy. American and British surveys covering 1888 to 1898 and 1925 to 1930 reported adhesions to be the cause of small bowel obstruction (SBO) in only 18%[82] and 7%,[218] respectively. To put this problem in perspective, Foster and colleagues reported in 2005 that during the year 1997 in the state of California, SBO accounted for 32,583 unscheduled admissions, and that approximately 85% of these were secondary to adhesions.[74] In a Canadian study, the etiology of SBO was reported in 552 patients.[147] They accounted for 1,001 admissions over 10 years: adhesions 74%, miscellaneous 11%, Crohn's disease 7%, cancer 5%, hernia 2%, and radiation 1%.[147] The development of adhesions leading to SBO has been universally recognized by surgeons ever since abdominal operations have been performed. However, laparotomy for the treatment of adhesive SBO seems paradoxical because a laparotomy is the most common cause of adhesive SBO. The reader is encouraged to review the extensive literature on this subject, a number of references for which are appended.[68,72,74,119,123,133,143,148,198,233]

Rationale

SBO was initially viewed as a relative contraindication for performing laparoscopy due to the frequent adhesions, the risk of performing enterotomies, and the decreased visualization as a consequence of the distended bowel. Although a substantial number of these patients can be treated nonoperatively, some require immediate surgery. As laparoscopic experience has increased and advances with instrumentation have been made, laparoscopic treatment of SBO has become possible, but nonetheless this approach is seldom used.

In 1991, Bastug and colleagues reported the first laparoscopic lysis of a single adhesive band that had caused an SBO.[14] Since then, case reports and small series have been published describing the use of laparoscopy in treating selected patients with this condition.[44,45,205] The postulated benefits over that of open laparotomy may include decreased postoperative pain, decreased ileus, lower rates of wound infection and incisional hernia, improved cosmetic appearance, and the decreased potential for additional adhesions. Despite these potential benefits, the surgical community has been slow to adopt laparoscopy in the treatment of this common disorder. The most likely reasons are the paucity of clinical reports, the overall absence of selection criteria, and perhaps the lack of experience in performing advanced laparoscopy in an emergency setting. In experienced hands, however, laparoscopy is a reasonable alternative to formal laparotomy. In the only two retrospective comparative studies in the literature, laparoscopic management of SBO appears to offer the advantages of decreased overall morbidity, earlier return of bowel function, decreased length of hospital stay, and faster return of full activity.[44,230]

Duron and coworkers reported a long-term follow-up investigating the risk factors of mortality and morbidity after surgery for adhesive postoperative SBO.[65] They concluded that there was no difference in mortality or morbidity between the open and laparoscopic approaches. Although the results from published, mostly retrospective, individual series vary significantly, pooled data from a review in 2007 show that laparoscopic management of SBO is successful in 66% of patients but with a conversion rate of 33.5%.[81] Conversion was most frequently due to dense adhesions (28%), followed by the need for bowel resection (23%) as a result of injury, ischemia, gangrene, and other causes.

More reliable are probably the results of the largest of these series over 8 years (308 patients from 35 centers).[127] The "successful" laparoscopy rate was 54.6%, and the conversion to laparotomy rate was 45.4%. There were significantly more successes among patients with a history of one or two laparotomies than among those with three or more (56% vs. 37%; $P < .05$). There were significantly more successes among patients who had undergone appendectomy only (67/94; 71%) than among patients who underwent other operations (33%; $P < .001$). The rate of success was significantly higher ($P < .001$) in patients operated on early (less than 24 hours) and in patients with adhesive bands (54%), than in those with matted adhesions (31%). Selection criteria for laparoscopy may be helpful: (1) proximal obstruction, (2) partial obstruction, (3) anticipated single band, (4) localized distension on radiography, (5) no sepsis, and (6) mild abdominal distension.[63] Some authors have determined a soft list of clinical parameters for the successful laparoscopic management of adhesive SBO: (1) SBOs that temporarily improve/resolve after placement of a nasogastric tube but recur or prevent the patient from tolerating an oral diet, (2) limited abdominal distension, (3) proximal obstruction, (4) previous operative treatment in a limited area of the abdomen, (5) previous operative note did not describe massive or severe adhesions, (6) ability to gain safe access into the peritoneal cavity, (7) obstructed segments not fixed to the retroperitoneum, and (8) widespread peritoneal cancer.[234] Complications included intraoperatively recognized enterotomy (6.5%). These complication rates compare favorably with the published results of open surgery for SBO, where morbidity and mortality rates are as high as 32% and 3.8%, respectively.[9,225]

Strickland and associates found that duration of surgery longer than 120 minutes, intraoperative perforation, bowel necrosis, and conversion to laparotomy were significant predictors of postoperative morbidity.[203] There are clinical data backed up by several animal studies supporting the hypothesis that laparoscopy leads to a decreased rate of adhesion formation when compared with laparotomy.[62,89] This should be the main rationale to offer laparoscopy to prospective patients. It is not clear, however, if laparoscopic adhesiolysis for SBO will lead to a decrease in recurrence rate.

As compared with laparotomy, no attempt is generally made during laparoscopy to free up the entire abdominal wall and interloop adhesions. Only adhesions impeding exposure and causing obstructions are divided. Ghosheh and colleagues reported early recurrence of SBO in 22 (2.1%) of 1,061 patients.[85] However, no conclusion can be drawn regarding the true rate of recurrence of SBO because adequate follow-up is lacking in most published studies.

Surgical Technique

Once the decision has been made to proceed surgically and laparoscopically, the patient should be informed of the possible risks and complications, including conversion to laparotomy, bowel resection, need for stoma, and provide appropriate informed consent. The patient should be placed in a modified lithotomy position for intraoperative endoscopy. Two monitors are ideal for this surgery. The site of first trocar placement should be carefully planned away from existing scars. Despite evolution of both laparoscopic instruments and techniques, injury to intra-abdominal structures continues to be a not uncommon, yet generally avoidable complication of laparoscopy. Many of these injuries are related to the blind placement of the Veress needle or sharp primary trocar into the abdomen when performing a technique referred to as "closed" laparoscopy. Although "open" laparoscopy (where the peritoneal cavity is opened before placing a blunt trocar into the abdomen) has been successful in avoiding major vessel injury, bowel injuries with this technique have not been eliminated.

Most authors recommend mandatory open insertion of the initial trocar, whereas others have not encountered bowel injuries after the use of the Veress needle. In response, trocars have been developed for laparoscopy, termed "optical access" trocars. These ports were designed to decrease the risk of injury to intra-abdominal structures by allowing the surgeon to visualize abdominal wall layers during placement. As of this writing, only two serious complications have been reported in the medical literature with their use. Two "optical access" trocar systems are available: one uses a blade that strikes the fascia and peritoneum under laparoscopic visualization, and the other system has a conical, clear tip that is rotated under laparoscopic vision as it penetrates the fascia and peritoneum. The 30-degree scope provides excellent visualization. The pneumoperitoneum should never exceed 15 mm Hg. Bowel should be examined for perforation and signs of ischemia. Free fluid should be aspirated and sent for gram staining, amylase, bilirubin, and culture. To facilitate exposure, table tilt and external manual compression of the abdominal wall should be used. Second and third ports can be added to avoid excessive tenting of the abdominal wall.

One of the most concerning complications in laparoscopic management of SBO is the creation of an inadvertent enterotomy. In a single comparative study, the risk of perforation was 27% in the laparoscopic group.[230] This was clearly higher than in the open group. As discussed earlier, the overwhelming concern is that the bowel injury may be missed at the time of operation, a complication that can have devastating consequences. Bowel graspers with nonlocking handles should be used to gently run the bowel. Exposure can be achieved by pushing with closed instruments rather than by grasping. The small bowel should be inspected in a retrograde fashion commencing at the cecum and/or decompressed bowel until the point of transition is identified. Cold scissors should be used to divide matted adhesions or a band. Energy-based devices should be avoided when dividing adhesions. There should be a low threshold for conversion. Although the incidence of conversion, itself, has not been shown to correlate with the number of prior operations, it may be predicted by the presence of bowel distension greater than 4 cm, a documented history of dense adhesions, or the presence of complete distal obstruction.

Laparoscopic Restorative Proctocolectomy for Ulcerative Colitis or Familial Adenomatous Polyposis

Introduction

Restorative proctocolectomy with ileal J-pouch anal anastomosis (IPAA) with loop ileostomy is a technically challenging procedure, whether it is performed open or laparoscopically. In the latter case, this is considered an advanced procedure and should only be offered to selected patients by surgeons who have extensive experience with conventional surgery for inflammatory bowel diseases and with advanced laparoscopic colorectal surgery. However, the benefits of laparoscopic restorative proctocolectomy have not been clearly established as of this date. In fact, as early as 1992 Wexner and colleagues reported no immediately recognizable benefits for patients undergoing laparoscopic total colectomy.[221] A Cochrane systematic review (2009) encompassing 253 patients who underwent laparoscopic restorative proctocolectomy from 11 studies reported no significant differences in postoperative outcome measures when compared with conventional surgery.[3] Technically speaking, laparoscopic restorative proctocolectomy has been described as laparoscopic-assisted in most case series and also as hand-assisted to a lesser extent.

Indications

Laparoscopic proctocolectomy with IPAA and protecting ileostomy may be considered as an option to its conventional counterpart with the same indications that currently apply to that of elective open surgery. All reasonable efforts should be made to ascertain whether the patient understands the concept and to the likelihood of conversion to conventional open surgery. Advantages and disadvantages of surgical treatment options must be comprehensively discussed with the patient. Conservative estimates of pouch failure rates must be shared, and alternative treatment plans discussed in the event the pouch would have to be subsequently excised.[219] Permanent ileostomy and possibly continent ileostomy are among the options one should discuss. Patients should ideally attend ostomy care classes before undergoing the operation (see Chapters 29 and 32). Appropriate timing for discontinuation of medications should also be evaluated for patients with ulcerative colitis. Conservative estimates of the possible impact of preoperative steroids and/or biologics upon postoperative septic complications should be included when counseling ulcerative colitis patients. The patient should understand the material facts, possible risks, complications, and alternatives to the planned surgery before the patient signs an informed consent.

Preoperative Care

In addition to the requisite preoperative studies, preoperative evaluation of the anal sphincters by means of manometry and ultrasound is reasonable, particularly in older women.

Operating Room Setup

The operating table needs to be capable of side tilt as well as maximum Trendelenburg and reverse Trendelenburg positionings. A Foley catheter and orogastric tube should be inserted. The patient is placed supine on the operating table with the lower limbs either in modified stirrups or abducted. Sequential compression devices are applied to the legs. Both arms should be tucked. The patient should be securely strapped to the table at the chest. The abdomen and perineum should be prepared and draped sterile. All equipment should be placed on the patient's right side in clear view of the surgeon. The surgeon stands on the patient's left side for most of the procedure. Mobile monitors need to be located on both sides of the patient. One assistant is required to operate the camera, and a second assistant aids with retraction, especially during the pelvic dissection.

Surgical Technique

The following is a description of a clockwise sequence, broken down into anatomical sections, and the steps of each section identified. The major difference between this procedure and standard segmental resections is that the vessels are divided close to the colon or where it is most convenient, not necessarily at their origin, because oncologic concerns are not relevant, and there is no need to remove all lymph-bearing tissue. The instruments used are a blunt 5-mm bowel grasper held in the surgeon's left hand and a 5-mm electrosurgical vessel-sealing device held in the surgeon's right hand. The latter may be used for both dissecting and cauterizing. If the surgeon prefers to employ an ultrasonic device, a vascular stapler should be used for securing the vascular pedicles. Additional instruments needed are scissors, long graspers, powered suction device, endoscopic staplers, and a 30-degree scope (10 mm in diameter). A pretied loop or clip applier should always be available to treat bleeding not controlled by the energy device. It is preferable to have a smoke filter attached to one of the ports in order to allow for safe venting of smoke. The choice of mode of access to the peritoneal cavity (open Hasson or Veress needle) should be based on the surgeon's experience and preference. Port placement includes five trocars: a 10-mm port placed supraumbilically, a 12-mm port on the right at the planned stoma site, a 5-mm port in the right lower quadrant, a 12-mm port placed suprapubically, and a 5-mm port in the left lower quadrant.

Step 1: Ileocolic Vessels

While placing the ports, the surgeon and assistant stand on opposite sides of the patient. They then both move to the patient's left side, and the right-sided monitor is placed below the patient's shoulder. The camera is placed at the number 1 port, and the surgeon uses port numbers 4 and 5. The table is turned into a moderate left tilt as well as into a slight Trendelenburg position. The peritoneal surfaces and liver are inspected for possible tumor growth. The omentum and small bowel are gently displaced into the left upper quadrant. The ileocolic vessels are identified by gentle traction applied to the mesentery of the cecum, and the superior mesenteric vein (SMV) and duodenum are located. A window beneath the ileocolic vessels is opened, incising the peritoneum close to the origin of the vessels. This gives access to the avascular space underneath the colonic mesentery, where the colon can be pealed off the retroperitoneum. The ileocolic vessels are gently dissected out and then divided as close to the colon as is comfortable.

Step 2: Medial Mobilization
The dissection continues medially along the mesentery from the point where the ileocolic vessels were divided and proceeds cephalad. The right ureter is identified and the duodenum kept in clear view. If present, the right colic vessels are divided. For now, the dissection ends at the origin of Henle's gastrocolic trunk from the SMV.

Step 3: Opening the Lesser Sac
The table is leveled from the Trendelenburg position but kept in a moderate left tilt; the gastrocolic ligament (omentum) is grasped with the left hand and retracted caudally and up toward the abdominal wall. It is then opened using the energy device and the lesser sac entered. The division of the gastrocolic ligament is performed in a medial-to-lateral direction toward the hepatic flexure, caudal to the right gastroepiploic vessels.

Step 4: The Hepatic Flexure
The hepatic flexure is mobilized in a medial-to-lateral direction. The lateral peritoneal reflection of the ascending colon is divided along the white line of Toldt in a caudal to cephalad direction, and the mesentery of the ascending colon is mobilized off the retroperitoneum.

Step 5: Terminal Ileum
The surgeon switches the instruments so the grasper is in port number 5 and the energy device in port number 4. The cecum and the terminal ileum are mobilized from the lateral side and the dissection continued until it meets the dissection from the medial side. The final attachments of the ascending colon are taken down, thus fully mobilizing the right colon.

Step 6: Middle Colic Vessels
The surgeon and assistant move to the patient's right side, and the left-sided monitor is placed at the patient's shoulder. The camera remains in port number 1, and the surgeon uses port number 2 for the grasper and number 3 for the energy device. The table is tilted to the right and in reverse Trendelenburg position in order to allow the right colon to fall out of the way. The transverse colon is gently elevated off the duodenum in order to identify the middle colic vessels. It is important to recognize the anatomic location of the SMV as well as the gastrocolic trunk of Henle. These vessels are quite short, and excessive traction can lead to profuse bleeding at the inferior border of the pancreas. The branches of the middle colic vessel are divided close to the colon while the transverse mesentery is held up. The mesentery is divided toward the splenic flexure.

Step 7: Splenic Flexure
Division of the greater omentum is continued toward the patient's left by grasping the gastrocolic ligament, thus fully opening the lesser sac, always avoiding traction on the spleen. The splenic flexure is mobilized laterally by retracting the colon gently medially and dividing the lateral attachments, as well as peeling the colon off of Gerota's fascia, carefully avoiding the tail of the pancreas.

Step 8: Repositioning
The patient is now placed in steep Trendelenburg position while maintaining the right tilt. The left-sided monitor is moved toward the patient's hip. The camera is moved to port number 2, and the surgeon uses port numbers 1 and 3. The previously mobilized right colon, along with the small bowel and omentum, are swept out of the pelvis and placed in the right upper quadrant.

Step 9: Inferior Mesenteric Vessels
The medial mobilization of the descending colon starts by opening the retroperitoneum at the sacral promontory, mobilizing underneath the mesentery of the colon and lifting it up, making sure that the left ureter and gonadal vessels are not included. The inferior mesenteric artery is identified and its branches dissected out, preserving the hypogastric nerves. The vessel branches are divided individually near the colon. The opening of the retroperitoneum is continued cephalad until the inferior mesenteric vein is located. This is dissected out and divided. The remaining mesentery is lifted off the retroperitoneum and divided.

Step 10: Lateral Mobilization
Following the peritoneal reflection of the white line of Toldt, while retracting the colon medially, the dissection from above and medial is connected, thereby completing the mobilization of the colon. It is important to be mindful of the position of the ureter from this side, especially as it courses across the pelvic brim.

Step 11: Rectal Mobilization
It is necessary to have a second assistant available in order to aid with the rectal mobilization, using ports 4 and 5 for retraction. In women, a bulky uterus can be elevated with a heavy suture placed through the fundus and the abdominal wall. First, the peritoneum is opened down both pararectal sulci and then anteriorly at the peritoneal reflexion (inferior aspect of the pouch of Douglas in women or rectovesical excavation in men). It is easier and safer to stay outside the mesorectal fascia because this is avascular and allows for sparing of the branches of the inferior hypogastric nerve plexus. The dissection is performed with a combination of blunt dissection and cautery. The surgeon places traction on the rectum while the assistant retracts the tissue along the pelvic walls laterally and anteriorly, thus maintaining three-way retraction. The middle rectal artery can be divided using the energy source instrument used before. The rectum is mobilized anteriorly below the level of the seminal vesicles in men and in women well below the cervix. Laterally and posteriorly, the mobilization is carried down to the levator muscles. The junction of the rectum and the anus is recognized where the mesorectum ends and is confirmed by digital examination of the rectum.

Step 12: Transecting the Rectum
An endoscopic stapler is brought in through port number 4 and the rectum transected where it meets the anus. Usually, at least two cartridges are needed because the longer staplers cannot be easily applied this low in the pelvis. The cut end is grasped with a locking grasper and the abdomen desufflated.

Step 13: Extraction of Specimen
In thin patients, the extraction of the specimen through the stoma site is a potential option. The stoma site can be opened

in the usual fashion. The stapled proximal end of the colon is brought to the stoma site and the specimen delivered. Alternatively, a short Pfannenstiel incision (4 to 5 cm) is performed, a wound protector placed, and the specimen retrieved.

Step 14: Creation of Pouch

The terminal ileum is transected with a linear stapler. A 15-cm long pouch is created extracorporeally in the usual fashion (see Chapter 29). The end of the pouch should reach at least 5 cm below the symphysis pubis to ensure a tension-free anastomosis. The anvil of the circular stapler is placed in the enterotomy and secured with a purse-string suture. The pouch is returned to the abdomen. If the specimen has been removed through a Pfannenstiel incision, the wound protector is removed, the fascia closed, and the abdomen reinsufflated. If the specimen has been removed through the stoma site, the wound protector is wrapped around itself and secured with towel clips so the abdomen can be reinsufflated.

Step 15: Anastomosis

A second assistant moves between the legs and irrigates the rectal stump with an iodine solution. If the staple line demonstrates no leak, a circular stapler is placed through the anus and the trocar brought out through the anal wall just anterior to the staple line. The anvil is connected to the trocar and the stapler closed, ensuring that no extra tissue has been incorporated. Once proper orientation of the pouch and lack of tension have been confirmed, the stapler is fired. The tissue rings from the stapler are examined to make certain they are both complete (full circle and full thickness). The anastomosis is not tested for leakage because insertion of an instrument may itself damage the very low ileoanal anastomosis. Final inspection for adequate hemostasis in all four quadrants is performed. A drain is placed in the pelvis and brought out through port 3.

Step 16: Creation of the Ileostomy

The small bowel is traced back from the pouch (at least 20 cm) to find a convenient loop for the stoma. At that level, the small bowel is grasped with a locking, nontraumatic grasper, noting the orientation of the bowel regarding the afferent and efferent limbs. The abdomen is desufflated and the chosen bowel loop grasped with a Babcock clamp and delivered. A rod is placed under the bowel loop, all trocars are removed, and the fascia at the 10- and 12-mm ports is closed. All skin incisions are closed and dressings applied. A loop ileostomy is created, everting the cut edges and making certain that the afferent limb is cephalad.

Postoperative Care

If a nasogastric or orogastric tube is used intraoperatively, this should be removed at the end of the procedure. A liquid diet may be started on postoperative day 1 if there are no clinical signs of ileus. Usually, oral pain medications are tolerated on postoperative day 1. The Foley catheter should also be removed on postoperative day 1 unless there are signs of hypovolemia. Most patients are ready for discharge from the hospital on postoperative days 3 to 4. Follow-up should be at 2 and 6 weeks and after that according to each individual surgeon's policy. Closure of the temporary stoma can usually be performed after 3 months, once the integrity of the pouch has been verified by contrast enema and by flexible endoscopy.

Laparoscopic Reoperative Surgery

Introduction

Complex reoperative cases can be defined as operations where one anticipates that intraoperative adverse events are likely to be encountered. Reasons may include difficult laparoscopic access due to multiple laparotomies, dense adhesions, risk of inadvertent organ injury secondary to altered anatomy, and risk of hemorrhage in patients on anticoagulation therapy (which cannot be discontinued). As laparoscopic experience has increased and instruments have improved, a large number of cases can be safely performed through a laparoscopic approach. Reoperative cases, once viewed as a contraindication for laparoscopy, are currently performed by this means by experienced surgeons.

Indications

The benefits of embarking on such procedures through a laparoscopic approach are several. Decreased postoperative pain, shorter duration of postoperative ileus, faster resumption of solid food, lower surgical site infection rates, reduced incisional hernia rates, fewer intra-abdominal adhesions, and improved cosmetic appearance are some of the advantages. Surgeons, however, should have a very low threshold for conversion. Such a decision should not be perceived as a failure but rather as good clinical judgment.

Operative Technique

Operated Abdomen

Most surgeons favor a cutdown technique in undertaking reoperative surgery. When dealing with a reoperation, it is advisable to avoid prior scars because the risk of inadvertent injury to intra-abdominal organs is increased. Assuming that the patient has a midline laparotomy, which is the most frequently encountered scenario, the initial trocar should be placed lateral to the rectus muscle sheath in the midpoint between the lower edge of the rib cage and the anterior superior iliac spine, along the anterior axillary line. The surgeon must also be careful not to place the trocar too far laterally because of the risk of injuring the descending colon and because of issues with regard to obtaining a horizon visualization of the operative field. Detailed awareness of the patient's previous abdominal surgeries will assist in determining on which side the first trocar should be placed. For example, if the patient had previously undergone a left colectomy, the first trocar should be inserted in the right abdominal quadrants. The observation is true for surgeries performed on the right side. New optical access trocar systems have been developed. These allow the surgeon to visualize the abdominal wall layers as the trocar enters the peritoneal cavity. These ports were made with the intention of minimizing organ injury while gaining laparoscopic access. There are currently two optical view trocars: one of them uses a blade and the other uses a rotating sharp plastic clear tip. Both are inserted under direct laparoscopic view. Regardless of what type of trocar the surgeon chooses, the insertion technique should involve minimal force with consistent direct visualization.

Burned Abdomen

Patients with extensive burns of the abdominal wall (third- and fourth-degree burns) represent a challenge for laparoscopic access. One must be aware that the omentum may be firmly adherent to the peritoneum of the anterior abdominal wall. One solution is to use a Hasson technique and to carefully introduce the first trocar in the most caudal portion (right or left) because these areas are more likely to be free of adhesions to the greater omentum. The surgeon must then dissect the omentum off the parietal peritoneum in order to provide access for inserting additional trocars.

Small Bowel Distention

As previously discussed, the development of adhesions is the leading cause of bowel obstruction and distention. Bowel obstruction at one time had been a contraindication for performing a laparoscopy. This is because distended bowel provides only limited visualization and increases the risk for inadvertent bowel injuries. Data on laparoscopic management of adhesive small bowel obstruction are limited and vary considerably. For example, in a large multicenter retrospective case series with 308 patients from 35 centers over 8 years, successful laparoscopic management was demonstrated in 54.6% with a conversion rate of 45.4%. There were also more successes in patients who underwent one or two previous laparotomies as opposed to three or greater (56% vs. 37%; $P < .05$).[127] Some authors have determined the following list of clinical parameters for the successful laparoscopic management of adhesive small bowel obstruction: (1) recurrent small bowel obstruction after placement of a nasogastric tube, (2) limited abdominal distention, (3) proximal obstruction, (4) previous surgery in a limited area of the abdomen, (5) previous operative note did not state the presence of dense adhesions, (6) ability to gain safe access to the peritoneal cavity, and (7) obstructed segments not fixed to the retroperitoneum.

Enterotomy

One of the most serious complications in undertaking laparoscopic reoperative surgery is causing a bowel injury. This chapter, however, will not address large bowel or rectal injuries. A life-threatening complication, however, is a missed enterotomy. Although as previously discussed such an adverse event can occur during conventional, open surgery, the risk of a missed enterotomy is greater when one performs laparoscopic surgery. It is critically important to again remind the reader that one of the most common causes of unrecognized small bowel injury is the use of energy-based devices for laparoscopic lysis of adhesions.

A retrospective matched-pair analysis comparing the outcomes of patients with small bowel obstruction treated laparoscopically and conventionally revealed a bowel perforation rate of 27% versus 13.5%, respectively.[230] Other studies have not shown a difference in overall morbidity and mortality between the two approaches.[65] Should an enterotomy occur and be recognized, I believe it is important to differentiate a perforation due to energy-based devices (monopolar, ultrasound, or bipolar) as opposed to mechanical perforations caused by cold scissors or extensive force applied with a grasper. In the latter circumstance, the surgeon can safely proceed to a hand-sewn repair. Whether this should be accomplished laparoscopically or open will depend on the surgeon's expertise and his or her familiarity with laparoscopic suturing and intracorporeal knot-tying. Extracorporeal knot-tying is not recommended, however, because of the risk of tearing the bowel wall. Should the enterotomy be the result of thermal injury, suture repair should *not* be considered. Under the circumstances, resection should be employed. In case of copious spillage of small bowel contents through the enterotomy site, we recommend that one consider applying a laparoscopic bulldog clamp proximal to the enterotomy.

Urinary Tract Injury

Although the rate of ureteral injuries during laparoscopic surgery remains unknown, they continue to occur, often during reoperative pelvic operations. I personally recommend the use of ureteral stents in every reoperative laparoscopic procedure. My preference is the use of lighted stents, which must be removed at the end of the operation because they are not hollow. Ureteral stents do not inevitably protect the ureter from harm but rather assist the surgeon in identifying the injury. This is particularly true when the patient has undergone prior radiation and/or multiple abdominal surgeries, distorting the anatomy. If the surgeon's preference is not to use stents and there is concern for possible injury, identification of the location can be facilitated through the intravenous injection of indigo carmine dye. The presence of blue dye in the abdominal cavity leaves no doubt that the urinary tract has been breached.

It is important to recognize and repair ureteral injuries immediately. The surgeon must differentiate between a partial and a complete transection. Although repair of a complete transection of the ureter can be accomplished laparoscopically, this should involve the expertise of a urologist and should not be attempted by the surgeon unless he or she feels experienced and confident.[84] Partial transections of the ureter can be repaired laparoscopically with interrupted 5–0 absorbable braided sutures. Stents are necessary to prevent a stricture, and placement of an intra-abdominal drain to avoid urinoma is advisable.

Bladder injuries are also a recognized complication but are generally less worrisome. The repair may be accomplished with 3–0 absorbable braided suture in two layers. The Foley catheter must remain in place until a voiding cystogram is performed that conclusively reveals a healed cystotomy site.

References

1. Agachan F, Joo JS, Sher M, et al. Laparoscopic colorectal surgery. Do we get faster? *Surg Endosc*. 1997;11(4):331–335.
2. Agarwal M. Nomenclature of abbreviated acronyms (Naa . . .)—caveamus surgeons. *Surg Endosc*. 2010;24(3):724–725.
3. Ahmed Ali U, Keus F, Heikens JT, et al. Open versus laparoscopic (assisted) ileo pouch anal anastomosis for ulcerative colitis and familial adenomatous polyposis. *Cochrane Database Syst Rev*. 2009;(1):CD006267.
4. Alamili M, Gögenur I, Rosenberg J. Acute complicated diverticulitis managed by laparoscopic lavage. *Dis Colon Rectum*. 2009;52(7):1345–1349.
5. Alexander RJ, Jaques BC, Mitchell KG. Laparoscopically assisted colectomy and wound recurrence. *Lancet*. 1993;341(8839):249–250.
6. Ambrosetti P, Chautems R, Soravia C, et al. Long-term outcome of mesocolic and pelvic diverticular abscesses of the left colon: a prospective study of 73 cases. *Dis Colon Rectum*. 2005;48(4):787–791.
7. American College of Surgeons. Statement on issues to be considered before new surgical technology is applied to the care of patients. Committee

on Emerging Surgical Technology and Education. *Bull Am Coll Surg.* 1995;80(9):46–47.

8. Arregui ME. Editorial comment to "Two-stage laparoscopic management of generalized peritonitis due to perforated sigmoid diverticula: eighteen cases." *Surg Laparosc Endosc Percutan Tech.* 2000;10(3): 139–141.

9. Asbun HJ, Pempinello C, Halasz NA. Small bowel obstruction and its management. *Int Surg.* 1989;74(1):23–27.

10. Atallah S, Albert M, Larach S. Transanal minimally invasive surgery: a giant leap forward. *Surg Endosc.* 2010;24(9):2200–2205.

11. Aydin HN, Remzi FH, Tekkis PP, et al. Hartmann's reversal is associated with high postoperative adverse events. *Dis Colon Rectum.* 2005;48(11):2117–2126.

12. Aziz O, Constantinides V, Tekkis PP, et al. Laparoscopic versus open surgery for rectal cancer: a meta-analysis. *Ann Surg Oncol.* 2006;13(3): 413–424.

13. Baik SH, Kwon HY, Kim JS, et al. Robotic versus laparoscopic low anterior resection of rectal cancer: short-term outcome of a prospective comparative study. *Ann Surg Oncol.* 2009;16(6):1480–1487.

14. Bastug DF, Trammell SW, Boland JP, et al. Laparoscopic adhesiolysis for small bowel obstruction. *Surg Laparosc Endosc.* 1991;1(4):259–262.

15. Basu A, Wexner SD, Bergamaschi R. Validity of current experimental evidence on laparoscopic surgery for colorectal cancer. *Surg Endosc.* 2003;17(2):179.

16. Bennett CL, Stryker SJ, Ferreira MR, et al. The learning curve for laparoscopic colorectal surgery. Preliminary results from a prospective analysis of 1194 laparoscopic-assisted colectomies. *Arch Surg.* 1997;132(1):41–44.

17. Bergamaschi R. Nonrestoration of pneumoperitoneum in laparoscopic-assisted left colon resection. *Am J Surg.* 2000;180(3):174–175.

18. Bergamaschi R. Farewell to see one, do one, teach one? *Surg Endosc.* 2001;15(7):637.

19. Bergamaschi R. What role, if any, for laparoscopic surgery in Crohn disease of the hindgut? *Scand J Gastroenterol.* 2001;36(7):673–676.

20. Bergamaschi R, Arnaud JP. Intracorporeal colorectal anastomosis following laparoscopic left colon resection. *Surg Endosc.* 1997;11(8): 800–801.

21. Bergamaschi R, Dicko A. Instruction versus passive observation: a randomized educational research study on laparoscopic suture skills. *Surg Laparosc Endosc Percutan Tech.* 2000;10(5):319–322.

22. Bergamaschi R, Essani R. Laparoscopic resection for rectal cancer: are we there yet? *Colorectal Dis.* 2008;11(1):1–2.

23. Bergamaschi R, Haughn C, Reed JF III, et al. Laparoscopic intracorporeal ileocolic resection for Crohn's disease: is it safe? *Dis Colon Rectum.* 2009;52(4):651–656.

24. Bergamaschi R, Lovvik K, Marvik R. Preserving the superior rectal artery in laparoscopic sigmoid resection for complete rectal prolapse. *Surg Laparosc Endosc Percutan Tech.* 2003;13(6):374–376.

25. Bergamaschi R, Myrvold HE. Laparoscopic surgery for cure of colorectal cancer. *Surg Endosc.* 1997;11(8):797–799.

26. Bergamaschi R, Pessaux P, Arnaud JP. Comparison of conventional and laparoscopic ileocolic resection for Crohn's disease. *Dis Colon Rectum.* 2003;46(8):1129–1133.

27. Bergamaschi R, Schochet E, Haughn C, et al. Standardized laparoscopic intracorporeal right colectomy for cancer: short-term outcome in 111 unselected patients. *Dis Colon Rectum.* 2008;51(9):1350–1355.

28. Bergamaschi R, Tuech JJ, Cervi C, et al. Re-establish pneumoperitoneum in laparoscopic-assisted sigmoid resection? Randomized trial. *Dis Colon Rectum.* 2000;43(6):771–774.

29. Bergamaschi R, Tuech JJ, Pessaux P, et al. Intracorporeal vs laparoscopic-assisted resection for uncomplicated diverticulitis of the sigmoid. *Surg Endosc.* 2000;14(6):520–523.

30. Bergamaschi R, Yavuz Y, Marvik R. Laparoscopic bowel resection: a comparison of three ultrasound activated devices. *JSLS.* 2003;7 (1):19–22.

31. Berguer R, Gerber S, Kilpatrick G, et al. An ergonomic comparison of in-line vs pistol-grip handle configuration in a laparoscopic grasper. *Surg Endosc.* 1998;12(6):805–808.

32. Bhoyrul S, Vierra MA, Nezhat CR, et al. Trocar injuries in laparoscopic surgery. *J Am Coll Surg.* 2001;192(6):677–683.

33. Bleday R, Babineau T, Forse RA. Laparoscopic surgery for colon and rectal cancer. *Semin Surg Oncol.* 1993;9(1):59–64.

34. Böhm B, Milsom JW, Kitago K, et al. Use of laparoscopic techniques in oncologic right colectomy in a canine model. *Ann Surg Oncol.* 1995;2(1):6–13.

35. Brannigan AE, De Buck S, Suetens P, et al. Intracorporeal rectal stapling following laparoscopic total mesorectal excision: overcoming a challenge. *Surg Endosc.* 2006;20(6):952–955.

36. Bretagnol F, Dedieu A, Zappa M, et al. T4 colorectal cancer: is laparoscopic resection contraindicated? *Colorectal Dis.* 2011;13(2): 138–143.

37. Breukink S, Pierie J, Wiggers T. Laparoscopic versus open total mesorectal excision for rectal cancer. *Cochrane Database Syst Rev.* 2006;(4):CD005200. doi:10.1002/14651858.CD005200.pub2.

38. Buess G, Theiss R, Günther M, et al. Transanal endoscopic microsurgery [in German]. *Leber Magen Darm.* 1985;15(6):271–279.

39. Butler CE, Gündeslioglu AO, Rodriguez-Bigas MA. Outcomes of immediate vertical rectus abdominis myocutaneous flap reconstruction for irradiated abdominoperineal resection defects. *J Am Coll Surg.* 2008;206(4):694–703.

40. Cesanek P, Uchal M, Uranues S, et al. Do hybrid simulator-generated metrics correlate with content-valid outcome measures? *Surg Endosc.* 2008;22(10):2178–2183.

41. Chang YJ, Marcello PW, Rusin LC, et al. Hand-assisted laparoscopic sigmoid colectomy: helping hand or hindrance? *Surg Endosc.* 2005;19(5):656–661.

42. Chapman J, Davies M, Wolff B, et al. Complicated diverticulitis: is it time to rethink the rules? *Ann Surg.* 2005;242(4):576–581.

43. Chen W, Sailhamer E, Berger DL, et al. Operative time is a poor surrogate for the learning curve in laparoscopic colorectal surgery. *Surg Endosc.* 2007;21(2):238–243.

44. Chopra R, McVay C, Phillips E, et al. Laparoscopic lysis of adhesions. *Am Surg.* 2003;69(11):966–968.

45. Chosidow D, Johanet H, Montariol T, et al. Laparoscopy for acute small-bowel obstruction secondary to adhesions. *J Laparoendosc Adv Surg Tech A.* 2000;10(3):155–159.

46. Chouillard E, Maggiori L, Ata T, et al. Laparoscopic two-stage left colonic resection for patients with peritonitis caused by acute diverticulitis. *Dis Colon Rectum.* 2007;50(8):1157–1163.

47. Christoforidis D, Cho HM, Dixon MR, et al. Transanal endoscopic microsurgery versus conventional transanal excision for patients with early rectal cancer. *Ann Surg.* 2009;249(5):776–782.

48. Church JM, Raudkivi PJ, Hill GL. The surgical anatomy of the rectum—a review with particular relevance to the hazards of rectal mobilisation. *Int J Colorectal Dis.* 1987;2(3):158–166.

49. Cohen SM, Clem MF, Wexner SD, et al. An initial comparative study of two techniques of laparoscopic colonic anastomosis and mesenteric defect closure. *Surg Endosc.* 1994;8(2):130–134.

50. Constantinides VA, Heriot A, Remzi F, et al. Operative strategies for diverticular peritonitis: a decision analysis between primary resection and anastomosis versus Hartmann's procedures. *Ann Surg.* 2007;245(1):94–103.

51. Constantinides VA, Tekkis PP, Senapati A; Association of Coloproctology of Great Britain Ireland. Prospective multicentre evaluation of adverse outcomes following treatment for complicated diverticular disease. *Br J Surg.* 2006;93(12):1503–1513.

52. Cotin S, Stylopoulos N, Ottensmeyer M, et al. Metrics for laparoscopic skills trainers: the weakest link! *Lect Notes Comptu Sci.* 2002;2478:35–43.

53. Cutait D. Sacro-promontory fixation of the rectum for complete prolapse. *J R Soc Med.* 1959;52(suppl):105.

54. Darzi A, Datta V, Mackay S. The challenge of objective assessment of surgical skill. *Am J Surg.* 2001;181(6):484–486.

55. Darzi A, Super P, Guillou PJ, et al. Laparoscopic sigmoid colectomy: total laparoscopic approach. *Dis Colon Rectum.* 1994;37(3):268–271.

56. den Dulk M, Marijnen CA, Putter H, et al. Risk factors for adverse outcome in patients with rectal cancer treated with an abdominoperineal resection in the total mesorectal excision trial. *Ann Surg.* 2007;246 (1):83–90.

57. DeSouza A, Domajnko B, Park J, et al. Incisional hernia, midline versus low transverse incision: what is the ideal incision for specimen extraction and hand-assisted laparoscopy? *Surg Endosc.* 2011;25(4):1031–1036.

58. Dharmarajan S, Hunt SR, Birnbaum EH, et al. The efficacy of nonoperative management of acute complicated diverticulitis. *Dis Colon Rectum.* 2011;54(6):663–671.

59. DiGiuro G, Ignjatovic D, Brogger J, et al; Rectal Prolapse Recurrence Study Group. How accurate are published recurrence rates after rectal prolapse surgery? A meta-analysis of individual patient data. *Am J Surg.* 2006;191(6):773–778.

60. Dinçler S, Koller MT, Steurer J, et al. Multidimensional analysis of learning curves in laparoscopic sigmoid resection: eight-year results. *Dis Colon Rectum.* 2003;46(10):1371–1378.

61. Doornebosch PG, Tollenaar RA, Gosselink MP, et al. Quality of life after transanal endoscopic microsurgery and total mesorectal excision in early rectal cancer. *Colorectal Dis.* 2007;9(6):553–558.

62. Duepree HJ, Senagore AJ, Delany CP, et al. Does means of access affect the incidence of small bowel obstruction and ventral hernia after

bowel resection? Laparoscopy versus laparotomy. *J Am Coll Surg.* 2003;197(2):177–181.

63. Duh QY. Small bowel obstruction. In: Toouli J, Gossot D, Hunter JG, eds. *Endosurgery.* New York, NY: Churchill Livingstone; 1998:425–431.

64. Dunker MS, Stiggelbout AM, van Hogezand RA, et al. Cosmesis and body image after laparoscopic-assisted and open ileocolic resection for Crohn's disease. *Surg Endosc.* 1998;12(11):1334–1340.

65. Duron JJ, du Montcel ST, Berger A, et al. Prevalence and risk factors of mortality and morbidity after operation for adhesive postoperative small bowel obstruction. *Am J Surg.* 2008;195(6):726–734.

66. Duthie GS, Bartolo DC. Abdominal rectopexy for rectal prolapse: a comparison of techniques. *Br J Surg.* 1992;79(2):107–113.

67. Egger B, Peter MK, Candinas D. Persistent symptoms after elective sigmoid resection for diverticulitis. *Dis Colon Rectum.* 2008;51(7): 1044–1048.

68. Ellis H. The clinical significance of adhesions: focus on intestinal obstruction. *Eur J Surg.* 1997;163:5–9.

69. Emam TA, Frank TG, Hanna GB, et al. Influence of handle design on the surgeon's upper limb movements, muscle recruitment, and fatigue during endoscopic suturing. *Surg Endosc.* 2001;15(7):667–672.

70. Essani R, Scriven RJ, McLarty AJ, et al. Simulated laparoscopic sigmoidectomy training: responsiveness of surgery residents. *Dis Colon Rectum.* 2009;52(12):1956–1961.

71. Etzioni CP. Discharge data—some words of caution. *Dis Colon Rectum.* 2011;54(7):769–770.

72. Fevang BT, Fevang J, Lie SA, et al. Long-term prognosis after operation for adhesive small bowel obstruction. *Ann Surg.* 2004;240(2):193–201.

73. Fleshman JW, Wexner SD, Anvari M, et al. Laparoscopic vs. open abdominoperineal resection for cancer. *Dis Colon Rectum.* 1999;42(7): 930–939.

74. Foster NM, McGory ML, Zingmond DS, et al. Small bowel obstruction: a population-based appraisal. *J Am Coll Surg.* 2006;203(2):170–176.

75. Fowler DL, White SA. Laparoscopic-assisted sigmoid resection. *Surg Laparosc Endosc.* 1991;1(3):183–188.

76. Fozard JB, Armitage NC, Schofield JB, et al; Association of Coloproctology of Great Britain and Ireland. ACPGBI position statement on elective resection for diverticulitis. *Colorectal Dis.* 2011;13(suppl 3):1–11. doi:10.1111/j.1463-1318.2010.02531.x.

77. Fusco MA, Paluzzi MW. Abdominal wall recurrence after laparoscopic-assisted colectomy for adenocarcinoma of the colon. *Dis Colon Rectum.* 1993;36(9):858–861.

78. Gallagher A, Satava RM, Seymour NE, et al. An ergonomic analysis of the effects of camera rotation on laparoscopic performance [published online ahead of print December 06, 2008]. *Surg Endosc.*

79. Gao F, Cao YF, Chen LS. Meta-analysis of short-term outcomes after laparoscopic resection for rectal cancer. *Int J Colorectal Dis.* 2006;21(7):652–656.

80. Gastinger I, Kockerling F, Schneider B, et al. Zum Problem der Praparatebergung im Rahmen del laparoskopischen kolorektalen Chirurgie. *Minimal Invasive Chirurgie.* 1992;1:73–75.

81. Ghosheh B, Salameh JR. Laparoscopic approach to acute small bowel obstruction: review of 1061 cases. *Surg Endosc.* 2007;21(11):1945–1949.

82. Gibson CL. A study of 1000 operations for acute intestinal obstructions 1888–1898. *Ann Surg.* 1900;32:486–490.

83. Gill IS, Advincula AP, Aron M, et al. Consensus statement of the consortium for laparoendoscopic single-site surgery. *Surg Endosc.* 2010;24(4):762–768.

84. Gözen AS, Cresswell J, Canada AE, et al. Laparoscopic ureteral reimplantation: prospective evaluation of medium-term results and current developments. *World J Urol.* 2010;28(2):221–226.

85. Grabham JA, Moran BJ, Lane RH. Defunctioning colostomy for low anterior resection: a selective approach. *Br J Surg.* 1995;82(10):1331–1332.

86. Graf W, Stefánsson T, Arvidsson D, et al. Laparoscopic suture rectopexy. *Dis Colon Rectum.* 1995;38(2):211–212.

87. Guerrieri M, Baldarelli M, de Sanctis A, et al. Treatment of rectal adenomas by transanal endoscopic microsurgery: 15 years' experience. *Surg Endosc.* 2010;24(2):445–449.

88. Guillou PJ, Quirke P, Thorpe H, et al; MRC CLASICC trial group. Short-term endpoints of conventional versus laparoscopic-assisted surgery in patients with colorectal cancer (MRC CLASICC trial): multicentre, randomised controlled trial. *Lancet.* 2005;365(9472):1718–1726.

89. Gutt CN, Oniu T, Schemmer P, et al. Fewer adhesions induced by laparoscopic surgery? *Surg Endosc.* 2004;18(6):898–906.

90. Halsted WS. The training of the surgeon. *Bull Johns Hopkins Hosp.* 1904;15:267–276.

91. Hartmann H. Nouveau procédé d'ablation des cancers de la partie terminate du colon pelvien [New procedure for the removal of cancers of the terminal part of the pelvic colon]. Strasbourg, France: Trentieme Congress de Chirurgie; 1932:411–413.

92. Hasegawa S, Nagayama S, Nomura A, et al. Multimedia article. Autonomic nerve-preserving total mesorectal excision in the laparoscopic era. *Dis Colon Rectum.* 2008;51(8):1279–1282.

93. Hasson HM. A modified instrument and method for laparoscopy. *Am J Obstet Gynecol.* 1971;110:886–887.

94. Haughn C, Ju B, Uchal M, et al. Complication rates following Hartmann's reversal: open vs. laparoscopic approach. *Dis Colon Rectum.* 2008;51(8):1232–1236.

95. Hays RD, Hadorn D. Responsiveness to change: an aspect of validity, not a separate dimension. *Qual Life Res.* 1992;1(1):73–75.

96. Heah SM, Hartley JE, Hurley J, et al. Laparoscopic suture rectopexy without resection is effective treatment for full-thickness rectal prolapse. *Dis Colon Rectum.* 2000;43(5):638–643.

97. Hunter JG. Laparoscopic pneumoperitoneum: the abdominal compartment syndrome revisited. *J Am Coll Surg.* 1995;181(5):469–470.

98. Ignjatovic D, Bergamaschi R. Rectal cancer: from outcomes of care to process of care. *Scand J Gastroenterol.* 2006;41(6):636–639.

99. Ignjatovic D, Stimec B, Finjord T, et al. Venous anatomy of the right colon: three-dimensional topographic mapping of the gastrocolic trunk of Henle. *Tech Coloproctol.* 2004;8(1):19–21; discussion 21–22.

100. Ito M, Sugito M, Kobayashi A, et al. Relationship between multiple numbers of stapler firings during rectal division and anastomotic leakage after laparoscopic rectal resection. *Int J Colorectal Dis.* 2008;23(7): 703–707.

101. Jacobs M, Verdeja JC, Goldstein HS. Minimally invasive colon resection (laparoscopic colectomy). *Surg Laparosc Endosc.* 1991;1(3): 144–150.

102. Jaspers JE, Breedveld P, Herder JL, et al. Camera and instrument holders and their clinical value in minimally invasive surgery. *Surg Laparosc Endosc Percutan Tech.* 2004;14(3):145–152.

103. Jayne DG, Guillou PJ, Thorpe H, et al. Randomized trial of laparoscopic-assisted resection of colorectal carcinoma: 3-year results of the UK MRC CLASICC Trial Group. *J Clin Oncol.* 2007;25(21):3061–3068.

104. Jordan JA, Gallagher AG, McGuigan J, et al. A comparison between randomly alternating imaging, normal laparoscopic imaging, and virtual reality training in laparoscopic psychomotor skill acquisition. *Am J Surg.* 2000;180(3):208–211.

105. Karanjia ND, Corder AP, Bearn P, et al. Leakage from stapled low anastomosis after total mesorectal excision for carcinoma of the rectum. *Br J Surg.* 1994;81(8):1224–1226.

106. Karanjia ND, Corder AP, Holdsworth PJ, et al. Risk of peritonitis and fatal septicemia and the need to defunction the low anastomosis. *Br J Surg.* 1991;78(2):196–198.

107. Karas JR, Uranues S, Altomare DF, et al. No rectopexy versus rectopexy following rectal mobilization for full-thickness rectal prolapse: a randomized controlled trial. *Dis Colon Rectum.* 2011;54(1):29–34.

108. Kaufman HH, Wiegand RL, Tunick RH. Teaching surgeons to operate—principles of psychomotor skills training. *Acta Neurochir (Wien).* 1987;87(1–2):1–7.

109. Keck JO, Collopy BT, Ryan PJ, et al. Reversal of Hartmann's procedure: effect of timing and technique on ease and safety. *Dis Colon Rectum.* 1994;37(3):243–248.

110. Kennedy JS, Stranahan PL, Taylor KD, et al. High-burst-strength, feedback-controlled bipolar vessel sealing. *Surg Endosc.* 1998;12(6): 876–878.

111. Khaikin M, Zmora O, Rosin D, et al. Laparoscopically assisted reversal of Hartmann's procedure. *Surg Endosc.* 2006;20(12):1883–1886.

112. Khanna AK, Misra MK, Kumar K. Simplified sutured sacral rectopexy for complete rectal prolapse in adults. *Eur J Surg.* 1996;162(2): 143–146.

113. Khoo RE, Montrey J, Cohen MM. Laparoscopic loop ileostomy for temporary fecal diversion. *Dis Colon Rectum.* 1993;36(10):966–968.

114. Kim HJ, Lee IK, Lee YS, et al. A comparative study on the short-term clinicopathologic outcomes of laparoscopic surgery versus conventional open surgery for transverse colon cancer. *Surg Endosc.* 2009;23(8): 1812–1817.

115. Klarenbeek BR, Veenhof AA, Bergamaschi R, et al. Laparoscopic sigmoid resection for diverticulitis decreases major morbidity rates: a randomized control trial: short-term results of the Sigma Trial. *Ann Surg.* 2009;249(1):39–44.

116. Kockerling F, Schneider I, Gastinger I, et al. Laparoskopische Tabaksbeutelnahtklemme fur die minimal invasive kolorektale Chirurgie. *Minimal Invasive Chirurgie.* 1993;2:68–75.

117. Köhler L, Sauerland S, Neugebauer E. Diagnosis and treatment of diverticular disease: results of a consensus development conference. The

Scientific Committee of the European Association for Endoscopic Surgery. *Surg Endosc*. 1999;13(4):430–436.

118. Kondraske GV, Hamilton EC, Scott DJ, et al. Surgeon workload and motion efficiency with robot and human laparoscopic camera control. *Surg Endosc*. 2002;16(11):1523–1527.

119. Kössi J, Salminen P, Rantala A, et al. Population-based study of the surgical workload and economic impact of bowel obstruction caused by postoperative adhesions. *Br J Surg*. 2003;90(11):1441–1444.

120. Kraft BM, Jager C, Kraft K, et al. The AESOP robot system in laparoscopic surgery: increased risk or advantage for surgeon and patient? *Surg Endosc*. 2004;18(8):1216–1223.

121. Kuroyanagi H, Oya M, Ueno M, et al. Standardized technique of laparoscopic intracorporeal rectal transection and anastomosis for low anterior resection. *Surg Endosc*. 2008;22(2):557–561.

122. Kuwabara K, Matsuda S, Fushimi H, et al. Quantitative comparison of the difficulty of performing laparoscopic colectomy at different tumor locations. *World J Surg*. 2010;34(1):133–139.

123. Landercasper J, Cogbill TH, Merry WH, et al. Long-term outcome after hospitalization for small-bowel obstruction. *Arch Surg*. 1993;128(7):765–770.

124. Lange V, Meyer G, Schardey HM, et al. Laparoscopic creation of a loop colostomy. *J Laparoendosc Surg*. 1991;1(5):307–312.

125. Leung KL, Kwok SP, Lam SC. Laparoscopic resection of rectosigmoid carcinoma: prospective randomised trial. *Lancet*. 2004;363(9416):1187–1192.

126. Leung KL, Lai PD, Ho RL, et al. Systemic cytokine response after laparoscopic-assisted resection of rectosigmoid carcinoma: a prospective randomized trial. *Ann Surg*. 2000;231(4):506–511.

127. Levard H, Boudet MJ, Msika S, et al. Laparoscopic treatment of acute small bowel obstruction: a multicentre retrospective study. *ANZ J Surg*. 2001;71(11):641–646.

128. Lin GL, Meng WC, Lau PY, et al. Local resection for early rectal tumours: comparative study of transanal endoscopic microsurgery (TEM) versus posterior trans-sphincteric approach (Mason's operation). *Asian J Surg*. 2006;29(4):227–232.

129. Lindsey I, Guy RJ, Warren BF, et al. Anatomy of Denonvilliers' fascia and pelvic nerves, impotence, and implications for the colorectal surgeon. *Br J Surg*. 2000;87(10):1288–1299.

130. Litwin DE, Darzi A, Jakimowicz J, et al. Hand-assisted laparoscopic surgery (HALS) with the HandPort system: initial experience with 68 patients. *Ann Surg*. 2000;231(5):715–723.

131. Madoff RD, Mellgren A. One hundred years of rectal prolapse surgery. *Dis Colon Rectum*. 1999;42(4):441–450.

132. Maggard MA, Zingmond D, O'Connell JB, et al. What proportion of patients with an ostomy (for diverticulitis) get reversed? *Am Surg*. 2004;70(10):928–931.

133. Mak SY, Roach SC, Sukumar SA. Small bowel obstruction: computed tomography features and pitfalls. *Curr Probl Diagn Radiol*. 2006;35(2):65–74.

134. Marcello PW. Single incision laparoscopic colectomy: boutique surgery or the new standard? *Dis Colon Rectum*. 2011;54(6):660–661.

135. Maslekar S, Pillinger SH, Sharma A, et al. Cost analysis of transanal endoscopic microsurgery for rectal tumours. *Colorectal Dis*. 2007;9(3):229–234.

136. Masoomi H, Buchberg BS, Magno C, et al. Trends in diverticulitis management in the United States from 2002 to 2007 [published online ahead of print December 20, 2010]. *Arch Surg*. doi:10.1001/archsurg.2010.276.

137. Matern U, Waller P. Instruments for minimally invasive surgery: principles of ergonomic handles. *Surg Endosc*. 1999;13(2):174–182.

138. Mayo WJ, Wilson LB, Giffin HZ. Acquired diverticulitis of the large intestine. *Surg Gynecol Obstet*. 1907;5:8.

139. McCloud JM, Waymont N, Pahwa N, et al. Factors predicting early recurrence after transanal endoscopic microsurgery excision for rectal adenoma. *Colorectal Dis*. 2006;8(7):581–585.

140. McDonnell Norms Group. Enhancing the use of clinical guidelines: a social norms perspective. *J Am Coll Surg*. 2006;202(5):826–836.

141. Meakins JL. Innovation in surgery: the rules of evidence. *Am J Surg*. 2002;183(4):399–405.

142. Mentges B, Buess G, Schäfer D, et al. Transanal endoscopic microsurgery and combined operations. In: Moreno-González E, Escartín P, Lygidakis NJ, eds. *Joint Meeting of Surgery, Gastroenterology and Endoscopy*. Madrid, Spain: Jarpyo; 1995:339–345.

143. Menzies D, Ellis H. Intestinal obstruction from adhesions—how big is the problem? *Ann R Coll Surg Engl*. 1990;72(1):60–63.

144. Merola S, Weber P, Wasielewski A, et al. Comparison of laparoscopic colectomy with and without the aid of a robotic camera holder. *Surg Laparosc Endosc Percutan Tech*. 2004;12(1):46–51.

145. Meshikhes AW. Controversy of hand-assisted laparoscopic colorectal surgery. *World J Gastroenterol*. 2010;16(45):5662–5668.

146. Millat B. Feasibility hazards. *Surg Endosc*. 2002;16(11):1511–1512.

147. Miller G, Boman J, Shrier I, et al. Etiology of small bowel obstruction. *Am J Surg*. 2000;180(1):33–36.

148. Miller G, Boman J, Shrier I, et al. Natural history of patients with adhesive small bowel obstruction. *Br J Surg*. 2000;87(9):1240–1247.

149. Moher D, Schulz KF, Altman DG; CONSORT Group. The CONSORT statement: revised recommendations for improving the quality of reports of parallel-group randomized trials. *Ann Intern Med*. 2001;134(8):657–662.

150. Monson JRT. Invited editorial. *Dis Colon Rectum*. 2000;43:271–272.

151. Moore JS, Cataldo PA, Osler T, et al. Transanal endoscopic microsurgery is more effective than traditional transanal excision for resection of rectal masses. *Dis Colon Rectum*. 2008;51(7):1026–1031.

152. Nakajima K, Lee SW, Sonoda T, et al. Intraoperative carbon dioxide colonoscopy: a safe insufflation alternative for locating colonic lesions during laparoscopic surgery. *Surg Endosc*. 2005;19(3):321–325.

153. Neary P, Makin GB, White TJ, et al. Transanal endoscopic microsurgery: a viable operative alternative in selected patients with rectal lesions. *Ann Surg Oncol*. 2003;10(9):1106–1111.

154. Nelson H, Sargent D, Wieand HS, et al; Clinical Outcomes of Surgical Therapy Study Group. A comparison of laparoscopically assisted and open colectomy for colon cancer. *N Engl J Med*. 2004;350(20):2050–2059.

155. Nelson R, Spitz J, Pearl RK, et al. What role does full rectal mobilization alone play in the treatment of rectal prolapse? *Tech Coloproctol*. 2001;5(1):33–35.

156. Nelson RS, Ewing BM, Wengert TJ, et al. Clinical outcomes of complicated diverticulitis managed nonoperatively. *Am J Surg*. 2008;196(6):969–972; discussion 973–974.

157. Neudecker J, Saucrland S, Neugebauer E, et al. The European Association for Endoscopic Surgery clinical practice guidelines on the pneumoperitoneum for laparoscopic surgery. *Surg Endosc*. 2002;16(7):1121–1143.

158. Nissan A, Guillem JG, Paty PB, et al. Abdominoperineal resection for rectal cancer at a specialty center. *Dis Colon Rectum*. 2001;44(1):27–35.

159. Okolica D, Bishawi M, Karas JR, et al. Factors influencing postoperative adverse events after Hartmann's reversal. *Colorectal Dis*. 2012;14(3):369–373. doi:10.1111/j.1463-1318.2011.02629.x.

160. O'Rourke N, Price PM, Kelly S, et al. Tumor inoculation during laparoscopy. *Lancet*. 1993;342(8867):368.

161. Papagrigoriadis S. Transanal endoscopic micro-surgery (TEMS) for the management of large or sessile rectal adenomas: a review of the technique and indications. *Int Semin Surg Oncol*. 2006;3:13.

162. Park JS, Choi GS, Kim HJ, et al. Natural orifice specimen extraction versus conventional laparoscopically assisted right hemicolectomy. *Br J Surg*. 2011;98(5):710–715. doi:10.1002/bjs.7419.

163. Parks TG. Natural history of diverticular disease of the colon. A review of 521 cases. *Br Med J*. 1969;4(5684):639–645.

164. Pearce NW, Scott SD, Karran SJ. Timing and method of reversal of Hartmann's procedure. *Br J Surg*. 1992;79(8):839–841.

165. Pezet D, Fondrinier E, Rotman N, et al. Parietal seeding of carcinoma of the gallbladder after laparoscopic cholecystectomy. *Br J Surg*. 1992;79(3):230.

166. Phillips EH, Franklin M, Carroll BJ, et al. Laparoscopic colectomy. *Ann Surg*. 1992;216(6):703–707.

167. Pigazzi A, Luca F, Patriti A, et al. Multicentric study on robotic tumor-specific mesorectal excision for the treatment of rectal cancer. *Ann Surg Oncol*. 2010;17(6):1614–1620.

168. Proske JM, Dagher I, Franco D. Comparative study of human and robotic camera control in laparoscopic biliary and colon surgery. *J Laparoendosc Adv Surg Tech A*. 2004;14(6):345–348.

169. Quah HM, Jayne DG, Eu KW, et al. Bladder and sexual dysfunction following laparoscopically assisted and conventional open mesorectal resection for cancer. *Br J Surg*. 2002;89(12):1551–1556.

170. Radcliffe A. Can the results of anorectal (abdominoperineal) resection be improved: are circumferential resection margins too often positive? *Colorectal Dis*. 2006;8(3):160–167.

171. Rafferty J, Shellito P, Hyman NH, et al; Standards Committee of American Society of Colon and Rectal Surgeons. Practice parameters for sigmoid diverticulitis. *Dis Colon Rectum*. 2006;49(7):939–944.

172. Raftopoulos I, Reed JF III, Bergamaschi R. Circumferential resection margin involvement after laparoscopic abdominoperineal excision for rectal cancer. *Colorectal Dis*. 2012;14(4):431–437.

173. Raftopoulos Y, Senagore AJ, Di Giuro G, et al; Rectal Prolapse Recurrence Study Group. Recurrence rates after abdominal surgery for

complete rectal prolapse: a multicenter pooled analysis of 643 individual patient data. *Dis Colon Rectum*. 2005;48(6):1200–1206.

174. Ramos JM, Gupta S, Anthone GJ, et al. Laparoscopy and colon cancer. Is the port site at risk? A preliminary report. *Arch Surg*. 1994;129(9):897–899.

175. Reichenbach DJ, Tackett AD, Harris J, et al. Laparoscopic colon resection early in the learning curve: what is the appropriate setting? *Ann Surg*. 2006;243(6):730–737.

176. Reissman P, Cohen S, Weiss EG, et al. Laparoscopic colorectal surgery: ascending the learning curve. *World J Surg*. 1996;20(3):277–281.

177. Reitsma AM, Moreno JD. Ethical regulations for innovative surgery: the last frontier? *J Am Coll Surg*. 2002;194(6):792–801.

178. Reznick RK, MacRae H. Teaching surgical skills—changes in the wind. *N Engl J Med*. 2006;355(25):2664–2669.

179. Rhodes RS. Quality in surgery: from outcomes to process—and back again. *Surgery*. 1999;126(1):76–77.

180. Rink AD, John-Enzenauer K, Haaf F, et al. Laparoscopic-assisted or laparoscopic-facilitated sigmoidectomy for diverticular disease? A prospective randomized trial on postoperative pain and analgesic consumption. *Dis Colon Rectum*. 2009;52(10):1738–1745.

181. Ritter FE, Schooler LJ. The learning curve. In: *International Encyclopedia of the Social and Behavioral Sciences*. Amsterdam, The Netherlands: Pergamon; 2002:8602–8605.

182. Roe AM, Prabhu S, Ali A, et al. Reversal of Hartmann's procedure: timing and operative technique. *Br J Surg*. 1991;78(10):1167–1170.

183. Rosen MJ, Cobb WS, Kercher KW, et al. Laparoscopic restoration of intestinal continuity after Hartmann's procedure. *Am J Surg*. 2005;189(6):670–674.

184. Rullier E, Laurent C, Bretagnol F, et al. Sphincter-saving resection for all rectal carcinomas: the end of the 2-cm distal rule. *Ann Surg*. 2005;241(3):465–469.

185. Salem L, Anaya DA, Roberts KE, et al. Hartmann's colectomy and reversal in diverticulitis: a population-level assessment. *Dis Colon Rectum*. 2005;48(5):988–995.

186. Salem L, Flum DR. Primary anastomosis or Hartmann's procedure for patients with diverticular peritonitis? A systematic review. *Dis Colon Rectum*. 2004;47(11):1953–1964.

187. Santaniello M, Bergamaschi R. Perforated diverticulitis: should the method of surgical access to the abdomen determine treatment? *Colorectal Dis*. 2007;9(6):494–495.

188. Sarker SK, Kumar I, Delaney C. Assessing operative performance in advanced laparoscopic colorectal surgery. *World J Surg*. 2010;34(7):1594–1603.

189. Sauerland S, Agresta F, Bergamaschi R, et al. Laparoscopy for abdominal emergencies: evidence-based guidelines of the European Association for Endoscopic Surgery. *Surg Endosc*. 2006;20(1):14–29.

190. Sayfan J, Pinho M, Alexander-Williams J, et al. Sutured posterior abdominal rectopexy with sigmoidectomy compared with Marlex rectopexy for rectal prolapse. *Br J Surg*. 1990;77(2):143–145.

191. Schiessel R, Karner-Hanusch J, Herbst F, et al. Intersphincteric resection for low rectal tumours. *Br J Surg*. 1994;81(9):1376–1378.

192. Schlachta CM, Mamazza J, Poulin EC. Are transverse colon cancers suitable for laparoscopic resection? *Surg Endosc*. 2007;21(3):396–399.

193. Schlinkert RT. Laparoscopic-assisted right hemicolectomy. *Dis Colon Rectum*. 1991;34(11):1030–1031.

194. Schunn CD, Wallach D. Evaluating goodness of fit in comparison of models to data. In: Tack W, ed. *Psychologie der Kognition: Reden und Vortrage anlasslich der Emeritierung von Werner Tack*. Saarbrueken, Germany: University of Saarland Press; 2005:115–154.

195. Schwesinger WH, Page CP, Gaskill HV III, et al. Operative management of diverticular emergencies: strategies and outcomes. *Arch Surg*. 2000;135(5):558–562; discussion 562–563.

196. Senagore AJ, Delaney CP, Brady KM, et al. Standardized approach to laparoscopic right colectomy: outcomes in 70 consecutive cases. *J Am Coll Surg*. 2004;199(5):675–679.

197. Senagore AJ, Duepree HJ, Delaney CP, et al. Results of a standardized technique and postoperative care plan for laparoscopic sigmoid colectomy: a 30-month experience. *Dis Colon Rectum*. 2003;46(4):503–509.

198. Seror D, Feigin E, Szold A, et al. How conservatively can postoperative small bowel obstruction be treated? *Am J Surg*. 1993;165(1):121–125.

199. Shukla PJ, Barreto SG, Hawaldar R, et al. Feasibility of laparoscopic abdomino-perineal resection for large-sized anorectal cancers: a single-institution experience of 59 cases. *Indian J Med Sci*. 2009;63(3):109–114.

200. Siewert B, Tye G, Kruskal J, et al. Impact of CT-guided drainage in the treatment of diverticular abscesses: size matters. *AJR Am J Roentgenol*. 2006;186(3):680–686.

201. Simons AJ, Anthone GJ, Ortega AE, et al. Laparoscopic-assisted colectomy learning curve. *Dis Colon Rectum*. 1995;38(6):600–603.

202. Soumian S, Thomas S, Mohan PP, et al. Management of Hinchey II diverticulitis. *World J Gastroenterol*. 2008;14(47):7163–7169.

203. Strickland P, Lourie DJ, Suddleson EA, et al. Is laparoscopy safe and effective for treatment of acute small-bowel obstruction? *Surg Endosc*. 1999;13(7):695–698.

204. Sturm L, et al. *Surgical Simulation for Training: Skills Transfer to the Operating Room*. Adelaide, South Australia: ASERNIP-S; 2007. ASERNIP-S Report No. 61.

205. Suter M, Zermatten P, Halkic N, et al. Laparoscopic management of mechanical small bowel obstruction: are there predictors of success or failure? *Surg Endosc*. 2000;14(5):478–483.

206. Tekkis PP, Senagore AJ, Delaney CP, et al. Evaluation of the learning curve in laparoscopic colorectal surgery: comparison of right-sided and left-sided resections. *Ann Surg*. 2005;242(1):83–91.

207. Terwee CB, Dekker FW, Wiersinga WM, et al. On assessing responsiveness of health-related quality of life instruments: guidelines for instrument evaluation. *Qual Life Res*. 2003;12(4):349–362.

208. Thaler K, Baig MK, Berho M, et al. Determinants of recurrence after sigmoid resection for uncomplicated diverticulitis. *Dis Colon Rectum*. 2003;46(3):385–388.

209. Tou S, Brown SR, Malik AI, et al. Surgery for complete rectal prolapse in adults. *Cochrane Database Syst Rev*. 2008;(4):CD001758. doi:10.1002/14651858.

210. Touzios JG, Dozois EJ. Diverticulosis and acute diverticulitis. *Gastroenterol Clin North Am*. 2009;38(3):513–525.

211. Uchal M, Brogger J, Rukas R, et al. In-line versus pistol-grip handles in a laparoscopic simulators. A randomized controlled crossover trial. *Surg Endosc*. 2002;16(12):1771–1773.

212. Uchal M, Haughn C, Raftopoulos Y, et al. Robotic camera holder as good as expert camera holder: a randomized crossover trial. *Surg Laparosc Endosc Percutan Tech*. 2009;19(3):272–275.

213. Uchal M, Raftopoulos Y, Tjugum J, et al. Validation of a six-task simulation model in minimally invasive surgery. *Surg Endosc*. 2004;19(1):109–116.

214. van de Wall BJ, Draaisma WA, Schouten ES, et al. Conventional and laparoscopic reversal of the Hartmann procedure: a review of literature. *J Gastrointest Surg*. 2010;14(4):743–752.

215. van der Linden W. Pitfalls in randomized surgical trials. *Surgery*. 1980;87(3):258–262.

216. van Veelen MA, Meijer DW. Ergonomics and design of laparoscopic instruments: results of a survey among laparoscopic surgeons. *J Laparoendosc Adv Surg Tech A*. 1999;9(6):481–489.

217. Veldkamp R, Kuhry E, Hop WC, et al; Colon cancer Laparoscopic or Open Resection Study Group (COLOR). Laparoscopic surgery versus open surgery for colon cancer: short-term outcomes of a randomised trial. *Lancet Oncol*. 2005;6(7):477–484.

218. Vick RM. Statistics of acute intestinal obstruction. *Br Med J*. 1932;2(3741):546–548.

219. Wassmuth HH, Myrvold HE, Bengtsson J, et al. Conversion of a failed pouch to a continent ileostomy: a controversy. *Colorectal Dis*. 2011;13(1):2–5.

220. Way LW, Stewart L, Gantert W, et al. Causes and prevention of laparoscopic bile duct injuries: analysis of 252 cases from a human factors and cognitive psychology perspective. *Ann Surg*. 2003;237(4):460–469.

221. Wexner SD, Johansen OB, Nogueras JJ, et al. Laparoscopic total abdominal colectomy. A prospective trial. *Dis Colon Rectum*. 1992;35(7):651–655.

222. Whitehouse PA, Tilney HS, Armitage JN, et al. Transanal endoscopic microsurgery: risk factors for local recurrence of benign rectal adenomas. *Colorectal Dis*. 2006;8(9):795–799.

223. Wibe A, Møller B, Norstein J, et al; Norwegian Rectal Cancer Group. A national strategic change in treatment policy for rectal cancer—implementation of total mesorectal excision as routine treatment in Norway. A national audit. *Dis Colon Rectum*. 2002;45(7):857–866.

224. Wibe A, Syse A, Andersen E, et al; Norwegian Rectal Cancer Group. Oncological outcomes after total mesorectal excision for cure for cancer of the lower rectum: anterior vs. abdominoperineal resection. *Dis Colon Rectum*. 2004;47(1):48–58.

225. Williams SB, Greenspon J, Young HA, et al. Small bowel obstruction: conservative vs. surgical management. *Dis Colon Rectum*. 2005;48(6):1140–1146.

226. Winde G, Nottberg H, Keller R, Schmid KW, Bunte H. Surgical cure for early rectal carcinomas (T1): Transanal endoscopic microsurgery vs. anterior resection. *Dis Colon Rectum* 1996;39:969-976.

227. Wolff BG, Michelassi F, Gerkin TM, et al; Alvimopan Postoperative Ileus Study Group. Alvimopan, a novel, peripherally acting mu opioid antagonist: results of a multicenter, randomized, double-blind, placebo-controlled, phase III trial of major abdominal surgery and postoperative ileus. *Ann Surg.* 2004;240(4):728–734; discussion 734–735.

228. Wolff GB, Ready RL, MacCarty RL, et al. Influence of sigmoid resection on progression of diverticular disease of the colon. *Dis Colon Rectum.* 1984;27(10):645–647.

229. Wong NY, Eu KW. A defunctioning ileostomy does not prevent clinical anastomotic leak after a low anterior resection: a prospective, comparative study. *Dis Colon Rectum.* 2005;48(11):2076–2079.

230. Wullstein C, Gross E. Laparoscopic compared with conventional treatment of acute adhesive small bowel obstruction. *Br J Surg.* 2003;90(9):1147–1151.

231. Yan J, Trencheva K, Lee SW, et al. Treatment for right colon polyps not removable using standard colonoscopy: combined laparoscopic-colonoscopic approach. *Dis Colon Rectum.* 2011;54(6):753–758.

232. Young-Fadok TM, Nelson H. Laparoscopic right colectomy. *Dis Colon Rectum.* 2000;43:267–273.

233. Zbar RI, Crede WB, McKhann CF, et al. The postoperative incidence of small bowel obstruction following standard, open appendectomy and cholecystectomy: a six-year retrospective cohort study at Yale-New Haven Hospital. *Conn Med.* 1993;57(3):123–127.

234. Zerey M, Sechrist CW, Kercher KW, et al. The laparoscopic management of small-bowel obstruction. *Am J Surg.* 2007;194(6):882–888.

235. Zorcolo L, Covotta L, Carlomagno N, et al. Safety of primary anastomosis in emergency colo-rectal surgery. *Colorectal Dis.* 2003;5:262–269.

20

Constipation, Disorders of Defecation, and Anal Pain

R. John Nicholls and Ian Lindsey

*I hav finally kum to the konklusion, that a good
reliable sett ov bowels iz wurth more tu a man,
than enny quantity of brains.*

—HENRY WHEELER SHAW (JOSH BILLINGS): *His Sayings*

*A man should always endeavor to keep his bowels lax;
they may even approach a diarrheal state. For this is
a leading rule in hygiene, as long as the bowels are
constipated or when they act with difficulty, serious
disease ensues.*

—SCHULCHAN ARUCH: *Code of Jewish Law*

► CONSTIPATION AND DISORDERS OF DEFECATION

Introduction

Patients who present with constipation may have a mechanical reason for it or the condition may be functional. In the latter case, the defect may be due to a slow transit issue or to difficulty in evacuation of the rectum. Frequently, both factors are present in the same individual. Constipation is a common reason for patients to visit their physician; the causes are myriad (Table 20-1).

Delayed transit can be present in bowel of normal caliber or with gross dilatation. In the latter circumstance, this is in the form of an aganglionic or idiopathic megabowel (usually chronic), or it may be acute as in pseudoobstruction (Ogilvie's syndrome—see later).[255] Normal caliber constipation occurs in patients who consume insufficient dietary fiber. The condition may also be caused by other factors, such as age, institutionalization, immobility, drugs, metabolic disorders

(hypothyroidism, hypercalcemia), depression, and neurologic disease.

Evacuation difficulty or obstructed defecation can be broken down into mechanical (anatomical) and functional (pathophysiologic) causes, although overlap is common, and occasionally multiple factors are involved. In the past 10 years, there has been a move away from surgery for those with functional constipation due to delayed transit, with a greater number of patients receiving behavioral treatments such as biofeedback and neuromodulation.

Epidemiology

In the United States alone, the cost of over-the-counter laxatives for 1991 was in excess of $400 million. Today, the outpatient medical care of American women who suffer with constipation is twice as costly as for those who do not.[56] The prevalence in the general community of the irritable bowel syndrome (IBS) and so-called functional constipation has been reported to be between 20% and 30% in each case.[146] Sandler and colleagues investigated the association between self-reported constipation and several demographic and dietary variables in 15,014 men and women 12 to 74 years of age who were examined between 1971 and 1975 at the time of the first National Health and Nutrition Examination Survey.[294] Overall, 12.8% reported constipation, but this correlated poorly with stool frequency. Nine percent of those with daily stools and 30.6% of those with four to six stools per week noted that they were "constipated." Constipation was more common in blacks (17%), in women (18%), in individuals older than 60 years of age (23%), and in those who were inactive, had low income, or of the lower socioeconomic class. Constipated individuals reported lower consumption of cheese, dry beans and peas, milk,

TABLE 20-1 Nonmechanical Causes of Constipation

Normal Caliber Bowel	Dilated Bowel
Dietary	Aganglionosis
Immobility	Hirschsprung's
Age	disease
Drugs	Chagas' disease
Metabolic and endocrine	Idiopathic megabowel
Psychological neurologic disease	Pseudoobstruction
Irritable bowel syndrome	
Slow-transit constipation	

Evacuation Disorder	Special Cases
Rectocele	Stercoral ulceration
Rectal prolapse	Melanosis coli
Descending perineum syndrome	
Solitary rectal ulcer syndrome	
Anismus	
Internal sphincter myopathy	

meat and poultry, beverages (sweetened, carbonated, and non-carbonated), and fruits and vegetables. They reported higher consumption of coffee or tea. They consumed fewer total calories even after controlling for body mass and for exercise.

Classification

Constipation may be mechanical or nonmechanical. The former can be caused by any obstructing lesion outside the bowel wall, within the wall, or inside the lumen. These conditions are dealt with in specific chapters on carcinoma, diverticular disease, volvulus, and other mechanical causes of obstruction. Painful anal disease may also result in constipation through the reluctance of the patient to defecate. This ultimately can lead to fecal impaction.

Nonmechanical causes of constipation are shown in Table 20-1. They include conditions that result in reduced intestinal transit. The causes of the various forms other than aganglionosis are unknown, but delayed transit appears to be divisible into involvement of the entire intestine (including gastric function) and involvement confined to the large bowel—so-called colonic inertia.[279] This distinction is usually established by isotope scintigraphy, a study that can measure gastric emptying as well as orocecal and colonic transit. Patients with reduced transit are divided into those with a normal caliber colon and those with a dilated colon or rectum or both (megabowel).

Obstructed defecation is a common cause of constipation. The etiology may be mechanical, such as from rectal carcinoma or stricture, or it may be functional. Functional, obstructed defecation may be caused by failure of the pelvic floor adequately to relax as in anismus. This may include the condition of the solitary rectal ulcer syndrome, or it may be due to laxity of the pelvic floor and be associated with perineal descent and/or rectocele.[369] The diagnosis may be based on the Rome III criteria,[199] and its severity can be assessed by the Cleveland Clinic Constipation Score.[1] Another scoring system, the KESS score was devised to distinguish

constipation from normal patients and to discriminate between those with slow-transit constipation (STC), obstructed defecation, or both.[171] In a study of 71 individuals with constipation and 20 asymptomatic controls, this scoring system is closely correlated with the Cleveland Clinic score ($r = 0.9$) and achieved a clear separation from patients with STC and defecation, although it was not able to distinguish those with a combined disorder. The common causes of nonmechanical constipation are shown in Table 20-1.

Pathophysiology

In constipation, there is a degree of colonic sensorimotor dysfunction. The colon demonstrates myoelectric activity, which can result in phasic and tonic contractile activity. In many cases, there is a reduction in the rate of colonic transit. Scintigraphy has shown that the motility disorder is more extensive in some patients who demonstrate delayed gastric emptying and delayed orocecal transit. This is referred to as *whole gut dysmotility*.[22,279] Degeneration and fibrosis of the intestinal muscle is seen in familial visceral myopathies. These involve genetic and mitochondrial abnormalities, which result in reduction in intestinal motility.[2] The genetic abnormality may be highly specific in, for example, alpha-actin deficiency.[176]

Motility

The physiology of colorectal sensorimotor activity is dealt with in Chapters 2 and 7. Research in intestinal physiology, however, is difficult and may explain why little is understood despite many attempts to record motility and measure sensation. One of the main reasons is that motor patterns such as the migrating motor complex or colonic mass action occur at a frequency over time base longer than the convenient recording of intraluminal pressure. It is very difficult to obtain recordings over many hours. Yet only by doing so is it possible to study the changes in intestinal motility with time.

The basic motility activities of the colon are a slow net distal propulsion, extensive kneading, and exposure of its contents to the mucosal surface.[295] Material in the bowel is moved along a pressure gradient, with the rate and volume related to the pressure differential, the diameter of the tube, and the viscosity of the contents.[188] It may take only 1 or 2 hours for a meal to traverse the small intestine, but it may frequently take up to 30 hours to pass through the colon. The length and diameter of the colon tend to favor prolonged contact between the contents and the absorptive mucosa; this increases the amount of water removed and, as a consequence, may yield hard stools.[193] Additionally, widening of the rectosigmoid can produce a capacious distal reservoir; hence, a larger fecal mass is required to stimulate elimination.[193]

The pathophysiology of constipation is still poorly understood. It is characterized by reduced colonic motility, dysfunctional rectal emptying, and rectal hyposensitivity.[298] The first of these may coexist with a panintestinal motility disorder evidenced by delayed gastric emptying and retarded orocecal transit time.[279] Neural connections of the rectum include pathways to the dorsal ganglia of the spinal cord, ascending spinothalamocortical tracts and projections to the insular and dorsal anterior cingulate cortex. Rectal neural function may also be influenced by psychological factors.[353] Additionally, impaired rectal sensation is frequently found in patients with idiopathic constipation.[12]

At the time of publication of the previous edition of this book, the normal range of colorectal motor activity and its variations in disease had yet to be clearly defined,[188] but there was evidence that chronic constipation might be associated with either increased or decreased colonic motility.[164] Colonic motility relies upon there being normal smooth muscle and a competent enteric nervous system modulated by the intact autonomic parasympathetic and sympathetic nerves. Smooth muscle cells are formed into a syncytium with interstitial cells of Cajal (ICC), which together result in a rhythmic myogenic activity. Peristalsis is the synchronized contraction of colorectal smooth muscle, which, when the muscle fibers shorten, results in propulsion. Research into colonic motility has mostly involved pressure recordings from multichannel catheters introduced at colonoscopy or via a nasogastric tube. The former requires bowel preparation that may affect the activity.[38]

Three forms of colonic motility patterns have been identified. They are as follows:

1. Nonpropagating. These are random waves of a frequency of 2 to 4 per minute. They comprise the majority of the activity and are suppressed at night.
2. Propagating sequences. These may be of high amplitude. They may be antegrade or retrograde. In the normal colon, the former outweigh the latter by about 3/1. These also are suppressed at night.
3. Colorectal motor complexes. These are periodic contractions in the sigmoid and rectum of unknown function. They are more prevalent at night and have an amplitude of 80 to 90 mm Hg, occurring every 3 to 30 minutes.[38]

Defecation

Defecation begins with involuntary filling of the rectum through caudally passing migratory contractions from the proximal colon. This leads to rectal sensory awareness through the sampling reflex, which in turn promotes urgency.[236] As the rectum continues to fill, the urgency increases and rectal contraction with relaxation of the internal sphincter follows. Inhibition of pelvic floor tone then occurs, and the pelvic floor descends with simultaneous contraction of the longitudinal muscle of the anal canal.[38,295]

If a voluntary effort is required to defecate, intra-abdominal pressure is increased by closure of the glottis and by contraction of the muscles of the pelvic floor (resisting the forward movement of stool and closing the lumen distally). The diaphragm descends, and the voluntary muscles of the abdominal wall are contracted, creating a closed system.[372] Relaxation of the pelvic muscles produces descent of the pelvic floor and straightening of the previously angulated rectum. Closure of the anal canal by the sphincters allows an increase of pressure within the rectum so that subsequent sphincteric inhibition results in expulsion of stool. When paradoxical contraction of the voluntary sphincter muscle occurs during attempts at evacuation, it is termed "obstructed defecation" or "anismus" (see later). The point at which complete inhibition of the external sphincter occurs can be demonstrated experimentally with an intrarectal balloon. When the volume reaches 150 to 200 mL of air, the intrarectal pressure achieves 45 to 55 mm Hg. At the end of defecation, when straining is discontinued, the pelvic floor rises to its normal position and again obliterates the lumen. A rebound contraction of the anal sphincter occurs; this has been termed the *closing reflex*.[262]

Berman and colleagues subdivided patients with disorders of defecation into three categories: those with motility (i.e., transit) problems, those with mural difficulties (e.g., internal procidentia), and those with musculoskeletal problems (e.g., obstructed defecation).[29] Kuijpers applied the colorectal laboratory in the diagnosis of 74 patients with so-called functional constipation.[186] Outlet obstruction was noted in approximately three-fourths, with abnormal transit times identified in two-thirds. These results imply that only after evacuation studies have been proved to be normal should the physician embark on transit studies. Karasick and Ehrlich also suggested based on their studies that constipation is often a disorder of defecation rather than an impairment of colonic motility.[159] However, Roe and colleagues believed that the most useful investigations were transit studies and defecography.[288] Grotz and coworkers performed a study to identify differences in rectal wall contractility between healthy volunteers and those with chronic severe constipation.[111] In response to feeding of a cholinergic agonist and a smooth muscle relaxant, rectal wall contractility was decreased in constipated patients. The authors concluded that these findings suggested the presence of an abnormality of rectal muscular wall contractility in constipated patients.[111] To identify the optimal regimen for the management of intractable constipation, Wexner and Dailey offered an algorithmic approach.[366]

Etiology

The classification of constipation in Table 20-1 shows that many factors can be responsible. Essentially, they all influence bowel function either by slowing intestinal transit or by inhibiting rectal evacuation.

In a useful review of the subject, Müller-Lissner and colleagues considered many issues that have been invoked as causes of constipation, some of which have been substantiated by evidence and some not.[244] The colon has three functions: absorption of water; the harboring of bacteria, which split fiber into absorbable nutrients; and the retention and expulsion of the residue when convenient to the individual. Among misconceptions that have been disproved, there is no evidence for the retention of stool in the large bowel causing "autointoxication" as propounded by Arbuthnot Lane in the early 20th century. Also, there is no evidence for a lengthened, nondilated colon, a so-called dolichocolon, as a cause for the condition.[228,324]

Dietary Fiber and Water Intake

Fiber binds water, but when split by bacteria, it no longer does so. No difference has been found in dietary fiber intake in constipated compared with nonconstipated individuals. In a study of various fiber preparations, an inverse relationship between fecal bulk and water holding has been identified, suggesting that dietary fiber does not have its effect on stool weight by increasing water retention in the intestine.[319] In another study, 9 constipated women were compared with 9 nonconstipated women in the third semester of pregnancy. There was no difference in the ingestion of fiber in the two groups. In a further 40 constipated women in the third trimester, dietary fiber manipulation had no effect on bowel function.[6] Müller-Lissner and colleagues concluded that a poor fiber diet should not be assumed to be the cause of constipation, but it may contribute to the issue.[244] Some are helped and others are made worse by fiber. The available data do not indicate that bowel frequency can be manipulated to a clinically useful degree by the ingestion of liquids. There is no evidence that constipation can be treated by increasing liquid intake unless the patient is dehydrated.

Immobility

During sleep, colonic motility is almost absent. There is no difference between constipated and nonconstipated individuals at these times.[21] There is, however, evidence that physical activity is associated with a higher stool frequency,[39] so an association can be quite marked in runners.[329]

In a survey of 201 elderly patients, the overall incidence of constipation was no different from that of younger patients, but within the groups, any association appeared to be related to immobility and to depression.[69] Bedbound elderly patients are more likely to have constipation than those who are able to walk with help and even more so than do patients who walk several hundred meters per day.[168]

Constipation is often due to fecal loading in the rectum. Impaction is commonly seen in institutions where immobility and constipating drugs are both factors delaying transit and evacuation. Exercise improves bowel function in normal sedentary men and women,[33] but not in patients who are already severely constipated.[231] There is evidence from institutional studies that exercise, adequate hydration, and fiber intake can reduce the need for laxatives.[158]

Drugs

Drugs that cause constipation include opiates, anticholinergics, antidepressants, iron, bismuth, antiparkinsonians, aluminum-containing antacids, antihypertensives (diuretics, ganglion blockers, calcium channel blockers), and anticonvulsants. Drug-induced constipation is very common (see Chapter 4). The bowel symptoms and even the radiologic findings of colonic dilatation may completely resolve after the medication responsible has been discontinued.[46]

Laxatives

There is a large literature on whether laxatives can affect the structure and function of the intestine. Stimulant laxatives have been thought to cause damage to the myenteric nerves or smooth muscle causing impaired motility.[77] Certainly, they can result in *melanosis coli* if used over time. This condition, first recognized by Cruveilhier in 1830, is caused by the deposition of pigment due to staining by anthraquinones of cell debris from colocytes ingested by macrophages in the submucosa (Figure 20-1).[92] The condition is of no clinical significance and disappears within weeks to months of stopping the laxative. The effect of purgation on the enteric nerves and smooth muscle of constipated individuals was reported by Smith.[310] He opined that any changes seen might have been due to the primary condition itself, rather than to secondary damage by the laxatives. Furthermore, ultrastructural changes seen in patients on long-term laxatives may also occur in amyloid, diabetic autonomic neuropathy, and inflammatory bowel disease.[284] Other studies have demonstrated reduced numbers of Cajal cells and enteric neurons in patients with severe colonic inertia.[122,364] These changes may be due to the disease and not to any laxative medication. When patients taking anthraquinones were compared with a control group of constipated patients not taking laxatives, there was no evidence in favor of laxatives causing any damage.[283] Thus, the evidence that laxatives can cause intestinal nerve and smooth muscle damage per se is poor.

Laxatives can cause electrolyte disturbances when taken in high doses. In a special article, Müller-Lissner discusses whether or not the cathartic colon exists.[243] In a series of 200 patients with diarrhea, the incidence of laxative abuse was 3.5%.[43] Review of the literature demonstrated 70 publications, including 240 patients in whom diarrhea was caused by sub rosa laxative administration. Of these, 95% were female; the laxative in question was phenolphthalein, and the metabolic disturbance was hypokalemia.[192]

Metabolic and Endocrine
Sex Hormones

In children, constipation is more common in boys than in girls, but after the age of 14, females vastly exceed males with this problem.[209] There is evidence that bowel function may be related to the menstrual cycle, but no difference in colonic transit was found during the follicular and luteal phases (48 and 51 hours).[130,150] There is, however, evidence that transit time is increased in pregnancy.[359] In another study, 26 female patients with severe constipation were compared with 23 age-matched, normal healthy women.[151] There were significant differences during the follicular phase in progesterone, hydroxyprogesterone, cortisol, and testosterone levels. Parenthetically, ultrasound studies have failed to demonstrate any abnormality in the female genital organs in constipated patients.[156]

LÉON JEAN BAPTISTE CRUVEILHIER (1791–1874)

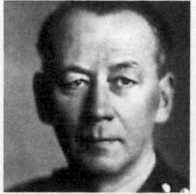

Cruveilhier was the son of a military surgeon who had planned to enter the priesthood, but he was denied this course by his father who wanted him to become his successor. He attended the University at Limoges and in 1810 moved to Paris to study medicine under Guillaume Dupuytren, a friend of his father. Dupuytren made him his protégé and aroused his interest in pathology. Cruveilhier received his doctorate in medicine in 1816 with a dissertation on a new classification of organs according to their pathologic changes. Stung by failure to secure an appointment as surgeon in Limoges, he returned to Paris and, supported by Dupuytren, was appointed professor agrégé of surgery at the Faculty of Medicine of Montpellier. In 1825, he accepted the position of professor of descriptive anatomy in Paris and the following year was named Médecin des Hôpitaux. In 1836, he was elected to the Académie de Médecine and became president in 1839. In 1836, he was offered the first chair of pathologic anatomy, which had been established with funds from his teacher, Dupuytren. He remained in this position for more than 30 years. The vast material from the deadhouse of the Salpêtrière, the establishment of the Musée Dupuytren, and the lectureship in morbid anatomy provided the impetus for his prolific writings. His best known work was *Anatomie pathologique du corps humain* in which he reports the first pathologic account of disseminated sclerosis. Cruveilhier devoted himself to his enormous practice, following the rules of a very strict ethic that he condensed in his *Des devoirs et de la moralité du médecin* (1837). He died on his country estate in Sussac near Limoges at the age of 83. (With appreciation to Faisal Aziz, MD.)

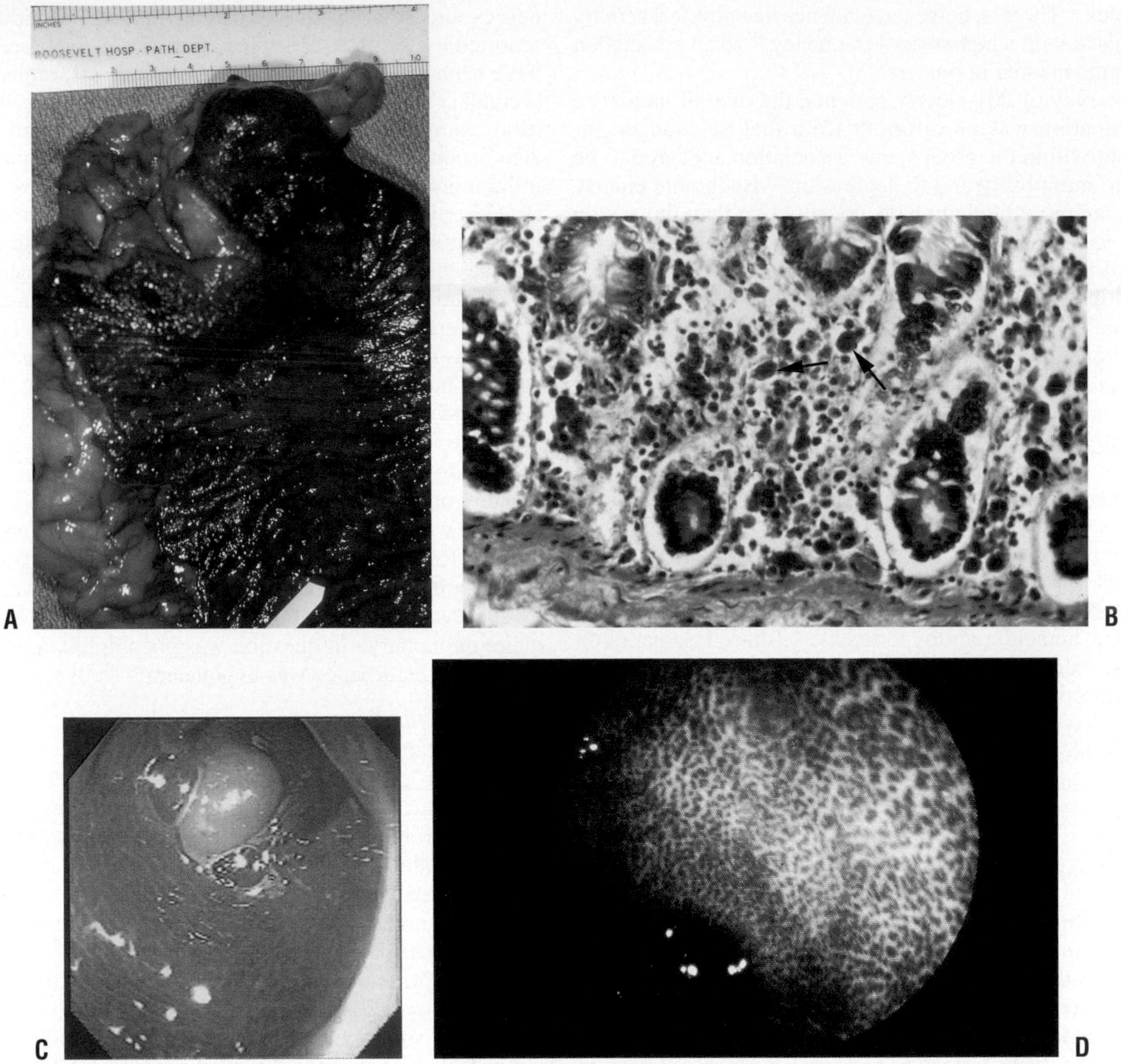

FIGURE 20-1. Melanosis coli. **A:** Note the dark black pigment characteristic of melanosis coli in a resected specimen. **B:** Pigmented macrophages (*arrows*) appear in the lamina propria. (Original magnification × 600; from Corman ML, Veidenheimer MC, Swinton NW. *Diseases of the Anus, Rectum and Colon. Part I: Neoplasms.* New York, NY: Mecom; 1972.) **C:** A polypoid lesion is clearly evident against a background of the darkly pigmented, otherwise normal mucosa. **D:** Characteristic appearance of melanosis coli as seen through a colonoscope.

Other Hormones

Gastrointestinal hormones have been studied in patients with constipation.[350] Twelve individuals with severe constipation were compared with 12 healthy normal women after taking a radioisotope-labeled meal. Circulating gastrointestinal hormones were measured over the following 180 postprandial minutes. Levels of somatostatin were increased in the constipated patients, but there was no correlation with upper gastrointestinal transit rates. Pancreatic glucagon and enteroglucagon levels were lower, but there were no significant differences in insulin, gastric inhibitory polypeptide (GIP), glucagon-like peptide 1 (GLP 1), cholecystokinin (CCK), gastrin, pancreatic polypeptide (PP), motilin, neurotensin, and peptide tyrosine-tyrosine (PYY).

Abnormal levels of thyroid hormones have been regarded as causes of constipation or diarrhea, but in a prospective study, there was a low prevalence of hypothyroidism in female patients with constipation.[11] The authors recommended testing for thyroid function if there were other features of thyroid underactivity.

Other

Hypercalcemia, hypokalemia, and porphyria can all be associated with constipation. In the case of hypokalemia, this may be the result of excessive intestinal losses by purgatives (see Laxatives).

Psychological

It is accepted that constipation may be associated with psychological abnormalities, particularly depression. In a study of 25 consecutive patient referrals who harbored severe constipation, 10 with normal transit had higher psychological distress than the 15 with increased transit. When compared with 25 normal controls, the authors concluded that different therapeutic approaches may be required based on behavioral and psychological assessment.[358] In a subsequent study of 38 patients with severe idiopathic constipation, the Hopkins Symptom Checklist (SCL-90-R) score was higher in 15 patients with normal transit compared with 23 in whom it was prolonged.[357] In addition, those with depression may develop constipation as a consequence of antidepressant drug treatment.

Neurologic Disease

Neurologic disease at almost any level of the nervous system can cause constipation. These include multiple sclerosis and diabetes mellitus, both leading to autonomic neuropathy.[101] The mechanisms of action are complex and not well understood. Autonomic dysfunction may reduce motor intestinal function and diminish the defecation reflex activity through impairment of anorectal sensation.[272] Intracranial diseases such as cerebrovascular accident, tumor, and Parkinson's disease can all be associated with problems of bowel elimination. Other contributing neurologic conditions include lesions of the spinal cord, cauda equina injury, meningomyelocele, spina bifida, and tertiary syphilis.

Smooth Muscle Dysmotility

Connective tissue disorders that may be associated with constipation include systemic lupus, dermatomyositis, and scleroderma.[55,213,292,302,315] In fact, most patients with scleroderma have intestinal involvement.[370] This leads to dysmotility, owing to the involvement of the smooth muscle. Muscular dystrophy and amyloid may cause a secondary incompetence of the intestinal muscle.

Assessment and Investigation

The most common causes of constipation encountered in practice include constipation-predominant IBS, drugs, depression, and inadequate consumption of fiber and liquid. Once a mechanical cause has been excluded, the likely reasons for constipation in patients with a normal colonic caliber include STC or an evacuation disorder.

Clinical Assessment

The words "constipation" or "diarrhea" when used by the patient may not truly be referring to bowel frequency and may therefore be misinterpreted by the physician. There are three elements that the clinician should take into account: frequency of defecation (expressed as the number of bowel actions per 24 hours or per week), the consistency of the stool, and the presence of urgency. The term *constipation* may be used by the patient when there is any difficulty with evacuation.

Some patients feel constipated because they have an unproductive urge to defecate or feelings of incomplete evacuation that prompt them to return to the bathroom and to continue further attempts at evacuation by straining at stool. The need for accurate symptom assessment requires the clinician to obtain details of straining, urgency, and incomplete evacuation, taking stool consistency into account.

Urgency is usually not applicable to constipation, but if present, it should be recorded as the number of minutes the patient requires in order to get to the bathroom when the desire to defecate comes on.

Patients with an evacuation disorder of the type seen in the solitary ulcer syndrome may make numerous fruitless visits to the bathroom where they may remain, stay straining for many minutes up to hours. Ten or more visits to the bathroom in a 24-hour period are not uncommon in this group of patients, and the time spent there may often be more than 30 minutes. In such cases, it is helpful to compute the total time per 24 hours spent in the bathroom. In exceptional cases, this may amount to several hours.

It is important to document the presence of abdominal symptoms such as pain, discomfort, and distension. The general well-being of the patient as judged by appetite, weight, and energy levels should also be assessed. A family and drug history should be obtained and a dietary assessment made. Any history of prior surgery, neurologic disease, and mental illness should be noted.

The examination should include a neurologic assessment. Any distension of the abdomen or mass suggesting a mechanical cause or fecal impaction should be noted. The anorectal examination should record the state of the rectum, whether capacious, empty, or full of feces. With a fecal impaction, the anal sphincter may be patulous. In Hirschsprung's disease and anismus, the sphincter may feel hypertonic. In patients with neurologic disease, including spinal cord injury, the sphincter is usually quite lax.

Investigations

Colorectal examination by means of colonoscopy or imaging is necessary in patients with symptoms suggestive of a mechanical cause or those with a family history of large bowel cancer. In individuals who do not need such investigation, it is reasonable to treat the patient in general terms before carrying out any further studies.

Most patients with constipation can be managed in a primary care setting with attention to likely causative factors and with simple targeted interventions. Withdrawal of medication, adjustment of diet, and other lifestyle changes such as exercise should be attempted, unless it is clear that these measures are unlikely to be successful. Thus, a patient with a long history of evacuation difficulties and who has tried laxatives without improvement is likely to require further investigation. This includes tests to estimate intestinal transit and to determine whether there is an evacuation disorder.

Specialist referral should be considered, but it is uncommonly undertaken given the vast number of patients attending primary care who harbor a constipation problem.

Colonic Function

Plain Abdominal X-ray and Barium Enema

Occasionally, a plain abdominal x-ray will show fecal loading of the large bowel (Figure 20-2), but this investigation is generally of limited value in the investigation of constipation. It may have some usefulness in determining whether the bowel is distended or not. In the past, a barium enema (Figure 20-3) would have been requested, but this investigation is performed less, often owing to the availability of computed tomography (CT) or magnetic resonance imaging (MRI).

If the colon or rectum is dilated, then aganglionic bowel disease, idiopathic megabowel (megacolon), or pseudoobstruction should be considered. The distinction between them is obvious and will be described later.

Intestinal Transit

Marker Studies. In clinical practice, transit is measured by following the intraluminal passage of a radiopaque or radioactive marker detected by conventional radiology and scintigraphy, respectively. Essentially, this will be normal or may be delayed, such as in STC.[68] The use of radiopaque markers was initially described by Hinton.[131] In this evaluation, 20 to 50 radiopaque gelatin capsules are given on day 0 and day 5. Delayed transit is inferred if more than 20% of the markers are still present at 5 days (Figure 20-4). Alternatively, capsules of different shape may be given on days 0, 1, and 2, followed by an abdominal x-ray on day 5.[233] It can be argued that this allows an assessment of transit through different segments of the colon (Figure 20-5), although regional

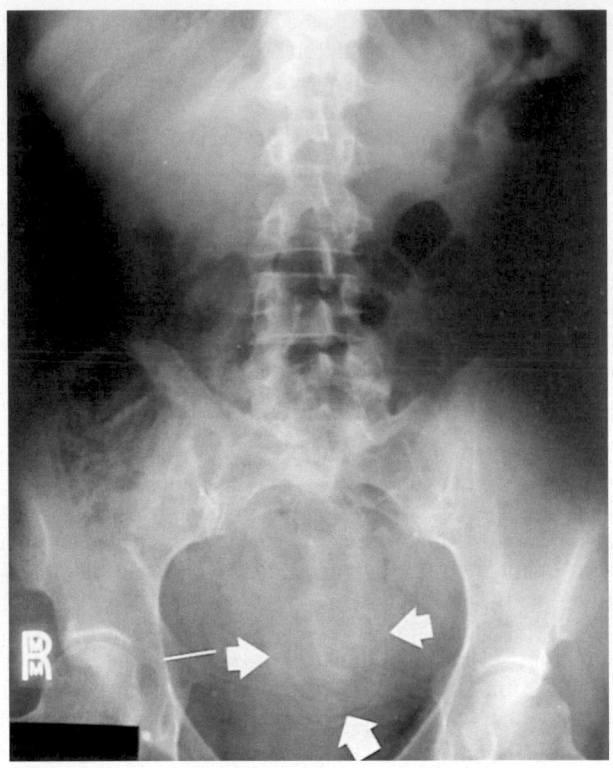

FIGURE 20-2. Fecal impaction. A large, laminated pelvic calcification (*arrows*) is indicative of a retained, massive fecaloma.

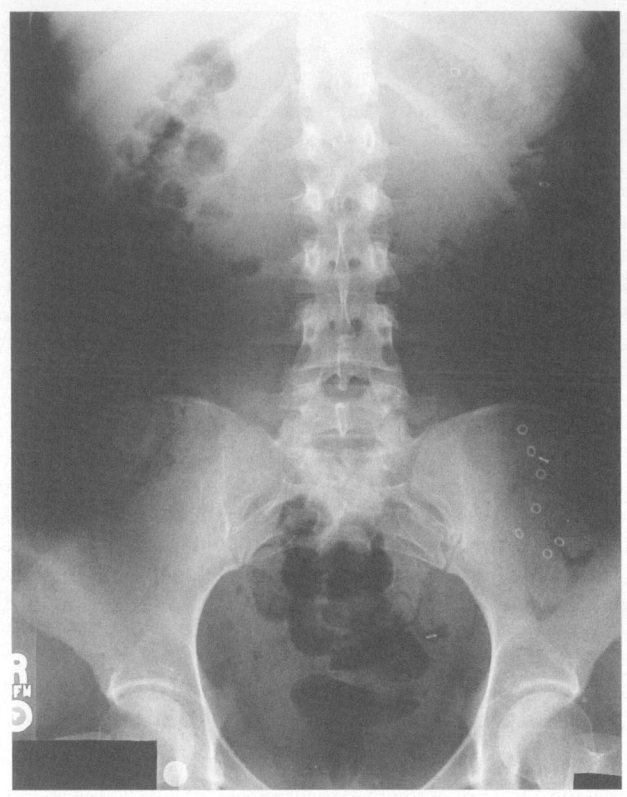

FIGURE 20-4. Plain abdominal radiograph showing radiopaque markers primarily in the sigmoid colon, a distribution consistent with hindgut inertia.

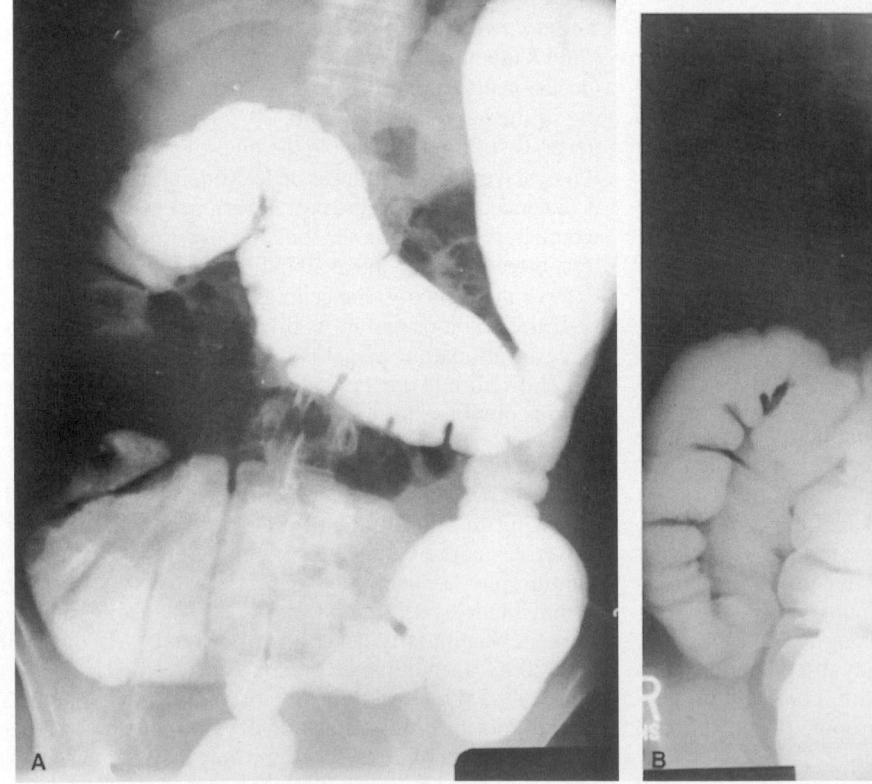

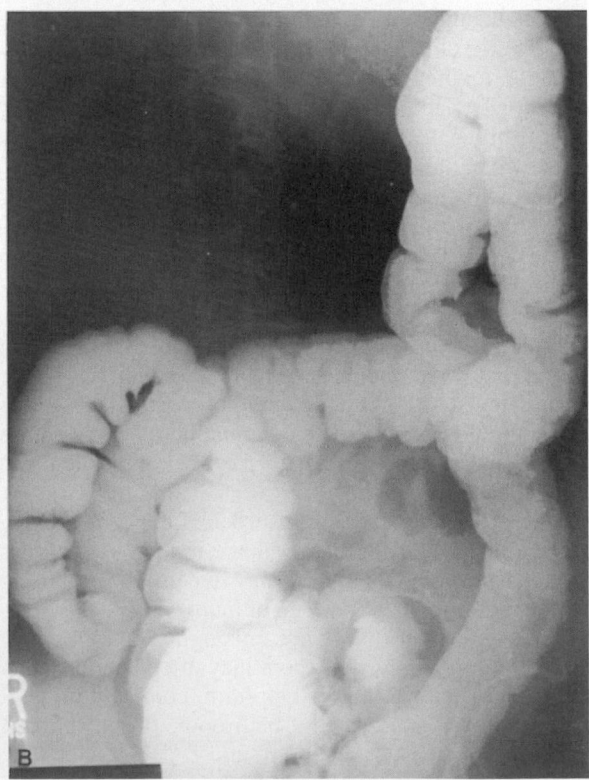

FIGURE 20-3. Barium enema studies of adult megacolon in patients with intractable constipation. **A:** A large-caliber bowel is especially notable in the proximal **(right)** colon. The patient moved her bowels once in 2 weeks. **B:** A markedly redundant colon leading to infrequent bowel action.

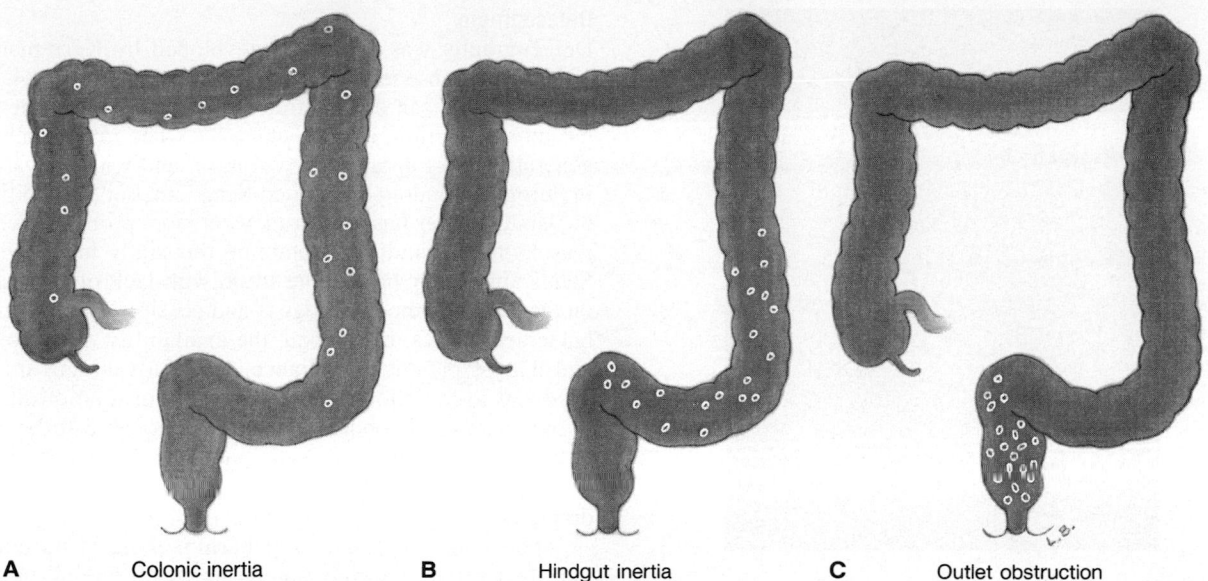

A   Colonic inertia   **B**   Hindgut inertia   **C**   Outlet obstruction

FIGURE 20 5. Artist's representation of three types of radiologic appearances that may be seen with radiopaque rings on the plain abdominal x-ray study. **A:** Colonic inertia: typical pattern of distribution throughout the colon. **B:** Hindgut inertia. Markers are clustered on the left side of the colon but not limited to the rectum. **C:** Outlet obstruction. Markers are clustered in the rectum, a classic pattern indicating obstructed defecation.

retardation of transit within the large bowel is not accepted by all workers in the field. The investigation will be positive in about one-half of the patients with STC.[175] Radiopaque markers are inexpensive, easy to use, and are widely available.[322] In the United States, the commercially produced rings, Sitzmarks, are generally employed for this purpose (Figure 20-6).

The second method of assessing transit is scintigraphy. Krevsky and colleagues gave oral ^{111}In bound to diethylene-triaminepentaacetic acid (DTPA) followed by a gamma scan at 72 and 96 hours and scanned the abdomen at intervals after ingestion.[183] Others have used ^{111}In mixed with charcoal in a methyl acrylate capsule, which is then broken down in the gut to release the radionuclide in the terminal ileum and cecum.[42,45,227] There is some variation in the technique, but all protocols share common aspects. Any constipating medications should be stopped 48 hours prior to undertaking the study. The patient should have fasted from the previous day.

A standard meal with contained carbohydrate, fat, and protein commensurate with the normal relative contents of these foodstuffs is then ingested. This contains a radionuclide label of ^{111}In of ^{99}Tc in solid and liquid phase. Imaging is started immediately by gamma scanner recording to estimate gastric emptying. This is continued for 6 hours and thereafter at 24, 48, and 72 hours.[37,222,301] The transit time is determined by the location of the center of the mass of radioactivity at the selected interval from ingestion (Figure 20-7).[68] This technique allows measurement of gastric emptying, orocecal transit, and colonic transit.

Colonic Manometry

Colonic manometry is another technique that has been used to estimate transit and has been advocated by some workers.[20,277] It involves the siting of open-tipped or balloon probes into the intestine via the anus or nasal orifice. This is often difficult to accomplish. Recording must be

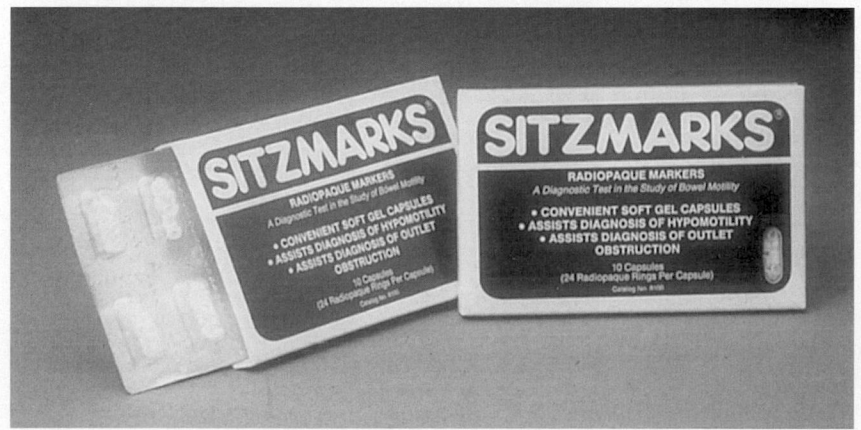

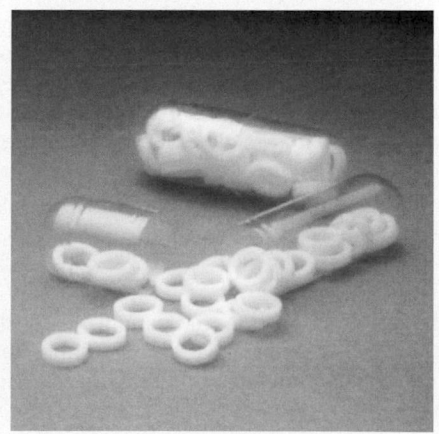

A   **B**

FIGURE 20-6. **A:** Bowel transit markers are commercially available in gelatin capsules (Sitzmarks). **B:** Each capsule contains 24 radiopaque markers.

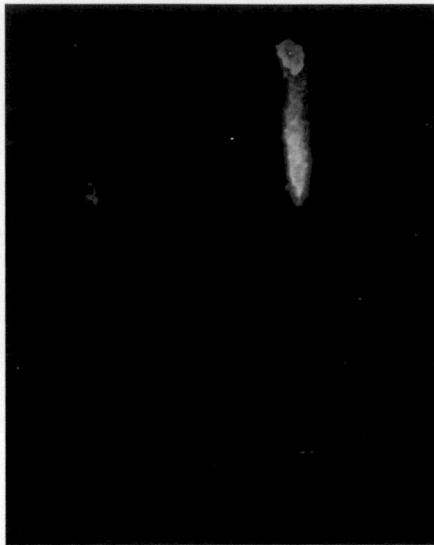

FIGURE 20-7. Scintigraphy in a patient with slow-transit constipation. There is concentration of radioactive nuclide in the splenic flexure and descending colon at 3 days.

maintained for many hours to give a meaningful picture of the motility of the intestine. There is much published in the literature, but owing to the methodologic difficulty and the individual variation of intestinal behavior, there is little standardization of the method. At the present time, manometry is more a research tool than a method of clinical investigation.

Rectal Evacuation

Many patients with STC will have evidence of impaired rectal evacuation. Thus, patients who have transit studies should also have investigations to determine whether there is impairment of evacuation. These include manometry, balloon expulsion, defecography, and magnetic imaging of the pelvic floor.[369] Measurement of perineal descent using the perineometer formed the subject of much research 30 years ago but has never become part of clinical practice.[125,145]

Anal Manometry

Anal manometry has a limited role in the investigation of obstructed defecation (see Chapter 7). Patients who have a lax pelvic floor may have reduced resting tone and impaired voluntary contraction, but such findings are not useful in management. In those with anismus, resting anal pressure may be increased. Attempts at defecation may be associated with paradoxical contraction of the puborectalis muscle, although the validity of this effect has been questioned. Ambulant manometry is technically difficult and is confined to research.

Balloon Expulsion

In this investigation, the patient lies in the left lateral position.[16,270] A catheter with an inflatable balloon is introduced into the rectum, and 50 mL of liquid (originally barium suspension) are injected into the balloon. The patient is then asked to evacuate. Failure to accomplish this is an indication of obstructed defecation.

Defecography

Defecography was originally developed by Kerremans in 1952[167] and subsequently modified by Mahieu in 1984.[209,210] The procedure can demonstrate a rectocele, enterocele, rectal intussusception, and anismus.[119,120] The investigation is generally well tolerated, inexpensive, and widely available in Europe, including the United Kingdom, but availability in the United States has been somewhat more problematic. The reasons for difficulty in obtaining this study in the United States apparently have more to do with lack of motivation on the part of some radiologists and possible financial reimbursement issues, rather than the availability of equipment and that of patient compliance. Its disadvantages include exposure to radiation and the inconsistent relationship between anatomical abnormality and functional disturbance as indicated by symptoms. Some patients experience embarrassment, but this issue should be avoidable through proper draping.

Approximately 120 mL of barium paste is introduced into the rectum, with the patient in the left lateral position. The patient then sits upright on a radiolucent commode (see Figure 7-13) after having taken 100 mL of barium sulfate suspension by mouth to opacify the small intestine (Figure 20-8). The examination includes imaging in three phases: at rest, during maximum voluntary contraction (squeeze), and expulsion (Figure 20-9). In the last of these, the patient makes three attempts at evacuation lasting 30 seconds to assess the ability of emptying. Digital fluoroscopy is used to minimize the radiation dosage.

In normal defecography, the anorectal angle is approximately 90 degrees, and the pelvic floor lies above the level of the ischial tuberosities. During squeeze, the pelvic floor rises, and the impression of the puborectalis muscle can be seen to be indenting the anorectal junction posteriorly. When the patient evacuates, the pelvic floor descends, and the anorectal angle opens to a wide angle. Barium is then expelled (Figure 20-10). This normally is complete in about 30 seconds (see also Figure 7-14).[83]

The radiologic signs must be interpreted with caution in light of the patient's symptoms. Abnormalities such as

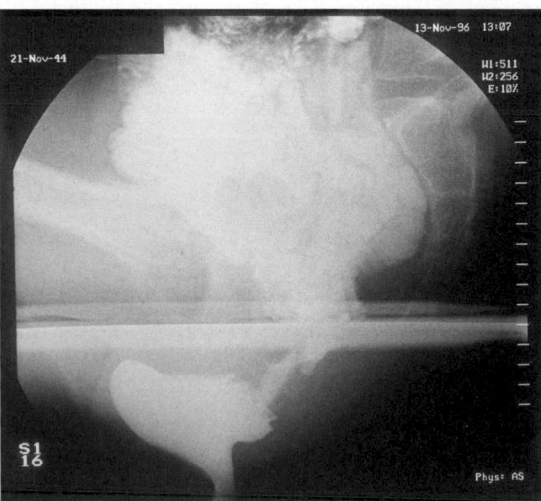

FIGURE 20-8. Defecography in a patient with difficulty in evacuation. Large rectocele and enterocele shown in the pouch of Douglas after administration of oral contrast.

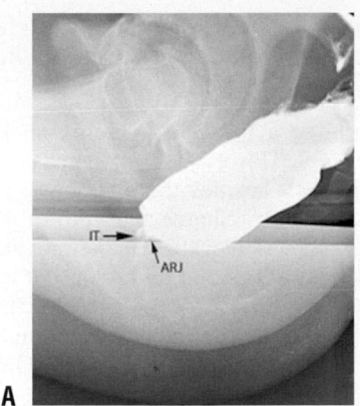 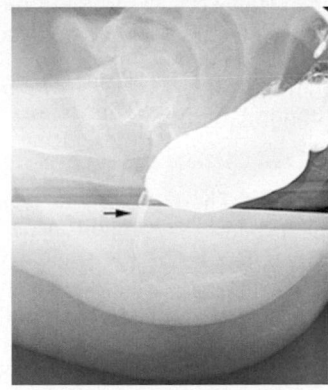 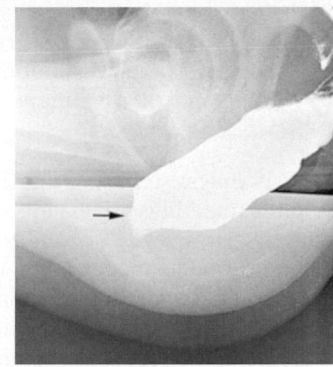

FIGURE 20-9. Defecogram at rest **(A)**, during contraction **(B)**, and during strain **(C)**. All are performed with lateral projections and with the patient seated. The position of the pelvic floor is taken as the lower aspect of the ischial tuberosity (IT). At rest, the anorectal junction (ARJ) is normally at or just above the level of the ischial tuberosities. During squeeze, it rises, and during straining, it descends below this level. The anorectal angle is clearly seen.

rectocele and rectal folds may be observed in nearly one-half of normal individuals.[304] Rectocele is a common incidental finding and is often associated with signs of anismus, intussusception, and enterocele (see Chapter 21). A significant rectocele is defined based on its size and the degree of barium retention (trapping).[118]

Magnetic Resonance Imaging

MRI began to be used for the assessment of the pelvic floor in the 1990s.[31,124] It has the advantage of not involving ionizing radiation, but it is expensive and not generally available. To date, it has been used more as a research than as a clinical tool.

Closed or open MR machines are employed.[31,291] No bowel preparation is necessary, and no vaginal or bladder contrast is required. The rectum is filled with a contrast resembling the consistency of soft feces for dynamic MRI defecography. Axial T2 images are followed by coronal and sagittal views at rest and during attempts at defecation. Views of the sequence from rest to straining back to rest are also obtained (Figure 20-11).

In a normal patient, the bladder neck and cervix lie above a line drawn from the inferior point of the pubic symphysis to the sacrococcygeal joint. During defecation, these structures move posteriorly and inferiorly but still remain above the line. The anal canal opens, and the impression of the puborectalis muscle is lost as the anorectal angle widens from its normal right angle to more than 120 degrees.

Clinical Forms
Normal Caliber Constipation
Irritable Bowel Syndrome

Definition. IBS is a functional gastrointestinal disorder (FGID) in which abdominal pain or discomfort is associated with defecation or a change in bowel habit and often with features of disordered defecation. There are no abnormal physical or radiologic signs, and there is no abnormal histopathology. The condition is identified by the presence of certain symptoms defined by the Rome III criteria (see later).[199]

Epidemiology. IBS, also known as functional bowel disease, mucous colitis, or spastic colon, is very common with an estimated prevalence in the general population worldwide of 10% to 20% and with a female predominance. The frequency of constipation varies according to how it is determined,

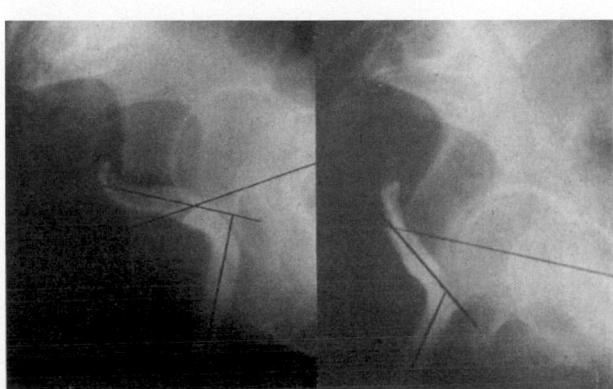

FIGURE 20-10. Defecogram showing descent of the pelvic floor and widening of the anorectal angle with emptying of the rectum.

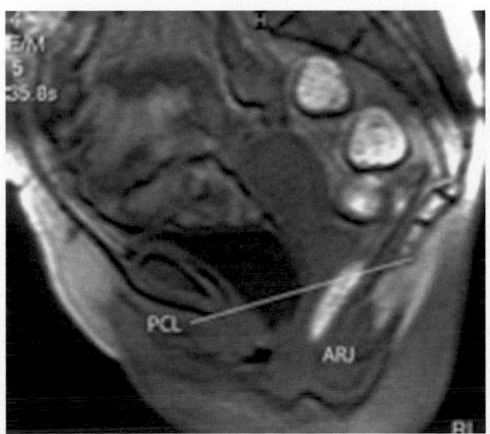

FIGURE 20-11. MRI showing a thick-section sagittal view during straining and with the bladder base and anorectal junction (ARJ) well below the pubococcygeal (PC) line.

whether from the patient herself, by application of Rome criteria, or by the Bristol scale for intestinal transit. In a study in which these approaches were compared, approximately 8% had constipation by each definition, but only 2% were constipated by all three.[254] This may lead to confusion of definitions.[199]

Diagno\sis. IBS is diagnosed using the Rome criteria. There have been three meetings of experts that have been reported: Rome I,[340] Rome II,[341,342] and Rome III.[199] The last two modifications divided patients into those with diarrhea-predominant and constipation-predominant IBS. Recurrent abdominal pain or discomfort at least 3 days per month in the last 3 months should be part of the symptomatology.[199] Pain has to be present, and this should be related to bowel function. Included also should be altered stool frequency, with straining another feature. The Rome II and III criteria have attempted to classify functional bowel disorders according to symptoms without investigation, but this approach is not very practical.[373] Supportive symptoms that are not part of the diagnostic criteria include abnormal stool frequency (less than or equal to three bowel movements per week or more than three bowel movements per day), abnormal stool form (lumpy/hard stool or loose/watery stool), defecation straining, urgency or a feeling of incomplete bowel movement, passing mucus, and bloating.

For a diagnosis of IBD according to the Rome III criteria, two or more of the following should be present:

- Straining during at least 25% of defecation
- Lumpy or hard stools in at least 25% of defecations
- Sensation of incomplete evacuation for at least 25% of defecations
- Sensation of anorectal obstruction/blockage for at least 25% of defecations
- Manual maneuvers to facilitate at least 25% of defecations (e.g., digital evacuation, support of the pelvic floor)
- Fewer than three defecations per week

The effectiveness of treatment has been reviewed by Trinkley and colleagues.[345] They identified 58 placebo-controlled clinical trials of various medications for IBS. They concluded that more studies with better design were necessary, but there was evidence of efficacy depending on the symptoms for the use of loperamide, fiber, selective serotonin receptor inhibitors (SSRIs) and tricyclic antidepressants, probiotics, octreotide, and antispasmodics.

Chronic Idiopathic Constipation

This is an example of a FGID in which constipation is present but pain is not. However, there must be a considerable overlap with IBS besides the absence of pain. In a meta-analysis conducted by Suares and Ford of 45 articles reporting 261,040 subjects worldwide, the prevalence was estimated to be 14% lower in Southeast Asia.[326] It was higher in women (odds ratio [OR] = 2.22; 95% confidence interval [CI], 1.87–2.62) with age, socioeconomic class, and in patients who also fulfilled the criteria for IBS (OR = 7.98; 95% CI, 4.58–13.92).

The large overlap of definitions and discrete clinical groupings of constipation is illustrated by McCallum and colleagues.[224] They prefer a more inclusive definition—that is, any patient experiencing persistent difficulty with defecation. This will therefore include most patients with a nonorganic cause.

Slow-Transit Constipation

A large number of diseases, including diabetes and flat feet, are due to autointoxication arising from chronic sepsis in the intestinal cesspool.
—WILLIAM ARBUTHNOT LANE (1900)

In 1908, Lane first offered a surgical alternative to the treatment of chronic constipation.[189] After initially performing ileocolonic bypass and then partial colectomy, he reported 38 patients who underwent subtotal colectomy for this complaint. However, it is only since the mid-1980s that publications have appeared to reconfirm the legitimacy of subtotal or total colectomy in the treatment of chronic constipation.

STC occurs almost exclusively in young women. It often starts in childhood or there may be an apparent trigger such as a pelvic operation or an episode of acute constipation.[174] The condition is likely to include various functional disorders and should therefore be regarded as a heterogeneous condition.[254]

The colon generally is of normal caliber, and there is delay in colonic transit as can be demonstrated by radiopaque markers or by scintigraphy.[19,155,322] In addition, there

WILLIAM ARBUTHNOT LANE (1856–1943)

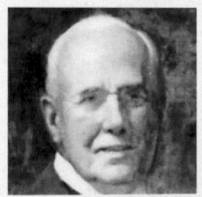

Lane was born at Fort George, Inverness, Scotland, the eldest son of a military surgeon. As a youth, Lane moved frequently with his parents—to South Africa, Ceylon, Nova Scotia, Malta, and Ireland. He entered Guy's Hospital in London in 1872 and achieved his fellowship of the Royal College of Surgeons in 1882. Following a period of travel in the Caribbean as a ship's surgeon, Lane was appointed to the staff of Guy's Hospital. He quickly became known as a master technician whose operations a patient could be expected to survive. There were three procedures for which he was renowned: the treatment of cleft palate, open reduction and internal fixation of fractures, and the surgical management of "chronic intestinal stasis." He wrote voluminously (313 articles) and produced a number of short books. During the First World War, Lane was consulting surgeon to the Aldershot Command, in addition to his responsibilities at Guy's Hospital and at the Hospital for Sick Children (Great Ormond Street). He received a baronetcy in 1913, and in 1917 he was named a Chevalier of the Legion of Honor. At the end of the war, he retired from Guy's, and shortly thereafter, he extended his views from the hospital to the whole world. In 1925, he founded the New Health Society, an organization dedicated to social concerns in medicine. (Photograph courtesy of Guy's Hospital, London.)

is evidence of low-amplitude propulsive waves of short duration.[18] The early postprandial colonic response is absent, and the response to bisacodyl is reduced.[155] There is evidence of a reduction of the ICC.[122] The results of studies up to the year 2000, which have investigated neuronal morphology, in vitro pharmacologic behavior of colonic smooth muscle, immunocytochemistry of neuronal antigens, and neurotransmitters, have been summarized by Knowles and Martin.[174]

Belsey and colleagues conducted a review of reports describing the quality of life in individuals with constipation.[27] They identified 13, of which 10 dealt with adults and 3 with children. Using the SF-36 (12 tools), there was consistent impairment of mental and physical domains, greater in the former. The degree of diminution was comparable to that seen in inflammatory bowel disease.

Treatment
Medical
Medical management includes the treatment of any underlying medical disorder and the suspension of constipating medication if this is being taken by the patient. The patient should be given dietary advice, and exercise should be encouraged. The efficacy of many commonly prescribed drugs, such as stool softeners, medications containing senna, and bisacodyl, remains to be defined.[224]

In a person with an evacuation disorder primarily responsible for symptoms, the condition should be explained, ideally with the use of diagrams. Suppositories may be prescribed to promote a strain-free defecation. Glycerine suppositories have a lubricant effect, but bisacodyl suppositories may be more reliable, owing to their pharmacologic action on the smooth muscle of the rectum. The patient should be exhorted to avoid straining, although this is very difficult to accomplish in practice.

Prucalopride is a selective high-affinity serotonin receptor antagonist, which has been applied to the management of constipation. There have been three controlled double-blinded clinical trials with author overlap, which show improved frequency of defecation and well-being in those taking the drug.[44,273,332,367] Of 1,974 patients pooled from these studies, more than 85% were female. Bowel frequency assessed at 12 weeks increased from less than two evacuations per week to three or more in the prucalopride group compared with 10% among those taking the placebo. The PAC quality-of-life score was 29% to 49% and 16% to 26% in the prucalopride and placebo groups. Despite these results, it was felt that the drug could not be recommended for constipation, owing to its cost and the incidence of the side effects of nausea, headache, and abdominal pain.[367] However, there will be cases so refractory that anything is reasonable to try if tolerated by the patient.

Biofeedback
This behavioral treatment was introduced for the treatment of fecal incontinence (see Chapter 16) but has also been applied to constipation. There is evidence that it is effective in patients with obstructed defecation as opposed to those with STC. In a study of 52 patients with delayed transit, 34 had simultaneous evidence of obstructed defecation.[52] Biofeedback improved in 71% of these patients but only in 8% of the 18 individuals with STC alone. Interestingly, colonic transit improved in those in the former group but not in the latter.

Other studies have demonstrated efficacy of biofeedback for the treatment of constipation or evacuation disorders in prospective, often randomized controlled trials.[23,53,54,81,128,182,229,276,348,365] Koh and colleagues reviewed the literature on biofeedback for pelvic floor dysfunction.[179] They included seven publications, and the authors concluded that high-quality studies were lacking. Despite this, they felt that biofeedback conferred a sixfold chance of successful treatment improvement. Others have published useful reviews on this issue.[275]

Biofeedback is free of complications and should be advised before any invasive treatment is considered. No trial of neuromodulation or surgical technique should be conducted without the patient having already tried and failed biofeedback.

Neuromodulation
Sacroneuromodilation. Following the report by Matzel and colleagues in 1995 of three patients treated for fecal incontinence by sacroneuromodulation, this approach began to be applied to patients with constipation.[10,220,247] Its effectiveness for incontinence and the technique, possible modes of action, and clinical results are described in Chapter 16.

Early reports of sacroneuromodulation for constipation include case reports and small series in which it became clear that some patients responded in the short and some in the intermediate term.[84,165,166,212] In a study of 19 patients with constipation, improvement was reported in 42%.[134]

The most important evaluation of sacroneuromodulation for constipation is the prospective multicenter European trial, which recruited 62 patients who had failed to respond to medical treatment and biofeedback.[149] Forty-five exhibited a positive peripheral nerve evaluation and thus went on to permanent implantation. Not only did bowel frequency and symptoms of evacuation difficulty improve, but abdominal symptoms of pain and bloating did also. Thus, the number of days of pain per week experienced by the patient fell from 5 (0–7) to 1.7 (0–7) and those for bloating from 5.7 (0–7) to 2.3 (0–7). The Cleveland Clinic Constipation Score (maximum 30 points) fell from 18 (11–27) to 10 (2–22), and the patients' visual analogue score rose from 8 (0–100) to 66 (11–100). There were improvements in frequency of defecation from 2.3 (0–20) times per week to 6.6 (1–16), time in the toilet fell from 10.5 (2.4–60) minutes to 5.7 (1–31), and the percentage of successful defecations followed by a sense of incomplete evacuation fell from 71% to 45%.

Several authors have demonstrated an increase in the rate of colonic transit after sacroneuromodulation for severe constipation.[66,67] This action is unlikely to be the only factor resulting in the clinical improvement as discussed in Chapter 16. In practice today, a patient who has not responded to medical or behavioral treatment should be considered for neuromodulation before contemplating a more invasive procedure.

Posterior Tibial Neuromodulation. There are now some preliminary data on this form of neuromodulation for constipation. In pilot study of 18 (17 females) patients, twelve 30-minute sessions were given over several weeks. The Cleveland Clinic score fell significantly from 18 (10–24) to 14 (7–22), and the patient assessment of constipation quality-of-life (PAC-QoL) score also improved.[60] A modest objective gain may be considered satisfactory by the patient.

Irrigation

Irrigation, either antegrade or retrograde, has also been used for the treatment of both incontinence and constipation. This has been described in Chapter 16. Retrograde irrigation has been made easier for self-administration by the development of closed systems. A rectal balloon can be used (Peristeen anal irrigation system; Coloplast A/S, Kokkedal, Denmark or Mallinckrodt, St. Louis, MO; see Figure 16-23), or a cone-shaped colostomy tip may be employed (Coloplast A/S, Humlebæk, Denmark; Qufora irrigation system; Allerød, Denmark; or Biotrol irrimatic pump; Braun; see Figure 31-25).

Antegrade. Access of antegrade irrigation is achieved via an appendicostomy (see Figure 16-23),[185,211,266,290] via a colonic conduit (see Figure 16-24),[137] or the sigmoid colon via a percutaneous endoscopic colostomy (PEC).[13,61,126,205] Successful medium-term irrigation results with this last procedure were achieved in 73% of 92 patients, but there were serious side effects, including peritonitis in up to 10% of cases. Furthermore, the dropout rate was high. Late erosion with perforation can also occur.

Retrograde. Retrograde irrigation is safer and has achieved "success" in 57% of 113 patients, but again, the dropout rate was high in some reports (ranging from 8% to 70%).[48,62,106,177] This has been demonstrated further by Chan and colleagues.[50] They reported the outcome of irrigation in 50 of 60 patients with constipation who attended follow-up (83%). Half had stopped irrigating. This was attributed to failure of improvement in symptoms; 7 ultimately underwent some form of surgery. The conclusion from these reports is that irrigation should be discussed with the patient. Retrograde irrigation appears preferable to antegrade, and the patient will need encouragement from the nurse/therapist to persist. The chance of success over 1 to 2 years appears to be about 50%. For those with spinal cord injury or spina bifida, the reader is referred to Chapter 16. The concept of the value of irrigation has also been reviewed by Tod and colleagues.[343]

Surgery

Since the last edition of this text, the use of surgery for constipation has declined markedly. Whether this is an entirely beneficial occurrence is a matter of debate, but there can be no question that fewer operations for constipation are performed in most units today compared with 10 years ago. To some extent, this is because the intermediate results of surgery are now known. First, there is significant morbidity, especially small bowel obstruction.[261,381] Although stool frequency and laxative consumption decrease in approximately 70% of patients, this effect may last for only a few years or less. In addition, about 10% of patients experience frequency, sometimes with urgency incontinence. Moreover, abdominal symptoms, such as pain and bloating, are often not improved, unlike with neuromodulation. Another reason for the reduced application of colectomy is the demonstration of the efficacy in many cases of neuromodulation. In Europe, it has become the first choice for an invasive treatment when the patient continues to be symptomatic despite medical and behavioral treatment.

There has clearly been considerable case selection in the studies reporting the results of surgery. In a series of 228 patients with constipation, 111 (38%) had a normal proctogram.[330] Of these, 21 had delayed transit of whom 18 underwent a total colectomy with ileorectal anastomosis. Of these patients, 19 had excellent function at 2 years. The authors suggested that using proctography to exclude those with a defecation disorder improved the case selection and the results of surgery. Similar evidence of case selection was apparent in a series of 277 patients (43 subtotal colectomy [STC], 38 colectomy),[261] and in another of 403 patients (STC 50, colectomy 50).[263] "Success" after colectomy ranged from 80% to 100% in three series, which together included approximately 200 patients.[261,263,330] When, however, the duration of follow-up was taken into account, 22 of 44 patients followed for 38 (3 to 168) months had relief of constipation as determined by frequency of defecation, but 6 had some degree of incontinence, 5 were still constipated, 17 had diarrhea, 30 still had pain, and 12 were still taking laxatives.[153] In another series of 54 patients followed for 42 months (range, 3 to 81), 6 experienced incontinence, 14 constipation, 2 diarrhea, 27 pain, and 5 continued laxative administration.[202] In a recent report from the Cleveland Clinic of 69 patients who underwent colectomy between 1983 and 1998, 11 (16%) developed early and 32 (46%) late complications.[381] Thirty-five out of a possible 64 responded to a questionnaire, which showed that abdominal, pelvic, and rectal pain were present in 13, 10, and 11 patients; bloating in 23 (66%); and nausea in 13 (37%). Nevertheless, 27 (77%) expressed satisfaction with the operation, although social function and mental vitality were low. In a report from the Mayo Clinic of 104 patients with STC treated by colectomy with ileorectal anastomosis at a median interval of 11 years previously, data were available on 85.[121] Constipation resolved in 98%, and 85% of patients were satisfied. Fifty-nine patients responded to a questionnaire. All reported improved frequency of defecation, and 83% were not taking any medication. The KESS score improved significantly. Restorative proctocolectomy has been used by our unit in highly selected patients.[250]

In an important paper, Redmond and colleagues used scintigraphy to distinguish between patients with colonic inertia and those with a generalized intestinal motility disorder in which gastric emptying as well as colonic transit was impaired. "Success" after colectomy was reported in 90% of 21 individuals with colonic inertia alone compared with 16% of 16 patients with generalized intestinal dysmotility.[279] It appears then that case selection based on proctography and scintigraphy may improve the results of surgery, but there remain disadvantages for the patient. These may have to be accepted in the uncommon individual who continues to have disabling symptoms despite medical, behavioral, and neurostimulatory treatment. The subject has been usefully reviewed by Levitt and colleagues.[195]

Dilated Bowel
Aganglionosis

Hirschsprung's Disease. Hirschsprung's disease was described in 1887 (see Chapter 3).[132] It occurs in 1 in 5,000 births and is four times more common in boys than girls. The clinical picture is due to a physiologic intestinal obstruction caused by lack of ganglion cells in the distal large bowel. The affected segment becomes spastic, causing failure of the normal transmission of stool. This results in constipation proximal to the aganglionic segment. This can vary in extent from the lowest part of the rectum (ultrashort segment) to any distance more proximally. Agangliosis of the entire large bowel is very rare; in most cases, the segment does not extend beyond

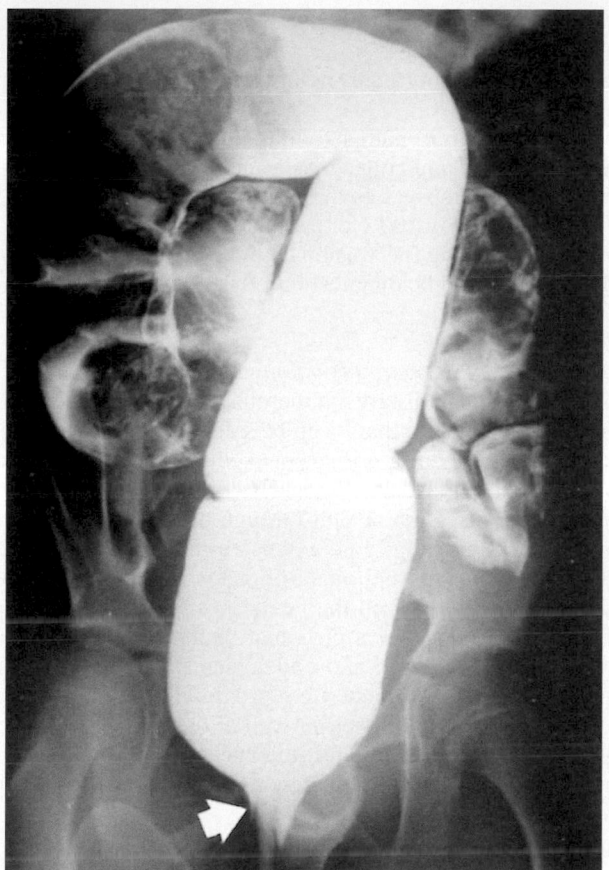

FIGURE 20-12. Short-segment Hirschsprung's disease is confirmed by the abrupt change in caliber from the normal-appearing distal rectum (*arrow*) to the dilated proximal bowel.

the rectosigmoid junction. It seems that the spastic segment can also occur above a normal distal rectum. There has been a case report of narrowing at the rectosigmoid junction with dilatation of the colon above and a normal rectum with a normal rectoanal inhibitory reflex (RAIR) below.[379]

In most cases, the diagnosis is made shortly after birth when there is failure to pass meconium in the first 24 to 48 hours of life. Depending on the extent of the aganglionic segment, the infant may be initially treated by repeated digital examination, laxatives, and enemas. If the aganglionic segment is long, medical management is not possible, and relief of obstruction by surgery will be necessary. Sometimes, the disease does not present early but may become apparent in childhood or even in adulthood. Hirschsprung's disease presenting in infancy is discussed in Chapter 3 (Pediatric Surgical Problems). It is noteworthy, however, that many of those who are treated in infancy continue to have intestinal symptoms into childhood and adult life.[139]

LATE-PRESENTATION HIRSCHSPRUNG'S DISEASE. Adult or late-onset Hirschsprung's disease is very uncommon, and yet it seems to command a place of importance beyond its frequency in clinical practice. Many articles in the literature are case reports or small case series. Doodnath and Puri, in a review of the English language literature between 1950 and 2009, found only 490 cases (341 males [70%]) of late-onset Hirschsprung's disease.[70] Of these, only 8 (1.6%) had extension of aganglionosis beyond the rectosigmoid. Nearly 80% had disease confined to

the rectum, and involvement to the rectosigmoid was present on only 12%. Major surgery was performed in approximately 80% of cases, and only 9% underwent myectomy.

It is likely that the more severe cases are treated in infancy. When Hirschsprung's disease presents in childhood or adulthood, the condition is often mild with short-segment involvement of 2 or 3 cm of the distal rectum. "Late-onset" Hirschsprung's disease is a misnomer because, being congenital, the disease has *always* been there. The late presentation is due to the interval during which the propulsive activity of the large bowel begins to become decompensated, owing to the chronic distal resistance to evacuation. The history will reveal constipation from birth in most cases.[112]

MANIFESTATIONS. Udassin and colleagues reported 39 children who underwent treatment for Hirschsprung's disease.[347] The authors distinguished the mild from the severe form on clinical grounds. In the former situation, patients were constipated, had abdominal distension, and exhibited soiling with stool in the rectum. The onset of symptoms tended to be late. In the severe form, the rectal ampulla was empty, soiling did not occur, and symptoms usually developed within the first month of life. Barnes and coworkers analyzed 65 patients and suggested that two subgroups with Hirschsprung's disease could be distinguished: one with onset of symptoms in childhood and the other developing after 10 years of age, often in adulthood.[17] Distinguishing features, according to the authors, were that fecal soiling was virtually universal in the former but rare in the latter, and that medical treatment was successful in most patients with early onset disease but unsuccessful in those with development later in life.

DIAGNOSIS. The diagnosis is based on the clinical, radiographic, manometric, and histologic studies. Contrast radiology in the form of a barium enema may demonstrate a short-segment involvement (Figure 20-12), or the spastic segment may extend more proximally (Figure 20-13). Demonstration of a lack of ganglion cells is regarded as diagnostic of the condition (see Figures 3-2 and 3-3). A full-thickness rectal biopsy should be taken, but it should come from a level above the

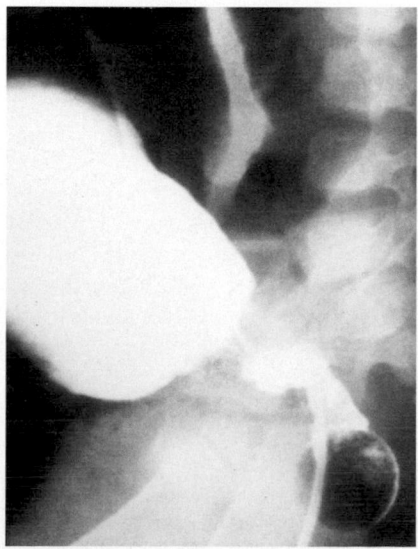

FIGURE 20-13. Hirschsprung's disease. Barium enema examination showing spastic segment in the rectum with dilatation of the proximal bowel.

anal canal because ganglion cells are not present in the internal sphincter. Ricciardi and colleagues have shown that the distance of physiologic aganglionosis is about 20 mm above the dentate line,[281] and Vorobyov and coworkers measured it to be 24 mm (range, 7.5 to 50).[356]

Absence of the RAIR has been thought to be diagnostic of Hirschsprung's disease, but failure of relaxation of the internal sphincter with rectal distension is not necessarily diagnostic, especially in instances of severe, long-standing, idiopathic constipation.[237] The reflex may also be apparently absent if resting anal canal pressure is low. False-positive readings may be obtained. It was weakly present in 36% of 90 patients with Hirschsprung's disease reported by Vorobyov and colleagues.[356]

Acetylcholinesterase histochemistry has been shown to be accurate for the diagnosis of Hirschsprung's disease especially in children and can obviate the need for a full-thickness rectal biopsy under a general anesthetic. Ikawa and colleagues achieved a 99% diagnostic accuracy, compared with a 61% rate using routine staining with hematoxylin and eosin.[140] A reliable diagnosis, even in adults, can be achieved by means of suction rectal biopsy and histochemical detection of acetylcholinesterase activity in the nerve fibers of the lamina propria and muscularis mucosae,[107] although others have found its diagnostic accuracy to be less than 90%.[356] Immunocytochemical staining using antibodies to neuron-specific enolase and S-100 protein has also been used,[115] as has been staining for neurofilament proteins that identify the hyperplastic axon bundles.[170] Moore and associates showed the absence of nitric oxide synthase–containing neurons in two of three patients with the disease.[240]

In a report of 90 patients with adult Hirschsprung's disease, Vorobyov and colleagues found that examination of a full-thickness biopsy was the most reliable investigation.[356] It was diagnostic in 100% of patients compared with anticholinesterase staining (86%), and absent RAIR in 64%. Barium enema was felt to be diagnostic in 84%.

Treatment

Anal Myectomy. *Anorectal myectomy* has been recommended for short-segment disease. Numerous reports have been published demonstrating that it can be safely and simply used in children, not only as a primary procedure for short-segment involvement but also as a secondary operation after a failed low anterior resection or pull-through procedure. Anorectal myectomy is essentially an extensive internal anal sphincterectomy. The internal anal sphincter is divided, or ideally, partially excised, in the lateral position from the level of the dentate line, for a proximal distance of 8 to 10 cm (Figure 20-14). Nissan and colleagues advise incising the mucosa transversely about 1 cm proximal to the mucocutaneous junction on the posterior wall of the anal canal.[253] The mucosa is elevated, and a full-thickness strip of muscularis, including the internal sphincter, is removed as proximally as possible.

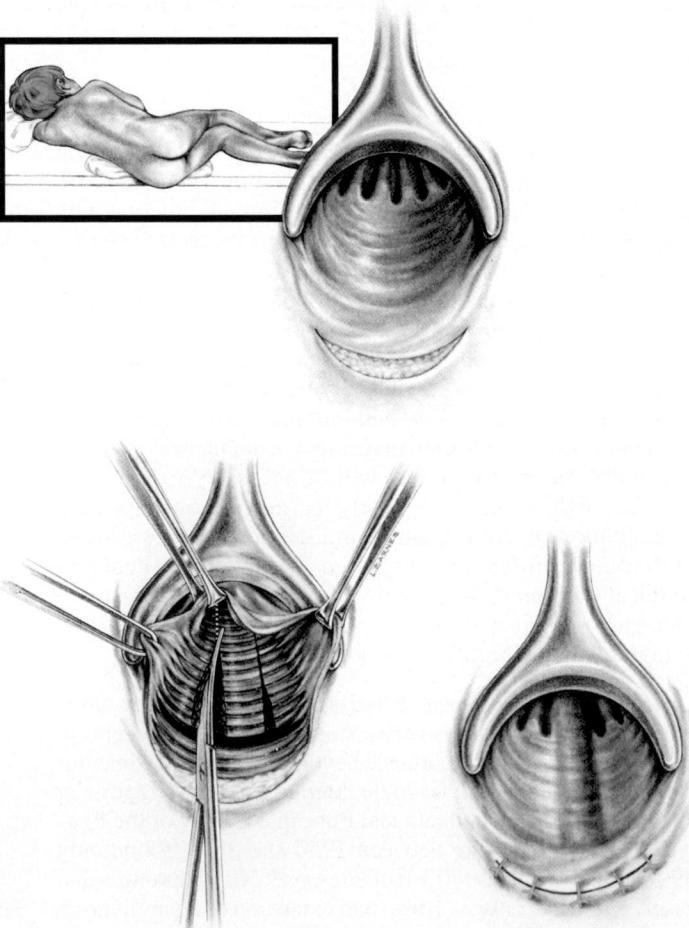

FIGURE 20-14. Treatment of short-segment Hirschsprung's disease by anorectal myectomy. **A:** Child in the left lateral position with an incision made outside the anal verge. **B:** Internal anal sphincterectomy performed for at least 8 cm, incorporating the muscularis propria of the rectum. **C:** Primary wound closure.

RESULTS. Udassin and coworkers described 30 children treated by a modification of internal anal sphincterectomy.[347] Their mean age at diagnosis was 6 years, and more than two-thirds were boys. Four of the 30 patients subsequently required a Duhamel operation. At long-term follow-up, 27 patients were essentially asymptomatic, 7 had a good result, and the result was equivocal in 1. Thomas and colleagues reported 11 patients with chronic constipation but without evidence of a long aganglionic segment on barium enema.[338] They performed a sphincterotomy and rectomyectomy through a posterior approach. Four of the 11 patients had previously undergone a Swenson procedure. The results were mixed and greatly depended on the length of the aganglionic segment—the shorter the segment, the more successful the myectomy.

Lynn and van Heerden reported the Mayo Clinic experience of 37 patients who underwent anorectal myectomy.[206] In 28 patients, myectomy was the definitive procedure; 20 had an excellent result, 6 were improved, and 2 were unchanged. Of the 4 patients who had had a previous operation, 3 had an excellent result and 1 was improved. Others have shown that anorectal myectomy is effective for older children with Hirschsprung's disease.[297] Yoshioka and Keighley reported 29 patients who underwent anorectal myectomy for Hirschsprung's disease.[377] None had been able to defecate spontaneously more than once a week. All had two of three features suggesting a diagnosis of "outlet obstruction." This included failure to expel a rectal balloon containing 80 mL of air, increased electrical activity of the puborectalis on attempted defecation, and failure to evacuate contrast during proctography. Following anorectal myectomy, 62% were able to eliminate spontaneously more than three times per week. There was a significant fall in maximum resting anal pressure after operation in those who had had a good result, but not in those who had not. The authors also performed a randomized trial comparing anorectal myectomy with a standard anal dilatation.[378] No patient was able to evacuate spontaneously prior to the procedure, but 7 of the 13 who underwent myectomy were able to do so more than three times a week, compared with none after anal dilatation ($P < .05$). Other reports from the same institution involving 63 patients revealed improvement in only 31%.[264,265] The results were independent of preoperative colonic transit or histologic evidence of aganglionosis.

Abdominal Resection. Once the colon has become very dilated and where the aganglionic segment is longer than a few centimeters, anorectal myectomy is no longer indicated, and a more extensive resection is needed. Of the many techniques described, all include a close rectal dissection in which the rectum is mobilized, dividing the blood vessels at their point of entry into the bowel muscular wall in order to avoid damage to the pelvic nerves. In their review of the literature from 1950 to 2009, Doodnath and Puri reported that 47% of the 490 cases had had a Duhamel procedure, 10% Swenson, 8% Soave, 6% low anterior resection, and 9% myomectomy only.[70] These operations all have one aim in common, which is to bring normally innervated bowel down to the upper anal canal. They differ in the mode of reconstruction, however. It should be remembered that these procedures were described in an era before the common use of low anastomosis, either hand-sutured coloanal or stapled.

The *Duhamel procedure*,[72] with or without a temporary proximal stoma,[204,249] has the advantage of being able to deal with a considerable discrepancy in size between the ganglionic and aganglionic segments. But when proximal dilatation is not marked, a low anterior resection with coloanal anastomosis is probably the operation of choice for the late form of the disease because surgeons are familiar with this procedure. The operation can be performed with or without an intervening pouch.[317] In patients with gross dilatation of the colon, some have recommended a two-stage strategy by which an initial operation is carried out to defunction the colon in order to allow it to recover its normal caliber. Once this has occurred, an abdominal restorative resection with distal anastomosis can be undertaken. If diversion is required, the stoma should always be made to the right of the middle colic vessels to avoid any damage to the marginal artery and vein. An ileostomy is preferred to that of a proximal transverse colostomy by most surgeons. Ricketts and Pettitt make several suggestions concerning technique when applied to adolescents and adults.[282] These include the use of rectal tube decompression. This may facilitate bowel preparation. Several applications of the linear stapler is advised to divide fully the septum between the aganglionic rectum anteriorly and the normal colon posteriorly (see Figure 3-9).

The Swenson[331] and Soave[312] operations as well as endoanal pull-through[36] are rarely performed in adults. The functional results may not be satisfactory.[238] These procedures may now be considered obsolete in the older individual, owing to the availability of low anterior resection in patients with a colon of near-normal caliber. An ileal pouch-anal anastomosis is a possible alternative but only in the rare patient with aganglionosis extending into the colon.

Fishbein and colleagues reported a series of eight adult patients with lifelong refractory constipation successfully treated by rectal myectomy, alone or in combination with anterior resection.[79] Bowel resection was performed when there was a more extensive aganglionic section, but the sphincterectomy limited the amount of pelvic dissection.

There are a few reports of larger series in the literature. Elliot and Todd of St. Mark's Hospital reviewed 39 adults with Hirschsprung's disease who were managed by the Duhamel procedure; all but 2 of whom gave a history of constipation since birth.[74] Thirty-six (92%) were believed to have had an excellent functional result. McCready and Beart reported the Mayo Clinic experience of surgery on 50 adult patients with so-called Hirschsprung's disease.[225] Numerous operations were employed including the Swenson procedure, anorectal myectomy, and a variety of bowel resections. Although morbidity was low, there was a high failure rate (38%). In the large series of 90 patients reported by Vorobyov and colleagues of the State Scientific Centre of Coloproctology, Moscow, a Duhamel procedure was performed in 91%. Complications occurred in 20 (22%) patients, 13 of whom required reoperation.[356] At a follow-up of nearly 6 years, 82% were said to have a good and 15% a satisfactory result. Wu and coworkers found that adult patients did not seem to benefit from anorectal myectomy.[375] However, those who underwent resection with a conventional anal anastomosis had excellent function. Wheatley and colleagues reviewed the literature in 199 patients with adult Hirschsprung's disease.[368] Even with a comprehensive assessment of this rare condition, no statistically significant differences could be determined because of the variety of procedures employed and the length of time encompassed by the study.

It is evident that there is no obvious best choice of operation for short-segment or adult Hirschsprung's disease, but anorectal myectomy, with or without low anterior resection; the endorectal pull-through; and the Duhamel procedure are all associated with reasonable long-term results.[368] Because untreated short-segment disease inevitably leads to intractable symptoms and to megacolon, it is wise to recommend surgery as soon as the diagnosis is confirmed.[204]

Chagas' Disease (See Chapter 33)
Idiopathic Megabowel

There is a group of patients with dilatation of the rectum or colon or both in whom there is no evident mechanical cause.[96] The condition is likely to occur in childhood but occasionally appears in adolescence for the first time. It is uncommon.[87] There were only 20 of 1,600 patients referred to a large teaching hospital over a 10-year period.[175] It may prove, however, that the condition is more prevalent but is not well recognized in some instances.[95,354,360]

Diagnosis. In many cases, dilatation of the bowel may be clinically obvious, but if not, it is likely to be demonstrated by plain and contrast radiography. In one of the first studies to examine this condition, Preston and colleagues[271] reported that a rectal dimension of 6.5 cm at the pelvic inlet was diagnostic, whereas in a more recent study, Gladman and coworkers, using volumetric distension of the rectum with simulated stool, defined idiopathic megarectum as a diameter of 8.3 cm.[95] Estimations by contrast radiography may underestimate the diameter of the bowel if the instillation pressure is too low or through the introduction of too little contrast.[76]

Estimation of the maximal tolerable volume (MTV) upon inflation of a balloon in the rectum has been used to diagnose megarectum.[308] The condition may be associated with rectal hyposensitivity. The position of the balloon is important. If it rides up into the colon, then the MTV may be lower, thereby giving a false reading.[208] Gladman and colleagues have recently reported a technique for the diagnosis of idiopathic megarectum in which the rectal diameter was measured at the minimal distension pressure of the rectum by the use of a barostat. A diameter up to 6.3 cm was within the normal range, with megarectum therefore being inferred at a diameter beyond this limit.[95]

Idiopathic megarectum is distinguished from Hirschsprung's disease by the presence of soiling, the absence of evident constipation at birth, the patulous anal sphincter, the dilated rectum, and the presence of the anorectal inhibition reflex. The rectal dilatation goes right down to the anorectal junction with no hint of a constricted segment (Figure 20-15).

Etiology

HISTOLOGIC CHANGES. The etiology of this condition is unknown. Many authors have reported histologic abnormalities, but these are variable and inconsistent, and it is not possible to say whether any change is primary or secondary. Several studies have reported no abnormality of the enteric nervous system,[26,230,311,317] whereas others have reported variable changes in the chemical composition of neurons.[86] Fibrosis in smooth muscle has been reported.[230] Two studies have noted decreased density of the ICC,[190] but this was not found by others.[230]

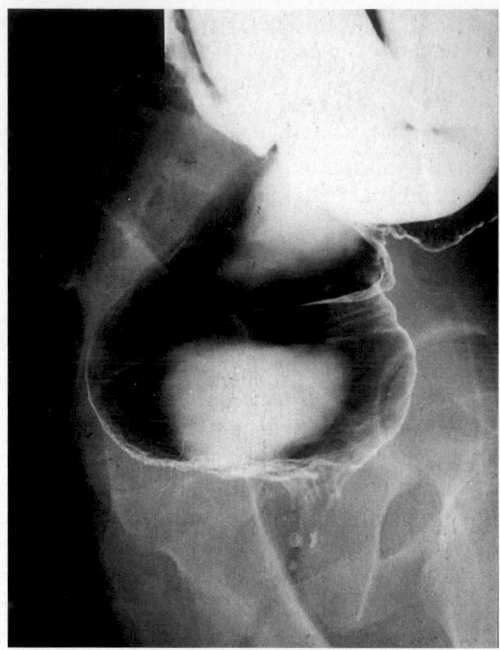

FIGURE 20-15. Idiopathic megabowel showing rectal distension to the level of the anorectal junction.

PHYSIOLOGIC ABNORMALITIES. Motor and sensory abnormalities have also been reported. There are several studies showing hypomotility[258] and impaired rectal evacuation.[87,99] Delayed colonic transit has been demonstrated.[88,371] Anal pressure is normal unless there is fecal impaction of the rectum. However, if this triggers the RAIR, anal pressure will be reduced.

Sensory testing of the rectum usually by balloon inflation uniformly demonstrates an apparent reduction in rectal sensitivity, with abnormally large volumes being required before the presence of the balloon is perceived. Barostat estimation of compliance appears to identify two groups of patient with megarectum: one with normal, the other with increased compliance.[94] These authors speculate that the former may follow rectal hyposensitivity, thus resulting in gradual distension of the rectum through chronic fecal filling.

CAUSATION. Some authors have asserted that the condition is acquired through poor defecation training in early childhood, perhaps combined with voluntary fecal retention through withholding of stool. This, it is argued, will lead to dilatation of the rectum with secondary damage to the organ and its regulatory control.[349,371] Others maintain that there is a primary rectal pathology, perhaps neuronal, in which hyposensitivity may result in gradual rectal dilatation.[94] No mutation or deletion of genes that are associated with murine megacolon have been found in families with patients affected with idiopathic megarectum,[172] and there is no consistent evidence for viral infection[85] or autoimmune disease.[51,173]

CLINICAL FEATURES. The condition usually starts in childhood with fecal soiling. This is associated with fecal loading in the rectum, which may present episodically with fecal impaction. Extension of the dilatation more proximally will lead to abdominal distension. Rarely, this may become so extreme that respiration is embarrassed by upward pressure on the diaphragm. The frequency of defecation is usually greatly reduced, sometimes to once every few weeks. Fecal impaction in the rectum or a fecaloma palpated abdominally may be evident (see Figure 20-2). Sigmoid volvulus may occur (see Chapter 28).[59,344] The patient may demonstrate a behavioral disorder, and there may be psychological tensions within the family.

Treatment

MEDICAL MANAGEMENT. The initial aim must be to treat the patient conservatively. In the child, careful assessment of one's psychological and social relationships should be made. It may be necessary to seek the advice of a child psychiatrist.

Management of the bowel disorder includes attempts with the help of the parents to establish a regular bowel habit with the aid of enemas or suppositories. Manual disimpaction may be required intermittently.

Even if medical treatment improves the frequency of defecation and soiling, the rectum is likely to remain dilated.[97] Moreover, there is little information in the literature on the effectiveness of medical treatment. O'Súilleabháin and colleagues described a series of 28 patients, mean age 21 years (range, 4 to 71), who were treated by laxatives and enemas for 6 months.[258] At the end of this period, 8 (28%) had responded successfully. Two were lost to follow-up and 1 died, leaving 17 patients who underwent surgery. In an article on the treatment of idiopathic megabowel, Kamm and Stabile do not give figures on the success of medical treatment, but they recommend magnesium sulfate as the most suitable laxative.[157]

SURGERY. The literature on surgery for idiopathic megabowel includes only small numbers of patients. Moreover, the preoperative assessment and quality of follow-up are often wanting. Owing to the infrequency of surgery for the condition, there are no examples of comparative trials. The results of any report should therefore be interpreted with caution. In a useful review, Gladman and colleagues reported the outcome from 27 published studies.[98] The quality of the submissions was poor; most were case series, and there were no comparative studies. The median number of patients per study was 12 (3 to 50), and the follow-up was 3 years (0.5 to 7).

Surgery aims either to remove the rectum or the colon. In the review, rectal procedures were said to be followed by success in about 70% of patients, but there was a high mortality (3% to 25%) and morbidity (6% to 29%), with early postoperative sepsis noted especially in patients having a coloanal anastomosis, including the Duhamel procedure. One might note a different experience if the surgery was performed today, but nevertheless, it is clear that this operation is no trivial undertaking.

In patients having a colonic resection, whether total or segmental, success rates were approximately 70% and 50%, respectively.[98] Subtotal colectomy was successful in 71.1% (0% to 100%) but was associated with significant morbidity related to small bowel obstruction (14.5%, range 0% to 29%). Kamm and Stabile reported 40 patients treated by subtotal colectomy, of whom 80% achieved normal bowel frequency with a high degree of relief of bloating and soiling.[157] There was a suggestion that total colectomy achieved better results than colectomy with cecorectal anastomosis or sigmoid colectomy. Segmental resection was successful in 48.4% (12.5% to 100%), and recurrent symptoms were common (23.8%).[98] Restorative proctocolectomy has been used for this indication with about a 70% success.[321]

All 17 of the 28 patients who did not respond to medical treatment reported by O'Súilleabháin and colleagues underwent a full-thickness biopsy.[258] Two improved simply by this procedure alone, leaving 15 who underwent major surgery. Thirteen had a "satisfactory" result by means of proctectomy with coloanal anastomosis, restorative proctocolectomy, or conventional proctocolectomy.

The Duhamel operation was associated with high morbidity. Stabile and associates reported a series of 20 patients undergoing this procedure over a 17-year period.[316] Three developed pelvic sepsis, 5 fecal fistula, and 1 rectovaginal fistula. Improvement in well-being and frequency of defecation was experienced in 10 patients. Vertical reduction rectoplasty resulted in benefit in 70% of 10 patients who underwent this procedure.[371]

In summary, many surgical options have been tried with variable results. Complications are indeed frequent. Patients should therefore be selected with great care, especially when one considers the small numbers that are reported in the literature.

Pseudoobstruction (Ogilvie's Syndrome)

Pseudoobstruction and Ogilvie's syndrome (see Biography) are terms used to denote a condition in which patients appear to have signs and symptoms suggestive of intestinal

WILLIAM HENEAGE OGILVIE (1887–1971)

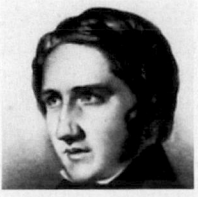

Ogilvie was born in Valparaíso, Chile; his father was an engineer from Dundee, Scotland, who had been in Chile for business reasons. He was educated at Clifton College and New College, Oxford, at which institution he gained first-class honors in physiology. He then entered Guy's Hospital in London for his medical training and obtained his fellowship of the Royal College of Surgeons in 1920. He was one of the very few medical men of his generation who served in three wars: the Balkan War and the two World Wars. He rose to the rank of major general and was the consultant surgeon to the East Africa Force in 1941. One of his most important admonitions was to require the performance of a colostomy for all wounds of the colon. It was for his military service that he was appointed Knight of the British Empire in 1946. He was considered a brilliant essayist and wrote several books, which provide some of the finest medical writing. He was also responsible for the first two editions of *Recent Advances in Surgery*. Ogilvie developed an international reputation, and many surgeons often visited his theater sessions. Among his many distinctions were honorary fellowships of the Royal College of Surgeons of Canada, the Royal Australasian College of Surgeons, and the American College of Surgeons. (Photograph courtesy of the Royal College of Surgeons of England.)

obstruction without an evident mechanical cause.[255] The differential diagnosis includes Hirschsprung's disease, especially short-segment involvement, toxic megacolon in ulcerative colitis and Crohn's disease, volvulus, fecal impaction, and a distal obstructing lesion.[73,296] Middle-aged males around 60 years old are most often affected.[352]

Etiology

The condition is usually seen in association with other diseases and occasionally complicates the postoperative course of patients after abdominal surgery. The individual is often elderly. Predisposing factors include electrolyte imbalance (potassium, sodium, phosphate, calcium, and magnesium), infection (e.g., Epstein–Barr and cytomegalovirus), organ failure (including renal, pulmonary, and cardiac), trauma such as operative (e.g., following orthopedic joint replacement), malignancy (such as small cell carcinoma), drugs, collagen diseases (scleroderma and disseminated lupus), and autoimmune disorders.[73] In a retrospective series of 400 patients, trauma, infection, and cardiac disease were the clinical associations in 11%, 10%, and 10%, respectively.[352] Those with pseudoobstruction can therefore present with a virtual textbook of medical and surgical ills.[7,9,14,102,200,234,246,256,278,320,333]

Pathophysiology

The condition may be associated with myogenic and neurogenic factors. In theory, there may be an autonomic imbalance of parasympathetic and sympathetic control.[219,318] The fasting migrating motor complex showed abnormal bursts of activity in a study in children.[362] There is some evidence of a diminution in the number of ICC.[141] ICC may be activated by nitric oxide (NO) to cause relaxation of smooth muscle fibers.[351] In pseudoobstruction, there is evidence that there is increased nitric oxide synthase activity, which results in increased production of nitric oxide.[361] Other possible factors include alpha-actin deficiency[176,305] and autoimmune disease, with the presence of antineuronal and anticalcium antibodies.[306]

In a communication of more than 20 years ago, pseudoobstruction was reported in 10% of patients following renal transplantation.[323] When this occurs, there is a small (5%) but very real chance of colonic perforation (see Chapter 27). Visceral myopathy may be a cause of pseudoobstruction. When this occurs, the pathology is in the myocytes, with atrophy leading to weakness. This situation may also be found in collagen disorders.[314]

Other factors including the underlying disease contribute to the development of the dilatation. Impairment of electrical activity of the intestine as well as a defect in intestinal motility may be precipitated by numerous intrinsic and extrinsic agents, such as secretin, glucagon, epinephrine, anticholinergics, and prostaglandins. Ravo and associates believed that involvement of the sacral parasympathetic nerve supply to the colon may be the explanation for the syndrome.[278] In an attempt to identify the functional abnormalities in the bowel and anal canal, Loening-Baucke and colleagues compared measurements of motility and anorectal pressure in 11 patients with pseudoobstruction with an equal number of control subjects.[197] Motility in the lower bowel was decreased, and rectal wall elasticity was increased, but no specific neural or muscular morphologic defect was identified in colonic transmural pathologic sections in individuals without preexisting colonic disease. Krishnamurthy and coworkers analyzed the clinical, radiographic, manometric, and pathologic features of 26 women with severe idiopathic constipation.[184] They identified an abnormality of the myenteric plexus that could be distinguished from the one described in intestinal pseudoobstruction. Koch and colleagues found that this condition was often associated with decreased colonic concentrations of vasoactive intestinal peptide.[178]

Clinical Features

The presenting features of pseudoobstruction are abdominal distension, with or without abdominal pain or constipation. Diarrhea can occasionally occur. The condition may present in the immediate postoperative period in elderly patients usually with comorbidity. If mild, the condition may resolve spontaneously, but in most cases, it does not. The distension can be massive. This can lead to cecal perforation, a complication that may occur in up to 15% of patients.

Diagnosis

The distinction between pseudoobstruction and mechanical obstruction is usually obvious.[309] But the need to exclude a mechanical obstruction means that pseudoobstruction is basically a radiologic diagnosis. CT will show the massively dilated bowel (Figure 20-16), but this is often demonstrated clearly by a plain abdominal x-ray. Endoscopy and contrast studies are necessary to confirm that there is no mechanical cause, but one must take care not to aggravate the condition by overinflation.

Pseudoobstruction should be suspected if it develops while the patient is in the hospital for another problem, whether surgical or nonsurgical. An antecedent history of colonic pseudoobstruction is a helpful clue. Chronic intestinal pseudoobstruction may be recurrent. The patient is often cachectic, with hypoactive or absent bowel sounds and a mildly tender, grossly distended abdomen.

In clinical practice, a patient with suspected pseudoobstruction should be considered for undergoing a water-soluble contrast enema.[376] This has a high chance of demonstrating the absence of mechanical obstruction. If this assessment reveals no obstruction, then careful colonoscopy should be carried out to examine the large bowel mucosa and to hopefully permit decompression. CT is unlikely to yield additional information, but in current practice, it is likely to be requested. Only if there is mechanical pathology proximal to the colon will it be likely to add to the diagnosis.

Treatment

Conservative Management. Initial management is medical, but as mentioned, it should include an attempt at decompression. Insertion of a rectal tube is an option, but if not effective, colonoscopy is the best means to accomplish this. Treatment includes nutritional support, rehydration, electrolyte replacement, the suppression of bacterial overgrowth, and the improvement of intestinal motility by prokinetics. Specific problems, such as infection, should be treated. Any underlying cause (e.g., endocrine) should be addressed. A nasogastric is advisable, and constipating drugs should be stopped. These measures may result in spontaneous resolution of the condition. Sloyer and colleagues, in an experience of 25 patients with pseudoobstruction, reported that all but one were successfully treated conservatively and by gentle attempts to decompress the bowel by enema, rectal tube placement, and decrease in narcotics.[309] There was no colonic perforation nor any obstruction-related death.

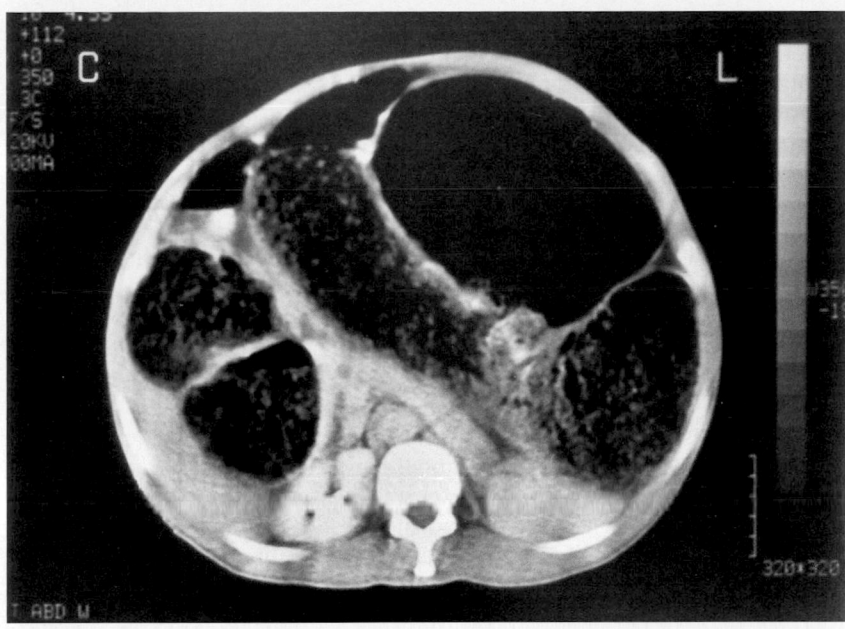

FIGURE 20-16. Computed tomography demonstrates a massively dilated colon. There is no evidence of perforation. Although not diagnostic, the radiologic picture is consistent with Ogilvie's syndrome.

Colonoscopy. Colonoscopy combines diagnosis with therapy. Most authorities regard colonic decompression by colonoscopy as the most effective treatment for selected patients.[35,40,89,103,285,325,352] The success rate is about 80%.[4]

Care should be taken to visualize the lumen adequately and to insufflate minimal volumes of air. Safety and ease of passage are facilitated by using carbon dioxide instead of air, or a water instillation system instead of gas.[241,245] A tap water enema of about 1,000 mL may be instilled prior to the procedure in order to allow the stool in the distal bowel to be aspirated.[245] Burke and Shellito advocate the use of a larger, flexible, fenestrated overtube (C tube), which permits continuous decompression after passage of a single-channel colonoscope.[41] This theoretically avoids the requirement for repeated colonoscopy for recurrent symptoms. Others have placed a catheter or have positioned a guidewire through the colonoscope and threaded the catheter over the guidewire.[30,58,232] Many endoscopists contend that the procedure is safer and easier than would be anticipated, perhaps because the colon is already dilated and filled with gas. Successful decompression should be verified by an abdominal radiograph.[262] Unresolved cecal distension greater than 12 cm may warrant operative decompression in order to limit the risk of perforation.[218] In a review of 400 patients, Vanek and Al-Salti correlated increased patient age, maximal cecal diameter, and delay in initiating colonic decompression with increased mortality.[352]

Strodel and colleagues reviewed 44 patients who underwent 52 colonoscopic examinations for colonic ileus.[325] In approximately a quarter, the condition developed during convalescence from recent surgery, whereas two-thirds had major systemic disorders. The mean cecal diameter before colonoscopy was approximately 13 cm. Based on radiographic or clinical criteria, 38 patients (86%) underwent successful decompression on the initial colonoscopic examination; perforation of the cecum occurred in 1 individual. The authors advocate at least one attempt at colonoscopic decompression before performing laparotomy or cecostomy. Vanek and Al-Salti performed colonoscopic decompression of 125 patients with a success rate of 82%

and a recurrence rate of 22%.[352] Bode and colleagues decompressed the colon in 20 of 22 patients (91%) by this technique, although 18% experienced a recurrence.[35] Gosche and coworkers noted an 89% rate of success, but 41% required repeated endoscopic decompression during their hospital stay,[103] Jetmore and associates reported a 6% success rate.[142]

Epidural Anesthesia. On the theory that pseudoobstruction is caused by excess sympathetic tone, Lee and colleagues performed splanchnic sympathetic blockade by means of epidural anesthesia in eight patients.[191] The epidural catheter is inserted in the T11–12 interspace and advanced cephalad; 0.25% bupivacaine is used with a loading dose of 5 to 10 mL, followed by continuous infusion at 3 mL/hour. Five of the patients (63%) were managed successfully.[191] Others have used the same technique, but whether this will ultimately prove to be a worthwhile therapeutic option remains to be determined.[219]

Drug Therapy. Drug treatment includes cholinesterase inhibitors, antibiotics, prokinetics, and somatostatin analogues. Neostigmine given intravenously results in rapid decompression through stimulating peristalsis.[64,260] In a randomized controlled trial, 10 of 11 patients who received neostigmine at a dose of 2 mg were successfully managed.[267] Others have reported similar success.[320] The clinician, however, should be aware of the possible side effects. These include cardiac arrhythmia; therefore, the patient should be monitored in the coronary care unit. Antibiotics such as metronidazole or ciprofloxacin will decrease bacterial concentrations, but they will not have a specific effect on colonic motility. This is not the case with prokinetic agents. Erythromycin acts as a motilin antagonist.[198] It may be useful in treating postoperative ileus as well as pseudoobstruction. Emmanuel and colleagues reported success in 40% of 15 consecutive patients.[75] Four of the six responders had a visceral myopathy. Cisapride has also been used but was suspended, owing to its side effects, including cardiac arrhythmia.[207]

Surgery. Surgical treatment is to be avoided if at all possible in these often severely ill patients. Clearly, it should never be performed simply to establish the diagnosis. Only when all reasonable attempts at medical treatment or endoscopic decompression have been implemented should it be considered. Pseudoobstruction is one of the few indications for performing a cecostomy. The operation may be carried out by an open technique or by a laparoscopically guided approach.[71] Percutaneous cecostomy under computed tomographic guidance has also been successfully employed as an alternative,[47] but another option is to perform percutaneous colonoscopic cecostomy.[274] This is analogous to that of percutaneous gastrostomy or colonoscopy.[268,339]

If the bowel is ischemic or perforated, resection with or without anastomosis is required. There is a mortality of more than 40% in those with perforation.[296]

▶ EVACUATION DISORDERS

Constipation may also occur as a result of impaired rectal evacuation. Conditions responsible include prolapsing disorders (see Chapter 21), internal sphincter hypertrophy, and anismus, which may be associated with the solitary rectal ulcer syndrome.

Anismus

Anismus is described as a functional disorder of the pelvic floor muscle in which straining or attempting to defecate leads to muscle contraction instead of relaxation, thereby causing a physiologic outlet obstruction and the inability to defecate.[187] It is an evacuation disorder in which the resistance to emptying of the rectum is due to the spastic action of the pelvic floor musculature. Other terms for the condition include spastic pelvic floor syndrome, paradoxical puborectalis muscle contraction, and obstructed defecation. Kuijpers and Bleijenberg evaluated 12 severely "constipated" individuals by defecography. They demonstrated that the anorectal angle did not increase during straining but remained at 90 degrees (see Figure 20-8).[187] Electromyogram (EMG) studies confirmed persistent contraction during defecation straining. Other authors have demonstrated an abnormal increase in the activity of the sphincter mechanism during evacuation on defecography, simultaneous measurement of the intrarectal pressure, and electrical activity of the external anal sphincter.[372] Jones and colleagues have suggested that paradoxical contraction of the puborectalis muscle is not a specific finding.[144] In their EMG analyses, they observed this phenomenon in patients with the solitary ulcer syndrome and in those with idiopathic perineal pain. Anismus is felt to be part of the solitary rectal ulcer syndrome.

Pathophysiology

The pathophysiology of anismus is poorly understood. It seems that the patient has simply forgotten how to defecate, although clearly, the disturbance is more complex than this. Predisposing or associated factors are often present, including physical and emotional stress, prior anal surgery, prior hysterectomy, and even sigmoidoscopy. Diminished rectal perception as determined by balloon distension has been reported, but its significance is unknown.[105] Rectal compliance has, however, been found to be normal.[104] Fucini and colleagues compared EMG findings with asymptomatic individuals and noted that there was a higher prevalence of coordinated inhibitory patterns in normal subjects and a lower frequency of pubococcygeus muscle inhibition in patients with anismus.[82]

Diagnosis

Most patients with anismus are women. The characteristic complaint is an inability to evacuate by straining. Despite this, the patient does not necessarily report that she or he is "constipated." It has been suggested that obstructed defecation may be diagnosed when two or more of the following symptoms are present: prolonged and unsuccessful straining at stool, a feeling of incomplete evacuation, the requirement for manual assistance, and the regular use of laxatives and enemas.[104]

Physical examination may demonstrate an associated rectocele and increased resting tone. Whether the presence of this anatomic abnormality predisposes to obstructed defecation is a matter of debate.

The balloon expulsion test is a simple and inexpensive method to simulate a patient's ability to expel stool.[25,80] As previously mentioned, cinedefecography (CD) and EMG have also been used to make the diagnosis of obstructed defecation.[148,287] Fleshman and colleagues compared balloon expulsion, defecography, colonic transit times, anal manometry, and EMG in 21 individuals with severe constipation.[80] Twelve were unable to expel a balloon. These investigators concluded that balloon expulsion was the most reliable way to diagnose pelvic floor outlet obstruction resulting from nonrelaxation of the puborectalis muscle.

A prospective study was undertaken by Jorge and colleagues, who assessed the correlation between EMG and CD for the diagnosis of nonrelaxing puborectalis syndrome.[148] Sensitivity, specificity, and predictive values of EMG and CD were considered suboptimal. The authors concluded that a combination of these two tests is suggested in order to make the diagnosis of anismus. Roberts and coworkers believe that the definition of anismus should be based on three criteria: demonstration of puborectalis EMG recruitment of greater than 50%, evidence of an adequate level of intrarectal pressure on straining (greater than 50 cm H_2O), and the presence of defective evacuation.[287]

The diagnosis of obstructed defecation is not difficult to make provided it is considered. Although simple balloon expulsion is very useful, the findings can be objectified through manometry and/or defecography. Figure 20-17 shows paradoxical elevation of the anal pressure when the patient tries to evacuate.

Treatment
Biofeedback
Biofeedback has been applied to patients with obstructed defecation. The aim is to achieve a sphincter response to rectal balloon insufflation to help the patient relax the pelvic floor and to allow expulsion of the balloon.

In one report, 90% of 56 patients were subjectively improved,[133] and others have had similar success in those suffering from anismus.[259] However, Keck and colleagues, at the Lahey Clinic, obtained disappointing results in the treatment of constipation.[163] Among 12 patients, all could be taught to relax the sphincter in response to biofeedback, but only 1 reported resolution of symptoms. McKee and coworkers found that 9 of their 30 patients improved on this regimen.[226] Lestàr and associates noted good improvement using a small volume balloon in an ambulatory method.[194]

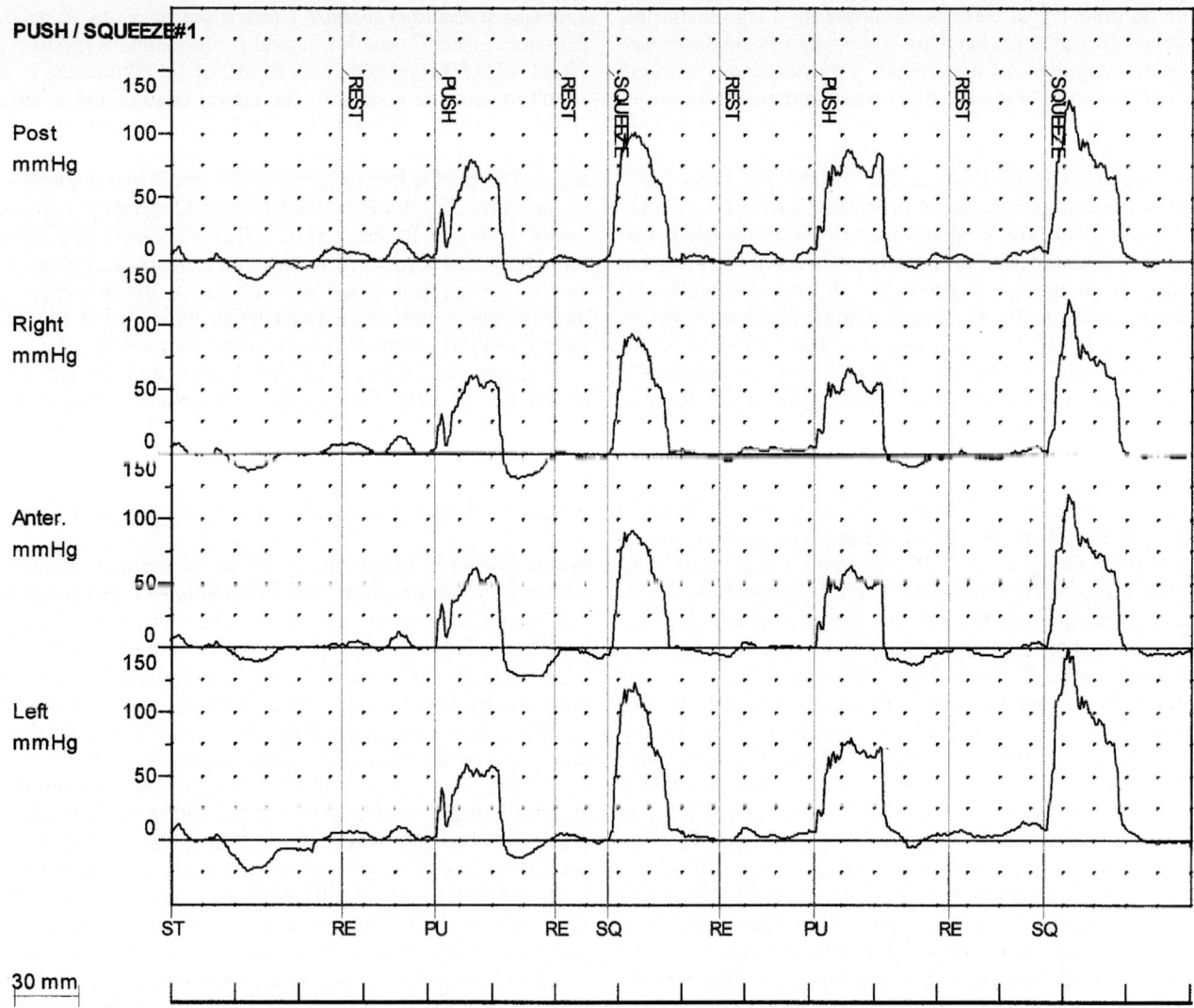

FIGURE 20-17. Paradoxical elevation of anal canal pressure when the patient tries to evacuate. Note that squeeze pressure and "push" pressures are quite similar.

Bleijenberg and Kuijpers reported a treatment regimen of EMG biofeedback followed by simulation of the defecation process by insertion of oatmeal porridge into the rectum.[34] Seven of their 10 patients achieved successful evacuation. Weber and colleagues also found that biofeedback was useful by conditioning the sphincter to relax in the presence of the desire to defecate.[363] Dahl and coworkers treated nine women and five children by means of an EMG biofeedback device connected to an anal probe with considerable success.[63] Kawimbe and colleagues used a self-applied biofeedback device that permitted EMG recording of the external anal sphincter.[162] Biofeedback training was maintained on a domiciliary basis for just over 3 weeks, with marked improvement noted. The clinical benefit persisted after a mean follow-up of more than 6 months.

Wexner and colleagues performed a mean of 8.9 1-hour EMG-based biofeedback sessions on 18 patients.[365] They reported an 89% success rate at a mean length of follow-up of approximately 9 months. Karlbom and associates prospectively studied EMG audiovisual biofeedback and noticed a 43% benefit sustained at 12 months.[160] Battaglia and coworkers reported 50% improvement at 12 months with EMG biofeedback, superior to patients with STC (20%).[23] However,

Loening-Baucke investigated the efficacy of biofeedback in 38 children with anismus and encopresis, with somewhat disappointing results.[196] Biofeedback was completely unsuccessful in approximately 25%, and of the remainder, only one-half recovered from their constipation.

Turnbull and Ritvo used biofeedback from a manometric anal sphincter probe in their patients.[346] Follow-up of up to 4.5 years showed continued improvement in bowel function and abdominal symptoms. Glia and associates compared EMG and manometric biofeedback and found them both equally effective.[100]

Fleshman and colleagues used a fluctuating light bar or an auditory signal.[81] Each day, three training sessions were scheduled in the morning and three in the afternoon. By using an electrode plug, the patient records the muscular activity at rest, during squeeze, and during straining in order to expel the plug. Subsequent sessions are directed toward attempting to control the activity of the sphincter mechanism during straining. A final step is the instillation of 120 mL of psyllium slurry to simulate an actual bowel movement.

The Cleveland Clinic Florida group compared four methods of biofeedback: intra-anal EMG; EMG plus intrarectal balloon; EMG plus home training; and EMG, balloon, and home training.[129] All were associated with a significant improvement in outcome, but there was no significant difference in results regardless of the method. Heymen and coworkers also performed a comprehensive review and meta-analysis of 38 studies in which biofeedback was used for the treatment of constipation.[127] They determined that there were no anatomic, physiologic, or demographic variables that could reasonably assist the physician in predicting success or failure.

It is not clear how long and how often biofeedback sessions are necessary, but all investigators seem to agree that booster treatments are suggested in those individuals who have a relapse. Ideally, training should be performed several times a day for 10 or 15 minutes at a time. This can be accomplished only with a home training device. Unfortunately, despite the availability of often elegant biofeedback devices, the results are less than ideal.

Botulinum Toxin

Joo and coworkers used botulinum toxin type A (BTX-A) for the treatment of anismus (see the discussion of botulinum toxin in Chapter 12).[147] Contingent on body mass, 6 to 15 U of BTX-A were injected bilaterally under EMG guidance into the external sphincter or the puborectalis muscle. Treatment was repeated as necessary for a maximum of three sessions during a 3-month period. Of four individuals who had failed to respond to conventional biofeedback, all improved. There was no morbidity or mortality. The success rate in the longer term was 50%.[147] Maria and colleagues used this approach for four patients, one of whom was lost to follow-up.[215] The results were mixed. The authors indicated that repeated injections may be necessary if clinical improvement is to persist because the drug effect wears off within 3 months. Ron and associates reported an overall satisfaction rate of 58% in their 25 patients but believe that there was a need for a prospective, double-blind study to determine the exact role of this approach.[289] These reports led to its being taken up in several units, and in larger studies, the success rate has been shown to be around 50% (Table 20-2).[117,135,216]

Technique of Botulinum Injection. Carried out as a day case, the patient is placed in the left lateral position, and a mixture of 20 mL of 0.5% marcaine and 10 mL of 1% lignocaine is injected toward the coccyx at the lateral edge of the external sphincter using a 21-gauge needle, directed posteriorly medially toward the coccyx and cranially. The local anesthetic is injected bilaterally into the ischiorectal spaces in order to block the anal branches of the pudendal nerve. One hundred units of Botox (Allergan, Irvine, CA) or 500 U of Dysport (Ipsen Ltd., Slough, United Kingdom) are then injected into the puborectalis and external sphincter. The botulinum toxin is then injected into the puborectalis and external sphincter in the left and right lateral positions in small aliquots along the muscle.

Patients are followed up at 6 weeks, and the presence or absence of a classic symptom response is noted. In our opinion, the former are treated with further botulinum injection for recurrent symptoms that reemerge between 6 and 12 weeks. The latter undergo a rectal examination under anesthetic (EUA) with a circular anal dilator (CAD) device.

Results. In a series of patients from Oxford, the success rate for botulinum toxin injection used in patients with proctographically diagnosed anismus was 39%.[135] Those who failed underwent EUA of the rectum with a CAD (Frankenman International Ltd., Hong Kong). Almost all (97%) were found to have another condition to explain their symptoms, and in most (94%), this was a high-grade internal rectal prolapse. Excluding these, the revised success rate of botulinum toxin was 96%.

Patients who responded to the first dose showed improvement of symptoms after 2 to 3 days, with a gradual relapse after 6 to 12 weeks. A repeat injection at that stage using the same dose lead to a sustained improvement in almost all patients (95%) at a median follow-up of 19 months. It seems that the second dose of botulinum toxin may lead to some kind of downregulation. This is useful because the first dose can be given as a diagnostic "test" dose. If it works, the second dose becomes therapeutic; if it fails, it wears off and an alternative diagnosis can be sought.

TABLE 20-2 Results of Botulinum Toxin Injection for Anismus

AUTHOR	NUMBER	IMPROVED %	DOSE[a]	REPEATED	FOLLOW-UP (MONTHS)
Hallan[117]	7	57	3 ng	No	12
Joo[147]	4	50	12 U	No	12
Maria[215]	4	100 ST 75 LT	30 U	Yes (75%)	24
Ron[289]	25	71	30 U	Yes	6
Maria[216]	24	71	60 U	Yes	39
Hompes[135]	56	39 ST	500 U[b]	Yes[135]	19

[a]Botox (Allergan) unless otherwise stated.
[b]Dysport (Ipsen).
ST, short term; LT, long term.

These data suggest several new and important concepts. First, botulinum toxin should be an ideal treatment for what is a disorder of the voluntary pelvic floor musculature. The range of responses in the literature probably reflects variable diagnostic criteria for anismus. Almost certainly, some patients with prolapse have been inadvertently included. Second, it suggests that the current proctographic diagnostic criteria for anismus (failure to empty more than 60% of paste at 30 seconds) are nonspecific. According to these data, about 20% of patients undergoing proctography fulfill these criteria, yet only about 40% of these (5% to 10% overall) respond to botulinum toxin. This means that about 60% of patients are overdiagnosed by traditional screening criteria. These results give a diagnostic explanation for this observation. They suggest that the proctographic findings in those individuals who ultimately receive another diagnosis have a "*radiologic pseudoanismus.*" Third, they show that prolapse is probably underdiagnosed by current proctographic methods and that EUA is a very useful diagnostic test.

Surgical Approaches
Puborectalis Muscle Division

Barnes and colleagues offered a radical alternative in the form of posterior division of the puborectalis muscle.[15] Incontinence for solid stool was not reported, but only 2 of 9 patients were improved. Kamm and coworkers performed lateral division of the puborectalis muscle in 15 patients with severe idiopathic constipation and three with megarectum (12 unilateral and 6 bilateral).[152] The operation caused a marked reduction in voluntary squeeze pressure. However, only 4 patients experienced symptomatic improvement, and this did not correlate with the ability to expel a balloon; 3 experienced mild mucous or urgency incontinence. No one was incontinent for formed stool, however.

Although botulinum toxin injection leads to a reversible weakening rather than a permanent and irreversible surgical division of the puborectalis, the latter procedure is a potentially hazardous undertaking.

Anal Dilatation

Maria and colleagues performed progressive anal dilatation in 13 patients with anismus by using three dilators of 20, 23, and 27 mm in diameter.[214] The dilators were inserted every day for 30 minutes. At 6 months, there was significant improvement of spontaneous defecation (from zero to six times per week), and the number of individuals with the requirement for laxatives decreased from 12 (with a weekly mean of 4.6) to 2 (with a requirement of once per week). No patient was incontinent for formed stool, and none experienced mucous discharge or fecal urgency.

Familial Internal Anal Sphincter Myopathy

There have been several reports describing this rare condition affecting the internal anal sphincter.[65,113,154,181,380] Familial internal anal sphincter myopathy is characterized by obstructed defecation, often associated with anal pain similar to that of proctalgia fugax. Suspicion should be raised by the finding on anal ultrasound of an internal anal sphincter thicker than 5 mm and sometimes as much as 8 to 9 mm. The hallmark is the presence of inclusion bodies on electron microscopy in the muscle fibers of the internal sphincter. The condition seems to run in families. The treatment includes the previously discussed strip myomectomy (see Figure 20-14), which seems to be effective in improving both the pain and the obstructed defecation.

Stercoral Ulceration

A hard, scybalous, inspissated fecal mass may cause ulceration of the large bowel by pressure necrosis. As the condition progresses, it may lead to perforation. The condition usually occurs in constipated, elderly bedridden patients. It often presents as an isolated lesion in the rectosigmoid along the antimesenteric margin, but the lesions may be multiple.[169,221] The condition can also occur in a more proximal location and even in an unobstructed bowel.[203] In 1972, Bauer and colleagues identified 25 patients from the literature and described 4 of their own.[24] Since that time, numerous reviews have been published.[90,114,221,300,303]

The frequency of stercoral ulceration is uncertain, but based on postmortem examinations, the incidence may be greater than 5%.[303] Those who harbor this condition and undergo an emergency operation for perforation may be labeled with the incorrect diagnosis of perforated diverticulitis (see Chapter 27). In fact, in one series, only 11% of patients were given a correct diagnosis with respect to cause prior to operation.[303] A less common clinical manifestation is hemorrhage, but the true cause may not be apparent during the investigation of a patient with lower gastrointestinal bleeding (see Chapter 28). It is certainly possible that someone presumed to be bleeding from an angiodysplastic lesion could actually be bleeding from a stercoral ulcer.

Maurer and coworkers undertook a study to determine the frequency of stercoral perforation of the colon and the criteria for establishment of the diagnosis.[223] In a 5-year period, 1,295 patients underwent a colonic surgical procedure, of whom 11% were considered emergencies. Thirty-nine percent of the emergency colon operations were a consequence of perforation. Seven patients were thought to have a stercoral perforation, which made up 0.5% of all colonic operations, 1.2% of colonic emergency procedures, and 3.2% of all colonic perforations. All were left sided or rectal perforations. The authors considered the following to be characteristic of stercoral perforation: a round or ovoid perforation exceeding 1 cm in diameter, the presence of a fecaloma protruding through the perforation site,[90] microscopic pressure necrosis, and no other apparent cause of perforation. They concluded that the incidence of stercoral perforation may be underestimated.[221]

Microscopically, the ulcer is nonspecific (Figure 20-18). The epithelium is denuded over a variable area, depending on the size of the fecal mass.[221]

Treatment depends on the degree of contamination, the condition of the patient, and other factors discussed in subsequent chapters. In the absence of a perforation, an attempt to evacuate "fecalomas" from the colon should reduce the risk of pressure necrosis or ulceration.[28] As with any perforation of the colon, irrespective of its cause, removal of the source of sepsis from the peritoneal cavity is essential. The involved bowel is resected, and the decision whether an anastomosis should be performed rests on the judgment of the surgeon.

In reviewing the literature, it is evident that the mortality rate associated with stercoral ulcer is very high. This can be attributed to several factors, not the least of which is the morbidity associated with colonic perforation and peritonitis. Additionally, these patients often are elderly and have major medical problems that place them at an increased risk. Serpell and Nicholls postulate that failure to resect, as opposed to simple closure and proximal colostomy, is responsible for the high mortality.[300] They emphasize that the disease involves a segment of colon and that merely addressing the focal point of perforation is inadequate.

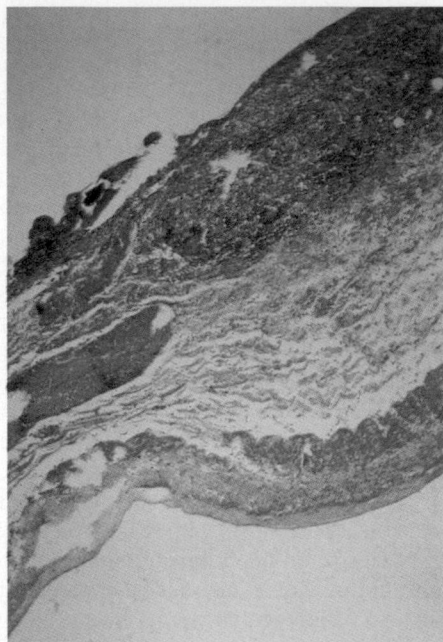

FIGURE 20-18. Stercoral ulcer, the floor of which is lined by inflammatory exudate. (Original magnification × 120; courtesy of Rudolf Garret, MD.)

Fecal Impaction

Fecal impaction is a common finding in surgical patients. The diagnosis is not usually difficult to make, unless the impaction is beyond the reach of the examining finger. Even under these circumstances, the patient's history and the plain abdominal radiograph are usually more than suggestive (see Figure 20-2). The condition is often associated with idiopathic megabowel.

There are numerous complications of fecal impaction, the most common of which is incontinence. Other more serious potential sequelae include stercoral ulceration; large bowel obstruction; perforation at some distance from the rectum, especially in the cecum; gangrene secondary to ischemia; autonomic dysreflexia; pneumothorax from straining; hypoxia; and associated colorectal problems (e.g., hemorrhoids, rectal prolapse, volvulus).[299,374]

Treatment usually requires manual disimpaction, laxatives, and large-volume or retention enemas. In the interest of patient safety and comfort, manual disimpaction ideally should be undertaken in the operating room with intravenous sedation or a general, local, or regional anesthetic. Double gloves are recommended to minimize the retention of the odor on the physician's hands. The stool is defragmented by finger manipulation, but in some cases, a large clamp may be necessary to accomplish this. When the bulk of the mass has been removed, high colonic irrigation with isotonic salt solution is performed using a large-bore catheter. The use of the standard setup for cystoscopy irrigation is helpful. At the conclusion of the procedure, the rectum should be checked by sigmoidoscopic examination.

Kokoszka and colleagues reported the use of a pulsed irrigation-enhanced evacuation device.[180] This is a mobile unit that can be transported throughout the hospital. It consists of two components: the reservoir and irrigation/drainage system. The former serves as a storage compartment for the irrigant and has a capacity of 20 L. The latter consists of two tubes that are connected to the reservoir, the drainage bag, and a rectal speculum. In an experience with 14 individuals

who had fecal impaction, the authors concluded that the pulsed irrigation technique is a simple, quick, and effective treatment for the management of severe fecal impaction.[180]

▶ ANAL PAIN

Proctalgia Fugax

Proctalgia fugax or levator spasm was recognized as a clinical entity as early as 1841 by Hall,[116,247] but it was not until 1935 that the term proctalgia fugax was coined by Thaysen.[334] Hall's description was of a "peculiar and severe pain of the rectum, which comes on in paroxysms, generally during sleep."[116] This complaint is heard frequently, yet most physicians fail to recognize the entity and will often classify the patient as hysterical and prescribe various sedatives or tranquilizers as treatment.

Characteristically, the individual complains of severe, episodic, often agonizing pain within the rectum. Its deep-seated location distinguishes proctalgia from a thrombosed hemorrhoid or an anal fissure, problems that are often limited to the anal or perianal area. The pain may awaken the individual from sleep and is not usually provoked by defecation, although sometimes it may be exacerbated by bowel action. The pain usually lasts only a few moments but occasionally may persist for several hours. Patients may sit on the toilet and strain, believing that this will give relief.

There is no unanimity of opinion on the etiology of proctalgia fugax. Numerous causes have been suggested (e.g., neuralgia, neurosis, infection, allergy, vasospasm, venous stasis, mechanical factors), but none can be supported by conclusive evidence.[161] There is, however, general agreement that the specific problem is a muscle spasm of the levators, analogous to a "charley horse" of the hamstring muscle. The condition often occurs in patients who spend a great deal of time on the toilet, whether straining, with diarrhea, or reading the newspaper. Other predisposing factors that have been suggested include trauma from riding a long distance, childbirth, low anterior resection or pelvic surgery, anal surgery, spinal surgery, psychiatric disorders, IBS, and the act of sexual intercourse.[293] A hereditary predisposition has also been reported.[49]

The psychological aspects of proctalgia were examined by Renzi and Pescatori in 20 patients.[280] Interviews and personality testings demonstrated that patients showed elevated depression and anxiety levels as well as a "strong tendency to use primitive defense mechanisms and showed a lack of personality formation."

Evaluation

Physical examination is usually negative. The characteristic discomfort may be duplicated when the physician presses on the sensitive area.

Christiansen and coworkers undertook a study to analyze whether anal ultrasound, physiologic evaluation, and histopathologic examination presented any specific abnormalities or common features.[57] None was found. However, Grimaud and colleagues studied 12 patients with proctalgia fugax by means of manometry and noted that the resting pressure in the anal canal of these individuals was significantly higher than that of controls.[110]

Treatment

Initial treatment should consist of instructions on bowel management and removing reading material from the toilet.

Sitz baths may offer some relief, but often the pain will cease before the bathwater can be drawn. Grant and colleagues believe that the syndrome is optimally treated by levator massage, with success reported in almost two-thirds of their patients.[109] We have not found this approach helpful and recommend instead perineal strengthening exercises (see Chapter 16). With a vigorous exercise program and assurance that the pain is not caused by neurosis, the symptoms usually abate within a few days or weeks.

Grimaud and colleagues assumed that their findings were caused by dysfunction of the external sphincter and observed that a biofeedback exercise regimen was very helpful in management.[110] Heah and coworkers studied the effects of biofeedback on pain relief in 16 consecutive patients with levator syndrome.[123] All underwent a course of biofeedback using a manometric balloon technique. After a mean follow-up of 1 year, all required fewer analgesics. Gilliland and associates used EMG-based biofeedback in 86 patients.[93] Thirty-four percent reported an improvement, with significant benefit observed in those individuals who completed the scheduled course of therapy and did not self-discharge.

In the intractable situation, muscle relaxants may be useful, but narcotic pain medication should not be given because of the risk for habituation. The teaching of self-hypnosis has been of benefit to some patients. Other alternatives that have been suggested are the administration of sublingual, topical, or controlled-release nitroglycerin and quinine sulfate.[201] Idiopathic proctalgia is often associated with an irritable bowel. These individuals should receive appropriate medical management for this condition. Adequate control of the irritable bowel symptom complex often leads to amelioration of the proctalgia fugax, especially with the use of antispasmodic medication such as hyoscyamine (Levsin) and dicyclomine (Bentyl).

Another alternative in the treatment of the levator syndrome was reported initially by Sohn and colleagues—the use of electrogalvanic stimulation by means of a specially designed rectal probe (Electro-Med Health Industries, Miami, FL; 800–232-EMHI; Figure 20-19).[313] The negative electrode is used, and the stimulator is set at 80 cycles/second. The machine is adjusted to deliver 150 to 400 V, depending on patient tolerance. The authors theorize that the technique may overstimulate and overcontract the levator muscle to

fatigue it. They reported their results with 80 patients to be excellent in 69%, good in 21%, and poor in 10%. Nicosia and Abcarian treated 45 patients by this method for 20 minutes every other day.[252] On average, five sessions were required for complete pain relief. Excellent results (i.e., total pain relief) were obtained in 36 patients, good results in 5, fair in 2, and no relief in 2. Other authors also report a favorable response to this modality in those individuals who failed to improve with conservative regimens.[257,293] Billingham and colleagues had less success, however.[32]

The effect of this treatment may not be maintained in the longer term. In a follow-up survey of 20 patients, only 5 (20%) remained symptom free. Hull and coworkers, reporting from the Cleveland Clinic, noted that only 19% had relief of symptoms with a mean follow-up of 28 months.[138] Partial relief was achieved in 24%, but 57% were unrelieved. When comparing three methods of treatment—electrogalvanic stimulation, biofeedback, and steroid caudal block—Ger and colleagues noted a success rate of 38%, 43%, and 18%, respectively.[91] More than half of the patients were refractory to all three therapeutic options.

A publication from Japan noted good or excellent results in 33 of 35 consecutive patients who complained of vague and deep pain in the anorectum treated by means of *linearly polarized near-infrared irradiation*.[235] This can penetrate the skin surface for a distance of more than 5 cm. Further experience and long-term follow-up are, of course, needed.

Approximately two-thirds of patients seem to benefit from three or more electrogalvanic treatments of 1 hour each, spaced over weekly intervals. In an occasional individual, one session may suffice. About one-third report no improvement. Unfortunately, the longer the patient has symptoms prior to implementation of this approach, the less likely will be the success. If all has been tried and these efforts fail, the surgeon's only recourse, in our opinion, is to refer the patient to a pain management center.

Coccygodynia (Coccydinia)

The term coccygodynia was coined by Simpson in 1859, when he initially recognized this entity.[307] Because of the failure of standard pain medications to relieve the symptoms of coccygodynia, the author suggested that coccygectomy

JAMES YOUNG SIMPSON (1811–1870)

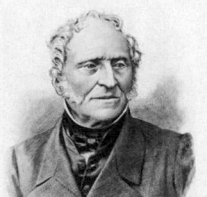

Simpson was born in Bathgate, Scotland, the youngest of seven sons of the village baker. His mother died when he was quite young, but because of James's obvious scholastic aptitude, his entire family agreed to do without to give him a higher education. Simpson entered Edinburgh University at the age of 14 and began his medical studies 2 years later, graduating with his MD in 1832. His extraordinary abilities were soon recognized. He was made president of the Royal Medical Society of Edinburgh in 1835 and was appointed to the chair of midwifery in 1839 at the age of 28. He was the first in Britain to employ ether as an anesthetic, and with his associates was the first to use chloroform as an anesthetic (1847). In addition to his achievements in the field of anesthesia, Simpson was responsible for laying a considerable part of the foundation of gynecology and obstetrics. He invented the uterine sound and the obstetric forceps. In 1866, Simpson was awarded a baronetcy, the first given to a doctor practicing in Scotland. When he died, his family declined the offer of a grave in Westminster Abbey, but a bust was placed there noting that to Simpson's "genius and benevolence the world owes the blessings derived from the use of chloroform for the relief of suffering." (Photo courtesy of the Royal College of Surgeons of England.)

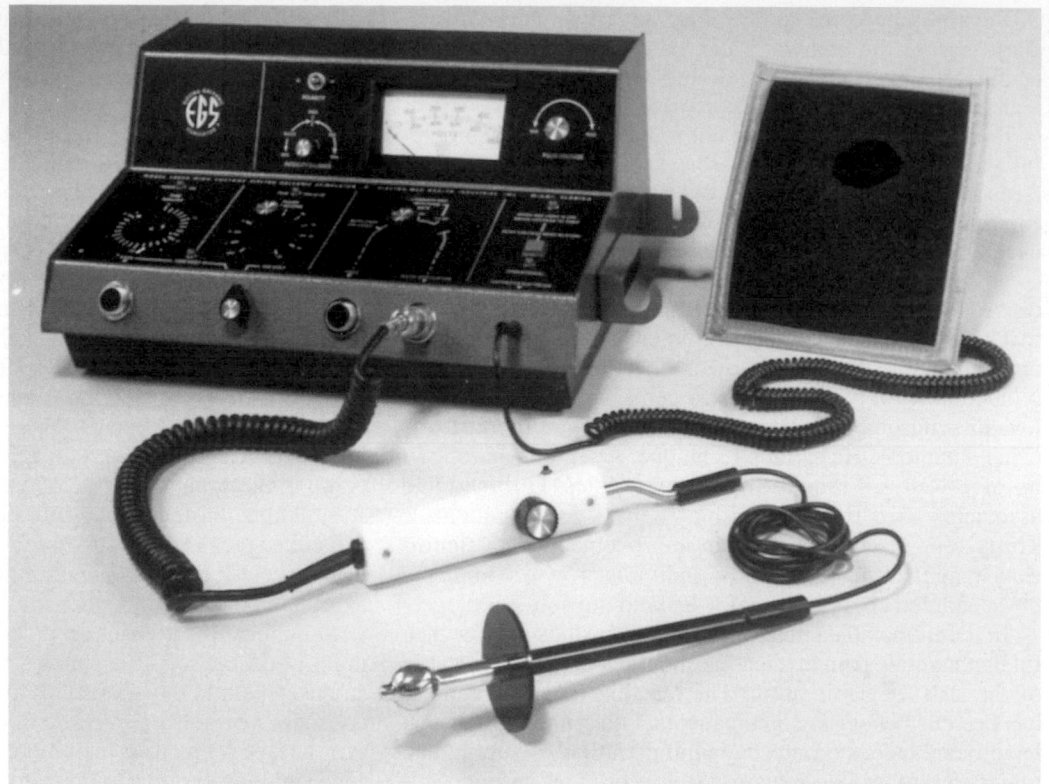

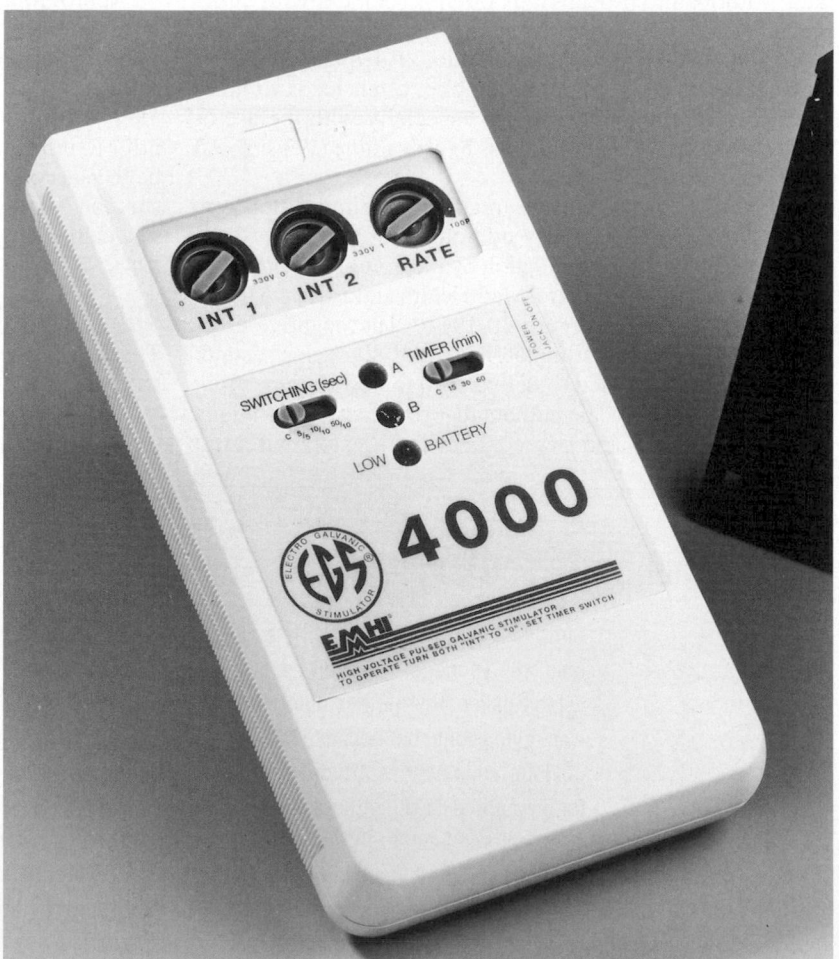

FIGURE 20-19. A: An electrogalvanic stimulator (Model 100–2) with Sohn's electrode rectal probe. **B:** EGS 4000 EGXtra portable unit for home use. (Courtesy of Electro-Med Health Industries, Miami, FL.)

was the optimal treatment. Several comprehensive reviews of the subject have been published by Thiele.[335–337]

The condition is part of the levator syndrome or another manifestation of proctalgia fugax, but the pain is directed to the coccyx. This is possibly caused by spasm of the pubococcygeal portion of the levator ani muscle. Classically, the pain is exacerbated when the person rises from a sitting position.

Maroy reported a study analyzing the association between coccygodynia and depression.[217] A highly significant correlation was found between pain evoked by rectal digital examination and depressive status in patients without coccygodynia and between coccygodynia and evoked pain. It has been speculated that although individuals usually do not appear depressed initially, subsequent follow-up evaluation suggests that they are.

To initiate proper therapy, it is important to recognize the clinical syndrome and the characteristic pain. Some authors advocate levator massage, but, as with proctalgia fugax, perineal strengthening exercises and appropriate bowel management are suggested. Electrogalvanic stimulation may be of value for selected individuals (see earlier discussion).

Coccygectomy was originally described by Nott to treat coccygodynia, usually by orthopedic surgeons, but this operation should not be performed for this condition unless the coccyx has been injured or is dislocated. Even under these circumstances, coccygectomy rarely alleviates the pain. Johnson suggests that injection of a local anesthetic and cortisone may be beneficial; he cautions, however, that the relief is usually only temporary.[143] Albrektsson evaluated the long-term effects of sacral rhizotomy in 24 patients with coccygodynia.[3] Only 6 responded well to the procedure; serious complications occurred in 25%. It is difficult to justify a surgical procedure of any kind in a patient with coccygodynia.

Chronic Idiopathic Perineal Pain

A recent study has looked at how often an anatomical abnormality is present in patients with chronic idiopathic perineal pain (CIPP), noting that underlying treatable structural abnormalities have been suspected but rarely objectively demonstrated.[136] The condition is frequently considered to be a psychological disorder. Patients seen in a pelvic floor clinic with chronic idiopathic pain (study group) underwent defecating proctography, anorectal physiology, and anal ultrasound, and some underwent rectal EUA. Those with obstructed defecation with or without fecal incontinence with advanced (external or high-grade internal) rectal prolapse served as controls. Fifty-nine patients were found to have CIPP (5% of all pelvic floor presentations), 33 without, and 26 (44%) obstructed defecation. Overall, 59% had an underlying high-grade internal rectal prolapse (73% CIPP + obstructed defecation vs. CIPP alone 48%, $P < .05$). Anorectal pain was present in 50% of 543 controls. The investigators concluded that advanced rectal prolapse commonly underlies CIPP, particularly when obstructed defecation is present. This condition is often missed by defecating proctography, but rectal examination under an anesthetic is helpful.

Although biofeedback is the mainstay of management, some newer treatments are becoming available for chronic anorectal pain, including botulinum toxin and sacral nerve stimulation.[8,108]

Pudendal Canal Syndrome

Clinical Presentation

This is an unusual and poorly recognized pain syndrome that arises from entrapment of the pudendal nerve in Alcock's canal with a subsequent neuropathy. About 5% of patients with a pelvic floor disorder complain primarily of severe chronic anorectal pain,[239] and about 5% of these will have pudendal canal syndrome.

The pain is typically perceived in the perineum from anus to clitoris/penis. However, a less specific pain distribution may occur, with a regional pain syndrome, and the musculoskeletal system may become involved, confusing the pain picture. Burning, crushing, and swelling or a feeling of a foreign body in the rectum or perineum, often described as a golf or tennis ball, are terms used by patients. Other complaints are discomfort and numbness. Classically, pain is worse on sitting, requiring these patients often to remain

JOSIAH CLARK NOTT (1804–1873)

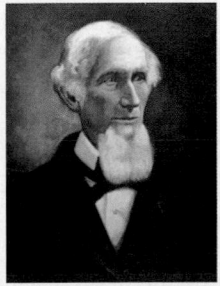

Born in 1804 to a South Carolina Federalist politician, Josiah Nott earned his medical degree at the University of Pennsylvania in 1827 and completed his postgraduate surgical training in Paris, France. Shortly thereafter, he started surgical practice in Mobile, Alabama. In 1858, he would help found the Medical College of Alabama in Mobile, where he served as professor of surgery and championed the school's cause in the state legislature. During his career, he opened a private infirmary for African American patients and served as a surgeon in the Confederate Army during the Civil War.

Among Dr. Nott's contributions to surgery was the "relief" of coccygeal neuralgia ("coccygodynia") by resection of the coccyx.

In this operation, admittedly among Dr. Nott's "most painful I ever performed," he "disarticulated the bone at the second joint, divided the muscular and ligamentous attachments, and without much difficulty dissected out the two terminating bones" to liberate the "exquisitely sensitive" nerves (from Rutkow IM. Moments in surgical history. *Arch Surg.* 1996;131(3):342). Unfortunately, his procedure fell into disrepute.

Dr. Nott's career accomplishments were not limited to surgery alone, however. He was among the first to attribute the spread of malaria and yellow fever (the latter claimed four of his children) to insect vectors, rejecting the *miasma* ("bad air") theory that was widely supported at the time. A follower of Samuel George Morton's theory of physical anthropology, Dr. Nott also maintained in his 1854 book of essays that each race of humanity represented discrete species with different biologic lineages. (Courtesy of Merrit M. DeBartolo, MD.)

standing. As a consequence, they can develop a wide range of other aches and pains. The discomfort may be exacerbated by bowel or bladder evacuation.

Pudendal nerve damage may be associated with paresthesia, dysesthesia (unpleasant sensory perceptions), allodynia (pain on light touch), and hyperalgesia (increased pain perception following a painful stimulus but also to hot and cold stimuli).

Being unable to sit is a major disability. Over time, patients struggle to stand and they often become bedbound. The immobility produces generalized muscle wasting because minimal activity hurts. As a consequence of the widespread pain and disability, patients will often experience emotional problems, in particular depression. Those with chronic pelvic pain are also often anxious and have the tendency to catastrophize. Depression, catastrophizing, and disability are all prognostic markers of a poor outcome.[327]

Clinical Examination

Often there is little to identify in patients with pudendal neuralgia. Frequently, the findings are nonspecific. The main pathognomonic features are signs of nerve injury in the appropriate distribution (e.g., allodynia or numbness). Tenderness brought on by pressure over the pudendal nerve may facilitate the diagnosis. Pain may be elicited by rectal or vaginal examination as well as by palpation in the region of the ischial spines and/or Alcock's canal.

Investigations

MRI scanning of the pelvis and spine is essential to help with the differential diagnosis. Electrophysiologic studies may reveal signs of perineal denervation, increased pudendal nerve latency, or impaired bulbocavernosus reflex.

Treatment

The approach to treating pudendal neuralgia is essentially the same as that for the treatment of any neuropathic pain. There is a suggestion that early treatment has a better prognosis.

Injection

An injection of local anesthetic with steroids at the site of nerve injury may produce a therapeutic action.[5] Another benefit of local infiltration is for diagnosis. Differential nerve blocks of the pudendal nerve will help to provide information in relation to the location where the nerve may be trapped. Infiltration at the ischial spine requires the use of a nerve stimulator/locator. Both motor (anal contraction) and sensory end points may be noted. The anatomical end point may be localized by fluoroscopy (the most frequently used technique), CT guidance (involves a significant amount of radiation), or ultrasound.

Surgery

The most traditional approach is transgluteal. However, a transperineal operation may be an alternative, particularly if the nerve damage is thought to be related to prior pelvic surgery.

Currently, there is only one prospective randomized study.[286] This report suggests that if the patient has had the pain for less than 6 years, 66% will see some improvement with surgery (compared to 40% if the pain has been present for greater than 6 years). Surgery is by no means the answer for all patients.

Clearly, surgeons involved in the management of these pain syndromes will do so in conjunction with a chronic pain specialist. Such an individual may employ one or more of the following approaches:

Drug Therapy

There are numerous texts on the application of neuropathic analgesics to reduce the pain associated with nerve injury. Most of the literature uses diabetic neuropathy or postherpetic neuralgia as the model. There is little published data on the use of neuropathic analgesics, specifically in pudendal neuralgia.

Antidepressants. The gold standard antidepressant is amitriptyline, taken at a mean analgesic dose of approximately 70 mg, and a number needed to treat (NNT) of about two to three. Other antidepressants are also used, including imipramine and duloxetine. Both may be helpful if there are significant irritable bladder symptoms. Mirtazapine and fluoxetine may have a particular role if depression is a significant feature.

Antiepileptic Drugs. Most of the research on antiepileptic drugs and neuropathic pain has been done with gabapentin, with NNT of about 3.8. Pregabalin is thought to be equally as effective. The starting dose for gabapentin is 300 mg a day; doses up to 3.6 g have been used. The maximum dose of pregabalin is 600 mg/day.

Opioids. The use of opioids in neuropathic pain is controversial. However, there is evidence that opioids can reduce neuropathic pain and, if appropriate, guidelines are instigated and followed.

Other Medications. There are a range of specialized neuropathic analgesics that are prescribed through pain centers. The availability of these drugs depends on local formulary regulations. These may include the cannabinoids, sodium channel blockers, and NMDA (*N*-methyl-D-aspartate) antagonists.

Management of Associated Symptoms

Patients with persistent pelvic pain are best managed within a center that can provide multidisciplinary and multispecialty care. In view of the effect of pudendal nerve damage on multiple systems, it is important to have access to a number of specialty clinics. In an ideal world, shared clinics among pain specialists, urologists, urogynecologists, and bowel specialists should occur. In the absence of this form of close collaboration, then detailed communication among specialists is important. Within any specialty, there will be found numerous disciplines, such as medical, physiotherapy, psychology, and nursing, all of which will have an important role to play.

Psychology and Physiotherapy

It is well established that mood, catastrophizing, and inappropriate resting are all associated with a poor prognosis in a chronic pain patient.[251,328] The best way to manage these conditions is through an appropriate program that is usually organized and run by chronic pain psychologists and physiotherapists. These programs are usually conducted on a one-on-one basis for individuals with chronic pelvic pain. More recently, group pain management programs have also been incorporated. These programs for the management of chronic pain have been well established. As such, there is reliable evidence that they can provide a major improvement in the quality of life of the patient.[78,239,355]

Neuromodulation

There is scientific evidence that spinal cord stimulation is helpful in reducing the pain associated with nerve injury.[248] For pain relief by means of spinal cord stimulation, it is necessary to have paresthesia perceived in the same area as the pain. In order to achieve this for pelvic pain, some specialists have turned the spinal cord stimulator electrode around so that it passes in a caudal direction, thereby stimulating the sacral nerve roots. Others have used S3 transforaminal approach. The beauty of this last technique is that efficacy trial is relatively easy to undertake. However, it must be noted that the action of a spinal cord stimulator on the nervous system is different from the action of stimulating the sacral nerve roots. This, in turn, is different from stimulating the dorsal root ganglia and peripheral nerves with sacral transforaminal stimulation.

References

1. Agachan F, Chen T, Pfeifer J, et al. A constipation scoring system to simplify evaluation and management of constipated patients. *Dis Colon Rectum.* 1996;39(6):681–685.
2. Ahlfors F, Linander H, Lindström M, et al. Familial intestinal degenerative neuropathy associated with chronic intestinal pseudo-obstruction. *Neurogastroenterol Motil.* 2011;23(4):347–355.
3. Albrektsson B. Sacral rhizotomy in cases of ano-coccygeal pain. A follow-up of 24 cases. *Acta Orthop Scand.* 1981;52(2):187–190.
4. Alwan MH, van Rij AM. Acute colonic pseudo-obstruction. *Aust N Z J Surg.* 1998;68(2):129–132.
5. Amarenco G, Kerdraon J, Bouju P, et al. [Treatments of perineal neuralgia caused by involvement of the pudendal nerve]. *Rev Neurol (Paris).* 1997;153(5):331–334.
6. Anderson AS. Dietary factors in the aetiology and treatment of constipation during pregnancy. *Br J Obstet Gynaecol.* 1986;93(3):245–249.
7. Anuras S. Clinical presentation: chronic intestinal pseudo-obstuction. *Pract Gastroenterol.* 1991;15:13.
8. Atkin GK, Suliman A, Vaizey CJ. Patient characteristics and treatment outcome in functional anorectal pain. *Dis Colon Rectum.* 2011;54(7):870–875.
9. Attiyeh FF, Knapper WH. Pseudo-obstruction of the colon (Ogilvie's syndrome). *Dis Colon Rectum.* 1980;23(2):106–108.
10. Baeten CG. Status of sacral neuromodulation for refractory constipation. *Colorectal Disease.* 2011;13(suppl 2):19–22.
11. Baker JT, Harvey RF. Bowel habit in thyrotoxicosis and hypothyroidism. *Br Med J.* 1971;1(5744):322–323.
12. Bampton PA, Dinning PG, Kennedy ML, et al. Spatial and temporal organization of pressure patterns throughout the unprepared colon during spontaneous defecation. *Am J Gastroenterol.* 2000;95(4):1027–1035.
13. Baraza W, Brown S, McAlindon M, et al. Prospective analysis of percutaneous endoscopic colostomy at a tertiary referral centre. *Br J Surg.* 2007;94(11):1415–1420.
14. Bardsley D. Pseudo-obstruction of the large bowel. *Br J Surg.* 1974; 61(12):963–969.
15. Barnes PR, Hawley PR, Preston DM, et al. Experience of posterior division of the puborectalis muscle in the management of chronic constipation. *Br J Surg.* 1985;72(6):476–477.
16. Barnes PR, Lennard-Jones JE. Balloon expulsion from the rectum in constipation of different types. *Gut.* 1985;26(10):1049–1052.
17. Barnes PR, Lennard-Jones JE, Hawley PR, et al. Hirschsprung's disease and idiopathic megacolon in adults and adolescents. *Gut.* 1986;27(5): 534–541.
18. Bassotti G, Chiaroni G, Imbimbo BP, et al. Impaired colonic motor response to cholinergic stimulation in patients with severe chronic idiopathic (slow transit type) constipation. *Dis Dig Sci.* 1993;38(6):1040–1045.
19. Bassotti G, Chiaroni G, Vantini I, et al. Anorectal manometric abnormalities and colonic propulsive impairment in patients with severe chronic idiopathic constipation. *Dig Dis Sci.* 1994;39(7):1558–1564.
20. Bassotti G, Gaburri M, Imbimbo BP, et al. Colonic mass movements in idiopathic chronic constipation. *Gut.* 1988;29(9):1173–1179.
21. Bassotti G, Germani U, Fiorella S, et al. Intact colonic motor response to sudden awakening from sleep in patients with chronic idiopathic (slow-transit) constipation. *Dis Colon Rectum.* 1998;41(2):1555–1555.
22. Bassotti G, Stanghellini V, Chiaroni G, et al. Upper gastrointestinal motor activity in patients with slow-transit constipation. Further evidence for an enteric neuropathy. *Dig Dis Sci.* 1996;41(10):1999–2005.
23. Battaglia E, Serra AM, Buonafede G, et al. Long-term study on the effects of visual biofeedback and muscle training as a therapeutic modality in pelvic floor dyssynergia and slow-transit constipation. *Dis Colon Rectum.* 2004;47(1):90–95.
24. Bauer JJ, Weiss M, Dreiling DA. Stercoraceous perforation of the colon. *Surg Clin North Am.* 1972;52(4):1047–1053.
25. Beck DE. Simplified balloon expulsion test. *Dis Colon Rectum.* 1992;35(6):597–598.
26. Belliveau P, Goldberg SM, Rothenberger DA, et al. Idiopathic acquired megacolon: the value of subtotal colectomy. *Dis Colon Rectum.* 1982;25(2):118–121.
27. Belsey J, Greenfield S, Candy D, et al. Systematic review: impact of constipation on quality of life in adults and children. *Aliment Pharmacol Ther.* 2010;31(9):938–949.
28. Berardi RS, Lee S. Stercoraceous perforation of the colon. Report of a case. *Dis Colon Rectum.* 1983;26(4):283–286.
29. Berman IR, Manning DH, Harris MS. Streamlining the management of defecation disorders. *Dis Colon Rectum.* 1990;33(9):778–785.
30. Bernton E, Myers R, Reyna T. Pseudo-obstruction of the colon. *Curr Surg.* 1983;40(1):30–31.
31. Bertschinger KM, Hetzer FH, Roos JE, et al. Dynamic MR imaging of the pelvic floor performed with patient sitting in an open-magnet unit versus with patient supine in a closed magnet unit. *Radiology.* 2002;223(2): 501–508.
32. Billingham RP, Isler JT, Friend WG, et al. Treatment of levator syndrome using high-voltage electrogalvanic stimulation. *Dis Colon Rectum.* 1987;30(8):584–587.
33. Bingham SA, Cummings JH. Effect of exercise and physical fitness on large intestinal function. *Gastroenterology.* 1989;97(6):1389–1399.
34. Bleijenberg G, Kuijpers HC. Treatment of the spastic pelvic floor syndrome with biofeedback. *Dis Colon Rectum.* 1987;30(2):108–111.
35. Bode WE, Beart RW Jr, Spencer RJ, et al. Colonoscopic decompression for acute pseudoobstruction of the colon (Ogilvie's syndrome). Report of 22 cases and review of the literature. *Am J Surg.* 1984;147(2): 243–245.
36. Boley SJ. An endorectal pull-through operation with primary anastomosis for Hirchsprung's disease. *Surg Gynecol Obstet.* 1968;127(2):353–357.
37. Bonapace ES, Maurer AH, Davidoff S, et al. Whole gut transit scintigraphy in the clinical evaluation of patients with upper and lower gastrointestinal symptoms. *Am J Gastroenterol.* 2000;95(10):2838–2847.
38. Brookes SJ, Dinning PG, Gladman MA. Neuroanatomy and physiology of colorectal function and defaecation: from basic science to human clinical studies. *Neurogastroenterol Motil.* 2009;21(suppl 2):9–19.
39. Brown WJ, Mishra G, Lee C, et al. Leisure time physical activity in Australian women: relationship with well being and symptoms. *Res Q Exerc Sport.* 2000;71(3):206–216.
40. Bullock PR, Thomas WE. Acute pseudo-obstruction of the colon. *Ann R Coll Surg Engl.* 1984;66(5):327–330.
41. Burke G, Shellito PC. Treatment of recurrent colonic pseudo-obstruction by endoscopic placement of a fenestrated overtube. Report of a case. *Dis Colon Rectum.* 1987;30(8):615–619.
42. Burton DD, Camilleri M, Mullan BP, et al. Colonic transit scintigraphy labeled activated charcoal compared with ion exchange pellets. *J Nucl Med.* 1997;38(11):1807–1810.
43. Bytzer P, Stokholm M, Andersen I, et al. Prevalence of surreptitious laxative abuse in patients with diarrhoea of uncertain oigin: a cost benefit analysis of a screening procedure. *Gut.* 1989;30(10):1379–1384.
44. Camilleri M, Kerstens R, Rykx A, et al. A placebo-controlled trial of prucalopride for severe chronic constipation. *N Engl J Med.* 2008; 358(22):2344–2354.
45. Camilleri M, Thompson WG, Fleshman JW, et al. Clinical management of intractable constipation. *Ann Intern Med.* 1994;121(7):520–528.
46. Campbell WL. Cathartic colon. Reversibility of roentgen changes. *Dis Colon Rectum.* 1983;26(7):445–448.
47. Casola G, Withers C, van Sonnenberg E, et al. Percutaneous cecostomy for decompression of the massively distended cecum. *Radiology.* 1986;158(3):793–794.
48. Cazemier M, Felt-Bersma RJ, Mulder CJ. Anal plugs and retrograde colonic irrigation are helpful in fecal incontinence or constipation. *World J Gastroenterol.* 2007;13(22):3101–3105.
49. Celik AF, Katsinelos P, Read NW, et al. Hereditary proctalgia fugax and constipation: report of a second family. *Gut.* 1995;36(4):581–584.
50. Chan DS, Saklani A, Shah PR, et al. Rectal irrigation: a useful tool in the armamentarium for functional bowel disorders [published online ahead of print August 29, 2011]. *Colorectal Dis.* doi:10.1111/j.1463-1318.2011.02797.x.

51. Chen B, Knowles CH, Scott M, et al. Idiopathic slow transit constipation and megacolon are not associated with neurturin mutations. *Neurogastroenterol Motil.* 2002;14(5):513–517.

52. Chiarioni G, Salandini L, Whitehead WE. Biofeedback benefits only patients with outlet dysfunction, not patients with isolated slow transit constipation. *Gastroenterology.* 2005;129(1):86–97.

53. Chiarioni G, Whitehead WE, Pezza V, et al. Biofeedback is superior to laxatives for normal transit constipation due to pelvic floor dyssynergia. *Gastroenterology.* 2006;130(3):657–664.

54. Chiotakakou-Faliakou E, Kamm MA, Roy AJ, et al. Biofeedback provides long-term benefit for patients with intractable, slow and normal transit constipation. *Gut.* 1998;42(4):517–521.

55. Chiou AW, Lin JK, Wang FM. Anorectal abnormalities in progressive systemic sclerosis. *Dis Colon Rectum.* 1989;32(5):417–421.

56. Choung RS, Branda ME, Chitkara D, et al. Longitudinal direct medical costs associated with constipation in women. *Aliment Pharmacol Ther.* 2011;33(2):251–260.

57. Christiansen J, Bruun E, Skjoldbye B, et al. Chronic idiopathic anal pain: analysis of ultrasonography, pathology, and treatment. *Dis Colon Rectum.* 2001;44(5):661–665.

58. Chung RS. A technique for rapid intubation of the sigmoid and left colon. *Surg Gynecol Obstet.* 1983;157(3):279–281.

59. Chung YF, Eu KW, Nyam DC, et al. Minimizing recurrence after sigmoid volvulus. *Br J Surg.* 1999;86(2):231–233.

60. Collins B, Norton C, Maeda Y. Percutaneous tibial nerve stimulation for slow transit constipation: a pilot study [published online ahead of print September 12, 2011]. *Colorectal Dis.* doi:10.1111/j.1463-1318.2011.02820.

61. Cowlam S, Watson C, Elltringham M, et al. Percutaneous endoscopic colostomy of the left side of the colon. *Gastrointest Endosc.* 2007;65(7):1007–1014.

62. Crawshaw AP, Pigott L, Potter MA, et al. A retrospective evaluation of rectal irrigation in the treatment of disorders of faecal continence. *Colorectal Dis.* 2004;6(3):185–190.

63. Dahl J, Lindquist BL, Tysk C, et al. Behavioral medicine treatment in chronic constipation with paradoxical anal sphincter contraction. *Dis Colon Rectum.* 1991;34(9):769–776.

64. De Giorgio R, Stanghellini V, Barbara G, et al. Prokinetics in the treatment of acute intestinal pseudo-obstruction. *IDrugs.* 2004;7(2):160–165.

65. de la Portilla F, Borrero JJ, Rafel E. Hereditary vacuolar internal anal sphincter myopathy causing proctalgia fugax and constipation: a new case contribution. *Eur J Gastroenterol Hepatol.* 2005;17(3):359–361.

66. Dinning PG. Colonic manometry and sacral nerve stimulation in patients with severe constipation. *Pelviperineology.* 2007;26(3):113–116.

67. Dinning PG, Fuentealba SE, Kennedy ML, et al. Sacral nerve stimulation induces pan-colonic propagating pressure waves and increases defecation frequency in patients with slow-transit constipation. *Colorectal Dis.* 2007;9(2):123–132.

68. Dinning PG, Smith TK, Scott SM. Pathophysiology of colonic causes of chronic constipation. *Neurogastroenterol Motil.* 2009;21(suppl 2):20–30.

69. Donald IP, Smith RG, Cruikshank JG, et al. A study of constipation in the elderly living at home. *Gerontology.* 1985;31(2):112–118.

70. Doodnath R, Puri P. A systematic review and meta-analysis of Hirschsprung's disease presenting after childhood. *Pediatr Surg Int.* 2010;26(11):1107–1110.

71. Duh QY, Way LW. Diagnostic laparoscopy and laparoscopic cecostomy for colonic pseudo-obstruction. *Dis Colon Rectum.* 1993;36(1):65–70.

72. Duhamel B. New operation for congenital megacolon: retrorectal and transanal lowering of the colon, and its possible application to the treatment of various other malformations [in French]. *Presse Med.* 1956;64(95):2249–2250.

73. Durai R. Colonic pseudo-obstruction. *Singapore Med J.* 2009;50(3):237–244.

74. Elliot MS, Todd IP. Adult Hirschsprung's disease: results of the Duhamel procedure. *Br J Surg.* 1985;72(11):884–885.

75. Emmanuel AV, Shand AG, Kamm MA. Erythromycin for the treatment of chronic intestinal pseudo-obstruction: description of six cases with a positive response. *Aliment Pharmacol Ther.* 2004;19(6):687–694.

76. Felt-Bersma RJ, Sloots CE, Poen AC, et al. Rectal compliance as a routine measurement: extreme volumes have direct clinical impact and normal volumes exclude rectum as a problem. *Dis Colon Rectum.* 2000;43(12):1732–1738.

77. Fioramonti J, Bueno L. Toxicity of laxatives: how to discriminate between myth and fact? *Eur J Gastroenterol Hepatol.* 1995;7(1):5–7.

78. Fishbain DA, Cutler R, Rosomoff HL, et al. Chronic pain-associated depression: antecedent or consequence of chronic pain? A review. *Clin J Pain.* 1997;13(2):116–137.

79. Fishbein RH, Handelsman JC, Schuster MM. Surgical treatment of Hirschsprung's disease in adults. *Surg Gynecol Obstet.* 1986;163(5):458–464.

80. Fleshman JW, Dreznik Z, Cohen E, et al. Balloon expulsion test facilitates diagnosis of pelvic floor outlet obstruction due to nonrelaxing puborectalis muscle. *Dis Colon Rectum.* 1992;35(11):1019–1025.

81. Fleshman JW, Dreznik Z, Meyer K, et al. Outpatient protocol for biofeedback therapy of pelvic floor outlet obstruction. *Dis Colon Rectum.* 1992;35(1):1–7.

82. Fucini C, Ronchi O, Elbetti C. Electromyography of the pelvic floor musculature in the assessment of obstructed defecation symptoms. *Dis Colon Rectum.* 2001;44(8):1168–1175.

83. Ganeshan A, Anderson EM, Upponi S, et al. Imaging of obstructed defecation. *Clin Radiol.* 2008;63(1):18–26.

84. Ganio E, Masin A, Ratto C, et al. Short-term sacral nerve stimulation for functional anorectal and urinary disturbances: results in 40 patients: evaluation of a new option for anorectal functional disorders. *Dis Colon Rectum.* 2001;44(9):1261–1267.

85. Gattuso JM, Debinski HS, Kangro HO, et al. Evaluation of specific herpes DNA viruses in idiopathic megarectum and idiopathic megacolon. *Int J Colorectal Dis.* 1998;13(3):131–133.

86. Gattuso JM, Hoyle CH, Milner P, et al. Enteric innervation in idiopathic megarectum and megacolon. *Int J Colorectal Dis.* 1996;11(6):264–271.

87. Gattuso JM, Kamm MA. Clinical features of idiopathic megarectum and idiopathic megacolon. *Gut.* 1997;41(1):93–99.

88. Gattuso JM, Kamm MA, Morris G, et al. Gastrointestinal transit in patients with idiopathic megarectum. *Dis Colon Rectum.* 1996;39(9):1044–1050.

89. Geelhoed GW. Colonic pseudo-obstruction in surgical patients. *Am J Surg.* 1985;149(2):258–265.

90. Gekas P, Schuster MM. Stercoral perforation of the colon: case report and review of the literature. *Gastroenterology.* 1981;80(5 pt 1):1054–1058.

91. Ger GC, Wexner SD, Jorge JM, et al. Evaluation and treatment of chronic intractable rectal pain—a frustrating endeavor. *Dis Colon Rectum.* 1993;36(2):139–145.

92. Ghadially FN, Walley VM. Melanoses of the gastrointestinal tract. *Histopathology.* 1994;25(3):197–207.

93. Gilliland R, Heymen JS, Altomare DF, et al. Biofeedback for intractable rectal pain: outcome and predictors of success. *Dis Colon Rectum.* 1997;40(2):190–196.

94. Gladman MA, Aziz Q, Scott SM, et al. Rectal hyposensitivity: pathophysiological mechanisms. *Neurogastroenterol Motil.* 2009;21(5):508–516.

95. Gladman MA, Dvorkin LS, Scott SM, et al. A novel technique to identify patients with megarectum. *Dis Colon Rectum.* 2007;50(5):621–629.

96. Gladman MA, Knowles CH. Novel concepts in the diagnosis, pathophysiology and management of idiopathic megabowel. *Colorectal Dis.* 2008;10(6):531–538.

97. Gladman MA, Lunniss PJ, Scott SM, et al. Rectal hyposensitivity. *Am J Gastroenterol.* 2006;101(5):1140–1151.

98. Gladman MA, Scott SM, Lunniss PJ, et al. Systematic review of surgical options for idiopathic megarectum and megacolon. *Ann Surg.* 2005;241(4):562–574.

99. Gladman MA, Williams NS, Scott SM, et al. Medium-term results of vertical reduction rectoplasty and sigmoid colectomy for idiopathic megarectum. *Br J Surg.* 2005;92(5):624–630.

100. Glia A, Gylin M, Gullberg K, et al. Biofeedback retraining in patients with functional constipation and paradoxical puborectalis contraction: comparison of anal manometry and sphincter electromyography for feedback. *Dis Colon Rectum.* 1997;40(8):889–895.

101. Glick ME, Meshkinpour H, Haldeman S, et al. Colonic dysfunction in multiple sclerosis. *Gastroenterology.* 1982;83(5):1002–1007.

102. Golladay ES, Byrne WJ. Intestinal pseudo-obstruction. *Surg Gynecol Obstet.* 1981;153(2):257–273.

103. Gosche JR, Sharpe JN, Larson GM. Colonoscopic decompression for pseudo-obstruction of the colon. *Am Surg.* 1989;55(2):111–115.

104. Gosselink MJ, Hop WC, Schouten WR. Rectal compliance in females with obstructed defecation. *Dis Colon Rectum.* 2001;44(7):971–977.

105. Gosselink MJ, Schouten WR. Rectal sensory perception in females with obstructed defecation. *Dis Colon Rectum.* 2001;44(9):1337–1344.

106. Gosselink MP, Darby M, Zimmerman DD, et al. Long-term follow-up of retrograde colonic irrigation for defaecation disturbances. *Colorectal Dis.* 2005;7(1):65–69.

107. Goto S, Ikeda K, Nagasaki A, et al. Hirschsprung's disease in an adult. Special reference to histochemical determination of the acetylcholinesterase activity. *Dis Colon Rectum.* 1984;27(5):319–320.

108. Govaert B, Melenhorst J, van Kleef M, et al. Sacral neuromodulation for the treatment of chronic functional anorectal pain: a single center experience. *Pain Pract.* 2010;10(1):49–53.

109. Grant SR, Salvati EP, Rubin RJ. Levator syndrome: an analysis of 316 cases. *Dis Colon Rectum.* 1975;18(2):161–163.

110. Grimaud JC, Bouvier M, Naudy B, et al. Manometric and radiologic investigations and biofeedback treatment of chronic idiopathic anal pain. *Dis Colon Rectum*. 1991;34(8):690–695.

111. Grotz RL, Pemberton JH, Levin KE, et al. Rectal wall contractility in healthy subjects and in patients with chronic severe constipation. *Ann Surg*. 1993;218(6):761–768.

112. Grover K, Ahlawat SK. Hirschsprung disease in adults. *South Med J*. 2009;102(2):127–128.

113. Guy RJ, Kamm MA, Martin JE. Internal anal sphincter myopathy causing proctalgia fugax and constipation: further clinical and radiological characterization in a patient. *Eur J Gastroenterol Hepatol*. 1997;9(2):221–224.

114. Guyton DP, Evans D, Schreiber H. Stercoral perforation of the colon. Concepts of operative management. *Am Surg*. 1985;51(9):520–522.

115. Hall CL, Lampert PW. Immunohistochemistry as an aid in the diagnosis of Hirschsprung's disease. *Am J Clin Pathol*. 1985;83(2):177–181.

116. Hall M. Severe pain in the rectum and its remedy. *Lancet*. 1841;1:838–854.

117. Hallan RI, Williams NS, Melling J, et al. Treatment of anismus in intractable constipation with botulinum A toxin. *Lancet*. 1988;2(8613):714–717.

118. Halligan S, Bartram C, Hall C, et al. Enterocele revealed by simultaneous evacuation proctography and perineography: does "defecation block" exist? *Am J Roentgenol*. 1996;167(2):461–466.

119. Halligan S, Bartram CI, Park HJ, et al. Proctographic features of anismus. *Radiology*. 1995;197(3):679–682.

120. Halligan S, Nicholls RJ, Bartram CI, et al. Evacuation proctography in patients with solitary rectal ulcer syndrome: anatomic abnormalities and frequency of impaired emptying and prolapse. *Am J Roentgenol*. 1995;164(1):91–95.

121. Hassan I, Pemberton JH, Young-Fadok TM, et al. Ileorectal anastomosis for slow transit constipation: long-term functional and quality of life results. *J Gastrointest Surg*. 2006;10(10):1330–1337.

122. He CL, Burgart L, Wang L, et al. Decreased interstitial cell of cajal volume in patients with slow-transit constipation. *Gastroenterology*. 2000;118(1):14–21.

123. Heah SM, Ho YH, Tan M, et al. Biofeedback is effective treatment for levator ani syndrome. *Dis Colon Rectum*. 1997;40(2):187–189.

124. Healy JC, Halligan S, Reznek RH, et al. Magnetic resonance imaging of the pelvic floor in patients with obstructed defaecation. *Br J Surg*. 1997;84(11):1555–1558.

125. Henry MM, Parks AG, Swash M. The pelvic floor musculature in the descending perineum syndrome. *Br J Surg*. 1982;69(8):470–472.

126. Heriot AG, Tilney HS, Simon JN. The application of percutaneous endoscopic colostomy to the management of obstructed defecation. *Dis Colon Rectum*. 2002;45(5):700–702.

127. Heymen S, Jones KR, Scarlett Y, et al. Biofeedback treatment of constipation: a critical review. *Dis Colon Rectum*. 2003;46(9):1208–1217.

128. Heymen S, Scarlett Y, Jones K, et al. Randomized, controlled trial shows biofeedback to be superior to alternative treatments for patients with pelvic floor dyssynergia-type constipation. *Dis Colon Rectum*. 2007;50(4):428–441.

129. Heymen S, Wexner SD, Vickers D, et al. Prospective, randomized trial comparing four biofeedback techniques for patients with constipation. *Dis Colon Rectum*. 1999;42(11):1388–1393.

130. Hinds JP, Stoney B, Wald A. Does gender or the menstrual cycle affect colonic transit? *Am J Gastroenterol*. 1989;84(2):123–126.

131. Hinton JM, Lennard-Jones JE, Young AC. A new method for studying gut transit times using radioopaque markers. *Gut*. 1969;10(10):842–847.

132. Hirschprung H. Stuhltragheit neugeborener in forge von diation und hypertropic des colons. *Jahrbuch fur Kinderkrankheiten*. 1887;27:1–7.

133. Ho YH, Tan M, Goh HS. Clinical and physiologic effects of biofeedback in outlet obstruction constipation. *Dis Colon Rectum*. 1996;39(5):520–524.

134. Holzer B, Rosen HR, Nove G, et al. Sacral nerve stimulation in patients with severe constipation. *Dis Colon Rectum*. 2008;51(5):524–529.

135. Hompes R, Harmston C, Wijffels N, et al. Excellent response rate of anismus to botulinum toxin if rectal prolapse misdiagnosed as anismus ("pseudoanismus") is excluded. *Colorectal Dis*. 2012;14(2):224–230.

136. Hompes R, Jones OM, Cunningham C, et al. What causes chronic idiopathic perineal pain? *Colorectal Dis*. 2010;13(9):1035–1039. doi:10.1111/j.1463-1318.2010.02422.x.

137. Hughes SF, Williams NS. Continent colonic conduit for the treatment of faecal incontinence associated with disordered evacuation. *Br J Surg*. 1995;82(10):1318–1320.

138. Hull TL, Milsom JW, Church J, et al. Electrogalvanic stimulation for levator syndrome: how effective is it in the long-term? *Dis Colon Rectum*. 1993;36(8):731–733.

139. Hyman PE. Adolescents and young adults with Hirschsprung's disease. *Curr Gastroenterol Rep*. 2006;8(5):425–429.

140. Ikawa H, Kim SH, Hendren WH, et al. Acetylcholinesterase and manometry in the diagnosis of the constipated child. *Arch Surg*. 1986;121(4):435–438.

141. Jain D, Moussa K, Tandon M, et al. Role of interstitial cells of Cajal in motility disorders of the bowel. *Am J Gastroenterol*. 2003;98(3):618–624.

142. Jetmore AB, Timmcke AE, Gathright JB Jr, et al. Ogilvie's syndrome: colonoscopic decompression and analysis of predisposing factors. *Dis Colon Rectum*. 1992;35(12):1135–1142.

143. Johnson PH. Coccygodynia. *J Ark Med Soc*. 1981;77(10):421–424.

144. Jones PN, Lubowski DZ, Swash M, et al. Is paradoxical contraction of puborectalis muscle of functional importance? *Dis Colon Rectum*. 1987;30(9):667–670.

145. Jones PN, Lubowski DZ, Swash M, et al. Relation between perineal descent and pudendal nerve damage in idiopathic faecal incontinence. *Int J Colorectal Dis*. 1987;2(2):93–95.

146. Jones R, Lydeard S. Irritable bowel syndome in the general population. *Br Med J*. 1991;304(6819):87–90.

147. Joo JS, Agachan F, Wolff B, et al. Initial North American experience with botulinum toxin type A for treatment of anismus. *Dis Colon Rectum*. 1996;39(10):1107–1111.

148. Jorge JM, Wexner SD, Ger GC, et al. Cinedefecography and electromyography in the diagnosis of nonrelaxing puborectalis syndrome. *Dis Colon Rectum*. 1993;36(7):668–676.

149. Kamm MA, Dudding TC, Melenhost J, et al. Sacral nerve stimulation for intractable constipation. *Gut*. 2010;59(3):333–340.

150. Kamm MA, Farthing MJ, Lennard-Jones JL. Bowel function and transit rate during the menstrual cycle. *Gut*. 1989;30(5):605–608.

151. Kamm MA, Farthing MJ, Lennard-Jones JE, et al. Steroid hormone abnormalities in women with severe idiopathic constipation. *Gut*. 1991;32(1):80–84.

152. Kamm MA, Hawley PR, Lennard-Jones JE. Lateral division of the puborectalis muscle in the management of severe constipation. *Br J Surg*. 1988;75(7):661–663.

153. Kamm MA, Hawley PR, Lennard-Jones JE. Outcome of colectomy for severe idiopathic constipation. *Gut*. 1988;29(7):969–973.

154. Kamm MA, Hoyle CH, Burleigh DE, et al. Hereditary internal anal sphincter myopathy causing proctalgia fugax and constipation. A newly identified condition. *Gastroenterology*. 1991;100(3):805–810.

155. Kamm MA, Lennard-Jones JE, Thompson DG, et al. Dynamic scanning defines a colonic defect in severe idiopathic constipation. *Gut*. 1988;29(8):1085–1092.

156. Kamm MA, McLean A, Farthing MJ, et al. Ultrasonography shows no abnormality of pelvic structures in women with severe idiopathic constipation. *Gut*. 1989;30(9):1241–1243.

157. Kamm MA, Stabile G. Management of idiopathic megarectum and megacolon. *Br J Surg*. 1991;78(8):899–900.

158. Karam SE, Nies DM. Student/staff collaboration: a pilot bowel management program. *J Gerontol Nurs*. 1994;20(3):32–40.

159. Karasick S, Ehrlich SM. Is constipation a disorder of defecation or impaired motility? Distinction based on defecography and colonic transit studies. *AJR Am J Roentgenol*. 1996;166(1):63–66.

160. Karlbom U, Hållden M, Eeg-Olofsson KE, et al. Results of biofeedback in constipated patients: a prospective study. *Dis Colon Rectum*. 1997;40(10):1149–1155.

161. Karras JD, Angelo G. Proctalgia fugax. Clinical observations and a new diagnostic aid. *Am J Surg*. 1951;82(5):616–625.

162. Kawimbe BM, Papachrysostomou M, Binnie NR, et al. Outlet obstruction constipation (anismus) managed by biofeedback. *Gut*. 1991;32(10):1175–1179.

163. Keck JO, Staniunas RJ, Coller JA, et al. Biofeedback training is useful in fecal incontinence but disappointing in constipation. *Dis Colon Rectum*. 1994;37(12):1271–1276.

164. Keighley MR, Henry MM, Bartolo DC, et al. Anorectal physiology measurement: report of a working party. *Br J Surg*. 1989;76(4):356–357.

165. Kenefick NJ, Nicholls RJ, Cohen RG, et al. Permanent sacral nerve stimulation for treatment of idiopathic constipation. *Br J Surg*. 2002;89(7):882–888.

166. Kenefick NJ, Vaizey CJ, Cohen CR, et al. Double-blind placebo-controlled crossover study of sacral nerve stimulation for idiopathic constipation. *Br J Surg*. 2002;89(12):1570–1571.

167. Kerremans R. Radio-cinematographic examination of the rectum and the anal canal in cases of rectal constipation. A radio-cinematographic and physical explanation of dyschezia. *Acta Gastroenterol Belg*. 1968;31(8):561–570.

168.   Kinnunen O. Study of constipation in a geriatric hospital, day hospital, old people's home and at home. *Aging (Milano)*. 1991;3(2):161–170.

169.   Kirshner R. Stercoraceous ulcer and perforation of the colon: a case report and review of the literature. *Contemp Surg*. 1985;26:57.

170.   Klück P, van Muijen GN, van der Kamp AW, et al. Hirschsprung's disease studied with monoclonal antineurofilament antibodies on tissue sections. *Lancet*. 1984;1(8378):652–654.

171.   Knowles CH, Eccersley AJ, Scott SM, et al. Linear discriminant analysis of symptoms in patients with chronic constipation: validation of a new scoring system (KESS). *Dis Colon Rectum*. 2000;43(10):1419–1426.

172.   Knowles CH, Gayther SA, Scott M, et al. Idiopathic slow-transit constipation is not associated with mutations of the RET proto-oncogene or GDNF. *Dis Colon Rectum*. 2000;43(6):851–857.

173.   Knowles CH, Lang B, Clover L, et al. A role for autoantibodies in some cases of acquired non-paraneoplastic gut dysmotility. *Scand J Gastroenterol*. 2002;37(2):166–170.

174.   Knowles CH, Martin JE. Slow transit constipation: a model of human gut dysmotility. Review of possible aetiologies. *Neurogastroenterol Motil*. 2000;12(2):181–196.

175.   Knowles CH, Scott SM, Rayner C, et al. Idiopathic slow-transit constipation: an almost exclusively female disorder. *Dis Colon Rectum*. 2003; 46(12):1716–1717.

176.   Knowles CH, Silk DB, Darzi A, et al. Deranged smooth muscle alpha-actin as a biomarker of intestinal pseudo-obstruction: a controlled multinational case series. *Gut*. 2004;53(11):1583–1589.

177.   Koch SM, Melenhorst J, van Gemert WG, et al. Prospective study of colonic irrigation for the treatment of defaecation disorders. *Br J Surg*. 2008;95(10):1273–1279.

178.   Koch TR, Carney JA, Go L, et al. Idiopathic chronic constipation is associated with decreased colonic vasoactive intestinal peptide. *Gastroenterology*. 1988;94(2):300–310.

179.   Koh CE, Young CJ, Young JM, et al. Systematic review of randomized controlled trials of the effectiveness of biofeedback for pelvic floor dysfunction. *Br J Surg*. 2008;95(9):1079–1087.

180.   Kokoszka J, Nelson R, Falconio M, et al. Treatment of fecal impaction with pulsed irrigation enhanced evacuation. *Dis Colon Rectum*. 1994; 37(2):161–164.

181.   König P, Ambrose NS, Scott N. Hereditary internal anal sphincter myopathy causing proctalgia fugax and constipation: further clinical and histological characterization in a patient. *Eur J Gastroenterol Hepatol*. 2000; 12(1):127–128.

182.   Koutsomanis D, Lennard-Jones JE, Roy AJ, et al. Controlled randomised trial of visual biofeedback versus muscle training without a visual display for intractable constipation. *Gut*. 1995;37(1):95–99.

183.   Krevsky B, Malmud LS, D'Ercole F, et al. Colonic transit scintigraphy. A physiologic approach to the quantitative measurement of colonic transit in humans. *Gastroenterology*. 1986;91(5):1102–1112.

184.   Krishnamurthy S, Schuffler MD, Rohrmann CA, et al. Severe idiopathic constipation is associated with a distinctive abnormality of the colonic myenteric plexus. *Gastroenterology*. 1985;88(1 pt 1):26–34.

185.   Krogh K, Laurberg S. Malone antegrade continence enema for faecal incontinence and constipation in adults. *Br J Surg*. 1998;85(7):974–977.

186.   Kuijpers HC. Application of the colorectal laboratory in diagnosis and treatment of functional constipation. *Dis Colon Rectum*. 1990;33(1): 35–39.

187.   Kuijpers HC, Bleijenberg G. The spastic pelvic floor syndrome. A cause of constipation. *Dis Colon Rectum*. 1985;28(9):669–672.

188.   Kumar D, Wingate DL. Colorectal motility. In: Henry MM, Swash M, eds. *Coloproctology and the Pelvic Floor. Pathophysiology and Management*. London, United Kingdom: Butterworths; 1985:47–61.

189.   Lane WA. Remarks on the results of the operative treatment of chronic constipation. *Br Med J*. 1908;1(2455):126–130.

190.   Lee JI, Park H, Kamm MA, et al. Decreased density of interstitial cells of Cajal and neuronal cells in patients with slow-transit constipation and acquired megacolon. *J Gastroenterol Hepatol*. 2005;20(8):1292–1298.

191.   Lee JT, Taylor BM, Singleton BC. Epidural anesthesia for acute pseudo-obstruction of the colon (Ogilvie's syndrome). *Dis Colon Rectum*. 1988; 31(9):686–691.

192.   Leng-Peschlow E. Senna and its rational use. *Pharmacology*. 1992; 44(suppl 1)1–52.

193.   Lennard-Jones JE. Pathophysiology of constipation. *Br J Surg*. 1985; 72(suppl):S7–S8.

194.   Lestàr B, Penninckx F, Kerremans R. Biofeedback defaecation training for anismus. *Int J Colorectal Dis*. 1991;6(4):202–207.

195.   Levitt MA, Mathis KL, Pemberton JH. Surgical treatment for constipation in children and adults. *Best Pract Res Clin Gastroenterol*. 2011; 25(1):167–179.

196.   Loening-Baucke V. Persistence of chronic constipation in children after biofeedback treatment. *Dig Dis Sci*. 1991;36(2):153–160.

197.   Loening-Baucke VA, Anuras S, Mitros FA. Changes in colorectal function in patients with chronic colonic pseudoobstruction. *Dig Dis Sci*. 1987; 32(10):1104–1112.

198.   Longo WE, Vernava AM III. Prokinetic agents for lower gastrointestinal motility disorders. *Dis Colon Rectum*. 1993;36(7):696–708.

199.   Longstreth GF, Thompson WG, Chey WD, et al. Functional bowel disorders. *Gastroenterology*. 2006;130(5):1480–1491.

200.   Lopez MJ, Memula N, Doss LL, et al. Pseudo-obstruction of the colon during pelvic radiotherapy. *Dis Colon Rectum*. 1981;24(3):201–204.

201.   Lowenstein B, Cataldo PA. Treatment of proctalgia fugax with topical nitroglycerin: report of a case. *Dis Colon Rectum*. 1998;41(5):667–668.

202.   Lubowski DZ, Chen FC, Kennedy ML, et al. Results of colectomy for severe slow transit constipation. *Dis Colon Rectum*. 1996;39(1):23–29.

203.   Lui RC, Herz B, Plantilla E, et al. Stercoral perforation of the colon: report of a new location. *Am J Gastroenterol*. 1988;83(4):457–459.

204.   Luukkonen P, Heikkinen M, Huikuri K, et al. Adult Hirschsprung's disease. Clinical features and functional outcome after surgery. *Dis Colon Rectum*. 1990;33(1):65–69.

205.   Lynch CR, Jones RG, Hilden K, et al. Percutaneous endoscopic cecostomy in adults: a case series. *Gastrointest Endosc*. 2006;64(2):279–282.

206.   Lynn HB, van Heerden JA. Rectal myectomy in Hirschsprung's disease: a decade of experience. *Arch Surg*. 1975;110(8):991–994.

207.   MacColl C, MacCannell KL, Baylis B, et al. Treatment of acute colonic pseudo-obstruction (Ogilvie's syndrome) with cisapride. *Gastroenterology*. 1990;98(3):773–776.

208.   Madoff RD, Orrom WJ, Rothenberger DA, et al. Rectal compliance: a critical reappraisal. *Int J Colorectal Dis*. 1990;5(1):37–40.

209.   Mahieu P, Pringot J, Bodart P. Defecography: I. Description of a new procedure and results in normal patients. *Gastrointest Radiol*. 1984; 9(3):247–251.

210.   Mahieu P, Pringot J, Bodart P. Defecography: II. Contribution to the diagnosis of defecation disorders. *Gastrointest Radiol*. 1984;9:253–261.

211.   Malone PS, Ransley PG, Kiely EM. Preliminary report: the antegrade continence enema. *Lancet*. 1990;336(8725):1217–1218.

212.   Malouf AJ, Wiesel PH, Nicholls T, et al. Short-term effects of sacral nerve stimulation for idiopathic slow transit constipation. *World J Surg*. 2002;26(2):166–170.

213.   Mapp E. Colonic manifestations of the connective tissue disorders. *Am J Gastroenterol*. 1981;75(5):386–393.

214.   Maria G, Anastasio G, Brisinda G, et al. Treatment of puborectalis syndrome with progressive anal dilation. *Dis Colon Rectum*. 1997;40(1):89–92.

215.   Maria G, Brisinda G, Bentivoglio AR, et al. Botulinum toxin in the treatment of outlet obstruction constipation caused by puborectalis syndrome. *Dis Colon Rectum*. 2000;43(3):376–380.

216.   Maria G, Cadeddu F, Brandara F, et al. Experience with type A botulinum toxin for treatment of outlet-type constipation. *Am J Gastroenterol*. 2006;101(11):2570–2575.

217.   Maroy B. Spontaneous and evoked coccygeal pain in depression. *Dis Colon Rectum*. 1988;31(3):210–215.

218.   Martin FM, Robinson AM Jr, Thompson WR. Therapeutic colonoscopy in the treatment of colonic pseudo-obstruction. *Am Surg*. 1988; 54(8):519–522.

219.   Mashour GA, Peterfreund RA. Spinal anesthesia and Ogilvie's syndrome. *J Clin Anesth*. 2005;17(2):122–123.

220.   Matzel KE, Stadelmaier U, Hohenfeller M, et al. Electrical stimulation of sacral spinal nerves for treatment of faecal incontinence. *Lancet*. 1995;346(8983):1124–1127.

221.   Maull KI, Kinning WK, Kay S. Stercoral ulceration. *Am Surg*. 1982; 48(1):20–24.

222.   Maurer AH, Krevsky B. Whole-gut transit scintigraphy in the evaluation of small-bowel and colon transit disorders. *Semin Nucl Med*. 1995;25(4):326–338.

223.   Maurer CA, Renzulli P, Mazzucchelli L, et al. Use of accurate diagnostic criteria may increase incidence of stercoral perforation of the colon. *Dis Colon Rectum*. 2000;43(7):991–998.

224.   McCallum IJ, Ong S, Mercer-Jones M. Chronic constipation in adults. *Br Med J*. 2009;338:b831.

225.   McCready RA, Beart RW Jr. Adult Hirschsprung's disease: results of surgical treatment at Mayo Clinic. *Dis Colon Rectum*. 1980;23(6):401–407.

226.   McKee RF, McEnroe L, Anderson JH, et al. Identification of patients likely to benefit from biofeedback for outlet obstruction constipation. *Br J Surg*. 1999;86(3):355–359.

227.   McLean RG, Smart RC, Lubowski DZ, et al. Oral colon transit scintigraphy using indium-111 DTPA: variability in healthy subjects. *Int J Colorectal Dis*. 1992;7(4):173–176.

228. McMahon JM, Underwood ES, Kirby WE. Colon spasm and pseudo-obstruction in an elongated colon secondary to physical exertion: diagnosis by stress barium enema. *Am J Gastroenterol.* 1999;94(11):3362–3364.

229. Meagher A, Sun WM, Kennedy ML, et al. Biofeedback for anismus: has placebo effect been overlooked? *Colorectal Disease.* 1999;1(2):80–87.

230. Meier-Ruge WA, Müeller-Lobeck H, Stoss F, et al. The pathogenesis of idiopathic megacolon. *Eur J Gastroenterol Hepatol.* 2006;18(11):1209–1215.

231. Meshkinpour H, Selod S, Movahedi H, et al. Effects of regular exercise in management of chronic idiopathic constipation. *Dig Dis Sci.* 1998;43(11):2379–2383.

232. Messmer JM, Wolper JC, Loewe CJ. Endoscopic-assisted tube placement for decompression of acute colonic pseudo-obstruction. *Endoscopy.* 1984;16(4):135–136.

233. Metcalf AM, Phillips SF, Zinsmeister AR, et al. Simplified assessment of segmental colonic transit. *Gastroenterology.* 1987;92(1):40–47.

234. Meyers MA. Colonic ileus. In: Greenbaum EI, ed. *Radiographic Atlas of Colon Disease.* Chicago, IL: Year Book; 1980:85.

235. Mibu R, Hotokezaka M, Mihara S, et al. Results of linearly polarized near-infrared irradiation therapy in patients with intractable anorectal pain. *Dis Colon Rectum.* 2003;46(suppl 10):S50–S53.

236. Miller R, Bartolo DC, Cervero F, et al. Anorectal sampling: a comparison of normal and incontinent patients. *Br J Surg.* 1988;75(1):44–47.

237. Mishalany HG, Woolley MG. Chronic constipation. Manometric patterns and surgical considerations. *Arch Surg.* 1984;119(11):1257–1259.

238. Miyamoto M, Egami K, Maeda S, et al. Hirschsprung's disease in adults: report of a case and review of the literature. *J Nihon Med Sch.* 2005;72(2):113–120.

239. Moffett JK, Torgerson D, Bell-Syer S, et al. Randomised controlled trial of exercise for low back pain patients: clinical outcomes, costs, and preferences. *Br Med J.* 1999;319(7205):279–283.

240. Moore BG, Singaram C, Eckhoff DE, et al. Immunohistochemical evaluations of ultrashort-segment Hirschsprung's disease. Report of three cases. *Dis Colon Rectum.* 1996;39(7):817–822.

241. Morrisey KP, Cahan AC. Colonoscopic decompression for nonobstructed colonic dilatation. *Curr Concepts Gastroenterol.* 1989;13:7–10.

242. Mowatt G, Glazener C, Jarrett M. Sacral nerve stimulation for fecal incontinence and constipation in adults: a short version Cochrane review. *Neurourol Urodyn.* 2008;27(3):155–161.

243. Müller-Lissner S. What has happened to the cathartic colon? *Gut.* 1996;39(3):486–488.

244. Müller-Lissner SA, Kamm MA, Scarpignato C, et al. Myths and misconceptions about chronic constipation. *Am J Gastroenterol.* 2005;100(1):232–242.

245. Nakhgevany KB. Colonoscopic decompression of the colon in patients with Ogilvie's syndrome. *Am J Surg.* 1984;148(3):317–320.

246. Nanni G, Garbini A, Luchetti P, et al. Ogilvie's syndrome (acute colonic pseudo-obstruction): review of the literature (October 1948 to March 1980) and report of four additional cases. *Dis Colon Rectum.* 1982;25(2):157–166.

247. Nathan BN. An early clinical account of proctalgia fugax. *Dis Colon Rectum.* 1990;33(6):539.

248. National Institute for Health and Clinical Excellence. Spinal cord stimulation for chronic pain of neuropathic or ischaemic origin. http://www.nice.org.uk/nicemedia/pdf/TA159Guidance.pdf. Issue date October 2008. Accessed.

249. Natsikas NB, Sbarounis CN. Adult Hirschsprung's disease. An experience with the Duhamel-Martin procedure with special reference to obstructed patients. *Dis Colon Rectum.* 1987;30(3):204–206.

250. Nicholls RJ, Kamm MA. Proctocolectomy with restorative ileoanal reservoir for severe idiopathic constipation. Report of two cases. *Dis Colon Rectum.* 1988;31(12):968–969.

251. Nickel JC, Tripp DA, Chuai S, et al. Psychosocial variables affect the quality of life in men diagnosed with chronic prostatitis/chronic pelvic pain syndrome. *BJU Int.* 2008;101(1):59–64.

252. Nicosia JF, Abcarian H. Levator syndrome. A treatment that works. *Dis Colon Rectum.* 1985;28(6):406–408.

253. Nissan S, Bar-Maor JA, Levy E. Anorectal myomectomy in the treatment of short segment Hirschsprung's disease. *Ann Surg.* 1969;170(6):969–977.

254. O'Donnell LJ, Virjee J, Heaton KW. Detection of pseudodiarrhoea by simple clinical assessment of intestinal transit rate. *Br Med J.* 1990;300(6722):439–440.

255. Ogilvie H. Large-intestine colic due to sympathetic deprivation: a new clinical syndrome. *Br Med J.* 1948;2(4579):671–673.

256. Ohri SK, Patel T, Desa L, et al. Drug-induced colonic pseudo-obstruction. Report of a case. *Dis Colon Rectum.* 1991;34(4):347–351.

257. Oliver GC, Rubin RJ, Salvati EP, et al. Electrogalvanic stimulation in the treatment of levator syndrome. *Dis Colon Rectum.* 1985;28(9):662–663.

258. O'Súilleabháin CB, Anderson JH, McKee RF, et al. Strategy for the surgical management of patients with idiopathic megarectum and megacolon. *Br J Surg.* 2001;88(10):1392–1396.

259. Papachrysostomou M, Smith AN. Effects of biofeedback on obstructive defecation—reconditioning of the defecation reflex? *Gut.* 1994;35(2):252–256.

260. Park CH, Joo YE, Kim HS, et al. Neostigmine for the treatment of acute hepatic encephalopathy with acute intestinal pseudo-obstruction in a cirrhotic patient. *J Korean Med Sci.* 2005;20(1):150–152.

261. Pemberton JH, Rath DM, Ilstrup DM. Evaluation and surgical treatment of severe chronic constipation. *Ann Surg.* 1991;214(4):403–411.

262. Pham TN, Cosman BC, Chu P, et al. Radiographic changes after colonoscopic decompression for acute pseudo-obstruction. *Dis Colon Rectum.* 1999;42(12):1586–1591.

263. Pikarsky AJ, Singh JJ, Weiss EG, et al. Long-term follow-up of patients undergoing colectomy for colonic inertia. *Dis Colon Rectum.* 2001;44(2):179–183.

264. Pinho M, Yoshioka K, Keighley MR. Long term results of anorectal myectomy for chronic constipation. *Br J Surg.* 1989;76(11):1163–1164.

265. Pinho M, Yoshioka K, Keighley MR. Long-term results of anorectal myectomy for chronic constipation. *Dis Colon Rectum.* 1990;33(9):795–777.

266. Poirier M, Abcarian H, Nelson R. Malone antegrade continent enema: an alternative to resection in severe defecation disorders. *Dis Colon Rectum.* 2007;50(1):22–28.

267. Ponec RJ, Saunders MD, Kimmey MB. Neostigmine for the treatment of acute colonic pseudo-obstruction. *N Engl J Med.* 1999;341(3):137–141.

268. Ponsky JL, Aszodi A, Perse D. Percutaneous endoscopic cecostomy: a new approach to nonobstructive colonic dilation. *Gastrointest Endosc.* 1986;32(2):108–111.

269. Preston DM, Lennard-Jones JE. Severe chronic constipation of young women: "idiopathic slow transit constipation." *Gut.* 1986;27(1):41–48.

270. Preston DM, Lennard-Jones JE, Thomas BM. The balloon proctogram. *Br J Surg.* 1984;71(1):29–32.

271. Preston DM, Lennard-Jones JE, Thomas BM. Towards a radiologic definition of idiopathic megacolon. *Gastrointest Radiol.* 1985;10(2):167–169.

272. Preziosi G, Emmanuel A. Neurogenic bowel dysfunction: pathophysiology, clinical manifestations and treatment. *Expert Rev Gastroenterol Hepatol.* 2009;3(4):417–423.

273. Quigley EM, Vandeplassche L, Kerstens R, et al. Clinical trial: the efficacy, impact on quality of life, and safety and tolerability of prucalopride in severe chronic constipation—a 12-week, randomized, double-blind, placebo-controlled study. *Aliment Pharmacol Ther.* 2009;29(3):315–328.

274. Ramage JI Jr, Baron TH. Percutaneous endoscopic cecostomy: a case series. *Gastrointest Endosc.* 2003;57(6):752–755.

275. Rao SS. Biofeedback therapy for constipation in adults. *Best Pract Res Clin Gastroenterol.* 2011;25(1):159–166.

276. Rao SS, Seaton K, Miller M, et al. Randomized controlled trial of biofeedback, sham feedback, and standard therapy for dyssernergic defecation. *Clin Gastroenterol Hepatol.* 2007;5(3):331–338.

277. Rao SS, Singh S. Clinical utility of colonic and anorectal manometry in chronic constipation. *J Clin Gastroenterol.* 2010;44(9):597–609.

278. Ravo B, Pollane M, Ger R. Pseudo-obstruction of the colon following caesarean section. A review. *Dis Colon Rectum.* 1983;26(7):440–444.

279. Redmond JM, Smith GW, Barofsky I, et al. Physiological tests to predict long-term outcome of total abdominal colectomy for intractable constipation. *Am J Gastroenterol.* 1995;90(5):748–753.

280. Renzi C, Pescatori M. Psychologic aspects in proctalgia. *Dis Colon Rectum.* 2000;43(4):535–539.

281. Ricciardi R, Counihan TC, Banner BF, et al. What is the normal aganglionic segment of anorectum in adults? *Dis Colon Rectum.* 1999;42(3):380–382.

282. Ricketts RR, Pettitt BJ. Management of Hirschsprung's disease in adolescents. *Am Surg.* 1989;55(4):219–225.

283. Riecken EO, Zeitz M, Emde C, et al. The effect of an anthraquinone laxative on colonic nerve tissue: a controlled trial in constipated women. *Z Gastroenterol.* 1990;28(12):660–664.

284. Riemann JF, Schmidt H. Ultrastructural changes in the gut autonomic nervous system following laxative abuse and in other conditions. *Scand J Gastroenterol Suppl.* 1982;71:111–124.

285. Robbins RD, Schoen R, Sohn N, et al. Colonic decompression of massive cecal dilatation (Ogilvie's syndrome) secondary to cesarean section. *Am J Gastroenterol.* 1982;77(4):231–232.

286. Robert R, Labat JJ, Bensignor M, et al. Decompression and transposition of the pudendal nerve in pudendal neuralgia: a randomized controlled trial and long-term evaluation. *Eur Urol.* 2005;47(3):403–408.

287. Roberts JP, Womack NR, Hallan RI, et al. Evidence from dynamic integrated proctography to redefine anismus. *Br J Surg.* 1992;79(11):1213–1215.

288. Roe AM, Bartolo DC, Mortensen NJ. Diagnosis and surgical management of intractable constipation. *Br J Surg.* 1986;73(10):854–861.

289. Ron Y, Avni Y, Lukovetski A, et al. Botulinum toxin type-A in therapy of patients with anismus. *Dis Colon Rectum.* 2001;44(12):1821–1826.

290. Rongen MJ, van der Hoop AG, Baeten CG. Cecal access for antegrade colon enemas in medically refractory slow-transit constipation: a prospective study. *Dis Colon Rectum.* 2001;44(11):1644–1649.

291. Roos JE, Weishaupt D, Wildermuth S, et al. Experience of 4 years with open MR defecofraphy: pictorial review of anorectal anatomy and disease. *Radiographics.* 2002;22(4):817–832.

292. Sacher P, Buchmann P, Burger H. Stenosis of the large intestine complicating scleroderma and mimicking a sigmoid carcinoma. *Dis Colon Rectum.* 1983;26(5):347–348.

293. Salvati EP. The levator syndrome and its variant. *Gastroenterol Clin North Am.* 1987;16(1):71–78.

294. Sandler RS, Jordan MC, Shelton BJ. Demographic and dietary determinants of constipation in the US population. *Am J Public Health.* 1990;80(2):185–189.

295. Sarna SK. Physiology and pathophysiology of colonic motor activity (1). *Dig Dis Sci.* 1991;36(6):827–862.

296. Saunders MD, Kimmey MB. Systematic review: acute colonic pseudo-obstruction. *Aliment Pharmacol Ther.* 2005;22(10):917–925.

297. Sawin R, Hatch E, Schaller R, et al. Limited surgery for lower-segment Hirschsprung's disease. *Arch Surg.* 1994;129(9):920–924.

298. Scott SM, van den Berg MM, Benninga MA. Rectal sensorimotor dysfunction in constipation. *Best Pract Res Clin Gastroenterol.* 2011;25(1):103–118.

299. Senati E, Coen LD. Massive gangrene of the colon—a complication of fecal impaction. Report of a case. *Dis Colon Rectum.* 1989;32(2):146–148.

300. Serpell JW, Nicholls RJ. Stercoral perforation of the colon. *Br J Surg.* 1990;77(12):1325–1329.

301. Shahid S, Ramzan Z, Maurer AH, et al. Chronic idiopathic constipation: more than a simple colonic transit disorder. *J Clin Gastroenterol.* 2012;46(2):150–154.

302. Shamberger RC, Crawford JL, Kirkham SE. Progressive systemic sclerosis resulting in megacolon. A case report. *JAMA.* 1983;250(8):1063–1065.

303. Shatila AH, Ackerman NB. Stercoraceous ulcerations and perforations of the colon: report of cases and survey of the literature. *Dis Colon Rectum.* 1977;20(6):524–527.

304. Shorvon PJ, McHugh S, Diamant NE, et al. Defecography in normal volunteers: results and implications. *Gut.* 1989;30(12):1737–1749.

305. Silk DB. Chronic idiopathic intestinal pseudo-obstruction: the need for a multidisciplinary approach to management. *Proc Nutr Soc.* 2004;63(3):473–480.

306. Simpson DA, Pawlak AM, Tegmeyer L, et al. Paraneoplastic intestinal pseudo-obstruction, mononeuritis multiplex, and sensory neuropathy/neuronopathy. *J Am Osteopath Assoc.* 1996;96(2):125–128.

307. Simpson JY. Clinical lectures on the diseases of women. Lecture XVII. Coccygodynia and diseases and deformities of the coccyx. *M Times Gaz.* 1859;40:1–7.

308. Siproudhis L, Le Gall R, Ropert A, et al. Does manometric megarectum have a symptomatic role in patients complaining of dyschezia? [in French]. *Gastroenterol Clin Biol.* 1993;17(3):162–167.

309. Sloyer AF, Panella VS, Demas BE, et al. Ogilvie's syndrome. Successful management without colonoscopy. *Dig Dis Sci.* 1988;33(11):1391–1396.

310. Smith B. Effect of irritant purgatives on the myenteric plexus in man and the mouse. *Gut.* 1968;9(2):139–143.

311. Smith B, Grace RH, Todd IP. Organic constipation in adults. *Br J Surg.* 1977;64(5):313–314.

312. Soave F. A new surgical technique for treatment of Hirschsprung's disease. *Surgery.* 1964;56:1007–1014.

313. Sohn N, Weinstein MA, Robbins RD. The levator syndrome and its treatment with high-voltage electrogalvanic stimulation. *Am J Surg.* 1982;144(5):580–582.

314. Sørhaug S, Steinshamn SL, Waldum HL. Octreotide treatment for paraneoplastic intestinal pseudo-obstruction complicating SCLC. *Lung Cancer.* 2005;48(1):137–140.

315. Soudah HC, Hasler WL, Owyang C. Effect of octreotide on intestinal motility and bacterial overgrowth in scleroderma. *N Engl J Med.* 1991;325(21):1461–1467.

316. Stabile G, Kamm MA, Hawley PR, et al. Results of the Duhamel operation in the treatment of idiopathic megarectum and megacolon. *Br J Surg.* 1991;78(6):661–663.

317. Stabile G, Kamm MA, Phillips RK, et al. Partial colectomy and coloanal anastomosis for idiopathic megarectum and megacolon. *Dis Colon Rectum.* 1992;35(2):158–162.

318. Stanghellini V, Cogliandro RF, De Giorgio R, et al. Natural history of chronic idiopathic intestinal pseudo-obstruction in adults: a single center study. *Clin Gastroenterol Hepatol.* 2005;3(5):449–458.

319. Stephen AM, Cummings JH. Water-holding by dietary fibre in vitro and its relationship to faecal output in man. *Gut.* 1979;20(8):722–729.

320. Stephenson BM, Morgan AR, Salaman JR, et al. Ogilvie's syndrome: a new approach to an old problem. *Dis Colon Rectum.* 1995;38(4):424–427.

321. Stewart J, Kumar D, Keighley MR. Results of anal or low rectal anastomosis and pouch construction for megarectum and megacolon. *Br J Surg.* 1994;81(7):1051–1053.

322. Stivland T, Camilleri M, Vassallo M, et al. Scintigraphic measurement of regional gut transit in idiopathic constipation. *Gastroenterology.* 1991;101(1):107–115.

323. Stratta RJ, Starling JR, D'Alessandro AM, et al. Acute colonic ileus (pseudo-obstruction) in renal transplant recipients. *Surgery.* 1988;104(4):616–623.

324. Strel'nikov BE, Tsarev NI. Treatment of dolichosigmoid and dolichocolon [in Russian]. *Vestn Khir Im I I Grek.* 1978;121(10):80–84.

325. Strodel WE, Nostrant TT, Eckhauser FE, et al. Therapeutic and diagnostic colonoscopy in nonobstructive colonic dilatation. *Ann Surg.* 1983;197(4):416–421.

326. Suares NC, Ford AC. Prevalence of, and risk factors for, chronic idiopathic constipation in the community: systemic review and meta-anaysis. *Am J Gastroenterol.* 2011;106(9):1582–1591.

327. Sullivan M, Bishop S, Pivik J. The pain catastrophizing scale: development and validation. *Psychol Assess.* 1995;7:524–532.

328. Sullivan MJ, Martel MO, Tripp D, et al. The relation between catastrophizing and the communication of pain experience. *Pain.* 2006;122(3):282–288.

329. Sullivan SN, Wong C, Heidenheim P. Does running cause gastrointestinal symptoms? A survey of 93 randomly selected runners compared with controls. *N Z Med J.* 1994;107(984):328–331.

330. Sunderland GT, Poon FW, Lauder J, et al. Videoproctography in selecting patients with constipation for colectomy. *Dis Colon Rectum.* 1992;35(3):235–237.

331. Swenson O, Rheinlander HF, Diamond I. Hirschsprung's disease: a new concept of the etiology: operative results in 34 patients. *N Engl J Med.* 1949;241(15):551–556.

332. Tack J, van Outryve M, Beyens G, et al. Prucalopride (Resolor) in the treatment of severe chronic constipation in patients dissatisfied with laxatives. *Gut.* 2009;58(3):357–365.

333. Tada S, Iida M, Yao T, et al. Intestinal pseudo-obstruction in patients with amyloidosis: clinicopathologic differences between chemical types of amyloid protein. *Gut.* 1993;34(10):1412–1417.

334. Thaysen TE. Proctalgia fugax: a little known form of pain in the rectum. *Lancet.* 1935;2:243–246.

335. Thiele G. Tonic spasm of the levator ani, coccygeus, and piriformis muscles: its relationship to coccygodynia and pain in the region of the hip and down the leg. *Trans Am Proctol Soc.* 1936;37:145–155.

336. Thiele GH. Coccygodynia and pain in the superior gluteal region and down the back of the thigh: causation by tonic spasm of the levator ani, coccygeus, and piriformis muscles and relief by massage of these muscles. *JAMA.* 1937;109(16):1271–1275.

337. Thiele G. Coccygodynia: the mechanism of its production and its relationship to anorectal disease. *Am J Surg.* 1950;79:110–116.

338. Thomas CG Jr, Bream CA, DeConnick P. Posterior sphincterotomy and rectal myotomy in the management of Hirschsprung's disease. *Ann Surg.* 1970;171(5):796–810.

339. Thompson AR, Pearson T, Ellul J, et al. Percutaneous endoscopic colostomy in patients with chronic intestinal pseudo-obstruction. *Gastrointest Endosc.* 2004;59(1):113–115.

340. Thompson WG, Creed FH, Drossman DA, et al. Functional bowel disorders and functional abdominal pain. *Gastroenterol Int.* 1992;5:75–91.

341. Thompson WG, Longstreth GF, Drossman DA, et al. C. functional bowel disorders and D. functional abdominal pain. In: Drossman DA, Corazziari E, Talley NJ, et al, eds. *Rome II: The Functional Gastrointestinal Disorders.* 2nd ed. Washington, DC: Degnon; 2000:351–432.

342. Thompson WG, Longstreth GF, Drossman SA, et al. Functional bowel disorders and functional abdominal pain. *Gut.* 1999;45(suppl 2):II43–II47.

343. Tod AM, Stringer E, Levery C, et al. Rectal irrigation in the management of functional bowel disorders: a review. *Br J Nurs*. 2007;16(14): 858–864.

344. Todd IP. Discussion on megacolon and megarectum with the emphasis on conditions other than Hirschsprung's disease. *Proc R Soc Med*. 1961;54:1035–1040.

345. Trinkley KE, Nahata MC. Treatment of irritable bowel syndrome. *J Clin Pharm Ther*. 2011;36(3):275–282.

346. Turnbull GK, Ritvo PG. Anal sphincter biofeedback relaxation treatment for women with intractable constipation symptoms. *Dis Colon Rectum*. 1992;35(6):530–536.

347. Udassin R, Nissan S, Lernau O, et al. The mild form of Hirschsprung's disease (short segment): fourteen-years experience in diagnosis and treatment. *Ann Surg*. 1981;194(6):767–770.

348. van der Plas RN, Benninga MA, Büller HA, et al. Biofeedback training in treatment of childhood constipation: a randomised controlled study. *Lancet*. 1996;348(9030):776–780.

349. van der Plas RN, Benninga MA, Staalman CR, et al. Megarectum in constipation. *Arch Dis Child*. 2000;83(1):52–58.

350. van der Sijp JR, Kamm MA, Nightingale JM, et al. Circulating gastrointestinal hormone abnormalities in patients with severe idiopathic constipation. *Am J Gastroenterol*. 1998;93(8):1351–1356.

351. Vanderwinden JM. Role of interstitial cells of Cajal and their relationship with the enteric nervous system. *Eur J Morphol*. 1999;37(4–5): 250–256.

352. Vanek VW, Al Salti M. Acute pseudo obstruction of the colon (Ogilvie's syndrome). An analysis of 400 cases. *Dis Colon Rectum*. 1986; 29(3):203–210.

353. Van Oudenhove L, Geeraerts B, Tack J. Limitations of current paradigms for visceral sensitivity testing. *Neurogastroenterol Motil*. 2008; 20(2):95–98.

354. Varma JS, Smith AN. Neurophysiological dysfunction in young women with intractable constipation. *Gut*. 1988;29(7):963–968.

355. Vlaeyen JW, Linton SJ. Fear-avoidance and its consequences in chronic musculoskeletal pain: a state of the art. *Pain*. 2000;85(3):317–332.

356. Vorobyov GI, Achkasov SI, Diryukov OM. Clinical features' diagnostics and treatment of Hirschsprung's disease in adults. *Colorectal Dis*. 2010;12(12):1242–1248.

357. Wald A, Burgio K, Holeva K, et al. Psychological evaluation of patients with severe idiopathic constipation: which instruments to use. *Am J Gastroenterol*. 1992;87(8):977–980.

358. Wald A, Hinds JP, Caruana BJ. Psychological and physiological characteristics of patients with severe idiopathic constipation. *Gastroenterology*. 1989;97(4):932–937.

359. Wald A, Van Thiel DH, Hoechstetter L, et al. Effect of pregnancy on gastrointestinal transit. *Dig Dis Sci*. 1982;27(11):1015–1018.

360. Waldron D, Bowes KL, Kingma YJ, et al. Colonic and anorectal motility in young women with severe idiopathic constipation. *Gastroenterology*. 1988;95(5):1388–1394.

361. Wang ZQ, Watanabe Y, Toki A, et al. Involvement of endogenous nitric oxide and c-kit-expressing cells in chronic intestinal pseudo-obstruction. *J Pediatr Surg*. 2000;35(4):539–544.

362. Watanabe Y, Ito T, Ando H, et al. Manometric evaluation of gastrointestinal motility in children with chronic intestinal pseudo-obstruction syndrome. *J Pediatr Surg*. 1996;31(2):233–238.

363. Weber J, Ducrotte P, Touchais JY, et al. Biofeedback training for constipation in adults and children. *Dis Colon Rectum*. 1987;30(11):844–846.

364. Wedel T, Spiegler J, Soellner S, et al. Enteric nerves and interstitial cells of Cajal are altered in patients with slow-transit constipation and megacolon. *Gastroenterology*. 2002;123(5):1459–1467.

365. Wexner SD, Cheape JD, Jorge JM, et al. Prospective assessment of biofeedback for the treatment of paradoxical puborectalis contraction. *Dis Colon Rectum*. 1992;35(2):145–150.

366. Wexner SD, Dailey TH. The diagnosis and surgical treatment of chronic constipation. *Contemp Surg*. 1988;32:59–70.

367. What role for prucalopride in constipation? [special article]. *Drug Ther Bull*. 2011;49(8):93–96.

368. Wheatley MJ, Wesley JR, Coran AG, et al. Hirschsprung's disease in adolescents and adults. *Dis Colon Rectum*. 1990;33(7):622–629.

369. Whitehead WE, Bharucha AE. Diagnosis and treatment of pelvic floor disorders: what's new and what to do. *Gastroenterology*. 2010;138(4): 1231–1235.

370. Wielosz E, Borys O, Zychowska I, et al. Gastrointestinal involvement in patients with systemic sclerosis. *Pol Arch Med Wewn*. 2010;120(4): 132–136.

371. Williams NS, Fajobi OA, Lunniss PJ, et al. Vertical reduction rectoplasty: a new treatment for idiopathic megarectum. *Br J Surg*. 2000; 87(9):1203–1208.

372. Womack NR, Williams NS, Holmfield JH, et al. New method for the dynamic assessment of anorectal function in constipation. *Br J Surg*. 1985; 72(12):994–998.

373. Wong RK, Palsson OS, Turner MJ, et al. Inability of the Rome III criteria to distinguish functional constipation from constipation-subtype irritable bowel syndrome. *Am J Gastroenterol*. 2010;105(10):2228–2234.

374. Wrenn K. Fecal impaction. *N Engl J Med*. 1989;321(10):658–662.

375. Wu JS, Schoetz DJ Jr, Coller JA, et al. Treatment of Hirschsprung's disease in the adult. Report of five cases. *Dis Colon Rectum*. 1995;38(6): 655–659.

376. Yokota T, Suda T, Tsukioka S, et al. The striking effect of hyperbaric oxygenation therapy in the management of chronic idiopathic intestinal pseudo-obstruction. *Am J Gastroenterol*. 2000;95(1):285–288.

377. Yoshioka K, Keighley MR. Anorectal myectomy for outlet obstruction. *Br J Surg*. 1987;74(5):373–376.

378. Yoshioka K, Keighley MR. Randomized trial comparing anorectal myectomy and controlled anal dilatation for outlet obstruction. *Br J Surg*. 1987;74(12):1125–1129.

379. Yüksel I, Ataseven H, Ertug;abrul I, et al. Adult segmental Hirschsprung disease. *South Med J*. 2009;102(2):184–185.

380. Zbar AP, de la Portilla F, Borrero JJ, et al. Hereditary internal anal sphincter myopathy: the first Caribbean family. *Tech Coloproctol*. 2007; 11(1):60–63.

381. Zutshi M, Hull TL, Trzcinski R, et al. Surgery for slow transit constipation: are we helping patients? *Int J Colorectal Dis*. 2007;22(3): 265–269.

21

Rectal Prolapse (Internal and External), Solitary Rectal Ulcer, Descending Perineum Syndrome, and Rectocele

Ian Lindsey and R. John Nicholls

Man should always strive to have his intestines relaxed all the days of his life and that bowel function should approximate diarrhea. This is a fundamental principle in medicine that whenever the stool is withheld or is extruded with difficulty, grave illnesses result.

—MOSES BEN MAIMON (MAIMONIDES):
Mishneh Torah, Hilchoth De'oth, 4.13

► EXTERNAL RECTAL PROLAPSE

Rectal prolapse (procidentia) or "falling down of the hindgut" has long fascinated surgeons. It was recognized in antiquity, having been described in the Ebers Papyrus of 1500 BC.[188] It usually occurs in persons at the extremes of life. The two types of presentations are a complete or full-thickness involvement of the bowel and a partial or incomplete type involving prolapse of the mucosa only. The latter may be circumferential or may be limited to only a portion of the rectal mucosa.

Anatomy and Physiology

The precise cause of rectal prolapse is not fully understood, but certain factors seem to be implicated in its development.[314] The normal spine with its curvature and the tilt of the pelvis serve to shift the weight of the abdominal organs forward, away from the pelvic floor and cause the rectum to follow a serpentine course through the pelvis.[234] The stability of the rectum is greatly aided by the support of the levator ani muscle. An extensive interweaving of the longitudinal fibers of the rectum with the levator fibers creates a stable attachment between the rectum and this muscle. This provides a firm fixation to the pelvic floor and is an important element in rectal stability; without it, the rectum would slip down through the muscle during defecation (Figure 21-1).[39,234–236]

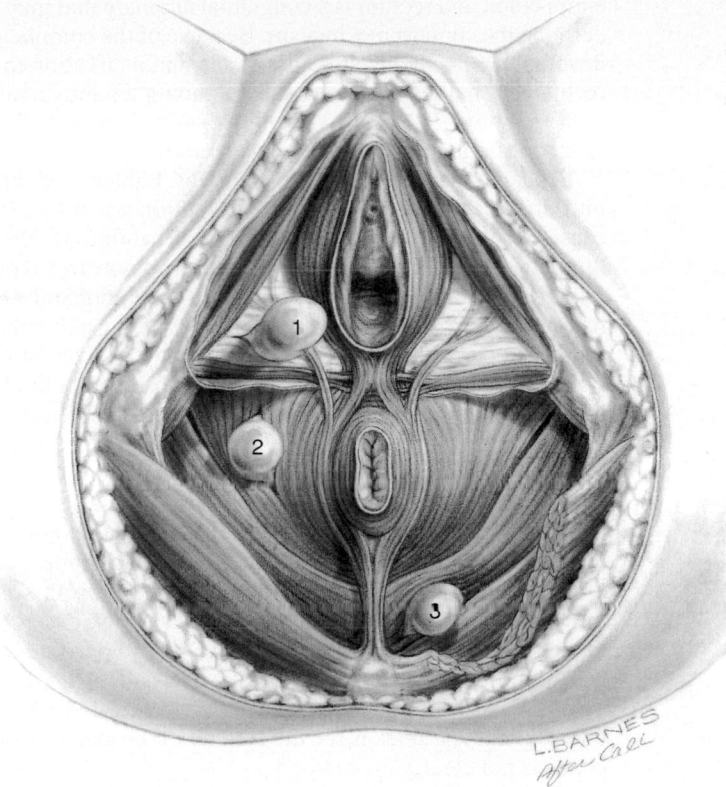

FIGURE 21-1. Muscles of the pelvic floor showing fixation of the rectum to the levator fibers. Weaknesses in the floor can lead to herniation as illustrated in several locations: (*1*) anterior perineal hernia through the urogenital diaphragm, (*2*) posterior perineal hernia through the levator ani muscle, and (*3*) posterior perineal hernia between the levator ani and coccygeus muscles. (Redrawn from Cali RL, Pitsch RM, Blatchford GJ, et al. Rare pelvic floor hernias. Report of a case and review of the literature. *Dis Colon Rectum.* 1992;35(6):604–612.)

The puborectalis sling forms the functional anorectal junction and tilts it forward toward the pubis creating an acute angle, which is important for fecal continence. Relaxation results in descent of the pelvic floor, widening the anorectal angle so that the rectum and anal canal comes to lie more in a direct line.

During defecation, intra-abdominal pressure is increased by contraction of the abdominal wall musculature and the diaphragm. Contraction of the levator ani muscle is inhibited, the puborectalis sling lengthens, and the pelvic floor descends, thereby obliterating the anorectal angle. The external sphincter muscle, which functionally forms a single unit with the puborectalis sling, relaxes at the same time. The rectum now occupies a vertical position, and the fecal mass is expelled by the contraction of the circular muscle of the rectum combined with the pressure from above (see also Chapters 2 and 16 for the discussions on defecation). The rectum is held in place by fixation of the levator muscle anteriorly and by the various ligamentous structures laterally when the rectum is in a vertical position. The levator sling returns to its usual support position after defecation.

Etiology

The etiologic factors believed to produce rectal prolapse may be congenital or acquired.

Predisposing and Associated Factors for the Development of Prolapse

The following list summarizes possible predisposing influences and associated conditions:

- Constipation, including evacuation disorder
- Neurologic disease (e.g., congenital anomaly, cauda equina lesion, spinal cord injury, senility)
- Patulous anus (i.e., weak internal sphincter)
- Diastasis of levator ani muscle (i.e., defect in the pelvic floor)
- Female gender
- Parity
- Redundant rectosigmoid
- Deep pouch of Douglas
- Lack of fixation of rectum to sacrum

The altered pelvic anatomy can be observed at laparotomy. This usually includes a redundant rectosigmoid and a deep rectovaginal or rectovesical pouch of Douglas.[206] This is associated with increased mobility of the rectum with a more extensively covered peritoneum than in the normal situation. Whether these are truly causative factors or merely frequently associated anatomic variables has been a subject of considerable debate. Similarly, it has been questioned whether the patulous anus and weak pelvic floor musculature, with diastasis of the levator ani muscle that produces a defect in the pelvic floor, is more the *result* of the prolapse than its cause (Figure 21-2). In the older patient, pelvic floor weakness often with associated incontinence is the usual finding, suggesting that reduced support of the pelvic organs may be an initiating factor. There is, however, evidence of improvement of resting anal pressure after rectopexy, thus favoring the idea that the prolapse causes secondary stretching of the sphincter.[279] Probably, weakness is partially causative and partially a consequence of prolapse once established. General neurologic diseases and traumatic lesions of the cauda equina may lead to rectal prolapse. Excessive pressure on the pelvic floor, particularly when related to attenuated muscle, is another etiologic factor.[314]

Many reports have confirmed the association between prolapse and pelvic floor muscular weakness.[94,116,134,136,147,236,290,295,335] Parks and colleagues suggested that because of stretch injury to pudendal and perineal nerves, loss of continence in individuals

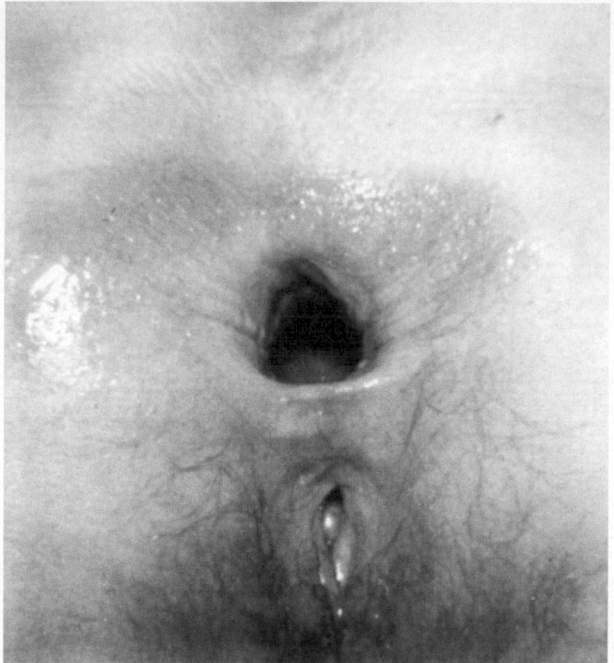

FIGURE 21-2. Patulous anus is seen after prolapse has been reduced. (From Corman ML, Veidenheimer MC, Coller JA. Managing rectal prolapse. *Geriatrics.* 1974;29(10):87–93, with permission.)

with rectal prolapse was secondary to prolonged protrusion.[238] They cite publications that demonstrate histologic abnormalities of small nerves supplying the anorectal musculature. Neill and associates reported electromyography (EMG) studies that showed reduced amplitude of action potentials in the external sphincter and puborectalis muscles in patients with fecal incontinence, but not in those with rectal prolapse without incontinence.[215] These findings indicate that denervation causes pelvic floor weakness, with prolapse and incontinence in some patients; in others, however, prolapse occurs without detectable abnormality of the pelvic musculature.

In infants, prolapse may be caused by a lack of skeletal support and by excessive intra-abdominal pressure (see Rectal Prolapse in Children). In adults, prolapse may result from incomplete skeletal development. A free mesentery to the entire colon and rectum is a congenital anomaly that may undermine the support mechanism. Because of the complicated development of the levator ani muscle and its fixation to the rectum, anomalies of this muscle including tenuous fixation to the rectum may occur more often than is realized and may also contribute to instability of the rectum.

Brodén and Snellman,[34] Ripstein and Lanter, and others introduced the concept of intussusception as the primary cause of rectal prolapse.[65–67,258,261,305,314] What initiates the intussusception is not exactly clear, but, as demonstrated cineradiographically, over a period the intussusception draws the rectum farther from the sacrum as it descends, and eventually the bowel presents at the anal verge.[34,258,305] Lack of fixation of the rectum to the sacrum can be observed both at the time of laparotomy and cineradiographically. When the act of defecation is viewed by this means or by defecography (see Defecography), the sequence of events is confirmed. A so-called colorectoanal intussusception may also occur in patients with a rectal tumor, which acts as a lead point.[346]

Patients in psychiatric hospitals, nursing homes, and other institutions are occasionally afflicted with this condition. Goligher, as a nonpsychiatrist, described one-third of his patients as being "rather odd," with approximately 3% "definitely psychotic."[96] Nearly one-half of the Lahey Clinic (Boston) patients demonstrated somewhat aberrant behavior.[139] The reason for the frequency of mental disturbance is not clearly understood.

By far, the most common group of patients with prolapse, however, are those in the sixth decade of life and older. In contrast to the younger age group, most (90%) are women.[139] Multiparity has sometimes been cited as an etiologic factor, but in the Lahey Clinic experience and in that of others, 40% to 60% are nulliparous.[139] Boutsis and Ellis reported that 58% of their patients with prolapse were childless, and Hughes reported an incidence of 39%.[32,128] Such rates of nulliparity are much higher than would be expected in the general population.

Clinical Features

Anorectal Assessment

It is important to determine the tone and contractility of the sphincter. If the resting tone is poor and the anus is patulous, and if the patient is unable to contract the external sphincter

---

JOHN CEDRIC GOLIGHER (1912–1998)

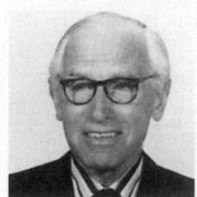

Goligher has been described as the preeminent clinical investigative surgeon in the world. He was born in Londonderry, Northern Ireland. He achieved his medical degree in 1934 from the University of Edinburgh, and after serving as a house officer at the Royal Infirmary in that city, he took the post of resident surgical officer at St. Mark's Hospital in London. Following a period as senior registrar at St. Mary's Hospital, he accepted a position as consultant surgeon to both St. Mary's and St. Mark's in 1947. In 1955, he assumed the chair of the University of Leeds, Department of Surgery, and at the General Infirmary, achieving emeritus status in 1978. Professor Goligher's papers represent a spectrum of accomplishment that is unparalleled in contemporary surgery. His individually authored text, *Surgery of the Anus, Rectum and Colon*, flourished through five editions. Others may continue to attempt to imitate his mastery of the field, but none can equal it. He has been responsible for more than 15 named lectures and has been recognized through honorary fellowship in as many societies throughout the world, including that of the American Society of Colon and Rectal Surgeons. His theatres in Leeds had been the center for every surgeon pursuing an interest in gastrointestinal disease. Professor Goligher was indeed the personification of the master surgeon.

and puborectalis voluntarily, the functional results after repair may be suboptimal. Conversely, if the patient has relatively good sphincter tone and contractility, good bowel control can be anticipated following successful repair. It is also important to specify the degree of prolapse and whether it is full thickness or mucosal.

A thorough endoscopic examination is necessary in individuals with any anorectal complaint, and this is especially true for patients with rectal prolapse. Occasionally, a polyp or carcinoma of the rectum or sigmoid colon may be the "lead point" for an intussusception. A high index of suspicion should be maintained, especially in a male patient with no evidence of neurologic disease. Total colonic evaluation by colonoscopy is mandatory. Flexible sigmoidoscopy or colonoscopy should exclude a tumor, and it may also reveal an intussusception if performed with the patient straining.[260] Evacuation proctography may be helpful if the diagnosis is in question.

Older Patients

In the older age group, the most frequent primary complaint is referable to the prolapse itself. Three-quarters of patients report a lump in the perineum. Problems with bowel regulation and incontinence are also common presenting features. At least 50% have a history of constipation.[139] Major bleeding is rare unless the prolapse is massive or irreducible. The patient may, however, complain of small amounts of blood and mucous soiling the underwear.

Fecal incontinence is frequently associated with prolapse. Indeed, among the one-quarter of patients who do not report a lump, many will complain of fecal incontinence as the main presenting problem. Rectal prolapse should be suspected whenever this symptom presents, especially in the elderly.[90] Incontinence becomes more severe as the protrusion increases in degree. Dilatation of the canal by the mass results in further relaxation of the sphincter muscles and further prolapse.[281] Protrusion may occur when the patient lifts or coughs, not necessarily solely upon defecation. Initially, the prolapse may retract spontaneously, but manual replacement, eventually, may become necessary. Ultimately, the mass may protrude most of the time. Infrequently, the prolapse may become incarcerated or even strangulated resulting in a surgical emergency (Figure 21-3). Transanal

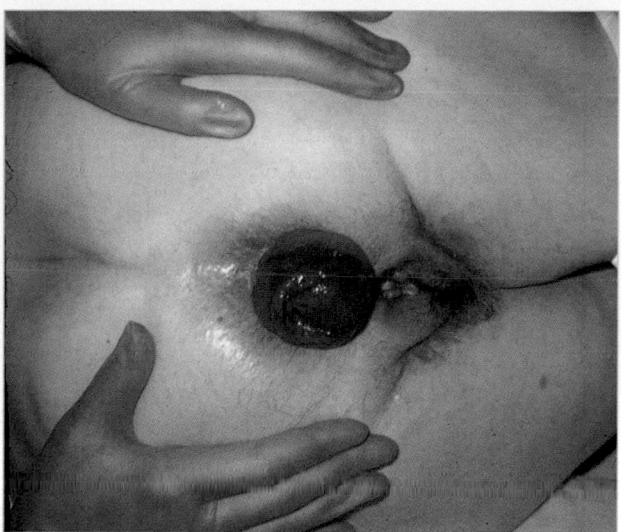

FIGURE 21-4. Standard, full-thickness rectal prolapse or procidentia. (From Corman ML, Veidenheimer MC, Coller JA. Managing rectal prolapse. *Geriatrics.* 1974;29(10):87–93, with permission.)

evisceration of the small bowel through a rent in the protruding rectum has also been reported.[97] Anorectal or pelvic pain is an underrecognized symptom of rectal prolapse. In one study, it was present at least some of the time in up to 50% of patients.[125]

The duration of symptoms before the patient seeks attention is often quite prolonged. This may be a reflection of the patient's psyche, but too often it represents failure of the family physician to recognize the entity and to recommend appropriate consultation.

Diagnosis

Usually, the diagnosis of a full-thickness prolapse is obvious on inspection of the perineum (Figure 21-4), but if it is not evident, the patient should be asked to go to the bathroom and to strain as in defecation. Once seen, the diagnosis is made. Rectal prolapse may be associated with uterine descensus (Figure 21-5) or prolapse (Figure 21-6) or with a cystocele (Figure 21-7).[56]

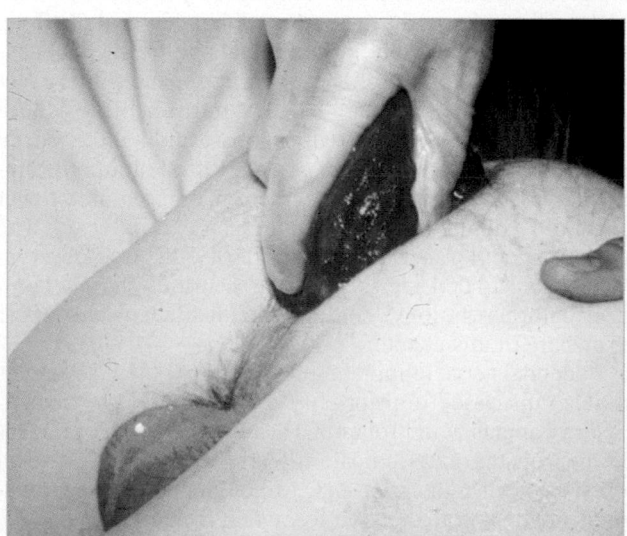

FIGURE 21-3. Manual replacement of incarcerated procidentia.

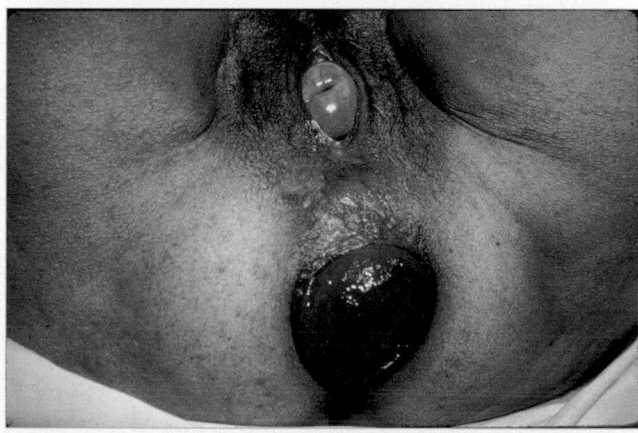

FIGURE 21-5. Rectal prolapse with uterine descensus. The cervical os appears at the introitus. (From Corman ML, Veidenheimer MC, Coller JA. Managing rectal prolapse. *Geriatrics.* 1974;29(10):87–93, with permission.)

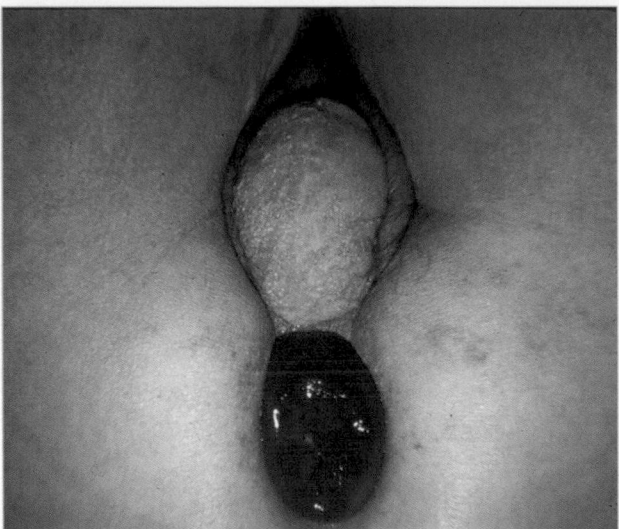

FIGURE 21-6. Rectal prolapse with uterine prolapse. (From Corman ML, Veidenheimer MC, Coller JA. Managing rectal prolapse. *Geriatrics.* 1974;29(10): 87–93, with permission.)

Younger Patients

These patients often have a pronounced functional disturbance of defecation. This may be characterized by frequent visits to the bathroom (e.g., more than 10 times per 24 hours), with long periods spent there on each occasion. In severe cases, the patient may be spending several hours in the bathroom straining. In these individuals, the gender ratio is approximately equal. Such patients may have psychiatric symptoms, whereas others may show obsessional features.

On clinical examination, the patient is usually young and healthy. There is often a degree of perineal descent, sometimes

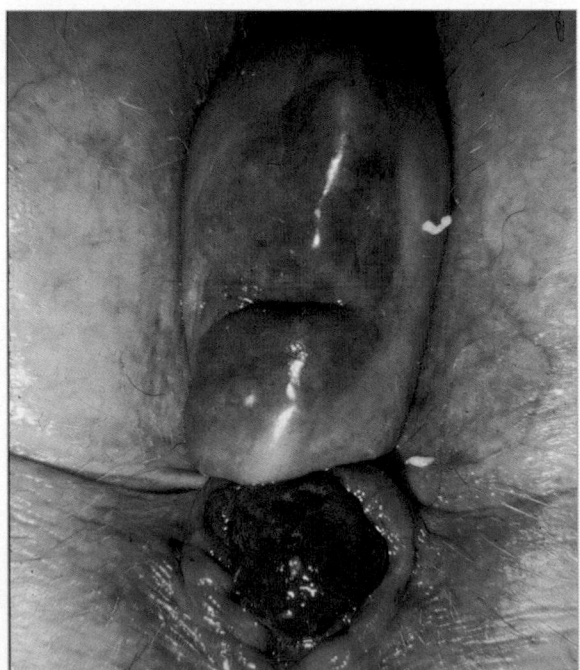

FIGURE 21-7. Rectal prolapse with fourth-degree cystocele. (From Corman ML, Veidenheimer MC, Coller JA. Managing rectal prolapse. *Geriatrics.* 1974;29(10):87–93, with permission.)

considerable. The sphincter may be patulous as may be appreciated in the older age group, but it may be normal and sometimes it is hypertonic. The prolapse usually requires straining to demonstrate. The mucous membrane of the rectum may appear irritated, and there may be free mucus in the rectum as well as mucosal changes suggestive of the solitary ulcer syndrome.

Differential Diagnosis

The condition that most often misleads the examiner into believing he or she is dealing with procidentia is prolapsed hemorrhoids (see Figure 11-8). A protruding mass of hemorrhoidal tissue tends to be lobular with a definite sulcus or groove between it and the perianal skin. With very large hemorrhoids that have become edematous and thrombosed, the enlarged size may give the incorrect impression that the entire rectal wall is protruding. However, in rectal prolapse, concentric rings of intact tissue are evident throughout the entire circumference.

The differential diagnosis includes any large rectal polypoid lesion prolapsing through the anus. The prolapsed lesion should be replaced, and the rectum should be examined manually and endoscopically. A polypoid tumor is usually mobile and can be separated from the lower part of the rectum and anal canal by digital examination. Proctosigmoidoscopic examination should clarify any differential diagnostic difficulty.

Anal deformity associated with hemorrhoidectomy, fistula surgery, and pull-through procedures may produce an ectropion or mucosal prolapse, but this should pose no difficulty in differential diagnosis. However, it is extremely important to distinguish full-thickness from mucosal prolapse because treatment of the two conditions is different. Unfortunately, some patients have undergone multiple anal operations because rectal prolapse has been mistaken for hemorrhoids.

Physiologic Studies

There is merit for performing certain physiologic studies, especially when there are symptoms of incontinence.[120,166] The various studies and techniques are discussed in Chapters 7 and 16. Sun and colleagues evaluated anorectal pressures at rest, during contraction, and during balloon distension of the rectum in individuals with full-thickness rectal prolapse, anterior mucosal prolapse, and solitary rectal ulcer.[302] When compared with control subjects, those with rectal prolapse, mucosal prolapse, and solitary rectal ulcer had lower anal pressures, demonstrated a higher incidence of repetitive rectal contraction, and required lower threshold volumes to stimulate a desire to defecate. The authors hypothesized that the similarity of these observations suggests that the three disease entities share a common pathophysiology. Solitary rectal ulcer is discussed elsewhere in this chapter.

Pudendal nerve terminal motor latency (PNTML) studies are also discussed in prior chapters and should be considered in patients with prolapse. The demonstration of pudendal neuropathy may indicate a worse outcome of surgical repair than when this is absent. Although pudendal neuropathy is not a contraindication for repair, it is helpful to know this in advance to be able to give the patient an idea of the prognosis. Others report that fecal continence after surgical correction of the prolapse can be predicted by postoperative measurement of the PNTML.[26]

Treatment of External Rectal Prolapse

In general, partial or incomplete (i.e., mucosal) prolapse should be treated by an anal operation. If only one quadrant is involved, simple excision, leaving the wound open, may be all that is required (see Figure 11-65). If the protruding area is circumferential, excision with an S-plasty may be considered (see Figures 11-75 and 11-79). Another suggestion for the management of mucosal prolapse is the use of the circular stapler, especially the so-called PPH modification (stapled hemorrhoidopexy; see Chapter 11).[10]

With respect to the management of acute, incarcerated (i.e., irreducible) rectal prolapse (Figure 21-3), some have recommended a local anesthetic to paralyze the sphincters and to effect reduction (see Figure 11-37). Others suggest a spinal or general anesthetic. The placement of ordinary table sugar or powdered sugar on the bowel mucosa can result in decreased edema and spontaneous or easily induced reduction from the desiccating effect. This is a well-recognized technique in the veterinary literature.[209] Emergency resection is occasionally indicated, usually because of compromised viability.[253]

Nonoperative Treatment of Rectal Prolapse

If surgical treatment for incomplete or complete prolapse is contraindicated, or if the patient refuses an operation, numerous noninvasive approaches and limited office procedures may be employed as follows:

- Adhesive strapping of buttocks
- Manual anal support during defecation
- Correction of constipation
- Establishment of workable time and method of defecation
- Perineal strengthening exercises
- Electronic stimulation
- Injection of sclerosing agent
- Rubber ring ligation
- Infrared coagulation

Although instructing the patient on proper bowel management and perineal exercises may be salutary, and other methods may offer some degree of palliation of symptoms, these measures cannot be expected to produce a cure.

Surgical Therapy for Rectal Prolapse

More than 50 operations have been designed for the treatment of complete rectal prolapse. Most are variations of a few basic modes of therapy and depend on the surgeon's concept of the anatomic defect. The options for treatment include narrowing of the anal orifice, obliteration of the peritoneal pouch of Douglas, restoration of the pelvic floor, resection of the bowel (by an abdominal, perineal, or transsacral approach), and suspension or fixation of the rectum to the sacrum or to other structures. Additional operations are listed that combine one or more of these approaches.

- Narrowing of the anal orifice
- Obliteration of the peritoneal pouch of Douglas
- Restoration of the pelvic floor
- Resection of bowel
  - Transabdominal
  - Perineal
  - Transsacral

- Suspension or fixation of the rectum
  - To sacrum
  - To pubis
  - To other structures
- Combinations of two or more of the operations[32]

Many of the techniques described are included for historical completeness only. The vast majority of procedures these days involve either an *abdominal rectopexy* (usually a posterior sutured rectopexy, with or without resection, or increasingly a laparoscopic ventral rectopexy) or a *perineal procedure* (either Delorme's or Altemeier's procedure). The decision making between the two approaches has generally hinged on the balance between recurrence and safety. Higher rates of recurrence are noted following perineal procedures (15% to 20%), but this may be considered an acceptable trade-off for the safety of avoiding a laparotomy in often elderly patients with benign disease, albeit, by an operation with a lower recurrence rate (less than 5%).[89,182] Undoubtedly, the advent of laparoscopy has made an abdominal approach safer, shifting the balance in favor of this approach even in the elderly (see Chapter 19).[10,111,222] The recurrence rates of the laparoscopic approach are and should be comparable to that of the open technique.

Perineal Procedures

Rectopexy is generally considered preferable by some surgeons for correction of rectal prolapse, owing to the lower recurrence rates (less than 5%) than after perineal procedures (pooled series, 18%).[182] This difference has, however, not been conclusively established. Recent Cochrane analyses have cited a lack of high-quality data.[18] For this reason, the PROSPER study was set up in the United Kingdom to compare perineal and abdominal surgery for rectal prolapse. Its findings are yet to be published, but early reports suggest recurrence rates of 20% and 10%, respectively. Generally, perineal procedures are advised for older, frailer patients.

Thiersch Repair

In the older, poor-risk patient, some surgeons preferred to use the Thiersch operation but this is now only rarely performed.[95,116,153] It can be carried out under local anesthetic, making it a satisfactory technique for these individuals. In the historic operation, silver wire was placed into the perianal space to encircle and narrow the anus. Today, surgeons have abandoned the use of wire because of the complications of breakage and ulceration. Other materials such as nylon, Mersilene, Dacron, polypropylene mesh (i.e., Marlex), Teflon, fascia lata, silicone rubber, Silastic, and Dacron-impregnated Silastic mesh have been used for the same purpose (Figure 21-8).[84,111,126,129,153,162,177,222,244,247,268,303]

Other Thiersch-Type Repairs (Historical)

Other approaches have been advocated as alternatives to the Thiersch operation. Marlex mesh has been employed by Lomas and Cooperman.[177] Despite their wound infection rate of 33%, they believe this to be a rapid, safe procedure for use in the elderly patient who is not a candidate for a more extensive surgical operation.

Notaras used a ribbon of Mersilene (approximately 4 cm wide), passing it around the anus as has been described with the other material, except that a more extensive mobilization is required, and the mesh is placed more deeply.[222] Notaras reported an experience with 18 patients with no

CARL THIERSCH (1822–1895)

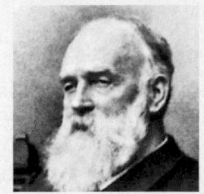

Thiersch was born in Munich, Germany, to a very educated family. His father held the Professorship of Classics in the university and was president of the Academy of Science. Following his graduation from the gymnasium, the young Thiersch entered the study of medicine in his home university. Then, after a period at a number of European medical centers, he joined the Munich faculty. At the age of 32, he achieved professorial status. Shortly thereafter, he accepted a position as professor of surgery in Erlangen, and after 14 years, Leipzig. Like most of his contemporaries, he was expected to be a general surgeon, but his work with children and his head and neck surgery were particularly well recognized. The operation for which he was most famous was the preparation of thin skin grafts (i.e., Thiersch grafts), founded on his earlier microscopic investigations of granulation tissue. His name is also associated with the field of colon and rectal surgery for his suggestion of the management of procidentia by means of the circumanal placement of a silver wire.

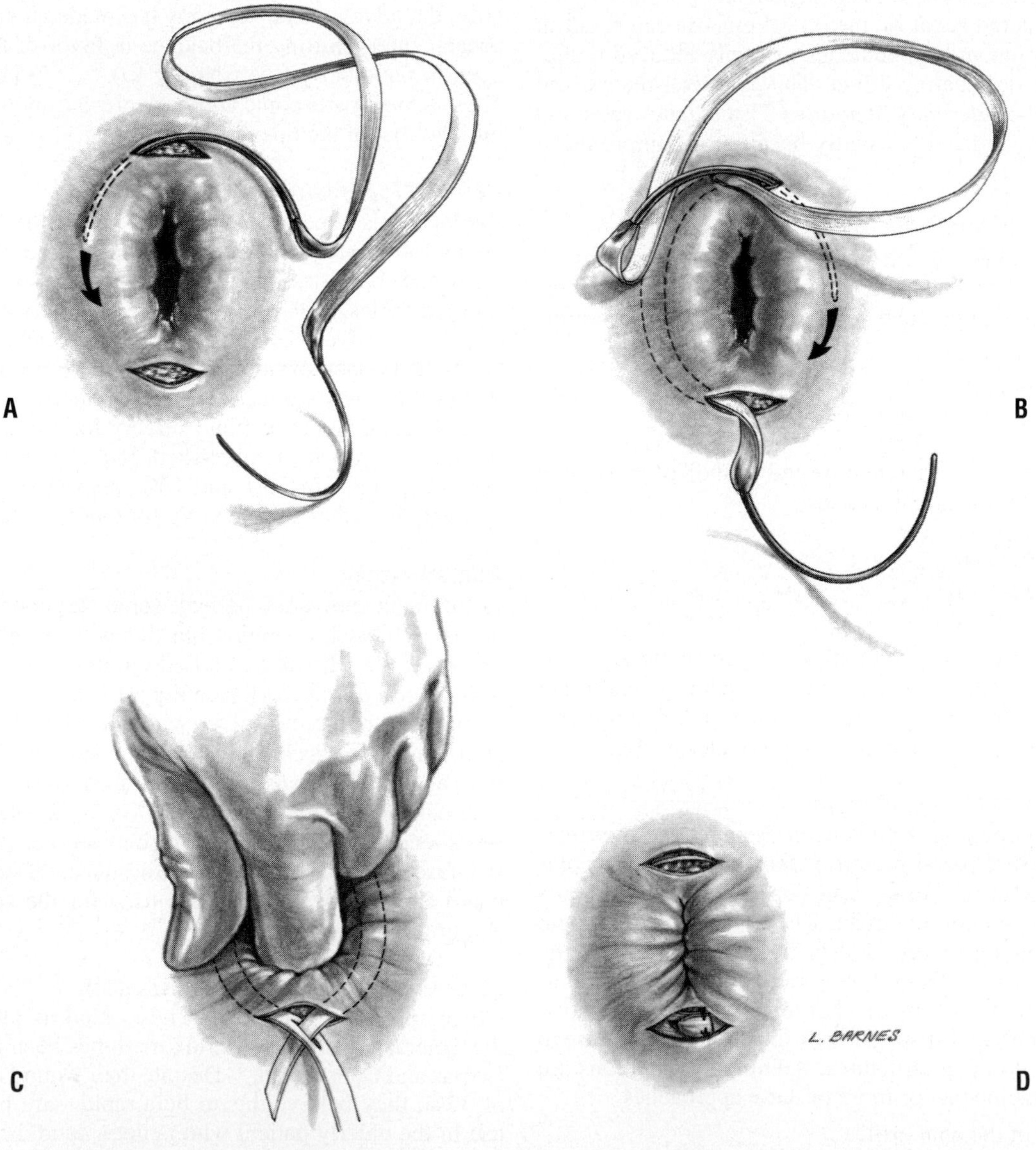

FIGURE 21-8. Thiersch repair with Mersilene tape. **A,B:** Each needle arm is passed from anterior to posterior. **C:** The tape is secured after tightening to the level of the proximal interphalangeal joint. An 18-French Hegar dilator is the preferred measuring device. **D:** The tape is sutured to itself rather than knotted.

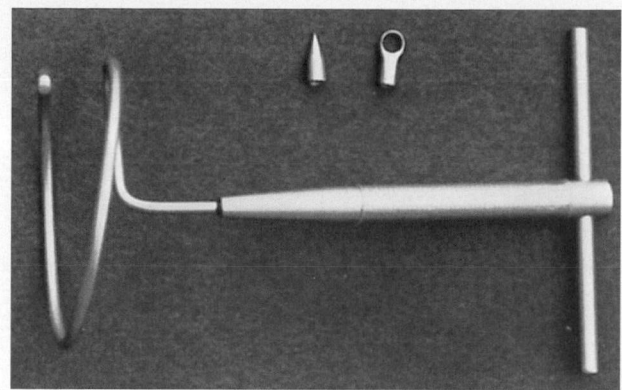

FIGURE 21-9. Encircler with a detachable mole and carrier tips. (Courtesy of Hyman Swerdlow, MD.)

infection, breakage, or erosion.[222] Sainio and colleagues reported 14 selected patients with prolapse who underwent anal encirclement with polypropylene mesh.[268] Although two had recurrences (15%), no breakage, erosion, or infection was observed. Labow and associates described the use of an elastic fabric sling, a Dacron-impregnated Silastic sheet (see Figures 16-64 through 16-66).[162] Hunt and colleagues treated 43 patients (mean age, 80 years) for full-thickness prolapse by implanting Silastic rods.[129] The authors reported adequate control of the prolapse in 71% of patients, with no operative mortality.

Swerdlow addressed the issue of performing the operation through only one incision.[303] He describes a helical rod (the Encircler)—a single loop having a diameter of 6 cm with an extension beyond 360 degrees—the end of which is adapted to accept varying tips (Figure 21-9). Khanduja and colleagues presented their experience with a compressible prosthesis composed of silicone elastomer surrounded by a silicone-coated Dacron tape.[153] Dacron mesh is embedded in the ends for reinforcement. Sixteen "extremely poor-risk" individuals were submitted to the procedure. Complications included breakage of the prosthesis in three, infection in one, and late sepsis in one individual. Ladha and colleagues employed the Angelchik antireflux prosthesis—a device that was introduced for the treatment of gastroesophageal reflux—for the repair of rectal prolapse in elderly patients.[163] The prosthesis is placed in a supralevator location around the rectum, a position that may help to restore the anorectal angle. The authors reported eight patients, with one death and one complication of wound sepsis.

Perineal Procedures

Perineal resection of the prolapse, or rectosigmoidectomy, is an operation that has been employed for more than 100 years. Indeed, it was the routine method of surgical treatment for many years, with the advantage of being simple and safer than abdominal procedures. Unfortunately, the high rate of recurrence (up to 25%) dissuaded many surgeons from adopting this approach.[128] However, this attitude has changed in recent years with improvements in surgical technique, such as that of the Altemeier's and Delorme's procedures. Perineal removal may be the safest approach in the rare circumstance of a strangulated, nonreducible prolapse where gangrene may occur. The functional results of perineal procedures are less predictable than with abdominal operations, particularly fecal continence.

Altemeier's Operation

Altemeier and Culbertson developed a modification of perineal resection.[6,7] They advocated the operation with the patient placed in the lithotomy stirrups. Although this is the position that is illustrated in this text, our own preference is to place the patient in the prone jackknife position on the operating table. This permits one's assistants to be involved in the procedure and to offer the needed help. The prolapse is exteriorized, and its apex is grasped with clamps (Figure 21-10A). A circumferential incision is made through all layers of the outer bowel wall 1 cm proximal to the mucocutaneous junction (Figure 21-10A). When the circumferential incision is completed, clamps are reapplied to the distal edge of rectum (Figure 21-10B), and the prolapse is delivered as a single loop of exteriorized bowel (Figure 21-10C). With a deep pouch of Douglas, it is usually quite straightforward to enter the peritoneal cavity by incising the peritoneum anteriorly (Figure 21-11A). The redundant colon is delivered through the defect (Figure 21-11B). The peritoneum is ultimately repaired using a continuous suture to obliterate the sac, excising redundant peritoneum (if necessary), analogous to that of the technique employed for a sliding hernia (Figure 21-12).

A modification of this procedure involves plication of the levator ani muscle. This maneuver is thought by some to be associated with a lower incidence of recurrence and may have an ameliorative effect on problems with bowel control.[50] The levator ani muscles are identified and plicated anterior or posterior to the bowel with interrupted long-term absorbable sutures (Figure 21-13). This eliminates the large defect in the pelvic diaphragm. The redundant intestine is then divided in half by anterior and posterior incisions carried to the point of the proposed resection (Figure 21-14). The intestine is

WILLIAM ARTHUR ALTEMEIER (1910–1983)

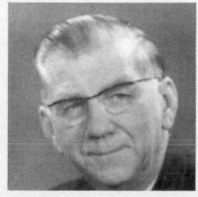

Altemeier was born in Cincinnati, Ohio, the son of a railroad employee. He attended the University of Cincinnati, receiving a bachelor of science degree in 1930 and his doctorate in medicine 3 years later. After a surgical residency at Henry Ford Hospital in Detroit, Michigan and a period as an associate surgeon, he returned to Cincinnati General Hospital as an instructor.

He rose to become professor and chairman of the department of surgery in 1952, positions he retained for 26 years. Altemeier was a member of at least 38 surgical societies, serving as president of 10 of them, including the American College of Surgeons and the American Surgical Association. He developed a special interest in surgical infections and became one of the world authorities in this discipline. However, it is the management of procidentia with which his name is eponymously associated.

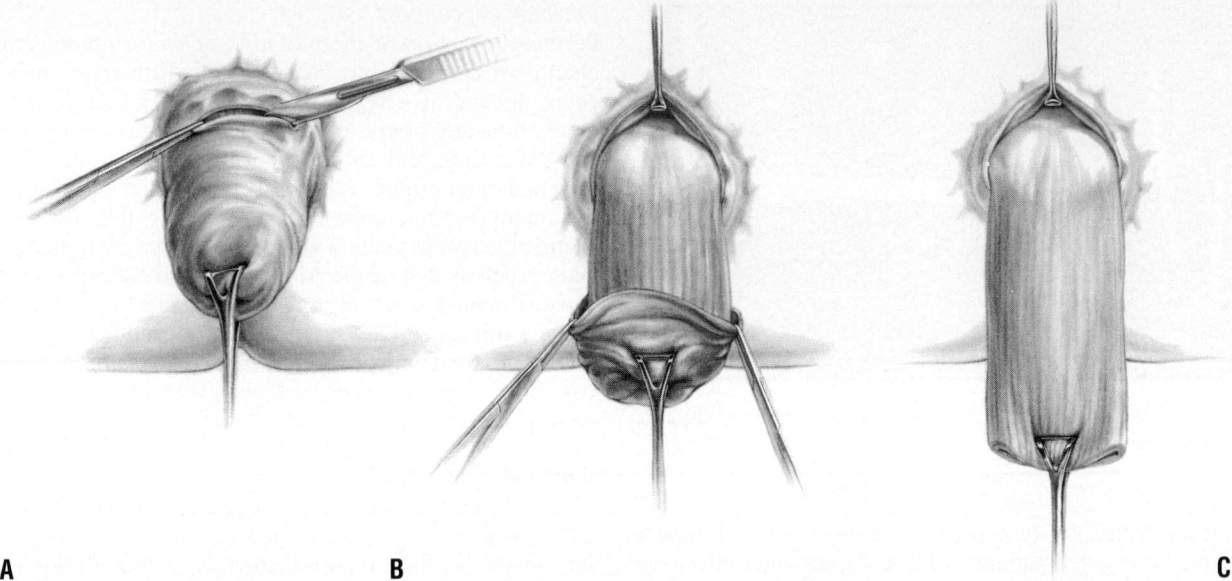

FIGURE 21-10. Altemeier procedure. **A:** An incision is made circumferentially in the anal canal, just above the dentate line. **B,C:** The rectum is mobilized and completely everted.

transected obliquely and progressively, completing the anastomosis of the intestinal wall to the distal rectum/anal ring in each quadrant (Figure 21-14). The anastomosis is fashioned with an interrupted long-term absorbable suture technique; no drains are used. Others have successfully used the circular stapler for reestablishment of continuity.[21] In principle, the pelvic pouch is obliterated, the levators are plicated, and the

redundant bowel is resected. The rectum is not usually fixed to the sacrum.

Despite the success experienced by some authors, the complex technique and the unfamiliar approach dissuade most surgeons from attempting the operation. Altemeier and colleagues reported the results in 106 patients, of whom three developed recurrence.[8] Gopal and colleagues noted only one failure with

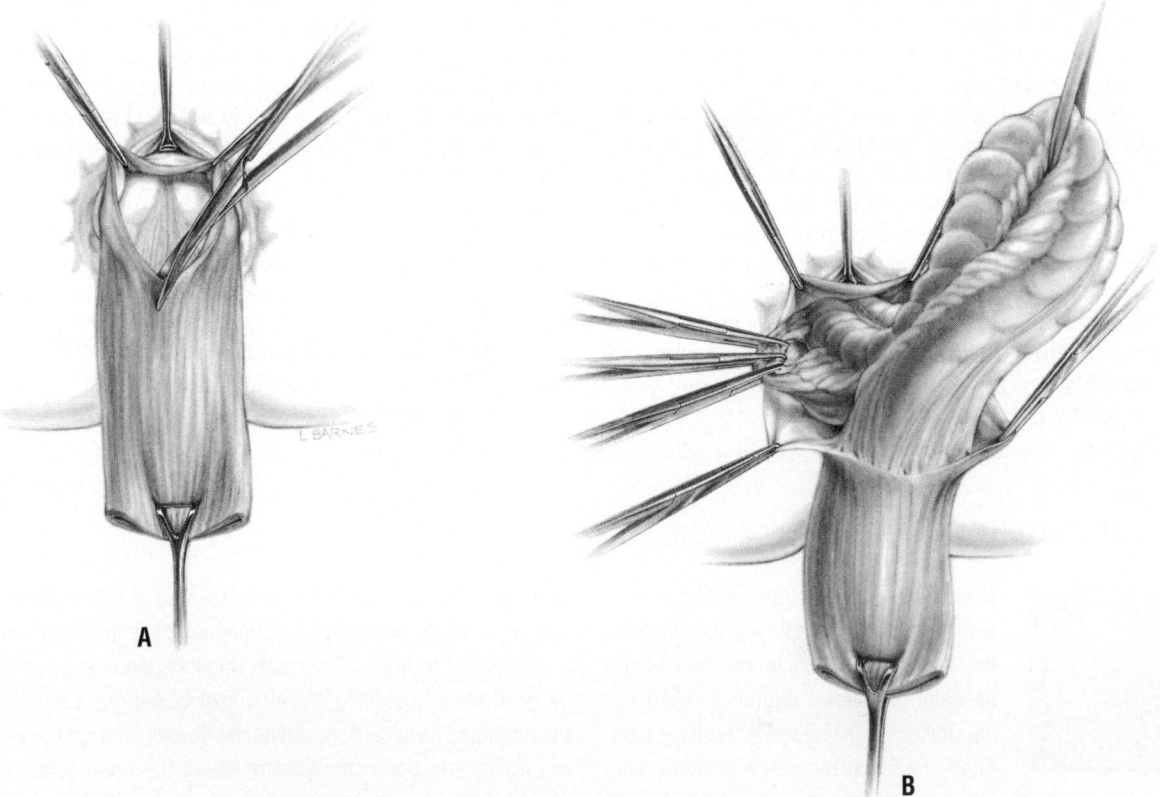

FIGURE 21-11. Altemeier procedure. **A:** The peritoneal reflection is identified and opened. **B:** Any redundant bowel is delivered through the peritoneal defect.

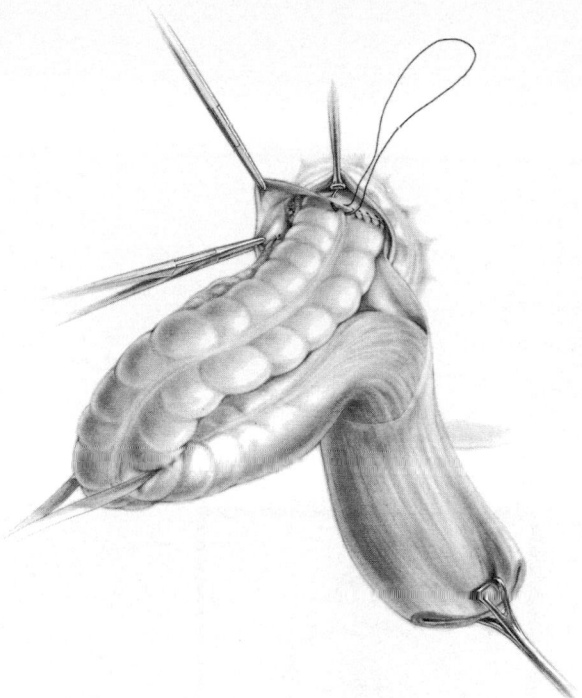

FIGURE 21-12. Altemeier procedure. The peritoneum is closed, and the sutures are anchored to the bowel wall as illustrated.

18 elderly, debilitated individuals so treated.[98] Kimmins and coworkers performed the modified Altemeier's procedure on 63 patients (mean age, 79 years), noting an overall recurrence rate of 6.4% (median follow-up, 20.8 months).[154] So benign is this operation for most patients that, in their experience, almost two-thirds were discharged the day of surgery.

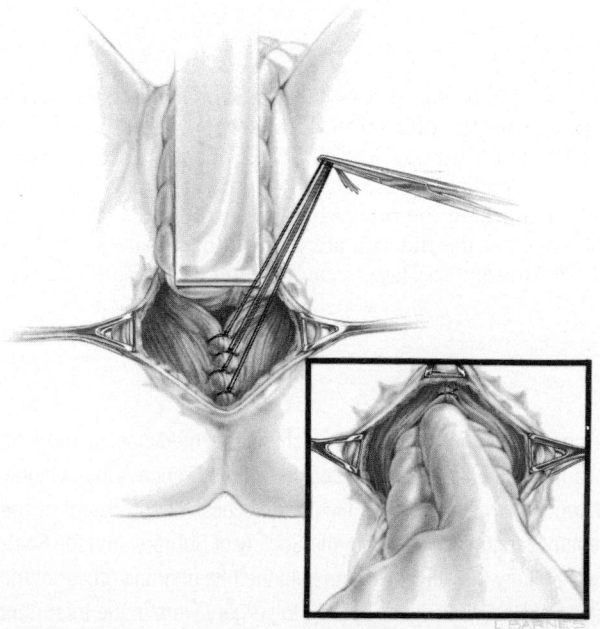

FIGURE 21-13. Altemeier procedure. The levator ani muscle is reefed anteriorly or, as illustrated, posteriorly, with long-term absorbable sutures. Care should be taken to avoid narrowing the rectum. A finger should be able to pass easily through the defect (*inset*).

Others have described similarly favorable results with the addition of a posterior levator plication.[250] The Cleveland Clinic Florida group compared the outcomes of perineal rectosigmoidectomy with and without levatorplasty in 109 patients.[50] Recurrence rates and mean time to recurrence were 20.6% and 13.3 months when rectosigmoidectomy alone was performed. When levatorplasty was added, the recurrence rate was 7.7%, and mean time to recurrence increased to 45.5 months. However, Friedman and associates considered the Altemeier's operation unsatisfactory.[92] In 27 patients, 50% experienced recurrence. When incontinence is discussed in publications, it seems that better functional results are achieved with concomitant levator plication than with proctosigmoidectomy alone.[2,51,254,334] The Cleveland Clinic Florida group noted that a prolonged PNTML was not shown to be an accurate predictor of postoperative incontinence nor was there a statistically significant difference In functional outcome, both groups having marked improvement in continence scores.[50,135] In the experience of the University of Minnesota group with 114 patients treated by perineal rectosigmoidectomy, a 10% incidence of recurrence was observed.[334] Ramanujam and coworkers performed this operation on 72 elderly, high-risk patients, 9 of whom presented with acute, incarcerated rectal prolapse.[254] Their recurrence rate was 5.5%. In another report from the same group, 8 elderly patients were treated for acute incarcerated prolapse, half of whom developed gangrene.[253] There were two (25%) cases of anastomotic leakage. There were, however, no deaths. Deen and colleagues performed a randomized trial, comparing anterior resection and rectopexy with perineal rectosigmoidectomy.[59] Pelvic floor repair was undertaken in both groups. There was no recurrence in 10 patients in the former group, but 1 occurred in the latter (10%). The abdominal operation was believed to be associated with better functional and physiologic results.

Vermeulen and associates reported another approach to perineal rectosigmoidectomy without levator plication by the use of the circular stapling device (Figure 21-15).[326] In nine women (mean age, 79 years), they noted no significant complications and no recurrences. They believed that this technique is the procedure of choice in the elderly, poor-risk patient.

Transtar

Occasional short reports have appeared describing the use of Transtar (Ethicon Endo-Surgery) to perform a form of perineal Altemeier's procedure (Figure 21-16). There are theoretic concerns using this technique, in particular the security of stapling the superior rectal artery within the mesorectum. Scherer reported on 15 patients who underwent this procedure.[278] In 14, perineal stapled prolapse resection was performed without complications, with a median operating time of 33 minutes (range, 22 to 52). One procedure was changed to an Altemeier because of a staple line disruption. Two patients required reintervention as a result of postoperative hemorrhage. No other serious complications occurred. At follow-up, all patients were well and showed no early recurrence of prolapse.

Delorme's Procedure

Since its original description by the French military surgeon Delorme in 1900,[64] this operation has reemerged in recent years as a good choice for mucosal prolapse and as an alternative to abdominal surgery for full-thickness rectal prolapse.[65,283,313] The dissection may be facilitated by employing the suggestions of Sullivan and Garnjobst and Berman and colleagues.[23,299] With the patient in the lithotomy or the prone jackknife position,

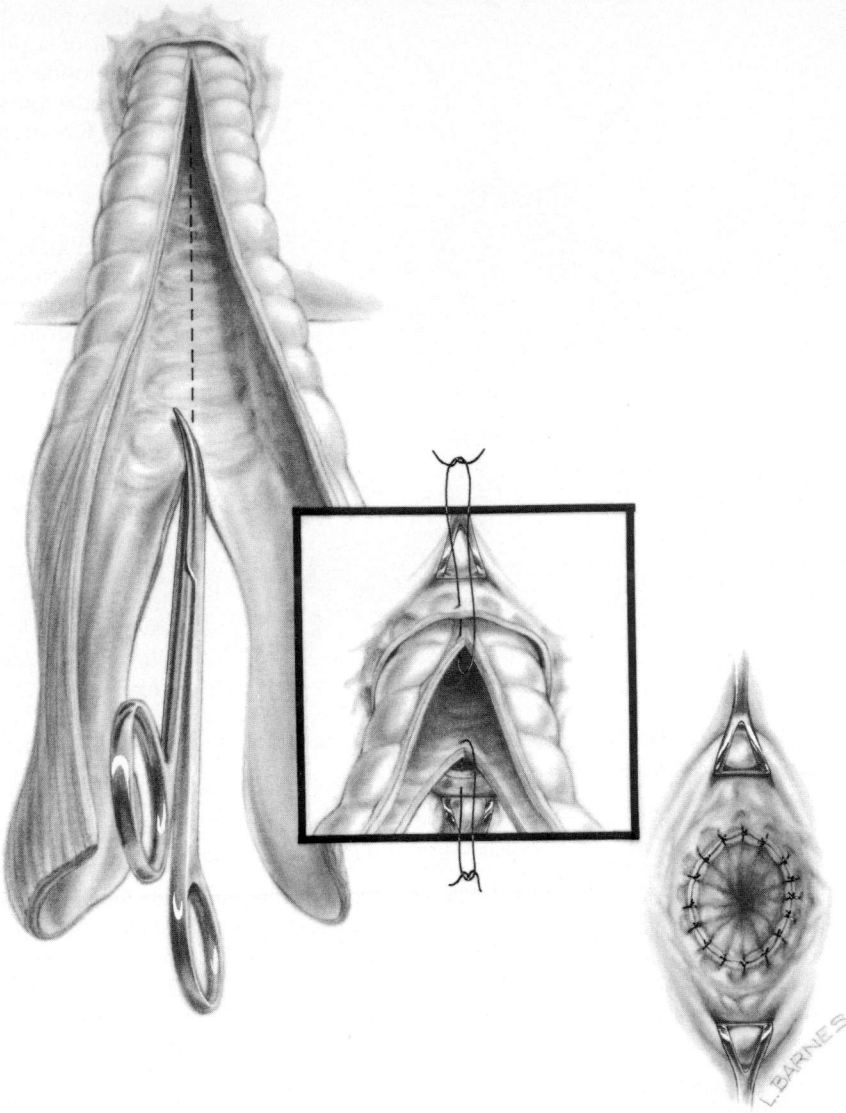

FIGURE 21-14. Altemeier procedure. The redundant bowel is incised longitudinally and sutured in the anterior and posterior midline to the residual cuff of the anal mucosa (*inset*). After the redundant bowel is trimmed, interrupted sutures are placed between the anal canal and the underlying internal sphincter to the full thickness of the rectum.

a circumferential incision is made 1 cm proximal to the dentate line, similar to that for the Altemeier's procedure (Figure 21-17A). The bowel is not divided, however. This is a submucosal dissection with a mucosal stripping (Figure 21-17B). Using electrocautery, the mucosa is stripped to the apex of the protruding bowel. Dissection may be facilitated by infiltrating the submucosa with saline or a dilute epinephrine solution. Some have advocated the use of the Cavitron Ultrasonic Surgical Aspirator for the dissection (Extracorporeal Medical Specialties, King of Prussia, PA).[105] The redundant mucosa is excised, and the denuded muscularis propria is pleated longitudinally, collapsing the bowel like an accordion (Figure 21-18). The edges of the mucosa are then sutured. Alternatively, the mucosa-muscularis layers can be directly reapproximated in

EDMOND DELORME (1847–1929)

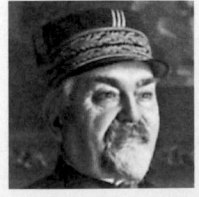

Delorme was born in Lunéville, France, the son of a cabinetmaker. He demonstrated an interest in military sciences and enrolled in the medical military school at Strasbourg in 1866. He followed the army in its battles throughout Europe and North Africa, and in 1877 Delorme was named professor of operative medicine at Val-de-Grâce, and ultimately, professor of clinical surgery. He was the director of a number of hospitals and introduced the concept of antisepsis into French military medicine. In 1903, he became head of all the health services of the French Army. A highly influential surgeon, he was elected successively president of the French Academy of Medicine, the Society of Surgery, and the Society of Military Medicine. He also held the title of grand officer of the Legion of Honor. His contributions to surgery were in the treatment of war injuries, fractures, lung decortication, and rectal surgery. In his publication of the operation for rectal prolapse that bears his name, Delorme reported three patients, one of whom died.

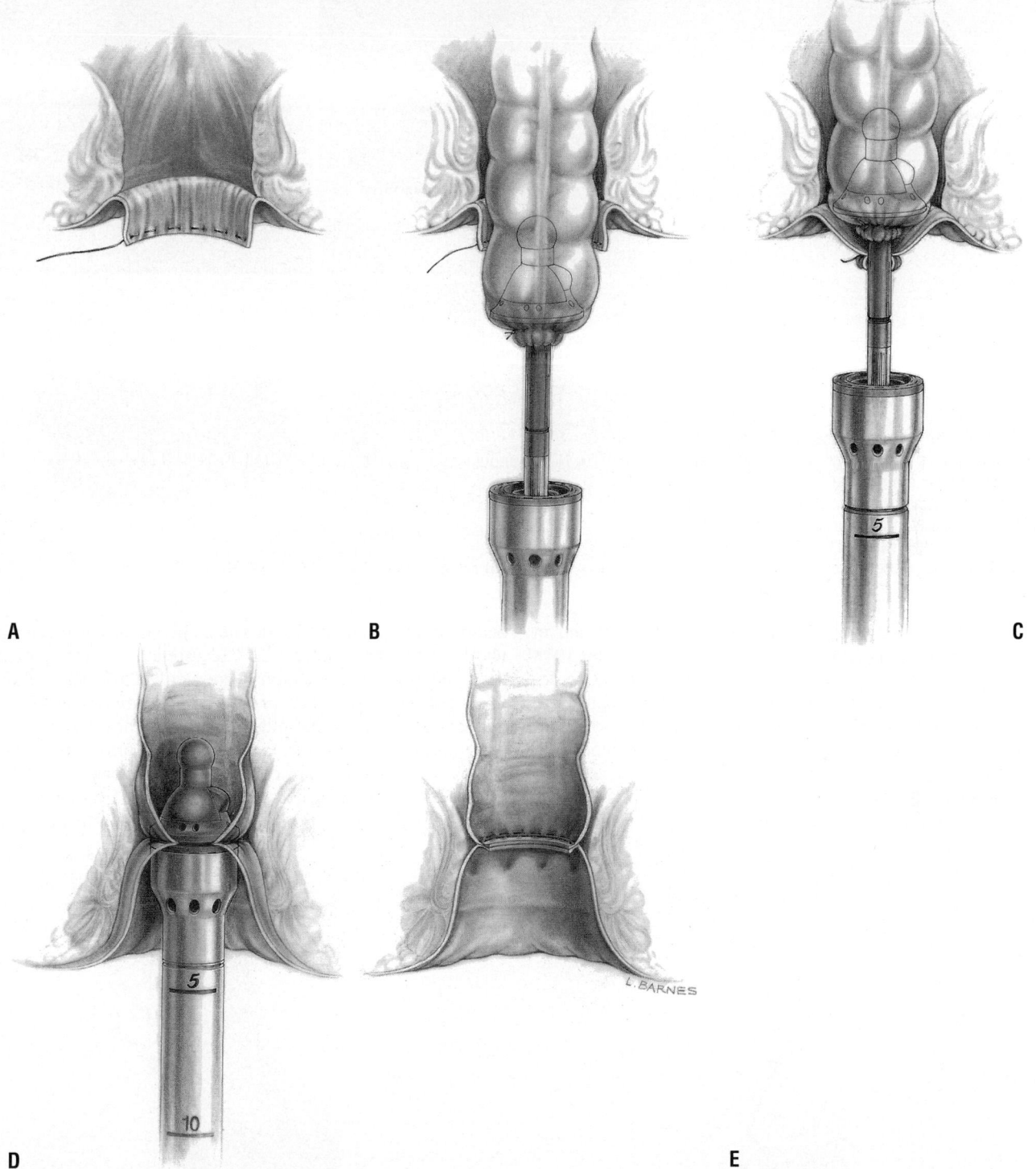

FIGURE 21-15. Perineal proctosigmoidectomy with circular stapler. **A:** Purse-string sutures to the proximal and distal bowel after perineal resection. **B:** The proximal segment is secured over the anvil. **C:** The distal segment is secured. **D:** The instrument is closed and fired. **E:** Completed anastomosis. (Adapted from Vermeulen FD, Nivatvongs S, Fang DT, et al. A technique for perineal rectosigmoidectomy using autosuture devices. *Surg Gynecol Obstet.* 1983;156(1):84–86, with permission.)

a circumferential fashion with multiple interrupted absorbable sutures.[105] Complications from this operation are common and include hemorrhage, hematoma, suture line dehiscence, stricture, incontinence, and, of course, recurrence.

In 30 patients treated by Nay and Blair, a 10% incidence of incontinence or recurrence was noted.[214] Uhlig and Sullivan have been quite enthusiastic about this technique, reporting only three failures in 44 patients, an incidence of less than 7%.[321] McCaffrey recommended this approach after a failed abdominal suspension operation.[193] He reported good results in 3 patients. Gundersen and colleagues noted "significant complications" in 17% of 18 patients so treated.[105]

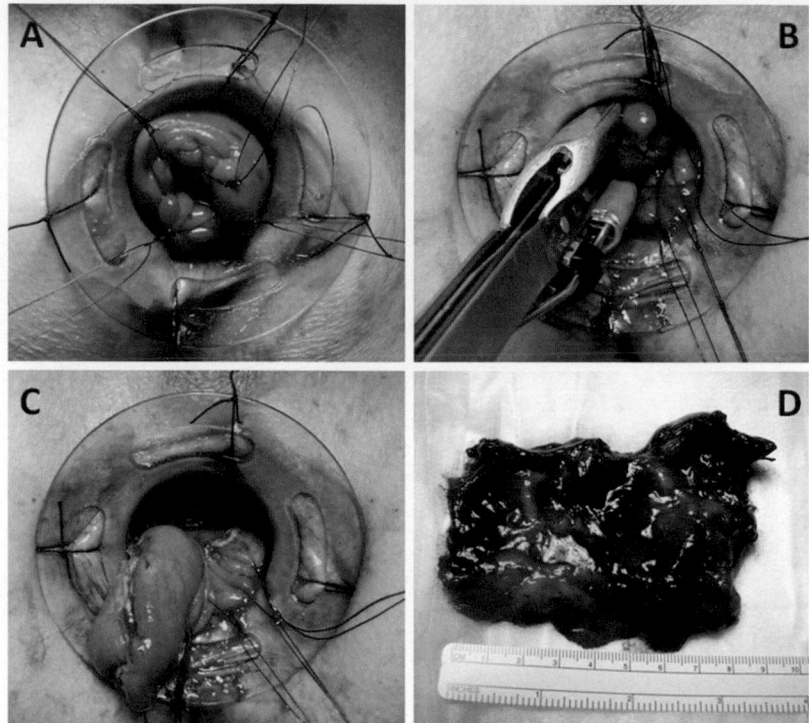

FIGURE 21-16. Transtar procedure. **A:** The prolapse is delivered with stay sutures. **B,C:** The prolapse is excised, and the residual rectum anastomosed full thickness by sequential firings of the Transtar stapler. **D:** This excises a significantly larger prolapse than conventional STARR, allowing the excision to potentially be tailored to the size of the prolapse, unlike STARR which excises a fixed amount of tissue.

The St. Mark's Hospital experience was published in 1994.[283] Only 32 operations were performed between 1978 and 1990. There was no mortality and one anastomotic dehiscence. With a mean follow-up of 24 months, there were four recurrences (12.5%). Approximately one-half noted improved bowel control. The operation was recommended on so-called unfit patients. Oliver and associates analyzed their experience of 41 individuals who underwent this procedure.[226] This operation was selected when advanced age and/or poor

health contraindicated an abdominal operation. The mean age was 82 years. They noted a 22% recurrence rate. One patient died, and minor complications were seen in 25%. The authors observed the importance of an adequate mucosectomy.[226] Others suggest also that elderly patients, those with failed prior prolapse procedures, and those with prior pelvic surgery or radiation should be considered for this procedure.[155,193]

Lechaux and coworkers reviewed their 85 patients who underwent this operation.[170] Their complication rate was

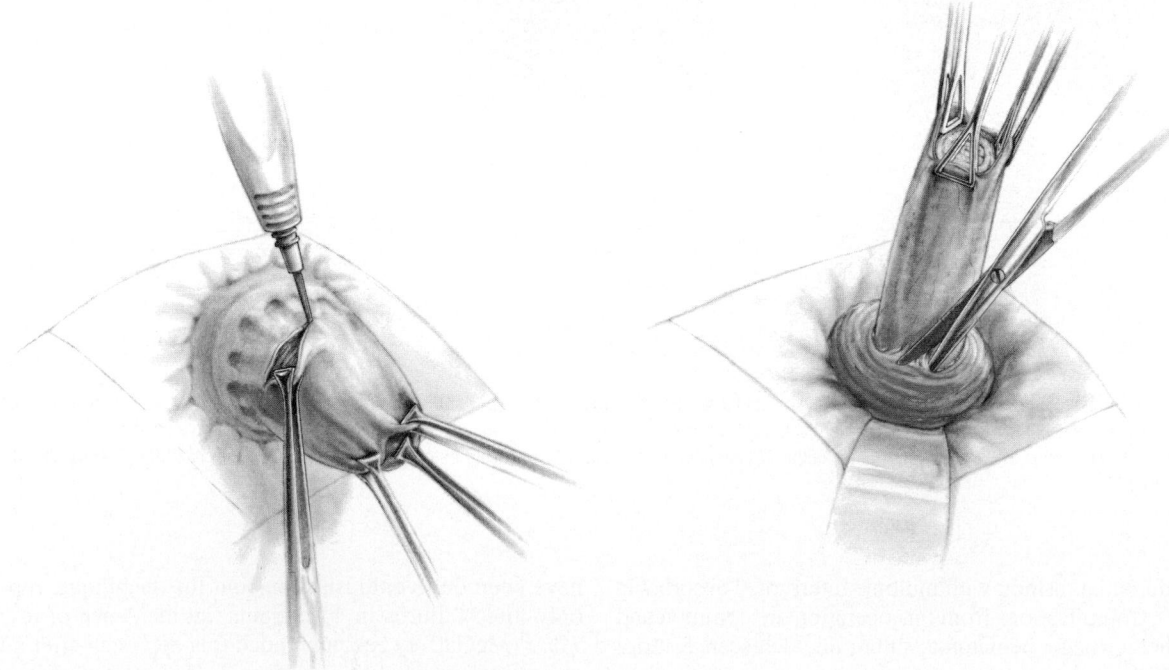

A   **B**

FIGURE 21-17. Delorme procedure. **A:** The mucosa is circumferentially incised above the dentate line. **B:** Submucosal stripping is carried out as far cephalad as is possible.

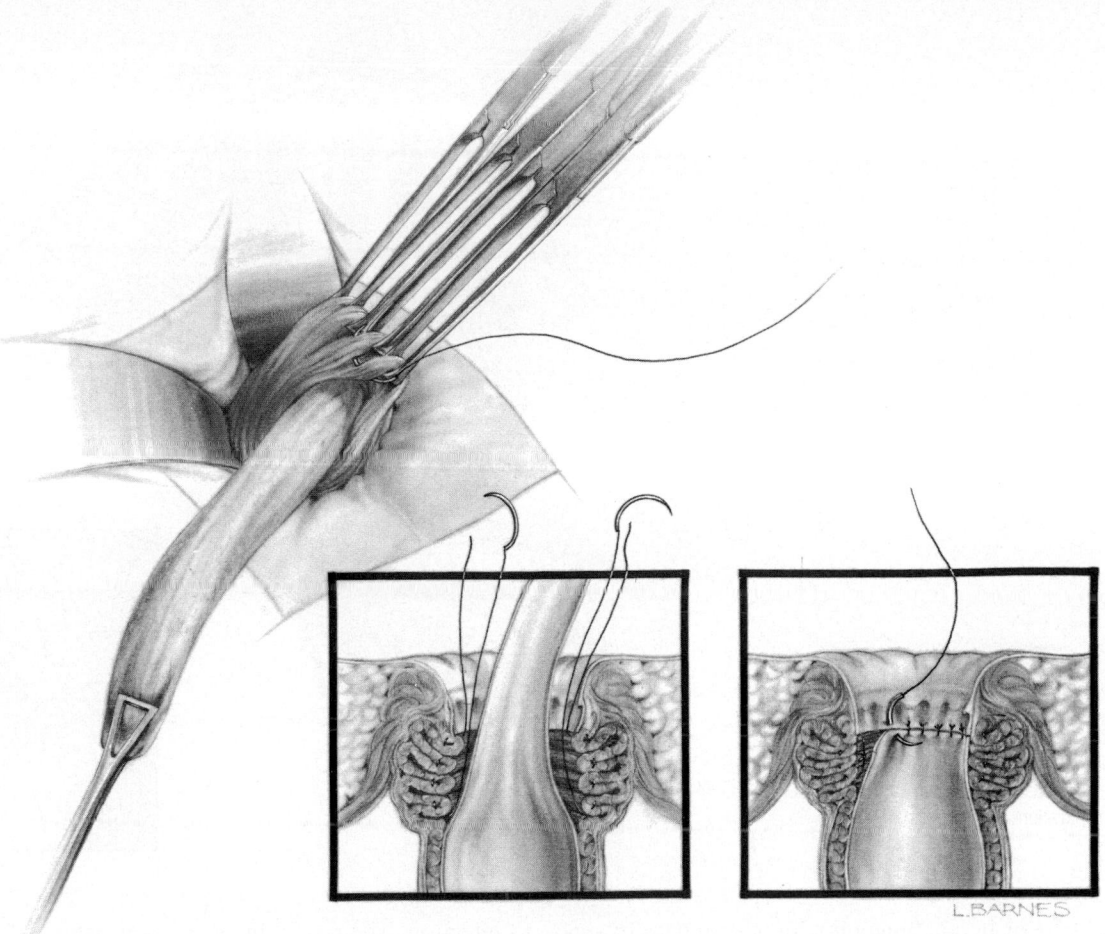

FIGURE 21-18. The circular muscle of the rectum is prepared for suturing by the placement of serial Allis clamps. Plication is carried out using 2–0 long-term absorbable sutures. The *insets* illustrate the completed "anastomosis" after the redundant mucosa has been amputated. (Adapted from Berman IR, Harris MS, Rabeler MB. Delorme's transrectal excision for internal prolapse. Patient selection, technique, and three-year follow-up. *Dis Colon Rectum.* 1990;33(7):573–580, with permission.)

14%, with one death. The recurrence rate was 13.5%, with approximately two-thirds achieving improved bowel control. Plusa and colleagues evaluated physiologic changes following this procedure in 19 women.[245] There were no significant changes in anal sphincter pressures, but there was an observed decrease in the volume required for first rectal sensation, as well as a decline in the maximum tolerated rectal volume. Furthermore, rectal compliance was reduced in addition to improved rectal sensation. Tsunoda and associates noted a 13% recurrence rate in their 31 patients (median follow-up, 39 months).[320] They also performed physiologic assessment and found a statistically significant improvement in squeeze pressures, volume at first sensation, and maximum tolerable volume. The preoperative incontinence score improved from 11.5 to 6.0 ($P < .0001$). Watts and Thompson performed the Delorme's procedure on 101 patients with "full-thickness rectal prolapse" and followed them for more than 1 year.[329] Thirty-eight had no recurrence, 33 died without recurrence, and 30 developed a recurrence (30%).

Restoration of the Pelvic Floor (Historical)

Restoration of the pelvic floor by means of plicating the levators and obliteration of the pouch of Douglas was initially described by Graham in 1942.[101] Others have advocated this

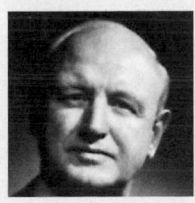

ROSCOE REID GRAHAM (1890–1948)

Graham was born in the village of Lobo, near London, Ontario, Canada, the son of a country physician. He received his medical degree at the University of Toronto, and after a year of internship went abroad to do postgraduate work in Great Britain and on the European continent. He served with the Royal Canadian Medical Corps in England during World War I and returned to resume his practice at Toronto General Hospital, ultimately becoming director of the Division of Surgery. He is credited with being the first to remove an islet cell tumor of the pancreas, and at the time was the youngest surgeon elected to the American Surgical Association.

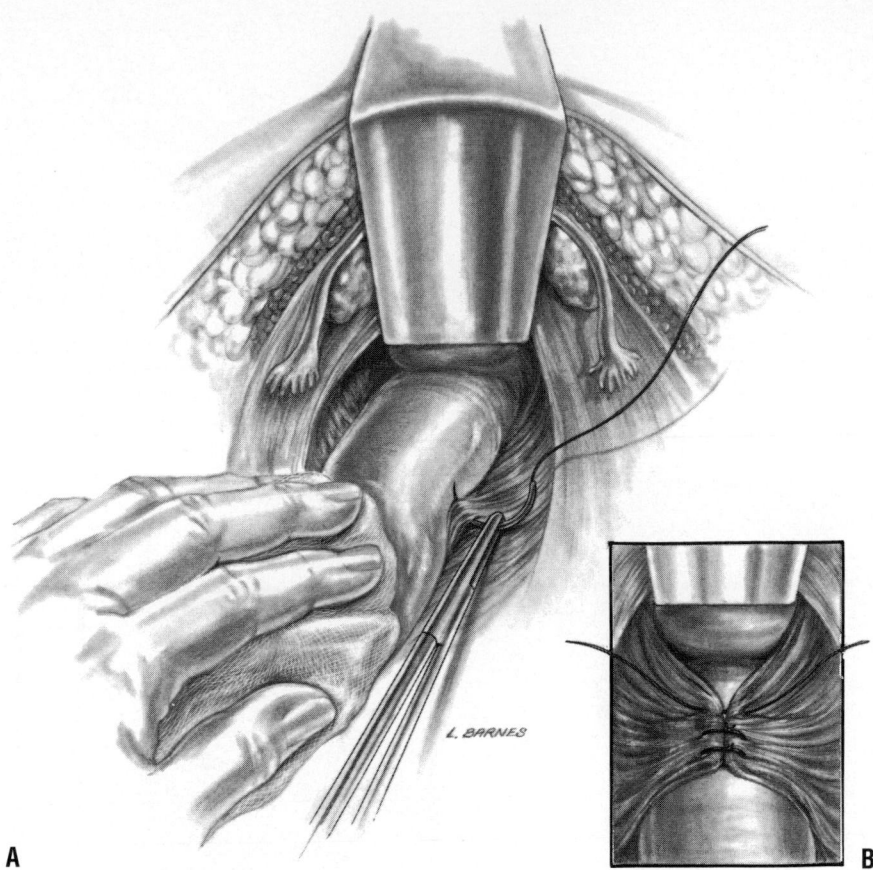

FIGURE 21-19. Roscoe Graham operation. **A:** Reefing of the levator ani muscle is performed transabdominally. A suture is placed into the muscle adjacent to the right lateral aspect of the rectum. **B:** Reefing or plication is accomplished anterior to the rectum.

A

B

operation alone or in combination with other modes of surgical therapy.[7,80,81,134,232] The procedure can be accomplished through the abdomen or the perineum (see also Chapter 16) or after removing the coccyx or lower sacrum.[134] Plicating the levators transabdominally can be performed anterior or posterior to the rectum, although the latter may be technically difficult to accomplish (Figure 21-19). If the surgeon were to use plication of the levators as the sole method of treatment for rectal prolapse, the incidence of recurrence would be prohibitively high.

Transsacral Resection (Historical)
The transsacral operation uses the approach to the rectum described by Kraske for resection of rectal cancer (see Chapter 24).[157] This procedure has been advocated by Davidian and Thomas and by Jenkins and Thomas.[58,134]

An incision is made overlying the sacrum and coccyx, and the latter is disarticulated and removed. The levator ani muscles are divided to expose the rectum. The peritoneum is incised anteriorly and the rectum fully mobilized. The redundant colon is liberated and delivered through the sacral wound (Figure 21-20A). The levator ani muscles are approximated anterior to the rectum (Figure 21-20B), the peritoneum is closed, and resection of the redundant bowel is carried out. After the anastomosis is completed, all wounds are primarily closed.

The theoretical advantages of this procedure are that the operation does not require a laparotomy and that the levator ani muscles are reconstituted, thus narrowing the defect in the pelvic floor. The pouch of Douglas is obliterated, and the rectum is secured posteriorly. The major disadvantage is that the patient has a painful sacrococcygeal wound that is subject

to infection. The possibility of a fecal fistula, although not noted by Davidian and Thomas, is well recognized when this procedure has been undertaken for other indications. The authors reported 30 patients who underwent this operative approach; neither mortality nor recurrence occurred.[58] There have been no published reports of this esoteric operation for many years.

Gant-Miwa Procedure
For an operative approach that is virtually unheard of in the West, it is interesting to note that the Gant-Miwa procedure has been the most common surgical option employed for the treatment of rectal prolapse in Japan.[343] The concept is simply the placement of 20 to 40 absorbable sutures that incorporate the mucosa and submucosa, thereby creating tags or lumps from the apex of the prolapsed rectum to 1 cm from the dentate line. The sutures should be placed at least 5 mm apart in order to avoid mucosal ulceration or necrosis. Gant introduced the procedure in Japan in the 1920s, but the recurrence rate was prohibitively high. Miwa suggested combining the operation with an anal encirclement to reduce the likelihood of recurrence. Still, even with the combined operation (i.e., the Gant-Miwa Procedure), recurrence rates in the range of approximately 15% are considered acceptable in Japan.

Abdominal Procedures
Historical
Teflon or Marlex Sling Repair (Ripstein Operation) (Historical). Arguably, this was the most common surgical approach for the treatment of rectal prolapse in the United States until the advent of sutured posterior rectopexy. The procedure was

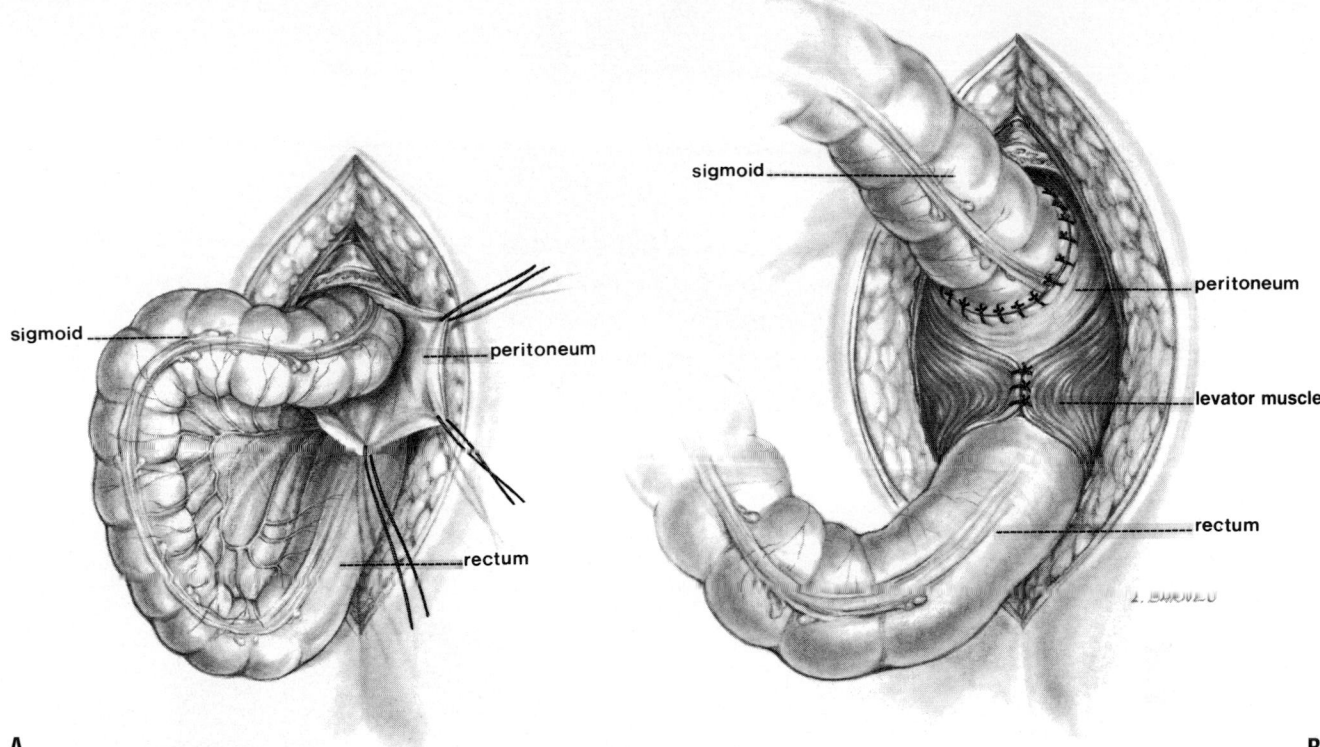

A   **B**

FIGURE 21-20. Thomas operation. **A:** The hernial sac is identified anteriorly and opened, and the redundant sigmoid is delivered. **B:** The hernial sac is excised and the floor of the pelvis reconstituted by suturing the seromuscular layer of the proximal bowel to the peritoneum. The levator ani muscle is plicated anterior to the rectum. The bowel is resected and an anastomosis is performed in the conventional way (not shown).

described initially by Ripstein in 1965.[259] After mobilization of the rectum, a rectopexy is carried out using a sling of Teflon, Marlex, or Gore-Tex placed around the anterior surface of the rectum and fixed to the sacrum on each side.

Securing the Teflon mesh (or Marlex or Gore-Tex) to the sacrum can be accomplished in one of three ways. Sutures can be placed into the periosteum of the sacrum approximately 1 cm to the right of the midline by using a half circle Mayo trocar point needle. Three or four nonabsorbable sutures are used (Figure 21-21A). The mesh is trimmed to approximately 4 cm wide and secured in place along the right side of

the sacrum (Figure 21-21B). At this point in the operation, it is important for the assistant to maintain proximal traction while the mesh is anchored to the muscularis propria of the rectum. If the rectum is not under cephalad tension and if redundant rectum is left below the mesh, a prolapse will recur. Nonabsorbable sutures are placed from the mesh into the rectal wall (Figure 21-21C). After the mesh has been laid around two-thirds of the bowel, the redundant material is appropriately trimmed so that it can be secured without tension (Figure 21-21D). Sutures are then anchored in the sacrum on the left side and placed into the mesh. An approximately 1-cm

CHARLES BENJAMIN RIPSTEIN (1913–2003)

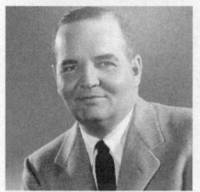

Charles Ripstein was born in Winnipeg, Manitoba, Canada, December 13, 1913, one of four children of a whiskey manufacturer. He wished to be an engineer but developed tuberculosis. He moved to Arizona to recuperate and while there attended the University of Tucson. Because of his own illness, he became interested in studying medicine. He then returned to Canada to enter medical school at McGill University, graduating first in his class. One of his classmates was Rupert Turnbull, his lifelong friend. Upon graduation in 1940, he enlisted in the Canadian Air Force as a flight surgeon and flew many bombing missions over Europe. Following the war, he returned to McGill for his surgical residency. His primary interest at that time was cardiothoracic surgery. He accepted a position as professor of thoracic surgery at Downstate Medical Center (Brooklyn, New York) in 1949. During this time, he developed an extensive clinical cardiac surgery, teaching, and research program. In 1955, he accepted the position as the first professor of surgery at the newly established Albert Einstein College of Medicine (New York) and chief of General Thoracic Surgery, Brookside and Jacobi Hospitals. During the following decade, he developed a particular interest in colon and rectal surgery and ultimately became a fellow of the American Society of Colon and Rectal Surgeons. In 1972, he moved to Miami, Florida, where he practiced colon and rectal surgery until he retired in his early 80s. (With appreciation to Linda Ripstein Dresnick, MD and Rene F. Hartmann, MD.)

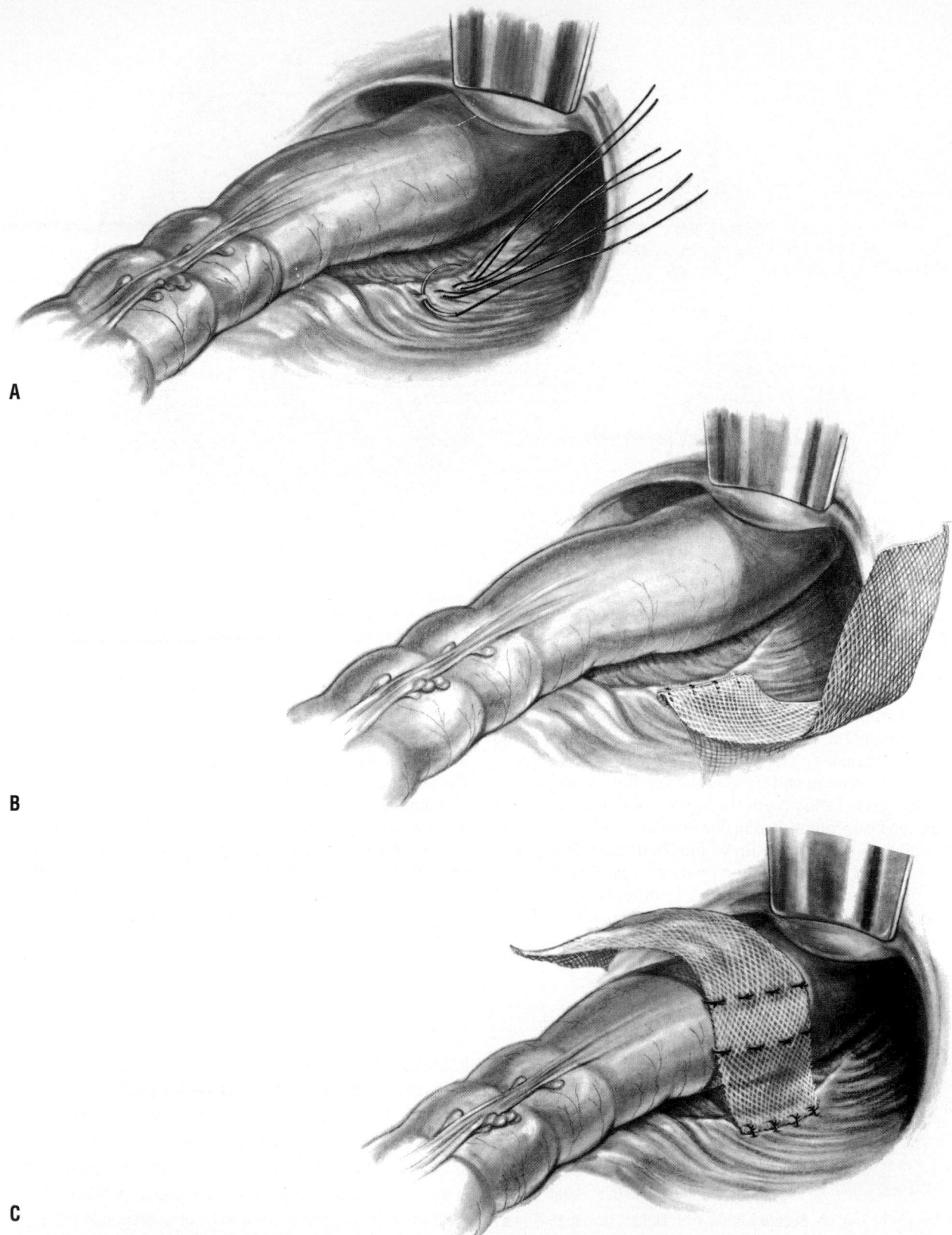

A

B

C

FIGURE 21-21. Teflon sling repair. **A:** Sutures are placed into the periosteum on the right side of the sacrum. **B:** The mesh is anchored into place after appropriate trimming. **C:** With the rectum held under tension, the mesh is sutured to the muscularis of the bowel. (*continued*)

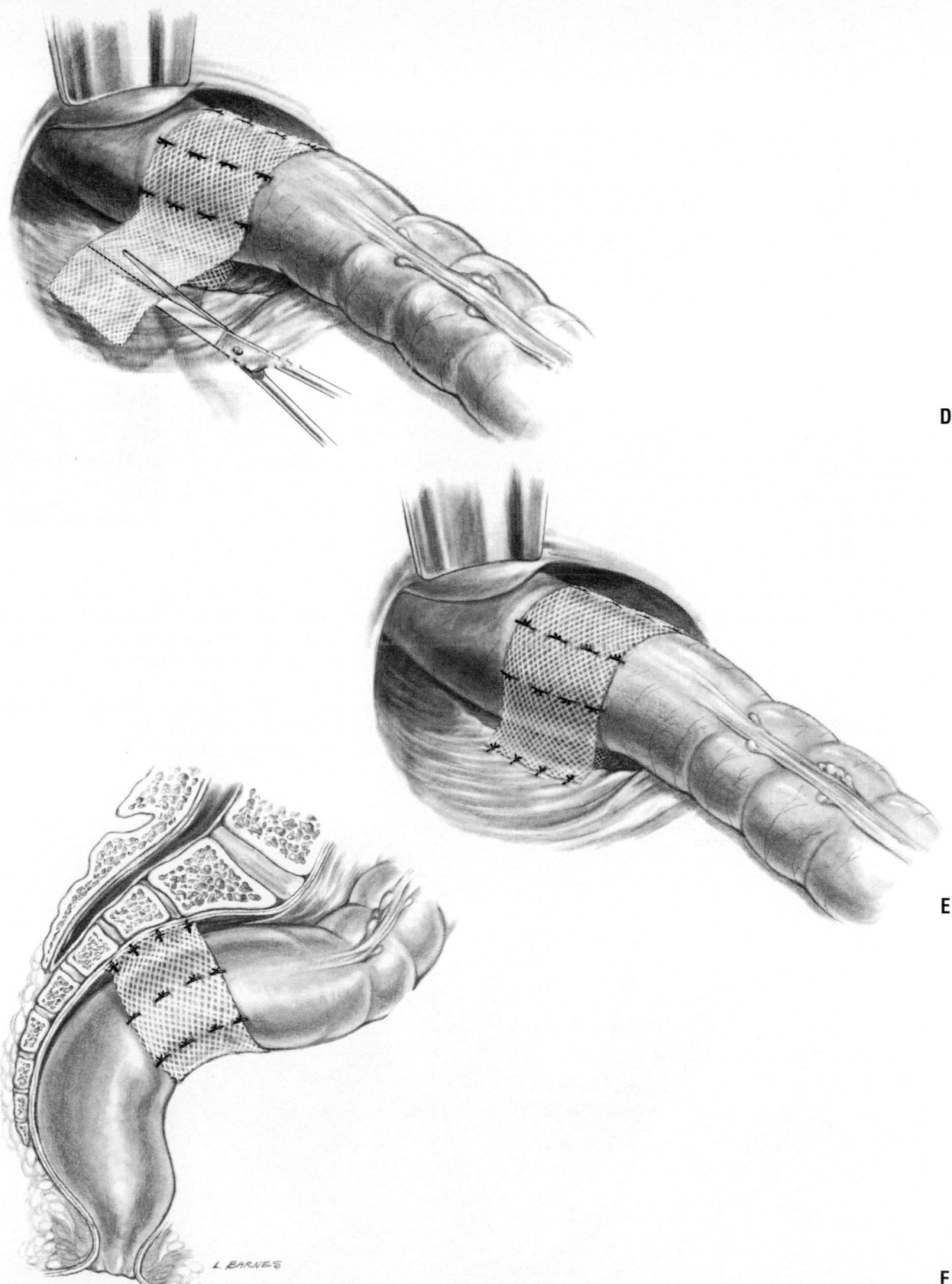

D

E

F

FIGURE 21-21. (*continued*) **D:** After the mesh has been placed approximately two-thirds of the way around the rectum, it is trimmed so that it can be sutured without tension to the contralateral side of the sacrum. **E:** The mesh is secured to the sacrum on the left side, leaving a defect of ~1 cm posteriorly. **F:** A lateral view shows the position of the mesh as secured to the sacrum.

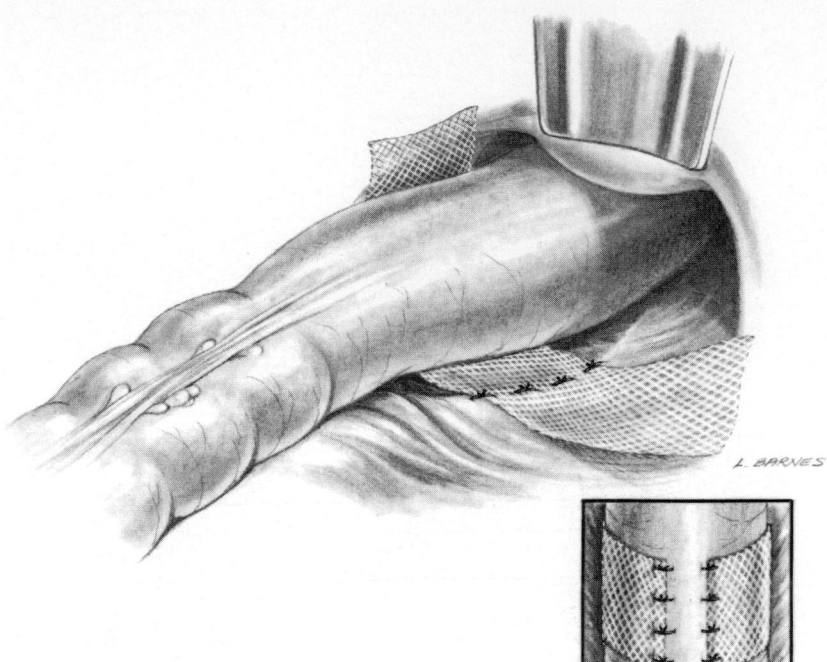

FIGURE 21-22. Alternative method of Teflon sling repair showing position of the mesh sutured in the midline. The mesh is brought around either side of the rectum and sutured to the anterior wall, leaving a defect of ~1 cm anteriorly (*inset*).

defect is present posteriorly (Figure 21-21E). The remaining sutures on the left side are placed through the mesh and in the muscularis of the bowel (Figure 21-21F). Another method of securing the mesh is to place a single row of sutures into the midline of the sacrum. The middle of the mesh is sutured into place and the material brought onto either side of the rectum (Figure 21-22). With proximal traction maintained on the rectum, the mesh is anchored, leaving a 1-cm defect anteriorly (Figure 21-22, *inset*). This is a simpler technique than the former, but it has the potential risk of leaving only a solitary row of sutures posteriorly with which to hold the rectum to the sacrum. A simpler modification for attaching the mesh to the sacrum has been proposed by Nicosia and Bass.[218] A fascial stapler was used successfully in 12 patients to accomplish fixation expeditiously and with essentially no risk of inducing hemorrhage (Figure 21-23).

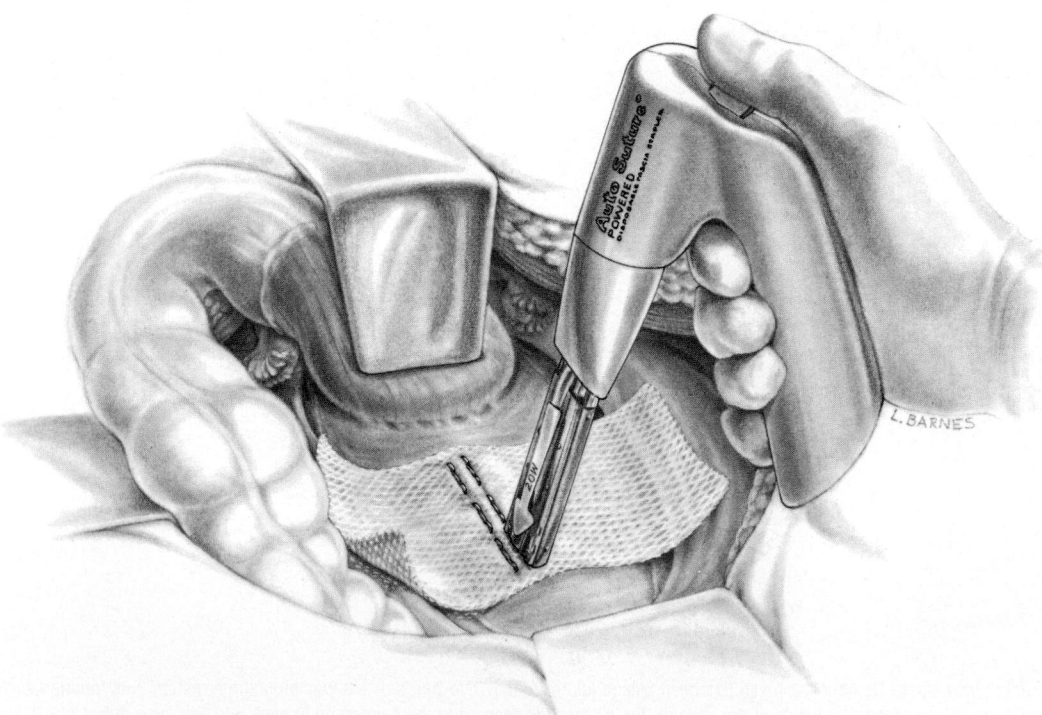

FIGURE 21-23. Securing Teflon mesh to sacrum with power fascial stapler. (Adapted from Nicosia JF, Bass NM. Use of the fascial stapler in proctopexy for rectal prolapse. *Dis Colon Rectum*. 1987;30(11):900–901, with permission.)

Following suspension, it is not necessary to reperitonealize the floor of the pelvis, but it can be done if the surgeon so wishes. If hemostasis is secured, pelvic drainage is not necessary, and with the foreign material, the presence of a drain can pose a particular hazard for infection. However, when venous bleeding has been encountered, a closed suction drain may be placed into the pelvis and brought out through a stab wound in the left lower quadrant. This is usually maintained for 2 to 3 days.

Kuijpers and Mollen routinely perform a rectovaginoplasty in patients with complete prolapse.[158] These surgeons believe that the incidence of concomitant genital prolapse is "at least 25%" or will surely develop later. They further emphasize that the pouch of Douglas should be obliterated.

Sepsis is an unusual complication of mesh repair, but when it occurs it is extremely difficult to treat. Removal of the mesh inevitably becomes necessary, a technical tour de force that may lead to the requirement for a bowel resection. It is primarily because of the risk of entering the bowel during some phase of the procedure that a mechanical preparation has been strongly suggested. If the lumen is breached, the surgeon is advised to carry on with a resection rather than risk insertion of foreign material in a contaminated field.

The mean follow-up period was 46 months in the Lahey Clinic series, with 35 patients available for evaluation more than 5 years later.[139] Bowel management and incontinence remained persistent problems after the prolapse was corrected. Approximately one-third complained of difficulty in regulating bowel function after the repair, and 11% reported incontinence or soiling. Of course, bowel function and incontinence problems are common complaints prior to surgery. The habits of excessive straining to pass stool and dependence on laxatives are often long-standing and not remedied by anatomic correction of the prolapse.

Gordon and Hoexter, in a study based on a questionnaire sent to members of the American Society of Colon and Rectal Surgeons, were able to gain information on 1,111 Teflon sling repairs performed by 129 surgeons.[99] The overall complication rate was 16.5%, with a recurrence of 2.3%. Fecal impaction was seen in 6.7%. It was the opinion of the authors that the complications seemed to be related primarily to applying the mesh too tightly around the rectum. The complication rate seems to diminish as the surgeon's experience increases.

Holmström and associates reported their initial experience with the Teflon sling repair in 59 patients.[121] The operative mortality was high (5%). However, in 2 of the 3 patients who died, the cause of death was coronary artery disease. The recurrence rate was 5.4% during a mean observation period of 5 years. A later report from the same institution included 108 patients, 97 of whom were available for evaluation.[122] The recurrence rate in this study was 4.1%. The proportion of continent patients increased from 33% preoperatively to 72% postoperatively. However, problems with defecation were a major source of dissatisfaction; difficulties increased from 27% preoperatively to 43% postoperatively.

Biehl and colleagues reported on their experience at the Ochsner Clinic and compared it with the Altemeier, sigmoidectomy, and Thiersch procedures that had been formerly used.[25] The Ripstein operation was associated with a lower recurrence rate and a lower morbidity rate. Launer and coworkers reported the Cleveland Clinic experience with the Teflon sling repair.[168] Although there was no operative mortality in 57 patients, there was a high morbidity rate (26%). Seven (14%) developed recurrent mucosal prolapse, and six patients (12%) had a full-thickness recurrence. Despite the somewhat disappointing results, the authors believed that the Ripstein procedure remained the treatment of choice for rectal prolapse. A later report from the same institution involved 142 patients.[310] The recurrence rate had fallen to 8%. About one-half experienced improvement in bowel control, but persistence or worsening of constipation was more common than after resection. Approximately one-third remained dissatisfied with the functional results despite anatomic correction of the prolapse.

It has also been pointed out that enterocele is observed in about one-third of patients with rectal prolapse.[198] Using the Ripstein rectopexy, none had recurrent prolapse or enterocele in the experience of the group from the Department of Surgery at the Karolinska Institute of Stockholm.[198]

Late Complications. Lescher and colleagues reported the late complications of Teflon sling repair, including when the original procedure was performed elsewhere.[173] Rectal stricture (Figure 21-24) developed in five patients. These individuals had in common a troublesome history of bowel management problems, specifically severe constipation that antedated insertion of the Teflon sling. Patients with rectal stricture also had a longer history of prolapse (79 vs. 37 months). Barium enema examination showed stenosis in all five of these individuals (Figure 21-25), ranging from a diameter of 3 to 19 mm. The presence of narrowing was also identified by proctosigmoidoscopy.

McMahan and Ripstein confirmed that difficulties have arisen with Teflon as the suspension material.[197] They recommend Gore-Tex as being ideal because of its inert properties and its porous structure, which allows tissue incorporation. They also place the sling posteriorly, leaving the anterior rectal wall free to distend. Others have reported the results of polypropylene mesh with no recurrences in a series of 23 patients.[177]

Clearly, constipation is not improved by the Teflon sling repair. On the contrary, abdominal pain, distension, and constipation may be exacerbated by the now-exaggerated redundancy of the sigmoid colon (Figure 21-26).[35,344] Sigmoid volvulus has been reported to occur under these circumstances. In some individuals who present with obstructive symptoms relatively soon after the operation, faulty technique must be assumed. However, fibrotic reaction secondary to the mesh must also be considered as a possible contributing factor. In any patient with chronic constipation, particularly with a history of long-standing rectal prolapse, serious consideration should be given to performing an anterior resection initially. At the very least, these individuals should undergo careful preoperative investigation to identify those who have associated disturbances of function (e.g., slow-transit constipation, obstructed defecation).[74]

Recurrent rectal prolapse after Teflon sling repair may be related to faulty surgical technique. The mesh may not be secured adequately to the presacral fascia or bone. In addition, as has been previously stated, when traction on the rectosigmoid is not maintained while the sling is inserted, the mesh will not be anchored sufficiently low on the rectum. The error is more likely to occur in a male whose pelvis is narrow and in whom mobilization and suture placement are more difficult.

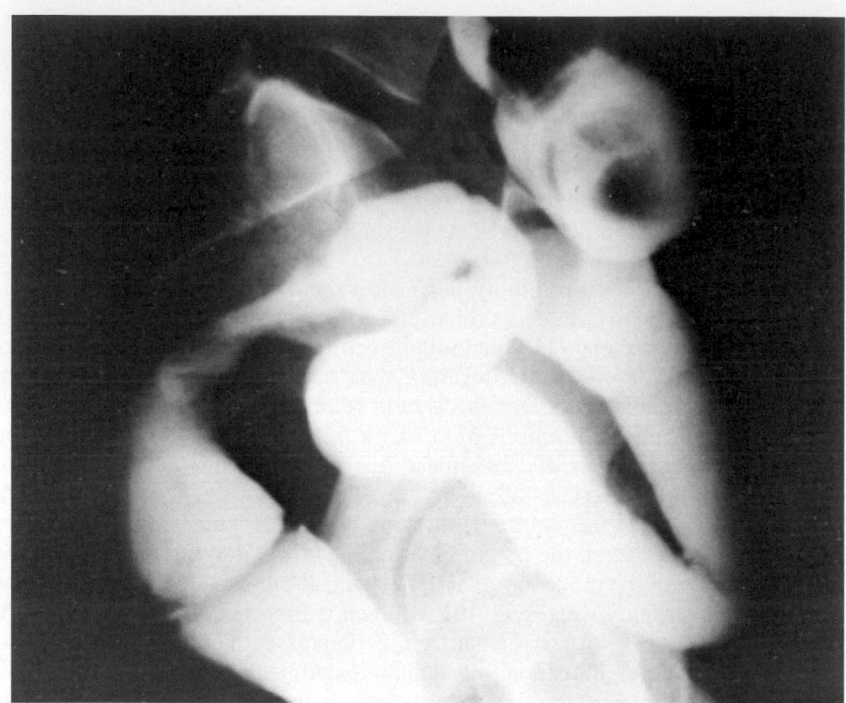

FIGURE 21-24. Barium enema study shows rectal stricture after Teflon sling repair. Note the redundant sigmoid colon. It is readily evident how this could predispose to volvulus. (From Lescher TJ, Corman ML, Coller JA, et al. Management of late complications of Teflon sling repair for rectal prolapse. *Dis Colon Rectum.* 1979;22(7):445–447, with permission.)

Ivalon Sponge Implant or the Wells Operation (Historical). The use of Ivalon sponge as a wrapping about the rectum was initially described by Wells in 1959[330]; it has been enthusiastically advocated, primarily by the British and the Canadians.[5,15,31,32,41,189,195,205,239,266,297] However, because polyvinyl alcohol (i.e., Ivalon) has not been approved for this purpose in the United States, there is no American experience. The Ivalon sponge implant operation basically consists of the implantation of a synthetic polymer around the rectum. After full mobilization of the rectum, the appropriately

tailored sponge is sutured to the sacrum in the posterior midline (Figure 21–27A,B), not unlike the modified Teflon sling operation. It is then wrapped around the rectum, leaving a defect in the anterior midline (Figure 21-27C).

Results of this procedure on 26 patients were reported by Boutsis and Ellis.[32] One operative death occurred, but no instance of pelvic sepsis or wound complication had developed. Follow-up study revealed nine mucosal recurrences—an incidence of 35%. Complete rectal prolapse developed in 11.5%. Stewart reported using this procedure in 41 patients;

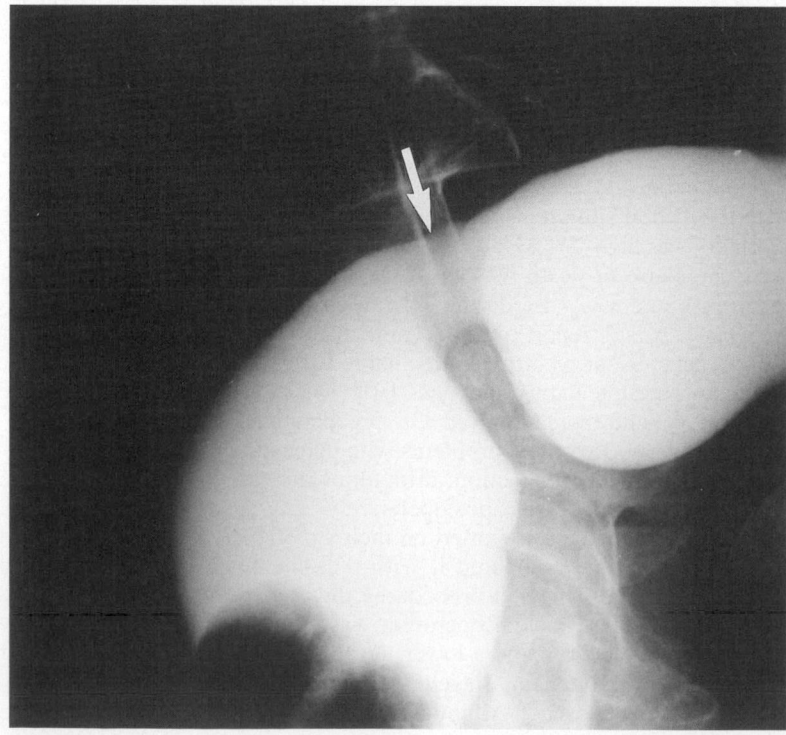

FIGURE 21-25. Profound rectal stricture (*arrow*) can be readily appreciated on this lateral film of the barium-filled rectum.

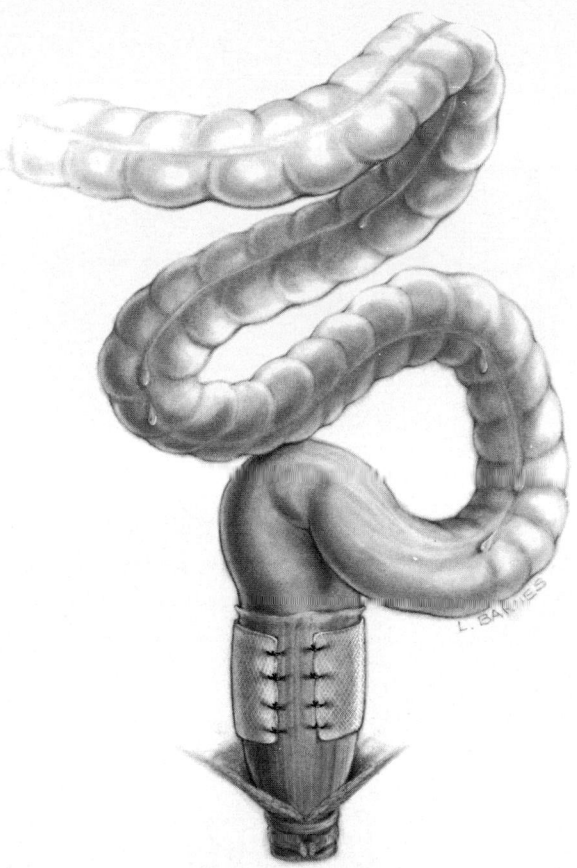

FIGURE 21-26. Rectal suspension procedures may exacerbate bowel management difficulties. Note the sigmoid redundancy that may result.

no operative deaths occurred, complete recurrence developed in 3 patients (7%), and a mucosal recurrence was noted in 10 individuals (24%).[297] McCue and Thomson identified two recurrences in 53 patients (3.8%).[194] Boulos and associates reported 25 patients younger than 40 years of age who were followed for at least 5 years.[31] Twenty percent were found to have recurrence. Mann and Hoffman, however, noted no recurrences after 2 years in 44 patients.[189] A conscientious effort was made to mobilize the rectum fully, to shorten the lateral ligaments, and to excise the redundant peritoneum. Despite the absence of recurrence, constipation (47%) and incontinence (19%) caused difficult management problems. Rogers and Jeffery evaluated 24 individuals who were treated by concomitant Ivalon sponge rectopexy and postanal repair.[263] There was one recurrence (4%), with a

maximum of 4 years of follow-up. Every patient was rendered continent in this uncontrolled study.

Allen-Mersh and colleagues noted a statistically significant increase in the prevalence of constipation following this operation.[5] One of the possible explanations that they suggest is the increased rectal wall thickness that occurs in some individuals. This may impede the passage of stool through the rectum and result in constipation.

Novell and coworkers performed a prospective, randomized trial of Ivalon sponge and sutured rectopexy (see later).[223] At a median follow-up of 47 months, prolapse had recurred in two patients (3%), one in each group; 22% suffered from incontinence, and 40% developed constipation. The authors concluded that the results of rectopexy by suture alone were equivalent to those obtained when Ivalon sponge was implanted, and they concluded that an implant was not necessary.

Although septic problems are not common, removal of the sponge may be quite difficult, particularly when the physician attempts to identify foreign material within an abscess cavity.[164] Symptoms of this complication include sacral, coccygeal, or lower abdominal pain, pus per rectum, pus per vaginam, rectal discharge, and fever. No instance of recurrence was reported by the St. Mark's Hospital group (eight cases) after removal of the implant.[266] They recommended that removal of the implant should be performed through the vagina or the rectum if at all possible. The apparent advantage of the Ivalon sponge implant operation is that fecal impaction has not been as great a problem.[205,239] However, the incidence of recurrence is higher than that generally reported for the Teflon sling repair and for resection.

Obliteration of the Pouch of Douglas (Historical). The Moschcowitz procedure was designed on the theory that the cause of rectal prolapse is a sliding hernia. The technique involves the placement of serial purse-string sutures into the floor of the pelvis to obliterate the pouch of Douglas (Figure 21-28). The recurrence rate, however, as reviewed by Theuerkauf and associates, was close to 50%. Although we have had no experience with this technique, the lack of success of others and the theoretical premise on which it is based would seem to imply that the procedure should be abandoned.

Teflon Halter Operation (Historical). A unique approach to rectal suspension has been suggested by Nigro (see Biography, Chapter 25).[220] He believed the most effective way to correct prolapse was to use a method that most closely simulated the normal anatomy. It was his contention that the most important factor is the angulation and fixation provided by the

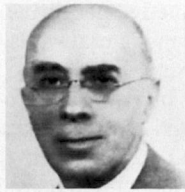

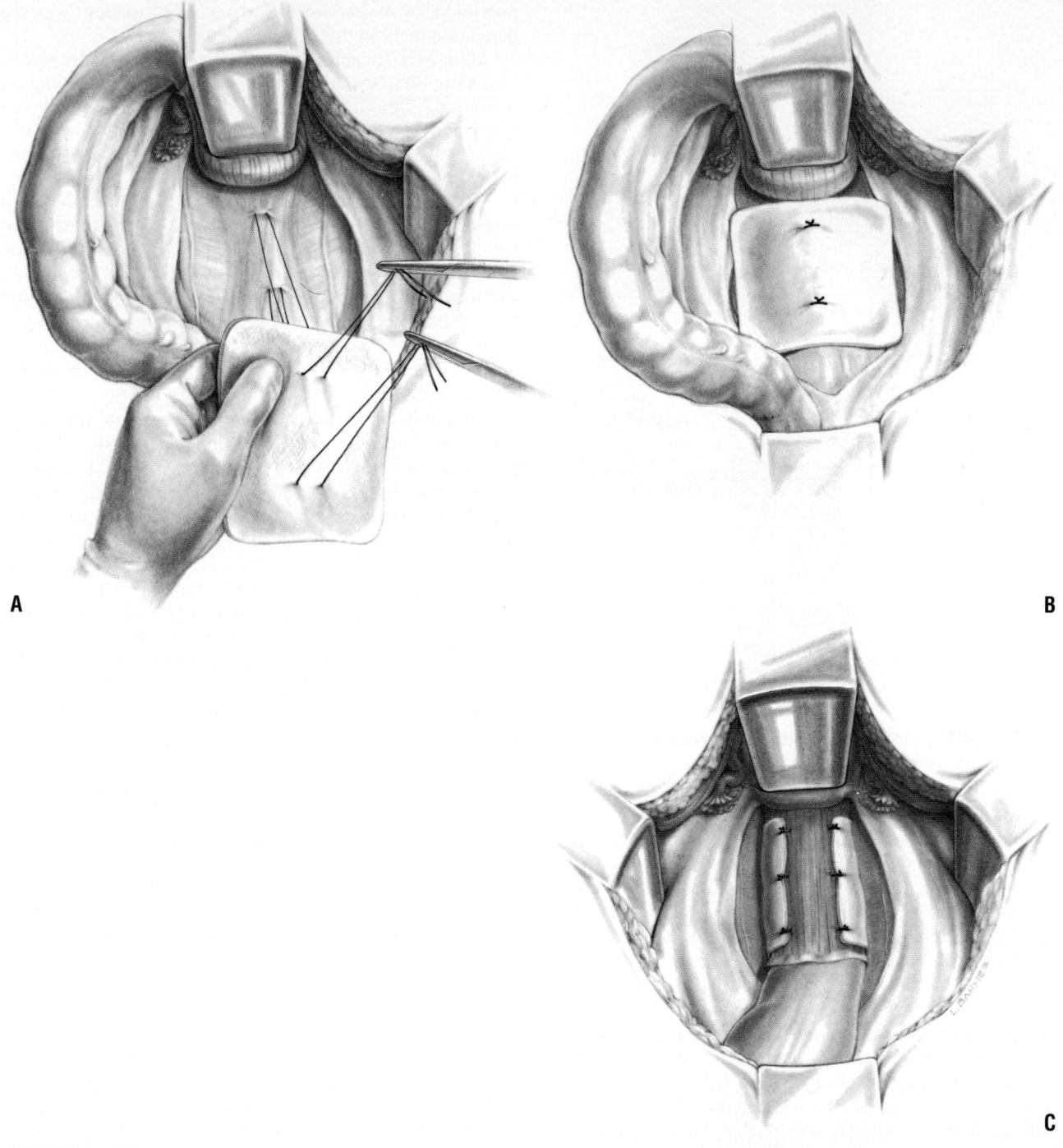

A

B

C

FIGURE 21-27. Technique of Ivalon sponge implant. **A,B:** Suturing of sponge and anchoring to sacrum. **C:** Suspension completed.

pelvic floor musculature, and that maximum support came with contraction of the muscle as it lifted the lower rectum and tilted it forward toward the pubis.[219] Accordingly, he designed an intra-abdominal sling approach that suspends the rectum from the pubis. Successful results were experienced in all six patients.

The patient is placed in the Trendelenburg position on the operating table. A midline incision is made in the lower abdomen, and the rectum is mobilized in the same manner as that for a Ripstein or Wells repair. Care is taken to avoid injury to the inferior mesenteric vessels. The dissection is

carried posteriorly down to the coccyx. The mesh is cut to be approximately 4 cm wide by 20 cm long. The central portion is secured to the rectum with interrupted nonabsorbable sutures. It is then sutured to the posterior and lateral walls of the rectum as low as possible.

The space of Retzius, in front of the bladder and close to the pubic rami, is opened. A long curved clamp is placed into this space and directed downward and posteriorly to the presacral space. The mesh is then grasped and pulled forward to lie on the pubic bone. The same is done on the contralateral side. Each end is then secured to the pubic ramus with

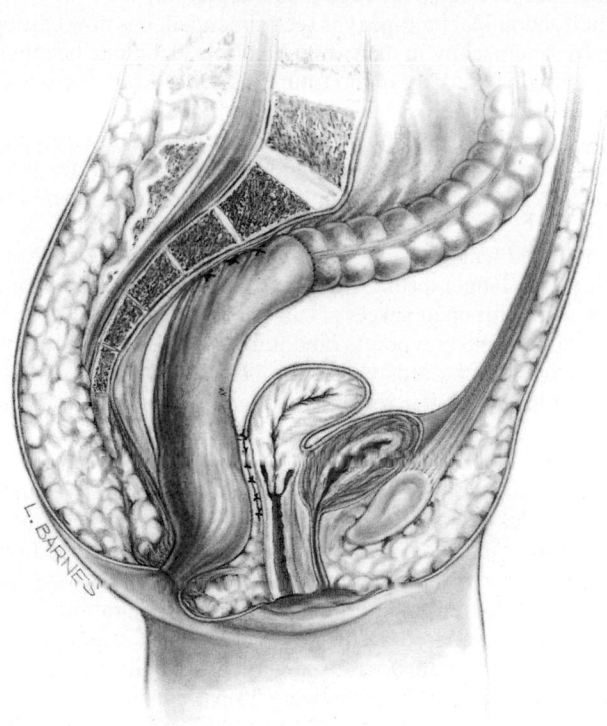

FIGURE 21-28. The Moschcowitz procedure involves the obliteration of the pouch of Douglas by serial purse-string sutures.

interrupted nonabsorbable sutures. The length of graft is determined by holding it to the pubic bone with just enough tension to prevent slack (Figure 21-29). The presacral space is left open, and the abdomen is closed without drainage. Postoperative care is essentially the same as that for the conventional operation.

Greene reported 15 patients who underwent this operation.[103] There was no mortality, no operative morbidity, and

no recurrence with a minimum follow-up of 6 months. Severe incontinence was corrected in all but one patient, and this person was improved. There were no problems with sexual function or micturition. Greene believed that the particular advantage of this operation was on the improvement in continence. This operation seems to be no longer performed.

Combined Abdominal and Perineal Operation (Historical). Dunphy reported a combined abdominal and perineal operation for rectal prolapse.[80] The perineal operation is essentially the same as that described by Altemeier and colleagues.[8] The abdominal operation, however, is accomplished several days later. Full mobilization of the rectum is carried out, and a plication of the ligamentous structures lateral to the rectum is performed. The pouch of Douglas is obliterated in the manner of Moschcowitz. Dunphy described this technique and results of treatment in four patients; no recurrence was noted.

Currently Used Procedures
Suture Rectopexy

In this prodecure, the rectum and rectosigmoid are mobilized, usually without difficulty, with care taken to avoid injury to the ureters. Mobilization of the rectum to the level of the levator ani muscle is usually easily accomplished. This maneuver facilitates adhesion or passive fixation of the rectum to the sacrum. One may reasonably ask whether rectal fixation is indeed important.

It was long suspected that if nothing more than mobilization were done, many patients would be cured by this maneuver alone. This question has been recently addressed by a multicenter controlled trial involving 41 tertiary centers in 21 countries, in which patients were randomly assigned to rectal mobilization with or without a posterior rectopexy.[143] The end point was recurrence of external full-thickness rectal prolapse. Sigmoid resection was not randomized and was added when constipation was present. One hundred and sixteen nonrectopexy patients were comparable to 136 rectopexy patients for age, body mass index (BMI), American Society of Anesthesiologists (ASA) grade, and previous

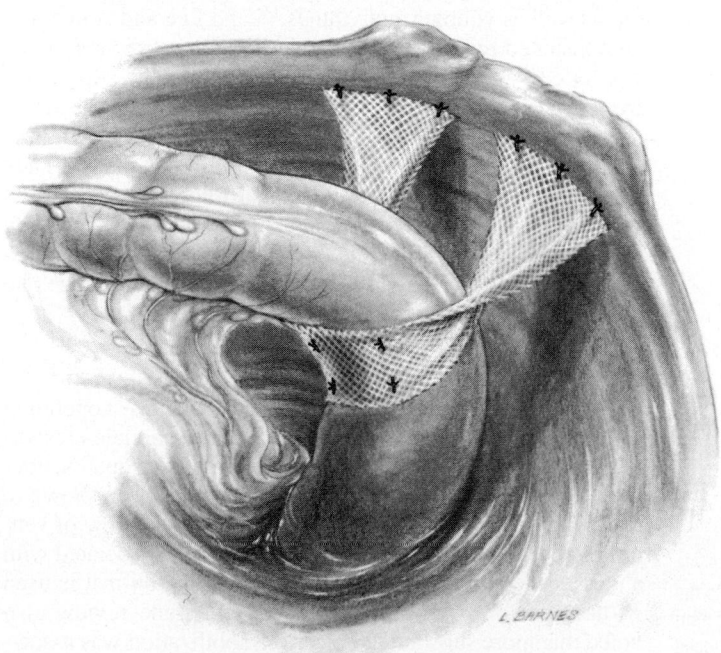

FIGURE 21-29. Nigro procedure. The mesh is suspended from the pubis and brought around the posterior wall of the rectum as a halter.

abdominal surgery, but not for sex ($P = .013$) and prolapse length (8 [1 to 25] cm vs. 5 [1 to 20] cm; $P = .026$). Sigmoid resection was performed more frequently in the nonrectopexy arm ($P < .001$). There was no significant difference in complication rates (11% vs. 18%; $P = .139$). The mortality rate was 0.8%, and the loss of patients at 5-year follow-up was 10%. Actuarial analysis demonstrated a significant difference in 5-year recurrence rates between study arms (8.6% vs. 1.5%) (log-rank, $P = .003$). The authors concluded that recurrence following no rectopexy was higher than when a rectal fixation had been performed.

Perhaps now the most popular and simplest abdominal approach for the treatment of rectal prolapse is suture rectopexy. The operation is also easily adapted to laparoscopic surgery. Simple sutured posterior rectopexy without resection has been especially advocated when preoperative constipation is present.[310] The operation consists of mobilizing the posterolateral rectum down to the levator ani muscle and securing the mesentery of the rectum and its muscularis propria to the presacral fascia (Figure 21-30). This can be performed using nonabsorbable interrupted sutures or staples.

Blatchford and colleagues undertook suture rectopexy on 43 patients.[27] Only one recurrence was noted at a mean follow-up of 28 months. Others reported two recurrences out of 46 patients, a rate comparable to that of standard suspension procedures.[86]

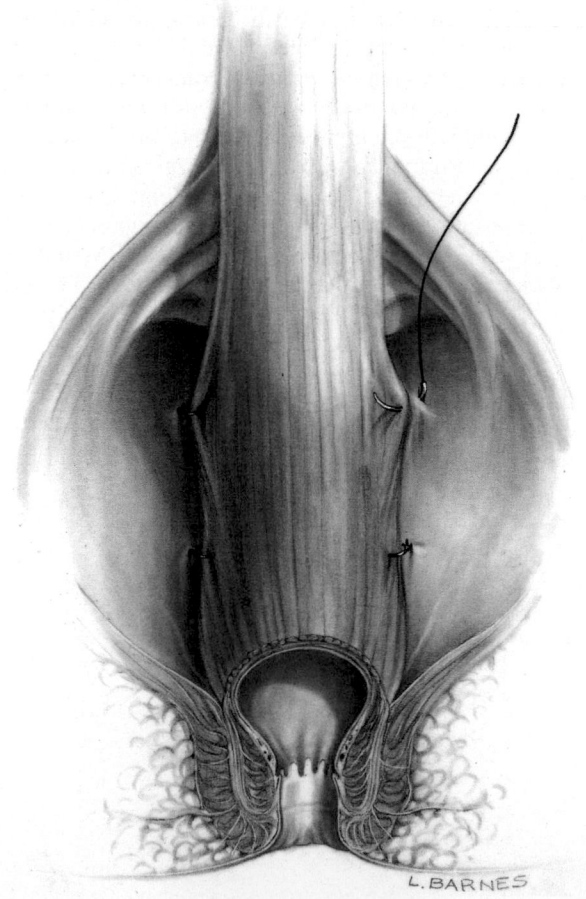

FIGURE 21-30. Suture rectopexy. The mobilized rectum is secured to the sacrum or presacral fascia with interrupted nonabsorbable sutures. (Redrawn from Blatchford GJ, Perry RE, Thorson AG, et al. Rectopexy without resection for rectal prolapse. *Am J Surg.* 1989;158(6):574–576.)

Laparoscopic Rectopexy (See also Chapter 19)

When abdominal rectopexy is recommended, it is now carried out by laparoscopy in many units. As this technique becomes more used, it is likely in the future that only a rare rectopexy will be performed using an open technique.[19,22,100,114,161,291,292] Many surgeons have now reported their results with laparoscopic posterior rectopexy, and the recurrence rates have matched the rates of less than 5% achieved with open surgery.[16,19,22,79,127,169,171,265,337] Most notable, however, has been the reduced length of stay and the low rates of surgical morbidity. The longer term results appear to be durable and compare well with open surgery.[38]

Solomon and coworkers randomized 40 patients to receive either open or laparoscopic rectopexy.[292] Their study was limited to in-hospital results as judged by their response to landmarks adopted through a clinical pathway regimen. The laparoscopic group was clearly superior in all areas (pain, diet advancement, bowel action) except for operative time. In a parallel health economic study, they also demonstrated that despite more expense associated with a prolonged operative time, overall costs in the laparoscopic arm were less because of the reduction in hospital stay.[271] Kairaluoma and colleagues compared a consecutive series of patients who underwent an open operation with those who underwent laparoscopic repair.[140] There were 53 patients in each group. Operating time was longer (210 vs. 117 minutes), but median postoperative hospital stay was shorter (5 vs. 7 days). There was no statistically significant difference in morbidity or mortality, rate of recurrence, and late complications. Day case laparoscopic rectopexy has also been reported.[327]

As of this writing, there have been two meta-analyses of open versus laparoscopic rectopexy.[251,270] Both have shown a significant reduction in length of stay as the major benefit, with no difference in function (constipation and incontinence), morbidity and mortality, and recurrence. The operating time was significantly longer.

It has also been shown that laparoscopic rectopexy is safe in the elderly. This is particularly important given the average age of patients with external rectal prolapse. In a small series, Kaiwa and associates showed that patients older than 70 did as well as younger individuals,[141] and Lee and colleagues demonstrated that in elderly patients, laparoscopic rectopexy was safe.[171] Wijffels and coworkers reported the experience from two centers in the United Kingdom involving 80 patients aged 80 years or older.[333] They noted a low morbidity (13%) and mortality (0%) and a median hospital stay of 2 days. They suggested that the safety profile of laparoscopic rectopexy was similar to that of a perineal approach, and because of the low recurrence rate (3%), a perineal procedure was difficult to justify simply based on age *alone*, given a pooled recurrence rate of 18% of the latter procedure.[333]

Laparoscopic Ventral Rectopexy

Laparoscopic ventral rectopexy (LVR) is the newest operation for rectal prolapse (Figure 21-31).[30,69,288] Its rationale is based on avoiding the well-documented problem of constipation after posterior rectopexy. A posterior dissection has been shown to denervate the rectum.[36,68,204,280,294] A systematic review of ventral rectopexy concluded that this operation is associated with a greater reduction in postoperative constipation if it is used without posterior mobilization.[272] A Cochrane review also noted that more substantial posterior mobilization was associated with lower recurrence but at a higher rate of constipation.[18]

serted, in addition to a left iliac fossa port in males (5 mm). If present, the uterus is hitched to the anterior abdominal using 2–0 silk on a straight needle. A very superficial peritoneal window is made using a hook dissector, with monopolar diathermy from the right sacral promontory over the right outer border of the mesorectum down toward the right side of the deep pouch of Douglas (Figure 21-32A). The right hypogastric nerve (deeper) and ureter (more lateral) are spared, avoiding mobilization of the mesorectum. At the deepest point of the right pouch of Douglas, the longitudinal incision is terminated. The overlying peritoneum just posterior to the apex of the rectovaginal septum is grasped and retracted posterocranially. A narrow Deaver retractor placed in the vagina is retracted antero-caudally, equal, and opposite. The areolar plane opens nicely with the first transverse incision in the peritoneum overlying the apex of the rectovaginal septum. A purely anterior rectal dissection is then undertaken in this areolar tissue to create a 4-cm wide pocket from the depth of the pouch of Douglas to the level of the pelvic floor. The distal limit is confirmed by digital rectal exam. A 3 by 20 cm strip of polypropylene or biologic collagen mesh is introduced and positioned as distally as possible on the anterior side of the rectum. The mesh is sutured to the anterior borders of the rectum in two parallel rows of interrupted nonabsorbable sutures (Ethibond Excel 00; Ethicon, Johnson & Johnson) (Figure 21-32B). The mesh is very slightly obliquely angled from the midline distally to the right sacral promontory to which it is secured using a ProTack device (Auto-Suture, Tyco Healthcare). The vaginal vault (or cervix) is fixed to the mesh without tension by two additional sutures. A shallow neo-pouch of Douglas is created by reefing the edges of the peritoneal incision in the midline with three "figure of eight" 2–0 Vicryl 75 cm sutures (Ethicon, Johnson & Johnson) to completely cover the repair and mesh with peritoneum (Figure 21-32C). We recommend that patients be covered with a single dose of cephalosporin and metronidazole at induction. Postoperative intravenous narcotic infusions and epidural anesthesia are avoided. Pain relief is provided by regular nonsteroidal analgesia within an enhanced recovery program. Postoperatively, patients are commenced on an osmotic laxative three times daily, reducing to once daily by the 6-week clinic review in order to avoid strain on the mesh.

There have been several published reports on laparoscopic ventral rectopexy for rectal prolapse.[30,69,288] At follow-up of between 29 and 62 months, these series reported recurrence rates between 0% and 5%, 0% mortality and major morbidity, and rates of minor morbidity ranging from 5% to 21%. Median hospital stay ranged from 2 to 5 days, and constipation improved in 72% to 84%, worsening in 2% to 5%.

Laparoscopic Orr-Loygue Rectopexy

In 1947, Orr described a suspension procedure by which the rectum is anchored to the sacrum with strips of fascia lata.[230] Loygue and coworkers and Orr modified the operation to include full rectal mobilization.[178] They reported their experience with 140 patients. Two operative deaths were noted, and the incidence of recurrent prolapse was 3.6%. Christiansen and Kirkegaard reported two recurrences in 24 patients (8%) who underwent this procedure.[49] Douard and associates assessed the functional results after the Orr-Loygue for complete rectal prolapse in 31 patients.[75] There were no recurrences at a mean follow-up of 28 months. Continence improved in 24 of the 25 who were incontinent preoperatively. Evacuation difficulties increased significantly, however.

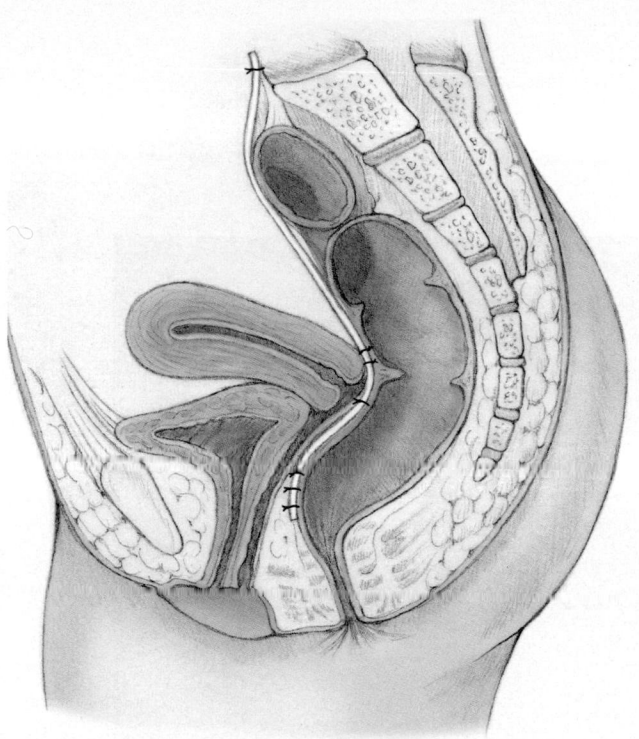

FIGURE 21-31. Laparoscopic ventral rectopexy. The attachments of the mesh to the anterior rectum, the vagina, and the sacral promontory.

Posterior mobilization has been used out of familiarity with the posterior surgical plane used for rectal cancer, but posterior rectopexy remains the only surgical procedure where the rectum is mobilized, denervated, and yet not resected. A ventral dissection avoids rectal denervation by restricting the dissection to the front of the rectum between the deepest limits of the pouch of Douglas and the pelvic floor (Figure 21-32). D'Hoore and Penninckx pioneered laparoscopic ventral rectopexy,[69] although a similar open version for internal rectal prolapse had been described by Silvis and colleagues in 1998.[286] D'Hoore reported a 5-year follow-up of 42 patients with low morbidity, acceptable recurrence, and short hospital stay.[69] Improvement in incontinence was seen in 90%, but most notable was the resolution of constipation in 16 of 19 patients (84%). The improvement in constipation and the rare (less than 5%) occurrence of deterioration of constipation or its de novo appearance is the great advantage of ventral rectopexy.

The nerve-sparing nature of ventral compared with posterior rectopexy has been demonstrated objectively. D'Hoore has shown that distal colorectal transit improved after ventral rectopexy.[68] In contrast, Mollen demonstrated that overall colorectal transit time increased; this was especially so in the distal third.[204] Another potential advantage over traditional posterior rectopexy is the simultaneous treatment of middle compartment prolapse.[9] This coexists with posterior compartment prolapse in a high proportion of cases.

Technique. The patient is positioned in the perineolithotomy position, with shoulder supports and a vacuum beanbag under the sacrum. A 30-degree scope is placed in the subumbilical position. After the creation of a pneumoperitoneum, right iliac fossa (5 mm) and right upper quadrant (5 mm) ports are in-

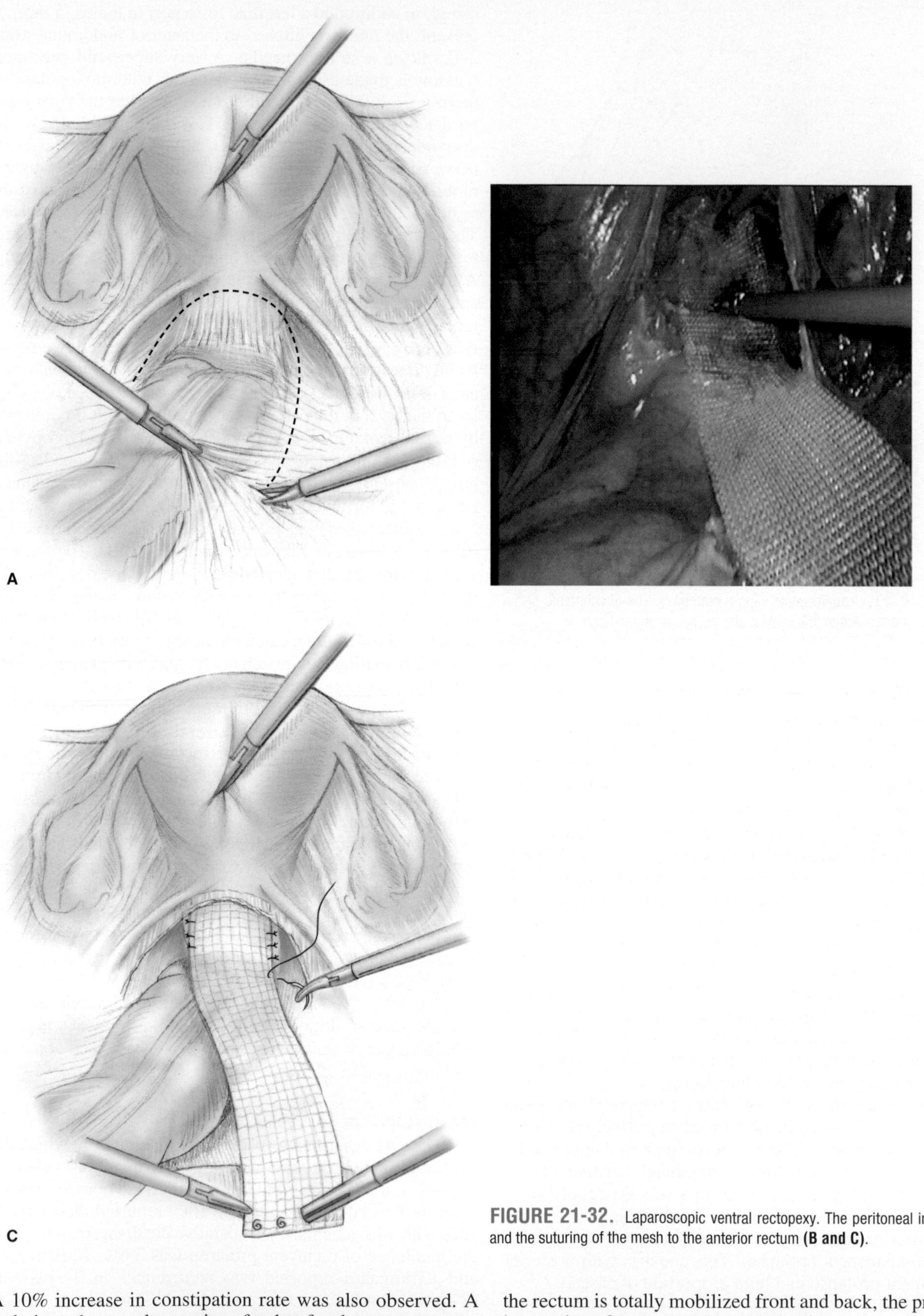

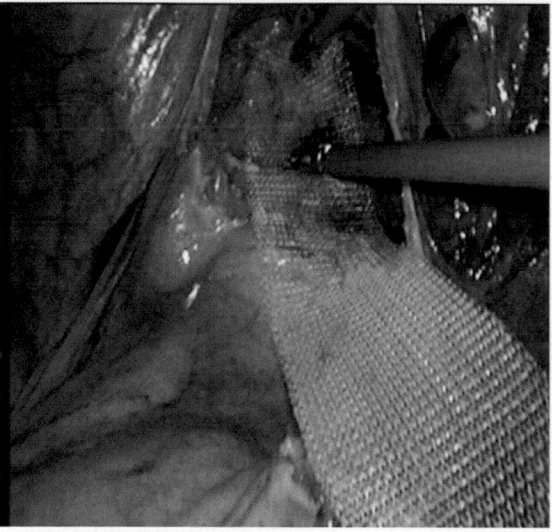

FIGURE 21-32. Laparoscopic ventral rectopexy. The peritoneal incision **(A)**, and the suturing of the mesh to the anterior rectum **(B and C)**.

A 10% increase in constipation rate was also observed. A technique that employs strips of nylon for the same purpose has been described. Loygue and colleagues reported 257 patients who underwent rectopexy by this technique.[179] There were two operative deaths. Recurrent rectal prolapse was observed in 4.3% at a minimum follow-up of 5 years. Because

the rectum is totally mobilized front and back, the procedure is notorious for aggravating constipation.

Robotic Rectopexy

Robotic rectopexy has been described in a few small series. Draaisma and colleagues reported on 15 consecutive patients with a rectal prolapse who underwent robot-assisted laparoscopic rectovaginopexy with the da Vinci robotic system (see Chapter 19).[77] The median age was 62 years, and median BMI, 24.9. The median robot setup time was 10 minutes, and operating time was 160 minutes. No conversions to open surgery were necessary. No in-hospital complications occurred, and there was no mortality. The median hospital stay was 4 days. Munz and coworkers reported six patients with rectal prolapse, all completed successfully using the robotic system.[207] There were no major complications and no deaths. The mean setup time was 28 minutes, mean operation time was 127 minutes, and mean hospital stay was 6 days. At 3 to 6 months follow-up, all were in good health, with no signs of recurrence and with no report of constipation.

A case-control study by de Hoog and associates was designed to evaluate recurrence and functional outcome of open, laparoscopic, and robot-assisted rectopexy for consecutive patients undergoing surgery for external rectal prolapse between 2000 and 2006.[60] Of 82 patients (71 females, mean age 56.4 years), 9 (11%) developed a recurrence. Robotic rectopexy demonstrated significantly higher recurrence rates when controlled for age and follow-up time compared with open surgery ($P = .027$). Functional results improved with all three operation types. Wong and colleagues reported their early experience with robotic-assisted ventral mesh rectopexy compared to a laparoscopic approach in terms of safety and short-term postoperative outcomes.[340] Of a cohort of 63 consecutive patients, 40 underwent laparoscopic and 23 robotic procedures. Both groups were of similar mean age (59 ± 13 vs. 61 ± 11; $P = .44$) and ASA status. Patients undergoing the robotic procedure had a significantly higher BMI (mean, 27 ± 4 vs. 24 ± 4; $P = .03$) and longer operative time (mean, 221 ± 39 minutes vs. 162 ± 60 minutes; $P = .0001$). Patients who underwent a laparoscopic procedure had slightly more blood loss (mean, 45 ± 91 mL vs. 6 ± 23 mL; $P = .05$). The conversion rate (10% vs. 5%; $P = .75$) and duration of hospitalization were similar (mean, 5 ± 2 days vs. 5 ± 1.6 days; $P = .87$). There was no mortality or recurrence at the 6-month postoperative review.

Rectopexy and Postoperative Constipation

All posterior rectopexy techniques—be they suture or mesh rectopexy, laparoscopic or open—involve a posterolateral mobilization of the rectum. The anatomical disturbance is corrected but is frequently traded for a functional one that can be more debilitating and certainly more difficult to treat than the prolapse itself. At least 50% and up to 80% of patients with rectal prolapse are constipated prior to surgery.[30,294] Preexisting hindgut neural abnormalities, postulated to be a traction injury from the loss of rectal support, disappear following correction of the prolapse, as do the reduced anal canal pressures and evidence of pelvic floor neuropathy.[88] There is no doubt that classical posterior rectopexy corrects constipation in some patients by stopping the rectum from intussuscepting, but it frequently worsens or induces new onset of constipation in others.

The mechanism for postoperative constipation has been the subject of debate. Some have suggested that rectopexy leaves a redundant sigmoid colon that might kink to produce a mechanical obstruction.[276] Others have postulated that posterolateral mobilization interrupts the autonomic sympathetic innervation of the rectum, causing a hindgut "denervation inertia" and distal slow transit (Figure 21-33).[58] Randomized studies have shown an improvement in constipation by avoiding division of the so-called lateral ligaments (i.e., full vs. partial lateral rectal mobilization),[204,294] This would explain why posterior rectopexy sometimes corrects and yet other times aggravates or induces constipation. The denervation inertia variably overrides any mechanical improvement from fixation of the intussuscepting prolapse. It also explains why resection-rectopexy reduces postoperative constipation, mitigating any hindgut denervation inertia by removing the neuropathic hindgut and reducing hindgut segmental transit.

Presacral Hemorrhage

Presacral hemorrhage is an uncommon but important intraoperative complication of rectal mobilization. Usually, it results from damage to a presacral vein. Diathermy coagulation may be tried, but all too often the basivertebral vein exits directly from the bone, and continuing hemorrhage can ensue as it retracts into the foramen. Application of direct pressure to the area with an abdominal pack will usually arrest it, especially if the surgeon leaves the operating room for 10 or 15 minutes while the assistant maintains compression. Dissecting the area in an attempt to visualize the bleeding point usually only worsens the bleeding. Local measures to secure hemostasis include suturing, application of hemoclips, cauterization, packing, microfibrillar collagen (Avitene), and absorbable gelatin sponges (Gelfoam).[33]

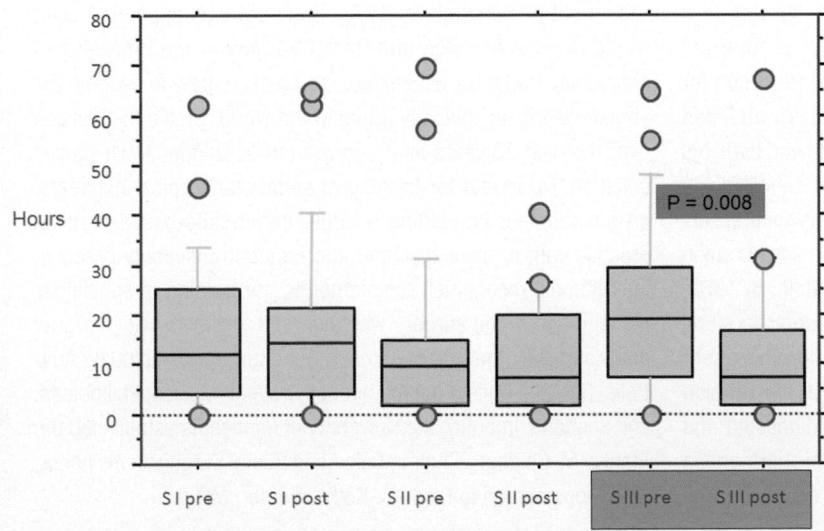

FIGURE 21-33. Influence of ventral rectopexy on distal colonic transit. (From D'Hoore A. Thesis, University of Leuven.)

HOWARD MARTIN FRYKMAN (1917–1969)

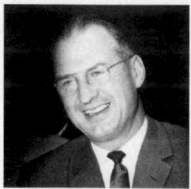

Howard Frykman was born on February 24, 1917 in North Dakota and received his undergraduate and medical school training at the University of Minnesota. He entered medical school but took time out to do research and to obtain a masters degree in neuroanatomy. After a 2-year stint in the U.S. Army, during which time he was wounded in the battle of Guadalcanal, he returned to Minnesota and received his MD degree in 1943. He completed his surgical residency at Minnesota and underwent additional training in proctology under the tutelage of Walter Fansler. He joined the University of Minnesota clinical faculty and ultimately achieved the rank of clinical professor of surgery in the Division of Colon and Rectal Surgery. Early in his career, he worked with Professor Clarence Dennis to study the role of vagotomy in the treatment of ulcerative colitis. In addition, he had an early interest in procidentia and popularized an intra-abdominal repair combining several other previously described techniques. He also studied sepsis associated with bowel surgery and was an early advocate of an intraluminal bowel preparation prior to colonic surgery. He modified the Fansler technique of hemorrhoidectomy by completely closing all anorectal wounds following a submucosal hemorrhoidectomy. Frykman died on October 2, 1969, of a renal tumor. In 1970, the Division of Colon and Rectal Surgery at the University of Minnesota established the Annual Howard M. Frykman Memorial Lecture to honor this pioneer in the specialty. (With appreciation to David A. Rothenberger, MD.)

Abcarian recommends harvesting a small piece of rectus muscle, placing it on the bleeding site, and coagulating the muscle onto the bone. An alternative is a titanium thumbtack inserted into the bone at the site of the bleeding (Figure 21-34),[152,221] but this method has lost favor. Other methods described include the use of an endoscopic stapling device, a Silastic tissue expander for tamponade, and a breast implant sizer.

The most reliable methods, however, are tamponade and heat coagulation at the highest setting of the diathermy of a fragment of rectus abdominis muscle pressed onto the bleeding point by a ball electrode ("muscle–fragment welding").[33,57,110,111,119,341] If one or two attempts to stop the bleeding by simple electrocoagulation or suturing are not effective, this approach should be abandoned. In this situation, the presacral region should be packed or muscle–fragment welding should be tried. It is safer to pack the pelvis and to close the abdomen, returning the following day. Upon removal of the pack, the bleeding will almost certainly have stopped, and the operation can be completed.

One-half of the patients with presacral bleeding in the Lahey Clinic's experience had undergone a prior colorectal operation.[139] Most had anorectal procedures, and 20% had multiple operations. With an experience of more than 100 such operations, the success rate was greater than 95%.[173] Four patients required reoperation: two because of recurrent rectal prolapse and two because of postoperative rectal stricture. There were no operative deaths in their experience. Based on the initial report of 55 patients, 48 (87%) had an uneventful postoperative course.[139]

Rectopexy with Sigmoid Resection

Resection-Rectopexy

This operation was described in the United States by Frykman and Goldberg and is often referred to as the Frykman-Goldberg procedure (Figure 21-35). The rectum is mobilized, and in addition the redundant sigmoid colon

STANLEY MORTON GOLDBERG (1932–PRESENT)

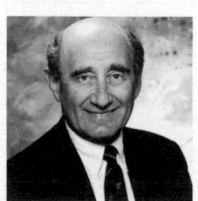

Stanley Goldberg was born May 20, 1932 in Minneapolis, Minnesota, the son of a physician. He has been at the forefront of colon and rectal surgical education for nearly half a century. Goldberg attended the University of Minnesota for both his undergraduate and medical school education. After an internship at the Minneapolis General Hospital, he completed his general surgical residency training under Owen H. Wangensteen and his colon and rectal surgery training under William C. Bernstein. In 1962, he obtained an American Cancer Society grant in order to study colorectal surgery at St. Mark's Hospital in London. Upon his return to Minnesota, Goldberg joined the clinical faculty in the Division of Colon and Rectal Surgery at the University of Minnesota and in the private practice of Howard M. Frykman. Their partnership led to the publication of the 1969 classic article describing the "Frykman-Goldberg repair" for rectal procidentia. Following the retirement of Bernstein in 1972, Goldberg was appointed chief of the Division of Colon and Rectal Surgery at the University of Minnesota. Under his leadership, the practice grew to become the largest colorectal specialty group in the world. He led the division over the next 20 years as it evolved into a unique "town-gown" collaborative model for training of colorectal surgical residents, an environment combining a large, community-based surgical practice with a major teaching and research university practice. International recognition for promoting the training of specialists in colon and rectal surgery was awarded to Stanley Goldberg by many surgical organizations from around the world, including Australia, Canada, Chile, England, France, Ireland, Mexico, Philippines, and Scotland. In 2000, the University of Minnesota established the Stanley M. Goldberg Chair in Colon and Rectal Surgery in his honor. (With appreciation to David A. Rothenberger, MD.)

is excised, and a colorectal anastomosis is performed. The operation has been shown to improve constipation but at the expense of the risk of an anastomotic complication.[59,93,196,276] In addition to a low rate of constipation, function is generally good, and with the higher anastomosis than is necessary for rectal cancer anastomotic leakage, rates are low.[13,137,151,167,342]

The technique also adapts well to a laparoscopic approach. Laubert and colleagues reported the largest experience of laparoscopic resection-rectopexy (152 patients), with a conversion rate of 0.7% and mean operative time of 204 (± 65.3) minutes. The mortality was 0.7%, and major and minor morbidity occurred in 4% and 19%, respectively. The mean length of stay was 11 days. At a follow-up of 48 months, the recurrence rate was 11%, and improvement or elimination of constipation and incontinence was 81% and 67%, respectively.

Rectal Prolapse and Fecal Incontinence

The majority of patients with a continence disturbance will experience improvement once the prolapse has been treated.[63,122] This is not surprising because in addition to the prolapse no longer stretching and attenuating the sphincter, perineal descent distance during attempted defecation usually decreases, and the anorectal angle becomes more acute.[345] Farouk and coworkers performed ambulatory recordings using a computerized anal EMG and anorectal manometry system on 32 patients with neurogenic fecal incontinence and rectal prolapse as well as on 33 controls.[88] They observed that recovery of

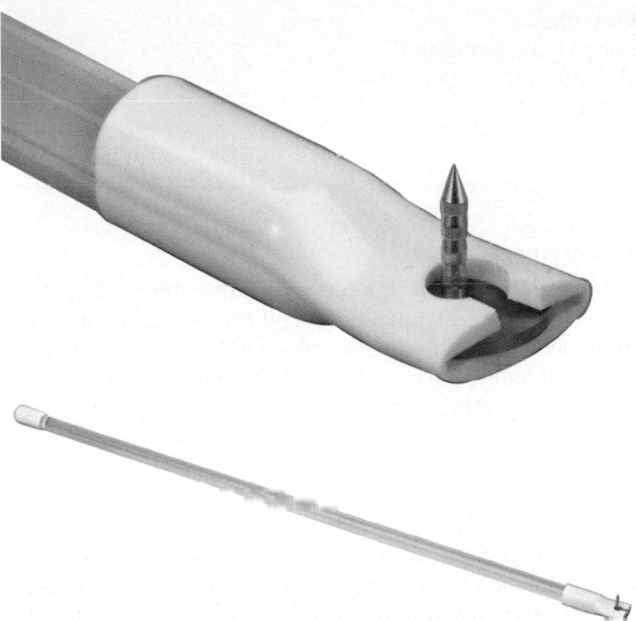

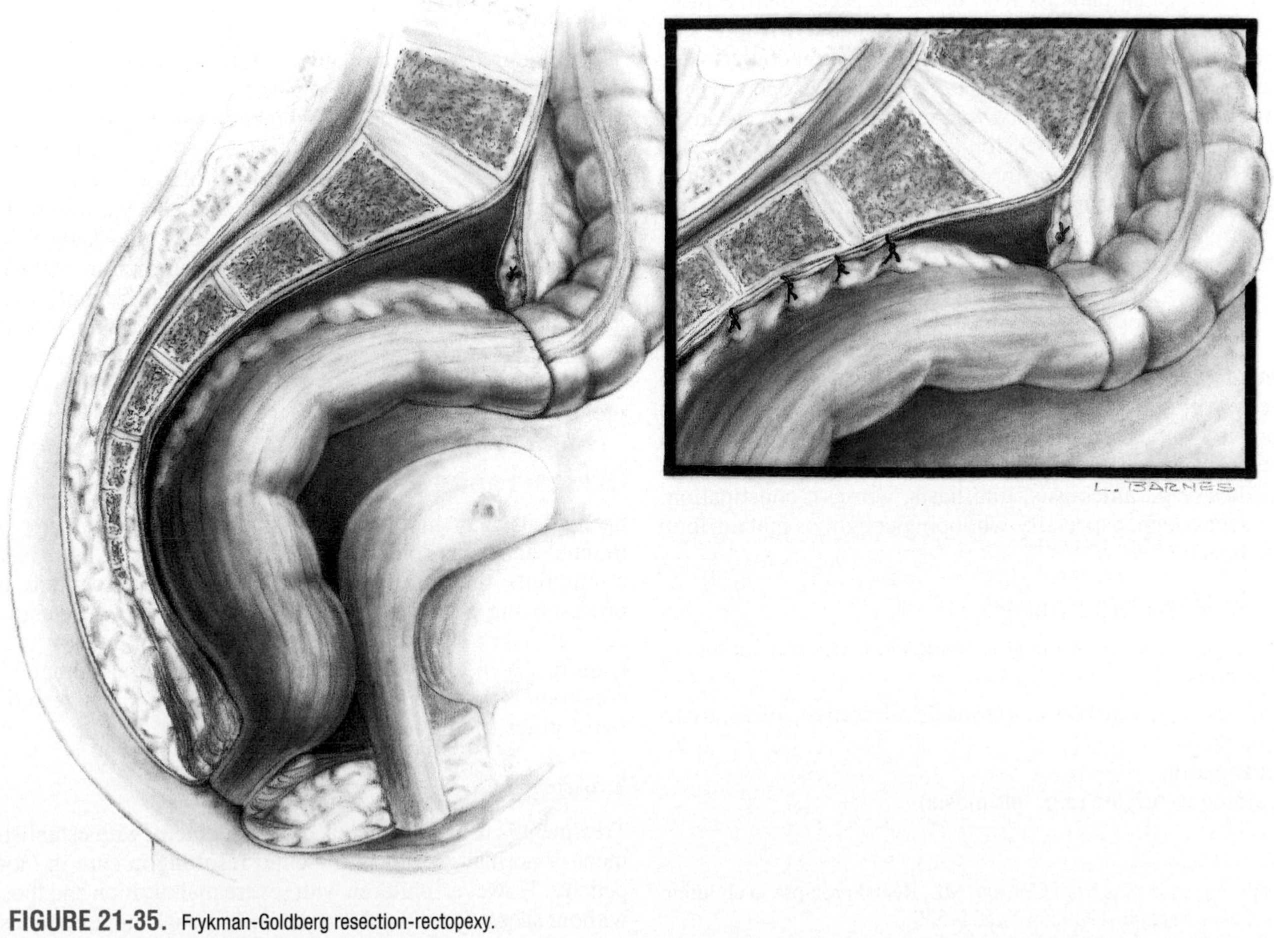

FIGURE 21-34. Titanium hemorrhage occluder pin with applicator. Fingertip pressure is applied to the flat head of the pin until pin is flush with the bony cortex. (Courtesy of Tools for Surgery, LLC, Stony Brook, NY.)

FIGURE 21-35. Frykman-Goldberg resection-rectopexy.

continence occurs by abolition of high-pressure rectal waves. These waves produce maximal inhibition of sphincter activity before the operation. Others have shown that improvement in continence is not accompanied by changes in rectal sensation or reflex function of the internal sphincter.[269]

Keighley and Matheson reported 20 patients with prolapse and anal incontinence. Rectopexy alone controlled the incontinence in all but four.[145] Blatchford and colleagues noted that the proportion of continent patients increased from 36% preoperatively to 74% postoperatively following simple suture rectopexy.[27] In the experience of Yoshioka and coworkers, incontinence was observed in 58% before surgery, but in only 16% after Marlex mesh repair.[344]

There is, however, a small group of people for whom anal incontinence may be disabling despite correction of the rectal prolapse. Parks advocated postanal repair of the pelvic floor muscles for these individuals (see Chapter 16).[237] Although his overall failure rate for patients with incontinence was a respectable 17%, many did not have a prolapse initially. In fact, the results following this procedure were much less satisfactory when carried out after prolapse repair. Furthermore, the more severe the prolapse, the worse the result. Sainio and associates suggest that their preoperative and postoperative physiologic investigations lead them to the opinion that recovery of the resting and voluntary functions of the sphincter muscles is the cause of the improvement in continence.[269] Because anal manometry was unable to predict the outcome, they believe that supplementary procedures for restoration of continence are not advisable and that rectopexy alone is as likely as rectopexy with the Parks operation to result in full restoration of bowel control. Williams and colleagues, however, have shown that patients who remained incontinent following surgery had a significantly lower preoperative resting anal pressure and lower maximum voluntary contraction pressure than those who improved.[335] Shafik described an operative approach for fecal incontinence with rectal prolapse by means of pudendal canal decompression by freeing the nerve on each side from the ischial spine through the pudendal canal.[284] In an uncontrolled study involving 13 patients, 7 improved with this operation. This is no better, however, than one would expect without this decompression procedure.

▶ RECTAL PROLAPSE IN CHILDREN*

Rectal prolapse in children is uncommon. It occurs in Western countries and most frequently in infants with cystic fibrosis, although it can be associated with malnutrition. The condition can also be associated with any illness that causes diarrhea (e.g., amebiasis, giardiasis, worms); constipation; frequent cough, especially whooping cough; or malnutrition (see later).[24,160,211,224,293,316]

Associated Disorders

Rectal prolapse in children is associated with the following conditions:

Diarrhea (e.g., amebiasis, giardiasis, ulcerative colitis, trichuriasis)
Constipation
Straining to urinate (e.g., phimosis)

Vomiting
Cough (e.g., pertussis)
Malnutrition
Cystic fibrosis
Polyp or tumor[131,165]
Ehlers-Danlos syndrome[76]
Myelomeningocele
Spina bifida
Hirschsprung's disease[315]

Malnutrition is by far the most common predisposing factor for the development of rectal prolapse in infancy and childhood in developing countries. Most of the reports in the current literature emanate from Africa and Asia. The reasons for this geographic distribution are probably attributable to the diarrhea, in addition to the loss of ischiorectal fat and the lack of support for the rectum experienced by children in these regions. In 1914, Lockhart-Mummery stated that "rectal prolapse is a comparatively common affliction among children, especially in that class which attends hospitals."[176] The implication of this remark is that in the "better classes," children are more well nourished and more quickly attended to if they become ill.

Soriano and colleagues reported 10 cases of rectal prolapse associated with *Trichuris trichiura* as the only intestinal parasite (see Chapter 33).[293] Stern and coworkers noted that rectal prolapse occurred in 112 of 605 patients with cystic fibrosis (18.5%).[296] In one-third of the patients, the prolapse preceded the diagnosis of cystic fibrosis. Kulczycki and Shwachman reported an incidence of almost 25% in 386 children afflicted with cystic fibrosis.[160]

Etiology

The etiology of rectal prolapse in infancy may be related to the loose attachment of the mucosa to the underlying muscularis. In this age group, the rectal mucosa may be normally redundant.[274] Other anatomic factors in the child that tend to predispose to the development of prolapse are the vertical course of the rectum, flat sacrum and coccyx, low rectal position in relation to other pelvic organs, and lack of levator support. Rectal prolapse is most common in children younger than 3 years of age, with the most frequent incidence being in the first year of life. In this age group, it is the mucosa that tends to prolapse, not the full thickness of the bowel. Most studies report an approximately equal gender incidence.[24,82,211]

Clinical Features

Symptoms may include protrusion, bleeding, passage of mucus, diarrhea, constipation, abdominal pain, and those complaints that may be referable to the associated or predisposing condition. Findings include the protrusion, lax sphincter tone and contractility, and, often, malnutrition (Figure 21-36). The most common differential diagnostic condition is that of a juvenile polyp. Distinction between the two entities should not be difficult, however.

Treatment

Treatment is usually by medical management, with establishment of normal growth of the child resulting in cure in most patients. However, children with severe malnutrition and those without access to medical care and nutritional support are less

---

*Reproduced in part from Corman ML. Rectal prolapse in children. *Dis Colon Rectum*. 1985;28(7):535–539.

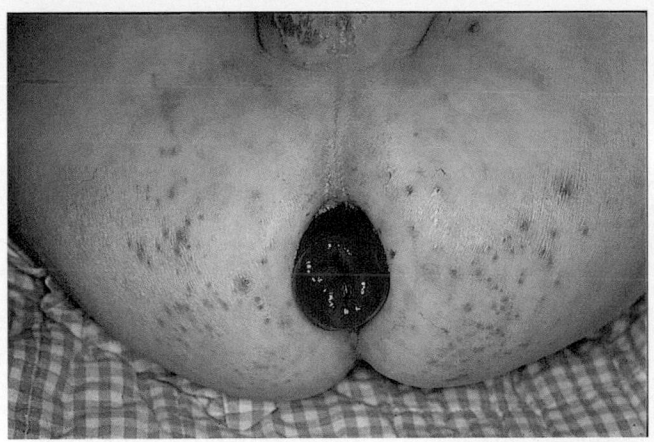

FIGURE 21-36. Rectal prolapse in an infant. (Courtesy of John Campbell, MD and Marvin W. Harrison, MD.)

likely to have spontaneous resolution of the prolapse. Medical management includes manual replacement of the prolapse, with sedation if necessary. Supporting the perineum during defecation is also beneficial as well as to have the child defecate in the recumbent position. It may be necessary to tape the buttocks to prevent the prolapse from recurring spontaneously. Stool softeners are suggested for constipation.

Surgical treatment has been advised for patients who do not respond to medical management. Recommended procedures include the following:

- Excision of the mucosal prolapse[274]
- Anal encirclement with Silastic[73] or with catgut[211]
- Use of a sclerosing solution such as 30% saline[82,144] or 70% alcohol[187] (Figure 21-37)
- Packing of the presacral space with gauze or Gelfoam[73,176,224]
- Linear cauterization of the anorectum[118] (Figure 21-38)
- Transsacral rectopexy with obliteration of the pouch of Douglas and puborectalis plication[45]
- Transcoccygeal rectopexy and puborectalis plication[14]
- Perineal proctosigmoidectomy[212]
- Transanal rectopexy with delayed suture removal[112]

Results

Kay and Zachary employed a sclerosing solution of 30% saline in 51 children.[144] They noted 100% success with up to three treatments; however, two abscesses complicated the procedure. Dutta and Das used the same technique in 30 children.[82] They reported an 83% cure rate with one treatment and a 100% cure rate with three treatments. Malyshev and Gulin reported a series of 353 children from the former Soviet Union with rectal prolapse treated by perirectal 70% alcohol.[187] Ninety-six percent were cured. The authors advised, however, that no more than 35 mL should be used, and that this treatment should be limited to those children who do not satisfactorily respond to medical measures.

Anal encirclement with Silastic has been recommended.[73] Narasanagi and colleagues performed anal encirclement using no. 1 chromic catgut in 30 patients.[211] There was one failure due to breakage of the suture. Subsequent treatment effectively cured the prolapse. Groff and Nagaraj advocate encirclement of the anus with a nonabsorbable suture (no. 0 or 1 Prolene) tightened over a Hegar dilator.[104] They observed that four patients required a repeat insertion and one required a third, but they believe that the safety and simplicity of the technique make it worthy of recommendation.

Packing the presacral space with gauze through a posterior approach, as well as excision of the prolapsed mucosa, have been recommended in the intractable case in Rudolph and Hoffman's textbook, *Pediatrics*.[274] Nwako packed the presacral space with Gelfoam in 100 patients and reported complete cure in every case.[224]

Hight and colleagues recommend a surgical approach for patients who do not respond to medical measures.[118] There were a total of 102 children in their series, 29 of whom responded adequately to medical treatment. The remaining 73 underwent linear cauterization of the anorectum; all but two were successfully treated by this approach. Heald, in a report of one child, secured the rectum by a transanal rectopexy, passing a suture through the full thickness of the rectum and skin overlying the coccyx.[112] The suture was removed at a later date.

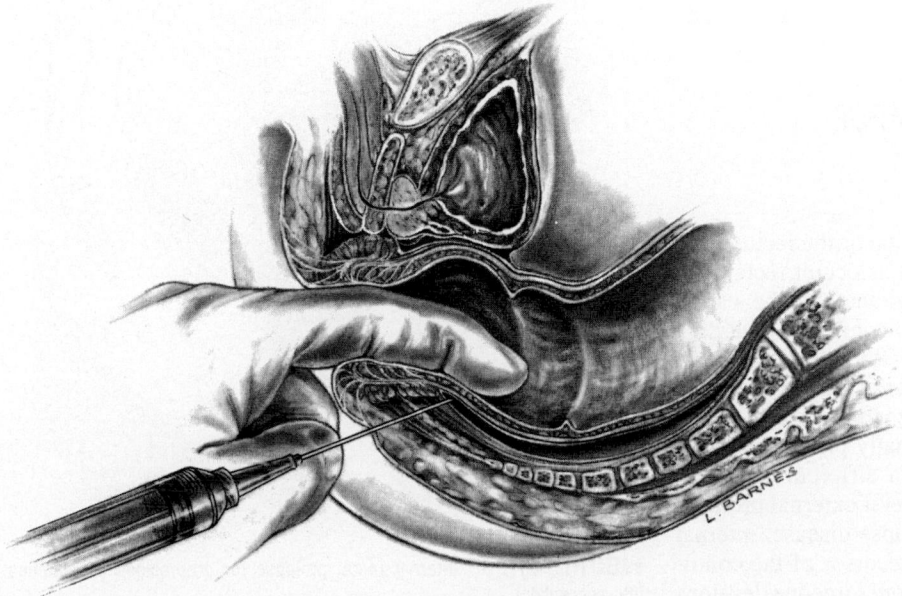

FIGURE 21-37. Injection technique. Sclerosing agent is infiltrated in the perirectal tissue posteriorly and laterally. The index finger is inserted into the rectum to confirm the position of the needle tip. (From Corman ML. Rectal prolapse in children. *Dis Colon Rectum*. 1985;28(7):535–539, with permission.)

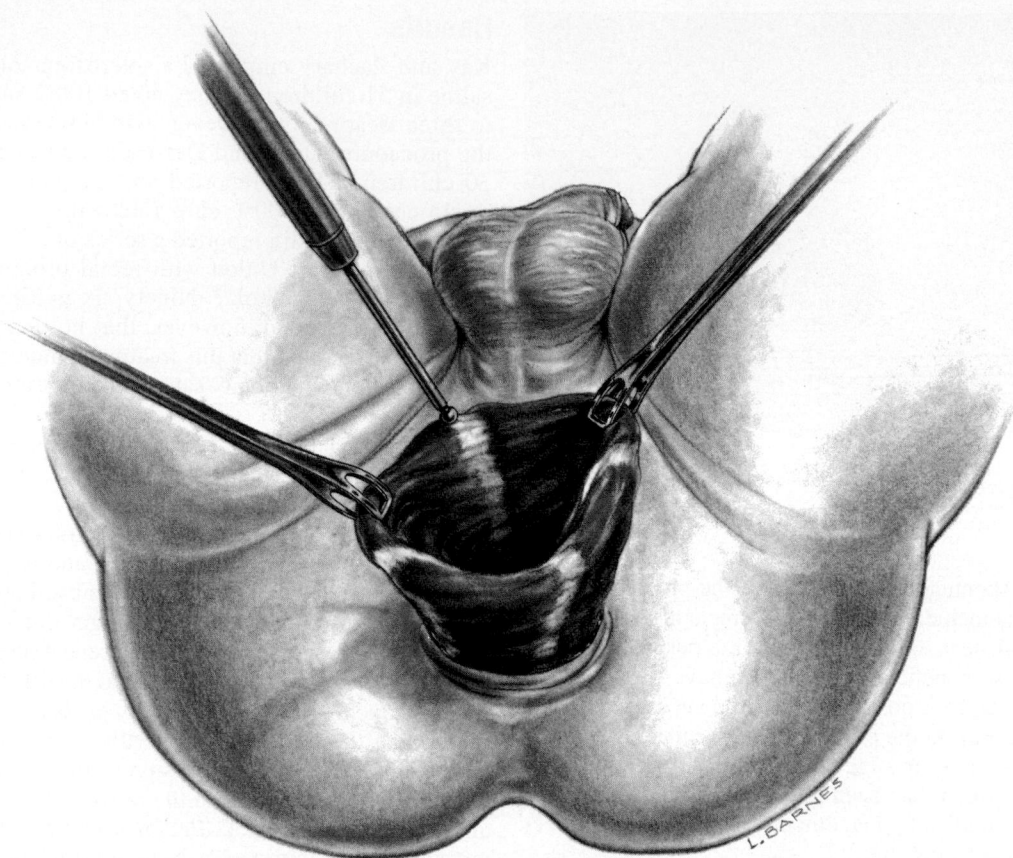

FIGURE 21-38. Linear cauterization. Four-quadrant electrocoagulation through the submucosa. (Adapted from Hight DW, Hertzler JH, Philippart AI, et al. Linear cauterization for the treatment of rectal prolapse in infants and children. *Surg Gynecol Obstet.* 1982;154(3):400–402; Corman ML. Rectal prolapse in children. *Dis Colon Rectum.* 1985;28(7):535–539, with permission.)

Perineal proctosigmoidectomy has been used in intractable situations in children who had developed rectal prolapse as a consequence of spina bifida.[212] Chino and Thomas suggested transsacral rectopexy with obliteration of the pouch of Douglas and puborectalis plication, the technique that has been used for adults, except that resection is not recommended.[45] Successful repair was noted in four patients. Transcoccygeal rectopexy and puborectalis plication have been suggested by Ashcraft and colleagues, who treated and cured four children by this technique.[14]

► INTERNAL RECTAL PROLAPSE (PREPROLAPSE, RECTAL INTUSSUSCEPTION)

Internal rectal prolapse is an invagination of the rectum into itself (Figure 21-39). It is also known as occult rectal prolapse or rectal intussusception. Unfortunately, the varied nomenclature may have contributed to confusion regarding its proper treatment. It is a condition with a chequered surgical experience. External rectal prolapse has always been regarded as an unquestioned surgical condition. Yet a rectal prolapse that invaginates without actually protruding from the anal verge has been regarded as a different condition not appropriate for surgical remedy. Yet if external prolapse represents an advanced stage of prolapse disease, internal rectal prolapse would seem to be a precursor of the condition. It is unimaginable that the day before someone develops

an external prolapse, the pelvic floor had been normal and that internal rectal prolapse was not present. Certainly at laparoscopy, the patients with external and internal prolapse have very similar pelvic anatomy, including a deep pouch of Douglas and a rectal mesentery. Therefore, it is reasonable

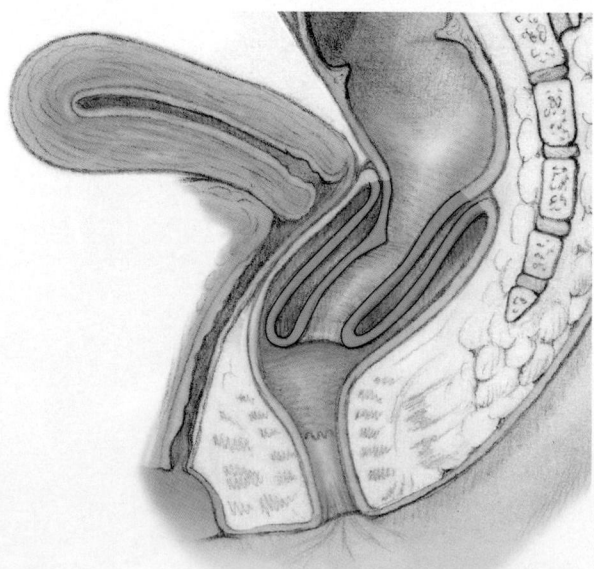

FIGURE 21-39. Internal rectal prolapse (or preprolapse or rectoanal intussusception).

to conclude that internal rectal prolapse must be related to external rectal prolapse, and its identification indicates that there exists a spectrum of prolapse disease.

Internal rectal prolapse is also part of the descending perineum syndrome (see later), a term first coined by Parks.[238] It included such demonstrable pathoanatomical entities as rectocele (with or without enterocele) and pelvic floor descent. Internal rectal prolapse may be the central component of a commonly coexisting triad of internal prolapse, rectocele, and perineal descent. Some units have focused on rectocele as being the main defect requiring treatment. Thus, the unit in Auckland, New Zealand, will offer a transanal rectocele repair by an anterior Delorme's procedure as the initial operation.[1] If symptoms are not improved, internal rectal prolapse is suspected and more extensive surgery may then be employed. Others including the authors take the view that rectocele usually coexists with internal rectal prolapse, although the latter may occasionally be seen on its own.

Proctographic Internal Rectal Prolapse: Normal Variant or Pathologic?

Several factors have lead to a historical widely held and still largely prevailing view that internal rectal prolapse is a variant of the normal. The proctographic studies of Shorvon and colleagues in the late 1980s demonstrated that 20% of asymptomatic normal volunteers had a high-grade internal rectal prolapse (intussusception impinging on or entering into the anal canal).[285] Two large proctographic series of symptomatic patients showed that internal rectal prolapse seldom progressed to external rectal prolapse[47,201] and that external prolapse rarely followed a diagnosis of mucosal prolapse.[4]

More recently, there has been a radiologic reevaluation of internal rectal prolapse in asymptomatic normal volunteers. Dvorkin and colleagues showed that internal rectal prolapse is morphologically more advanced in symptomatic patients, with significantly more full-thickness and anal intussusceptions, rather than mucosal, shallower, and rectal intussusceptions in asymptomatic individuals.[83] These findings are supported by Pomerri and coworkers who showed that the rectal fold thickness and the ratio between the diameter of the intussusciplens and the lumen of the intussusceptum were significantly greater in the symptomatic than in asymptomatic volunteers.[246]

These proctographic studies can also be criticized. In one series, the most advanced prolapses were operated upon,

leaving those of lesser degree of severity for follow-up.[201] It is unsurprising that patients in this second group, highly selected and biased, rarely progressed to external prolapse. These studies were also limited in their follow-up of patients. A study of the natural history of internal rectal prolapse suggests that progression to external prolapse is variable and slow.[332] The time line of progression of internal rectal prolapse to external prolapse is beyond the ability and duration of most surgical studies to capture (Figure 21-40). Males and nulliparous women appear to develop symptoms at a younger age and progress to higher grades of prolapse faster than parous females.[332]

Classification Systems

There have been several classifications of internal rectal prolapse, but few have become generally accepted. The key to the usefulness of any classification is simplicity. The Oxford Prolapse Grading system divides internal rectal prolapse into four grades according to the most caudal descent of the lead point of the intussusceptum relative to the rectocele and anal sphincter[69] (Figure 21-41). This can be resolved into high and low rectal and anal intussusception. Grade 5 prolapse is external rectal prolapse. Generally speaking, patients with prolapse grades 3 to 5 are suitable for surgery. Other grading systems include that used by Shorvon and colleagues (7 grades),[285] Pescatori and colleagues,[242] and the system used in Leuven, Belgium (grades 1 to 3).[70]

Symptoms

Previous proctographic studies have overestimated the numbers in this group, but undoubtedly some patients have high-grade prolapse without functional disturbance. When these patients develop an external rectal prolapse, they do so without a functional prodrome. The proportion of external rectal prolapse patients who present without a functional prodrome is about 20% (unpublished personal series).[90] It is not clear why some patients with internal rectal prolapse remain asymptomatic. One theory is that some are susceptible to developing symptoms associated with their structural anatomical abnormalities. Those with so-called *visceral hypersensitivity* are commonly seen with functional disorders.[328] Such patients have been noted to frequently have a heavy burden of psychological symptoms. This has given rise to a temptation to provide a psychological explanation for such

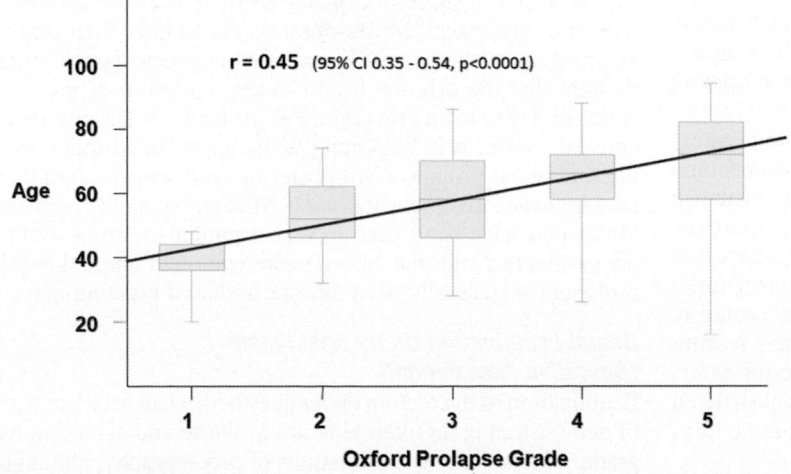

FIGURE 21-40. The relationship between age and Oxford Prolapse Grade (From Wijffels NA, Collinson R, Cunningham C, et al. What is the natural history of internal rectal prolapse? *Colorectal Dis.* 2010;12(8):822–830.)

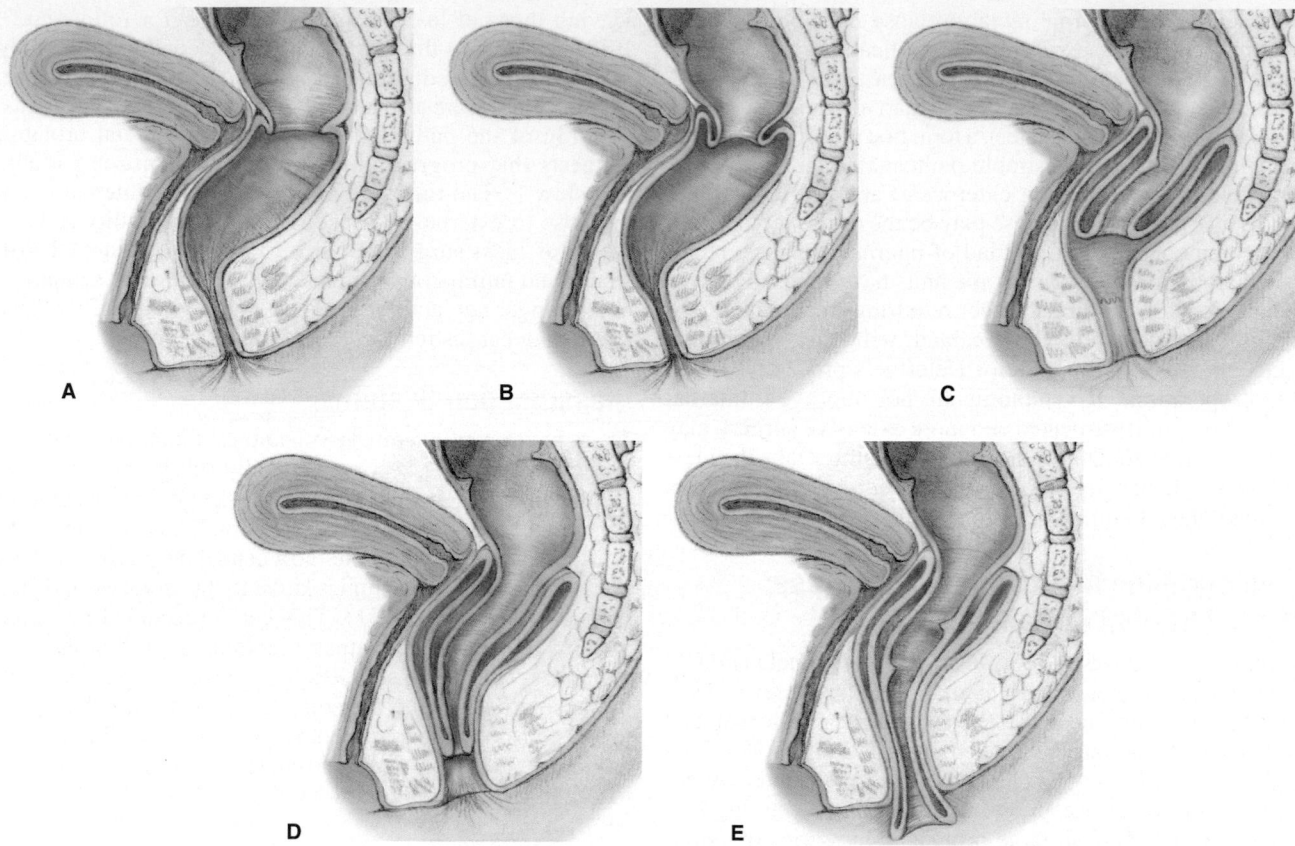

FIGURE 21-41. Oxford Rectal Prolapse Grade: grade 1 **(A)**, grade 2 **(B)**, grade 3 **(C)**, grade 4 **(D)**, and grade 5 (external rectal prolapse) **(E)**.

symptoms. It might also explain the apparent psychological overlay in many of these individuals.[203]

When internal rectal prolapse gives rise to symptoms, patients can present in several different ways. Classically recognized symptoms are obstructed defecation (frequent ineffective evacuatory attempts), stool infrequency in a pattern more usually attributed to slow-transit constipation, or a variable pattern between both. Fecal incontinence is undoubtedly underrecognized as a symptom of internal rectal prolapse. It coexists with obstructed defecation in about 60% of patients with high-grade internal prolapse who come to surgery.[331] The remaining complain of either isolated obstructed defecation (20%) or isolated fecal incontinence (20%). There is a high incidence of high-grade internal rectal prolapse found on proctography in patients presenting with fecal incontinence, with no significant structural or functional disturbance found on anorectal physiology and anal ultrasound.[52] These patients were previously labeled as having idiopathic fecal incontinence.

Other presentations include chronic idiopathic perineal pain and solitary rectal ulcer syndrome.[87,125] It has become apparent that in some patients, internal rectal prolapse underlies more common proctologic complaints, particularly chronic anal fissure and hemorrhoids. It appears that there is a relationship between internal anal sphincter function and the mode of presentation of internal rectal prolapse. Those with poorer function and lower maximal resting pressures tend to present with fecal incontinence (or external prolapse), and those with higher pressures, obstructed defecation, or solitary rectal ulcer tend to have chronic idiopathic perineal pain.[125]

Assessment

Clinical Assessment

Internal rectal prolapse can be suggested by clinical assessment during straining, including digital rectal examination, rigid rectoscopy (high takeoff), and proctoscopy (low takeoff). It is most evident anteriorly and is distinguishable from mucosal prolapse by the smoothing out of the wrinkled mucosa as the prolapse descends to the anal canal.

Radiologic Assessment

The gold standard for diagnosing internal rectal prolapse remains proctography (Figures 21-42 to 21-44). It provides a very important objective record of the degree of internal rectal prolapse that can be referred back to. The intussusception can be seen as a space-occupying lesion in the contrast-filled rectum or anal canal. Most intussusceptions have their origin anteriorly, and this is best appreciated at proctoscopy.[34] It is thought that the original lesion in the evolution of internal rectal prolapse is anterior mucosal prolapse.[302] Despite their anterior origin, it is beginning to be appreciated that some internal rectal prolapses are posterior-predominant, and this may influence treatment approach. MRI and dynamic perineal ultrasound have been used to assess patients with descending perineum syndrome, but characterization of internal rectal prolapse has generally been inferior to that of proctography.

Rectal Examination Under Anesthesia (Operative Assessment)

Examination of the rectum under anesthetic is an accurate way of demonstrating an internal rectal prolapse and assessing its grade. It overcomes the limitations of proctography, although

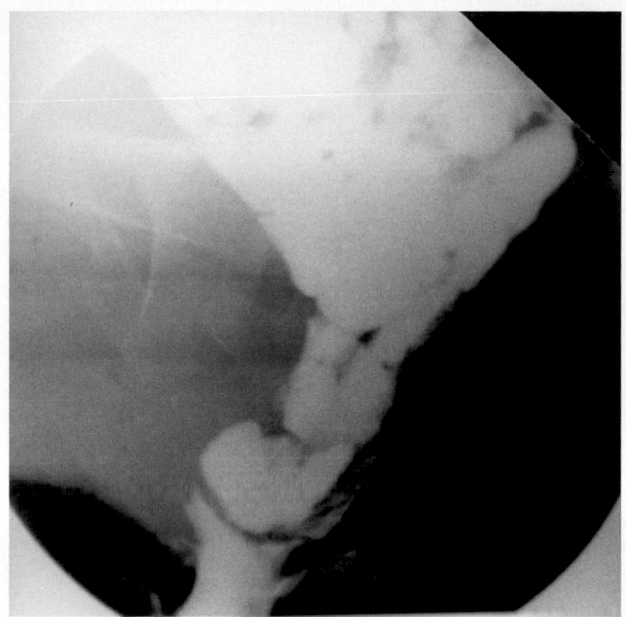

FIGURE 21-42. Defecogram with concomitant small bowel follow-through demonstrates a rectocele with a deep pouch of Douglas. An enterocele is also noted.

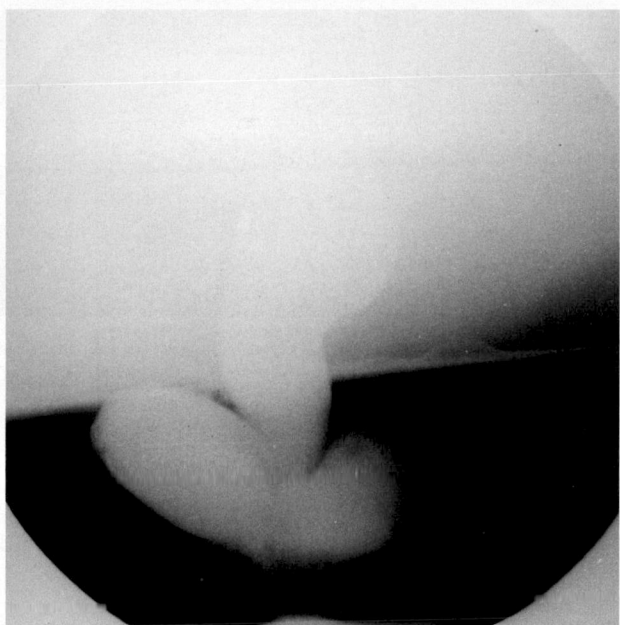

FIGURE 21-44. Defecogram. Colorectal intussusception (internal rectal prolapse).

at the inconvenience of a general anesthetic.[208] It is of particular use when an internal rectal prolapse is suspected but cannot be confirmed on proctography. It is important that typical instrumentation such as an Eisenhammer retractor not be used because the long blades tend to splint the internal rectal prolapse and prevent it from descending to allow proper assessment. A circular anal dilator (CAD) device is used (Figure 21-45), which allows the prolapse to descend as far as possible (Figure 21-46). Anterior or posterior predominance is noted.

Diagnostic Laparoscopy

Occasionally, the diagnosis of internal rectal prolapse is elusive and cannot be demonstrated during examination under anesthetic (EUA). In this circumstance (always due to high takeoff internal rectal prolapse), diagnostic laparoscopy and assessment of the shape of the pelvis and depth of the pouch of Douglas will enable a diagnosis to be made.

Treatment

Conservative Measures Including Biofeedback

A conservative approach is recommended at the outset. This includes laxatives, dietary advice and biofeedback, or pelvic floor retraining (see Chapter 16). A diagnostic workup should be carried out before committing the patient to a full 6-month course of biofeedback or pelvic floor retraining. This is because proctography may reveal an external rectal prolapse not demonstrated on clinical assessment, which is an obvious indication for surgical intervention.

It is unclear how successful biofeedback is for treating internal rectal prolapse because patients have generally not been

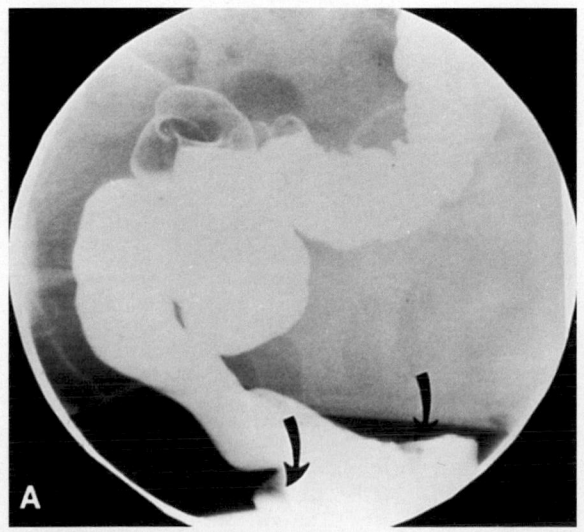

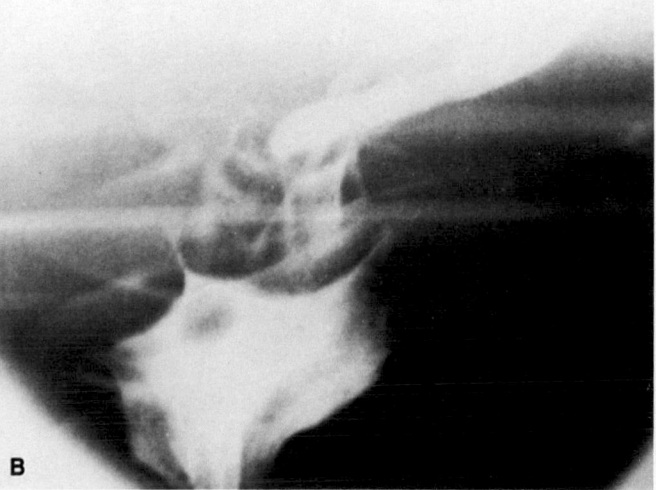

FIGURE 21-43. Defecogram of internal rectal prolapse. **A:** A ring pocket (*arrows*) is demonstrated. **B:** Intussusception is clearly evident.

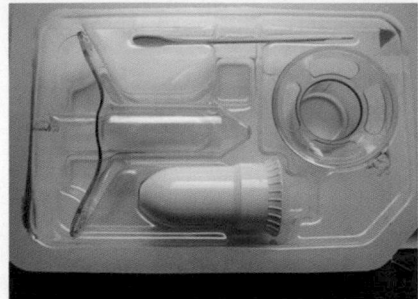
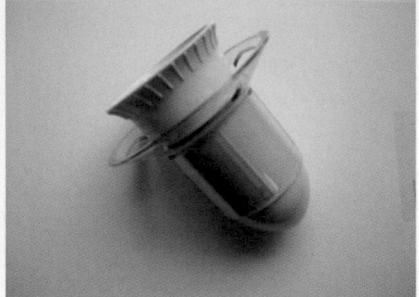
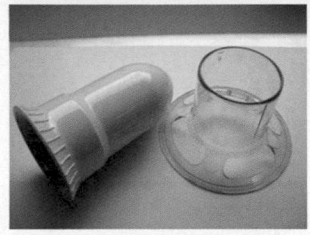

FIGURE 21-45. Circular anal dilator (CAD) device. (Frankenman International Ltd., Hong Kong.)

investigated or well stratified in the past. This was because 10 to 15 years ago, there were limited surgical options. Biofeedback was used as the primary treatment for all patients with chronic constipation and for whom there was no specific etiology. Often, no special investigations were undertaken. It is now known that biofeedback works less well for chronic constipation than for fecal incontinence.[156] Much is not understood, and there is little data on biofeedback specifically for the treatment of internal rectal prolapse.[130]

Surgery

The principles of surgery for internal rectal prolapse are to eliminate the intussusception, either by reduction and fixation from above (rectopexy) or excision from below (STARR procedure). However, despite ignorance about the precise physiologic mechanisms involved, sacral neuromodulation may have a significant future role.

Posterior Rectopexy with or without Resection

A Cochrane review, including randomized, controlled studies, concluded that posterior rectal mobilization for *external* rectal prolapse leads to autonomic rectal denervation and a hindgut neuropathy, with worsened or new onset constipation in about 50% of patients.[18] Not surprisingly, posterior rectopexy has also largely become discredited for the management of *internal* rectal prolapse because inducing a similar neural lesion and worsening constipation (the very indication for surgery) is not acceptable.[231] Some of these drawbacks can be offset by a resection-rectopexy, and published results demonstrate reasonably good functional outcomes.[318] However, resected denervated hindgut makes a virtue out of a necessity, risks an anastomotic complication, and provides no direct treatment of middle compartment prolapse. Given that there is a nerve-sparing alternative not requiring an anastomosis, we believe a posterior approach, even with resection, cannot be recommended.

Laparoscopic Ventral Rectopexy

Laparoscopic ventral rectopexy for external prolapse was pioneered by D'Hoore and Penninckx from Leuven, Belgium.[69] Recurrence rates are low (less than 5%), and constipation (75% to 80%) and fecal incontinence usually

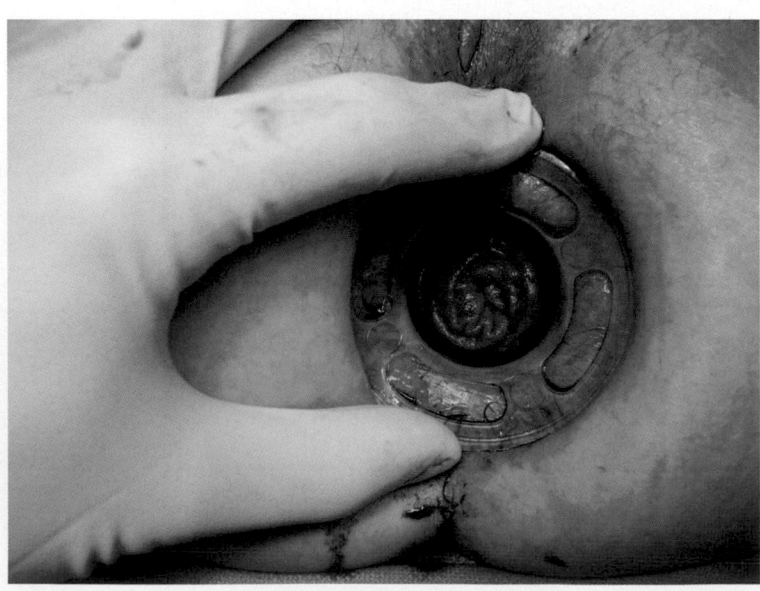

FIGURE 21-46. CAD rectal examination under anesthetic (EUA).

improve (85% to 90%) and rarely worsen. Exclusive to a ventral approach, middle compartment prolapse is concurrently treated with ease. Mortality (0%), morbidity (5% to 10%, mostly minor), and hospital stay (median, 2 days) are extremely low, and reassuringly the results are reproducible.[30,288]

The features of laparoscopic ventral rectopexy that make it attractive for internal rectal prolapse are autonomic nerve-sparing and cotreatment of a range of prolapse-related pathoanatomical entities, such as rectocele, middle compartment prolapse, and enterocele.[272] The functional results of ventral rectopexy for internal rectal prolapse seem to generally mirror those for external prolapse, with an improvement in about 75% to 80% of patients with obstructed defecation.[53] This underlines the concept of it as a true autonomic nerve-sparing "antiprolapse procedure." It also supports the notion that internal rectal prolapse and external prolapse share many properties and, therefore, exist in a spectrum of rectal prolapse disease. This concept had never truly been accepted in the past.[332]

What about those with colonic slow-transit *and* outlet obstruction? About 30% of all patients attending the clinic in Oxford with chronic constipation will have slow-transit constipation as demonstrated by transit study.[252] Approximately 85% of such individuals will have a significant associated outlet obstruction (high-grade internal rectal prolapse), whereas 15% (about 5% of all patients) will have classical isolated slow-transit constipation and a normal proctogram. Therefore, about one-third of patients with outlet obstruction and high-grade internal rectal prolapse will have, in addition, colonic slow transit (often in the second or third segments of the colorectum), and two-thirds will have normal colonic transit. It had been policy to regard outlet obstruction with slow transit as a contraindication to performing internal rectal prolapse surgery. However, with the good results of ventral rectopexy for internal rectal prolapse with normal transit plus the pressure of referrals, mainly from gastroenterologists, these criteria were gradually relaxed. We expected these more complex patients to benefit less from surgery and counseled them accordingly. However, when their outcomes were reviewed, counterintuitively they appeared to benefit as much as those with normal colonic transit.[108] In other words, the additional finding of colonic slow transit did not adversely impact the results of surgery for internal rectal prolapse. D'Hoore has shown that laparoscopic ventral rectopexy improves colonic transit time in the distal segment of the colorectum (see Figure 21-32).[68]

Interestingly, fecal incontinence with internal rectal prolapse improves more reliably than constipation.[53] It is probable that internal rectal prolapse underlies many cases of fecal incontinence and may account for much of so-called idiopathic fecal incontinence. In Oxford, proctography is a routine part of the workup for those presenting with fecal incontinence.[52] This complaint is now an indication (with or without obstructed defecation) for advising ventral rectopexy.[249]

Persistent Symptoms After Ventral Rectopexy: Posterior STARR

We use the STARR procedure mainly for failed ventral rectopexy. About 75% to 80% of patients with obstructed defecation secondary to internal rectal prolapse are improved, leaving 20% to 25% of patients who do not respond. Initially, it was thought that these individuals had an underlying

neural rather than a mechanical etiology and that sacral neuromodulation might be useful. Postoperative proctography can sometimes be useful if it discloses residual or recurrent posterior internal rectal prolapse. More often, however, it is not helpful, and rectal EUA (with a CAD device) is probably the preferred assessment after failed ventral rectopexy (see Figures 21-45 and 21-46). Why these patients behave differently to the 80% whose anterior and posterior internal rectal prolapse component both reduces and remains reduced is unclear. This is currently the subject of research, and it is our impression that some patients have a posterior-predominant internal rectal prolapse from the outset. In most individuals (80%), ventral mesh placement will support a posterior prolapse, but in this group it probably will not. It appears that those with a more vertical rather than horizontal rectum at proctography have a greater chance of improvement in their symptoms with a ventral rectopexy.[262] In this setting, a posterior STARR can be performed either at the time of a diagnostic EUA or later if informed consent had not been given preoperatively. This approach of complimentary posterior STARR improves about one-half to two-thirds of patient with persistent symptoms and a posterior prolapse. Again, it is our impression that patients suffer less of the urgency that is typical of STARR when only a posterior hemicircumferential staple line is made.

Modified Orr-Loygue Rectopexy

The original description of the Orr-Loygue rectopexy includes a full anterior and posterior rectal mobilization and support. Unfortunately, high rates of constipation ensued.[178,179] This could be predicted with our current understanding of posterior rectal mobilization and autonomic rectal denervation. The procedure had since fell out of favor except for French surgeons.[216] However, the approach recognizes the ventral origin of internal rectal prolapse, and with a modified, restricted central posterior dissection, Lazorthes appears to have achieved good functional results.[248] It may be that this modified incarnation of Orr-Loygue will come back into vogue. Nicholls and Simson at St. Mark's Hospital employed an anterior/posterior rectopexy for a small group of patients with solitary rectal ulcer, a condition believed to be secondary to internal rectal prolapse (see later).[216] Excellent rates of good functional outcome with ulcer healing were achieved (86%).

More recently, Lazorthes and colleagues have attempted to consolidate the data on ventral and posterior rectopexy, refining and advancing the case for a modified Orr-Loygue rectopexy by undertaking a partial nerve-sparing limited posterior dissection.[248,249] This technique provides ventral support and preserves the left autonomic nerve pedicle while sacrificing the right. No subsequent exacerbation of constipation similar to that of posterior or traditional Orr-Loygue rectopexy was seen, confirming the importance of at least unilateral nerve preservation. However, a small group of patients did experience worsening of evacuatory function (5%).

In Oxford, we are moving toward using primary modified posterior rectopexy, in addition to ventral rectopexy, to try to improve outcomes of surgery for internal rectal prolapse. We use a somewhat different technique than Lazorthes, with a restricted 3- to 4-cm wide midline posterior mobilization to the level of the coccyx tip. The dissection is, therefore, between the autonomic nerve pedicles, thus preserving both. We employ this primarily in patients with a more horizontal-

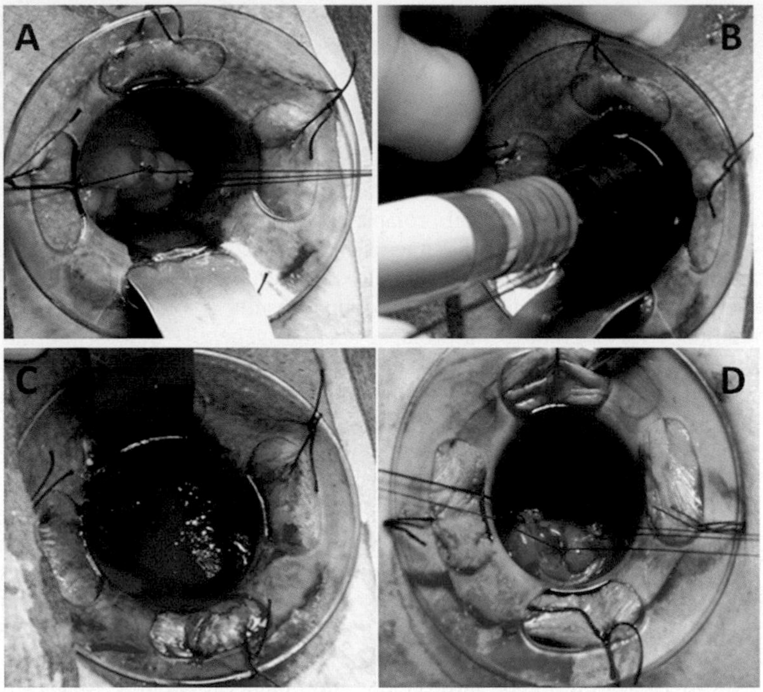

FIGURE 21-47. STARR procedure (PPH-03). **A:** The posterior "half" of the prolapse is delivered with stay sutures. **B:** The PPH-03 STARR stapler excises a fixed amount of prolapse from the posterior hemi-rectum, with a protective spatula in place **(C)**. The posterior prolapse has been resected, leaving the anterior hemi-prolapse for the second firing **(D)**. The sutures are placed to deliver the anterior hemi-prolapse for subsequent stapling.

lying rectum, a cohort with a higher failure rate when ventral surgery alone is performed. In an unpublished series of 50 patients with short follow-up, there was a negligible rate of worse function. Improvement of obstructed defecation appears to be somewhat superior to that for ventral surgery alone. Since employing this technique, our rate of completion posterior STARR has fallen from about 15% to 10% to 4% to 3%. Patients relapsing following previous ventral rectopexy are able to be offered a conversion to a modified Orr-Loygue rectopexy by the addition of a limited posterior mobilization without great technical difficulty. No outcome data are available at this time.

STARR Procedure

The other new surgical treatment for internal rectal prolapse is a stapled transanal rectal resection (STARR) (Figure 21-47). This approach treats internal rectal prolapse by excision rather than reduction of the intussusception. Although the success rates are generally similar, it has some advantages over laparoscopic ventral rectopexy. It is a perineal procedure and can be undertaken under spinal anesthesia. It is also relatively easy to learn and to perform. There are, however, disadvantages. STARR takes a longer time for one to obtain a good functional result when compared with ventral rectopexy. Most patients complain of urgency. This can be debilitating and may persist for several months. After ventral rectopexy, once patients are weaned from their postoperative laxative regime, they notice a marked functional benefit by 4 weeks if the procedure has been successful. With STARR, the potential for complications is greater, although the risk of bleeding, anastomotic leak, sepsis, and rectovaginal fistula appears to be low in well-trained hands. The PPH-01 stapler removes a standardized amount of prolapsed. Therefore, the prolapse must not be too great in order for it to be completely excised by the stapler. Because of this limitation, a Contour Transtar curved cutting stapling technique has been used as a second-generation procedure (Figure 21-48). This

can remove an internal rectal prolapse of various sizes and even an external prolapse. STARR is not suitable for high takeoff internal rectal prolapse, although most are of the low takeoff variety. It is also less suitable for the globally failing pelvic floor. Complex combinations of pelvic floor descent, internal rectal prolapse, and enterocele should preferentially be treated by an abdominal approach.

Boccasanta described the potential benefits of STARR.[29] His study included 90 patients who had failed biofeedback therapy. There was a significant improvement in obstructed defecation at a mean follow-up of 16.3 months, with patient satisfaction reported as either good or excellent in 90%. Complications included urgency (18%) and flatus incontinence (9%). There were no major complications or mortality. Other small series have reported good outcomes in approximately 90% of patients, although follow-up was limited.[228,257,282]

Guidelines for the use of the STARR procedure were published following a Consensus Conference attended by a group of experts in Rome in 2005.[55] Shortly thereafter, the National Institute for Health and Clinical Excellence in the United Kingdom published its guidelines for STARR. It concluded as follows: "*Current evidence on the safety and efficacy of stapled transanal rectal resection (STARR) for obstructed defaecation syndrome (ODS) does not appear adequate for*

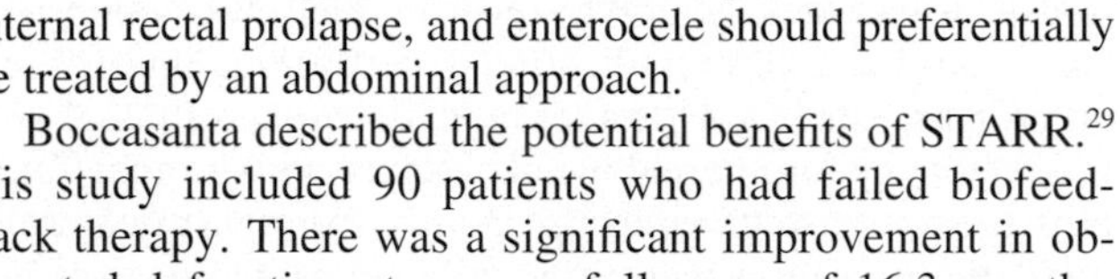

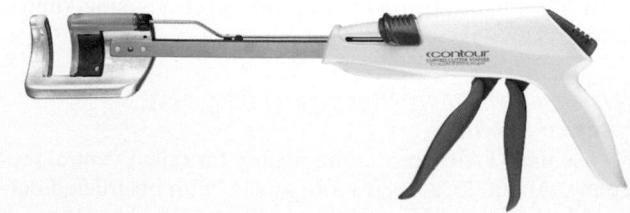

FIGURE 21-48. Contour curved cutter stapler. (Courtesy Ethicon Endo-Surgery, Inc.)

this procedure to be used without special arrangements for consent and for audit or research."[213] In response to this statement, a European STARR Registry was established as a mechanism for accumulating data on the short-term safety and efficacy of the procedure. Between 2006 and 2008, almost 3,000 PPH-01 STARR cases were registered, mostly from Italy (77%). The results demonstrated similar trends across the countries involved (Italy, Germany, and United Kingdom). A significant reduction in ODS score, symptom severity score, and quality of life (PAQ-QoL and EQ-5D) were observed. In addition, incontinence for the cohort as a whole was improved. Complications were reported in 36% of patients. These included pain (7%), urinary retention (7%), bleeding (5%), septic events (4%), and staple line complications (4%). Postoperative defecatory urgency was noted in 20%, and postoperative fecal incontinence was observed in 2%. There was no incident of rectovaginal fistula, although a single serious adverse event of rectal necrosis necessitating colostomy was reported. The final publication of the European STARR Registry (12-month follow-up data) was published in 2009 and concluded that STARR for obstructed defecation was safe and effective, at least in the short term, with significant improvements in obstructed defecation symptoms and in one's quality of life.[133]

There have been few studies comparing STARR with other treatment modalities.[109] One controlled trial by Lehur and colleagues randomized 119 patients to either STARR or biofeedback.[172] One-half of patients in the biofeedback arm failed to complete the course of treatment, and some were subsequently treated with STARR. The morbidity was higher in the STARR group (15%), although this was relatively minor. A significant improvement in ODS score was observed in both the STARR group and in those that completed biofeedback, but satisfaction was considerably higher following STARR than biofeedback (82% vs. 33%).

Delorme's Procedure (for Internal Prolapsed)

Internal prolapse has been treated using an endoanal approach in which the redundant internal prolapse is removed in the same manner as is performed for the convention Delorme indication.[23,72,317] This has the advantages over abdominal rectopexy of avoiding pelvic nerve damage and surgery-related constipation. Symptoms of tenesmus and evacuation difficulty are relieved in 70% to 80%, with overall improvement in the incontinence and constipation scores. However, new instances of constipation and incontinence may occur.

Sacral Nerve Stimulation (for Obstructed Defecation)

The role of sacral nerve stimulation (SNS) for obstructed defecation caused by internal rectal prolapse is unclear. Data are available primarily for fecal incontinence, but there is some information of its application for the management of chronic constipation.[123] The technique is described in Chapters 16 and 20. Unfortunately, the causes for chronic constipation are commingled, and the therapeutic outcome for subgroups including internal prolapse is unknown. It is unclear exactly how SNS would improve function in obstructed defecation, but presumably some hindgut neural mechanism may be involved.

▶ SOLITARY RECTAL ULCER SYNDROME

Solitary rectal ulcer syndrome (SRUS) is an unusual condition that was initially described by Madigan and subsequently by

Madigan and Morson; they collected a series of 68 cases.[183,184] Unfortunately, the term is bewildering because the syndrome does not necessarily have to be solitary, nor does it have to be confined to the rectum; in fact, it may be polypoid rather than ulcerating. The condition may be confused with nonspecific inflammatory bowel disease, villous adenoma, colitis cystica profunda, and other inflammatory and neoplastic diseases affecting the colon and rectum.

Etiology

A lack of consensus exists as to the cause of SRUS. Physiologic and histologic studies have illustrated a spectrum of findings suggesting a possible variety of causes.[3,142,255,302] Some believe that the victims are "unusual personalities, similar to that which is often ascribed to an individual with procidentia."[308] A possible mechanism is the failure of inhibition of puborectalis muscle contraction. This may result in a repeated desire to defecate and cause the persistent need to strain to pass stool. Most agree that patients with SRUS harbor an internal or external rectal prolapse. A simultaneous opposing force on the rectal mucosa—the downward force of defecation countered by upward force from the pelvic floor—generates the trauma required for the formation of SRUS. These forces may lead to mucosal ischemia and subsequent ulceration. In addition, the prolapsed mucosa may be traumatized by the closed anal canal.[78,159,175,216,238] Although the presence of rectal prolapse, external or internal, is understood, the nature of the opposing upward physiologic force is unclear. Some believe this to be a paradoxical contraction of the pelvic floor, anismus, or paradoxical puborectalis contraction. Current radiologic criteria for anismus are such that misinterpretation of the diagnosis (so-called radiologic pseudoanismus) may occur.[124] It seems likely that the upward force of the internal anal sphincter (IAS) opposes the downward force of the prolapse. Endoanal ultrasound reveals characteristically marked thickening of IAS in SRUS.[107,191] This thickening of the IAS is also seen in obstructed defecation associated with internal rectal prolapse without SRUS, but less prominently so. Patients with SRUS are known to have higher maximum resting pressures than those with prolapse without SRUS. It is possible that the response of the IAS to the prolapse leads to the development of the SRUS. If prolapse and anismus coexisted in SRUS, one would expect to see poor results following nerve-sparing ventral rectopexy. This operation treats only the prolapse, and biofeedback or botulinum toxin treatment postoperatively is necessary (see Chapter 20).

We and others believe that rectal prolapse and SRUS are different conditions caused by the same pathologic process.[302] Others think the two conditions occur separately with different etiologies. It is clear, however, that the two conditions coexist in many patients.[142]

Clinical Features

Solitary rectal ulcer syndrome is usually seen in women, especially those who harbor the bowel management problems previously described. However, in the St. Mark's Hospital experience of 119 patients, the condition occurred in men and women equally.[188] Symptoms usually consist of a variety of bowel complaints: constipation, diarrhea, passage of mucus, tenesmus, rectal bleeding, and proctalgia fugax. A classic history is one of blood and mucus per rectum associated with straining and a feeling of incomplete evacuation.[322]

Martin and coworkers reviewed 51 patients with the syndrome and noted that 98% presented with rectal bleeding, 96% with the passage of mucus, and 93% with tenesmus.[192] Approximately one-half of the patients were constipated. Bleeding was severe enough to require transfusion in three individuals. Chiang reported bleeding in 91%, mucous discharge in 77%, rectal pain in 61%, excessive straining in 63%, tenesmus in 64%, digitation in 29%, incontinence in 38%, constipation in 47%, and diarrhea in 18%.[43] In the experience at the Cleveland Clinic in Ohio, the principal symptoms were rectal bleeding (84%) and a disturbance of bowel function (56%).[311] Patients often present long after the onset of symptoms, sometimes more than 5 years.[322]

Examination

Examination demonstrates combinations of perineal descent with straining, rectoanal incoordination with straining, palpable prolapse, and features of the SRUS itself, induration/ulceration and fibrosis. In established fibrosis, it may not be possible to digitalize the narrowed rectal lumen. Classically, sigmoidoscopic examination reveals an ulcer with hyperemic edges and surrounding induration. Alternatively, exophytic lesions may be seen. A combination of ulcerating and polypoid lesions are often noted on the anterior rectal wall, usually at a level of 6 to 8 cm. Thomson and associates, in their report of six patients, found that the lesions were not necessarily solitary nor ulcerated.[307]

Histopathology

There are numerous characteristic features that permit the pathologist to distinguish solitary rectal ulcer from other lesions. Inflammatory changes may consist of replacement of the normal lamina propria by fibroblasts arranged at right angles to the muscularis mucosae (Figures 21-49 and 21-50).[267,275] The microscopic appearance, however, is quite variable and can include loss of normal polarity of the glandular epithelial cells, shortening of the crypts, mucin depletion, mucosal thickening, and inflammatory reaction in the submucosa. Many of the manifestations are those that have been described in patients with inflammatory bowel disease. Electron microscopic changes have also been identified; these include dense collagen deposition within the lamina propria as well as numerous fibroblasts.[42]

Franzin and colleagues reported a follow-up study of 27 patients with solitary ulcer of the rectum.[91] The authors noted a striking change in the histologic pattern. Although the patient's symptoms may have improved, the histologic appearance seemed to suggest chronic ischemia and an evolution to a transitional mucosa.

Chiang summarized the histologic findings of 158 cases. Fifty-six percent demonstrated an ulcerated pattern, 24% a polypoid, and 20% a flat lesion (also called erythematous lesion).[43] Glandular crypt abnormalities were seen in 91%, fibromuscular obliteration of the lamina propria in 98%, hypertrophied and splayed muscularis mucosae upward into

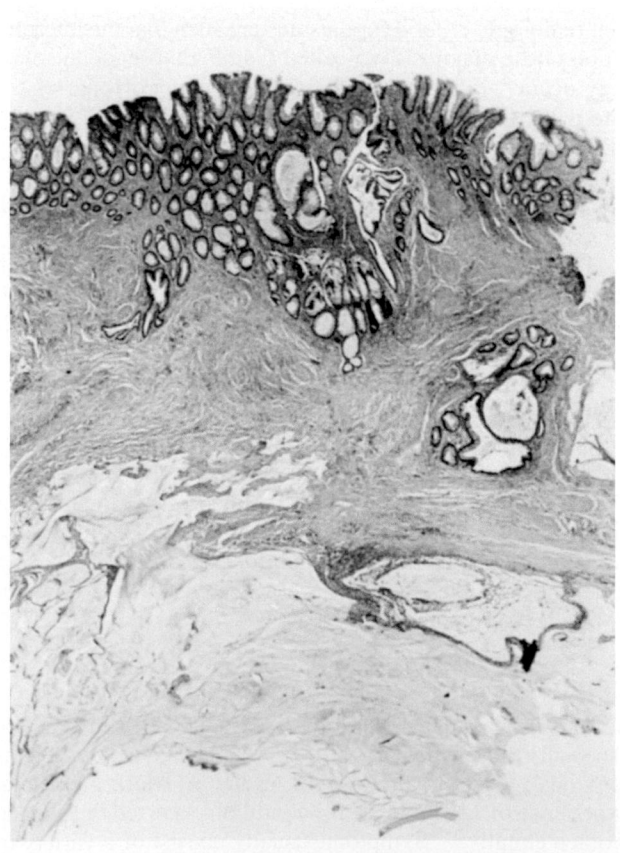

FIGURE 21-49. The submucosa of a solitary rectal ulcer contains a large mucous lake **(bottom)** and a group of glands in the submucosa between the lake and the overlying mucosa. (Original magnification × 20; courtesy of Rodger C. Haggitt, MD.)

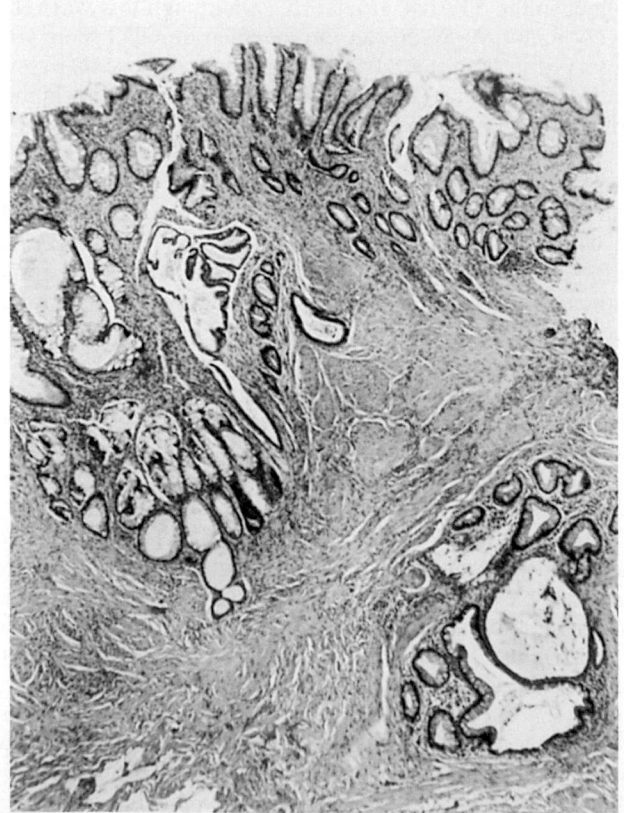

FIGURE 21-50. Solitary rectal ulcer. Markedly hyperplastic muscularis mucosa separates a group of glands in the submucosa **(lower right)** from the overlying mucosa. Fibers of muscularis mucosa extend into and obliterate the lamina propria between crypts. (Original magnification × 40; courtesy of Rodger C. Haggitt, MD.)

lamina propria in 96%, inflammatory cells and granulation tissue infiltration in the lamina propria in 75%, mucosal capillary abnormalities in 48%, hemosiderin deposition in the lamina propria in 53%, surface erosion with fully mature and normal epithelium in 56%, and misplaced glands in the submucosa in 7%.

Physiologic Evaluation and Contrast Studies

The diagnosis is made predominantly based on symptoms, endoscopic appearance, and results of biopsy. Anorectal physiologic evaluation and radiologic studies of patients with solitary rectal ulcer has been reported but is of limited value.[322] Defecography has frequently revealed an occult rectal prolapse (see previous discussion). Other findings that have been noted include failure of the sphincter to relax on defecation, high intrarectal pressure, increased anorectal angle, perineal descent, and impaired sensation on balloon inflation of the rectum.[106,146,241,336,339] It has been suggested that a high evacuation pressure may cause mucosal ulceration by exposing the rectal wall to a high transmural pressure gradient.[338] Goei and colleagues performed conventional barium enema studies on 15 individuals with histologically proven solitary rectal ulcer syndrome.[94] Findings included rectal stricture, granularity of the mucosa, and thickened rectal folds in 60%, but the remainder showed no abnormalities. Defecography demonstrated an intussusception in eight, and in four the puborectalis muscle failed to relax. There is general agreement on a high incidence and association of "rectoanal lack of coordination," perineal descent, and pudendal neuropathy in these individuals.[322]

Transrectal Ultrasound

Transrectal ultrasonography has been used in an attempt to understand the pathogenesis of solitary rectal ulcer syndrome. In a study by van Outryve and associates involving 15 patients, a rigid linear endorectal probe was used.[324] All but two demonstrated a thickened rectal wall. Poor relaxation of the puborectalis muscle during straining was noted in 11 of the 15. The authors opined that thickening of the muscularis propria suggests a chronic mechanical load on the rectal wall, and that ulcerations are formed as a consequence of this phenomenon.[324] They concluded that nonrelaxation of the puborectalis muscle is an important element in the pathogenesis of this condition. The St. Mark's Hospital group performed *anal* endosonography on 20 patients with solitary rectal ulcer syndrome.[191] Thirteen were found to have an abnormally thick internal anal sphincter. The investigators observed that these individuals were significantly more likely to have defecographic evidence of internal prolapse and opined that this study (when positive) has a high predictive value for this association.

Management

Treatment of solitary rectal ulcer syndrome has been regarded as rather problematic. Some individuals' symptoms may be ameliorated by a high-fiber diet and bowel management instructions.[323] Some have observed marked improvement of symptoms through the use of sucralfate retention enemas although histologic changes persisted.[347] Fibrin sealant has also been suggested.[85] Rarely, a colostomy may be indicated for the treatment of symptoms and complications, such as massive rectal bleeding.

Biofeedback has been used both as the primary therapy and to supplement surgery, especially in individuals with obstructed defecation.[322] Transanal excision of localized lesions has been performed with mixed results; some recur, others do not. Because operations designed for the treatment of rectal prolapse have been reported to be of benefit in patients with the solitary ulcer syndrome (suspension, rectopexy, and resection), a high index of suspicion for the presence of sigmoidorectal intussusception (i.e., preprolapse, internal prolapse) should be maintained if the examiner perceives the characteristic changes in the rectal mucosa.[146,216,336] Anorectal physiologic evaluation, specifically defecography, is strongly encouraged under these circumstances.

Results

The St. Mark's group reported their results of behavioral treatment (biofeedback) in 13 patients with solitary ulcer syndrome.[186] Approximately one-half improved, but there was significant deterioration over time (median follow-up, 36 months). In the experience of the Cleveland Clinic group, intractable symptoms led to surgery in 60% of their patients, with symptomatic improvement noted in more than two-thirds.[311] They further observed that the optimal surgical procedure is still indeterminate, but rectopexy, local excision, and fecal diversion seemed to achieve improvement in the majority of patients. The authors were rather circumspect regarding recommendation of resective surgery for this condition. van Tets and Kuijpers performed rectopexy on 18 patients with solitary rectal ulcer syndrome.[325] All lesions healed, and patients became significantly less symptomatic. The authors believe that characteristic defecographic features and the presence of solitary rectal ulcer syndrome are indications for surgery, provided that pelvic floor function during straining is normal—in other words, if there is no suggestion of obstructed defecation. In the experience of the St. Mark's Hospital group with 16 patients who remained symptomatic following rectopexy, they concluded that a prolonged preoperative evacuation time (obstructed defecation) may predict a poor surgical outcome.[106] A more recent publication from the same institution involved 81 patients who underwent surgery for this condition.[287] The ultimate stomal rate was 30%. Nicholls and Simson had success with a ventral-posterior rectopexy in patients without external prolapse (86%).[216] Choi reported about 70% success with use of a combination of perineal and abdominal approaches.[46] Marchal described 60% success in a small cohort of 13 patients undergoing a similar combination of approaches.[190]

Some of the newer surgical treatments have shown promise in the treatment of solitary rectal ulcer. Boccasanta treated 10 patients with a STARR.[28] At a mean follow-up of 27 months, 80% were noted to have excellent or good results, and none of the 10 patients developed a recurrence of rectal ulcer. These data would support the view that internal prolapse is the etiology of solitary rectal ulcer syndrome.

Posterior rectopexy has been the primary method of "pexing" for solitary rectal ulcer. The results, unfortunately, have been quite variable. Recent use of a nerve-sparing ventral rectopexy has been more promising, with 13 of 15 (87%) patients responding successfully to surgery.[87] Significant improvement of obstructed defecation ($P = .04$) and fecal incontinence ($P = .03$) scores at 3 months, with sigmoidoscopic healing of the ulcer, was found in all 15 patients.

Surgery has a role in the treatment of solitary rectal ulcer. However, it should be reserved for those individuals with intractable symptoms, in whom behavioral therapy has failed, and/or who have incontrovertible evidence of internal prolapse.[322]

DESCENDING PERINEUM SYNDROME

When a healthy person increases intra-abdominal pressure and relaxes the pelvic floor muscles, no significant change can be observed in the concavity of the perineum. However, in patients with chronic illness, malnutrition, and internal prolapse, perineal descent may be observed, the normal concavity being obliterated when the patient strains.[238] In those with this syndrome, either the anal canal is situated several centimeters below a line drawn between the pubis and coccyx, or it de-

scends 3 or 4 cm during straining.[238] The perineum can even descend 5 or 6 cm in some individuals (Figure 21-51). A "perineometer" has been described that can measure the amount of descent,[115] but some authors question its accuracy and advise instead, standard defecography for this determination.[12,225,304] The Cleveland Clinic Florida group studied the reproducibility of measuring the anorectal angle and pelvic floor descent by two different methods.[48] The investigators concluded that both methods were consistently reliable.

A descending perineum is the result of injury to the pelvic floor muscles, especially the levators. Patients usually complain of tenesmus, difficulty evacuating, and incontinence. The problem with bowel control may be due to excessive straining with defecation, which stretches the pudendal nerves and results in anorectal muscular atrophy. Jorge and coworkers at the Cleveland Clinic Florida performed a prospective study

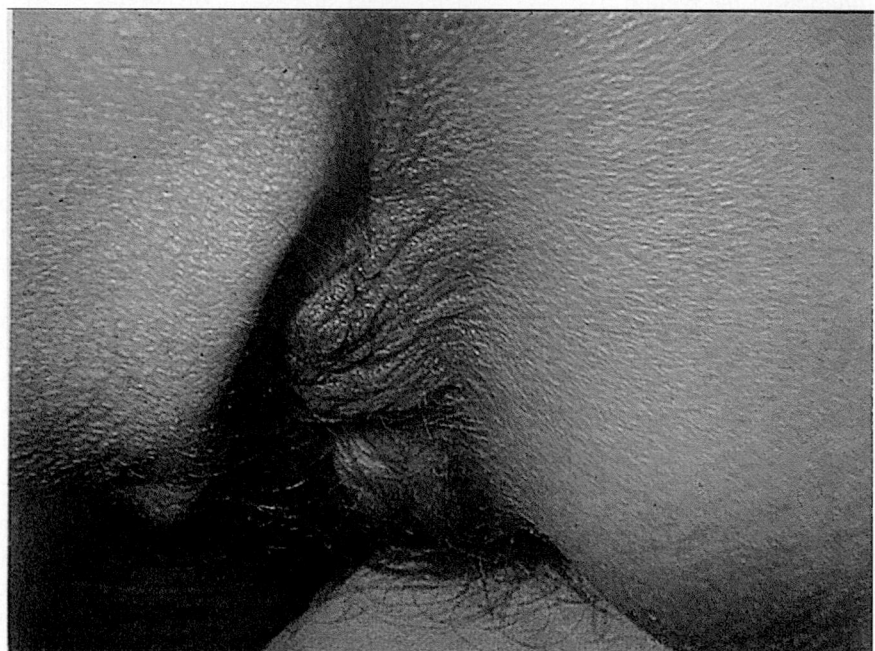

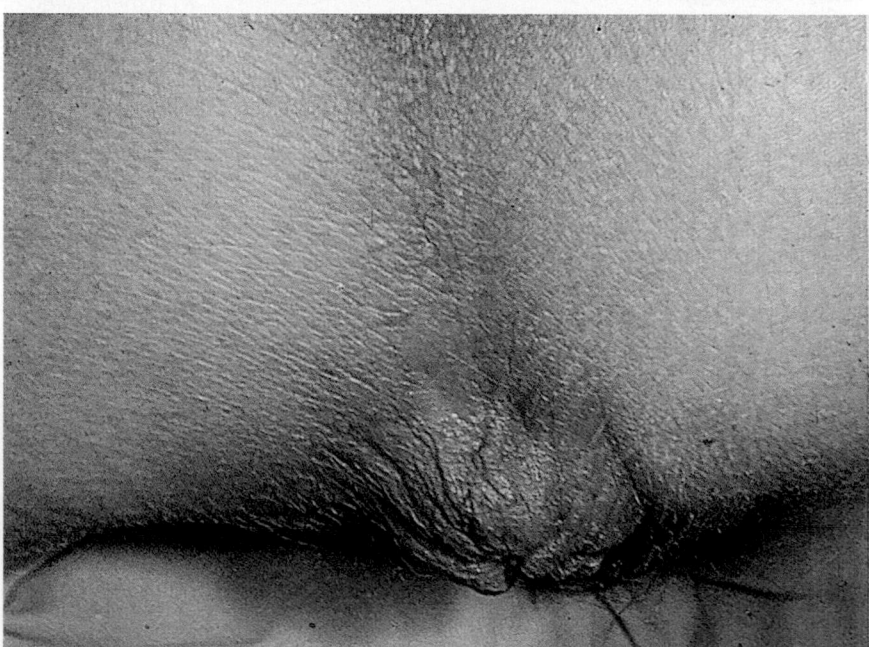

FIGURE 21-51. Descending perineum (perineal descensus). **A:** At rest. **B:** During straining. (From De los Rios Margrina E. *Color Atlas of Anorectal Diseases.* Philadelphia, PA: WB Saunders; 1980, with permission.)

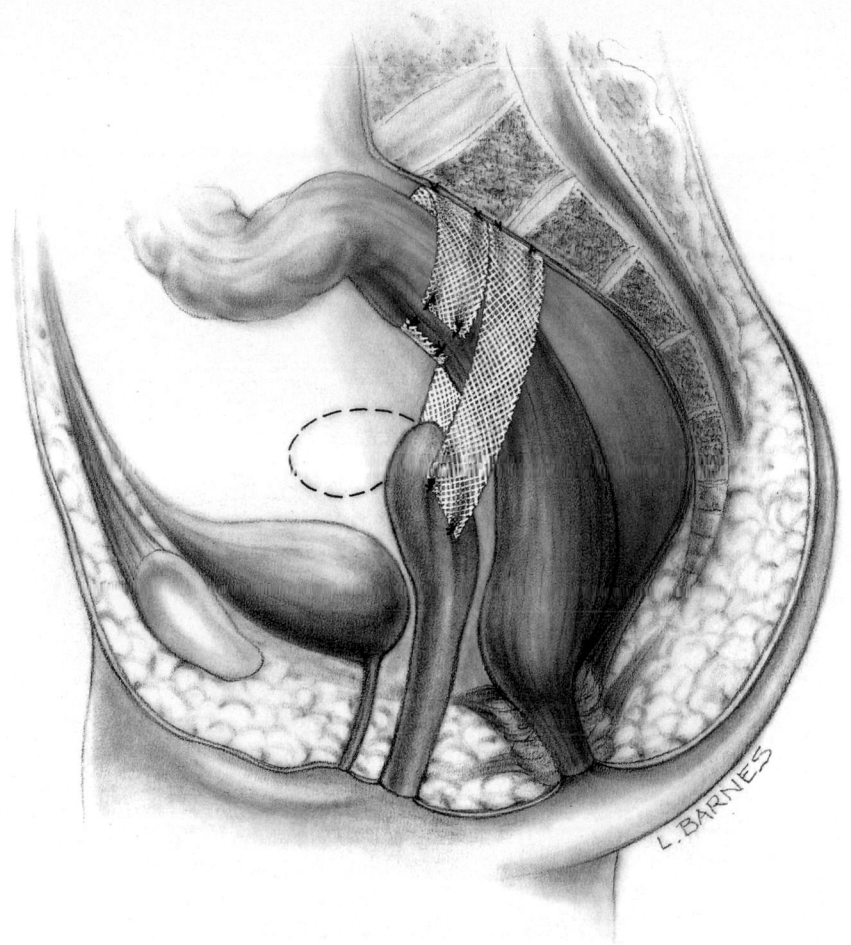

L. BARNES

FIGURE 21-52. Abdominal colporectopexy with pelvic cul-de-sac closure. Lateral view of the completed procedure. Note that mesh is secured to the sacrum, to the rectum, and to the apex of the anatomically restored vagina. The *dotted line* indicates the obliterated cul-de-sac. (Redrawn from Collopy BT, Barham KA. Abdominal colporectopexy with the pelvic cul-de-sac closure. *Dis Colon Rectum*. 2002;45(4):522–526.)

to assess the correlation between perineal descent and pudendal neuropathy in 213 consecutive patients.[138] There was no relationship found, leading the authors to conclude that these may represent independent findings despite being frequently observed in those with disordered defecation.

Treatment

Treatment is usually directed toward bowel management (e.g., diet, laxatives, suppositories) and to education (e.g., avoiding straining). When incontinence is the major complaint, restoration of the pelvic floor, with possible implantation of mesh, and resection or suspension of the rectum may be necessary. One approach is shown in Figure 21-52. An alternative, suggested by Nichols, is to hitch the posterior wall of the rectum to the sacrum through a transcoccygeal approach (Figure 21-53).[217] The operation can be combined with plication of the levators as well as an anterior perineorrhaphy. Unfortunately, almost irrespective of the various options that may be implemented, results are less than ideal.

Another innovation for the surgical treatment of pelvic floor laxity (including enterocele, rectocele, and cystocele) has been through the use of what Sullivan and Lee call a total pelvic Marlex mesh repair.[301] This is a most complicated operation that involves stripping of the parietal and visceral peritoneum from the floor of the pelvis, separating the posterior vaginal wall from the rectum all the way down to the perineal body, and then implanting a trapezoid-shaped Marlex mesh with two additional strips—securing the mesh at the introitus, at the adjacent endopelvic fascia, and to the upper sacrum. In addition, the Marlex is secured to Cooper's ligament on each side as part of the anterior fixation. The authors have reported their considerable experience (236 women) with this operation.[300] The median age was 64 years. The primary complaints were bladder protrusion, vaginal protrusion, or both (54%), but almost two-thirds were found to have perineal descent. More than one-third required additional surgery for persistent or new complaints, but there were no recurrences of rectal or vaginal prolapse. As one may appreciate, this is an esoteric operation indeed, the application of which thus far seems to be confined to one center.

Collopy and colleagues reported a group of patients with rectal prolapse and posthysterectomy vaginal wall prolapse in whom they performed rectopexy, abdominal closure of the pelvic cul-de-sac, and a colpopexy (attaching forward extensions of the same mesh to the apex of the anatomically restored and reinforced vaginal vault).[54] Eighty-nine were provided considerable relief of symptoms without evident recurrent rectal or vaginal vault prolapse.

▶ RECTOCELE

Rectocele is defined as a herniation or bulging of the anterior rectal wall and posterior vaginal wall into the vagina. Others extend the definition to encompass the pathophysiology, a defective rectovaginal septum. Figure 21-54 demonstrates an artist's conception of a typical rectocele.

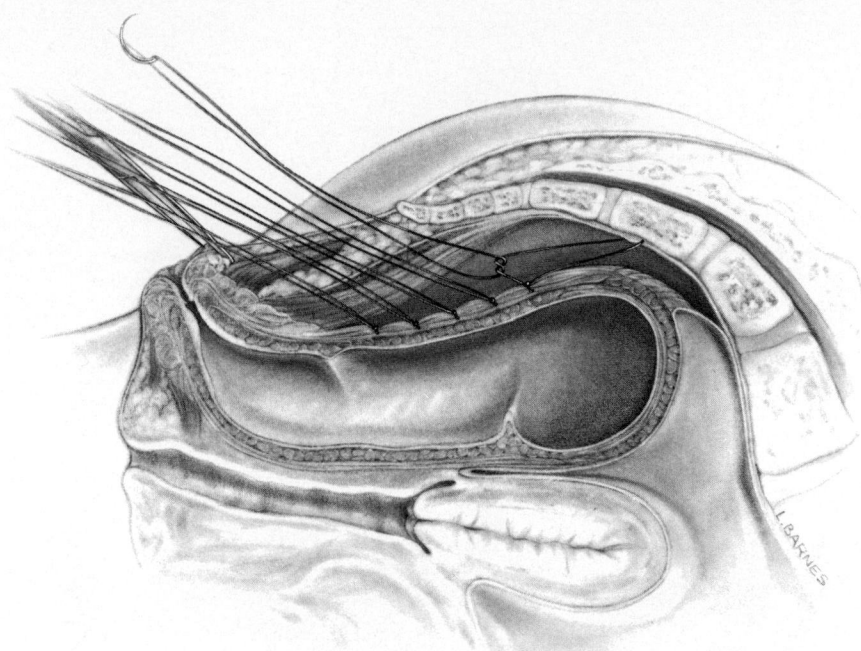

FIGURE 21-53. Series of plication sutures are placed 1 cm apart in the posterior wall of the rectum. Sutures are then sewn individually to the anterior periosteum of the sacrum. (Adapted from Nichols DH. Retrorectal levatorplasty for anal and perineal prolapse. *Surg Gynecol Obstet.* 1982;154(2):251–254, with permission.)

Pathophysiology

It is likely that this problem is related to a deficiency of, or damage to, the supportive layer of fascia lying between the rectum and vagina, a fascia analogous to Denonvilliers' fascia in the male. Others describe it as a specialized condensation of the visceral endopelvic fascia.[61] This fascia exists as a component of a more confluent connective tissue package enveloping the pelvic organs (endopelvic fascia) and is, therefore, intimately related to organ mobility and support.

The rectovaginal fascia is a diaphragm-like sheet with several points of fixity. It is a fibromuscular elastic layer composed of dense collagen, smooth muscle, and coarse elastic fibers with associated small blood vessels.[62,210] DeLancey divides it into thirds: the upper third (level I) blending with the peritoneum of the cul-de-sac, the uterosacral ligaments,

and the base of the cardinal ligaments. In its middle third (level II), the rectovaginal fascia extends laterally out to the fascia overlying the levator ani muscle. Here, it is a component of the endopelvic fascia that provides lateral support to the level II structures. In the distal third of the vagina/rectum (level III), it blends with the perineal body.

Etiology and Demographics

A symptomatic rectocele rarely exists in isolation, often coexisting with varying degrees of cystocele, uterovaginal prolapse, enterocele, excessive perineal descent, and rectal intussusception.[306] Hence, the major risk factors in its development are those causing pelvic organ prolapse. The condition can exist in both parous and nulliparous patients as well as males, although parous women constitute the most affected group. The major risk factor is vaginal delivery. This may cause a multicomponent injury to the musculoaponeurotic pelvic floor, endopelvic connective tissue, the levator ani, and pudendal nerves.[277] This varies in severity according to duration of labor, the use of epidural anesthesia, whether forceps are applied, and the size of the newborn. The end result may be attenuation or tearing of the rectovaginal fascia. Widening of the genital hiatus affects vaginal closure, meaning that the posterior vaginal wall is subjected to a high-pressure gradient from transmitted intra-abdominal pressure.[62] Interestingly, cesarean delivery is not protective.[181]

Age is also associated with rectocele development, probably representative of a complex interplay of age-related connective tissue degeneration, postmenopausal hypoestrogenism, expression of the patient's collagen phenotype, and the onset of organic diseases.[150] A BMI of greater than 25 correlates with a higher stage of rectocele.[113] A first-degree relative with pelvic organ prolapse confers a threefold relative risk increase, and there is also a racial influence.[150] Risk factors for the development of rectocele are as follows:

- Female gender
- Vaginal childbirth
- Pregnancy

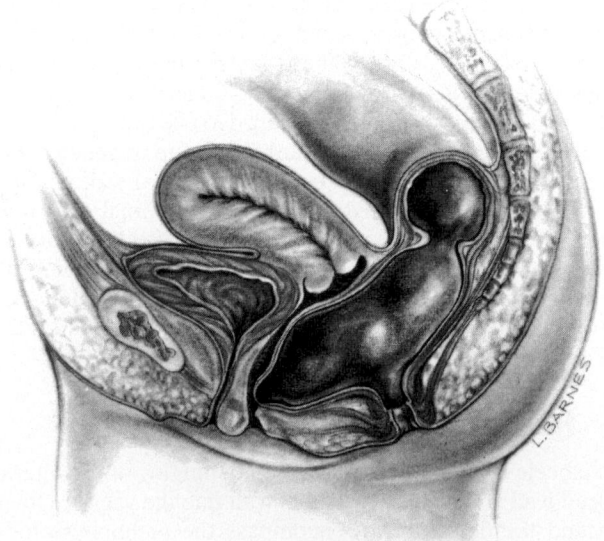

FIGURE 21-54. Sagittal view of a typical rectocele deformity.

- Aging
- Menopause/hypoestrogenism
- Genetic factors

A small rectocele in a woman is a common finding and should not be regarded as abnormal. In Shorvon's widely quoted study, of 46 nulliparous volunteers younger than 35 years of age with no defecation symptoms, small rectoceles (i.e., less than 2 cm) were found in 81% of female and 13% of male volunteers; only one had a rectocele greater than 2 cm in size. Rectoceles greater than 2 cm are uncommon in otherwise asymptomatic young nulliparous women. The condition is frequently found in patients presenting to gynecologists and pelvic floor clinics with a variety of symptoms. In one observational population study, pelvic organ prolapse was diagnosed in more than 50% of women older than 50 years, with an incidence of 31% in those aged 20 to 60 years.[273] Rectocele was diagnosed in more than 30% of the patients with any stage of pelvic organ prolapse. However, most were morphologically at an early stage. In the United States, 1 in 10 women will have surgery for symptomatic pelvic organ prolapse, with up to one-third of operations being revisions.[227] Seventy-six percent undergo surgery for documented pelvic organ prolapse with a rectocele. In a cost analysis, 22% of American women undergoing surgery for pelvic organ prolapse also underwent a rectocele repair.[298] It is estimated that the rate of women seeking care for pelvic floor disorders will double in the next 30 years.[180]

Symptoms, Signs, and Investigations

Patients present with a variety of gynecologic and bowel symptoms: obstructed defecation, fecal incontinence (especially postdefecation), pruritus ani, dyspareunia, pelvic pressure, and vaginal bulge. However, few of these symptoms can be directly attributed to the rectocele. This is important for two reasons. First, it is a reminder that symptomatic rectocele is often the reflection of a more global pelvic floor dysfunction issue, and second, that symptoms generally direct the treatment.[243] For colorectal surgeons, the most reliable symptoms are the need to self-digitalize and/or a sense of incomplete evacuation.[71] A "rectocele-specific" symptom scoring system has recently been reported, but it has not been validated.[70] It remains to be seen whether it offers any advantage over an established but less specific scoring system, such as the Obstructed Defecation Score.[11]

Physical examination characterizes the rectocele and the coexistent pelvic floor findings. The perineum may be descended at or below the ischial tuberosities at rest, or may be obviously ballooned outward. Further descent (greater than 3 cm) may be noticed on straining. Note should be made of any evidence of cystocele or vaginal vault prolapse. Asking the patient to bear down during digital rectal examination may unmask a nonrelaxing puborectalis. The same maneuver may reveal uterine prolapse or a rectal intussusception. The integrity of the perineal body and anal sphincter can also be assessed. Proctoscopy may demonstrate mucosal prolapse overlying the rectocele. The important differential diagnostic concern is an enterocele. This can also present as a posterior vaginal protrusion. Simultaneous rectal and vaginal palpation while the patient performs a Valsalva maneuver may help in the differentiation. The negative predictive value of clinical examination is low, and ultimately, the differential diagnosis may need to be excluded radiologically.[149]

Mellgren observed that patients with enterocele rarely have a coexistent rectocele and hypothesized that the two conditions may be mutually exclusive.[199]

Colorectal surgeons describe rectocele size as the amount of protrusion into the vaginal lumen beyond the expected normal contour of the rectum, similar to the radiologic measurement at defecating proctography.[285] A clinical classification of rectoceles by the International Continence Society, the American Urogynecologic Society, and the Society of Gynecological Surgeons was proposed in 1996.[37] This is also known as the "POP-Q" system of assessment of the anatomical grade of gynecologic prolapse, including that of rectocele. Rectocele severity is expressed as stages I to IV. This classification depends on the maximal protrusion inferiorly, with reference to the hymenal ring when the patient is examined in the semi-upright lithotomy position during the Valsalva maneuver.

Defecating Proctography

Rectal contrast study can provide useful radiologic information. The size of the rectocele can be measured by the extent of protrusion anteriorly beyond the normal contour of the rectum. Extent of perineal descent at rest or straining can be quantitated, and anismus confirmed if present. Coexistent mucosal or internal rectal prolapse will also be evident. Contrast trapping is thought to occur because of a low-pressure zone occurring within the rectocele when one strains. Although trapping has been reported to be associated with a larger rectocele and the symptom of vaginal digitalization, it does not appear to be predictive of treatment outcome. In a variation of standard proctography, it has been proposed that a further radiograph be taken after the patient has eliminated much of the contrast. This may offer a clearer representation of the degree of rectocele emptying.[102]

Magnetic Resonance Defecography

This is a new and attractive modality, especially because there is no exposure to radiation and there is the ability to visualize all pelvic viscera. Two methods exist: supine closed-configuration magnet and the newer open-configuration magnet. A criticism of the former is that the patient position is nonphysiologic, and asking the patient to bear down in the supine position is likely to underestimate the degree of pelvic organ prolapse. A solution to this problem is to use intrarectal contrast (usually sonographic transmission gel) that the patient is required to evacuate. Using this technique, Kelvin and associates found that MR compared favorably with triphasic fluoroscopic cystocolpoproctography in estimating rectocele size, but that it underestimated the extent of cystoceles and enteroceles.[148]

Dynamic Perineal Ultrasound

This is an emerging alternative diagnostic approach. Using the translabial technique, Perniola and colleagues found a positive predictive value for rectocele of 0.82 when blindly compared with standard fluoroscopy, but the procedure had a low negative predictive value.[240] The authors concluded that as a screening test it may be useful, but a negative result may necessitate further investigation with fluoroscopic proctography. Beer-Gabel and coworkers reported promising results in a similar study with evacuated intrarectal gel.[20]

Management and Surgery

A discussion of the role of biofeedback is truly the recognition of the frequent coexistence of anismus (pelvic floor dyssynergia). In a defecographic and electromyographic study of 112 patients with obstructed defecation, Mellgren and associates found that 60% of patients with rectocele had paradoxical anal sphincter activity.[200] This compared with 24% of those without rectocele.

Biofeedback is an effective therapy for pelvic floor dyssynergia,[256] with a recent study showing it to be more beneficial than laxatives.[44] Concurrent presence of a rectocele does not affect the likelihood of success.

Patients with symptomatic rectocele in the presence of anismus should have a trial of biofeedback before operative options are pursued. However, whether failure of biofeedback is a contraindication to proceeding with repair is not clear. Two case series report a worse subjective outcome in those with untreated anismus who underwent transanal repair.[1,312]

Transanal Sutured Repair

This is usually performed with the patient in the prone jackknife position. The procedure consists of the placement of reinforcing sutures into the anterior rectal wall following mucosectomy overlying the rectocele (Figure 21-55). It is well tolerated with major morbidity rare. Minor perioperative complications include urinary tract infection, urinary retention, secondary hemorrhage, and fecal impaction. Rectovaginal fistula is rare with this approach.

In follow-up studies at 6 to 24 months, subjective measures of symptoms note "cure" or improvement in 75% to 93% of patients.[132,312] In reports with greater than 2 years follow-up, this figure falls to 62% to 50%, suggesting some diminution of efficacy with time.[1,117,264] As discussed earlier, it has been shown that coexistent anismus predicts a poor subjective outcome. Other parameters that appear to benefit from repair are rectal distension sensation and efficacy of evacuation.[117,132] Whether the transanal approach adversely affects anal sphincter function is unclear. Whereas some have shown a significant decrease in mean anal resting pressure following transanal repair,[132] others have demonstrated no such effect.[117] A beneficial result of transanal rectocele repair on preoperative fecal incontinence symptoms has also been demonstrated.[1,132] A selective operative approach has been advocated, whereby patients with significant preoperative incontinence issues as a consequence of a sphincter defect undergo a transperineal or transvaginal repair, and those with incontinence thought due to mucosal prolapse undergo a transanal repair.[17,319] Transanal repair has not been shown to affect sexual function adversely.[117]

Transvaginal Repair

Gynecologists usually perform a transvaginal repair using one of three types of approaches: plication of the deficient rectovaginal septum (posterior colporrhaphy), a defect-specific repair of identified tears in the rectovaginal septum, or a prosthetic reinforcement of the rectovaginal septum. A randomized trial of all three has shown similar anatomic and improved functional outcomes.[233] For transvaginal prosthetic reinforcement of the rectovaginal septum, nonbiologic, nonabsorbable mesh (e.g., polypropylene); nonbiologic, absorbable mesh (e.g., polyglactin); and biologic mesh (e.g., porcine small intestine submucosa) have all been reported. Although

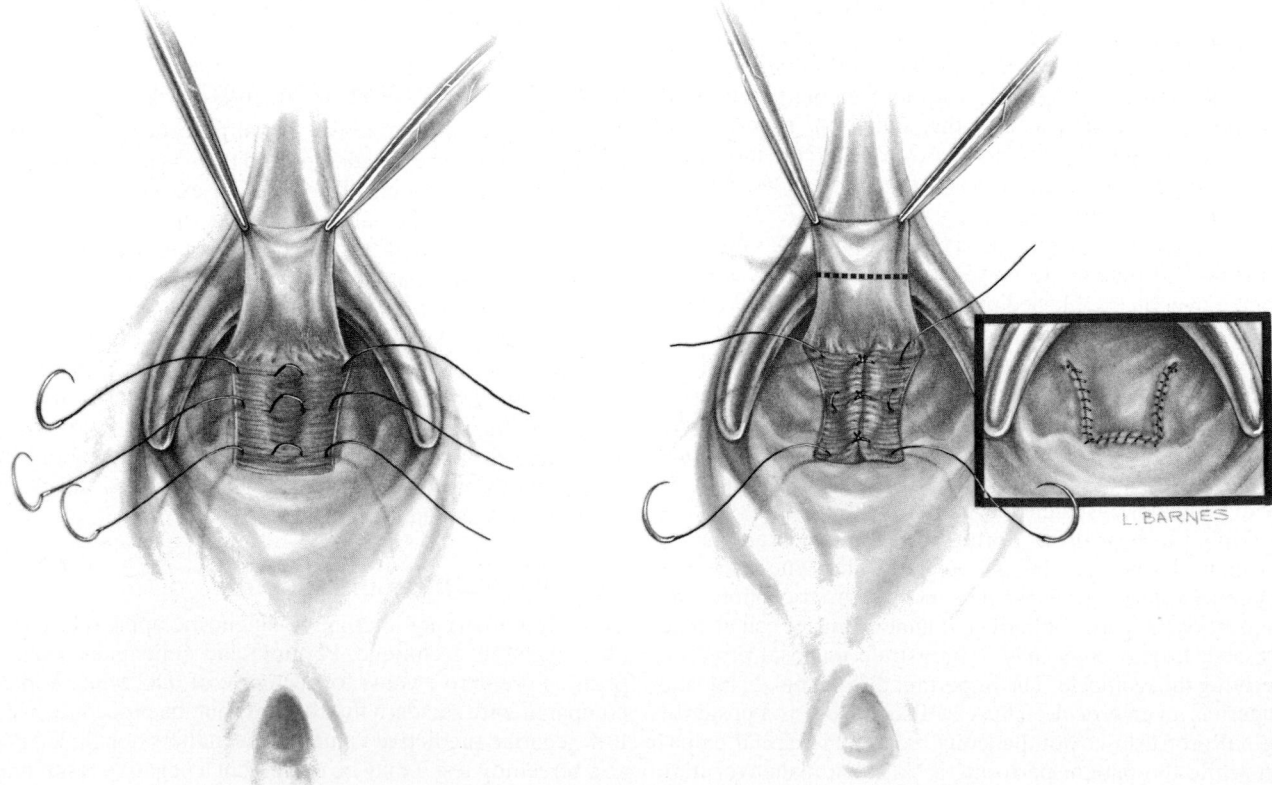

A   **B**

FIGURE 21-55. Transanal rectocele repair. Plication in layers of the lax rectovaginal septum.

there are proponents of all of the aforementioned operations, high-quality comparative data in this area are lacking. Enthusiasm for which technique to employ is usually dictated by subspecialty interest. However, a recent Cochrane review found that posterior vaginal wall repair had a significantly lower recurrence rate than transanal repair, despite higher blood loss and greater use of pain medication.[185] The data were too limited to determine clinical outcomes of flatus or fecal incontinence, or dyspareunia.

Transperineal Repair

Repair via a transperineal incision has been reported using nonbiologic, absorbable mesh[174]; nonbiologic, nonabsorbable mesh[202]; and biologic mesh.[289] This approach is attractive as it avoids anal sphincter stretching and facilitates concurrent anal sphincter repair where indicated. It may also minimize the risk of new-onset dyspareunia by avoiding a vaginal incision. Wound morbidity is a concern, however, with wound infection, hematoma, and mesh infection necessitating removal all described. Although the results of these studies are generally encouraging, they are small case series with short follow-up, and as such longer term comparative data are needed.

Transabdominal Repair

This involves dissection of the rectovaginal septum to the pelvic floor and reinforcement of the anterior rectal wall with prosthetic mesh. Results are variable and seem to be related to technique. Anterolateral mesh placement has produced disappointing results.[229] However, solely anterior mesh placement with a perineal incision to bring the mesh down onto the perineal body has been more encouraging.[70] A retrospective matched cohort study favored transanal repair over that of laparoscopic surgery for alleviation of obstructed defecation symptoms, although the authors noted a nonsignificant trend toward anal sphincter morbidity in the transanal group.[309] The approach appears to be safe and well tolerated. Transabdominal rectocele repair is more likely considered in the situation of global pelvic floor dysfunction, such as uterovaginal prolapse (e.g., sacrocolpopexy) or rectal prolapse/intussusception (e.g., ventral mesh rectopexy).[53,288] In these situations, the rectocele is more an incidental concern.

Stapled Transanal Rectal Resection

The STARR procedure consists of a transanal resection of rectal redundancy using either a circular or curved stapling device (see earlier discussion). As with transabdominal repair, the rectocele correction should be viewed as incidental. There is little justification for performing the procedure simply for rectocele in the absence of rectal intussusception or mucosal prolapse.

References

1. Abbas SM, Bissett IP, Neill ME, et al. Long-term results of the anterior Délorme's operation in the management of symptomatic rectocele. *Dis Colon Rectum.* 2005;48(2):317–322.
2. Agachan F, Pfeifer J, Joo JS, et al. Results of perineal procedures for the treatment of rectal prolapse. *Am Surg.* 1997;63(1):9–12.
3. Alexander-Williams J. Solitary–ulcer syndrome of the rectum. Its association with occult rectal prolapse. *Lancet.* 1977;1(8004):170–171.
4. Allen-Mersh TG, Henry MM, Nicholls RJ. Natural history of anterior mucosal prolapse. *Br J Surg.* 1987;74(8):679–682.
5. Allen-Mersh TG, Turner MJ, Mann CV. Effect of abdominal Ivalon rectopexy on bowel habit and rectal wall. *Dis Colon Rectum.* 1990;33(7):550–553.
6. Altemeier WA. One-stage perineal surgery for complete rectal prolapse. *Hosp Pract.* 1972;7:102–108.
7. Altemeier WA, Culbertson WR. Technique for perineal repair of rectal prolapse. *Surgery.* 1965;58:758–764.
8. Altemeier WA, Culbertson WR, Schowengerdt C, et al. Nineteen years' experience with the one-stage perineal repair of rectal prolapse. *Ann Surg.* 1971;173(6):993–1006.
9. Altman D, Zetterstrom J, Schultz I, et al. Pelvic organ prolapse and urinary incontinence in women with surgically managed rectal prolapse: a population-based case-control study. *Dis Colon Rectum.* 2006;49(1):28–35.
10. Altomare DF, Rinaldi M, Chimarulo C, et al. Treatment of external anorectal mucosal prolapse with circular stapler: an easy and effective new surgical technique. *Dis Colon Rectum.* 1999;42(8):1102–1105.
11. Altomare DF, Spazzafumo L, Rinaldi M, et al. Set-up and statistical validation of a new scoring system for obstructed defaecation syndrome. *Colorectal Dis.* 2008;10(1):84–88.
12. Ambrose S, Keighley MR. Outpatient measurement of perineal descent. *Ann R Coll Surg Engl.* 1985;67(5):306–308.
13. Ashari LH, Lumley JW, Stevenson AR, et al. Laparoscopically-assisted resection rectopexy for rectal prolapse: ten years' experience. *Dis Colon Rectum.* 2005;48(5):982–987.
14. Ashcraft KW, Amoury RA, Holder TM. Levator repair and posterior suspension for rectal prolapse. *J Pediatr Surg.* 1977;12(2):241–245.
15. Atkinson KG, Taylor DC. Wells procedure for complete rectal prolapse. A ten-year experience. *Dis Colon Rectum.* 1984;27(2):96–98.
16. Auguste T, Dubreuil A, Bost R, et al. Technical and functional results after laparoscopic rectopexy to the promontory for complete rectal prolapse. Prospective study in 54 consecutive patients. *Gastroenterol Clin Biol.* 2006;30(5):659–663.
17. Ayabaca SM, Zbar AP, Pescatori M. Anal continence after rectocele repair. *Dis Colon Rectum.* 2002;45(1):63–69.
18. Bachoo P, Brazzelli M, Grant A. Surgery for complete rectal prolapse in adults. *Cochrane Database Syst Rev.* 2000 (update 2008) (2):CD001758 and (4):CD001758.
19. Baker R, Senagore AJ, Luchtefeld MA. Laparoscopic-assisted vs. open resection. Rectopexy offers excellent results. *Dis Colon Rectum.* 1995;38(2):199–201.
20. Beer-Gabel M, Teshler M, Schechtman E, et al. Dynamic transperineal ultrasound vs. defecography in patients with evacuatory difficulty: a pilot study. *Int J Colorectal Dis.* 2004;19(1):60–67.
21. Bennett BH, Geelhoed GW. A stapler modification of the Altemeier procedure for rectal prolapse. Experimental and clinical evaluation. *Am Surg.* 1985;51(2):116–120.
22. Berman IR. Sutureless laparoscopic rectopexy for procidentia. Technique and implications. *Dis Colon Rectum.* 1992;35(7):689–693.
23. Berman IR, Harris MS, Rabeler MB. Delorme's transrectal excision for internal prolapse. Patient selection, technique, and three-year follow-up. *Dis Colon Rectum.* 1990;33(7):573–580.
24. Bhandari B, Ameta DK. Etiology of prolapse rectum in children with special reference to amoebiasis. *Indian J Pediatr.* 1977;14(8):635–637.
25. Biehl AG, Ray JE, Gathright JB Jr. Repair of rectal prolapse: experience with the Ripstein sling. *South Med J.* 1978;71(8):923–925.
26. Birnbaum EH, Stamm L, Rafferty JF, et al. Pudendal nerve terminal motor latency influences surgical outcome in treatment of rectal prolapse. *Dis Colon Rectum.* 1996;39(11):1215–1221.
27. Blatchford GJ, Perry RE, Thorson AG, et al. Rectopexy without resection for rectal prolapse. *Am J Surg.* 1989;158(6):574–576.
28. Boccasanta P, Venturi M, Calabro G, et al. Stapled transanal rectal resection in solitary rectal ulcer associated with prolapse of the rectum: a prospective study. *Dis Colon Rectum.* 2008;51(3):348–354.
29. Boccasanta P, Venturi M, Stuto A, et al. Stapled transanal rectal resection for outlet obstruction: a prospective, multicenter trial. *Dis Colon Rectum.* 2004;47(8):1285–1296.
30. Boons P, Collinson R, Cunningham C, et al. Laparoscopic ventral rectopexy for external rectal prolapse improves constipation and avoids de novo constipation. *Colorectal Dis.* 2009;12(6):526–532.
31. Boulos PB, Stryker SJ, Nicholls RJ. The long-term results of polyvinyl alcohol (Ivalon) sponge for rectal prolapse in young patients. *Br J Surg.* 1984;71(3):213–214.
32. Boutsis C, Ellis H. The Ivalon-sponge-wrap operation for rectal prolapse: an experience with 26 patients. *Dis Colon Rectum.* 1974;17(1):21–37.
33. Braley SC, Schneider PD, Bold RJ, et al. Controlled tamponade of severe presacral venous hemorrhage: use of a breast implant sizer. *Dis Colon Rectum.* 2002;45(1):140–142.
34. Brodén B, Snellman B. Procidentia of the rectum studied with cineradiography. A contribution to the discussion of causative mechanism. *Dis Colon Rectum.* 1968;11(5):330–347.

35. Brodén G, Dolk A, Holmström B. Evacuation difficulties and other characteristics of rectal function associated with procidentia and the Ripstein operation. *Dis Colon Rectum*. 1988;31(4):283–286.

36. Brown AJ, Nicol L, Anderson JH, et al. Prospective study of the effect of rectopexy on colonic motility in patients with rectal prolapse. *Br J Surg*. 2005;92(11):1417–1422.

37. Bump RC, Mattiasson A, Bø K, et al. The standardization of terminology of female pelvic organ prolapse and pelvic floor dysfunction. *Am J Obstet Gynecol*. 1996;175(1):10–17.

38. Byrne CM, Smith SR, Solomon MJ, et al. Long-term functional outcomes after laparoscopic and open rectopexy for the treatment of rectal prolapse. *Dis Colon Rectum*. 2008;51(11):1597–1604.

39. Cali RL, Pitsch RM, Blatchford GJ, et al. Rare pelvic floor hernias. Report of a case and review of the literature. *Dis Colon Rectum*. 1992;35(6):604–612.

40. Carpelan-Holmström M, Kruuna O, Scheinin T. Laparoscopic rectal prolapse surgery combined with short hospital stay is safe in elderly and debilitated patients. *Surg Endosc*. 2006;20(9):1353–1359.

41. Carter AE. Rectosacral suture fixation for complete rectal prolapse in the elderly, the frail and the demented. *Br J Surg*. 1983;70(9):522–523.

42. Chanvitan A, Nopanitaya W. Solitary rectal ulcer. Electron microscopy study of two cases. *Dis Colon Rectum*. 1986;29(6):421–425.

43. Chiang JM, Changchien CR, Chen JR. Solitary rectal ulcer syndrome: an endoscopic and histological presentation and literature review. *Int J Colorectal Dis*. 2006;21(4):348–356.

44. Chiarioni G, Whitehead WE, Pezza V, et al. Biofeedback is superior to laxatives for normal transit constipation due to pelvic floor dyssynergia. *Gastroenterology*. 2006;130(3):657–664.

45. Chino ES, Thomas CG Jr. Transsacral approach to repair of rectal prolapse in children. *Am Surg*. 1984;50(2):70–75.

46. Choi HJ, Shin EJ, Hwang YH, et al. Clinical presentation and surgical outcome in patients with solitary rectal ulcer syndrome. *Surg Innov*. 2005;12(4):307–313.

47. Choi JS, Hwang YH, Salum MR, et al. Outcome and management of patients with large rectoanal intussusception. *Am J Gastroenterol*. 2001;96(3):740–744.

48. Choi JS, Wexner SD, Nam YS, et al. Intraobserver and interobserver measurements of the anorectal angle and perineal descent in defecography. *Dis Colon Rectum*. 2000;43(8):1121–1126.

49. Christiansen J, Kirkegaard P. Complete prolapse of the rectum treated by modified Orr operation. *Dis Colon Rectum*. 1981;24(2):90–92.

50. Chun SW, Pilarsky AJ, You SY, et al. Perineal rectosigmoidectomy for rectal prolapse: role of levatorplasty. *Dis Colon Rectum*. 2001;44:A5–A26.

51. Chun SW, Pikarsky AJ, You SY, et al. Perineal rectosigmoidectomy for rectal prolapse: role of levatorplasty. *Tech Coloproctol*. 2004;8(1):3–9.

52. Collinson R, Cunningham C, D'Costa H, et al. Rectal intussusception and unexplained faecal incontinence: findings of a proctographic study. *Colorectal Dis*. 2009;11(1):77–83.

53. Collinson R, Wijffels N, Cunningham C, et al. Laparoscopic ventral rectopexy for internal rectal prolapse: short-term functional results. *Colorectal Dis*. 2010;12(2):97–104.

54. Collopy BT, Barham KA. Abdominal colporectopexy with pelvic cul-de-sac closure. *Dis Colon Rectum*. 2002;45(4):522–526.

55. Corman ML, Carriero A, Hager T, et al. Consensus conference on the stapled transanal rectal resection (STARR) for disordered defaecation. *Colorectal Dis*. 2006;8(2):98–101.

56. Corman ML, Veidenheimer MC, Coller JA. Managing rectal prolapse. *Geriatrics*. 1974;29(10):87–93.

57. Cosman BC, Lackides GA, Fisher DP, et al. Use of tissue expander for tamponade of presacral hemorrhage. Report of a case. *Dis Colon Rectum*. 1994;37(7):723–726.

58. Davidian VA Jr, Thomas CG Jr. Trans-sacral repair of rectal prolapse. Efficacy of treatment in thirty consecutive patients. *Am J Surg*. 1972;123(2):231–235.

59. Deen KI, Grant E, Billingham C, et al. Abdominal resection rectopexy with pelvic floor repair versus perineal rectosigmoidectomy and pelvic floor repair for full-thickness rectal prolapse. *Br J Surg*. 1994;81(2):302–304.

60. de Hoog DE, Heemskerk J, Nieman FH, et al. Recurrence and functional results after open versus conventional laparoscopic versus robot-assisted laparoscopic rectopexy for rectal prolapse: a case–control study. *Int J Colorectal Dis*. 2009;24(10):1201–1206.

61. DeLancey JO. Anatomic aspects of vaginal eversion after hysterectomy. *Am J Obstet Gynecol*. 1992;166(6 pt 1):1717–1724.

62. DeLancey JO. Structural anatomy of the posterior pelvic compartment as it relates to rectocele. *Am J Obstet Gynecol*. 1999;180(4):815–823.

63. Delemarre JB, Gooszen HG, Kruyt RH, et al. The effect of posterior rectopexy on fecal continence. A prospective study. *Dis Colon Rectum*. 1991;34(4):311–316.

64. Delorme R. Sur le traitment des prolapsus de la muqueuse rectale ou recto colique. *Bull Soc Chir Paris*. 1900;26:459.

65. Devadhar DS. A new operative treatment for complete prolapse rectum. *J Christ Med Assoc India*. 1961;36:18–23.

66. Devadhar DS. New thoughts on the mechanism and treatment of rectal procidentia. *J Int Coll Surg*. 1964;42:672–681.

67. Devadhar DS. A new concept of mechanism and treatment of rectal procidentia. *Dis Colon Rectum*. 1965;8:75–77.

68. D'Hoore A. New surgical techniques to correct rectal prolapse syndromes. *Acta Biomedica Lovansiensia*. 2007;395:1–208. Leuven University Press.

69. D'Hoore A, Cadoni R, Penninckx F. Long-term outcome of laparoscopic ventral rectopexy for total rectal prolapse. *Br J Surg*. 2004;91(11): 1500–1505.

70. D'Hoore A, Vanbeckevoort D, Penninckx F. Clinical, physiological and radiological assessment of rectovaginal septum reinforcement with mesh for complex rectocele. *Br J Surg*. 2008;95(10):1264–1272.

71. Dietz HP, Korda A. Which bowel symptoms are most strongly associated with a true rectocele? *Aust N Z J Obstet Gynaecol*. 2005;45(6): 505–508.

72. Dippolito A, Esser S, Reed J III. Anterior modification of Delorme procedure provides equivalent results to Delorme procedure in treatment of rectal outlet obstruction. *Curr Surg*. 2005;62(6):609–612.

73. Doershuk C, Boat TF. Infectious croup (Acute nondiptheritic infections). In: Behrman RE, Vaughan VC, eds. *Nelson's Textbook of Pediatrics*. 12th ed. Philadelphia, PA: WB Saunders; 1983:1097.

74. Dolk A, Brodén G, Holmström B, et al. Slow transit of the colon associated with severe constipation after the Ripstein operation. A clinical and physiologic study. *Dis Colon Rectum*. 1990;33(9):786–790.

75. Douard R, Frileux P, Brunel M, et al. Functional results after the Orr-Loygue transabdominal rectopexy for complete rectal prolapse. *Dis Colon Rectum*. 2003;46(8):1089–1096.

76. Douglas BS, Douglas HM. Rectal prolapse in the Ehlers-Danlos syndrome. *Aust Paediatr J*. 1973;9(2):109–110.

77. Draaisma WA, Nieuwenhuis DH, Janssen LW, et al. Robot-assisted laparoscopic rectovaginopexy for rectal prolapse: a prospective cohort study on feasibility and safety. *J Robotic Surg*. 2008;1(4):273–277.

78. Duff JH, Wright FF. Acute and chronic ulcers of the rectum. *Surg Gynecol Obstet*. 1981;153(3):398–400.

79. Dulucq JL, Wintringer P, Mahajna A. Clinical and functional outcome of laparoscopic posterior rectopexy (Wells) for full-thickness rectal prolapse. A prospective study. *Surg Endosc*. 2007;21(12):2226–2230.

80. Dunphy JE. A combined perineal and abdominal operation for the repair of rectal prolapse. *Surg Gynecol Obstet*. 1948;86(4):493–498.

81. Dunphy JE, Botsford TW, Savlov E. Surgical treatment of procidentia of the rectum: an evaluation of combined abdominal and perineal repair. *Am J Surg*. 1953;86(5):605–607.

82. Dutta BN, Das AK. Treatment of prolapse rectum in children with injections of sclerosing agents. *J Indian Med Assoc*. 1977;69(12): 275–276.

83. Dvorkin LS, Hetzer F, Scott SM, et al. Open-magnet MR defaecography compared with evacuation proctography in the diagnosis and management of patients with rectal intussusception. *Colorectal Dis*. 2004;6(1):45–53.

84. Earnshaw JJ, Hopkinson BR. Late results of silicone rubber perianal suture for rectal prolapse. *Dis Colon Rectum*. 1987;30(2):86–88.

85. Ederle A, Bulighin G, Orlandi PG, et al. Endoscopic application of human fibrin sealant in the treatment of solitary ulcer syndrome [letter]. *Endoscopy*. 1992;24(8):736–737.

86. Ejerblad S, Krause U. Repair of rectal prolapse by rectosacral suture fixation. *Acta Chir Scand*. 1988;154(2):103–105.

87. Evans C, Jones OM, Cunningham C, et al. Managing solitary rectal ulcer syndrome: Ignore the ulcer, treat the underlying posterior compartment prolapse. *Colorectal Dis*. 2010;12(suppl 1):16.

88. Farouk R, Duthie GS, MacGregor AB, et al. Rectoanal inhibition and incontinence in patients with rectal prolapse. *Br J Surg*. 1994;81(5): 743–746.

89. Fleming FJ, Kim MJ, Gunzler D, et al. It's the procedure not the patient: the operative approach is independently associated with an increased risk of complications after rectal prolapse repair. *Colorectal Dis*. 2012;14(3):362–368.

90. Franchelli L, Jones OM, Cunningham C, et al. No difference in patients with external rectal prolapse with and without bowel functional disturbance (unpublished). 2009.

91. Franzin G, Dina R, Scarpa A, et al. "The evolution of the solitary ulcer of the rectum"—an endoscopic and histopathological study. *Endoscopy*. 1982;14(4):131–134.

92. Friedman R, Muggia-Sulam M, Freund HR. Experience with the one-stage perineal repair of rectal prolapse. *Dis Colon Rectum.* 1983;26(12):789–791.

93. Frykman HM, Goldberg SM. The surgical treatment of rectal procidentia. *Surg Gynecol Obstet.* 1969;129(6):1225–1230.

94. Goei R, van Engelshoven J, Schouten H, et al. Anorectal function: defecographic measurement in asymptomatic subjects. *Radiology.* 1989;173(1):137–141.

95. Goldman J. Über Mastdarmvorfall mit besonderer berücksichtigung der Thierschschen Operation. Inaugural dissertation before the Faculty of Medicine at Kaiser-Wilhelms University, Strassburg. Strassburg: BC Goelle. *Dis Colon Rectum.* 1892;31(154).

96. Goligher JC. Rectal prolapse. In: Goligher JC, Duthie HL, Nixon HH, eds. *Surgery of the Anus, Rectum and Colon.* 3rd ed. London, United Kingdom: Balliere Tindall; 1975:293.

97. Gooley NA, Kuhnke M, Eusebio EB. Acute transanal ileal evisceration. *Dis Colon Rectum.* 1987;30(6):479–481.

98. Gopal KA, Amshel AL, Shonberg IL, et al. Rectal procidentia in elderly and debilitated patients. Experience with the Altemeier procedure. *Dis Colon Rectum.* 1984;27(6):376–381.

99. Gordon PH, Hoexter B. Complications of the Ripstein procedure. *Dis Colon Rectum.* 1978;21(4):277–280.

100. Graf W, Stefánsson T, Arvidsson D, et al. Laparoscopic suture rectopexy. *Dis Colon Rectum.* 1995;38(2):211–212.

101. Graham RR. The operative repair of massive rectal prolapse. *Ann Surg.* 1942;115(6):1007–1014.

102. Greenberg T, Kelvin FM, Maglinte DD. Barium trapping in rectoceles: are we trapped by the wrong definition? *Abdom Imaging.* 2001;26(6):587–590.

103. Greene FL. Repair of rectal prolapse using a puborectal sling procedure. *Arch Surg.* 1983;118(4):398–401.

104. Groff DB, Nagaraj HS. Rectal prolapse in infants and children. *Am J Surg.* 1990;160(5):531–532.

105. Gundersen AL, Cogbill TH, Landercasper J. Reappraisal of Delorme's procedure for rectal prolapse. *Dis Colon Rectum.* 1985;78(10):721–724.

106. Halligan S, Nicholls RJ, Bartram CI. Proctographic changes after rectopexy for solitary rectal ulcer syndrome and preoperative predictive factors for a successful outcome. *Br J Surg.* 1995;82(3):314–317.

107. Halligan S, Sultan A, Rottenberg G, et al. Endoscopy of the anal sphincters in solitary rectal ulcer syndrome. *Int J Colorectal Dis.* 1995;10(2):79–82.

108. Harmston C, Wijffels NA, Cunningham C, et al. Colonic slow transit has no impact on the results of laparoscopic anterior rectopexy for internal rectal prolapse [abstract]. *Colorectal Dis.* 2009;11(suppl 1):7.

109. Harris MA, Ferrara A, Gallagher J, et al. Stapled transanal rectal resection vs. transvaginal rectocele repair for treatment of obstructive defecation syndrome. *Dis Colon Rectum.* 2009;52(4):592–597.

110. Harrison JL, Hooks VH, Pearl RK, et al. Muscle fragment welding for control of massive presacral bleeding during rectal mobilization: a review of eight cases. *Dis Colon Rectum.* 2003;46(8):1115–1117.

111. Haskell B, Rovner H. A modified Thiersch operation for complete rectal prolapse using a Teflon prosthesis. *Dis Colon Rectum.* 1963;6:192–195.

112. Heald C. A simple, bloodless operation for anorectal prolapse in children. *Surg Gynecol Obstet.* 1926;42:840.

113. Hendrix SL, Clark A, Nygaard I, et al. Pelvic organ prolapse in the Women's Health Initiative: gravity and gravidity. *Am J Obstet Gynecol.* 2002;186(6):1160–1166.

114. Henry LG, Cattey RP. Rectal prolapse. *Surg Laparosc Endosc.* 1994;4(5):357–360.

115. Henry MM, Parks AG, Swash M. The pelvic floor musculature in the descending perineum syndrome. *Br J Surg.* 1982;69(8):470–472.

116. Henschen C. Ueber den Ersatz des Thierschschen Drahtringes bei der Operation des Mastdarmvorfalls durch geflochtene Seidenriemen, frei überpflanzte gefäss-sehnenperiost-oder Faszien Stücke. *Munchen Med Wochenschr.* 1912;59:128.

117. Heriot AG, Skull A, Kumar D. Functional and physiological outcome following transanal repair of rectocele. *Br J Surg.* 2004;91(10):1340–1344.

118. Hight DW, Hertzler JH, Philippart AI, et al. Linear cauterization for the treatment of rectal prolapse in infants and children. *Surg Gynecol Obstet.* 1982;154(3):400–402.

119. Hill AD, Menzies-Gow N, Darzi A. Methods of controlling presacral bleeding. *J Am Coll Surg.* 1994;178(2):183–184.

120. Hiltunen KM, Matikainen M, Auvinen O, et al. Clinical and manometric evaluation of anal sphincter function in patients with rectal prolapse. *Am J Surg.* 1986;151(4):489–492.

121. Holmström B, Ahlberg J, Bergstrand O, et al. Results of the treatment of rectal prolapse operated according to Ripstein. *Acta Chir Scand.* 1978;482:51–52.

122. Holmström B, Brodén G, Dolk A, et al. Increased anal resting pressure following the Ripstein operation. A contribution to continence? *Dis Colon Rectum.* 1986;29(8):485–487.

123. Holzer B, Rosen HR, Novi G, et al. Sacral nerve stimulation in patients with severe constipation. *Dis Colon Rectum.* 2008;51(5):524–529.

124. Hompes R, Harmston C, Wijffels N, et al. Excellent response rate of anismus to Botulinum toxin if rectal prolapse misdiagnosed as anismus on proctography ('pseudoanismus') is excluded. *Colorectal Dis.* 2011;14(2):224–230.

125. Hompes R, Jones OM, Cunningham C, et al. What causes chronic idiopathic perineal pain? *Colorectal Disease.* 2010;13(9):1035–1039. doi:10.1111/j.1463-1318.2010.02422.x.

126. Hopkinson BR, Hardman J. Silicone rubber perianal suture for rectal prolapse. *Proc R Soc Med.* 1973;66(11):1095–1098.

127. Hsu A, Brand MI, Saclarides TJ. Laparoscopic rectopexy without resection: a worthwhile treatment for rectal prolapse in patients with prior constipation. *Am Surg.* 2007;73(9):858–861.

128. Hughes E. Discussion on rectal prolapse of the rectum. *Proc R Soc Med.* 1949;421:1007.

129. Hunt TM, Fraser IA, Maybury NK. Treatment of rectal prolapse by sphincteric support using silastic rods. *Br J Surg.* 1985;72(6):491–492.

130. Hwang YH, Person B, Choi JS, et al. Biofeedback therapy for rectal intussusception. *Tech Coloproctol.* 2006,10(1).11 16.

131. Impieri M, Zambarda E. Rectal prolapse in a child with Peutz-Jeghers syndrome. *Acta Gastroenterol Belg.* 1982;45(9–10):429–433.

132. Janssen LW, van Dijke CF. Selection criteria for anterior rectal wall repair in symptomatic rectocele and anterior rectal wall prolapse. *Dis Colon Rectum.* 1994;37(11):1100–1107.

133. Jayne D, Schwandner O, Stuto A. Stapled transanal rectal resection for obstructed defecation syndrome: one-year results of the European STARR Registry. *Dis Colon Rectum.* 2009;52(7):1205–1212.

134. Jenkins SG Jr, Thomas CG Jr. An operation for the repair of rectal prolapse. *Surg Gynecol Obstet.* 1962;114:381–383.

135. Johansen OB, Wexner SD, Daniel N, et al. Perineal rectosigmoidectomy in the elderly *Dis Colon Rectum.* 1993;36(8):767–772.

136. Johansson C, Ihre T, Ahlbäck SO. Disturbances in the defecation mechanism with special reference to intussusception of the rectum (internal procidentia). *Dis Colon Rectum.* 1985;28(12):920–924.

137. Johnson E, Stangeland A, Johannessen HO, et al. Resection rectopexy for external rectal prolapse reduces constipation and anal incontinence. *Scand J Surg.* 2007;96(1):56–61.

138. Jorge JM, Wexner SD, Ehrenpreis ED, et al. Does perineal descent correlate with pudendal neuropathy? *Dis Colon Rectum.* 1993;36(5):475–483.

139. Jurgeleit HC, Corman ML, Coller JA, et al. Procidentia of the rectum: teflon sling repair of rectal prolapse, Lahey Clinic experience. *Dis Colon Rectum.* 1975;18(6):464–467.

140. Kairaluoma MV, Viljakka MT, Kellokumpu, IH. Open vs. laparoscopic surgery for rectal prolapse: a case-controlled study assessing short-term outcome. *Dis Colon Rectum.* 2003;46(3):353–360.

141. Kaiwa Y, Kurokawa Y, Namiki K, et al. Outcome of laparoscopic rectopexy for complete rectal prolapse in patients older than 70 years versus younger patients. *Surg Today.* 2004;34(9):742–746.

142. Kang YS, Kamm MA, Nicholls RJ. Solitary rectal ulcer and complete rectal prolapse: one condition or two? *Int J Colorectal Dis.* 1995;10(2):87–90.

143. Karas JR, Uranues S, Altomare DF, et al. No rectopexy versus rectopexy following rectal mobilization for full-thickness rectal prolapse: a randomized controlled trial. *Dis Colon Rectum.* 2011;54(1):29–34.

144. Kay NR, Zachary RB. The treatment of rectal prolapse in children with injections of 30 percent saline solutions. *J Pediatr Surg.* 1970;5(3):334–337.

145. Keighley MR, Matheson DM. Results of treatment for rectal prolapse and fecal incontinence. *Dis Colon Rectum.* 1981;24(6):449–453.

146. Keighley MR, Shouler P. Clinical and manometric features of the solitary rectal ulcer syndrome. *Dis Colon Rectum.* 1984;27(8):507–512.

147. Keighley MR, Shouler PJ. Abnormalities of colonic function in patients with rectal prolapse and faecal incontinence. *Br J Surg.* 1984;71(11):892–895.

148. Kelvin FM, Maglinte DD, Hale DS, et al. Female pelvic organ prolapse: a comparison of triphasic dynamic MR imaging and triphasic fluoroscopic cystocolpoproctography. *AJR Am J Roentgenol.* 2000;174(1):81–88.

149. Kelvin FM, Maglinte DD, Hornback JA, et al. Pelvic prolapse: assessment with evacuation proctography (defecography). *Radiology.* 1992;184(2):547–551.

150. Kerkhof MH, Hendriks L, Brölmann HA. Changes in connective tissue in patients with pelvic organ prolapse—a review of the current literature. *Int Urogynecol J Pelvic Floor Dysfunct.* 2009;20(4):461–474.

151. Kessler H, Hohenberger W. Laparoscopic resection rectopexy for rectal prolapse. *Dis Colon Rectum.* 2005;48(9):1800–1801.

152. Khan FA, Fang DT, Nivatvongs S. Management of presacral bleeding during rectal resection. *Surg Gynecol Obstet.* 1987;165(3):274–276.

153. Khanduja KS, Hardy TG Jr, Aguilar PS, et al. A new silicone prosthesis in the modified Thiersch operation. *Dis Colon Rectum.* 1988;31(5):380–383.

154. Kimmins MH, Evetts BK, Isler J, et al. The Altemeier repair: outpatient treatment of rectal prolapse. *Dis Colon Rectum.* 2001;44(4):565–570.

155. Kling KM, Rongione AJ, Evans B, et al. The Delorme procedure: a useful operation for complicated rectal prolapse in the elderly. *Am Surg.* 1996;62(10):857–860.

156. Koh CE, Young CJ, Young JM, et al. Systematic review of randomized controlled trials of the effectiveness of biofeedback for pelvic floor dysfunction. *Br J Surg.* 2008;95(9):1075–1087.

157. Kraske P. Zur Exstirpation hochsitzender Mastdarmkrebse. *Verh Dtsch Ges Chir.* 1885;14:464.

158. Kuijpers HC, Mollen M. Invited commentary. *Dis Colon Rectum.* 2002;45:526.

159. Kuijpers HC, Schreve RH, ten Cate Hoedemakers H. Diagnosis of functional disorders of defecation causing the solitary ulcer syndrome. *Dis Colon Rectum.* 1986;29(2):126–129.

160. Kulczycki LL, Shwachman H. Studies in cystic fibrosis of the pancreas: occurrence of rectal prolapse. *N Engl J Med.* 1958;259(9):409–412.

161. Kwok SP, Carey DP, Lau WY, et al. Laparoscopic rectopexy. *Dis Colon Rectum.* 1994;37(9):947–948.

162. Labow S, Rubin RJ, Hoexter B, et al. Perineal repair of rectal procidentia with an elastic fabric sling. *Dis Colon Rectum.* 1980;23(7):467–469.

163. Ladha A, Lee P, Berger P. Use of Angelchik Anti-Reflux Prosthesis for repair of total rectal prolapse in elderly patients. *Dis Colon Rectum.* 1985;28(1):5–7.

164. Lake SP, Hancock BD, Lewis AA. Management of pelvic sepsis after Ivalon rectopexy. *Dis Colon Rectum.* 1984;27(9):589–590.

165. Lamesch AJ. An unusual hamartomatous malformation of the rectosigmoid presenting as an irreducible rectal prolapse and necessitating rectosigmoid resection in a 14-week-old infant. *Dis Colon Rectum.* 1983;26(7):452–457.

166. Lane RH. Clinical application of anorectal physiology. *Proc R Soc Med.* 1975;68(1):28–30.

167. Laubert T, Kleemann M, Schorcht A, et al. Laparoscopic resection rectopexy for rectal prolapse: a single-center study during 16 years. *Surg Endosc.* 2010;24(10):2401–2406.

168. Launer DP, Fazio VW, Weakley FL, et al. The Ripstein procedure: a 16-year experience. *Dis Colon Rectum.* 1982;25(1):41–45.

169. Lechaux D, Trebuchet G, Siproudhis L, et al. Laparoscopic rectopexy for full-thickness rectal prolapse: a single-institution retrospective study evaluating surgical outcome. *Surg Endosc.* 2005;19(4):514–518.

170. Lechaux JP, Lechaux D, Perez M. Results of Delorme's procedure for rectal prolapse. Advantages of a modified technique. *Dis Colon Rectum.* 1995;38(3):301–307.

171. Lee SH, Lakhtaria P, Canedo J, et al. Outcome of laparoscopic rectopexy versus perineal rectosigmoidectomy for full-thickness rectal prolapse in elderly patients. *Surg Endosc.* 2011;25(8):2699–2702.

172. Lehur PA, Stuto A, Fantoli M, et al. Outcomes of stapled transanal rectal resection vs. biofeedback for the treatment of outlet obstruction associated with rectal intussusception and rectocele: a multicenter, randomized, controlled trial. *Dis Colon Rectum.* 2008;51(11):1611–1618.

173. Lescher TJ, Corman ML, Coller JA, et al. Management of late complications of Teflon sling repair for rectal prolapse. *Dis Colon Rectum.* 1979;22(7):445–447.

174. Leventog;ablu S, Mentes BB, Akin M, et al. Transperineal rectocele repair with polyglycolic acid mesh: a case series. *Dis Colon Rectum.* 2007;50(12):2085–2092.

175. Levine DS. "Solitary" rectal ulcer syndrome. Are "solitary" rectal ulcer syndrome and "localized" colitis cystica profunda analogous syndromes caused by rectal prolapse? *Gastroenterology.* 1987;93(1):243–253.

176. Lockhart-Mummery P. *Diseases of the Rectum and Anus.* New York, NY: William Wood; 1914.

177. Lomas MI, Cooperman H. Correction of rectal procidentia by use of polypropylene mesh (Marlex). *Dis Colon Rectum.* 1972;15(6):416–419.

178. Loygue J, Huguier M, Malafosse M, et al. Complete prolapse of the rectum. A report on 140 cases treated by rectopexy. *Br J Surg.* 1971;58(11):847–848.

179. Loygue J, Nordlinger B, Cunci O, et al. Rectopexy to the promontory for the treatment of rectal prolapse. Report of 257 cases. *Dis Colon Rectum.* 1984;27(6):356–359.

180. Luber KM, Boero S, Choe JY. The demographics of pelvic floor disorders: current observations and future projections. *Am J Obstet Gynecol.* 2001;184(7):501–503.

181. MacLennan AH, Taylor AW, Wilson DH, et al. The prevalence of pelvic floor disorders and their relationship to gender, age, parity and mode of delivery. *BJOG.* 2000;107(12):1460–1470.

182. Madiba TE, Baig MK, Wexner SD. Surgical management of rectal prolapse. *Arch Surg.* 2005;140(1):63–73.

183. Madigan M. Solitary ulcer of the rectum. *Proc R Soc Med.* 1964;57:403.

184. Madigan MR, Morson BC. Solitary ulcer of the rectum. *Gut.* 1969;10(11):871–881.

185. Maher C, Baessler K, Glazener CM, et al. Surgical management of pelvic organ prolapse in women. *Cochrane Database Syst Rev.* 2007;(3):CD004014.

186. Malouf AJ, Vaizey CJ, Kamm MA. Results of behavioral treatment (biofeedback) for solitary rectal ulcer syndrome. *Dis Colon Rectum.* 2001;44(1):72–76.

187. Malyshev YI, Gulin VA. Our experience with the treatment of rectal prolapse in infants and children. *Am J Proctol.* 1973;24(6):470–472.

188. Mann CV. Rectal prolapse. In: Morson BC, ed. *Diseases of the Colon, Rectum and Anus.* New York, NY: Appleton-Century-Crofts; 1969:238.

189. Mann CV, Hoffman C. Complete rectal prolapse: the anatomical and functional results of treatment by an extended abdominal rectopexy. *Br J Surg.* 1988;75(1):34–37.

190. Marchal F, Bresler L, Brunaud L, et al. Solitary rectal ulcer syndrome: a series of 13 patients operated with a mean follow-up of 4.5 years. *Int J Colorectal Dis.* 2001;16(4):228–233.

191. Marshall M, Halligan S, Fotheringham T, et al. Predictive value of internal anal sphincter thickness for diagnosis of rectal intussusception in patients with solitary rectal ulcer syndrome. *Br J Surg.* 2002;89(10):1281–1285.

192. Martin CJ, Parks TG, Biggart JD. Solitary rectal ulcer syndrome in Northern Ireland. 1971–1980. *Br J Surg.* 1981;68(10):744–747.

193. McCaffrey J. Delorme repair for prolapse of the rectum following "failed" Ripstein operation. *Am J Proctol Gastroenterol Colon Rectal Surg.* 1983;34:5.

194. McCue JL, Thomson JP. Rectopexy for internal rectal intussusception. *Br J Surg.* 1990;77(6):632–634.

195. McCue JL, Thomson JP. Clinical and functional results of abdominal rectopexy for complete rectal prolapse. *Br J Surg.* 1991;78(8):921–923.

196. McKee RF, Lauder JC, Poon FW, et al. A prospective randomized study of abdominal rectopexy with and without sigmoidectomy in rectal prolapse. *Surg Gynecol Obstet.* 1992;174(2):145–148.

197. McMahan JD, Ripstein CB. Rectal prolapse. An update on the rectal sling procedure. *Am Surg.* 1987;53(1):37–40.

198. Mellgren A, Dolk A, Johansson C, et al. Enterocele is correctable using the Ripstein rectopexy. *Dis Colon Rectum.* 1994;37(8):800–804.

199. Mellgren A, Johansson C, Dolk A, et al. Enterocele demonstrated by defaecography is associated with other pelvic floor disorders. *Int J Colorectal Dis.* 1994;9(3):121–124.

200. Mellgren A, López A, Schultz I, et al. Rectocele is associated with paradoxical anal sphincter reaction. *Int J Colorectal Dis.* 1998;13(1):13–16.

201. Mellgren A, Schultz I, Johansson C, et al. Internal rectal intussusception seldom develops into total rectal prolapse. *Dis Colon Rectum.* 1997;40(7):817–820.

202. Mercer-Jones MA, Sprowson A, Varma JS. Outcome after transperineal mesh repair of rectocele: a case series. *Dis Colon Rectum.* 2004;47(6):864–868.

203. Miliacca C, Gagliardi G, Pescatori M. The "Draw-the-Family Test" in the preoperative assessment of anorectal diseases and psychological distress: a prospective controlled study. *Colorectal Dis.* 2010;12(8):792–798.

204. Mollen RM, Kuijpers JH, van Hoek F. Effects of rectal mobilization and lateral ligaments division on colonic and anorectal function. *Dis Colon Rectum.* 2000;43(9):1283–1287.

205. Morgan CN, Porter NH, Klugman DJ. Ivalon (polyvinyl alcohol) sponge in the repair of complete rectal prolapse. *Br J Surg.* 1972;59(11):841–846.

206. Moschcowitz AV. The pathogenesis, anatomy, and cure of prolapse of the rectum. *Surg Gynecol Obstet.* 1912;15:7–21.

207. Munz Y, Moorthy K, Kudchadkar R, et al. Robotic assisted rectopexy. *Am J Surg.* 2004;187(1):88–92.

208. Myers A, Hompes R, Jones OM, et al. Rectal examination under anaesthetic (EUA) with a CAD device is superior to defaecating proctography in the assessment of rectal prolapse. *Colorect Dis.* 2011;13(suppl 2).

209. Myers JO, Rothenberger DA. Sugar in the reduction of incarcerated prolapsed bowel. Report of two cases. *Dis Colon Rectum*. 1991;34(5):416–418.

210. Nagata I, Murakami G, Suzuki D, et al. Histological features of the rectovaginal septum in elderly women and a proposal for posterior vaginal defect repair. *Int Urogynecol J Pelvic Floor Dysfunct*. 2007;18(8):863–868.

211. Narasanagi SS. Rectal prolapse in children. *J Indian Med Assoc*. 1974;62(11):378–380.

212. Nash DF. Bowel management in spina bifida patients. *Proc R Soc Med*. 1972;65(1):70–71.

213. National Institute for Health and Clinical Excellence. Stapled transanal rectal resection for obstructed defaecation syndrome: understanding NICE guidance—information for people considering the procedure, and for the public. *Interventional Procedure Guidance*. 2006;169.

214. Nay HR, Blair CR. Perineal surgical repair of rectal prolapse. *Am J Surg*. 1972;123(5):577–579.

215. Neill ME, Parks AG, Swash M. Physiological studies of the anal sphincter musculature in faecal incontinence and rectal prolapse. *Br J Surg*. 1981;68(8):531–536.

216. Nicholls RJ, Simson JN. Anteroposterior rectopexy in the treatment of solitary rectal ulcer syndrome without overt rectal prolapse. *Br J Surg*. 1986;73(3):222–224.

217. Nichols DH. Retrorectal levatorplasty for anal and perineal prolapse. *Surg Gynecol Obstet*. 1982;154(2):251–254.

218. Nicosia JF, Bass NM. Use of the fascial stapler in proctopexy for rectal prolapse. *Dis Colon Rectum*. 1987;30(11):900–901.

219. Nigro ND. An evaluation of the cause and mechanism of complete rectal prolapse. *Dis Colon Rectum*. 1966;9(6):391–398.

220. Nigro ND. A sling operation for rectal prolapse. *Proc R Soc Med*. 1970;63(suppl):106–107.

221. Nivatvongs S, Fang DT. The use of thumbtacks to stop massive presacral hemorrhage. *Dis Colon Rectum*. 1986;29(9):589–590.

222. Notaras MJ. The use of Mersilene mesh in rectal prolapse repair. *Proc R Soc Med*. 1973;66(7):684–686.

223. Novell JR, Osborne MJ, Winslet MC, et al. Prospective randomized trial of Ivalon sponge versus sutured rectopexy for full-thickness rectal prolapse. *Br J Surg*. 1994;81(6):904–906.

224. Nwako F. Rectal prolapse in Nigerian children. *Int Surg*. 1975;60(5):284–285.

225. Oettle GJ, Roe AM, Bartolo DC, et al. What is the best way of measuring perineal descent? A comparison of radiographic and clinical methods. *Br J Surg*. 1985;72(12):999–1001.

226. Oliver GC, Vachon D, Eisenstat TE, et al. Delorme's procedure for complete rectal prolapse in severely debilitated patients. An analysis of 41 cases. *Dis Colon Rectum*. 1994;37(5):461–467.

227. Olsen AL, Smith VJ, Bergstrom JO, et al. Epidemiology of surgically managed pelvic organ prolapse and urinary incontinence. *Obstet Gynecol*. 1997;89(4):501–506.

228. Ommer A, Albrecht K, Wenger F, et al. Stapled transanal rectal resection (STARR): a new option in the treatment of obstructive defecation syndrome. *Langenbecks Arch Surg*. 2006;391(1):32–37.

229. Oom DM, Gosselink MP, van Wijk JJ, et al. Rectocele repair by anterolateral rectopexy: long-term functional outcome. *Colorectal Dis*. 2008;10(9):925–930.

230. Orr T. A suspension operation for prolapse of the rectum. *Ann Surg*. 1947;126(5):833–837.

231. Orrom WJ, Bartolo DC, Miller R, et al. Rectopexy is an ineffective treatment for obstructed defecation. *Dis Colon Rectum*. 1991;34(1):41–46.

232. Palmer JA. Prolapse of the rectum: treatment by the Moschcowitz-Graham operation. *Can J Surg*. 1969;12(1):116–123.

233. Paraiso MF, Barber MD, Muir TW, et al. Rectocele repair: a randomized trial of three surgical techniques including graft augmentation. *Am J Obstet Gynecol*. 2006;195(6):1762–1771.

234. Paramore RH. The supports-in-chief of the female pelvic viscera. *J Obstet Gynaecol*. 1908;1(obstet gynaecol sect):195–214.

235. Paramore RH. The pelvic floor aperture: with an appendix. *J Obstet Gynaecol*. 1910;18(2):95–114.

236. Paramore RH. The Hunterian lecture on the intra-abdomino-pelvic pressure in man. *Lancet*. 1911;2:1677.

237. Parks A. Royal Society of Medicine, Section of Proctology: Meeting 27 November 1974. President's Address. Anorectal incontinence. *Proc R Soc Med*. 1975;68(11):681–690.

238. Parks AG, Porter NH, Hardcastle J. The syndrome of the descending perineum. *Proc R Soc Med*. 1966;59(6):477–482.

239. Penfold JC, Hawley PR. Experience of Ivalon-sponge implant for complete rectal prolapse at St. Mark's Hospital, 1960–1970. *Br J Surg*. 1972;59(11):846–848.

240. Perniola G, Shek C, Chong CC, et al. Defecation proctography and translabial ultrasound in the investigation of defecatory disorders. *Ultrasound Obstet Gynecol*. 2008;31(5):567–571.

241. Pescatori M, Maria G, Mattana C, et al. Clinical picture and pelvic floor physiology in the solitary rectal ulcer syndrome. *Dis Colon Rectum*. 1985;28(11):862–867.

242. Pescatori M, Quondamcarlo C. A new grading of rectal internal mucosal prolapse and its correlation with diagnosis and treatment. *Int J Colorectal Dis*. 1999;14(4–5):245–249.

243. Pescatori M, Spyrou M, Pulvirenti d'Urso A. A prospective evaluation of occult disorders in obstructed defecation using the 'iceberg diagram.' *Colorectal Dis*. 2006;8(9):785–789.

244. Plumley P. A modification to Thiersch's operation for rectal prolapse. *Br J Surg*. 1966;53(7):624–625.

245. Plusa SM, Charig JA, Balaji V, et al. Physiological changes after Delorme's procedure for full-thickness rectal prolapse. *Br J Surg*. 1995;82(11):1475–1478.

246. Pomerri F, Zuliani M, Mazza C, et al. Defecographic measurements of rectal intussusception and prolapse in patients and in asymptomatic subjects. *AJR Am J Roentgenol*. 2001;176(3):641–645.

247. Poole GV Jr, Pennell TC, Myers RT, et al. Modified Thiersch operation for rectal prolapse. Technique and results. *Am Surg*. 1985;51(4):226–229.

248. Portier G, Iovino F, Lazorthes F. Surgery for rectal prolapse: Orr-Loygue ventral rectopexy with limited dissection prevents postoperative-induced constipation without increasing recurrence. *Dis Colon Rectum*. 2006;49(8):1136–1140.

249. Portier G, Kirzin S, Cabarrot P, et al. The effect of abdominal ventral rectopexy on faecal incontinence and constipation in patients with internal intra-anal rectal intussusception. *Colorectal Dis*. 2011;13(8):914–917.

250. Prasad ML, Pearl RK, Abcarian H, et al. Perineal proctectomy, posterior rectopexy, and postanal levator repair for the treatment of rectal prolapse. *Dis Colon Rectum*. 1986;29(9):547–552.

251. Purkayastha S, Tekkis P, Athanasiou T, et al. A comparison of open vs. laparoscopic abdominal rectopexy for full-thickness rectal prolapse: a meta-analysis. *Dis Colon Rectum*. 2005;48(10):1930–1940.

252. Ragg J, McDonald R, Hompes R, et al. Isolated colonic inertia is not usually the cause of chronic constipation. *Colorectal Dis*. 2011;13(11):1299–1302.

253. Ramanujam PS, Venkatesh KS. Management of acute incarcerated rectal prolapse. *Dis Colon Rectum*. 1992;35(12):1154–1156.

254. Ramanujam PS, Venkatesh KS, Fietz MJ. Perineal excision of rectal procidentia in elderly high-risk patients. A ten-year experience. *Dis Colon Rectum*. 1994;37(10):1027–1030.

255. Rao SS, Ozturk R, De Ocampo S, et al. Pathophysiology and role of biofeedback therapy in solitary rectal ulcer syndrome. *Am J Gastroenterol*. 2006;101(3):613–618.

256. Rao SS, Seaton K, Miller M, et al. Randomized controlled trial of biofeedback, sham feedback, and standard therapy for dyssynergic defecation. *Clin Gastroenterol Hepatol*. 2007;5(3):331–338.

257. Renzi A, Izzo D, Di Sarno G, et al. Stapled transanal rectal resection to treat obstructed defecation caused by rectal intussusception and rectocele. *Int J Colorect Dis*. 2006;21(7):661–667.

258. Ripstein CB. The repair of massive rectal prolapse. *Surg Proc*. 1965;2:2.

259. Ripstein CB. Surgical care of massive rectal prolapse. *Dis Colon Rectum*. 1965;8:34–38.

260. Ripstein CB. Symposium: procidentia of the rectum: internal intussusception of the rectum (Stage I rectal prolapse). *Dis Colon Rectum*. 1975;18(6):458–460.

261. Ripstein CB, Lanter B. Etiology and surgical therapy of massive prolapse of the rectum. *Ann Surg*. 1963;157:259–264.

262. Ris F, Ragg J, Slater A, et al. Can proctographic criteria help predict the outcome of laparoscopic ventral rectopexy for internal rectal prolapse [abstract]? *Colorectal Dis*. 2011;13(suppl 2):x.

263. Rogers J, Jeffery PJ. Postanal repair and intersphincteric Ivalon sponge rectopexy for the treatment of rectal prolapse. *Br J Surg*. 1987;74(5):384–386.

264. Roman H, Michot F. Long-term outcomes of transanal rectocele repair. *Dis Colon Rectum*. 2005;48(3):510–517.

265. Rose J, Schneider C, Scheidbach H, et al. Laparoscopic treatment of rectal prolapse: experience gained in a prospective multicenter study. *Langenbecks Arch Surg*. 2002;387(3–4):130–137.

266. Ross AH, Thomson JP. Management of infection after prosthetic abdominal rectopexy (Wells' procedure). *Br J Surg*. 1989;76(6):610–612.

267. Rutter KR, Riddell RH. The solitary ulcer syndrome of the rectum. *Clin Gastroenterol*. 1975;4(3):505–530.

268. Sainio AP, Halme LE, Husa AI. Anal encirclement with polypropylene mesh for rectal prolapse and incontinence. *Dis Colon Rectum*. 1991;34(10):905–908.

269. Sainio AP, Voutilainen PE, Husa AI. Recovery of anal sphincter function following transabdominal repair of rectal prolapse: cause of improved continence? *Dis Colon Rectum*. 1991;34(9):816–821.

270. Sajid MS, Siddiqui MR, Baig MK. Open vs laparoscopic repair of full-thickness rectal prolapse: a re-meta-analysis. *Colorectal Dis*. 2010;12(6):515–525.

271. Salkeld G, Bagia M, Solomon MJ. Economic impact of laparoscopic versus open abdominal rectopexy. *Br J Surg*. 2004;91(9):1188–1191.

272. Samaranayake CB, Luo C, Plank AW, et al. Systematic review on ventral rectopexy for rectal prolapse and intussusception. *Colorectal Dis*. 2009;12(6):504–512.

273. Samuelsson EC, Victor FT, Tibblin G, et al. Signs of genital prolapse in a Swedish population of women 20 to 59 years of age and possible related factors. *Am J Obstet Gynecol*. 1999;180(2 pt 1):299–305.

274. Santulli T. Rectal prolapse. In: Rudolph AM, Hoffman JI, eds. *Pediatrics*. 17th ed. Norwalk, CT: Appleton-Century-Crofts; 1983:990.

275. Saul SH, Sollenberger LC. Solitary rectal ulcer syndrome. Its clinical and pathological underdiagnosis. *Am J Surg Pathol*. 1985;9(6):411–421.

276. Sayfan J, Pinho M, Alexander-Williams J, et al. Sutured posterior abdominal rectopexy with sigmoidectomy compared with Marlex rectopexy for rectal prolapse. *Br J Surg*. 1990;77(2):143–145.

277. Schaffer JI, Wai CY, Boreham MK. Etiology of pelvic organ prolapse. *Clin Obstet Gynecol*. 2005;48(3):639–647.

278. Scherer R, Marti L, Hetzer F. Perineal stapled prolapse resection: a new procedure for external rectal prolapse. *Dis Colon Rectum*. 2008;51(11):1727–1730.

279. Schultz I, Mellgren A, Dolk A, et al. Continence is improved after the Ripstein rectopexy. Different mechanisms in rectal prolapse and rectal intussusception? *Dis Colon Rectum*. 1996;39(3):300–306.

280. Schultz I, Mellgren A, Oberg M, et al. Whole gut transit is prolonged after Ripstein rectopexy. *Eur J Surg*. 1999;165(3):242–247.

281. Schuster MM. The riddle of the sphincters. *Gastroenterology*. 1975;69(1):249–262.

282. Schwandner O, Farke S, Bruch HP. Stapled transanal rectal resection (STARR) for obstructed defecation caused by rectocele and rectoanal intussusception. *Viszeralchirurgie*. 2005;40:331–341.

283. Senapati A, Nicholls RJ, Thomson JP, et al. Results of Delorme's procedure for rectal prolapse. *Dis Colon Rectum*. 1994;37(5):456–460.

284. Shafik A. Pudendal canal decompression for the treatment of fecal incontinence in complete rectal prolapse. *Am Surg*. 1996;62(5):339–343.

285. Shorvon PJ, McHugh S, Diamant NE, et al. Defecography in normal volunteers: results and implications. *Gut*. 1989;30(12):1737–1749.

286. Silvis R, Gooszen HG, Kahraman T, et al. Novel approach to combined defaecation and micturition disorders with rectovaginovesicopexy. *Br J Surg*. 1998;85(6):813–817.

287. Sitzler PJ, Kamm MA, Nicholls RJ, et al. Long-term clinical outcome of surgery for solitary rectal ulcer syndrome. *Br J Surg*. 1998;85(9):1246–1250.

288. Slawik S, Soulsby R, Carter H, et al. Laparoscopic ventral rectopexy, posterior colporrhaphy and vaginal sacrocolpopexy for the treatment of recto-genital prolapse and mechanical outlet obstruction. *Colorectal Dis*. 2008;10(2):536–539.

289. Smart NJ, Mercer-Jones MA. Functional outcome after transperineal rectocele repair with porcine dermal collagen implant. *Dis Colon Rectum*. 2007;50(9):1422–1427.

290. Snooks SJ, Henry MM, Swash M. Anorectal incontinence and rectal prolapse: differential assessment of the innervation to puborectalis and external anal sphincter muscles. *Gut*. 1985;26(5):470–476.

291. Solomon MJ, Eyers AA. Laparoscopic rectopexy using mesh fixation with a spiked chromium staple. *Dis Colon Rectum*. 1996;39(3):279–284.

292. Solomon MJ, Young CJ, Eyers AA, et al. Randomized clinical trial of laparoscopic versus open abdominal rectopexy for rectal prolapse. *Br J Surg*. 2002;89(1):35–39.

293. Soriano LR, Del Mundo F, Naguit-Sim L. Rectal prolapse in children with trichuriasis. *J Philipp Med Assoc*. 1966;42(12):843–848.

294. Speakman CT, Madden MV, Nicholls RJ, et al. Lateral ligaments division during rectopexy causes constipation but prevents recurrence: results of a prospective randomized study. *Br J Surg*. 1991;78(12):1431–1433.

295. Spencer RJ. Manometric studies in rectal prolapse. *Dis Colon Rectum*. 1984;27(8):523–525.

296. Stern RC, Izant RJ Jr, Boat TF, et al. Treatment and prognosis of rectal prolapse in cystic fibrosis. *Gastroenterology*. 1982;82(4):707–710.

297. Stewart R. Long-term results of Ivalon wrap operation for complete rectal prolapse. *Proc R Soc Med*. 1972;65(9):777–778.

298. Subak LL, Waetjen LE, van den Eeden S, et al. Cost of pelvic organ prolapse surgery in the United States. *Obstet Gynecol*. 2001;98(4):646–651.

299. Sullivan ES, Garnjobst WM. Advantage of initial transanal mucosal stripping in ileo-anal pull-through procedures. *Dis Colon Rectum*. 1982;25(2):170–171.

300. Sullivan ES, Longaker CJ, Lee PY. Total pelvic mesh repair: a ten-year experience. *Dis Colon Rectum*. 2001;44(6):857–863.

301. Sullivan ES, Stranburg CO, Sandoz IL, et al. Repair of total pelvic prolapse: an overview. *Perspect Colon Rectal Surg*. 1990;3:119–131.

302. Sun WM, Read NW, Donnelly TC, et al. A common pathophysiology for full thickness rectal prolapse, anterior mucosal prolapse and solitary rectal ulcer. *Br J Surg*. 1989;76(3):290–295.

303. Swerdlow H. The encircler. A new instrument for the performance of the Thiersch procedure for rectal procidentia. *Dis Colon Rectum*. 1986;29(2):145–147.

304. Takano M, Hamada A. Evaluation of pelvic descent disorders by dynamic contrast roentgenography. *Dis Colon Rectum*. 2000;43(10 suppl):S6–S11.

305. Theuerkauf FJ Jr, Beahrs OH, Hill JR. Rectal prolapse. Causation and surgical treatment. *Ann Surg*. 1970;171(6):819–835.

306. Thompson JR, Chen AH, Pettit PD, et al. Incidence of occult rectal prolapse in patients with clinical rectoceles and defecatory dysfunction. *Am J Obstet Gynecol*. 2002;187(6):1494–1499.

307. Thomson G, Clark A, Handyside J, et al. Solitary ulcer of the rectum—or is it? A report of 6 cases. *Br J Surg*. 1981;68(1):21–24.

308. Thomson H, Hill D. Solitary rectal ulcer: always a self-induced condition? *Br J Surg*. 1980;67(11):784–785.

309. Thornton MJ, Lam A, King DW. Laparoscopic or transanal repair of rectocele? A retrospective matched cohort study. *Dis Colon Rectum*. 2005;48(4):792–798.

310. Tjandra JJ, Fazio VW, Church JM, et al. Ripstein procedure is an effective treatment for rectal prolapse without constipation. *Dis Colon Rectum*. 1993;36(5):501–507.

311. Tjandra JJ, Fazio VW, Petras RE, et al. Clinical and pathologic factors associated with delayed diagnosis in solitary rectal ulcer syndrome. *Dis Colon Rectum*. 1993;36(2):146–153.

312. Tjandra JJ, Ooi BS, Tang CL, et al. Transanal repair of rectocele corrects obstructed defecation if it is not associated with anismus. *Dis Colon Rectum*. 1999;42(12):1544–1550.

313. Tobin SA, Scott IH. Delorme operation for rectal prolapse. *Br J Surg*. 1994;81(11):1681–1684.

314. Todd IP. Etiological factors in the production of complete rectal prolapse. *Postgrad Med J*. 1959;35(400):97–100.

315. Traisman E, Conlon D, Sherman JO, et al. Rectal prolapse in two neonates with Hirschprung's disease. *Am J Dis Child*. 1983;137(11):1126–1127.

316. Traynor LA, Michener WM. Rectal procidentia—a rare complication of ulcerative colitis. Report of two cases in children. *Cleve Clin Q*. 1966;33(3):115–117.

317. Trompetto M, Clerico G, Realis Luc A, et al. Transanal Delorme procedure for treatment of rectocele associated with rectal intussusception. *Tech Coloproctol*. 2006;10(4):389.

318. Tsiaoussis J, Chrysos E, Athanasakis E, et al. Rectoanal intussusception: presentation of the disorder and late results of resection rectopexy. *Dis Colon Rectum*. 2005;48(4):838–844.

319. Tsujinaka S, Tsujinaka Y, Matsuo K, et al. Changes in bowel function following transanal and transvaginal rectocele repair. *Dig Surg*. 2007;24(1):46–53.

320. Tsunoda A, Yasuda N, Yokoyama N, et al. Delorme's procedure for rectal prolapse: clinical and physiological analysis. *Dis Colon Rectum*. 2003;46(9):1260–1265.

321. Uhlig BE, Sullivan ES. The modified Delorme operation: its place in surgical treatment for massive rectal prolapse. *Dis Colon Rectum*. 1979;22(8):513–521.

322. Vaizey CJ, van den Bogaerde JB, Emmanuel AV, et al. Solitary rectal ulcer syndrome. *Br J Surg*. 1998;85(12):1617–1623.

323. van den Brandt-Grädel V, Huibregtse K, Tytgat GN. Treatment of solitary rectal ulcer syndrome with high-fiber diet and abstention of straining at defecation. *Dig Dis Sci*. 1984;29(11):1005–1008.

324. van Outryve MJ, Pelckmans PA, Fierens H, et al. Transrectal ultrasound study of the pathogenesis of solitary rectal ulcer syndrome. *Gut*. 1993;34(10):1422–1426.

325. van Tets WF, Kuijpers JH. Internal rectal intussusception—fact or fancy? *Dis Colon Rectum*. 1995;38(10):1080–1083.

326. Vermeulen FD, Nivatvongs S, Fang DT, et al. A technique for perineal rectosigmoidectomy using autosuture devices. *Surg Gynecol Obstet*. 1983;156(1):84–86.

327. Vijay V, Halbert J, Zissimopoulos A, et al. Day case laparoscopic rectopexy is feasible, safe, and cost effective for selected patients. *Surg Endosc.* 2008;22(5):1237–1240.

328. Walter S, Bodemar G, Hallbook O, et al. Sympathetic (electrodermal) activity during repeated maximal rectal distensions in patients with irritable bowel syndrome and constipation. *Neurogastroenterol Motil.* 2008;20(1):43–52.

329. Watts AM, Thompson MR. Evaluation of Delorme's procedure as a treatment for full-thickness rectal prolapse. *Br J Surg.* 2000;87(2):218–222.

330. Wells C. New operation for rectal prolapse. *Proc R Soc Med.* 1959;52:602–603.

331. Wijffels NA, Collinson R, Cunningham C, et al. Internal rectal prolapse: occult by name, occult by nature [abstract]. *Colorectal Dis.* 2008;10(suppl 2):16.

332. Wijffels N, Collinson R, Cunningham C, et al. What is the natural history of internal rectal prolapse. *Colorectal Dis.* 2010;12(8):822–830.

333. Wijffels N, Cunningham C, Dixon A, et al. Laparoscopic ventral rectopexy for external rectal prolapse is safe and effective in the elderly. Does this make perineal procedures obsolete? *Colorectal Dis.* 2011;13(5). 561–566.

334. Williams JG, Rothenberger DA, Madoff RD, et al. Treatment of rectal prolapse in the elderly by perineal rectosigmoidectomy. *Dis Colon Rectum.* 1992;35(9):830–834.

335. Williams JG, Wong WD, Jensen L, et al. Incontinence and rectal prolapse: a prospective manometric study. *Dis Colon Rectum.* 1991;34(3):209–216.

336. Williams NS. Impact of new technology on anorectal disorders. *Br J Surg.* 1987;74(4):235–236.

337. Wilson J, Engledow A, Crosbie J, et al. Laparoscopic nonresectional suture rectopexy in the management of full-thickness rectal prolapse: substantive retrospective series. *Surg Endosc.* 2011;25(4):1062–1064.

338. Womack NR, Williams NS, Holmfield JH, et al. Pressure and prolapse—the cause of solitary rectal ulceration. *Gut.* 1987;28(10):1228–1233.

339. Womack NR, Williams NS, Mist JH, et al. Anorectal function in the solitary rectal ulcer syndrome. *Dis Colon Rectum.* 1987;30(5):319–323.

340. Wong MT, Meurette G, Rigaud J, et al. Robotic versus laparoscopic rectopexy for complex rectocele: a prospective comparison of short-term outcomes. *Dis Colon Rectum.* 2011;54(3):342–346.

341. Xu J, Lin J. Control of presacral hemorrhage with electrocautery through a muscle fragment pressed on the bleeding vein. *J Am Coll Surg.* 1994;179(3):351–352.

342. Xynos E, Chrysos E, Tsiaoussis J, et al. Resection rectopexy for rectal prolapse. The laparoscopic approach. *Surg Endosc.* 1999;13(9):862–864.

343. Yamana T, Iwadare J. Mucosal plication (Gant-Miwa procedure) with anal encircling for rectal prolapse—a review of the Japanese experience. *Dis Colon Rectum.* 2003;46(10 suppl):S94–S99.

344. Yoshioka K, Heyen F, Keighley MR. Functional results after posterior abdominal rectopexy for rectal prolapse. *Dis Colon Rectum.* 1989;32(10):835–838.

345. Yoshioka K, Hyland G, Keighley MR. Anorectal function after abdominal rectopexy: parameters of predictive value in identifying return of continence. *Br J Surg.* 1989;76(1):64–68.

346. Zainea GG, Szilagy EJ. Perineal repair of colorectoanal intussusception. Report of a case and review of the literature. *Dis Colon Rectum.* 1996;39(12):1434–1437.

347. Zargar SA, Khuroo MS, Mahajan R. Sucralfate retention enemas in solitary rectal ulcer. *Dis Colon Rectum.* 1991;34(6):455–457.

22

Colorectal Polyps

James M. Church and Matthew F. Kalady

If people are falling over the edge of a cliff and sustaining injuries, the problem could be dealt with by stationing ambulances at the bottom or erecting a fence at the top. Unfortunately, we put far too much effort into the provision of ambulances and far too little into the simple approach of erecting fences.

—DENIS BURKITT

A *polyp* is an abnormal projection above an epithelial surface. Polyps project from the surface of epithelium in many different organs, but this chapter discusses colorectal polyps and associated diseases. Colorectal polyps are diverse in appearance and histology. They may be pedunculated, sessile, or even depressed lesions with size varying from 1 to 2 mm to more than 10 cm. Polyp is merely a descriptive term and not a histologic diagnosis. Histologically, any of the tissues present in the colon can appear as a polyp including fat (lipoma), nerve (ganglioneuroma, schwannoma), muscle (leiomyoma), lymphoid tissue, and fibrous tissue (fibroma). Normal mucosa can look like a polyp, either just because it is raised or because it is made to be raised by peristalsis (mucosal prolapse), surrounding inflammation (pseudopolyp), or suction. Inflammation can cause polyps to form, in particular the very vascular granulation polyps that are found at recent anastomoses and in chronic colitis. Repeated trauma can also produce polypoid mucosa, as seen in variants of the solitary rectal ulcer syndrome. However, this chapter is dedicated to a discussion of the three most common and most important types of polyps found in the large intestine—those arising from overgrowth of epithelium. These include serrated (hyperplastic or metaplastic), hamartomatous, and adenomatous. Each polyp type has unique morphologic, clinical, and histologic traits and is associated with its own polyposis syndrome. These will be addressed later in this chapter.

▶ SERRATED POLYPS

In 1934, Westhues described a nonneoplastic mucosal lesion that came to be known in the United States as a hyperplastic polyp.[343] In England, polyps of similar histology were called metaplastic, a term introduced by Morson in 1962.[226] For the next 70 years, hyperplastic polyps were widely believed to be completely benign with no malignant potential. A few authors were suspicious of the role for hyperplastic polyps in colorectal carcinogenesis,[165] however, and in 1988 Fenoglio-Preiser and Longacre introduced the term *serrated adenoma* to describe polyps in which hyperplastic and adenomatous epithelium coexisted.[99,210] Since then, "serrated" has been increasingly used to refer to a family of lesions in which the crypt epithelium is thrown into serrations, as in a sawtooth pattern. Serrated polyps of the colon and rectum include all that were previously known as "hyperplastic." The World Health Organization (WHO) classification describes three main types of serrated lesions in the large intestine: hyperplastic polyp (HP), sessile serrated adenoma (also called sessile serrated polyp—SSA/P), and traditional serrated adenoma (TSA).[303] All of these polyps feature serrated epithelium but are distinguished based on crypt architecture and abnormalities of proliferation. HPs have normal-appearing crypts and a restricted basal proliferative zone (Figure 22-1), whereas SSA/Ps show distorted crypts and an irregular proliferative zone, which can be expanded or contracted (Figure 22-2). TSAs show ectopic or budded crypts with proliferation within the buds, but also feature adenomatous type dysplasia.[302] Although HPs are generally not precursors of cancer in themselves, they may serve as markers of a colon at risk for developing colorectal cancer. SSA/P and TSA, however, are definitely precursors of cancer. This changes the clinical approach to these lesions from "ignore" to "remove and follow."

BASIL MORSON (1921–PRESENT)

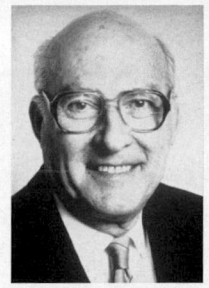

Basil Morson was born November 13, 1921. He enrolled in Oxford University in 1939 with the intent of studying medicine. However, in 1943 he deferred his degree and joined the British Royal Navy as an ordinary seaman. Within 6 months, he was promoted to sublieutenant. Upon demobilization, Morson returned to Oxford and qualified as a physician in 1949 before gaining his doctorate in 1955 with his thesis on intestinal metaplasia of the gastric mucosa. He ultimately succeeded Cuthbert Dukes as consultant histopathologist at St. Mark's Hospital, London, and served in that position for 30 years, 1956 to 1986. Among his notable academic achievements are a detailed description of the adenoma-carcinoma sequence (with Tetsuichiro Muto), the first description of large bowel Crohn's disease (with Sir Hugh Lockhart-Mummery), and the standard book of British gastrointestinal pathology, known colloquially as Morson and Dawson, now on its fifth edition. He is recognized throughout the world as the father of the specialty of gastrointestinal pathology. A prolific writer, he has been honored by both colleges and medical societies. He was made a fellow both of the Royal College of Surgeons of England and the Royal College of Physicians. He was awarded the John Hunter Medal of the Royal College of Surgeons in 1987 and served as president of the Proctology Section of the Royal Society of Medicine, president of the British Society of Gastroenterology, (BSG—the first pathologist so to be honored), and both vice president and honorary treasurer of the Royal College of Pathologists. He was made CBE (Commander of the British Empire) just after his retirement in 1987. More recently, he received the President's Medal of the British Division of the International Academy of Pathology (2005), a new award that has been introduced to honor a member of the division who has made an outstanding contribution to pathology education. The inaugural recipient was Basil Morson. Morson has left an indelible mark in gastrointestinal education in both pathology and clinical circles, the latter exemplified by the fact that he was the first pathologist to be elected as president of the British Society of Gastroenterology. Even though he has been retired officially for more than 20 years as of this writing, he continues to be active in gastrointestinal pathology education and is a regular attendee at the BSG meetings. At that gathering, there is an annual Basil Morson Lecture, given in his honor by eminent gastrointestinal pathologists from the United Kingdom and abroad. (Courtesy of Robin K.S. Phillips.)

Genetics

Serrated polyps have a different genetic origin from that of adenomas and lead to cancers with a different and specific genetic makeup. Although every colorectal cancer is genetically unique, there are three basic genetic mechanisms by which they arise: chromosomal instability (CIN), DNA mismatch repair deficiency, and DNA promoter hypermethylation. Methylation underlies serrated polyps. DNA methylation is a normal mechanism by which gene expression is controlled. Methylation inhibits expression, so hypermethylation suppresses gene expression, and hypomethylation amplifies it. DNA is normally methylated at CpG dinucleotides, which tend to be concentrated in promoter regions of genes. Promoter methylation abrogates gene expression, and if the gene is a tumor suppressor gene, it encourages carcinogenesis. Widespread DNA hypermethylation is evidence of the CpG island methylator phenotype (CIMP)[341] and is involved in about 23% of all colorectal cancer.[287] CIMP cancers arise from serrated polyps, in particular SSA/P. Figure 22-3 shows one suggested genetic pathway causing serrated lesions in which the early event is a mutation in *BRAF*, leading to the formation of HPs. The addition of methylation produces an SSA/P that can also develop dysplasia. Promoter methylation of the mismatch repair gene *MLH1* seems to be the final step leading to CIMP cancer in SSA/Ps. This creates an overlap between the mismatch repair (MMR) dysfunction and methylator mechanisms of carcinogenesis because some CIMP cancers do not express *MLH1* and are microsatellite unstable.[7] An alternative, albeit less prevalent serrated pathway, involves a *KRAS* mutation as the initiating event with a traditional serrated adenoma as an intermediate lesion. This pathway is believed to yield a microsatellite stable colorectal cancer.

Clinical Profiles

The three types of serrated polyps have different clinical profiles. Hyperplastic polyps are usually found in the rectum and sigmoid colon, often at the summit of mucosal folds and on the apex of the valves of Houston. At least one HP is found in 12% of colonoscopic examinations, although this

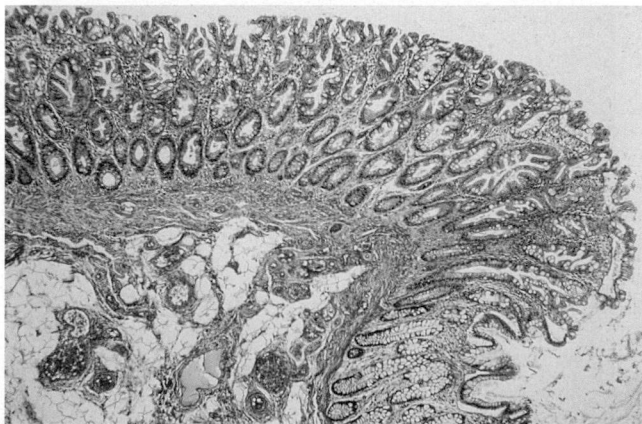

FIGURE 22-1. Hyperplastic (metaplastic) polyp. Note the hyperplastic changes in the mucosa and the serrated glands near the surface with papillary projections. (Original magnification × 240; from Corman ML, Veidenheimer MC, Swinton NW. *Diseases of the Anus, Rectum, and Colon. Part I: Neoplasms.* New York, NY: Medcom; 1972, with permission.)

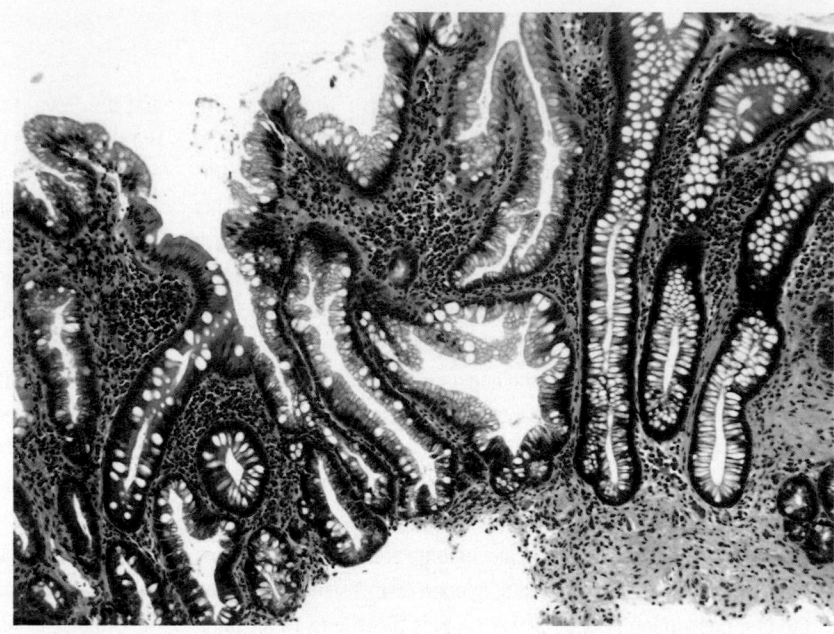

FIGURE 22-2. Sessile serrated adenoma/polyp (SSA/P). Note the branching irregular crypts and distorted proliferative zone that characterize this lesion. (Original magnification × 100.)

is likely to be an underestimate because they can be difficult to see and often may be ignored.[140] There are few data on detection rates or endoscopic recognition of any of the serrated polyps, and those that are available generally do not distinguish between HP, SSA/P, or TSA. HPs are often multiple. More than 20 polyps qualify for the diagnosis of serrated polyposis.[303] The majority of HPs are usually small (2 to 5 mm), are often pale or whitish, and sometimes have a translucent appearance that causes them to disappear when the colon is insufflated with air (Figure 22-4).

In contrast, SSA/Ps are more commonly located in the right colon. They are less numerous than HPs but are also often associated with synchronous polyps, including other serrated polyps and adenomas. They are often more than 1 cm in diameter and sometimes more than 3 cm. They can be difficult to see because they have an indistinct border and have the same coloring as the surrounding mucosa. They have an innocent crypt pattern that sometimes suggests an edematous fold (Figure 22-5). Many SSA/Ps have a "cap" of tenacious mucus that is characteristic and provides a clue to their presence (Figure 22-6).

TSA is much less common than either HP or SSA/P, being found in less than 1% of colonoscopies. They are generally difficult to pick out endoscopically and, therefore, are usually an unsuspected finding for endoscopists when the pathology report is received. Morphologically, they tend to be more polypoid than SSA/Ps and more discrete.

Evaluation and Management

The approach to serrated lesions of the colon and rectum has changed considerably over the last 10 years. This change has

```
Normal Colorectal Mucosa
        |
  BRAF  |
 mutation
        ↓
      MVHP
        |
  DNA   |
 methylation
        ↓
      SSA/P
        ↓
 SSA/P with cytologic dysplasia
        |
   Methylation of MLH1 or
   other tumorigenic targets
        ↓
 MSI-H Colorectal Cancer
```

FIGURE 22-3. The "serrated" pathway to colorectal cancer. One suggested paradigm of genetic and epigenetic changes in the serrated pathway to colorectal cancer. The inciting event is a mutation in the *BRAF* oncogene, which may lead to a microvesicular hyperplastic polyp (MVHP) or to a sessile serrated adenoma/polyp (SSA/P). Further changes over time can result in cytologic dysplasia. It is proposed that methylation of the mismatch repair gene, *MLH1*, leads to the formation of a microsatellite instability high (MSI-H) colorectal cancer.

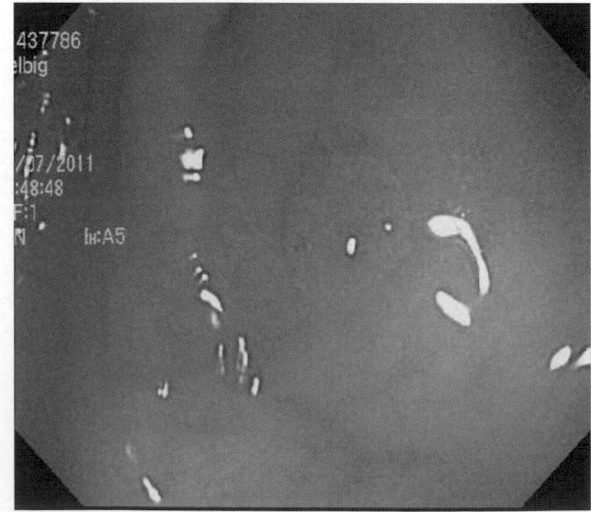

FIGURE 22-4. Hyperplastic (metaplastic) polyp with a translucent appearance. This sort of polyp is prone to disappear on insufflation of the bowel.

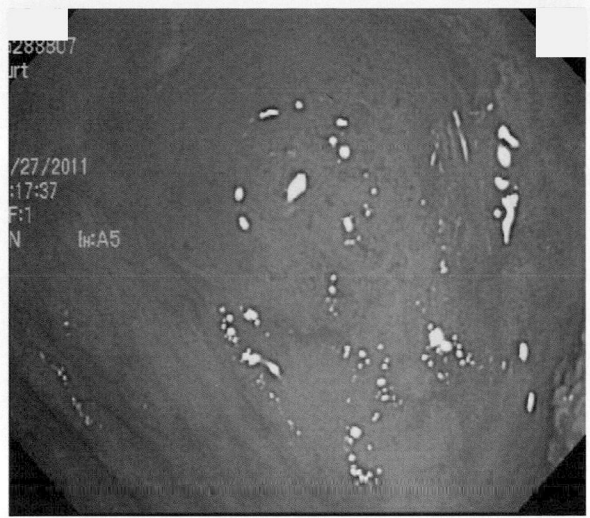

FIGURE 22-5. Sessile serrated adenoma/polyp in the cecum. It is difficult to see and may be ignored as an edematous fold.

been caused by a realization that serrated polyps have important implications for cancer risk and prevention. Although some serrated polyps can be diagnosed endoscopically, the accuracy rate is relatively low. Clearly, there is no substitute for accurate histologic assessment. Moreover, there is a lack of uniformity among pathologists in diagnosing the different subtypes of serrated polyps. Because most large right-sided lesions are SSA/Ps, if a large (more than 1 cm) right-sided polyp is reported to be hyperplastic, the slides should be reviewed by a gastrointestinal pathologist and the lesions treated as high risk.[115,187,288]

Current approaches to serrated colorectal polyps are based on expert opinion. Small (less than 5 mm), left-sided hyperplastic polyps should be sampled to confirm the diagnosis but need not be completely removed. They may be a marker of risk for proximal adenomas but are unlikely to be dangerous in themselves. Church and colleagues, reporting from the Cleveland Clinic, found that small *colonic* polyps are usually neoplastic, but even if hyperplastic, they are associated

with adenomas elsewhere in 75% of cases.[70] Small rectal polyps were usually hyperplastic but still were associated with metachronous neoplasms elsewhere in the colon in 63% of the patients in their report.[70] The authors, therefore, recommended total colonoscopy even if only hyperplastic polyps were found at flexible proctosigmoidoscopy. Ansher and associates found that almost one-third of their patients in whom an isolated hyperplastic polyp was found in the left colon harbored a proximal adenomatous polyp.[9] They opined that hyperplastic colonic polyps *do* serve as a marker for adenomatous colonic neoplasms. Conversely, Provenzale and colleagues, in reviewing the records of 1,836 consecutive colonoscopies, found that distal hyperplastic polyps were *not* strong predictors of the risk for concomitant proximal benign or malignant neoplasms.[14] The authors advocated biopsy, however, to confirm the true nature of the lesion. Others also have concluded that small adenomatous and hyperplastic polyps cannot reliably be distinguished by their endoscopic appearance.[239]

Tonooka and coworkers reported a case of carcinoma in a 12-mm hyperplastic polyp in the cecum diagnosed by a magnifying colonoscope.[319] When the lesion was seen in the magnified view, an irregularly shaped pit was evident in the center. Biopsy confirmed malignant change at that location.

SSA/Ps are premalignant lesions and should be completely removed. Recent reports describe a high incidence of colon cancer in patients with large serrated polyps and high rates of synchronous and metachronous serrated lesions and advanced adenomas.[222] Removal of serrated polyps can be accomplished by snare excision. Although the margins of the polyps can be indistinct and thus predispose to possible recurrence, serrated polyps seem less strongly attached to the underlying mucosa than adenomas and easier to coax into the snare. Polypectomy complication rates are no higher than that for adenomas and may even be lower. Appropriate recognition and detection are as important as resection in their management. Serrated polyps, especially SSA/Ps, can be difficult to see. They are generally the same color as the surrounding mucosa, flatter than adenomas, and with a benign looking crypt pattern that appears like edematous mucosa (see Figure 22-5). The mucus cap is an important clue to their presence, but once this is washed off, the underlying polyp can be almost invisible. The combination of a lack of awareness of the existence of these lesions, the failure to recognize their clinical significance, and an inability to detect them combine to produce a coherent explanation why they pose such a problem in colon cancer screening programs.[20] Serrated polyp detection rates, measured in two early studies, reflect these difficulties because of considerable variation between endoscopists.[140,178]

Surveillance of Patients with Serrated Polyps

Once a patient has a large (more than 1 cm) SSA/P or TSA, he or she is identified as having a high-risk colon. The first aim of surveillance is to make sure that the index lesion is completely removed, and the second aim is to ensure that missed synchronous or rapidly growing metachronous lesions are identified. Therefore, an early follow-up is needed for very large lesions where completeness of excision is in question, with repeat colonoscopy in 6 months. Once a well-healed scar is seen at the site of the polypectomy, and the colon is cleared of any previously missed synchronous lesions,

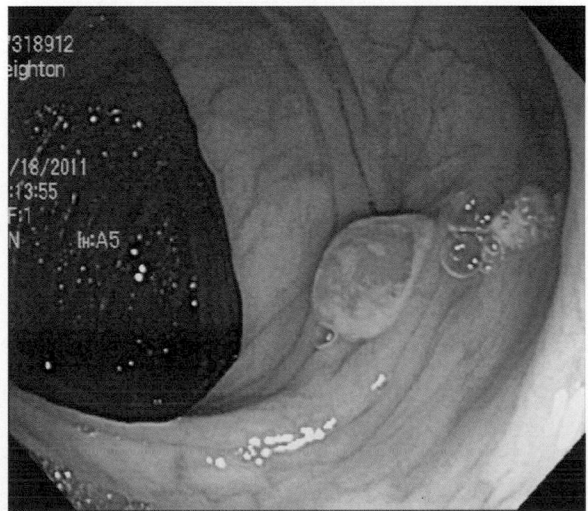

FIGURE 22-6. Sessile serrated adenoma/polyp with a mucus cap in the transverse colon. The cap is an important clue to its presence and its diagnosis.

regular surveillance can start. There are no data upon which to base guidelines, but regimens should be stricter than those that apply to similar sized adenomas, given the increased difficulty in recognizing SSA/Ps. For a single large lesion that was completely removed, a 2-year colonoscopy is reasonable. For several large lesions, a yearly examination is appropriate.

Serrated lesions of the colon and rectum are not harmless. Every polyp seen at colonoscopy must be either biopsied or removed, except in cases where there are multiple small hyperplastic polyps in the rectum and sigmoid or in those with polyposis. Colonoscopists must be alert to the possible presence of SSA/Ps and make certain that the right side of every colon is carefully inspected. If a lesion suspicious for SSA/P is seen (mucus cap—see Figure 22-6), it must be completely removed and a sharp lookout maintained for likely synchronous lesions. Such a patient has a high-risk colon, and surveillance must be frequent and meticulous.

Serrated Polyposis Syndrome

Background

Serrated polyposis syndrome (SPS), formerly called hyperplastic polyposis syndrome, is characterized by multiple or large serrated colorectal polyps. Because serrated polyps have been viewed as benign lesions without malignant potential, serrated polyposis has been overlooked as a significant clinical identity. However, increasing understanding of the serrated pathway of colorectal oncogenesis has shed light on this syndrome. In the 1990s, molecular observations demonstrated that some serrated lesions can transform into colorectal adenocarcinoma.[44] Before the molecular mechanisms were elucidated, there were multiple reports of colorectal cancer arising in colons affected with multiple hyperplastic polyps. In 2000, Jass described molecular evidence of malignant transformation of serrated polyps via the serrated pathway in a patient with serrated polyposis.[166] Recent reports of relatively large case series support an association between serrated polyposis and colorectal cancer,[34,37,181] and this is now an accepted entity.

Diagnosis

Although thought to be hereditary, an underlying germ line mutation has not yet been identified. Thus, SPS is a clinical diagnosis based on criteria defined by the WHO initially in 2000[45] and revised in 2010.[303] Diagnostic criteria include (1) at least five serrated polyps proximal to the sigmoid colon with two or more of these being more than 10 mm, (2) any number of serrated polyps proximal to the sigmoid colon in an individual who has a first-degree relative with serrated polyposis, or (3) more than 20 serrated polyps of any size, but distributed throughout the colon.[303] For a definition of SPS, any of the serrated polyps (HP, SSA/P, TSA) qualify, and polyp counts may be cumulative.[143] The newer nomenclature has been adopted in recognition of the fact that many of the serrated polyps in this syndrome are actually sessile serrated polyps/adenomas rather than solely traditional hyperplastic polyps.

Clinical Presentation

As implied by the varied definitions, SPS is a phenotypically diverse disease. These broad and diverse criteria make it difficult to summarize specific patient characteristics of the

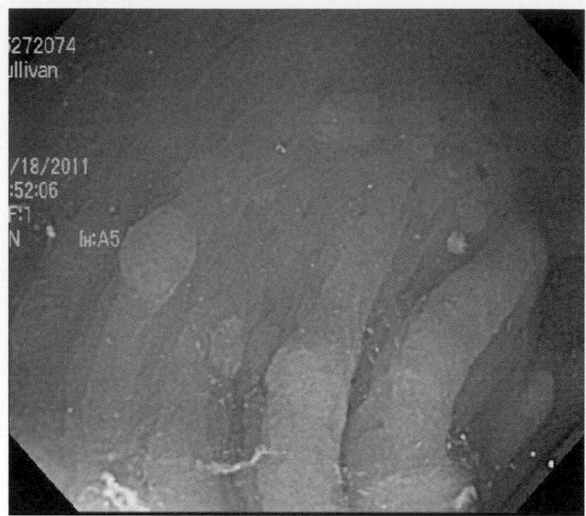

FIGURE 22-7. Multiple small hyperplastic polyps in the left colon in a patient with serrated polyposis syndrome.

condition, and different SPS phenotypes have been suggested. Some patients have multiple small polyps throughout the colon (Figure 22-7), whereas others have a few large, right-sided polyps[181] as demonstrated in Figure 22-8. In addition to serrated polyps, the majority of patients with SPS also harbor adenomas.[34,48,58,181]

Serrated polyposis mainly affects individuals with white European ancestry; this population accounts for approximately 95% of cases.[37,181,353] It affects both genders and has been diagnosed across age groups. Larger series report an equal gender distribution or a slight male predominance,[34,48,181] but one series notes a majority (55%) being women.[58] Median age at diagnosis ranges from 44 to 62 years, with extremes of age including SPS in a 10-year-old and a man in his 80s.[34,48,58,181] SPS is usually asymptomatic, but bleeding may arise from colorectal cancer or from large polyps.

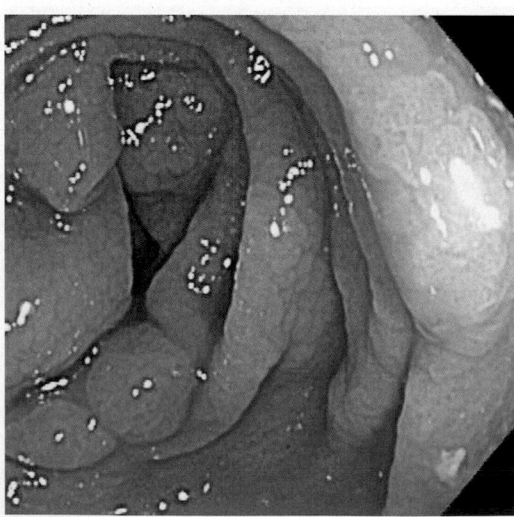

FIGURE 22-8. Larger, right-sided polyps in a patient with serrated polyposis syndrome.

Association with Malignancy

Based on multiple case series, the incidence of colorectal cancer in SPS is approximately 25% to 50%, although the precise risk is still uncertain.[48,58,101,151,181,197,201,271,281,353] The natural history is not well defined because the initial diagnosis is often made when a cancer is detected.[34,181] In a retrospective study reporting on 77 SPS patients who were followed for a mean of 5.6 years, 27 (35%) developed colorectal cancer—22 at initial endoscopy and 5 during follow-up. The cumulative risk of colorectal cancer was calculated to be 7% at 5 years while under a surveillance program.[34] Cancer risk seems to be similar regardless of the polyp phenotype.[181] The true incidence of colorectal cancer risk will only be determined when the disease is defined genetically, and longitudinal long-term observational studies are conducted.

Colorectal cancers seem to be more prevalent within SPS families because approximately 40% to 50% of patients have a family history of colorectal cancer.[58,181] A recent study noted a relative risk of 5.4 for the incidence of colorectal cancer in first-degree relatives of those with SPS compared with the general population.[34] These numbers may be overestimates because the data are likely to be affected by ascertainment bias, with patients having a family history more likely to be recognized and pursued in the clinics.

There have not been any proven associations with extracolonic cancers, although some studies have suggested an increased risk.[162,181,327] The data are not sufficiently meaningful to suggest surveillance for extracolonic malignancies.

Clinical Management
Surveillance and Colonoscopy

The goal of colorectal surveillance in SPS is to prevent colorectal cancer by detection and removal of premalignant lesions. Management guidelines are based on clinical experience and expert opinion and continue to evolve.[237,181,303] For those with an established clinical diagnosis, suggested protocols include colonoscopy every 1 to 2 years. The interval to subsequent colonoscopy depends on the number and histologic characteristics of the polyps. All single polyps larger than 5 mm should be removed and examined histologically. For clusters of small (3 to 4 mm) left-sided polyps, which are likely benign hyperplastic polyps, representative biopsies should be performed. The interval to the next examination may be extended to 2 to 3 years if the colon remains clear of polyps on successive annual colonoscopies, but this should be considered on a case-by-case basis. Surgical consultation is necessary when endoscopic management cannot control the polyp burden, if histologic high-grade dysplasia is found, or if patients are not compliant with the surveillance regimen.

Because there is a suggested increased risk of colorectal cancer in first-degree relatives of patients with SPS, colonoscopy screening should be offered to first-degree relatives, particularly those older than 40 years. Endoscopic findings and polyp histology should guide the interval to the next colonoscopy. Patients with a normal colonoscopy may reasonably be evaluated every 5 years. Prospective longitudinal studies with regular surveillance protocols for SPS patients and first-degree relatives are necessary in order to determine the true natural history of the disease and to guide clinical management.

Surgical Management

Indications for surgery include the inability to adequately control the polyp burden endoscopically, uncontrolled symptoms such as bleeding, and the development of colorectal cancer. The risk of neoplasia affects the entire colorectum, and so subtotal or total colectomy should be considered. This should be determined on an individual basis considering medical comorbidities and anal sphincter function. For patients who cannot tolerate an extended surgery or who have focal disease (e.g., a few large right-sided polyps), a segmental colectomy may be performed. Regardless of surgical treatment, the remaining colorectum should be surveyed endoscopically every year. There are no prospective studies evaluating this management plan. It is simply based on our opinion.

► HAMARTOMAS

A hamartoma is defined as a nonneoplastic growth that is composed of an abnormal mixture of tissue normally found at the site. In the colon, this includes juvenile and Peutz–Jeghers polyps.

Juvenile Polyps

The solitary juvenile polyp (congenital polyp, retention polyp, juvenile adenoma) is usually found in children younger than 10 years of age, but it is also seen in older children and in adults at any age.[227] It is an uncommon condition, occurring in approximately 1% of asymptomatic children.[108] The age distribution has been reported to have a bimodal pattern.[280] According to Roth and Helwig, the childhood group has a modal age of 4 years, whereas the adult group has a modal age of 18 years. The incidence is twice as frequent in boys, and there is a 13:1 ratio of men to women in adults.[200]

Although juvenile polyps are the most common colorectal tumor in children, benign and malignant neoplasms can present at virtually any age.[24,195] Billingham and colleagues observed that solitary adenomas accounted for 7.4% of all polyps found in patients younger than 20 years of age.[29]

Appearance

Juvenile polyps are usually round or oval, with a smooth, continuous surface, in contrast to the papillary surface that characterizes the adenomatous polyp.[194] They are usually pedunculated, and in juvenile polyposis, the stalks can be long with secondary polyps developing like branches on a tree. Juvenile polyps are characteristically cherry red. Their cut surface demonstrates numerous cystic spaces filled with mucus (Figure 22-9).

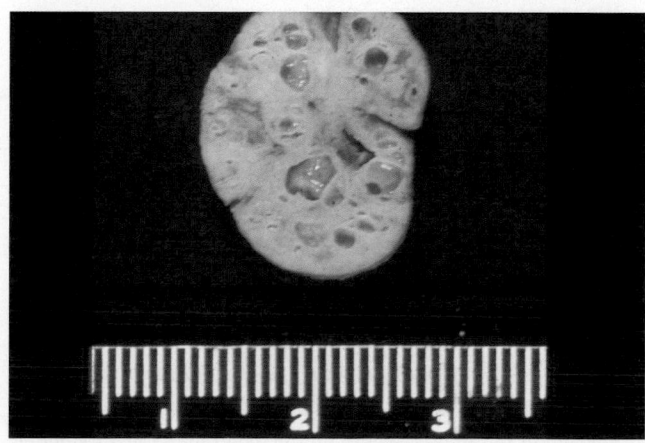

FIGURE 22-9. Juvenile polyp. Note the characteristic cystic spaces in cross section. (Courtesy of Rudolf Garret, MD.)

Histology

Microscopic examination reveals that juvenile polyps are due to an overgrowth of the lamina propria. They are composed of an epithelial and a connective tissue element, with the latter contributing the bulk of the tumor mass (Figure 22-10).[176] Mucin-filled spaces are characteristic, and acute and chronic inflammatory cells are frequently seen. This may lead to their being labeled as "inflammatory polyps," a label that can lead to a delay in diagnosis.

Etiology

Alexander and colleagues noted that a frequent microscopic finding is infiltration by eosinophils.[5] They postulated that because eosinophils usually connote an allergic response, the polyps are the result of allergy. In support of this theory is the observation that there was a statistically significant increased incidence of allergy in children with polyps and in the families of those children. Despite the suggestion by some that juvenile polyps may be neoplastic, most pathologists today agree with Morson that the lesion is a hamartoma.[227] Morson based his conclusion on the observations that there is an abnormality of the mucosal connective tissue or lamina propria and that this connective tissue stroma bears a resemblance to primitive mesenchyme. This concept lends support to the contention that the lesion is a malformation rather than a neoplasm. One theory proposes that the polyp is a form of retention cyst that takes on a polypoid form from traction as a result of peristalsis.

Symptoms and Signs

The most common presenting complaint is rectal bleeding, followed by prolapse or protrusion of the mass, passing of tissue, and abdominal pain. Autoamputation is noted in up to 10% of patients. Diarrhea, mucus, proctalgia, tenesmus, and rectal prolapse have also been reported, although are unlikely to happen with solitary polyps and are symptoms more typical of juvenile polyposis.

Distribution

Mazier and associates reported 258 patients with juvenile polyps.[219] Sixty percent of the polyps were located within 10 cm of the anal verge. Only 10% were located farther away than 20 cm, but these were scattered throughout the colon. Approximately 75% were greater than 1 cm in diameter. Jalihal and colleagues found that 80% of the more than 100 colonoscopic polypectomies performed for juvenile polyps were in the rectosigmoid region.[160]

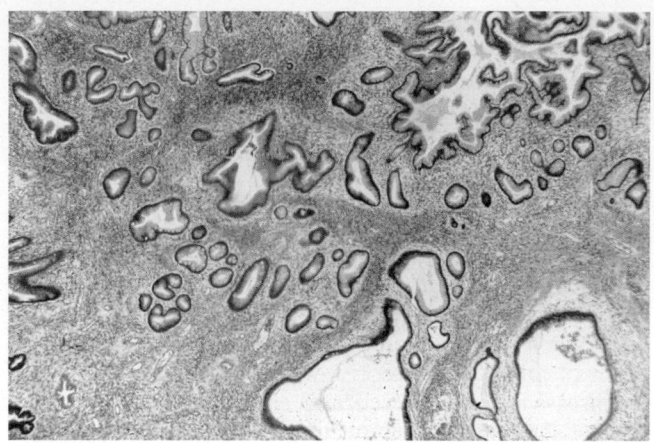

FIGURE 22-10. Juvenile polyp. Note the cystically dilated glands lined by normal-appearing epithelium. (Original magnification × 170; courtesy of Rudolf Garret, MD.)

Diagnosis and Management

Diagnosis is usually made at proctosigmoidoscopy or colonoscopy, and the lesion should be removed. Full colonoscopy is performed to exclude the possibility of juvenile polyposis. Five or more synchronous juvenile polyps, or a family history of juvenile polyposis in a patient with one polyp, are enough to make the diagnosis.[167] One solitary juvenile polyp, itself, is neither a neoplasm nor a premalignant condition. Once the polyp is removed, no further follow-up is required.[184,243]

Peutz–Jeghers Polyps

In 1921, Peutz reported a familial syndrome of polyps of the gastrointestinal tract with pigmentation of the mouth and other parts of the body.[261] Later, Jeghers and his colleagues established the syndrome by describing a number of cases.[169] The disease appears to be transmitted in an autosomal dominant fashion, but de novo cases have been reported without any suggestive family history.

Pathology of Peutz–Jeghers Polyps

Although hamartomas, Peutz–Jeghers polyps are histologically distinct from juvenile polyps. The main difference is that they are due to an overgrowth of the muscularis mucosae, rather than the lamina propria. The arborizing muscle of

JOHANNES LAURENTIUS AUGUSTINUS PEUTZ (1886–1957)

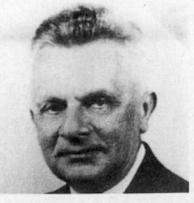

Johannes Peutz was born in Holland and educated at Rolduc, where he began the study of medicine in 1905. After qualification in 1914, Peutz trained in internal medicine at the Coolsingel Hospital in Rotterdam, as well as at clinics in Germany, Italy, and Belgium. In 1917, he became principal physician to the hospital of St. Joannes de Deo, a Roman Catholic hospital at the Hague, where he remained for 34 years until his retirement in 1951. He is credited with the establishment of an independent department of internal medicine and a laboratory with electrocardiographic facilities built to his specifications. Peutz was a dedicated clinician and a keen observer, with broad scientific and humanitarian interests. In 1921, he was conferred the degree of doctor of medicine for his thesis involving the diagnosis and treatment of disorders of the pancreas. In recognition of his many contributions, Peutz was awarded the Pro Ecclesia et Pontifice Medal, the Order of St. Gregorius the Great, and the Order of Orange-Nassau. (Courtesy of Faisal Aziz. Photograph courtesy of Udo Rudloff, MD.)

HAROLD JOSEPH JEGHERS (1904–1990)

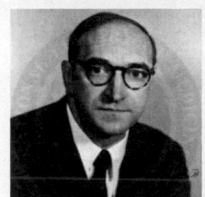

Harold Jeghers was born September 26, 1904. He received his bachelor of science degree in 1928 from the Rensselaer Polytechnic Institute in Troy, New York and then attended the Case Western Reserve University Medical School in Cleveland, Ohio, graduating in 1932. There followed training in internal medicine at the Evans Memorial Institute for Clinical Research in Boston and at the Boston City Hospital. He then became consultant physician to the Boston City Hospital, where he held a teaching post from 1937 to 1946. In 1946, he was appointed professor of medicine and physician-in-chief at Georgetown University School of Medicine in Washington, DC while also serving as consultant to the Walter Reed Army Medical Center and the National Naval Hospital. Jeghers returned to Boston as professor of medicine at Tufts University Medical School in 1966 and retired in 1974. Jeghers was active as a visiting lecturer at a large number of American institutions and English universities. In 1935, Jeghers began building a medical library based on his own method of indexing, which today is known as the Jeghers Medical Index System. (With appreciation to Faisal Aziz.)

the muscularis mucosae makes a longitudinal polyp section look like a tree. There is less mucin and less inflammatory infiltrate than found with juvenile polyps. As with juvenile polyps, solitary Peutz–Jeghers polyps are occasionally found during routine colonoscopy. In the absence of a family history of Peutz–Jeghers polyposis or any of the other phenotypic characteristics of this syndrome, solitary Peutz–Jeghers polyps carry no increased risk of cancer and no surveillance is required.[249]

Hamartomatous Polyposis Syndromes

The hereditary hamartomatous polyposis syndromes are represented by a variety of rare autosomal dominant conditions characterized by the presence of gastrointestinal hamartomatous polyps. The various diseases include juvenile polyposis syndrome (JPS), Peutz–Jeghers syndrome (PJS), and the PTEN hamartoma tumor syndrome (PHTS) of which Cowden syndrome and Bannayan-Riley-Ruvalcaba syndrome (BRRS) are subsets. Each of the hamartomatous syndromes has a unique clinical picture and associated cancer risks. Taken together, hamartomatous polyposis syndromes are responsible for less than 1% of cases of colon cancer in North America.[235]

Juvenile Polyposis Syndrome

JPS occurs in approximately 1 in 100,000 individuals[43] and is characterized by the development of multiple juvenile polyps throughout the gastrointestinal tract. The term "juvenile" is indicative of the type of polyp rather than to the age of onset. Histologically, juvenile polyps are characterized by a normal epithelial component and an abundant lamina propria, but lack smooth muscle. Approximately 2% of children and adolescents will have a solitary juvenile polyp. This manifestation does not carry an increased risk of malignancy and is distinct from JPS.

Genetics

JPS is an autosomal dominantly inherited disease. Approximately 60% of cases of JPS are considered familial, whereas the remaining 40% are believed to occur sporadically.[290] Germ line alterations in three genes—BMPR1A, SMAD4, and ENG1—are associated with JPS. SMAD4 is a tumor suppressor gene in the transforming growth factor-beta (TGF-β) signal transduction pathway, and approximately 20% of patients will have detectable SMAD4 mutations.[148] BMPR1A

is a type I receptor of the TGF-β superfamily that regulates BMP intracellular signaling through SMAD4. Gene sequence analysis will identify BMPR1A mutations in 20% of cases,[148] and an additional 4% will be detected by analysis of large deletions in BMPR1A.[12,330] Patients with JPS may also have mutations in ENG1.[312]

Diagnosis

JPS remains a clinical diagnosis made by endoscopy with confirmation of a germ line mutation in approximately 50% of cases. Clinical criteria for a JPS diagnosis include the following: (1) more than five juvenile polyps of the colon or rectum, (2) juvenile polyps in the extracolonic gastrointestinal tract, or (3) any number of juvenile polyps and a positive family history.[167] Patients who satisfy any of these criteria should be offered genetic counseling and genetic testing. After identification of a specific mutation, at-risk family members should also be tested for that mutation. Approximately 75% of patients will have an affected parent, and if the mutation is detected in such an individual, testing should be offered to siblings of the proband because they have a 50% chance of also being affected. Offspring of the proband also have a 50% chance of inheriting the mutation and should be tested accordingly. After appropriate genetic counseling, at-risk family members should be tested in their teenage years.

Clinical Presentation

Gastrointestinal juvenile polyps are the cornerstone of this disease with variable expression leading to different severity of disease. Polyps occur throughout the gastrointestinal tract, including the colon and rectum, stomach, and small bowel. The majority of patients develop polyps by their teen years, with the polyp burden varying from a few to hundreds. Symptoms are related to the polyps and most commonly include acute or chronic gastrointestinal bleeding, iron-deficiency anemia, prolapsed rectal polyps, abdominal pain, or diarrhea. Hypoproteinemia, hypokalemia, anergy, finger clubbing, and a failure to thrive may also be seen.[88,221] Extracolonic congenital and acquired manifestations have also been associated with JPS, including abnormalities of the heart and cranium, double renal pelvis and ureter, cleft palate, polydactyly, and malrotation of the gut.[88,167]

Recently, JPS has been linked to hereditary hemorrhagic telangiectasia (HHT) via a mutation in SMAD4. HHT is an autosomal dominant condition that is characterized by skin and mucosal telangiectasias; cerebral, pulmonary, and hepatic arteriovenous malformations; and an increased risk of associated hemorrhage. JPS patients with an *SMAD4* mutation are also at risk for the visceral manifestations of HHT, and any HHT patient with *SMAD4* mutation is at risk for early onset gastrointestinal cancer.[105,156]

Association with Malignancy

Patients with JPS have approximately a 50% lifetime risk of developing colorectal cancer with a wide range between 17% and 68%.[1,147,164] Colorectal cancer is diagnosed at a mean age of 43 years,[36] but there is a report of cancer developing in a 15-year-old.[167] Cancers also may develop in the stomach, duodenum, pancreas, and jejunum. The risk of gastric or duodenal cancer is 15% to 21%.[147,291] Neoplastic degeneration is more likely to occur in patients with the generalized form of polyposis compared with those who have colorectal polyposis only.[1]

Clinical Management
Surveillance

Colonoscopic surveillance for patients with JPS is recommended to begin at age 15 or earlier if symptoms develop.[47,237] Colonoscopy is preferred to that of flexible sigmoidoscopy because the right colon is also prone to developing polyps and cancer. If the examination reveals no polyps, repeat colonoscopy is recommended in 2 to 3 years. If any polyps are found, they should be removed endoscopically and sent for pathologic examination. When polyps are detected and removed, repeat examinations should be performed annually until the colon is free of polyps. At this time, the screening interval may revert to every 2 to 3 years. Colectomy is recommended if the polyp burden cannot be managed endoscopically or if high-grade dysplasia is seen. Upper gastrointestinal surveillance is recommended to begin between ages 15 and 25 or earlier if symptoms develop. Endoscopic management principles follow those as given for adenomas, although juvenile polyps are almost always pedunculated and tend to have longer stalks.

Surgery

Surgery is an important part of treating JPS patients. Despite a known significant cancer risk, there is no evidence that prophylactic colectomy reduces cancer development when compared with colonoscopy with polypectomy. Prophylactic colectomy may be considered for patients with significant symptoms, those whose polyp burden cannot be managed endoscopically, those whose family history includes colorectal cancer, and for those with poor compliance. A colectomy is also warranted when a patient develops dysplasia in the polyps. A resected colon with diffusely distributed juvenile polyps is shown in Figure 22-11.

Surgical options for colonic disease include colectomy with ileorectal anastomosis, subtotal colectomy with ileosigmoid anastomosis, or total proctocolectomy. The authors prefer to leave the rectum in place and perform total abdominal colectomy with ileorectal anastomosis unless there is cancer in the rectum or if symptoms are being caused by rectal disease. This operation avoids the potential complications of pelvic surgery and yields better bowel function, an issue that is particularly important for younger patients. In a retrospective study from the Cleveland Clinic, 10 patients with JPS underwent colectomy with preservation of the rectum.[248] Five of these individuals eventually required a proctectomy

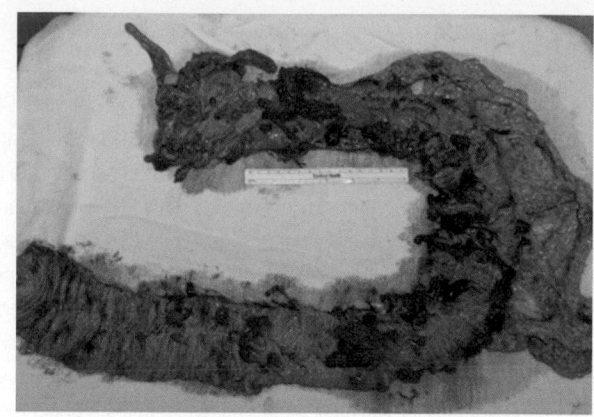

FIGURE 22-11. Colon resection from patient with juvenile polyposis syndrome.

at a median time of 9 years (range, 6 to 34 years). It is also important to note continued surveillance is still required regardless of the surgery performed because polyps may develop in the remaining rectum or ileal pouch.[248]

Cancer risk is lower in the upper gastrointestinal tract compared to the colon, and the need for surgery is determined by symptoms, development of malignant change, or the presence of protein-losing gastropathy/enteropathy. Subtotal gastrectomy is usually the procedure of choice for disease in the stomach, and segmental resection is performed for small bowel disease.

Peutz–Jeghers Syndrome

PJS was first reported in 1895 as a familial syndrome of gastrointestinal polyps with characteristic pigmentation of the mouth and other parts of the body.[261] It was not recognized as a distinct entity until 1949 when Jeghers reported two additional cases.[170] PJS occurs in approximately 1 in 25,000 to 1 in 280,000 people. Peutz–Jeghers polyps have a characteristic frond-like branching structure, with smooth muscle proliferation and appropriate epithelium of the gastrointestinal tract (Figure 22-12).

Genetics

PJS is autosomal dominantly inherited, and germ line mutations in *STK11* are the underlying cause.[138] It is believed that a somatic loss of the second allele results in manifestations of the disease. Gene sequence analysis uncovers approximately 40% to 70% of mutations.[8,11,334]

Diagnosis

PJS is a clinical diagnosis based on meeting one of the following WHO criteria: (1) three or more histologically confirmed Peutz–Jeghers polyps; (2) any number of Peutz–Jeghers polyps with a family history of PJS; (3) characteristic, prominent, mucocutaneous pigmentation with a family history of PJS; or (4) any number of Peutz–Jeghers polyps and characteristic prominent, mucocutaneous pigmentation.[112]

Genetic counseling should be offered to any patient meeting the aforementioned criteria. After identification of a specific mutation, at-risk family members can be tested for this family-specific mutation. Approximately half of cases will have an affected parent, and parents should be carefully evaluated for features of PJS. If one of the parents is affected, then testing should be offered to the siblings of

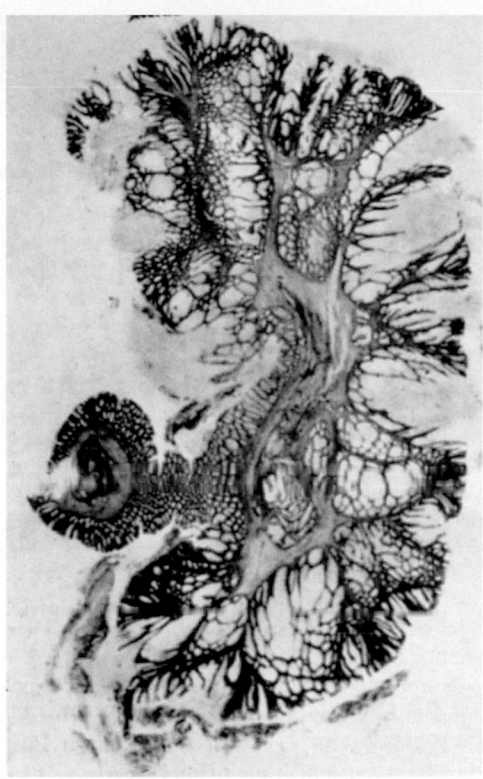

FIGURE 22-12. Peutz–Jeghers polyp of the large intestine. Note the treelike muscular framework. (From Morson BC. Some peculiarities in the histology of intestinal polyps. *Dis Colon Rectum.* 1962;5:337, with permission.)

the proband. Additionally, all children of the proband have a 50% risk of inheriting the mutation and should be tested accordingly. Genetic testing for at-risk family members may be performed at age 8 after appropriate genetic counseling and informed consent.[113]

Clinical Presentation

Gastrointestinal hamartomatous polyps coupled with the unique, distinctive mucocutaneous pigmentation are the key features of PJS. The classic PJS pigmentation is seen in approximately 95% of cases and most commonly detected on the vermillion border of the lips (94%), buccal mucosa (66%), hands (74%), and feet (62%), but has also been reported in the periorbital, perianal, and genital areas.[112,355] The usual appearance is that of small, dark brown or blue-brown macules in infancy, which may fade in late adolescence.

Approximately 88% of patients with PJS will develop hamartomatous polyps,[324] with the small bowel as the most common site, followed by colon, stomach, and rectum. Polyps vary in size from a few millimeters to several centimeters, and with increasing size, they tend to become pedunculated. Most patients will have fewer than 20 polyps, but these will often cause symptoms such as obstruction, abdominal pain, gastrointestinal bleeding, polyp prolapse per anus, or recurrent small bowel intussusception (Figures 22-13 and 22-14).[324] Symptoms usually develop by the second or third decade of life. Rare cases of polyps developing in the renal pelvis, urinary bladder, lungs, and nares have been reported.

Association with Malignancy

Patients with PJS have an increased risk of developing various malignancies. A meta-analysis of 210 patients reported a 93% estimated lifetime risk of developing cancer.[109] The risk for developing breast, colon, pancreatic, and gastric cancer is 54%, 39%, 36%, and 29%, respectively. Cancers in the reproductive organs have also been rarely associated with PJS. Men are at risk for testicular tumors of sex cord and Sertoli cell type, and women are at risk for the development of sex cord tumors with annular tubules of the ovary and adenoma malignum of the cervix.

Clinical Management
Surveillance and Endoscopic Intervention

Regular surveillance of multiple organs is necessary for PJS patients. Randomized controlled trials have not been performed to evaluate the efficacy of cancer surveillance protocols, and published recommendations are based on expert opinion. Specific testing depends on the patient's age and gender. For patients with a diagnosis of PJS, the National Comprehensive Cancer Network (NCCN) recommends screening starting at age 8 to 10 years, with evaluation of the small bowel. The interval to the next examination is based on the findings of that exam. If it is normal, repeat evaluation is recommended at age 18 at the latest, then at 2 to 3 years

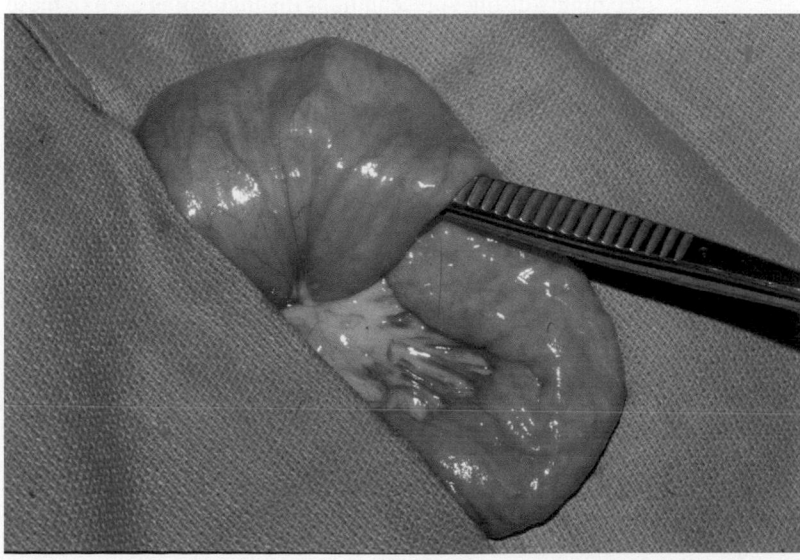

FIGURE 22-13. Ileal intussusception in teenager with Peutz–Jeghers syndrome.

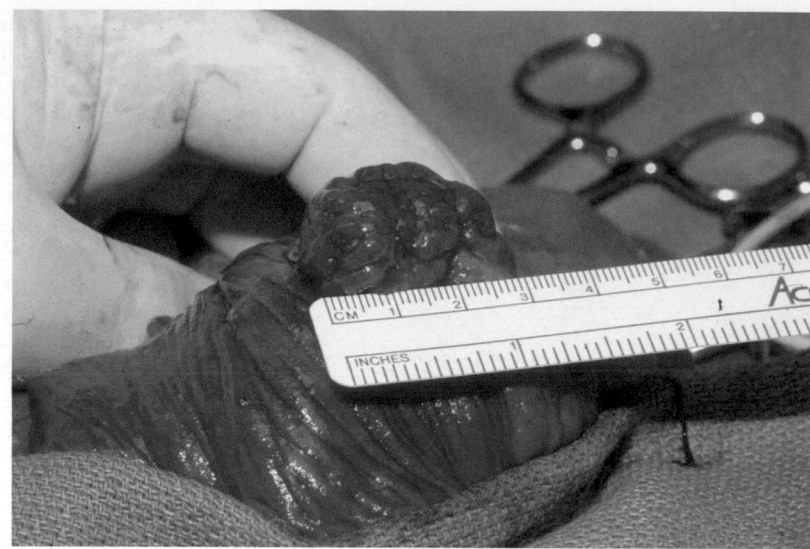

FIGURE 22-14. The ileal hamartoma that was causing the intussusception.

intervals.[237] Males should undergo annual testicular physical examination starting at age 10 years, and females should undergo annual pelvic examination and Papanicolaou stain starting at age 18 to 20 years. Women should also have breast physical examinations every 6 months and annual mammogram and breast MRI starting at age 25 years. Both genders should undergo colonoscopy and upper endoscopy beginning in their late teens and repeated every 2 to 3 years based on findings. To detect early pancreatic cancer, endoscopic ultrasound or magnetic resonance cholangiopancreatography (MRCP) along with serum CA19-9 every 1 to 2 years starting at age 25 to 30 years is recommended. Other screening regimens have been proposed by other authors.[46,113,355]

Evaluation of small bowel polyposis is technically difficult because much of the small bowel is not easily evaluated by endoscopy. Capsule endoscopy and double-balloon enteroscopy are more commonly being used to identify jejunal and ileal polyps.[42,57,193] However, the true impact that these tests have on surveillance and treatment remains inadequately defined.

Endoscopic management of PJS can be considered both prophylactic, as in polypectomy on asymptomatic polyps found during surveillance, and treatment of polyp-related complications. Similar to the surveillance guidelines, intervention recommendations are from expert opinion rather than through controlled studies. Asymptomatic gastric or colonic polyps larger than 1 cm should be removed endoscopically. For small bowel polyps, those larger than 1 to 1.5 cm or those that are rapidly growing (based on prior examinations) should be removed to decrease future complications. The most common complications are bleeding and intussusception. For slowly bleeding polyps causing anemia, endoscopic resection is the first option. However, polyps may be located beyond the reach of conventional endoscopic techniques. An endoscopic approach combined with laparoscopy or laparotomy, which allows the surgeon to guide the endoscope, may be employed to reach the lesion of interest.[306,326]

Surgery

Obstruction and bleeding are the most common indications for surgical intervention. Although most intussusceptions resolve spontaneously, if the obstruction does not resolve in a few hours, surgery is required. The affected area should be resected with sparing as much bowel as possible because there will likely be future surgery, and resection may be needed. Removing all polyps at the time of surgery to achieve a "clean sweep" is advocated to reduced the need for future operations.[250] The search for polyps may be accomplished through the open resection ends of the bowel or via an enterotomy. An operative endoscopy by means of an enterotomy (intraoperative enteroscopy) can also facilitate this search. Edwards used this method on 25 patients and identified 350 polyps not detectable by palpation or transillumination.[92]

PTEN Hamartoma Tumor Syndrome

The term PHTS was introduced to group the clinically described syndromes that are caused by germ line *PTEN* mutations.[215,216] Both Cowden syndrome and BRRS are characterized by colonic hamartomatous polyps and are caused by mutation in the *PTEN* gene. Cowden syndrome was first recognized in 1962 and was named for the patient who had the disease.[208] In 1971, Bannayan reported the first case of what later became known as BRRS.[17] Despite the seemingly distinct presentations distinguishing each of these hamartomatous polyposis syndromes, making the correct diagnosis for these conditions can be challenging because significant overlap exists.

Genetics

Cowden syndrome and BRRS are both autosomally dominant inherited disorders. Germ line mutations in *PTEN* were identified in patients and families with Cowden syndrome in 1996[203,215] and also in patients with BRRS in 1997.[217] *PTEN* is a tumor suppressor gene that encodes a phosphatase, which is involved in the PI3K/AKT signaling pathway. It plays a key role in apoptosis. Approximately 80% of patients who meet the diagnostic criteria for Cowden syndrome and 60% of patients with BRRS have *PTEN* mutations.[215,216]

Diagnosis and Clinical Presentation

A PHTS diagnosis can be considered based on clinical findings, but definitive diagnosis is made by identification of a germ line *PTEN* mutation. The International Cowden

Consortium has proposed operational clinical diagnostic criteria for Cowden syndrome, including both major and minor criteria.[127,355] Major criteria include breast cancer, thyroid cancer (especially follicular), macrocephaly, endometrial cancer, and Lhermitte-Duclos disease. Minor features include benign thyroid changes (such as a goiter), mental retardation, hamartomatous intestinal polyps, fibrocystic changes in the breast, lipomas, fibromas, genitourinary tumors (such as kidney cancer or uterine fibroids), or malformations. Cowden's syndrome is diagnosed if a patient has either macrocephaly or Lhermitte-Duclos disease and one other major feature. A diagnosis of Cowden is also made when a person has one major feature and three minor features, or at least four minor features.

Consensus diagnostic criteria for BRRS are not established, but a diagnosis should be considered in patients with the key features of macrocephaly, hamartomatous colonic polyposis, lipomas, and pigmented macules of the glans penis.[118] Approximately half of the patients with BRRS will have hamartomatous polyps in the digestive tract, particularly in the ileum and colon.[118] These can cause intussusception and rectal bleeding but are not believed to increase the risk of colon cancer.

Association with Malignancy

PHTS syndromes carry mainly a risk of extracolonic cancers. Women have a 50% lifetime risk of developing breast cancer and a 5% to 10% lifetime risk of developing endometrial cancer. Men and women with Cowden syndrome have a 10% lifetime risk of developing epithelial thyroid cancer. Hamartomatous polyps have been reported in patients with Cowden syndrome, although they have not yet been recognized as a major or minor component of the condition. One recent report identified colorectal cancer in 13% of *PTEN* mutation carriers. All cancers occurred before the age of 50 years. The adjusted standardized incidence ratio was 224 (95% confidence interval [CI], 109.3–411.3; $P < .0001$).[135] This is the first report of an association with Cowden syndrome and colorectal cancer.

Patients with BRRS by virtue of a *PTEN* mutation carry similar extracolonic malignancy risks as those with Cowden syndrome. Approximately half of the patients with BRRS will have hamartomatous polyps in the digestive tract, particularly in the ileum and colon.[118] These polyps can become symptomatic but are not believed to increase the risk of colon cancer.

Surveillance and Clinical Management

There are no specific recommendations for colon cancer or polyposis surveillance because data are limited about the true prevalence of colon cancer in Cowden syndrome. A Cleveland Clinic study reported an adjusted standardized incidence ratio for colorectal cancer of 224 (95% CI, 109.3–411.3; $P < .0001$). All cancers occurred before the age of 50. The authors of that study recommended baseline colonoscopy at age 35 for patients with Cowden syndrome, with subsequent follow-up dependent on the polyp burden but no less frequent than every 5 years. This is a fairly new conclusion, and the recommendation has not been adopted into any published professional guidelines.[135] In BRRS, although there is not believed to be a cancer risk, the colorectal polyp burden may be significant and cause symptoms such as bleeding or obstruction. Treatment is based on symptoms. Extracolonic cancer surveillance focuses on more prevalent cancers, such as breast, thyroid, and endometrium.[237]

Cronkhite-Canada Syndrome

In 1955, Cronkhite and Canada described a nonfamilial syndrome of gastrointestinal polyposis, hyperpigmentation, alopecia, and nail dystrophy.[81] The syndrome is thought to be a variant of juvenile polyposis with ectodermal changes, but this is not believed to be an inherited or genetically transmitted disease.[270] Gastrointestinal polyps are found in 52% to 96% of patients and may be located along the alimentary tract from the stomach to the rectum.[83] These are hamartomatous polyps with similar histology to that of juvenile polyps, but the intervening mucosa between polyps is histologically abnormal, characterized by inflammation and edema. These polyps may contain adenomatous changes. The finding of dysplasia in a polyp should encourage the endoscopist to pursue an aggressive surveillance program. The polyps may be seen in association with neoplasms of the colon and are considered by some authors to represent a premalignant condition.[214,270]

Presentation

Cronkhite-Canada syndrome usually presents as an acute illness with rapid progress of protein-losing enteropathy and unique extraintestinal manifestions. Anemia and rectal bleeding are commonly reported.[83] The mean age at diagnosis is 62 years. Morbidity is caused by the physiologic effects of severe diarrhea, weight loss, and complications of malnutrition.[83]

Association with Malignancy

The risk of colorectal cancer is approximately 9%, and the risk of colorectal adenomas or adenomatous change is 40%.[46] Because there is also an increased risk of gastric cancer in this syndrome, screening of the colon and stomach should be considered.

Management

Overall prognosis is poor because there is no effective specific treatment. Most patients have been treated symptomatically by means of nutritional support.[100] If possible, enteral feeding is preferred, but it is more likely that parenteral feeding will be necessary with supplemental calories, nitrogen, and lipids, in addition to appropriate fluids, electrolytes, and vitamins. Symptomatic remission occasionally may occur with supportive care. Glucocorticoids, anabolic steroids, antibiotics, and surgical resections have been successful in some patients, but the variety of approaches makes it difficult to identify the most effective intervention. Surgical therapy is risky in these malnourished patients and, therefore, has a limited role. Resection is indicated when involvement is confined to a segment amenable to excision, whether it be stomach, small bowel, or colon.[78] The causes of death are subsequent to the disease complications, such as cachexia, malnutrition, septicemia, and shock.[83] Specific management awaits a better understanding of this perplexing syndrome.

Hereditary Mixed Polyposis Syndrome

Hereditary mixed polyposis syndrome was described in 1997 in a family with a number of polyps with different histology, including atypical juvenile polyps, hyperplastic polyps, adenomas, and even carcinoma.[346] This disease follows autosomal dominant inheritance. Linkage to chromosome 15q14-q22 in a region of a potential colonic cancer gene, *CRAC1*, has been reported.[158,317] This is a rare disease, but the usual presentation includes less than 15 colonic polyps at presentation. There are no extracolonic manifestations. The median age of onset of symptoms is 40 years. The mean age of colorectal cancer diagnosis is 47 years, and the risk is believed to increase compared with the general population. Surveillance colonoscopy has been recommended every 1 to 2 years for patients with this disease.[46]

▶ ADENOMAS

Polyps in the large bowel keep bad company.
—RUPERT B. TURNBULL

An adenoma is a benign neoplasm of glandular origin and the most common neoplasm of the colon and rectum. Adenocarcinoma, the most common cancer of the colon and rectum and the third most common cancer of solid organs in the human body, arises from an adenoma. Thus, adenomas are significant because they are cancers "in the making." Although only 1 in every 100 to 200 adenomas will ever become malignant, all adenocarcinomas of the large bowel arise in dysplastic epithelium. Their significance lies in the fact that we have access to these precursor lesions containing dysplasia via colonoscopy and the opportunity to prevent cancer by removing them.

Genetic Basis of Adenomas

A common question asked by patients is "Why did I get these polyps?" A simple answer is "It's in your genes." All colorectal neoplasia is genetic, the result of an accumulation of genetic abnormalities in the colorectal mucosa that begins in early childhood and progresses throughout life. These genetic abnormalities predispose to loss of function in key pathways controlling cell growth, differentiation, and death. In 1988, Vogelstein proposed a sequence of genetic abnormalities that could be associated with progressively higher risk adenomas, providing a genetic mechanism for a polyp-cancer sequence (Figure 22-15).[332] It may seem that this observation had been well established, but it has been less than 40 years since the validity of the polyp-cancer sequence has been generally accepted. It was in 1939 that Swinton and Warren published their seminal article on the subject, and then it was roundly criticized.[313] At the time, most physicians believed cancers of the colon arose de novo, in otherwise normal bowel.

Since then, the "Vogelgram" has been confirmed and labeled as a chromosomal instability mechanism for the development of colorectal cancer. It involves early loss of *APC*, setting the stage for multiple chromosomal abnormalities that in turn cause loss of gene expression by loss of heterozygosity. Global hypomethylation causes an overall instability of DNA expression. Mutations in *SMAD4* and *P53* are later events as larger adenomas become cancers.[332] Sanchez and associates showed that this mechanism causes 70% of colorectal cancers,[287] whereas Kalady and colleagues refined its role, describing participation in 90% of rectal cancer and approximately 60% of colon cancers.[182] There are two other main genetic mechanisms by which colorectal cancer develops. The mutator mechanism is caused by deficient DNA mismatch repair. When this is due to an inherited mutation in a mismatch repair gene (Lynch syndrome), the precursor lesion to cancer is an adenoma.[31] Some of these mutator adenomas are microsatellite unstable, with the proportion depending on size.

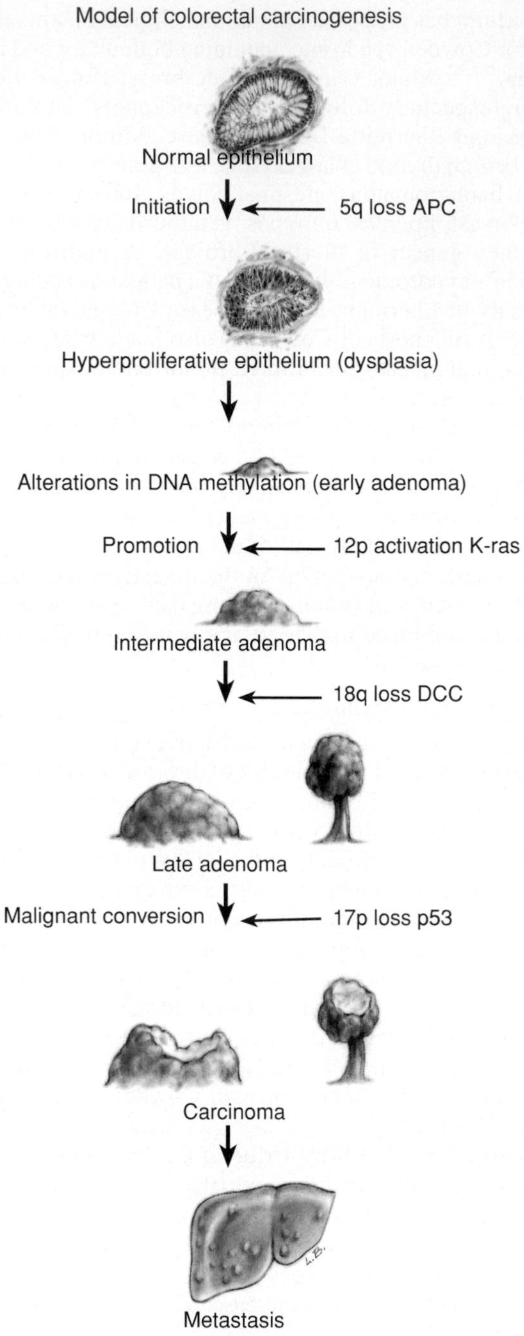

Model of colorectal carcinogenesis

FIGURE 22-15. Model of colorectal carcinogenesis. (Redrawn from Fearon ER, Vogelstein B. A genetic model of colorectal cancer tumorigenesis *Cell*. 1990;61(5):759–767.)

Sporadic mutator cancers due to promoter methylation of the mismatch repair gene *MLH1* have serrated polyps as precursor lesions.[51,166,255,320]

Epidemiology

The fact that all colorectal neoplasia is genetic begs the question as to what causes the genetic abnormalities that lead to polyps and cancer. The answer to this is undoubtedly multifactorial, but Lichtenstein in a study of 4,000 sets of Scandinavian twins was able to conclude that 65% of all colorectal cancer is from environmental influences, whereas 35% has some hereditary component.[204] The environmental influences

NEIL WILLIAMS SWINTON (1907–1980)

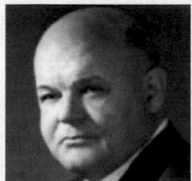

Swinton was born in Ontonagon, Michigan and spent his early years in Marquette. He attended Lehigh University and the University of Michigan, and he obtained his medical degree from the latter institution in 1929. Following postgraduate training in the department of surgery at the university, he became a fellow in surgery at the Lahey Clinic in Boston. He volunteered for duty at the start of World War II and served with distinction as commanding officer in a portable surgical hospital in the Southwest Pacific Theatre. Following the war, he returned to the Lahey Clinic as a staff surgeon and ultimately became one of the leaders in the field of proctology in the United States. Swinton wrote or co-authored 144 scientific papers, including the paper quoted that he wrote with his colleague, Shields Warren, chairman of the Department of Pathology at the New England Deaconess Hospital. Swinton was recognized by his colleagues through serving as president of the American Proctologic Society, now the American Society of Colon and Rectal Surgeons. He was an honorary fellow of the Section of Proctology of the Royal Society of Medicine. After 40 years as a surgeon at the clinic, he retired to Arizona, where he died.

SHIELDS WARREN (1898–1980)

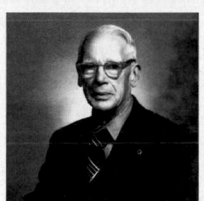

Shields Warren was born in Cambridge, Massachusetts on February 26, 1898, the grandson of the first president of Boston University. He received a classical Greek and Latin education and entered Boston University, from which he graduated in 1918. Following a period of ill health and travel, he was admitted to Harvard Medical School, where he developed a lifelong interest in pathology. He received an appointment to the then world-renowned Pathology Department at Boston City Hospital. In 1927, he went to the New England Deaconess Hospital in Boston and established their Department of Pathology, remaining as chairman until 1963. Warren was recognized by his clinical peers as the "pathologist to the living" because of their reliance on his expertise in the decision-making process for the care of their patients. In 1948, he was appointed professor at Harvard Medical School. His interest in radiation and radiation injuries resulted in his involvement in the shipment of uranium ore during the Second World War. From 1047 until 1052, he assumed the post of head of the Division of Biology and Medicine at the Atomic Energy Commission. He died on July 1, 1980 on Cape Cod, Massachusetts. (Abstracted from Corman ML. Landmark articles of the 20th century. *Semin Colon Rectal Surg.* 1999;10:209.)

include diet, lifestyle, and exposure to other carcinogens such as nicotine. Dietary factors associated with a predisposition to cancer include red meat, animal fats, and alcohol, whereas fresh fruit and fiber have a protective effect.[4,186,269,295] Estrogen is a protective factor as shown by the reduced rate of polyps and cancer in women on hormone replacement therapy.[173,279] Obesity, smoking, and a sedentary lifestyle have also been incriminated in increasing neoplasia risk.[189] In a Japanese study, cigarette smoking was found to be a risk factor for the development of colorectal adenoma.[234] Naveau and colleagues reported that cirrhosis is an independent risk factor for colorectal adenomatous polyps and confirmed that alcoholism increases this risk.[238] Immunodeficiency has also been suggested to play a possible role in the pathogenesis, but Parikshak and coworkers noted that transplant recipients are not more likely to develop metachronous polyps than the general population.[253]

Underlying these risk factors is the basic genotype that each individual inherits from his or her parents, and the occasional sporadic mutation or loss of heterozygosity that inevitably occurs in the course of life. Only 5% of colorectal neoplasia is associated with germ line mutations of a key gene that causes a syndrome of hereditary colorectal cancer (familial adenomatous polyposis, *MYH*-associated polyposis, Lynch syndrome). However, about 30% of colorectal cancers have less obvious forms of inheritance of colorectal cancer predisposition. These may include cancer-predisposing polymorphisms or poorly penetrant mutations that have not been characterized.

Geographic Distribution

Carcinoma of the colon and rectum is primarily a disease of Western civilization. The incidence of adenomatous polyps parallels the geographic distribution: high in Western societies (e.g., Europe, the United States, Australia, New Zealand), in other countries with high meat consumption, and in urban populations. The epidemiology of colorectal carcinoma is discussed in Chapter 23.

Anatomic Distribution

The distribution of colonic adenomas is similar to that of cancers: more frequent in the distal bowel, with a relatively high incidence in the cecum. In an autopsy study, Ekelund found that more than one-half of people had adenomas in the rectum and sigmoid colon, slightly fewer than those who were found to have a carcinoma.[93] Nineteen percent of the benign lesions were in the right colon, virtually the same as the distribution for cancer. In Helwig's series, the sigmoid colon was the most common site of adenomas, adenomas with malignant transformation, and carcinomas.[137] Other studies have demonstrated a more uniform distribution for adenomas than for carcinomas, anticipating a future trend to more proximal cancers. Greene noted that a left-to-right shift was apparent in the decade from 1971 to 1980 in comparison with the prior 10-year period.[120] Thirty-two percent of adenomas were found in the rectum in the former decade and 13% in the latter.

Age

The National Polyp Study estimated that adenomatous polyps antedate cancer by an average of 10 years,[350] a figure also suggested by Basil Morson.[226] Corman reports the mean age of his patients who underwent colonoscopy-polypectomy was 55 years, compared with patients with colorectal cancer, whose mean age was 62 years. Adenomas occurring to those younger than the age of 40 are unusual and should raise a suspicion for an inherited syndrome. An adenoma in a patient younger than age 40 was one of the original Bethesda criteria, suggesting microsatellite instability (MSI) testing would be appropriate in this setting.[32]

Gender

Men and women have an approximately equal frequency of colorectal cancer; the same observation is true for adenomas. Women have a slightly greater number of right-sided lesions (both benign and malignant), and men have a tendency to rectal neoplasia.

Family History

Relatives of patients with adenomatous polyps have an increased risk of developing colorectal cancer, with an odds ratio that approaches 2.[172] Winawer and colleagues interviewed a random sample of participants in the National Polyp Study who had newly diagnosed adenomatous polyps with respect to the history of colorectal cancer in parents and siblings.[350] There were 1,031 patients with adenomas, 1,865 parents, and 2,381 siblings. The authors concluded that siblings and parents of patients with adenomatous polyps are at an increased risk for the development of colorectal cancer, particularly if the adenomas were diagnosed prior to the age of 60 years, or in the case of siblings, when a parent has had a colorectal cancer.[350]

Natural History of Adenomas

There are three situations in which the "natural" history of the adenoma-carcinoma sequence can be demonstrated: first, in the unusual circumstance where a patient with a benign polyp refuses removal of the lesion and subsequently develops a carcinoma at the same site; second, in familial polyposis, a condition that always results in a bowel cancer if the colon is not resected (see later); and third, in hereditary nonpolyposis colorectal cancer (see Lynch Syndromes, Chapter 23). Because the histologic nature of the polyps in the familial polyposis condition is no different from that seen in the common solitary adenoma, one must infer that there is a cause and effect relationship. The huge number of polyps present in the bowel implies that the risk is multiplied many times.

Muto and coworkers reported four patients who had untreated adenomatous polyps.[233] In one, cancer was diagnosed at the same site after 5 years; in the second, cancer was found after 6 years. The third patient had cancer of the rectum that developed 13 years after the original observation of a benign polyp. In the fourth case, after 11 years the tumor was still benign. The authors concluded that the life history of the adenoma-cancer sequence is probably at least 5 years and may in some cases be more than 10 years.

A retrospective review of Mayo Clinic records from a 6-year period prior to the development of colonoscopy revealed 226 patients with colonic polyps at least 1 cm in diameter for whom periodic radiographic examination was elected rather than colotomy and polypectomy.[309] Actuarial analysis revealed that the cumulative risk of diagnosis of cancer at the polyp site at 5, 10, and 20 years was 2.5%, 8%, and 24%, respectively.

Patients with large, sessile, villous adenomas represent a special situation. Although rectal bleeding is the most frequent presenting complaint for both adenomatous conditions, change in bowel habits and mucous discharge are much more frequent concerns in a patient with a large villous adenoma. In fact, there is a unique symptom complex associated with villous adenoma that today has become quite rare: hypokalemia and dehydration. The syndrome was originally reported

TETSUICHIRO MUTO (1938–PRESENT)

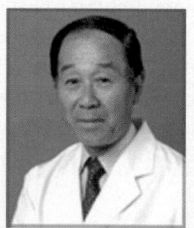

Muto attended the University of Tokyo where he received his medical degree in 1963 and his PhD in 1968. He was an early user and advocate of the fiberoptic colonoscope. In a 1972 paper with Christopher Williams, he described the colonoscopy of the entire length of the colon in 50 patients. This paper showed the utility of colonoscopy to investigate cases of unexplained rectal bleeding, but the authors predicted that in the future, colonoscopy would likely be limited to specialized centers. They stated, "It seems likely that colonoscopy will be a specialist service provided in a few centres." However, in the next year, 1973, he began to advocate for the spread of colonoscopic techniques to more hospitals. In that year, he published an early study on the safety of colonoscopic snare polypectomy with researchers at St. Mark's Hospital in England. In that paper, the authors advocated the replacement of colotomy with colonoscopic polypectomy because of the lower risk of complications with the colonoscopic technique and recommended that hospitals "set up local facilities" for colonoscopy. In 1987, he published a retrospective study on 1,000 polyps removed colonoscopically. In the 1990s, screening colonoscopy for colorectal cancer became widespread. The flat adenoma of Muto was first characterized in his 1985 paper as an adenoma less than 1 cm in diameter, either flat or slightly raised, which often showed severe atypia. Since then, this entity has been the subject of many investigations. Tetsuichiro Muto also studied Crohn's disease, diverticulosis, and cancer. He was the 10th director of the Cancer Institute Hospital of the Japanese Foundation for Cancer Research. He has been active in international conferences and societies and was the president of the International Society of University Colon and Rectal Surgeons in 2004. (Biography courtesy of Thomas Gregg, MD.)

LELAND STERLING MCKITTRICK (1893–1978)

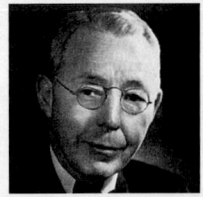

Leland McKittrick was born in Thorp, Wisconsin, the son of a town physician. He attended the University of Wisconsin and graduated from Harvard Medical School in 1918. McKittrick began his surgical experience at the University of Minnesota but then transferred to the Massachusetts General Hospital in Boston. Following the completion of his training, he joined the surgical practice of a preeminent Boston surgeon, Daniel Fiske Jones. McKittrick was a thoughtful and innovative clinician. He introduced synchronous resection with ileostomy for ulcerative colitis, rather than employ the multistaged approach that had been in vogue, and he was also an advocate of side-to-end anastomoses in the bowel. In addition to his technical mastery, he was an authority on gastrointestinal pathophysiology. He was the first to recognize the electrolyte imbalance and fluid loss associated with villous adenomas of the large bowel. McKittrick took on a leadership role in surgery, not only in New England, but also nationally. He was elected president of the American Surgical Association in 1965. He retired from surgical practice at the age of 78 but pursued an active life until his death at age 85. (Reproduced in part from Drazan KE. Leland Sterling McKittrick. *Dis Colon Rectum.* 1997;40:1494. Photograph courtesy of John McKittrick, MD.)

by McKittrick and Wheelock in 1954 and is attributed to the loss of copious fluid and electrolytes from the mucus-secreting tumor (Figure 22-16).[220] Since this original article, many other reports have been published. Jeanneret-Grosjean and Thompson noted that sodium loss is as frequently seen and may actually be the dominant feature of this syndrome in some cases.[168]

The lesions are frequently removed locally by a transanal approach and have a tendency to recur. Muto and associates observed the long-term follow-up in 10 such patients (5 to 30 years).[233] All had periodic evaluation and further treatment as necessary for recurrence. Two patients subsequently developed cancers: one after 10 years and the other at 28 years.

Histology

Adenomas are neoplasms: a tumor characterized by new (and by implication disordered) growth. All adenomas have dysplastic epithelium, where the cells lining the colorectal crypts show nuclear stratification, hyperchromasia, and frequent mitoses (Figures 22-17 and 22-18). Although the degree of dysplasia can differ from one adenoma to another, and severe or high-grade dysplasia means that the cells are similar to those found in invasive cancer, all adenomas are dysplastic to some degree (Figures 22-19 and 22-20). Most adenomas show low-grade dysplasia but the term "dysplastic adenoma" is a redundancy.

Pseudocarcinomatous Invasion

Benign-appearing glandular tissue has been described deep to the muscularis mucosae. This condition has been termed pseudocarcinomatous invasion.[233] It is believed to be associated with larger tumors, those with a long pedicle, and lesions of the sigmoid colon.[84] Day and Morson suggested that the histologic appearance is the result of trauma, possibly secondary to repeated twisting of the stalk.[84] Histologic examination reveals gland-like or cyst-like structures in the submucosa that show a cytologic appearance similar to that of the overlying benign tumor (Figure 22-21).

Differentiation of pseudocarcinomatous invasion from invasive cancer is important. In the St. Mark's Hospital series of 56 patients, no one developed a recurrence or metastasis following local excision.[77]

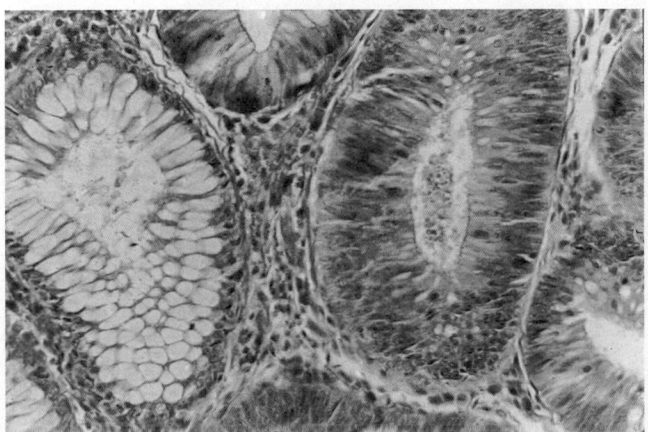

FIGURE 22-16. A large villous adenoma. This huge lesion produced electrolyte depletion. (From Corman ML, Veidenheimer MC, Swinton NW. *Diseases of the Anus, Rectum, and Colon. Part I: Neoplasms.* New York, NY: Medcom; 1972, with permission.)

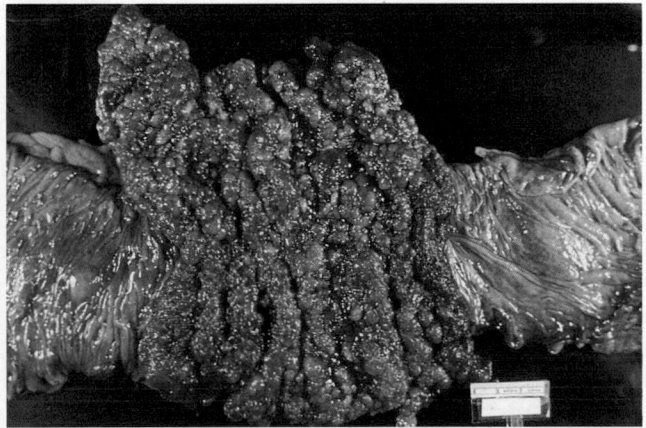

FIGURE 22-17. This section from the edge of a polypoid adenoma illustrates a neoplastic and a normal gland, side by side. Note the crowding of cells, piling up of nuclei, and the loss of ability to produce mucus in the neoplastic gland **(right)**. (From Corman ML, Veidenheimer MC, Swinton NW. *Diseases of the Anus, Rectum, and Colon. Part I: Neoplasms.* New York, NY: Medcom; 1972, with permission.)

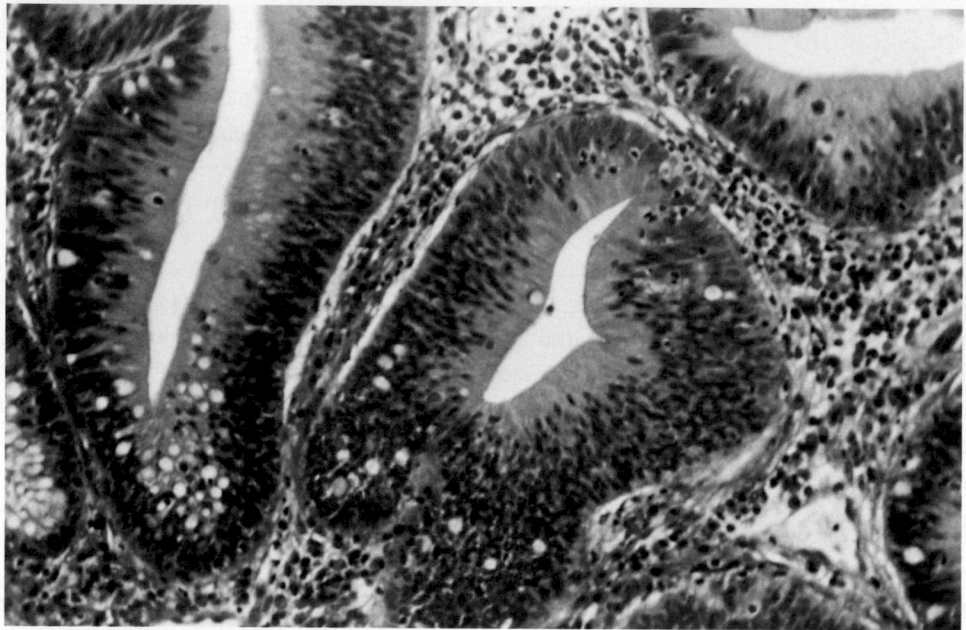

FIGURE 22-18. Adenomatous polyp. Note the dysplasia characterized by loss of polarity with some mitotic figures. (Original magnification × 600; courtesy of Rudolf Garret, MD.)

When Does an Adenoma Become a Cancer?

As long as dysplastic cells are confined to the colorectal epithelium, they cannot reach the blood and lymphatic vessels that allow them to metastasize, and so the lesion is not a cancer. Once the dysplastic cells invade out of the epithelium into the submucosa, metastasis is possible and the lesion *is* a cancer. Malignant cells confined to the epithelium by the basement membrane of the crypt are referred to as "carcinoma in situ" or simply "high-grade dysplasia." These terms are synonymous. Adenomas containing carcinoma in situ are cured by complete polypectomy but are an indication of high risk. Incomplete removal of such lesions means that progression to invasive dysplasia, or cancer, may occur. If dysplastic cells penetrate the basement membrane of the crypt but are confined to the lamina propria of the epithelium and do not penetrate the muscularis mucosa into the submucosa, the lesion is referred to as "intramucosal carcinoma." Although metastasis is theoretically possible under these circumstances, this lesion to all intents and purposes benign, and a complete polypectomy is sufficient for cure. It is unfortunate

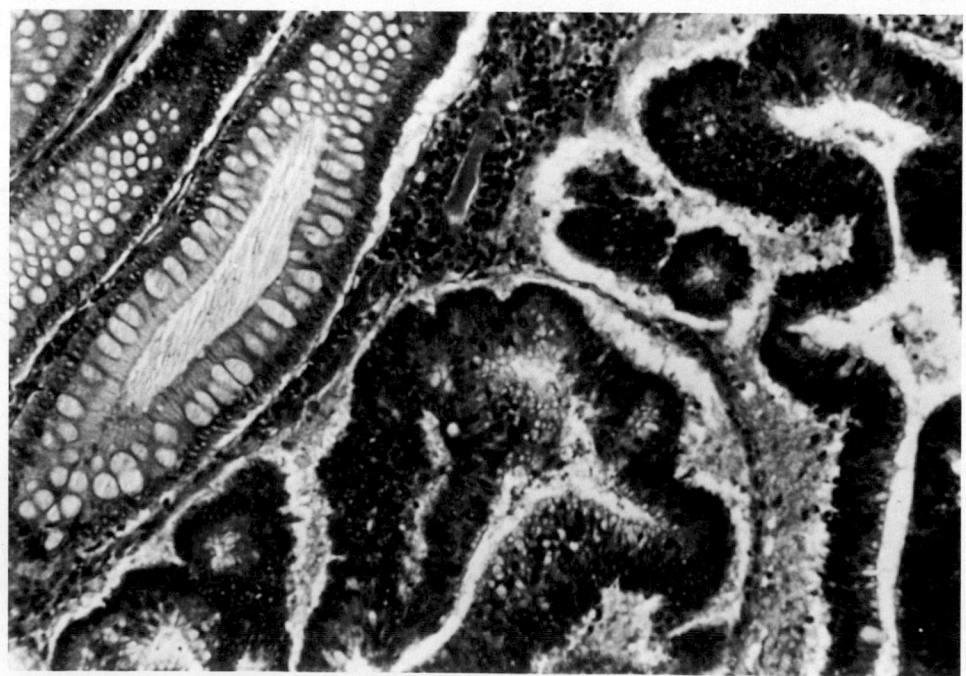

FIGURE 22-19. Adenomatous polyp with severe dysplasia **(right)**; normal glands **(left)**. (Original magnification × 600; courtesy of Rudolf Garret, MD.)

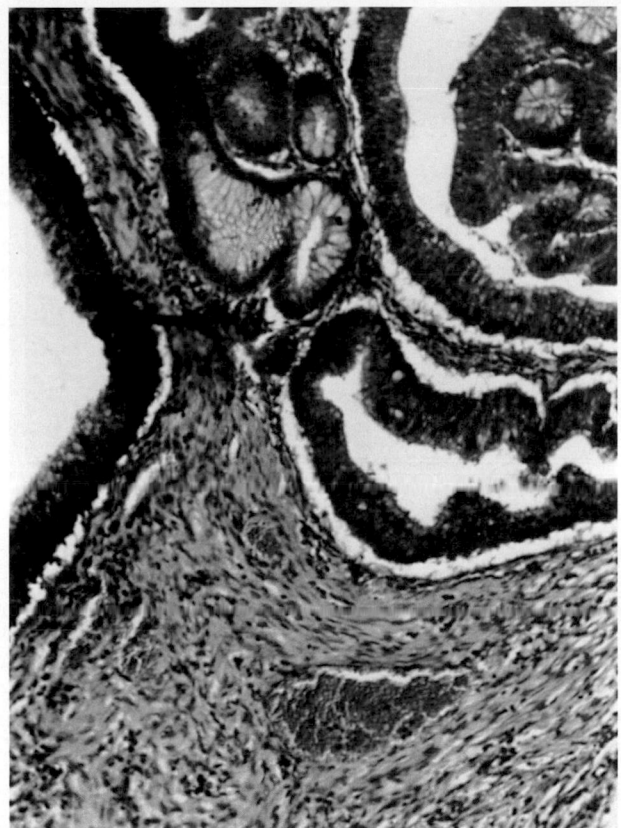

FIGURE 22-20. Adenomatous polyp with severe dysplasia; the whole thickness of the glandular epithelium shows total loss of polarity. (Original magnification × 600; courtesy of Rudolf Garret, MD.)

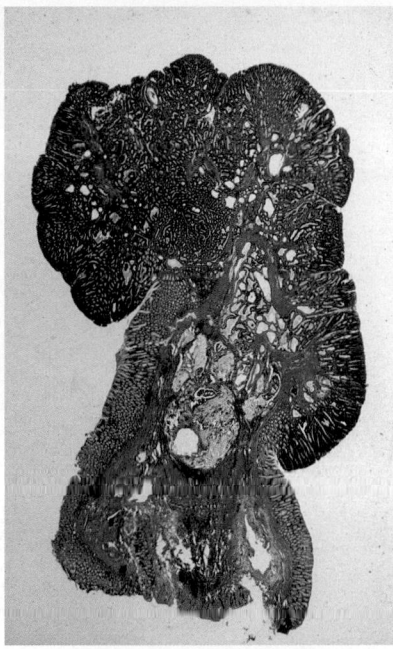

FIGURE 22-21. Adenomatous polyp with pseudoinvasion of the pedicle. The glands are cystically dilated and look identical to those in the polyp. The glands in the stalk are lined by normal-appearing epithelium. (Original magnification × 80; from Corman ML, Veidenheimer MC, Swinton NW. *Diseases of the Anus, Rectum, and Colon. Part I: Neoplasms.* New York, NY: Medcom; 1972, with permission.)

that in both the terms "carcinoma in situ" and "intramucosal carcinoma" the word "carcinoma" is used. This may lead to unnecessarily aggressive treatment. Therefore, it is wise to have such lesions reviewed by an independent pathologist because histologic diagnosis is somewhat subjective, and crucial management decisions are made based on the report.

Classification of Adenomas

Adenomas can be classified by size, shape, histology, degree of dysplasia, number, and location in the colon. Each of these properties allows stratification of adenomas in one or more of a number of considerations: cancer risk, complications of polypectomy, and the need for surgery. The most common and the most clinically applicable classification of adenomas is simply by high risk and low risk. Here the word "risk" refers to the risk of metachronous cancer. It also carries the connotation that the "high-risk" adenoma would probably have become malignant had it not been removed, whereas "low-risk" adenomas probably would not. The basic definitions of high-risk and low-risk adenomas are derived from a seminal paper by Atkin and colleagues from St. Mark's Hospital in which the data were derived from follow-up of patients with polyps removed by flexible sigmoidoscopy.[14] Criteria for defining high-risk adenomas are the following

- Size ≥1 cm
- Histology ≥25% villous component
- Dysplasia: any adenoma with high-grade dysplasia
- Number greater than or equal to three synchronous adenomas

In general, the criteria move together, so that the larger the adenoma, the longer it has been present, and the higher the chance of there being villous histology and severe dysplasia. All of these criteria confer an increased risk of metachronous adenomas and imply that surveillance should be more aggressive.

Classifying Adenomas by Shape

A "polyp" can be defined as a "lump" on an epithelial lining. Therefore, adenomatous polyps should protrude into the lumen to a certain extent. Certainly, these are the most common sorts of adenomas: pedunculated (with a stalk) or sessile (no stalk—Figures 22-22 and 22-23). However, adenomas

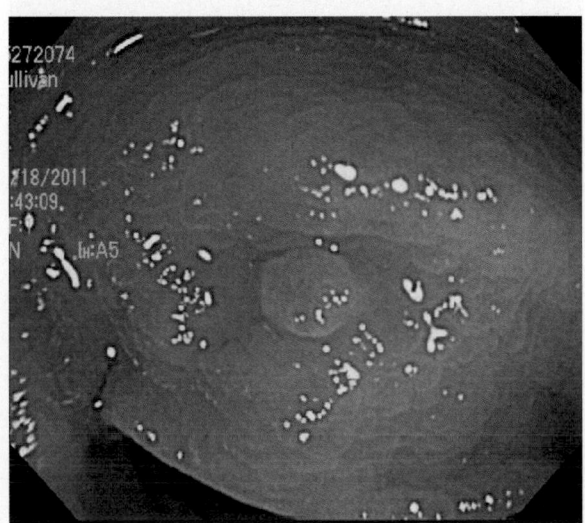

FIGURE 22-22. 3-mm sessile adenoma.

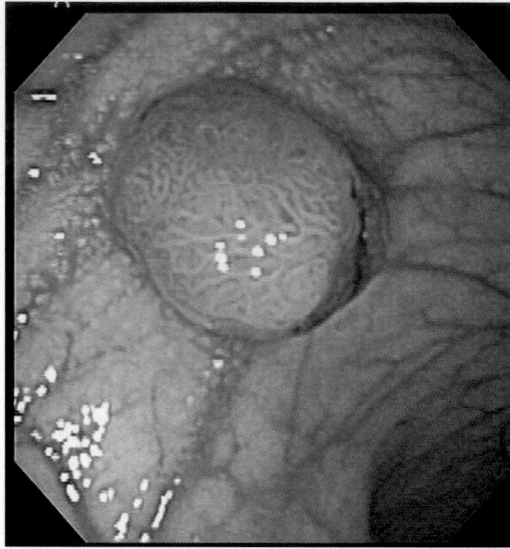

FIGURE 22-23. 1-cm pedunculated adenoma with a short stalk.

may be flat or even depressed (Figures 22-24 through 22-26). It is, therefore, more correct to refer to adenomatous lesions because this includes the nonpolypoid varieties. A system of classifying adenomas by shape is used by some endoscopists. The Paris classification includes four types (I, II, III, IV) and up to three subtypes (a, b, c, d).[254] Recent data show that polyp appearance can predict the presence of malignancy within the polyp.[231] "Flat" adenomas have become a controversial topic as they apparently occur quite commonly in Japan and China and other Eastern countries, but much less frequently in the West. This may be due to differences in recognition and definition, rather than in biology and epidemiology.[72] In 2,659 colonoscopies, Church removed 5,749 colorectal lesions from 2,003 patients. There were

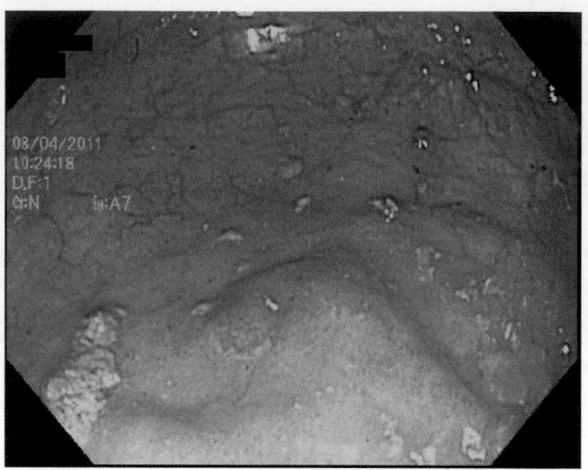

FIGURE 22-25. 1-cm irregular flat adenoma in the cecum.

3,115 adenomas (54% of lesions): 315 were flat (10.1%); 23 (0.8%) were depressed; 2,575 were sessile (82.7%); and 200 were pedunculated (6.4%). Two hundred twelve patients had flat adenomas (10.6% of patients): 172 patients had one, and 40 had multiple (two to eight) flat adenomas. Eight patients with flat adenomas had more flat adenomas on follow-up.[117]

Implications for Diagnosis

Flat or depressed lesions are difficult to see even when the bowel preparation is good. When the preparation is suboptimal, they are very difficult to identify.[179]

Implications for Treatment

Pedunculated polyps are easy to snare completely; thus, persistence rates should be close to zero. They are also easily evaluated histologically. When they contain cancer, the need for subsequent bowel resection can be more accurately assessed (see later). Sessile polyps are more difficult to snare because the snare may slip off of the polyp. Large sessile polyps are often removed piecemeal. Flat adenomas and especially depressed adenomas are the most difficult to remove endoscopically. They may be raised by an injection of saline or by some other agent into the submucosa below the lesion, but remain a challenge to endoscopists.

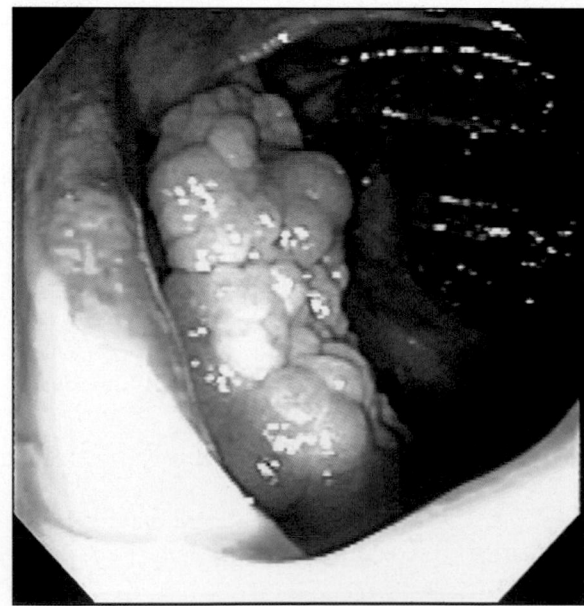

FIGURE 22-24. 3-cm sessile adenoma on a fold in the ascending colon.

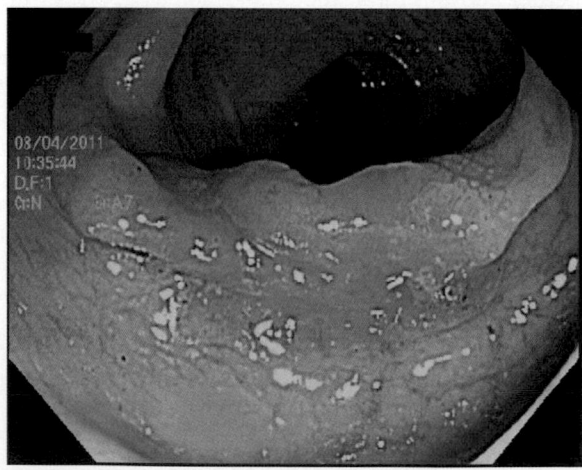

FIGURE 22-26. 20-mm flat adenoma on a fold in the sigmoid colon.

Classifying Adenomas by Size

The size of adenomas is a crude reflection of the duration they have been present, although growth rates vary between patients and presumably between genotypes. However, the risk of containing a cancer is at least partially related to maximum diameter. Size also influences resectability in that the risk of complication of snare polypectomy is higher with larger lesions. This is understandable because as more tissue is pulled into the snare, the chance of pulling muscularis propria along with mucosa and submucosa increases. Waye and others have recommended that no more than 2 cm of tissue be snared at one application. Polyps greater than 2 cm in diameter must, therefore, be removed piecemeal or by endoscopic submucosal dissection (ESD).[340]

Conventionally, polyps less than 6 mm in diameter are called "diminutive." Although dismissed as clinically insignificant by some (especially radiologists involved in virtual colonoscopy),[190] there is a rate of advanced adenomas or cancer that approaches 5%. Church divided 5,722 adenomas into three groups by size: 4,381 were less than 6 mm and included 2 cancers and 91 with high-risk histology (4.4%), 666 (11.6%) were 6 to 10 mm in diameter and included 1 cancer and 15.6% with high-risk histology; and 675 (11.8%) were more than 10 mm in diameter, including 21 invasive cancers and 326 (57.8%) with unfavorable histology. There was no effect of age, family history, or site of the polyp on the proportion that were high risk.[69] At the other end of the spectrum, the risk of cancer in an adenoma is associated with size and degree of villous change.[244] Gschwantler and associates found that the percentage of diminutive adenomas with severe dysplasia or cancer was 3.4%; for adenomas 5 to 10 mm, it was 13.5%, and for adenomas more than 10 mm, it was 38.5%.[125]

The ability to detect, or at least to be suspicious of cancer in a polyp, is helpful because it can be an indication for tattooing the lesion in order to facilitate resection should this be required. Obvious cancers should not be resected endoscopically (except with transanal endoscopic microsurgery) because invasion into the submucosa increases the risk of perforation and because surgery is likely to be needed even after polypectomy. Polyps that are ulcerated, hard, irregular, and fragile are likely to contain cancer. In addition, a "nonlifting" sign in the absence of past attempts at polypectomy or biopsy is a sign of cancer.

Classifying Adenomas by Histology

All adenomas are neoplastic and dysplastic. However, the architecture of the epithelium may be tubular or villous. Tubular epithelium shows parallel straight crypts, whereas villous demonstrates proliferative crypts like a fern frond (Figure 22-27). Adenomas with less than 25% villous component are considered tubular; with 25% to 75% villous component, tubulovillous; and those with more than 75% villous component are villous. Villous adenomas are uncommon but are more likely to contain severe dysplasia or cancer. In patients with villous adenomas, the incidence of malignant change has been reported to be 10% in polyps less than 2 cm and 53% in polyps greater than 2 cm in diameter.[233] Stulc and colleagues, reporting from the Roswell Park Memorial Institute (Buffalo, NY), identified 65 villous and tubulovillous adenomas ≥4 cm.[310] They noted that 85% contained invasive adenocarcinoma.

Classifying Adenomas by Pit Pattern

Some 25 years ago, studies of the ability of the endoscopist to distinguish adenomas from hyperplastic polyps showed that endoscopic guesses were inaccurate.[52,239] Since then, endoscopic technology has advanced and now includes chromoendoscopy, magnifying colonoscopy with high-definition imaging, and narrow band imaging.[95,188,337] Tissue spectroscopy is still experimental, but the combination of a very

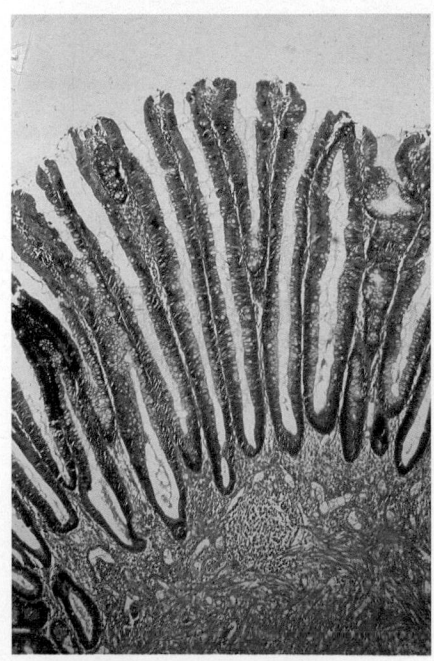
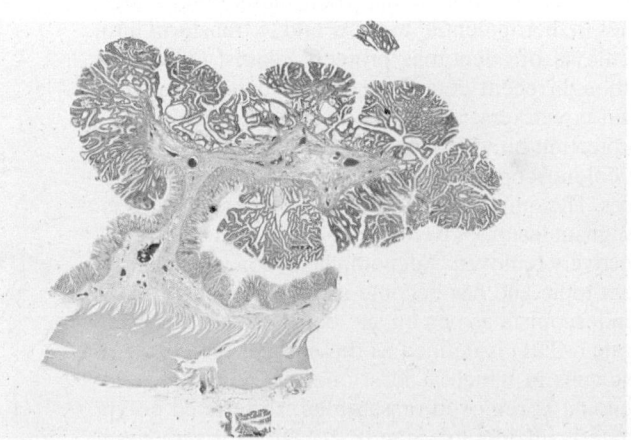

FIGURE 22-27. Villous adenoma. Papillary fronds extend from the mucosa **(A)**. (Original magnification × 280; from Corman ML, Veidenheimer MC, Swinton NW. *Diseases of the Anus, Rectum, and Colon. Part I: Neoplasms*. New York, NY: Medcom; 1972, with permission.) **B:** Villous adenoma (whole mount specimen). Note the papillary projections with transition between the normal large bowel mucosa and the polyp. Villoglandular polyp. (Courtesy of Rudolf Garret, MD.)

detailed look at the epithelium of polyps with a pit pattern classification system, such as that devised by Kudo,[196] allows a much more accurate diagnosis of lesions by inspection alone. However, as technology has improved, the clinical premise has changed in that "nonneoplastic" lesions such as hyperplastic polyps are no longer viewed as clinically insignificant and harmless (see earlier discussion).

Classifying Adenomas by Number

In general terms, the number of adenomas reflects the stability of the colorectal epithelium in any individual patient. One who never develops an adenoma has a favorable balance of colorectal genotype, environment, and host defense. A patient with multiple adenomas has an unfavorable balance, and a patient with a cancer has no balance at all. Church reported on patients who were "polyp resistant" and "polyp prone" after removal of an index lesion, showing the extremes of colorectal fertility.[66] Not surprisingly, female gender and a single index lesion favored neoplasia resistance, whereas male gender and multiple index lesions favored a predisposition to neoplasia.

The number of adenomas is important in that three synchronous adenomas is an indication of a significantly higher risk of metachronous lesions and should stimulate different, more aggressive surveillance.[240] More than 10 adenomas suggest adenomatous polyposis and is a trigger for genetic testing for *APC* and *MYH* mutations.

Classifying Adenomas by Location

The right side of the colon is conventionally defined as proximal to the splenic flexure. This is the site of preference for hereditary nonpolyposis colorectal cancer (HNPCC)-associated neoplasia and for serrated neoplasia. Sporadic adenomas occur throughout the large intestine, however, and their malignant potential is the same wherever they are found. Right-sided adenomas are more difficult to remove because the bowel wall is thinner, and complications such as bleeding and perforation are harder to avoid. More right-sided adenomas are likely to be flat than those on the left, and, therefore, right-sided lesions are more difficult to detect and to remove.

Adenoma Detection

Most adenomas are asymptomatic. Their major clinical significance lies in their potential to grow and to transform into cancer. Removal of adenomas protects against colorectal cancer, although recent data from Baxter and colleagues, Brenner and coworkers, and Mulder and associates show that this protection only applies to left-sided cancers.[20,35,232] Screening colonoscopy fails to protect against right-sided colon cancer. The only explanation for these observations is that premalignant lesions are either not being seen or, if seen, are not effectively removed. Adenoma detection is, therefore, an important topic and has become as much a quality indicator for endoscopists as percentage completion. Adenoma detection rate (ADR) is defined as the number (percentage) of colonoscopies in which at least one histologically confirmed adenoma is removed or sampled.[224] Serrated polyp detection rate is analogous. Standard ADRs for screening colonoscopy in average risk patients are 25% for men and 15% for women. ADR is related strongly to withdrawal time and withdrawal technique[199,224] and varies considerably among endoscopists.[178,224] Although the application of ADR

as a quality indicator for the performance of colonoscopy may be considered somewhat controversial,[60] it is now an established principle.[183]

Diagnosis and Evaluation

Most colorectal adenomas are found during colonoscopy. Occasionally, a polyp prolapses through the anus (Figure 22-28) or may be seen incidentally on a CT scan or barium enema (Figure 22-29), but the vast majority are found during colonoscopy performed for screening, surveillance, or for the cause of symptoms. Once a polyp is found, it should be removed. Attempts at estimating polyp histology by endoscopic appearance are often incorrect.[52,239] However, advances in colonoscopic technology offer magnifying scopes and high definition and may increase accuracy. It is reasonable to leave polyps untreated if they are typical hyperplastic polyps in a cluster in the rectum and sigmoid. Even so, some of the cluster should be sampled to confirm the endoscopic diagnosis. Otherwise, every individual polyp should be removed. Some polyps are not removable endoscopically, such as flat lesions on the ileocecal valve or recurrent lesions with submucosal fibrosis from prior attempts at polypectomy.[68] In the year 2011, the techniques of ESD and endoscopic mucosal resection (EMR) offer the prospect of making almost all benign colorectal polyps removable without surgery.[2,76,97,102,145,231,311,314] If surgery is required, minimally invasive techniques have made even

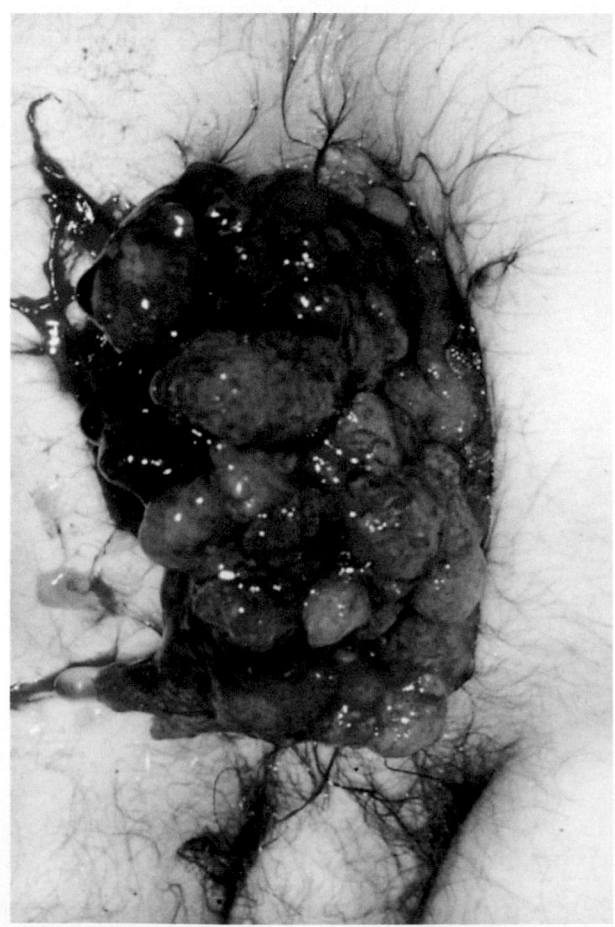

FIGURE 22-28. Villous adenoma presenting outside the anus. (Courtesy of Rudolf Garret, MD.)

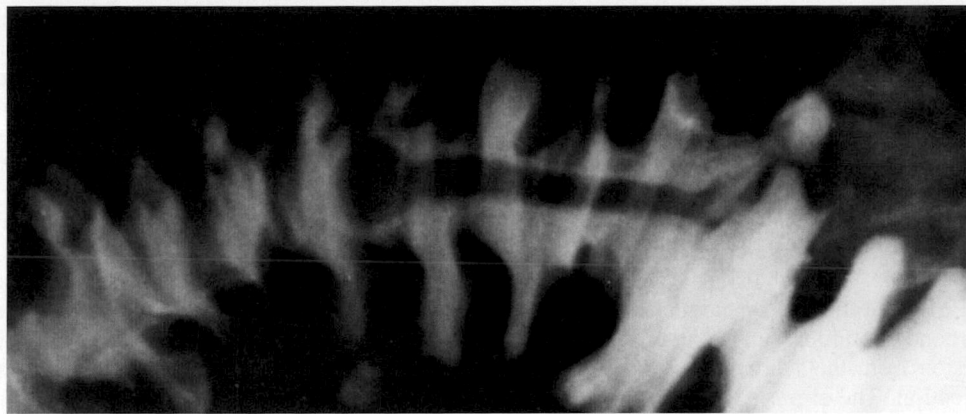

FIGURE 22-29. Adenomatous polyp. Barium enema demonstrates a 1.5-cm lesion on a very long pedicle.

surgery a relatively minor and usually straightforward experience.[133,263,356] Laparoscopy can be used with endoscopy to optimize polypectomy and limit risk.[174] Size and location rarely make a polyp unremovable. In several series of polyps referred for surgery, up to 74% were able to be resected endoscopically.[67,335] Therefore, when patients have an apparently unsnareable polyp or if the colonoscopist is concerned or inexperienced in performing polypectomy, the first step in treatment is to refer the patient to a more experienced therapeutic endoscopist.[207] In someone with a short life expectancy and/or a high morbidity, polyps should not necessarily be removed. In these patients, colonoscopy, itself, should not even be performed.

When polyps are found during colonoscopy, correct labeling of each lesion according to size, shape, and location is essential. It is easy for reports to become confused, but in the interests of appropriate surveillance and communication with referring and consulting doctors, a clear and accurate picture of the findings at colonoscopy is required. When polyps are treated, a clear description of the technique used, the specimen recovered, the completeness of resection, and the occurrence of immediate complications are necessary.

Treatment and Surveillance

Medical Treatment

Although the preferred treatment of colorectal adenomas is excision, there may be a role for medical and dietary treatment for prevention of adenomas and cancer. In fact, chemoprevention studies using adenomas as a surrogate end point for cancer abound.[134] The role for a diet high in vegetables and fruits and low in red meats is dubious, however, because the chance of reversing the molecular changes in the mucosa that have accumulated over a lifetime are miniscule.[157] Dietary therapy is better directed to the young, those whose colons are relatively pure genetically. There has been a particular interest in supplementary antioxidant vitamins to prevent colorectal cancer because these are present in more "wholesome" food groups. A clinical trial of such antioxidant vitamins (β-carotene, vitamin C, and vitamin E) was undertaken to determine their efficacy in prevention of colorectal adenomas. In the experience of Greenberg and his associates in the Polyp Prevention Study Group in which 751 patients completed a 4-year clinical trial, there was no demonstrable benefit with the use of supplemental β-carotene and vitamins C and E.[119] However, in a publication by Whelan and

colleagues, the use of multivitamins, vitamin E, and calcium supplements was found to be associated with a lower incidence of *recurrent* adenomas.[345]

Nonsteroidal anti-inflammatory drugs are effective in reducing both risks of colorectal cancer and of recurrent adenomas. Aspirin and sulindac have been shown to be effective, and the combination of sulindac and difluoromethylornithine (DFMO) has been the most effective chemopreventive regimen for sporadic adenomas ever reported.[223] Calcium has also been shown to be effective in reducing the development of metachronous adenomas after initial colectomy. Epidemiologic evidence suggests that vitamin D levels may also be related to neoplasia risk in the colon.[19] There are several newer agents that may be effective as chemoprevention for adenomas and cancer. These include folate, curcumin, and statins.[18,134,257]

Colonoscopic Polypectomy

The technique of colonoscopic polypectomy is discussed in detail in Chapter 6. Almost all colorectal polyps should be able to be excised, with a specimen recovered for histology (Figure 22-30). Recently, EMR and ESD have been used increasingly frequently for removal of large, sessile, or flat lesions. EMR relies on a sublesional injection of saline or

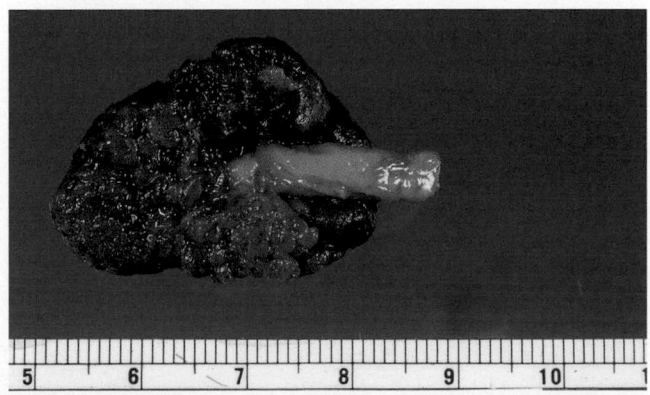

FIGURE 22-30. Colonoscopy-polypectomy of villoglandular polyp. This pedunculated lesion has areas of varied coloration that, on microscopic examination, showed both villous and adenomatous changes. (From Corman ML, Veidenheimer MC, Swinton NW. *Diseases of the Anus, Rectum, and Colon. Part I: Neoplasms.* New York, NY: Medcom; 1972, with permission.)

other fluid to raise the polyp and facilitate piecemeal excision with a snare. Usually, the injected fluid contains weak (1:10,000) adrenaline and a small amount of a stain (methylene blue or indigo carmine). The technique is safe, with perforation rates less than 2% and acceptable polyp persistence rates less than 15%.[231] A specialized therapeutic endoscopy center is the ideal place for this technique to be practiced because it generally applies to lesions larger than 3 cm.

ESD is a technique originally described in Japan for removal of gastric lesions. The sublesional injection is the same as that for EMR, but then the technique involves making an incision around the tumor with a diathermy knife and dissecting the lesion from the submucosa in the plane enlarged by the injection. The aim is to remove the lesion in one piece to allow better histologic examination and a more complete excision. Data show less polyp recurrence, but the technique is time consuming and associated with perforation rates of 5% or more.[146,245] This procedure should be reserved for specialist endoscopists.

Operative Techniques and Polypectomy

Open polypectomy, making a colotomy for the purposes of polyp excision, is uncommonly employed today. Almost all polyps can be reached endoscopically and managed endoscopically. However, if colonoscopy is unavailable, if the lesion is believed to be beyond the limit of the endoscopist's ability, if the instrument cannot be passed to the level of the lesion, or if adequate control cannot be obtained during an attempt at polypectomy, abdominal operation may be justified. Even with one of these criteria fulfilled, however, a second opinion from another endoscopist would be the prudent alternative. Figure 22-31 illustrates the classic technique of colotomy-polypectomy for a pedunculated lesion.

The major concerns for laparotomy as the method for removing the lesion are, of course, the operative morbidity and mortality, hospital costs, and time lost from work. These issues have been minimized by the routine use of minimally invasive techniques. The combination of laparoscopy and polypectomy is now commonly reported. Grünhagen and colleagues reported successful polypectomy facilitated by laparoscopic mobilization of the colon in 9 of 11 patients. In the other two, segmental resection was performed.[124] Franklin and Portillo had excellent long-term outcomes in 209 cases of laparoscopic-monitored colonoscopic polypectomy. There was no case of polyp recurrence.[103] Wilhelm and coworkers used all possible combinations of laparoscopy and colonoscopy in 146 consecutive patients with 154 lesions.[348] One hundred twenty (82%) underwent local excision (including laparoscopy-assisted endoscopic resection, endoscopy-assisted wedge resection, and endoscopy-assisted transluminal resection), whereas 26 (18%) had endoscopy-assisted segmental colon resection. Conversion rate was 5%. Intraoperative complications occurred in two patients (1%), and major postoperative complications occurred in five (3%). There was a local recurrence rate of 0.9%.[348] Delaney and associates reported the first experience with a "tissue apposition system" that allows an endoscopic closure of large defects created by EMR.[87] Five of seven patients were successfully managed using laparoscopy to monitor safety, thus showing that advances in both endoscopy and surgery apply to the management of colorectal polyps.[87]

Polyp Follow-up

There are two concerns for the endoscopist contemplating follow-up of a colorectal adenoma. The first is to make certain that the resected polyp is completely treated. The second is to make sure that missed synchronous polyps and metachronous polyps

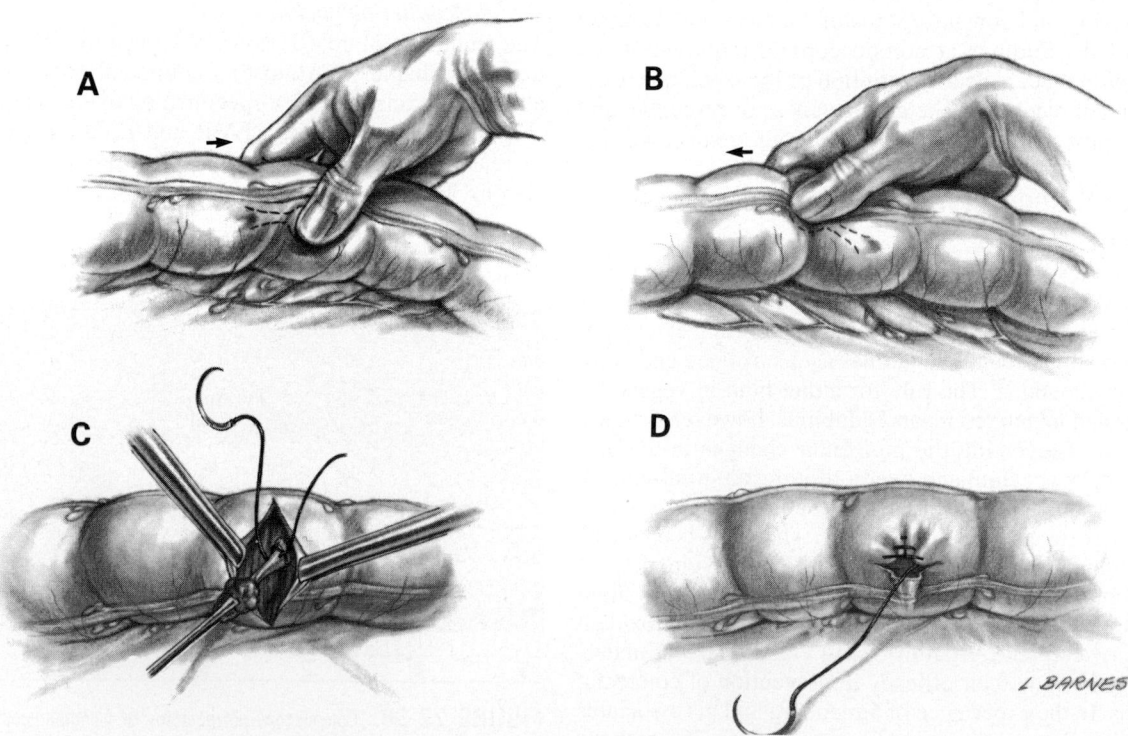

FIGURE 22-31. Colotomy and polypectomy. The base of the pedicle is determined by traction to create dimpling (**A**), or the polyp is moved in both directions (**B**), with the site (**C**) for colotomy determined by splitting the difference. Transverse colotomy is preferred, and the base is suture ligated. Longitudinal enterotomy (**D**) with transverse closure to avoid luminal narrowing is also acceptable.

are diagnosed and removed prior to the development of malignant change. The first concern arises from the colonoscopist's own assessment of how the polypectomy went. A clean snare through the stalk of a pedunculated polyp guarantees complete removal. Piecemeal removal of a large sessile polyp does not. Follow-up of the first scenario can be dictated by the risk of new lesions: missed synchronous or metachronous polyps. Follow-up of the latter occurs soon after mucosal healing to allow a check of the polypectomy site (about 6 months is reasonable). The stakes are higher when the index lesion contains severe dysplasia.

Follow-up of lesions treated by cold or hot biopsy, or cold snare, depends on their size and the colonoscopist's feeling about completeness of excision. In general, these are small, less significant tumors, and so the presence of residual adenoma is not a calamity. Surveillance can be designed without concern for recurrence, and recurrent lesions are picked up in the same way as missed synchronous lesions.

Missed Synchronous Polyps

It is difficult to design a surveillance program to guard against missed adenomas because adenoma miss rates have been reported only by a small number of expert endoscopists. However, miss rates can be extrapolated as the obverse of adenoma detection rates and so calculated by each endoscopist based on a review of their own experience. In a review of six tandem colonoscopy studies, van Rijn and associates found a pooled miss rate for polyps of any size of 22% (95% CI, 19–26). Adenoma miss rate by size was 2.1% for adenomas more than 10 mm, 13% for adenomas 5 to 10 mm, and 26% for adenomas 1 to 5 mm.[331] There are obviously multiple factors that apply to polyp and adenoma detection rates,[62] and the following society recommendations apply to most competent colonoscopists after examination of a clean colon.

Recommendations for surveillance colonoscopy intervals are based on guidelines issued by the various professional organizations. The most recent guidelines come from the U.S. Multisociety Task Force on Colorectal Cancer and the American Cancer Society. They are based on the presence of high-risk adenomas at index examination.[10,349] Patients with three or more adenomas or high-grade dysplasia, or villous features, or an adenoma ≥1 cm in size should have a 3-year follow-up colonoscopy. Those with one or two small (less than 1 cm) tubular adenomas with no high-grade dysplasia can have a follow-up in 5 to 10 years. Patients with only small hyperplastic polyps should have a 10-year follow-up,

the same as patients with a normal colon. These baseline recommendations can be tempered by other factors such as poor preparation or incomplete colonoscopy. Their success will also depend on patients receiving a thorough, well-performed examination, something that clearly cannot be guaranteed given the range of ADRs that has been reported. In addition, the recommendation of 10-year surveillance for hyperplastic polyps is out of date and oversimplified. A discussion of serrated polyps is discussed earlier in this chapter.

Management of Malignant Polyp

The situation of invasive carcinoma found in a polypectomy specimen can be difficult to judge and to advise (Figure 22-32).[21,25,79,228,277,294,297,351] Options include observation, attempts at resecting more polyp or stalk, or surgical resection of the segment of bowel containing the malignant polyp. Most advise resection selectively, separating patients into those at high risk of having residual cancer from those at low risk. The clinical sequelae of a colon resection are important, even in the age of minimally invasive surgery, and removal of a colon containing no residual cancer, while reassuring, is in retrospect an unnecessary operation.

Most authors advise the use of criteria to define lesions as high risk and low risk, or unfavorable and favorable. Wolff and Shinya have encapsulated the most important criteria for surgical resection: cancer close to the plane of excision, tumor in the lymphatics, or if the lesion is poorly differentiated.[351] The definition of "close to the plane of excision" has been interpreted differently by various authors. At the Cleveland Clinic, a 2-mm margin is required. Others are content with 1 mm, whereas some do not specify a distance. All studies see poor differentiation as an ominous prognostic indicator, which generally overlaps lymphovascular invasion.

Haggitt and colleagues determined the prognostic significance of invasion at different levels in 129 colorectal carcinomas arising in adenomas (Figure 22-33).[129] The level of invasion was defined according to the following criteria:

Level 1: carcinoma invading through the muscularis mucosae into the submucosa but limited to the head of the polyp

Level 2: carcinoma invading to the level of the junction between adenoma and stalk

Level 3: carcinoma invading any part of the stalk

Level 4: carcinoma invading into the submucosa of the bowel wall but above the muscularis propria[129]

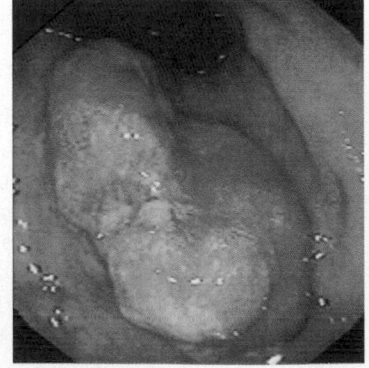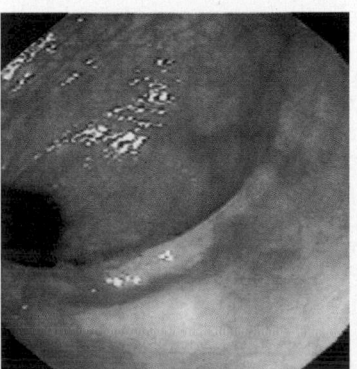

FIGURE 22-32. **A:** A large adenomatous polyp was found to contain invasive carcinoma. **B:** The postpolypectomy site appeared relatively benign. Resection revealed lymph node involvement with adenocarcinoma.

RODGER C. HAGGITT (1942–2000)

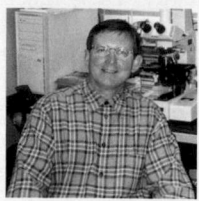

Rodger Haggitt was born in Detroit, Michigan on August 28, 1942. At the age of 11, he and his family moved to Tennessee. At age 16, he was introduced to what would become a lifelong passion while assisting a local pathologist with an autopsy. By the time he entered medical school, literally hundreds of autopsies later, he took pride in his finely honed autopsy skills and knack for making visual observations. He began his formal pathology training at the Baptist Memorial Hospital in Memphis and completed it at the New England Deaconess Hospital in Boston with Shields Warren (see the biography in this chapter), William Meissner, and Merle Lagg. After fulfilling his military obligation at Tripler Army Medical Center in Honolulu, he returned to Boston and the Deaconess Hospital as one of pathology's rising stars. In 1977, Haggitt returned to the University of Tennessee and the Baptist Memorial Hospital, where he directed the Division of Surgical Pathology. In 1984, he moved to the University of Washington in Seattle as director of the Division of Gastrointestinal Pathology. Haggitt's interest in this specialty developed when the era of colonoscopy and of gastrointestinal endoscopic biopsy began. Because of his desire to combine clinical relevance with pathologic interpretation, he enjoyed a close interaction with his gastrointestinal medical and surgical colleagues. His study of prognostic factors for adenocarcinoma arising in endoscopically resected colonic adenomas has come to be known as the Haggitt Classification. His collaboration with the late Warren Nugent, chief of gastroenterology at the Lahey Clinic in Boston, resulted in the publication of one of the first long-term,

prospective, follow-up studies of neoplastic progression in ulcerative colitis. They showed that endoscopic surveillance reduced mortality from colorectal cancer. At Tripler in Hawaii, while fulfilling his military obligation, Haggitt worked with Larry Johnson and Tom DeMeester to establish esophageal 24-hour pH monitoring as the gold standard for investigating gastroesophageal reflux disease. In 1978, he and his colleagues at the Deaconess Hospital published a landmark study documenting that dysplasia was the precursor of adenocarcinoma in Barrett's esophagus and suggested that its detection by endoscopic biopsy could lead to earlier surgical intervention in order to prevent cancer in these patients. Haggitt also made important contributions to hepatic pathology, including the first American description of nonalcoholic steatohepatitis and, with James Williams at the University of Tennessee, the initial implementation of hepatic allograft biopsies. These protocol biopsies are now standard practice in many transplant centers. Dr. Haggitt was a dedicated and generous mentor to a generation of pathology residents and fellows. Through his activities with the American Society of Clinical Pathologists, he taught more practicing pathologists and had more influence on the practice of gastrointestinal pathology than any other person working with that organization. Haggitt was an active member of the national society, the Gastrointestinal Pathology Club. In 2001, after his tragic and untimely death on June 28, 2000, at the hands of a disturbed pathology resident, the name of the society was officially changed to the Rodger C. Haggitt Gastrointestinal Pathology Society. (With special appreciation to the Departments of Pathology and Gastroenterology, University of Washington, Seattle.)

Level 0 lesions are not defined as carcinomas because the muscularis mucosae is not breached. Level 4 invasion and rectal location were the only statistically significant adverse prognostic factors. The Haggit levels apply only to pedunculated polyps. Sessile lesions containing cancer generally need surgical resection because the piecemeal nature of the polypectomy makes assessment of margin status impossible. There are exceptions, however, such as when the focus of cancer is tiny and has clearly been encapsulated by the polypectomy.

There are two keys to proper management of malignant polyps. The first is accurate identification of the site of the polyps, and the second is competent interpretation of the microscopic findings. If the polyp location has been tattooed, if it is located close to a permanent landmark such as the ileocecal valve, or if it is clearly visible on follow-up colonoscopy, there is no problem with resection. Sometimes, however, polyp location is given as a number of centimeters form the anal verge. This is particularly unhelpful and dangerous in that the wrong section of colon can be removed. If the polypectomy site cannot be recognized and the referring endoscopist's report is not exact in defining polyp location, it is difficult to plot a course of action. A more extensive colectomy may be needed to make sure that the

cancer-containing section of bowel is removed. Repeat colonoscopy by the surgeon preoperatively or intraoperatively may need to be done to precisely localize the lesion.

Review of histology is the second key to effective management of the malignant polyp. Severe dysplasia, adenoma with atypia, carcinoma in situ, and intramucosal carcinoma must be excluded because none of these lesions require surgery.[278] The surgeon is well advised to look at the slides with the pathologist in order to determine whether there is need for an aggressive approach.

Management of Benign Rectal Tumors

Large benign neoplasms of the rectum are a particularly challenging issue in that they are relatively common, and there are multiple options for their management. They are usually villous adenomas, and because of this histology and their size, they have an increased likelihood of malignant degeneration when compared with polypoid adenomas. Biopsy is not very accurate for excluding cancer, so the tumor should be inspected and, where possible, palpated carefully. Ulceration or fixity raises the suspicion of invasion.

Taylor and colleagues reported their experience with preoperative assessment of villous adenomas.[315] Forty-four

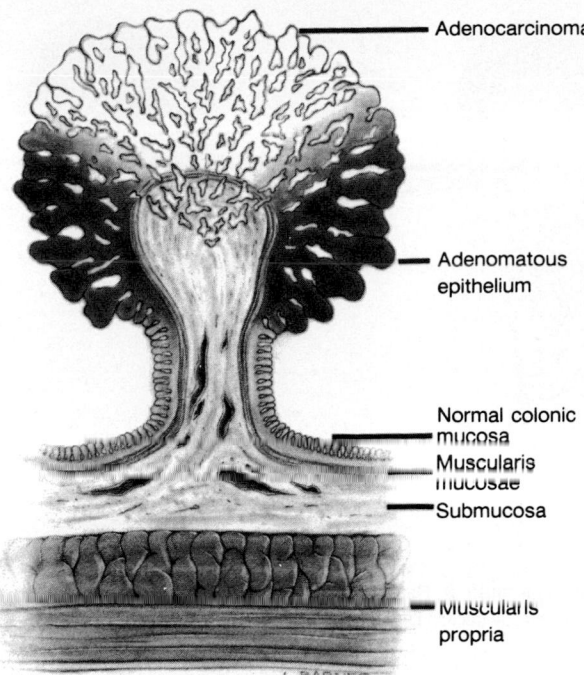

FIGURE 22-33. A pedunculated adenoma has various structures that determine the significance of invasion at different levels. (Adapted from Haggitt RC, Glotzbach RE, Soffer EE, et al. Prognostic factors in colorectal carcinomas arising in adenomas: implications for lesions removed by endoscopic polypectomy. *Gastroenterology* 1985;89(2):328–336, with permission.)

percent of the biopsy reports were misleading when compared with the interpretation when the specimen was completely excised. Most disturbing was a 10% false-positive incidence. Therefore, the most important criterion for determining the type of operative approach is the clinical impression gained by palpation and inspection. Transrectal ultrasound and MRI may be helpful when the surgeon suspects a malignant growth. If one is convinced that the lesion harbors no invasive cancer, every effort should be made to perform a sphincter-saving operation.

Techniques

There are basically three methods of removing rectal tumors: endoscopic mucosal resection/endoscopic submucosal dissection, transanal excision, and rectal resection with or without restoration of intestinal continuity. These methods are discussed in Chapter 24, but transanal excision is reviewed here.

Transanal Excision

Transanal excision can be performed by snare electrocoagulation, by laser therapy, by conventional excision with some type of retractor, or by means of transanal endoscopic microsurgery (TEM). It is helpful to have the specimen removed intact, pinned out, and submitted for pathologic evaluation. This can usually be easily accomplished with a small lesion but is difficult with larger tumors. EMR and ESD are currently the preferred ways of removing larger benign rectal lesions. For smaller lesions (up to 3 cm), endoscopic snare polypectomy can result in complete removal. If the tumor is in the lower third of the rectum and is flat or depressed, transanal excision through the use of an anal retractor and electrocautery provides a better opportunity for excision. A margin of 5 mm around the lesion is marked initially, and the dissection can be undertaken as a full-thickness dissection through the rectal wall (Figure 22-34).

It is helpful to infiltrate the submucosa with saline solution or possibly dilute epinephrine in order to facilitate dissection and to limit blood loss. The rectal defect may be closed sequentially as the dissection proceeds with each suture held for traction. It is important to place the suture distally initially. Traction can also be effected by elevating a flap of

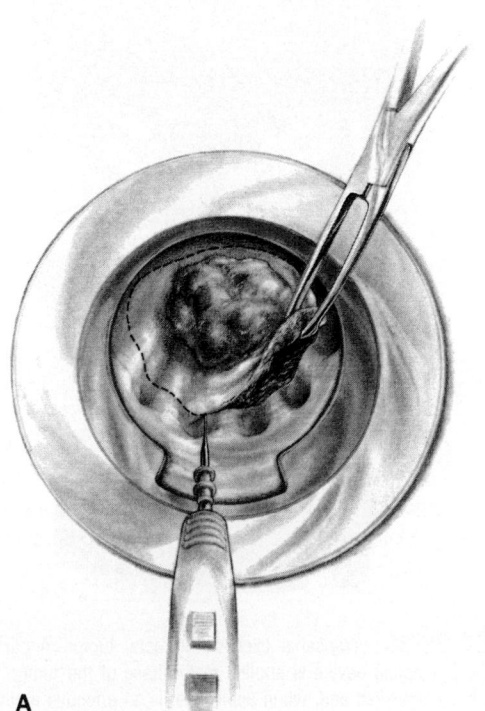

A

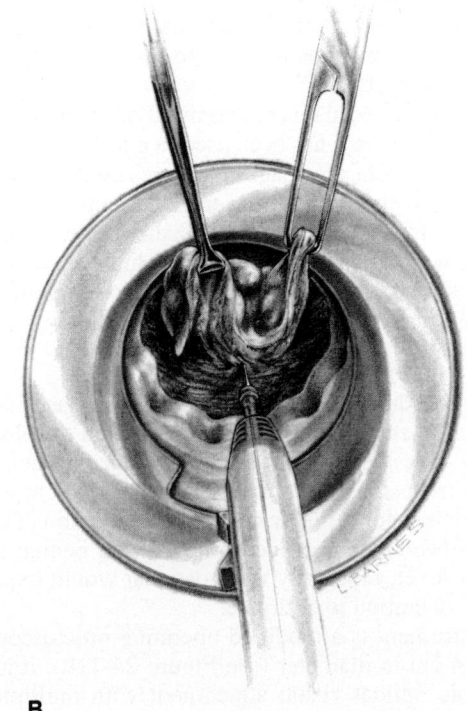

B

FIGURE 22-34. Transanal excision of rectal tumor by means of electrocautery. **A:** The tumor is outlined with the needle-tip electrode with an adequate margin. **B:** Complete excision of lesion with good hemostatic control.

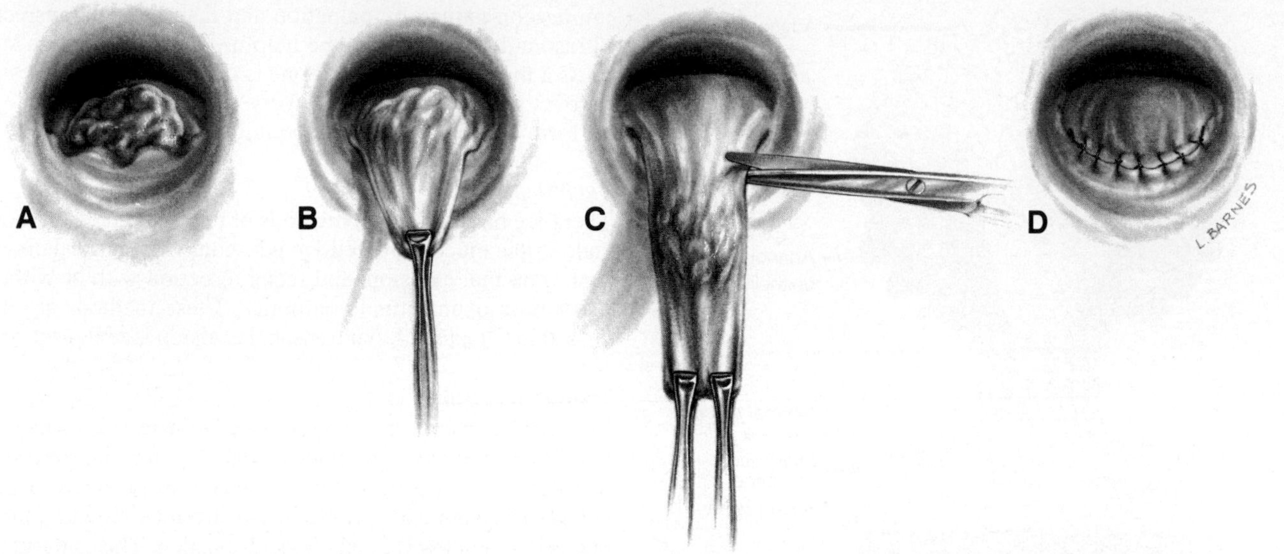

FIGURE 22-35. Transanal excision of tumor using mucosa for traction. **A:** Lesion identified. **B:** Flap mobilization with tumor. **C:** Excision. **D:** Closure. (Adapted from Pello MJ. Transanal excision of large sessile villous adenomas using an endorectal traction flap. *Surg Gynecol Obstet.* 1987;164(3):280–282, with permission.)

mucosa somewhat distal to the tumor (Figure 22-35).[259] However, closure of the defect is not necessary unless required for hemostasis. Other approaches have been described. In one, a pseudostalk composed of normal mucosa and submucosa is created by traction on the tumor with Allis or Babcock forceps, and a stapling device is applied across the base (Figure 22-36).[225] Another option is to use a laparoscopic stapler to excise the lesion and to maintain hemostasis (Figure 22-37).[86,266] The tumor is then removed. Even if the muscularis is incorporated by the staple line, bowel closure should still be secure. A further alternative is to use an endoscopic clipping apparatus as one excises the polyp in order to maintain hemostasis.[153]

The concept of rectal mucosectomy, as adapted from restorative proctocolectomy, has been used to manage large benign tumors of the rectum. Keck and colleagues used this approach in 12 patients with lesions, on average 8.5 cm in diameter.[185] After a mean follow-up of 47 months, the incidence of tumor persistence was 17% in this group, with a high recurrence rate. This technique is recommended for large or circumferential benign lesions and is illustrated in Figure 22-38.

Transanal Endoscopic Microsurgery

TEM is a procedure that has been available primarily through its German inventors since 1983.[218,283] It is an endoluminal, minimally invasive technique that permits transanal excision of rectal lesions up to a level of about 20 cm without the requirement for a major abdominal operation. The procedure has been recommended primarily for benign tumors at a higher level, especially for those that would require an abdominal operation to extirpate.

The instrument is a modified operating proctoscope that measures 4 cm in diameter (see Figure 24-119). It holds a stereoscopic optical visual attachment with multiple gastight ports to allow simultaneous use of up to four instruments. Carbon dioxide is constantly infused, and various instruments such as tissue graspers, a high-frequency knife,

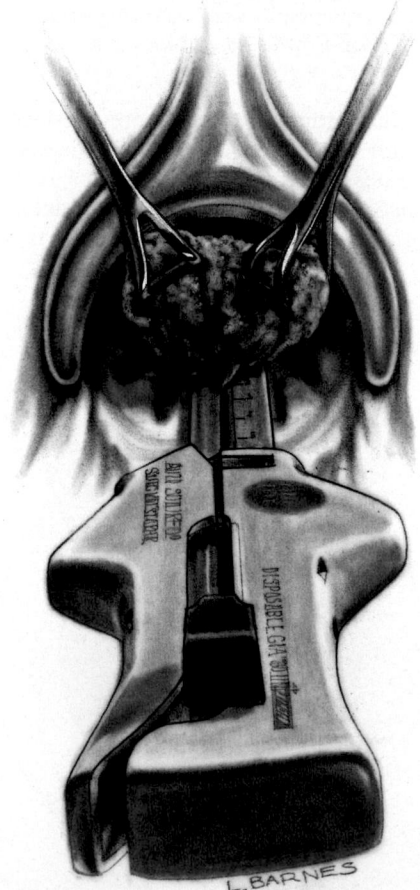

FIGURE 22-36. Transanal excision of rectal tumor. A gastrointestinal anastomosis stapling device is applied to the base of the tumor. The normal mucosa is incorporated and, when applicable, is an effective method for excision while maintaining hemostasis. (Redrawn from Miskowiak J, Lindenberg S. Excision of rectal villous adenoma using a TA or GIA stapler. *Br J Surg.* 1986; 73(8):630.)

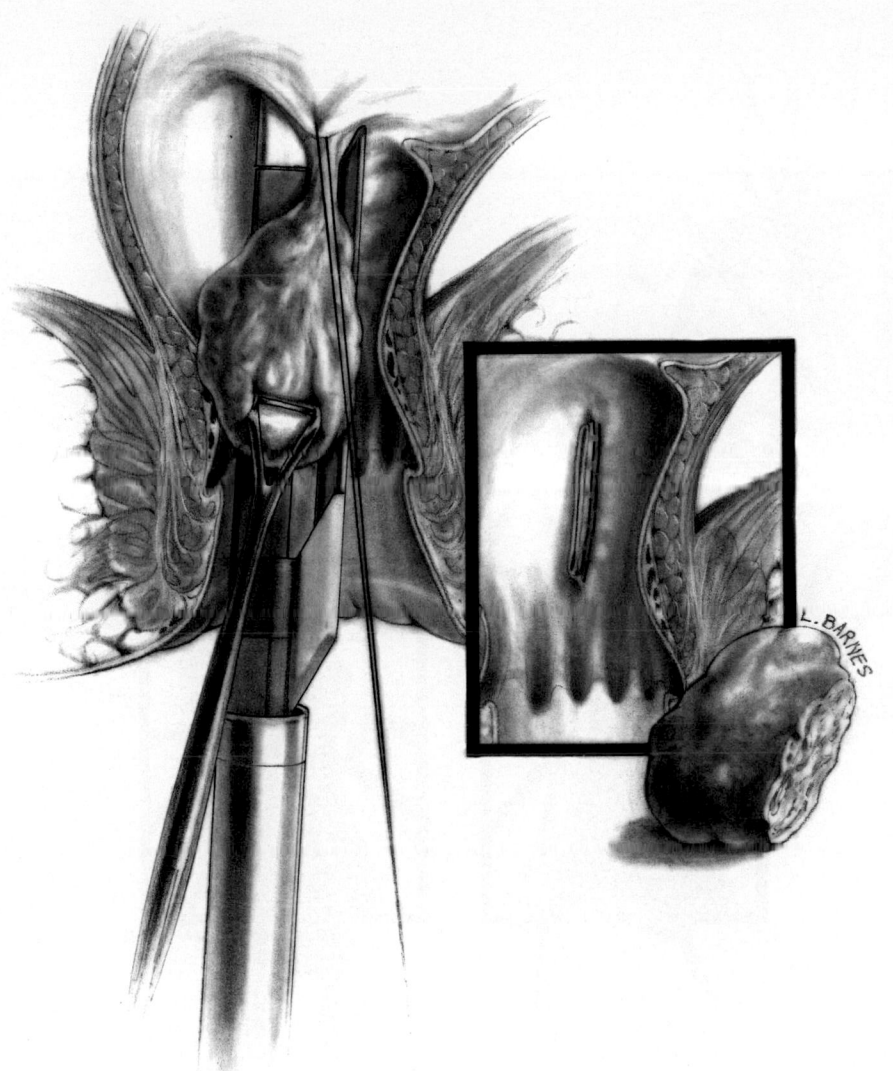

FIGURE 22-37. Transanal excision of rectal tumor using a principle similar to that outlined in Figure 22-36. A laparoscopic stapling device is employed. (Redrawn from De Gennaro VA, Lescher TC. Transanal excision of rectal tumors using a laparoscopic stapler. *Dis Colon Rectum.* 1995;38(3):327–328.)

suction devices, and needle holders are inserted through the facepiece.[283] Circumferential adenomas as well as selected early stage carcinomas can be removed with TEM.

Results

There are no meaningful (i.e., prospective, randomized, controlled) studies of the results of surgical treatment of benign rectal tumors by means of transanal excision, snare excision, electrocoagulation, or any other method. This is perhaps because there is the perception that the results are satisfactory, the complications minimal, and the rates of recurrence low, irrespective of the method of treatment.

Chiu and Spencer reported the Mayo Clinic experience of 331 villous adenomas treated over a 10-year period.[55] Patients with synchronous carcinomas were excluded. Numerous methods were employed, depending on the location and size of the tumors. Only three individuals underwent abdominoperineal resection. Sixty-nine electrocoagulations were associated with four recurrences, whereas 26 transanal excisions yielded seven patients who developed recurrences. The authors reiterated the importance of nonradical resection for lesions without invasive carcinoma.

Sakamoto and colleagues reviewed the experience from the Ferguson Clinic (Grand Rapids, MI), involving 118 individuals with villous adenoma treated by transanal excision.[285] With a mean follow-up period of 55 months, 30% developed recurrences. Important complications included 10 instances of hemorrhage and 2 instances of perforation (complication rate, 10%).

In the Memorial Sloan-Kettering (New York) experience, 72 patients underwent local excision, and 9 developed recurrences.[265] The authors advocated local excision by means of cautery snare for all benign-appearing villous adenomas. Because of the 12% recurrence rate, frequent follow-up examination was recommended. The recurrence rate in 24 patients who underwent transanal excision as reported by Jahadi and Bailey was also 12%.[159] Other investigators confirmed general satisfaction with the standard approaches used for complete removal of benign rectal tumors.[91,284,354]

Westbrook and colleagues reported 19 patients who underwent transsacral (transcoccygeal) or transsphincteric operations; 9 had villous adenomas.[342] Although there were no recurrences, in this series the technique was associated with significant morbidity, including four fecal fistulas, two wound dehiscences, one rectal stricture, and one sacrococcygeal hernia.

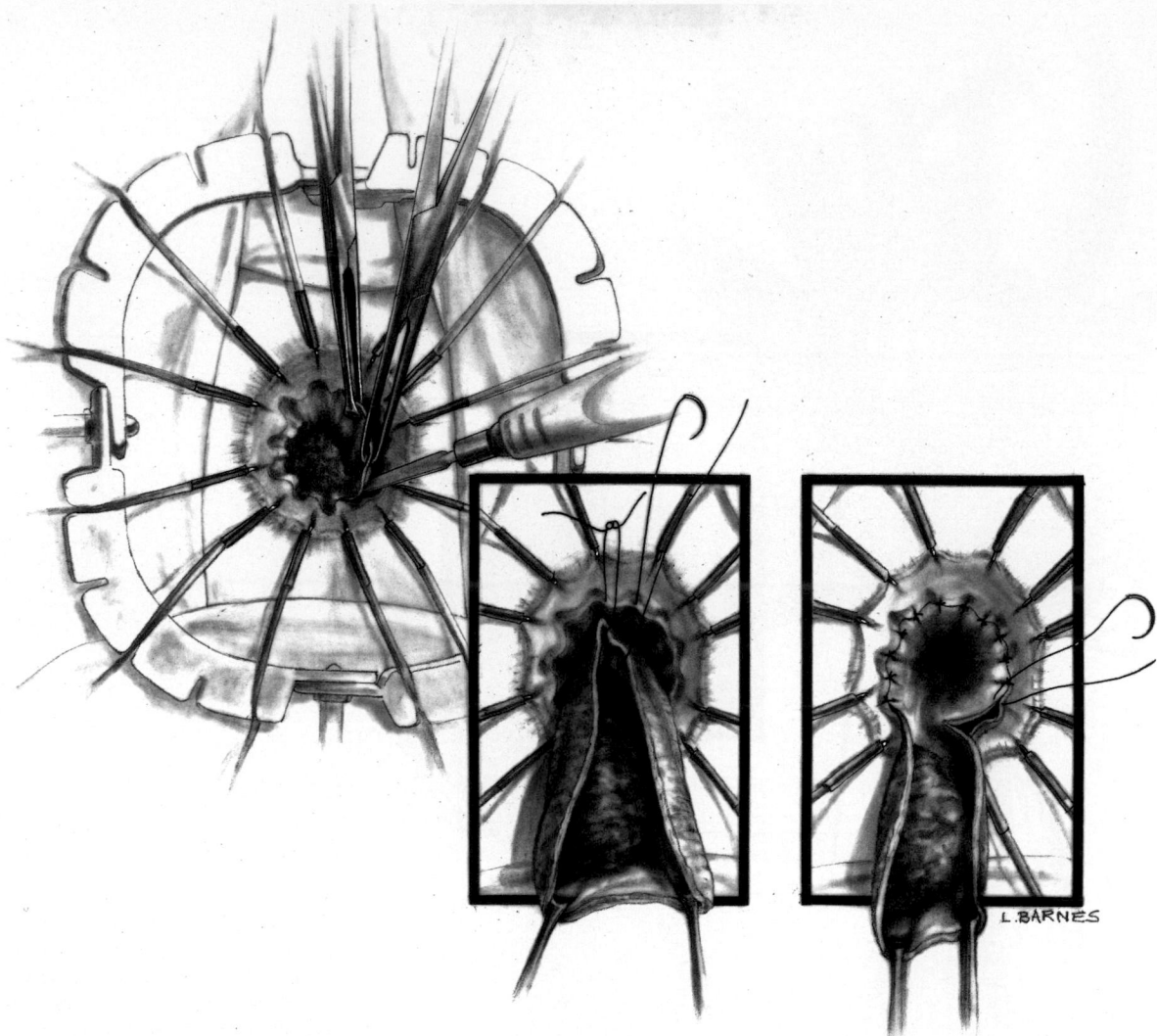

FIGURE 22-38. Excision of a large rectal tumor. **A:** A Lone Star self-retaining retractor provides exposure of the anal canal and lower rectum. A circumferential incision is made distal to the tumor, just above the dentate line. **B:** Following dissection and freeing of the rectal mucosa circumferentially, including the tumor, the rectal mucosal sleeve is incised. Sutures are placed between the proximal rectal mucosa and the dentate line to prevent retraction. **C:** The rectal mucosa above the tumor is progressively divided, and the anastomosis is completed with interrupted sutures as the tumor is being excised. (Redrawn from Keck JO, Schoetz DJ Jr, Roberts PL, et al. Rectal mucosectomy in the treatment of giant rectal villous tumors. *Dis Colon Rectum.* 1995;38(3):233–238.)

Familial Adenomatous Polyposis

Introduction

Familial adenomatous polyposis (FAP) is an autosomal dominant hereditary syndrome caused by a germ line mutation in the adenomatous polyposis coli (*APC*) gene on chromosome 5q. The disease is primarily characterized by diffuse colorectal adenomas with a risk of colorectal cancer in untreated patients near 100%. It accounts for about 1% of all colorectal cancers.[158] FAP is also a multisystem disease with important extracolonic malignant and benign manifestations. Approximately 1 in 8,000 to 1 in 20,000 live births will develop FAP.[89,96] It affects both genders and all races.

The first definitive reported cases of colonic adenomatous polyposis were noted in 1859 by Chargelaigue when he described a 21-year-old male and a 16-year-old female with this condition.[53] Cripps later described adenomatous polyposis in two young siblings in 1882.[80] Increasing numbers of

observations eventually led to the establishment of family registries to study and learn about polyposis syndromes. The first FAP registry was established by Sir Lockhart-Mummery at St. Mark's Hospital in London, England (see Biography, Chapter 12). Organized registries have facilitated scientific and clinical advances that have enhanced understanding and treatment of this disease, leading to the decreased incidence of colon cancer and to improved survival.[40,230,276] Important collaborations continue to evolve as evidenced by international alliances among registries and centers as exemplified by the Collaborative Group of the Americas on Inherited Colorectal Cancer (CGA-ICC) and the International Society for Gastrointestinal Hereditary Tumors (InSiGHT).

Genetics

FAP is caused by a germ line mutation in the *APC* gene located on chromosome 5q21.[192,258,267] The majority of mutations occur in a section of the gene between exons 1286 and 1585, but mutations also occur outside this region. More than 850 different mutations have been described, most of which produce a "stop" codon that halts translation and results in a truncated *APC* protein. This truncated protein may still have some biologic effect, depending on its size and the domains that are intact. This likely contributes to a "genotype-phenotype" association where the effects of the mutation are partly determined by its location. About 25% of patients with FAP have a "de novo" mutation and thus have no family history. This means that they are unaware of their risk and do not present for screening.

The *APC* gene encodes a protein that binds to the β-catenin complex and causes its phosphorylation. This prevents β-catenin transportation into the cell nucleus where it would normally stimulate cellular proliferation. Mutations in *APC* result in the inability of the gene product to bind β-catenin, and thus increases the number of β-catenin molecules in the cell cytoplasm. This abundance allows for transfer of β-catenin into the nucleus where it activates several downstream pathways, including c-myc and cyclin D1 that results in cell proliferation. Because *APC* acts as a tumor suppressor gene, spontaneous loss of the second allele leads to increased cellular proliferation that results in the characteristic adenomas and eventually cancers.

Genetic Testing and Counseling

Patients with a clinical diagnosis of FAP should be referred for genetic counseling and potential genetic testing. All first-degree relatives of someone with FAP are at risk for also having the disease (a 50% chance). Pretest genetic counseling is important so that families understand the implications of both negative or positive results. Therefore, all immediate family members in an FAP kindred should undergo counseling and testing. The first step in the process is to test an affected family member. If a mutation in *APC* is identified in the patient's germ line DNA, the immediate family and other branches of the family can be encouraged to come forward for genetic counseling and to learn their risk status if they so choose. More important, if no mutation is detected, genetic testing for *APC* mutations in the family is not indicated. However, that does not mean that a family does not have FAP. The clinical diagnosis guides surveillance and treatment recommendations. More than 90% of patients with classical FAP have a mutation identified.

Clinical Presentation and Manifestations

Familial adenomatous polyposis is a broad term that encompasses a number of related syndrome subtypes. The different subtypes share the same common underlying etiology, which is a mutation in *APC*; however, the clinical phenotypes differ between the subtypes. Classical FAP is characterized by hundreds to thousands of colorectal adenomas. An example of multiple clustered adenomas is shown in Figure 22-39. Patients with 100 to 1,000 colorectal adenomas are considered to have mild polyposis, whereas those patients with more than 1,000 adenomas have severe (profuse) disease (Figure 22-40). Patients with fewer than 100 adenomas are considered to have attenuated FAP. Gardner's syndrome is FAP with extracolonic manifestations of desmoid tumors, osteomas, epidermoid cysts, or extranumerary teeth.[292] The syndrome is caused by mutations in the *APC* gene and is a variant of FAP associated with mutations 3' of codon 1400. Turcot's syndrome is FAP associated with malignant tumors of the central nervous system.[154]

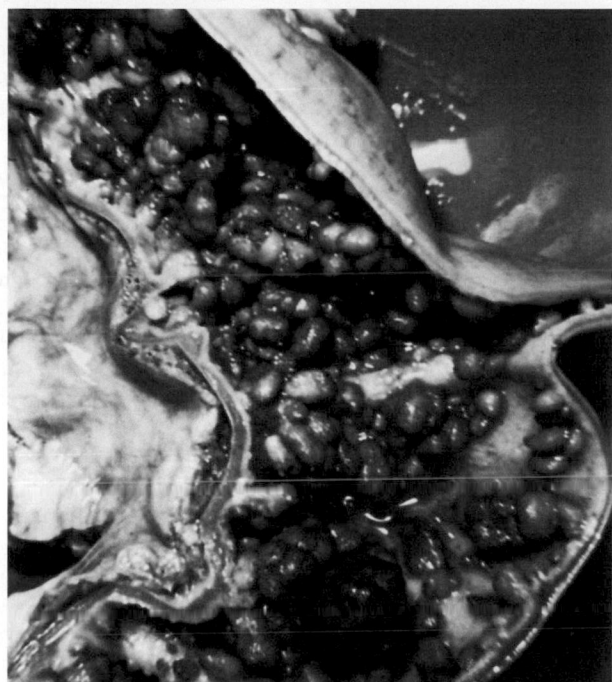

FIGURE 22-39. Familial adenomatous polyposis. This portion of a sigmoid colon demonstrates numerous, variable-sized polypoid excrescences throughout the bowel. (From Corman ML, Veidenheimer MC, Swinton NW. *Diseases of the Anus, Rectum, and Colon. Part I: Neoplasms*. New York, NY: Medcom; 1972, with permission.)

FAP patients are typically identified in one of two ways: by screening or by evaluation of symptoms. Despite the well-recognized inheritance pattern, approximately 20% to 30% of patients have no family history,[282] and the disease presumably arises from spontaneous genetic mutations.

Because colorectal penetrance is 100%, the most common symptoms relate to colorectal polyps. The mean age of the

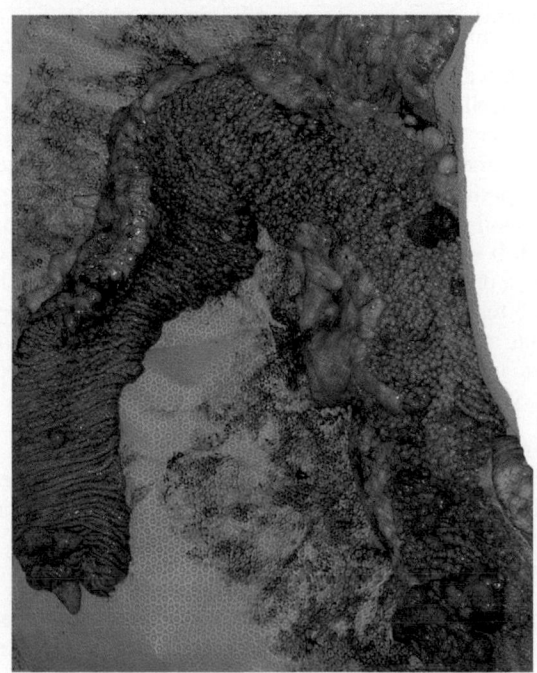

FIGURE 22-40. Profuse polyposis in familial adenomatous polyposis.

appearance of polyps in a series from St. Mark's Hospital was 22 years, but polyps develop at a much earlier age and may exist for a long time before causing symptoms to trigger evaluation.[45] Symptoms may develop as the polyp burden increases or if individual polyps become large enough to cause problems. Bleeding is the most common complaint (80%), followed by diarrhea (70%), abdominal pain, and mucous discharge. Weight loss, anemia, and intestinal obstruction are ominous signs, implying the presence of cancer. In a series of 115 patients from the Mount Sinai Medical Center in New York, 27% of patients had colorectal cancer at presentation.[161]

The clinical phenotype can often be confusing based on appearance of the colon alone. Diseases in the differential diagnosis include serrated polyposis, lymphoid polyposis, and inflammatory polyposis. Polyp histology on biopsy allows for easy differentiation of the polyp types. *MYH*-associated polyposis, which is also characterized by adenomas, can be distinguished from FAP with germ line genetic mutation testing. Although colorectal adenomas and cancer dominate the FAP phenotype, it is a multisystem disease with significant extracolonic manifestations. These include gastroduodenal adenomas and carcinoma, adrenal adenomas and carcinomas, desmoid disease, osteomas, epidermoid cysts, papillary thyroid carcinoma, small bowel polyps and carcinoma, congenital hyperplasia of the retinal pigment epithelium (CHRPE), and dental anomalies. These extracolonic manifestations and their management recommendations are discussed later.

Management of Colorectal Disease
Screening
Flexible endoscopy is considered the gold standard screening tool for evaluation of potential FAP patients. This allows for evaluation of the entire colorectum and provides the ability to intervene by biopsy and/or polypectomy. Screening and treatment must be preceded by counseling about the nature of the syndrome, extracolonic manifestations, natural history of the disease, and the need for compliance.[61] The National Comprehensive Cancer Network recommends flexible sigmoidoscopy or colonoscopy beginning at age 10 to 15 years for patients at risk based on family history or germ line *APC* mutation.[237] If no polyps are found, they recommend annual exam until age 24, then every 2 years until age 34, then every 3 years until age 44, and every 3 to 5 years thereafter.[237] Once polyposis is detected on screening, the colonoscopy should be accomplished annually until a decision is made for surgery.

For patients who are screened based on family history alone (without genetic testing) and no polyps are found by age 40, it is safe to assume that the patient is not affected. This is a practical approach for patients who do not undergo genetic testing and for those with a clinical phenotype but without a known germ line mutation. For families with a known mutation, at-risk individuals can be screened by endoscopy or genetic testing at puberty.

Surgery
The two main goals of surgery in FAP are to decrease the risk of colorectal cancer and to preserve quality of life. Quality of life is particularly important in this patient population, who are generally young and healthy.

Timing of Surgery. The timing of surgery impacts both cancer risk as well as quality of life. Cancer is rare before the age of 20,[67] and as long as an effective surveillance program is in place, it is reasonable to defer operation until the late teen years, when physical, emotional, and social maturity have been reached. Patients often consider the impact on time away from school or work, and it is common for students to wait until their transition from high school to college. Genotype, phenotype, and family history may also help stratify cancer risk to that particular individual and to the impact and the timing of surgery. Symptomatic patients have an increased risk of cancer already being present,[39] and treatment at the time of symptoms is recommended.

There are certain situations when surgery may be deferred beyond the teen years. These are not absolute recommendations but are considerations in the overall approach to surgery in FAP. Young women who wish to have children may defer an ileal-pouch-anal anastomosis (IPAA) until after their childbearing is complete. Patients at risk for desmoid disease may defer surgery as long as possible given that surgery seems to stimulate desmoid formation. Obesity is another complicating factor that makes IPAA surgery technically difficult or even impossible to accomplish. In this situation, surgery may be delayed until hopefully weight loss can be achieved. Again, these are only some considerations. This approach can only be done in the absence of symptoms and in a patient who is compliant with his or her colonoscopy schedule.

Type of Surgery. There are three main surgical options in the treatment of FAP: colectomy with ileorectal anastomosis, restorative proctocolectomy with IPAA, and proctocolectomy (with end ileostomy or continent ileostomy). With the exception of continent ileostomy formation, these surgeries may be performed laparoscopically. Each option impacts cancer risk and quality of life. The first major surgical decision point is determining the fate of rectum, that is, to perform a colectomy alone or to do a proctocolectomy. While leaving the rectum in place means a risk of developing rectal cancer, the surgery is simpler, does not involve a temporary stoma, and quality of life is better than with proctocolectomy. The data to be considered in making decisions are presented next.

Colectomy versus Proctocolectomy
Cancer Risk
Cancer risk following surgical management of FAP must be viewed in a historical perspective given the impact of the introduction of the ileal pouch. In the prepouch era, surgical options were essentially limited to colectomy and ileorectal anastomosis (IRA) or proctocolectomy and end ileostomy. As might be expected, most patients opted for an IRA because of an aversion to having a permanent ileostomy. In a study comparing the risk of developing rectal cancer in patients treated by IRA before and after 1983, the year when IPAA became a generally available alternative, there was a large decrease in the rectal cancer risk after 1983.[63] At a single institution, 62 IRA operations were performed in the prepouch era (median follow-up, 212 months), and 135 in the pouch era (median follow-up, 60 months). Almost one-third of the prepouch era patients underwent subsequent proctectomy compared with only 2% in the pouch era. The authors concluded that the improved results probably are based in part on the ability to select patients appropriately for IRA and by offering IPAA to those with severe polyposis.[63] Practice patterns have changed since the availability of the IPAA option, and there is better selection of patients for an IRA. In fact, a lower percentage of patients are being treated

by IRA, but they are selected more carefully, representing a group that is at lower risk for rectal cancer.[82]

Several authors have shown that a colectomy and IRA may be performed safely and leaves a reasonable rectal cancer risk if done in properly selected patients. Patient selection depends on the colon and rectal polyp phenotype and the perceived risk of cancer developing in the residual rectum.[293] Colectomy and ileorectal anastomosis for FAP is the preferred operation if the rectum is relatively spared.[62,82,94] The preoperative rectal polyp burden serves as a good predictor of future rectal cancer risk.[62] Valuable information can be obtained by simple office proctoscopy. Finding fewer than five rectal adenomas at presentation almost always predicts mild disease, and these patients do well with an ileorectal anastomosis. Finding 20 or more rectal adenomas implies severe disease, and proctectomy is, therefore, recommended.[62] Consideration should also be given to the colon polyp burden. For 95 patients with less than 20 rectal adenomas and fewer than 1,000 colon polyps, none required proctectomy at a 12-year median follow-up. In contrast, of 33 patients with significant colon and rectal polyp burden (> 1,000, > 20 polyps, respectively) who underwent an IRA, 56% required proctectomy.[62]

In a series reported from St. Mark's Hospital in London, only 2 of 89 patients surviving colectomy and IRA for FAP subsequently developed rectal carcinoma. Because these individuals had been followed closely, at the time of subsequent proctectomy all were found to have early stage cancers. Bussey computed the cumulative risk of the development of cancer in the retained rectum at 3.6%.[45] The Cleveland Clinic group reported 10 of 133 patients to have developed cancer in the rectal remnant.[289] Others reported a similar relatively favorable experience.[155,241,299]

If the rectum does need to be removed after colectomy and ileorectal anastomosis, IPAA can still be safely performed.[30] Björk and colleagues presented the Swedish experience of IPAA in FAP (120 patients) and compared this operation with IPAA as a secondary procedure after an initial IRA. Complications occurred in 40% of the patients who underwent IPAA initially and in 56% who underwent IPAA as a secondary procedure. Functional outcome did not differ between an initial IPAA and IPAA as a secondary procedure.[30]

Although some authors recommend IPAA as the initial surgery for patients who are prone to desmoid formation due to potential difficulty with proctectomy or subsequent pouch formation, we do not agree. Recent data presented from Cleveland Clinic suggests that IPAA is more likely than IRA to result in clinically significant desmoid disease (Table 22-1). Furthermore, in a series of 67 patients needing proctectomy for progressive neoplasia after initial IRA, all were able to have a proctectomy, and a secondary IPAA was possible in 57 of the 62 patients in which it was planned (unpublished author's data).

Regression of Rectal Polyps after Colectomy

Another factor influencing the decision to perform an ileorectal anastomosis is the phenomenon of rectal polyp regression following total colectomy.[75,98,209] Spontaneous regression occurs in up to 64% of patients after colectomy and seems to happen in the first decade after surgery. It appears that the trend is reversed in the second decade.[45,98] It is important to note that initial polyp regression does not prevent the subsequent development of rectal cancer, and continued

TABLE 22-1	Clinical Staging System for Intra-abdominal Desmoid Disease[64]
STAGE	**FINDINGS**
Stage I	Asymptomatic disease, and not growing, and <10 cm in maximum diameter
Stage II	Minimally symptomatic, and not growing, or >10 cm in maximum diameter
Stage III	Symptomatic disease, or slowly growing, or obstructive complications
Stage IV	Symptomatic disease, and rapidly growing, or severe complications (e.g., fistula)

follow-up is necessary in order to remove or ablate recurrent polyps and to screen for the development of cancer.[98] Although the regression may be only temporary, avoiding an IPAA or an ileostomy with close follow-up makes colectomy and ileorectal anastomosis an appealing surgical option for many patients.

Pouch and Ileostomy Neoplasia after Proctocolectomy

The risk of adenomatous neoplasia remains in an ileal pouch or terminal ileum after proctocolectomy in patients with FAP. Theoretically, chronic changes in the epithelium induced by fecal stasis combined with a germ line *APC* mutation promotes adenoma formation. The risk of neoplasia is time dependent, and there is an estimated 42% rate of pouch polyposis at 7 years after proctectomy.[316,352] Some series report an incidence as high as 57%.[122,323] Adenomas have also been observed in the ileum following colectomy and ileorectal anastomosis.[152] In addition, adenocarcinomas have been found in an IPAA as well as in end ileostomies.[59,114,141,308] Because of the risk of neoplasia, annual endoscopic surveillance of the reservoir itself and the terminal ileum, not just the anastomotic area, is recommended with interval adjustment depending on findings.[150]

Functional Results

Functional outcomes should be considered in surgical decision making in FAP. Conflicting data exists in the literature, but most evidence weighs in favor of IRA. A large study from the Netherlands reported on 161 patients who underwent IRA and 118 patients who underwent IPAA. IRA patients had significantly better outcomes for stool frequency, soiling, occasional passive incontinence, flatus and feces discrimination, stool consistency, and need for antidiarrheal medication. IRA patients also fared significantly better based on the aggregate score of the Gastrointestinal Functional Outcome Scale.[328] Madden reported on the St. Mark's experience on 99 FAP patients between 1979 and 1989. There was little difference in bowel function between the operations, but IPAA had significantly more morbidity. IPAA resulted in a longer hospital stay, higher percentage of complications, higher reoperation rate, and longer return to normal activities.[213]

Aziz and coworkers conducted a meta-analysis including 1,002 patients from 12 studies. Patients in the ileorectal group had reduced bowel frequency, less nighttime defecation, and less use of incontinence pads compared to the IPAA group. In their analysis, there was no significant difference between the techniques in terms of sexual dysfunction, dietary restriction, or postoperative complications.[15]

Effect on Fecundity

All women with FAP should be counseled regarding the effects of surgery on fecundity. Fecundity, defined as the ability to become pregnant and give birth, is decreased following proctocolectomy. This exact decrease is difficult to interpret based on inherent flaws and confounding factors in the published literature, but fecundity may be decreased to nearly 50% compared with the general population based on a report of 230 Scandinavian women with FAP.[247] This is believed to be associated with pelvic surgery, and there is little effect following colectomy and ileorectal anastomosis.[247] For these reasons, a woman wishing to have children may consider an IRA with close surveillance of the rectum even if the polyp burden is unfavorable. This is only recommended if there is not severe polyposis in the rectum, there are no symptoms referable to the rectum, and the patient is compliant with endoscopic surveillance. The rectum can be removed after childbearing is completed. In one study, 23% of women with FAP chose not to have children because they did not want to pass the disease to the next generation.[247]

Other Considerations

Other patient factors must also be considered in surgical decision making. Obesity portends a worse outcome and often limits the technical ability to create an IPAA. In certain circumstances, an IRA may be done with a plan of future weight loss so that when a complication develops in the rectum, an IPAA may be more feasible as opposed to that of an end ileostomy. Patients with weakened sphincter function also will not have a good quality of life with an IPAA and may consider an IRA or end ileostomy. A recommendation may also be offered to have an IRA as a bridge for women wishing to have children. Avoiding pelvic surgery obviates the risk of decreased fecundity as described next.

Technical Considerations
Laparoscopy versus Laparotomy

There are an increasing number of colorectal surgery cases being performed laparoscopically in the United States, and this includes surgery for FAP. Both total colectomy and IRA, as well as restorative proctocolectomy, can be done safely laparoscopically with similar results in terms of complications and functional outcomes. Cosmetic appearance seems to be the biggest advantage of the laparoscopic approach, and this factor may be important for this relatively younger patient population.

A Cochrane review included 607 patients from 11 trials in which open and laparoscopic IPAA for either FAP or ulcerative colitis were compared. Two hundred fifty-three (41%) were treated laparoscopically, but only one of the trials included was randomized controlled. The review found no significant differences between the two groups with respect to postoperative recovery outcomes. The total incision length was significantly shorter in the laparoscopic group, and cosmesis favored the laparoscopic group. The authors concluded that large, high-quality trials studying

differences regarding specific postoperative complications, cosmesis, and quality of life and costs are needed.[3]

One theoretical advantage of laparoscopy is decreased postoperative adhesions. Because laparoscopy generally is associated with less handling of the bowel, less bleeding, and less contamination by foreign bodies, some claim laparoscopy reduces postoperative adhesions. This translates into a lower incidence of postoperative bowel obstruction.[107,128,344] Using a similar rationale, decreased adhesions after laparoscopy may ameliorate the detrimental effect on fertility. These claims are not yet confirmed by data and will only be validated through appropriate trials.

On a technical note, it is often difficult to dissect the rectum to the level of the anal canal laparoscopically. This surgical aspect is crucial so that minimal rectal mucosa remains. This principle should not be compromised. If it cannot be achieved laparoscopically, alternative approaches should be used. Several centers and surgeons have adopted a laparoscopic approach to the colectomy portion of the restorative proctocolectomy, but then make a Pfannenstiel incision for the proctectomy.

Anastomosis: Stapled versus Mucosectomy and Hand-Sewn

The choice of mucosectomy and hand-sewn versus stapled pouch-anal anastomosis has been a subject of debate. Removal of the anal transition zone by mucosectomy theoretically prevents cuff neoplasia and has been argued as an essential component of proctocolectomy and IPAA in FAP patients. However, this is a controversial topic, and opposing views are supported by cases of neoplasia and worse functional outcomes after mucosectomy.

In a series of 119 patients who underwent IPAA at a single institution, 77 underwent a stapled anastomosis, and 42 underwent a mucosectomy and hand-sewn IPAA.[274] The stapled group had superior outcomes in terms of incontinence, daytime and nighttime seepage, and pad usage. However, 28% of patients in the stapled group developed adenomas in the anal transition zone compared with a 14% neoplasia rate in the mucosectomy group. The authors concluded that the functional advantages of stapled IPAA outweighed the increase in neoplasia (which could be managed by local procedures). In a later report from the same center, two patients who were operated on at referring institutions and followed at the tertiary care center developed anal transitional zone cancer. One case occurred after a double-stapled anastomosis and one after a mucosectomy.[251]

Conversely, a single surgeon prospective, randomized trial evaluated function in 14 patients with mucosectomy and 14 individuals with a stapled anastomosis. There was no difference in terms of number of bowel movements per 24 hours, frequency of nighttime evacuation, or episodes of incontinence.[56]

A meta-analysis was undertaken, evaluating studies that compared hand-sewn to stapled IPAA, between the years 1988 and 2003. Twenty-one studies involving 4,183 patients (2,699 hand-sewn and 1,484 stapled) were included in the analysis. No significant difference was noted in postoperative complications, but functional results favored the stapled IPAA. Patients with IPAA had a lower incidence of nocturnal seepage and pad usage, but there was not a difference in the number of daily bowel movements nor the need for antimotility agents. On anorectal physiology, the hand-sewn group had a significant reduction in resting and squeeze pressures compared with the stapled group. The stapled IPAA group had a higher incidence of dysplasia in the anal transition zone, but this did not reach statistical significance.[211] The reported range of anal transition zone adenomas after hand-sewn IPAA is 10% to 19% compared to 28% to 38% after a stapled IPAA.[274,275,329,336] There are eight reported cases of cancer developing at the anastomosis: four of which occurred after a mucosectomy and hand-sewn anastomosis, and four after stapled anastomosis.[59] This underscores the fact that anal neoplasia happens even after mucosectomy. The surgical approach to mucosectomy is challenging, and islands of mucosa may be left behind.

The authors generally perform a stapled IPAA but recommend mucosectomy in the setting of rectal cancer or blanketing/carpeted anal canal or the presence of rectal polyps.

Management of Extracolonic Disease

Because prophylactic colectomy has increased life expectancy of patients with FAP, extracolonic manifestations, both benign and malignant, have become more evident.[22] After colorectal cancer, desmoid disease and duodenal adenocarcinoma are the leading causes of mortality in FAP.[13,22,242] Cancers of the thyroid, pancreas, liver, and adrenal glands have all been reported but occur much less frequently. Benign lesions such as lipomas, fibromas, sebaceous and epidermoid cysts, osteomas, and congenital hypertrophy of the retinal pigment epithelium (CHRPE) are also common.[94] Clinicians must be aware of these extracolonic manifestations in order to provide appropriate surveillance, diagnosis, and intervention.

Upper Gastrointestinal Polyps

The majority of patients with FAP will develop gastric and duodenal polyps[71] as shown in Figures 22-41 to 22-43. Approximately 50% of patients grow primarily nonneoplastic, fundic gland polyps in the stomach.[338] Despite the regular finding of low-grade dysplasia in biopsies, fundic gland polyps have a minimal risk of malignancy,[78,144] and the incidence of gastric cancer associated with FAP in Western societies is low. About 10% of FAP patients develop antral adenomas, and these may contribute to the occasional case of gastric cancer.

In contrast, approximately 90% of patients with FAP develop duodenal adenomas. These carry a significant malignancy risk as precursor lesions to duodenal cancer.[136,305]

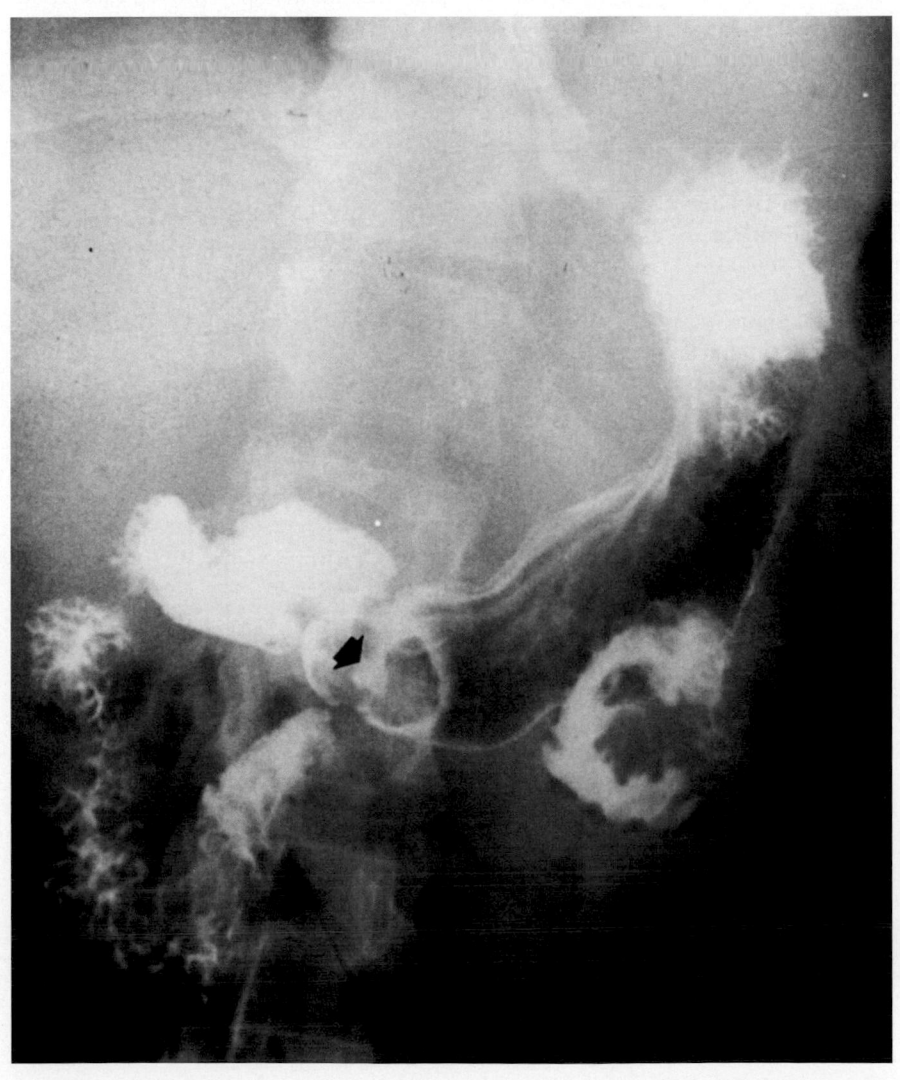

FIGURE 22-41. Antral polypoid lesion with central ulceration (*arrow*) on an upper gastrointestinal series in a patient with familial adenomatous polyposis.

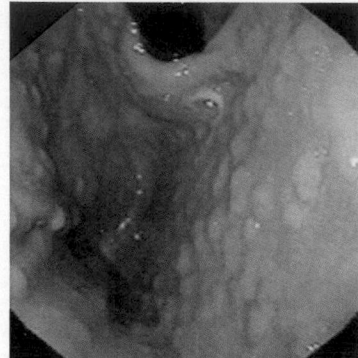

FIGURE 22-42. Upper gastrointestinal endoscopy in a patient with familial adenomatous polyposis reveals a gastric fundus showing a sheet of polyps.

About 3% to 14% of patients with FAP will be diagnosed with periampullary carcinoma, the third most frequent cause of death with FAP.[13,22] Twelve percent of patients in the St. Mark's Hospital series who survived for 5 years after colectomy developed carcinoma of the duodenum, ampulla of Vater, or pancreas.[45] de Vos tot Nederveen Cappel and associates calculated that the lifetime risk of developing duodenal cancer in FAP is 5%.[90]

Management

Upper gastrointestinal endoscopic surveillance is essential in the management of FAP. This normally begins at age 20 to 25 and is done with both end-viewing and side-viewing endoscopes in order to allow broader inspection and biopsy of the ampulla of Vater. Burke and colleagues showed that rapid progression from adenoma to carcinoma in duodenal adenomas occurred in only 11% of cases at 7 years follow-up.[41] Thus, complete polypectomy of all duodenal polyps is not necessary, but representative polyp biopsies should be obtained for staging according to the Spigelman staging system.[307] The American Society of Colon and Rectal Surgeons' guidelines state that all high-risk adenomas, those defined as greater than 1 cm in size or containing high-grade dysplasia, should be removed.[65] The Spigelman staging system can be used to estimate cancer risk based on characteristics of the adenomas as shown in Tables 22-2 and 22-3. Patients with early stage disease have a low risk for developing periampullary cancer (2%), but those with Spigelman stage IV

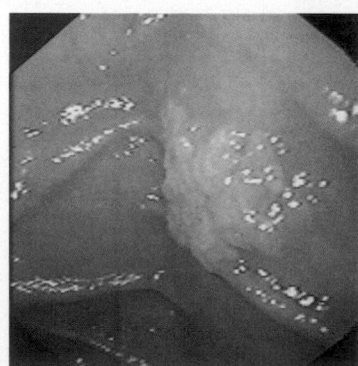

FIGURE 22-43. Duodenoscopy reveals a sessile villous tumor of the duodenum in a patient with familial adenomatous polyposis.

TABLE 22-2 Scoring of Duodenal Adenoma Features According to Spigelman

DUODENAL DISEASE GRADING SCALE (POINTS ASSIGNED)

	1	2	3
Number of polyps	1–4	5–20	>20
Size of polyps (mm)	1–4	5–10	>10
Histology	Tubular	Tubulovillous	Villous
Dysplasia	Mild	Moderate	Severe

From Spigelman AD, Williams CB, Talbot IC, et al. Upper gastrointestinal cancer in patients with familial adenomatous polyposis. *Lancet.* 1989;2(8666):783–785.

disease have a 36% risk of adenocarcinoma.[123] Surgery is required to treat adenocarcinoma or persistent or recurrent high-grade dysplasia.[65] Pancreaticoduodenectomy (Whipple's procedure) is preferred for a biopsy-proven cancer, but for benign disease, pancreas-preserving duodenectomy can be performed with reasonably low morbidity and good functional outcomes.[85,104,174,180]

Desmoid Disease

Desmoid disease is an overgrowth of fibroblasts that can manifest as flat sheetlike lesions or defined masses (Figures 22-44 and 22-45). It affects approximately 5% of patients with FAP,[301] with a prevalence much higher than that of the general population.[273] The absolute risk of desmoids in patients with FAP is 2.56/1,000 person-years, with the comparative risk 852 times that of the general population. Most FAP-associated desmoid disease in FAP is within the abdominal cavity (50%) or in the abdominal

TABLE 22-3 Spigelman Score-Based Recommendations

TOTAL POINTS	SPIGELMAN STAGE	RECOMMENDATION
0	0	Repeat endoscopy in 5 years
1–4	I	Repeat endoscopy in 5 years
5–6	II	Repeat endoscopy in 2–3 years
7–8	III	Repeat endoscopy in 6–12 months
9–12	IV	Surgical evaluation

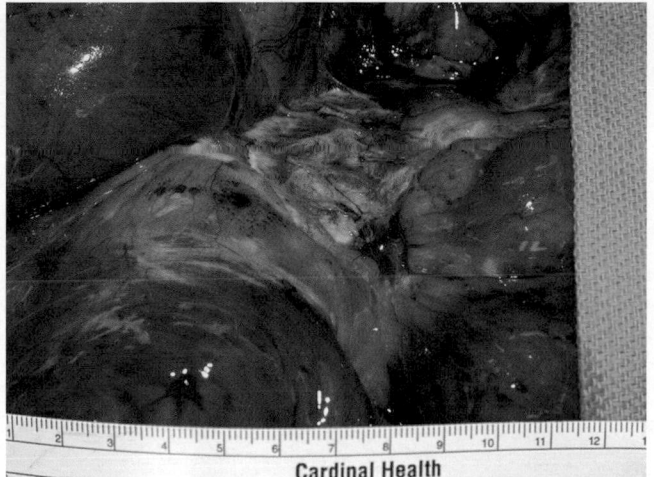

FIGURE 22-44. Sheetlike lesion in a patient with desmoid disease. It lines the small bowel mesentery and can pucker and kink adjacent bowel.

wall (40%—Figure 22-46). A small percentage present in extra-abdominal locations, such as the back, neck, or limbs. Approximately 3% of FAP patients have intra-abdominal desmoids at the time of their first surgery,[132] but the majority develop within 5 years after abdominal surgery.[73,304]

Desmoid disease has been associated with female gender,[132] the presence of extracolonic manifestations of Gardner's syndrome, a family history of desmoids, and an *APC* mutation at the 3' end of codon 1440.[27,94,298] Desmoid risk influences the timing of surgery because patients at increased risk may opt to delay colectomy as long as possible, as long as the colorectal polyp burden is controlled. Church has proposed a desmoid risk factor (DRF) score to delineate desmoid risk.[94]

Management

Clinically, desmoid disease ranges from asymptomatic to severe complications such as pain, obstruction, fistulization, or obstruction, and approximately 7% of patients die from complications of desmoid disease.[73,177,304] The symptoms may be cyclical because desmoids often undergo cycles of growth and regression with different treatments. Approximately

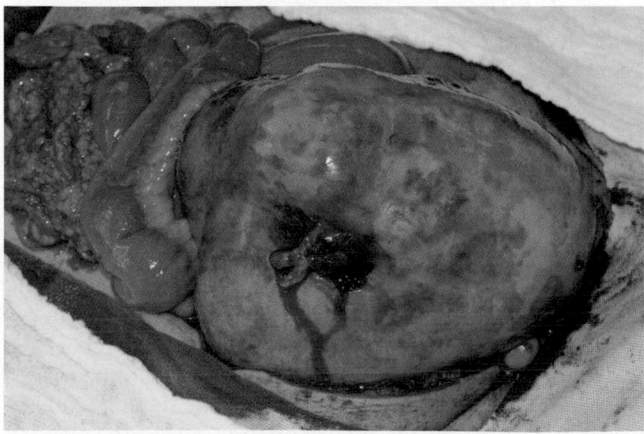

FIGURE 22-45. Mesenteric desmoid tumor surrounded by attached loops of small intestine.

10% of desmoids completely disappear spontaneously or following treatment.[212] A proposed surveillance protocol based on stage is shown in Table 22-4.[302]

Treatment decisions are based on the location of the tumor, extent of disease, and symptoms caused by the desmoids. Various approaches including medicine, radiation, and surgery have been employed alone or in combination. Desmoid tumors are radiosensitive, but the close proximity to the small bowel in intra-abdominal desmoids tumors hinders its use. The Cleveland Clinic approach is described next. Stage I desmoids are either observed or treated with the nonsteroidal anti-inflammatory drug, sulindac (150 to 200 mg twice daily).[322] Stage II desmoids may be treated with sulindac and an estrogen-blocking agent, such as raloxifene (60 mg twice daily).[318] Stage III desmoids are more advanced and are generally treated with chemotherapy (methotrexate and vinorelbine or doxil),[16,26] whereas stage IV desmoids usually require antisarcoma chemotherapy (doxil or adriamycin).[264] Other agents such as Gleevec, interferon, and pirfenidone have been used with limited data on efficacy.[131,205,272]

Surgery for intra-abdominal desmoids is reserved for well-defined tumors that can be safely resected to negative margins. Indications for surgery for abdominal desmoids are related to complications from the disease and include bowel obstruction, enterocutaneous fistula, and ureteric obstruction. Tumors located at the root of the small bowel mesentery are often not resectable, and attempts may lead to complications of compromised blood supply to the small bowel as well as the need for extensive small bowel resection. A bypass procedure is often the wiser alternative. Desmoid disease in the pelvis or in the small bowel mesentery may make proctectomy and IPAA technically challenging or even impossible.[260] Intestinal transplantation for desmoid disease is a growing field, and there have been reports of success.[54]

Symptomatic abdominal wall desmoids should be resected with grossly negative margins of 1 cm. The resulting defect usually needs closure with the construction of tissue flaps or the assistance of prosthetic or bioprosthetic mesh.

Thyroid Cancer

Patients with FAP have an approximately 2% incidence of thyroid cancer, a risk that is increased compared to the general population. Papillary carcinoma is the predominant type.[111,163,262] It tends to affect women more commonly than men (17:1 ratio) and strikes at a relatively young mean age (27 years). FAP women younger than 35 years old have a 160 times relative risk of developing thyroid cancer compared with the general population.[262] Thyroid cancer in FAP is correlated with mutations in the 5' end of exon 15.[50]

The Cleveland Clinic reported 192 asymptomatic FAP patients who were prospectively screened by thyroid ultrasound annually. Seventy-two (38%) had thyroid nodules and 5 (2.6%) had thyroid cancer. Four of the five cancers were multifocal papillary carcinoma, with a mean size of 15 mm. More important, neither history nor clinical neck examination were able to detect any of these cancers.[163] Because the cancer risk is relatively high and an ultrasound screening test is noninvasive and rather simple, the authors support annual screening for thyroid malignancy by means of ultrasound. Nodules larger than 1 cm should undergo fine needle aspiration. Identification of a thyroid cancer warrants total thyroidectomy and radioiodine ablation because these lesions tend to be multifocal.[23,38] Adjuvant medical suppression

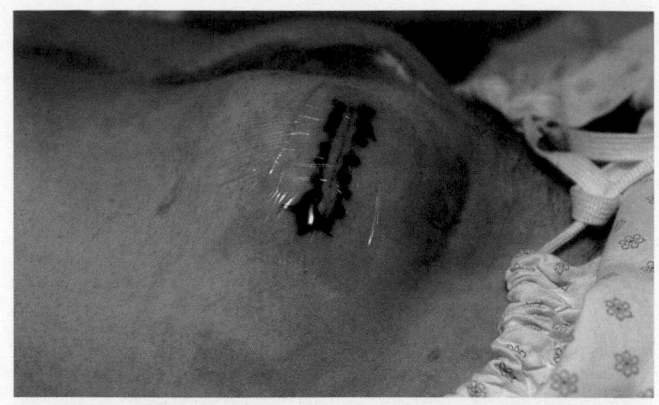

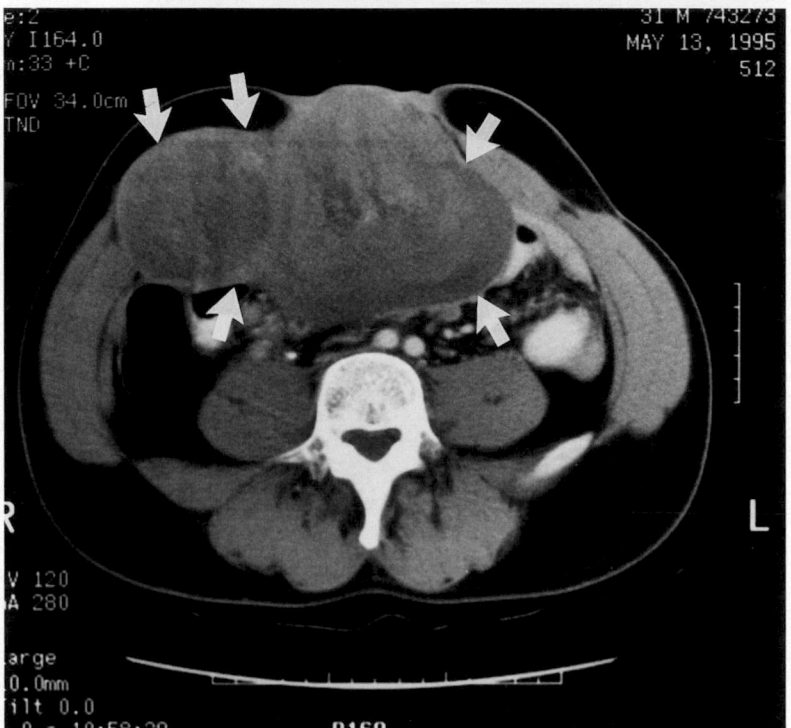

FIGURE 22-46. Desmoid tumor of the abdomen in a young man who had previously undergone total colectomy for familial adenomatous polyposis. **A:** Massive tumor can be appreciated in the mid-abdomen. Note the broad scar from the prior surgical procedure. An excisional biopsy was performed in the left side of the abdomen to confirm the diagnosis. (Note the adhesive dressing.) **B:** Computed tomography demonstrates huge mass involving the abdominal wall (*arrows*).

TABLE 22-4 Proposed Desmoid Surveillance Protocol Based on Desmoid Disease Stage for Patients with Familial Adenomatous Polyposis

DESMOID STAGE	SURVEILLANCE METHOD	INTERVAL
I	Physical exam, abdominal imaging[a]	Every 12 months
II	Physical exam, abdominal imaging[a]	Every 6 months
III–IV	Physical exam, abdominal imaging[a]	Every 3 months

[a]CT scan is the preferred abdominal imaging technique, but MRI is also used.

of thyroid-stimulating hormone with levothyroxine is recommended.[7] FAP patients with papillary thyroid cancer generally do well with appropriate treatment and can expect a normal life expectancy.[38,206]

Other Malignant Tumors

FAP is also associated with several rare extracolonic malignancies that have an increased incidence relative to the general population. The relative risk of developing pancreatic adenocarcinomas is 4.5 times higher than in the general population, with a lifetime risk of approximately 1.7% in the FAP population.[111] The absolute risk of hepatoblastoma in children is 2%, but this is 750 to 7,500 times higher than the general population.[110,149] Similarly, the absolute risk of developing medulloblastoma is approximately 1:4,000 in FAP patients,[130] but the relative risk is 7-fold for all FAP patients and 23-fold for patients before the age of 29.[130] Routine imaging or surveillance, looking for these tumors, is not justified due to the overall low incidence. Specific examinations may be considered in FAP patients with a strong family history of specific extra-intestinal manifestations or to evaluate patients with symptoms that may be attributed to these cancers.

Other Benign Lesions

Congenital hypertrophy of the retinal pigment epithelium (CHRPE) is the most common benign extracolonic manifestation in FAP and can be found in 60% to 85% of patients.[325] These lesions are well-demarcated gray-brown to black ovoid spots, which are usually bilateral and may be multiple in number (Figure 22-47).[321] It is a good diagnostic sign but does not require treatment. The Cleveland Clinic group has shown that the existence of a total of four or more CHRPE lesions involving both eyes is a congenital marker for FAP in about two-thirds of families.[142] Morton and colleagues undertook an evaluation of this manifestation as a disease marker in a defined population with FAP.[229] Indirect ophthalmoscopy was performed on 75 individuals from 25 known families with FAP. Using a combined set of diagnostic criteria, CHRPE identified affected patients with a specificity of at least 94% and a sensitivity of 84%. Absence of this ophthalmologic finding, however, does not guarantee that an individual is unaffected.

Mandibular and cranial osteomas and dental abnormalities occur in about 20% of FAP patients. These findings should alert clinicians to a potential diagnosis of FAP as these lesions often exist before colonic polyps develop.[43,121] The combination of these bony lesions with adenomatous polyposis, epidermoid cysts, and desmoids are the hallmarks of Gardner's syndrome. This particular phenotype has been associated with mutations at the 3' end of the *APC* gene. Dental abnormalities take the form of supernumerary teeth, dentigerous cysts, and secondary retention of teeth.[45,106] Surgical removal is often necessary because these abnormalities can prevent the eruption of normal teeth. Early intervention reduces morbidity.[268] No formal guidelines for screening have been established,

but some groups recommend a panorama x-ray be done at least every 2 years in a developing child until the teeth have erupted.[121,347] This usually occurs by age 18 years.

Epidermoid cysts, lipomas, and fibromas are benign cutaneous lesions associated with FAP. The association of epidermoid (sebaceous) cysts with FAP has been termed Oldfield's syndrome.[246] Although these lesions are common in the general population, the distribution in young patients with FAP is more frequently seen on the face, scalp, and extremities rather than on the back.[198] Because these tumors are rarely identified before puberty in the general population, the presence of epidermoid cysts in this age group should alert the physician to pursue colorectal investigation for potential FAP.[202] These benign lesions are treated by simple surgical excision if they cause symptoms or cosmetic concerns. No particular surveillance other than routine physical examination during regular follow-up is indicated.

Attenuated Familial Adenomatous Polyposis

Attenuated FAP (aFAP) is part of a spectrum that includes FAP but is caused by *APC* mutations at either the 5' or the 3' end of the gene.[139] These patients typically develop fewer than 100 colorectal polyps and present at a later age than classical FAP, usually in the 30s and 40s. The mean age of cancer development is also delayed and has been reported to be 56 years.[139] The distribution of polyps is more commonly right sided instead of pancolonic, but the distribution and the number of polyps vary among family members, suggesting incomplete penetrance. The phenotype may make the diagnosis difficult, and it can often be confused with *MYH*-associated polyposis or HNPCC. The management is similar to patients with classical FAP except that the polyp burden is less, and cancer risk is delayed. A colectomy with ileorectal anastomosis is usually the preferred surgical procedure.

Turcot's Syndrome

Turcot's syndrome is described as the association of colorectal adenomatous polyposis and tumors of the central nervous system. In contrast to classical FAP, the colorectal polyp burden differs in Turcot's syndrome. It is believed that there are fewer polyps present (20 to 100), there is a higher frequency of larger polyps (greater than 3 cm), and there is an earlier development of colon cancer (70% to 100% during the second or third decade).[154]

About two-thirds of families with a clinical definition of Turcot's syndrome have a mutation in *APC*.[252] These patients have an increased incidence of medulloblastoma.[198,252] Families without an *APC* mutation are said to have brain tumor polyposis type 1 and tend to have glioma and colorectal adenomas without polyposis. These patients also have an increased incidence of skin lesions (e.g., café au lait spots).[198,252] Genetic analysis of these tumors show DNA replication errors, which suggests a relationship with hereditary nonpolyposis colorectal cancer rather than FAP.[252]

MYH-Associated Polyposis

In 2002, biallelic mutations in the *MutYH* (also called *MYH*) gene were described in a family with multiple colorectal adenomas and adenocarcinomas and a normal *APC* gene.[6] This newly described autosomal recessive condition was later called *MYH*-associated polyposis (MAP). The syndrome, which is primarily characterized by multiple colorectal adenomas and an increased risk of colorectal

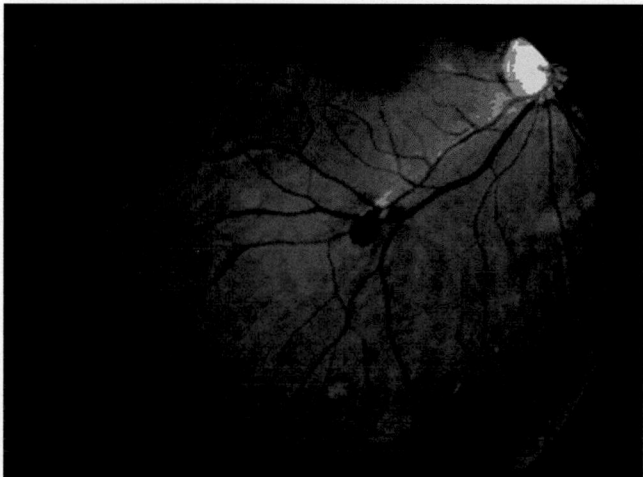

FIGURE 22-47. Congenital hypertrophy of the retinal pigment epithelium (CHRPE). This is a darker CHRPE lesion. More typical lesions are lighter with a halo. (From Tiret A, Taiel-Sartral M, Tiret E, et al. Diagnostic value of fundus examination in familial adenomatous polyposis. *Br J Ophthalmol.* 1997;81[9]:755–758, with permission.)

adenocarcinoma, has variable phenotypes. The spectrum of disease continues to be defined. MAP is responsible for approximately 0.3% of colorectal cancers.

Genetics

MYH is located on the short arm of chromosome 1, between p32.1 and p34.3.[300] It is 7.1 kilobase (kb) long and encodes a protein of 535 amino acid protein that is critical to DNA base excision repair mechanisms.[191] The gene product, *MYH* glycosylase, is a base excision repair protein needed for repair of DNA damage caused by guanine oxidation. Guanine oxidation results in DNA G:C to T:A transversions.[175] The base excision repair system recognizes and repairs the oxidized guanine, preventing or correcting the transversions and resulting mutations.[256] Mutation in *MYH*, therefore, results in decreased or lost base excision repair function and subsequently the accumulation of unrepaired G:C to T:A transversions. Genes that contain an abundance of guanine nucleotides, such as *APC* and *KRAS*, are particularly susceptible to unrepaired oxidative damage. This explains why the phenotype of MAP is similar to that of familial adenomatous polyposis. When a DNA mismatch repair gene is inactivated by G:C to T:A transversions, the mismatch repair mechanism can be inactivated, leading to a mutator phenotype, and microsatellite unstable neoplasia.[126] If a gene involved in control of methylation is predominantly affected by the transversions, a methylated tumor may develop.[33,49]

There are more than 80 *MYH* germ line variants,[116] but within Northern European ancestry, two common mutations, Y165C and G382D, account for more than 80% of all mutations.[286,296]

Clinical Presentation

Because of the recessive inheritance pattern of the disease, patients are often not diagnosed with MAP until they are evaluated for the development of symptoms, such as bleeding per anum, constipation, or abdominal pain. The symptoms are nonspecific but may be caused by colorectal polyps or cancer. Colonoscopy may reveal adenomatous polyposis, but the clinical phenotype varies. Typically, MAP is associated with early onset of multiple colorectal adenomas distributed throughout the colon and rectum. The polyps are usually small tubular or tubulovillous adenomas. The polyp burden varies considerably. Approximately 40% of patients will have 10 to 100 adenomas, and up to 29% will have more than 100 adenomas. Thus, MAP is often diagnosed as attenuated or even classical familial adenomatous polyposis. MAP should be considered in the differential diagnosis for patients with polyposis who do not have an *APC* mutation. More important, approximately 35% of patients will not have adenomas at the time of diagnosis.[74] A suspicion should be raised for those with a family tree suggestive of a recessive pattern of inheritance or those with young onset colorectal cancer.

Biallelic *MYH* mutations do not always cause adenomatous polyposis. Other syndromes of hereditary colorectal cancer may be mimicked, and there may even be no hint at all of hereditary risk when *MYH* mutations give rise to apparently sporadic colorectal cancers. MAP has been reported to present as Lynch syndrome[126,200] or serrated polyposis.[33,49]

Association with Malignancy

The cumulative lifetime risk of developing colorectal cancer for patients with biallelic *MYH* mutations is estimated at 80% by age 70.[171] Onset of cancer is earlier than sporadic colorectal cancer, with the mean age at diagnosis reported between 45 and 56 years old.[116,286,296,339]

Associations with extracolonic malignancies remain incompletely defined due to small cohorts, but data suggests an increased risk of upper gastrointestinal polyps and cancers.[296,333] One retrospective European multicenter study evaluated 276 MAP cases for extracolonic tumors. The cumulative lifetime risk was determined and compared to that of the general population to determine standardized incidence ratios and relative risk. The study reported a nearly twofold incidence of extracolonic malignancies in MAP patients (38%) compared with the general population. The relative risk of duodenal cancer was 129, with a lifetime risk of 4%. There was also a smaller, but significant risk for bladder, ovarian, and skin cancers with standard incidence ratios of 7.2, 5.7, and 2.8, respectively.[333]

Clinical Management
Diagnosis

The diagnosis of MAP is based on the detection of germ line biallelic mutations in the *MYH* gene. Due to the recessive pattern of inheritance and the variable clinical presentation, clinicians must have a high suspicion for MAP. Several clinical situations warrant referral to genetic counseling for discussion of genetic testing such as the following: (1) presence of more than 100 synchronous colorectal adenomas, with or without a family history, in whom *APC* mutation testing is negative; (2) presence of multiple (more than 10 cumulative but less than 100) adenomas where FAP is unlikely, especially when the family history suggests recessive inheritance; (3) development of early age onset (less than 50 years) colorectal cancer, with or without a family history of colorectal neoplasia; (4) familial clustering of colorectal cancer that does not fulfill Amsterdam criteria for HNPCC, where tumors are microsatellite stable; (5) diagnosis of HNPCC by Amsterdam criteria with a microsatellite stable tumor (i.e., familial colorectal cancer type X); (6) diagnosis of HNPCC by Amsterdam criteria with microsatellite unstable tumors but no mismatch repair gene mutation identified; and (7) the presence of "mixed polyposis" of adenomas and serrated polyps.

Once biallelic pathogenic mutations are identified in a proband, genetic counseling and screening should be offered to the family. Siblings have a 25% chance of also having biallelic mutations. Children of affected patients are not at increased risk unless the other parent also is a carrier. Therefore, the partner of the affected patient should be tested to assign risk to the offspring. If the partner is a monoallelic mutation carrier, each offspring has a 50% chance of being MAP. If the partner has two normal *MYH* alleles, then the children are not at risk for developing MAP, but they are obligate carriers of a monoallelic *MYH* mutation, and thus there is a future risk to their children. The family tree should also be evaluated back in time because each parent of an affected child is likely to be a monoallelic mutation carrier. This has implications for aunts and uncles, cousins, nephews, and nieces.

Surveillance

Optimal times to begin screening and screening intervals are not completely defined. According to the National Comprehensive Cancer Network screening recommendations,[237] patients with known biallelic mutation carriers without symptoms should begin screening by means of colonoscopy at age 25 to 30 years. If the screening colonoscopy is negative for adenomas, one should repeat the examination every 3 to 5 years with consideration for decreasing the interval with advancing age. If polyps are found during the screening colonoscopy, polypectomy should be performed. When technically possible, the adenoma burden should be controlled endoscopically by means of repeated colonoscopies every 1 to 2 years. The interval between examinations may be shortened, depending on the polyp burden and the comfort of the endoscopist. For patients with dense polyposis or large polyps that cannot be controlled endoscopically, referral to a colorectal surgeon is warranted.

Upper gastrointestinal polyp surveillance is achieved via esophagoduodenoscopy with side-viewing gastroscope starting at age 30 to 35 years and repeated every 3 to 5 years after normal examinations. For patients with duodenal adenomas, surveillance and management parallels the recommendations for similar patients with FAP.

Surgical Management

Patients with MAP are treated similarly to those with other polyposis syndromes. The role of prophylactic colectomy has not been prospectively studied and is not recommended in routine cases. The development of cancer obviously warrants surgical referral. Patients whose polyp burden cannot be effectively managed endoscopically should also be referred for surgical consultation. For example, dense or carpeted polyposis may not be effectively managed endoscopically.

Surgical options include total or subtotal colectomy, or in certain circumstances, segmental colectomy. Because the entire colon is at risk, a total colectomy and ileorectal anastomosis should be considered as the first choice, although there is no prospective data that demonstrates this intervention reduces the risk of subsequent colorectal cancers. If the disease is limited to a confined segment of the colon and there are medical reasons to avoid an extended resection, a segmental colectomy may be performed. In this situation, it is recommended that the remaining colorectum be surveyed annually with removal of subsequent polyps.

There are little long-term natural history data following surgical management of MAP. One small study retrospectively reviewed 11 patients with biallelic *MYH* mutations and polyposis who underwent total proctocolectomy and ileorectal anastomosis. Endoscopic findings of the remaining rectum using a yearly surveillance regimen were reported. At a median follow-up of 5 years (range, 2 to 23 years), no patient developed rectal cancer. The mean number of adenomas removed per proctoscopy was 1.23 ± 2.19 (range, 0 to 10 adenomas per proctoscopy).[236]

References

1. Agnifili A, Verzaro R, Gola P, et al. Juvenile polyposis: case report and assessment of the neoplastic risk in 271 patients reported in the literature. *Dig Surg.* 1999;16(2):161–166.
2. Agrawal D, Chak A, Champagne BJ, et al. Endoscopic mucosal resection with full-thickness closure for difficult polyps: a prospective clinical trial. *Gastrointest Endosc.* 2010;71(6):1082–1088.
3. Ahmed Ali U, Keus F, Heikens JT, et al. Open versus laparoscopic (assisted) ileo pouch anal anastomosis for ulcerative colitis and familial adenomatous polyposis. *Cochrane Database Syst Rev.* 2009;(1):CD006267.
4. Alexander DD, Cushing CA. Red meat and colorectal cancer: a critical summary of prospective epidemiologic studies. *Obes Rev.* 2011;12(5): e472–e493.
5. Alexander RH, Beckwith JB, Morgan A, et al. Juvenile polyps of the colon and their relationship to allergy. *Am J Surg.* 1970;120(2):222–225.
6. Al-Tassan N, Chmiel NH, Maynard J, et al. Inherited variants of MYH associated with somatic G:C→T:A mutations in colorectal tumors. *Nat Genet.* 2002;30(2):227–232.
7. American Thyroid Association Guidelines Taskforce on Thyroid Nodules and Differentiated Thyroid Cancer, Cooper DS, Doherty GM, et al. Revised American Thyroid Association management guidelines for patients with thyroid nodules and differentiated thyroid cancer. *Thyroid.* 2009;19(11):1167–1214.
8. Amos CI, Keitheri-Cheteri MB, Sabripour M, et al. Genotype-phenotype correlations in Peutz-Jeghers syndrome. *J Med Genet.* 2004;41(5):327–333.
9. Ansher AF, Lewis JH, Fleischer DE, et al. Hyperplastic colonic polyps as a marker for adenomatous colonic polyps. *Am J Gastroenterol.* 1989;84(2):113–117.
10. Arditi C, Gonvers JJ, Burnand B, et al. Appropriateness of colonoscopy in Europe (EPAGE II). Surveillance after polypectomy and after resection of colorectal cancer. *Endoscopy.* 2009;41(3):209–217.
11. Aretz S, Stienen D, Uhlhaas S, et al. High proportion of large genomic STK11 deletions in Peutz-Jeghers syndrome. *Hum Mutat.* 2005;26(6):513–519.
12. Aretz S, Stienen D, Uhlhaas S, et al. High proportion of large genomic deletions and a genotype phenotype update in 80 unrelated families with juvenile polyposis syndrome. *J Med Genet.* 2007;44(11):702–709.
13. Arvanitis ML, Jagelman DG, Fazio VW, et al. Mortality in patients with familial adenomatous polyposis. *Dis Colon Rectum.* 1990;33(8):639–642.
14. Atkin WS, Morson BC, Cuzick J. Long-term risk of colorectal cancer after excision of rectosigmoid adenomas. *N Engl J Med.* 1992;326(10):658–662.
15. Aziz O, Athanasiou T, Fazio VW, et al. Meta-analysis of observational studies of ileorectal versus ileal pouch-anal anastomosis for familial adenomatous polyposis. *Br J Surg.* 2006;93(4):407–417.
16. Azzarelli A, Gronchi A, Bertulli R, et al. Low-dose chemotherapy with methotrexate and vinblastine for patients with advanced aggressive fibromatosis. *Cancer.* 2001;92(5):1259–1264.
17. Bannayan GA. Lipomatosis, angiomatosis, and macrencephalia. A previously undescribed congenital syndrome. *Arch Pathol.* 1971;92(1):1–5.
18. Baron JA. Statins and the colorectum: hope for chemoprevention? *Cancer Prev Res (Phila).* 2010;3(5):573–575.
19. Baron JA, Beach M, Mandel JS, et al. Calcium supplements and colorectal adenomas. Polyp Prevention Study Group. *Ann N Y Acad Sci.* 1999;889:138–145.
20. Baxter NN, Goldwasser MA, Paszat LF, et al. Association of colonoscopy and death from colorectal cancer. *Ann Intern Med.* 2009;150(1):1–8.
21. Behringer GE. Polypoid lesions of the colon. Which should be removed? *Surg Clin North Am.* 1974;54(3):699–712.
22. Belchetz LA, Berk T, Bapat BV, et al. Changing causes of mortality in patients with familial adenomatous polyposis. *Dis Colon Rectum.* 1996;39(4):384–387.
23. Bell B, Mazzaferri EL. Familial adenomatous polyposis (Gardner's syndrome) and thyroid carcinoma. A case report and review of the literature. *Dig Dis Sci.* 1993;38(1):185–190.
24. Belliveau P, Graham AM. Mesenteric desmoid tumor in Gardner's syndrome treated by sulindac. *Dis Colon Rectum.* 1984;27(1):53–54.
25. Berci G, Panish J, Morgenstern L. Diagnostic colonoscopy and colonoscopic polypectomy. *Arch Surg.* 1973;106(6):818–819.
26. Bertagnolli MM, Morgan JA, Fletcher CDM, et al. Multimodality treatment of mesenteric desmoid tumours. *Eur J Cancer.* 2008;44(16):2404–2410.
27. Bertario L, Russo A, Sala P, et al. Genotype and phenotype factors as determinants of desmoid tumors in patients with familial adenomatous polyposis. *Int J Cancer.* 2001;95(2):102–107.
28. Bianchi LK, Burke CA, Bennett AE, et al. Fundic gland polyp dysplasia is common in familial adenomatous polyposis. *Clin Gastroenterol Hepatol.* 2008;6(2):180–185.
29. Billingham RP, Bowman HE, MacKeigan JM. Solitary adenomas in juvenile patients. *Dis Colon Rectum.* 1980;23(1):26–30.
30. Björk J, Akerbrant H, Iselius L, et al. Outcome of primary and secondary ileal pouch-anal anastomosis and ileorectal anastomosis in patients with familial adenomatous polyposis. *Dis Colon Rectum.* 2001;44(7):984–992.
31. Boland CR, Goel A. Microsatellite instability in colorectal cancer. *Gastroenterology.* 2010;138(6):2073–2087.e3.
32. Boland CR, Thibodeau SN, Hamilton SR, et al. A National Cancer Institute Workshop on Microsatellite Instability for cancer detection and familial predisposition: development of international criteria for the determination of microsatellite instability in colorectal cancer. *Cancer Res.* 1998;58(22):5248–5257.
33. Boparai KS, Dekker E, Van Eeden S, et al. Hyperplastic polyps and sessile serrated adenomas as a phenotypic expression of MYH-associated polyposis. *Gastroenterology.* 2008;135(6):2014–2018.

34. Boparai KS, Mathus-Vliegen EM, Koornstra JJ, et al. Increased colorectal cancer risk during follow-up in patients with hyperplastic polyposis syndrome: a multicentre cohort study. *Gut.* 2010;59(8):1094–1100.

35. Brenner H, Hoffmeister M, Arndt V, et al. Protection from right- and left-sided colorectal neoplasms after colonoscopy: population-based study. *J Natl Cancer Inst.* 2010;102(2):89–95.

36. Brosens LA, van Hattem A, Hylind LM, et al. Risk of colorectal cancer in juvenile polyposis. *Gut.* 2007;56(7):965–967.

37. Buchanan DD, Sweet K, Drini M, et al. Phenotypic diversity in patients with multiple serrated polyps: a genetics clinic study. *Int J Colorectal Dis.* 2010;25(6):703–712.

38. Bulow C, Bulow S. Is screening for thyroid carcinoma indicated in familial adenomatous polyposis? The Leeds Castle Polyposis Group. *Int J Colorectal Dis.* 1997;12(4):240–242.

39. Bulow C, Bulow S, Nielsen TF, et al. Prognosis in familial adenomatous polyposis. Results from the Polyposis Registry. *Ugeskr Laeger.* 1996;158(29):4188–4190.

40. Bulow S. Results of national registration of familial adenomatous polyposis. *Gut.* 2003;52(5):742–746.

41. Burke CA, Beck GJ, Church JM, et al. The natural history of untreated duodenal and ampullary adenomas in patients with familial adenomatous polyposis followed in an endoscopic surveillance program. *Gastrointest Endosc.* 1999;49(3 pt 1):358–364.

42. Burke CA, Santisi J, Church J, et al. The utility of capsule endoscopy small bowel surveillance in patients with polyposis. *Am J Gastroenterol.* 2005;100(7):1498–1502.

43. Burt RW, Bishop DT, Lynch HT, et al. Risk and surveillance of individuals with heritable factors for colorectal cancer. WHO Collaborating Centre for the Prevention of Colorectal Cancer. *Bull World Health Organ.* 1990;68(5):655–665.

44. Burt RW, Jass JR. Hyperplastic polyposis. In: Hamilton SR, Aaltonen LA, eds. *Pathology and Genetics of Tumors of the Digestive System.* Vol 2. Lyon, France: IARC Press; 2000:135–136.

45. Bussey H. *Familial Polyposis Coli.* Baltimore, MD: Johns Hopkins University Press; 1975.

46. Calva D, Howe JR. Hamartomatous polyposis syndromes. *Surg Clin North Am.* 2008;88(4):779–817, vii.

47. Calva D, Howe JR. Juvenile polyposis. In: Riegert-Johnson DL, Boardman LA, Hefferon T, et al, eds. *Cancer Syndromes* [Internet]. Bethesda, MD: National Center for Biotechnology Information; 2009.

48. Carvajal-Carmona LG, Howarth KM, Lockett M, et al. Molecular classification and genetic pathways in hyperplastic polyposis syndrome. *J Pathol.* 2007;212(4):378–385.

49. Castells A. MYH-associated polyposis: adenomas and hyperplastic polyps, partners in crime? *Gastroenterology.* 2008;135(6):1857–1859.

50. Cetta F, Montalto G, Gori M, et al. Germline mutations of the APC gene in patients with familial adenomatous polyposis-associated thyroid carcinoma: results from a European cooperative study. *J Clin Endocrinol Metab.* 2000;85(1):286–292.

51. Chan TL, Zhao W, Leung SY, et al. BRAF and KRAS mutations in colorectal hyperplastic polyps and serrated adenomas. *Cancer Res.* 2003;63(16):4878–4881.

52. Chapuis PH, Dent OF, Goulston KJ. Clinical accuracy in the diagnosis of small polyps using the flexible fiberoptic sigmoidoscope. *Dis Colon Rectum.* 1982;25(7):669–672.

53. Chargelaigue A. *Des polyps du rectum* [in French]. Paris, France; 1859.

54. Chatzipetrou MA, Tzakis AG, Pinna AD, et al. Intestinal transplantation for the treatment of desmoid tumors associated with familial adenomatous polyposis. *Surgery.* 2001;129(3):277–281.

55. Chiu YS, Spencer RJ. Villous lesions of the colon. *Dis Colon Rectum.* 1978;21(7):493–495.

56. Choen S, Tsunoda A, Nicholls RJ. Prospective randomized trial comparing anal function after hand sewn ileoanal anastomosis with mucosectomy versus stapled ileoanal anastomosis without mucosectomy in restorative proctocolectomy. *Br J Surg.* 1991;78(4):430–434.

57. Choi H, Choi KY, Eun CS, et al. Korean experience with double balloon endoscopy: Korean Association for the Study of Intestinal Diseases multi-center study. *Gastrointest Endosc.* 2007;66(3 suppl):S22–S25.

58. Chow E, Lipton L, Lynch E, et al. Hyperplastic polyposis syndrome: phenotypic presentations and the role of MBD4 and MYH. *Gastroenterology.* 2006;131(1):30–39.

59. Church J. Ileoanal pouch neoplasia in familial adenomatous polyposis: an underestimated threat. *Dis Colon Rectum.* 2005;48(9):1708–1713.

60. Church J. Adenoma detection rate and the quality of colonoscopy: the sword has two edges. *Dis Colon Rectum.* 2008;51(5):520–523.

61. Church J. Familial adenomatous polyposis. *Surg Oncol Clin N Am.* 2009;18(4):585–598.

62. Church J, Burke C, McGannon E, et al. Predicting polyposis severity by proctoscopy: how reliable is it? *Dis Colon Rectum.* 2001;44(9):1249–1254.

63. Church J, Burke C, McGannon E, et al. Risk of rectal cancer in patients after colectomy and ileorectal anastomosis for familial adenomatous polyposis: a function of available surgical options. *Dis Colon Rectum.* 2003;46(9):1175–1181.

64. Church J, Lynch C, Neary P, et al. A desmoid tumor-staging system separates patients with intra-abdominal, familial adenomatous polyposis-associated desmoid disease by behavior and prognosis. *Dis Colon Rectum.* 2008;51(6):897–901.

65. Church J, Simmang C. Practice parameters for the treatment of patients with dominantly inherited colorectal cancer (familial adenomatous polyposis and hereditary nonpolyposis colorectal cancer). *Dis Colon Rectum.* 2003;46(8):1001–1012.

66. Church JM. Men tend to be neoplasia prone and women neoplasia resistant. *Surg Endosc.* 2000;14(12):1162–1166.

67. Church JM. Avoiding surgery in patients with colorectal polyps. *Dis Colon Rectum.* 2003;46(11):1513–1516.

68. Church JM. Experience in the endoscopic management of large colonic polyps. *ANZ J Surg.* 2003;73(12):988–995.

69. Church JM. Clinical significance of small colorectal polyps. *Dis Colon Rectum.* 2004;47(4):481–485.

70. Church JM, Fazio VW, Jones IT. Small colorectal polyps. Are they worth treating? *Dis Colon Rectum.* 1988;31(1):50–53.

71. Church JM, McGannon E, Hull-Boiner S, et al. Gastroduodenal polyps in patients with familial adenomatous polyposis. *Dis Colon Rectum.* 1992;35(12):1170–1173.

72. Church JM, Muto T, Appau K. Flat lesions of the colorectal mucosa: differences in recognition between Japanese and American endoscopists. *Dis Colon Rectum.* 2004;47(9):1462–1466.

73. Clark SK, Neale KF, Landgrebe JC, et al. Desmoid tumours complicating familial adenomatous polyposis. *Br J Surg.* 1999;86(9):1185–1189.

74. Cleary SP, Cotterchio M, Jenkins MA, et al. Germline MutY human homologue mutations and colorectal cancer: a multisite case-control study. *Gastroenterology.* 2009;136(4):1251–1260.

75. Cole JW, Holden WD. Postcolectomy regression of adenomatous polyps of the rectum. *Arch Surg.* 1959;79:385–392.

76. Conio M, Blanchi S, Filiberti R, et al. Cap-assisted endoscopic mucosal resection of large polyps involving the ileocecal valve. *Endoscopy.* 2010;42(8):677–680.

77. Corman ML, Veidenheimer MC, Swinton NW. *Diseases of the Anus, Rectum, and Colon. Part I: Neoplasms.* New York, NY: Medcom; 1972.

78. Cotterill JA, Hughes JP, Day JL, et al. The Cronkhite-Canada syndrome. *Postgrad Med J.* 1973;49(570):268–273.

79. Coutsoftides T, Sivak MV Jr, Benjamin SP, et al. Colonoscopy and the management of polyps containing invasive carcinoma. *Ann Surg.* 1978;188(5):638–641.

80. Cripps W. Two cases of disseminated polyps of the rectum. *Tr Path Society London.* 1882;33:165–168.

81. Cronkhite LW Jr, Canada WJ. Generalized gastrointestinal polyposis; an unusual syndrome of polyposis, pigmentation, alopecia and onychotrophia. *N Engl J Med.* 1955;252(24):1011–1015.

82. da Luz Moreira A, Church JM, Burke CA. The evolution of prophylactic colorectal surgery for familial adenomatous polyposis. *Dis Colon Rectum.* 2009;52(8):1481–1486.

83. Daniel ES, Ludwig SL, Lewin KJ, et al. The Cronkhite-Canada Syndrome. An analysis of clinical and pathologic features and therapy in 55 patients. *Medicine (Baltimore).* 1982;61(5):293–309.

84. Day D, Morson B. The polyp problem. In: Hunt R, Waye J, eds. *Colonoscopy: Techniques, Clinical Practice and Colour Atlas.* London, United Kingdom: Chapman & Hall; 1981.

85. de Castro SMM, van Eijck CHJ, Rutten JP, et al. Pancreas-preserving total duodenectomy versus standard pancreatoduodenectomy for patients with familial adenomatous polyposis and polyps in the duodenum. *Br J Surg.* 2008;95(11):1380–1386.

86. De Gennaro VA, Lescher TC. Transanal excision of rectal tumors using a laparoscopic stapler. *Dis Colon Rectum.* 1995;38(3):327–328.

87. Delaney CP, Champagne BJ, Marks JM, et al. Tissue apposition system: new technology to minimize surgery for endoscopically unresectable colonic polyps. *Surg Endosc.* 2010;24(12):3113–3118.

88. Desai DC, Neale KF, Talbot IC, et al. Juvenile polyposis. *Br J Surg.* 1995;82(1):14–17.

89. Desai TK, Barkel D. Syndromic colon cancer: lynch syndrome and familial adenomatous polyposis. *Gastroenterol Clin North Am.* 2008;37(1):47–72, vi.

90. de Vos tot Nederveen Cappel WH, Jarvinen HJ, Bjork J, et al. Worldwide survey among polyposis registries of surgical management of severe duodenal adenomatosis in familial adenomatous polyposis. *Br J Surg.* 2003;90(6):705–710.

91. Dickinson AJ, Savage AP, Mortensen NJ, et al. Long-term survival after endoscopic transanal resection of rectal tumours. *Br J Surg.* 1993;80(11):1401–1404.

92. Edwards DP, Khosraviani K, Stafferton R, et al. Long-term results of polyp clearance by intraoperative enteroscopy in the Peutz-Jeghers syndrome. *Dis Colon Rectum.* 2003;46(1):48–50.

93. Ekelund G. On cancer and polyps of colon and rectum. *Acta Pathol Microbiol Scand.* 1963;59:165–170.

94. Elayi E, Manilich E, Church J. Polishing the crystal ball: knowing genotype improves ability to predict desmoid disease in patients with familial adenomatous polyposis. *Dis Colon Rectum.* 2009;52(10):1762–1766.

95. Emura F, Saito Y, Taniguchi M, et al. Further validation of magnifying chromocolonoscopy for differentiating colorectal neoplastic polyps in a health screening center. *J Gastroenterol Hepatol.* 2007;22(11):1722–1727.

96. Evans DG, Howard E, Giblin C, et al. Birth incidence and prevalence of tumor prone syndromes: estimates from a UK family genetic register service. *Am J Med Genet A.* 2010;152A(2):327–332.

97. Farhat S, Chaussade S, Ponchon T, et al. Endoscopic submucosal dissection in a European setting. A multi-institutional report of a technique in development. *Endoscopy.* 2011;43(8):664–670.

98. Feinberg SM, Jagelman DG, Sarre RG, et al. Spontaneous resolution of rectal polyps in patients with familial polyposis following abdominal colectomy and ileorectal anastomosis. *Dis Colon Rectum.* 1988;31(3):169–175.

99. Fenoglio-Preiser CM. Hyperplastic polyps, adenomatous polyps, and mixed hyperplastic adenomatous polyps of the colon: definitions. *Prog Clin Biol Res.* 1988;279:3–12.

100. Ferney DM, DeSchryver-Kecskemeti K, Clouse RE. Treatment of Cronkhite-Canada syndrome with home total parenteral nutrition. *Ann Intern Med.* 1986;104(4):588.

101. Ferrandez A, Samowitz W, DiSario JA, et al. Phenotypic characterization and risk of cancer development in hyperplastic polyposis: case series and literature review. *Am J Gastroenterol.* 2004;99(10):2012–2018.

102. Ferrara F, Luigiano C, Ghersi S, et al. Efficacy, safety and outcomes of "inject and cut" endoscopic mucosal resection for large sessile and flat colorectal polyps. *Digestion.* 2010;82(4):213–220.

103. Franklin ME Jr, Portillo G. Laparoscopic monitored colonoscopic polypectomy: long-term follow-up. *World J Surg.* 2009;33(6):1306–1309.

104. Gallagher MC, Shankar A, Groves CJ, et al. Pylorus-preserving pancreaticoduodenectomy for advanced duodenal disease in familial adenomatous polyposis. *Br J Surg.* 2004;91(9):1157–1164.

105. Gallione CJ, Repetto GM, Legius E, et al. A combined syndrome of juvenile polyposis and hereditary haemorrhagic telangiectasia associated with mutations in MADH4 (SMAD4). *Lancet.* 2004;363(9412):852–859.

106. Gardner EJ, Plenk HP. Hereditary pattern for multiple osteomas in a family group. *Am J Hum Genet.* 1952;4(1):31–36.

107. Garrard CL, Clements RH, Nanney L, et al. Adhesion formation is reduced after laparoscopic surgery. *Surg Endosc.* 1999;13(1):10–13.

108. Gelb AM, Minkowitz S, Tresser M. Rectal and colonic polyps occurring in young people. *N Y State J Med.* 1962;62:513–518.

109. Giardiello FM, Brensinger JD, Tersmette AC, et al. Very high risk of cancer in familial Peutz-Jeghers syndrome. *Gastroenterology.* 2000;119(6):1447–1453.

110. Giardiello FM, Offerhaus GJ, Krush AJ, et al. Risk of hepatoblastoma in familial adenomatous polyposis. *J Pediatr.* 1991;119(5):766–768.

111. Giardiello FM, Offerhaus GJ, Lee DH, et al. Increased risk of thyroid and pancreatic carcinoma in familial adenomatous polyposis. *Gut.* 1993;34(10):1394–1396.

112. Giardiello FM, Trimbath JD. Peutz-Jeghers syndrome and management recommendations. *Clin Gastroenterol Hepatol.* 2006;4(4):408–415.

113. Giardiello FM, Trimbath JD, Giardiello FM, et al. Peutz-Jeghers syndrome and management recommendations. *Clin Gastroenterol Hepatol.* 2006;4(4):408–415.

114. Gilson TP, Sollenberger LL. Adenocarcinoma of an ileostomy in a patient with familial adenomatous polyposis. Report of a case. *Dis Colon Rectum.* 1992;35(3):261–265.

115. Glatz K, Pritt B, Glatz D, et al. A multinational, internet-based assessment of observer variability in the diagnosis of serrated colorectal polyps. *Am J Clin Pathol.* 2007;127(6):938–945.

116. Goodenberger M, Lindor NM. Lynch syndrome and MYH-associated polyposis: review and testing strategy. *J Clin Gastroenterol.* 2011;45(6):488–500.

117. Gorgun E, Church J. Flat adenomas of the large bowel: a single endoscopist study. *Dis Colon Rectum.* 2009;52(5):972–977.

118. Gorlin RJ, Cohen MM Jr, Condon LM, et al. Bannayan-Riley-Ruvalcaba syndrome. *Am J Med Genet.* 1992;44(3):307–314.

119. Greenberg ER, Baron JA, Tosteson TD, et al. A clinical trial of antioxidant vitamins to prevent colorectal adenoma. Polyp Prevention Study Group. *N Engl J Med.* 1994;331(3):141–147.

120. Greene FL. Distribution of colorectal neoplasms. A left to right shift of polyps and cancer. *Am Surg.* 1983;49(2):62–65.

121. Groen EJ, Roos A, Muntinghe FL, et al. Extra-intestinal manifestations of familial adenomatous polyposis. *Ann Surg Oncol.* 2008;15(9):2439–2450.

122. Groves CJ, Beveridge G, Swain DJ, et al. Prevalence and morphology of pouch and ileal adenomas in familial adenomatous polyposis. *Dis Colon Rectum.* 2005;48(4):816–823.

123. Groves CJ, Saunders BP, Spigelman AD, et al. Duodenal cancer in patients with familial adenomatous polyposis (FAP): results of a 10 year prospective study. *Gut.* 2002;50(5):636–641.

124. Grünhagen DJ, van Ierland MC, Doornebosch PG, et al. Laparoscopic-monitored colonoscopic polypectomy: a multimodality method to avoid segmental colon resection. *Colorectal Dis.* 2011;13(11):1280–1284.

125. Gschwantler M, Kriwanek S, Langner E, et al. High-grade dysplasia and invasive carcinoma in colorectal adenomas: a multivariate analysis of the impact of adenoma and patient characteristics. *Eur J Gastroenterol Hepatol.* 2002;14(2):183–188.

126. Guillen-Ponce C, Castillejo A, Barbera VM, et al. Biallelic MYH germline mutations as cause of Muir-Torre syndrome. *Fam Cancer.* 2010;9(2):151–154.

127. Gustafson S, Zbuk KM, Scacheri C, et al. Cowden syndrome. *Semin Oncol.* 2007;34(5):428–434.

128. Gutt CN, Oniu T, Schemmer P, et al. Fewer adhesions induced by laparoscopic surgery? *Surg Endosc.* 2004;18(6):898–906.

129. Haggitt RC, Glotzbach RE, Soffer EE, et al. Prognostic factors in colorectal carcinomas arising in adenomas: implications for lesions removed by endoscopic polypectomy. *Gastroenterology.* 1985;89(2):328–336.

130. Hamilton SR, Liu B, Parsons RE, et al. The molecular basis of Turcot's syndrome. *N Engl J Med.* 1995;332(13):839–847.

131. Hardell L, Breivald M, Hennerdal S, et al. Shrinkage of desmoid tumor with interferon alfa treatment: a case report. *Cytokines Cell Mol Ther.* 2000;6(3):155–156.

132. Hartley JE, Church JM, Gupta S, et al. Significance of incidental desmoids identified during surgery for familial adenomatous polyposis. *Dis Colon Rectum.* 2004;47(3):334–338; discussion 339–340.

133. Hauenschild L, Bader FG, Laubert T, et al. Laparoscopic colorectal resection for benign polyps not suitable for endoscopic polypectomy. *Int J Colorectal Dis.* 2009;24(7):755–759.

134. Hawk ET, Umar A, Viner JL. Colorectal cancer chemoprevention—an overview of the science. *Gastroenterology.* 2004;126(5):1423–1447.

135. Heald B, Mester J, Rybicki L, et al. Frequent gastrointestinal polyps and colorectal adenocarcinomas in a prospective series of PTEN mutation carriers. *Gastroenterology.* 2010;139(6):1927–1933.

136. Heiskanen I, Kellokumpu I, Jarvinen H. Management of duodenal adenomas in 98 patients with familial adenomatous polyposis. *Endoscopy.* 1999;31(6):412–416.

137. Helwig EB. Adenomas and the pathogenesis of cancer of the colon and rectum. *Dis Colon Rectum.* 1959;2(1):5–17.

138. Hemminki A, Markie D, Tomlinson I, et al. A serine/threonine kinase gene defective in Peutz-Jeghers syndrome. *Nature.* 1998;391(6663):184–187.

139. Hernegger GS, Moore HG, Guillem JG. Attenuated familial adenomatous polyposis: an evolving and poorly understood entity. *Dis Colon Rectum.* 2002;45(1):127–134; discussion 134–126.

140. Hetzel JT, Huang CS, Coukos JA, et al. Variation in the detection of serrated polyps in an average risk colorectal cancer screening cohort. *Am J Gastroenterol.* 2010;105(12):2656–2664.

141. Heuschen UA, Heuschen G, Autschbach F, et al. Adenocarcinoma in the ileal pouch: late risk of cancer after restorative proctocolectomy. *Int J Colorectal Dis.* 2001;16(2):126–130.

142. Heyen F, Jagelman DG, Romania A, et al. Predictive value of congenital hypertrophy of the retinal pigment epithelium as a clinical marker for familial adenomatous polyposis. *Dis Colon Rectum.* 1990;33(12):1003–1008.

143. Higuchi T, Jass JR. My approach to serrated polyps of the colorectum. *J Clin Pathol.* 2004;57(7):682–686.

144. Hofgartner WT, Thorp M, Ramus MW, et al. Gastric adenocarcinoma associated with fundic gland polyps in a patient with attenuated familial adenomatous polyposis. *Am J Gastroenterol.* 1999;94(8).2275–2281.

145. Honma K, Kobayashi M, Watanabe H, et al. Endoscopic submucosal dissection for colorectal neoplasia. *Dig Endosc.* 2010;22(4):307–311.

146. Hotta K, Oyama T, Shinohara T, et al. Learning curve for endoscopic submucosal dissection of large colorectal tumors. *Dig Endosc.* 2010;22(4):302–306.

147. Howe JR, Mitros FA, Summers RW. The risk of gastrointestinal carcinoma in familial juvenile polyposis. *Ann Surg Oncol.* 1998;5(8):751–756.

148. Howe JR, Sayed MG, Ahmed AF, et al. The prevalence of MADH4 and BMPR1A mutations in juvenile polyposis and absence of BMPR2, BMPR1B, and ACVR1 mutations. *J Med Genet.* 2004;41(7):484–491.

149. Hughes LJ, Michels VV. Risk of hepatoblastoma in familial adenomatous polyposis. *Am J Med Genet.* 1992;43(6):1023–1025.

150. Hurlstone DP, Saunders BP, Church JM. Endoscopic surveillance of the ileoanal pouch following restorative proctocolectomy for familial adenomatous polyposis. *Endoscopy.* 2008;40(5):437–442.

151. Hyman NH, Anderson P, Blasyk H. Hyperplastic polyposis and the risk of colorectal cancer. *Dis Colon Rectum.* 2004;47(12):2101–2104.

152. Iida M, Itoh H, Matsui T, et al. Ileal adenomas in postcolectomy patients with familial adenomatosis coli/Gardner's syndrome. Incidence and endoscopic appearance. *Dis Colon Rectum.* 1989;32(12):1034–1038.

153. Iida Y, Miura S, Munemoto Y, et al. Endoscopic resection of large colorectal polyps using a clipping method. *Dis Colon Rectum.* 1994;37(2):179–180.

154. Itoh H, Hirata K, Ohsato K. Turcot's syndrome and familial adenomatous polyposis associated with brain tumor: review of related literature. *Int J Colorectal Dis.* 1993;8(2):87–94.

155. Iwama T, Mishima Y. Factors affecting the risk of rectal cancer following rectum-preserving surgery in patients with familial adenomatous polyposis. *Dis Colon Rectum.* 1994;37(10):1024–1026.

156. Iyer NK, Burke CA, Leach BH, et al. SMAD4 mutation and the combined syndrome of juvenile polyposis syndrome and hereditary haemorrhagic telangiectasia. *Thorax.* 2010;65(8):745–746.

157. Jacobs ET, Thompson PA, Martinez ME. Diet, gender, and colorectal neoplasia. *J Clin Gastroenterol.* 2007;41(8):731–746.

158. Jaeger EE, Woodford-Richens KL, Lockett M, et al. An ancestral Ashkenazi haplotype at the HMPS/CRAC1 locus on 15q13-q14 is associated with hereditary mixed polyposis syndrome. *Am J Hum Genet.* 2003;72(5):1261–1267.

159. Jahadi MR, Bailey W. Papillary adenomas of the colon and rectum: a twelve-year review. *Dis Colon Rectum.* 1975;18(3):249–253.

160. Jalihal A, Misra SP, Arvind AS, et al. Colonoscopic polypectomy in children. *J Pediatr Surg.* 1992;27(9):1220–1222.

161. Jang YS, Steinhagen RM, Heimann TM. Colorectal cancer in familial adenomatous polyposis. *Dis Colon Rectum.* 1997;40(3):312–316.

162. Jarrar AM, Church JM, Fay S, et al. Is the phenotype mixed or mistaken? Hereditary nonpolyposis colorectal cancer and hyperplastic polyposis syndrome. *Dis Colon Rectum.* 2009;52(12):1949–1955.

163. Jarrar AM, Milas M, Mitchell J, et al. Screening for thyroid cancer in patients wtih familial adenomatous polyposis. *Ann Surg.* 2011;253(3):515–521.

164. Jass J. *Juvenile Polyposis.* London, United Kingdom: Edward Arnold; 1994.

165. Jass JR. Relation between metaplastic polyp and carcinoma of the colorectum. *Lancet.* 1983;1(8314-5):28–30.

166. Jass JR, Iino H, Ruszkiewicz A, et al. Neoplastic progression occurs through mutator pathways in hyperplastic polyposis of the colorectum. *Gut.* 2000;47(1):43–49.

167. Jass JR, Williams CB, Bussey HJ, et al. Juvenile polyposis—a precancerous condition. *Histopathology.* 1988;13(6):619–630.

168. Jeanneret-Grosjean AJ, Tse GN, Thompson WG. Villous adenoma with hyponatremia and syncope: report of a case. *Dis Colon Rectum.* 1978;21(2):118–119.

169. Jeghers H. Pigmentation of skin. *N Engl J Med.* 1944;231:88.

170. Jeghers H, McKusick VA, Katz KH. Generalized intestinal polyposis and melanin spots of the oral mucosa, lips and digits; a syndrome of diagnostic significance. *N Engl J Med.* 1949;241(25):993, illust; passim.

171. Jenkins MA, Croitoru ME, Monga N, et al. Risk of colorectal cancer in monoallelic and biallelic carriers of MYH mutations: a population-based case-family study. *Cancer Epidemiol Biomarkers Prev.* 2006;15(2):312–314.

172. Johns LE, Houlston RS. A systematic review and meta-analysis of familial colorectal cancer risk. *Am J Gastroenterol.* 2001;96(10):2992–3003.

173. Johnson JR, Lacey JV Jr, Lazovich D, et al. Menopausal hormone therapy and risk of colorectal cancer. *Cancer Epidemiol Biomarkers Prev.* 2009;18(1):196–203.

174. Johnson MD, Mackey R, Brown N, et al. Outcome based on management for duodenal adenomas: sporadic versus familial disease. *J Gastrointest Surg.* 2010;14(2):229–235.

175. Jones S, Emmerson P, Maynard J, et al. Biallelic germline mutations in MYH predispose to multiple colorectal adenoma and somatic G:C→T:A mutations. *Hum Mol Genet.* 2002;11(23):2961–2967.

176. Joslyn G, Carlson M, Thliveris A, et al. Identification of deletion mutations and three new genes at the familial polyposis locus. *Cell.* 1991;66(3):601–613.

177. Joyce M, Mignanelli E, Church J. Ureteric obstruction in familial adenomatous polyposis-associated desmoid disease. *Dis Colon Rectum.* 2010;53(3):327–332.

178. Kahi CJ, Hewett DG, Norton DL, et al. Prevalence and variable detection of proximal colon serrated polyps during screening colonoscopy. *Clin Gastroenterol Hepatol.* 2011;9(1):42–46.

179. Kahi CJ, Hewett DG, Rex DK. Relationship of non-polypoid colorectal neoplasms to quality of colonoscopy. *Gastrointest Endosc Clin N Am.* 2010;20(3):407–415.

180. Kalady MF, Clary BM, Tyler DS, et al. Pancreas-preserving duodenectomy in the management of duodenal familial adenomatous polyposis. *J Gastrointest Surg.* 2002;6(1):82–87.

181. Kalady MF, Jarrar A, Leach B, et al. Defining phenotypes and cancer risk in hyperplastic polyposis syndrome. *Dis Colon Rectum.* 2011;54(2):164–170.

182. Kalady MF, Sanchez JA, Manilich E, et al. Divergent oncogenic changes influence survival differences between colon and rectal adenocarcinomas. *Dis Colon Rectum.* 2009;52(6):1039–1045.

183. Kaminski MF, Regula J, Kraszewska E, et al. Quality indicators for colonoscopy and the risk of interval cancer. *N Engl J Med.* 2010;362(19):1795–1803.

184. Kapetanakis AM, Vini D, Plitsis G. Solitary juvenile polyps in children and colon cancer. *Hepatogastroenterology.* 1996;43(12):1530–1531.

185. Keck JO, Schoetz DJ Jr, Roberts PL, et al. Rectal mucosectomy in the treatment of giant rectal villous tumors. *Dis Colon Rectum.* 1995;38(3):233–238.

186. Key TJ. Fruit and vegetables and cancer risk. *Br J Cancer.* 2011;104(1):6–11.

187. Khalid O, Radaideh S, Cummings OW, et al. Reinterpretation of histology of proximal colon polyps called hyperplastic in 2001. *World J Gastroenterol.* 2009;15(30):3767–3770.

188. Kiesslich R, Jung M, DiSario JA, et al. Perspectives of chromo and magnifying endoscopy: how, how much, when, and whom should we stain? *J Clin Gastroenterol.* 2004;38(1):7–13.

189. Kikendall JW, Bowen PE, Burgess MB, et al. Cigarettes and alcohol as independent risk factors for colonic adenomas. *Gastroenterology.* 1989;97(3):660–664.

190. Kim DH, Pickhardt PJ. Colorectal cancer: managing diminutive polyps-what is the optimal approach? *Nat Rev Gastroenterol Hepatol.* 2011;8(3):129–131.

191. Kim IJ, Ku JL, Kang HC, et al. Mutational analysis of OGG1, MYH, MTH1 in FAP, HNPCC and sporadic colorectal cancer patients: R154H OGG1 polymorphism is associated with sporadic colorectal cancer patients. *Hum Genet.* 2004;115(6):498–503.

192. Kinzler KW, Nilbert MC, Su LK, et al. Identification of FAP locus genes from chromosome 5q21. *Science.* 1991;253(5020):661–665.

193. Kita H, Yamamoto H, Nakamura T, et al. Bleeding polyp in the mid small intestine identified by capsule endoscopy and treated by double-balloon endoscopy. *Gastrointest Endosc.* 2005;61(4):628–629.

194. Knox WG, Miller RE, Begg CF, et al. Juvenile polyps of the colon. A clinicopathologic analysis of 75 polyps in 43 patients. *Surgery.* 1960;48:201–210.

195. Kottmeier PK, Clatworthy HW Jr. Intestinal polyps and associated carcinoma in childhood. *Am J Surg.* 1965;110(5):709–716.

196. Kudo S, Rubio CA, Teixeira CR, et al. Pit pattern in colorectal neoplasia: endoscopic magnifying view. *Endoscopy.* 2001;33(4):367–373.

197. Lage P, Cravo M, Sousa R, et al. Management of Portuguese patients with hyperplastic polyposis and screening of at-risk first-degree relatives: a contribution for future guidelines based on a clinical study. *Am J Gastroenterol.* 2004;99(9):1779–1784.

198. Lal G, Gallinger S. Familial adenomatous polyposis. *Semin Surg Oncol.* 2000;18(4):314–323.

199. Lee RH, Tang RS, Muthusamy VR, et al. Quality of colonoscopy withdrawal technique and variability in adenoma detection rates (with videos). *Gastrointest Endosc.* 2011;74(1):128–134.

200. Lefevre JH, Colas C, Coulet F, et al. MYH biallelic mutation can inactivate the two genetic pathways of colorectal cancer by APC or MLH1 transversions. *Fam Cancer.* 2010;9(4):589–594.

201. Leggett BA, Devereaux B, Biden K, et al. Hyperplastic polyposis: association with colorectal cancer. *Am J Surg Pathol.* 2001;25(2):177–184.

202. Leppard BJ. Epidermoid cysts and polyposis coli. *Proc R Soc Med.* 1974;67(10):1036–1037.

203. Liaw D, Marsh DJ, Li J, et al. Germline mutations of the PTEN gene in Cowden disease, an inherited breast and thyroid cancer syndrome. *Nat Genet.* 1997;16(1):64–67.

204. Lichtenstein P, Holm NV, Verkasalo PK, et al. Environmental and heritable factors in the causation of cancer—analyses of cohorts of twins from Sweden, Denmark, and Finland. *N Engl J Med*. 2000;343(2):78–85.

205. Lindor NM, Dozois R, Nelson H, et al. Desmoid tumors in familial adenomatous polyposis: a pilot project evaluating efficacy of treatment with pirfenidone. *Am J Gastroenterol*. 2003;98(8):1868–1874.

206. Links TP, van Tol KM, Jager PL, et al. Life expectancy in differentiated thyroid cancer: a novel approach to survival analysis. *Endocr Relat Cancer*. 2005;12(2):273–280.

207. Lipof T, Bartus C, Sardella W, et al. Preoperative colonoscopy decreases the need for laparoscopic management of colonic polyps. *Dis Colon Rectum*. 2005;48(5):1076–1080.

208. Lloyd KM II, Dennis M. Cowden's disease. A possible new symptom complex with multiple system involvement. *Ann Intern Med*. 1963;58:136–142.

209. Localio SA. Spontaneous disappearance of rectal polyps following subtotal colectomy and ileoproctostomy for polyposis of the colon. *Am J Surg*. 1962;103:81–82.

210. Longacre TA, Fenoglio-Preiser CM. Mixed hyperplastic adenomatous polyps/serrated adenomas. A distinct form of colorectal neoplasia. *Am J Surg Pathol*. 1990;14(6):524–537.

211. Lovegrove RE, Constantinides VA, Heriot AG, et al. A comparison of hand-sewn versus stapled ileal pouch anal anastomosis (IPAA) following proctocolectomy: a meta-analysis of 4183 patients. *Ann Surg*. 2006;244(1):18–26.

212. Lynch AC, Ozuner G, Church JM. The clinical course of desmoid tumors in familial adenomatous polyposis. *Dis Colon Rectum*. 2003;46:A53.

213. Madden MV, Neale KF, Nicholls RJ, et al. Comparison of morbidity and function after colectomy with ileorectal anastomosis or restorative proctocolectomy for familial adenomatous polyposis. *Br J Surg*. 1991;78(7):789–792.

214. Malhotra R, Sheffield A. Cronkhite-Canada syndrome associated with colon carcinoma and adenomatous changes in C-C polyps. *Am J Gastroenterol*. 1988;83(7):772–776.

215. Marsh DJ, Dahia PL, Caron S, et al. Germline PTEN mutations in Cowden syndrome like families. *J Med Genet*. 1998;35(11):881–885.

216. Marsh DJ, Dahia PL, Coulon V, et al. Allelic imbalance, including deletion of PTEN/MMAC1, at the Cowden disease locus on 10q22-23, in hamartomas from patients with Cowden syndrome and germline PTEN mutation. *Genes Chromosomes Cancer*. 1998;21(1):61–69.

217. Marsh DJ, Dahia PL, Zheng Z, et al. Germline mutations in PTEN are present in Bannayan-Zonana syndrome. *Nat Genet*. 1997;16(4):333–334.

218. Mayer J, Mortensen NJ. Transanal endoscopic microsurgery: a forgotten minimally invasive operation. *Br J Surg*. 1995;82(4):435–437.

219. Mazier WP, MacKeigan JM, Billingham RP, et al. Juvenile polyps of the colon and rectum. *Surg Gynecol Obstet*. 1982;154(6):829–832.

220. McKittrick LS, Wheelock FC Jr. *Carcinoma of the Colon*. Springfield, IL: Charles C Thomas; 1954.

221. Merg A, Howe JR. Genetic conditions associated with intestinal juvenile polyps. *Am J Med Genet C Semin Med Genet*. 2004;129(1):44–55.

222. Messick CA, Church J, Casey G, et al. Identification of the methylator (serrated) colorectal cancer phenotype through precursor serrated polyps. *Dis Colon Rectum*. 2009;52(9):1535–1541.

223. Meyskens FL Jr, McLaren CE, Pelot D, et al. Difluoromethylornithine plus sulindac for the prevention of sporadic colorectal adenomas: a randomized placebo-controlled, double-blind trial. *Cancer Prev Res (Phila)*. 2008;1(1):32–38.

224. Millan MS, Gross P, Manilich E, et al. Adenoma detection rate: the real indicator of quality in colonoscopy. *Dis Colon Rectum*. 2008;51(8):1217–1220.

225. Miskowiak J, Lindenberg S. Excision of rectal villous adenoma using a TA or GIA stapler. *Br J Surg*. 1986;73(8):630.

226. Morson BC. Precancerous lesions of the colon and rectum. Classification and controversial issues. *JAMA*. 1962;179:316–321.

227. Morson BC. Some peculiarities in the histology of intestinal polyps. *Dis Colon Rectum*. 1962;5:337.

228. Morson BC, Whiteway JE, Jones EA, et al. Histopathology and prognosis of malignant colorectal polyps treated by endoscopic polypectomy. *Gut*. 1984;25(5):437–444.

229. Morton DG, Gibson J, Macdonald F, et al. Role of congenital hypertrophy of the retinal pigment epithelium in the predictive diagnosis of familial adenomatous polyposis. *Br J Surg*. 1992;79(7):689–693.

230. Morton DG, Macdonald F, Haydon J, et al. Screening practice for familial adenomatous polyposis: the potential for regional registers. *Br J Surg*. 1993;80(2):255–258.

231. Moss A, Bourke MJ, Williams SJ, et al. Endoscopic mucosal resection outcomes and prediction of submucosal cancer from advanced colonic mucosal neoplasia. *Gastroenterology*. 2011;140(7):1909–1918.

232. Mulder SA, van Soest EM, Dieleman JP, et al. Exposure to colorectal examinations before a colorectal cancer diagnosis: a case-control study. *Eur J Gastroenterol Hepatol*. 2010;22(4):437–443.

233. Muto T, Bussey HJ, Morson BC. The evolution of cancer of the colon and rectum. *Cancer*. 1975;36(6):2251–2270.

234. Nagata C, Shimizu H, Kametani M, et al. Cigarette smoking, alcohol use, and colorectal adenoma in Japanese men and women. *Dis Colon Rectum*. 1999;42(3):337–342.

235. Nagy R, Sweet K, Eng C. Highly penetrant hereditary cancer syndromes. *Oncogene*. 2004;23(38):6445–6470.

236. Nascimbeni R, Pucciarelli S, Di Lorenzo D, et al. Rectum-sparing surgery may be appropriate for biallelic MutYH-associated polyposis. *Dis Colon Rectum*. 2010;53(12):1670–1675.

237. National Comprehensive Cancer Network. *NCCN Clinical Practice Guidelines in Oncology*. Fort Washington, PA: Author.

238. Naveau S, Chaput JC, Bedossa P, et al. Cirrhosis as an independent risk factor for colonic adenomas. *Gut*. 1992;33(4):535–540.

239. Norfleet RG, Ryan ME, Wyman JB. Adenomatous and hyperplastic polyps cannot be reliably distinguished by their appearance through the fiberoptic sigmoidoscope. *Dig Dis Sci*. 1988;33(9):1175–1177.

240. Noshirwani KC, van Stolk RU, Rybicki LA, et al. Adenoma size and number are predictive of adenoma recurrence: implications for surveillance colonoscopy. *Gastrointest Endosc*. 2000;51(4 pt 1):433–437.

241. Nugent KP, Phillips RK. Rectal cancer risk in older patients with familial adenomatous polyposis and an ileorectal anastomosis: a cause for concern. *Br J Surg*. 1992;79(11):1204–1206.

242. Nugent KP, Spigelman AD, Phillips RK. Life expectancy after colectomy and ileorectal anastomosis for familial adenomatous polyposis. *Dis Colon Rectum*. 1993;36(11):1059–1062.

243. Nugent KP, Talbot IC, Hodgson SV, et al. Solitary juvenile polyps: not a marker for subsequent malignancy. *Gastroenterology*. 1993;105(3):698–700.

244. O'Brien MJ, O'Keane JC, Zauber A, et al. Precursors of colorectal carcinoma. Biopsy and biologic markers. *Cancer*. 1992;70(5 suppl):1317–1327.

245. Oka S, Tanaka S, Kanao H, et al. Current status in the occurrence of postoperative bleeding, perforation and residual/local recurrence during colonoscopic treatment in Japan. *Dig Endosc*. 2010;22(4):376–380.

246. Oldfield MC. The association of familial polyposis of the colon with multiple sebaceous cysts. *Br J Surg*. 1954;41(169):534–541.

247. Olsen KO, Juul S, Bulow S, et al. Female fecundity before and after operation for familial adenomatous polyposis. *Br J Surg*. 2003;90(2):227–231.

248. Oncel M, Church JM, Remzi FH, et al. Colonic surgery in patients with juvenile polyposis syndrome: a case series. *Dis Colon Rectum*. 2005;48(1):49–55; discussion 55–56.

249. Oncel M, Remzi FH, Church JM, et al. Course and follow-up of solitary Peutz-Jeghers polyps: a case series. *Int J Colorectal Dis*. 2003;18(1):33–35.

250. Oncel M, Remzi FH, Church JM, et al. Benefits of "clean sweep" in Peutz-Jeghers patients. *Colorectal Dis*. 2004;6(5):332–335.

251. Ooi BS, Remzi FH, Gramlich T, et al. Anal transitional zone cancer after restorative proctocolectomy and ileoanal anastomosis in familial adenomatous polyposis: report of two cases. *Dis Colon Rectum*. 2003;46(10):1418–1423; discussion 1422–1413.

252. Paraf F, Jothy S, Van Meir EG. Brain tumor-polyposis syndrome: two genetic diseases? *J Clin Oncol*. 1997;15(7):2744–2758.

253. Parikshak M, Pawlak SE, Eggenberger JC, et al. The role of endoscopic colon surveillance in the transplant population. *Dis Colon Rectum*. 2002;45(12):1655–1660.

254. The Paris endoscopic classification of superficial neoplastic lesions: esophagus, stomach, and colon: November 30 to December 1, 2002. *Gastrointest Endosc*. 2003;58(6 suppl):S3–S43.

255. Park SJ, Rashid A, Lee JH, et al. Frequent CpG island methylation in serrated adenomas of the colorectum. *Am J Pathol*. 2003;162(3):815–822.

256. Parker AR, Eshleman JR. Human MutY: gene structure, protein functions and interactions, and role in carcinogenesis. *Cell Mol Life Sci*. 2003;60(10):2064–2083.

257. Patel BB, Majumdar AP. Synergistic role of curcumin with current therapeutics in colorectal cancer: minireview. *Nutr Cancer*. 2009;61(6):842–846.

258. Paul P, Jagelman DG, Fazio VW, et al. Evaluation of polymorphic genetic markers for linkage to the familial adenomatous polyposis locus on chromosome 5. *Dis Colon Rectum*. 1990;33(9):740–744.

259. Pello MJ. Transanal excision of large sessile villous adenomas using an endorectal traction flap. *Surg Gynecol Obstet*. 1987;164(3):280–282.

260. Penna C, Tiret E, Parc R, et al. Operation and abdominal desmoid tumors in familial adenomatous polyposis. *Surg Gynecol Obstet.* 1993;177(3):263–268.

261. Peutz J. Very remarkable case of familial polyposis of mucous membrane of intestinal tract and nasopharynx accompanied by peculiar pigmentations of skin and mucous membrane. *Ned Maandschr Geneeskd.* 1921;10:134.

262. Plail RO, Bussey HJ, Glazer G, et al. Adenomatous polyposis: an association with carcinoma of the thyroid. *Br J Surg.* 1987;74(5):377–380.

263. Pokala N, Delaney CP, Kiran RP, et al. Outcome of laparoscopic colectomy for polyps not suitable for endoscopic resection. *Surg Endosc.* 2007;21(3):400–403.

264. Poritz LS, Blackstein M, Berk T, et al. Extended follow-up of patients treated with cytotoxic chemotherapy for intra-abdominal desmoid tumors. *Dis Colon Rectum.* 2001;44(9):1268–1273.

265. Quan SH, Castro EB. Papillary adenomas (villous tumors): a review of 215 cases. *Dis Colon Rectum.* 1971;14(4):267–280.

266. Qureshi MA, Monson JR, Lee PW. Transanal MULTIFIRE ENDO GIA technique for rectal polypectomy. *Dis Colon Rectum.* 1997;40(1):116.

267. Rabelo R, Foulkes W, Gordon PH, et al. Role of molecular diagnostic testing in familial adenomatous polyposis and hereditary nonpolyposis colorectal cancer families. *Dis Colon Rectum.* 2001;44(3):437–446.

268. Ramaglia L, Morgese F, Filippella M, et al. Oral and maxillofacial manifestations of Gardner's syndrome associated with growth hormone deficiency: case report and literature review. *Oral Surg Oral Med Oral Pathol Oral Radiol Endod.* 2007;103(6):e30–e34.

269. Randi G, Edefonti V, Ferraroni M, et al. Dietary patterns and the risk of colorectal cancer and adenomas. *Nutr Rev.* 2010;68(7):389–408.

270. Rappaport LB, Sperling HV, Stavrides A. Colon cancer in the Cronkhite-Canada syndrome. *J Clin Gastroenterol.* 1986;8(2):199–202.

271. Rashid A, Houlihan PS, Booker S, et al. Phenotypic and molecular characteristics of hyperplastic polyposis. *Gastroenterol.* 2000;119(2):323–332.

272. Ravaioli A, Nicoletti S, Tamburini E, et al. Control of aggressive fibromatosis by treatment with imatinib mesylate: a step forward? *J Cancer Res Clin Oncol.* 2009;135(2):325–326.

273. Reitamo JJ, Hayry P, Nykyri E, et al. The desmoid tumor. I. Incidence, sex-, age- and anatomical distribution in the Finnish population. *Am J Clin Pathol.* 1982;77(6):665–673.

274. Remzi FH, Church JM, Bast J, et al. Mucosectomy vs. stapled ileal pouch-anal anastomosis in patients with familial adenomatous polyposis: functional outcome and neoplasia control. *Dis Colon Rectum.* 2001;44(11):1590–1596.

275. Remzi FH, Fazio VW, Delaney CP, et al. Dysplasia of the anal transitional zone after ileal pouch-anal anastomosis: results of prospective evaluation after a minimum of ten years. *Dis Colon Rectum.* 2003;46(1):6–13.

276. Reyes Moreno J, Ginard Vicens D, Vanrell M, et al. Impact of a registry on survival in familial adenomatous polyposis. *Med Clin (Barc).* 2007;129(2):51–52.

277. Richards WO, Webb WA, Morris SJ, et al. Patient management after endoscopic removal of the cancerous colon adenoma. *Ann Surg.* 1987;205(6):665–672.

278. Riddell RH. Hands off "cancerous" large bowel polyps. *Gastroenterology.* 1985;89(2):432–435.

279. Rossouw JE, Anderson GL, Prentice RL, et al. Risks and benefits of estrogen plus progestin in healthy postmenopausal women: principal results from the Women's Health Initiative randomized controlled trial. *JAMA.* 2002;288(3):321–333.

280. Roth SI, Helwig EB. Juvenile polyps of the colon and rectum. *Cancer.* 1963;16:468–479.

281. Rubio CA, Stemme S, Jaramillo E, et al. Hyperplastic polyposis coli syndrome and colorectal carcinoma. *Endoscopy.* 2006;38(3):266–270.

282. Rustin RB, Jagelman DG, McGannon E, et al. Spontaneous mutation in familial adenomatous polyposis. *Dis Colon Rectum.* 1990;33(1):52–55.

283. Saclarides TJ, Smith L, Ko ST, et al. Transanal endoscopic microsurgery. *Dis Colon Rectum.* 1992;35(12):1183–1191.

284. Said S, Huber P, Pichlmaier H. Technique and clinical results of endorectal surgery. *Surgery.* 1993;113(1):65–75.

285. Sakamoto GD, MacKeigan JM, Senagore AJ. Transanal excision of large, rectal villous adenomas. *Dis Colon Rectum.* 1991;34(10):880–885.

286. Sampson JR, Dolwani S, Jones S, et al. Autosomal recessive colorectal adenomatous polyposis due to inherited mutations of MYH. *Lancet.* 2003;362(9377):39–41.

287. Sanchez JA, Krumroy L, Plummer S, et al. Genetic and epigenetic classifications define clinical phenotypes and determine patient outcomes in colorectal cancer. *Br J Surg.* 2009;96(10):1196–1204.

288. Sandmeier D, Seelentag W, Bouzourene H. Serrated polyps of the colorectum: is sessile serrated adenoma distinguishable from hyperplastic polyp in a daily practice? *Virchows Arch.* 2007;450(6):613–618.

289. Sarre RG, Jagelman DG, Beck GJ, et al. Colectomy with ileorectal anastomosis for familial adenomatous polyposis: the risk of rectal cancer. *Surgery.* 1987;101(1):20–26.

290. Sayed MG, Ahmed AF, Ringold JR, et al. Germline SMAD4 or BMPR1A mutations and phenotype of juvenile polyposis. *Ann Surg Oncol.* 2002;9(9):901–906.

291. Scott-Conner CE, Hausmann M, Hall TJ, et al. Familial juvenile polyposis: patterns of recurrence and implications for surgical management. *J Am Coll Surg.* 1995;181(5):407–413.

292. Sener SF, Miller HH, DeCosse JJ. The spectrum of polyposis. *Surg Gynecol Obstet.* 1984;159(6):525–532.

293. Setti-Carraro P, Nicholls RJ. Choice of prophylactic surgery for the large bowel component of familial adenomatous polyposis. *Br J Surg.* 1996;83(7):885–892.

294. Shatney CH, Lober PH, Gilbertsen VA, et al. The treatment of pedunculated adenomatous colorectal polyps with focal cancer. *Surg Gynecol Obstet.* 1974;139(6):845–850.

295. Shin A, Kim J. Effect modification of meat intake by genetic polymorphisms on colorectal neoplasia susceptibility. *Asian Pac J Cancer Prev.* 2010;11(2):281–287.

296. Sieber OM, Lipton L, Crabtree M, et al. Multiple colorectal adenomas, classic adenomatous polyposis, and germ-line mutations in MYH. *N Engl J Med.* 2003;348(9):791–799.

297. Silverberg SG. Focally malignant adenomatous polyps of the colon and rectum. *Surg Gynecol Obstet.* 1970;131(1):103–114.

298. Sinha A, Tekkis PP, Rashid S, et al. Risk factors for secondary proctectomy in patients with familial adenomatous polyposis. *Br J Surg.* 2010;97(11):1710–1715.

299. Skinner MA, Tyler D, Branum GD, et al. Subtotal colectomy for familial polyposis. A clinical series and review of the literature. *Arch Surg.* 1990;125(5):621–624.

300. Slupska MM, Baikalov C, Luther WM, et al. Cloning and sequencing a human homolog (hMYH) of the Escherichia coli mutY gene whose function is required for the repair of oxidative DNA damage. *J Bacteriol.* 1996;178(13):3885–3892.

301. Smith WG. Desmoid tumors in familial multiple polyposis. *Proc Staff Meet Mayo Clin.* 1959;34(2):31–38.

302. Snover DC. Update on the serrated pathway to colorectal carcinoma. *Hum Pathol.* 2011;42(1):1–10.

303. Snover DC, Ahnen D, Burt R, et al. Serrated polyps of the colon and rectum and serrated polyposis. In: Bosman FT, Carneiro F, Hruban RH, eds. *WHO Classification of Tumours of the Digestive System (IARC WHO Classification of Tumours).* 4th ed. Lyon, France: IARC Press; 2010.

304. Soravia C, Berk T, McLeod RS, et al. Desmoid disease in patients with familial adenomatous polyposis. *Dis Colon Rectum.* 2000;43(3):363–369.

305. Spigelman AD, Talbot IC, Penna C, et al. Evidence for adenoma-carcinoma sequence in the duodenum of patients with familial adenomatous polyposis. The Leeds Castle Polyposis Group (Upper Gastrointestinal Committee). *J Clin Pathol.* 1994;47(8):709–710.

306. Spigelman AD, Thomson JP, Phillips RK. Towards decreasing the relaparotomy rate in the Peutz-Jeghers syndrome: the role of peroperative small bowel endoscopy. *Br J Surg.* 1990;77(3):301–302.

307. Spigelman AD, Williams CB, Talbot IC, et al. Upper gastrointestinal cancer in patients with familial adenomatous polyposis. *Lancet.* 1989;2(8666):783–785.

308. Starke J, Rodriguez-Bigas M, Marshall W, et al. Primary adenocarcinoma arising in an ileostomy. *Surgery.* 1993;114(1):125–128.

309. Stryker SJ, Wolff BG, Culp CE, et al. Natural history of untreated colonic polyps. *Gastroenterology.* 1987;93(5):1009–1013.

310. Stulc JP, Petrelli NJ, Herrera L, et al. Colorectal villous and tubulovillous adenomas equal to or greater than four centimeters. *Ann Surg.* 1988;207(1):65–71.

311. Swan MP, Bourke MJ, Alexander S, et al. Large refractory colonic polyps: is it time to change our practice? A prospective study of the clinical and economic impact of a tertiary referral colonic mucosal resection and polypectomy service (with videos). *Gastrointest Endosc.* 2009;70(6):1128–1136.

312. Sweet K, Willis J, Zhou XP, et al. Molecular classification of patients with unexplained hamartomatous and hyperplastic polyposis. *JAMA.* 2005;294(19):2465–2473.

313. Swinton NW, Warren S. Polyps of the colon and rectum and their relation to malignancy. *JAMA.* 1939;113:1927.

314. Tanaka S, Oka S, Chayama K, et al. Knack and practical technique of colonoscopic treatment focused on endoscopic mucosal resection using snare. *Dig Endosc.* 2009;21 suppl 1:S38–S42.

315. Taylor EW, Thompson H, Oates GD, et al. Limitations of biopsy in preoperative assessment of villous papilloma. *Dis Colon Rectum.* 1981;24(4):259 262.

316. Thompson-Fawcett MW, Marcus VA, Redston M, et al. Adenomatous polyps develop commonly in the ileal pouch of patients with familial adenomatous polyposis. *Dis Colon Rectum.* 2001;44(3):347–353.

317. Tomlinson I, Rahman N, Frayling I, et al. Inherited susceptibility to colorectal adenomas and carcinomas: evidence for a new predisposition gene on 15q14-q22. *Gastroenterology.* 1999;116(4):789–795.

318. Tonelli F, Ficari F, Valanzano R, et al. Treatment of desmoids and mesenteric fibromatosis in familial adenomatous polyposis with raloxifene. *Tumori.* 2003;89(4):391–396.

319. Tonooka T, Sano Y, Fujii T, et al. Adenocarcinoma in solitary large hyperplastic polyp diagnosed by magnifying colonoscope: report of a case. *Dis Colon Rectum.* 2002;45(10):1407–1411.

320. Toyota M, Ahuja N, Ohe-Toyota M, et al. CpG island methylator phenotype in colorectal cancer. *Proc Natl Acad Sciences USA.* 1999;96(15):8681–8686.

321. Traboulsi EI. Familial adenomatous polyposis. *Dis Colon Rectum.* 1989;32(7):633–634.

322. Tsukada K, Church JM, Jagelman DG, et al. Noncytotoxic drug therapy for intra-abdominal desmoid tumor in patients with familial adenomatous polyposis. *Dis Colon Rectum.* 1992;35(1):29–33.

323. Tulchinsky H, Keidar A, Strul H, et al. Extracolonic manifestations of familial adenomatous polyposis after proctocolectomy. *Arch Surg.* 2005;140(2):159–163; discussion 164.

324. Utsunomiya J, Gocho H, Miyanaga T, et al. Peutz-Jeghers syndrome: its natural course and management. *Johns Hopkins Med J.* 1975;136(2):71–82.

325. Valanzano R, Cama A, Volpe R, et al. Congenital hypertrophy of the retinal pigment epithelium in familial adenomatous polyposis. Novel criteria of assessment and correlations with constitutional adenomatous polyposis coli gene mutations. *Cancer.* 1996;78(11):2400–2410.

326. van Coevorden F, Mathus-Vliegen EM, Brummelkamp WH. Combined endoscopic and surgical treatment in Peutz-Jeghers syndrome. *Surg Gynecol Obstet.* 1986;162(5):426–428.

327. Vandrovcova J, Lagerstedt-Robinsson K, Pahlman L, et al. Somatic BRAF-V600E mutations in familial colorectal cancer. *Cancer Epidemiol Biomarkers Prev.* 2006;15(11):2270–2273.

328. van Duijvendijk P, Slors JF, Taat CW, et al. Functional outcome after colectomy and ileorectal anastomosis compared with proctocolectomy and ileal pouch-anal anastomosis in familial adenomatous polyposis. *Ann Surg.* 1999;230(5):648–654.

329. van Duijvendijk P, Vasen HF, Bertario L, et al. Cumulative risk of developing polyps or malignancy at the ileal pouch-anal anastomosis in patients with familial adenomatous polyposis. *J Gastrointest Surg.* 1999;3(3):325–330.

330. van Hattem WA, Brosens LA, de Leng WW, et al. Large genomic deletions of SMAD4, BMPR1A and PTEN in juvenile polyposis. *Gut.* 2008;57(5):623–627.

331. van Rijn JC, Reitsma JB, Stoker J, et al. Polyp miss rate determined by tandem colonoscopy: a systematic review. *Am J Gastroenterol.* 2006;101(2):343–350.

332. Vogelstein B, Fearon ER, Hamilton SR, et al. Genetic alterations during colorectal-tumor development. *N Engl J Med.* 1988;319(9):525–532.

333. Vogt S, Jones N, Christian D, et al. Expanded extracolonic tumor spectrum in MUTYH-associated polyposis. *Gastroenterology.* 2009;137(6):1976–1985.e1-10.

334. Volikos E, Robinson J, Aittomaki K, et al. LKB1 exonic and whole gene deletions are a common cause of Peutz-Jeghers syndrome. *J Med Genet.* 2006;43(5):e18.

335. Voloyiannis T, Snyder MJ, Bailey RR, et al. Management of the difficult colon polyp referred for resection: resect or rescope? *Dis Colon Rectum.* 2008;51(3):292–295.

336. von Roon AC, Tekkis PP, Clark SK, et al. The impact of technical factors on outcome of restorative proctocolectomy for familial adenomatous polyposis. *Dis Colon Rectum.* 2007;50(7):952–961.

337. Wada Y, Kashida H, Kudo SE, et al. Diagnostic accuracy of pit pattern and vascular pattern analyses in colorectal lesions. *Dig Endosc.* 2010;22(3):192–199.

338. Wallace MH, Phillips RK. Upper gastrointestinal disease in patients with familial adenomatous polyposis. *Br J Surg.* 1998;85(6):742–750.

339. Wang L, Baudhuin LM, Boardman LA, et al. MYH mutations in patients with attenuated and classic polyposis and with young-onset colorectal cancer without polyps. *Gastroenterology.* 2004;127(1):9–16.

340. Waye JD. Advanced polypectomy. *Gastrointest Endosc Clin N Am.* 2005;15(4):733–756.

341. Weisenberger DJ, Siegmund KD, Campan M, et al. CpG island methylator phenotype underlies sporadic microsatellite instability and is tightly associated with BRAF mutation in colorectal cancer. *Nat Genet.* 2006;38(7):787 793.

342. Westbrook KC, Lang NP, Broadwater JR, et al. Posterior surgical approaches to the rectum. *Ann Surg.* 1982;195(6):677–685.

343. Westhues M. *Die pathologisch-anatomischen Grundlagen der Chirurgie des Rektumkarzinoms.* Leipzig, Germany: Georg Thieme Verlag; 1934.

344. Wexner SD, Cera SM. Laparoscopic surgery for ulcerative colitis. *Surg Clin North Am.* 2005;85(1):35–47, viii.

345. Whelan RL, Horvath KD, Gleason NR, et al. Vitamin and calcium supplement use is associated with decreased adenoma recurrence in patients with a previous history of neoplasia. *Dis Colon Rectum.* 1999;42(2):212–217.

346. Whitelaw SC, Murday VA, Tomlinson IP, et al. Clinical and molecular features of the hereditary mixed polyposis syndrome. *Gastroenterology.* 1997;112(2):327–334.

347. Wijn MA, Keller JJ, Brand HS. Oral and maxillofacial manifestations of familial adenomatosis polyposis. Gardner's syndrome. *Ned Tijdschr Tandheelkd.* 2005;112(9):340–344.

348. Wilhelm D, von Delius S, Weber L, et al. Combined laparoscopic-endoscopic resections of colorectal polyps: 10-year experience and follow-up. *Surg Endosc.* 2009;23(4):688–693.

349. Winawer SJ, Zauber AG, Fletcher RH, et al. Guidelines for colonoscopy surveillance after polypectomy: a consensus update by the US Multi-Society Task Force on Colorectal Cancer and the American Cancer Society. *Gastroenterology.* 2006;130(6):1872–1885.

350. Winawer SJ, Zauber AG, Gerdes H, et al. Risk of colorectal cancer in the families of patients with adenomatous polyps. National Polyp Study Workgroup. *N Engl J Med.* 1996;334(2):82–87.

351. Wolff WI, Shinya H. Definitive treatment of "malignant" polyps of the colon. *Ann Surg.* 1975;182(4):516–525.

352. Wu JS, McGannon EA, Church JM. Incidence of neoplastic polyps in the ileal pouch of patients with familial adenomatous polyposis after restorative proctocolectomy. *Dis Colon Rectum.* 1998;41(5):552–556.

353. Yeoman A, Young J, Arnold J, et al. Hyperplastic polyposis in the New Zealand population: a condition associated with increased colorectal cancer risk and European ancestry. *N Z Med J.* 2007;120(1266):U2827.

354. Yokota T, Sugihara K, Yoshida S. Endoscopic mucosal resection for colorectal neoplastic lesions. *Dis Colon Rectum.* 1994;37(11):1108–1111.

355. Zbuk KM, Eng C. Hamartomatous polyposis syndromes. *Nat Clin Pract Gastroenterol Hepatol.* 2007;4(9):492–502.

356. Zmora O, Benjamin B, Reshef A, et al. Laparoscopic colectomy for colonic polyps. *Surg Endosc.* 2009;23(3):629–632.

23
Carcinoma of the Colon

Neil H. Hyman

There is a tremendous literature on cancer, but what we know for sure about it can be printed on a calling card.

—AUGUST BIER

Excluding cancer of the skin, colorectal carcinoma is the second most common malignancy found in most Western countries. In women, lung and breast cancers are more common, whereas in men, lung and prostate cancers are more frequently observed. In 2010, the American Cancer Society estimated that 141,210 new cases would be diagnosed in the United States, and 49,380 deaths would occur.[941] The chance of colorectal carcinoma developing during the life of an infant born in the United States today is approximately 5%.

The incidence of colorectal cancer had been relatively stable for the 40 years before the last two decades, even as death rates were falling. However, the incidence now appears to be decreasing significantly, with an approximately 3% drop observed in the past 10 years alone. This largely reflects increased screening, with adenoma detection and removal.[209,792] Further, the death rate from colorectal cancer has dropped by more than 30% since 1990, owing to earlier detection and better treatment.[941] The trends in cancer incidence, mortality, and patient survival in the United States are derived from the SEER Program (Survey of Epidemiology and End Results) of the National Cancer Institute.[941]

▶ ETIOLOGY AND EPIDEMIOLOGY

The epidemiology of large bowel cancer has become a major area of investigative interest. Interpopulation and nationality differences were the inspiration for Burkitt's hypothesis on the contributory role of a low-residue, high-carbohydrate diet in causing colorectal cancer.[134,137] His observations generated additional reports about the incidence and mortality of large bowel cancer, and other hypotheses have been suggested.[92,396,398,402,442,742]

Distribution and Nationality

The mortality rates for colorectal cancer in Western European countries are generally high.[265,846] Scotland is the leader in the world, with rates much higher than even those of England.[912] Spain and Portugal, conversely, have relatively low rates, more consistent with those of Eastern Europe.[265] The two populations with risks similar to those of Western Europe are the people of Israel and the Chinese in Singapore. In Israel, a considerable difference has existed between Israelis born in Europe and those born in North Africa or Asia. The incidence in the former is 2.5 times that of the latter. With the exception of Singapore, Asia has a low incidence. African countries generally have a very low frequency of colorectal cancer; in Latin American countries, the incidence rates vary.[207,443,1071]

In addition to the differences in the incidence of colorectal cancer from one population to another, observations have been made concerning the variations in the distribution within the colon and rectum. It has been postulated that low-risk populations have a relatively increased incidence of right-sided cancers, whereas relatively high-risk communities have an increased risk of left-sided malignancies.[109,134,137,399]

A difference in the incidence of cancer has been observed from country to country when urban populations are compared with rural populations.[93,186,254,573,729,964,1012] The nature of the urban-rural gradient with respect to risk has been extensively investigated in the United States. By comparing metropolitan and nonmetropolitan counties, Haenszel and Dawson showed that in the United States, increased risk for large bowel cancer is found in urban populations in each major region of the country.[401]

With respect to immigrants, colorectal cancer is less common among Japanese Americans than among white Americans.[945] However, the rates for Japanese Americans are higher than those for Japanese living in Japan. The children of these immigrants have an incidence approximating that of native white Americans.[402] A similar phenomenon has been seen in other populations.[963]

Race

African American men and women have a higher incidence of colorectal cancer than that of Whites, although African Americans and Whites within the same community and region of the country may have a similar rate.[220,1135] The risk for large bowel cancer in Asian American and Pacific Islander, Native American, Alaska native, and Hispanic/Latino appears to be lower than Whites.[941] There is a higher death rate among African American men and women because they are less likely to be diagnosed at a localized stage, often have more comorbidities and may have diminished access to quality health care.[941] Studies suggest that African Americans who receive medical and oncologic treatment comparable to that of Whites appear to achieve the same outcomes.

▶ SOCIOECONOMIC STATUS AND OCCUPATION

Some studies have shown a higher death rate for colorectal cancer in more affluent people.[187,752] Colombia, a country with a low incidence, reported a higher rate in this group.[400] However, the vast majority of reports suggest worsened cancer survival in patients with a lower socioeconomic status, typically attributed to patient comorbidities, advanced stage at diagnosis, and diminished access to high-quality care.[1126] Two large studies performed in the United States found that patients of lower socioeconomic status were more likely to have advanced cancer at diagnosis.[143,185] Interestingly, a publication from Ontario demonstrated that significant disparities in survival persist even without a difference in stage at presentation, suggesting other factors are playing a role, such as tumor biology and comorbidities.[106] Elevated body mass index (BMI), obesity, and low physical activity appear to increase the risk of colorectal cancer and may be important confounding variables.[499] Occupation has been investigated as a possible causative factor.[684,752] The relative affluence associated with some occupations appears to be the reason why certain professionals have a higher incidence of colorectal cancer.

▶ RELIGION

In studies of the religion of patients, Jews have a higher incidence than people of other religions.[396,397,737,913] Members of the Church of Jesus Christ of Latter-Day Saints (Mormons) have a low incidence.[131,282,613] Their religion prohibits the use of tobacco, alcohol, tea, and coffee. Seventh-Day Adventists have a significantly lower rate of colorectal cancer; their church proscribes tobacco and alcohol.[568,569,794]

▶ ALCOHOL AND TOBACCO

The data regarding alcohol as an independent risk factor for colorectal cancer is conflicting.[175,323,592,781] For example, a prospective study of Japanese men in Hawaii revealed an association between the consumption of alcohol and rectal cancer, attributable to a monthly consumption of beer of 500 oz (15 L) or more.[805] On the other hand, moderate alcohol intake (especially wine) has been found to be protective against the development of distal colorectal cancer.[210] Two meta-analyses on cigarette smoking and colorectal cancer have demonstrated an increased risk among cigarette smokers; the pooled risk estimate ranged from 1.07 to 1.25.[107,575] Current smokers have been shown to have a relative risk of 1.7 for adenomas when compared with nonsmokers. This effect was even more pronounced for advanced or multiple adenomas in a "dose-dependent" relationship, suggesting a direct role in colorectal carcinogenesis.[721] A report from Quebec, Canada evaluated the effects of smoking on the risk of colorectal cancer according to anatomic subsite.[923] A positive association with cigar smoking and rectal cancer was observed. There was no statistically significant association with cigarette smoking, but there was a "positive association" with proximal colon cancer.

Diet

Diet is the epidemiologic area that has received the most attention since the mid-1980s 20 years, especially since Burkitt's observations (see Biography, Chapter 27).[133-137] He and Painter postulated that a high content of fiber was the primary factor responsible for the low incidence of colorectal cancer in African natives.[777] In essence, their theory states that whatever carcinogen is ingested or produced should be present in a relatively diluted form, and when the transit time is decreased, it is excreted rapidly. Fleiszer and colleagues and Chen and coworkers found that parenteral administration of dimethylhydrazine, a known colon carcinogen, conferred great protection on rats, provided their dietary fiber was increased.[173,303]

Other studies have demonstrated correlations between colorectal cancer and additional dietary factors. For example, Nigro (see Biography, Chapter 25) and colleagues demonstrated that cancer in the animal model can be inhibited by an increased fiber intake only when the fat content is relatively low.[742-744] They presented a program for possible prevention of colorectal cancer: a 10% reduction in fat consumption, the addition of 25 g of dietary fiber per day, and plant sterols.[742] These substances have been shown to inhibit the cancer that can be induced by carcinogens. One theory holds that inositol hexaphosphate (phytic acid), an abundant plant seed component present in many fiber-rich diets, is one of the specific agents responsible for suppression of colon carcinogenesis.[362]

The mechanism by which increased dietary fiber achieves protection from the development of large bowel cancer remains speculative. Fiber may provide protection by increasing stool bulk and dilution of putative carcinogens in the colonic lumen, by more rapid transit with diminished exposure to injurious agents, and by fermentation of fiber to short-chain fatty acids.[582] Because fiber is heterogeneous, its mechanism of action within the gut may vary. McIntyre and colleagues studied the effects of three types of dietary fiber in fermentative production of butyrate in the distal colon to ascertain the influence on tumor mass in a rat model of bowel cancer.[663] They observed that the fiber associated with high butyrate concentrations in the distal large bowel is protective against large bowel cancer, whereas soluble fibers that do not raise distal butyrate concentrations are not protective.

Sengupta and coworkers conducted a literature search on the effect of dietary fiber on tumor incidence through the use of the MEDLINE database of all case-control, longitudinal, and randomized, controlled studies published in English between 1988 and 2000, as well as animal model studies in the period, 1986 to 2000.[917] Thirteen of 24 case-control studies demonstrated a protective effect of dietary fiber against colorectal neoplasms; conversely, only 3 of 13 longitudinal studies in various cohorts demonstrated a protective effect of fiber. The animal studies were more impressive; 15 of 19 demonstrated protection against tumor induction when compared with controls. A meta-analysis of 25 prospective studies concluded that a high intake of dietary fiber (in particular, cereal fiber and whole grains) was associated with a modest reduction in the risk of colorectal cancer.[41]

Fecal Bile Acids

Population-based studies have demonstrated that a Western diet is associated with high levels of fecal secondary bile acids, primarily deoxycholic acid and lithocholic acid, the same trend as has been observed in patients with colon carcinoma.[46,662] Elevated secondary bile acid concentrations exert detrimental effects both on colonic epithelial structure and function.[235] Fecal bile acid concentration is increased by dietary fat and decreased by dietary cereal fiber. Others have shown an unambiguous connection between the fecal bile acid level and the incidence of dimethylhydrazine-induced colon cancer.[716] Hill and associates determined that the feces of people in Western countries exhibit a high concentration of bile acids when compared with the feces of residents of African and Eastern countries.[444]

Cholesterol

Some investigators have demonstrated a strong correlation between colorectal cancer and a high intake of animal fat and protein.[28,455,456] Others opine that the consumption of red meat, or total or saturated fat, has only a weak association with the development of colorectal cancer.[1020] Populations with a high consumption of beef generally have the highest incidence of bowel cancer.[253,254] The epidemiologic evidence is conflicting, but there seems to be an inconsistent relationship of colorectal cancer with respect to fat and sugar consumption, serum cholesterol, and serum β-lipoprotein.[119,633,736,1028,1092] Winawer and colleagues performed a time-trend, case-control study in which serum cholesterol was determined at several intervals before the diagnosis of colon cancer.[1102] They concluded that although individuals in whom colorectal cancer

developed had the same levels of serum cholesterol as the general population initially, during the 10 years before the diagnosis of cancer was established, they demonstrated a decline in cholesterol values. This took place in a population of "control" individuals whose serum cholesterol levels tended to increase with age.

A nested case-control study of 520,000 Western Europeans was performed to examine the association between serum levels of total cholesterol and its constituent lipoproteins and colorectal cancer. This included 1,238 incident cases of colorectal cancer during the study period. High concentration of high-density lipoprotein (HDL) was inversely related to the risk of colon cancer (but not rectal cancer); there was no robust association between other blood lipid concentrations and the risk of colorectal cancer.

Bacteria

Bacteria are thought to play a role in the causation of colorectal cancer; their action on ingested fat or metabolites may be a critical factor. Hill and associates demonstrated that people in the United States and Great Britain have a higher colony count of anaerobic flora and a lower count of aerobic bacteria.[444] Others have confirmed this observation.[26] The similarity between the chemical structure of bile salts and the carcinogen, methylcholanthrene, has been observed. It is not unreasonable to hypothesize that the action of bacteria on bile salts may produce a substance capable of inducing malignant degeneration. Burkitt, in fact, postulated that one of the reasons for the preponderance of carcinoma in the distal bowel is the higher concentration of bacteria in this location.[134] Nonpathogenic bacteria play an important role in preserving the function and integrity of the gut's mucosal barrier. Other bacteria produce toxic metabolites that can cause cell mutations and affect intracellular signal transduction. As such, the intestinal microflora may be a modifiable target for diminishing the risk of colorectal cancer. For example, colorectal cancer patients have higher bacterial counts in the *Bacteroides/Prevotella* group.[929] Probiotics continue to receive attention as potential chemoprotective agents, but there remains little convincing evidence of efficacy to date. Limited studies have suggested a possible increase in colorectal cancer in patients with *Helicobacter pylori* infection.[1138]

Cholecystectomy

Because of the clinical evidence for an increased quantity of secondary bile acids in the feces of patients with bowel cancer and experimental studies demonstrating that secondary bile acids promote chemical carcinogenesis, cholecystectomy has been implicated as a possible precipitating factor.[1037,1056] This operation increases secondary bile acids in the enterohepatic circulation.[1037] Other reports have failed to confirm a relationship between gallbladder removal and the subsequent development of colorectal cancer.[2,6,95,504] There is, however, some opposing evidence to suggest that more than 10 years following cholecystectomy older women may have an increased risk, especially for right-sided lesions.[632,706] Johansen and coworkers evaluated 40,000 patients with gallstones identified in the Danish Hospital Discharge Register.[495] A borderline significant association was seen between gallstones and cancer of the colon. Jorgensen and Rafaelsen believe that cholecystectomy per se is not responsible for the apparent association, but rather that gallstone disease itself accounts for the relationship.[501] A meta-analysis of 33 case-control studies showed a pooled relative risk with cholecystectomy of 1.34 for the development of colorectal cancer; the risk for proximal colon cancer was the most significant.[336]

Jejunoileal Bypass

With respect to jejunoileal bypass, an operation that in animals promotes the development of chemically induced bowel cancers, there has been no evidence to date to suggest an increased risk in humans,[661] despite profound alterations in transit time, bile salt metabolism, and fecal flora. In a long-term follow-up study (up to 17 years), Sylvan and associates examined these patients postoperatively by means of colonoscopy and biopsy as well as by flow cytometric DNA analysis.[991] These investigators were not able to verify any colorectal malignant transformation.

Ulcer Surgery

An association has been reported between colorectal cancer and prior peptic ulcer surgery, specifically truncal vagotomy.[717] Mullan and colleagues observed increased proportions of chenodeoxycholic acid and lithocholic acid as well as decreased proportions of cholic acid in the duodenal bile of these individuals.[717] They proposed that abnormalities in bile acid metabolism as a consequence of vagotomy could explain the increased risk for the development of colorectal cancer. The cancer risk associated with peptic ulcer surgery was assessed in a cohort of 1,992 surgical patients who were seen in a peptic ulcer clinic in Glasgow, most of whom had undergone vagotomy and a drainage procedure. The risk of colorectal cancer in long-term follow-up was no greater than the general population, irrespective of procedure.[490]

▶ ASPIRIN

There is considerable evidence to suggest that regular use of aspirin and other nonsteroidal anti-inflammatory agents reduces the risk for the development of colorectal cancer.[1000,1020,1021] Giovannucci and colleagues determined the rates of colorectal cancer among women in the Nurses' Health Study who reported regular aspirin use, comparing the rates in this group with those of women who stated that they did not use aspirin.[337] They concluded that the risk for colorectal cancer is reduced only after 10 or more years of aspirin use. Thun and coworkers found that dietary consumption of vegetables and grains and regular use of aspirin were the only factors having an independent and statistically significant association with prevention of colon cancer.[1020] An overall analysis of four studies assessing the impact of aspirin in the general population (n = 69,535) showed no protective effect for the first 10 years of follow-up.[197] However, analysis of the studies involving higher dose aspirin (300 to 1,500 mg/daily) demonstrated a 26% reduction in the incidence of colorectal cancer over a 23-year follow-up period.[197]

Estrogen

Most epidemiologic studies have reported an inverse association between postmenopausal hormone (PMH) therapy and colorectal cancer risk.[162] In a report by Paganini-Hill of 7,701 women who were initially free of cancer and used estrogen replacement therapy, there was a statistically significant reduction in the incidence of colorectal cancer and colorectal cancer deaths compared with those individuals who did not take this replacement medication.[775] The impact of hormone replacement therapy may be more pronounced based on the molecular pathway of carcinogenesis. In the Iowa Women's Health Study, PMH reduced colorectal cancer incidence by 18% overall.[580] The relative risk for microsatellite unstable-low (MSI-L)/MSS tumors was 0.6 when PMH use exceeded 5 years, whereas there was no protection afforded for microsatellite unstable-high (MSI-H) tumors.[580]

Inflammatory Bowel Disease

Patients with inflammatory bowel disease, either ulcerative colitis (UC) or Crohn's colitis, are at increased risk for the development of colorectal cancer; the estimates of this risk has varied considerably in different studies but appears to accrue beginning 8 to 10 years after the onset of symptoms (see Chapters 29 and 30).[614,682] It seems clear that the duration and extent of disease are key risk factors.[494,552,1053,1109] A Swedish population-based study of 3,000 UC patients found a relative risk of colorectal cancer of 1.7 for proctitis, 2.8 for left-sided disease, and 14.8 for pancolitis.[173] With respect to Crohn's disease, some reports have been published implicating an association between regional enteritis and small bowel carcinoma.[578,712,875,927] The relationship between granulomatous colitis and large bowel cancer is perhaps less emphasized but appears to be real (see Chapter 30).[1141]

Radiation

There have been considerable differences of opinion about the risk for the development of colorectal cancer following pelvic irradiation. One report demonstrated an increased risk for women who were irradiated for gynecologic cancer.[888] Additional studies are required for an accurate assessment of any relationship, especially in light of the increased application of neoadjuvant therapy.

Immunosuppression

Immunosuppressive therapy, especially following organ transplantation, is associated with an increased risk for the development of malignant tumors, possibly including that of the colon and rectum. Renal transplant patients may have up to twice the risk of colon cancer but do not seem to have an increased risk of rectal cancer. A surveillance colonoscopy program for these individuals is recommended.

Appendectomy

McVay reported an appreciably increased incidence of colorectal carcinoma in patients who had undergone appendectomy.[668] He suggested that the relationship could be explained by immunologic factors. Others have failed to substantiate this relationship.[383,457,467] However, a prior history of appendectomy has been found to be an independent risk factor for decreased survival, worsening the prognosis for those in whom carcinoma of the cecum subsequently developed.[29]

Ureterosigmoidostomy

Numerous authors have recognized the relationship between ureterosigmoidostomy and carcinoma of the colon at the site of the ureteral implant into the colon.[394,411,543,616,681,962,981,1042,1082] The incidence of carcinoma ranges from 2% to 15%, with a lag time in the 20-year range.[45] The cause may be related to

HENRY T. LYNCH (1928–PRESENT)

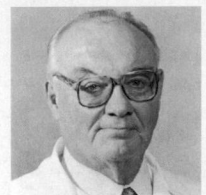

Henry Lynch was born in Lawrence, Massachusetts on January 4, 1928 and grew up in New York. Although underage, he enlisted in the U.S. Navy in March of 1944 and served in the European and South Pacific theaters. He received his bachelor's degree from the University of Oklahoma, a master's degree in clinical psychology from Denver University, and was nearing completion of a PhD in human genetics when he entered medical school at the University of Texas Medical Branch in Galveston, from which he received his MD degree in 1960. He completed several post-degree medical training programs and was on the faculty of the University of Texas: MD Anderson Cancer Center in Houston before coming to Creighton University School of Medicine in Omaha, Nebraska in 1967. Since that time, he has been Chairman of Preventive Medicine and Public Health at Creighton, advancing to full professor in 1972. During the 1960s, when cancer was considered an almost solely environmentally caused disease, Lynch demonstrated mendelian inheritance patterns for a previously unrecognized form of colon cancer (hereditary nonpolyposis colorectal cancer, now known as Lynch syndrome) and for the hereditary breast-ovarian cancer syndrome, which he subsequently helped link to the *BRCA1* and *BRCA2* genes. In addition, he provided some of the first findings of hereditary malignant melanoma and of familial aspects of prostate and pancreatic cancer. The purpose of this work has been to enable physicians to identify high-risk patients more quickly and accurately, leading to earlier and more effective surveillance, management, and treatment. Henry Lynch's contributions to cancer research have been recognized by many awards from such groups as the American Cancer Society, Bristol-Myers Squibb, the American Association for Cancer Research, the Susan G. Komen Breast Cancer Foundation, the American Society of Clinical Oncology, and the Jacqueline Seroussi Memorial Foundation for Cancer Research.

bathing of the colonic mucosa by urine, the presence of a carcinogen in the urine, the by-products of the interaction of colonic bacteria, and urine or the effects of the ureter, itself, implanted into the colon. Alterations in the mucus glycoproteins in the surrounding mucosa has been described.[934]

It is suggested that this type of diversion of the urinary tract be abandoned, especially in young patients with benign disease.[922] Periodic endoscopic evaluation of the bowel is required. Consideration should be given to resecting that area of the colon, with conversion to another diversionary procedure.[283,533,962]

Congenital Urinary Tract Anomalies

Atwell and coworkers believed they had recognized an association between a family history of congenital anomalies of the urinary tract and the development of colorectal cancer at a young age.[38] Their observations should be taken with caution because the numbers reported were small.

Extracolonic Tumors

With respect to the incidence and risk for the development of a metachronous colorectal cancer following an extracolonic primary tumor, one study demonstrates that a patient with breast cancer has the same risk for a colorectal malignancy as for a second primary tumor in the opposite breast.[11]

An association between sebaceous gland tumors and internal malignancies has been called the *Muir-Torre syndrome*. The incidence of colorectal malignancies is estimated to be almost 50%.[1059] Muir-Torre syndrome appears to be a variant of Lynch syndrome, necessitating genetic evaluation, counseling, and appropriate workup for associated malignancies as described next.[608]

Genetic Predisposition

Genetic influences have been known for some time to be an independent risk factor for the development of colorectal cancer. Of all colorectal cancer cases, 2% to 5% can be attributed to known genetic disorders, such as hereditary nonpolyposis colorectal cancer (Lynch syndrome) or familial adenomatous polyposis (FAP).[484] However, another 25% of colorectal cancer patients have at least one first-degree relative with colorectal cancer, without a known, defined genetic predisposition.[1095] These individuals appear to have double the risk of colorectal cancer when compared with the general population.[142]

This observation could conceivably be a consequence of common environmental exposures, primary genetic factors, the interaction of environment and heredity, or simply of chance.[606] However, in a prospective study, Rozen and colleagues confirmed the relationship of the family history, even when one member harbors a large bowel neoplasm.[866] As a consequence, they and others have advocated a screening program for such family members.[727] Conversely, there is no evidence to suggest a greater frequency of bowel tumors in spouses of colorectal cancer victims. Fuchs and coworkers conducted a prospective study of almost 120,000 patients who had not been previously examined by colonoscopy or sigmoidoscopy and who provided data on first-degree relatives with colorectal cancer.[318] The relative risk of cancer in persons with affected first-degree relatives, compared with those without a family history, was 1.72 for one relation and 2.75 for two or more. This increased risk for disease was especially evident among younger individuals (5.37).

Rapid advances in the identification of genetic events that are important in colonic carcinogenesis have been made in the past few years.[13] Specifically inherited abnormalities such as that for familial adenomatous polyposis have been discussed in Chapter 22. Both acquired and genetic anomalies (*ras* gene point mutations; c-*myc* gene amplification; allelic deletion at specific sites on chromosomes 5, 17, and 18) seem to be capable of mediating steps in the progression from normal to malignant colonic mucosa (see Figure 22-15 and Chapter 22).[13] Chromosomal studies have succeeded in identifying a gene on chromosome 18q that is altered in colorectal cancers.[291] Allelic deletions have been found to occur in more than 70% of such tumors. These are thought to signal the existence of a tumor suppressor gene in the affected region.[291] Specifically, an abnormality of the *p53* tumor suppressor gene, the most commonly mutated gene in human cancer, is thought to be critical to the development of the majority of human tumors.[967] In essence, the presence of the gene through its product (the p53 protein) acts to induce cell cycle arrest or apoptosis in response to DNA damage.[967]

Lynch Syndromes

Excluding the polyposis syndromes, carcinoma of the colon has been reported in cancer families, the so-called cancer family syndrome or hereditary nonpolyposis colorectal cancer (HNPCC).[394,601,603,604,806] This hereditary predisposition has been reported to account for at least 3% of colorectal cancer cases worldwide.[409] In a prospective multicenter study from Finland, Mecklin and coworkers investigated family history and other risk factors during a 1-year period for all new patients in whom colorectal cancer was diagnosed.[673] Lynch and colleagues estimate that the risk for development of colorectal cancer is three times greater than that of the general population if one has a first-degree relative with this condition.[606] Familial colorectal cancer, however, requires the presence of the disease in two or more first-degree relatives. Itoh and colleagues noted a sevenfold increased risk for colon cancer.[475] Unfortunately, it has been shown that although family cancer history is commonly obtained during the initial surgical consultation of patients with colorectal cancer, there is a tendency to underestimate the extent and its implications.[871]

Based on early observations by Warthin,[1068] Lynch and colleagues have defined two clinical variants: Lynch syndrome I or HNPCC and Lynch syndrome II or hereditary site-specific nonpolyposis colonic cancer (HSSCC).[600]

Lynch syndrome I is characterized by the following features:

- Autosomal dominance
- Early age at onset
- Predominance of proximal bowel involvement
- Multiple primary colon tumors

Lynch syndrome II is characterized by the same features but, additionally, shows an excess of other adenocarcinomas, particularly involving the endometrium and the ovary.[604,606,612] Others have added stomach, small bowel, and urinary tract cancers to the spectrum.[602,611,1051] Itoh and coworkers noted that the risk for breast cancer was increased fivefold, and the lifetime risk was estimated at 1 in 3.7 for first-degree relatives of persons with Lynch syndrome II.[475] Even carcinoma of the larynx has been suggested to be associated.[605]

In the era of molecular genetics, Lynch syndrome is defined in terms of a germ line mutation in a DNA mismatch repair (MMR) gene.[101] The clinical distinctions originally described are largely arbitrary, and the list of associated extracolonic malignancies continues to grow.[608] These include endometrium, ovary, stomach, hepatobiliary tract, pancreas, upper tract urothelial tumors, brain (Turcot's syndrome), and sebaceous adenomas (Muir-Torre syndrome).

It is useful at this point to define three terms that have entered the literature in this field: Amsterdam criteria, Bethesda guidelines, and microsatellite instability. These criteria are useful in identifying patients who should undergo MSI testing and/or molecular genetic testing to identify germ line mutation in one of the four MMR genes (*MLH1*, *MSH2*, *MSH6*, and *PMS2*).

Amsterdam Criteria

In 1991, the following clinical criteria (*Amsterdam criteria*) were established to facilitate consistency in research and are often applied in diagnosing HNPCC[1051]:

- Three or more cases of colorectal cancer in a minimum of two generations
- One affected individual a first-degree relative of the others with colorectal cancer
- One case of colorectal cancer diagnosed before age 50 years
- Exclusion of a diagnosis of familial adenomatous polyposis

The criteria have since been modified as follows:

- Two cases of colorectal cancer when families are small (one younger than 55 years old)
- Two cases of colorectal cancer and one of endometrial cancer or other early-onset cancer

Bethesda Guidelines

The Bethesda guidelines were developed in 1997 from the results of a National Cancer Institute workshop on HNPCC.[854] These guidelines include all of the criteria described in Amsterdam I and Amsterdam II. Because it was believed that the Amsterdam criteria alone led to an underestimation of the true incidence of HNPCC, additional criteria were added. These include histopathologic (signet ring cell, poorly differentiated), morphologic (right-sided), and less selective clinical criteria. Additionally, the guidelines were proposed to assist in the selection of patients whose tumors should be analyzed for microsatellite instability.[1129]

Microsatellite Instability

Colorectal cancers demonstrate increased rates of intragenic mutation, characterized by generalized instability of short, tandemly repeated DNA sequences known as microsatellites.[385] A high frequency of microsatellite instability (defined as 40% or more of the microsatellite loci) has been found in most patients with HNPCC. This is because of the inactivation of MMR function by the subsequent loss of the second allele that results in length variations of short sequences in HNPCC colorectal cancers.[1129] This alteration of dinucleotide repeats in microsatellite sequences, MSI or replication error, is used as a diagnostic criterion of MMR deficiency.[755] Early-age-at-onset colorectal cancer has been demonstrated to be correlated with high-frequency microsatellite instability tumor status.[813] It has also been shown to be a marker for predicting development of metachronous colorectal carcinoma after surgery.[937]

Specific findings of the patients in accordance with Lynch and coworkers were as follows: mean age at the initial colon cancer diagnosis was 44.6 years; of first colon cancers, 72.3% were located in the right side of the colon and only 25.0% were in the sigmoid and rectum; 18.1% of the patients had synchronous colon cancer, with a risk for metachronous lesions at 10 years of 40.0%.[606] Studies have shown the existence of a genetic defect with a population frequency of 19.0% that is transmitted in a mendelian, dominant mode.[266] This defect may predispose the bowel epithelium to the effects of fecal carcinogens.

What clinical clues should lead a physician to suspect the diagnosis of HNPCC? The following have been determined:

- Early onset of carcinoma of the colon, especially in the proximal bowel (in the absence of multiple colonic polyps)
- Presence of multiple primary cancers (e.g., of the colon, endometrium, ovary)
- Having a first-degree relative with early-onset cancers integral to Lynch syndrome II[610]

It must be remembered, however, that in the experience of Mecklin and Järvinen, only 40% of patients had a positive family history at the time the tumor was diagnosed.[671] Some have suggested that the flat adenoma, a slightly raised lesion with adenomatous tubules concentrated near the luminal surface, or even a small, flat carcinoma may represent markers for the syndrome (see Chapter 21).[104,465,549] When cancers do develop, the incidence of the mucinous type is high.[3,606,674] Svenden and colleagues suggest that young individuals with metachronous colorectal cancer developing after a previous diagnosis of colorectal carcinoma could in fact have HNPCC.[987] The possibility of HNPCC should certainly be considered in adolescents in whom colorectal cancer is diagnosed.[622] Such consideration would inevitably lead the surgeon to make a recommendation concerning the nature of the operation. For example, some have suggested that because there is a high risk for the development of a metachronous colorectal cancer following a limited resection, a total colectomy may be indicated.[1047] Others concur that close relatives of early-onset cases warrant more intensive colonoscopic screening at an earlier age than do relatives of patients in whom disease is diagnosed at an older age.[404,405]

Screening

The American Society of Colon and Rectal Surgeons (ASCRS) established a task force that led to the publication of *Practice Parameters* for the identification and testing of patients at risk for dominantly inherited colorectal cancer. The following are the conclusions of that collaborate group[958,959]:

- Take a family history.
- Document a suspicious pedigree. Request medical records to confirm the diagnosis.
- Identify criteria for genetic testing (Amsterdam, Bethesda, microsatellite instability in tumors).
- Offer surveillance to families not meeting the aforementioned criteria for genetic testing.
- Adhere to all protocols for genetic testing, including institutional review board, informed consent, and counseling.

Surveillance

Because the lifetime risk for the development of colorectal cancer approaches 80% in HNPCC, a surveillance program is recommended. In Lynch syndrome I, the surveillance approach is directed to the bowel exclusively. However, with Lynch syndrome II, one must also be aware of the increased risk for the development of extracolonic tumors. Annual colonoscopy is generally believed to be the preferred screening modality for bowel cancer in these individuals, although some believe that this is too frequent; evaluation of the stool for occult blood is unsatisfactory for this purpose.[453,548,606] Because of the increased risk for harboring benign and malignant tumors, colonoscopy is recommended for screening asymptomatic individuals with first-degree relatives having colon cancer, even in the absence of one

of the Lynch syndromes.[389,978] Indeed, colonoscopy has superceded prophylactic surgery in those with an inherited mutation.[557] Lynch and associates point out the potential for adverse medicolegal consequences because of failure to diagnose colorectal cancer.[609]

Green and colleagues performed colonoscopic screening on 61 asymptomatic individuals with an affected first-degree relative who had HNPCC.[372] Neoplasms were found in 15% and malignancies in 3%. Because of the high incidence of multiple lesions, consideration should be given to the performance of subtotal or total colectomy if surgery becomes necessary for colon cancer.[154] A regular, annual endoscopic follow-up of the residual rectum is still necessary, of course.[672] The risk for development of rectal cancer has been estimated to be 3% every 3 years after abdominal colectomy for the first 12 years.[855] There is no doubt that the familial cancer risk associated with early-onset disease outside of the recognized cancer predisposition syndromes is markedly increased.[496]

With respect to Lynch syndrome II patients, annual pelvic examinations are recommended beginning at age 25, including endometrial aspiration biopsy and ovarian ultrasonography.[606] Prophylactic hysterectomy with bilateral salpingo-oophorectomy should be considered in postmenopausal women and in those who have completed childbearing.[606]

Lynch and Lynch have made a plea for the establishment of computerized registries, such as have been developed for familial adenomatous polyposis, to transmit information about the diagnosis, surveillance, and management of hereditary colon cancer syndromes.[599,607] Recognizing high-risk families and individuals who would benefit from surveillance should help reduce the incidence of this common malignancy.[112]

In the Netherlands, families with HNPCC are monitored in an intensive surveillance program. Of the 35 cancers detected while patients were on the program, all but 2 were reported as identified at a local stage.[245]

Genetic Testing and Counseling

It is known that HNPCC is caused by germ line mutations in one of four DNA MMR genes: *hMSH2*, *hMLH1*, *hPMS1*, or *hPMS2* (see also Chapter 22). It is estimated that defects in two of the known MMR genes, *hMSH2* and *hMLH1*, account for 90% of mutations found in HNPCC families.[69,815] Although many mutations in these genes have been found in HNPCC kindreds, thereby complying with the so-called Amsterdam criteria, little is known about the involvement of these genes in families not satisfying these criteria but showing clear-cut familial clustering of colorectal cancer and other cancers.[1087] Wijnen and colleagues found *hMSH2* and *hMLH1* mutations in 49% of the kindreds that fully complied with the Amsterdam criteria, whereas a disease-causing mutation could be identified in only 8% of the families in which the criteria were not satisfied fully.[1087] These results imply that there are significant consequences to genetic testing and counseling in the management of colorectal cancer families.

Once the diagnosis has been established, the importance of genetic counseling has been strongly emphasized by Lynch and colleagues and by others.[611,975] It is recommended that all families with suggestive pedigrees should be referred to a geneticist for genetic testing. If the test result is negative for carrying the gene, the family member's cancer risk drops to that of the general population.[677] Conversely, the lifetime cancer risk for a gene carrier is approximately 90%. However, individuals need to know the implications and consequences of genetic test results before acquiescing to the testing.[1122]

Commercial testing is available in the United States through OncorMed.* The company has produced a protocol for testing. People who meet the following inclusion criteria should be tested:

- A person with colorectal cancer who has three relatives with colorectal cancer (at least one being a first-degree relative to the other two)
- A person with colorectal cancer who has two or more first- or second-degree blood relatives with colorectal cancer
- A person with colorectal cancer with onset before 30 years of age
- A person with colorectal cancer with onset between 30 and 50 years who has at least one other first- or second-degree relative with colorectal cancer
- A person with colorectal cancer with multiple colon primary tumors
- A person with colorectal cancer and another related primary cancer
- A relative of an individual with a documented *MSH2* or *MLH1* mutation

The following people should not be tested:

- A person younger than 18 years old
- A person with a known diagnosis of ulcerative colitis for 7 or more years, familial adenomatous polyposis/Gardner's syndrome, hereditary flat adenoma syndrome, Peutz-Jeghers syndrome, familial juvenile polyposis syndrome, or hereditary discrete polyp-carcinoma syndrome
- A cognitively impaired person or one unable to provide informed consent
- Someone who has a psychological condition precluding testing

Treatment

The Standards Task Force of the American Society of Colon and Rectal Surgeons established practice parameters for the treatment of patients with dominantly inherited colorectal cancer (HNPCC).[960] The following guidelines have been published:

- Treatment must be preceded by thorough counseling about the nature of the syndrome, its natural history, its extracolonic manifestations, and the need for compliance with all recommendations for management and surveillance.
- When patients with HNPCC as defined by genotype or compliance with Amsterdam I criteria are diagnosed with more than one advanced adenoma or a colon cancer, they should be offered the options of prophylactic total colectomy and ileorectal anastomosis or hemicolectomy plus yearly colonoscopy.
- Patients with HNPCC who have *rectal cancer* should be offered the options of total proctocolectomy and ileopouch anal anastomosis or anterior proctosigmoidectomy, assuming that the sphincters can be saved.
- Female patients with HNPCC and uterine cancer in their families may be offered prophylactic hysterectomy once childbearing is complete or when they undergo surgery for other intra-abdominal conditions.

---

*OncorMed, 205 Perry Parkway, Gaithersburg, MD 208777; 301-208-1888.

▶ AGE AND GENDER

The incidence of carcinoma of the colon and rectum increases with age, but the progression also varies by anatomic site, population, and sex. In our experience, the mean age at diagnosis for men was 63 years, and for women, 62 years.[204] Cook and associates computed the slopes of the logarithm of the incidence against the logarithm of the age from a number of cancer registries and demonstrated that the slopes of the curves for colon and rectal cancer for men were consistently higher than the slopes of curves for women in almost every population.[196] They noted, furthermore, that this variation in male–female difference was greater for colon than for rectal carcinoma.

In women, colorectal cancer ranks third in the United States in number of cancer deaths, 9%. Lung (26%) and breast (15%) are first and second, respectively.[041] The 2011 estimated cancer incidence is third, after breast and lung (30%, 14%, and 9%, respectively).

In men, colorectal cancer (8%) ranks third, after lung (28%) and prostate (11%), for deaths. Prostate cancer is now the single most common cancer (29%); lung is second (14%), and colorectal, third (9%). Men have a preponderance of rectal cancer and a slight excess of cancer of the descending and transverse colon. The incidence of cancer of the ascending colon and cecum is essentially the same for both sexes according to one report,[160] but according to another, women were found to have more right-sided tumors.[980]

▶ SYMPTOMS AND SIGNS

Change in Bowel Habits

Change in bowel habits is the most frequent complaint of patients with colorectal cancer. The change may be as insignificant as that from a bowel movement every other day to one daily. All too often, people place little emphasis on this observation until a profound alteration occurs. Generally, a more distal lesion creates more obvious symptoms than a proximal one. The reasons for this are threefold: first, it is more "difficult" for formed stool in the distal colon to pass through an area of narrowing than for the relatively liquid stool present in the proximal bowel; second, the lumen of the bowel itself is larger proximally than distally; and third, because of the presence of other symptoms (bleeding, pain, discharge), the patient is more likely to pay attention when a distal tumor produces a change in bowel habits.

Bleeding

Bleeding is the second most common symptom of colorectal cancer. It may be overt or occult. The blood may be bright red, purple, mahogany, black, or inapparent. The more distal the location of the lesion, the less altered the blood will be, and the redder it will appear. Although bleeding can represent a relatively early sign of cancer of the bowel, it is often a neglected symptom. Helfand and colleagues performed a prospective cohort study of 201 individuals who mentioned rectal bleeding as part of their review of systems evaluation and then determined whether such a complaint merits investigation for significant pathology.[434] They identified 24% with "serious disease," including benign and malignant neoplasms and inflammatory bowel disease. The authors concluded that physicians should ask all adults about visible rectal bleeding and should visualize the entire colon in those who manifest such symptoms. Individuals frequently attribute bleeding to hemorrhoids, particularly if they have had prior difficulty with hemorrhoids. For this reason, it is important to treat bleeding hemorrhoids, so that the presence of this symptom succeeds in alerting the patient to seek medical attention.

Conversely, the physician may mistakenly attribute the bleeding to hemorrhoids. Nothing is more tragic than the misdiagnosis of a potentially curable cancer because of inadequate examination or investigation. Too often, patients are managed with suppositories, creams, and laxatives, and only when symptoms become severe enough is proper investigation undertaken.

Mucus

The presence of mucus, either as a discharge (implying a distal lesion) or mixed with the stool, is another symptom; it often accompanies bleeding. The presence of mucus and bleeding should be considered a highly suggestive combination that necessitates bowel investigation.

Pain

Rectal pain is an unlikely presenting symptom of cancer. The most common reasons for anorectal pain are thrombosed hemorrhoids, anal fissure, abscess, and proctalgia fugax. When rectal cancer produces pain, the lesion usually is very distal or very large. Pain may result from infiltration of the sensitive anal canal or from sphincteric invasion. Such invasion may produce tenesmus, a painful urgency to defecate.

Abdominal pain resulting from tumor implies an obstructing or partially obstructing lesion. This pain is usually colicky in nature and may be associated with abdominal distension, nausea, or vomiting. Intestinal obstruction is a presenting complaint in 5% to 15% of individuals with colorectal cancer. Back pain from retroperitoneal extension of a tumor of the ascending or descending colon is an unusual and late sign.

Mass

A palpable or visible abdominal mass in the absence of other signs and symptoms implies a slow-growing, infiltrative process that may be much more amenable to surgical extirpation than might otherwise be anticipated. Such tumors often metastasize quite late in the course of disease.

Weight Loss

Weight loss, in the absence of other symptoms, is a poor prognostic sign. Inanition and loss of strength and appetite suggest metastatic disease, most commonly to the liver. Presentation with symptoms of metastatic disease occurs in approximately 5% of patients with colorectal cancer. Hepatomegaly is a frequent observation, but pulmonary, cerebral, and osseous metastases as isolated findings may reveal an occult colorectal primary on investigation.

Peritonitis

Perforation with peritonitis is an unusual presentation today (except in certain hospitals that serve an indigent population). Differentiating carcinoma from perforated diverticulitis, particularly with a sigmoid lesion, may be extremely difficult (see Surgical Treatment).

"Appendicitis"

Rarely, carcinoma of the cecum can obstruct the lumen of the appendix and cause signs and symptoms of acute appendicitis.[745] An even more uncommon phenomenon is perforation of the appendix from obstructing carcinoma of the more distal bowel.[986] The development of a fecal fistula after appendectomy should lead the physician to suspect an underlying malignancy. Although such presentations are uncommon, any individual older than 50 years old with a presentation of acute appendicitis should be evaluated carefully at the time of surgery for underlying carcinoma.

Inguinal Hernia

It has been thought that inguinal hernia in older men is associated with colorectal carcinoma, especially if the hernia is of relatively short duration.[226,650,812,1013] Because of this observation, some have advised routine colonic examination for all patients before herniorrhaphy. However, Brendel and Kirsh reported no such association.[114] The high incidence of colorectal neoplasms in the general population suggests that the theoretical relationship is more likely to be coincidental. That said, it is known that carcinoma of the colon can present, albeit rarely, as an incarcerated hernia.[451] It is therefore prudent to perform colonoscopic examination prior to undertaking hernia repair in patients experiencing a change in bowel habits or other symptoms suggestive of underlying bowel pathology.

Septicemia

Septicemia from *Streptococcus bovis* is associated with gastrointestinal neoplasms, especially colonic neoplasms.[75] Kline and colleagues prospectively studied individuals with sepsis caused by this organism.[527] Eight of 15 who completed gastrointestinal evaluation, including colonoscopy, were found to harbor colon carcinoma. The differential diagnosis of a fever of unknown origin includes colorectal cancer and demands appropriate evaluation.[665] Additionally, fevers of undetermined origin in individuals with known colorectal carcinoma should lead one to investigate the possibility of bacterial endocarditis.[861] Secondary infections of hepatic metastases in an individual with a known primary tumor of the colon are well recognized. However, it is much less appreciated that colonic cancer can be an underlying cause of pyogenic liver abscesses in the absence of metastases. After the usual causes have been excluded, an asymptomatic colon cancer should be considered in the differential diagnosis.[1005] The presence of an organism normally found in the colon should heighten the clinician's suspicion.

Cutaneous Manifestations

Nonmetastatic cutaneous presentations of colorectal cancer have been reviewed by Rosato and associates.[859] They noted a number of conditions associated with gastrointestinal malignancy, including acanthosis nigricans, dermatomyositis, pemphigoid, and others (see Chapter 9). Such manifestations are rare, but any disseminated skin condition that is unresponsive to conventional therapy should encourage the physician to consider gastrointestinal investigation.

Cutaneous metastases from colorectal carcinoma are extremely unusual except, of course, in the incision or port site (see later). Even rarer is the individual who presents with skin lesions as the initial complaint.[225] Certainly, the incidence must be less than 1%. Biopsy will usually clarify any confusion as to the diagnosis.

Intussusception

Intussusception in the adult is always a condition that requires surgical treatment. This is in contradistinction to children, for whom medical management (e.g., reduction by barium enema) may result in cure. Patients usually present with signs and symptoms of intestinal obstruction.

Nagorney and associates reviewed the Mayo Clinic experience with 144 cases of adult intussusception treated at that institution since 1910.[724] Almost 9 in 10 were associated with a definitive pathologic process: malignant neoplasm, benign tumor, metastatic lesion, or Meckel's diverticulum (Figures 23-1 and 23-2). Two-thirds of the colonic intussusceptions were associated with primary carcinoma of the colon, whereas only one-third of the intussusceptions of the small intestine were associated with an underlying cancer; most of those malignancies were metastatic. Others have also recognized the association between colonic intussusception and the presence of underlying tumors in the adult.[117,293,734,887,1079] The importance of resection without reduction is discussed later.

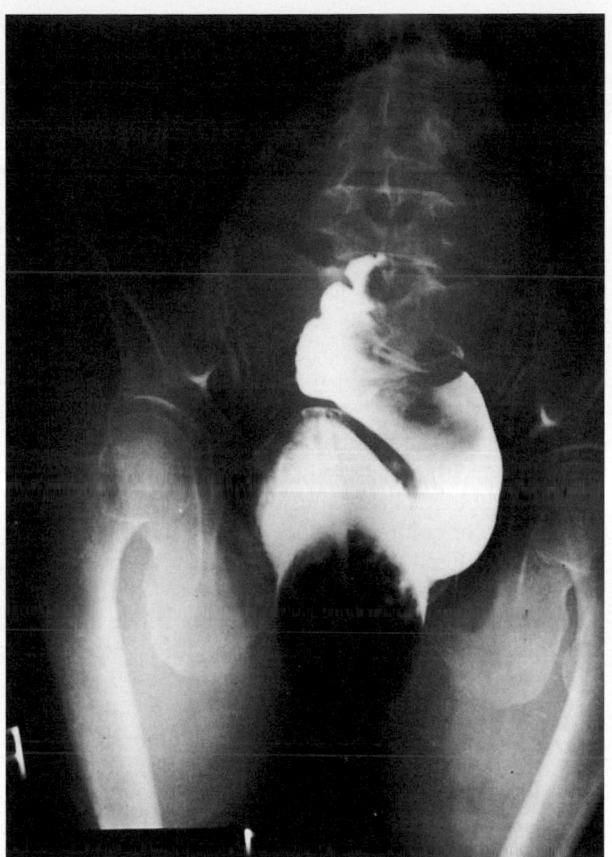

FIGURE 23-2. Partial colonic obstruction secondary to carcinoma of the sigmoid with intussusception. Note the characteristic coiled-spring appearance of the intussusceptum.

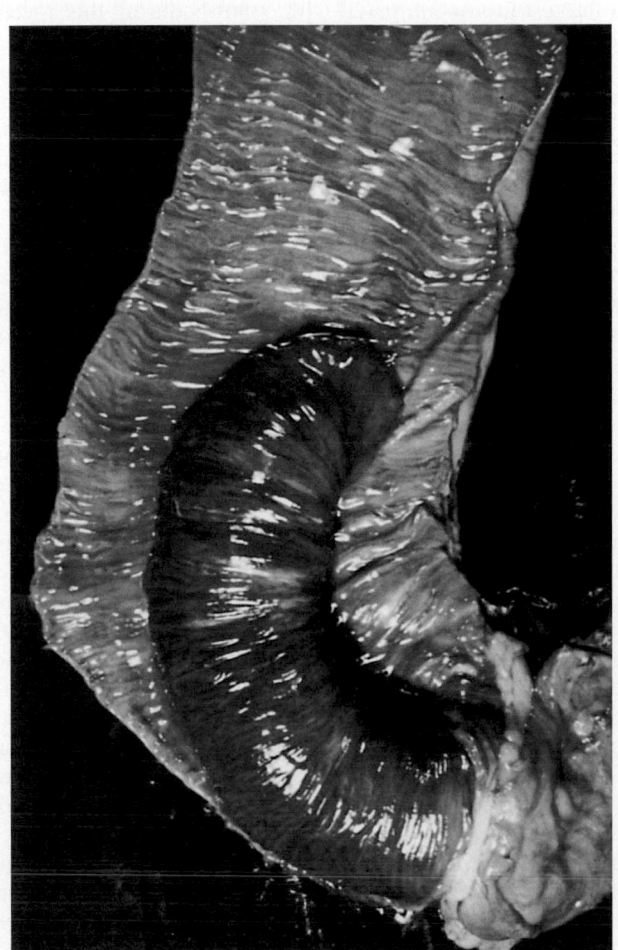

FIGURE 23-1. Ileocecal intussusception from cecal carcinoma producing intestinal obstruction. (Courtesy of Rudolf Garret, MD.)

Duration of Symptoms

Unfortunately, one continues to be impressed by the long history of symptoms reported by many patients who come to surgery for colorectal cancer. However, those with a short history of symptoms do not have a better prognosis. Individuals with symptoms of less than 5 months' duration have a higher incidence of resection for cure, but the actual long-term survival has not been shown to be improved.[473,897]

▶ EVALUATION

Practice Parameters for the Detection of Colorectal Neoplasms

Colorectal cancer screening is relatively inexpensive compared with screening for breast and cervical cancer, with cost estimates suggesting that the amount necessary to prevent one cancer is essentially equivalent to that required to treat a symptomatic patient.[425] Although the most cost-effective approach has yet to be identified, screening can decrease mortality by making possible the identification of tumors at an earlier stage and the removal of benign lesions before they become malignant, thus preventing the subsequent development of cancer.[1027] Several protocols have been established by a number of organizations for the detection of colorectal neoplasms at the earliest possible stage.

Clinical guidelines and a rationale for colorectal screening have been endorsed by the American Cancer Society, the American College of Gastroenterology, the American Gastroenterological Association, the American Society of Colon and Rectal Surgeons, the American Society for Gastrointestinal Endoscopy, the Crohn's and Colitis Foundation of America, the Oncology Nursing Society, and the Society of American Gastrointestinal and Endoscopic Surgeons (SAGES). Guidelines from the United States Multi-Society Task Force were published in 2003 and updated in 2008.[572,1103] The following general recommendations have been proposed:

- People with symptoms that suggest the presence of colorectal cancer or polyps should have appropriate diagnostic evaluation and fall outside of screening recommendations.
- Personal and familial risk factors need to be evaluated when screening is being considered.
- Screening for colorectal cancer and adenomatous polyps should be offered to all men and women without risk factors beginning at age 50.
- Physicians should recommend a diagnostic evaluation of the colon to follow up a positive result of a screening test.
- Follow-up surveillance should be considered after treatment of colorectal cancer or removal of adenomatous polyps or in the presence of underlying premalignant conditions such as inflammatory bowel disease.
- Health care providers who perform the tests should have appropriate proficiency, and the tests should be performed correctly.
- Screening should be accompanied by efforts to optimize the participation of both patients and health care providers in screening tests and appropriate diagnostic follow-up.
- People who are candidates for screening should be given adequate information on the risks and benefits of the various screening procedures.

In 2006, the American Society of Colon and Rectal Surgeons published guidelines for the detection of colorectal neoplasms based on the recommendations described earlier.[528]

Determination of Occult Blood

The stool guaiac or orthotoluidine test has been the subject of a number of reports (see Chapter 5). In fact, fecal occult blood tests are the only colorectal screening tests with supporting evidence from prospective, randomized trials, with demonstrated reductions in colorectal cancer mortality of 15% to 33%. Greegor studied patients with known asymptomatic colorectal cancers and found the presence of blood in at least one of three stool specimens.[370] Because of the relatively high false-positive rate, he recommended a special diet that succeeded in reducing this rate to approximately 1%. The diet is free of meat, fish, and chicken and is relatively high in roughage (fiber) to stimulate bleeding from an existing lesion. Norfleet's study, however, failed to demonstrate any benefit with respect to sensitivity or specificity from this diet.[747] Ostrow and associates studied healthy volunteers and found that the test slide preparation gave consistently positive results after the administration of 25 mL of blood and usually gave positive results with only 10 mL.[769]

A study from the United Kingdom by Tate and colleagues compared three fecal occult tests—Hemoccult, Fecatwin, and E-Z Detect—to determine which is best suited for use in asymptomatic patients.[1004] The test most sensitive for blood was Fecatwin; it found 93% of cancers and 69% of other mucosal diseases, but the incidence of false-positive results was three times that of Hemoccult. Home testing methods have thus far demonstrated no advantage through increased compliance to outweigh the lower sensitivity.[814]

In Gilbertsen's study, guaiac testing revealed that cancer was responsible for positive test results in 5.1% of patients, and benign tumors in 24%, with no evidence of gastrointestinal neoplasms in 68%.[333] A later report from this center evaluated 48,000 asymptomatic patients during a period of approximately 4 years.[746] Invasive carcinoma was found in 113; more than one-half of the tumors had not breached the seromuscular surface of the bowel wall. Hardcastle and Pye believe that the predictive value of a positive test result for invasive cancer is 11% to 17%, and for adenomas, 36% to 41%.[413] In another report from the Minnesota Colon Cancer Control Study, annual fecal occult blood testing with rehydration of the samples decreased the 13-year cumulative mortality from colorectal cancer by 33%.[631]

In a prospective randomized trial, Kewenter and coworkers investigated a number of new colorectal neoplasms that developed during the first 7 years after the end of a rescreening program by means of occult blood determination.[516] One hundred one carcinomas were diagnosed in the screened group and 128 in the control group during the follow-up period. The results indicated that screening and rescreening of a population had little influence on the stage of the cancers in the test group compared with controls during this 7-year period.

Robinson and colleagues reported the use of an immunologic fecal occult blood test called Hemeselect, comparing this with standard guaiac testing in almost 1,500 patients who completed both evaluations.[850] Hemeselect had a much higher positive predictive value for cancer and adenomas than did Hemoccult.

Evaluation of a patient with a positive occult blood determination can be expensive, but other pathologic entities that may be of significance are worth identifying.[272] Although the cost versus the benefit of a massive screening program is debatable, no one doubts the value of early diagnosis, especially before a malignancy supervenes.[18,333,517,621,630,1100,1105] Scudamore showed that when a patient has no gastrointestinal symptoms, a 100% possibility of curative resection can be expected, with an 88% 5-year survival.[909] Mapp and coworkers found that screening by means of occult blood determination improved survival in a randomized, controlled study.[634] Others challenge the concept of unsupervised mass screening from the point of view of cost-effectiveness, but because of voluntary services and supplies, such projects are probably useful in educating the public about colon and rectal cancer and the value of early detection.[163,520] Lieberman suggests that screening with fecal occult blood testing and sigmoidoscopy, as recommended by the American Cancer Society, may not be as cost effective as screening with colonoscopy.[576] The guidelines previously mentioned, as published under the auspices of multiple societies, recommend fecal occult blood test screening on an annual basis.[1103] Testing of two samples from each of three consecutive stools for the presence of occult blood, followed by colonoscopy, has been demonstrated to reduce the risk of death from colorectal cancer. Average-risk people with an abnormal screening test result by fecal occult blood testing (i.e., a trace-positive or positive test result from any sample) require an accurate examination of the entire colon and rectum, ideally by colonoscopy.[1103] The other option would be to perform a double-contrast barium enema, preferably with flexible sigmoidoscopy (see later and Chapter 5). Newer approaches to screening and additional data are also discussed in Chapter 5.

Digital Rectal Examination

William J. Mayo remarked, "The physician often hesitates to make the necessary examination because it involves soiling the finger."[653] Or, simply stated, if you do not put your finger in, you'll put your foot in. The index finger has also been termed "God's bioprobe." However, the efficacy of digital examination today for identifying cancer of the rectum is less compelling than previously thought. Only 10% of colorectal cancers are potentially within reach of the examiner's finger. Even when the cancer is palpable, the physician may not be sufficiently cautious and diligent to permit discovery of a lesion. The risks of the examination, however, are nonexistent, and no one can argue the cost versus the benefit.

Digital examination will identify the location of the tumor, anterior or posterior, and whether it occupies part or the whole of the circumference. The tumor may be fixed or movable, ulcerated or scirrhous, exophytic or invasive. Careful palpation of the presacral space may reveal hard lymph nodes suggestive of tumor metastases; this may be a valuable prognostic sign. The fact that the tumor is palpable will often suggest the type of operation possible or whether the lesion is indeed resectable. Fixity may indicate a need for supplemental treatment, such as neoadjuvant therapy. Therefore, despite the numerous, often esoteric studies available to evaluate today's patient, digital examination of the rectum is still a very important adjunct.

Proctosigmoidoscopy

The rigid sigmoidoscope is one of the most valuable diagnostic tools used (see also Chapter 5). Examination with this instrument may reveal mucosal excrescences, polyps, polypoid lesions, cancer, inflammatory changes, strictures, vascular malformation, and anatomic distortion from extraluminal masses. It may also detect numerous anal conditions, such as fistulas, hemorrhoids, fissures, and abscesses. When the instrument is passed to its full length of 25 cm, perhaps one-half to two-thirds of all cancers of the colon and rectum may be identified. Unfortunately, with the rigid instrument, insertion to its full length is possible in only about 50% of patients, the average penetration being approximately 20 cm.

Many investigators have advocated routine proctosigmoidoscopy for early diagnosis,[150,183,332,441,493,808,921,989] but others have questioned the need for this procedure on an annual basis.[259,260,700] The American Cancer Society encourages physicians to search for colorectal cancer before the onset of symptoms. Optimally, an annual proctosigmoidoscopic examination for all patients 40 years of age and older would be recommended. However, with more than 90 million such persons in the United States, this is indeed an awesome task. It was estimated in 1980 that annual sigmoidoscopic examination on all people more than 40 years old in the United States would cost approximately $2.75 billion.[272] Corman and colleagues studied 2,500 consecutive asymptomatic patients with the rigid sigmoidoscope as part of a general examination. Excluded from the study were symptomatic patients and those with a prior history of colorectal disorders. The proctoscope was inserted to a mean length of 20 cm. Adenocarcinoma was found in eight patients, and in two of these, carcinoma developed in polypoid adenomas. A total of 432 benign polypoid lesions were found in 228 patients (9.1%).[199]

In this study, all lesions found in patients younger than 50 years old were benign; no cancers were detected before the sixth decade of life. This is not surprising because only 5% of colorectal cancers occur in patients younger than 45 years old.[43] Although bowel cancer can develop in a person at any age, because of the limitations of time, space, and personnel, they suggested that routine proctosigmoidoscopic examination be performed in those age groups most likely to benefit from the procedure: patients 50 years old and older.[199] If this criterion were met, 30% fewer examinations would need to be performed.

Selby and colleagues provided the strongest possible evidence of the value of screening rigid sigmoidoscopy.[914] In a case-control study, they determined that individuals who had undergone one or more screening sigmoidoscopic examinations in the preceding 10 years had a 60% to 70% reduction in the risk of death from rectal or distal colon cancer in comparison with those who had not undergone such an examination. Furthermore, their finding that the risk for death from these cancers was markedly reduced for 10 years *following* a single examination is of considerable interest.[571] The authors concluded that screening once every 10 years may be nearly as efficacious as more frequent examinations.[914]

The flexible sigmoidoscope has virtually replaced the rigid instrument for screening purposes (see later and Chapter 6). Flexible sigmoidoscopy every 5 years is one of the recommended options for average risk colorectal cancer screening.[572] Although no one can argue against the value of screening a greater colonic surface, it is a sad commentary that many surgical residents coming out of training programs today do not know how to use the rigid instrument. There is no question that the rigid instrument is far superior to the flexible one for determining the level of the lesion when a cancer is identified in the rectum or rectosigmoid. It is also generally superior for evaluating the state of the anastomosis as part of a follow-up protocol or when the patient experiences symptoms following resective surgery.

Biopsy

Obviously when a patient has symptoms, a proctosigmoidoscopic examination, at least, is mandatory. When a tumor is identified, a biopsy of the lesion should be performed. This is usually a simple office procedure requiring no anesthetic and the very minimum of special tools. For polypoid, exophytic lesions, appreciable bleeding is rarely a concern after a biopsy. If electrocoagulation equipment is not readily available and bleeding is encountered, pressure with a long, cotton-tip applicator soaked in a topical solution of adrenaline will usually suffice.

The sample for biopsy should be taken from the edge of the lesion at the junction of the tumor and the normal-appearing bowel, and placed in a fixative solution. Notation should be made of the distance from the anal verge to the lower level of the lesion. The size, macroscopic appearance (ulcerated or polypoid), and location should also be recorded.

Flexible Sigmoidoscopy and Colonoscopy

The flexible sigmoidoscope has been recommended as the preferred initial screening tool for colorectal cancer (see also Chapter 6).[1027,1052,1106] Its primary advantage is that it allows more proximal evaluation of the bowel. It remains to be seen whether the relatively high cost of the instrument and the time spent in examination are justified by the increased yield. It must be remembered, however, that the rectum is evaluated better by the rigid sigmoidoscope than by the flexible instrument.

The examiner must be wary of performing such procedures as biopsy-cautery and snare excision with the flexible instrument in an inadequately prepared colon. With the limited cleansing regimen commonly employed for this instrument examination, there is a serious risk for explosion when electrical equipment is used for tumor biopsy or removal.

The place of colonoscopy as a screening tool in the asymptomatic, low-risk population has been somewhat controversial. Lieberman and coworkers reported the Veterans Cooperative Study Group experience with 3,197 patients who had been enrolled.[577] In this group of almost exclusively men, colonoscopic examination demonstrated one or more neoplasms in 37.5% of the patients. As a consequence of this and other studies, the United States government insurance program, Medicare, will pay for colonoscopy as a screening test every decade beginning at age 50. Furthermore, colonoscopic screening for neoplasms in asymptomatic first-degree relatives of patients with colon cancer is strongly recommended.[388,669,773] The aforementioned multiorganizational cancer screening guideline protocol recommends that close relatives (e.g., siblings, parents, and children) of a person who has had colorectal cancer or an adenomatous polyp should be offered the same options as average-risk people, but beginning at the age of 40 years.[1103] If colorectal cancer has been diagnosed in the close relative before the age of 55 years, or an adenomatous polyp before the age of 60, special effort should be made to ensure that screening takes place. Interestingly, transplant patients have the same risk for the development of colorectal neoplasms as the general population.[780] In the absence of risk factors, consideration should be given to offering a colonoscopy every 10 years.

Estimates have indicated that up to 14 million colonoscopies are performed in the United States each year, most often for colorectal cancer screening. The rationale for screening colonoscopy is that identification and removal of adenomatous polyps will prevent later colorectal cancer (or at least detect malignancies at an early stage). Yet, there are no prospective randomized trials attesting to a reduction in either the incidence or mortality associated with colorectal cancer. In the National Polyp Study, the incidence of colorectal cancer after a clearing colonoscopy was reduced by 76% to 90%, as compared to three reference populations.[1107] However, subsequent studies have not suggested a level of protection anywhere close to this magnitude.[14,849,893]

Colonoscopy has been of demonstrable value for the patient with a known neoplasm by identifying a synchronous tumor (Figure 23-3). Herbst and associates, in a retrospective study of 55 patients, found that 9 (16%) harbored another lesion.[437] This discovery caused the operation to be modified. In the report of Reilly and associates, 7.6% of 92 patients had a synchronous cancer.[838] All were missed on barium enema examination, and none was more invasive than the index lesion. Other studies have demonstrated that 2% to 8% of patients will have a synchronous carcinoma elsewhere in the colon.[474,546,771,774,838,1019,1074] When polyps are present, the risk

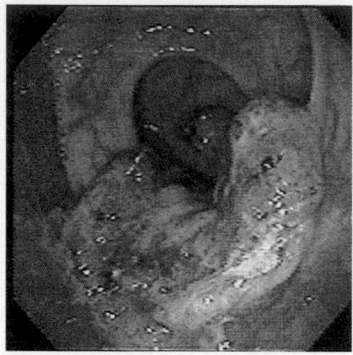

FIGURE 23-3. Colonoscopic examination reveals an ulcerating tumor of the sigmoid colon. The tumor encompasses approximately one-third of the bowel circumference. There is a small polyp proximal to the tumor that should emphasize the importance of total colonoscopic evaluation.

is even higher. Conversely, perhaps as many as 50% of patients with colon cancer harbor one or more colon polyps.[771]

Because many symptomatic patients undergo proctosigmoidoscopy and barium enema sequentially, Winawer suggests that the colonoscope be used if small-to-moderate tumors are present because the instrument can usually slip past the lesion.[1101] He believes that the procedure is more valuable in evaluating patients with known right-sided tumors of the colon. The yield is higher, and the distal bowel can be more easily examined. These studies confirm what has long been suspected: often, the metachronous tumor actually represents the missed synchronous one.

Gilbertsen and coworkers believe that barium enema examination is not sufficiently reliable in evaluating patients for suspected colorectal cancer and have abandoned the routine use of this modality in favor of colonoscopy for patients in whom a colorectal lesion is suspected.[334] They hold that barium enema examination often need not be performed if colonoscopy is diagnostic. Others have recommended the technique as a valuable screening tool for those who are at an increased risk for development of colon cancer (e.g., with a positive family history).[386,593] Most concur, however, that the detection rate of colon cancer is about the same with both studies, provided that they are competently performed and bowel preparation is adequate. Colonoscopy, though, is believed to be superior to barium enema in detecting rectal carcinoma.[835] One must remember that even colonoscopy is imperfect. Byrd and colleagues noted a 97% correlation with the resected specimen, but in 3%, lesions were missed.[144] Blind areas in the colon plus misjudgment that the instrument had been inserted to the perceived level were responsible for the majority of colonoscopic errors. Recognizing the limits of this procedure, colonoscopy should be the initial examination that is performed on anyone who presents with signs and symptoms suggestive of a large bowel problem.[944]

Complete visualization of the colon must be accomplished within a reasonable time following identification of a bowel neoplasm. Optimally, this should be performed preoperatively because it may alter the type of operation.[454] Many patients are submitted to this investigation the day before or the day of colon resection in order to obviate the need for a second bowel preparation. Preoperative barium enema is used only when the size of the lesion precludes passage of the instrument. If total colonoscopy is not undertaken before surgery, it should be carried out by the sixth postoperative week.

Comment

From the economic and manpower perspective, *frequent colonoscopy* as a screening test cannot be justified in an asymptomatic individual who is not in a high-risk group. The procedure often requires sedation and is not without complication (e.g., a perforation rate of 0.1% to 0.5%). In any event, the reality is that there are insufficient resources for performing total colonoscopy on everyone older than 50 years old, even if this were accomplished every 5 years. The real question is how much is a human life worth, or putting it in another way, how much "good medicine" can one afford!

Cytology

Establishing the diagnosis of carcinoma of the colon by means of cytologic evaluation, washing out the colon with saline solution, has been advocated by some authors (see Chapter 5).[174,819] Winawer and colleagues performed brush cytology and lavage on selected patients with colonic neoplasms.[1104] They and others believe that brush cytology improves the yield of tissue diagnosis when combined with biopsy, but lavage cytology alone does not seem to be as useful.[714,1104] Chen suggests that cell brushings may be of particular value when colonic stricture and obstruction prevent the colonoscope from reaching the lesion for biopsy.[174]

Stool DNA

Because of the utility of identification of mutations in oncogenes and tumor suppressor genes, it has been suggested that this observation may have a demonstrable advantage over such indirect studies of the stool, such as occult blood determination.[12,570,1032] Some studies have been reported which use purified DNA from stool samples in individuals known to harbor colorectal cancer and have detected these mutations.[538,1032] Additional work is needed to determine the specificity of these genetic tests in asymptomatic patients and to define more precisely the prevalence of the mutations and the sensitivity of the assay.[257] A commercially available, stool-based, DNA colorectal cancer screening test, Pre-Gen, can be obtained in the United States through EXACT Sciences (http://www.exactsciences.com). Testing stool for molecular markers is a promising and rapidly evolving area.

Barium Enema: Air-Contrast Enema Examination

There are no studies evaluating whether screening double-contrast (air-contrast) barium enema alone reduces the incidence or mortality of colorectal cancer in individuals who are at average risk for development of the disease.[1103] The previously mentioned cooperative recommendation on colorectal cancer screening suggests that an individual be offered this radiologic study every 5 to 10 years.

The barium enema has traditionally been the most commonly employed investigative study for evaluation of carcinoma of the large bowel, but for screening and preoperative assessment, it has been replaced by colonoscopy. Most people believe that despite meticulous double-contrast technique, the examination cannot be performed with the accuracy of colonoscopy (see Chapter 5). Even the most careful and competent of radiologists can overlook a colon carcinoma through failure to observe such subtle points as missing haustral folds; disharmony of interhaustral fold patterns; small,

radiolucent filling defects; local contractions; and residue-like masses.[307] Also, the absence of any therapeutic potential relegates this examination to a second choice.

When barium enema is performed in the presence of a known rectal carcinoma, it should be accomplished with great care (Figure 23-4). After the procedure, the rectum must be cleansed vigorously by multiple enemas to avoid the possibility of obstruction from inspissated barium.

Figure 23-5 demonstrates a typical apple-core lesion at the rectosigmoid juncture. This segment is fairly long; the normal mucosal pattern is lost in the involved bowel, and characteristically the mucosa overhangs the lesion. Another frequent appearance of carcinoma of the sigmoid is shown in Figure 23-6.

The presence of a pedicle (Figure 23-7) does not rule out the diagnosis of carcinoma. In fact, the illustration shows a polypoid carcinoma on a stalk measuring more than 2 cm in length. However, the radiologist is not in a position to comment whether a polyp is benign or malignant.[206]

Barium enema study (Figure 23-8) reveals complete retrograde obstruction to the flow of barium at the level of the mid-sigmoid colon. Retrograde obstruction, although an impressive radiologic finding, is not necessarily indicative

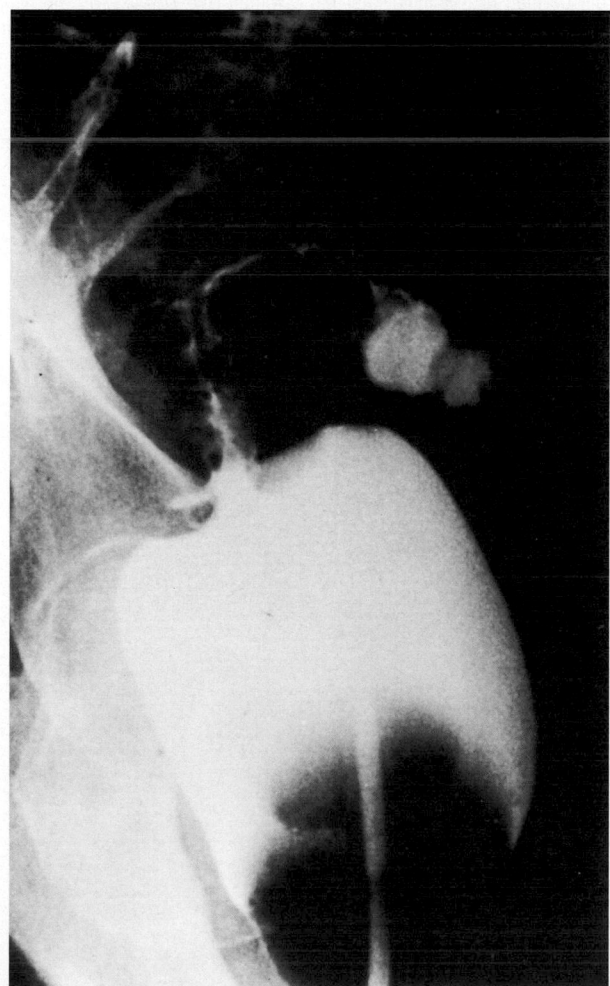

FIGURE 23-4. Barium enema study of a patient with known rectal carcinoma invites the hazard of inspissated barium precipitating colonic obstruction. The physician must weigh the value of screening the proximal bowel against this risk. (From Corman ML, Veidenheimer MC, Swinton NW. *Diseases of the Anus, Rectum, and Colon. Part I: Neoplasms.* New York, NY: Medcom; 1972, with permission.)

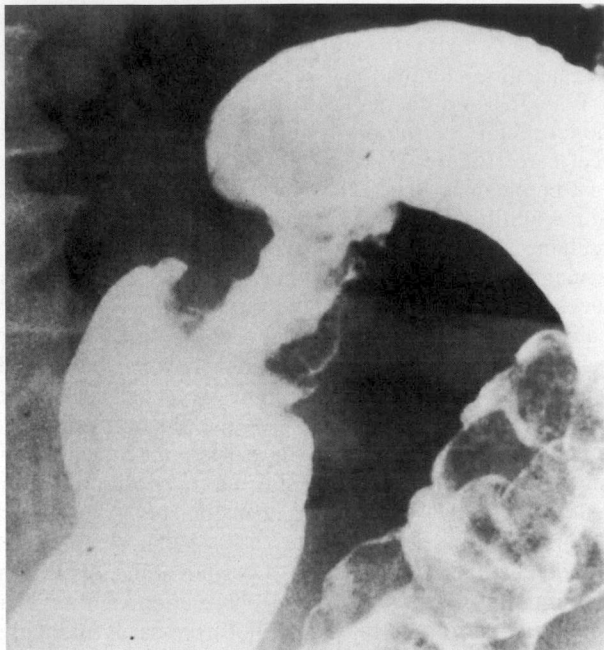

FIGURE 23-5. Apple-core carcinoma at the rectosigmoid juncture. (From Corman ML, Veidenheimer MC, Swinton NW. *Diseases of the Anus, Rectum, and Colon. Part I: Neoplasms.* New York, NY: Medcom; 1972, with permission.)

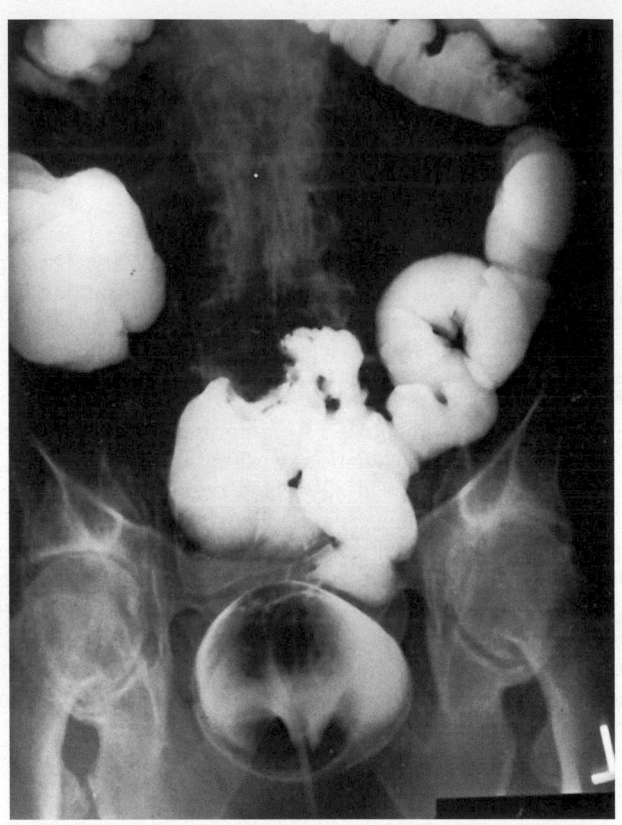

FIGURE 23-6. Carcinoma of the sigmoid. An irregularly marginated mass projecting into the lumen of the colon shows the characteristic shoulders of a malignancy.

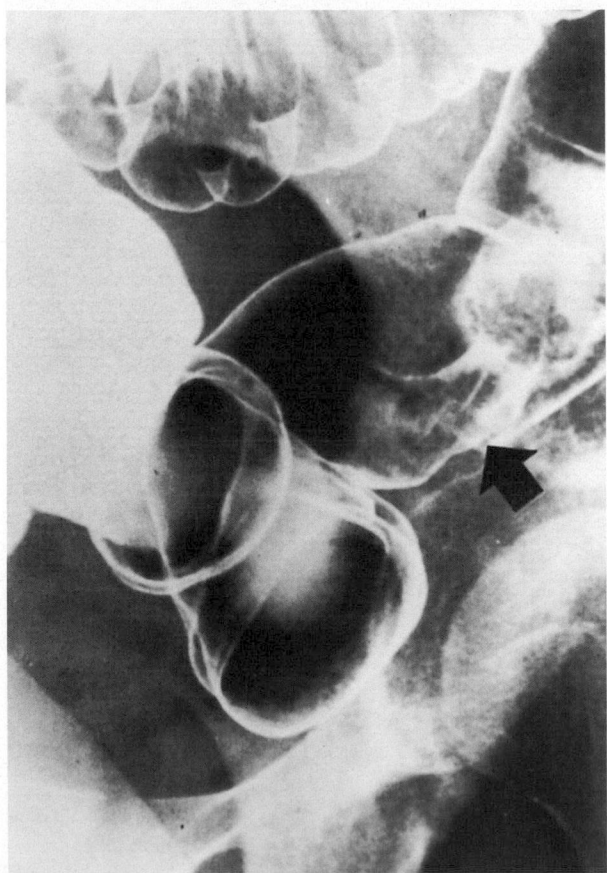

FIGURE 23-7. The presence of a pedicle (*arrow*) does not exclude carcinoma. This lesion was entirely malignant. (From Corman ML, Veidenheimer MC, Swinton NW. *Diseases of the Anus, Rectum, and Colon. Part I: Neoplasms.* New York, NY: Medcom; 1972, with permission.)

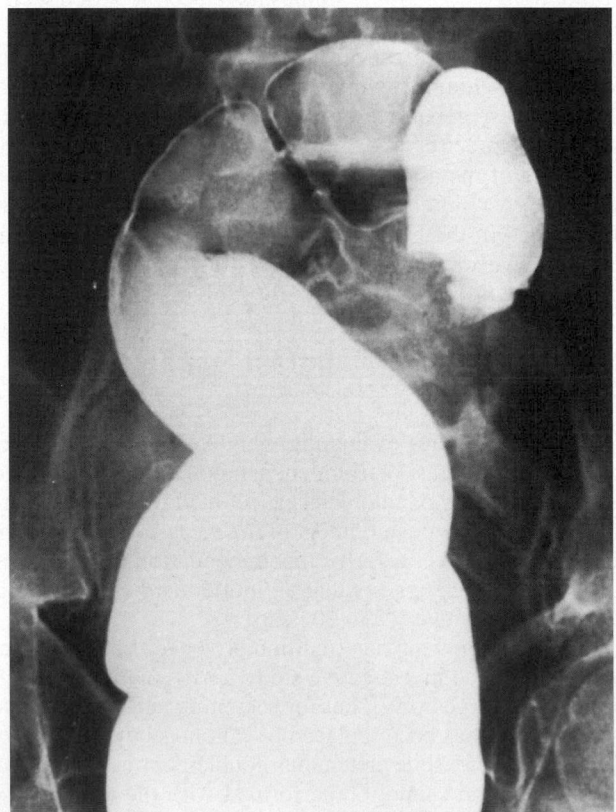

FIGURE 23-8. Retrograde obstruction to the flow of barium from a carcinoma may or may not be associated with significant obstructive symptoms clinically. (From Corman ML, Veidenheimer MC, Swinton NW. *Diseases of the Anus, Rectum, and Colon. Part I: Neoplasms.* New York, NY: Medcom; 1972, with permission.)

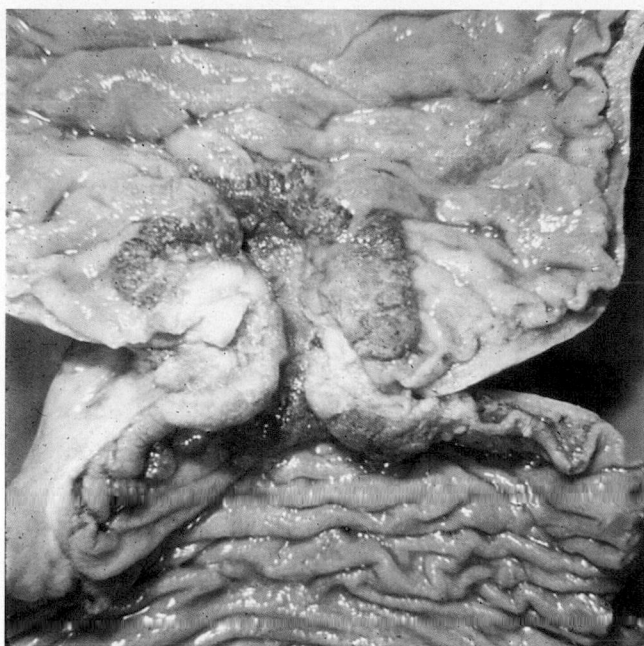

FIGURE 23-9. String stricture. Resected specimen of the carcinoma causing obstruction shown in Figure 23-8. (From Corman ML, Veidenheimer MC, Swinton NW. *Diseases of the Anus, Rectum, and Colon. Part I: Neoplasms.* New York, NY: Medcom; 1972, with permission.)

of antegrade obstruction. Occasionally, patients will report minimal change in bowel habits, even with this radiologic picture. The resected specimen is shown in Figure 23-9.

The barium enema study shown in Figure 23-10 demonstrates carcinoma of the sigmoid colon with associated diverticular disease. Differentiating between these two conditions is often difficult. It is sometimes said that the presence of diverticula, as seen in this patient, excludes the diagnosis of carcinoma. This is certainly not true. The most important radiologic distinction is that the mucosal pattern usually is maintained in diverticular disease, whereas in carcinoma the mucosa is destroyed or the pattern is lost. In some patients, however, it is impossible to distinguish between the two conditions, and without further information a resection must be performed.

Carcinoma of the sigmoid colon with perforation is shown in Figure 23-11. Under such circumstances, differentiation between carcinoma and diverticular disease is virtually impossible. Another complication of colon cancer is fistulization. Figure 23-12 demonstrates reflux of barium into the upper intestinal tract from a carcinoma near the hepatic flexure.

Figure 23-12 demonstrates carcinoma involving one wall of the cecum in a patient who presented with anemia. Careful bowel preparation is necessary for evaluation of cecal tumors because fecal matter frequently obscures this area.

It is important to remember that not all tumors of the colon originate within the bowel. Metastases of cancers from an ovary, breast, or other sites, as well as direct extension from adjacent organs, can produce a radiologic picture virtually identical to that of an intrinsic lesion. For example, the transverse colon is involved in 8% of pancreatic malignancies (Figure 23-13).[277] This is another area in which colonoscopy with biopsy has a particular advantage. Despite the plethora of illustrative radiologic material shown, colonoscopy has indeed become the standard for evaluation and interpretation of colonic tumors. The use of barium enema as a diagnostic tool, particularly for screening, continues to decline rather markedly.[280,849] In fact, a barium enema for neoplastic disease is almost a historical curiosity, so effectively has colonoscopy replaced this examination. There is so little interest in gastrointestinal radiology on the part of radiologists today that it is virtually impossible to recruit such an individual with this expertise to any radiology department. Although there is no denying that colonoscopy is a superior study for the evaluation of mucosal disease, barium enema is much preferred for understanding colonic anatomy, extrinsic compression, and identification of intramural lesions. Even in this area, however, barium enema has been relegated to a secondary role because of the advent of computed tomography (CT).

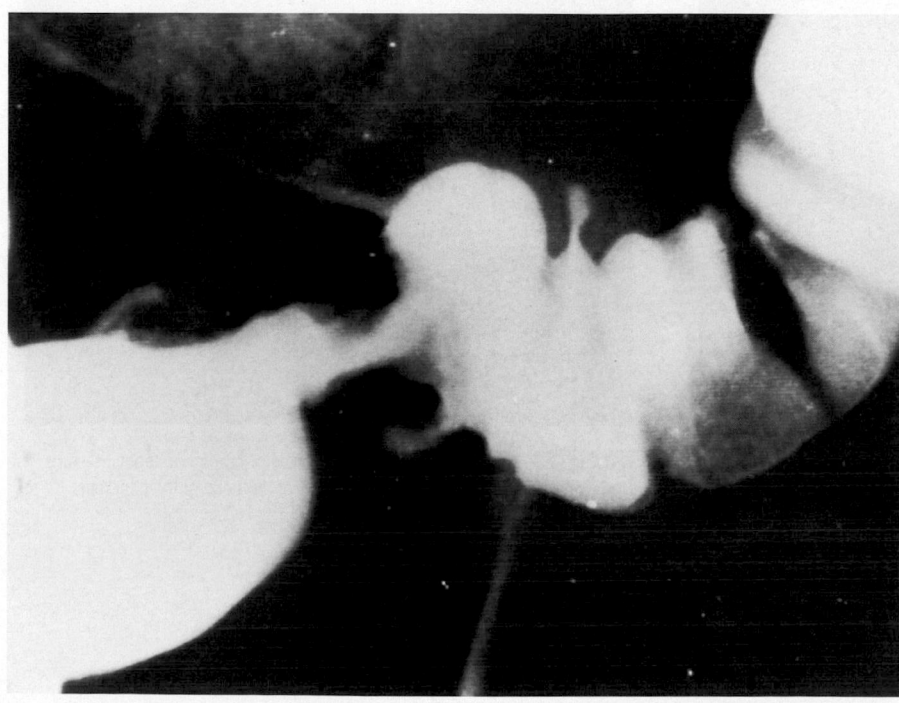

FIGURE 23-10. Carcinoma of the sigmoid with diverticular disease. Because of the relative frequency of both conditions, this is not an uncommon picture. (From Corman ML, Veidenheimer MC, Swinton NW. *Diseases of the Anus, Rectum, and Colon. Part I: Neoplasms.* New York, NY: Medcom; 1972, with permission.)

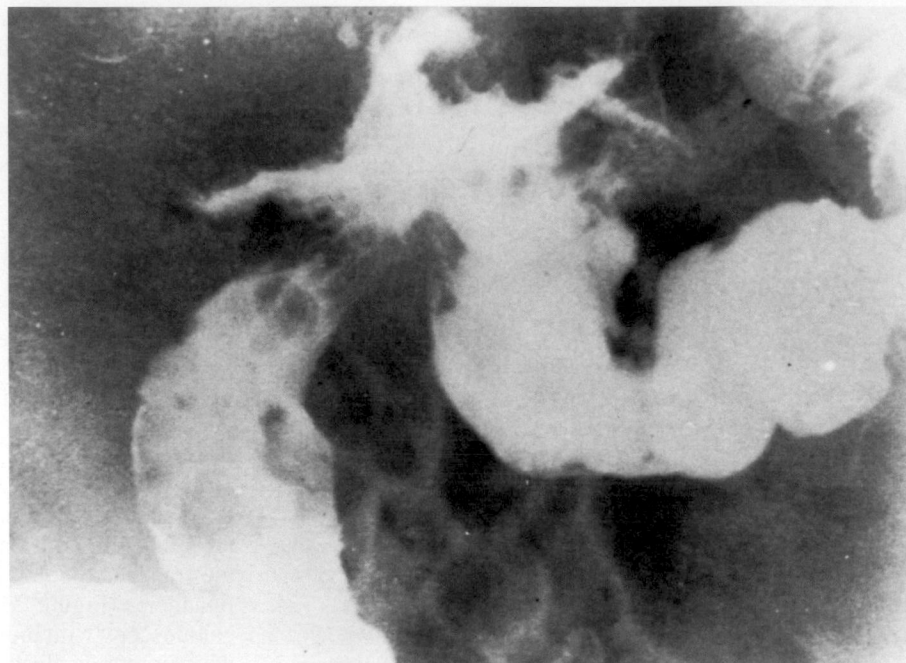

FIGURE 23-11. Perforated carcinoma may be indistinguishable from diverticulitis. (From Corman ML, Veidenheimer MC, Swinton NW. *Diseases of the Anus, Rectum, and Colon. Part I: Neoplasms.* New York, NY: Medcom; 1972, with permission.)

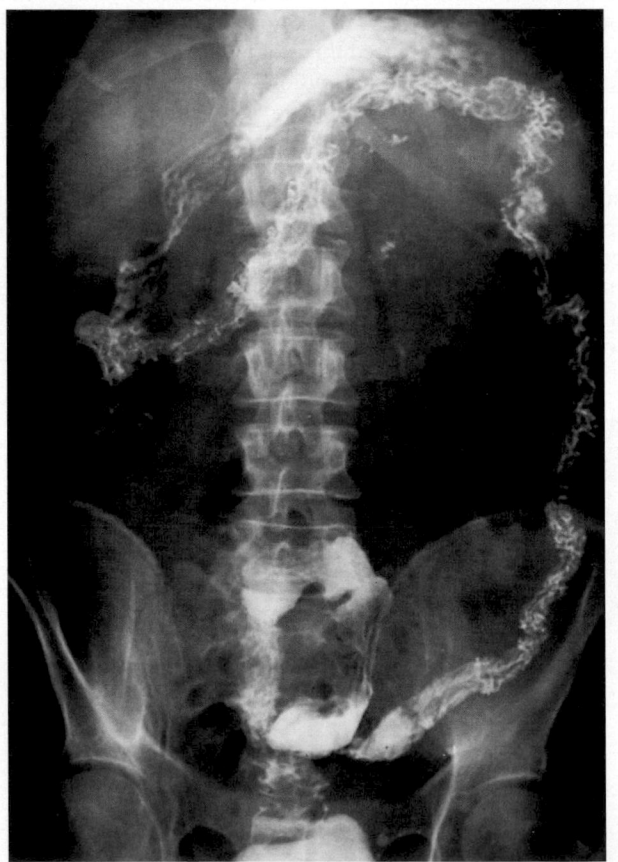

FIGURE 23-12. Carcinoma with fistula. Note the reflux of barium into the duodenum and stomach through a fistula from a hepatic flexure lesion.

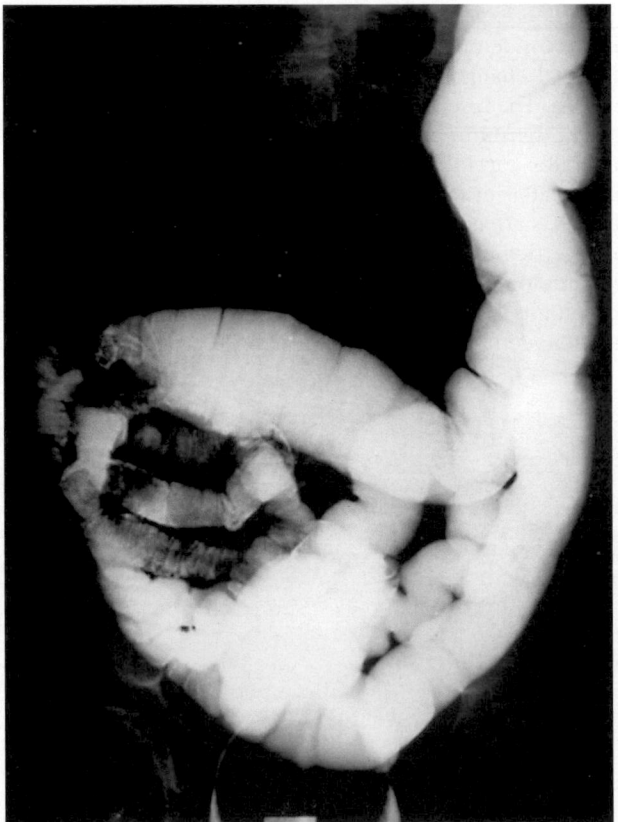

FIGURE 23-13. Partial obstruction to flow of barium at hepatic flexure. The lesion was caused by an invasive carcinoma of the head of the pancreas.

Urologic Evaluation

For many surgeons in the past, an integral part of the preoperative evaluation of a patient about to undergo bowel surgery was intravenous pyelography (IVP).[1057] Unexpected findings are often identified through its use. In the experience of Prager and coworkers, ureteral duplication was seen in 2.2% of patients, in addition to a number of other congenital anomalies and serendipitous findings.[810] Moreover, the course of the ureters and the presence of ureteral obstruction can be ascertained, and the postvoiding residual may be estimated. However, in a retrospective study of more than 500 individuals, the incidence of complications was the same in patients with normal and abnormal IVP results as well as in patients who did not undergo IVP.[1002] Because most injuries occur after low anterior resection or abdominoperineal resection, it seems reasonable to apply the technique to the preoperative evaluation of those whose surgical procedure predisposes them to an increased risk. However, with the ubiquitous application of CT with intravenous contrast in the preoperative assessment of individuals with colorectal cancer, IVP is unnecessary. The urinary tract is well visualized by means of this investigation.

Virtual Colonoscopy

See Chapters 5 and 6.

Computed Tomography

Sophisticated radiologic studies may be worthwhile if they can help in therapeutic decision making before the operation. However, it has been said that CT is not useful in this respect because the presence of metastases does not, in and of itself, contraindicate palliative surgery.[767] Still, although useful information may be obtained, it rarely causes the proposed colon surgery to be altered (Figures 23-14 and 23-15). Kerner and colleagues studied 158 consecutive patients who underwent CT as part of the preoperative evaluation for

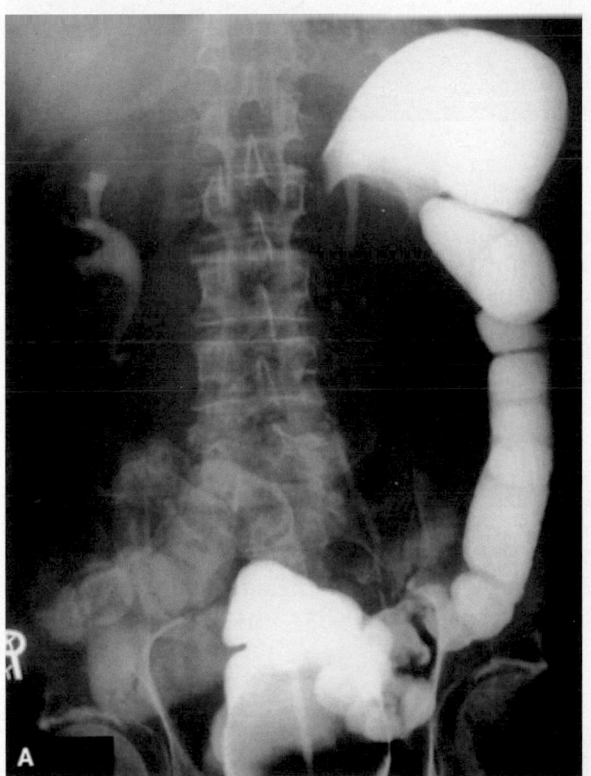

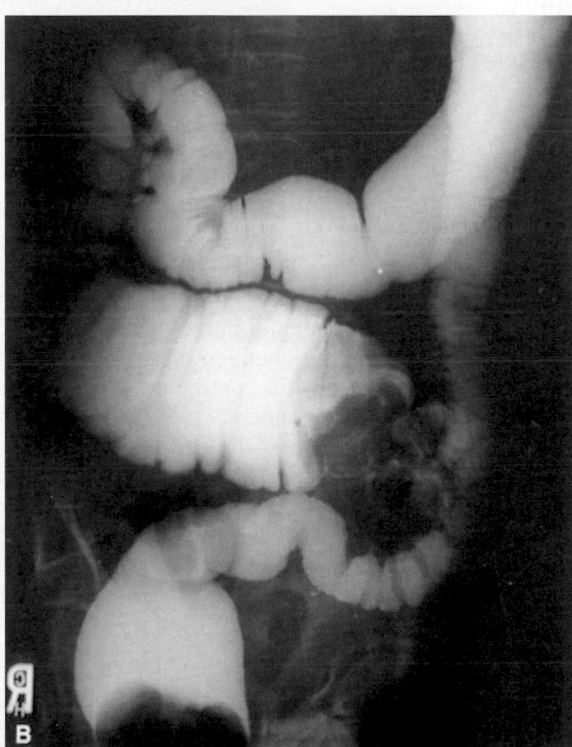

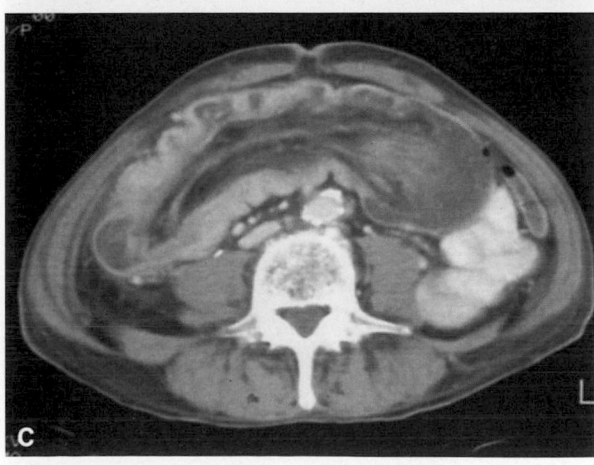

FIGURE 23-14. Carcinoma of the cecum presenting with bowel obstruction. **A:** Note retrograde obstruction to the flow of barium by the rounded mass. The radiologic picture is that of an intussusception. **B:** Following reduction by the enema, the polypoid tumor can be seen to fill the cecum. **C:** Computed tomography reveals the transverse position of the right colon, with a soft tissue mass in the cecum.

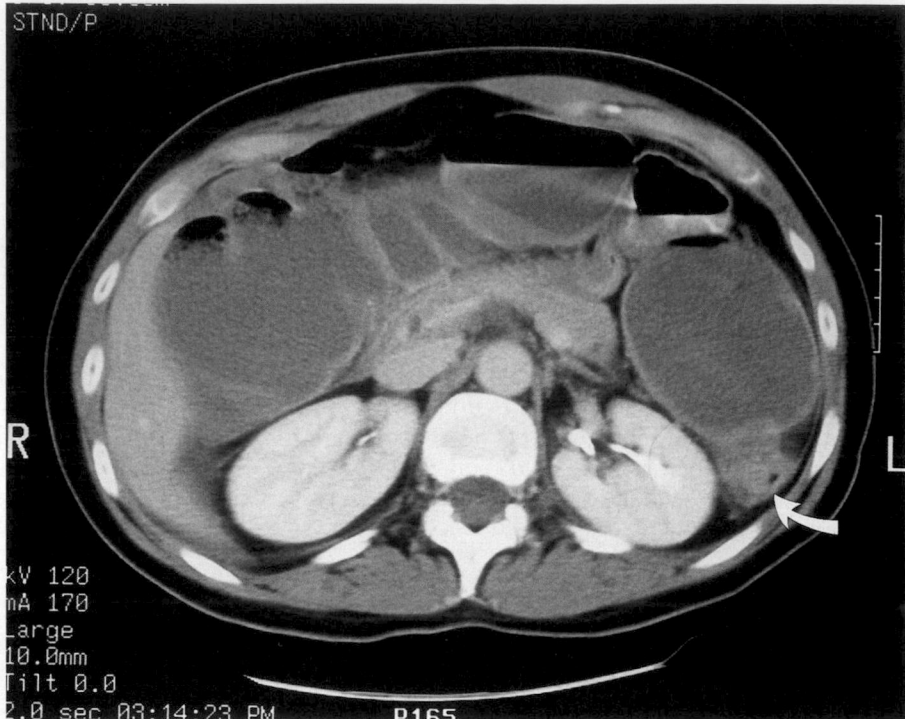

FIGURE 23-15. Computed tomography demonstrates profound colonic dilatation secondary to an obstructing carcinoma of the descending colon (*arrow*).

primary colorectal carcinoma.[515] Fifty-six percent had unsuspected findings, of which 35% were considered clinically important. These observations caused the surgeon to alter the proposed operative procedure, or they added additional technical information that was meaningful in the preoperative assessment. Still, the single most common finding was liver metastasis, with abdominal wall or contiguous organ invasion as the second most common finding.

The issue of performing closed liver biopsy with the potential risk of dissemination of tumor was addressed by Rodgers and colleagues.[852] The investigators undertook a multicenter, retrospective review that involved 43 individuals who underwent preoperative biopsy. The authors concluded that there is a significant risk of local dissemination of the tumor, but there was no demonstrated effect on resectability or survival.[852] Liver surgeons uniformly recommend against percutaneous biopsy if surgery is contemplated.

The accuracy of CT scan for liver evaluation has improved considerably with the incorporation of methods that can assess volume—that is, injection of contrast medium in order to permit visualization of the parenchyma in the arterial, portal, and delayed phases.[24] CT has also been used to assess the stage of the *primary tumor*, but studies have failed to demonstrate that the technique is sufficiently accurate (Figure 23-16).[316] Hypodense contrast media (air or 1,000 to 1,200 mL of water) by retrograde administration (CT enteroclysis) immediately before scanning allow the entire

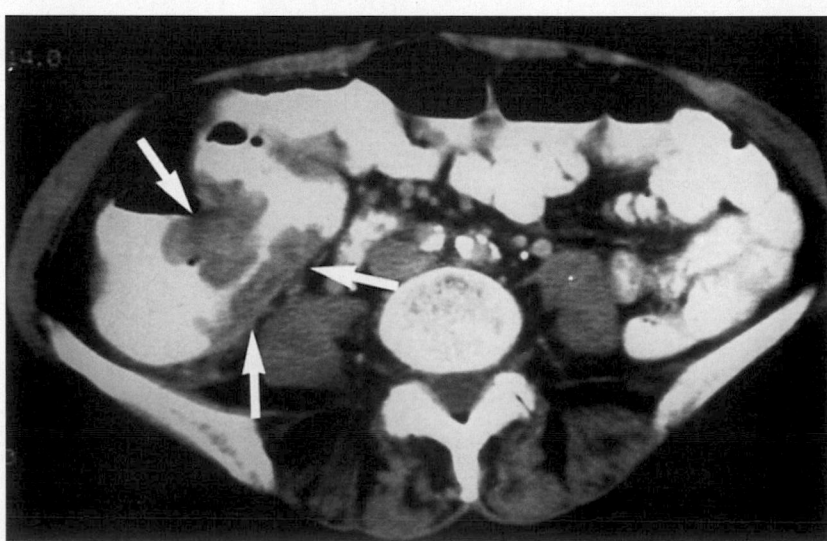

FIGURE 23-16. Computed tomography demonstrates polypoid mass filling part of the ascending colon, consistent with the subsequently demonstrated apple-core lesion observed on barium enema study (*arrows*).

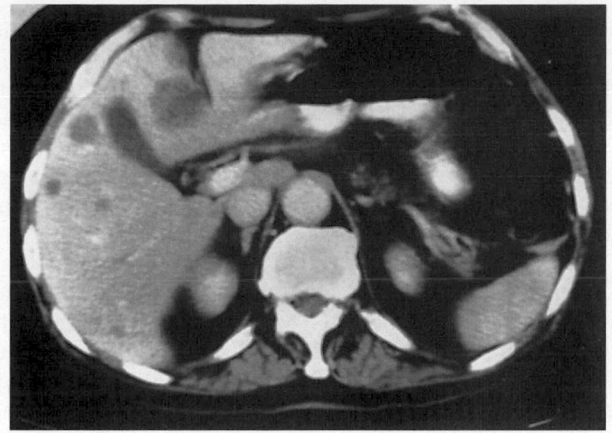

FIGURE 23-17. Computed tomography demonstrates multiple defects in the liver parenchyma, consistent with metastases.

Ultrasonography

Ultrasonographic examination has become well established for the evaluation of a host of conditions within the abdominal cavity—most commonly, assessment of gallstones or gallbladder disease. With the use of sonography alone, however, it has been considered impossible to detect lesions of the colon with any reliability. Figure 23-18 illustrates a classic ultrasonographic finding in a patient with carcinoma of the colon, the "pseudokidney," or "target" sign. Limberg studied this modality and compared it with hydrocolonic sonography in the diagnosis and staging of colonic tumors.[579] The latter method consisted of instillation of up to 1,500 mL of water into the colon following the injection of a bowel relaxant. Continuous transabdominal sonographic examination of the large intestine was then carried out beginning at the time of water instillation. In every case, colonoscopy was performed following the examination. With the instillation of water into the colon, it was possible to display the bowel sonographically from the rectosigmoid to the cecum in 97% of the patients examined.[579] A further advantage was the fact that the layers of the colonic wall could be seen in detail so that the depth of invasion by tumor could be determined. The authors confirmed the lack of value of conventional abdominal sonography. Hydrocolonic sonography is certainly an interesting diagnostic procedure that merits further evaluation.

Transcolorectal endosonography has been suggested to offer an important advantage. The application of this modality for assessing rectal cancers is well established and is discussed in Chapters 5, 7, and 24. Tio and colleagues performed echoendoscopy in some cases with newer instruments that were prototypes being developed.[1024] The accuracy of staging rectal and colonic carcinomas was 81% and 93%, respectively. Although the potential for benefit in managing patients with rectal cancer is genuine (there may be other surgical options besides resection), the alternatives to colon resection constitute a less valid proposition.

large bowel to be visualized for such lesions.[24] The density of the tumor with respect to the adjacent wall markedly increases following injection of the contrast. CT scans have a reported sensitivity of 19% to 67% for the detection of regional lymphadenopathy[464,654] and 90% to 95% for liver lesions more than 1 cm in diameter.[1067]

The main advantage of preoperative CT is that it provides a means for comparison should the patient require subsequent evaluation for the possibility of recurrent tumor.[341] Depending on the timing of planned surgery, one should always try to obtain a preoperative CT scan. This study is a requisite, however, if one plans to remove the bowel by a laparoscopic technique (Figure 23-17; see Chapter 19). The place of CT and ultrasonographic evaluation of an individual with known or suspected metastatic disease is discussed later in this chapter.

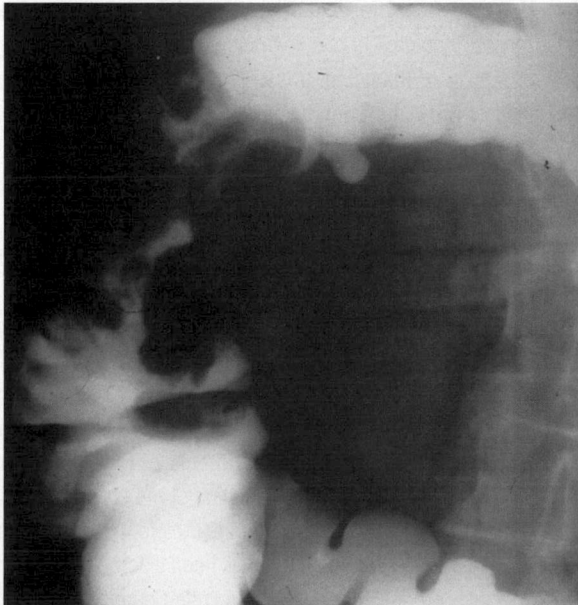

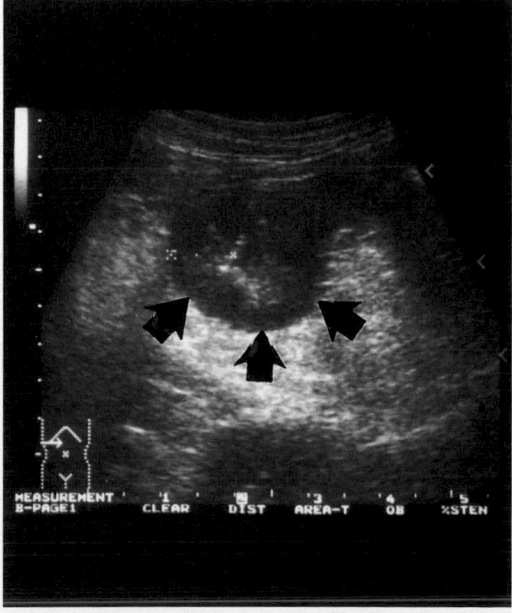

A   **B**

FIGURE 23-18. Carcinoma of the colon. **A:** Barium enema study reveals classic napkin ring tumor with destruction of the mucosa. **B:** Ultrasonography demonstrates so-called pseudokidney or target sign. A hypoechoic mass can be seen (*arrows*) with an echogenic center. The echogenic portion represents the "bull's-eye" of the target. This is the narrowed lumen. The thickened bowel wall, a consequence of tumor, can be clearly seen. (Courtesy of Cynthia Withers, MD.)

Carcinoembryonic Antigen

Attention to the immunologic aspects of bowel cancer has been stimulated by the findings of Gold and Freedman, who identified an antigen in extracts from colon cancer tissue.[343,344] This antigen is a glycoprotein absent from normal adult intestinal mucosa but present in primitive endoderm. It was therefore called carcinoembryonic antigen (CEA). Thomson and associates described a radioimmunoassay for CEA in the serum and reported positive results in 97% of patients with colon cancer.[1015] However, the high accuracy of CEA as a diagnostic test for bowel cancer reported in earlier articles apparently resulted from the fact that most of the patients studied had advanced disease with extensive metastases. In such individuals, CEA is not only frequently detected but also is present at very high levels in the blood, especially when the liver is involved. In cancer localized to the mucosa and submucosa, without invasion into the muscularis propria, the percentage of patients with an elevated test result falls to between 30% and 40%. Even when recurrence is confined to the bowel wall, the results of the test are usually negative. Therefore, the use of CEA as a screening technique for the asymptomatic population cannot be justified.[342,436,844]

Despite this admonition, levels of CEA can be applied usefully in assessing the prognosis of individuals with colorectal cancer. If the tumor has been completely excised, any elevated level preoperatively should return to normal within a few days. A limited fall to an intermediate, albeit elevated, level is indicative of incomplete excision. Subsequent elevation after return to normal implies recurrence of tumor (see later). There have been many articles attesting to the fact that preoperative and postoperative assessment of the serum CEA level is extremely helpful in determining whether tumor has been left behind after operation. This is true not only after resection of the primary cancer but also after resection for recurrent tumor.[448] Specifically, by determining preoperative and postoperative CEA levels, one can identify patients in a poorer prognostic group who may benefit from early introduction of adjuvant therapy.[178]

The preoperative CEA level in and of itself also has some prognostic significance. Patients with localized disease (as evaluated by clinical methods) have a higher recurrence rate when a high preoperative CEA level is noted than when the preoperative level is low.[424] Such an elevation may be suggestive of inapparent spread of the tumor. Wiratkapun and coworkers noted that CEA levels about 15 ng/mL predicted an increased risk of metastatic recurrence in potentially curative colonic cancer.[1111] This suggests undetected disseminated disease. Ashton and colleagues demonstrated a statistically significant association between survival and a high preoperative CEA level.[35] Others have demonstrated a relationship between the preoperative CEA level and the depth of invasion according to Dukes' classification (see later).[1119] Tumor fixation has also been correlated with the level of CEA elevation.[268] Sener and colleagues showed, through the use of a cancer registry system in a retrospective analysis, that the preoperative serum CEA level can be an indicator of survival that is independent of the stage of disease at diagnosis.[916]

CEA is of limited value in the search for a primary site if metastatic carcinoma is noted. The antigen is detected

PHIL GOLD (1936–PRESENT)

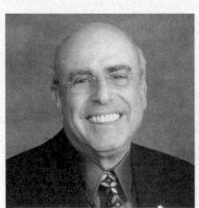

Phil Gold was born in Montreal, Canada and attended McGill University in that city, where he obtained four degrees. He received a bachelor of science in physiology in 1957 and his doctorate in medicine as well as master of science in 1961. Medical graduation was accompanied by the Wood Gold Medal, the J. Francis Williams Scholarship in Medicine and Clinical Medicine, the Women's Pavilion Prize in Obstetrics and Gynecology, and the Prize of the College of Physicians and Surgeons of the Province of Quebec in Pathology and Medicine. After a year of rotating internship and another of residency in internal medicine, the next 2 years were spent in the laboratories of the Montreal General Hospital Research Institute; he obtained a PhD for his thesis *Carcinoembryonic Antigens of the Human Digestive System*. Gold's discovery of the carcinoembryonic antigen (CEA), along with the description of α-fetoprotein at about the same time, ushered in the modern era of human tumor marker research. The radioimmunoassay for circulating serum CEA has become the most frequently used marker for human cancer. During training at the Public Health Research Institute of New York City in 1967 and 1968 as a Centennial Fellow of the Medical Research Council of Canada, Gold acquired the concepts and technology for electromicroscopy, tissue culture, virology, and cell biology. He then returned to the Montreal General Hospital, its Research Institute, and McGill University as an assistant professor of medicine and a medical research council career investigator. In 1972, he was appointed professor of medicine. In 1977, he became Director of the Division of Clinical Immunology and Allergy at the Montreal General Hospital, and the following year he assumed the position as the first Director of the McGill Cancer Centre, now the Department of Oncology of McGill's Faculty of Medicine. In 1980, Gold returned to the Montreal General Hospital as Physician-in-Chief and served as the Chairman of the Department of Medicine at McGill University for the statutory 5-year period between 1985 and 1990. In 1995, he became Executive Director of the Clinical Research Centre of the Research Institute of the McGill University Health Centre. The other positions he holds include Douglas G. Cameron Professor of Medicine and Professor, Departments of Physiology and Oncology, McGill University. In recognition of the scientific contributions made by Phil Gold, he has been the recipient of numerous international awards and honors and has been elected to a wide variety of scientific organizations. These include Companion of the Order of Canada, Officer of the L'Ordre Nationale du Québec, and recipient of the Gold Medal Award of Merit of the Graduate Society of McGill University. (Courtesy of Faisal Aziz.)

in about 50% of tumors of the breast, stomach, lung, and in other solid tumors. Levels higher than normal have also been found in heavy smokers and in persons with cirrhosis, pancreatitis, uremia, peptic ulcer, intestinal metaplasia of the stomach, as well as ulcerative colitis. The antigen has been reported in tissue of intestinal polyps, colonic inflammatory mucosa, and normal intestinal mucosa of children. CEA has also been found in cancerous tissue from the breast, liver, and lung, as well as in body fluids exposed to cancer. In colonic washings, high levels of CEA have been found in patients with colon cancer and colon polyps, intermediate levels in those with ulcerative colitis, and lower levels in normal subjects.[1099] Yeatman and colleagues demonstrated an elevated CEA in gallbladder bile in some individuals who showed no evidence of hepatic metastasis at the time of surgery for the primary tumor.[1133] They suggested that those with slight increases should be followed closely for the possible subsequent appearance of such lesions.

Nuclear Medicine Studies

Positron Emission Tomography

Positron emission tomography (PET) scan is a functional imaging technique that uses short-lived radioisotopes attached to tracers to examine abnormal biochemical processes associated with disease. PET scans typically use fluorine-18-labelled deoxyglucose (FDG) to identify tissues with increased glucose metabolism and transport, such as cancer cells. PET scans are particularly useful in distinguishing indeterminate lesions identified on conventional imaging studies such as CT scan.[952] Such distinctions are especially valuable for excluding occult metastases in patients being considered for resection of metastatic disease or in the detection of disease recurrence.[116]

Liver Scan

The liver scan has been abandoned for the evaluation of this organ in patients with colorectal cancer, either preoperatively or postoperatively. The study has been supplanted by CT.

Pelvic Lymphoscintigraphy

Pelvic lymphoscintigraphy has been used to try to discriminate between normal and diseased large bowel and to determine the extent of nodal uptake, but it has no demonstrable value in the diagnosis or staging of colorectal cancer.[829] Angiography of the mesenteric arteries likewise has not been proved useful in the preoperative evaluation of colon carcinoma.[509]

Radiolabeled Antibody Imaging
Anti-Carcinoembryonic Antigen

A modification of the CEA assay involves the use of radiolabeled antibodies to the antigen followed by an external photoscan.[347-349] Goldenberg and coworkers evaluated 50 patients by injecting antibody against CEA labeled with ^{131}I and performing total body scans.[348] In this study, 83% of the preoperative group and approximately 90% of the postoperative group were found to have the tumors correctly localized. The authors conclude that among other potential benefits, this technique can help to stage the tumor preoperatively and complement other methods used to assess tumor response to therapy.

Beatty and colleagues studied 100 patients with known or suspected colorectal cancer by radioimmunoscintigraphy, using murine monoclonal anti-CEA antigen labeled with indium.[62] Sensitivity was 76% for primary tumors, 44% for hepatic metastases, 38% for extrahepatic abdominal metastases, and 78% for extra-abdominal metastases.

Lechner and coworkers submitted 47 patients to radioimmunoscintigraphic investigations for primary or recurrent colorectal cancer by means of technetium-99m ([99mTc])-fab' fragment (Immu 4).[559] The advantage of this particular commercially available product is that it has a short half-life with high photon abundance. It can be administered at high doses and permits early imaging with a gamma camera. The overall accuracy of this study was 93.75% in primary and 91.60% in recurrent colorectal cancer. The investigators concluded that immunoscintigraphy had a decisive influence on treatment planning in one-third of patients with primary colorectal cancer and was superior to CT in the detection of early recurrences (see the later discussion under follow up evaluation).[559]

Gastrointestinal Cancer Antigen

Gastrointestinal cancer antigen (CA 19–9) is a monoclonal antibody produced against human colorectal carcinoma cell line SW1116.[476,822] However, this antigen is not specific for cancer and has been found in certain normal tissues, most notably pancreas, gallbladder, and gastric mucosa.[476] There is no evidence to suggest that CA 19–9 is superior to CEA in predicting recurrence, although there may be some advantage in screening high-risk patients for colorectal cancer.[822]

Other Antibody Imaging Options

Yiu and colleagues used the same concept through the application of monoclonal antibodies that react with epithelial membrane antigen.[1134] Indium-111 (^{111}In)-M8 detected 13 of 16 tumor sites, whereas In[111]–77–1 detected 10 of 15 tumor sites. The implication again is that these monoclonal antibodies may have a role in the preoperative immunolocalization of colorectal cancers. Additionally, others have shown unsuspected tumor sites using a similar technique, a method that directly affected treatment in 18% of patients.[250]

Yamaguchi and colleagues used another tumor marker, NCC-ST 439, in the preoperative and postoperative evaluation of individuals with colorectal cancer.[1131] This is a monoclonal antibody obtained using ST-4, a cell line derived from poorly differentiated stomach cancer. The authors demonstrated results comparable to those obtained with the other markers, especially when it was used in combination with CEA.

Shibata and coworkers studied circulating anti-p53 antibodies in patients with known colorectal carcinoma to evaluate the clinical application of this technique.[932] Circulating anti-p53 antibodies were detected in 68% of their patients.[932] The authors concluded that this particular analysis may become an important diagnostic indicator of colorectal malignancies (see earlier discussion).

Carpelan-Holmström and associates investigated whether there are differences in serum levels of CA 242, a tumor marker demonstrated to have a high preoperative sensitivity for colorectal cancer and CEA.[157] The authors concluded that the two studies supplement each other, in that the two markers together show a higher sensitivity than either one alone.

van Kamp and coworkers assessed CA M43, a serum marker for colorectal cancer, to determine its clinical utility.[1049] This monoclonal antibody study identifies tumor-associated mucin. The investigators concluded that this marker shows a positivity rate equivalent to that of CEA, and as was demonstrated with CA 242, it appears to complement CEA. Together, they reached 87% positivity in the presence of metastatic disease.[1049]

Vasoactive Intestinal Peptide Receptor Imaging

Vasoactive intestinal peptide (VIP) is a major regulator of water and electrolyte secretion in the gut. Various endocrine tumors, as well as intestinal adenocarcinomas, express large numbers of high-affinity receptors for VIP. Virgolini and associates evaluated the usefulness of scanning with VIP-labeled ^{123}I to localize gastrointestinal tumors.[1061] Among those with colorectal cancer, primary recurring tumors were visualized in all 10 patients, liver metastases were seen in 15 of 18, and lung metastases were detected in 2 of 3. All four patients with lymph node metastases were identified with this technique. It appears that scanning with radiolabeled VIP permits visualization of intestinal tumors and metastases, provided, of course, that they express receptors for VIP.

Comment

The advent of monoclonal antibody technology has permitted the development of a number of radiolabeled tumor-reactive probes. These can be used in conjunction with gamma camera imaging equipment to identify the anatomic distribution of colorectal cancer within an individual. The reader is referred to the discussion on the postoperative application of these techniques in the section on follow-up evaluation. The real excitement will occur when it will be possible to attach a therapeutic agent to the monoclonal antibody to treat the primary or metastatic cancer.

Serum Gastrin

Kameyama and colleagues evaluated the relationship between serum gastrin levels and liver metastases in colorectal cancer to determine whether serum gastrin can be used as a predictor of liver metastases, independent of other prognostic variables.[505] In a series of 140 patients who underwent surgery for colorectal cancer, the fasting serum gastrin level was determined preoperatively. The incidence of liver metastases was statistically significantly higher in those patients with a serum gastrin level of 150 pg/mL or greater than in those with a serum gastrin level less than this number.[505] These results suggest that serum gastrin serves as a useful predictor of liver metastases that correlates well with the pathologic determination of venous invasion.

Leukocyte Adherence Inhibition

The leukocyte adherence inhibition assay is an in vitro test based on the observation that, following incubation with tumor extracts from the same organ, leukocytes from cancer patients lose their ability to adhere to glass surfaces.[44] Reports have demonstrated relatively consistent identification of malignant processes.[384,1003,1016] Theoretically, it may be possible to use this phenomenon to improve the detection rate of colorectal cancer.[583] However, the lack of specificity for localization of the growth and inconsistencies in the performance of the technique relegate the procedure at this time to the status of a research tool.

▶ PATHOLOGY

By far the most common malignant lesion affecting the colon and rectum is adenocarcinoma. The tumor arises from the glandular epithelium, and it can invade microscopic blood vessels as well as metastasize to distant organs, most commonly the liver. It can spread by way of the lymphatics to regional lymph nodes and ultimately pass into the systemic circulation. The tumor may also extend locally into adjacent organs (e.g., posterior vaginal wall, uterus, bladder, small bowel, stomach, and retroperitoneal structures).

Microscopic Appearance

Histologically, the cancer may appear well differentiated (Figure 23-19), moderately differentiated (Figure 23-20), or poorly differentiated (Figure 23-21). The tumor may produce so much mucin that the nucleus is pushed to one side of the cell, creating a signet ring appearance (Figure 23-22). This last type has been the subject of some debate with respect to its prognostic implications. Minsky has observed that the incidence of this manifestation in patients with colorectal cancer is approximately 17%.[686] He found that colloid carcinoma was not an independent prognostic factor for survival, but believed that it should be reported separately from other histologic patterns in order to achieve a better understanding of its natural history. Generally, the more poorly differentiated tumors are more invasive at the time of diagnosis, and the more invasive the tumor, the poorer the prognosis.

Macroscopic Appearance

In addition to degree of differentiation, tumor morphology—whether polypoid, infiltrative, or ulcerated—has been found to be an important prognostic variable. It, too, should be reported as part of a comprehensive pathologic evaluation of the patient.[972] Macroscopically, the tumor can display a number of forms (Figures 23-23 through 23-32).

Factors Affecting Rates of Growth and Spread of Tumor

Carcinomas of the colon and rectum are relatively slow-growing tumors. Symptoms usually appear early in the development of the disease, and metastases occur relatively late. Tumor growth and spread display considerable variation, depending partly on histologic grade (based on cellular

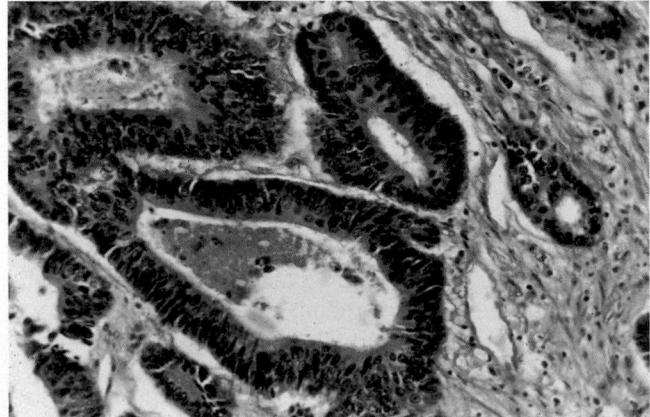

FIGURE 23-19. Well-differentiated adenocarcinoma. The neoplastic glands display somewhat oriented epithelium and resemble crypts in their overall architecture. (Original magnification × 250; courtesy of Rudolf Garret, MD.)

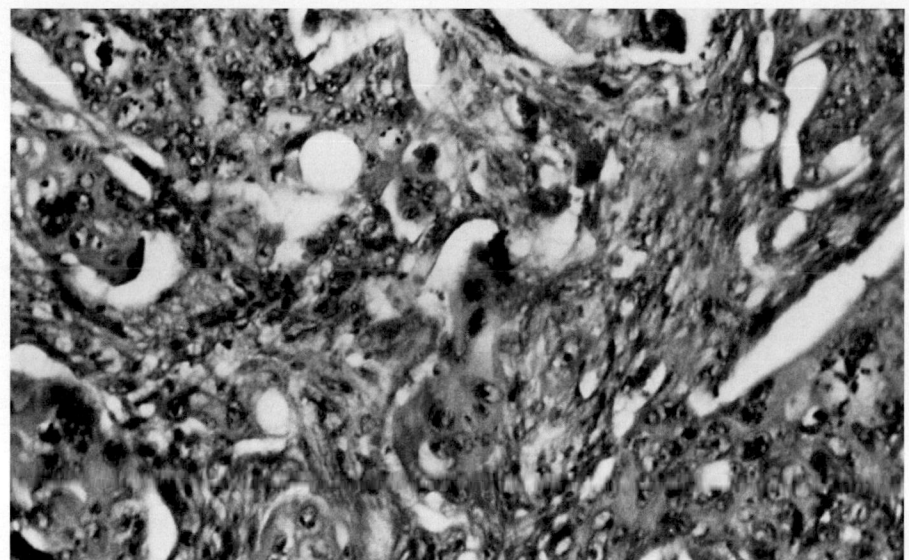

FIGURE 23-20. Moderately differentiated adenocarcinoma. The glands are more irregular and exhibit less orientation of the epithelium. (Original magnification × 250; courtesy of Rudolf Garret, MD.)

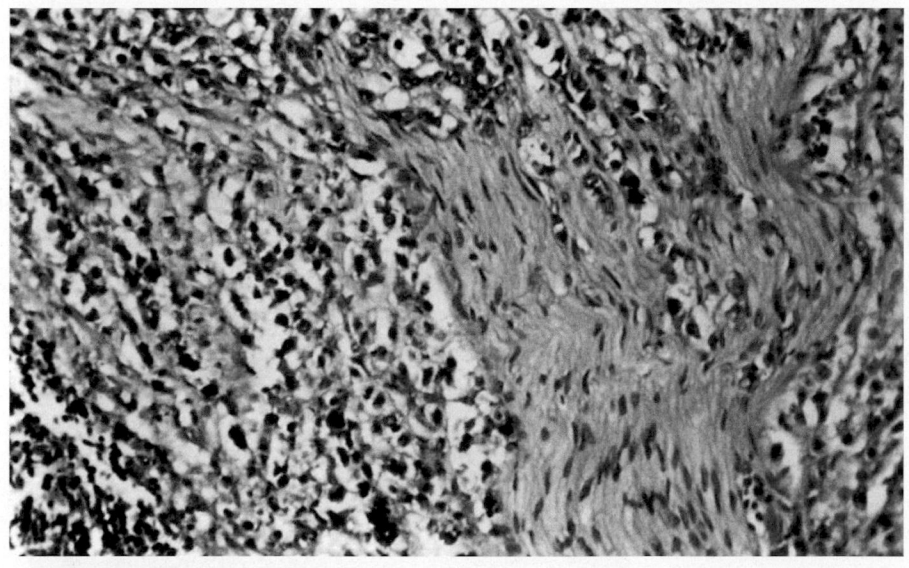

FIGURE 23-21. Poorly differentiated (undifferentiated) adenocarcinoma. There is no definite formation of glands. (Original magnification × 250; courtesy of Rudolf Garret, MD.)

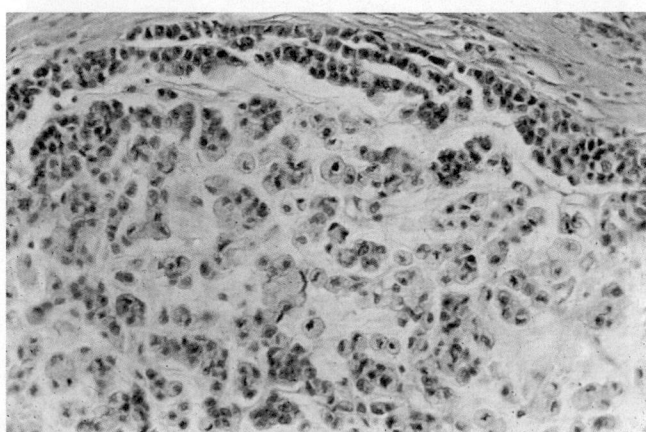

FIGURE 23-22. Signet ring carcinoma. In this malignant variant, mucin displaces the nucleus to one side. This is occasionally seen in lesions of the right side and when carcinoma arises in ulcerative colitis. (Original magnification × 600; from Corman ML, Veidenheimer MC, Swinton NW. *Diseases of the Anus, Rectum, and Colon. Part I: Neoplasms.* New York, NY: Medcom; 1972, with permission.)

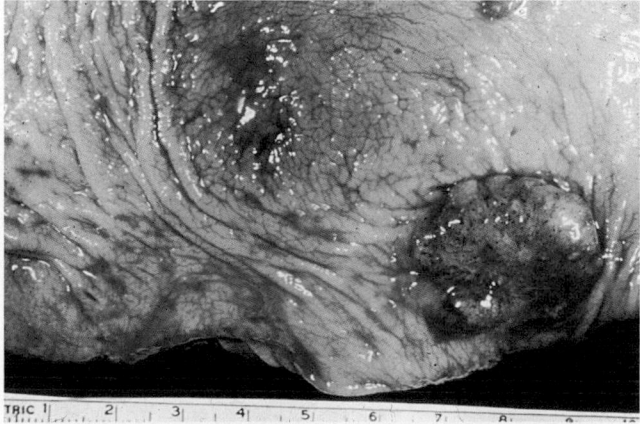

FIGURE 23-23. Relatively small polypoid carcinoma. (From Corman ML, Veidenheimer MC, Swinton NW. *Diseases of the Anus, Rectum, and Colon. Part I: Neoplasms.* New York, NY: Medcom; 1972, with permission.)

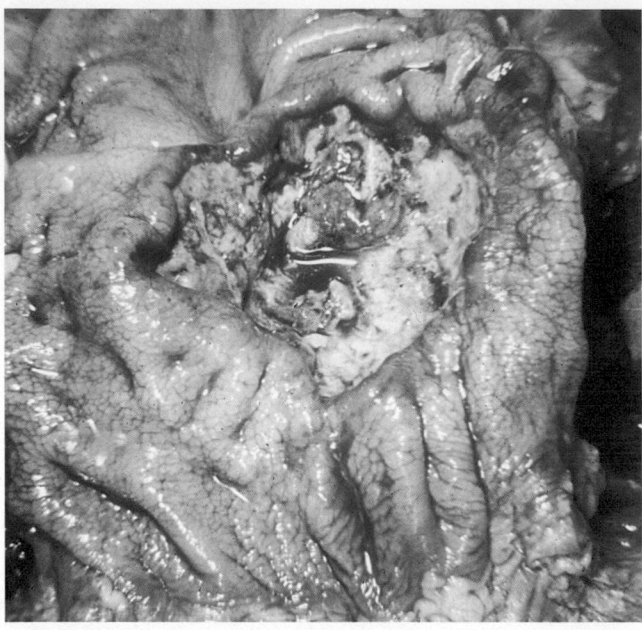

FIGURE 23-24. Ulcerating carcinoma. (From Corman ML, Veidenheimer MC, Swinton NW. *Diseases of the Anus, Rectum, and Colon. Part I: Neoplasms.* New York, NY: Medcom; 1972, with permission.)

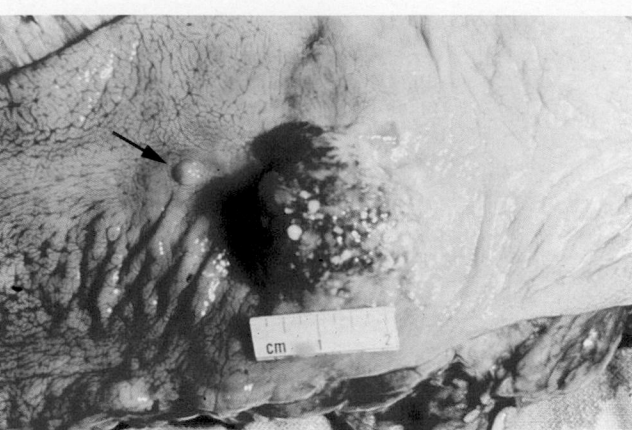

FIGURE 23-26. Polypoid carcinoma with mucosal hyperplasia (*arrow*). This association is commonly seen. (From Corman ML, Veidenheimer MC, Swinton NW. *Diseases of the Anus, Rectum, and Colon. Part I: Neoplasms.* New York, NY: Medcom; 1972, with permission.)

arrangement and differentiation), increased ameboid action of some cancer cells, enzymes such as hyaluronidase, decreased adhesiveness of the tumor cells, size of the lesion at the primary site, and length of time the tumor has been present.[379,990] Daneker and colleagues showed the interaction of the tumor with the basement membrane to be an important factor in predicting spread.[222] They noted that in general, more poorly differentiated cancers tend to adhere and therefore to invade much more readily. Additional variables include location of the tumor, indeterminate host

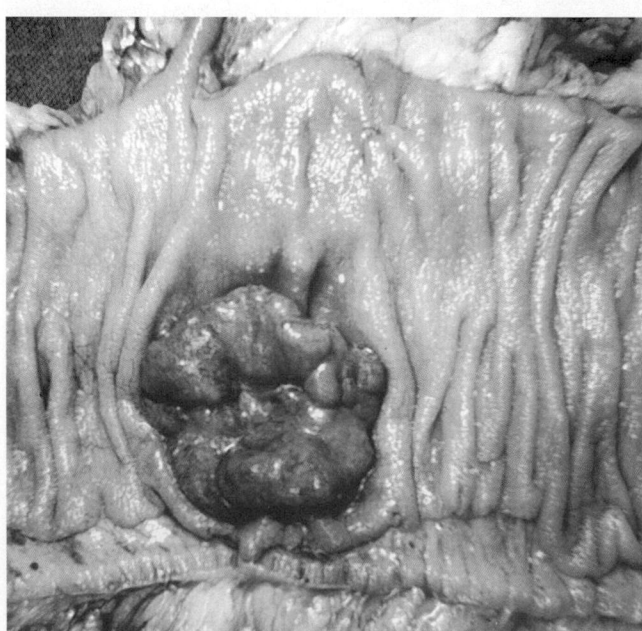

FIGURE 23-25. Polypoid carcinoma with ulceration. (From Corman ML, Veidenheimer MC, Swinton NW. *Diseases of the Anus, Rectum, and Colon. Part I: Neoplasms.* New York, NY: Medcom; 1972, with permission.)

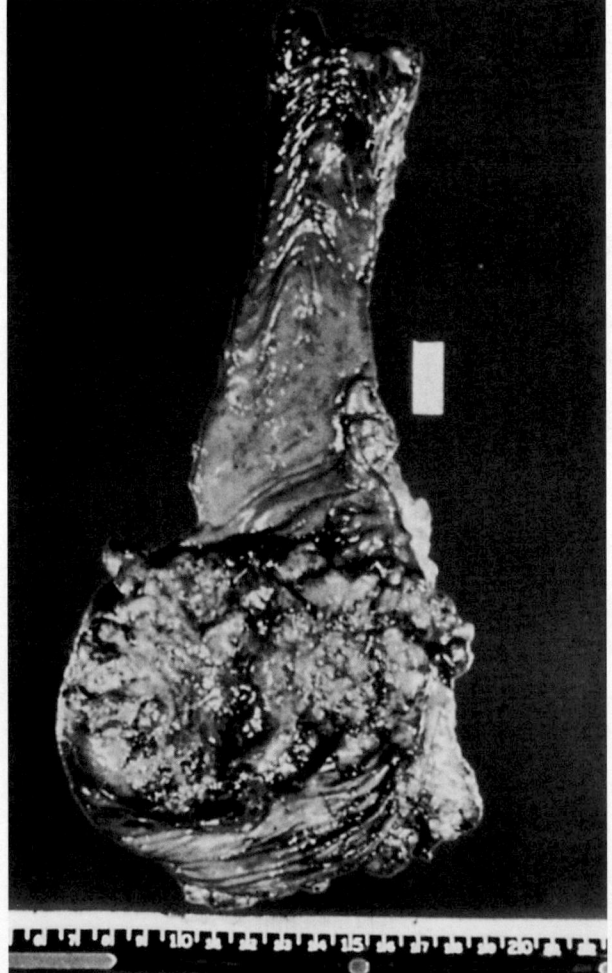

FIGURE 23-27. Large polypoid carcinoma. Despite its size, the prognosis is better with this tumor than with a smaller, invasive lesion. (From Corman ML, Veidenheimer MC, Swinton NW. *Diseases of the Anus, Rectum, and Colon. Part I: Neoplasms.* New York, NY: Medcom; 1972, with permission.)

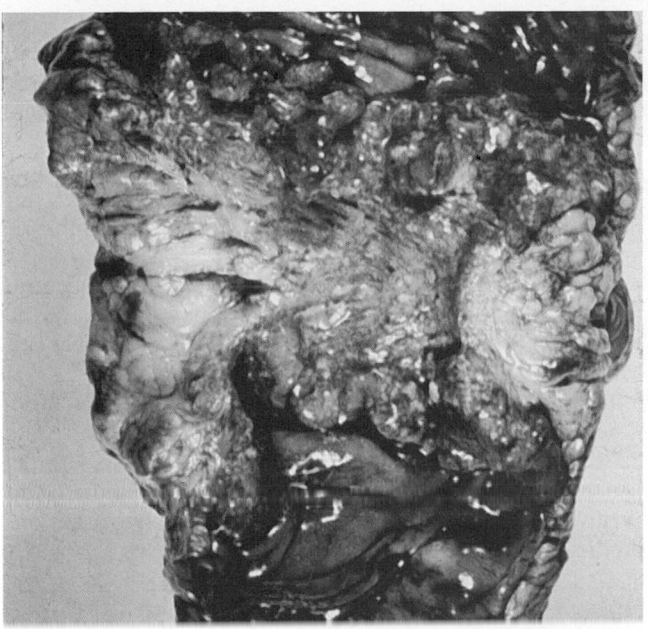

FIGURE 23-28. Scirrhous or infiltrating carcinoma is associated with a poorer prognosis. (From Corman ML, Veidenheimer MC, Swinton NW. *Diseases of the Anus, Rectum, and Colon. Part I: Neoplasms*. New York, NY: Medcom; 1972, with permission.)

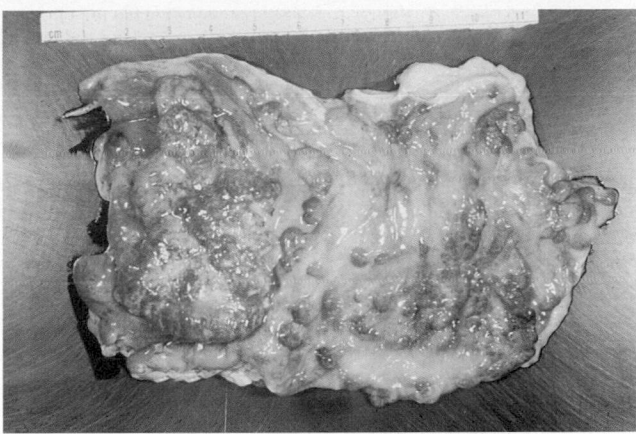

FIGURE 23-30. Colloid carcinoma. Prognosis has generally been believed to bo pooror with thio variant of carcinoma. Note the gelatinous appearance. (From Corman ML, Veidenheimer MC, Swinton NW. *Diseases of the Anus, Rectum, and Colon. Part I: Neoplasms*. New York, NY: Medcom; 1972, with permission.)

factors, manipulation at surgery, and the age and sex of the person.[40,189,270,440,889]

Histochemical studies assess those factors that contribute to tumor growth and spread. These include changes in sialomucin in the distal resection margin and the presence of human chorionic gonadotropin.[229,938] For example, Dawson and colleagues showed that sialomucin adjacent to a primary colorectal cancer provides a crude assessment of tumor invasiveness and therefore the risk for local recurrence.[228]

Ideally, as more information is developed about prognostic factors, more meaningful recommendations with respect to supplementary therapy will be made.

The first opportunity to measure the growth of colonic cancer at its site of origin was reported in 1961 by Spratt and Ackerman.[955] In this study, nine air-contrast enemas were performed during a period of 7.5 years.[954] Radiographic measurements of the tumor were taken, and by appropriate plotting on a graph, the growth curve was shown to conform to an exponential increase in volume. The tumor was calculated to have a doubling time of 636.5 days. When desquamation from the surface was taken into account, it was postulated that a net increase of only one cell per 1,000 cells per day was adequate to account for the observed rate of growth. Another study demonstrated the mean doubling time of tumor volume to be only 130 days.[103] The authors believed that this high rate of growth could be attributed to the large

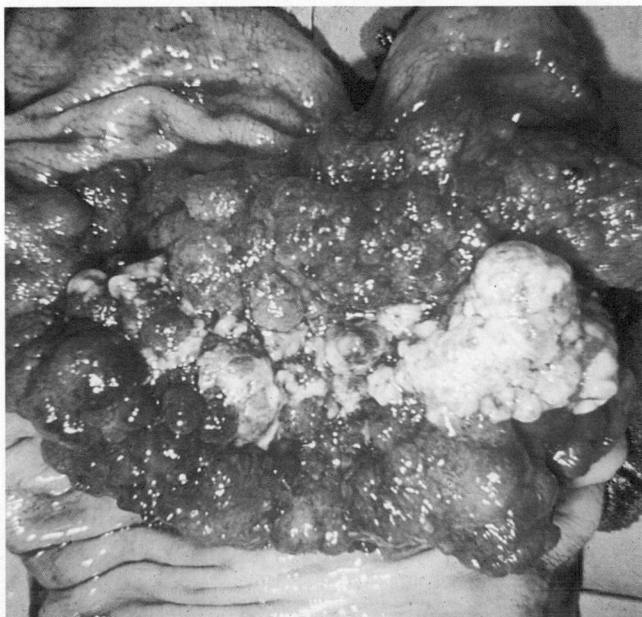

FIGURE 23-29. Carcinoma (*light area*, **center**) arising in villous adenoma. (From Corman ML, Veidenheimer MC, Swinton NW. *Diseases of the Anus, Rectum, and Colon. Part I: Neoplasms*. New York, NY: Medcom; 1972, with permission.)

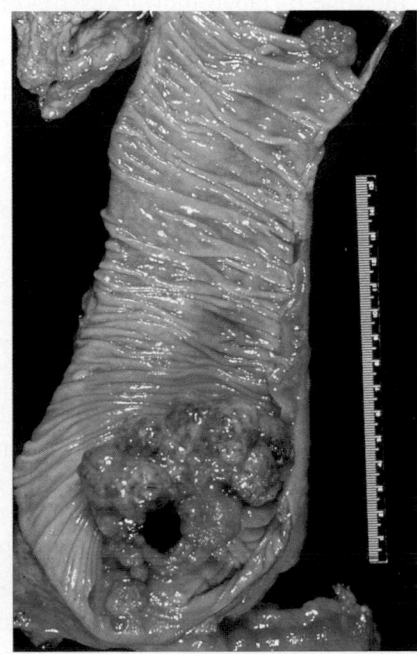

FIGURE 23-31. Perforated cecal carcinoma.

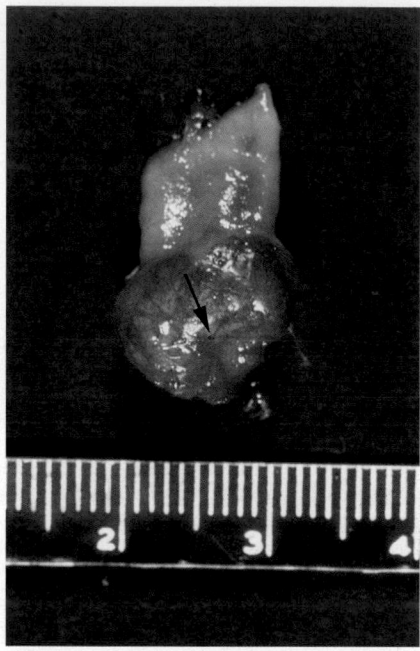

FIGURE 23-32. A polypoid adenoma with carcinoma at the tip. An ulcer is shown (*arrow*). (Courtesy of Rudolph Garret, MD.)

size of the tumors and therefore their greater likelihood of being malignant at the initial examination.

Doubling time of pulmonary metastases from colon and rectal carcinomas has been calculated radiographically and found to be 109 days.[953] Metastatic tumors increase their cellular complement six times faster than primary cancers.[954] It is theorized that the absence of desquamation in the metastatic site accounts for this observed difference.

Finlay and colleagues studied the growth rate of hepatic metastases by means of serial CT.[299] They discovered that the mean doubling time for obvious metastases (those discovered at the time of laparotomy) was 155 days, compared with 86 days for occult metastases. By means of extrapolation, the authors concluded that the mean age of the former lesions was 3.7 years, and the latter was 2.3 years.

The metastatic behavior of neoplasms varies. According to Spratt, examination of the cancer-host interface is helpful in determining the behavioral pattern of the tumor.[953] One that is less likely to metastasize exhibits a well-circumscribed, intact margin. The tumor that is more likely to metastasize to lymph nodes has a loose or infiltrating margin with little inflammatory reaction. Sacchi and coworkers looked at the border between normal tissue and tumor in colorectal cancer and opined that it is the mast cell, probably influenced by the inflammatory infiltrate and/or colorectal cancer cells themselves, which destroy lymphatic vessels, thereby preventing spread into the lymphatic system.[874]

Some investigators have suggested that the concentration of circulating C-reactive protein may play a role in predicting recurrence and survival in colorectal cancer. McMillan and colleagues studied the presence of a systemic inflammatory response as measured by circulating C-reactive protein in 174 patients who were believed to have undergone a curative resection.[666] C-reactive protein concentration was found to be an independent predictor for survival—that is, the presence of elevated concentrations predicts a poor outcome.

Delay in Diagnosis: Legal Implication

The one article by Spratt and Ackerman has been responsible for more confusion, misinterpretation, and misrepresentation in the sphere of medical litigation with respect to the accusation of delay in diagnosis than all other variables combined. A question asked by attorneys in medicolegal actions is when an earlier diagnosis will make a difference with respect to prognosis (see Chapter 34). Clearly, the issue of tumor doubling time does not provide the answer. In an unofficial poll of the Chicago Society of Colon and Rectal Surgeons (1997), all but 2 of the more than 50 surgeons who were in attendance responded "6 months." For the record, the concept of cancer doubling time is without merit in considering the likelihood of survival and its applicability to earlier diagnosis and prognosis in the individual patient.

Staging and Prognosis—History and Current Status

Classifications

The importance of tumor invasion and its prognostic implications was postulated by Dukes in 1930 and was subsequently revised by him in 1932.[262,263] This has come to be known as Dukes' classification (not Duke's). The classification was originally directed toward rectal cancer (Table 23-1). After performing numerous meticulous dissections of resected specimens to identify metastases to lymph nodes, Dukes

CUTHBERT ESQUIRE DUKES (1890–1977)

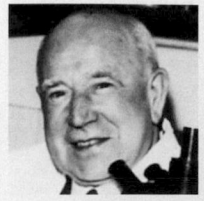

Cuthbert Dukes was born in Bridgwater, Somerset, England and graduated in medicine from Edinburgh University in 1914. He served in World War I in the Royal Army Medical Corps, receiving the Order of the British Empire. After the war, he became a demonstrator in bacteriology at University College, London, and he joined the staff of St. Mark's Hospital in 1922 as its first pathologist.

It was there that he produced his classification of cancer of the rectum that became invaluable as a guide to prognosis. His many writings include the pioneering work on familial polyposis (and the Polyposis Registry at St. Mark's Hospital) as well as several books. He became successively presidents of the Royal Society of Medicine (1944), the section of urology (1957), and the section of the history of medicine (1959), and was elected to honorary fellowship in the Royal College of Surgeons and the American Society of Colon and Rectal Surgeons.

TABLE 23-1 Dukes' Classification of Rectal Cancer (1932)

STAGE	CLASSIFICATION
A	Carcinoma limited to wall of rectum
B	Carcinoma spread by direct continuity to extrarectal tissues; no lymph node metastases
C	Metastases present in regional lymph nodes

TABLE 23-3 Modified Dukes' Clinicopathologic Classification of Colorectal Cancer

STAGE	CLASSIFICATION
A	Carcinoma confined to wall of bowel
B	Carcinoma spread by direct continuity to perirectal or pericolonic tissue; no lymph node metastasis
C	Metastasis present in regional lymph node
D	Omental implant; peritoneal seeding; metastasis beyond the confines of surgical resection

further modified his classification in 1944.[264] Those tumors with lymph node involvement but with a negative node at the ligation of the inferior mesenteric artery he called C_1. Lesions classified as C_2 had metastases to the node at the level of the ligature (Table 23-2). The addition of the D category has been generally accepted as representative of tumor spread beyond the reach of potential surgical cure but was not included in his classification (Table 23-3).

Others have introduced their own classifications, expanding and subdividing Dukes' system and broadening it to include colon cancer and disseminated metastases; degree of differentiation; tumor morphology; and histogram pattern, among others.[36,295,523,785,1036,1140] Jass and colleagues suggested a classification based on prognosis[485].

I.   Excellent prognosis
II. Good
III. Fair
IV. Poor

A scoring system was developed based on several factors that appear to influence survival—number of lymph nodes with metastatic tumor, character of the invasive margin, presence of peritumoral lymphocytic infiltration, and local spread. Most observers believe that the classification of Dukes is of greater prognostic value and more reproducible than that of Jass.[233]

Figure 23-33 illustrates other staging systems. In theory, the more one "substages," the greater the refinement potential to predict tumor behavior, and therefore to gain more information about the possible outcome.[738] There is even a Japanese classification that subdivides vertical invasion of

the submucosa into Sm1 (upper third of the submucosa), Sm2 (middle third), and Sm3 (invasion near the "inner surface of the muscularis propria"). The question, however, is whether this is really important, especially in the absence of adjuvant therapy specific to disease-invasion subsets. The TNM system has become the most popular classification in use in the United States and indeed in the world (Tumor-Node-Metastasis). The American Joint Committee on Cancer (AJCC) seventh edition staging system is shown in Table 23-4.

Fisher and colleagues compared the relative prognostic value of the Dukes, Astler-Coller, and TNM staging systems in 745 pathologically evaluable individuals with rectal cancer.[301] They concluded that the Dukes method was the simplest and most consistent algorithm related to prognosis. They observed, however, that the Astler-Coller C1 and C2 designations were a uniquely valuable contribution to prognostic discrimination. The same is probably true of the TNM classification.

Goligher's Commentary

John Cedric Goligher (see Biography, Chapter 21) wrote that the various classifications proposed can create only confusion and mislead the reader interpreting the surgical results from one institution to another. He observed,

> It is the unalienable right of every pathologist and surgeon to evolve his own system for categorizing the extent of spread of cancers of the colon and rectum . . . [but] I suggest that it would be more useful to restrain his urge to classify and accept Dukes' categorization exactly as it was defined by him.[351]

Despite this suggestion, since 1991 the Council of the American Society of Colon and Rectal Surgeons endorsed the TNM staging classification. More's the pity, for I believe that the clinicopathologic classification of Dukes fulfills all reasonable criteria for prognostication. Other studies comparing the various staging classifications concur with this conclusion.[166,233,300,301,581,728] Sadly, the plea for romance and historical precedent has inevitably fallen on deaf ears—the TNM classification has become the benchmark that we all must accept and adopt.

Lymphatic Invasion

The importance of lymph node involvement by tumor has been well established through providing important prognostic

TABLE 23-2 Dukes' Classification of Rectal Cancer (1944)

STAGE	CLASSIFICATION
A	Carcinoma confined to wall of rectum
B	Carcinoma spread by direct continuity to perirectal tissue; no lymph node metastasis
C_1	Metastasis present in nodes but not to ligature
C_2	Metastasis present in nodes to level of ligature

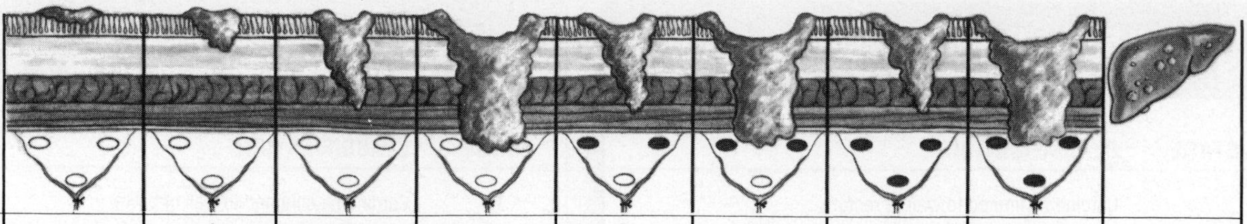

Dukes	–	A	A	B	C₁	C₁	C₂	C₂	D
Astler-Coller	A	A	B₁	B₂	C₁	C₂	C₁	C₂	–
TNM *	T$_{is}$ N$_0$	T$_1$N$_0$	T$_2$ N$_0$	T$_3$ N$_0$	T$_2$ N$_1$	T$_3$N$_1$	T$_2$ N$_1$	T$_3$N$_1$	M$_1$

* T = Tumor · N = Nodes · M = Metastases (M$_0$= none)

FIGURE 23-33. Comparison of staging classifications for colorectal carcinoma.

information.[331,335,368,382] It seems reasonable, therefore, that if one were to use special clearing techniques, a greater number of lymph nodes will be identified, thereby improving the ability to prognosticate.[382,468,796] Koren and colleagues proposed the use of a lymph node–revealing solution composed of various traditional fixatives and fatty solvents to clear the mesentery and identify more lymph nodes.[535] In 30 problematic cases, in which an unsatisfactory number of lymph nodes were found by the traditional method, this approach resulted in upstaging a number of tumors from N0 to N1. The number of positive nodes has been shown in one study to be a more accurate predictor of survival than depth of tumor penetration.[1118] Very few pathology laboratories employ a clearing technique, but if all pathologists vigorously pursued lymph node identification, a greater consistency in reporting the results of treatment would be achieved.

Tsakraklides and colleagues evaluated the histologic morphology of lymph nodes in an attempt to improve prognostic ability.[1035] They found a higher rate of survival (which was not statistically significant) in patients whose nodes showed germinal center predominance compared with those whose nodes showed lymphocyte predominance, the "unstimulated pattern."

Cutait and coworkers demonstrated that by using immunoperoxidase staining of CEA and cytokeratins of lymph nodes previously considered free of disease, restaging of 22 nodes became necessary.[217] However, follow-up at 5 years failed to show any statistically significant difference in survival.

Numerous studies have appeared in the literature in recent years attesting to the impressive survival advantage for patients with more lymph nodes identified in their surgical specimens.[171,499,574] The implication is that low node counts are markers for inadequate surgical technique and/or suboptimal pathologic examination, often falsely "downstaging" patients who harbor undetected lymph node metastases. The need to find 12 or more nodes has even been specified as a quality indicator for colon cancer surgery. However, it should be clear that this is a marked oversimplification of the relationship between lymph node counts and prognosis because studies using node clearing techniques to identify dozens of additional nodes have shown only a minimal frequency of upstaging.[123,906] Indeed, even when surgical and pathologic factors are controlled for, the number of lymph nodes identified in the specimen continues to be strongly associated with improved prognosis.[705] It may be that a greater number of nodes is a surrogate for a more immunogenic tumor or a more immunocompetent host.

Blood Vessel Invasion

Compared with lymph node involvement, the importance of blood vessel invasion (Figure 23-34) has been emphasized to a much lesser extent.[115,122,302] However, the prognostic implication of blood vessel invasion has been well established,[203,936] a fact that has stimulated different approaches to the technique of surgical removal of the tumor (see later).[53,302,882,1036] It should be axiomatic that the pathologist seek to identify and report invasion of blood vessels with the same concern applied to identifying involvement of lymph nodes.

Neural Invasion

As with blood vessel invasion, neural invasion has prognostic import—that is, the presence of perineural invasion implies a more ominous prognosis than if such invasion were not present.

DNA Content or DNA Ploidy

Some studies have suggested that tumor DNA content, as determined by flow cytometry, can provide valuable information about the biologic behavior of neoplastic cells and is therefore an important prognostic factor in determining survival.[27,51,531,908,1093] Aneuploid (nondiploid) tumors contain a population of cells that exhibit a DNA content distinctly different from the DNA noted in "normal" (diploid) malignant cells. For example, Scott and colleagues reported that DNA nondiploid rectal carcinomas were associated with a statistically significant increased incidence of vascular invasion, tumor fibrosis, and advanced Dukes' stage.[907] In another study from the same unit, these cancers also were associated with a significantly poorer prognosis in patients with unresectable disease.[908] Kokal and colleagues demonstrated that in comparison with diploid tumors, tumors with abnormal DNA content tended to be less well differentiated, to invade the serosa or extend beyond, and to have lymph node metastases.[532] It should be remembered, however, that tumor cell DNA content, although it can be an independent prognostic factor, is not as accurate as Dukes' classification in this respect.[108,433,902] Deans and associates performed flow cytometry on 312 patients with adenocarcinoma of the colon and rectum and found by univariate survival analysis that no flow cytometric variable was statistically significantly related to survival.[234] They concluded that Dukes' stage, patient age, and tumor differentiation are the variables most closely related to survival, and that conventional histologic variables remain the best predictors of prognosis for this condition.[234] Others believe, however, that tumor DNA content

TABLE 23-4 Tumor Staging with Tumor-Node-Metastasis (TNM) System

STAGE	DESCRIPTION
Tumor (T)	
TX	Primary tumor cannot be assessed
T0	No evidence of primary tumor
Tis	Carcinoma in situ: intraepithelial or invasion of lamina propria
T1	Tumor invades submucosa
T2	Tumor invades muscularis propria
T3	Tumor invades through the muscularis propria into pericolorectal tissues
T4a	Tumor penetrates to the surface of the visceral peritoneum
T4b	Tumor directly invades or is adherent to other organs or structures
Regional Lymph Nodes (N)	
NX	Regional lymph nodes cannot be assessed
N0	No regional lymph node metastasis
N1	Metastasis in one to three regional lymph nodes
N1a	Metastasis in one regional lymph node
N1b	Metastasis in two to three regional lymph nodes
N1c	Tumor deposit(s) in the subserosa, mesentery, or nonperitonealized pericolic or perirectal tissues without regional nodal metastasis
N2	Metastasis in four or more regional lymph nodes
N2a	Metastasis in four to six regional lymph nodes
N2b	Metastasis in seven or more regional lymph nodes
Distant Metastasis (M)	
M0	No distant metastasis
M1	Distant metastasis
M1a	Metastasis confined to one organ or site (e.g., liver, lung, ovary, nonregional node)
M1b	Metastases in more than one organ/site or the peritoneum

is the single most important prognostic factor among all the clinical and pathologic variables available.[232,532,533] Although there may be some controversy in this respect, there is no disagreement that nondiploid lesions are generally associated with a greater level of invasion and therefore a more advanced Dukes' stage.

Oncogene Analysis
Rowley and colleagues compared DNA ploidy and nuclear-expressed p62 c-*myc* oncogene in the prognosis of colorectal cancer.[863] As discussed earlier, oncogenes exist in the normal human genome as proto-oncogenes but may be activated by various means in tumors, including overexpression and mutation (see also Chapter 22).[863] The authors could not suggest a replacement for Dukes' staging system for prognostication but observed that the combination of ploidy status and oncogene expression predicted survival better than ploidy alone.

Nucleolar Organizer Regions
Nucleolar organizer regions are loops of ribosomal DNA in nuclei that direct ribosome and protein formation.[708] Moran and colleagues studied the prognostic implication of these regions, as well as ploidy, in individuals with advanced colorectal cancer.[708] They concluded that nucleolar organizer regions are the most important individual variable for predicting survival, whereas ploidy values are equivalent to histologic differentiation.

Nuclear Morphology
Mitmaker and coworkers studied nuclear shape as a possible factor in determining prognosis.[693] The nuclear shape factor was defined as the degree of circularity of the nucleus, with a perfect circle recorded as 1.0. A shape value greater than 0.84 was associated with a poor outcome and indeed was the most significant predictor of survival even when corrections were made for sex, age, histologic grade, and Dukes' classification.

Doppler Perfusion Index
Leen and associates assessed the relative value of Dukes' staging and the Doppler perfusion index (DPI) as prognostic indices in individuals who underwent apparently curative surgery for colorectal cancer.[561] This index, the ratio of hepatic arterial to total liver blood flow, was measured before resection by means of duplex/color Doppler sonography. The authors observed that the DPI identified two groups of individuals—78% of those with an abnormally elevated DPI value had recurrent disease or died, whereas 97% of those with a normal DPI value survived. The implications concerning the suitability for adjuvant therapy following apparent curative resection are clear.

Tumor Budding
Tumor "budding" refers to the presence of microscopic clusters of undifferentiated cancer cells ahead of the invasive front of the lesion. This has been believed to have prognostic significance with respect to cure rates following resection for colon and rectal cancer. Hase and colleagues analyzed all surgical specimens for this phenomenon in 663 patients who underwent curative resection.[427] The presence of severe budding was associated with a poorer prognosis and paralleled a more invasive Dukes' classification.

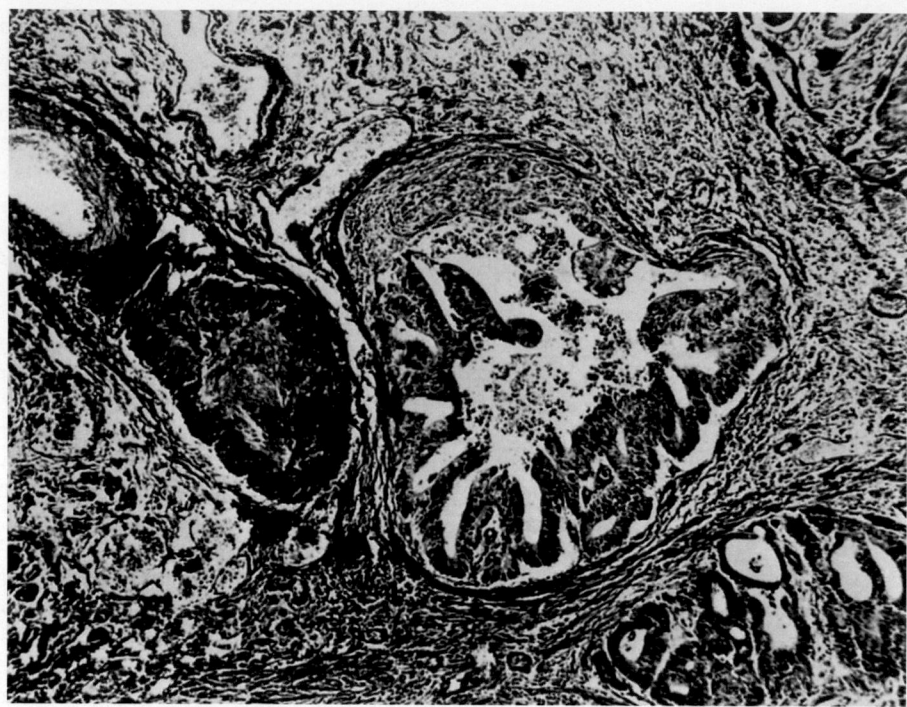

FIGURE 23-34. Blood vessel invasion by colonic adenocarcinoma. Note the extensive growth of tumor inside the vein that has thin, black elastica in its wall and fibrous thickening of the intima in the artery **(left)**. (Original magnification × 80; from Corman ML, Swinton NW Sr, O'Keefe DD, et al. Colorectal carcinoma at the Lahey Clinic, 1962–1966. *Am J Surg.* 1973;125:424.)

Miscellaneous

Lindmark and coworkers, in an attempt to identify better prognostic predictors than Dukes' classification, studied 212 patients by means of clinical, histopathologic, cellular, and serologic tumor characteristics.[581] Dukes' stage was the most powerful variable. Others found significant survival associations with erythrocyte sedimentation rate, leukocyte blood count, alkaline phosphatase level, aspartate aminotransferase level, number of small blood vessels, age of the patient, and six different serum tumor markers.

Proliferating Cell Nuclear Antigen Expression

Cellular proliferative activity has been shown to be a useful indicator of biologic aggressiveness in colorectal carcinoma. Choi and associates investigated the correlation between proliferative activity and malignancy potential in colorectal cancers to determine whether the proliferative index of cancer cells has prognostic significance.[176] Using immunohistochemical methods involving a monoclonal antibody to proliferating cell nuclear antigen (PCNA), they obtained 86 pathologic sections and compared PCNA with conventional clinicopathologic factors as well as other prognostic parameters. The authors determined that PCNA at the invasive tumor margin was a valuable predictor for determining those individuals with a higher potential for metastasis or recurrence.[176]

Anatomic Distribution

Numerous reports have demonstrated a change in the distribution of colorectal carcinoma.[1,148,211,356,374,710,943] It had long been thought that 75% of colorectal cancers were within the range of the rigid proctosigmoidoscope. More recent data suggest that the figure should be closer to 60%.

Cady and associates reviewed almost 6,000 resected specimens of the large bowel that had been removed during a 40-year period (1928 to 1967).[148] During this time, the incidence of cancer of the right side of the colon increased from 7% to

22%, and the incidence of rectosigmoid, sigmoid, and rectal carcinomas fell from 80% to 62%. These changes represented statistically significant differences. A trend to smaller tumors was also evident, with less frequent lymph node involvement of the distal lesions, possibly reflecting an improvement in early detection. Beart and colleagues reviewed the Mayo Clinic experience by studying the new cases diagnosed among residents of Rochester, Minnesota, between 1940 and 1979.[60] They found an increase in the incidence of proximal lesions (from 15.1/100,000 person-years in 1940 to 1959 to 17.3/100,000 in 1960 to 1979). This coincided with a fall in distal lesions (from 35.5/100,000 person-years to 28.2/100,000 person-years). In a 2002 report from the Netherlands, the incidence of colorectal cancer has almost doubled from 1981 to 1996, whereas the proportion of proximal cancers increased from 25% to 37%.[678] Gonzalez and colleagues found that increased age, female gender, Black non-Hispanic race, and the presence of comorbid illnesses were factors associated with a greater likelihood of developing colorectal cancer in a proximal location.[356] In a Veterans Administration study, black race was likewise shown to be associated with a higher incidence of right-sided tumors than that of whites.[211]

A possible explanation for the observed increase in the proportion of more proximal colon cancers is the "search and destroy" concept for the management of colorectal polyps. By clearing the rectum through electrocoagulation, biopsy excision, and snare excision, one essentially prevents the subsequent development of a distal malignancy. Another obvious implication is the limitation of proctoscopy or flexible sigmoidoscopy as a screening tool.

▶ SURGICAL TREATMENT

Historical Perspective

Resection of the bowel with intestinal anastomosis is a relatively recent operation. In 1818, Zang declared that "every intestinal suture is a mighty procedure in a highly vulnerable organ, and therefore a dangerous, yes, a very dangerous undertaking."[314] Exteriorization was the method of treatment for intestinal disease and injury, a technique that had remained essentially unchanged for more than two millennia.

Reybard of Lyons in 1833 was the first to perform a successful resection of the sigmoid colon; for this he was criticized by the Paris Academy of Medicine.[221,843] Colostomy was advocated as a palliative procedure as early as 1839. Before this time, an occasional obstructing carcinoma of the colon was relieved by the spontaneous formation of a fecal fistula, when it was relieved at all. Before 1889, the mortality rate for colonic resection was 60%, but this figure had been reduced to 37% by 1900.[709] Because of the high mortality for intra-abdominal resection and anastomosis, the staged extraperitoneal operations of Paul,[784] von Mikulicz,[683] and Bloch[97] (exteriorization-resection) were usually employed.

The initial attempts to coapt ends of intestine involved insertion of various objects into the lumina of the cut ends of the bowel, with or without the addition of sutures. These procedures involved the use of a reed pipe, goose trachea, cardboard smeared with sweet oil, a cylin-

JEAN-FRANÇOIS REYBARD (1790–1863)

Reybard was born in Cloisia (Jura) in France near the Swiss border. His parents were farmers. His father was also the mayor of the community and was therefore able to send his son to college at Nantes and then to Lyons for the completion of his studies. Reybard developed an interest in medicine while at the university and became an assistant at the Hôtel-Dieu in 1813 when he was 18 years old. While at the Charity Hospital, he had the opportunity of seeing the horrible consequences of war injuries, the result of Napoleon's campaigns. When the city of Lyons was occupied by the Austrians, Reybard treated the wounds of both sides. In 1816, he was appointed to the Faculty of Medicine at Lyons. In 1827, he reported the results of his experiments on intestinal suturing. In May 1833, he successfully performed a resection of the sigmoid colon with a primary anastomosis on a 28-year-old man, although the tumor recurred 6 months later. Because of skepticism by the academy, he offered to repeat the procedure on dogs, but all seven died. While performing an operation for anal fistula, he stuck himself, developed septicemia, and succumbed 5 days later.

FRANK THOMAS PAUL (1851–1941)

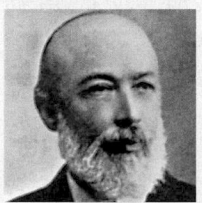

Paul was born at Pentney, Norfolk, England and was educated at the Yarmouth grammar school. In 1869, he entered Guy's Hospital and qualified as a member of the Royal College of Surgeons in 1873. After a year as resident house surgeon, he left London for Liverpool, where he practiced for the rest of his professional life. In 1875, he was made the first resident medical officer at the Liverpool Royal Infirmary. He became successively pathologist, lecturer in dental surgery, professor of medical jurisprudence, and surgeon to the Royal Infirmary. His 1891 article on exteriorization-resection, using "Paul's tube," antedated the modification described by von Mikulicz by a dozen years. Although he wrote little else, he was considered a masterful technician. Lord Moynihan of Leeds often visited his theater, observing that Paul was "the neatest operator he had ever seen." Another visitor stated, "Paul, operating in the heyday of his manual efficiency, always made me think that he did with his hands what Pavlova did with her feet, only Paul's work was much more useful." He retired to grow orchids and died in his 90th year. (Photo from Paul FT. Frank T. Paul—his life. *Br J Surg.* 1951;39:195, with permission.)

JOHANN VON MIKULICZ-RADECKI (1850–1905)

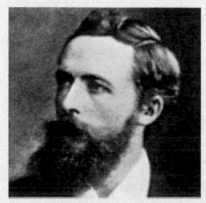

Mikulicz was born in Cernowicz in the Balkan Peninsula, then a part of the Austro-Hungarian Empire. He was educated at Hermannstadt and earned his way through the university by giving piano lessons and playing the organ. He achieved the MD degree in Vienna in 1875 and became an assistant to Billroth. At the age of 32, he was appointed director and professor of surgery at Kraków, Poland. While there, he performed the first esophageal resection and introduced lateral pharyngotomy for excision of malignant tumors of the tonsillar region. In 1887, Mikulicz became director of the clinic and professor of surgery at Konigsburg. At the age of 40 (1890), he moved to Breslau as professor of surgery, a position he held until his death. One of the great innovative minds of 19th-century surgery, Mikulicz's name has been used eponymously for various conditions and procedures, including Mikulicz's cells, disease, drain, line, mask, ointment, and at least 10 operations (e.g., exteriorization-resection of the colon).

der of fish glue, a wax ring, and a silver ring, to name a few.[314,545] Balfour suggested the use of a tube stent.[49] Probably the most famous internal stent was the Murphy "button" (Figure 23-35).[720] Introduced in 1892, it quickly became the primary method of anastomosing bowel.

Until the 19th century, most surgeons regarded wounds of the intestine as a *noli me tangere* (do not touch), believing that nature would be more successful in the healing process than any artificial attempt to effect closure.[918] Travers (1812) is believed to be the pioneer in the use of sutures to perform intestinal anastomoses.[1031] Lembert (1826) is eponymously associated with a type of intestinal suturing that produced a serosa-to-serosa apposition.[566] As he was with so many other operative innovations, Billroth was also one of the leaders of intestinal anastomotic surgery. In 1887, Halsted reported an experimental study demonstrating the submucosa to be the primary layer responsible for a safe and secure anastomosis and emphasized the importance of inversion of the intestinal suture line.[406] This was confirmed in a subsequent report.[407] Later, Connell described his continuous inverting suture.[194] Allis simplified the technique of suturing intestine when he introduced his tenaculum forceps in 1901.[17] For an excellent, comprehensive review of the history and evolution of the diverse anastomotic techniques developed prior to the 20th century, one should read Senn's classic article on the subject.[918] A wonderful, contemporary perspective can be gleaned from the article by Steichen and Ravitch.[968]

In the 20th century, resection of the colon and primary anastomosis did not become generally used until the antibiotic era. In fact, in many centers, resection of the sigmoid colon was not attempted without a diversionary colostomy until the 1950s. Dixon, among others, is regarded as one of the advocates of primary anastomosis without colostomy.[247] Numerous articles have been written that address the means to avoid fecal contamination with bowel resection (closed anastomosis with noncrushing clamps; rubber-shod clamps) and to avoid inverting too much tissue (e.g., the Gambee suture).[322] To complicate the issue further, Getzen and associates advocated the use of eversion, concluding that it produces a more secure anastomosis than inversion.[329] Although this contention was supported by some studies,[152,408,431,587] other reports refuted the observation.[355,873] The hand-sewn eversion technique is in disfavor and should never be used. Suturing has historically been the true surgeons' art form. But today, surgeons-in-training have only a limited opportunity to sew. Maintaining this skill, however, is critically important because there are times that one cannot employ a stapling technique.

de Petz was not the first person to describe a stapling device, but he is generally credited with having produced the initial practical instrument, employing it for gastrectomy.[244] Stapling techniques, however, were developed as early as 1908 by Hültl and Fischer.[969] However, the real credit must be given to the Russians for producing the contemporary

DONALD CHURCH BALFOUR (1882–1963)

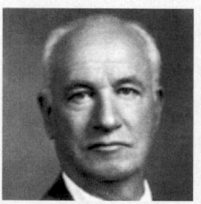

Donald Balfour was born in Toronto, Canada and obtained his undergraduate education at the Hamilton Collegiate Institute. He graduated from the University of Toronto Medical School in 1906. In 1907, Balfour became an assistant in pathology at the Mayo Clinic in Rochester, Minnesota and was appointed successively a junior surgeon and, in 1912, head of a section of general surgery. In 1937, he became director of the department of surgery. In 1910, he married Carrie Mayo, daughter of William J. Mayo. Balfour wrote on varied subjects, including tonsillectomy and thyroid and biliary procedures, but he gradually focused his research and writings on gastrointestinal surgery. He devised a number of instruments—an abdominal retractor, an operating table, and an operating room mirror. Among his many offices and honorary fellowships, he was one of the founders of the World Medical Organization and a charter member of the World Health Organization.

JOHN B. MURPHY (1857–1916)

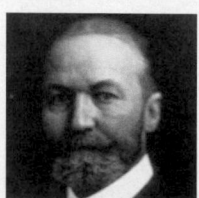

John Murphy was born in Appleton, Wisconsin, the son of Irish immigrant pioneers. He entered the Rush Medical College in Chicago and graduated in 1879, winning the "first place" position as intern at the Cook County Hospital. In 1882, following 2 years of medical practice, he traveled for 18 months throughout Europe and came under the direction of Billroth in Vienna. On his return to practice in Chicago, he became known as a bold, brilliant surgeon and teacher, an indefatigable worker, and an innovator. Although he was often the subject of controversy ("the stormy petrel of surgery"), he was always greatly respected. In succession, he became Chief Surgeon at Chicago's Mercy Hospital; Professor of Surgery at the Northwestern University Medical School; Chief of the Editorial Staff of the *Journal of Surgery, Gynecology and Obstetrics*; and President of the American Medical Association. He was a founder and regent of the American College of Surgeons and a recipient of numerous honorary titles. His writings were diverse and numerous and included treatises on the following: gunshot wounds of the abdomen; appendicitis; ileus; and vascular, pulmonary, neurologic, and orthopedic surgery. His interests in experimental surgery inspired the anastomotic button. Although controversial even in his day, it is still appreciated and indeed has been imitated as an ingenious method of possibly circumventing the risks of conventional suture technique.

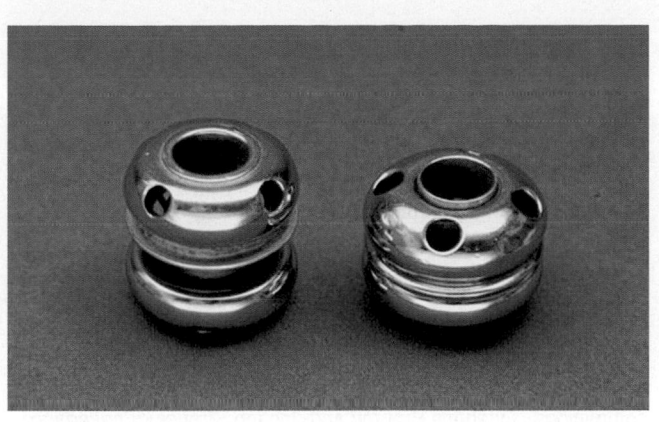
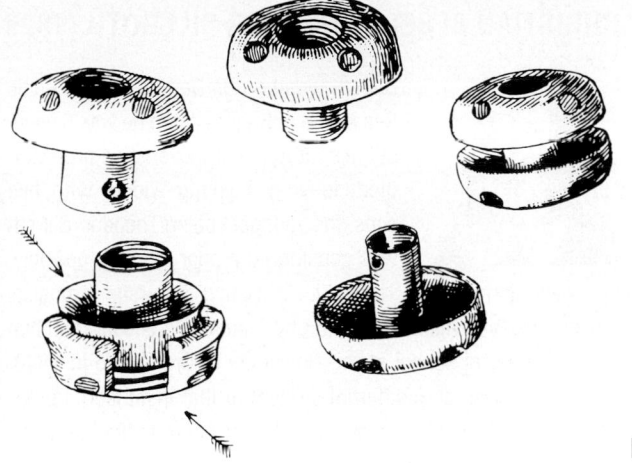

A   D

FIGURE 23-35. Murphy button (A) with and without spring cup attachment (B). (From Murphy JB. Cholecysto-intestinal, gastro-intestinal and entero-intestinal anastomosis, and approximation without sutures. *Med Rec N Y.* 1892;42:665.)

BENJAMIN TRAVERS (1783–1858)

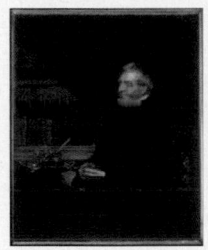

Benjamin Travers was born in London, the second of 10 children of Joseph Travers, sugar broker. After receiving a classical education at the Grammar School of Cheshunt, Hertfordshire, he was taught privately until he was put into his father's countinghouse at the age of 16. He evinced a decided dislike for commercial life, and since his father frequently attended the surgical lectures of Henry Cline and Astley Cooper, he was articled to Cooper in 1800 for a term of 6 years. During the last year of his apprenticeship, Travers gave occasional lectures on anatomy to his fellow students and established a Clinical Society, meeting weekly. Travers spent most of the year 1807 at Edinburgh, and on his return began to practice. He was appointed Demonstrator of Anatomy at Guy's Hospital and was elected in 1809 to the lucrative office of surgeon to the East India Company's warehouses and brigade. The following year he was appointed surgeon to the London Infirmary for Diseases of the Eye. He is justly described as the first general hospital surgeon in England to devote himself specially to the treatment of diseases of the eye. Travers became a fellow of the Royal Society in 1813, and on May 1, 1815, was elected a surgeon to St. Thomas' Hospital. He became president of the Hunterian Society in 1827 and in the same year was elected president of the Royal Medico-Chirurgical Society. Travers was a good pathologist, inheriting the best traditions of the Hunterian School. He was a man of cultivated mind and of a strong personality. As an operator, he was considered nervous and clumsy. Tradition assigns to him an exquisite polish of manners and states that he took off his hat and acknowledged salutes more elegantly than any contemporary dandy. He died at his home in Grosvenor Square, London, March 6, 1858. (From Power D, Spencer WG, Gask GE. *Plarr's Lives of the Fellows of the Royal College of Surgeons of England.* London, United Kingdom: John Wright & Sons Ltd., Simpkin Marshall Ltd.; 1930:2 and with appreciation to Muath M. Bishawi, MD.)

ANTOINE LEMBERT (1802–1851)

Lembert was born April 19, 1802 in Nancy, France. Very little is known about his life, and no rendering of his likeness has been found. He studied under Guillaume Dupuytren in Paris, where he was epidemiologist to the Seine-Départment. In 1828, he won a 5,000-franc prize from the Académie des Sciences for his essay, *la Méthode Endermique*. He is particularly remembered for his intestinal suture, an inverting technique used in circular enterorrhaphy that was published in 1826 (*Mémoire sur l'entéroraphie avec la description d'un procédé nouveau pour pratiquer cette opération chirurgicale*). What has come to be known as Lembert's suture ensures serosa-to-serosal apposition, the cornerstone of contemporary gastric and intestinal suturing. Johann Dieffenbach is credited with being the first person to employ his method successfully. Lembert died of stomach cancer at the age of 49.

CHRISTIAN ALBERT THEODOR BILLROTH (1829–1894)

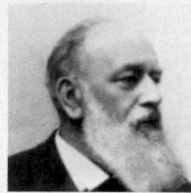

Billroth was born in Bergen, on the Baltic Sea island of Rügen. When he was 5 years old, his father, an impoverished preacher, died, leaving a young widow with five sons, the youngest being Theodor. Billroth was considered a poor student, possibly, by today's terminology, dyslexic. He wished to pursue a musical career; however, his mother and physician uncle encouraged him to enter medical school at the University of Greifswald in 1848. Although he was an indifferent student at that institution, he became inspired when he followed Professor Baum to the University of Göttingen. After 3 years of physiologic and pathologic investigations in a number of areas, he completed his studies in Berlin under von Langenbeck. After a year and a half of military service, travel, and failure to establish a general practice, Billroth fortunately obtained a position as assistant in the Langenbeck Clinic, his entrée into surgery. In 1859, he was appointed professor of surgery in Zurich. It was there that he wrote his famous textbook, *General Surgical Pathology and Therapy*, which ran through 11 editions. He also wrote a number of musical pieces. In 1867, Billroth accepted a professorship of surgery in Vienna. He was the first surgeon to resect the stomach for cancer, the first to resect the esophagus, and the first to perform a laryngectomy. Billroth declined many offers of other positions, including the chair in Berlin, preferring to remain in his adopted Austrian homeland with his close musical companions, Johannes Brahms and Johann Strauss. (Concerning enterorrhaphy. *Dis Colon Rectum*. 1986;29:284–287 [Über enterorraphie. *Wien Med Wochenschr*. 1879;1:1–6]).

WILLIAM STEWART HALSTED (1852–1922)

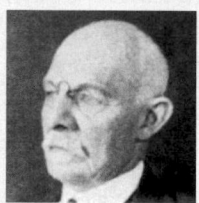

William Halsted was born in New York City to a prominent, affluent family. He attended Phillips Academy in Andover, Massachusetts and received his AB degree from Yale University in 1874. He entered medical school at the Columbia University College of Physicians and Surgeons in New York and graduated first in his class in 1877. After a time at Bellevue Hospital in New York, he became the first house physician at New York Hospital. In 1878, he went to Europe to study at the great institutions of the day. It was through his association with the German, Austrian, and Swiss masters that he developed his passionate interest in clinical and laboratory investigation. Returning to New York in the fall of 1880, he began his practice of surgery. Within a period of 6 years, he held appointments, including chief surgeon, in at least eight hospitals. His clinical duties were awesome, but he still managed to be actively involved in teaching and research. When an infected finger became complicated by painful neuritis, Halsted sought relief by the use of cocaine and became habituated. As an invalid unable to carry on his practice, he came to Baltimore in 1887, having been attracted to the university under the leadership of William Welch. It was there that his genius for investigation flourished. In 1899, Halsted was elected surgeon-in-chief of the Johns Hopkins Hospital, subsequently leading that department for 33 years. He laid the foundation for a model training school for surgeons and introduced numerous instruments and techniques: rubber gloves, hemostat, "mosquito" forceps, and "cigarette" drain, to mention only a few. He was an advocate of fine silk sutures, as opposed to catgut. His study of a comparison of suture techniques to effect intestinal anastomosis is generally regarded as the best example of the importance of laboratory investigation to the clinical setting. Halsted can with justification be called the father of American surgery.

OSCAR HUNTINGTON ALLIS (1836–1921)

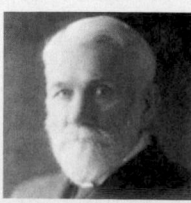

Oscar Allis was born in Holley, New York, a direct descendant of a Puritan settler of the first colony at Salem, Massachusetts. He attended Lafayette College, receiving an MA degree in 1864, and graduated from Jefferson Medical College in 1866. Following an internship at the Philadelphia General Hospital, he ultimately became one of the original surgeons at the Presbyterian Hospital of Philadelphia. Allis acquired a special interest in orthopedic surgery and was recognized as an authority on fractures and dislocations. Relaxation of the fascia between the iliac crest and the greater trochanter, a sign of fracture of the neck of the femur, is Allis' sign. Among his many valuable contributions to surgery were his dissector, his ether inhaler, and his splint—all called by his name. Today, Allis forceps continues to be one of the standard instruments in any general kit.

NICHOLAS SENN (1844–1908)

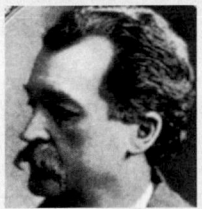

Nicholas Senn was born in the canton of St. Gall in Switzerland. In 1852, he came with his parents to the United States and settled in the frontier town of Ashford, Wisconsin. Following 2 years at a local country school, he attended Northwestern University. In 1865, he entered the Chicago Medical College, and on completing the course of study there, he won the competitive examination for residency at the Cook County Hospital. He practiced for 5 years in the small town of Elmore, Wisconsin, and in 1877 he traveled to Munich, where he spent a year studying bacteriology. Returning to Milwaukee, he was called to the chair in surgery at the College of Physicians and Surgeons in Chicago. In 1888, he became professor of surgical pathology at the Rush Medical College. Senn was a prolific writer, his manuscripts comprising 160 volumes. His personal library was believed to be the best private medical collection in America. Senn was one of the first surgeons in the Western hemisphere to recognize the importance of the animal laboratory as a resource for improving and modifying surgical technique. In association with Connell, it was said that he "constructed the arch and placed the keystone in the structure of intestinal anastomosis."

CLAUDE F. DIXON (1893–1968)

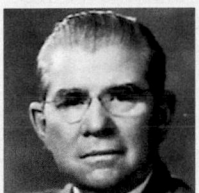

Claude Dixon was born in Piedmont, Kansas and received his doctor of science degree from the University of Kansas in 1919 and his medical degree from the same institution in 1921. Following an internship at the University of Kansas Hospital, he entered the Mayo Graduate School in Rochester, Minnesota as a resident in surgery. In 1928, he became a member of the Mayo Clinic staff and head of the section of general surgery, a post he held until he retired in 1957. With a special interest in abdominal surgery, particularly surgery of the colon, Dixon became one of the leaders in the development of anterior resection. He was also a recognized authority in surgery of the head and neck and contributed more than 300 articles to the surgical literature.

stapling instruments.[314] They, as well as others, performed stapled anastomoses that were sometimes everting and sometimes inverting.[23,823,824] Ultimately, the Russian SPTU gun was described. It produced an inverting end-to-end anastomosis by means of a circular row of staples placed within the lumen of the bowel. The United States Surgical Corporation (Tyco; Covidien, Inc., Norwalk, CT) was the initial developer of stapling instruments in this country, and other American companies produced further modifications. Reports of their successful application are myriad.[352,354,429,825,836] The latest major innovations involve the application to laparoscopic bowel surgery (see Chapter 19).

Preoperative Preparation

For elective colon resection in the United States, patients are usually admitted to the hospital the day of surgery, depending on the likelihood of achieving an adequate bowel cleansing if the preparation is undertaken on an outpatient basis. A more prolonged hospitalization to prepare the bowel or to perform preoperative testing is generally not believed to be necessary and, in the era of cost containment, can rarely be justified to insurance carriers, even when the indications are reasonable.

Several studies have been published comparing inpatient and outpatient preparation for elective colorectal surgery.[315,410,560,791] Results of both approaches are certainly comparable with respect to surgical complications. However, individuals with medical problems may not tolerate extensive fluid shifts and may require intravenous supplementation and monitoring.[560] Certainly, if the preoperative preparation cannot be performed with safety because of medical conditions (cardiac, renal, hepatic) or because of certain logistic concerns, the procedure should be undertaken in a hospital setting.

Mechanical Preparation

A bowel preparation regimen consists of appropriate dietary restriction and mechanical cleansing. Generally, the patient is placed on a clear liquid diet 24 hours before the operation. Ideally, the mechanical preparation begins at noon the day before surgery. A vigorous cathartic is administered at this time so that its effect will have dissipated in time for the patient to have a reasonable night of sleep. The choice of laxative is a matter of the surgeon's personal experience or prejudice because when adjusted for dosage, most laxatives have a comparable effect.[65–67,261,304,420,479] Whole gut irrigation has become (at least for surgeons if not patients) the most commonly used option. Another alternative that has achieved some converts is the use of Visicol tablets (sodium phosphate monobasic monohydrate, USP, sodium phosphate dibasic anhydrous, USP). This has the advantage of the patient consuming virtually tasteless tablets with comparable cleansing efficacy in clinical trials. At least of equal or perhaps greater importance than the administration of the cathartic itself, according to many surgeons, is the use of enemas until the returns are clear on the morning of the operation. The fact is that most surgeons base their protocol in this area on their subjective experience and habit.[1143]

Wolters and colleagues undertook a prospective, randomized study of preoperative bowel cleansing using three different methods—gut irrigation with Ringer's lactate, Prepacol (a combined preparation comprising bisacodyl tablets and sodium phosphate solution), and polyethylene glycol (PEG).[1120] All were equally effective in cleansing the bowel. However, the postoperative complication rate was significantly increased in the Prepacol group despite its being tolerated better. Overall, the authors observed that PEG is the recommended bowel preparation for individuals undergoing elective colorectal surgery. Oliveira and coworkers also performed a randomized, controlled study in which sodium phosphate and PEG-based oral lavage solutions were compared.[762] Although the two were equally effective and safe, patient tolerance was much greater with the sodium phosphate.

The question has been posed whether mechanical bowel preparation is truly necessary. This seems counterintuitive, suggesting that one turn back the clock to those bad old days of a high incidence of septic complications following elective colon surgery. But intraoperative spillage of bowel contents has been reported to occur in 14% of cases, increasing the rate of postoperative infectious complications. In one study, spillage was more likely to occur in patients receiving a mechanical bowel preparation owing to the liquid content.[623] All surgeons agree that it is preferable to deal with formed stool in the bowel rather than to have watery feces spilling into the peritoneal cavity as a consequence of an incomplete preparation.

van Geldere and colleagues prospectively analyzed 250 consecutive operations without a mechanical bowel preparation, with no deleterious consequences observed.[1048] Burke and coworkers also reported whether a mechanical bowel preparation for elective colorectal surgery was indeed required.[132] Patients were randomized to receive a standard mechanical preparation or none. The overall morbidity rate (18%) was similar in the two groups. The two deaths that occurred were both in individuals who had received bowel preparations. The authors concluded that bowel preparation does not affect the outcome after elective colorectal surgery.[132] Zmora and associates randomized patients undergoing elective colon surgery into two groups: ethylene glycol bowel preparation and no mechanical preparation.[1142] Almost 200 patients were allocated to each group. There were no statistically significant differences between the two with respect to overall septic complications (10.2% vs. 8.8%), wound infection (6.4% vs. 5.7%), anastomotic leak (3.7% vs. 2.1%), and abdominal abscess (1.1% vs. 1.0%). In a meta-analysis of randomized trials, Wille-Jørgensen and colleagues found no evidence in the literature for any beneficial effects from the use of bowel cleansing.[1091]

Antibiotics

The nonabsorbable antibiotic regimen advocated by Nichols and coworkers has been believed to reduce the incidence of infectious complications.[739] This consists of neomycin (1 g) and an erythromycin base (1 g) at 1 p.m., 2 p.m., and 11 p.m. the day before surgery. The use of a broad-spectrum systemic antibiotic immediately preoperatively, intraoperatively, and for one or two doses postoperatively has been suggested in numerous experimental regimens to reduce the incidence of infection following elective colon resection.[240,286,360,660,676,1073,1096] In a survey of 352 colon and rectal

surgeons, all favored some antibiotic preparation.[948] Eighty-eight percent preferred a combined regimen with oral and systemic antibiotics. Condon and associates, as well as others, have demonstrated no discernible benefit from adding parenteral antibiotic prophylaxis in elective colon surgery if mechanical cleansing and neomycin and erythromycin are employed.[193,974] However, other investigators have found that the addition of perioperative parenteral cefoxitin, in comparison with oral antimicrobial agents alone, greatly reduces the incidence of wound infections in patients undergoing elective colorectal surgery.[553] Corman and coworkers showed that single preoperative doses of cefuroxime and metronidazole are as effective in the prevention of postoperative infections associated with colorectal surgery as standard therapy with four doses of cefoxitin, but single doses of either cefuroxime or cefoxitin were less effective than the combination regimen.[202] Others reached a similar conclusion with the use of a single 2-g dose of cefotetan, given preoperatively and 12 hours postoperatively.[480,715] Favorable results were reported with a single intravenous dose of Timentin (ticarcillin-clavulanic acid),[94,219,1041] metronidazole-netilmicin,[94] ceftizoxime,[1108] and mezlocillin.[1041] Still others have found that oral ciprofloxacin offers advantages in efficacy and ease of administration and is as effective as other parenteral antibiotics.[656] Jensen and colleagues concluded, based on their prospective, randomized trial, that a single dose of an appropriate antibiotic in acute or elective colorectal surgery is as protective for infection as a triple-dose regimen.[492]

Song and Glenny used several databases and found 147 relevant trials in order to assess the relative efficacy of antimicrobial prophylaxis for the prevention of postoperative wound infection in patients undergoing elective colorectal surgery.[949] Although they confirmed that antibiotic prophylaxis is indeed effective, they could not demonstrate statistically significant benefit with one or another regimen. Still, they were able to show that certain regimens are *inadequate*. These include metronidazole alone, doxycycline alone, piperacillin alone, and *oral neomycin and erythromycin the day before surgery* (note the earlier discussion). Furthermore, they concluded that a single dose administered immediately (or within 1 hour) before the operation is as effective as long-term postoperative antimicrobial prophylaxis.[949]

Opinion and Recommendations

It is clear that systematic antibiotic prophylaxis is indicated for elective colon surgery. Surgeons by now should have accepted the favorable results reported in many studies by using preoperative intravenous antibiotics within 1 hour of making the incision. Furthermore, there is no good evidence to suggest that the oral preparations administered the day before add any benefit. Therefore, the so-called Nichols-Condon preparation should be abandoned. All studies that determine effective blood levels with systemically administered antibiotics indicate that the drug should be circulating within 1 hour before making the incision, ideally less. The likely pathogens when performing colorectal surgery are enteric gram-negative bacilli, anaerobes, and enterococci. Therefore, the most beneficial and cost-effective drugs for elective, uncomplicated colorectal surgery are cefotetan, cefmetazole, or cefoxitin. Another alternative is cefazolin plus metronidazole. In the individual who is allergic to penicillin, fluoroquinolone plus clindamycin is preferred (Medicare Quality Improvement Project, 2002). When there has been gross fecal contamination, in the presence of obstruction, perforation, abscess, and when there has been a prolonged operative time or excessive blood loss, antibiotics should be reasonably continued beyond the prophylactic regimen. A patient with valvular heart disease and immunocompromised individuals may require special consideration with respect to antibiotics (see Chapter 5).

Urinary Catheter

An indwelling urinary catheter should be placed for all bowel operations in my opinion. It may be removed the day after surgery. For an abdominoperineal resection or low pelvic operation, the urinary catheter should remain in place for a longer time in order to minimize the likelihood of subsequent urinary retention.

Ureteral Catheters

The routine placement of ureteral catheters before colonic surgery has been advised by some surgeons. However, most surgeons limit their use selectively, especially to those individuals who are to have reoperative pelvic surgery, who underwent radiation, and when the dissection is anticipated to be difficult. Indications are generally broadened for laparoscopic surgery (see Chapter 19). One must remember, however, that although they may aid in identifying the ureters (by palpation), care must be taken not to rely too much on them. The precaution of seeking and carefully dissecting the ureters away from the area of the surgical dissection should be taken, regardless of the ease or difficulty of the operation or the presence or absence of ureteral catheters. Lighted catheters, of course, permit easier visualization without the need to palpate, but they are quite expensive. Darkening the operating room to facilitate identification by these means is a nuisance. Ureteral catheters are not harmless—ureteral edema, oliguria, and anuria, as well as ureteral injury itself, are potential consequences.[926] However, one unquestioned benefit is that there is no doubt as to the location or nature of the injury when the catheter is divided. It is suggested that the reader peruse an excellent article on ureteral stents by Saltzman.[886]

It is wise to remove one catheter at a time. Generally, the first may be taken out at the end of the operation. The second can usually be removed the following day. Still, prudence suggests that one use the services of the urologist in determining the timing of withdrawal—after all, he or she is the individual responsible for inserting the catheter in the first place and should be given the opportunity to provide an opinion.

Hydration

Overnight intravenous hydration before operation is advisable for any patient who may be prone to adverse cardiac or renal consequences of excessive fluid loss. Oral hydration during catharsis is also helpful and is one of the reasons why a PEG preparation may be the better mechanical cleansing for high-risk individuals.

Hyperalimentation and Nutritional Assessment

Hyperalimentation has been advocated before operation for the nutritionally depleted patient in order to prepare for the assault on the patient's metabolic processes. Many individuals with colorectal cancer have lost weight, are anemic and hypoalbuminemic, or have a variety of fluid and electrolyte problems. With the exception of weight loss, however, laboratory abnormalities can usually be corrected by 2 or 3 days of appropriate therapy. Delaying surgical intervention for a week or more to administer hyperalimentation is an expensive, time-consuming extravagance that has in itself an associated morbidity.

Nutritional assessment has also been advised because of its potential in anticipating postoperative morbidity and mortality. In the experience of Thompson and colleagues, subnormal findings for triceps skinfold thickness and percentage of ideal body weight were associated with a higher complication rate, but these occurred so infrequently that the routine use of such tests was not recommended.[1014] Ondrula and coworkers identified a number of preoperative factors that increased the risk of colon resection: emergency operation, age older than 75 years, congestive heart failure, prior abdominal or pelvic radiation therapy, corticosteroid use, serum albumin less than 2.7 g/dL, chronic obstructive pulmonary disease, previous myocardial infarction, diabetes, cirrhosis, and renal insufficiency.[764]

Opinion

One is impressed by the salutary effects of surgery and the consequent improvement in the nutritional status after the expeditious removal of colonic pathology. The patient can usually commence a diet rather quickly. Therefore, I am not an advocate of the use of hyperalimentation in the preoperative management of patients who need surgery for malignant disease.

Nasogastric Intubation

The routine use of a nasogastric tube is discouraged for colon resections. It does not protect the anastomosis and merely causes patient discomfort. In a prospective study by Colvin and colleagues comparing the preoperative use of a long intestinal tube (Cantor), a nasogastric tube, and no tube, there were no significant differences in the lengths of hospital stay, duration of postoperative ileus, adequacy of intraoperative intestinal decompression, gastric dilatation, and postoperative complications.[191] Wolff and coworkers counsel that even though there is an increase in the rate of minor symptoms of nausea, vomiting, and abdominal distension when nasogastric decompression is not employed, nasogastric intubation still is not warranted prophylactically.[1115] The only caveat with respect to advocating the prophylactic use of a nasogastric tube is the patient who is obtunded or who is at serious risk for aspiration. Obviously, on a therapeutic basis (intestinal obstruction, postoperative vomiting), gastric drainage is indicated.

Thrombophlebitis Prophylaxis

There has been a tendency for many surgeons to eschew deep vein thrombosis prophylaxis because of the fear of bleeding and to a lesser extent because of the misconception that their patients are not at risk for this complication. The likelihood of bleeding is small, about 1%, whereas the risk of a hematoma is approximately 3%. The fact is that the highest risk patients are the ones that are being discussed in this chapter—major surgery, older than 40 years, and cancer—each is an independent variable for increased thromboembolism risk. The use of anti-embolism stockings has been of proven value in the prevention of postoperative thrombophlebitis and pulmonary embolism. It has been suggested that these be worn before surgery, ideally placed on the night before (an impossible criterion if the patient is admitted the day of surgery). Both the use of low-dose heparin and low-molecular-weight heparin have been shown to significantly reduce the incidence of deep vein thrombosis and pulmonary embolism in the moderate- and high-risk patient. Specific guidelines with supporting evidence are available in the ASCRS Practice Parameters for the Prevention of Venous Thrombosis.[957]

Operative Technique

Surgeons must be careful when they take their knife,
Underneath their fine incisions stirs the culprit—life!
—EMILY DICKINSON

General Principles of Open Colectomy
Incision

Most surgeons prefer to perform colon operations through a midline incision. This permits ready access to both sides of the abdomen and allows rapid entry into the peritoneal cavity. Furthermore, it leaves both sides of the abdomen free should a colostomy or ileostomy be required. The wound heals strongly and is easily closed in a single layer. Some surgeons use a right-sided oblique incision for right colon resections. These wounds heal well and are perhaps associated with less discomfort, but one may compromise on the exposure.

Older surgeons have been trained through the adage, "a big surgeon means a big incision." However, the advent of minimally invasive surgery has resulted in earlier return of bowel function, the ability to feed patients sooner, less discomfort, and a shortened hospital stay (see Chapter 19). This has stimulated some surgeons to perform open colon resections through a much smaller incision, the so-called minilaparotomy. Minilaparotomy has been defined as complete resection performed through a skin incision less than 7-cm long. Nakagoe and coworkers in Japan reported that this exposure could be successfully accomplished for colonic cancer in 72 out of 84 patients.[725] Using historical controls,

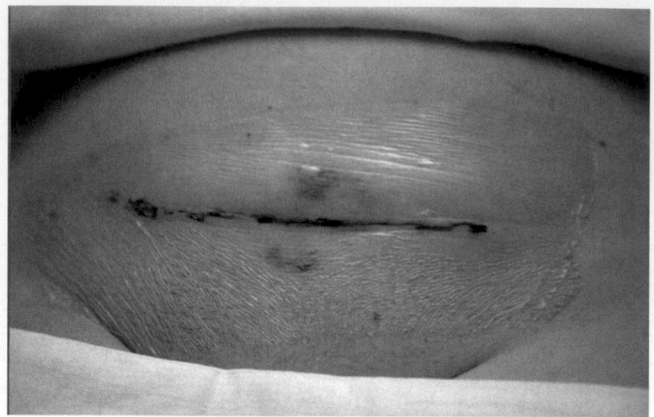

FIGURE 23-36. Maylard incision for a total colectomy. Note the small infra-umbilical incision from prior port site for a laparoscopic cholecystectomy.

they found statistically significant shorter hospitalizations and lower analgesia requirements. However, some surgeons may argue that the body habitus of the average Japanese patient is more conducive to minilaparotomy than that of the frequently large and obese Western patient.

A Pfannenstiel incision can be used for its cosmetic benefit, but exposure may be limited. The rectus muscles, however, can be divided in order to permit better visualization (Maylard incision; Figure 23-36), an operative approach that has merit especially in pelvic surgery (e.g., low anterior resection). Furthermore, this incision may be easily extended, if necessary, to facilitate taking down the splenic flexure. A self-retaining (e.g., Balfour, Bookwalter, protractor) retractor is often inserted for retraction of the abdominal wall. In actuality, Weitlaner was the inventor of the first self-retaining retractor.

Exploration

The abdominal contents are examined carefully for the presence of metastatic disease and any incidental lesion. The cancer itself is evaluated last. It is important to determine whether the tumor is freely movable or fixed, whether abscess or perforation is present, whether the mesentery is

JOHN R. BOOKWALTER (1938–PRESENT)

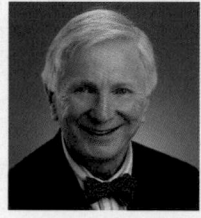

John Bookwalter was born and raised in Columbiana, Ohio. His mother was a nurse and his father and grandfather were physicians. He attended Amherst College and Harvard Medical School, followed by surgical residency on the Harvard (Fifth) Surgical Service at the Boston City Hospital. Following 2 years as a major in the Army Medical Corps at Fort Bragg, North Carolina, he returned to the New England Deaconess Hospital in Boston for a year of training in cardiothoracic surgery. He then moved to Brattleboro, Vermont, where he has practiced surgery since 1973. Subsequently, he rejoined the Army Reserves, ultimately achieving the rank of full colonel. Widely recognized as an innovator in the field of modern surgery, he is best known for inventing the "Bookwalter Retractor," a table-fixed, surgical retractor, the most commonly employed in the world today. It was developed during the early years of his practice in Vermont and was created in order to ameliorate the problem of lack of availability of assistants during the performance of major surgery. He is a fellow of the American College of Surgeons, the New England Vascular Society, and the New England Surgical Society. John Bookwalter is known for his warmth, his enthusiasm, his generosity, his "humanistic" approach to patient care, and his lifelong interest in disease prevention.

FRANZ WEITLANER (1872–1944)

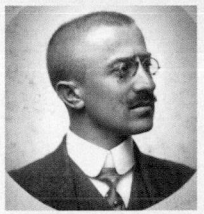

Born in Welsberg, Italy near the Italy-Austria border, Franz Weitlaner (pronounced VIGHT-lahn-er) studied theology and philosophy at a local Catholic seminary before ultimately choosing medicine over the priesthood. Thanks to a scholarship valued at nearly twice his father's salary, Weitlaner studied medicine at Innsbruck Medical University in Austria. After remaining there as an assistant hospital doctor, he became a "Schiffsarzt" or shipboard surgeon for the Austrian Lloyd shipping company. After returning, he married a classically trained Viennese pianist and moved to the small town of Ottenthal in Northeast Austria. As the "Gemeindearzt" or community doctor of Ottenthal, Weitlaner became increasingly frustrated with the Broz Wound Dilator. The most advanced self-retaining retractor available at the time. The Broz Wound Dilator functioned via a screw mechanism, required use of both hands, and was notoriously difficult to sterilize. To address these issues, in 1905, Weitlaner developed *Ein Automatischer Wundspreizer* (the automatic wound-spreader), his now-ubiquitous self-retaining retractor. Unfortunately, in failing to secure a patent for this ingenious device, Weitlaner forfeited his right to all monetary rewards from the invention and maintained only the right to name the device. Even then, the device's name has come to be misspelled as "Wheatlander." Nevertheless, by any name, self-retaining retractors have revolutionized surgical exposure, have taken a prominent place in the surgeon's inventory, and saved the arm strength of medical students the world over. In 1944, 10 days before his 72nd birthday, he died of a myocardial infarction. (Reference: Sharma A, Swan KG. Franz Weitlaner: the great spreader of surgery. *J Trauma Inj Inf Crit Care*. 2009;67:1431 and with appreciation to Merrit M. DeBartolo.)

---

invaded by tumor, and whether seeding of the peritoneal cavity has occurred. It is often difficult to determine by inspection alone whether lymph nodes contain tumor or are uninvolved. Large, firm nodes may prove to be inflammatory when examined under the microscope.

Tumoricidal Agents

The use of topical tumoricidal agents has been suggested to minimize the risk for implantation metastases, especially with respect to resection of the rectum (see Chapter 24). Long and Edwards instilled dilute formalin (as a cancericidal agent) into the lumen of the bowel in 40 patients before opening it.[591] A statistically significant difference in actuarial survival was observed in comparison with historical controls. Most, however, remain unconvinced as to the merits of this technique and do not use it.

Drains

In the absence of pus, no drains are employed. Some studies have demonstrated that the prophylactic use of drains is at best ineffective and poses a potential hazard for further complications, especially an anastomotic leak.[447]

Wound Closure

For midline wound closure, a single-layer of interrupted long-term absorbable sutures placed through all layers except the skin is the only requirement absent in special wound-healing concerns. In a controlled trial by Corman and colleagues involving three different suture materials for abdominal wound closure (a nonabsorbable monofilament suture, a nonabsorbable multifilament suture, and a long-term absorbable suture), no statistically significant difference was seen in the incidence of wound infection, wound dehiscence, and incisional hernia.[205] They believe that closure of the abdominal wall with long-term absorbable suture is the preferred method. Another alternative is to use a continuous suturing technique, such as looped no. 1 polydioxanone suture (PDS). Carlson and Condon performed a prospective, randomized comparison of nylon versus polyglyconate (Maxon), using a looped suture in a running mass closure of midline abdominal incisions in 225 patients.[156] There was no significant difference in the overall rate of ventral hernia and dehiscence between the two groups with a 2-year follow-up. Needless to say, other surgeons involved in many varied trials conclude that different materials and methods are preferred.[287,353,645,846]

The general or trauma surgeon may be faced with a situation wherein abdominal wound closure may not be possible without tension. Numerous methods are available, including the use of polyglycolic acid (Vicryl) mesh, Marlex, Gore-Tex, "Bogota bag," and sandwich-vacuum pack, just to name a few.[732] Fortunately, it is unusual that one cannot close the abdomen in colon and rectal surgery in an elective situation, but such an occasion may arise, especially in the presence of bowel obstruction, perforation, an anastomotic leak, with intra-abdominal packing, following abdominal radiation, with the abdominal compartment syndrome, or when tumor invades the abdominal wall.

Operations

As with all operations for malignancy, the objective of surgical treatment for carcinoma of the colon is to remove the growth with an adequate margin through the performance of a wide excision of the tumor-bearing area and associated lymphatics, with attention to the blood supply to that segment (see Figure 1-15) and the creation of an anastomosis without tension. What the actual distance is between the tumor margin and the cut edge of bowel may be somewhat problematic. Depending on when it is measured, a margin of 5 cm unstretched in situ has been noted to shrink to under 2 cm.[1076]

The operations that are generally employed for cancer above the rectum include right colectomy, transverse colectomy, left colectomy, sigmoid colectomy, high anterior resection, subtotal colectomy, and total colectomy. Other, more limited resections are occasionally performed for palliation, but these generally should be avoided because of the potential for inadequate blood supply, insufficient mesenteric removal, and tension on the anastomosis.

Right Hemicolectomy

Lesions of the cecum, ascending colon, and hepatic flexure usually are treated by right hemicolectomy because the blood supply to this area comes from the ileocolic and right colic arteries. The dissection may be expedited if the surgeon stands on the patient's left side, although this is a matter of personal preference. Resectability of the tumor is evaluated with a minimum of manipulation. The small bowel is retracted into the left half of the abdominal cavity, and the root of the mesentery and the base of the transverse mesocolon are exposed. Many surgeons ligate the right colic and right branch of the middle colic arteries and veins as the initial maneuver (Figure 23-37). This procedure is not difficult unless the patient is obese, in which case preliminary ligation of the blood vessels may be neither convenient nor safe. The small incision in the root of the mesentery required for this preliminary main trunk ligation is now extended to the point on the transverse colon and ileum where division of the bowel is to take place. The vessels in the mesentery and mesocolon are ligated, and the entire blood supply to the tumor is divided. An alternative to ligating the mesenteric blood supply is to employ a vessel-sealing device, such as the LigaSure vessel-sealing system. This approach can be used in place of clips, sutures, and other energy-based ligation methods. In essence, it produces within a few seconds a consistent seal of vessels up to 7 mm in diameter without dissection or isolation.

Although there is no data to support the concept of a no-touch technique, especially when one considers hand-assisted laparoscopy as an alternative (see later and Chapter 19), it certainly makes sense not to manipulate the bowel or handle the tumor unnecessarily. One may still adhere to this principle and yet expedite the operation by initially mobilizing the colon. The terminal ileum and right colon are elevated from the retroperitoneal structures by dividing the peritoneum along the lateral gutter, at the so-called white line of Toldt (Figure 23-38). Included in the resected specimen is any lateral peritoneum involved by serosal tumor. Care must

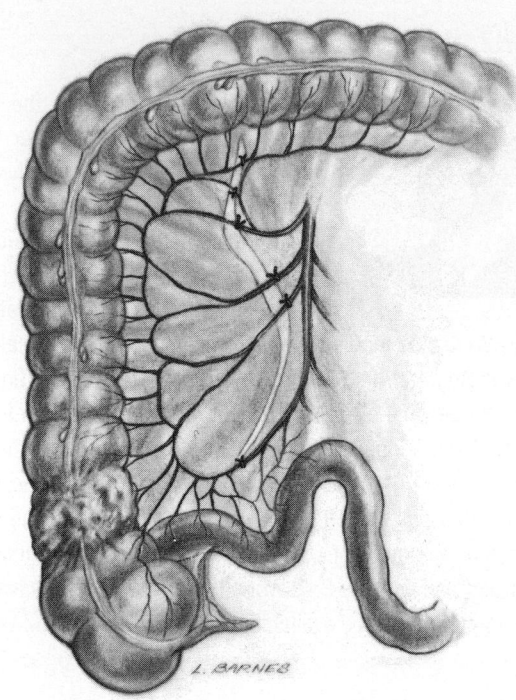

FIGURE 23-37. Right hemicolectomy. Early ligation of the vascular supply to the right colon is illustrated.

be taken to avoid injury to the ureter, spermatic or ovarian vessels, and inferior vena cava. The terminal ileum is prepared by incising the antimesenteric fold of Treves.

The next structure of concern is the second portion of the duodenum. This must be displaced carefully as the colon is freed from its retroperitoneal attachments. The developmental adhesions from the gallbladder and liver to the hepatic flexure are incised. When the head of the pancreas is in view (Figure 23-39), the duodenum is sufficiently clear from the dissection so that clamping of the blood supply can be accomplished with safety. This can be performed by passing a hand around the vessels through the avascular plane (Figure 23-40).

It is often advisable to enter the lesser sac, dividing the gastrocolic omentum as far to the left as possible. This

CARL FLORIAN TOLDT (1840–1920)

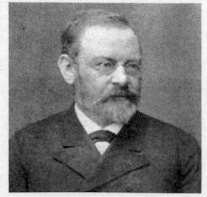

Carl Toldt was born May 3, 1840 in Bruneck, Austria, the second of 10 children. As a young man, he spent much of his free time learning to assemble and repair clocks with a local clockmaker. He believed that this experience was beneficial to both his analytical skills and to his manual dexterity. Toldt attended medical school at Joseph's University in Vienna, from which he received his doctorate in 1864. His expertise encompassed a number of areas in medicine, but he held a special interest for anatomy. He was first appointed professor of anatomy at the University of Vienna in 1875, then went on to become professor of anatomy at the German University in Prague. In 1884, he returned to Vienna where he created the Anatomy Institute of Vienna together with his colleague, Langer. Toldt was responsible for many publications on histology, tissue growth, forensic medicine, and anatomy. His best-known work is his anatomic atlas, *Anatom Atlas fur Studierende und Aerzte*, which was translated into English and last published in New York in 1926. In addition to his writing, Toldt showed his creative nature by inventing an electrical lighting system for dissecting rooms. Toldt died of pneumonia in Vienna on November 13, 1920. (With appreciation to Brian de Rubertis.)

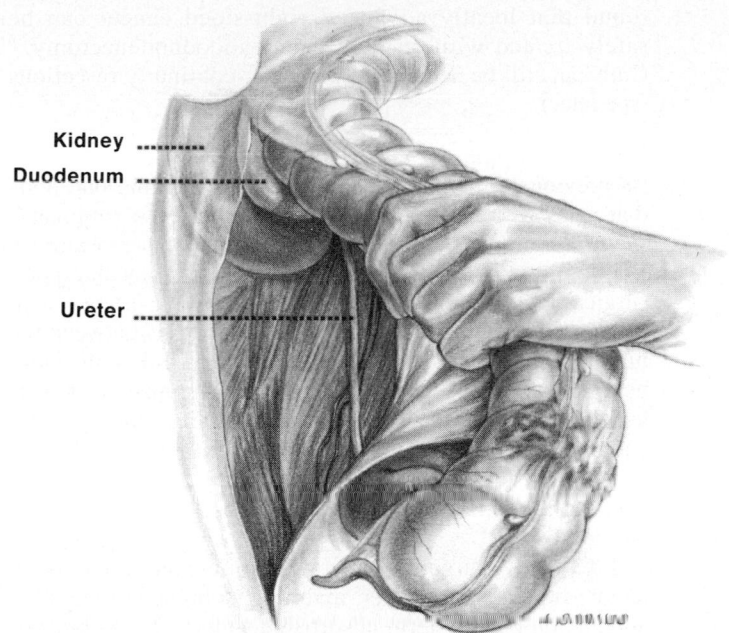

Kidney
Duodenum

Ureter

FIGURE 23-38. Right hemicolectomy. The dissection proceeds along the right paracolic gutter, and the retroperitoneal structures are identified and preserved.

maneuver expedites entrance into the sac and permits the posterior wall of the stomach to be retracted out of harm's way. The remainder of the gastrocolic omentum is then divided until the hepatic flexure is no longer tethered. The omentum is incised to the point where the anastomosis will be performed. With all the blood supply divided to the segment, the bowel is resected (Figure 23-41).

Bokey and coworkers emphasize as in rectal surgery that mobilization of the colon along anatomic planes is an important principle and an independent prognostic factor that influences outcome.[100] Curley and colleagues comment that fixation may occur to the duodenum or pancreas, albeit rarely.[214] They reported en bloc pancreaticoduodenectomy or lateral duodenectomy in 12 individuals. Others have

FREDERICK TREVES (1853–1923)

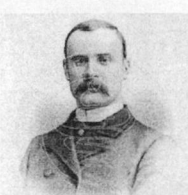

Frederick Treves was born in Dorchester, Dorset, England on February 15, 1853. He received his medical education at the London School of Medicine, and in 1879 he became surgical registrar and assistant surgeon at the London Hospital. For a time, he worked as a lecturer of practical anatomy and demonstrator in anatomy at that hospital and became, in 1883, surgeon as well as head of the department of anatomy. Later in this year, he met Joseph Merrick, known as the "elephant man." Treves rescued Merrick from destitution and created a home for him in the attic of the London Hospital until Merrick died in 1890. Treves was a prolific author as well as a brilliant investigator and observer. In 1883, the Royal College of Surgeons awarded him the Jacksonian Prize for his dissertation, *Pathology, Diagnosis and Treatment of Obstruction of the Intestine*. His best-recognized works are his Hunterian lectures, delivered to the Royal College of Surgeons, on *The Anatomy of the Intestinal Canal and Peritoneum* (1885). In 1884, Treves, at the age of 31, became full surgeon to the London Hospital. He was one of the first to devote special attention to diseases of the appendix. He concluded that the disease, then known as perityphlitis, involved the appendix and not the cecum. His consulting rooms at 6 Wimpole Street became among the best known in England. In 1899, upon the outbreak of the Boer War, he was called to serve as consulting surgeon to the field forces. The following year he published an account of his experiences in charge of No. 4 Field Hospital and being present at the relief of Ladysmith, in his *Tale of a Field Hospital*. Treves was a brilliant lecturer and a very able surgeon who made original contributions to surgical anatomy, peritonitis, intestinal obstruction, and appendicitis. He was knighted by King Edward VII, on whom he performed an appendectomy in June 1902. Later that year, Treves retired from medical practice to become an author, moving in 1918 to Lake Geneva, Switzerland because of poor health. Treves had by this time become quite a successful travel writer through the publication of a series of books based on his experiences. His last book was devoted to recollections of his medical experiences and was entitled *The Elephant Man and Other Reminiscences* (1923). He died of peritonitis on December 7, 1923 in Lausanne, Switzerland. His lifelong friend, the author and poet, Thomas Hardy, arranged for and spoke at the funeral in Dorset. (Photograph courtesy of the Wellcome Library, London.)

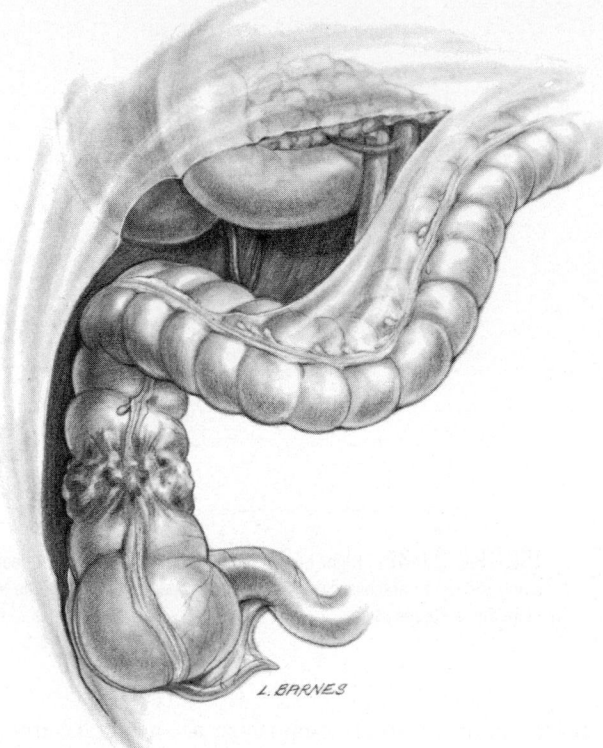

FIGURE 23-39. Right hemicolectomy. The hepatic flexure is mobilized, exposing the duodenum and the head of the pancreas.

found that locally advanced right-sided cancer can be safely treated with en bloc pancreaticoduodenectomy.[80] Cure can still be achieved by such in-continuity resections (see later).

Suturing Principles

As previously mentioned, in this era of stapling, one finds that many residents have little or no experience with hand-sewn techniques. Although it is clear that performing a side-to-side stapled ileocolic anastomosis is easy and rapid, surgical residents often wish to gain more experience with sewing. Not uncommonly a discrepancy exists between the luminal sizes of the ileum and the transverse colon, the latter being considerably larger. Under such circumstances, it is usually advisable to make a Cheatle cut into the antimes-enteric portion of the ileum when performing a hand-sewn anastomosis (Figure 23-42A). Another alternative is to perform a hand-sewn ileocolic side-to-end or end-to-side anastomosis.

Frequently, surgeons undertake colonic anastomoses by an interrupted, single-layer, inverting technique through the application of long-term absorbable sutures. Small bites of mucosa are taken, with a relatively deeper passage through the seromuscular layer. Although the submucosal layer is the most important, there is little consequence of incorporating a small amount of mucosa. The use of a second row of seromuscular sutures is not necessary but is preferred by some surgeons. However, it adds nothing to the security of the anastomosis, inverts more tissue, and further narrows

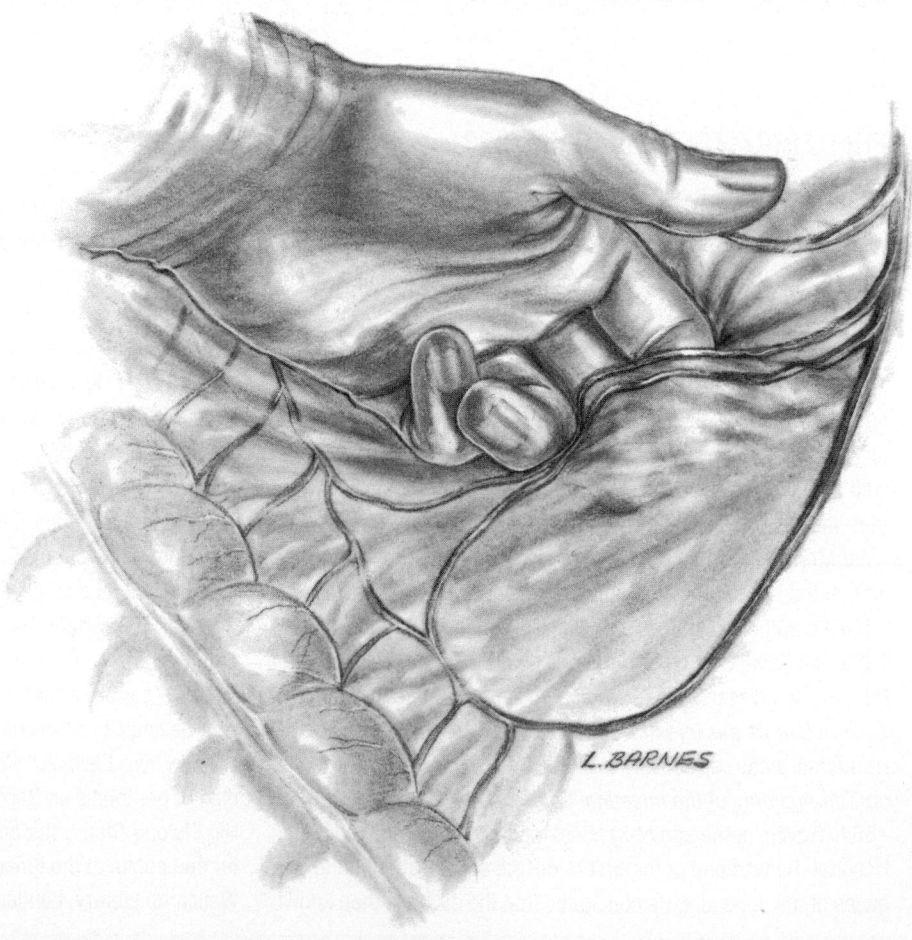

FIGURE 23-40. Right hemicolectomy. Technique of identification and manual isolation of major blood supply to the right colon.

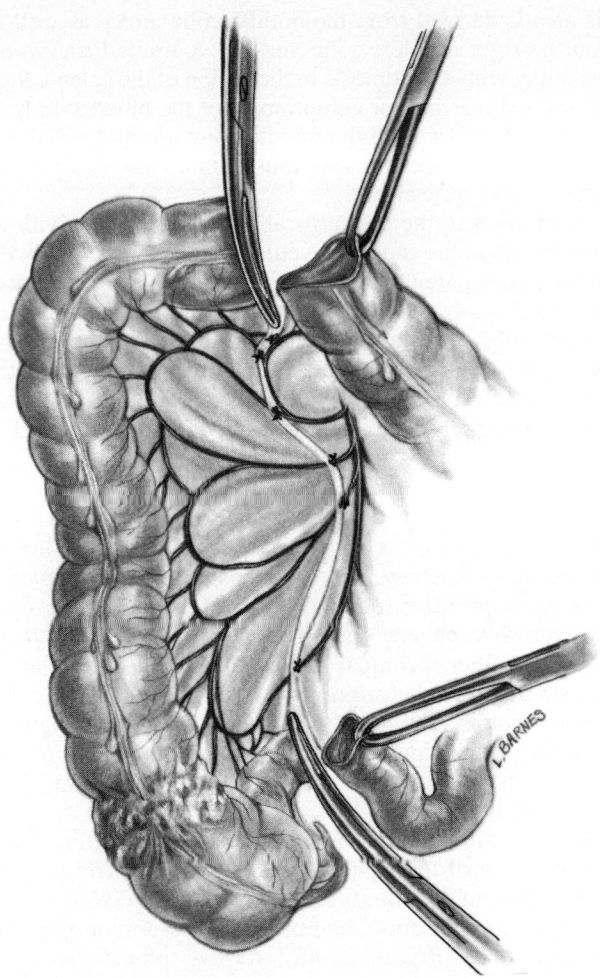

FIGURE 23-41. Right hemicolectomy. After ligation of the vascular supply and mobilization of the bowel, crushing clamps are applied to the ileum and transverse colon, and the bowel is divided with a scalpel, leaving the ends open for anastomosis.

the lumen. The fact is that we are talking about a subject that is pervaded by prejudice and dogma and is always a reflection of an individual's training, experience, and personal preference. The reality is that a surgeon has the right to use whatever technique with which he or she is comfortable.

Every suture material has been used, and everything works reasonably well. Logically, one cannot blame the suture material if an anastomosis fails, but this excuse is still postulated. Prolene and wire work but they are tedious to tie, and braided, nonabsorbable material creates more tissue reaction, which, theoretically, can serve as a nidus for infection. Catgut is acceptable, but objectively it has no advantage over a long-term absorbable suture. Reasonable people have differences of opinion with respect to choice of suture material and technique (whether a single- or a double-layer is preferable, interrupted, or continuous), but there is little disagreement that an inverting approach is the proper one for all colonic anastomoses when a conventional hand-sewn technique is used.

After a satisfactory anastomosis has been achieved, the mesenteric defect may be closed with either an interrupted or a continuous technique. Theoretically, this may prevent herniation of small bowel through the defect in the mesentery, but there is no evidence to support this claim. Many surgeons always leave the defect open, but it is probably prudent to close a small opening. It is also useful to place omentum around all colonic anastomoses to protect further against the possibility of leakage (see later).

Suture Technique: Study Results

Max and colleagues prefer a single-layer continuous technique, using polypropylene (Figure 23-43); they reported a successful experience with 1,000 intestinal anastomoses.[649] Carty and coworkers advocate a single-layer extramucosal approach.[158] Thomson and Robinson also prefer a one layer continuously sutured anastomosis, using a double-ended absorbable monofilament suture placed in an extramucosal fashion.[1018] Clark and coworkers performed a randomized trial of polyglycolic acid sutures and catgut in colonic anastomoses, but with a double-layer approach.[182] Interrupted silk was used as a seromuscular suture, and a continuous inverting mucosal suture was employed with either of the two materials. Although clinical evidence of anastomotic breakdown occurred with equal frequency in the two groups studied, radiologic evidence of anastomotic leak was twice as common with the catgut.[182]

Some investigators are of the opinion that the type of suture material may have an effect on the risk for anastomotic recurrence. In an experimental study, Hubens and colleagues

GEORGE LENTHAL CHEATLE (1865–1951)

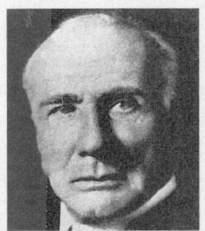

George Cheatle was born in Belvedere, Kent, England on June 13, 1865. He was educated at King's College, London. Following graduation and while awaiting his house appointment at King's College Hospital, he acted as assistant demonstrator of anatomy. He was the last to serve as Lord Lister's Assistant in Surgery. In 1900, he became full surgeon to King's while also teaching surgical pathology. In the South African War (Boer War), he served as consulting surgeon, and in the First World War, he held the rank of surgeon rear admiral in the Royal Navy, receiving the honor of Knight Commander of the Bath for his services. In his obituary in the *Lancet* (1951;1:115), the following statement was made about him: "The accumulation of a large, consulting practice was inevitable to a man of such distinction, but he remained a keen and conscientious teacher and a rabid research-worker." In 1931, he was awarded the Walker Prize for his work on cancer. Among his many recognitions were honorary fellow of the American College of Surgeons, chevalier of the French Legion of Honor, and officer of the Grand Cross of Italy. He was so esteemed that in order to lecture at Hines Hospital, Chicago, a privilege accorded to none but American nationals, he was granted American citizenship for 1 week. Sir Lenthal died at his home in London on January 3, 1951, at the age of 85. (Photograph from the journal, *Cancer.* 1951;4:220, with permission.)

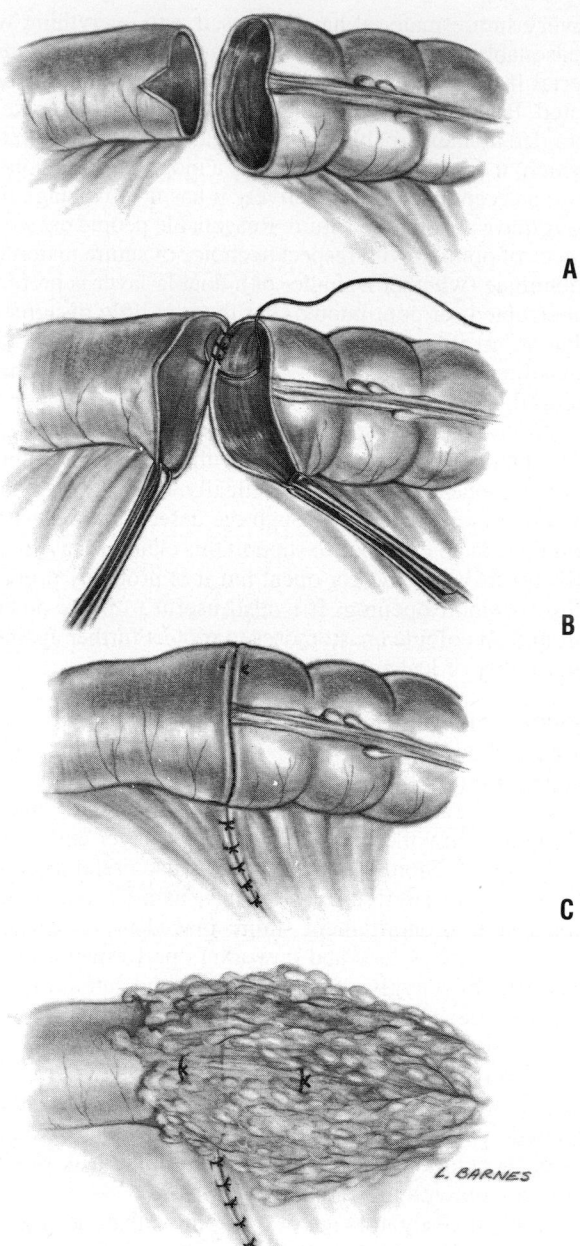

FIGURE 23-42. Right hemicolectomy. **A:** Any disparity between the luminal ends can be corrected by dividing the smaller segment of bowel along its antimesenteric border. **B:** The anastomosis is accomplished using a single layer of interrupted sutures. **C:** Note the single mattress suture used to effect final closure. The rent in the mesentery is closed. **D:** Omentum is placed around the anastomosis.

found that persisting suture material at a colonic anastomosis affected the distribution of tumor formation when a chemical carcinogen was administered.[459] They opined that the actual elimination process of such material may influence the crypt cell proliferation rate. In view of these observations, the authors suggest that either inert suture material be used or sutureless anastomotic techniques be applied.[459]

Surgery for Carcinoma of the Transverse Colon

Carcinoma of the transverse colon often presents a challenge in the choice of operative procedure. The blood supply to

this area is derived from the middle colic artery as well as from the right and left colic vessels. A limited transverse colectomy with anastomosis in the region of the splenic flexure poses some risk for compromise of the blood supply to the bowel because with the middle colic artery divided, the blood supply to the left side must come entirely from the inferior mesenteric artery.

In addition to the concerns about blood supply with an anastomosis in the transverse colon, another problem is the lymph-bearing area. Carcinoma in this location can spread to regional lymphatics through the middle colic, right colic, and left colic branches. Because of this risk, subtotal colectomy has been advocated as the optimal approach to the treatment of carcinoma of the transverse colon. For proximal lesions, right hemicolectomy is generally advised. For distal transverse colon lesions, left partial or left hemicolectomy is reasonable (Figure 23-44) with anastomosis of the transverse colon to the sigmoid colon (Figure 23-45). However, for lesions of the mid-transverse colon, limited transverse colectomy may be considered for palliation or as a compromise for other indications. As mentioned, however, as a cancer operation it may be inadequate. If tension or other technical difficulty prevents a safe anastomosis between the proximal and distal transverse colon (Figure 23-46), subtotal or total colectomy and ileosigmoid or ileorectal anastomosis is strongly recommended. A consequence of tension on a transverse colon anastomosis is illustrated in Figure 23-47.

Mobilization of the splenic flexure is facilitated by, first, division of the gastrocolic omentum to within a few centimeters of the flexure and, second, incision of the lateral peritoneal attachments along the descending and sigmoid colon (Figure 23-48). As the splenic flexure is approached, the spleen is seen, and the lienocolic and phrenocolic ligaments are divided (Figure 23-49). Only one clamp should be used to avoid tearing the splenic capsule. The splenic flexure is delivered into the wound, and any back-bleeding can be clamped at this point without concern about injury to the spleen (Figure 23-50). The technique of anastomosis does not differ from that already described.

Splenectomy

Locally invasive tumors of the splenic flexure may not be amenable to wide excision unless the spleen and tail of the pancreas are also removed. Removal of the spleen, whether intentional or inadvertent in conjunction with a colonic resection, is associated with a high morbidity and an increased mortality rate (Figure 23-51).[181,223,526,547,864] Langevin and colleagues reviewed 993 consecutive colon and rectal operations and found that the spleen was injured in 8.[547] Splenectomy was required in 3. Therefore, the incidence of splenectomy during splenic flexure mobilization is approximately 1%. Varty and colleagues reviewed the experience of splenectomy concomitant with resections for colon and rectal cancer at University College, London, comparing the patients with individually matched controls.[1050] There was no influence on long-term survival, although there was an increased incidence of postoperative sepsis.

Because most injuries to the spleen are capsular tears caused by inadequate exposure and too vigorous traction, every effort should be made to conserve the organ. Topical hemostatic agents such as Avitene, Surgicel, Helistat, and Gelfoam have been recommended as well as primary su-

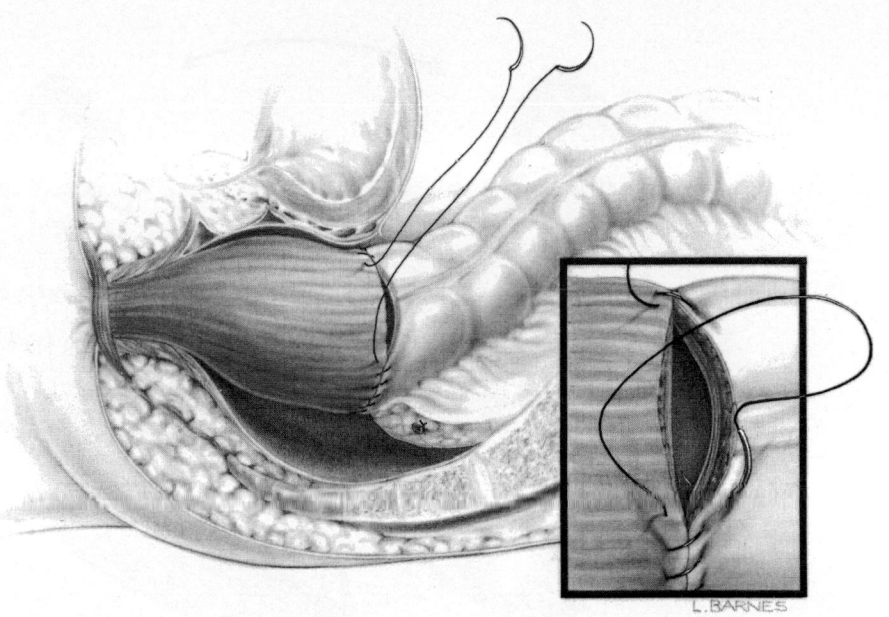

FIGURE 23-43. Colorectal anastomosis by continuous suturing, incorporating minimal mucosa. The method illustrated uses a no. 4–0, double-armed polypropylene suture, as advocated by Max and colleagues.[649]

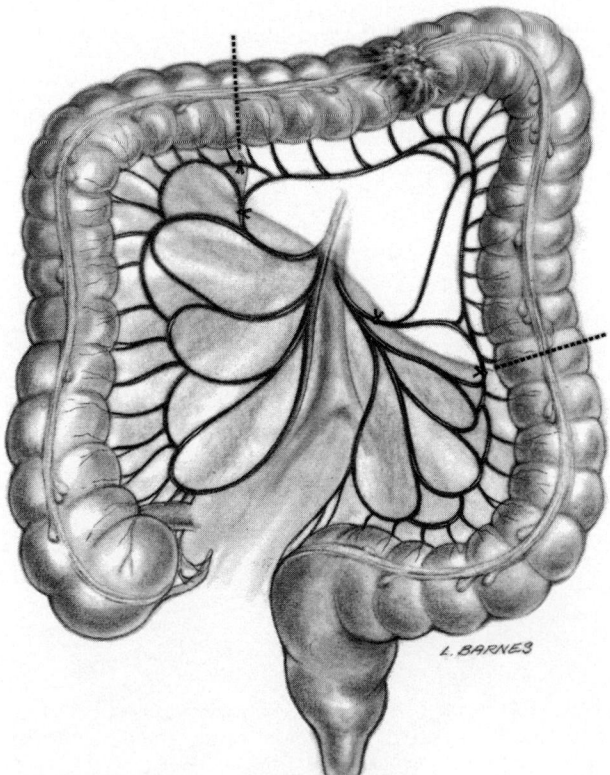

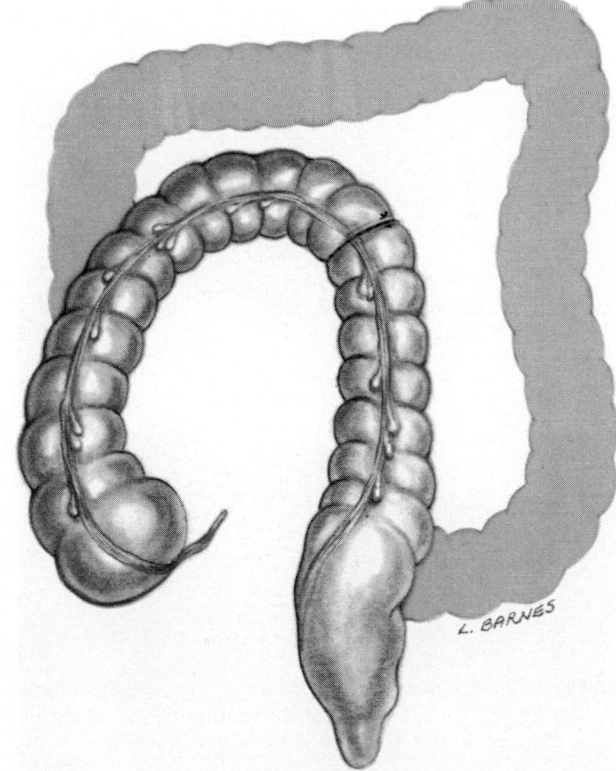

FIGURE 23-44. Left partial colectomy. With tumors of the left portion of the transverse colon, resection of the descending colon is required to obtain a safe anastomosis while removing lymphatic drainage areas.

FIGURE 23-45. Left partial colectomy. Anastomosis between the mid-transverse colon and the upper sigmoid is usually possible without difficulty, except in very obese patients.

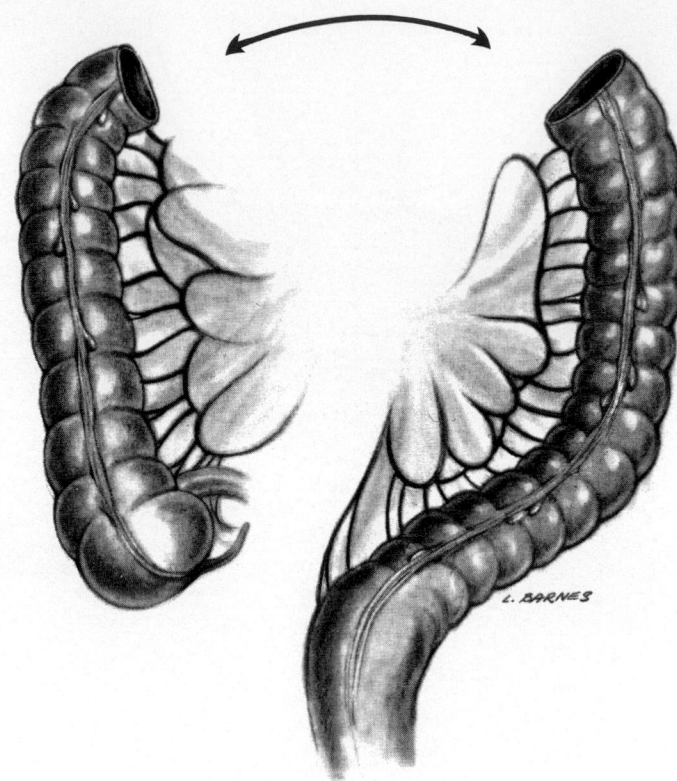

FIGURE 23-46. Transverse colon resection. Anastomosis may not be feasible because of tension.

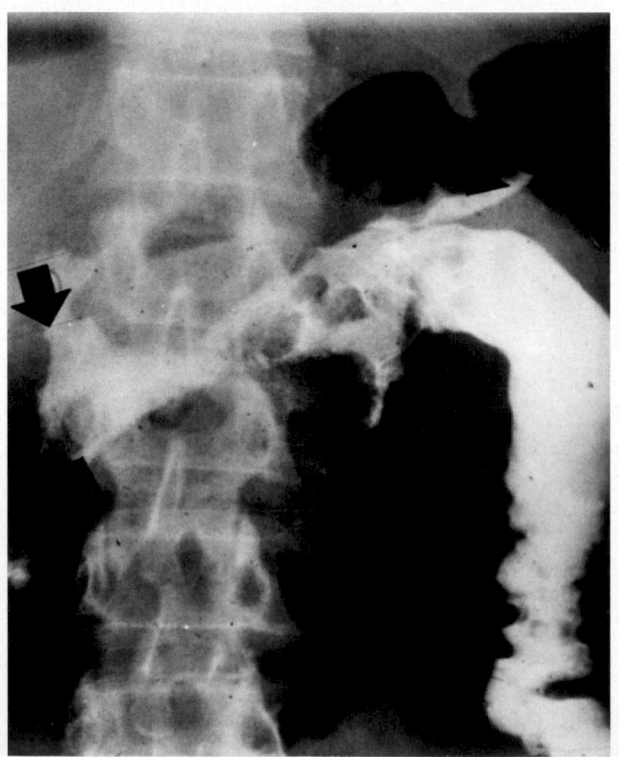

FIGURE 23-47. Anastomotic leak (*arrows*) demonstrated on a postoperative barium enema study 2 weeks after transverse colectomy for carcinoma. At the second operation, the ends of the bowel were found to have separated completely.

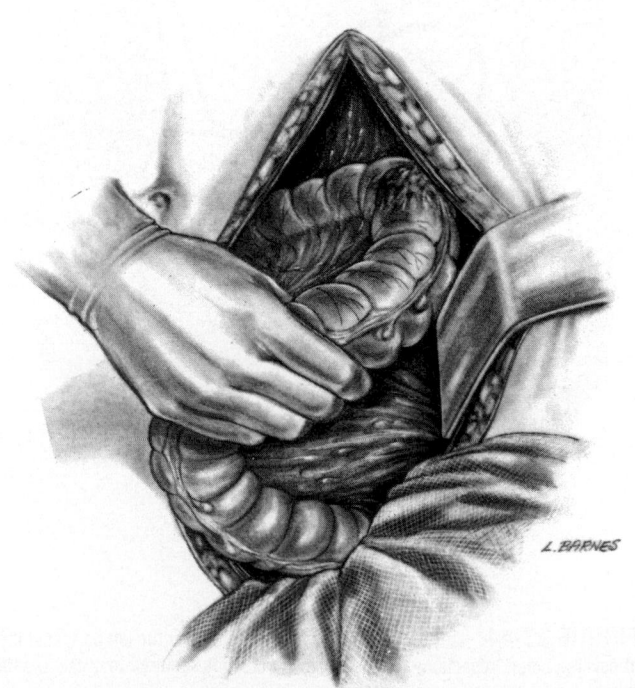

FIGURE 23-48. Mobilization of the splenic flexure is facilitated by freeing the descending colon.

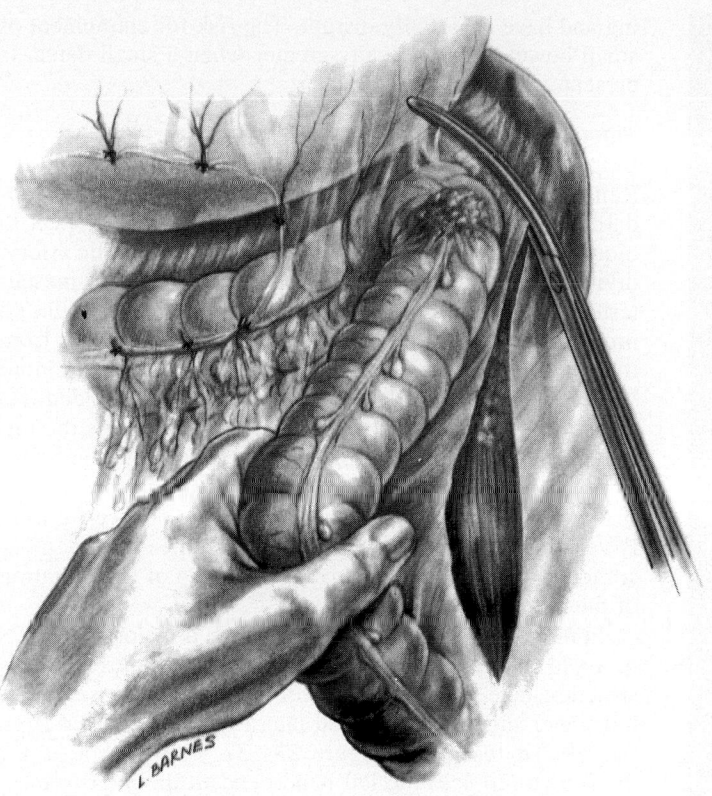

FIGURE 23-49. The lienocolic ligament is divided. Back-bleeding can be dealt with as the splenic flexure is brought into the wound.

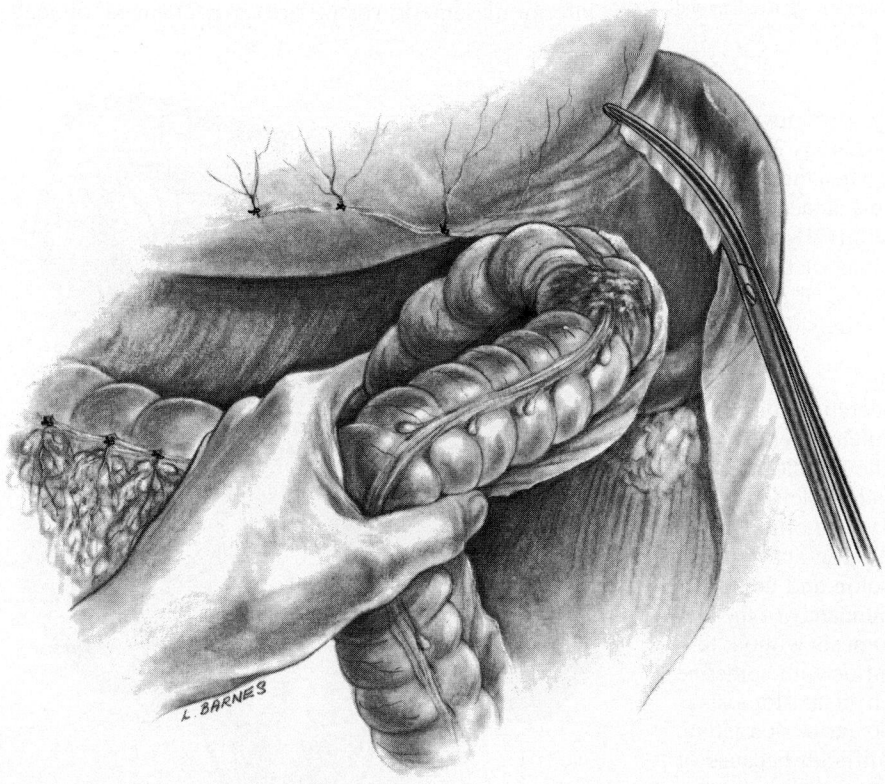

FIGURE 23-50. With traction on the transverse colon and descending colon, the splenic flexure is delivered from its retroperitoneal attachments.

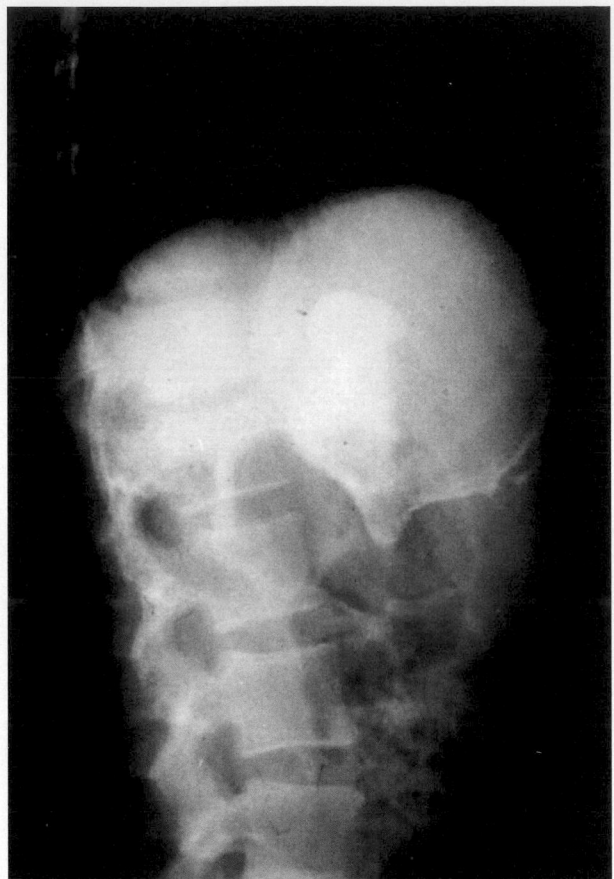

FIGURE 23-51. Subphrenic abscess that developed following colectomy and splenectomy.

ing and have it partially disrupt. The risk for entrapment of small bowel is theoretically greater when a small defect is present.

Sigmoid Colectomy and High Anterior Resection (Anastomosis into the Upper Rectum)

Removal of the sigmoid colon for carcinoma is the standard operation for tumors in this location. With respect to blood supply, this operation preserves the left colic artery, dividing only the sigmoid branches of the inferior mesenteric artery. Viability of the distal bowel should present no problem because of the usually excellent blood supply from the middle hemorrhoidal arteries and the upper sigmoid vessels. The proximal blood supply is usually adequate through the left colic artery. Some surgeons stress the importance of high ligation of the inferior mesenteric artery (on the aorta).[381] Outside of the implications for staging, if a node at this level harbors cancer, the chance for cure is very remote indeed. At least three studies have demonstrated that there is no survival advantage of high ligation of the inferior mesenteric artery.[530]

In mobilization of the sigmoid colon, a major concern is to avoid traumatizing the left ureter. Most injuries to this structure take place at the level of the iliac vessels. The left ureter should be retracted laterally and displaced from the area of resection (Figure 23-53). One method is for the surgeon to pass the left hand beneath the inferior mesenteric vessels, and the peritoneum is incised on the right side (Figure 23-54). The left hand is then withdrawn and passed around the vessels and through the defect between the left colic artery and the sigmoid vessels (Figure 23-55). The inferior mesenteric vessels are cross-clamped, divided,

ture repair and even partial splenectomy. If removal is required, the incidence of septic complications is increased. Drains should not be used except perhaps when there is gross contamination. Under such circumstances, closed drainage with sump suction is preferred. Postoperatively, appropriate counseling concerning the implications of the loss of the spleen is advised, and the administration of polyvalent pneumococcal vaccine (Pneumovax) is a requisite.

Left Partial Colectomy or Hemicolectomy

Left partial colectomy is the preferred operation for tumors involving the distal transverse colon, splenic flexure, and descending colon. The right branch of the middle colic artery should be kept intact proximally, and the left colic artery is ligated, care being taken to preserve the origin of the inferior mesenteric artery (Figure 23-52). The anastomosis is effected between the midtransverse colon and the upper sigmoid. In most instances, sufficient redundancy of the sigmoid colon is present to permit an anastomosis without tension. Occasionally, with an obese patient or with someone who has undergone a prior resection, such an anastomosis is not possible. A left hemicolectomy is a potential alternative, but attempts at an anastomosis may be difficult because of inadequate length and tension. Under these circumstances, total or subtotal colectomy is a reasonable alternative.

Whereas one can virtually always close the defect in the mesentery following a right hemicolectomy, it is often not possible to accomplish such a closure on the left side. One prefers to leave a large opening rather than to attempt sutur-

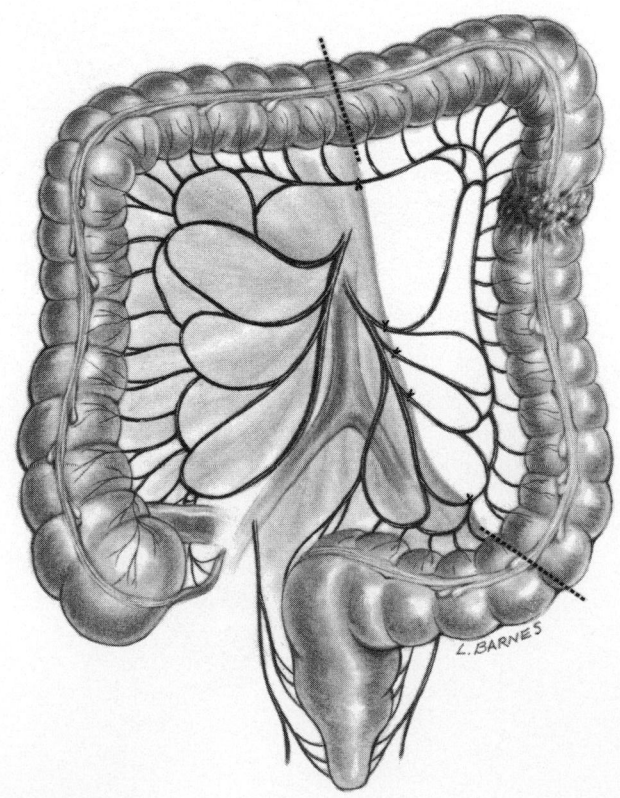

FIGURE 23-52. Left partial colectomy. Area of resection for a lesion of the descending colon, with preservation of sigmoid and rectal vessels.

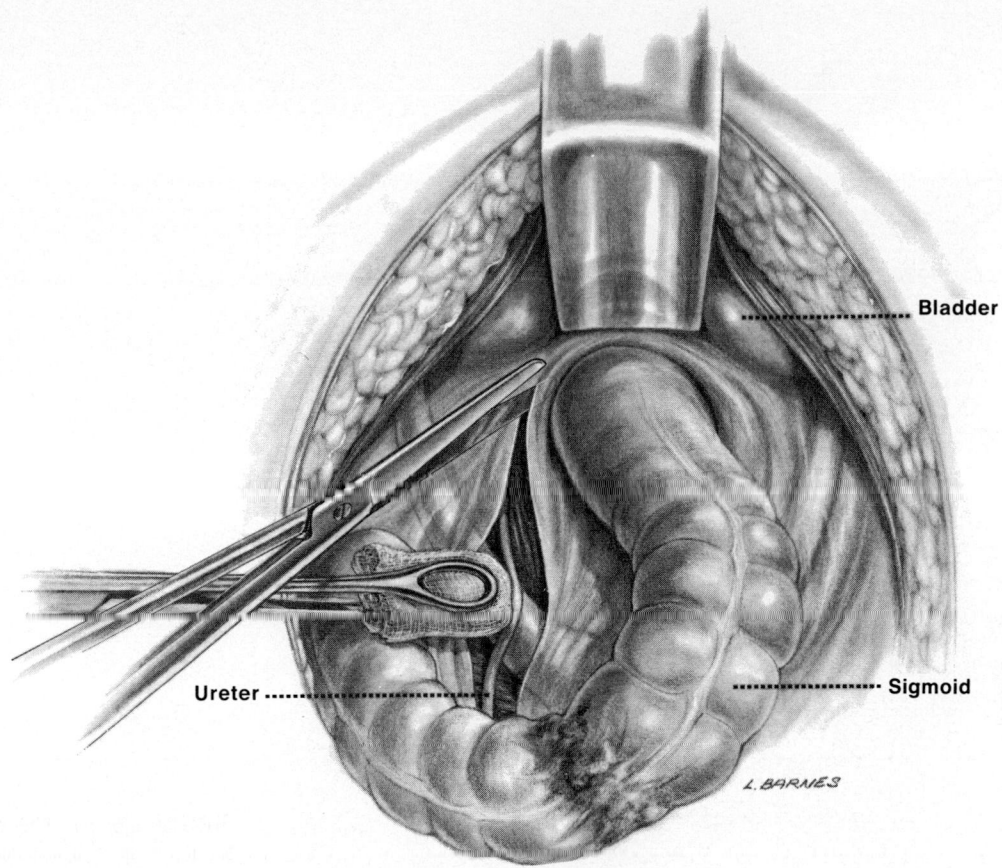

FIGURE 23-53. High anterior resection. The sigmoid colon is mobilized, with care taken to avoid injury to the ureter.

and ligated, and the arcade vessels to the upper sigmoid are divided. Rather than perform an anastomosis between the upper sigmoid and lower sigmoid (because of a potential problem with distal sigmoid blood supply), it is often preferable to do a high anterior resection, anastomosing the bowel to the upper rectum at or just below the peritoneal reflection. For distal sigmoid lesions, it may be necessary to mobilize the rectum somewhat and preserve a portion of proximal sigmoid to effect a safe anastomosis without tension. Conversely, for proximal sigmoid lesions, it may be prudent to preserve the distal sigmoid and perform an anastomosis between the lower descending colon and the distal sigmoid colon rather than to mobilize the splenic flexure. This allows adequate length without tension. One of the advantages of

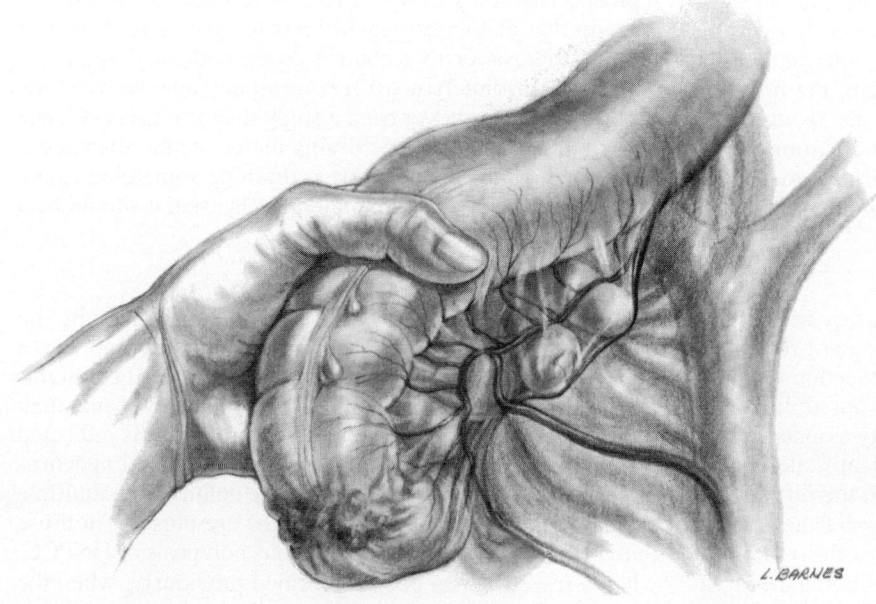

FIGURE 23-54. High anterior resection. The left hand is passed behind the bowel and beneath the vessels.

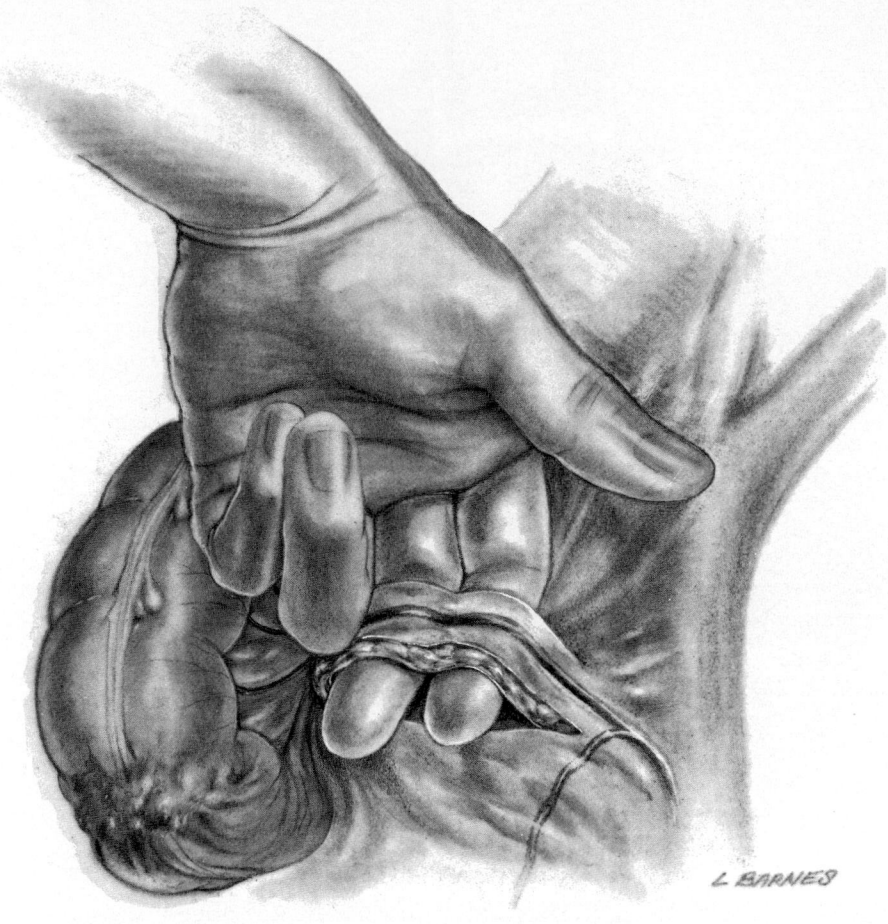

FIGURE 23-55. High anterior resection. The left hand is repositioned to pass around the mesenteric vessels. The vascular pedicle is clamped as it is held by the left hand.

beginning the operation laparoscopically is to mobilize the splenic flexure, even if the surgeon plans ultimately to perform an open operation. While one can, of course, mobilize the splenic flexure by the open technique, this may require a longer incision and be more difficult to accomplish with safety. The technique that many surgeons use for dividing the mesorectum is often unnecessarily nitpicking. A single right-angle clamp can be placed into the mesorectum; by vigorous exertion of proximal traction, the mesentery is divided (Figure 23-56). This maneuver effectively strips the bowel in preparation for the anastomosis. Alternatively, a finger or a large clamp can be passed along the posterior rectal wall, separating the mesentery of the rectum. The mesorectum is then clamped with the large instrument, and the rectum is "stripped" of its mesentery in one maneuver. One may elect also to use the LigaSure or another alternative of the surgeon's preference.

Left Hemicolectomy

Left hemicolectomy should rarely be necessary for sigmoid colon lesions. Despite the potential advantage of radical removal of the lymphatics, the additional dissection required, the prolongation of the operative time, the possibility of injury to the spleen, and the technical difficulty associated with a transverse colon-rectal anastomosis all militate against this approach. Le and Gathright recognized the difficulty in reestablishing rectal continuity following a left hemicolectomy and developed an anastomotic approach to facilitate this maneuver.[558] The procedure involves bringing the proxi-

mal ascending colon or transverse colon through a distal ileal mesenteric defect in order to reach the rectum without tension (Figure 23-57).

Use of Drains

The application of intra-abdominal drains following elective colon resection has traditionally been a subject for debate at surgical meetings. Johnson and colleagues reported a prospective study of 49 patients who were randomized to a group that had a corrugated Silastic drain placed next to the anastomosis or to a control group without drainage.[497] There was absolutely no difference in outcome between the groups. There has never been a study that provides evidence in support of prophylactic drains under the circumstances mentioned. Conversely, if one is draining something (pus). Parenthetically, if an abdominal drain is used, it should be a closed-suction system.

Subtotal or Total Colectomy

Removal of all or most of the colon and anastomosing the bowel to the upper rectum or sigmoid colon comprises a more extensive operation but permits a technically straightforward anastomosis. It also has the advantage of maximal removal of lymph-bearing tissue. The procedure is indicated or should be considered when tumors are found synchronously on the left and right sides of the colon, when multiple tumors (benign or malignant or both) are present, in those individuals with familial adenomatous polyposis or HNPCC, when a resection has been performed previously, when the

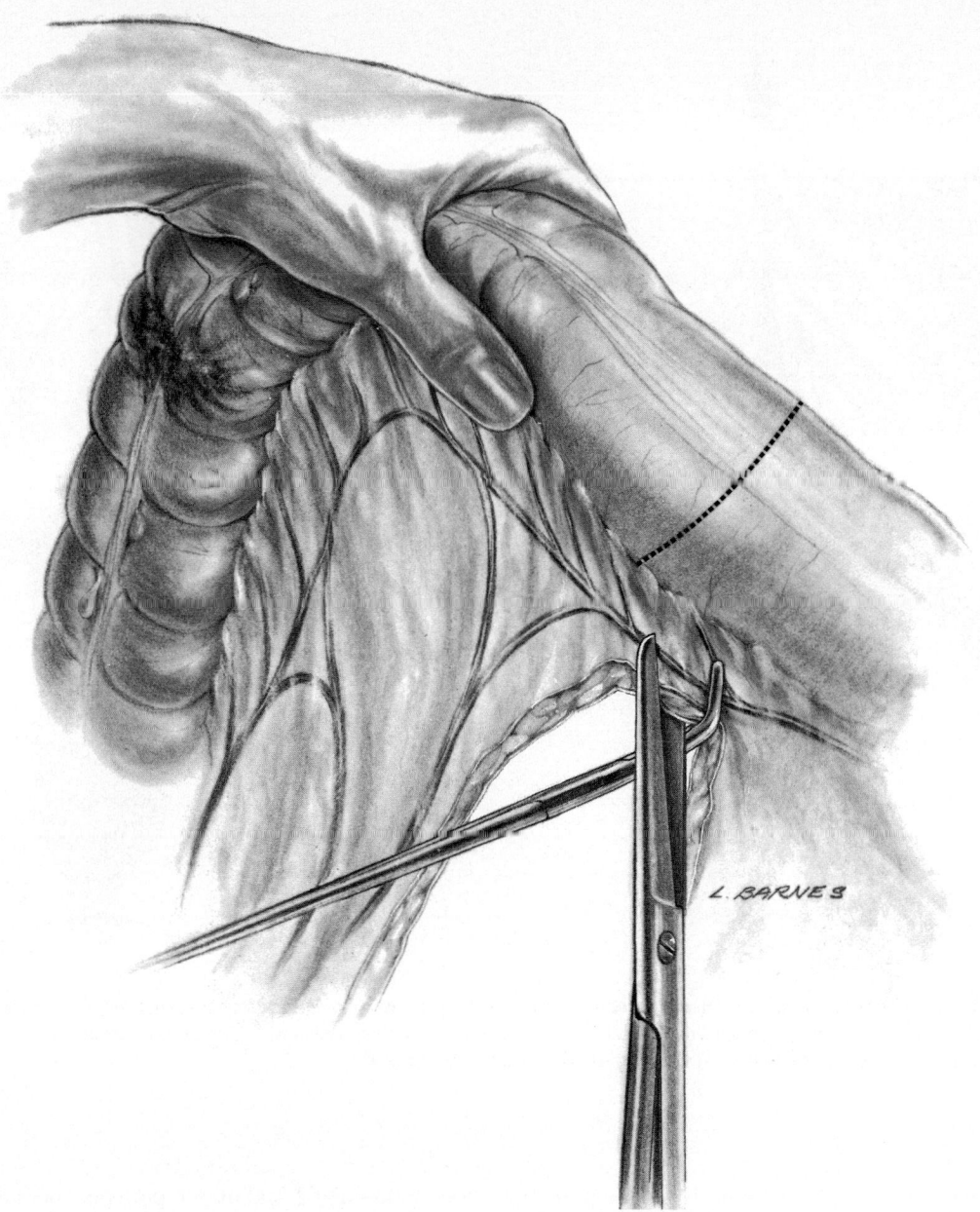

FIGURE 23-56. High anterior resection. The mesentery is clamped with vigorous cephalad traction as the mesocolon is divided.

distal colon is obstructed (see the discussion of management of obstruction), or when technical factors preclude a limited bowel resection.[115,339,380,460,942] Although synchronous resections of two bowel segments with two intestinal anastomoses can be relatively safely performed without a diversionary procedure if the bowel preparation is satisfactory, with minimal fecal soilage and with lack of tension on the suture lines,[1081] this is generally a less attractive alternative except when part or most of the rectum must be resected.

Usually, an end-to-end anastomosis between the ileum and the rectum or sigmoid colon can be accomplished easily, but occasionally, because of discrepancy between the bowel lumina or because of the angulation of the mesentery when the ileum is turned down onto the rectum, a side-to-end anastomosis may be usefully applied (Figure 23-58). Some surgeons always prefer a side-to-end anastomosis under these circumstances, often by a stapling technique.

Some of the expressed concerns of subtotal or total colectomy, as opposed to the so-called lesser alternatives, are the morbidity and mortality rates, and the patient's quality of life. Walsh and colleagues reviewed 107 consecutive total abdominal colectomies performed for a number of indications.[1063] There were two anastomotic leaks leading to deaths (1.8%). These were attributable to a failure to divert the fecal stream. In other words, no anastomosis should have been performed. Morbidity was 10.3%, with only 5% complaining of debilitating diarrhea. Beckwith and colleagues reported the experience with this operation in 32 patients older than 60 years of age at the Mayo Clinic.[71] The average increase in number of bowel movements immediately following surgery was 3.6 per day, and this gradually decreased over time. After 5 years, the average number was only 1.5 times the preoperative number. One should, however, be circumspect before contemplat-

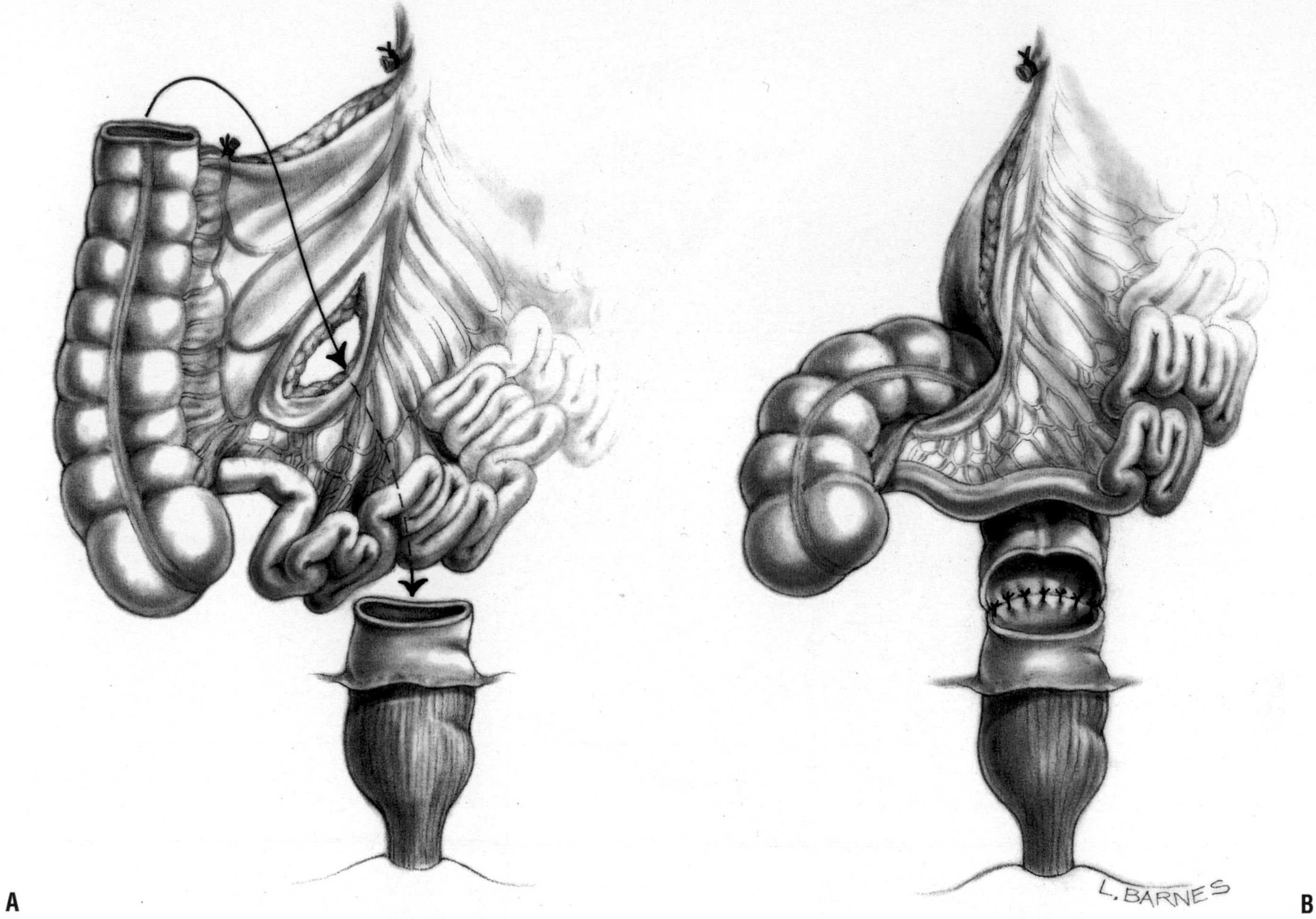

FIGURE 23-57. Reconstitution of intestinal continuity following extended left colectomy. **A:** A mesenteric defect is created following resection. **B:** The proximal ascending or transverse colon stump is brought through the ileal mesenteric defect to reach the rectum without tension. (Adapted from Le TH, Gathright JB Jr. Reconstitution of intestinal continuity after extended left colectomy. *Dis Colon Rectum.* 1993;36:197.)

ing the procedure on a prophylactic basis for the potential development of a metachronous cancer.[115] Surveillance by means of colonoscopy may be appropriate depending on the circumstances.

No-Touch Technique

In 1954, the studies of Cole and associates with respect to circulating cancer cells and others prompted Turnbull and colleagues to ligate the vascular pedicle before mobilizing the colon and to develop the method known as the no-touch technique.[190,302,487,1036] In Turnbull's operation, the cancer-bearing segment is mobilized last.

Although the theoretical value of early ligation of the vascular pedicle seems reasonable, it is difficult to understand how the excellent cure rates reported by the Cleveland Clinic (Ohio) group are achieved solely by this maneuver. Many patients already harbor inapparent tumor above the ligature. They obviously would not be cured by this technique. One possible explanation for Turnbull's results is that a somewhat different classification was used for staging cancers of the colon. However, in a prospec-

tive, randomized trial of 236 patients operated on for colon cancer, Jeekel reported that liver metastases appeared later, particularly where there was evidence of blood vessel invasion in the resected specimen.[488,1086] Fielding comments that modest gains in prognosis for colon cancer can be expected in some individuals if this method is used.[296] García-Olmo and associates studied whether "conventional" surgery could provoke the circulation of tumor cells as detected by genetic technology.[324] They used the reverse transcriptase-polymerase chain reaction to analyze tumor biopsy specimens and blood samples obtained from the antecubital vein before and after surgery, as well as from the main drainage vein of the tumor when the tumor had been removed. The investigators concluded that there was no evidence to suggest detachment of cells from the tumor at surgery.[324] Bessa and colleagues found that neither intraoperative nor postoperative detection of blood circulating tumor cells had prognostic significance in patients with colorectal cancer operated on for cure.[82] Others have concluded that there is no statistically significant advantage in the no-touch technique.[530]

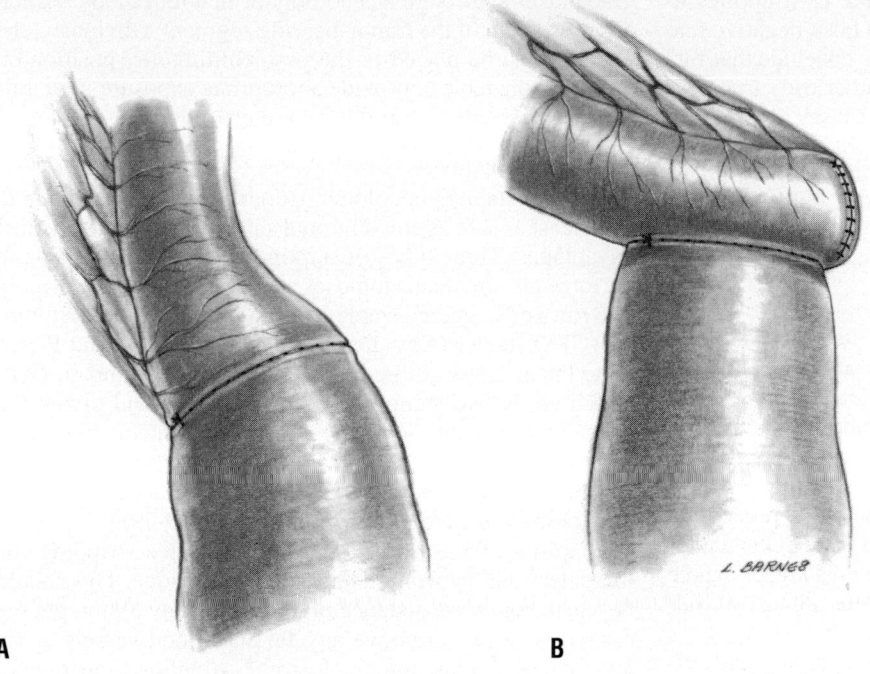

FIGURE 23-58. Ileorectal anastomosis can usually be accomplished end to end (**A**), with or without a Cheatle cut of the ileum, or as a side-to-end anastomosis (**B**).

A   **B**

Radical Lymphadenectomy

As has been mentioned previously, the concepts of high ligation of the inferior mesenteric artery and of radical lymphadenectomy have failed to show any survival benefit. With respect to radical lymphadenectomy, the complications far outweigh the theoretical advantages.[530] That stated, if there are only a small number of lymph nodes identified in the resected specimen, there is the real possibility that the patient's tumor extent will be understaged.[811] This may have implications for adjuvant therapy (see the following discussion on Sentinel Lymph Nodes and Mapping).

Sentinel Lymph Nodes and Mapping

If one were to ask the question, "what is the single most important variable for determining prognosis in colorectal cancer?" most surgeons and oncologists would state, "the presence or absence of lymph node involvement." An improved understanding of the likelihood of harboring such metastases would, therefore, seem to have merit. The first possible sites of metastasis along the route of lymphatic drainage from the primary lesion are known as sentinel nodes.[524] These are, therefore, the lymph nodes that are most likely to harbor metastases. Beside sentinel node evaluation, the concept of "ultrastaging" by serial sectioning, combined with immunohistochemical techniques, improves one's ability to detect lymph node micrometastases (smaller than 2 mm).[513,718]

Technique

"Mapping" may be performed in vivo at the time of laparotomy or following removal of the specimen. Typically, lymphatic mapping is performed intraoperatively through the subserosal injection of blue dye. Regional nodes take up the dye in about 5 minutes. Another technique is to employ colloidal antimony sulfide in blue dye or other agents, with detection by the use of a gamma probe. This may be accomplished by endoscopic injection or by injection directly around the tumor. One may then perform a standard lymphadenectomy or remove additional mesentery containing lymphatics and nodes when there appears to be atypical drainage.

Ex vivo mapping involves the injection of blue dye around the tumor and then massaging the mesentery to propel the dye through the lymphatics and into the nodes. Such identified nodes are then harvested for microscopic sectioning.

Results

Kitagawa and colleagues enrolled 56 patients with curatively resectable colorectal carcinoma in order to test the feasibility of performing the technique and the accuracy of radioactivity-guided mapping of the first lymph nodes found in draining the primary tumor site.[524] They used a technique that involved preoperative endoscopic injection of ^{99m}Tc-labeled tin colloid. Diagnostic accuracy according to sentinel node status was determined to be 92%.[524] As expected, the incidence of metastasis in the sentinel node (22%) was significantly higher than that in the nonsentinel nodes (3%). Joosten and associates injected blue dye around the tumor in 50 patients.[500] Routine pathologic assessment was made of all nodes, with the blue-stained ones additionally tested immunohistochemically. A false-negative rate of 60% was observed, leading the authors to conclude that the concept of lymph node mapping and sentinel node identification is not valid for colorectal cancer.[500] Esser and colleagues injected 31 colorectal cancers with lymphazurin blue dye, reporting a sensitivity of 67%, a specificity and positive predictive value of 100%, and a negative predictive value of 94%.[284] Trocha and associates emphasize that dual-agent lymphatic mapping (radiotracer plus blue dye) more accurately identifies sentinel node metastases than blue dye alone and allows a more focused histopathologic examination.[1034] Mulsow and coworkers in 2003 reviewed the literature as it applies to mapping of colorectal cancer and noted a false-negative rate of approximately 10%.[718] They and others conclude that further follow-up studies are necessary in order truly to assess the prognostic significance of micrometastases and staging benefits with respect to therapeutic implications.[513,1125] A multicenter cooperative trial concluded that sentinel nodes did not accurately predict the presence of either conventionally defined lymph node metastases or micrometastatic disease.[832]

Radioimmunoguided Surgery

Radioimmunoguided surgery (RIGS) uses a handheld gamma-detecting probe to identify radioactivity following injection of one of a number of radiolabeled monoclonal antibodies. This approach is discussed later in this chapter, especially as it applies to second-look operations. Some, however, have explored the use of RIGS in the management of colorectal cancer at the time of the initial procedure. Through this technique, it has been shown that RIGS enables surgeons to define lymphatic metastases with a higher degree of sensitivity and specificity than can be determined by clinical assessment alone (see later discussion).[387]

As with the discussion on sentinel node mapping, the critical issue is whether these applications improve cure rates. That is unlikely. However, such techniques are potentially useful in improving the staging of colorectal cancer.

Peritoneal Cytology

Intraoperative peritoneal washings have been performed in order to examine whether the presence or absence of positive cytology has prognostic implications. Kanellos and colleagues undertook 110 such examinations by placing 100 mL of saline over the tumor site and then aspirating the fluid for cytologic assessment.[506] Patients with positive cytology were found to have a significantly higher rate of recurrence, but the survival rate did not correlate with the findings.

Intraoperative Colonoscopy

The importance of complete evaluation of the colon before undertaking a colectomy for cancer cannot be overestimated. However, there are instances when such an evaluation may not be feasible. Under such circumstances, one may consider using intraoperative colonoscopy. Various clinical settings have been suggested—assessment of a new anastomosis to determine whether any air leakage is present or to identify any suture line defects, identification of a prior polypectomy site, inability to do a complete or adequate preoperative colonoscopy, detection of a source of intestinal bleeding, and detection of a colon lesion that cannot be palpated.[879] With respect to resection of colon tumors, however, the primary indications are identification of a nonpalpable lesion and an incomplete or inadequate preoperative colonoscopy. The relatively poor reliability for colonoscopy in providing accurate anatomic localization of colorectal cancer has been highlighted.[800]

Although the procedure may be somewhat awkward and generally requires a skilled endoscopist as well as the operating surgeon, it can be performed safely as the instrument is guided through the bowel by the surgeon, but not necessarily easily or expeditiously. Clamping the region of the distal ileum is important to avoid reflux of air back into the small bowel; this can result in dilatation. When an obstructing tumor is present, the procedure can be undertaken in an ante-grade fashion through a cecotomy or in a retrograde fashion after resection of the tumor-bearing segment. Obviously, the patient must be placed in the perineolithotomy position on the operating table to provide appropriate exposure. Still, this is not necessarily a straightforward procedure.

Stapling Techniques

The use of staplers in colonic operations has been proven to be at least as safe as conventional suturing and offers distinct advantages. Three types of stapling devices are available to perform intestinal anastomoses: linear staplers, which apply two rows of staggered staples; the gastrointestinal anastomosis (GIA) stapler (Covidien, Inc., Norwalk, CT) and Proximate linear cutter (Ethicon Endo-Surgery, Cincinnati, OH), which apply two staggered rows of staples and divide the tissue by means of a contained knife; and the circular, end-to-end anastomosis stapler, which secure two rows of staples from within the lumen of the bowel to produce an inverting anastomosis in a circular fashion (Figure 23-59).

Stapling of the bowel generally requires stripping the mesentery and fat from the ends of the intestine. This should be carried out for a distance of approximately 5 mm, but the critical issue is to remove any fat and blood vessels at the level where the instrument closes.[836] Attention to that detail minimizes the risk of bleeding.

Anastomosis of the bowel can be accomplished by a number of methods. Figure 23-60 demonstrates the application of the linear stapler by a triangulation technique. The staple lines should cross each other. This produces an everting anastomosis that, although contraindicated when used with conventional suturing, does not seem to be a problem with the stapling device. An alternative approach is to invert the posterior row, everting the two anterior limbs (Figure 23-61). Venkatesh and colleagues used the triangulation stapling technique to perform colorectal anastomoses in 259 patients.[1054] The incidence of anastomotic leak was certainly comparable with that of the circular stapled anastomoses performed for this purpose (1.1%). Still, these methods are rarely employed, having been replaced by the following.

The GIA or linear cutter stapler creates a side-to-side anastomosis, but the tissue is divided, producing a functional end-to-end anastomosis. Figure 23-62 illustrates the closed technique and subsequent closure of the enterotomies (Figure 23-63). Alternatively, an open method can be employed (Figures 23-64 and 23-65). Other variations include division of the bowel with a linear stapler (Figure 23-66) or with the GIA/linear cutter stapler (Figure 23-67). A final modification to effect right hemicolectomy has been suggested by Meagher and Wolff, using the GIA stapler or linear cutter (Figure 23-68).[670]

The circular stapling devices can also be used to create colonic anastomoses. Figure 23-69 demonstrates this procedure. Additionally, an ileocolic anastomosis can be accomplished with the circular stapler (Figure 23-70). Other methods of application are illustrated in Chapter 24.

A newer concept on circular stapling is called the Surg-ASSIST (Power Medical Interventions, New Hope, PA; http://www.pmi2.com). This is a long, flexible power source that is passed through the anus and guided by the surgeon to effect a circular stapled anastomosis higher up in the colon than may be achieved by the conventional circular stapling instruments. The device consists of a computer-mediated clo-

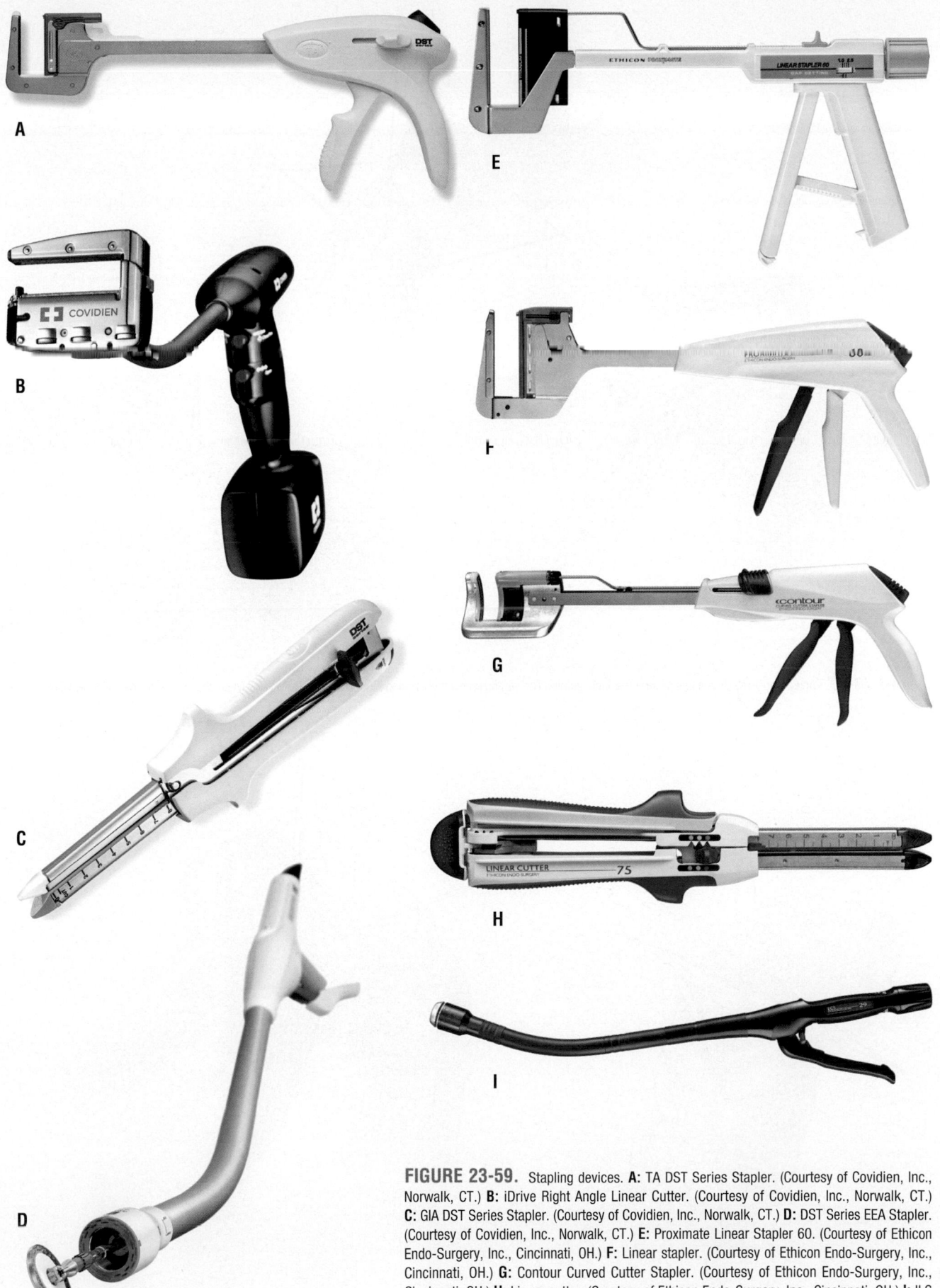

FIGURE 23-59. Stapling devices. **A:** TA DST Series Stapler. (Courtesy of Covidien, Inc., Norwalk, CT.) **B:** iDrive Right Angle Linear Cutter. (Courtesy of Covidien, Inc., Norwalk, CT.) **C:** GIA DST Series Stapler. (Courtesy of Covidien, Inc., Norwalk, CT.) **D:** DST Series EEA Stapler. (Courtesy of Covidien, Inc., Norwalk, CT.) **E:** Proximate Linear Stapler 60. (Courtesy of Ethicon Endo-Surgery, Inc., Cincinnati, OH.) **F:** Linear stapler. (Courtesy of Ethicon Endo-Surgery, Inc., Cincinnati, OH.) **G:** Contour Curved Cutter Stapler. (Courtesy of Ethicon Endo-Surgery, Inc., Cincinnati, OH.) **H:** Linear cutter. (Courtesy of Ethicon Endo-Surgery, Inc., Cincinnati, OH.) **I:** ILS Intraluminal Stapler—29. (Courtesy of Ethicon Endo-Surgery, Inc., Cincinnati, OH.)

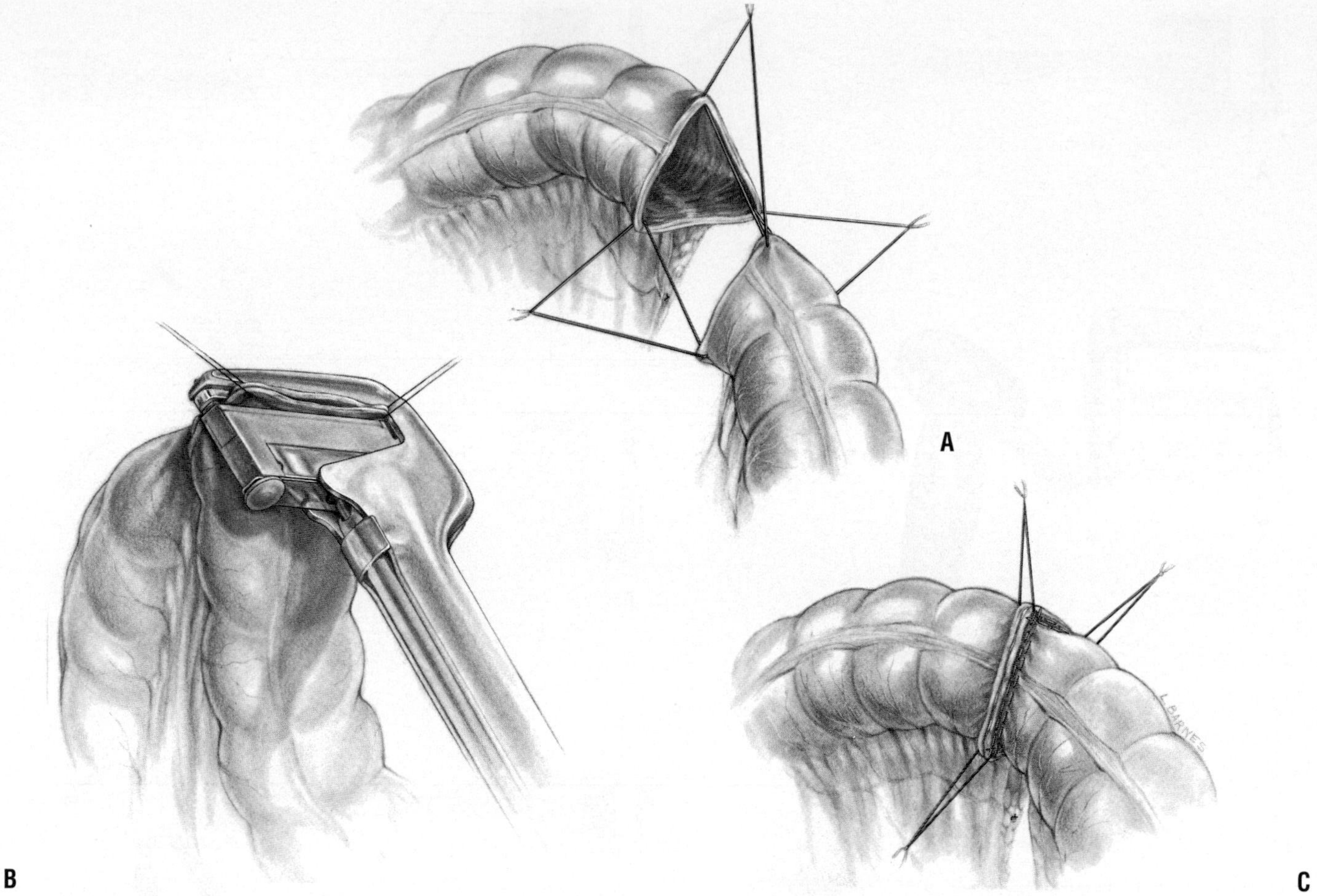

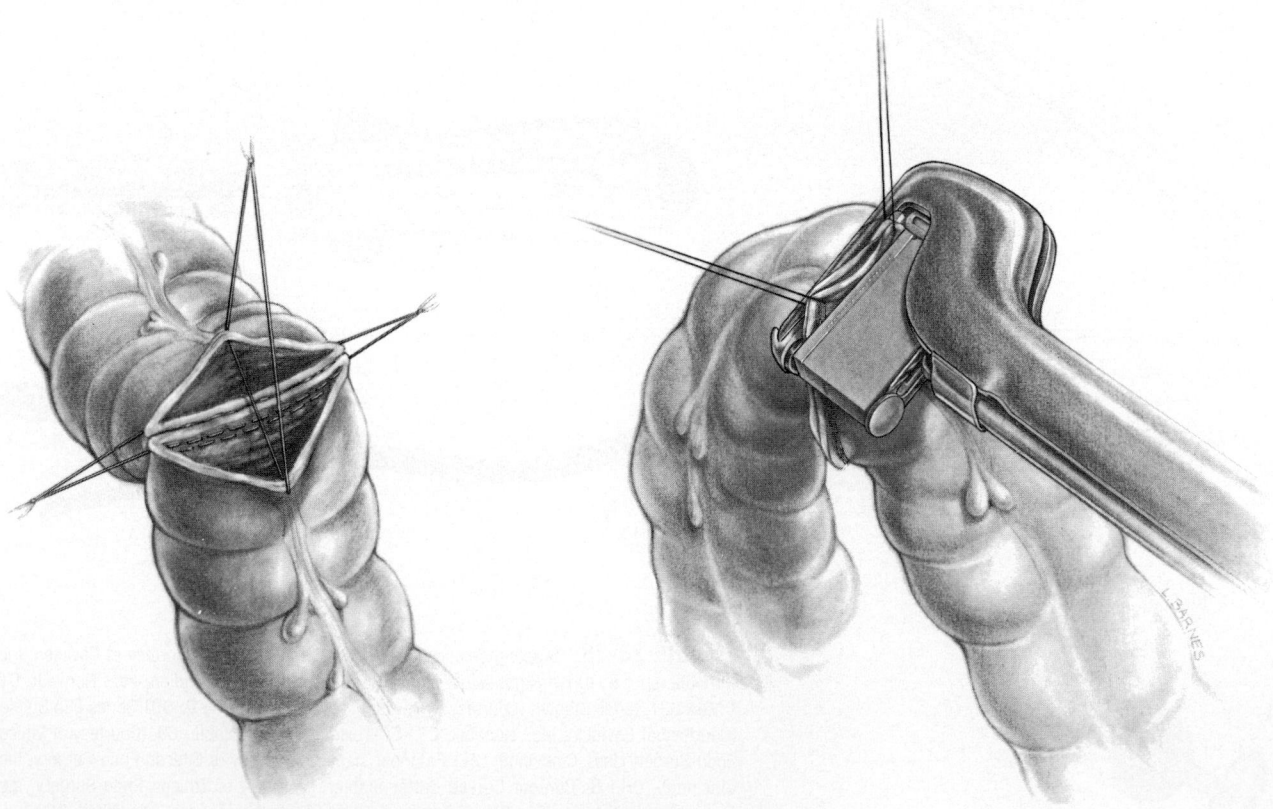

FIGURE 23-60. Anastomosis by triangulation using the linear stapler. **A:** Everting anastomosis using three stay sutures. **B:** The TA stapler. **C:** Eversion of all three applications.

FIGURE 23-61. Triangulation anastomosis by inversion of the posterior (mesenteric) wall **(A)** and eversion of the anterior walls **(B)**.

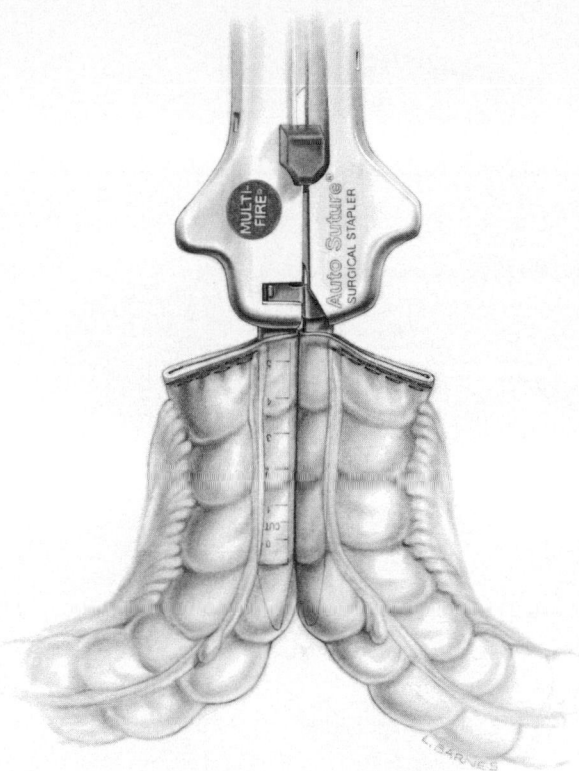

FIGURE 23-62. Functional end-to-end anastomosis by the closed technique after creation of two enterotomies for insertion of the separate limbs of the gastrointestinal anastomosis stapler.

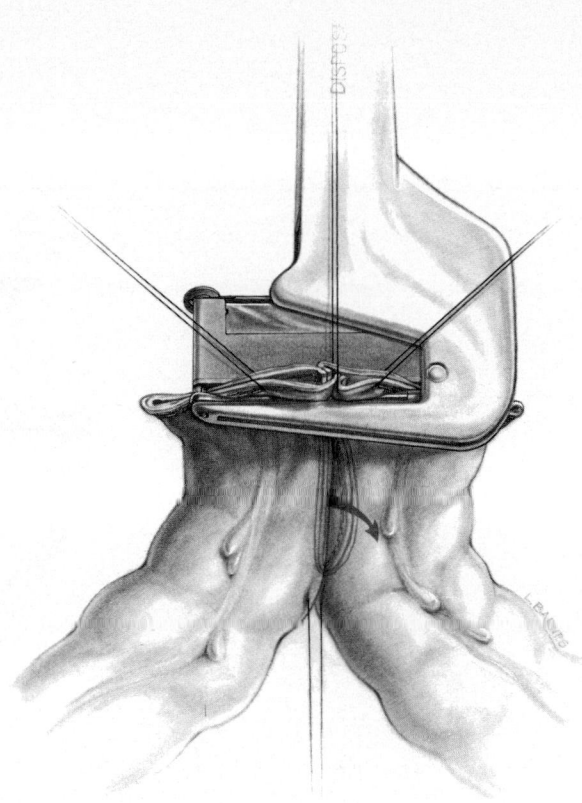

FIGURE 23-63. Closure of the enterotomies using the TA stapler.

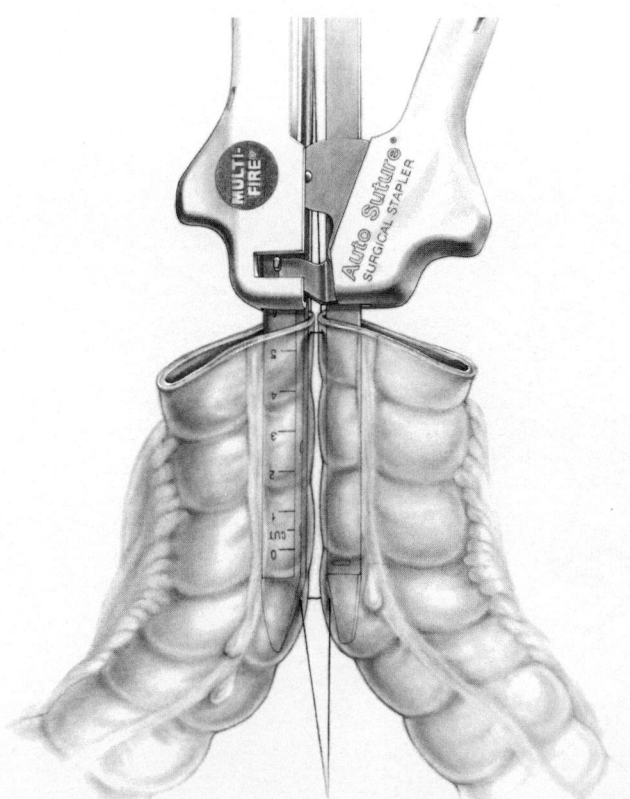

FIGURE 23-64. Functional end-to-end anastomosis by the open technique with the gastrointestinal anastomosis stapler.

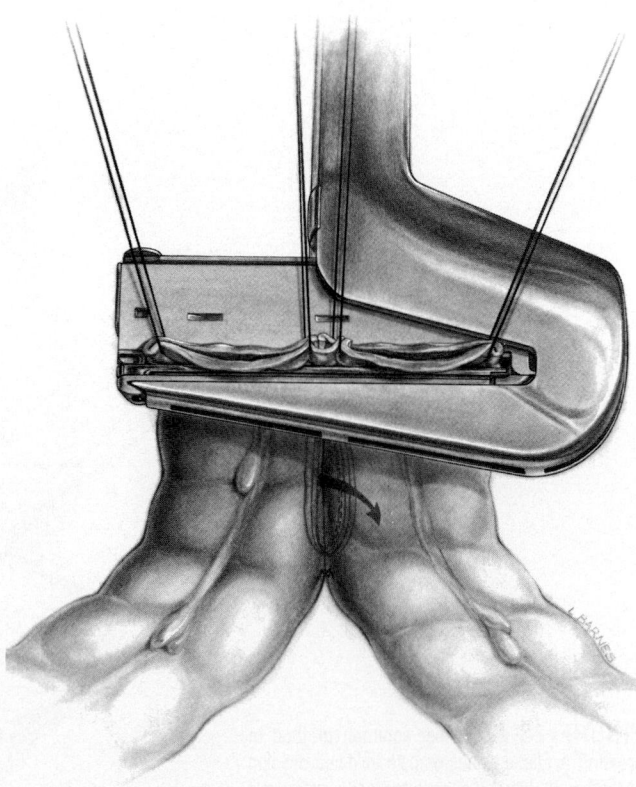

FIGURE 23-65. Closure of the bowel ends with the TA stapler and open functional end-to-end anastomosis.

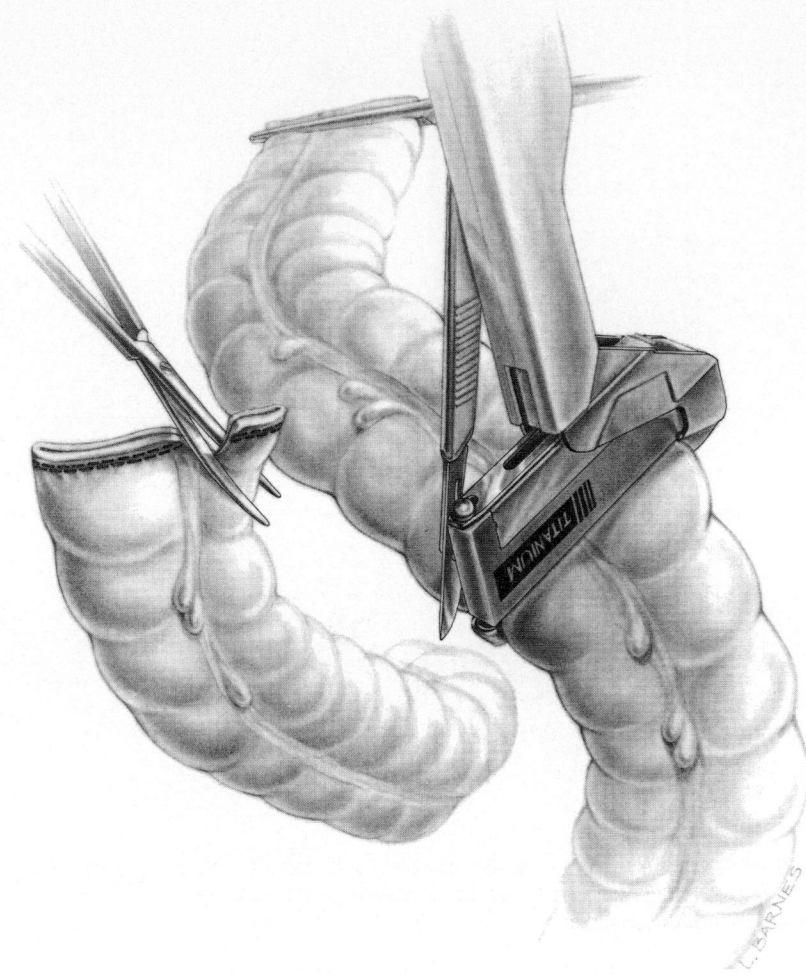

FIGURE 23-66. One option for resection and division of the bowel in preparation for the anastomosis is to use the linear stapler.

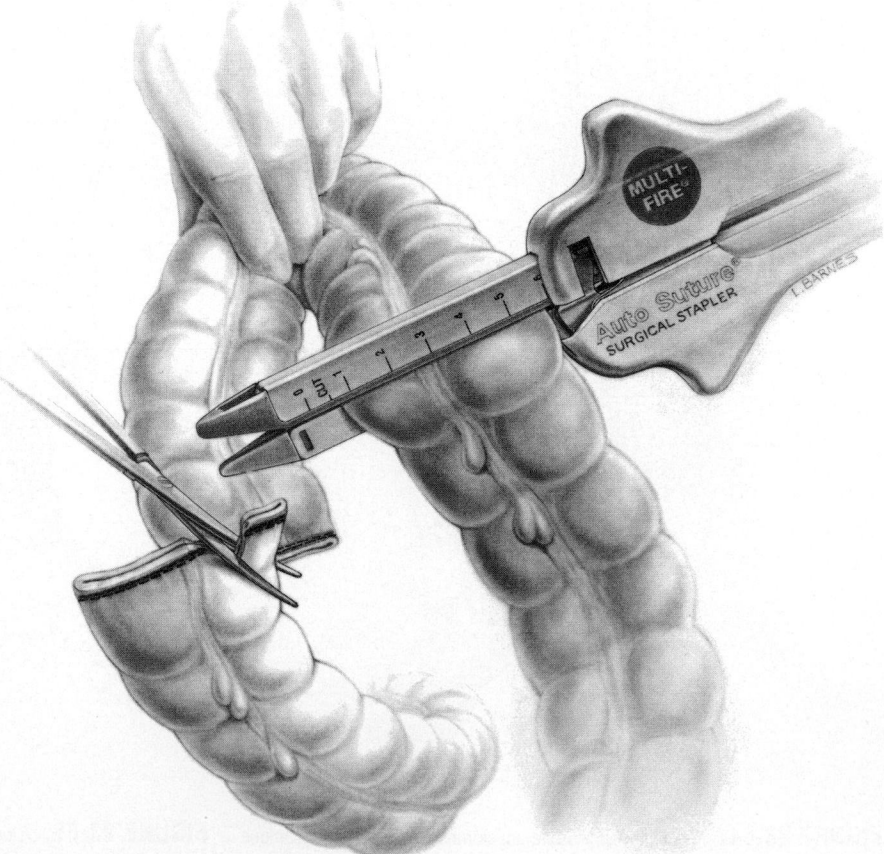

FIGURE 23-67. Most common method of creating a stapled anastomosis involves division of the bowel with the gastrointestinal anastomosis stapler and anastomosis through several firings of the instrument. Linear closure of the created defect is then accomplished.

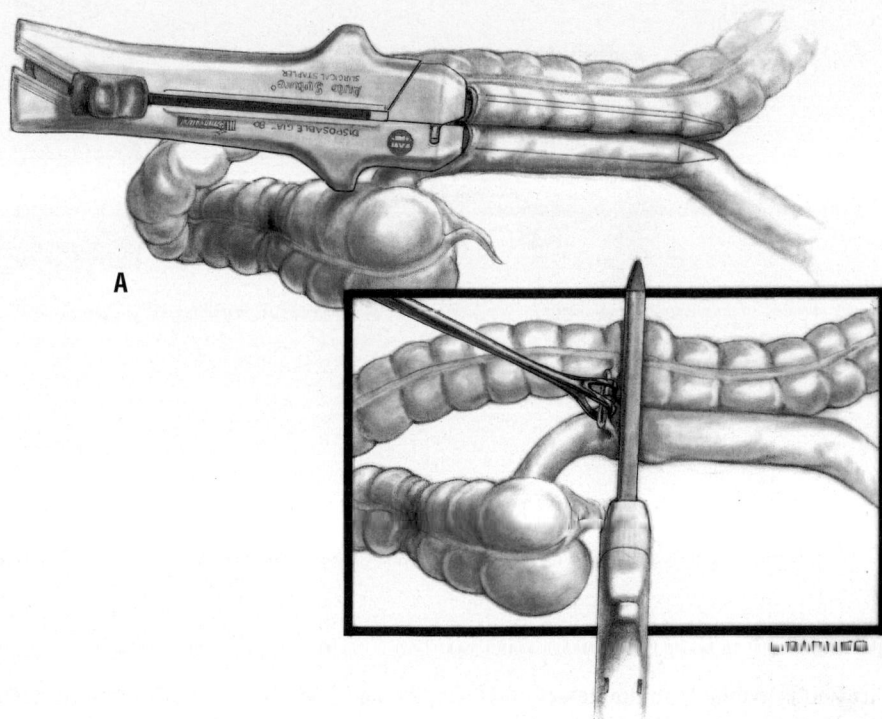

FIGURE 23-68. Colon anastomosis is facilitated following mobilization of the right colon by use of the gastrointestinal anastomosis stapling device to create a functional end-to-end anastomosis (**A**) and simultaneous firing of the instrument across both the ileum and colon (**B**). (Adapted from Meagher AP, Wolff BG. Right hemicolectomy with a linear cutting stapler. *Dis Colon Rectum*. 1994;37:1043.)

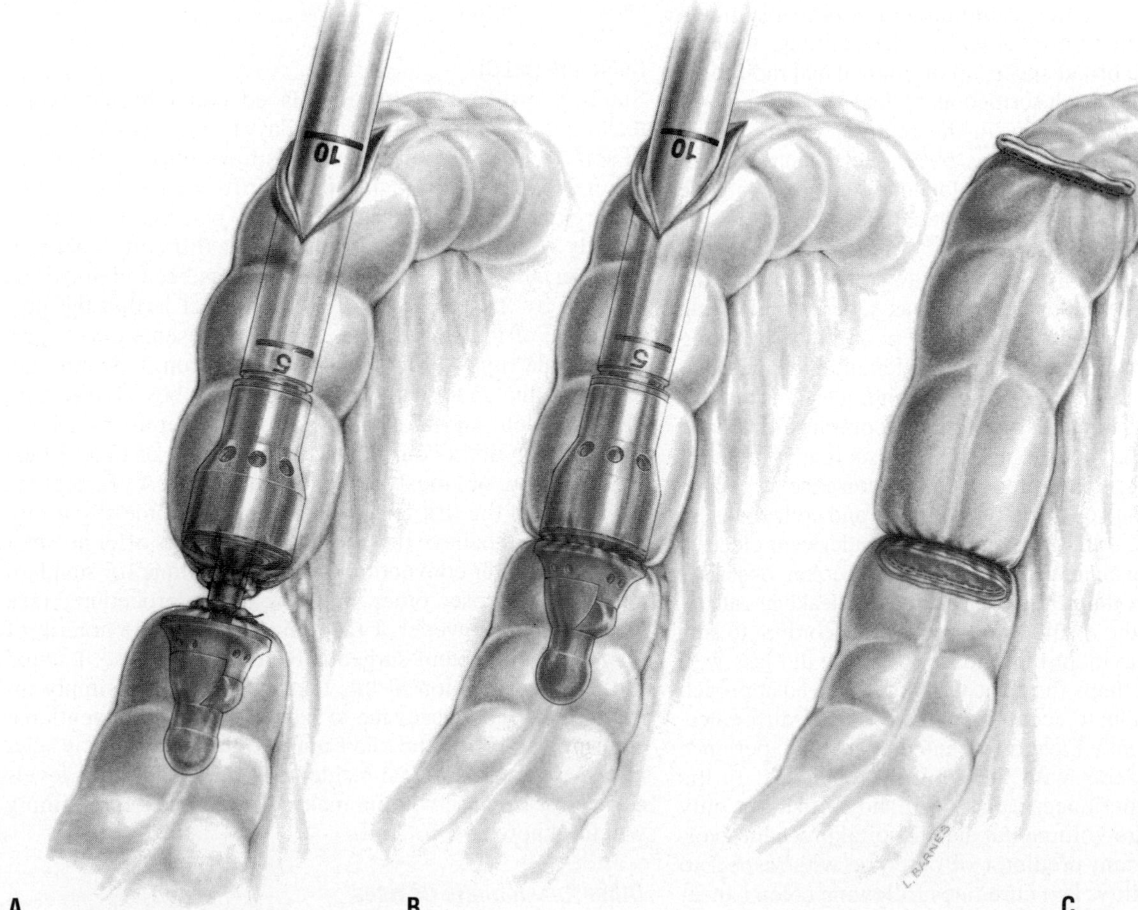

A

B

A   **B**   **C**

FIGURE 23-69. **A,B:** Steps of circular end-to-end anastomosis stapler used in colonic anastomosis through a proximal colotomy. **C:** Note the stapled closure of the colotomy converting the longitudinal incision to a transverse closure.

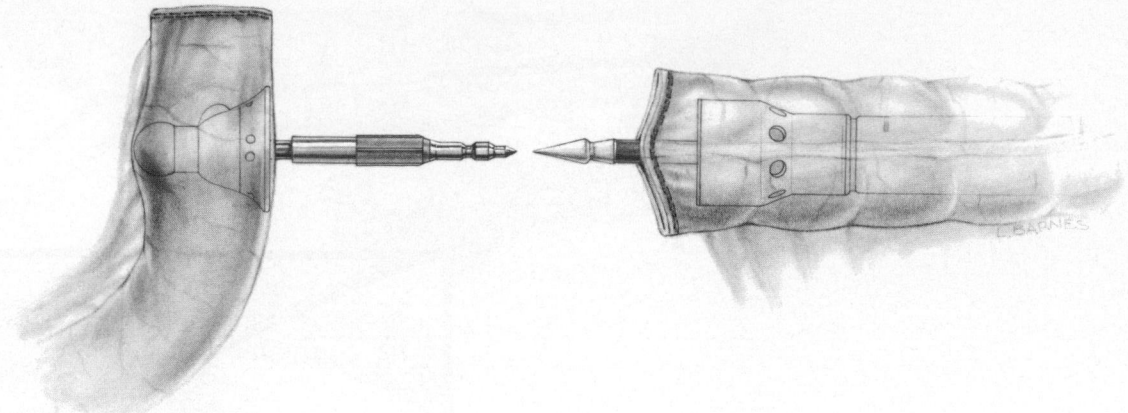

FIGURE 23-70. Anastomosis of the distal ileum to the transverse colon by means of the circular stapler. The proximal anvil can be placed either in the end of the ileum or in the side (as illustrated). The stapling device is placed through an enterotomy in the colon with anastomosis shown by a double-stapling technique (note the trocar). A purse-string suture is another option. There are several possible variations on this theme.

sure and is available in diameters of 21, 25, 29, and 33 mm. The loading unit is disposable. All instrument movements are automated and executed via push-button remote control.

Complications and Results of Anastomoses

Disruption of the suture or staple line is clinically apparent in approximately 5% of all colonic anastomoses, but the true incidence of this complication is probably much higher.[904] Definitions are critical in determining the leak rate, owing to the broad spectrum of clinical and radiologic scenarios that may be described as a "leak."[469] The rate of anastomotic disruption low in the rectum, when studied thoroughly, may be as high as 69% (see Chapter 24).[904] Irrespective of the technique employed to reapproximate the bowel, the rates of complications (fecal fistula, hemorrhage, stricture) are about the same.[169,249,285,519,837,1069,1072] However, Dunn and colleagues, in a study on dogs, believed that the one-layer, hand-sewn anastomosis was superior.[267] Reiling and associates, in a controlled trial, reported that operating time, nasogastric intubation, and total length of hospitalization were about the same for both techniques.[837] This implies that the variables responsible for complications have less to do with the method of anastomosis than with other factors, such as tension, blood supply, presence of sepsis, and nutritional state of the patient. Friend and colleagues, in a randomized trial of 250 patients who underwent elective surgery involving an anastomosis in the left colon, observed no differences in the clinical or radiologic leakage rate.[317] However, when the results were analyzed according to surgeon, it became evident that those in training did less well with suturing. Perhaps the relatively standardized approach to stapling was able to account for the observed difference. Alternatively, it may have represented a lack of experience by surgical residents with the suturing technique. In the area of one's experience, it has been shown that not only surgeon procedure volume but also hospital procedure volume is an important predictor of outcome with respect to morbidity, mortality, and cure rates following colon cancer resection.[903]

A problem that appears to be more specific with stapled intestinal anastomoses is bleeding. Many surgeons make a conscientious effort to visualize the staple line before final closure in a functional end-to-end anastomosis. Any bleeding point can be managed with a simple suture ligature. Atabek and colleagues have successfully employed vasopressin to control bleeding from a stapled intestinal anastomosis in the postoperative period.[37] This method of treatment is frightening, however, because of the risk of causing ischemia.

Comment (MLC)

Stapling instruments have replaced conventional suture techniques for many surgeons today. In fact, as mentioned, in some teaching centers residents have only minimal exposure to the traditional approach. It is true that as one gains experience, an anastomosis may be constructed more quickly with a stapling instrument. It is difficult to believe, however, that operative time can, as has been claimed, be reduced by 25% and even 50%. The fact is that the performance of the anastomosis, itself, represents only a part of the time invested in the whole operation. Opening and exploring the abdomen, dissecting out the bowel, resecting the specimen, and closing the abdomen represent efforts that may require a considerable expenditure of time. Intestinal stapling, obviously, fails to expedite these. Except for avoidance of the risk for needle injury and some slight savings in time, I believe that the stapling devices offer no great advantages over conventional suture technique for standard colon anastomoses other than low pelvic procedures (see Chapter 24). However, I recognize that a large coterie of respected, competent surgeons believes otherwise. I stated in the second edition of this text, "Perhaps it is simply intransigence that causes me to persist in using conventional suturing, but if truth be told I must confess that I enjoy sewing." Moreover, surgical residents at the most senior levels ask to sew because without making this request they simply will not know how to do it.

Other Anastomotic Devices

Biofragmentable Ring (Valtrac)

In 1985, Hardy and colleagues described a biofragmentable ring for sutureless intestinal anastomosis.[417] The ring is composed of two segments containing polyglycolic acid (Dexon) and 12% barium sulfate. The major advantage when compared with the classic Murphy button (see Figure 23-35) is that it does not produce necrosis but fragments during the third week following implantation. The procedure is probably somewhat more rapid than conventional suturing and has the advantage of applicability to all parts of the intestine. However, it is quite limiting with respect to low rectal anastomoses, especially when compared with the circular stapling device, although an adapter for transanal placement has been reported from Taiwan.[172] It is at least as safe as other anastomotic alternatives. The rings are available in six sizes represented by the outside diameter, inside diameter, and closed position gap. The outside diameters are 28, 31, and 34 mm, and the gap width varies between 1.5 and 2.5 mm.

Technique. Figure 23-71 illustrates the bowel anastomosis ring in the open position with the holder in place. The method of performing the anastomosis is as follows: After the bowel has been mobilized, a purse-string suture is placed (Figures 23-72 and 23-73). As with the placement of a purse string for the circular stapling instrument, a monofilament suture, preferably absorbable, is recommended. Three Allis clamps are triangulated on the proximal limb if a colorectal anastomosis is contemplated. A sizing device is available to determine which diameter ring is applicable (Figure 23-74). It is important to place the device into the proximal end first because it is easier to pull the rectum onto the ring rather than to push the proximal bowel down (Figure 23-75). It does not matter whether the proximal or distal end is secured initially if the anastomosis is well out of the pelvis. The purse-string suture is then secured (Figure 23-76). With the use of a triangulation technique, the ring is inserted into the distal bowel (Figure 23-77). A "holding" device is available that may make this maneuver easier to accomplish (Figure 23-78). The second purse-string suture is then tied (Figure 23-79). The ring is then snapped shut with an audible and tactile click, and an inverted serosa-to-serosa anastomosis is created (Figure 23-80). The security of the closure needs to be checked by the application of gentle pressure between the two anvils, to make certain that they cannot be separated (Figure 23-81).[161]

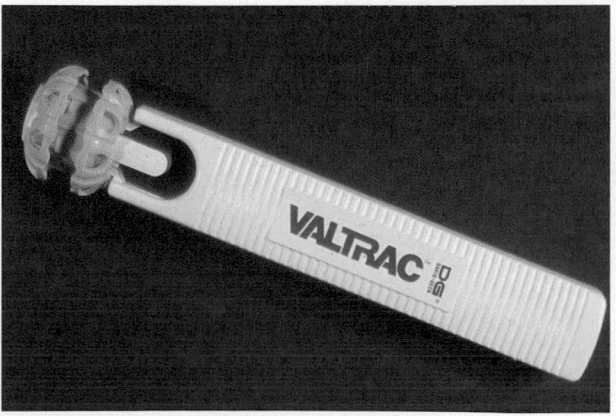

FIGURE 23-71. Valtrac biofragmentable ring. (Courtesy of Covidien, Inc., Norwalk, CT.)

Results. Because the ring is impregnated with barium, it is radiopaque and can be seen on a plain abdominal x-ray film (Figure 23-82). Fragmentation usually takes place between 17 and 21 days (Figure 23-83). The material at this time is soft and is rarely noted by the patient when it is passed during defecation.

Since the original publication of the experimental reports, hundreds of patients have undergone resection and anastomosis by this method.[288,306,415,419] In randomized, multicenter, prospective clinical trials that compared the biofragmentable ring with suture technique and with stapling, there was no significant difference in morbidity, mortality, or clinical course of the patients.[126,390] The safety and efficacy of this device were confirmed in several other trials.[153,201,1124] Gullichsen and colleagues studied the late results after colonic anastomosis performed with the biofragmentable ring in 30 patients at a mean of 2 years.[391] One had undergone reoperation because of a stricture. Endoscopic and radiology examination could not identify the anastomotic site in approximately half of the patients.

Comment (MLC). The Valtrac device is indeed still available, but no one seems motivated to write about it. There are apparently only a very few surgeons who continue to employ it, however. Along these same lines, there has also been a virtual absence of publications in the last few years on the whole subject of stapling and suturing. Perhaps everything has been said, taught, and learned regarding the technical aspects of reestablishing intestinal continuity—I hope not.

Circular Compression Device
In 1988, Rosati and colleagues described a mechanical device for creating a circular anastomosis through compression.[857] This is much more like the Murphy button, in that both innovations effect an anastomosis by means of compression. The apparatus consists of three molded polypropylene rings carried by a gun that introduces them into the bowel. For a colorectal anastomosis, transanal insertion is undertaken in the same way that the conventional circular stapling instruments are employed. Firing of the gun causes simultaneous assemblage of the rings, expulsion of the entire anastomotic apparatus, and disengagement of the gun, with the creation of two tissue rings.[857] The rings are evacuated between the 9th and 13th postoperative days. In contrast to the circular stapler, it leaves no staples or foreign material within the bowel.

Results. Malthaner and colleagues employed the device experimentally in dogs and compared it with the circular stapler.[628] They noted that the button was easier to use; caused less ulceration, fibrosis, and inflammation; and was associated with better reepithelialization at the anastomotic site. Rebuffat and colleagues used the technique for 56 patients in diverse colon operations.[830] There was one operative death (myocardial infarction) and one anastomotic leak.

Magnetic Ring Anastomosis
A modification of the Murphy button has been described by Jansen and colleagues.[483] An anastomotic apparatus consisting of two magnetic rings embedded in polyester progressively compresses and causes necrosis in the intervening bowel through increasing magnetic force while healing takes place. After 7 to 12 days, the magnets cut through and are eliminated through the stool.

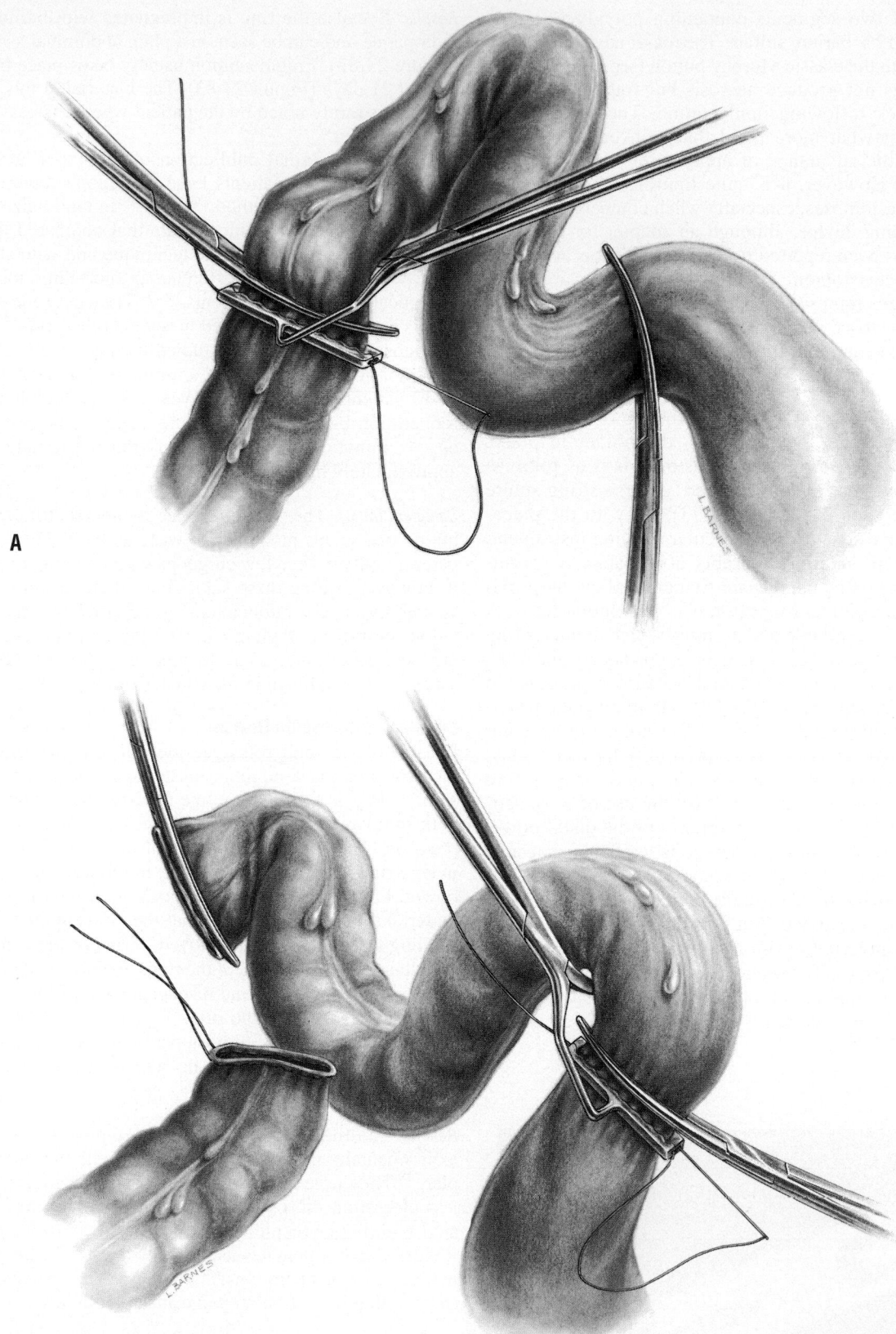

FIGURE 23-72. **A,B:** Anastomosis by biofragmentable ring. Purse-string technique with an applicator.

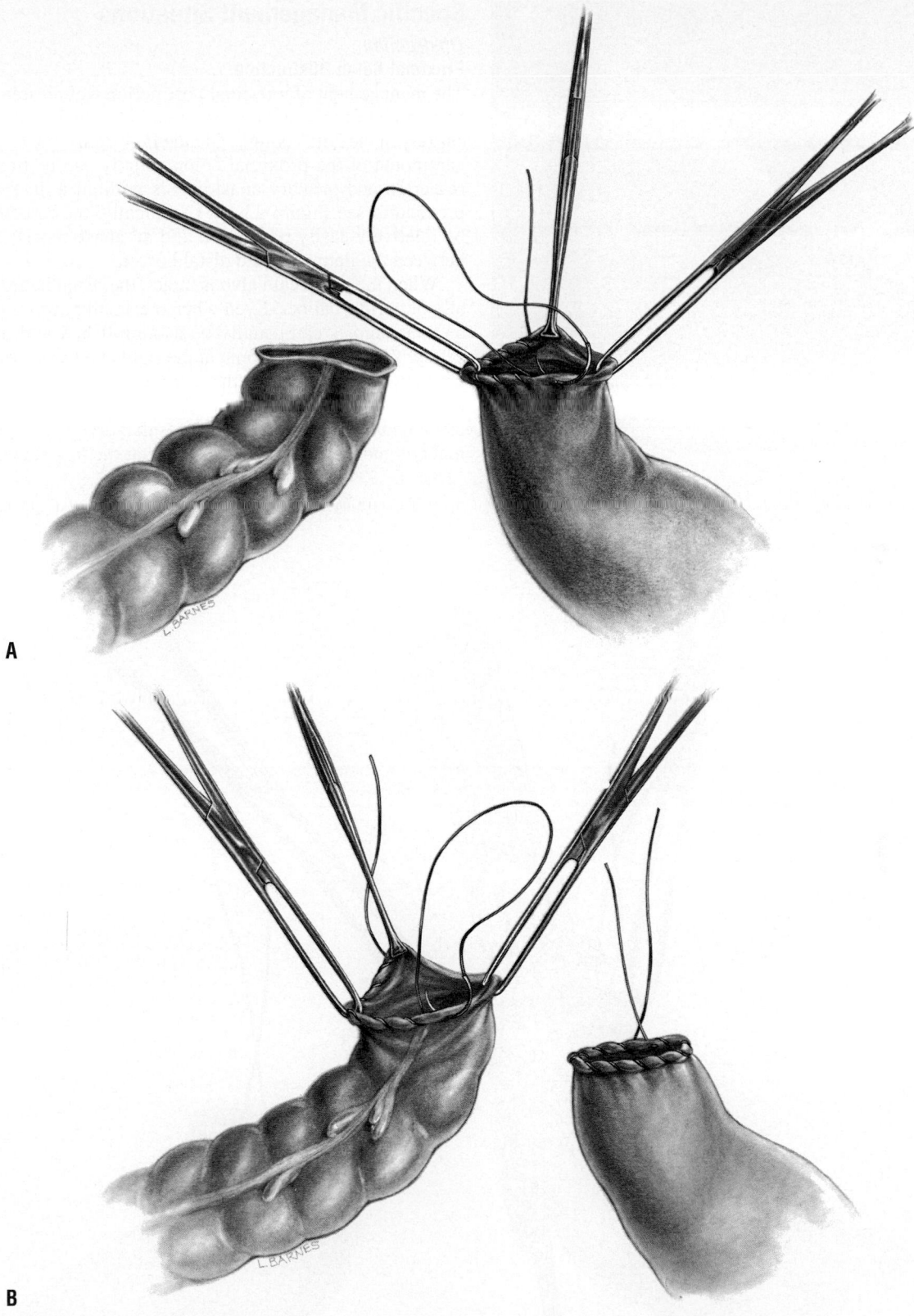

A

B

FIGURE 23-73. **A,B:** Anastomosis by biofragmentable ring. Hand-sewn purse string.

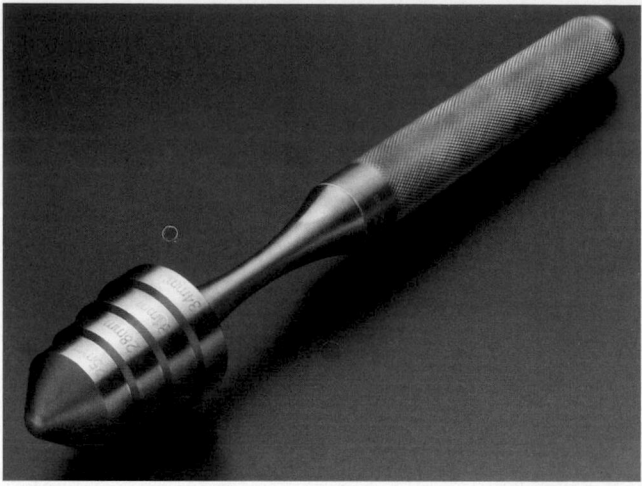

FIGURE 23-74. Sizing device for determining which diameter Valtrac ring is appropriate. (Courtesy of Covidien, Inc., Norwalk, CT.)

Specific Management Situations

Obstruction

Proximal Colon Obstruction

The management of intestinal obstruction was an area of particular interest for one of the singular individuals in American surgery in the 20th century, Claude E. Welch.[1080] Obstructing carcinoma of the proximal colon usually can be treated by resection and primary anastomosis without a diversionary procedure (see Figure 23-1). Technically, the resection can be relatively easily performed and an anastomosis effected between the ileum and the distal bowel.

When the ileocecal valve is intact, the distal ileum is usually of normal caliber. Even when the small bowel is dilated, an anastomosis can usually be accomplished with relative safety. Whenever carcinoma of the right and transverse colon presents with obstruction, the resected bowel proximal to the lesion should always include the colon to the level of the distal ileum. If the surgeon believes that diversion of a proximal colonic obstruction is necessary at the first stage, or if a

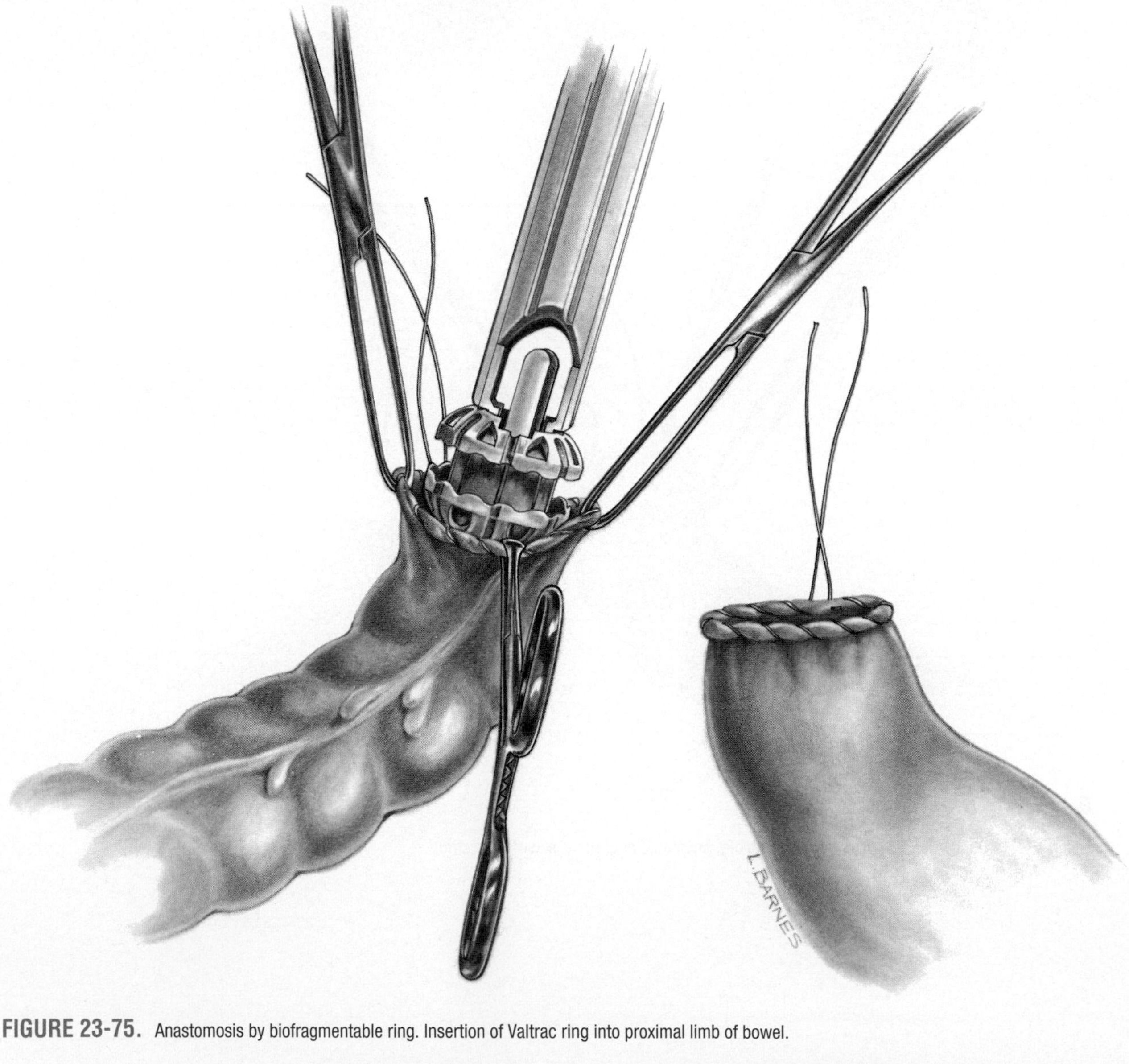

FIGURE 23-75. Anastomosis by biofragmentable ring. Insertion of Valtrac ring into proximal limb of bowel.

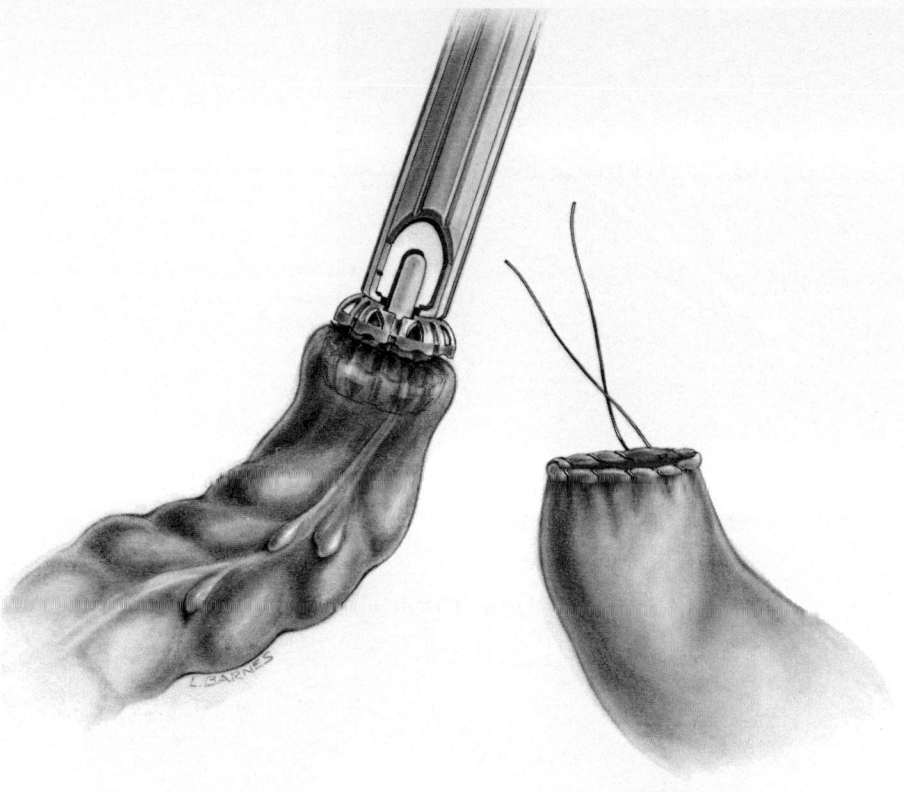

FIGURE 23-76. Anastomosis by biofragmentable ring. A purse-string suture is secured around the device.

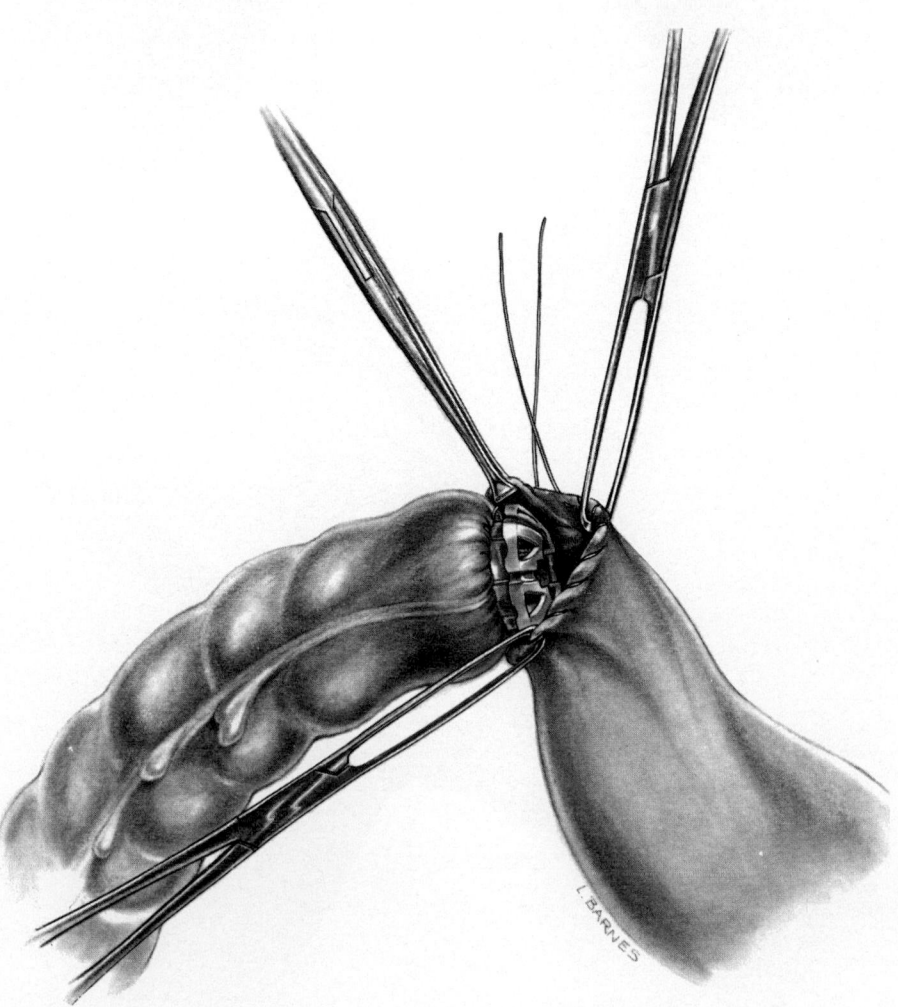

FIGURE 23-77. Anastomosis by biofragmentable ring. The ring is inserted into the distal bowel.

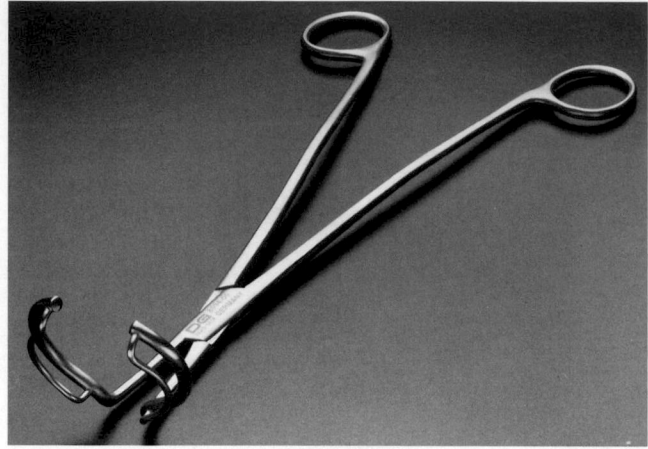

FIGURE 23-78. Device for holding the biofragmentable ring while the distal bowel is pulled upward. (Courtesy of Covidien, Inc., Norwalk, CT.)

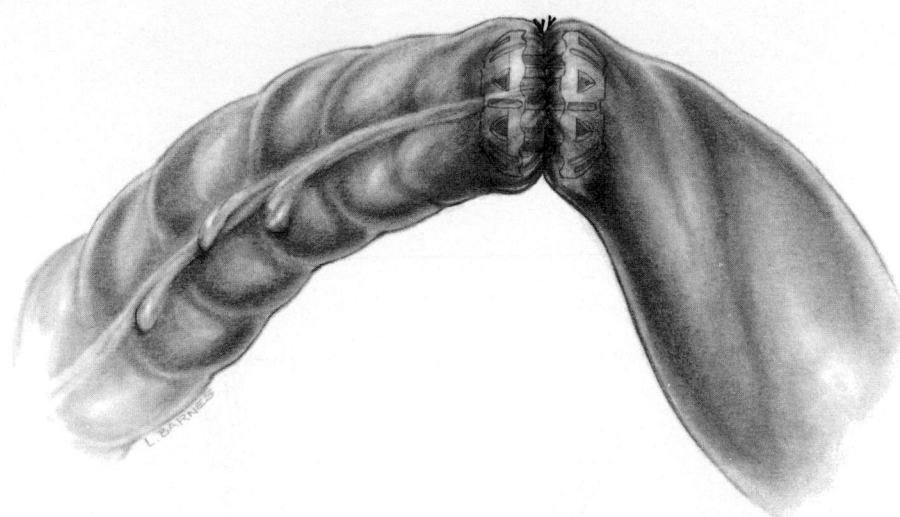

FIGURE 23-79. Anastomosis by biofragmentable ring. The distal purse-string suture is now tied.

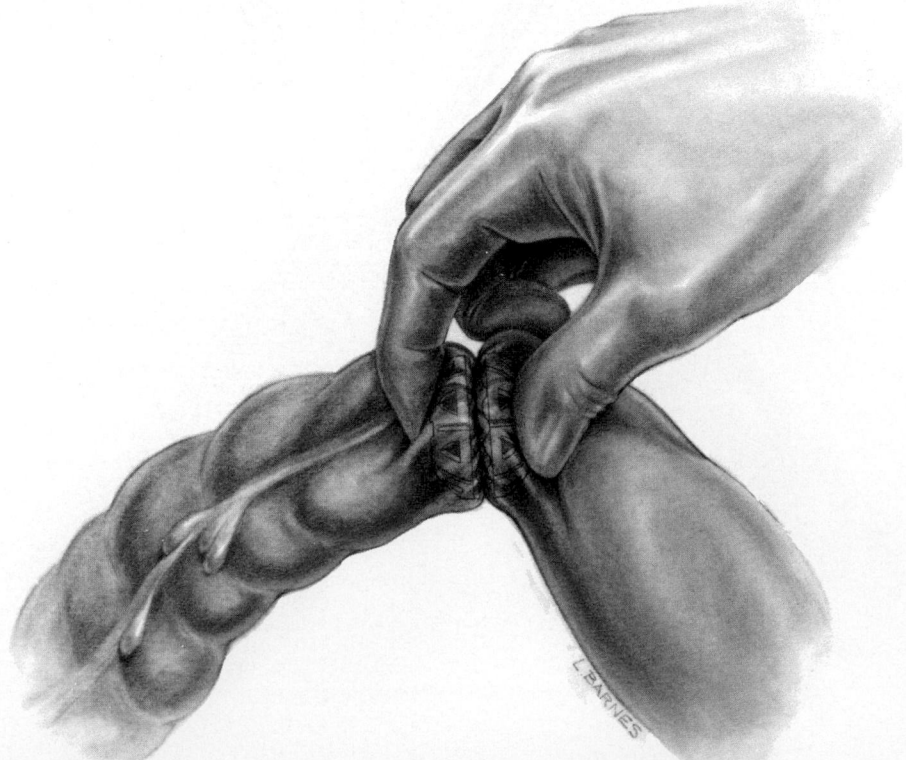

FIGURE 23-80. Anastomosis by biofragmentable ring. The ring is closed.

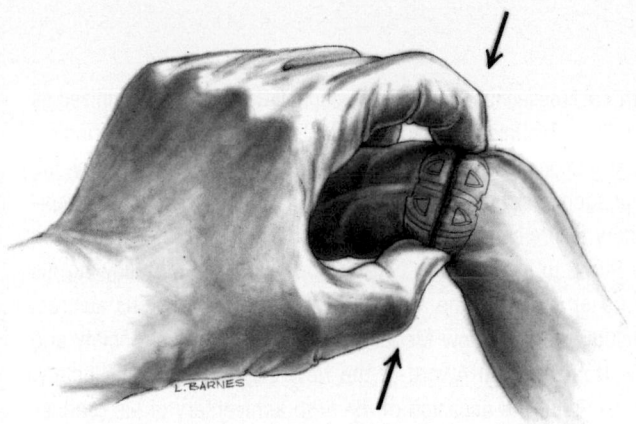

FIGURE 23-81. Testing the security of the Valtrac biofragmentable anastomotic ring by attempted distraction of the anvils through gentle pressure. (Adapted from Celoria G, Falco E, Nardini A, et al. Intraoperative testing of the Valtrac biofragmentable anastomotic ring. *Br J Surg.* 1993;80:618.)

protective stoma after ileocolonic anastomosis is indicated, loop ileostomy is the preferred option (see Figures 31-67 through 31-69).

Left Colon Obstruction

Ninety percent of colonic obstructions occur distal to the splenic flexure. When carcinoma precipitates a left-sided obstruction, the surgeon faces a more difficult decision. Should primary resection be undertaken? Should an anastomosis be performed? Should a diversion be created? It is difficult to answer these questions dogmatically because nuances in the presentation or in the findings may lead the surgeon to take an alternative course of action. One of the important considerations is to note whether the obstruction is complete or partial (see Figures 23-2 and 23-84). If the patient continues to have bowel movements or to pass flatus or is seen to have gas distal to the site of obstruction on a plain film of the abdomen, the obstruction is incomplete. Conversely, if the patient has not passed flatus or defecated for many hours or even days, and no gas

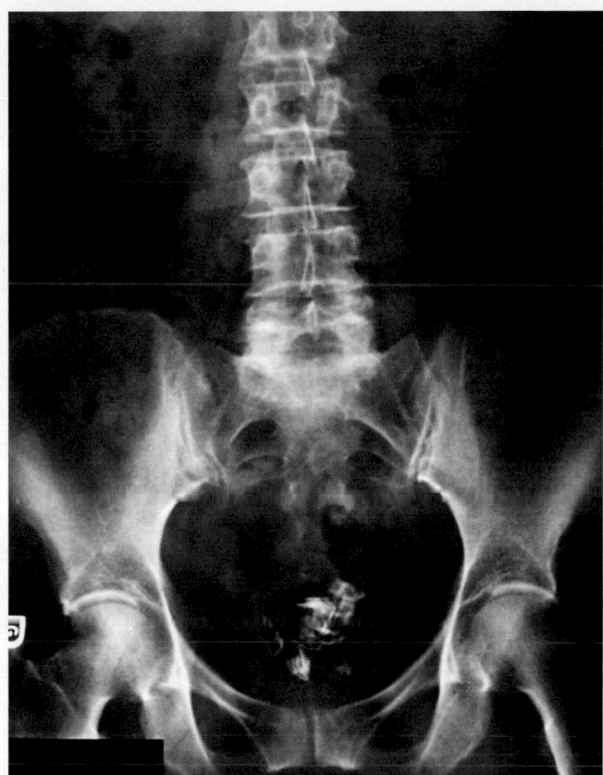

FIGURE 23-83. Fragmented ring apparent on a plain abdominal x-ray film just prior to its passing.

is visible distally, the obstruction is probably complete. At exploratory laparotomy, the degree of dilatation of the proximal bowel can be assessed and the choice of operation determined. Obstruction as a result of a malignancy does not necessarily mandate an exploratory operation. For example, when carcinomatosis is known to be present, it may be prudent to observe the patient and to treat the condition nonoperatively in the hope that the obstruction may resolve. In any event, it is reasonable to at least consider this alternative under these circumstances.

For a primary tumor, if the dilatation is minimal or moderate and removal can be accomplished without an extensive dissection (as for a sigmoid lesion), resection is advisable. It is always preferred to extirpate a mass initially and obtain a definitive pathology report. An anastomosis may then be considered. If a limited distal colon resection is accomplished, however, a proximal diversion should be performed. Not to do so in a situation in which the bowel is unprepared and the colon is dilated invites disaster. In the experience of Phillips and coworkers, immediate anastomosis in the obstructed left colon was associated with a high rate of clinical leakage (18%).[793] Another report demonstrated an operative mortality of 12% and a wound infection rate of 40%.[19] Emergency surgery for colon carcinoma has been shown to have a strong negative influence on immediate surgical morbidity and mortality.[946] Setti Carraro and colleagues reported 528 patients who underwent colonic resection over a 10-year period (1980 to 1989), wherein 179 presented with obstructing tumors.[920] There was a statistically significant increased risk of the development of metastases and death in the obstructed group.

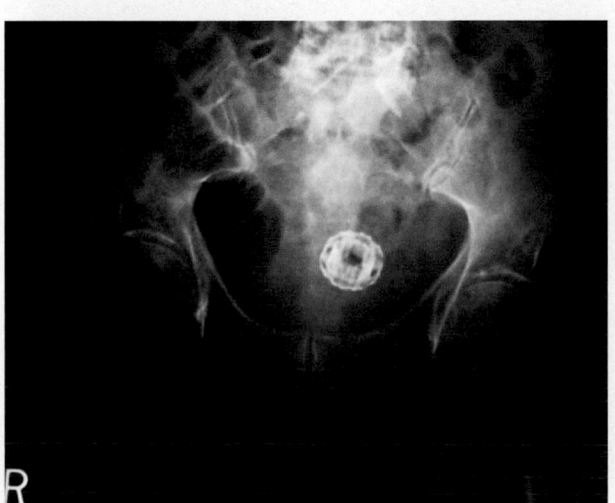

FIGURE 23-82. Plain abdominal roentgenogram reveals radiopaque ring at the site of rectal anastomosis.

CLAUDE E. WELCH (1907–1996)

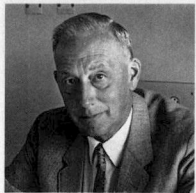

Claude Welch was born in Stanton, Nebraska, February 25, 1907. He attended Doane College in Crete, Nebraska and graduated in 1927. He then obtained a master's degree in chemistry from the University of Missouri. He entered medical school at Harvard and graduated in 1932. There followed a residency in pathology at Boston City Hospital and a residency in surgery at Pondville Hospital in suburban Boston and at the Massachusetts General Hospital. He joined the faculty at Harvard in 1937 and remained there for the rest of his life. His role model was Arthur Allen, Chief of the East Service at the General. In 1942, Welch joined the Harvard medical group in North Africa and then in Italy, returning in 1945. That same year, he performed the first vein graft at Massachusetts General Hospital. He became recognized as a brilliant technical surgeon and clinical investigator. His principal contributions were the introduction of catheter duodenostomy, the management of intestinal obstruction, and the treatment of respiratory failure concomitant with peritonitis. In 1981, he was called to Rome to assist in the care of Pope John Paul II following his gunshot wound to the abdomen. Welch won numerous awards, including the Bigelow Medal of the Boston Surgical Society and the Nathan Smith Award of the New England Surgical Society. In 1992, on the occasion of the 60th anniversary of his graduation from Harvard Medical School, the university established an endowed chair of surgery in his honor. He died on March 9, 1996 of a cerebrovascular accident. (With appreciation to Harvard Medical School. Photograph courtesy of Dr. Welch.)

Fecal Diversion. The surgeon may elect to decline an anastomosis in favor of, for example, a colostomy or ileostomy (see Chapter 31)—safe, acceptable alternatives. It should be remembered, however, that a dilated stoma (especially a sigmoid colostomy) tends to retract. An extra length should be delivered to avoid this complication. Ten days to 2 weeks later, elective resection can be undertaken, or the stoma may be allowed to remain. The stoma may or may not be closed or resected at the same time. However, there is an increased risk when two anastomoses are closed synchronously.

A loop ileostomy is often preferred if resection cannot be performed. It is always easier to make an ileal stoma than a transverse colostomy. It is also easier to manage the appliance (see Chapter 31). With respect to end- versus loop-ostomy, one must be circumspect regarding a distal obstruction. There is the theoretical possibility that an end stoma will result in a blown stump in the distal bowel, thus

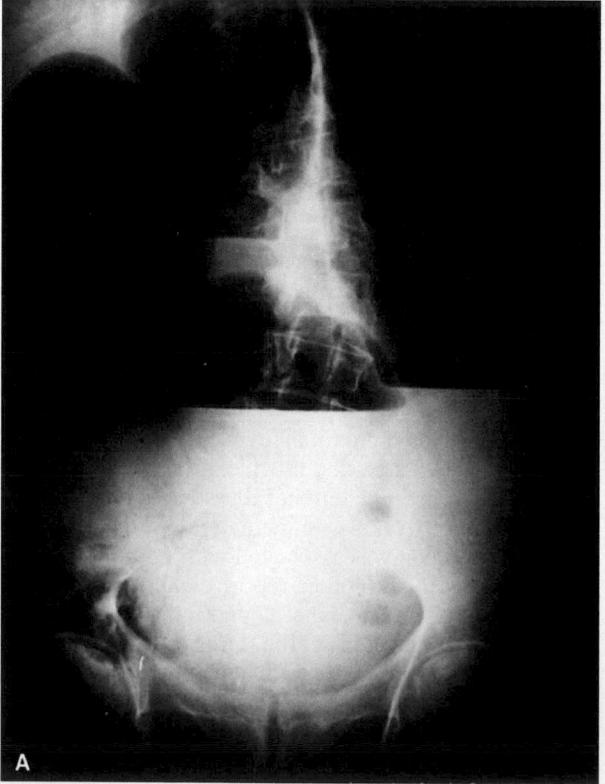
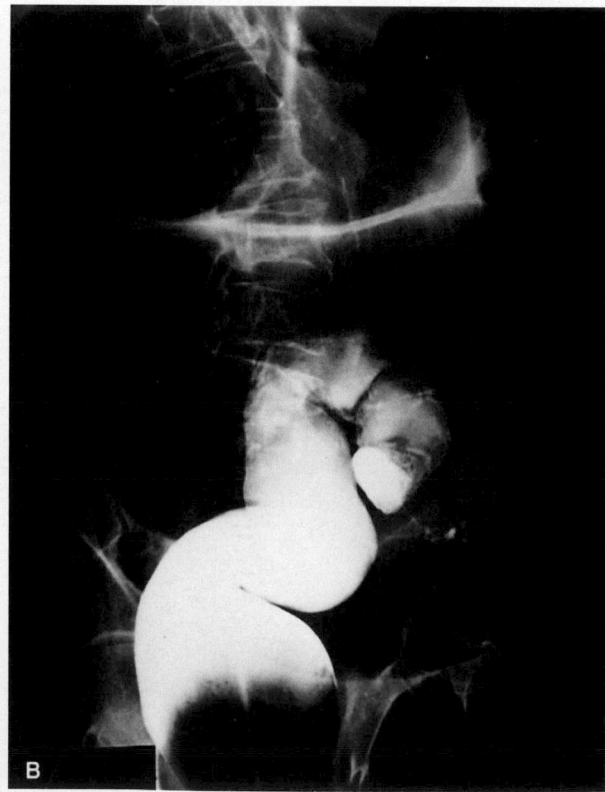

FIGURE 23-84. Complete colonic obstruction. **A:** Huge gas- and fluid-filled loops of colon are characteristic of mechanical obstruction. **B:** Barium enema demonstrates complete retrograde obstruction to the flow of barium.

exposing the patient to the risk of fecal contamination and peritonitis. One can avoid this problem by creating an end-loop colostomy (see Figure 31-36) or a loop ileostomy (see Figures 31-67 through 31-69). However, creating separate openings for a stoma and a mucus fistula is generally a poor idea. Often, this will lead to intolerable mucus drainage that may even require separate appliances. Furthermore, it may be more difficult to manage than the functioning stoma itself.

de Almeida and colleagues compared two methods of dealing with a left colon acutely obstructed by cancer in a retrospective fashion.[230] Colostomy alone was associated with 10% mortality and 30% morbidity. Subtotal colectomy (see later) was associated with a 9% mortality but only an 18% morbidity.

Cecostomy. Tube cecostomy has been recommended by some as a conservative option for the patient believed to be at a prohibitively high risk for a more major procedure.[351,446] This operation, however, although it may succeed in venting the bowel, truly does not divert the fecal stream. If the obstruction can be relieved by enemas or by endoscopic decompression, thereby permitting the surgeon sufficient time to prepare the bowel, this may be optimal.[565]

Salim performed percutaneous decompression and irrigation through a small cecostomy tube in 28 individuals, in preparation for elective operation.[880] This is not the same technique as colonoscopically assisted cecostomy, performed for the treatment of Ogilvie's syndrome (see Chapter 20). This procedure cannot be undertaken with the use of a colonoscope because of the distal obstruction. This is a risky concept indeed, with the possible consequences of precipitating a perforation, in addition to the obstruction.

There are, however, several other options that permit resection and ultimate reestablishment of intestinal continuity in the first instance for malignant left-sided colonic obstruction.

Colonic Stenting. Nonoperative alternatives to relieving colonic obstruction have been attempted with indifferent results. These include balloon dilation, placement of a plastic non-expandable rectal tube, cryosurgical destruction, electrocoagulation, and laser ablation. Most apply to the palliative management of rectal cancer (see Chapter 24). The concept of using a self-expandable metal stent to relieve obstruction in an occluded lumen was first introduced in 1985, when Wright and coworkers successfully placed stents in the canine jugular vein and abdominal aorta.[224] Dohmoto was the first to describe this application in the colon.[252] The procedure may be performed as a bridge to elective surgery, for palliation, and it may be successfully maintained through neoadjuvant therapy until resection is undertaken.[7]

The endoluminal Wallstent enteral endoprosthesis (Boston Scientific/Microvasive, Natick, MA; http://www.bsci.com) is a metal self-expanding stent with an internal diameter of 20 mm and a column length of 80 mm (Figure 23-85). It is placed endoscopically, usually under fluoroscopic guidance, to palliate colon obstruction (Figure 23-86). Figure 23-87 demonstrates the stent in place in the sigmoid colon on a plain film of the abdomen, and Figure 23-88 is an artist's concept of the stent in position. The resected specimen, incorporating the stent, is illustrated in Figure 23-89. A technical precaution that should be mentioned is the attention necessary for performing the resection without unnecessarily handling the area of the stent placement. There is a real concern for the possibility that the sharp metal ends may have penetrated the bowel sufficiently to cause a laceration if one is not careful.

Numerous articles have been published on the use of this device.[624,625,842,1006,1007] One of the largest experiences has been reported from Spain by Tejero and colleagues.[1006] Thirty-eight patients underwent insertion of the stent for malignant obstruction of the left colon. The obstruction was relieved in 35 (92%), and in 13 individuals the stent constituted definitive palliative treatment. In approximately two-thirds, definitive elective surgery was successfully concluded. Dauphine and coworkers reported their experience with 26 patients.[224] In 14, the stents were placed for palliation, whereas in 12, they were placed as a bridge to ultimate resection. In 22 individuals (85%), stent placement was successful initially, and in 1, subsequently. The remaining 4 required emergency surgery. Nine of the 12 patients (75%) in the bridge-to-surgery group underwent elective colon resection. In the palliative group, 4 (29%) developed recurrent obstruction, and in 1 (9%), the stent migrated. In the remaining 9 (64%), the stent was patent until the patient expired or until the end of the follow-up (median, 156 days).[224] Martinez-Santos and coworkers assigned patients to either preoperative stenting followed by elective resection or palliative stenting versus emergency surgery.[644] Obstruction was relieved in 41 of 43 patients after stent placement (95%). Eighty-five percent ultimately underwent resection and primary anastomosis without a stoma. Only 41% avoided a stoma when emergency resection was performed. Others report comparable success.[56,556,878,994] Endoscopic transanal decompression with a drainage tube has also been described for acute colonic obstruction.[999]

On-Table Lavage. The literature abounds, especially from the United Kingdom, with various approaches that attempt to prepare the bowel for primary anastomosis.[256,312,414,418,537,542,719,804,816,935,942,1017] The technique is particularly applicable to obstructing rectal cancers, but it

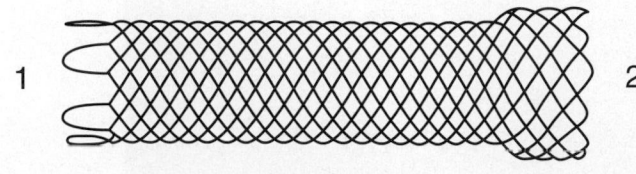

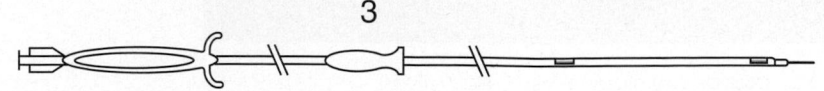

FIGURE 23-85. WallFlex colonic stent. *1:* Proximal end. *2:* Flared distal end. *3:* TTS/OTW delivery system. (Courtesy of Boston Scientific Corporation, Natick, MA.)

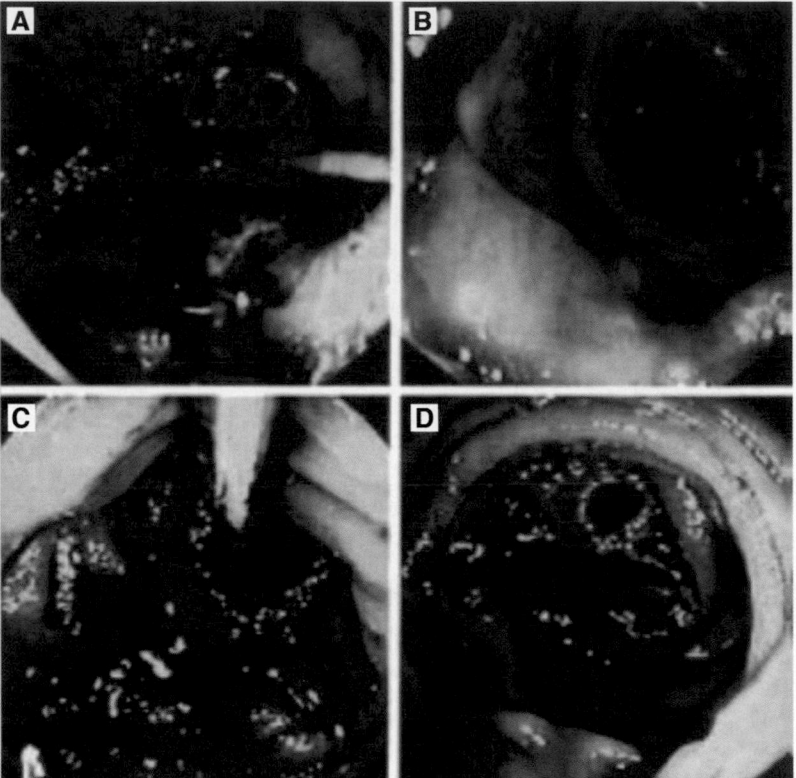

FIGURE 23-86. Obstructing sigmoid colon cancer. Insertion of endoluminal colonic stent. **A:** Guidewire inserted through the obstruction. **B:** Stent negotiated through the obstruction. **C:** Stent inserted with guidewire in place. **D:** Stent in position. (From Aziz SA, Afifi A, Auf K. Endoluminal colonic wall stents for the management of malignant recto-sigmoid obstruction. *J Egypt Nat Canc Inst.* 2001;13:43.)

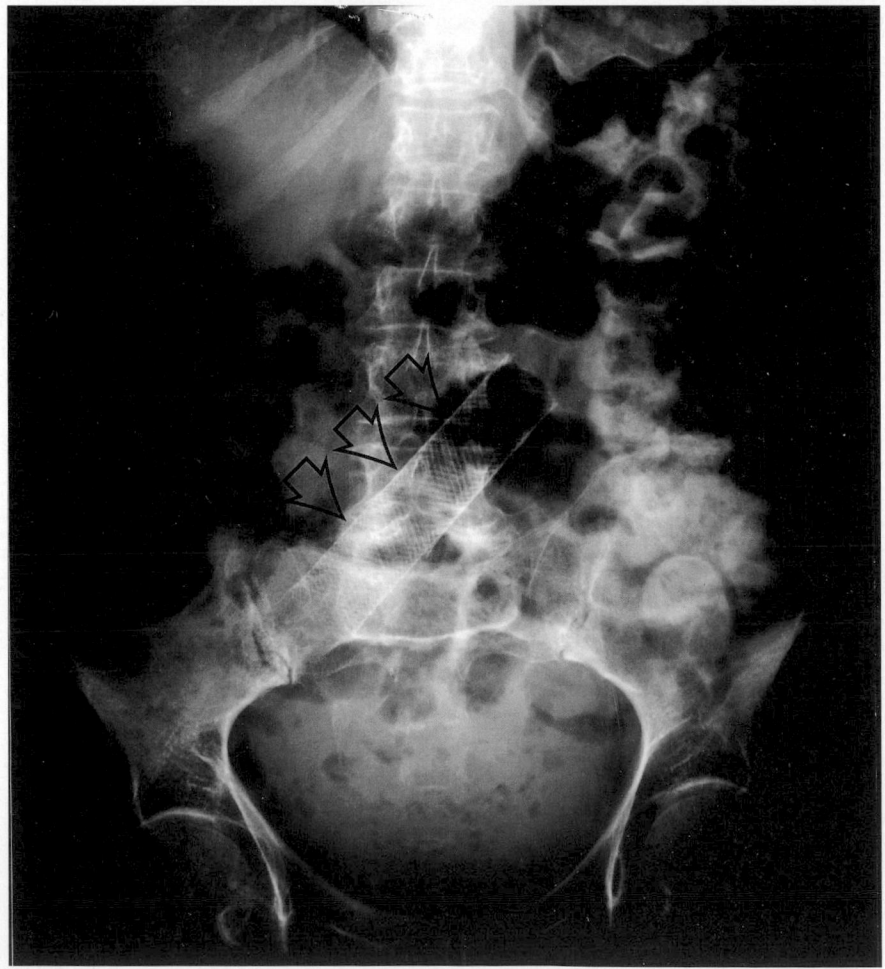

FIGURE 23-87. Plain film of the abdomen demonstrates the stent in place (*arrows*).

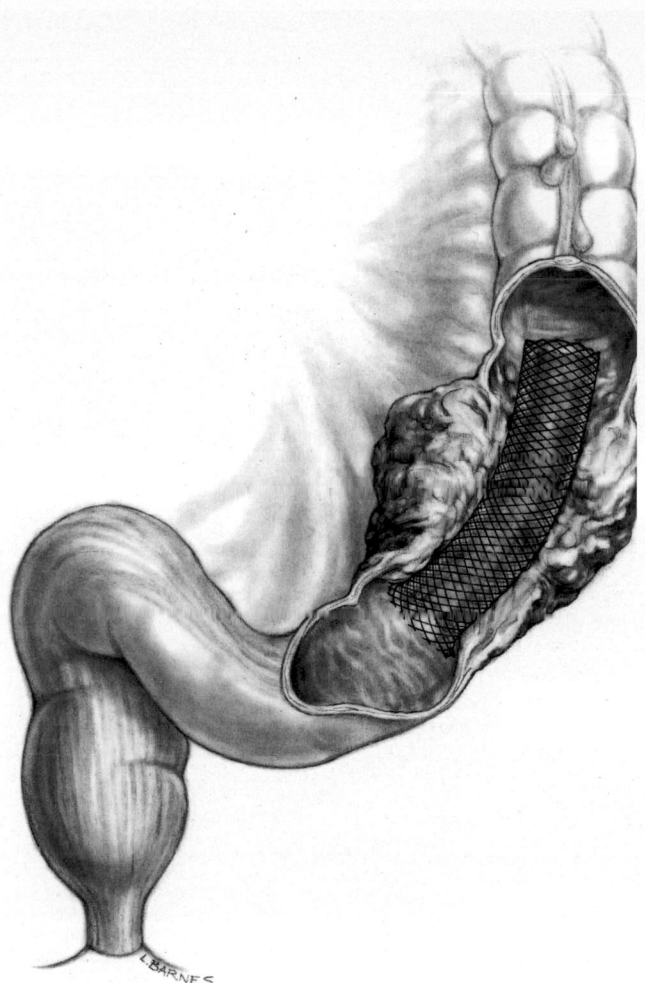

FIGURE 23-88. Artist's concept of a Wallstent in place through an obstructing carcinoma of the sigmoid colon.

has been recommended as an alternative for left-sided colon lesions as well. The irrigation can be accomplished in an antegrade or retrograde fashion, either before or after the tumor has been removed, through the open bowel, a cecotomy, or an appendicostomy (Figure 23-90).[110,1098] Some authors report relatively good results (a clinical anastomotic leak rate of 5% to 7%),[366,537,816,979,1017] but others note a clinical and radiologic leak rate of 10% to 14% and a mortality rate of up to 17%.[804] The SCOTIA Study Group, reporting from Aberdeen, Scotland, developed a prospective, randomized trial comparing subtotal colectomy with segmental resection and primary anastomosis and the use of intraoperative irrigation for malignant left-sided colonic obstruction.[905] Hospital mortality and complication rates did not differ significantly, but 4 months after operation, increased bowel frequency was significantly more common in the subtotal colectomy group. Because of this complaint, the authors concluded that segmental resection following intraoperative irrigation is the preferred alternative for uncomplicated left-sided bowel obstruction. Tan and colleagues noted an operative mortality of 13% and a wound infection rate of 30%.[996] Nonetheless, all who describe their experiences are quite enthusiastic.

COMMENT. One may be rather surprised that this procedure has been welcomed with such enthusiasm. Despite modifications designed to simplify the method, it involves insertion of a catheter into the cecum (thus necessitating at least an additional enterotomy), the instillation of several liters of saline solution, and the evacuation of the contents through a large-bore tube (into a collecting bag, it is hoped, rather than onto the floor of the operating room). The other problem one has is interpreting the definition of a "large bowel obstruction." Surgeons often find articles and verbal presentation examples of alleged large bowel obstruction that merely represent mild dilatation. In many cases, these individuals could in all probability have undergone bowel preparation and elective surgery. Still, one must respect the opinions of well-recognized surgeons. Most, however, prefer subtotal or total colectomy for this indication (see later).

Intracolonic or Intraluminal Bypass. In 1985, Ravo and Ger described a unique approach to effecting re-establishment of intestinal continuity in situations in which one would hesitate to undertake such a procedure, the intracolonic bypass.[826] The procedure, which involves only a limited resection, is theoretically applicable to obstruction and to perforation.[858] Because the product is not available in the United States, it has been dropped from this edition.

Subtotal or Total Colectomy. Generally, the optimal way of dealing with an obstructed colon is to perform subtotal or total colectomy and ileosigmoid or ileorectal anastomosis.[115,128,339,403] This operation has the additional merit of removing any synchronous lesions, especially if unsuspected.[56] The procedure is technically somewhat more difficult, but results indicate that the morbidity and mortality do not exceed, and in most series are considerably better, than those of staged operations.[297,461,525,976,1083] Following the procedure, virtually all patients can tolerate a normal diet, and those with an ileorectal anastomosis usually stabilize at about two or three bowel movements per day.[403] Occasionally, an individual may have to resort to one of the "slowing" medications. This procedure is also preferred for the management of perforation, in which situation it is of paramount importance to remove the bowel in the first instance (see later).

Colitis Proximal to a Partially Obstructing Carcinoma of the Colon

A nonspecific type of ulcerative colitis proximal to a partially obstructing carcinoma is an uncommon condition. It is a clinical and pathologic entity that must be distinguished from idiopathic ulcerative colitis, from which a carcinoma may subsequently develop.[292,876,1023,1084,1116] The location of the colitis is invariably proximal to the tumor, with the bowel distal to the tumor normal. In almost all reported cases, a short segment of normal mucosa separates the area of colitis from the tumor. The pathologic description of the colitis varies from involvement of the entire bowel wall with hemorrhagic necrosis to superficial mucosal ulcerations only.

The colitis is frequently unsuspected and discovered only at the time of surgery for the colonic tumor. Although often apparent from the macroscopic appearance of the proximal intestine and mesentery, the extent of the inflammatory process may not be fully appreciated until the bowel is opened. The limits of resection will be dictated not only by the requirement of an adequate cancer operation but also by the length of the inflamed bowel.

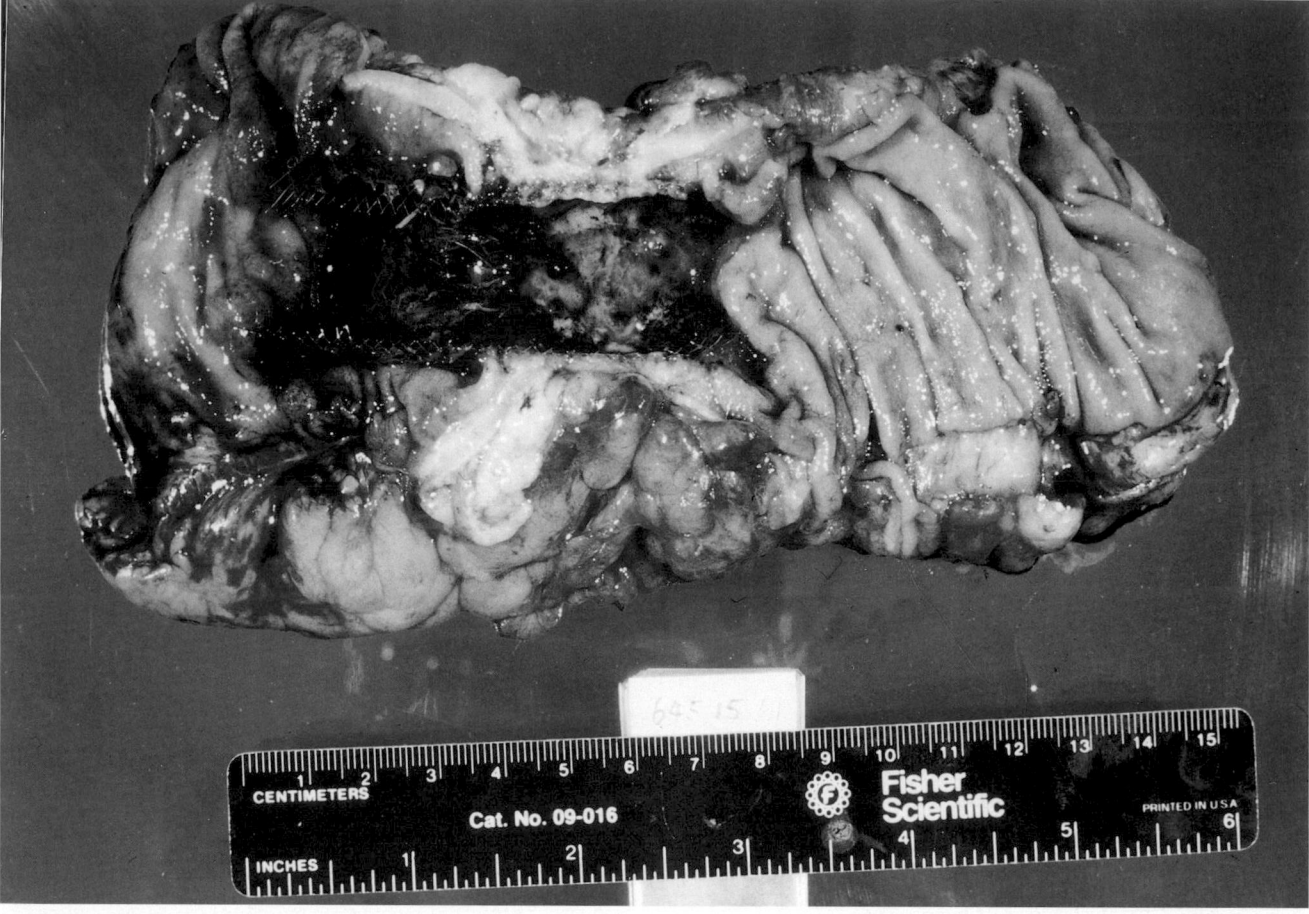

FIGURE 23-89. Resected, opened sigmoid colon specimen showing an incised stent in place with transmural invasion by cancer. Note that there is very little difference in luminal size between the proximal and distal bowel.

Bypass

As mentioned earlier, resection of right-sided obstructing lesions can generally be performed with reestablishment of intestinal continuity, even with unprepared bowel and small bowel dilatation. Obviously, clinical judgment remains the primary criterion. The alternative is resection and ileostomy.

Enteroenterostomy is a reasonably safe alternative for patients with obstructing tumors and for those unresectable cancers that are likely to obstruct (Figure 23-91). To effect a safe bypass, the enterostomy should ideally be at least 20 cm from the lesion proximally and distally, and the anastomosis should be free of areas of tumor implantation if this is possible. A colocolostomy is the preferred approach whenever it can be accomplished, in order to save as much useful bowel as possible and to decrease the likelihood of diarrhea (Figure 23-91B). For right-sided lesions, an ileocolostomy is usually very effective (Figure 23-91A), but if the entire colon is in jeopardy for recurrent tumor, ileorectal or ileosigmoid bypass is suggested (Figure 23-91C).

Perforation

Carcinoma of the colon with perforation is another challenging surgical problem. All too often, the pathologic diagnosis is not clearly established preoperatively or even intraoperatively. The patient often presents with a rigid abdomen, generalized peritonitis, and a pneumoperitoneum. Surgery may be required without benefit of gastrointestinal investigation or even a meaningful history from the patient. Even though extravasation is demonstrated on a limited water-soluble enema, the differential diagnosis (especially for a sigmoid lesion) always includes diverticulitis. Colonoscopy will usually fail to define the nature of the lesion because of inadequate bowel preparation, the general condition of the patient, and the inflammatory reaction in the area.[231] Failure to demonstrate a carcinoma by means of colonoscopy at or near the site of a known perforation does not exclude cancer. Realistically, if one makes an attempt to perform a colonoscopy in the presence of free gas within the peritoneal cavity, it is not merely an exercise in futility, but it is likely to increase the amount of contamination and certainly to expand the pneumoperitoneum. Performing a flexible instrument examination under the circumstances is poor judgment.

The establishment of the diagnosis can usually be confirmed with certainty only by an exploratory laparotomy and resection of the involved segment of bowel. It should be emphasized repeatedly to all surgical trainees that limited exploration and blind diversionary procedures for suspected colonic perforation are to be condemned. Passing the hand into the pelvis to attempt diagnosis in the presence of inflammatory reaction, adhesions, pus, or feces is a gesture in futility. A transverse colostomy for a perforated cecal carcinoma is a totally preventable tragedy. The lesion should be clearly demonstrable before definitive treatment is undertaken.

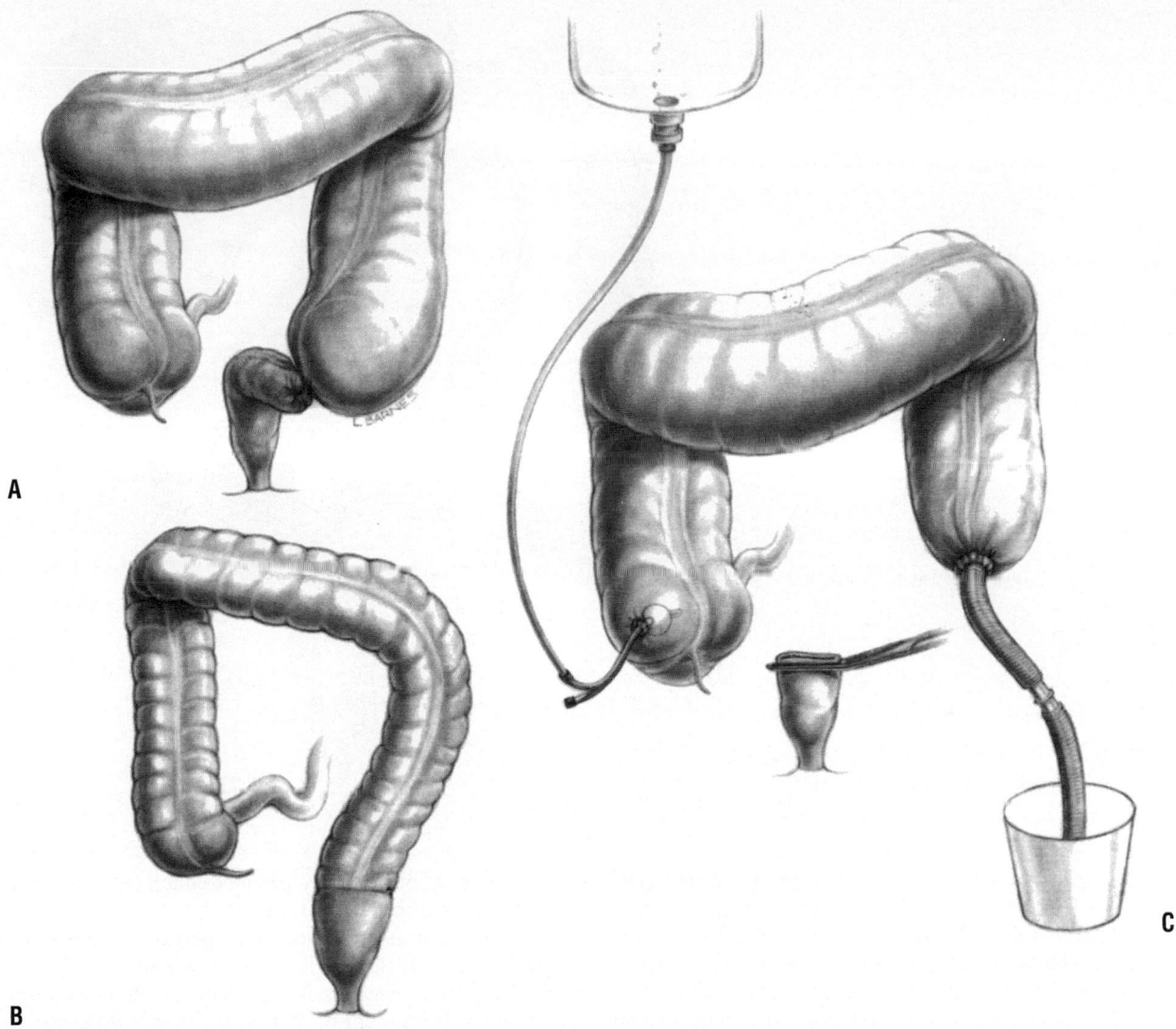

FIGURE 23-90. Technique of on-table lavage for bowel obstruction. **A:** Profound large bowel obstruction from cancer is conceptually illustrated. **B:** Lavage is performed by insertion of a large-bore catheter into the cecum, with drainage from the distal end effected by means of corrugated anesthetic gas tubing. **C:** Anastomosis is completed by the usual means, without a diversionary procedure and without removing the entire colon.

Parenthetically, it is important to evaluate the rectum before the incision is made. It is more than embarrassing to perform a resection and leave behind a synchronous carcinoma of the rectum. It is virtually impossible to evaluate the extraperitoneal rectum through an exploratory laparotomy without full mobilization, much less with a laparoscopic approach. By simply passing a rigid sigmoidoscope with the patient on the operating table, the surgeon should be able to confirm adequately that the rectum is spared of disease.

Treatment

The surgical options in the treatment of perforation are somewhat more limited than those for obstruction. The goal should be to remove the diseased segment. As mentioned, if a colostomy and drainage procedure is performed for a sigmoid lesion, the actual histology may not be defined for several weeks. However, if a carcinoma is diagnosed but not removed, resection should be undertaken in 10 to 14 days unless neoadjuvant therapy is planned. If diverticular disease is the cause, resection

theoretically may be deferred for 6 weeks to many months (see Chapter 27).

Another reason for initially resecting the lesion is to remove the septic process. Even with drainage and proximal diversion, the contamination will continue because a foot or more of stool-filled bowel may be situated between the stoma and the perforation. In addition, desquamated cells from the tumor itself may continue to seed the abdomen and further worsen the already grim prognosis.

Surgical alternatives for removal of a perforated bowel include resection of the disease-bearing segment, anastomosis if appropriate, *always* a protective colostomy or ileostomy, and drainage of the area of contamination. With a right-sided perforation, the surgeon may elect to perform an end-ileostomy and adjacent mucous fistula of the colon (at the same site), ileocolic anastomosis with protective loop ileostomy, or an end-ileostomy with closure of the colonic stump. With more distal lesions, the surgeon can attempt an anastomosis with protective loop colostomy or loop ileostomy, end-stoma with adjacent mucous fistula, or end-stoma with closure of the distal stump.

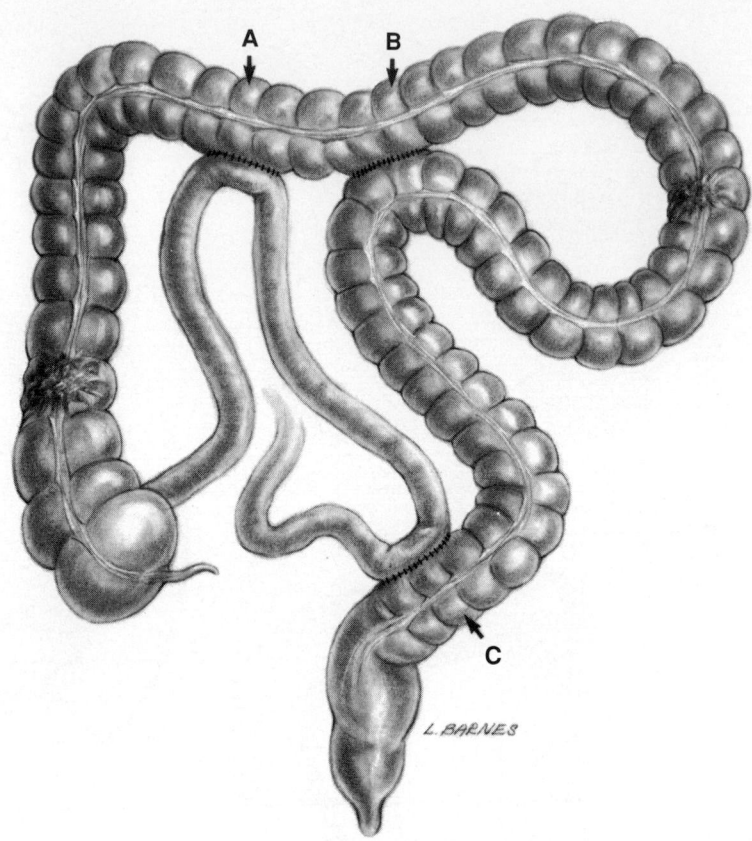

FIGURE 23-91. Bypass procedures. **A:** Ileotransverse colostomy. **B:** Colocolostomy. **C:** Ileosigmoidostomy.

Subtotal or total colectomy with ileosigmoid or ileorectal anastomosis is another alternative for the treatment of perforation. It fulfills the criterion of removing the disease, and it permits a relatively safe anastomosis for left-sided perforations. It also treats synchronous lesions that could otherwise be overlooked. However, dissection in the upper part of the abdomen in the presence of a hypogastric perforation increases the risk for spreading the septic process under the diaphragms and below the liver. Even with a technically secure anastomosis, loop ileostomy should be considered when contamination has occurred. Although possibly applicable to a number of situations, concomitant loop ileostomy is the procedure of choice in one circumstance—when obstructing carcinoma of the left colon produces perforation of the right colon. Under these circumstances, subtotal or total colectomy is preferred despite the more extensive dissection required.

When an emergency resection is performed, blunt dissection should be employed as often as possible. Unless invasion by the tumor has caused fixation of the bowel, sharp dissection invites injury to the ureter and other retroperitoneal structures. If unusual difficulty is encountered, the area should be drained, with proximal diversion of the fecal stream. Although this is not the optimal course of action, it is an acceptable alternative under these circumstances. In addition, because of the poor prognosis of perforating carcinomas of the colon and the high risk for local recurrence, clips should be applied to serve as markers for subsequent radiotherapy. Generally, adjuvant postoperative radiotherapy should be initiated for the perforated tumor (see later). Metallic clips (e.g., stainless steel), although readily visible on plain radiographs, often distort and interfere with the interpretation of CT scans. Plastic clips cannot be seen on the plain film, but because they produce much less artifact than steel, titanium clips are preferred.[1077]

Finally, vigorous irrigation of the peritoneal cavity should be performed with many liters of saline solution.[42,491,664,685] Continuous postoperative lavage may also be helpful for up to 72 hours. Placement of antibiotics or povidone-iodine in the irrigating solution is not advised. This opinion is based on the absence of literature to support its application, although many surgeons like to use this method. Perioperative mortality, especially with free perforation, is very high, even in the modern era.[1139]

Prevention of Adhesions

There has been concern and considerable therapeutic effort regarding the prevention of intestinal adhesions. The magnitude of the problem is not insignificant. In a prospective analysis of 210 patients undergoing a laparotomy, Menzies and Ellis found that 93% had intra-abdominal adhesions that were the result of prior surgery.[680] This compared with 115 first-time laparotomies in which only 10.4% were found to have adhesions. The authors noted that approximately 1% of adult general surgical admissions to the hospital were for intestinal obstruction. Furthermore, 3.3% of laparotomies were for adhesive obstruction.[680] The majority of the surgical procedures that produced intestinal obstruction principally involved the colon. It is obvious that the economic consequences of such a formidable incidence are considerable. Ray and colleagues noted, in an article published in 1993, that hospitalizations in which adhesiolysis was performed in the United States in 1988 were responsible for expenditures of more than $1 billion.[827] Cox and coworkers performed a retrospective analysis of all patients admitted with a diagnosis of acute adhesive small bowel obstruction during a 9-year period in Victoria, Australia.[208] The following was the breakdown of the prior operations: appendectomy, 23.3%; colorectal resection, 20.8%; gynecologic surgery, 11.7%; upper gastrointestinal and biliary surgery, 9.2%; small bowel surgery, 8.3%; and more than one prior abdominal operation, 23.6%.[208]

Ellis and associates used data from the Scottish National Health Service from patients who underwent abdominal or pelvic surgery in 1986 and followed them for up to 10 years.[279] Overall, 34.6% of the 29,790 patients who underwent surgery were readmitted a mean of 2.1 times over 10 years for adhesions or for abdominal surgery that could be complicated by adhesions.[279] Beck and colleagues, in the United States, used Health Care Financing Administration data to evaluate a random 5% sample of all Medicare patients who underwent open colorectal and general surgery in 1993.[68] *Within 2 years* of the surgery for incision, excision, and anastomosis of intestine (*International Classification of Diseases, Ninth Revision* [ICD-9] code 45), 14.3% developed intestinal obstruction, 2.6% required adhesiolysis, and 12.9% underwent additional colorectal or general surgery. Furthermore, of those with *ICD-9* code 46 (other operations on the intestine), 17% developed obstruction (3.1 having to undergo adhesiolysis), and 20.2% underwent additional colorectal or general surgery. Numerous other articles have been published attesting to the enormity of the problem.[679,703,766]

Physical barriers have been developed to prevent adhesion formation by limiting tissue apposition during the early stages of mesothelial repair.[248] Although certain agents have been proposed, including solutions and physical barriers, none has been demonstrated to be consistently effective. However, hyaluronic acid has indeed been shown to protect tissue from injury and to prevent adhesion development. A bioresorbable membrane has been developed to provide a mechanical barrier for this purpose.[138] The product, Seprafilm, is composed of a sodium salt of hyaluronic acid, sodium hyaluronate, combined with another polyanionic polysaccharide, carboxymethyl cellulose. This membrane is produced by Genzyme Corp. (Cambridge, MA; http://www.genzyme.com). Other available products that have been demonstrated to reduce adhesion formation are Interceed (Johnson & Johnson Medical Co., Arlington, TX) and Gore-Tex Surgical Membrane (W.L. Gore, Flagstaff, AZ).[248]

Results and Recommendations

Seprafilm has been shown to decrease adhesion formation and has been recommended as a potentially safe adjuvant for preventing postoperative abdominal adhesions through both clinical and animal studies.[63,675] A randomized, controlled, blinded, prospective multicenter study was performed involving 183 patients who underwent restorative proctocolectomy and ileal J-pouch anastomosis with diverting ileostomy.[63] All patients would have subsequently required closure of the ileostomy, so that the patients were ideal candidates for reassessment of the magnitude of the adhesion formation with and without the bioresorbable membrane. It was found that Seprafilm decreased the rate of adhesion formation by nearly 50%.[63] Fifty-one percent of recipients were adhesion free compared with only 6% of untreated patients. There were no adverse reactions that could be attributed to the product. A similar multicenter study was reported by Becker and coworkers.[70] Eleven centers enrolled 183 patients

with ulcerative colitis or familial polyposis who were scheduled for colectomy and ileo-pouch anal anastomosis with loop ileostomy. Only 6% of control patients were found to be without adhesions, whereas 51% with Seprafilm were free of adhesions. There was no increased incidence of complications attributable to the use of the bioresorbable membrane.

A large, prospective, randomized, multicenter, controlled study was published on the safety of Seprafilm (Adhesion Study Group Steering Committee) and involved 1,791 patients.[64] Just prior to closure, patients were randomized to receive Seprafilm or no treatment. Complications within the first month were evaluated. This report concluded that there were no increased risks related to abdominal abscess, pelvic abscess, and pulmonary embolism. However, the authors commented that wrapping the suture or staple line of a new bowel anastomosis with Seprafilm is unwise because the data suggested that it may increase the risk of an anastomotic leak. A subsequent follow-up of 1,701 patients who underwent intestinal resection demonstrated no difference in the overall rate of postoperative bowel obstruction, although a very small decrease in the rate of reoperation was suggested in the Seprafilm group.[290] Another study by Oikonomakis and associates showed that Seprafilm did not adversely affect the short-term recurrence rate after curative resection of colorectal cancer.[760]

Technique

Depending on the amount of surface that one would hope to treat prophylactically will determine how many sheets of Seprafilm to apply. Generally, the full length of the incision, the floor of the pelvis, and the stoma, itself, are the most critical areas. The raw retroperitoneal surfaces where the bowel has been mobilized as well as any sites that required excessive handing are recommended for application. It is easier and preferable to wrap the stoma before it is brought through the abdominal wall (see Figure 31-69). Furthermore, it is important to keep the sheet dry, applying it to the areas to be treated by means of a dry sponge-stick rather than the surgeon's fingers.

Comment

Most experienced surgeons have been impressed with the reduction in the amount and the severity of adhesions whenever tone must reoperate on the patient, especially when closing a stoma that had been previously wrapped with Seprafilm. Whether its application will inevitably prevent the development of subsequent intestinal obstruction continues to be part of a prospective, randomized, long-term, follow-up evaluation.

Liver Metastases

What to do with metastatic liver disease at the time of colon resection is a problem that often confronts the surgeon. CT will usually provide adequate evaluation of the liver to determine the presence or absence of metastases. However, as mentioned previously, this rarely changes the approach to the management of the primary tumor. There are a number of options for treatment when a known or unsuspected hepatic metastatic tumor is identified preoperatively or intraoperatively (see later). What is actually accomplished, however, may depend on the availability of specialized equipment.

Intraoperative Ultrasonography

Numerous articles have been published attesting to the value of intraoperative ultrasonography for identifying tumor in the

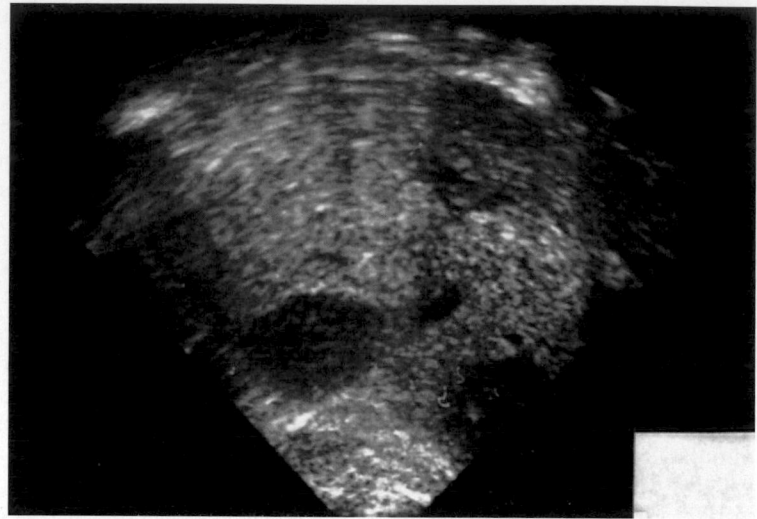

FIGURE 23-92. Intra-abdominal ultrasonography demonstrates multiple filling defects in the liver, consistent with metastatic disease.

liver that may not be apparent by means of palpation alone (Figure 23-92).[184,618,763,820,1033] Often, the equipment employed is an ordinary real-time, linear-array, B-mode scanner not specifically designed for operative use.[1033] A smaller probe is preferred, however, if available. The sterile probe is placed directly on the liver surface by the surgeon who performs the examination. A technician or radiologist may facilitate interpretation of the visual picture. A complete examination consists of identifying the vascular landmarks (three hepatic veins and inferior vena cava) and assessing the liver parenchyma segment by segment.

Olsen performed intraoperative ultrasonography on 213 patients with carcinoma of the colon and rectum and compared preoperative ultrasonography and inspection of the liver during surgery with this technique.[763] Intraoperative ultrasonography detected 116 previously unrecognized metastatic lesions. The authors concluded that the procedure is safe and more accurate than either standard exploratory methods or preoperative imaging.

Intraoperative ultrasonography is particularly applicable for assessment of the liver when a resection of metastastic tumor is planned, and it is an excellent substitute for manual palpation in someone who is undergoing laparoscopically assisted colectomy for cancer (see Chapter 19).

General Principles of Management

Surgical resection is the only potentially curative treatment for colorectal liver metastases, but only 20% to 25% of such lesions are considered resectable.[326] If a small focus of disease is present on the margin of the liver and no other lesion can be palpated or identified by means of operative ultrasonography, it is reasonable to remove it. For any other situation, resection is not advised. The location and size of the residual tumor or tumors are determined, and the patient is re-evaluated following the operation. A CT scan (Figure 23-17) is obtained during the postoperative convalescence, although many surgeons prefer to learn whether there is CT evidence of metastatic disease preoperatively, especially if the CEA is elevated. A PET scan is another screening option. If multiple or bilobar tumors are confirmed, no attempt is made to perform a resection. If solitary or unilobar disease is seen on the first scan, the study is repeated in 3 weeks. If only localized disease persists, the patient is admitted to the hospital for

selective hepatic angiography. If there is still no evidence of extension, exploratory laparotomy and resection are recommended in accordance with the protocol discussed in Liver Metastases in the section Treatment of Recurrence.

Weber and colleagues, however, emphasize that the surgical strategy for treatment of synchronous colorectal liver metastases is still controversial.[1075] They were able to simultaneously resect 36% of 97 patients from 1987 to 2000, and the remainder underwent delayed resection. The morbidity with the synchronous resection did not differ from that of the delayed resection, nor did the extent of liver resection. The overall survival rate was 94%, 45%, and 21% at 1, 3, and 5 years, respectively, after simultaneous resection, and 92%, 45%, and 22% after delayed resection.[1075] Geoghegan and Scheele, following an extensive MEDLINE literature search, concluded that patients with colorectal liver metastases should be assessed in units that can offer all of the specialized techniques necessary in order to deliver optimal care.[326]

As chemotherapeutic agents continue to improve and new ablative techniques are developed, the optimal management strategy continues to be reassessed. Simultaneous resection (or ablation) of the liver metastases at the time of colon resection is becoming increasingly commonplace.[643,998] Considerable judgment and multidisciplinary involvement is typically required for optimal outcomes.

Resection of Other Organs
Excision in Continuity

Resection of adjacent small or large intestine, bladder wall, uterus, tubes and ovaries, stomach, spleen, tail of pancreas, duodenum, kidney, and portions of the abdominal wall may be performed for cure or to offer better palliation.[544] Because of the differences in the biologic nature of neoplasms, occasionally a tumor will invade locally and not metastasize until late in the course of the disease. If this locally invasive tumor is not removed, the patient may experience many months or years of pain. Intestinal obstruction or a visible protrusion of the tumor may develop—all situations that may be preventable by a more aggressive attempt at extirpation at the time of the initial operation. In the experience of Gall and Altendorf, operative mortality following multivisceral resections was 12%, as compared with a 6% mortality with bowel resection alone.[321] En bloc resection, removal in continuity with adjacent organs, is preferable to individual organ resection, with the recognition that adhesions may be inflammatory rather than neoplastic. However, the risk of seeding viable tumor cells justifies this approach. Eisenberg and colleagues have shown that survival in locally advanced colorectal carcinoma depends more on lymph node status than on the extent of local invasion.[274] Others have confirmed that the most important predictors of survival are lymph node status and involvement of the resection margins by tumor.[596,802]

Therefore, the importance of obtaining tumor-free margins, even if radical resection is required for locally advanced colorectal cancer, should be emphasized. However, major resections of the abdominal wall, alloplasty, hemicorporectomy, and total pelvic exenteration, in the hope of improving the likelihood of cure for colorectal cancer, should be discouraged except in highly selected instances. The morbidity and mortality rates associated with these operations are so high that they almost preclude the possibility of a meaningful lifestyle.

Oophorectomy

A Krukenberg tumor refers to a malignancy in the ovary that metastasizes from a primary site, classically the gastrointestinal tract, although it can arise in other tissues such as the breast. Gastric adenocarcinoma, especially at the pylorus, is the most common source. Krukenberg described this manifestation in 1896, observing that tumors are often found in both ovaries, consistent with its metastatic nature. However, Paget had described the condition in 1854 (see Biography, Chapter 9). The ovary may be the only site of macroscopic spread of disease; it is the site of metastases in 3% to 5% of patients.

Bilateral oophorectomy has been recommended on a prophylactic basis in all postmenopausal women who have colorectal cancer because of the risk for harboring a metastatic focus as well as for the prevention of primary ovarian carcinoma. There is no question as to the advisability of therapeutic oophorectomy when macroscopic tumor is evident in the adnexa.

The incidence of such involvement, usually found in younger, premenopausal women, often concomitantly found with diffuse intra-abdominal metastases, is approximately 6%.[50,90,713] Ovarian metastases make up 5% to 10% of colorectal metastases; overall median survival is 27 months.[761] The incidence of carcinoma of the ovary in women with carcinoma of the colon and rectum is approximately five times that of a primary ovarian malignant neoplasm.[751]

The ovarian tumor may produce symptoms in advance of the colon cancer.[438,646] These include abdominal or pelvic pain, bloating, ascites, and pain during sexual intercourse. Krukenberg tumors can occasionally provoke a reaction of the ovarian stroma, which leads to hormone production that results in vaginal bleeding, a change in menstrual habits, hirsutism, and occasionally virilization.

There has been some debate over the exact mechanism of metastasis from the stomach, appendix, or colon to the ovaries. Classically, it was thought that direct seeding across the abdominal cavity accounted for this phenomenon, but lymphatic spread is now considered more likely. The average earlier age of diagnosis of Krukenberg tumors may be related to the relatively increased vascularity of the ovaries.

In the past, women were not uncommonly submitted to panhysterectomy for an ovarian tumor only to discover subsequently that the histologic nature of the lesion was consistent with a colonic primary tumor. A cure is only rarely obtained even when all the obvious visual disease is removed. Even so, unremoved ovarian tumors may grow to such an enormous size that symptoms may dictate an additional operation.

The question of the role of *prophylactic oophorectomy* has been a matter of some controversy. Blamey and colleagues noted that only 1.4% of 882 women who underwent resection for colorectal cancer subsequently required an operation for ovarian recurrence.[95] The low incidence of clinical recurrence indicated to these authors that

FRIEDRICH ERNST KRUKENBERG (1871–1946)

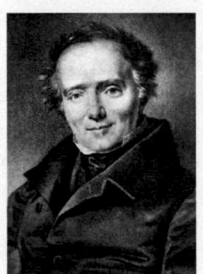

Krukenberg was a German gynecologist and pathologist, born in 1871 in Halle, Germany, the youngest of seven children. Although his father was not a physician (he was a lawyer), notable physicians in his family included his brother Hermann (1863–1935), an orthopedic surgeon, and another brother, Georg Heinrich Peter Krukenberg (1855–1899), a professor of gynecology. The Krukenberg's were also grandchildren to Peter Krukenberg (1788–1865) and great-grandchildren to Johann Christian Reil (1759–1813), a neuropathologist. After studying in Halle, Germany, Krukenberg continued his education at the University of Marburg under the German ophthalmologist, Karl Theodor Paul Polykarpus Axenfeld (1867–1930). He also worked with Felix Jacob Marchand (1846–1928) who was the pathology department chief. In 1879, Marchand described a peculiar form of ovarian cancer and later he gave his student (Krukenberg) six cases of ovarian tumors that he could subsequently use to form his doctoral thesis. At the time, none of these tumors was thought to be metastatic. In 1896, Krukenberg described his findings of what he called *fibrosarcoma ovarii mucocellulare carcinomatodes* in an article entitled "Über das Fibrosarcoma ovarii mucocellulare (carcinomatodes)." This later became known as a *Krukenberg tumor*. This refers to a metastatic ovarian cancer arising from a primary lesion in the gastrointestinal (GI) tract. Krukenberg also made contributions to the field of ophthalmology when he discovered a congenital, vertical, spindle-shaped symmetrical deposition of brown pigment in the deep layers of the cornea. This was later aptly named a Krukenberg spindle. After his studies, he returned to his birthplace of Halle, Germany, where he went into private practice. He died in 1946 at the age of 75. (References: http://www.dsog.dk/files/krugen.htm; http://www.whonamedit.com/doctor.cfm/620.html.) (Courtesy of Seth A. Stein, MD.)

prophylactic oophorectomy could not be supported. Young-Fadok and coworkers undertook a prospective, randomized trial to evaluate the influence of oophorectomy on recurrence and survival in patients with Dukes' B and C cancers.[1136] No patient had evidence of gross or microscopic metastatic disease among the 77 individuals randomized to oophorectomy. Others, however, have reported the occasional cure of a patient found to have micrometastases and strongly recommend prophylactic oophorectomy.[363,620] Still, others believe that these successes are merely anecdotal, but they continue to recommend prophylactic oophorectomy in postmenopausal women if for no other reason than to prevent primary ovarian cancer.[90,218]

Rozario and colleagues found, depending on the age of the patient, that prophylactic oophorectomy results in a 4% to 11% reduction in the incidence of ovarian carcinoma, a rate that increases to 16.6% to 26.9% if general surgery procedures in which access could be more difficult are considered.[865] The additional procedure adds minimal risk and increases operative time only slightly. However, in the premenopausal patient, replacement estrogen therapy is required, and the operation will obviously precipitate early menopause.[90] To date, therefore, there are no objectives, compelling data to support prophylactic oophorectomy in premenopausal woman. However, the need for closer follow-up by means of pelvic ultrasonography or CT has been suggested for these individuals.[271]

Incidental Cholecystectomy

The risk of additional intra-abdominal procedures at the time of colectomy was reviewed by Biggers and colleagues.[84] In a series of 242 patients from the Mayo Clinic in whom an adequate bowel preparation had been performed, the risk was minimal. Cholecystectomy represented the most frequently applied incidental operation (81 patients; 33%). There were two deaths and one complication in this group. The morbidity and mortality did not differ significantly from those previously reported following colon resections without cholecystectomy. Others have confirmed the relative merit of incidental, simultaneous cholecystectomy.[930] It is usually preferred that one perform a cholecystectomy during elective colon resection when cholelithiasis is present, unless the operative time would be inappropriately prolonged or the incision (in an open operation) would need to be extended for an unreasonable length.

Appendectomy

It has been advocated in the past that appendectomy should be performed concomitantly with cholecystectomy, gynecologic procedures, and bowel resections. However, the incidence of acute appendicitis in the older population—that is, the patient population most likely to require surgery for colon cancer—is extremely small. It has been estimated that to prevent a single lifetime case of acute appendicitis in someone 60 years of age, 166 incidental appendectomies would be required.[1114] Based on a number of actuarial studies, it has been concluded that appendectomy as a preventive measure in individuals more than 40 years old is not cost-effective. Furthermore, although the morbidity associated with the appendectomy itself is extremely low, the differential diagnostic concerns may be increased when an intra-abdominal septic problem develops in a patient following colectomy. Therefore, incidental appendectomy is not considered advisable.

Meckel's Diverticulectomy

Meckel's diverticulum is the most common congenital abnormality of the small intestine. When symptomatic, it may lead to rectal bleeding, intussusception, and Meckel's diverticulitis. Abdominal pain and lower gastrointestinal hemorrhage are the usual presentations (see Chapter 28 and Figure 28-10). Children most often present with bowel obstruction and/or bleeding, whereas in adults intestinal obstruction is more likely to develop. After a thorough review of the literature, Wolff concluded that, as with appendectomy, Meckel's diverticulum in the older patient should be left alone.[1114]

Incidental Abdominal Aortic Aneurysmectomy

The incidence of colonic cancer coexisting with an aneurysm of the abdominal aorta is approximately 2%.[586] As a general surgeon or colon and rectal surgeon, one rarely gives consideration to the potential dilemma of being confronted with an unsuspected abdominal aortic aneurysm. Generally, the preoperative plan would not waiver; the aneurysm would be duly noted and dealt with by a vascular surgeon at the appropriate interval.

Lobbato and colleagues reported the opinions of 46 professors of general and vascular surgery.[586] Whenever the preoperative diagnosis was clearly established, approximately one-third favored excision of the carcinoma first, one-third stated that priority should be given to the aneurysm, and the remaining one-third stated that they would make a decision at the time of the laparotomy. Only two individuals believed that simultaneous operations should be attempted. Because of risk for sepsis in the graft and the potentially catastrophic consequences of such a complication, there should be real concern about adopting the last position.

However, Minu and colleagues reported the clinical courses of three patients who concomitantly underwent resection for colorectal cancer and wrapping of the aneurysm with a Dacron or Teflon mesh.[690] With a follow-up in excess of 2 years, no complications relative to the procedures or to the subsequent development of symptoms referable to the aneurysm were encountered. The authors concluded that in the absence of an impending rupture of the aneurysm, the tumor can be resected and an interim aneurysmal wrapping performed. Baxter and coworkers retrospectively reviewed the Mayo Clinic experience with colorectal cancer and concomitant abdominal aortic aneurysm.[58] Eighty-three such patients were identified between the years 1986 and 2000. In 64, the colorectal cancer was treated initially (44 with aneurysms less than 5 cm in diameter). No complication referable to the aneurysm was encountered in the postoperative period. Twenty patients had an aneurysm 5 cm or greater in diameter and underwent solely colorectal cancer resection. In 2, the aneurysms ruptured in the postoperative period. Twelve patients underwent treatment of both conditions concomitantly without graft complication (median follow-up, 3.2 years). Seven patients underwent graft repair before colon resection. There was a highly significant delay in resection of the colon cancer (median, 122 days) when compared with the other groups. The authors conclude that patients requiring aneurysm surgery for smaller lesions, less than 5 cm, should undergo colon resection first. Larger aneurysms present a risk of rupture and therefore can be reasonably treated concomitantly with the cancer. Treating the aneurysm without resecting the colon leads to an unacceptable delay in cancer therapy for many patients. However, the newer modality of endovascular repair may be considered, followed by colon resection shortly thereafter.[58]

POSTOPERATIVE CARE

The relative merits of postoperative antibiotics and the use of an indwelling urinary catheter have been previously discussed. The relative lack of benefit of a nasogastric tube has also been addressed.

Pain Control

One of the most important concerns to the patient and to the surgeon is the ability to control pain. The use of an epidural catheter or a patient-controlled intravenous analgesic regimen is usually preferred.[856] However, Petros and colleagues found that patient-controlled analgesia after uncomplicated colectomy increases the risk for postoperative ileus.[790] However, in those patients in whom meperidine (Demerol) is the agent employed for pain control, delayed transit time does not appear to be an issue.

The use of continuous epidural analgesia is discussed in Chapter 8. Lehman and Wiseman studied the effect of epidural analgesia and the return of peristalsis and length of stay following elective colorectal surgery.[563] No statistically significant difference was found between this modality and traditional analgesia with respect to either variable. Furthermore, there was no increased complication rate and, specifically, no increased incidence of anastomotic leaks. Certainly, any individual who poses a risk because of pulmonary difficulties will benefit from epidural analgesia.[113] Despite the foregoing conclusions, continuous epidural analgesia is not the panacea that many people believe. Reasons for problems in management include inconsistent dosing, catheter migration, and inability to adjust the medication or to supply additional medications without the advice and consent of the anesthesiology department (or pain management center). Clearly, success with this technique is very much dependent on the skill of the individual performing the procedure.

Diet

It has been generally believed that patients who undergo colon resection should be given only minimal oral alimentation until flatus has passed, at which time a progressive diet is instituted. Since the advent of laparoscopic surgery, the concept of early feeding has been explored. Based on the experience of early postoperative feeding in patients who have undergone laparoscopic surgery, the principles have been applied to open colon resection. Numerous articles have confirmed that early feeding, if tolerated, decreases the length of hospital stay and may not be uniquely applicable to laparoscopy.[86,129,177,426,489,839]

Some have observed in a prospective, randomized, controlled study that gum-chewing aids in the early recovery from abdominal surgery by limiting ileus, and it is an inexpensive means for stimulating the return of intestinal activity.[34] In an experience from the Kaiser Permanente Medical Center, when a protocol consisting of a clear liquid diet on the second postoperative day and a regular diet on the third was used, two-thirds of patients who underwent colon resection were able to be discharged home by the fourth

postoperative day.[177] Such reports have led many surgeons to introduce oral alimentation sooner, with progression more quickly advanced in those individuals who seem to tolerate it.

Holte and Kehlet pointed out that the pathogenesis of ileus involves inhibitory neural reflexes and inflammatory mediators released from the site of injury.[450] They strongly encouraged a multimodal rehabilitation strategy in order to minimize this problem. This may include epidural analgesia, avoidance of nasogastric tubes, immediate enforced oral nutrition, early mobilization, protein drinks, laxatives, and planned early discharge.[54,55,242,511]

Without doubt, the use of opioids contributes to the prolongation of ileus. In 1972, opioid receptors were discovered in the gut, on presynaptic nerve terminals in the myenteric plexus.[510] These receptors are believed to send signals that decrease propulsive contractions when bound with opioids. There are pharmacologic agents that block the peripheral or so-called mu (μ) receptors in the bowel wall and yet simultaneously allow the central analgesic effects.[510,1094] Alvimopan (Entereg), a peripherally acting mu antagonist, has been associated with a moderate acceleration in GI recovery after colectomy.[241] In the United States, it has been approved for in-hospital use in patients who are to undergo a colon resection (Adolor Corporation, Exton, PA).

COMPLICATIONS

The complications of rectal surgery, especially as applied to cancer, are discussed in Chapter 24.

MORTALITY AND RECURRENCE AFTER RESECTION

Considerable difficulty is encountered in analyzing the survival results after resection for colorectal carcinoma from various institutions. Many reports use actuarial methods, correcting the data for the age of the patient, thereby theoretically giving more accurate survival statistics. However, confusion may still arise. For example, only a few patients who are older than 90 years old and whose disease is cured survive 5 years. If a patient in this age group dies of carcinoma of the colon 4 years after resection, this is still considered a cure. Another method commonly employed to analyze results divides patients who have undergone surgery into two categories: those who have had resection and in whom the surgeon believes the disease is potentially curable and those whose disease is considered incurable and for whom the operation is palliative.

A third method of analysis is to determine the "crude" survival rate. This is calculated based on the number of patients alive 5 years after treatment. Obviously, this may not be a true estimate of the number of deaths from cancer because the patient may have died of another cause during the interim. Determinate survivors are those individuals who die within 5 years with no evidence of recurrent disease. Some institutions employ this means for reporting data. The obvious implication is that the survival figures are improved if patients are considered cured even if they die, albeit free of disease, before 5 years have elapsed. A need exists for uniformity in reporting the results of treatment for colorectal cancer as well as for the use of consistently comparable classifications of staging. What is more, there seems to be less interest in reporting overall survival statistics, at least for colon cancer. Moreover, what data exist, often combine colon and rectal cancer mortalities when there is a recognized difference in survival between the two areas, especially in light of the fact that the confines of the pelvis tend to limit the ability for one to widely resect the tumor. In the literature, there is much greater attention to survival with rectal cancer, especially with respect to, for example, neoadjuvant therapy, total mesorectal excision, and palliative treatment. Therefore, one may infer that surgery has accomplished all it can for colon cancer stage for stage.

In order better to evaluate and compare the morbidity and mortality rates associated with major surgery, a scoring system has been developed. The *Physiologic* and *Operative Severity Score* for the en*U*meration of *Mortality* and morbidity (POSSUM) and Portsmouth (P-POSSUM) equations were derived from a heterogeneous general surgical population in order to provide this information.[77,1008] Tekkis and colleagues evaluated these scoring systems in patients undergoing colorectal surgery and found that both overpredicted mortality in young patients and underpredicted mortality in the elderly.[1008] Emergency surgical deaths were also underpredicted.

Mitry and coworkers studied specifically operative mortality after colorectal cancer surgery over a 20-year period (1976 to 1995).[695] Overall mortality decreased from 17.7% to 8.1%, whereas rates after curative resection fell from 12.6% to 6.2%. These still seem very high numbers, the consequence of which has been the dramatic improvement in overall survival based on this criterion alone. Survival rates are often based on previous outcomes of large numbers of people who had the disease, but they cannot predict what will happen in any particular person's case. Knowing the type and the stage of a person's cancer is important in estimating his or her outlook. But many other factors may also affect a person's prognosis, such as the grade of the cancer, the genetic changes in the cancer cells, and how well the cancer responds to treatment (see earlier discussion). Even when taking these and other factors into account, survival rates are at best approximations.

Survival Rates for Colon Cancer by Stage

The numbers below come from a study of the National Cancer Institute's SEER database, looking at more than 28,000 people diagnosed with colon cancer between 1998 and 2000. These are *observed* survival rates. They include people diagnosed with colon cancer who may have later died from other causes, such as heart disease.

Stage	*5-Year Survival Rate*
I	74%
IIA	67%
IIB	59%
IIC	37%
IIIA	73%*
IIIB	46%*
IIIC	28%
IV	6%

---

*In this study, survival was better for some stage III cancers than for some stage II cancers. The reasons for this are not clear.

The Conundrum of Lymph Nodes

Survival rates generally correlate with the extent of lymph node involvement. In an older study, Corman and colleagues illustrated the survival rate based on the number of lymph nodes found to be positive (Table 23-5). If more than three nodes were positive, the overall survival rate was only 18%. These results lend some support to the contention that ultraradical resection for colorectal carcinoma is probably not justifiable for improving cure rates.

The number of positive nodes in the specimen appears to be as important as the level of nodes involved by tumor. Others have also concluded that the location rather than the number of nodal metastases has a greater impact on prognosis in colorectal cancer patients.[933] This is not to say that involvement of an apical lymph node is not an important criterion for survival (see earlier discussion on the Sentinel Lymph Nodes). Wong and associates conducted a study on 345 patients with M0 disease to determine whether increasing the number of *negative* nodes recovered would better stage the patient and more accurately predict disease-free survival.[1121] When compared with a national registry (OncoPool), they observed a significantly greater number of lymph nodes sampled in their study population and a statistically significantly improved survival between their patients and the National Cancer Registry population.[1121] Komuta and coworkers noted that the identification of extracapsular invasion of metastatic lymph nodes has a negative effect on survival when compared with lymph node invasion that does not extend outside the capsule.[534]

Malassagne and colleagues explored the relationships between a host of pathologic parameters, including the location and number of lymph nodes involved, blood vessel invasion, depth of tumor penetration, and metastases.[627] The 5-year survival rates were 45% and 17% for patients without and with apical lymph node involvement, respectively, and 44% and 6% with four or fewer nodes involved and more than four involved, respectively. These differences were statistically significant.

It has become increasingly important to remove and examine a sufficient number of lymph nodes at the time of resection for colon and rectal cancers. The implication is that more extensive nodal resection has been associated with lower rates of cancer recurrence. Moreover, such a search allows for more accurate cancer staging and possibly more appropriate use of adjuvant chemotherapy. Many factors affect the number of lymph nodes examined, including extent of surgical resection, patient age, tumor location, and pathology techniques. A 12-node minimum has been endorsed as a consensus standard for hospital-based performance of colectomy for colon cancer. However, using the number of lymph nodes examined may not significantly influence staging or patient survival. Although there remains little controversy about the prognostic importance of higher lymph node counts for individual patients, it is not clear that node counts are useful indicators of hospital's, surgeon's, or pathologist's quality.

Regardless, there has been a high level of interest in lymph node counts and survival rates of patients with colon and rectal cancers. Over the years, several studies using retrospective cohort data and administrative claims data have demonstrated improved survival among colon cancer patients in whom a higher number of nodes was examined after resection. Several observational studies found an association

TABLE 23-5 Survival versus Number of Lymph Nodes Involved (1962–1971)

NUMBER OF POSITIVE LYMPH NODES	TOTAL	DEATHS	5-YEAR SURVIVAL NUMBER	PERCENTAGE
1	71	39	32	45
2	47	33	14	30
3	30	15	15	50
4	20	16	4	20
5	11	9	2	18
6	8	6	2	25
7	7	6	1	14
8 or more	9	8	1	11
Total	203	132	71	35

From Corman ML, Veidenheimer MC, Coller JA. Colorectal carcinoma: a decade of experience at the Lahey Clinic. *Dis Colon Rectum.* 1979;22:477, with permission.

between the evaluation of an "adequate" number of lymph nodes and improved survival.[350,988] In many studies, the benefit was seen across nodal staging groups, noting improved survival with an increasing number of lymph nodes removed among those with node-negative and node-positive colon cancers.[170,574] Because increased survival was seen in those with known lymph node involvement, a therapeutic benefit was suggested for higher lymph node retrieval.

A recent systematic review examined whether the number of lymph nodes retrieved following colon resection was related to survival.[164] Sixteen of 17 studies, including a total of 61,371 patients, showed a positive association between the number of lymph nodes examined and survival in stage II and III colon cancer patients. The data are convincing. There is general agreement about the prognostic implications of this variable for long-term survival for individual colon cancer patients.

However, the association between lymph node counts and survival in rectal cancer is not as uniform. An analysis of 1,664 patients from a national intergroup trial of adjuvant therapy for rectal cancer found an association between higher number of nodes examined and survival only in node-negative patients.[1010] Although such results may support the role of adequate nodal retrieval for staging, a causal link between extent of resection, number of nodes examined, and survival could not be made because that association was not seen in node-positive patients.

The International Union Against Cancer, the American Joint Committee on Cancer, and a National Cancer Institute consensus panel have all recommended evaluation of at least

12 nodes to ensure adequate sampling.[733,947,1112] The College of American Pathologists has, for many years, recommended pathologic examination of at least 12 nodes in order to accurately predict node negativity.[192] If fewer than 12 nodes are found after thorough gross examination, there are recommendations for use of additional visual enhancement techniques.

Nevertheless, population-based data suggest that only 37% of colon cancer patients have adequate lymph node evaluation (i.e., at least 12 nodes examined).[59] In fact, concern for widespread understaging of patients led to the development of recommendations for consideration of adjuvant chemotherapy in colon cancer patients with a small number of examined nodes.[78]

In the recent systematic review of lymph node counts, a wide range of cutpoints was reported for the number of nodes necessary to have an associated improvement in survival.[164] Findings ranged from 6 nodes[155] to 40 nodes.[502] The 12-node minimum has been endorsed by many groups because there was a suggestion of "diminishing returns" beyond examination of 12 to 17 nodes.[164] However, it is unclear if a higher lymph node retrieval rate improves staging of colon cancer, and the causal mechanism between lymph node counts and survival remains unclear.

Many factors affect the number of lymph nodes examined, including extent of surgical resection, patient age, tumor location, and pathologic techniques. Patient factors must also be taken into account; for example, older age and obesity are associated with decreased lymph node recovery.[59,358] Tumor location may play a role because right-sided tumors are generally associated with higher numbers of lymph nodes examined.[164] The number of lymph nodes involved may also reflect a patient's improved immune response; as such, the relationship between node counts and survival may be confounded by the tumor-host response because a stronger immunologic response leads to improved survival.[776]

Surgeon-dependent factors must also be taken into account. Certainly, the extent of resection is determined by the surgeon in the operating room. Accepted oncologic principles for surgical resection include resection of the involved segment of colon and proximal ligation of the feeding vascular pedicle, with en bloc lymphadenectomy of associated draining lymph nodes. If a tumor is found between two draining vessels, it is important to include the distribution of both of those vessels. Pathologic evaluation following surgical resection is critical for determining subsequent treatment because adjuvant chemotherapy is indicated for patients with lymph node metastases. There are variations in extent of pathologic examination to be considered as well. Studies have shown that variation in number of lymph nodes examined can be attributed to pathology assistants who process the specimens[768] or to practice patterns of the pathologists themselves.[567] Furthermore, laparoscopic colon resections must be held to the same standards as that of open procedures.[305]

Resection of *rectal cancers*, because of anatomic considerations, requires an adequate circumferential margin. Performance of a total mesorectal excision (TME) assures that the fat, vessels, and lymphatics contained within the visceral pelvic fascia are removed en bloc with the rectal cancer (see Chapter 24). Tumor involvement of the circumferential margin is the most critical factor in predicting local recurrence and independently increases the risk of death from disease.[89]

Rectal cancer, especially in the context of neoadjuvant therapies, deserves special consideration in this discussion of lymph node examination rates. Preoperative radiotherapy appears to decrease the number of nodes examined.[57] It is unknown if preoperative chemoradiation decreases lymph node numbers more than radiation alone. Because of the increasing use of preoperative radiotherapy in patients with intermediate- and high-risk rectal cancers, the prognostic significance of lymph node counts in rectal cancers is less clear.

While staging is dependent on the number of positive nodes, a higher number of nodes examined does not necessarily predict having more nodes involved. To help adjust for the problem of low lymph node counts, the use of "lymph node ratios" has been proposed to help stratify risk in stage III patients. Studies show that a lower ratio of the number of positive nodes to the total number of nodes examined (calculated as a proportion) is associated with both disease-free survival and overall survival in colon cancer.[79]

As previously discussed, the National Quality Forum, in conjunction with major stakeholders in cancer care, such as the American Society of Clinical Oncology (ASCO), the American College of Surgeons Commission on Cancer (CoC), and the National Comprehensive Cancer Network (NCCN), endorsed a minimum 12-lymph node count as a quality measure for improving outcome for colon cancer patients.[730] Although there is an accepted association between a higher number of lymph nodes retrieved and improved long-term survival for individual patients, the mechanism underlying this association is unknown. The quality indicator is meant to be applied at a hospital level, which seems appropriate given the multiple variables that can affect the outcome. However, it is unclear if this metric will ultimately lead to improved survival in patients with colon cancer.

Based on recent hospital level analyses, it appears that the majority of hospitals do not meet the minimal 12-node count.[85,1123] The number of lymph nodes that hospitals examine in colon cancer resection specimens does not appear to significantly influence staging, use of adjuvant chemotherapy, or patient survival.[1123] It is likely that unmeasured patient- or hospital-related factors are confounding the relationship. Although there is consensus that the quality of cancer care can be improved, it is unclear whether enforcing a minimum number of lymph nodes is the correct quality measure to use.

Although a 12-node minimum is commonly accepted as necessary for accurate staging, evidence to support this measure as a quality indicator for cancer care is lacking on a hospital level. Numerous studies and sufficient data support that retrieval of more lymph nodes is associated with improved survival for individual patients, but the causality underlying this relationship is unknown. It is important to adhere to strict oncologic principles for cancer resections, including high vascular ligation and complete en bloc resection of the mesocolon, lymphadenectomy, and circumferential margins (for rectal cancer). In addition, it is important for pathologists to perform diligent examination of resected specimens.

Blood Vessel Invasion

In addition to lymph node involvement, there is interest in the presence or absence of blood vessel invasion as an independent prognostic indicator (see Figure 23-34). In this same older study, Table 23-6 shows the uncorrected survival rate in patients with Dukes' C lesions (stage III) with and without blood vessel invasion. The survival rate of patients with blood vessel invasion was 31%, compared with 43% in those without blood vessel invasion. These differences are not statistically significant, but they do suggest that the combination of blood vessel invasion and lymph node involvement is associated with a poorer prognosis for survival than lymph node involvement alone. The importance of blood vessel invasion is further evident in Table 23-7. With Dukes' B lesions, 5-year survival was 70% in those without blood vessel invasion but only 55% in those with such invasion. This difference is statistically significant ($P < .05$). The mean ages of patients with and without blood vessel invasion, alive or dead, were identical. Oh-e and associates opine that intratumor microvessel count at the site of deepest penetration of the cancer is a predictor for the presence of lymph node metastasis.[758]

Gervaz and coworkers studied Dukes' B colorectal cancers with respect to p53 protein expression and determined that it is an independent factor for survival.[328] Furthermore, this also correlated with tumor location; 86% of p53-positive tumors were located in the distal colon and rectum.

TABLE 23-6 Uncorrected Survival Rates, Dukes' Classification C Colorectal Carcinoma (1962–1966)

BLOOD VESSEL INVASION	5-YEAR SURVIVAL	DEATHS	LIVING TOTAL	LIVING PERCENTAGE
Present	19	43	62	31
Absent	24	32	56	43

From Corman ML, Veidenheimer MC, Coller JA. Colorectal carcinoma: a decade of experience at the Lahey Clinic. *Dis Colon Rectum.* 1979;22:477, with permission.

TABLE 23-7 Uncorrected Survival Rates, Dukes' Classification B Colorectal Carcinoma (1962–1966)

BLOOD VESSEL INVASION	LIVING	DEATHS	TOTAL	LIVING (%)
Present	32	26	58	55
Absent	82	35	117	70
Total	**114**	**61**	**175**	**65**

From Corman ML, Swinton NW Sr, O'Keefe DD, et al. Colorectal carcinoma at the Lahey Clinic, 1962–1966. *Am J Surg.* 1973;125:424, with permission.

Galandiuk and colleagues reviewed the patterns of recurrence after curative resection for carcinoma of the colon and rectum.[320] As expected, colon cancer had a better prognosis than rectal cancer (52% vs. 40%). The most frequent sites for recurrence were hepatic (33%), pulmonary (22%), local or regional (21%), intra-abdominal (18%), retroperitoneal (10%), and peripheral lymph nodes (4%). There was a much higher incidence of local recurrence in rectal sites than in colonic, a fact that is attributable to the difficulties with the technique of wide excision within the confines of the pelvis. This has been confirmed in a number of reports.[750]

Mzabi and colleagues undertook a retrospective study to determine the factors associated with mortality and survival after resection for colonic cancer.[722] As could be expected, patients who presented for operation with no symptoms had a significantly better rate of survival than those who presented with symptoms. Furthermore, these investigators and others demonstrated that rectal bleeding as a symptom was a better prognostic sign than the other presenting complaints of colonic cancer.[722,971] Other variables, ranked according to their relative importance independent of stage according to one study, were as follows: histologic grade, level of direct spread, presence of venous invasion, age and sex of the patient, and presence of obstruction.[165] The Cleveland Clinic surgeons reported their observations on the factors affecting local recurrence in colon cancer and concluded that the location of the tumor is not relevant.[421] In their experience, fixity to another viscus, perforation or fistulization, advanced stage of disease, and dedifferentiation of tumor increase the risk of recurrence following curative resections.[421] In the Mayo Clinic experience, whereas the grade of anaplasia and ploidy had a strong influence on the rate of recurrence, these factors did not influence the timing or the pattern.[320] Goodman and Irvin studied the effect of a delay of diagnosis on prognosis following resection of carcinoma of the right side of the colon.[357] The authors observed that a delayed presentation was not associated with a different rate of survival than an early presentation.

Significance of Gender

Some reports suggest that survival after colorectal cancer surgery is better in women when controlled for tumor stage. The previously alluded to anatomic differences between the male and female pelvis may play an important factor with respect to rectal cancer resection from the technical perspective, but that does not account for improved survival with colon cancer. McArdle and colleagues noted in their 3,200 patients that overall survival at 5 years was higher in women, better in women with colonic tumors, in those who underwent elective surgery, and in those who underwent apparently curative resection.[655] It has been suggested that immunologic factors may play a role.[1085]

Significance of Blood Transfusion

Perioperative blood transfusion, possibly because of the potential for immunosuppression, may be associated with an increased risk for recurrence according to some studies, even when this variable is controlled for age, sex, TNM stage, and histologic differentiation.[83,782,1000] Wobbes and colleagues noted a statistically significant worsening of disease-free survival when more than six units of blood were administered in comparison with a lesser amount.[1113] Marsh and colleagues found that the risk for recurrence in patients who received a transfusion of plasma was twice that in patients who did not receive any.[637] These investigators were not able to show a harmful effect of transfusion with packed cells. These data suggest that the plasma protein rather than the cellular component of whole blood mediates the accelerated tumor recurrence.[637] However, others have found no relationship between transfusion status and tumor recurrence, tumor behavior, or patient survival.[179,313,939,1078] Conversely, Houblers and colleagues found that their patients had a lower 3-year survival than those who were not transfused, but this poor survival was not related to recurrent cancer.[452] Busch and coworkers opine that the association between blood transfusions and prognosis in colorectal cancer is a result of circumstances that necessitate the transfusions in the first place.[140] Furthermore, the association may be greater with the development of local recurrence than with distant metastases.[140]

Obstructing and Perforating Carcinoma

Patients who present with obstruction or perforation have a poorer prognosis than other individuals with colorectal carcinoma.[972] The operative morbidity and mortality are also much higher.[870] Often, patients have evidence of metastatic disease at the time of presentation.[1039,1058] As previously mentioned, perforated carcinoma should be treated by primary resection whenever possible. In addition, primary resection should be carried out for proximal obstructing lesions. The concept of intraoperative colonic lavage with primary anastomosis in the presence of perforation (even peritonitis in certain instances) and obstruction has been advocated by a number of investigators (see earlier discussion).[87]

Some studies suggest that operative mortality and even prognosis are better when primary resection with anastomosis is performed rather than a staged approach. Umpleby and Williamson reported a 48% 5-year survival in curative resections with anastomosis, compared with an 18% survival rate with a staged resection.[1039] Gennaro and Tyson noted an overall operative mortality of 14% for obstructing carcinoma.[325] The uncorrected survival rate at 5 years was approximately 9%, whereas only 18% of patients who underwent curative resection survived 5 years. Glenn and McSherry reported an operative mortality of 13% in patients with obstruction and a 5-year survival rate of approximately 20%.[340] Their experience with perforated carcinoma revealed an equally poor prognosis. The operative mortality was 15%, and the 5-year survival rate, 28%.[340] Serpell and colleagues reviewed 148 patients with colonic obstruction and found a significantly higher incidence of recurrence after curative resection and a lower survival rate.[919] Kriwanek and coworkers commented on the recognized high postoperative mortality for malignant perforation, concluding that it is the cumulative effect of the malignancy and sepsis that is responsible.[539]

Carcinoma in Younger Patients

Colorectal carcinoma has been believed to be associated with a poor prognosis when it develops in young patients. Only a small percentage of these individuals will have a predisposing factor, such as familial adenomatous polyposis. Although the incidence is much lower in the younger group, it is imperative for the physician at least to consider investigating anyone who presents with symptoms suggestive of a bowel tumor (vague abdominal pain, nausea and vomiting, weight loss, rectal bleeding, or change in bowel habits). Determination of occult blood in the stool may be helpful. Because of the symptoms at presentation and the difficulty in interpreting their significance, delay in diagnosis and treatment is one of the major factors responsible for the poor survival rates. In the experience of Palmer and colleagues, no Dukes' A or B lesions were seen in individuals younger than 20 years of age, and only 11% were observed in those in their 20s.[778]

Even for the same stage of lesion, however, younger persons have been believed to do less well when compared with older individuals. This may be because younger patients have a higher incidence of mucinous and poorly differentiated tumors.[8,507,801] Recalde and associates reported a 13% 5-year survival rate in 40 patients 35 years of age or younger.[831] Furthermore, they noted that no 5-year survivors were found among individuals who had lymph node metastases, visceral metastases, or tumors larger than 5 cm in diameter. Sanfelippo and Beahrs reported on 118 patients younger than 40 years of age who underwent resection for colorectal carcinoma.[890] Their overall 5-year survival rate was 39%. Patients with Dukes' C lesions had a 5-year survival rate of 21%.

Carcinoma of the colon is extremely uncommon in children. In contrast to the presentation in adults, the most frequent symptom is abdominal pain, often with vomiting. The diagnosis was delayed for more than 1 year in more than one-half of the adolescents reviewed by Steinberg and coworkers.[970] Pemberton reported on the cure of a 9-year-old child and stated that no other report was found in the literature of a survivor in whom the disease developed at such an early age.[787] He further observed that in children, the colon is affected more frequently by cancer than any other part of the digestive system.

Fundamentally, three factors contribute to the increased mortality in these individuals: delay in diagnosis, advanced stage of disease, and poorly differentiated histology.[124,216] Mitry and colleagues emphasized that inadequate screening and treatment of young people with familial adenomatous polyposis or a family history of early-age-at-onset colorectal cancer are the primary factors contributing to poorer prognosis rather than young age itself.[694]

Carcinoma in the Elderly

Simply stated, there is no justification for avoiding needed surgery based on a patient's age. Generally, there are no differences with respect to presentation, location, Dukes' classification, and prognosis in comparison with younger individuals. All studies confirm that there are no statistically significant differences in age-corrected survival curves.[472] However, emergency operations are associated with a higher morbidity and mortality in this age group.[76]

Carcinoma in Pregnancy

Colorectal carcinoma in pregnancy is extremely unusual. Nesbitt and colleagues reported their experience with five patients and reviewed the literature.[735] As with carcinoma in young patients, and for essentially the same reasons, prognosis is poor. Management is determined by the gestational age of the fetus at the time of diagnosis, as well as by religious and ethical considerations. The question of concomitant oophorectomy is problematic, especially during the first trimester, because of the risk for spontaneous abortion.[735]

Palliative Resection

Because carcinoma of the colon is a relatively slow-growing tumor, palliative resection should be performed whenever

possible, subject to a few relative contraindications. Even with extensive metastatic disease, patients may live a relatively long time and be free of the often miserable sequelae associated with an untreated primary lesion.

Cady and coworkers reported that during the years from 1941 to 1960, patients with liver metastases diagnosed at operation survived a mean of 13 months.[146] Factors that adversely influenced survival included weight loss, intestinal symptoms, ascites, peritoneal seeding, extension of the primary cancer to other viscera, histologic involvement of lymph nodes or blood vessels, and extent of surgical treatment.[146] Takaki and associates noted a mean survival time of approximately 12 months in 59 patients who underwent palliative resection.[993] Goslin and colleagues reported a similar median survival.[359] With the newer adjuvant approaches to the treatment of metastatic cancer (see later), patients now live longer, especially with liver metastases. Those whose tumors are poorly differentiated or who have weight loss of greater than 10% at presentation (with metastases) survive a median of only 6 months.[359]

Contraindications to performing palliative resection include the presence of ascites, massive peritoneal seeding, jaundice, and severe debilitation. Jayne and colleagues found that the median survival with peritoneal carcinomatosis from colorectal cancer for synchronous disease was 7 months.[486] Liu and coworkers found that palliative resection of primary colon cancers is associated with a relatively high postoperative mortality but that it should be performed as long as hepatic metastases occupy less than 50% of liver volume.[584] Obviously, the decision to carry out such a procedure is a matter of surgical judgment.

The decision to perform a palliative resection in someone with bleeding, a profound anemia, perforation, or obstruction is usually not difficult. However, when a relatively asymptomatic colorectal cancer is found in someone with metastastic disease, one must consider whether the primary tumor should be removed. Sarela and colleagues identified 24 such patients and managed them with systemic chemotherapy without surgery.[892] Four patients developed bowel obstructions requiring operative management in two and stents in two. Additionally, three subsequently underwent right hemicolectomy for abdominal pain with poor relief. One other patient was downstaged and underwent a curative resection. The overall median survival was 10.3 months. The problem clearly is that some patients live longer than one anticipates. Ruo and coworkers reported the experience of the Memorial Sloan-Kettering Cancer Center in New York with patients with asymptomatic stage IV disease who underwent *elective* resection (127 individuals) and compared the results with 103 patients with stage IV disease who did not undergo resection.[872] Resected patients had longer median (16 vs. 9 months) and 2-year survivals (25% vs. 6%). The investigators concluded that patients with stage IV disease who were selected for elective palliative resection of asymptomatic primary colorectal cancers had a substantial postoperative survival that was significantly better than those not submitted to resection.[872] Case selection clearly plays a major role in the reported outcomes of these series. The optimal management of patients with asymptomatic primary colonic tumors remains to be defined.[195]

Follow-up Evaluation

How to follow patients who have undergone resection for carcinoma of the colon is a subject worthy of some discussion. Methods of evaluation include physical examination, fecal occult blood testing, proctosigmoidoscopy, colonoscopy, barium enema examination, chest radiography, determination of CEA levels, liver function studies, liver scan, ultrasonographic evaluation, CT, MRI, PET-CT, and exploratory laparotomy at an interval after operation, among others.[289,1055]

Besides the variety of examinations, tests, and procedures that are available to follow the patient with cancer postoperatively, the frequency with which such evaluation should be undertaken is also the subject of debate. One school of thought postulates that the patient should be discharged after recovery from surgery and report only if symptoms develop, so nihilistic is the attitude of many physicians and surgeons that earlier diagnosis and treatment of recurrent disease fail to result in a sufficiently improved survival rate to justify the cost and the effort.

Moertel and colleagues contributed an article in 1993 that stimulated considerable debate about the value of monitoring patients following resection of colon cancer.[698] The authors concluded that cancer cures attributable to monitoring of CEA are, at best, infrequent. Therefore, they question whether this small gain justifies the substantial cost and physical and emotional stress that this intervention usually causes patients. Obviously, cost is a major issue today, with no indication that higher cost strategies increase the survival or quality of life.[1060] Clearly, an intensive follow-up program is associated with, at best, only a minimally increased survival rate, but for those individuals fortunate enough to have recurrent tumors that are amenable to curative re-resection, it would seem very important.[98,276,595,626,772,860,877,900,1029] Bruinvels and colleagues found that patients with an intensive follow-up regimen noted a 9% better 5-year survival than those with minimal or no follow-up.[125] The fact is that few patients are salvaged in whom a recurrence of cancer develops. However, there is a group of individuals for whom a cure can still be achieved, or at least for whom lifestyle can be improved and long-term survival made possible, if recurrent tumor is recognized early. These include those with a longer disease-free interval between initial resection and recurrence, with negative margins of resection, and smaller recurrent tumor size.[931]

In one area, at least, there appears to be no controversy: that is, the acknowledged increased risk for the development of a metachronous lesion. The calculated annual incidence for metachronous tumors was determined by Cali and colleagues to be 0.35%.[151] The cumulative incidence at 18 years was 6.3%. If for no other reason than this observation, the patient should never be discharged from follow-up study but should be evaluated periodically for the development of a second primary tumor in the bowel.

Heald and Lockhart-Mummery showed that the chance of cure was much improved in those patients who attended a follow-up clinic at the time of the occurrence of a second growth.[430] It has also been shown that metachronous cancers are diagnosed at earlier stages than the index cancers.[151] Ovaska and colleagues compared the results of 368 individuals who underwent regular follow-up evaluation with 139 who did not.[771] The cancer-related 5-year survival rate was 72% in the former group and 62% in the latter. Curative reoperations were performed in 21% of the former, but in only 7% of the latter. These investigators concluded that regular follow-up detects more recurrent tumors, enabling radical reoperations to be performed significantly more often than when this is not undertaken.

Physical Examination

Physical examination is quite unrewarding for identifying an early recurrence. By the time palpation of the abdomen reveals a tumor in the liver or a recurrent lesion in the peritoneal cavity, the cancer is virtually always nonresectable. Therefore, palpation of the abdomen, pelvic examination, and evaluation of supraclavicular and inguinal nodes serve primarily to reassure the patient and the physician. The primary value of such examinations and findings is to follow the response to adjuvant treatment once an obvious tumor has been identified.

Occult Blood Determination

The importance of examination of the stool for occult blood has been emphasized earlier in this chapter and in Chapter 5. As with the early identification of a primary tumor, the main purpose of performing this test is to look for a second (metachronous) lesion. It has been suggested that a lifelong follow-up regimen following resection of colorectal carcinoma for cure should include an annual occult blood determination.[130]

Proctosigmoidoscopy and Flexible Sigmoidoscopy

On an annual basis, or even more frequently, proctosigmoidoscopy is of particular value if the anastomosis can be seen with the instrument. Recurrence at the suture line, which most often results from inward growth of the tumor from the pelvis and not from residual cancer within the bowel wall or mucosa, can be identified, so that re-resection for possible cure may be performed. Flexible sigmoidoscopy serves the same purpose if the anastomosis can be seen within range of this instrument. If the anastomosis is above this level, the only purpose of either examination is to identify a metachronous lesion within the limitations of the instrument.

Colonoscopy

Colonoscopy should be employed to evaluate the residual colon following resection if the procedure was not performed preoperatively or if visualization of the entire bowel had not been accomplished. Many studies have demonstrated the high incidence of benign and malignant lesions harbored in the residual colon, presumably missed at the time of resection.[319,521,540,551,555,731,1040] Harris and colleagues described the colonoscopic features of anastomoses in 117 postoperative patients.[422] The following were identified:

- Neovascularity (89.7%)
- White anastomotic edge (54.7%)
- Disruption of haustral pattern (54.7%)
- Radial suture tracks (38.0%)
- Exposed suture (11.9% of those sutured)
- Exposed staples (24% of those stapled)
- Scar tissue adjacent to anastomotic line (6.8%)
- Nondistensibility (4.3%)
- Blind colonic pouch (8.5%)

The site of seven anastomoses (5.5%) could not be identified.[422]

Reilly and associates performed perioperative colonoscopy on 92 patients.[838] Synchronous cancers were found in almost 8%. Approximately 3 or more years following treatment of the index cancer, a metachronous malignancy was demonstrated in an additional 8%.

The procedure is also of value in identifying recurrent disease at the anastomosis, although the incidence appears quite low in individuals following resection of a colon cancer. Colonoscopy is advised by some authors every 3 years once the bowel has been demonstrated to be completely free of neoplasm,[130] but others believe that an annual evaluation with this instrument for the first 4 years after curative resection is preferable.[551,771] Leggett and coworkers performed colonoscopy within 6 months of surgery and then at intervals of 3 years thereafter on 433 individuals.[562] They calculated the rate of development of metachronous cancer at 0.61% annually. Juhl and colleagues performed annual colonoscopy in their surveillance program of 174 patients.[503] The combined findings of anastomotic recurrences, metachronous colon cancers, and polyps represented an interval yield of 3% to 5% annually. Based on these results, they suggest an annual colonoscopy for at least the initial 6 years after resection.

Recent studies have shown a surprisingly high incidence of "metachronous" colorectal cancer at a relatively short interval after curative resection.[371,575a,869] In one study of 432 patients, 10% had one to two adenomas, 3.7% had three or more adenomas, 3.7% had an advanced adenoma, and 2.3% had a "new" cancer within 1 year of a supposed clearing colonoscopy prior to resection.[470] The incidence of intraluminal recurrence was 0.23%. The yield of surveillance colonoscopy for the detection of metachronous carcinoma compares very favorably with the rate of prevalent cancers detected during screening colonoscopy.[841]

A common preference is to perform an annual colonoscopic examination until the bowel is clear; then colonoscopy is performed every 3 years. It must be remembered that endoscopy is a poor tool for evaluating extramucosal, locally recurrent disease. Any follow-up program must, therefore, address this concern through alternative studies.[52]

Barium Enema Examination

The barium enema examination is of limited benefit in the follow-up evaluation of the patient with colorectal cancer. It is unlikely that recurrent disease at the suture line will be identified more readily by this technique than by colonoscopy. A possible exception to this dictum, however, is that extrinsic compression might be perceived more readily with a barium enema study than by means of colonoscopy. As suggested, in the follow-up evaluation of the bowel of patients who have undergone resection for colorectal cancer, colonoscopy appears to be the preferred technique, certainly for identifying a mucosal lesion.

Chest Radiography

Chest radiography should be performed annually to identify patients with possible pulmonary metastases; some of these individuals may still be operated on for cure (see Pulmonary Metastases in the section Treatment of Recurrence). Resectable disease is identified in ~1% to 2% of patients who have a follow-up chest x-ray.[345,365,786] The yield of chest radiography is clearly higher in those with rectal cancer, where the probability of isolated lung metastases is greater. The data regarding the utility of routine chest radiography in the

follow-up of patients after colon resection has been considered inconclusive.[25]

Liver Function Studies

Liver function studies have traditionally been considered useful in the follow-up evaluation of patients with colorectal cancer. In the experience of most physicians, the alkaline phosphatase determination has been about as effective in diagnosing liver metastases as has the CEA determination, but the most sensitive overall test for detecting occult metastases has been CEA. One study has demonstrated that if patients with elevated serum alkaline phosphatase values are not found to have metastases to the liver at the time of laparotomy, then these individuals are at no greater risk for the development of liver tumors than those with normal serum levels.[1001] Rocklin and colleagues believe that liver function tests should be deleted from follow-up of cancer patients because the CEA heralds the onset of liver metastases much more frequently.[851] The ASCRS Practice Parameter recommendations concur, citing a yield for potentially resectable disease of only 2 to 3 patients per 1,000.[25]

Liver Scan

Postoperatively, in a patient with known liver metastases, the liver scan is useful to confirm the location and presence of the lesion or lesions. However, in the absence of a positive CEA determination or elevated level of alkaline phosphatase, this study has no place in postoperative screening. CT has replaced this study in the evaluation of colorectal cancer patients.

Computed Tomography

CT offers a simple, noninvasive method for the evaluation of metastatic colon tumor by enabling visualization of the liver, pelvis, retroperitoneum, and adrenal glands (see Figures 23-17 and 23-93). Some clinicians and investigators suggest that it be employed as a baseline study after surgery and then used at intervals to detect local recurrence.[278] It has also proved valuable in the evaluation of patients for supplemental therapy. Most studies confirm that both postoperative baseline

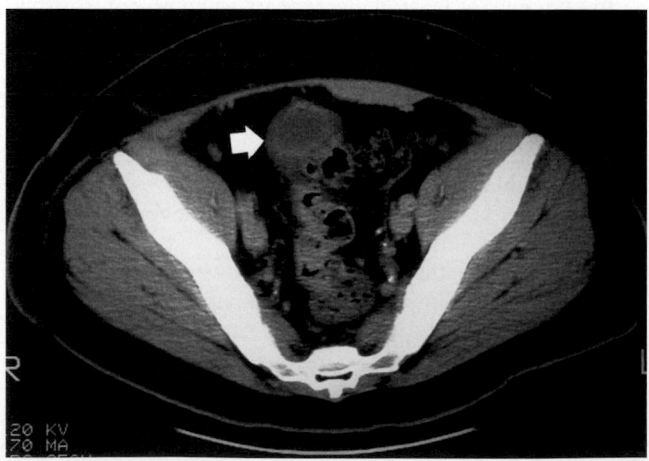

FIGURE 23-93. Computed tomography of the abdomen reveals tumor mass adjacent to the colon (*arrow*). The radiologic study was pursued because of an elevation in the carcinoembryonic antigen determination. Because no other site of spread was identified, the patient underwent re-exploration with resection of this solitary recurrence.

CEA values and CT of the abdomen have the highest positive predictive rate when metastases or persistent disease is suspected.[330] In addition, the CT-guided aspiration technique is useful for obtaining cytologic confirmation of malignancy.

Glover and colleagues prospectively assessed the accuracy of a number of imaging techniques in 100 patients who were considered free of liver metastases after colorectal cancer resections.[341] These included CT, magnetic resonance imaging (MRI), ultrasound, isotope assessment, and serum CEA. The most sensitive technique was CT. CT and MRI (but not ultrasound) were completely accurate in differentiating liver metastases from other hepatic lesions, but only two-thirds of affected patients were identified. The role of routine CT scanning after colon resection remains controversial. Whereas medical oncology guidelines tend to recommend periodic surveillance scans based on the appreciable rate of identifying asymptomatic lesions,[901] the ASCRS guidelines recommend against routine imaging because other less costly modalities (i.e., CEA) may pick up these lesions, noting further that the ultimate cure rate attributable directly to the CT scan is probably quite low.[25] As the options and outcomes for the treatment of recurrent disease continue to be modified and evolve, this issue will require ongoing assessment.

Magnetic Resonance Imaging

MRI is a promising modality that has certain advantages in comparison with CT, even replacing it as the diagnostic study of choice for lesions of the central nervous system. However, this advantage does not translate as well to the evaluation of tumor in other organs. CT is still the preferred alternative for the detection and follow-up of metastatic liver tumors, although MRI has a role in characterizing indeterminate lesions.

Tumor Markers

The primary role of tumor markers today is in the postoperative surveillance of individuals who, theoretically, underwent surgery for cure and therefore are at risk for recurrence.[1128] The most frequently employed such marker is serum CEA. In addition, monoclonal antibodies labeled with radioisotopes are being used to identify possible sites of recurrent disease.

Carcinoembryonic Antigen

Although the studies of Gold and Freedman demonstrated that elevated titers of CEA preceded clinical signs of disease by 2 weeks to 10 months, Moertel and coworkers opined that the CEA test is grossly insensitive in the diagnosis of recurrent colorectal carcinoma.[343,344,701] They tested 36 patients with histologically demonstrable recurrent or residual malignant disease after resection but with no clinical evidence of distant metastases. Only nine patients (25%) had abnormal CEA levels even though most of them had had symptoms of recurrence for several months. Sugarbaker and colleagues studied the serial monthly CEA determinations of 33 individuals after resection for large bowel cancer.[984] Confirmed recurrent malignant disease subsequently developed in 12 of these patients. A rising titer was the first evidence of recurrence in only 4 of these 12, and all 4 had distant metastases.

Despite objections about the lack of specificity of CEA and the question whether it is a sufficiently early diagnostic marker of recurrent disease to make cure possible, most researchers generally agree that increasing levels are found with more advanced disease. A failure of elevated levels of CEA to return to normal after resection is associated with a poor prognosis, and elevated levels usually appear before any clinical evidence of recurrence.[30,367,585,589,595,639–641,740,747,748,757,950,1090,1137] Chu and colleagues further showed that the preoperative and postoperative levels were predictive of recurrence and survival independently of tumor stage.[178] Many asymptomatic patients suspected of having recurrent colorectal cancer based on an elevated CEA will be spared unnecessary surgery if strict attention is paid to the preoperative assessment.[757] McCall and coworkers found that CEA was the first indicator of recurrent disease in 58% of their patients and in 80% of those with liver metastases.[657] At least three meta-analyses have suggested a benefit for scheduled follow-up, including CEA determinations.[125,840,860] CEA is the only blood test/tumor marker recommended for routine follow-up in the ASCRS Practice Parameter publication.[75]

Carcinoembryonic Antigen Concentration Gradient

Another possible application of the CEA determination has been reported by Patt and coworkers.[783] By means of selective angiographic techniques, a CEA concentration gradient can be determined by sampling from appropriate vessels. Identification of the site of recurrence may be possible with this method.

CA 19–9

CA 19–9 has been a widely used tumor marker for colorectal cancer, especially in Japan. Morita and coworkers undertook a retrospective investigation of 118 patients who underwent curative colorectal cancer surgery, analyzing and comparing CEA with CA 19–9 as indicators of prognosis for recurrent disease.[711] This study failed to demonstrate evidence to support the use of CA 19–9 to predict prognosis or to detect recurrence of colorectal cancer.

CA 242

CA 242 is a mucin tumor marker of interest in colorectal cancer. In a prospective study comparing it with CEA, Engarås found that CEA is preferred for postoperative surveillance.[281]

Messenger RNA of a Tumor-Specific Antigen (L6)

Schiedeck and colleagues compared CEA levels with the detection of messenger RNA (mRNA) coding for the tumor-associated antigen L6 in patients with colorectal cancer.[895] These investigators concluded that L6 is more sensitive and precise than CEA in diagnosing and monitoring colorectal cancer.

Acute-Phase Response

It has been postulated that measurement of acute-phase proteins in serum may serve as a useful marker for tumor recurrence. McMillan and coworkers examined this phenomenon in 36 patients with colorectal cancer who had undergone an apparently curative resection.[667] The authors found a significantly higher recurrence rate in individuals with an acute-phase response (11 of 15) than in those with no such response (2 of 21). The place of this particular study in the postoperative assessment of persons who have undergone resection for colorectal cancer needs further exploration.

Radiolabeled Imaging

The advent of monoclonal antibody technology has permitted the development of radiolabeled tumor reactive probes, which can be used in conjunction with gamma camera imaging equipment to identify the presence of a malignancy within a patient.[702] Some studies have been published concerning the value of radioimmunolocalization with radiolabeled antibody to CEA in individuals with no physical signs of local recurrence but with elevated CEA levels.[74] Generally, these tests can distinguish between localized and disseminated disease and often are more accurate than conventional radiologic studies, including CT. For example, an antibody fragment (Fab′) specific to CEA and labeled with [99m]Tc (CEA-Scan, Arcitumomab, Immunomedics, Morris Plains, NJ) is a nuclear imaging test for clinical use. Although this nuclear medicine study depends on the presence of the same antigen as the serum CEA test, it is apparently more sensitive than the serum evaluation.

Other monoclonal antibodies have been developed.[992] One such agent, monoclonal antibody B72.3 (Oncoscint CR/OV, Cytogen Corp., Princeton, NJ), has been the focus of study because of its pattern of extensive reactivity with a wide variety of mucin-producing adenocarcinomas. Because of its well-documented selectivity in binding to such tumors, it has been a useful target for patients with colorectal carcinoma. Monoclonal antibody B72.3 is a murine monoclonal antibody of the immunoglobulin G1 subclass that detects a glycoprotein, TAG-72, associated with high-molecular-weight tumors. This glycoprotein is expressed on certain human colon and breast carcinoma cell lines. To serve as a useful diagnostic agent, however, it must be coupled or conjugated to a radionuclide for imaging purposes. Corman and associates have reported the use of this monoclonal antibody conjugate, termed CYT-103, labeled with ^{111}In for diagnostic imaging of colorectal carcinoma in 103 patients.[200] Enrollment was restricted to cases in which standard diagnostic modalities did not provide sufficient information for patient management decisions. Forty-nine of these individuals had rising CEA levels with no evidence of a site for recurrence. The antibody imaging study detected occult (inapparent) disease in 70%, a finding responsible for altering or canceling the planned procedure (Figure 23-94). A total of 83% of the patients was found to have benefited from the study. Others have demonstrated that monoclonal antibody labeled with ^{111}In is safe and can be helpful in the detection of extrahepatic abdominal and pelvic tumors.[251,255,633,788,795,1110] Because this is a physiologic study, it has proved to be more sensitive than CT in the detection of disease in the pelvis and extrahepatic abdomen.[636] Confusion with radiation changes or postoperative scarring may be resolved in many instances through the use of radioimaging techniques.

Numerous factors influence the success of imaging, including the experience of the individual interpreting the scan as well as the level of tissue antigen expression.[1009] Problems may arise with certain studies, such as the use of monoclonal antibody B72.3, in that murine antibodies may produce human antimouse antibody (HAMA) response, which can lead to allergic reactions and difficulty in interpreting findings of subsequent studies, including CEA determination. Of course, there is the concern for false-positive and false-negative imaging.

Comment. Radiolabeled imaging techniques that have been applied to the follow-up management of patients who have undergone resection for colorectal cancer certainly have added much to our knowledge of the pathologic processes. Questions remain, however, as to the sensitivity and whether there is a tangible survival benefit. For the present, these modalities are of value in only two scenarios—that of an individual who will be submitted to re-exploration for a presumed isolated recurrence and that of someone with a rising CEA in whom other evaluations fail to identify the site of recurrence. That stated, PET scan has largely replaced monoclonal antibody studies for this purpose. It is axiomatic that prior to embarking on a second-look procedure (see later), an imaging study should be undertaken. In some instances, the tumor will be localized, and in others, one may be able to identify cancer beyond the limits of surgical cure. In both instances, the operative procedure would be changed. As the technology improves, it is hoped that the sensitivity and specificity will be high enough so that the surgeon can make an appropriate recommendation to the patient concerning the advisability of re-exploration.

Other Markers

Other markers that have been employed in an attempt to increase the sensitivity of monitoring for tumor recurrence include serum protein hexose, transferrin, and ceruloplasmin.[367] More work must be done, however, before the true value of all these newer techniques can be accurately assessed.

Positron Emission Tomography

Initially developed for brain evaluation in the 1970s and unlike conventional nuclear medicine technology, PET uses unique radiopharmaceuticals or "tracers" labeled with isotopes that are the basic elements of biologic substrates. These isotopes mimic natural substrates such as sugars, water, proteins, and oxygen. The technique uses CT imaging equipment and rings of detectors surrounding the patient to record gamma radiation produced when positrons (positively charged particles) emitted by the tracer collide with electrons. As a result, PET will often reveal more about the cellular-level metabolic status of a disease than other types of imaging modalities. Furthermore, PET images can be acquired quantitatively to reflect the actual amounts of tracer in the regions of interest. Therefore, recurrent disease may be diagnosed before structural changes become detectable by anatomic imaging techniques, such as CT.

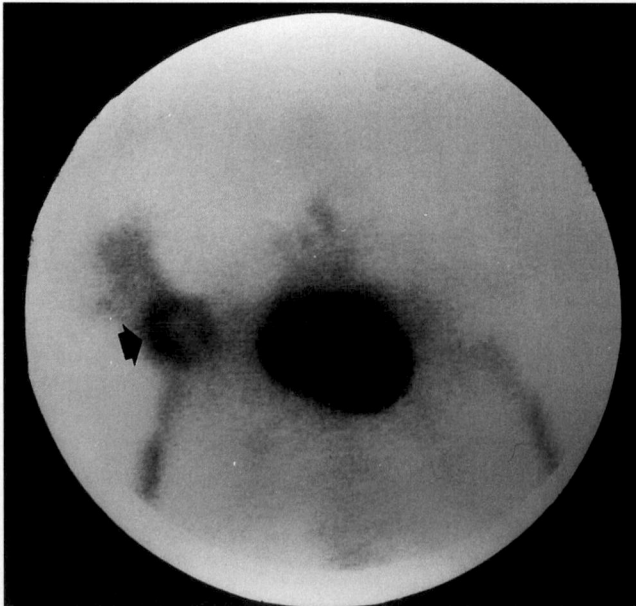

FIGURE 23-94. Oncoscint scan demonstrating uptake in the right hip, which on subsequent biopsy proved to be metastatic adenocarcinoma consistent with a colon primary tumor (*arrow*). The patient had been asymptomatic. Results of all other studies were negative, except for a rising carcinoembryonic antigen value.

As with radiolabeled imaging, PET may be helpful for localizing tumor recurrence following resection of colorectal cancer. Beets and colleagues performed a prospective study to evaluate the clinical impact of this whole-body imaging technique using fluoride-18fluorodeoxyglucose.[73] The investigators found that whole-body PET affected management in 14 of the 35 patients who were studied. Johnson and coworkers correlated CT and PET scan with operative findings in 41 patients with metastatic colorectal cancer.[498] PET scanning was found to be more sensitive for the liver, for the extrahepatic region, and within the abdomen, but results were comparable in the pelvis.

The main disadvantages of PET are the cost and the limited availability. As with radiolabeled imaging, the indications for the use of this modality are limited: an equivocal evaluation or a presumed isolated recurrence. As described previously, the main value of PET seems to be in clarifying the nature of indeterminate lesions on conventional imaging studies and searching for occult disease in patients being considered for resection of metastases. PET may be of particular usefulness in the evaluation of the resectability of a presacral mass of equivocal nature on CT or MRI.[73]

Second-Look Operation (Re-exploration of the Abdomen)

When recurrence of tumor is discovered, surgical resection offers the best possible chance for cure in those patients who have localized disease. Wangensteen first proposed the second-look procedure in the management of colorectal cancer in 1949 in an attempt to increase the cure rate for patients with nodal disease at the time of resection.[1066] Patients were subjected to an exploratory laparotomy 6 months to 1 year after operation. Obviously, this meant that some patients underwent exploration who had no evidence of recurrent disease. Only 15% of Wangensteen's patients actually had recurrence at the time of exploratory laparotomy. For this reason, the second-look concept was abandoned until the advent of the CEA determination. Since the mid-1950s, we have sought less invasive and more sensitive ways of detecting early recurrence.

Minton and associates reoperated 36 patients based on progressive elevation of the CEA determination and found recurrent tumor in 30 of them.[689] The last 11 patients were able to have the tumor removed. They attributed their later improved results to a decrease in the time delay between identification of an appreciable rise in CEA and reoperation.

They recommended serial CEA determination every 2 months, but whether these patients have been cured is another matter. Many studies fail to report 5-year follow-up evaluations after re-resection. Steele and associates reported on 75 patients with Dukes' B and C lesions followed for a median of 24 months.[966] Of 15 individuals found to have a tumor at a second-look operation (based on successive increased elevations of the CEA value), four underwent resection. Tong and colleagues performed a laparotomy on 64 patients with known recurrent disease.[1026] Seventeen percent underwent attempted curative resection; "prolonged" survival was achieved in three. Some reports suggest that second-look surgical procedures appear to be beneficial in selected patients.[243,1065] However, as conventional and functional imaging studies continue to improve, the role for empiric second-look surgery has few indications.

Gamma-Guided Surgery; Radioimmunoguided Surgery

It is axiomatic that accurate assessment of the extent and location of tumor within the abdomen is necessary if one is to perform a truly useful exercise by reoperation. Standard methods of visual examination and palpation at the time of surgery are, of course, supplemented by the information gleaned through the preoperative methods previously discussed. It has been suggested that radioimmunolocalization using labeled monoclonal antibodies potentially may complement the traditional approaches.[31,33,188,227,445,541,638,642,741,891,973,1022]

Technique

One of the monoclonal antibody tumor markers previously discussed, such as anti-CEA labeled with [111]In (^{111}In-MoAb), is injected preoperatively. At the time of laparotomy, a handheld gamma-detecting probe is used to locate foci of malignancy (e.g., C-Trak Galaxy System—Figure 23-95). Depending on the location of the tumor or tumors, an en bloc excision or "tumorectomy" is performed. If one is dealing with lymph nodes that are producing the uptake seen on the imager, the operation may become little more than "cherry picking."

Results

The results of studies with the various gamma-guided alternatives are still preliminary. Whether there will truly be long-term benefits, represented by a decreased incidence of recurrence and a higher cure rate, remains to be determined with longer follow-up. Martin and colleagues used labeled

---

OWEN H. WANGENSTEEN (1899–1981)

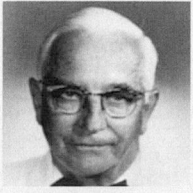

Owen Wangensteen was born on a farm in Lake Park, Minnesota and received all his degrees (AB, MB, MD, and PhD) from the University of Minnesota. In addition, he pursued virtually his entire surgical training there and became chairman of the department of surgery, a post he held for 37 years. His surgical "progeny" included more than 60 professors of surgery or heads of departments. Wangensteen was a great believer in the importance of the laboratory in the training of surgeons. He stated, "The laboratory trains the surgeon's hand while it schools him in the disciplines of observation, thinking and reasoning." Among his many recognitions were the American Medical Association's Distinguished Service Award, the American Cancer Society's Award, and the Samuel D. Gross Award of the Philadelphia Academy of Surgery. His many writings and books cover the spectrum of surgery, including gastric freezing, open heart surgery, the "conservative" management of bowel obstruction, and the "second-look" operation. He was made an honorary fellow of the Royal College of Surgeons of Edinburgh, served as president of the American Surgical Association, and president of the American College of Surgeons.

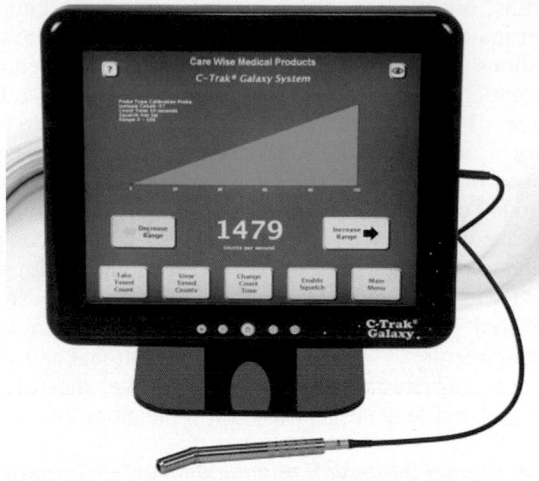

FIGURE 23-95. C-Trak Galaxy System with probe for gamma detection of recurrent tumor. (Courtesy of Care Wise Medical Products Corp., Morgan Hill, CA.)

monoclonal antibody B72.3 in 66 individuals with tissue-proven tumor.[642] Positive probe counts were detected in 83% with primary colon cancer and in 79% with recurrent tumor. The technique failed to identify known tumor in 20%. The authors suggest that improvements in specificity and sensitivity will depend on the availability of higher affinity, newer generation antibodies, alternate routes of antibody administration, other radionuclides, and more sophisticated, bioengineered antibodies and antibody combinations.[642]

Using the same antibody, Cohen and coworkers noted an overall sensitivity of 77% and a predictive value of a positive detection of 78%.[188] They concluded that the antibody study provided unique data that contraindicated resection in 10 individuals (9.6%), and in another 8 (7.7%), it extended the potentially curative procedure. Others have also found that the gamma-guided system is more dependable in localizing clinically inapparent metastases than are other methods.[891] It is stated by the advocates of this technique that the RIGS system has the advantage of providing immediate staging information that may affect therapeutic decision making and upstaging of tumors, even in the initial management of a primary colorectal cancer.[32,629]

Lunniss and associates used RIGS in 40 patients with recurrent colorectal cancer and noted that 25% were "benefited."[598] For the majority of their patients, however, accurate detection of recurrent disease was not associated with the possibility of cure. The authors believed that there is a need for a prospective, randomized trial to confirm the utility of this technique.

In the opinion of all investigators, RIGS is of particular value in the accurate selection of patients with disease deemed potentially resectable at second-look surgery for recurrent colorectal cancer.[31,227,445,522,541,638,741] It has also been successfully applied to patients with recurrent tumor or suspected recurrent tumor who have negative results on intra-abdominal exploration and by all other radiographic criteria for identification of "micrometastases."[246] Finally, in patients who are to be submitted to exploration and resection of liver metastases, the use of the RIGS system may be a valuable adjunct for the detection of periportal lymph node metastases.[899]

Opinion

The problem that one may reasonably have with RIGS is that therapeutic efforts to remove lymph nodes by identification through radiolocalization are not consistent with the concepts of cancer operative technique. In other words, "cherry picking" lymph nodes adds nothing to the survival benefit for an individual with metastatic disease at that focus. This has been discussed previously with respect to apical nodes in the resected specimen. Still, there is value in the technique, particularly with respect to upstaging. The pathologist can identify tumor only within the specimen submitted for examination. The surgeon, conversely, may be able to identify tumor beyond the reach of surgical excision. This obviously might possibly have an influence on subsequent management decisions (e.g., adjuvant therapy). One must weigh the theoretical benefit of changing the classification of the patient's tumor against the additional cost in terms of both equipment and increased operative time.

The philosophical issue of the relative merits of an aggressive follow-up regimen must focus on the unanswerable question, "How much is a human life worth?" A pragmatic, if rhetorical question in response would be, "How much *good medicine* can one afford?" I do not pretend to know the answer to either of these questions. Obviously, cost-effectiveness is inversely correlated with the frequency of screening. As mentioned previously, Moertel and colleagues opined that CEA assay could not be justified in colorectal cancer follow-up.[698] Their rationalization was that the cost of evaluation (including other studies when the CEA was elevated) turned out to be $1,415 per patient, whereas the cost per patient saved was $62,500 and change. Frankly, that may be reasonably considered to be cheap, but we can be even more perspicacious in our testing, and, therefore, we can reduce costs even further.

One can calculate approximately how much it costs to perform annual occult blood determinations to save one life—the Minnesota Group computed it to be $24,660. The same principle obtains for sigmoidoscopy and colonoscopy. Annual sigmoidoscopy starting at age 60 costs about $4,800 per life-year saved (1998 dollars). In a Norwegian follow-up program involving CEA, ultrasound, chest radiography, and colonoscopy, the cost of the program was $3,200 per patient, and the cost per life saved was $26,720.[749] For many years, no one seemed to question the value and cost of annual Papanicolaou testing for cervical cancer; in 1999, Brown and Garber determined that the cost per life saved was $166,000.[121]

It is useful to put the costs of screening for colorectal cancer in proper perspective. To do so requires that one examine the costs and the benefits of other governmental screening and safety programs. There is little question about the value of a mass media antismoking campaign for adolescents. The cost per student exposed has been determined to be $41, the cost per student smoker averted is $754, the cost per life saved is $969, and the cost per year of cigarettes at one pack per day is $1,460 (1997 dollars).[911] One is able to compute the cost per life saved with the use of motorcycle helmets, automobile shoulder harnesses, and air bags. Driver's-side air bags cost $24,000 per life saved, and passenger-side air bags cost $61,000 per life saved (1997 dollars).[364,550] The cost of head injury avoided with the use of bicycle helmets has been determined to be $144,500, and the cost per life saved in primary school children is $100,000; secondary school children, $750,000; and adults, $900,000 (1995 dollars).[412,428] Would anyone not advocate bicycle helmets for children? And what of the cost per human life saved of earthquake retrofitting—who knows?

Some suggest that potentially curative recurrences are detected primarily by liver imaging and colonoscopy.[96] The inference is that the yields of CEA measurements, chest radiography, and physical examination are so low that they should not be part of a routine program. Clearly, there must be some rationale or an algorithm that one can apply to a follow-up protocol for individuals who underwent curative colorectal cancer surgery. The issue of the metachronous lesion and the requirement for all patients to undergo follow-up on that basis alone has been discussed previously. However, there is no point in pursuing further investigations if the physician will do nothing in response to an abnormal test. Therefore, it is only a patient in whom one would perform additional surgery or adjuvant treatment that testing should be performed.

The following regimen is suggested:

- For stage I tumors, no testing for recurrent disease is necessary.
- For stage II and III tumors, CEA determination should be done every 3 months for 2 years. If the test is elevated, repeat the CEA study; if it is still elevated, complete the full workup, including chest x-ray, colonoscopy, CT scan, and PET scan (or antibody scan). If localized (resectable) disease is identified, one should perform a complete medical and preoperative workup and attempt surgical extirpation, having available intraoperative ultrasound for the liver and possibly consider the application of RIGS.

The burden of proof that there is no recurrence once the CEA level remains persistently elevated must rest with the surgeon. Some studies have demonstrated prolonged survival after re-resection with and without objective preoperative evidence of localized or definitive disease.[641,956] However, there appears to be a relative consistency with respect to the salvage rates in those who are identified as having recurrent disease, and that is about 2%.[276,772,860,877,1029] Most cures are in patients with isolated liver metastases. In a study from Sweden in which patients who underwent curative resection for colorectal cancer were randomized either to no follow-up or *intense* follow-up, one-third developed recurrent disease in each group.[759] Three patients in the "no follow-up group" were submitted to re-resection, but none was cured. Conversely, five individuals in the "intense follow-up group" underwent re-resection, and two were cured. Despite the small numbers, these differences were statistically significant.[759] Even more impressive results were described in a study from the University of Parma, Italy.[798] In a randomized trial involving 207 patients who were submitted to either conventional or intensive follow-up, curative re-resection was possible in only 10% of those conventionally followed, but was 65% in those who underwent intensive follow-up. The survival rates were 2.5% and 12.2%, respectively ($P = .0004$). Whether the morbidity, mortality, and cost of a second-look procedure are justified remains unanswered.[748]

▶ TREATMENT OF RECURRENCE

Anastomotic Recurrence

Anastomotic recurrence following resection for colon carcinoma is much less commonly seen than after resection for rectal cancer. It is usually much more feasible to perform an adequate, wide excision of the cancer-bearing segment than when limitations are imposed by the confines of the pelvis.

Symptoms of recurrence include abdominal pain, anorexia, nausea, vomiting, weight loss, change in bowel habits, and rectal bleeding. If a tumor is identified in the bowel, an aggressive surgical attitude should be adopted because the so-called recurrence may, in reality, be a missed synchronous lesion. Excluding this possibility, in contrast to recurrence following rectal resection in which an inadequate lateral or distal margin is often the precipitating factor, anastomotic recurrence that develops after a more proximal bowel resection is usually a result of initial retroperitoneal fixation by that tumor. In one series, the median survival following "curative" re-resection was 23 months.[982] A few patients are actually cured, but this is quite unusual.[896,979,1066] However, surgical alternatives such as re-resection, bypass, and diversion are recommended for palliation whenever possible.

The specific problems of anastomotic recurrence and local recurrence following rectal excision are discussed in Chapter 24.

Pulmonary Metastases

Solitary lung metastases from colorectal cancer have been resected for cure more often than metastases to all other sites combined.[868] Cahan and coworkers reported that in a patient with a history of colorectal carcinoma, a solitary lung lesion will be metastatic from that primary one-half of the time.[149] It still should be remembered, however, that primary lung cancer is the most common visceral malignancy when both sexes are combined. An isolated pulmonary metastasis should not contraindicate radical surgical removal of the bowel tumor. In fact, the chance of a cure is better for resection of a solitary lung lesion that has metastasized from a primary colon carcinoma than when the lesion is a primary bronchogenic carcinoma.

Bronchoscopy, mediastinoscopy, and sputum cytology are useful in identifying the histologic nature of the neoplasm. Lung tomograms are essential to rule out the presence of additional nodules.

In the experience of McCormack and Attiyeh, the 5-year survival rate following excision was 22% and was significantly improved when the primary colonic cancer was a Dukes' A or B lesion.[658] Wilking and colleagues reported a 14% 5-year survival for patients with solitary lesions.[1089] Brister and associates found a 5-year survival of 21%.[118] McCormack and colleagues found that the overall 5- and 10-year survival rates in 144 patients who underwent resection for pulmonary metastases at the Memorial Sloan-Kettering Cancer Center were 40% and 30%, respectively.[659] Watanabe and coworkers noted a 5-year survival rate of 56% in their 49 patients.[1070] Pihl and coworkers noted that lung recurrence is significantly more common after potentially curative resection of rectal than of colonic carcinoma.[799] Scheele and associates, however, noted no difference between colon and rectal primaries in this respect.[894] Several studies have found that the only factor that appears to be significant is the disease-free interval—the longer the interval, the better the survival rate.[118,471,928]

Yano and colleagues investigated whether *multiple pulmonary metastases* from colorectal cancer preclude surgical resection.[1132] The rate of disease-free survival at 5 years was 62% for solitary lesions, 35% for two metastases, and 0% for four or more. Additionally, the incidence of local recurrence at the primary site increased with the number of lesions identified in the lung. The authors concluded that one should search for the presence of a local recurrence at the primary site when multiple pulmonary metastases are identified.[1132]

Wedge resection, preserving as much lung tissue as possible, is usually performed, although resection of the lobe is sometimes necessary to remove the lesion completely.

Ovarian Metastases (See Earlier Discussion)

Liver Metastases

As has been discussed earlier, the overall mean survival of patients with untreated metastatic colorectal cancer to the liver has been approximately 16 months.[779] However, with contemporary adjuvant therapy protocols (see later), this may be too low a figure. Stangl and colleagues prospectively analyzed 566 patients with unresectable hepatic metastases from colorectal cancer who received no treatment.[961] They were able to identify six independent determinants of survival in the following order: percentage of liver volume replaced by tumor, grade of malignancy of the primary tumor, presence of extrahepatic disease, mesenteric lymph node involvement, serum CEA determination, and age. They were able to provide a prognostic tree that displayed median survival times for a number of subgroups of these variables.[961]

The poor prognosis has stimulated a number of approaches that have yielded successful results, including neoadjuvant chemotherapy prior to resection.[10,39,141,145,310,311,463,478,536,588,789,817,997] Fortner and associates estimated that 15% to 25% of individuals with metastatic disease are candidates.[309] Before embarking on such an effort, however, it is imperative to determine the extent of disease and the surgical anatomy. This can be accomplished by several preoperative and intraoperative methods. Radiolabeled imaging, CT, and the gamma-guided approach have already been discussed. It has been estimated that standard CT will detect approximately two-thirds of all tumors (12% of lesions smaller than 1 cm).[1062] The characterization of liver metastases by CT is the single most important independent prognostic factor in patients undergoing curative hepatic resection.[723]

Computed Tomography with Arterial Portography

Although CT is important in the preliminary assessment of an individual who is being evaluated for a rising CEA, particularly with respect to identification of liver metastases, it is not as sensitive as one would wish. Still, with the resolution of modern multidetector helical CT scans, the sensitivity for the detection of liver metastases may approach 90%.[88,691] CT undertaken during arterial portography (CTAP) is the most sensitive preoperative imaging technique for the detection of hepatic metastases from colorectal cancer.[951] Knowledge of the extent of the metastases is important not only in intraoperative decision making, but also in determining which patients are not candidates for a resective approach. Karl and colleagues compared CTAP with conventional CT in 109 consecutive patients who had evidence of hepatic tumors.[508] They, too, observed that CTAP is the most sensitive test for assessing the distribution of intrahepatic disease. Soyer and associates undertook a prospective study to compare the sensitivities of intraoperative ultrasonography (see later) and CTAP.[951] Fifty-one of the 56 metastases were preoperatively identified by means of CTAP (91%), whereas intraoperative ultrasonography identified 54 of the 56 metastases (96%). It is clear, therefore, that the two studies are complementary. Vogel and coworkers attempted to predict the surgical resectability of hepatic colorectal metastases by comparing conventional CT, CTAP, and hepatic artery perfusion scintigraphy.[1062] As previously implied, 64% of

all lesions greater than 1 cm were identified by standard CT. These investigators found that of the 40 patients who had resection for possible cure, CTAP and hepatic artery scintigraphy falsely predicted *unresectability* in 15% and 25% of patients, respectively. The positive predictive value for unresectability of the two studies was 73% and 60%, respectively. The authors concluded that false-positive results by the two evaluations may limit the ability to predict accurately unresectability before surgery and may actually deny patients the chance for surgical resection and cure.[1062]

Matsui and colleagues compared the total detection rate (sensitivity) of liver metastases with a number of modalities and discovered the following: ultrasonography (58% success), CT (63%), selective celiac arteriography (27%), infusion hepatic angiography (50%), and CTAP (84%).[647] Others have also found that CTAP is the most accurate technique for identifying hepatic neoplasms and suggest that it be employed preoperatively for all individuals who are being considered for liver resection.[432,1130] Although certainly not perfect, CT scans have improved to the extent that they are usually the only imaging modality that is necessary preoperatively.

Hepatic Angiography

Liver angiography has been believed to be a useful guide in the preoperative assessment of known hepatic metastatic tumor as well as in the evaluation of vascular anatomy, particularly if a major hepatic resection is contemplated. Lundstedt and coworkers, however, showed that based on the findings at laparotomy, angiography adequately demonstrated tumor growth in the right lobe of the liver but repeatedly failed to do so in the left.[597] CT was believed to be more accurate.

The primary roles of angiography are in the accurate assessment of the sources of blood supply to the liver and of vascular anomalies and as a method of visualizing the conduit for intra-arterial chemotherapy. Again, modern CT scanning with its ability to delineate the hepatic vasculature has made angiography largely unnecessary.

Hepatic Resection

The precise steps in the performance of the various hepatic resection maneuvers are not within the purview of this text. Options include right hepatic lobectomy, right trisegmentectomy, left hepatectomy, left lateral segmentectomy, wedge resection, extended left hepatectomy (left trisegmentectomy), and segmental resections.

Results

Many studies confirm that hepatic resection for colorectal metastatic disease can be undertaken in a number of individuals for cure.[376,435,462,688,833,985] The Mayo Clinic group was among the early advocates of resection and reported 60 patients with hepatic metastases from colorectal cancer.[9,1097] Two-thirds of the lesions were solitary. The results were "unexpectedly favorable." Forty-two percent of the individuals with apparent solitary lesions survived 5 years, although a later report revealed that the overall 5-year survival rate was 25%.[10] Contrary to the earlier observations, this later study justified removal of some multiple hepatic metastases. A later publication from the Mayo Clinic, involving 280 consecutive individuals who underwent hepatic resection for colorectal cancer metastases, revealed an overall 5-year survival of 27%.[482] Rees and associates found that 37% of their patients survived 5 years.[834] Wanebo and coworkers advise that resection of bilobar disease should generally be avoided, especially in medically compromised patients.[1064] Steele and Ravikumar have concluded that major liver resection can be performed safely, with less than a 5% operative mortality, and a cure rate between 20% and 25%.[965]

An early Dukes' stage initially, absence of extrahepatic metastases, and female sex are relatively favorable prognostic findings.[10] In reports from the National Cancer Institute in Bethesda, Maryland, and from other institutions, however, the Dukes' stage of the primary lesion was not predictive of survival after resection.[39,789] Other factors reported to improve the outcome include resection margins of at least 1 cm and fewer than four metastatic nodules.[111,145,377,463,478] Rodgers and McCall note that there are few 5-year survivors after liver resection, with or without lymph node dissection for colorectal hepatic metastases involving the hepatic lymph nodes.[853]

The biologic behavior of the tumor is probably the vital criterion that determines survival, not the timing of the resection or perhaps even the vigor and frequency with which one pursues the CEA level.[39,145] Geoghegan and Scheele undertook a literature review based on a MEDLINE search from 1970 to 1998 on the treatment of colorectal liver metastases.[328] They concluded that with the use of multimodality regimens, 5-year survival rates of patients with lesions that were even *unresectable* are being reported.

Fortner observed a median survival time of 31 months after complete removal of a *second hepatic recurrence*, considerably greater than the median of 14 months when excision was not possible.[308] Others confirm that repeat hepatic resection for isolated metastases can result in long-term survival in selected patients.[3,91,378,1043] Advances in preoperative and postoperative chemotherapy, portal vein embolization, ablative techniques, staged resections, and reoperative surgery are rapidly changing and extending the frontier I and indications for liver resection in the management of colorectal metastases. Because hepatic resection is really the only treatment that can permit long-term survival, many centers will offer resection if all of the disease can be encompassed and sufficient parenchyma left to allow for adequate function, irrespective of size, number, location, and distribution.[691]

Intraoperative Ultrasonography

The area of occult hepatic metastases has been emphasized earlier with respect to the application of intraoperative ultrasonography (see Figure 23-92).[102,160,298,361,617,820] Many centers are recommending its routine use during surgery for colorectal cancer. Charnley and colleagues found that more metastases were diagnosed by intraoperative ultrasonography than by palpation, abdominal ultrasonography, or CT.[168]

Operative ultrasonography has certain advantages that are of particular importance in hepatic surgery: (1) because no energy is lost in passage through the abdominal wall, greater resolution is possible and smaller lesions can be detected; (2) landmarks on the liver parenchyma can be easily correlated with the position of the probe; and (3) ultrasonographic guidance can facilitate biopsy as well as other hepatobiliary procedures.[160] The technique can be used to confirm the presence of tumor in the liver that was suspected based on preoperative evaluation. It can prevent the surgeon from embarking on an ill-advised resection when cure is unattainable (e.g., when multiple lesions are involved). Finally, it can establish the relationship between tumor and intrahepatic vessels, thus possibly preventing vascular injury and perhaps making radical hepatic resection safer.[361]

Rifkin and colleagues evaluated 49 patients with suspected liver disease by means of intraoperative ultrasonography.[848] In 19%, new information was gathered that changed the operative approach. Finlay and McArdle demonstrated unsuspected hepatic metastases in 17 of 24 patients (24%) by this technique.[298] It was their contention that the presence or absence of occult metastases predicts the majority of deaths from disseminated cancer following apparently curative resections. Other articles attest to the better accuracy of intraoperative ultrasonography in diagnosing liver metastases in comparison with other screening methods.[184,618]

Cryosurgery and Radiofrequency Ablation

Intraoperative ultrasonography has been employed not only to identify the location of hepatic metastases, but also to direct the application of treatment, specifically cryotherapy and radiofrequency ablation (RFA). In situ destruction of tumors by means of freezing has been applied to the management of skin, rectal, prostatic, gynecologic, and head and neck cancers, so it is not surprising that some centers have begun to use this approach in the treatment of primary and metastatic lesions of the liver.[820] The cryoprobe, which uses circulating liquid nitrogen and produces a spherical ball of ice around each treated metastatic site, is controlled by the imaging technique.[167] A method has also been described that uses cryosurgery in combination with hepatic resection, in essence excising the ice ball.[803]

Cryodestruction can accomplish a number of possibilities:

- Treat multiple areas of involvement focally.
- Preserve a maximal amount of normal liver tissue.
- Destroy tumors deep in the liver parenchyma without the need for major resection.
- Avoid large vessels or vital structures.
- Minimize blood loss.
- Cause lower morbidity and mortality than resection.
- Combine with other modalities—for example, resection of one lobe and cryosurgical destruction in other areas.[764]

Ravikumar and colleagues used this approach in the treatment of multiple unresectable hepatic metastases from colorectal carcinoma.[820] There were no significant complications. One patient subsequently underwent repeated laparotomy and resection of the frozen lesions; there was no residual tumor. A later report from the same group involved 32 patients, 28% of whom remained disease-free after a follow-up period of 5 to 60 months.[821] Onik and coworkers treated 18 patients with unresectable tumors, 14 of whom had bilobar disease.[765] Mean survival of the 14 cases with recurrence was 21.4 months, with two individuals still living. Adam and coworkers reported their experience with 25 patients who had nonresectable metastases from colorectal cancer.[4] At a mean follow-up of 16 months, the local recurrence rate was 44%. The survival rate was 52% at that time, with 20% free of disease.

Radiofrequency ablation is also used alone or in combination with hepatic resection to achieve complete eradication of disease.[215,518] Resection appears to be preferable when feasible and appropriate because of a lower local recurrence rate.[477] Other ablative techniques and more precise localization technologies continue to be investigated actively.

Osseous Metastases

Osseous metastases from colonic and rectal cancer are relatively uncommon, occurring in up to 9% of reported series.[127]

The usual locations correspond to the areas where there is active hematopoiesis, but involvement of the phalanges has also been described.[127] In the experience of the Memorial Sloan-Kettering Cancer Center, 6.9% of patients with disseminated colorectal carcinoma had osseous metastases.[53,81] Most of these tumors had spread to bone in association with widespread metastases elsewhere. In a study from the Roswell Park Memorial Institute, 19 of 47 patients (40%) had osseous metastases only.[105] The median survival time from establishment of the diagnosis was 7 months.

Bone scanning is believed to be more sensitive for diagnosing metastases than is radiography.[105] Palliative treatment by means of radiation therapy for the bone pain is usually quite effective.

Cerebral Metastases

Metastatic carcinoma to the brain is uncommon and is usually associated with metastatic disease elsewhere, especially in the lung. Rarely will a metastatic focus be present in the brain with no other evidence of disease. Ko and colleagues found that brain metastases are more common with rectal cancer.[529] Craniotomy is indicated to remove the metastatic lesion, with the expectation that good palliation of neurologic signs and symptoms can be accomplished. Nakajima and associates reported on a patient who had removal of a metastatic lesion of the brain; at postmortem examination 2 years later, no evidence of intracranial metastases was found.[726]

Occasionally, a patient will present with neurologic signs and symptoms as the initial manifestation of colorectal cancer. Subsequent gastrointestinal investigation may be stimulated by the histologic interpretation after the intracranial tumor has been removed.

Penile Metastases

Metastatic tumors to the penis are uncommon. More than 80% of them originate in the bladder, prostate, rectum, sigmoid colon, and kidney.[809] Direct invasion, retrograde venous extension, retrograde lymphatic extension, perineural spread, and arterial embolism are proposed mechanisms for the spread.[395,809]

Extent of involvement of the urethra may be determined by urethrography, but cavernosography may be able to give a more precise definition of the size and extent of the nodule or nodules.[395] Surgical excision with or without chemoradiation therapy is the primary treatment. Prognosis for long-term survival is poor.

Chemotherapy

In light of the extraordinarily rapid changes in the chemotherapeutic approaches to the management of colorectal cancer, I have asked Herbert M. Dean, a board-certified hematologist and medical oncologist, Assistant Professor of Medicine at the University of Massachusetts Medical School, to provide this completely rewritten and contemporary perspective. MLC

Major advances in the treatment of colorectal cancer have occurred through the combination of two chemotherapeutic agents, either irinotecan or oxaliplatin, to 5-fluorouracil (FU)/leucovorin (LV), or its oral substitute, capecitabine.

In addition, biologic response modifiers are being used, which unlike conventional chemotherapeutic agents that act as cellular poisons and effect DNA synthesis and growth of cancer cells, have different mechanisms of action. These include interference with membrane receptors, alteration of signal pathways necessary for tumor growth, and inhibition of tumor-supported angiogenesis to promote cancer cell death. Two have demonstrated efficacy in phase III clinical trials, cetuximab and bevacizumab (BV), and have been introduced into clinical practice.[72,213,466,867,1045] This section reviews advances in the adjuvant treatment of stage III metastatic colorectal cancer.

Studies have identified effectiveness of the drugs cited earlier, resulting in the incorporation of these drugs in combination with FU/LV (so-called triplets). This has given rise to a new nomenclature—IFL (FU/LV and irinotecan), FOLFOX (FU/LV and oxaliplatin), CAPOX, and FOLFIRI, which have become the standard for treating patients with metastatic disease. Furthermore, these new agents in a variety of combinations have been evaluated in the adjuvant and in the neoadjuvant settings, together with radiation for colorectal cancers that present with advanced local stage (large tumors, those adherent to adjacent structures), in order to shrink and downstage the malignancy and, therefore, to increase the likelihood of surgical resection.[22,258,885,995] Even in the setting of unresectable metastatic disease, neoadjuvant chemotherapy with FOLFOX, FOLFOX/cetuximab or FOLFIRI, FOLFIRI/cetuximab has produced response rates of 36% to 50%, with up to 10% able to go on to surgery and up to 2.5% to 5% achieving resections with no residual disease (R0).[99,1044]

5-Fluorouracil/Leucovorin

Since the 1950s, intravenous FU, biomodulated with LV, has been the most effective of all the chemotherapeutic regimens employed in treating colon cancer, both in the metastatic or advanced disease setting and as adjuvant chemotherapy.[652,697] In an attempt to improve the results, the FU/LV regimen has been administered in various dose schedules, including the Mayo Clinic regimen developed by Moertel and colleagues.[807] This involves the intravenous administration of FU/LV daily for 5 days as a bolus at 425 mg/m^2 along with LV at 20 mg/m^2 for 5 days each 4-week cycle; or on a weekly schedule at doses of between 600 and 750 mg/m^2 along with LV at doses between 20 mg/m^2 (low dose) up to using 500 mg/m^2 (high dose) weekly for six cycles every 8 weeks; or as infusional FU, usually at 300 mg/m^2 per 24-hour period for several days up to 20 days depending on toxicity.[139,590,704,807] The use of intraperitoneal chemotherapy has not been shown to prolong survival and is considered investigational.[635]

Bolus FU has been more commonly used for simplicity and the avoidance of a catheter, usually a requisite in infusional FU schedules. Comparable median survival data are reported with infusional FU, although there are generally higher response rates. Different toxicities are seen with the bolus programs, including bone marrow suppression with neutropenia and thrombocytopenia, along with mucositis, nausea, vomiting, and diarrhea. The hand-foot syndrome is the main side effect seen with prolonged infusional treatment.

In stage III colon cancer, FU/LV administered as adjuvant chemotherapy (after surgery) has demonstrated improved disease-free and overall survival, but in the metastatic setting, results have generally been disappointing—that is, only slight improvement in survival when compared with optimal supportive care.[554,619,704] A meta-analysis of

18 randomized studies of metastatic colon cancer, using the combination of FU/LV versus FU alone, demonstrated a doubling of the response rate from 11% to 23% with the "doublet" but no difference in the median survival (11.5 vs. 11 months).[797] A small, statistically significant increase in the 1-year survival of 48% versus 43% was noted. A European study compared the Mayo Clinic schedule with that which is commonly referred to as the de Gramont schedule.[237] This latter protocol consisted of bimonthly intravenous LV, 200 mg/m^2, as a 2-hour infusion, followed by bolus FU, 400 mg/m^2; then a 22-hour infusion of FU at 600 mg/m^2 was given for 2 consecutive days every 2 weeks until disease progression demonstrated a statistically significant improvement in response rate. The de Gramont schedule, combining infusional and bolus FU, had a response rate of 33% versus only a 14% response with the bolus arm alone. A progression-free interval of 28 versus 22 weeks was noted, but there was no significant survival benefit (62 vs. 57 weeks).[237]

Irinotecan (Camptosar)

Based on the results of a randomized, multicenter, three-arm trial, IFL, consisting of irinotecan and FU/LV (Saltz regimen), was approved as first-line treatment for metastatic colon cancer in March 2000. Six hundred eighty-three patients were randomized to irinotecan, 125 mg/m^2 weekly for 4 weeks every 6 weeks; FU/LV administered by the Mayo schedule (control arm); or irinotecan as administered as a single agent combined with weekly FU, 500 mg/m^2 for 4 weeks every 6 weeks. The control arm (FU/LV) showed a response rate, time to progression, and overall survival of 21%, 4.2 months, and 12 months, respectively, essentially the same as that of the single agent, irinotecan. With IFL, the response rate was 39%, the time to progression was 7 months, and the overall survival was 14.4 months.[885] A European study of 387 patients compared FU/LV with IFL, employing the de Gramont schedule of FU/LV and irinotecan, either 80 mg/m^2 for 6 weeks every 7 weeks or 180 mg/m^2 day 1 every 2 weeks. This showed similar results to the Saltz study, with a response rate, time to progression, and median survival in the FU/LV arm of 23%, 4.4 months, and 14 months, respectively, with 59% alive at 1 year. The IFL arm demonstrated a 41% response rate, a time to progression of 6.7 months, and a median survival of 16.8 months, with 69% alive at 1 year.[258]

Toxicity with irinotecan includes both an acute and delayed diarrhea that can cause significant fluid loss. This is associated with an increased 60-day mortality rate, a fact that led to a manufacturer's alert and increased efforts to control the diarrhea with anticholinergic drugs during and after the administration of the agent. Close monitoring of fluids and electrolytes is a requisite.[862] The FDA has recommended testing for the UGT1A1 mutation (the same one that accounts for the elevation of bilirubin in Gilbert's syndrome) in order to identify patients who experience increased toxicity with this agent.

Oxaliplatin (Eloxatin)

Unlike other platinum compounds, oxaliplatin demonstrates activity in human tumor xenografts and in cisplatinum and carboplatin-resistant colon cancer cell lines.[828] de Gramont compared FU/LV, the control arm using the de Gramont schedule, versus the addition of oxaliplatin, 85 mg/m^2, given 1 day every 2 weeks (FOLFOX). The response rate was 49% compared with 22% for the control arm. Progression-free survival was 8.9 versus 5.9 months, and median survival was 15.9 months compared with 14.7 months.[238]

An intergroup study was undertaken that ultimately became a three-arm trial: IFL, FOLFOX, and irinotecan combined with oxaliplatin (IROX). The following were the results of that effort[346,1088] (Table 23-8).

The interpretation of the results is impacted by the crossover design that led to 60% of patients who were on the FOLFOX arm to subsequently receive irinotecan because of disease progression. However, only 24% of patients who received IFL received oxaliplatin because that agent had not yet been approved for second-line treatment in the United States. Although FOLFOX appeared to be a superior regimen to IFL and IROX for first-line treatment of metastatic disease and is less toxic, except for peripheral neuropathy, differences with respect to those who received second-line treatment in the IFL arm with the crossover drug create difficulty in the interpretation of the results.

Oxaliplatin is associated with neurosensory side effects, including acute dysesthesia that occurs in up to 80% of patients, with numbness and tingling of the distal extremities. This is usually mild and brief and aggravated by cold, including chilled beverages. Oral and perioral pharyngolaryngeal tingling occurs in fewer than 2% of patients, but this can be quite distressing. Chronic sensory neuropathy that is dose related can cause grade 3 or 4 toxicity when doses greater than 850 mg/m^2 are administered. This generally improves

TABLE 23-8 Results of Intergroup N9741 Trial of First-line IFL versus FOLFOX versus IROX

	IFL	IROX	FOLFOX
Response rates	31%	34%	45%
Medium time to progression (mo)	6.9	6.5	8.7
Overall survival (mo)	14.8	17.4	19.5

	GRADE III TOXICITY (%)		
	IFL	IROX	FOLFOX
Neutropenia	40	36	50
Febrile neutropenia	15	11	4
Nausea	16	19	6
Vomiting	14	22	3
Diarrhea	28	24	12
Paresthesia	3	7	18

FOLFOX, 5-fluorouracil, leucovorin, and oxaliplatin; IFL, irinotecan, 5-fluorouracil, and leucovorin; IROX, irinotecan and oxaliplatin.

over several months with discontinuance of the drug, but in some cases, residual chronic peripheral neuropathy may persist indefinitely to varying degrees.[346,1088]

Capecitabine (Xeloda)

FU/LV given in various schedules often requires the placement of an indwelling, long-term, intravenous access catheter, with frequent office visits for treatment and for catheter care as well as complications related to the device.[48,180,416,818,977,1127] Oral fluoropyrimidine, capecitabine (Xeloda), undergoes a three-step conversion to FU and can achieve blood levels and efficacy comparable to that obtained with infusional chemotherapy while offering greater patient convenience and a more acceptable side effect profile.[564] The main toxicity is the hand-foot syndrome, the same as seen with infusional FU. However, the frequency of this side effect has greatly diminished because the initial recommended dose of 2,500 mg/m^2 in two divided daily doses has been reduced to 2,000 mg/m^2.

A trial of combined capecitabine, 1,000 mg/m^2 twice daily for 14 days, followed by 7 days off, combined with oxaliplatin, 130 mg/m^2, as a 2-hour infusion on day 1 at 3-week intervals, achieved in a trial of 96 patients a response rate of 45%, progression-free survival of 7.6 months, and an overall survival of 19.5 months.[1046] Grade 3 toxicities included neutropenia in 7%, nausea and vomiting in 13%, diarrhea in 16%, and neuropathy in 16%.

Bevacizumab (Avastin)

Since the pioneering work of Judah Folkman, which demonstrated that tumor growth requires the cancer to induce the host to provide new blood vessels (angiogenesis) by means of chemical mediators secreted by the tumor, efforts to develop antiangiogenesis agents have been sought to inhibit new blood vessel formation and tumor growth.[294,481] Tumor angiogenesis can be assessed noninvasively by measuring angiogenic cytokine concentrations in peripheral circulation and by dynamic contrast-enhanced MRI.[327] Bevacizumab is a humanized monoclonal antibody developed against vascular endothelial growth factor.[369] A trial involving 815 patients comparing IFL/placebo with IFL/bevacizumab (BV) as first-line therapy in metastatic colorectal cancer demonstrated in the BV arm a response rate of 45% versus a 35% response in the IFL, progression free survival of 10.6 months versus 6.3 months, and a median survival of 20.3 months versus 15.6 months.[466] Grade III hypertension was noted in 10.9% of those in the BV arm versus 2.3% in the IFL arm. Another study comparing the addition of bevacizumab to FOLFOX4 or XELOX showed an improvement in progression-free survival (9 months vs. 8 months), but no improvement in overall survival (21.3 months vs. 19.4 months) or response rate (47% vs. 49%).[883]

Cetuximab (Erbitux)

Cetuximab was FDA approved in 2004 for the treatment of epidermal growth factor receptor (EGFR)-expressing metastatic colorectal cancer alone or in combination with irinotecan in patients no longer responsive to oxaliplatin-based chemotherapy. Cetuximab is a chimeric monoclonal antibody to the EGFR. By attaching to the receptor on the cancer cell, this drug inhibits the binding and signal activity of epidermal growth factor and is synergistic with chemotherapy and radiation.[756] A trial in irinotecan-refractory, EGFR-positive patients with metastatic colorectal disease compared cetuximab alone versus cetuximab combined with irinotecan.[212] Cetuximab was given at an initial dose of 400 mg/m^2, intravenously, followed by 250 mg/m^2 weekly, and combined with irinotecan at the same dose the patient was on while the disease had progressed. A partial response was seen in 11% on cetuximab alone, and 23% in the combined arm. Time to progression was noted to be 1.5 and 4.1 months, respectively, and overall survival was 6.9 versus 9.4 months.

Another EGFR inhibitor, panitumumab (Vectibix), was approved as second-line treatment for metastatic colorectal cancer. Both agents manifest unique skin side effects, including rash, hives, and, in severe cases, desquamation with some suggestion that those who exhibit these findings are more likely to achieve clinical benefit.[692] Clinical benefit with either of the currently approved EGFR inhibitors is guided by the presence of the KRAS oncogene, present in 40% of colorectal cancers, with tumors expressing the wild type having a higher likelihood of response than those who harbor the mutated KRAS gene.[940]

COX-2 Inhibitors

Epidemiologic studies have suggested that aspirin and cyclo-oxygenase-2 (COX-2) inhibitors reduce the risk of polyps, colon cancer, and mortality, and COX-2 inhibitors and aspirin have demonstrated activity in reducing polyp formation in patients with familial adenomatous polyps.[373,983] A study of 47,900 male health care professionals showed that those taking at least two aspirin tablets per week over 20 years reduced their risk of cancer by 50%.[338]

COX-2 expression demonstrated by immunochemistry has been shown to be present in colorectal carcinomas, with greater staining noted in larger tumors and in those with advanced stage (e.g., nodal involvement).[924] This observation supports a possible therapeutic role for COX-2 inhibitors. Trials have incorporated the COX-2 inhibitors previously described in both the adjuvant and metastatics.[707,910]

New Directions

Further attempts to improve the results with chemotherapy and biologic response modifiers have led to additional trials using various combinations of agents. These include sequencing or combining FOLFOX and FOLFIRI and additional trials that incorporate EGFR inhibitors, BV, and COX-2 inhibitors with the various doublets and triplets as well as substituting capecitabine for FU/LV.[21,369,898,1030,1038,1046] Combining two of the therapies that are target-directed, bevacizumab and cetuximab, together with irinotecan in the BOND-2 trial in patients not previously exposed to either of the two agents, demonstrated modest improvement in response rate, time to progression, and overall survival without overlapping toxicities.[884] Other attempts to combine a vascular endothelial growth factor (VEGF) inhibitor along with an EGFR agent in first-line setting of metastatic disease have generally been disappointing in improving disease-free or overall survival.[651,1025]

Many other chemotherapeutic agents too numerous to include and various biologic modifiers, including tyrosine kinase inhibitors, have been tested with disappointing results, such as gefitinib (Iressa), erlotinib (Tarceva), and sunitinib (Sutent).

Adjuvant Chemotherapy

The TNM classification system for colon cancer has replaced the Dukes' classification and its modification, Astler-Coller, for oncologists, especially. Published series have reported a range of survival in Dukes' C patients from 44% to 70%, and in Dukes' B, 58% to 88%.[273] Dukes' classification fails to distinguish the differences in prognosis and risk for metastatic disease stratified according to the number of involved nodes, nor does it take into account the size of the primary tumor. The TNM classification improves one's ability to predict the course and survival more accurately because it stratifies stage by tumor penetration and size as well as the number of involved nodes.

The latest revision of the seventh edition of the American Joint Committee on Cancer's staging manual includes several modifications.[273] Stage II is now subdivided into IIA if the primary tumor is T3 and into IIB or IIC for T4 lesions. Stage III is now split into IIIA, IIIB, or IIIC based both on tumor and nodal characteristics. The surgeon is asked to define the completeness of his resection as follows: R0 for complete resection and negative margins, R1 for incomplete resection because of a positive microscopic margin, or R2 with nonresected gross residual tumor.[375] Pathology reports have been expanded and standardized over recent years to increase precision and uniformity of both reporting and specimen handling. Further, they include potential quality measures, such as radial margins and the adequacy of mesorectal dissection in the case of rectal cancer, highlighting the need for surgeons and pathologists to work together to achieve optimal results.

Adjuvant chemotherapy for stage III colorectal cancer as previously discussed has been shown to be effective in overall survival, initially using FU/LV regimens with the doublet and triplet combinations.[704,753,754] Stage II patients who exhibit some unfavorable pathologic characteristics such as lymphovascular invasion, circumferential obstructing lesions, and perforation are also felt to benefit from adjuvant chemotherapy.[699] Radiation treatment, preoperatively or after surgery, should be considered along with chemotherapy for lesions adherent to adjacent structures, in those with perforation, and especially in T3 and T4 lesions of the rectum and lower sigmoid (see Chapter 24).[687,1011]

Several adjuvant trials for colorectal cancer have been cited comparing the newer regimens to FU/LV, including the Mosaic trial of FU/LV compared with FOLFOX. This demonstrated an overall risk reduction of 23% with the FOLFOX regimen.[236] The FOLFOX regimen has generally been employed as the treatment of choice for adjuvant chemotherapy, although certain patients, such as those with preexisting neuropathies, including diabetics should be considered for FOLFIRI.[20] Attempts to further improve outcome by the addition of some of the newer agents in an attempt to improve results have been disappointing. Adding bevacizumab to FOLFOX or XELOX as adjuvant treatment of stage III colorectal cancer did not improve disease-free or overall survival at a median follow-up of 4 years.[239] However, another adjuvant study from the Mayo Clinic with a limited number of patients *did* show a significant improved disease-free and overall survival by combining cetuximab with FOLFIRI versus FOLFIRI alone. This included some patients with mutated *KRAS*.[458]

Summary and Conclusions

Chemotherapy in both the metastatic setting and as adjuvant treatment has shown modest improvement in response rates, time to progression, and overall survival with FU/LV. The addition of either irinotecan or oxaliplatin and the ability to administer an oral fluoropyrimidine, capecitabine, comparable to FU/LV, providing a more convenient outpatient program for patients, has led to at least a 50% increase in response rates, time to progression, and doubling in overall survival in the metastatic setting and improved survival in adjuvant treatment of stage III cancer. Oxaliplatin combinations (FOLFOX) may have a better side effect profile than IFL.

The era of personalized medicine has been trumpeted since the entire human genome was determined in 2003. Certain information such as the presence of the *KRAS* mutation distinguishes patients more likely to respond to EGFR inhibitors, and in the field of pharmacogenetics, the ability to predict the UGT1A1 mutation identifies those for whom irinotecan may cause lethal toxicities. Attempts to use genetic information that will lead to new drug development, identification of new targets for treatment, and improvement in selecting agents to treat cancer with the appropriate therapeutic agent have proven disappointing. The complexity of tumorigenesis within malignancies is caused by multiple mutational cellular events in most cases (up to 80 in colorectal cancer) that unfold even as therapy proceeds.

Author's Comment

It is self-evident that despite the high rate of resectability and the improvement in the surgical management of patients with colorectal cancer, almost one-half die of recurrent disease. Although chemotherapeutic agents have doubled survival duration with the newer agents, the diagnosis of metastatic disease, except in certain clinical presentations (liver metastases or isolated spread), is not curable. Chemotherapy has been ineffectual in the treatment of peritoneal seeding.[120]

In addition to long-term survival or even cure, tumor response, defined as clinical or radiologic tumor shrinkage, is the primary objective of chemotherapy. Allen-Mersh and colleagues assessed whether a fall in the serum CEA concentration after chemotherapy is a predictor of prolonged survival and compared it with "tumor response."[16] They observed that monitoring the serum CEA, especially during the first 2 months of treatment, appears to provide a sensitive and economical means for identifying those individuals whose survival is likely to be prolonged by the treatment.[16] Others have shown that FU-based adjuvant chemotherapy benefited patients with stage II or stage III colon cancers with microsatellite-stable tumors or tumors exhibiting low-frequency microsatellite instability, but not those with tumors exhibiting high-frequency microsatellite instability.[845]

One must remember that chemotherapy is not innocuous. The potential complications are myriad, a partial list of which includes bone marrow depression, alopecia, sepsis, renal and hepatic toxicity, gastrointestinal hemorrhage, mutagenesis, typhlitis, and bowel wall necrosis.[512] Obviously, the toxicity and expense of chemotherapy must be weighed against the potential benefits. Drug resistance is the principal reason why chemotherapy often fails. However, as one may appreciate from Dean's contribution, patients today no longer have limited treatment options. Furthermore, one even has the possibility of identifying drug resistance through an in vitro test, the tumor stem cell assay (clonogenic chemosensitivity test—Oncotech, Tustin, CA—http://www.oncotech.com).[881,915] Although surgery has been and continues to be the mainstay in the treatment of colorectal cancer, it is exciting to contemplate the day when this cancer and all cancers may be either prevented or completely eliminated without the need for operation.

Hepatic Artery Infusion, Ligation, Dearterialization; Portal Vein Infusion

Hepatic artery infusion is sometimes recommended for the treatment of metastatic disease to the liver that is unresectable. In the opinion of some authors, it produces higher regression rates and slightly longer remissions than other techniques.[147,514] However, these advantages are at the cost of increased morbidity, time in the hospital, and technical difficulties, which may make this route less than desirable. Because of the risk for inducing chemical cholecystitis by this approach, some authors recommend elective cholecystectomy at the time of the placement of the arterial catheter.[770]

Usually, hepatic artery infusion is applied to those individuals who have failed to show improvement with more conventional systemic techniques. Miyanari and colleagues assessed the value of hepatic arterial infusion chemotherapy, noting that it was possible to perform resection of metastatic liver disease in those who responded.[696] The survival rate for all patients was about two-thirds after 1 year and 10% after 5 years. Of the 25% who responded (16 of 64 patients), however, 35.1% were alive after 5 years.

Hepatic artery ligation and hepatic dearterialization also have been employed, but similarly have not been shown to produce worthwhile benefit either in terms of palliation or survival.[910] Portal vein infusion has also been performed, with mixed results.[61] Allen-Mersh and colleagues employed continuous hepatic artery infusion with floxuridine in a randomized study of 100 patients, who were compared with patients receiving conventional palliation only.[15] A significant prolongation of survival was noted in the former group, as well as a qualitative and quantitative improvement in a host of other variables.

Newer modalities to treat hepatic metastases from colorectal cancer, either at presentation or that developed subsequent to treatment, include thermal ablation, infusional chemotherapy, and radioactive ^{90}Y embedded spheres. The primary thermal modalities use RFA, microwave, and cryoablation techniques. Transarterial chemoembolization (TACE) uses chemotherapeutic agents such as cisplatin, doxorubicin (Doxil), and mitomycin C, all through the use of hepatic artery perfusion. These agents may also be incorporated into drug-eluting spheres.

These therapies are effective in causing tumor shrinkage and increasing progression-free survival while also providing effective palliation. In some cases, significant tumor regression to complete response can be seen. This may allow surgical resection in what had previously been considered an inoperable condition.

Immunotherapy

Chemotherapeutic agents, especially FU, have been used in combination with other modalities of treatment, such as surgery, radiation, and immunotherapy. The value of chemoimmunotherapy has been studied, and in reports from the MD Anderson Hospital and the Southwest Oncology Group, FU plus bacille Calmette-Guérin (BCG) has been shown to produce a longer disease-free period with increased survival in some patients.[47,393] These studies have not yet been confirmed by randomized, controlled trials from other institutions.

Immunotherapy with BCG is most effective when the tumor mass is reduced to a minimum, when it is administered directly into or close to the tumor, when the patient is able to respond to BCG, and when a large enough dose is given. Routes of administration include direct insertion into the tumor; administration may also be intradermal (by skin scarification), intracavitary, or oral.[439,615]

Although the number of patients with reported colorectal cancer for whom BCG immunotherapy has been used is still small, this regimen has occasionally produced increased survival, most striking in those individuals with liver metastases. Mavligit and coworkers reported on 83 patients with Dukes' C colorectal carcinoma who received postoperative BCG alone or in combination with orally administered FU.[648] The BCG was administered by the scarification method at weekly intervals. Patients were followed for as long as 30 months, with an appreciable prolongation of both disease-free interval and overall survival. The conclusion of these observers is that adjuvant immunotherapy without chemotherapy improves the prognosis of patients with surgically treated Dukes' C colorectal carcinoma. Wolmark and colleagues compared patients who received postoperative BCG with controls and with patients given chemotherapy (FU, semustine, and vincristine) in a randomized trial involving individuals with Dukes' B and C colon cancer.[1117] The authors found no significant difference in survival advantage with the use of BCG.

Another study employed adjuvant immunochemotherapy with PSKR, an immunomodulator comprising a protein-bound polysaccharide extracted from mycelia of *Coriolus versicolor*.[198] The PSKR group received this agent orally over 3 years, in addition to mitomycin C and FU. The median follow-up time was 4 years. When the PSKR patients were compared with the control group (chemotherapy alone), a statistically significant improvement was noted in the disease-free survival curve.

Immunotherapy with agents such as interferon alfa-2a, monoclonal antibody 17–1, and autologous tumor vaccines is also under investigation, and preliminary results suggest improved survival.[159] The German Cancer Aid 17–1A study group designed a protocol in which a monoclonal antibody (17–1A) was used to target minimal residual disease (i.e., Dukes' C patients).[847] Patients were randomly assigned to an observation regimen or to postoperative treatment with this antibody, infused each month. Antibody treatment reduced the overall death rate by 30% and decreased the recurrence rate by 27%.[847]

Gene Therapy

Note: the following information is abstracted from the United States Office of Biological and Environmental Research, Human Genome Program.

Gene therapy is a research technique for correcting defective genes responsible for causing diseases. Investigators may use several approaches for accomplishing this:

- A normal gene may be inserted into a nonspecific location within the genome to replace a nonfunctional gene.
- An abnormal gene may be swapped for a normal gene through homologous recombination.
- The abnormal gene may be repaired through selective reverse mutation, which returns the gene to its normal function.
- The regulation (the degree to which a gene is turned on or off) of a particular gene may be altered.

In most gene therapy studies, a "normal" gene is inserted into the genome to replace an "abnormal," disease-causing gene. A carrier molecule, called a vector, must be used to deliver the therapeutic gene to the patient's target cells. Currently, the most common vector is a virus that has been genetically altered to carry normal human DNA. Viruses have evolved a method of encapsulating and delivering their genes to human cells in a pathogenic manner. Target cells, such as the patient's liver, are infected with the viral vector. The vector then unloads its genetic material containing the therapeutic human gene into the target cell. The generation of a functional protein product from the therapeutic gene restores the target cell to a normal state. Some of the different types of viruses used as gene therapy vectors are the following:

- Retroviruses: A class of viruses that can create double-stranded DNA copies of their RNA genomes. These copies of its genome can be integrated into the chromosomes of host cells. Human immunodeficiency virus is a retrovirus.
- Adenoviruses: A class of viruses with double-stranded DNA genomes that cause respiratory, intestinal, and eye infections in humans. The virus that causes the common cold is an adenovirus.
- Adeno-associated viruses: A class of small, single-stranded DNA viruses that can insert their genetic material at a specific site on chromosome 19.
- Herpes simplex viruses: A class of double-stranded DNA viruses that infect neurons.

Besides virus-mediated gene-delivery systems, there are several nonviral options for gene delivery. The simplest method is the direct introduction of therapeutic DNA into target cells. This approach is limited in its application because it can be used only with certain tissues and requires large amounts of DNA. Another nonviral approach involves the creation of an artificial lipid sphere with an aqueous core. This liposome, which carries the therapeutic DNA, is capable of passing the DNA through the target cell's membrane.

Therapeutic DNA also can get inside target cells by chemically linking the DNA to a molecule that will bind to special cell receptors. Once bound to these receptors, the therapeutic DNA constructs are engulfed by the cell membrane and passed into the interior of the target cell. This delivery system tends to be less effective than other options.

Sheen and coworkers applied gene therapy principles through the use of patient-derived T lymphocytes to target and eradicate hepatic metastases.[925] The T lymphocytes that had been isolated preoperatively were modified genetically with recombinant retroviruses and tested for functional activity against freshly isolated harvested autologous tumor cells. The potential for this approach to therapy was believed to be encouraging.

Radiotherapy

Radiotherapy has been applied primarily in the treatment of rectal cancer (see Chapter 24). However, conventional external radiation therapy should still be considered when macroscopic tumor remains or when fixity of the lesion precludes complete excision. Usually, 45 to 60 Gy (4,500 to 6,000 rad) is administered over a period of 5 to 6 weeks. There is evidence to suggest that this reduces the likelihood of local recurrence and improves survival rates.[269]

Gunderson and associates reported the administration of radiation therapy for colon carcinoma by an intraoperative technique.[392] For treatment of inoperable, residual, or recurrent cancer, doses in excess of 60 Gy (6,000 rad) were given by this means at the time of laparotomy. This required transporting the patient, while anesthetized and with the abdomen open, to a different area of the hospital for radiation therapy. The authors postulated that if this technique proved feasible, it could be possible to ablate the tumor by radiation therapy, a result that could not be expected with a lower dose, externally applied method. Other institutions are employing this approach and have designed operating room suites to accommodate the requisite radiation therapy equipment.[423] Results of further experience are awaited.

When FU is combined with radiation therapy, a modest improvement takes place in length of remission and survival compared with survival after radiation therapy alone in patients with local, inoperable, or recurrent disease.

Holt and colleagues have used intraoperative interstitial radiation therapy in the treatment of hepatic metastases from colorectal carcinomas.[449] It is premature to assess the results of this concept.

Comment

In reviewing the experience with colon carcinoma since the 1960s, it is evident that no significant improvements in operative mortality and cure rate have taken place. It appears, then, that surgery has accomplished all it possibly can for this condition. Any further improvement in survival rates will depend on bringing patients to operation earlier and on the effectiveness of other modalities of therapy.

References

1. Abrams JS. Elective resection for colorectal cancer in Vermont: 1971–1975. *Am J Surg*. 1980;139:78.
2. Abrams JS, Anton JR, Dreyfuss DC. The absence of a relationship between cholecystectomy and the subsequent occurrence of cancer of the proximal colon. *Dis Colon Rectum*. 1983;26:141.
3. Abusamra H, Maximova S, Bar-Meir S, et al. Cancer family syndrome of Lynch. *Am J Med*. 1987;83:981.
4. Adam R, Akpinar E, Johann M, et al. Place of cryosurgery in the treatment of malignant liver tumors. *Ann Surg*. 1997;225:39.
5. Adam R, Bismuth H, Castaing D, et al. Repeat hepatectomy for colorectal liver metastases. *Ann Surg*. 1997;225:51.
6. Adami HO, Krusemo UB, Meirik O. Unaltered risk of colorectal cancer within 14–17 years of cholecystectomy: updating of a population-based cohort study. *Br J Surg*. 1987;74:675.
7. Adler DG, Young-Fadok TM, Smyrk T, et al. Preoperative chemoradiation therapy after placement of a self-expanding metal stent in a patient with an obstructing rectal cancer: clinical and pathologic findings. *Gastrointest Endosc*. 2002;55:435.
8. Adloff M, Arnaud JP, Schloegel M, et al. Colorectal cancer in patients under 40 years of age. *Dis Colon Rectum*. 1986;29:322.
9. Adson MA, van Heerden JA. Major hepatic resections for metastatic colorectal cancer. *Ann Surg*. 1980;191:576.
10. Adson MA, van Heerden JA, Adson MH, et al. Resection of hepatic metastases from colorectal cancer. *Arch Surg*. 1984;119:647.
11. Agarwal N, Cayten CG, Ulahannan MJ, et al. Increased risk of colorectal cancer following breast cancer. *Ann Surg*. 1986;203:307.
12. Ahlquist DA, Skoletsky JE, Boynton KA, et al. Colorectal cancer screening by detection of altered human DNA in stool: feasibility of a multitarget assay panel. *Gastroenterology*. 2000;119:1219.
13. Ahnen DJ. Genetics of colon cancer. *West J Med*. 1991;154:700.
14. Alberts DS, Martínez ME, Roe DJ, et al. Lack of effect of a high-fiber cereal supplement on the recurrence of colorectal adenomas. Phoenix Colon Cancer Prevention Physicians' Network. *N Engl J Med*. 2000;342:1156.
15. Allen-Mersh TG, Earlam S, Fordy C, et al. Quality of life and survival with continuous hepatic-artery floxuridine infusion for colorectal liver metastases. *Lancet*. 1994;344:1255.
16. Allen-Mersh TG, Kemeny N, Niedzwiecki D, et al. Significance of a fall in serum CEA concentration in patients treated with cytotoxic chemotherapy for disseminated colorectal cancer. *Gut*. 1987;28:1625.

17. Allis OH. Intestinal anastomosis with suturing of the entire thickness of the intestinal wall. *Am J Obstet*. 1902;60.

18. Allison JE, Feldman R. Cost benefits of hemoccult screening for colorectal carcinoma. *Dig Dis Sci*. 1985;30:860.

19. Amsterdam E, Krispin M. Primary resection with colocolostomy for obstructive carcinoma of the left side of the colon. *Am J Surg*. 1985;150:558.

20. Andre T, Boni C, Mounedju-Boudiiaf L, et al. Oxaliplatin, fluorouracil and leucovorin as adjuvant treatment for colon cancer. *N Eng J Med*. 2004;350:2343.

21. Andre T, Figer A, Cervantes A, et al. FOLFOX7 compared to FOLFOX4: preliminary results of the randomized optimox study [abstract]. *Proc ASCO*. 2003;22.

22. Andre T, Louvet C, Raymond E, et al. Bimonthly high-dose leucovorin, 5-fluorouracil 48 hour infusion and oxaliplatin (FOLFOX) for metastatic colorectal cancer resistant to the same LV-5FU regimen. *Ann Oncol*. 1998;9:1251.

23. Androsov PI. Experience in the application of instrumental suture in surgery of the stomach and rectum. *Acta Chir Scand*. 1970;136:57.

24. Angelelli G, Stabile Ianora AA, Scardapane A, et al. Role of computerized tomography in the staging of gastrointestinal neoplasm's. *Semin Surg Oncol*. 2001;20:109.

25. Anthony T, Simmang C, Hyman N, et al; Standards Practice Task Force, The American Society of Colon and Rectal Surgeons. Practice parameters for the surveillance and follow-up of patients with colon and rectal cancer. *Dis Colon Rectum*. 2004;47:807.

26. Aries V, Crowther JS, Drasar BS, et al. Bacteria and the aetiology of cancer of the large bowel. *Gut*. 1969;10:334.

27. Armitage NC, Robins RA, Evans DF, et al. The influence of tumour cell DNA abnormalities on survival in colorectal cancer. *Br J Surg*. 1985;72:828.

28. Armstrong B, Doll R. Environmental factors and cancer incidence and mortality in different countries, with special reference to dietary practices. *Int J Cancer*. 1975;15:617.

29. Armstrong CP, Ahsan Z, Hinchley G, et al. Appendicectomy and carcinoma of the caecum. *Br J Surg*. 1989;76:1049.

30. Arnaud JP, Koehl C, Adloff M. Carcinoembryonic antigen (CEA) in diagnosis and prognosis of colorectal carcinoma. *Dis Colon Rectum*. 1980;23:141.

31. Arnold MW, Schneebaum S, Berens A, et al. Intraoperative detection of colorectal cancer with radioimmunoguided surgery and CC49, a second-generation monoclonal antibody. *Ann Surg*. 1992;216:627.

32. Arnold MW, Schneebaum S, Berens A, et al. Radioimmunoguided surgery challenges traditional decision making in patients with primary colorectal cancer. *Surgery*. 1992;112:624.

33. Arnold MW, Young DC, Hitchcock CL, et al. Radioimmunoguided surgery in primary colorectal carcinoma: an intraoperative prognostic tool and adjuvant to traditional staging. *Am J Surg*. 1995;170:315.

34. Asao T, Kuwano H, Nakamura JI, et al. Gum chewing enhances early recovery from postoperative ileus after laparoscopic colectomy. *J Am Coll Surg*. 2002;195:30.

35. Ashton WS, Sariego J, Byrd M, et al. A multivariate analysis of colon cancer, preoperative carcinoembryonic antigen levels, and patient survival. *Contemp Surg*. 1993;43:11.

36. Astler VB, Coller FA. Prognostic significance of direct extension of carcinoma of colon and rectum. *Ann Surg*. 1954;139:846.

37. Atabek U, Pello MJ, Spence RK, et al. Arterial vasopressin for control of bleeding from a stapled intestinal anastomosis: report of two cases. *Dis Colon Rectum*. 1992;35:1180.

38. Atwell JD, Taylor I, Cruddas M. Increased risk of colorectal cancer associated with congenital anomalies of the urinary tract. *Br J Surg*. 1993;80:785.

39. August DA, Sugarbaker PH, Ottow RT, et al. Hepatic resection of colorectal metastases. Influence of clinical factors and adjuvant intraperitoneal 5-fluorouracil via Tenckhoff catheter on survival. *Ann Surg*. 1985;201:210.

40. Ault GW. Carcinoma of rectum: factors responsible for recurrent or residual disease. *Am Surg*. 1953;19:1035.

41. Aune D, Chan DS, Lau R, et al. Dietary fibre, whole grains, and risk of colorectal cancer: systematic review and dose-response meta-analysis of prospective studies. *BMJ*. 2011;343:d6617. doi:10.1136/bmj.d6617.

42. Aune S, Norman E. Diffuse peritonitis treated with continuous peritoneal lavage. *Acta Chir Scand*. 1970;136:401.

43. Axtell LM, Cutler SJ, Myers MH, eds. *End Results in Cancer*. Bethesda, MD: US Department of Health, Education, and Welfare; 1972:217. Report No. 4. NIH publication 73–272.

44. Ayeni AO, Thomson DMP, MacFarlane JK. A comparison of tube leukocyte adherence inhibition assay and standard physical methods for diagnosing colorectal cancer. *Cancer*. 1981;48:1855.

45. Azimuddin K, Khubchandani IT, Stasik JJ, et al. Neoplasia after ureterosigmoidostomy. *Dis Colon Rectum*. 1999;42:1632.

46. Bajor A, Gillberg PG, Abrahamsson H. Bile acids: short and long term effects in the intestine. *Scand J Gastroenterol*. 2010;45:645.

47. Baker LH, Matter R, Talley R, et al. 5-FU vs. 5-FU and Me CCNU in gastrointestinal cancers: a phase III study of the South West Oncology Group [abstract]. *Proc Am Assoc Cancer Res*. 1975;16:229.

48. Balch CM, Urist MM, McGregor ML. Continuous regional chemotherapy for metastatic colorectal cancer using a totally implantable infusion pump: a feasibility study in 50 patients. *Am J Surg*. 1983;145:285.

49. Balfour DC. A method of anastomosis between sigmoid and rectum. *Ann Surg*. 1910;51:239.

50. Ballantyne GH, Reigel MM, Wolff BG, et al. Oophorectomy and colon cancer. *Ann Surg*. 1985;202:209.

51. Banner BF, Tomas de la Vega JE, Roseman DL, et al. Should flow cytometric DNA analysis precede definitive surgery for colon carcinoma? *Ann Surg*. 1985;202:740.

52. Barkin JS, Cohen ME, Flaxman M, et al. Value of a routine follow-up endoscopy program for the detection of recurrent colorectal carcinoma. *Am J Gastroenterol*. 1988;88:1355.

53. Barringer PL, Dockerty MB, Waugh JM, et al. Carcinoma of the large intestine: a new approach to the study of venous spread. *Surg Gynecol Obstet*. 1954;98:62.

54. Basse L, Billesbølle P, Kehlet H. Early recovery after abdominal rectopexy with multimodal rehabilitation. *Dis Colon Rectum*. 2002;45:195.

55. Basse L, Jacobsen DH, Billesbølle P, et al. Colostomy closure after Hartmann's procedure with fast-track rehabilitation. *Dis Colon Rectum*. 2002;45:1661.

56. Bat L, Neumann G, Shemesh E. The association of synchronous neoplasms with occluding cancer. *Dis Colon Rectum*. 1985;28:149.

57. Baxter NN, Morris AM, Rothenberger DA, et al. Impact of preoperative radiation for rectal cancer on subsequent lymph node evaluation: a population-based analysis. *Int J Radiat Oncol Biol Phys*. 2005;61:426.

58. Baxter NN, Noel AA, Cherry K, et al. Management of patients with colorectal cancer and concomitant abdominal aortic aneurysm. *Dis Colon Rectum*. 2002;45:165.

59. Baxter NN, Virnig DJ, Rothenberger DA, et al. Lymph node evaluation in colorectal cancer patients: a population-based study. *J Natl Cancer Inst*. 2005;97:219.

60. Beart RW, Melton JL III, Maruta M, et al. Trends in right- and left-sided colon cancer. *Dis Colon Rectum*. 1983;26:393.

61. Beart RW Jr, Moertel CG, Wieand HS, et al. Adjuvant therapy for resectable colorectal carcinoma with fluorouracil administered by portal vein infusion: a study of the Mayo Clinic and the North Central Cancer Treatment Group. *Arch Surg*. 1990;125:897.

62. Beatty JD, Hyams DM, Morton BA, et al. Impact of radiolabeled antibody imaging on management of colon cancer. *Am J Surg*. 1989;157:13.

63. Beck DE. The role of Seprafilm bioresorbable membrane in adhesion prevention. *Eur J Surg*. 1997;577:49.

64. Beck DE, Cohen Z, Fleshman JW, et al. A prospective, randomized multicenter, controlled study of the safety of Seprafilm adhesion barrier in abdominopelvic surgery of the intestine. *Dis Colon Rectum*. 2003;46:1310.

65. Beck DE, Fazio VW. Current preoperative bowel cleansing methods: results of a survey. *Dis Colon Rectum*. 1990;33:12.

66. Beck DE, Fazio VW, Jagelman DG. Comparison of oral lavage methods for preoperative colonic cleansing. *Dis Colon Rectum*. 1986;29:699.

67. Beck DE, Harford FJ, DiPalma JA, et al. Bowel cleansing with polyethylene glycol electrolyte lavage solution. *South Med J*. 1985;78:1414.

68. Beck DE, Opelka FG, Bailey HR, et al. Incidence of small-bowel obstruction and adhesiolysis after open colorectal and general surgery. *Dis Colon Rectum*. 1999;42:241.

69. Beck NE, Tomlinson IPM, Homfray T, et al. Genetic testing is important in families with a history suggestive of hereditary non-polyposis colorectal cancer even if the Amsterdam criteria are not fulfilled. *Br J Surg*. 1997;84:233.

70. Becker JM, Dayton MT, Fazio VW, et al. Prevention of postoperative abdominal adhesions by a sodium hyaluronate-based bioresorbable membrane: a prospective, randomized, double-blind multicenter study. *J Am Coll Surg*. 1996;183:297.

71. Beckwith PS, Wolff BG, Frazee RC. Ileorectostomy in the older patient. *Dis Colon Rectum*. 1992;35:301.

72. Becouam Y, Ychou M, Ducreux M, et al. Oxaliplatin as first line chemotherapy in metastatic colorectal patients. *J Clin Oncol*. 1998;8:2739.

73.   Beets G, Penninckx F, Schiepers C, et al. Clinical value of whole-body positron emission tomography with [^{18}F]fluorodeoxyglucose in recurrent colorectal cancer. *Br J Surg.* 1994;81:1666.

74.   Begent RHJ, Keep PA, Searle F, et al. Radioimmunolocalization and selection for surgery in recurrent colorectal cancer. *Br J Surg.* 1986;73:64.

75.   Bclinkic SA, Narayanan NC, Russell JC, et al. Splenic abscess associated with *Streptococcus bovis* septicemia and neoplastic lesions of the colon. *Dis Colon Rectum.* 1983;26:823.

76.   Bender JS, Magnuson TH, Zenilman ME, et al. Outcome following colon surgery in the octagenerian. *Am Surg.* 1996;62:276.

77.   Bennett-Guerrero E, Hyam JA, Shaefi S, et al. Comparison of P-POSSUM risk-adjusted mortality rates after surgery between patients in the USA and the UK. *Br J Surg.* 2003;90:1593.

78.   Benson AB, Schrag D, Somerfield MR, et al. American Society of Clinical Oncology recommendations on adjuvant chemotherapy for stage II colon cancer. *J Clin Oncol.* 2004;22:3408.

79.   Berger AC, Sigurdson ER, LeVoyer T, et al. Colon cancer survival is associated with decreasing ratio of metastatic to examined lymph nodes. *J Clin Oncol.* 2005;23:8706.

80.   Berrospi F, Celis J, Ruiz E, et al. En bloc pancreaticoduodenectomy for right colon cancer invading adjacent organs. *J Surg Oncol.* 2002;79:194.

81.   Besbeas S, Stearns MW Jr. Osseous metastases from carcinomas of the colon and rectum. *Dis Colon Rectum.* 1978;21:266.

82.   57A. Bessa X, Piñol V, Castellví-Bel S, et al. Prognostic value of postoperative detection of blood circulating tumor cells in patients with colorectal cancer operated on for cure. *Ann Surg.* 2003;237:368.

83.   Beynon J, Davies PW, Billings PJ, et al. Perioperative blood transfusion increases the risk of recurrence in colorectal cancer. *Dis Colon Rectum.* 1989;29:975.

84.   Biggers OR, Ready RL, Beart RW Jr. Risk of additional intra-abdominal procedures at the time of colectomy. *Dis Colon Rectum.* 1982; 15:185.

85.   Bilimoria KY, Bentrem DJ, Stewart AK, et al. Lymph node evaluation as a colon cancer quality measure: a national hospital report card. *J Natl Cancer Inst.* 2008;100:1310.

86.   Binderow SR, Cohen SM, Wexner SD, et al. Must early postoperative oral intake be limited to laparoscopy? *Dis Colon Rectum.* 1994;37:584.

87.   Biondo S, Jaurrieta E, Jorba R, et al. Intraoperative colonic lavage and primary anastomosis in peritonitis and obstruction. *Br J Surg.* 1997;84:222.

88.   Bipat S, van Leeuwen MS, Comans EF, et al. Colorectal liver metastases: CT, MR imaging, and PET for diagnosis—meta-analysis. *Radiology.* 2005;237:123.

89.   Birbeck KF, Macklin CP, Tiffin NJ, et al. Rates of circumferential margin involvement vary between surgeons and predict outcomes in rectal cancer surgery. *Ann Surg.* 2002;235:449.

90.   Birnkrant A, Sampson J, Sugarbaker PH. Ovarian metastasis from colorectal cancer. *Dis Colon Rectum.* 1986;29:767.

91.   Bismuth H, Adam R, Lévi F, et al. Resection of nonresectable liver metastases from colorectal cancer after neoadjuvant chemotherapy. *Ann Surg.* 1996;224:509.

92.   Bjelke E. Epidemiologic studies of cancer of the stomach, colon, and rectum: with special emphasis on the role of diet. *Scand J Gastroenterol Suppl.* 1974;9:1.

93.   Bjelke E. *Epidemiologic Studies of Cancer of the Stomach, Colon, and Rectum: With Special Emphasis on the Role of Diet: Abstracts and Literature Review.* Oslo, Norway: Universitets Forlaget; 1974.

94.   Blair JE, McLeod RS, Cohen Z, et al. Ticarcillin/clavulanic acid (Timentin) compared to metronidazole/netilmicin in preventing postoperative infection after elective colorectal surgery. *Can J Surg.* 1987; 30:120.

95.   Blamey SL, McDermott FT, Pihl E, et al. Resected ovarian recurrence from colorectal adenocarcinoma: a study of 13 cases. *Dis Colon Rectum.* 1981;24:272.

96.   Bleeker WA, Mulder NH, Hermans J, et al. Value and cost of follow-up after adjuvant treatment of patients with Dukes' C colonic cancer. *Br J Surg.* 2001;88:101.

97.   Bloch OT. Om extra-abdominal behandlung af cancer intestinalis (rectum derfra undtaget) med en frem stilling af de for denne sygdom foretagne operationer og deres resultater. *Nord Med Ark.* 1892;24:1.

98.   Böhm B, Schwenk W, Hucke HP, et al. Does methodic long-term follow-up affect survival after curative resection of colorectal carcinoma? *Dis Colon Rectum.* 1993;36:280.

99.   Bokemeyer C, Bondarenko I, Makhson A, et al. Fluorouracil, leucovorin, and oxaliplatin with and without cetuximab in the first line treatment of metastatic colorectal cancer. *J Clin Oncol.* 2009;27:663.

100.   Bokey EL, Chapuis PH, Dent OF, et al. Surgical technique and survival in patients having a curative resection for colon cancer. *Dis Colon Rectum.* 2003;46:860.

101.   Boland CR. Evolution of the nomenclature for the hereditary colorectal cancer syndromes. *Fam Cancer.* 2005;4:211.

102.   Boldrini G, de Gaetano AM, Giovannini I, et al. The systematic use of operative ultrasound for detection of liver metastases during colorectal surgery. *World J Surg.* 1987;11:622.

103.   Bolin S, Nilsson E, Sjödahl R. Carcinoma of the colon and rectum: growth rate. *Ann Surg.* 1984;198:151.

104.   Boman B, Fitzgibbons RJ, Lanspa SJ, et al. Hereditary nonpolyposis colon cancer (Lynch syndrome I and II): a challenge for the clinician. *Nebr Med J.* 1989;74:2.

105.   Bonnheim DC, Petrelli NJ, Herrera L, et al. Osseous metastases from colorectal carcinoma. *Am J Surg.* 1986;151:457.

106.   Booth CM, Li G, Zhang-Salomons J, et al. The impact of socioeconomic status on stage of cancer at diagnosis and survival: a population-based study in Ontario, Canada. *Cancer.* 2010;116:4160.

107.   Botteri E, Iodice S, Bagnardi V, et al. Smoking and colorectal cancer: a meta-analysis. *JAMA.* 2008;300:2765.

108.   Bottger TC, Gabbert HE, Stöckle M, et al. DNA image cytometry: a prognostic tool in rectal cancer? *Dis Colon Rectum.* 1992;35:436.

109.   Boyd JT, Langman M, Doll R. The epidemiology of gastrointestinal cancer with special reference to causation. *Gut.* 1964;5:196.

110.   Bradnock B. Speeding up colonic lavage. *Br J Surg.* 1987;74:464.

111.   Bradpiece HA, Benjamin IS, Halevy A, et al. Major hepatic resection for colorectal metastases. *Br J Surg.* 1987;74:324.

112.   Bralow SP, Green S. Forewarned is forearmed: some colorectal cancer is hereditary. *Contemp Gastroenterol.* 1990;3:57.

113.   Bredtmann RD, Herden HN, Teichmann W, et al. Epidural analgesia in colonic surgery: results of a randomized prospective study. *Br J Surg.* 1990;77:638.

114.   Brendel TH, Kirsh IE. Lack of association between inguinal hernia and carcinoma of the colon. *N Engl J Med.* 1971;284:369.

115.   Brief DK, Brener BJ, Goldenkranz R. An argument for increased use of subtotal colectomy in the management of carcinoma of the colon. *Am Surg.* 1983;49:66.

116.   Briggs RH, Chowdhury FU, Lodge JP, et al. Clinical impact of FDG PET-CT in patients with potentially operable metastatic colorectal cancer. *Clin Radiol.* 2011;66:1167.

117.   Brisson PA, Morere D. Colorectal intussusception. *Contemp Surg.* 1990;36:30.

118.   Brister SJ, de Varennes B, Gordon PH, et al. Contemporary operative management of pulmonary metastases of colorectal origin. *Dis Colon Rectum.* 1988;31:786.

119.   Bristol JB, Emmett PM, Heaton KW, et al. Sugar, fat, and the risk of colorectal cancer. *BMJ.* 1985;291:1467.

120.   Brodsky JT, Cohen AM. Peritoneal seeding following potentially curative resection of colonic carcinoma: implications for adjuvant therapy. *Dis Colon Rectum.* 1991;34:723.

121.   Brown AD, Garber AM. Cost-effectiveness of three methods to enhance the sensitivity of Papanicolaou testing. *JAMA.* 1999;281:347.

122.   Brown CE, Warren S. Visceral metastasis from rectal carcinoma. *Surg Gynecol Obstet.* 1938;66:611.

123.   Brown HG, Luckasevic TM, Medich DS, et al. Efficacy of manual dissection of lymph nodes in colon cancer resections. *Mod Pathol.* 2004; 17:402.

124.   Brown RA, Rode H, Millar AJW, et al. Colorectal carcinoma in children. *J Pediatr Surg.* 1992;27:919.

125.   Bruinvels DJ, Stiggelbout AM, Kievit J, et al. Follow-up of patients with colorectal cancer: a meta-analysis. *Ann Surg.* 1994;219:174.

126.   Bubrick MP, Corman ML, Cahill CJ, et al. Prospective, randomized trial of the biofragmentable anastomosis ring. *Am J Surg.* 1991;161:136.

127.   Buckley N, Brown DAP. Metastatic tumors in the hand from adenocarcinoma of the colon. *Dis Colon Rectum.* 1987;30:141.

128.   Buechter KJ, Boustany C, Caillouette R, et al. Surgical management of the acutely obstructed colon. A review of 127 cases. *Am J Surg.* 1988;156:163.

129.   Bufo AJ, Feldman S, Daniels GA, et al. Early postoperative feeding. *Dis Colon Rectum.* 1994;37:1260.

130.   Bülow S, Svendsen LB, Mellemgaard A. Metachronous colorectal carcinoma. *Br J Surg.* 1990;77:502.

131.   Burbank F. Patterns in cancer mortality in the United States: 1950–1967. *Natl Cancer Inst Monogr.* 1971;33:1.

132.   Burke P, Mealy K, Gillen P, et al. Requirement for bowel preparation in colorectal surgery. *Br J Surg.* 1994;81:907.

133.   Burkitt DP. Relationship as a clue to causation. *Lancet.* 1970;2:1237.

134. Burkitt DP. Epidemiology of cancer of the colon and rectum. *Cancer.* 1971;28:3.

135. Burkitt DP. Some neglected leads to cancer causation. *J Natl Cancer Inst.* 1971;47:913.

136. Burkitt DP. An approach to the reduction of the most common Western cancers: the failure of therapy to reduce disease. *Arch Surg.* 1991;126:345.

137. Burkitt DP, Walker AR, Painter NS. Effect of dietary fibre on stools and the transit times, and its role in the causation of disease. *Lancet.* 1972;2:1408.

138. Burns JW, Skinner K, Colt J, et al. Prevention of tissue injury and postsurgical adhesions by precoating tissues with hyaluronic acid solutions. *J Surg Res.* 1995;59:644.

139. Buroker TR, O'Connell MJ, Wieand HS, et al. Randomized comparison of two schedules of fluorouracil and leucovorin in the treatment of advanced colorectal cancer. *J Clin Oncol.* 1994;12:14.

140. Busch ORC, Hop WCJ, Marquet RL, et al. Blood transfusions and local tumor recurrence in colorectal cancer: evidence of a noncausal relationship. *Ann Surg.* 1994;220:791.

141. Butler J, Attiyeh FF, Daly JM. Hepatic resection for metastases of the colon and rectum. *Surg Gynecol Obstet.* 1986;162:109.

142. Butterworth AS, Higgins JP, Pharoah P. Relative and absolute risk of colorectal cancer for individuals with a family history: a meta-analysis. *Eur J Cancer.* 2006;42:216.

143. Byers TE, Wolf HJ, Bauer KR, et al; Patterns of Care Study Group. The impact of socioeconomic status on survival after cancer in the United States: findings from the National Program of Cancer Registries Patterns of Care Study. *Cancer.* 2008;113:582.

144. Byrd RL, Boggs HW Jr, Slagle GW, et al. Reliability of colonoscopy. *Dis Colon Rectum.* 1989;32:1023.

145. Cady B, McDermott WV. Major hepatic resection for metachronous metastases from colon cancer. *Ann Surg.* 1985;201:204.

146. Cady B, Monson DO, Swinton NW Sr. Survival of patients after colonic resection for carcinoma with simultaneous liver metastases. *Surg Gynecol Obstet.* 1970;131:697.

147. Cady B, Oberfield RA. Regional infusion chemotherapy of hepatic metastases from carcinoma of the colon. *Am J Surg.* 1974;127:220.

148. Cady B, Persson AV, Monson DO, et al. Changing patterns of colorectal carcinoma. *Cancer.* 1974;33:422.

149. Cahan WG, Castro El B, Hajdu SI. The significance of a solitary lung shadow in patients with colon carcinoma. *Cancer.* 1974;33:414.

150. Cahill CJ, Betzler M, Gruwez J, et al. Sutureless large-bowel anastomosis: European experience with the biofragmentable anastomosis ring. *Br J Surg.* 1989;76:344.

151. Cali RL, Pitsch RM, Thorson AG, et al. Cumulative incidence of metachronous colorectal cancer. *Dis Colon Rectum.* 1993;36:388.

152. Cameron BH, William G, Fitzgerald N, et al. Hereditary site-specific colon cancer in a Canadian kindred. *Can Med Assoc J.* 1989;140:41.

153. Camp TF Jr, Connolly JM. Colorectal polypoid lesions. *Arch Surg.* 1966;93:625.

154. Canalis F, Ravitch MM. Study of healing of inverting and everting intestinal anastomoses. *Surg Gynecol Obstet.* 1968;126:109.

155. Caplin S, Cerottini JP, Bosman FT, et al. For patients with Dukes' B (TNM stage II) colorectal carcinoma, examination of six or fewer lymph nodes is related to poor prognosis. *Cancer.* 1998;83:666.

156. Carlson MA, Condon RE. Polyglyconate (Maxon) versus nylon suture in midline abdominal incision closure: a prospective randomized trial. *Am Surg.* 1995;61:980.

157. Carpelan-Holmström MA, Haglund CH, Roberts PJ. Differences in serum tumor markers between colon and rectal cancer: comparison of CA 242 and carcinoembryonic antigen. *Dis Colon Rectum.* 1996;39:799.

158. Carty NJ, Keating J, Campbell J, et al. Prospective audit of an extramucosal technique for intestinal anastomosis. *Br J Surg.* 1991;78:1439.

159. Casillas S, Pelley RJ, Milsom JW. Adjuvant therapy for colorectal cancer: present and future perspectives. *Dis Colon Rectum.* 1997;40:977.

160. Castaing D, Emond J, Bismuth H, et al. Utility of operative ultrasound in the surgical management of liver tumors. *Ann Surg.* 1986;204:600.

161. Celoria G, Falco E, Nardini A, et al. Intraoperative testing of the Valtrac biofragmentable anastomotic ring. *Br J Surg.* 1993;80:618.

162. Chan AT, Giovannucci EL. Primary prevention of colorectal cancer. *Gastroenterology.* 2010;138:2029e10.

163. Chang FC, Jackson TM, Jackson CR. Hemoccult screening for colorectal cancer. *Am J Surg.* 1988;156:457.

164. Chang GJ, Rodriguez-Bigas MA, Skibber JM, et al. Lymph node evaluation and survival after curative resection of colon cancer: systematic review. *J Natl Cancer Inst.* 2007;99:433.

165. Chapuis PH, Dent OF, Fisher R, et al. A multivariate analysis of clinical and pathological variables in prognosis after resection of large-bowel cancer. *Br J Surg.* 1985;72:698.

166. Chapuis PH, Dent OF, Newland RC, et al. An evaluation of the American Joint Committee (pTMN) staging method for cancer of the colon and rectum. *Dis Colon Rectum.* 1986;29:6.

167. Charnley RM, Doran J, Morris DL. Cryotherapy for liver metastases: a new approach. *Br J Surg.* 1989;76:1040.

168. Charnley RM, Morris DL, Dennison AR, et al. Detection of colorectal liver metastases using intraoperative ultrasonography. *Br J Surg.* 1991;78:45.

169. Chassin JL, Rifkind KM, Sussman B, et al. The stapled gastrointestinal tract anastomosis: incidence of postoperative complications compared with the sutured anastomosis. *Ann Surg.* 1978;188:689.

170. Chen SL, Bilchik AJ. More extensive nodal dissection improves survival for stages I to III colon cancer. *Ann Surg.* 2006;244:602.

171. Chen SL, Bilchik AJ. More extensive nodal dissection improves survival for stages I to III of colon cancer: a population-based study. *Ann Surg.* 2006;244:602.

172. Chen TC, Ding KC, Yang MJ, et al. New device for biofragmentable anastomotic ring in low anterior resection. *Dis Colon Rectum.* 1994;37:834.

173. Chen WF, Patchefsky AS, Goldsmith HS. Colonic protection from dimethylhydrazine by a high-fiber diet. *Surg Gynecol Obstet.* 1978; 147:503.

174. Chen YL. The diagnosis of colorectal cancer with cytologic brushings under direct vision at fiberoptic colonoscopy: a report of 59 cases. *Dis Colon Rectum.* 1987;30:342.

175. Cho E, Smith-Warner SA, Ritz J, et al. Alcohol intake and colorectal cancer: a pooled analysis of 8 cohort studies. *Ann Intern Med.* 2004; 140:603.

176. Choi HJ, Jung IK, Kim SS, et al. Proliferating cell nuclear antigen expression and its relationship to malignancy potential in invasive colorectal carcinomas. *Dis Colon Rectum.* 1997;40:51.

177. Choi J, O'Connell TX. Safe and effective early postoperative feeding and hospital discharge after open colon resection. *Am Surg.* 1996;62:853.

178. Chu DZJ, Erickson CA, Russell MP, et al. Prognostic significance of carcinoembryonic antigen in colorectal carcinoma. *Arch Surg.* 1991;126:314.

179. Chung M, Steinmetz OK, Gordon PH. Perioperative blood transfusion and outcome after resection for colorectal carcinoma. *Br J Surg.* 1993;80:427.

180. Cioffiro W, Schein CJ, Gliedman ML. Splenic injury during abdominal surgery. *Arch Surg.* 1976;11:167.

181. Clark CG. Implantable vascular access devices in the treatment of colorectal liver metastases. *Br J Surg.* 1986;73:419.

182. Clark CG, Harris J, Elmasri S, et al. Polyglycolic acid sutures and catgut in colonic anastomoses: a controlled clinical trial. *Lancet.* 1972;2:1006.

183. Clark TW, Schor SS, Elsom KE, et al. The periodic health examination: evaluation of routine tests and procedures. *Ann Intern Med.* 1961;54:1209.

184. Clarke MP, Kane RA, Steele GS Jr, et al. Prospective comparison of preoperative imaging and intraoperative ultrasonography in the detection of liver tumors. *Surgery.* 1989;106:849.

185. Clegg LX, Reichman ME, Miller BA, et al. Impact of socioeconomic status on cancer incidence and stage at diagnosis: selected findings from the surveillance, epidemiology, and end results: National Longitudinal Mortality Study. *Cancer Causes Control.* 2009;20:417.

186. Clemmesen J. Statistical studies in the aetiology of malignant neoplasms. *Acta Pathol Microbiol Scand Suppl.* 1974;247:1.

187. Clemmesen J, Nielsen A. Social distribution of cancer in Copenhagen, 1943 to 1947. *Br J Cancer.* 1951;5:159.

188. Cohen AM, Martin EW Jr, Lavery I, et al. Radioimmunoguided surgery using iodine 125 B72.3 in patients with colorectal cancer. *Arch Surg.* 1991;126:349.

189. Cohn I Jr. Implantation in cancer of the colon. *Surg Gynecol Obstet.* 1967;124:501.

190. Cole WH, Packard D, Southwick HW. Carcinoma of the colon with special reference to prevention of recurrence. *JAMA.* 1954;155:1549.

191. Colvin DB, Lee W, Eisenstat TE, et al. The role of nasointestinal intubation in elective colonic surgery. *Dis Colon Rectum.* 1986;29:295.

192. Compton CC, Fielding LP, Burgart LJ, et al. Prognostic factors in colorectal cancer: College of American Pathologists consensus statement 1999. *Arch Pathol Lab Med.* 2000;124:979.

193. Condon RE, Bartlett JG, Greenlee H, et al. Efficacy of oral and systemic antibiotic prophylaxis in colorectal operations. *Arch Surg.* 1983; 118:496.

194. Connell ME. Intestinal anastomosis—by a new method, without plates and with but two knots—either silk or catgut sutures may be used. *JAMA.* 1893;21:150.

195. Cook AD, Single R, McCahill LE. Surgical resection of primary tumors in patients who present with stage IV colorectal cancer: an analysis of surveillance, epidemiology, and end results data, 1988 to 2000. *Ann Surg Oncol.* 2005;12:637.

196. Cook PJ, Doll R, Fellingham SA. A mathematical model for the age distribution of cancer in man. *Int J Cancer.* 1969;4:93.

197. Cooper K, Squires H, Carroll C, et al. Chemoprevention of colorectal cancer: systematic review and economic evaluation. *Health Technol Assess.* 2010;14:1.

198. The Cooperative Study Group of Surgical Adjuvant Immunochemotherapy for Cancer of Colon and Rectum (Kanagawa). Mitomi T, Tsuchiya S, Ijima N, et al. Randomized controlled study on adjuvant immunochemotherapy with PSKR in curatively resected colorectal cancer. *Dis Colon Rectum.* 1992;35:123.

199. Corman ML, Coller JA, Veidenheimer MC. Proctosigmoidoscopy: age criteria for examination in the asymptomatic patient. *CA Cancer J Clin.* 1975;24:286.

200. Corman ML, Galandiuk S, Block GE, et al. Immunoscintigraphy with ^{111}In-Satumomab pendetide in patients with colorectal adenocarcinoma: performance and impact on clinical management. *Dis Colon Rectum.* 1994;37:129.

201. Corman ML, Prager ED, Hardy TG Jr, et al. Comparison of the Valtrac biofragmentable anastomosis ring with conventional suture and stapled anastomosis in colon surgery: results of a prospective, randomized clinical trial. *Dis Colon Rectum.* 1989;32:183.

202. Corman ML, Robertson WG, Lewis TH, et al. A controlled clinical trial: cefuroxime, metronidazole, and cefoxitin as prophylactic therapy for colorectal surgery. *Contemp Surg.* 1993;12:36.

203. Corman ML, Swinton NW Sr, O'Keefe DD, et al. Colorectal carcinoma at the Lahey Clinic, 1962–1966. *Am J Surg.* 1973;125:424.

204. Corman ML, Veidenheimer MC, Coller JA. Colorectal carcinoma: a decade of experience at the Lahey Clinic. *Dis Colon Rectum.* 1979;22:477.

205. Corman ML, Veidenheimer MC, Coller JA. Controlled clinical trial of three suture materials for abdominal closure after bowel resections. *Am J Surg.* 1981;141:510.

206. Corman ML, Veidenheimer MC, Swinton NW. *Diseases of the Anus, Rectum, and Colon. Part I: Neoplasms.* New York, NY: Medcom; 1972.

207. Correa P, Llanos G. Morbidity and mortality from cancer in Cali, Colombia. *J Natl Cancer Inst.* 1966;36:717.

208. Cox MR, Gunn IF, Eastman MC, et al. The operative aetiology and types of adhesions causing small-bowel obstruction. *Aust N Z J Surg.* 1993;63:848.

209. Cress RD, Morris C, Ellison GL, et al. Secular changes in colorectal cancer incidence by subsite, stage at diagnosis, and race/ethnicity, 1992-2001. *Cancer.* 2006;107(5 suppl):1142.

210. Crockett SD, Long MD, Dellon ES, et al. Inverse relationship between moderate alcohol intake and rectal cancer: analysis of the North Carolina Colon Cancer Study. *Dis Colon Rectum.* 2011;54:887.

211. Cucino C, Buchner AM, Sonnenberg A. Continued rightward shift of colorectal cancer. *Dis Colon Rectum.* 2002;45:1035.

212. Cunningham D, Humblet Y, Siena S, et al. Cetuximab (C225) alone or in combination with irinotecan (CPT-11) in patients with epidermal growth factor receptor (EGFR)-positive, irinotecan-refractory metastatic colorectal cancer (MCRC) [abstract 1012]. *Proc ASCO.* 2003;22.

213. Cunningham D, Purhonen S, James RD, et al. Randomized trial of irinotecan plus supportive care versus supportive care alone after fluorouracil failure for patients with metastatic colorectal cancer. *Lancet.* 1998;352:1413.

214. Curley SA, Evans DB, Ames FC. Resection for cure of carcinoma of the colon directly invading the duodenum or pancreatic head. *J Am Coll Surg.* 1994;179:587.

215. Curley SA, Izzo F, Delrio P, et al. Radiofrequency ablation of unresectable primary and metastatic hepatic malignancies: results in 123 patients. *Ann Surg.* 1999;230:1.

216. Cusack JC, Giacco GG, Cleary K, et al. Survival factors in 186 patients younger than 40 years old with colorectal adenocarcinoma. *J Am Coll Surg.* 1996;183:105.

217. Cutait R, Alves VAF, Lopes LC, et al. Restaging of colorectal cancer based on the identification of lymph node micrometastases through immunoperoxidase staining of CEA and cytokeratins. *Dis Colon Rectum.* 1991;34:917.

218. Cutait R, Less ML, Enker WE. Prophylactic oophorectomy in surgery for large-bowel cancer. *Dis Colon Rectum.* 1983;16:6.

219. Cuthbertson AM, McLeish AR, Penfold CB, et al. A comparison between single- and double-dose intravenous Timentin for the prophylaxis of wound infection in elective colorectal surgery. *Dis Colon Rectum.* 1991;34:151.

220. Cutler SJ, Young JL Jr, eds. The third national cancer survey: incidence data: cancer morbidity. *Natl Cancer Inst Monogr.* 1975;41:1.

221. d'Allaines F, Morgan CN, Lloyd-Davies OV. Discussion on conservative resection in carcinoma. *Proc R Soc Med.* 1950;43:697.

222. Daneker GW Jr, Piazza AJ, Steele GD Jr, et al. Interactions of human colorectal carcinoma cells with basement membranes: analysis and correlation with differentiation. *Arch Surg.* 1989;124:183.

223. Danforth DN Jr, Thorbjarnarson B. Incidental splenectomy: a review of the literature and the New York Hospital experience. *Ann Surg.* 1976;183:124.

224. Dauphine CE, Tan P, Beart RB Jr, et al. Placement of self-expanding metal stents for acute malignant large-bowel obstruction: a collective review. *Ann Surg Oncol.* 2002;9:574.

225. Davis TP, Knollmann-Ritschel B, DeNobile JW. An unusual cutaneous presentation of metastatic colon cancer. *Dis Colon Rectum.* 1995;38:670.

226. Davis WC, Jackson FC. Inguinal hernia and colon carcinoma. *CA Cancer J Clin.* 1968;18:143.

227. Dawson PM, Blair SD, Begent RHJ, et al. The value of radioimmunoguided surgery in first- and second-look laparotomy for colorectal cancer. *Dis Colon Rectum* 1991;34:217.

228. Dawson PM, Habib NA, Fanc J, et al. Association between extent of colonic mucosal sialomucin change and subsequent local recurrence after curative excision of primary colorectal cancer. *Br J Surg.* 1990;77:1279.

229. Dawson PM, Habib NA, Rees HC, et al. Mucosal field change in colorectal cancer. *Am J Surg.* 1987;153:281.

230. de Almeida ACM, Gracias CW, dos Santos NM, et al. One-stage colectomy in the management of acutely obstructed left colon cancer. *Dig Surg.* 1992;9:155.

231. Dean ACB, Newell JP. Colonoscopy in the differential diagnosis of carcinoma from diverticulitis of the sigmoid colon. *Br J Surg.* 1973;60:633.

232. Dean PA, Vernava AM III. Flow cytometric analysis of DNA content in colorectal carcinoma. *Dis Colon Rectum.* 1992;35:95.

233. Deans GT, Heatley M, Anderson N, et al. Jass' classification revisited. *J Am Coll Surg.* 1994;179:11.

234. Deans GT, Williamson K, Heatley M, et al. The role of flow cytometry in carcinoma of the colon and rectum. *Surg Gynecol Obstet.* 1993;177:377.

235. Degirolamo C, Modica S, Palasciano G, et al. Bile acids and colon cancer: solving the puzzle with nuclear receptors. *Trends Mol Med.* 2011;17:564.

236. de Gramont A, Banzi M, Navarro M, et al. Oxaliplatin/5FU/LV in adjuvant colon cancer: results of the international randomized Mosaic trial [abstract 1015]. *Proc ASCO.* 2003;22.

237. de Gramont A, Bosset JF, Milan C, et al. Randomized trial comparing monthly low-dose leucovorin and fluorouracil bolus with bimonthly high-dose leucovorin and fluorouracil bolus plus continuous infusion for advanced colorectal cancer: a French intergroup study. *J Clin Oncol.* 1997;15:808.

238. de Gramont A, Figer A, Seymour M, et al. Leucovorin and fluorouracil with or without oxaliplatin as first line treatment in advanced colorectal cancer. *J Clin Oncol.* 2000;18:2938.

239. Degramont E, Van Cutsem J, Tabernero J, et al. AVANT: results from a randomized, three-arm multinational phase III study to investigate bevacizumab with either XELOX or FOLFOX4 versus FOLFOX4 alone as treatment for colon cancer [abstract 362]. *J Clin Oncol.* 2011;29:(suppl 4).

240. de la Hunt MN, Karran SJ. Sulbactam/ampicillin compared with cefoxitin for chemoprophylaxis in elective colorectal surgery. *Dis Colon Rectum.* 1986;29:157.

241. Delaney CP, Weese JL, Hyman NH, et al; Alvimopan Postoperative Ileus Study Group. Phase III trial of alvimopan, a novel, peripherally acting, mu opioid antagonist, for postoperative ileus after major abdominal surgery. *Dis Colon Rectum.* 2005;48:1114; discussion 1125; author reply 1127.

242. Delaney CP, Zutshi M, Senagore AJ, et al. Prospective, randomized, controlled trial between a pathway of controlled rehabilitation with early ambulation and diet and traditional postoperative care after laparotomy and intestinal resection. *Dis Colon Rectum.* 2003;46:851.

243. Delpero JR, Pol B, Le Treut YP, et al. Surgical resection of locally recurrent colorectal adenocarcinoma. *Br J Surg.* 1998;85:372.

244. de Petz A. Aseptic technic of stomach resections. *Ann Surg.* 1927;83:388.

245. de Vos tot Nederveen Cappel WH, Nagengast FM, Griffioen G, et al. Surveillance for hereditary nonpolyposis colorectal cancer: a long-term study on 114 families. *Dis Colon Rectum.* 2002;45:1588.

246. Di Carlo V, Badellino F, Stella M, et al. Role of B72.3 iodine in 125-labeled monoclonal antibody in colorectal cancer detection by radioimmunoguided surgery. *Surgery.* 1994;115:190.

247. Dixon CF. Anterior resection for malignant lesions of the upper part of the rectum and lower part of the sigmoid. *Ann Surg.* 1948;128:425.

248. diZerega GS. Contemporary adhesion prevention. *Fertil Steril.* 1994;61:219.

249.   Docherty JG, McGregor JR, Akyol AM, et al. Comparison of manually constructed and stapled anastomoses in colorectal surgery. *Ann Surg*. 1995;221:176.

250.   Doerr RJ, Abdel-Nabi H, Baker JM, et al. Detection of primary colorectal cancer with indium 111 monoclonal antibody B72.3. *Arch Surg*. 1990;125:1601.

251.   Doerr RJ, Kulaylat MN, Bumpers H, et al. The role of immunoscintigraphy in the staging and management of colorectal cancer. *Am Surg*. 1996;62:956.

252.   Dohmoto M. New method: endoscopic implantation of rectal stent in palliative treatment of malignant stenosis. *Endosc Digest*. 1991;3:1507.

253.   Doll R. The geographical distribution of cancer. *Br J Cancer*. 1969;23:1.

254.   Doll R, Muir C, Waterhouse J, eds. *Cancer Incidence in Five Continents: Technical Reports of the International Union Against Cancer*. New York, NY: Springer-Verlag; 1970.

255.   Dominguez JM, Wolff BG, Nelson H, et al. ^{111}In-CYT-103 scanning in recurrent colorectal cancer: does it affect standard management? *Dis Colon Rectum*. 1996;39:514.

256.   Donaldson DR, Hughes LE. Notes on "on table" lavage. *Br J Surg*. 1987;74:465.

257.   Dong SM, Traverso G, Johnson C, et al. Detecting colorectal cancer in stool with the use of multiple genetic targets. *J Natl Cancer Inst*. 2001;93:858.

258.   Douillard JY, Cunningham D, Roth AD, et al. Irinotecan combined with fluorouracil compared with fluorouracil alone as first line treatment for metastatic colorectal cancer: a multicenter randomized trial. *Lancet*. 2000;355:1041.

259.   Drexler J. Asymptomatic polyps of the colon and rectum. 3. Proximal and distal polyp relationships. *Arch Intern Med*. 1971;127:466.

260.   Drexler J. Proctosigmoidoscopy: when and why? *N Engl J Med*. 1972;286:668.

261.   Dueholm S, Rubinstein E, Reipurth G. Preparation for elective colorectal surgery: a randomized blinded comparison between oral colonic lavage and whole-gut irrigation. *Dis Colon Rectum*. 1987;30:360.

262.   Dukes CE. The spread of cancer of the rectum. *Br J Surg*. 1930; 17:643.

263.   Dukes CE. The classification of cancer of the rectum. *J Pathol Bacteriol*. 1932;35:323.

264.   Dukes CE. The surgical pathology of rectal cancer (President's address). *Proc R Soc Med*. 1944;37:131.

265.   Dunham LJ, Bailar JC III. World maps of cancer mortality rates and frequency ratios. *J Natl Cancer Inst*. 1968;41:155.

266.   Dunlop MG. Inheritance of colorectal cancer susceptibility. *Br J Surg*. 1990;77:245.

267.   Dunn DH, Robbins P, Decanini C, et al. A comparison of stapled and hand-sewn anastomoses. *Dis Colon Rectum*. 1978;21:636.

268.   Durdey P, Williams NS, Brown DA. Serum carcinoembryonic antigen and acute-phase reactant proteins in the preoperative detection of fixation of colorectal tumours. *Br J Surg*. 1984;71:881.

269.   Duttenhaver JR, Hoskins RB, Gunderson LL, et al. Adjuvant postoperative radiation therapy in the management of adenocarcinoma of the colon. *Cancer*. 1986;57:955.

270.   Dwight RW, Higgins GA, Keehn RJ. Factors influencing survival after resection in cancer of the colon and rectum. *Am J Surg*. 1969; 117:512.

271.   Dwyer WA Jr. The role of the ovary in colon cancer management. *Contemp Surg*. 1991;38:15.

272.   Eddy D. Cancer of the colon and rectum. *CA Cancer J Clin*. 1980;30:208.

273.   Edge SB, Byrd DR, Compton CC, et al. *AJCC Cancer Staging Manual*. 7th ed. Philadelphia, PA: Springer; 2010:143–164.

274.   Eisenberg SB, Kraybill WG, Lopez MJ. Long-term results of surgical resection of locally advanced colorectal carcinoma. *Surgery*. 1990;108:779.

275.   Ekbom A, Helmick C, Zack M, et al. Ulcerative colitis and colorectal cancer. A population-based study. *N Engl J Med*. 1990;323:1228.

276.   Ekman CA, Gustavson J, Henning A. Value of a follow-up study of recurrent carcinoma of the colon and rectum. *Surg Gynecol Obstet*. 1977;145:895.

277.   Eldar S, Meguid MM. Pancreatic cancer presenting as colonic obstruction. *Contemp Surg*. 1984;25:36.

278.   Ellert J, Kreel L. The value of CT in malignant colonic tumors. *CT*. 1980;4:225.

279.   Ellis H, Moran BJ, Thompson JN, et al. Adhesion-related hospital readmissions after abdominal and pelvic surgery: a retrospective cohort study. *Lancet*. 1999;353:1476.

280.   El-Serag HB, Petersen L, Hampel H, et al. The use of screening colonoscopy for patients cared for by the Department of Veterans Affairs. *Arch Intern Med*. 2006;166:2202.

281.   Engarås B. Individual cutoff levels of carcinoembryonic antigen and CA 242 indicate recurrence of colorectal cancer with high sensitivity. *Dis Colon Rectum*. 2003;46:313.

282.   Enstrom JE. Cancer mortality among Mormons. *Cancer*. 1975; 36:825.

283.   Eraklis AJ, Folkman MJ. Adenocarcinoma at the site of ureterosigmoidostomies for exstrophy of the bladder. *J Pediatr Surg*. 1978;13:730.

284.   Esser S, Reilly WT, Riley LB, et al. The role of sentinel lymph node mapping in staging of colon and rectal cancer. *Dis Colon Rectum*. 2001; 44:850.

285.   Everett WG, Friend PJ, Forty J. Comparison of stapling and hand-suture for left-sided large bowel anastomosis. *Br J Surg*. 1986;73:345.

286.   Fabian TC, Mangiante EC, Boldreghini SJ. Prophylactic antibiotics for elective colorectal surgery or operation for obstruction of the small bowel: a comparison of cefonicid and cefoxitin. *Rev Infect Dis*. 1984;6:896.

287.   Fagniez PL, Hay JM, Lacine F, et al. Abdominal midline incision closure: a multicentric randomized prospective trial of 3,135 patients, comparing continuous versus interrupted polyglycolic acid sutures. *Arch Surg*. 1985;120:1351.

288.   Fansler RF, Mero K, Steinberg SM, et al. Utility of the biofragmentable anastomotic ring in traumatic small-bowel injury. *Am Surg*. 1994;60:379.

289.   Fantani GA, De Cosse JJ. Surveillance strategies after resection of carcinoma of the colon and rectum. *Surg Gynecol Obstet*. 1990;171:267.

290.   Fazio VW, Cohen Z, Fleshman JW, et al. Reduction in adhesive small-bowel obstruction by Seprafilm adhesion barrier after intestinal resection. *Dis Colon Rectum*. 2006;49:1.

291.   Fearon ER, Cho KR, Nigro JM, et al. Identification of a chromosome 18q gene that is altered in colorectal cancers. *Science*. 1990;247:49.

292.   Feldman PS. Ulcerative disease of the colon proximal to partially obstructive lesions: report of two cases and review of the literature. *Dis Colon Rectum*. 1975;8:601.

293.   Felix EL, Cohen MH, Bernstein AD, et al. Adult intussusception: case report of recurrent intussusception and review of the literature. *Am J Surg*. 1976;131:758.

294.   Fernando N, Hurwitz H. Inhibition of vascular endothelial growth factor in the treatment of colorectal cancer. *Semin Oncol*. 2003;30(suppl 6):39.

295.   Fielding LP. Clinical-pathologic staging of large-bowel cancer: a report of the ASCRS Committee. *Dis Colon Rectum*. 1988;31:204.

296.   Fielding LP. The portal vein and colorectal cancer. *Br J Surg*. 1988; 75:402.

297.   Fielding LP, Stewart-Brown S, Blesovsky L. Large-bowel obstruction caused by cancer: a prospective study. *BMJ*. 1979;2:515.

298.   Finlay IG, McArdle CS. Occult hepatic metastases in colorectal carcinoma. *Br J Surg*. 1986;73:732.

299.   Finlay IG, Meek D, Brunton F, et al. Growth rate of hepatic metastases in colorectal carcinoma. *Br J Surg*. 1988;75:641.

300.   Fisher ER, Robinsky B, Sass R, et al. Relative prognostic value of the Dukes and the Jass systems in rectal cancer: findings from the National Surgical Adjuvant Breast and Bowel Projects (Protocol R-01). *Dis Colon Rectum*. 1989;32:944.

301.   Fisher ER, Sass R, Palekar A, et al. Dukes' classification revisited: findings from the National Surgical Adjuvant Breast and Bowel Projects (Protocol R-01). *Cancer*. 1989;64:2354.

302.   Fisher ER, Turnbull RB Jr. The cytologic demonstration and significance of tumor cells in the mesenteric venous blood in patients with colorectal carcinoma. *Surg Gynecol Obstet*. 1955;100:102.

303.   Fleiszer D, MacFarlane J, Murray D, et al. Protective effect of dietary fibre against chemically induced bowel tumours in rats. *Lancet*. 1978;2:552.

304.   Fleites RA, Marshall JB, Eckhauser ML, et al. The efficacy of polyethylene glycol-electrolyte lavage solution versus traditional mechanical bowel preparation for elective colonic surgery: a randomized, prospective, blinded clinical trial. *Surgery*. 1985;98:708.

305.   Fleshman J, Sargent DJ, Green E, et al. Laparoscopic colectomy for cancer is not inferior to open surgery based on 5-year data from the COST Study Group trial. *Ann Surg*. 2007;246:655.

306.   Forde KA, McLarty A, Tsai J, et al. Murphy's button revisited: clinical experience with the biofragmentable anastomotic ring. *Ann Surg*. 1993;217:78.

307.   Fork FT. Radiographic findings in overlooked colon carcinomas. *Acta Radiol*. 1988;29:331.

308.   Fortner JG. Recurrence of colorectal cancer after hepatic resection. *Am J Surg*. 1988;155:378.

309. Fortner JG, Kim DK, Barrett MK, et al. Eight years' experience with surgical management of 321 patients with liver tumors. In: Fox BW, ed. *Advances in Medical Oncology Research and Education: Basis for Cancer Therapy I*. Vol 5. Oxford, NY: Pergamon Press; 1979:257.

310. Foster JH. Survival after liver resection for secondary tumors. *Am J Surg*. 1978;135:389.

311. Foster JH, Berman M. *Solid Liver Tumors*. Philadelphia, PA: WB Saunders; 1977.

312. Foster ME, Johnson CD, Billings PJ, et al. Intraoperative antegrade lavage and anastomotic healing in acute colonic obstruction. *Dis Colon Rectum*. 1986;29:255.

313. Fowler DL, White SA. Laparoscopy-assisted sigmoid resection. *Surg Laparosc Endosc*. 1991;1:183.

314. Fraser I. An historical perspective on mechanical aids in intestinal anastomosis. *Surg Gynecol Obstet*. 1982;155:566.

315. Frazee RC, Roberts J, Symmonds R, et al. Prospective, randomized trial of inpatient versus outpatient bowel preparation for elective colorectal surgery. *Dis Colon Rectum*. 1992;35:223.

316. Freeny PC, Marks WM, Ryan JA, et al. Colorectal carcinoma evaluation with CT: preoperative staging and detection of postoperative recurrence. *Radiology*. 1986;158:347.

317. Friend PJ, Scott R, Everett WG, et al. Stapling or suturing for anastomoses of the left side of the large intestine. *Surg Gynecol Obstet*. 1990;171:373.

318. Fuchs CS, Giovannucci EL, Colditz GA, et al. A prospective study of family history and the risk of colorectal cancer. *N Engl J Med*. 1994; 331:1669.

319. Gabrielsson N, Grangvist S, Ohlsn H. Recurrent carcinoma of the colon in the anastomosis diagnosed by roentgen examination and colonoscopy. *Endoscopy*. 1976;8:47.

320. Galandiuk S, Wieand HS, Moertel CG. Patterns of recurrence after curative resection of carcinoma of the colon and rectum. *Surg Gynecol Obstet*. 1992;174:27.

321. Gall FP, Altendorf JT. Multivisceral resections in colorectal cancer. *Dis Colon Rectum*. 1987;30:337.

322. Gambee LP. Single layer open intestinal anastomosis applicable to small as well as large intestine. *West J Surg*. 1951;59:1.

323. Gapstur SM, Potter JD, Folsom AR. Alcohol consumption and colon and rectal cancer in postmenopausal women. *Int J Epidemiol*. 1994;23:50.

324. García-Olmo D, Ontañón J, García-Olmo DC, et al. Experimental evidence does not support use of the "no-touch" isolation technique in colorectal cancer. *Dis Colon Rectum*. 1999;42:1449.

325. Gennaro AR, Tyson RR. Obstructive colonic cancer. *Dis Colon Rectum*. 1978;21:346.

326. Geoghegan JG, Scheele J. Treatment of colorectal liver metastases. *Br J Surg*. 1999;86:158.

327. George ML, Dzik-Jurasz ASK, Padhani AR, et al. Non-invasive methods of assessing angiogenesis and their value in predicting response to treatment in colorectal cancer. *Br J Surg*. 2001;88:1628.

328. Gervaz P, Bouzourene H, Cerottini JP, et al. Dukes B Colorectal cancer: distinct genetic categories and clinical outcome based on proximal or distal tumor location. *Dis Colon Rectum*. 2001;44:364.

329. Getzen LC, Roe RD, Holloway CI. Comparative study of intestinal anastomotic healing in inverted and everted closures. *Surg Gynecol Obstet*. 1966;123:1219.

330. Gianola FJ, Dwyer A, Jones AE, et al. Prospective studies of laboratory and radiologic tests in the management of colon and rectal cancer patients: I. Selection of useful preoperative tests through an analysis of surgically occult metastases. *Dis Colon Rectum*. 1984;27:811.

331. Gilbertsen VA. Improving the prognosis for patients with intestinal cancer. *Surg Gynecol Obstet*. 1967;124:1253.

332. Gilbertsen VA. Proctosigmoidoscopy and polypectomy in reducing the incidence of rectal cancer. *Cancer*. 1974;34(suppl):936.

333. Gilbertsen VA. The detection of colorectal cancers. Paper presented at: International Symposium on Colorectal Cancer; March 1979; New York, NY.

334. Gilbertsen VA, Williams SE, Schuman L, et al. Colonoscopy in the detection of carcinoma of the intestine. *Surg Gynecol Obstet*. 1979;149:877.

335. Gilchrist RK, David VC. A consideration of pathological factors influencing 5 year survival in radical resection of the large bowel and rectum for carcinoma. *Ann Surg*. 1947;126:421.

336. Giovannucci E, Colditz GA, Stampfer MJ. A meta-analysis of cholecystectomy and risk of colorectal cancer. *Gastroenterology*. 1993;105:130.

337. Giovannucci E, Egan KM, Hunter DJ, et al. Aspirin and the risk of colorectal cancer in women. *N Engl J Med*. 1995;333:609.

338. Giovannucci E, Rimm E, Stampfer M, et al. Aspirin use and the risks for colorectal cancer and adenoma in male health professionals. *Ann Intern Med*. 1994;121:241.

339. Glass RL, Smith LE, Cochran RC. Subtotal colectomy for obstructing carcinoma of the left colon. *Am J Surg*. 1983;145:335.

340. Glenn F, McSherry CK. Obstruction and perforation in colorectal cancer. *Ann Surg*. 1971;173:983.

341. Glover C, Douse P, Kane P, et al. Accuracy of investigations for asymptomatic colorectal liver metastases. *Dis Colon Rectum*. 2002;45:476.

342. Go VLW. Carcinoembryonic antigen: clinical application. *Cancer*. 1976;37:562.

343. Gold P, Freedman SO. Demonstration of tumor-specific antigens in human colonic carcinomata by immunological tolerance and absorption techniques. *J Exp Med*. 1965;121:439.

344. Gold P, Freedman SO. Specific carcinoembryonic antigens of the human digestive system. *J Exp Med*. 1965;122:467.

345. Goldberg RM, Fleming TR, Tangen CM, et al. Surgery for recurrent colon cancer: strategies for identifying resectable recurrence and success rates after resection. Eastern Cooperative Oncology Group, the North Central Cancer Treatment Group, and the Southwest Oncology Group. *Ann Intern Med*. 1998;129:27.

346. Goldberg RN, Sargent DJ, Morton RF, et al. A randomized controlled trial of fluorouracil plus leucovorin, irinotecan, and oxaliplatin combinations in patients with previously untreated metastatic colorectal cancer. *J Clin Oncol*. 2004;22:23.

347. Goldenberg DM, DeLand FH, Kim E, et al. Use of radiolabeled antibodies to carcinoembryonic antigen for the detection and localization of diverse cancers by external photoscanning. *N Engl J Med*. 1978; 298:1384.

348. Goldenberg DM, Kim EE, Bennett SJ, et al. Carcinoembryonic antigen radioimmunodetection in the evaluation of colorectal cancer and in the detection of occult neoplasms. *Gastroenterology*. 1983;84:524.

349. Goldenberg DM, Kim EE, DeLand FH, et al. Radioimmunodetection of cancer with radioactive antibodies to carcinoembryonic antigen. *Cancer Res*. 1980;40:2984.

350. Goldstein NS. Lymph node recoveries from 2427 pT3 colorectal resection specimens spanning 45 years: recommendations for a minimum number of recovered lymph nodes based on predictive probabilities. *Am J Surg Pathol*. 2002;26:179.

351. Goligher JC. The Dukes' A, B and C categorization of the extent of spread of carcinomas of the rectum. *Surg Gynecol Obstet*. 1976;143:793.

352. Goligher JC. Use of circular stapling gun with peranal insertion of anorectal purse-string suture for construction of very low colorectal or coloanal anastomoses. *Br J Surg*. 1979;66:501.

353. Goligher JC, Irvin TT, Johnston ID, et al. A controlled clinical trial of three methods of closure of laparotomy wound. *Br J Surg*. 1975; 62:823.

354. Goligher JC, Lee PWR, Macfie J, et al. Experience with the Russian Model 249 suture gun for anastomosis of the rectum. *Surg Gynecol Obstet*. 1979;148:517.

355. Goligher JC, Morris C, McAdam WAF, et al. A controlled trial of inverting versus everting intestinal suture in clinical large-bowel surgery. *Br J Surg*. 1970;57:817.

356. Gonzalez EC, Roetzheim RG, Ferrante JM, et al. Predictors of proximal vs. distal colorectal cancer. *Dis Colon Rectum*. 2001;44:251.

357. Goodman D, Irvin TT. Delay in the diagnosis and prognosis of carcinoma of the right colon. *Br J Surg*. 1993;80:1327.

358. Gorog D, Nagy P, Peter A, et al. Influence of obesity on lymph node recovery from rectal resection specimens. *Pathol Oncol Res*. 2003;9:180.

359. Goslin R, Steele G, Zamcheck N, et al. Factors influencing survival in patients with hepatic metastases from adenocarcinoma of the colon or rectum. *Dis Colon Rectum*. 1982;25:749.

360. Gottrup F, Diederich P, Sorensen K, et al. Prophylaxis with whole-gut irrigation and antimicrobials in colorectal surgery. *Am J Surg*. 1985;149:317.

361. Gozzetti G, Mazziotti A, Bolundi L, et al. Intraoperative ultrasonography in surgery for liver tumors. *Surgery*. 1986;99:523.

362. Graf E, Easton JW. Dietary suppression of colonic cancer: fiber or phytate? *Cancer*. 1985;56:717.

363. Graffner HOL, Alm POA, Oscarson JEA. Prophylactic oophorectomy in colorectal carcinoma. *Am J Surg*. 1983;146:233.

364. Graham JD, Thompson KM, Goldie DJ, et al. The cost-effectiveness of air bags by seating position. *JAMA*. 1997;278:1148.

365. Graham RA, Wang S, Catalano PJ, et al. Postsurgical surveillance of colon cancer: preliminary cost analysis of physician examination, carcinoembryonic antigen testing, chest x-ray, and colonoscopy. *Ann Surg*. 1998;228:59.

366. Gramegna A, Saccomani G. On-table colonic irrigation in the treatment of left-sided large-bowel emergencies. *Dis Colon Rectum*. 1989; 32:585.

367.   Gray BN, Walker C. Monitoring of patients with carcinoma of the large intestine by use of acute-phase proteins and carcinoembryonic antigen. *Surg Gynecol Obstet.* 1983;156:777.

368.   Gray JH. The relation of lymphatic vessels to the spread of cancer. *Br J Surg.* 1939;26:462.

369.   Gray R, Giantonio BJ, O'Dwyer PJ, et al. The safety of adding angiogenesis inhibition into treatment for colorectal, breast, and lung cancer: the Eastern Cooperative Oncology Group's (ECOG) experience with bevacizumab (anti-VEGF) [abstract 825]. *Proc ASCO.* 2003;22.

370.   Greegor DH. Occult blood testing for detection of asymptomatic colon cancer. *Cancer.* 1971;28:131.

371.   Green RJ, Metlay JP, Propert K, et al. Surveillance for second primary colorectal cancer after adjuvant chemotherapy: an analysis of Intergroup 0089. *Ann Intern Med.* 2002;136:261.

372.   Green SE, Chapman PD, Burn J, et al. Clinical impact of colonoscopic screening in first-degree relatives of patients with hereditary nonpolyposis colorectal cancer. *Br J Surg.* 1995;82:1338.

373.   Greenberg E, Baron J, Freeman D, et al. Reduced risks of large bowel adenomas among aspirin users: the Polyp Prevention Study Group. *J Natl Cancer Inst.* 1993;85:912.

374.   Greene FL. Distribution of colorectal neoplasms. *Am Surg.* 1983; 49:62.

375.   Greene FL, Page D, Fleming T, et al. *AJCC Cancer Staging Manual.* 6th ed. New York, NY: Springer-Verlag; 2002.

376.   Greenwald P, Korns RF, Nasca PC, et al. Cancer in United States Jews. *Cancer Res.* 1975;35:3507.

377.   Greenway B. Hepatic metastases from colorectal cancer: resection or not. *Br J Surg.* 1988;75:513.

378.   Griffith KD, Sugarbaker PH, Change AE. Repeat hepatic resections for colorectal metastases. *Surgery.* 1990;107:101.

379.   Grinnell RS. The spread of carcinoma of the colon and rectum. *Cancer.* 1950;3:641.

380.   Grinnell RS. The rationale of subtotal and total colectomy in the treatment of cancer and multiple polyps of the colon. *Surg Gynecol Obstet.* 1958;106:288.

381.   Grinnell RS. Results of ligation of inferior mesenteric artery at the aorta in resections of carcinoma of the descending and sigmoid colon and rectum. *Surg Gynecol Obstet.* 1965;120:1031.

382.   Grinnell RS. Lymphatic block with atypical and retrograde lymphatic metastasis and spread in carcinoma of the colon and rectum. *Ann Surg.* 1966;163:272.

383.   Gross L. Incidence of appendectomies and tonsillectomies in cancer patients. *Cancer.* 1966;19:849.

384.   Grosser N, Thomson DMP. Cell-mediated anti-tumor immunity in breast cancer patients evaluated by antigen-induced leukocyte adherence inhibition in test tubes. *Cancer Res.* 1975;35:2571.

385.   Gryfe R, Kim H, Hsieh ETK, et al. Tumor microsatellite instability and clinical outcome in young patients with colorectal cancer. *N Engl J Med.* 2000;342:69.

386.   Gryska PVR, Cohen AM. Screening asymptomatic patients at high risk for colon cancer with full colonoscopy. *Dis Colon Rectum.* 1987; 30:18.

387.   Gu J, Zhao J, Li Z, et al. Clinical application of radioimmunoguided surgery in colorectal cancer using ^{125}I-labeled carcinoembryonic antigen-specific monoclonal antibody submucosally. *Dis Colon Rectum.* 2003;46:1659.

388.   Guillem JG, Forde KA, Treat MR, et al. Colonoscopic screening for neoplasms in asymptomatic first-degree relatives of colon cancer patients: a controlled, prospective study. *Dis Colon Rectum.* 1992;35:523.

389.   Guillem JG, Neugut AI, Forde KA, et al. Colonic neoplasms in asymptomatic first-degree relatives of colon cancer patients. *Am J Gastroenterol.* 1988;83:271.

390.   Gullichsen R, Havia T, Ovaska J, et al. Colonic anastomosis using the biofragmentable anastomotic ring and manual suture: a prospective, randomized study. *Br J Surg.* 1992;79:578.

391.   Gullichsen R, Ovaska J, Havia T, et al. What happens to the Valtrac anastomosis of the colon? A follow-up study. *Dis Colon Rectum.* 1993;36:362.

392.   Gunderson LL, Cohen AM, Welch CE. Interaction of surgery and radiotherapy. *Am J Surg.* 1980;139:518.

393.   Gutherman JU, Mavligit GM, Blumenshein G, et al. Immunotherapy of human solid tumors with Bacillus Calmette-Guérin: prolongation of disease-free interval and survival in malignant melanoma, breast and colorectal cancer. *Ann N Y Acad Sci.* 1976;277:135.

394.   Guy RJ, Handa A, Traill Z, et al. Rectosigmoid carcinoma at previous uterosigmoidostomy in a renal transplant patient. *Dis Colon Rectum.* 2001;44:1534.

395.   Haddad FS, Manne RK. Involvement of the penis by rectocolic adenocarcinoma: report of a case and review of the literature. *Dis Colon Rectum.* 1987;30:123.

396.   Haenszel W. Cancer mortality among the foreign-born in the United States. *J Natl Cancer Inst.* 1961;26:37.

397.   Haenszel W. Cancer mortality among U.S. Jews. *Isr J Med Sci.* 1971;7:1437.

398.   Haenszel W, Berg JW, Segi M, et al. Large-bowel cancer in Hawaiian Japanese. *J Natl Cancer Inst.* 1973;51:1765.

399.   Haenszel W, Correa P. Cancer of the colon and rectum and adenomatous polyps: a review of epidemiological findings. *Cancer.* 1971;28:14.

400.   Haenszel W, Correa P, Cuello C. Social class in differences among patients with large-bowel cancer in Cali, Colombia. *J Natl Cancer Inst.* 1975;54:1031.

401.   Haenszel W, Dawson EA. A note on the mortality from cancer of the colon and rectum in the United States. *Cancer.* 1965;18:265.

402.   Haenszel W, Kurihara M. Studies of Japanese migrants. I. Mortality from cancer and other diseases among Japanese in the United States. *J Natl Cancer Inst.* 1968;40:43.

403.   Halevy A, Levi J, Orda R. Emergency subtotal colectomy: a new trend for treatment of obstructing carcinoma of the left colon. *Ann Surg.* 1989;210:220.

404.   Hall NR, Bishop DT, Stephenson BM, et al. Hereditary susceptibility to colorectal cancer: relatives of early-onset cases are particularly at risk. *Dis Colon Rectum.* 1996;39:739.

405.   Hall NR, Finan PJ, Ward B, et al. Genetic susceptibility to colorectal cancer in patients under 45 years of age. *Br J Surg.* 1994;81:1485.

406.   Halsted WS. Circular suture of the intestine: an experimental study. *Am J Med Sci.* 1887;94:436.

407.   Halsted WS. Intestinal anastomosis. *Bull Johns Hopkins Hosp.* 1891;2:1.

408.   Hamilton JE. Reappraisal of open intestinal anastomoses. *Ann Surg.* 1967;165:917.

409.   Hampel H, Frankel WL, Martin E, et al. Feasibility of screening for Lynch syndrome among patients with colorectal cancer. *J Clin Oncol.* 2008;26:5783.

410.   Handelsman JC, Zeiler S, Coleman J, et al. Experience with ambulatory preoperative bowel preparation at the Johns Hopkins Hospital. *Arch Surg.* 1993;128:441.

411.   Haney MJ, McGarity WC. Ureterosigmoidostomy and neoplasms of the colon: report of a case and review of the literature. *Arch Surg.* 1971; 103:69.

412.   Hansen P, Scuffham PA. Cost-effectiveness of compulsory bicycle helmets in New Zealand. *Aust J Pub Health.* 1995;19:450.

413.   Hardcastle JD, Pye G. Screening for colorectal cancer: a critical review. *World J Surg.* 1989;13:38.

414.   Hardy TG Jr, Aguilar PS, Stewart WRC. Complete obstruction of the sigmoid colon treated by primary resection and anastomosis: an improved technique (preliminary report): report of three cases. *Dis Colon Rectum.* 1989;32:528.

415.   Hardy TG Jr, Aguilar PS, Stewart WRC, et al. Initial experience with a biofragmentable ring for sutureless bowel anastomosis. *Dis Colon Rectum.* 1987;30:55.

416.   Hardy TG Jr, Hartmann RF, Samson RB, et al. Percutaneous intrahepatic chemotherapy via indwelling portal vein catheter and subcutaneous injection reservoir. *Dis Colon Rectum.* 1982;25:292.

417.   Hardy TG Jr, Pace WG, Maney JW, et al. A biofragmentable ring for sutureless bowel anastomosis. *Dis Colon Rectum.* 1985;28:484.

418.   Hardy TG Jr, Stewart WRC, Aguilar PS. Prevention of colostomy in partial colonic obstruction by intraoperative rectal tube irrigation. *Dis Colon Rectum.* 1985;28:122.

419.   Hardy TG Jr, Stewart WRC, Aguilar PS, et al. Biofragmentable ring for sutureless bowel anastomosis: early clinical experience. *Contemp Surg.* 1987;31:39.

420.   Hares MM, Alexander-Williams J. The effect of bowel preparation on colonic surgery. *World J Surg.* 1982;6:175.

421.   Harris CGJ, Church JM, Senagore AJ, et al. Factors affecting local recurrence of colonic adenocarcinoma. *Dis Colon Rectum.* 2002;45:1029.

422.   Harris MT, Laudito A, Waye JD. Colonoscopic features of colonic anastomoses. *Gastrointest Endosc.* 1994;40:554.

423.   Harrison LB, Enker WE, Anderson LL. High-dose-rate intraoperative radiation therapy for colorectal cancer. *Oncology.* 1995;9:679.

424.   Harrison LE, Guillem JG, Paty P, et al. Preoperative carcinoembryonic antigen predicts outcomes in node-negative colon cancer patients: a multivariate analysis of 572 patients. *J Am Coll Surg.* 1997;185:55.

425.   Hart AR, Wicks ACB, Mayberry JF. Colorectal cancer screening in asymptomatic populations. *Gut.* 1995;36:590.

426. Hartsell PA, Frazee RC, Harrison JB, et al. Early postoperative feeding after elective colorectal surgery. *Arch Surg.* 1997;132:518.

427. Hase K, Shatney C, Johnson D, et al. Prognostic value of tumor "budding" in patients with colorectal cancer. *Dis Colon Rectum.* 1993;36:627.

428. Hatziandreu EJ, Sacks JJ, Brown R, et al. The cost-effectiveness of three programs to increase use of bicycle helmets among children. *Public Health Rep.* 1995;110:251.

429. Heald RJ, Leicester RJ. The low stapled anastomosis. *Br J Surg.* 1981;68:333.

430. Heald RJ, Lockhart-Mummery HE. The lesion of the second cancer of the large bowel. *Br J Surg.* 1972;59:16.

431. Healey JE Jr, McBride CM, Gallagher HS. Bowel anastomosis by inverting and everting techniques. *J Surg Res.* 1967;7:299.

432. Heiken JP, Weyman PJ, Lee JKT, et al. Detection of focal hepatic masses: prospective evaluation with CT, delayed CT, CT during arterial portography, and MR imaging. *Radiology.* 1989;171:47.

433. Heimann TM, Martinelli G, Szporn A, et al. Prognostic significance of DNA content abnormalities in young patients with colorectal cancer. *Ann Surg.* 1989;210:792.

434. Helfand M, Marton KI, Zimmer-Gembeck MJ, et al. History of visible rectal bleeding in a primary care population: initial assessment and 10-year follow-up. *JAMA.* 1997;277:44.

435. Hemming AW, Scudamore CH, Davidson A, et al. Evaluation of 50 consecutive segmental hepatic resections. *Am J Surg.* 1993;165:621.

436. Herberman RB. Immunologic approaches to the diagnosis of cancer. *Cancer.* 1976;37:549.

437. Herbst CA Jr, Sessions JT, Lapis JL. Fiberoptic colonoscopic examination in surgical patients with colorectal cancer. *South Med J.* 1980;73:548.

438. Herrera-Ornelas L, Natarajan N, Tsukada Y, et al. Adenocarcinoma of the colon masquerading as primary ovarian neoplasia: an analysis of ten cases. *Dis Colon Rectum.* 1983;26:377.

439. Hersh EM, Gutterman JU, Mavligit GM, et al. BCG vaccine and its derivatives: potential, practical considerations, and precautions in human cancer immunotherapy. *JAMA.* 1976;235:246.

440. Herter FP, Slanetz CF Jr. Preoperative intestinal preparation in relation to the subsequent development of cancer at the suture line. *Surg Gynecol Obstet.* 1968;127:49.

441. Hertz RE, Deddish MR, Day E. Value of periodic examinations in detecting cancer of the rectum and colon. *Postgrad Med.* 1960;27:290.

442. Higginson J. Etiology of gastrointestinal cancer in man. *Natl Cancer Inst Monogr.* 1967;25:191.

443. Higginson J, Oettle AG. Cancer incidence in the Bantu and "Cape Colored" races of South Africa: report of a cancer survey for the Transvaal (1953–1955). *J Natl Cancer Inst.* 1960;24:589.

444. Hill MJ, Drasar BS, Aries V, et al. Bacteria and aetiology of cancer of large bowel. *Lancet.* 1971;1:95.

445. Hitchcock CL. Radioimmunoguided surgery and the staging of colorectal carcinoma. *Semin Colon Rectal Surg.* 1995;6:207.

446. Hoffmann J, Jensen HE. Tube cecostomy and staged resection for obstructing carcinoma of the left colon. *Dis Colon Rectum.* 1984;27:24.

447. Hoffmann J, Shokouh-Amiri M, Damm P, et al. A prospective, controlled study of prophylactic drainage after colonic anastomoses. *Dis Colon Rectum.* 1987;30:449.

448. Hohenberger P, Schlag PM, Gerneth T, et al. Pre- and postoperative carcinoembryonic antigen determinations in hepatic resection for colorectal metastases: predictive value and implications for adjuvant treatment based on multivariate analysis. *Ann Surg.* 1994;219:135.

449. Holt RW, Nauta RJ, Lee TC, et al. Intraoperative interstitial therapy for hepatic metastases from colorectal carcinomas. *Am Surg.* 1988;54:231.

450. Holte K, Kehlet H. Postoperative ileus: a preventable event. *Br J Surg.* 2000;87:1480.

451. Horowitz J, Tessier J, Rodriguez-Bigas M, et al. Sigmoid carcinoma presenting in an inguinal hernia sac. *Contemp Surg.* 1995;47:78.

452. Houblers JGA, Brand A, van de Watering LMG, et al. Randomised controlled trial comparing transfusion of leucocyte-depleted or buffy-coat-depleted blood in surgery for colorectal cancer. *Lancet.* 1994;344:573.

453. Houlston RS, Murdey V, Harocopos C, et al. Screening and genetic counselling for relatives of patients with colorectal cancer in a family cancer clinic. *BMJ.* 1990;301:366.

454. Howard ML, Greene FL. The effect of preoperative endoscopy on recurrence and survival following surgery for colorectal carcinoma. *Am Surg.* 1990;56:124.

455. Howell MA. Factor analysis of international cancer mortality data and per capita food consumption. *Br J Cancer.* 1974;29:328.

456. Howell MA. Diet as an etiological factor in the development of cancer of the colon and rectum. *J Chronic Dis.* 1975;28:67.

457. Howie JGR, Timperley WR. Cancer and appendectomy. *Cancer.* 1966;19:1138.

458. Huang J. Adjuvant FOLFIRI with or without Cetuximab in patients with resected Stage III colon cancer; NCCTG Intergroup phase III trial No 147 [abstract 363]. *J Clin Oncol.* 2011;29(suppl 4).

459. Hubens G, Totté E, Verhulst A, et al. The influence of the interaction of sutures with the mucosa on tumour formation at colonic anastomoses in rats. *Eur Surg Res.* 1993;25:213.

460. Hughes ESR, Cuthbertson AM. Subtotal colectomy for obstructing carcinoma of the upper left colon. *Dis Colon Rectum.* 1965;8:411.

461. Hughes ESR, McDermott FT, Polglase AL, et al. Total and subtotal colectomy for colonic obstruction. *Dis Colon Rectum.* 1985;28:162.

462. Hughes KS, Rosenstein RB, Songhorabodi S, et al. Resection of the liver for colorectal carcinoma metastases: a multi-institutional study of long-term survivors. *Dis Colon Rectum.* 1988;31:1.

463. Hughes KS, Simon R, Songhorabodi S, et al. Resection of the liver for colorectal carcinoma metastases: a multi-institutional study of patterns of recurrence. *Surgery.* 1986;100:278.

464. Hundt W, Braunschweig R, Reiser M. Evaluation of spiral CT in staging of colon and rectum carcinoma. *Eur Radiol.* 1999;9:78.

465. Hunt DR, Chorian M. Endoscopic diagnosis of small flat carcinoma of the colon: report of three cases. *Dis Colon Rectum.* 1990;33:143.

466. Hurwitz H, Fehrenbacher L, Cartwright T, et al. Bevacizumab (a monoclonal antibody to vascular endothelial growth factor) prolongs survival in first-line colorectal cancer (CRC): results of a phase III trial of bevacizumab in combination with bolus IRL (irinotecan, 5-fluorouracil, leucovorin) as first line therapy in subjects with meta-static CRC [abstract 3646]. *Proc ASCO.* 2003;23.

467. Hyams L, Wynder EL. Appendectomy and cancer risk: an epidemiological evaluation. *J Chronic Dis.* 1968;21:391.

468. Hyder JW, Talbott TM, Maycroft TC. A critical review of chemical lymph node clearance and staging of colon and rectal cancer at Ferguson Hospital, 1977 to 1982. *Dis Colon Rectum.* 1990;33:923.

469. Hyman N, Manchester TL, Osler T, et al. Anastomotic leaks after intestinal anastomosis: it's later than you think. *Ann Surg.* 2007;245:254.

470. Hyman N, Moore J, Cataldo P, et al. The high yield of 1-year colonoscopy after resection: is it the handoff? *Surg Endosc.* 2010;24:648.

471. Ike H, Shimada H, Ohki S, et al. Results of aggressive resection of lung metastases from colorectal carcinoma detected by intensive follow-up. *Dis Colon Rectum.* 2002;45:468.

472. Irvin TT. Prognosis of colorectal cancer in the elderly. *Br J Surg.* 1988;75:419.

473. Irvin TT, Greaney MG. Duration of symptoms and prognosis of carcinoma of the colon and rectum. *Surg Gynecol Obstet.* 1977;144:883.

474. Isler JT, Brown PC, Lewis FG, et al. The role of preoperative colonoscopy in colorectal cancer. *Dis Colon Rectum.* 1987;30:435.

475. Itoh H, Houlston RS, Harocopos C, et al. Risk of cancer death in first-degree relatives of patients with hereditary non-polyposis cancer syndrome (Lynch type II): a study of 130 kindreds in the United Kingdom. *Br J Surg.* 1990;77:1367.

476. Itzkowitz SH, Kim YS. New carbohydrate tumor markers [editorial]. *Gastroenterology.* 1986;92:491.

477. Iwatsuki S, Dvorchik I, Madariaga JR, et al. Hepatic resection for metastatic colorectal adenocarcinoma: a proposal of a prognostic scoring system. *J Am Coll Surg.* 1999;189:291.

478. Iwatsuki S, Esquivel CO, Gordon RD, et al. Liver resection for metastatic colorectal cancer. *Surgery.* 1986;100:804.

479. Jacobs M, Verdeja JC, Goldstein HS. Minimally invasive colon resection (laparoscopic colectomy). *Surg Laparosc Endosc.* 1991;1:144.

480. Jagelman DG, Fazio VW, Lavery IC, et al. A prospective, randomized, double-blind study of 10 percent mannitol mechanical bowel preparation, combined with oral neomycin and short-term, perioperative, intravenous Flagyl as prophylaxis in elective colorectal operations. *Surgery.* 1985;98:861.

481. Jain RK. Tumor angiogenesis and accessibility: role of vascular endothelial growth factor. *Semin Oncol.* 2002;29(suppl 16):3.

482. Jamison RL, Donohue JH, Nagorney DM, et al. Hepatic resection for metastatic colorectal cancer results in cure for some patients. *Arch Surg.* 1997;132:505.

483. Jansen A, Brummelkamp WH, Davies GAG, et al. Clinical applications of magnetic rings in colorectal anastomosis. *Surg Gynecol Obstet.* 1981;153:537.

484. Jasperson KW, Tuohy TM, Neklason DW, et al. Hereditary and familial colon cancer. *Gastroenterology.* 2010;138:2044.

485. Jass JR, Love SB, Northover JMA. A new prognostic classification of rectal cancer. *Lancet.* 1987;1:1303.

486. Jayne DG, Fook S, Loi C, et al. Peritoneal carcinomatosis from colorectal cancer. *Br J Surg.* 2002;89:1545.

487. Jeekel J. Curative resection of primary colorectal cancer. *Br J Surg.* 1986;73:687.

488. Jeekel J. Can radical surgery improve survival in colorectal cancer? *World J Surg.* 1987;11:412.

489. Jeffery KM, Harkins B, Cresci GA, et al. The clear liquid diet is no longer a necessity in the routine postoperative management of surgical patients. *Am Surg.* 1996;62:167.

490. Jenkins JT, Duncan JR, Hole D, et al. Malignant disease in peptic ulcer surgery patients after long term follow-up: a cohort study of 1992 patients. *Eur J Surg Oncol.* 2007;33:706.

491. Jennings WC, Wood CD, Guernsey JM. Continuous postoperative lavage in the treatment of peritoneal sepsis. *Dis Colon Rectum.* 1982;25:641.

492. Jensen LS, Andersen A, Fristrup SC, et al. Comparison of one dose versus three doses of prophylactic antibiotics, and the influence of blood transfusion, on infectious complications in acute and elective colorectal surgery. *Br J Surg.* 1990;77:513.

493. Jenson CB, Shahon DB, Wangensteen OH. Evaluation of annual examinations in the detection of cancer: special reference to cancer of the gastrointestinal tract, prostate, breast, and female generative tract. *JAMA.* 1960;174:1783.

494. Jess T, Loftus EV Jr, Velayos FS, et al. Incidence and prognosis of colorectal dysplasia in inflammatory bowel disease: a population-based study from Olmsted County, Minnesota. *Inflamm Bowel Dis.* 2006;12:669.

495. Johansen C, Chow WH, Jörgensen T, et al. Risk of colorectal cancer and other cancers in patients with gall stones. *Gut.* 1996;39:439.

496. Johns LE, Kee F, Collins BJ, et al. Colorectal cancer mortality in first-degree relatives of early-onset colorectal cancer cases. *Dis Colon Rectum.* 2002;45:681.

497. Johnson CD, Lamont PM, Orr N, et al. Is a drain necessary after colonic anastomoses? *J R Soc Med.* 1989;82:661.

498. Johnson K, Bakhsh A, Young D, et al. Correlating computed tomography and positron emission tomography scan with operative findings in metastatic colorectal cancer. *Dis Colon Rectum.* 2001;44:354.

499. Johnson PM, Porter GA, Ricciardi R, et al. Increasing negative lymph node count is independently associated with improved long-term survival in stage IIIB and IIIC colon cancer. *J Clin Oncol.* 2006;24:3570.

500. Joosten JJA, Strobbe LJA, Wauters CAP, et al. Intraoperative lymphatic mapping and the sentinel node concept in colorectal carcinoma. *Br J Surg.* 1999;86:482.

501. Jorgensen T, Rafaelsen S. Gallstones and colorectal cancer: there is a relationship, but it is hardly due to cholecystectomy. *Dis Colon Rectum.* 1992;35:24.

502. Joseph NE, Sigurdson ER, Hanlon AL, et al. Accuracy of determining nodal negativity in colorectal cancer on the basis of the number of nodes retrieved on resection. *Ann Surg Oncol.* 2003;10:213.

503. Juhl G, Larson GM, Mullins R, et al. Six-year results of annual colonoscopy after resection of colorectal cancer. *World J Surg.* 1990;14:255.

504. Kaibara N, Wakatsuki T, Mizusawa K, et al. Negative correlation between cholecystectomy and the subsequent development of large-bowel carcinoma in a low-risk Japanese population. *Dis Colon Rectum.* 1986;29:644.

505. Kameyama M, Fukuda I, Imaoka S, et al. Level of serum gastrin as a predictor of liver metastasis from colorectal cancer. *Dis Colon Rectum.* 1993;36:497.

506. Kanellos I, Demetriades H, Zintzaras E, et al. Incidence and prognostic value of positive peritoneal cytology in colorectal cancer. *Dis Colon Rectum.* 2003;46:535.

507. Kanemitsu Y, Kato T, Hirai T, et al. Survival after curative resection for mucinous adenocarcinoma of the colorectum. *Dis Colon Rectum.* 2003;46:160.

508. Karl RC, Morse SS, Halpert RD, et al. Preoperative evaluation of patients for liver resection: appropriate CT imaging. *Ann Surg.* 1993;217:226.

509. Karlsson S, Jonsson K, Rosengren JE, et al. Angiography in colonic carcinoma. *Dis Colon Rectum.* 1984;27:648.

510. Kehlet H, Holte K. Review of postoperative ileus. *Am J Surg.* 2001;182(suppl):3S.

511. Kehlet H, Mogensen T. Hospital stay of 2 days after open sigmoidectomy with a multimodal rehabilitation programme. *Br J Surg.* 1999;86:227.

512. Keidan RD, Fanning J, Gatenby RA, et al. Recurrent typhlitis: a disease resulting from aggressive chemotherapy. *Dis Colon Rectum.* 1989;32:206.

513. Kell MR, Winter DC, O'Sullivan GC, et al. Biological behaviour and clinical implications of micrometastases. *Br J Surg.* 2000;87:1629.

514. Kemeny N, Daly J, Reichman B, et al. Intrahepatic or systemic infusion of fluorodeoxyuridine in patients with liver metastases from colorectal carcinoma: a randomized trial. *Ann Intern Med.* 1987;107:459.

515. Kerner BA, Oliver GC, Eisenstat TE, et al. Is preoperative computerized tomography useful in assessing patients with colorectal carcinoma? *Dis Colon Rectum.* 1993;36:1050.

516. Kewenter J, Brevinge H, Engarås B, et al. Follow-up after screening for colorectal neoplasms with fecal occult blood testing in a controlled trial. *Dis Colon Rectum.* 1994;37:115.

517. Kewenter J, Engars B, Haglind E, et al. Value of retesting subjects with a positive hemoccult in screening for colorectal cancer. *Br J Surg.* 1990;77:1349.

518. Khatri VP, Chee KG, Petrelli NJ. Modern multimodality approach to hepatic colorectal metastases: solutions and controversies. *Surg Oncol.* 2007;16:71.

519. Khoury GA, Waxman BP. Large-bowel anastomoses. I. The healing process and sutured anastomoses: a review. *Br J Surg.* 1983;70:61.

520. Khubchandani IT, Karamchandani MC, Kleckner FS, et al. Mass screening for colorectal cancer. *Dis Colon Rectum.* 1989;32:754.

521. Kiefer PJ, Thorson AG, Christensen MA. Metachronous colorectal cancer: time interval to presentation of a metachronous cancer. *Dis Colon Rectum.* 1986;29:378.

522. Kim JA, Triozzi PL, Martin EW Jr. Radioimmunoguided surgery for colorectal cancer. *Oncology.* 1993;7:55.

523. Kirklin JW, Dockerty MB, Waugh JM. Role of peritoneal reflection in prognosis of carcinoma of rectum and sigmoid colon. *Surg Gynecol Obstet.* 1949;88:326.

524. Kitagawa Y, Watanabe M, Hasegawa H, et al. Sentinel node mapping for colorectal cancer with radioactive tracer. *Dis Colon Rectum.* 2002;45:1476.

525. Klatt GR, Martin WH, Gillespie JT. Subtotal colectomy with primary anastomosis without diversion in the treatment of obstructing carcinoma of the left colon. *Am J Surg.* 1981;141:577.

526. Klaue P, Eckert P, Kern E. Incidental splenectomy: early and late postoperative complications. *Am J Surg.* 1979;138:296.

527. Kline RS, Catalano MT, Edberg SC, et al. *Streptococcus bovis* septicemia and carcinoma of the colon. *Ann Intern Med.* 1979;91:560.

528. Ko C, Hyman NH; Standards Committee of The American Society of Colon and Rectal Surgeons. Practice parameter for the detection of colorectal neoplasms: an interim report (revised). *Dis Colon Rectum.* 2006;49:299.

529. Ko FC, Liu JM, Chen WS, et al. Risk and patterns of brain metastases in colorectal cancer: 27-year experience. *Dis Colon Rectum.* 1999;42:1467.

530. Köhler L, Eypasch E, Paul A, et al. Myths in management of colorectal malignancy. *Br J Surg.* 1997;84:248.

531. Kokal WA, Duda RB, Azumi N, et al. Tumor DNA content in primary and metastatic colorectal carcinoma. *Arch Surg.* 1986;121:1434.

532. Kokal WA, Gardine RL, Sheibani K, et al. Tumor DNA content in resectable, primary colorectal carcinoma. *Ann Surg.* 1989;209:188.

533. Kokal WA, Sheibani K, Terz J, et al. Tumor DNA content in the prognosis of colorectal carcinoma. *JAMA.* 1986;255:3123.

534. Komuta K, Okudaira S, Haraguchi M, et al. Identification of extracapsular invasion of the metastatic lymph nodes as a useful prognostic sign in patients with resectable colorectal cancer. *Dis Colon Rectum.* 2001;44:1838.

535. Koren R, Siegal A, Klein B, et al. Lymph node-revealing solution: simple new method for detecting minute lymph nodes in colon carcinoma. *Dis Colon Rectum.* 1997;40:407.

536. Kortz WJ, Meyers WC, Hanks JB, et al. Hepatic resection for metastatic cancer. *Ann Surg.* 1984;199:182.

537. Koruth NM, Krukowski ZH, Youngson GG, et al. Intraoperative colonic irrigation in the management of left-sided large-bowel emergencies. *Br J Surg.* 1985;72:708.

538. Koshiji M, Yonekura Y, Saito T, et al. Microsatellite analysis of fecal DNA for colorectal cancer detection. *J Surg Oncol.* 2002;80:34.

539. Kriwanek S, Armbruster C, Dittrich K, et al. Perforated colorectal cancer. *Dis Colon Rectum.* 1996;39:1409.

540. Kronborg O, Hage F, Deichgraeber E. The remaining colon after radical surgery for colorectal cancer: the first three years of a prospective study. *Dis Colon Rectum.* 1983;26:172.

541. Kuhn JA, Corbisiero RM, Buras RR, et al. Intraoperative gamma detection probe with presurgical antibody imaging in colon cancer. *Arch Surg.* 1991;126:1398.

542. Kwok SPY, Varma JS, Li AKC. Quicker intraoperative colonic irrigation. *Br J Surg.* 1989;76:604.

543. Labow SB, Hoexter B, Walrath DC. Colonic adenocarcinomas in patients with ureterosigmoidostomies. *Dis Colon Rectum.* 1979;22:157.

544. Landercasper J, Stolee RT, Steenlage E, et al. Treatment and outcome of right colon cancers adherent to adjacent organs or the abdominal wall. *Arch Surg.* 1992;127:841.

545. Lanfranco of Milan. *Science of chirurgerie.* Fleischhaker R, trans. London, United Kingdom: Early English Text Society, Kegan Paul, Trench, Trubner and Co; 1894.

546. Langevin JM, Nivatvongs S. The true incidence of synchronous cancer of the large bowel. *Am J Surg.* 1984;147:330.

547. Langevin JM, Rothenberger DA, Goldberg SM. Accidental splenic injury during surgical treatment of the colon and rectum. *Surg Gynecol Obstet.* 1984;159:139.

548. Lanspa SJ, Lynch HT, Smyrk TC, et al. Colorectal adenomas in the Lynch syndrome. *Gastroenterology.* 1990;98:1117.

549. Lanspa SJ, Smyrk TC, Lynch HT. The colonoscopist and the Lynch syndromes. *Gastrointest Endosc.* 1990;36:156.

550. Larkin GL, Weber JE. Cost-effectiveness of air bags in motor vehicles. *JAMA.* 1998;279:506.

551. Larson GM, Bond SJ, Shallcross C, et al. Colonoscopy after curative resection of colorectal cancer. *Ann Surg.* 1986;121:331.

552. Lashner BA, Silverstein MD, Hanauer SB. Hazard rates for dysplasia and cancer in ulcerative colitis. Results from a surveillance program. *Dig Dis Sci.* 1989;34:1536.

553. Lau WY, Chu KW, Poon GP, et al. Prophylactic antibiotics in elective colorectal surgery. *Br J Surg.* 1988;75:782.

554. Laurie JA, Moertel CG, Fleming TR, et al. Surgical adjuvant therapy of large-bowel carcinoma: an evaluation of levamisole and the combination of levamisole and fluorouracil. *J Clin Oncol.* 1989;7:1447.

555. Lautenbach E, Forde KA, Neugut AI. Benefits of colonoscopic surveillance after curative resection of colorectal cancer. *Ann Surg.* 1994;220:206.

556. Law WL, Choi HK, Chu KW. Comparison of stenting with emergency surgery as palliative treatment for obstructing primary left-sided colorectal cancer. *Br J Surg.* 2001;90:1429.

557. Lawes DA, SenGupta SB, Boulos PB. Pathogenesis and clinical management of hereditary non-polyposis colorectal cancer. *Br J Surg.* 2002;89:1357.

558. Le TH, Gathright JB Jr. Reconstitution of intestinal continuity after extended left colectomy. *Dis Colon Rectum.* 1993;36:197.

559. Lechner P, Lind P, Binter G, et al. Anticarcinoembryonic antigen immunoscintigraphy with a ^{99m}Tc-Fab' fragment (Immu 4) in primary and recurrent colorectal cancer. *Dis Colon Rectum.* 1993;36:930.

560. Lee EC, Roberts PL, Taranto R, et al. Inpatient versus outpatient bowel preparation for elective colorectal surgery. *Dis Colon Rectum.* 1996;39:369.

561. Leen E, Angerson WG, Cooke TG, et al. Prognostic power of Doppler perfusion index in colorectal cancer: correlation with survival. *Ann Surg.* 1996;223:199.

562. Leggett BA, Cornwell M, Thomas LR, et al. Characteristics of metachronous colorectal carcinoma occurring despite colonoscopic surveillance. *Dis Colon Rectum.* 1997;40:603.

563. Lehman JF, Wiseman JS. The effect of epidural analgesia on the return of peristalsis and the length of stay after elective colonic surgery. *Am Surg.* 1995;61:1009.

564. Leichman C, Lyman G, Remedios P, et al. Molecular biologic correlates with continuous infusion 5-FU (CIFU) or capecitabine(C) in disseminated colorectal cancer (CRC) [abstract 1720]. *Proc ASCO.* 2002.

565. Lelcuk S, Klausner JM, Merhav A, et al. Endoscopic decompression of acute colonic obstruction: avoiding staged surgery. *Ann Surg.* 1986;203:292.

566. Lembert A. Mémoire sur l'enterorrhaphie avec la description d'un procédé nouveau pour pratiquer cette opération chirurgicale. *Rep Gen Anat Physiol Pathol.* 1826;2:100.

567. Lemmens VE, van Lijnschoten I, Janssen- Heijnen ML, et al. Pathology practice patterns affect lymph node evaluation and outcome of colon cancer: a population-based study. *Ann Oncol.* 2006;17:1803–1809.

568. Lemon FR, Walden RT. Death from respiratory system disease among Seventh-Day Adventist men. *JAMA.* 1966;198:117.

569. Lemon FR, Walden RT, Woods RW. Cancer of the lung and mouth in Seventh-Day Adventists: preliminary report on a population study. *Cancer.* 1964;17:486.

570. Lev Z, Kislitsin D, Rennert G, et al. Utilization of *k*-ras mutations identified in stool DNA for the early detection of colorectal cancer. *J Cell Biochem Suppl.* 2000;34:35.

571. Levin B. Screening sigmoidoscopy for colorectal cancer. *N Engl J Med.* 1992;326:700.

572. Levin B, Lieberman DA, McFarland B, et al; American Cancer Society Colorectal Cancer Advisory Group; US Multi-Society Task Force; American College of Radiology Colon Cancer Committee. Screening and surveillance for the early detection of colorectal cancer and adenomatous polyps, 2008: a joint guideline from the American Cancer Society, the US Multi-Society Task Force on Colorectal Cancer, and the American College of Radiology. *Gastroenterology.* 2008;134:1570.

573. Levin ML, Haenszel W, Carroll BE, et al. Cancer incidence in urban and rural areas of New York State. *J Natl Cancer Inst.* 1960;24:1243.

574. LeVoyer TE, Sigurdson ER, Hanlon AL, et al. Colon cancer survival is associated with increasing number of lymph nodes analyzed: a secondary survey of Intergroup trial INT-0089. *J Clin Oncol.* 2003;21:2912.

575. Liang PS, Chen TY, Giovannucci E. Cigarette smoking and colorectal cancer incidence and mortality: systematic review and meta-analysis. *Int J Cancer.* 2009;124:2406.

576. Lieberman DA. Cost-effectiveness of colon cancer screening. *Am J Gastroenterol.* 1991;86:1789.

577. Lieberman DA, Weiss DG, Bond JH, et al. Use of colonoscopy to screen asymptomatic adults for colorectal cancer. *N Engl J Med.* 2000;343:162.

578. Lightdale CJ, Sternberg SS, Posner G, et al. Carcinoma complicating Crohn's disease: report of seven cases and review of the literature. *Am J Med.* 1975;59:262.

579. Limberg B. Diagnosis and staging of colonic tumors by conventional abdominal sonography as compared with hydrocolonic sonography. *N Engl J Med.* 1992;327:65.

580. Limsui D, Vierkant RA, Tillmans LS, et al. Postmenopausal hormone therapy and colorectal cancer risk by molecularly defined subtypes among older women [published online ahead of print October 24, 2011]. *Gut.*

581. Lindmark G, Gerdin B, Påhlman L, et al. Prognostic predictors in colorectal cancer. *Dis Colon Rectum.* 1994;37:1219.

582. Lipkin M, Reddy B, Newmark H, et al. Dietary factors in human colorectal cancer. *Ann Rev Nutr.* 1999;19:545.

583. Liu HP, Yan ZS, Zhang SS. The application of leukocyte adherence inhibition assay to patients with colorectal cancer: comparison with serum level of carcinoembryonic antigen and sialic acid. *Dis Colon Rectum.* 1989;32:210.

584. Liu SKM, Church JM, Lavery IC, et al. Operation in patients with incurable colon cancer: is it worthwhile? *Dis Colon Rectum.* 1997;40:11.

585. Livingstone AS, Hampson LG, Shuster J, et al. Carcinoembryonic antigen in the diagnosis and management of colorectal carcinoma: current status. *Arch Surg.* 1974;109:259.

586. Lobbato VJ, Rothenberg RE, LaRaja RD, et al. Coexistence of abdominal aortic aneurysm and carcinoma of the colon: a dilemma. *J Vasc Surg.* 1985;2:724.

587. Loeb MJ. Comparative strength of inverted, everted and end-on-intestinal anastomoses. *Surg Gynecol Obstet.* 1967;125:301.

588. Logan SE, Meier SJ, Ramming KP. Hepatic resection of metastatic colorectal carcinoma. *Arch Surg.* 1982;117:25.

589. Lo Gerfo P, Herter FP. Carcinoembryonic antigen and prognosis in patients with colon cancer. *Ann Surg.* 1975;181:81.

590. Lokich J, Ahlgren J, Gullo J, et al. A prospective randomized comparison of continuous infusion fluorouracil with a conventional bolus schedule in metastatic colorectal cancer: a Mid-Atlantic Oncology Program Study. *J Clin Oncol.* 1989;7:425.

591. Long RTL, Edwards RH. Implantation metastasis as a cause of local recurrence of colorectal carcinoma. *Am J Surg.* 1989;157:194.

592. Longnecker MP, Orza MJ, Adams ME, et al. A meta-analysis of alcoholic beverage consumption in relation to risk of colorectal cancer. *Cancer Causes Control.* 1990;1:59.

593. Love RR, Morrissey JF. Colonoscopy in asymptomatic individuals with a family history of colorectal cancer. *Arch Intern Med.* 1984;144:2209.

594. Lovett E. Family studies in cancer of the colon and rectum. *Br J Surg.* 1976;63:13.

595. Lucha PA Jr, Rosen L, Olenwine JA, et al. Value of carcinoembryonic antigen monitoring in curative surgery for recurrent colorectal carcinoma. *Dis Colon Rectum.* 1997;40:145.

596. Luna-Pérez P, Rodríguez-Ramírez SE, Gutiérez de la Barrera M, et al. Multivisceral resection for colon cancer. *J Surg Oncol.* 2002;80:100.

597. Lundstedt C, Ekberg H, Halldorsdottir A, et al. Angiography as diagnostic, prognostic and therapeutic tool in liver metastases from a colorectal primary tumor. *Acta Radiol Diagn.* 1985;4:373.

598. Lunniss PJ, Skinner S, Britton KE. Effect of radioimmunoscintigraphy on the management of recurrent colorectal cancer. *Br J Surg.* 1998;86:244.

599. Lynch HT. Frequency of hereditary nonpolyposis colorectal carcinoma (Lynch syndromes I and II). *Gastroenterology.* 1986;90:486.

600. Lynch HT. The surgeon and colorectal cancer genetics: case identification, surveillance, and management strategies. *Arch Surg.* 1990;125:698.

601. Lynch HT, Bronson EK, Strayhorn PC, et al. Genetic diagnosis of Lynch syndrome II in an extended colorectal cancer-prone family. *Cancer.* 1990;66:2233.

602. Lynch HT, Ens JA, Lynch JF. The Lynch syndrome II and urological malignancies. *J Urol.* 1990;143:24.

603. Lynch HT, Guirgis H, Swartz M, et al. Genetics and colon cancer. *Arch Surg.* 1973;106:669.

604. Lynch HT, Kimberling W, Albano WA, et al. Hereditary nonpolyposis colorectal cancer (Lynch syndromes I and II). I. Clinical description of recurrence. *Cancer.* 1985;56:934.

605. Lynch HT, Kriegler M, Christiansen TA, et al. Laryngeal carcinoma in a Lynch syndrome II kindred. *Cancer.* 1988;62:1007.

606. Lynch HT, Lanspa SJ, Boman BM, et al. Hereditary nonpolyposis colorectal cancer: Lynch syndromes I and II. *Gastroenterol Clin North Am.* 1988;17:679.

607. Lynch HT, Lynch J. Genetic predictability and minimal cancer clues in Lynch syndrome II. *Dis Colon Rectum.* 1987;30:243.

608. Lynch HT, Lynch PM, Lanspa SJ, et al. Review of the Lynch syndrome: history, molecular genetics, screening, differential diagnosis, and medicolegal ramifications. *Clin Genet.* 2009;76:1.

609. Lynch HT, Paulson J, Severin M, et al. Failure to diagnose hereditary colorectal cancer and its medicolegal implications. *Dis Colon Rectum.* 1999;42:31.

610. Lynch HT, Smyrk TC, Lynch PM, et al. Adenocarcinoma of the small bowel in Lynch syndrome II. *Cancer.* 1989;64:2178.

611. Lynch HT, Watson P, Lanspa SJ, et al. Natural history of colorectal cancer in hereditary nonpolyposis colorectal cancer (Lynch syndromes I and II). *Dis Colon Rectum.* 1988;31:439.

612. Lynch PM, Lynch HT, Harris RE. Hereditary proximal colonic cancer. *Dis Colon Rectum.* 1977;20:662.

613. Lyons JL, Klauber MR, Gardner JW, et al. Cancer incidence in Mormons and non-Mormons in Utah, 1966–1970. *N Engl J Med.* 1976;294:129.

614. MacDougall IPM. The cancer risk in ulcerative colitis. *Lancet.* 1964;2:655.

615. MacGregor AB, Falk RE. Immunotherapy of malignant disease: part 2. *J R Coll Surg Edinb.* 1976;21:43.

616. MacGregor AMC. Mucus-secreting adenomatous polyp at the site of ureterosigmoidostomy: a case report and review of the literature. *Br J Surg.* 1968;55:591.

617. Machi J, Isomoto H, Kurohiji T, et al. Detection of unrecognized liver metastases from colorectal cancers by routine use of operative ultrasonography. *Dis Colon Rectum.* 1986;29:405.

618. Machi J, Isomoto H, Kurohiji T, et al. Accuracy of intraoperative ultrasonography in diagnosing liver metastasis from colorectal cancer: evaluation with postoperative follow-up results. *World J Surg.* 1991;15:551.

619. Machover D, Diaz-Rubio E, de Gramont A, et al. Modulation of fluorouracil by LV in patients with advanced colorectal cancer: evidence in terms of response rate: Advanced Colorectal Cancer Meta-Analysis Project. *J Clin Oncol.* 1992;10:896.

620. MacKeigan JM, Ferguson JA. Prophylactic oophorectomy and colorectal cancer in premenopausal patients. *Dis Colon Rectum.* 1979;22:401.

621. Macrae F, St John DJB. Hemoccult tests. *Dig Dis Sci.* 1987;32:947.

622. Madlensky L, Bapat B, Redston M, et al. Using genetic information to make surgical decisions: report of a case of a 13-year-old boy with colon cancer. *Dis Colon Rectum.* 1997;40:240.

623. Mahajna A, Krausz M, Rosin D, et al. Bowel preparation is associated with spillage of bowel contents in colorectal surgery. *Dis Colon Rectum.* 2005;48:1626.

624. Mainar A, de Gregorio Ariza MA, Tejero E, et al. Acute colorectal obstruction: treatment with self-expandable metal stents before scheduled surgery: results of a multicenter study. *Radiology.* 1999;210:65.

625. Mainar A, Tejero E, Maynar M, et al. Colorectal obstruction: treatment with metallic stents. *Radiology.* 1996;198:761.

626. Mäkelä JT, Laitinen SO, Kairaluoma MI. Five-year follow-up after radical surgery for colorectal cancer: results of a prospective randomized trial. *Arch Surg.* 1995;130:1062.

627. Malassagne B, Valleur P, Serra J, et al. Relationship of apical lymph node involvement to survival in resected colon carcinoma. *Dis Colon Rectum.* 1993;36:645.

628. Malthaner RA, Hakki FZ, Saini N, et al. Anastomotic compression button: a new mechanical device for sutureless bowel anastomosis. *Dis Colon Rectum.* 1990;33:291.

629. Manayan RC, Hart MJ, Friend WG. Radioimmunoguided surgery for colorectal cancer. *Am J Surg.* 1997;173:386.

630. Mandel JS, Bond JH, Bradley M. Sensitivity, specificity, and positive predictivity of the Hemoccult test in screening for colorectal cancers. *Gastroenterology.* 1989;97:597.

631. Mandel JS, Bond JH, Church TR, et al. Reducing mortality from colorectal cancer by screening for fecal occult blood. *N Engl J Med.* 1993;328:1365.

632. Mannes AG, Weinzierl M, Stellaard F, et al. Adenomas of the large intestine after cholecystectomy. *Gut.* 1984;25:863.

633. Mannes GA, Maier A, Thieme C, et al. Relation between the frequency of colorectal adenoma and the serum cholesterol level. *N Engl J Med.* 1986;315:1634.

634. Mapp TJ, Hardcastle JD, Moss SM, et al. Survival of patients with colorectal cancer diagnosed in a randomized controlled trial of faecal occult blood screening. *Br J Surg.* 1999;86:1286.

635. Markman M. Intraperitoneal chemotherapy in the management of colon cancer. *Semin Oncol.* 1999;26:536.

636. Markowitz A, Saleemi K, Freeman LM. Role of In-111-labeled CYT-103 immunoscintigraphy in the evaluation of patients with recurrent colorectal carcinoma. *Clin Nucl Med.* 1993;18:685.

637. Marsh J, Donnan PT, Hamer-Hodges DW. Association between transfusion with plasma and the recurrence of colorectal carcinoma. *Br J Surg.* 1990;77:623.

638. Martin EW Jr, Carey LC. Second-look surgery for colorectal cancer: the second time around. *Ann Surg.* 1991;214:321.

639. Martin EW Jr, James KK, Hurtubise PE, et al. The use of CEA as an early indicator for gastrointestinal tumor recurrence and second-look procedures. *Cancer.* 1977;39:440.

640. Martin EW Jr, Kibbey WE, DiVecchia L, et al. Carcinoembryonic antigen: clinical and historical aspects. *Cancer.* 1976;37:62.

641. Martin EW Jr, Minton JP, Carey LC. CEA-directed second-look surgery in the asymptomatic patient after primary resection of colorectal carcinoma. *Ann Surg.* 1985;202:310.

642. Martin EW Jr, Mojzisik CM, Hinkle GH Jr, et al. Radioimmunoguided surgery using monoclonal antibody. *Am J Surg.* 1988;156:386.

643. Martin R, Paty P, Fong Y, et al. Simultaneous liver and colorectal resections are safe for synchronous colorectal liver metastasis. *J Am Coll Surg.* 2003;197:233; discussion 241.

644. Martinez-Santos C, Lobato RF, Fradejas JM, et al. Self-expandable stent before elective surgery vs. emergency surgery for the treatment of malignant colorectal obstructions: comparison of primary anastomosis and morbidity rates. *Dis Colon Rectum.* 2002;45:401.

645. Martyak SN, Curtis LW. Abdominal incision and closure, a systems approach. *Am J Surg.* 1976;131:476.

646. Mason MH III, Kovalcik PJ. Ovarian metastases from colon carcinoma. *J Surg Oncol.* 1981;17:33.

647. Matsui O, Takashima T, Kadoya M, et al. Liver metastases from colorectal cancers: detection with CT during arterial portography. *Radiology.* 1987;165:65.

648. Mavligit GM, Burgess MA, Seibert GB, et al. Prolongation of postoperative disease-free interval and survival in human colorectal cancer by B.C.G. or B.C.G plus 5-fluorouracil. *Lancet.* 1976;1:171.

649. Max E, Sweeney WB, Bailey HR, et al. Results of 1,000 single-layer continuous polypropylene intestinal anastomoses. *Am J Surg.* 1991;162:461.

650. Maxwell JW Jr, Davis WC, Jackson FC. Colon carcinoma and inguinal hernia. *Surg Clin North Am.* 1965;45:1165.

651. Mayer RJ. Targeted therapy for advanced colorectal cancer—more is not necessarily better [editorial]. *N Eng J Med.* 2009;360:623.

652. Mayer RJ. Moving beyond fluorouracil for colorectal cancer. *N Engl J Med.* 2000;343:963.

653. Mayo WJ. The cancer problem. *Lancet.* 1915;35:339.

654. McAndrew MR, Saba AK. Efficacy of routine preoperative computed tomography scans in colon cancer. *Am Surg.* 1999;65:205.

655. McArdle CS, McMillan DC, Hole DJ. Male gender adversely effects survival following surgery for colorectal cancer. *Br J Surg.* 2003;90:711.

656. McArdle CS, Morran CG, Pettit L, et al. Value of oral antibiotic prophylaxis in colorectal surgery. *Br J Surg.* 1995;82:1046.

657. McCall JL, Black RB, Rich CA, et al. The value of serum carcinoembryonic antigen in predicting recurrent disease following curative resection of colorectal cancer. *Dis Colon Rectum.* 1994;37:875.

658. McCormack PM, Attiyeh FF. Resected pulmonary metastases from colorectal cancer. *Dis Colon Rectum.* 1979;22:553.

659. McCormack PM, Burt ME, Bains MS, et al. Lung resection for colorectal metastases: 10-year results. *Arch Surg.* 1992;127:1403.

660. McCulloch PG, Blamey SL, Finlay IG, et al. A prospective comparison of gentamicin and metronidazole and moxalactam in the prevention of septic complications associated with elective operations of the colon and rectum. *Surg Gynecol Obstet.* 1986;162:521.

661. McFarland RJ, Talbot RW, Woolf N, et al. Dysplasia of the colon after jejuno-ileal bypass. *Br J Surg.* 1987;74:21.

662. McGarr SE, Ridlon JM, Hylemon PB. Diet, anaerobic bacterial metabolism, and colon cancer: a review of the literature. *J Clin Gastroenterol.* 2005;39:98.

663. McIntyre A, Gibson PR, Young GP. Butyrate production from dietary fibre and protection against large-bowel cancer in a rat model. *Gut.* 1993;34:386.

664. McKenna JP, Currie DJ, MacDonald JA. The use of continuous postoperative peritoneal lavage in the management of diffuse peritonitis. *Surg Gynecol Obstet.* 1970;130:254.

665. McMahon AJ, Auld CD, Dale BAS, et al. *Streptococcus bovis* septicaemia associated with uncomplicated colonic carcinoma. *Br J Surg.* 1991;78:883.

666. McMillan DC, Canna K, McArdle CS. Systemic inflammatory response predicts survival following curative resection of colorectal cancer. *Br J Surg.* 2003;90:215.

667. McMillan DC, Wotherspoon HA, Fearon KCH, et al. A prospective study of tumor recurrence and acute-phase response after apparently curative colorectal cancer surgery. *Am J Surg.* 1995;170:319.

668. McVay JR Jr. The appendix in relation to neoplastic disease. *Cancer.* 1964;17:929.

669. Meagher AP, Stuart M. Colonoscopy in patients with a family history of colorectal cancer. *Dis Colon Rectum.* 1992;35:315.

670. Meagher AP, Wolff BG. Right hemicolectomy with a linear cutting stapler. *Dis Colon Rectum.* 1994;37:1043.

671. Mecklin JP, Järvinen HJ. Clinical features of colorectal carcinoma in cancer family syndrome. *Dis Colon Rectum.* 1986;29:160.

672. Mecklin JP, Järvinen HJ. Treatment and follow-up strategies in hereditary nonpolyposis colorectal carcinoma. *Dis Colon Rectum.* 1993;36:927.

673. Mecklin JP, Järvinen HJ, Hakkiluoto A, et al. Frequency of hereditary nonpolyposis colorectal cancer: a prospective multicenter study in Finland. *Dis Colon Rectum.* 1995;38:588.

674. Mecklin JP, Sipponen P, Järvinen HJ. Histopathology of colorectal carcinomas and adenomas in cancer family syndrome. *Dis Colon Rectum.* 1986;29:849.

675. Medina M, Paddock HN, Connolly RJ, et al. Novel antiadhesion barrier does not prevent anastomotic healing in a rabbit model. *J Invest Surg.* 1995;8:179.

676. Menaker GJ. The use of antibiotics in surgical treatment of the colon. *Surg Gynecol Obstet.* 1987;164:581.

677. Menko FH, Wijnen JT, Vasen HFA, et al. Genetic counseling in hereditary nonpolyposis colorectal cancer. *Oncology.* 1996;10:71.

678. Mensink PBF, Kolkman JJ, van Baarlen J, et al. Change in anatomic distribution and incidence of colorectal carcinoma over a period of 15 years: clinical considerations. *Dis Colon Rectum.* 2002;45:1393.

679. Menzies D. Peritoneal adhesions: incidence, cause, and prevention. *Surg Ann.* 1992;24:27.

680. Menzies D, Ellis H. Intestinal obstruction from adhesions: how big is the problem? *Ann R Coll Surg Engl.* 1990;72:60.

681. Metzger PP. Adenocarcinoma developing in a rectosigmoid conduit used for urinary diversion: report of a case. *Dis Colon Rectum.* 1989;32:247.

682. Michener WM, Gage RP, Sauer WG, et al. The prognosis of chronic ulcerative colitis in children. *N Engl J Med.* 1961;265:1075.

683. Mikulicz J von. Chirurgische erjahrun ber das Darmcarcinom [Surgical experience with intestinal carcinoma]. *Arch Klin Chir Berl.* 1903;69:28. (Translated in *Med Classics.* 1937–1938;2:210 and reproduced in *Dis Colon Rectum.* 1980;23:513.)

684. Milham S Jr. *Occupational mortality in Washington State, 1950–1971.* Vols 2–3. Cincinnati, OH: United States Dept of Health, Education and Welfare, Public Health Service; Centers for Disease Control; and National Institute for Occupational Safety and Health, Division of Surveillance, Hazard Evaluation, and Field Studies; 1976.

685. Minervini A, Bentley S, Young D. Prophylactic saline peritoneal lavage in elective colorectal operations. *Dis Colon Rectum.* 1980;23:392.

686. Minsky BD. Clinicopathologic impact of colloid in colorectal carcinoma. *Dis Colon Rectum.* 1990;33:714.

687. Minsky BD. Adjuvant therapy of rectal cancer. *Semin Oncol.* 1999;26:540.

688. Minton JP, Hamilton WB, Sardi A, et al. Results of surgical excision of one to 13 hepatic metastases in 98 consecutive patients. *Arch Surg.* 1989;124:46.

689. Minton JP, James KK, Hurtubise PE, et al. The use of serial carcinoembryonic antigen determinations to predict recurrence of carcinoma of the colon and the time for a second-look operation. *Surg Gynecol Obstet.* 1978;147:208.

690. Minu AR, Takemura K, Iwai T, et al. Role of wrapping in concomitant intra-abdominal aneurysm and colorectal carcinoma: report of three cases. *Dis Colon Rectum.* 1992;35:991.

691. Misiakos EP, Karidis NP, Kouraklis G. Current treatment for colorectal liver metastases. *World J Gastroenterol.* 2011;17:4067.

692. Mitchell E, Piperdi B, Le Coutre PD, et al. The efficacy and safety of panitumumab administered concomitantly with FOLFIRI or irinotecan in second line therapy for metastatic colorectal cancer; the secondary analysis from STEPP (skin toxicity evaluation of protocol with panitumumab) by KRAS status. *Clin Colorectal Cancer.* 2011;10:333.

693. Mitmaker B, Begin LR, Gordon PH. Nuclear shape as a prognostic discriminant in colorectal carcinoma. *Dis Colon Rectum.* 1991;34:249.

694. Mitry E, Benhamiche AM, Jouve JL, et al. Colorectal adenocarcinoma in patients under 45 years of age: comparison with older patients in a well-defined French population. *Dis Colon Rectum.* 2001;44:380.

695. Mitry E, Bouvier AM, Esteve J, et al. Benefit of operative mortality reduction on colorectal cancer survival. *Br J Surg.* 2002;89:1557.

696. Miyanari N, Mori T, Takahashi K, et al. Evaluation of aggressively treated patients with unresectable multiple liver metastases from colorectal cancer. *Dis Colon Rectum.* 2002;45:1503.

697. Moertel CG, Fleming TR, MacDonald JS, et al. Levamisole and fluorouracil for adjuvant therapy of resected colon carcinoma. *N Engl J Med.* 1990;322:352.

698. Moertel CG, Fleming TR, MacDonald JS, et al. An evaluation of the carcinoembryonic antigen (CEA) for monitoring patients with resected colon cancer. *JAMA.* 1993;270:943.

699. Moertel CG, Fleming TR, MacDonald JS, et al. Intergroup study of fluorouracil plus levamisole adjuvant therapy for stage III Dukes' B2 colon cancer. *J Clin Oncol.* 1995;13:2936.

700. Moertel CG, Hill JR, Dockerty MB. The routine proctoscopic examination: a second look. *Mayo Clin Proc.* 1966;41:368.

701. Moertel CG, Schutt AJ, Go VLW. Carcinoembryonic antigen test for recurrent colorectal carcinoma. *JAMA.* 1978;239:1065.

702. Moffat FL Jr, Pinsky CM, Hammershaimb L, et al. Clinical utility of external immunoscintigraphy with IMMU-4 technetium-99m Fab' antibody fragment in patients undergoing surgery for carcinoma of the colon and rectum: results of a pivotal, phase III trial. *J Clin Oncol.* 1996;14:2295.

703. Monk BJ, Berman ML, Montz FJ. Adhesions after extensive gynecologic surgery: clinical significance, etiology, and prevention. *Am J Obstet Gynecol.* 1994;170:1396.

704. Moore HC, Haller DG. Adjuvant therapy of colon cancer. *Semin Oncol.* 1999;59:545.

705. Moore J, Hyman N, Callas P, et al. Staging error does not explain the relationship between the number of lymph nodes in a colon cancer specimen and survival. *Surgery.* 2010;147:358.

706. Moorehead RJ, Kernohan RM, Patterson CC, et al. Does cholecystectomy predispose to colorectal cancer? A case-control study. *Dis Colon Rectum.* 1986;29:36.

707. Morabito A, Gattuso D, Sarmiento R, et al. Rofecoxib associated with an antiangiogenic schedule of weekly irinotecan and infusional 5-fluorouracil as second line treatment of patients with metastatic colorectal cancer: results of a dose-finding study [abstract 1311]. *Proc ASCO.* 2003;22.

708. Moran K, Cooke T, Forster G, et al. Prognostic value of nucleolar organizer regions and ploidy values in advanced colorectal cancer. *Br J Surg.* 1989;76:1152.

709. Morgan CN. The management of carcinoma of the colon. *Ann R Coll Surg Engl.* 1952;10:305.

710. Morgenstern L, Lee SE. Spatial distribution of colonic carcinoma. *Arch Surg.* 1978;113:1142.

711. Morita S, Nomura T, Fukushima Y, et al. Does serum CA 19–9 play a practical role in the management of patients with colorectal cancer? *Dis Colon Rectum.* 2004;47:227.

712. Morowitz DA, Block GE, Kirshner JB. Adenocarcinoma of the ileum complicating chronic regional enteritis. *Gastroenterology.* 1968;55:397.

713. Morrow M, Enker WE. Late ovarian metastases in carcinoma of the colon and rectum. *Arch Surg.* 1984;119:1385.

714. Mortensen NJ, Eltringham WK, Mountford RA, et al. Direct vision brush cytology with colonoscopy: an aid to the accurate diagnosis of colonic strictures. *Br J Surg.* 1984;71:930.

715. Morton AL, Taylor EW, Lindsay G, et al. A multicenter study to compare cefotetan alone with cefotetan and metronidazole as prophylaxis against infection in elective colorectal operations. *Surg Gynecol Obstet.* 1989;169:41.

716. Morvay K, Szentlleki K, Trk G, et al. Effect of change of fecal bile acid excretion achieved by operative procedures on 1,2-dimethylhydrazine induced colon cancer in rats. *Dis Colon Rectum.* 1989;32:860.

717. Mullan FJ, Wilson HK, Majury CW, et al. Bile acids and the increased risk of colorectal tumours after truncal vagotomy. *Br J Surg.* 1990;77:1085.

718. Mulsow J, Winter DC, O'Keane JC, et al. Sentinel lymph node mapping in colorectal cancer. *Br J Surg.* 2003;90:659.

719. Munro A, Steele RJC, Logie JRC. Technique for intraoperative colonic irrigation. *Br J Surg*. 1987;74:1039.

720. Murphy JB. Cholecysto-intestinal, gastro-intestinal and enterointestinal anastomosis, and approximation without sutures. *Med Rec N Y*. 1892;42:665.

721. Murphy TK, Rodriguez C, Kahn HS, et al. Body mass index and colon cancer mortality in a large prospective study. *Am J Epidemiology*. 2000;152:847.

722. Mzabi R, Himal HS, Demers R, et al. A multiparametric computer analysis of carcinoma of the colon. *Surg Gynecol Obstet*. 1976;143:959.

723. Nagakura S, Shirai Y, Hatakeyama K. Computed tomographic features of colorectal carcinoma liver metastases predict posthepatectomy patient survival. *Dis Colon Rectum*. 2001;44:1148.

724. Nagorney DM, Sarr MG, McIlrath DC. Surgical management of intussusception in the adult. *Ann Surg*. 1981;193:230.

725. Nakagoe T, Sawai T, Tsuji T, et al. Use of minilaparotomy in the treatment of colonic cancer. *Br J Surg*. 2001;88:831.

726. Nakajima N, Ramadan H, Lapi N, et al. Rectal carcinoma with solitary cerebral metastasis: report of a case and review of the literature. *Dis Colon Rectum*. 1979;22:252.

727. Narod SA, Ginsburg O, Jothy S. Family history and colorectal cancer. *N Engl J Med*. 1995;332:1578.

728. Nathanson SD, Schultz L, Tilley B, et al. Carcinomas of the colon and rectum: a comparison of staging classifications. *Am Surg*. 1986;52:428.

729. National Board of Health and Welfare. *Cancer Incidence in Sweden, 1959–1965*. Stockholm, Sweden: Swedish Cancer Registry; 1971.

730. National Quality Forum. Specifications of the national voluntary consensus standards for breast and colon cancer. http://www.qualityforum.org/pdf/cancer/txAppA-Specifications_web.pdf. Accessed October 1, 2008.

731. Nava HR, Pagana TJ. Postoperative surveillance of colorectal carcinoma. *Cancer*. 1982;49:1043.

732. Navsaria PH, Bunting M, Omoshoro-Jones J, et al. Temporary closure of open abdominal wounds by the modified sandwich-vacuum pack technique. *Br J Surg*. 2003;90:718.

733. Nelson H, Petrelli N, Carlin A, et al. Guidelines 2000 for colon and rectal cancer surgery. *J Natl Cancer Inst*. 2001;93:583.

734. Nesbakken A, Haffner J. Colo-recto-anal intussusception: case report. *Acta Chir Scand*. 1989;155:201.

735. Nesbitt JC, Moise KJ, Sawyers JL. Colorectal carcinoma in pregnancy. *Arch Surg*. 1985;120:636.

736. Neugut AI, Johnsen CM, Finl DJ. Serum cholesterol levels in adenomatous polyps and cancer of the colon: a case-control study. *JAMA*. 1986;255:365.

737. Newill VA. Distribution of cancer mortality among ethnic subgroups of the white population of New York City, 1953–1958. *J Natl Cancer Inst*. 1961;26:405.

738. Newland RC, Chapuis PH, Smyth EJ. The prognostic value of substaging colorectal carcinoma: a prospective study of 1117 cases with standardized pathology. *Cancer*. 1987;60:852.

739. Nichols RL, Broido P, Condon RE, et al. Effect of preoperative neomycin-erythromycin intestinal preparation on the incidence of infectious complications following colon surgery. *Ann Surg*. 1973;178:453.

740. Nicholson JR, Aust JC. Rising carcinoembryonic antigen titers in colorectal carcinoma: an indication for the second-look procedure. *Dis Colon Rectum*. 1978;21:163.

741. Nieroda CA, Mojzisik C, Sardi A, et al. The impact of radioimmunoguided surgery (RIGS) on surgical decision making in colorectal cancer. *Dis Colon Rectum*. 1989;32:927.

742. Nigro ND. A strategy for prevention of cancer of the large bowel. *Dis Colon Rectum*. 1982;25:755.

743. Nigro ND, Bull AW. Experimental intestinal carcinogenesis. *Br J Surg*. 1985;72(suppl):S36.

744. Nigro ND, Bull AW, Klopfer BA, et al. Effect of dietary fiber on azoxymethane-induced intestinal carcinogenesis in the rat. *J Natl Cancer Inst*. 1979;62:1097.

745. Nitschke J, Richter H, Herguth D, et al. Acute appendicitis and postoperative fecal fistula: symptoms of an unrecognized carcinoma of the colon. *Dis Colon Rectum*. 1976;19:605.

746. Nivatvongs S, Gilbertsen VA, Goldberg SM, et al. Distribution of large-bowel cancers detected by occult blood test in asymptomatic patients. *Dis Colon Rectum*. 1982;25:420.

747. Norfleet RG. Effect of diet on fecal occult blood testing in patients with colorectal polyps. *Dig Dis Sci*. 1986;31:498.

748. Northover J. Carcinoembryonic antigen and recurrent colorectal cancer. *Gut*. 1986;27:117.

749. Norum J, Olsen JA. Cost-effectiveness approach to the Norwegian follow-up programme in colorectal cancer. *Ann Oncol*. 1997;8:1081.

750. Obrand DI, Gordon PH. Incidence and patterns of recurrence following curative resection for colorectal carcinoma. *Dis Colon Rectum*. 1997;40:15.

751. O'Brien PH, Newton BB, Metcalf JS, et al. Oophorectomy in women with carcinoma of the colon and rectum. *Surg Gynecol Obstet*. 1981;153:827.

752. *Occupational mortality. Decennial Supplement England and Wales. Population Censuses and Surveys Office, 1970–1972*. London, United Kingdom: HM Stationery Office; 1978.

753. O'Connell M, Laurie J, Kahn M, et al. Prospective randomized trial of postoperative adjuvant therapy in patients with high risk colon cancer. *J Clin Oncol*. 1998;16:295.

754. O'Connell M, Malliard J, MacDonald J, et al. An Intergroup trial of intensive 5-FU and low dose leucovorin as surgical adjuvant for high-risk colon cancer [abstract 190]. *Proc ASCO*. 1993;12.

755. Oda S, Oki E, Maehara Y, et al. Precise assessment of microsatellite instability using high resolution fluorescent microsatellite analysis. *Nucl Acids Res*. 1997;25:3415.

756. O'Dwyer PJ, Benson A. Epidermal growth factor receptor targeted therapy in colorectal cancer. *Semin Oncol*. 2002;29(suppl 14):10.

757. O'Dwyer PJ, Mojzisik C, McCabe DP, et al. Reoperation directed by carcinoembryonic antigen level: the importance of a thorough preoperative evaluation. *Am J Surg*. 1988;155:227.

758. Oh-e H, Tanaka S, Kitadai Y, et al. Angiogenesis at the site of deepest penetration predicts lymph node metastasis of submucosal colorectal cancer. *Dis Colon Rectum*. 2001;44:1129.

759. Ohlsson B, Breland U, Ekberg H, et al. Follow-up after curative surgery for colorectal carcinoma: randomized comparison with no follow-up. *Dis Colon Rectum*. 1995;38:619.

760. Oikonomakis I, Wexner SD, Gervaz P, et al. Seprafilm: a retrospective preliminary evaluation of the impact on short-term oncologic outcome in colorectal cancer. *Dis Colon Rectum*. 2002;45:1376.

761. Ojo J, De Silva S, Han E, et al. Krukenberg tumors from colorectal cancer: presentation, treatment and outcomes. *Am Surg*. 2011;77:1381.

762. Oliveira L, Wexner SD, Daniel N, et al. Mechanical bowel preparation for elective colorectal surgery: a prospective, randomized, surgeon-blinded trial comparing sodium phosphate and polyethylene glycol-based oral lavage solutions. *Dis Colon Rectum*. 1997;40:585.

763. Olsen AK. Intraoperative ultrasonography and the detection of liver metastases in patients with colorectal cancer. *Br J Surg*. 1990;77:998.

764. Ondrula DP, Nelson RL, Prasad ML, et al. Multifactorial index of preoperative risk factors in colon resections. *Dis Colon Rectum*. 1992;35:117.

765. Onik G, Rubinsky B, Zemel R, et al. Ultrasound-guided hepatic cryosurgery in the treatment of metastatic colon carcinoma: preliminary results. *Cancer*. 1991;67:901.

766. Operative Laparoscopy Study Group. Postoperative adhesion development after operative laparoscopy: evaluation at early second-look procedures. *Fertil Steril*. 1991;55:700.

767. Oren JW, Folse R, Kraudel KL, et al. The preoperative liver scan and surgical decision making in patients with colorectal cancer. *Am J Surg*. 1986;151:452.

768. Ostadi MA, Harnish JL, Stegienko S, et al. Factors affecting the number of lymph nodes retrieved in colorectal cancer specimens. *Surg Endosc*. 2007;21:2142.

769. Ostrow JD, Mulvaney CA, Hansell JR, et al. Sensitivity and reproducibility of chemical tests for fecal occult blood with an emphasis on false-positive reactions. *Am J Dig Dis*. 1973;18:930.

770. Ottery FD, Scupham RK, Weese JL. Chemical cholecystitis after intrahepatic chemotherapy. The case for prophylactic cholecystectomy during pump replacement. *Dis Colon Rectum*. 1986;29:187.

771. Ovaska J, Järvinen H, Kujari H, et al. Follow-up of patients operated on for colorectal carcinoma. *Am J Surg*. 1990;159:593.

772. Ovaska J, Järvinen HJ, Mecklin JP. The value of a follow-up programme after radical surgery for colorectal carcinoma. *Scand J Gastroenterol*. 1989;24:416.

773. Overholt BF. Colonoscopy and colon cancer: current clinical practice. *CA Cancer J Clin*. 1982;32:180.

774. Pagana TJ, Ledesma EJ, Mittelman A, et al. The use of colonoscopy in the study of synchronous colorectal neoplasms. *Cancer*. 1984;53:356.

775. Paganini-Hill A. Estrogen replacement therapy and colorectal cancer risk in elderly women. *Dis Colon Rectum*. 1999;42:1300.

776. Pages F, Berger A, Camus M, et al. Effector memory T cells, early metastasis, and survival in colorectal cancer. *N Engl J Med*. 2005;353:2654.

777. Painter NS, Burkitt DP. Diverticular disease of the colon: a deficiency disease of Western civilization. *BMJ*. 1971;2:450.

778. Palmer ML, Herrera L, Petrelli NJ. Colorectal adenocarcinoma in patients less than 40 years of age. *Dis Colon Rectum*. 1991;34:343.

779. Palmer M, Petrelli NJ, Herrera L. No treatment option for liver metastases from colorectal adenocarcinoma. *Dis Colon Rectum*. 1989;32:698.

780. Parikshak M, Pawlak SE, Eggenberger JC, et al. The role of endoscopic colon surveillance in the transplant population. *Dis Colon Rectum.* 2002;45:1655.

781. Park JY, Mitrou PN, Dahm CC, et al. Baseline alcohol consumption, type of alcoholic beverage and risk of colorectal cancer in the European Prospective Investigation into Cancer and Nutrition-Norfolk study. *Cancer Epidemiol.* 2009;33:347.

782. Parrott NR, Lennard TWJ, Taylor RMR, et al. Effect of perioperative blood transfusion on recurrence of colorectal cancer. *Br J Surg.* 1986;73:970.

783. Patt YZ, Mavligit G, Chuang VP, et al. Arteriovenous carcinoembryonic antigen gradient: determination by selective angiography for localization of metastatic colorectal cancer. *Arch Surg.* 1980;115:1122.

784. Paul FT. Colectomy. *BMJ.* 1895;1:1136.

785. Payne JE. International colorectal carcinoma staging and grading. *Dis Colon Rectum.* 1989;32:282.

786. Peethambaram P, Weiss M, Loprinzi CL, et al. An evaluation of postoperative follow-up tests in colon cancer patients treated for cure. *Oncology.* 1997;54:287.

787. Pemberton M. Carcinoma of the large intestine with survival in a child of nine and in his father; a study of carcinoma of the colon with particular reference to children. *Br J Surg.* 1970;57:841.

788. Petersen BM Jr, Bass BL, Bates HR, et al. Use of radiolabeled murine monoclonal antibody, ^{111}In-CYT-103, in the management of colon cancer. *Am J Surg.* 1993;165:137.

789. Petrelli NI, Nambisan RN, Herrera L, et al. Hepatic resection for isolated metastasis from colorectal carcinoma. *Am J Surg.* 1985;149:205.

790. Petros JG, Realica R, Ahmad S, et al. Patient-controlled analgesia and prolonged ileus after uncomplicated colectomy. *Am J Surg.* 1995; 170:371.

791. Philip RS. Efficacy of preoperative bowel preparation at home. *Am Surg.* 1995;61:368.

792. Phillips KA, Liang SY, Ladabaum U, et al. Trends in colonoscopy for colorectal cancer screening. *Med Care.* 2007;45:160.

793. Phillips RKS, Hittinger R, Fry JS, et al. Malignant large-bowel obstruction. *Br J Surg.* 1985;72:296.

794. Phillips RL. Role of life-style and dietary habits in risk of cancer among Seventh-Day Adventists. *Cancer Res.* 1975;35(suppl 2):3513.

795. Philpott GW, Siegel BA, Schwarz SW, et al. Immunoscintigraphy with a new indium-111-labeled monoclonal antibody (Mab 1A3) in patients with colorectal cancer. *Dis Colon Rectum.* 1994;37:782.

796. Pickren JW. Nodal clearance and detection. *JAMA.* 1975;231:969.

797. Piedbois P, Michiels S. Survival benefit of 5FU/LV over 5FU bolus in patients with advanced colorectal cancer: an updated meta-analysis based on 2,751 patients [abstract 1180]. *Proc ASCO.* 2003;22.

798. Pietra N, Sarli L, Costi R, et al. Role of follow-up in management of local recurrences of colorectal cancer: a prospective, randomized study. *Dis Colon Rectum.* 1998;41:1127.

799. Pihl E, Hughes ESR, McDermott FT, et al. Lung recurrence after curative surgery for colorectal cancer. *Dis Colon Rectum.* 1987;30:417.

800. Piscatelli N, Hyman N, Osler T. Localizing colorectal cancer by colonoscopy. *Arch Surg.* 2005;140:932.

801. Pitluk H, Poticha SM. Carcinoma of the colon and rectum in patients less than 40 years of age. *Surg Gynecol Obstet.* 1983;157:335.

802. Poeze M, Houbiers JGA, van de Velde CJH, et al. Radical resection of locally advanced colorectal cancer. *Br J Surg.* 1995;82:1386.

803. Polk W, Fong Y, Karpeh M, et al. A technique for the use of cryosurgery to assist hepatic resection. *J Am Coll Surg.* 1995;180:171.

804. Pollack AV, Playforth MJ, Evans M. Peroperative lavage of the obstructed left colon to allow safe primary anastomosis. *Dis Colon Rectum.* 1987;30:171.

805. Pollack ES, Nomura AMY, Heilbrun LK, et al. Prospective study of alcohol consumption and cancer. *N Engl J Med.* 1984;310:617.

806. Ponz de Leon M, Sassatelli R, Sacchetti C, et al. Familial aggregation of tumors in the three-year experience of a population-based colorectal cancer registry. *Cancer Res.* 1989;49:4344.

807. Poon M, O'Connell M, Moertel C, et al. Biochemical modulation of fluorouracil: evidence of significant improvement of survival and quality of life in patients with advanced colorectal cancer. *J Clin Oncol.* 1989;7:1407.

808. Portes C, Majarakis JD. Proctosigmoidoscopy: incidence of polyps in 50,000 examinations. *JAMA.* 1957;163:411.

809. Powell BL, Craig JB, Muss HB. Secondary malignancies of the penis and epididymis: a case report and review of the literature. *J Clin Oncol.* 1985;3:110.

810. Prager E, Swinton NW, Corman ML, et al. Intravenous pyelography in colorectal surgery. *Dis Colon Rectum.* 1973;16:479.

811. Prandi M, Lionetto R, Bini A, et al. Prognostic evaluation of stage B colon cancer patients is improved by an adequate lymphadenectomy: results of a secondary analysis of a large scale adjuvant trial. *Ann Surg.* 2002;235:458.

812. Pratt SM, Weaver FA, Potts JR III. Preoperative evaluation of patients with inguinal hernia for colorectal disease. *Surg Gynecol Obstet.* 1987;165:53.

813. Pucciarelli S, Agostini M, Viel A, et al. Early-age-at-onset colorectal cancer and microsatellite instability as markers of hereditary nonpolyposis colorectal cancer. *Dis Colon Rectum.* 2003;46:305.

814. Pye G, Jackson J, Thomas WM, et al. Comparison of Coloscreen Self-Test and haemoccult faecal occult blood tests in the detection of colorectal cancer in asymptomatic patients. *Br J Surg.* 1990;77:630.

815. Rabelo R, Foulkes W, Gordon PH, et al. Role of molecular diagnostic testing in familial adenomatous polyposis and hereditary nonpolyposis colorectal cancer families. *Dis Colon Rectum.* 2001;44:437.

816. Radcliffe AG, Dudley HAF. Intraoperative antegrade irrigation of the large intestine. *Surg Gynecol Obstet.* 1983;156:721.

817. Rajpal S, Dasmahapatra KS, Ledesma EJ, et al. Extensive resections of isolated metastasis from carcinoma of the colon and rectum. *Surg Gynecol Obstet.* 1982;155:813.

818. Ramming KP, O'Toole K. The use of the implantable chemoinfusion pump in the treatment of hepatic metastases of colorectal cancer. *Arch Surg.* 1986;121:1440.

819. Raskin HF, Pleticka S. The cytologic diagnosis of cancer of the colon. *Acta Cytol (Baltimore).* 1964;8:131.

820. Ravikumar TS, Kane R, Cady B, et al. Hepatic cryosurgery with intraoperative ultrasound monitoring for metastatic colon carcinoma. *Arch Surg.* 1987;122:403.

821. Ravikumar TS, Kane R, Cady B, et al. A 5-year study of cryosurgery in the treatment of liver tumors. *Arch Surg.* 1991;126:1520.

822. Ravikumar TS, Steele G Jr. Conventional and new tumor markers in the diagnosis and therapy of colorectal cancer. *Surg Rounds.* 1987;10:30.

823. Ravitch MM, Lane R, Cornell WP, et al. Closure of duodenal, gastric and intestinal stumps with wire staples: experimental and clinical studies. *Ann Surg.* 1966;163:573.

824. Ravitch MM, Steichen FM. Technics of staple suturing in the gastrointestinal tract. *Ann Surg.* 1972;175:815.

825. Ravitch MM, Steichen FM. A stapling instrument for end-to-end inverting anastomoses in the gastrointestinal tract. *Ann Surg.* 1979;189:791.

826. Ravo B, Ger R. Temporary colostomy: an outmoded procedure? A report on the intracolonic bypass. *Dis Colon Rectum.* 1985;28:904.

827. Ray NF, Larsen JW Jr, Stillman RJ, et al. Economic impact of hospitalizations for lower abdominal adhesiolysis in the United States in 1988. *Surg Gynecol Obstet.* 1993;176:271.

828. Raymond E, Faivre S, Waynarowski, et al. Oxaliplatin: mechanisms of action and anti-neoplastic activity. *Semin Oncol.* 1998;25(suppl 5):4.

829. Reasbeck PG, Manktelow A, McArthur AM, et al. An evaluation of pelvic lympphoscintigraphy in the staging of colorectal carcinoma. *Br J Surg.* 1984;71:936.

830. Rebuffat C, Rosati R, Montorsi M, et al. Clinical application of a new compression anastomotic device for colorectal surgery. *Am J Surg.* 1990;159:330.

831. Recalde M, Holyoke ED, Elias EG. Carcinoma of the colon, rectum, and anal canal in young patients. *Surg Gynecol Obstet.* 1974;139:909.

832. Redston M, Compton CC, Miedema BW, et al; Leukemia Group B Trial 80001. Analysis of micrometastatic disease in sentinel lymph nodes from resectable colon cancer: results of Cancer and Leukemia Group B Trial 80001. *J Clin Oncol.* 2006;24:878.

833. Redwine DB, Sharpe DR. Laparoscopic segmental resection of the sigmoid colon for endometriosis. *J Laparoendosc Surg.* 1991;1:217.

834. Rees M, Plant G, Bygrave S. Late results justify resection for multiple hepatic metastases from colorectal cancer. *Br J Surg.* 1997;84:1136.

835. Registry of Hepatic Metastases. Resection of the liver for colorectal carcinoma metastases: a multi-institutional study of indications for resection. *Surgery.* 1988;103:278.

836. Reiling RB. Staplers in gastrointestinal surgery. *Surg Clin North Am.* 1980;60:381.

837. Reiling RB, Reiling WA Jr, Bernie WA, et al. Prospective controlled study of gastrointestinal stapled anastomoses. *Am J Surg.* 1980;139:147.

838. Reilly JC, Rusin LC, Theuerkauf FJ Jr. Colonoscopy: its role in cancer of the colon and rectum. *Dis Colon Rectum.* 1982;25:532.

839. Reissman P, Teoh TA, Cohen SM, et al. Is early oral feeding safe after elective colorectal surgery? A prospective randomized trial. *Ann Surg.* 1995;222:73.

840. Renehan AG, Egger M, Saunders MP, et al. Impact on survival of intensive follow up after curative resection for colorectal cancer: systematic review and meta-analysis of randomised trials. *BMJ.* 2002;324:813.

841. Rex DK, Kahi CJ, Levin B, et al. Guidelines for colonoscopy surveillance after cancer resection: a consensus update by the American Cancer Society and US Multi-Society Task Force on Colorectal Cancer. *CA Cancer J Clin*. 2006;56:160; quiz 185.

842. Rey JF, Romanczyk T, Greff M. Metal stents for palliation of rectal carcinoma: a preliminary report on 12 patients. *Endoscopy*. 1995;27:501.

843. Reybard JF. Mémoire sur une tumeur cancéreuse affectant l'iliaque du colon: ablation de la tumeur et de l'intestin. *Bull R Med*. 18833;296.

844. Reynoso G, Chu TM, Holyoke D, et al. Carcinoembryonic antigen in patients with different cancers. *JAMA*. 1972;220:361.

845. Ribic CM, Sargent DJ, Moore MJ, et al. Tumor microsatellite-instability status as a predictor of benefit from fluorouracil-based adjuvant chemotherapy for colon cancer. *N Engl J Med*. 2003;349:247.

846. Richards PC, Balch CM, Aldrete JS. Abdominal wound closure: a prospective study of 571 patients comparing continuous versus interrupted suture techniques. *Ann Surg*. 1983;197:238.

847. Riethmüller G, Schneider-Gädicke E, Schlimok G, et al. Randomised trial of monoclonal antibody for adjuvant therapy of resected Dukes' C colorectal carcinoma. *Lancet*. 1994;343:1177.

848. Rifkin MD, Rosato FE, Branch HM, et al. Intraoperative ultrasound of the liver: an important adjunctive tool for decision making in the operating room. *Ann Surg*. 1987;205:466.

849. Robertson DJ, Greenberg ER, Beach M, et al. Colorectal cancer in patients under close colonoscopic surveillance. *Gastroenterology*. 2005;129:34.

850. Robinson MHE, Marks CG, Farrands PA, et al. Population screening for colorectal cancer: comparison between guaiac and immunological faecal occult blood tests. *Br J Surg*. 1994;81:448.

851. Rocklin MS, Senagore AJ, Talbott TM. Role of carcinoembryonic antigen and liver function tests in the detection of recurrent colorectal carcinoma. *Dis Colon Rectum*. 1991;34:794.

852. Rodgers MS, Collinson R, Desai S, et al. Risk of dissemination with biopsy of colorectal liver metastases. *Dis Colon Rectum*. 2003;46:454.

853. Rodgers MS, McCall JL. Surgery for colorectal liver metastases with hepatic lymph node involvement: a systematic review. *Br J Surg*. 2000;87:1142.

854. Rodríguez-Bigas MA, Boland CR, Hamilton SR, et al. A National Cancer Institute workshop on hereditary nonpolyposis colorectal cancer syndrome: meeting highlights and Bethesda guidelines. *J Natl Cancer Inst*. 1997;89:1758.

855. Rodríguez-Bigas MA, Vasen HFA, Pekka-Mecklin J, et al. Rectal cancer risk in hereditary nonpolyposis colorectal cancer after abdominal colectomy. *Ann Surg*. 1997;225:202.

856. Rogers DA, Dingus D, Stanfield J, et al. A prospective study of patient-controlled analgesia: impact on overall hospital course. *Am Surg*. 1990;56:86.

857. Rosati R, Rebuffat C, Pezzuoli G. A new mechanical device for circular compression anastomosis. *Ann Surg*. 1988;207:245.

858. Rosati R, Smith L, Deitel M, et al. Primary colorectal anastomosis with the intracolonic bypass tube. *Surgery*. 1992;112:618.

859. Rosato FE, Shelley WB, Fitts WT Jr, et al. Non-metastatic cutaneous manifestations of cancer of the colon. *Am J Surg*. 1969;117:277.

860. Rosen M, Chan L, Beart RW Jr, et al. Follow-up of colorectal cancer: a meta-analysis. *Dis Colon Rectum*. 1998;41:1116.

861. Roses DF, Richman H, Localio SA. Bacterial endocarditis associated with colorectal carcinoma. *Ann Surg*. 1973;179:190.

862. Rothenberg M, Meropol N, Poplin E, et al. Mortality associated with irinotecan plus bolus fluorouracil/leucovorin: summary findings of an independent panel. *J Clin Oncol*. 2001;19:3801.

863. Rowley S, Newbold KM, Gearty J, et al. Comparison of deoxyribonucleic acid ploidy and nuclear expressed p62 c-*myc* oncogene in the prognosis of colorectal cancer. *World J Surg*. 1990;14:545.

864. Roy M, Geller JS. Increased morbidity of iatrogenic splenectomy. *Surg Gynecol Obstet*. 1974;139:392.

865. Rozario D, Brown I, Fung MFK, et al. Is incidental prophylactic oophorectomy an acceptable means to reduce the incidence of ovarian cancer? *Am J Surg*. 1997;173:495.

866. Rozen P, Fireman Z, Figer A, et al. Family history of colorectal cancer as a marker of potential malignancy within a screening program. *Cancer*. 1987;60:248.

867. Rubin MS, Shin DM, Pasmantier M, et al. Monoclonal antibody (MoAb) IMC-C225. An epidermal growth factor (EGFr) for patients with EGFr positive tumors refractory to or in relapse from previous therapeutic regimens [abstract 1860]. *Proc ASCO*. 2000;19.

868. Rubin P, Green J. *Solitary Metastases*. Springfield, IL: Charles C Thomas; 1968.

869. Rulyak SJ, Lieberman DA, Wagner EH, et al. Outcome of follow-up colon examination among a population-based cohort of colorectal cancer patients. *Clin Gastroenterol Hepatol*. 2007;5:470; quiz 407.

870. Runkel NS, Schlag P, Schwarz V, et al. Outcome after emergency surgery for cancer of the large intestine. *Br J Surg*. 1991;78:183.

871. Ruo L, Cellini C, La-Calle JP Jr, et al. Limitations of family cancer history assessment at initial surgical consultation. *Dis Colon Rectum*. 2001;44:98.

872. Ruo L, Gougoutas C, Paty PB, et al. Elective bowel resection for incurable stage IV colorectal cancer: prognostic variables for asymptomatic patients. *J Am Coll Surg*. 2003;196:722.

873. Rusca JA, Bornside GH, Cohn I. Everting versus inverting gastrointestinal anastomoses: bacterial leakage and anastomotic disruption. *Ann Surg*. 1969;169:727.

874. Sacchi G, Weber E, Aglianó M, et al. Lymphatic vessels in colorectal cancer and their relation with inflammatory infiltrate. *Dis Colon Rectum*. 2003;46:40.

875. Saeed W, Kim S, Burch BH, et al. Development of carcinoma in regional enteritis. *Arch Surg*. 1974;108:376.

876. Saegesser F, Sandblom P. Ischemic lesions of the distended colon. *Am J Surg*. 1975;129:309.

877. Safi F, Link KH, Beger HG. Is follow-up of colorectal cancer patients worthwhile? *Dis Colon Rectum*. 1993;36:636.

878. Saida Y, Sumiyama Y, Nagao J, et al. Long-term prognosis of preoperative "bridge to surgery" expandable metallic stent insertion for obstructive colorectal cancer: comparison with emergency operation. *Dis Colon Rectum*. 2003;46(suppl):S44.

879. Sakanoue Y, Nakao K, Shoji Y, et al. Intraoperative colonoscopy. *Surg Endosc*. 1993;7:84.

880. Salim AS. Percutaneous decompression and irrigation for large-bowel obstruction. New approach. *Dis Colon Rectum*. 1991;34:973.

881. Salmon SE, Hamburger AW, Soehnlen B, et al. Quantitation of differential sensitivity of human tumor stem cells to anticancer drugs. *N Engl J Med*. 1978;298:1321.

882. Salsbury AJ, McKinna JA, Griffiths JD, et al. Circulating cancer cells during excision of carcinomas of the rectum and colon with high ligation of the inferior mesenteric vein. *Surg Gynecol Obstet*. 1965;120:1266.

883. Saltz L, Clark S, Diaz-Rubio E, et al. Bevacizumab (Bev) in combination with XELOX or FOLFOX4: updated efficacy results from XELOX-1/ NO16966, a randomized phase III trial in first-line metastatic colorectal cancer. *J Clin Oncol*. 2007;25:107s.

884. Saltz L, Lenz H, Kindler H, et al. Randomized phase II trial of cetuximab, bevacizumab, and irinotecan compared with cetuximab and bevacizumab alone in irinotecan refractory colorectal cancer: the BOND-2 study. *J Clin Oncol*. 2007;25:4487.

885. Saltz LB, Cox JV, Blanke C, et al. Irinotecan Study Group. Irinotecan plus fluorouracil and leucovorin for metastatic colorectal cancer. *N Engl J Med*. 2000;343:905.

886. Saltzman B. Ureteral stents: indications, variations and complications. *Urol Clin North Am*. 1988;15:481.

887. Sanders GB, Hagan WH, Kinnaird DW. Adult intussusception and carcinoma of the colon. *Ann Surg*. 1958;147:796.

888. Sandler RS, Sandler DP. Radiation-induced cancers of the colon and rectum: assessing the risk. *Gastroenterology*. 1983;84:51.

889. Sanfelippo PM, Beahrs OH. Factors in the prognosis of adenocarcinoma of the colon and rectum. *Arch Surg*. 1972;104:401.

890. Sanfelippo PM, Beahrs OH. Carcinoma of the colon in patients under forty years of age. *Surg Gynecol Obstet*. 1974;138:169.

891. Sardi A, Workman M, Mojzisik C, et al. Intra-abdominal recurrence of colorectal cancer detected by radioimmunoguided surgery (RIGS system). *Arch Surg*. 1989;124:55.

892. Sarela AI, Guthrie JA, Seymour MT, et al. Non-operative management of the primary tumour in patients with incurable stage IV colorectal cancer. *Br J Surg*. 2001;88:1352.

893. Schatzin A, Lanza E, Corle D, et al. Lack of effect of a high-fiber cereal supplement on the recurrence of colorectal adenomas. Polyp Prevention Trial Study Group. *N Engl J Med*. 2000;342:1149.

894. Scheele J, Altendorf-Hofmann A, Stangl R, et al. Pulmonary resection for metastatic colon and upper rectum cancer: is it useful? *Dis Colon Rectum*. 1990;33:745.

895. Schiedeck THK, Wellm C, Roblick UJ, et al. Diagnosis and monitoring of colorectal cancer by L6 blood serum polymerase chain reaction is superior to carcinoembryonic antigen-enzyme-linked immunosorbent assay. *Dis Colon Rectum*. 2003;46:818.

896. Schiessel R, Wunderlich M, Herbst F. Local recurrence of colorectal cancer: effect of early detection and aggressive surgery. *Br J Surg*. 1986;73:342.

897. Schillaci A, Cavallaro A, Nicolanti V, et al. The importance of symptom duration in relation to prognosis of carcinoma of the large intestine. *Surg Gynecol Obstet.* 1984;158:423.

898. Schmoll H, Cartwright T, Tabernero J, et al. Phase III trial of capecitabine plus oxaliplatin as adjuvant therapy for stage III colon cancer: a planned safety study analysis in 1864 patients. *J Clin Oncol.* 2007;25:102.

899. Schneebaum S, Arnold MW, Houchens DP, et al. The significance of intraoperative periportal lymph node metastasis identification in patients with colorectal carcinoma. *Cancer.* 1995;75:2809.

900. Schneebaum S, Arnold MW, Young D, et al. Role of carcinoembryonic antigen in predicting resectability of recurrent colorectal cancer. *Dis Colon Rectum.* 1993;36:810.

901. Schoemaker D, Black R, Giles L, et al. Yearly colonoscopy, liver CT, and chest radiography do not influence 5-year survival of colorectal cancer patients. *Gastroenterology.* 1998;114:7.

902. Schoetz DJ Jr, Roberts RL, Murray JJ, et al. Addition of parenteral cefoxitin to regimen of oral antibiotics for elective colorectal operations: a randomized prospective study. *Ann Surg.* 1990;212:209.

903. Schrag D, Panageas KS, Riedel E, et al. Surgeon volume compared to hospital volume as a predictor of outcome following primary colon cancer resection. *J Surg Oncol.* 2003;83:68.

904. Schrock TR, Deveney CW, Dunphy JE. Factors contributing to leakage of colonic anastomoses. *Ann Surg.* 1973;177:513.

905. SCOTIA Study Group. Single-stage treatment for malignant left-sided colonic obstruction: a prospective randomized clinical trial comparing subtotal colectomy with segmental resection following intraoperative irrigation. *Br J Surg.* 1995;82:1622.

906. Scott KW, Grace RH. Detection of lymph node metastases in colorectal carcinoma before and after fat clearance. *Br J Surg.* 1989;76:1165.

907. Scott NA, Rainwater LM, Weiand HS, et al. The relative prognostic value of flow cytometric DNA analysis and conventional clinicopathologic criteria in patients with operable rectal carcinoma. *Dis Colon Rectum.* 1987;30:513.

908. Scott NA, Weiand HS, Moertel CG, et al. Colorectal cancer: Dukes' stage, tumor site, preoperative plasma CEA pattern. *Arch Surg.* 1987;122:1375.

909. Scudamore HH. Cancer of the colon and rectum — general aspects, diagnosis, treatment, and prognosis: a review. *Dis Colon Rectum.* 1969;12:105.

910. Searle/Pharmacia Corporation. Data on File.

911. Secker-Walter RH, Worden JK, Holland RR, et al. A mass media programme to prevent smoking among adolescents: costs and cost effectiveness. *Tobacco Control.* 1997;6:207.

912. Segi M. *Cancer Mortality for Selected Sites in 24 Countries: 1950–1957.* Sendai, Japan: Department of Public Health, Tohoku University School of Medicine; 1960.

913. Seidman H. Cancer death rates by site and sex for religious and socioeconomic groups in New York City. *Environ Res.* 1970;3:234.

914. Selby JV, Friedman GD, Quesenberry CP Jr, et al. A case-control study of screening sigmoidoscopy and mortality from colorectal cancer. *N Engl J Med.* 1992;326:653.

915. Selby P, Buick RN, Tannock I. A critical appraisal of the human tumor stem-cell assay. *N Engl J Med.* 1983;308:129.

916. Sener SF, Imperato JP, Chmiel J, et al. The use of cancer registry data to study preoperative carcinoembryonic antigen level as an indicator of survival in colorectal cancer. *CA Cancer J Clin.* 1989;39:50.

917. Sengupta S, Tjandra JJ, Gibson PR. Dietary fiber and colorectal neoplasia. *Dis Colon Rectum.* 2001;44:1016.

918. Senn N. Enterorrhaphy: its history, technique and present status. *JAMA.* 1893;21:215.

919. Serpell JW, McDermott FT, Katrivessis H, et al. Obstructing carcinomas of the colon. *Br J Surg.* 1989;76:965.

920. Setti Carraro PG, Segala M, Cesana BM, et al. Obstructing colonic cancer: failure and survival patterns over a ten-year follow-up after a one-stage curative surgery. *Dis Colon Rectum.* 2001;44:243.

921. Shahon DB, Wangensteen OH. Early diagnosis of cancer of the gastrointestinal tract. *Postgrad Med.* 1960;27:306.

922. Shapiro A, Berlatsky Y, Lijovetsky G, et al. Carcinoma of colon after ureteric anastomosis. *Urology.* 1979;13:617.

923. Sharpe CR, Siemiatycki JA, Rachet BP. The effects of smoking on the risk of colorectal cancer. *Dis Colon Rectum.* 2002;45:1041.

924. Sheehan KM, Sheahan K, O'Donoghue D, et al. The relationship between cyclooxygenase-2 expression and colorectal cancer. *JAMA.* 1999;282:1254.

925. Sheen AJ, Irlam J, Kirillova N, et al. Gene therapy of patient-derived T lymphocytes to target and eradicate colorectal hepatic metastases. *Dis Colon Rectum.* 2003;46:793.

926. Sheikh FA, Khubchandani IT. Prophylactic ureteric catheters in colon surgery: how safe are they? *Dis Colon Rectum.* 1990;33:508.

927. Sheil FO, Clark CG, Goligher JC. Adenocarcinoma associated with Crohn's disease. *Br J Surg.* 1968;55:53.

928. Sheiner NM, Brister SJ, Gordon PH. Management of pulmonary metastases of colorectal origin. *Surg Rounds.* 1988;11:29.

929. Shen XJ, Rawls JF, Randall T, et al. Molecular characterization of mucosal adherent bacteria and associations with colorectal adenomas. *Gut Microbes.* 2010;1:138.

930. Shennib H, Fried GM, Hampson LG. Does simultaneous cholecystectomy increase the risk of colonic surgery? *Am J Surg.* 1986;151:266.

931. Shibata D, Paty PB, Guillem JG, et al. Surgical management of isolated retroperitoneal recurrences of colorectal carcinoma. *Dis Colon Rectum.* 2002;45:795.

932. Shibata Y, Kotanagi H, Andoh H, et al. Detection of circulating anti-p53 antibodies in patients with colorectal carcinoma and the antibody's relation to clinical factors. *Dis Colon Rectum.* 1996;39:1269.

933. Shida H, Ban K, Matsumoto M, et al. Prognostic significance of location of lymph node metastases in colorectal cancer. *Dis Colon Rectum.* 1992;35:1046.

934. Shimamoto C, Hirata I, Takao Y, et al. Alteration of colonic mucin after ureterosigmoidostomy. *Dis Colon Rectum.* 2000;43:526.

935. Shimotsuma M, Takahashi T, Yamane T, et al. Intraoperative cleansing of the impacted colon using an endotracheal tube. *Dis Colon Rectum.* 1990;33:241.

936. Shirouzu K, Isomoto H, Kakegawa T. A prospective clinicopathologic study of venous invasion in colorectal cancer. *Am J Surg.* 1991;162:216.

937. Shitoh K, Konishi F, Miyakura Y, et al. Microsatellite instability as a marker in predicting metachronous multiple colorectal carcinomas after surgery: a cohort-like study. *Dis Colon Rectum.* 2002;45:328.

938. Shousha A, Chappell R, Matthews J, et al. Human chorionic gonadotrophin expression in colorectal adenocarcinoma. *Dis Colon Rectum.* 1986;29:558.

939. Sibbering DM, Locker AP, Hardcastle JD, et al. Blood transfusion and survival in colorectal cancer. *Dis Colon Rectum.* 1994;37:358.

940. Siddiqui A, Piperdi B. KRAS mutation in colon cancer: a marker of resistance to EGFR-1 therapy. *Ann Surg Oncol.* 2010;17:1168.

941. Siegel R, Ward E, Brawley O, et al. Cancer statistics, 2011: The impact of eliminating socioeconomic and racial disparities on premature cancer deaths. *CA Cancer J Clin.* 2011;61:212.

942. Slater G, Aufses AH Jr, Szporn A. Synchronous carcinoma of the colon and rectum. *Surg Gynecol Obstet.* 1990;171:283.

943. Slater GI, Haber RH, Aufses AH Jr. Changing distribution of carcinoma of the colon and rectum. *Surg Gynecol Obstet.* 1984;158:216.

944. Smith GA, Oien KA, O'Dwyer PJ. Frequency of early colorectal cancer in patients undergoing colonoscopy. *Br J Surg.* 1999;86:1328.

945. Smith RL. Recorded and expected mortality among the Japanese of the United States and Hawaii, with special reference to cancer. *J Natl Cancer Inst.* 1956;17:459.

946. Smothers L, Hynan L, Fleming J, et al. Emergency surgery for colon carcinoma. *Dis Colon Rectum.* 2003;46:24.

947. Sobin LH, Greene FL. TNM classification: clarification of number of regional nodes for pN0. *Cancer.* 2001;92:452.

948. Solla JA, Rothenberger DA. Preoperative bowel preparation: a survey of colon and rectal surgeons. *Dis Colon Rectum.* 1990;33:154.

949. Song F, Glenny AM. Antimicrobial prophylaxis in colorectal surgery: a systematic review of randomized controlled trials. *Br J Surg.* 1998;85:1232.

950. Sorokin JJ, Sugarbaker PH, Zamcheck N, et al. Serial carcinoembryonic antigen assays: use in detection of cancer recurrence. *JAMA.* 1974;228:49.

951. Soyer P, Levesque M, Elias D, et al. Detection of liver metastases from colorectal cancer: comparison of intraoperative US and CT during arterial portography. *Radiology.* 1992;183:541.

952. Soyka JD, Veit-Haibach P, Strobel K, et al. Staging pathways in recurrent colorectal carcinoma: is contrast-enhanced 18F-FDG PET/CT the diagnostic tool of choice? *J Nucl Med.* 2008;49:354.

953. Spratt JS Jr. The rates and patterns of growth of neoplasms of the large intestine and rectum. *Surg Clin North Am.* 1965;45:1103.

954. Spratt JS Jr. Gross rates of growth of colonic neoplasms and other variables affecting medical decisions and prognosis. In: Burdette WJ, ed. *Carcinoma of the Colon and Antecedent Epithelium.* Springfield, IL: Charles C Thomas; 1970:66.

955. Spratt JS Jr, Ackerman LV. The growth of a colonic adenocarcinoma. *Am Surg.* 1961;27:23.

956. Staab HJ, Anderer FA, Stumpf E, et al. Eighty-four potential second-look operations based on sequential carcinoembryonic antigen determinations and clinical investigations in patients with recurrent gastrointestinal cancer. *Am J Surg.* 1985;149:198.

957. Stahl TJ, Gregorcyk SG, Hyman NH, et al; Standards Practice Task Force of The American Society of Colon and Rectal Surgeons. Practice parameters for the prevention of venous thrombosis. *Dis Colon Rectum.* 2006;49:1477.

958. Standards Task Force of the American Society of Colon and Rectal Surgeons. Practice parameters for the identification and testing of patients at risk for dominantly inherited colorectal cancer. *Dis Colon Rectum.* 2001;44:1403.

959. Standards Task Force of the American Society of Colon and Rectal Surgeons. Practice parameters for the identification and testing of patients at risk for dominantly inherited colorectal cancer: supporting documentation. *Dis Colon Rectum.* 2001;44:1404.

960. Standards Task Force of the American Society of Colon and Rectal Surgeons. Practice parameters for the treatment of patients with dominantly inherited colorectal cancer (familial adenomatous polyposis and hereditary nonpolyposis cancer). *Dis Colon Rectum.* 2003;46:1001.

961. Stangl R, Altendorf-Hofmann A, Charnley RM, et al. Factors influencing the natural history of colorectal liver metastases. *Lancet.* 1994;343:1405.

962. Starling JR, Uehling DT, Gilchrist KW. Value of colonoscopy after ureterosigmoidoscopy. *Surgery.* 1984;96:784.

963. Staszewski J, McCall MG, Stenhouse NS. Cancer mortality in 1962–66 among Polish migrants to Australia. *Br J Cancer.* 1971;25:599.

964. *Statistical Review of England and Wales. Supplement on Cancer, 1968–1970.* London, United Kingdom: HM Stationery Office; 1975.

965. Steele G Jr, Ravikumar TS. Resection of hepatic metastases from colorectal cancer. *Ann Surg.* 1989;210:127.

966. Steele G Jr, Zamcheck N, Wilson R, et al. Results of CEA-initiated second-look surgery for recurrent colorectal cancer. *Am J Surg.* 1980;139:544.

967. Steele RJC, Thompson AM, Hall PA, et al. The p53 tumour suppressor gene. *Br J Surg.* 1998;85:1460.

968. Steichen FM, Ravitch MM. History of mechanical devices and instruments for suturing. *Curr Probl Surg.* 1982;19:1.

969. Steichen FM, Ravitch MM. Contemporary stapling instruments and basic mechanical suture techniques. *Surg Clin North Am.* 1984;64:425.

970. Steinberg JB, Tuggle DW, Postier RG. Adenocarcinoma of the colon in adolescents. *Am J Surg.* 1988;156:460.

971. Steinberg SM, Barkin JS, Kaplan RS, et al. Prognostic indicators of colon tumors: the Gastrointestinal Tumor Study Group experience. *Cancer.* 1986;57:1866.

972. Steinberg SM, Barwick KW, Stablein DM. Importance of tumor pathology and morphology in patients with surgically resected colon cancer: findings from the Gastrointestinal Tumor Study Group. *Cancer.* 1986;58:1340.

973. Stella M, De Nardi P, Paganelli G, et al. Avidin-biotin system in radioimmunoguided surgery for colorectal cancer: advantages and limits. *Dis Colon Rectum.* 1994;37:335.

974. Stellato TA, Danziger LH, Gordon N, et al. Antibiotics in elective colon surgery: a randomized trial of oral, systemic, and oral/systemic antibiotics for prophylaxis. *Am Surg.* 1990;56:251.

975. Stephenson BM, Finan PJ, Gascoyne J, et al. Frequency of familial colorectal cancer. *Br J Surg.* 1991;78:1162.

976. Stephenson BM, Shandall AA, Farouk R, et al. Malignant left-sided large bowel obstruction managed by subtotal/total colectomy. *Br J Surg.* 1990;77:1098.

977. Sterchi JM, Fulks D, Cruz J, et al. Operative technique for insertion of a totally implantable system for venous access. *Surg Gynecol Obstet.* 1986;163:381.

978. Stevenson GW, Hernandez C. Single-visit screening and treatment of first-degree relatives: colon cancer pilot study. *Dis Colon Rectum.* 1991;34:1120.

979. Stewart J, Diament RH, Brennan TG. Management of obstructing lesions of the left colon by resection, on-table lavage, and primary anastomosis. *Surgery.* 1993;114:502.

980. Stewart RJ, Stewart AW, Turnbull PRG, et al. Sex differences in subsite incidence of large bowel cancer. *Dis Colon Rectum.* 1983;26:658.

981. Strachan JR, Woodhouse CRJ. Malignancy following ureterosigmoidoscopy in patients with exstrophy. *Br J Surg.* 1991;178:1216.

982. Stule JP, Petrelli NJ, Herrera L, et al. Anastomotic recurrence of adenocarcinoma of the colon. *Arch Surg.* 1986;121:1077.

983. Sub O, Mettlin C, Petrelli N. Aspirin use, cancer, and polyps of the large bowel. *Cancer.* 1993;72:1171.

984. Sugarbaker PH, Zamcheck N, Moore FD. Assessment of serial carcinoembryonic antigen (CEA) assays in postoperative detection of recurrent colorectal cancer. *Cancer.* 1976;38:2310.

985. Sugihara K, Hojo K, Moriya Y, et al. Pattern of recurrence after hepatic resection for colorectal metastases. *Br J Surg.* 1993;80:1032.

986. Sumpio BE, Ballantyne GH, Zdon MJ, et al. Perforated appendicitis and obstructing colonic carcinoma in the elderly. *Dis Colon Rectum.* 1986;29:688.

987. Svenden LB, Blow S, Mellemgaard A. Metachronous colorectal cancer in young patients: expression of the hereditary nonpolyposis colorectal cancer syndrome? *Dis Colon Rectum.* 1991;34:790.

988. Swanson RS, Compton CC, Stewart AK, et al. The prognosis of T3N0 colon cancer is dependent on the number of lymph nodes examined. *Ann Surg Oncol.* 2003;10:65.

989. Swinton NW Sr, Nahra KS, Khazei AM, et al. The evolution of colorectal cancer. *Dis Colon Rectum.* 1968;11:413.

990. Swinton NW Sr, Scherer WP. The value of proctosigmoidoscopic examinations. *CA Cancer J Clin.* 1968;18:88.

991. Sylvan A, Sjölund B, Janunger KG, et al. Colorectal cancer risk after jejunoileal bypass: dysplasia and DNA content in longtime follow-up of patients operated on for morbid obesity. *Dis Colon Rectum.* 1992;35:245.

992. Takahashi H, Carlson R, Ozturk M, et al. Radioimmunolocation of hepatic and pulmonary metastasis of human colon adenocarcinoma. *Gastroenterology.* 1989;96:1317.

993. Takaki HS, Ujiki GT, Shields TS. Palliative resections in the treatment of primary colorectal cancer. *Am J Surg.* 1977;133:548.

994. Tamin WZ, Ghellai A, Counihan TC, et al. Experience with endoluminal colonic wall stents for the management of large bowel obstruction for benign and malignant disease. *Arch Surg.* 2000;135:434.

995. Tan B, Thomas F, Myerson RJ, et al. Thymidylate synthesis genotype-directed neoadjuvant chemoradiation for patients with rectal cancer. *J Clin Oncol.* 2011;29:875.

996. Tan SG, Nambiar R, Rauff A, et al. Primary resection and anastomosis in obstructed descending colon due to cancer. *Arch Surg.* 1991;126:748.

997. Tanaka K, Adam R, Shimada H, et al. Role of neoadjuvant chemotherapy in the treatment of multiple colorectal metastases to the liver. *Br J Surg.* 2003;90:963.

998. Tanaka K, Shimada H, Matsuo K, et al. Outcome after simultaneous colorectal and hepatic resection for colorectal cancer with synchronous metastases. *Surgery.* 2004;136:650.

999. Tanaka T, Furukawa A, Murata K, et al. Endoscopic transanal decompression with a drainage tube for acute colonic obstruction. *Dis Colon Rectum.* 2001;44:418.

1000. Tartter PI. The association of perioperative blood transfusion with colorectal cancer recurrence. *Ann Surg.* 1992;216:633.

1001. Tartter PI, Slater G, Papatestas AE, et al. The prognostic significance of elevated serum alkaline phosphatase levels preoperatively in patients with carcinoma of the colon and rectum. *Surg Gynecol Obstet.* 1984;158:569.

1002. Tartter PI, Steinberg BM. The role of preoperative intravenous pyelogram in operations performed for carcinoma of the colon and rectum. *Surg Gynecol Obstet.* 1986;163:65.

1003. Tataryn DN, MacFarlane JK, Murray D, et al. Tube leukocyte adherence inhibition (LAI) assay in gastrointestinal (GIT) cancer. *Cancer.* 1979;43:898.

1004. Tate JJT, Northway J, Royle GT, et al. Faecal occult blood testing in symptomatic patients: comparison of three tests. *Br J Surg.* 1990;77:523.

1005. Teitz S, Guidetti-Sharon A, Manor H, et al. Pyogenic liver abscess: warning indicator of silent colonic cancer: report of a case and review of the literature. *Dis Colon Rectum.* 1995;38:1220.

1006. Tejero E, Fernández-Lobato R, Mainar A, et al. Initial results of a new procedure for treatment of malignant obstruction of the left colon. *Dis Colon Rectum.* 1997;40:432.

1007. Tejero E, Mainar A, Fernández L, et al. New procedure for the treatment of colorectal neoplastic obstructions. *Dis Colon Rectum.* 1994;37:1158.

1008. Tekkis PP, Kessaris N, Kocher HM, et al. Evaluation of POSSUM and P-POSSUM scoring systems in patients undergoing colorectal surgery. *Br J Surg.* 2003;90:340.

1009. Tempero M. Pitfalls in antibody imaging in colorectal cancer. *Cancer.* 1993;71:4248.

1010. Tepper JE, O'Connell MJ, Niedzwiecki D, et al. Impact of number of nodes retrieved on outcome in patients with rectal cancer. *J Clin Oncol.* 2001;19:157.

1011. Tepper JE, O'Connell M, Niedzwiecki D, et al. Adjuvant therapy in rectal cancer: analysis of stage, sex and local control-Final Report of Intergroup 0114. *J Clin Oncol.* 2002;20:1744.

1012. Teppo L, Hakamd M, Hakulinen T, et al. *Cancer in Finland, 1953–1970: Incidence, Mortality, Prevalence.* Copenhagen, Denmark: Munksgaard; 1975.

1013. Terezis NL, Davis WC, Jackson FC. Carcinoma of the colon associated with inguinal hernia. *N Engl J Med.* 1963;268:774.

1014.   Thompson JS, Beart RW Jr, Anderson CF. Limitations of nutritional assessment in predicting the outcome of colorectal operations. *Dis Colon Rectum.* 1986;29:488.

1015.   Thomson DMP, Krupey J, Freedman SO, et al. The radioimmunoassay of circulating carcinoembryonic antigen of the human digestive system. *Proc Natl Acad Sci USA.* 1969;64:161.

1016.   Thomson DMP, Tataryn DN, Lopez M, et al. Human tumor-specific immunity assayed by a computerized tube leukocyte adherence inhibition. *Cancer Res.* 1979;39:638.

1017.   Thomson WHF, Carter SS. On-table lavage to achieve safe restorative rectal and emergency colonic resection without covering colostomy. *Br J Surg.* 1986;73:61.

1018.   Thomson WHF, Robinson MHE. One-layer continuously sutured colonic anastomosis. *Br J Surg.* 1993;80:1450.

1019.   Thorsen AG, Christensen MA, Davis SJ. The role of colonoscopy in the assessment of patients with colorectal cancer. *Dis Colon Rectum.* 1986;29:306.

1020.   Thun MJ, Calle EE, Namboodiri MM, et al. Risk factors for fatal colon cancer in a large prospective study. *J Natl Cancer Inst.* 1992;84:1491.

1021.   Thun MJ, Namboodiri MM, Health CW Jr. Aspirin use and reduced risk of fatal colon cancer. *N Engl J Med.* 1991;323:1393.

1022.   Thurston MO, Kaehr JW, Martin EW III, et al. Radionuclide of choice for use with an intraoperative probe. *And Immun Radio.* 1991;4:595.

1023.   Tietjen GW, Markowitz AM. Colitis proximal to obstructing colonic carcinoma. *Arch Surg.* 1975;110:1133.

1024.   Tio TL, Coene PPLO, van Delden OM, et al. Colorectal carcinoma: preoperative TNM classification with endosonography. *Radiology.* 1991;179:165.

1025.   Tol J, Koopman M, Cats A, et al. Chemotherapy, bevacizumab, and cetuximab in metastatic colorectal cancer. *N Eng J Med.* 2009;360:563.

1026.   Tong D, Russell AH, Dawson LE, et al. Second laparotomy for proximal colon cancer: sites of recurrence and implications for adjuvant therapy. *Am J Surg.* 1983;145:382.

1027.   Toribara NW, Sleisenger MH. Screening for colorectal cancer. *N Engl J Med.* 1995;332:861.

1028.   Tornberg SA, Holm LE, Cartensen JM, et al. Risks of cancer of the colon and rectum in relation to serum cholesterol and beta-lipoprotein. *N Engl J Med.* 1986;315:1629.

1029.   Tornqvist A, Ekelund G, Leandoer L. The value of intensive follow-up after curative resection for colorectal carcinoma. *Br J Surg.* 1982;69:725.

1030.   Tournigand C, Louvet C, Quinaux E, et al. FOLFIRI followed by FOLFOX versus FOLFOX followed by FOLFIRI in metastatic colorectal cancer (MCRC): final results of a phase III study [abstract 494]. *Proc ASCO.* 2001;20.

1031.   Travers B. *An Inquiry into the Process of Nature in Repairing Injuries of the Intestine.* London, United Kingdom: Longmans, Green and Co; 1812.

1032.   Traverso G, Shuber A, Levin B, et al. Detection of *APC* mutations in fecal DNA from patients with colorectal tumors. *N Engl J Med.* 2002;346:311.

1033.   Traynor O, Castaing D, Bismuth H. Peroperative ultrasonography in the surgery of hepatic tumours. *Br J Surg.* 1988;75:197.

1034.   Trocha SD, Nora DT, Saha SS, et al. Combination probe and dye-directed lymphatic mapping detects micrometastases in early colorectal cancer. *J Gastrointest Surg.* 2003;7:340.

1035.   Tsakraklides V, Wanebo HJ, Sternberg SS, et al. Prognostic evaluation of regional lymph node morphology in colorectal cancer. *Am J Surg.* 1975;129:174.

1036.   Turnbull RB Jr, Kyle K, Watson FR, et al. Cancer of the colon: the influence of the no-touch isolation technic on survival rates. *Ann Surg.* 1967;166:420.

1037.   Turunen MJ, Kivilaakso EO. Increased risk of colorectal cancer after cholecystectomy. *Ann Surg.* 1981;194:639.

1038.   Twelves C, Wong A, Nowacki MP, et al. Improved safety results of a phase III trial of capecitabine vs. bolus 5-FU/leucovorin (LV) as adjuvant therapy for colon cancer (the X-ACT Study) [abstract 1182]. *Proc ASCO.* 2003;22.

1039.   Umpleby HC, Williamson RCN. Survival in acute obstructing colorectal carcinoma. *Dis Colon Rectum.* 1984;27:299.

1040.   Unger SW, Wanebo HJ. Colonoscopy: an essential monitoring technique after resection of colorectal cancer. *Am J Surg.* 1983;145:71.

1041.   University of Melbourne Colorectal Group. A comparison of single-dose systemic Timentin with mezlocillin for prophylaxis of wound infection in elective colorectal surgery. *Dis Colon Rectum.* 1989;32:940.

1042.   Urdaneta LF, Duffell D, Creevy CD, et al. Late development of primary carcinoma of the colon following ureterosigmoidostomy: report of three cases and literature review. *Ann Surg.* 1966;164:503.

1043.   Valliant JC, Balladur P, Nordlinger B, et al. Repeat liver resection for recurrent colorectal metastases. *Br J Surg.* 1993;80:340.

1044.   Van Cutsem E, Kohne C, Hitre E, et al. Cetuximab and chemotherapy as initial treatment for metastatic colorectal cancer. *N Eng J Med.* 2009;360:1408.

1045.   Van Cutsem E, Twelves C, Cassidy J, et al. Oral capecitabine compared with intravenous fluorouracil plus leucovorin in patients with metastatic colorectal cancers: results of a large phase III study. *J Clin Oncol.* 2001;19:4097.

1046.   Van Cutsem E, Twelves C, Taberno J, et al. XELOX: mature results of a multinational, phase 11 trial of capecitabine plus oxaliplatin, an effective 1st line option for patients (pts) with metastatic colorectal cancer (MCRC) [abstract 1023]. *Proc ASCO.* 2003;22.

1047.   van Dalen R, Church J, McGannon E, et al. Patterns of surgery in patients belonging to Amsterdam-positive families. *Dis Colon Rectum.* 2003;46:617.

1048.   van Geldere D, Fa-Si-Oen P, Noach LA, et al. Complications after colorectal surgery without mechanical bowel resection. *J Am Coll Surg.* 2002;194:40.

1049.   van Kamp GJ, von Mensdorff-Pouilly S, Kenemans P, et al. Evaluation of colorectal cancer-associated mucin CA M43 assay in serum. *Clin Chem.* 1993;39:1029.

1050.   Varty PP, Linehan IP, Boulos PB. Does concurrent splenectomy at colorectal cancer resection influence survival? *Dis Colon Rectum.* 1993;36:602.

1051.   Vasen HFA, Mecklin JP, Khan PM, et al. Hereditary non-polyposis colorectal cancer. *Lancet.* 1991;338:877.

1052.   Vellacott KD, Smith JHF, Mortensen NJ. Rising detection rate of symptomatic Dukes' A colorectal cancers. *Br J Surg.* 1987;74:18.

1053.   Venkataraman S, Mohan V, Ramakrishna BS, et al. Risk of colorectal cancer in ulcerative colitis in India. *J Gastroenterol Hepatol.* 2005;20:705.

1054.   Venkatesh KS, Morrison N, Larson DM, et al. Triangulating stapling technique: an alternative approach to colorectal anastomosis. *Dis Colon Rectum.* 1993;36:73.

1055.   Verne JECW, Northover JMA. Screening strategies for the secondary prevention of colorectal cancer. *Gastroenterology J Club.* 1990;2:6.

1056.   Vernick LJ, Kuller LH, Lohsoonthorn P, et al. Relationship between cholecystectomy and ascending colon cancer. *Cancer.* 1980;45:392.

1057.   Vezeridis MP, Petrelli NJ, Mittelman A. The value of routine preoperative urologic evaluation in patients with colorectal carcinoma. *Dis Colon Rectum.* 1987;30:758.

1058.   Vigder L, Tzur N, Huber M, et al. Management of obstructive carcinoma of the left colon: comparative study of staged and primary resection. *Arch Surg.* 1985;120:825.

1059.   Vigo FC, Pardo R, Saenz D, et al. Muir-Torre syndrome with multiple neoplasia. *Br J Surg.* 1992;79:1161.

1060.   Virgo KS, Vernava AM, Longo WE, et al. Cost of patient follow-up after potentially curative colorectal cancer treatment. *JAMA.* 1995;273:1837.

1061.   Virgolini I, Raderer M, Kurtaran A, et al. Vasoactive intestinal peptide-receptor imaging for the localization of intestinal adenocarcinomas and endocrine tumors. *N Engl J Med.* 1994;331:1116.

1062.   Vogel SB, Drane WE, Ros PR, et al. Prediction of surgical resectability in patients with hepatic colorectal metastases. *Ann Surg.* 1994;219:508.

1063.   Walsh RM, Aranha GV, Freeark RJ. Mortality and quality of life after total abdominal colectomy. *Arch Surg.* 1990;125:1564.

1064.   Wanebo HJ, Chu QD, Vezeridis MP, et al. Patient selection for hepatic resection of colorectal metastases. *Arch Surg.* 1996;131:322.

1065.   Wanebo HJ, Llaneras M, Martin T, et al. Prospective monitoring trial for carcinoma of colon and rectum after surgical resection. *Surg Gynecol Obstet.* 1989;169:479.

1066.   Wangensteen OH. Cancer of the colon and rectum: with special reference to (1) earlier recognition of alimentary tract malignancy; (2) secondary delayed re-entry of the abdomen in patients exhibiting lymph node involvement; (3) subtotal primary excision of the colon; (4) operation in obstruction. *Wis Med J.* 1949;48:591.

1067.   Ward D, Naik KS, Guthrie JA, et al. Hepatic lesion detection: comparison of MR imaging after the administration of superparamagnetic iron oxide with dual-phase CT by using alternative-free response receiver operating characteristic analysis. *Radiology.* 1999;210:459.

1068.   Warthin AS. Heredity with reference to carcinoma. *Arch Intern Med.* 1913;12:546.

1069.   Wassner JD, Yohai E, Heimlich HJ. Complications associated with the use of gastrointestinal stapling devices. *Surgery.* 1977;82:395.

1070.   Watanabe I, Arai T, Ono M, et al. Prognostic factors in resection of pulmonary metastasis from colorectal cancer. *Br J Surg.* 2003;90:1436.

1071.   Waterhouse J, Muir C, Correa P, et al, eds. *Cancer Incidence in Five Continents*. Vol 3. New York, NY: Springer-Verlag; 1976.

1072.   Waxman BP. Large-bowel anastomoses. II. The circular staplers. *Br J Surg*. 1983;70:64.

1073.   Weaver M, Burdon DW, Youngs DJ, et al. Oral neomycin and erythromycin compared with single-dose systemic metronidazole and ceftriaxone prophylaxis in elective colorectal surgery. *Am J Surg*. 1986; 151:437.

1074.   Weber CA, Deveney KE, Pellegrini CA, et al. Routine colonoscopy in the management of colorectal carcinoma. *Am J Surg*. 1986;152:87.

1075.   Weber JC, Bachellier P, Oussoultzoglou E, et al. Simultaneous resection of colorectal primary tumour and synchronous liver metastases. *Br J Surg*. 2003;90:956.

1076.   Weese JL, O'Grady MG, Ottery FD. How long is the five-centimeter margin? *Surg Gynecol Obstet*. 1986;163:101.

1077.   Weese JL, Rosenthal MS, Gould H. Avoidance of artifacts on computerized tomograms by selection of appropriate surgical clips. *Am J Surg*. 1984;147:684.

1078.   Weiden PL, Bean MA, Schultz P. Perioperative blood transfusion does not increase the risk of colorectal cancer recurrence. *Cancer*. 1987;60:870.

1079.   Weilbaecher D, Bolin JA, Hearn D, et al. Intussusception in adults: review of 160 cases. *Am J Surg*. 1971;121:531.

1080.   Welch CE. The treatment of combined intestinal obstruction and peritonitis by refunctionalization of the intestine. *Ann Surg*. 1955; 142:739.

1081.   Whelan RL, Wong WD, Goldberg SM, et al. Synchronous bowel anastomoses. *Dis Colon Rectum*. 1989;32:365.

1082.   Whitaker RH, Pugh RC, Dowe D. Colonic tumours following uretero-sigmoidostomy. *Br J Urol*. 1971;43:562.

1083.   White CM, Macfie J. Immediate colectomy and primary anastomosis for acute obstruction due to carcinoma of the left colon and rectum. *Dis Colon Rectum*. 1985;28:155.

1084.   Whitehouse GH, Watt J. Ischemic colitis associated with carcinoma of the colon. *Gastrointest Radiol*. 1977;2:31.

1085.   Wichmann MW, Müller C, Hornung HM, et al. Gender differences in long-term survival of patients with colorectal cancer. *Br J Surg*. 2001;88:1092.

1086.   Wiggers T, Jeekel J, Arends JW, et al. No-touch isolation technique in colon cancer: a controlled prospective trial. *Br J Surg*. 1988;75:409.

1087.   Wijnen J, Khan PM, Vasen H, et al. Hereditary nonpolyposis colorectal cancer families not complying with the Amsterdam criteria show extremely low frequency of mismatch-repair-gene mutations. *Am J Hum Genet*. 1997;61:329.

1088.   Wilkes G. Oxaliplatinin: third-generation platinum analog. *Clin J Oncol Nurs*. 2003;7:353.

1089.   Wilking N, Petrelli NJ, Herrera L, et al. Surgical resection of pulmonary metastases from colorectal adenocarcinoma. *Dis Colon Rectum*. 1985;28:562.

1090.   Wilking N, Petrelli NJ, Herrera L, et al. Abdominal exploration for suspected recurrent carcinoma of the colon and rectum based upon elevated carcinoembryonic antigen alone or in combination with other diagnostic methods. *Surg Gynecol Obstet*. 1986;162:465.

1091.   Wille-Jørgensen P, Guenaga KF, Castro AA, et al. Clinical value of preoperative mechanical bowel cleansing in elective colorectal surgery: a systematic review. *Dis Colon Rectum*. 2003;46:1013.

1092.   Willett WC, MacMahon B. Diet and cancer: an overview (second of two parts). *N Engl J Med*. 1984;310:697.

1093.   Williams NN, Daly JM. Flow cytometry and prognostic implications in patients with solid tumors. *Surg Gynecol Obstet*. 1990;171:257.

1094.   Wilmore DW. Can we minimize the effects of opioids on the bowel and still achieve adequate pain control? *Am J Surg*. 2001; 182(suppl):1S.

1095.   Wilschut JA, Steyerberg EW, van Leerdam ME, et al. How much colonoscopy screening should be recommended to individuals with various degrees of family history of colorectal cancer? *Cancer*. 2011;117:4166. doi:10.1002/cncr.26009.

1096.   Wilson SE, Sokol T. Antimicrobials in elective colon surgery. *Infect Surg*. 1985;4:609.

1097.   Wilson SM, Adson MA. Surgical treatment of hepatic metastases from colorectal cancers. *Arch Surg*. 1976;111:330.

1098.   Wimpson AHRW, Thomson WHF. Technical modifications making on-table washout easier. *Br J Surg*. 1987;74:464.

1099.   Winawer SJ. The role of CEA in the diagnosis of colonic cancer and other lesions. *Natl Large-Bowel Cancer Project Newslett*. 1975;3:7.

1100.   Winawer SJ. Screening for colorectal cancer. Presented at: International Symposium on Colorectal Cancer; March 1979, New York, NY.

1101.   Winawer SJ. Colon cancer. In: Hunt RH, Waye JD, eds. *Colonoscopy: Techniques, Clinical Practice and Colour Atlas*. London, United Kingdom: Chapman & Hall; 1981:327.

1102.   Winawer SJ, Flehinger BJ, Buchalter J, et al. Declining serum cholesterol levels prior to diagnosis of colon cancer: a time-trend case-control study. *JAMA*. 1990;263:2083.

1103.   Winawer S, Fletcher R, Rex D, et al; Gastrointestinal Consortium Panel. Colorectal cancer screening and surveillance: clinical guidelines and rationale-Update based on new evidence. *Gastroenterology*. 2003;124:544.

1104.   Winawer SJ, Leidner SD, Hajdu SI, et al. Colonoscopic biopsy and cytology in the diagnosis of colon cancer. *Cancer*. 1978;42:2849.

1105.   Winawer SJ, Leidner SD, Miller DG, et al. Results of a screening program for the detection of early colon cancer and polyps using fecal occult blood testing [abstract A127]. *Gastroenterology*. 1977;72:1150.

1106.   Winawer SJ, Miller C, Lightdale C, et al. Patient response to sigmoidoscopy: a randomized, controlled trial of rigid and flexible sigmoidoscopy. *Cancer*. 1987;60:1905.

1107.   Winawer SJ, Zauber AG, Ho MN, et al. Prevention of colorectal cancer by colonoscopic polypectomy. The National Polyp Study Workgroup. *N Engl J Med*. 1993;329:1977.

1108.   Winslet MC, Youngs D, Burdon DW, et al. Short-term chemoprophylaxis with ceftizoxime versus five-day aminoglycoside with metronidazole in "contaminated" lower gastrointestinal surgery. *Dis Colon Rectum*. 1990;33:878.

1109.   Winther KV, Jess T, Langholz E, et al. Long-term risk of cancer in ulcerative colitis: a population-based cohort study from Copenhagen County. *Clin Gastroenterol Hepatol*. 2004;2:1088.

1110.   Winzelberg GG, Grossman SJ, Rizk S, et al. Indium-111 monoclonal antibody B72.3 scintigraphy in colorectal cancer: correlation with computed tomography, surgery, histopathology, immunohistology, and human immune response. *Cancer*. 1992;69:1656.

1111.   Wiratkapun S, Kraemer M, Seow-Choen F, et al. High preoperative serum carcinoembryonic antigen predicts metastatic recurrence in potentially curative colonic cancer: results of a five-year study. *Dis Colon Rectum*. 2001;44:231.

1112.   Wittekind CH, Wagner G, eds. Colon and rectum. In: *TNM-Classification of Malignant Tumors*. New York, NY: Springer; 1997:64–67.

1113.   Wobbes T, Joosen KHG, Kuypers HHC, et al. The effect of packed cells and whole-blood transfusions on survival after curative resection for colorectal carcinoma. *Dis Colon Rectum*. 1989;32:743.

1114.   Wolff BG. Current status of incidental surgery. *Dis Colon Rectum*. 1995;38:435.

1115.   Wolff BG, Pemberton JH, van Heerden JA, et al. Elective colon and rectal surgery without nasogastric decompression. *Ann Surg*. 1989;209:670.

1116.   Wolloch Y, Zer M, Lurie M, et al. Ischemic colitis proximal to obstructing carcinoma of the colon. *Am J Proctol*. 1979;30:17.

1117.   Wolmark N, Fisher B, Rockette H, et al. Postoperative adjuvant chemotherapy or BCG for colon cancer: results from NSABP protocol C-01. *J Natl Cancer Inst*. 1988;80:30.

1118.   Wolmark N, Fisher B, Wieand HS. The prognostic value of the modifications of the Dukes' C class of colorectal cancer: an analysis of the NSABP clinical trials. *Ann Surg*. 1986;203:115.

1119.   Wolmark N, Fisher B, Wieand HS, et al. The prognostic significance of preoperative carcinoembryonic antigen levels in colorectal cancer. *Ann Surg*. 1984;199:375.

1120.   Wolters U, Keller HW, Sorgatz S, et al. Prospective randomized study of preoperative bowel cleansing for patients undergoing colorectal surgery. *Br J Surg*. 1994;81:598.

1121.   Wong JH, Bowles BJ, Bueno R, et al. Impact of the number of negative nodes on disease-free survival in colorectal cancer patients. *Dis Colon Rectum*. 2002;45:1341.

1122.   Wong N, Lasko D, Rabelo R, et al. Genetic counseling and interpretation of genetic tests in familial adenomatous polyposis and hereditary nonpolyposis colorectal cancer. *Dis Colon Rectum*. 2001;44:271.

1123.   Wong SL, Ji H, Hollenbeck BK, et al. Hospital lymph node examination rates and survival after resection for colon cancer. *JAMA*. 2007; 298:2149.

1124.   Wood JS, Frost DB. Results using the biofragmentable anastomotic ring for colon anastomosis. *Am J Surg*. 1993;59:642.

1125.   Wood TF, Nora DT, Morton DL, et al. One hundred consecutive cases of sentinel lymph node mapping in early colorectal carcinoma: detection of missed micrometastases. *J Gastrointest Surg*. 2002;6:322.

1126.   Woods LM, Rachet B, Coleman MP. Origins of socio-economic inequalities in cancer survival: a review. *Ann Oncol*. 2006;17:5.

1127.   Wool NL, Straus AK, Roseman DL. Hickman catheter placement simplified. *Am J Surg*. 1983;145:283.

1128.   Woolfson K. Tumor markers in cancer of the colon and rectum. *Dis Colon Rectum*. 1991;34:506.

1129.   Wüllenweber HP, Sutter C, Autschbach F, et al. Evaluation of Bethesda guidelines in relation to microsatellite instability. *Dis Colon Rectum*. 2001;44:1281.

1130.   Yamaguchi A, Ishida T, Nishimura G, et al. Detection by CT during arterial portography of colorectal cancer metastases to liver. *Dis Colon Rectum*. 1991;34:37.

1131.   Yamaguchi A, Kurosaka Y, Ishida T, et al. Clinical significance of tumor markers NCC-ST 439 in large bowel cancers. *Dis Colon Rectum*. 1991;34:921.

1132.   Yano T, Fukuyama Y, Yokoyama H, et al. Failure in resection of multiple pulmonary metastases from colorectal cancer. *J Am Coll Surg*. 1997;185:120.

1133.   Yeatman TJ, Bland KI, Copeland EM III, et al. Relationship between colorectal liver metastases and CEA levels in gallbladder bile. *Ann Surg*. 1989;210:505.

1134.   Yiu CY, Baker LA, Boulos PB. Anti-epithelial membrane antigen monoclonal antibodies and radioimmunolocalization of colorectal cancer. *Br J Surg*. 1991;78:1212.

1135.   Young JL Jr, Devesa SS, Cutler SJ. Incidence of cancer in United States blacks. *Cancer Res*. 1975;35:3523.

1136.   Young-Fadok TM, Wolff BG, Nivatvongs S, et al. Prophylactic oophorectomy in colorectal carcinoma: preliminary results of a randomized prospective trial. *Dis Colon Rectum*. 1998;41:277.

1137.   Zamcheck N, Moore TL, Dhar P, et al. Immunologic diagnosis and prognosis of human digestive-tract cancer: carcinoembryonic antigens. *N Engl J Med*. 1972;286:83.

1138.   Zhao YS, Wang F, Chang D, et al. Meta-analysis of different test indicators: *Helicobacter pylori* infection and the risk of colorectal cancer. *Int J Colorectal Dis*. 2008;23:875.

1139.   Zielinski MD, Merchea A, Heller SF, et al. Emergency management of perforated colon cancers: how aggressive should we be? *J Gastrointest Surg*. 2011;15:2232.

1140.   Zinkin LD. A critical review of the classifications and staging of colorectal cancer. *Dis Colon Rectum*. 1983;26:37.

1141.   Zinkin LD, Brandwein C. Adenocarcinoma in Crohn's colitis. *Dis Colon Rectum*. 1980;23:115.

1142.   Zmora O, Mahajna A, Bar-Zakai B, et al. Colon and rectal surgery without mechanical bowel preparation: a randomized prospective trial. *Ann Surg*. 2003;237:363.

1143.   Zmora O, Pikarsky AJ, Wexner SD. Bowel preparation for colorectal surgery. *Dis Colon Rectum*. 2001;44:1537.

24
Carcinoma of the Rectum

E. Leslie Bokey

*Doctors without anatomy are like moles: they work in
the dark and their daily tasks are mole hills.*
—FRIEDRICH TIEDEMANN (1781–1861)

The management of patients with rectal cancer is very much
a team effort, and I would like to thank three members of
my team who have assisted me with the preparation of this
chapter: Professor Pierre Chapuis, who has maintained our
database; our statistician, Professor Owen Dent; and senior
lecturer, Dr. Scott MacKenzie.

Colorectal cancer is the second most common cancer among women worldwide and the third most common
among men.[173] In high-incidence countries, approximately
25% of colorectal cancers are located in the rectum; 21%
among women and 30% among men. Surgical technique is
important in the treatment of rectal cancer, and a clear understanding of the anatomy of the rectum and its fascial relationships is therefore essential.

Over the past 30 years or so, many advances have been
made in the management of rectal cancer. These include
earlier diagnosis, improved preoperative assessment, implementation of adjuvant therapy, better surgical technique,
enhanced operating room lighting, and upgraded instruments. A better understanding of fecal continence and the
importance of the levator muscle in that regard has enabled
a profound increase in sphincter-saving procedures, whereas
in those patients requiring a permanent colostomy signal
advances in enterostomal care have improved their quality
of life.

SYMPTOMS AND SIGNS OF RECTAL CANCER

Many patients with rectal cancer are asymptomatic and are
discovered after having a positive fecal occult blood test.
Some lesions are found on "routine" endoscopy, whereas
others are identified while undergoing a screening colonoscopy for a family history of colorectal cancer or a history
of inflammatory bowel disease. Occasionally, a patient may

present with a CT scan or an ultrasound, which may have been performed for another reason, showing an abnormality in the pelvis or liver or other site of metastases.

The most common symptoms of rectal cancer include bleeding per rectum, mucous discharge, unexplained weight loss, a feeling of incomplete evacuation from the rectum, or a persisting change in bowel habit, the last often taking the form of spurious diarrhea. Rectal or pelvic pain that radiates is often a symptom of a locally advanced tumor.

▶ DIAGNOSIS

The diagnosis is usually suspected on rectal examination and is confirmed by proctoscopy, flexible sigmoidoscopy, or colonoscopy and biopsy.

▶ TRENDS IN THE MANAGEMENT OF RECTAL CANCER

The history of the surgical management of rectal cancer will be outlined later. Briefly, there has been a trend away from abdominoperineal resection (APR) of the rectum toward that of restorative procedures. Furthermore, there has been a trend for these procedures to be performed by specialist colorectal surgeons because it has become clear that surgical technique[65,248] and volume of work[12,460] can influence outcome.

There is good evidence that neoadjuvant radiotherapy and chemoradiotherapy can reduce the risk of local recurrence. Therefore, close collaboration with medical and radiation oncologists is essential in the management of each individual patient.[298] In fact, a wider range of experts is now required to treat patients with rectal cancer. These include enterostomal therapists, psychologists, radiologists, anatomical pathologists, as well as radiation and medical oncologists. Most centers now conduct regular multidisciplinary meetings to canvas opinions and to plan treatment options for each patient.

In this chapter, I will deal mainly with open surgery, but I will also include current views on laparoscopic and robotically assisted surgery for rectal cancer. Although there is evidence that laparoscopic surgery is as satisfactory as open surgery for colon cancer,[26,378] the evidence for its value with rectal cancer is not yet at hand.[503,530]

▶ DECIDING THE BEST OPTIONS FOR PATIENTS WITH RECTAL CANCER

There are many options that can be considered in the management of patients with rectal cancer. In many individuals, a decision must be made whether to recommend a restorative or a nonrestorative procedure and whether to recommend preoperative (neoadjuvant) therapy. In a smaller number of patients, other procedures may need to be considered, such as local operations and that of palliative care. Before taking a final decision, several clinical and histopathologic features, as well as certain specific investigations, can be used to help both the surgeon and the patient to decide on the best option. I believe that treating a patient with rectal cancer is analogous to ordering a hand-tailored suit rather than accepting an off-the-rack product.

▶ INVESTIGATIONS

If the entire colon cannot be visualized at colonoscopy, then occasionally a contrast study may be useful in order to exclude synchronous lesions, provided there is no obstruction.

A CT scan of the chest and abdomen should also be performed to document distant metastases. A pelvic MRI is now considered essential in assessing the extent of local tumor invasion and, in particular, in assessing whether the tumor extends beyond the perirectal fascia to potentially involve a postoperative circumferential margin (CRM). This information is important when the patient is a candidate for preoperative chemoradiotherapy. Logically, preoperative MRI cannot validly predict an involved circumferential margin, but it should guide the surgeon in determining patients at risk and in choosing the appropriate operation. Indeed, a patient with a positive MRI margin, if properly managed, should have a negative histologic CRM.[144]

Endoluminal ultrasound assessment of low tumors is also useful in determining local invasion and is described in full later. Other investigations include a complete blood count, liver and renal function tests, baseline carcinoembryonic antigen (CEA), and cardiac and respiratory assessment.

▶ FACTORS INFLUENCING THE CHOICE OF OPERATION

To save or not to save the sphincter is a perennial question. Is there a level below which an anastomosis should not be attempted? When is an APR inappropriate or an anterior resection the operation of choice? Unfortunately, there is no reliable answer to these questions. Some may even advise with the simple adage, "if you can feel the lesion you should not perform a sphincter-saving operation"—the rule of the index finger. However, this is much too simplistic an approach and may prejudice the surgeon to embark upon an inappropriate proctectomy.

Conversely, surgeons, in a zealous effort to avoid a colostomy and to reestablish intestinal continuity, may compromise the margins of resection. The consequences can be tragic: recurrent disease, anastomotic obstruction, unremitting pelvic pain, and the requirement for subsequent surgery, including a colostomy. An important factor that may influence the choice of operation is the experience of the surgeon. In most developed countries, there are centers that specialize in colorectal surgery. Moreover, there is evidence that volume of work[12,460] and technique[65,248] are independent factors that affect outcomes. Variables that are helpful in determining the choice of operation for cancer in the rectum are summarized as follows:

- Level of the tumor
- Macroscopic appearance (ulcerated, polypoid)
- Extent of circumferential involvement
- Fixity
- Degree of differentiation (histologic appearance)
- Endorectal ultrasound
- CT scanning
- Magnetic resonance imaging
- Positron emission tomography (PET) scanning
- Presacral adenopathy
- Body habitus
- Gender
- Age
- Metastatic disease

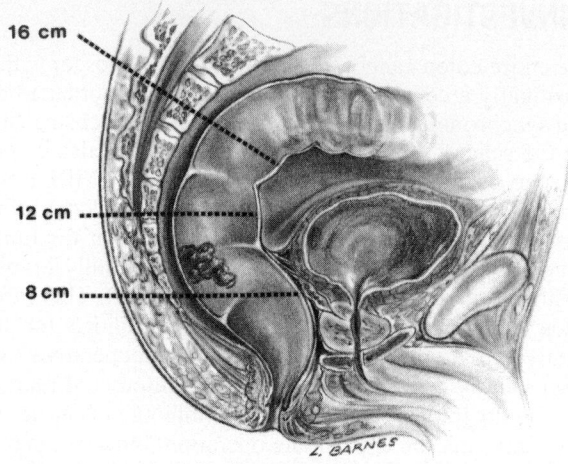

FIGURE 24-1. Distance of tumor from anal verge measured by rigid sigmoidoscopy.

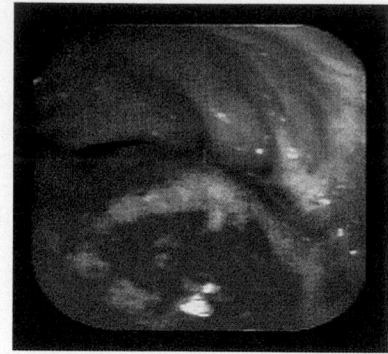

FIGURE 24-2. Endoscopy demonstrates macroscopic appearance of exophytic malignant tumor.

- Other systemic disease
- Other conditions that may affect one's ability to manage a colostomy (e.g., blindness, severe arthritis, mental incapacity)

The reader is referred to a publication by the American Society of Colon and Rectal Surgeons. This organization has established practice parameters for the preoperative evaluation and treatment of rectal cancer.[611]

Level of the Lesion

The distance of the lower edge of the tumor from the anal verge is probably the single most important variable that aids the surgeon in the choice of operation. This distance should be carefully measured using the rigid proctosigmoidoscope, and the result should be recorded (Figure 24-1). The flexible sigmoidoscope is not as accurate for this determination. When measuring, care must be taken to spread the buttocks, so that the instrument can be seen emerging from the anus, not from the contour of the buttocks. The preconceived notion that a tumor 7 cm from the anal verge requires APR but one at 8 cm can be treated by anterior resection is erroneous. Other factors may prove the opposite to be true in both cases (e.g., fixity, size, pelvic anatomy).

Macroscopic Appearance and Level of the Tumor

Ascertaining the appearance of the lesion, whether ulcerated, scirrhous (infiltrative), or polypoid, is very helpful in aiding the surgeon in the choice of operation (Figure 24-2). Generally, the distal margin of resection should be at least 1 cm; but for infiltrative carcinomas, 1 cm may not be sufficient to avoid local recurrence, even if the tumor is at or above 7 cm from the anal verge. The length of distal intramural spread of tumor in resected specimens is extremely variable, with three-fourths of the rectal tumors in one study demonstrated to have no intramural spread.[655] A small, exophytic, well-differentiated lesion may be adequately removed with a 1-cm cuff of normal distal bowel.

Extent of Circumferential Involvement

Usually, more highly aggressive tumors tend to involve a greater circumference of the bowel wall. Anteriorly, located lesions have a higher incidence of local recurrence,[94] and this should be taken into account when deciding whether or not to include neoadjuvant therapy in the management plan. The depth of local anterior invasion also has to be considered when planning the extent of surgical excision. For example, in females, one may have to include an en bloc hysterectomy or an en bloc disk excision of the posterior wall of the vagina. In selected male patients with anterior invasion of the prostate gland, consideration may be given to prostatectomy, and in those with invasion of the bladder, consideration should be given to partial or total cystectomy after consultation with and seeking the assistance of a specialist urologist.

Fixity

Fixity is best assessed by an examination under anesthesia (EUA). Fixity of the tumor in the pelvis implies locally advanced disease, a greater likelihood of residual tumor following resection, and hence local recurrence. Under these circumstances, an APR may offer a better chance of avoiding local recurrence. The presence of a fixed tumor usually signals the need for neoadjuvant therapy (see later).

Histologic Appearance

A biopsy is, of course, mandatory and is done routinely, usually at the time of initial discovery of the lesion. Ideally, the material obtained should be from the edge of the lesion because much useful information can be achieved. For example, an "expanding" margin implies that the area of invasion is pushing or reasonably well circumscribed, whereas an "infiltrating" margin suggests diffuse or widespread penetration of normal tissue.[289] All too often, however, the surgeon pays scant attention to the details of the report, except for noting whether the tumor is indeed malignant. However, it is important to be aware of the specific histologic appearance of a malignant tumor. Is it poorly differentiated, moderately well-differentiated, or well-differentiated (see Figures 23-19 through 23-22)? Generally, tumors regarded as poorly differentiated have highly irregular glands or no glandular differentiation.[289] The more anaplastic, the more aggressive is the lesion; the more aggressive, the greater is the resection margin that would be required. The chance of local recurrence is much higher with a poorly differentiated cancer than with one that is well-differentiated. It is axiomatic that one must choose the most favorable cancers for performing less than a radical resection (see later). Therefore, one cannot overestimate the importance of degree of differentiation (Broders' classification), the depth of penetration, and the

ALBERT C. BRODERS (1885–1964)

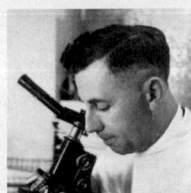

Albert Broders was born on August 8, 1885, in Fairfax County, Virginia. He received his MD degree in 1910 from the Medical College of Virginia (Richmond). After his internship, he trained at the Mayo Clinic in surgical pathology and became head of the section in 1922. Broders first began his microscopic grading (lip) in 1920. This was followed by an application of his classification (grading) to tumors of the skin, genitourinary organs, and head and neck. By 1925, he had completed his studies and presented his final classification. A numerical microscopic grading is used in Broders' classification (1935): grade 1, lesions in which between 100% and 50% of the cells are differentiated; grade 2, lesions in which between 75% and 50% of the cells are differentiated; grade 3, lesions in which between 50% and 25% of the cells are differentiated; and grade 4, lesions in which between 25% and none of the cells are differentiated. It has been said that in some respects, Broders' classification is more valuable than Dukes' because it is more versatile and applied more universally. In 1935, Broders was granted a 1-year leave of absence to become professor of surgical pathology and director of cancer research at the Medical College of Virginia. He returned to the Mayo Clinic as Chairman of the Department of Surgical Pathology. When he retired in 1950, he had been in surgical pathology at the Mayo Clinic for 37 years. Following his retirement, Broders joined the Scott and White Clinic in Temple, Texas, as senior consultant in surgical pathology. He worked in Texas for 10 years, and on March 26, 1964, at the age of 78 years, he died of a stroke in Temple. (Biography courtesy of the Mayo Clinic and Classic articles in colonic and rectal surgery. Albert Compton Broders 1885–1964. Prognosis in carcinoma of the rectum. A comparison of the Broders and Dukes methods of classification. *Dis Colon Rectum.* 1985;28:687. Photograph courtesy of Mayo Foundation for Medical Education and Research.)

presence or absence of venous or perineural invasion (PNI) in making the appropriate choice. Shirouzu and colleagues evaluated whether PNI is an independent prognostic factor in individuals who underwent curative surgery.[566] There was a significant difference in local recurrence rates between those individuals with stage III lesions who were found to have PNI and those without PNI. In addition, the investigators found that patients with PNI and stage III lesions had a significantly lower survival rate. Nevertheless, the importance of PNI as an independent prognostic factor needs further evaluation (see also Chapter 23).

Gagliardi and colleagues studied the effect of microacinar growth patterns on survival following radical surgery for rectal cancer in 138 consecutive patients.[192] They found that acinar size (whether microacinar or macroacinar) had independent prognostic value. Patients with microacinar tumors had a significantly reduced 5-year survival rate compared with those with macroacinar lesions. Saclarides and colleagues attempted to determine which features were predictors of nodal metastases.[536] They used 9 histologic and morphologic features of 62 radically excised rectal cancers to determine which were associated with nodal disease. Statistically significant variables were worsening differentiation, increasing depth of penetration, microtubular configuration of 20% or more, the presence of venous invasion or PNI, and, of course, lymphatic invasion. Exophytic tumor morphology, mitotic count, and tumor size were not significant predictors.[536] In an analysis of all the variables or combination of factors, Broders' classification was the strongest predictor of nodal disease.

A particularly useful microscopic variable to identify is the extent of lymphocytic infiltration at the border of the tumor.[288] Jass and colleagues regarded this observation as "conspicuous" when there is a distinctive and delicate connective tissue mantle or cap at the invasive margin of the growth.[289] Patients who harbor tumors that demonstrate pronounced lymphocytic infiltration have a better prognosis than those who do not. If the pathologist fails to supply this information, he or she should be asked to review the slides and to amend the report. Optimally, the surgeon should view the histologic evidence himself or herself in order to make the most reasoned recommendation to the patient.

Presacral Adenopathy

By careful palpation of the rectum with the patient in the knee-chest position, the surgeon can occasionally identify a hard lesion outside the rectal wall, presumably a lymph node with metastasis. This should be taken into account when formulating a treatment plan. Endorectal ultrasound is much more accurate for identifying enlarged and presumably involved lymph nodes in this area, but this does not diminish the importance of careful palpation.

Imaging Techniques

Several imaging modalities exist today for preoperative staging of rectal cancer, including endorectal ultrasonography, CT, MRI, and PET.[451,576,662] All of these modalities are complementary, and each has a specific role.

Computed Tomography

CT is of great value in the diagnosis of metastatic disease, especially in the liver (see Figure 23-17) and elsewhere within the abdomen (Figure 24-3) or the chest.

Magnetic Resonance Imaging

MRI is used for preoperative assessment of local invasion. It allows accurate assessment of size and relationship of the tumor to the perirectal fascia.[477] Brown and coworkers used high-resolution MRI and compared their stagings with the pathologic specimens.[77] There was a 94% weighted agreement between MRI and pathology assessment of T stage.

An improvement in MRI technique is the use of powerful gradient coil systems and high-resolution surface coils to allow a higher definition of obtainable image with a smaller field of view.[317]

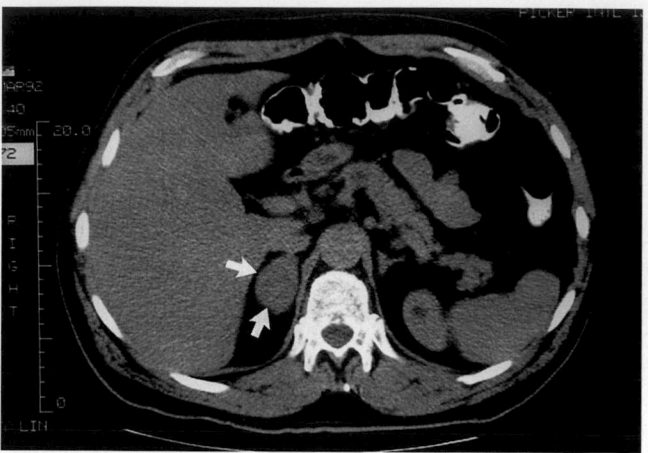

FIGURE 24-3. **A:** Computed tomography demonstrates a tumor in the wall of the rectum (*arrows*). **B:** Metastatic tumor to the adrenal gland in this same patient can be appreciated (*arrows*).

Endorectal or Transrectal Ultrasound Examination

Endorectal ultrasound (Brüel & Kjær Instruments, Inc., North Billerica, MA) (see Figure 7-18) was first described by Beynon in 1986.[51] Since then, both the technique and the equipment have improved, and the method has developed into an extremely useful tool for the preoperative assessment of patients with rectal cancer.[40,619] After a small enema is administered, the probe is introduced into the rectum beyond the tumor (Figure 24-4). A balloon is filled with approximately 50 mL of water, and an acoustic contact is produced between the rotating part of the transducer and the rectal wall.[257] During withdrawal, the monitor is observed and the findings recorded.

Each of the layers of the rectum can be sonographically visualized, with a tumor usually appearing as a hypoechoic disruption of the rectal wall. The procedure may also reveal whether underlying lymph nodes are affected. Detection of invasive carcinoma within an otherwise villous lesion can be achieved with this technique.[5,337] In the experience of Hildebrandt and colleagues, lymph node metastases can be predicted with an accuracy of 72% and inflammatory lymph nodes with a specificity of 83%.[258] Many investigators, however, have expressed concern about the lack of specificity in distinguishing benign from malignant nodes.[293,529] The Memorial Sloan-Kettering Cancer Center group observed

that the overall risk of undetected and untreated (if a local procedure is embarked upon) is 15%.[64]

Accurate preoperative assessment of local invasion with endorectal ultrasound implies the patients may be selected for a less than radical operation (see Other Local Procedures for Rectal Cancer).[206] There is uniformity of agreement that optimal results can only be obtained if there is consistency in technique and in interpretation. Certainly, accuracy improves considerably with experience.[469] MacKay and colleagues emphasized that one needs to undertake 50 or more ultrasound procedures before optimal accuracy is achieved.[382] It is therefore preferable for the surgeon to be the individual responsible for performing and evaluating the study. Some investigators have commented that tumors of the lower rectum are incorrectly assessed much more frequently than those of the middle and upper rectum.[253]

Technique

The late Douglas Wong was regarded as an international authority on TRUS and in its interpretation. He previously had been kind enough to provide me a narrative of his technique, and I thought it would be useful to reproduce it here:

> The patient is instructed to take a small volume enema
> 1 hour prior to the examination. The procedure is

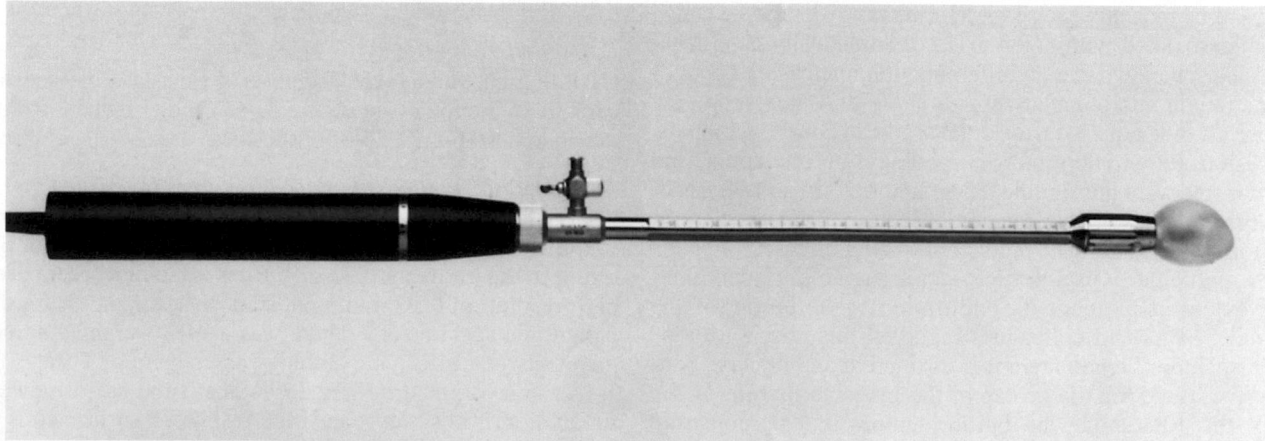

FIGURE 24-4. Ultrasound probe. (Courtesy of Brüel & Kjær Instruments, Inc., North Billerica, MA.)

W. DOUGLAS WONG (1948–2011)

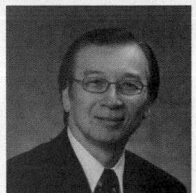

Doug, as he was known to his friends, was born in Brandon, Canada, a small town in Manitoba. It had been settled in part by Chinese immigrants after completion of the Canadian Pacific Railway in 1885. He often spoke of his family's roots and recounted with justifiable pride their history of overcoming discrimination and difficult times for them to succeed in Canada. The love of Doug's life was Sola. As a young nursing student, she had emigrated from her home in Hong Kong to Canada. Sola and Doug met in Winnipeg where he was then a first year medical student at the University of Manitoba. They were married in 1970. After obtaining his MD degree in 1972, he completed his internship and general surgical training also at the University of Manitoba in Winnipeg. Doug established a general surgical practice in 1977 in Steinbach, Manitoba. As the first surgeon in the town of 7,000 people with a drawing area of 20,000, he was soon extremely busy and constantly in demand. He decided to pursue further training in colorectal surgery and enrolled in the University of Minnesota colon and rectal surgery residency training program in 1983, after which he practiced in Calgary until 1987. He then returned to Minnesota to join the faculty of the Division of Colon and Rectal Surgery at the University of Minnesota. Wong quickly established himself as a world expert in colorectal surgery and was a pioneer in staging rectal cancer by the use of endorectal ultrasonography. He developed a large practice in St. Paul, pursued his many academic interests, and assumed leadership positions in the American Society of Colon and Rectal Surgeons (ASCRS) and other professional societies, including that of president. He especially enjoyed teaching and served as the residency program director for the Division of Colon and Rectal Surgery at the University of Minnesota from 1992 to 1997. After being offered a leadership position at Memorial Sloan-Kettering Cancer Center (MSKCC), he moved to New York City. Doug was awarded the Stuart H. Q. Quan Chair in Colorectal Surgery at MSKCC, and the next 10 years had been the much respected and beloved chief of the colorectal surgery service. His colorectal surgical colleagues at MSKCC offered this tribute to their leader as follows: "Doug Wong was a strong force in the ASCRS; an admired leader in the international community of surgeons; a proud husband, father and grandfather; and a man of unshakeable goodness, quiet grace, and true wisdom. He was a magnificent teacher, a trusted friend, and a superb doctor. His dedication to the things he loved—his work, his friends, and his family—was inspiring to us all." He died on January 20, 2011, as a result of a progressive degenerative neurologic illness. (From the Memorial Tribute by David A. Rothenberger, January 23, 2011, American Society of Colon and Rectal Surgeons Newsletter.)

carefully explained to the patient and pertinent questions answered. The assistant enters the demographic data in the ultrasound computer as well as the frequency of the ultrasound probe and its focal range. The patient is placed in the left lateral position on the examining table. The study is preceded by a digital rectal examination to evaluate the size, fixation, location, and morphology of the rectal lesion. In most instances the use of a large-bore proctoscope serves several purposes. It allows visual examination of the rectal tumor with exact determination of its location both with respect to circumferential involvement of the rectal wall and the distance from the anal verge. Secondly, it allows suctioning of any residual stool or enema fluid that might interfere with the acoustic pathways of the ultrasound waves that may distort the image. Most important, however, it allows easy passage of the probe above the tumor to ensure that the transducer is advanced above the rectal lesion to allow complete imaging. This is significant since the lower border of a rectal cancer can differ in the depth of invasion than the center or upper portions of the cancer and lymph nodes in the perirectal region are often seen just above the level of the tumor. They will be missed if complete imaging is not obtained. Small distal lesions can be adequately imaged with the ultrasound inserted blindly and advanced above the lesion, but for most midrectal, bulky tumors the use of a proctoscope will facilitate the passage of the transducer.

The probe is prepared by placing a condom over the transducer head followed by a metal ring or rubber band that secures the base of the balloon. The assistant holds the probe with the balloon in the most dependent position and fills the balloon with about 50 mL of water via the connector at the base of the metal shaft. Any air in the system is aspirated through the syringe and expelled. A water-soluble lubricant is liberally applied to the outside of the balloon. The probe is now ready for insertion. The proctoscope is then advanced above the rectal lesion, and water-soluble lubricant is inserted into the lumen of the proctoscope to facilitate passage of the probe. The probe is then gently introduced through the proctoscope and advanced such that the transducer is sited above the rectal cancer. Once the 20 cm mark on the shaft of the probe is at the proximal end of the proctoscope, the proctoscope is then pulled back on the probe as far as possible, thus exposing the transducer for 7 cm beyond the end of the instrument and positioned about the rectal cancer. The balloon is then instilled with 30 to 60 mL of water; this is the volume required to obtain optimal imaging. The transducer is activated by depressing the button on the proximal end of the probe, and the image on the screen is visualized.

When the connector for introducing the water into the balloon is pointing upwards (towards the ceiling), by convention the anterior aspect of the rectum will be on the superior part of the screen, the right lateral rectum will be on the examiner's left, the left lateral wall will be on the examiner's right, and the posterior rectum will be in the lower screen. The tip of the ultrasound probe should be maintained in the center of the rectal lumen in order to achieve optimal imaging of the rectal wall and perirectal structures. Some adjustments may have to be made on the *gain* of the ultrasound unit in order to provide better imaging. Occasionally, it is possible to perfectly depict all five layers of the rectum circumferentially, but usually only a portion of the rectal wall at a time will be optimally imaged. Minor adjustments will have to be made in the location of the probe relative to the rectal wall at various locations to optimally image all five layers clearly. Once optimal imaging of the rectal wall and surrounding structures has been achieved, the ultrasound probe is gradually withdrawn while carefully observing the screen and the images obtained. Several hard-copy images should be obtained for future reference through the use of a Polaroid image recorder. These images can be obtained by stopping the rotation of the transducer by depressing the activation/deactivation button and holding it longer, thus activating the recorder.

When a critical area of the tumor needs to be visualized at a higher magnification, the window can be activated which gives a large image of the area being examined. The entire length of the rectal tumor is evaluated. It is not uncommon for one to perform several passes along the full length of the tumor in order to acquire all the relevant information.

Attention must also be focused on the perirectal tissues in order to search for potentially involved lymph nodes. In general, normal lymph nodes are not visualized with the ultrasound, and, therefore, any hypoechoic structure in the surrounding perirectal tissue should be suspected of harboring metastatic disease. Lymph nodes often exhibit hypoechoic echogenicity comparable to that of the primary tumor, are more often round than oval, and are frequently irregular in appearance. Lymph nodes can be distinguished from blood vessels that are also circular hypoechoic areas, but when followed distally and proximally, they seem to extend further and may be seen to elongate and to branch. Once the study is completed, the balloon is deflated, and the probe is removed. Figure 24-5 illustrates the five layers of the rectal wall seen schematically and in the TRUS image of the normal rectum. The *inner white*

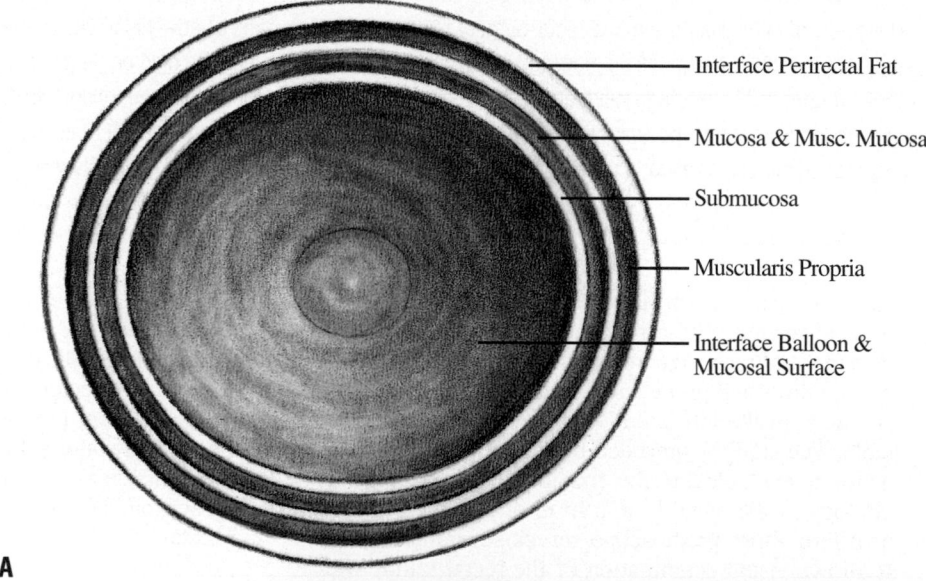

Interface Perirectal Fat

Mucosa & Musc. Mucosa

Submucosa

Muscularis Propria

Interface Balloon &
Mucosal Surface

A

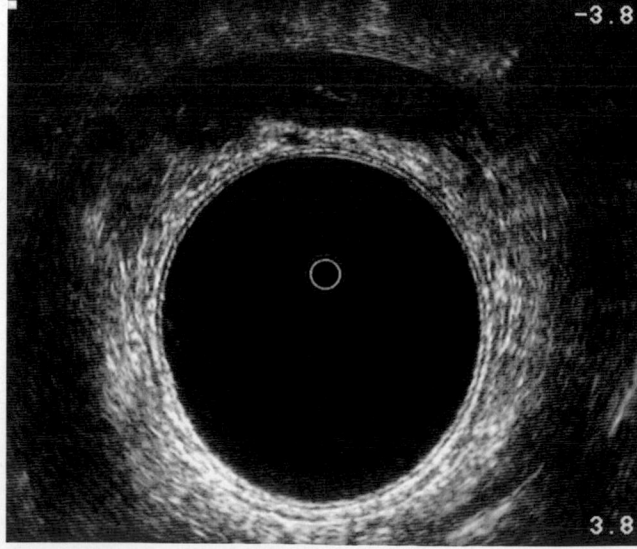

FIGURE 24-5. Endorectal ultrasound. **A:** Schematic diagram of normal rectal wall anatomic layers. **B:** Endorectal ultrasound imaging of normal rectum.

B

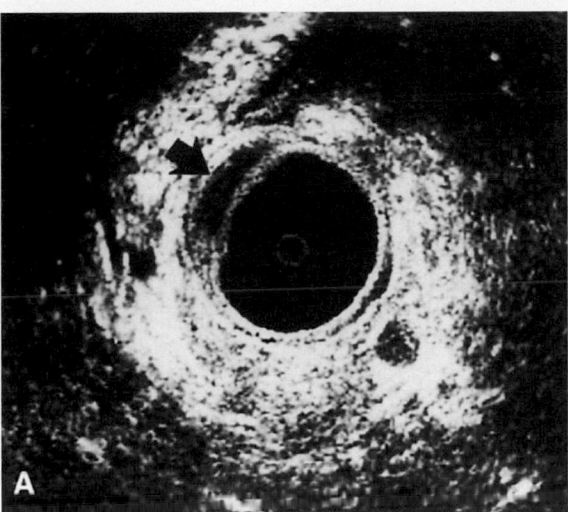
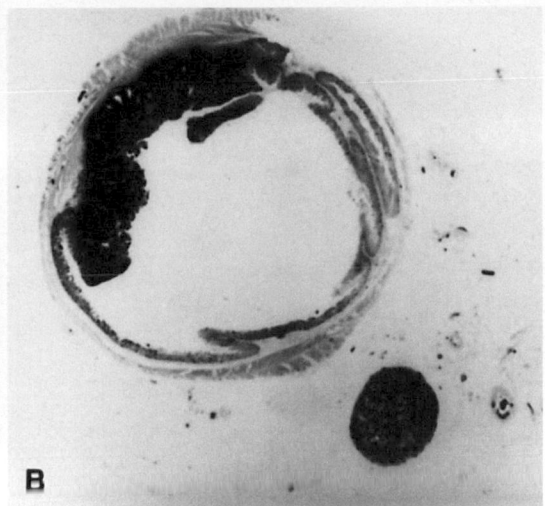

FIGURE 24-6. Endorectal ultrasound. **A:** Sonogram of a rectal cancer confined to wall of the bowel (*arrow*). The *black cavity* is the water-filled balloon with the *white circle in the center* corresponding to the transducer. A hyperechoic lymph node can be seen in the **lower right**. **B:** Corresponding photomicrograph of the excised specimen confirms the depth of invasion by tumor. The lymph node in the **lower right** was free of tumor. (Courtesy of Ulrich Hildebrandt, MD.)

line represents the interface of the balloon with the mucosal surface of the rectal wall. The *inner black line* represents the mucosa and muscularis mucosa, whereas the *middle white line* corresponds to the submucosa. It is this *middle white line* that is the most crucial layer to visualize in order to determine whether the tumor is invasive.[292] The *outer black line* corresponds to the muscularis propria, whereas the *outer white line* represents the interface between the muscularis propria and the perirectal fat. Once it has been ascertained that the *middle white line* is broken, then the presence of an invasive tumor has been confirmed. It is then a matter of determining the depth of invasion. Figure 24-6 demonstrates an ultrasound of a minimally invasive cancer with the corresponding resected, microscopic area. Figure 24-7 shows transmural involvement by tumor.

The TNM (tumor, node, metastasis) classification is used with a *u* modifier to describe depth of invasion and the presence or absence of metastatic lymph nodes as described by Beynon and coworkers[51,53]:

T Stage	Ultrasound Characteristics
uT$_0$	Noninvasive lesion. Hyperechoic submucosal interface is intact.
uT$_1$	Invasion of submucosa only. Hyperechoic middle white line is stippled and irregular but not disrupted.
uT$_2$	Breaching of hyperechoic *middle white line* indicates invasion of **hypo**echoic muscularis

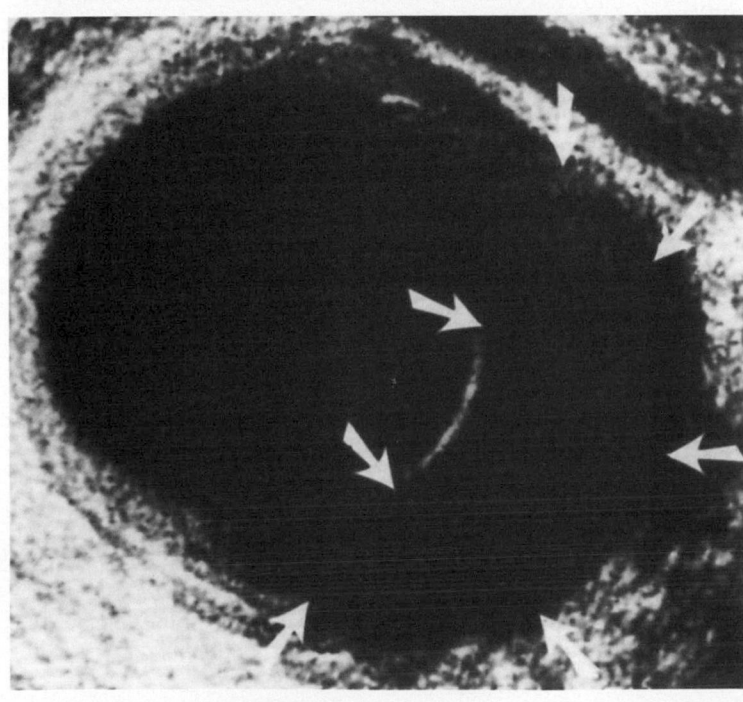

FIGURE 24-7. Endorectal ultrasound. Sonogram of a rectal cancer that penetrates into perirectal fat. Note the hypoechoic area (*arrows*). The outermost layer of the bowel wall has been interrupted. (Courtesy of Ulrich Hildebrandt, MD.)

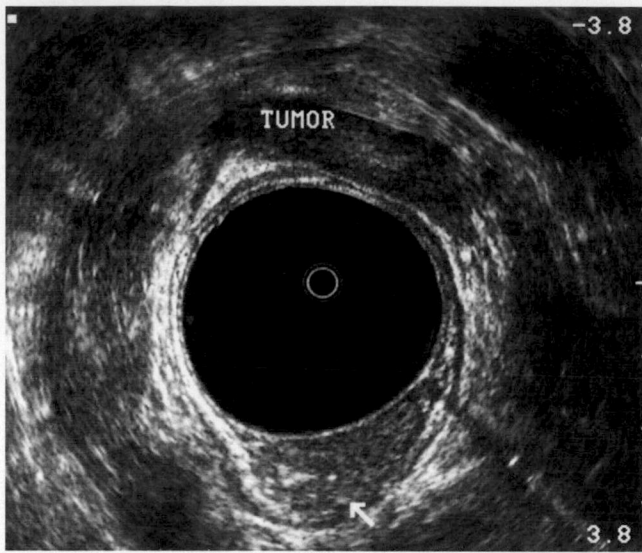

FIGURE 24-8. Endorectal ultrasound scan of a uT₂ tumor. Note disruption of the *middle white line* with the intact *outer white line*.

	propria (Figure 24-8). *Outer white line* is intact. Deep uT₂ lesions have a scalloped appearance.
uT₃	Invasion through muscularis propria into perirectal fat (Figure 24-7). Outer (hyperechoic) white line (junction of muscularis propria with perirectal fat) is disrupted.
uT₄	Extension into adjacent organ or structure (e.g., vagina, prostate, bladder, cervix, seminal vesicles). Plane between any of these structures and the rectum is obliterated.

In the foregoing, uN₀ represents evidence of lymph nodes, uN₁ represents lymph nodes positive for tumor, MX indicates metastatic tumor status unknown, M0 represents no evidence of metastatic tumor, and M1 means that metastatic tumor is present.

In addition to the cited indications, this technique offers the opportunity for clear visualization of the full thickness of an anastomotic area in those patients who have undergone restoration of rectal continuity, especially with respect to the possibility of early detection of recurrent cancer and for assessing the effects of preoperative radiotherapy.[52,102,296,400,454,519] Further information can be obtained by means of ultrasonographically guided biopsy and histologic determination of lymph node status.[562,664]

Published Experience and Comparative Results

The Creighton University group in Omaha, Nebraska, performed preoperative ultrasound staging on 107 patients with rectal cancer.[4] TRUS identified 18 of 19 patients with uT₃ tumors and 44 of 51 individuals with less invasion than uT₃ (86.3%). Garcia-Aguilar and colleagues reported the University of Minnesota group's experience of 1,184 patients with rectal adenocarcinoma or villous adenoma who underwent TRUS, comparing their assessment with pathologic specimens obtained by either resection or transanal excision without neoadjuvant treatment.[198] Somewhat disappointingly, overall accuracy in assessing the degree of rectal wall invasion was only 69%, with 18% overstaged and 13% understaged. Overall accuracy in assessing nodal involvement

in those who underwent radical surgery (238 patients) was 64%, with 25% overstaged and 11% understaged. The primary benefits appear to have been in determining which tumors were benign and those that either went completely through the rectal wall and those that did not.[198]

Positron Emission Tomography

As yet, there is no evidence base for preoperative PET "T and N" staging of rectal cancer, and the technique is not routinely used for this purpose.[451,662] However, PET may assist in identifying systemic distant metastases when CT results are equivocal.[565]

Rectal Endoscopic Lymphoscintigraphy

Endoscopic lymphoscintigraphy is not in routine practice and is still being evaluated.[42] Arnaud and colleagues performed preoperative evaluation of patients with known rectal cancer in order to identify evidence of lymphatic spread.[13] The procedure involves the endoscopic injection of 0.1 mL of radiocolloid (rhenium sulfur marked with ^{99m}Tc) into the submucosa of the extraperitoneal rectum bilaterally. The diffusion of the tracer along the lymphatics was registered by means of a computerized gamma camera. In 10 control subjects and in a series of 85 patients with rectal cancer, the technique was found to have a sensitivity rate of 85%, a specificity of 68%, an overall accuracy of 76%, a positive predictive value of 71%, and a negative predictive value of 71%. The authors concluded that rectal endoscopic lymphoscintigraphy represented the only currently available method for evaluating lymphatic spread in rectal cancer.[13]

Other Factors That May Influence Management Plan and Surgical Procedure

The previously discussed methods of evaluation concern the tumor itself. The following factors are patient related and may also influence the choice of operation.

Body Habitus

A rectal resection carried out on an asthenic patient usually permits a technically lower anastomosis than does an operation for the same level of lesion in an obese individual. Body habitus is an important factor to consider when deciding whether or not a restorative procedure is possible. As a rule, however, I try to make that decision with the patient before the operation rather than at the time of surgery.

Gender

An anastomotic procedure is more likely to be possible in women than in men. A broad pelvis, furthermore, usually permits a wider resection, whereas a narrow pelvis tends to impede dissection, potentially limiting the adequacy of tumor margins and the use of conventional anastomotic techniques. This is especially true when one performs a low anterior resection.

Age

Age is not a contraindication to a restorative procedure. However, one has to take into account continence and bowel dysfunction in an elderly patient after a low or ultralow restorative procedure. In some elderly and frail patients, it may be more prudent to perform an APR or even a low Hartmann procedure rather than a restorative operation. A radical resection is not contraindicated in patients solely because of advanced age. However, some elderly patients may be better suited to a local approach to treatment.

Metastatic Disease

If metastatic disease is present at the time of diagnosis, then the extent has to be carefully evaluated. This is preferentially accomplished by means of PET scanning. A multidisciplinary team approach is very useful. If there is significant intra-abdominal metastatic disease, a restorative procedure aimed at avoiding a colostomy may not be the ideal solution because there is a high risk of developing bowel obstruction that may require further operation and a stoma. In some patients with extensive metastatic disease at the time of operation, a Hartmann procedure or even a defunctioning loop stoma may be preferable. Alternatively, a local procedure or other nonsurgical form of therapy may suffice to palliate the individual's symptoms.

Comorbidities at the Time of Surgery

Patients, regardless of age, are at increased surgical risk if comorbidities are present (e.g., cardiovascular, pulmonary, renal). In those with significant or multiple comorbidities, a procedure that does not involve an anastomosis may be considered safer.

Ondrula and colleagues analyzed the predictive value of a number of preoperative risk factors on operative outcomes in 825 patients.[466] Those factors that were found to be statistically significant in predicting a greater risk were emergency operation, age greater than or equal to 75 years, congestive heart failure, prior abdominal or pelvic radiation therapy, corticosteroid use, serum albumin less than 2.7 g/dL, chronic obstructive pulmonary disease, prior myocardial infarction, diabetes, cirrhosis, and renal insufficiency. The authors assigned a "risk score" for each category in order to determine a strategy for management based on the sum total of the risks.

Other Conditions

Avoiding a colostomy in a patient who cannot cope with an appliance or a stoma is an unusual, albeit legitimate, reason for choosing an alternative procedure. This can happen if the individual is blind, has severe impairment in the use of hands (e.g., arthritis), or cannot be taught, or if there is no family or community support.

Preoperative Assessment Under Anesthesia

Examination under anesthesia is very useful for assessing patients with a low rectal cancer. Valuable information can be gathered about the circumferential location of the tumor, the distance of the tumor from the anal verge, and the presence and extent of tumor tethering or fixity. All of these are important in determining the choice of operation and whether preoperative adjuvant therapy is appropriate.

Multidisciplinary Meetings

Although such meetings are not mandatory, they are very useful in canvassing the opinions of other specialist nursing and medical staff. The final decision, however, should remain between the surgeon and patient.[420,429] One of the main advantages of multidisciplinary meetings is the opportunity to discuss the appropriateness of neoadjuvant therapy.

Neoadjuvant Therapy

Over the past 30 years, there has been considerable debate over the use of neoadjuvant therapy for rectal cancer. In particular, there has been debate whether radiotherapy is useful at all, whether it should be given preoperatively or

postoperatively, and whether it is applicable for all rectal cancers or for only those in the lower third of the rectum and for those that are locally advanced. There has been debate whether a long course is superior to that of short-course preoperative radiotherapy[82,425,432] and whether adjuvant chemotherapy is useful for rectal cancer.[114,447]

In this section, I include a brief historical review of the subject and conclude with a summary of current practice.

Historical Review

The rationale for neoadjuvant radiation therapy in the management of rectal cancer is to alter the viability of cancer cells so that they are no longer capable of local implantation.[570] When the concept was first proposed, however, there was concern that delay in initiating surgical treatment could increase the risk of tumor spread, but there is no evidence today to suggest that this is in fact the case. The primary issue is identifying those patients in advance who would most likely benefit from neoadjuvant radiotherapy. How can one make this determination? Clinical assessment is probably the gold standard, but endorectal ultrasound, CT, and MRI may also be quite helpful. Staging laparotomy has been suggested in order to determine mobility, resectability, staging, and the possibility of constructing a diversionary stoma before embarking on radiotherapy.[81] Some authors believe that every rectal cancer should be treated by preoperative radiation, but most surgeons are selective in their approach. The following variables are generally considered appropriate indications for performing preoperative radiation:

- Fixed tumor
- Evidence of ureteric obstruction
- Invasion of adjacent structures (e.g., bladder, seminal vesicles, vagina)
- Presacral adenopathy
- Anal canal invasion
- Ultrasound uT_3 or uT_4 lesion
- Poorly differentiated histology

The impetus for the application of preoperative radiotherapy can be attributed to the reports by Jean Papillon in Lyon[483] and by Quan and Stearns and their colleagues at the Memorial Sloan-Kettering Cancer Center in New York.[346,582,585-587] Although their initial studies indicated improved survival, a prospective evaluation demonstrated that the overall survival rate was not better, but that the incidence of failure because of local recurrence was reduced.[587] At that institution, Stearns and colleagues used external radiation through opposing anterior and posterior portals, 2.5 Gy daily to 20 Gy. The resection was carried out 2 days to 6 weeks following treatment.

The classic article that evaluated preoperative radiation was reported by Dwight and Higgins and their colleagues from the Veterans Administration (VA).[157] This study randomly allocated 700 men either to surgery or to preoperative radiotherapy plus surgery. These investigators found a statistically significant decreased incidence of positive nodes in the irradiated group and a lower incidence of recurrent disease in those who died. Roswit and associates used 20 Gy over 2 weeks, with a booster dose of 5 Gy if the tumor was less than 9 cm from the anal verge.[527]

Since these initial reports, there have been numerous papers that attest to the success of radiotherapy in reducing the size of the tumor, downstaging the degree of invasion, and decreasing

JEAN PAPILLON (1914–1993)

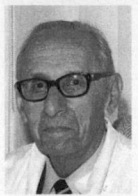

Jean Papillon was born in Lyons, France, September 18, 1914, the city in which he resided for his entire life. He graduated from the Medical School in 1936 and entered the Internship Program at Lyons Hospital. He completed his training in radiology at the University of Lyons in 1944 with his thesis *Radiological Studies of Bronchial Obstruction*. In 1946, he became radiologist physician to the Hôpitaux de Lyons. In 1943, he also worked at the Centre Léon Bérard, a well-recognized institution devoted to oncology. Through these auspices, he contributed more than 500 articles and lectures on a variety of tumor problems, such as Hodgkin's disease, head and neck malignancies, and thoracic, gynecologic, and osseous tumors. In 1950, he became interested in the management of cancer of the anus and rectum. Using the concepts initially advocated by Lamarque in Montpellier, Papillon developed the techniques of intrarectal contact x-ray therapy and anal cancer curietherapy. As a consequence of his initial observations, he formulated the protocol of treatment using radiation therapy alone or in combination with surgery for the management of anal and rectal cancers in order to effect sphincteric preservation. Papillon was appointed head of radiotherapy at the Centre Léon Bérard in 1951 and in 1955 became professor of radiotherapy at Lyons University. Author of a text dedicated to Rupert Turnbull, *Conservative Treatment by Irradiation—An Alternative to Radical Surgery*, he received international recognition for his contributions through honorary fellowship in the Royal College of Radiologists, the Canadian College of Radiologists, and the American College of Radiologists.

STUART H. Q. QUAN (1920–PRESENT)

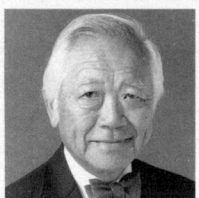

Stuart Quan was born in Oakland, California on July 4, 1920, the youngest of 10 children and the son of a physician from China who practiced Chinese medicine in San Francisco. Although Quan was only 3 years old when his father passed away, he knew as early as 6 years old that he wished to become a doctor. He completed his undergraduate education at Stanford University and graduated from Harvard Medical School in Boston in 1945. There followed 3 years of residency in Boston before his initial visit to New York. In 1949, his interest in oncologic surgery took him to the Memorial Hospital for Cancer and Allied Diseases as an assistant resident in surgery. Except for 2 years serving with the U.S. Air Force as a flight surgeon in France and Libya, he has been continuously on the surgical staff at the Memorial Sloan-Kettering Cancer Center in New York to this day. Quan has contributed extensively to his chosen field, that of colorectal cancer surgery. As such, he has been recognized through numerous awards and honors, including presidency of the American Society of Colon and Rectal Surgeons and an endowed chair in his honor at Memorial-Sloan Kettering. He and his colleagues were pioneers in promoting preoperative irradiation for cancer of the rectum. After 51 years of caring for a huge number of patients, he retired from the practice of surgery, but not from his academic pursuits.

MAUS W. STEARNS (1914–2009)

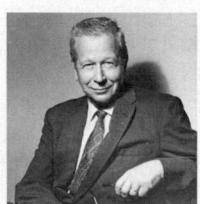

Maus Stearns was born in Schenectady, New York. He accomplished his premedical studies at Union College in that city and graduated from the Albany Medical College in 1939. Following his internship in Port Chester, New York, he began his long association with the Memorial Hospital from resident surgeon to chief of the rectal and colon service. In 1942, his training was interrupted by World War II. Stearns served 3 years in the China-Burma-India theater, and he helped to operate on 25,000 Chinese patients and cared for such legendary soldiers as Merrill's Marauders and others under the command of General Stillwell. Following his demobilization, he received a National Cancer Institute fellowship through the Memorial Hospital for 3 years. Stearns then joined the Colon and Rectal Service, which had been organized by George Binkley, a man who had been recruited by James Ewing to treat rectal cancer with radium. This experience led to the comprehensive evaluation of radiation by Stearns and his colleagues at that institution. Many important publications were the result of his leadership of the department, with Stearns being the prime motivator for accumulating and publishing the Memorial Hospital's experience. In response to Turnbull's description of the "no-touch" technique, Stearns opined that the time-honored tenet of sound surgical technique to encompass radical en bloc excision of the primary tumor with the lymphatics was the critical issue and that it is the radical treatment and completeness of the resection responsible for optimal results—not the so-called no-touch approach. Stearns received many honors and recognitions, including presidency of the Society of Surgical Oncology (now the James Ewing Society) and presidency of the American Society of Colon and Rectal Surgeons. He passed away in Pacific Grove, California, June 3, 2009. (Photograph courtesy of Blackstone-Shelburne, New York.)

GEORGE ALFRED HIGGINS (1917–1994)

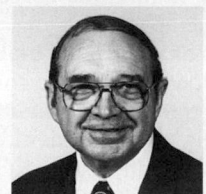

George Higgins was born in Towanda, Kansas, but grew up in Mountainair, New Mexico, where he attended the University of New Mexico. Following graduation, he entered Harvard Medical School in Boston in 1942 and then pursued a residency in surgery at the Boston City Hospital. His training was interrupted by World War II. Following his service as a battalion surgeon at Fort Hood, Texas and at the Walter Reed Hospital in Washington, DC, he completed his surgical training at the Veterans Administration (VA) Hospital in Washington, DC. Following appointments as chief of surgery at the Wichita, Kansas and Kansas City, Missouri VA Hospitals, he accepted the position as chief of surgery at the Washington, DC, VA. Certified in general and thoracic surgery, he achieved the rank of professor of surgery at both Georgetown University and the George Washington University Medical Schools. At the age of 65, he retired from the VA and embarked on a new career—that of director of surgical education at the Santa Barbara Cottage Hospital in California. He remained in that position until his death. Higgins was the quintessential academician, holding numerous research grants and writing or stimulating the writing of hundreds of peer-reviewed papers and three books. However, his greatest love and commitments were to the training of surgical residents. Higgins assumed the position of chairman of the VA Surgical Adjuvant Chemotherapy Study Group and provided the leadership and inspiration for the 34 clinical research protocols that were developed for the neoadjuvant and adjuvant treatments of cancer of the lung, stomach, colon, rectum, and pancreas. Among his many honors and recognitions were the Gold Medal Paper Award of the Southeastern Surgical Congress, the Arthur Shipley Award of the Southern Surgical Association, and the Lucy Wortham James Clinical Research Award of the Society of Surgical Oncology. He died on September 3, 1994. (With appreciation to Elliot D. Prager, MD and to the American Surgical Association.)

the risk of local recurrence.[69,73,84,101,118–120,128,152,174,178,194,197,200,201,224,254,280,286,303,322,399,413,414–418,427,474,483,521,524,526,571,574,577,615,626]

Some have stated that survival rates are better.[181,605] Kandioler and coworkers observe that a tumor with a normal p53 genotype is predictive for response to preoperative short-term radiotherapy and increased patient survival.[300] However, there remains disagreement whether preoperative radiation therapy has any effect on survival.[204]

Methods

Minsky commented about the weaknesses of the prospective, randomized trials.[523] He stated that none uses standard dosages of radiation therapy. He also opined that the interval between the completion of radiation and surgery is generally considered to be inadequate. The Memorial Sloan-Kettering Cancer Center group demonstrated a trend toward an increased pathologic response rate and downstaging when an interval between completing the radiotherapy and surgery is at least 44 days.[434] Most recommend 4 to 6 weeks following completion of the treatment in order to achieve maximum downstaging and tissue recovery. Moreover, he affirmed that using anterior-posterior/posterior-anterior portals, rather than multiple-field techniques, predisposes to increased morbidity associated with the radiation.[424] Others confirmed that the morbidity and mortality of both preoperative and postoperative radiotherapy are higher when two-portal rather than three-portal or four-portal radiation technique is employed.[467] This is especially true for elderly patients who may have an increased risk of impairment for blood supply. Stein and colleagues concluded in the analysis of their patients that a longer time interval (beyond 8 weeks) between completion of neoadjuvant chemoradiation and surgical resection did not increase the tumor response rate or reduce the morbidity associated with the surgery.[591]

There is considerable controversy as to what the optimal dose for preoperative radiation treatment should be. Some have recommended a short course of high-dose therapy, whereas most centers in the United States suggest 40 to 45 Gy, delivered in 4 to 6 weeks. Surgery is recommended approximately 4 to 6 weeks after the completion of the treatment because tumoricidal benefits may continue for some time. Data show no increased morbidity or mortality associated with supplementary treatment.[155,504]

Results

The largest prospective, randomized trials come from Sweden—actually a combination of two Swedish protocols (the Stockholm Rectal Cancer Study Group and the Swedish Rectal Cancer Trial).[185,266,267,269,270,603–605] In the Stockholm trial, the most recent publication analyzed postoperative morbidity, mortality, local recurrence, and death from rectal cancer in 1,399 patients who were prospectively randomized to preoperative radiotherapy or no radiotherapy.[267] Those allocated to preoperative radiotherapy received a total dose of 35 Gy in five fractions over 1 week, with surgery performed within 1 week thereafter. Interestingly, patients operated on by surgeons who were certified specialists for at least 10 years had a lower risk of local recurrence and death from rectal cancer.[267] A significantly reduced risk of local recurrence was observed, but there was no clear improvement in survival. However, the investigators also found that the postoperative mortality rate may be increased in the radiotherapy group.[269]

In the Swedish Rectal Cancer Trial involving 1,168 patients (as of the most recent date), preoperative radiation was accomplished through 25 Gy and five fractions in 1 week, also followed by operation within 1 week.[604] In this randomized, prospective study, the local recurrence rate during a period of 2 years was reduced by approximately 65%. Furthermore, this short-term regimen of high-dose preoperative radiotherapy was found to improve survival.[605] The overall 5-year survival rate was 58% in the radiotherapy plus surgery group and 48% in the surgery-alone group ($P = .004$). This appears to be truly the first clear demonstration of improved survival by means of preoperative radiotherapy. In another report from the Uppsala, Sweden group involving patients who underwent preoperative radiotherapy followed by low anterior resection using historical controls, there was strong evidence for improved long-term survival.[130] In still another prospective, randomized trial that was undertaken by the Medical Research Council Rectal Cancer Working Party in Birmingham, England, investigators used 40 Gy given in 20 fractions of 2 Gy over 4 weeks in those individuals randomized to preoperative radiotherapy.[412] At 5-year follow-up, those who were randomized to radiation therapy had a statistically significantly lower incidence of local recurrence as well as fewer distant metastases. However, survival results were equivocal.

There is an inherent problem concerning a well-controlled, randomized trial with this group of patients. Stratification by the usual criterion, namely, depth of invasion (e.g., Dukes' classification), cannot be applied. One must use other, less well-defined criteria such as clinical judgment. Endorectal ultrasound is of help for staging the depth of penetration,[454,553] and DNA ploidy seems to be an independent factor for predicting response to radiotherapy,[250] but for the present time, one must await the results of the studies currently in progress.

Complications and Functional Results

Wichmann and associates concluded based on their evaluation of 30 patients who underwent preoperative chemoradiotherapy that this treatment results in significant immune dysfunction as indicated by depression of lymphocyte subpopulations, monocytes, granulocytes, and proinflammatory cytokine release.[651] They believed that these observations are important in contributing to the increased perioperative morbidity that is seen as a consequence of neoadjuvant therapy. Experienced surgeons are well aware of the problem of delayed healing of the perineal wound after proctectomy when preoperative radiation is performed.[513] The safety of performing anastomosis in the rectum following radiation therapy has been a matter of conjecture. Some studies, however, have demonstrated that colorectal anastomoses can be performed without concern for an increased risk of complications if the radiation dose does not exceed 45 Gy.[110,112,180, 271,397,428,431,517,648] Still, preoperative radiotherapy may have an adverse effect on long-term anorectal function.[648] For example, the Cleveland Clinic group reviewed anal canal specimens following pelvic radiation and noted damage to the myenteric plexus of the internal anal sphincter.[131] A tendency to increased collagen deposition was also observed. Birnbaum and colleagues prospectively evaluated the acute effect of preoperative radiation (45 Gy) on anal function in 20 individuals.[55] These investigators concluded that preoperative radiation therapy has minimal immediate effect on the anal sphincter and is not a major contributing factor to postoperative incontinence after sphincter-saving operations for rectal cancer. However, preoperative radiotherapy alters endosonographic staging and interferes with the endosonographic interpretation of the anastomotic area.[454] Others have observed that preoperative radiotherapy may have a pejorative effect on male sexual and urinary function.[66]

Dahlberg and coworkers ascertained the long-term effects on bowel function by means of a questionnaire of 171 patients who could be evaluated and who were included in the Swedish Rectal Cancer Trial.[129] Mean bowel frequency per week, incontinence for loose stool, urgency, and emptying difficulties were statistically significantly more common

following preoperative radiation when compared with those operated on without radiation. This serves to emphasize the importance of patient selection in order to limit the consequences of nonbeneficial neoadjuvant therapy.

A recent trial that is often referred to as the "Dutch trial" has demonstrated a clear reduction in local recurrence following "TME" surgery and short-course preoperative radiotherapy, but there was no survival benefit.[301,498] The addition of chemotherapy is noteworthy in the German CAO/ARO/A10 94 trial in which all patients had "TME" surgery and postoperative adjuvant chemotherapy. The study compared patients having preoperative and postoperative chemoradiotherapy plus "TME" surgery (see later). Results showed a lower local recurrence rate in the preoperative treated group (6% vs. 12%) and a reduction in toxicity, but again no effect on overall survival.[551]

My current practice is to discuss patients with rectal cancer at a multidisciplinary meeting. Patients with a cancer in the lower third of the rectum are considered suitable for neoadjuvant therapy as are many with tumors in the middle third. Those in the upper third are not felt to be suitable. Those who have a locally advanced tumor (as determined by digital examination, MRI, endoanal ultrasonography) and considered likely candidates (provided they are younger than 80 years of age and do not have significant comorbidities, especially serious cardiovascular comorbidities), are included. Treatment should be individualized to meet the needs of the patient, and if the risk of local recurrence is significant, then the use of radiotherapy is justified. I recommend this treatment for the following:

1. Patients with low bulky tumors
2. Those in whom the tumor is tethered or fixed
3. Patients whose preoperative ultrasound suggests extensive direct spread beyond the rectal wall and/or the presence of suspicious nodes
4. Where biopsy indicates a poorly differentiated or high-grade tumor

I use postoperative radiotherapy rarely and only where there is histologic confirmation of an incomplete excision or circumferential resection margin involvement.[95] I favor a course of long-term chemoradiotherapy followed by a rest period of at least 6 weeks prior to resection. Once all wounds are healed, patients complete a course of postoperative chemotherapy.

Preoperative Preparation

In my practice, the patient is assessed in a preadmission clinic and admitted on the day of surgery. An orthograde bowel preparation is administered at home. The patient is assessed by an enterostomal nurse preoperatively, and possible stoma is sited appropriately. Perioperative broad-spectrum intravenous antimicrobials and subcutaneous heparin are administered.

▶ SURGICAL MANAGEMENT OF RECTAL CANCER

Historical Notes

Colostomy as a diverting procedure has its origins in antiquity. Praxagoras (c. 400 BC) was alleged to have employed some form of decompression maneuver for ileus. Alexis Littre (1710) is usually credited with the concept

ALEXIS LITTRE (1658–1726)

Alexis Littre's name is often confused with that of another eminent French anatomist, Emile Littré, who lived about a century later (note the accent over the "e"). Littre was born on July 21, 1658, at Cordes, Tarn-et-Garonne, France. He studied in Montpellier and in Paris. In 1690, he became licensed in medicine and received a doctorate in 1691. As an anatomist and surgeon, Littre lectured extensively and is credited with numerous advances in surgical techniques. He was the first to suggest that a deliberate colostomy could be successfully performed when he examined the body of a 6-day-old infant born with an imperforate anus. His concept was extraordinarily prescient. His many papers were published in *L'Histoire de l'Académie des Sciences*. Littre's name is associated with the mucus glands of the male urethra and the diverticular hernia. He died on February 3, 1726.

JEAN ZULEMA AMUSSAT (1796–1855)

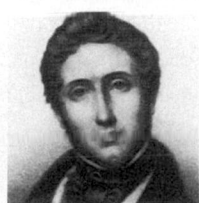

Amussat was born at St. Maixent in the Poitou, France. He was the son of a physician, and he received his basic tutelage at the hands of his father and from another surgeon in the town. At the age of 17, Amussat joined the army in a position equivalent to today's medic and performed many battlefield operations during the Napoleonic Wars. He became quite knowledgeable in anatomy through his wartime experiences and by dissecting the corpses of Russian soldiers. Following the war, he went to Paris to complete his medical studies. While there, he developed an interest in neurologic disease and is credited with having invented the rachitome. In 1822, he described a technique for removing foreign bodies from the bladder and for dilating urethral strictures. In 1826, he described the different kinds of groin hernias as they related to the inferior epigastric artery. In 1835, he published an experimental technique of intestinal anastomosis. He also presented classic works on experimental air embolism in animals, surgery for uterine fibroids, surgery for strabismus, and hemorrhoidectomy. He is believed to be the first person to perform a colostomy for an obstructing carcinoma of the rectum and was considered one of the most ingenious and innovative surgeons of his time. He was recognized by his colleagues through his elevation to membership in the Imperial Academy of Medicine and was a Chevalier of the French Legion of Honor.

JAMES LUKE (1799–1881)

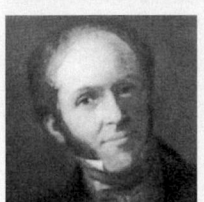

Luke was born at Exeter, England, the son of a merchant and banker. At the age of 17, and upon the death of his father, he became attached to John Andrews of the London Hospital. He attended the lectures and, 3 years later, was appointed Demonstrator of Anatomy. In 1827, he was elected assistant surgeon and ultimately achieved the position of consulting surgeon in 1861. At the Royal College of Surgeons, Luke was a member of the council for 20 years and was president in 1853 and again in 1862. He was a Hunterian Orator in 1852. Luke was a tall man who was said to harbor an irascible temper. A rapid surgeon, he once amputated a leg at the hip and removed the limb in 27 seconds. He was particularly interested in the treatment of cleft palate and of fractures and in the repair of groin hernias. He is believed to have been the first surgeon to perform a pararectus incision for bowel obstruction, bringing the proximal colon out in this location. He recommended this approach in preference to Amussat's suggestion, particularly when the site of the obstruction had not been clearly delineated preoperatively. Luke retired to Buckinghamshire, where he lived as a country gentleman, employing himself in woodcarving until his death.

of ultimately performing a colostomy when he undertook a postmortem examination on an infant who died with an imperforate anus. He is quoted as stating, ". . . it would be necessary to make an incision into the belly, open the two ends of the closed bowel, . . . bring the bowel to the surface of the body wall where it would never close, but perform the function of an anus."[360] Colostomy, however, did not achieve an important role until Amussat (1839),[9] a French surgeon, urged that it be the routine procedure for obstructing rectal cancer.[386] For most of the 19th and into the 20th century, the stoma was placed in the inguinal or iliac region. This avoided entering the peritoneal cavity. Luke,[379] however, was an exception. He was the first to bring the bowel out in the area of the rectus muscle, whereas Deaver[134] was an advocate of lumbar colostomy.

The treatment of carcinoma of the rectum by some form of excisional or amputative procedure dates back more than 250 years, but it was not until 1826 that Lisfranc successfully

JOHN BLAIR DEAVER (1855–1931)

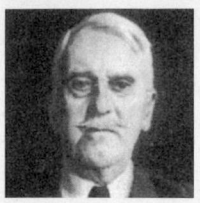

Deaver was born in Lancaster County, Pennsylvania, the son of a country physician. He attended Nottingham Academy near his home and matriculated in America's first medical school, the University of Pennsylvania in Philadelphia, graduating in 1878. Following internship at the German Hospital and Children's Hospital of Philadelphia, he embarked in clinical practice. In 1886, he joined the staff of the German Hospital and developed an enormous personal practice in surgery. His Saturday afternoon operative clinics were attended by surgeons throughout the world while he performed as many as 25 operations in an afternoon. It was, in fact, at the German Hospital that he achieved his greatest recognition, although he was called to the post of Professor of the Practice of Surgery at the University of Pennsylvania in 1911 and assumed the Chair 7 years later. Deaver was considered an aggressive and radical surgeon—a great "slasher." He was among the early advocates of immediate appendectomy for acute appendicitis. He often stated, "An inch and a half, a minute and a half, a week and a half," to mean respectively the length of the incision, the time it took to perform the operation, and the duration of the hospital stay. "Cut well, get well, stay well," was another of his favorite aphorisms. He was also responsible for using the word "pathology" to mean pathologic finding or lesion rather than the study (e.g., "What is the pathology?"). Deaver's name is well recognized by every medical student and surgical house officer who has had the displeasure of holding "his" retractor. He, in fact, never permitted his assistants to perform any aspect of the operation. He insisted that all be done by his own hand. Although he was accorded many honors, including that of President of the American College of Surgeons, the practice of surgery was his total commitment—this, and the writing of five books and almost 250 articles.

JACQUES LISFRANC (1790–1847)

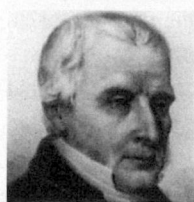

Lisfranc was born in Saint-Paul-Jarrest (Loire), France, the son of a physician. He accomplished his preliminary studies at the Lyceum in Lyons and then went to Paris to continue his medical training at the Hôtel-Dieu. It was there that he came under the tutelage of Dupuytren. Later, however, the two became rivals and developed a vigorous animosity toward each other. Lisfranc received his doctorate in medicine in 1812 at a time when France was involved in the Napoleonic Wars. He was commissioned as a surgeon and distinguished himself in campaigns in Saxony and in France. Following the wars, he established his practice in Paris. Fortuitously, one day Lisfranc rescued a magistrate who fell from a horse, and through this serendipitous meeting, he was invited to join the Faculty of Medicine at the Hospital of Pity. He rose rapidly to become chief of surgery. For more than 20 years, he was affiliated with this institution and wrote numerous articles on such diverse subjects as shoulder disarticulation, the application of the stethoscope in the diagnosis of fractures, and diseases of the uterus. It has been generally attributed that Lisfranc was the first person to remove a cancerous tumor from the rectum, essentially by means of a transanal operation. A man of formidable reputation, Lisfranc was a founding member and ultimately president of the French Academy of Medicine and a Chevalier of the Legion of Honor.

RICHARD VON VOLKMANN (1830–1889)

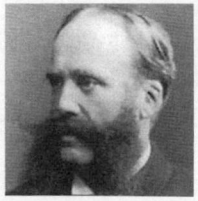

von Volkmann was born at Leipzig, Germany, the son of the Professor of Anatomy and Physiology at the University of Halle. All of his life he was associated with the university at which his father taught. In 1856, he was appointed Deputy to the Surgical Clinic of Professor Blasius, and in 1867, von Volkmann achieved the Chair in Surgery. After a time in military service during the Franco-Prussian War, he returned to his own hospital to confront the ravages of sepsis, having become familiar with Lister's work. He was so successful in applying listerian principles that it was to Volkmann's unit rather than to Britain that surgeons came from throughout the world to learn these methods. A visitor to the clinic he designed would be impressed with the terrazzo paving, constructed in such a manner as to permit efficient drainage. This was extremely important because flushing the wounds with carbolic solution from gardening pots was always employed during a procedure, given that sepsis was such a pervasive problem. Volkmann's primary interests were orthopedics and general surgery. He emphasized the importance of open drainage and widening of wounds and made other contributions to the management of hydatid cyst of the liver, intra-abdominal abscess, ulcer disease, tuberculous arthritis, joint dislocation, and compound fractures. His "improved" operation for excision of the rectum is less familiar than that of his pupil, Kraske. In fact, his name is recognized today primarily because of his description of the pathophysiology of ischemic muscle contracture. Besides being a master surgeon with an enormous private practice, von Volkmann was a superb orator. He could lecture fluently in several languages, including Latin. He was also well recognized and extremely popular throughout Germany as a published author of poems and fairy tales for children.

excised the rectum for this condition.[359] His was a transanal approach and, as such, was of necessity, used only for low-lying rectal lesions. This procedure and merely supportive care were the only available options. Modifications were introduced by von Volkmann,[631] Cripps,[116] and others, but the results of the perineal operation were poor. There was frequent incontinence, a high recurrence rate, and a high mortality rate.[512]

In 1885, Kraske removed the coccyx and part of the sacrum (a maneuver that had been accomplished many times as an extension of the perineal proctectomy), but he preserved the anus and sphincters to effect an anastomosis.[325,326] Often, however, continuity of the bowel could not be restored, either because of too much tension on the upper segment, impairment of the blood supply, or both, and the procedure was often completed by the establishment of a sacral anus. The operation was quite popular for a time but ultimately fell into disrepute because of the complications of sepsis, anastomotic leak, and recurrent disease.

In 1894, Czerny was unable to remove a rectal cancer and combined the extirpation with an abdominal operation, thus

WILLIAM HARRISON CRIPPS (1850–1923)

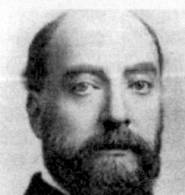

Cripps was born in Gloucestershire, England, of a prominent family. He received his medical education at St. Bartholomew's Hospital, obtaining his membership in the Royal College of Surgeons in 1872. He was attached to St. Bartholomew's for the remainder of his professional life. In 1876, he was awarded the Jacksonian Prize by the Royal College of Surgeons for his monograph, *Carcinoma of the Rectum*. Cripps was not a particular enthusiast for Listerian methods. For example, he did not operate under the carbolic spray, which was then in vogue. He was, however, the only surgeon at the hospital at that time who would make a complete change of clothes before surgery. Cripps was one of the early British advocates of inguinal colostomy, often employing the procedure both for palliation and before perineal and transsacral excision for rectal cancer.

PAUL KRASKE (1851–1930)

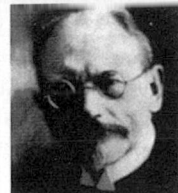

Kraske was born in Berg, near Muskau, Germany, and obtained his surgical training in Halle under the tutelage of Richard von Volkmann, whom he assisted from 1876 through 1883. For several years, Kraske demonstrated a particular interest in colorectal cancer and produced a number of papers on the subject. It was this, the foundation for his fame, that caused him to be selected as Director of the Surgical Clinic in Freiburg at the age of 32 years. In 1885, he presented a lecture at the Fourteenth Congress of the German Society of Surgery on the subject of the transsacral approach to the removal of rectal cancer. His experience was based on cadaver dissections and the treatment of two patients. Kraske was also considered a great patriot, having volunteered as a soldier in the Franco-Prussian War of 1870 to 1871 and as a medical officer in the beginning of the First World War. His particular interest in his later years was in the value of early laparotomy for abdominal wounds. Kraske remained faithful to the University of Freiburg until his death and led the clinic for 36 years until he retired in 1919.

VINCENZ CZERNY (1842–1916)

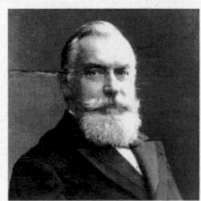

Vincenz Czerny was born in Trautenau, Bohemia, on November 19, 1842, the son of a pharmacist. Having become fascinated with the microscope, he became quite interested in the study of botany and zoology. He entered the University of Prague in 1860 to study medicine. He continued his education at the University of Vienna and achieved his medical degree, summa cum laude, in 1866. In 1868, he was appointed assistant to the great Theodor Billroth. He soon developed an abiding commitment to general surgery, especially the performance of pioneering work in gastric and esophageal surgery. In addition, he was the first to remove the larynx. In 1870 and 1871, he served with the German army in France and upon his return was appointed Professor of Surgery at the University of Freiburg, at the remarkable age of 29. At this time, his writings were numerous and diverse, including those on tuberculosis, intestinal suturing, embolism, and tumor transplantation, to name only a few. In 1877, Czerny was appointed professor of surgery at Heidelberg, where he served for 25 years. It was there that he performed the first vaginal hysterectomy and, in 1884, the first abdominoperineal resection. In 1906, he established the Institute of Cancer Research in Heidelberg following an international tour, which included a visit to the New York State Institute for the Study of Malignant Disease in Buffalo. Czerny was recognized with numerous honors and awards, including Honorary Fellowship in the American Surgical Association (1885) and Presidency of the International Association for Cancer Research.

W. ERNEST MILES (1869–1947)

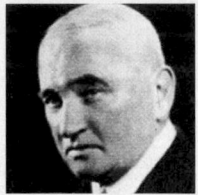

The name Miles is probably the best-recognized eponym in surgery of the colon and rectum. Miles was born in Trinidad, British West Indies, and trained at St. Bartholomew's Hospital, but the area of rectal surgery attracted him, and he became house surgeon to St. Mark's Hospital in London. Within a few years, he was appointed to the Gordon Hospital for Diseases of the Rectum and attained the senior honorary staff at the Royal Cancer Hospital in 1903. Much of his early training he owed to David Goodsall, to whose memory he dedicated his own book, *Rectal Surgery*, in 1939, and with whom he collaborated 40 years earlier on a two-volume work entitled *Diseases of the Rectum and Anus*.

Miles did much to clarify the pathologic anatomy of hemorrhoids and their operative treatment; he classified and had unique success in the treatment of anal fistula, but his pecten band failed to endure. It is, however, in connection with the operation of abdominoperineal resection of the rectum that posterity will forever honor him. It was an operation that, as he planned it in 1906, required unswerving conviction and remarkable courage. A master surgeon and a brilliant and dexterous craftsman, he eventually was able to perform the entire operation in less than 30 minutes. He was the recipient of numerous honors, not only from his own country, but also from Ireland, the United States, France, and Greece. (Adapted from Burghard FF. In memorium: W. Ernest Miles. *Br J Surg.* 1947;35:320.)

becoming the first person to perform an APR.[127] In 1908, Miles described his modification of Czerny's operation, placing emphasis on meticulous dissection and removing the zone of upward spread of the cancer (Figure 24-9).[421] He concluded as follows:

(1) that an abdominal anus is a necessity; (2) that the whole of the pelvic colon, with the exception of the part from which the colostomy is made, must be removed because its blood-supply is contained in the zone of upward spread; (3) that the whole of the pelvic mesocolon below the point where it crosses the common iliac artery, together with a strip of peritoneum at least one-inch wide on either side of it, must be cleared

away; (4) that the group of lymph nodes situated over the bifurcation of the common iliac artery are in all instances to be removed; and lastly (5) that the perineal portion of the operation should be carried out as widely as possible so that the lateral and downward zones of spread may be effectively extirpated.

Although initially presenting 12 patients, with an operative mortality of 42%, Miles believed that with improved technique and further experience, the operation could be performed relatively safely. Later, as performed by him, it was a most impressive display of operative technique—one of the noted sites of London surgery in the 1920s and 1930s.[210] The abdominal phase, carried out with the patient lying flat on the table and

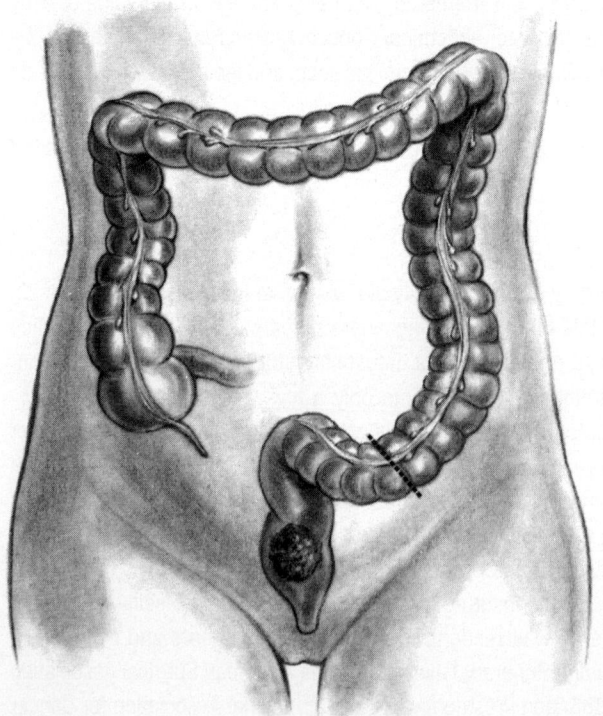

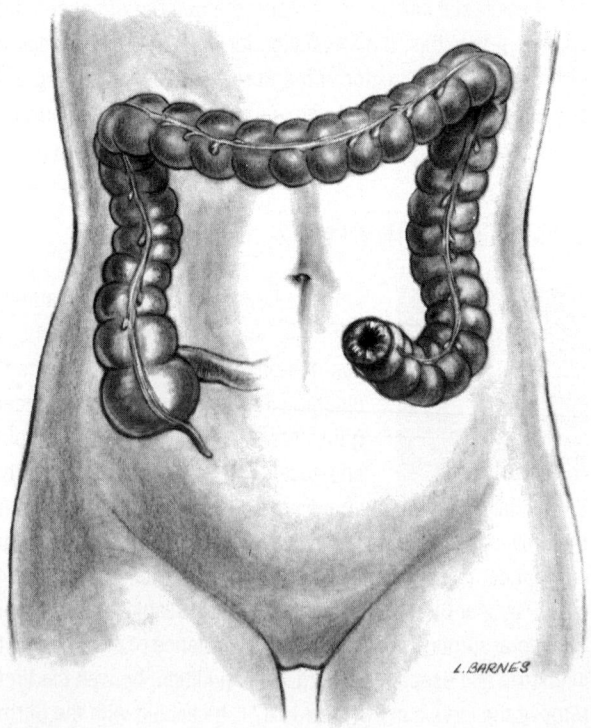

A   **B**

FIGURE 24-9. Carcinoma of the rectum. **A:** Extent of removal in classic abdominoperineal resection. **B:** The sigmoid colostomy is created in the left iliac fossa.

in a steep Trendelenburg tilt, seldom took more than 35 to 40 minutes. Miles was quite prescient: the Miles resection has become the standard operation for the treatment of cancers of the low rectum. A presumably less radical but perhaps safer procedure was the attitude taken by Miles' rival, Percy Lockhart-Mummery (see Biography, Chapter 12), who favored a perineal excision, preceded 2 or 3 weeks earlier by a minilaparotomy to determine that the growth was resectable.[210] When this was the case, a loop-iliac colostomy was established.

Another option was proposed by Gabriel, an assistant to Lockhart-Mummery for many years.[188] Gabriel started out as a perineal excisionist, but after careful study of the lymphatic spread of rectal cancer, he switched to his version of proctectomy, the perineoabdominal excision.

In 1939, Lloyd-Davies[361] reaffirmed the value of the synchronous-combined (two-team) APR that had been originally proposed by Mayo as early as 1904.[408] Mayo suggested that the synchronous-combined approach be considered "if the

WILLIAM BASHALL GABRIEL (1893–1975)

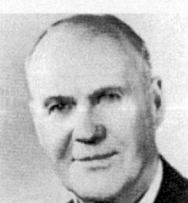

Gabriel was born in Oulton Broad, Suffolk, England, the son of an engineer. He attended Epsom College and distinguished himself as a very capable athlete. In 1912, he entered the Middlesex Hospital Medical School in London as the Freer Lucas Scholar. He was an outstanding student, winning a medal and scholarship for proficiency in surgery and another medal for theoretical and practical medicine. Following graduation, he served in World War I on a destroyer in the Mediterranean. In 1919, he became House Surgeon at St. Mark's Hospital in London, subsequently joining Sir Charles Gordon-Watson, J. P. Lockhart-Mummery, and Lionel Norbury. One of his most outstanding achievements was the establishment of a cancer follow-up department, the first of its kind in Great Britain. From this evolved the cumulative data of survival statistics for cancer treatment at St. Mark's. Gabriel was best known for his advocacy of the so-called perineoabdominal excision, a procedure that he performed more than 1,000 times. He was also renowned as the author of a major textbook that went through five editions, *Principles and Practice of Rectal Surgery*.

OSWALD VAUGHAN LLOYD-DAVIES (1905–1987)

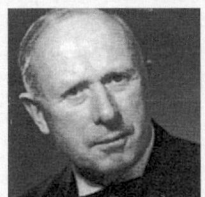

Lloyd-Davies was born the son of a Welsh clergyman and was educated at Caterham School. He received his medical education at the Middlesex Hospital in London. In 1935, at the age of 30, he was appointed to the staff of St. Mark's Hospital. Lloyd-Davies was regarded as a slow and meticulous surgeon. He was also an original thinker and designer of instruments for colon and rectal surgery. Among these was a small-bore sigmoidoscope with a proximal light source that he produced to permit outpatient and bedside evaluation of the lower bowel. His best-recognized contribution, however, was the development of specially designed leg supports as a means for providing access to the abdomen and to the perineum in the abdominoperineal resection. As a consequence, the lithotomy-Trendelenburg position has come to be associated with his name. Lloyd-Davies was a modest and self-effacing man. In spite of his international reputation, few surgeons outside the United Kingdom knew him personally. He was, however, recognized as President by the Section of Proctology of the Royal Society of Medicine and was an Honorary Fellow of the American Society of Colon and Rectal Surgeons. (Adapted from Obituary. *BMJ.* 1987;295:676; Obituary. *Lancet.* 1987;1:465.)

CHARLES HORACE MAYO (1865–1939)

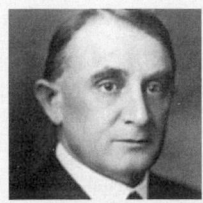

Charles Mayo was born in Rochester, Minnesota, the son of William Worrall Mayo, a native of England and a general practitioner of medicine who had settled in the Territory of Minnesota in 1855. The young boy accompanied his father and elder brother, William J. Mayo, on numerous trips throughout the area as the father ministered to his patients. Charles Mayo studied in the public schools of Rochester and took the degree of doctor of medicine from Northwestern University in 1888. He returned to Rochester and joined his father and brother in their practice. In about 1903, what has come to be known as the Mayo Clinic had acquired sufficient form to warrant the use of that term by persons who sought the services of the brothers and their associates. Charles Mayo was considered, at least by his brother, to be the better surgeon. He could master a difficult situation with exceptional speed, and he had a facility for performing a variety of challenging operations (e.g., excision of a knee joint, sectioning the gasserian ganglion). Honors of every description were conferred upon Charles Mayo, as they were upon his brother. He was elected president of numerous medical organizations, including the Western Surgical Association, the Society of Clinical Surgery, the American Medical Association, the American College of Surgeons, and the American Surgical Association.

FRANK HOWARD LAHEY (1880–1953)

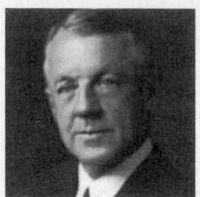

Lahey was born in Haverhill, Massachusetts, the only child of a bridge-building contractor. An outstanding athlete, Lahey attended Harvard University both as an undergraduate and as a medical student. Following graduate training at Boston City Hospital, he joined the staffs of Harvard and Tufts Medical Schools, when World War I interrupted his career. He became a Major in the Medical Corps and went to France to be the chief of surgery at an evacuation hospital. Following the war, he opened an office and shortly thereafter was joined by a surgeon and then an anesthesiologist. It was at this time that he conceived the idea of developing a multiple-specialty clinic, a practice that had been successful in the Midwest, but not in New England. The concept of staged operations was vigorously applied at the Lahey Clinic for many conditions—thyrotoxicosis, esophageal diverticulum, subphrenic and subhepatic abscess, pancreatic cancer, and diverticular disease. By staging the operation, Lahey and others were able to reduce the operative mortality considerably. The two-stage operation for cancer of the rectum was the procedure employed by surgeons on the staff of the Lahey Clinic until the early 1940s, more than 30 years after Miles' original publication. Lahey was a master surgeon; he was consistent and thorough. He often cautioned, "Be not the first to adopt a new technique nor the last to discard an old one." His most cherished award, the Bigelow Medal of the Boston Surgical Society, stated in part, ". . . superlative surgeon, doctor who teaches doctors, redoubtable administrator, advisor of Presidents in war and peace and, above all, a man who has the courage to be honest with himself. . . ."

surgeon has a good assistant." By 1963, the Lloyd-Davies technique was the most commonly employed alternative at the St. Mark's Hospital, and the operative mortality had been reduced to less than 3%.[439] It is particularly helpful when one is confronted with a bulky or fixed tumor or a patient with a narrow pelvis. With all appropriate deference to Miles and to his statement that the operation takes no more than 1 hour and that his patients suffer "no more shock than after an ordinary perineal excision,"[421] blood loss can be reduced and operative time decreased by using a two-team method. Interestingly, Miles' resection as performed by Richard Cattell of the Lahey Clinic in Boston (see Biography, Chapter 31) was called by his assistants "the *hour* of charm."

Others (e.g., Lahey) believed that if the operation were divided into two stages, it could be better tolerated by the patient.[339] The first stage consisted of making a median incision, dividing the sigmoid colon, and creating a left iliac colostomy with a mucous fistula of the distal segment delivered through the lower part of the abdominal incision. Care was taken to preserve the superior hemorrhoidal artery to the distal bowel. In the second stage, the proctectomy was carried out. An alternative operation for treatment of cancer of the middle to upper rectum or of the rectosigmoid was proposed by Hartmann in 1923.[240] This procedure succeeded in removing the tumor following establishment of a colostomy, but avoided the perineal dissection. However, the operation was useful for higher lesions only and, of course, was not designed for eventual reestablishment of intestinal continuity, although the Hartmann resection is frequently applied today in the initial surgical management of complicated sigmoid diverticulitis. The original article probably is worth reproducing in translation. It must represent a record for the briefest paper leading to one's eponymous immortality because Hartmann's fame is based on only two paragraphs of narrative:

It is the rule that, in order to remove cancers of the distal pelvic colon, it is necessary to perform a very serious operation when removing the rectum by means of an abdominoperineal excision. In two patients who underwent colostomy for intestinal obstruction, at the second operation I limited resection to the intermediate portion of the colon between the artificial anus and the rectum, including the corresponding area of innervation. Following this, I closed the upper end of the rectum and reperitonealized it, without reconstructing the perineal floor. Following the operation both cases

HENRI ALBERT HARTMANN (1860–1952)

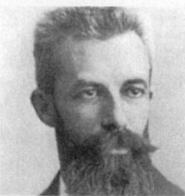

Hartmann was born in Paris. He apparently developed an early interest in pursuing a medical career, becoming a prosector in anatomy in 1884 at the University of Paris. Following graduation from the Medical School in 1887, he continued on the staff of the Hôtel-Dieu and ultimately became professor and chairman of the department of surgery in 1909. Hartmann developed a huge clinical practice, performing in excess of 1,000 operations each year for 20 years. He took meticulous notes of each procedure and of the postoperative course. Most of his writings were in the areas of breast, gastric, and biliary surgery, but he also wrote books on gynecology, war injuries, and cancer. Hartmann achieved international recognition, and his clinic at the Hôtel-Dieu became a mecca for surgeons from all over the world. He was accorded tributes in many countries, including honorary fellowship in the American Surgical Association and the Royal College of Surgeons of England and of Ireland. In his own country, he was a grand officer of the Legion of Honor. He died in Paris, January 2, 1952, at the age of 91.

HENRY WIDENHAM MAUNSELL (1847–1895)

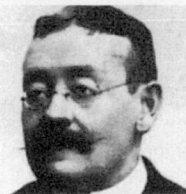

Maunsell was born in Dublin in 1847 and obtained his degree from the College of Surgeons in 1867. He moved to Melbourne, Australia, the following year and became resident medical officer at the Melbourne Hospital. Following this appointment, he took a similar post in Hokitika, New Zealand. After achieving his MD degree from the College of Surgeons in Dublin, he returned to New Zealand and settled in Dunedin. In 1892, he re-emigrated to the South Kensington section of London and devoted his efforts to writing, lecturing, and illustrating. He was quite well known as a fine artist who supplemented his surgical tutorials with his own beautiful drawings. The Maunsell method, the abdominoanal pull-through procedure, became for many surgeons the sphincter-saving operation of choice for the treatment of carcinoma of the rectum. He was an innovative surgeon and is credited with original concepts in the technique of intra-abdominal hysterectomy. He was elected to fellowship of the British Gynaecological Society in 1889 and was appointed a councilor in 1893. Maunsell died of bronchitis following a bout of influenza.

JULIUS VON HOCHENEGG (1859–1940)

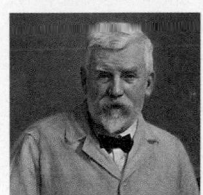

von Hochenegg was born to a family from the Tyrol on August 2, 1859. He was educated in Vienna and obtained his doctorate in 1884. He was a surgical apprentice under Christian Albert Theodor Billroth and became assistant at the surgical clinic under Eduard Albert. He ultimately became head of the department (Abteilungsvorstand) at the Wiener Allgemeine Poliklinik. He was appointed professor extraordinary in 1894 and was promoted to Ordinarius in 1904. At the time of his retirement in 1920, he was also head of the second surgical clinic. Hochenegg's career reached its zenith on November 12, 1914, when he was raised to the nobility by Emperor Franz Josef, becoming Julius von Hochenegg. On May 9, 1915, his only son was killed on the Russian front during the First World War. His international reputation grew remarkably, as attested to by the following article in the *New York Times* that was published on May 10, 1908: "American surgeons, who by the reluctant consent of their European confrères are now ranked at the top of their profession, will be interested in the brilliant achievement reported at last week's surgical congress in Berlin by Prof. Hochenegg of Vienna. The professor told how he operated successfully on a case of acromegaly, a disease which causes strange and enormous enlargements of the bones of the hands, feet, and face. The patient on whom the operation was performed was a young girl. She showed the usual symptoms of brain tumors and a marked disturbance of vision. The diagnosis having been confirmed by means of x-rays, Prof. Hochenegg moved the girl's nose to one side, cut through the thin floor of the skull, and then removed the tumor from the hypophysis or gland-like body that is suspended like a cherry from the base of the brain. It is said that none of the operations reported prior to last week was successful; but the Vienna girl left the hospital six weeks after Prof. Hochenegg's operation, fully restored to health." He was also the first to perform a total excision of the rectum with preservation of the anal sphincter. Hochenegg's ulcer (ulcus callosum recti) is a rare, firm type of rectal tumor with central ulceration that is associated with stenosis, difficulty passing stool, blood and mucus in the feces, colic, meteorism, and loss of appetite. Von Hochenegg died in Vienna in 1940.

were as uneventful as an operation for a cold appendix. The conservation of a small cul-de-sac of the rectum above the sphincters did not present a particular problem, and follow-up 9 and 10 months later revealed the patients to be quite well.[240]

The first documented attempt at abdominal resection with restoration of continuity is generally attributed to Reybard of Lyons (see Biography, Chapter 23).[515] He performed a partial sigmoid resection; the patient survived approximately 10 months. The fear of sepsis and anastomotic leak inspired Murphy, in 1892, to create his "button" (see Biography, Chapter 23; see Figure 23-35).[450] The same year, Maunsell[407] reported a technique using an anastomotic method employed by Hochenegg[263] in what has come to be called the "pull-through" procedure. A more practical modification of this approach was suggested by Weir[644] in 1901.

During the first half of the 20th century, restoration of continuity by means of primary anastomosis evolved through abdominosacral resection and the familiar operation of anterior resection. The introduction of newer suture materials, the advocacy by some of interrupted suture technique, and the application of the stapling devices all indicate that the operation can nevertheless be improved and that the risk of complications can still be diminished.

The Anatomy of the Rectum and Its Fascial Relationships

Surgical technique is an important predictor of outcome for rectal cancer and is intimately related to a clear understanding of the anatomy of the rectum and its fascial relationships. Therefore, before proceeding with a description of operative details, a précis of this subject is presented.

ROBERT FULTON WEIR (1838–1927)

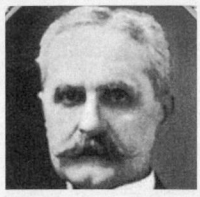

Weir was born in New York City, the son of a prominent pharmacist. His early education was in public school, and in 1854 he graduated, the youngest in his class, from the College of the City of New York, then known as the Free Academy. In 1857, he earned the degree of master of arts from the same institution. By clerking for his father and through contacts with local physicians, he developed an interest in surgery. In 1859, he received his degree in medicine from the New York College of Physicians and Surgeons and became a pupil and assistant to Gurdon Buck (who originated Buck's extension). In 1861, Weir entered the army and for most of the Civil War was in charge of the general hospital at Frederick, Maryland. Following the war, he practiced in New York City, ultimately becoming chief of the surgical service at Roosevelt Hospital and professor of surgery at Women's Medical College and at the College of Physicians and Surgeons. Weir was one of the first in the United States to adopt Lister's technique of antisepsis; he was among the early workers in surgery of the brain and was one of the first persons to recognize duodenal ulcer as a distinct pathologic entity. Weir went on to become president of the American Surgical Association, the New York Surgical Society, and the New York Academy of Medicine. He was made an honorary fellow of the Royal College of Surgeons of England and was one of five surgeons honored by the American College of Surgeons at its initial convocation.

THOMA IONESCU (1860–1926)

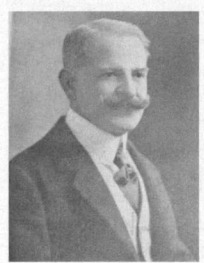

Thoma Ionescu was born in Ploiesti, Romania. He came to Paris in 1878 to further his education and simultaneously enrolled in the Faculty of Medicine and the Faculty of Law. He followed these studies at both colleges until 1882. In 1886, he was installed as resident (Interne des Hôpitaux de Paris) and spent 4 years of training in surgery. In 1887, he obtained through competition the title of anatomy assistant (aide d'anatomie) and was ranked first in that year. Following this he was named prosector of the Faculty of Medicine. In 1892, Ionescu obtained a PhD in medicine with his thesis *Evolution of Intrauterine Pelvic Colon*. In that same year, France's Ministry of Public Instruction delegated Ionescu to study and report on the anatomical education in universities in Germany and Austria. In 1894, together with Paul Poirier, then head of anatomical works (Chef des Travaux Anatomiques) of the Faculty of Medicine in Paris; Adrien Charpy, Professor at the Faculty of Medicine of Toulouse; and Nicolas of the Faculty of Medicine of Nancy, Ionescu collaborated in drafting the first installment of the most important anatomical treatise written in France to that date (*Traité D'anatomie Humaine*). Thoma Ionescu was the anatomist who first described in detail the sigmoid colon, called by him the "pelvic colon." Also in 1894, a special law created the Institute of Topographical Anatomy and Experimental Surgery in Bucharest, and the jury's decision was that the chair would be occupied by Professor Thoma Ionescu. Thus, in February 1895, Professor Thoma Ionescu took the directorate of the Institute of Topographical Anatomy and Experimental Surgery and of the Surgical Clinic of the Coltea Hospital. Ionescu introduced rigorous aseptic techniques and made numerous contributions to general surgery, gynecology, orthopedics, and neurosurgery. These included surgery of the cervical sympathetic chain, maxillary nerve interruption, Meckel's ganglion resection, optic nerve tumor ablation with preservation of the eye, decompression hemicraniectomy, and probably most famous, the practice of spinal anesthesia, especially for abdominal surgery. The anesthetic used was stovaine (a cocaine-related substance) in combination with strychnine (to overcome the effects of depression) and, later, with caffeine. He demonstrated his technique in London, New York (at the Mount Sinai Hospital), Philadelphia (at Pennsylvania University), Chicago, and also at the Mayo Clinic. In recognition of his achievements in advancing surgical science, he was received at the White House in 1909 by President William Howard Taft, who thanked him for his tireless work in his purpose of alleviating human suffering. Professor Thoma Ionescu passed away on March 28, 1926. (From Ciurea AV, Palade CL. Professor Thoma Ionescu—founder of modern surgical practice in Romania. *Romanian Neurosurg.* 2010;17(2):137.)

Anatomists generally agree that the rectum commences opposite the sacral promontory and is approximately 15 cm in length, extending from the rectosigmoid junction proximally to the palpable, lower, anorectal ring. If one includes the length of the anal canal (2 to 3 cm), then the rectosigmoid junction is identified approximately at 16 cm from the anal verge when examining an anesthetized patient in the left lateral position with a rigid sigmoidoscope.[275] The rectum is usually described as having three segments: an upper, a middle, and a lower.

Although there are excellent contemporary reviews of the surgical anatomy of the rectum and its fascial planes,[58,106,199,542,667] the description by the little-known Romanian surgeon-anatomist, Thoma Ionescu (Thomas Jonnesco), is generally considered the "most graphic and complete."[30] In particular, his original description in French of the perirectal fascia in the first edition of *Poirier and Charpy's Traité d'Anatomie Humaine* in 1896 has not been surpassed. His description was adopted by Waldeyer in 1899 in his classic text, *Das Becken*, and remains essentially unchanged in

RICHARD JOHN (BILL) HEALD (1936–PRESENT)

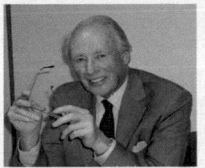

Bill Heald (as he prefers to be called) was born on May 11, 1936 and studied medicine at Gonville and Caius College, at the prestigious Cambridge University, United Kingdom. He received his FRCS from Edinburgh in 1964 and from England in 1965. He developed an interest in colon and rectal surgery and established himself as a specialist in colorectal cancer surgery and as an international teacher of surgical technique. He has performed more than 400 television-based live operative demonstrations in more than 30 countries. He is a former vice president and currently a member of the Council at the Royal College of Surgeons of England, past president of the Section of Coloproctology at the Royal Society of Medicine and of the Association of Coloproctology, and president of the Colostomy Association. He has received honorary degrees and professorships from numerous institutions throughout the world, including from such countries as Sweden, the Netherlands, Switzerland, Yugoslavia, Italy, Austria, France, Poland, Russia, and Germany. He has been recognized as a recipient of the Order of the British Empire. In 1988, Heald wrote as follows: "In developing these planes there are thus three basic principles: (1) recognition of mobility between tissues of different embryological origins. (2) sharp dissection under direct vision in a good light. And (3), gentle opening of the plane by continuous traction with no actual tearing. The job of the assistant is to put the tissues on stretch. In my view the fascia itself is 'impenetrable' only in the sense of being an avascular interface between viscus and soma—it is indeed the 'Holy Plane.'" Bill's main interest for the past 25 years has been the research and development of the total mesorectal excision (TME) technique for rectal cancer. The TME operation has now become the "gold standard" for rectal cancer surgery. His current position is director of surgery at the Pelican Cancer Foundation, Basingstoke, United Kingdom. He continues to operate and to lecture around the world.

contemporary anatomy textbooks.[96] Knowledge and understanding of this anatomy is the key to identifying the correct plane of mobilization when resecting the rectum for cancer. Indeed, this anatomy has been rediscovered by many surgeons over the past century who were unaware of Ionescu's singular contribution. For example, Heald rediscovered this anatomy for himself and renamed and popularized the "retrorectal space" and plane as the "holy plane" in his operation of total mesorectal excision or TME.[248] However, some would describe Heald's use of the term "mesorectum" as a misnomer[438] or simply incorrect.[621] These authors reinforce the key feature, as described by Ionescu, that the perirectal fascia per se takes its origin from the endopelvic parietal fascia off the pelvic side walls to encapsulate the rectum and not from the peritoneum.[621] In this manner, surrounded by loose lobulated fat, the rectum is cushioned and cocooned in a serofibrous fascial envelope, together with its lymphatics, vessels, and nodes. Superiorly, the perirectal fascia is continuous with the peritoneum of the pelvic mesocolon at the level of S3 and where there is abundant fat enclosed within. Inferiorly, at its lower third, there is only minimal fat present, and a plane exists between the perirectal fascia and Denonvilliers' fascia, separating the rectum from the prostate and seminal vesicles. This plane must be recognized in order to avoid unnecessary bleeding from the prostatic venous plexus or damage to the cavernous nerves when mobilizing the rectum anteriorly.[358] The key is to dissect behind Denonvilliers' fascia whenever possible, unless there is strong suspicion of direct involvement by tumor.[358]

Very likely the term "mesorectum" was introduced by Maunsell in 1892 (see earlier Biography) when describing his pull-through operation[407] and was probably based on a misunderstanding of the term "meso" as used by Ionescu in his thesis on the pelvic colon that was published in same year.[297] It should be noted that the term "meso" in gross anatomy pertains to two layers of peritoneum that suspend an organ, but as Ionescu quite rightly argued, because the rectum is not suspended but rather lies nestled and closely applied to the sacral hollow, there is no need for "meso," and

the term is therefore inappropriate. For this reason, it does not appear in *Nomina Anatomica* but is restricted to the *Nomina Embryologica*. More important, the proper emphasis should be on the precise recognition of the perirectal fascia to mobilize the rectum in the appropriate anatomical plane rather than to perform a TME when resecting the rectum.

Brief Description of the Anatomy of the Pelvic Nerves

In a recent review of the subject, Moszkowicz and colleagues present a summary of the innervation of the pelvis based on anatomy and highlighting where pelvic nerve injury occurs.[448] Pelvic innervation is described as comprising supralevator and infralevator compartments. The supralevator pathways consist of the superior hypogastric (SHP) and inferior hypogastric plexuses (IHP). The infralevator compartment is essentially the pudendal nerve. The supralevator compartment consists of the superior hypogastric plexus and hypogastric nerves. These are a continuation of the preaortic sympathetic trunks. They can be readily identified and preserved as has been discussed in Operative Technique.

The parasympathetic nerves (pelvic splanchnic or erectile nerves), however, are not as easily identifiable as the hypogastric nerves. They arise from the ventral roots of S2–4, and they enter the pelvis through the sacral foramina. Small branches of these nerves have been reported in the lateral ligaments.[548] Moszkowicz describes the *inferior hypogastric plexus* as a network of sympathetic and parasympathetic fibers that lie outside the fascia propria. It is located laterally and retroperitoneally on either side of the rectum. Damage to this plexus can cause urogenital and sexual dysfunction.

▶ RESTORATIVE PROCEDURE: ANTERIOR RESECTION

Indications

The most important factor that determines the likelihood of performing an anastomosis is the level of the lesion, although

TABLE 24-1 Options for Low-Lying Rectal Cancer

Exposure of distal rectum
    Abdominal
    Abdominotransanal
    Abdominosacral
    Abdominotranssphincteric

Resection
    Ultralow anterior resection
    Intersphincteric resection
    Transanal endoscopic microsurgery
    Abdominoperineal resection and neosphincter

Reconstruction
    Straight (end-to-end, side-to-end, end-to-side)
    J-Pouch
    Coloplasty

Level of anastomosis
    Distal rectum
    Pelvic floor (anorectal ring)
    Anal canal

Type of anastomosis
    Hand-sewn
        Perianal
        Eversion of stump
    Stapled
        Single
        Double
        Triple

Adapted from Tytherleigh MG, Mortensen NJ. Options for sphincter preservation in surgery for low rectal cancer. *Br J Surg.* 2003;90:922.

if one is strongly motivated to reestablishing intestinal continuity, it can virtually always be accomplished. The obvious question is not can you put the bowel together, but should you. Table 24-1 summarizes the various procedures and the method of reconstruction.

Favorable indices such as good differentiation, limited bowel wall penetration with endorectal ultrasound, small size, and polypoid configuration may safely reduce the distal margin of resection to 1 or 2 cm. The only absolute contraindications to performing a low colorectal or coloanal anastomosis are invasion into the anal canal and invasion of the sphincter mechanism.

Today, low and ultralow anterior resections are the most common method of restoring continuity. Other methods have been described and are included later in this chapter, but they are rather esoteric and not commonly performed.

Open Anterior Resection

Technique
The technique that I use has been developed over many years (since 1980). Although it differs from the traditional method of mobilizing the rectum in that I start the dissection on the right side of the mid-pelvis, it is essentially a separation of the rectum along well-defined and previously described anatomical planes. I choose this approach because at that level the retrorectal space is totally avascular, and the risk of obscuring the view with minor bleeding is minimal. The technique incorporates many elements adapted from laparoscopic colorectal surgery (see Chapter 19).

Instruments
The instruments that I commonly use are listed next and are shown in Figure 24-10.

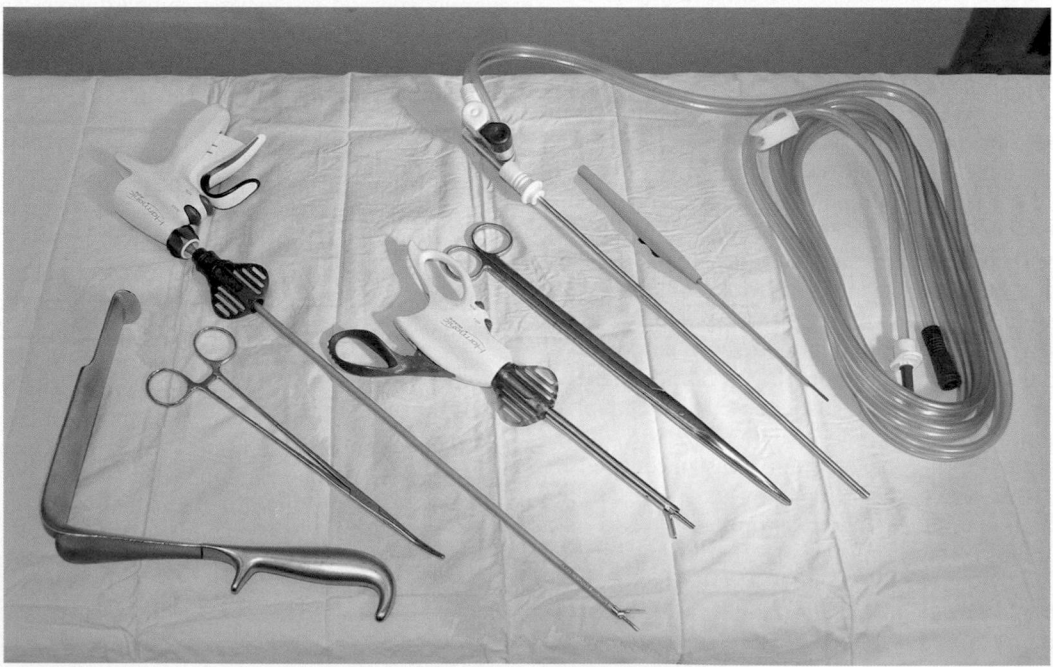

FIGURE 24-10. Instrument tray for anterior resection. From left to right: St. Mark's retractor, Zenker forceps, Harmonic scalpel, Wave Harmonic scalpel, Abel scissors, sucker irrigation, and long diathermy.

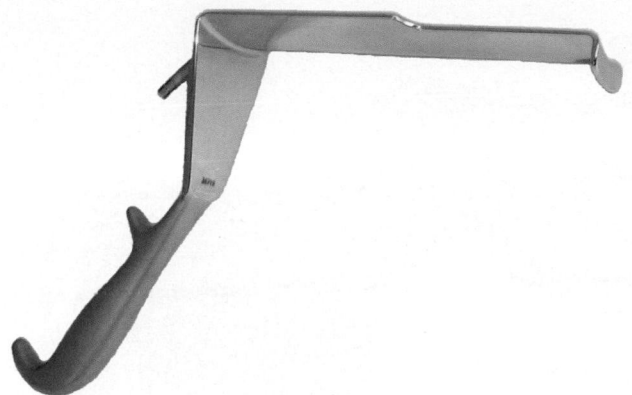

FIGURE 24-11. St. Mark's pattern retractor.

Long Sucker/Irrigator

I prefer this instrument to the traditional Yankauer suction because of its length and also because I frequently use high-pressure water irrigation to open up planes, especially in redo surgery. Once an incision is made in the correct plane, water irrigation can develop the plane with ease. Furthermore, the long sucker does not have a bend in it. I find that an angled sucker can interfere with the line of vision deep in the pelvis, whereas straight suction permits a clear line of view.

Long Diathermy

A long diathermy is essential because sharp dissection is used throughout the procedure. I do not use hands or fingers for mobilizing.

Harmonic Scalpel

For the past 3 years, I have increasingly adapted the use of different energy sources for open as well as for laparoscopic surgery. I have found the long Harmonic scalpel and the Wave Harmonic scalpel particularly useful; they have complemented, and in some steps of the operation, they have replaced the use of diathermy.

St. Mark's Pattern Retractor

This is essential for dissection in the pelvis (Figure 24-11).

Renal Vein Retractor

This retractor has the same shape as a St. Mark's retractor but is much narrower (Figure 24-12). It is very useful in patients with a narrow pelvis or in those with a bulky tumor in whom it may be difficult to accommodate the width of a St. Mark's retractor.

Lighting

Good lighting is essential for pelvic surgery. There are numerous battery-operated, fiberoptic, cable-connected headlights that provide excellent illumination.

Assistant

Teamwork is essential. Therefore, I strongly recommend having an experienced surgeon or a senior trainee assist with this operation.

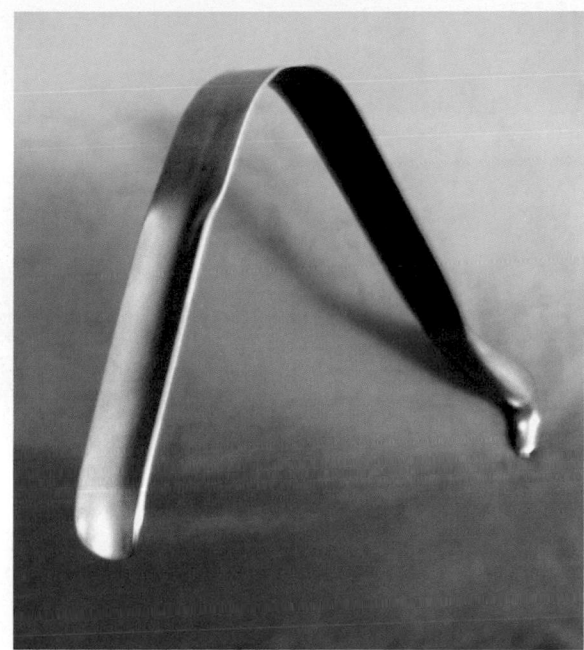

FIGURE 24-12. Wylie renal vein retractor.

Anterior Resection Technique (Total Anatomical Dissection of the Rectum)

The basic principles underpinning a successful restorative procedure for rectal cancer are as follows:

1. A total anatomical dissection (TAD) with mobilization along anatomical planes[65]
2. Achieving a distal clearance margin of at least 1 cm
3. Mobilizing the proximal colon, including the splenic flexure, and division and ligation of the inferior mesenteric vein at the lower border of the pancreas to ensure a tension-free anastomosis
4. Ensuring a good arterial blood supply to the segment of proximal colon that will be anastomosed to the rectum
5. Ligation and division of the inferior mesenteric artery close to its origin from the aorta
6. An anastomotic technique that ensures circumferential seromuscular bites

Positioning the Patient

The patient is placed in the Yellowfins stirrups (Allen Medical Systems, Acton, MA—Figures 24-13 and 24-14). Calf compressors are used to minimize the risk of deep

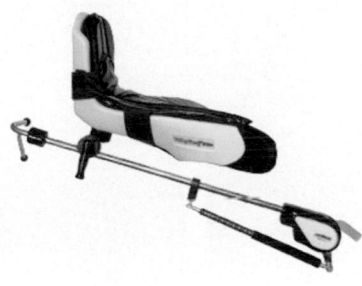

FIGURE 24-13. Yellowfins stirrups. (Courtesy of Allen Medical Systems, Acton, MA.)

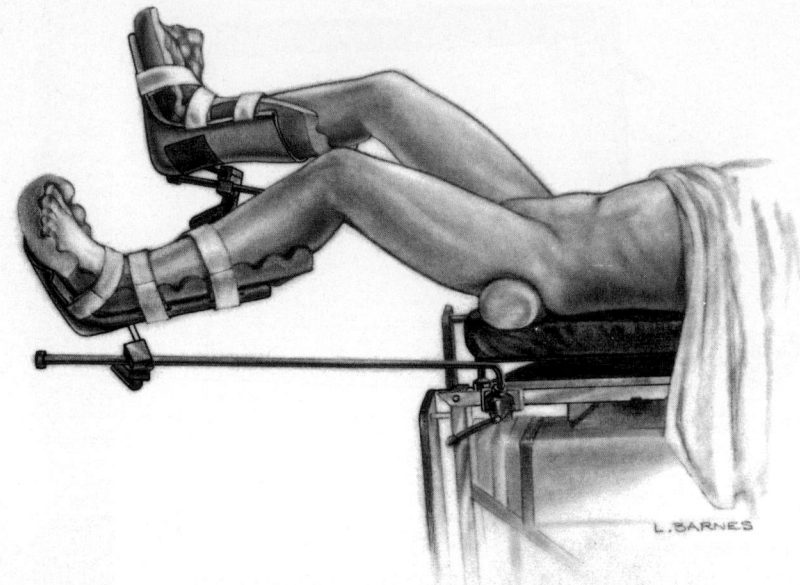

FIGURE 24-14. Perineolithotomy position with Allen's stirrups (earlier version). The thighs are abducted and extended.

vein thrombosis. The abdomen is shaved. A urinary catheter is inserted, and when indicated, cystoscopy with insertion of ureteric catheters is performed by a urologist. The surgeon stands on the left side and the assistant stands opposite. A second assistant may stand between the legs.

A midline incision is made (Figure 24-15), and after an exploratory laparotomy is performed, the small bowel is exteriorized in a wet pack (Figure 24-16). The technique

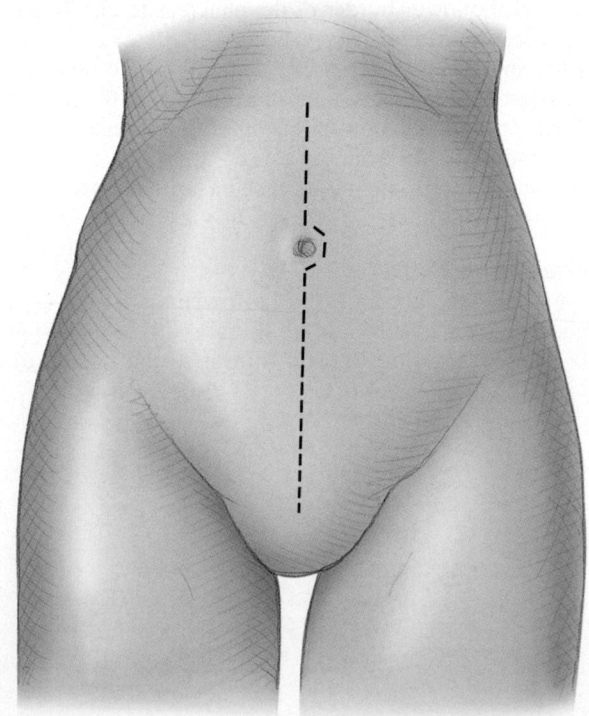

FIGURE 24-15. Midline incision.

used for mobilizing the rectum differs from that which is traditionally described, in that the dissection starts in the mid-pelvis on the right side rather than by mobilizing the sigmoid colon. Figure 24-17 shows a panoramic view of the pelvis in preparation for mobilization. A small diathermy incision is made strictly in the line of reflection of the visceral peritoneum covering the right anterolateral aspect of the rectum and carried onto the parietal peritoneum lining the right pelvic wall (Figure 24-18A). As soon as this is made, air is allowed into the retrorectal space as described by Ionescu earlier (Figure 24-18B). Once the retrorectal space is entered, the right branch of the hypogastric nerve is identified (Figure 24-19). This nerve is an important landmark. It lies anterior to the parietal fascia that lines the sacrum and lateral pelvic wall. The plane of dissection must stay anterior and medial to the nerve. Sharp diathermy or Harmonic scalpel is used to continue the dissection into the pelvis along the retrorectal space down to the floor of the pelvis (Figure 24-20). By remaining in that space, the surgeon avoids injury both to the nerve and to the presacral venous plexus.

A St. Mark's retractor is used to retract the rectum anteriorly. Sharp dissection from right to left along the retrorectal space separates the rectum (encapsulated in its intact fascial envelope) from the hypogastric nerves and the parietal fascia covering the anterior surface of the sacrum Figure 24-21).

Attention is then directed to the sigmoid colon. The assistant holds the sigmoid colon up. The peritoneal attachments of the mesocolon to the lateral wall are dissected by sharp diathermy dissection (Figure 24-22). A diathermy incision is then made in the line of reflection of the peritoneum covering the mesocolon and the posterolateral abdominal wall peritoneum. The gonadal vessels are identified, and medial to them is the left ureter (Figure 24-23). The sigmoid colon is retracted anteriorly, and the areolar plane between the posterior aspect of the superior rectal artery and branches of the hypogastric nerves is identified. That plane is dissected by diathermy into the pelvis to join the retrorectal space.

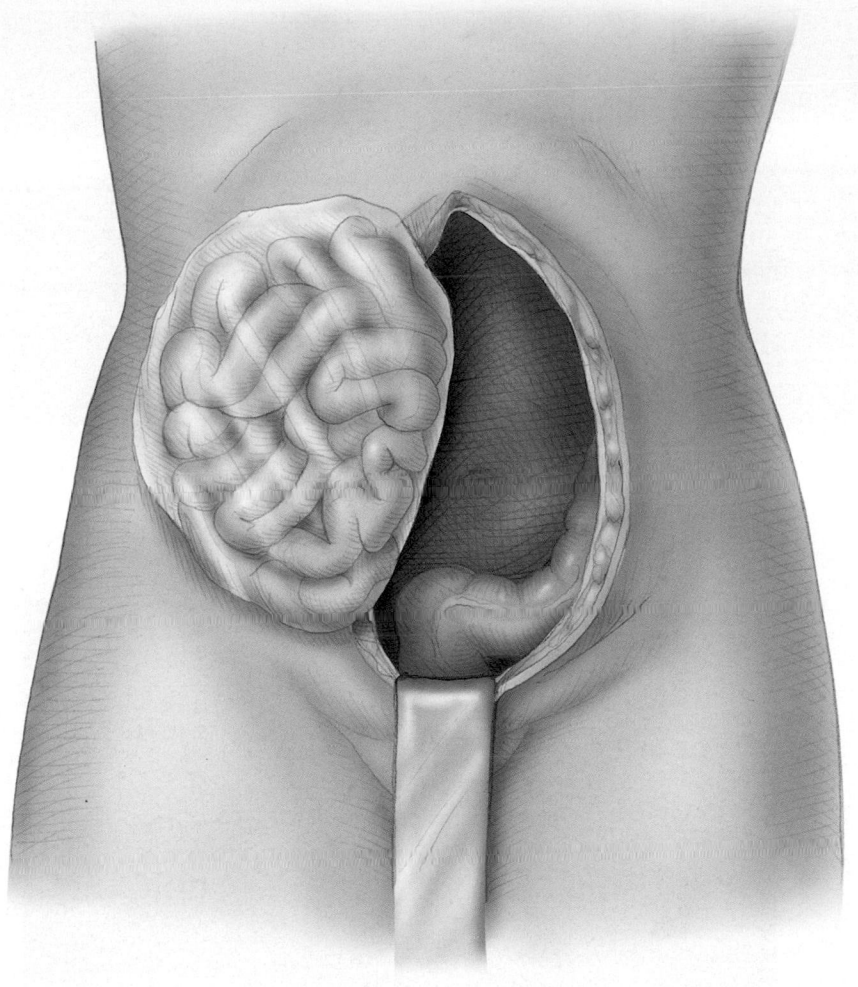

FIGURE 24-16. Small bowel exteriorized in a wet pack.

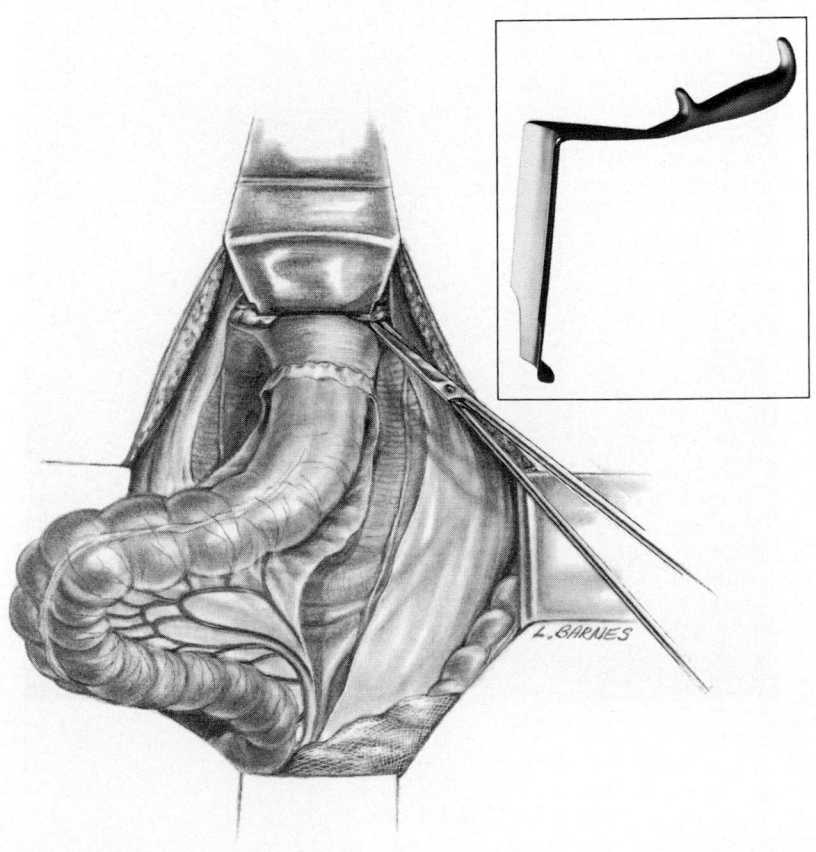

FIGURE 24-17. Panoramic view of the pelvis. St. Mark's retractor is seen anteriorly.

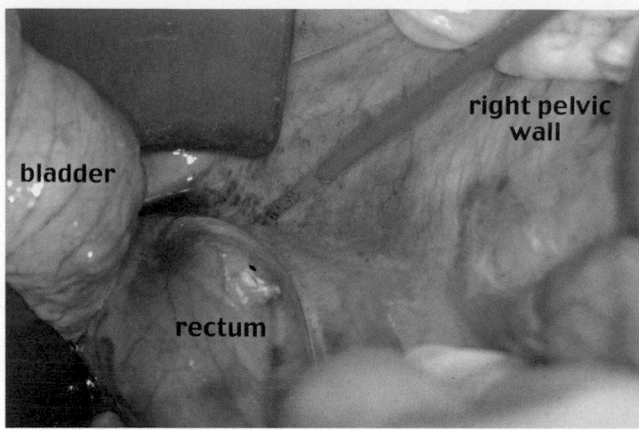

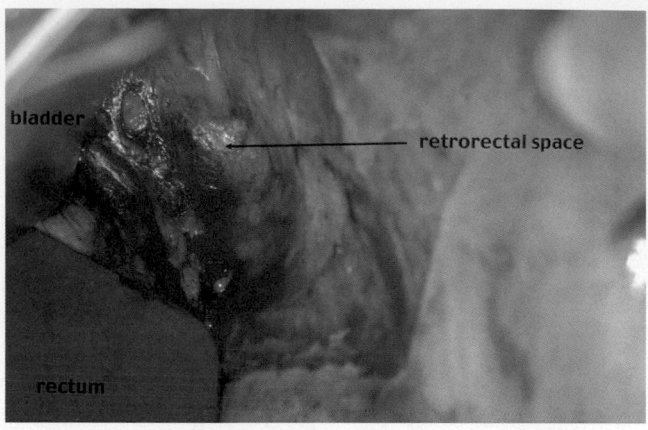

FIGURE 24-18. An incision is made along the line of reflection of visceral onto parietal peritoneum in the right mid-pelvis **(A)**. Air is introduced into the retrorectal space **(B)**.

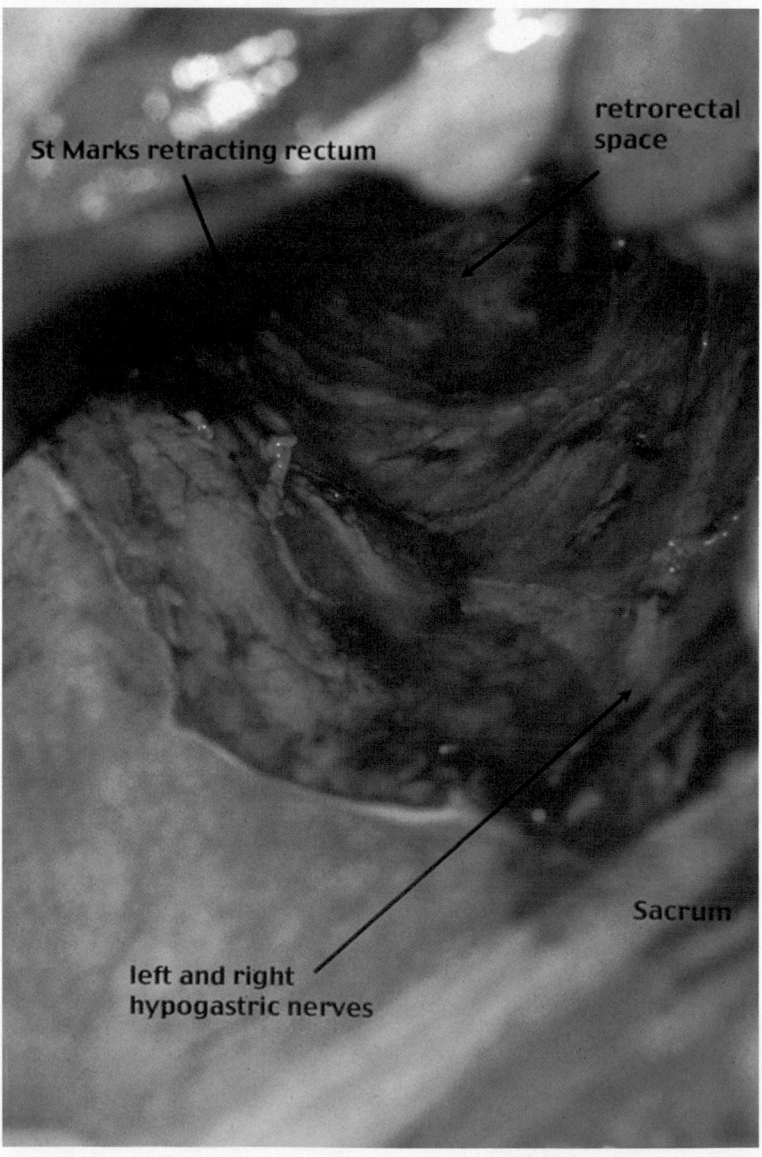

FIGURE 24-19. The hypogastric nerves are identified.

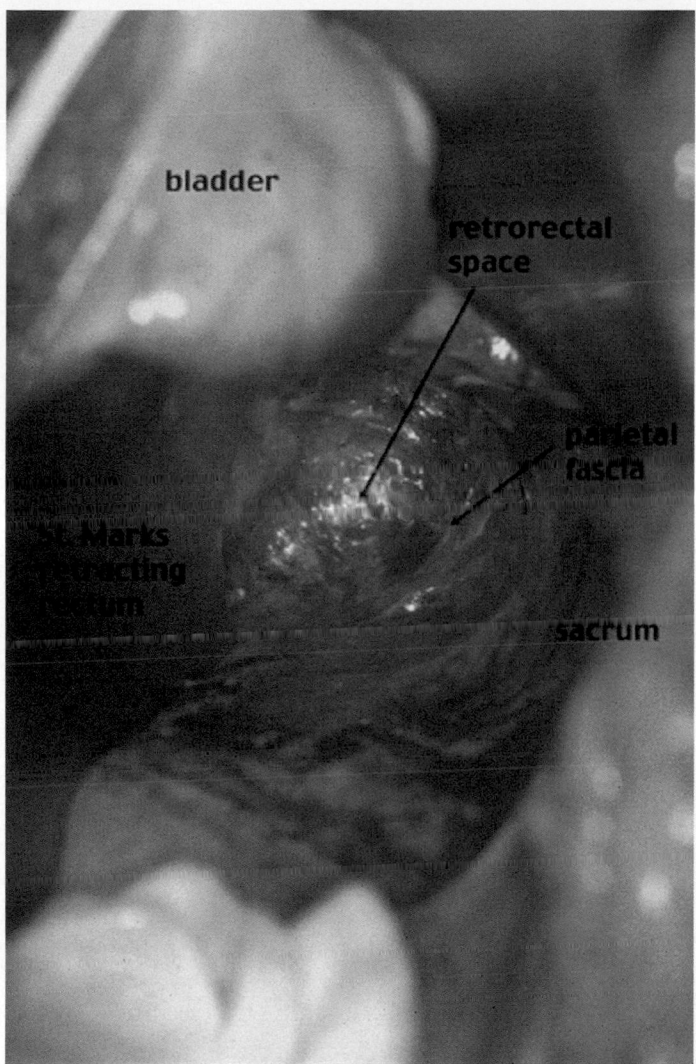

FIGURE 24-20. Dissection in the retrorectal space down to the pelvic floor.

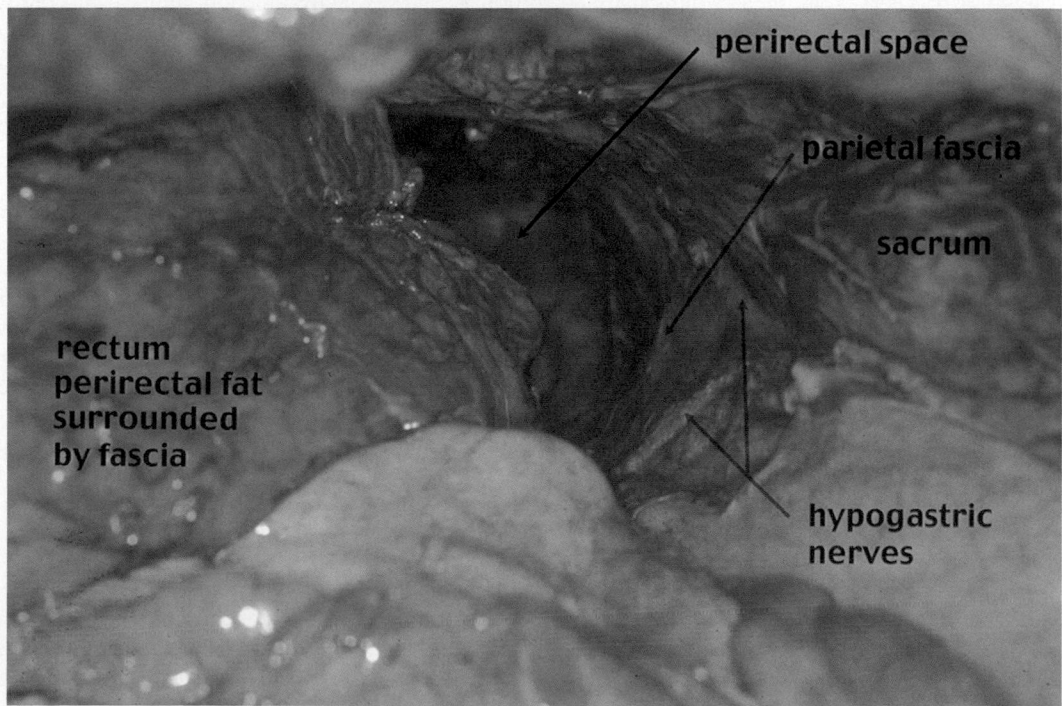

FIGURE 24-21. Pelvic dissection. Hypogastric nerves are clearly seen. Rectum, perirectal fat (with intact perirectal fascia) are separated from sacral parietal fascia.

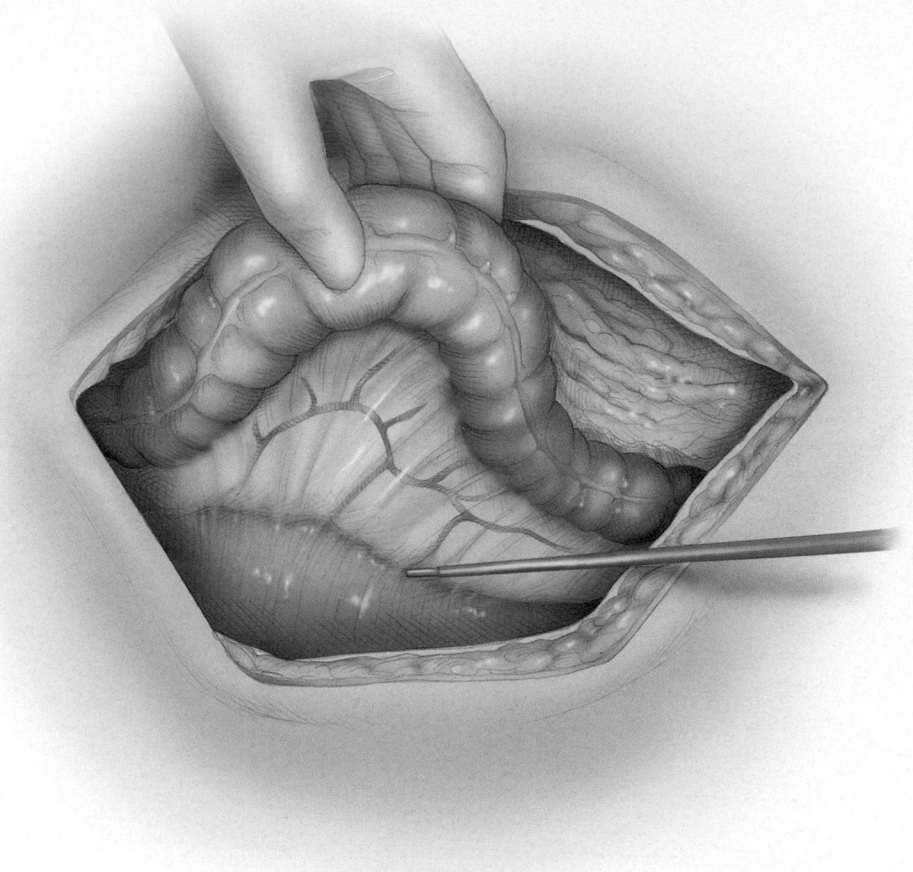

FIGURE 24-22. Congenital adhesions between the sigmoid mesocolon and left lateral wall are dissected.

Figure 24-24 shows the retrorectal dissection completed; the left and right hypogastric nerves are clearly demonstrated, and the perirectal fat is seen anteriorly, surrounded by an intact fascial layer.

Attention is then directed to the anterior part of the dissection. A small wet sponge under the left hand is used to retract the rectum upward and backward. The headlight is directed to the reflection of the visceral peritoneum onto the back of the vagina or prostate, and a small diathermy incision is made strictly in that line of reflection (Figure 24-25). This will open up the areolar avascular plane posterior to Denonvilliers' fascia. A St. Mark's retractor or a renal vein retractor is used to elevate the prostate or vagina, and the areolar plane is further developed using either diathermy or Harmonic scalpel. The anterior plane is developed as low as possible to enable a full mobilization of the rectum down to its lower third, where it is devoid of perirectal fat and consists only of a tubular muscular structure. Attention is then directed to the lateral ligaments and the middle hemorrhoidal and neurovascular bundles on the left and right anterolateral aspects of the midrectum. The left hand or a St. Mark's retractor is used to retract the rectum anteriorly and to the left. This puts the lateral ligaments and neurovascular bundles under tension. The lateral ligaments are often avascular and are not ligaments at all. However, the neurovascular bundles containing the middle hemorrhoidal vessels and branches of the inferior hypogastric plexus need to be specifically attended to. This step of the dissection is important because injury to that

plexus of sympathetic and parasympathetic nerves can result in urinary and sexual dysfunction. Injury can occur when the tissue in which it is contained is dissected too close to the parietal pelvic fascia. There is no need to do so; the dissection can remain close to the anterior and posterolateral aspects of the fascia enveloping the rectum. The Harmonic scalpel is used for this part of the dissection. It can seal vessels up to 7 mm in diameter and has simplified this step of the procedure (Figure 24-26A).

On the left side, the assistant retracts the rectum anterolaterally to the right and the same step is performed (Figure 24-26B). Once this is accomplished, there is usually more mobilization to be performed posteriorly. It is important to note that in the lower third of the pelvis, the parietal peritoneum covering the lower segments of the sacrum is reflected anteriorly to fuse with the encapsulating perirectal fascia. This fusion can be demonstrated by lifting the lower rectum upward and forward using a lipped St. Mark's retractor. The fused fascia is divided by the Harmonic scalpel, and the dissection continues posteriorly to the levator muscle.

Transection of the Rectum
Tumors of the Upper Third of the Rectum

If the tumor is in the upper third of the rectum, the perirectal fat is divided 3 to 5 cm distal to the lower end of the tumor. This is usually straightforward in thin patients. However, in obese individuals, this can be a difficult step, and I have found the following technique useful and reproducible.

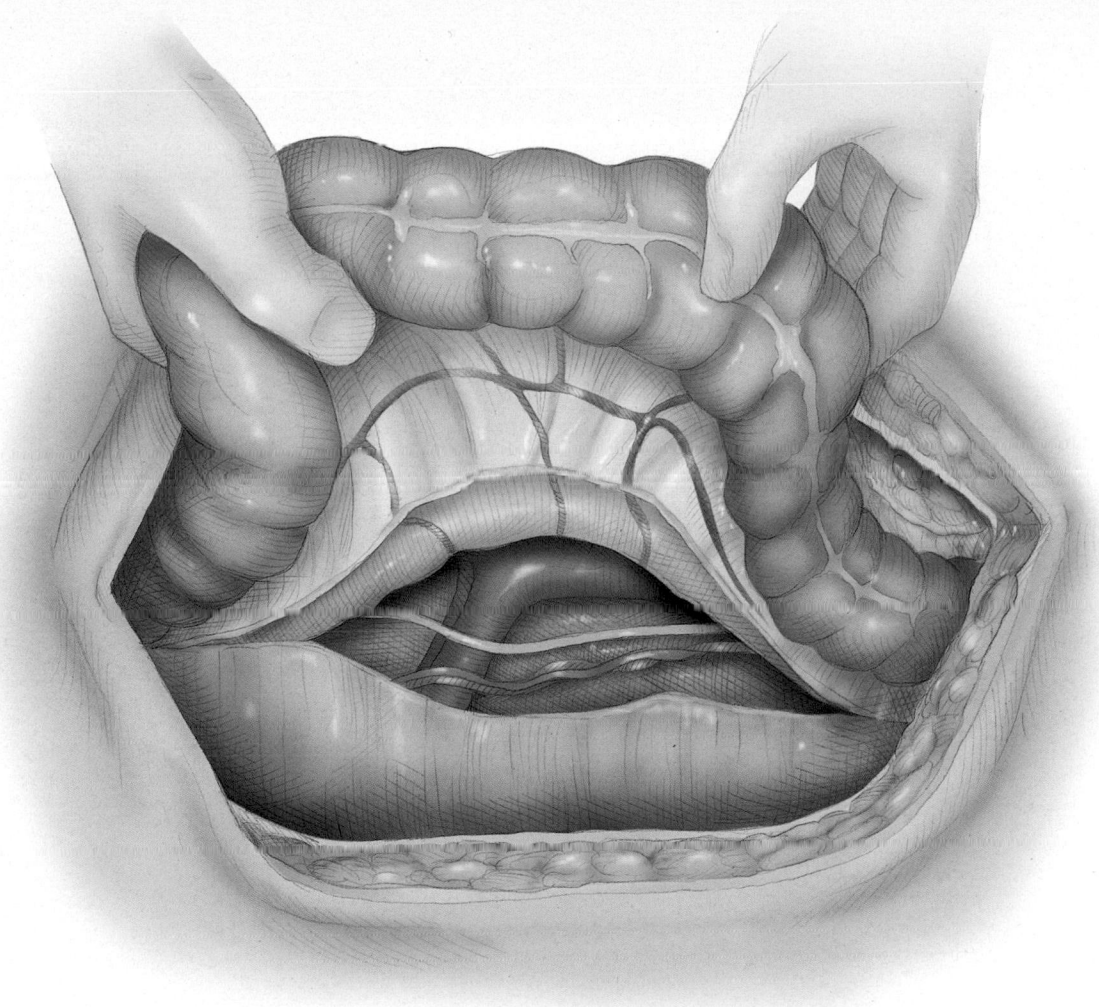

FIGURE 24-23. Gonadal vessels and left ureter identified.

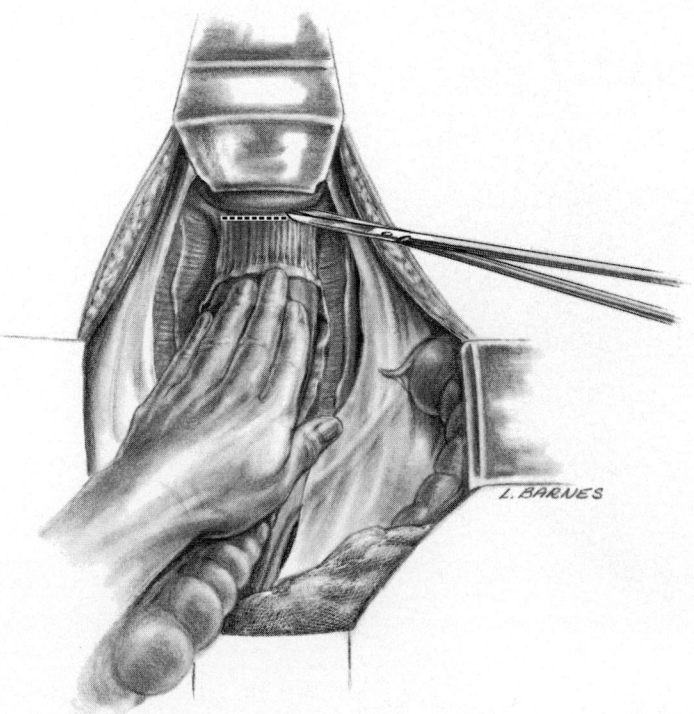

L. BARNES

FIGURE 24-24. Anterior dissection. Incision is made strictly along the line of reflection of the rectal visceral peritoneum onto the peritoneum, covering posterior vagina or prostate.

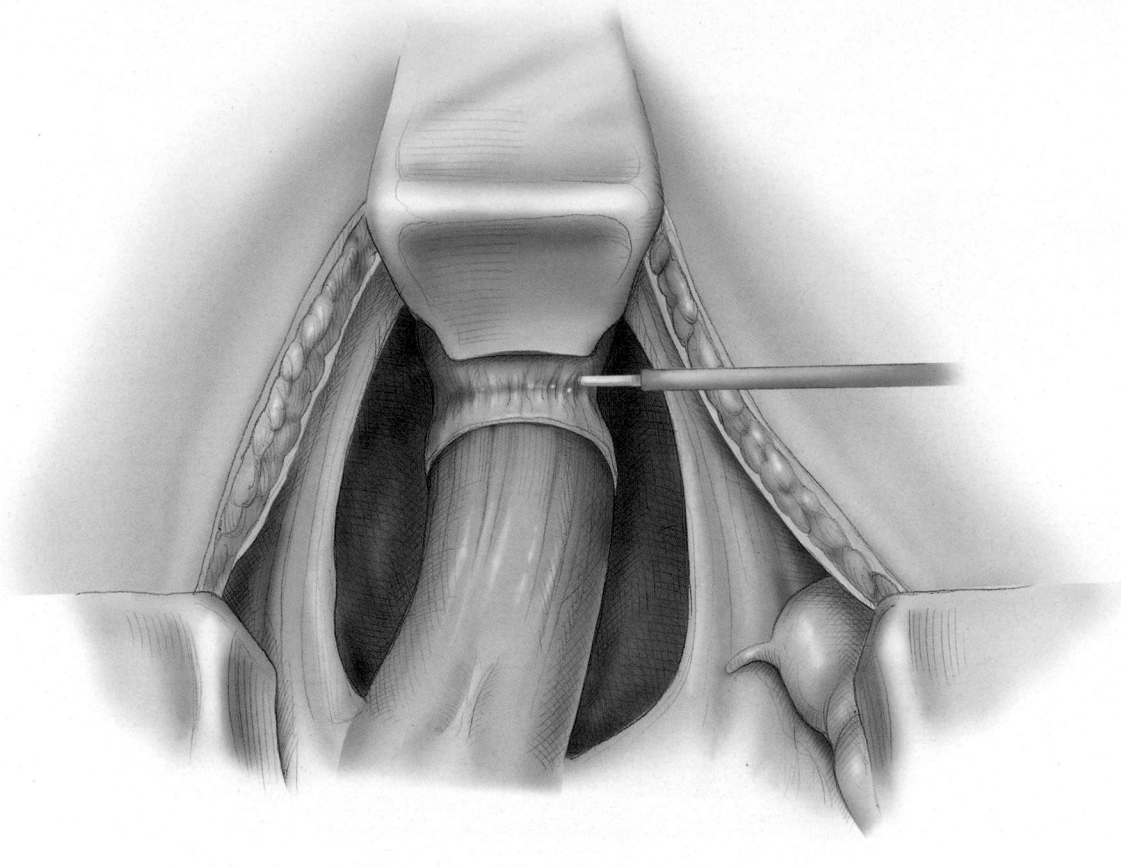

A

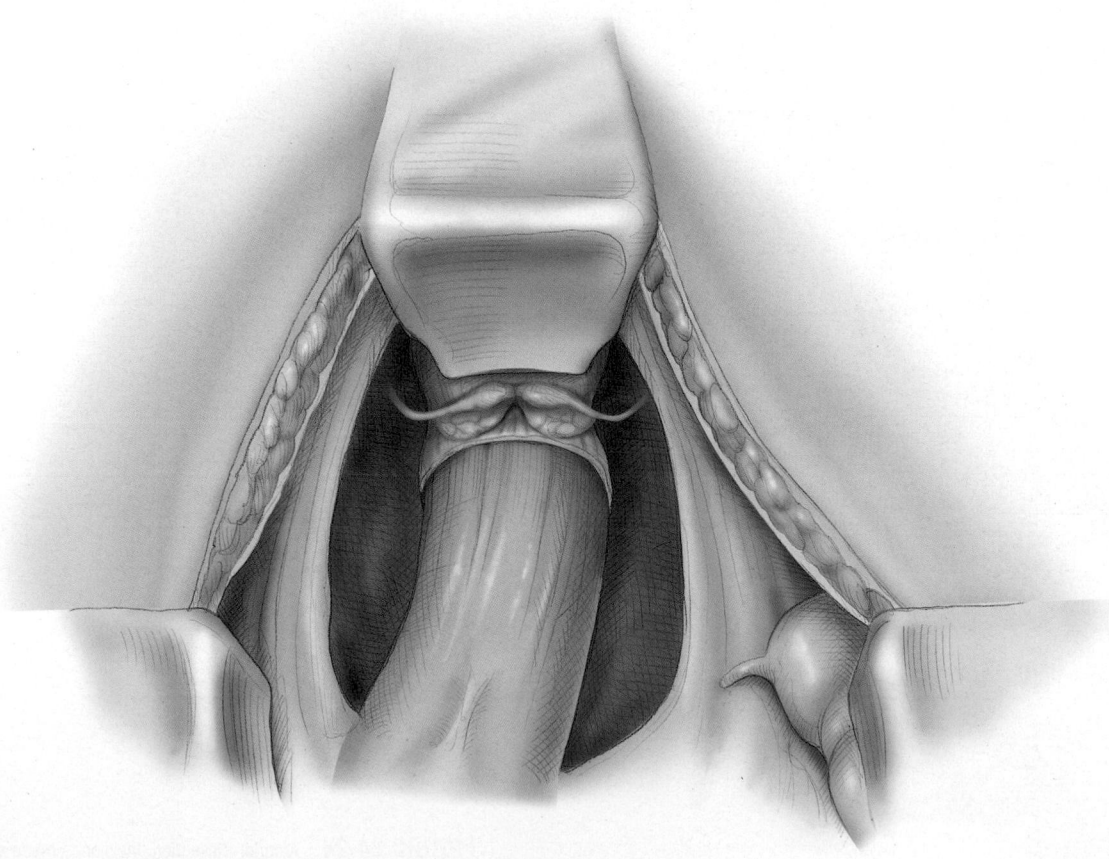

B

FIGURE 24-25. Anterior dissection behind the vagina **(A)** or prostate **(B)** posterior to Denonvilliers' fascia.

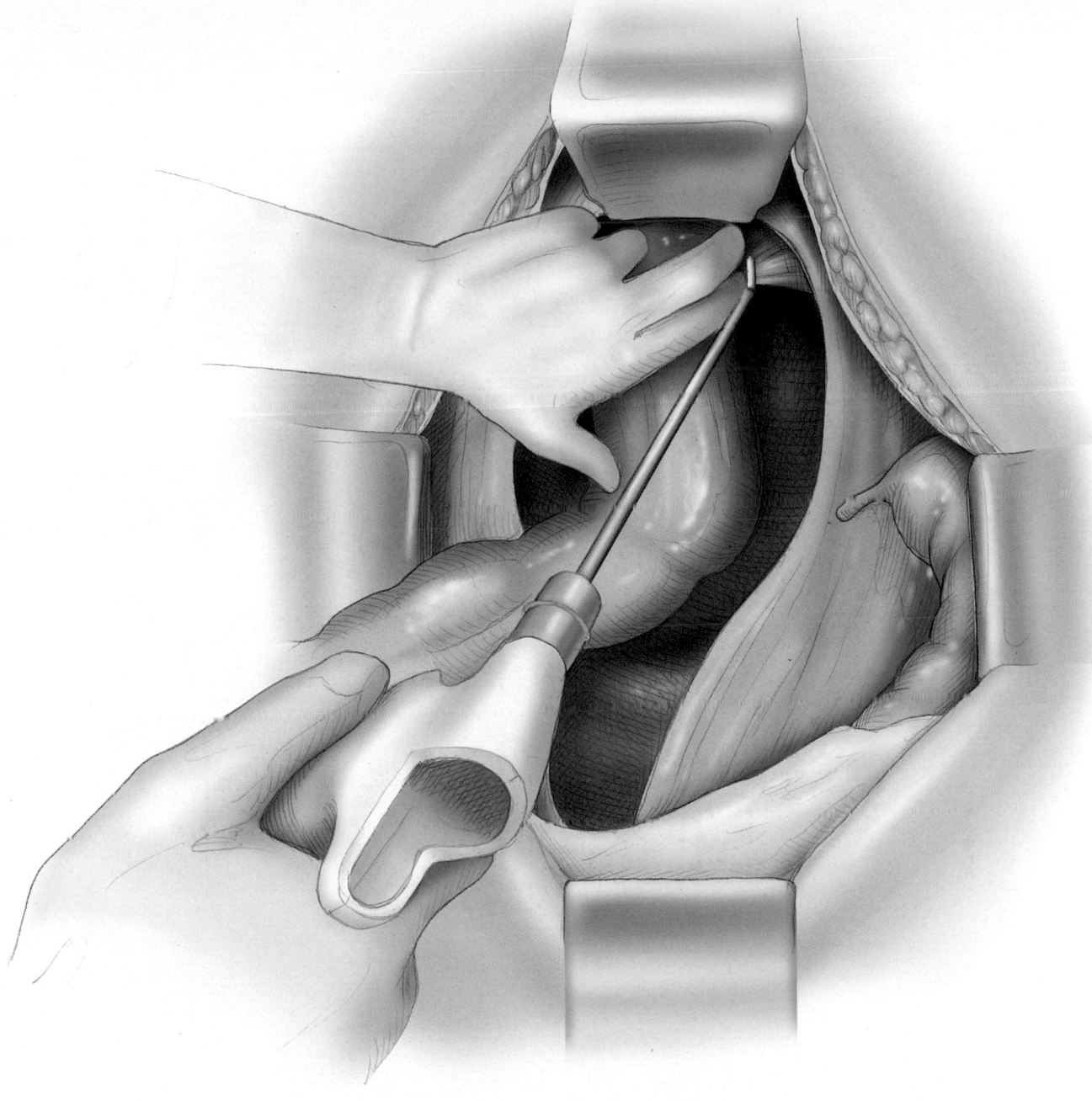

A

FIGURE 24-26. Harmonic scalpel is used to divide the "lateral ligaments" and neurovascular bundles on the right **(A)** and on the left **(B)**. *(continued)*

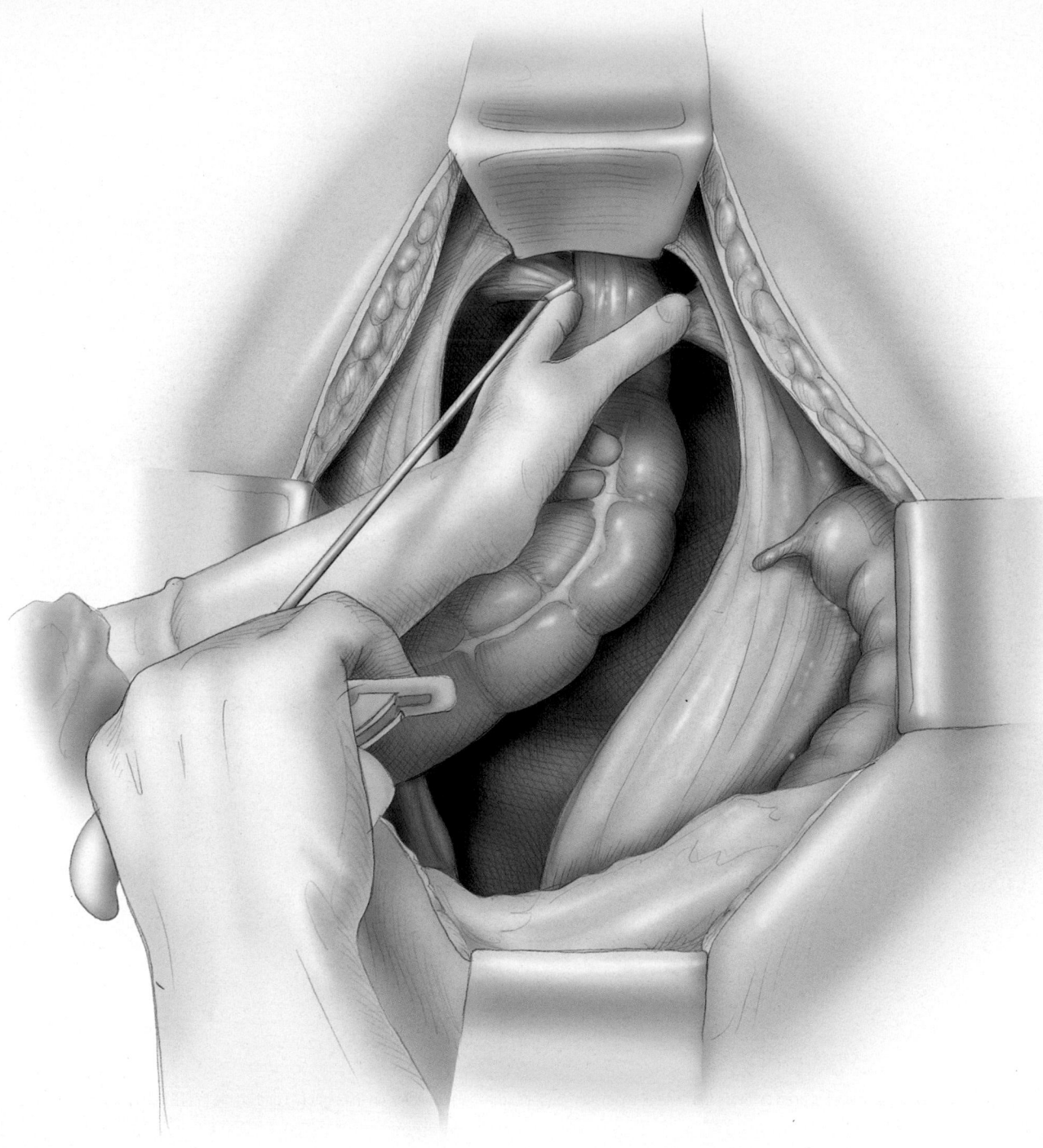

B

FIGURE 24-26. *(continued)*

The visceral peritoneum is divided by diathermy on either side of the rectum at the required level. The rectum is held up between the left index finger and thumb to palpate the antimesenteric border of the rectum. While keeping the index finger in place, the thumb is replaced by a long pair of straight scissors and pushed through from left to right. This opens up the plane between the posterior longitudinal muscle wall of the rectum and the perirectal fat. The perirectal fat is taken in two portions, the larger of which contains the superior rectal artery. Straight Kocher clamps are used for that purpose, and ligation is performed using a heavy suture

ligature (Figure 24-27). The back of the rectum can then be inspected to ensure that there is an intact layer of longitudinal muscle, and the rectum is stapled and divided between two double rows of staples with a stapling device. I prefer to use the Contour stapler because its curved shape fits well into the pelvis and also because the rectum can be divided between two rows of staples on either side, thus avoiding any spillage (Figure 24-28). Alternatively, the rectum can be divided between a crushing clamp and a Furness clamp, which can then be used to apply a purse string to the rectum (Figure 24-29). I no longer use the Furness clamp because in a narrow pelvis,

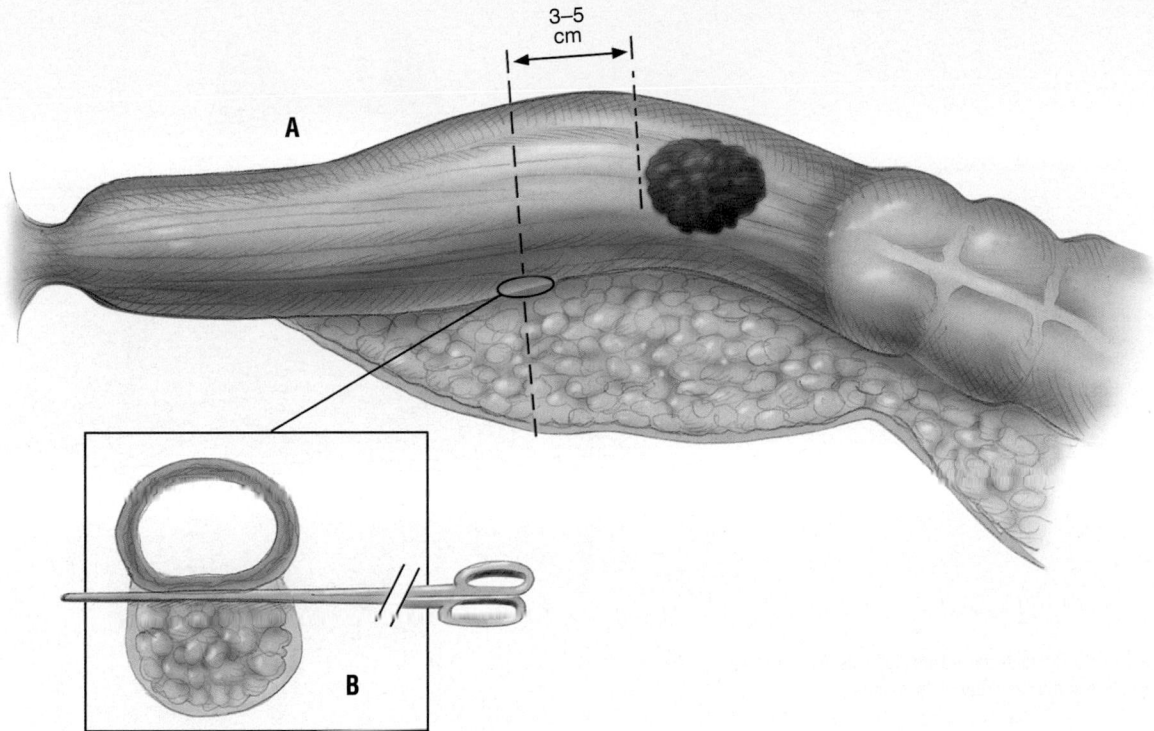

FIGURE 24-27. Division of perirectal fat for a tumor in the upper third of rectum. *Inset:* Opening the plane between the rectum and the perirectal fat.

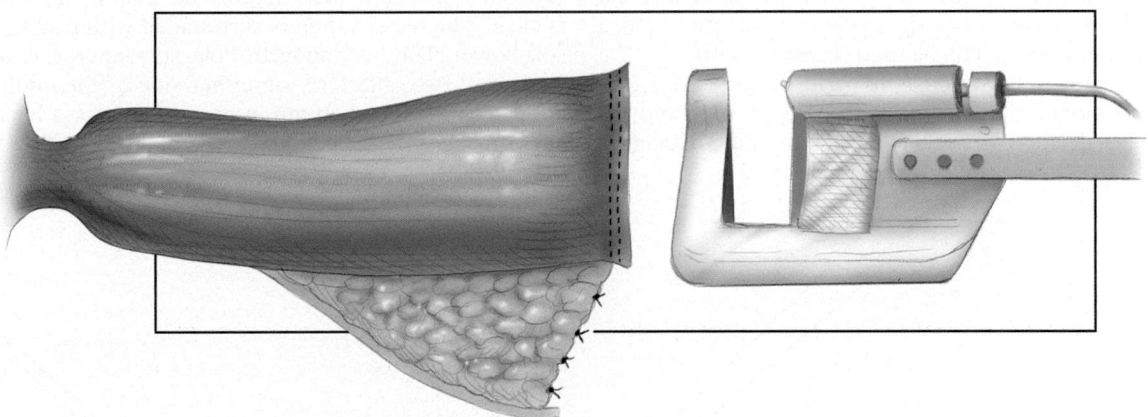

FIGURE 24-28. Transecting the rectum with Contour stapling device.

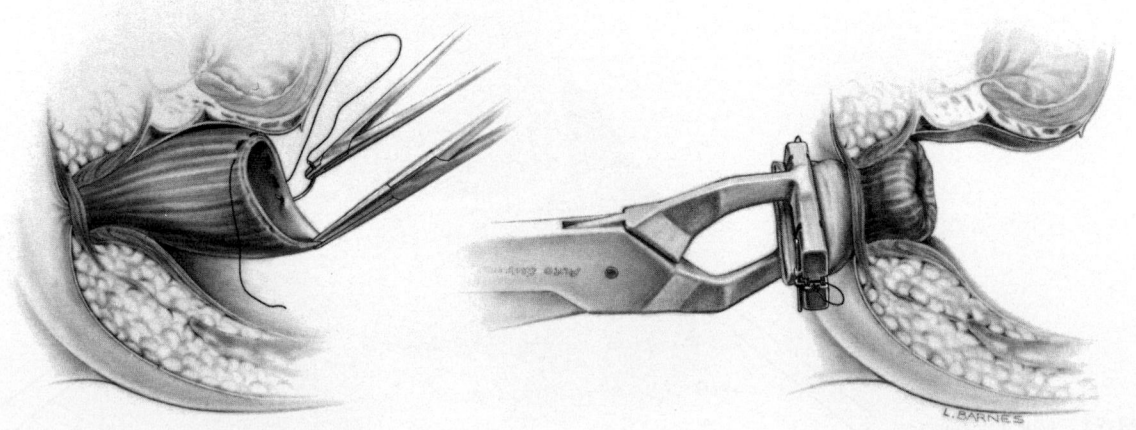

FIGURE 24-29. Circular-stapled anastomosis. **A:** Hand-sewn purse-string suture placed using "weaving" technique. **B:** Purse-string applicator employed on an inverted rectal stump.

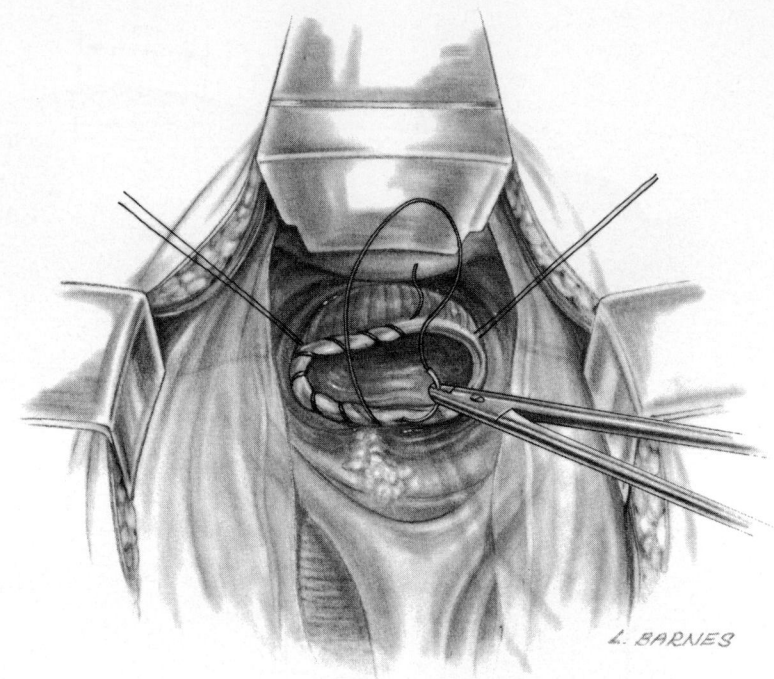

FIGURE 24-30. Circular-stapled anastomosis. A hand-sewn purse-string suture is placed in the rectal stump.

there is the risk of a straight needle injuring structures on the lateral walls as it enters or exits the clamp. Alternatively, a hand-sewn purse string can be used (Figure 24-30).

If a hand-sewn anastomosis is performed, then a right-angled soft bowel clamp is applied to the rectum, and the specimen is divided between that clamp and a Kocher's clamp. An assistant then irrigates the rectum until the return is clear. The rectal stump is surrounded with packs, and the soft bowel clamp is removed. Four stay sutures, two posteriorly and two anteriorly on either side of the midline, are applied to the rectal stump in preparation for a hand-sewn anastomosis as described later (Figure 24-31).

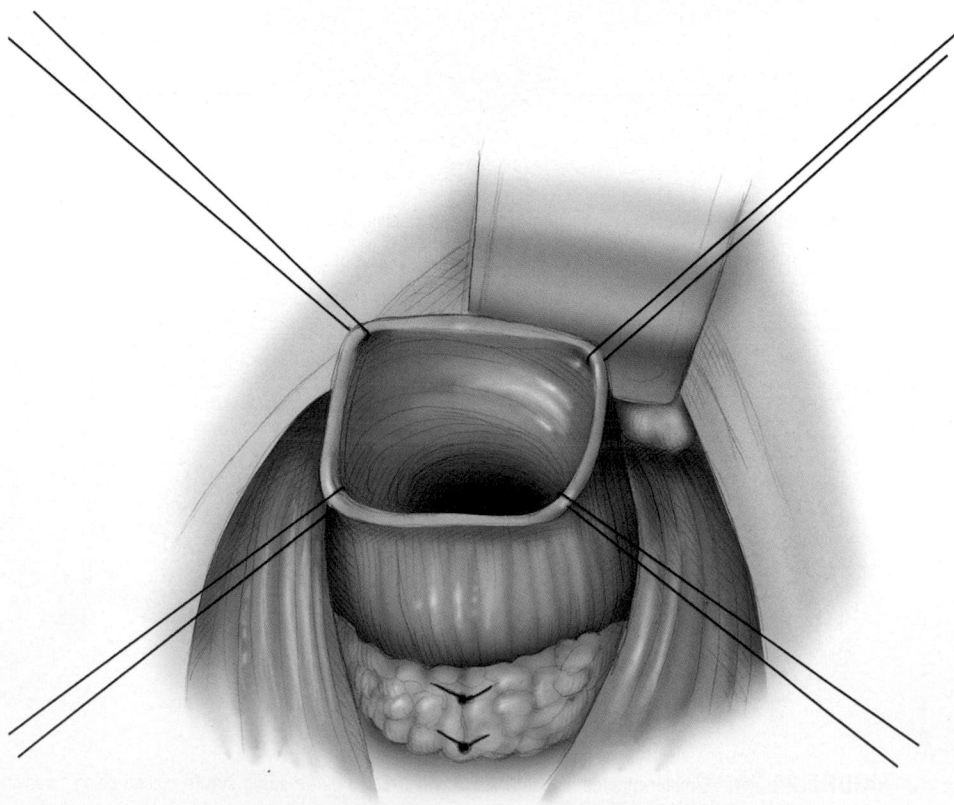

FIGURE 24-31. Four stay sutures applied to rectal stump in preparation for hand-sewn anastomosis.

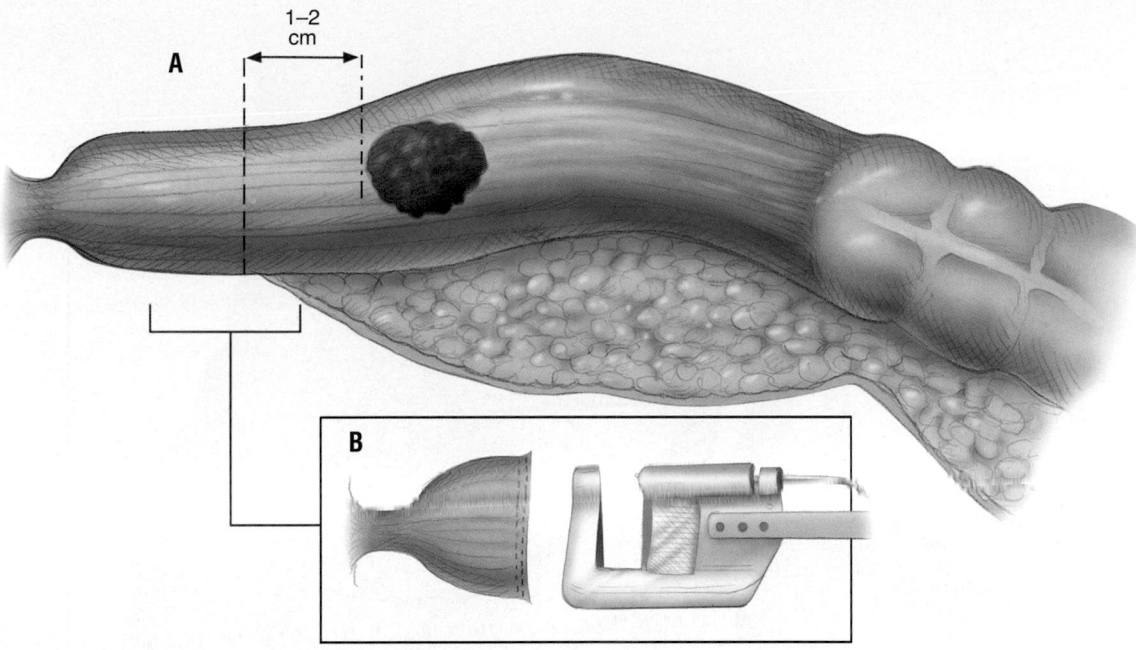

FIGURE 24-32. Tumor in the lower third of the rectum transected with Contour.

Tumors of the Middle or Lower Thirds of the Rectum

When the tumor is in the midportion or lower portion of the rectum, the dissection has to proceed in the retrorectal space to the pelvic floor, and the anterior plane of dissection should be as low as possible. The tubular lower end of the rectum is thus fully mobilized. There is little or no perirectal fat at this level, and the rectum can be transected using the Contour stapling device (Figure 24-32).

In obese patients and males with narrow pelvis, it is sometimes useful to ask an assistant to apply pressure to the perineum. This can often push the lower rectum into the pelvis and facilitate stapling and transection (Figure 24-33).

Dividing the Inferior Mesenteric Artery

Once the rectum has been transected, the inferior mesenteric artery is doubly ligated and divided (Figure 24-34). I usually perform a high ligation close to the origin of the artery on the aorta. Before doing so, the position of the ureter is again noted to avoid injury.

Mobilization of the Splenic Flexure

Several factors contribute to anastomotic leakage. These include poor blood supply, tension, and inadequate seromuscular apposition. Many patients in Western societies are obese and have concomitant sigmoid diverticular disease with a fat laden and shortened mesentery. In these individuals, the proximal descending colon must be mobilized to reach the lower rectum. Tension is avoidable by performing the following three steps:

1. Mobilizing the splenic flexure
2. Ligating and dividing the inferior mesenteric vein at the lower border of the pancreas
3. Unfolding the splenic mesentery

The method of mobilizing the splenic flexure must be reproducible and has to protect against injuries to the spleen.

In order to minimize the risk of splenic injury, the plane of dissection has to be strictly in the lesser sac.

The surgeon stands on the patient's right with an assistant between the patient's legs and another retracting the left abdominal wall. The head of the operating table is elevated, and the table is rotated to the right. The surgeon wears a headlight. The dissection is performed by diathermy, or a long Harmonic scalpel is used.

The greater omentum is retracted vertically out of the wound and lifted caudally. The surgeon should resist the temptation of retracting the greater omentum across to the right

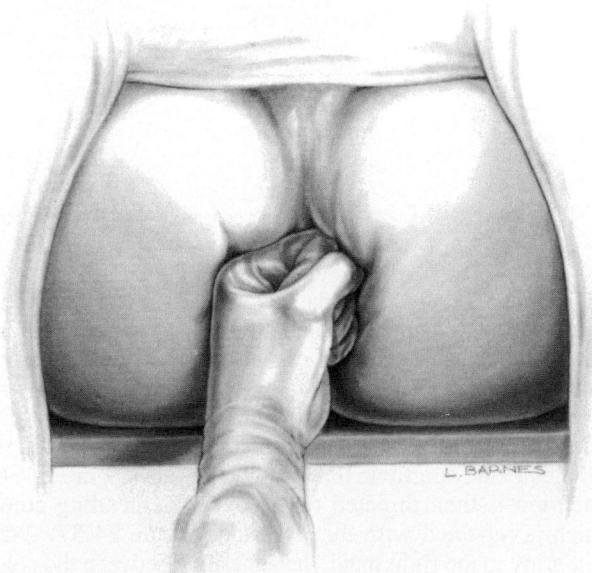

FIGURE 24-33. Pressure on the perineum by the fist or some other blunt object facilitates the placement of sutures into the rectal remnant.

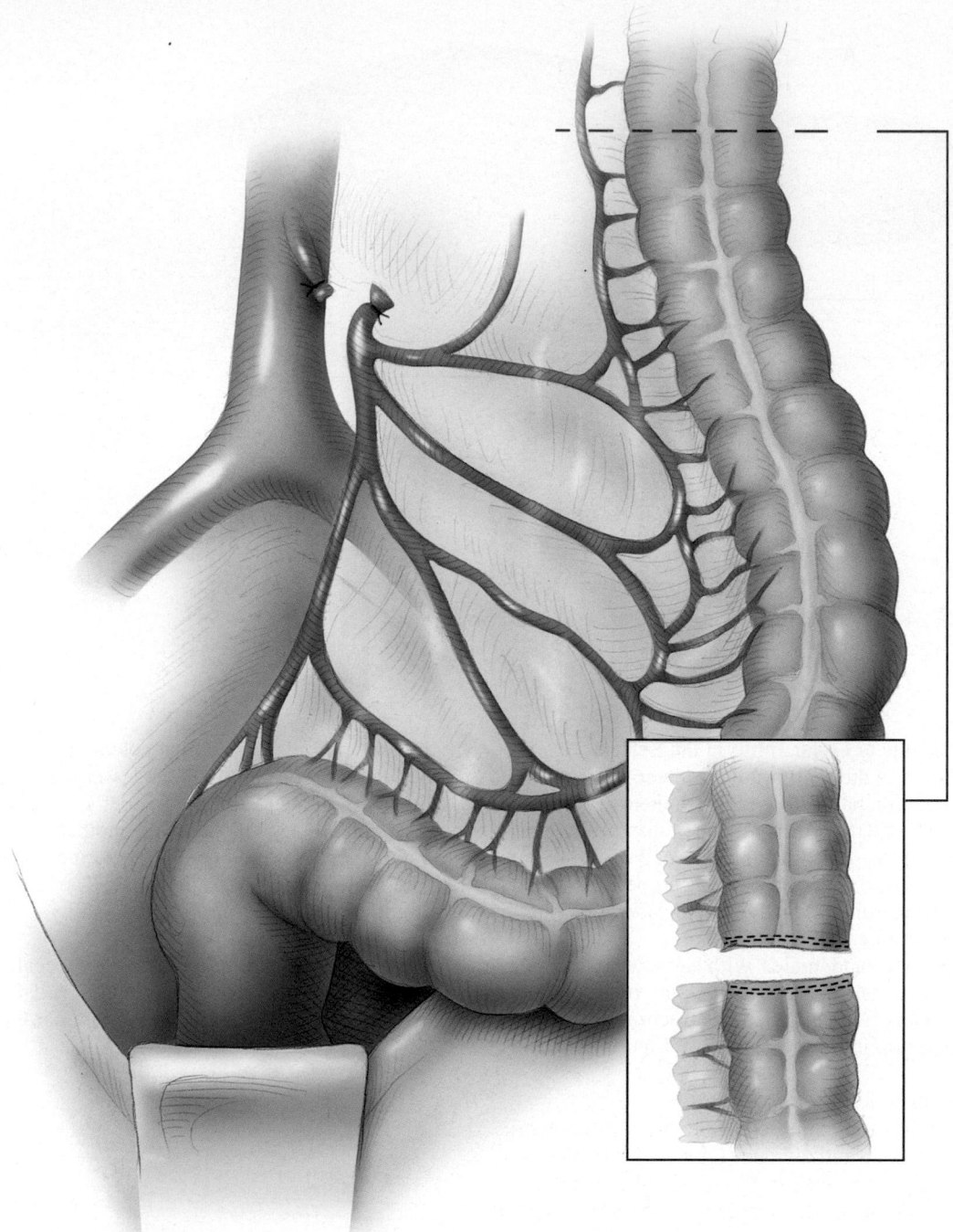

FIGURE 24-34. Author's preference of ligating the inferior mesenteric artery on the aorta.

side. This is a dangerous maneuver that can tear fine adhesions between the omentum and the splenic capsule, resulting in injury to the spleen. The assistant gently retracts the distal transverse colon downward, and the greater omentum is retracted caudally (Figure 24-35). Sharp dissection then allows access into the lesser sac. The dissection continues toward the splenic flexure strictly in that avascular plane (Figure 24-36). Attention is then directed to the upper descending colon, which is retracted with the left hand (Figure 24-37). With diathermy in the right hand, the adhesions between the colon and the lateral abdominal wall are divided to meet the line of dissection of the distal transverse colon. The descending colon is thus mobilized to the midline.

Dividing the Inferior Mesenteric Vein
It is important to understand that even after the flexure has been fully mobilized, the mesentery is still not sufficiently free. This is because it is held back by the inferior mesenteric vein at the inferior border of the pancreas (Figure 24-38). The vein should be ligated and divided at that level.

Unfolding the Splenic Flexure Mesentery
Once the flexure is mobilized, further length can be obtained by unfolding the splenic flexure mesentery to the marginal vessels as shown in Figure 24-39. The colon is now fully mobilized and can reach the low rectum deep in the pelvis without tension.

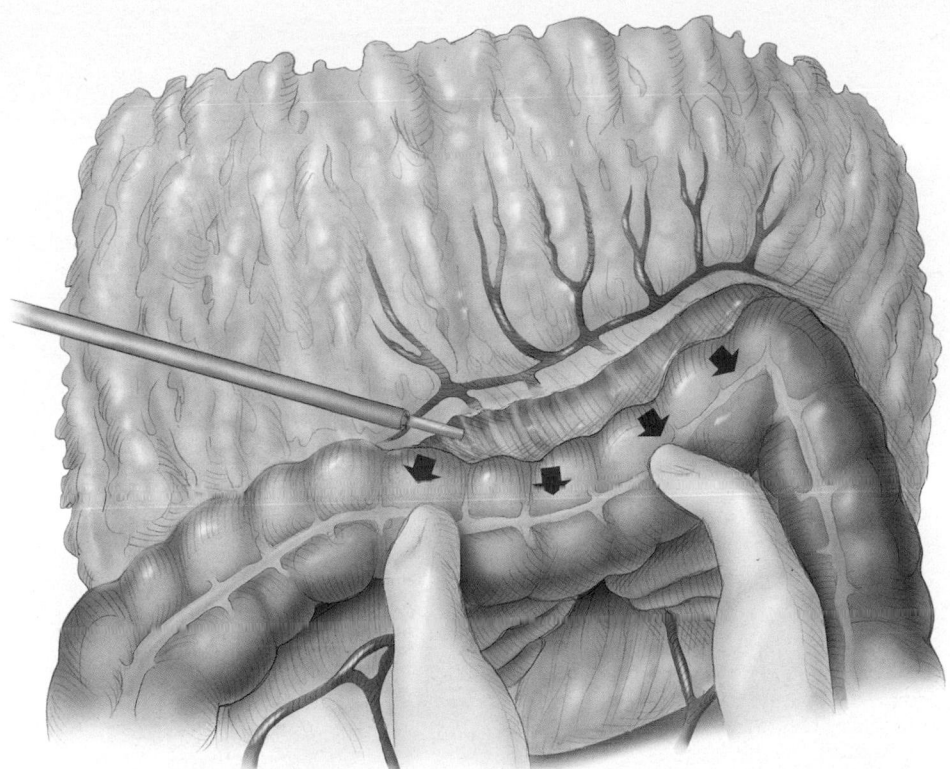

FIGURE 24-35. Mobilization of splenic flexure. The assistant holds the distal transverse colon down, and the lesser sac is entered.

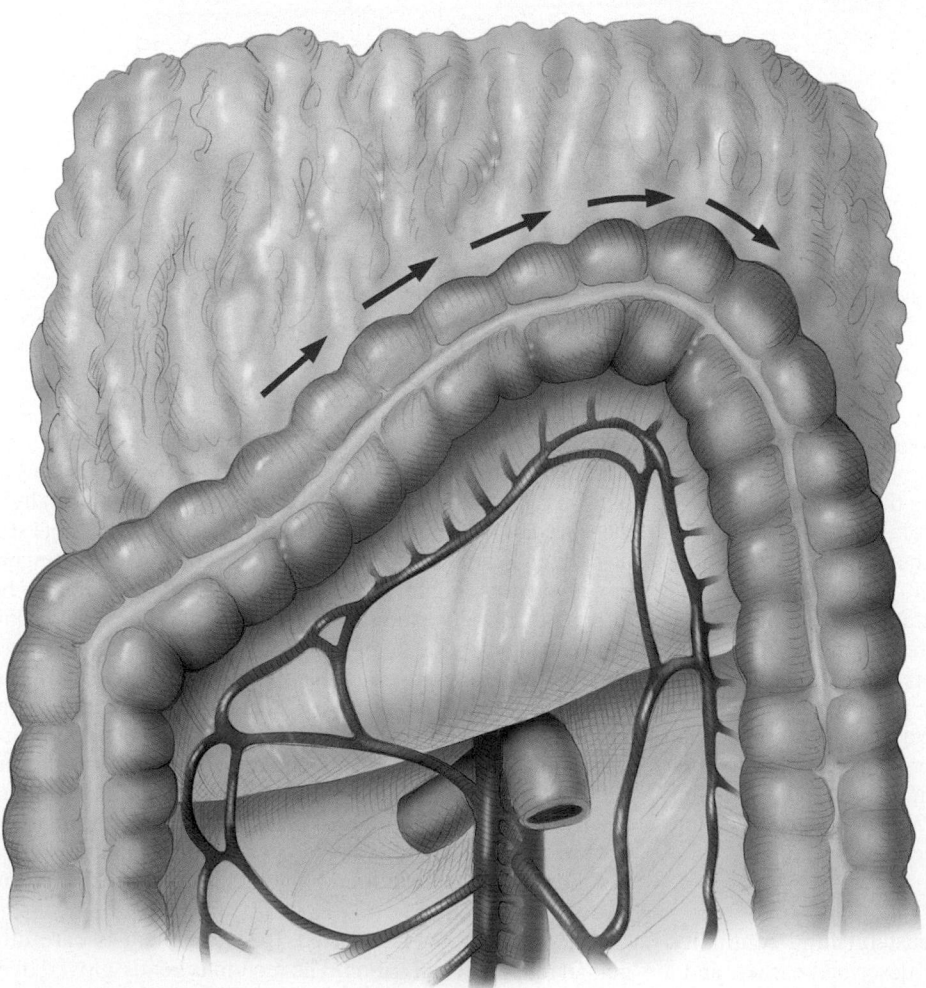

FIGURE 24-36. Line of dissection during mobilization of splenic flexure.

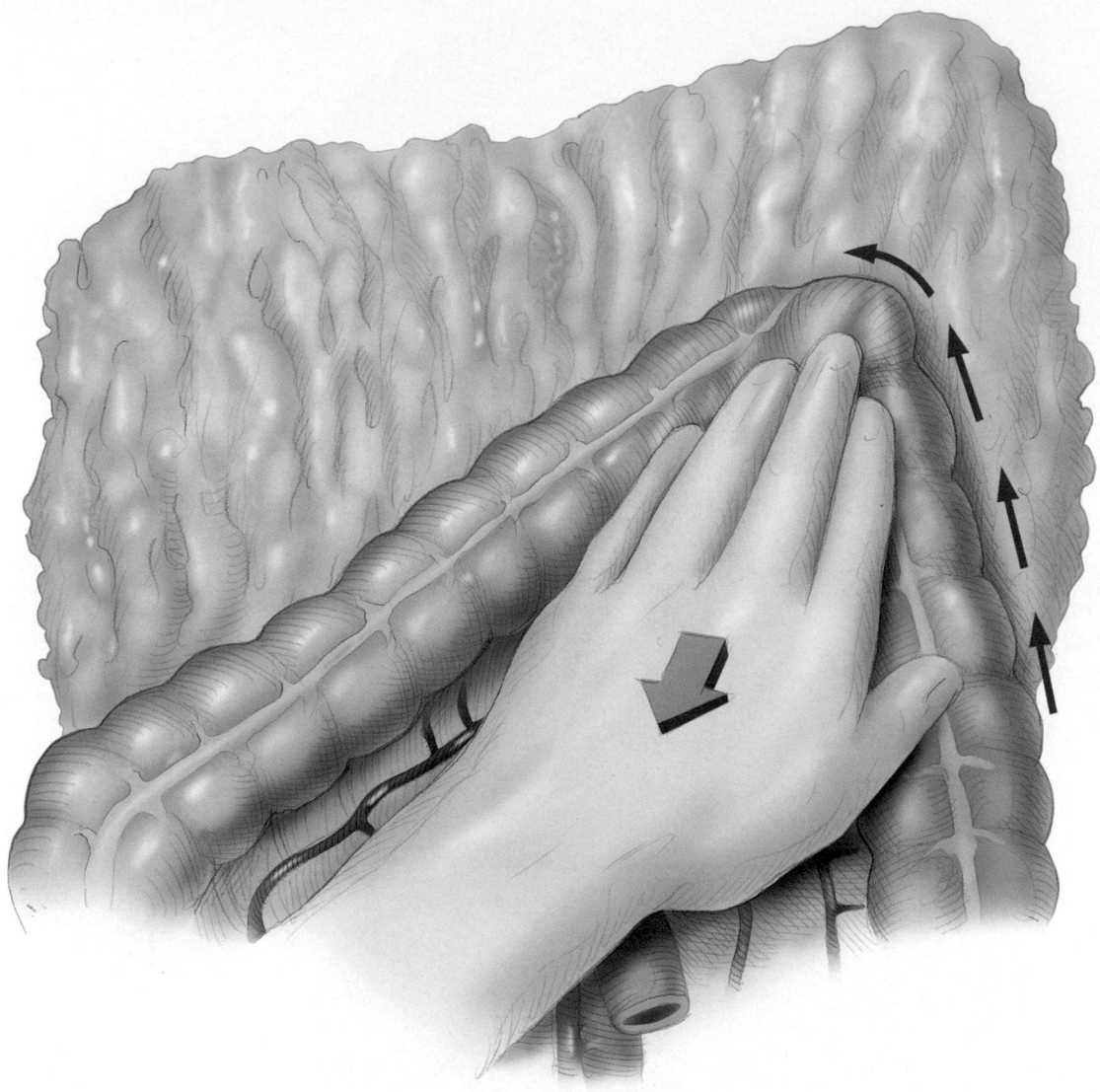

FIGURE 24-37. Mobilization of upper descending colon.

Testing the Blood Supply of the Proximal Colon

The proximal colon is now ready to be divided at an appropriate level after ligating and dividing the marginal vessels. It is advisable to test the blood supply of the proximal colon by observing pulsatile bleeding from the marginal artery prior to ligation.

The colon is then divided. If a stapled anastomosis is to be performed (and that is the preferred method), a purse string is applied before the colon is divided. This can either be performed by a disposable purse-string applicator (Figure 24-40), a Furness clamp, or a hand-sewn technique. I prefer to use a disposable applicator because I have found it to be accurate and less time consuming. The anvil of stapling instrument (Figures 24-41 and 24-42) is now introduced into the colon, and the purse string is tied.

Staple-on-Staple (Double-Stapled) Anastomosis

This is my preferred method of reestablishing continuity. The rectum has been stapled off as described earlier, and a purse string has been applied to the proximal colon.

Insertion of Stapling Instrument into the Rectal Stump

An assistant then washes out the rectal stump and inserts the stapling instrument. This step can at times be difficult, especially if there is anal stenosis or if the patient is obese. If there is anal stenosis, then gentle dilatation may be performed with the fingers or with dilators (Figure 24-43). If the patient is obese, it may be difficult to introduce the stapling instrument. The perianal skin can get caught by the lip of the instrument and pushed in, making insertion even more difficult. Occasionally, the rectum can be injured if an inexperienced assistant forces the instrument in.

Whenever there is difficulty in inserting the stapling instrument, I take charge of the situation and perform the insertion myself. I have used a simple technique to facilitate insertion under these circumstances. A Lone Star retractor is used to retract the anal skin and open the anal canal as shown in Figure 24-44. I have found that this is particularly helpful in obese patients.

Once the stapler is inserted, the instrument is carefully guided into the rectal stump. The rectum is gently gloved over the instrument, and the instrument is fully opened. I prefer to

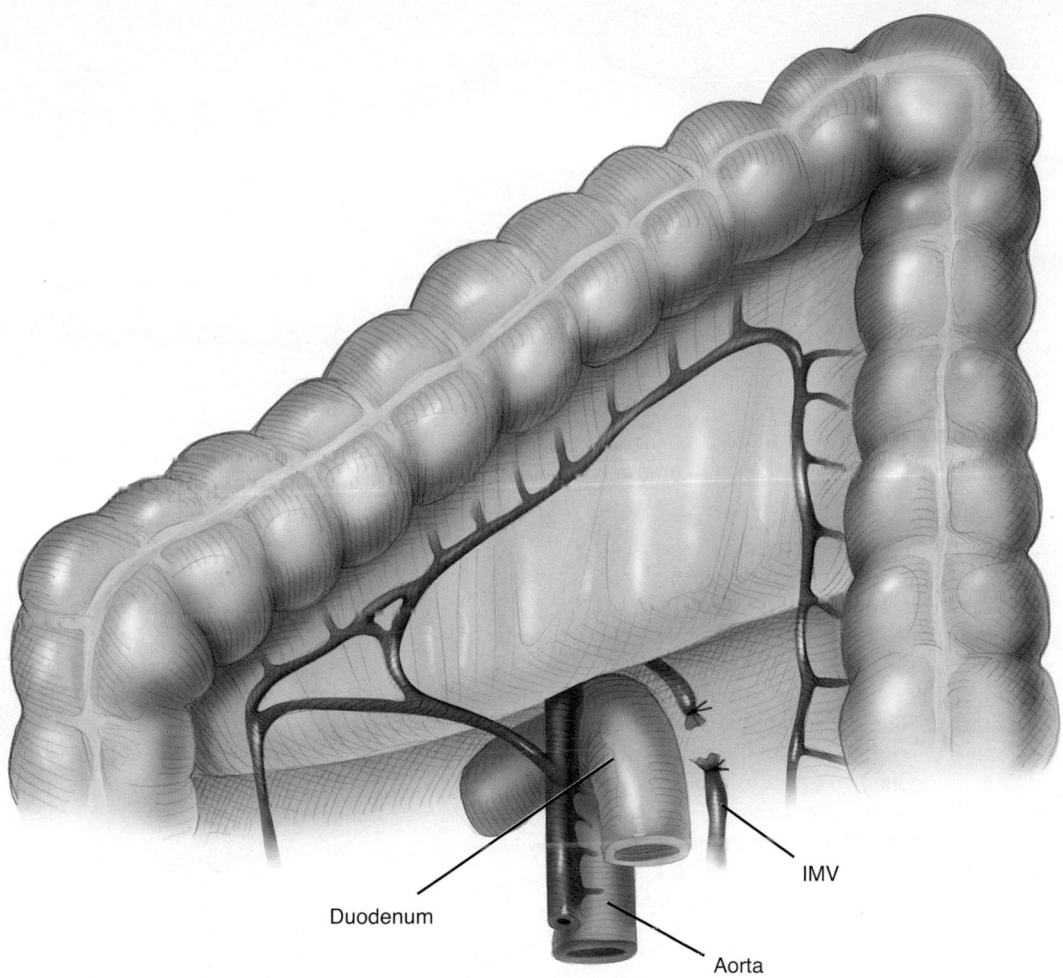

FIGURE 24-38. Inferior mesenteric vein divided at the inferior border of the pancreas.

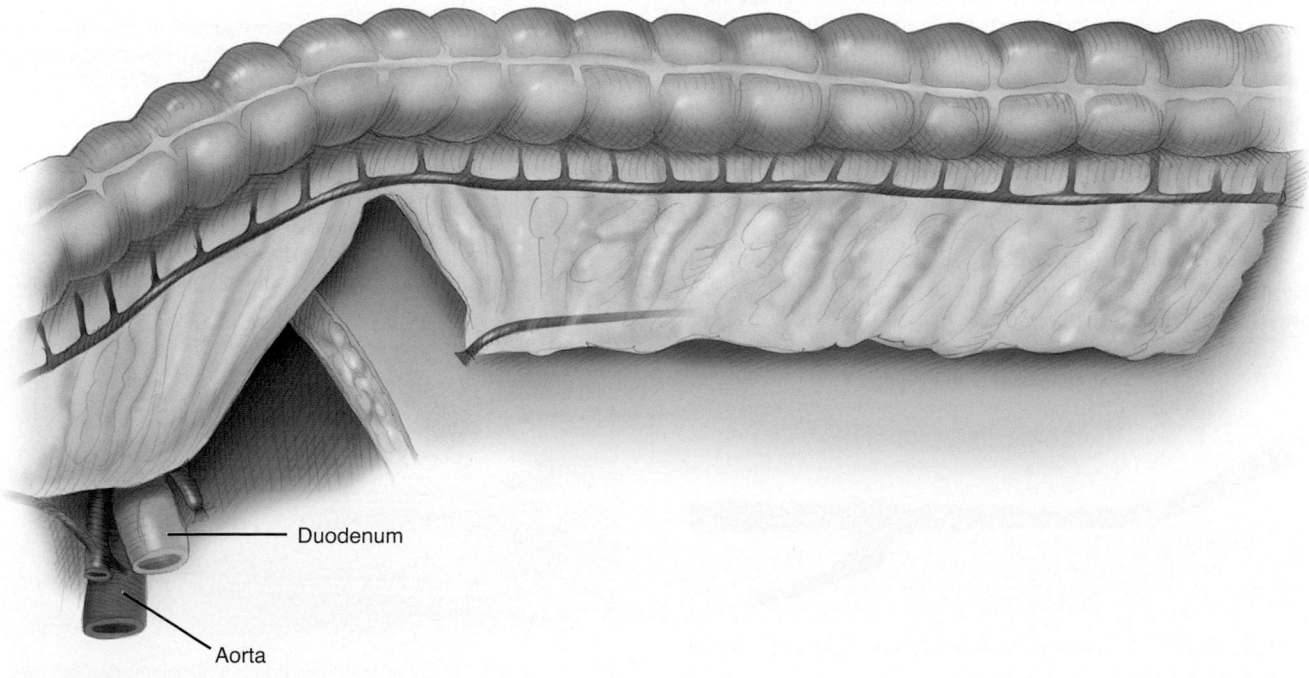

FIGURE 24-39. Splenic flexure unfolded to avoid tension on anastomosis.

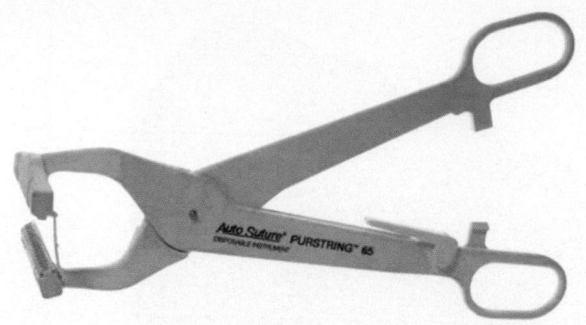

FIGURE 24-40. The Purstring 65 single-use instrument places a circumferential strand of 2–0 MONOSOF nonabsorbable monofilament nylon surgical suture (United States Pharmacopeia [USP]) held in place by stainless steel staples. (Courtesy of Covidien, Inc., Norwalk, CT.)

advance the trocar tip through the staple line (Figure 24-45), but some surgeons like to penetrate the adjacent bowel. It is critical, however, to incorporate the linear staple line.

The proximal colon with the anvil is then pulled down into the pelvis. Care is taken to ensure that the mesentery is not twisted. The proximal anvil is pushed into the pin, and the assistant closes the mechanism so that the anvil and head are fully approximated (Figure 24-46). After the staples are fired, the instrument is opened three turns, and the stapler is gently withdrawn. The tissue rings (donuts) are carefully assessed for completeness and for an intact muscle coating.

Following this, the anastomosis is tested for leakage (Figure 24-47). Provided there is no leak, I use a drain in the retrorectal space, and the abdomen is then closed.

Temporary Proximal Loop Stoma

The decision whether to construct a proximal stoma is one that the surgeon must consider at surgery. It is preferable to forewarn the patient that a temporary stoma may be necessary and to always site a stoma preoperatively (see Chapter 31). As a rule, the lower the anastomosis, the more likely it is that a temporary stoma will be advisable. Other relative indications include a technically difficult procedure, unexpected intraoperative pelvic hemorrhage, significant comorbidities, obesity, and those in whom the donuts were incomplete even though there was no leakage on air testing. If there was a leak on testing, even though the site of leakage may have been identified and oversewn, this is another possible indication for fecal diversion.

If a decision is made to construct a temporary stoma, a temporary loop ileostomy rather than a loop colostomy is preferred. There are three reasons for this: no tension is

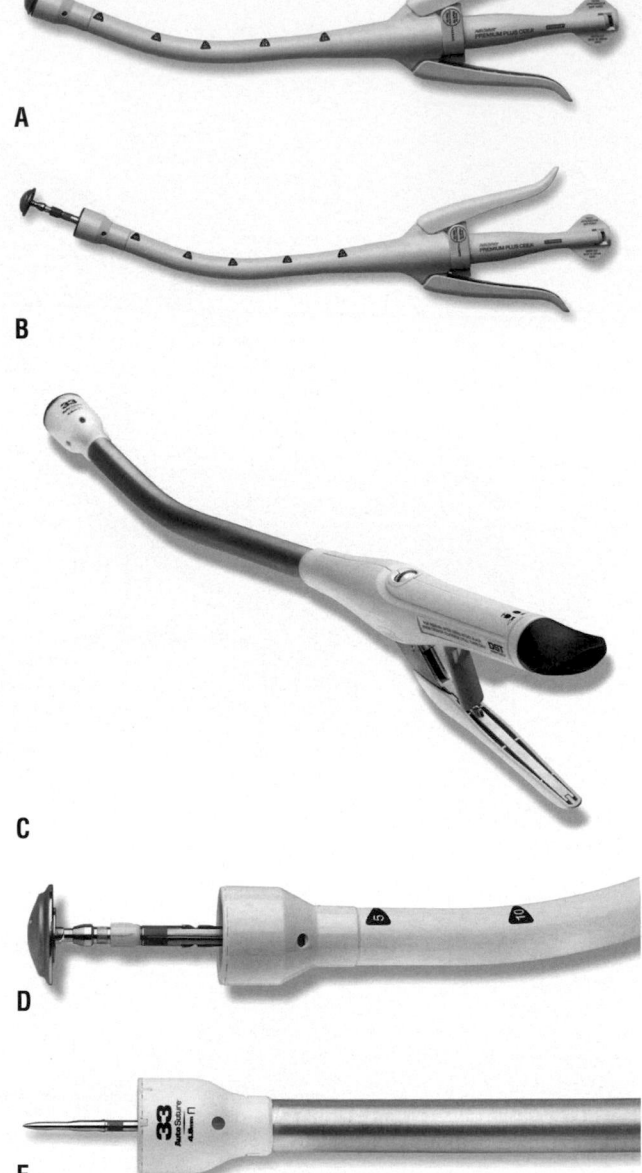

FIGURE 24-42. Multiple options are available in the circular instruments. Disposable curved CEEA (end-to-end circular stapler) with integrated flip-top anvil. This permits a low profile for ease of insertion and removal. **A:** Closed instrument. **B:** Opened instrument. **C:** End-to-end anastomosis (EEA) Open/XL—available in two shaft lengths, ergonomic handle and knob, and one-handed firing. **D:** Close-up view of open instrument. **E:** Distal anvil removed. (Courtesy of Covidien, Inc., Norwalk, CT.)

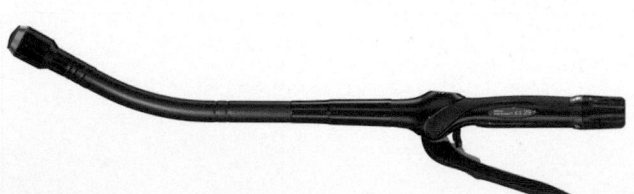

FIGURE 24-41. Proximate ILS curved intraluminal stapler with detachable head and with low-profile anvil. This is available in sizes 21, 25, 29, and 33 mm. (Courtesy of Ethicon Endo-Surgery, Inc., Cincinnati, OH.)

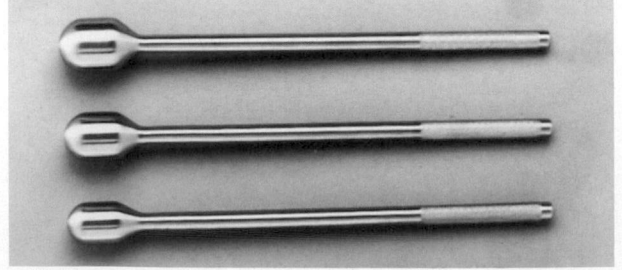

FIGURE 24-43. Sizers in three diameters. (Courtesy of Covidien, Inc., Norwalk, CT.)

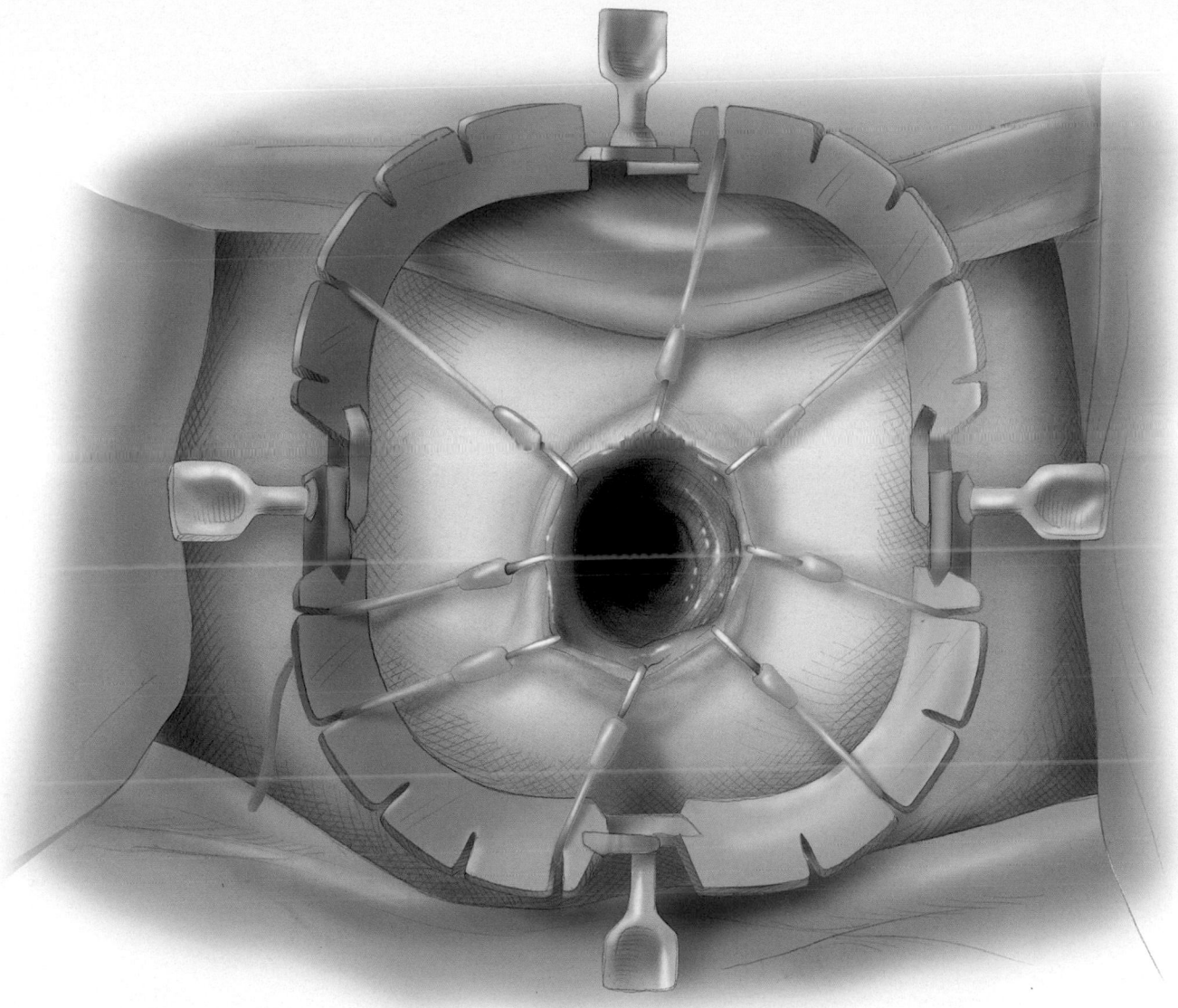

FIGURE 24-44. Lone Star retractor used to expose the anus and facilitate insertion of the stapling instrument.

put on the proximal colon by exteriorizing the transverse colon; there is no risk of injuring the vital marginal vessels of the proximal colon either when the colostomy is being constructed or when it is closed; and if a planned temporary stoma needs to be permanent, a loop ileostomy is easier to manage. Moreover, there is a lesser incidence of prolapse and parastomal herniation with a loop ileostomy.

Hand-Sewn Anastomosis

Although I prefer to use a staple-on-staple (double-stapled) anastomosis as described earlier, occasionally one needs to perform a hand-sewn anastomosis. When doing so, the rectum is transected as described, and four stay sutures are inserted in the rectal stump (see Figure 24-31). I use a single layer of interrupted 2 0 Vicryl sutures. The posterior layer is inserted first, including at least 1 cm of the muscle layer (Figure 24-48). The corners are turned, and then an interrupted seromuscular sutures are applied to the anterior row of the anastomosis (Figure 24-49).

Total Mesorectal Excision

This term was coined by Heald in the late 1970s (see earlier Biography).[246] Heald and others[163] had rediscovered the retrorectal space that Heald renamed the "holy plane." Furthermore, he described the perirectal fat as the mesorectum even though the rectum has no true mesentery. He also came to understand that the rectum and its perirectal fat were covered by an intact layer of fascia, and that the specimen could be removed within an intact fascial envelope to reduce the risk of local recurrence by ensuring clear surgical margins.

When the term TME was first introduced, many colorectal surgeons were already mobilizing the rectum along well-defined and well-described anatomical planes, preserving an intact perirectal fascial envelope[163,259,312,358,442,616]; so there was some confusion as to what exactly was meant by the term TME.

Many general surgeons who performed few rectal dissections per year were keen to adopt this technique and

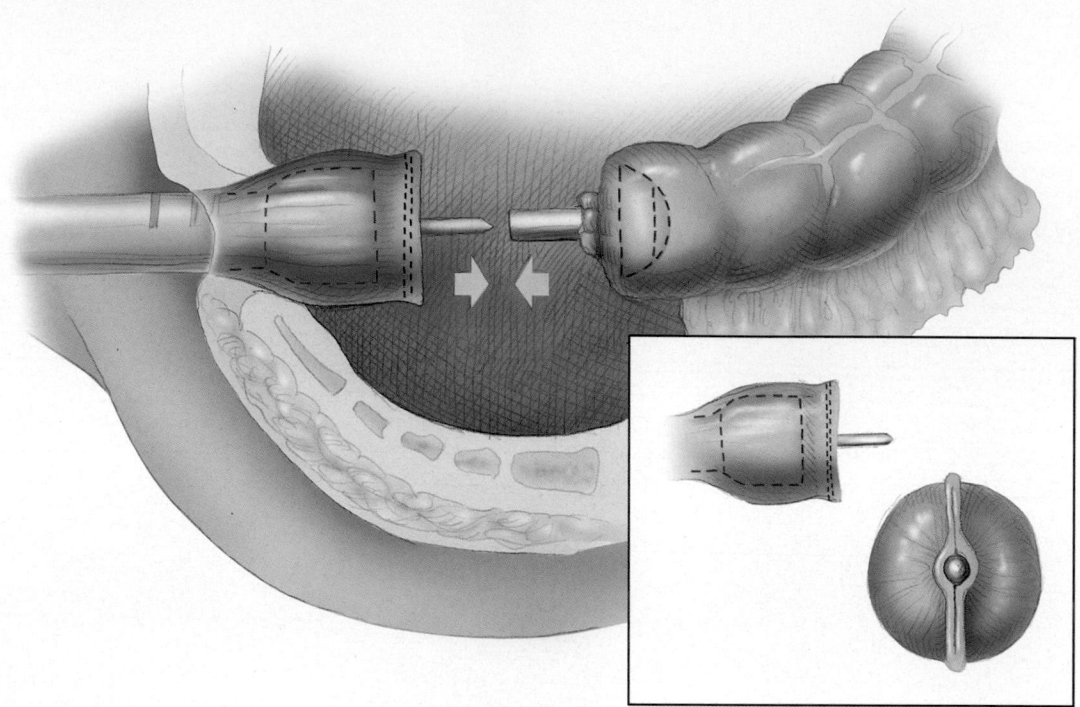

FIGURE 24-45. Tip of stapling instrument is opened through the linear staple line.

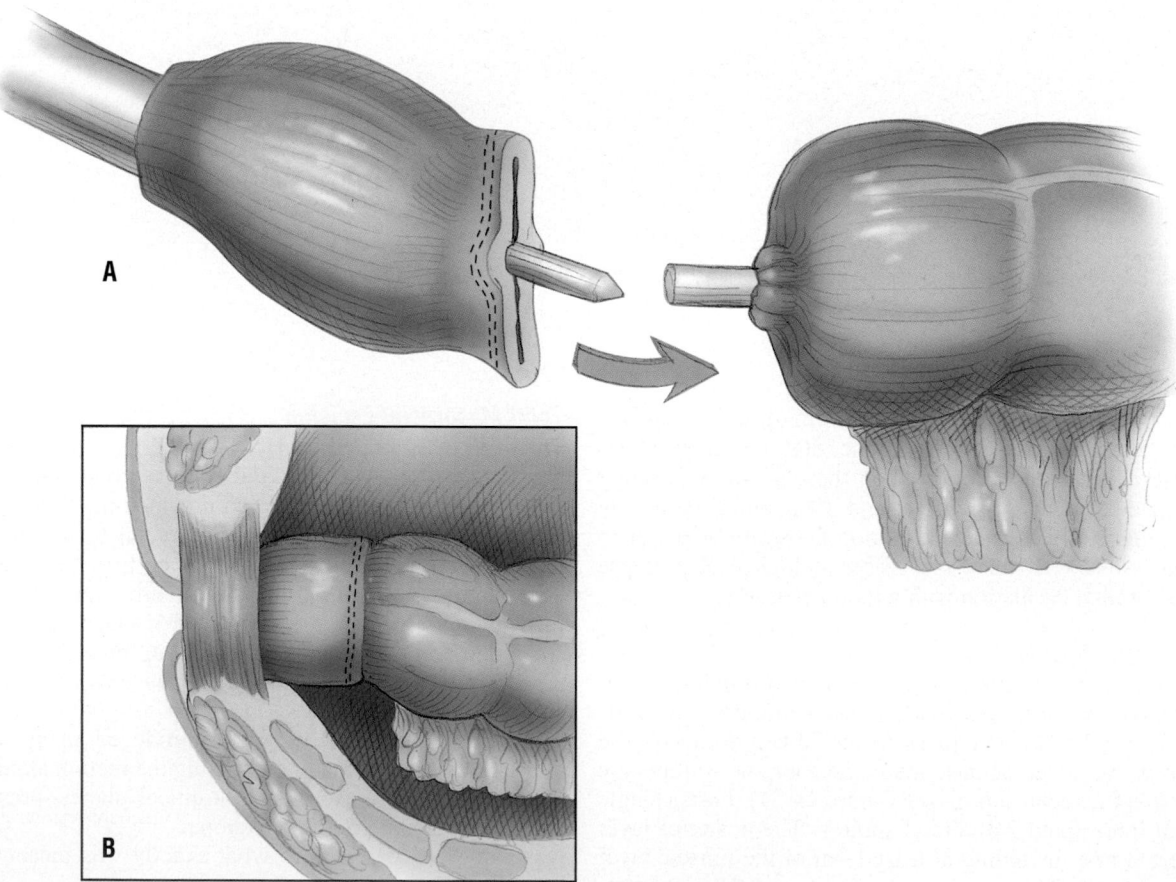

FIGURE 24-46. The anvil and head are approximated, and the staples are fired to form the anastomosis (*inset*).

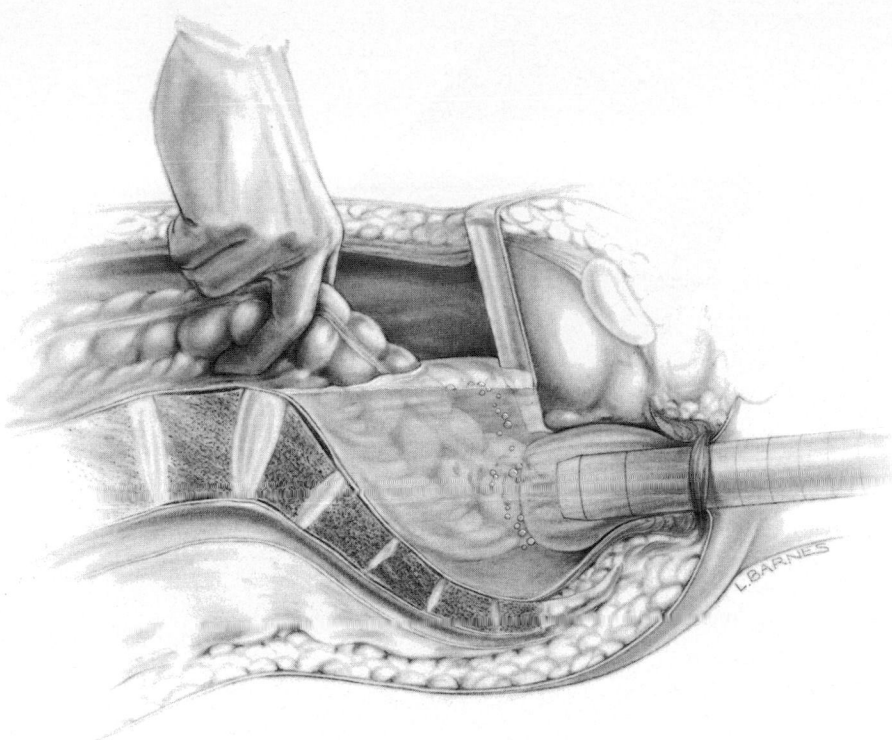

FIGURE 24-47. Method of testing for integrity of rectal anastomosis. Inspection can be achieved by means of the rigid sigmoidoscope. By compression of the proximal bowel with the fingers or a noncrushing clamp and by the insufflation of air with saline in the pelvis, bubbles may be seen to escape from a leak. The site can then be identified and possibly repaired.

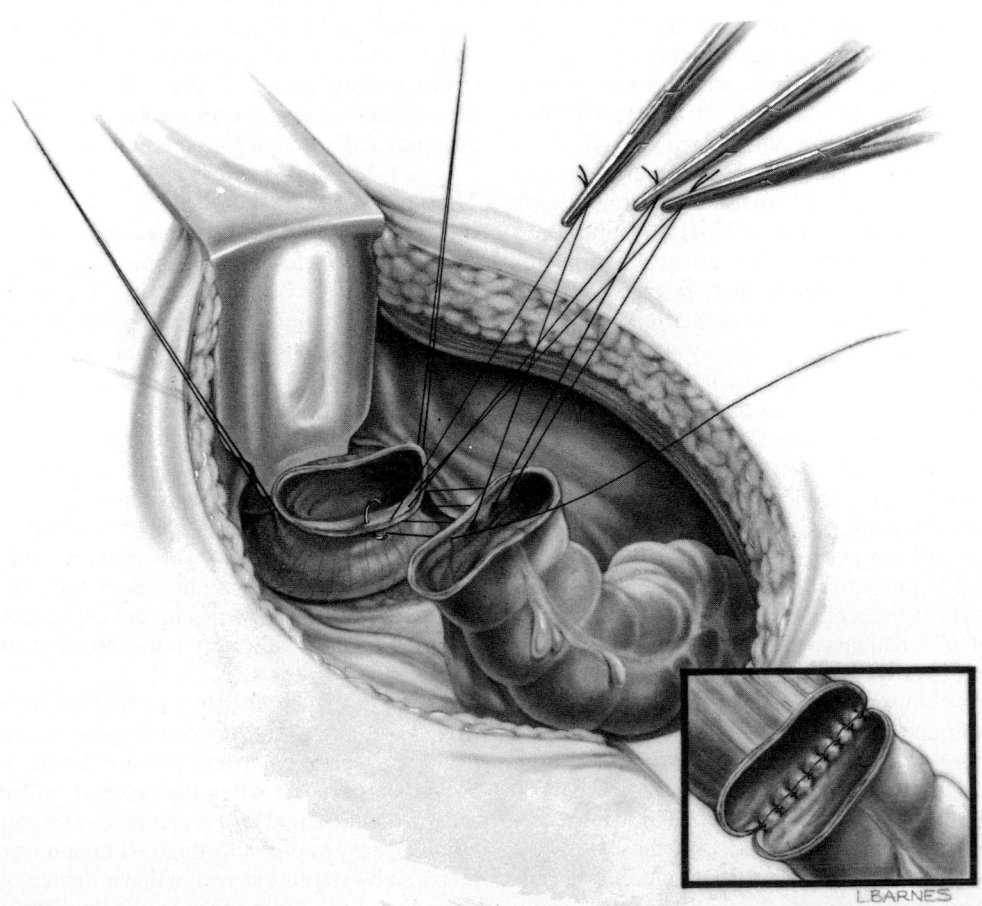

FIGURE 24-48. Hand-sewn rectal anastomosis. Sutures are initially placed in the posterior row but not secured. The *inset* demonstrates the posterior row completed.

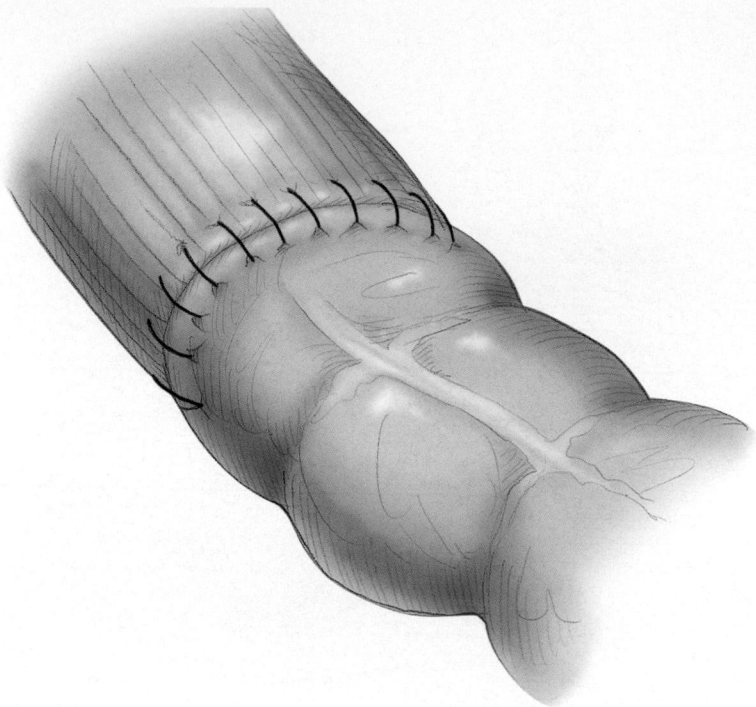

FIGURE 24-49. Hand-sewn rectal anastomosis. Interrupted sutures applied to anterior row.

took the word "total" in TME quite literally, performing unnecessary low and ultralow anterior resections when a high anterior resection would have sufficed. This resulted in a number of avoidable complications after low anastomoses, of which anastomotic leakage was the most worrisome. Karanjia and colleagues reported on the Basingstoke experience of 219 patients who underwent a TME for a tumor between 3.5 and 15.0 cm from the anal verge; an anastomotic leak rate of 17.4% resulted.[302] Hainsworth and coworkers questioned the use of TME for upper third tumors in view of the high morbidity rate following this operation in their patients.[233] The term TME has, however, taken hold. Today, it tends to refer to dissection of the rectum along the same anatomical planes as were originally described by Jonnesco (see earlier Biography), although many would now question the need to perform a TME for cancers of the upper rectum or rectosigmoid.[352,372] From this concern has arisen the terms "partial" or "tailored" TME, wherein the mesorectum is divided 3 to 5 cm below the tumor. This shifts the emphasis to clearly identifying the retrorectal space and the perirectal fascia and not to the complete removal of the perirectal fat or "mesorectum" for tumors at all levels of the rectum.

In a study of 622 patients who underwent an anterior resection for cancer at the Queen Mary Hospital in Hong Kong, the authors compared the results of patients who had a TME for middle and lower third tumors with those who had a partial mesorectal excision (PME) for tumors in the upper rectum (this group constituted, in our experience, 30% of rectal cancers).[342] There was no difference in local recurrence or survival between the two groups, but those who had a TME had a higher rate of complications, including anastomotic leakage. This study supports the view that what really matters in rectal cancer surgery is the anatomical nature of the mobilization rather than the total excision of the "mesorectum." Moreover, it is noteworthy that TME has never

been subjected to rigorous testing by a randomized, controlled trial. Indeed, some would argue that the recurrence rates claimed by Heald are the results of patient selection and/or case mix and the method of statistical analysis used to interpret the data.[282–284] Nevertheless, the concept of TME has contributed to a greater awareness of the need for precise anatomical dissection for rectal cancer surgery.

Side-to-End and Side-to-Side Anastomoses
Baker advocated side-to-end anastomosis of the colon to the rectum in order to deal with the disparity between the two lumina.[28] Others have also found this to be a useful technique.[310] In my opinion, the anastomosis can be more readily accomplished in an end-to-end fashion, with the circular stapling device.

Coloanal Hand-Sewn Anastomosis
An alternative technique for reestablishing intestinal continuity is the coloanal anastomosis. Pulling the colon through the anus was first described by Cutait and Turnbull in 1961 (see later), and in 1972, Parks described a hand-sewn coloanal anastomosis.[124,487,622] Circumstances where it is indicated include very low rectal cancers and on occasions when there has been a failure of a very low-stapled anastomosis.

Author's Technique for Coloanal Hand-Sewn Technique
It is essential that the proximal colon be completely mobilized as described earlier. There must be no tension at all on the anastomosis when the colon is pulled through. As a rule, if the proximal colon can reach the patient's left knee, it will be easy to pull it through without tension. The colon is prepared by stapling it with a linear device. A small incision is made in the middle of the staple line, and a Foley catheter is inserted into the colon; the catheter balloon is inflated. The catheter will be used to pull the colon down through the anal canal.

JOEL W. BAKER (1905–1999)

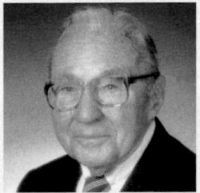

Joel Baker was born in Shenandoah, Virginia. Thanks to the influence of his uncle, the town physician, Baker always wanted to pursue medicine. He graduated from the University of Virginia Medical School in 1928 and went to Seattle, Washington for his internship, having been recruited by the founder of the Virginia Mason Hospital, James Mason. He continued his training under Mason and remained as a member of the medical staff. Concomitantly, Baker went on to train at the Mayo Clinic in Rochester, Minnesota and at the Lahey Clinic in Boston. Returning to Seattle, he became chief of surgery at the Virginia Mason Clinic,

a position he held for 34 years. He was a champion of medical education and research and founded the department's general surgery residency program. He published 136 papers, including landmark articles on techniques and new instruments that carry his name (e.g., Baker tube and anastomosis). He served as president of the American College of Surgeons and was awarded honorary fellowship in the Royal College of Surgeons of England and Scotland. In his capacity as Inspector General of the U.S. Army, Navy, and Air Force, he was awarded the Outstanding Civilian Service Medal by the U.S. Army. Baker died on July 4, 1999. (With appreciation to Richard C. Thirlby, MD and to John Baker; photograph courtesy of Virginia Mason Medical Center, Seattle, WA.)

When the rectum is fully mobilized to the pelvic floor, it is transected by diathermy at least 1 cm below the tumor. A Lone Star retractor is then used for exposure, and eight sutures (at regular round-the-clock intervals) are inserted into it using 2–0 Vicryl on a 26 needle. The sutures are placed from outside in. The needles are not cut off, and the sutures are pulled out and clipped to the rim of the retractor (Figure 24-50). The proximal colon is then pulled through using the Foley catheter as a guide and for traction (Figure 24-51). The staple line is excised, and the colon is sutured to the anal canal by each of the individual sutures that had been preserved. After this has been accomplished, each suture is tied and divided. The suture line disappears out of sight into the anal canal.

Alternative Techniques for a Coloanal Hand-Sewn Anastomosis

A Parks' self-retaining, three-bladed anal retractor (Figure 24-52); Gelpi retractors place at right angles to each other (Figure 24-53); a Lone Star retractor (Figure 24-54); or a Bookwalter rectal kit (Figure 24-55) can facilitate exposure for a hand-sewn transanal anastomosis (Figure 24-56). A ⅝-circle needle is particularly helpful for placing the sutures—for example, a round-bodied modification of a Turner-Warwick urethroplasty needle or a long-term absorbable suture. This is the technique employed for reestablishing continuity after colectomy, proctectomy, and ileal pouch for inflammatory bowel disease (see Chapter 29). The sutures incorporate the full thickness of the colon with the anal canal and the underlying internal sphincter. An alternative approach is to use a double-stapling technique.

Results

Parks reported 76 patients who underwent rectal excision for carcinoma with restoration of bowel continuity by coloanal anastomosis.[488] Ten developed pelvic sepsis, 2 with anastomotic breakdown. Sixty-nine of 70 patients reviewed had a good functional result. Although not all were followed for 5 years, Parks believed that the preliminary survival data were comparable to that for patients treated by APR.

Enker and colleagues reported their experience with 41 individuals treated by this anastomotic technique.[162]

The mean distance of the tumor from the anal verge was 6.7 cm. At the time of their publication, the median follow-up period was only 31 months, with 73% free of disease. The authors recommend that every patient undergo a temporary diverting colostomy and that the left colon be completely mobilized to avoid tension on the anastomosis. A more recent report from the same institution (Memorial Sloan-Kettering Cancer Center) involved 134 patients.[490] Actuarially, corrected 5-year survival for all patients was 73%. Mesenteric implants, positive microscopic resection margin, T3 tumor, positive nodal involvement, blood vessel invasion, and high tumor grade were associated with increased risk for pelvic recurrence. Gamagami and coworkers performed coloanal anastomoses on 174 patients.[195] Mean follow-up was 66 months. The mean anastomotic height was 2.3 cm, and the overall recurrence rate was 7.9%. The 5-year survival was comparable to that of APR. Others report at least as satisfactory results in terms of both bowel function and recurrent disease.[89,110,162,244,532,606,629]

In the experience of the Memorial Sloan-Kettering Cancer Center, the median stool frequency was two per day, with 22% of patients reporting four or more stools in 24 hours.[489] Stool frequency tended to decrease with time, with the use of postoperative adjuvant radiotherapy influencing the frequency and difficulty with evacuation. Poor sphincter function has been found to be significantly more common in women than in men.[423] All agree that the surgical morbidity is significantly higher than that of low anterior resection.

Handling and Examination of the Surgical Specimen and Tumor Staging

The information provided by the surgeon to the patient must include details of the operative findings as well as details of the histopathologic features of the tumor. Without this information, the patient's prognosis and the potential need for adjuvant therapy cannot be meaningfully discussed. Accurate reporting (classification and tumor staging) is essential for quality patient care when dealing with rectal cancer. To achieve this, there is an onus on the surgeon and the pathologist to collaborate closely to produce a comprehensive

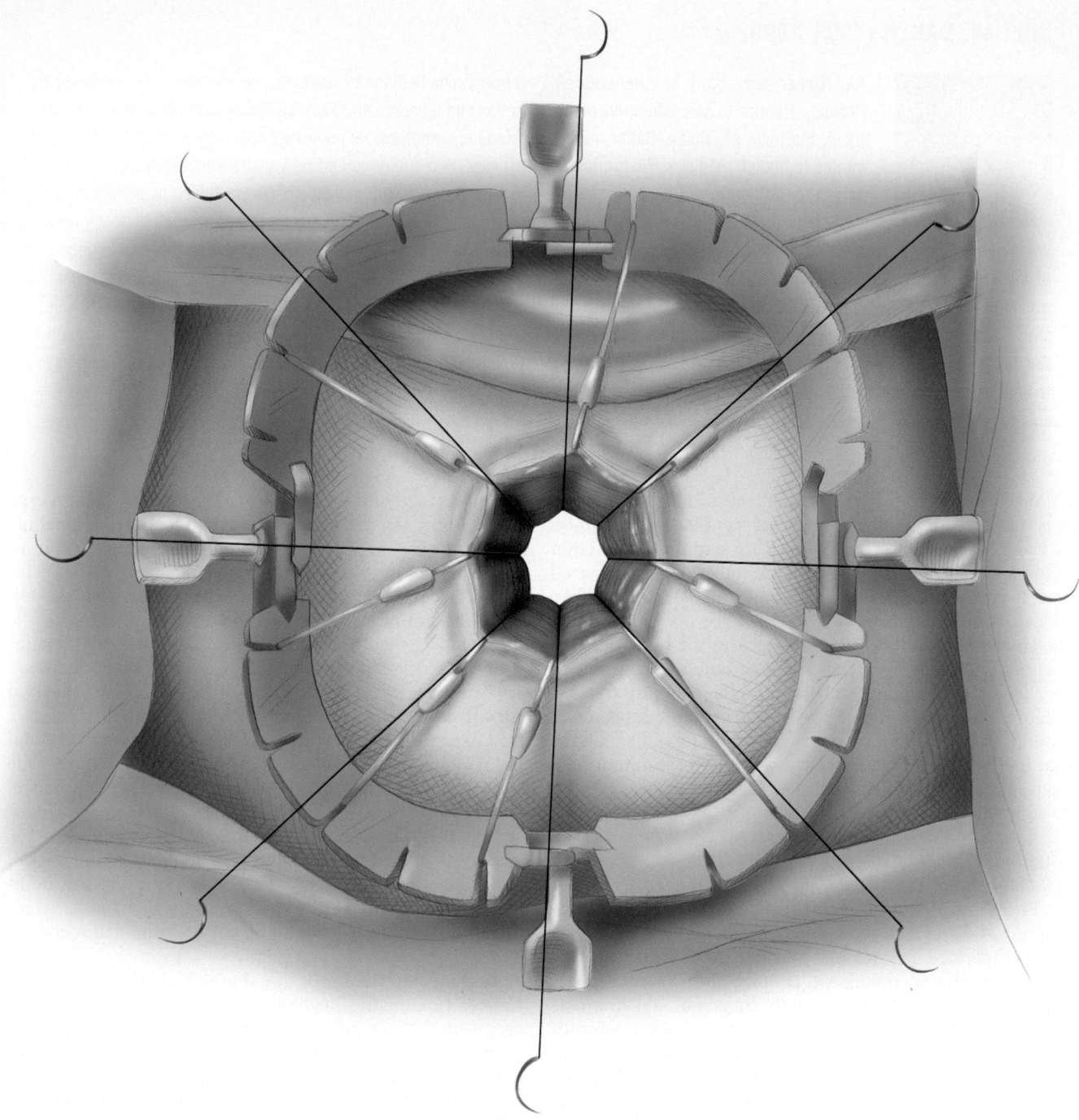

FIGURE 24-50. Lone Star retracting anus. Sutures are applied from outside in, and needles are kept.

report incorporating key clinical and pathologic features from the findings at operation and the examination of the surgical specimen as a basis for appropriate multimodality treatment for the individual patient.[98]

The traditional method of staging rectal cancer is that of Dukes (see Chapter 23). This classification is based on the extent of sequential direct spread of tumor through successive layers of the rectal wall and the presence or absence of locoregional lymph node metastases in the operative specimen.[154] In this strictly pathologic approach, there is no information provided that addresses the issue of "residual tumor," whether local due to tumor transection (involved margin) or the presence of known distant metastases outside the operative field. This information is only available when tumors are staged using a *clinicopathological* system, now internationally adopted as a preferred method of cancer staging.[97] I have adopted this approach, and I support the use of generic reporting to ensure that all relevant information is captured using a standardized, structured template.[71,531] Although the majority of my published results have been reported using the Australian Clinicopathological System, one of the six internationally

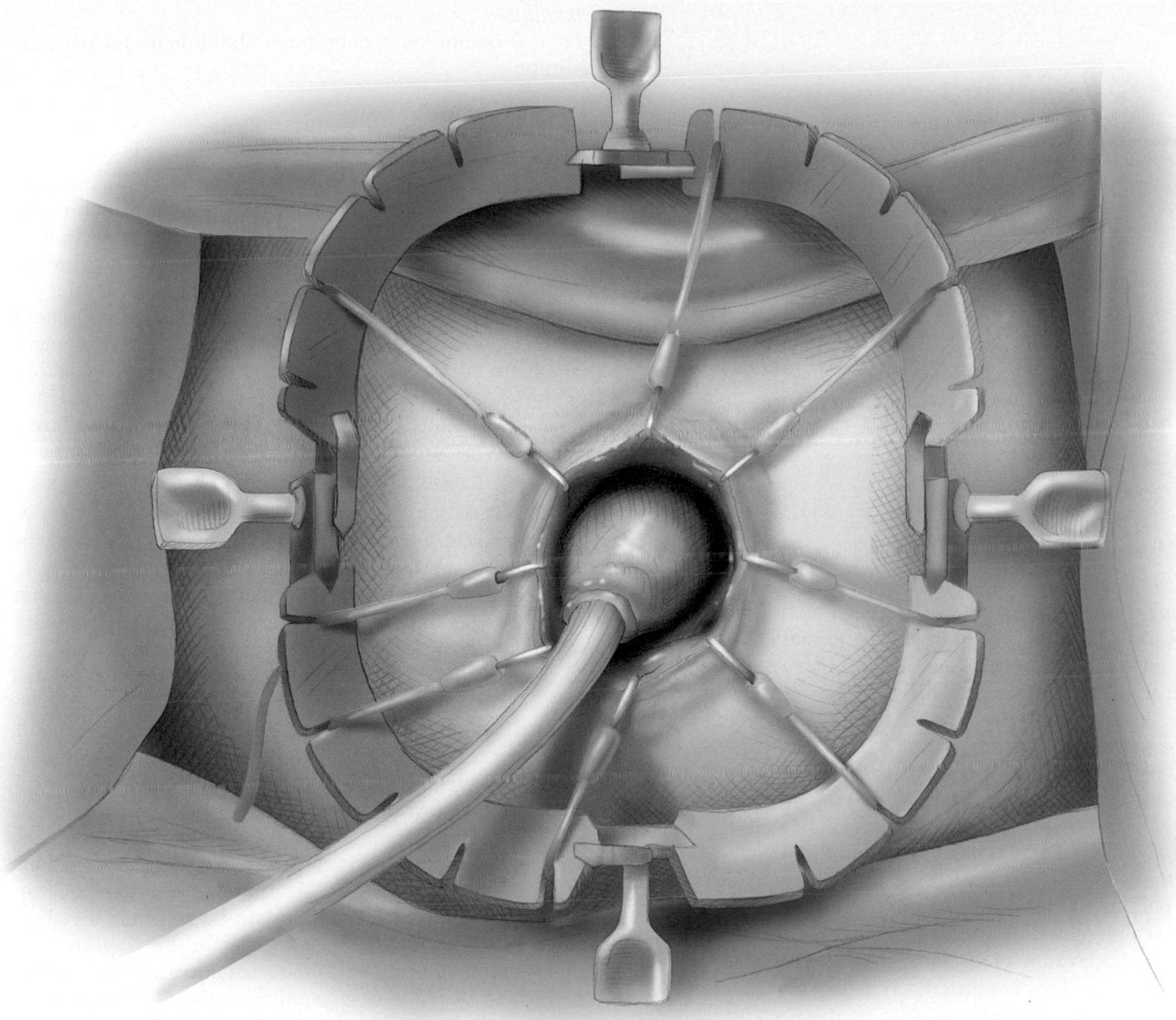

FIGURE 24-51. Foley catheter in proximal colon with balloon inflated, pulling colon down to anus to complete the coloanal anastomosis.

recognized staging classifications,[133] for the purpose of this chapter, the results tabulated are summarized using the TNM system.[143]

The surgeon must also take responsibility for prompt delivery of the correctly labeled and orientated specimen, preferably transported fresh and unopened to the laboratory. The pathologist should be provided with a precise but clinically relevant history, including a brief description of the important observations made at laparotomy. In particular, the surgeon should provide information about the type of resection, the site of the tumor, and the presence or otherwise of distant metastases or local residual tumor in order to enable the pathologist to determine the final clinicopathologic stage. In turn, the pathologist is responsible for preparing a thorough report, noting all key

diagnostic (macroscopic and microscopic) and prognostic indicators. These should include the presence of extramural venous invasion, serosal surface involvement, clearance of all resection margins (proximal, distal, and circumferential), and presence of perforation in the specimen.[97] Certainly, specimen handling, sampling, and dissection should be standardized to allow meaningful comparisons between treatment centers and for entering patients into clinical trials.[507] Ideally, the final report should include representative images of key macroscopic and histologic features of the tumor. This will greatly assist discussion of prognosis and in counseling patients and their relatives. In this regard, the essential standardized protocol favored by the author over many years is that recommended by the Australian National Health and Medical Research Council.[456]

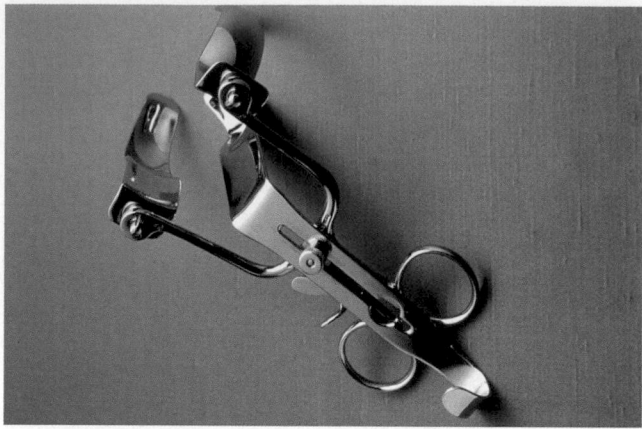

FIGURE 24-52. Parks retractor.

Abdominoperineal Resection

Indications

As mentioned earlier, there has been a trend away from APR to restorative procedures. Traditionally, APR was indicated when the lower edge of the tumor was at or below 8 cm from the anal verge. This view has now changed, and lower lesions including those in the middle third and many in the lower third of the rectum can be satisfactorily managed by low or ultralow anterior resections with restoration of continuity by any number of methods, including colo-anal anastomoses. APR is, however, indicated when there is invasion of the anal canal and invasion of the sphincter mechanism (i.e., levators). APR should also be considered as a palliative procedure, even in the presence of metastatic disease that may limit life expectancy. Greater comfort can often be achieved with resection than by a diversionary procedure alone. This is particularly true when the tumor invades the sphincter mechanism to produce tenesmus, when it extends to the perineum, or when bleeding is a major concern.

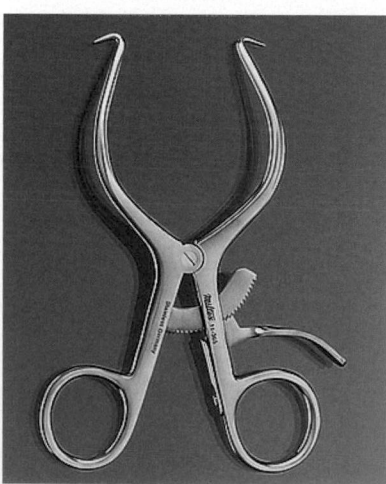

FIGURE 24-53. Gelpi retractor. (Courtesy of Milltex Instruments, York, PA; http://www.Milltex.com.)

Technique

I favor a combined synchronous abdominal and perineal resection.

Abdominal Procedure

The mobilization of the rectum is the same as has been described earlier for a low anterior resection. The rectum is mobilized along anatomical planes all the way down to the pelvic floor. I aim to perform as much of the dissection as possible during the abdominal dissection before proceeding with the perineal operation. The inferior mesenteric artery is ligated and divided as previously described, and the sigmoid mesentery is divided at an appropriately selected segment (see Figure 24-34). I always test the marginal artery before ligation and division to ensure a good blood supply. Once the mesentery is divided, the colon is transected with a linear stapling device.

Perineal Dissection

General Comments. Various techniques have been described for the perineal dissection. In the first instance, the "traditional" method of dissection will be described. Other techniques that involve a wider and more radical approach will be dealt with later in this text.

I consider the perineal dissection as important, if not more important, than the abdominal procedure. It can be technically demanding, and I strongly recommended that it should be performed either by the principal surgeon or by another experienced colorectal surgeon or by senior-level resident or a fellow under direct supervision. It should not be left to a junior or inexperienced resident. The perineum is prepared and draped. I prefer to have instruments, including diathermy and the Wave Harmonic scalpel, placed on a small perineal table. There should be no leads dangling off the patient's leg drapes; they get in the way and obstruct the view. The table is tilted head down and the stirrups are elevated. A purse-string suture is applied to the anus to prevent fecal contamination. An elliptical incision is made with the diathermy (Figure 24-57), and a Lone Star retractor is used to retract the skin. In the past, the rest of the dissection was performed using diathermy; however, over the past 3 years, I have used the Wave Harmonic scalpel. This instrument is useful in preventing bleeding during the procedure and an almost bloodless dissection can be achieved (Figure 24-58). The Wave Harmonic scalpel is used to deepen the incision through the ischiorectal adipose tissue. The index finger of the left hand is then used as a guide to locate the tip of the coccyx, and the anococcygeal ligament is divided (Figure 24-59). The finger is then inserted anterior to the coccyx. The abdominal operator lifts the rectum in his left hand and inserts his right hand deep into the retrorectal space until both operators can feel each other's fingers as separated by Waldeyer's fascia (Figure 24-60). The perineal surgeon then uses a pair of Abel scissors to break through this layer into the retrorectal space (see also Figure 24-60). Usually, a small amount of blood that has collected at the lower end of that space needs to be sucked out. Attention is then directed to dividing the iliococcygeus part of the levator muscles on either side. The left index finger is inserted into the opening, which has been made in the presacral space, and the finger is hooked under the left levator muscle. The Wave Harmonic scalpel is used to

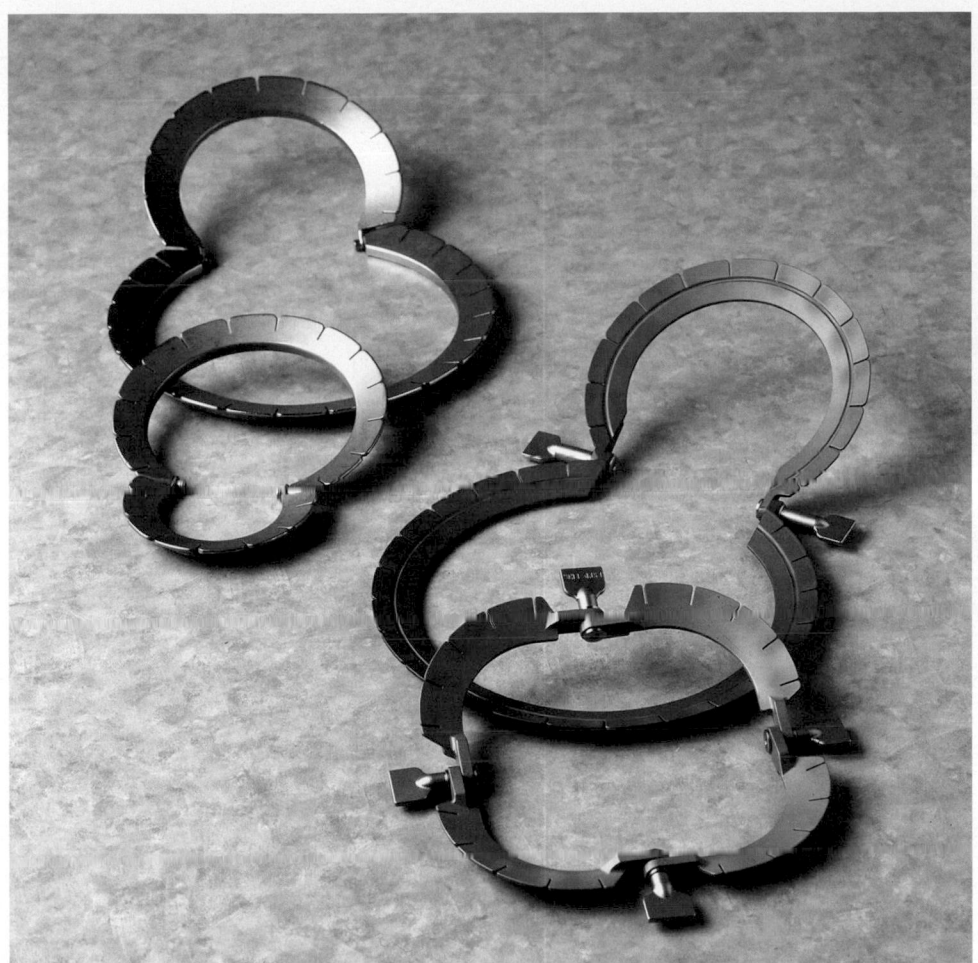

A

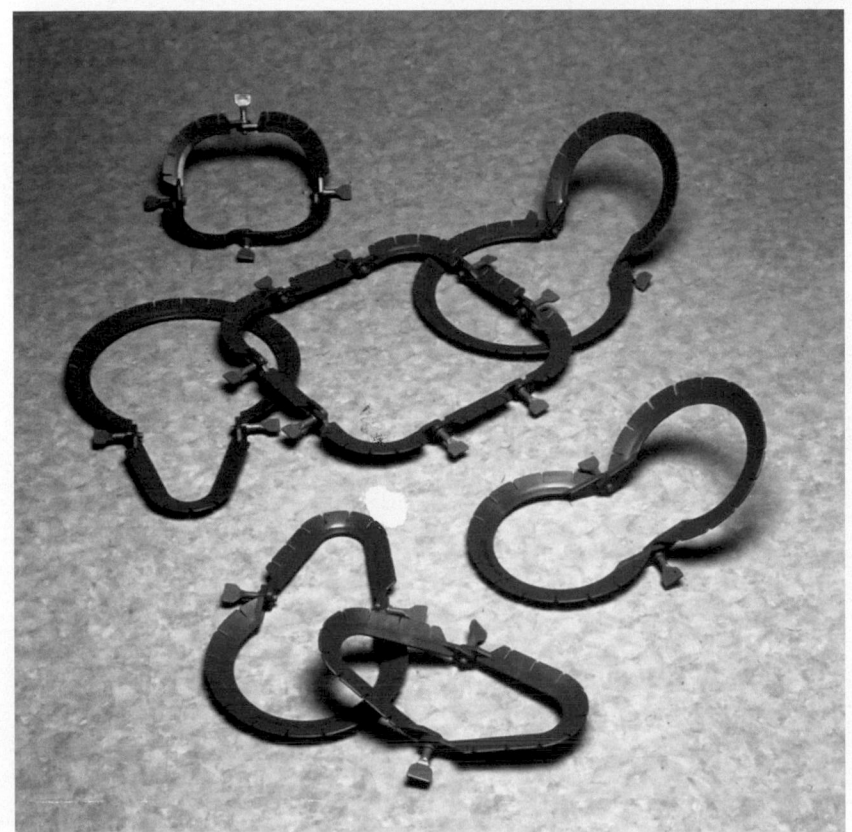

B

FIGURE 24-54. Loan Star retractors.

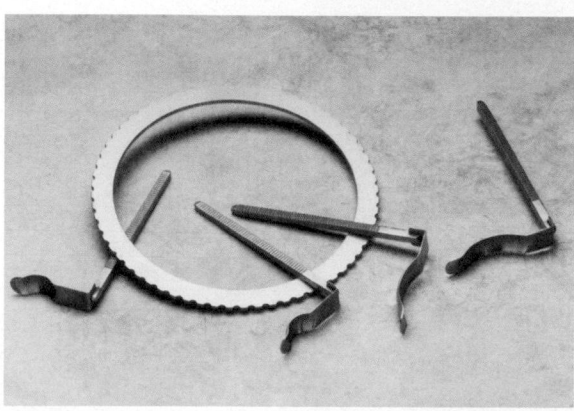

FIGURE 24-55. Bookwalter rectal kit. (Courtesy of Codman & Shurtleff, Inc., Raynham, MA.)

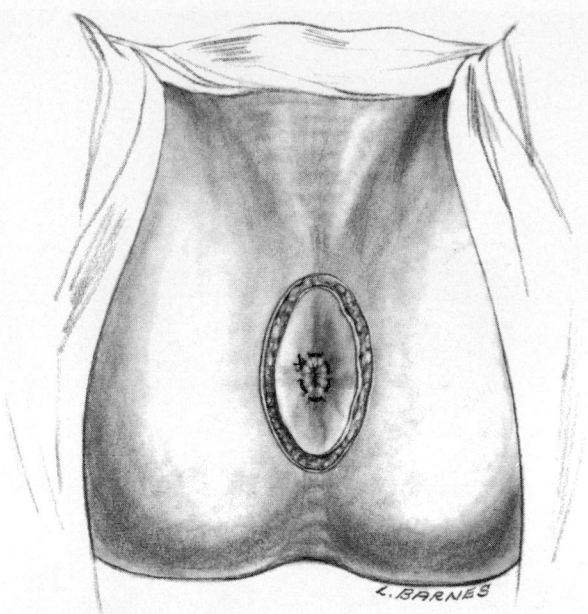

FIGURE 24-57. Perineal dissection. An elliptical incision is made outside the anus.

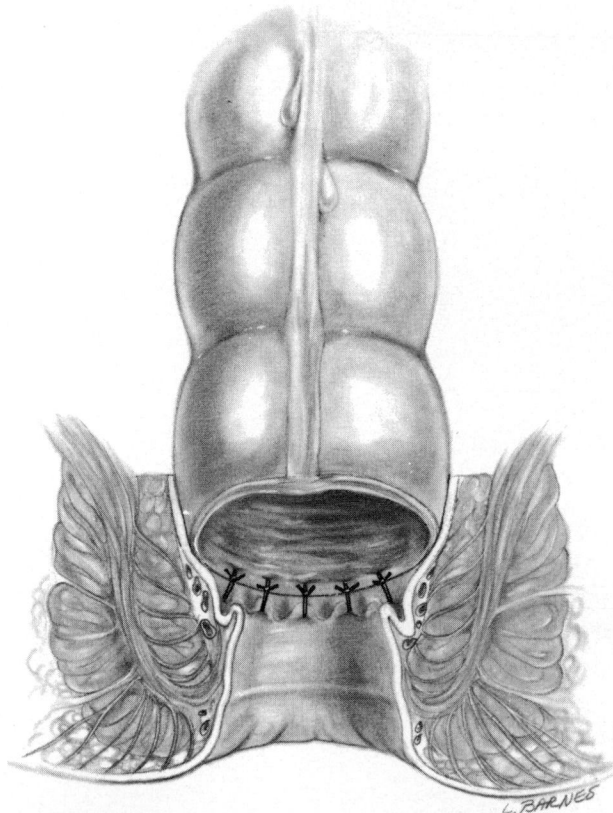

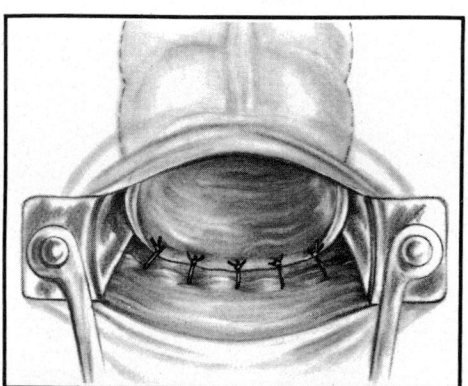

FIGURE 24-56. A Parks retractor facilitates the insertion of sutures (*inset*) in creating a coloanal anastomosis.

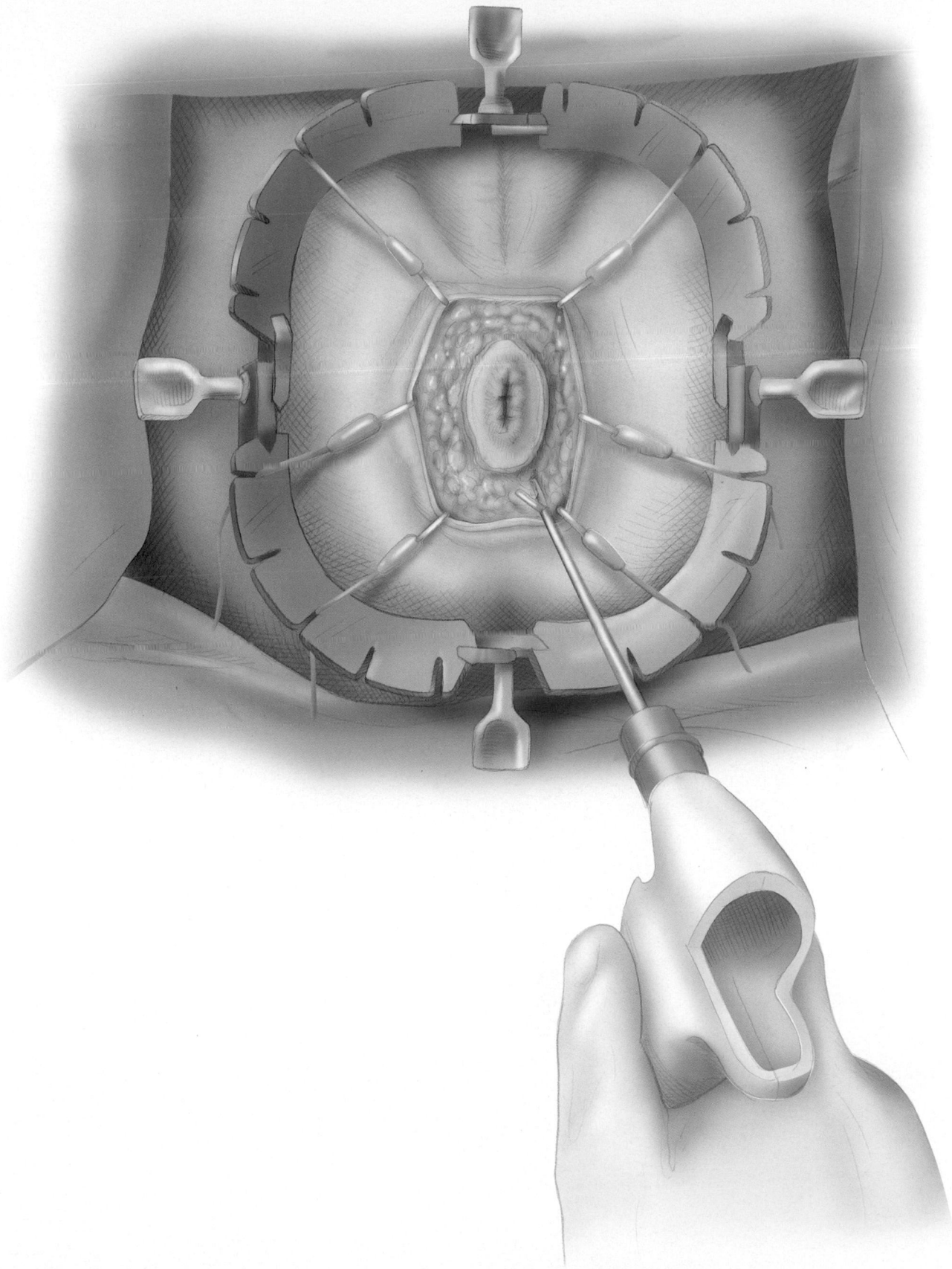

FIGURE 24-58. Perineal dissection. Lone Star retractor in place. Wave Harmonic scalpel is used to deepen incision.

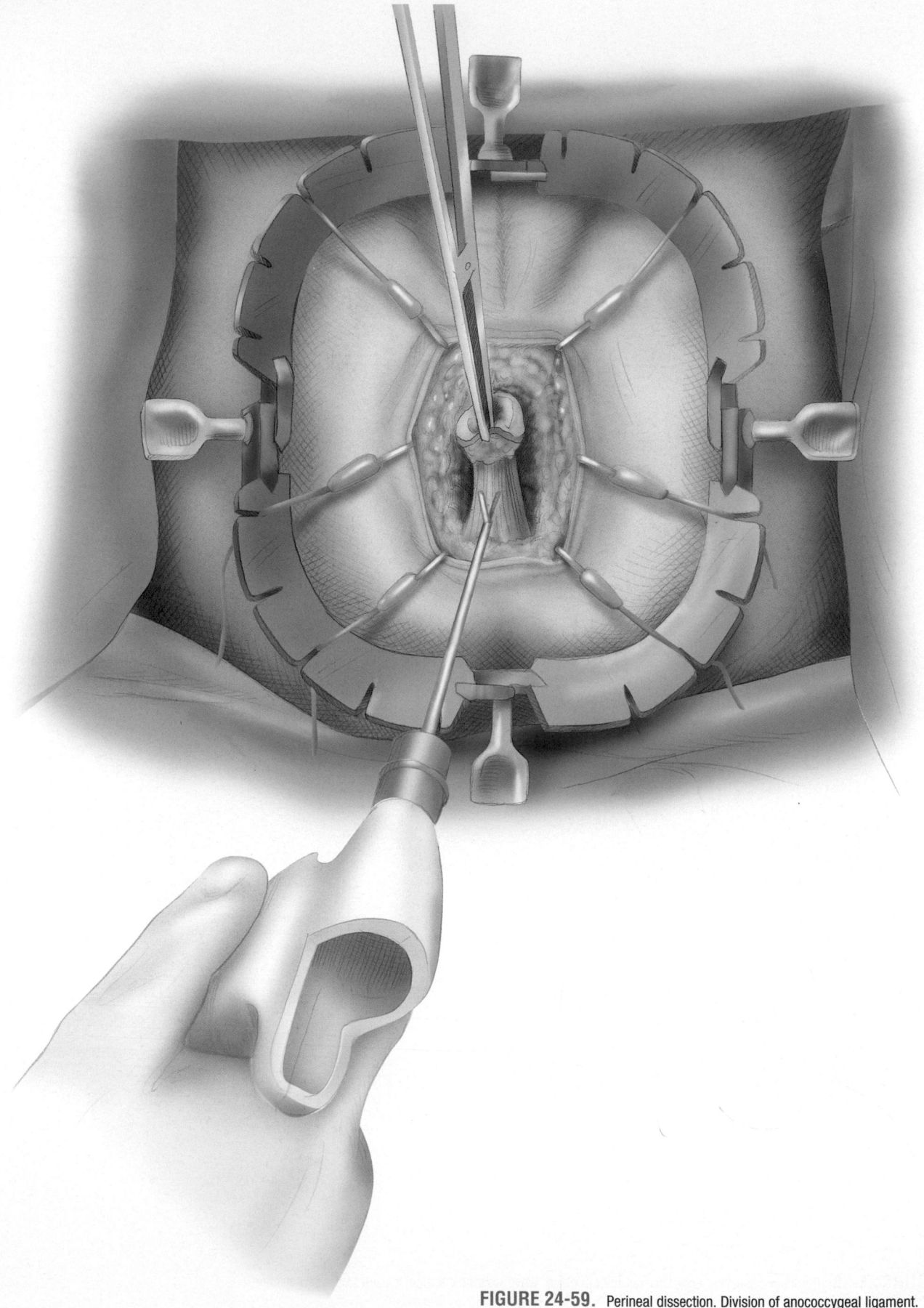

FIGURE 24-59. Perineal dissection. Division of anococcygeal ligament.

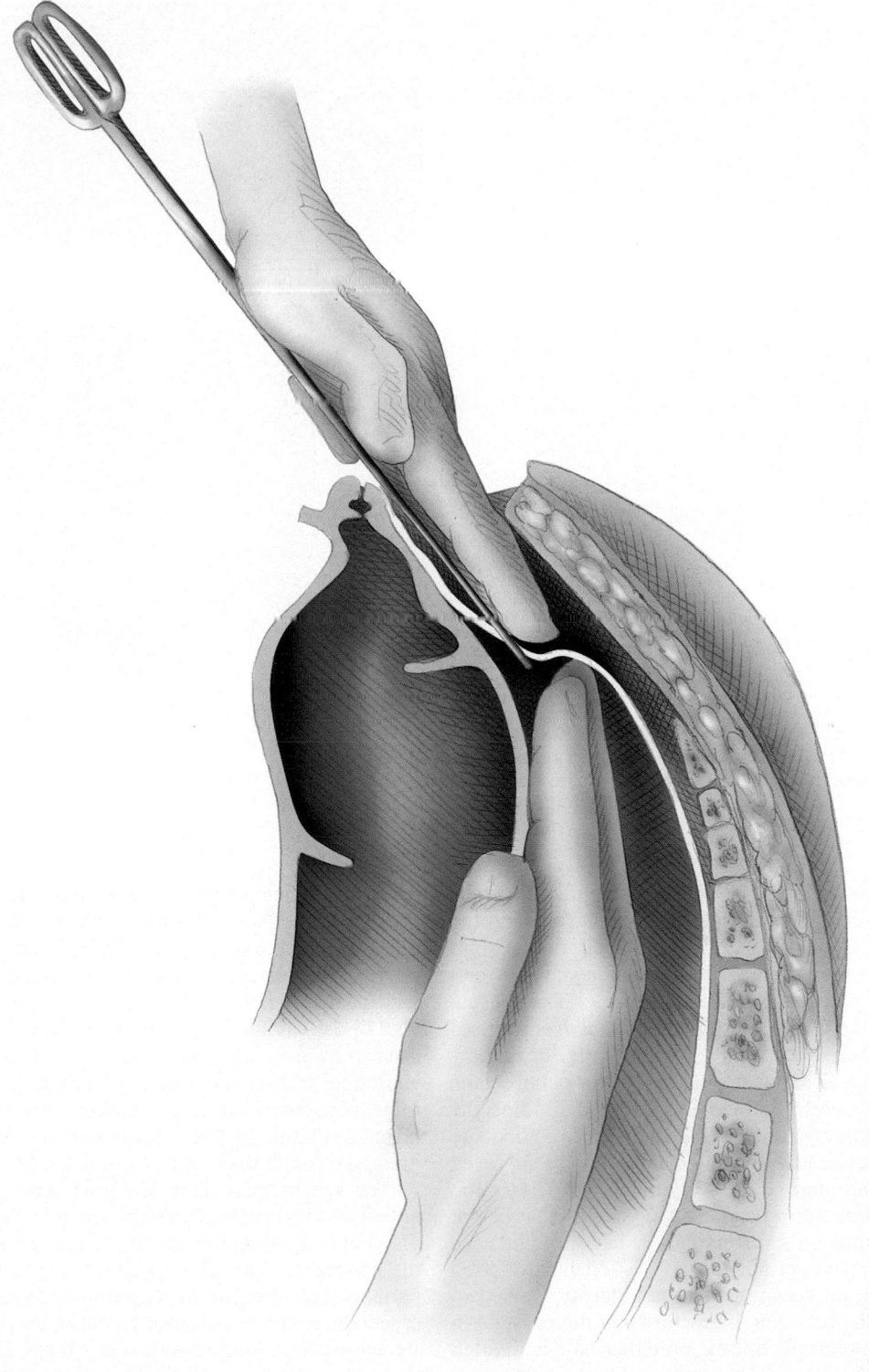

FIGURE 24-60. Perineal dissection. Identifying Waldeyer's fascia and confirmation of the plane of dissection as the two surgeons' fingers touch. The scissors facilitates their joining.

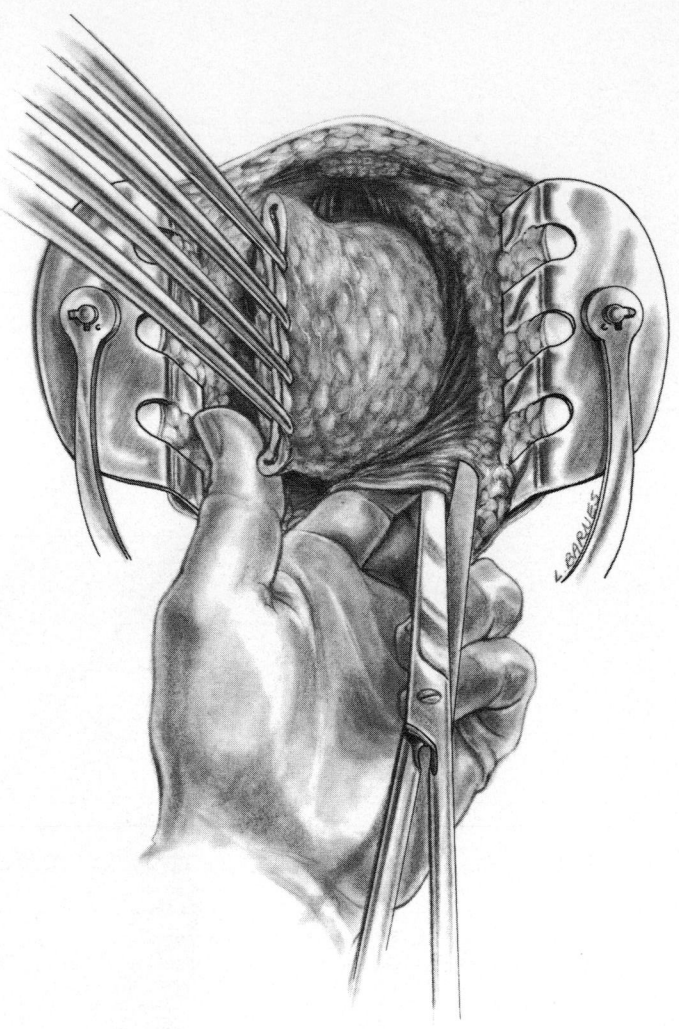

FIGURE 24-61. Perineal dissection. Left index finger hooked under right levator muscle, which is divided by Wave Harmonic scalpel (the illustration shows it being accomplished with scissors—not my personal preference).

divide the muscle (Figure 24-61). The left index finger is similarly used to identify the right levator muscle, and the wave instrument is used to divide the muscle on the right side. Attention is then directed to the pubococcygeus and the puborectalis parts of the levator muscle. The muscle is divided with the Wave Harmonic scalpel from lateral to medial on either side. Branches of the inferior hemorrhoidal vessels are in close proximity to the puborectalis and can cause troublesome bleeding. Simply dividing the muscle with diathermy usually does not achieve adequate hemostasis. However, I have found that this can be achieved with the Wave Harmonic scalpel (Figure 24-62). Dissection between the rectum and prostate or vagina can now begin. The abdominal surgeon's fingers can be used to guide the perineal surgeon. The perineal surgeon's left hand is used to retract the rectum down, and the diathermy is used to dissect in the plane between the rectum and the prostate in males. The rectourethralis muscle on either side is divided (Figure 24-63); the dissection continues until the abdominal surgeon's fingers are met, posterior to Denonvilliers' fascia; and the dissection breaks into the pelvic cavity. By remaining in this plane, injury to the urethra is avoided. Another method of performing the anterior part of the dissection is to deliver the specimen through the perineum; once the posterolateral part of the dissection is performed, the

specimen can be passed to the perineal surgeon who then retracts the specimen downward to better identify the anterior plane of dissection (Figure 24-64). In females, the anterior plane of dissection is between the rectum and the posterior wall of the vagina. If the tumor has invaded the posterior wall of the vagina, then the Wave Harmonic scalpel can be used to excise en bloc a portion of the vaginal wall. If the Harmonic scalpel is not available, then the vaginal wall has to be oversewn with an interlocking suture to prevent hemorrhage (Figure 24-65). The wound is closed in layers and drained through the vagina (Figure 24-66).

The specimen is then delivered through the perineum, although sometimes if the specimen is bulky and the pelvis is narrow, then the specimen can be delivered through the abdomen. Once the specimen has been delivered, the perineal wound is carefully examined to ensure hemostasis, especially from the posterior aspect of the prostate or vagina. Because I have started to use the Wave Harmonic scalpel to perform the perineal dissection, there has been a noticeable reduction in blood loss. Once hemostasis is secured, the wound is closed in layers around a drain (Figure 24-67). Occasionally, if there is a bulky tumor with a significant anterior component, the perineal dissection can be performed with the patient in the jackknife position. In order to do so, the colostomy must be exteriorized and the abdomen closed

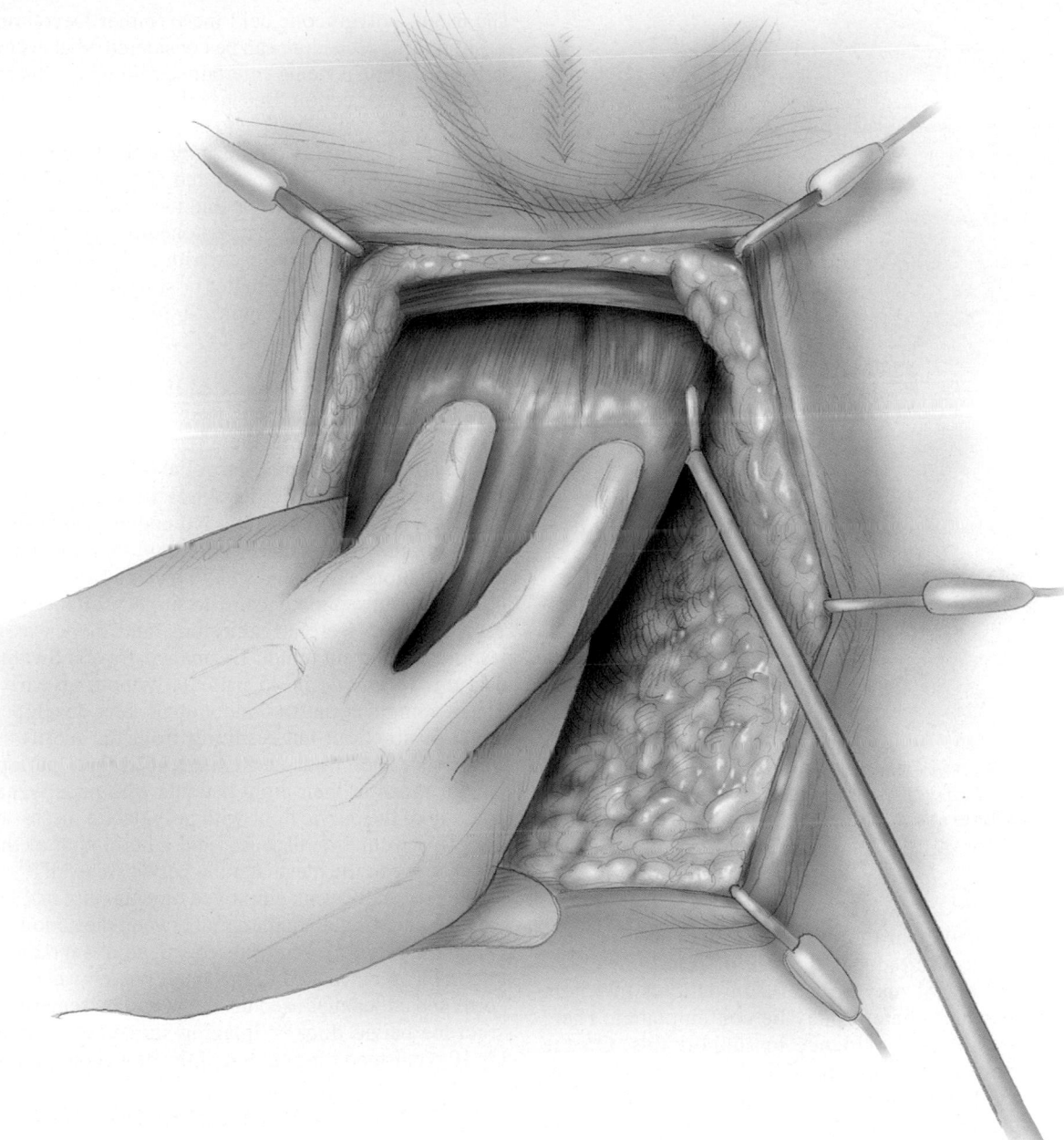

FIGURE 24-62. Perineal dissection. Division of puborectalis muscle.

before the patient is turned over for the perineal dissection. Although repositioning the patient is cumbersome, this position can achieve better exposure and access to the perineal anatomy. It is also more comfortable for both surgeon and assistant. Although I have occasionally used this technique, it is not routine in my practice.

▶ EXTERIORIZING THE COLOSTOMY

The colostomy site would have been carefully selected and marked preoperatively by an enterostomal therapist. A disk of skin is excised and deepened to the anterior rectus sheath (Figure 24-68). The sheath is divided transversely and to a lesser extent vertically. The assistant retracts the skin as well as anterior and posterior rectus sheaths to the right of the incision. With hand protected by a sponge, the assistant pushes the posterior

rectus sheath forward. The surgeon exposes the underlying rectus muscle, its fibers are separated, and the posterior rectus sheath is divided by diathermy onto the assistant's fingers, which are protected by the sponge. The opening is enlarged to admit two fingers. The colostomy exit site is carefully inspected to ensure that there is no bleeding from the inferior epigastric vessels. These are suture ligated if they have been torn. It is best to inspect for bleeding from the posterior aspect of the colostomy exit wound as shown in Figure 24-69. The stapled sigmoid colon is then exteriorized through the opening, and when the abdomen is closed, the stoma is matured (Figure 24-70).

Closing the Pelvic Floor

Some surgeons advocate closure of the pelvic floor by mobilizing the peritoneum on either side and suturing the

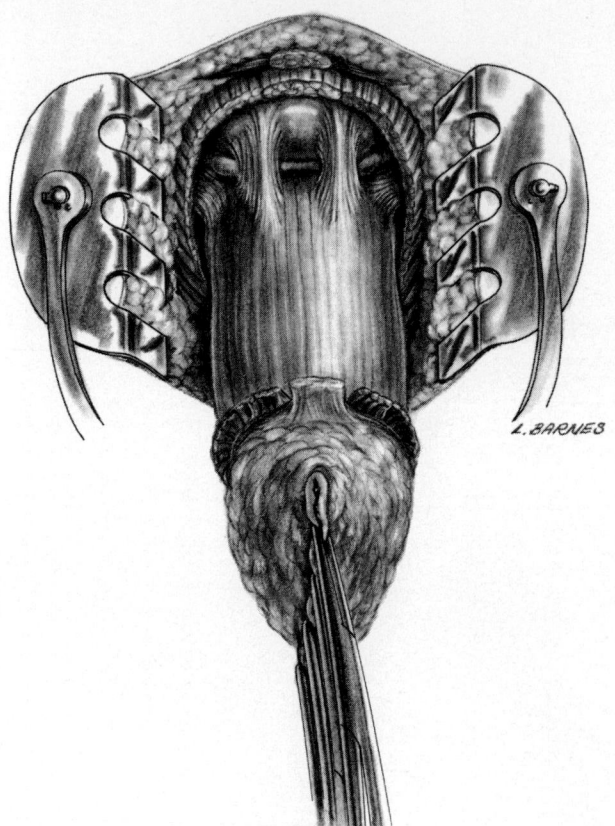

FIGURE 24-63. Perineal dissection. The rectourethralis muscle has been divided, exposing the prostate. With the division of the fascia of Denonvilliers, the peritoneal cavity can be entered anteriorly.

two leaves together in the midline (Figure 24-71). It is thought that closure reduces the risk of small bowel obstruction and that it may be useful in patients in whom postoperative radiotherapy may be contemplated. There is, however, no clear evidence to support this. On the contrary, there is a theoretical risk that a gap can occur in the suture line through which a loop of small bowel may herniate and cause obstruction. Furthermore, during mobilization of the parietal peritoneum from the lateral pelvic wall, the ureters could be injured. However, in the few patients in whom postoperative radiotherapy is contemplated, there is a potential risk of radiotherapy injury to the small intestine if it were to fall into the dissected pelvis. For this reason, several techniques have been proposed to reconstruct the pelvic floor. In view of the fact that adjuvant therapy is now mainly given preoperatively, closing the pelvic floor is not essential nor is it practiced routinely.

They are described here, although I do not use them in my practice. These include suturing the terminal ileum and its mesentery around the linea terminalis[632]; construction of an omental envelope; the use of the rectus abdominis muscle; and placement of a synthetic absorbable or nonabsorbable mesh sling, a breast prosthesis, and a synthetic polymer mold.[79,139,146–148,156,166,220,225,324,347,560,601] The possibility of infection with nonabsorbable material is, of course, a concern, as well as the inconvenience if one must remove it.

Technique

The use of polyglycolic acid mesh (either Dexon or Vicryl mesh) for this procedure can be considered whenever postoperative radiation is being entertained following either APR or even anterior resection. Because the mesh that is provided is not usually of sufficient size to create the sling, two are used and sutured together. Commencing at the level of the sacral promontory, the mesh is anchored (Figure 24-72). Using a continuous, locking suture technique, one anchors the mesh laterally on each side to the peritoneum (Figure 24-73). The mesh is then brought to the anterior abdominal wall and secured in place, creating a halter or sling that keeps the small bowel out of the pelvis (Figure 24-74).

Results

Devereux and colleagues reported 19 patients who underwent resection with simultaneous use of the sling procedure.[148] Postoperatively, all received contrast-simulation studies that documented the small bowel above the sacral promontory. Fractional tumoricidal doses ranging from 5,200 to 5,800 cGy were administered. No patient demonstrated obstruction, infection, nausea, vomiting, cramps, diarrhea, or acute radiation–associated small bowel injury.[148] When three individuals subsequently came to surgery, all mesh had been resorbed, there were no adhesions, and there was no suggestion of recurrent tumor. Dasmahapatra and Swaminathan used this technique in 45 patients without an early mesh-related complication (two individuals later developed small bowel obstruction, not resulting from the mesh).[132] However, Sener and colleagues experienced three perioperative complications in their eight patients who underwent reconstruction of the pelvic floor with polyglactin mesh—a pelvic abscess, a wound dehiscence, and a herniation of the small bowel between the mesh and the pelvic sidewall.[560]

Lechner and Cesnik employed omentopexy in 43 patients to create an artificial diaphragm between the abdominal cavity and the pelvis.[347] With subsequent adjuvant radiotherapy, no complication related to the small bowel was recognized. Voros and colleagues used the ileum and mesentery to reconstruct the pelvic floor.[632] Imaging studies on postoperative day 10 confirmed the position of the bowel out of the pelvis.

Extralevator Abdominoperineal Resection

In recent years, several authors have questioned the perineal technique described earlier. There have been concerns that the perineal dissection may not be sufficiently wide. It is thought that this can result in a higher rate of involvement of the circumferential margins, a higher rate of perforation, and, subsequently, a higher rate of local recurrence and ultimately poorer survival. These surgeons advocate a wider excision, an extralevator abdominoperineal resection (ELAPR). The theory is that this operation will result in a cylindrical specimen rather than a "waisted" one.[646,647] The philosophy behind ELAPR is that the wider the resection margins, the better the outcome. Some surgeons have recommended the inclusion of the coccyx as part of the wider excision.[37] ELAPR is not dissimilar to the original procedure that Miles described in 1908.[421] He recommended that ". . . the perineal portion of the operation should be carried out as widely as possible so that the lateral and downward zones of spread may be effectively extirpated." To date, there is no randomized trial evidence that an ELAPR is any better than a conventional APR, and the evidence advanced by its proponents is based

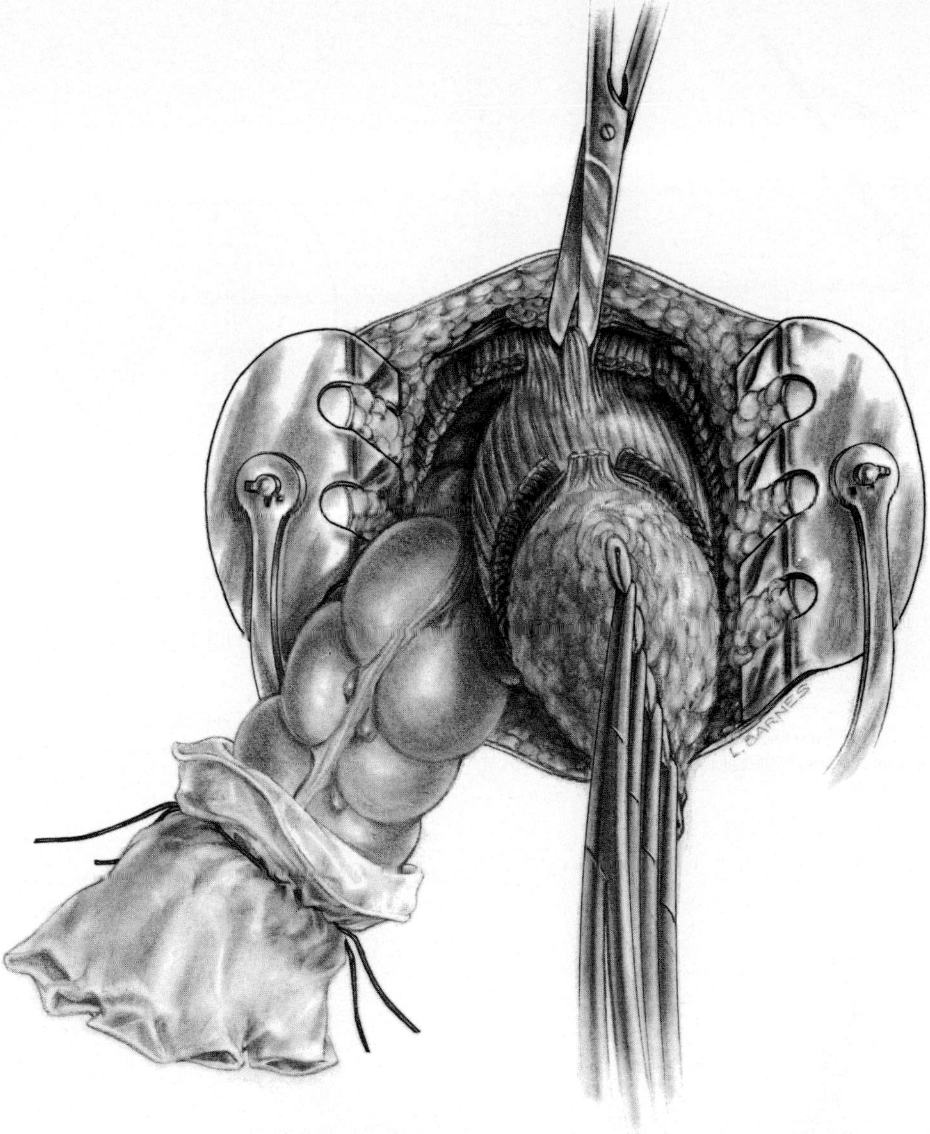

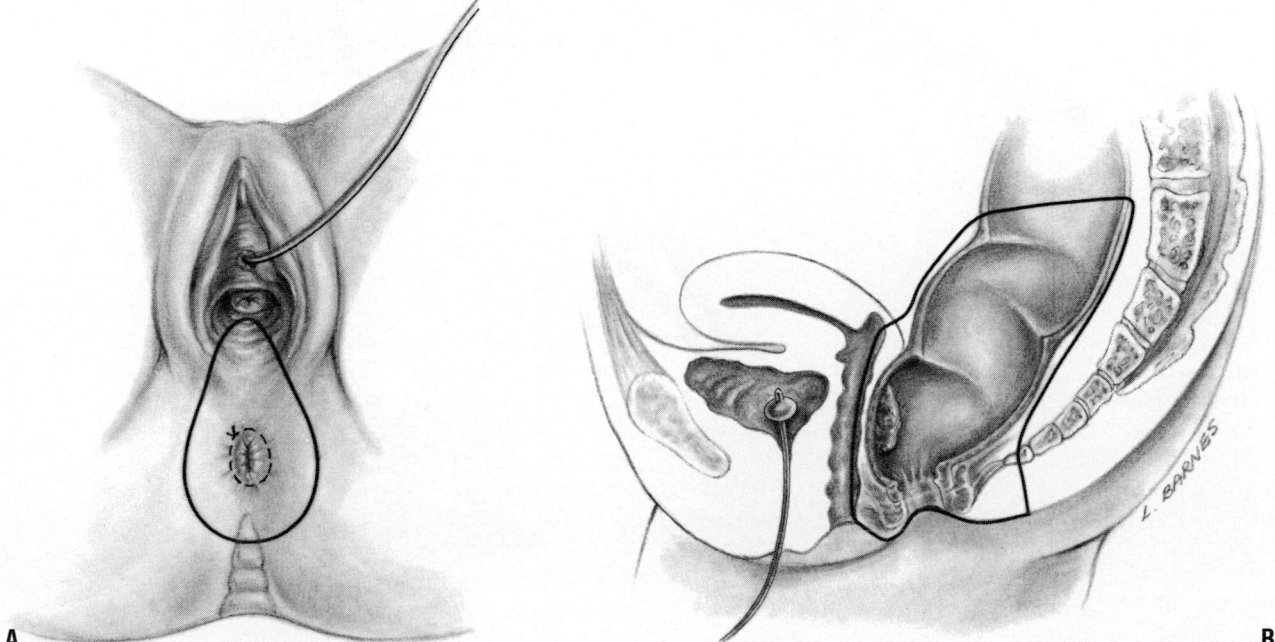

FIGURE 24-64. Perineal dissection. The proximal colon has been delivered through the pelvic defect. The rectourethralis muscle and the visceral fascia are the only structures remaining to be divided.

A

B

FIGURE 24-65. Perineal dissection in women. **A:** Outline of the incision for excising the posterior vaginal wall. **B:** Lateral view showing the extent of removal.

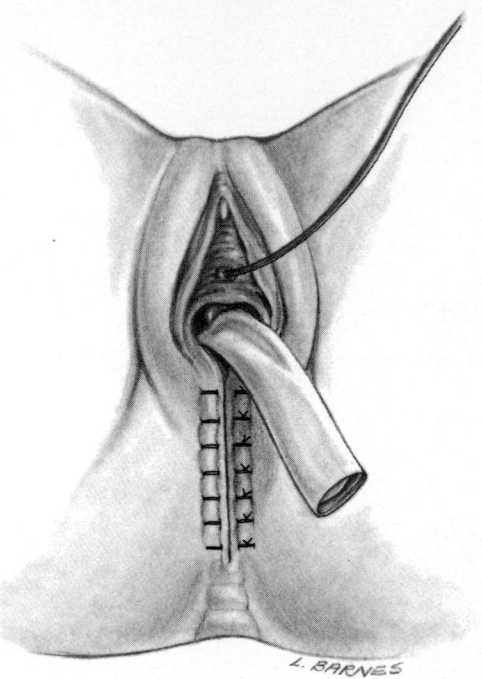

FIGURE 24-66. Perineal dissection in women. The skin wound is completely closed, and the perineal body is reconstructed. The drain is placed in the pelvis and brought out through the defect in the posterior vaginal wall.

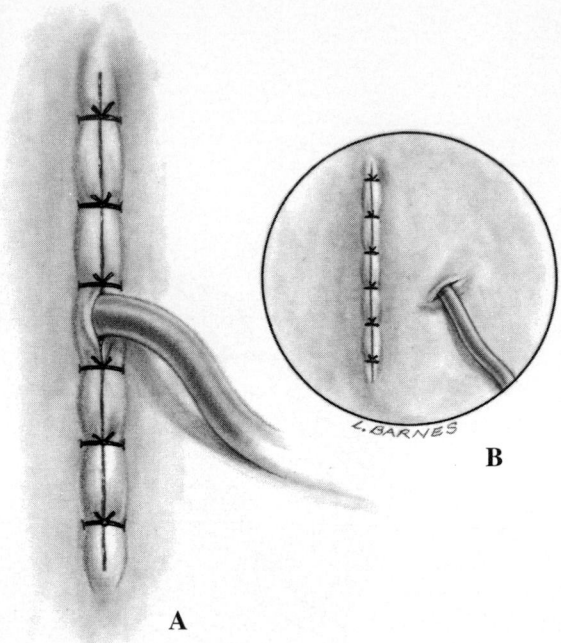

FIGURE 24-67. Perineal dissection. The wound is closed primarily, and the pelvis is drained, either through the incision **(A)** or through a stab wound **(B)**.

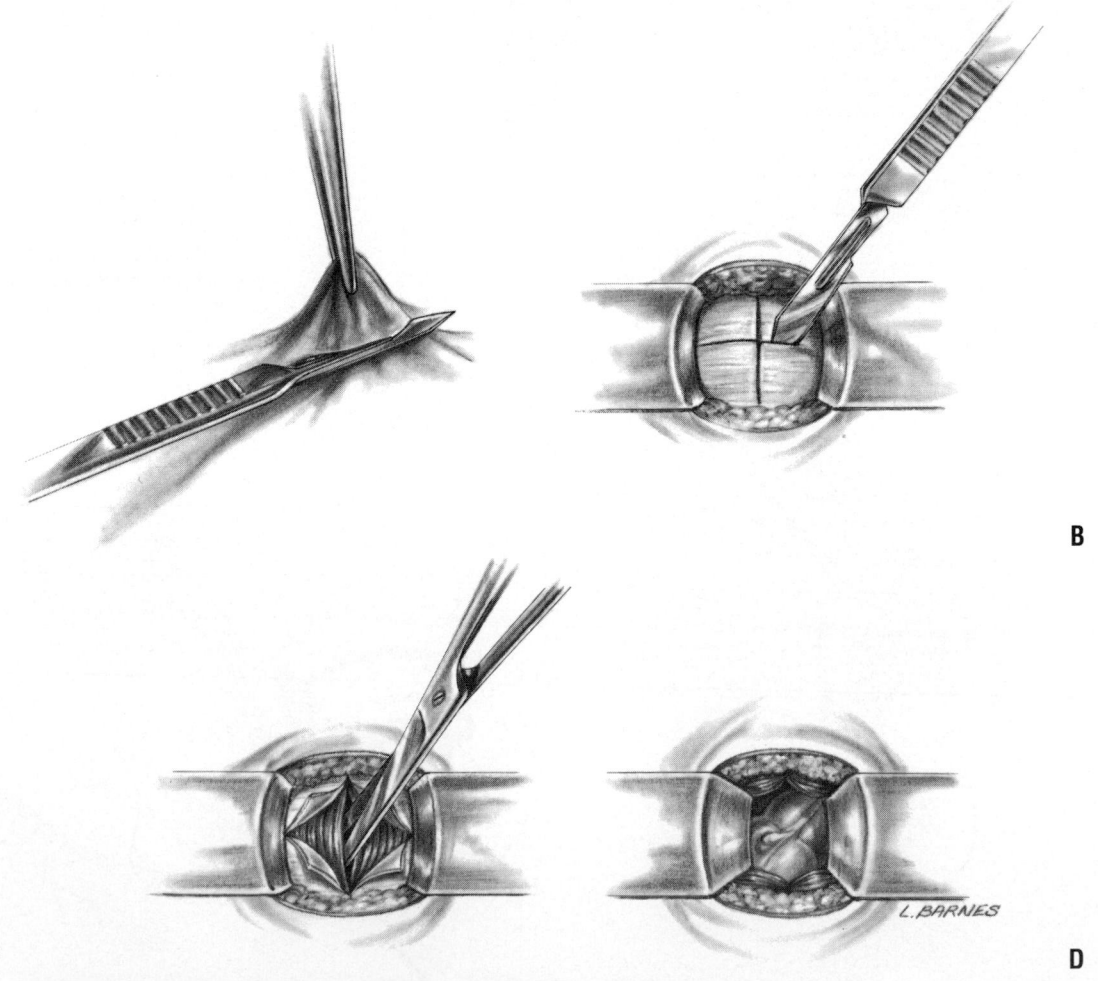

FIGURE 24-68. Abdominoperineal resection. Creating the abdominal wall opening for the colostomy. **A:** A disk of skin is excised. **B:** A cruciate incision is made in the anterior rectus fascia. **C:** The rectus muscle is split longitudinally. **D:** The completed abdominal wall opening.

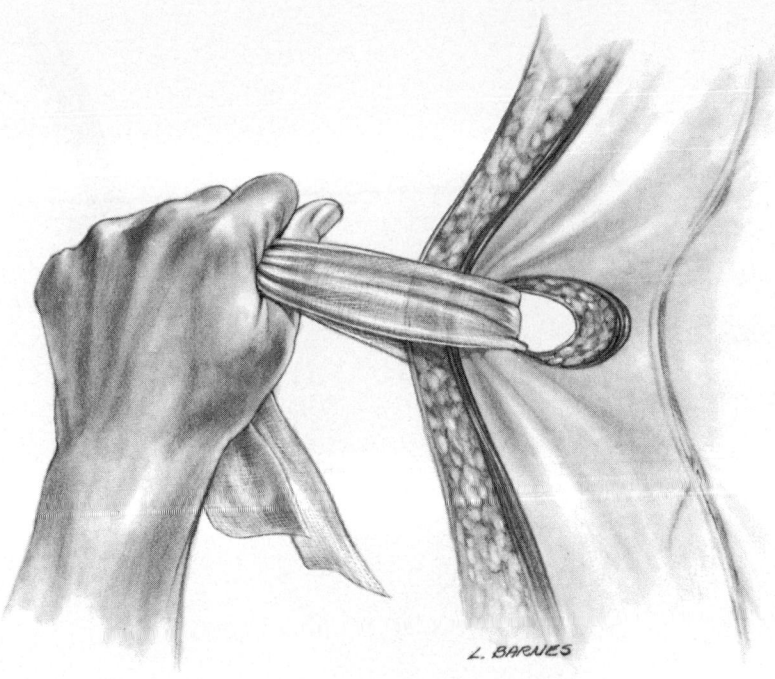

L. BARNES

FIGURE 24-69. Abdominoperineal resection. Exposure of the epigastric vessels by sponge retraction.

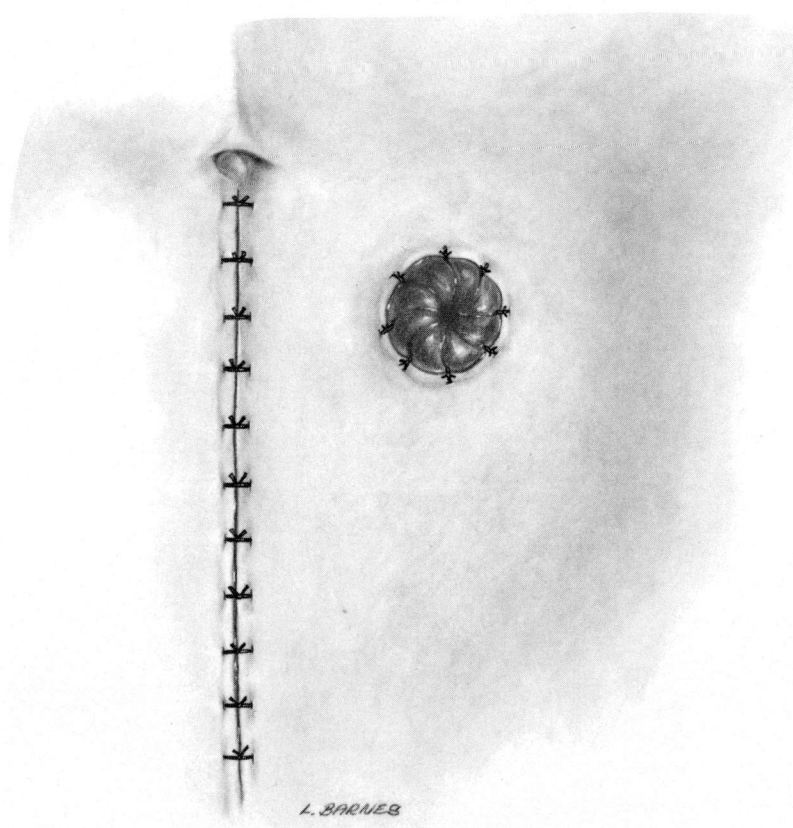

L. BARNES

FIGURE 24-70. Abdominoperineal resection. The wound is closed and the colostomy matured.

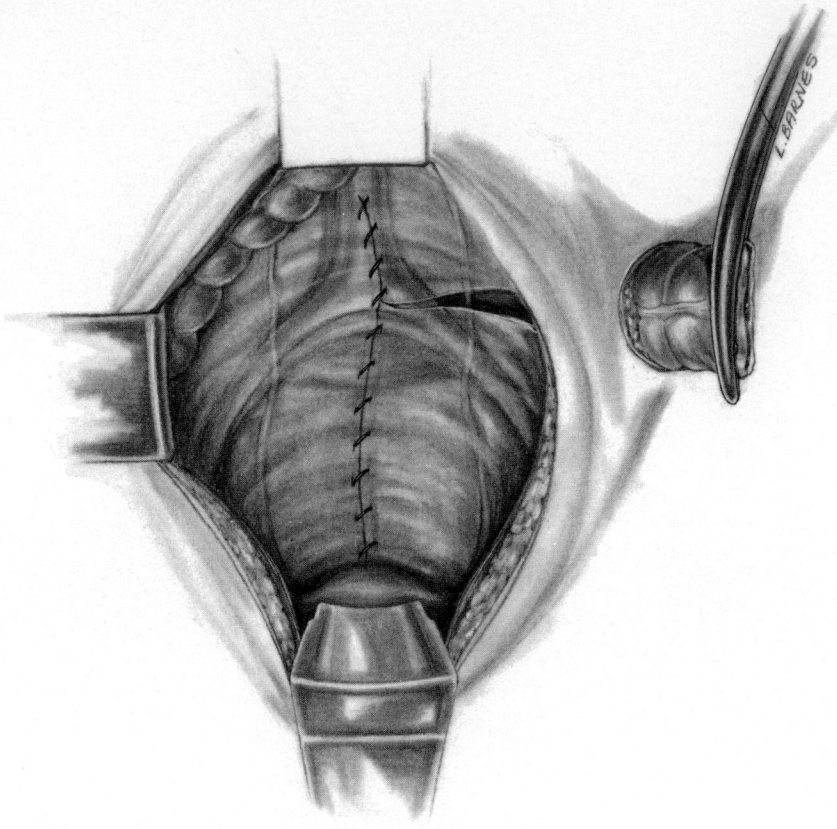

FIGURE 24-71. Abdominoperineal resection. The floor of the pelvis has been reconstituted.

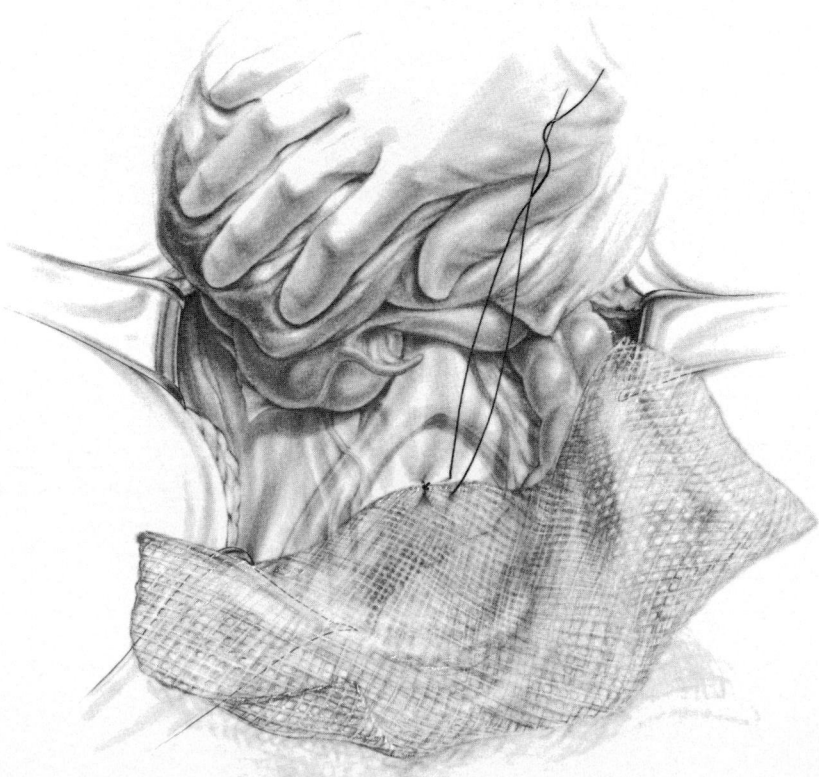

FIGURE 24-72. Implantation of mesh for postoperative radiation. The mesh is anchored to the sacral promontory.

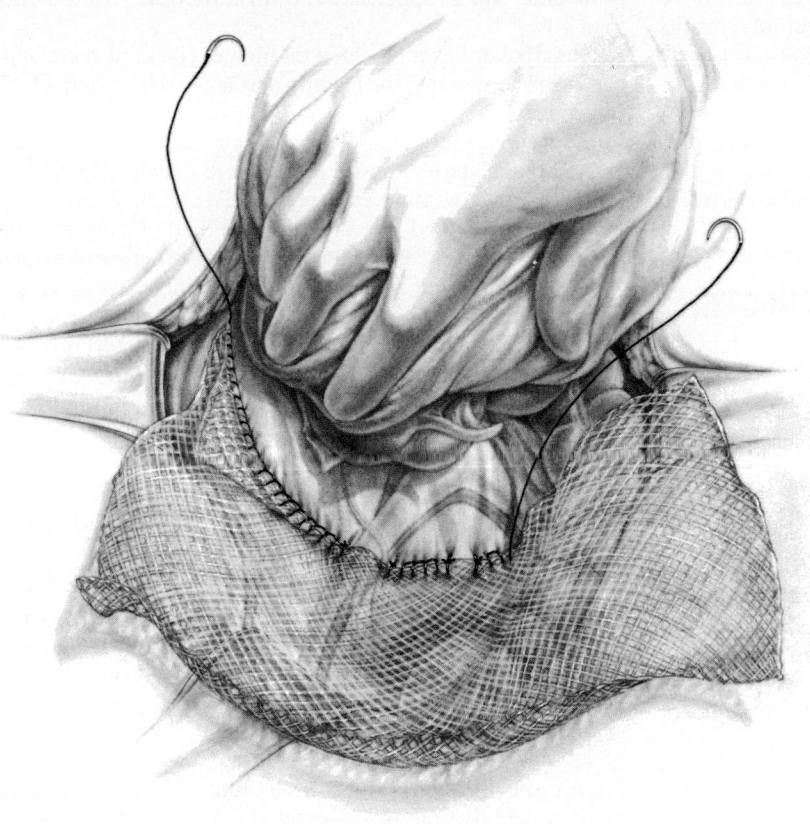

FIGURE 24-73. Implantation of mesh for post-operative radiation. Using a continuous, interlocking suture technique, the mesh is anchored to the posterior and lateral peritoneal surfaces. Two pieces of mesh may be required to effect this maneuver.

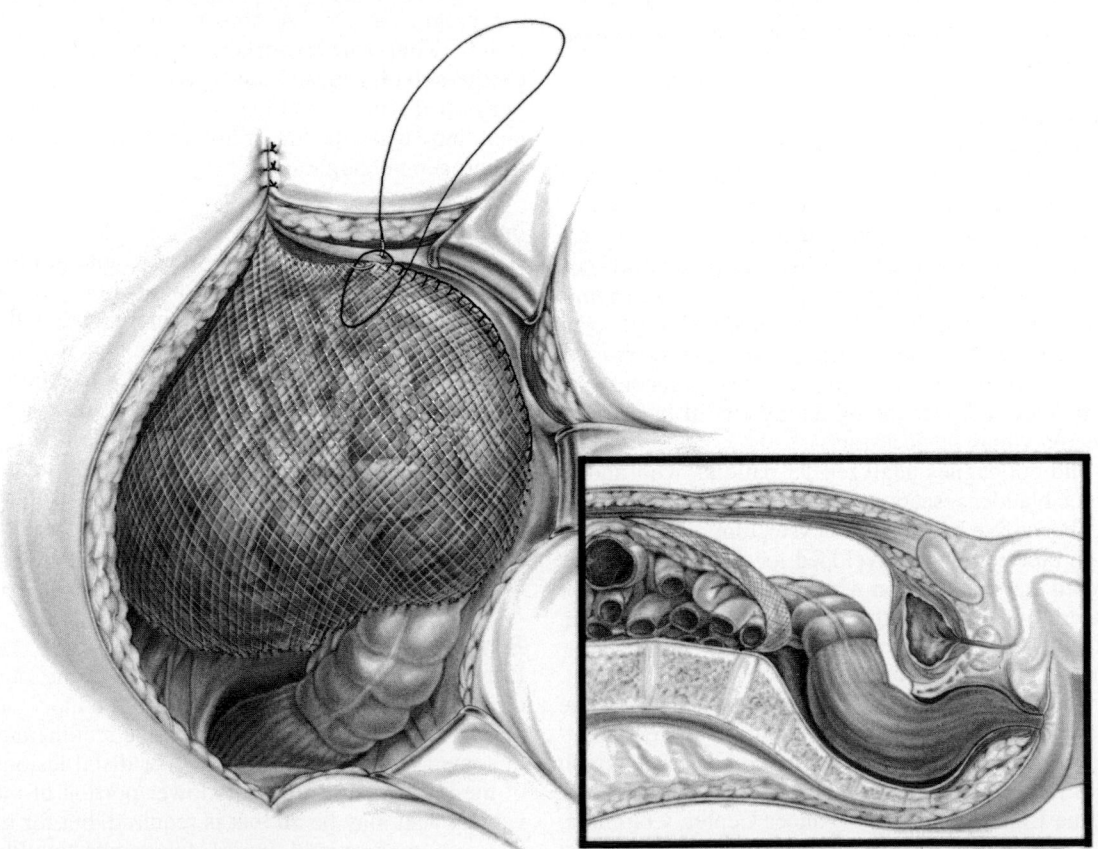

FIGURE 24-74. Implantation of mesh for postoperative radiation. The completed suspension requires the mesh to be anchored to the anterior abdominal wall. Care must be taken not to impede the exit of the bowel for the stoma. The abdominal wound should be closed without incorporating the mesh, but anterior fixation can be achieved to the peritoneum. Final position of the fixation in an individual who has undergone an anterior resection (*inset*).

on limited, selected patient series. Furthermore, it has to be recognized that ELAPR, with or without sacrectomy, results in a larger perineal wound. This may require various plastic surgical procedures to close, potentially leading to a higher risk of perineal wound complications.[37,268]

Before adopting ELAPR as a standard, it would be prudent to conduct a randomized study to determine among other things whether the procedure is beneficial in terms of local recurrence and survival.

► LAPAROSCOPIC SURGERY FOR RECTAL CANCER (SEE CHAPTER 19)

Other Procedures That May Accompany Resection of the Rectum

En Bloc Resection of Adjacent Organs

It is not unusual for another organ to be involved with a rectal cancer mass. Most commonly, the bladder, the vagina, the uterus, or a loop of small bowel are involved. Occasionally, the sigmoid colon, especially if it is on a long mesentery, may fall into the pelvis and become involved. It is sometimes difficult to know at the time of operation whether these structures are adherent to the cancer by an inflammation or by the tumor invasion. Whenever possible, the involved organ (or part of it) should be resected en bloc. Some of these procedures are described next.

Incidental Appendectomy

Incidental appendectomy is unnecessary and not indicated at the time of rectal resection, unless the appendix is involved in the tumor mass.

Bladder Resection

The urinary bladder is not uncommonly directly invaded by rectal cancer. If the dome of the bladder is invaded, an en bloc resection is recommended. It is difficult to know exactly whether the involvement is neoplastic invasion or inflammatory. It is better to assume that it is neoplastic and proceed with en bloc resection of the dome. However, if the trigone is involved, then a specialist urologist should be invited to attend and assist. Under these circumstances, the ureters must be protected from injury, and complex ureteric reconstruction may be required. Depending on the site of invasion, a total cystectomy may be necessary.

Carne and colleagues analyzed 53 patients who underwent en bloc bladder resection for colorectal cancer in New Zealand.[87] Forty-five had a partial cystectomy. All who did not have en bloc resection developed local recurrence. The authors noted that the decision whether to perform partial or total cystectomy depends on the site of the bladder invasion.

Sacrectomy and Pelvic Exenteration

Total pelvic exenteration is defined as the removal of the distal colon and rectum, along with the lower ureters, bladder, internal reproductive organs, perineum, draining lymph nodes, and pelvic peritoneum.[370] In a highly selected series from the Ellis Fischel State Cancer Center, Columbia, Missouri involving 24 patients over a 30-year period, Lopez and colleagues reported an operative mortality of about 20% (9% during the last decade).[370] The overall survival rate was a remarkable 42%. A review by Williams and colleagues summarizing the results of several series concluded that the

procedure can be carried out with a mortality rate of less than 10%.[654]

Sugarbaker has advocated en bloc excision of rectal cancer with sacrectomy for lesions that are fixed posteriorly.[600] In reporting his experience with six patients, he noted that four survived more than 3 years. Pearlman and colleagues carried out 12 pelvic and 7 sacropelvic exenterations.[493] Of the 15 patients without extrapelvic disease, there was 1 operative death, 2 died free of disease, 3 died of cancer, 1 was alive with recurrence, and the remainder were free of disease (none had achieved 5 years). Shirouzu and coworkers performed total pelvic exenteration on 26 patients for locally advanced colorectal cancer.[567] The operative mortality was 8%. In those with stage II primary disease, the recurrence rate after curative surgery was three of seven, but the mean survival time was 58 months, with a 5-year survival of 71%. Those with stage IV disease had a mean survival time of only 5 months. Others have demonstrated that pelvic exenteration (APR and cystectomy) in selected patients may produce a 25% to 50% 5-year survival.[117,281,316]

Jiminez and colleagues reported the Memorial Sloan-Kettering Cancer Center experience with total pelvic exenteration in the treatment of rectal cancer.[291] Fifty-five patients were identified—71% with recurrent disease and 29% for the primary tumor. At the time of the procedure, 49% received intraoperative radiation treatment and 20% required sacrectomy. The perioperative mortality was 5.5%. Median disease-specific survival was 48.9 months. Univariate analysis identified five factors associated with decreased survival: male gender, recurrent disease, prior APR, positive surgical margins, and the administration of intraoperative radiation.[291] Koda and coworkers commented that total pelvic exenteration for locally advanced cancers can be selectively performed with reestablishment of both bowel and urinary continuity when the tumor invades neither the anal canal nor the urogenital diaphragm.[320]

Comment

It is often difficult to interpret the results of this procedure from the literature because the indications are variable and may include a large percentage of individuals with carcinoma of the uterine cervix.[327] Furthermore, a major problem with most published studies is that in order to report more than an anecdotal experience, authors tend to supplement their reports with patients who have limited follow-up. It is well advised that optimal care is facilitated by specialist urologic consultation.[411] It certainly seems appropriate that evaluation of potential candidates for this operation and the procedure itself (if indicated) should be undertaken by individuals who have a particular interest and experience with this operation.

Perineal Dissection in Women

If the tumor invades the posterior wall of the vagina, a posterior vaginectomy may be performed en bloc. One must remember that the distance between the rectum and vagina is, in some areas, less than 1 mm. For distal lesions, excision of the lower one-third or the lower portion of the posterior vaginal wall may be all that is required, but for more extensive or more proximal tumors, the vagina should be excised to the level of the posterior cul-de-sac (see Figure 24-65). Alternatively, a transverse incision can be made at the cephalad limit of the dissection in the vagina, and the two lateral incisions connected.

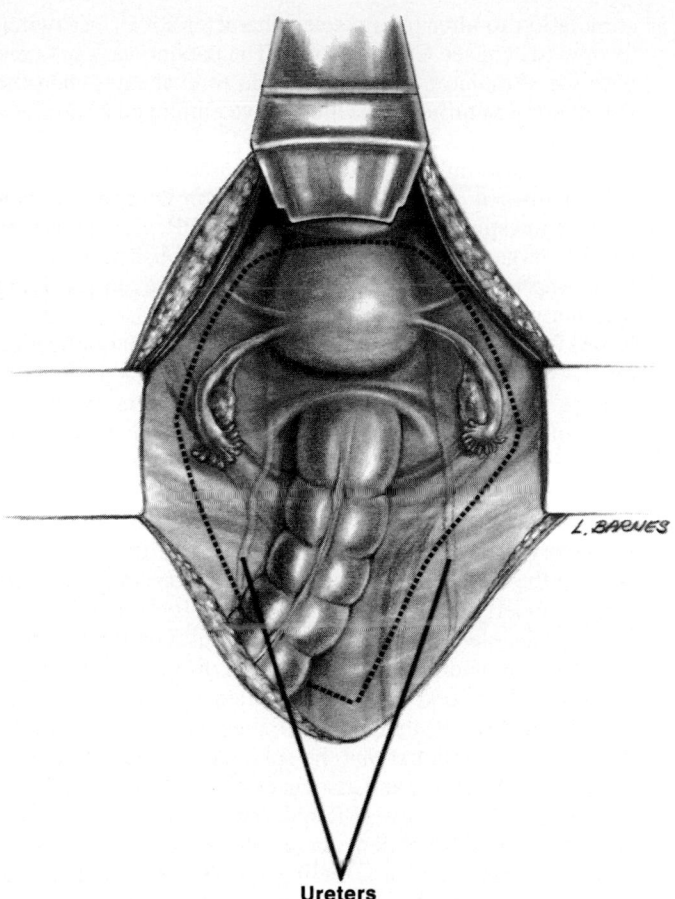

Ureters

FIGURE 24-75. Hysterectomy concomitant with abdominoperineal resection. Peritoneal incision (*dotted line*) must be quite wide to incorporate the uterus and rectum for removal in continuity.

Following posterior vaginectomy, the perineal skin closure is carried out until the forchette has been reconstituted. The vagina will eventually heal with minimal or no narrowing, depending on the extent of the vaginectomy. Obviously, if much of the vagina is removed, stenosis will result.

Concomitant Hysterectomy

En bloc hysterectomy concomitant with APR or anterior resection is occasionally required if the uterus or vagina are invaded. The incision of the peritoneum in the floor of the pelvis must be wider than that for APR (Figure 24-75). Both ureters are in greater danger of injury when this operation is performed. They should therefore be clearly identified virtually throughout their lengths. If invasion is predicted preoperatively, then cystoscopy and ureteric catheters are helpful in minimizing the risk of ureteric injury.

The peritoneum is swept off the uterus, and the bladder is bluntly pushed away from the cervix and vaginal wall. The infundibulopelvic and round ligaments are cross clamped, divided, and ligated (Figure 24-76). The broad ligament is dissected away from the pelvic wall, exposing the uterine artery. By retraction of the uterus to the contralateral side, the uterine artery is cross clamped, divided, and ligated. Division of the cardinal ligament poses the greatest threat to the ureter. If the tumor approaches this area, the cardinal ligament should be clamped close to the pelvic wall; thus, the ureter must be clearly visualized (Figure 24-77). I prefer to use a single curved Kocher clamp, dividing the tissue on the medial aspect, a maneuver analogous to the technique employed

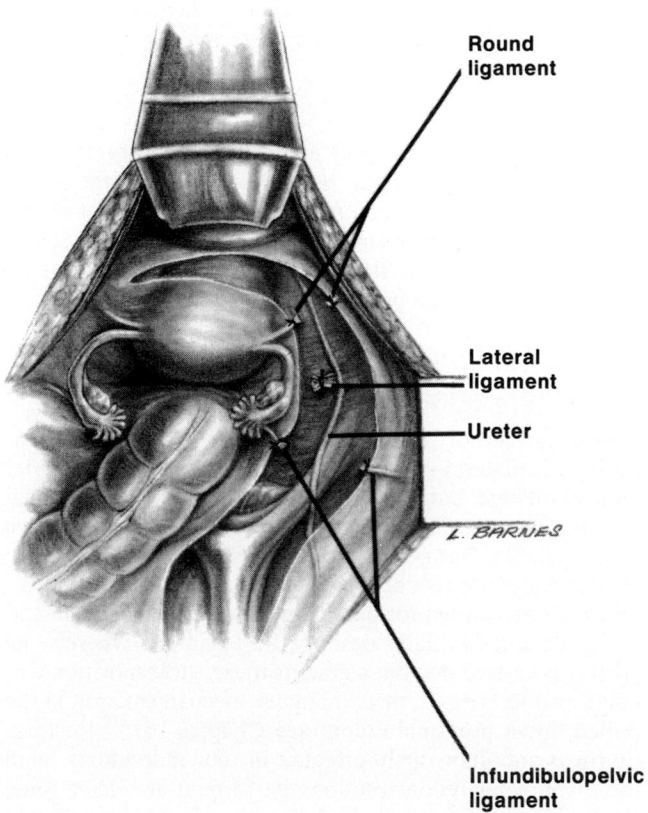

Round ligament

Lateral ligament

Ureter

Infundibulopelvic ligament

FIGURE 24-76. Concomitant hysterectomy. The uterus and rectum are mobilized on the right side by division of the round, infundibulopelvic, and lateral ligaments.

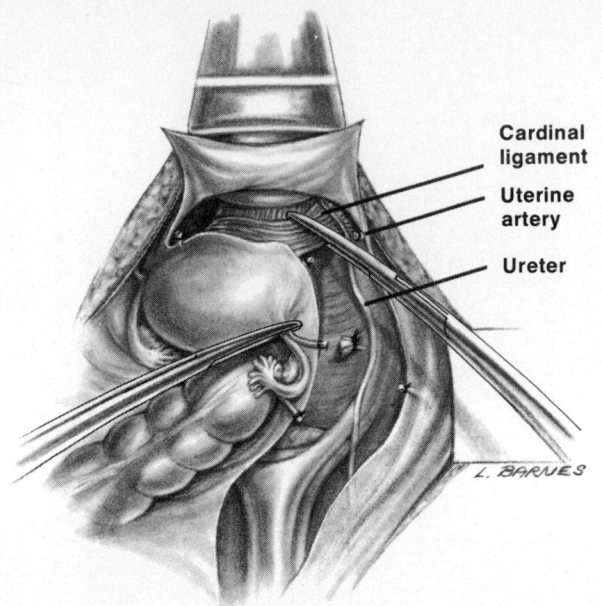

FIGURE 24-77. Concomitant hysterectomy. The uterine artery has been divided, and the cardinal ligament is clamped. The ureter is quite vulnerable to injury at this point.

for division of the lateral ligaments. The clamp is replaced more distally after each suture ligature is tied.

When the dissection has been completed on both sides, the anterior vaginal wall is incised and the posterior vaginal wall removed with the proctectomy specimen. The vagina may be closed or left open in order to facilitate drainage, depending on how much of the posterior vaginal wall has been excised.

Oophorectomy

Metastatic disease apparent at the time of surgery is an indication for therapeutic oophorectomy, but the value of prophylactic oophorectomy has been the subject of debate.[11,48,61,62,318] It appears that the prevention of primary ovarian cancer is probably the main benefit,[125] and there is no reason to recommend prophylactic oophorectomy.

Reconstruction with a Neosphincter following Abdominoperineal Resection

This technique of reconstruction with a neosphincter consisting of bilateral graciloplasties has only attracted a brief clinical interest, but it is of sufficient research and historical importance to be included in this chapter. The results have been variable, but on the whole disappointing. One must also consider the risk of local recurrence when these procedures are performed for patients with rectal cancer. Mercati and colleagues initially described a technique whereby an APR was carried out, but a gracilis muscle transposition was employed to create a new sphincter mechanism around the pulled down proximal colon (see Chapter 16).[419] Restoration was simultaneously effected in four individuals, with three sphincter reconstructions performed at a later time. Williams and colleagues described a similar operation in which neorectum and neoanal sphincters are constructed by means of the gracilis muscle and by using low-frequency

stimulation to alter the muscles characteristics (fast twitch to slow twitch; see Chapter 16).[656] The patient was continent with the stimulator on and was able to evacuate when the stimulator was turned off. Others have employed a seromuscular graft for this purpose.[618]

Since these initial contributions, numerous articles have been published concerning reconstruction with reestablishment of intestinal continuity following APR. Cavina has the world's largest experience and in 1996 published a 10-year follow-up report with 81 patients.[92] Thirty-seven surviving patients who underwent APR with graciloplasty were followed for a mean of 78.6 months. The overall complication rate was 37%, with a 5-year survival rate of 58%. Fecal continence was achieved in 90%, with apparently no pejorative effect on survival. Others, too, confirm that total anorectal reconstruction is possible in selected patients without adverse consequences for survival.[1] Geerdes and colleagues used double dynamic graciloplasty with and without an intervening reservoir.[203] The authors caution that further modifications in the technique will be required before the procedure can be undertaken with minimal morbidity. Of the 15 patients evaluable, 53% were continent, but 5 underwent conversion to an abdominal stoma (33%). In the experience of Santoro and coworkers, of the 11 patients available for long-term evaluation, 8 demonstrated adequate stool control.[546] The authors concluded that the sphincter is really an elastic stenosis. Abercombie and associates measured anorectal sensory function following APR and total anal reconstruction in six individuals.[2] No patient appreciated neorectal distension, a desire to defecate, or a feeling of passage of flatus. The authors concluded that the loss of rectal sensation suggests that the prime sensors of rectal feeling probably lie within the rectum itself.[2]

Romano and coworkers performed anorectal reconstruction with the artificial bowel sphincter (Acticon; see Chapter 16).[520] Eight underwent reconstruction—five with a synchronous operation and three as a delayed procedure. All but one achieved a good incontinence score (Cleveland Clinic Score). Sato and colleagues have explored the possibility of a perineal colostomy with pudendal nerve anastomosis to a reconstructed gluteus muscle as a staged procedure.[549,550]

▶ INTRAOPERATIVE COMPLICATIONS FOLLOWING EXCISION OF THE RECTUM FOR CANCER

Hemorrhagic Complications during the Pelvic Dissection

Hemorrhagic complications can occur during the pelvic procedure. This is usually associated with dissection in the plane posterior to the parietal fascia in front of the sacrum. By doing so, the presacral venous plexus can be injured resulting in catastrophic hemorrhage. The use of blunt hand dissection in the pelvis can be a contributing factor.[642]

The best way to deal with bleeding is to avoid it in the first place. This can be accomplished by identifying the hypogastric nerves anterior to the parietal fascia and by keeping anterior and medial to them in the avascular retrorectal space during the rectal mobilization. Hemorrhage can also occur during the posterior dissection of the lowermost portion of the rectum. At that level, the fascia covering the lower sacrum is reflected off the sacrum onto the posterior aspect of the rectum to fuse with the perirectal fascia. The dissection at that level must be along that line of fusion and not posterior to it. Inadvertent dissection posterior to that line can lead to injury to the lower portion of the median sacral vein.

If massive bleeding occurs, it is usually difficult to control. In the first instance, avoid diathermy or suturing. They make matters worse. It is better to pack and apply pressure, ensure that there is good lighting and suction, alert the anesthetist, and, if possible, use a thumbtack to control the bleeding (see Figure 21-34).[593] If this fails, tightly pack the pelvis and wait for a while before reexamining. On some occasions, the rectal resection may need to be aborted, and the pelvis tightly packed with surgical sponges. Other methods of applying pressure in the pelvis have been described. They include using a breast prosthesis and a Bakri balloon that can be introduced through a divided rectal stump into the pelvis and inflated.[29] The patient is then taken to intensive care and reexamined several hours later when hopefully the bleeding has abated.

Injury to the Small Bowel

Inadvertent injury to the small bowel during surgery is uncommon and readily dealt with providing it is recognized at the time of surgery.

Ureteric Injuries

Injuries to the ureter are rare in the hands of experienced pelvic surgeons. In our experience, only 1 out of 884 patients undergoing APR or anterior resection had a ureteric injury. The best way to avoid injury is by knowing the status of the urinary tract preoperatively by performing a CT scan and by having a high index of suspicion in those who may have a complex tumor. In such patients, cystoscopy and the insertion of ureteric catheters is very useful.

The left ureter is most at risk. Care must be taken to identify it clearly at operation. It is important to make certain that the left ureter is not included in the ligature around the inferior mesenteric artery. Both ureters are at risk at the pelvic brim and also at the level of the middle hemorrhoidal vessels.

In patients who have had previous pelvic surgery (e.g., hysterectomy) or in those who have a bulky and locally invasive tumor, the ureters are especially vulnerable. Similarly, tumors that have invaded the trigone pose a threat to the ureters. The ureters are at risk during mobilization of the parietal peritoneum in patients in whom the surgeon chooses to close the pelvic floor—a technique that the author does not recommend.

If there is concern that the ureter has been injured, one should enlist the help of a specialist urologist. Identification of the injury site may be revealed by injecting 12.5 g of mannitol intravenously followed by the intravenous administration of 5 mL of indigo carmine dye. The presence of a blue stain in the operative field is diagnostic of injury. If the distal ureter cannot be identified, a cystotomy should be made and a ureteric catheter placed through the ureteric orifice until it presents in the operative field. If ligation without penetration is suspected, a proximal linear ureterotomy permits antegrade insertion of a ureteric catheter to test the patency.[669]

Many ureteric injuries go unrecognized and may remain so if only one of the ureters has been ligated. Flank pain, fever, leukocytosis, and tenderness are the most frequent presenting signs and symptoms of ureteric ligation during the early postoperative period. Urinary fistula can be suspected if there is copious serous or serosanguineous perineal wound drainage in the early postoperative period. A blue stain appearing on the perineal or abdominal wound dressing after intravenous administration of indigo carmine confirms the diagnosis. When there is no perineal wound, such as after low anterior resection, it often takes a number of days before the presence of urine within the abdominal cavity is appreciated.

Late urinary fistula can occur because of ureteric necrosis from devascularization injury, from the membranous urethra, or from the base of the bladder.

Treatment

With crush injury from a hemostat or with partial ligation, removing the ligature and stenting the ureter may be all that is required. However, careful patient selection is mandatory in order to avoid postoperative complications. If the ureter at the site of the injury is considered nonviable, a formal repair with excision of the devascularized portion of the ureter may need to be performed. Under these circumstances, a urologist must be involved. Proximal ureteric ligation with the expectation of renal death in the poor risk patient who has a limited life expectancy is generally to be condemned because of the risks of sepsis and fistula formation.[669] One also must be concerned about the function of the contralateral kidney.

Injury to the Lower Ureter

Ureteroneocystotomy is the preferred procedure for injuries of the pelvic ureter. Injuries within 5 cm of the bladder and often at greater distances are suitable for this approach. The technique has been described by Politano and Leadbetter and by others.[355,356,502] The procedure achieves an antirefluxing ureteric anastomosis. The following operations have been advocated by Libertino et al.[355,356]

A midline cystotomy is made, and 3 mL of saline solution is injected through a 23-gauge needle, raising a small bleb of mucosa (Figure 24-78). An ellipse of mucosa is excised, and a 3-cm submucosal tunnel is created with a right-angle clamp (Figure 24-79). The clamp is then rotated to point through the bladder wall, and the detrusor muscle is pierced. The distal ureter is pulled through the tunnel with the aid of traction sutures and spatulated for approximately 1 cm.[356] A no. 6 or 8 French catheter is inserted to make certain that the ureter pursues a direct course. The ureter is then sutured to the bladder with interrupted 5–0 chromic catgut sutures or 5–0 long-term absorbable sutures. Deep bites of detrusor must be included in the two distal sutures at the 5 and 7 o'clock positions to help restore normal ureterovesical function.[355] A no. 5 or 8 feeding tube is used as a ureteric stent and is brought out alongside a suprapubic cystotomy catheter. This is removed on the seventh day.

Ureteric Reimplantation

Ureteric reimplantation into the bladder is the best method for restoring continuity following ureteric injury. Therefore, every effort should be made to accomplish this. If the ureter cannot be brought down without tension, a Boari bladder flap tube technique can be employed, or preferably a so-called psoas bladder hitch maneuver can be used.[47,57,624] These techniques are best accomplished by a urologist who

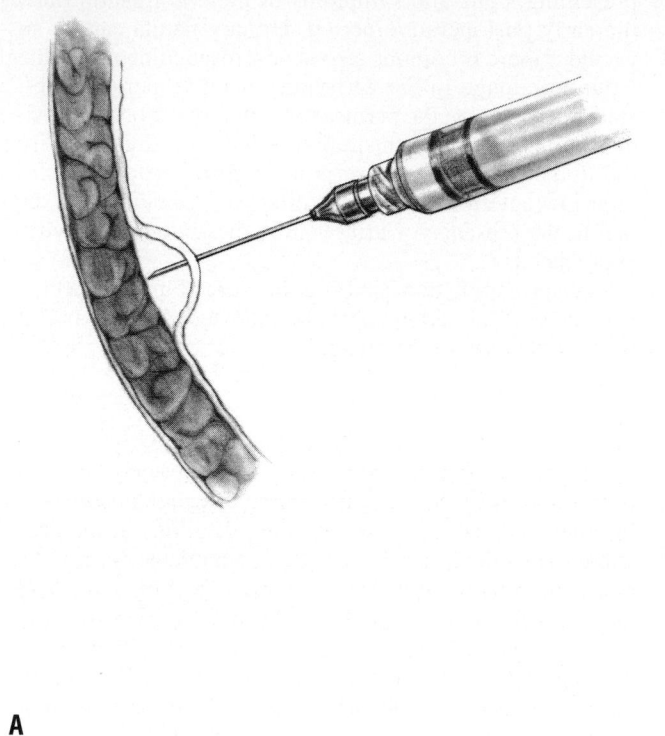
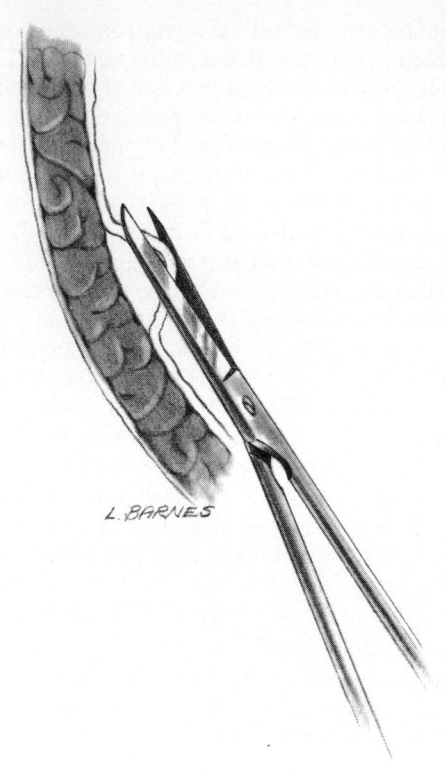

A

B

FIGURE 24-78. Ureteroneocystotomy. **A:** Submucosal injection of saline. **B:** A small ellipse of bladder mucosa is excised to allow creation of a submucosal tunnel. (Adapted from Libertino JA, Zinman L. Technique for uretero-neocystotomy in renal transplantation and reflux. *Surg Clin North Am.* 1973;53:459, with permission.)

is familiar with the specialized approaches to ureterovesical surgery. It is always wise to take advantage of the availability of urologic consultation when injury to the urinary tract has occurred.

Injury to the Middle and Upper Ureter

Injuries to the proximal ureter are the most difficult and least satisfactory to treat. Fortunately, this is a rare complication of bowel surgery. Because of the distance, reimplantation into the bladder is not possible, and the blood supply is less adequate. Direct repair by *end-to-end ureteroureterostomy* is the treatment of choice. With loss of ureteric length from excision or necrosis, defects of up to 8 cm can be traversed by this method if one uses a renal-lowering technique.[356] If direct repair is impossible, one can consider the highly specialized techniques of *transureteroureterostomy*, *ileal interposition*, or *autotransplantation*. Benson and colleagues reported success with ureteric reconstruction in 17 of their 18 patients by the selective application of psoas hitch, Boari bladder tube, ileal interposition, or autotransplantation.[47] *Nephrectomy* may be used if the surgeon is satisfied that contralateral kidney function is adequate and calculus disease or other conditions that may affect the kidney are not present.

Transureteroureterostomy

Transureteroureterostomy is another alternative that may be employed for the injured ureter. Hodges and colleagues reported a large, successful experience with this technique,[264] but because of the possibility of injury to the recipient ureter, it should be used only sparingly and only by a specialist urologist and limited to injuries of the upper pelvic ureter when

reimplantation cannot be accomplished.[356] The technique is shown in Figure 24-80. The injured ureter should be resected at a point of certain viability, with care being taken to preserve the adventitia and blood supply. The recipient ureter should not be mobilized from its bed. Ureteric stents are advised to provide proximal drainage of the kidneys while the anastomosis takes time to heal.

Whenever a direct repair of a ureteric injury is performed, proximal diversion is advised. Zinman and colleagues recommend a no. 7 French polyurethane double pigtail ureteric stent (Figure 24-81A).[669] The cut edges of the ureter are debrided and spatulated, and the kidney, ureter, or both are adequately mobilized.[356] The ureter is spatulated on opposing sides of each end to prevent stricture (Figure 24-81B). Anastomosis is effected with interrupted 5–0 chromic catgut or long-term absorbable sutures placed full thickness, with the knots on the outside inverting the mucosa (Figure 24-81C). Noncrushing vascular forceps can be used to grasp the tissue, whereas the presence of a catheter within the lumen facilitates the procedure. A continuous suture should never be employed. The ureter can be wrapped in omentum if the anastomosis is believed to be precarious. A suitable drain (e.g., Jackson-Pratt or Blake drain) is placed at the site of the ureteroureterostomy and brought out through a stab wound. The drain is removed when the drainage has reduced to less than 50 mL of fluid per day and if it is shown, by biochemical analysis, not to be urine. The stent is usually removed by cystoscopy at approximately 4 to 6 weeks.

Bladder Injury

Bladder injury that is recognized at the time of surgery can usually be repaired by means of a layered closure of 2–0

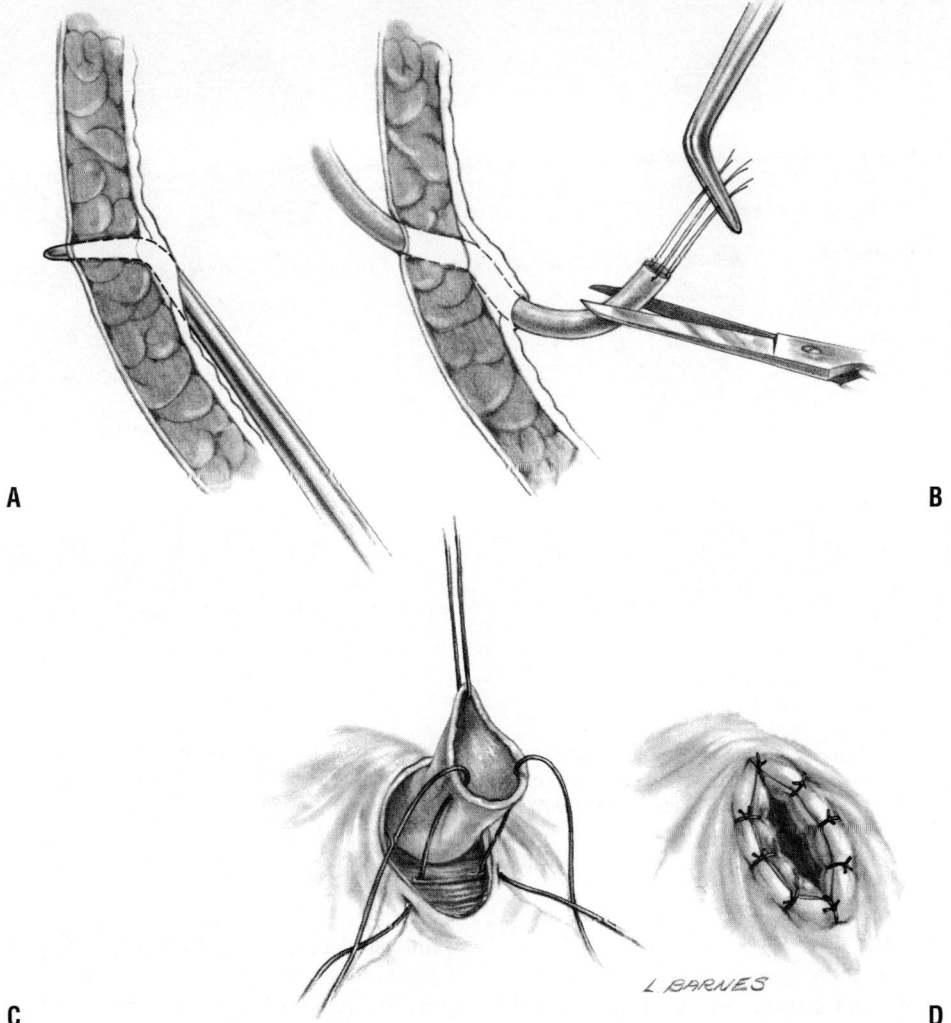

FIGURE 24-79. Ureteroneocystotomy. **A:** A right-angle clamp pierces the detrusor muscle. **B:** The ureter is pulled through the submucosal tunnel; the distal ureter is cut at a 45-degree angle, creating a new ureteral meatus. **C:** The ureter is anchored to the bladder detrusor muscle. **D:** Completion of the anastomosis to the bladder mucosa. (Adapted from Libertino JA, Zinman L. Technique for uretero-neocystotomy in renal transplantation and reflux. *Surg Clin North Am.* 1973;53:459, with permission.)

chromic catgut or long-term absorbable suture. When injury to the bladder neck or trigone has occurred, great care must be taken to avoid incorporating the distal ureters in the suture. A cystotomy with insertion of small ureteric catheters, or infant feeding tubes, in a retrograde fashion through the ureteric orifices is useful in preventing this complication. Drainage of the area is advised. Suprapubic cystotomy is prudent when the injury is to the bladder neck or trigone.

Urethral Injury

Injury to the urethra occurs most often as a result of dissecting in the wrong plane while performing the anterior part of the perineal dissection. In addition, tumor may invade the prostate, and in an attempt to perform a curative resection, the prostatic urethra may be entered. External trauma can cause a delayed urethral stricture, which may require catheterization or subsequent reconstruction. If injury to this area is recognized at the time of proctectomy, direct repair or urethroplasty may be indicated. A urologist should be consulted if the surgeon is not experienced with reparative approaches.

Urethral stricture may require dilatation, internal urethrotomy, or reconstructive urethroplasty.[668] Here again, one should seek the advice of someone who has expertise in the management of such a complication.

Seminal Vesicle Injury

Injury to the seminal vesicles probably occurs much more frequently than is generally suspected. This may be responsible for some problems related to fertility but should otherwise be of no consequence. However, a case of seminal vesicle–rectal fistula has been reported.[208] Moreover, a fistula to the perineum following an APR has been seen.[323] Treatment in this case included percutaneous drainage of the abscess, antibiotics, and oral administration of finasteride (Proscar).

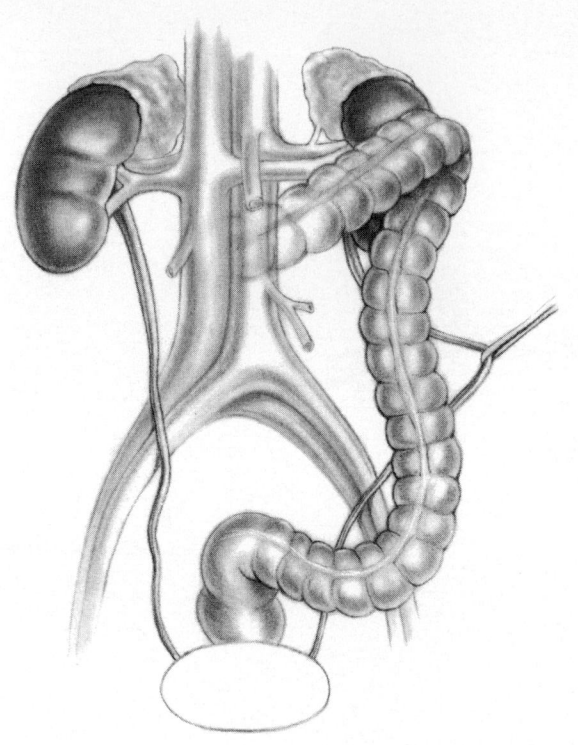
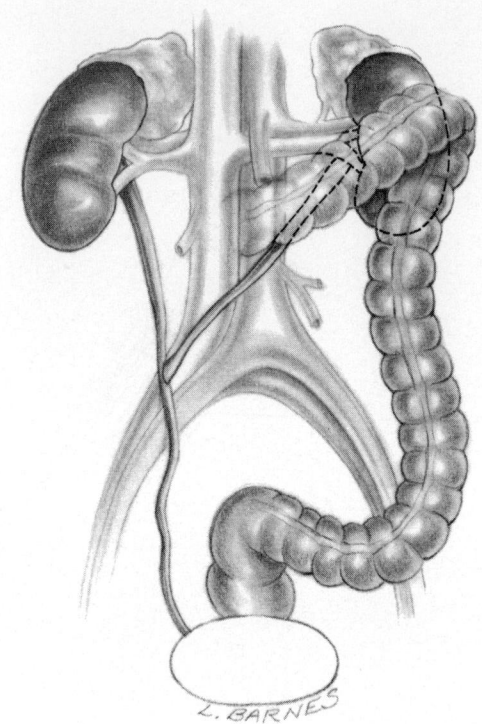

A

B

FIGURE 24-80. Transureteroureterostomy. **A:** A tunnel is developed by retroperitoneal dissection after exposure of the upper ureter lateral to the colon. **B:** The ureter is brought across the retroperitoneal space and is anastomosed. (Adapted from Libertino JA, Zinman L. Technique for ureteroneocystotomy in renal transplantation and reflux. *Surg Clin North Am.* 1973;53:459, with permission.)

Postoperative Complications

Urinary Retention and Infection or Bladder Dysfunction

Urinary tract infection and urinary retention are the most common complications following abdominoperineal or low anterior resection. Marks and Ritchie reported an incidence of 34%.[395] Janu and colleagues noted that 25% of their patients developed a urinary tract infection, whereas bladder dysfunction occurred in 22%.[287] In the experience of Cunsolo and colleagues, urinary retention occurred in 41% of men and 35% of women.[122] Wide iliopelvic lymphadenectomy increases the risk of voiding difficulties.[83,265] Urinary retention may be the result of injury to the sympathetic or parasympathetic nerves to the bladder, postoperative distension, local trauma, prostatic hypertrophy, or prolapse of the bladder into the pelvis.

The most important preventive maneuver that one may employ is to retain a Foley catheter in place for 5 to 7 days. The effects of direct trauma to the bladder necessitate a period of recovery. The catheter is removed at 6:00 a.m. and the voiding pattern carefully observed. If the patient is unable to void or urinates frequently in small amounts, a residual urine determination should be made. If it is more than 300 mL, the catheter should be reinserted and left for an additional 2 or 3 days. During this interval, it is reasonable to place the patient on bethanechol chloride (Urecholine), 25 to 50 mg, four times daily. This is suggested in an effort to improve detrusor tone. Urodynamic studies are advised if the patient is unable to void after removal of the catheter.

A cystometrogram usually will demonstrate a flaccid type of bladder, but the urethral pressure profile will probably be normal. What is important is to determine the external sphincter electromyogram (EMG). Very often after an APR, the internal pudendal nerve is compromised, and the patient loses the innervation of the external sphincter. Continence, therefore, is maintained by the internal sphincter or bladder neck mechanism only. The cystometrogram, urethral pressure profile, and external sphincter EMG should be correlated with the anatomic findings of cystourethroscopy. If the patient has an obstructed prostate and a normal sphincter EMG, then it is reasonable to carry out a transurethral resection. If the external sphincter EMG shows a flaccid external sphincter, one would be loath to carry out a transurethral resection of the prostate or any form of prostatectomy for fear of making the patient incontinent. Under these circumstances, it is advisable to leave the catheter in place for a period of 6 weeks to 2 months or to instruct the patient in the use of intermittent catheterization. Hopefully, this respite will allow the bladder residual urine to be of small enough volume to avoid overdistension of the bladder and decompensation of the detrusor musculature. Intermittent catheterization is preferable to the patient's incontinence. Current urologic practice discourages clamping and unclamping the catheter in an attempt to restore detrusor tone. If the goal of keeping the bladder empty is achieved, the detrusor tone will ultimately return.

By evaluating preoperatively the urologic situation in a systematic way, Leadbetter and Leadbetter believed that they could selectively perform prostatectomy at the time of the APR and decrease the incidence of postoperative urinary retention.[345] From a limited experience with this approach, I believe that such a combined operation should be condemned. There is an associated high incidence of urinary

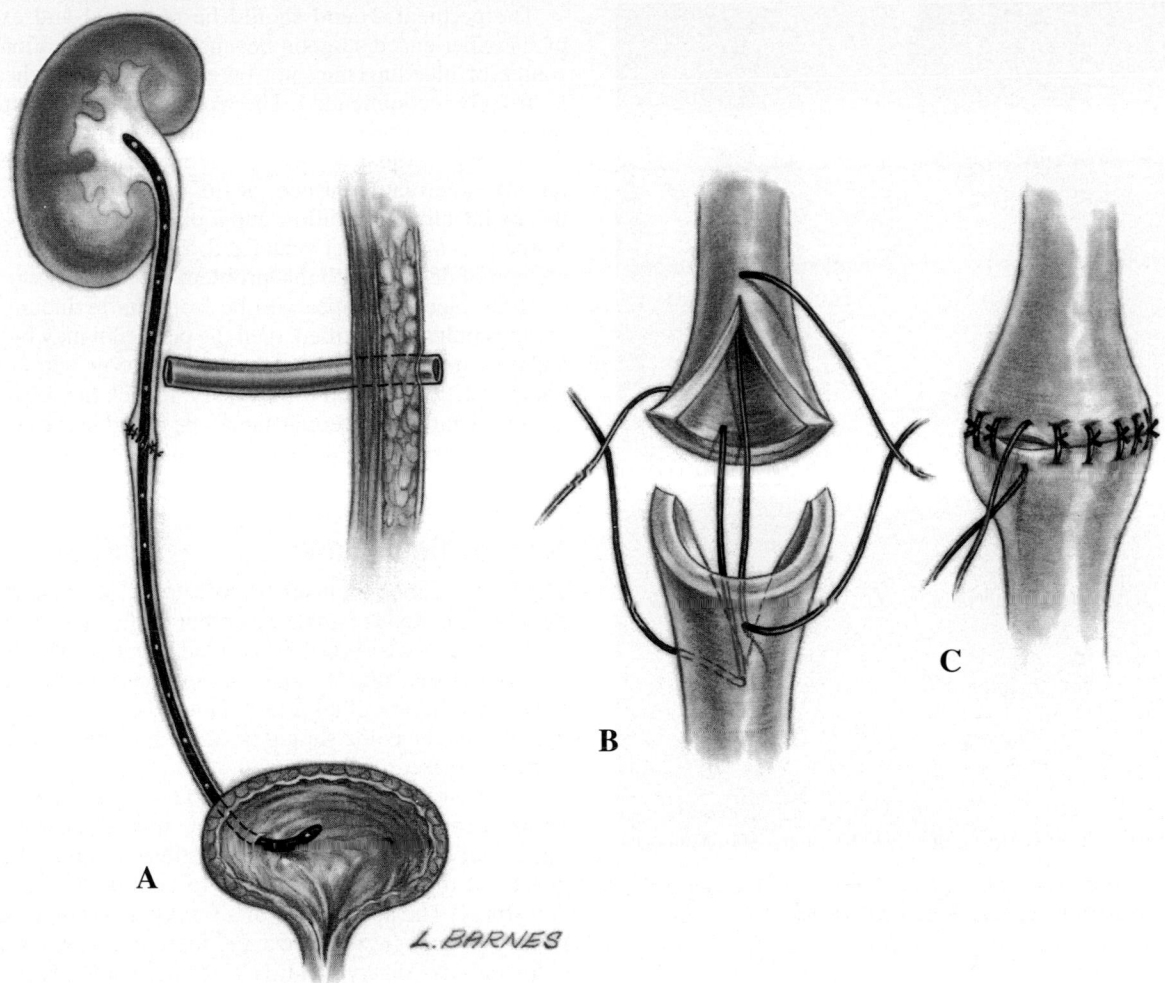

FIGURE 24-81. Ureteroureterostomy. **A:** Midureteroureterostomy is diverted by a Silastic double-J stent. **B:** The ureters are spatulated on opposing sides of each end to achieve oblique anastomosis. **C:** The edges are approximated with interrupted fine catgut sutures placed through the full thickness of the ureteral wall, thus inverting the mucosa. (Adapted from Libertino JA, Zinman L. Technique for ureteroneocystotomy in renal transplantation and reflux. *Surg Clin North Am*. 1973;53:459, with permission.)

tract infection, pelvic sepsis, and urinary-perineal fistula (Figure 24-82).

In women, the procedure should be essentially the same as that described earlier. If the woman has difficulty voiding after an additional period of catheter drainage and treatment with bethanechol, she should be taught the technique of intermittent self-catheterization until the bladder tone returns and normal voiding occurs. Self-catheterization is an option in men also.

▶ POSTOPERATIVE MORTALITY FOLLOWING EXCISION OF THE RECTUM FOR CANCER

The rate of postoperative mortality following either anterior resection or APR is low. Between the years 1995 and 2010, the 30-day mortality in 977 patients operated on by myself and colleagues in the colorectal unit at Concord Hospital was 1%, with no differences between anterior resection, APR, and Hartmann's operations. In a recent systematic review of

75 series, the mortality rate was 2%. The ability of patient and operative features to predict postoperative mortality in colorectal surgery has been evaluated using a risk-adjusted scoring system.[612]

▶ POSTOPERATIVE COMPLICATIONS AFTER EXCISION OF THE RECTUM COMMON TO BOTH ANTERIOR RESECTION AND ABDOMINOPERINEAL RESECTION

Many complications can occur after either APR or anterior resection. Most are not specific to excision of the rectum and can eventuate after any major abdominal procedures. These include urinary tract infection; cardiac complications, of which atrial fibrillation is the most common; and respiratory complications, of which basal atelectasis is the most common.

Abdominal wound infection can occur but has become less common following the introduction of perioperative

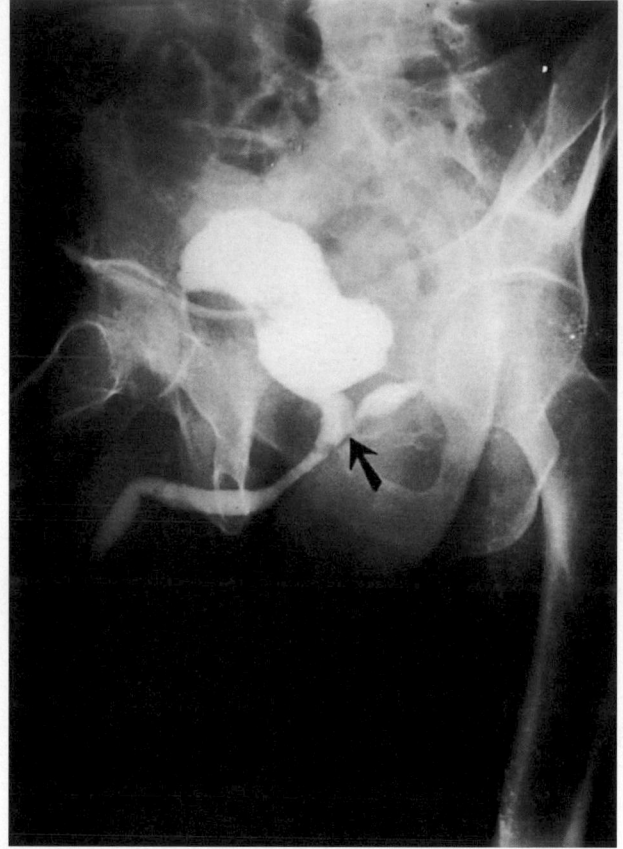

FIGURE 24-82. Urethroperineal fistula (*arrow*) is a serious consequence of an ill-advised concomitant proctectomy and prostatectomy.

antimicrobial prophylaxis. Table 24-2 lists the complications after excision of the rectum for 884 patients treated by myself and members of the colorectal unit at Concord Hospital over the past 16 years.

► POSTOPERATIVE COMPLICATIONS SPECIFIC TO ABDOMINOPERINEAL RESECTION

Hemorrhage from the Perineal Wound

This is an important but infrequent complication. It has occurred in 2.3% of our patients. Bleeding can either be from the abdominal (pelvic) or perineal dissection. Blood trickles out of the perineal drain. It is important to understand that the amount of blood seeping through may only represent a fraction of the actual bleeding. A significant amount of blood may be lying hidden in the abdomen or pelvis. Because of this, any undue bleeding from the perineal drain should be regarded with concern. The vital signs and urine output should be closely observed, and hemoglobin levels should be determined at regular intervals if necessary.

If the patient becomes hemodynamically compromised, if the hemoglobin level drops significantly, or if the patient is in shock, prompt resuscitation is indicated. Blood should be urgently crossmatched, and the patient should be returned to the operating room.

The perineal wound should be reopened and explored by an experienced surgeon because the identification of the source of bleeding may not be easy. Wearing a headlight is strongly recommended. The wound should be thoroughly washed out. On many occasions, the bleeding is from the inferior hemorrhoidal vessels. These may have retracted deep into the anterolateral aspect of the dissection. I have found that by kneeling on a pillow and looking upward, this area of dissection can be better visualized. Suture ligature is the best method of dealing with this problem.

If the bleeding appears to be from the perineum but no obvious point is identified, then the perineum may be packed and the patient returned to the operating room within several hours to reexplore, and if necessary, repack the wound.

If the source of bleeding cannot be found in the perineum, then the abdomen should be explored to identify and control the source of hemorrhage.

Necrotic Colostomy

The most common causes of colostomy necrosis are poor blood supply and tension, or as often occurs, tension leading to ischemia. Necrosis can be avoided by meticulous attention to detail at the time of constructing the colostomy. Blood flow from the marginal artery should be tested before it is ligated, and the colon should be under no tension at all when it is exteriorized.

In patients who have a short and fatty mesentery, it may be necessary to fully mobilize the splenic flexure and to ligate and divide the inferior mesenteric vein at the lower border of the pancreas in order to achieve a tension-free colostomy. The appearance of a frankly necrotic colostomy is easy to recognize. However, there are times when the colostomy is "dusky" and its viability is uncertain. A submucosal hematoma can also mimic a necrotic stoma, and in some patients, melanosis coli can cause confusion. If there is any doubt about the viability of the stoma, an easy way of resolving the dilemma is to use a sterile needle to pinprick the mucosa. A viable stoma bleeds readily. In addition, a proctoscope or pediatric sigmoidoscope can be used to examine the stoma and determine if there is any evidence of ischemia.

A patient with a necrotic stoma should undergo urgent laparotomy. The ischemic segment should be resected. The proximal colon should be fully mobilized as described earlier, and a new colostomy should be exteriorized. It is important not to delay laparotomy in the hope that the colostomy will "pink up"; it never does, and if untreated, ischemic bowel can be life threatening.

Intestinal Obstruction

Small bowel obstruction due to adhesions has occurred in 3.4% of our patients. The most common site of adherence is in the freshly dissected pelvis. As discussed, some surgeons advocate closing the pelvic floor by reperitonealizing. However, this can cause small bowel obstruction if a defect occurs in the peritoneal suture line and a loop of bowel herniates through (Figure 24-83). Harshaw recommends not closing the pelvic floor for that reason.[239]

Occasionally, herniation of the small bowel can occur through the defect in the paracolostomy gutter.[213] This can theoretically be avoided by closing the paracolostomy gutter or by an extraperitoneal exteriorization of the colon. I choose

TABLE 24-2 Postoperative complications after anterior resection and abdominoperineal resection performed by members of the colorectal unit at Concord Hospital, Sydney, NSW, Australia, from 1995 to 2010.

COMPLICATION	ANTERIOR RESECTION PERCENTAGE n = 665	ABDOMINOPERINEAL RESECTION PERCENTAGE n = 219	TOTAL PERCENTAGE n = 884
Prolonged ileus	15.6	13.7	15.2
Respiratory	12.3	16.4	13.3
Cardiac	13.8	10.5	13.0
Urinary	11.8	14.7	11.8
Organic confusional state >24 hours	6.6	7.8	6.9
Pelvic hematoma	4.4	8.7	5.4
Pelvic abscess	3.8	4.1	3.8
Small bowel obstruction	3.5	3.2	3.4
Deep vein thrombosis	1.7	0.5	1.4
Pulmonary embolus	1.4	0.9	1.2
Hemorrhage	0.9	2.3	1.2
Fistula	1.1	0.9	1.0

to leave the gutter open because there is no evidence that closing it makes any difference.

If bowel obstruction occurs, it should be managed expectantly in the first instance, and the surgeon should be guided by the patient's clinical signs and progress. However, it is important to understand that if the site of obstruction is in the pelvis, the signs and symptoms may be different from those of an obstruction due to intra-abdominal adhesions. In these patients, abdominal tenderness is an important clinical sign of ischemia that can influence the need for urgent laparotomy. In patients with an obstruction in the pelvis, abdominal tenderness may not be a prominent feature and cannot be relied on to signal impending ischemia.

A postoperative CT scan with oral contrast is very useful in demonstrating the site of obstruction. If the patient does not respond to initial conservative measures, then laparotomy becomes necessary.

Perineal Wound Sepsis

Perineal sepsis is not uncommon following APR. This complication may be caused by contamination at the time of proctectomy from injury to the rectal wall, fecal spillage, the presence of a perforated carcinoma, an infected hematoma, or the presence of perineal disease (e.g., fistula or abscess).

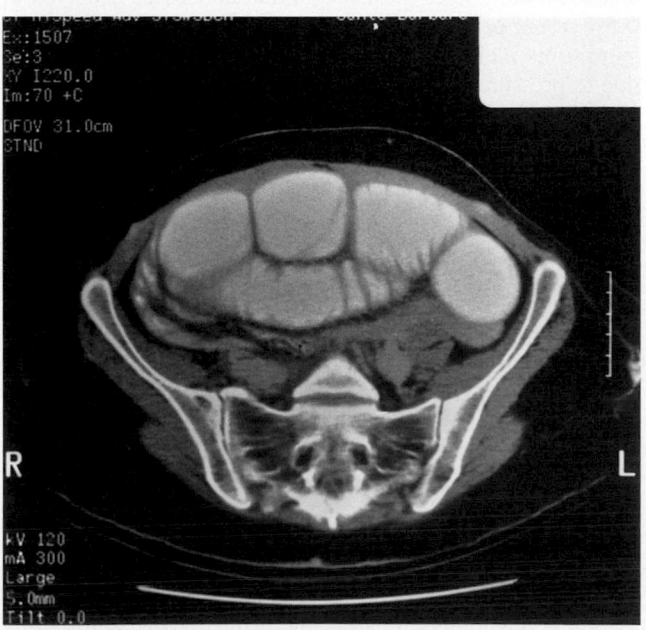

FIGURE 24-83. Computed tomography demonstrates small bowel obstruction. This was secondary to herniation through a defect in the pelvic floor, which had been initially closed. Note the decompressed small bowel.

Characteristically, the patient develops a low-grade fever on the third or fourth postoperative day, which progresses to a higher spiking fever elevation. In the absence of another obvious source for pyrexia, the perineal wound should be carefully explored with a gloved finger. Loculations should be broken and, if necessary, the wound reopened. Irrigating with one-half strength Dakin's solution (using a rubber catheter) is important to remove clot and debris. A sitz bath, even with the wound wide open, is inadequate for treating or preventing perineal sepsis.

Some perineal abscesses are really an extension of a pelvic abscess. The most appropriate way of dealing with this is to perform a CT scan and drain the abscess percutaneously under CT guidance.

Perineal wound sepsis can be avoided by leaving the wound wide open to heal by second intention. The disadvantage of a prolonged healing time (not infrequently for more than 4 months) makes this alternative inadvisable. Conversely, primary closure without drainage is contraindicated because of the high likelihood of sepsis. A satisfactory compromise is to close the skin and to bring a drain through the wound or through a separate incision (see Figure 24-67). I have also tried another method of draining the perineal wound—namely, by closing the perineal wound completely and inserting suction drains into the pelvis from the abdomen. I have not been impressed by this method of drainage and have now abandoned its use.

Abdominal Wound Infection and Intra-abdominal Sepsis

Since the introduction of systemic prophylactic antibiotics in the perioperative period, these complications have become less common. Five percent of our patients developed a wound infection. Nevertheless, wound infection can be quite debilitating and can delay the patient's discharge. Managing a wound infection in the presence of a nearby colostomy can be challenging and requires the expertise of an experienced enterostomal nurse. Intra-abdominal abscesses occurred in 0.5% of our patients after an APR, mainly in the pelvis. The symptoms include malaise, rigors, and urinary symptoms due to pressure on the bladder.

Pelvic abscesses usually discharge spontaneously through the perineal wound, but pelvic and other intra-abdominal abscesses can be identified by CT scan and drained percutaneously under CT guidance.

Neurologic and Vascular Complications

The perineolithotomy position has been associated with a number of intraoperative and postoperative complications, especially as related to the compartment syndrome. It is for this reason that special care needs to be taken in positioning the patient to minimize the risk of vascular injury. Another complication that has been noted has been related to the self-retaining retractor, that of femoral neuropathy. This complication has been reported to be a consequence of a number of operations, most commonly inguinal hernia repair. However, three instances have been associated with the use of the self-retaining Bookwalter retractor.[72] In a slender patient, the same phenomenon can occur if the Balfour retractor is used or if the O'Connor-O'Sullivan instrument is employed. Brasch and colleagues attribute risk factors to be as follows: a transverse incision, anticoagulation, uremia, diabetes, and those patients of thin, short stature or those who have poorly developed rectus muscles.[72] With careful attention to the location of the retractor blades, this complication should be preventable.

Acute arterial occlusion is a rare complication of low pelvic surgery. Underlying peripheral vascular disease may contribute to the development of this complication, but the use of the perineolithotomy position, the common hypercoagulable state of many patients with cancer, and the prolonged use of sequential compression devices all may be factors.[88]

Impotence, Infertility, and Dyspareunia

Impotence following proctectomy for carcinoma of the rectum is very common, especially in the older age group, and particularly when a wide iliopelvic lymphadenectomy is performed.[31,265,314,340,643] This complication must be discussed in detail preoperatively with the patient. Although one might think that it is a concern primarily for younger patients, I have found that individuals of all ages are equally concerned about their sexual function. A man may choose to "bank" his sperm prior to undergoing this operation or he may elect alternative therapy (e.g., local excision).

Cunsolo and colleagues reported that 59% of the preoperatively sexually active men who underwent APR became impotent.[122] The resection requires extensive pelvic dissection, which may result in injury to the parasympathetic nerves (nervi erigentes). Additionally, the patient's preoperative sexual function may have been less than adequate, and even minimal trauma may be sufficient to precipitate impotence. This may be an important explanation for why young people who undergo proctectomy for inflammatory bowel disease rarely have such difficulty when compared with older patients with cancer. In other words, preoperative libido may be the critical issue with respect to postoperative sexual function.

Women seem less likely to experience problems with orgasms, although most reports include a high number of widowed, elderly women who have no sexual partners. Retained menstrual blood, colpitis, chronic discharge from the vagina, and dyspareunia are not uncommon symptoms after proctectomy.[575] In one study, the incidence of dyspareunia was 50%.[122] Sjödahl and colleagues recommend an operation for this complaint that they attribute to dorsocaudal dislocation of the posterior vaginal wall (the horizontal vagina syndrome).[575] This involves coccygectomy, separation of the posterior fornix from the lower part of the sacrum, and interposition of muscle flaps from the right and left gluteus maximus muscle.

In men, infertility can result even if tumescence is not impaired because of injury to the sympathetic nerves and the consequence of retrograde ejaculation. Injury to the vas or seminal vesicles has also been reported and may be associated with infertility.[350]

In the past, organic impotence was reported to be rather unsuccessfully treated with drugs, but in order that the patient may satisfy a sexual partner and gain an element of self-satisfaction, penile prosthetic implants have been used.[41,172,202,366,495,496] However, Lindsey and colleagues found that sildenafil (Viagra) improved erectile dysfunction in 79% of their patients.[357] They further observed that nocturnal penile tumescence, although diminished, is not always ablated by surgical dissection, suggesting that some of the cavernous nerves that govern inflow to the corpora cavernosa are intact, and that the nerve injury responsible for erectile dysfunction is partial. This helps to explain the response to sildenafil. Penile implantation should not be performed for at least 1 year after APR because of the possibility of return of this function.

Unhealed Perineal Wound and Persistent Perineal Sinus

The problem of delayed healing following proctectomy for cancer is quite unusual. This is in contradistinction to the frequency of the complication in individuals who undergo proctectomy for inflammatory bowel disease (see Chapter 29). However, with the use of preoperative and postoperative radiation therapy, the incidence of perineal wound breakdown and delayed healing is significantly increased. This is a particular concern if the radiation dose approaches 60 Gy. Techniques have been employed to ameliorate the condition and to effect healing, including reoperation and curettage, excision and grafting, muscle transposition,[10,27,332] and the use of fibrin adhesive fibrinogen concentrate and thrombin.[260] Radice and coworkers found that immediate myocutaneous flap closure in patients who underwent extended resection for locally advanced malignancy (including chemoradiation) achieved complete healing with reduced requirement for readmission and reoperation than those who underwent primary skin closure.[508] Numerous articles have been published concerning recommendations for managing sacral and perineal defects following APR, often with the use of muscle flaps.[567]

Perineal Hernia

Symptomatic perineal hernia is a rare, late complication of APR (Figure 24-84). Only a handful of cases have been reported.[38,76,93,221] The condition is much more common in women. Symptoms may include perineal pressure, fullness, pain, or feeling as if sitting on a lump. The hernia may produce skin breakdown or may be associated with an evisceration. Two patients who were reported from the Cleveland Clinic had symptoms of partial small bowel obstruction.[38]

So and colleagues identified 13 patients who underwent APR and developed a perineal hernia postoperatively, an

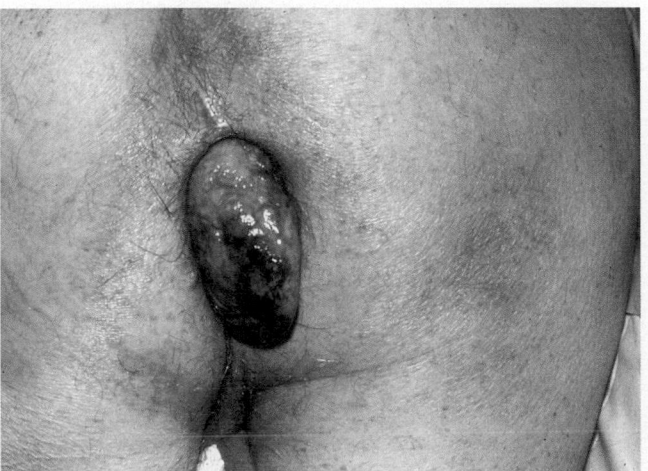

FIGURE 24-84. Perineal hernia developing 6 months following abdominoperineal resection. Treatment requires laparotomy and reconstruction of the pelvic floor.

incidence of 0.62%.[579] No definitive predisposing factors could be clearly identified. The authors emphasized the importance of the standard surgical principles for repairing a hernia in any other location—mobilization of the sac, reduction of its contents, excision of the sac, and repair of the defect—usually with mesh.

Treatment should be directed to an abdominal or a combined abdominal and perineal approach. Attempting repair from the perineum alone is unlikely to be successful. In principle, the bowel must be delivered out of the pelvis and the pelvic floor reconstituted, usually with mesh.[38,547] The pelvis should be drained, and if necessary, the redundant skin excised. Brotschi and colleagues reported a successful result after two operations using the gracilis muscle following a failed Marlex mesh repair.[76]

Phantom Sensations after Abdominoperineal Resection

Phantom sensations are quite common after amputation of extremities, so it is not surprising that patients may experience feelings of an urge to defecate or to pass flatus after excision of the rectum. In a review by Lubbers of 40 patients who underwent proctectomy, 65% reported the presence of these sensations.[375] Theoretically, such feelings are a normal response to removal of the rectum because innervation is still represented at the level of the cerebral cortex. Reassurance and the passage of time usually alleviate patient anxiety.

Perineal Pain

Intractable pain in the perineum in an individual who has undergone proctectomy for carcinoma of the rectum is indicative of recurrent tumor until proved otherwise. However, patients may occasionally complain bitterly of severe, deep-seated pain that is analogous to that of levator spasm (proctalgia fugax; see Chapter 20).

Entrapped Ovary Syndrome

Matthews and colleagues reported retroperitoneal cysts with entrapped ovaries in the retroperitoneal pelvis of six patients who had undergone proctectomies.[406] Patients may present with abdominal pain, a mass, or distension. If the ovary is to be preserved, excision of the cyst and oophoropexy is advised.[406] Care should be taken at the time of the initial operation to be certain that the ovary remains as an intraperitoneal structure if the pelvic floor is closed.

Stomal Problems

Colostomy retraction, stenosis, prolapse, and hernia, as well as peristomal dermatitis and appliance management problems, are discussed in Chapters 31 and 32.

▶ POSTOPERATIVE COMPLICATIONS SPECIFIC TO RESTORATIVE PROCEDURES FOR RECTAL CANCER

Anastomotic Bleeding

Hemorrhage from the anastomosis is a rare complication. This may be the result of inadequate hemostasis at the suture line itself. The problem may be managed expectantly, but occasionally, bleeding from the anastomosis persists and has to be dealt with formally in the operating room. If the anastomosis is very low, then it may be possible to identify the bleeding point and oversew it from below. This is by no means an easy task. It should be performed in the operating room and with the patient in stirrups. Good access and vision are essential, and I recommend wearing a headlight and using a Lone Star retractor. This permits better access and vision. When oversewing a very low anastomosis, a long needle holder is necessary. If the anastomosis is not within easy reach, colonoscopy may be useful. I prefer to use an endoscopic clip rather than electrocoagulation, especially if the anastomosis is intraperitoneal. Anastomotic hemorrhage was at one time thought to be a problem with the single row of staples associated with the early Russian instrument. However, with the double row of interlocking staples, bleeding is an unusual complication.[247]

Cirocco and Golub reviewed the literature and identified 17 patients with postoperative hemorrhage from a combined total of 775 (1.8%) after stapled colorectal anastomosis that required blood transfusion and/or emergency surgery.[108] Nonoperative therapy was successful in 82%. The frequency of this complication is probably more common than is evident from the literature, but the fact that most spontaneously cease and do not go on to anastomotic leak implies that this is a relatively minor concern.

Postoperative Intra-abdominal Hemorrhage

This is a rare complication and should be treated on its merits. The management of postoperative bleeding should include immediate resuscitation. If the patient is stable, then conservative treatment may be initially indicated. However, if there is any evidence of hemodynamic decompensation, then urgent laparotomy should be performed. The threshold for reoperation should be very low.

Prolonged Ileus

The failure of postoperative ileus to resolve within a few days after major abdominal surgery leads to significant medical consequences for the patient, including continuing discomfort, pain, loss of confidence, possible admission to a high dependency unit, delayed resumption of normal diet and mobility, prolonged hospital stay, elevated risk of other complications and nosocomial infections, and increased postoperative mortality (Figure 24-85). Increased length of hospital stay also generates considerable costs for both the patient and the hospital system.[304] The pathophysiology and treatment has been reviewed thoroughly by Person and Wexner.[500] The frequency of prolonged ileus was 15.3% in 17,876 patients undergoing colectomy in more than 500 hospitals in the United States in 2004, and this high level of morbidity has persisted despite the widespread adoption of a range of preventive policies for which there is relatively little conclusive evidence of efficacy.[500] These include avoidance of opiate analgesia, early postoperative feeding, avoidance or early removal of the nasogastric tube, and early ambulation. Laparoscopic surgery is widely believed to reduce the likelihood of a prolonged ileus, but this remains to be established in a randomized controlled trial.

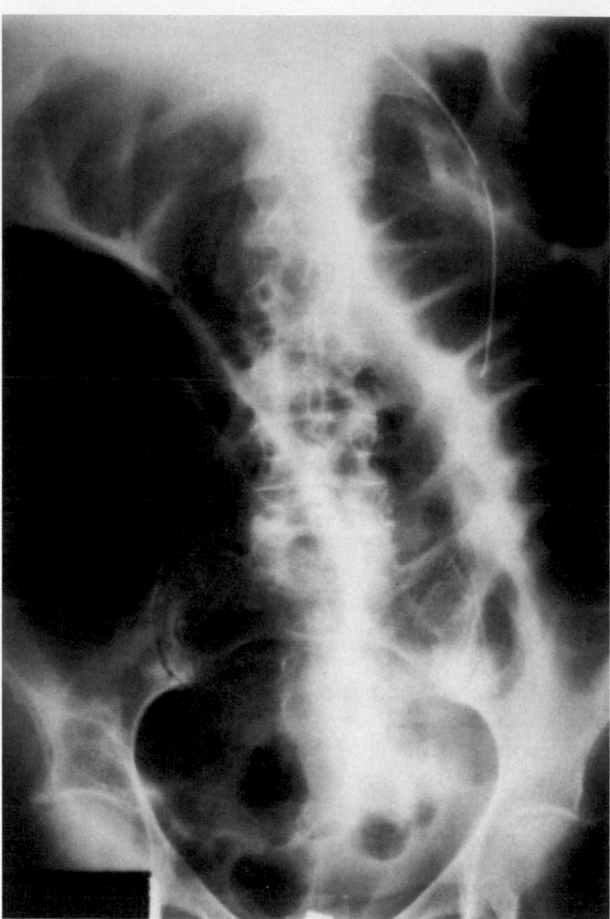

FIGURE 24-85. Colonic ileus. A massively dilated colon in a patient who underwent a low anterior resection. With an "intact" ileocecal valve, there is a high risk of perforation.

Anastomotic Leakage

Anastomotic leakage is one of the most feared complications following colorectal anastomosis (Figure 24-86). Its consequences can be fatal, and if not fatal, it can result in significant short- and long-term morbidity.

There are three principal factors that can contribute to anastomotic leakage: tension, poor blood supply, and inadequate full-thickness bites during the anastomosis. That is why so much care is required in preparing both the colon and the rectum before finally joining them. Tension is entirely preventable by fully mobilizing the proximal colon, dividing the inferior mesenteric vein at the lower border of the pancreas, and unfolding the splenic flexure as described earlier. Poor blood supply is often caused by tension. If there is tension on the proximal colon, its blood supply, which may have appeared to be satisfactory when tested in the abdomen, becomes compromised when an inadequately mobilized colon is forcibly stretched down into the pelvis. The anastomosis must not resemble a dog on a tight leash.

Anastomotic leakage is often referred to as clinical (overt) or subclinical. The reported incidence varies between 1% and 29%, with an average of 11%.[485,486,492] The frequency is higher after low and ultralow colorectal anastomoses. The anastomotic leak rates in our patients are shown in Table 24-3.

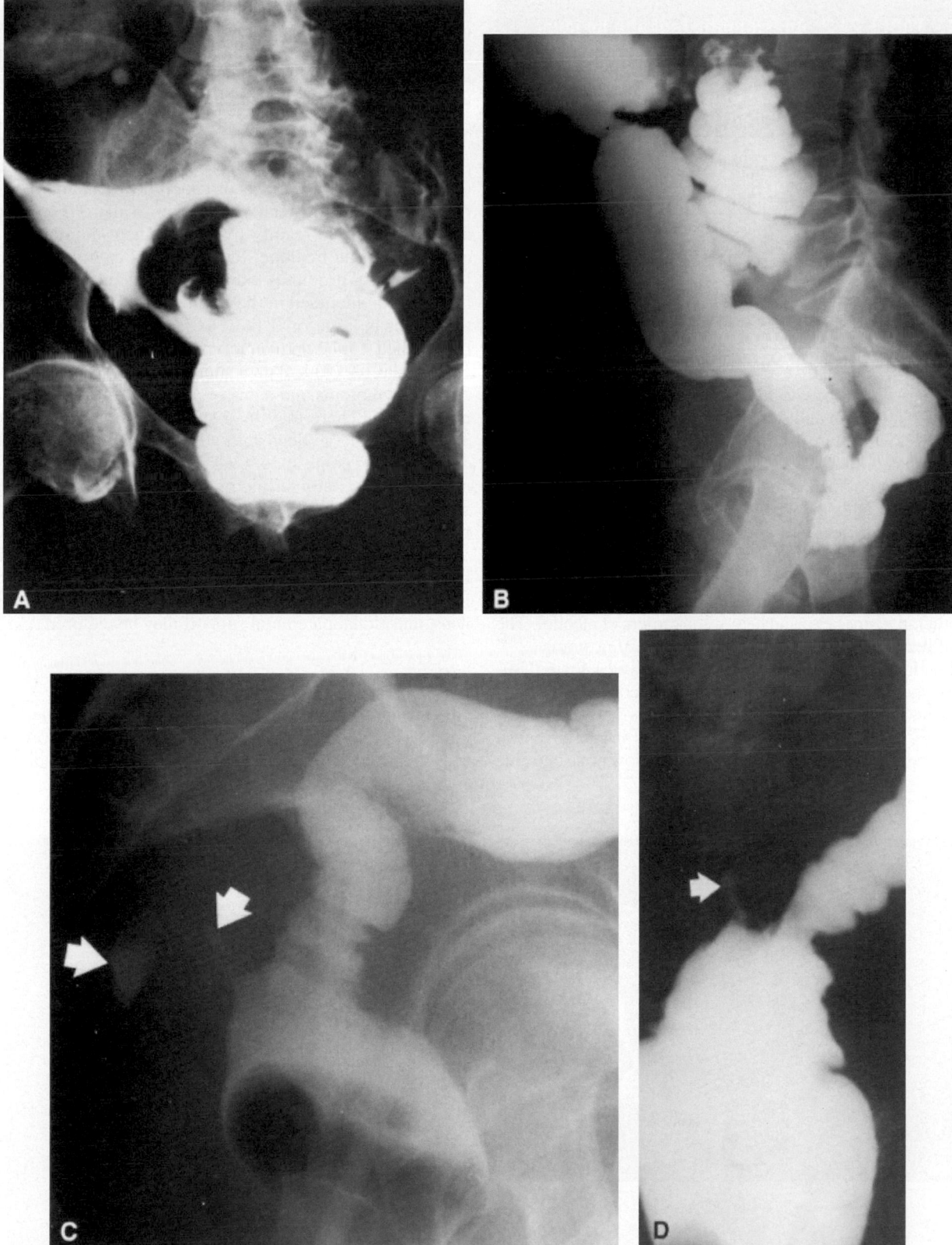

FIGURE 24-86. Anastomotic leaks. **A:** Gastrografin enema demonstrates extravasation into the pelvis 1 week following anterior resection. **B:** Large, abscess cavity in presacral space. **C:** Fistula tract with abscess (*arrows*). **D:** Short anastomotic sinus tract (*arrow*).

TABLE 24-3 Anastomotic leakage by level of tumor following anterior resections performed by members of the Concord Hospital Colorectal Unit (Sydney, Australia) between 1995 and 2010.

	0–7 cm n = 135	8–11 cm n = 256	≥12 cm n = 274
Clinical leak	4%	1%	1%
Subclinical leak	8%	4%	2%

There is no evidence to suggest that there is any difference between hand-sewn and stapled anastomoses, although most surgeons now prefer a stapled technique. Several risk factors for anastomotic leak have been identified, although not all have been confirmed as having an independent effect in multivariable analyses. The two factors having the strongest association with leak are nodal involvement and height of the anastomosis above the anal verge; the higher the site, the lower the risk. Leaks are reported as being more common in males; older patients; obese patients; after short-course radiotherapy; smokers; and heavy consumers of alcohol. The risk of leak is decreased by temporary diverting stoma.[141,436]

The clinical picture of overt leakage is well known. Usually, on the fourth or fifth day, the patient becomes unwell and complains of abdominal pain and tenderness. The abdomen is frequently distended with rebound tenderness and absent bowel sounds. Fever, tachycardia, hypotension, and low urine outcome are common. An abdominal x-ray usually shows dilated loops of small bowel and there may be gas under the diaphragm. The diagnosis can be confirmed either by an urgent limited gastrograffin enema or a CT scan (see Figure 24-86). In some patients, there may be a gas or fecal discharge through the drain.

Overt clinical leakage is a medical emergency. The patient needs to be resuscitated urgently and reoperated as soon as possible. At laparotomy, a decision has to be made whether to maintain the anastomosis or take it down and convert the procedure to a Hartmann's operation. If there is a discreet defect that can be readily oversewn, then maintaining the anastomosis can be done; the peritoneal cavity thoroughly lavaged and a proximal loop ileostomy constructed if that had not been included in the original operation. If, however, the defect is large or if there is ischemia of the proximal bowel, then it is better to convert to a Hartmann's procedure.

Whereas the clinical presentation of an overt leak is obvious, the symptoms and signs of a subclinical leak are much more subtle. There may be a slight fever and tachycardia. There is usually an ileus with varying degrees of abdominal distension and some abdominal discomfort with mild tenderness. If there is any suspicion, a gastrograffin enema may show a very small leak, and this may or may not be confirmed by CT scan (Figure 24-87).

Patients with a subclinical leak are often treated expectantly by keeping them fasting and administering broad-spectrum intravenous antibiotics. In some patients with a prolonged ileus, nutritional parenteral support may be required.

Consequences of Anastomotic Leakage

Apart from the clinical consequences discussed earlier, anastomotic leakage is often associated with one or more other complications. These include cardiovascular, respiratory,

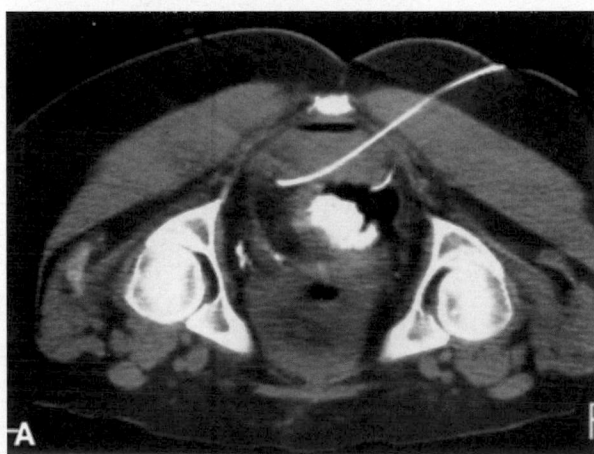
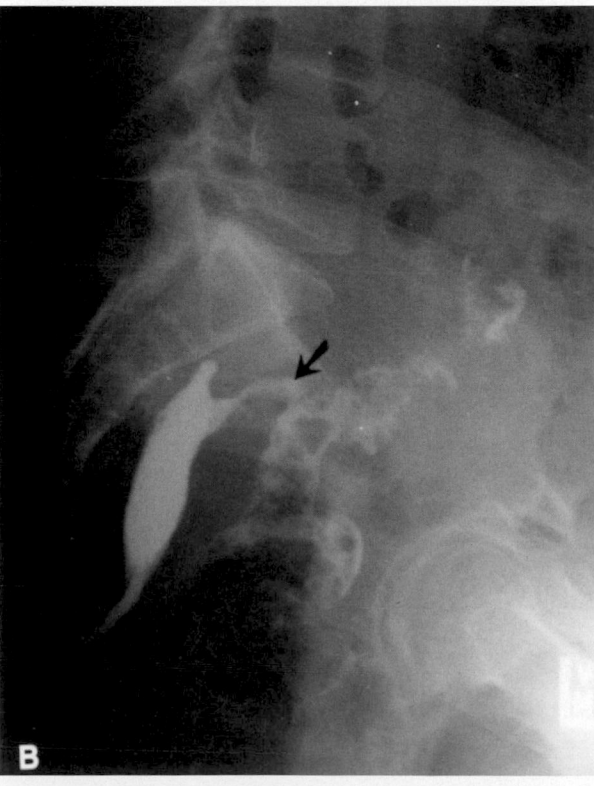

FIGURE 24-87. Anastomotic leak. **A:** Computed tomography–guided transgluteal drainage. **B:** Lateral view demonstrates contrast material in the presacral cavity and communication with rectum (*arrow*).

and thromboembolic complications. This is equally true of both clinically overt and subclinical leakage. There is a misconception that subclinical leakage is a minor and relatively unimportant complication, whereas in fact we have found that it can be associated with as much additional morbidity as that of clinically overt leakage.[627]

Apart from the septic complications associated with anastomotic leakage, we have found that there is a significant increase in length of stay, an increase in use of hospital resources (including high dependency and intensive care), and an increase demand for cross consultation with other physicians from other disciplines.[184] Unfortunately, there are other serious consequences of anastomotic leakage.[141,393,430,436,485,486] We have also found that leakage is associated with a significantly higher rate of local recurrence.[43] Furthermore, our group has reported that survival is diminished in patients who develop a leak.[634]

Pelvic Abscess and Hematoma

Pelvic abscess and hematoma can develop after a restorative procedure. The symptoms include a fever, tachycardia, pelvic discomfort, an urge to defecate, urinary frequency, and dysuria. The white cell count is usually raised, and the patient looks septic. A CT scan can readily identify the abscess that is often located posteriorly and close to the anastomosis.

The treatment is percutaneous CT-guided drainage. A hematoma can be treated expectantly in the hope that it does not develop into an abscess.

Pelvic abscesses can spontaneously drain through the back wall of the anastomosis in which case an anastomotic leak becomes established (see Figure 24-87). If a loop ileostomy has already been performed, then no further surgical treatment may be indicated. If, however, a loop ileostomy had not been constructed and the patient develops symptoms and signs of an overt anastomotic dehiscence, then laparotomy with peritoneal lavage and the establishment of a loop ileostomy may be necessary.

Fecal Fistula

Fecal fistula may develop in the postoperative period as a consequence of an anastomotic leak (see earlier discussion). Usually, this complication requires abdominal drainage and a diversionary procedure. However, if the fistula arises at a later time, perhaps following drainage of an intra-abdominal or pelvic abscess, it can often be treated expectantly if there is absence of overt intraperitoneal sepsis and the patient continues to have bowel movements. Without distal obstruction, sepsis, or persistent tumor, the fistula may close spontaneously. If drainage is excessive, a stomal appliance may be used (see Chapters 31 and 32).

There is no need to limit dietary intake for a colonic fistula. This will not expedite the healing process, and moreover, outputs generally are not excessive. Total parenteral nutrition and an elemental diet are both costly and unhelpful for individuals with a fistula in this location. If the patient does experience quite a bit of drainage, one must be certain of the location of the fistula and that the small bowel is not involved. A fistulogram and CT scan may be helpful in locating the site of the fistula. One can limit the amount of drainage through the use of a "slowing" regimen, including codeine, deodorized tincture of opium, and diphenoxylate with atropine (Lomotil) or loperamide (Imodium).

Failure to heal suggests the formation of an epithelialized tract or recurrent tumor. The presence of foreign material is another possibility, and an obstructed anastomosis must be ruled out. Reoperation for an established fistula from a colorectal anastomosis can be very challenging. The patient is best served by an expert team in a well-resourced tertiary referral hospital.

Rectovaginal Fistula

Rectovaginal fistula following low anterior resection may result from pelvic sepsis and an anastomotic leak, with spontaneous drainage through the vagina, especially in patients who have had a hysterectomy. Occasionally, the cause of a rectovaginal fistula is the inadvertent inclusion of the vagina in a stapled anastomosis, a complication that is more likely to occur if the patient had a prior hysterectomy. Transvaginal drainage of a pelvic collection may ultimately yield feculent material. Unfortunately, rectovaginal fistulas will rarely heal spontaneously, and fecal diversion as an initial procedure is required. Several months later, consideration can be given to dealing with this complex situation. Major reoperative surgery is required, usually involving a redo ultralow anterior resection or a coloanal pull-through procedure, and in some patients, a permanent stoma.

Psychological Support for Patients with Anastomotic Leakage and Fistulae

Patients who develop these complications are especially at risk of developing depression, frustration, and anger. They and their families need to be informed openly and honestly about these complications, and competent psychological support should be provided. There should be no hesitation in seeking wide consultation and offering a second opinion. These complications are trying for both patient and surgeon.

Stomal Closure after Low Anterior Resection

If a loop ileostomy has been performed at the time of anterior resection, then closure is usually performed 6 to 8 weeks after the initial operation. Before closing the stoma, a limited gastrograffin enema and a flexible sigmoidoscopy are performed to ensure that the anastomosis is patent and not leaking. Closure of a loop ileostomy can be technically demanding and should be performed with meticulous attention to detail (see Chapter 31).

Closure of the Stoma in Patients Who Have Had an Anastomotic Leak

Several months need to elapse before closing a stoma under these circumstances. The gastrograffin enema should be repeated to ensure that there is no free leakage into the peritoneal cavity. Ideally, there should be no leakage at all, but if the anastomoses is very low and there is a small posterior and well-confined leak, the stoma may be closed.

If a significant leak persists, consideration should be given to reoperating at a later date and to resect the anastomosis or to refashion it. This is a very complex procedure requiring considerable expertise in redo pelvic surgery.

Late Complications of Anterior Resection
Rectal Stricture

Rectal stricture has been defined by members of the American Society of Colon and Rectal Surgeons as one's inability to

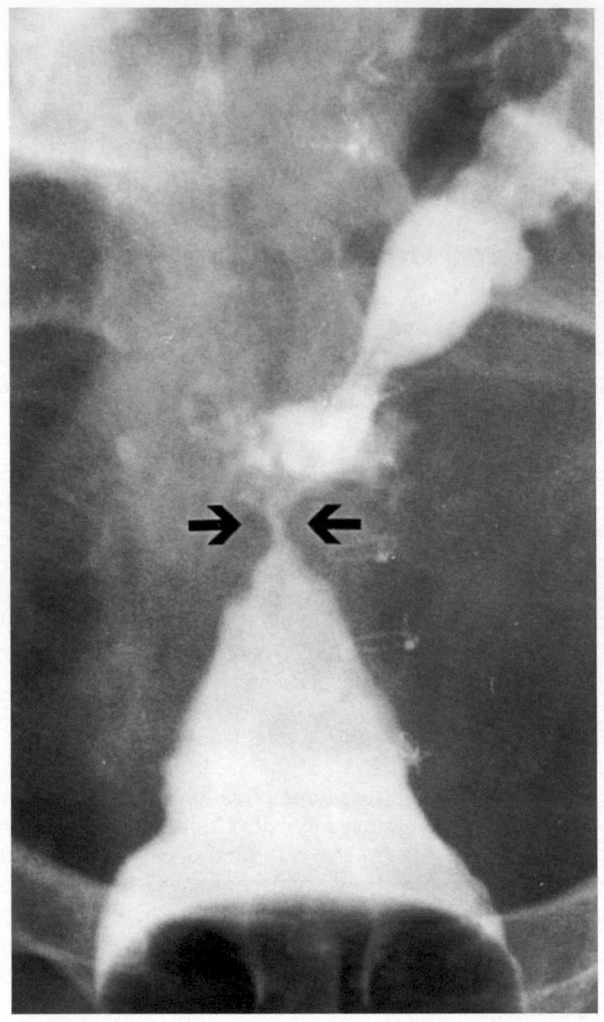

FIGURE 24-88. Contrast enema reveals rectal stricture (*arrows*) following anastomotic leak. This proved to be benign.

Many colorectal strictures can be dealt with simply by endoscopic balloon dilatation or other straightforward methods. A significant proportion, however, are much more complicated. This group is usually a consequence of such complex issues as ischemia of the proximal colon, anastomotic leakage, pelvic sepsis, the effects of radiation, and recurrent disease. These are much more difficult to diagnose and to treat. The patients require considerable expertise in reoperative pelvic surgery. It is important to determine early whether one is dealing with a simple or a complex stricture, and this issue requires careful evaluation.

Management

Nonsurgical treatment of an anastomotic stricture consists of the use of stool softeners, enemas, or suppositories. Dilatation can be performed manually if it is within reach of the finger. For higher strictures (i.e., at a level of 8 to 12 cm), a double-ended Hegar's dilator (17 to 18 mm) or a flexible bougie may be used (Figure 24-89). Another alternative is to pass a narrow (1.1 cm) sigmoidoscope with its obturator through the stricture, gradually dilating the opening with serial passage of instruments of increasing diameter. For higher level strictures, Hood and Lewis recommend a curved metal dilator, modeled after the Lister urethral dilator, because the curvature of the sacrum and the angulation of the bowel may make passage impossible.[270] The application of the technique of endoscopic balloon dilatation, with or without the use of a guidewire, has also been reported (Figure 24-90).[16,35,39,410,457,471] Most patients require two to four dilatations, repeated at 3-month intervals.[313] There is a risk, of course, of perforating the bowel, a particular concern if the stricture is above the level of the peritoneal reflection. One must weigh the morbidity of the procedure itself against the alternative of a major abdominal operation.

If a symptomatic stricture persists, transanal lysis with knife or electrocautery in the posterior midline may ameliorate the condition (Figure 24-91A). The use of the optical urethrotome knife has also been described[105] as well as a device called a "staple cutter" (a variation of a bone cutter).[564] Another option is the use of an endostapler (Figure 24-92).[103,473] Endoscopic laser has also been use to deal with this complication.[377] The application of the technique used for endoscopic papillotomy has also been suggested for the treatment of stricture,[3] as has the Eder-Puestow dilatation over a guidewire, the technique employed for the management of esophageal strictures.[658]

Following the procedure, frequent office visits with dilatation as necessary is recommended for a number of weeks. This requirement may be obviated if it is possible to perform a proctoplasty, closing a proctotomy in a transverse fashion

pass a 12-mm diameter sigmoidoscope through the narrowed area.[376] Symptoms are quite variable, however, and do not necessarily parallel the degree of narrowing. These may include constipation, tenesmus, fecal soiling, urgency, diarrhea, and signs and symptoms of large bowel obstruction. Much depends on stool consistency and the level of the anastomosis, not only the degree narrowing. Benign stricture following anterior resection is usually a consequence of an anastomotic breakdown with subsequent fibrosis (Figure 24-88).

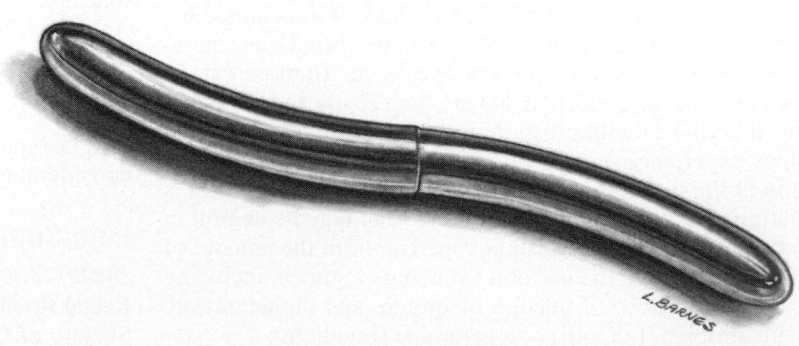

FIGURE 24-89. The double-ended Hegar's dilator is a useful tool in the treatment of strictures in the middle and upper rectum.

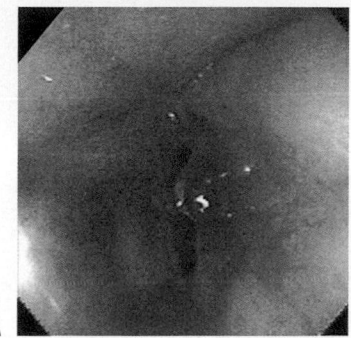
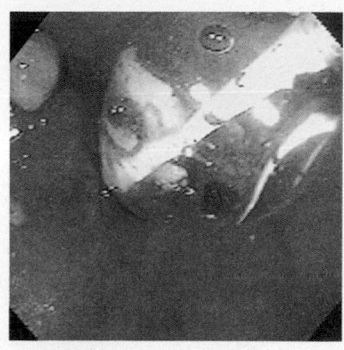

FIGURE 24-90. A benign rectal stricture is discovered following high anterior resection. **A:** Marked narrowing can be seen through the flexible endoscope. **B:** The stricture is dilated by the insertion of an endoscopic balloon.

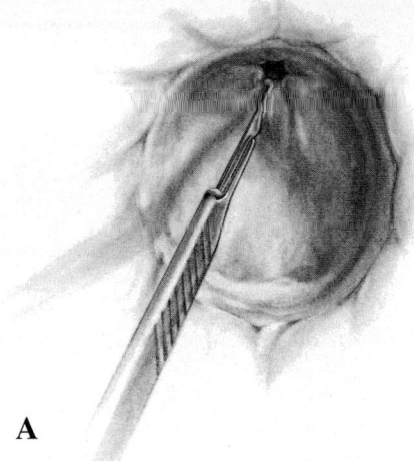

A

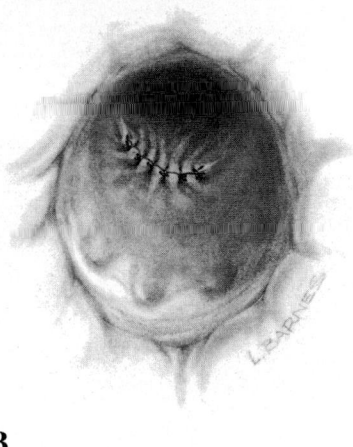

B

FIGURE 24-91. Rectal stricture at the site of a low colorectal anastomosis. **A:** Lysis is performed posteriorly. **B:** Ideally, a proctoplasty is accomplished by means of transverse closure of the longitudinal proctotomy.

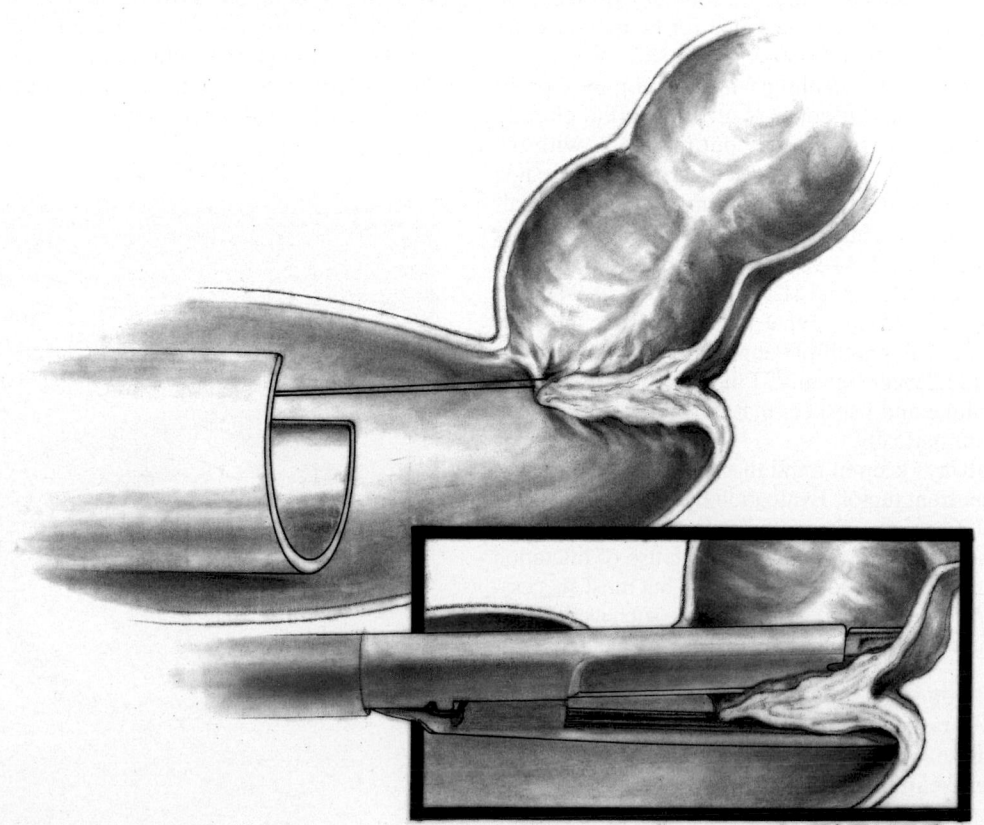

FIGURE 24-92. Technique of division of anastomotic stricture as performed through a Fansler rectoscope using the endo-GIA stapler. (Adapted from Pagni S, McLaughlin CM. Simple technique for the treatment of strictured colorectal anastomosis. *Dis Colon Rectum.* 1995;38:433.)

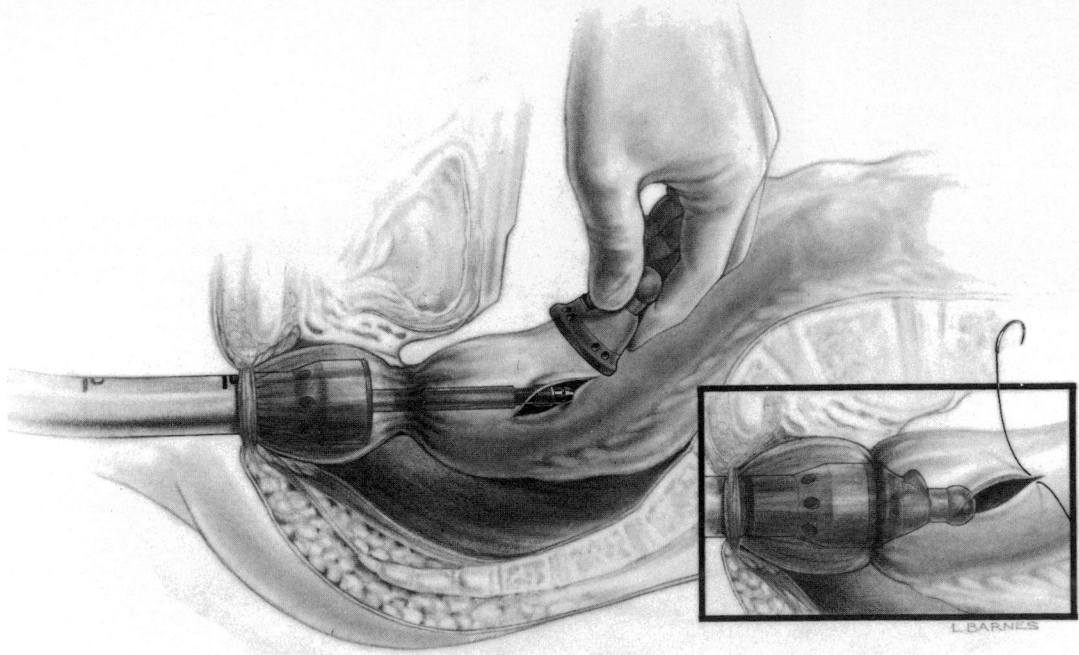

FIGURE 24-93. Excision of strictured anastomosis with circular stapler. Enterotomy in proximal bowel permits replacement of anvil. The enterotomy is then closed (*inset*).

(Figure 24-91B). Analogous to the Heineke-Mikulicz pyloroplasty as applied to the rectum, it is hoped that the diameter can be maintained without recurrent stenosis. The Wallstent prosthesis has also been advocated for relieving obstruction, not only for malignant tumors but also for benign stricture (see Figures 23-85 through 23-89).[543]

Another technique for dealing with this complex problem has been described. It consists of passing the circular stapling instrument transanally without the anvil, with the center rod traversing the stricture. An enterotomy is created proximal to the strictured anastomosis, and the rod is visualized (Figure 24-93). The anvil is replaced, and the instrument closed and fired (Figure 24-93, *inset*). A single tissue ring is created, which is the actual stricture (Figure 24-94). The enterotomy is then closed. Ovnat and colleagues describe the same method, using multiple applications of the circular stapler to create a larger lumen.[470] I have had no experience with this technique and I suspect that it is not as simple as it appears diagrammatically.

One must always keep in mind that the cause of the stricture may be recurrent tumor. Evaluation by means of CT scan may be helpful, but biopsy or cytologic study is mandatory for establishing the diagnosis.[653] Obviously, the use of dilatation as a palliative measure has some merit,[594,620] but most successful reports employ cutting and ablating tools, such as the laser and electrocoagulator, for malignant disease (see later).[471]

Redo Pelvic Surgery for Anastomotic Strictures

If conservative measures fail, then redo surgery should be considered. These are complex procedure that requires considerable expertise in redo pelvic surgery.

Virtually, all of the reports concerning the management of rectal strictures are essentially individual case studies. The long-term effectiveness of the various modalities has not been subjected to critical analysis. One exception is the

publication of Johansson in a prospective study of 18 patients with rectal stricture.[294] Through the use of endoscopic balloon dilatation, two-thirds had complete relief of their obstructive symptoms. Two of the patients considered the results to be poor, and four were not subjected to follow-up evaluation. One perforation developed as a consequence of the procedure. Schlegel and colleagues in Paris identified 13 patients who had been referred for surgical treatment of

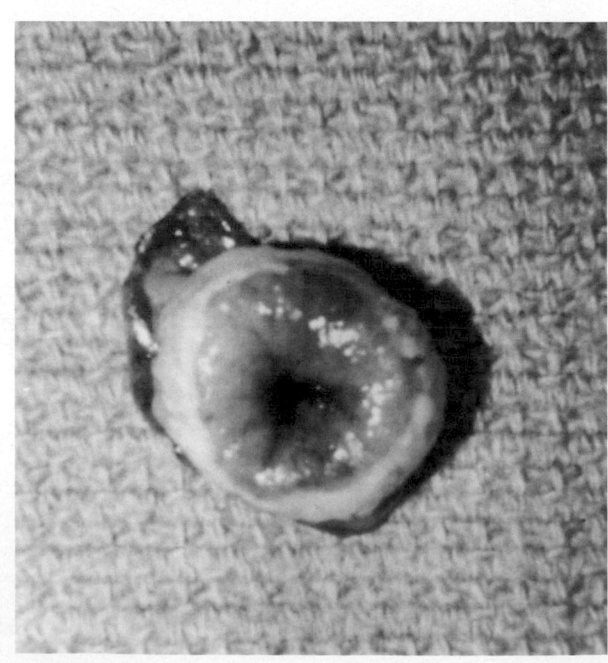

FIGURE 24-94. Single "doughnut" demonstrates marked luminal narrowing following stapler resection of a stricture.

rectal anastomotic strictures whose original procedure was for rectal cancer.[556] Repeat resection was performed using various techniques for reestablishment of anal continuity without recurrence and with satisfactory functional results.

Incontinence and Irregular Bowel Function

Low anterior resection, irrespective of anastomotic technique, may be associated with varying degrees of incontinence for flatus, feces, or both.[209,212] After closure of a loop ileostomy, many patients experience a period of erratic bowel function that usually settles within 6 to 12 months. It is worthwhile forewarning patients of this likelihood before closing the stoma.

One concern about the stapling technique is that sphincter disruption can occur from dilatation associated with the passage of the instrument. The issue of stretching the internal and external sphincters is addressed in Chapter 12. Injury to the sphincters during transanal instrumentation has been demonstrated by a number of techniques, including endorectal ultrasound, and has been found to be associated with reduced resting and squeeze pressures when compared with patients who underwent hand-sewn anastomoses.[168,261,433] Long-term functional impairment may also be a consequence of anastomotic leakage and pelvic sepsis.[235]

Studies by Pedersen and colleagues of anorectal function following low anterior resection revealed that most patients demonstrate an abnormal rectoanal inhibitory reflex.[497] Rectal compliance was also lower 3 months after operation but had returned to normal in every individual by 12 months. Nakahara and coworkers found that all of their patients who underwent low anterior resection with anastomosis by the circular stapling device suffered from frequent bowel actions and soiling.[453] These symptoms improved to a virtually normal state by 6 months, as did rectal sensation and reservoir capacity. However, abnormal rectoanal inhibitory reflex, anal canal resting pressure, and maximum squeeze pressure persisted. O'Riordain and colleagues found that in the majority of patients who underwent low anterior resection, the rectoanal inhibitory reflex was abolished and remained absent throughout the first year.[468] However, in their experience, this reflex had recovered by the end of the second postoperative year in all patients. Lewis and associates opined that continence after anterior resection is related to the sampling response that the anal sphincter develops to activity within the neorectum.[353,354] The length of the residual rectum is believed to be of critical importance in maintaining effective function. Yamana and coworkers performed preoperative and postoperative physiologic studies on patients who underwent low anterior resection.[661] They found that a longer preoperative high-pressure zone, a larger preoperative maximum tolerable volume, and a lower sensory threshold were associated with better postoperative defecatory function. Older age has been thought by some to be an independent prognostic factor for increased incontinence risk. When patients older than 75 years were asked at 1 year following some form of restorative proctectomy, Phillips and colleagues found that 78 of their 92 patients (85%) denied "significant problems."[501]

Inflammatory reaction, narrowing at the anastomosis, sensory impairment, and bowel denervation all may contribute to impairment of control and irregular bowel habits. However, as long as the anal canal and sphincter muscles have been preserved and there is no anastomic abnormality, the symptoms usually resolve in a matter of a few months. Most patients are able to regulate themselves by paying more attention to their diet than had been their custom. Eventually, for most patients, dietary restrictions become unnecessary.

▶ LOCAL RECURRENCE AFTER EXCISION OF THE RECTUM FOR CANCER

The term "local recurrence" after potentially curative resection (M0, R0) of the rectum for cancer has been variously described as recurrence at an anastomotic line (if a restorative procedure has been performed), recurrence in the pelvis alone, or recurrence in the pelvis with distant metastases. However, the actual definition of local recurrence after potentially curative resection of rectal cancer varies among studies but is most appropriately defined as histologically confirmed recurrence anywhere in the pelvis, either occurring alone or in the presence of newly diagnosed distant metastasis.[145] These specifications are important in order to enable meaningful comparisons between series and for testing different treatment modalities.

The reported frequency of local recurrence varies widely in the literature, partly because of different definitions, different staging systems, differences in the follow-up period, different follow-up protocols, and different statistical analytic methods. In our hospital series (Concord, Sydney, NSW, Australia) analyzing 1,084 anterior resections, abdominoperineal excisions, and Hartmann's operations between 1980 and 2004, 80% of recurrences were diagnosed within 3 years and 97% within 5 years. The rate of local recurrence in an operative series is conventionally quoted for a given time period (e.g., a 3-year rate or a 5-year rate). It is essential that all patients who have not died nor lost to follow-up should be followed for the full time period of the specified rate. The local recurrence rate should not be given as a crude rate; rather, a time-to-event method of calculation should be used (e.g., the Kaplan-Meier method or competing risks method).

In the Concord Hospital series from 1980 to 2004 and in patients who had a potentially curative resection (no tumor in any margin histologically), there were 87 local recurrences within 5 years (a K-M rate of 9.7). As in other studies,[164,338] by far the strongest factor influencing the local recurrence rate was tumor stage, particularly the distinction between stage I/II and stage III. In the Concord Hospital series, the 5-year rate for stage I tumors was 3.5%; for stage II, 7.0%; and for stage III, 17.6%. There was no significant difference in rates between anterior resection, abdominoperineal excision, and Hartmann's operation. Other factors that were not related to local recurrence were patient age, preoperative chemoradiotherapy, tumor level, tumor size, histologic type, surgical perforation, distal margin ≤ 1 cm, and the length of time for the operation. Factors that had a univariate association with local recurrence are shown in Table 24-4. For simplicity of presentation, each factor is given in binary form as the risk group (e.g., high histologic grade) versus the reference group (average grade or low grade). Despite the broad range of factors having a univariate association with local recurrence, a multivariable Cox regression model showed that only lymph node metastasis, T3/T4 direct spread, male sex, and anastomotic leak were independently associated with local recurrence. Anterior position of the tumor has also been shown as independently associated with local recurrence.[94]

TABLE 24-4 Features associated with local recurrence in 1,048 patients who had a potentially curative resection for rectal cancer at Concord Hospital between 1995 and 2010 inclusive.

	UNIVARIATE HAZARD RATIO	UNIVARIATE P VALUE	MULTIVARIABLE HAZARD RATIO	MULTIVARIABLE P VALUE
Male sex	1.6	.059	1.7	.042
Direct spread beyond muscularis propria	3.3	<.001	2.0	.023
Lymph node metastasis	3.6	<.001	2.3	.002
Apical node involved	1.4	.005	—	n.s.
≥4 nodes involved	3.5	<.001	—	n.s.
Venous invasion	2.2	<.001	—	n.s.
High grade	2.6	<.001	—	n.s.
Adjacent organ or structure infiltrated	3.6	.030	—	n.s.
Free serosal surface involved	3.1	.002	—	n.s.
Anastomotic leak	2.1	.024	2.2	.024

n.s., not significant.

There is an extensive literature on the association between local recurrence and tumor clearance from the circumferential resection margin, and although it is clear that tumor actually transected at the resection margin must carry a high risk of recurrence, there is less clarity on the risk associated with tumor in a defined marginal zone but not actually in the line of resection.[145] Thus, apart from these clinical and histopathologic variables, the only other factor that has been found to be associated with a significantly lower prevalence of local recurrence is *surgical technique*. In particular, an anatomical extrafascial technique of rectal mobilization, as has been described earlier in this chapter, and other similar approaches have proven effective.[43,68]

In the past, local recurrence has been regarded as an important outcome variable in studies assessing the quality of surgical and other treatments for rectal cancer; but more recently, it has been appreciated that from the patient's point of view, neither local recurrence, overall recurrence, nor cancer-specific survival are as important as overall survival. Hence, contemporary studies, particularly randomized controlled trials of treatment, are increasingly accepting overall survival as the principal outcome variable.

Circumferential Resection Margins and Local Recurrence

In recent literature, the importance of assessing circumferential margins has been stressed by both surgeons and pathologists as a prognostic indicator of local recurrence (LR), survival, and quality assurance.[305,452,505,506,652] There is great variability in the rate of circumferential margin involvement in published reports (1% to 33%).[452] Assessing the evidence for an association between circumferential resection margin involvement (CRMI) and the development of LR is complex and variable. This is due to the impact of a large number of factors, including the nature of the patient series (prospective vs. retrospective), surgical technique, curative versus palliative resection, pathology, the definition of CRMI as transected tumor versus tumor within a specified marginal zone, the use of radiotherapy, definition and ascertainment of LR, length of follow-up, and methods of statistical analysis.[145] In view of these factors, a simple objective definition of CRMI as histologic confirmation of tumor transected in a surgical margin is preferable.[145] Emphasizing the use of CRMI as a measure of quality of surgery without taking into consideration the impact of the varying prevalence of numerous risk factors is of concern and an important source of bias.[99] The role of preoperative MRI in predicting CRMI should be interpreted with some caution. Although MRI is undoubtedly a useful tool for providing accurate assessment of the extent of spread of tumor within the pelvis and therefore assists the multidisciplinary team in planning neoadjuvant therapy and surgery, logically it cannot predict validly histologic CRMI. Indeed, patients with a positive MRI margin, correctly managed, should have a negative resection margin.[144]

▶ SURVIVAL AFTER EXCISION OF THE RECTUM FOR CANCER

Overall survival—that is, patient survival from the time of resection to the time of death from any cause—is the principal survival measure for assessing outcome following excision of the rectum for cancer. Disease-specific survival is computed in some studies, but this fails to take account of treatment-related (iatrogenic) mortality. Also, from the patient's point of view, what matters is foreshortened life span from any cause rather than death directly attributable to cancer. Because disease-specific survival does not take account deaths due to causes other than rectal cancer, survival rates in studies reporting such survival will be lower than in studies reporting overall survival. This needs to be taken into account when comparing different patient series.

Clinicopathologic stage, incorporating the extent of direct tumor spread within the bowel wall, local or regional lymph node involvement, and systemic metastasis, is by far the strongest predictor of overall survival. In the Concord Hospital consecutive series of all rectal cancer resections from 1980 to 2004 (n = 1,297), all with follow-up to 2009, the overall 5-year survival rates according to the TNM staging system were stage I, 81%; stage II, 65%; stage III, 44%; and stage IV, 4% (Figure 24-95). Apart from stage, many other patient characteristics, operative variables, pathology features, and potential genetic or proteomic tumor markers have been investigated regarding their independent prognostic power—that is, their ability to predict survival after adjustment for other

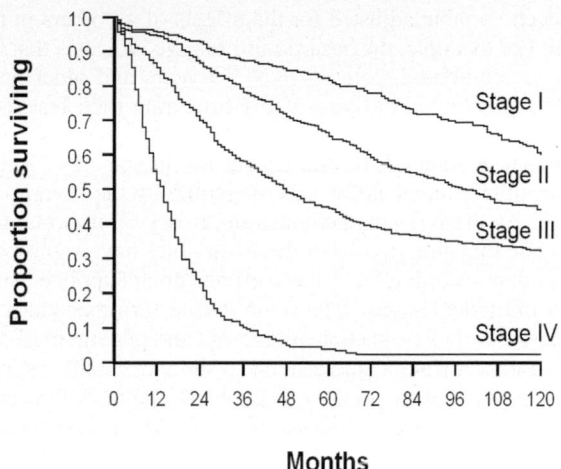

FIGURE 24-95. Survival according to stage in 1,297 patients with rectal cancer treated at Concord Hospital (Sydney, NSW, Australia).

already well-understood prognostic features, such as stage. Examples include histologic grade, venous invasion, perineural involvement, distal and circumferential clearance margins, anastomotic leakage, the position of the tumor (anterior, posterior, etc.), surgical technique, numbers of rectal cancer surgery performed, neoadjuvant and adjuvant therapy, and many other factors. Table 24-5 shows the results of multivariable modeling of such variables in the Concord Hospital series,

TABLE 24-5 Association between prognostic features and overall survival in 1,297 patients who had a resection for rectal cancer at Concord Hospital between 1980 and 2004, with follow-up to end of 2009.

FEATURES	ALL PATIENTS n = 1,297 HR, P	STAGE I n = 287 HR, P	STAGE II n = 374 HR, P	STAGE III n = 447 HR, P	STAGE IV n = 189 HR, P
Age ≥75 years	2.1, <.001	3.9, <.001	2.5, <.001	1.9, <.001	n.s.
Direct spread beyond muscularis propria	1.5, <.001	n.a.	n.a.	1.5, .028	n.s.
Apical node involved	1.9, <.001	n.a.	n.a.	1.9, .005	n.s.
≥4 nodes involved	1.8, <.001	n.a.	n.a.	1.4, .009	n.s.
High grade	1.3, .001	n.s.	n.s.	n.s.	1.5, .020
Venous invasion	1.5, <.001	n.s.	n.s.	1.6, <.001	n.s.
Distal margin ≤1 cm	1.6, .003	n.s.	n.s.	2.5, .003	n.s.
Free serosal surface involved	1.5, .002	n.a.	n.s.	n.s.	n.s.
Tumor in a line of resection	2.3, <.001	n.a.	2.7, <.001	2.1, <.001	1.7, .013
Nonrestorative operation[a]	1.3, <.001	.028	n.s.	n.s.	n.s.

[a]Abdominoperineal resection or Hartmann's operation. HR, hazard ratio; n.s., not significant; n.a., not applicable.

with each variable adjusted for the effects of all others in the model. For example, the hazard ratio for age indicates that for all stages combined, patients aged 75 years and older have 2.1 times likelihood of dying at any time after their resection as compared with younger patients. This effect is statistically significant in stages I, II, and III but not in stage IV, where any possible influence of age is overcome by the severity of disease. As these results demonstrate, it is very important to appreciate that although all of these variables have significant independent overall effects, these effects do not apply equally within individual stages. The same is true for other kinds of prognostic variables, such as proteomic and genetic markers. Furthermore, different studies tend to show different survival results because of the range of variables analyzed, the stage mix of included patients, and sample size. Despite the already very extensive literature on factors influencing survival after excision of rectal cancer, considerable investigative work remains to be completed in this area of interstage differences.

▶ TREATMENT OF LOCAL RECURRENCE

The treatment of metastatic disease following resection of colorectal carcinoma is presented in Chapter 23. The discussion that follows is limited to the specific problem of recurrence in the pelvis following either APR or a restorative procedure for cancer.

Symptoms and Diagnosis of Perineal Recurrence

Perineal recurrence is seldom perineal alone. It is often a manifestation of systemic disease. The patient may complain of a painful mass (Figure 24-96). This may be the result of implantation in the skin, but more commonly, it is a consequence of downward extension of pelvic tumor. Biopsy usually confirms the diagnosis. With pelvic recurrence, an individual may be asymptomatic, but usually the patient will report perineal,

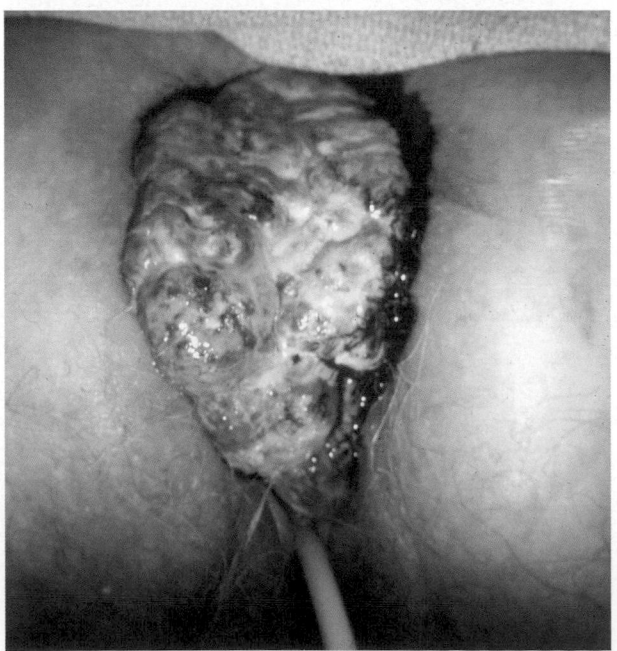

FIGURE 24-96. Fungating recurrent carcinoma of the perineum following abdominoperineal resection.

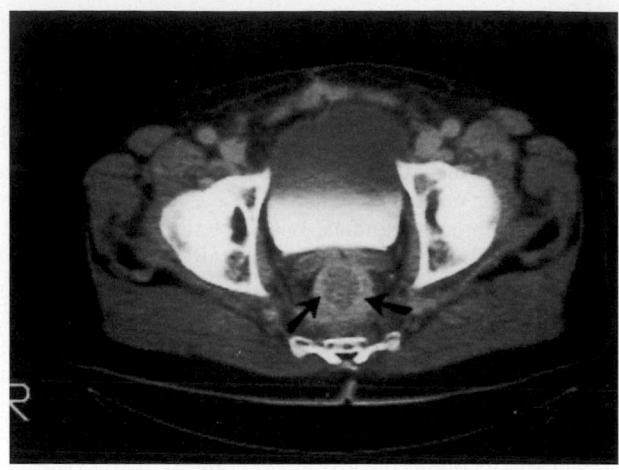

FIGURE 24-97. Computed tomography scan of pelvis. Recurrent pelvic carcinoma following abdominoperineal resection. Note the tumor mass with central necrosis (*arrows*). The seminal vesicles can be clearly seen.

pelvic, or low abdominal pain or the sensation of "sitting on a lump." The pain may radiate to the back, to the buttock, or have a sciatic distribution. If the tumor involves the bladder, prostate, or urethra, urinary symptoms (including hematuria) may develop. Urethral obstruction can supervene, but the most troubling, indeed disabling, complaint is the pain.

A mass may be felt in the perineum or in the vagina. CT and MRI have been used successfully to delineate both the presence of a tumor mass and the extent of pelvic spread, as well as evidence of ureteric obstruction (Figures 24-97 and 24-98).[279] These studies have also been suggested as potentially valuable adjuncts for follow-up evaluation in order to anticipate recurrence before symptoms appear. CT-guided percutaneous biopsy has been demonstrated to be a particularly useful tool for establishing the histologic diagnosis of recurrent carcinoma in the pelvis.[85,349,459,665] Still, one should not need histologic confirmation in order to implement therapy. Elevation of the CEA level is certainly suggestive of recurrent disease, but the CEA may be within the normal range if the recurrence is confined to the pelvis. This is in contradistinction to those patients who have involvement of the liver or another organ (see Chapter 23). A CT with intravenous and oral contrast or an intravenous pyelogram may be performed, especially if there is concern for impingement on the ureters on the basis (Figure 24-99). An elevated serum creatinine is obviously an ominous finding. Treatment, at least initially, requires decompression by means of an internal stent.

Surgical Treatment

The surgical treatment of pelvic recurrence is complex. It requires careful assessment to determine the extent of the recurrence, the degree of local invasion and invasion into vital pelvic structures, and the elimination of metastatic disease. A multidisciplinary approach is often needed involving several surgical and oncologic specialties.

V. W. Fazio (personal communication) has described a number of technical tips for reoperative abdominal and pelvic surgery for cancer. Extensive preoperative investigation is mandatory, including CT. T1- and T2-weighted imaging is important to exclude bony erosion or pelvic side wall involvement. The presence of such tumor extension implies nonresectability and contraindication to adventuresome

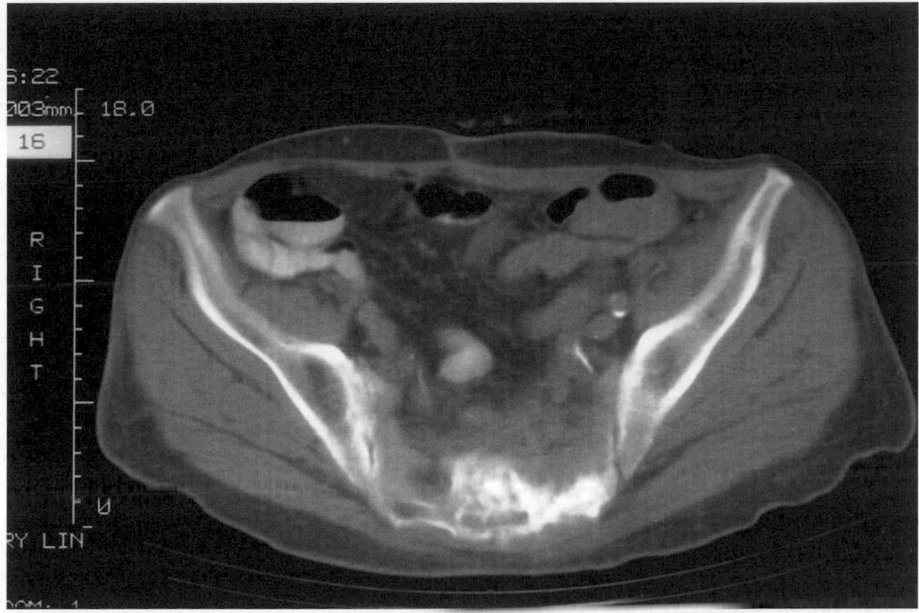

FIGURE 24-98. Computed tomography demonstrates erosion of the sacral bone from recurrent rectal cancer.

surgery. It is wise to begin this type of surgery first thing in the morning and to not schedule any other difficult operations during that day. One should anticipate the need for specialty help, such as urology, orthopedics, and neurosurgery. The list of recommendations made by V. W. Fazio includes the following:

- Conduct a colon study for local and remote metastases.
- Provide ureteric stents.

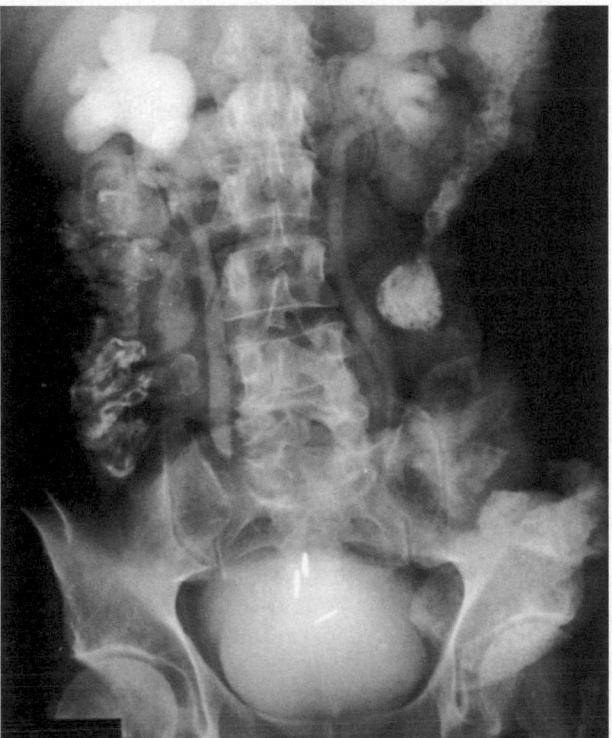

FIGURE 24-99. Intravenous pyelogram demonstrates hydroureters with marked dilatation of the renal pelvices and calyces, a consequence of recurrent rectal cancer.

- Schedule the case early in the day.
- Anticipate the need for other specialists.
- Ensure the availability of experienced assistance.
- Plan the incision carefully.
- Allow for a steep Trendelenburg position.
- Position the patient's arms at the sides.
- Use lighted instruments and/or headlights.
- Anticipate excessive blood loss.

The foregoing list is only a means for preoperatively reminding the surgeon of the magnitude of reoperative cancer surgery. It is by no means exhaustive.

Results

Unfortunately, there is no truly satisfactory treatment for perineal or pelvic recurrence. There is, however, the rare instance when perineal (the equivalent of suture line) recurrence develops secondary to implantation or to an inadequate skin excision (Figure 24-100). It still may be possible to cure the condition by reexcising the perineal wound. With recurrent pelvic malignancy, rarely can resection be successfully effected. Stearns in a 1980 report of the experience from the Memorial Sloan-Kettering Cancer Center stated, "Pelvic recurrence, in our experience, has not been curable by surgical excision or by any other modality of treatment."[584] Others concur that a surgical procedure can offer more effective palliation than other options and may prolong life in selected instances, but even the most radical resection rarely cures this disease.[236,387,422,463,538]

In the experience of Cunningham and colleagues, the only patients who had a survival benefit from reoperative pelvic surgery for rectal cancer were those whose disease could be completely resected (an uncommon situation).[121] Gagliardi and colleagues showed that recurrent tumor diameter was the only prognostic variable, in that a diameter of less than 5 cm in the resected specimen achieved local control in 47% of their patients.[191] Others have shown that independent variables for resectability include younger age at diagnosis, earlier stage of the primary tumor, and initial treatment by a sphincter-saving approach.[196] In a report from the Mayo Clinic published in 1996, 224 patients with a preoperative

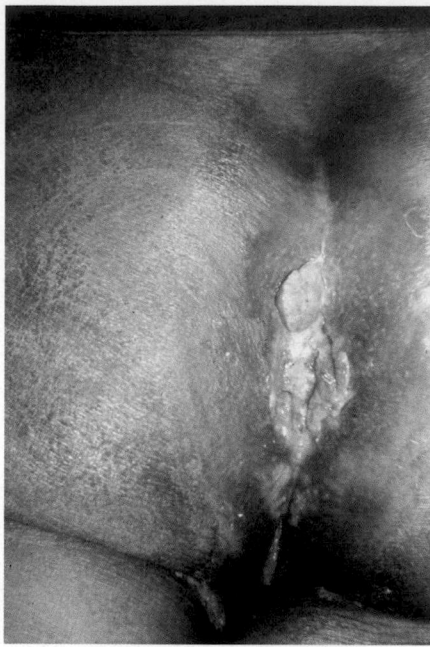

FIGURE 24-100. Perineal recurrence following APR. This was attributed to inadequate margins at the time of skin excision.

diagnosis of recurrent rectal cancer underwent additional surgery.[602] Of these, 65 underwent surgery with the hope of cure. Three-year, 5-year, and median survival were 57.0, 34.0, and 44.7 months, respectively. Survival tended to be greater in women and those without pain. Cumulative probability of local treatment failure was 24%, 41%, and 47% at 1, 3, and 5 years, respectively. The authors concluded that complete excision of locally recurrent rectal cancer can provide meaningful survival benefits.[602] Wanebo and colleagues, reporting from Brown University in Rhode Island, observed that pelvic recurrence can be safely resected with expectation of long-term survival in approximately one-third.[637] Salvage surgery for properly selected patients based on known risk factors is recommended and may lead to long-term palliation and the improving length of disease-free survival.[371] There is little disagreement, however, that unilateral or bilateral hydronephrosis appears to be a contraindication for potentially curative surgical resection for recurrent rectal carcinoma.[518]

Radiotherapy

Surgical extirpation for pelvic recurrence has been used for palliation.[635,638] However, radiation therapy has been and continues to be the most effective treatment for palliating symptoms of locally recurrent disease (see later, Radiotherapy). Wang and Schulz, for example, reported a palliative benefit lasting from several months up to 10 years.[639] This may imply an increased survival rate, but our patients survived a median of only 15 months following radiotherapy for pelvic recurrence, the same as the median survival rate of those reported by Moossa and colleagues, with no radiotherapy.[435,511] There is, however, little controversy concerning improvement of symptoms. Radiation therapy is effective in the treatment of pain for approximately three-fourths of patients. It may also decrease the size of a mass and, for an ulcerating lesion, the amount of perineal or vaginal drainage.

Radiotherapy can be administered to a total of 60 Gy (depending on whether the patient received preoperative treatment; see later). The Memorial Sloan-Kettering group recommends short treatments of 20 Gy when symptoms develop rather than a large-dose course.[584,589] In the experience of Villalon and Green with 85 patients who developed pelvic recurrence following APR, 92% with pain and 80% with a mass responded to 45 to 50 Gy.[630] Symptomatic relief was achieved in 80% of 143 patients reported by Pacini and colleagues.[472] They noted no significant difference in response to the three dose levels: 40, 50, and 60 Gy. Others reported comparable results.[149] Those who are severely debilitated may be treated by the so-called hypofractionation—the delivery of a single large dose (10 Gy) once a month for 3 months.[570]

One of the burdens that the patient and the surgeon may be forced to deal with is the radionecrosis that develops after high-dose radiation therapy for extensive primary or recurrent rectal cancer. Managing this type of problem often presents extraordinary challenges for the surgeon. Associated complications, such as enterocutaneous fistula, urinary fistula, pelvic abscess, osteomyelitis, and persistent sinuses, further complicate the picture. Treating the foul-smelling discharge, alleviating the pain, and addressing the need for frequent dressing changes are of paramount concern.

Intraoperative Radiotherapy

Intraoperative radiotherapy (IORT) is a technique by which a fundamentally resectable lesion is removed and the remaining cancer cells "sterilized" at the time of the operation, with the patient's abdomen open.[569] The procedure may be of value for those who are found to have fixed, unresectable rectal or rectosigmoid primary or recurrent tumors.[226,569,614] According to Sischy, in 1986 there were approximately 40 institutions in the United States employing this modality.[569] He suggested that the following criteria be used to identify patients who may be suitable for IORT:

- Tumor must be localized.
- Tumor must be accessible to treatment applicator and in an area from which normal tissue may be displaced.
- The condition must be potentially curable, yet the tumor is unable to be controlled by surgery alone.

Usually, the patient receives external beam radiation of 45 to 50 Gy. Four to 6 weeks following completion of this treatment and after CT evaluation is performed to ascertain that there is no evidence of disseminated disease, the patient undergoes re-exploration and resection. If there is microscopic residual tumor as determined by frozen-section examination or if it is believed that cure is unlikely, an appropriate-sized Lucite "radiation applicator" is selected.[614] Few institutions have dedicated IORT operating suites, so it may be necessary to transport the patient to the radiation therapy unit for "booster therapy." A dose of 15 to 20 Gy is then delivered as a single treatment.

It is difficult to offer firm conclusions about the relative merits of this approach. According to Sischy, 3- to 5-year results from a number of centers for marginally resectable disease are approximately 50% and, for recurrent disease, approximately 40%.[569] Farouk and colleagues reviewed the evidence to support aggressive preoperative chemoradiation followed by surgical resection and IORT.[169] An overall 5-year survival of 42% was reported, even in those with locally unresectable primary rectal cancer. Some reports indicate that better local control and palliation of individuals with locally recurrent disease is achieved with IORT in combination with multimodality treatment.[334,391] Hashiguchi and coworkers concluded that those with nonresectable distant metastasis, those with pain, elevated preoperative CA19–9, fixed tumors, or gross residual tumor after surgical resection are not suitable candidates for IORT.[242] The Memorial Sloan-Kettering Cancer Center group performed IORT with curative intent for recurrent rectal cancer in 111 patients.[568] Median disease-free survival was 31.2 months for complete resection compared with 7.9 months when the patient had microscopic or grossly positive margins. The presence of vascular invasion was also an independent variable for a poorer outcome. Numerous articles have been published that support the concept of combined sacropelvic resection with intraoperative radiation therapy to effect palliation and possible cure in selected patients with locally advanced or recurrent disease.[238,243,374,388,580]

Sadahiro and coworkers used IORT in 78 individuals for "curatively resected" rectal cancer.[537] The electron beam was administered as uniformly as possible to the entire dissected surface of the pelvis. Using historical controls, these investigators found that survival, disease-free survival, and local recurrence-free survival in the IORT group were all significantly more favorable than in the non-IORT group.

Radiofrequency Ablation

A limited approach, that of CT-guided, percutaneous radiofrequency ablation, has been described for nonresectable recurrence.[464]

Chemotherapy

Other treatment modalities for recurrence include radium implantation and chemotherapy (see Chapter 23). The reader is referred to the prior chapter for the current status of chemotherapy.

Pain Management

For pain that cannot be effectively treated by radiotherapy and that is no longer responsive to narcotic analgesics, neurosurgical consultation is advised. Placement of epidural, intrathecal, and intraventricular catheters for narcotic drug delivery as well as the use of intrathecal alcohol or chordotomy may be appropriate alternatives in an intractable situation.[176]

Management of Recurrence following Anterior Resection

When anastomotic recurrence develops, it usually presents within 5 years following resection. The patient may be without symptoms, but a suspicious mass may be noted either by palpation (digital examination) or by proctosigmoidoscopy as part of the cancer follow-up regimen. Unfortunately, anastomotic recurrence usually implies incurable disease because the presentation is virtually always a consequence of pelvic recurrence. Many patients who present with recurrent cancer in the pelvis do not have disseminated disease, and under these circumstances, the CEA is often not elevated. When symptoms develop, they may include bleeding; change in the caliber of the stool; and pelvic, abdominal, or sacral pain. Biopsy or scrapings for cytologic examination usually will confirm the diagnosis, but MRI and CT also may be helpful (Figure 24-101). Positron emission tomography has been used to follow-up individuals with colorectal malignancy to differentiate between recurrent tumor and scar (see Chapter 23).[15] The method employs the injection of fluorine-18-labelled deoxyglucose (FDG) to assess tumor metabolism. In the experience of Schlag and Strauss and their colleagues, nonmalignant lesions had a low-FDG accumulation as compared with the high levels seen with recurrent cancer.[555,599] Based on subsequent histologic confirmation, the test was 100% accurate in their hands.

The only hope for cure is repeat resection. This usually involves an APR but sometimes continuity may again reestablished (Figure 24-102). Before undertaking reoperation, however, it is imperative to determine whether the patient has evidence of disseminated disease. Because of the possibility of retroperitoneal extension of the tumor and the likelihood of urinary tract involvement (ureteric obstruction is common; Figure 24-103), a CT scan is mandatory.

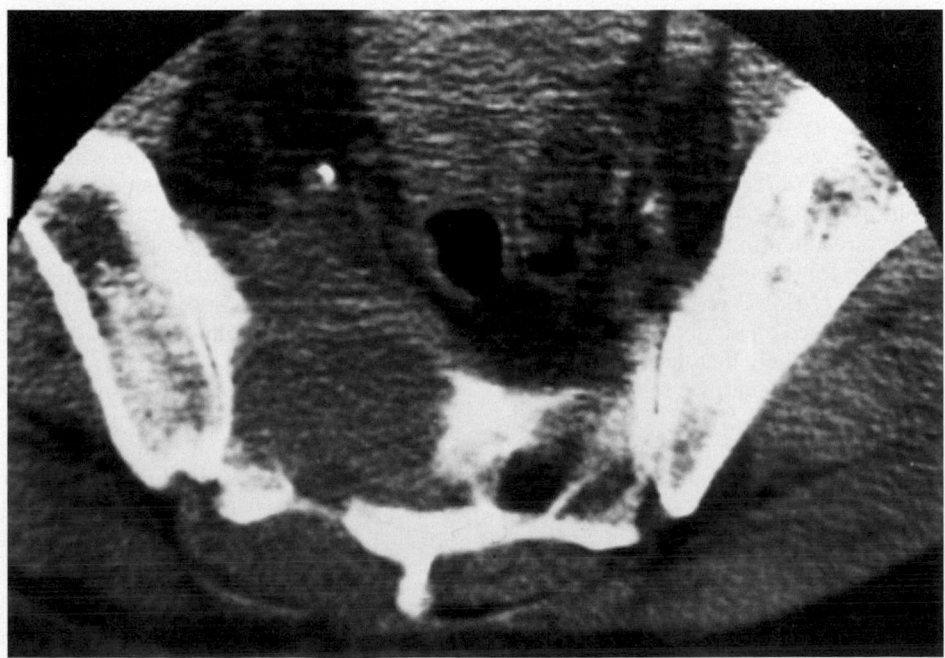

FIGURE 24-101. Recurrent rectal cancer. Computed tomography scan shows marked bony erosion.

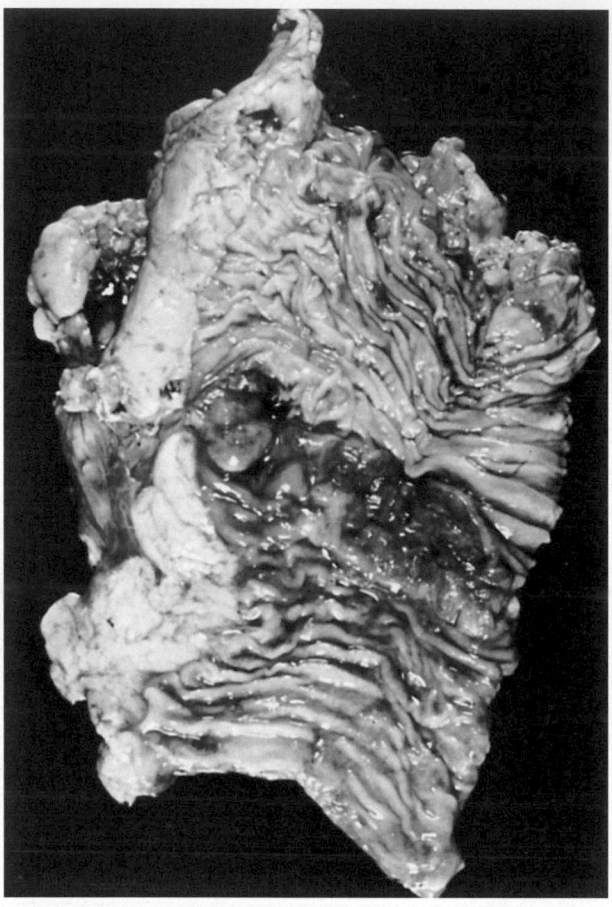

FIGURE 24-102. A portion of resected specimen showing suture line recurrence of tumor.

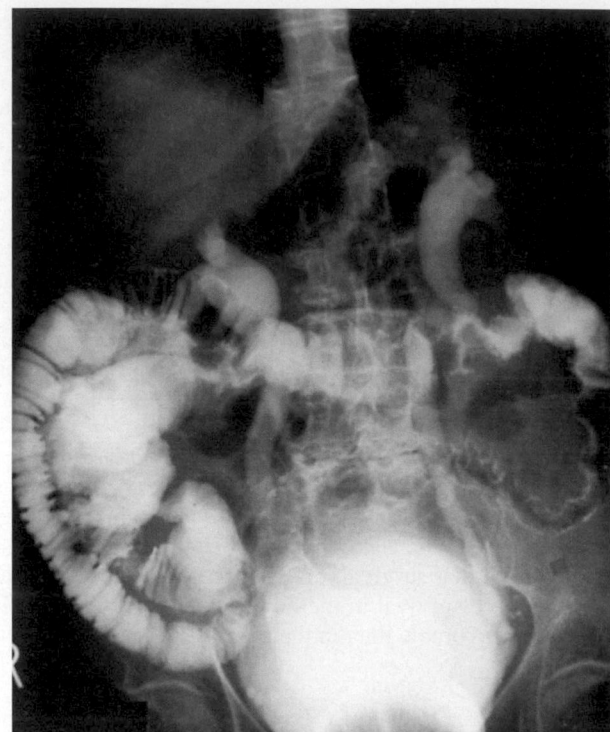

FIGURE 24-103. Recurrent rectal cancer with ureteral obstruction.

Results of Reoperation

Studies of APR following anastomotic recurrence have limited numbers of patients and are difficult to interpret.[559] Overall cure rates are certainly less than 25% in those considered resectable for cure. Wanebo and colleagues reported limited success with a combined abdominosacrectomy, with more than one-half of the patients requiring a bladder resection.[636] The operative mortality was 12%.

Recently, there have been more encouraging reports following pelvic exenteration for pelvic recurrence. A combination of a multidisciplinary approach and improved surgical techniques have resulted in more hopeful results[18] and a better quality of life for selected patients undergoing this form of major surgery.[19] However, it must be emphasized that these reports are based on highly selected patients.

Despite all the efforts, it is likely that the best chance for cure is restricted to patients in whom the recurrence is confined to, but does not breach, the bowel wall. This may be the rare circumstance when mucosal seeding produces the recurrence rather than an inward growth of residual pelvic disease.

▶ OTHER PROCEDURES FOR RECTAL CANCER

So far I have dealt with the three most common surgical operations for the management of rectal cancer. There are, however, several other approaches, some of which are limited to that of historical value and others which are occasionally employed today. These are summarized next.

Palliative Abdominoperineal Resection

Palliative APR in patients with advanced or metastatic disease has been advocated by a number of authors.[25,67,365] Others have suggested that alternative forms of therapy should be considered because of the high surgical morbidity and mortality rates.[306,437,511] Individuals who have extensive liver metastases, lung metastases, or disseminated disease (e.g., bone, brain) are poor candidates. Those with ascites or multiple peritoneal implants are also extremely high operative risks. Because the mean survival time in patients with metastatic disease is limited, certain patients should be considered for a palliative resection; these include those with perineal pain, tenesmus, or hemorrhage. If the tumor can be extirpated, a better quality of life may be anticipated. In the experience of Moran and colleagues with 125 patients who underwent palliative surgical treatment, the median survival was 6.4 months for those treated by diverting colostomy, 14.8 months for abdominal resection, and 14.7 months for transanal excision.[437]

The fact that there are long-term survivors when so-called palliative procedures are performed implies that some individuals may still be well managed surgically, even though they have locally advanced disease. Extended resection in these patients, if feasible, has the potential of providing excellent palliation and even occasionally a cure.[348,494]

Pelvic Lymphadenectomy

Lateral pelvic lymph node dissection has been believed, especially by the Japanese, to be a requisite for proper rectal resection, especially of advanced cancer. Yamakoshi and coworkers found metastases to lymph nodes or lymphatic permeation in the tissue around the autonomic nerves in 14.3% of lower rectal cancers.[659] They, therefore, cautioned about the use of nerve-sparing techniques that fail to remove these nodes. Fujita and colleagues noted that individuals with lymph node metastases had an overall 5-year disease-free survival rate of 73.3% for those who underwent lateral pelvic lymph node dissection compared with a 35.3% survival rate for those who did not ($P = .013$).[186] The authors caution, however, that what is needed is a randomized clinical trial. Moriya and colleagues reported a 5-year survival rate of 69% in their patients who did not undergo extended lymphadenectomy, as compared with a rate of 76% for those who did.[441]

I have had no experience with en bloc pelvic lymphadenectomy, and I am not convinced that there is sufficient data to support its use.

Inguinal Node Metastases

Inguinal node metastases with rectal cancer are an ominous prognostic finding. Graham and Hohn found no 5-year survivors irrespective of the method of management.[219] They still recommend therapeutic node dissection for purposes of local control and "possible cure." However, these unfortunate individuals indeed have surgically incurable disease. Therefore, one should endeavor to employ adjuvant measures, such as chemotherapy and radiotherapy, rather than to attempt a major resection. Depending on the findings and symptoms associated with the primary tumor, it may not be possible to achieve adequate palliation other than by operation. In 21 patients so observed by Tocchi and associates, the mean survival was 14.8 months (range, 2 to 42).[617]

Nerve-Preserving Operation

Urinary dysfunction and sexual dysfunction are common sequelae of excision of the rectum for cancer. Impotence is directly related to the extent of lateral pelvic dissection, hence my reluctance to perform the so-called radical lymphadenectomy as a routine in the treatment of rectal cancer. Injury to the parasympathetic nerves, especially in relation to the lateral ligaments where their course may be quite variable, is a clear risk (see Figure 1-20).[161,358] In recent years, there have been a number of publications that addressed the issue of autonomic nerve-preserving pelvic wall dissection, which theoretically combines the benefits of en bloc parietal pelvic dissection with nerve preservation.

In an attempt to minimize the risk of nerve injury, I make it a rule to identify and preserve the hypogastric nerves as a first step in rectal mobilization. When performing the anterolateral aspect of the mobilization, the dissection must remain in an extrafascial plane, but there is no need to dissect lateral to the parietal pelvic fascia where the inferior hypogastric plexus can be injured. For the same reason, during the anterior mobilization, the dissection should be posterior to Denonvilliers' fascia unless there is local invasion anteriorly.[358]

Enker has reported autonomic nerve-preservation in 42 men undergoing sphincter-saving operations for the treatment of rectal cancer—not APR.[161] The incidence of potency was 86.7%, with 87.8% having normal ejaculation. Others report equally favorable results with this approach.[299,380,404,659]

Hartmann's Procedure

A Hartmann's procedure should be seriously considered in patients with high-volume metastatic disease and in those with significant comorbidities in whom an anastomosis is preferably avoided (Figure 24-104). I have found this procedure especially useful in frail and elderly patients who already have poor continence and in whom a low anastomosis would result in a very poor functional outcome.

Transanal or Coloanal Anastomosis with Colonic Reservoir

In 1986, Lazorthes and colleagues and Parc and associates developed the concept of restoration of continuity by means of a colonic reservoir in order to address the functional concerns associated with a straight coloanal anastomosis.[344,484] However, this "problem" would appear to be a nonissue if one reviews the references in the earlier section.[277] The technique is essentially the same as that for a J-pouch ileal reservoir (see Chapter 29), except that the colon is used (Figure 24-105). Banerjee and Parc attempted to develop a model for appropriate pouch size.[34] According to the authors, ideal pouch dimensions should be 6 to 7 cm of nondistended bowel circumference, with limb lengths of 8 to 10 cm. Others suggest that a shorter limb is satisfactory, and that there is no justification for creating a limb of 10 or more cm. Ho and coworkers, in fact, demonstrated in a randomized, controlled trial by means of scintigraphy that a small colonic J-pouch improves retention of liquid stool.[262] All investigators emphasized the importance of mobilizing the splenic flexure and preserving the first branch of the inferior mesenteric artery.

A theoretical advantage of the J-reservoir when compared with a straight coloanal anastomosis is that the blood supply

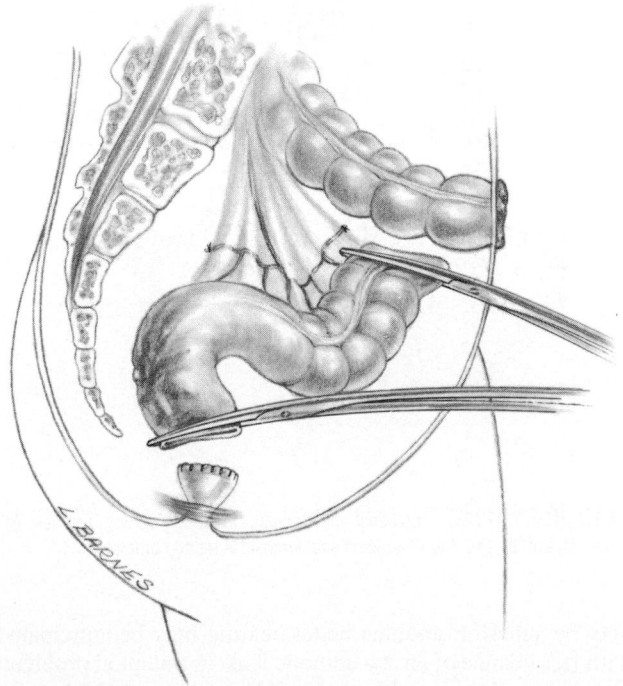

FIGURE 24-104. Hartmann's resection. The rectal stump is inverted by conventional suture technique or is closed with a linear stapler distal to the tumor. A sigmoid colostomy is created.

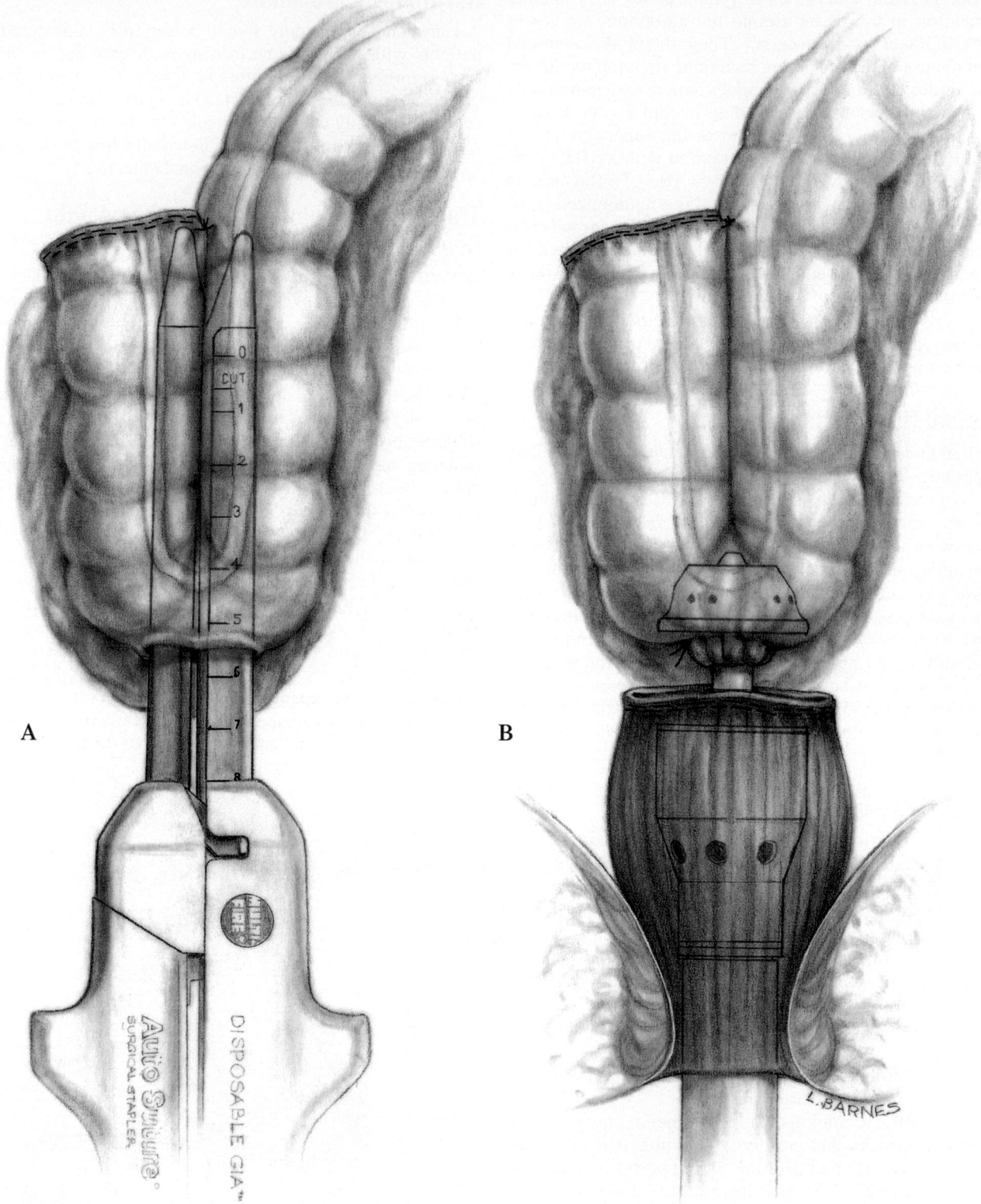

A

B

FIGURE 24-105. Coloanal anastomosis using intervening J-pouch. **A:** The pouch is constructed either by a hand-sewn technique or by using a stapler (as shown). **B:** The double-stapled anastomosis is being completed.

may be superior, and that better healing may be anticipated with less chance of an anastomotic leak. A potential problem, however, is that a narrow, male pelvis may preclude the possibility of creating a reservoir. Likewise, a thickened, fatty mesentery may cause the operation to be technically nonfeasible. Finally, some surgeons selectively recommend the use of the descending colon rather than to create a reservoir with a thickened sigmoid colon, but others have found that pouches made from sigmoid or descending colon provide similar bowel function.[245] The same principle of fecal diversion applies to the colonic J-pouch as it does to the straight coloanal anastomosis—namely, diversion, in my opinion, is a requisite. In the experience of Dehni and colleagues, there was a clinical anastomotic leak rate of 17% in those without a defunctioning stoma.[138]

Results

Drake and colleagues reported the Mayo Clinic experience with 29 individuals suffering from either benign or malignant disease.[153] Anastomotic stricture was found in 28.0%, and a 3.4% leak rate was noted. Fourteen percent could not have their colostomy or ileostomy closed. A later report incorporating the experience from both Mayo and Cleveland Clinics, involving 117 patients most of whom had undergone a straight coloanal anastomosis, satisfactory fecal continence was achieved in 78%.[91] No J-pouch recipient had frequent incontinence. Five-year survival was 69%, but 62% had complications (anastomotic leak, 18%). Some institutions have found that stool frequencies are fewer with this method, especially during the first year,[46,137,142,255,256,351,446,510,561,641] than with patients who undergo reconstruction procedures without a reservoir, but others note that approximately 25% of individuals must evacuate with a small enema.[344,484,499] This is the primary reason for limiting the size of the reservoir and, furthermore, to use this option only for anastomoses at the level of the anal canal or very low rectum. Evacuation problems are more likely to occur with an intact lower rectum.

Sailer and associates, in Würzburg, Germany, performed a prospective trial in which 64 patients were randomized to either a straight (n = 32) or coloanal J-pouch (n = 32).[541] These investigators found that patients who underwent pouch reconstruction had better functional results as well as an improved quality of life in the early months. Nicholls and colleagues compared the St. Mark's Hospital experience with the colonic reservoir and straight coloanal anastomoses.[458] They found no significant difference in balloon expulsion testing, defecation proctography, or methylcellulose evacuation in the two groups. Frequency of defecation and daytime soiling were inversely correlated with the maximal tolerable volume.[336] Hallböök and colleagues performed a randomized comparison of straight and J-pouch anastomoses in 100 consecutive patients with rectal cancer in whom a sphincter-saving procedure was considered appropriate.[234] The incidence of symptomatic anastomotic leakage was lower in the pouch group (2% vs. 15%). At 1 year, the patients who had undergone the pouch procedure had significantly fewer bowel movements in 24 hours and less nocturnal evacuation, urgency, and incontinence.[234] Those familiar with the technique report no increase in morbidity or mortality attributable to the reservoir itself. Machado and coworkers in Stockholm showed that either a colonic J-pouch or a side-to-end anastomosis performed in the descending colon, in a prospective randomized trial, can be used with the expectation of similar functional and surgical results.[381]

The Cleveland Clinic group identified seven reasons why the J-pouch could not be constructed and stipulated that coloplasty has reduced the frequency of these problems (see the following section).[237] They were as follows:

- Narrow pelvis
- Bulky sphincters or mucosectomy
- Diverticulosis
- Insufficient colon length
- Pregnancy
- Complex surgery
- Distant metastases

One of the concerns for any operation that restores continuity in the patient with rectal cancer is the impact of adjuvant or neoadjuvant chemoradiotherapy. The Cleveland Clinic group assessed individuals who underwent either preoperative or postoperative treatment and concluded that chemoradiation therapy adversely affects continence and evacuation in those who underwent colonic J-pouches.[205] The authors expressed concern over long-term functional results with radiation of the anal canal, sphincter mechanism, and neorectum (in the adjuvant patient) and offered the suggestion that consideration should be given to excluding the anal canal from the field of irradiation in those with stage II and III rectal cancer whenever a sphincter-preserving operation is contemplated.[205] Others have found that preoperative radiotherapy significantly increases the frequency of nocturnal defecation and diarrhea when compared with nonirradiated patients.[136]

Initially, I was impressed by the results that were reported for this technique. However, although the reports suggest an improvement in bowel function in the first year, it is becoming apparent that after 12 months the functional results are not all that different. Furthermore, I am concerned at long-term complications that include an inability to spontaneously empty the pouch. It must be remembered that the construction of any pouch results in the apposition of a peristaltic and an antiperistaltic segment. This may result in an atonic pouch that is difficult to empty. I am yet to be convinced on the usefulness of creating a J-pouch for my patients.

Coloanal Anastomosis with Coloplasty

Following a series of experimental studies, Z'graggen and coworkers in Bern, Switzerland conceptually explored whether a coloplasty, equivalent to a very small pouch, could decrease stool frequency without the technical and functional problems associated with the J-pouch.[666] Forty-three patients were so treated, all with a proximal stoma. The early results were comparable to that of the J-pouch reservoir procedure.

Technique

Z'graggen's group used a segment of descending colon for the coloplasty. The procedure is analogous to that of the Heineke-Mikulicz pyloroplasty as applied to the colon—that is, a linear colostomy with a transverse closure. After the anvil is secured in the colon, an 8-cm incision is made longitudinally between the tenia, 2 cm proximal to the rim of the anvil (Figure 24-106). Lateral traction by stay sutures develops the appearance of the reservoir. The colostomy is closed in two layers (their preference), with the stapled anastomosis performed in the usual manner. The procedure can also be accomplished with a hand-sewn coloanal anastomosis. All patients require fecal diversion.

Results

Besides Z'graggen and colleagues, other surgeons have expressed satisfaction with this procedure. Fürst and coworkers randomized 40 consecutive patients to either a J-pouch or coloplasty.[187] The construction of a coloplasty pouch was possible in every instance, but 4 of 20 (20%) in the J-pouch group could not undergo the procedure because of a fatty mesentery. At 6 months, there was no significant difference in stool frequency and no significant difference in resting and squeeze pressures, as well as neorectal volume. However,

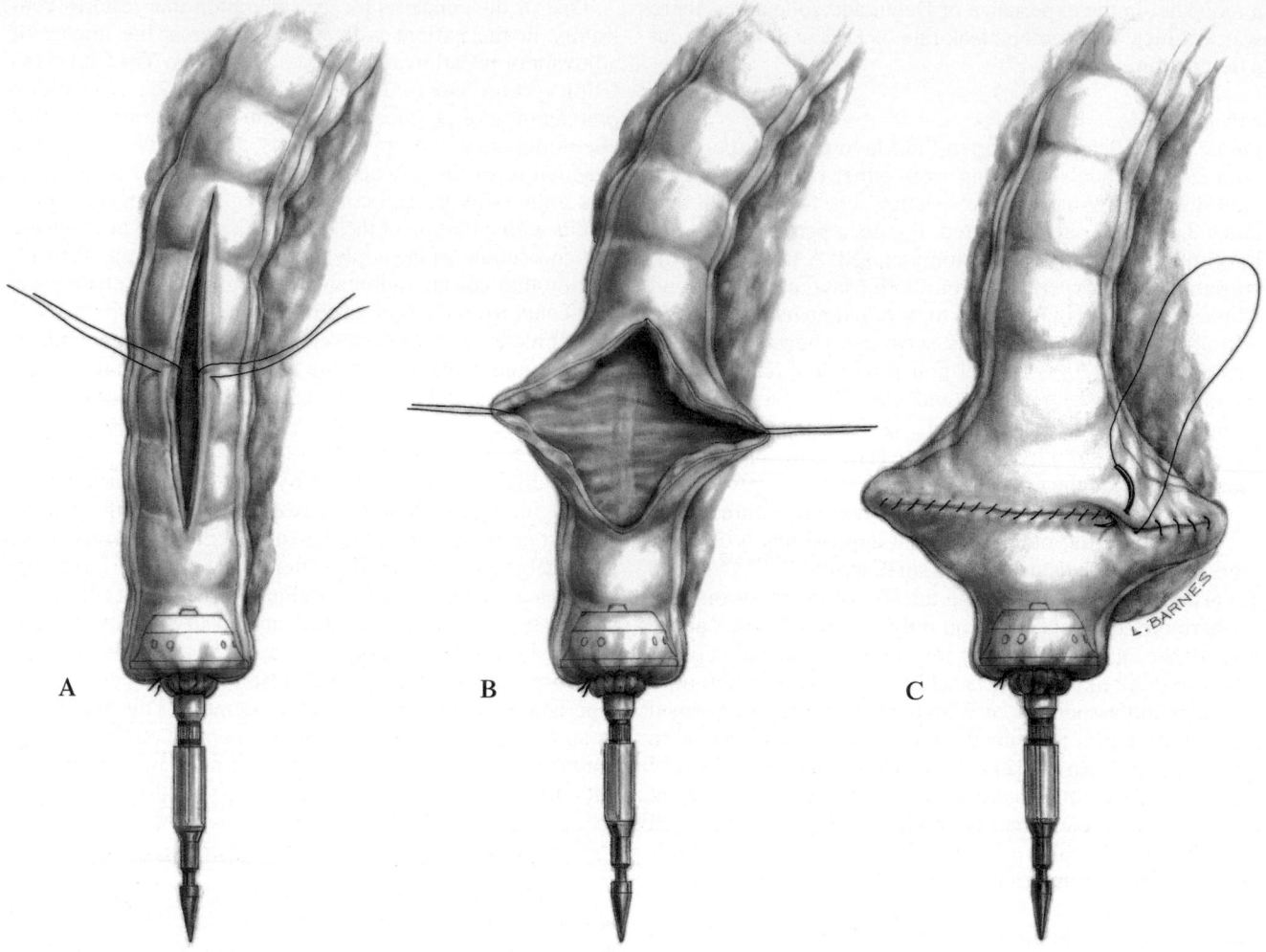

FIGURE 24-106. Coloplasty. **A:** Linear incision is made between the taeniae. **B:** Guide sutures are placed in preparation for transverse closure. **C:** Pouch is completed.

there was an increased neorectal sensitivity in the coloplasty group. The authors concluded the coloplasty is a particularly attractive alternative because of its simplicity and one's ability to apply it for all patients. The Cleveland Clinic group members were of like opinion, based on their report of 20 patients.[392]

Coloanal Anastomosis with Intersphincteric Resection

In an effort to restore intestinal continuity in those patients who have even invasion of the anal canal, some have suggested restoration by incorporating intersphincteric resection. By this means, the anal canal and internal sphincter are removed with preservation of the external sphincter mechanism. In other words, if the tumor has low rectal transmural infiltration without invasion of the levator ani or external sphincter, this operation may be undertaken.[533,628] Others have suggested that tumors close to the anal canal, not infiltrating the external sphincter, and with good to moderate differentiation may be removed by intersphincteric resection and coloanal reconstruction.[514] This removes, at least theoretically in the minds of some individuals, one of the

absolute contraindications to restoration of bowel continuity, namely, invasion of the anal canal. Figure 24-107 illustrates the concept of the extent of resection.

Rullier and colleagues in Bordeaux, France prospectively studied 16 patients with infiltrating T2 and T3 rectal tumors located between 2.5 and 4.5 cm from the anal verge.[533] Six underwent partial resection of the internal sphincter and 10 complete resection. A colonic J-pouch was performed in one-half of their patients. Twelve had undergone neoadjuvant radiation therapy. There were no deaths. No local recurrence developed (median, 44 months). Two required proctectomy for complications and two died of metastatic disease. Continence was normal in one-half of the patients.

Clearly, the concept of sphincter-sparing by this new approach will require a larger series before accepting the premise that this procedure can be performed without compromising the possibility for cure.

Other Methods for Restoring Intestinal Continuity

Abdominoanal pull-through procedures,[407,644] eversion techniques,[113,622] and delayed union techniques[21,22,24,60] are

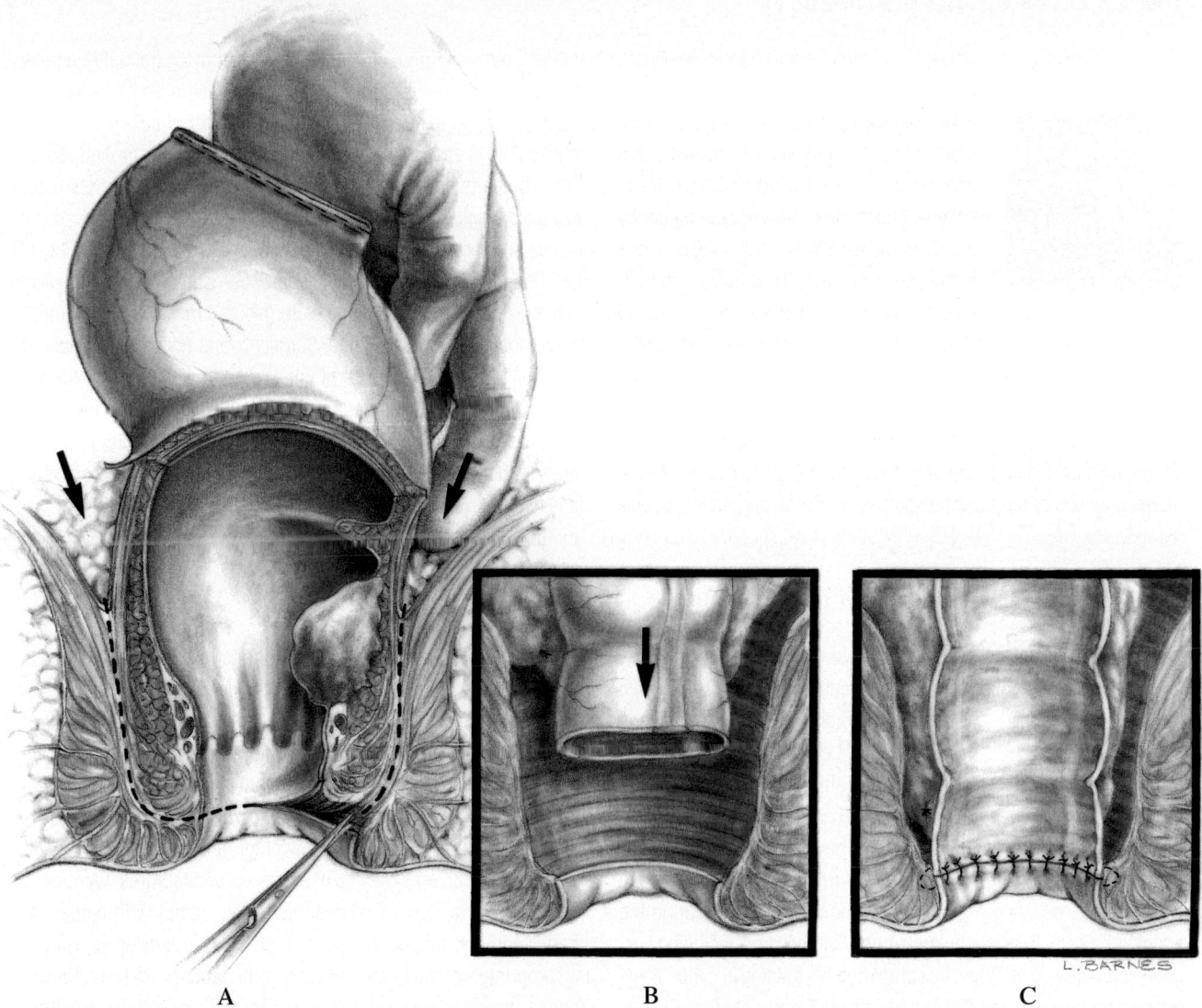

A   B   C

FIGURE 24-107. Intersphincteric resection. **A:** The *dashed line* indicates the extent of resection in the intersphincteric plane. Note the artist's conception of a small tumor invading the internal sphincter at the top of the anal canal. **B:** The external sphincter is intact, and the proximal colon is pulled through. **C:** Completed anastomosis.

other methods of restoring intestinal continuity. Alternative methods have been described by Maunsell and Weir (see earlier Biographies), Cutait, Turnbull (see Biography, Chapter 31), Babcock, Bacon, and others. However, they are no longer in common practice and are included here only to be referenced for the occasional application.

Results

Cutait and colleagues had considerable experience with the various pull-through operations; in 1985, they reported a total of 728 patients treated by several methods.[123] Only 57 individuals, however, underwent the operation for rectal cancer. These investigators noted that the incidence of leakage was 31.9% in immediate anastomoses and only 2.2% in delayed anastomoses. Likewise, the incidence of septic complications was much less when the delayed technique was used (6.8% vs. 27.9%). Operative mortality was also less with the delayed method (2.2% vs. 6.1%).

Rosen and colleagues and Khubchandani and coworkers reported the results of 28 patients with respect to defecation, to continence, and to survival after the Bacon-type of pull-through operation had been performed.[309,523] Although these individuals all were continent, 83% failed to defecate spontaneously and required an enema. Rather than abstract the results of the moderately extensive earlier literature on the subject, I have appended a list of references.[23,44,45,59,211,315,328,329,341,583,622] All studies are uncontrolled or, at best, relate only to historical controls. Morbidity is generally higher than with APR, as is the length of hospitalization. Mortality rates generally are also higher with the pull-through procedures. Cure rates and problems with pelvic recurrence are comparable, however.

Transsacral or Transcoccygeal Resection

Sacral excision had been performed by Theodor Kocher as early as 1875.[319] However, it has been associated with the

DAHER ELIAS CUTAIT (1913–2001)

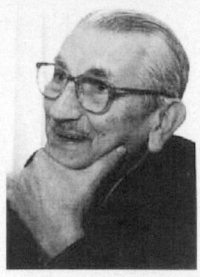

Daher Cutait was born in São Paulo, Brazil, where he attended the University of São Paulo Medical School, graduating in 1939. From 1941 to 1943, as the recipient of a scholarship provided by the Institute of International Education of New York and later by the Kellogg Foundation (Michigan), he came to the United States to the Presbyterian Hospital of Columbia University. From there, he went to the University of Michigan Hospital, where Frederick Coller trained him in colorectal surgery. Upon his return to Brazil, Cutait initiated an active career at the University of São Paulo Hospital das Clínicas. In 1947, he was appointed Head of Colo-Proctology, a position he held until his retirement in 1983. During his tenure of service, he became one of the most prestigious colorectal surgeons, not only in Brazil, but also throughout Latin America, having trained hundreds of surgeons. He published more than 120 papers and 3 books. His unique technical abilities were applied to a host of colorectal conditions, but he is eponymously remembered for his pull-through procedure, an operation that was designed for the treatment of chagasic megacolon (see Chapter 33). Cutait received numerous international awards and recognitions. He was president of the Brazilian Society of Colo-Proctology, the Brazilian College of Surgeons, and the Brazilian Chapter of the American College of Surgeons; a member of the American Society of Colon and Rectal Surgeons; and honorary member of the Royal College of Surgeons of England and Ireland and the French Society of Medicine, to name only a few. In the early 1960s, he established the Hospital Sírio Libanês, a referral center for surgery in São Paulo. He directed this hospital until his last days. Daher Cutait died on June 6, 2001. (With appreciation to his son, Raul Cutait, MD.)

WILLIAM WAYNE BABCOCK (1872–1963)

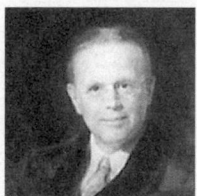

Babcock was born in East Worcester, New York. After 2 years as a preceptee, when he studied medicine and the classics, he enrolled in the College of Physicians and Surgeons in Baltimore, graduating with honors in 1895. After 1 year as a resident physician in Salt Lake City, Utah, he matriculated for an additional year of medical training at the University of Pennsylvania in Philadelphia, receiving his second MD degree in 1895. During the ensuing 7 years, Babcock held a number of positions, including surgeon and pathologist. When he completed his training in gynecology, he was offered the Chair in this specialty at Temple Medical College of Philadelphia. However, he elected to accept the Chair of Surgery at the same school when he was only 31 years of age. He served as professor and head of the department for 40 years and was one of America's most renowned surgeons. His textbook, *Principles of Surgery*, was highly regarded through several revisions. His list of accomplishments was extraordinary. He was the first person in the United States to employ a spinal anesthetic. He is eponymously associated with an operation for stripping varicose veins and for inguinal herniorrhaphy. He was the inventor of the acorn-shaped vein stripper; he introduced the use of alloy steel wire sutures, wire mesh in hernia repairs, and, of course, his bowel clamp. With respect to his pull-through procedure, he was often criticized for applying it inappropriately or too often. Certainly, with Babcock and with Bacon, Temple University became the center for this particular procedure. (Photograph courtesy of the Department of Surgery, Temple University School of Medicine, Philadelphia.)

HARRY ELLICOTT BACON (1900–1981)

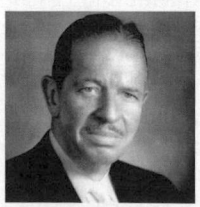

Harry Bacon was born in Philadelphia on August 25, 1900, the son of a professor of surgery at Temple University Medical School. He received his bachelor of science degree from Villanova University and his doctorate in medicine from Temple University in 1925. Following an internship in surgery at the Philadelphia General Hospital, he became interested in proctology. He pursued further training at the Graduate Hospital in that city, St. Mark's Hospital in London, St. Antoine in Paris, and the Algemeine Krankenhuis in Vienna. Returning to Philadelphia, he became associate professor of proctology at the University of Pennsylvania and subsequently professor of surgery and chairman of the Department of Colon and Rectal Surgery at Temple University, a position he held until 1972, when he achieved emeritus status. Bacon was a prolific writer, with six books plus numerous scientific articles to his credit. Additionally, he published three volumes of poetry as well as musical arrangements for the piano and organ. He played a principal role in the establishment of the journal *Diseases of the Colon and Rectum* and served in an editorial capacity from its inception until his death. He received numerous awards and recognitions throughout his life, including a silver medallion from Pope Pius XII and a gold medallion from Pope John XXIII. He was the founder of the Pennsylvania Society of Colon and Rectal Surgery, a founding member of the International Society of University Colon and Rectal Surgeons, and president of the American Proctologic Society (he was instrumental in changing the name to the American Society of Colon and Rectal Surgeons), and he received honorary degrees from 8 universities and honorary fellowships from 18 international surgical organizations. Bacon died on May 12, 1981. (With appreciation to Indru T. Khubchandani, MD.)

EMIL THEODOR KOCHER (1841–1917)

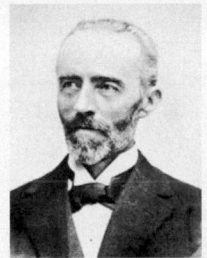

Emil Kocher was born in Switzerland on August 25, 1841 and graduated from medical school, summa cum laude, from the University of Bern. He visited distinguished professors such as Billroth, Lister, Pasteur, and Nelaton and settled in Bern in 1866. He was awarded the Chair of Surgery at this university in 1875 and held the position for the next 45 years. He was the first to excise the thyroid for goiter (1876) and ultimately performed more than 5,000 thyroid operations. In 1909, Kocher won the Nobel Prize for physiology or medicine for his work on the physiology, pathology, and surgery of the thyroid gland. He has been described as a calm and imperturbable operator, while also maintaining total asepsis in an era of frequent infections. His name is eponymously associated with numerous techniques and instruments—an incomplete list includes his incisions (abdominal and thyroid), his maneuver, his methods (uterine fixation, inguinal herniorrhaphy, shoulder dislocation), his reflex, his sign, his syndrome (for thyrotoxicosis), his forceps, his clamp, his drain, and his probe. He even has a verb named after him—every surgeon knows what it means to kocherize the duodenum. Kocher contributed extensively to the literature in general surgery, endocrine surgery, urology, gynecology, neurosurgery, and war-related injuries. His lifelong efforts were compiled in his textbook, *Operative Surgery* (*Chirurgische Operationslehre*, 1892), a monumental tome that was published in a number of editions and translations. He was named the first president of the International Surgical Society. In 1909, the Kocher Institute in Bern was established as a permanent memorial to him. He retired as professor of surgery in 1911 and died on July 25, 1917. (Photograph courtesy of Archiv fur Kunst und Geschichte, Berlin.)

GEORGE GREY TURNER (1877–1951)

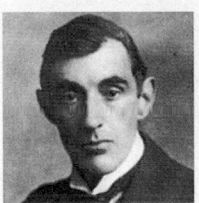

Turner was born in Tynemouth, the county of Northumberland, England. He was educated at a private school and graduated from the Newcastle Medical School of Durham University with first-class honors in 1898. He obtained his MS in 1901 and his FRCS in 1903. After holding resident surgical posts at Newcastle, Turner went to London and continued his postgraduate studies at King's College Hospital. After visiting a number of surgical clinics on the continent, he returned to Newcastle and to the staff of the Royal Victoria Infirmary. Because of his dexterity, daring, and extraordinary capacity for work, his operating theater became a center for visitors comparable to that of the great Lord Moynihan. In 1927, he was named professor of surgery at the University of Durham, and in the following year was made president of the Association of Surgeons of Great Britain and Ireland. Grey Turner was more of a "generalist" and was considered one of the boldest individuals because of his aggressive treatment of malignant disease. His point of view with respect to the anal sphincter was perhaps somewhat less radical, however. Preservation of the "wonderful sphincteric apparatus" did appear to be a priority concern. Grey Turner was recognized through numerous awards and honors. He was Hunterian Professor on two occasions and honorary fellow of the American and Royal Australasian Colleges of Surgeons. He was elected president of the Proctologic and General Surgical Sections of the Royal Society of Medicine. He delivered the John B. Murphy Oration in Philadelphia and received the Bigelow Medal in Boston for the advancement of surgery. His name is eponymously associated with the sign that produces local discoloration of the skin of the flank in acute pancreatitis. (Photograph courtesy of the Royal College of Surgeons of England.)

name of Kraske (see earlier Biography) ever since he described the technique in detail to the Fourteenth Congress of the German Association of Surgeons in 1884 (see earlier history).[325] Interestingly, in the classic description of the procedure, the bowel was brought out by establishing a sacral anus at the posterior end of the wound, amputating the entire distal rectum. This, in essence, was a sacral colostomy. Others, such as Turner, modified the operation by performing an anastomosis to the residual anorectum.[623]

Technique
Routine bowel preparation is carried out as if for an anterior resection. The operation is performed with the patient in the prone position and with the buttocks taped. Some surgeons prefer the lateral position, but the prone jackknife position is easier. An incision is made in the midline from just above the anal verge to the lower sacrum and carried through the subcutaneous tissue to expose the levator ani muscle and coccyx (Figure 24-108). The levator ani muscle is then divided, exposing the posterior wall of the rectum. The coccyx is then freed from its muscular attachments, disarticulated, and removed. If it is apparent that sufficient exposure has been achieved, then no part of the sacrum is removed. However, if further exposure is necessary, the lower portion (two sacral segments) is excised using a Gigli saw. It is imperative when dividing the sacrum that the third sacral nerve on one side be preserved in order to avoid problems with incontinence. Figures 24-109 and 24-110 show this approach for usually benign conditions.

The rectum is then completely mobilized. Care must be taken to avoid injuring the anterior rectum where it is adherent to the vagina or to the prostate. A Penrose drain is

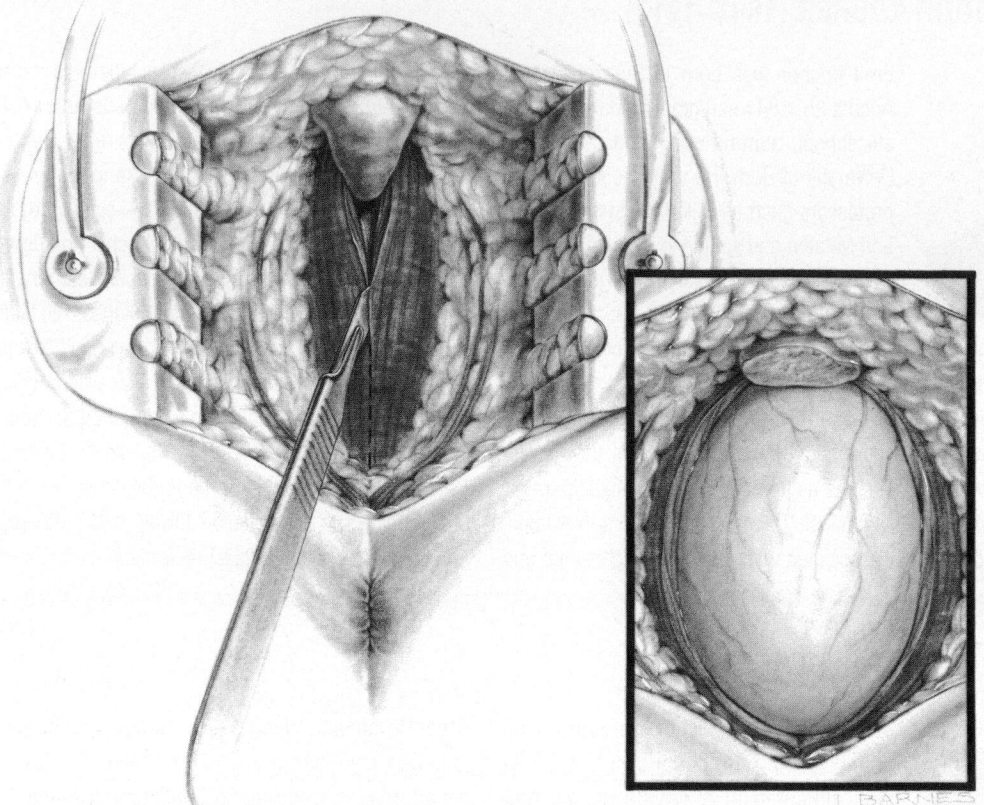

FIGURE 24-108. Transcoccygeal approach to removal of rectal tumors. A midline incision is made, and the levator ani muscle is divided. The coccyx is excised, and the posterior wall of the rectum is exposed (*inset*).

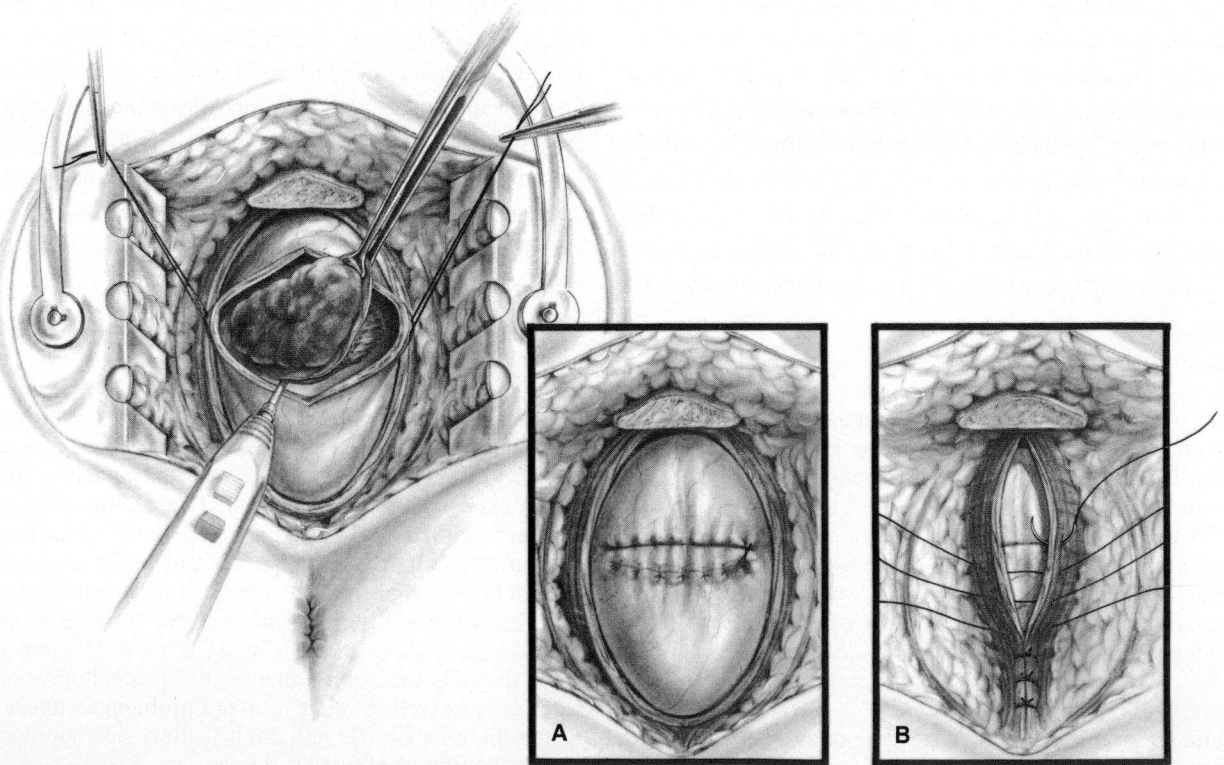

FIGURE 24-109. Transcoccygeal approach to removal of rectal tumors. A posterior proctotomy reveals a tumor on the anterior wall. This is excised by means of electrocautery. Tumor excision alone or full-thickness excision of the bowel wall can be accomplished. **A:** The enterotomy wounds can be closed separately. **B:** Repair of the sphincter muscles is accomplished in a layered fashion.

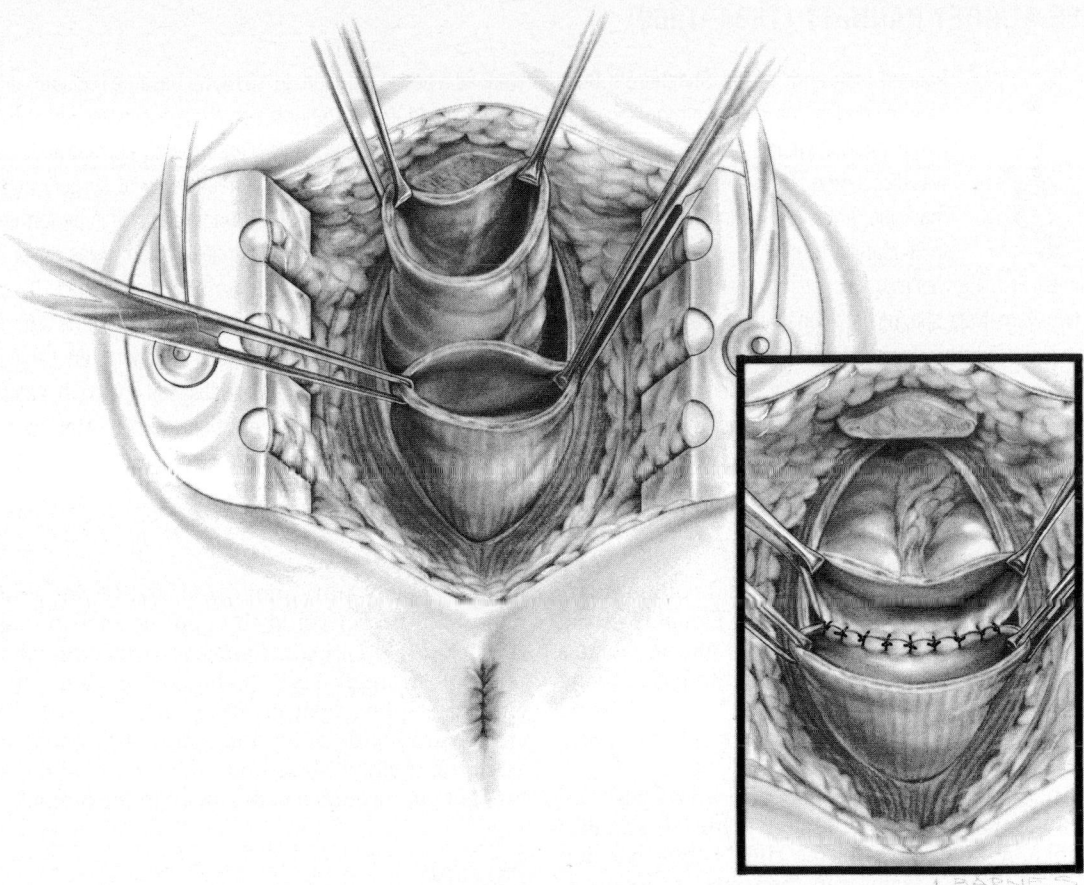

FIGURE 24-110. Transcoccygeal approach to removal of rectal tumors. Sleeve resection can be performed, if necessary, but additional length may be required through the floor of the pelvis. Anastomosis is shown by means of an interrupted suture technique (*inset*).

placed around the rectum for traction, and the dissection is completed. The peritoneum may be opened on the anterior rectal surface. The bowel is then drawn downward as far as possible, and the superior hemorrhoidal vessels divided. The bowel is divided at the desired level and an anastomosis is effected with interrupted 3–0 long-term absorbable sutures as a single layer. A Silastic drain is placed through a stab wound of the buttock into the presacral space and connected to suction. It is usually left in place for 48 to 72 hours or until drainage ceases.

Postoperatively, management is essentially the same as that for a low anterior resection. When flatus is passed, a progressive diet is instituted. During the time of convalescence, the patient is instructed on perineal strengthening exercises (see Chapter 16). A degree of incontinence occurs for several days to a few weeks, but in all cases virtually normal control will be restored eventually, assuming that there has been preservation of the nerve supply.

Results
Results of this operation in contemporary writings are essentially anecdotal. However, Sweeney and Deshmukh performed the procedure on 11 patients, but in only 1 was primary rectal carcinoma the diagnosis.[608] These investigators reported no morbidity or mortality. McCready and colleagues used this approach combined with radiotherapy as a means for effecting a local excision of selected patients

with rectal cancer (see later).[409] Wound infection or a fistula was noted in 29%. Although no recurrences were identified, follow-up was only 13 months.

Sacral excision rapidly had become the most popular modality of treatment for carcinoma of the rectum by the end of the 19th century, but the problems of anastomotic breakdown, fecal fistula, wound sepsis, and tumor recurrence have since caused the procedure to fall into disrepute. The Kraske operation usually permits resection of 8 to 10 cm of rectum without difficulty. However, by contemporary standards, the operation must be regarded as inadequate for the management of rectal cancer because it fails to remove the "zone of upward spread."

Some surgeons, however, still recommend this alternative for small malignant tumors, but there are preferred local procedures for such conditions (see later). The operation does, however, have application in carefully selected patients for benign disease: villous adenoma, benign rectal stricture, rectovaginal fistula, and rectoprostatic fistula (see Chapters 15 and 22).

Abdominosacral Resection

Kraske was the first to suggest a combined abdominosacral resection to overcome the disadvantage of failure to remove the lymphatics of the rectum and rectosigmoid. In the early 1930s, Goetz[207] and Pannett[478] resected the

CHARLES AUBREY PANNETT (1884–1969)

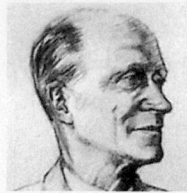

Pannett was born in the Shepherd's Bush area of London, the only surviving son of an ironmonger. Coming from a poor family, he was discouraged from attempting a career in medicine; however, having gained entrance to St. Mary's Hospital, he obtained a scholarship. Alexander Fleming was also a scholarship recipient in the same class. The two were rivals, sharing between them all the medical school prizes. Pannett obtained his degree of doctor of medicine in 1907 with a gold medal and his fellowship in the Royal College of Surgeons in 1910. Shortly thereafter, he contracted tuberculosis and was forced to spend most of the ensuing 4 years in a sanitorium, performing light work as a house surgeon. In 1914, he became registrar at St. Mary's. During World War I, Pannett served as a surgeon on a hospital ship and in the Middle East. Following the war, he returned to St. Mary's and ultimately achieved the professorship of surgery in the University of London. He was best known for his skill in performing a partial gastrectomy at a time when gastrojejunostomy was the preferred and safer procedure for ulcer disease. In 1929, he reported 100 consecutive operations without a death, a remarkable achievement for that or any time. He was the first British surgeon to perform the sphincter-saving operation by means of the abdominosacral approach. Later, he abandoned the operation in favor of anterior resection. A master surgeon, his motto was "cut well, see well, and your patients will get well."

rectum and were able to reestablish intestinal continuity by the sacral approach. In the United States, Donaldson and colleagues, Localio and Stahl, and Marks and associates revived interest in this operation for the treatment of rectal cancer.[150,364,396]

Technique

In the modification described by Localio and Stahl, access to the abdomen and the sacrum is achieved simultaneously by placing the patient in the right lateral position (Figure 24-111).[364] Two teams can then operate independently on the abdomen and over the sacrum. I have found this approach cumbersome, however, and much prefer the patient to be placed in the perineolithotomy position. The abdominal phase is completed as if for a low anterior resection. The lateral stalks are divided, and the surgeon then decides on the advisability of reestablishing continuity and the choice of operation to accomplish this. If the sacral approach is elected, the abdomen is closed. It is important fully to mobilize the entire left colon and splenic flexure so that the bowel can be easily delivered and so that there is no tension on the subsequent anastomosis. The bowel is not divided during the abdominal phase of the procedure. A transverse colostomy or, preferably, a loop ileostomy is routinely performed.

The patient is then placed in the prone jackknife position, and Kraske's approach is used (see above). With the rectum already fully mobilized, the bowel containing the tumor can be delivered through the incision and resected (Figure 24-112). Anastomosis is accomplished with an interrupted single-layer technique or alternatively by the circular stapling instrument (Figure 24-113). The muscles are repaired with heavy long-term absorbable sutures, and a Silastic drain is placed into the hollow of the sacrum and brought out through a stab wound in the buttock.

Results

Localio and colleagues had probably the largest experience with this operation, reporting the results of 427 patients with carcinoma of the rectum.[362,363] Preoperative assessment was made to determine the type of operation that the patient would require: APR, anterior resection, or abdominosacral resection. A total of 100 abdominosacral resections were performed. Although recurrence rates and mortality rates were comparable for the three procedures, the morbidity of abdominosacral resection was much higher. Twelve percent of the patients developed either a fecal fistula or peritonitis (Figure 24-114). Because of these complications, the authors advised that a colostomy should always be performed.

Marks and colleagues reported the results of this operation as performed following radiotherapy.[396] Only those presumed to have locally unfavorable disease were selected.

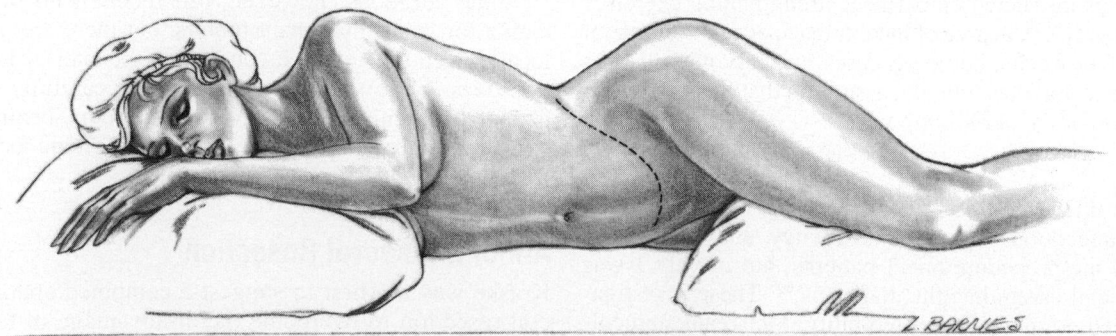

FIGURE 24-111. Position of the patient for synchronous abdominosacral resection and anastomosis (not recommended).

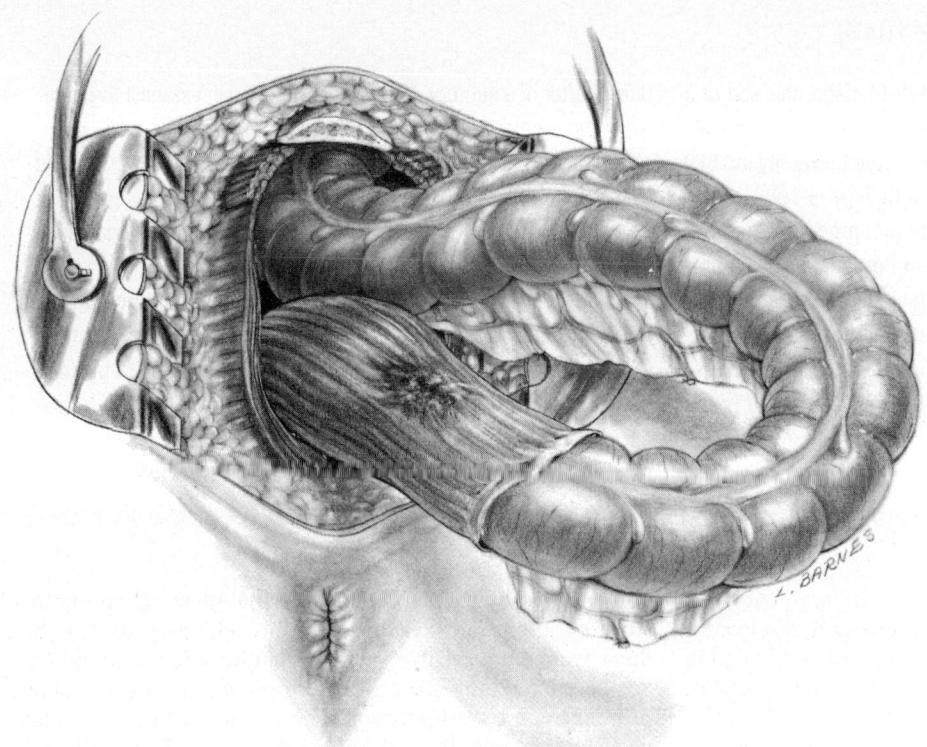

FIGURE 24-112. Abdominosacral resection. The colon is delivered through the sacral defect and is resected. Anastomosis is readily performed through the sacral wound.

The tumors were located 3 to 7 cm from the anal verge. Twenty-four patients were followed from 20 to 84 months with no evidence of pelvic or perineal recurrence.[396] This is probably attributable to the use of preoperative radiation (see later), rather than to the choice of operation. In fact, the radiotherapy was undoubtedly responsible for "downgrading" of the depth of invasion as determined by the subsequent pathology report (see later). However, the authors succeeded in demonstrating that preoperative radiation therapy (40 to 50 Gy) permitted the safe application of this anastomotic alternative.

Transsphincteric Excision

Interest was stimulated in transsphincteric excision as a method for removal of selected, low-lying cancers of the rectum by Mason in 1970.[402] The procedure, however, is not new, having been advocated by Bevan in 1917 for "small carcinomas of the rectum without any radial involvement."[50] Interestingly, however, the author did not seem to repair the sphincter, simply stating, "I do not hope to attain anything like complete continence," nor did he comment about the risk of the development of a fistula.

AUBREY YORK MASON (1910–1993)

York Mason was born in Pietermaritzburg, South Africa. His father was a farmer. Mason attended Ladysmith High School and received a BSc from the University of Witwatersrand in Johannesburg in 1933. While there, he developed an interest in archeology and published a paper on South African cave paintings. He received an MBBCh (MD equivalent) at the same university in 1935 and a medal for being the most distinguished medical graduate. He entered residency in surgery at Johannesburg General Hospital in 1936 and registered as a surgeon in South Africa. However, he left the country, first spending time as a fellow at the Mayo Clinic, then emigrating to England in 1939. He served in the Royal Army Medical Corps in India during World War II. He began operating at St. Helier Hospital in Carshalton, England, in 1949. His wife Margaret, an Australian, was one of the first female anesthetists in the United Kingdom. Mason practiced and publicized the transsphincteric approach to the rectum, now known as the York Mason procedure. He first used this operation in 1960, and by 1970 he began publishing articles advocating the technique in selected cases. He applied this method for the excision of rectal cancer and low rectal anastomosis, and operations for rectourethral and rectoprostatic fistulas. He ultimately applied the technique to almost 100 patients and claimed to achieve good functional outcomes in every instance. Mason was an early advocate of breast-conserving operations for cancer and published the first study comparing radical mastectomy with local excision and radiation. He advocated thorough physical examination including rectal exams for all patients and was a consistent advocate for a multidisciplinary approach to cancer. He was an expert in the diagnosis and treatment of rectal cancer and devised a clinical classification system for this disease. (With appreciation to Thomas R. Gregg, MD.)

ARTHUR DEAN BEVAN (1861–1943)

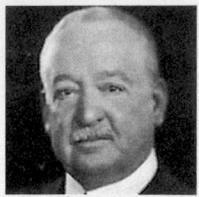

Bevan was born in Chicago, the son of a physician. He graduated from the Sheffield Scientific School of Yale University in 1879 and Rush Medical College in 1883. Bevan began his medical career at the U.S. Marine Hospital in Portland and as a professor of anatomy at Oregon State University. In 1888, he returned to Chicago as professor of anatomy at Rush Medical College, holding the Chair until 1902, when he assumed the position of professor of surgery. Seven years later, he was appointed head of the department, succeeding Nicholas Senn. As chairman of the Council of Medical Education of the American Medical Association for one-quarter of a century, he was instrumental in establishing minimum requirements for admission to medical school and for virtually eliminating the so-called homeopathic and eclectic schools in the United States. Bevan was the first to perform an operation using ethylene anesthesia. His lateral rectus approach for gallbladder surgery is known as the Bevan incision. He devised operations for undescended testis and for the repair of ventral hernia. During World War I, Bevan became director of the Surgical Division of the Office of the Surgeon General of the U.S. Army. He took an active part in organizing physicians for the war effort, for which he received the French Legion of Honor. In 1932, he served as president of the American Surgical Association.

Technique

With the patient in the prone jackknife position, the levator ani and external sphincter muscles are completely divided in the posterior midline. The bowel is opened, offering excellent exposure of the low and middle rectum (Figure 24-115). Although tumors on the anterior wall are the easiest to demonstrate, those on the posterior or lateral walls can be brought into view by fully mobilizing the rectum.

In an experience with 14 patients, Mason reported a recurrence rate of 13%.[401] Allgöwer and colleagues reported 36 patients with rectal cancers treated by a sphincter-splitting approach.[6,7] There were no operative deaths, but there were nine recurrences. The authors recommend frozen-section examination of the surgical margins and depth of penetration by the tumor. The results of the experience with 116 patients from the same unit are rather difficult to interpret.[273] The authors reported this application for many indications, approximately one-half of which were for malignancy.

Abdomino-Transsphincteric Resection

Mason also reported the foregoing technique as an alternative means for effecting an anastomosis following an abdominoanal pull-through.[403] By dividing the sphincter muscles as described in the preceding section, an anastomosis can be performed quite readily at the anal verge.

Lazorthes and colleagues undertook this operation in 65 patients.[343] More than one-half received preoperative radiotherapy. In 57 cases, a diverting colostomy was performed. There were no operative deaths, but six patients (9%) developed pelvic sepsis or an anastomotic leak. Of those surviving 1 year, 91% reported normal control for feces.

Other Local Procedures for Rectal Cancer

In addition to transsacral (transcoccygeal) excision and transsphincteric excision, there are a number of other local procedures that can be used both for palliation and as curative approaches for the management of carcinoma of the rectum. With respect to cure, extensive preoperative evaluation should be obtained to be certain that a curative approach can be reasonably achieved through some form of local treatment. This includes clinical assessment, biopsy, degree of differentiation, CT or MRI, endorectal ultrasound, and a number of other possible studies—all of which are addressed earlier in this chapter and in Chapter 23. Individuals who are poor candidates for curative attempt at local excision include those with transmural involvement (T3 lesions), those with poorly differentiated tumors, those with evident lymph node metastases, those in whom a sphincter-saving operation can be carried out by conventional means, and those who can tolerate a major operation. Hase and colleagues identified five

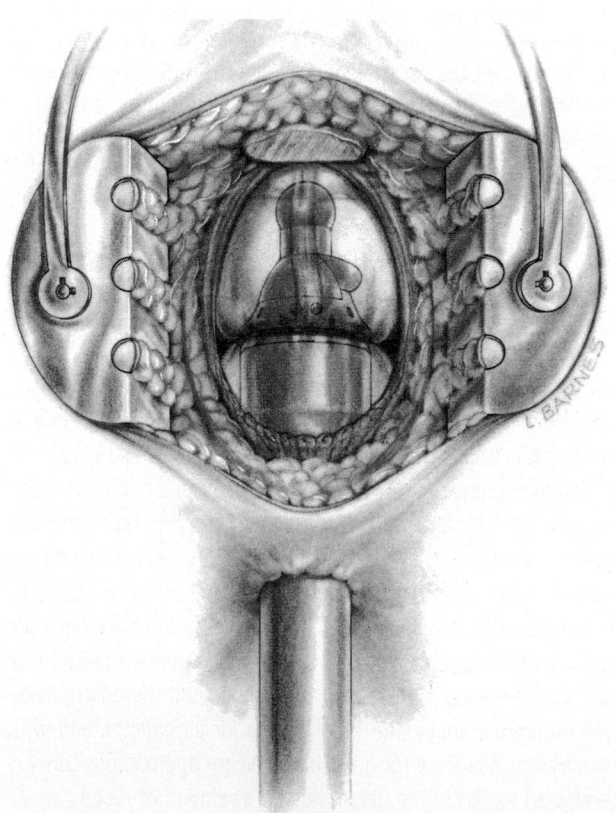

FIGURE 24-113. Circular-stapled anastomosis by transcoccygeal approach. Note the coccyx has been removed.

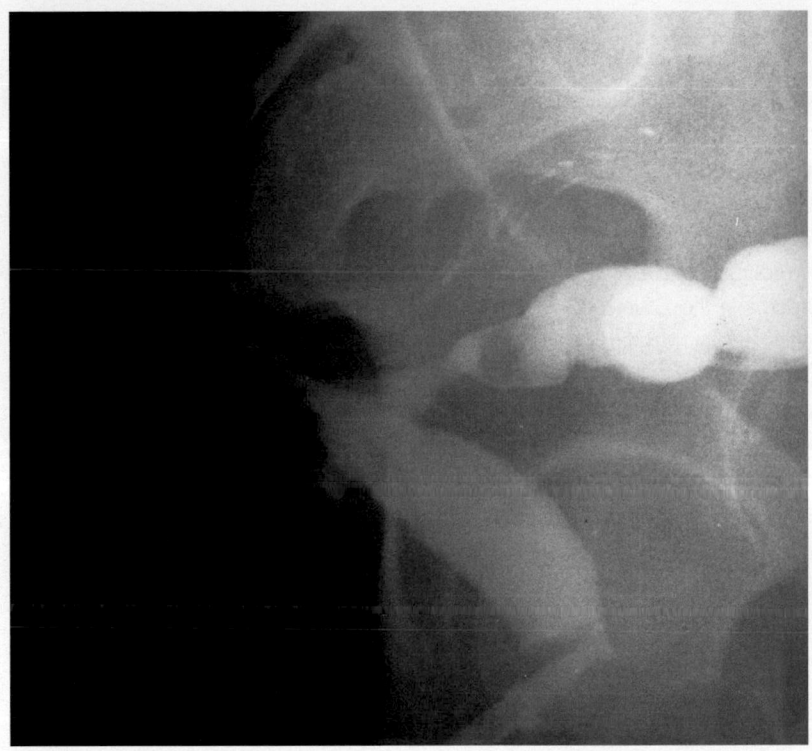

FIGURE 24-114. Anastomotic fistula following an abdominosacral procedure. Note the absence of the coccyx and lower sacrum, which have been resected.

histopathologic characteristics as risk factors for lymph node metastases[241]:

- Small clusters of undifferentiated cancer cells ahead of the invasive front of the lesion ("tumor budding")
- A poorly demarcated invasive front
- Moderately or poorly differentiated cancer cells in the invasive front

- Extension of the tumor to the middle or deep submucosal layer
- Cancer cells in the lymphatics

The investigators concluded that those individuals with three or fewer risk factors had no nodal spread, whereas the rate of lymph node involvement with four or more risk factors was 33% and 67%, respectively.[241] Such a classification

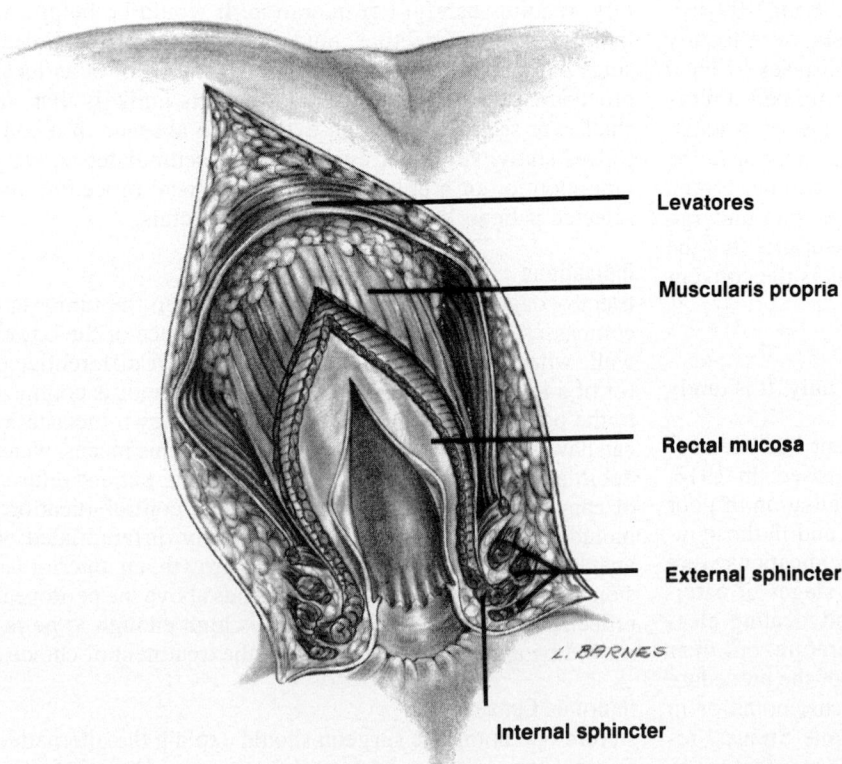

Levatores

Muscularis propria

Rectal mucosa

External sphincter

L. BARNES

Internal sphincter

FIGURE 24-115. Transsphincteric excision. The rectum is opened like a book, posteriorly.

JOHN LEO MADDEN (1912–1999)

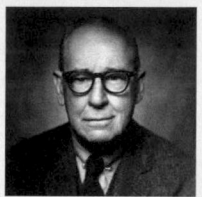

John Madden was born in Washington, DC, and received his medical degree from the George Washington University in 1937. He completed his surgical residency training at the Long Island College Hospital-Kings County Hospital in New York. During World War II, Madden served in the Army Medical Corps in the Pacific theater. Upon returning to New York City, he joined the staff of St. Clare's hospital and in 1948 was appointed director of surgery, a position he held until 1975. He was also on the staff of New York Hospital/Cornell University Medical Center as well as clinical professor of surgery at Cornell. Madden was a prolific author and innovative thinker. His contributions were varied and numerous. In 1952, he received the Ludwig Hektoen gold medal from the American Medical Association for his work illustrating blood vessels. Madden was a true pioneer in the emerging field of vascular surgery. He also has been credited with singular approaches to the treatment of breast and colorectal disease, especially that of diverticulitis and rectal cancer. He was also an innovator in video teaching. The American College of Surgeons' video library contains almost 50 of his procedures. Madden received numerous recognitions and awards during his long and fruitful career, including president of the New York Academy of Medicine, chairman of the Section on Surgery of the American Medical Association, president of the International Cardiovascular Society, and membership in the French Academy of Surgery. He died on March 25, 1999. (With appreciation to Keith P. Meslin, MD; photograph courtesy of the New York Academy of Medicine.)

may be useful in determining those individuals who may be preferred candidates for local excision. Others suggest that the incidence of lymph node metastases is higher for lesions greater than 1 cm in diameter, for those showing "massive" submucosal invasion, and for moderately differentiated adenocarcinomas.[609]

It has been noted that lymph node–clearing techniques may demonstrate tumor in lymph nodes as small as 1 mm, suggesting that even the best methods for preoperative assessment may miss tumors that are theoretically beyond surgical curability through local excision.[252] The implication of this observation is that one should consider supplementary radiotherapy, either preoperatively or postoperatively, whenever a local procedure is recommended or performed. In a study by Huddy and colleagues, involving 109 rectal excision specimens in which the tumors were locally confined to the bowel wall, 20% had metastases to local lymph nodes.[274] Although less well-differentiated tumors were more likely to have metastasized, there was no statistically significant difference in the size of tumors or in the depth of invasion between patients with or without lymph node metastases. The reality is that patients who undergo local procedures do so without complete assurance that the operation is as effective in curing cancer as is the conventional, radical approach.

Electrocoagulation

This section is included for reference value only. It is rarely practiced today.

Destruction of tumors by electric current has been reported virtually since electricity was harnessed. In 1913, Strauss advocated electrocoagulation for palliation in poor risk patients with carcinoma of the rectum and in those individuals with extensive lesions.[595–598] His indications were gradually broadened to include almost all stages of carcinoma of the rectum. Subsequent reports advocating electrosurgical destruction have dotted the literature, but their authors emphasized that the primary value of the procedure was in those patients who had incurable carcinoma or in those who refused colostomy.[285,308,525] Despite Strauss' results, which were reported to be at least as satisfactory as those for surgically resected carcinomas, the value of this technique failed to have any significant impact on surgical thinking until Madden and Kandalaft reported their series in 1967.[383] They believed electrocoagulation to be the preferred treatment for carcinoma of the rectum. Subsequently, they updated their study in 1971, and Crile and Turnbull reported a series with favorable results in 1972.[115,384] As a consequence, others have been encouraged to selectively apply this technique.[330,544,657] Because of these reports, many surgeons had begun to use this treatment not only for palliation, but also for the potentially curable lesion.

The decision of attempting to avoid APR, a surgical procedure that has been reasonably successful in the primary treatment of carcinoma of the rectum for more than a century, requires careful consideration. It would be helpful if there were a prospective, randomized, controlled clinical study comparing APR with electrocoagulation or other local procedures for that matter. However, it is unlikely that we shall ever see one, although even in the absence of a controlled study, sufficient evidence has accumulated to warrant adoption of a policy of advising a local procedure for selected patients with carcinoma of the rectum.

Indications

Electrocoagulation may be considered when the tumor encompasses less than 50% of the circumference of the bowel wall, when the lesion is exophytic and well differentiated (or of a low-grade malignancy), when the tumor is confined to the bowel wall, when the patient with known metastases can have symptoms effectively palliated by this means, when debilitating disease is present, or when the patient refuses or cannot manage a colostomy. Relative contraindications include a circumferential lesion, a poorly differentiated or anaplastic tumor, a deeply ulcerating growth, an anterior lesion in a woman, or a tumor that extends above the peritoneal reflection. Certainly, if the growth is high enough to be removed by anterior resection, this is the treatment of choice.

Informed Consent

Before operation, the surgeon should explain the alternative forms of therapy available and the pros and cons of each procedure. If electrocoagulation is contemplated, the importance of close follow-up examination and the possibility of readmission to the hospital must be stressed. This places a considerable emotional burden on both the patient and the surgeon, and this clearly must be recognized at the outset. It is much easier for a surgeon to perform an abdominoperineal excision knowing that there is little more to offer the patient from the surgical point of view if the tumor recurs. However, if tumor recurs following electrocoagulation, it is extremely difficult to judge when this approach should be abandoned and when abdominoperineal excision should be undertaken. Even after unsuccessful electrocoagulation, the patient may be cured by radical surgery many months after the initial therapy.

Technique

All individuals are treated in the hospital, not as outpatients, unless one is dealing with a very small lesion. Regional or general anesthesia is required. The technique has been described by Madden and Kandalaft.[383] The patient is placed in the prone position if the tumor is primarily anterior and in the lithotomy position if the tumor is essentially posterior. Following sphincter stretch, a plastic-operating anal retractor (Ferguson Clinic, Grand Rapids, MI) of appropriate diameter and length is inserted (Figure 24-116). These instruments were initially advocated by Schultz and Muldoon and by Muldoon and Capehart for use in excision of polyps of the colon and rectum.[449,557] Other retractors may, of course, be used. Salvati and Rubin suggested the use of local infiltration with bupivacaine and epinephrine to improve anal relaxation and to limit the depth of anesthesia required.[544]

The goal of electrocoagulation is to destroy by coagulating current the entire tumor and a margin of normal tissue both deep to and around it. A standard electrocautery unit is used with the needle-tip adapter, and only coagulating current is employed. The area for electrocoagulation is outlined by means of the needle (Figure 24-117A). The tip is then plunged into the tumor while the current is applied, and the process is repeated until the entire area has been treated[44] (Figure 24-117B). Necrotic tissue is removed by scraping with the aid of an electrified wire loop or endometrial curette (Figure 24-117C). When normal tissue is encountered (muscular wall or perirectal adipose tissue), the procedure

is terminated. It is helpful to have available special lighting. This may include a headlamp, fiberoptic light source, or lighted retractor. A Frazier-tip suction is helpful for smoke as well as bleeding because it is quite small and is not as likely to impede the already limited view. Frequent irrigation with a bulb syringe is also a requisite. Operative time varies according to the size of the lesion and the degree of penetration; it may be as long as 2 hours (Figure 24-118). By no means should this procedure be considered a minor undertaking. For larger tumors, more than one session may be required, each necessitating hospitalization and an anesthetic.

After a large tumor has been ablated, the patient, ideally, is confined in the hospital for several days, at which time further biopsies are taken, and a repeat coagulation is performed if necessary. Unfortunately, ideal (i.e., in-hospital) management is often not possible because of economic constraints. As a consequence, one must be willing to assume the risks of sepsis and delayed hemorrhage with the individual's having been discharged. The patient is seen at monthly intervals for the first 6 months and is readmitted to the hospital (if possible) for biopsy and electrocoagulation if a recurrent tumor is suspected. After 6 months without evidence of tumor, the intervals between office visits are gradually lengthened to approximately four times a year.

Complications

The most common postoperative complication is pyrexia. An oral temperature of 103° F (39.4° C) on the evening after surgery is not uncommon. It is because of this problem that broad-spectrum antibiotic treatment is recommended preoperatively and postoperatively for at least 24 hours. Pelvic peritonitis may occur without rectal perforation, but abdominal exploration, drainage, and colostomy are rarely indicated.

Hemorrhage at the time of surgery may necessitate multiple blood transfusions. All patients should have blood available when electrocoagulation is performed for large lesions. This can be a time-consuming operation, a procedure during which blood loss may appear to be minimal, but it can be persistent and ultimately not inconsequential. Late hemorrhage can occur up to several weeks after the procedure, probably secondary to sloughing of the eschar. This often requires readmission to the hospital and transfusion, and it has been reported to occur in as many as 22% of patients who

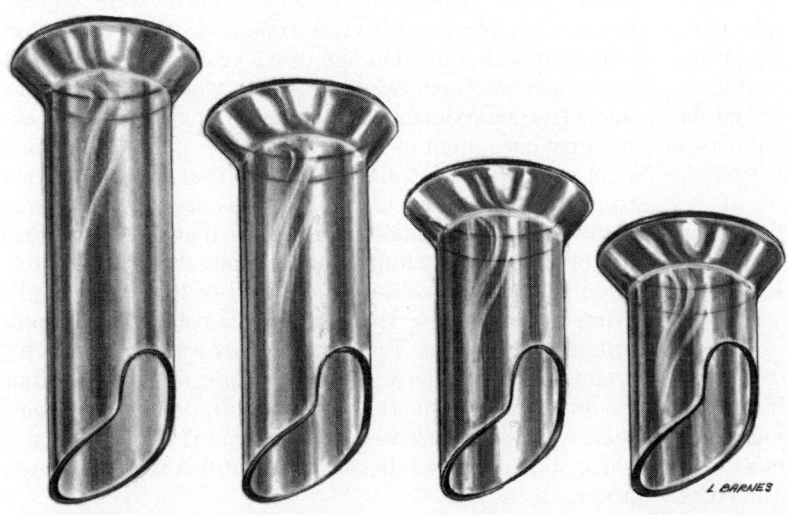

FIGURE 24-116. Plastic retractors of varied lengths and diameters permit excellent visualization for electrocoagulation.

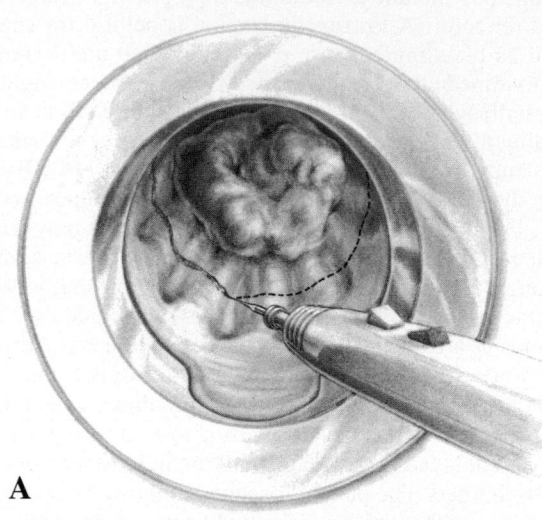

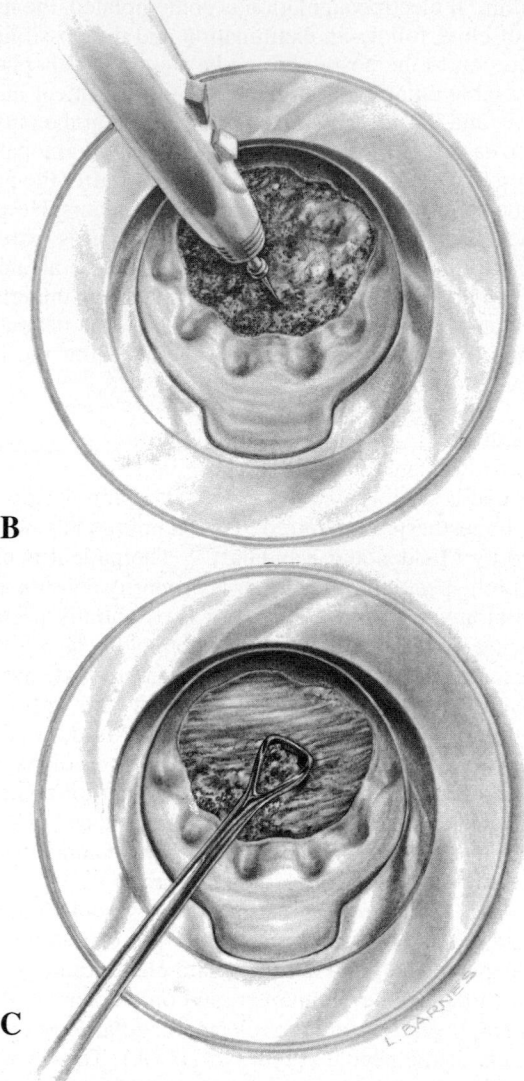

FIGURE 24-117. Electrocoagulation of rectal cancer. **A:** The area of excision/ electrocoagulation is outlined with the needle-tip electrode. **B:** Using the needle, the entire tumor mass is electrocoagulated. **C:** With an endometrial curette, the coagulum is scraped off and the process repeated. When only normal tissue remains, the operation is complete.

undergo electrocoagulation.[384] Five of 48 patients (10%) had hemorrhage sufficiently severe to require transfusion in the early experience of Hughes and colleagues.[276]

Rectal stricture may result from electrocoagulation if more than 50% of the bowel wall is involved by tumor. Repeated procedures increase the risk of this complication. Furthermore, the development of a stricture may impede the ability of the surgeon to visualize the area for possible recurrence. Benign stricture may be treated by lysis and the frequent insertion by the patient of a Hegar's dilator (see Figure 24-89). Strictures occurred in 8% of the Lahey Clinic (Boston) series.[276]

In women, rectovaginal fistula may result from vigorous burning of an anterior lesion. Electrocoagulation, therefore, should be performed only for small, exophytic lesions when they occur in this location.

Results

Madden and Kandalaft updated their experience in 1983 to include a total of 204 patients treated by electrocoagulation.[385] Their 5-year survival rates even with ulcerating tumors were very impressive (57% with lesions larger than 3 cm and 63%

if smaller than 3 cm). Patients with polypoid tumors had a 70% 5-year survival rate for the smaller tumors and a 64% rate for the larger ones.

In the Lahey Clinic experience, 39 patients were operated on for cure.[276] Twenty-one were men, and 18 were women. The median age was 70 years (range, 48 to 89 years), as compared with a median age of 62 years for the group of individuals who underwent APR. Ten were 80 years old or older. The approximate sizes of the lesions were up to 2 cm in 14 patients, 3 cm in 13 patients, 4 cm in 8 patients, and 6 cm or larger in 4 patients. Twenty-four individuals had exophytic tumors, and 15 had ulcerative lesions. Only three of the exophytic tumors were greater than 3 cm, whereas nine of the ulcerating tumors were greater than 3 cm. Thirty-seven patients had well-differentiated or moderately well-differentiated tumors. The remaining 2 patients had poorly differentiated lesions. Ten required only a single session for treatment. Nine underwent two sessions, 4 underwent four sessions, and 4 patients underwent six or more sessions. There were two operative deaths related to cardiac problems, which should remind the surgeon that this is not a benign procedure.

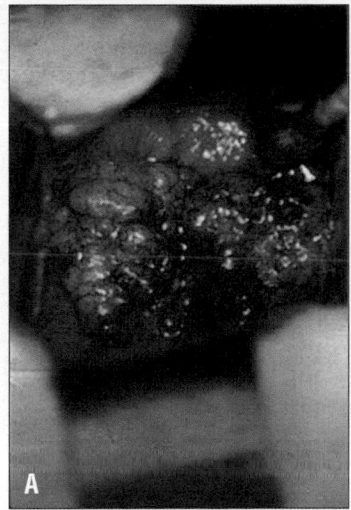
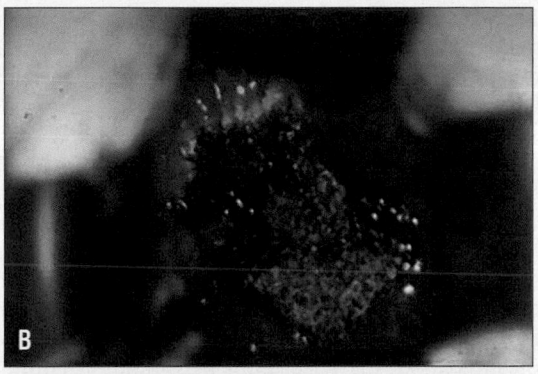
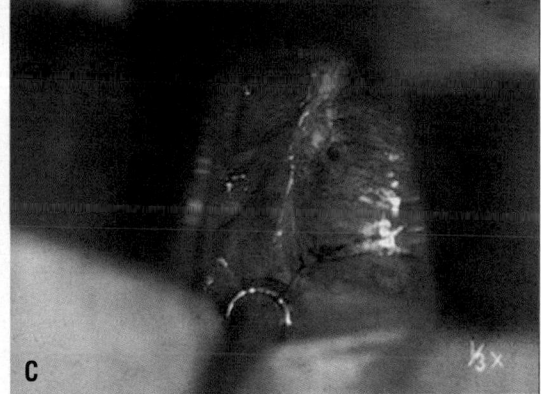

FIGURE 24-118. Electrocoagulation. **A:** Rectal cancer is exposed. **B:** The tumor has been completely electrocoagulated. **C:** Only the scar remains 2 months following treatment. (Courtesy of John L. Madden, MD.)

In 27 of the 39 patients (69%), no evidence of disease was apparent at the end of the follow-up period. Twenty patients were alive, and 7 had died of causes unrelated to the rectal cancer. Of the 24 patients with exophytic tumors, 22 (92%) had no evidence of the disease. However, only 5 of the 15 patients with ulcerative tumors (33%) had no evidence of disease. Forty percent of patients who initially had ulcerative lesions could not have their local disease controlled by electrocoagulation; 27% required APR.

Salvati and colleagues reported 81 patients who underwent electrocoagulation for cure and in whom at least a 5-year follow-up was available.[545] The criteria for selection were essentially the same as those previously discussed. The overall 5-year survival rate was 47%, but 38% required conversion to an APR. This last group had a 29% 5-year survival. The morbidity rate for electrocoagulation was 21%. Others had also become advocates of the judicious application of this technique.[649] The subsequent colostomy rate, however, has been reported to be as high as 25%.[33]

Palliation by Electrocoagulation

Christiansen and Kirkegaard employed electrocoagulation after recurrence developed following low anterior resection in an attempt to avoid colostomy.[107] Of 15 patients so treated, 9 were alive without colostomy 8 to 16 months after the first treatment, and 3 had died without a stoma. There was one death, a consequence of the procedure. Kurz and colleagues reported the use of the urologic resectoscope for palliating symptoms from obstructing and bleeding lesions.[335] They emphasize the unique benefit of cutting current with continuous fluid irrigation to provide excellent visibility. Berry and coworkers used the same technique both for benign and malignant lesions.[49] Salvati and Rubin reported that colostomy

was avoided in all but 3 of the 19 patients they treated for palliation.[544]

Sequential Treatment (Electrocoagulation Followed by Resection)

Eisenberg combined electrocoagulation with subsequent resection in the treatment of 250 patients.[159] The author preferred to perform low anterior resection, which calls into question the issue of performing this sphincter-saving alternative in the first instance. The survival results were exceptionally good: 85% following low anterior resection and 61% after APR. Despite these favorable results, no one else has been motivated to report their experience.

Transanal Excision

Transanal excision has been advocated by a number of surgeons for the definitive treatment of small (less than 3 cm), exophytic, movable, well-differentiated lesions.[54,126,135,311,390,444,588,650] As with electrocoagulation, the preoperative evaluation should include, among all of the other criteria, histopathologic confirmation, especially the degree of differentiation, as well as endorectal ultrasound (see prior discussion). The policy of less than resection is based on the knowledge that there is only a 10% risk of synchronous metastasis to regional lymph nodes when the cancer is confined to the rectal wall.[443] Conversely, the Mayo Clinic group observed that the risk of harboring lymph nodes metastases with T1 low rectal cancers that have lymphovascular invasion on biopsy or invasion into the lower third of the submucosa was sufficiently high as to mandate either radical resection or adjuvant therapy.[455]

The singular advantage of local excision over that of electrocoagulation is that it offers the opportunity for histologically evaluating a "total biopsy." Theoretically, if local excision is judged by the pathologist to be "complete" and the tumor is well-differentiated or moderately well-differentiated, then one may reasonably recommend that no additional surgical treatment is required.[443] The essential variables, therefore, are the capability and the interest of the pathologist. It is also extremely important to orient the specimen for histologic examination accurately. Sweeney suggests that one use 25-gauge needles to pin the specimen onto a cautery cleansing pad for this purpose.[607] Whether one is truly satisfied with the margins of the excision and whether there is evidence of lymphatic, or blood vessel invasion may create additional concerns about the wisdom of performing a limited procedure. Guillem and colleagues at Memorial Sloan-Kettering Cancer Center suggested using the following criteria in order to determine which tumors are theoretically suitable for transanal excision[223]:

- Size less than 4 cm
- Tumor confined to less than one quadrant
- Site less than 9 cm from anal verge
- Mobility
- Well-differentiated appearance
- Absence of lymphovascular invasion
- Absence of nodal involvement
- Ultrasonographic T1, T2, N0 lesion
- On CT scan, no metastases

Unfortunately, there are no statistically meaningful studies available concerning the risk of harboring additional tumor, and there have been no prospective randomized clinical trials.

Technique

The procedure can be performed through an operating proctoscope (depending on the location and the size of the lesion), but more commonly it is accomplished by dilating the anus and inserting retractors. The technique is essentially the same as that illustrated in Figure 22-34 for benign lesions. As with electrocoagulation, proper positioning is crucial. Anterior lesions are best managed with the patient in the prone jackknife position, and posterior lesions are optimally treated with the patient in the lithotomy position. Ideally, one attempts to achieve a 1-cm margin, but lesser margins may be as satisfactory. The tumor is outlined with an adequate margin by means of the needle-tip electrocautery. Some individuals prefer injection of saline with or without epinephrine to facilitate hemostasis and to aid in the dissection. Generally, it is easier to begin the dissection from below the tumor using a clamp to hold the specimen as the dissection proceeds cephalad. A full-thickness rectal wall excision is performed; one should not attempt to preserve part of the bowel wall. The wound may be closed if the size of the opening permits or left open, provided it is posterior and below the peritoneal reflection. Other minimally invasive techniques are described in Chapter 19.

Results

Hager and associates reported 95 patients treated by local excision.[231] The 5-year survival rate for tumors confined to the mucosa and submucosa was 90%, and 78% when the cancer invaded the muscularis propria. Biggers and colleagues reported the Mayo Clinic experience of 234 patients.[54] Of these, 180 never developed a recurrence, 5 developed metastases, and 49 had local recurrences. Although it may seem that the overall failure rate is excessive (23%), many patients who had undergone this treatment would today not fulfill the previously mentioned criteria for selection. For example, if one limits the indications for this treatment to those tumors that have a pedicle or pseudopedicle, Grigg and colleagues reported that 100% of their 16 patients survived for 5 years.[222]

Graham and colleagues identify three pathologic features that correlate with a high risk of recurrence and a poor outcome: positive surgical margins, poorly differentiated histology, and increasing depth of bowel wall invasion.[218] Coco and associates employed local excision in 36 patients, adding postoperative radiation therapy if the tumor unexpectedly had breached the rectal wall.[109] The complication rate was 9.3%. The results were not sufficiently long term to give meaningful cure or recurrence rates. Close follow-up examination is emphasized. Bleday and colleagues noted an 8% recurrence rate with local excision and concluded that either a positive margin or lymphatic invasion were believed to be indications for resection.[63] Faivre and coworkers noted a 28% incidence of recurrence in their 126 patients.[167] Vascular invasion and a mucinous component were believed to be poor prognostic factors. Rouanet and associates opined that local control should improve if postoperative radiotherapy is given for more invasive tumors and those greater than 3 cm in diameter.[528] Others reported a reasonably satisfactory experience in a highly selected group of patients.[179,193,272]

Mellgren and colleagues reported the University of Minnesota experience.[415] One hundred eight patients with T1 and T2 rectal cancers treated by local excision were compared with 153 individuals with T1N0 and T2N0 rectal cancers managed by radical resection. Mean follow-up was greater than 4 years in each group. The estimated 5-year recurrence rate was 18% for T1 and 47% for T2 tumors. The rate following radical resection was 9% for T1 and 16% for T2 cancers. The authors concluded that local excision carries with it a much greater risk of recurrence than radical resection, and despite salvage surgery (see the following), local excision for T2 tumors especially may compromise overall survival.[415]

Löhnert and coworkers, as part of their follow-up routine, evaluated by means of endorectal ultrasound all of their 116 patients who had undergone local excision, in addition to the usual clinical and laboratory investigations.[368] Evidence of local recurrence suggested by endorectal ultrasound was confirmed by ultrasound-guided needle biopsy. All 25 patients who were found to have occult rectal cancer recurrences were alive at the end of the study period (four with recurrences). Because endoluminal ultrasound can apparently detect local recurrence at an earlier and subclinical stage, the authors encourage the routine application of this modality as part of the follow-up regimen.

Local Excision and Radiotherapy

Downstaging with neoadjuvant therapy followed by local excision is another controversial issue. Schell and coworkers found that some of their patients with T3 lesions experienced significant downstaging and submitted 11 to local excision.[554] There were no local recurrences in these individuals (median follow-up, 47.9 months). Marks and colleagues reported their experience of 20 patients with preoperative radiation (45 Gy) followed by full-thickness local excision 4 to 6 weeks later.[398] They found a recurrence rate of 21%.

As a consequence, they believed that this approach is of value only for the individual who cannot tolerate a standard resection.

Ellis and colleagues performed local excision of favorable rectal cancers followed by radiotherapy (45 Gy).[160] They found no evidence of disease in their eight patients, with a mean of 67 months of follow-up. The obvious question, however, is whether the patients would have been equally served without the radiation. A less successful experience was noted by others.[426]

Salvage Resection after Local Treatment

Baron and colleagues retrospectively reviewed 155 patients who were submitted to initial curative treatment by a local procedure.[36] A total of 21 patients underwent radical resection because of an unfavorable pathology report, either APR or low anterior resection immediately following the local treatment. An additional 21 patients underwent a so-called salvage resection for local recurrence. The disease-free survival for those who had undergone immediate resection was 94.1% as compared with the delayed group survival rate of 55.5%. The authors recommended that when adverse pathologic features are present in the excision specimen, immediate resection should be performed.[36] The 5-year survival rate as reported by Rouanet and colleagues was 30% for those individuals subjected to resection for recurrent disease.[528]

The aforementioned University of Minnesota group identified 24 of 27 patients with recurrence after local excision who underwent salvage surgery.[116] The estimated 5-year survival rate was 72% for T1 tumors and 65% after salvage surgery for what was initially T2 lesions. Another report from the same institution revealed that the stage of recurrent tumor was more advanced than that of the primary in 93%.[182] The authors emphasized the importance of appropriate selection for those offered local excision. In still another publication from the Memorial Sloan-Kettering Cancer Center involving 125 patients, the investigators concluded that two-thirds of the patients who developed recurrence have local treatment failure, implicating inadequate excision.[491] Furthermore, neither adjuvant radiotherapy nor salvage surgery was believed to be reliable in controlling or preventing local recurrence.

Comment

Local excision of early rectal cancer, even in the ideal candidate, is followed by a much higher recurrence rate than **had earlier been believed**. Although **many** patients in whom local recurrence develops can be **theoretically** salvaged by radical resection, the long-term outcome remains **problematical**. Pelvic recurrence following transanal excision of early rectal cancer is often locally advanced, requiring an extended pelvic dissection with en bloc resection of adjacent pelvic organs to achieve salvage. **The fact is that** long-term outcome in patients undergoing resection is less than expected, considering the early stage of their initial disease. When contemplating local excision for early rectal cancer, the risk of recurrence, the extent and morbidity of surgery required for salvage, and the modest cure rate following salvage should all be considered.[645]

Transanal Endoscopic Microsurgery

Transanal endoscopic microsurgery (TEMS) was developed by Buess and colleagues as a technique for treating adenomas of the rectum.[80,509] TEMS has been slow to gain popularity for reasons of cost and the steep learning curve. Over the last two decades, TEMS has become an established minimally invasive procedure carrying lesser morbidity and mortality risks, particularly in elderly and unfit patients. Although radical resection represents the best curative procedure, it comes at significant potential morbidity, particularly in an aging patient population.

The perioperative risk of death is 0.5% for healthy patients undergoing radical rectal surgery who are classified as American Society of Anesthesiologists (ASA) grade I. This risk increases to more than 25% for patients with poorly controlled comorbidities (ASA grade IV). Patients older than the age of 80 undergoing rectal resection have a 15% risk of perioperative death.[8,171,612] Local procedures offer an alternative with less morbidity and mortality. Local excision, or transanal resection, is a minimally invasive procedure limited to lesions lying within 5 cm of the anal verge. In comparison, TEMS is able to access the upper rectum and permits a stereoscopic, magnified view of the gas-filled rectum, facilitating precise surgery in an otherwise inaccessible area.

The role of TEMS has not been clearly defined. Significant heterogeneity limits conclusions from the current literature. A review of available studies found oncologic outcomes in TEMS similar to those achieved with radical resection in highly selected cases, but with far less mortality, morbidity, blood loss, and hospital stay.[140] TEMS alone may be sufficient for "favorable" T1 tumors. "Unfavorable" T1 or T2 tumors require adjuvant therapies. TEMS should only be used for palliation in T3+ lesions.

The equipment required to perform TEMS includes a 4 cm in diameter operating proctoscope, with lengths available in either 12 or 20 cm and the 0-degree telescope (Figure 24-119). Instruments are designed for laparoscopic work and consist of

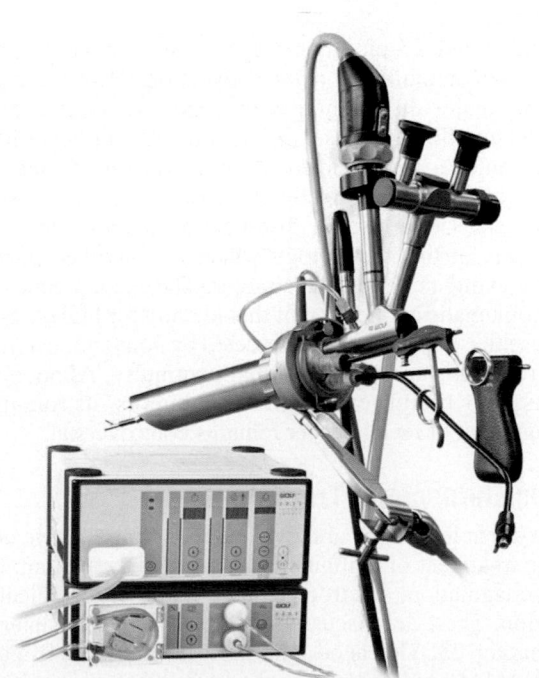

FIGURE 24-119. Transanal endoscopic microsurgery (TEM) system. Up to four surgical instruments can be inserted at the same time. The assistant can follow the procedure through the use of a fiberoptic channel or through a video monitor. (Courtesy of Richard Wolf Medical Instruments, Inc., Vernon Hills, IL.)

angled atraumatic grasping forceps, laparoscopic diathermy or hemostatic device, scissors, clip applicators, needle holder, and irrigation-suction device.

Full bowel preparation is required preoperatively. Under general anesthesia, the patient is placed in the lithotomy position. Following the procedure, patients may drink and eat immediately. In most cases, simple oral non-opiate analgesia provides adequate pain relief, and discharge occurs within 24 hours.

Temporary minor urge incontinence may occur for several days. Despite short-term alterations in laboratory measurements of anorectal function, there are no reported long-term detrimental effects on fecal continence.[251,307,331,640] One study found no difference between preoperative and postoperative function as measured by ability to defer defecation, number of bowel movements per 24 hours, the Fecal Incontinence Severity Index, and Fecal Incontinence Quality of Life Survey.[90] Another report demonstrated improvement in perceived quality of life due to excision of the tumor.[151]

The height of the tumor from the anal verge is important; TEMS is considered safe only when lesions are located in the extraperitoneal colon. Resection of tumors of the distal sigmoid carry a higher risk of intra-abdominal perforation and possibly the need for laparotomy. Bleeding is common and difficult to control. However, in all series, the incidence of complications during TEMS is lower than that of major rectal surgery.[20,140,445,535,539,540,552] Thus far, there has been no reported mortality from TEMS.

When TEMS is used for a presumed adenoma, the final histopathology may demonstrate the presence of malignancy, in which case the report should be discussed in detail with the pathologist and a decision made about further treatment. This could include repeat TEMS,[581] salvage resectional surgery, or additional treatment with radiotherapy or chemotherapy or both.[578,590]

Comment

Transanal endoscopic microsurgery can obviously accomplish what amounts to a local excision. However, there are two major disadvantages or concerns. First, the cost is considerable. Because of the limited applicability of this technique, it is doubtful whether very many surgeons or institutions can justify the expense associated with this investment. Certainly, for distal rectal lesions, there is no advantage of this technology when one has the option of merely using an anorectal retractor. The second concern is the problematic application of this method for higher lesions because these can usually be resected by conventional means with reestablishment of intestinal continuity. Although the technique is useful for benign rectal tumors, its role in the management of rectal cancer remains controversial.

Other Endoscopic Treatment

There are at least three ablative methods for palliative endoscopic treatment of malignant strictures of the rectum: laser photocoagulation, electrocoagulation, and cryosurgical destruction. These are discussed previously in this chapter and in Chapter 23. The neodymium:yttrium-aluminum-garnet (Nd:YAG) laser has been applied by many groups for the palliative treatment of rectal cancer.[70,78,104,369,373,389,405,558] No one, however, is advocating this approach for the management of curable cancers of the rectum. For the unresectable tumor or when bleeding is a problem, the laser can restore luminal patency and achieve at least temporary hemostasis.[405] When compared with other local procedures, laser therapy is unique in that it is of equal applicability to tumors above the peritoneal reflection as it is to those below. Eckhauser and colleagues employed the Nd:YAG laser as a preresective treatment for obstructing rectal carcinoma.[158] They found that recanalization by this method permitted primary resection and anastomosis to be accomplished.

The procedure may be performed selectively on an outpatient basis, but it usually requires hospitalization. Standard bowel preparation is employed; sedation alone may be adequate. Concern has been expressed that the energy delivered by the laser can be quite misleading. The actual tissue effect is as much related to the technique of application as it is to the laser power settings.[373] Although laser endoscopy permits change of these settings to enhance a hemostatic or vaporizing effect, this must be recognized if one is to avoid excessive cavitation.[373]

Initial relief of symptoms has been reported to be approximately 90% in several published series, but after a few months, individuals may require an additional treatment.[70,78,104,369,405,462,633] The primary aim is to avoid a colostomy, and this is usually successful because patients are not expected to survive for very long. Perirectal abscess and bowel perforation are reportedly infrequent complications. Mandava and coworkers experienced a 15% complication rate in their 27 patients.[389]

Escudero-Fabre and Sack have proposed what seems to me to be reasonable indications for this technique[165]:

- For palliation of malignant neoplasms in individuals with extensive local disease, disseminated disease, high operative risk, or refusal to undergo surgery
- As a temporizing measure to improve preoperative status in those individuals with lesions complicated by obstruction or bleeding
- As an alternative approach for the management of benign lesions

Farouk and colleagues reported that laser treatment offered adequate palliation for 78% of their 41 patients.[170] They further observed that those who survived more than 2 years were more likely to require surgical intervention.

Bright and associates had a less favorable experience with this approach in their report of 38 patients.[74] Two-thirds of those with large tumors required an alternative surgical approach. Furthermore, the overall mortality rate within 1 month of treatment was 21%. The authors concluded those tumors that are circumferential or those involving the anal sphincters are better managed by approaches other than laser therapy.[74]

Laser photocoagulation may be used in combination with either implantation of a plastic prosthesis or a self-expanding metal stent (see Chapter 23).[534] The advantage of stent placement is to maintain luminal patency in order to prevent the need for repetitive laser treatments. Rupp successfully used self-expanding metal stents in combination with palliative laser therapy.[534] Serious complications or signs of reobstruction were not observed until the patient's death, with survival time up to 25 months. The novel use of combined endoscopic laser and radiotherapy in patients with advanced recurrent rectal cancer who have a limited life expectancy is a useful alternative to stenting and considered by some as preferable to stenting with its attendant complications. The laser treatment is administered under conscious sedation with effective control of bleeding and mucus discharge by vaporization of protuberant tumor, and this effect is maintained by additional radiotherapy administered either by standard external beam or by brachytherapy.[100]

Cryosurgery

Gage reported the use of cryotherapy for palliation of symptoms in seven patients with inoperable rectal cancer and one with perineal recurrence after APR.[189] Bleeding was controlled, obstruction was relieved, and colostomy was not required. These benefits were believed to be related to the reduction of tumor bulk. Gage believed that cryotherapy can compete successfully with radiation and electrocoagulation in the management of selected cases of inoperable rectal cancer.[190]

Fritsch and colleagues treated 219 patients with this technique but only for palliation.[183] At 6 months to 7 years following treatment, local tumor was eradicated in 30% and reduced in size sufficiently to relieve symptoms in 24%. Fourteen percent of patients experienced hemorrhage, and 26% developed stenoses. Other major complications (e.g., peritonitis) were seen in 8%. Disadvantages included frequent discharge of necrotic tissue and malodorous secretions, as well as rather costly equipment. Heberer and coworkers used cryosurgery for palliation in 268 patients.[249] A colostomy was avoided in 80% (mean observation time, 2.3 years). The experience of others suggests that the cryosurgical technique provides therapeutic benefits for selected patients with advanced rectal cancer and for those who cannot tolerate a major operation.[660]

Endocavitary Irradiation

The use of radium needles and radiation therapy has been employed in the palliative treatment of incurable or recurrent rectal cancer for more than 50 years. In fact, Sir Charles Gordon-Watson presented a paper on the use of radium in the treatment of rectal cancer as early as 1927.[214] Although he recognized in several publications in the 1930s that in most cases the results were somewhat less than gratifying, he believed that there was indeed a place for this method, especially in the nonresectable situation.[215–217] However, it was not until Papillon reported his experience in 1973 that radiation was applied as an alternative to surgery for a potentially curable lesion.[479]

Technique

The procedure requires a special device that can be inserted through a large-diameter proctoscope. The contact unit, manufactured by Phillips (Eindhoven, the Netherlands; Figure 24-120), develops a high-radiation output (10 to 20 Gy/minute) with low-voltage (50-kV) x-rays. The effective area is approximately 3 cm in diameter, with absorption of the x-rays essentially limited to a depth of 2 cm. Papillon recommended 25 to 40 Gy at each treatment, administered within 3 minutes.[481] The procedure is repeated from 1 to 3 weeks later, for a total dose of between 80 and 150 Gy over a period of 4 to 10 weeks. Most patients can be managed outside of a hospital setting, and no anesthesia is usually required.

In a later publication, Papillon suggested that in patients younger than 60 years old, a perirectal lymphadenectomy be considered.[482] He also added a combination of external beam radiation (30 Gy in 12 days), followed by ^{192}Ir implant 2 months later, to extend the field of radiation in the poor risk patient in whom one wishes to use a "conservative" treatment.[482]

Patient Selection

According to Papillon, certain criteria must be met if a patient is to be considered for this treatment[480]:

- Accessibility of the entire lesion
- Small size (<4.5 cm)
- Noninfiltrating status
- Histologically well-differentiated status
- Palpability
- Mobility
- Absence of palpable mesorectal nodes

Results

Papillon reported initially 106 patients, 70% of whom were alive and free of disease after 5 years.[480] Local recurrence developed in 14 individuals (13%). Sixteen patients (15%) died of malignant disease. A later report from his center included 245 patients followed for more than 5 years.[482] A local failure rate of 5.3% was noted. The death rate from cancer was 8.9%, and the 5-year survival rate, 76%.

Sischy and Remington reported 23 of 25 patients to have responded to treatment and to be free of disease, but the follow-up period was considerably shorter.[572,573] Fleshman

SIR CHARLES GORDON-WATSON (1874–1949)

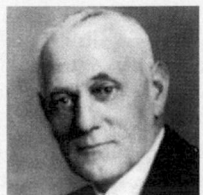

Gordon-Watson was born 1 of 12 children who survived into adulthood, the fifth son of a Buckinghamshire (England) vicar. His youthful ambition was to become a soldier, but because life in the army during those days was impossible for a man without means, he endeavored to establish himself in country life by becoming apprenticed to a land agent. When a position failed to materialize, with no science background and upon a whim, he applied and was accepted to St. Bartholomew's Medical College and Hospital in London. Following his qualification in 1898 and a period as house surgeon, he volunteered to serve as a civil surgeon in the Boer War. After 2 years, he returned to England and became a fellow of the Royal College of Surgeons. In 1908, he joined the staff of St. Mark's Hospital in London, and in 1910 he was elected assistant surgeon to St. Bartholomew's. When World War I broke out, he joined the expeditionary forces in France, and while there, he received many tributes for field military service. He was the first person to describe the syndrome of trench foot. In 1919, he had conferred upon him a Knighthood of the Order of the British Empire. In 1931, he was made an honorary fellow of the American College of Surgeons. He is remembered for his numerous contributions to coloproctology through his association with St. Mark's Hospital.

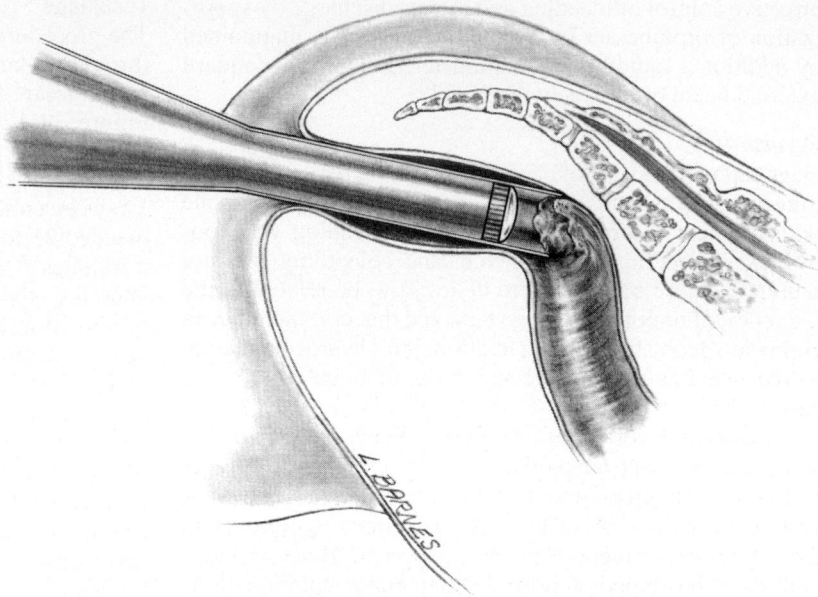

FIGURE 24-120. Endocavitary irradiation. The unit is introduced by means of a rectoscope.

and colleagues noted one failure in treating eight patients (13%).[175] From the Cleveland Clinic came a report of 199 patients treated by means of endocavitary radiation, 126 of whom were managed with curative intent.[278] Twenty-nine percent developed a recurrence. With additional treatment, 11% were rendered free of disease. With more than 5 years of follow-up, 91% had no evidence of disease with additional treatment, but only 68% were cured based on endocavitary irradiation alone.

Birnbaum and colleagues reported the Washington University (St. Louis, MO) experience with combined external and endocavitary radiation in order to identify factors predictive for recurrence of rectal cancer.[56] Seventy-two patients underwent pretreatment assessment by means of endorectal ultrasound staging. After a median follow-up of 31 months, there were no recurrences in the uT_1 group, a 22% recurrence rate in the uT_2 individuals, and a 51% recurrence for uT_3 lesions.

Complications

Very few complications are attributable to the treatment. Jelden reported mild proctitis of short duration and occasional bleeding.[290] Rectovaginal fistula has also been seen. Deaths directly related to the therapy have not been reported.

Comment

As with all local procedures, it is difficult to assess the results of endocavitary radiation by comparison with standard resection treatment. Only those who have the most favorable prognoses are selected. A patient who undergoes APR for a T1 or T2 tumor has a chance of cure that approaches 90%, so that claiming a cure rate less than this figure does not represent a great breakthrough in the treatment of cancer of the rectum. Furthermore, as with any local treatment, one wonders whether some patients are being deprived of the only possibility for cure if they harbor lymph node metastases. As previously discussed, even with careful patient selection, the decision whether to employ any local procedure requires a dedication to preoperative counseling and to close follow-up.

▶ RADIOTHERAPY

The use of external beam radiotherapy in the management of rectal cancer has received considerable attention in recent years as an adjunctive treatment to surgery, either preoperatively or postoperatively. There is good evidence that preoperative treatment (neoadjuvant) may decrease the size and the extent of tumor invasion and permit complete removal as well as to minimize the risk of local recurrence. Preoperative treatment may also limit the likelihood of dissemination of viable tumor cells during surgical manipulation.

Postoperative therapy offers the distinct advantage of one having the availability of a pathology report. Thus, the known extent of disease determines the field of treatment. In the postoperative patient who is known to have a less favorable lesion, radiotherapy may reduce the risk of pelvic recurrence. The downside of postoperative radiotherapy is the likelihood of adverse functional consequences because one will inevitably be radiating the neorectum if continuity has been reestablished.

Preoperative Radiotherapy (Neoadjuvant Radiation Therapy)

Background and Indications

The rationale for neoadjuvant radiation therapy in the management of rectal cancer is to alter the viability of cancer cells so that they are no longer capable of local implantation.[570] When the concept was first proposed, however, there was concern that delay in initiating surgical treatment could increase the risk of tumor spread, but there is no evidence today to suggest that this is in fact the case. The primary issue is identifying those patients in advance who would most likely benefit from neoadjuvant radiotherapy. How can one make this determination? Clinical assessment is probably the gold standard, but endorectal ultrasound, CT, and MRI are also quite helpful. Staging laparotomy has been suggested in order to determine mobility, resectability, staging, and the possibility of constructing a diversionary stoma before embarking on radiotherapy.[81] Some authors believe that every rectal cancer should be treated by preoperative radiation, but most surgeons are selective in their approach. The following variables are generally considered appropriate indications for performing preoperative radiation:

- Fixed tumor
- Evidence of ureteral obstruction
- Invasion of adjacent structures (e.g., bladder, seminal vesicles, vagina)
- Presacral adenopathy
- Anal canal invasion
- Ultrasound uT_3 or uT_4 lesion
- Poorly differentiated histology

The impetus for the application of preoperative radiotherapy can be attributed to the reports by Quan and Stearns and their colleagues that emanated from the Memorial Sloan-Kettering Cancer Center in New York.[446,57,675,37] Although their initial studies indicated improved survival, a prospective evaluation demonstrated that the overall survival rate was not better, but that the incidence of failure because of local recurrence was reduced.[587] At that institution, Stearns and colleagues used external radiation through opposing anterior and posterior portals, 2.5 Gy daily to 20 Gy. The resection was carried out 2 days to 6 weeks following treatment.

The classic article that evaluated preoperative radiation was reported by Dwight and Higgins and their colleagues from the Veterans Administration (VA).[157] This study randomly allocated 700 men either to surgery or to preoperative radiotherapy plus surgery. These investigators found a statistically significant decreased incidence of positive nodes in the irradiated group and a lower incidence of recurrent disease in those who died. Roswit and associates used 20 Gy over 2 weeks, with a booster dose of 5 Gy if the tumor was less than 9 cm from the anal verge.[527]

Since these initial reports, there have been numerous papers that attest to the success of radiotherapy in reducing the size of the tumor, downstaging the degree of invasion, and decreasing the risk of local recurrence.[69,73,84,101,118–120,128,152,174,178,194,197,200,201,224,254,280,286,303,322,399,413,414–418,427,474,483,521,524,526,571,574,577,615,626] Some have stated that survival rates are better.[181,605] Kandioler and coworkers observe that a tumor with a normal p53 genotype is predictive for response to preoperative short-term radiotherapy and increased patient survival.[300] In one meta-analysis of patients with resectable rectal cancer, preoperative radiotherapy significantly improved overall and cancer-specific survival compared with surgery alone.[86] The magnitude of the benefit was relatively small, however. In a *New England Journal of Medicine* lead article published in 2006, Bosset and colleagues concluded that in patients with rectal cancer who received preoperative radiotherapy, adding fluorouracil-based chemotherapy preoperatively or postoperatively had no significant effect on survival.[68] However, they noted that chemotherapy, regardless of whether it is administered before or after surgery, confers a significant benefit with respect to local control. There remains disagreement whether preoperative radiation therapy has any effect on survival.[204]

Methods

Minsky commented about the weaknesses of the prospective, randomized trials.[424] He stated that none uses standard dosages of radiation therapy. In addition, he opined that the interval between the completion of radiation and surgery is generally considered to be inadequate. The Memorial Sloan-Kettering Cancer Center group demonstrated a trend toward an increased pathologic response rate and downstaging when an interval between completing the radiotherapy and surgery is at least 44 days.[434] Moreover, he affirmed that using anterior-posterior/posterior-anterior portals, rather than multiple-field techniques, predisposes to increased morbidity associated with the radiation.[424] Others confirm that the morbidity and mortality of both preoperative and postoperative radiotherapy are higher when two-portal rather than three-portal or four-portal radiation technique is employed.[467] This is especially true for elderly patients who may have an increased risk of impairment for blood supply. Stein and colleagues concluded in the analysis of their patients that a longer time interval (beyond 8 weeks) between completion of neoadjuvant chemoradiation and surgical resection did not increase the tumor response rate or reduce the morbidity associated with the surgery.[591] Most recommend 6 to 8 weeks following completion of the treatment in order to achieve maximum downstaging and tissue recovery, although that interval has been gradually increasing. Some advise waiting as long as 3 months.

There is considerable controversy as to what the optimal dose for preoperative radiation treatment should be. Some have recommended a short course of high-dose therapy, whereas most centers in the United States suggest 40 to 45 Gy, delivered in 4 to 6 weeks. Data show no increased morbidity or mortality associated with supplementary treatment.[155,504]

Results

The largest prospective, randomized trials come from Sweden—actually a combination of two Swedish protocols (the Stockholm Rectal Cancer Study Group and the Swedish Rectal Cancer Trial).[185,266,267,269,270,603–605] In the Stockholm trial, the most recent publication analyzed postoperative morbidity, mortality, local recurrence, and death from rectal cancer in 1,399 patients who were prospectively randomized to preoperative radiotherapy or no radiotherapy.[267] Those allocated to preoperative radiotherapy received a total dose of 35 Gy in five fractions over 1 week, with surgery performed within 1 week thereafter. Interestingly, patients operated on by surgeons who were certified specialists for at least 10 years had a lower risk of local recurrence and death from rectal cancer.[267] A significantly reduced risk of local recurrence was observed, but there was no clear improvement in survival. However, the investigators also found that the postoperative mortality rate may be increased in the radiotherapy group.[269]

In the initial report of Swedish Rectal Cancer Trial involving 1,168 patients, preoperative radiation was accomplished through 25 Gy and five fractions in 1 week, also followed by operation within 1 week.[604] In this randomized, prospective study, the local recurrence rate during a period of 2 years was reduced by approximately 65%. Furthermore, this short-term regimen of high-dose preoperative radiotherapy was found to improve survival.[605] The overall 5-year survival rate was 58% in the radiotherapy plus surgery group and 48% in the surgery-alone group ($P = .004$). This appears to have been the first clear demonstration of improved survival by means of preoperative radiotherapy. In a later report (2005), the overall survival rate in the irradiated group was 38% versus 30% in the nonirradiated group ($P = .008$).[177] The cancer-specific survival rate in the irradiated group was 72% versus 62% in the nonirradiated group ($P = .03$), and the local recurrence rate was 9% versus 26% ($P < .001$), respectively. The reduction of local recurrence rates was observed at all tumor heights, although it was not statistically significant for tumors greater than 10 cm from the anal verge. The study concluded that preoperative radiotherapy with 25 Gy in 1 week before curative surgery for rectal cancer is beneficial for overall and cancer-specific survival and local recurrence rates after long-term follow-up.

There is an inherent problem concerning a well-controlled, randomized trial with this group of patients. Stratification by the usual criterion, namely, depth of invasion (e.g., TNM classification), cannot be applied. One must use other, less well-defined criteria such as clinical judgment. Endorectal ultrasound is of help for staging the depth of penetration,[454,553] and DNA ploidy seems to be an independent factor for predicting response to radiotherapy,[250] but it does appear that neoadjuvant therapy for more advanced lesions has become the standard approach.

Complications and Functional Results

Wichmann and associates concluded based on their evaluation of 30 patients who underwent preoperative chemoradiotherapy that this treatment results in significant immune dysfunction as indicated by depression of lymphocyte subpopulations, monocytes, granulocytes, and proinflammatory cytokine release.[651] They believed that these observations are important in contributing to the increased perioperative morbidity that is seen as a consequence of neoadjuvant therapy. Experienced surgeons are well aware of the problem of delayed healing of the perineal wound after proctectomy when preoperative radiation is performed.[513] The safety of performing anastomosis in the rectum following radiation therapy has been a matter of some conjecture. Some studies, however, have demonstrated that colorectal anastomoses can be performed without concern for an increased risk of complications if the radiation dose does not exceed 45 Gy.[110,112, 180,271,397,428,431,517,648] Still, preoperative radiotherapy may have an adverse effect on long-term anorectal function.[648] For example, the Cleveland Clinic group reviewed anal canal specimens following pelvic radiation and noted damage to the myenteric plexus of the internal anal sphincter.[131] A tendency to increased collagen deposition was also observed. Birnbaum and colleagues prospectively evaluated the acute effect of preoperative radiation (45 Gy) on anal function in 20 individuals.[55] These investigators concluded that preoperative radiation therapy has minimal immediate effect on the anal sphincter and is not a major contributing factor to postoperative incontinence after sphincter-saving operations for rectal cancer. However, preoperative radiotherapy alters endosonographic staging and interferes with the endosonographic interpretation of the anastomotic area.[454] Others have observed that preoperative radiotherapy may have a pejorative effect on male sexual and urinary function.[66]

Dahlberg and coworkers ascertained the long-term effects on bowel function by means of a questionnaire of 171 patients who could be evaluated and who were included in the Swedish Rectal Cancer Trial.[129] Mean bowel frequency per week, incontinence for loose stool,

urgency, and emptying difficulties were statistically significantly more common following preoperative radiation when compared with those operated on without radiation. This serves to emphasize the importance of patient selection in order to limit the consequences of nonbeneficial neoadjuvant therapy.

Management following Complete Tumor Regression

It has for some time been a principle of treatment that neoadjuvant therapy should not change the subsequent operation—whether APR or sphincter preservation. This concept has been challenged in recent years by the work of Habr-Gama and coworkers in São Paulo, Brazil.[227–230] The observation of complete tumor regression led to the proposition of nonoperative management of selected patients. This is analogous to the observational method elected with complete responders following neoadjuvant therapy for anal cancer (see Chapter 25). The absence of residual cancer cells in the resected specimen of patients undergoing radical surgery after neoadjuvant treatment had raised the issue of whether surgery is appropriate if it does not remove a single cancer cell.[229] A proportion of these patients present with a complete clinical response, an entity defined by the group as absence of any residual scar, mass, or ulcer after clinical and radiologic assessment. This includes absence of symptoms and negative results on digital rectal examination, CT or endorectal ultrasonography, as well as normal CEA levels. For these highly selected patients with no detectable residual tumor, a strategy of close observation without immediate surgery has been suggested by the authors as an initial approach.[228] Also added were those with suspicious, small, residual, and excisable lesions who underwent full-thickness local excision with negative pathologic results. Such patients were all offered a strict surveillance program, with regular and frequent visits to an experienced colorectal surgeon. Such an approach requires several features[229]:

- The tumor location must be accessible to the examining surgeon's finger
- Timing should be taken into account relative to residual nodal involvement
- Both patient and surgeon must be aware that disease recurrence or tumor regrowth may occur at any time
- Establishment of a strict follow-up regimen

By applying an individualized management strategy for highly selected patients with distal rectal cancer, Habr-Gama was able to avoid more extensive operation in more than 120 patients over a period of 15 years. Those individuals who sustained a complete clinical response for at least 12 months did no worse than those who had surgery over the same period, with no residual cancer at pathologic evaluation.[228] Local recurrence developed in 11% of patients not operated on immediately and who had a sustained complete clinical response, and all were amenable to salvage therapy. Patients who eventually required surgery after an initially suspected complete clinical response or who experienced early tumor regrowth during the initial 12-month period did not seem to have any worse oncologic outcome than those not considered to have a complete clinical response.[230] Although the authors' data suggest that this nonoperative approach is safe

ANGELITA HABR-GAMA (1931–PRESENT)

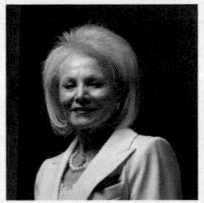

Angelita Habr-Gama was born into a family of Lebanese immigrants in the north of Brazil, where she spent her early years, and grew up in São Paulo, where she had moved with her family. She has spent her entire professional career at São Paulo University. Her surgical performance excelled, and she became the first woman general surgeon in Brazil. After deciding to pursue coloproctology, then an emerging subspecialty, Angelita successfully applied for a program in England, supported by the British Council. She spent a number of months at St. Mark's Hospital in London and also in Oxford and Leeds. On her return to the University of São Paulo and Hospital das Clínicas, her career was marked by a series of major accomplishments. She pioneered the field of research into anorectal physiology in Brazil and set up the country's first anorectal physiology laboratory. In 1966, she presented her doctoral thesis on *Motility of the Sigmoid and Rectum in Chagasic Megacolon*. In 1972, she presented her thesis on *Rectosigmoidectomy with Delayed Coloanal Anastomosis for the Treatment of Mid-Rectal Cancer*, which qualified her as associate professor. She has introduced in Brazil many new technologies and techniques, such as colonoscopy, mechanical sutures, PPH for treating hemorrhoids, and the artificial anal sphincter. Her main interest has long been the management of rectal cancer with sphincter preservation. Having been in practice for over 40 years, Angelita has earned her reputation for excellence in digestive tract and particularly in colorectal surgery. She has received numerous national and international prizes and awards and has been honored as honorary fellow of the Brazilian Society of Coloproctology, American Surgical Association, American College of Surgeons, European Surgical Association, the Italian Society of Surgery, and the Latin American Association of Coloproctology. She has been the only woman president of the Latin American Association of Coloproctology and the first woman president of the Brazilian Society of Coloproctology. In addition, Habr-Gama has served as governor of the American College of Gastroenterology in Brazil and she has been a member of the editorial boards of many prestigious international journals. She has been head of the Gastroenterological Department in the University of São Paulo Medical School and, for 22 years, was the head of the Surgery of Colon, Rectum, and Anus Department at the Hospital das Clínicas of the University of São Paulo Medical School. As a distinguished educator, professor, and director of the Department of Gastroenterology and of the Colorectal Unit at the University of São Paulo Medical School, Angelita has given more than 1,000 invited lectures and has nurtured the careers of hundreds of trainees, graduate and postgraduate students, residents, and fellows, not only from Brazil but also from many other Latin American countries. She worked hard to establish residency training in coloproctology in Brazil, a goal which was achieved in 1994. She has been dedicated to research in neoadjuvant chemoradiation therapy for rectal cancer. In fact, 31 of her published 160 papers are related to this subject. A refined, soft-spoken, and gentle woman, she is a true leader in the field of coloproctology in Brazil and in the world.

---

for appropriately selected patients, randomized controlled clinical trials are necessary.

Postoperative Radiotherapy (Adjuvant Therapy)

In 1991, Krook and colleagues demonstrated encouraging results with postoperative chemoradiation therapy.[333] A total of 204 patients with rectal carcinoma that was either deeply invasive or metastatic to lymph nodes was randomly assigned to postoperative radiation alone (45 to 50 Gy) or to radiation plus 5 FU, which was both preceded and followed by a cycle of systemic therapy with 5 FU plus semustine (methyl-CCNU).[333] After a median follow-up of more than 7 years, the combined regimen reduced the recurrence rate by 34%. Initial local recurrence was reduced by 46% and distant metastasis by 37%. Additionally, the combined treatment reduced the rate of cancer-related deaths by 36% and the overall death rate by 29%.

O'Connell and colleagues, reporting from the Mayo Clinic, administered 5 FU by protracted infusion throughout the duration of radiation therapy in 660 patients with Dukes' B and C tumors.[461] With a median follow-up of 46 months among surviving patients, those who received the infusion had a significantly increased time before relapse as well as an improved survival. Others confirmed that 5 FU combined with irradiation appears to maximize control of both local and distant metastatic disease.[516] A 1-month protocol reported on behalf of the Norwegian Adjuvant Rectal Cancer Project Group, using 5 FU, revealed a reduced local recurrence rate and increased recurrence-free survival and overall survival, without serious side effects when compared with those who did not undergo such treatment.[625] More recent studies of adjuvant protocols incorporate the newer chemotherapeutic agents discussed in the prior chapter.

As previously stated, the primary advantage of postoperative radiotherapy is that selected patients may be submitted to this additional treatment based on their "unfavorable" pathology reports. Conversely, disadvantages of this alternative include the risk that cells may be seeded outside the treatment area, wound healing may be delayed, and the physiology of residual tumor may be altered by reduction in the vascular supply.[570] Furthermore, there is the concern for the possibility of prolonged delay in initiating the therapy when postoperative complications arise, such as wound infection, the need for reoperation, medical problems, and other issues.

Romsdahl and Withers delivered a total of 55 Gy following APR to patients who were found to have Dukes' B and C lesions.[522] The local recurrence rate was 8%, as compared with a 27% rate in historical controls. According to Brizel and Tepperman, among 51 patients who received at least 45 Gy of pelvic irradiation, only five tumors recurred (10%) when there was no gross residual disease at the time of resection.[75] Arnaud and colleagues undertook a prospective, randomized trial involving 172 patients who had previously undergone resection for either a Dukes' B or C rectal cancer.[14] Patients received 46 Gy for 5 days per week within a 30- to 38-day period. This trial failed to demonstrate any improvement in overall survival or local control when postoperative radiation was given compared with those who did not receive radiation therapy. Tang and associates, using historic controls, also treated patients with Dukes' B and C rectal cancer and likewise found no improvement in survival or local recurrence.[610] Others believe that prophylactic postoperative adjuvant radiotherapy is not justified because the incidence of local recurrence in the absence of disseminated disease is relatively low.[17] In two studies, that figure was approximately 10%.[32,476] Several prospective randomized trials are currently in progress, but as of this writing, 5-year follow-up conclusions are not available.[474,526]

Problems

Generally, there is the perception that postoperative radiotherapy is not as well tolerated as preoperative treatment.[476,563] Anastomotic strictures have been reported to occur as a consequence of this regimen.[475] In the long term, small bowel complications are of most concern (see Chapter 28).[394] Ooi and colleagues, in their MEDLINE and literature search, noted that with postoperative radiotherapy, small bowel obstruction occurs in 5% to 10%; delay in commencing radiotherapy because of wound healing problems, 6%; postoperative fatigue, 14%; and toxicities precluding completion of adjuvant therapy, 49% to 97%.[467] Other symptoms and complications include abscess and fistula formation, mucus discharge, urgency, tenesmus, and bleeding.[295] Therefore, before embarking on such treatment one must consider other factors, such as the age of the patient and the anticipated quality of life.

General Recommendations

Until the results of controlled studies are available, one should advise adjuvant chemoradiation therapy for patients who are at a high risk of tumor recurrence: those with poorly differentiated tumors, those with T3 or T4 lesions, and those with positive regional lymph nodes. Treatment should begin not sooner than 1 month following the operation (in order to avoid problems with wound healing) or later than 2 months (in order to limit the likelihood of spread). The dosage to the tumor bed (in total) should be approximately 60 Gy.

Palliative Radiotherapy

Radiotherapy can be uniquely beneficial in the treatment of patients with recurrent disease who have pelvic pain. This is discussed earlier in this chapter. It has also been suggested for use in those patients with locally advanced lesions, in

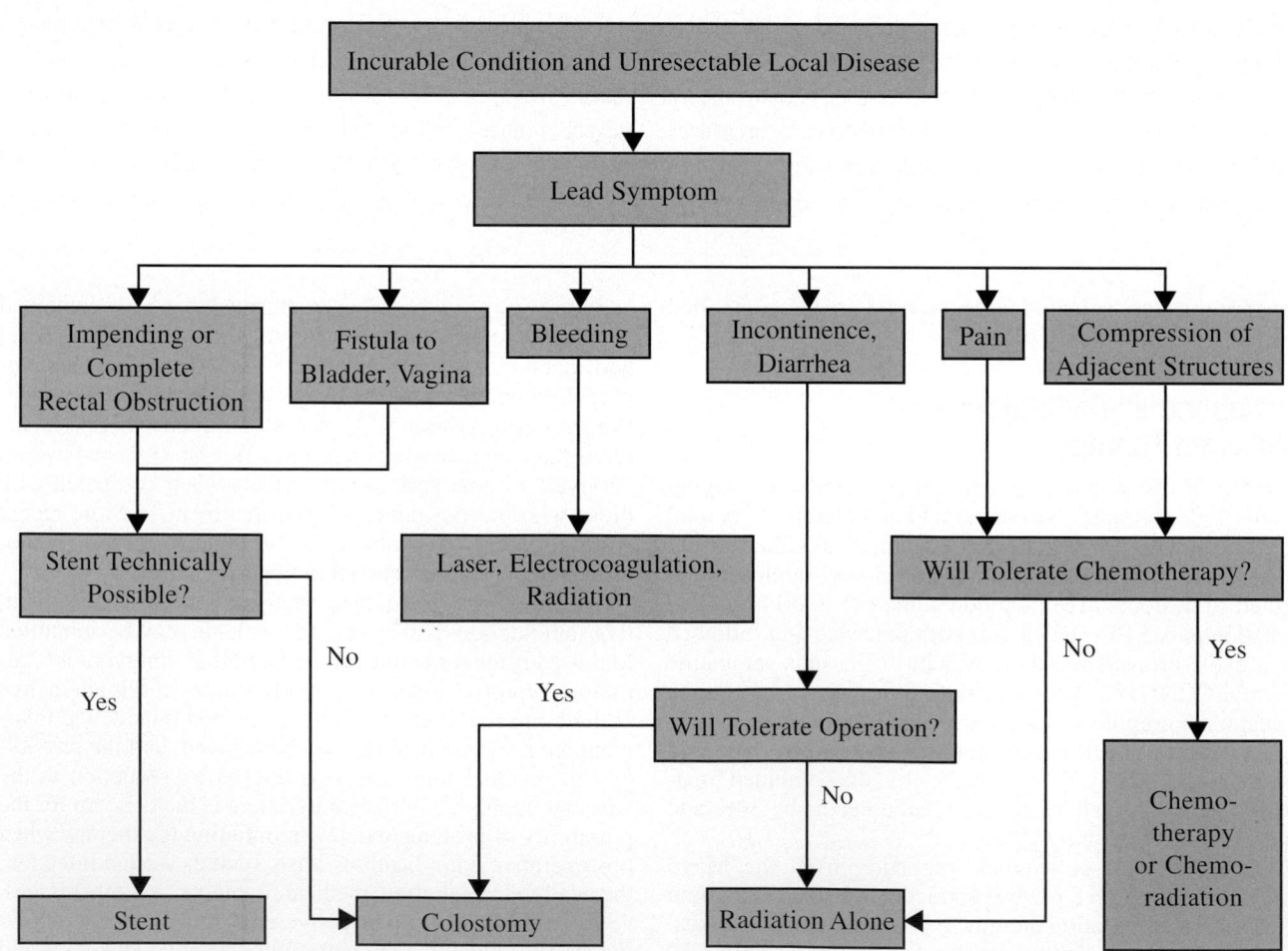

FIGURE 24-121. Algorithm for palliative care of patients with locally unresectable rectal cancer. (From Stelzner M. Palliative therapy of rectal cancer: summary statement. *J Gastrointest Surg.* 2004;8:253, with permission.)

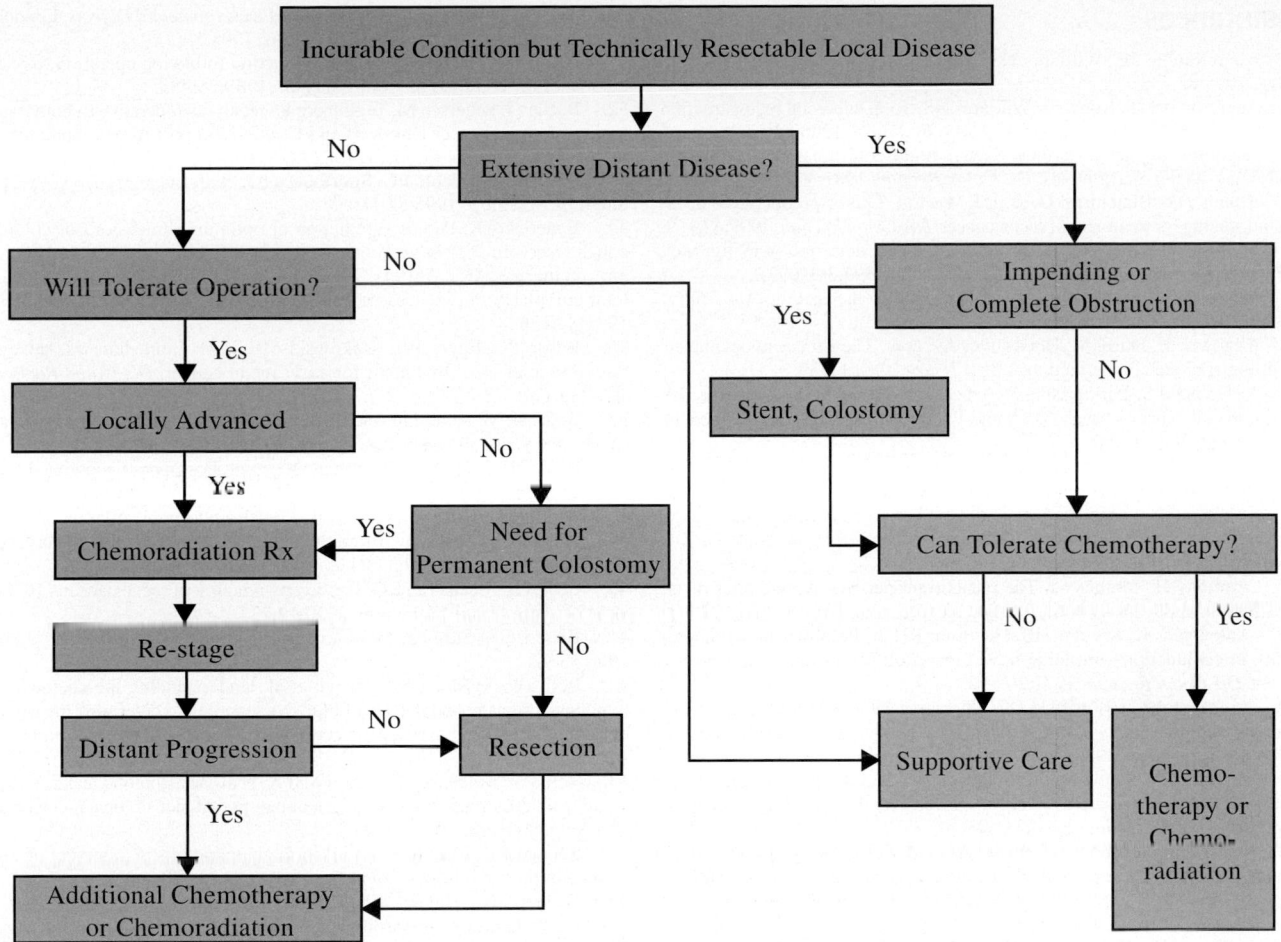

FIGURE 24-122. Algorithm for palliative care of patients with locally resectable rectal cancer. (From Stelzner M. Palliative therapy of rectal cancer: summary statement. *J Gastrointest Surg.* 2004;8:253, with permission.)

combination with chemotherapy and/or surgery.[111,613] Kodner and colleagues definitively treated by means of external radiation 84 patients with invasive rectal carcinoma.[321] The use of external radiation before endocavitary radiation achieved local control in 93% of patients with favorable lesions. However, the investigators found that there was little place for nonresective management of aggressive rectal cancers, even for palliation, unless an individual's life expectancy was less than 6 months. Still, Zacherl and coworkers opined that partial sacral resection as a means for achieving palliation of perineosacral pain is justified "even though cure can very rarely be achieved."[663] Others have demonstrated that many patients with locally recurrent rectal cancer can benefit from multimodality therapy.[232]

The implications of these studies are such that any individual with pathologic confirmation of a Dukes' B or C (T3, T4, or N1) lesion should be considered for a postoperative protocol.

Intraoperative Radiotherapy

See the earlier discussion.

► CHEMOTHERAPY

The role of chemotherapy in colorectal cancer is discussed in Chapter 23.

Hyperthermochemoradiotherapy

Mori and colleagues have reported the application of a multimodality approach in the management of patients with rectal cancer, that of hyperthermochemoradiotherapy.[440] This consists of a preoperative combination of hyperthermia at 42° to 45° C for 40 minutes (twice per week for 2 weeks), 5 FU intravenously, and a total of 30 Gy irradiation. Reduction in tumor size was evident in their 11 patients with either no or only a few viable cancer cells present in the resected specimen. A later report from the same institution involving 36 patients revealed that 5-year survival rates were 91% compared with historical controls of 74% in those not receiving hyperthermochemoradiotherapy.[465] Whether this approach will prove to have merit in the management of patients with rectal cancer remains to be determined.

Palliative Therapy: An Algorithmic Approach

At the 2003 Annual Meeting of the Society for Surgery of the Alimentary Tract, Stelzner suggested an algorithmic approach to the palliative management of nonresectable and resectable rectal cancer.[592] They are included here for reference purposes and as a point for stimulating further discussion (Figures 24-121 and 24-122).

References

1. Abercrombie JE, Williams NS. Total anorectal reconstruction. *Br J Surg.* 1995;82:438.

2. Abercrombie JF, Rogers J, Williams NS. Total anorectal reconstruction results in complete anorectal sensory loss. *Br J Surg.* 1996;83:57.

3. Accordi F, Sogno O, Carniato S, et al. Endoscopic treatment of stenosis following stapler anastomosis. *Dis Colon Rectum.* 1987;30:647.

4. Adams DR, Blatchford GJ, Lin KM, et al. Use of preoperative ultrasound staging for treatment of rectal cancer. *Dis Colon Rectum.* 1999;42:159.

5. Adams WJ, Wong WD. Endorectal ultrasonic detection of malignancy within rectal villous lesions. *Dis Colon Rectum.* 1995;38:1093.

6. Allgöwer M. Sphincter-splitting approach to the rectum. *Am J Surg.* 1983;145:5.

7. Allgöwer M, Dürig M, Hochstetter AV, et al. The parasacral sphincter-splitting approach to the rectum. *World J Surg.* 1982;6:539.

8. Al-Homoud S, Purkayastha S, Aziz O, et al. Evaluating operative risk in colorectal cancer surgery: ASA and POSSUM-based predictive models. *Surg Oncol.* 2004;13:83.

9. Amussat JZ. *Mémoire sur la possibilité d'établir un anus artificiel dans la région lombaire sans pénétrer dans le péritoine* [Notes on the possible establishment of an artificial anus in the lumbar region without entering the peritoneal cavity]. Paris, France: Germer-Bailliére; 1839. Translated in *Dis Colon Rectum.* 1983;26:483.

10. Anthony JP, Mathes SJ. The recalcitrant perineal wound after rectal extirpation: applications of muscle flap closure. *Arch Surg.* 1990;125:1371.

11. Antoniades K, Spector HB, Hecksher RH Jr. Prophylactic oophorectomy in conjunction with large-bowel resection for cancer: report of two cases. *Dis Colon Rectum.* 1977;20:506.

12. Archampong D, Borowski DW, Dickinson HO. Impact of surgeon volume on outcomes of rectal cancer surgery: a systematic review and meta-analysis. *Surgeon.* 2010;8:341.

13. Arnaud JP, Bergamaschi R, Schloegel M, et al. Progress in the assessment of lymphatic spread in rectal cancer: rectal endoscopic lymphoscintigraphy. *Dis Colon Rectum.* 1990;33:398.

14. Arnaud JP, Nordlinger B, Bosset JF, et al. Radical surgery and postoperative radiotherapy as combined treatment in rectal cancer: final results of a phase III study of the European Organisation for Research and Treatment of Cancer. *Br J Surg.* 1997;84:352.

15. Arulampalam THA, Costa DC, Loizidou M, et al. Positron emission tomography and colorectal cancer. *Br J Surg.* 2001;88:176.

16. Aston NO, Owen WJ, Irving JD. Endoscopic balloon dilatation of colonic anastomotic strictures. *Br J Surg.* 1989;76:780.

17. Auld RM, Chapman S, Kuster GGR, et al. Local recurrence of adenocarcinoma of the rectosigmoid: is postoperative adjuvant radiotherapy justified? *Dis Colon Rectum.* 1986;29:326.

18. Austin-Kirk KS, Solomon M. Pelvic exenteration with iliac vessel resection for lateral pelvic wall involvement. *Dis Colon Rectum.* 2009;52:1223–1233.

19. Austin-Kirk KS, Young JM, Solomon M. Quality of life of survivors after pelvic exenteration for rectal cancer. *Dis Colon Rectum.* 2010;53:1121.

20. Azimuddin K, Riether RD, Stasik JJ, et al. Transanal endoscopic microsurgery for excision of rectal lesions: technique and initial results. *Surg Laparosc Endosc Percutan Tech.* 2000;10:372.

21. Babcock WW. Experiences with resection of the colon and the elimination of colostomy. *Am J Surg.* 1939;4:186.

22. Babcock WW. Radical single-stage extirpation for cancer of the large bowel, with retained functional anus. *Surg Gynecol Obstet.* 1947;85:1.

23. Bacon HE. Abdominoperineal proctosigmoidectomy with sphincter preservation: five-year and ten-year survival after "pull-through" operation for cancer of rectum. *JAMA.* 1956;160:628.

24. Bacon HE. Evaluation of sphincter muscle preservation and re-establishment of continuity in the operative treatment of rectal and sigmoidal cancer. *Surg Gynecol Obstet.* 1945;81:113.

25. Bacon HE, Martin PV. The rationale of palliative resection for primary cancer of the colon and rectum complicated by liver and lung metastasis. *Dis Colon Rectum.* 1964;7:211.

26. Bai HL, Chen B, Zhou Y, et al. Five-year long-term outcomes of laparoscopic surgery for colon cancer. *World J Gastroenterol.* 2010;16:4992.

27. Baird WL, Hester TR, Nahai F, et al. Management of perineal wounds following abdominoperineal resection with inferior gluteal flaps. *Arch Surg.* 1990;125:1486.

28. Baker JW. Low end to side rectosigmoidal anastomosis: description of technique. *Arch Surg.* 1950;61:143.

29. Bakri YN, Amri A, Abdul-Jabbar F. Tamponade-balloon for obstetrical bleeding. *Int J Gynaecol Obstet.* 2001;74:139.

30. Ball C. *The Rectum. Its Diseases and Developmental Defects.* London, United Kingdom: Oxford University Press; 1908:1.

31. Balslev I, Harling H. Sexual dysfunction following operation for carcinoma of the rectum. *Dis Colon Rectum.* 1983;26:785.

32. Balslev I, Pedersen M, Teglbjaerg PS, et al. Postoperative radiotherapy in rectosigmoid cancer Dukes' B and C: interim report from a randomized multicentre study. *Br J Cancer.* 1982;46:551.

33. Banerjee AK, Jehle EC, Shorthouse AJ, et al. Local excision of rectal tumours. *Br J Surg.* 1995;82:1165.

34. Banerjee AK, Parc R. Prediction of optimum dimensions of colonic pouch reservoir. *Dis Colon Rectum.* 1996;39:1293.

35. Banerjee AK, Walters TK, Wilkins R, et al. Wire-guided balloon coloplasty: a new treatment for colorectal strictures. *J R Soc Med.* 1991;84:136.

36. Baron PL, Enker WE, Zakowski MF, et al. Immediate vs. salvage resection after local treatment for early rectal cancer. *Dis Colon Rectum.* 1995;38:177.

37. Bebenek M. Abdominosacral amputation of the rectum for low rectal cancer: ten years of experience. *Ann Surg Oncol.* 2009;16:2211.

38. Beck DE, Fazio VW, Jagelman DG, et al. Postoperative perineal hernia. *Dis Colon Rectum.* 1987;30:21.

39. Bedogni G, Ricci E, Pedrazzoli C, et al. Endoscopic dilation of anastomotic colonic stenosis by different techniques: an alternative to surgery? *Gastrointest Endosc.* 1987;33:21.

40. Beets GL, Beets-Tan RG. Pretherapy imaging of rectal cancers: ERUS or MRI? *Surg Oncol Clin N Am.* 2010;19:733.

41. Beheri GE. Surgical treatment of impotence. *Plast Reconstr Surg.* 1966;38:92.

42. Bell SW, Sasaki J, Singlair G, et al. Understanding the anatomy of lymphatic drainage and the use of blue dye mapping to determine the extent of lymphadenectomy in rectal cancer surgery: unresolved issues. *Colorectal Dis.* 2009;11:443.

43. Bell SW, Walker KG, Rickard MJFX, et al. Anastomotic leakage after curative anterior resection results in a higher prevalence of local recurrence. *Br J Surg.* 2003;90:1261.

44. Bennett RC. The place of pull-through operations in treatment of carcinoma of the rectum. *Dis Colon Rectum.* 1976;19:420.

45. Bennett RC, Hughes ES, Cuthbertson AM. Long-term review of function following pull-through operations of the rectum. *Br J Surg.* 1972;59:723.

46. Benoist S, Panis Y, Boleslawski E, et al. Functional outcome after coloanal versus low colorectal anstomosis for rectal carcinoma. *J Am Coll Surg.* 1997;185:114.

47. Benson MC, Ring KS, Olsson CA. Ureteral reconstruction and bypass: experience with ileal interposition, the Boari flap-psoas hitch and renal autotransplantation. *J Urol.* 1990;143:20.

48. Bernard HR, Cole WR. The prophylaxis of surgical infection: the effect of prophylactic antimicrobial drugs on the incidence of infection following potentially contaminated operations. *Surgery.* 1964;56:151.

49. Berry AR, Souter RG, Campbell WB, et al. Endoscopic transanal resection of rectal tumours-a preliminary report of its use. *Br J Surg.* 1990;77:134.

50. Bevan AD. Carcinoma of the rectum: treatment by local excision. *Surg Clin Chicago.* 1917;1:1233.

51. Beynon J, Foy DMA, Roe AM, et al. Endoluminal ultrasound in the assessment of local invasion in rectal cancer. *Br J Surg.* 1986;73:474.

52. Beynon J, Mortensen NJMC, Foy DMA, et al. The detection and evaluation of locally recurrent rectal cancer with rectal endosonography. *Dis Colon Rectum.* 1989;32:509.

53. Beynon J, Mortensen NJMC, Foy DMA, et al. Preoperative assessment of mesorectal lymph node involvement in rectal cancer. *Br J Surg.* 1989;76:276.

54. Biggers OR, Beart RW Jr, Ilstrup DM. Local excision of rectal cancer. *Dis Colon Rectum.* 1986;29:374.

55. Birnbaum EH, Dreznik Z, Myerson RJ, et al. Early effect of external beam radiation therapy on the anal sphincter: a study using anal manometry and transrectal ultrasound. *Dis Colon Rectum.* 1992;35:757.

56. Birnbaum EH, Ogunbiyi OA, Gagliardi G, et al. Selection criteria for treatment of rectal cancer with combined external and endocavitary radiation. *Dis Colon Rectum.* 1999;42:727.

57. Bischoff PF. Boari-plasty and vesicorenal reflux. In: Whitehead ED, ed. *Current Operative Urology.* New York, NY: Harper & Row; 1975:708.

58. Bissett IP, Chan KY, Hill GL. Extra fascial excision of the rectum. Surgical anatomy of the fascia propria. *Dis Colon Rectum.* 2000;43:903.

59. Black BM, Botham RJ. Combined abdominoendorectal resection: a critical reappraisal based on 91 cases. *Surg Clin North Am.* 1957;37:989.

60. Black BM, Kelly AH. Recurrent carcinoma of the rectum and rectosigmoid: results of treatment after continence preserving procedures. *Arch Surg.* 1955;72:538.

61. Blamey SL, McDermott FT, Pihl E, et al. Ovarian involvement in adenocarcinoma of the colon and rectum. *Surg Gynecol Obstet.* 1981;153:42.

62. Blamey SL, McDermott FT, Pihl E, et al. Resected ovarian recurrence from colorectal adenocarcinoma. *Dis Colon Rectum.* 1981;24:272.

63. Bleday R, Breen E, Jessup JM, et al. Prospective evaluation of local excision for small rectal cancers. *Dis Colon Rectum.* 1997;40:388.

64. Blumberg D, Paty PB, Guillem JG, et al. All patients with small intramural rectal cancers are at risk for lymph node metastasis. *Dis Colon Rectum.* 1999;42:881.

65. Bokey EL, Ojerskog B, Chapuis PH, et al. Local recurrence after curative excision of the rectum for cancer without adjuvant therapy: the role of total anatomical dissection. *Br J Surg.* 1999;86:1164.

66. Bonnel C, Parc YR, Pocard M, et al. Effects of preoperative radiotherapy for primary resectable rectal adenocarcinoma on male sexual and urinary function. *Dis Colon Rectum.* 2002;45:934.

67. Bordos DC, Baker RR, Cameron JL. An evaluation of palliative abdominoperineal resection for carcinoma of the rectum. *Surg Gynecol Obstet.* 1974;139:731.

68. Bosset JF, Collette L, Calais G, et al. Chemotherapy with preoperative radiotherapy in rectal cancer. *N Engl J Med.* 2006;355:1114.

69. Botti C, Cosimelli M, Ambesi Impiombato F, et al. Improved local control and survival with the sandwich technique of pelvic radiotherapy for resectable rectal cancer: a retrospective, multivariate analysis. *Dis Colon Rectum.* 1994;37:S6.

70. Bown SG, Barr H, Matthewson K, et al. Endoscopic treatment of inoperable colorectal cancers with the Nd YAG laser. *Br J Surg.* 1986;73:949.

71. Branston LK, Greening S, Newcombe RG, et al. The implementation of guidelines and computerized forms improve the completeness of cancer pathology reporting. The CROPS project: a randomized trial in pathology. *Eur J Cancer.* 2002;38:764.

72. Brasch RC, Bufo AJ, Kreienberg PF, et al. Femoral neuropathy secondary to the use of a self-retaining retractor: report of three cases and review of the literature. *Dis Colon Rectum.* 1995;38:1115.

73. Brierley JD, Cummings BJ, Wong CS, et al. Adenocarcinoma of the rectum treated by radical external radiation therapy. *Int J Radiat Oncol.* 1995;31:255.

74. Bright N, Hale P, Mason R. Poor palliation of colorectal malignancy with the neodymium yttrium-aluminium-garnet laser. *Br J Surg.* 1992;79:308.

75. Brizel HE, Tepperman BS. Postoperative adjuvant irradiation for adenocarcinoma of the rectum and sigmoid. *Am J Clin Oncol.* 1984;7:679.

76. Brotschi E, Noe JM, Silen W. Perineal hernias after proctectomy. *Am J Surg.* 1985;149:301.

77. Brown G, Radcliffe AG, Newcombe RG, et al. Preoperative assessment of prognostic factors in rectal cancer using high-resolution magnetic resonance imaging. *Br J Surg.* 2003;90:355.

78. Brunetaud JM, Maunoury V, Ducrotte P, et al. Palliative treatment of rectosigmoid carcinoma by laser endoscopic photoablation. *Gastroenterology.* 1987;92:663.

79. Buchsbaum HJ, Christopherson W, Lifshitz S, et al. Vicryl mesh in pelvic floor reconstruction. *Arch Surg.* 1985;120:1389.

80. Buess G, Mentges B, Manncke K, et al. Technique and results of transanal endoscopic microsurgery in early rectal cancer. *Am J Surg.* 1992;163:63.

81. Buhre LM, Verschueren RCJ, Mehta DM, et al. Staging laparotomy for inoperable or borderline operable cancer of the rectum. *Dis Colon Rectum.* 1987;30:352.

82. Bujko K, Bujko M. Point: short course radiation therapy is preferable to the neoadjuvant treatment of rectal cancer. *Semin Radiat Oncol.* 2011;21:220.

83. Burgos FJ, Romero J, Fernandez E, et al. Risk factors for developing voiding dysfunction after abdominoperineal resection for adenocarcinoma of the rectum. *Dis Colon Rectum.* 1988;31:682.

84. Buroker T, Nigro N, Correa J, et al. Combination preoperative radiation and chemotherapy in adenocarcinoma of the rectum: a preliminary report. *Dis Colon Rectum.* 1976;19:660.

85. Butch RJ, Wittenberg J, Mueller PR, et al. Presacral masses after abdominoperineal resection for colorectal carcinoma: the need for needle biopsy. *AJR Am J Roentgenol.* 1985;144:309.

86. Cammà C, Giunta M, Fiorica F, et al. Preoperative radiotherapy for resectable rectal cancer: a meta-analysis. *JAMA.* 2000;284:1008.

87. Carne PWG, Frye JNR, Kennedy-Smith A, et al. Local invasion of the bladder with colorectal cancers: surgical management and patterns of local recurrence. *Dis Colon Rectum.* 2004;47:44.

88. Casillas S, Nicholson JD. Aortic thrombosis after low anterior resection for rectal cancer: report of a case. *Dis Colon Rectum.* 2002;45:829.

89. Castrini G, Toccaceli S. Cancer of the rectum sphincter-saving operation: a new technique of coloanal anastomosis. *Surg Clin North Am.* 1988;68:1383.

90. Cataldo PA, O'Brien S, Osler T. Transanal endoscopic microsurgery: a prospective evaluation of functional results. *Dis Colon Rectum.* 2005;48:1366.

91. Cavaliere F, Pemberton JH, Cosimelli M, et al. Coloanal anastomosis for rectal cancer: long-term results at the Mayo and Cleveland Clinics. *Dis Colon Rectum.* 1995;38:807.

92. Cavina E. Outcome of restorative perineal graciloplasty with simultaneous excision of the anus and rectum for cancer: a ten-year experience with 81 patients. *Dis Colon Rectum.* 1996;39:182.

93. Cawkwell I. Perineal hernia complicating abdominoperineal resection of the rectum. *Br J Surg.* 1963;50:431.

94. Chan CLH, Bokey EL, Chapuis PH, et al. Local recurrence after resection for rectal cancer is associated with anterior position of the tumour. *Br J Surg.* 2006;93:105.

95. Chapuis PH, Bokey EL, Yuile P. Radiotherapy in rectal cancer. *Aust N Z J Surg.* 1994;64:455.

96. Chapuis PH, Bokey L, Fahrer M, et al. Mobilization of the rectum: anatomic concepts and the bookshelf revisited. *Dis Colon Rectum.* 2002;45:1.

97. Chapuis PH, Chan C, Dent OF. Clinicopathological staging of colorectal cancer: evolution and consensus—an Australian perspective. *J Gastroenterol Hepatol.* 2011;26(suppl 1):58.

98. Chapuis PH, Chan C, Lin BPC, et al. Pathology reporting of resected colorectal cancer in New South Wales in 2000. *ANZ J Surg.* 2007;77:963.

99. Chapuis PH, Lin BPC, Chan C, et al. Risk factors for tumour in a circumferential line of resection after excision of rectal cancer. *Br J Surg.* 2006;93:860.

100. Chapuis PH, Yuile P, Dent OF, et al. Combined endoscopic laser and radiotherapy palliation of advanced rectal cancer. *ANZ J Surg.* 2002;72:95.

101. Chari RS, Tyler DS, Anscher MS, et al. Preoperative radiation and chemotherapy in the treatment of adenocarcinoma of the rectum. *Ann Surg.* 1995;221:778.

102. Charnley RM, Pyf G, Amar SS, et al. The early diagnosis of recurrent rectal carcinoma by rectal endosonography. *Br J Surg.* 1988;75:1232.

103. Chew SSB, King DW. Use of endoscopic titanium stapler in rectal anastomotic stricture. *Dis Colon Rectum.* 2002;45:283.

104. Chia YW, Ngoi SS, Goh PMY. Endoscopic Nd:YAG laser in the palliative treatment of advanced low rectal carcinoma in Singapore. *Dis Colon Rectum.* 1991;34:1093.

105. Chia YW, Ngoi SS, Tung KH. Use of the optical urethrotome knife in the treatment of a benign low rectal anastomotic stricture. *Dis Colon Rectum.* 1991;34:717.

106. Church JM, Randkivi PJ, Hill GL. The surgical anatomy of the rectum—a review of particular relevance to the hazards of rectal mobilisation. *Int J Colorectal Dis.* 1987;2:158.

107. Christiansen J, Kirkegaard P. Treatment of recurrent rectal cancer by electroresection/coagulation after low anterior resection. *Dis Colon Rectum.* 1983;26:656.

108. Cirocco WC, Golub RW. Endoscopic treatment of postoperative hemorrhage from a stapled colorectal anastomosis. *Am Surg.* 1995;61:460.

109. Coco C, Magistrelli P, Granone P, et al. Conservative surgery for early cancer of the distal rectum. *Dis Colon Rectum.* 1992;35:131.

110. Cohen AM, Enker WE, Minsky BD. Proctectomy and coloanal reconstruction for rectal cancer. *Dis Colon Rectum.* 1990;33:40.

111. Cohen AM, Minsky BD. Aggressive surgical management of locally advanced primary and recurrent rectal cancer. *Dis Colon Rectum.* 1990;33:432.

112. Cohen AM, Minsky BD. A phase I trial of preoperative radiation, proctectomy, and endoanal reconstruction. *Arch Surg.* 1990;125:247.

113. Cooperman M, Pace WG, Martin EW Jr, et al. Determination of viability of ischemic intestine by Doppler ultrasound. *Surgery.* 1978;83:705.

114. Craven I, Sebag-Montefiore D. Is there a role for radiotherapy in operable rectal cancer? *Clin Oncol.* 2007;19:687.

115. Crile G Jr, Turnbull RB Jr. The role of electrocoagulation in the treatment of carcinoma of the rectum. *Surg Gynecol Obstet.* 1972;135:391.

116. Cripps WH. *Cancer of the Rectum: Its Pathology, Diagnosis and Treatment (Including a Portion of the Jacksonian Prize Essay for 1876).* London, United Kingdom: Churchill; 1880.

117. Crowe PJ, Temple WJ, Lopez MJ, et al. Pelvic exenteration for advanced pelvic malignancy. *Semin Surg Oncol.* 1999;17:152.

118. Cummings BJ. Adjuvant radiation therapy for rectal adenocarcinomas. *Dis Colon Rectum*. 1984;27:826.

119. Cummings BJ. A critical review of adjuvant preoperative radiation therapy for adenocarcinoma of the rectum. *Br J Surg*. 1986;73:332.

120. Cummings BJ, Rider WD, Harwood AR, et al. Radical external beam radiation therapy for adenocarcinoma of the rectum. *Dis Colon Rectum*. 1983;26:30.

121. Cunningham JD, Enker W, Cohen A. Salvage therapy for pelvic recurrence following curative rectal cancer resection. *Dis Colon Rectum*. 1997;40:393.

122. Cunsolo A, Bragaglia RB, Manara G, et al. Urogenital dysfunction after abdominoperineal resection for carcinoma of the rectum. *Dis Colon Rectum*. 1990;33:918.

123. Cutait DE, Cutait R, Ioshimoto M, et al. Abdominoperineal endoanal pull-through resection. *Dis Colon Rectum*. 1985;28:294.

124. Cutait DE, Figliolini FJ. A new method of colorectal anastomosis in abdominoperineal resection. *Dis Colon Rectum*. 1961;4:335.

125. Cutait R, Enker WE. Prophylactic oophorectomy in surgery for large-bowel cancer. *Dis Colon Rectum*. 1983;26:6.

126. Cuthbertson AM, Kaye AH. Local excision of carcinomas of the rectum, anus and anal canal. *Aust N Z J Surg*. 1978;48:412.

127. Czerny V. Casuistische Mittheilungen aus der Chirurg. Klin zu Heidelberg. *Munch Med Wochenschr*. 1894:11.

128. Dahl O, Horn A, Morild I, et al. Low-dose preoperative radiation postpones recurrences in operable rectal cancer: results of a randomized multicenter trial in western Norway. *Cancer*. 1990;66:2286.

129. Dahlberg M, Glimelius B, Graf W, et al. Preoperative irradiation affects functional results after surgery for rectal cancer: results from a randomized study. *Dis Colon Rectum*. 1998;41:543.

130. Dahlberg M, Påhlman L., Bergström R, et al. Improved survival in patients with rectal cancer: a population-based register study. *Br J Surg*. 1998;85:515.

131. da Silva GM, Berho M, Wexner SD, et al. Histologic analysis of the irradiated anal sphincter. *Dis Colon Rectum*. 2003;46:1492.

132. Dasmahapatra KS, Swaminathan AP. The use of a biodegradable mesh to prevent radiation-associated small-bowel injury. *Arch Surg*. 1991;126:366.

133. Davis NC, Newland RC. Terminology and classification of colorectal cancer: the Australian clinico-pathological staging system. *Aust N Z J Surg*. 1983;53:211.

134. Deaver JB. Lumbar versus iliac colotomy. *J Phila County Med Soc*. 1891;12:97.

135. Deddish MR. Local excision. *Surg Clin North Am*. 1974;54:877.

136. Dehni N, McNamara DA, Schlegel RD, et al. Clinical effects of preoperative radiation therapy on anorectal function after proctectomy and colonic J-pouch-anal anastomosis. *Dis Colon Rectum*. 2002;45:1635.

137. Dehni N, Parc R. Colonic J-pouch-anal anastomosis for rectal cancer. *Dis Colon Rectum*. 2003;46:667.

138. Dehni N, Schlegel RD, Cunningham C, et al. Influence of a defunctioning stoma on leakage rates after low colorectal anastomosis and colonic J pouch-anal anastomosis. *Br J Surg*. 1998;85:1114.

139. DeLuca FR, Ragins H. Construction of an omental envelope as a method of excluding the small intestine from the field of postoperative irradiation to the pelvis. *Surg Gynecol Obstet*. 1985;160:365.

140. Demartines N, von Flue MO, Harder FH. Transanal endoscopic microsurgical excision of rectal tumors: indications and results. *World J Surg*. 2001;25:870.

141. den Dulk M, Marijnen CA, Collette L, et al. Multicentre analysis of oncological and survival outcomes following anastomotic leakage after rectal cancer surgery. *Br J Surg*. 2009;96:1066.

142. Dennett ER, Parry BR. Misconceptions about the colonic J-pouch: what the accumulating data show. *Dis Colon Rectum*. 1999;42:804.

143. Denoix PF. Tumour, node and metastasis (TNM). *Bull Inst Nat Hyg (Paris)*. 1954;1:1.

144. Dent OF, Chapuis PH, Haboubi N, et al. Magnetic resonance imaging cannot predict histological tumor involvement of a circumferential surgical margin in rectal cancer. *Colorectal Dis*. 2011;13:974.

145. Dent OF, Haboubi N, Chapuis PH, et al. Assessing the evidence for an association between circumferential tumor clearance and local recurrence after resection of rectal cancer. *Colorectal Dis*. 2007;9:112.

146. Deutsch AA, Stern HS. Technique of insertion of pelvic Vicryl mesh sling to avoid postradiation enteritis. *Dis Colon Rectum*. 1989;32:628.

147. Devereux DF, Chandler JJ, Eisenstat T, et al. Efficacy of an absorbable mesh in keeping the small bowel out of the human pelvis following surgery. *Dis Colon Rectum*. 1988;31:17.

148. Devereux DF, Eisenstat T, Zinkin L. The safe and effective use of postoperative radiation therapy in modified Astler Coller stage C3 rectal cancer. *Cancer*. 1989;63:2393.

149. Dobrowsky W, Schmid AP. Radiotherapy of presacral recurrence following radical surgery for rectal carcinoma. *Dis Colon Rectum*. 1985;28:917.

150. Donaldson GA, Rodkey GV, Behringer GE. Resection of the rectum with anal preservation. *Surg Gynecol Obstet*. 1966;123:571.

151. Doornebosch PG, Gosselink MP, Neijenhuis PA, et al. Impact of transanal endoscopic microsurgery on functional outcome and quality of life. *Int J Colorectal Dis*. 2008;23:709.

152. Dosoretz DE, Gunderson LL, Hedberg S, et al. Preoperative irradiation for unresectable rectal and rectosigmoid carcinomas. *Cancer*. 1983;52:814.

153. Drake DB, Pemberton JH, Beart RW Jr, et al. Coloanal anastomosis in the management of benign and malignant rectal disease. *Ann Surg*. 1987;206:600.

154. Dukes CE. The classification of cancer of the rectum. *J Pathol*. 1932;35:323.

155. Duncan W. Adjuvant radiotherapy in rectal cancer: the MRC trials. *Br J Surg*. 1985;72:59.

156. Dürig M, Steenblock U, Herberer M, et al. Prevention of radiation injuries to the small intestine. *Surg Gynecol Obstet*. 1984;159:162.

157. Dwight RW, Higgins GA, Roswit B, et al. Preoperative radiation and surgery for cancer of the sigmoid colon and rectum. *Am J Surg*. 1972;123:93.

158. Eckhauser ML, Imbembo AL, Mansour EG. The role of pre-resectional laser recanalization for obstructing carcinomas of the colon and rectum. *Surgery*. 1989;106:710.

159. Eisenberg HW. Sequential electrocoagulation and resection for carcinoma of the rectum. *Surg Gynecol Obstet*. 1984;159:471.

160. Ellis LM, Mendenhall WM, Bland KI, et al. Local excision and radiation therapy for early rectal cancer. *Am Surg*. 1988;54:217.

161. Enker WE. Potency, cure, and local control in the operative treatment of rectal cancer. *Arch Surg*. 1992;127:1396.

162. Enker WE, Stearns MW Jr, Janov AJ. Perianal coloanal anastomosis following low anterior resection for rectal carcinoma. *Dis Colon Rectum*. 1985;28:576.

163. Enker WE, Thaler HT, Cranor ML, et al. Total mesorectal excision in the operative treatment of carcinoma of the rectum. *J Am Coll Surg*. 1995;181:334.

164. Enriquez-Navascués JM, Borda N, Lizerazu A, et al. Patterns of local recurrence in rectal cancer after a multidisciplinary approach. *World J Gastroenterol*. 2011;17:1674.

165. Escudero-Fabre A, Sack J. Endoscopic laser therapy for neoplastic lesions of the colorectum. *Am J Surg*. 1992;163:260.

166. Evans DB, Shumate CR, Ames FC, et al. Use of Dexon mesh for abdominal partitioning above the peritoneal reflection. *Dis Colon Rectum*. 1991;34:833.

167. Faivre J, Chaume JC, Pigot F, et al. Transanal electroresection of small rectal cancer: a sole treatment? *Dis Colon Rectum*. 1996;39:270.

168. Farouk R, Drew PJ, Duthie GS, et al. Disruption of the internal anal sphincter can occur after transanal stapling. *Br J Surg*. 1996;83:1400.

169. Farouk R, Nelson H, Gunderson LL. Aggressive multimodality treatment for locally advanced irresectable rectal cancer. *Br J Surg*. 1997;84:741.

170. Farouk R, Ratnaval CD, Monson JRT, et al. Staged delivery of Nd:YAG laser therapy for palliation of advanced rectal carcinoma. *Dis Colon Rectum*. 1997;40:156.

171. Fazio VW, Tekkis PP, Remzi F, et al. Assessment of operative risk in colorectal cancer surgery: the Cleveland Clinic Foundation cancer model. *Dis Colon Rectum*. 2004;47:2015.

172. Fein RL, Needell MH, Winton L. An orderly approach to the impotent male and the dorsal approach for insertion of the Jonas penile prosthesis. *Contemp Surg*. 1983;23:93.

173. Ferlay J, Shin HR, Bray F, et al. Estimates of worldwide burden of cancer in 2008: GLOBCAN 2008. *Int J Cancer*. 2010;127:2893.

174. Fisher B, Wolmark N, Rockette H, et al. Postoperative adjuvant chemotherapy or radiation therapy for rectal cancer: results from NSABP Protocol R-01. *J Natl Cancer Inst*. 1988;80:21.

175. Fleshman JW, Kodner IJ, Fry RD, et al. Adenocarcinoma of the rectum: results of radiotherapy and resection, endocavitary irradiation, local excision, and preoperative clinical staging. *Dis Colon Rectum*. 1985;28:810.

176. Foley KM. The treatment of cancer pain. *N Engl J Med*. 1985;313:84.

177. Folkesson J, Helgi Birgisson H, Pahlman L, et al. Swedish Rectal Cancer Trial: long lasting benefits from radiotherapy on survival and local recurrence rate. *J Clin Oncol*. 2005;23:5644.

178. Fortier GA, Constable WC. Preoperative radiation therapy for rectal cancer. *Arch Surg*. 1986;121:1380.

179. Frazee RC, Patel R, Belew M, et al. Transanal excision of rectal carcinoma. *Am Surg*. 1995;61:714.

180. Friedmann P, Garb JL, McCabe DP, et al. Intestinal anastomosis after preoperative radiation therapy for carcinoma of the rectum. *Surg Gynecol Obstet.* 1987;164:257.

181. Friedmann P, Garb JL, Park WC, et al. Survival following moderate-dose preoperative radiation therapy for carcinoma of the rectum. *Cancer.* 1985;55:967.

182. Friel CM, Cromwell JW, Marra C, et al. Salvage radical surgery after failed local excision for early rectal cancer. *Dis Colon Rectum.* 2002;45:875.

183. Fritsch A, Seidl W, Walzel C, et al. Palliative and adjunctive measures in rectal cancer. *World J Surg.* 1982;6:569.

184. Frye J, Bokey EL, Chapuis PH, et al. Anastomotic leakage after resection of colorectal cancer generates prodigious use of hospital resources. *Colorectal Dis.* 2009;11:917.

185. Frykholm GJ, Glimeluis B, Påhlman L. Preoperative or postoperative irradiation in adenocarcinoma of the rectum: final treatment results of a randomized trial and an evaluation of late secondary effects. *Dis Colon Rectum.* 1993;36:564.

186. Fujita S, Yamamoto S, Akasu T, et al. Lateral pelvic lymph node dissection for advanced lower rectal cancer. *Br J Surg.* 2003;90:1580.

187. Fürst A, Suttner S, Agha A, et al. Colonic J-pouch vs. coloplasty following resection of distal rectal cancer: early results of a prospective, randomized, pilot study. *Dis Colon Rectum.* 2003;46:1161.

188. Gabriel WB. Perineal-abdominal excision of the rectum in one stage. *Lancet.* 1934;2:69.

189. Gage AA. Cryotherapy for inoperable rectal cancer. *Dis Colon Rectum.* 1968;11:36.

190. Gage AA. Cryosurgery in the treatment of cancer. *Surg Gynecol Obstet.* 1992;174:73.

191. Gagliardi G, Hawley PR, Hershman MJ, et al. Prognostic factors in surgery for local recurrence of rectal cancer. *Br J Surg.* 1995;82:1401.

192. Gagliardi G, Stepniewska KA, Hershman MJ, et al. New grade-related prognostic variable for rectal cancer. *Br J Surg.* 1995;82:599.

193. Gall FP, Hermanek P. Cancer of the rectum-local excision. *Surg Clin North Am.* 1988;68:1353.

194. Galloway DJ, Cohen AM, Shank B, et al. Adjuvant multimodality treatment of rectal cancer. *Br J Surg.* 1989;76:440.

195. Gamagami RA, Liagre A, Chiotasso P, et al. Coloanal anastomosis for distal third rectal cancer: prospective study of oncologic results. *Dis Colon Rectum.* 1999;42:1272.

196. Garcia-Aguilar J, Cromwell JW, Marra C, et al. Treatment of locally recurrent rectal cancer. *Dis Colon Rectum.* 2001;44:1743.

197. Garcia-Aguilar J, Hernandez de Anda E, Sirivongs P, et al. A pathologic complete response to preoperative chemoradiation is associated with lower local recurrence and improved survival in rectal cancer patients treated by mesorectal excision. *Dis Colon Rectum.* 2003;46:298.

198. Garcia-Aguilar J, Pollack J, Lee SH, et al. Accuracy of endorectal ultrasonography in preoperative staging of rectal tumors. *Dis Colon Rectum.* 2002;45:10.

199. Garcia-Armengol J, Garcia-Botello S, Martinez-Soriano F, et al. Review of the anatomic concepts in relation to the retro-rectal space and the endopelvic fascia: Waldeyer's fascia and the retrosacral fascial. *Colorectal Dis.* 2008;10:298.

200. Gastrointestinal Tumor Study Group. Prolongation of the disease-free interval in surgically treated rectal carcinoma. *N Engl J Med.* 1985;312:1465.

201. Gastrointestinal Tumor Study Group. Survival after postoperative combination treatment of rectal cancer. *N Engl J Med.* 1986;315:1294.

202. Gee WF, McRoberts JW, Ansell JS. Penile prosthetic implant for the treatment of organic impotence. *Am J Surg.* 1973;126:698.

203. Geerdes BP, Zoetmulder FAN, Heineman E, et al. Total anorectal reconstruction with a double dynamic graciloplasty after abdominoperineal reconstruction for low rectal cancer. *Dis Colon Rectum.* 1997;40:698.

204. Gérard A, Buyse M, Nordlinger B, et al. Preoperative radiotherapy as adjuvant treatment in rectal cancer: final results of a randomized study of the European Organisation for Research and Treatment of Cancer (EORTC). *Ann Surg.* 1988;208:606.

205. Gervas P, Rotholtz N, Wexner SD, et al. Colonic J-pouch function in rectal cancer patients: impact of adjuvant chemoradiotherapy. *Dis Colon Rectum.* 2001;44:1667.

206. Glaser F, Kuntz C, Schlag P, et al. Endorectal ultrasound for control of preoperative radiotherapy of rectal cancer. *Ann Surg.* 1993;217:64.

207. Goetz O. Das Rektumkarzinom als Exstirpationsobjekt; Vorschläge zur sakralen und abdominosakralen Operation. *Zentralbl Chir.* 1931;58:1746.

208. Goldman HS, Sapkin SL, Foote RF, et al. Seminal vesicle-rectal fistula: report of a case. *Dis Colon Rectum.* 1989;32:67.

209. Goligher JC. Further reflections on preservation of the anal sphincters in the radical treatment of rectal cancer. *Proc R Soc Med.* 1962;55:341.

210. Goligher JC. Ernest Miles: the rise and fall of abdominoperineal excision in the treatment or carcinoma of the rectum. *J Pelv Surg.* 1996;2:53.

211. Goligher JC, Duthie HL, DeDombal FT, et al. Abdominoanal pull-through excision for tumors of the mid-third of the rectum: a comparison with low anterior resection. *Br J Surg.* 1965;52:323.

212. Goligher JC, Hughes ESR. Sensibility of the rectum and colon: its role in the mechanism of anal continence. *Lancet.* 1951;1:543.

213. Goligher JC, Lloyd-Davies OV, Robertson CT. Small-gut obstructions following combined excision of rectum, with special reference to strangulation around the colostomy. *Br J Surg.* 1951;38:467.

214. Gordon-Watson C. Treatment of cancer of the rectum with radium by open operation. *Proc R Soc Med.* 1927;21:309.

215. Gordon-Watson C. The treatment of carcinoma of the rectum with radium. *Br J Surg.* 1930;17:649.

216. Gordon-Watson C. How far can radium replace radical surgery for cancer of the rectum? *Ann Surg.* 1931;93:467.

217. Gordon-Watson C. Discussion on the radium treatment of malignant disease of the rectum and anus. *Proc R Soc Med.* 1935;28:1251.

218. Graham RA, Garnsey L, Jessup JM. Local excision of rectal carcinoma. *Am J Surg.* 1990;160:306.

219. Graham RA, Holm DC. Management of inguinal lymph node metastases from adenocarcinoma of the rectum. *Dis Colon Rectum.* 1990;33:212.

220. Granai CO, Gajewski W, Madoc-Jones H, et al. Use of the omental J flap for better delivery of radiotherapy to the pelvis. *Surg Gynecol Obstet.* 1990;171:71.

221. Gregory JS, Muldoon JP. Perineal herniation—a late complication of abdominoperineal resection of the rectum: report of a case. *Dis Colon Rectum.* 1969;12:33.

222. Grigg M, McDermott FT, Pihl EA, et al. Curative local excision in the treatment of carcinoma of the rectum. *Dis Colon Rectum.* 1984;27:81.

223. Guillem JG, Paty PB, Cohen AM. Surgical treatment of colorectal cancer. *CA Cancer J Clin.* 1997;47:113.

224. Guillem JG, Puig-La Calle J Jr, Akhurst T, et al. Prospective assessment of primary rectal cancer response to preoperative radiation and chemotherapy using 18-fluorodeoxyglucose positron emission tomography. *Dis Colon Rectum.* 2000;43:18.

225. Gunderson LL, Cohen AM, Welch CE. Residual, inoperable or recurrent colorectal cancer: interaction of surgery and radiotherapy. *Am J Surg.* 1980;139:518.

226. Gunderson LL, Martin JK, Beart RW, et al. Intraoperative and external beam irradiation for locally advanced colorectal cancer. *Ann Surg.* 1988;207:52.

227. Habr-Gama A, Perez RO. Non-operative management of rectal cancer after neoadjuvant chemoradiation. *Br J Surg.* 2009;96:125.

228. Habr-Gama A, Perez RO, Nadalin W, et al. Operative versus nonoperative treatment for stage 0 distal rectal cancer following chemoradiation therapy: long-term results. *Ann Surg.* 2004;240:711.

229. Habr-Gama A, Perez RO, Proscurshim I, et al. Patterns of failure and survival for nonoperative treatment of stage c0 distal rectal cancer following neoadjuvant chemoradiation therapy. *J Gastrointest Surg.* 2006;10:1319.

230. Habr-Gama A, Perez RO, Proscurshim I, et al. Interval between surgery and neoadjuvant chemoradiation therapy for distal rectal cancer: does delayed surgery have an impact on outcome? *Int J Radiat Oncol Biol Phys.* 2008;71:1181.

231. Hager TH, Gall FP, Hermanek P. Local excision of cancer of the rectum. *Dis Colon Rectum.* 1983;26:149.

232. Hahnlosser D, Nelson H, Gunderson LL, et al. Curative potential of multimodality therapy for locally recurrent rectal cancer. *Ann Surg.* 2003;237:502.

233. Hainsworth PJ, Egan MJ, Cunliffe WJ. Evaluation of a policy of total mesorectal excision for rectal and sigmoid cancer. *Br J Surg.* 1997;84:652.

234. Hallböök O, Påhlman L, Krog M, et al. Randomized comparison of straight and colonic J pouch anastomosis after low anterior resection. *Ann Surg.* 1996;224:58.

235. Hallböök O, Sjödahl R. Anastomotic leakage and functional outcome after anterior resection of the rectum. *Br J Surg.* 1996;83:60.

236. Harris GJC, Church JM, Senagore AJ, et al. Factors affecting local recurrence of colonic adenocarcinoma. *Dis Colon Rectum.* 2002;45:1029.

237. Harris GJC, Lavery IJ, Fazio VW. Reasons for failure to construct the colonic J-pouch. What can be done to improve the size of the neorectal reservoir should it occur? *Dis Colon Rectum.* 2002;45:1304.

238. Harrison LB, Enker WE, Anderson LL. High-dose-rate intraoperative radiation therapy for colorectal cancer. *Oncology.* 1995;9:737.

239. Harshaw DH, Gardner B, Vives A, et al. The effect of technical factors upon complications from abdominal perineal resections. *Surg Gynecol Obstet.* 1974;139:756.

240. Hartmann H. Nouveau procédé d'ablation des cancers de la partie terminale du colon pelvien. In: *Trentième Congrès de Chirurgie.* Strasbourg, France: 1923:411.

241. Hase K, Shatney CH, Mochizuki H, et al. Long-term results of curative resection of minimally invasive colorectal cancer. *Dis Colon Rectum.* 1995;38:19.

242. Hashiguchi Y, Sekine T, Kato S, et al. Indicators for surgical resection and intraoperative radiation therapy for pelvic recurrence of colorectal cancer. *Dis Colon Rectum.* 2003;46:31.

243. Hashiguchi Y, Sekine T, Sakamoto H, et al. Intraoperative irradiation after surgery for locally recurrent rectal cancer. *Dis Colon Rectum.* 1999;42:886.

244. Hautefeuille P, Valleur P, Perniceni T, et al. Functional and oncologic results after coloanal anastomosis for low rectal carcinoma. *Ann Surg.* 1988;207:61.

245. Heah SM, Seow-Choen F, Eu KW, et al. Prospective, randomized trial comparing sigmoid vs. descending colonic J-pouch after total rectal excision. *Dis Colon Rectum.* 2002;45:322.

246. Heald RJ, Husband EM, Ryall RDH. The mesorectum in rectal cancer surgery—the clue to pelvic recurrence. *Br J Surg.* 1982;69:613.

247. Heald RJ, Leicester RJ. The low stapled anastomosis. *Dis Colon Rectum.* 1981;24:437.

248. Heald RJ, Moran BJ, Rydall RD, et al. Rectal cancer—the Basingstoke experience of total meso-rectal excision 1978–1997. *Arch Surg.* 1998;133:894.

249. Heberer G, Denecke H, Demmel N, et al. Local procedures in the management of rectal cancer. *World J Surg.* 1987;11:499.

250. Heimann TM, Miller F, Martinelli G, et al. Significance of DNA content abnormalities in small rectal cancers. *Am J Surg.* 1990;159:199.

251. Herman RM, Richter P, Walega P, et al. Anorectal sphincter function and rectal barostat study in patients following transanal endoscopic microsurgery. *Int J Colorectal Dis.* 2001;16:370.

252. Herrera L, Villarreal JR. Incidence of metastases from rectal adenocarcinoma in small lymph nodes detected by a clearing technique. *Dis Colon Rectum.* 1992;35:783.

253. Herzog U, von Flüe M, Tondelli P, et al. How accurate is endorectal ultrasound in the preoperative staging of rectal cancer? *Dis Colon Rectum.* 1993;36:127.

254. Hickey RC, Romsdahl MM, Johnson DE, et al. Recurrent cancer and metastases. *World J Surg.* 1982;6:585.

255. Hida JI, Yasutomi M, Fujimoto K, et al. Functional outcome after low anterior resection with low anastomosis for rectal cancer using the colonic J-pouch. *Dis Colon Rectum.* 1996;39:986.

256. Hida JI, Yasutomi M, Maruyama T, et al. Indications for colonic J-pouch reconstruction after anterior resection for rectal cancer: determining the optimum level of anastomosis. *Dis Colon Rectum.* 1998;41:558.

257. Hildebrandt U, Feifel G, Scherr O. Endorectal ultrasound: instrumentation and clinical aspects. *Int J Colorect Dis.* 1986;1:203.

258. Hildebrandt U, Klein T, Feifel G, et al. Endosonography of pararectal lymph nodes. In vitro and in vivo evaluation. *Dis Colon Rectum.* 1990;33:863.

259. Hill GL, Rafique M. Extrafascial excision of the rectum for rectal cancer. *Br J Surg.* 1998;85:809.

260. Hjortrup A, Moesgaard F, Kjaergård J. Fibrin adhesive in the treatment of perineal fistulas. *Dis Colon Rectum.* 1991;34:752.

261. Ho YH, Tsang C, Tang CL, et al. Anal sphincter injuries from stapling instruments introduced transanally: randomized, controlled study with endoanal ultrasound and anorectal manometry. *Dis Colon Rectum.* 2000;43:169.

262. Ho YH, Yu S, Ang ES, et al. Small colonic J-pouch improves colonic transit of liquids: randomized, controlled trial with scintigraphy. *Dis Colon Rectum.* 2002;45:76.

263. Hochenegg J. Die Sakrale Methode der Exstirpation von Mastdarmkrebsen nach Prof. Kraske. *Wien Klin Wochenschr.* 1888;1:254.

264. Hodges CV, Moore RJ, Lehman TH, et al. Clinical experiences with transureteroureterostomy. *J Urol.* 1963;90:552.

265. Hojo K, Sawada T, Moriya Y. An analysis of survival and voiding, sexual function after wide iliopelvic lymphadenectomy in patients with carcinoma of the rectum, compared with conventional lymphadenectomy. *Dis Colon Rectum.* 1989;32:128.

266. Holm T, Cedermark B, Rutqvist LE. Local recurrence of rectal adenocarcinoma after curative surgery with and without preoperative radiotherapy. *Br J Surg.* 1994;81:452.

267. Holm T, Johansson H, Cedermark B, et al. Influence of hospital- and surgeon-related factors on outcome after treatment of rectal cancer with or without preoperative radiotherapy. *Br J Surg.* 1997;84:657.

268. Holm T, Ljung A, Haggmark T, et al. Extended abdominoperineal resection with gluteus maximus flap reconstruction of the pelvic floor for rectal cancer. *Br J Surg.* 2007;94:232.

269. Holm T, Rutqvist LE, Johansson H, et al. Postoperative mortality in rectal cancer treated with or without preoperative radiotherapy: causes and risk factors. *Br J Surg.* 1996;83:964.

270. Hood K, Lewis A. Dilator for high rectal strictures. *Br J Surg.* 1986;73:633.

271. Horn A, Halvorsen JF, Dahl O. Preoperative radiotherapy in operable rectal cancer. *Dis Colon Rectum.* 1990;33:823.

272. Horn A, Halvorsen JF, Morild I. Transanal extirpation of early rectal cancer. *Dis Colon Rectum.* 1989;32:769.

273. Huber A, von Hockstetter A, Allgöwer M. Anatomy of the pelvic floor for translevatoric-transsphincteric operations. *Am Surg.* 1987;53:247.

274. Huddy SPJ, Husband EM, Cook MG, et al. Lymph node metastases in early rectal cancer. *Br J Surg.* 1993;80:1457.

275. Hughes E, Cuthbertson AM, Killingback MK. *Colorectal Surgery.* Edinburgh, United Kingdom: Churchill Livingstone; 1983:chap 1.

276. Hughes EP, Veidenheimer MC, Corman ML, et al. Electrocoagulation of rectal cancer. *Dis Colon Rectum.* 1982;25:215.

277. Huguet C, Harb J, Bona S. Coloanal anastomosis after resection of low rectal cancer in the elderly. *World J Surg.* 1990;14:619.

278. Hull TL, Lavry IC, Saxton JP. Endocavitary irradiation: an option in select patients with rectal cancer. *Dis Colon Rectum.* 1994;37:1266.

279. Husband JE, Hodson NJ, Parsons CA. The use of computed tomography in recurrent rectal tumors. *Radiology.* 1980;134:677.

280. Hyams DM, Mamounas EP, Petrelli N, et al. A clinical trial to evaluate the worth of preoperative multimodality therapy in patients with operable carcinoma of the rectum: a progress report of national surgical adjuvant breast and bowel project protocol R-03. *Dis Colon Rectum.* 1997;40:131.

281. Ike H, Shimada H, Yamaguchi S, et al. Outcome of total pelvic exenteration for primary rectal cancer. *Dis Colon Rectum.* 2003;46:474.

282. Isbister WH. Basingstoke revisited. *Aust N Z J Surg.* 1990;60:243.

283. Isbister WH. Food for thought: Basingstoke revisited again. *Aust N Z J Surg.* 1999;69:85.

284. Isbister WH. Basingstoke: the final word. *Aust N Z J Surg.* 2000; 70:675.

285. Jackman RJ. Conservative management of selected patients with carcinoma of the rectum. *Dis Colon Rectum.* 1961;4:429.

286. James RD, Schofield PF. Resection of "inoperable" rectal cancer following radiotherapy. *Br J Surg.* 1985;72:279.

287. Janu NC, Bokey EL, Chapuis PH, et al. Bladder dysfunction following anterior resection for carcinoma of the rectum. *Dis Colon Rectum.* 1986;29:182.

288. Jass JR. Lymphocytic infiltration and survival in rectal cancer. *J Clin Pathol.* 1986;39:585.

289. Jass JR, Love SB, Northover JMA. A new prognostic classification of rectal cancer. *Lancet.* 1987;1:1303.

290. Jelden GL. Presentation to American Society of Therapeutic Radiologists, Miami Beach (as reported in *Medical News*). *JAMA.* 1981;246:2419.

291. Jiminez RE, Shoup M, Cohen AM, et al. Contemporary outcomes of total pelvic exenteration in the treatment of colorectal cancer. *Dis Colon Rectum.* 2003;46:1619.

292. Jin Kim H, Wong WD. Role of endorectal ultrasound in the conservative management of rectal cancers. *Semin Surg Oncol.* 2000;19:358.

293. Jochem RJ, Reading CC, Dozois RR, et al. Endorectal ultrasonographic staging of rectal carcinoma. *Mayo Clin Proc.* 1990;65:1571.

294. Johansson C. Endoscopic dilation of rectal strictures: a prospective study of 18 cases. *Dis Colon Rectum.* 1996;39:423.

295. Johnston MJ, Robertson GM, Frizelle FA. Management of late complications of pelvic radiation in the rectum and anus: a review. *Dis Colon Rectum.* 2003;46:247.

296. Jones DJ, Zaloudik J, James RD, et al. Predicting local recurrence of carcinoma of the rectum after preoperative radiotherapy and surgery. *Br J Surg.* 1989;76:1172.

297. Jonnesco T. *Le côlon pelvien pendant la vie intra-utérine* [thesis]. Havre: Lemale et Cie; 1892.

298. Julien LA, Thorson AG. Current neoadjuvant strategies in rectal cancer. *J Surg Oncol.* 2010;101:321.

299. Junginger T, Kneist W, Heintz A. Influence of identification and preservation of pelvic autonomic nerves in rectal cancer surgery on bladder dysfunction after total mesorectal excision. *Dis Colon Rectum.* 2003;46:621.

300. Kandioler D, Zwrtek R, Ludwig C, et al. TP53 genotype but not p53 immunohistochemical result predicts response to preoperative short-term radiotherapy in rectal cancer. *Ann Surg.* 2002;235:493.

301. Kapiteijn E, Marijnen CA, Nagtegaal ID, et al. Preoperative radiotherapy combined with total mesorectal excision for resectable rectal cancer. *N Engl J Med.* 2001;345:638.

302. Karanjia ND, Corder AP, Bearn P, et al. Leakage from stapled low anastomosis after total mesorectal excision for carcinoma of the rectum. *Br J Surg.* 1994;81:1224.

303. Katin MJ, Dosoretz DE, Gunderson L. The role of radiation therapy in the treatment of unresectable, residual, or recurrent colorectal carcinoma. *Contemp Surg.* 1984;24:25.

304. Kehlet H, Holte K. Review of postoperative ileus. *Am J Surg.* 2001; 182(5A suppl):3S.

305. Kelly SB, Mills SJ, Bradburn DM, et al. Effect of circumferential resection margin on survival following rectal cancer surgery. *Br J Surg.* 2011;98:573.

306. Kelly SR, Nugent KP. Formalin instillation for control of rectal hemorrhage in advanced pelvic malignancy: report of two cases. *Dis Colon Rectum.* 2002;45:121.

307. Kennedy ML, Lubowski DZ, King DW. Transanal endoscopic microsurgery excision: is anorectal function compromised? *Dis Colon Rectum.* 2002;45:601.

308. Kergin FG. Diathermy fulgurization in treatment of certain cases of rectal carcinoma. *Can Med Assoc J.* 1953;69:14.

309. Khubchandani IT, Karamchandani MC, Sheets JA, et al. The Bacon pull-through procedure. *Dis Colon Rectum.* 1987;30:540.

310. Khubchandani IT, Trimpi HD, Sheets JA. Low end-to-side rectoenteric anastomosis with single-layer wire. *Dis Colon Rectum.* 1975;18:308.

311. Killingback MJ. Indications for local excision of rectal cancer. *Br J Surg.* 1985;72:54.

312. Killingback M, Barron P, Dent OF. Local recurrence after curative resection of cancer of the rectum without total mesorectal excision. *Dis Colon Rectum.* 2001;44:473.

313. Kingsley AN. Colonic strictures: management by endoscopic balloon dilation. *Contemp Surg.* 1991;38:50.

314. Kinn AC, Öhman U. Bladder and sexual function after surgery for rectal cancer. *Dis Colon Rectum.* 1986;29:43.

315. Kirwan WO, Turnbull RB Jr, Fazio VW, et al. Pull-through operation with delayed anastomosis for rectal cancer. *Br J Surg.* 1978;65:695.

316. Kiselow M, Butcher HR Jr, Bricker EM. Results of the radical surgical treatment of advanced pelvic cancer: a fifteen-year study. *Ann Surg.* 1967;166:428.

317. Klessen C, Rogalla P, Taupitz M. Local staging of rectal cancer: the current role of MRI. *Eur Radiol.* 2007;17:379.

318. Knoepp LF, Ray JE, Overby I. Ovarian metastases from colorectal carcinoma. *Dis Colon Rectum.* 1973;16:305.

319. Kocher T. Quoted in: Rankin FW, Bargen JA, Buie LA, eds. *The Colon, Rectum and Anus.* Philadelphia, PA: WB Saunders; 1932.

320. Koda K, Tobe T, Takiguchi N, et al. Pelvic exenteration for advanced colorectal cancer with reconstruction of urinary and sphincter functions. *Br J Surg.* 2002;89:1286.

321. Kodner IJ, Gilley MT, Shemesh EI, et al. Radiation therapy as definitive treatment for selected invasive rectal cancer. *Surgery.* 1993;114:850.

322. Kodner IJ, Shemesh EI, Fry RD, et al. Preoperative irradiation for rectal cancer: improved local control and long-term survival. *Ann Surg.* 1989;209:194.

323. Kollmorgen TA, Kollmorgen CF, Lieber MM, et al. Seminal vesicle fistula following abdominoperineal resection for recurrent adenocarcinoma of the rectum. *Dis Colon Rectum.* 1994;37:1325.

324. Kouraklis G. Reconstruction of the pelvic floor using the rectus abdominis muscles after radical pelvic surgery. *Dis Colon Rectum.* 2002;45:836.

325. Kraske P. Ueber die Entstehung sek undarer Krebsqeschwüre durch Impfung. *Zentralbl Chir.* 1884;11:801.

326. Kraske P. Zur exstirpation hochsitzender Mastdarmkrebse [Extirpation of high carcinomas of the large bowel]. *Arch Klin Chir (Berl).* 1886;33:563. Translated in *Dis Colon Rectum.* 1984;27:499.

327. Kraybill WG, Lopez MJ, Bricker EM. Total pelvic exenteration as a therapeutic option in advanced malignant disease of the pelvis. *Surg Gynecol Obstet.* 1988;166:259.

328. Kratzer GL. The pull-through operation. *Dis Colon Rectum.* 1967; 10:112.

329. Kratzer GL. Modification of the pull-through operation. *Dis Colon Rectum.* 1972;15:288.

330. Kratzer GL, Onsanit T. Fulguration of selected cancers of the rectum. *Dis Colon Rectum.* 1972;15:431.

331. Kreis ME, Jehle EC, Haug V, et al. Functional results after transanal endoscopic microsurgery. *Dis Colon Rectum.* 1996;39:1116.

332. Kroll SS, Pollock R, Jessup JM, et al. Transpelvic rectus abdominis flap reconstruction of defects following abdomino-perineal resection. *Am Surg.* 1989;55:632.

333. Krook JE, Moertel CG, Gunderson LL, et al. Effective surgical adjuvant therapy for high-risk rectal carcinoma. *N Engl J Med.* 1991;324:709.

334. Kuehne H, Kleisli T, Biernacki P, et al. Use of high-dose-rate brachytherapy in the management of locally recurrent rectal cancer. *Dis Colon Rectum.* 2003;46:895.

335. Kurz KR, Pitts WR, Speer D, et al. Palliation of carcinoma of the rectum and pararectum using the urologic resectoscope. *Surg Gynecol Obstet.* 1988;166:60.

336. Kusunoki M, Shoji Y, Yanagi H, et al. Function after anoabdominal rectal resection and colonic J pouch-anal anastomosis. *Br J Surg.* 1991;78:1434.

337. Kusunoki M, Yanagi H, Gondoh N, et al. Use of transrectal ultrasonography to select type of surgery for villous tumors in the lower two thirds of the rectum. *Arch Surg.* 1996;131:714.

338. Lahaye MJ, Engelen SM, Nelemans PJ, et al. Imaging for predicting risk factors—the circumferential resection margin and nodal disease—of local recurrence in rectal cancer: a meta-analysis. *Semin Ultrasound CT MR.* 2005;26:259.

339. Lahey FH. Two-stage abdominoperineal removal of cancer of the rectum. *Surg Gynecol Obstet.* 1930;51:622.

340. La Monica G, Audisio RA, Tamburini M, et al. Incidence of sexual dysfunction in male patients treated surgically for rectal malignancy. *Dis Colon Rectum.* 1985;28:937.

341. Lane RHS, Parks AG. Function of the anal sphincters following colo-anal anastomosis. *Br J Surg.* 1977;64:596.

342. Law WL, Chu KW. Anterior resection for rectal cancer with mesorectal excision. *Ann Surg.* 2004;240:260.

343. Lazorthes F, Fages P, Chiotasso P, et al. Synchronous abdominotranssphincteric resection of low rectal cancer: new technique for direct colo-anal anastomosis. *Br J Surg.* 1986;73:573.

344. Lazorthes F, Fages P, Chiotasso P, et al. Resection of the rectum with construction of a colonic reservoir and colo-anal anastomosis for carcinoma of the rectum. *Br J Surg.* 1986;73:136.

345. Leadbetter GW, Leadbetter WF. A new approach to the problem of urinary retention following abdominoperineal resection for carcinoma of the rectum. *Surg Gynecol Obstet.* 1958;107:333.

346. Leaming RH, Stearns MW, Deddish MR. Preoperative irradiation in rectal carcinoma. *Radiology.* 1961;77:257.

347. Lechner P, Cesnik H. Abdominopelvic omentopexy: preparatory procedure for radiotherapy in rectal cancer. *Dis Colon Rectum.* 1992;35:1157.

348. Lee PH, Khauli RB, Baker S, et al. Prognostic and therapeutic observations of manifestations in the genitourinary tract of adenocarcinoma of the colon and rectum. *Surg Gynecol Obstet.* 1989;169:511.

349. Leer JWH, Scholten RE, Heslinga T, et al. Role of computed tomography in the diagnosis and radiotherapy planning of recurrent rectal carcinoma. *Diagn Imaging.* 1980;49:208.

350. Lelcuk S, Yavez H, Klausner JM, et al. "Spermatocele" following abdominoperineal resection and radiotherapy. *Dis Colon Rectum.* 1986;29:355.

351. Leo E, Belli F, Baldini MT, et al. New perspective in the treatment of low rectal cancer: total rectal resection and coloendoanal anastomosis. *Dis Colon Rectum.* 1994;37:S62.

352. Leong AF. Selective total mesorectal excision for rectal cancer. *Dis Colon Rectum.* 2000;43:1237.

353. Lewis WG, Holdsworth PJ, Stephenson BM, et al. Role of the rectum in the physiological and clinical results of coloanal and colorectal anastomosis after anterior resection for rectal carcinoma. *Br J Surg.* 1992;79:1082.

354. Lewis WG, Martin IG, Williamson MER, et al. Why do some patients experience poor functional results after anterior resection of the rectum for carcinoma? *Dis Colon Rectum.* 1995;38:259.

355. Libertino JA, Rote AR, Zinman L. Ureteral reconstruction in renal transplantation. *Urology.* 1978;12:641.

356. Libertino JA, Zinman L. Technique for uretero-neocystotomy in renal transplantation and reflux. *Surg Clin North Am.* 1973;53:459.

357. Lindsey I, George B, Kettlewell M, et al. Randomized, double-blind, placebo-controlled trial of sildenafil (Viagra) for erectile dysfunction after rectal excision for cancer and inflammatory bowel disease. *Dis Colon Rectum.* 2002;45:727.

358. Lindsey I, Mortensen NJ. Iatrogenic impotence and rectal dissection. *Br J Surg.* 2002;89:1493.

359. Lisfranc J. Mémoire sur l'excision de la partie inférieure du rectum devenue carcinomateuse [Observation on a cancerous condition of the rectum treated by excision]. *Rev Med Franc.* 1826;2:380. Translated in *Dis Colon Rectum.* 1983;26:694.

360. Littre A. *Mémoire de l'academie des sciences.* 1710;10:36.

361. Lloyd-Davies OV. Lithotomy-Trendelenburg position for resection of rectum and lower pelvic colon. *Lancet.* 1939;2:74.

362. Localio SA, Baron B. Abdominotranssacral resection and anastomosis for midrectal cancer. *Ann Surg.* 1973;178:540.

363. Localio SA, Eng K, Gouge TH, et al. Abdominosacral resection for carcinoma of the mid-rectum: ten years experience. *Ann Surg.* 1978;188:475.

364. Localio SA, Stahl WH. Simultaneous abdominotranssacral resection and anastomosis for midrectal cancer. *Am J Surg.* 1969;117:282.

365. Lockhart-Mummery HE. Surgery in patients with advanced carcinoma of the colon and rectum. *Dis Colon Rectum*. 1959;2:36.

366. Loeffler RA, Sayegh ES. Perforated acrylic implants in the management of organic impotence. *J Urol*. 1960;84:559.

367. Loessin SJ, Meland NB, Devine RM, et al. Management of sacral and perineal defects following abdominoperineal resection and radiation with transpelvic muscle flaps. *Dis Colon Rectum*. 1995;38:940.

368. Löhnert MSS, Doniec JM, Henne-Bruns D. Effectiveness of endoluminal sonography in the identification of occult local rectal cancer recurrences. *Dis Colon Rectum*. 2000;43:483.

369. Loizou LA, Grigg D, Boulos PB, et al. Endoscopic Nd:YAG laser treatment of rectosigmoid cancer. *Gut*. 1990;31:812.

370. Lopez MJ, Kraybill WG, Downey RS, et al. Exenterative surgery for locally advanced rectosigmoid cancers: is it worthwhile? *Surgery*. 1987;102:644.

371. Lopez-Kostner F, Fazio VW, Vignali A, et al. Locally recurrent cancer predictors and success of salvage surgery. *Dis Colon Rectum*. 2001;44:173.

372. Lopez-Kostner F, Lavery IC, Hool GR, et al. Total mesorectal excision is not necessary for cancer of the upper rectum. *Surgery*. 1998;124:612.

373. Low DE, Kozarek RA, Ball TJ, et al. Colorectal neodymium-YAG photoablative therapy. *Arch Surg*. 1989;124:684.

374. Lowy AM, Rich TA, Skibber JM, et al. Preoperative infusional chemoradiation, selective intraoperative radiation, and resection for locally advanced pelvic recurrence of colorectal adenocarcinoma. *Ann Surg*. 1996;223:177.

375. Lubbers EJC. Phantom sensations after excision of the rectum. *Dis Colon Rectum*. 1984;27:777.

376. Luchtefeld MA, Milsom JW, Senagore A, et al. Colorectal anastomotic stenosis: results of a survey of the ASCRS membership. *Dis Colon Rectum*. 1989;32:733.

377. Luck A, Chapuis PH, Sinclair G, et al. Endoscopic laser stricturotomy and balloon dilatation for benign colorectal strictures. *ANZ J Surg*. 2001;71:594.

378. Luglio G, Nelson H. Laparoscopy for colon cancer: state of the art. *Surg Oncol Clin N Am*. 2010;19:777.

379. Luke J. A case of obstruction of the colon relieved by an operation performed at the groin. *Med Chir Trans*. 1850;34:263.

380. Maas CP, Moriya Y, Steup WH, et al. Radical and nerve-preserving surgery for rectal cancer in the Netherlands: a prospective study on morbidity and functional outcome. *Br J Surg*. 1998;85:92.

381. Machado M, Nygren J, Goldman S, et al. Similar outcome after colonic pouch and side-to-end anastomosis in low anterior resection for rectal cancer: a prospective randomized trial. *Ann Surg*. 2003;238:214.

382. MacKay SG, Pager CK, Joseph D, et al. Assessment of the accuracy of transrectal ultrasonography in anorectal neoplasia. *Br J Surg*. 2003;90:346.

383. Madden JL, Kandalaft S. Electrocoagulation: a primary and preferred method of treatment for cancer of the rectum. *Ann Surg*. 1967;166:413.

384. Madden JL, Kandalaft S. Clinical evaluation of electrocoagulation in the treatment of cancer of the rectum. *Am J Surg*. 1971;122:347.

385. Madden JL, Kandalaft SI. Electrocoagulation as a primary curative method in the treatment of carcinoma of the rectum. *Surg Gynecol Obstet*. 1983;157:164.

386. Maeda K, Hashimoto M, Katai H, et al. Peranal introduction of the stapler in colorectal anastomosis with a double-stapling technique. *Br J Surg*. 1994;81:1057.

387. Maetani S, Nishikawa T, Iijima Y, et al. Extensive en bloc resection of regionally recurrent carcinoma of the rectum. *Cancer*. 1992;69:2876.

388. Magrini S, Nelson H, Gunderson LL, et al. Sacropelvic resection and intraoperative electron irradiation in the management of recurrent anorectal cancer. *Dis Colon Rectum*. 1996;39:1.

389. Mandava N, Petrelli N, Herrera L, et al. Laser palliation for colorectal carcinoma. *Am J Surg*. 1991;162:212.

390. Mann CV. Techniques of local surgical excision for rectal carcinoma. *Br J Surg*. 1985;72:57.

391. Mannaerts GHH, Rutten HJT, Martijn H, et al. Comparison of intraoperative radiation therapy-containing multimodality treatment with historical treatment modalities for locally recurrent rectal cancer. *Dis Colon Rectum*. 2001;44:1749.

392. Mantyh CR, Hull TL, Fazio VW. Coloplasty in low colorectal anastomosis: manometric and functional comparison with straight and colonic J-pouch anastomosis. *Dis Colon Rectum*. 2001;44:37.

393. Mantzoros I. Oncologic impact of anastomotic leakage after low anterior resection for rectal cancer. *Tech Coloproctol*. 2010;14(suppl 1):S39.

394. Marijnen CAM, van de Velde CJH. Preoperative radiotherapy for rectal cancer. *Br J Surg*. 2001;88:1556.

395. Marks CG, Ritchie JK. The complications of synchronous combined excision for adenocarcinoma of the rectum at St. Mark's Hospital. *Br J Surg*. 1975;62:901.

396. Marks G, Mohiuddin M, Borenstein BD. Preoperative radiation therapy and sphincter preservation by the combined abdominotranssacral technique for selected rectal cancers. *Dis Colon Rectum*. 1985;28:565.

397. Marks G, Mohiuddin M, Eitan A, et al. High-dose preoperative radiation and radical sphincter-preserving surgery for rectal cancer. *Arch Surg*. 1991;126:1534.

398. Marks G, Mohuiddin M, Masoni L, et al. High-dose preoperative radiation and full-thickness local excision: a new option for patients with select cancers of the rectum. *Dis Colon Rectum*. 1990;33:735.

399. Marsh PJ, James RD, Schofield PF. Adjuvant preoperative radiotherapy for locally advanced rectal carcinoma: results of a prospective, randomized trial. *Dis Colon Rectum*. 1994;37:1205.

400. Mascagni D, Corbellini L, Urciuoli P, et al. Endoluminal ultrasound for early detection of local recurrence of rectal cancer. *Br J Surg*. 1989;76:1176.

401. Mason AY. The place of local resection in the treatment of rectal carcinoma. *Proc R Soc Med*. 1970;63:1259.

402. Mason AY. Surgical access to the rectum-a transsphincteric exposure. *Proc R Soc Med*. 1970;63:91.

403. Mason AY. Trans-sphincteric exposure for low rectal anastomosis. *Proc R Soc Med*. 1972;65:974.

404. Masui H, Ike H, Yamaguchi S, et al. Male sexual function after autonomic nerve-preserving operation for rectal cancer. *Dis Colon Rectum*. 1996;39:1140.

405. Mathus-Vliegen EMH, Tytgat GNJ. Laser photocoagulation in the palliation of colorectal malignancies. *Cancer*. 1986;57:2212.

406. Matthews JM, Kodner IJ, Fry RD, et al. Entrapped ovary syndrome. *Dis Colon Rectum*. 1986;29:341.

407. Maunsell HW. A new method of excising the two upper portions of the rectum and the lower segment of the sigmoid flexure of the colon. *Lancet*. 1892;2:473.

408. Mayo CH. Cancer of the large bowel. *Med Sent*. 1904;12:37.

409. McCready DR, Ota DM, Rich TA, et al. Prospective phase I trial of conservative management of low rectal lesions. *Arch Surg*. 1989;124:67.

410. McLean GK, Cooper GS, Hartz WH, et al. Radiologically guided balloon dilation of gastrointestinal strictures. Part I. Technique and factors influencing procedural success. *Radiology*. 1987;165:35.

411. McNamara DA, Fitzpatrick JM, O'Connell PR. Urinary tract involvement by colorectal cancer. *Dis Colon Rectum*. 2003;46:1266.

412. Medical Research Council Rectal Cancer Working Party. Randomised trial of surgery alone versus radiotherapy followed by surgery for potentially operable locally advanced rectal cancer. *Lancet*. 1996;348:1605.

413. Medich D, McGinty J, Parda D, et al. Preoperative chemoradiotherapy and radical surgery for locally advanced distal rectal adenocarcinoma: pathologic findings and clinical implications. *Dis Colon Rectum*. 2001;44:1123.

414. Mella O, Dahl O, Horn A, et al. Radiotherapy and resection for apparently inoperable rectal adenocarcinoma. *Dis Colon Rectum*. 1984;27:663.

415. Mellgren A, Sirivongs P, Rothenberger DA, et al. Is local excision adequate therapy for early rectal cancer? *Dis Colon Rectum*. 2000;43:1064.

416. Mendenhall WM, Bland KI, Copeland EM III, et al. Does preoperative radiation therapy enhance the probability of local control and survival in high-risk distal rectal cancer? *Ann Surg*. 1992;215:696.

417. Mendenhall WM, Bland KI, Pfaff WW, et al. Initially unresectable rectal adenocarcinoma treated with preoperative irradiation and surgery. *Ann Surg*. 1987;205:41.

418. Mendenhall WM, Million RR, Bland KI, et al. Preoperative radiation therapy for clinically resectable adenocarcinoma of the rectum. *Ann Surg*. 1985;202:215.

419. Mercati U, Trancanelli V, Castagnoli GP, et al. Use of the gracilis muscle for sphincteric construction after abdominoperineal resection: technique and preliminary results. *Dis Colon Rectum*. 1991;34:1085.

420. Meredith KL, Koffe SE, Shibata D. The multidisciplinary management of rectal cancer. *Surg Clin North Am*. 2009;89:177.

421. Miles WE. A method of performing abdomino-perineal excision for carcinoma of the rectum and the terminal portion of the pelvic colon. *Lancet*. 1908;2:1812.

422. Miller AR, Cantor SB, Peoples GE, et al. Quality of life and cost effectiveness analysis of therapy for locally recurrent rectal cancer. *Dis Colon Rectum*. 2000;43:1695.

423. Miller AS, Lewis WG, Williamson MER, et al. Factors that influence functional outcome after coloanal anastomosis for carcinoma of the rectum. *Br J Surg*. 1995;82:1327.

424. Minsky BD. Preoperative combined modality treatment for rectal cancer. *Oncology*. 1994;8:53.

425. Minsky BD. Counterpoint: long-course chemoradiation is preferable in the neoadjuvant treatment of rectal cancer. *Semin Radiat Oncol*. 2011;21:228.

426. Minsky BD, Cohen AM, Enker WE, et al. Sphincter preservation in rectal cancer by local excision and postoperative radiation therapy. *Cancer.* 1991;67:908.

427. Minsky B, Cohen A, Enker W, et al. Preoperative 5-fluorouracil, low-dose leucovorin, and concurrent radiation therapy for rectal cancer. *Cancer.* 1994;73:273.

428. Minsky BD, Cohen AM, Enker WE, et al. Sphincter preservation with preoperative radiation therapy and coloanal anastomosis. *Int J Radiat Oncol.* 1995;31:553.

429. Minsky BD, Guillem JG. Multidisciplinary management of resectable rectal cancer. New developments and controversies. *Oncology.* 2008;15:1430.

430. Mirnezami AH, Mirnezami R, Chandrakumaran K, et al. Increased local recurrence and reduced survival from colorectal cancer following anastomotic leak: systematic review and meta-analysis. *Ann Surg.* 2011;253:890.

431. Mohiuddin M, Marks G. Patterns of recurrence following high-dose preoperative radiation and sphincter-preserving surgery for cancer of the rectum. *Dis Colon Rectum.* 1993;36:117.

432. Mohiuddin M, Marks J, Marks G. Management of rectal cancer: short- vs. long-course preoperative radiation. *Int J Radiat Oncol Biol Phys.* 2000;1:636.

433. Molloy RG, Moran KT, Coulter J, et al. Mechanism of sphincter impairment following low anterior resection. *Dis Colon Rectum.* 1992;35:462.

434. Moore HG, Gittleman AE, Minsky BD, et al. Rate of pathologic complete response with increased interval between preoperative combined modality therapy and rectal cancer resection. *Dis Colon Rectum.* 2004;47:279.

435. Moossa AR, Ree PC, Marks JE, et al. Factors influencing local recurrence after abdominoperineal resection for cancer of the rectum and rectosigmoid. *Br J Surg.* 1975;62:727.

436. Moran BJ. Predicting the risk and diminishing the consequences of anastomotic leakage after anterior resection for rectal cancer. *Acta Chir Iugosl.* 2010;57:47.

437. Moran MR, Rothenberger DA, Lahr CJ, et al. Palliation for rectal cancer. Resection? Anastomosis? *Arch Surg.* 1987;122:640.

438. Morgado PJ. Total mesorectal excision: a misnomer for a sound surgical approach. *Dis Colon Rectum.* 1998;41:120.

439. Morgan CN. Carcinoma of the rectum. *Ann R Coll Surg Engl.* 1965;36:73.

440. Mori M, Sugimachi K, Matsuda H, et al. Preoperative hyperthermochemoradiotherapy for patients with rectal cancer. *Dis Colon Rectum.* 1989;32:316.

441. Moriya Y, Hojo K, Sawada T, et al. Significance of lateral node dissection for advanced rectal carcinoma at or below the peritoneal reflection. *Dis Colon Rectum.* 1989;32:307.

442. Moriya Y, Sugihara K, Akasu T, et al. Nerve-sparing surgery with lateral node dissection for advanced low rectal cancer. *Eur J Cancer.* 1995;31A:1229.

443. Morson BC. Histological criteria for local excision. *Br J Surg.* 1985;72:53.

444. Morson BC, Bussey HJ, Samoorian S. Policy of local excision for early cancer of the colorectum. *Gut.* 1977;18:1045.

445. Morschel M, Heintz A, Bussmann M, et al. Follow-up after transanal endoscopic microsurgery or transanal excision of large benign rectal polyps. *Langenbecks Arch Surg.* 1998;383:320.

446. Mortensen NJM, Ramirez JM, Takeuchi N, et al. Colonic J pouch-anal anastomosis after rectal excision for carcinoma: functional outcome. *Br J Surg.* 1995;82:611.

447. Moser L, Ritz JP, Hinkelbein W, et al. Adjuvant and neoadjuvant chemoradiation in rectal cancer—a review focusing on open questions. *Int J Colorect Dis.* 2008;23:227.

448. Moszkowicz D, Alsaid B, Bessede T, et al. Where does pelvic nerve injury occur during rectal surgery for cancer? *Colorectal Dis.* 2011;13:1326.

449. Muldoon JP, Capehart RJ. Two scope technique for the transrectal removal of lesions high in the rectum and sigmoid colon. *Surg Gynecol Obstet.* 1973;137:1019.

450. Murphy JB. Cholecysto-intestinal, gastro-intestinal, entero-intestinal anastomosis, and approximation without sutures. *Med Rec.* 1892;42:665.

451. Muthusamy VR, Chang KJ. Optimal methods for staging rectal cancer. *Clin Cancer Res.* 2007;13(suppl 22):6877s.

452. Nagtegaal ID, Quirke P. What is the role for circumferential margin in the modern treatment of rectal cancer? *J Clin Oncol.* 2008;26:303.

453. Nakahara S, Itoh H, Mibu R, et al. Clinical and manometric evaluation of anorectal function following low anterior resection with low anastomotic line using an EEATM stapler for rectal cancer. *Dis Colon Rectum.* 1988;31:762.

454. Napoleon B, Pujol B, Berger F, et al. Accuracy of endosonography in the staging of rectal cancer treated by radiotherapy. *Br J Surg.* 1991;78:785.

455. Nascimbeni R, Burgart LJ, Nivatvongs S, et al. Risk of lymph node metastasis in T1 carcinoma of the colon and rectum. *Dis Colon Rectum.* 2002;45:200.

456. National Health and Medical Research Council. Clinical practice guidelines for the prevention, early detection and management of colorectal cancer. Canberra, Australia: National Health and Medical Research Council; 1999.

457. Neufeld DM, Shemesh EI, Kodner IJ, et al. Endoscopic management of anastomotic colon strictures with electrocautery and balloon dilation. *Gastrointest Endosc.* 1987;33:24.

458. Nicholls RJ, Lubowski DZ, Donaldson DR. Comparison of colonic reservoir and straight colo-anal reconstruction after rectal excision. *Br J Surg.* 1988;75:318.

459. Nielsen MB, Pedersen JF, Hald J, et al. Recurrent extraluminal rectal carcinoma: transrectal biopsy under sonographic guidance. *AJR Am J Roentgenol.* 1992;158:1025.

460. Nugent E, Neary P. Rectal cancer surgery: volume-outcome analysis. *Int J Colorectal Dis.* 2010;25:1389.

461. O'Connell MJ, Martenson JA, Wieand HS, et al. Improving adjuvant therapy for rectal cancer by combining protracted-infusion fluorouracil with radiation therapy after curative surgery. *N Engl J Med.* 1994;331:502.

462. O'Connor JJ. Endoscopic palliative management of rectal cancer. *South Med J.* 1991;84:472.

463. Ogunbiyi OA, McKenna K, Birnbaum EH, et al. Aggressive surgical management of recurrent rectal cancer: is it worthwhile? *Dis Colon Rectum.* 1997;40:150.

464. Ohhigashi S, Nishio T, Watanabe F, et al. Experience with radiofrequency ablation in the treatment of pelvic recurrence in rectal cancer: report of two cases. *Dis Colon Rectum.* 2001;44:741.

465. Ohno S, Tomoda M, Tomisaki S, et al. Improved surgical results after combining preoperative hyperthermia with chemotherapy and radiotherapy for patients with carcinoma of the rectum. *Dis Colon Rectum.* 1997;40:401.

466. Ondrula DP, Nelson RL, Prasad ML, et al. Multifactorial index of preoperative risk factors in colon resections. *Dis Colon Rectum.* 1992;35:117.

467. Ooi BS, Tjandra JJ, Green MD. Morbidities of adjuvant chemotherapy and radiotherapy for resectable rectal cancer: an overview. *Dis Colon Rectum.* 1999;42:403.

468. O'Riordain MG, Molloy RG, Gillen P, et al. Rectoanal inhibitory reflex following low stapled anterior resection of the rectum. *Dis Colon Rectum.* 1992;35:874.

469. Orrom WJ, Wong WD, Rothenberger DA, et al. Endorectal ultrasound in the preoperative staging of rectal tumors. *Dis Colon Rectum.* 1990;33:654.

470. Ovnat A, Peiser J, Avinoah E, et al. A new approach to rectal anastomotic stricture. *Dis Colon Rectum.* 1989;32:351.

471. Oz MC, Forde KA. Endoscopic alternatives in the management of colonic strictures. *Surgery.* 1990;108:513.

472. Pacini P, Cionini L, Pirtoli L, et al. Symptomatic recurrences of carcinoma of the rectum and sigmoid: the influence of radiotherapy on the quality of life. *Dis Colon Rectum.* 1986;29:865.

473. Pagni S, McLaughlin CM. Simple technique for the treatment of strictured colorectal anastomosis. *Dis Colon Rectum.* 1995;38:433.

474. Påhlman L, Glimelius B. Pre- or postoperative radiotherapy in rectal and rectosigmoid carcinoma: report from a randomized multicenter trial. *Ann Surg.* 1990;211:187.

475. Påhlman L, Glimelius B, Frykholm G. Ischaemic strictures in patients treated with a low anterior resection and perioperative radiotherapy for rectal carcinoma. *Br J Surg.* 1989;76:605.

476. Påhlman L, Glimelius B, Graffman S. Pre- versus postoperative radiotherapy in rectal carcinoma: an interim report from a randomized multicentre trial. *Br J Surg.* 1985;72:961.

477. Påhlman L, Torkzad MR. Rectal cancer staging: is there an optimal method? *Future Oncol.* 2011;7:93.

478. Pannett CA. Resection of the rectum with restoration of continuity. *Lancet.* 1935;2:423.

479. Papillon J. Endocavitary irradiation of early rectal cancers for cure: a series of 123 cases. *Proc R Soc Med.* 1973;66:1179.

480. Papillon J. Endocavitary irradiation in the curative treatment of early cancers. *Dis Colon Rectum.* 1974;17:172.

481. Papillon J. Intracavitary irradiation of early rectal cancer for cure: a series of 186 cases. *Cancer.* 1975;36:696.

482. Papillon J. New prospects in the conservative treatment of rectal cancer. *Dis Colon Rectum.* 1984;27:695.

483. Papillon J. The future of external beam irradiation as initial treatment of rectal cancer. *Br J Surg.* 1987;74:449.

484. Parc R, Tiret E, Frileux P, et al. Resection and colo-anal anastomosis with colonic reservoir for rectal carcinoma. *Br J Surg.* 1986;73:139.

485. Park IJ. Influence of anastomotic leak on oncological outcome in patients with rectal cancer. *J Gastrointest Surg.* 2010;14:1190.
486. Park YA, Kim JM, Kim SA, et al. Totally robotic surgery for rectal cancer: from splenic flexure to pelvic floor in one step. *Surg Endosc.* 2010;24:715.
487. Parks AG. Transanal technique in low rectal anastomosis. *Proc R Soc Med.* 1972;65:975.
488. Parks AG. Per-anal anastomosis. *World J Surg.* 1982;6:531.
489. Paty PB, Enker WE, Cohen AM, et al. Long-term functional results of coloanal anastomosis for rectal cancer. *Am J Surg.* 1994;167:90.
490. Paty PB, Enker WE, Cohen AM, et al. Treatment of rectal cancer by low anterior resection with coloanal anastomosis. *Ann Surg.* 1994;219:365.
491. Paty PB, Nash GM, Baron P, et al. Long-term results of local excision for rectal cancer. *Ann Surg.* 2002;236:522.
492. Paun BC, Cassie S, MacLean AR, et al. Postoperative complications following surgery for rectal cancer. *Ann Surg.* 2010;251:807.
493. Pearlman NW, Donohue RE, Steigmann GV, et al. Pelvic and sacropelvic exenteration for locally advanced or recurrent anorectal cancer. *Arch Surg.* 1987;122:537.
494. Pearlman NW, Stiegmann GV, Donohue RE. Extended resection of fixed rectal cancer. *Cancer.* 1989;63:2438.
495. Pearman RO. Treatment of organic impotence by implantation of a penile prosthesis. *J Urol.* 1967;97:716.
496. Pearman RO. Insertion of a Silastic penile prosthesis for the treatment of organic sexual impotence. *J Urol.* 1972;107:802.
497. Pedersen IK, Hint K, Olsen J, et al. Anorectal function after low anterior resection for carcinoma. *Ann Surg.* 1986;204:133.
498. Peeters KC, Marijnen CA, Nagtegaal ID, et al. The TME trial after a median follow-up of 6 years: increased local control of but no survival benefit in irradiated patients with rectal carcinoma. *Ann Surg.* 2007;246:693.
499. Pélissier EP, Blum D, Bachour A, et al. Functional results of coloanal anastomosis with reservoir. *Dis Colon Rectum.* 1992;35:843.
500. Person B, Wexner SD. The management of postoperative ileus. *Curr Probl Surg.* 2006;43:6065.
501. Phillips PS, Farquharson SM, Sexton R, et al. Rectal cancer in the elderly: patients' perception of bowel control after restorative surgery. *Dis Colon Rectum.* 2004;47:287.
502. Politano VA, Leadbetter WF. An operative technique for the correction of vesicoureteral reflux. *J Urol.* 1958;79:932.
503. Poon JT, Law WL. Laparoscopic resection for rectal cancer: a review. *Ann Surg Oncol.* 2009;16:3038.
504. Porter NH, Nicholls RJ. Pre-operative radiotherapy in operable rectal cancer: interim report of a trial carried out by the Rectal Cancer Group. *Br J Surg.* 1985;72:62.
505. Quirke P, Dixon MF. The prediction of local recurrence in rectal adenocarcinoma by histopathological examination. *J Colorect Dis.* 1988;3:127.
506. Quirke P, Durdey P, Dixon MF, et al. Local recurrence of rectal adenocarcinoma due to inadequate surgical resection. *Lancet.* 1986;2:996.
507. Quirke P, Williams GT, Ectors N, et al. The future of the TNM staging system in colorectal cancer: time for a debate? *Lancet Oncol.* 2007;7:651.
508. Radice E, Nelson H, Mercill S, et al. Primary myocutaneous flap closure following resection of locally advanced pelvic malignancies. *Br J Surg.* 1999;86:349.
509. Raestrup H, Manncke K, Mentges B, et al. Indications and technique for TEM (transanal endoscopic microsurgery). *Endosc Surg Allied Technol.* 1994;2:241.
510. Ramirez JM, Mortensen NJM, Takeuchi N, et al. Colonic J-pouch rectal reconstruction is it really a neorectum? *Dis Colon Rectum.* 1996;39:1286.
511. Ramsey WH. Treatment of inoperable cancer of the rectum by fulguration. *Dis Colon Rectum.* 1963;6:114.
512. Rankin FW, Graham AS. *Cancer of the Colon and Rectum.* Springfield, IL: Charles C Thomas; 1939.
513. Reed WP, Garb JL, Park WC, et al. Long-term results and complications of preoperative radiation in the treatment of rectal cancer. *Surgery.* 1988;103:161.
514. Renner K, Rosen HR, Novi G, et al. Quality of life after surgery for rectal cancer: do we still need a permanent colostomy? *Dis Colon Rectum.* 1999;42:1160.
515. Reybard JF. Mémoire sur une tumeur cancéreuse affectant l'iliaque du colon; ablation de la tumeur et de l'intestin: réunion directe et immédiate des deux bouts de cet organe. *Bull Acad Med Paris.* 1843–1844;9:1031.
516. Rich TA. Infusional chemoradiation for operable rectal cancer: post-, pre-, or nonoperative management? *Oncology.* 1997;11:295.
517. Roberson SH, Heron HC, Kerman HD, et al. Is anterior resection of the rectosigmoid safe after preoperative radiation? *Dis Colon Rectum.* 1985;28:254.
518. Rodriguez-Bigas MA, Herrera L, Petrelli NJ. Surgery for recurrent rectal adenocarcinoma in the presence of hydronephrosis. *Am J Surg.* 1992;164:18.

519. Romano G, de Rosa P, Vallone G, et al. Intrarectal ultrasound and computed tomography in the pre- and postoperative assessment of patients with rectal cancer. *Br J Surg.* 1985;72:117.
520. Romano G, La Torre F, Cutini G, et al. Total anorectal reconstruction with the artificial bowel sphincter: report of eight cases. A quality-of-life assessment. *Dis Colon Rectum.* 2003;46:730.
521. Rominger CJ, Gelber RD, Gunderson LL, et al. Radiation therapy alone or in combination with chemotherapy in the treatment of residual or inoperable carcinoma of the rectum and rectosigmoid or pelvic recurrence following colorectal surgery. *Am J Clin Oncol.* 1985;8:118.
522. Romsdahl M, Withers H. Radiotherapy combined with curative surgery: its use as therapy for carcinoma of the sigmoid colon and rectum. *Arch Surg.* 1978;113:446.
523. Rosen L, Khubchandani IT, Sheets JA, et al. Clinical and manometric evaluation of continence after the Bacon two-stage pull-through procedure. *Dis Colon Rectum.* 1985;28:232.
524. Rosenberg SA. Combined-modality therapy of cancer: what is it and when does it work? *N Engl J Med.* 1985;312:1512.
525. Rosenthal II, Turell R. Surgical diathermy (electrothermia) of cancer of the rectum. *JAMA.* 1958;167:1602.
526. Rosenthal SA, Trock BJ, Coia LR. Randomized trial of adjuvant radiation therapy for rectal carcinoma: a review. *Dis Colon Rectum.* 1990;33:335.
527. Roswit B, Higgins G, Keehn R. Preoperative irradiation for carcinoma of the rectum and rectosigmoid colon: report of a National Veterans Administration randomized study. *Cancer.* 1975;35:1597.
528. Rouanet P, Saint Aubert B, Fabre JM, et al. Conservative treatment for low rectal carcinoma by local excision with or without radiotherapy. *Br J Surg.* 1993;80:1452.
529. Roubein LD, David C, DuBrow R, et al. Endoscopic ultrasonography in staging rectal cancer. *Am J Gastroenterol.* 1990;85:1391.
530. Row D, Weiser MR. An update on laparoscopic resection for rectal cancer. *Cancer Control.* 2010;17:16.
531. The Royal College of Pathologists. *Standards and Datasets for Reporting Cancers—Dataset for Colorectal Cancer.* 2nd ed. London, United Kingdom: The Royal College of Pathologists; 2007.
532. Rudd WWH. The transanal anastomosis: a sphincter-saving operation with improved continence. *Dis Colon Rectum.* 1979;22:102.
533. Rullier E, Zerbib F, Laurent C, et al. Intersphincteric resection with excision of internal anal sphincter for conservative treatment of very low rectal cancer. *Dis Colon Rectum.* 1999;42:1168.
534. Rupp KD, Dohmoto M, Meffert R, et al. Cancer of the rectum palliative endoscopic treatment. *Eur J Surg Oncol.* 1995;21:644.
535. Saclarides TJ. Transanal endoscopic microsurgery: a single surgeon's experience. *Arch Surg.* 1998;133:595.
536. Saclarides TJ, Bhattacharyya AK, Britton-Kuzel C, et al. Predicting lymph node metastases in rectal cancer. *Dis Colon Rectum.* 1994;37:52.
537. Sadahiro S, Suzuki T, Ishikawa K, et al. Intraoperative radiation therapy for curatively resected rectal cancer. *Dis Colon Rectum.* 2001;44:1689.
538. Sagar PM, Pemberton JH. Surgical management of locally recurrent rectal cancer. *Br J Surg.* 1996;83:293.
539. Said S, Stippel D. Transanal endoscopic microsurgery in large, sessile adenomas of the rectum. A 10-year experience. *Surg Endosc.* 1995;9:1106.
540. Said S, Stippel D. 10 years experiences with transanal endoscopic microsurgery. Histopathologic and clinical analysis. *Chirurg.* 1996;67:139.
541. Sailer M, Fuches KH, Fein M, et al. Randomized clinical trial comparing quality of life after straight and pouch coloanal reconstruction. *Br J Surg.* 2002;89:1108.
542. Salerno G, Sinnatamby C, Branagan G, et al. Defining the rectum: surgically, radiologically and anatomically. *Colorectal Dis.* 2006;8(suppl 3):5.
543. Salinas JC, Quintana J, De Gregorio MA, et al. Management of benign rectal stricture by implantation of a self-expanding prosthesis. *Br J Surg.* 1997;84:674.
544. Salvati EP, Rubin RJ. Electrocoagulation as primary therapy for rectal carcinoma. *Am J Surg.* 1976;132:583.
545. Salvati EP, Rubin RJ, Eisenstat TE, et al. Electrocoagulation of selected carcinoma of the rectum. *Surg Gynecol Obstet.* 1988;166:393.
546. Santoro E, Tirelli C, Scutari F, et al. Continent perineal colostomy by transposition of gracilis muscles: technical remarks and results in 14 cases. *Dis Colon Rectum.* 1994;37:S73.
547. Sarr MG, Stewart JR, Cameron JC. Combined abdominoperineal approach to repair of postoperative hernia. *Dis Colon Rectum.* 1982;25:597.
548. Sato K, Sato T. The vascular and neural composition of the lateral ligament of the rectum and the rectosacral fascia. *Surg Radiol Anat.* 1991;13:17.
549. Sato T, Konishi F, Kanazawa K. Anal sphincter reconstruction with a pudendal nerve anastomosis following abdominoperineal resection: report of a case. *Dis Colon Rectum.* 1997;40:1497.

550. Sato T, Konishi F, Kanazawa K. Functional perineal colostomy with pudendal nerve anastomosis following anorectal resection: a cadaver operation study on a new procedure. *Surgery*. 1997;121:569.

551. Sauer R, Beeker H, Hohenberger W, et al. Preoperative versus postoperative chemoradiotherapy for rectal cancer. *New Engl J Med*. 2004;351:1731.

552. Schafer H, Baldus SE, Holscher AH. Giant adenomas of the rectum: complete resection by transanal Endoscopic microsurgery (TEM). *Int J Colorectal Dis*. 2005;20:1.

553. Schaldenbrand JD, Siders DB, Zainea GG, et al. Preoperative radiation therapy for locally advanced carcinoma of the rectum: clinicopathologic correlative review. *Dis Colon Rectum*. 1992;35:16.

554. Schell SR, Zlotecki RA, Mendenhall WM, et al. Transanal excision of locally advanced rectal cancers downstaged using neoadjuvant chemoradiotherapy. *J Am Coll Surg*. 2002;194:584.

555. Schlag P, Lehner B, Strauss LG, et al. Scar or recurrent rectal cancer: positron emission tomography is more helpful for diagnosis than immunoscintigraphy. *Arch Surg*. 1989;124:197.

556. Schlegel RD, Dehni N, Parc R, et al. Results of reoperations in colorectal anastomotic strictures. *Dis Colon Rectum*. 2001;44:1464.

557. Schultz PE, Muldoon JP. A transrectal approach to the high-lying lesion in the rectosigmoid. *Dis Colon Rectum*. 1969;12:417.

558. Schulze S, Lyng KM. Palliation of rectosigmoid neoplasms with Nd:YAG laser treatment. *Dis Colon Rectum*. 1994;37:882.

559. Segall MM, Nivatvongs S, Balcos E, et al. Abdominoperineal resection for recurrent cancer following anterior resection. *Dis Colon Rectum*. 1981;24:80.

560. Sener SF, Imperato JP, Blum MD, et al. Technique and complications of reconstruction of the pelvic floor with polyglactin mesh. *Surg Gynecol Obstet*. 1989;168:475.

561. Seow-Choen F. Colonic pouches in the treatment of low rectal cancer. *Br J Surg*. 1996;83:881.

562. Shami VM, Parmar KS, Waxman I. Clinical impact of endoscopic ultrasound and endoscopic ultrasound-guided fine-needle aspiration in the management of rectal carcinoma. *Dis Colon Rectum*. 2004;47:59.

563. Shehata WM, Meyer RL, Jazy FK, et al. Total abdominopelvic irradiation and a boost for cancer of the colon: a pilot study. *Appl Radiol*. 1989;26.

564. Shimada S, Matsuda M, Uno K, et al. A new device for the treatment of coloproctostomic stricture after double stapling anastomoses. *Ann Surg*. 1996;224:603.

565. Shin SS, Jeong YY, Min JJ, et al. Preoperative staging of colorectal cancer: CT vs. integrated FDG PET/CT. *Abdom Imaging*. 2008;33:270.

566. Shirouzu K, Isomoto H, Kakegawa T. Prognostic evaluation of perineural invasion in rectal cancer. *Am J Surg*. 1993;165:233.

567. Shirouzu K, Isomoto H, Kakegawa T. Total pelvic exenteration for locally advanced colorectal carcinoma. *Br J Surg*. 1996;83:32.

568. Shoup M, Guillem JG, Alektiar KM, et al. Predictors of survival in recurrent rectal cancer after resection and intraoperative radiotherapy. *Dis Colon Rectum*. 2002;45:585.

569. Sischy B. Intraoperative electron beam radiation therapy with particular reference to the treatment of rectal carcinomas-primary and recurrent. *Dis Colon Rectum*. 1986;29:714.

570. Sischy B. The role of radiation therapy in the management of carcinoma of the rectum. *Contemp Surg*. 1987;30:13.

571. Sischy B, Graney MJ, Hinson EJ, et al. Preoperative radiation therapy with sensitizers in the management of carcinoma of the rectum. *Dis Colon Rectum*. 1985;28:56.

572. Sischy B, Remington JH. Treatment of carcinoma of the rectum by intracavitary irradiation. *Surg Gynecol Obstet*. 1975;141:562.

573. Sischy B, Remington JH, Sobel SH. Treatment of rectal carcinomas by means of endocavity irradiation. *Cancer*. 1978;42:1073.

574. Sischy B, Remington JH, Sobel SH, et al. Treatment of carcinoma of the rectum and squamous carcinoma of the anus by combination chemotherapy, radiotherapy and operation. *Surg Gynecol Obstet*. 1980;151:369.

575. Sjödahl R, Nyström PO, Olaison G. Surgical treatment of dorsocaudal dislocation of the vagina after excision of the rectum: the Kylberg operation. *Dis Colon Rectum*. 1990;33:762.

576. Skandarajah AR, Tjandra JJ. Preoperative loco-regional imaging in rectal cancer. *ANZ J Surg*. 2006;76:497.

577. Smith DE, Muff NS, Shetabi H. Combined preoperative neoadjuvant radiotherapy and chemotherapy for anal and rectal cancer. *Am J Surg*. 1986;151:577.

578. Smith LE, Ko ST, Saclarides T, et al. Transanal endoscopic microsurgery. Initial registry results. *Dis Colon Rectum*. 1996;39:S79.

579. So JB, Palmer MT, Shellito PC. Postoperative perineal hernia. *Dis Colon Rectum*. 1997;40:954.

580. Sofo Luigi, Ratto C, Doglietto GB, et al. Intraoperative radiation therapy in integrated treatment of rectal cancers: results of phase II study. *Dis Colon Rectum*. 1996;39:1396.

581. Spinelli P, Calarco G, Gallo C, et al. Endoscopic treatment of carpet-like adenomas of the rectum. *Tumori*. 1999;85:265.

582. Stearns MW Jr. Preoperative radiation in carcinoma of the rectum. *Proc Natl Cancer Conf*. 1964;5:489.

583. Stearns MW Jr. The choice among anterior resection, the pull-through, and abdominoperineal resection of the rectum. *Cancer*. 1974;34:969.

584. Stearns MW Jr. Diagnosis and management of recurrent pelvic malignancy following combined abdominoperineal resection. *Dis Colon Rectum*. 1980;23:359.

585. Stearns MW Jr, Bert JW, Deddish MR. Preoperative irradiation of cancer of the rectum. *Dis Colon Rectum*. 1961;4:403.

586. Stearns MW Jr, Deddish MR, Quan SIIQ. Preoperative roentgen therapy for cancer of the rectum. *Surg Gynecol Obstet*. 1959;109:225.

587. Stearns MW Jr, Deddish MR, Quan SHQ, et al. Preoperative roentgen therapy for cancer of the rectum and rectosigmoid. *Surg Gynecol Obstet*. 1974;138:584.

588. Stearns MW Jr, Sternberg SS, DeCosse JJ. Treatment alternatives: localized rectal cancer. *Cancer*. 1984;54:2691.

589. Stearns MW Jr, Whiteley HW Jr, Leaming RH, et al. Palliative radiation therapy in patients with localized cancer of the colon and rectum. *Dis Colon Rectum*. 1970;13:112.

590. Steele RJ, Hershman MJ, Mortensen NJ, et al. Transanal endoscopic microsurgery—initial experience from three centres in the United Kingdom. *Br J Surg*. 1996;83:207.

591. Stein DE, Mahmoud NN, Anné PR, et al. Longer time interval between completion of neoadjuvant chemoradiation and surgical resection does not improve downstaging of rectal carcinoma. *Dis Colon Rectum*. 2003;46:448.

592. Stelzner M. Palliative therapy of rectal cancer: summary statement. *J Gastrointest Surg*. 2004;8:253.

593. Stolfi VM, Milsom JW, Lavery IC, et al. Newly designed occluder pin for presacral hemorrhage. *Dis Colon Rectum*. 1992;35:166.

594. Stone JM, Bloom RJ. Transendoscopic balloon dilatation of complete colonic obstruction. An adjunct in the treatment of colorectal cancer: report of three cases. *Dis Colon Rectum*. 1989;32:429.

595. Strauss AA. *Immunologic Resistance to Carcinoma Produced by Electrocoagulation: Based on Fifty-seven Years of Experimental and Clinical Results*. Springfield, IL: Charles C Thomas; 1969.

596. Strauss AA, Appel M, Saphir O, et al. Immunologic resistance to carcinoma produced by electrocoagulation. *Surg Gynecol Obstet*. 1965;121:989.

597. Strauss AA, Strauss SF, Crawford RA, et al. Surgical diathermy of carcinoma of rectum: its clinical end results. *JAMA*. 1935;104:1480.

598. Strauss AA, Strauss SF, Strauss HA. New method and end results in treatment of carcinoma of stomach and rectum by surgical diathermy (electrical coagulation). *South Surg*. 1936;5:348.

599. Strauss LG, Clorius JH, Schlag P, et al. Recurrence of colorectal tumor: PET evaluation. *Radiology*. 1989;170:329.

600. Sugarbaker PH. Partial sacrectomy for en bloc excision of rectal cancer with posterior fixation. *Dis Colon Rectum*. 1982;25:708.

601. Sugarbaker PH. Intrapelvic prosthesis to prevent injury of the small intestine with high dosage pelvic irradiation. *Surg Gynecol Obstet*. 1983;157:269.

602. Suzuki K, Dozois RR, Devine RM, et al. Curative reoperations for locally recurrent rectal cancer. *Dis Colon Rectum*. 1996;39:730.

603. Swedish Rectal Cancer Trial. Initial report from a Swedish multicentre study examining the role of preoperative irradiation in the treatment of patients with resectable rectal carcinoma. *Br J Surg*. 1993;80:1333.

604. Swedish Rectal Cancer Trial. Local recurrence rate in a randomised multicentre trial of preoperative radiotherapy compared with operation alone in resectable rectal carcinoma. *Eur J Surg*. 1996;162:397.

605. Swedish Rectal Cancer Trial. Improved survival with preoperative radiotherapy in resectable rectal cancer. *N Engl J Med*. 1997;336:980.

606. Sweeney JL, Ritchie JK, Hawley PR. Resection and sutured peranal anastomosis for carcinoma of the rectum. *Dis Colon Rectum*. 1989;32:103.

607. Sweeney WB. Local excision of rectal tumors: specimen orientation. *Dis Colon Rectum*. 1992;35:204.

608. Sweeney WB, Deshmukh N. Modified Kraske approach for disease of the mid-rectum. *Am J Gastroenterol*. 1991;86:75.

609. Tanaka S, Yokota T, Saito D, et al. Clinicopathologic features of early rectal carcinoma and indications for endoscopic treatment. *Dis Colon Rectum*. 1995;38:959.

610. Tang R, Wang JY, Chen JS, et al. Postoperative adjuvant radiotherapy in Astler-Coller stages B2 and C rectal cancer. *Dis Colon Rectum*. 1992;35:1057.

611. Task Force. American Society of Colon and Rectal Surgeons. Practice parameters for the treatment of rectal carcinoma. *Dis Colon Rectum*. 1993;36:989.

612. Tekkis PP, Prytherch DR, Kocher HM, et al. Development of a dedicated risk-adjusted scoring system for colorectal surgery (colorectal POSSUM). *Br J Surg.* 2004;91:1174.

613. Temple WJ, Ketcham AS. Surgical palliation for recurrent rectal cancers ulcerating in the perineum. *Cancer.* 1990;65:1111.

614. Tepper JE, Cohen AM, Wood WC, et al. Intraoperative electron beam radiotherapy in the treatment of unresectable rectal cancer. *Arch Surg.* 1986;121:421.

615. Theodoropoulos G, Wise WE, Padmanabhan A, et al. T-level downstaging and complete pathologic response after preoperative chemoradiation for advanced rectal cancer result in decreased recurrence and improved disease-free survival. *Dis Colon Rectum.* 2002;45:895.

616. Tiret E, Pocard M. Exérèse totale du mesorectum et conservation del l'innervation à dessinée genito-urinaire dans la chirurgie du cancer do rectum. *Ann Chir.* 1999;53:507.

617. Tocchi A, Lepre L, Costa G, et al. Rectal cancer and inguinal metastases: prognostic role and therapeutic indications. *Dis Colon Rectum.* 1999;42:1464.

618. Torres RA, González MA. Perineal continent colostomy: report of a case. *Dis Colon Rectum.* 1988;31:957.

619. Torricelli P. Rectal cancer staging. *Surg Oncol.* 2007;16(suppl 1):S49.

620. Triadafilopoulos G, Sarkisian M. Dilatation of radiation-induced sigmoid stricture using sequential Savary-Guilliard dilators: a combined radiologic-endoscopic approach. *Dis Colon Rectum.* 1990;33:1065.

621. Tufano A,Tufano G, Brusciano L, et al. Mesorectum, is it an appropriate term? *Int J Colorectal Dis.* 2007;22:1127.

622. Turnbull RB Jr, Cuthbertson A. Abdominorectal pull-through resection for cancer and for Hirschsprung's disease: delayed posterior colorectal anastomosis. *Cleve Clin Q.* 1961;28:109.

623. Turner GG. Conservative resection of the rectum by the lower route: the after results in seventeen cases. *Acta Chir Scand.* 1932;72:519.

624. Turner-Warwick R, Worth PH. The psoas bladder-hitch procedure for the replacement of the lower third of the ureter. *Br J Urol.* 1969;41:701.

625. Tveit KM, Guldvog I, Hagen S, et al. Randomized controlled trial of postoperative radiotherapy and short-term time-scheduled 5-fluorouracil against surgery alone in the treatment of Dukes B and C rectal cancer. *Br J Surg.* 1997;84:1130.

626. Twomey P, Burchell M, Strawn D, et al. Local control in rectal cancer: a clinical review and meta-analysis. *Arch Surg.* 1989;124:1174.

627. Tytherleigh MG, Bokey L, Chapuis PH, et al. Is a minor clinical anastomotic leak significant after resection of colorectal cancer? *J Am Coll Surg.* 2007;205:648.

628. Tytherleigh MG, Mortensen NJ. Options for sphincter preservation in surgery for low rectal cancer. *Br J Surg.* 2003;90:922.

629. Vernava AM III, Robbins PL, Brabbee GW. Restorative resection: coloanal anastomosis for benign and malignant disease. *Dis Colon Rectum.* 1989;32:690.

630. Villalon AH, Green D. The use of radiotherapy for pelvic recurrence following abdominoperineal resection for carcinoma of the rectum: a 10-year experience. *Aust N Z J Surg.* 1981;51:149.

631. von Volkmann R. *Ueber den Mastdarmkrebs und die Exstirpatio recti* [Concerning rectal cancer and the removal of the rectum]. *Sammlung klinischer vorträge in verbindung mit deutschen klinikern* [Collection of clinical lectures in cooperation with German clinicians] Nos. 29–53. Leipzig, Germany: Breitkopf and Hartel. Translated in *Dis Colon Rectum.* 1986;29:679.

632. Voros D, Fragoulidis G, Theodosopoulos T, et al. Pelvic floor reconstruction after major cancer surgery. *Dis Colon Rectum.* 1996;39:1232.

633. Walfisch S, Stern H, Ball S. Use of Nd-Yag laser ablation in colorectal obstruction and palliation in high-risk patients. *Dis Colon Rectum.* 1989;32:1060.

634. Walker KG, Bell SW, Rickard MJ, et al. Anastomotic leakage is predictive of diminished survival after potentially curative resection for colorectal cancer. *Ann Surg.* 2004;240:255.

635. Wanebo HJ. Resection of pelvic recurrence of rectal cancer. *Contemp Surg.* 1982;21:21.

636. Wanebo HJ, Gaker DL, Whitehill R, et al. Pelvic recurrence of rectal cancer: options for curative resection. *Ann Surg.* 1987;205:482.

637. Wanebo HJ, Koness RJ, Vezeridis MP, et al. Pelvic resection of recurrent rectal cancer. *Ann Surg.* 1994;220:586.

638. Wanebo HJ, Marcove RC. Abdominal sacral resection of locally recurrent rectal cancer. *Ann Surg.* 1981;194:458.

639. Wang CC, Schulz MO. The role of radiation therapy in the management of carcinoma of the sigmoid, rectosigmoid, and rectum. *Radiology.* 1962;79:1.

640. Wang HS, Lin JK, Yang SH, et al. Prospective study of the functional results of transanal endoscopic microsurgery. *Hepatogastroenterology.* 2003;50:1376.

641. Wang JY, You YT, Chen HH, et al. Stapled colonic J-pouch-anal anastomosis without a diverting colostomy for rectal carcinoma. *Dis Colon Rectum.* 1997;40:30.

642. Wang QY, Shi WJ, Zhao YR, et al. New concepts in severe presacral hemorrhage during proctectomy. *Arch Surg.* 1985;120:1013.

643. Weinstein M, Roberts M. Sexual potency following surgery for rectal carcinoma. *Ann Surg.* 1977;185:295.

644. Weir RF. An improved method of treating high-seated cancers of the rectum. *JAMA.* 1901;37:801.

645. Weiser MR, Landmann RG, Wong WD, et al. Surgical salvage of recurrent rectal cancer after transanal excision. *Dis Colon Rectum.* 2005;48:1169.

646. West NP, Anderin C, Smith KJE, et al. Multicentre experience with extralevator abdominoperineal excision for low rectal cancer. *Br J Surg.* 2010;97:588.

647. West NP, Finan PJ, Andrin C. Evidence of the oncologic superiority of cylindrical abdominoperineal excision for low rectal cancer. *J Clin Oncol.* 2008;26:3517.

648. Wheeler JMD, Warren BF, Jones AC, et al. Preoperative radiotherapy for rectal cancer: implications for surgeons, pathologists and radiologists. *Br J Surg.* 1999;86:1108.

649. Whelan CS, Deckers PJ. Electrocoagulation: its value in treating skin, internal, and rectal cancers. *Contemp Surg.* 1988;33:35.

650. Whiteway J, Nicholls RJ, Morson BC. The role of surgical local excision in the treatment of rectal cancer. *Br J Surg.* 1985;72:694.

651. Wichmann MW, Meyer G, Adam M, et al. Detrimental immunologic effects of preoperative chemoradiotherapy in advanced rectal cancer. *Dis Colon Rectum.* 2003;46:875.

652. Wiggers T,van de Velde CJ. The circumferential margin in rectal cancer. Recommendation based on the Dutch Total Mesorectal Excision Study. *Eur J Cancer.* 2002;38:973.

653. Williams JG, Williams LA. Colonoscopy and brush cytology in the diagnosis of colonic strictures. *J R Coll Surg Edinb.* 1988;33:119.

654. Williams LF Jr, Huddleston CB, Sawyers JL, et al. Is total pelvic exenteration reasonable primary treatment for rectal carcinoma? *Ann Surg.* 1988;207:670.

655. Williams NS, Dixon MF, Johnston D. Reappraisal of the 5 centimetre rule of distal excision for carcinoma of the rectum: a study of distal intramural spread and of patients' survival. *Br J Surg.* 1983;70:150.

656. Williams NS, Hallan RI, Koeze TH, et al. Restoration of gastrointestinal continuity and continence after abdominoperineal excision of the rectum using an electrically stimulated neoanal sphincter. *Dis Colon Rectum.* 1990;33:561.

657. Wilson E. Local treatment of cancer of the rectum. *Dis Colon Rectum.* 1973;16:194.

658. Woodward A, Tydeman G, Lewis MH. Eder Puestow dilatation of benign rectal stricture following anterior resection. *Dis Colon Rectum.* 1990;33:79.

659. Yamakoshi H, Ike H, Oki S, et al. Metastasis of rectal cancer to lymph nodes and tissues around the autonomic nerves spared for urinary and sexual function. *Dis Colon Rectum.* 1997;40:1079.

660. Yamamoto Y, Sano K, Kimoto M. Cryosurgical treatment for anorectal cancer: a method of palliative or adjunctive management. *Am Surg.* 1989;55:252.

661. Yamana T, Oya M, Komatsu J, et al. Preoperative anal sphincter high pressure zone, maximum tolerable volume, and anal mucosal electrosensitivity predict early postoperative defecatory function after low anterior resection for rectal cancer. *Dis Colon Rectum.* 1999;42:1145.

662. Yeung JM, Ferris NJ, Lynch AC, et al. Preoperative staging of rectal cancer. *Future Oncol.* 2009;5:1295.

663. Zacherl J, Scheissel R, Windhager R, et al. Abdominosacral resection of recurrent rectal cancer in the sacrum. *Dis Colon Rectum.* 1999;42:1035.

664. Zainea GG, Lee F, McLeary RD, et al. Transrectal ultrasonography in the evaluation of rectal and extrarectal disease. *Surg Gynecol Obstet.* 1989;169:153.

665. Zelas P, Haaga JR, Fazio VW. The diagnosis by percutaneous biopsy with computed tomography of a recurrence of carcinoma of the rectum in the pelvis. *Surg Gynecol Obstet.* 1980;151:525.

666. Z'graggen K, Maurer CA, Birrer S, et al. A new surgical concept for rectal replacement after low anterior resection: the transverse coloplasty pouch. *Ann Surg.* 2001;234:780.

667. Zhang C, Ding ZH, Li GX, et al. Perirectal fascial and spaces: annular distribution pattern around the mesorectum. *Dis Colon Rectum.* 2010;53:1315.

668. Zinman LM, Libertino JA. Surgical management of urethral strictures. *Surg Clin North Am.* 1973;53:465.

669. Zinman LM, Libertino JA, Roth RA. Management of operative ureteral injury. *Urology.* 1978;12:290.

25

Malignant Tumors of the Anal Canal

Gerald A. Isenberg

While there are several chronic diseases more destructive to life than cancer, none is more feared.
—CHARLES H. MAYO

Carcinomas of the anal canal and perianal skin are uncommon clinical entities, accounting for only 2% or fewer of all colorectal carcinomas. At the Memorial Sloan-Kettering Cancer Center in New York between 1929 and 1974, approximately 400 uncommon neoplasms were found in this area, as compared with almost 10,000 adenocarcinomas of the rectum.[126] This is an incidence of 4% in a specialized referral center. The National Cancer Institute (NCI) estimated 5,820 new cases of anal cancer with 770 deaths in 2011.[100]

Anal canal cancer is almost three times more common than carcinoma of the anal margin.[96] If the dentate line is taken as the distal limit of the anal canal, approximately 70% of all anal tumors will occur in the anal canal.[37] However, if the anal canal is assumed to extend from the anorectal ring to the anal verge (the junction of modified squamous epithelium with the hair-bearing, keratinized perianal skin), 85% of anal tumors will arise in the anal canal.[37] Anal canal tumors are more frequently seen in women (3:2), whereas carcinoma of the anal margin is more common in men (4:1). Morson and Pang noted the same median age for both genders at presentation (57 years).[96]

▶ ANATOMY AND HISTOLOGY

There is some controversy about the anatomic limits of the anal canal, although it is generally agreed that the proximal extent corresponds to the anorectal ring.[58] The distal end has been variously proposed to be the dentate line, Hilton's line, and the anal verge.[56,58] My interpretation of the anal canal is that portion of the distal segment of the intestinal tract that lies between the termination of the rectal mucosa above and the beginning of the perianal skin below (i.e., the mucocutaneous junction; Figure 25-1). It is divided into a proximal transitional zone encompassing the columns and sinuses of Morgagni and a distal zone lined by squamous epithelium (Figure 25-2). The transition zone is derived from the embryonic cloaca and separates the rectal mucosa from the squamous epithelium of the distal anal canal. The anal glands and ducts arise from this area and are lined by stratified columnar epithelium (Figure 25-3). The median number of anal glands is six, with 80% extending to the submucosa, 8% to the circular internal sphincter, 8% to the longitudinal internal sphincter, 2% to the intersphincteric space, and only 1% penetrating the external anal sphincter.[140] The implications of the depth of penetration of the anal glands concerning the etiology of fistula-in-ano are discussed in Chapter 14. The anal glands have definite secretory activity and are presumed to be responsible for lubricating the anal canal.

The transitional zone contains epithelium resembling that found in the urethra, but much variability exists in the region. Patches of squamous epithelium are frequently present, especially over the crests of the columns of Morgagni. The junction between the transitional zone and squamous mucosa lies at the inferior limit of the columns of Morgagni and has been referred to as the dentate or pectinate line.

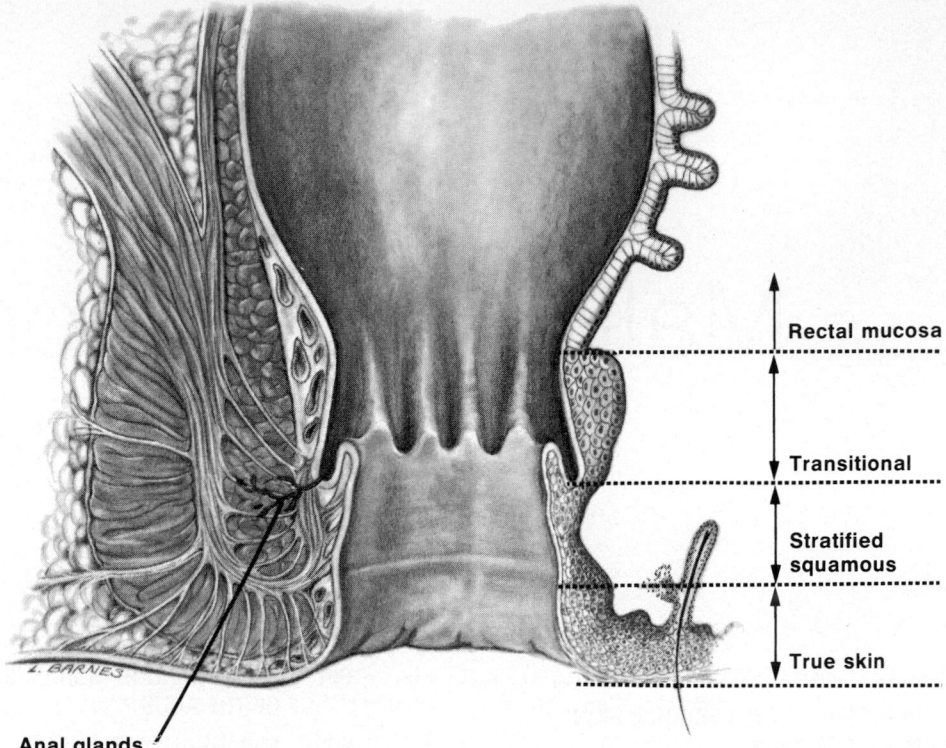

FIGURE 25-1. Anatomy of the anus with histologic pattern schematically illustrated.

Anal glands

However, some authors place the dentate line at the proximal limit of the anal canal, at the junction between the rectal mucosa and transitional zone.[60,78] The more distal zone of the anal canal is lined by stratified squamous epithelium and can be differentiated histologically from perianal skin by the absence of the epidermal appendages found in the skin. Thus, a finger examining the anal canal first passes the perianal skin, the squamous epithelium of the distal anal canal, the transition zone, and finally reaches the rectal mucosa. Separating tumors that arise in the anal canal from those of the perianal skin is important because their biologic behavior and, consequently, the treatments are distinctly different.

▶ CARCINOMA OF THE PERIANAL SKIN AND ANAL MARGIN

Neoplasms of the anal margin and perianal skin include squamous cell carcinoma, Bowen's disease, Paget's disease, and basal cell carcinoma. It is generally accepted that wide surgical excision is an adequate treatment for lesions of the

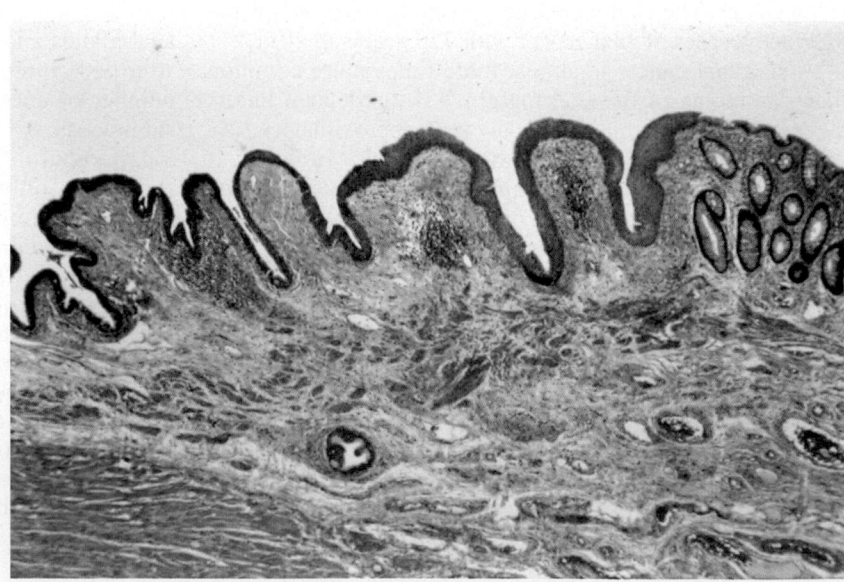

FIGURE 25-2. Normal anal canal. The epithelium of the transition zone **(center, right)** resembles the transitional epithelium of the lower genitourinary tract. (Original magnification × 100.)

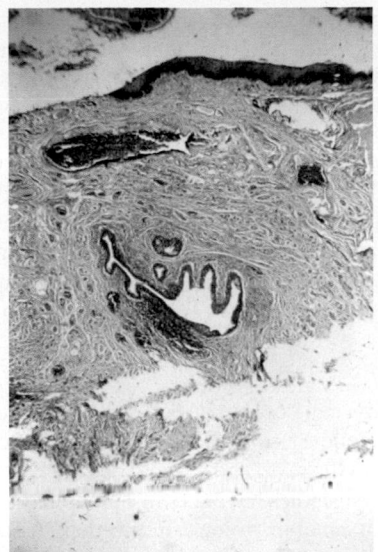
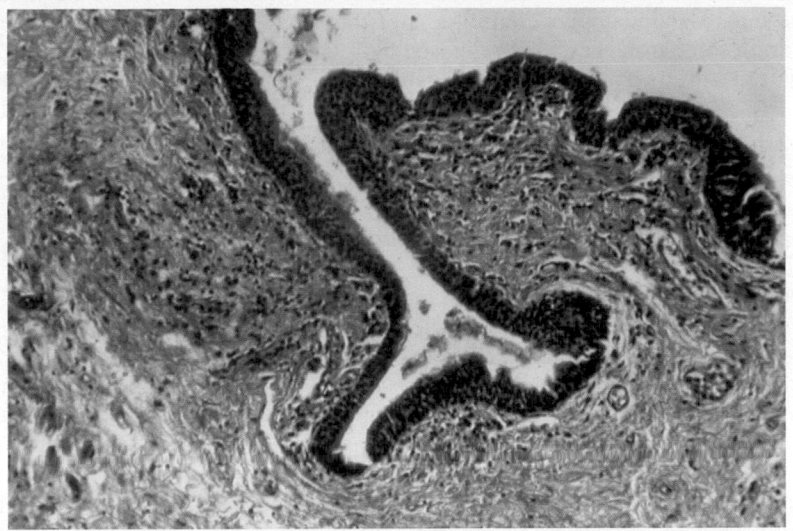

FIGURE 25-3. Cross section of a normal gland **(A)** and an anal duct **(B)**. (Original magnification × 250; courtesy of Rudolf Garret, MD.)

perianal skin (Figure 25-4).[119] Management of these conditions is discussed in Chapter 9. Carcinomas of the anal margin have a better prognosis than that of tumors of the anal canal. Mendenhall and colleagues reviewed the experience at the University of Florida, Gainesville, of squamous cell carcinoma of the anal margin.[95] They concluded that superficial, well to moderately differentiated T1 cancers of the anal margin may be successfully treated with radiotherapy alone or by local excision. However, because stage T2 lesions have an increased risk for lymph node metastases to the groin, they recommended radiotherapy to the primary tumor in conjunction with elective inguinal lymph node radiation. Concurrent chemotherapy may also be prudent for T2 or greater tumors.[5] Abdominoperineal resection (APR) is reserved for those who

have complications secondary to the radiation therapy or locally recurrent disease.[5,95] Greenall and coworkers reported the results of treatment of 48 patients with anal margin lesions.[57] Local excision was associated with a corrected 5-year survival rate of 88%, but 46% of these individuals developed a local or regional recurrence. Additional treatment contributed to the satisfactory results, but APR did not improve survival.

Recommendation

It is self-evident that any suspicious finding around the anus should be examined by biopsy. If the lesion is confirmed to be a malignant neoplasm, the usual treatment is to perform wide local excision because these lesions tend not to

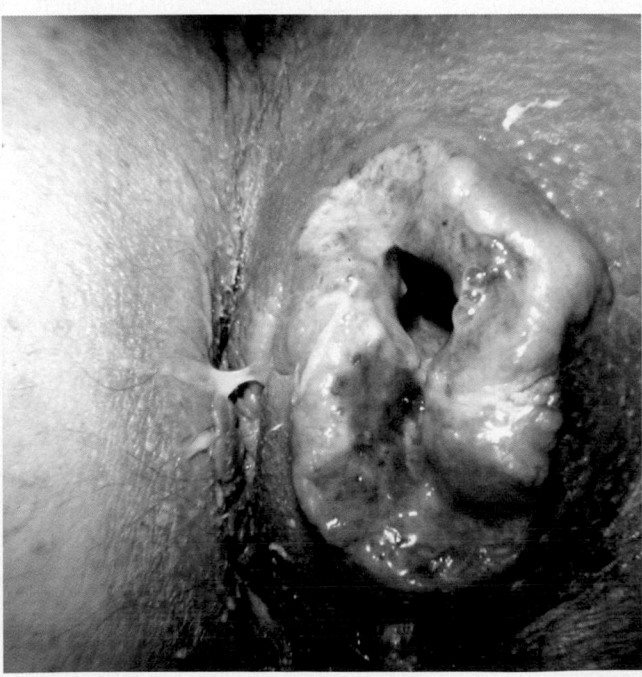
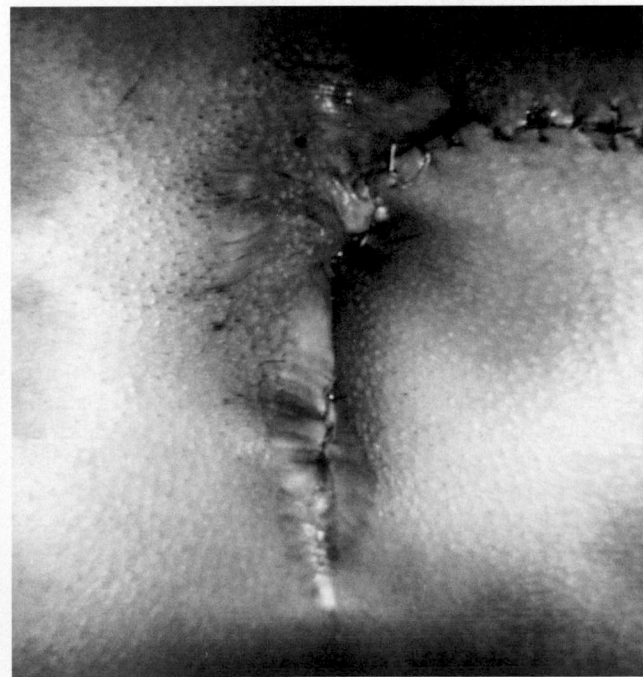

FIGURE 25-4. Ulcerating squamous cell carcinoma of the buttock. **A:** The lesion has been excised. **B:** A rotation flap of full-thickness skin covers the defect.

metastasize (see Figure 9-75). The defect created by excision can be left to granulate, covered by a split-thickness skin graft or, in some instances, may be closed by rotating a flap of adjacent skin such as described in Chapter 11.

▶ CLASSIFICATION OF ANAL CANAL TUMORS

Several histologic types of tumors are identified in the anal canal: epidermoid (squamous cell) and mucoepidermoid carcinoma, transitional-cloacogenic carcinoma, adenocarcinoma, and malignant melanoma. Some physicians regard transitional-cloacogenic carcinoma as a manifestation of epidermoid carcinoma,[109,113] whereas others believe it is a separate entity that arises from the transition zone of the anal canal with different morphologic and clinical features.[47,78] Although it is true that transitional-cloacogenic carcinomas are generally recognizable as a distinct group of tumors, there is some overlap with standard epidermoid carcinomas. They, therefore, form one part of a spectrum that ranges from pure transitional-cloacogenic tumors through lesions with mixtures of squamous elements to those with purely squamous differentiation. The Memorial Sloan-Kettering Cancer group recommends that tumors be classified as squamous or basaloid (transitional-cloacogenic) according to the predominant cell type, although the authors recognize that this may be quite subjective and dependent on tissue sampling.[56] With the exception of melanoma, the clinical behavior of carcinoma of the anal canal appears to be relatively independent of the morphologic subtype when compared stage for stage and grade for grade.

Epidermoid (squamous cell) carcinoma accounted for the majority of the tumors of the anal canal in that reported by Corman and Haggitt (almost two-thirds), whereas transitional-cloacogenic carcinomas comprised approximately one-fourth, and melanomas made up the remainder (14%).[27]

▶ EPIDERMOID OR SQUAMOUS CELL CARCINOMA OF THE ANUS

Incidence

Epidermoid carcinoma of the anus is a rare condition. It can be multifocal in the anal canal as well as in the perianal skin, perineum, and vulvar areas. Most published articles describe each institution's rather limited experience. Failes and Morgan reported 59 patients over a 20-year period; Sawyers and colleagues reported 42 patients over a period of 35 years (2.4% of cancers of the colon, rectum, and anus); and Cattell and Williams reported a 1.7% incidence of epidermoid carcinoma in 600 rectal and anal neoplasms.[19,41,137] Grinnell noted a 1.8% incidence of epidermoid carcinoma in colorectal cancers.[59] Golden and Horsley reported on 26 patients, an incidence of 1.8% of all colorectal cancers.[49] Beahrs and Wilson at the Mayo Clinic in Rochester, Minnesota, reported on 113 patients with epidermoid carcinoma, an incidence of approximately 1% of all colorectal carcinomas seen during the 20-year review.[9] Stearns and Quan (see biographies in Chapter 24) identified 234 epidermoid carcinomas, which represented approximately 3.9% of all malignant tumors detected in the terminal 18 cm of the alimentary tract.[148] The annual incidence of anal cancer among men in the United States is 1.4 per 100,000, but in men who have sex with men the incidence has been estimated to be as high as 37 in 100,000.[123]

As of the publication of this text, the NCI SEER database (November 2011) includes 5,820 patients with anal cancer, 2,140 men and 3,680 women.[101] This data, based on patients from 2004 to 2008, found the median age to be 60 years. The incidence is highest in white women and black men, and there is an increasing trend in both men and women. Overall survival from 2001 to 2007 was 65%. However, African American men had the lowest survival (50%). Half of the anal cancers were localized and one-third had spread to regional lymph nodes at the time of diagnosis. The incidence by race and stage at diagnosis are shown in Tables 25-1 and 25-2.

Age and Gender

Epidermoid carcinoma can occur at almost any age, but absent human immunodeficiency virus (HIV)–positivity, the condition is usually found in the sixth and seventh decades. As mentioned previously, most studies have shown a preponderance of carcinoma of the anal canal in women. In Sweden, the annual age-adjusted incidence per 100,000 population for squamous cell carcinoma is 1.40 for women and 0.68 for men. However, where there are centers with a large patient population of men at high risk, the female-to-male ratio may approach unity.[37]

Predisposing Conditions and Etiology

An increased incidence of anal cancer is seen with a number of anorectal inflammatory conditions, such as chronic anal fistula (see Chapter 14) and anal condylomata, as well as in those with HIV infection (see Chapters 9 and 10). This includes patients with Crohn's disease (see Chapter 30). An association

TABLE 25-1 Incidence Rates by Race

RACE/ETHNICITY	MALE	FEMALE
All races	1.4 per 100,000 men	1.8 per 100,000 women
White	1.5 per 100,000 men	2.0 per 100,000 women
Black	1.9 per 100,000 men	1.7 per 100,000 women
Asian/Pacific Islande	0.5 per 100,000 men	0.5 per 100,000 women
American Indian/ Alaska Native[a]	^	1.5 per 100,000 women
Hispanic[b]	0.9 per 100,000 men	1.3 per 100,000 women

[a]Incidence data for American Indians/Alaska Natives is based on the CHSDA (Contract Health Service Delivery Area).
[b]Incidence date for Hispanics is based on NHIA and excludes cases from Alaska Native Registry.
^Statistics not shown. Rate based on less than 16 cases for the time interval.
From National Cancer Institute. SEER stat fact sheets: anal cancer. 2011. http://seer.cancer.gov/statfacts/html/anus.html.

TABLE 25-2 Stage Distribution and 5-Year Relative Survival by Stage at Diagnosis for 2001–2007, All Races, Both Sexes

STAGE AT DIAGNOSIS	STAGE DISTRIBUTION (%)	5-YEAR RELATIVE SURVIVAL (%)
Localized (confined to primary site)	50	79.0
Regional (spread to regional lymph nodes)	30	58.5
Distant (cancer has metastasized)	12	20.6
Unknown (unstaged)	8	54.7

From National Cancer Institute. SEER stat fact sheets: anal cancer. 2011. http://seer.cancer.gov/statfacts/html/anus.html.

with smoking, anoreceptive intercourse, and immunosuppression has also been described. A relationship with human papillomavirus (HPV) types that are known to be associated with cervical and other genital cancers has been established. Individuals who engage in anal intercourse and who are infected with HPV type 16 have a relative risk of developing anal canal cancer as high as 33% over the general population.[76] Palmer and colleagues affirmed that both HPV types 16 and 18 are involved in the development of anal and genital squamous cell carcinoma.[108] Youk and associates identified HPV type 16 in all 21 of their patients with anal cancer.[166] High-risk HPV is found in 85% of patients with anal squamous cancer, depending on the assay used. Holmes and associates found associations between positive herpes simplex virus 2 titer, cigarette smoking, a prior positive or questionable cervical Papanicolaou smear, and an increasing number of sexual partners with the development of anal cancer.[65] An increased incidence of cancers in the anogenital region has also been observed in patients who have undergone renal transplantation, presumably as a consequence of immunosuppression.[117] Anal cancers have occurred following radiation therapy for pruritus.[37]

Several reports have suggested a significantly higher incidence in patients with Crohn's disease.[145] Although it is unlikely that a patient with an anal fistula or with condylomata would be treated with expectant observation, individuals with Crohn's disease are often managed in this way. Therefore, it is important to perform a biopsy of any unusual lesion. It may even be good counsel to suggest random anal biopsies or biopsy of the fistula/sinus tract at intervals for patients with this condition.

Frisch and colleagues examined the risk of anal cancer developing in individuals who harbored benign anal lesions, including fissures, fistulas, perianal or perirectal abscesses, and hemorrhoids.[46] Whereas these investigators concluded that there was a strong temporal association between the diagnosis of benign anal lesions and that of anal cancer, their data did not support the view that there was an association for these diagnoses.

Melbye and coworkers compared the numbers of observed cases and expected cases of anal cancer among patients with acquired immunodeficiency syndrome (AIDS) by using registries in seven health departments in the United States.[94] These investigators found that there was a strikingly increased risk for the development of this malignancy in individuals with AIDS. Lorenz and associates retrospectively reviewed six patients with squamous cell carcinoma treated between 1985 and 1988.[89] All were homosexual men; five had AIDS, and one was HIV positive. Because of the increased incidence of venereal disease in the homosexual population, there is increasing evidence to suggest that homosexual men are at a particular risk for the development of anal cancer.[84] Piketty and colleagues found an increased incidence of anal cancer in HIV patients despite their treatment with antiretroviral therapy from this French database of HIV-positive patients.[121] In addition, the incidence was higher in men who have sex with men. Even in the absence of AIDS, anal canal carcinoma, Kaposi's sarcoma, and anorectal lymphoma are seen in younger patients and much more frequently than would be expected.[34,38,69,81,99]

Daling and colleagues demonstrated that two correlates of homosexual behavior, unmarried status and positive serologic test result for syphilis, are related to an increased incidence of anal cancer.[33,34] Because having had syphilis and being single are associated with the practice of anal intercourse in men, but not in women, the authors suggest that this act is an independent risk factor for the development of anal cancer. Goldstone and associates recommend that all men who have sex with men with presumed benign anorectal disease undergo high-resolution anoscopy and multiple biopsies of all abnormal areas in order to look for high-grade, squamous intraepithelial lesions that represent precursors of invasive carcinoma (see Chapter 10).[55] Place and coworkers opined that anal squamous cell carcinoma in an HIV-positive patient should be considered an AIDS-defining illness.[123]

It can be appreciated, therefore, that certain predisposing conditions are associated with the development of malignant anal canal tumors. This implies that the etiology probably represents an interaction between genetic and environmental factors.[37] The genetic aspect may be related to changes in chromosome 11 (11q22) or the short arm of chromosome 3 (3p22).[98]

In summary, the following variables are related to the development of anogenital carcinoma:

- Prior radiotherapy
- Chronic anal fistula
- Crohn's disease
- Smoking
- Positive Papanicolaou smear
- Cervical carcinoma
- HPV infection
- Hodgkin's disease
- Renal transplantation
- Multiple partners
- Positive herpes simplex virus 2 titer
- HIV infection
- Male homosexuality
- Anoreceptive intercourse
- Immunosuppression
- Positive serologic test for syphilis
- Anal condylomata
- Anal intraepithelial neoplasia (AIN)

Current evidence indicates that the etiology of anal cancer is a multifactorial interaction among environmental factors, HPV infection, immune status, and suppressor genes.[37]

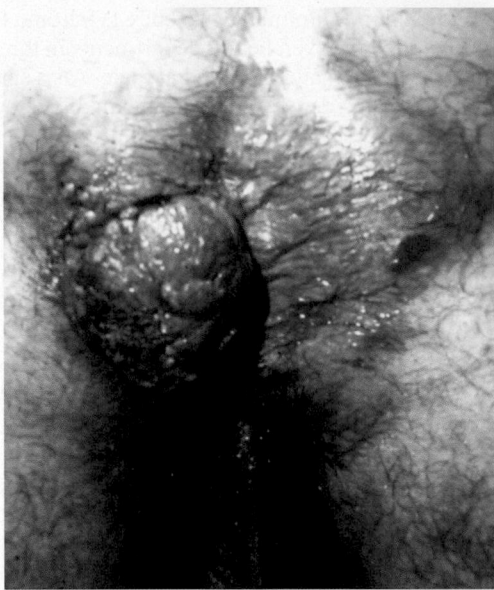

FIGURE 25-5. Squamous cell carcinoma. The patient complained of a lump. (From Corman ML, Veidenheimer MC, Swinton NW. *Diseases of the Anus, Rectum and Colon. Part I: Neoplasms.* New York, NY: Medcom; 1972, with permission.)[28]

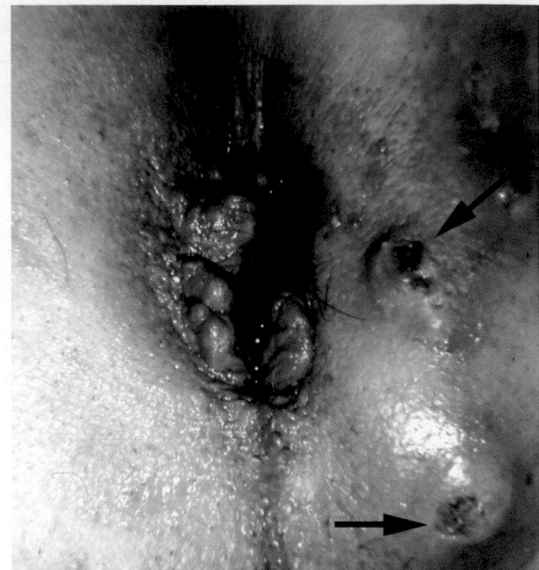

FIGURE 25-6. Two fistulous openings (*arrows*) from anal canal carcinoma. Biopsy of the tracts confirmed the presence of tumor. (From Corman ML, Veidenheimer MC, Swinton NW. *Diseases of the Anus, Rectum and Colon. Part I: Neoplasms.* New York, NY: Medcom; 1972, with permission.)

Signs and Symptoms

Symptoms of anal canal carcinoma include rectal bleeding, anal pain, pruritus, mucous discharge, tenesmus, the sensation of a lump in the anus, and a change in bowel habits (Figure 25-5). Rectal bleeding occurs in more than one-half of individuals. The duration of symptoms is of little prognostic significance.[56] Complaints such as discharge, incontinence, change in bowel habits, pelvic pain, or the passage of stool or gas through the vagina suggest an advanced lesion.[37] Tenesmus, the painful urgency to defecate, implies invasion of the sphincter mechanism. Presentation is often late, with the mean size of tumor at diagnosis between 3 and 4 cm.[37] Occasionally, a patient may present with a mass in the groin, a manifestation of a metastasis before the primary tumor causes significant symptoms. The condition may also be identified incidentally upon review of the histology of a hemorrhoidectomy specimen (see later).

Examination and Biopsy

Rectal examination may reveal an ulcerating, hard, tender, bleeding mass in the anal canal or lower rectum. Examination of an advanced lesion may be excruciatingly tender and may require evaluation using an anesthetic to identify the accurate extent and to perform a biopsy of the lesion. The tumor may fungate through the anal canal and appear on the perianal skin, or it may present through a chronic draining anal fistula (Figure 25-6). The lesion can be confused with other anorectal conditions, such as an ulcerated hemorrhoid or an ulceration as a consequence of an infection.

Proctosigmoidoscopic examination usually shows that the tumor is confined to the anal canal. However, in far-advanced cases, the lesion may extend upward to involve the rectum. Conversely, a carcinoma that seems to arise within the anal canal may occasionally be a rectal cancer that has spread downward (Figure 25-7). Another possibility is implantation from a colon tumor, a particular concern if hemorrhoidectomy is performed at the time of a colectomy for cancer.

Scott and colleagues demonstrated by flow cytometric DNA analysis that an anal malignancy was actually the result of a "dropped" metastasis from a sigmoid colon carcinoma.[139] Biopsy of the lesion will establish its histologic nature.

Pathology

Epidermoid Carcinoma

Epidermoid carcinoma originates from the stratified squamous epithelium of the distal anal mucosa and therefore

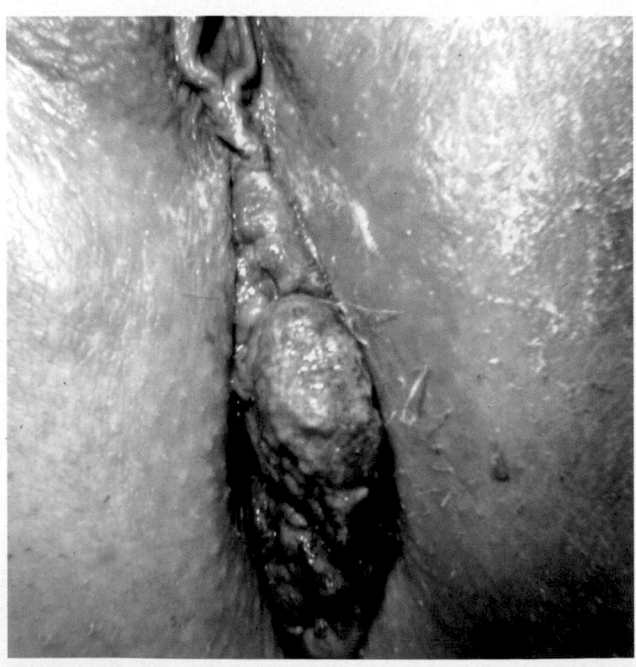

FIGURE 25-7. Adenocarcinoma of the rectum fungating through the anal canal. (From Corman ML, Veidenheimer MC, Swinton NW. *Diseases of the Anus, Rectum and Colon. Part I: Neoplasms.* New York, NY: Medcom; 1972, with permission.)

morphologically resembles carcinoma arising from the buccal mucosa, esophagus, uterine cervix, and so forth. The tumor is composed of squamous epithelial cells that resemble normal anal mucosa to a varying extent, depending on the degree of differentiation. The more differentiated tumors have readily apparent keratin formation, either as pearls or as individual cell keratinization (Figure 25-8). The lesions can be graded based on the degree of keratinization and the nuclear morphology, and this grade correlates with the behavior of the tumor, that is, well-differentiated tumors tend to be less deeply invasive and are less likely to metastasize. More than 50% of anal canal tumors are nonkeratinizing, whereas 80% are poorly differentiated.[37] This is in contrast to anal margin tumors, with 80% demonstrating keratinization and 85% being well differentiated.[37]

Goldman and colleagues examined 15 patients with anal carcinoma by means of percutaneous and transanorectal fine needle aspiration cytology, confirming the diagnosis by this means.[54] Interestingly, despite the predominance in women, neither estrogen receptors nor progesterone receptors could be detected. Surawicz and coworkers used anal cytology and biopsy to determine the presence of anal dysplasia (anal intraepithelial neoplasia) in 90 homosexual men with abnormalities of the anal canal.[150] Eighty-six percent had HPV-associated abnormalities, including condylomata. Dysplasia was detected by cytology in 36% and by biopsy in 92% (27% high grade).[150] The authors concluded that further studies are indicated to determine the clinical significance of the dysplastic phenomenon and its rate of progression to cancer (see also Chapter 10). Obviously, this has implications with respect to screening and to treatment.

A careful search using mucin stains may disclose a focus of mucin-producing cells in as many as 10% to 15% of patients (Figure 25-9).[97] Such tumors have been classified separately as mucoepidermoid carcinomas, but little evidence exists that differences in the behavior of this subgroup warrant its separation. A case of mucoepidermoid carcinoma of the anal canal with special reference to immunohistochemical analysis of the tumor to clarify its histogenesis has been reported.[79] The staining patterns were different from those of anal squamous epithelium, confirming that mucoepidermoid carcinoma of the anus may arise from the anal transitional zone, and that it is biologically different from squamous cell carcinoma of the anus. A spindle cell carcinoma (pseudosarcoma) has been reported to be another variant.[74]

Squamous cell carcinoma tumor-associated antigen (SCC antigen) has been shown to be a tumor marker that seems to be related to the histologic characteristics of differentiated epidermoid tumors rather than to tumor site.[120] Fontana and colleagues measured SCC antigen in epidermoid carcinoma of the anal canal in 66 patients at diagnosis, before treatment, and during follow-up.[44] There did not appear to be a correlation with the primary tumor, itself, except with respect to nodal involvement. These investigators concluded that there was no prognostic value of this study at the time of diagnosis, but that the level of SCC antigen correlated well with the development of recurrence.

Transitional-Cloacogenic Carcinoma

In 1956, Grinvalsky and Helwig published a study of the anatomy of the anal canal in which they detailed the features

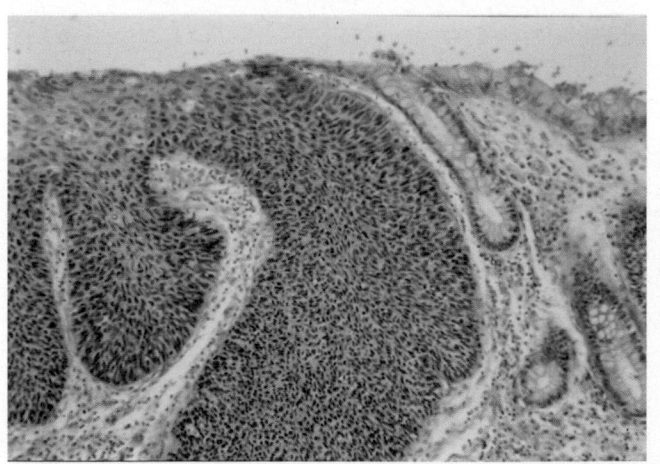

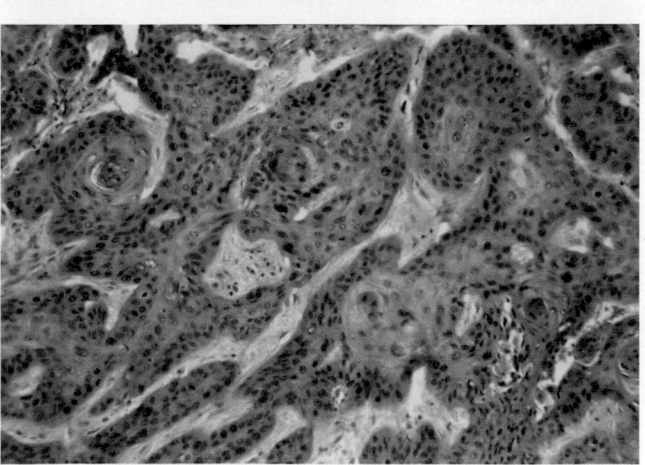

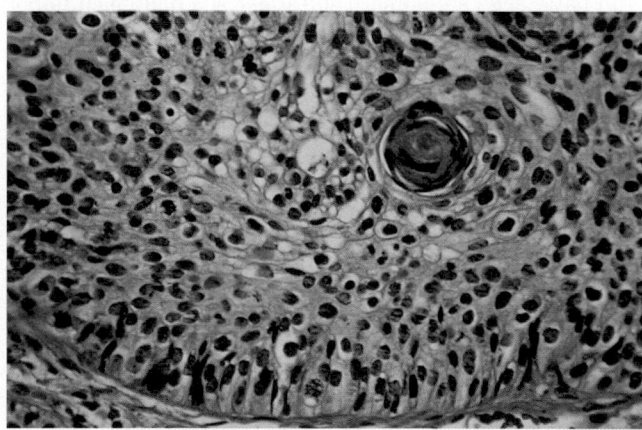

FIGURE 25-8. Squamous cell carcinoma of the anus. **A:** Carcinoma in situ. Note that there is no invasion. **B:** This well-differentiated squamous cell carcinoma resembles normal squamous epithelium and is producing a keratin pearl. **C:** Less well-differentiated lesions lose their resemblance to squamous epithelium, lack keratin pearls, and behave more aggressively.

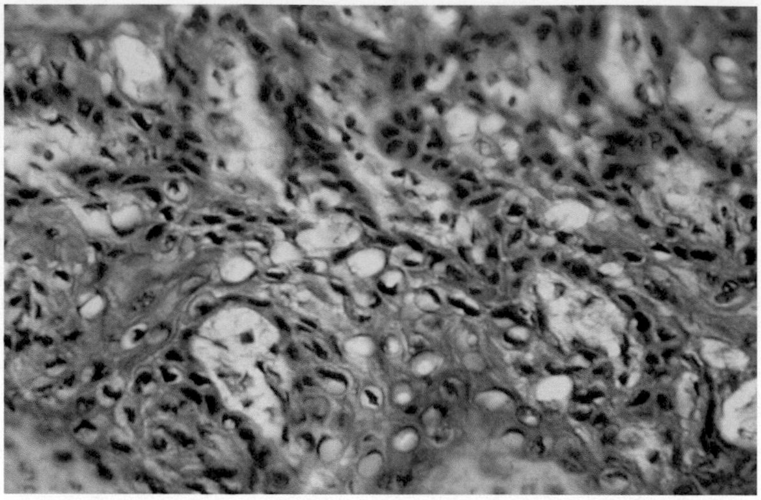

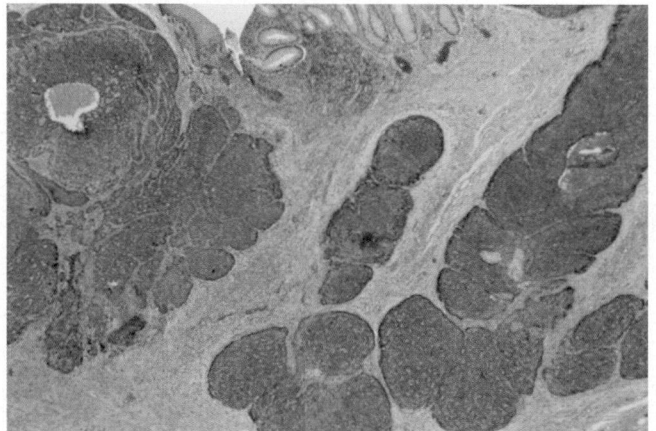

FIGURE 25-9. Mucoepidermoid cell pattern in an anal canal cancer. (Original magnification × 260.)

of the transitional or "cloacogenic" zone and suggested that tumors, which arise in this area, differ from the usual epidermoid carcinomas originating in the squamous epithelium of the distal anal canal.[60] They proposed the term transitional-cloacogenic for these lesions. Subsequent studies have confirmed the morphologic difference from that of the usual squamous carcinomas.[78,109]

Transitional-cloacogenic carcinomas may resemble carcinomas of urothelium to a certain extent, or they may have patterns similar to that of basal cell carcinoma of skin—hence the term basaloid because the cells at the periphery are arranged in an orderly, palisade fashion (Figure 25-10). However, this variation in cell pattern must not be confused with basal cell carcinoma. The former is a malignant tumor that frequently metastasizes, whereas the latter is relatively benign (see Chapter 9).

Those tumors resembling urothelial carcinomas are composed of islands or nests of cells that have indistinct borders and oval nuclei (Figure 25-11). A focus of keratinization is often present. As stated previously, varying amounts of squamous elements produce a spectrum of lesions ranging from purely transitional through mixed varieties to purely squamous tumors. Some examples of transitional-cloacogenic

carcinoma appear to arise in the lower part of the rectum above the transitional zone, whereas others may not even involve the mucosa. The probable explanation for these phenomena is that such tumors may originate from the transitional epithelium that lines the anal ducts deep to the mucosa or in proximal ramifications of the ducts beneath the rectal mucosa.

Transitional-cloacogenic tumors form a histologically recognizable subgroup of anal canal carcinomas, but based on the grade and stage of the lesions, their behavior appears to be

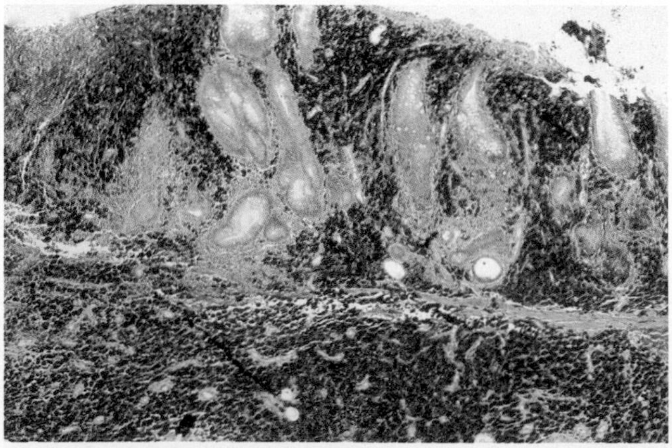

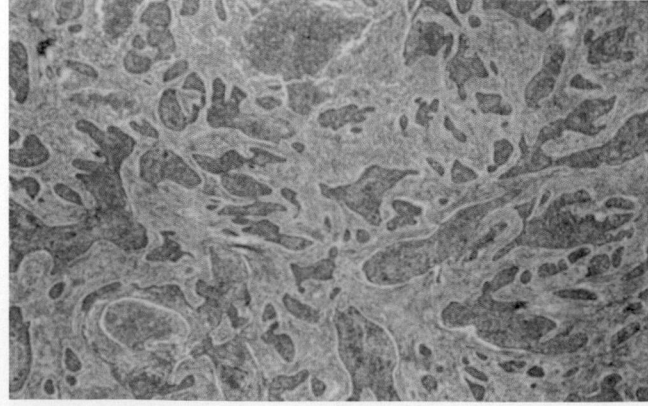

FIGURE 25-10. Transitional-cloacogenic carcinoma. In this tumor, the cells at the periphery tend to arrange themselves in a palisade, thus resembling basal cell carcinoma of the skin. This variant of transitional-cloacogenic carcinoma is sometimes called basaloid carcinoma. (Original magnification × 80.)

FIGURE 25-11. Transitional-cloacogenic carcinoma. **A:** The tumor has an in situ component resembling a transitional cell carcinoma of the urinary bladder, hence its name. **B:** A poorly differentiated lesion. (Original magnification × 125.)

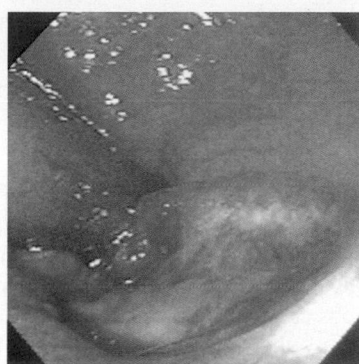

FIGURE 25-12. Retroflexion with the endoscope in the rectum reveals an ulcerating lesion in the transitional zone at the top of the anal canal and lower rectum. Biopsy confirmed the presence of a cloacogenic carcinoma.

comparable to that of epidermoid carcinomas of similar grade and stage (Figure 25-12). There are fewer published studies of transitional-cloacogenic tumors than that of epidermoid carcinoma, but evidence suggests that there is sufficient overlap in the epidemiology (e.g., an increased incidence in anal-receptive homosexual men),[25] the clinical presentation, and the results of treatment that, for the purposes of management, one should consider the two entities identical.

Melanoma

The histopathology of malignant melanoma is discussed later in this chapter.

Adenocarcinoma

Adenocarcinoma of the anus is sometimes seen as a downward extension of a primary rectal tumor. However, glandular epithelium may be found on biopsy from ectopic glands of the anal wall, from sebaceous glands of the perineum, from anal fistulas, or from tumors arising in anal glands or ducts (Figure 25-13). Hobbs and colleagues found that a useful and discriminating definition of anal gland carcinoma is an anal tumor composed of "haphazardly dispersed, small glands with scant mucin production invading the wall of the anorectal area without an intraluminal component" (see later).[64] As discussed

in Chapter 9, the association with an underlying mucinous adenocarcinoma and Paget's disease has been well documented.

Staging

No completely satisfactory method for staging anal canal tumors has been developed. Dukes' classification is not applicable because invasion to groin nodes may occur when lymph node involvement is not evident in the resected specimen. The TNM system has been criticized because it is difficult to distinguish tumor invasion limited to the internal sphincter from that involving the external sphincter and because extension into the rectum or perianal skin does not necessarily imply a poorer prognosis.[56,58] That stated, however, the staging system for anal canal cancer that has been described by the American Joint Committee on Cancer (AJCC) and the International Union Against Cancer, the system that is currently used by pathologists, tumor boards, oncologic centers, and therefore most colorectal surgeons is presented in Table 25-3.

Goldman and colleagues examined specimens from 47 cases of squamous cell carcinoma of the anus with respect to clinical stage, histologic grade, and DNA content of the tumor cells.[50] Because most tumors were aneuploid, no statistically significant difference could be demonstrated with respect to DNA content and survival. The authors affirmed that histologic grade and clinical stage seem to be the best predictors of patient outcome.

Treatment

Until the middle to late 1970s, APR was believed by most surgeons to be the only curative approach to the management of anal canal carcinoma.[134] Before the advent of neoadjuvant therapy, selective application of local excision could also be considered.[51] The choice of treatment depended on the stage of the tumor as determined by depth of invasion. The current approach relies heavily on the success of neoadjuvant therapy. However, other modalities are first discussed in order to provide some perspective.

Local Excision

For carcinoma confined to the mucosa and submucosa or carcinoma in situ, wide local excision with or without an

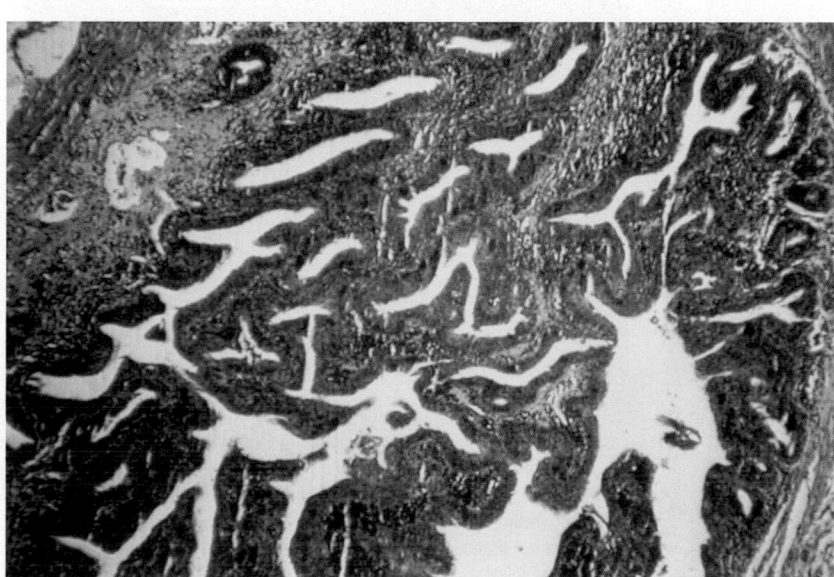

FIGURE 25-13. Adenocarcinoma arising from an anal gland. (Original magnification × 200.)

TABLE 25-3 The AJCC Staging System for Anal Canal Cancer

Primary Tumor (T)[a]

TX	Primary tumor cannot be assessed.
T0	No evidence of primary tumor.
Tis	Carcinoma in situ (i.e., Bowen disease, high-grade squamous intraepithelial lesion, and anal intraepithelial neoplasia II–III.)
T1	Tumor ≤2 cm in greatest dimension.
T2	Tumor >2 cm but ≤5 cm in greatest dimension.
T3	Tumor >5 cm in greatest dimension.
T4	Tumor of any size invades adjacent organ(s), e.g., vagina, urethra, and bladder.[b]

Regional Lymph Nodes (N)[a]

NX	Regional lymph nodes cannot be assessed.
N0	No regional lymph node metastasis.
N1	Metastases in perirectal lymph node(s).
N2	Metastases in unilateral internal iliac and/or inguinal lymph node(s).
N3	Metastases in perirectal and inguinal lymph nodes and/or bilateral internal iliac and/or inguinal lymph nodes.

Distant Metastasis (M)[a]

M0	No distant metastasis.
M1	Distant metastasis.

Anatomic Stage/Prognostic Groups [a]

Stage	T	N	M
0	Tis	N0	M0
I	T1	N0	M0
II	T2	N0	M0
	T3	N0	M0
IIIA	T1	N1	M0
	T2	N1	M0
	T3	N1	M0
	T4	N0	M0
IIIB	T4	N1	M0
	Any T	N2	M0
	Any T	N3	M0
IV	Any T	Any N	M1

[a]Reprinted with permission from Edge SB, Byrd DR, Compton CC, et al, eds. Part III digestive system: anus. In: *AJCC Cancer Staging Manual.* 7th ed. New York, NY: Springer; 2010:165–173.
[b]Direct invasion of the rectal wall, perirectal skin, subcutaneous tissue, or the sphincter muscle(s) is not classified as T4.

anoplasty will usually be curative (see Chapter 11). For more deeply invading tumors such as those that invade the internal sphincter, local excision including the internal sphincter may also achieve cure. However, for tumors that invade more deeply than the internal sphincter, APR has, historically, been the preferred alternative. These differences in therapy based on the stage of the tumor require precise preoperative evaluation, including careful digital examination to assess the depth of invasion and endoanal ultrasound. Tarantino and Bernstein evaluated 13 consecutive patients with biopsy-proven squamous cell carcinoma of the anal canal by means of endoanal ultrasound.[152] These investigators proposed the following staging system:

uT_1 = Tumor confined to the submucosa
uT_{2a} = Tumor invaded internal sphincter
uT_{2b} = Tumor invades external sphincter
uT_3 = Tumor invades through sphincter complex into perianal tissues
uT_4 = Tumor invades adjacent structures

The authors concluded that endoanal ultrasound can accurately determine the depth of penetration and can also be used to determine the efficacy of neoadjuvant therapy.[152]

The preferred modality for staging remains controversial. Comparisons of anal ultrasound and MRI often demonstrate similar results for "T" diagnosis; however, MRI is obviously better for nodal status (Figures 25-14 through 25-16).[107] Parikh and colleagues compared these two methods and suggest that MRI may be preferred, especially following treatment because of changes in signal intensity.[114] But positron emission tomography (PET) imaging may offer the best results. Winton and coworkers compared PET imaging with other diagnostic tests and found improved nodal staging as well as changed treatment intent (such as radiation fields) in

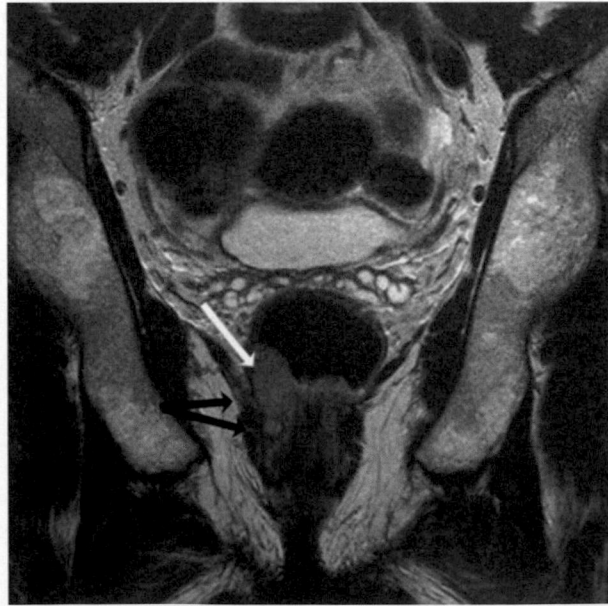

FIGURE 25-14. Primary staging of an anal carcinoma on MRI—T2N0M0: Coronal T2-weighted MRI demonstrating a 4-cm long intermediate signal intensity mass arising from the upper right anterolateral anal canal. T2-weighted MRI clearly delineates the tumor (*white arrow*) from the low signal intensity right EAS/levator plate (*black arrows*). (From Parikh J, Shaw A, Grant LA, et al. Anal carcinomas: the role of endoanal ultrasound and magnetic resonance imaging in staging, response evaluation and follow-up. *Eur Radiol.* 2011;21(4):776–785.)

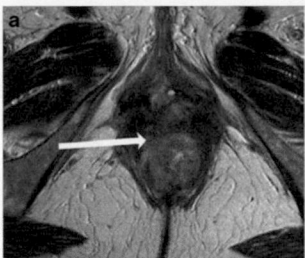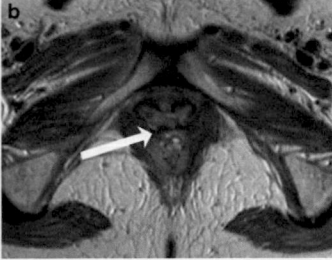

FIGURE 25-15. Primary staging and restaging of anal carcinoma on MRI—T4N0M0. **A:** Axial T2-weighted MRI demonstrating a bulky intermediate signal intensity mass filling the anal canal and extending anteriorly to invade the posterior wall of the vagina with loss of the low signal intensity outline of the posterior vaginal wall (*white arrow*). **B:** Axial T2-weighted image of the same patient 8 months following treatment. There has been a complete radiologic response with restoration of the low signal intensity outline of the vagina wall (*white arrow*). (From Parikh J, Shaw A, Grant LA, et al. Anal carcinomas: the role of endoanal ultrasound and magnetic resonance imaging in staging, response evaluation and follow-up. *Eur Radiol.* 2011;21(4):776–785.)

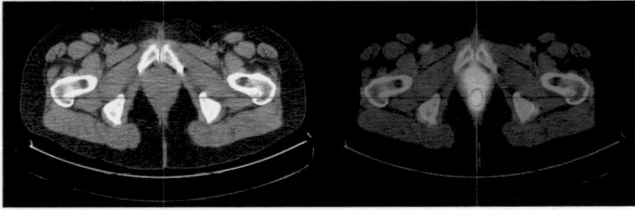

FIGURE 25-16. A 56-year-old woman with a T2 squamous cell carcinoma of the anal canal not appreciated on CT **(left)** but clearly visualized by PET-CT **(right)**. (From Nguyen BT, Joon DL, Khoo V, et al. Assessing the impact of FDG-PET in the management of anal cancer. *Radiother Oncol.* 2008;87(3):376–382.)

a significant number of patients.[165] Preliminary results show that PET/CT may be still better.[151]

Scholefield and associates reported the management of 70 patients with anal intraepithelial neoplasia.[138] In concert with the foregoing recommendations, the authors performed local excision and in some cases skin grafting to those larger lesions that were more invasive. Chang and coworkers performed excision and cauterization directed by high-resolution anoscopy in HIV-negative and HIV-positive patients with high-grade intraepithelial lesions.[21] No HIV-negative patient developed recurrence (mean follow-up, 32 months), but 23 of 29 individuals who were HIV positive had persistent or recurrent lesions.

Other options in the management of small, superficial, or minimally invasive anal canal cancers include cryosurgery, laser vaporization, and possibly the use of chemical or immuno-ablational topical agents (especially for intraepithelial neoplasia).[138] Hamdan and colleagues reported the use of photodynamic therapy for the treatment of this condition.[63] This consists of a two-step process that involves the topical or systemic application of a photosensitizer followed by illumination of the treatment area with a nonthermal laser or nonlaser light of a specific wavelength.[63] The effect is to create a local cytotoxic action.

Abdominoperineal Resection

The technique of APR is described in Chapter 24. An important principle to remember is that when the anal margin is involved by tumor, a wider excision of perianal skin is required than is customary for adenocarcinoma of the rectum (Figures 25-17 and 25-18).

Results of Conventional, Nonneoadjuvant Abdominoperineal Resection, and Local Excision ("Historical" Data)

Five-year survival after APR has been reported to be between 20% and 70% and depends on tumor size, histologic grading, and depth of invasion.[53,56,58,125] Pelvic or perineal recurrence accounts for 50% to 70% of failures, with only 10% of patients dying of disseminated disease.[56] Welch and Malt noted a 30% recurrence rate in the perineum of 37 patients who underwent APR.[161] Carcinoma was present in 20% of the resection margins. The authors, therefore, caution the surgeon to perform posterior vaginectomy in women as well as wide excision of the perianal skin. Madden and colleagues reported a 21% survival rate in 29 patients after 5 years.[90]

Singh and associates reported 65 patients from Roswell Park Memorial Institute in Buffalo, New York, two-thirds of whom had epidermoid carcinoma of the anal canal.[143]

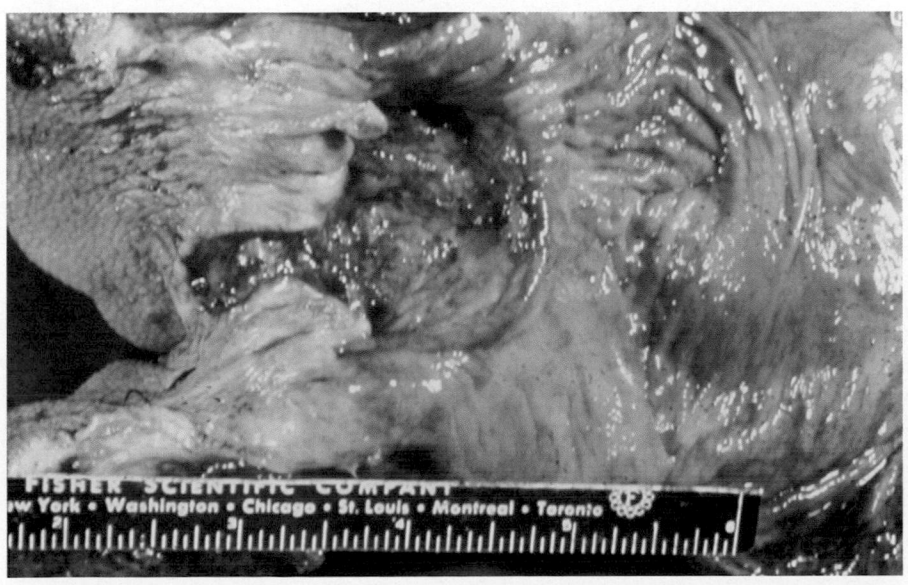

FIGURE 25-17. Proctectomy specimen of squamous cell carcinoma of the anus infiltrating the pectinate line. (Courtesy of Rudolf Garret, MD.)

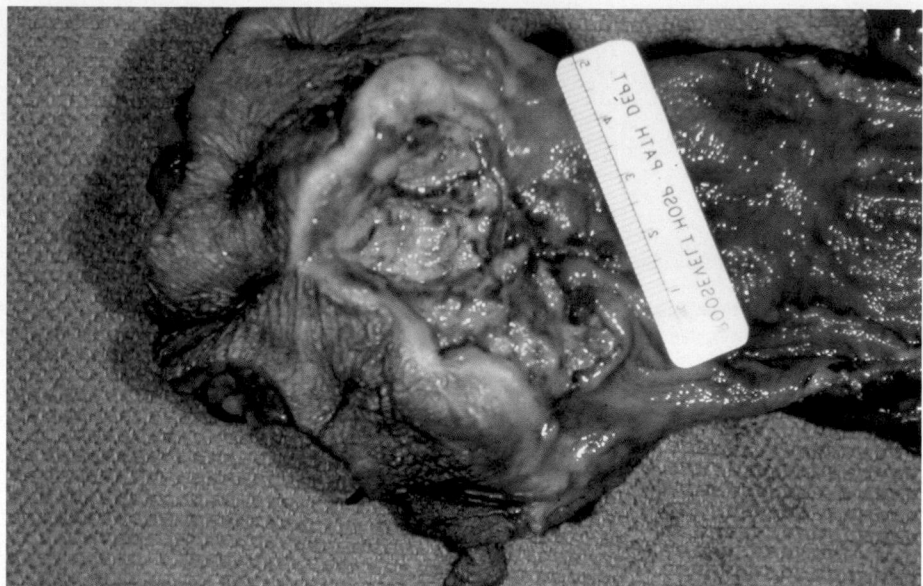

FIGURE 25-18. Cloacogenic carcinoma. Resected specimen of an ulcerated tumor impinging on the pectinate line. (Courtesy of Rudolf Garret, MD.)

The remainder harbored cloacogenic cancers. The overall survival rate depended on the depth of invasion, but it was approximately 50% in both groups. Wide local excision for tumors that invaded through the submucosa was accompanied by a recurrence rate of 100%. Of all surgical approaches, APR with posterior exenteration had the lowest recurrence rate.

The Memorial Sloan-Kettering Cancer group observed that they had treated very few patients with epidermoid cancer of the anal canal by local excision, and interpretation of the results may be somewhat confusing because these individuals may be combined with those who had tumors of the anal margin.[56] The fact is that fewer than 10% of tumors were suitable for local excision, and more than 60% of these patients developed recurrence.[56]

In the experience of Corman and Haggitt, all patients who had disease confined to the mucosa or submucosa were cured by local excision or by APR.[27] Likewise, all who had APR were cured (without supplemental therapy) when the disease was confined to muscle. However, with mesorectal lymph node involvement or invasion into the perirectal or perianal fat, the prognosis was much less optimistic. With lymph node involvement, they observed a 29% 5-year survival rate.[27] It is generally agreed that the depth of invasion and the presence or absence of lymph node involvement are the major criteria for determining length of survival. The prognosis after resection for transitional-cloacogenic carcinoma is essentially the same as that for epidermoid carcinoma for the same depth of invasion. In analyzing survival with respect to cell differentiation, no relationship is apparent except that the more poorly differentiated lesions tend to present at a more advanced stage.

To all intents and purposes, the foregoing results are of historical interest only. Today it is not within the standard of care to go directly to APR for carcinoma of the anal canal. This is because of the advances made with the application of neoadjuvant therapy.

Groin Dissection

Radical groin dissection was advocated in the past as a valuable adjunctive procedure in the primary treatment of carcinoma of the anal canal because of the possibility of spread to inguinal nodes. Later reports have been highly critical of this approach, however.[9,27,148,149] Because of its high morbidity and because it is an unnecessary operation in most patients, radical groin dissection as a therapeutic modality should be employed only when adenopathy is subsequently discovered.[136] For diagnostic and staging purposes, it seems reasonable to excise a large inguinal mass. Even though the cure rate is still low, some authors believe that this procedure reduces the risk of groin complications from tumor growth.[136] It is unlikely that radical inguinal node dissection will lead to the cure of a patient with groin node involvement by tumor. However, one should consider chemotherapy and radiotherapy for these individuals in light of the responsiveness of this tumor to such an approach (see later).

Sentinel Node Biopsy

Damin and colleagues, in 2003, undertook a study to assess the feasibility of inguinal sentinel node biopsy and staging in 14 patients with anal canal cancer and with no evident inguinal node involvement.[35] The procedure consisted of a combination of preoperative lymphoscintigraphy with ^{99m}Tc dextran 500 injected around the tumor and intraoperative detection of the sentinel node with a gamma probe. Patent blue V dye was also injected to permit identification of the blue-stained node. The investigators were able to detect and remove sentinel nodes in all patients and found one individual with a metastatic node. The authors opined that the results of a sentinel lymph node procedure may have a role in directing a different approach to management.

Perera and coworkers used injections of antimony sulfide around the tumor with gamma scanning of the inguinal area in order to identify sentinel nodes in 12 patients.[118] The sentinel node was found in 8 (67%). In two individuals, metastases were histologically confirmed.

Pelvic Lymphadenectomy

Pelvic lymphadenectomy in conjunction with APR may be performed relatively easily in some patients. The value of obtaining lymph nodes to determine the prognosis and the advisability of adding other treatment may justify this approach, but it should not be performed if the dissection is difficult.

Wade and colleagues accomplished a retrospective study of 29 patients who underwent potentially curative APR and whose surgical specimens were treated by a clearing technique of the lymph nodes.[158] These investigators found a lack of association between the size of the primary tumor and the lymph nodes and noted that metastasis to small nodes (less than 5 mm) was a common occurrence. This perhaps is an explanation for understaging of some patients.

Neoadjuvant (Combined Modality) Therapy (Nigro Protocol)

In 1974, Nigro and associates reported dramatic results in the treatment of epidermoid carcinoma of the anus by means of preoperative radiation therapy and chemotherapy.[105] Subsequent reports from Nigro's unit at Wayne State University School of Medicine in Detroit revealed continued enthusiasm.[15,16,82,103,104] Its remarkable success in the management of even locally extensive tumors or in individuals with regional node metastases has revolutionized the approach to the management of this condition.

The protocol initially consisted of preoperative radiation (a total of 30 Gy) to the tumor and to the pelvic and inguinal nodal areas in 15 treatments over a 3-week period (2 Gy per day, 5 days a week). The first day that radiotherapy is commenced the patient was administered 5-fluorouracil (5-FU) in 5% glucose, 1,000 mg/m² per day, for 4 days as a continuous 24-hour infusion, and again from days 29 through 32. In addition, the patient was given mitomycin-C, 15 mg/m², as a single bolus on the first day. This protocol is usually associated with only a mild degree of thrombocytopenia and leukopenia. The most frequent side effects are low-grade stomatitis and moderate diarrhea.[82]

There are now numerous variations on this radiation-chemotherapy scheme in terms of both drugs used and radiation dosage and frequency. For example, Löhnert and colleagues in Kiel, Germany, use a three-dimensional, endosonographic-based radiation target simulation method, using an afterloading needle application.[87] The anal cancer is restaged following external beam radiation with 45 Gy. The Memorial Sloan-Kettering group suggested that in patients who are selected to undergo an initial excisional biopsy followed by combined-modality therapy, 30 Gy may be an adequate radiation dose.[67]

Results

Analysis of 45 patients treated at Wayne State University School of Medicine revealed that 38 of 45 patients (84%) were rendered free of cancer.[82] Although the follow-up period of many was less than 5 years, 34 (89%) were alive and free of disease. All patients with residual tumor, even after APR had been performed, died of disseminated disease. The initial median size of those with persistent tumor was 5 cm, as compared with 3.5 cm for those lesions with no residual tumor.

Others have reported favorable experiences.[11,24,31,40,42,61,122,127,144,147] Enker and colleagues noted that 59% of their patients had no residual tumor at the time of proctectomy.[40] Seventy-seven percent were free of disease at follow-up. Sischy and coworkers reported 15 patients who received chemotherapy and radiotherapy with a complete response, thereby avoiding APR.[144] Cummings and associates achieved tumor control in all six patients by the protocol, and Wancho and colleagues had good results even in patients with recurrent and locally advanced disease.[31,159]

Cummings and coworkers compared the results of treatment by radical external beam radiation alone with the combined-modality approach.[30] Although the uncorrected 5-year survival rate for the two groups was approximately 70%, control of the primary tumor was much better with combination treatment (93%) than with radiation therapy alone (60%). Almost one-half of the patients who underwent chemoradiation therapy developed hematologic toxicity, and in one-third the course was complicated by enterocolitis that did not respond to antidiarrheal agents. This is a higher complication rate than that reported by the Nigro group and caused the authors to recommend interrupting the course of therapy for 1 week. None of those who underwent combination therapy required a colostomy for uncontrolled tumor, but 4 of 30 had treatment complications that necessitated a stoma.

Intensity-modulated radiation therapy (IMRT) with chemotherapy is currently being used by some centers to help focus the radiation beam and to reduce the toxicity of the treatment.[73,133] Salama and colleagues reported a multicenter trial with 53 patients using this technique.[133] Preliminary results showed this method to be effective and tolerated well compared to controls.

NORMAN D. NIGRO (1912–2009)

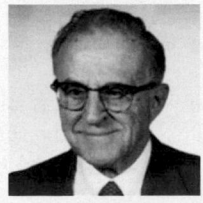

Norman Nigro was born in Syracuse, New York, but moved to Detroit for his early education. He returned to attend Syracuse University, graduating Phi Beta Kappa with a liberal arts degree in 1934 and a doctorate in medicine in 1937. Following internship at Syracuse, he became a preceptee in surgery in Detroit under the tutelage of L. J. Hirshmann. During World War II, he was assigned to the Seventeenth Army General Hospital with the Fifth Army in Italy. At the conclusion of the war, he returned to Wayne State University in Detroit, where he remained for his entire distinguished career. His experiences with Hirshmann led him to develop an interest in colon and rectal surgery, and eventually he achieved the position of secretary to the American Proctologic Society. In 1965, Nigro was elected president of this organization, now known as the American Society of Colon and Rectal Surgeons. He also served as secretary to the American Board of Colon and Rectal Surgery from 1972 to 1986. As a consequence of his work on the combined therapy for anal canal cancer, numerous honors have been bestowed on him, including an honorary lectureship in his name at the annual convention of the American Society of Colon and Rectal Surgeons. His papers have been among the most requested and quoted, according to the National Library of Medicine. In later years, he made notable contributions to the understanding of the role of nutrition in the etiology of cancer of the large bowel. Norman Nigro retired from active practice in 1989 and died in retirement in Scottsdale, Arizona, in his 98th year.

The United Kingdom Coordinating Committee on Cancer Research trial compared the results of treatment, randomizing radiation therapy alone versus radiotherapy and chemotherapy (5-fluorouracil and mitomycin).[156] A total of 585 individuals participated in the protocol. Clinical responses were assessed 6 weeks following initial treatment. Good responders were recommended for boost radiotherapy, whereas poor responders were submitted to "salvage surgery." After a median follow-up of 42 months, patients receiving radiation therapy alone had a local treatment failure rate of 59%, whereas those receiving combined-modality therapy had a local failure rate of only 36%. These differences were highly statistically significant. The only downside was that early morbidity was significantly more frequent with the combined treatment, but late morbidity was about the same. The working party concluded that standard treatment should be a combined approach. They further recommended that surgery should be reserved for patients in whom this regimen fails.[156]

Das and coworkers from MD Anderson Cancer Center examined their data with 167 patients treated by chemoradiation in order to determine patterns of recurrence.[36] Of note is that the majority of patients were administered 5-FU and Cisplatin, not mitomycin C. They found that a higher T or N stage predicted locoregional failure. A higher N stage or basaloid histopathology revealed a greater number of more distant metastases. Overall survival was worse with a higher N stage or a positive HIV status. They suggested that different (more aggressive) therapy is warranted for those individuals with more advanced disease. Also, because of local pelvic recurrences, they recommended that the radiation field should include up to L5/S1.[C]

Doci and colleagues treated 56 consecutive patients with a modified protocol, emphasizing that because of variable toxicity it may be necessary to suspend or alter treatment for certain individuals.[39] A complete response was noted in 87%, 8 of whom had evidence of positive nodes. The actuarially corrected 5-year survival was 81%.

Flam and associates reported that 26 of 30 patients were rendered free of disease as a result of initial combined-modality treatment.[42] The 4 patients with demonstrable residual tumor were subjected to additional treatment with radiation and chemotherapy. None underwent an operation, and none had evidence of recurrence, although follow-up for many was relatively short. The authors counsel that a salvage regimen, such as 5-fluorouracil infusion and cisplatin or sequential methotrexate–5-fluorouracil–leucovorin with radiotherapy, should be instituted before consideration of radical resective measures.[42]

The Radiation Therapy Oncology Group (RTOG) compared cisplatin with mitomycin-based chemoradiation.[3] They concluded that cisplatin did not improve disease-free survival. Furthermore, cisplatin-based therapy led to a higher requirement for a colostomy. However, a study from the United Kingdom (ACT II) showed equivalent results with cisplatin and mitomycin, but less hematologic toxicities in the cisplatin group.[1,20] Willett presented the most recent data from the RTOG 98-11 study and demonstrated an improved survival with mitomycin.[163] The best regimen remains unclear although most centers prefer mitomycin-based therapy as of this writing.

It would clearly be advantageous if one could predict which patients were more likely to recur or not respond to treatment. Roohipour and colleagues (Memorial Sloan-Kettering Cancer Center) looked at predictors of treatment outcomes from their database of 131 patients with stages 1 to 3 disease.[130] They concluded that more advanced stage and incomplete radiation treatment were significant risk factors for failure. Tomaszewski and coworkers reviewed their 25-year Australian experience and found that a higher T stage and male sex led to more local failure.[154] A higher N stage indicated a greater risk for distant metastases. They suggest that groin irradiation could be omitted but only for T1 lesions.[154]

It has been thought that HIV-positive patients do less well with anal cancer than HIV-negative individuals. Kim and coworkers tested this hypothesis by analyzing 98 patients in accordance with their HIV status.[76] The HIV-positive and HIV-negative groups differed by age (42 vs. 62 years), gender (92% vs. 42% males), and homosexuality (46% vs. 15%). Acute treatment toxicities also differed significantly (positive, 80% vs. negative, 30%). Finally, only 62% of HIV-positive patients were disease free after initial therapy as compared with 85% of HIV-negative persons. Median time to cancer-related death was also statistically significantly shorter in HIV-positive patients (1.4 as compared with 5.3 years).[76]

However, Chiao and associates presented data from a large Veterans Administration (VA) study.[22] Almost 1,200 patients with anal squamous cancer were studied, and 175 were HIV positive. They found that HIV infection did not affect survival. Age, sex, metastatic disease at diagnosis, and comorbidities were adverse factors. Survival was the same at 2 years in both groups.

In the previously mentioned population-based study that used data from the Surveillance, Epidemiology, and End Results Cancer Registry, the overall 5-year relative survival for the entire cohort (5,820 patients) was 64.9%.[101]

Treatment and Results of Cloacogenic Carcinoma

As with all invasive anal canal cancers, classical treatment had been APR (Figure 25-18). Results following resection (without chemoradiation) have been essentially the same as that reported for epidermoid carcinoma, the 5-year survival rate being approximately 50%.[29,66,75,141] However, the applicability of the combined-modality approach is as valid for this histologic type as it is for epidermoid carcinoma, and this should be the objective of management. As has been established by a number of authors, survival rates should be the same.

Posttherapy Evaluation and Treatment

The question of how to address posttherapy evaluation is still a matter of some debate. Biopsy or local excision of the scar site *may* be performed 6 to 12 weeks after completion of the regimen. If no tumor is found, the patient is observed at intervals, perhaps every 2 to 3 months. Any suspicious area is subsequently examined by biopsy. Some surgeons prefer observation without biopsy if no suspicious area is evident. Most clinicians believe that recurrent or persistent tumor following chemoradiation therapy mandates radical resection. Others assert that an additional course of chemoradiation therapy may be warranted.[42]

Recent studies indicate the use of PET/CT for posttreatment assessment.[102,157] Vercellino and colleagues demonstrated PET/CT to be an accurate staging modality, but also found it to helpful in the posttreatment evaluation phase. As more studies are undertaken, this may become the standard of care and replace the need for subsequent biopsies.

It is not unusual to develop radiation-induced injury after combined-modality treatment. Problems such as stricture, fistula, and ulceration may supervene. Oral vitamin A therapy has been anecdotally suggested for those with symptomatic postradiation anal ulceration (see Chapter 28).[83]

Petrelli and colleagues reported the application of SCC antigen as a tumor marker for the follow-up of patients with carcinoma of the anal canal.[119] The procedure was initially developed and used primarily for women with carcinoma of the uterus, but its applicability for epidermoid carcinoma of the anal canal has been proposed. In the report from the Roswell Park Cancer Institute, 33 patients with histologic documentation of squamous cell carcinoma of the anal canal underwent serial collection for radioimmunoassay of SCC antigen.[119] In the 33 individuals analyzed, the sensitivity of this antigen was 76%, specificity 86%, and positive predictive value 62%. The implication of this is that with longer follow-up and greater accumulation of patients, SCC antigen may prove to be a valuable tumor marker in the long-term follow-up of individuals with squamous cell carcinoma of the anal canal. Additionally, there are preliminary studies evaluating epidermal growth factor targeting with cetuximab, a monoclonal antibody.[1,132] This and other markers may impact diagnosis and treatment in the future.

Salvage Surgery

There are now numerous articles reporting the results of so-called salvage surgery following chemoradiation therapy—that is, APR. In the experience of Longo and colleagues, 53% of those who underwent APR for persistent tumor were alive.[88] Not all achieved a 5-year follow-up, however. Zelnick and coworkers analyzed 30 patients who underwent APR for treatment failures.[167] The mean follow-up was 35 months. In their experience and that of others, the mortality rate within 3 years was 71%.

Pocard and associates (Paris) identified 21 patients with residual or recurrent anal canal carcinoma following radiotherapy on whom an APR had been performed.[124] Of these, 11 had residual disease following treatment, and 10 subsequently developed recurrence. With a mean follow-up of 40 months, the overall survival was 58%. However, 60% of those with residual disease were alive at 5 years, whereas there were no survivors in the group that developed recurrences.[124] Clearly, there is a need for adjuvant treatment in addition to APR for those who develop recurrence.

Nilsson and colleagues in Stockholm analyzed 35 individuals from the Stockholm Health Care Region who had locoregional failure after multimodality treatment and who underwent APR.[106] There were no postoperative deaths. However, there was considerable morbidity associated with healing of the perineal wound. The crude 5-year survival was 52% (median follow-up, 33 months). The issue of management of the perineal wound is discussed in Chapter 24. Tei and coworkers advocated the use of a transpelvic rectus abdominis musculocutaneous flap concomitant with APR that is undertaken following radiation therapy for anal cancer.[153] Primary healing occurred in all 14 patients so managed.

Overview Opinion

The following protocol is recommended for the management of carcinoma of the anal canal:

- *Local excision* may be an adequate operation for patients with invasion into the submucosa or the internal sphincter only. Endoanal ultrasound, MRI, or PET/CT may be useful for staging the tumor. Close follow-up evaluation should be pursued, and biopsies of suspicious areas should be undertaken. Chemoradiation therapy should be considered for recurrent tumor, with APR reserved for those in whom this therapy fails.
- Those with *suspected invasion into the muscle, perirectal, or perianal soft tissue* should undergo preoperative combined-modality therapy in accordance with the Nigro protocol.
- *Persistent tumor* following chemoradiation therapy should be managed by APR and with the possible addition of chemoradiation therapy. *Recurrent tumor* that develops during follow-up after combined-modality treatment requires APR with adjuvant therapy to the level of tolerance.
- If *metastatic inguinal nodes persist or subsequently develop* following chemoradiation therapy, interval radical groin dissection should be considered.

The Nigro protocol or one of his modifications has clearly become the standard for the treatment of anal canal cancer against which all other options must be compared. However, the optimal dosage for radiation and the timing and choices of chemotherapeutic regimens are still evolving. Because there are now sufficient numbers of patients from many centers who have undergone combined-modality treatment for this condition, one is justified in making a dogmatic statement. Results are so impressive that unless otherwise contraindicated, contemporary medical treatment mandates that this approach be used initially for all patients with invasive anal canal cancer.

Radiation Therapy Alone

As previously discussed, squamous cell carcinoma is a radiosensitive tumor. The application of external beam radiation therapy as the sole method for the treatment of carcinoma of the anal canal, without chemotherapy, therefore, still has relevance. In a retrospective review of 51 patients who were treated with radiation therapy alone, with surgery reserved for those with residual carcinoma, Cummings and associates noted a survival rate of 59%.[32] More than one-half of the patients' tumors were controlled by this approach. Twenty-three of 30 long-term survivors did not require a colostomy.

Following treatment with 45 to 50 Gy, 183 patients at the Curie Institute in Paris were examined by both the radiotherapist and the surgeon.[109] When there was evidence to suggest a lack of response, the patient underwent excisional surgery. Otherwise, the radiation treatment was carried to 60 or 65 Gy. An operation was performed only for persistent tumor or for recurrence. One hundred fifty-eight patients received curative radiotherapy, 115 of whom did not undergo operation. Eighty were alive with no evidence of disease with a minimum of 3 years of follow-up. Five-year survival was 56% for squamous cancers and 62% for cloacogenic cancers.[135]

Experience from the Mayo Clinic using external radiation therapy without chemotherapy revealed that the overall 5-year survival rate was in excess of 90%.[92] However, most of these patients had very favorable initial lesions, some of which were completely excised before radiation. Still, in this group of individuals especially, a radiation therapeutic approach without chemotherapy seems reasonable. Touboul and colleagues advocated a treatment protocol that differentiates the approach according to tumor stage and tumor size.[155] They recommended radiation therapy alone for those individuals who harbor a tumor of 4 cm or smaller and limit chemoradiation therapy to those with larger tumors or those that are fixed. One thing is clear: chemotherapy when combined with radiation reduces the amount of radiation required. Hence, fewer late complications may be anticipated.

As with chemoradiation therapy, the options following recurrence with radiation therapy alone are essentially the same—additional nonsurgical treatment, radical resection, and local excision. Zoetmulder and Baris performed local excision with reconstitution of the anal canal by means of myocutaneous flaps.[168] The advantage of this approach is that it theoretically brings nonirradiated tissue into the field, thereby increasing the likelihood of effecting primary healing.

Interstitial Curie Therapy

In 1974, Papillon (see Chapter 24) reported 98 epidermoid carcinomas treated by interstitial Curie therapy over a 20-year period.[110] This was usually accomplished with the patient under general anesthesia and by using radium needles inserted either through the skin or the anal mucosa. The dose was less than 40 Gy in 2 or 3 days. A second implant was usually performed for residual tumor 2 months after the first implant, and external irradiation could also be given coincident with the implantation. Sixty-four patients were followed for more than 5 years, 44 of whom were alive and free of disease (68%).

James and colleagues reported their experience from Manchester, England, with 74 patients who underwent this treatment.[70] Thirty-five developed recurrences (47%), of whom 26 underwent surgery (28 with curative intent). The local control rate for patients with tumors smaller than 5 cm and with negative inguinal nodes was significantly better than that for patients with more advanced disease.

Papillon cautioned that treatment must be planned carefully to avoid radionecrosis. Later, he and Montbarbon suggested a split course of irradiation with ^{60}Co and ^{192}Ir, and they have been adding chemotherapy during the first few days.[112]

Although selective in the choice of patients for this procedure, including only those with the most favorable prognosis, the results are encouraging and imply that this approach is worthy of further study. In a still later report from Papillon's center in Lyon, France, the following conclusion was reached: "The treatment of carcinoma of the anal margin is not as simple as it may seem to be at first sight. It should be conceived as a team effort by surgeons, radiotherapists, and medical oncologists to define the most appropriate treatment strategy."[111]

Carcinoma in a Hemorrhoidectomy Specimen

The problem of what to do when the pathologist reports a focus of carcinoma in a hemorrhoidectomy specimen is one of the quandaries that occasionally confronts the surgeon (Figures 25-19 and 25-20). Some have criticized the technique of rubber ring ligation for hemorrhoids because it fails to obtain a specimen that could harbor an occult neoplasm. However, the surgeon often wishes that he or she were not aware of the focus of carcinoma because it carries with it the burden of having to make some sort of recommendation. Some have suggested that hemorrhoid tissue should not be submitted for pathologic evaluation in order to avoid any confusion, so rare is malignant change observed and so favorable the prognosis with no treatment (see Chapter 11). However, if one is unfortunate enough to obtain a pathology report that describes the presence of *invasive* carcinoma, the microscopic appearance should at least be confirmed and the depth of invasion ascertained. This underscores the rationale for sending hemorrhoidectomy specimens separately, thereby identifying the exact location. It is usually not helpful to examine the patient until the wounds are healed. Parenthetically, the presence of carcinoma in situ does not require further evaluation or treatment. The following protocol is recommended for invasive cancer:

- Reexamine the patient under anesthesia in 4 to 6 weeks when the wounds are healed, and perform multiple biopsies.
- If results of the biopsies are negative, follow the patient's status at 3-month intervals for 1 year, and perform a biopsy of any suspicious areas.
- If no recurrence develops by 1 year, the patient is considered cured. If a recurrence is identified, the patient may be considered for local excision or the standard therapy protocol for anal canal carcinoma.

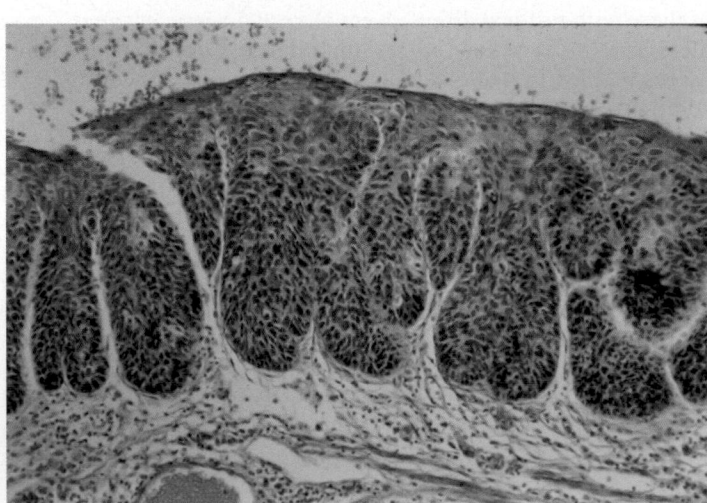

FIGURE 25-19. Squamous cell carcinoma in situ. Note the complete destruction of the architecture of the squamous epithelium with absence of maturation and preserved basement membrane. (Original magnification × 250; courtesy of Rudolf Garret, MD.)

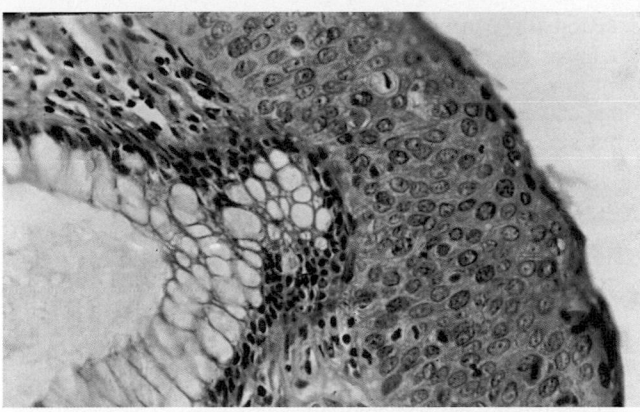

FIGURE 25-20. Squamous cell carcinoma in situ discovered in a hemorrhoidectomy specimen. Note the atypical squamous cells occupying the full thickness of the epithelium. Normally, surface mucosa consists of columnar cells, as in the gland seen here. (Original magnification × 250; from Corman ML, Veidenheimer MC, Swinton NW. *Diseases of the Anus, Rectum and Colon. Part I: Neoplasms.* New York, NY: Medcom; 1972, with permission.)

▶ MALIGNANT MELANOMA

Although the anal canal represents the most common site for the development of malignant melanoma in the alimentary tract, and the third most common overall, it is an extremely rare condition, accounting for only 0.2% of all melanomas and 0.5% of tumors of the anorectum.[13] The tumor is presumed to arise from melanocytes present in the squamous mucosa of the lower anal canal. Mason and Helwig reviewed 17 cases seen at the Armed Forces Institute of Pathology in Washington, DC, and concluded that all the evidence argued against any melanoma arising from the rectal mucosa.[93] Other authors, however, have claimed that melanoma may be primary in the lower rectum as well as in the anal canal.[4] Cooper and associates analyzed 255 cases and added 12 of their own, but fewer than 500 cases had been reported as of 1982.[26] The largest series from one institution is from the Memorial Sloan-Kettering Cancer Center.[6,128] The most recent paper, presented in 1994 and published in 1995, reviewed their experience from 1929 to 1993.[13] A total of 85 patients was identified: 46 females and 39 males. Others have shown a higher incidence of female predominance (2.4:1).[146] Goldman and colleagues analyzed the total Swedish population between 1970 and 1984 and found 49 people with this disease.[52]

Cagir and associates of Jefferson Medical College in Philadelphia used the NCI Surveillance, Epidemiology, and End Results database covering the period 1973 through 1992.[18] They identified 117 patients. This represents 0.048% of all colorectal malignancies. The male-to-female ratio was 1:1.72, and the mean age at diagnosis was 66 years, but men tended to be younger. There is a suggestion from this study that there is an increased predisposition for the development of malignant melanoma perhaps in a less virulent form in the HIV-positive population, but these observations require more data.

Ragnarsson-Olding and associates reviewed the 40-year Swedish national data (1960 to 1999) and found the incidence was also higher in women. Prognosis was poor, but female patients did fare better (10.6% vs. 15.7% 5-year survival).[129] The incidence increased with age for both sexes.

Symptoms

Rectal bleeding is the most common complaint, 54% in the Memorial Sloan-Kettering Cancer Center series.[6,13] Anorectal pain and change in bowel habits are also frequently reported. Many patients note a feeling of a lump or a "hemorrhoid," with its attendant discomfort. A mass in the groin may also be the initial complaint. In the experience of the Memorial Sloan-Kettering Cancer Center, 8% had the melanoma discovered upon pathologic review of hemorrhoidectomy specimens.[13]

Physical Findings

Findings on physical examination vary from a small, hemorrhoid-like, pigmented lesion to a deeply ulcerating or polypoid mass at or near the anorectal junction (Figure 25-21). Pigment may be readily apparent, but Quan and associates reported that 29% of these lesions were histologically amelanotic, an incidence similar to that noted by Cooper and colleagues.[13,26,128] In the Memorial Sloan-Kettering experience, an indication of the advanced stage of the disease and, therefore, the poor prognosis was reflected by the fact that 75% of individuals harbored tumors greater than 1 cm in diameter (average, 4 cm). A later report revealed the median tumor size in individuals undergoing APR to be 3.0 cm.[13] This compared with a median tumor size of 3.3 cm in individuals undergoing local procedures.[6]

Histology

Cells comprising the lesion usually assume either a polygonal or a spindle shape (Figure 25-22) and are often arranged in nests to produce an alveolar pattern. If the mucosa overlying the lesion is not ulcerated, evidence of a junctional

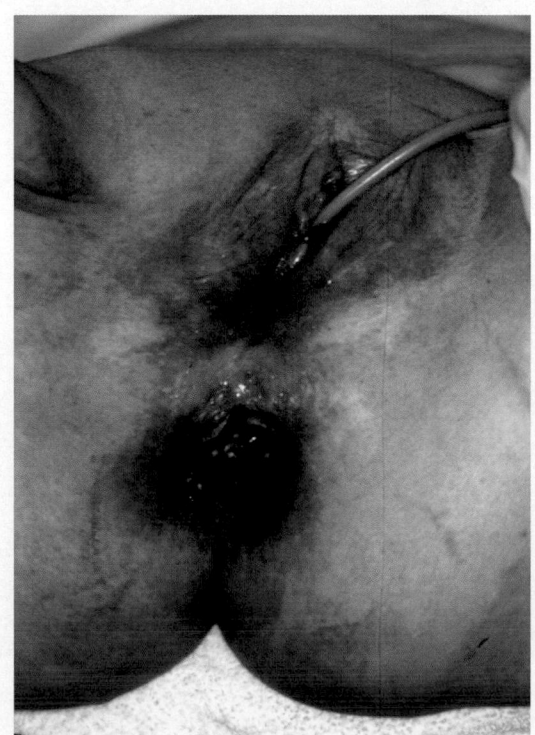

FIGURE 25-21. Malignant melanoma of the anus. A pigmented polypoid mass can be seen outside the anal verge.

component, such as nests of melanoma cells within the squamous epithelium, may be found. This finding confirms the squamous mucosa of the anal canal as the primary site of origin. Identification of melanin within the tumor cells permits diagnosis of the lesion as a melanoma rather than as a poorly differentiated carcinoma. Melanin pigmentation was readily apparent in 11 of the 17 tumors reported by Mason and Helwig and was demonstrable by special staining techniques in four additional lesions.[93] Electron microscopy can be of value in identifying apparently amelanotic melanomas by demonstrating melanosomes within the tumor cells.

Treatment and Results

Because anorectal melanoma is more likely to metastasize to mesenteric lymph nodes than squamous cell carcinoma of the anus, APR (Figure 25-23) has been the standard of treatment. This and radical groin lymph node dissection had been the mainstays of surgical therapies for this condition. However, because the prognosis has been so grim, a case has been made for either no treatment at all or simply local excision.[131] Several reports have noted no statistically significant difference in survival rate of patients treated for cure by local excision versus APR.[14,26,68,77,146] As a consequence, wide local

excision for a tumor that can be removed by this method has been suggested.[14,91] The major benefit of radical resection may be for controlling local and regional disease.[52,146] Quan and associates reported one survivor (5%),[128] and most other series report either none or only the occasional cure at 5 years.[8,12,23,27,45,131,142,146,160] Bullard and Tuttle in Minneapolis, Minnesota, noted that two patients out of seven (29%) were alive at 5 years.[14] Based on the Memorial Sloan-Kettering experience, two conclusions were set forth[13]:

- Most patients with anorectal melanoma will die of their disease regardless of therapy.
- There is a small subset of patients with localized, relatively early disease or favorable tumor biology in whom a surgical cure can be achieved.

The Memorial Sloan-Kettering group, therefore, opined that APR with pelvic lymphadenectomy is a reasonable alternative for those individuals without locally advanced tumors or evidence of regional lymph node involvement. In these patients, they emphasize the importance of pelvic lymphadenectomy. One pertinent observation was that all of their long-term survivors were women. It appears that female sex was a favorable prognostic factor in individuals with cutaneous melanoma as well. Women with operable

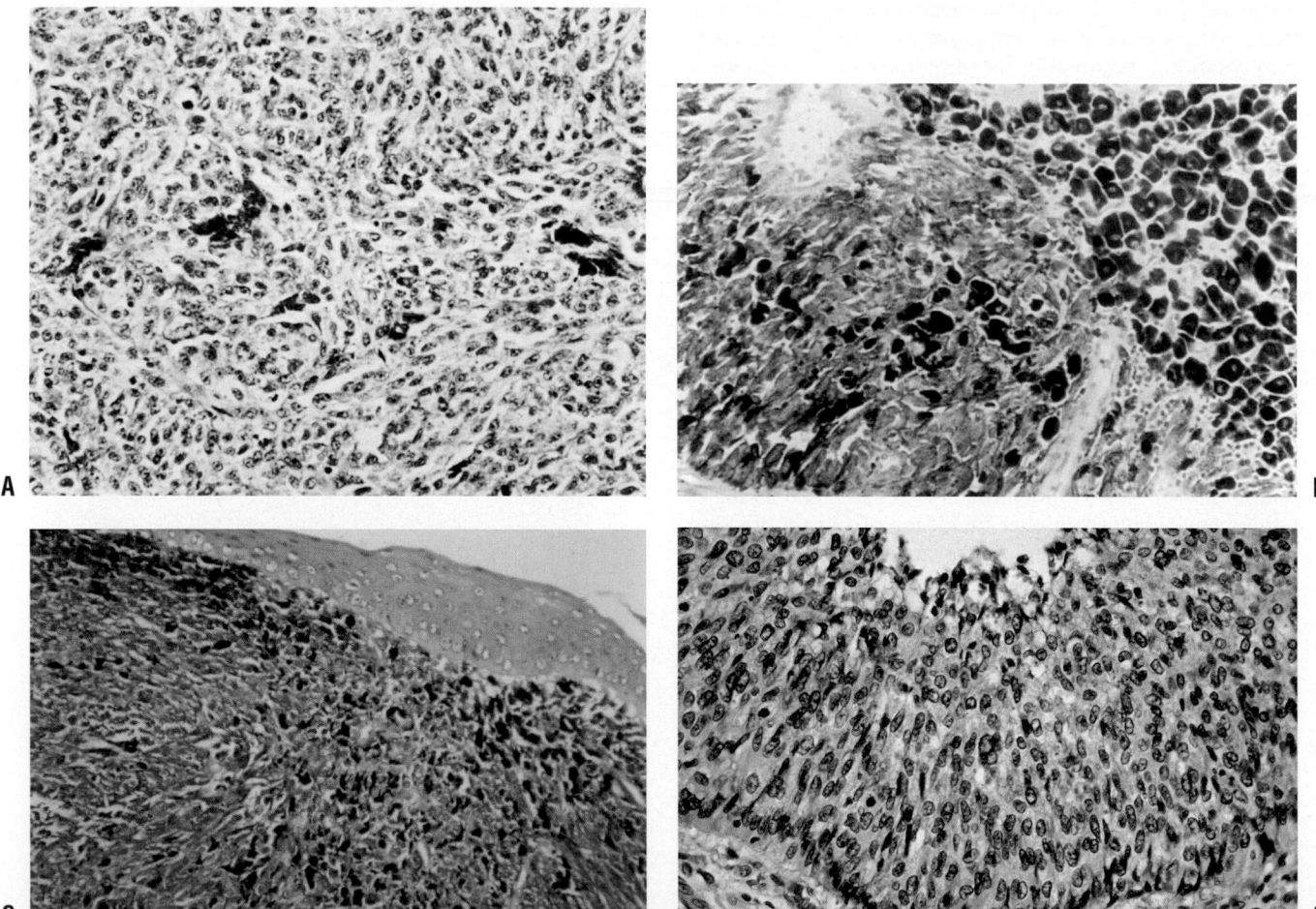

FIGURE 25-22. Melanoma of the anus. **A:** This very poorly differentiated tumor is recognizable as a melanoma only because of the black pigment being produced. (Original magnification × 250.) **B:** Melanoma of the anal canal. Another variant displaying an epithelioid pattern with extensive melanin pigment present. (Original magnification × 360.) **C:** Brown pigment of melanoma in poorly differentiated lesion; note overlying squamous/transitional epithelium. **D:** Malignant melanoma of the anus reveals sheets of melanin-pigmented cells infiltrating the mucosa and submucosa of the lower rectum. Foci of residual glands may still be seen. (Original magnification × 250.)

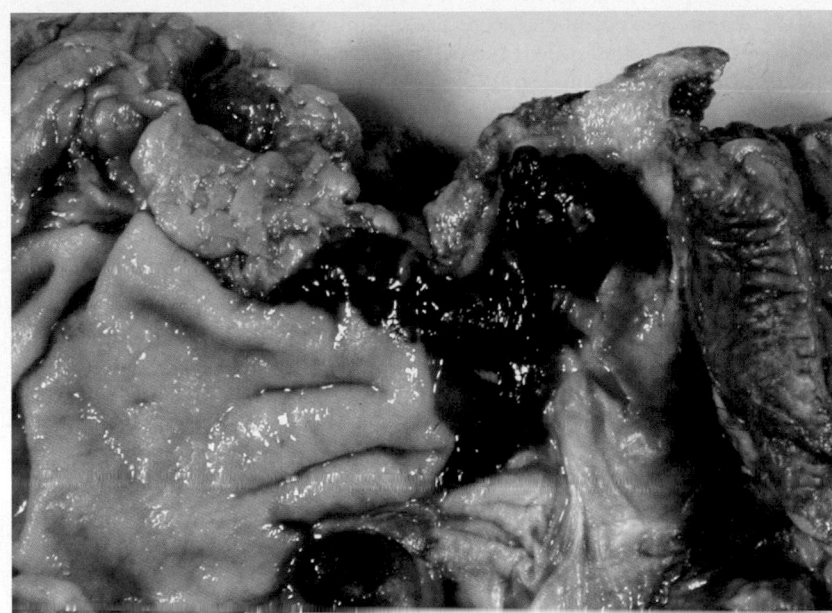

FIGURE 25-23. Proctectomy specimen reveals densely melanotic pigmentation of a practically circumferential lesion of the anal canal.

melanoma of the anus according to the criteria set forth by the Memorial Sloan-Kettering Cancer group have a 29% survival following APR. However, the previously mentioned report by Cagir and coworkers, based on 117 patients in the NCI registry, found that male patients (especially young and positive for HIV) do better than females, but it appears that age rather than sex is the more important variable.[18] The overall survival rate in both sexes was less than 20% at 5 years.

Supplementary treatment with radiotherapy has been of no consistent benefit nor have the various chemotherapeutic agents uniformly helped. Immunotherapy, usually with bacille Calmette–Guérin vaccine, has been employed for malignant melanoma in other sites, but recommendations concerning its value with malignant melanoma of the anal canal have been anecdotal and discouraging. Most investigators, however, recommend an aggressive multimodality approach, but there has been no consistency in the patient selection, pathologic extent, or treatment employed with the relatively few long-term survivors reported.

► MISCELLANEOUS ANAL CONDITIONS

Verrucous Squamous Carcinoma

A very rare tumor, verrucous squamous carcinoma, has come to be known as the tumor of Buschke and Löwenstein because of their description of it in 1925.[17] The lesion is frequently confused with benign anal conditions, especially condyloma (see Chapter 9). It may appear as a pale, pink, cauliflower-like mass on the perianal skin or in the anal canal (see Figure 9-61).

Histologically, the tumor is so well differentiated that it closely resembles benign proliferative lesions of squamous epithelium, and it may not be recognizable as a carcinoma until invasion of underlying structures can be identified. For this reason, superficial biopsies of verrucous squamous cell carcinomas are frequently not diagnosed as carcinoma. Biopsies should be taken from the base of the lesion to demonstrate invasion.

Classical treatment consists of wide local excision or APR for invasive tumors.[48,86,149] However, the value of combined-modality therapy needs to be explored (for additional discussion, see Chapter 9).

Keratoacanthoma

Keratoacanthoma is an exophytic, benign skin tumor, usually with a central crater, 0.5 to 2.0 cm in diameter, that is most often associated with exposure to the sun.[72] Only three cases involving the perianal skin and one in the anal canal have been reported.[72] Local excision or electrocoagulation should be curative, although the histologic appearance may mimic that of squamous cell carcinoma.

Pseudosarcomatous Carcinoma

Pseudosarcoma has been described in the esophagus, larynx, oral cavity, and other areas, but Kuwano and associates reported the first and only case of such a tumor in the anal canal.[80] The patient presented with a pedunculated 4-cm mass. Microscopic examination of the locally excised specimen revealed epithelial elements in sarcoma-like areas. No recurrence was noted after a 25-month follow-up.

Carcinoma of the Anal Glands and Ducts

Colloid or mucinous adenocarcinoma of anal glandular or ductal origin is a rare entity.[62,162,164] Parks stated, however, that although the condition is extremely uncommon, it may not be as infrequent as the literature suggests.[115] This, he postulated, is explained by the fact that the site of origin is destroyed early by the malignant growth. Jensen and colleagues identified 21 individuals treated from Denmark from 1943 to 1982.[71] Nine lesions were found in a perianal location, seven within the anal canal, and five in anal fistulas. Three were found serendipitously in hemorrhoidectomy specimens. The presence of Paget's disease may be a consequence of an underlying carcinoma, such as can arise from the anal ducts (see Chapter 9).

Abel and colleagues surveyed the members of the American Society of Colon and Rectal Surgeons and identified 52 cases for analysis.[2] Symptoms of anal pain were found in 58% and rectal bleeding in 40%. Thirty-seven percent perceived a mass, whereas more than half presented with a fistula.

Treatment

Because this is a highly malignant variant, APR is usually recommended. Local excision, however, may be considered for early lesions, but radical resection is generally required to control disease.[2] The place of chemoradiation therapy is probably similar to that of conventional adenocarcinoma of the rectum, but this has not been clearly defined. The Memorial Sloan-Kettering Cancer Center group in 2003 treated 13 patients with primary adenocarcinoma of the anal canal with three operative and chemoradiation therapy alternatives.[10] In a relatively short-term follow-up and with a small number of patients with this unusual tumor, the authors concluded that a combined-therapy approach is reasonable.

Results

Basik and coworkers reviewed the prognosis of anal adenocarcinoma from the Roswell Park Cancer Institute.[7] Eight patients underwent radical resection and two local excision. Median survival was 29 months, with seven patients developing recurrence. It is evident that anal adenocarcinoma is associated with a poor prognosis despite radical surgery.

Adenosquamous Carcinoma

This rare tumor of the large bowel composing both squamous and glandular malignant features can even more rarely affect the anal canal. The condition is discussed in Chapter 26.

Merkel Cell (Neuroendocrine) Carcinoma

Merkel cell tumors are rare neuroendocrine, small cell malignancies usually found on the skin, most commonly on exposed surfaces. These tumors behave aggressively when found in less typical areas.[116] A single example of this condition affecting the anal canal has been reported.[116] In this one instance that was treated by local excision, the patient died 13 months later of metastatic disease. Neuroendocrine tumors affecting the colon and rectum are discussed in Chapter 26.

Malignant Fibrous Histiocytoma

Malignant fibrous histiocytoma is a pleomorphic sarcoma that classically arises in the extremities and metastasizes to the lungs and regional lymph nodes, but it also can occur rarely in the gastrointestinal tract.[43] Flood and colleagues identified the first and only case involving the anal canal.[43] This was managed by APR and radiotherapy.

Inflammatory Cloacogenic Polyp

Inflammatory cloacogenic polyp is a nonneoplastic anal tumor that may be analogous to a prolapse in the area of the transitional zone. Lobert and Appelman identified eight such cases and noted that the primary complaint is usually rectal bleeding.[85] The polyp in their experience was found primarily on the anterior wall of the anal canal, not unlike the distribution seen in solitary rectal ulcer (see Chapter 20). However, in the eight cases identified by Lobert and Appelman, instead of the usual female predominance, there were five men.[85] The etiology of the condition is uncertain, but theories include ischemia, trauma (manual, stercoral), congenital, and early prolapse. Histologically, the lesion is characterized by a tubulovillous pattern of growth, superficial ulceration, displaced crypts, and extension of chronically inflamed fibromuscular stroma into the lamina propria (Figure 25-24).[85] Treatment consists simply of local excision.

Basal Cell Carcinoma, Bowen's Disease, and Paget's Disease

See Chapter 9.

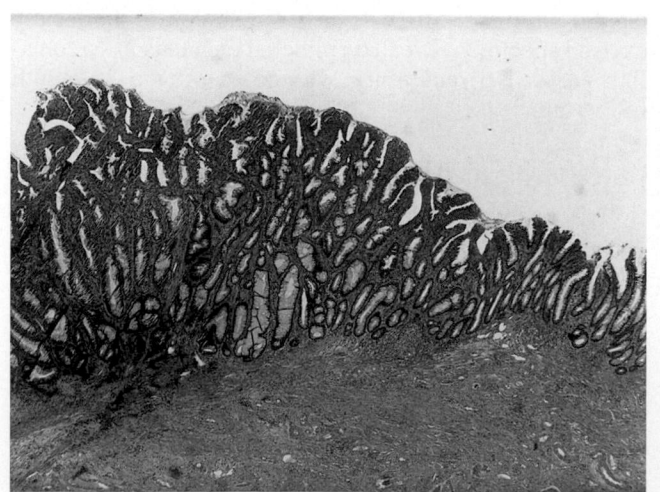
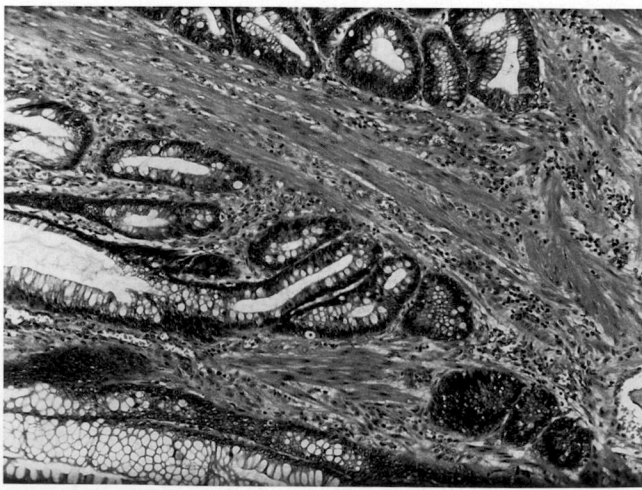

A

B

FIGURE 25-24. Inflammatory cloacogenic polyp. **A:** Nonulcerated surface showing glandular hyperplasia with a thickened submucosa. (Original magnification × 20.) **B:** Higher power demonstrates colonic glands and inflammatory cells with muscle bundles extending between the glands into the submucosa. (Original magnification × 100.)

References

1. Abbas A, Yang G, Fakih M, et al. Management of anal cancer in 2010. Part 2: current treatment standards and future directions. *Oncology (Williston Park).* 2010;24(5):417–424.
2. Abel ME, Chiu YS, Russell TR, et al. Adenocarcinoma of the anal glands. Results of a survey. *Dis Colon Rectum.* 1993;36(4):383–387.
3. Ajani JA, Winter KA, Gunderson LL, et al. Fluorouracil, mitomycin, and radiotherapy vs fluorouracil, cisplatin, and radiotherapy for carcinoma of the anal canal: a randomized controlled trial. *JAMA.* 2008;299(16):1914–1921.
4. Alexander RM, Cone LA. Malignant melanoma of the rectal ampulla: report of a case and review of the literature. *Dis Colon Rectum.* 1977;20(1):53–55.
5. Balamucki CJ, Zlotecki RA, Rout WR, et al. Squamous cell carcinoma of the anal margin: the university of Florida experience. *Am J Clin Oncol.* 2011;34(4):406–410.
6. Banner WP, Quan SHQ, Woodruff JM. Malignant melanoma of the anorectum. *Surg Rounds* 1990;13:28–32.
7. Basik M, Rodriguez-Bigas MA, Penetrante R, et al. Prognosis and recurrence patterns of anal adenocarcinoma. *Am J Surg.* 1995;169(2):233–237.
8. Baskies AM, Sugarbaker EV, Chretien PB, et al. Anorectal melanoma. The role of posterior pelvic exenteration. *Dis Colon Rectum.* 1982;25(8):772–777.
9. Beahrs OH, Wilson SM. Carcinoma of the anus. *Ann Surg.* 1976;184(4):422–428.
10. Beal KP, Wong D, Guillem JG. Primary adenocarcinoma of the anus treated with combined modality therapy. *Dis Colon Rectum.* 2003;46(10):1320–1324.
11. Beck DE, Karulf RE. Combination therapy for epidermoid carcinoma of the anal canal. *Dis Colon Rectum.* 1994;37(11):1118–1125.
12. Braastad FW, Dockerty MB, Dixon CF. Melano-epithelioma of anus and rectum: report of cases and review of literature. *Surgery.* 1949;25(1):82–90.
13. Brady MS, Kavolius JP, Quan SH. Anorectal melanoma. A 64-year experience at Memorial Sloan-Kettering Cancer Center. *Dis Colon Rectum.* 1995;38(2):146–151.
14. Bullard KM, Tuttle TM, Rothenberger DA, et al. Surgical therapy for anorectal melanoma. *J Am Coll Surg.* 2003;196(2):206–211.
15. Buroker TR, Nigro N, Bradley G, et al. Combined therapy for cancer of the anal canal: a follow-up report. *Dis Colon Rectum.* 1977;20(8):677–678.
16. Buroker TR, Nigro N, Correa J, et al. Combination preoperative radiation and chemotherapy in adenocarcinoma of the rectum: preliminary report. *Dis Colon Rectum.* 1976;19:660.
17. Buschke A, Löwenstein L. Condylomata acuminata simulating cancer on penis. *Klin Wochenschr.* 1925;4:1726–1728.
18. Cagir B, Whiteford MH, Topham A, et al. Changing epidemiology of anorectal melanoma. *Dis Colon Rectum.* 1999;42(9):1203–1208.
19. Cattell RB, Williams AC. Epidermoid carcinoma of the anus and rectum. *Arch Surg.* 1943;46:336.
20. Chakravarthy AB, Catalano PJ, Martenson JA, et al. Long-term follow-up of a Phase II trial of high-dose radiation with concurrent 5-fluorouracil and cisplatin in patients with anal cancer (ECOG E4292). *Int J Radiat Oncol Biol Phys.* 2011;81(4):e607–e613.
21. Chang GJ, Berry JM, Jay N, et al. Surgical treatment of high-grade anal squamous intraepithelial lesions: a prospective study. *Dis Colon Rectum.* 2002;45(4):453–458.
22. Chiao EY, Giordano TP, Richardson P, et al. Human immunodeficiency virus-associated squamous cell cancer of the anus: epidemiology and outcomes in the highly active antiretroviral therapy era. *J Clin Oncol.* 2008;26(3):474–479.
23. Chiu YS, Unni KK, Beart RW Jr. Malignant melanoma of the anorectum. *Dis Colon Rectum.* 1980;23(2):122–124.
24. Cho CC, Taylor CW III, Padmanabhan A, et al. Squamous-cell carcinoma of the anal canal: management with combined chemo-radiation therapy. *Dis Colon Rectum.* 1991;34(8):675–678.
25. Cooper HS, Patchefsky AS, Marks G. Cloacogenic carcinoma of the anorectum in homosexual men: an observation of four cases. *Dis Colon Rectum.* 1979;22(8):557–558.
26. Cooper PH, Mills SE, Allen MS Jr. Malignant melanoma of the anus: report of 12 patients and analysis of 255 additional cases. *Dis Colon Rectum.* 1982;25(7):693–703.
27. Corman ML, Haggitt RC. Carcinoma of the anal canal. *Surg Gynecol Obstet.* 1977;145(5):674–676.
28. Corman ML, Veidenheimer MC, Swinton NW. *Diseases of the Anus, Rectum and Colon. Part I: Neoplasms.* New York, NY: Medcom; 1972.
29. Cullen PK Jr, Pontius EE, Sanders RJ. Cloacogenic anorectal carcinoma. *Dis Colon Rectum.* 1966;9(1):1–12.
30. Cummings B, Keane T, Thomas G, et al. Results and toxicity of the treatment of anal canal carcinoma by radiation therapy or radiation therapy and chemotherapy. *Cancer.* 1984;54(10):2062–2068.
31. Cummings BJ, Harwood AR, Keane TJ, et al. Combined treatment of squamous cell carcinoma of the anal canal: radical radiation therapy with 5-fluorouracil and mitomycin-C, a preliminary report. *Dis Colon Rectum.* 1980;23(6):389–391.
32. Cummings BJ, Thomas GM, Keane TJ, et al. Primary radiation therapy in the treatment of anal canal carcinoma. *Dis Colon Rectum.* 1982;25(8):778–782.
33. Daling JR, Weiss NS, Hislop TG, et al. Sexual practices, sexually transmitted diseases, and the incidence of anal cancer. *N Engl J Med.* 1987;317(16):973–977.
34. Daling JR, Weiss NS, Klopfenstein LL, et al. Correlates of homosexual behavior and the incidence of anal cancer. *JAMA.* 1982;247(14):1988–1990.
35. Damin DC, Rosito MA, Gus P, et al. Sentinel lymph node procedure in patients with epidermoid carcinoma of the anal canal: early experience. *Dis Colon Rectum.* 2003;46(8):1032–1037.
36. Das P, Bhatia S, Eng C, et al. Predictors and patterns of recurrence after definitive chemoradiation for anal cancer. *Int J Radiat Oncol Biol Phys.* 2007;68(3):794–800.
37. Deans GT, McAleer JJ, Spence RA. Malignant anal tumors. *Br J Surg.* 1994;81(4):500–508.
38. DeGennaro VA, Grossi C, Nealon T Jr. Anorectal malignancy in male homosexuals. *Surg Rounds.* 1986;9:82.
39. Doci R, Zucali R, Bombelli L, et al. Combined chemoradiation therapy for anal cancer. A report of 56 cases. *Ann Surg.* 1992;215(2):150–156.
40. Enker WE, Heilwell M, Janov AJ, et al. Improved survival in epidermoid carcinoma of the anus in association with preoperative multidisciplinary therapy. *Arch Surg.* 1986;121(12):1386–1390.
41. Failes D, Morgan BP. Squamous-cell carcinoma of the anus. *Dis Colon Rectum.* 1973;16(5):397–401.
42. Flam MS, John MJ, Mowry PA, et al. Definitive combined modality therapy of carcinoma of the anus. A report of 30 cases including results of salvage therapy in patients with residual disease. *Dis Colon Rectum.* 1987;30(7):495–502.
43. Flood HD, Salman AA. Malignant fibrous histiocytoma of the anal canal. Report of a case and review of the literature. *Dis Colon Rectum.* 1989;32(3):256–259.
44. Fontana X, Lagrange JL, Francois E, et al. Assessment of "squamous cell carcinoma antigen" (SCC) as a marker of epidermoid carcinoma of the anal canal. *Dis Colon Rectum.* 1991;34(2):126–131.
45. Freedman LS. Malignant melanoma of the anorectal region: two cases of prolonged survival. *Br J Surg.* 1984;71(2):164–165.
46. Frisch M, Olsen JH, Bautz A, et al. Benign anal lesions and the risk of anal cancer. *N Engl J Med.* 1994;331(5):300–302.
47. Gillespie JJ, MacKay B. Histogenesis of cloacogenic carcinoma. Fine structure of anal transitional epithelium and cloacogenic carcinoma. *Hum Pathol.* 1978;9(5):579–587.
48. Gingrass PJ, Bubrick MP, Hitchcock CR, et al. Anorectal verrucose squamous carcinoma: report of two cases. *Dis Colon Rectum.* 1978;21(2):120–122.
49. Golden GT, Horsley JS III. Surgical management of epidermoid carcinoma of the anus. *Am J Surg.* 1976;131(3):275–280.
50. Goldman S, Auer G, Erhardt K, et al. Prognostic significance of clinical stage, histologic grade, and nuclear DNA content in squamous-cell carcinoma of the anus. *Dis Colon Rectum.* 1987;30(6):444–448.
51. Goldman S, Glimelius B, Glas U, et al. Management of anal epidermoid carcinoma—an evaluation of treatment results in two population-based series. *Int J Colorectal Dis.* 1989;4(4):234–243.
52. Goldman S, Glimelius B, Påhlman L. Anorectal malignant melanoma in Sweden. Report of 49 patients. *Dis Colon Rectum.* 1990;33(10):874–877.
53. Goldman S, Ihre T, Seligson U. Squamous-cell carcinoma of the anus. A follow-up study of 65 patients. *Dis Colon Rectum.* 1985;28(3):143–146.
54. Goldman S, Skoog L, Wilking N. Immunocytochemical analysis of receptors for estrogen and progesterone in fine needle aspirates from anal epidermoid carcinoma. *Dis Colon Rectum.* 1992;35(2):163–165.
55. Goldstone SE, Winkler B, Ufford LJ, et al. High prevalence of anal squamous intraepithelial lesions and squamous-cell carcinoma in men who have sex with men as seen in a surgical practice. *Dis Colon Rectum.* 2001;44(5):690–698.
56. Greenall MJ, Quan SH, DeCosse JJ. Epidermoid cancer of the anus. *Br J Surg.* 1985;72 suppl:S97–S103.
57. Greenall MJ, Quan SH, Stearns MW, et al. Epidermoid cancer of the anal margin. Pathologic features, treatment, and clinical results. *Am J Surg.* 1985;149(1):95–101.

58. Greenall MJ, Quan SH, Urmacher C, et al. Treatment of epidermoid carcinoma of the anal canal. *Surg Gynecol Obstet.* 1985;161(6):509–517.
59. Grinnell RS. An analysis of fortynine cases of squamous cell carcinoma of the anus. *Surg Gynecol Obstet.* 1954;98(1):29–39.
60. Grinvalsky HT, Helwig EB. Carcinoma of the anorectal junction. I. Histological considerations. *Cancer.* 1956;9(3):480–488.
61. Habr-Gama A, da Silva e Sousa Júnior AH, Nadalin W, et al. Epidermoid carcinoma of the anal canal. Results of treatment by combined chemotherapy and radiation therapy. *Dis Colon Rectum.* 1989;32(9):773–777.
62. Hagihara P, Vazquez MD, Parker JC Jr, et al. Carcinoma of anal-ductal origin: report of a case. *Dis Colon Rectum.* 1976;19(8):694–701.
63. Hamdan KA, Tait IS, Nadeau V, et al. Treatment of grade III anal intraepithelial neoplasia with photodynamic therapy: report of a case. *Dis Colon Rectum.* 2003;46(11):1555–1559.
64. Hobbs CM, Lowry MA, Owen D, et al. Anal gland carcinoma. *Cancer.* 2001;92(8):2045–2049.
65. Holmes F, Borek D, Owen-Kummer M, et al. Anal cancer in women. *Gastroenterology.* 1988;95(1):107–111.
66. Hsu YH, Guzman LG. Cloacogenic carcinoma of the anal canal: experience in eight cases and review of the literature. *Am J Proctol Gastroenterol Colon Rectal Surg.* 1984;35:5–16.
67. Hu K, Minsky BD, Cohen AM, et al. 30 Gy may be an adequate dose in patients with anal cancer treated with excisional biopsy followed by combined-modality therapy. *J Surg Oncol.* 1999;70(2):71–77.
68. Iddings DM, Fleisig AJ, Chen SL, et al. Practice patterns and outcomes for anorectal melanoma in the USA, reviewing three decades of treatment: is more extensive surgical resection beneficial in all patients? *Ann Surg Oncol.* 2010;17(1):40–44.
69. Ioachim HL, Weinstein MA, Robbins RD, et al. Primary anorectal lymphoma. A new manifestation of the acquired immune deficiency syndrome (AIDS). *Cancer.* 1987;60(7):1449–1453.
70. James RD, Pointon RS, Martin S. Local radiotherapy in the management of squamous carcinoma of the anus. *Br J Surg.* 1985;72(4):282–285.
71. Jensen SL, Shokouh-Amiri MH, Hagen K, et al. Adenocarcinoma of the anal ducts. A series of 21 cases. *Dis Colon Rectum.* 1988;31(4):268–272.
72. Jensen SL, Sjølin KE. Keratoacanthoma of the anus. Report of three cases. *Dis Colon Rectum.* 1985;28(10):743–745.
73. Kachnic LA, Tsai HK, Coen JJ, et al. Dose-painted intensity-modulated radiation therapy for anal cancer: a multi-institutional report of acute toxicity and response to therapy. *Int J Radiat Oncol Bio Phys.* 2012;82(1):153–158.
74. Kalogeropoulos NK, Antonakopoulos GN, Agapitos MB, et al. Spindle cell carcinoma (pseudosarcoma) of the anus: a light, electron microscopic and immunocytochemical study of a case. *Histopathology.* 1985;9(9):987–994.
75. Kheir S, Hickey RC, Martin RG, et al. Cloacogenic carcinoma of the anal canal. *Arch Surg.* 1972;104(4):407–415.
76. Kim JH, Sarani B, Orkin BA, et al. HIV-positive patients with anal carcinoma have poorer treatment tolerance and outcome than HIV-negative patients. *Dis Colon Rectum.* 2001;44(10):1496–1502.
77. Kiran RP, Rottoli M, Pokala N, et al. Long-term outcomes after local excision and radical surgery for anal melanoma: data from a population database. *Dis Colon Rectum.* 2010;53(4):402–408.
78. Klotz RG Jr, Pamukcoglu T, Souilliard DH. Transitional cloacogenic carcinoma of the anal canal. Clinicopathologic study of three hundred seventy-three cases. *Cancer.* 1967;20(10):1727–1745.
79. Kondo R, Hanamura N, Kobayashi M, et al. Mucoepidermoid carcinoma of the anal canal: an immunohistochemical study. *J Gastroenterol.* 2001;36(7):508–514.
80. Kuwano H, Iwashita A, Enjoji M. Pseudosarcomatous carcinoma of the anal canal. *Dis Colon Rectum.* 1983;26(2):123–128.
81. Lee MH, Waxman M, Gillooley JF. Primary malignant lymphoma of the anorectum in homosexual men. *Dis Colon Rectum.* 1986;29(6):413–416.
82. Leichman L, Nigro N, Vaitkevicius VK, et al. Cancer of the anal canal. Model for preoperative adjuvant combined modality therapy. *Am J Med.* 1985;78(2):211–215.
83. Levitsky J, Hong JJ, Jani AB, et al. Oral vitamin a therapy for a patient with a severely symptomatic postradiation anal ulceration: report of a case. *Dis Colon Rectum.* 2003;46(5):679–682.
84. Li FP, Osborn D, Cronin CM. Anorectal squamous carcinoma in two homosexual men. *Lancet.* 1982;2(8294):391.
85. Lobert PF, Appelman HD. Inflammatory cloacogenic polyp. A unique inflammatory lesion of the anal transitional zone. *Am J Surg Pathol.* 1981;5(8):761–766.
86. Lock MR, Katz DR, Samoorian S, et al. Giant condyloma of the rectum: report of a case. *Dis Colon Rectum.* 1977;20(2):154–157.

87. Löhnert M, Doniec JM, Kovács G, et al. New method of radiotherapy for anal cancer with three-dimensional tumor reconstruction based on endoanal ultrasound and ultrasound-guided afterloading therapy. *Dis Colon Rectum.* 1998;41(2):169–176.
88. Longo WE, Vernava AM III, Wade TP, et al. Recurrent squamous cell carcinoma of the anal canal. Predictors of initial treatment failure and results of salvage therapy. *Ann Surg.* 1994;220(1):40–49.
89. Lorenz HP, Wilson W, Leigh B, et al. Squamous cell carcinoma of the anus and HIV infection. *Dis Colon Rectum.* 1991;34(4):336–338.
90. Madden MV, Elliot MS, Botha JB, et al. The management of anal carcinoma. *Br J Surg.* 1981;68(4):287–289.
91. Malik A, Hull TL, Milsom J. Long-term survivor of anorectal melanoma: report of a case. *Dis Colon Rectum.* 2002;45(10):1412–1415.
92. Martenson JA Jr, Gunderson LL. External radiation therapy without chemotherapy in the management of anal cancer. *Cancer.* 1993;71(5):1736–1740.
93. Mason JK, Helwig EB. Ano-rectal melanoma. *Cancer.* 1966;19(1):39–50.
94. Melbye M, Coté TR, Kessler L, et al. High incidence of anal cancer among AIDS patients. The AIDS/Cancer Working Group. *Lancet.* 1994;343(8898):636–639.
95. Mendenhall WM, Zlotecki RA, Vauthey JN, et al. Squamous cell carcinoma of the anal margin. *Oncology (Williston Park).* 1996;10(12):1843–1848.
96. Morson BC, Pang LS. Pathology of anal cancer. *Proc R Soc Med.* 1968;61:623–624.
97. Morson BC, Volkstädt H. Muco-epidermoid tumours of the anal canal. *J Clin Pathol.* 1963;16(3):200–205.
98. Muleris M, Salmon RJ, Girodet J, et al. Recurrent deletions of chromosome 11q and 3p in anal canal carcinoma. *Int J Cancer.* 1987;39(5):595–598.
99. Nash G, Allen W, Nash S. Atypical lesions of the anal mucosa in homosexual men. *JAMA.* 1986;256(7):873–876.
100. National Cancer Institute. Anal cancer treatment (PDQ): General information about anal cancer. http://www.cancer.gov/cancertopics/pdq/treatment/anal/patient. Updated December 09, 2011. Accessed.
101. National Cancer Institute. SEER stat fact sheets: anal cancer. 2011. http://seer.cancer.gov/statfacts/html/anus.html. Accessed.
102. Nguyen BT, Joon DL, Khoo V, et al. Assessing the impact of FDG-PET in the management of anal cancer. *Radiother Oncol.* 2008;87(3):376–382.
103. Nigro ND. An evaluation of combined therapy for squamous cell cancer of the anal canal. *Dis Colon Rectum.* 1984;27(12):763–766.
104. Nigro ND, Vaitkevicius VK, Buroker T, et al. Combined therapy for cancer of anal canal. *Dis Colon Rectum.* 1981;24(2):73–75.
105. Nigro ND, Vaitkevicius VK, Considine B Jr. Combined therapy for cancer of the anal canal: a preliminary report. *Dis Colon Rectum.* 1974;17(3):354–356.
106. Nilsson PJ, Svensson C, Goldman S, et al. Salvage abdominoperineal resection in anal epidermoid cancer. *Br J Surg.* 2002;89(11):1425–1429.
107. Otto SD, Lee L, Buhr HJ, et al. Staging anal cancer: prospective comparison of transanal endoscopic ultrasound and magnetic resonance imaging. *J Gastrointest Surg.* 2009;13(7):1292–1298.
108. Palmer JG, Scholefield JH, Coates PJ, et al. Anal cancer and human papillomaviruses. *Dis Colon Rectum.* 1989;32(12):1016–1022.
109. Pang LS, Morson BC. Basaloid carconoma of the anal canal. *J Clin Pathol.* 1967;20(2):128–135.
110. Papillon J. Radiation therapy in the management of epidermoid carcinoma of the anal region. *Dis Colon Rectum.* 1974;17(2):181–187.
111. Papillon J, Chassard JL. Respective roles of radiotherapy and surgery in the management of epidermoid carcinoma of the anal margin. Series of 57 patients. *Dis Colon Rectum.* 1992;35(5):422–429.
112. Papillon J, Montbarbon JF. Epidermoid carcinoma of the anal canal. A series of 276 cases. *Dis Colon Rectum.* 1987;30(5):324–333.
113. Paradis P, Douglass HO Jr, Holyoke ED. The clinical implications of a staging system for carcinoma of the anus. *Surg Gynecol Obstet.* 1975;141(3):411–416.
114. Parikh J, Shaw A, Grant LA, et al. Anal carcinomas: the role of endoanal ultrasound and magnetic resonance imaging in staging, response evaluation and follow-up. *Eur Radiol.* 2011;21(4):776–785.
115. Parks TG. Mucus-secreting adenocarcinoma of anal gland origin. *Br J Surg.* 1970;57(6):434–436.
116. Paterson C, Musselman L, Chorneyko K, et al. Merkel cell (neuroendocrine) carcinoma of the anal canal: report of a case. *Dis Colon Rectum.* 2003;46(5):676–678.
117. Penn I. Cancers of the anogenital region in renal transplant recipients. Analysis of 65 cases. *Cancer.* 1986;58(3):611–616.
118. Perera D, Pathma-Nathan N, Rabbit P, et al. Sentinel node biopsy for squamous-cell carcinoma of the anus and anal margin. *Dis Colon Rectum.* 2003;46(8):1027–1029.

119. Petrelli NJ, Cebollero JA, Rodriguez-Bigas M, et al. Photodynamic therapy in the management of neoplasms of the perianal skin. *Arch Surg.* 1992;127(12):1436–1438.

120. Petrelli NJ, Palmer M, Herrera L, et al. The utility of squamous cell carcinoma antigen for the follow-up of patients with squamous cell carcinoma of the anal canal. *Cancer.* 1992;70(1):35–39.

121. Piketty C, Selinger-Leneman H, Grabar S, et al. Marked increase in the incidence of invasive anal cancer among HIV-infected patients despite treatment with combination antiretroviral therapy. *AIDS.* 2008;22(10):1203–1211.

122. Pintor MP, Northover JM, Nicholls RJ. Squamous cell carcinoma of the anus at one hospital from 1948 to 1984. *Br J Surg.* 1989;76(8):806–810.

123. Place RJ, Gregorcyk SG, Huber PJ, et al. Outcome analysis of HIV-positive patients with anal squamous cell carcinoma. *Dis Colon Rectum.* 2001;44(4):506–512.

124. Pocard M, Tiret E, Nugent K, et al. Results of salvage abdominoperineal resection for anal cancer after radiotherapy. *Dis Colon Rectum.* 1998;41(12):1488–1493.

125. Pyper PC, Parks TG. The results of surgery for epidermoid carcinoma of the anus. *Br J Surg.* 1985;72(9):712–714.

126. Quan SH. Anal and para-anal tumors. *Surg Clin North Am.* 1978;58(3):591–603.

127. Quan SH, Magill GB, Leaming RH, et al. Multidisciplinary preoperative approach to the management of epidermoid carcinoma of the anus and anorectum. *Dis Colon Rectum.* 1978;21(2):89–91.

128. Quan SH, White JE, Deddish MR. Malignant melanoma of the anorectum. *Dis Colon Rectum.* 1959;2(3):275–283.

129. Ragnarsson-Olding BK, Nilsson PJ, Olding LB, et al. Primary anorectal malignant melanomas within a population-based national patient series in Sweden during 40 years. *Acta Oncol.* 2009;48(1):125–131.

130. Roohipour R, Patil S, Goodman KA, et al. Squamous-cell carcinoma of the anal canal: predictors of treatment outcome. *Dis Colon Rectum.* 2008;51(2):147–153.

131. Ross M, Pezzi C, Pezz T, et al. Patterns of failure in anorectal melanoma. A guide to surgical therapy. *Arch Surg.* 1990;125(3):313–316.

132. Saif MW, Kontny E, Syrigos KN, et al. The role of EGFR inhibitors in the treatment of metastatic anal canal carcinoma: a case series. *J Oncol.* 2011. doi:10.1155/2011/125467.

133. Salama JK, Mell LK, Schomas DA, et al. Concurrent chemotherapy and intesity-modulated radiation therapy for anal canal cancer patients: a multicenter experience. *J Clin Oncol.* 2007;25(29):4581–4586.

134. Salmon RJ, Fenton J, Asselain B, et al. Treatment of epidermoid anal canal cancer. *Am J Surg.* 1984;147(1):43–48.

135. Salmon RJ, Zafrani B, Labib A, et al. Prognosis of cloacogenic and squamous cancers of the anal canal. *Dis Colon Rectum.* 1986;29(5):336–340.

136. Sawyers JL. Current management of carcinoma of the anus and perianus. *Am Surg.* 1977;43(7):424–429.

137. Sawyers JL, Herrington JL Jr, Main FB. Surgical considerations in the treatment of epidermoid carcinoma of the anus. *Ann Surg.* 1963;157:817–824.

138. Scholefield JH, Ogunbiyi OA, Smith JH, et al. Treatment of anal intraepithelial neoplasia. *Br J Surg.* 1994;81(8):1238–1240.

139. Scott NA, Taylor BA, Wolff BG, et al. Perianal metastasis from a sigmoid carcinoma—objective evidence of a clonal origin. Report of a case. *Dis Colon Rectum.* 1988;31(1):68–70.

140. Seow-Choen F, Ho JM. Histoanatomy of anal glands. *Dis Colon Rectum.* 1994;37(12):1215–1218.

141. Shindo K, Bacon HE. Transitional-cell cloacogenic carcinoma of the perianal region, anal canal, and rectum: report of seven cases. *Dis Colon Rectum.* 1971;14(3):222–225.

142. Sinclair DM, Hannah G, McLaughlin IS, et al. Malignant melanoma of the anal canal. *Br J Surg.* 1970;57(11):808–811.

143. Singh R, Nime F, Mittleman A. Malignant epithelial tumors of the anal canal. *Cancer.* 1981;48(2):411–415.

144. Sischy B, Remington JH, Hinson EJ, et al. Definitive treatment of anal-canal carcinoma by means of radiation therapy and chemotherapy. *Dis Colon Rectum.* 1982;25(7):685–688.

145. Slater G, Greenstein A, Aufses AH Jr. Anal carcinoma in patients with Crohn's disease. *Ann Surg.* 1984;199(3):348–350.

146. Slingluff CL Jr, Vollmer RT, Seigler HF. Anorectal melanoma: clinical characteristics and results of surgical management in twenty-four patients. *Surgery.* 1990;107(1):1–9.

147. Smith DE, Muff NS, Shetabi H. Combined preoperative neoadjuvant radiotherapy and chemotherapy for anal and rectal cancer. *Am J Surg.* 1986;151(5):577–580.

148. Stearns MW Jr, Quan SH. Epidermoid carcinoma of the anorectum. *Surg Gynecol Obstet.* 1970;131(5):953–957.

149. Sturm JT, Christenson CE, Uecker JH, et al. Squamous-cell carcinoma of the anus arising in a giant condyloma acuminatum: report of a case. *Dis Colon Rectum.* 1975;18(2):147–151.

150. Surawicz CM, Kirby P, Critchlow C, et al. Anal dysplasia in homosexual men: role of anoscopy and biopsy. *Gastroenterology.* 1993;105(3):658–666.

151. Sveistrup J, Loft A, Berthelsen AK, et al. Positron emission tomography/computed tomography in the staging and treatment of anal cancer [published online ahead of print October 12, 2011]. *Int J Radiat Oncol Biol Phys.* doi:10.1016/j.ijrobp.2011.06.1955.

152. Tarantino D, Bernstein MA. Endoanal ultrasound in the staging and management of squamous cell carcinoma of the anal canal. *Dis Colon Rectum.* 2002;45(1):16–22.

153. Tei TM, Stolzenburg T, Buntzen S, et al. Use of transpelvic rectus abdominis musculocutaneous flap for anal cancer salvage surgery. *Br J Surg.* 2003;90(5):575–580.

154. Tomaszewski JM, Link E, Leong T, et al. Twenty-five year experience with radical chemoradiation for anal cancer [published online ahead of print October 21, 2011]. *Int J Radiation Oncol Biol Phys.* doi:10.1016/j.ijrobp.2011.07.007.

155. Touboul E, Schlienger M, Buffat L, et al. Epidermoid carcinoma of the anal canal. Results of curative-intent radiation therapy in a series of 270 patients. *Cancer.* 1994;73(6):1569–1579.

156. UKCCCR Anal Cancer Trial Working Party. Epidermoid anal cancer: results from the UKCCCR randomised trial of radiotherapy alone versus radiotherapy, 5-fluorouracil, and mitomycin. UK Co-ordinating Committee on Cancer Research. *Lancet.* 1996;348(9034):1049–1054.

157. Vercellino L, Montravers F, de Parades V, et al. Impact of FDG PET/CT in the staging and the follow-up of anal carcinoma. *Int J Colorectal Dis.* 2011;26(2):201–210.

158. Wade DS, Herrera L, Castillo NB, et al. Metastases to the lymph nodes in epidermoid carcinoma of the anal canal studied by a clearing technique. *Surg Gynecol Obstet.* 1989;169(3):238–242.

159. Wanebo HJ, Futrell W, Constable W. Multimodality approach to surgical management of locally advanced epidermoid carcinoma of the anorectum. *Cancer.* 1981;47(12):2817–2826.

160. Wanebo HJ, Woodruff JM, Farr GH, et al. Anorectal melanoma. *Cancer.* 1981;47(7):1891–1900.

161. Welch JP, Malt RA. Appraisal of the treatment of carcinoma of the anus and anal canal. *Surg Gynecol Obstet.* 1977;145(6):837–841.

162. Wellman KF. Adenocarcinoma of anal duct origin. *Can J Surg.* 1962;5:311–318.

163. Willett C. Long-term update of U.S. GI Intergroup RTOG 98-11 phase III trial for anal carcinoma: comparison of concurrent chemoradiation with 5 FU-mitomycin versus 5FU-cisplatin for disease-free and overall survival. In: 2011 Gastrointestinal Cancers Symposium. Oral Abstract Session: Cancers of the Colon and Rectum. Abstract 367.

164. Winkleman J, Grosfeld J, Bigelow B. Colloid carcinoma of anal-gland origin. Report of a case and review of the literature. *Am J Clin Pathol.* 1964;42:395–401.

165. Winton ED, Heriot AG, Ng M, et al. The impact of 18-fluorodeoxyglucose positron emission tomography on the staging, management and outcome of anal cancer. *Br J Cancer.* 2009;100(5):693–700.

166. Youk EG, Ku JL, Park JG. Detection and typing of human papillomavirus in anal epidermoid carcinomas: sequence variation in the E7 gene of human papillomavirus Type 16. *Dis Colon Rectum.* 2001;44(2):236–242.

167. Zelnick RS, Haas PA, Ajlouni M, et al. Results of abdominoperineal resections for failures after combination chemotherapy and radiation therapy for anal canal cancers. *Dis Colon Rectum.* 1992;35(6):574–577.

168. Zoetmulder FA, Baris G. Wide resection and reconstruction preserving fecal continence in recurrent anal cancer. Report of three cases. *Dis Colon Rectum.* 1995;38(1):80–84.

26

Less Common Tumors and Tumorlike Lesions of the Colon, Rectum, and Anus

Michael H. Polcino and Marvin L. Corman

To pathology we owe the realization that the contrast between health and disease is not to be sought in a fundamental difference of two kinds of life, nor in an alteration of essence, but only in an alteration of conditions.

—RUDOLF VIRCHOW:
Disease, Life, and Man

Although adenoma and adenocarcinoma constitute the most commonly seen neoplasms of the colon, rectum, and anus, many other tumors and tumorlike conditions in this anatomic region have been described.[514] Of these, some represent extraordinarily rare lesions and may thus be the source of difficult decisions in the therapeutic approach to the patient. Others are important because they represent benign conditions that may be mistaken for malignant processes. Many lesions present a similar clinical picture despite their diverse pathologic natures. Understanding the biology of each is vital to sound therapeutic intervention. The importance of adequate pathologic examination, therefore, cannot be overstressed.

The following classification scheme organizes diseases essentially by their tissue of origin.

► CLASSIFICATION OF UNUSUAL TUMORS AND TUMORLIKE CONDITIONS

Tumors of Epithelial Origin

Neuroendocrine carcinoma
Carcinoid tumor
Bowen's disease
Perianal Paget's disease
Basal cell carcinoma
Cloacogenic carcinoma
Malignant melanoma
Squamous cell carcinoma
Adenosquamous carcinoma or adenoacanthoma
Stem cell carcinoma

Tumors of Lymphoid Origin

Lymphoid hyperplasia, benign lymphoma, and lymphoid polyp
Malignant lymphoma
Extramedullary plasmacytoma

Mesenchymal Tumors

Fibrous tissue origin
    Fibroma
        Inflammatory fibroid polyp or eosinophilic granuloma

Fibrosarcoma
Malignant fibrous histiocytoma
Stromal origin
Gastrointestinal stromal tumors
Smooth muscle origin
Colonic leiomyoma
Rectal leiomyoma
Leiomyosarcoma
Rhabdomyosarcoma
Adipose tissue origin
Lipoma
Lipomatosis

Tumors of Neural Origin

Neurofibroma
Ganglioneuromatosis
Neurilemoma or schwannoma
Granular cell tumor

Vascular Lesions

Hemangioma
Lymphangioma
Hemangiopericytoma
Malignant vascular tumors (angiosarcoma, Kaposi's sarcoma)

Heterotopias and Hamartomas

Endometriosis
Perineal endometrioma
Hamartoma
Retrorectal (presacral) cysts (developmental cysts, including dermoid cyst, epidermoid cyst, tailgut cyst, enteric cyst, rectal duplication, neurenteric cyst, and teratoma)
Colitis cystica profunda or enterogenous cysts
Ectopic tissue

Exogenous, Extrinsic, and Miscellaneous Conditions

Extraskeletal osteosarcoma
Choriocarcinoma
Metastatic tumor
Barium granuloma
Oleoma, eleoma, oil granuloma, and paraffinoma
Sarcoidosis
Wegener's granulomatosis
Amyloidosis
Amyloid tumor
Malacoplakia
Sacrococcygeal chordoma
Ependymoma
Extramedullary (extraadrenal myelolipoma or angiomyelolipoma)
Anterior sacral meningocele
Extramedullary hematopoiesis
Pneumatosis cystoides intestinalis or pneumatosis coli
Duplication

► TUMORS OF EPITHELIAL ORIGIN

Neuroendocrine Carcinoma

Colorectal neuroendocrine (NE) tumors are classified as either low-grade carcinoid tumors or high-grade neuroendocrine carcinomas.[54] This type of NE malignancy is usually found in the lung (oat cell carcinoma, small cell carcinoma), but it has on occasion been reported in extrapulmonary sites, including the colon and rectum.[93,422,463] The so-called NE system includes endocrine cells distributed throughout the gastrointestinal (GI) tract, pancreas, lung, thyroid, adrenal gland, skin, and elsewhere, with intestinal NE cells being the largest component. Staren and colleagues defined NE carcinoma as a malignant epithelial neoplasm of predominantly NE differentiation and reserved the term carcinoid for their benign or very low-grade malignant counterparts (see the following section).[478] The recognition that a neuroendocrine neoplasm is high grade (as opposed to a well-differentiated neuroendocrine neoplasm, such as a carcinoid tumor) is reasonably well standardized, with a mitotic cutoff of 10 per 10 high power fields (HPFs). This concept is widely used to separate these two groups, irrespective of the organ of origin.[455] Neoplastic proliferation of these cells occurs primarily in the appendix, ileum, and rectum, although tumors occur at other sites as well.[432] NE carcinomas can be further divided into small cell carcinoma and large cell carcinoma.[455] A case of presacral NE carcinoma arising in a tailgut cyst has been reported.[361] Another NE tumor, the very rare Merkel cell carcinoma, has been described in the anal canal.[390]

Associated Concerns

It is important to remember that there are certain colorectal manifestations of endocrine diseases that are not primary to the GI tract. Symptoms such as constipation are frequently observed in diabetic patients. Unexplained diarrhea should alert the clinician to the possibility of a pancreatic endocrine tumor.[453] Furthermore, thyroid disorders may be associated with refractory constipation, diarrhea, or steatorrhea, and hyperparathyroidism often presents with constipation.[453] In short, endocrine diseases can and often do present or are associated with intestinal symptoms.

Diagnosis

NE tumors may be identified by immunohistochemical stains with application of a limited battery of available antibodies. Robidoux and colleagues suggested that electron microscopic examination is essential for diagnosis of the poorly differentiated tumor.[422] Many of the so-called poorly differentiated GI malignancies are probably NE tumors, but through the application of appropriate markers the true incidence and distribution may become apparent.[478] Saclarides and coworkers found that NE differentiation occurred in at least 3.9% of colon and rectal cancers.[432] Many were initially diagnosed as carcinoids, but the diagnosis was altered to NE carcinoma after appropriate immunohistochemical staining. In the experience of New York's Memorial Sloan-Kettering Cancer Center involving 38 patients, 22 were categorized as small cell carcinomas and 16 large cell.[54] Eighty percent of these tumors stained positive by means of immunohistochemistry including chromogranin, synaptophysin, and/or neuron-specific enolase. These cancers must be differentiated from other small cell cancers such as lymphoma.

Slooter and coworkers opined that somatostatin receptor scintigraphic imaging with ^{111}In octreotide is essential in the diagnostic evaluation.[469] Moreover, they believe that such expression in vivo predicts the outcome with somatostatin analogue treatment.

Results

Generally, these tumors are extremely aggressive and are associated with a very poor prognosis. Extensive preoperative workup is suggested because there is a high rate of concomitant metastases, with the bone marrow frequently involved. In spite of the aggressive clinical behavior that is characteristic of the tumor in the lung, the Mayo Clinic of

Rochester, Minnesota, reported that more than one-half of the patients whose records were available survived 5 years.[93] In the Memorial Sloan-Kettering Cancer Center experience, metastatic disease was detected at the time of diagnosis in more than two-thirds of their patients.[54]

There was no significant difference in survival found among pathologic subtypes. Chemotherapy is often the same as that used for oat cell carcinoma of the lung.[78,422]

Carcinoid Tumor

Carcinoids are slow-growing tumors of neuroectodermal origin that belong to the *a*mine *p*recursor *u*ptake and *d*ecarboxylation system (APUD). They are the most common of the NE neoplasms of the GI tract. ***APUD cells*** constitute a group of apparently unrelated endocrine cells, which were named by the scientist A.G.E. Pearse, who developed the APUD concept in the early 1960s. These cells share the common function of secreting a low-molecular-weight polypeptide hormone. There are several different types that secrete the hormones secretin, cholecystokinin, and several others. Lubarsch, in 1888, was the first to describe a clinical case of carcinoid disease.[313] The term *Karzinoid*, meaning carcinoma-like, was introduced by Oberndorfer in 1907.[374] It was believed that the tumor was similar to carcinoma because metastases could develop, but the clinical course often tended to be relatively benign. Although carcinoids occur most commonly as primary tumors of the GI tract, they can also be found in such diverse locations as the bronchus, ovary, and kidney.

Carcinoids arise from Kulchitsky's or basogranular enterochromaffin cells located in the crypts of Lieberkühn (Figure 26-1). A report of a patient with multiple carcinoid tumors of the rectum demonstrated numerous proliferations of extraglandular endocrine cells with no increase in intraglandular cell production.[329] In the past few decades, numerous investigators have suggested that the histochemical, chemical, and clinical characteristics vary depending on the site of origin.[58,383,540]

Classification and Diagnosis

The current classification relates to both the anatomic site of the tumor and the reactivity to silver incorporation by cytoplasmic granules.[62] A positive argentaffin reaction (argentaffinity) involves the reduction of silver salts to metallic silver by strong endogenous reducing substances.[499] Argentaffinity usually

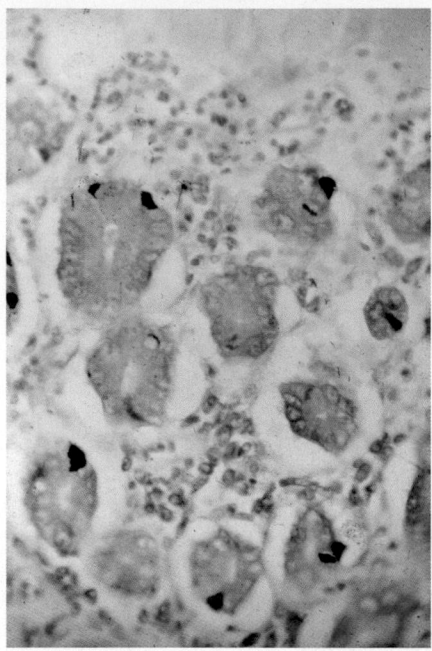

FIGURE 26-1. Normal bowel showing dark-staining argyrophilic granules (in Kulchitsky cells) from which carcinoid tumors arise. (Original magnification × 600; courtesy of Rudolf Garret, MD.)

implies that the argyrophil reaction will be positive, but the mechanism for the latter reaction is unknown.[499] A positive argyrophil reaction occurs when metallic silver added in solution is precipitated on the cytoplasmic granules of the carcinoid cells. Two distinctive types of neurosecretory granules have been observed by electron microscopy.[556] A relatively small granule appears to be associated with argyrophil carcinoids and a larger one with argentaffin (Figure 26-2).

Midgut carcinoids (mid-duodenum to mid-transverse colon) are usually both argyrophil and argentaffin positive, are frequently multicentric in origin, and often are associated with the carcinoid syndrome. The syndrome is characterized by a complex of symptoms thought to be related to overproduction of serotonin (5-hydroxytryptamine), but fewer than 10% of all patients with carcinoid tumors exhibit this manifestation. Hindgut carcinoids have been reported to be rarely

SIEGFRIED OBERNDORFER (1876–1944)

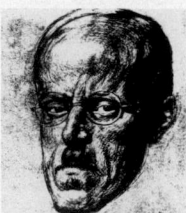

Siegfried Oberndorfer was born in Munich, Germany, on June 24, 1876. He attended medical school in Munich and finished his studies in 1900. After an internship in pathology with Hellers, he entered a residency at the Pathological Institute of the University of Munich. Subsequently, he joined the faculty and accomplished his thesis in 1906, focusing on appendicitis. In 1910, he became professor of pathology at the University of Munich. In World War I, he worked as a military pathologist, but after the rise of the Third Reich, he was dismissed from his position because he was a Jew. He emigrated to Turkey and soon became chair of the Department of Pathology at the University of Istanbul. Oberndorfer's first publication (1900) concerned the gastrointestinal manifestations of congenital syphilis. He was the first to describe carcinoid tumor of small bowel in 1907 in a presentation before the German Congress of Pathology (*Karzinoide Tumoren des Dünndarms*). He also precisely described the pathology of the male genital tract in his textbook, *Prostata, Hoden, Geschwülste* (1931). He also wrote a handbook of pathology in the Turkish language and published a German textbook on cancer, *Allgemeine Geschwülstlehre*. Oberndorfer died March 1, 1944 in Istanbul at the age of 68. (With appreciation to Oliver Pfaar and Udo Rudloff for the biographic sketch and to Udo Rudloff for the drawing.)

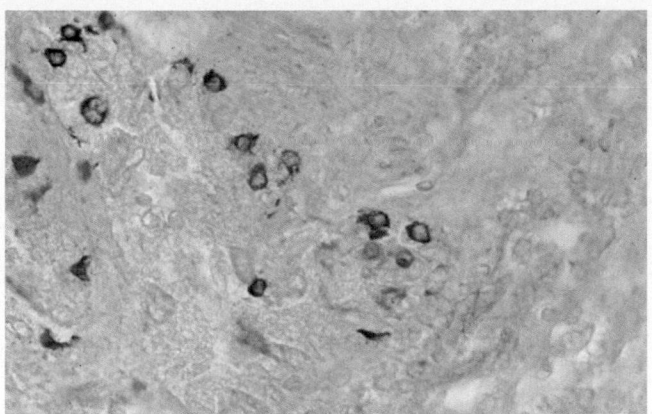

FIGURE 26-2. Carcinoid tumor showing argyrophilic granules in the cytoplasm. (Fontana stain; original magnification × 800, courtesy of Rudolf Garret, MD.)

argyrophil or argentaffin positive, are usually unicentric, and are not associated with the carcinoid syndrome.[383] Saegesser and Gross, however, reported the carcinoid syndrome in an individual with carcinoid of the rectum, and Taxy and associates noted, in 23 patients, that most rectal carcinoids are argyrophilic if the more sensitive Grimelius method is employed.[433,499] In this same group of patients, only three were argentaffin positive. The authors concluded that the Grimelius argyrophil stain is the most accurate light-microscopic means for confirming the diagnosis of a rectal carcinoid.

Determination of urine 5-hydroxyindoleacetic acid (5-HIAA) excretion is not helpful in defining metastatic disease in rectal tumors because hindgut lesions are generally argentaffin negative and do not produce a detectable increase in tryptophan metabolites.[58] Table 26-1 summarizes the classic differences between carcinoids based on gut location.

Incidence, Distribution, and Associated Conditions

The incidence of GI carcinoid tumors increases from duodenum to ileum, with more than 80% located in the distal small bowel. They arise most commonly in the appendix and are found in 0.26% of appendectomy specimens.[84] The next most common location is the small intestine, followed by the rectum and stomach. Colonic involvement is infrequent, comprising 2.5% of GI carcinoids.[84] Orloff collected 3,000 cases of such carcinoids from the literature and noted 38 patients with rectal tumors.[383] Morson reported only 21 cases of rectal carcinoids seen at St. Mark's Hospital in London in 25 years.[359]

In a collective review, Neary and colleagues analyzed the results of a number of studies.[366] For example, in the United Kingdom, an incidence of 0.7 per 100,000 population was found. This is consistent with other reports from both the United States and Spain.

Modlin and associates evaluated 10,878 carcinoid tumors that were identified by the Surveillance, Epidemiology, and End Results (SEER) Program of the National Cancer Institute (NCI) from 1973 to 1999 in addition to 2,837 carcinoid tumors that were registered previously by two earlier NCI programs.[351] Two-thirds were found in the GI tract and about 25% in the bronchopulmonary system. The following was the distribution within the GI tract:

- Small intestine (41.8%)
- Gastric (20.5%)
- Colonic (20.0%)
- Appendiceal (18.2%)

Carcinoid tumors, irrespective of their site of origin, are associated with an increased incidence of other malignant tumors, especially those of the GI tract. Moreover, an increased incidence of breast and uterine malignancies, as well as cancer of the hematopoietic system, has been described. The reported rates of the development of a second primary malignancy with

TABLE 26-1 Classic Differences among Foregut, Midgut, and Hindgut Carcinoids

	Foregut	Midgut	Hindgut
Location	Lungs, stomach, first part of duodenum	Duodenum through right colon, appendix	Transverse or left colon, rectum
Staining	Nonargentaffin but argyrophilic	Argentaffin + argyrophilic	Nonargentaffin but argyrophilic
Bioactivity	5-Hydroxytryptophan, ACTH, tachykinins, neurotensin, HCG; gastrin; low 5-HT content; high MAO activity without DAO activity	5-HT, tachykinins, rarely ACTH or 5-hydroxytryptophan; lower MAO activity than foregut carcinoids but higher DAO activity	Low 5-HT or ACTH content; may secrete somatostatin, tachykinins, glicentin, PYY, 5-hydroxytryptophan, neurotensin, pancreatic polypeptide, dopamine
Metastasis	25%, particularly to bone; metastases not required for systemic symptoms	60%–80% (proportional to tumor size) to liver; rarely to bone	5%–40% to bone
Presentation	Pulmonary obstruction, atypical neurohumoral symptoms	Bowel obstruction, classic carcinoid syndrome (diarrhea and flushing) if metastatic	Usually discovered by chance; rarely cause humoral symptoms

ACTH, adrenocorticotropic hormone; DAO, diamine oxidase; HCG, human chorionic gonadotropin; 5-HT, serotonin; MAO, monoamine oxidase; PYY, peptide YY.
From Basson MD, Ahlman H, Wangberg B, et al. Biology and management of the midgut carcinoid. *Am J Surg.* 1993;165(2):288–297, with permission.

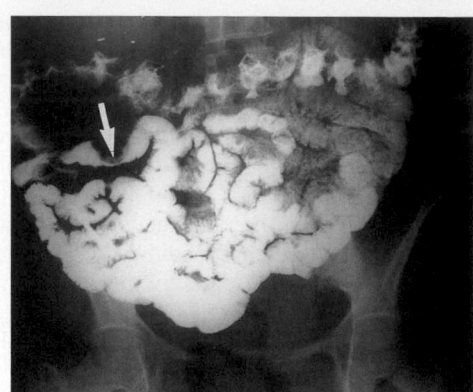 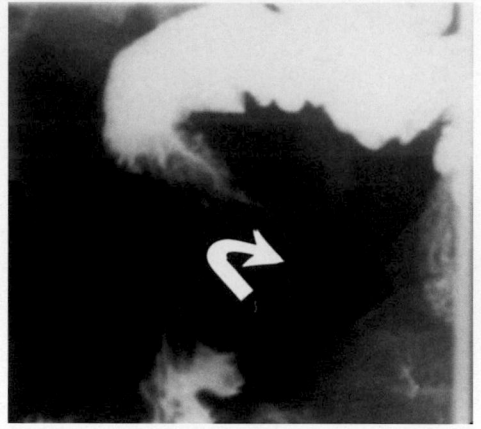

FIGURE 26-3. Carcinoid of the small bowel. Small bowel series. A right upper quadrant mass can be seen infiltrating the mesentery of the small bowel and proximal colon. **A:** Note the filling defect (*arrow*). **B:** Spot film of the same patient reveals another lesion producing a profound stricture (*arrow*).

GI carcinoid tumors is as high as 55%.[206] This includes an increased risk for synchronous colorectal, small bowel, gastric and esophageal cancers, as well as metachronous lung, prostate, and urinary tract neoplasms.[507] Because of the possible association with myelofibrosis, evaluation of the bowel in an individual with hematologic disease may be a useful exercise.[368] An association between ulcerative colitis and rectal carcinoid tumors has also been postulated.[445] The reason for the predisposition to develop other cancers may be due to the tumorigenic properties of the peptides secreted by NE cells, such as secretin, gastrin, bombesin, cholecystokinin, and vasoactive intestinal peptide.[206]

Age, Gender, and Race

The condition occurs most commonly in individuals in their sixth and seventh decades.[366] The mean age in Orloff's series was 55,[383] and the previously mentioned SEER study showed the mean age to be 61.4 years.[351] Appendiceal tumors had been seen most frequently in women at a 2:1 ratio,[426] but this has decreased to 57% in current reports. The male-to-female ratio is 0.93 for colonic carcinoids and 1.0 to 1.11 for rectal carcinoids.[351] For all sites, age-adjusted incidence rates are highest in black male patients.[351]

Signs, Symptoms, and Diagnosis
Appendix

The presentation is usually that of an individual with right lower quadrant abdominal pain and signs and symptoms of appendicitis. The identification of the tumor, itself, usually awaits pathologic confirmation. This often is a fortuitous finding that presents somewhat of a controversy in subsequent management (see later). The prevalence of carcinoids has been estimated to be 0.32% based on a series of more than 34,000 appendectomies.[355] Most are present at the tip (67%), with the body comprising 21%, and only 7% seen at the base.[355]

Small Bowel

Carcinoid tumors in the small bowel are frequently asymptomatic.[46] In those who are symptomatic, change in bowel habits, weight loss, and abdominal pain are the most frequent complaints. Moertel and colleagues advised that the presence of an abdominal mass on the right side and a long history of weight loss and diarrhea should raise suspicion of a carcinoid in the small intestine.[354] The frequency of metastases at diagnosis depends on the clinical presentation and ranges from

33% to 64%. In asymptomatic individuals, 93% who are diagnosed with small bowel carcinoids harbor metastases.[354]

The ileum is second only to the appendix as the site of origin of foregut carcinoid tumors.[65] Quantification of 5-hydroxytryptamine and its metabolites, especially 24-hour urinary 5-HIAA, have been found to detect up to 84% of carcinoid tumors.[65] Unfortunately, small bowel carcinoids commonly present late because of the nonspecific signs and symptoms that occur. This leads to failure to pursue investigative studies that could identify the lesion at an earlier stage. The single most common presenting complaint is that of small bowel obstruction, but most patients have nonspecific GI symptoms.

The most rewarding diagnostic study for the evaluation of a suspected small bowel carcinoid is enteroclysis (see Chapter 5). However, a routine small bowel series is usually sufficient (Figure 26-3). It is important to remember that small carcinoids are frequently multiple. The use of computed tomography (CT) scan to evaluate the small bowel has also been recommended (Figure 26-4), but knowledge gleaned is often ex post facto, the diagnosis of metastatic disease having already been established. Pilleul and colleagues concluded that contrast- and water-enhanced multidetector CT enteroclysis allows depiction of small bowel neoplasms with an accuracy of 84.7%.[398] Magnetic resonance imaging (MRI) has also been used for the evaluation of GI carcinoid tumors. In the experience of Bader and coworkers, the primary tumor could be identified in 8 of 12 of their patients.[32] The appearance is usually that of a nodular mass or bowel wall thickening with moderate enhancement on postgadolinium imaging. Liver metastases are commonly hypervascular and may be demonstrable only on immediate postgadolinium images.[32]

Colon

Colonic carcinoids usually grow to a large size before they become symptomatic. Even then, they are less likely to cause obstruction or rectal bleeding than adenocarcinoma of the colon. Thirty-two percent of Orloff's patients were asymptomatic, and an additional 21% had symptoms that were the result of another condition.[383] When the lesion does produce symptoms, they are indistinguishable from those caused by adenocarcinoma (e.g., bleeding, change in bowel habits, abdominal pain). Colonic carcinoids have a similar 5-year survival to that of adenocarcinoma.

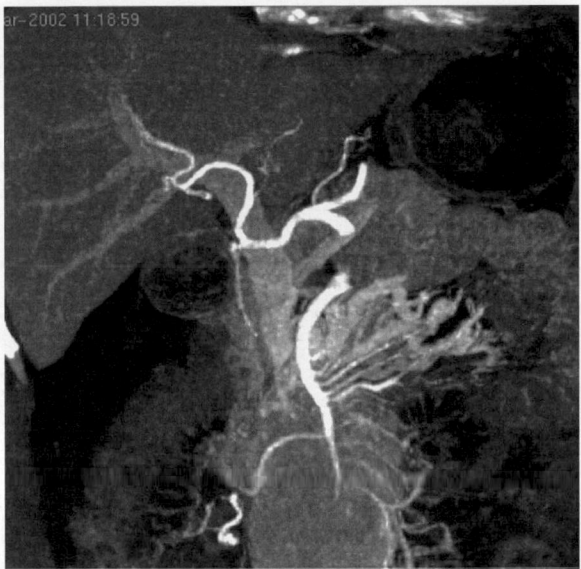

FIGURE 26-4. Coronal contrast-enhanced CT scan shows large mesenteric mass encasing superior mesenteric artery and its branches. Mass was carcinoid tumor. (From Horton KM, et al. Carcinoid tumors of the small bowel: a multitechnique imaging approach. *AJR Am J Roentgenol.* 2004;182(3):559–567, with permission.)

Radiologic evaluation of colonic carcinoids reflects the appearance of the clinically seen lesion (Figure 26-5). For larger tumors, it is virtually impossible to distinguish the pathology from that of an adenocarcinoma. This is true even on colonoscopy or direct visualization. In the experience of Ballantyne and colleagues, 48% of the colon carcinoids were

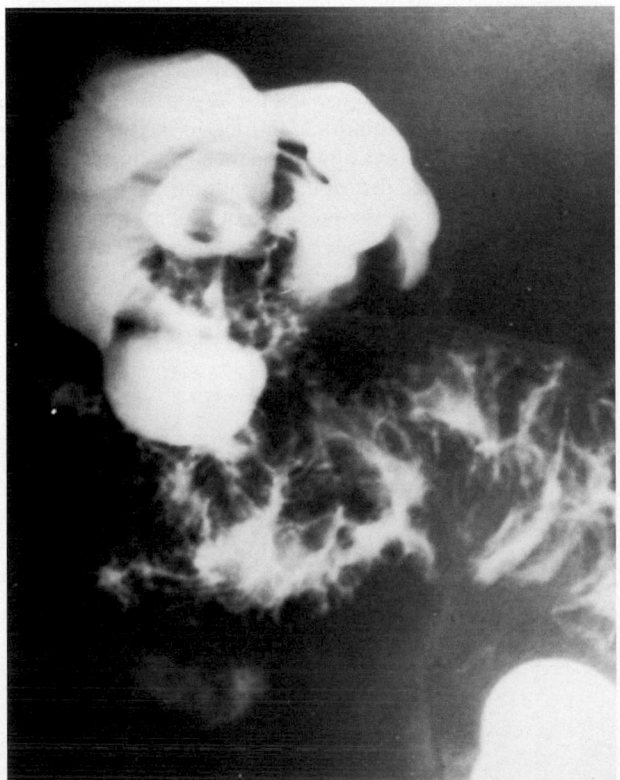

FIGURE 26-5. Carcinoid tumor of the hepatic flexure. Spot film on barium enema reveals distension of the colon with thickened folds. This appearance is caused by an intense fibrosis and desmoplastic response produced by the carcinoid tumor.

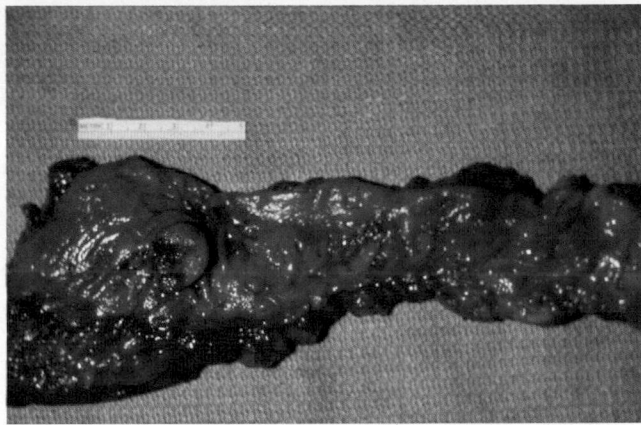

FIGURE 26-6. Carcinoid tumor. An ulcerated nodule protruding from the rectum in a resected specimen. (Courtesy of Rudolf Garret, MD.)

located in the cecum, 16% in the ascending colon, 6% in the transverse colon, 11% in the descending colon, and 13% in the sigmoid.[38] The remainder were not assigned. As previously mentioned, patients with carcinoid tumors have an increased incidence of GI adenocarcinoma.[38,47,72,407] Thorough evaluation of the entire GI tract is therefore essential.

Rectum

In the rectum, a carcinoid tumor usually is observed as a small, circumscribed, yellowish, submucosal nodule, 1 cm or less in diameter. It is often found incidentally, either at the time of pathologic examination of an excised rectum for another condition or in the course of clinical assessment for other complaints (Figures 26-6 and 26-7). In the Ochsner Clinic experience in New Orleans, one-half of rectal carcinoids were discovered at the time of anorectal examination of asymptomatic individuals.[249] The remainder were found primarily by evaluation of patients whose symptoms were the result of other benign conditions. In a review by Mani and coworkers, the most common finding at the time of presentation was described as "nonspecific."[323] The most common complaint was that of anorectal discomfort, with rectal bleeding being the second most common. Other complaints included constipation, weight loss, change in bowel habits, rectal obstruction, "hemorrhoids," diarrhea, and the presence

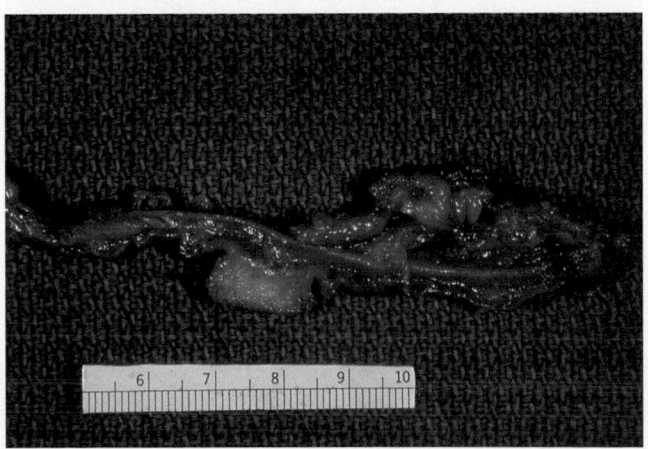

FIGURE 26-7. Longitudinal section of the specimen shown in Figure 26-6. Note the absence of infiltration of muscularis. (Courtesy of Rudolf Garret, MD.)

of an abdominal mass.[323] Endoscopic ultrasonography has been found to be applicable for determining depth of invasion, a useful consideration if one were to consider performing a local excision.

Presacral Lesion

The presentation of presacral lesions is discussed later in this chapter. It is of interest to note here, however, that an unusual presentation of carcinoid has been described within the presacral space.[136] In the absence of a demonstrable primary mucosal lesion, the authors concluded that the tumor arose from an enterochromaffin cell or teratoma within the presacral space or possibly a metastatic lymph node from an unknown primary.

Histopathology and DNA Ploidy

Microscopically, it is very difficult to differentiate between benign and malignant carcinoid. The usual criteria for malignancy such as mitotic activity or pyknotic nuclei are often lacking. The incidence of malignancy varies from 8% to 40%, with the evidence based on the presence of local extension or metastasis.[537] The tumor is composed of uniform, small, round, or polygonal cells with prominent, round nuclei and eosinophilic cytoplasmic granules (Figures 26-8 through 26-10). Johnson and colleagues suggest that there are five generally accepted carcinoid histologic growth patterns: insular, trabecular, glandular, undifferentiated, and mixed.[253] They further observed differences in median survival times in 138 patients based on these patterns and recommend the use of such stratification in future studies. Of the patients with carcinoid tumors, Bowen and coworkers reported that there was a trend to increased expression of vascular endothelial growth factor receptor (VEGFR) and insulin-like growth factor receptor (IGFR), particularly in the foregut and midgut carcinoids.[64]

Tsioulias and coworkers studied the nuclear DNA pattern of 22 rectal carcinoids, finding that the three with metachronous or synchronous metastatic disease had an aneuploid pattern.[513] Conversely, all of the 19 tumors with no metastases exhibited a diploid pattern. The authors concluded that DNA ploidy is an important, independent prognostic indicator. Others have confirmed the association of aneuploidy with stage, size, and invasion by tumor, but in one study the data suggested that a near-hypertriploid pattern was the most

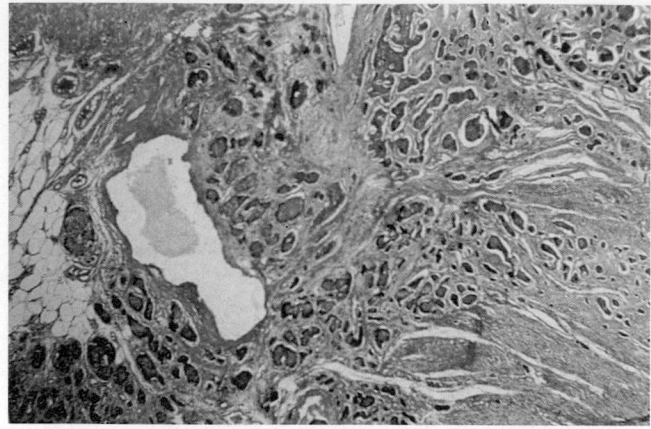

FIGURE 26-9. Malignant carcinoid infiltrating the whole wall of the rectum and invading adipose tissue. Note the cluster of tumor cells in tissue spaces and lymphatics. (Original magnification × 80; courtesy of Rudolf Garret, MD.)

precise and reliable parameter for predicting the prognosis of colorectal carcinoid tumors.[87]

Management
Appendix

Moertel and associates recommended appendectomy alone as an adequate treatment for appendiceal carcinoids of less than 2 cm in diameter, even if lymphatic invasion is noted on subsequent histologic examination (Figures 26-11 and 26-12).[353] These investigators found no recurrence in a group of more than 100 patients who had microscopic evidence of lymphatic invasion who were so treated. A later report involving 150 patients revealed no other recurrences with the same criterion.[353] The authors further suggest that if the individual is elderly or at high operative risk, appendectomy alone is appropriate for even larger lesions.

A right colectomy is suggested for larger lesions in young patients and for those tumors identified to have vascular involvement or to have invasion of the mesoappendix.[353] Gouzi and coworkers opined that a further indication for secondary right hemicolectomy is the presence of mucinous-producing cells.[192]

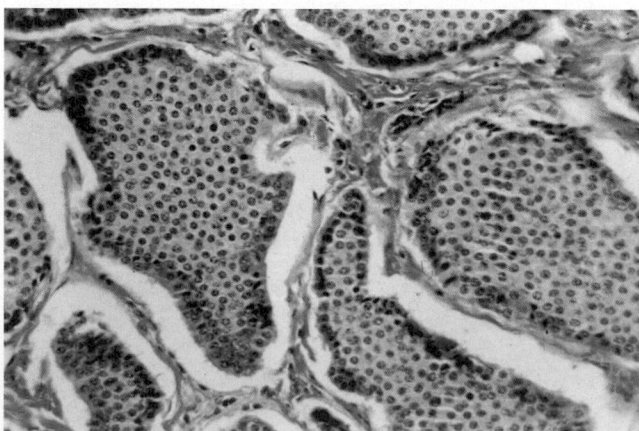

FIGURE 26-8. Carcinoid. Uniform cells with minimal variation of cell nuclei in clusters within the lymphatic spaces. (Original magnification × 280; from Corman ML, Veidenheimer MC, Swinton NW. *Diseases of the Anus, Rectum and Colon. Part I: Neoplasms.* New York, NY: Medcom; 1972.)

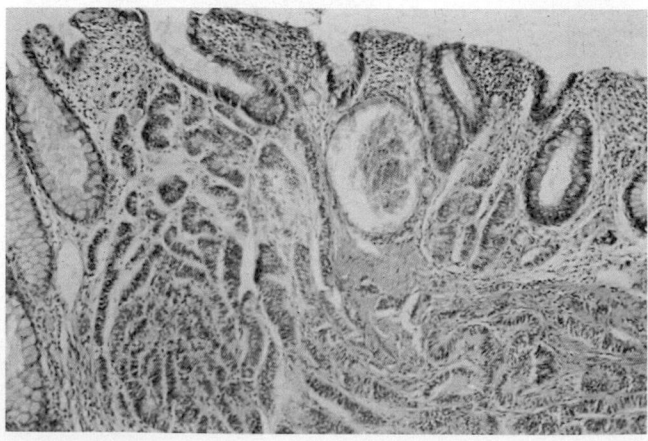

FIGURE 26-10. Malignant carcinoid. Uniform cells in tissue spaces, some forming abortive glandular structures. (Original magnification × 280; courtesy of Rudolf Garret, MD.)

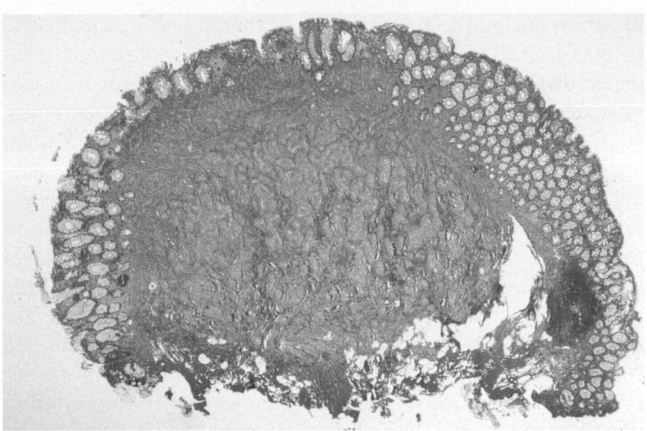

FIGURE 26-11 Carcinoid tumor of the appendix clearly seen histologically as a submucosal nodule. (Original magnification × 80.)

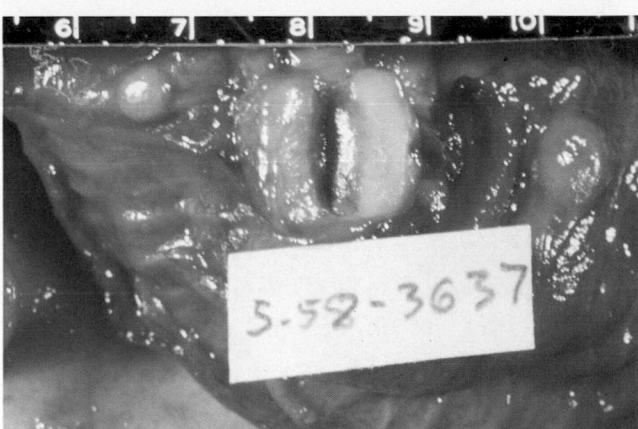

FIGURE 26-13. Resected specimen of ileum showing opened bowel with incised carcinoid demonstrating yellowish hue. This was one of multiple lesions within the jejunum and ileum.

Small Bowel

As suggested earlier, the major difficulty in managing patients with small bowel carcinoid is the fact that these individuals present quite late. There is a concern to which one must be sensitive, that of limiting the resection when the root of the mesentery is involved in order to minimize the risk of causing short-bowel problems. It is extremely important to examine the entire small bowel, looking for the presence of synchronous lesions (Figure 26-13). If at all possible, resection of obvious nodal involvement is encouraged, including removal of superficial hepatic metastases as well as performing a cholecystectomy. This last procedure is advised if prolonged somatostatin analogue therapy is anticipated.[65]

Colon

Treatment of colonic carcinoid is resection. Because these tumors are relatively slow growing, metastatic disease is not a contraindication to resection of the primary lesion. Metastases occur more frequently with carcinoids of the large bowel than with carcinoids of the small intestine. Perhaps this can be explained by the fact that carcinoid tumors may attain a considerable size in the colon before they become symptomatic.

Rectum

In the rectum, the size of the carcinoid is the distinguishing feature that determines treatment. Most tumors less than

2 cm in diameter require only local, transanal excision. In the experience of Shirouzu and associates, rectal carcinoids of less than 2 cm in diameter had neither muscle invasion nor lymph node metastases.[458] Other investigators confirm the appropriateness of transanal excision for smaller lesions.[249] However, those that are demonstrably invasive or are 2 cm in diameter or greater should probably be treated by a cancer type of resection.[323] Laparoscopic excision of a proximal rectal carcinoid has also been described.[298]

Carcinoid Syndrome

With the exception of tumors that originate outside of the intestinal tract, the carcinoid syndrome develops only in those individuals whose cancers have spread to the liver (Figure 26-14). The classic symptoms and signs are those of skin flushing, diarrhea, and a heart murmur (most commonly that of tricuspid insufficiency—Figure 26-15). The flushing may involve only the face or may involve the entire body. It may last anywhere from a few minutes to several hours. There may be excessive tearing, salivation, and facial edema, and the condition may be associated with respiratory symptoms such as wheezing. With increased involvement of the liver, the symptoms often become disabling. Pellagra is a vitamin deficiency disease most commonly caused by a chronic lack of niacin (vitamin B_3) in the diet. It may also result from alterations in

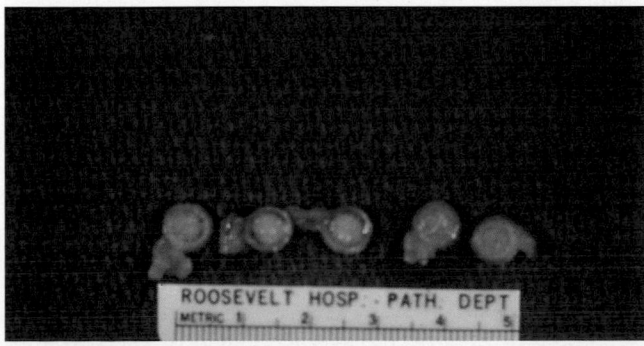

FIGURE 26-12. Carcinoid tumor of the appendix. Multiple cuts through resected specimen demonstrate macroscopic confinement of the tumor to the submucosa. (Courtesy of Rudolf Garret, MD.)

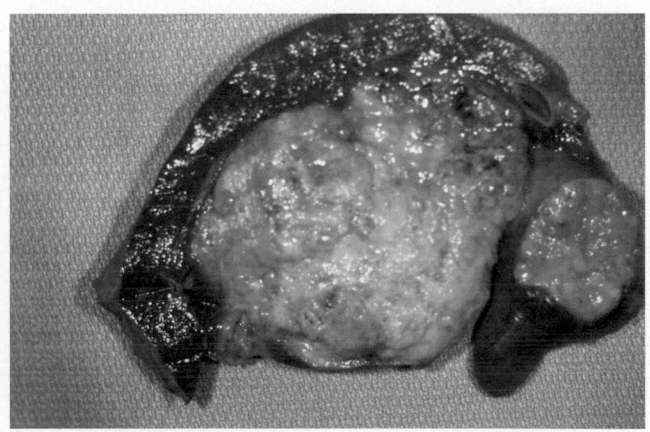

FIGURE 26-14. Liver showing large metastatic carcinoid tumor.

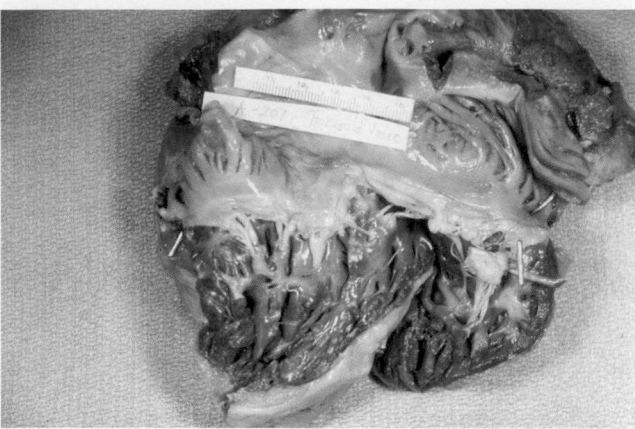

FIGURE 26-15. Heart removed at autopsy showing leaflet thickening and fibrosis, along with thickening of the chordae tendineae and papillary muscle. This resulted in massive regurgitation of the tricuspid valve.

protein metabolism in disorders such as carcinoid syndrome (Figure 26-16). The likelihood of developing the syndrome is dependent on the site of the cancer. Up to 60% of those with metastatic small bowel carcinoids will develop symptoms, whereas only about 1% of those with appendiceal primary disease will develop the syndrome. With the exception of the rare "case report," virtually no one with a rectal carcinoid will ultimately develop the symptoms of carcinoid syndrome.

Because of the secretion of serotonin, the diagnosis is made through its by-product, 5-HIAA, which is excreted in the urine. Some individuals with carcinoid syndrome may have normal urinary 5-HIAA levels. In such instances, the serum serotonin level must be measured in order to establish the diagnosis.

Treatment of the Carcinoid Syndrome. Treatment of symptoms of diarrhea include loperamide, diphenoxylate/atropine, cyproheptadine, and methysergide. For flushing, management includes antihistamines (e.g., diphenhydramine) and antiulcer medications such as ranitidine. Phenoxybenzamine has also been recommended for the flushing.

In addition to chemotherapy, which is often offered but usually unhelpful, a somatostatin, octreotide (Sandostatin), is advised because it inhibits the severe diarrhea and flushing episodes associated with the disease. The suggested daily

program during the first 2 weeks of therapy ranges from 100 to 600 μg/day, in two to four divided, subcutaneously injected doses. Along these lines, the resected specimen should be tested for somatostatin receptors. Somatostatin analogues, such as octreotide, lanreotide, and Somatuline, have shown variable inhibition of tumor growth and therapeutic tolerance.[65] Lanreotide requires injection every 10 days compared with twice daily injections of octreotide—therefore, the former may be preferred.[384] An antiproliferative effect of octreotide on metastatic carcinoid, with regression of the tumors, has been reported to occasionally occur.[300] The addition of interferon-α has also been successfully employed for controlling symptoms and possibly retarding tumor growth.[279] Adjuvant chemotherapeutic and biomodulating therapies are under clinical investigation.[65]

The most efficacious program for the treatment of the carcinoid syndrome is surgically to remove (debulk) as much of the primary and secondary tumors as is possible in order to limit production of the polypeptides. Other options include hepatic artery embolization, radiation therapy, and selective hepatic artery infusion chemotherapy.

Radiotherapy and chemotherapy have not proved to be effective in the treatment of carcinoid tumors of the colon and rectum. Adequate surgical excision remains the quintessential treatment. With respect to metastatic disease to the liver, drug combinations of 5-fluorouracil and streptozotocin have achieved high, albeit brief, response rates, whereas hepatic dearterialization and embolization are also useful palliative approaches.[28,505]

Results
Appendix
Anderson and Bergdahl reported results of treatment of carcinoid of the appendix in 25 children younger than the age of 15 years.[14] All underwent appendectomy, but 1 patient was subjected to right hemicolectomy because of tumor in the margin of the resected appendix. Despite serosal extension in 9 children and lymph node metastases in 1, no signs of recurrence were seen with a mean follow-up period of 12 years.

Gouzi and colleagues reviewed the records of 181 patients with carcinoid tumor of the appendix seen during a 10-year period ending in 1987.[192] Appendectomy was the sole treatment in 146 individuals, with right hemicolectomy performed on the remainder. None of those treated by appendectomy alone developed recurrent tumor. However, there were five instances of residual tumor upon re-exploration, with one death at 2 years and one patient alive with metastatic disease.

Small Bowel
Cure following resection of carcinoid of the small bowel is quite unusual because of the frequent late stage at presentation. In the unusual circumstance of disease confined to the bowel itself, without lymph node involvement or metastatic disease, the likelihood of cure is excellent.[65] For tumors of 1 to 2 cm in diameter, 18% to 44% have been found to be metastatic to the liver, with spread to the lymph nodes in up to 85% of cases reported by Box and colleagues.[65] Size appears to be the variable that correlates most well with survival.

Colon
According to Berardi, the average length of survival after resection of colonic carcinoids is 26 months.[51] Welch and Donaldson stated that the 5-year survival rate for patients with colonic carcinoids is similar to that of those with carcinoma

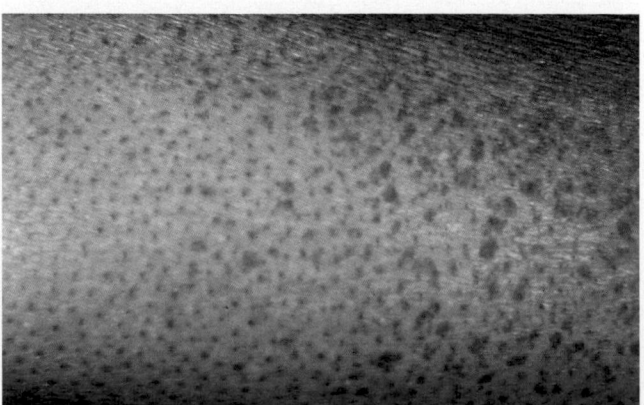

FIGURE 26-16. Pellagra dermatitis in a patient with carcinoid syndrome.

of the colon and rectum.[538] When a distinction is made between cecal and other colonic sites, the former is found to be associated with a 71% incidence of metastasis, whereas the latter has a 33% incidence.[441] Ballantyne and coworkers noted a 5-year survival rate of 37% in their 54 patients.[38] Tumors larger than 2 cm had metastasized in approximately three-quarters of their patients, whereas only one in six less than 2 cm metastasized. Spread and colleagues noted that survival for carcinoids of the colon was significantly lower when compared with carcinoids of the rectum or appendix or with colonic adenocarcinomas.[477] They, however, believed that size and tumor invasion were not the major prognostic factors. Rather, tumor stage, histologic pattern, tumor differentiation, nuclear grade, and mitotic rate were found to influence the survival rate significantly.[477]

Rectum

Orloff applied his therapeutic principle to the management of rectal carcinoids.[383] All 23 of his patients with lesions less than 2 cm survived 5 years. The survival rate of 15 patients with lesions measuring 2 cm or greater in diameter was 40%. However, the report from St. Mark's Hospital was less encouraging.[69] All with malignant tumors died irrespective of radical surgical treatment, but there were only 4 such individuals. Sauven and colleagues observed that rectal carcinoid tumors were cured only when they were discovered before the T3 stage, measured less than 2 cm in diameter, and when lymph nodes were not involved.[445] These investigators concluded that if local excision permits complete removal, radical resection provides little benefit. Others opined that extensive surgery offers no survival advantage over local excision.[283] Additional studies confirm that the two criteria, tumor size and depth of invasion, complement each other as prognostic indicators.[323]

Bowen's Disease, Perianal Paget's Disease, and Basal Cell Carcinoma

See Chapter 9.

Cloacogenic Carcinoma and Primary Malignant Melanoma

See Chapter 25.

Squamous Cell Carcinoma

Primary squamous cell carcinoma of the colon and rectum is an extremely rare tumor; approximately 75 cases have been reported.[68,99,175,301,521,541] The incidence of this tumor is believed to be 1 per 3,000 malignant tumors of the bowel.[99,521] These lesions tend to be distributed uniformly throughout the colon.[342]

Numerous theories have been postulated about the etiology and pathogenicity. These include metaplasia of glandular epithelium, embryonal rests, squamous metaplasia of existing adenoma or adenocarcinoma, damaged epithelium from toxic substances, and basal cell anaplasia.[52,99,316,521] Balfour believed that this entity is either a metastatic lesion or degeneration of a poorly differentiated adenocarcinoma.[36] Others suggest that this condition may represent an adenoacanthoma with primarily squamous elements (see later). Specific predisposing factors that have been associated are ulcerative colitis, radiotherapy, colonic duplication, and schistosomiasis.

Gelas and coworkers identified certain criteria that must be satisfied before one can definitively establish the diagnosis of primary squamous cell carcinoma of the *rectum*.[175] They are as follows:

- Metastases from another site must be excluded.
- A squamous-lined fistula tract must *not* involve the affected bowel.
- Squamous cell carcinoma of the anus with proximal extension must be excluded.

Symptoms are the same as those of adenocarcinoma, especially bleeding and change in bowel habits. Evaluation of the patient should proceed in the manner outlined in Chapters 23 and 24. Total colonoscopy is suggested because of the not uncommon association of synchronous benign and malignant tumors.

Histologic examination may demonstrate squamous metaplasia of the colonic mucosa as well as the carcinoma (Figure 26-17).

In the absence of metastases, the lesion should be treated in the same manner as that of adenocarcinoma. However, consideration should be given to implementing the neoadjuvant therapy described in Chapter 25, especially if abdominoperineal resection appears to be the surgical alternative.[294] It has been described as the primary treatment for rectal

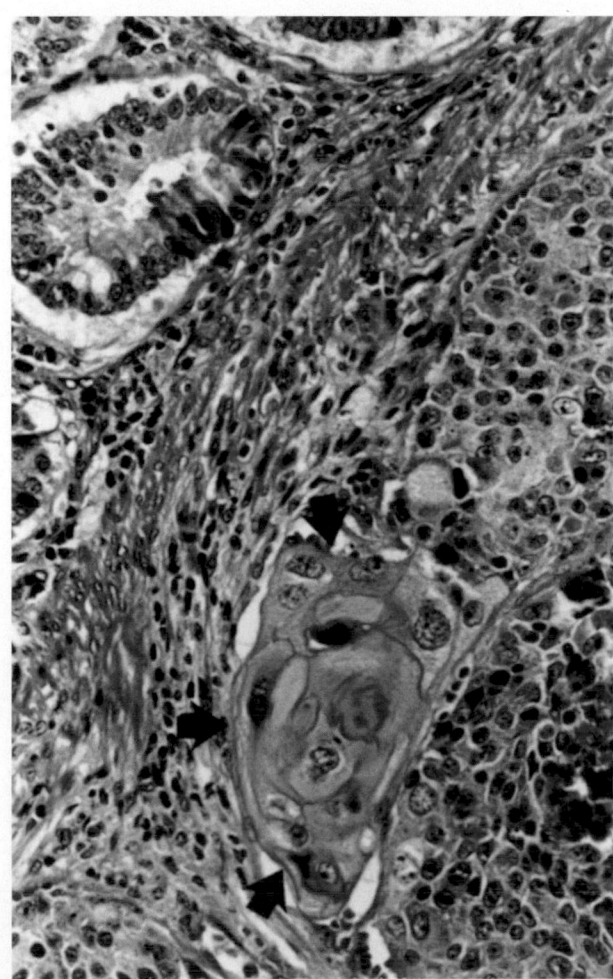

FIGURE 26-17. Squamous cell carcinoma of the cecum. Note the island of malignant squamous cells (*arrows*) near benign colonic glandular mucosa. (Original magnification × 50; courtesy of Rodger C. Haggitt, MD.)

squamous cell carcinoma.[413] A case report of squamous cell carcinoma of the sigmoid colon with metastatic disease to the liver has been reported that responded well to systemic chemotherapy.[258]

Adenosquamous Carcinoma or Adenoacanthoma

Adenosquamous carcinoma of the colon is an extremely rare tumor. In 1987, Chevinsky and colleagues identified 35 cases in the literature and also noted 25 reports of squamous carcinoma primary to the colon.[88] However, some authors believe that if careful review of the histologic pattern of tumors thought to be squamous carcinomas are undertaken, some of the lesions would prove to be adenosquamous cancers (adenoacanthomas), a mixture of both glandular and squamous features (Figure 26-18).[92] Petrelli and colleagues retrospectively reviewed the experience at the Roswell Park Cancer Institute in Buffalo, New York, between the years 1971 and 1994.[395] Seven patients were identified, representing 0.18% of the adenocarcinomas at that institution. Cagir and associates identified 145 patients with adenosquamous carcinoma of the colon, rectum, and anus in the NCI's SEER database for the years 1973 through 1992.[71] The mean age was 67 years. Twenty-eight percent of the lesions were in the right colon.

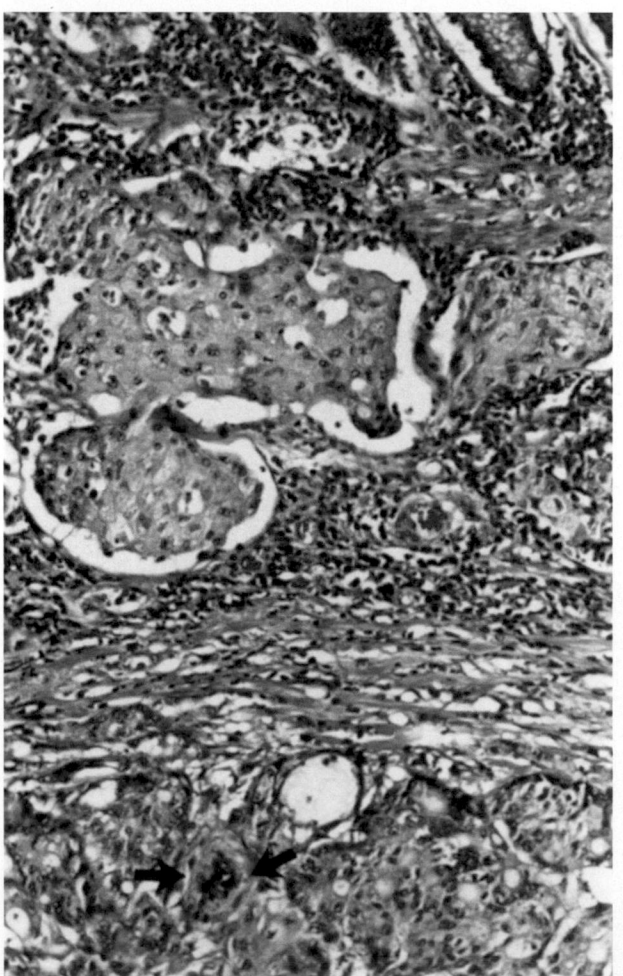

FIGURE 26-18. Adenoacanthoma of the colon. Islets of malignant squamous epithelium immediately underneath the mucosa and gland-forming tumor below that (*arrows*). (Original magnification × 40; courtesy of Rodger C. Haggitt, MD.)

Theoretical causes of this histologic manifestation include embryonal rests, indeterminate basal cells, squamous metaplasia, and a germ or pluripotential stem cell.[88] An increased association with ulcerative colitis has been suggested.[343]

Adenosquamous cancers in general are very aggressive tumors and are associated with a less favorable prognosis than is adenocarcinoma.[79] Because the squamous component may have a greater potential for metastasizing and can do so as an undifferentiated carcinoma, Cerezo and colleagues as well as others suggest that all such lesions be carefully evaluated by means of immunoperoxidase stains and/or electron microscopy in order to identify squamous features.[79,281] This would also imply that evidence of metastatic squamous cell carcinoma does not preclude the possibility of the source being the colon. In the Roswell Park experience, all patients had stage III or IV disease upon presentation.[355] Median survival was only 23 months. In three individuals, the tumor was associated with ulcerative colitis. All died of their disease.

An assessment of the Mayo Clinic experience revealed a total of 31 patients with adenosquamous cancers of the colon and rectum and 11 pure squamous cell carcinomas.[168] They did not separate the two groups but reported an overall 5-year survival of 34% with a 65% survival for stage I to stage III disease. When there was nodal involvement, the survival rate was 23%, whereas without nodal involvement it was 85%. In Cagir and associates' SEER report, the overall adjusted 5-year survival rate was 30.7%.[71] The survival rate for tumors that did not demonstrate nodal involvement was comparable to that of adenocarcinoma, but more advanced lesions were associated with a poorer survival rate than adenocarcinoma stage for stage.

Stem Cell Carcinoma

Another highly aggressive tumor of the colon and rectum may be a variant of adenoacanthoma, the so-called *stem cell carcinoma*. In theory, there may be a pluripotential stem cell in the mucosa of the GI tract capable of differentiation in several directions.[386] Only a few cases have been reported. Palvio and colleagues reviewed tumors with adenosquamous and carcinoid elements in one patient and exocrine, NE, and squamous differentiation in another.[386]

▶ TUMORS OF LYMPHOID ORIGIN

Lymphoid Hyperplasia, Benign Lymphoma, and Lymphoid Polyp

Lymphoid hyperplasia is a benign, focal, or diffuse condition that occurs typically where clusters of lymphoid follicles are present (terminal ileum, rectum).[106,107,133,219] Although the etiology is unknown, the possibility of an inflammatory reaction as well as a hereditary predisposition has been suggested. In children, an infectious process is thought to precipitate the acute form of the disease.[256]

One of the earliest reports of benign lymphoid hyperplasia was by Cohnheim who, in 1865, introduced the term *gastrointestinal pseudoleukemia*.[96] He described a hyperplasia of the lymphoid follicles of the GI tract with polyp formation but without the blood picture of lymphatic leukemia. In 1940, Ewing stated that "the gastrointestinal tract is the seat of a remarkable form of primary lymphoid hyperplasia which lacks the destructive character of lymphosarcoma and fails to give lymphocytosis in the blood."[147] He pointed out that lesions of the GI tract may be limited or diffuse and sometimes are associated with widespread lymphoid hyperplasia but never with leukemia. Symmers confirmed these findings in 1948.[495] Since that time, isolated cases have been reported sporadically, all of which confirm the benign nature of the disease.[70,98,108,242,256]

In 1961, Cornes and colleagues reviewed 100 such patients.[107] The tumors were described as usually single and most frequently found in the lower one-third of the rectum. They may be seen in an individual at any age, but in adults they are most commonly noted during the third and fourth decades.[70,107,405] In children, the peak incidence is between 1 and 3 years and is twice as common in boys as in girls.[12,256]

Gruenwald suggested that the lesions are congenital malformations or hamartomas, a hypothesis that is supported by their occasional familial occurrence.[202] Granet reported solitary benign lymphomas in identical twins.[195] Beatty and Keeling noted the lesions in three siblings, ages 6, 7, and 9 years.[48] Others have observed an association with familial polyposis.[199,520]

Lymphoid hyperplasia is characterized radiographically by small, uniform, localized, or generalized polypoid lesions (Figure 26-19). A fleck of barium may be seen in the center of the polyp on contrast study, representing umbilication at the apex of the lymphoid nodule. A central dimple in the nodule is considered good evidence for making the diagnosis.[254] Endoscopic examination with biopsy confirms the nature of the lesion. The nodules are usually small, firm, and sessile but occasionally may be large and can become pedunculated (Figure 26-20). When removed and sectioned, the tumors are found to be composed of well-differentiated lymphoid tissue, with follicles separated by white fibrous bands and covered by a rather thin mucous membrane. The macroscopic and microscopic appearance may resemble malignant lymphoma or Hodgkin's disease. In fact, the condition has been regarded by some as a form of malignant lymphoma and has even been designated as pseudolymphoma.[495] However, the lesion lacks the infiltrating and destructive characteristics of malignant lymphoma and does not become disseminated. In the benign lymphoid polyp, a follicular pattern with a clearly defined germinal center is seen (Figure 26-21), whereas malignant lymphoma shows a poorly defined and irregular pattern with no germinal centers.[405] The condition also can resemble leukemic infiltration of the bowel, but in leukemia the lesion tends to have a segmental distribution (Figure 26-22). In addition, evidence of the disease is usually apparent in the peripheral blood smear.

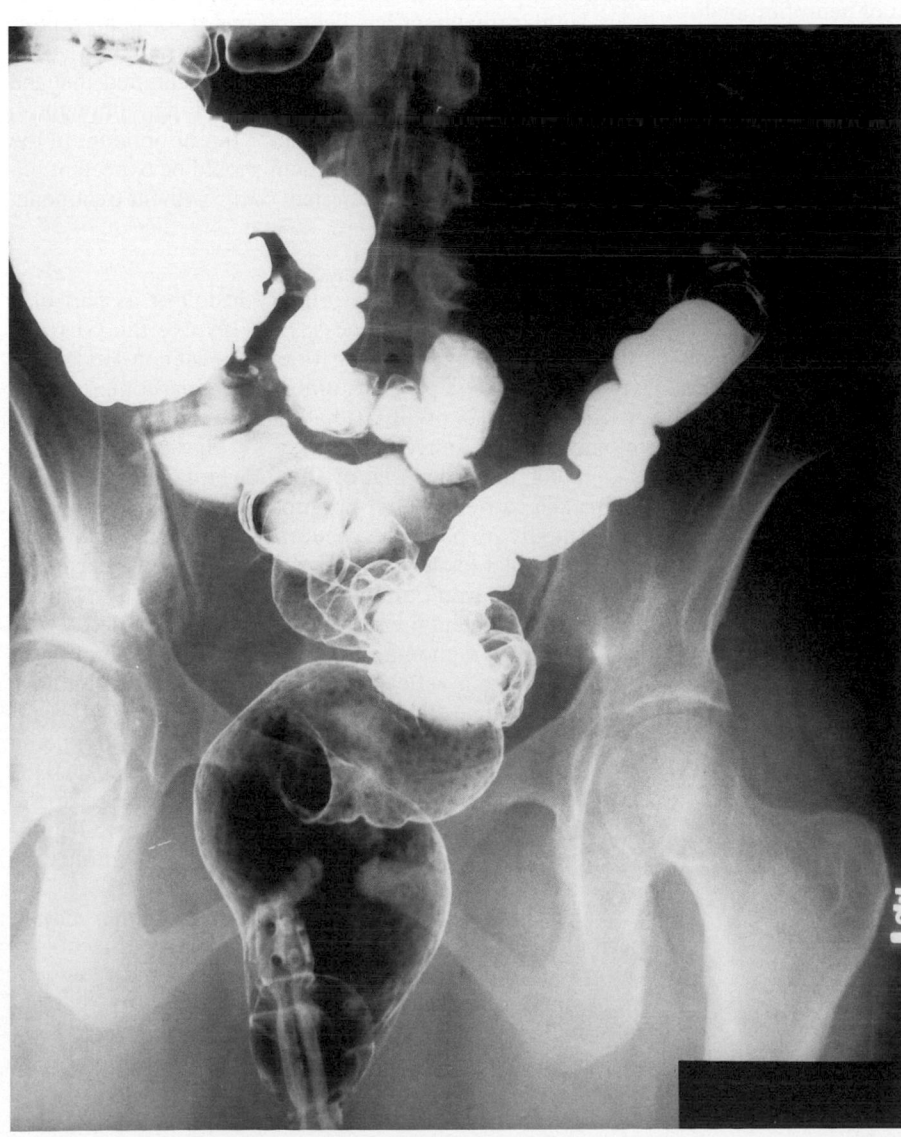

FIGURE 26-19. Lymphoid hyperplasia. Numerous small filling defects are evident in the rectum on this air-contrast barium enema study.

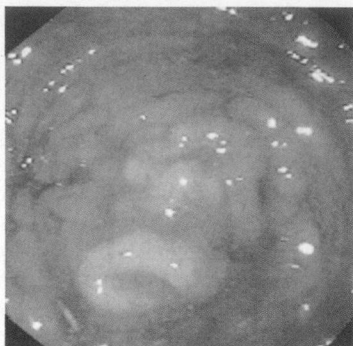

FIGURE 26-20. Colonoscopy reveals numerous confluent, sessile, mucosal nodules. Biopsy was consistent with nodular lymphoid hyperplasia.

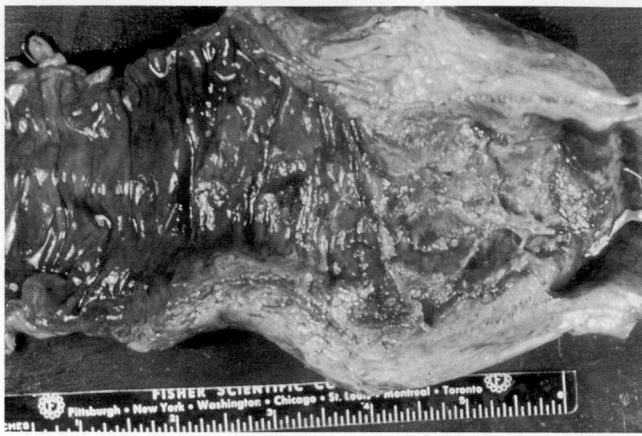

FIGURE 26-22. Autopsy specimen showing leukemic infiltration of the bowel wall simulating scirrhous carcinoma. (Courtesy of Rudolf Garret, MD.)

Symptoms

Although it may produce no symptoms if located in the rectum, a lymphoid polyp may cause considerable pain when it occurs in the anal canal. Colonic lesions may cause bleeding, abdominal pain, change in bowel habits, and symptoms related to intussusception, the last especially in children.[12,256] Anemia and weight loss may be seen in the chronic form. Collins and associates have reported a case in which the clinical presentation was identical to that of neurofibromatosis with neurovisceral involvement.[98] However, no similarity exists between the bowel lesions of lymphoid hyperplasia and neurofibromatosis.

Treatment

Local excision is indicated and is adequate for isolated or scattered lesions.[107,215,231] Removal is important in order to differentiate the condition from other neoplasms. In 100 patients so treated by Cornes and associates, only 5 developed recurrences, even though some polyps were incompletely removed.[107]

When the condition mimics acute appendicitis, a common presentation in children, appendectomy is performed. With chronic symptoms and extensive involvement of the terminal ileum, an ileocecal resection may be advisable.[256] Adults with lymphoid polyposis have been treated by colectomy with and without ileorectal anastomosis.[98,108] In other instances, less extensive bowel resections have been performed

in those with lymphoid hyperplasia who were misdiagnosed preoperatively.[166,491] It is crucial that one is aware of this entity and differentiates it from multiple polyposis.

Because radiotherapy and cytotoxic agents are often beneficial in the treatment of malignant lymphomas of the GI tract, similar treatment has been proposed for benign lymphoid polyposis.[106,161] Symmers stated that radiation is the accepted method of treatment.[495] Cosens claimed that the lesions may respond well to roentgen therapy, although no response occurred in his own case.[108] In our opinion, in the absence of symptoms, management should be expectant because spontaneous regression may occur without treatment.

Malignant Lymphoma

Malignant lymphoma, as a primary lesion or as part of a generalized malignant process, may involve the GI tract. This is the most common site for extranodal non-Hodgkin's lymphomas.[437] As a primary tumor lymphoma comprises between 1% and 4% of all GI malignancies, but only 0.5% of colonic and 0.1% of rectal cancers.[335,454] Gastric involvement is more common than that of small or large intestinal lymphoma and carries a better prognosis.[102] Colonic lymphoma preferentially involves the cecum and the rectum with 60% to 74% of colorectal lymphomas occurring in the cecum.[548] However, concurrent tumors elsewhere in the large bowel, the small bowel, and the stomach have been reported.

Malignant lymphoma of the colon has been reported in association with a variety of other entities, especially those of altered immune status (e.g., AIDS; see Chapter 10).[8,125,148,240,262,271,299,302,369,379,393,490,526] A high-grade B-cell lymphoma in an individual infected with HIV is considered an AIDS-defining condition.[434] Most intestinal lymphomas in the AIDS population are of the non-Hodgkin's type. GI non-Hodgkin's lymphoma represents 17% of those with extranodal involvement.[434]

Waldenström pointed out considerable overlap among macroglobulinemia, lymphoma, and lymphocytic leukemia.[526] This was exemplified by a case reported by Levy and coworkers in which cecal lymphoma developed in an 81-year-old individual while the patient was receiving immunosuppressive therapy for macroglobulinemia.[302] Associations with chronic ulcerative colitis, Crohn's disease, and celiac disease have also been observed.[304] With the concern for possible

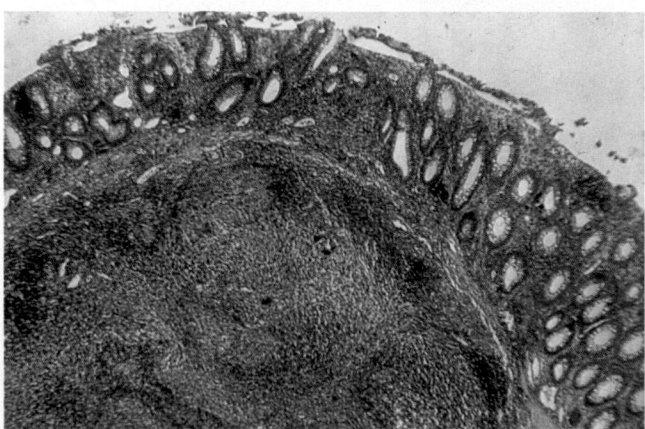

FIGURE 26-21. Lymphoid polyp of the rectum. Lymphocytic infiltration with irregular germinal centers in the submucosa. (Original magnification × 250; courtesy of Rudolf Garret, MD.)

concomitant leukemia, total and differential white blood cell counts are mandated as part of an evaluation.[544]

In most series, the incidence is greater in men than in women by a ratio of almost two to one.[550] Most patients are older than 50 years of age at diagnosis, but the condition can occur at any age.

Signs and Symptoms

Many individuals complain of abdominal pain that is usually cramping and localized to the area of the tumor. Other prominent symptoms include weight loss, change in bowel habits, diarrhea, weakness, nausea, vomiting, anorexia, bleeding, and fever. Discrete intra-abdominal masses are generally not appreciated until late in the course of the disease. The breakdown of signs and symptoms according to Fan and coworkers (37 patients) is as follows[149]:

- Abdominal pain (65%)
- Abdominal mass (54%)
- Weight loss (43%)

The symptoms produced by *rectal involvement* are variable and largely depend on whether the growth has become ulcerated. In early stages, with an intact mucosa, symptoms consist of a bearing-down sensation or a feeling of fullness in the rectum, with some rectal irritability and low backache. When ulceration of the overlying mucosa has developed, bleeding and mucous discharge may be noticed. Later, pain and soreness are described if the growth begins to encroach on the anal canal. A high index of suspicion must be maintained in homosexual patients, and obviously if AIDS is known or suspected. Obstructive symptoms are unlikely to occur because the primary growth often remains fairly localized to one quadrant and does not usually extend in an annular fashion as seen with carcinoma.

Pathogenesis

It is thought that malignant lymphoma starts in the submucosal lymphoid tissue, which in places extends into the mucosa. It is not known whether it begins multicentrically or arises from a single area and later spreads by direct extension or through lymphatic channels. At presentation, a large segment of colon may be involved in a uniform and continuous fashion. Submucosal infiltration often extends beyond the area of obvious involvement, and additional lesions may be found apart from that region. Marked involvement is most common in the ileocecal or the rectosigmoid area, where tumors sometimes become confluent and form a large conglomerate mass. This may cause intussusception and intestinal obstruction. In the ileocecal region, the process usually extends into the appendix and into the ileum for a variable distance. When the rectum is the site of the tumor, inguinal nodes may be enlarged and palpable. Extensive serosal or retroperitoneal involvement is not characteristic of diffuse lymphoma.

Endoscopy and Radiology

Clinical and radiographic diagnosis of colonic and rectal lymphoma may be obscured by the variety of appearances it may assume. Usher reported 10 patients with rectal lymphoma from the Mayo Clinic and observed that in all cases the lesion was visualized on proctoscopic examination.[517] In no instance could a definite diagnosis of lymphoma be made by the appearance of the lesion. Usually, it was described as a polypoid tumor, diffuse proctitis, a submucosal nodule, or carcinoma (Figure 26-23). The endoscopic appearance may resemble that of Crohn's disease, such as has been described for the extremely rarely reported cases of granulocytic sarcoma and malignant histiocytosis.[77,436]

From the radiologic point of view, diffuse lymphoma of the colon must be differentiated from familial polyposis, ulcerative colitis with pseudopolyposis, granulomatous colitis, nodular lymphoid hyperplasia, and schistosomiasis. Although radiologic differentiation from carcinoma may be impossible, Halls pointed out that certain presentations strongly suggest lymphoma: presence of a bulky extracolonic component, concentric dilatation of the lumen, and a polypoid filling defect of the terminal ileum and ileocecal valve (Figures 26-24 and 26-25).[209]

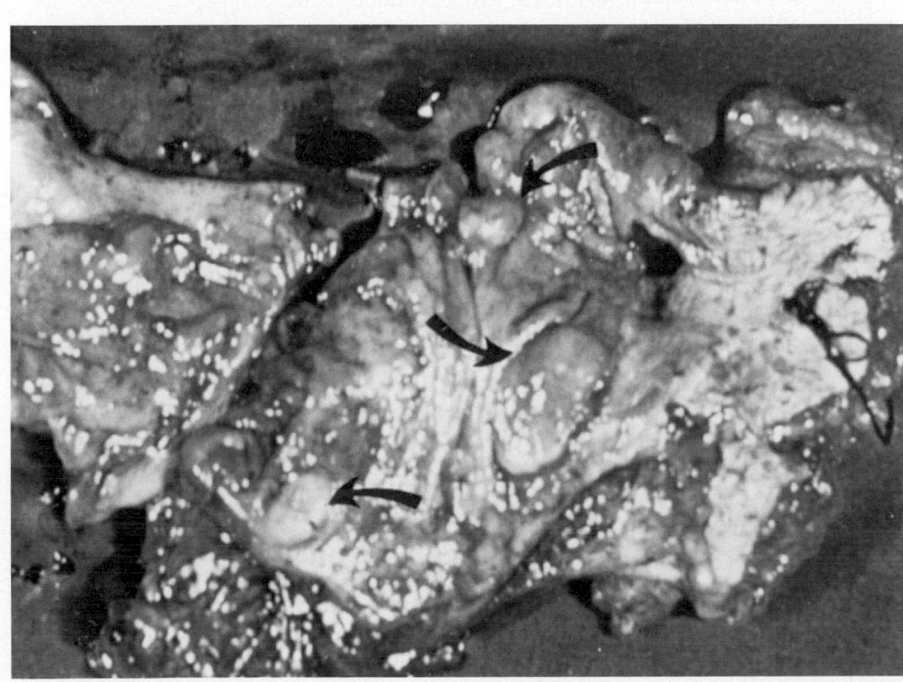

FIGURE 26-23. Lymphomatous infiltration of the rectum treated by abdominoperineal resection. Multiple lesions (*arrows*) are noted. (Courtesy of Rudolf Garret, MD.)

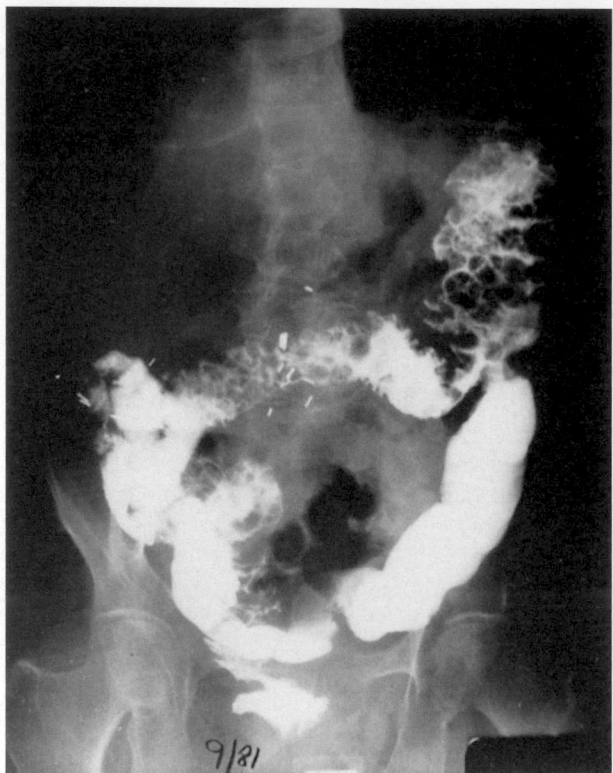

FIGURE 26-24. Malignant lymphoma. Postevacuation barium enema demonstrates multiple polypoid filling defects of varying size with areas of ulceration.

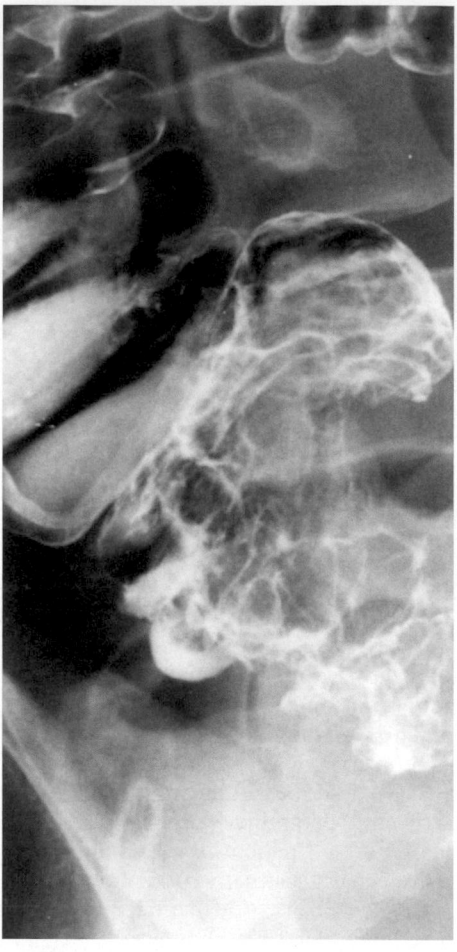

FIGURE 26-25. Malignant lymphoma of the cecum. Note the large, lobulated mass.

Pathology

Macroscopic examination of the tumor reveals a polypoid or ulcerated mass resembling carcinoma or a diffuse process extending over a large segment of colon, sometimes with numerous polypoid intraluminal excrescences. The bowel wall is thickened and rubbery in consistency, and its cut surface demonstrates a greatly thickened mucosa, often with prominent convoluted folds resembling the surface of brain and reaching a thickness of 1 or 2 cm (Figure 26-26). The submucosa is markedly thickened as a result of infiltration by closely packed tumor cells. In contrast to disease in the small bowel, deep ulceration and perforation are uncommon. However, superficial ulceration and necrosis may be seen.

The presence of a nonulcerated, submucous tumor in the rectal wall requires differentiation from benign lesions, such as lipoma, myoma, and nodular lymphoid hyperplasia, and also from an inflammatory condition, such as an intramuscular abscess. Thus, biopsy and histologic examination are crucial to the evaluation of such lesions (Figures 26-27 and 26-28). Microscopic examination usually readily distinguishes lymphoma from other malignancies.[519] However, a nonspecific lymphoid infiltrate in the mucosa and submucosa may present a problem with differential diagnosis. Under these circumstances, some investigators have recommended immunocytochemical studies as well as gene rearrangement analysis with DNA probes to elucidate the precise nature of the process.[378]

Regional lymph nodes are involved in approximately one-half of the patients at the time of laparotomy. The presence of enlarged nodes may, however, represent reactive lymphoid hyperplasia and must be carefully examined histologically

to document the presence of tumor. Because involvement beyond a single segment of bowel and its regional nodes excludes the diagnosis of primary lymphoma, a careful search for additional diseased nodes is necessary.

Classification

Malignant lymphoma is classified based on its cellular morphology and immunologic surface markers. Included are

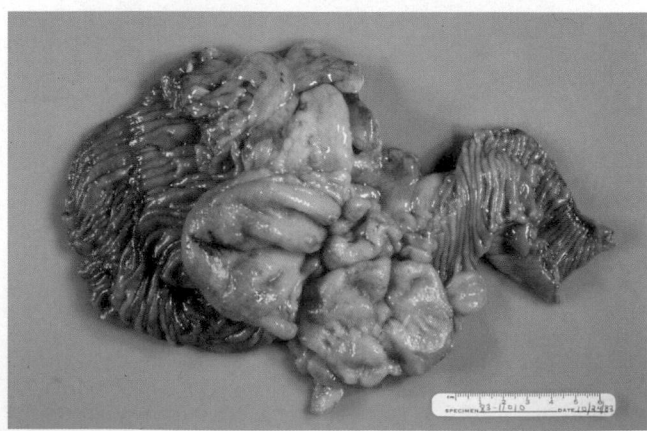

FIGURE 26-26. Resected specimen showing lymphoma of the cecum. Note the convoluted folds.

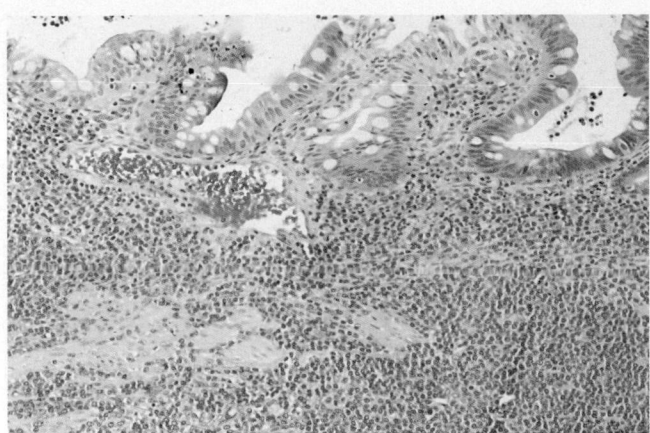

FIGURE 26-27. Lymphoma of the sigmoid colon. Note the heavy infiltrate of lymphocytic tumor cells involving the mucosa and submucosa. (Original magnification × 80; courtesy of Rudolf Garret, MD.)

the following histologic types: lymphocytic lymphoma, lymphosarcoma, reticulum cell sarcoma, giant follicular lymphoma, and Hodgkin's disease. Hodgkin's disease of the colon or rectum is the rarest.

Tumors are also classified based on the extent of involvement:

Class I: confined to bowel wall

Class II: regional node involvement within the drainage area of the bowel primary tumor

Class III: para-aortic node involvement; direct extension to adjacent viscera

As pointed out by Wychulis and associates and by others, the prognosis of primary extranodal lymphoma in the colon or rectum is not clearly related to cell type but is affected by stage.[149,304,438,550]

Treatment

Most agree that resection is preferred whenever malignant lymphoma is confined to the bowel (including regional nodes).[25] The Mayo Clinic group recommended that if lymphoma is confined to the rectum and the tumor is resectable, surgical excision should be followed by radiation therapy.[122] In those tumors considered unresectable, radia-

tion therapy is of definite benefit. A combined program with chemotherapy is recommended for systemic disease. Adjuvant therapy may include cyclophosphamide, doxorubicin (or epirubicin), vincristine, prednisone, and bleomycin.[25,548] Another approach uses mitoxantrone, chlorambucil, and prednisone.[437]

Results

Contreary and colleagues reported a 50% 5-year survival in those patients operated upon for cure.[102] When the tumor was confined to the bowel or involved only local nodes, the survival rate in both situations was also 50%. When regional nodes were involved, 5-year survival fell to 12%. Although this was not a controlled study, the difference in survival rates between those patients operated upon for cure with supplementary radiotherapy and without it was 83% versus 16%. Moertel reported an overall 5-year survival rate of 55%.[352]

The treatment of non-Hodgkin's lymphoma in the setting of HIV infection has been much less effective than in individuals without immunodeficiency (see Chapter 10). The use of cytotoxic agents exacerbates the already existing immune impairment and leaves the person with prolonged neutropenia and at further risk for opportunistic infection.[434] Survival times are generally less than 1 year.

Extramedullary Plasmacytoma

Primary plasmacytoma is a localized plasma cell tumor that is most commonly found in the nasopharynx, although it has been described in many other parts of the body. Plasma cell neoplasms are classified in five categories: multiple myeloma, solitary myeloma, extramedullary plasmacytoma (with multiple myeloma), plasma cell leukemia, and primary plasmacytoma.[460]

The condition involves the colon extremely rarely with fewer than 10 cases having been reported as a primary disease. Some have involved the bowel secondarily. Primary tumors elsewhere in the GI tract have also been noted.[189,212,218] Disseminated multiple myeloma is often diagnosed in patients who have a localized plasmacytoma if these patients are followed for a sufficiently long period. Therefore, a bone marrow examination should be performed at some point once an extramedullary plasmacytoma has been diagnosed. Primary and secondary colorectal plasmacytoma is more common in men than in women by a ratio of 3:2.

Presenting symptoms include abdominal pain, bleeding, anorexia, nausea, vomiting, and weight loss. The tumor can be single or multiple and may consist of diffuse cellular infiltrates or of polypoid or nodular protrusions. Microscopic examination demonstrates the characteristic population of plasma cells (Figure 26-29). Identification by means of immunoperoxidase staining has also been advised.[183]

Treatment ideally consists of total excision when possible. If, for example, a GI lesion has been excised for purposes of diagnosis and the entire tumor was removed, no additional treatment would in all probability be indicated. Of the cases reviewed by Sidani and associates, none metastasized to any organ other than lymph nodes.[460] Plasmacytomas that are not readily resectable may be responsive to radiotherapy. The use of chemotherapy is restricted to disseminated disease.

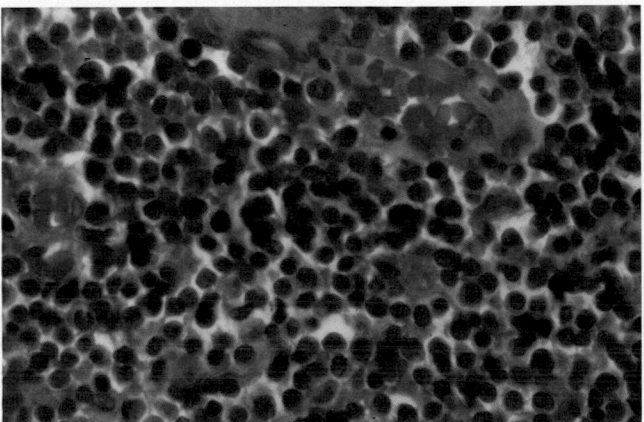

FIGURE 26-28. Lymphoma of the cecum. Note the lymphoblasts in the wall of the bowel. (Original magnification × 600; courtesy of Rudolf Garret, MD.)

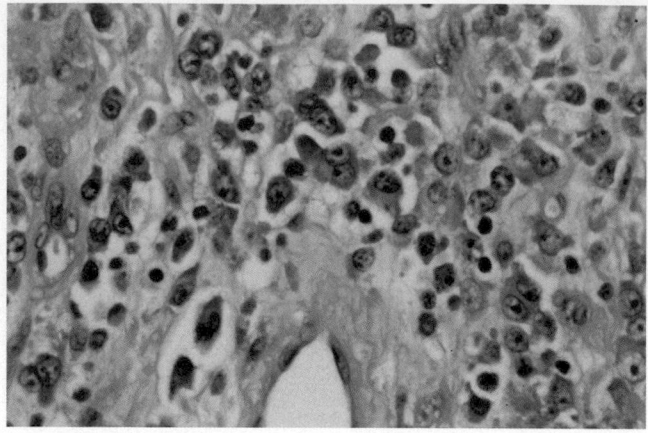

FIGURE 26-29. Extramedullary plasmacytoma. **A:** Colonic gland surrounded by atypical, infiltrative plasma cells. (Original magnification × 100.) **B:** Many plasma cells, some of which demonstrate hyperchromatic and eccentric nuclei. Note the apophyllic cytoplasm, a characteristic feature of plasma cells. There are also binucleate forms with discernible nucleoli. (Original magnification × 400.)

► MESENCHYMAL TUMORS

Fibrous Tissue Origin

Fibroma

Fibroma of the colon is a very rare tumor that belongs to the uncommon spindle cell group of benign tumors that also includes leiomyomas.[479] Its incidence is only one-tenth that of leiomyoma, however.[66]

Although many authors use the terms fibroma, leiomyoma, and fibromyoma interchangeably, Rose emphasized that differential histologic tissue staining techniques distinguish the true fibroma from other spindle cell tumors.[424] According to Aird, the tumor may originate in any layer of the bowel wall but arises most frequently in the submucosa.[6] Fibromas have been reported in the appendicular stump and near the mesentery.[154,511] Reports of fibroma of the colon are few.[23,150,381,424] Abdominal pain and distension may be noted, and resection is the treatment of choice.

Fibroma of the anorectal region is very rare. It may arise from a hypertrophied papilla or by fibrous infiltration of a large prolapsing internal hemorrhoid, generally as a result of repeated attacks of thrombosis and strangulation without sloughing. It is encapsulated, firm, slightly movable, ovoid, of small to moderate size, and has little tendency to ulcerate. It is usually situated in the wall. In time, the covering of columnar epithelium becomes converted into squamous epithelium. A smooth, pale fibrous polyp results. The tumor may remain in the wall of the rectum or become polypoid and extend into the lumen. In general, it is single and of slow growth. However, fibrous polyps may be multiple, so a careful proctoscopy is essential.

Symptoms include tenesmus and a sense of heaviness in the rectum. If ulceration has occurred (an exception), bleeding may be noted. The diagnosis is seldom made without microscopic examination. Transanal excision is the appropriate treatment.

Inflammatory Fibroid Polyp or Eosinophilic Granuloma

Inflammatory fibroid polyp is a rare, focal lesion occurring in the submucosa of the GI tract, least commonly in the colon.[255,305,400] Only a few cases have been reported.[334,338,387,523]

Another term for the condition is eosinophilic granuloma. Although the etiology is uncertain, the observation of the proliferation of submucosal mesenchymal fibrous tissue as well as variable eosinophilic infiltration suggests the effect of an inflammatory stimulus (Figure 26-30).[305]

Rectal bleeding, tenesmus, change in bowel habits, and diarrhea are the most common symptoms. Obstruction resulting from intussusception has also been reported.[305] Radiographically, the impression may be that of a carcinoma.[338] Because malignant degeneration has not been noted, however, endoscopic removal is suggested. A concern is that lesions may be sessile and submucosal and have a tendency to bleed readily. If colonoscopic resection is unsuccessful or inadvisable, colectomy or colotomy and polypectomy should be performed.

Fibrosarcoma

Of the sarcomas involving the GI tract, fibrosarcoma is one of the rarest. Stoller and Weinstein reported 21 cases of fibrosarcoma of the rectum in the literature from 1927 until 1954 and added 2 cases of their own.[483] The mean age of the patients in this series was 51 years. All tumors were situated in the rectum within 10 cm of the dentate line. Only 2 cases of fibrosarcoma of the colon have been reported.[45,228] Espinosa and Quan identified the only case of anal fibrosarcoma.[145] The lesion apparently arose at the site of a previous fistulectomy incision.

The most common presenting symptom of fibrosarcoma of the rectum is difficulty with defecation. Pain is the second most common symptom, and bleeding, third.[483] Proctosigmoidoscopic examination may reveal the tumor to be consistent with an adenocarcinoma, and only histologic determination can establish the definitive diagnosis.

Microscopically, the tumor is characterized by strands of fibrous tissue that infiltrate the adjacent structures of the bowel wall but tend to spare the mucosa until late in the disease (Figures 26-31).[483] The presence of mitoses is helpful in confirming the malignant nature of the lesion.

Treatment is essentially the same as that for adenocarcinoma: radical resection of the involved bowel with or without a sphincter-saving approach. Neither radiotherapy nor chemotherapy has been helpful in the management of this rare condition.

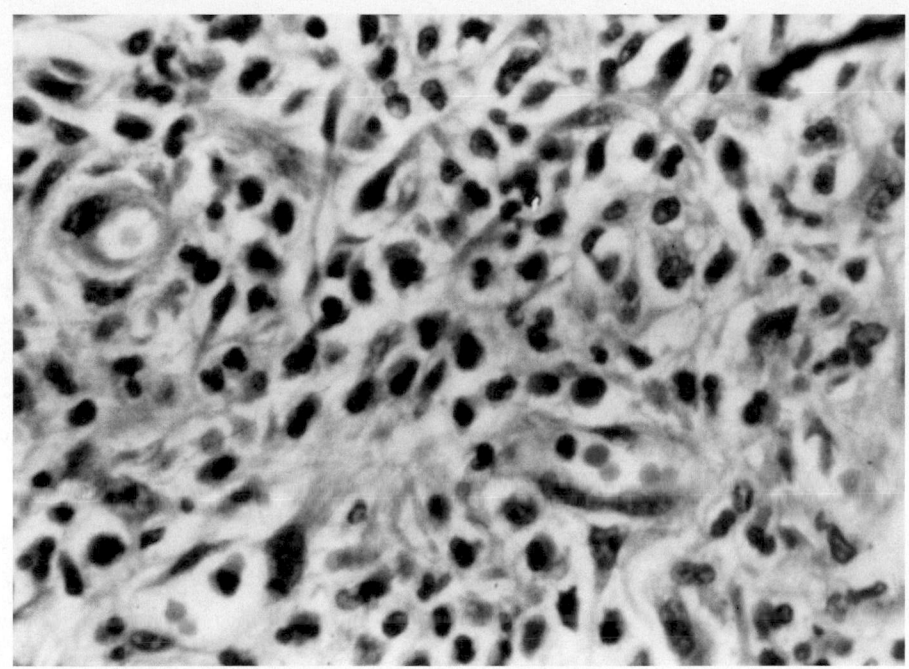

FIGURE 26-30. Inflammatory fibroid polyp. The bowel wall is infiltrated by many eosinophils. Note some fibroblasts and small blood vessels lined by prominent endothelial cells (Original magnification × 280; courtesy of Rudolf Garret, MD.)

Malignant Fibrous Histiocytoma

Malignant fibrous histiocytoma is an extremely rare fibrosarcoma variant in which histiocyte-like cells are present.[39,452,530] The term was originally proposed by O'Brien and Stout to describe tumors composed of both fibroblasts and histiocytes (Figure 26-32).[376] The lesion is usually found in the lower extremity.

It is difficult to present a meaningful evaluation of the signs, symptoms, diagnosis, therapy, and prognosis with such an uncommon condition. Tumors tend to be large, present with obstructive symptoms, and are thought clinically to be adenocarcinomas. Treatment is radical resection, but prognosis is presumably poor. A partial response has been reported with chemotherapy.[210]

Stromal Origin

Gastrointestinal Stromal Tumors

Gastrointestinal stromal tumors (GISTs) are sarcomas arising from mesenchymal tissue. They are believed to represent the most common nonepithelial sarcoma of the GI tract, comprising approximately 0.1% to 3% of all GI cancers and approximately 5% of soft tissue sarcomas. GISTs can occur anywhere in the GI tract but most commonly arise in the stomach (65%) or small intestine (25%); about 5% to 10% of GISTs are located in the colon and rectum.[185] GISTs are related to the muscle-like nerve cells, the interstitial cells of Cajal, which coordinate the autonomic movements of the GI tract. Although the exact incidence is still somewhat unclear, it is now estimated that between 5,000 and 10,000 people each year develop GISTs. GISTs have a slight male predominance with the median age of diagnosis approximately 60 years.[185] There appears to be an association with neurofibromatosis, and there have also been reports of germ line mutations in the KIT proto-oncogene.

Symptoms

Often, patients experience no symptoms from these tumors, but when symptomatic, complaints include rectal bleeding (50%), abdominal pain (30% to 40%), vomiting (from

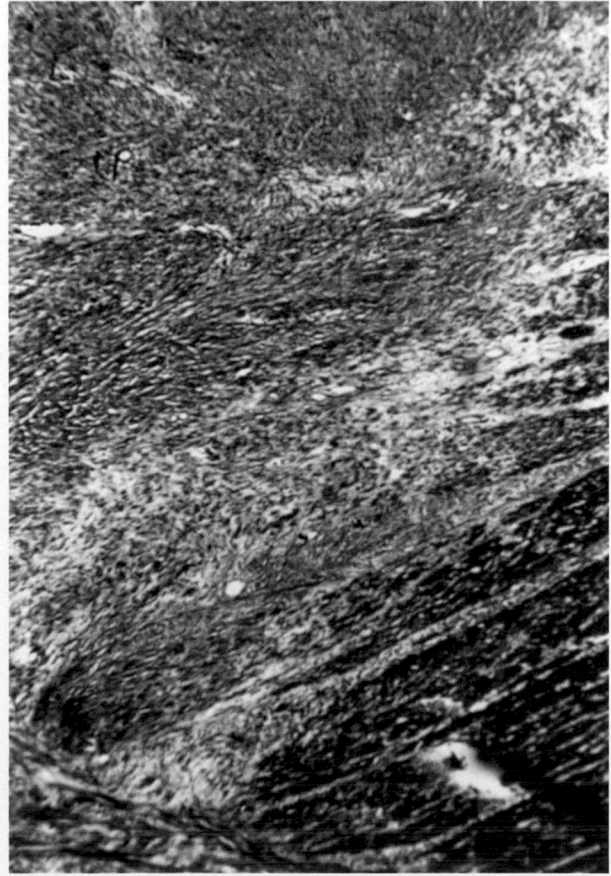

FIGURE 26-31. Fibrosarcoma. A well-differentiated tumor infiltrating the wall of the bowel. (Trichrome stain; original magnification × 80; courtesy of Rudolf Garret, MD.)

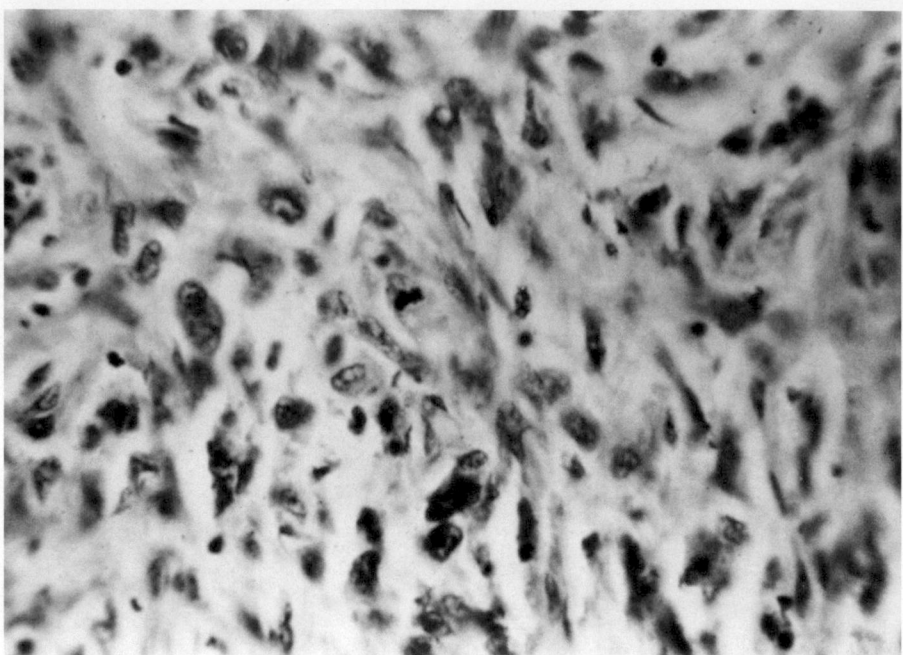

FIGURE 26-32. Malignant fibrous histiocytoma. Elongated cells with hyperchromatic nuclei and some mitotic figures. Some cells demonstrate large amounts of cytoplasm suggesting histiocytic origin. (Original magnification × 600; courtesy of Rudolf Garret, MD.)

obstruction), and fatigue (from anemia). About one-half have metastatic disease at the time of presentation.[159]

Diagnosis and Tumor Behavior

The diagnosis of GIST is usually made on biopsy or, more commonly, at the time of exploratory laparotomy that was performed for an unknown mass. However, the diagnosis of GIST may be suggested by preoperative CT through the presence of a large mass *without* adenopathy.[101] An incidental extrarectal mass may be felt or seen at the time of routine digital examination, proctoscopy, or colonoscopy (Figure 26-33).

In GIST, a specific DNA mutation causes the tyrosine kinase enzyme, known as KIT proto-oncogene, to be switched "on" all the time. KIT encodes for a transmembrane receptor tyrosine kinase signaling molecule, which is responsible for sending growth and survival signals inside the cell. If it is "on," the cell stays alive and grows or proliferates. The overactive mutant KIT enzyme triggers the uncontrolled growth of GIST tumor cells. KIT can be identified by looking for a portion of the enzyme, the CD117 antigen. The presence of CD117 is, in fact, a defining feature of GIST and is widely used to confirm the diagnosis. GIST tumors have also been found to contain a

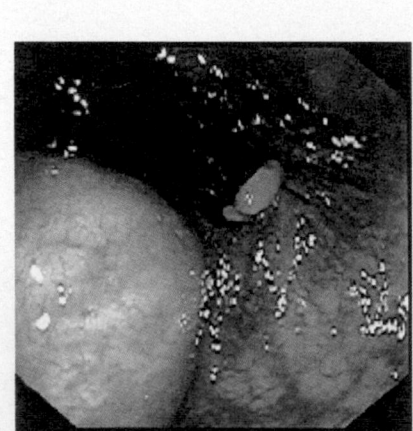

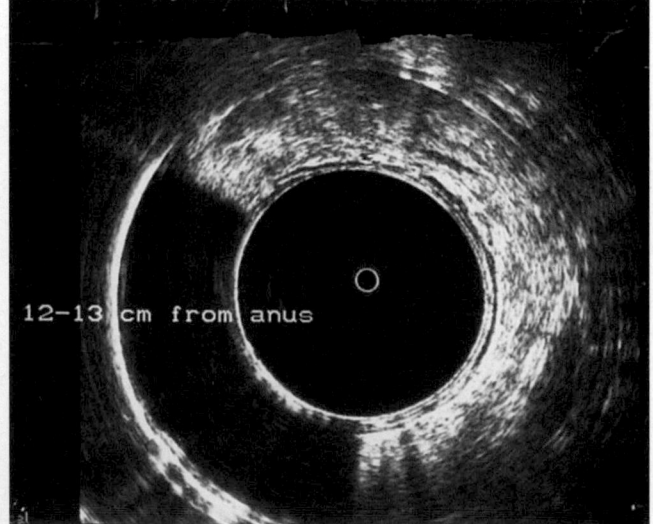

FIGURE 26-33. Malignant gastrointestinal stromal tumor (GIST). **A:** Extrarectal mass seen on retroflexion of colonoscope demonstrating mucosal preservation. **B:** Endorectal ultrasound shows a posterior mass of mixed echogenicity that upon excision proved to be a GIST.

ARTHUR PURDY STOUT (1885-1967)

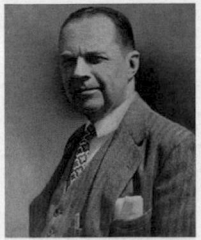

Arthur Purdy Stout was born in New York City on November 30, 1985. He graduated from Yale University with a baccalaureate degree in 1907 and was awarded his medical degree in 1912 from Columbia College of Physicians and Surgeons. He was a surgical intern at Roosevelt Hospital between 1912 and 1914. His first appointments were at Columbia Presbyterian Hospital as an instructor in surgery and as assistant attending surgical pathologist. He also served overseas during WWI as a first lieutenant in the United States Army Medical Corps. Stout returned to Columbia after the war in 1919 and remained there for the rest of his remarkable career. He was known best for his role in advancing the field of surgical pathology, authoring hundreds of scientific articles as well as several books, including *Human Cancer* (1932). His primary interest was the histologic classification of neoplasms and its correlation with prognosis. In the field of colorectal surgery, he was the first person to describe the histologic difference between the more common small bowel/appendiceal carcinoid tumor and large bowel/rectal carcinoids (*American Journal of Pathology*, 1942). He had a formidable impact on our understanding of a host of neoplastic conditions. His memory lives on through the Arthur Purdy Stout Society that supports advancements in the field of surgical pathology. Arthur Stout passed away at his home in New York in 1967 at the age of 82. (With appreciation to Brett T. Phillips, MD.)

mutation in platelet-derived growth factor receptor alpha (PDGFRA).[186]

Distinguishing benign from malignant tumors may be quite difficult. It is important to recognize that the current concept is that all GISTs are at risk for malignancy (Figure 26-34). The location of the tumor seems to affect behavior, but the most important prognostic factors for malignant risk are tumor size at diagnosis and mitotic count.[346] Still, a small GIST in the small intestine may grow more quickly and be more likely to spread than a large gastric tumor. When a GIST metastasizes, it usually spreads to the liver or peritoneal cavity but rarely spreads to the lymph nodes.

Treatment
Traditionally, the only treatment for GIST had been wide surgical resection. However, surgery alone for larger GISTs or for GISTs that have spread yields disappointing results. Unfortunately, conventional chemotherapy or radiation after surgery has not been demonstrably effective. However, imatinib mesylate (formerly known to as ST1571) manufactured as Gleevec in the United States and Glivec in Europe has been demonstrated to be an effective inhibitor of tyrosine kinases.[101] Imatinib is considered first-line treatment for metastatic GIST.[185]

Results
There is a very wide range in survival rates reported for these tumors, a fact that makes interpretation of published data quite difficult. As many as perhaps 90% of patients who have undergone resection for GIST develop recurrence.[117] Connolly and coworkers performed a MEDLINE literature search and concluded that the 5-year survival rate after complete excision is approximately 50%.[101] Langer and colleagues reviewed their experience with GISTs in 39 patients.[296] As one would expect, failure to extirpate the tumor completely had an adverse consequence on survival when compared with those lesions that could be completely removed. Tumor size of 5 cm or greater, mitotic count of two or more, and proliferative activity greater than 10% were significantly associated with a shorter recurrence-free survival. These investigators also found that patients did better if the tumors demonstrated significantly fewer genetic alterations.

Smooth Muscle Origin
Colonic Leiomyoma
Smooth muscle tumors of the alimentary tract are rare, and benign smooth muscle tumors of the colon are exceedingly uncommon. Stout conducted a 50-year study in which he found 30 leiomyomas in 200 benign neoplasms.[484] In a 15-year study, Ferguson and Houston reported 2 leiomyomas from a total of 67 benign tumors.[152] Skardalakis and Gray reviewed 59 cases of leiomyomas, and MacKenzie and coworkers collected reports of 19 cases from the literature and added 8 of their own.[318,464]

Smooth muscle tumors are found in patients of all ages, with a gradual increase in frequency and malignant degeneration up to the sixth decade.[270] The tumor is classified according to its appearance and direction of growth. The intracolonic type may be pedunculated or sessile. The extracolonic type grows away from the lumen of the bowel and lies in the abdominal cavity attached to the wall. The dumbbell type grows into the lumen and into the abdominal cavity simultaneously. This type of tumor accounts for 4% of all smooth muscle tumors of the GI tract. These usually reach a much larger size than those with unilateral spread. The constrictive type encircles a variable length of bowel. Lookanoff and Tsapralis observed that the sigmoid and transverse colon seemed to be the most common sites and that very few leiomyomas were found in the cecum.[309]

The tumor may be an incidental finding in an asymptomatic individual, or the patient may present with pain or a lump. Perforation, intestinal obstruction (secondary to the tumor itself or to intussusception), and hemorrhage have been reported.[85,362]

Macroscopically, the tumor appears well encapsulated. On cross section, leiomyomas have a fleshy appearance;

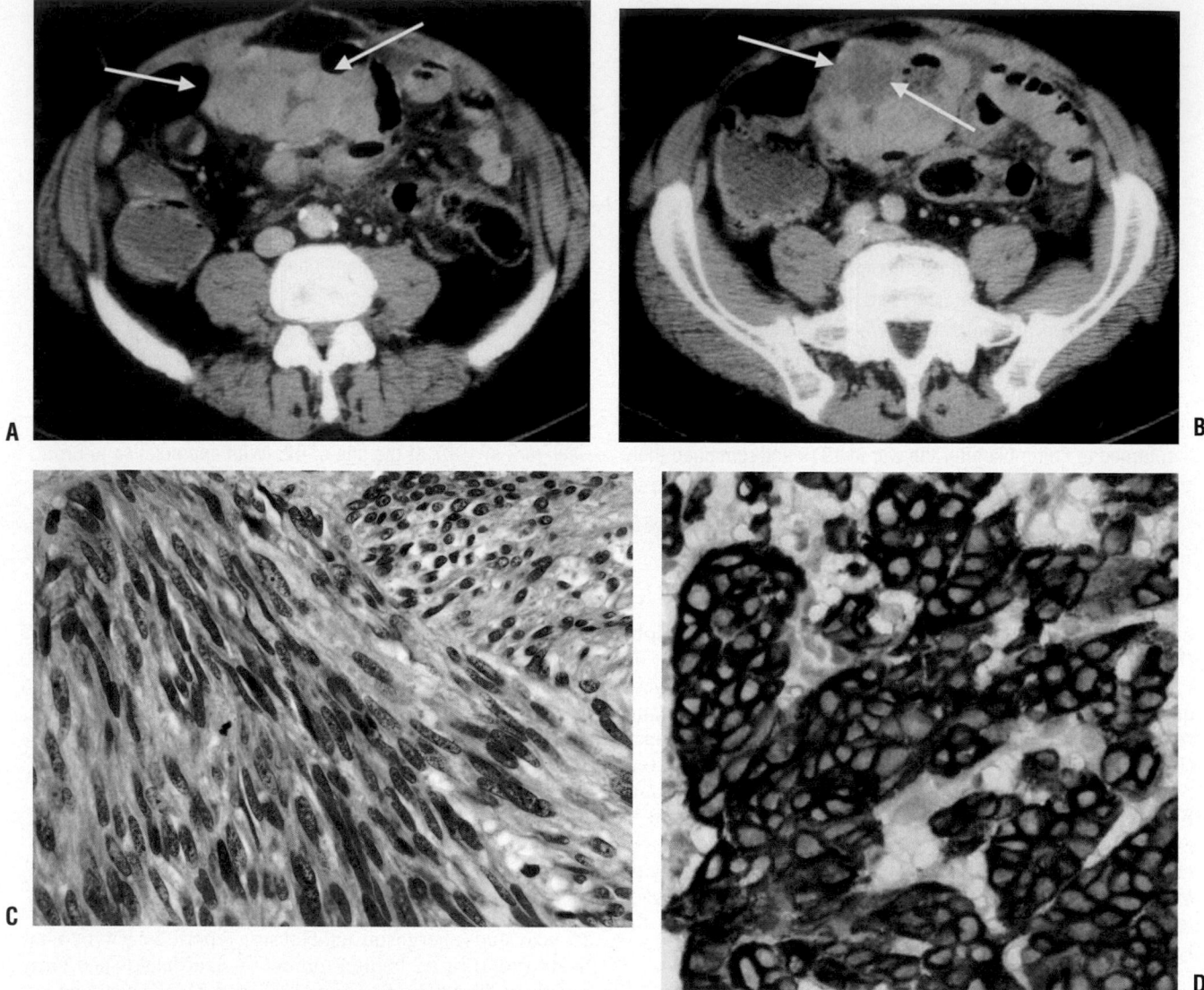

FIG. 26-34 A: Small-bowel gastrointestinal stromal tumor with a diffusely thickened bowel wall. **B:** Gastrointestinal stromal tumor. Image obtained in the same patient as in the previous image. A more caudal portion of the tumor has areas of necrosis (*arrows*), with air present within the necrotic cavity that communicates with the lumen of the small bowel. **C:** Spindle cell GIST shows uniform cigar-shape cells with elongated nuclei (H-E stain X40). **D:** Formalin-fixed, paraffin-embedded human gastrointestinal stromal tumor stained with peroxidase-conjugate and DAB chromogen. Note cytoplasmic/membranous staining.

because the tumor is under pressure, it tends to protrude (Figures 26-35 through 26-38).

Histologically, a typical spindle cell neoplasm can be observed (Figure 26-39). Most investigators believe that the mitotic rate is the single most important criterion for diagnosis of malignancy.[53,63,146,485] Other indicators are a variation in nuclear size and shape, hyperchromasia, frequent bizarre cells, and difficulty in identification of longitudinal myofibrils.[53,63,146] If the mitotic rate is high, if the growth is rapid, if an ulcer is present, or if the lesion is greater than 2.5 cm in diameter, malignant degeneration should be suspected. Smooth muscle tumors are usually locally invasive, but metastasis from a primary tumor in the GI tract has been described.[63]

Radiologic features vary depending on whether the tumor is intramural, submucosal, subserosal, or dumbbell shaped.[35]

Treatment

Surgical excision results in cure unless the tumor is extraperitoneal or rectal (see later). Complete removal should be attempted regardless of the radiologic appearance or of probable inoperability. Swerdlow and colleagues reported a case of an elderly individual with a benign leiomyoma of the cecum that had ulcerated and perforated the bowel wall.[493] The patient presented with an acute abdomen. Because it is generally not possible to distinguish benign from malignant lesions preoperatively, a standard cancer operation should be performed under such circumstances.

Rectal Leiomyoma

Only a few cases of rectal leiomyomas have been reported.[16,372,442,451] Vorobyov and colleagues reported their

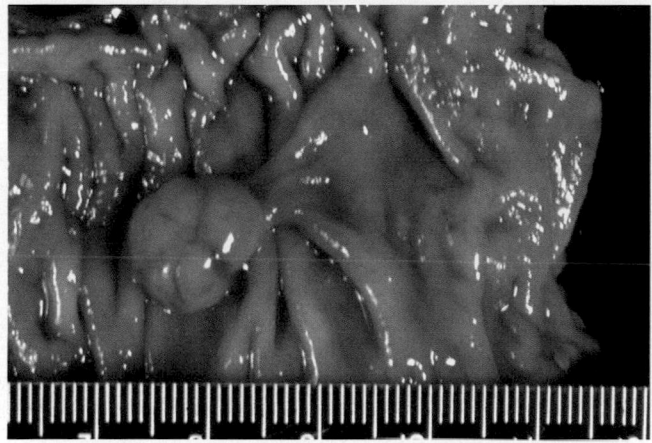

FIGURE 26-35. Pedunculated leiomyoma.

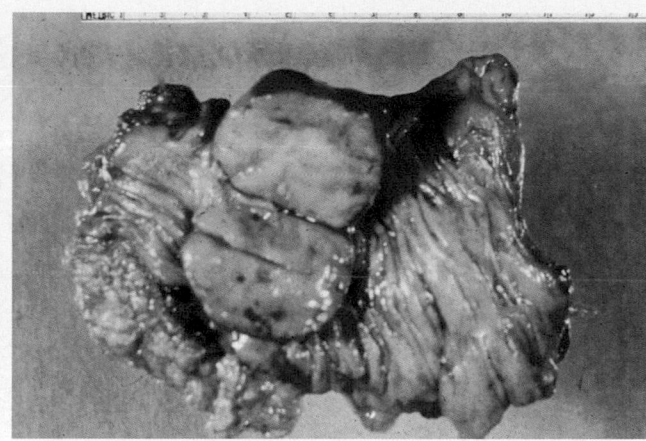

FIGURE 26-37. A leiomyoma resected from the hepatic flexure reveals a fleshy tumor on cross section. (From Corman ML, Veidenheimer MC, Swinton NW. *Diseases of the Anus, Rectum and Colon. Part I: Neoplasms.* New York, NY: Medcom; 1972.)

experience at the Research Institute of Proctology in Moscow.[525] Thirty-six patients with benign leiomyoma of the rectum underwent surgery between the years 1972 and 1990. Approximately one-third were male. In this experience, the tumors often tended to arise from the internal anal sphincter. Some investigators have found that endorectal ultrasound is helpful in determining the limits of the lesion.[451] A homogeneous hypoechoic tumor without invasion of the perirectal tissue may be noted.[236]

Smaller myomas usually cause no symptoms, can be found on routine rectal examination, and are usually removed with a diathermy snare or by transanal excision. Large lesions may cause interference with defecation, a sense of fullness in the rectum, and a frequent desire to defecate. Because of these distressing symptoms and the possibility of obstruction and malignant degeneration, removal of the growth is indicated.

When the tumor is essentially extrarectal, it is best to excise it by means of an extrarectal approach rather than transanally. Even large tumors may be treated by local excision, but if clinical suspicion of malignancy exists, such as ulceration,

hemorrhage, or extrarectal fixation, radical surgical treatment by excision of the rectum is indicated. Biopsies may be difficult to interpret in such cases. In the experience of the group from the Research Institute of Proctology, one-third of their patients (n = 12) harbored lesions less than 1 cm in diameter, and these were all removed by means of transanal excision.[525] An additional 10 patients with tumors from 2.5 to 5 cm also were treated by this approach. Six other individuals underwent excision by means of a perirectal operation, whereas abdominoperineal resection or abdominoanal operations were performed in those with tumors measuring from 8 to 20 cm. Recurrence was found in 9 patients, all of whom had local procedures. In 7, malignant transformation was the reason.

Leiomyosarcoma
Colon

Leiomyosarcoma of the large bowel is a very rare lesion. The total number of published cases is probably fewer than 150, although many would today probably be classified as GIST

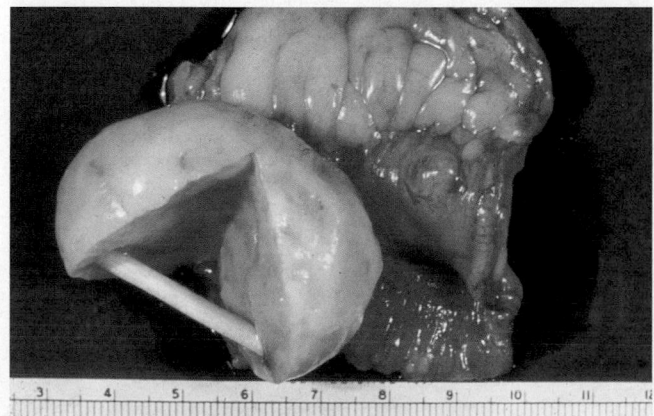

FIGURE 26-36. Leiomyoma. A well-encapsulated mass in the bowel wall. (Courtesy of Rudolf Garret, MD.)

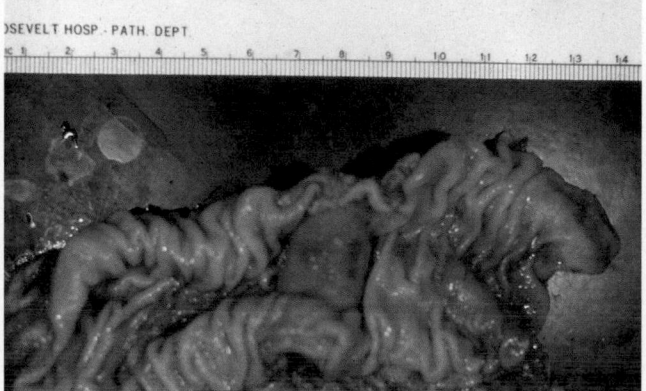

FIGURE 26-38. Sigmoid colectomy reveals characteristic leiomyoma in the bowel wall.

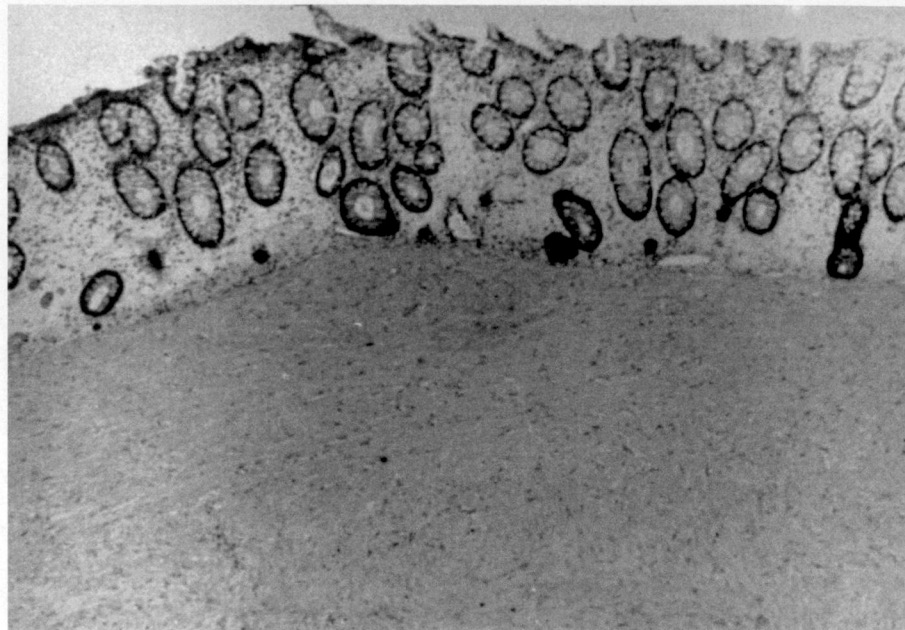

FIGURE 26-39. Leiomyoma of the colon. Spindle cell neoplasm filling the submucosa with thinning of the overlying mucosa. Nuclei are blunted at ends with surrounding vacuoles. There is no evidence of mitoses or pleomorphism. (Original magnification × 100.)

tumors (see earlier discussion).[21,30,35,73,90,119,234,412,449,480] No age predilection for this disease is apparent. It affects the genders equally and is more than twice as common in the rectum as it is in the rest of the colon.

Leiomyosarcoma arises from the smooth muscle of the bowel wall (Figure 26-40). A very insidious disease, it can remain asymptomatic for a long period. Weight loss is almost never recorded, but pain is a common symptom. Tarry stools and the sequelae of anemia are the most frequent presentations (Figure 26-41). A palpable tumor is almost always present when the lesion occurs in the rectum, and in some instances, obstruction is also seen.

Diagnosis of this lesion preoperatively is extremely difficult because it resembles carcinoma of the colon in its radiographic appearance. The tumor may project into the lumen of the bowel, grow outward, or present as a dumbbell-type

tumor.[120] An interesting radiologic finding may be demonstrated when tracts of barium extend into a subserosal tumor.[73] Sonographic features may include a thick echogenic rim with central cavitation.[259] Colonoscopy and biopsy are useful in confirming the diagnosis.

An attempt to stage the disease for the sake of better management was reported by Astarjian and colleagues as follows[21]:

Stage I: tumor confined to the intestinal wall; no invasion, no ulceration
  A. Submucosal tumor
  B. Subserosal tumor
Stage II: tumor extending beyond the wall of the colon
  A. Intraluminal ulceration
  B. Infiltration into adjacent extracolonic tissues
Stage III: tumor with distant metastases

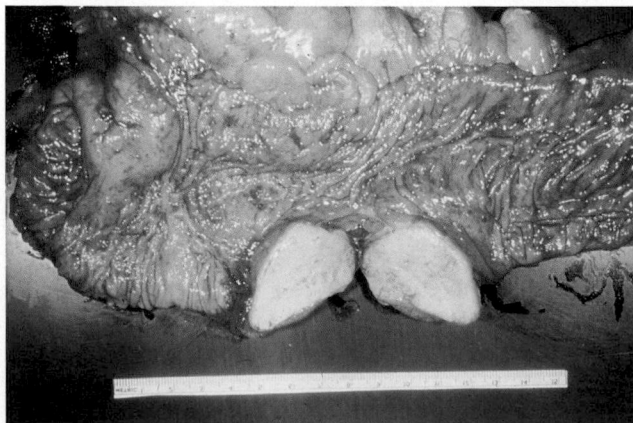

FIGURE 26-40. Leiomyosarcoma. This tumor of the bowel wall looks well encapsulated, but histologic examination revealed frequent mitotic figures. (From Corman ML, Veidenheimer MC, Swinton NW. *Diseases of the Anus, Rectum, and Colon. Part I: Neoplasms.* New York, NY: Medcom; 1972.)

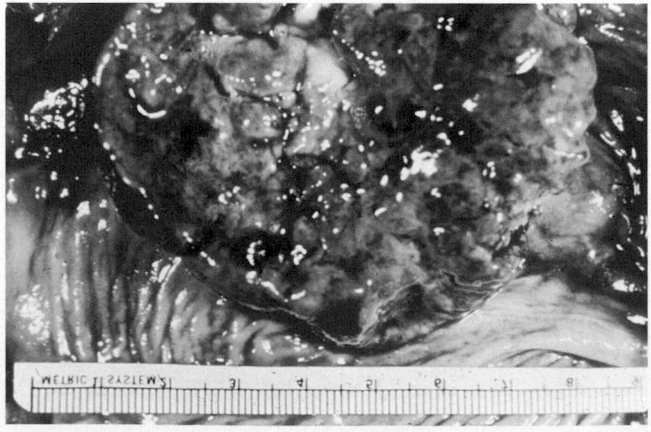

FIGURE 26-41. Ulcerating leiomyosarcoma producing hematochezia. The absence of infiltrating margins indicates that it is less likely to be an adenocarcinoma. (From Corman ML, Veidenheimer MC, Swinton NW. *Diseases of the Anus, Rectum, and Colon. Part I: Neoplasms.* New York, NY: Medcom; 1972.)

Based on this staging and on the slow-growing nature of colonic leiomyosarcoma, these investigators suggested that the prognosis for patients with this tumor is as follows:

Stage I-A and I-B: excellent
Stage II-A: excellent
Stage II-B: fair
Stage III: poor

The accuracy of prognosis based on the degree of differentiation has been described by the Mayo Clinic group.[7] Grade 1 tumors have a greater abundance of cells than leiomyomas; mitotic activity is minimal with no pleomorphism or anaplasia. With grade 2 tumors, mitoses are noted in one of five high-power fields. In grade 3 leiomyosarcoma, a mitosis is seen in every high-power field. Grade 4 lesions demonstrate marked cellularity, pleomorphism, and three or more mitoses per high power field.

Most of the reported cases have been managed by resection of the tumor-bearing portion of the colon. Leiomyosarcoma is usually a tumor of low-grade malignancy. Patients who have been treated by resection have lived many years despite residual tumor or metastases.[187] The lungs and regional lymph nodes are rarely involved, but the tumor does have a tendency to metastasize to the liver.

Rectum

More than 200 cases of rectal leiomyosarcoma have been recorded in the literature.[16,22,55,123,139,160,269,360,408,440,458,470,475,492,506,554,557] The tumor arises in the smooth muscle of the rectal wall. Most are seen in the lower one-third of the rectum and are more commonly found in men than in women. The tumor may present as a nodular or protuberant swelling with some central ulceration that appears to arise in the deeper layers of the bowel wall. Most are large and consist microscopically of interlacing bands of smooth muscle fibers that are well differentiated and histologically of a low-grade malignancy (Figures 26-42 and 26-43). Extensive direct spread into the perirectal tissue is a characteristic feature. This may make surgical removal so difficult that local recurrence even after excision of the rectum is not uncommon.

Smooth muscle sarcomas of the rectum do not usually metastasize to regional lymph nodes unless they are poorly differentiated. An exception was described by Thorlakson and Ross in a case with lymphatic spread to one hemorrhoidal lymph node and with venous involvement.[506]

As with colonic leiomyosarcoma, radical resection is generally the preferred approach. Local excision is liable to be followed by recurrence, even though this may be delayed for some years.[125,151,554] The tumor is not generally considered radiosensitive. Luna-Pérez and colleagues suggested that in rectal sarcoma, surgery plus radiotherapy may reduce the incidence of local recurrence and, in selected patients, allow for anal sphincter preservation.[314] Chemotherapy with vincristine, cyclophosphamide, actinomycin D, and doxorubicin (Adriamycin) has also been advocated.[18]

Results of Treatment of Leiomyosarcoma. Morson pointed out that although most leiomyosarcomas are of a low-grade malignancy, the ultimate prognosis is very poor.[360] This is essentially because of late diagnosis and extensive local spread by the time of surgery. In the experience of the Memorial Sloan-Kettering Cancer Center, a high-grade tumor and,

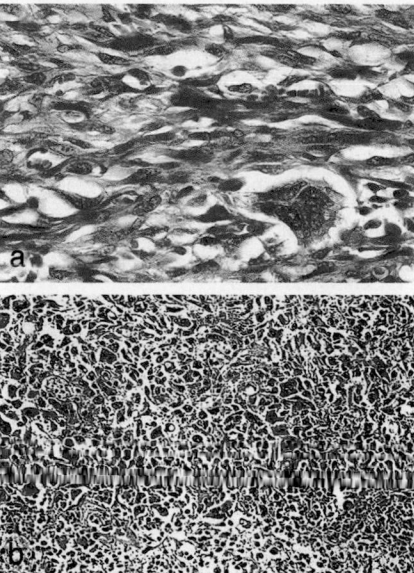

FIGURE 26-42. Histologic features of spindle and epithelioid cell leiomyosarcoma. **A:** Spindle cells arranged in a fascicular pattern with evident osteoclast-like giant cells (OGCs) (hematoxylin-eosin; original magnification × 400). **B:** Epithelioid cells growing in a diffuse pattern with abundant OGCs (hematoxylin-eosin, original magnification × 250; courtesy of *Archives of Pathology*.)

obviously, the presence of metastases were the two unfavorable characteristics that had independent prognostic value.[336] Rectal disease has been shown to have an overall survival rate of 20%.[139] In the experience of Yeh and associates in Taipei, Taiwan involving 40 patients with rectal tumors, the 5-year, disease-free survival was 46%, but 75% were alive at that time.[554] In addition to high histologic grade, younger age was a significant poor prognostic factor. Apart from local recurrence, metastasis to the liver and lungs is the most common cause of death.

Many of these patients give a rather long history of symptoms before coming to treatment.[7] Their general clinical course confirms the histologic observation that these smooth muscle tumors are mostly well differentiated and of a low-grade malignancy.

Rhabdomyosarcoma

Rhabdomyosarcoma is the most common soft tissue sarcoma in children; it occurs most frequently in the head and neck, genitourinary tract, extremity, and trunk.[348] A few cases have been reported in the perirectal area.[347,444] Horn and Enterline classified rhabdomyosarcoma into four types: pleomorphic,

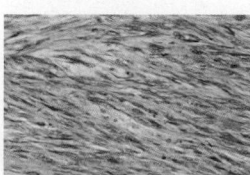

FIGURE 26-43. Leiomyosarcoma. Smooth muscle fibers showing at least six mitotic figures. (Original magnification × 600; from Corman ML, Veidenheimer MC, Swinton NW. *Diseases of the Anus, Rectum, and Colon. Part I: Neoplasms.* New York, NY: Medcom; 1972.)

alveolar, embryonal, and botryoid.[233] However, the histologic diagnosis may be confused with other mesenchymal lesions.[347]

The patient usually presents with a mass in the perianal area. Current therapy should include adequate local excision or resection followed by chemotherapy (vincristine, actinomycin D, and cyclophosphamide).[347,444] Prognosis is generally poor.

Adipose Tissue Origin

Lipoma

Excluding hyperplastic polyps, lipoma is the second most common benign tumor of the colon (after adenomatous polyp) and the most common intramural tumor. However, it is still a relatively rare entity. Weinberg and Feldman reviewed more than 60,000 autopsy reports and found only 135 lipomas of the colon (0.2%).[534] Haller and Roberts found 11 lipomas in more than 3,400 autopsies (0.3%).[208]

Colonic lipomas are well-differentiated, benign fatty tumors arising from deposits of adipose connective tissue in the bowel wall. Malignant change has not been reported. Approximately 90% are submucosal and 10% subserosal. The submucosal lipoma is covered by mucosa and occasionally by muscularis mucosae and grows toward the intestinal lumen (Figures 26-44 and 26-45). The mucosa covering the tumor may become atrophic, congested, ulcerated, or even necrotic, or it may retain its normal yellowish appearance. The subserosal type usually originates from the appendices epiploicae and grows toward the peritoneal cavity.

Colonic lipomas usually occur in patients between the ages of 50 and 70 years with about an equal gender distribution. The average age is similar to that of individuals with colonic carcinoma. Patients with colonic lipoma do not appear ill nor do they experience anorexia, weight loss, or anemia. Most colonic lipomas are asymptomatic and are found at autopsy or incidentally during an operation for some other problem. However, with size in excess of 2 cm, approximately one-third will give rise to some symptom.[344] This may include constipation, diarrhea, abdominal pain, and rectal bleeding (Figure 26-46).[423] The presence of a palpable mass may be the lipoma itself, impaction of fecal material, or intussuscepted bowel.[344]

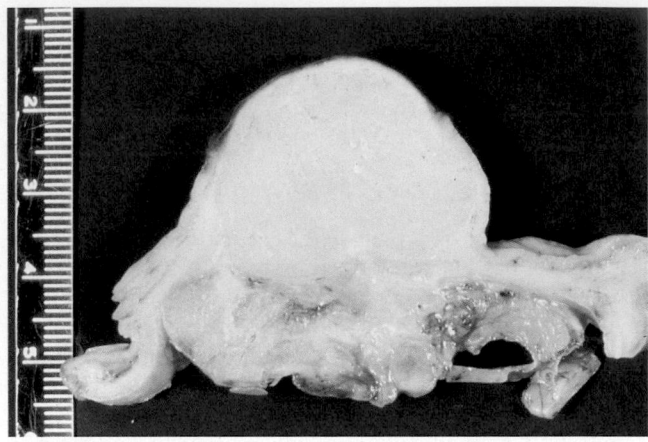

FIGURE 26-45. Lipoma. A formalin-fixed specimen of a well-circumscribed mass in the wall of the large bowel. (Courtesy of Rudolf Garret, MD.)

The most common sites for lipoma are the cecum, ascending colon, and sigmoid colon. Lipoma or lipomatosis of the ileocecal valve is characterized by diffuse submucosal adipose infiltration of the valve.[509] Pemberton and McCormack found 50 tumors in the right colon, 15 in the transverse colon, and 37 in the left colon and rectum.[392] Castro and Stearns reported 45 tumors, 31 of which were in the right colon (69%).[76] Eleven of their patients (26%) had two or

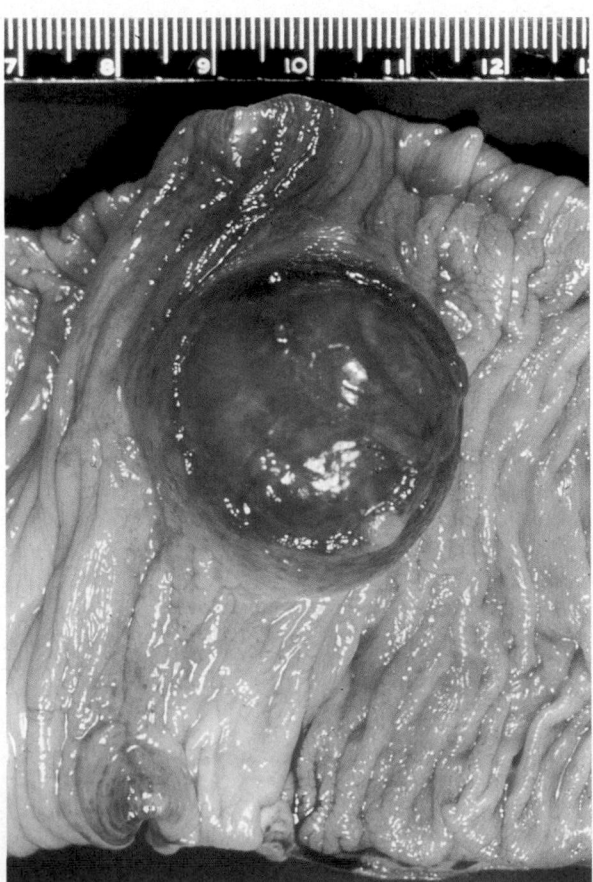

FIGURE 26-46. Submucosal lipoma of the transverse colon. Rectal bleeding is explained by the hemorrhagic appearance of the lesion. (Courtesy of Rudolf Garret, MD.)

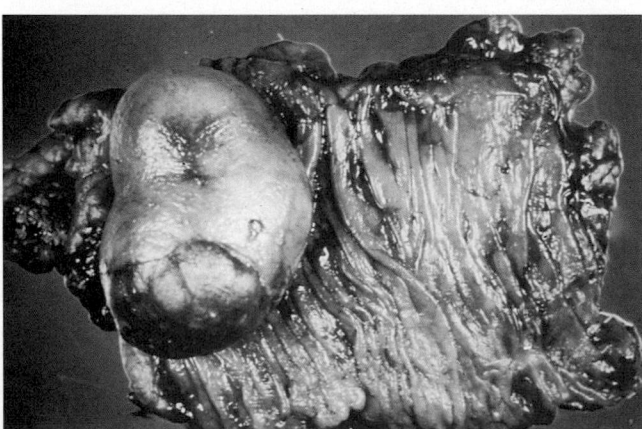

FIGURE 26-44. Submucosal lipoma in the region of the ileocecal valve. (From Corman ML, Veidenheimer MC, Swinton NW. *Diseases of the Anus, Rectum, and Colon. Part I: Neoplasms.* New York, NY: Medcom; 1972.)

more lipomas, and 4 had three or more. All multiple lipomas were found in the right half of the colon.

Barium enema examination can usually distinguish a lipoma from that of another type of tumor (Figures 26-47 through 26-49). A water enema with low-kilovoltage technique may take advantage of the different absorption coefficients of fat and water: fat-containing lesions will appear relatively radiolucent.[326] The shape of the mass may be observed to change during fluoroscopic examination as a consequence of peristalsis or of manual pressure, the so-called squeeze sign.[344] CT appearance is that of a homogeneous mass consistent with the density of fat.

Mucosal lipomas can also be diagnosed with the colonoscope (Figure 26-50).[116,509] Certain endoscopic features suggesting lipoma have been described, including the "cushion sign" (identification of the lipoma with pressure from a biopsy forceps), the "tenting sign" (elevation of the overlying mucosa with the biopsy forceps), and the "naked fat sign" (extrusion of fat following biopsy).[423] Not uncommonly, they may be removed by means of this instrument.[42,531] However, this approach is usually limited to symptomatic patients and those in whom the lesion is somewhat pedunculated (Figures 26-51 and 26-52).

The microscopic appearance is that of mature adipose tissue surrounded by a fibrous capsule (Figure 26-53).

Colonic lipomas do not require treatment except when they ulcerate. Once the diagnosis has been established and

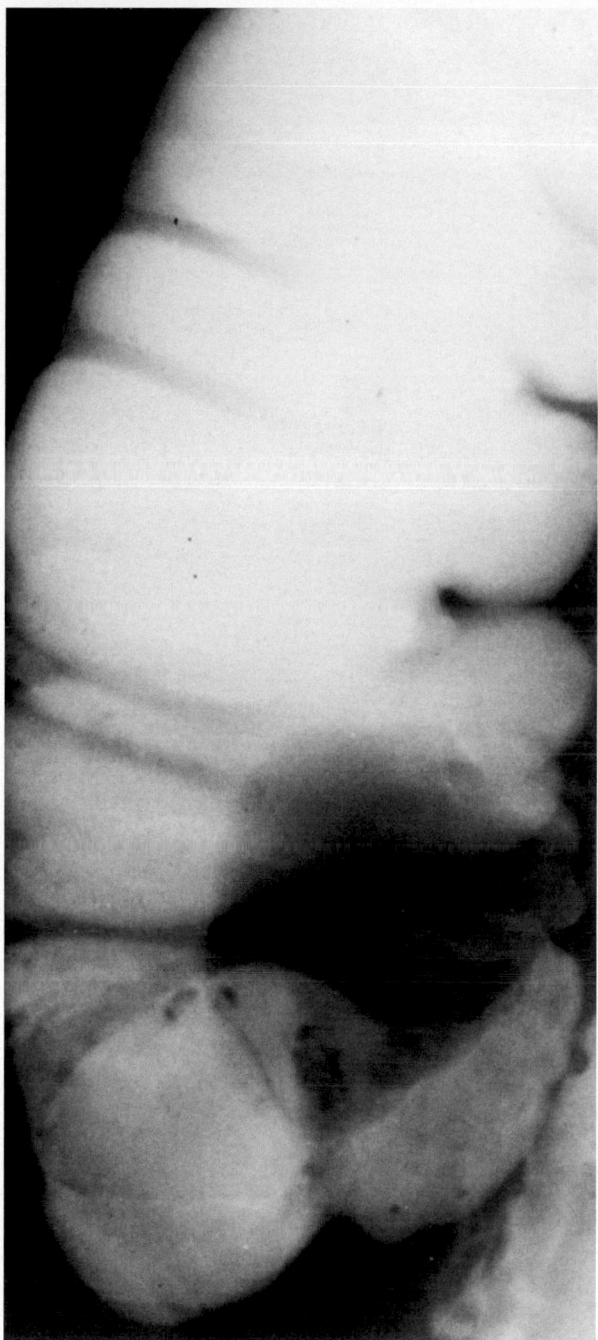

FIGURE 26-48. A lipoma of the ileocecal valve that produced abdominal pain and vomiting.

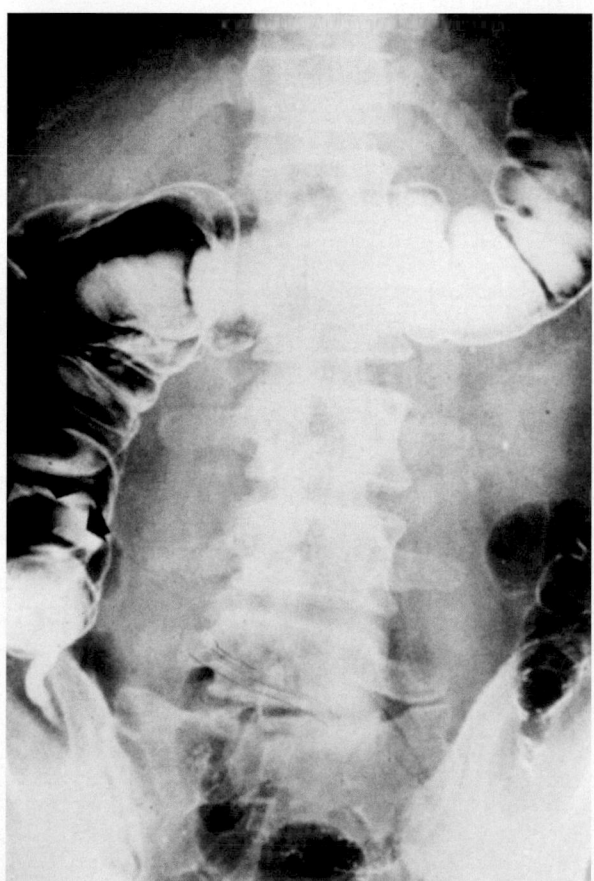

FIGURE 26-47. Barium enema demonstrates a characteristic filling defect in the proximal ascending colon (*arrows*). The smooth, spherical outline is practically pathognomonic of this disease. (From Corman ML, Veidenheimer MC, Swinton NW. *Diseases of the Anus, Rectum and Colon. Part I: Neoplasms.* New York, NY: Medcom; 1972.)

carcinoma has been ruled out, the patient need only be reassured. However, in the symptomatic patient, a limited resection or colotomy and lipomectomy will usually be advised. Laparoscopic removal has also been reported.[431] The requirement for resection because of confusion with a malignant process should be a rare occurrence today, with the availability of colonoscopy and CT (Figure 26-54).[235,260,428]

Lipoma of the *rectum* is extremely rare. When it can be reached with the finger, it is usually felt as a soft, smooth, lobulated mass. Pedunculated lesions may prolapse and present a slight problem of differential diagnosis, especially if it is hemorrhagic or necrotic. Tenesmus may result when the growth is in the lower rectum and involves the internal sphincter. When

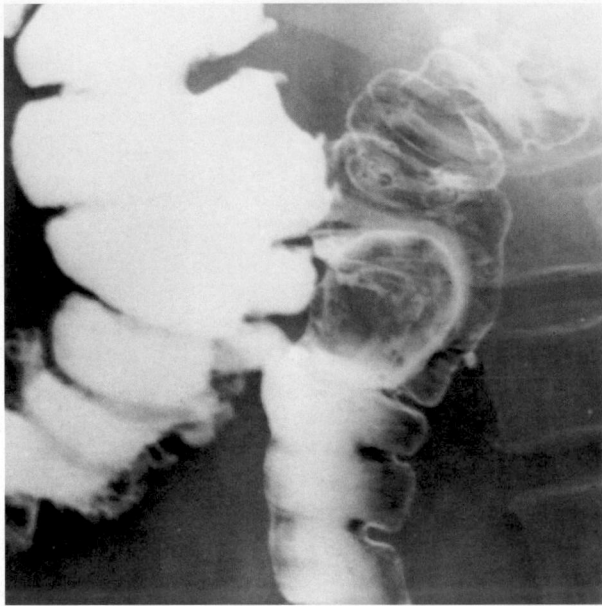

FIGURE 26-49. Lipoma of the descending colon. A submucosal polypoid mass without mucosal irregularity or destruction. The patient complained of left upper abdominal pain.

situated in the rectum or the sigmoid, it may produce symptoms because of its size or when traumatized. If seen with the aid of a proctoscope, the yellow color of the fat of which it is composed is usually apparent through the mucosa.

The most frequent site in the rectal area is the perianal region in which case the tumor develops from the subcutaneous tissue. A lipoma in this area or buttock usually causes no symptoms unless it becomes quite large, and the overlying skin becomes irritated.

Ligation of the base and removal may be performed when the tumor is pedunculated. Incision and enucleation may be employed if the lipoma is confined to the rectal wall.

Lipomatosis

Swain and coworkers reported a child with lipomatous polyposis throughout the entire colon, and Ling and associates resected the colon of a 60-year-old woman with 107 lipomas.[306,489] Radiographically, colonic lipomatosis must be differentiated from numerous benign and malignant conditions. These include familial polyposis,[327] juvenile polyposis,[461] Gardner syndrome,[559] Cronkhite–Canada syndrome,[109]

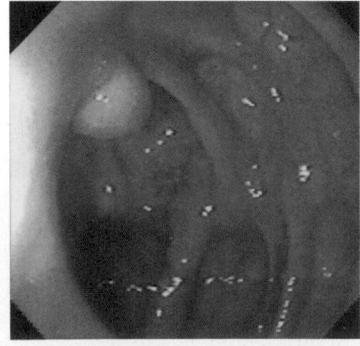

FIGURE 26-50. Lipoma of the ileocecal valve can be seen through the colonoscope.

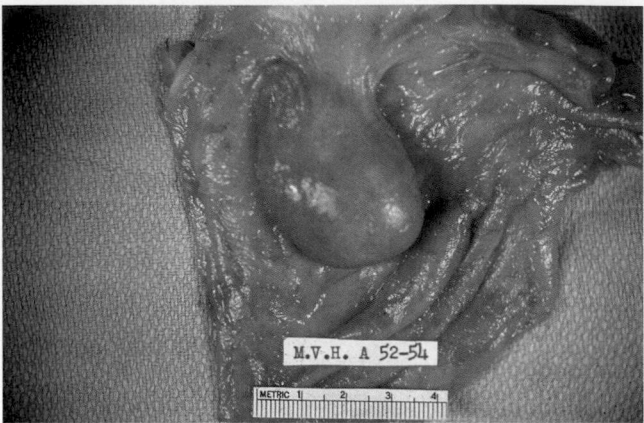

FIGURE 26-51. Pedunculated lipoma treated by bowel resection. (Courtesy of Rudolf Garret, MD.)

Peutz–Jeghers syndrome,[184] nodular lymphoid hyperplasia,[165] inflammatory bowel disease with pseudopolyposis, lymphosarcoma,[545] ganglioneurofibromatosis,[67] malacoplakia,[430] pneumatosis coli, and colitis cystica profunda.[532]

In 1985, Snover and colleagues described 24 cases of mucosal "pseudolipomatosis."[473] The lesions were removed through the colonoscope, but the absence of adipocytes led the authors to conclude that the condition was due to entrapment of gas in the lamina propria.

► TUMORS OF NEURAL ORIGIN

Neurofibroma

Neurofibromas are benign nerve sheath tumors. von Recklinghausen first described multiple subcutaneous neurofibromas

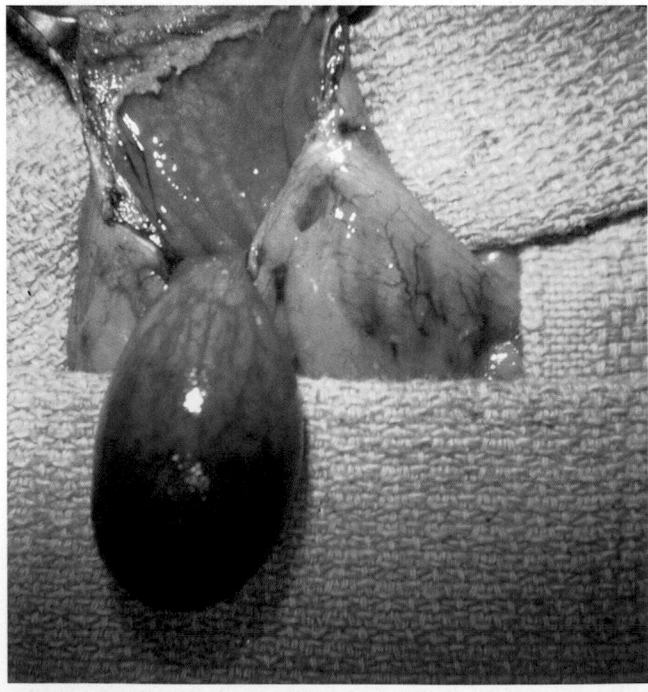

FIGURE 26-52. Pedunculated lipoma at laparotomy, treated by colotomy and lipomectomy. Attempt at colonoscopic removal was unsuccessful.

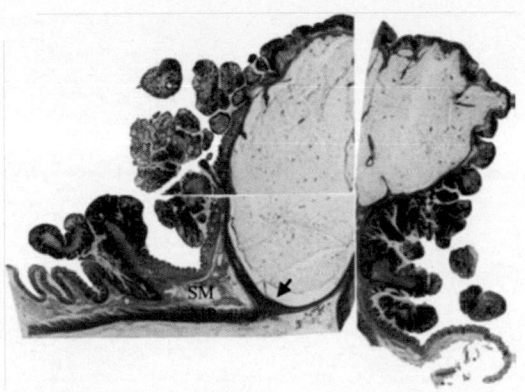

FIGURE 26-53. Histologic section demonstrates atypical location of a lipoma within the muscularis propria. The *arrow* shows the split of the muscularis propria. MP, muscularis propria; SM, submucosal layer. (From Adachi S, Hamano R, Shibata K, et al. Colonic lipoma with florid vascular proliferation and nodule-aggregating appearance related to repeated intussusception. *Pathol Int.* 2005;55(3):160–164.)

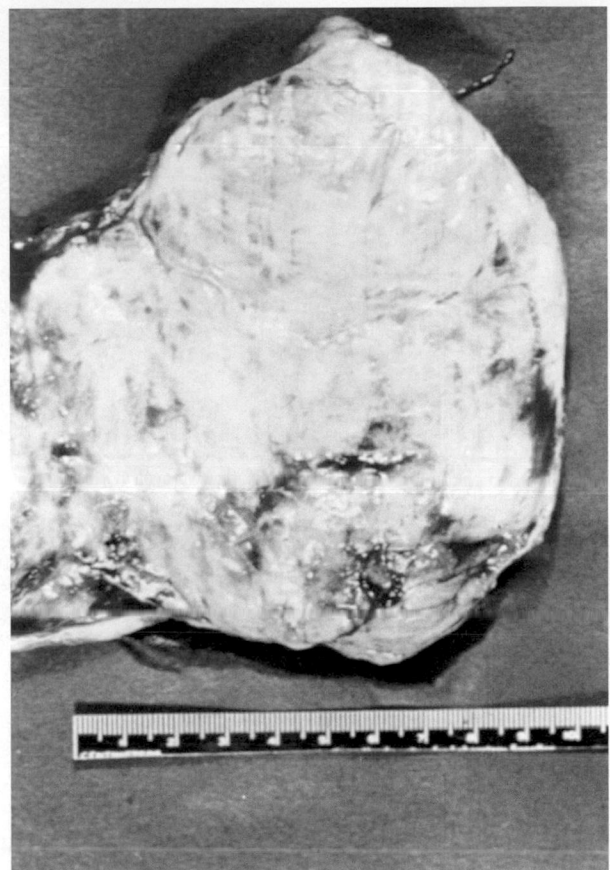

FIGURE 26-55. Neurofibroma. A firm, fleshy, whitish tumor attached to wall of the bowel. (Courtesy of Rudolf Garret, MD.)

(neurofibromatosis) in 1882.[521] The condition has since come to be known as von Recklinghausen's disease. Visceral involvement in disseminated neurofibromatosis is considered rare, yet reports appeared as early as 1930.[132] The possibility of this disease should be considered if GI bleeding or intestinal obstruction occurs in a patient known to have generalized neurofibromatosis.[43,197,301,324,401] It may, however, be seen in the alimentary tract and nowhere else.

The lesions in the intestinal tract arise in the submucosa or muscularis (Figures 26-55 and 26-56).[179] As the tumor enlarges, the overlying mucosa becomes ulcerated and bleeds. Intussusception can produce intestinal obstruction, and sarcomatous degeneration is a recognized complication.[272,301] Three cases of solitary neurofibromas have been confirmed in the anal canal.[167]

Local excision is preferred unless a large cluster is noted in one segment. Under these circumstances, resection may be advisable.

Ganglioneuromatosis

Ganglioneuromas are neuroectodermal tumors that are rarely found in the colon. They are composed of nerve fibers, Schwann sheath elements, and ganglion cells (Figures 26-57 through 26-59).[56] When solitary, they may resemble a carcinoma radiologically. Donnelly and colleagues reported a 9-year-old boy who underwent total colectomy because of multiple colonic polyps that caused severe rectal bleeding.[128]

Of the two kinds of polyps found, one was largely composed of groups of ganglion cells and nerve fibers in trunks and networks, and the other resembled retention polyps. Ganglion cells, nerve fiber networks, or both were also found in the nonpolypoid colonic mucosa and in the mucosa of the stalks of the retention polyps. These authors selected the term ganglioneuromatosis for its descriptive value and suggested that this lesion is probably akin to neurofibromatosis and should be distinguished from ganglioneuroma, although its precise relationship to the former is not definitely established. Normann and Otnes reported a case of diffuse intestinal ganglioneuromatosis in which severe diarrhea was the predominant symptom.[373] Kanter and colleagues described a 40-year-old man with the disease in association with a

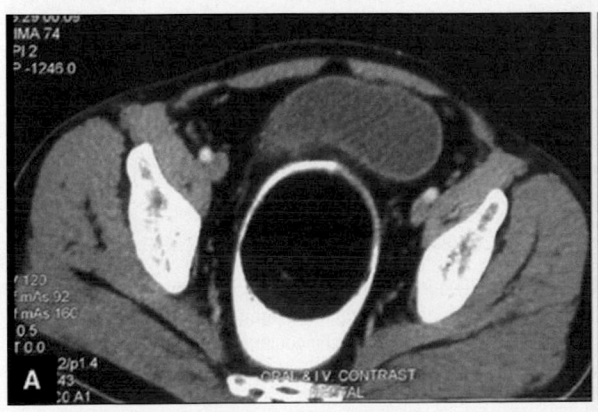
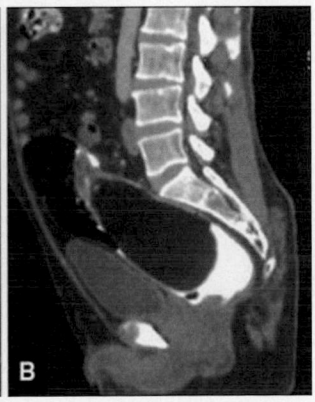

FIGURE 26-54. Axial **(A)** and sagittal reformatted **(B)** contrast-enhanced CT images of the pelvic region show the fat density hypodense intraluminal lesion within the rectum, which has been distended by per-rectal contrast. (From Arora R, Kumar A, Bansal V. Giant rectal lipoma. *Abdom Imaging.* 2011;36(5):545–547.)

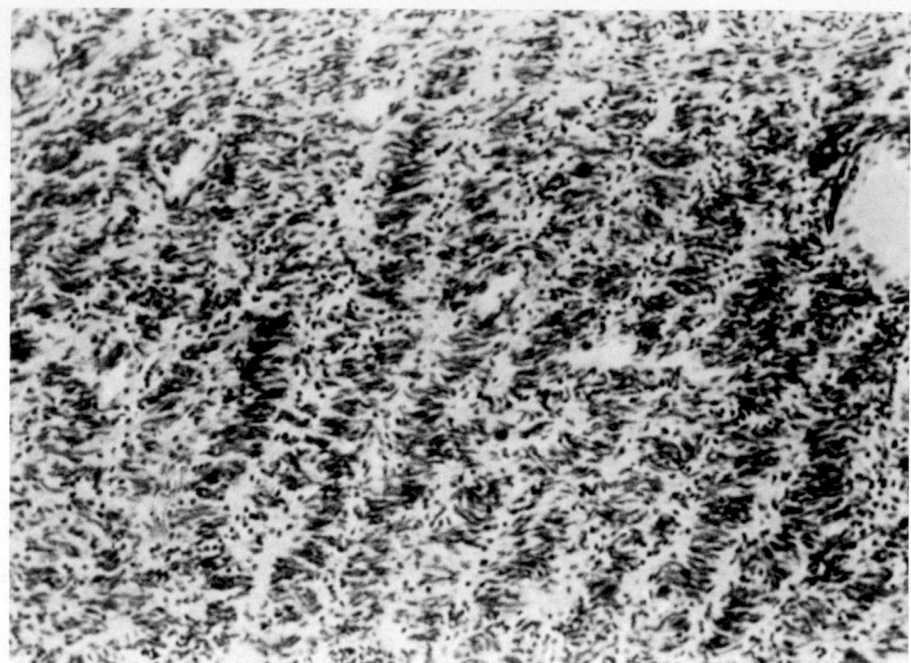

FIGURE 26-56. Neurofibroma, showing the herringbone appearance characteristic of nerve tissue tumor. (Original magnification × 260; courtesy of Rudolf Garret, MD.)

colorectal cancer.[261] They opined that ganglioneuromatous polyposis should be considered a premalignant condition.

Treatment is local excision or resection.

Neurilemoma or Schwannoma

Neurilemoma is a rare neoplasm that originates from Schwann cells. When it occurs in the GI tract, the colon is the least

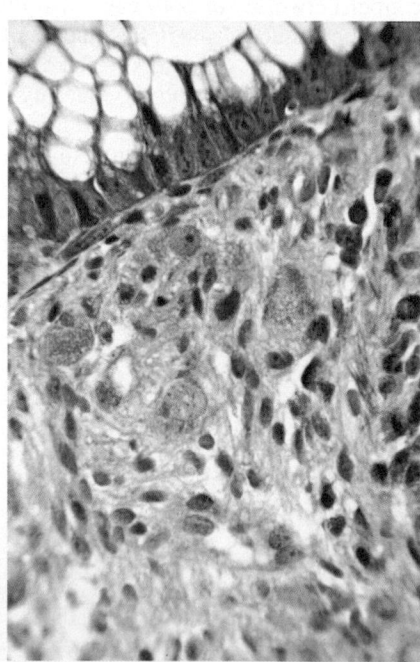

FIGURE 26-57. Ganglioneuroma. Interlacing bundles of nerve cells mixed with ganglion cells (*arrows*). (Original magnification × 280; courtesy of Lauren M. Monda, MD.)

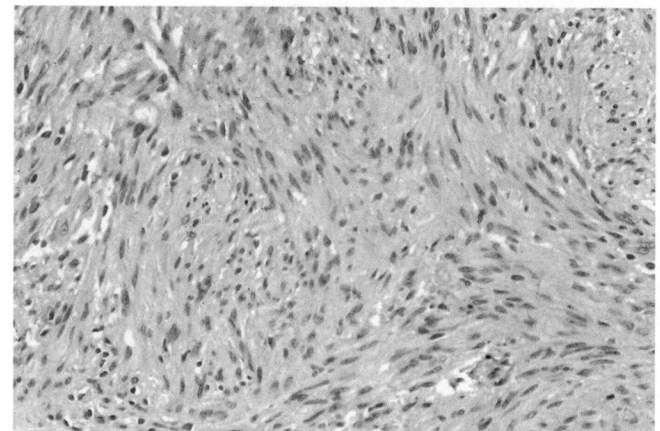

A

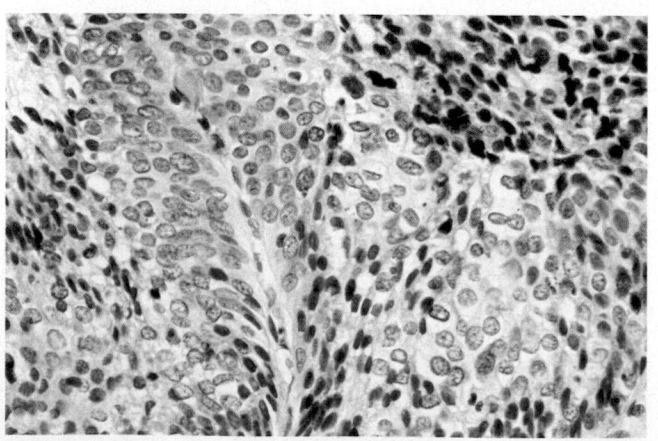

B

FIGURE 26-58. Neurilemoma. **A:** Edematous cells (Antoni A pattern) characteristic of schwannoma. (Original magnification × 260; courtesy of Rudolf Garret, MD.) **B:** Section of a multinodular tumor characterized by bland spindle-shaped cells arranged in a palisading pattern (Antoni B). (Original magnification × 260.)

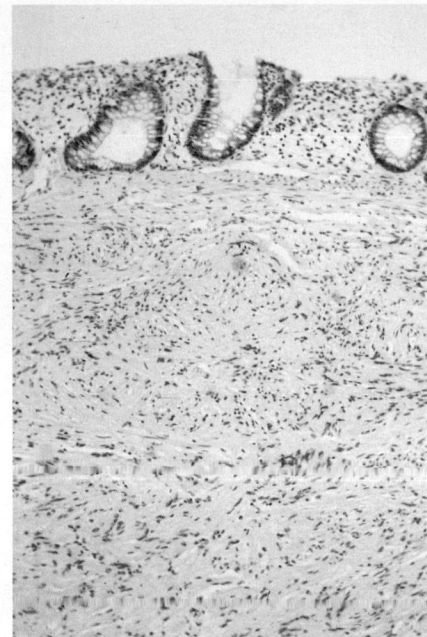

FIGURE 26-59. Schwannoma (perineural fibroblastoma). Well-delineated tumor replacing the submucosa. Interlacing bundles of cells with elongated nuclei of Antoni A pattern. (Original magnification × 80.)

likely site. Fewer than 10 cases have appeared in the literature.[465] Neurogenic tumors have also been reported to be the cause of masses in the presacral space. They may be identified by palpation on rectal examination and confirmed by CT (Figure 26-60). Treatment is local excision or resection, usually by a transcoccygeal approach (Figure 26-61; see later). Kovalcik and colleagues removed a 13-cm neurilemoma by means of a combined abdominotranssacral approach.[285] Anorectal neurilemoma has been reported uncommonly and also should be adequately treated by excisional biopsy.[2]

Granular Cell Tumor

Granular cell tumor is an uncommon tumor of uncertain histogenesis. It was first described in 1926 by Abrikossoff who named the tumor because of its resemblance to primitive myoblasts and its proximity to striated muscle.[4] He believed that neoplastic cells were formed from damaged adult muscle cells in the process of regeneration. Willis regarded the process as nonneoplastic and regenerative in nature.[542] However, Klinge suggested that the tumor could arise from heterotopic rests of myoblasts, a theory that was later accepted by Abrikossoff and Murray.[5,275,364]

Fisher and Wechsler, using electron microscopy and histochemical studies, concluded that the tumor had a definite neural pattern most closely resembling a damaged Schwann cell.[157] They believed that it was not similar to muscular tissue and noted that the tumor had a more histiocytic than neoplastic nature (Figure 26-62). We have elected to place this tumor in the classification under neural origin for these reasons.

Usually, the tumor involves the tongue (33%), skin and subcutaneous soft tissues (10%), and skeletal muscle (5%). About 50% of the tumors occur in the oral cavity and nasopharynx.[97] However, the lesion has also been reported in most other organ systems. Involvement of the GI tract is rare. Yanai-Inbar and associates, in their review of the literature, found 17 cases involving the large intestine, mainly in the proximal portion of the colon.[552] Only two tumors were identified in the rectum. Anal and perianal lesions have also been reported.[95,317,417,425,543]

In the colon, granular cell tumors appear as yellowish white submucosal nodules, usually less than 2 cm in diameter. Most are found incidentally, but abdominal pain and bleeding can occur. Malignant degeneration may result, but this is unusual, and the possibility of such an association is still controversial.

Treatment is local excision when possible or resection. Success with colonoscopic removal may prove to be the optimal therapy for most lesions.[319]

▶ VASCULAR LESIONS

Hemangioma

Vascular malformations of the GI tract have been reported since 1839 with Phillips' initial description of a lesion in the rectum.[397] The Armed Forces Institute of Pathology in Washington, DC, has included venous angiomas in its list

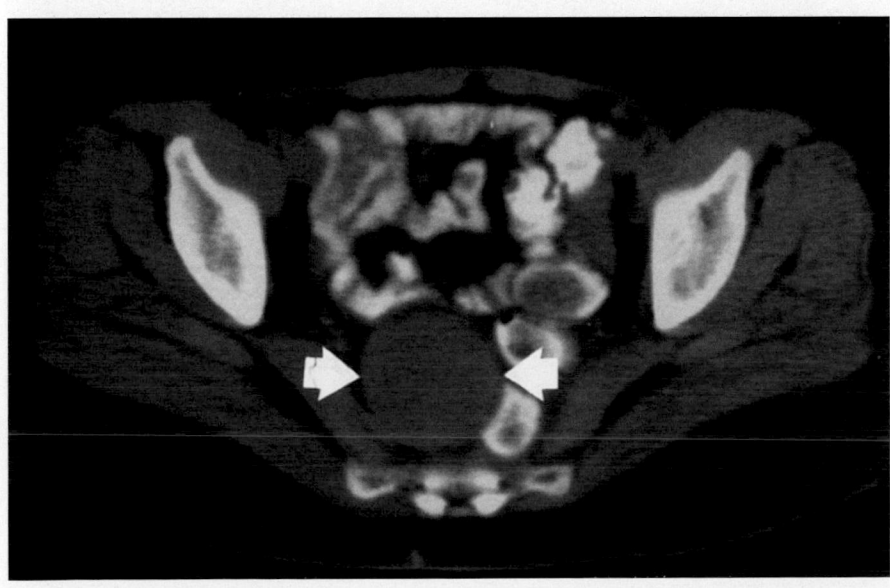

FIGURE 26-60. Computed tomography of the pelvis demonstrates a well-defined, presacral mass (*arrows*), which proved to be the lesion shown in Figure 26-63. (Courtesy of William G. Robertson, MD.)

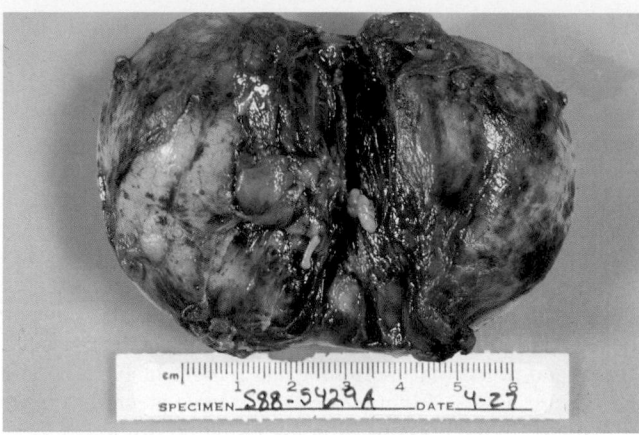
A

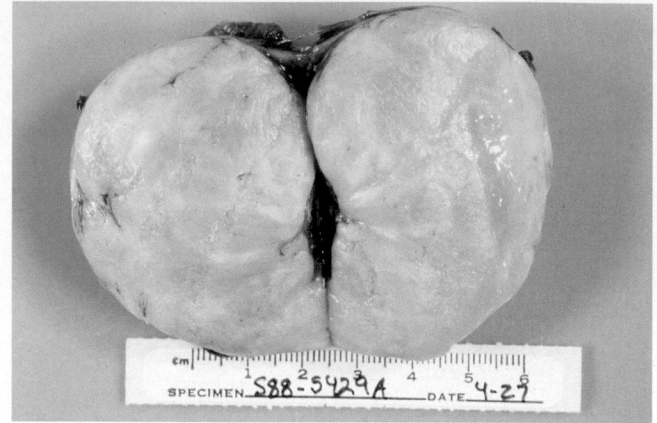
B

FIGURE 26-61. Schwannoma. Well-circumscribed, resected presacral tumor identified on prior CT **(A)**, which when opened reveals a homogeneous encapsulated mass with gray-white stroma and with small cystic foci and focal gelatinous areas characteristic of this type of tumor **(B)**. (Courtesy of William G. Robertson, MD.)

of benign vascular malformations as well as arteriovenous angiomas (racemose aneurysms), plexiform angiomas, and several other variants of hemangiomas.[294]

For the purposes of this chapter, this section deals only with hemangiomas. The vascular lesion that has come to be known as an arteriovenous malformation or vascular ectasia is discussed in Chapter 28. Hemangiomas are found in virtually every organ of the body, with the skin a particularly common location. However, it is one of the rarest tumors found in the colon. Gentry and associates reviewed the world literature through 1945 and found reports of 283 benign vascular tumors of the GI tract.[178] Only 31 of these were hemangiomas of the colon. Rissier reviewed 18 cases in 1960.[418] Thirteen additional reports appeared in the literature between 1957 and 1971.[135,156,188,274,337,358,380,388,415,427,459,482,515]

The pathogenesis of these tumors is not well defined. However, they are generally agreed to be congenital, with their origin in embryonic sequestrations of mesodermal tissue. Enlargement occurs by projection of budding endothelial cells. Whether these growths are neoplastic or congenital is a matter of some controversy.

The capillary hemangioma consists of small, thin-walled, closely packed vessels with a well-differentiated, hyperplastic endothelial lining. These tumors are distributed equally throughout the GI tract. They represent 6% of benign vascular tumors, arise from the submucosal vascular plexus, and are often encapsulated. Mucosal ulceration occurs in one-half of these lesions.

The cavernous hemangioma is composed of large, thin-walled vessels that are much larger than those of the capillary hemangioma. The supporting stroma contains scant connective tissue and may contain smooth muscle fibers (Figures 26-63 and 26-64). These lesions may be of the "multiple phlebectasia" type, characterized by a multitude of discrete tumors less than 1 cm in diameter. Although they represent one-third of all the benign vascular tumors of the GI tract, they are frequently overlooked. The simple polypoid type of cavernous hemangioma constitutes 10% of benign vascular intestinal malformations

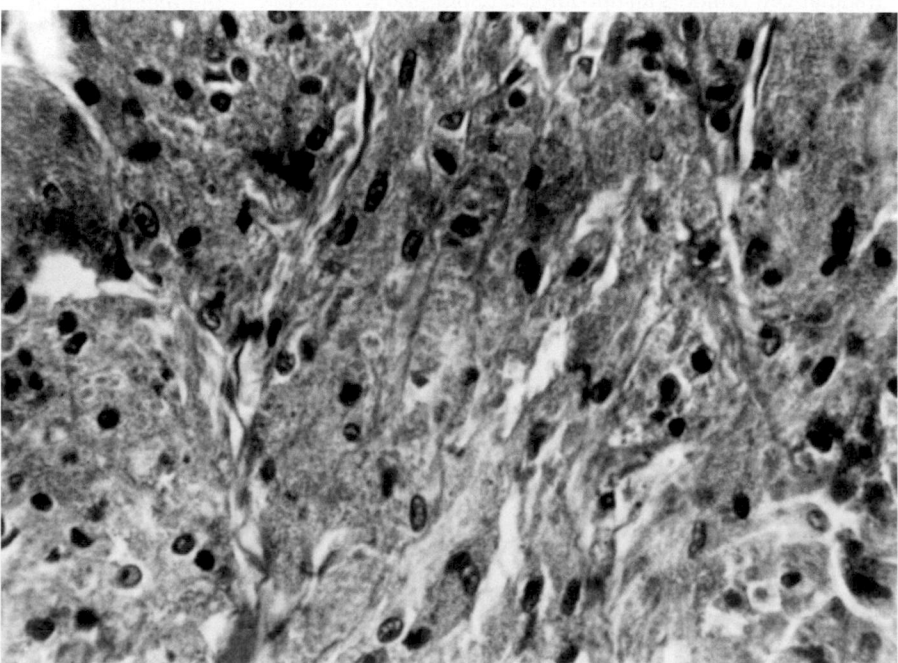

FIGURE 26-62. Granular cell tumor. Granular cells with uniform nuclei and granular cytoplasm. (Original magnification × 280; courtesy of Rudolf Garret, MD.)

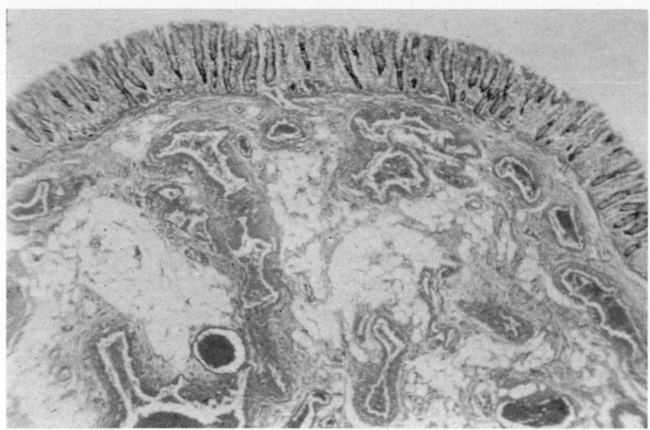

FIGURE 26-63. Hemangioma. Irregularly shaped arteries and veins in the areolar tissue of the submucosa. (From Corman ML, Veidenheimer MC, Swinton NW. *Diseases of the Anus, Rectum and Colon. Part I: Neoplasms.* New York, NY: Medcom; 1972.)

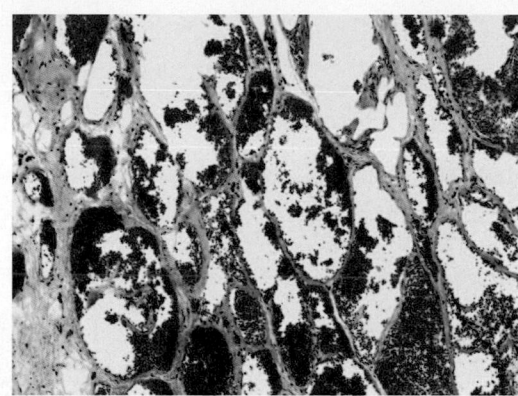

FIGURE 26-64. Histologic appearance of cavernous hemangioma of the rectum (hematoxylin and eosin, original magnification × 10; from Zurakowski J, Cwioroz P, Wroblewski T, et al. Diffuse cavernous hemangioma of the sigmoid colon treated with *n*-butyl-2-cyanoacrylate injections. *Endoscopy.* 2008;40(suppl 2): E120–E121.)

and is usually of sufficient size to produce such symptoms as obstruction and hemorrhage. The diffuse, expansive type varies widely in shape and size, and often involves 20 to 30 cm of intestine, occasionally in multiple locations. Diffuse cavernous hemangiomas, which produce severe symptoms at a relatively early age, account for 20% of intestinal angiomas.

Venous angiomas are often confused with cavernous hemangiomas. Both are composed of large, thin-walled vessels with large lumens. However, the walls of venous angiomas contain varying amounts of smooth muscle and usually resemble veins. Many of these tumors are extensive, especially those found in the extremities. Thrombosis is common in venous as well as in cavernous hemangiomas, and calcification frequently occurs in these thrombi as well as in the surrounding interstitial tissue.

Enlarged hemangiomas may produce symptoms of obstruction or hemorrhage. The obstructive symptoms may be caused by the tumor, by volvulus, or by intussusception. Intussusception has most frequently been reported from Eastern Europe. Additionally, invasion of adjacent structures has been described, including ureter and iliac vessels.[497]

The most common complication of hemangioma of the colon is bleeding (60% to 90%). Early onset and frequency of hemorrhage often lead to a diagnosis in adolescence or early adulthood. Characteristically, colonic hemangiomas bleed episodically, slowly, and persistently. Other symptoms include melena and the results of anemia: fatigue and weakness. Cavernous hemangiomas tend to bleed massively much more frequently than capillary hemangiomas (Figure 26-65). Melena begins in childhood, is recurrent throughout adolescence, and results in intermittent symptomatic anemia. Bleeding tends to become more severe with each recurrent episode. Although early onset of bleeding with recurrence usually leads to a definitive diagnosis and treatment during adolescence, hemangiomas of the colon may be difficult to confirm before laparotomy. A positive family history may be helpful.

Physical examination is often unremarkable, but the presence of hemangiomas of the skin or mucous membrane should raise a suspicion that a similar lesion could be present in the colon.

Barium enema may reveal a filling defect, and phleboliths may be noted within the filling defect (Figure 26-66). Hollingsworth first documented the association of narrowing of the sigmoid colon on barium enema examination with an area of surrounding phleboliths.[229] The occurrence of multiple, calcified, well-circumscribed densities is probably

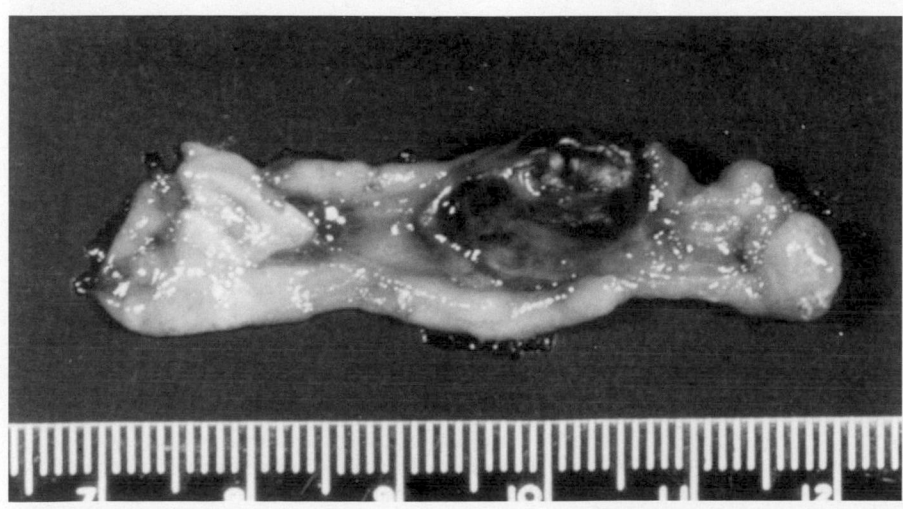

FIGURE 26-65. Cavernous hemangioma of the sigmoid colon with ulceration. Bleeding necessitated a resection. (Courtesy of Rudolf Garret, MD.)

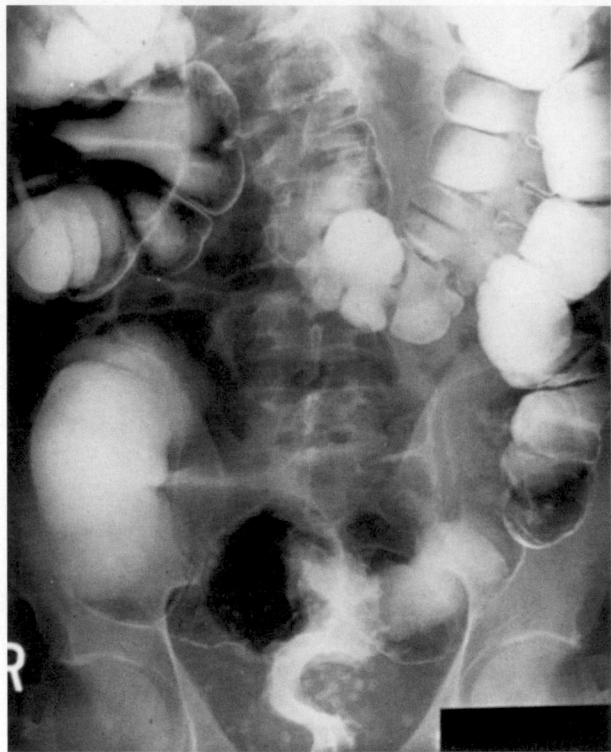

FIGURE 26-66. Hemangioma. Barium enema reveals extrinsic compression of the left wall of the rectum and irregularity of the rectosigmoid wall. The surrounding soft tissue mass contains multiple calcifications.

related to thrombosis within the tumor and is seen particularly with cavernous hemangioma of the colon.[34,229,380] CT has been shown to demonstrate certain characteristic findings—a thickened mesentery containing large vacuoles and transmural thickening of the involved segment (Figure 26-67).[26] Selective angiography may also reveal a vascular malformation, particularly in the late vascular phase (see Figures 28-14

and 28-15), although the differential diagnosis between angioma and arteriovenous malformation is often confusing. Injection of the resected specimen with contrast material may be useful for ensuring adequacy of the margins.[103]

Skovgaard and Sorensen reported an 8-year-old boy with a hemangioma of the sigmoid colon whose tumor was diagnosed by colonoscopy.[466] These investigators believed that because hemangioma can be diagnosed radiographically only if it is large and can easily be overlooked at exploratory laparotomy, colonoscopy should be used in evaluating all children with lower intestinal hemorrhage of unknown cause. Endoscopic diagnosis usually is not difficult; the tumor will appear deep red or purple. Hasegawa and colleagues performed colonoscopic polypectomy for a polypoid lesion, but their article was followed by an editorial comment cautioning the reader to be wary of the possibility of inducing uncontrolled hemorrhage.[213]

Resection of a bleeding colonic hemangioma is the optimal treatment.[103,315,402] If the benign nature of the tumor can be determined at laparotomy and confirmed by adequate frozen-section examination, local excision of the hemangioma is sufficient. If malignancy cannot be excluded, resection of the involved segment should be undertaken.

Only 75 cases of hemangioma of the rectum had been reported in the world literature prior to 1978.[247] However, in 2010, Wang and coworkers reported 17 patients with diffuse cavernous hemangioma of the rectum.[529] Treatments that have been proposed include sclerosing agents,[137] ligation of the feeding vessels,[169] local excision,[216] abdominoperineal resection,[217] and resection with coloanal anastomosis.[244,308,528] It seems reasonable to attempt a sphincter-saving operation, if hemorrhage can be controlled and there is no evidence for malignant change.[26,112,416,529]

Because radiation has been reported to be a successful treatment for hemangiomas of the neck and face,[227,447] Chaimoff and Lurie applied this technique in a woman who presented with a low-lying perirectal hemangioma.[80] Nearly 2 years after treatment consisting of five successive sessions of 3 Gy each (for a total of 15 Gy), the patient was asymptomatic.

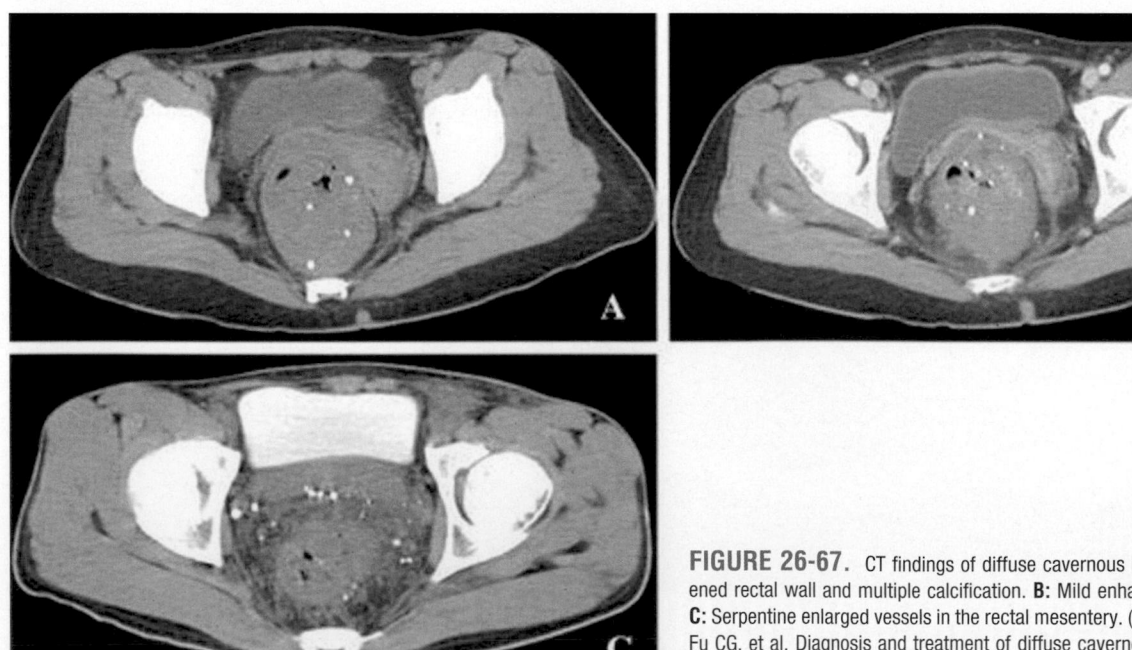

FIGURE 26-67. CT findings of diffuse cavernous hemangioma. **A:** Thickened rectal wall and multiple calcification. **B:** Mild enhancement of rectal wall. **C:** Serpentine enlarged vessels in the rectal mesentery. (From Wang HT, Gao XH, Fu CG, et al. Diagnosis and treatment of diffuse cavernous hemangioma of the rectum: report of 17 cases. *World J Surg.* 2010;34(10):2477–2486.)

Lymphangioma

Lymphangioma of the GI tract is a very rare lesion, and the colon is the least frequent site involved. Fleming and Carlson reported on nine lymphatic cysts of the abdomen diagnosed at the Mayo Clinic between 1959 and 1968.[158] Of these, three arose submucosally in the GI tract, and one originated in the colon. Only a few other cases have been published.[13,20,181,196,225,277,289,290,377,404] However, with increasing use of endoscopy to visualize the GI tract, this submucosal lesion is being observed with increased frequency.[404]

The lesion originates in the lymphatic plexus within the submucosa into which the lacteals of the villi empty. In 1958, Willis noted the frequent association of lymphangioma with smooth muscle and believed that these cysts, like angiomas, are hamartomas rather than true tumors.[542]

Another theory considers lymphangiomas to be secondary to obstructed mesenteric lymph nodes, with subsequent stasis and dilatation caused by a rise in pressure in the nodes, a mechanism similar to the production of postoperative lymphocysts.[126] If this theory were valid, one would expect an increased incidence of such lymphangiomatous cysts after laparotomy and abdominal node dissection. This finding has not been reported.

Lymphangiomas of the colon may be submucosal or pedunculated. The small number of documented submucosal lymphangiomas of the GI tract does not permit satisfactory analysis of the radiologic characteristics. However, Kuramoto and colleagues suggested that it is possible to diagnose these lesions endoscopically.[289] Because the tumors are lustrous and smooth on the surface, pliable on compression, and frequently have a stalk or a "waist" at the base, these investigators suggested that lesions less than 20 mm in diameter can be safely removed via the colonoscope. On other occasions, however, the mucosa may appear quite nodular. The example shown in Figure 26-68 reveals such a nodular mucosa.

The first report of lymphangioma of the rectum in an English language journal was that of Chisholm and Hillkowitz in 1932.[89] In 1973, we reported the case of a woman with rectal bleeding who had previously undergone a hemorrhoidectomy for this complaint.[104] Proctosigmoidoscopy revealed numerous extramucosal cystic masses scattered from the anorectal ring to approximately 9 cm from the anal verge and appearing to contain clear fluid.

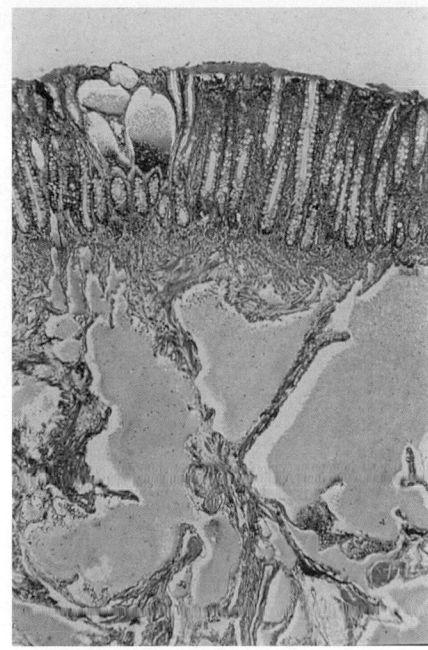

FIGURE 26-69. Lymphangioma. Endothelial-lined, irregular spaces in the submucosa of the bowel. (Original magnification × 80; from Corman ML, Veidenheimer MC, Swinton NW. *Diseases of the Anus, Rectum, and Colon. Part I: Neoplasms.* New York, NY: Medcom; 1972.)

After a GI investigation produced negative findings, the cystic masses were excised through the operating proctoscope. Pathologically, a noncapsulated, poorly circumscribed mass of cavernous, thin-walled vascular channels occupied the submucosa. These channels were irregular in size and shape. They had walls or septa formed of fibrous tissue and were lined by a single layer of flattened endothelium. Although the mucosal surface was intact throughout, focal discontinuities in the muscularis mucosa permitted some of the dilated lymphatic vessels to extend into the lamina propria. Homogeneous pink material, presumably lymph, filled most of the vessels (Figure 26-69). A few contained erythrocytes. Accumulations of lymphocytes were present both within the lymphatic channels and in the thin septa between them. The diagnosis of lymphangioma was made because of the presence of lymphocytes within the vessel and septa, the scarcity of elastic tissue, and the predominance of lymphatic elements (Figure 26-70).

The presence of blood vessels within many lesions designated as lymphangiomas is well recognized and has been taken as evidence that these lesions actually represent vascular malformations or hamartomas rather than true neoplasms. Differentiation from hemangioma may be impossible in those lesions that lack abundant intraluminal and interstitial lymphocytes as evidence of their lymphatic origin.

Apart from lymphangioma, the histologic differential diagnosis includes lesions that may produce cystic spaces in the submucosal region of the bowel. The epithelial lining of colitis cystica profunda usually permits its easy recognition. However, the giant cell lining that remains behind after dissolution of the oils in an oil granuloma (oleoma) may be more difficult to recognize. Gas cysts of recent origin may lack a lining. When they are chronic, they are lined by giant cells similar to those of the oil granuloma.

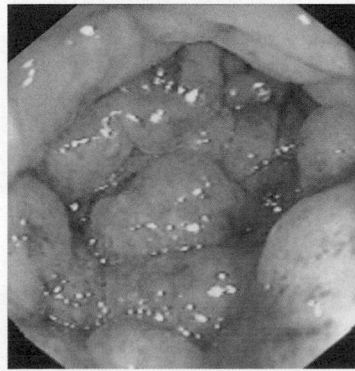

FIGURE 26-68. Submucosal cystic nodules were proven on biopsy to be lymphatic cysts.

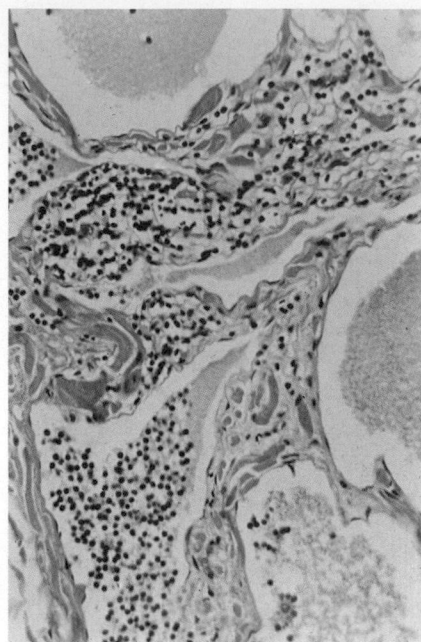

FIGURE 26-70. Lymphangioma. Endothelial-lined spaces, some of which contain lymphocytes. (Original magnification × 300; from Corman ML, Veidenheimer MC, Swinton NW. *Diseases of the Anus, Rectum, and Colon. Part I: Neoplasms.* New York, NY: Medcom; 1972.)[105]

None of the reported lymphangiomas of the colon and rectum had infiltrated the muscularis propria. However, such infiltration did occur in a lymphangioma of the small bowel reported by Wood.[549]

Excision biopsy with careful visualization under suitable anesthesia is the recommended procedure for rectal lesions. Colonoscopy is a valuable adjunct in the diagnosis of more proximal lesions. A cystic lymphangioma of the colon has been diagnosed by means of catheter endosonography.[241]

The typical image is that of an anechoic, septated lesion within the submucosa. Colonoscopic polypectomy for pedunculated lymphangiomas appears to be a satisfactory treatment, but a limited resection should be considered for all sessile or infiltrative tumors.

Hemangiopericytoma

Hemangiopericytoma is an extremely rare tumor that arises from pericytes and is usually found in the soft tissue of the trunk and extremities. Review of English language publications revealed only two cases involving the colon, the small intestine being the most common GI site.[24,176] Abdominal pain, intestinal obstruction, intussusception, and rectal bleeding are associated with intestinal tumors. Malignant degeneration is usually based on the clinical course (recurrence or metastases) rather than the histologic picture. Microscopically, the tumor is characterized by multiple endothelial-lined capillaries or capillary buds (Figure 26-71). Resection is the preferred treatment, although preoperative embolization has been suggested for large, highly vascular pelvic tumors because of the concern for bleeding.[131,176]

Malignant Vascular Tumors

Malignant vascular tumors include hemangioendothelioma, angiosarcoma, Kaposi's sarcoma, and benign metastasizing hemangioma. They represent approximately 13% of all vascular lesions of the colon and rectum, but with the epidemic of AIDS and the association of this condition with Kaposi's sarcoma, many more cases may be anticipated.[50,57,100,140,142,164,263,293,311,367,403,409,474,527,533,539]

Angiosarcoma

Angiosarcoma is a malignant tumor of the vascular endothelium that is thought to arise from a hemangioma. The histology is characterized by varying degrees of endothelial proliferation and the formation of anastomosing vascular

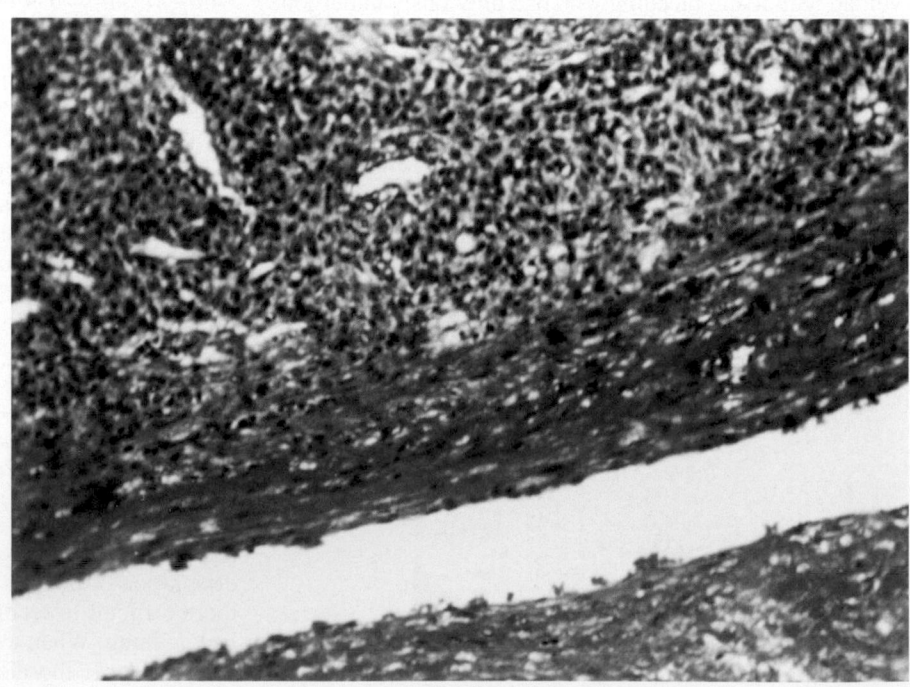

FIGURE 26-71. Hemangiopericytoma. Uniform cells derived from Zimmerman's pericytes surrounding the vascular spaces. (Original magnification × 260; courtesy of Rudolf Garret, MD.)

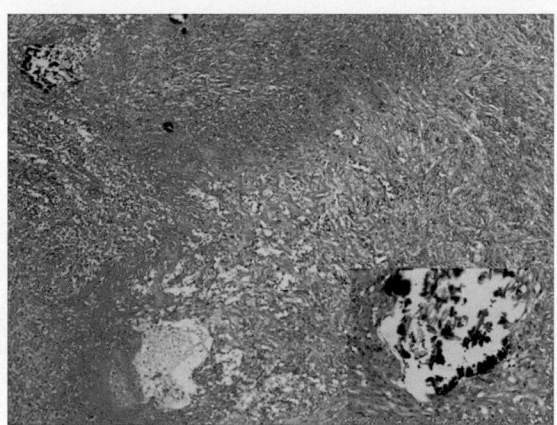

FIGURE 26-72. Angiosarcoma. Microscopic findings in the anteromedial aspect of ascending colon. Proliferation of malignant blood vessels was seen in the periphery of the abscess **(left upper corner)** (H&E, × 40). *Inset:* Malignant epithelioid tumor cells proliferating around the calcified foreign material, which is found in the periphery of the abscess (H&E, × 200). (From Joo YT, Jeong CY, Jung EJ, et al. Intra-abdominal angiosarcoma developing in a capsule of a foreign body: report of a case with associated hemorrhagic diathesis. *World J Surg Oncol.* 2005;3:60.)

channels (Figure 26-72). Fewer than a dozen of these tumors have been described involving the colon and rectum.[471] Treatment is resection, but the prognosis is poor.

Kaposi's Sarcoma

See Chapter 10.

▶ HETEROTOPIAS AND HAMARTOMAS

Endometriosis

Endometriosis is a disorder resulting from the presence of actively growing and functioning endometrial tissue, both glandular and stromal, in sites outside the uterus. In 1897, Pfannenstiel reported the case of a patient with aberrant endometrium that involved the rectovaginal septum.[396] In 1909, Meyer described the first instance of bowel endometriosis; the patient ultimately required resection.[339] In 1922, Blair Bell, in noting a series of cases of aberrant endometrium, first used the terms endometriosis and endometrioma, the former for the disease, the latter for the individual cystic lesion.[59]

Pathogenesis

The pathogenesis of this common disorder is not clearly understood. Many theories have been proposed to explain the disease. Sampson believed that fragments of endometrium regurgitated with the menstrual blood through the oviducts in a retrograde fashion and implanted onto peritoneal surfaces and pelvic and abdominal structures.[439] They would then erode into the subserosal tissues with viable cells growing and functioning and would ultimately lead to further implantation. This is the theory of tubal reflux and implantation.

Another proposal is that of coelomic epithelial metaplasia. This assumes that dormant, immature cellular elements of müllerian origin are known to persist into adult life, particularly throughout the central region of the pelvis. After menarche, repeated cyclic ovarian stimulation of these elements, with their totipotential capacities for differentiation, could result in the metaplastic formation of functioning endometrial tissue in ectopic sites.

Other theories have been suggested, including lymphatic dissemination of endometrial cells and deportation of normal endometrium by way of venous channels. These do not seem to offer a satisfactory explanation for the pathologic features.

Incidence

Endometriosis occurs almost exclusively in women. In 75% the condition develops between the ages of 20 and 40 years, and in 25% up to the age of menopause. Isolated case reports of endometriosis in men with prostatic cancer who are receiving estrogen therapy have also appeared.[399] The incidence of intestinal endometriosis among patients known to have endometriosis has been reported to be 5.4%.[406]

Symptoms and Signs

The classic history is one of acquired or secondary dysmenorrhea. The pain is related to, but does not necessarily occur simultaneously with each menstrual period. Pelvic discomfort associated with endometriosis is more likely to begin a day or two before the onset of menstrual flow, although its intensity may increase during the early days of menstruation. It tends to be a deep-seated ache or bearing-down pain in the lower part of the abdomen, posterior pelvis, vagina, or back, and it often radiates into the rectal and perineal areas with tenesmus and symptoms suggestive of an irritable bowel. When, as is often the case, an endometrioma of one or both ovaries is present, dull unilateral or bilateral lower abdominal pain, often with radiation to the thighs, may be noted.

The discomfort tends to abate after 2 or 3 days, subsiding completely toward the end of or just after the menstrual period. The patient will then be comfortable once more until a day or two before the onset of the next menstrual flow. However, as the disease progresses, pain tends to increase in severity and may last most of each cycle.

Not all patients with endometriosis have pain, however. Despite extensive disease that may be palpable on pelvic examination or found at laparotomy, 15% to 20% of patients report no discomfort whatsoever. They may harbor other manifestations of the pathologic process, notably infertility or the presence of a mass. Other symptoms include dyspareunia, cyclic bowel disturbances with painful defecation, rectal bleeding, and intestinal obstruction. Although rectal bleeding is an uncommon presenting symptom of endometriosis, colon endometriosis should be considered when bleeding is associated with the menses.

Leakage or rupture of an enlarging ovarian endometrioma may produce generalized peritonitis and an acute abdominal problem. Spillage of the contents of a "chocolate" endometrial cyst produces an intense local irritation and inflammatory response that results in chemical peritonitis.

A characteristic, almost diagnostic physical finding is the hard, fixed, fibrotic nodule in the uterosacral ligaments, culde-sac, or posterior surface of the lower uterine wall and cervix. This nodularity is almost universally present in patients with endometriosis and is pathognomonic for the disease. In endometriosis of the rectovaginal septum, bidigital rectovaginal examination helps to define the pathologic condition.

Diagnostic Studies

If the history is characteristic but the physical findings are minimal or equivocal, laparoscopy or culdoscopy may prove valuable in establishing a definitive diagnosis. When a trial of medical therapy is being considered, pelvic endoscopy using the laparoscope or culdoscope will usually provide a precise diagnosis before initiating treatment.

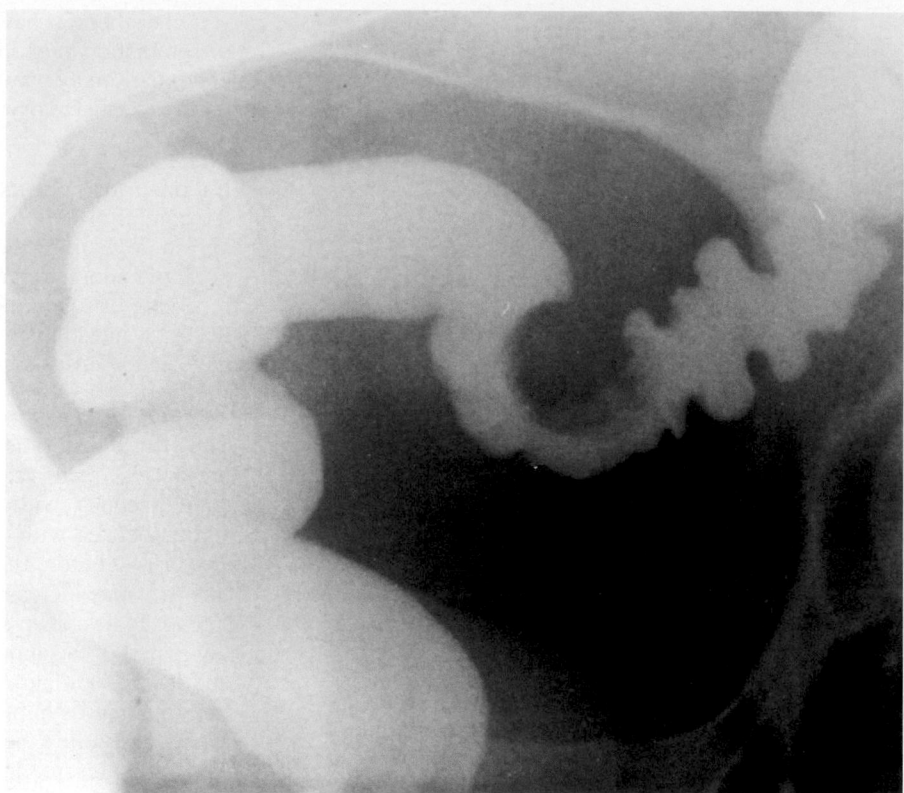

FIGURE 26-73. Endometrioma. Barium enema reveals a well-demarcated sigmoid mass. Confusion with carcinoma should not occur because the lesion demonstrated here has an intact overlying mucosa.

Other diagnostic tests include barium enema and CT (Figures 26-73 and 26-74). CT is especially useful for determining the location and degree of obstruction (if involvement of the ureters or periurethral tissue is suspected), and cystoscopy (during the menstrual period) to reveal the characteristic

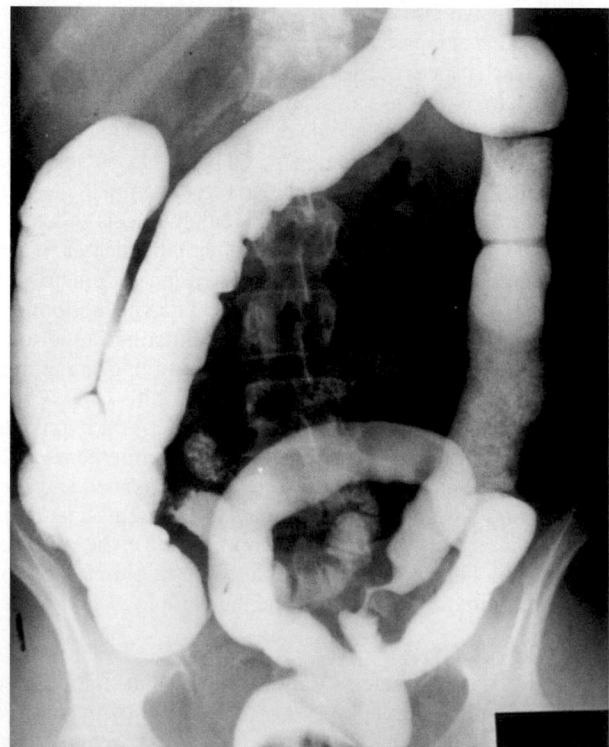

FIGURE 26-74. Endometrioma. Annular lesion of the proximal sigmoid. Because there is no mucosal abnormality, the lesion is either intramural or extrinsic.

bluish black, submucosal, cystic lesions if endometriosis of the bladder is suspected. Ileal endometriosis, especially, may present some confusion in differential diagnosis with Crohn's disease. Both conditions produce local inflammation and stricture.[74]

Schröder and colleagues evaluated 16 patients with suspected fixation of endometriomas to the rectal wall by means of endorectal ultrasound.[448] In 6 individuals, rectal wall involvement was diagnosed. In 2, endometriomas were found adjacent to the rectal wall, and in 8, rectal wall involvement was able to be excluded. Preoperative diagnosis was confirmed in all patients during the operation. Laparotomy was limited to those individuals with preoperatively assessed rectal wall involvement, whereas the remaining patients were treated by means of laparoscopic excision.[448] The authors concluded that preoperative endorectal ultrasound is reliable for assessing rectal wall involvement, thereby determining the type of operative approach that would appear to be best for the individual. Others have confirmed the high sensitivity and specificity of endorectal ultrasound for rectal endometriosis as well as its impact on operative decision making.[127]

Often, endometriosis is first discovered at the time laparotomy is performed for some other reason. In the experience of Keane and Peel, none of their patients with intestinal or abdominal wall endometriosis was helped by preoperative investigations.[267] However, these investigators did not have the benefit of endorectal ultrasound.

Histopathology

The three diagnostic histologic features of endometriosis are endometrial glands, endometrial stroma (Figure 26-75), and evidence of fresh hemorrhage (red cells and hemosiderin pigment) or old hemorrhage (hemosiderin-laden macrophages).

Because of its microscopic resemblance to normal endometrium and its known response to ovarian hormonal

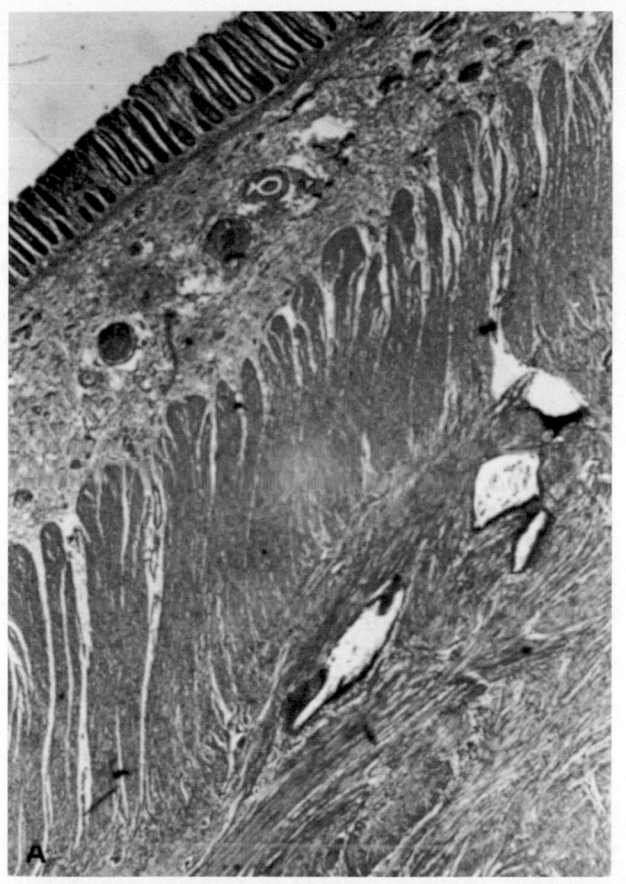

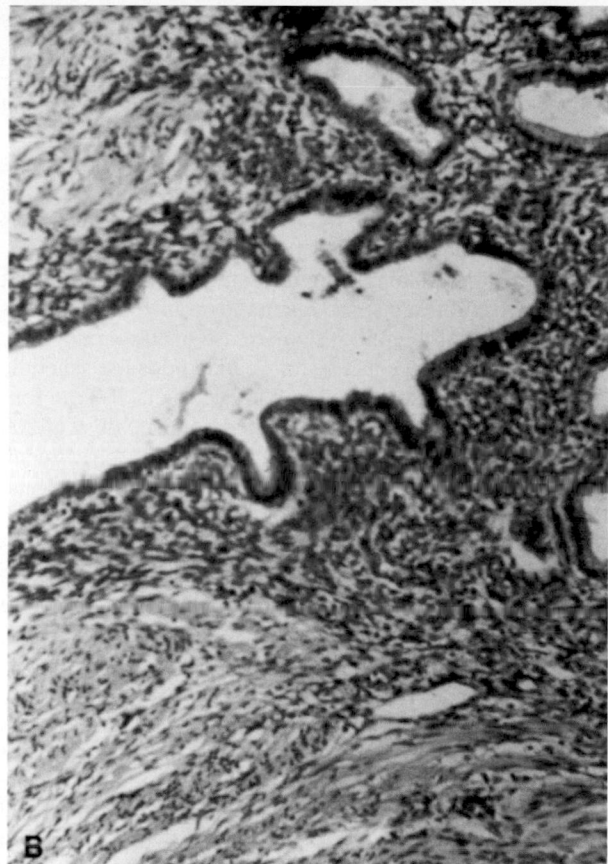

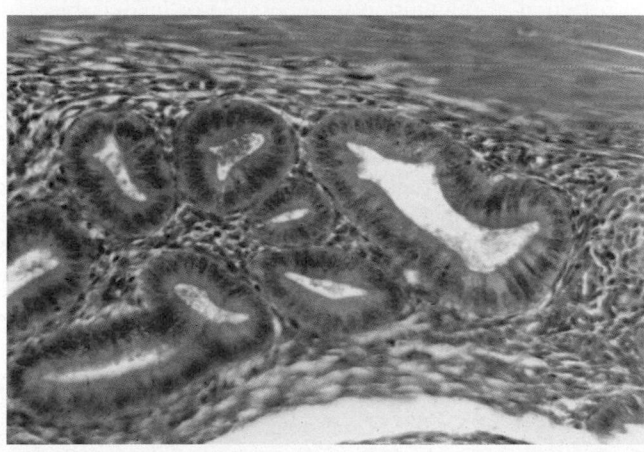

FIGURE 26-75. Endometrial glands and stroma within the wall of the bowel. **A:** Original magnification × 80. **B:** Original magnification × 260. **C:** Original magnification × 400.

stimulation, the functioning epithelium of an endometrioma sometimes closely duplicates phases of the normal intrauterine endometrium, showing proliferative changes in the preovulatory or progestational phase. However, more often, the ectopic endometrial tissues are out of phase with the normal endometrium and are found in the proliferative stage even during the secretory phase of the normal menstrual cycle. This may result from the difference in blood supply and the effects of increasing tissue fibrosis surrounding the endometriosis. Malignant transformation to adenocarcinoma has been reported.[321]

In the ovary, the process is almost always bilateral. The tendency is for the formation of cystic structures varying from tiny bluish or dark brown blisters to large "chocolate" cysts. Usually present are considerable fibrosis and puckering of the ovarian surface in the region of the cyst and adherence to neighboring structures.

Treatment

Treatment of endometriosis is often based on the patient's age, severity of symptoms, hormonal status, and desire for childbearing.[406]

Medical Treatment

Kistner observed that endometrial implants disappear after administration of large doses of progestins and estrogen.[273] Riva and associates likewise reported the beneficial effects of these compounds as observed by culdoscopy but cautioned about the rapidity of recurrence in some instances.[419] Gunning and Moyer, after using medroxyprogesterone acetate (Depo-Provera), demonstrated by culdoscopy and laparoscopy the shrinkage of endometrial tissue and confirmed microscopically that the endometriosis had disappeared.[204] The mechanism of action of these therapies has not been completely elucidated. Endometriosis disappears, but follow-up studies have shown considerable variation in the rate of reappearance. The use of progestin alone or in combination with estrogen has become the standard method of hormonal treatment of endometriosis.

Another medication for the management of endometriosis is danazol (Danocrine).[195] Its efficacy is based on the fact that it creates a hypoestrogenic-hyperandrogenic state, which is detrimental to the growth and function of endometrial tissue.[40] In doses of 200 to 800 mg/day, studies have shown that the pituitary inhibiting action results in suppression of ovulation, abolition of the midcycle increase of luteinizing hormone, and amenorrhea. The recommended dosage schedule for danazol in the treatment of endometriosis is 200 mg four times a day for at least 6 months. A maintenance dose of 200 to 400 mg daily may control pain after the initial treatment. Menstruation ceases with the commencement of therapy and returns promptly after the treatment has been discontinued. The pain of endometriosis is usually relieved in at least 80% of patients. Unfortunately, danazol has major side effects in approximately 85% of women treated with the drug.[40] These include weight gain, edema, acne, hirsutism, oily skin, deepening of the voice, clitoromegaly, and menometrorrhagia.

Most recently, the use of gonadotropin-releasing hormone (GRH) agonists has proved to be beneficial for the treatment of endometriosis. GRH is a hypothalamic decapeptide that controls pituitary secretion of luteinizing hormone and follicle-stimulating hormone.[40] Henzl and colleagues employed such a GRH agonist, nafarelin, to inhibit ovarian function reversibly and to induce hypoestrogenemia.[223] When administered by nasal spray (400 to 800 μg/day) and compared with danazol, the authors concluded that the drug was as effective as danazol and had fewer side effects, other than hypoestrogenism.

Surgical Treatment

When endometriosis involves the small or large bowel, it may be preferentially excised. Certainly, resection and anastomosis of the bowel is advisable for obstructing lesions or when malignancy cannot be excluded (Figure 26-76).[406] However, caution is suggested against extensive dissection beneath the peritoneal reflection, in the posterior cul-de-sac, or in the rectovaginal septum. Fistula complicating low anterior resection for endometriosis is not an uncommon occurrence. Laparoscopic management has been suggested, but with a cautionary note—while deep pelvic involvement can be successfully approached by this technique, it is technically challenging with a high rate of conversation to an open operation.[118] Bailey and colleagues reported 130 women who had undergone intestinal resection for endometriosis.[33] Most had had a history of previous surgical procedures and hormonal therapy before their intestinal surgery. Operations included low anterior resection with anastomosis to the extraperitoneal rectum (n = 109), sigmoid resection (n = 10), disc excision of the rectum (n = 7), ileocecal resection (n = 2), and small bowel resection (n = 2). There were no clinically apparent anastomotic leaks. With respect to fertility, of those who tried to become pregnant following resection, almost 50% went on to successful delivery. After a mean follow-up of 60 months, 100% noted relief with respect to cyclic bleeding, and 91% were free of rectal pain. It is evident from these authors' experience that a resectional approach to all visible colorectal endometriosis is a reasonable option for women with advanced disease.[33] Urbach and coworkers undertook low anterior resection for all but 7% of their 29 patients.[516] Everyone reported subjective improvement, but only 46% were "cured" based on not requiring additional medical or surgical treatment. The only variable that was associated with "cure" was concomitantly performed total abdominal hysterectomy and bilateral salpingo-oophorectomy. Laparoscopic resection has also been described.[173,414]

If pelvic endometriosis is so extensive that complete resection or fulguration is impossible or inadvisable and if childbearing has been completed, bilateral oophorectomy is curative because recurrence or progression depends on cyclic ovarian hormone production. Natural menopause, if imminent, may also be relied on to cure the process.

After surgical castration for relief of endometriosis, estrogen replacement therapy to prevent menopausal symptoms should be considered. Medroxyprogesterone acetate used for the first 6 to 9 months after operation alleviates menopausal symptoms and promotes further necrobiosis of any residual endometriosis.

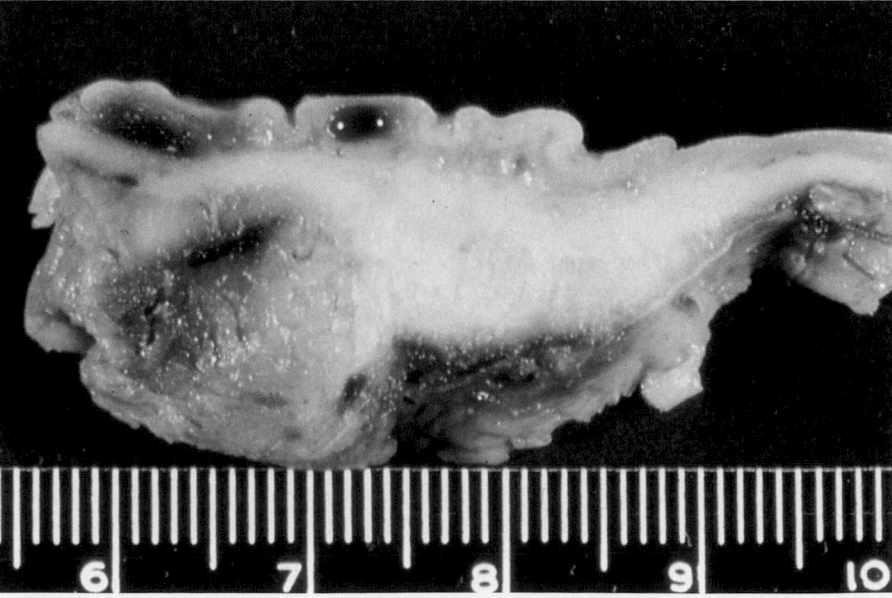

FIGURE 26-76. Endometriosis. Longitudinal section of the sigmoid colon showing blood-filled cysts.

Management to Maintain Reproductive Capacity

The most difficult therapeutic decisions arise when young women with extensive disease would like to retain reproductive capability. Reasonable efforts should be made to eradicate the disease surgically in these individuals. Postoperatively, patients should be advised to commence childbearing as soon as possible. Because pregnancy eliminates menstruation for a period of 9 months, some therapeutic benefit may be expected. When childbearing is completed, definitive surgical therapy is less traumatic.

If childbearing is not a practical alternative, the patient should be given hormone therapy designed to prevent menstruation. Oral contraceptive pills given in a cyclic manner to allow intermittent withdrawal bleeding are not beneficial therapeutically. Birth control pills given daily and in sufficient potency to prevent breakthrough bleeding will result in softening, resorption, and necrobiosis of the endometrial glands. Medroxyprogesterone acetate, 100 to 150 mg, given by intramuscular injection every 2 to 3 months, will suppress menstruation. Its main disadvantages are occasional troublesome breakthrough bleeding requiring the addition of estrogen for control and, in a small percentage of women, permanent anovulation and resultant sterility. Medroxyprogesterone acetate is not generally recommended in patients who are interested in further childbearing. Danazol is the treatment of choice.

In the experience of most physicians, hormone therapy does not always cure the process, but it gives the patient time to consider alternatives and to complete childbearing before progression of the disease or before increased symptoms and complications require the absolutely successful therapy: bilateral oophorectomy with hysterectomy.[94,110]

Perineal Endometrioma

Perineal endometrioma is a special situation in which implantation of viable endometrial cells occurs in episiotomy incisions. A tender nodule producing cyclic symptoms at the site of an episiotomy is highly suggestive of the diagnosis.[211] As with other benign and malignant conditions in the area, endoanal ultrasound has been employed for its assessment.[224] Local excision is the preferred treatment, although suppressive therapy may be employed. Patients harboring involvement of the anal sphincter have been managed successfully by wide excision and sphincteroplasty.[129,446]

Hamartoma

Albrecht introduced the term hamartoma to describe tumorlike malformations that result from inborn errors of tissue development.[9] These malformations are characterized by abnormal mixtures of mature tissue indigenous to that area. Hamartomas may be derived from any of the germinal layers, and any type of tissue may predominate.

According to Willis, the term hamartoma should be applied only to lesions for which evidence of a developmental anomaly is definite.[543] This includes either actual malformation with tissue excess present at birth or an inborn tissue anomaly that manifests itself by excessive growth continuing until puberty. The nomenclature depends on the tissue type that predominates: with vascular predominance, it is angiomatous; with fatty tissue, it is lipomatous; and with lymphoid tissue, it is lymphomatous.

Eichel and Hallberg differentiated hamartomas from teratomas and dermoids.[138] The term teratoma describes a spontaneous, autonomous new growth derived from pluripotential tissues. It is foreign to the region in which it occurs and is composed of elements of all three germinal layers. A dermoid tumor has the same histogenesis but differs in that it is usually cystic. Unlike a teratoma, it originates from only two germinal layers: the ectoderm and the mesoderm. Clinically, it is difficult to differentiate between teratomas, dermoids (especially when small), and hamartomas.

Suspicion of hamartoma may be aroused by a small but definite funnel-shaped dimple in the posterior midline at the anal margin or the midanal level. This anal dimple, associated with a higher lesion, has been reported only once, although it must have been encountered many times.[504]

Complete surgical removal is the only effective treatment for retrorectal cystic hamartoma. The surgical approach may be either through the anal canal or posteriorly, that is, transcoccygeally. However, when a large cyst lies at a very high level, an abdominal approach is indicated.

Retrorectal (Presacral) Cysts (Developmental Cysts, Including Dermoid Cyst, Epidermoid Cyst, Tailgut Cyst, Enteric Cyst, Rectal Duplication, Neurenteric Cyst, and Teratoma)

Retrorectal cystic lesions in adults are rare and are most commonly congenital. There are two types of enteric cysts: tailgut cysts (retrorectal cyst-hamartomas or mucin-secreting cysts) and cystic rectal duplication. Neurenteric cysts have also been reported.[114] Developmental cysts are defined by their histologic components and retrorectal location, lying anterior to the sacrum and posterior to the rectum. The most important complications of these cysts are infection and malignant degeneration. The differential diagnosis includes a wide variety of conditions that occur in the retrorectal space: cystic sacrococcygeal teratoma, anterior sacral meningocele, anal duct or gland cyst, abscess, neurogenic cyst, and sacral chordoma.[114]

Epidermoid cysts are benign unilocular lesions filled with clear fluid. These cysts are lined with stratified squamous epithelium. *Dermoid cysts* can be differentiated from epidermoid cysts with both gross and microscopic analysis because they contain skin appendages (e.g., hair follicles, sweat glands, and tooth buds). They are lined with stratified squamous epithelium and filled with dense muddy or fatty material. *Enteric cysts* are partially or completely lined with intestinal mucosa. They are grouped into tailgut cysts and cystic rectal duplication.

Dermoid cysts are tumors of epithelial origin believed to be caused by faulty inclusion of ectoderm when the embryo coalesces. They generally do not appear until adult life and are more common in women than in men.[243,370,494]

Galletly published a report in 1924 in which he stated, "Simple presacral cysts, lined by squamous or columnar epithelium, probably originate from cells of the neurenteric canal."[172] He included in his study 17 cases reported by Skutsch, all alleged to be dermoids.[467] Thomason reported one patient with a deep suppurating sinus extending from an anal dimple into the presacral region who required three operations.[504] Microscopic section showed a cyst lined with columnar epithelium and mucous glands in its wall. Robertson and Wride reported a patient who had a tumor with a draining sinus at the base of the spine with a foul-smelling discharge.[421] The sinus had a convoluted pattern, was anterior to the sacrum and coccyx, and was lined with columnar epithelium of a mucous type. Gius and Stout reported two patients, one of whom had three operations for multilocular lesions; the other underwent operation for an asymptomatic cystic tumor situated anterior to the coccyx.[182] Jackman and associates recognized the possibility that recurrent fistula may be associated with an infected dermoid cyst.[243] They believed that the cyst arose from remnants of the neurenteric canal. Landmann and Lewis reported a patient with a benign cystic ovarian teratoma who presented with a bleeding rectal lesion.[295] In a report from the Mayo Clinic, 49 congenital cystic lesions were identified: 15 epidermoid cysts, 16 mucus-secreting cysts, 15 teratomas, and 3 teratocarcinomas.[245] Others have also reported malignant changes in cysts.[37,111]

Currarino and colleagues described a syndrome of sacral agenesis and anorectal and presacral anomalies.[113] Others have confirmed the validity of this observation, the so-called Currarino triad, observing a high incidence of presacral teratomas.[382] The most common sacral anomaly was believed to be meningocele. Thambidorai and associates identified 200 cases of Currarino triad from the literature, but in only 22 did the presacral mass contain both meningocele and teratoma.[503]

Patients may be asymptomatic but are usually found to have an extrarectal mass as an incidental finding on rectal examination. Endoscopic examination is usually unrewarding. As mentioned, a cyst may become infected and mimic an anorectal abscess or fistula. Cysts may also prove to be of anal duct or gland origin.[287] A plain abdominal radiograph may be helpful, but CT should be employed if there is any question of malignancy. Preoperative biopsy is unnecessary and should *not* be performed.

Resection of the mass can frequently be accomplished by means of a posterior approach, with or without removal of the coccyx (see later).[3] An abdominal or abdominosacral operation may be required for a more extensive or more proximal lesion. Prognosis is excellent. Recurrence after surgery, however, is possible if the lesion is incompletely removed.

Dermoid cysts can also occur within the rectum, but this is even more unusual than the postanal or presacral locations. In this situation, intraluminal cysts may produce varied rectal symptoms, including hair protruding from the anus. Aldridge and colleagues identified only 12 such cases.[10] Their patient developed rectal bleeding and prolapse of the mass. With this type of presentation, transanal excision is the recommended approach. Endoscopic resection has also been described.[194]

Colitis Cystica Profunda or Enterogenous Cysts

Colitis cystica profunda is a rare, nonneoplastic condition characterized by the presence of mucous cysts deep to the muscularis mucosa and usually confined to the sigmoid colon and rectum. The most common symptoms are rectal bleeding, passage of mucus, diarrhea, and rectal pain.[41,328] The primary diagnosis from which it must be differentiated is mucus-producing adenocarcinoma.

Wayte and Helwig categorized colitis cystica profunda into two groups: localized, in which the cysts are confined to a distinct area of the rectum, and diffuse, in which the cysts are located in extensive areas.[532] The histogenesis of this benign condition remains in dispute. Based on differences in the evaluation of clinical and pathologic findings, the following descriptive terms have been used at one time or another:

Colitis cystica profunda[143,532]
Solitary ulcer of the rectum (see Chapter 21)[214,244,320]
Syndrome of the descending perineum (see Chapter 21)[389]
Enterogenous cysts of the rectum[496]
Hamartomatous inverted polyp of the rectum[11]

Colitis cystica profunda of the localized type may protrude slightly into the lumen of the bowel as a polypoid mass and can thus mimic carcinoma of the rectum. Because it is usually located on the anterior rectal wall, the most common site for solitary ulcer, considerable confusion may exist.

The etiology of the condition is unknown. However, some patients give a history of prior rectal trauma, especially the removal of a large polyp. Madigan and Morson described the correlation between anorectal dysfunction and this disease.[320] Epstein and associates theorized that the most probable primary factor was a weakness or defect in the muscularis mucosa resulting in mucosal herniation.[143] Certainly, the fact that resolution has followed the successful management of internal procidentia and rectal prolapse implies a causative or an associative role with these conditions.[203] Peterkin and colleagues identified three patients with paraplegia who developed proctitis cystica profunda.[394] This particular population may be at an increased risk because of digital stimulation applied to effect evacuation. One patient required a colostomy for recurrent symptoms.

Differentiation by biopsy may be difficult.[11] In order to establish the diagnosis with certainty, adequate tissue must be obtained in order to reveal submucosal cyst formation.[198] In Madigan and Morson's series, 31 of 51 patients had lesions with histologic appearances suggestive of both solitary ulcer and colitis cystica profunda (Figures 26-77 and 26-78).[320]

Although successful medical management through the use of steroid enemas has been reported, transanal excision of the lesion is the optimal therapy if it can be accomplished. A transcoccygeal approach is another alternative. Martin and associates reviewed the Mayo Clinic experience of 66 patients

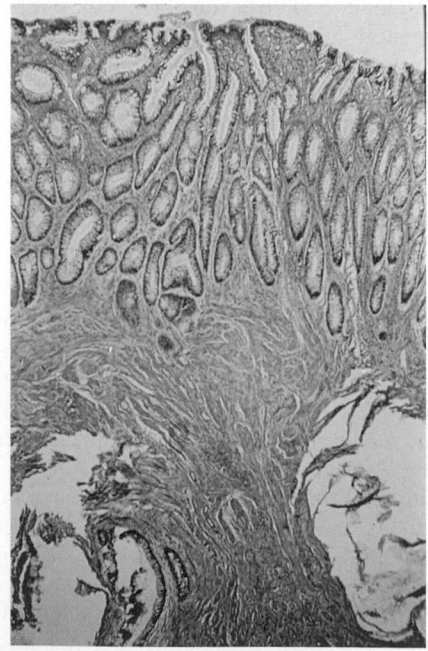

FIGURE 26-77. Colitis cystica profunda. Cystic structures in the wall of the bowel, one of which is lined by columnar epithelium. The other cyst has lost epithelium. (Original magnification × 80; from Corman ML, Veidenheimer MC, Swinton NW. *Diseases of the Anus, Rectum, and Colon. Part I: Neoplasms.* New York, NY: Medcom; 1972.)

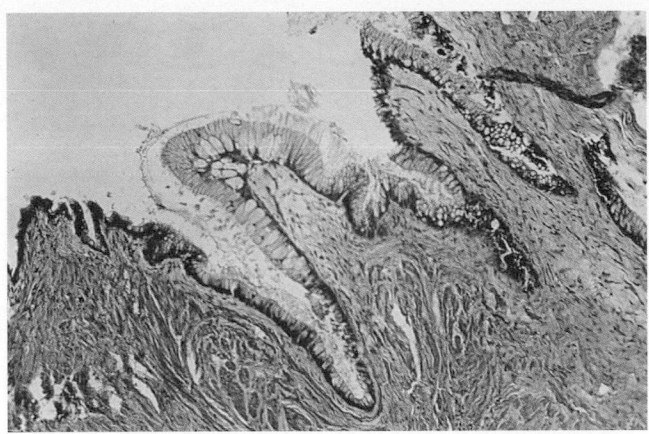

FIGURE 26-78. Colitis cystica profunda. The lining of the cyst shows columnar epithelium. (Original magnification × 260; from Corman ML, Veidenheimer MC, Swinton NW. *Diseases of the Anus, Rectum, and Colon. Part I: Neoplasms.* New York, NY: Medcom; 1972.)

with this condition.[328] Fewer than three-fourths were asymptomatic after local excision. Not uncommonly, the lesion is unresectable except by radical abdominoperineal resection. Such treatment is contraindicated, however, for this benign condition. Another option that has been described is mucosal sleeve excision with coloanal pull-through.[205] Reassurance and periodic proctosigmoidoscopy are suggested for those not amenable to complete removal of the lesion.

Ectopic Tissue

Besides ectopic gastric or pancreatic mucosa in a Meckel's diverticulum, ectopic tissue in the intestine or colon is very unusual. The two types that have been reported are gastric mucosal replacement of the rectal mucosa and salivary gland tissue in the submucosa.[310,371,457,488,536,546] It has been suggested that the cells lining the primitive gut have the capacity to differentiate into any epithelial type that would normally be present at another level. This would not, however, explain the presence of salivary gland tissue. Perhaps the presence of stem cells lining the cloacal zone may account for this rare observation.[457]

Testart and colleagues reviewed the literature on heterotopic gastric mucosa producing rectal "peptic" ulceration.[502] Analysis of 28 cases revealed the main features to be as follows:

All but one were diagnosed in infants or in adults younger than 26 years of age.
Rectal peptic ulceration was identified in only one-half, but almost all exhibited rectal bleeding.
Rectal duplication was present in 21%.
Limited excision is generally successful.[502]

Protrusion of tissue may occur in a child, thus causing one to suspect the presence of a juvenile polyp. Patients may be asymptomatic or complain of mucous discharge, change in bowel habits, or rectal bleeding.

The true pathologic nature of the lesion is usually not suspected at the time of removal but is confirmed by histologic examination (Figure 26-79). Carlei and colleagues were able to show different types of endocrine cells in the rectal and heterotopic mucosa by means of immunocytochemistry.[75] They could affirm that the heterotopic event also involved the differentiation of the endocrine elements into gastric-type endocrine cells. In their case, they were able to demonstrate that the activities of the heterotopic mucosa, such as endocrine system and mucin and acid production, were almost identical to those of the normal stomach.[75]

Transanal local excision is the appropriate treatment (Figure 26-80).

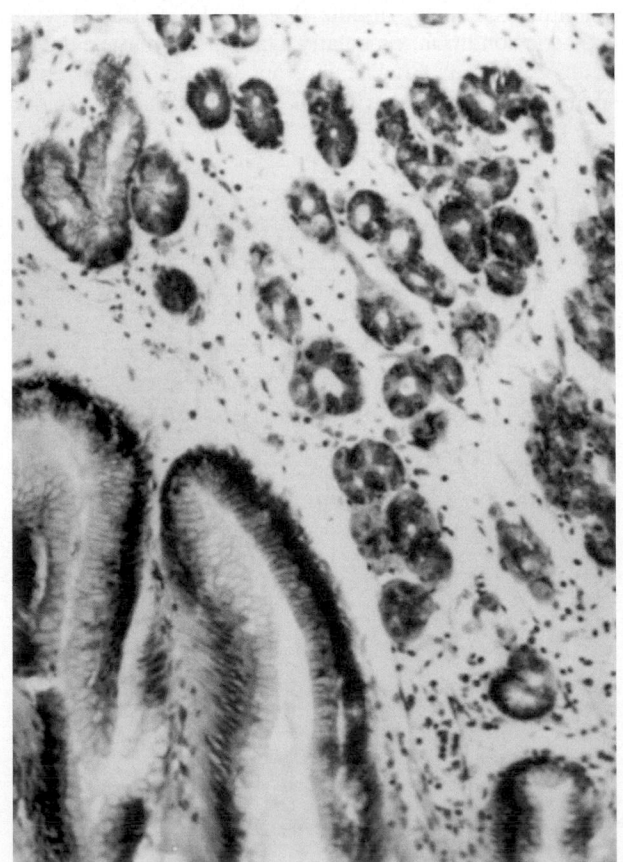

FIGURE 26-79. Heterotopic gastric mucosa in the rectum. Colonic mucosa on the left with gastric cells on the right. Special stains showed the presence of chief and parietal cells. (Original magnification × 260.)

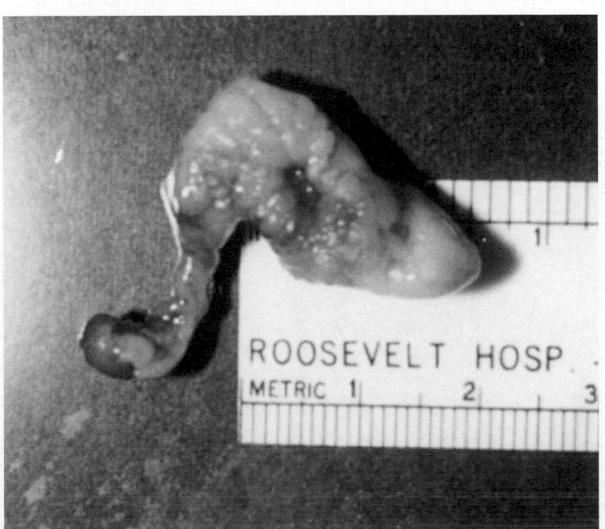

FIGURE 26-80. Heterotopic gastric mucosa in the rectum. Polypoid mass with 3-mm ulceration. The ulcer was found to contain the gastric glands seen in Figure 26-83.

There has been a total of six documented cases of heterotopic gastric mucosa occurring in the large bowel, proximal to the rectum. Most have been managed by resection because bleeding identified by means of angiography or radioisotope scan leads to surgery. It is only when the lesion has been submitted to histologic evaluation that the true cause is confirmed. There are now reports of successful management in individuals by means of a histamine (H_2) antagonist.[75,363]

EXOGENOUS, EXTRINSIC, AND MISCELLANEOUS TUMORS

Extraskeletal Osteosarcoma

Extraskeletal osteosarcoma is a rare, malignant tumor arising from soft tissue *without* attachment to bone or to periosteum. A single case that was primary to the colon has been reported.[456]

Choriocarcinoma

Choriocarcinoma primary to the colon is an exceedingly rare tumor, with only seven cases reported in the literature according to a review by Le and colleagues.[297] The etiology has been thought by some to be dedifferentiation of an adenocarcinoma, but there is also the possibility that the lesion may arise de novo. Treatment is resection, but prognosis is poor.

Metastatic Tumor

Metastatic tumor to the colon and rectum can cause symptoms of abdominal pain, bleeding, and change in bowel habits. Life-threatening emergencies in the form of massive GI hemorrhage, obstruction, and perforation have been reported.[472] Although usually it produces extrinsic compression of the bowel on barium enema examination or on CT, ulceration may mimic primary carcinoma of the colon (Figure 26-81). Tumors of adjacent organs that may invade the colon and rectum include prostate, uterus (Figures 26-82 and 26-83), ovary (Figure 26-84), kidney, stomach, duodenum, and pancreas.

Metastatic disease to the colon can occur from breast tumors, hypernephroma, lung tumors, malignant melanoma, and

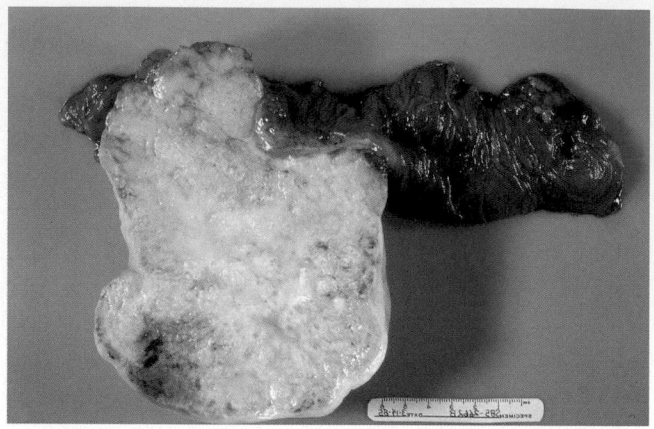

FIGURE 26-82. Tumor invading the serosa of the sigmoid colon from a uterine cancer.

even a Merkel cell carcinoma (Figure 26-81).[237,239,268,332,462,472] The Mayo Clinic group identified 24 patients treated for metastatic malignant melanoma.[501] The median interval between diagnosis of the primary lesion and the development of metastatic disease was more than 7 years. The most common presentation was bleeding. The 5-year survival for those who were resected was 21%. Palliative resection or bypass is usually advised for symptomatic tumors, but perforation or obstruction implies a poor prognosis.[239,268,501]

Barium Granuloma

A submucosal rectal nodule that can be confused with a neoplastic condition, especially a carcinoid, may be due to a barium granuloma. Such lesions appear in the lower rectum, usually as submucosal white or yellowish plaques, and are

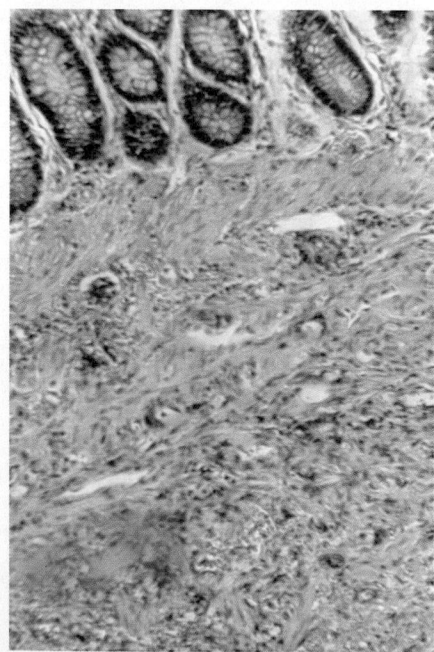

FIGURE 26-83. Metastatic adenocarcinoma from the uterine cervix. Note the normal overlying colonic epithelium. The wall is infiltrated by tumor cells forming small glandular structures. (Original magnification × 260; courtesy of Rudolf Garret, MD.)

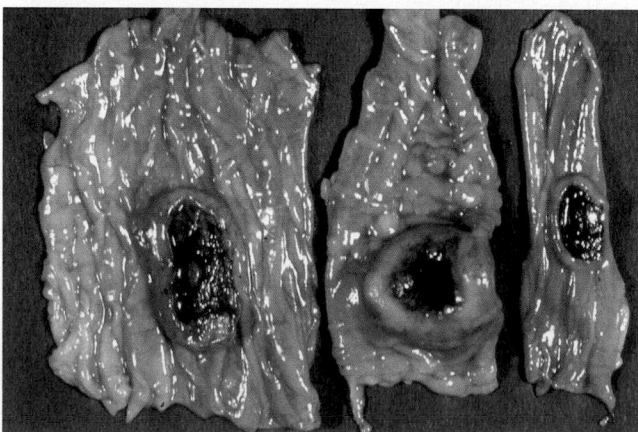

FIGURE 26-81. Multiple lesions of metastatic melanoma from the skin to the bowel mucosa; normal mucosa surrounds the deep ulcer in the center. (Courtesy of Rudolf Garret, MD.)

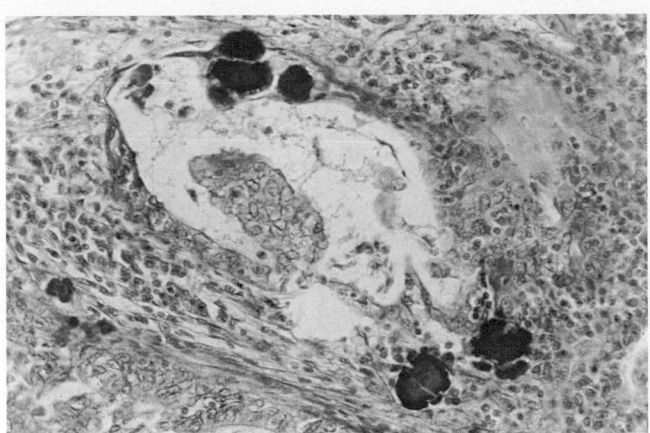

FIGURE 26-84. Metastatic tumor consisting of undifferentiated cells forming abortive glands with psammoma bodies. The tumor was metastatic from an ovary. (From Corman ML, Veidenheimer MC, Swinton NW. *Diseases of the Anus, Rectum, and Colon. Part I: Neoplasms.* New York, NY: Medcom; 1972.)

frequently asymptomatic. A break in the continuity of the rectal mucosa is the probable initiating factor. Transanal excision is mandatory for diagnosis.

Rand studied the effects of injection of barium in the rectal wall of dogs.[411] He produced a granulomatous ulcer that healed spontaneously despite retained barium in the tissues. Histologically, the presence of barium produces a typical foreign body granulomatous reaction (Figure 26-85). The barium crystals lie in a pool in the submucosa in early lesions, but macrophages rapidly accumulate and phagocytose in the crystalline barium sulfate. Care in the introduction of the enema catheter and caution with the use of the balloon tip are clearly indicated for prevention of barium granuloma.

Numerous cases of rupture of the bowel with barium peritonitis have been reported when barium enema examination has followed rectal biopsy.[221] Margulis and Burhenne stated that double-contrast examination of the colon should not be performed for at least 2 weeks after rectal biopsy.[325] Optimally, if a polyp excision or electrocoagulation is contemplated on an individual who is to have barium enema examination, the patient should complete the contrast study and then return for the other procedure (see Chapter 5). Barium granuloma of the more proximal colon is usually related to inflammatory bowel disease.[191]

Oleoma, Eleoma, Oil Granuloma, and Paraffinoma

Oleoma, also known as oleogranuloma or paraffinoma, is a rare entity that occurs in the GI tract or skin as a result of an injection of mineral oil (paraffin) for the treatment of hemorrhoids or enema or vegetable oil in the management of constipation. The lesion seen may be defined as an intramural pseudotumor that develops as a foreign body reaction. The "tumor" is occasionally cystic and may be termed an oleocyst. The differential diagnosis must be confirmed by biopsy to rule out other neoplastic and inflammation conditions.

The clinical manifestations may develop very rapidly or may not present for many years after oil enters the tissue. The injection site usually appears as one or more irregular, firm

nodules. In the GI tract, oleomas are usually found proximal to the dentate line in the lower portion of the rectum.

An oleoma is usually localized to the submucosa. However, considerable inflammation of the mucosa and even the perianal skin may be present. The appearance of the lesion depends on the oil present. Vegetable oils produce the least reaction, animal oils a greater one, and mineral oils the most severe changes.[207]

Histologically, oleomas are typified by large mononuclear phagocytes, epithelioid cells, eosinophilic leukocytes, and multinucleated giant cells of the foreign body type, surrounding large, clear spaces that give the tissue a swiss cheese or spongiform appearance under low-power amplification. Histologic staining with oil red O verifies the presence of the lipid. The reaction usually remains localized to the submucosa, but not infrequently involves the lamina propria of the mucosa and may actually extend into the perirectal fat (Figure 26-86).[207]

Mazier and associates reported four cases of oleoma.[331] All patients recovered after simple excision of the lesion.

Sarcoidosis

Sarcoidosis is a generalized granulomatous disease with protean manifestations. The condition usually creates restrictive lung disease but can occasionally involve the GI tract. In the limited number of cases, reported patients usually do not have symptoms referable to the bowel.[280,510] Proctosigmoidoscopic examination may reveal mild inflammatory changes or a submucosal rectal nodule.

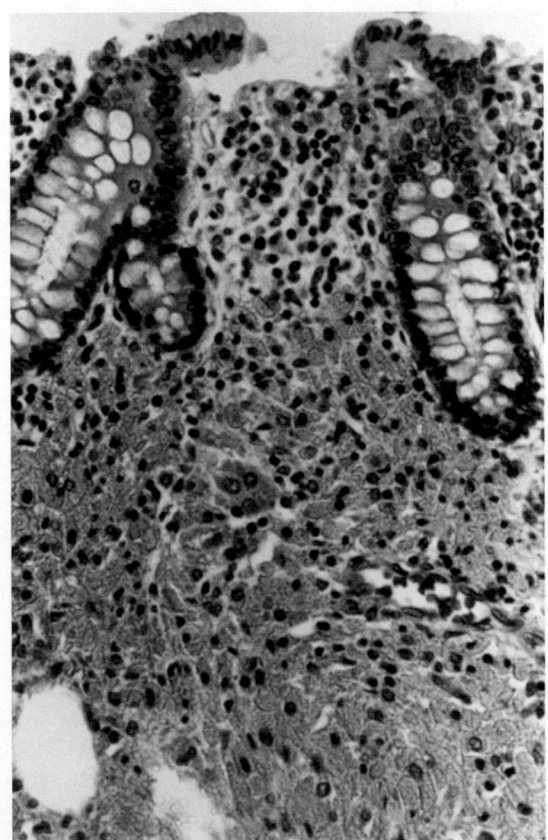

FIGURE 26-85. Barium granuloma. Normal glandular mucosa overlying plump, foamy histiocytes filled with refractile material when visualized under polarized light. (Original magnification × 80; courtesy of Rodger C. Haggitt, MD.)

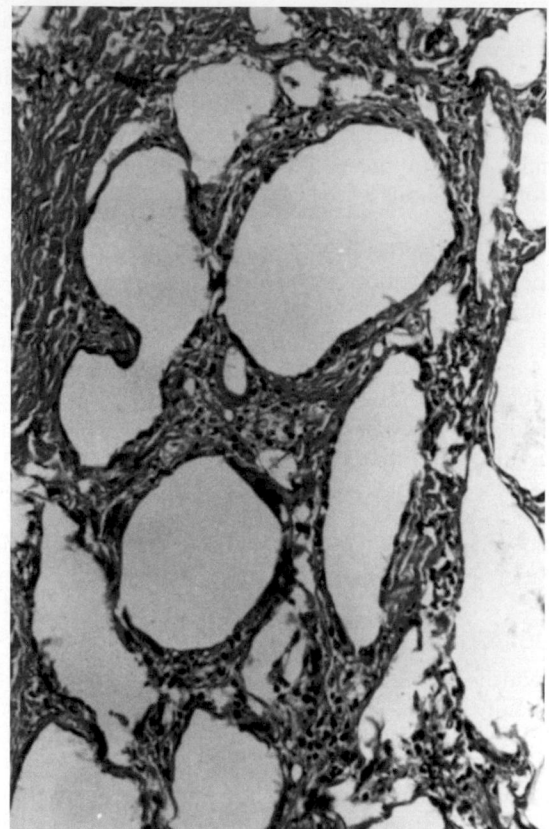

FIGURE 26-86. Oleogranuloma. Submucosal cysts of varied size with surrounding foreign body giant cell reaction and granulomatous change. The diagnosis is confirmed with oil red O stain. (Original magnification × 50; courtesy of Rodger C. Haggitt, MD.)

The characteristic noncaseating granuloma of sarcoidosis may be seen on biopsy or excision of a lesion (Figure 26-87). Histologic examination may confirm a granuloma composed primarily of histiocytes, but there is no evidence of caseous necrosis.

The clinical patterns produced by intestinal sarcoidosis are not well established, but anorexia, nausea, vomiting, abdominal pain, and GI bleeding have all been described.[207] Differential diagnosis must include Crohn's disease, but the presence of a lesion in the lung will usually clarify any possible confusion.

Wegener's Granulomatosis

Wegener's granulomatosis, a necrotizing vasculitis associated with granulomatous lesions of the upper and lower respiratory tract and the kidney, was reported in one instance to present as a perianal ulcer.[27] Treatment was by immunosuppressive therapy.

Amyloidosis

Amyloidosis is a pathologic condition caused by the deposition within tissues of a fibrillar protein known as amyloid.[498] Virchow misnamed the substance because he thought it resembled starch or cellulose. The Third International Symposium on Amyloidosis recommended the following classification[248]:

Primary amyloidosis: no evidence of preceding or coexisting disease except multiple myeloma
Secondary amyloidosis: coexistence of other conditions

Localized amyloid: single organ rather than generalized involvement
Familial
Senile amyloid

It is not within the purview of this text to undertake an assessment of the disease itself. Under the circumstances, the reader is advised to seek out any of a number of comprehensive reviews on the subject.[291]

Involvement of the GI tract is reported in 70% of patients with primary amyloidosis and 55% of those with the secondary form.[248,251] Amyloidosis not uncommonly affects the colon in association with a number of systemic diseases, particularly pulmonary, renal, hematologic, and arthritic. Symptoms include malabsorption, diarrhea, bleeding, vomiting, abdominal pain, and, rarely, signs of peritonitis, but the condition is usually asymptomatic. Ischemic colitis as a consequence of vascular involvement of the bowel is a well-recognized complication of the disease.[420]

Rectal Biopsy

The value of rectal biopsy for establishing the diagnosis of systemic amyloid has been a matter of controversy. Biopsies of the liver, spleen, or oral tissue (particularly gingiva) have been suggested as alternative sites.[450] Dinges and associates performed an autopsy study of 100 cases and took biopsy specimens of the rectum and gingiva.[124] In this unselected study, there was a higher incidence of amyloid detected in the gingival and buccal mucosa than in the rectal mucosa. Three-fourths of the biopsies taken from the mouth yielded positive results, as compared with one-third of the rectal mucosal specimens. The authors concluded that in view of the frequently found extensive amyloid deposits present in the mouth, biopsy should be obtained from the rectal mucosa. The theory behind this recommendation is that amyloid found on gingival biopsy is of less significance than if it were found on rectal biopsy.

Gafni and Sohar performed rectal biopsy on 30 patients with known amyloidosis, and a positive result was found in 26.[170] Blum and Sohar found that rectal biopsy yielded a 75% positive result in those with amyloidosis.[61] This was exceeded only by renal biopsy (87% positive). Biopsy of the liver gave positive results in fewer than one-half of the patients, and gingival biopsy in less than 20%.

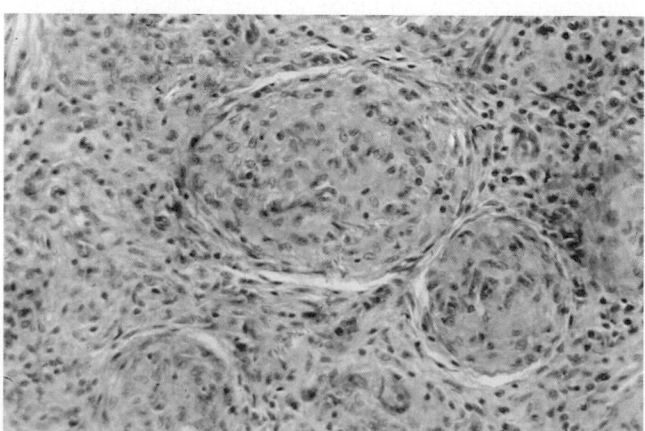

FIGURE 26-87. Sarcoidosis. Granuloma without caseous necrosis. Note the characteristic epithelioid cells. (Original magnification × 360; from Corman ML, Veidenheimer MC, Swinton NW. *Diseases of the Anus, Rectum, and Colon. Part I: Neoplasms.* New York, NY: Medcom; 1972.)

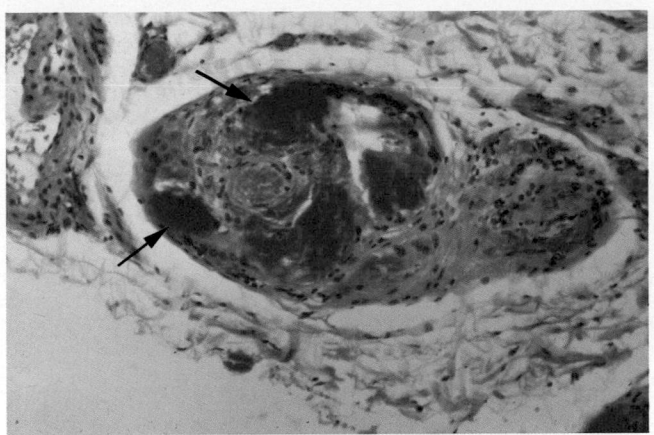

FIGURE 26-88. Amyloidosis. Congo red stain, which produces green color under polarized light, reveals homogeneous material (*arrows*) within the wall of an artery in the submucosa of the rectum. (Original magnification × 280.)

In a study by Kyle and coworkers, 17 of 20 patients with primary systemic amyloidosis were found to have positive rectal biopsies for amyloid.[292] In 2 of the 3 remaining individuals, the specimen did not contain submucosal tissue.

This is an important point. It is imperative that adequate submucosal tissue be obtained in order to confirm the diagnosis. Although some authors have advocated a suction biopsy forceps, our own preference is to employ the ordinary rectal biopsy instrument. Because one is not taking a sample of tissue from an exophytic lesion, the biopsy should be obtained from a valve of Houston or from the posterior rectal wall. If bleeding is encountered, pressure with an epinephrine-soaked cotton swab is advised. Electrocoagulation should be avoided because of the risk of perforating the bowel.

An interesting point was made by Slagel and Lupton concerning the observation of "postproctoscopic periorbital purpura."[468] The hydrostatic forces imposed on the delicate periorbital vasculature when the patient is placed in the prone jackknife position for biopsy may precipitate rupture of the vessels whose walls are compromised by amyloid deposition.

Special stains are important for identification of amyloid. A homogeneous eosinophilic substance can be seen by means of Congo red stain. This material may be overlooked if the standard hematoxylin and eosin technique is used (Figure 26-88).

Response to Treatment

Another purpose of rectal biopsy is to evaluate the success of different modalities of treatment. Bacon and colleagues performed repeated rectal biopsies in a group of patients who underwent penicillamine therapy.[31] Improvement could be observed by serial histologic examinations. Melphalan and prednisone have been employed with limited benefit. The mechanism is to decrease immunoglobulin production and prevent progressive amyloid deposition.[498] Colchicine has also been reported to have some therapeutic value as well as autologous hematopoietic stem cell transplantation.

Amyloid Tumor

Localized amyloid tumors of the GI tract are extremely unusual. All reported cases involving the large bowel presented with lower GI bleeding.[248] A colonic perforation has also been observed.[190] Rarely, amyloidosis of the colon may produce a mass lesion or obstructive symptoms.[252,288] Resection should be considered for a symptomatic, well-defined tumor.

Malacoplakia

In 1902, Michaelis and Gutmann described malacoplakia as a rare chronic inflammatory disorder most commonly affecting the urinary bladder and other portions of the genitourinary tract.[341] In 1965, Terner and Lattes reported the first case of colonic involvement.[500] This was followed by the publication of reports of several other patients.[410]

Clinical presentation is varied, but rectal bleeding, diarrhea, and obstructive symptoms are most commonly described. The lesion may be observed as an incidental finding. There is a preponderance of women among patients with the genitourinary lesion, but this is not the case with those who have colonic involvement.

There are no characteristic radiologic changes of malacoplakia. The barium enema may be indistinguishable from carcinoma or from granulomatous colitis.[257]

The macroscopic lesion appears as a mucosal thickening or plaque and may assume a polypoid configuration. Histologically, one observes a proliferation of eosinophilic, coarsely granular histiocytes (Hansemann's cells) of granular periodic acid–Schiff–positive inclusions often containing laminated calcific concretions, the so-called Michaelis-Gutmann bodies that are virtually pathognomonic of this entity (Figure 26-89).[330] The histiocytic proliferation is accompanied by a chronic inflammatory infiltrate and sometimes by fibrosis (Figure 26-90).

Although the pathogenesis is not fully understood, ultrastructural evidence suggests that altered heat response to certain species of gram-negative bacteria may be involved.[83,303] Abdou and colleagues have demonstrated a reversible lysosomal defect that could impair lysosomal bacterial killing in this disorder.[1] Sound ultrastructural evidence implies that the Michaelis-Gutmann body is a morphologic by-product of impaired lysosomal function.[312] There may be an immunologic association as well because the condition has been identified in a patient with hypogammaglobulinemia.[350] A genetic predisposition has also been observed.[141]

In 1981, McClure reviewed the world literature of malacoplakia of the GI tract.[333] There were 34 recorded cases with 86 sites involved, most commonly in the rectum and colon.

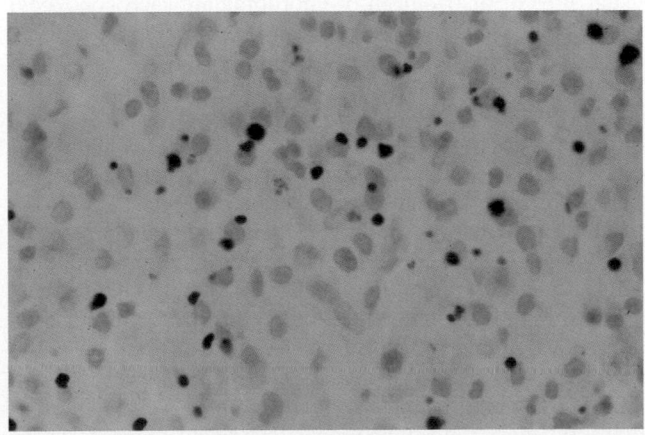

FIGURE 26-89. Malacoplakia. Von Kossa stain showing Michaelis-Gutmann bodies. (Original magnification × 600; courtesy of Rudolf Garret, MD.)

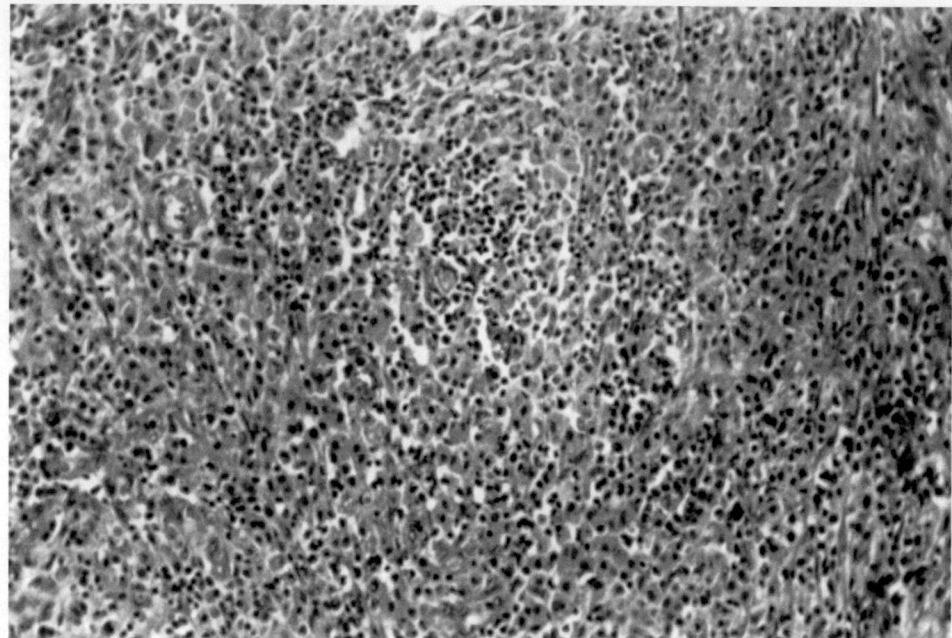

FIGURE 26-90. Malacoplakia. Many macrophages and lymphocytes are evident. (Original magnification × 260; courtesy of Rudolf Garret, MD.)

Although the lesions are for the most part self-limited or responsive to antibiotic therapy, occasionally resection is necessary because of bleeding, the development of nonhealing fistulas, or localized anatomic complications.[257] Biopsy and histologic examination are necessary to differentiate this lesion from carcinoma, which it may resemble clinically. It is of interest that malacoplakia has been associated as an incidental finding with colonic carcinoma that may actually cause the surgeon to overestimate the extent of the invasion by tumor.[330,333,410]

Sacrococcygeal Chordoma

Sacrococcygeal chordoma, a rare tumor of the fetal notochord, is characterized by a slow but inexorably progressive growth that usually spans a period of years. It invades by direct extension. Irrespective of the method of treatment chosen, the prognosis is poor. This tumor, thought by many to remain a local disease, has been reported to demonstrate distant metastases in more than 40% of patients.[177,226] The usual sites of distribution of chordoma are sacrococcygeal (50%), spheno-occipital (35%), and vertebral (15%). There are rare examples of extranotochordal origin.[209]

Signs, Symptoms, and Findings

Symptoms are produced as the tumor proliferates; the lesion often reaches considerable size before the diagnosis is made. Surrounding soft tissue and viscera are at first simply displaced, but eventually adjacent bone is gradually eroded (Figure 26-91). The most common initial symptom is pain. This is often so gradual in onset and of such indefinite character that patients with this complaint often experience a delay in diagnosis of months to years. Constipation is the second most common presenting complaint.[481]

The most significant physical finding is a firm, smooth, presacral mass with overlying intact rectal mucosa. There may be a history of prior treatment for a neurologic, orthopedic, or urologic disorder.

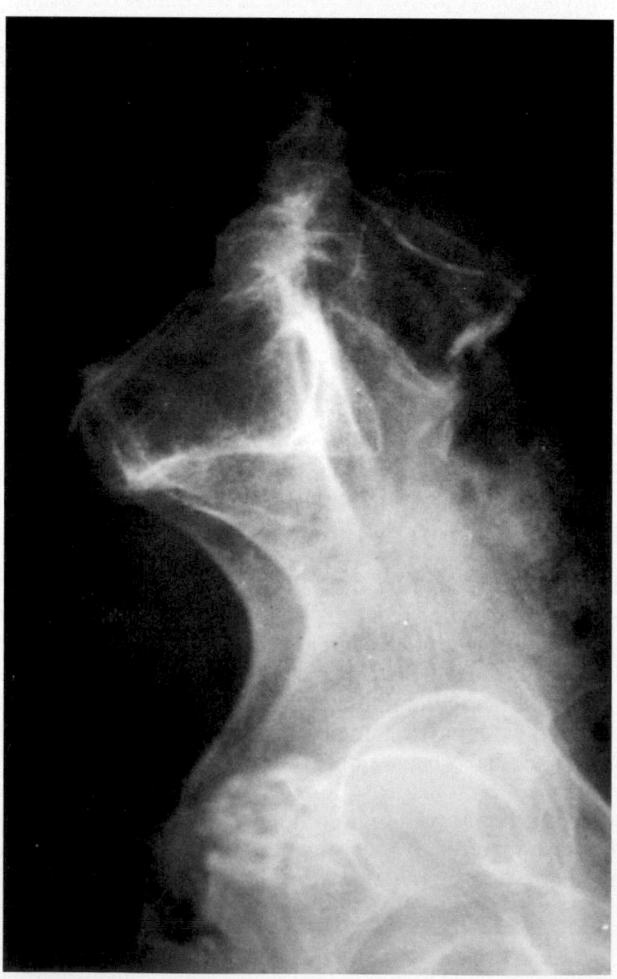

FIGURE 26-91. Sacrococcygeal chordoma. Invasion of the sacrum produces complete destruction as seen on lateral projection.

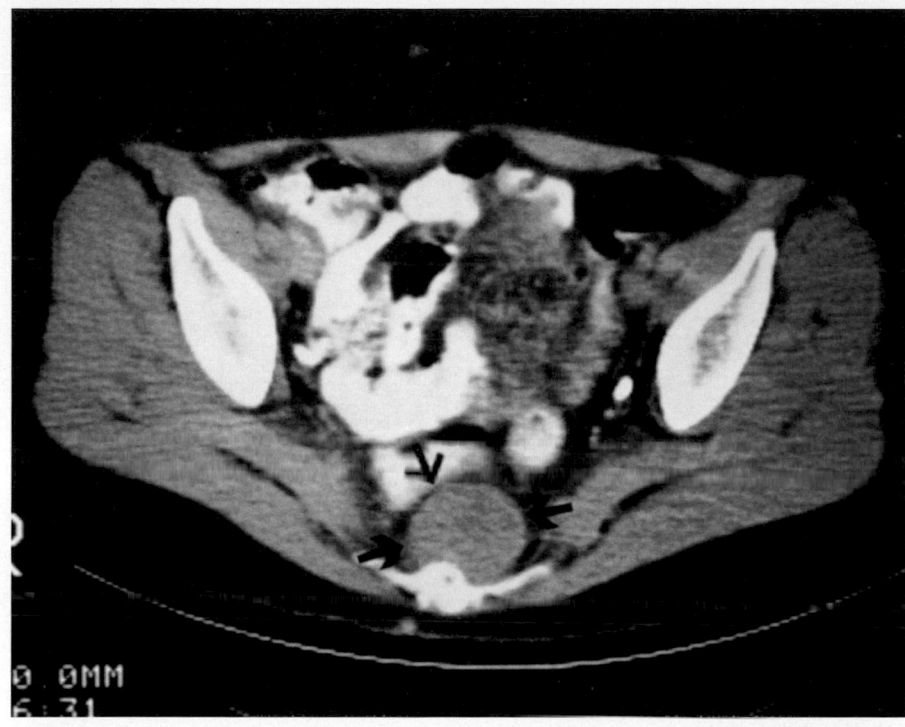

FIGURE 26-92. Sacrococcygeal chordoma. This computed tomography scan demonstrates a well-circumscribed mass invading the sacrum (*arrow*).

Evaluation

Bone destruction, soft tissue mass, and anterior displacement of the rectum are the characteristic radiographic signs. These tumors often involve far more soft tissue than the osseous deformity would imply, and at operation bone destruction is likely to be more extensive than had been evident from the radiographic studies.[259]

Radiographic examination, including CT scan and MRI (Figure 26-92), is the only investigative procedure necessary for making the diagnosis of chordoma. Suga and colleagues evaluated four patients with primary sacrococcygeal chordoma by means of bone scintigraphy with ^{99m}Tc hydroxymethylene diphosphonate and gallium scintigraphy.[487] All demonstrated photon-deficient or cold lesions corresponding to the tumor on scintigraphy. The findings led the authors to conclude that a tumor consistent with a chordoma demonstrates a cold lesion on scintigraphy with no increased accumulation on gallium scan. This finding is much more consistent with a chordoma as opposed to a malignant neoplasm.[487] Needle biopsy is to be condemned because of the likelihood of implanting viable tumor cells, although theoretically one may be able to excise skin and needle tract along with the ultimately resected specimen. The diagnosis should be able to be made on clinical and radiologic grounds without pathologic confirmation. Moreover, there may be confusion in the interpretation of limited material for histologic evaluation (Figures 26-93 and 26-94).

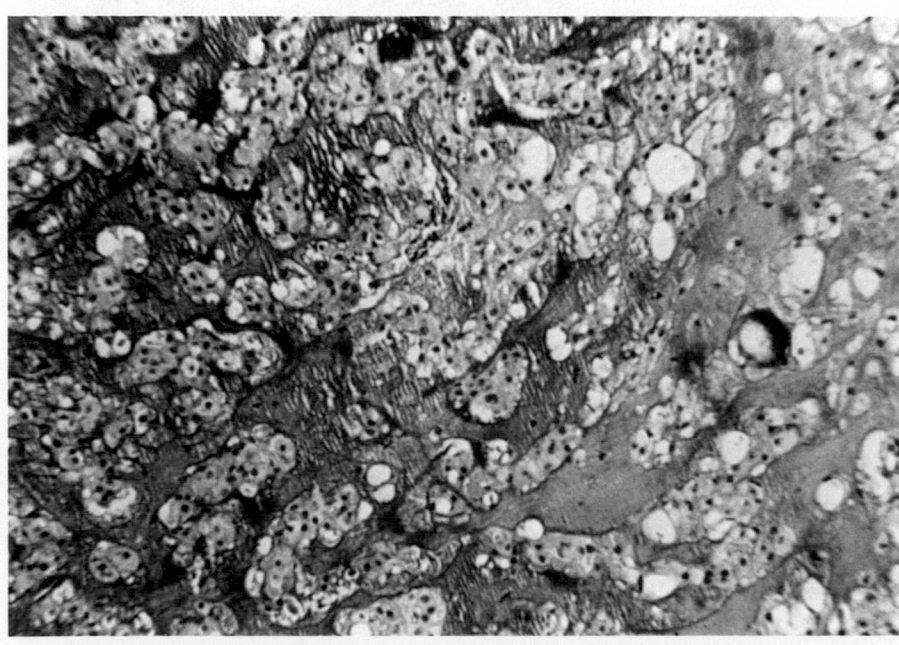

FIGURE 26-93. Sacrococcygeal chordoma. Cells with vacuolated cytoplasm resembling chondrocytes. (Original magnification × 280; courtesy of Rudolf Garret, MD.)

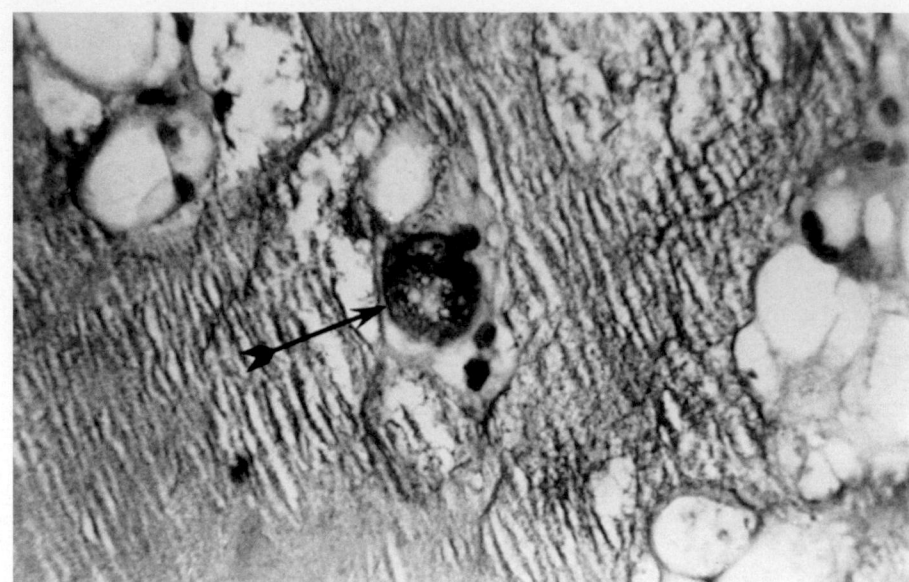

FIGURE 26-94. Sacrococcygeal chordoma. A physaliphorous cell (*arrow*), a large cell with a lobulated, large nucleus, is evident in this chordoma. (Original magnification × 600; courtesy of Rudolf Garret, MD.)

Treatment

Cure of sacrococcygeal chordoma depends on complete extirpation of the tumor, ideally by en bloc removal of the lesion with the coccyx and, if limited, the lower sacral segments (Figures 26-95 through 26-97).[435] The critical factor with respect to the extent of resection is the need to preserve the S2 nerve roots because their removal will lead to permanent neurologic damage and fecal and urinary incontinence.[19,365] However, a report of normal continence was observed in a patient with preservation of only one S2 root.[17] In addition to neurologic impairment, resections more extensive than the lower three sacral segments may result in instability and collapse of the pelvis and descent of the lumbar spine.[49,391]

The patient must understand that there is significant risk of impairment in spite of all precautions. Furthermore, it is strongly suggested that neurosurgical consultation be available in the operating room for all procedures involving the removal of a sacral chordoma.

Some surgeons favor a radical approach, including abdominosacral resection or even posterior exenteration and sacrectomy.[238,264,265,307] Clearly, this should only be considered for chordomas that cannot be removed by a more limited operation. Exposure of the sciatic and pudendal nerves is required if one must extirpate a large growth that extends into the buttocks.[264] High sacral resections may be performed by dividing the fused sacral laminae with fine rongeurs, opening the sacral canal, exposing the dural sac and sacral roots, and dividing the sacral bodies with an osteotome.[264,266]

Radiation therapy is controversial because the tumor has not been proved to be radiosensitive. It is often used, however, when surgical excision is impossible. Chemotherapy has not been proven to be beneficial.[29] However, there are current phase II trials that are attempting to determine the effect of Gleevec on locally advanced and metastatic chordomas.[155]

If recurrence develops following resection, debulking may palliate pain symptoms. If radiotherapy has been employed, subsequent healing may be considerably delayed, or the wound may not heal at all. For unremitting pain uncontrolled by medication, chordotomy may be necessary.

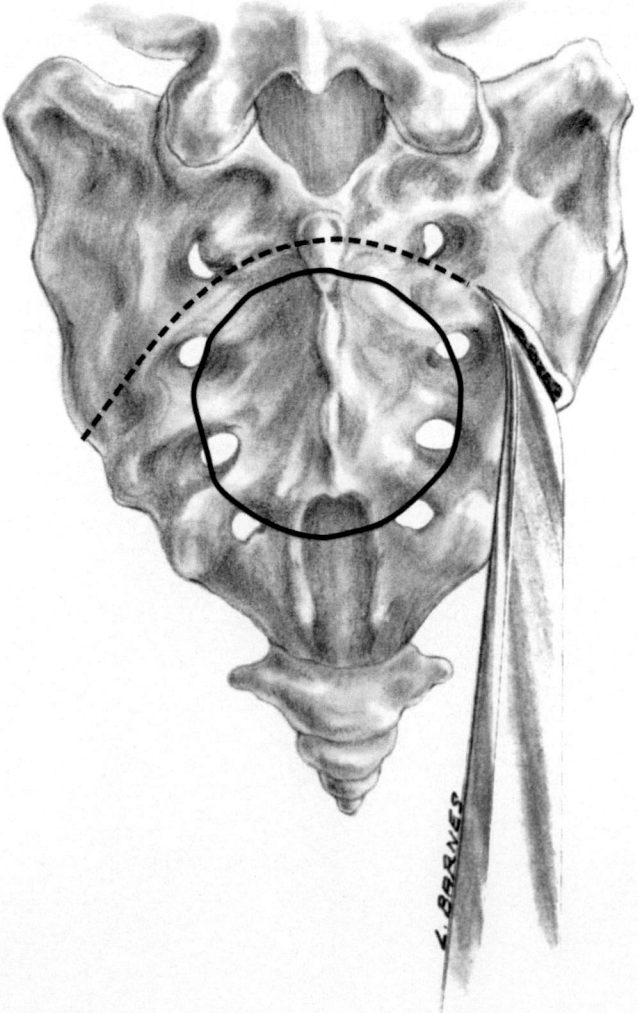

FIGURE 26-95. Technique of removing the sacrum with an osteotome.

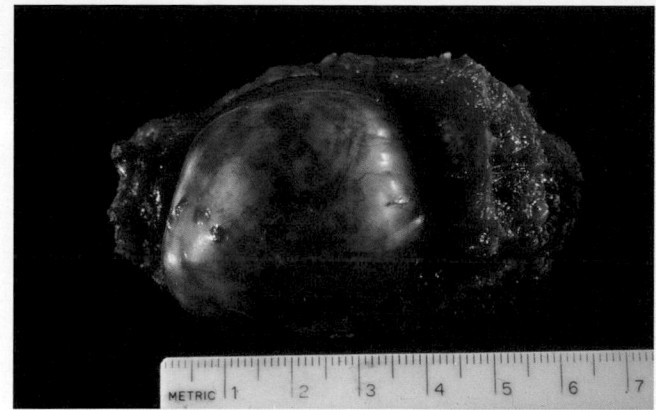

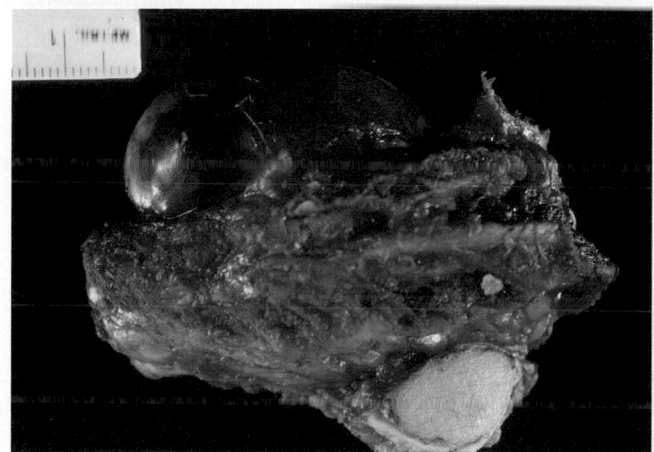

FIGURE 26-96. Sacrococcygeal chordoma. A well-encapsulated mass adherent to the sacrum **(A)**, with lateral view **(B)**.

Results

Results of surgical treatment for chordoma are difficult to interpret because patients often live a long time, even with persistent localized or disseminated disease. Furthermore, many publications are based on small numbers, with only a few months of follow-up.[81,115,226,385,512,555] The overall 5-year survival in the Mayo Clinic series of 30 patients was 75%.[245] However, only 30% were considered cured. Chandawarkar reviewed a 50-year experience with 50 consecutive patients.[82] All underwent partial sacrococcygectomy. Postoperative complications included the following:

Urinary incontinence (14%)
Anal incontinence (6%)
Hemorrhage (4%)
Rectal injury (2%)[82]

In his reported experience, the average disease-free survival was 63 months.

Ependymoma

Ependymomas are the most common tumors of glial origin in the spinal cord, especially in the region of the cauda equina.[508] Clinically, a mass thought to be a pilonidal cyst or sinus is a common presenting feature.[15] These lesions occur mainly in patients during the third decade of life and present either in the soft tissue posterior to the rectum or in the pelvis.[357] Those whose tumors are pelvic in location present with sphincter dysfunction attributable to sacral nerve involvement. The recognition of this entity has generally been attributed to Mallory in his 1902 presentation at the Harvard Medical School in Boston.[322]

Histologic examination reveals a papillary neoplasm with cells containing relatively regular nuclei without significant

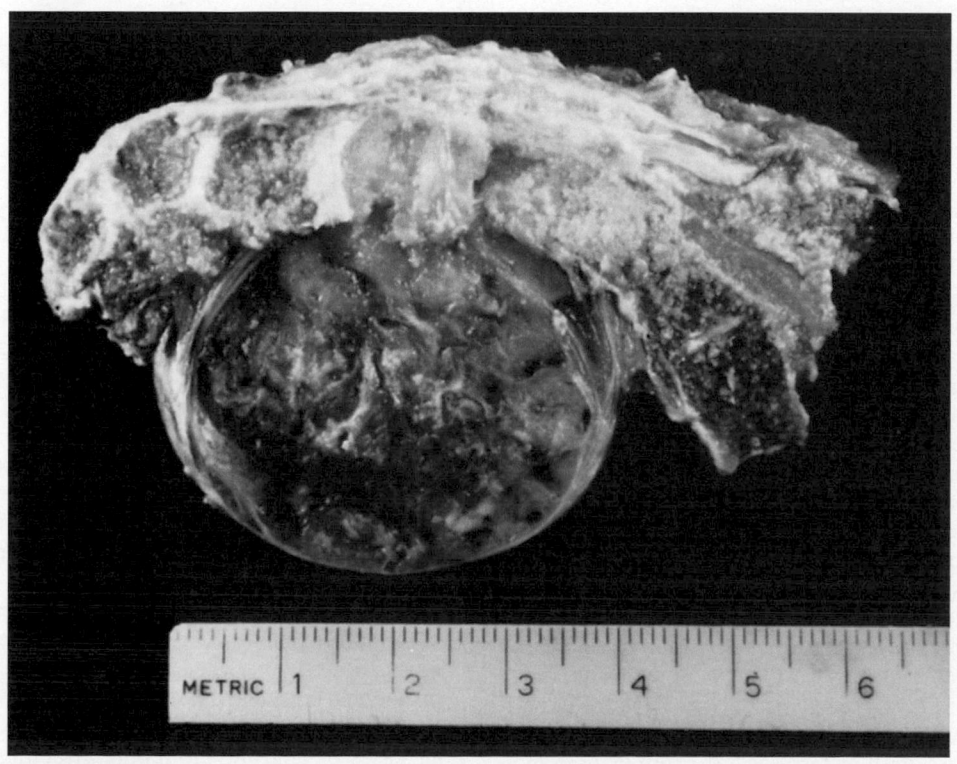

FIGURE 26-97. Sacrococcygeal chordoma. Cut section reveals the gelatinous appearance of the tumor.

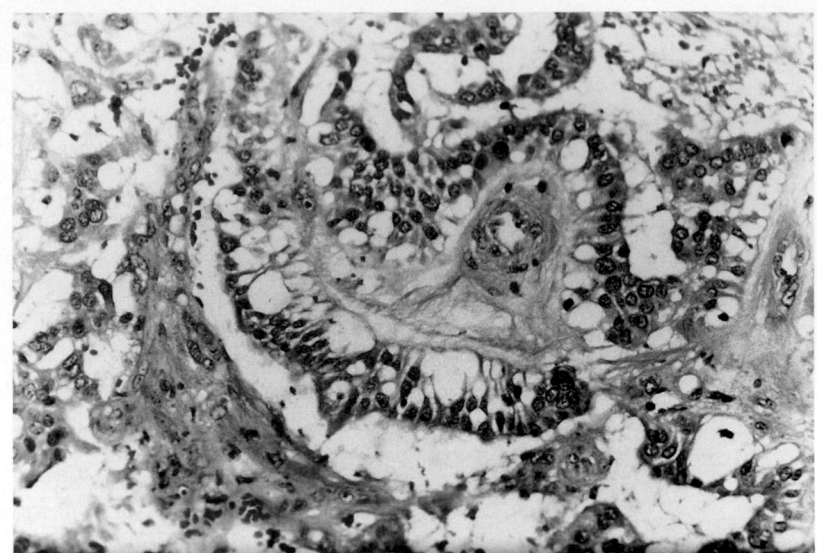

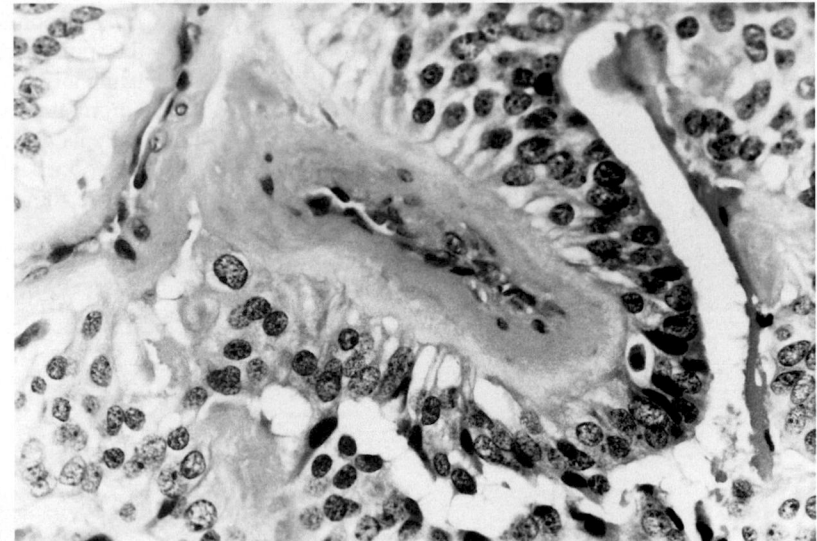

FIGURE 26-98. Malignant ependymoma. This tumor demonstrates papillary structures with fibrovascular cores lined by low epithelial cells displaying rather monotonous nuclei. Note the characteristic perivascular clearing. **A:** Original magnification × 180. **B:** Original magnification × 560. The patient subsequently developed pulmonary metastases. (Courtesy of David W. Kolegraff, MD and Peter L. Morris, MD.)

mitotic activity (Figure 26-98). Timmerman and Bubrick reviewed the literature and reported a patient with postsacral extraspinal ependymoma, the 17th such case.[508] In addition, there were 28 reports in a presacral location.[508] According to the authors, a postsacral tumor is most likely to present with an obvious mass, but in the presacral location, the signs and symptoms are similar to those of chordoma. Conventional and CT studies may reveal erosion of the sacrum, and myelography will demonstrate an extradural mass indenting the thecal sac from below.[357]

Wide excision is the preferred treatment, but as with chordoma, recurrence is common. A combined posterior and anterior approach with the goal of complete tumor removal (as is sometimes necessary with chordoma) is ideal when possible.[357] If this is not feasible, radiation therapy should be considered as palliative treatment.[15] Because of the increased incidence of systemic metastases, the average postoperative survival is approximately 10 years.[222,357,518,547] In the experience of Helwig and Stern with 23 patients, 6 were followed for at least 15 years, with metastases occurring in 4 (an incidence of 17%).[220]

Extramedullary (Extraadrenal Myelolipoma or Angiomyelolipoma)

Myelolipomas are usually found in the adrenal glands, but rarely they can be seen in other sites. These include intrathoracic, paravertebral, retroperitoneal, intracranial, and presacral locations, as well as the liver, stomach, and iliac fossa. The most frequent extraadrenal sight is the presacral area.

Symptoms include low back pain, rectal fullness, pain on sitting, and urinary symptoms. Rectal examination may reveal an anterior sacral mass. Because of the benign nature of the disease, radiologic studies do not demonstrate bony invasion (Figure 26-99).

Myelolipoma is characterized histologically by the presence of active hematopoietic elements intermixed with fat (Figure 26-100).[134,553]

Treatment consists of a standard transcoccygeal approach. One can anticipate a complete cure for this benign process. Four cases of angiomyelolipoma affecting the colon have been described.[86] Treatment is resection.

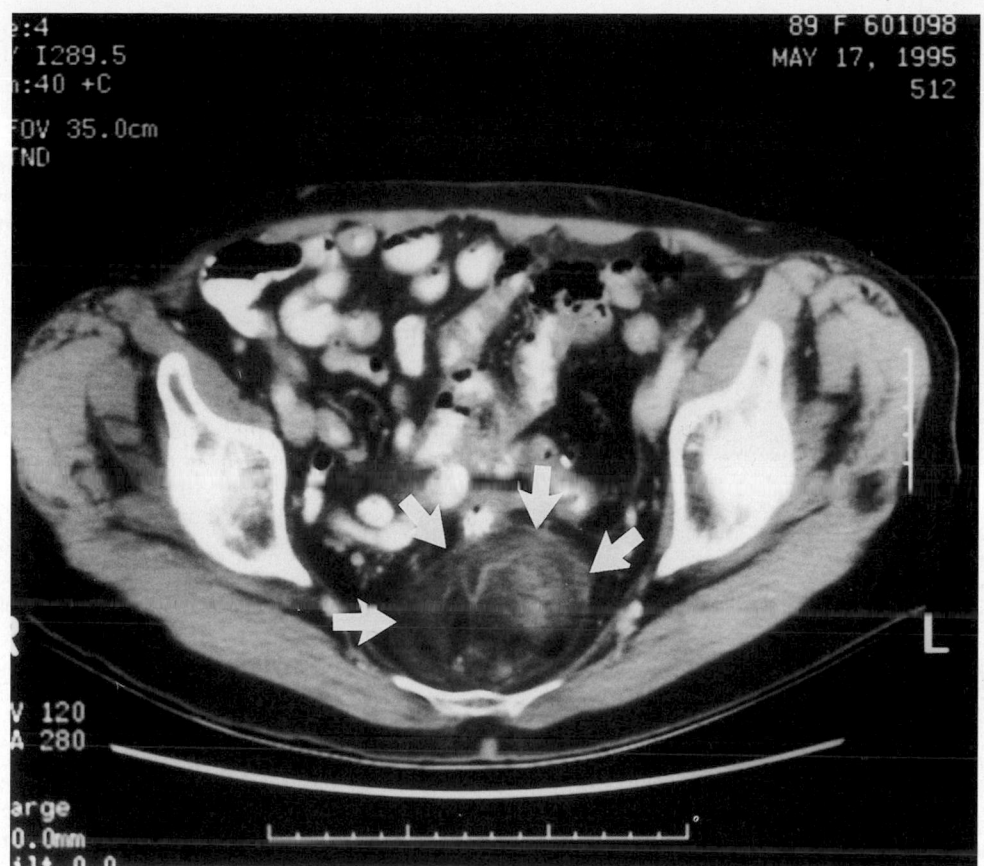

FIGURE 26-99. Extramedullary myelolipoma. Computed tomography scan demonstrates a presacral mass (*arrows*) without evident bony invasion.

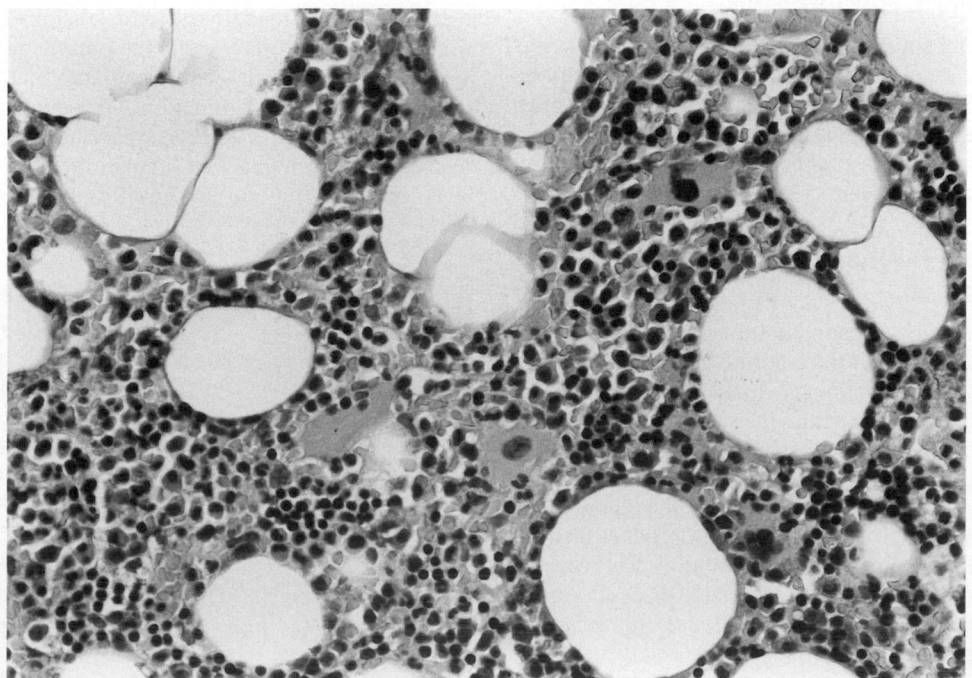

FIGURE 26-100. Extra-adrenal myelolipoma. Maturing hematopoietic elements are scattered in the background of benign adipose tissue. (Original magnification × 600.) This is the histologic specimen obtained from the patient whose computed tomography scan is demonstrated in Figure 26-103. (Courtesy of James T. Dunn, MD.)

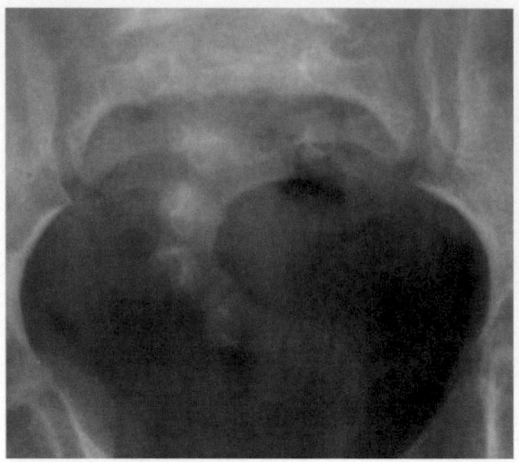

FIGURE 26-101. Anterior sacral meningocele. Radiography of the pelvis demonstrates a sacral deformity or "scimitar sign" that is pathognomonic for anterior sacral meningocele. A scimitar is an oriental sword with a curved blade broadening toward the point.

Anterior Sacral Meningocele

Anterior sacral meningocele is a congenital cystic structure that may appear as a presacral mass. Herniation of the dura through bony defects most often occurs posteriorly in the lumbar area, and if it contains neural elements, it is called a myelomeningocele. Located in the presacral space, it communicates with the dural sac through a narrow neck that passes through a much larger, smooth, sacral bony defect.[284] Radiography of the pelvis may demonstrate the characteristic "scimitar sign" (Figure 26-101).[284]

The treatment approach is via a posterior sacral laminectomy.

Extramedullary Hematopoiesis

Another retrorectal (presacral) mass that has been described in a solitary case report is asymptomatic extramedullary hematopoiesis.[443] The diagnosis was established by CT-guided biopsy, which revealed hematopoietic tissue and fatty bone marrow. The patient was treated nonoperatively, with no change in the mass at 1 year.[443]

Pneumatosis Cystoides Intestinalis or Pneumatosis Coli

Pneumatosis cystoides intestinalis (pneumatosis coli, when the condition is confined to the colon) is a relatively uncommon disease of unknown etiology. It is characterized by the presence of gas-filled cysts within the wall of portions of the GI tract. Koss reported an extensive review of the condition and noted that it most commonly occurs in the jejunum and ileum, with only 6% of cases being seen in the colon.[282] The disease is noted usually in the older population, but it can occur at any age. Its relationship with other conditions has been well documented. The most frequently associated diseases are pulmonary (e.g., chronic obstructive lung disease), but it can also be seen with peptic ulcer, pyloric stenosis, collagen disease, acute gastroenteritis, nontropical sprue, intestinal obstruction, mesenteric occlusion, ischemic colitis, inflammatory bowel disease, systemic sclerosis, carcinoma of the colon, following abdominal trauma, as a result of endoscopic maneuvers (especially colonoscopy), with steroid therapy, with exposure to organic solvents (e.g., trichloroethylene), following organ transplantation, and after surgical procedures on the bowel.[15] [3,171,174,201,232,251,278,340,345,486,551]

Etiology

The reasons for the occurrence in association with such diverse entities are unclear. One possibility is that increased intraluminal pressure may force the gas into the wall of the bowel. This may account for its association with certain primary diseases of the GI tract. However, on close inspection of the bowel in such patients, it does not appear that the integrity of the mucosa is breached.

The theory for the condition's occurring in association with chronic obstructive pulmonary disease is that a pulmonary bleb ruptures and dissects retroperitoneally along the vessels, reaching the bowel wall. In support of this postulate is the fact that segmental distribution of the blebs usually is often observed (Figure 26-102). A third theory, which may be more relevant in infants with severe gastroenteritis, speculates that gas-forming bacteria account for the formation of the cysts.[200]

Another possible implicating factor is the suggestion that the condition may result from abnormal hydrogen metabolism. Christl and colleagues measured hydrogen and methane levels in patients with pneumatosis cystoides intestinalis and found that these patients excrete more hydrogen than controls.[91] They further observed that the activity of methanogenic and sulfate-reducing bacteria is virtually absent in these individuals, possibly explaining the observed gas accumulation.

Symptoms and Findings

Many patients who harbor this condition do so without symptoms. The lesions may be noted on radiographic examination or at the time of endoscopy. When symptoms are present, they may be vague or they may include abdominal pain, diarrhea, and the passage of mucus and blood in the stool.

Physical examination is usually unrewarding. Rarely is there abdominal tenderness or distension. Digital examination of the rectum may reveal the presence of an extramucosal mass if the cysts indeed extend into that area.

Barium enema examination will usually reveal well-demarcated, lucent wall defects of varying size, usually grouped in clusters with an intact overlying mucosa (Figure 26-103).[60] The condition may be confused with inflammatory bowel

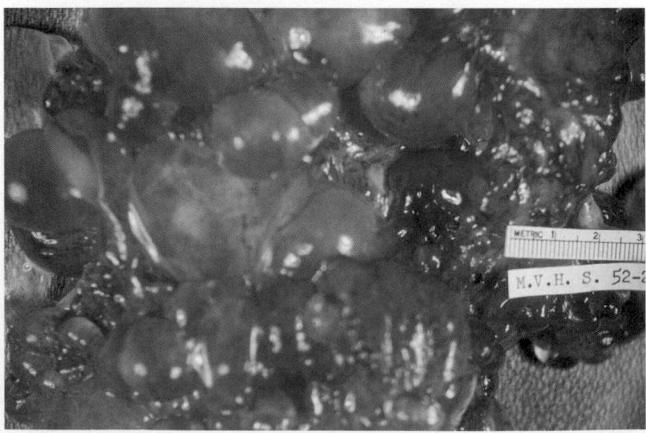

FIGURE 26-102. Pneumatosis coli. Cysts filled with gas, measuring up to 3 cm in diameter, occupy the sigmoid colon. (Courtesy of Rudolf Garret, MD.)

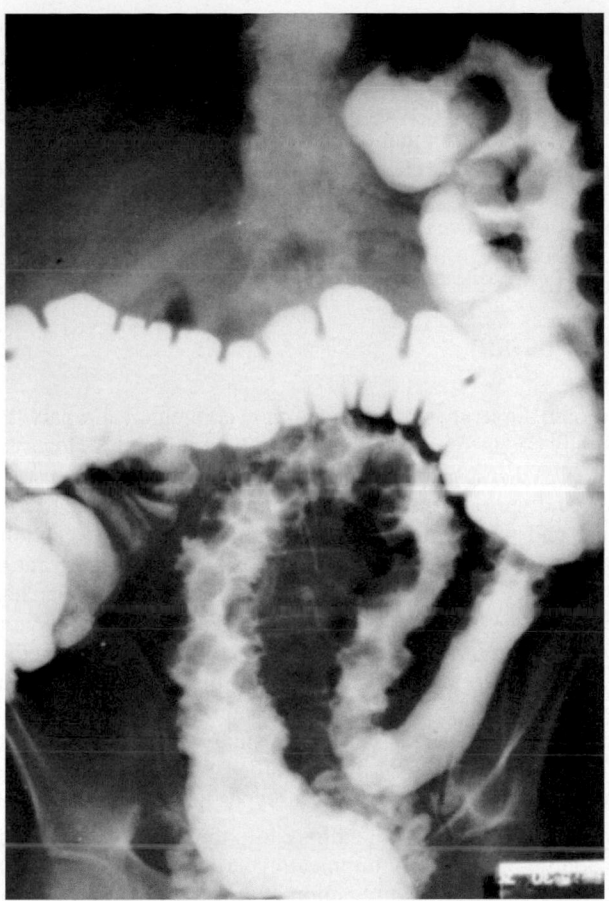

FIGURE 26-103. Pneumatosis coli. Multiple lucent cystlike defects throughout the left colon.

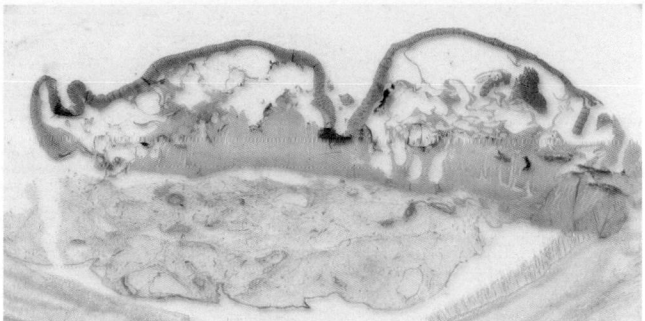

FIGURE 26-105. Pneumatosis cystoides intestinalis. Whole-mount specimen showing air-filled spaces in the submucosa of the colon. Some of the spaces are separating the bundles of the muscularis propria. (Courtesy of Rudolf Garret, MD.)

mild inflammatory infiltrate. Multinucleated giant cells are noticed frequently (Figures 26-106 and 26-107).

Treatment

It is important to recognize this entity and to differentiate it from neoplasms. Spigelman and colleagues suggested that needle deflation may be helpful if gross appearances are suggestive of cysts rather than of polyps.[476]

In 1973, Forgacs and colleagues proposed replacement of the gas (which consists mainly of nitrogen) with oxygen.[163] By administering oxygen at relatively high concentration, resorption of the gas in the cysts should occur. Although there is no consistent recommendation about its administration, most authors believe that it is necessary to reach an arterial oxygen tension in excess of 300 mm Hg to achieve the desired results. A concentration of oxygen between 55% and 75% is generally used in the inhaled gas.[349] A minimum of 48 hours of therapy is recommended for up to 5 days. Holt

disease, multiple polyposis, or carcinoma. Definitive diagnosis can be established by means of colonoscopy, with some clinicians advocating this technique for confirming the presence of the benign cysts (Figure 26-104).[121,162]

Pathology

Histologic examination of the biopsy specimen reveals normal mucosa beneath which cystic spaces are seen to be lined by endothelium (Figure 26-105).[191] There may be a

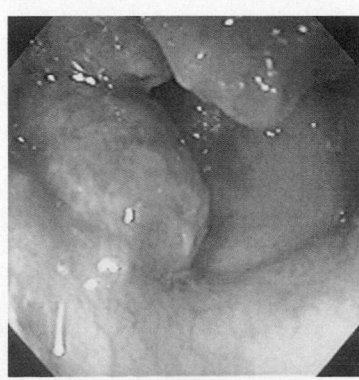

FIGURE 26-104. Pneumatosis cystoides intestinalis. Colonoscopy demonstrates cystic masses that pose a potential problem in differential diagnosis. Biopsy, however, will reveal the histologic picture consistent with this condition.

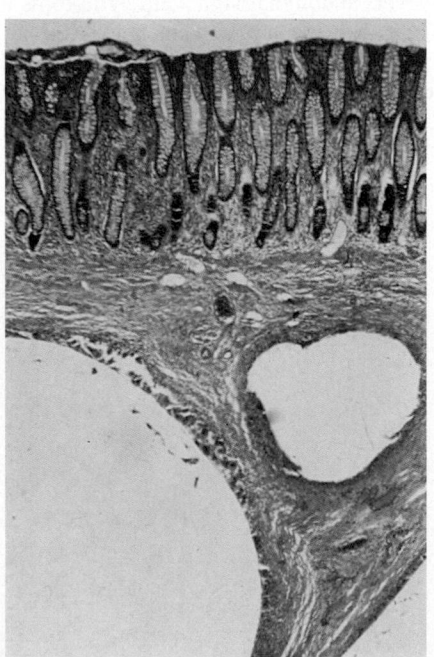

FIGURE 26-106. Pneumatosis coli. Cystic spaces occupy the submucosa. (Original magnification × 120; from Corman ML, Veidenheimer MC, Swinton NW. *Diseases of the Anus, Rectum, and Colon. Part I: Neoplasms*. New York, NY: Medcom; 1972.)

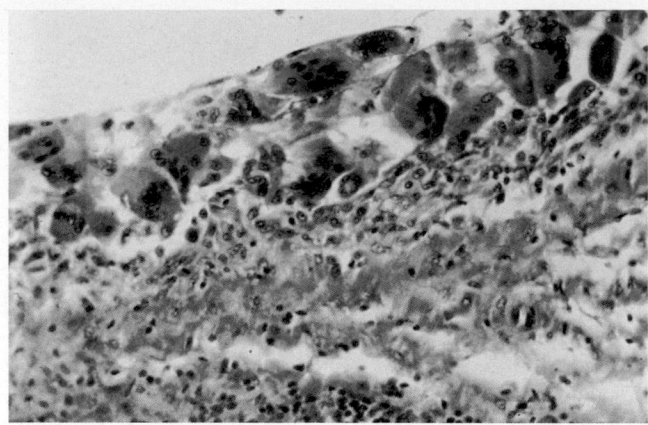

FIGURE 26-107. Pneumatosis coli. The cyst lining consists of multinucleated giant cells, which probably represent a reaction to the gaseous material trapped within the cyst. (From Corman ML, Veidenheimer MC, Swinton NW. *Diseases of the Anus, Rectum, and Colon. Part I: Neoplasms.* New York, NY: Medcom; 1972.)

and colleagues suggested a standardized regimen of intermittent high-flow oxygen therapy.[230] One must be concerned, however, about the possibility of oxygen toxicity. In these individuals, the ameliorative effect of oxygen therapy usually is apparent within 1 or 2 days. A report of successful treatment with metronidazole lends credence to the theory that anaerobic bacteria may in some manner be responsible.[246]

Surgery is usually reserved for those with symptomatic localized disease and when hemorrhage, obstruction, or perforation supervenes.[276,522] Treatment of obstruction by means of endoscopic puncture and sclerotherapy of the cyst walls has been described.[250]

Management of Pneumoperitoneum

Pneumoperitoneum can supervene in a patient with pneumatosis. However, abdominal signs and symptoms are usually minimal or absent. If the patient has been known to harbor cysts, a trial of conservative therapy is advocated. Usually, no communication with the GI tract is found to exist even at operation. Therefore, one should endeavor not to surgically treat what would usually be considered an operative condition

based on the radiographic findings alone. Expectant management will almost inevitably be followed by gradual disappearance of the free gas. If one embarks on an exploratory laparotomy for this presentation, it is probably better to close the abdomen rather than to undertake a resection. However, as implied, in the rare situation in which the disease continues to cause symptoms and the cysts are localized to a limited segment of the bowel, resection should be considered. Unusual complications, such as volvulus, intestinal obstruction, or massive bleeding, will also necessitate operative intervention.

Duplication

Colon

Colonic duplication is an uncommon congenital anomaly that usually occurs during infancy or early childhood.[44] However, occasional cases can present in the older age groups. Obstruction and the presence of an abdominal mass are usually the signs and symptoms apparent in infancy. Progressive abdominal pain, bleeding, an abdominal mass, and rarely perforation are characteristics of childhood or adult onset.[429] Diarrhea, constipation, distension, and obstruction are additional symptoms, and an intussusception may sometimes be observed.

True intestinal duplications must be distinguished from enteric cysts. Characteristics of this anomaly include intimate attachment to some part of the alimentary tract, a smooth muscle coat, and a mucosal lining similar to that of the stomach, small bowel, or colon.[44] Four subtypes have been described:

A tubular duplication branching into the mesenteric leaves
A double-barreled, communicating structure (Figure 26-108)
A free-lying, cystic duplication connected to the alimentary tract by a thin mesenteric stalk
A cystic duplication attached to the bowel by a common wall[429]

Plain abdominal x-ray films may demonstrate a soft tissue mass, evidence of small or large bowel obstruction, and the presence of a gas-filled structure with an air-fluid level on the erect film.[44] Barium enema examination may demonstrate displacement of the bowel, compression by the mass, or, in the case of a communicating lesion, an irregular double lumen.[144] The condition is not uncommonly associated with other congenital anomalies, such as malrotation, Meckel's diverticulum, lumbosacral spine deformities (e.g., double

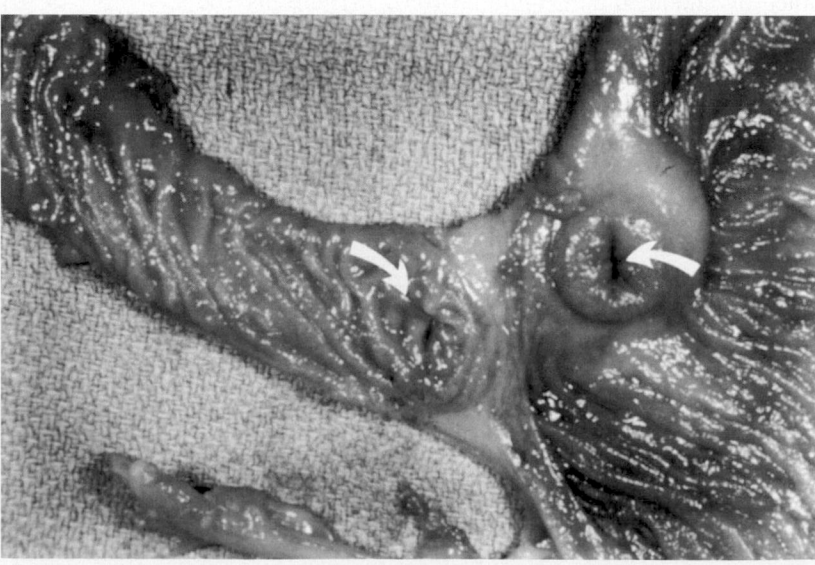

FIGURE 26-108. Colonic duplication. Note two distinct lumina (*arrows*). (Courtesy of Rudolf Garret, MD.)

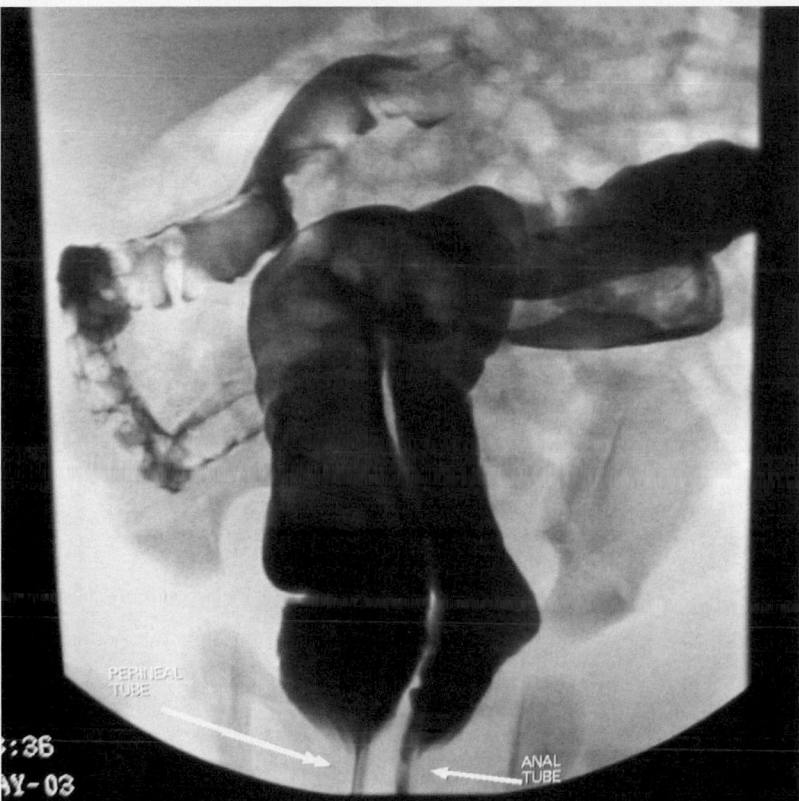

PERINEAL TUBE   **ANAL TUBE**

FIGURE 26-109. Rectal duplication. Barium study demonstrates two perineal openings communicating with two separate rectums that merge in the lower sigmoid colon. (Courtesy of Umut Sarpel, MD.)

vertebrae), and genitourinary abnormalities (double uterus, double vagina, double bladder, and double urethra).[558] CT and an intravenous pyelogram should be part of the evaluation of any individual found to harbor a colon or rectal duplication.

Treatment may involve excision of the mass with preservation of the normal colon (a communication is usually not demonstrable), although ischemia of the bowel wall and perforation are potential hazards if this approach is employed. Alternatively, an en bloc resection with anastomosis may be required when there is a double-barreled, communicating lesion.

Rectum

As suggested, all regions of the gut may be associated with a duplication, but the rectum is the least common location. Only about 70 cases have been reported.[356] It is likely that many patients remain asymptomatic, unless the situation is complicated by infection, bleeding, or malignant degeneration.[130] A painless buttock mass was described as the presenting manifestation in one report.[356] Numerous publications have addressed the issue of carcinoma arising in a rectal duplication, a finding suggesting that all such duplications should be treated by surgical excision, even if they appear benign.[130,180,535] The diagnosis can usually be made based on the examination of the rectum and confirmed on radiologic study, especially MRI, and by endosonography (Figure 26-109).[375] There is little diagnostic problem when there are two openings in the perineum or when a double-lumen appearance is noted on proctosigmoidoscopy. However, when there is no communication, the impression is that of a retrorectal mass compressing the rectum. Under these circumstances, the definitive diagnosis may not become evident until surgery.

Care must be taken to remove the duplication or cyst and still preserve integrity of the rectum, but the possibility of recurrence resulting from multiple satellites in the wall of the duplication should be recognized.[286]

References

1. Abdou NI, Napombejara C, Sagawa A, et al. Malakoplakia: evidence for monocyte lysosomal abnormality correctable by cholinergic antagonist in vitro and in vivo. *N Engl J Med*. 1977;297(26):1413–1419.
2. Abel ME, Kingsley AE, Abcarian H, et al. Anorectal neurilemomas. *Dis Colon Rectum*. 1985;28(12):960–961.
3. Abel ME, Nelson R, Prasad ML, et al. Parasacrococcygeal approach for the resection of retrorectal developmental cysts. *Dis Colon Rectum*. 1985;28(11):855–858.
4. Abrikossoff AI. Über Myome, ausgehend von der quergestreiften willkürlichen Muskalatur. *Virchows Arch Pathol Anat Physiol*. 1926;260:215–233.
5. Abrikossoff AI. Weiter Untersuchunger über Myoblast-emyome. *Virchows Arch*. 1931;280:723–740.
6. Aird I. *A Companion in Surgical Studies*. 2nd ed. Edinburgh, Scotland: E & S Livingstone; 1957.
7. Akwari OE, Dozois RR, Weiland LH, et al. Leiomyosarcoma of the small and large bowel. *Cancer*. 1978;42(3):1375–1384.
8. Albin J, Lewis E, Eftekhari F, et al. Computed tomography of rectal and perirectal disease in AIDS patients. *Gastrointest Radiol*. 1987;12(1):67–70.
9. Albrecht E. Ueber Hamartome. *Verh Dtsch Ges Pathol*. 1904;7:153–157.
10. Aldridge MC, Boylston AW, Sim AJ. Dermoid cyst of the rectum. *Dis Colon Rectum*. 1983;26(5):333–334.
11. Allen MS Jr. Hamartomatous inverted polyps of the rectum. *Cancer*. 1966;19(2):257–265.
12. Alvear DT. Localized lymphoid hyperplasia: an unusual cause of rectal bleeding. *Contemp Surg*. 1984;25:29.
13. Alvich JP, Lepow HI. Cystic lymphangioma of hepatic flexure of colon. Report of a case. *Ann Surg*. 1960;152:880–884.
14. Anderson A, Bergdahl L. Carcinoid tumors of the appendix in children. A report of 25 cases. *Acta Chir Scand*. 1977;143(3):173–175.

15. Anderson MS. Myxopapillary ependymomas presenting in the soft tissue over the sacrococcygeal region. *Cancer.* 1996;19(4):585–590.

16. Anderson PA, Dockerty MB, Buie LA. Myomatous tumors of the rectum (leiomyomas and myosarcomas). *Surgery.* 1950;28(4):642–650.

17. Andreoli F, Balloni F, Bigiotti A, et al. Anorectal continence and bladder function. Effects of major sacral resection. *Dis Colon Rectum.* 1986;29(10):647–652.

18. Angerpointner TA, Weitz H, Haas RJ, et al. Intestinal leiomyosarcoma in childhood—case report and review of the literature. *J Pediatr Surg.* 1981;16(4):491–495.

19. Anson KM, Byrne PO, Robertson ID, et al. Radical excision of sacrococcygeal tumors. *Br J Surg.* 1994;81(3):460–461.

20. Arnett NL, Friedman PS. Lymphangioma of the colon: roentgen aspects: a case report. *Radiology.* 1956;67(6):882–885.

21. Astarjian NK, Tseng CH, Keating JA, et al. Leiomyosarcoma of the colon: report of a case. *Dis Colon Rectum.* 1977;20(2):139–143.

22. Asuncion CM. Leiomyosarcoma of the rectum: report of two cases. *Dis Colon Rectum.* 1969;12(4):281–287.

23. Atlay RD, Cuschieri A. Torsion of a colonic fibroma complicating pregnancy. *Aust N Z J Obstet Gynaecol.* 1969;9(4):262–263.

24. Ault GW, Smith RS, Castro CF. Hemangiopericytoma of the sigmoid colon: case report. *Surgery.* 1951;30(3):523–527.

25. Avilés A, Neri N, Huerta-Guzmán J. Large bowel lymphoma: an analysis of prognostic factors and therapy in 53 patients. *J Surg Oncol.* 2002;80(2):111–115.

26. Aylward CA, Orangio GR, Lucas GW, et al. Diffuse cavernous hemangioma of the rectosigmoid—CT scan, a new diagnostic modality, and surgical management using sphincter-saving procedures. Report of three cases. *Dis Colon Rectum.* 1988;31(10):797–802.

27. Aymard B, Bigard MA, Thompson H, et al. Perianal ulcer: an unusual presentation of Wegener's granulomatosis. Report of a case. *Dis Colon Rectum.* 1990;33(5):427–430.

28. Azizkhan RG, Tegtmeyer CJ, Wanebo HJ. Malignant rectal carcinoid: a sequential multidisciplinary approach for successful treatment of hepatic metastases. *Am J Surg.* 1985;149(2):210–214.

29. Azzarelli A, Quagliuolo V, Cerasoli S, et al. Chordoma: natural history and treatment results in 33 cases. *J Surg Oncol.* 1988;37(3):185–191.

30. Bacon HE. *Cancer of the Colon, Rectum and Anal Canal.* Philadelphia, PA: JB Lippincott; 1964.

31. Bacon PA, Tribe CR, Harrison P, et al. Rheumatoid disease, amyloidosis, and its treatment with penicillamine [abstract]. *Arthritis Rheum.* 1981;44:454.

32. Bader TR, Semelka RC, Chiu VC, et al. MRI of carcinoid tumors: spectrum of appearances in the gastrointestinal tract and liver. *J Magn Reson Imaging.* 2001;14(3):261–269.

33. Bailey HR, Ott MT, Hartendorp P. Aggressive surgical management for advanced colorectal endometriosis. *Dis Colon Rectum.* 1994;37(8):747–753.

34. Bailey JJ, Barrick CW, Jenkinson EL. Hemangioma of the colon. *J Am Med Assoc.* 1956;160(8):658–659.

35. Baker HL Jr, Good CA. Smoothmuscle tumors of the alimentary tract: their roentgen manifestations. *Am J Roentgenol Radium Ther Nucl Med.* 1955;74(2):246–255.

36. Balfour TW. Does squamous carcinoma of the colon exist? *Br J Surg.* 1972;59(5):410–412.

37. Ballantyne EN. Sacrococcygeal tumors: adenocarcinoma of a cystic congenital embryonal remnant. *Arch Pathol.* 1932;14:1–9.

38. Ballantyne GH, Savoca PE, Flannery JT, et al. Incidence and mortality of carcinoids of the colon. Data from the Connecticut Tumor Registry. *Cancer.* 1992;69(10):2400–2405.

39. Baratz M, Ostrzega N, Michowitz M, et al. Primary inflammatory malignant fibrous histiocytoma of the colon. *Dis Colon Rectum.* 1986;29(7):462–465.

40. Barbieri RL. New therapy for endometriosis. *N Engl J Med.* 1988;318(8):512–514.

41. Barcia PJ, Washburn ME. Colitis cystica profunda: an unusual surgical problem. *Am Surg.* 1979;45(1):61–66.

42. Bar-Meir S, Halla A, Baratz M. Endoscopic removal of colonic lipoma. *Endoscopy.* 1981;13(3):135–136.

43. Barton AD, Inglis K. Neurofibromatosis with both cutaneous and visceral lesions. *J Coll Surg Australas.* 1931;3:397.

44. Bass EM. Duplication of the colon. In: Greenbaum EI, ed. *Radiographic Atlas of Colon Disease.* Chicago, IL: Year Book Medical; 1980:153.

45. Bassler A, Peter AG. Fibrosarcoma, an unusual complication of ulcerative colitis: report of a case. *Arch Surg.* 1949;59(2):227–231.

46. Basson MD, Ahlman H, Wangberg B, et al. Biology and management of the midgut carcinoid. *Am J Surg.* 1993;165(2):288–297.

47. Bates HR Jr. Carcinoid tumors of the rectum. *Dis Colon Rectum.* 1962;5:270–280.

48. Beatty GL, Keeling WM. Lymphoid polyps of the rectum; report of three cases in siblings. *AMA Arch Surg.* 1956;73(5):753–756.

49. Beaugié JM, Mann CV, Butler EC. Sacrococcygeal chordoma. *Br J Surg.* 1969;56(8):586–588.

50. Beral V, Peterman TA, Berkelman RL, et al. Kaposi's sarcoma among persons with AIDS: a sexually transmitted infection? *Lancet.* 1990;335(8682):123–128.

51. Berardi RS. Carcinoid tumors of the colon (exclusive of the rectum): review of the literature. *Dis Colon Rectum.* 1972;15(5):383–391.

52. Berardi RS, Chen HP, Lee SS. Squamous cell carcinoma of the colon and rectum. *Surg Gynecol Obstet.* 1986;163(5):493–496.

53. Berg J, McNeer G. Leiomyosarcoma of the stomach: a clinical and pathological study. *Cancer.* 1960;13:25–33.

54. Bernick PE, Klimstra DS, Shia J, et al. Neuroendocrine carcinomas of the colon and rectum. *Dis Colon Rectum.* 2004;47(2):163–169.

55. Bhargava KS, Lahiri B, Gupta RC, et al. Leiomyosarcoma of the rectum. *J Indian Med Assoc.* 1964;42:228–230.

56. Bibro MC, Houlihan RK, Sheahan DG. Colonic ganglioneuroma. *Arch Surg.* 1980;115(1):75–77.

57. Biggs VA, Crowe SM, Lucas CR, et al. AIDS-related Kaposi's sarcoma presenting as ulcerative colitis and complicated by toxic megacolon. *Gut.* 1987;28(10):1302–1306.

58. Black WC III. Enterochromaffin cell types and corresponding carcinoid tumors. *Lab Invest.* 1968;19(5):473–486.

59. Blair Bell W. Endometrioma and endometriomyoma of the ovary. *J Obstet Gynaecol Br Emp.* 1922;29(3):443–446.

60. Bloch C. The natural history of pneumatosis coli. *Radiology.* 1977;123(2):311–314.

61. Blum A, Sohar E. The diagnosis of amyloidosis. Ancillary procedures. *Lancet.* 1962;1(7232):721–724.

62. Bluth I. Gastrointestinal carcinoid tumors: roentgen features. *Radiology.* 1960;74:573–580.

63. Botting AJ, Soule EH, Brown AL Jr. Smooth muscle tumors in children. *Cancer.* 1965;18:711–720.

64. Bowen KA, Silva SR, Johnson JN, et al. An analysis of trends and growth factor receptor expression of GI carcinoid tumors. *J Gastrointest Surg.* 2009;13(10):1773–1780.

65. Box JC, Watne AL, Lucas GW. Small bowel carcinoid: review of a single institution experience and review of the literature. *Am Surg.* 1996;62(4):280–286.

66. Braasch JW, Denbo HE. Tumors of the small intestine. *Surg Clin North Am.* 1964;44:791–809.

67. Brodey PA, Hoover HC. Polypoid ganglioneurofibromatosis of the colon. *Br J Radiol.* 1974;47(560):494–495.

68. Burgess PA, Lupton EW, Talbot IC. Squamous-cell carcinoma of the proximal colon: report of a case and review of the literature. *Dis Colon Rectum.* 1979;22(4):241–244.

69. Burke M, Shepherd N, Mann CV. Carcinoid tumours of the anus and rectum. *Br J Surg.* 1987;74(5):358–361.

70. Byrne WJ, Jiminez JF, Euler AR, et al. Lymphoid polyps (focal lymphoid hyperplasia) of the colon in children. *Pediatrics.* 1982;69(5):598–600.

71. Cagir B, Nagy MW, Topham A, et al. Adenosquamous carcinoma of the colon, rectum and anus: epidemiology, distribution, and survival characteristics. *Dis Colon Rectum.* 1999;42(2):258–263.

72. Caldarola VT, Jackman RJ, Moertel CG, et al. Carcinoid tumors of the rectum. *Am J Surg.* 1964;107:844–849.

73. Calem SH, Keller RJ. Leiomyosarcoma of the sigmoid colon. *Mt Sinai J Med.* 1973;40(6):818–824.

74. Capell MS, Friedman D, Mikhail N. Endometriosis of the terminal ileum simulating the clinical roentgenographic, and surgical findings in Crohn's disease. *Am J Gastroenterol.* 1991;86(8):1057–1062.

75. Carlei F, Pietroletti R, Lomanto D, et al. Heterotopic gastric mucosa of the rectum—characterization of endocrine and mucin-producing cells by immunochemistry and lectin histochemistry. Report of a case. *Dis Colon Rectum.* 1989;32(2):159–164.

76. Castro EB, Stearns MW. Lipoma of the large intestine: a review of 45 cases. *Dis Colon Rectum.* 1972;15(6):441–444.

77. Catalano MF, Levin B, Hart RS, et al. Granulocytic sarcoma of the colon. *Gastroenterology.* 1991;100(2):555–559.

78. Cebrian J, Larach SW, Ferrara A, et al. Small-cell carcinoma of the rectum: report of two cases. *Dis Colon Rectum.* 1999;42(2):274–277.

79. Cerezo L, Alvarez M, Edwards O, et al. Adenosquamous carcinoma of the colon. *Dis Colon Rectum.* 1985;28(8):597–603.

80. Chaimoff C, Lurie H. Hemangioma of the rectum: clinical appearance and treatment. *Dis Colon Rectum.* 1978;21(4):295–296.

81. Chambers PW, Schwinn CP. Chordoma. A clinicopathologic study of metastasis. *Am J Clin Pathol.* 1979;72(5):765–776.

82. Chandawarkar RY. Sacrococcygeal chordoma: review of 50 consecutive patients. *World J Surg.* 1996;20(6):717–719.

83. Chaudhry AP, Saigal KP, Intengan M, et al. Malakoplakia of the large intestine found incidentally at necropsy: light and electron microscopic features. *Dis Colon Rectum.* 1979;22(2):73–81.

84. Cheek RC, Wilson H. Carcinoid tumors. *Curr Probl Surg.* 1970:4–31.

85. Chen CW, Jao SW, Wu CC, et al. Massive lower gastrointestinal hemorrhage caused by a large extraluminal leiomyoma of the colon: report of a case. *Dis Colon Rectum.* 2008;51(6):975–978.

86. Chen JS, Kuo LJ, Lin PY, et al. Angiomyolipoma of the colon: report of a case and review of the literature. *Dis Colon Rectum.* 2003;46(4): 547–549.

87. Cheng JY, Lin JC, Yu DS, et al. Flow cytometric DNA analysis of colorectal carcinoid. *Am J Surg.* 1994;168(1):29–32.

88. Chevinsky AH, Berelowitz M, Hoover HC Jr. Adenosquamous carcinoma of the colon presenting with hypercalcemia. *Cancer.* 1987;60(5):1111–1116.

89. Chisholm AJ, Hillkowitz P. Lymphangioma of the rectum. *Am J Surg.* 1932;17:281–282.

90. Cho KC, Smith TR. Multiple leiomyosarcoma of the transverse colon: report of a case and discussion. *Dis Colon Rectum.* 1980;23(2):118–121.

91. Christl SU, Gibson GR, Murgatroyd PR, et al. Impaired hydrogen metabolism in pneumatosis cystoides intestinalis. *Gastroenterology.* 1993;104(2):392–397.

92. Chulia F, Camps C, Rodriguez A, et al. Epidermoid carcinoma of the colon. Description of a lesion located in the hepatic flexure. *Dis Colon Rectum.* 1986;29(10):665–667.

93. Clery AP, Dockerty MB, Waugh JM. Small cell carcinoma of the colon and rectum. A clinicopathologic study. *Arch Surg.* 1961;83:164–172.

94. Cobb CF. Endometriosis in the general surgery patient. *Surg Rounds.* 1985;8:66.

95. Cohen MG, Greenwald ML, Garbus JE, et al. Granular cell tumor—a unique neoplasm of the internal anal sphincter: report of a case. *Dis Colon Rectum.* 2000;43(10):1444–1446.

96. Cohnheim J. Ein Fall von Pseudoleukämie. *Virchows Arch.* 1865; 33:451.

97. Colberg JE. Granular cell myoblastoma. *Surg Gynecol Obstet.* 1962; 115:205.

98. Collins JO, Falk M, Guibone R. Benign lymphoid polyposis of the colon. A case report. *Pediatrics.* 1966;38(5):897–899.

99. Comer TP, Beahrs OH, Dockerty MB. Primary squamous cell carcinoma and adenoacanthoma of the colon. *Cancer.* 1971;28(5):1111–1117.

100. Cone LA, Woodard DR, Potts BE, et al. An update on the acquired immunodeficiency syndrome (AIDS). Associated disorders of the alimentary tract. *Dis Colon Rectum.* 1986;29(1):60–64.

101. Connolly EM, Gaffney E, Reynolds JV, et al. Gastrointestinal stromal tumours. *Br J Surg.* 2003;90(10):1178–1186.

102. Contreary K, Nance FC, Becker WF. Primary lymphoma of the gastrointestinal tract. *Ann Surg.* 1980;191(5):593–598.

103. Coppa GF, Localio SA. Surgical management of diffuse cavernous hemangioma of the colon, rectum and anus. *Surg Gynecol Obstet.* 1984;159(1):17–22.

104. Corman ML, Haggitt RC. Lymphangioma of the rectum: report of a case. *Dis Colon Rectum.* 1973;16(6):524–529.

105. Corman ML, Veidenheimer MC, Swinton NW. *Diseases of the Anus, Rectum, and Colon. Part I: Neoplasms.* New York, NY: Medcom; 1972.

106. Cornes JS. Multiple lymphomatous polyposis of the gastrointestinal tract. *Cancer.* 1961;14:249–257.

107. Cornes JS, Wallace MH, Morson BC. Benign lymphomas of the rectum and anal canal: a study of 100 cases. *J Pathol Bacteriol.* 1961;82: 371–382.

108. Cosens CG. Gastro-intestinal pseudoleukemia: a case report. *Ann Surg.* 1958;148(1):129–133.

109. Cronkhite LW Jr, Canada WJ. Generalized gastrointestinal polyposis: unusual syndrome of polyposis, pigmentation, alopecia and onychotropia. *N Engl J Med.* 1955;252(24):1011–1015.

110. Croom RD III, Donovan ML, Schwesinger WH. Intestinal endometriosis. *Am J Surg.* 1984;148(5):660–667.

111. Crowley LV, Page HG. Adenocarcinoma arising in presacral enterogenous cyst. *Arch Pathol.* 1960;69:64–66.

112. Cunningham JA, Garcia VF, Quispe G. Diffuse cavernous rectal hemangioma—sphincter-sparing approach to therapy: report of a case. *Dis Colon Rectum.* 1989;32(4):344–347.

113. Currarino G, Coln D, Votteler T. Triad of anorectal, sacral, and presacral anomalies. *AJR Am J Roentgenol.* 1981;137(2):395–398.

114. Dahan H, Arrivé L, Wendum D, et al. Retrorectal developmental cysts in adults: clinical and radiologic-histopathologic review, differential diagnosis, and treatment. *Radiographics.* 2001;21(3):575–584.

115. Dahlin DC, MacCarty CS. Chordoma. A study of fifty-nine cases. *Cancer.* 1952;5:1170–1178.

116. De Beer RA, Shinya H. Colonic lipomas. An endoscopic analysis. *Gastrointest Endosc.* 1975;22(2):90–91.

117. DeMatteo RP, Lewis JJ, Leung D, et al. Two hundred gastrointestinal stromal tumors: recurrence patterns and prognostic factors for survival. *Ann Surg.* 2000;231(1):51–58.

118. De Nardi P, Osman N, Ferrai S, et al. Laparoscopic treatment of deep pelvic endometriosis with rectal involvement. *Dis Colon Rectum.* 2009;52(3):419–424.

119. de Roo T. Leiomyosarcoma of the colon, a rare tumor. Three case reports and review. *Radiol Clin Biol.* 1974;43(2):187–195.

120. de Roo T, Vaas F. Leiomyosarcoma of the transverse and descending colon. Two case reports and review. *Am J Gastroenterol.* 1969;52(2): 150–156.

121. Desbaillets LG, Mangla JC. Pneumatosis cystoides intestinalis diagnosed by colonoscopy. *Gastrointest Endosc.* 1974;20(3):120–122.

122. Devine RM, Beart RW Jr, Wolff BG. Malignant lymphoma of the rectum. *Dis Colon Rectum.* 1986;29(12):821–824.

123. Diamante M, Bacon HE. Leiomyosarcoma of the rectum: report of a case. *Dis Colon Rectum.* 1967;10(5):347–351.

124. Dinges HP, Werner R, Watzek G. The incidence and significance of amyloid deposits in gingival, buccal and rectal mucous membranes [in German]. *Wien Klin Wochenschr.* 1978;90(12):431–435.

125. Doak PB, Montgomerie JZ, North JD, et al. Reticulum cell sarcoma after renal homotransplantation and azathioprine and prednisone therapy. *Br Med J.* 1968;4(5633):746–748.

126. Dodd GD, Rutledge R, Wallace S. Postoperative pelvic lymphocysts. *AJR Am J Roentgenol Radium Ther Nucl Med.* 1970;108(2):312–323.

127. Doniec JM, Kahlke V, Peetz F, et al. Rectal endometriosis: high sensitivity and specificity of endorectal ultrasound with an impact for the operative management. *Dis Colon Rectum.* 2003;46(12):1667–1673.

128. Donnelly WH, Sieber WK, Yumis EJ. Polypoid ganglioneurofibromatosis of the large bowel. *Arch Pathol.* 1969;87(5):537–541.

129. Dougherty LS, Hull T. Perineal endometriosis with anal sphincter involvement: report of a case. *Dis Colon Rectum.* 2000;43(8): 1157–1160.

130. Downing R, Thompson H, Alexander-Williams J. Adenocarcinoma arising in a duplication of the rectum. *Br J Surg.* 1978;65(8):572–574.

131. Dozois EJ, Malireddy KK, Bower TC, et al. Management of a retrorectal lipomatous hemangiopericytoma by preoperative vascular embolization and a multidisciplinary surgical team: report of a case. *Dis Colon Rectum.* 2009;52(5):1017–1020.

132. Dudley GS. Visceral neurofibroma. *Surg Clin North Am.* 1930;10: 539–542.

133. Dukes C, Bussey HJR. The number of lymphoid follicles of the human large intestine. *J Pathol Bacteriol.* 1926;29(1):111–116.

134. Dusenbery D. Extra-adrenal myelolipoma. Intraoperative cytodiagnosis on touch preparations. *Acta Cytol.* 1990;34(1):89–91.

135. Dzioba H, Kabza R. Naczyniaki jelita grubego. *Pol Tyg Lek.* 1965;20:147–148.

136. Edelstein PS, Wong WD, La Valleur J, et al. Carcinoid tumor: an extremely unusual presacral lesion. Report of a case. *Dis Colon Rectum.* 1996;39(8):938–942.

137. Edgerton MT. The treatment of hemangiomas: with special reference to the role of steroid therapy. *Ann Surg.* 1976;183(5):517–532.

138. Eichel BS, Hallberg OE. Hamartoma of the middle ear and eustachian tube. Report of a case. *Laryngoscope.* 1966;76(11):1810–1815.

139. Eitan N, Auslander L, Cohen Y. Leiomyosarcoma of the rectum: report of three cases. *Dis Colon Rectum.* 1978;21(6):444–446.

140. Ell C, Matek W, Gramatzki M, et al. Endoscopic findings in a case of Kaposi's sarcoma with involvement of the large and small bowel. *Endoscopy.* 1985;17(4):161–164.

141. el-Mouzan MI, Satti MB, al-Quorain AA, et al. Colonic malacoplakia—occurrence in a family. Report of cases. *Dis Colon Rectum.* 1988;31(5):390–393.

142. Endean ED, Ross CW, Strodel WE. Kaposi's sarcoma appearing as a rectal ulcer. *Surgery.* 1987;101(6):767–769.

143. Epstein SE, Ascari WQ, Ablow RC, et al. Colitis cystica profunda. *Am J Clin Pathol.* 1966;45(2):186–201.

144. Espalieu P, Balique JG, Cuilleret J. Tubular colonic duplications. A case report and literature review. *Anat Clin.* 1985;7(2):125–130.

145. Espinosa MH, Quan SH. Anal fibrosarcoma: report of a case and review of literature. *Dis Colon Rectum.* 1975;18(6):522–527.

146. Evans N. Malignant myomas and related tumors of the uterus. (Report of seventy-two cases occurring in a series of 4000 operations for uterine fibromyomas.) *Coll Papers Mayo Clin.* 1919;11:349.

147. Ewing J. *Neoplastic Diseases: A Treatise on Tumors.* 4th ed. Philadelphia, PA: WB Saunders; 1940.

148. Fahey JL. Cancer in the immunosuppressed patient. *Ann Intern Med.* 1971;75(2):310–312.

149. Fan CW, Changchien CR, Wang JY, et al. Primary colorectal lymphoma. *Dis Colon Rectum.* 2000;43(9):1277–1282.

150. Fayemi AO, Toker C. Gastrointestinal fibroma. A clinicopathological study. *Am J Gastroenterol.* 1974;62(3):250–254.

151. Feldtman RW, Oram-Smith JC, Teears RJ, et al. Leiomyosarcoma of the rectum: the military experience. *Dis Colon Rectum.* 1981;24(5):402–403.

152. Ferguson EF Jr, Houston CH. Benign and malignant tumors of the colon and rectum. *South Med J.* 1972;65(10):1213–1220.

153. Fernandes C, Bungay P, O'Driscoll BR, et al. Mixed connective tissue disease presenting with pneumonitis and pneumatosis intestinalis. *Arthritis Rheum.* 2000;43(3):704–707.

154. Ferrarese R. Fibroma semplice del mesentere in sede ileocecale. *Arch Ostet Ginecol.* 1968;73(1):94–103.

155. Ferraresi V, Nuzzo C, Zoccali C, et al. Chordoma: clinical characteristics, management and prognosis of a case series of 25 patients. *BMC Cancer.* 2010;10:22.

156. Figliolini FJ, Cutait DE, de Oliveria MR, et al. Rectosigmoidal hemangioma: report of two cases. *Dis Colon Rectum.* 1961;4:349–355.

157. Fisher ER, Wechsler H. Granular cell myoblastoma—a misnomer. Electron microscopic and histochemical evidence concerning its Schwann cell derivation and nature (granular cell schwannoma). *Cancer.* 1962;15:936–954.

158. Fleming MP, Carlson HC. Submucosal lymphatic cysts of the gastrointestinal tract: a rare cause of submucosal mass lesion. *AJR Am J Roentgenol Radium Ther Nucl Med.* 1970;110(4):842–845.

159. Fletcher CD, Berman JJ, Corless C, et al. Diagnosis of gastrointestinal stromal tumors: a consensus approach. *Hum Pathol.* 2002;33(5):459–465.

160. Fontaine R, Suhler A, Babin S, et al. A propos de deux nouveaux cas de leiomyosarcome du rectum: revue de la littérature. *Ann Chir.* 1965;19:1353.

161. Foo M, Chao MW, Gibbs P, et al. Successful treatment of mucosa-associated lymphoid tissue lymphoma of the rectum with radiation therapy: report of a case. *Dis Colon Rectum.* 2008;51(11):1719–1723.

162. Forde KA, Whitlock RT, Seaman WB. Pneumatosis and cystoides intestinalis. Report of a case and colonoscopic findings of inflammatory bowel disease. *Am J Gastroenterol.* 1977;68(2):188–190.

163. Forgacs P, Wright PH, Wyatt AP. Treatment of intestinal gas cysts by oxygen breathing. *Lancet.* 1973;1(7803):579–582.

164. Frager DH, Frager JD, Brandt LJ, et al. Gastrointestinal complications of AIDS: radiologic features. *Radiology.* 1986;158(3):597–603.

165. Franken EA Jr. Lymphoid hyperplasia of the colon. *Radiology.* 1970;94(2):329–334.

166. Freeman FJ. Lymphoid hyperplasia and gastrointestinal bleeding in children. *Guthrie Clin Bull.* 1964;33:175–179.

167. Frick EJ Jr, Lapos L, Vargas HD. Solitary neurofibroma of the anal canal: report of two cases. *Dis Colon Rectum.* 2000;43(1):109–112.

168. Frizelle FA, Hobday KS, Batts KP, et al. Adenosquamous and squamous carcinoma of the colon and upper rectum: a clinical and histopathologic study. *Dis Colon Rectum.* 2001;44(3):341–346.

169. Gabriel WB. *The Principles and Practice of Rectal Surgery.* 5th ed. Springfield, IL: Charles C. Thomas; 1963.

170. Gafni J, Sohar E. Rectal biopsy for the diagnosis of amyloidosis. *Am J Med Sci.* 1960;240:332–336.

171. Galanduik S, Fazio VW. Pneumatosis cystoides intestinalis. A review of the literature. *Dis Colon Rectum.* 1986;29(5):358–363.

172. Galletly A. Presacral tumours of congenital origin. *Proc R Soc Med.* 1924;17(Obstet Gynaecol Sect):105–122.

173. Garcha IS, Perloe M, Strawn EY, et al. Laparoscopic resection of sigmoid endometrioma. *Am Surg.* 1996;62(4):274–275.

174. Gefter WB, Evers KA, Malet PF, et al. Nontropical sprue with pneumatosis coli. *AJR Am J Roentgenol.* 1981;137(3):624–625.

175. Gelas T, Peyrat P, Francois Y, et al. Primary squamous-cell carcinoma of the rectum: report of six cases and review of the literature. *Dis Colon Rectum.* 2002;45(11):1535–1540.

176. Genter B, Mir R, Strauss R, et al. Hemangiopericytoma of the colon: report of a case and review of literature. *Dis Colon Rectum.* 1982;25(2):149–156.

177. Gentil F, Coley BL. Sacrococcygeal chordoma. *Ann Surg.* 1948;127(3):432–455.

178. Gentry RW, Dockerty MB, Clagett OT. Vascular malformations and vascular tumors of the gastrointestinal tract [abstract]. *Surg Gynecol Obstet.* 1949;88(4):281–323.

179. Ghrist TD. Gastrointestinal involvement in neurofibromatosis. *Arch Intern Med.* 1963;112:357–362.

180. Gibson TC, Edwards JM, Shafiq S. Carcinoma arising in a rectal duplication cyst. *Br J Surg.* 1986;73(5):377.

181. Girdwood TG, Philip LD. Lymphatic cysts of the colon. *Gut.* 1971;12(11):933–935.

182. Gius JA, Stout P. Perianal cysts of vestigial origin. *Arch Surg.* 1938;37:268–287.

183. Gleason TH, Hammar SP. Plasmacytoma of the colon: case report with lambda light chain, demonstrated by immunoperoxidase studies. *Cancer.* 1982;50(1):130–133.

184. Godard JE, Dodds WF, Phillips JC, et al. Peutz-Jeghers syndrome: clinical and roentgenographic features. *AJR Am J Roentgenol Radium Ther Nucl Med.* 1971;113(2):316–324.

185. Gold JS, Dematteo RP. Combined surgical and molecular therapy: the gastrointestinal stromal tumor model. *Ann Surg.* 2006;244(2):176–184.

186. Gold JS, Gonen M, Gutierrez A, et al. Development and validation of a prognostic nomogram for recurrence-free survival after complete surgical resection of localised primary gastrointestinal tumour: a retrospective analysis. *Lancet Oncol.* 2009;10(11):1045–1052.

187. Golden T, Stout AP. Smooth muscle tumors of the gastrointestinal tract and retroperitoneal tissues. *Surg Gynecol Obstet.* 1941;73:784–810.

188. Goldlust D, Chalut J, Rault JJ, et al. L'hémangiomatose rectosigmoidienne. *J Radiol Electrol Med Nucl.* 1971;52(1):108–111.

189. Goldstein WB, Poker N. Multiple myeloma involving the gastrointestinal tract. *Gastroenterology.* 1966;51(1):87–93.

190. González Sánchez JA, Martin Molinero R, Dominguez Sayans J, et al. Colonic perforation by amyloidosis. Report of a case. *Dis Colon Rectum.* 1989;32(5):437–440.

191. Goodall RJR. Pneumatosis coli: report of two cases. *Dis Colon Rectum.* 1978;21(1):61–65.

192. Gouzi JL, Laigneau P, Delalande JP, et al. Indications for right hemicolectomy in carcinoid tumors of the appendix. The French Associations for Surgical Research. *Surg Gynecol Obstet.* 1993;176(6):543–547.

193. Granet E. Simple lymphoma of the sphincteric rectum in identical twins. *J Am Med Assoc.* 1949;141(14):990.

194. Green JB, Timmcke AE, Mitchell WT Jr. Endoscopic resection of primary rectal teratoma. *Am Surg.* 1993;59(4):270–272.

195. Greenblatt RB, Dmowski WP, Mahesh VB, et al. Clinical studies with an antigonadotropin-Danazol. *Fertil Steril.* 1971;22(2):102–112.

196. Greene EI, Kirshen MM, Greene JM. Lymphangioma of the transverse colon. *Am J Surg.* 1962;103:723–726.

197. Grill J, Kuzma JF. Recklinghausen's disease with unusual symptoms from intestinal neurofibroma. *Arch Pathol.* 1942;34:902.

198. Grotz RL, Macaulay WP. Colitis cystica profunda. *Contemp Surg.* 1989;35:57.

199. Gruenberg J, Mackman S. Multiple lymphoid polyps in familial polyposis. *Ann Surg.* 1972;175(4):552–554.

200. Gruenberg JC, Batra SK, Priest RJ. Treatment of pneumatosis cystoides intestinalis with oxygen. *Arch Surg.* 1977;112(1):62–64.

201. Gruenberg JC, Grodsinksy C, Ponka JL. Pneumatosis intestinalis: a clinical classification. *Dis Colon Rectum.* 1979;22(1):5–9.

202. Gruenwald P. Abnormal accumulation of lymph follicles in the digestive tract. *Am J Med Sci.* 1942;203:823–829.

203. Guest CB, Reznick RK. Colitis cystica profunda. Review of the literature. *Dis Colon Rectum.* 1989;32(11):983–988.

204. Gunning JE, Moyer D. The effect of medroxyprogesterone acetate on endometriosis in the human female. *Fertil Steril.* 1967;18(6):759–774.

205. Guy PJ, Hall M. Colitis cystica profunda of the rectum treated by mucosal sleeve resection and colo-anal pullthrough. *Br J Surg.* 1988;75(3):289.

206. Habal N, Sims C, Bilchik AJ. Gastrointestinal carcinoid tumors and second primary malignancies. *J Surg Oncol.* 2000;75(4):310–316.

207. Haggitt RC. Granulomatous diseases of the gastrointestinal tract. In: Ioachim HL, ed. *Pathology of Granulomas.* New York, NY: Raven Press; 1983:257.

208. Haller JD, Roberts TW. Lipomas of the colon. A clinicopathologic study of 20 cases. *Surgery.* 1964;55:773–781.

209. Halls JM. Lymphomas of the large intestine. In: Greenbaum EI, ed. *Radiographic Atlas of Colon Disease.* Chicago, IL: Year Book Medical; 1980:303.

210. Halpern J, Kopolovic J, Catane R. Malignant fibrous histiocytoma developing in irradiated sacral chordoma. *Cancer.* 1984;53(12):2661–2662.

211. Hambrick E, Abcarian H, Smith D. Perineal endometrioma in episiotomy incisions: clinical features and management. *Dis Colon Rectum.* 1979;22(8):550–552.

212. Hampton JM, Gandy JR. Plasmacytoma of the gastro-intestinal tract. *Ann Surg.* 1957;145(3):415–422.

213. Hasegawa K, Lee WY, Noguchi T, ct al. Colonoscopic removal of hemangiomas. *Dis Colon Rectum.* 1981;24(2):85–89.

214. Haskell B, Rovner H. Solitary ulcer of the rectum. *Dis Colon Rectum.* 1965;8(5):333–336.

215. Hayes HT, Burr HB. Benign lymphomas of the rectum. *Am J Surg.* 1952;84(5):545–550.

216. Head HD, Baker JQ, Muir RW. Hemangioma of the colon. *Am J Surg.* 1973;126(5):691–694.

217. Hellstrom J, Hultborn KA, Engstedt L. Diffuse cavernous hemangioma of the rectum. *Acta Chir Scand.* 1955;109(3–4):277–283.

218. Hellwig CA. Extramedullary plasma cell tumors as observed in various locations. *Arch Pathol.* 1943;36:95–111.

219. Helwig EB, Hansen J. Lymphoid polyps (benign lymphoma) and malignant lymphoma of the rectum and anus. *Surg Gynecol Obstet.* 1951;92(2):233–243.

220. Helwig EB, Stern JB. Subcutaneous sacrococcygeal myxopapillary ependymoma. A clinicopathologic study of 32 cases. *Am J Clin Pathol.* 1984;81(2):156–161.

221. Hemley SD, Kanick V. Perforation of the rectum: a complication of barium enema following rectal biopsy. Report of 2 cases. *Am J Dig Dis.* 1963;8:882–884.

222. Hendren TH, Hardin CA. Extradural metastatic ependymoma. *Surgery.* 1963;54:880–882.

223. Henzl MR, Corson SL, Moghissi K, et al. Administration of nasal nafarelin as compared with oral danazol for endometriosis. A multicenter double-blind comparative clinical trial. *N Engl J Med.* 1988;318(8):485–489.

224. Hernández-Magro PM, Villanueva Sáenz E, Alvarez-Tostado Fernández F, et al. Endoanal sonography in the assessment of perianal endometriosis with external anal sphincter involvement. *J Clin Ultrasound.* 2002;30(4):245–248.

225. Higgason JM. Lymphatic cyst of the transverse colon: report of a case. *AJR Am J Roentgenol Radium Ther Nucl Med.* 1958;79(5):850–853.

226. Higinbotham NL, Phillips RF, Farr HW, et al. Chordoma. Thirty-five year study at Memorial Hospital. *Cancer.* 1967;20(11):1841–1850.

227. Hoehn JG, Farrow GM, Devine KD, et al. Invasive hemangioma of the head and neck. *Am J Surg.* 1970;120(4).495–500.

228. Hoehn JL, Hamilton GH, Beltaos E. Fibrosarcoma of the colon. *J Surg Oncol.* 1980;13(3):223–225.

229. Hollingsworth G. Haemangiomatous lesions of the colon. *Br J Radiol.* 1951;24(280):220–222.

230. Holt S, Gilmour HM, Buist TA, et al. High-flow oxygen therapy for pneumatosis coli. *Gut.* 1979;20(6):493–498.

231. Holtz F, Schmidt LA III. Lymphoid polyps (benign lymphoma) of the rectum and anus. *Surg Gynecol Obstet.* 1958;106(6):639–642.

232. Honne K, Maruyama A, Onishi S, et al. Simultaneous pneumatosis cystoides intestinalis and pneumomediastinum in a patient with systemic sclerosis. *J Rheumatol.* 2010;37(10):2194–2195.

233. Horn RC Jr, Enterline HT. Rhabdomyosarcoma: a clinicopathological study and classification of 39 cases. *Cancer.* 1958;11(1):181–199.

234. Horowitz J, Spellman JE Jr, Driscoll DL, et al. An institutional review of sarcomas of the large and small intestine. *J Am Coll Surg.* 1995;180(4):465–471.

235. Howerton RA, Bonello JC. A lipoma simulating colon cancer. *Contemp Surg.* 1989;35:20–22.

236. Hsieh JS, Huang CJ, Wang JY, et al. Benefits of endorectal ultrasound for management of smooth-muscle tumor of the rectum: report of three cases. *Dis Colon Rectum.* 1999;42(8):1085–1088.

237. Huang WS, Lin PY, Lee IL. Metastatic Merkel cell carcinoma in the rectum: report of a case. *Dis Colon Rectum.* 2007;50(11):1992–1995.

238. Huth JF, Dawson EG, Eilber FR. Abdominosacral resection for malignant tumors of the sacrum. *Am J Surg.* 1984;148(1):157–161.

239. Ihde JK, Coit DG. Melanoma metastatic to stomach, small bowel, or colon. *Am J Surg.* 1991;162(3):208–211.

240. Immunology and cancer [annotation]. *Lancet.* 1968;1:1298.

241. Irisawa A, Bhutani MS. Cystic lymphangioma of the colon: endosonographic diagnosis with through-the-scope catheter miniprobe and determination of further management. Report of a case. *Dis Colon Rectum.* 2001;44(7):1040–1042.

242. Jackman RJ, Beahrs OH. *Tumors of the Large Bowel. Major Problems in Clinical Surgery.* Vol 8. Philadelphia, PA: WB Saunders; 1968.

243. Jackman RJ, Clark PL III, Smith ND. Retrorectal tumors. *J Am Med Assoc.* 1951;145(13):956–962.

244. Jalan KN, Brunt PW, Maclean N, et al. Benign solitary ulcer of the rectum—a report of 5 cases. *Scand J Gastroenterol.* 1970;5(2):143–147.

245. Jao SW, Beart RW Jr, Spencer RJ, et al. Retrorectal tumors. Mayo Clinic experience, 1960-1979. *Dis Colon Rectum.* 1985;28(9):644–652.

246. Jauhonen P, Lehtola J, Karttunen T. Treatment of pneumatosis coli with metronidazole. Endoscopic follow-up of one case. *Dis Colon Rectum.* 1987;30(10):800–801.

247. Jeffery PJ, Hawley PR, Parks AG. Colo-anal sleeve anastomosis in the treatment of diffuse cavernous haemangioma involving the rectum. *Br J Surg.* 1976;63(9):678–682.

248. Jensen K, Raynor S, Rose SG, et al. Amyloid tumors of the gastrointestinal tract: a report of two cases and review of the literature. *Am J Gastroenterol.* 1985;80(10):784–786.

249. Jetmore AB, Ray JE, Gathright JB Jr, et al. Rectal carcinoids: the most frequent carcinoid tumor. *Dis Colon Rectum.* 1992;35(8):717–725.

250. Johansson K, Lindström E. Treatment of obstructive pneumatosis coli with endoscopic sclerotherapy: report of a case. *Dis Colon Rectum.* 1991;34(1):94–96.

251. John A, Dickoy K, Fenwick J, et al. Pneumatosis intestinalis in patients with Crohn's disease. *Dig Dis Sci.* 1992;37(6):813–817.

252. Johnson DH, Guthrie TH, Tedesco FJ, et al. Amyloidosis masquerading as inflammatory bowel disease with a mass lesion simulating a malignancy. *Am J Gastroenterol.* 1982;77(3):141–145.

253. Johnson LA, Lavin P, Moertel CG, et al. Carcinoids: the association of histologic growth pattern and survival. *Cancer.* 1983;51(5): 882–889.

254. Johnson RC, Bleshman MH, DeFord JW. Benign lymphoid hyperplasia manifesting as a cecal mass: report of a case. *Dis Colon Rectum.* 1978;21(7):510–513.

255. Johnstone JM, Morson BC. Inflammatory fibroid polyp of the gastrointestinal tract. *Histopathology.* 1978;2(5):349–361.

256. Jona JZ, Belin RP, Burke JA. Lymphoid hyperplasia of the bowel and its surgical significance in children. *J Pediatr Surg.* 1976;11(6):997–1006.

257. Joyeuse R, Lott JV, Michaelis M, et al. Malakoplakia of the colon and rectum: report of a case and review of the literature. *Surgery.* 1977;81(2):189–192.

258. Juturi JV, Francis B, Koontz PW, et al. Squamous-cell carcinoma of the colon responsive to combination chemotherapy: report of two cases and review of the literature. *Dis Colon Rectum.* 1999;42:102.

259. Kaftori JK, Aharon M, Kleinhaus U. Sonographic features of gastrointestinal leiomyosarcoma. *J Clin Ultrasound.* 1981;9(1):11–15.

260. Kang JY, Chan-Wilde C, Wee A, et al. Role of computed tomography and endoscopy in the management of alimentary tract lipomas. *Gut.* 1990;31(5):550–553.

261. Kanter AS, Hyman NH, Li SC. Ganglioneuromatous polyposis: a premalignant condition. Report of a case and review of the literature. *Dis Colon Rectum.* 2001;44(4):591–593.

262. Kaplan LD, Abrams DI, Feigal E, et al. AIDS-associated non-Hodgkin's lymphoma in San Francisco. *JAMA.* 1989;261(5):719–724.

263. Kaplan LD, Wofsy CB, Volberding PA. Treatment of patients with acquired immunodeficiency syndrome and associated manifestations. *JAMA.* 1987;257(10):1367–1374.

264. Karakousis CP. Sacral resection with preservation of continence. *Surg Gynecol Obstet.* 1986;163(3):270–273.

265. Karakousis CP, Park JJ, Fleminger R, et al. Chordomas: diagnosis and management. *Am Surg.* 1981;47:497.

266. Karakousis CP, Wabnitz RC. Tumor involving the sacrum. In: Karakousis CP, ed. *Atlas of Operations for Soft Tissue Tumors.* St Louis, MO: McGraw-Hill; 1985:301.

267. Keane TE, Peel AL. Endometrioma. An intra-abdominal troublemaker. *Dis Colon Rectum.* 1990;33(11):963–965.

268. Khadra MH, Thompson JF, Milton GW, et al. The justification for surgical treatment of metastatic melanoma of the gastrointestinal tract. *Surg Gynecol Obstet.* 1990;171(5):413–416.

269. Khalifa AA, Bong WL, Rao VK, et al. Leiomyosarcoma of the rectum. Report of a case and review of the literature. *Dis Colon Rectum.* 1986;29(6):427–432.

270. Khanna KK, Chandra RK, Veliath AJ, et al. Leiomyoma of the cecum. *Am J Dis Child.* 1968;116(6):675–677.

271. Kim HH, Williams TJ. Endometrioid carcinoma of the uterus and ovaries associated with immunosuppressive therapy and anticoagulation: report of a case. *Mayo Clin Proc.* 1972;47(1):39–41.

272. Kim HR, Kim YJ. Neurofibromatosis of the colon and rectum combined with other manifestations of von Recklinhausen's disease: report of a case. *Dis Colon Rectum.* 1998;41(9):1187–1192.

273. Kistner RW. The use of newer progestins in the treatment of endometriosis. *Am J Obstet Gynecol.* 1958;75(2):264–278.

274. Kitoraga NF. Hemangioma of the large intestine causing profuse hemorrhage. *Vestn Khir Im I I Grek*. 1962;88:125–126.

275. Klinge F. Ueber die sogenannten ureifen, nicht guergestreiften Myoblastenmyome. *Verh Dtsch Ges Pathol*. 1928;23:376.

276. Knechtle SJ, Davidoff AM, Rice RP. Pneumatosis intestinalis. Surgical management and clinical outcome. *Ann Surg*. 1990;212(2): 160–165.

277. Koenig RR, Claudon DB, Byrne RW. Lymphatic cyst of the transverse colon: report of a case radiographically simulating neoplastic polyp. *AMA Arch Pathol*. 1955;60(4):431–434.

278. Koep LJ, Peters TG, Starzl TE. Major colonic complications of hepatic transplantation. *Dis Colon Rectum*. 1979;22(4):218–220.

279. Kölby L, Persson G, Franzén S, et al. Randomized clinical trial of the effect of interferon on survival in patients with disseminated midgut carcinoid tumours. *Br J Surg*. 2003;90(6):687–693.

280. Konda J, Ruth M, Sassaris M, et al. Sarcoidosis of the stomach and rectum. *Am J Gastroenterol*. 1980;73(6):516–518.

281. Kontozoglou TE, Moyana TN. Adenosquamous carcinoma of the colon—an immunocytochemical and ultrastructural study. Report of two cases and review of the literature. *Dis Colon Rectum*. 1989;32(8): 716–721.

282. Koss LG. Abdominal gas cysts (pneumatosis cystoides intestinorum hominis): an analyis with a report of a case and a critical review of the literature. *AMA Arch Pathol*. 1952;53(6):523–549.

283. Koura AN, Giacco GG, Curley SA, et al. Carcinoid tumors of the rectum: effect of size, histopathology, and surgical treatment on metastasis free survival. *Cancer*. 1997;79(7):1294–1298.

284. Kovalcik PJ, Burke JB. Anterior sacral meningocele and the scimitar sign. Report of a case. *Dis Colon Rectum*. 1988;31(10):806–807.

285. Kovalcik PJ, Simstein NL, Cross GH. Benign neurilemmoma manifesting as a presacral (retrorectal) mass: report of a case. *Dis Colon Rectum*. 1978;21(3):199–202.

286. Kraft RO. Duplication anomalies of the rectum. *Ann Surg*. 1962;155:230–232.

287. Kulaylat MN, Doerr RJ, Neuwirth M, et al. Anal duct/gland cyst: report of a case and review of the literature. *Dis Colon Rectum*. 1998;41(1):103–110.

288. Kumar SS, Appavu SS, Abcarian H, et al. Amyloidosis of the colon. Report of a case and review of the literature. *Dis Colon Rectum*. 1983;26(8):541–544.

289. Kuramoto S, Sakai S, Tsuda K, et al. Lymphangioma of the large intestine. Report of a case. *Dis Colon Rectum*. 1988;31(11):900–905.

290. Kuroda Y, Katoh H, Ohsato K. Cystic lymphangioma of the colon. Report of a case and review of the literature. *Dis Colon Rectum*. 1984;27(10):679–682.

291. Kyle RA, Bayrd ED. Amyloidosis: review of 236 cases. *Medicine (Baltimore)*. 1975;54(4):271–299.

292. Kyle RA, Spence RJ, Dahlin DC. Value of rectal biopsy in the diagnosis of primary systemic amyloidosis. *Am J Med Sci*. 1966;251(5): 501–506.

293. Laine L, Amerian J, Rarick M, et al. The response of symptomatic gastrointestinal Kaposi's sarcoma to chemotherapy: a prospective evaluation using an endoscopic method of disease quantification. *Am J Gastroenterol*. 1990;85(8):959–961.

294. Landing BH, Farber S. Tumors of the cardiovascular system. In: *Atlas of Tumor Pathology*. 1st series. Sect. 3. Fasc. 7. Washington, DC: United States Armed Forces Institute of Pathology; 1956:45.

295. Landmann DD, Lewis RW. Benign cystic ovarian teratoma with colorectal involvement. Report of a case and review of the literature. *Dis Colon Rectum*. 1988;31(10):808–813.

296. Langer C, Gunawan B, Schüler P, et al. Prognostic factors influencing surgical management and outcome of gastrointestinal stromal tumours. *Br J Surg*. 2003;90(3):332–339.

297. Le DT, Austin RC, Payne SNP, et al. Choriocarcinoma of the colon: report of a case and review of the literature. *Dis Colon Rectum*. 2003;46(2):264–266.

298. Leach SD, Modlin IM, Goldstein L, et al. Laparoscopic local excision of a proximal rectal carcinoid. *J Laparoendosc Surg*. 1994;4(1): 65–70.

299. Lee MH, Waxman M, Gillooley JF. Primary malignant lymphoma of the anorectum in homosexual men. *Dis Colon Rectum*. 1986;29(6): 413–416.

300. Leong WL, Pasieka JL. Regression of metastatic carcinoid tumors with octreotide therapy: two case reports and a review of the literature. *J Surg Oncol*. 2002;79(3):180–187.

301. Levy D, Khatib R. Intestinal neurofibromatosis with malignant degeneration: report of a case. *Dis Colon Rectum*. 1960;3:140–144.

302. Levy M, Stone AM, Platt N. Reticulum cell sarcoma of the cecum and macroglobulinemia: a case report. *J Surg Oncol*. 1976;8(2):149–153.

303. Lewin KJ, Harell GS, Lee AS, et al. Malacoplakia. An electron-microscopic study: demonstration of bacilliform organisms in malacoplakic macrophages. *Gastroenterology*. 1974;66(1):28–45.

304. Lewin KJ, Ranchod M, Dorfman RF. Lymphomas of the gastrointestinal tract: a study of 117 cases presenting with gastrointestinal disease. *Cancer*. 1978;42(2):693–707.

305. Lifschitz O, Lew S, Witz M, et al. Inflammatory fibroid polyp of sigmoid colon. *Dis Colon Rectum*. 1979;22(8):575–577.

306. Ling CS, Leagus C, Stahlgren LH. Intestinal lipomatosis. *Surgery*. 1959;46:1054–1059.

307. Localio SA, Francis KC, Rossaro PG. Abdominosacral resection of sacrococcygeal chordoma. *Ann Surg*. 1967;166(3):394–402.

308. Londono-Schimmer EE, Ritchie JK, Hawley PR. Coloanal sleeve anastomosis in the treatment of diffuse cavernous haemangioma of the rectum: long-term results. *Br J Surg*. 1994;81(8):1235–1237.

309. Lookanoff VA, Tsapralis PC. Smooth-muscle tumors of the colon. Report of a case involving the cecum and ascending colon. *JAMA*. 1966; 198(1):206–207.

310. Lord PH, Tribe CR. Gastric tissue in the rectum. *Lancet*. 1970; 1(7646):566–567.

311. Lorenz HP, Wilson W, Leigh B, et al. Kaposi's sarcoma of the rectum in patients with the acquired immunodeficiency syndrome. *Am J Surg*. 1990;160(6):681–682.

312. Lou Ty, Teplitz C. Malakoplakia: pathogenesis and ultrastructural morphogenesis. A problem of altered macrophage (phagolysosomal) response. *Hum Pathol*. 1974;5(2):191–207.

313. Lubarsch O. Ueber den primaren Krebs des Ileum, nebst Bemerhunge uber das gleichzeitge Vorkommen von Krebs und Tuberculose. *Virchows Arch*. 1888;111:280–317.

314. Luna-Pérez P, Rodríguez DF, Luján L, et al. Colorectal sarcoma: analysis of failure patterns. *J Surg Oncol*. 1998;69(1):36–40.

315. Lyon DT, Mantia AG. Large-bowel hemangiomas. *Dis Colon Rectum*. 1984;27(6):404–414.

316. Lyttle JA. Primary squamous carcinoma of the proximal large bowel. Report of a case and review of the literature. *Dis Colon Rectum*. 1983;26(4):279–282.

317. Ma WH. Myoblastoma: report of a case with review of 287 cases collected from the literature. *Chin Med J*. 1952;70(1–2):35–46.

318. MacKenzie DA, McDonald JR, Waugh JM. Leiomyoma and leiomyosarcoma of the colon. *Ann Surg*. 1954;139(1):67–75.

319. Madiedo G, Komorowski RA, Dhar GJ. Granular cell tumor (myoblastoma) of the large intestine removed by colonoscopy. *Gastrointest Endosc*. 1980;26(3):108–109.

320. Madigan MR, Morson BC. Solitary ulcer of the rectum. *Gut*. 1969; 10(11):871–881.

321. Magtibay PM, Heppell J, Leslie KO. Endometriosis-associated invasive adenocarcinoma involving the rectum in a postmenopausal female: report of a case. *Dis Colon Rectum*. 2001;44(10):1530–1533.

322. Mallory FB. Three gliomata of ependymal origin: two in the fourth ventricle, one subcutaneous over the coccyx. *J Med Res*. 1902;8(1):1–10.

323. Mani S, Modlin IM, Ballantyne G, et al. Carcinoids of the rectum. *J Am Coll Surg*. 1994;179(2):231–248.

324. Manley KA, Skyring AP. Some heritable causes of gastrointestinal disease. Special reference to hemorrhage. *Arch Intern Med*. 1961;107: 182–203.

325. Margulis AR, Burhenne HJ, eds. *Alimentary Tract Roentgenology*. Vol 2. St Louis, MO: CV Mosby; 1967.

326. Margulis AR, Jovanovich A. The roentgen diagnosis of submucous lipomas of the colon. *AJR Am J Roentgenol Radium Ther Nucl Med*. 1960;84:1114–1120.

327. Marshak RH, Moseley JE, Wolf BS. The roentgen findings in familial polyposis with special emphasis on differential diagnosis. *Radiology*. 1963;80:374–382.

328. Martin JK Jr, Culp CE, Weiland LH. Colitis cystica profunda. *Dis Colon Rectum*. 1980;23(7):488–491.

329. Maruyama M, Fukayama M, Koike M. A case of multiple carcinoid tumors of the rectum with extraglandular endocrine cell proliferation. *Cancer*. 1988;6l(1):131–136.

330. Matter MJ, Gygi C, Gillet M, et al. Malacoplakia simulating organ invasion in a rectosigmoid adenocarcinoma: report of a case. *Dis Colon Rectum*. 2001;44(9):1371–1371.

331. Mazier WP, Sun KM, Robertson WG. Oil-induced granuloma (eleoma) of the rectum: report of four cases. *Dis Colon Rectum*. 1978;21(4):292–294.

332. McClenathan JH. Metastatic melanoma involving the colon. Report of a case. *Dis Colon Rectum*. 1989;32(1):70–72.

333. McClure J. Malakoplakia of the gastrointestinal tract. *Postgrad Med J.* 1981;57(664):95–103.

334. McGee HJ Jr. Inflammatory fibroid polyps of the ileum and cecum. *Arch Pathol.* 1960;70:203–207.

335. McSwain B, Beal JM. Lymphosarcoma of the gastrointestinal tract: report of 20 cases. *Ann Surg.* 1944;119(1):108–123.

336. Meijer S, Peretz T, Gaynor JJ, et al. Primary colorectal sarcoma. A retrospective review and prognostic factor study of 50 consecutive patients. *Arch Surg.* 1990;125(9):1163–1168.

337. Mendoza CC. Arteriovenous angioma of the colon. *South Med J.* 1962;55:40–41.

338. Merkel IS, Rabinovitz M, Dekker A. Cecal inflammatory fibroid polyp presenting with chronic diarrhea. A case report and review of the literature. *Dig Dis Sci.* 1992;37(1):133–136.

339. Meyer R. Ueber entzündliche heterotope Epithel vucherungen im weiblichen Genitalgebiete und ueber eine bis in die Wurzel des Mesocolon ausgedehnte benigne Wucherung des Darmepithels. *Virchows Arch.* 1909;195:487.

340. Meyers MA, Ghahremani GG. Pneumatosis coli. In: Greenbaum EI, ed. *Radiographic Atlas of Colon Disease*, Chicago, IL: Year Book Medical; 1980:389.

341. Michaelis L, Gutmann C. Ueber Einschlusse in Blasentumoren. *Klin Med (Mosk).* 1902;47:208–215.

342. Michelassi F, Mishlove LA, Stipa F, et al. Squamous-cell carcinoma of the colon. Experience at the University of Chicago, review of the literature, report of two cases. *Dis Colon Rectum.* 1988;31(3):228–235.

343. Michelassi F, Montag AG, Block GE. Adenosquamous-cell carcinoma in ulcerative colitis. Report of a case. *Dis Colon Rectum.* 1988;31(4):323–326.

344. Michowitz M, Lazebnik N, Noy S, et al. Lipoma of the colon. A report of 22 cases. *Am Surg.* 1985;51(8):449–454.

345. Miercort RD, Merrill FG. Pneumatosis and pseudo-obstruction in scleroderma. *Radiology.* 1969;92(2):359–362.

346. Miettinen M, El-Rifai WE, H L Sobin L, et al. Evaluation of malignancy and prognosis of gastrointestinal stromal tumors: a review. *Hum Pathol.* 2002;33(5):478–483.

347. Mihara S, Yano H, Matsumoto H, et al. Perianal alveolar rhabdomyosarcoma in a child. Report of a long-term survival case. *Dis Colon Rectum.* 1983;26(11):728–731.

348. Miller RW, Dalager NA. Fatal rhabdomyosarcoma among children in the United States, 1960–1969. *Cancer.* 1974;34(6):1897–1900.

349. Miralbés M, Honojosa J, Alonso J, et al. Oxygen therapy in pneumatosis coli. What is the minimum oxygen requirement? *Dis Colon Rectum.* 1983;26(7):458–460.

350. Mir-Madjlessi SH, Tavassolie H, Kamalian N. Malakoplakia of the colon and recurrent colonic strictures in a patient with primary hypogammaglobulinemia: an association not previously described. *Dis Colon Rectum.* 1982;25(7):723–727.

351. Modlin IM, Lye KD, Kidd M. A 5-decade analysis of 13,715 carcinoid tumors. *Cancer.* 2003;97(4):934–959.

352. Moertel CG. Large bowel. In: Holland JF, Frei E III, eds. *Cancer Medicine.* Philadelphia, PA: Lea & Febiger; 1973:1597.

353. Moertel CG, Dockerty MB, Judd ES. Carcinoid tumors of the veriform appendix. *Cancer.* 1968;21(2):270–278.

354. Moertel CG, Sauer WG, Dockerty MB, et al. Life history of the carcinoid tumor of the small intestine. *Cancer.* 1961;14:901–912.

355. Moertel CG, Weiland LH, Nagorney DM, et al. Carcinoid tumor of the appendix: treatment and prognosis. *N Engl J Med.* 1987;317(27):1699–1701.

356. Monek O, Martin L, Heyd B, et al. Rectal duplication in an adult: unusual cause of a buttock mass. Report of a case. *Dis Colon Rectum.* 1999;42(6):816–818.

357. Morantz RA, Kepes JJ, Batnitzky S, et al. Extraspinal ependymomas. Report of three cases. *J Neurosurg.* 1979;51(3):383–391.

358. Morl FK, Dortenmann J. Hämangiome des Dickdarms. *Med Welt.* 1968;45:2483–2485.

359. Morson BC. Pathology of carcinoid tumours. In: Jones FA, ed. *Modern Trends in Gastroenterology.* London, United Kingdom: Butterworth; 1958:107.

360. Morson BC. In: Dukes CE, ed. *Cancer of the Rectum.* Vol 3. Edinburgh, Scotland: E & S Livingstone; 1960:92.

361. Mourra N, Caplin S, Parc R, et al. Presacral neuroendocrine carcinoma developed in a tailgut cyst: report of a case. *Dis Colon Rectum.* 2003;46(3):411–413.

362. Murphy B. Leiomyoma of intestine. *J Ir Med Assoc.* 1973;66(6):153–154.

363. Murray FE, Lombard M, Dervan P, et al. Bleeding from multifocal heterotopic gastric mucosa in the colon controlled by an H_2 antagonist. *Gut.* 1988;29(6):848–851.

364. Murray MR. Cultural characteristics of three granular-cell myoblastomas. *Cancer.* 1951;4(4):857–865.

365. Nakahara S, Itoh H, Mibu R, et al. Anorectal function after high sacrectomy with bilateral resection of S2–S5 nerves. Report of a case. *Dis Colon Rectum.* 1986;29(4):271–274.

366. Neary PC, Redmond PH, Houghton T, et al. Carcinoid disease: review of the literature. *Dis Colon Rectum.* 1997;40(3):349–362.

367. Neff R, Kremer S, Voutsinas L, et al. Primary Kaposi's sarcoma of the ileum presenting as massive rectal bleeding. *Am J Gastroenterol.* 1987;82(3):276–277.

368. Nelson RL. The association of carcinoid tumors of the rectum with myelofibrosis: report of two cases. *Dis Colon Rectum.* 1981;24(7):548–549.

369. Neoplasms. A complication of organ transplants? *JAMA.* 1968;206:246–247.

370. Nigam R. A case of dermoid arising from the rectal wall. *Br J Surg.* 1947;35(138):218.

371. Nigro ND, Hiratzka T. Aberrant gastric mucosa in the rectum: a case report. *Dis Colon Rectum.* 1961;4:275–276.

372. Norbury L. Specimen of post-rectal fibro-leiomyoma. *Proc R Soc Med.* 1934;27(7):930–931

373. Normann I, Otnes B. Intestinal ganglioneuromatosis, diarrhoea and medullary thyroid carcinoma. *Scand J Gastroenterol.* 1969;4(7):553–559.

374. Oberndorfer S. Karzinoide Tumoren des Dünndarms. *Frank Z Pathol.* 1907;1:426–432.

375. Oberwalder M, Tschmelitsch J, Conrad F, et al. Endosonographic image of a retrorectal bowel duplication: report of a case. *Dis Colon Rectum.* 1998;41(6):802–803.

376. O'Brien JE, Stout AP. Malignant fibrous xanthomas. *Cancer.* 1964;17:1445–1455.

377. Ochsner SF, Ray JE, Clark WH Jr. Lymphangioma of the colon: a case report. *Radiology.* 1959;72(3):423–425.

378. Ohri SK, Keane PF, Sackier JM, et al. Primary rectal lymphoma and malignant lymphomatous polyposis. Two cases illustrating current methods in diagnosis and management. *Dis Colon Rectum.* 1989;32(12):1071–1074.

379. Okano H, Azar HA, Osserman EF. Plasmacytic reticulum cell sarcoma. Case report with electron microscopic studies. *Am J Clin Pathol.* 1966;46(5):546–555.

380. Olnick HM, Woodhall JP Jr, Clay CB Jr. Hemangioma of the colon. *J Med Assoc Ga.* 1957;46(8):383–384.

381. Orda R, Bawnik JB, Wiznitzer T, et al. Fibroma of the cecum: report of a case. *Dis Colon Rectum.* 1976;19(7):626–628.

382. O'Riordain DS, O'Connell PR, Kirwan WO. Hereditary sacral agenesis with presacral mass and anorectal stenosis: the Currarino triad. *Br J Surg.* 1991;78(5):536–538.

383. Orloff MJ. Carcinoid tumors of the rectum. *Cancer.* 1971;28(1):175–180.

384. O'Toole D, Ducreux M, Bommelaer G, et al. Treatment of carcinoid syndrome: a prospective crossover evaluation of lanreotide versus octreotide in terms of efficacy, patient acceptability, and tolerance. *Cancer.* 2000;88(4):770–776.

385. Ozaki T, Hillmann A, Winkelmann W. Surgical treatment of sacrococcygeal chordoma. *J Surg Oncol.* 1997;64(4):274–279.

386. Palvio DHB, Sorensen FB, Klove-Mogensen M. Stem cell carcinoma of the colon and rectum. Report of two cases and review of the literature. *Dis Colon Rectum.* 1985;28(6):440–445.

387. Pardo MV, Rodriquez TI. Eosinophilic granuloma of the colon. *Arch Hosp Univ.* 1952;4(2):248–253.

388. Paris J, Goudemand M, Leduc M, et al. Angiome isolé du colon droit avec hemorragies digestives repetées pendant 15 ans. *Lille Med.* 1967;12(5):592–594.

389. Parks AG, Porter NH, Hardcastle J. The syndrome of the descending perineum. *Proc R Soc Med.* 1966;59(6):477–482.

390. Paterson C, Musselman L, Chorneyko K, et al. Merkel cell (neuroendocrine) carcinoma of the anal canal: report of a case. *Dis Colon Rectum.* 2003;46(5):676–678.

391. Pearlman AW, Friedman M. Radical radiation therapy of chordoma. *AJR Am J Roentgenol Radium Ther Nucl Med.* 1970;108(2):332–341.

392. Pemberton J, McCormack CJ. Submucous lipomas of colon and rectum. *Am J Surg.* 1937;37:205–218.

393. Penn I, Starzl TE. Immunosuppression and cancer. *Transplant Proc.* 1973;5(1):943–947.

394. Peterkin GA III, Moroz K, Kondi ES. Proctitis cystica profunda in paraplegics: report of three cases. *Dis Colon Rectum.* 1992;35(12):1174–1176.

395. Petrelli NJ, Valle AA, Weber TK, et al. Adenosquamous carcinoma of the colon and rectum. *Dis Colon Rectum.* 1996;39(11):1265–1268.

396. Pfannenstiel J. Über die Adenomyome des Genitalstrangs. *Verh Dtsch Ges Gynaekol.* 1897;7:195.

397. Phillips B. Lectures on the principles and practices of surgery. *London Med Gaz.* 1840;26:881–892.

398. Pilleul F, Penigaud M, Milot L, et al. Possible small-bowel neoplasms: contrast-enhanced and water-enhanced multidetector CT enteroclysis. *Radiology.* 2006;241(3):796–801.

399. Pinkert TC, Catlow CE, Straus R. Endometriosis of the urinary bladder in a man with prostatic carcinoma. *Cancer.* 1979;43(4):1562–1567.

400. Pitchumoni CS, Dearani AC, Burke AV, et al. Eosinophilic granuloma of the gastrointestinal tract. *JAMA.* 1970;211(7):1180–1182.

401. Poate H, Inglis K. Ganglioneuromatosis of the alimentary tract. *Br J Surg.* 1928;16(62):221–225.

402. Pontecorvo C, Lombardi S, Mottola L, et al. Hemangiomas of the large bowel. Report of a case. *Dis Colon Rectum.* 1983;26(12):818.

403. Port JH, Traube J, Winans CS. The visceral manifestations of Kaposi's sarcoma. *Gastrointest Endosc.* 1982;28(3):179–181.

404. Poulos JE, Presti ME, Phillips N, et al. Presentation and management of lymphatic cyst of the colon. *Dis Colon Rectum.* 1997;40(3):366–369.

405. Price AB. Benign lymphoid polyps and inflammatory polyps. In: Morson BC, ed. *The Pathogenesis of Colorectal Cancer.* Philadelphia, PA: WB Saunders; 1978:33.

406. Prystowsky JB, Stryker SJ, Ujiki GT, et al. Gastrointestinal endometriosis. Incidence and indications for resection. *Arch Surg.* 1988;123(7):855–858.

407. Quan SH, Bader G, Berg JW. Carcinoid tumors of the rectum. *Dis Colon Rectum.* 1964;7:197–206.

408. Quan SH, Berg JW. Leiomyoma and leiomyosarcoma of the rectum. *Dis Colon Rectum.* 1962;5:415–425.

409. Quinn TC. Gastrointestinal manifestations of AIDS. *Pract Gastroenterol.* 1985;9:23–24.

410. Ranchod M, Kahn LB. Malacoplakia of the gastrointestinal tract. *Arch Pathol.* 1972;94(1):90–97.

411. Rand AA. Barium granuloma of the rectum. *Dis Colon Rectum.* 1966;9(1):20–32.

412. Rao BK, Kapur MM, Roy S. Leiomyosarcoma of the colon: a case report and review of literature. *Dis Colon Rectum.* 1980;23(3):184–190.

413. Rasheed S, Yap T, Zia A, et al. Chemo-radiotherapy: an alternative to surgery for squamous cell carcinoma of the rectum—report of six patients and literature review. *Colorectal Dis.* 2008;11(2):191–197.

414. Redwine DB, Koning M, Sharpe DR. Laparoscopically assisted transvaginal segmental resection of the rectosigmoid colon for endometriosis. *Fertil Steril.* 1996;65(1):193–197.

415. Reiss H, Ryc K. Roxlegly naczyniak jelita grubego i odbytnicy o mieszenej budowie. *Pol Przegl Chir.* 1971;43:115.

416. Richardson JD. Vascular lesions of the intestines. *Am J Surg.* 1991;161(2):284–293.

417. Rickert RR, Larkey IG, Kantor EB. Granular-cell tumors (myoblastomas) of the anal region. *Dis Colon Rectum.* 1978;21(6):413–417.

418. Rissier HL Jr. Hemangiomatosis of the intestine. Discussion, review of the literature and report of two new cases. *Gastroenterologia.* 1960;93:357–385.

419. Riva HL, Kawasaki DM, Messinger AJ. Further experience with norethynodrel in treatment of endometriosis. *Obstet Gynecol.* 1962;19:111–117.

420. Rives S, Pera M, Rosiñol L, et al. Primary systemic amyloidosis presenting as a colonic stricture: successful treatment with left hemicolectomy followed by autologous hematopoietic stem-cell transplantation: report of a case. *Dis Colon Rectum.* 2002;45(9):1263–1266.

421. Robertson FN, Wride GE. A case of persistent cyst of post-anal gut origin in an adult. *Can Med Assoc J.* 1934;31(5):535–537.

422. Robidoux A, Monte M, Heppel J, et al. Small-cell carcinoma of the rectum. *Dis Colon Rectum.* 1984;28(8):594–596.

423. Rodriguez DI, Drehner DM, Beck DE, et al. Colonic lipoma as a source of massive hemorrhage. Report of a case. *Dis Colon Rectum.* 1990;33(11):977–979.

424. Rose TF. True fibroma of the caecum. *Med J Aust.* 1972;1(11):532–533.

425. Rosenberg I. Perianal granular cell myoblastoma. Report of a case. *J Int Coll Surg.* 1960;33:346–349.

426. Rosenberg JM, Welch JP. Carcinoid tumors of the colon. A study of 72 patients. *Am J Surg.* 1985;149(6):775–779.

427. Ruiz-Moreno F. Hemangiomatosis of the colon: report of a case. *Dis Colon Rectum.* 1962;5:453–456.

428. Ryan J, Martin JE, Pollock DJ. Fatty tumours of the large intestine: a clinicopathological review of 13 cases. *Br J Surg.* 1989;76(8):793–796.

429. Ryckman FC, Glenn JD, Moazam F. Spontaneous perforation of a colonic duplication. *Dis Colon Rectum.* 1983;26(4):287–289.

430. Rywlin AM, Ravel R, Hurwitz A. Malakoplakia of the colon. *Am J Dig Dis.* 1969;14(7):491–419.

431. Saclarides TJ, Ko ST, Airan M, et al. Laparoscopic removal of a large colonic lipoma. Report of a case. *Dis Colon Rectum.* 1991;34(11):1027–1029.

432. Saclarides TJ, Szeluga D, Staren ED. Neuroendocrine cancers of the colon and rectum. Results of a ten-year experience. *Dis Colon Rectum.* 1994;37(7):635–642.

433. Saegesser F, Gross M. Carcinoid syndrome and carcinoid tumours of the rectum. *Am J Proctol.* 1969;20(1):27–32.

434. Safai B, Diaz B, Schwartz J. Malignant neoplasms associated with human immunodeficiency virus infection. *CA Cancer J Clin.* 1992;42(2):74–95.

435. Sahakitrungruang C, Chantra K, Dusitanond N, et al. Sacrectomy for primary sacral tumors. *Dis Colon Rectum.* 2009;52(5):913–918.

436. Sakanoue Y, Kusunoki M, Shoji Y, et al. Malignant histiocytosis of the intestine simulating Crohn's disease. Report of a case. *Dis Colon Rectum.* 1992;35(3):266–269.

437. Sallach S, Schmidt T, Pehl C, et al. Primary low-grade B cell non-Hodgkin's lymphoma of MALT type simultaneously arising in the colon and in the lung: report of a case. *Dis Colon Rectum.* 2001;44(3):448–452.

438. Saltzstein SL. Extranodal malignant lymphomas and pseudolymphomas. *Pathol Annu.* 1969;4:159–184.

439. Sampson JA. Intestinal adenomas of endometrial type. *Arch Surg.* 1922;5:217.

440. Sanders RJ. Leiomyosarcoma of the rectum: report of six cases. *Ann Surg.* 1961;154(6 suppl):150–154.

441. Sanders RJ, Axtell HK. Carcinoids of the gastrointestinal tract. *Surg Gynecol Obstet.* 1964;119:369–380.

442. Sanger BJ, Leckie BD. Plain muscle tumours of the rectum. *Br J Surg.* 1959;47:196–198.

443. Sarmiento JM, Wolff BG. A different type of presacral tumor: extramedullary hematopoiesis: report of a case. *Dis Colon Rectum.* 2003;46(5):683–685.

444. Sasajima K, Okawa K, Sasamoto Y, et al. Pararectal rhabdomyosarcoma: report of a case. *Dis Colon Rectum.* 1980;23(8):576–577.

445. Sauven P, Ridge JA, Quan SH, et al. Anorectal carcinoid tumors. Is aggressive surgery warranted? *Ann Surg.* 1990;211(1):67–71.

446. Sayfan J, Benosh L, Segal M, et al. Endometriosis in episiotomy scar with anal sphincter involvement. Report of a case. *Dis Colon Rectum.* 1991;34(8):713–716.

447. Schlernitzauer DA, Font RL. Sebaceous gland carcinoma of the eyelid. *Arch Ophthalmol.* 1976;94(9):1523–1525.

448. Schröder J, Löhnert M, Doniec JM, et al. Endoluminal ultrasound diagnosis and operative management of rectal endometriosis. *Dis Colon Rectum.* 1997;40(5):614–617.

449. Schumann F. Leiomyosarcoma of the colon: report of a case and review of treatment and prognosis. *Dis Colon Rectum.* 1972;15(3):211–216.

450. Selikoff IJ, Robitzek EH. Gingival biopsy for the diagnosis of generalized amyloidosis. *Am J Pathol.* 1947;23(6):1099–1111.

451. Serra J, Ruiz M, Lloveras B, et al. Surgical outlook regarding leiomyoma of the rectum. Report of three cases. *Dis Colon Rectum.* 1989;32(10):884–887.

452. Sewell R, Levine BA, Harrison GK, et al. Primary malignant fibrous histiocytoma of the intestine: intussusception of a rare neoplasm. *Dis Colon Rectum.* 1980;23(3):198–201.

453. Sharma S, Longo WE, Baniadam B, et al. Colorectal manifestations of endocrine disease. *Dis Colon Rectum.* 1995;38(3):318–323.

454. Sherlock P, Winawer SJ, Goldstein MJ, et al. Malignant lymphoma of the gastrointestinal tract. In: Jerzy Glass GB, ed. *Progress in Gastroenterology.* Vol 2. New York, NY: Grune & Stratton; 1970:367.

455. Shia J, Tang LH, Weiser MR, et al. Is nonsmall cell type high-grade neuroendocrine carcinoma of the tubular gastrointestinal tract a distinct disease entity? *Am J Surg Pathol.* 2008;32(5):719–731.

456. Shimazu K, Funata N, Yamamoto Y, et al. Primary osteosarcoma arising in the colon: report of a case. *Dis Colon Rectum.* 2001;44(9):1367–1370.

457. Shindo K, Bacon HE, Holmes EJ. Ectopic gastric mucosa and glandular tissue of a salivary type in the anal canal concomitant with a diverticulum in hemorrhoidal tissue: report of a case. *Dis Colon Rectum.* 1972;15(1):57–62.

458. Shirouzu K, Isomoto H, Kakegawa T, et al. Treatment of rectal carcinoid tumors. *Am J Surg.* 1990;160(3):262–265.

459. Shklovskii GS, Kadyrov FA. Gemangioma tolst oi kishki s invaginatsiei. *Vestn Khir.* 1964;93:114.

460. Sidani MS, Campos MM, Joseph JI. Primary plasmacytomas of the colon. *Dis Colon Rectum.* 1983;26(3):182–187.

461. Silverberg SG. "Juvenile" retention polyps of the colon and rectum. *Am J Dig Dis.* 1970;15(7):617–625.

462. Silverman JM, Hamlin JA. Large melanoma metastases to the gastrointestinal tract. *Gut.* 1989;30(12):1783–1785.

463. Simon SR, Fox K. Neuroendocrine carcinoma of the colon. Correct diagnosis is important. *J Clin Gastroenterol.* 1993;17(4):304–307.

464. Skardalakis JE, Gray SW. *Smooth Muscle Tumors of the Alimentary Tract: Leiomyomas and Leiomyosarcomas, a Review of 2525 Cases.* Springfield, IL: Charles C. Thomas; 1962:155.

465. Skopelitou AS, Mylonakis EP, Charchanti AV, et al. Cellular neurilemoma (schwannoma) of the descending colon mimicking carcinoma: report of a case. *Dis Colon Rectum.* 1998;41(9):1193–1196.

466. Skovgaard S, Sorensen FH. Bleeding hemangioma of the colon diagnosed by coloscopy. *J Pediatr Surg.* 1976;11(1):83–84.

467. Skutsch. Quoted in: Galletly A. *Z Gebutschulfe Gunakol.* 1899;11:353.

468. Slagel GA, Lupton GP. Postproctoscopic periorbital purpura. Primary systemic amyloidosis. *Arch Dermatol.* 1986;122(4):464–465.

469. Slooter GD, Mearadji A, Breeman WA, et al. Somatostatin receptor imaging, therapy and new strategies in patients with neuroendocrine tumours. *Br J Surg.* 2001;88(1):31–40.

470. Smith G. Leiomyosarcoma of the rectum. *Br J Surg.* 1963;50: 603–605.

471. Smith JA, Bhathal PS, Cuthbertson AM. Angiosarcoma of the colon. Report of a case with long-term survival. *Dis Colon Rectum.* 1990;33(4):330–333.

472. Smith JL, Painter RW, Berman MM. Breast carcinoma: colonic metastases with perforation—report of two cases. *Contemp Surg.* 1989;35: 47–52.

473. Snover DC, Sandstad J, Hutton S. Mucosal pseudolipomatosis of the colon. *Am J Clin Pathol.* 1985;84(5):575–580.

474. Sohn N. Surgical conditions of the anus and rectum in male homosexuals. *Pract Gastroenterol.* 1985;9:46.

475. Somervell JL, Mayer PF. Leiomyosarcoma of the rectum. *Br J Surg.* 1971;58(2):144–146.

476. Spigelman AD, Williams CB, Ansell JK, et al. Pneumatosis coli: a source of diagnostic confusion. *Br J Surg.* 1990;77(2):155.

477. Spread C, Berkel H, Jewell L, et al. Colon carcinoid tumors. A population based study. *Dis Colon Rectum.* 1994;37(5):482–491.

478. Staren ED, Gould VE, Warren WH, et al. Neuroendocrine carcinomas of the colon and rectum: a clinicopathologic evaluation. *Surgery.* 1988;104(6):1080–1089.

479. Starr GF, Dockerty MB. Leiomyomas and leiomyosarcomas of the small intestine. *Cancer.* 1955;8(1):101–111.

480. Stavorovsky M, Jaffa AJ, Papo J, et al. Leiomyosarcoma of the colon and rectum. *Dis Colon Rectum.* 1980;23(4):249–254.

481. Steckler RM, Martin RG. Sacrococcygeal chordoma. *Am Surg.* 1974;40(10):579–581.

482. Stening SG, Heptinstall DP. Diffuse cavernous haemangioma of the rectum and sigmoid colon. *Br J Surg.* 1970;57(3):186–189.

483. Stoller R, Weinstein JJ. Fibrosarcoma of the rectum: a review of the literature and the presentation of two additional cases. *Surgery.* 1956;39(4):565–573.

484. Stout AP. Tumors of the colon and rectum (excluding carcinoma and adenoma). *Surg Clin North Am.* 1955;35:1283–1238.

485. Stout AP, Hill WT. Leiomyosarcoma of the superficial soft tissues. *Cancer.* 1958;11(4):844–854.

486. Stuart M. Pneumatosis coli complicating carcinoma of the colon. Report of a case. *Dis Colon Rectum.* 1984;27(4):257–259.

487. Suga K, Tanaka N, Nakanishi T, et al. Bone and gallium scintigraphy in sacral chordoma. Report of four cases. *Clin Nucl Med.* 1992;17(3):206–212.

488. Sugarman GI, Weitzman JJ, Isaacs H Jr, et al. Rectal bleeding from gastric tissue in the rectum. *Lancet.* 1970;1(7640):251.

489. Swain VA, Young WF, Pringle EM. Hypertrophy of the appendices epiploicae and lipomatous polyposis of the colon. *Gut.* 1969;10(7):587–589.

490. Swanson MA, Schwartz RS. Immunosuppressive therapy. The relation between clinical response and immunologic competence. *N Engl J Med.* 1967;277(4):163–170.

491. Swartley RN, Stayman JW Jr. Lymphoid hyperplasia of the intestinal tract requiring surgical intervention. *Ann Surg.* 1962;155:238–240.

492. Swartzlander FC. *A Clinico-Pathological Review of Submucosal Rectal Nodules* [thesis]. Minneapolis, MN: University of Minnesota; 1955.

493. Swerdlow DB, Pecora C, Gardone F. Leiomyoma of the cecum presenting as an acute surgical abdomen: report of a case. *Dis Colon Rectum.* 1975;18(5):438–440.

494. Swinton NW, Lehman G. Presacral tumors. *Surg Clin North Am.* 1958;38(3):849–857.

495. Symmers D. Lymphoid disease: Hodgkin's granuloma, giant follicular lymphadenopathy, lymphoid leukemia, lymphosarcoma and gastrointestinal pseudoleukemia. *Arch Pathol (Chic).* 1948;45(1):73–131.

496. Talerman A. Enterogenous cysts of the rectum (colitis cystica profunda). *Br J Surg.* 1971;58(9):643–647.

497. Tan TCF, Wang JY, Cheung YC, et al. Diffuse cavernous hemangioma of the rectum complicated by invasion of pelvic structures. Report of two cases. *Dis Colon Rectum.* 1998;41(8):1062–1066.

498. Tarver R, Smith GF, Kukora JS. Intestinal amyloidosis. *Contemp Surg.* 1985;26:69.

499. Taxy JB, Mendelsohn G, Gupta PK. Carcinoid tumors of the rectum. Silver reactions, fluorescence, and serotonin content of the cytoplasmic granules. *Am J Clin Pathol.* 1980;74(6):791–795.

500. Terner R, Lattes R. Malakoplakia of colon and retroperitoneum. Report of a case with a histochemical study of the Michaelis-Gutman inclusion bodies. *Am J Clin Pathol.* 1965;44:20–31.

501. Tessier DJ, McConnell EJ, Young-Fadok T, et al. Melanoma metastatic to the colon: case series and review of the literature with outcome analysis. *Dis Colon Rectum.* 2003;46(4):441–447.

502. Testart J, Maupas JL, Metayer J, et al. Rectal peptic ulceration—a rare cause of rectal bleeding. Report of a case. *Dis Colon Rectum.* 1988;31(10):803–805.

503. Thambidorai CR, Muin I, Razman J, et al. Currarino triad with dual pathology in the presacral mass: report of a case. *Dis Colon Rectum.* 2003;46(7):974–977.

504. Thomason TH. Cysts and sinuses of the sacrococcygeal region. *Ann Surg.* 1934;99(4):585–592.

505. Thompson GB, van Heerden J, Martin JK Jr, et al. Carcinoid tumors of the gastrointestinal tract: presentation, management, and prognosis. *Surgery.* 1985;98(6):1054–1063.

506. Thorlakson RH, Ross HM. Leiomyosarcoma of the rectum. *Ann Surg.* 1961;154:979–984.

507. Tichansky DS, Cagir B, Borrazzo E, et al. Risk of second cancers in patients with colorectal carcinoids. *Dis Colon Rectum.* 2002;45(1): 91–97.

508. Timmerman W, Bubrick MP. Presacral and postsacral extraspinal ependymoma. Report of a case and review of the literature. *Dis Colon Rectum.* 1984;27(2):114–119.

509. Tinkoff GH, Yum KY. Endoscopic diagnosis of lipomatosis of the ileocecal valve. *Contemp Surg.* 1987;30:69.

510. Tobi M, Kobrin I, Ariel I. Rectal involvement in sarcoidosis. *Dis Colon Rectum.* 1982;25(5):491–493.

511. Toti A, Tedeschi M. Fibroma cecale insorto su monocone appendicolare invaginato. *Minerva Chir.* 1952;7(11):420–422.

512. Touran T, Frost DB, O'Connell TX. Sacral resection. Operative technique and outcome. *Arch Surg.* 1990;125(7):911–913.

513. Tsioulias G, Muto T, Kubota Y, et al. DNA ploidy pattern in rectal carcinoid tumors. *Dis Colon Rectum.* 1991;34(1):31–36.

514. Turell R. *Diseases of the Colon and Anorectum.* 2nd ed. Philadelphia, PA: WB Saunders; 1969.

515. Upson JF, Bunnell I, Kokkinopoulis E. Hemangioma of the cecum—diagnosis by angiography. *JAMA.* 1971;217(8):1104–1105.

516. Urbach DR, Reedijk M, Richard CS, et al. Bowel resection for intestinal endometriosis. *Dis Colon Rectum.* 1998;41(9):1158–1164.

517. Usher FC. *Lymphosarcoma of the Intestines* [thesis]. Minneapolis, MN: University of Minnesota; 1940.

518. Vagaiwala MR, Robinson JS, Galicich JH, et al. Metastasizing extradural ependymoma of the sacrococcygeal region: case report and review of literature. *Cancer.* 1979;44(1):326–333.

519. Vanden Heule B, Taylor CR, Terry R, et al. Presentation of malignant lymphoma in the rectum. *Cancer.* 1982;49(12):2602–2607.

520. Venkitachalam PS, Hirsch E, Elguezabal A, et al. Multiple lymphoid polyposis and familial polyposis of the colon: a genetic relationship. *Dis Colon Rectum.* 1978;21(5):336–341.

521. Vezeridis MP, Herrera LO, Lopez GE, et al. Squamous-cell carcinoma of the colon and rectum. *Dis Colon Rectum.* 1983;26(3):188–191.

522. Viamonte M III, Viamonte ME. Pneumatosis cystoides intestinalis: case presentation and review of the literature. *Contemp Surg.* 1990; 37:37.

523. Vitolo RE, Rachlin SA. Inflammatory fibroid polyp of large intestine: report of a case. *J Int Coll Surg.* 1955;23(6, section 1):700–709.

524. Von Recklinghausen FH. *Ueber die multiplen Fibrome der Haut und ihre Beziehung zu den multiplen Neuromen.* Berlin, Germany: A Hirschwald; 1882.

525. Vorobyov GI, Odaryuk TS, Kapuller LL, et al. Surgical treatment of benign, myomatous rectal tumors. *Dis Colon Rectum.* 1992;35(4): 328–331.

526. Waldenström JG. Studies on conditions associated with disturbed gamma globulin formation (gammapathies). *Harvey Lect.* 1960–1961;56: 211–231.

527. Wall SD, Friedman SL, Margulis AR. Gastrointestinal Kaposi's sarcoma in AIDS: radiographic manifestations. *J Clin Gastroenterol.* 1984;6(2):165–171.

528. Wang CH. Sphincter-saving procedure for treatment of diffuse cavernous hemangioma of the rectum and sigmoid colon. *Dis Colon Rectum.* 1985;28(8):604–607.

529. Wang HT, Gao XH, Fu CG, et al. Diagnosis and treatment of diffuse cavernous hemangioma of the rectum: report of 17 cases. *World J Surg.* 2010;34(10):2477–2486.

530. Waxman M, Faegenburg D, Waxman JS, et al. Malignant fibrous histiocytoma of the colon associated with diverticulitis. *Dis Colon Rectum.* 1983;26(5):339–343.

531. Waye JD, Frankel A. Removal of pedunculated lipoma by colonoscopy. *Am J Gastroenterol.* 1974;62(3):221–222.

532. Wayte DM, Helwig EB. Colitis cystica profunda. *Am J Clin Pathol.* 1967;48:159–169.

533. Weber JN, Carmichael DJ, Boylston A, et al. Kaposi's sarcoma of the bowel—presenting as apparent ulcerative colitis. *Gut.* 1985;26(3): 295–300.

534. Weinberg T, Feldman M Sr. Lipomas of the gastrointestinal tract. *Am J Clin Pathol.* 1955;25(3):272–281.

535. Weitzel RA, Breed JR. Carcinoma arising in a rectal duplication (enterocystoma). *Ann Surg.* 1963;157:476–480.

536. Weitzner S. Ectopic salivary gland tissue in submucosa of rectum. *Dis Colon Rectum.* 1983;26(12):814–817.

537. Welch CE, Hedberg SE. *Polypoid Lesions of the Gastrointestinal Tract.* 2nd ed. Philadelphia, PA: WB Saunders; 1975:121.

538. Welch JP, Donaldson GA. Recent experience in the management of cancer of the colon and rectum. *Am J Surg.* 1974;127(3):258–266.

539. Weprin L, Zollinger R, Clausen K, et al. Kaposi's sarcoma: endoscopic observations of gastric and colon involvement. *J Clin Gastroenterol.* 1982;4(4):357–360.

540. Williams ED, Sandler M. The classification of carcinoid tumours. *Lancet.* 1963;1(7275):238–239.

541. Williams GT, Blackshaw AJ, Morson BC. Squamous carcinoma of the colorectum and its genesis. *J Pathol.* 1979;129(3):139–147.

542. Willis RA. *The Borderland of Embryology and Pathology.* London, United Kngdom: Butterworth; 1958.

543. Willis RA. *Pathology of Tumours.* 3rd ed. London, United Kingdom: Butterworth; 1960.

544. Wilson JAP. Richter's syndrome mimicking chronic colitis: a patient with diffuse histiocytic lymphoma complicating chronic lymphocytic leukemia. *Dis Colon Rectum.* 1986;29(3):191–195.

545. Wolf BS, Marshak RH. Roentgen features of diffuse lymphosarcoma of the colon. *Radiology.* 1960;75:733–740.

546. Wolff M. Heterotopic gastric epithelium in the rectum: a report of three new cases with a review of 87 cases of gastric heterotopia in the alimentary canal. *Am J Clin Pathol.* 1971;55(5):604–616.

547. Wolff M, Santiago H, Duby MM. Delayed distant metastasis from a subcutaneous sacrococcygeal ependymoma. Case report, with tissue culture, ultrastructural observations, and review of the literature. *Cancer.* 1972;30(4):1046–1067.

548. Wong MT, Eu KW. Primary colorectal lymphomas. *Colorectal Dis.* 2006;8(7):586–591.

549. Wood DA. Tumors of the intestines. In: *Atlas of Tumor Pathology.* 2nd series. Sect. 6. Fasc. 22. Washington, DC: Armed Forces Institute of Pathology; 1967:52.

550. Wychulis AR, Beahrs OH, Woolner LB. Malignant lymphoma of the colon. A study of 69 cases. *Arch Surg.* 1966;93(2):215–225.

551. Yamaguchi K, Shirai T, Shimakura K, et al. Pneumatosis cystoides intestinalis and trichloroethylene exposure. *Am J Gastroenterol.* 1985;80(10):753–757.

552. Yanai-Inbar I, Odes HS, Krugliak P, et al. Granular cell myoblastoma of the sigmoid colon. *Dig Dis Sci.* 1981;26(9):852–854.

553. Yang GCH, Coleman B, Daly JM, et al. Presacral myelolipoma. Report of a case with fine needle aspiration cytology and immunohistochemical and histochemical studies. *Acta Cytol.* 1992;36(6):932–936.

554. Yeh CY, Chen HH, Tang R, et al. Surgical outcome after curative resection of rectal leiomyosarcoma. *Dis Colon Rectum.* 2000;43(11):1517–1521.

555. Yonemoto T, Tatezaki S, Takenouchi T, et al. The surgical management of sacrococcygeal chordoma. *Cancer.* 1999;85(4):878–883.

556. Yoshida A, Yano M, Fujinaga Y, et al. Argentaffin carcinoid tumor of the rectum. *Cancer.* 1981;48(9):2103–2106.

557. Yoshikawa O. A case of leiomyosarcoma of the rectum. *Nihon Geka Hokan.* 1969;38(2):342–345.

558. Yousefzadeh DK, Bickers GH, Jackson JH, et al. Tubular colonic duplication—review of 1876–1981 literature. *Pediatr Radiol.* 1983;13(2): 65–71.

559. Ziter FM Jr. Roentgenographic findings in Gardner's syndrome. *JAMA.* 1965;192:1000–1002.

27

Diverticular Disease

R. John Nicholls

Diet cures more than the lancet.

—SPANISH PROVERB

Man shall not live by bread alone.

—MATTHEW 4:4; LUKE 4:4

Diverticulum (a; pl); Latin = a wayside inn, presumably of ill repute

Diverticular disease is a very common condition, and in an aging population it will become even more so. Most patients with diverticula have no symptoms, but about 20% have complaints and of these a minority develops a complication. These can be divided into septic or nonseptic, acute or chronic. Acute inflammation of a diverticulum results in the condition of acute diverticulitis. This can lead to a local or to a free perforation. Most patients with acute diverticular disease are managed medically but those with local abscess formation or free perforation may require intervention, either drainage of a localized abscess or surgery for peritonitis. Those who respond to medical measures have been usually often advised to consider a subsequent elective surgical resection of the diseased segment after the inflammation had settled.

In the last 5 years, important changes in practice have taken place. First, it is apparent from follow-up studies that the possibility of a recurrent acute attack (thought to have been 10% to 25% over the following few years) is lower than previously believed. This has led to a revision in the guidelines regarding further surgery. Those published by the American Society of Colon and Rectal Surgeons (ASCRS) in 2006 are currently in the process of revision.[242] The view of the Association of Coloproctology of Great Britain and Ireland expressed in a position statement in 2011 is that elective resection should be recommended based on the particular circumstances of the patient.[96] Thus, the number of prophylactic resections is likely to diminish. The second development is a consequence of the development of laparoscopic surgery whereby peritoneal lavage may now be favored over open surgery in patients with purulent peritonitis (Hinchey stage III).[129,208,301,311] At the present time, it is not known whether such patients should be advised to have a subsequent elective resection.

Chronic diverticular disease can take the form of fistulization from a diverticulum into an adjacent organ or of stricture formation that may cause obstruction, or it can simply be associated with symptoms of lower abdominal pain and a tendency to constipation. The indication for surgery in patients with a fistula or symptomatic stricture is usually straightforward. It is much more difficult to decide whether surgery will benefit patients with symptomatic noncomplicated disease. This is due to the overlapping of symptoms with that of an irritable bowel syndrome (IBS).

► HISTORY AND INCIDENCE

Diverticular disease was a rare condition prior to the beginning of the 20th century. It had been described by Littre in 1700 (see Biography, Chapter 24),[92] but further reports were not seen until the 19th century when Cruveilhier (see Biography, Chapter 20) included the disease in his beautifully illustrated book on pathology published in 1849 shortly before the introduction of photography.[71] Painter and Burkitt described further contributions by Rokitansky, Cripps, and Virchow but until the 20th century, the condition was regarded as a surgical curiosity.[222] The term peridiverticulitis was introduced by Graser in 1899.[111] He suggested that the diverticula were due to herniation through the bowel wall. Beer considered that the inflammation was the result of obstruction of the orifices of the diverticula by feces.[31] In reports by Telling and Gruner, the complications of acute diverticular disease were described including abscess and fistula formation.[303,304]

The disease had thus become progressively more pervasive in the 20th century and is virtually epidemic in Western countries today.[275] A person's risk for the development of diverticular disease by age 60 in the United States approximates 50%. By the age of 80 years, virtually all Americans have the condition. Yet, not more than 20% of persons with colonic diverticula have symptoms, and only a few of these ever require surgery.[229] Of the 10% to 15% of individuals with diverticula who go on to develop diverticulitis, 75% are uncomplicated in the sense of not having features of perforation, localized or general. However, 25% have an abscess, obstruction, perforation, or fistula. Perforation is uncommon, occurring at about the rate of 4 per 100,000 per year, with women having about half the incidence of men.[275]

In the United States, diverticular disease accounts for approximately 450,000 annual hospitalizations, 2 million office visits, and 112,000 disability cases, and it claims approximately 3,000 lives per year.[162] Diverticulosis of the colon is most common in the sigmoid in the United States, whereas the location is primarily right-sided in Asian populations. In recent years, there has been a marked increase in the number of hospital admissions for diverticular disease (see next).

► CLASSIFICATION

Diverticular disease is defined by the presence of diverticula. Most patients with diverticular disease are asymptomatic and are referred to as having diverticulosis or asymptomatic diverticular disease. About 20% complain of symptoms and are said to have symptomatic diverticular disease. A proportion of these develops a complication and are said to have complicated diverticular disease. Complications result from local sepsis causing acute diverticulitis; local contained perforation (paracolic abscess) or free perforation causing purulent or fecal peritonitis; or from chronic inflammation causing fistula formation, stricture formation, or secondary hemorrhage (Table 27-1).

In the report of the working party appointed by the ASCRS entitled "Practice Parameters for Sigmoid Diverticulitis," Rafferty and colleagues refer to diverticulitis without any abscess or other septic complication as "uncomplicated diverticulitis" and use the term "complicated diverticulitis" to include patients with abscess formation or perforation.[242] The reader needs to be aware of minor differences in terminology by careful reading of the text in question.

TABLE 27-1 Classification of Diverticular Disease

Asymptomatic (diverticulosis)	Symptomatic
Uncomplicated	Complicated
Acute diverticulitis ► (uncomplicated)	Acute diverticulitis (complicated)
Chronic symptomatic diverticular disease	Local abscess
	Perforation
	Purulent Fecal
	Stricture
	Hemorrhage

► EPIDEMIOLOGY

Diverticular disease is an important source of morbidity and mortality. As previously mentioned, there is evidence that it is becoming more prevalent. In the United States, the National Hospital Discharge Survey in the year 2004, it was demonstrated that diverticular disease was responsible for 312,000 admissions and 1.5 million days of inpatient care per year at an annual cost of $2.6 billion.[162,263] In a recent article, Etzioni and colleagues, using the Nationwide Inpatient Sample (NIS) from 1998 to 2005, showed a 26% increase in admissions for acute diverticulitis from 1998 (121,000) to 2005 (152,000).[86] They showed a reduction in age from 64.8 to 61.8 years during this period and also demonstrated that there was an increase in admissions in the age groups 18 to 44 and 45 to 64 years, whereas the figure for 65 to 74 years remained stable and that for older than 75 years fell. Mäkelä and colleagues have estimated the annual incidence of perforated diverticulitis in Finland to have increased from 2.4/100,000 per year to 3.8/100,000 per year from 1986 to 2000.[181] In England between 1989/1990 and 1999/2000, information from the Department of Health Hospital Episode Statistics showed that from 1989/1990 to 1999/2000 there had been an increase in admissions by 16% for males (20.1 to 23.2/100,000 population) and by 12% for females (28.6 to 31.9/100,000 population).[150] The proportions of admissions undergoing surgery also increased for males, from 22.9% to 24.1% (16%), and for females, 19.7% to 22.3% (14%). In a recent study using the Scottish national linkage database between 1996 and 2010, the number of hospital admissions increased from 5,284 to 10,935. Most of these were for endoscopy, but 26% were attributed to admissions for treatment of acute disease.[25]

It is difficult to measure the prevalence because most patients are asymptomatic. Most of the information comes from autopsy and barium enema series with rates varying between 2% and 10%.[222] The prevalence of diverticula increases with age, from less than 10% in those younger than age 40 years to 50% to 66% in patients older than age 80 years, with no apparent sex difference.[222,228]

Burkitt was the initiator of the theory that diverticular disease is a disease of Western industrialized societies such as in the United States, Europe, and Australia. The hypothesis was supported by the low prevalence of the condition in East Africans. Even within a given country the incidence can vary between ethnic groups, such as in Singapore where the frequency among the Chinese and European populations has been reported to be 0.14 and 5.41 cases per million

DENIS PARSONS BURKITT (1911–1993)

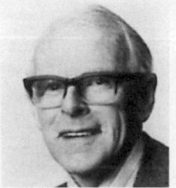

Denis Burkitt was born February 28, 1911, in Enniskillen, Northern Ireland, the son of an engineer. Without any particular interest in medicine, he followed in his father's footsteps to engineering school at Dublin University. An indifferent student, he learned of a letter the don had written to his father in which he expressed doubt as to Denis's ability to obtain a university degree and warned about the risk of forfeiting the £10 enrollment fee. It is therefore ironic that many years later he received the university's highest award, an honorary fellowship of Trinity College, Dublin. Interestingly, in light of Burkitt's subsequent career, the British Colonial Office rejected his offer for service in Africa because he had lost an eye in an accident at the age of 11. He abandoned the course he had initiated, instead seeking and obtaining admission to medical school, an act he attributed to a commitment to the highest ideals and principles of his Christian faith. Burkitt completed medical school at Dublin in 1936, received his fellowship in the Royal College of Surgeons in Edinburgh in 1938, and his doctorate in 1946. Through the Second World War, he served with the Royal Army Medical Corps, and in 1946 he joined His Majesty's Colonial Service in Uganda as a government surgeon and lecturer at the Makerere University College Medical School. He became committed to serving less privileged people than himself. The rest is medical history. In 1957, he treated a child with swellings in both maxillae and mandibles, a condition that ultimately came to be known as Burkitt's lymphoma. This led to the discovery of the cause and to the subsequent identification of the Epstein–Barr virus. His keen sense of observation and knowledge of epidemiology helped him to recognize that the most common diseases of Western civilization were virtually unknown in rural populations of developing countries. Modestly, he stated that were it not for the reputation of his eponymous association with a lymphoma, no one would have listened to his thoughts concerning the epidemiology of colon cancer. Numerous honors came to Burkitt, including the Harrison Prize of the Royal Society of Medicine, the Stewart Prize of the British Medical Association, and the Walker Prize of the Royal College of Surgeons. Honorary degrees and fellowships were awarded to him by numerous universities and organizations throughout the world. The author of six books and more than 300 scientific publications, he actively wrote from his home in Gloucester, England, until the end of his life. When autographing a book, he always penned these thoughts: "Attitudes are more important than abilities; motives are more important than methods; character is more important than cleverness; and stick-to-it-iveness is more important than the starting place."

population. There is evidence that in low-risk communities, the incidence is rising. For example, its prevalence in Singapore was reported to be 19% by Lee in 1986 and also in Africa.[170,213,330] With economic development, affluence, and westernization of diet, an increased incidence of diverticular disease has been noted among native Africans.[312] Other studies have demonstrated an increased incidence in immigrants to Western countries from less developed nations in comparison with persons remaining in the country of origin. Complicated diverticulitis has increased in Finland by 50% in the past two decades.[181]

Painter and Burkitt are the two individuals most responsible for our current concepts of the etiology and epidemiology of diverticular disease.[48,49,219–221,223] Because the condition was extremely rare in the 19th century and began to be relatively commonly observed in Western countries only after 1920, the authors postulated that a change in the dietary habits in those countries was the incriminating factor. During the years 1870 and 1880, the grist mills for grinding wheat into wholemeal flour were replaced by the much more efficient roller mills. This new process succeeded in crushing the grain so effectively that a very pure white flour was produced. At about the same time, with the advent of effective refrigeration and canning, consumption of refined sugar, fat, and protein increased. Painter and Burkitt stated that the greatest change in our diet in the past 100 years has been a reduction in the amount of cereal fiber consumption to as little as one-tenth of that previously eaten.[223] Because of this sudden change within a matter of approximately 40 years, diverticular disease had become epidemic.

Fiber increases stool weight, decreases whole-gut transit time, and lowers colonic intraluminal pressure.[24,68] A high-fiber diet produces a large, bulky stool that requires less "effort" for the bowel to expel its contents. Bran increases stool weight by virtue of its water-retentive properties. Bowel wall muscular hypertrophy does not occur, and segmentation is much less likely to develop. Burkitt and colleagues compared the transit times and stool weights of various ethnic groups.[49,219] They were particularly interested in the low incidence of colorectal disease in rural African natives. Ugandan villagers passed more than 400 g of stool within 35 hours, whereas shore-based United Kingdom naval personnel produced 100 g of constipated stool, with a transit time of approximately 5 days.

Gear and colleagues reported the results of barium enema examination in vegetarians and nonvegetarians.[105] The mean intake of dietary fiber was twice as great in the former group. Vegetarians were found to have a 12% incidence of diverticular disease, compared with 33% among nonvegetarians. Others have confirmed the importance of diet in the pathogenesis of diverticulosis.[127,183]

▶ PATHOGENESIS AND PATHOLOGY

Diverticular disease affects the sigmoid colon in almost all cases. Diverticula may extend proximally to a varying degree and rarely may be present throughout the whole colon. The rectum is not affected. In the East, right-sided diverticular disease is the more common form.[209] The bowel wall may be thickened with smooth muscular hypertrophy

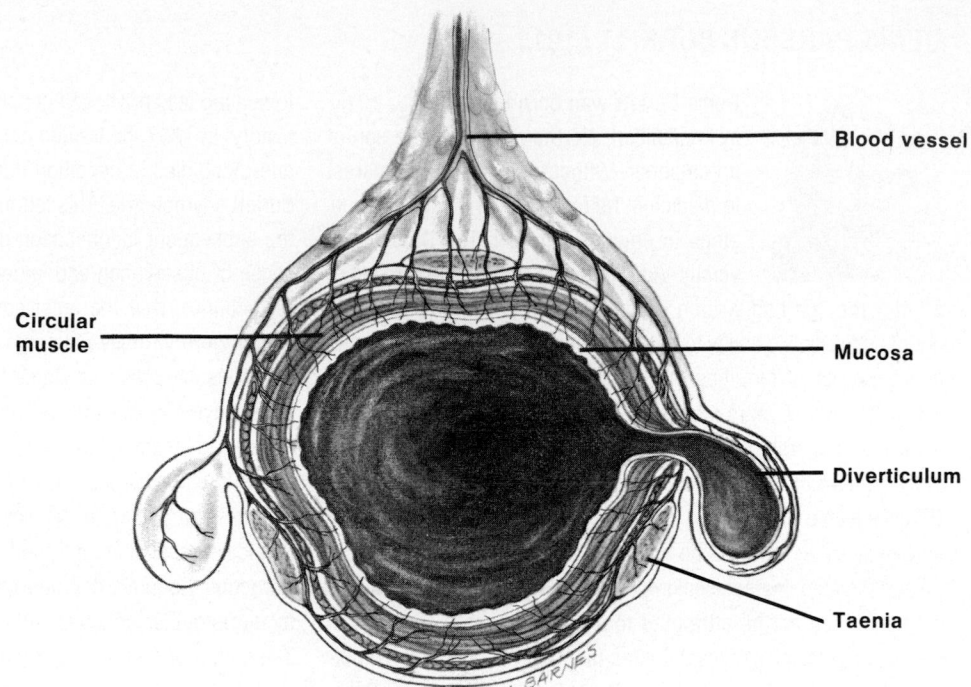

FIGURE 27-1. Cross section of colon showing areas of weakness through which the diverticula become manifest.

and degeneration when it may be replaced by elastic tissue. In an anatomic study, Slack examined 141 autopsy and 36 surgical resection specimens, including blood vessel injection by latex or barium paste.[287] He found that diverticula were consistently located to the points of penetration of the bowel wall by the circumferential branches of the mesenteric artery, which run symmetrically around the colon from the mesenteric to the antimesenteric border on each side. These vessels penetrate the circular muscle of the wall on the mesenteric side of the antimesenteric taenia where they then continue submucosally to anastomose with each other in the antimesenteric area (Figure 27-1). There was no case of a diverticulum emerging through a taenia. A branch of the circumferential artery was seen supplying the mucosa at this point, which may be relevant to the complication of hemorrhage (see Chapter 28).[199] In addition, he found that there was hypertrophy of the circular muscle resulting in a foldlike deformity of the lumen. The taeniae were also hypertrophied and the bowel length contracted (Figure 27-2).

The diverticula are of the pulsion type and are produced by herniation of mucous membrane through the weak points

of entry of the vessels as a result of raised intraluminal pressure (Figure 27-3).

In the absence of complications, particularly inflammation, the lining is entirely normal except for an increase in the size and number of lymphoid follicles.[199] The muscle shows thickening but no evidence of cellular hypertrophy or hyperplasia.[200] In an autopsy study, Hughes found abnormalities in the arrangement of muscle fibers.[136] These were more frequently seen with more extensive diverticular disease (from 30%, with disease limited to the sigmoid, to 86%, with total colonic involvement). Studies have found evidence of abnormal collagen when compared with normal controls.[298] Others have also found abnormal collagen.[333] Whiteway and Morson showed a marked increase in the elastin content of the bowel wall.[335] Antimesenteric diverticula have only a very thin layer of investing tissue, that is, mucous membrane and muscularis mucosae, separating the fecal contents of the bowel from the peritoneal cavity (Figure 27-4).

In the last few years, it has become apparent that there is an association between diverticular disease and that of segmental inflammation, so-called segmental colitis.[98,205,320] Study of the physiology of the normal colon by means of

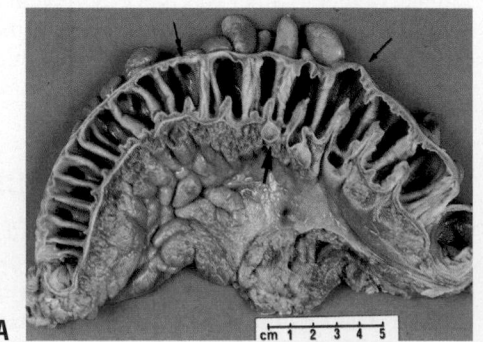
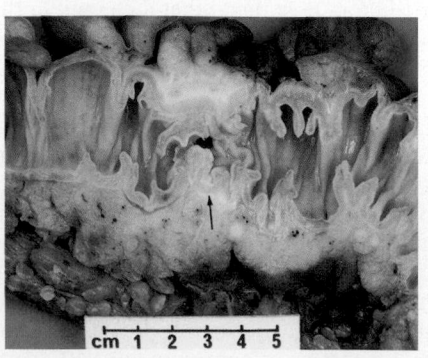

FIGURE 27-2. Segmentation with circular muscle hypertrophy and contraction of the bowel length.

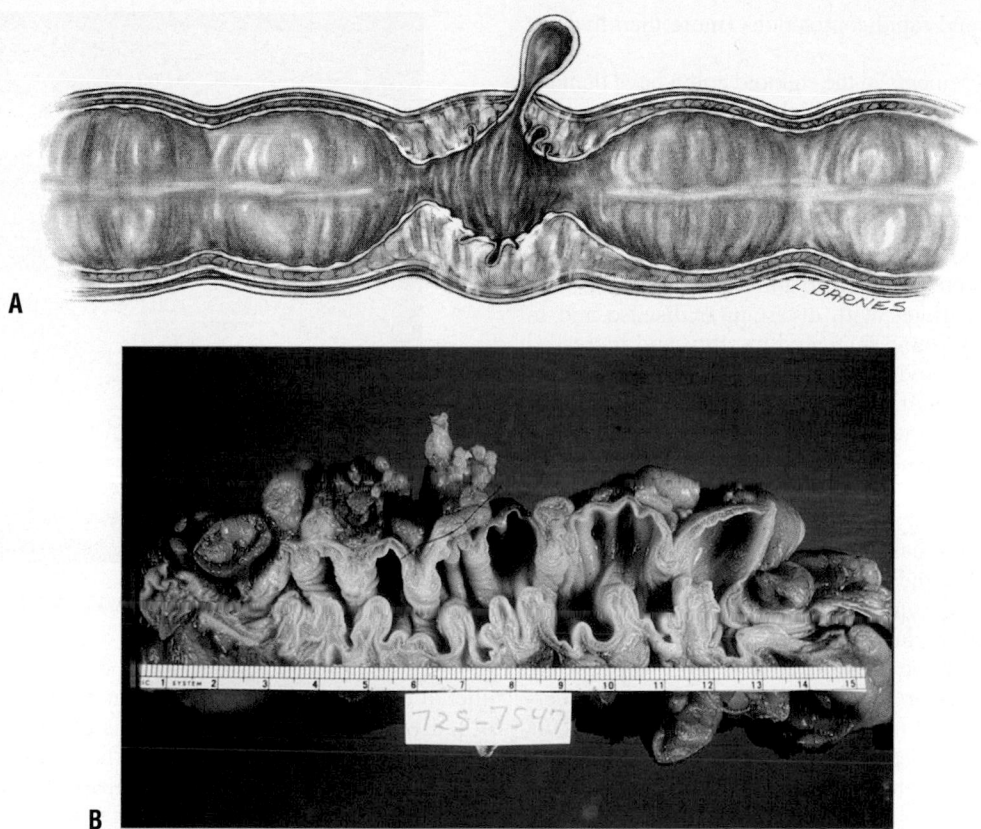

FIGURE 27-3. **A:** Mechanism of segmental contraction associated with elevated, localized intracolonic pressure and resultant diverticulum. **B:** Resected portion of the sigmoid colon demonstrating multiple "little bladders" or "rooms" resulting from hypertrophy and segmentation.

pressure tracings reveals that the principal waveform, that of "segmental contraction," is shown as a slow change of pressure, waxing, and waning during about 30 seconds.[62] Complete quiescence may normally be present for several hours. Usually, the waves are not transmitted to adjacent areas of the colon, but occasionally the transport of material over a considerable distance does occur, during a so-called mass contraction.[62] Radiologically, this is seen as a loss of haustration succeeded by movement of the contents through a number of centimeters. Motor studies in patients with diverticular disease reveal an exaggerated response to pharmacologic stimuli, increased intraluminal pressure, and faster

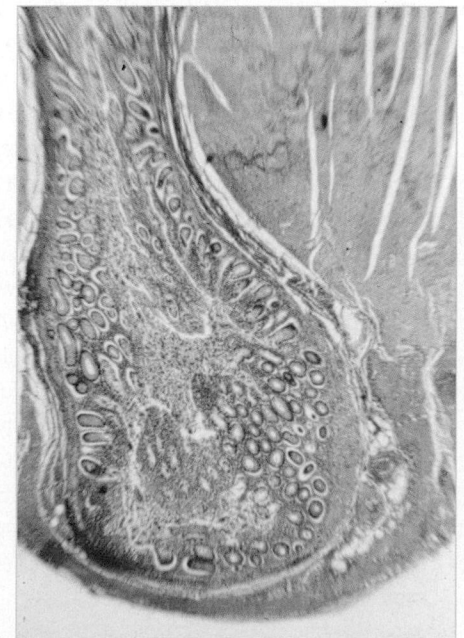

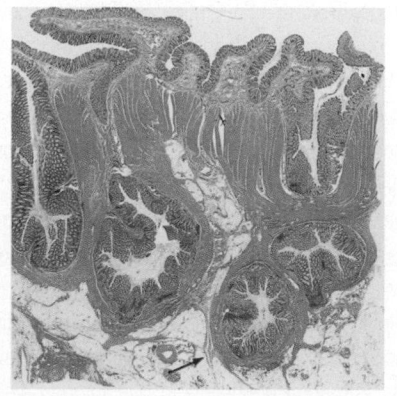

FIGURE 27-4. **A,B:** Diverticulum demonstrating only mucous membrane, muscularis mucosae, and peritoneum separating the lumen from the peritoneal cavity (hematoxylin and eosin).

frequency waves and rapid contractions (more than five per minute).[62]

Pressure measurements in the sigmoid colon have demonstrated a higher motility index or higher intraluminal pressure in patients with symptoms compared with those who harbor asymptomatic diverticular disease.[24,67,80,82] A correlation between low abdominal colicky pain and raised intraluminal pressure following neostigmine was found in patients with diverticular disease compared to those without disease.[332] Bassotti and colleagues performed 24-hour manometry measurements in 10 patients with diverticular disease and in 16 controls.[29] They found increased motility and increased forceful propulsive activity in the former group.

The points of penetration by the blood vessels create weaknesses in the muscle wall. Raised intraluminal pressure occurring during segmentation movements then results in the formation of diverticula.[24,221] When contraction occurs in a segment that is relatively narrowed, considerable intraluminal pressure develops, causing the colon to hypertrophy. The pressure is related to the narrowness or spasticity of the involved segment. According to the law of Laplace, the tension in the wall of an elastic hollow spheroid is proportional to its radius multiplied by the pressure within. This implies that the intraluminal pressure is greater when the lumen is narrowed and explains the increased likelihood that diverticula will develop in the sigmoid colon, the narrowest segment.

The increased pressure results in herniation of mucosa through the weak parts of the bowel wall (see Figure 27-1).[221] The problem is exacerbated by the fact that the tensile strength and elasticity of the colon decline with age; this is most marked on the left side.[331] The colonic muscle becomes thickened, and smooth muscle fibers may become replaced by elastic tissue.[335]

Chronic thickening of the colonic wall with contraction of the musculature explain the symptoms of pain and

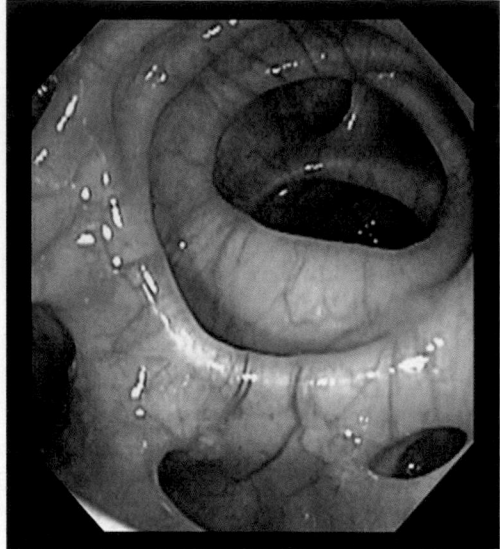

FIGURE 27-5. Colonoscopic view of diverticular orifices.

altered bowel habit. When seen on endoscopy, the orifice of a diverticulum is clear cut and is often accompanied by circular ridges indicative of circular muscle hypertrophy (Figure 27-5). An orifice can become occluded by a fecolith with resultant inflammation. This may lead to a contained or open perforation. In acute diverticulitis, there is evidence of acute inflammation around a diverticulum, with often only one being involved. This is associated with a peritoneal reaction. There may be adhesion to a neighboring structure, such as the bladder in males or the uterus or vagina in females. Local perforation, if contained, will cause abscess formation either in the immediate paracolic region or in the pelvis if

PIERRE-SIMON, THE MARQUIS DE LAPLACE (1749–1827)

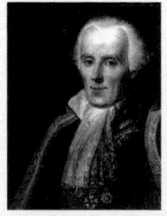

Pierre-Simon Laplace was born at Beaumont-en-Auge, in Normandy, France. Very little is known about his early life, but it is speculated that his father was either a laborer or a farmhand. Laplace sought a life in education and did so initially by becoming an usher in the school at Beaumont. He then moved to Paris after the paper he wrote on the principles of mechanics caught the attention of Jean le Rond D'Alembert, then at the height of his fame. With D'Alembert's support, Laplace obtained a position as professor of mathematics in the École Militaire de Paris, continuing his investigations in the field and writing papers on integral calculus, finite differences, and differential equations. He described his astronomical findings in *Mécanique Céleste* [celestial mechanics] and ultimately came to be regarded as the Isaac Newton of France. He became a member of the Academy of Science in 1785. Laplace built on the work initiated by Young; the Young–Laplace equation explains why the cecum is the part of the colon most susceptible to perforation because it has the greatest diameter. The formula states that the tension on the wall is directly proportional to the diameter, and the pressure within is inversely proportional to the wall's thickness. Laplace also had a need for recognition. He briefly held the post of Minister of the Interior under Napoleon Bonaparte, but after 6 weeks he was dismissed from the court and joined the Senate. During his later years, Laplace lived most of the time at Arcueil, where he had a country house. In this peaceful retirement he pursued his studies, receiving distinguished visitors from all parts of the world. He died in Paris on March 5, 1827, just short of his 78th birthday. His last words were, "Ce que nous connaissons est peu de chose; ce que nous ignorons est immense" [what we know is little; what we are ignorant of is immense]. He is remembered for his contributions to mathematics, astronomy, and medicine. His works in these fields became the cornerstone for a multitude of principles and other further research. (http://en.wikipedia.org/wiki/File:Pierre-Simon_Laplace.jpg; http://www.maths.tcd.ie/pub/HistMath/People/Laplace/RouseBall/RB_Laplace.html; http://en.wikipedia.org/wiki/Young%E2%80%93Laplace_equation; Bayless, Theodore M. Advanced therapy in gastroenterology and liver disease. Hamilton, Ontario; BC Decker Inc; 2005:503; with appreciation to Seth A. Stein, MD.)

the sigmoid loop is located in the pouch of Douglas. Alternatively, an abscess may erode into a neighboring structure and cause a fistula. A free perforation or perforation of an already formed paracolic abscess will lead to a generalized peritonitis—fecal in the former circumstance and purulent in the latter. The severity of septic complications has been categorized for clinical purposes by Hinchey (see later).[129] The bacterial picture is complex and there are no meaningful data on causation in this respect. In a study of 110 specimens from the peritoneal cavity after perforation and of 22 intra-abdominal abscesses, Brook and Frazier isolated many species.[47] Not surprisingly the majority included *Escherichia coli*, *Streptococcus* spp., *Bacteroides*, *Peptostreptococcus*, *Clostridium*, and *Fusobacterium*.

► ETIOLOGIC FACTORS

Various factors that may be important with respect to causation and clinical significance are considered later.

Age

From a historical standpoint, diverticulitis in younger patients (younger than the age of 50 years) has been described as more virulent and more likely to be associated with complications and more likely to require resection.[67,68,217] Young individuals have been variably defined as younger than 50 years in some series and younger than 40 or 45 years old in other reports. Despite the definition of what age defines "young patients," all series of so-called younger patients with acute diverticulitis have noted a striking male predominance in contrast to those who are older. Also, the older patients have a slight female predominance.[69] Earlier series of young persons in the precomputed tomography scan era have shown a large percentage of patients who underwent resection, presumably because they were frequently diagnosed preoperatively as having appendicitis. These individuals then underwent laparotomy and subsequent resection when diverticulitis and not appendicitis was encountered. Currently, such patients would most likely be correctly diagnosed as having acute diverticulitis on computed tomography (CT) scan preoperatively and treated with initial medical management of bowel rest and antibiotics. The current management of young patients with diverticulitis continues to be a source of considerable controversy and is discussed later in this chapter.

Sex and Heredity

Most studies report that diverticular disease is more common in women, the incidence increasing with advancing age.[228] Results of postmortem examinations usually place the frequency at about 50%. However, the correlation between the incidence of the condition and the presence or duration of symptoms is less clear. For example, young men are more likely to require surgical intervention for complications than are elderly patients, some even during the initial attack.[99] According to the Mayo Clinic experience (Rochester, MN), women tend to present about one-half decade after men with complications requiring surgery.[188] An inheritable tendency may also be a factor. Resection has been performed for acute disease in identical twins,[101] and Corman reported operating upon three siblings with acute, complicated diverticulitis.[66]

Anti-inflammatory Drugs

Numerous studies have suggested an association between steroidal and nonsteroidal anti-inflammatory drugs (NSAIDs) and the development of complications of diverticular disease.[50,65,197,337] Possible explanations include a direct effect on the bowel wall through inhibition of prostaglandin synthesis itself, or the inhibitory effect of leukocyte function with failure of the immune system to localize the process. In case-controlled studies, it has been consistently found that more individuals with complicated diverticulitis were taking NSAIDs than were randomly selected other groups.[50,337] In addition to NSAIDs, opioid analgesics and corticosteroids are positively associated with the risk of complications in individuals with diverticular disease.[197] The effect of drugs on acute diverticulitis is considered further later.

Immunocompromised

An immunocompromised patient is predisposed to infection, and someone with diverticular disease is at an increased risk for the development of diverticulitis. Such patients often mask typical symptoms and signs of an acute inflammatory process of the abdomen. Those with connective tissue disorders are often immunocompromised because of corticosteroids, but they appear to have an additional risk of complicated diverticulitis related to the underlying disorder (see later). Uncomplicated diverticular disease does not appear to be causally related to the immunocompromised condition.

Smoking, Alcohol, Caffeine, and Exercise

Aldoori and colleagues studied a population of 47,678 American males over a 4-year period. During this time, there were 382 newly diagnosed cases of diverticular disease.[9] There was no significant difference in alcohol or caffeine consumption when compared with the general population. Others have shown, however, that the risk of diverticulitis was significantly increased in patients with alcoholism.[310] Another study from Aldoori's group, smoking was found to be a modest risk factor in patients with symptomatic disease.[9] In a small report in which 45 patients requiring admission to hospital for diverticular disease were compared with 35 asymptomatic individuals, smoking was related to complications (odds ratio [OR] = 2.9).[224] There is also evidence that diverticular disease may be associated with lack of exercise.[8]

► DIFFERENTIAL DIAGNOSIS

The specific forms of presentation of diverticular disease will be discussed later after a consideration of the differential diagnosis. In all cases, it is important to exclude other possible causes of symptoms that might simulate diverticular disease. To do so, colonoscopy and CT scan with or without contrast are now the most frequently requested investigations. Conventional barium enema is still a useful test, but radiologists are generally hesitant to perform it, preferring CT. This is unfortunate because barium enema is capable of visualizing a small perforation not demonstrated on CT (Figure 27-6).

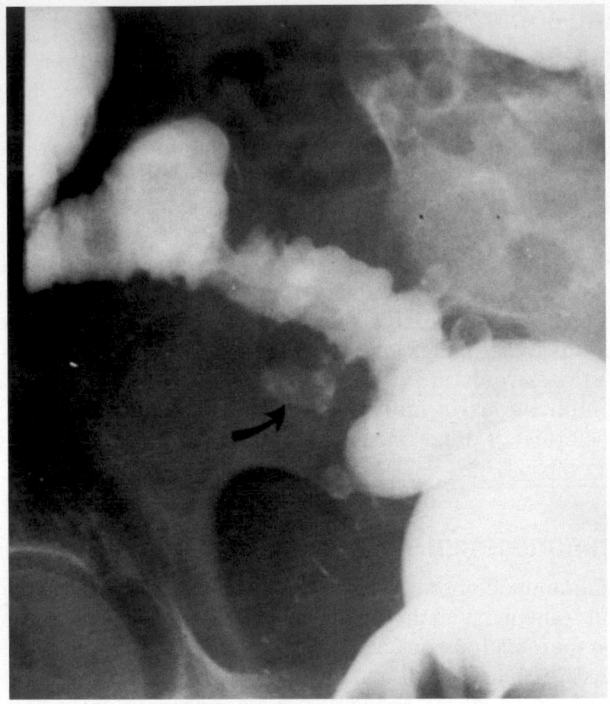

FIGURE 27-6. Perforation of diverticulum demonstrated by contrast enema (*arrow*) in a renal transplant patient. No symptoms were apparent except that the patient felt a mass.

Carcinoma

Colonoscopy

The possibility of carcinoma is likely to be considered more in the elective investigation of the patient. In most cases, this is easily excluded by colonoscopy, but when there is a degree of inflammation and thickening of the bowel wall or a stricture, it may not be possible to enter the sigmoid colon with the instrument.[73,95,186,336] Even in the noninflamed bowel, the sigmoid colon may be quite narrow because of thickening of the muscularis propria. Dean and Newell reported 36 patients in whom barium enema examination had suggested the possibility of carcinoma, but it was possible to visualize the diseased segment in only half the cases, although they were able to diagnose carcinoma in 4 patients and to exclude it in 5.[73] Max and Knutson performed colonoscopy in 26 patients with an inflammatory stricture in whom radiologic examination had shown an area that raised a suspicion of carcinoma.[185] In 19, the questionable area was completely visualized, and in every individual successfully examined, the diagnosis was proven correct.

The surgeon can feel assured only if the entire mucosa has been visualized and appears intact. Erythema and edema of the bowel wall may be seen (Figure 27-7), and occasionally pus may be observed to exude from one of the orifices. In such cases, CT or magnetic resonance imaging (MRI) colonography may be helpful. In acute diverticulitis, the clinical picture and the findings on CT will usually be sufficient to exclude a carcinoma. The poor correlation for barium enema of approximately 30% between radiologists reported by Parks and coworkers now 30 years on is no longer relevant.[231]

Colonoscopy is not without hazard. Overt perforation through a thin-walled diverticulum or walled-off abscess in a patient with acute diverticulitis is possible.[336] Examination

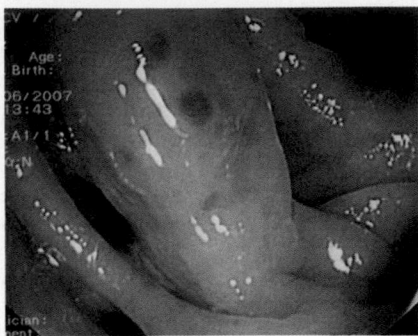

FIGURE 27-7. Erythema and edema of the bowel around the orifice of a diverticulum seen on colonoscopy. (From Tursi A, Elisei W, Giorgetti GM, et al. Inflammatory manifestations at colonoscopy in patients with colonic diverticular disease. *Aliment Pharmacol Ther.* 2011;33(3):358–365.)

under such a circumstance is probably contraindicated, but as the individual's symptoms improve, colonoscopy should be performed if the differential diagnosis is still in question. Very rarely carcinoma can arise in a diverticulum.[56]

Computed Tomography

CT is the imaging modality of choice to distinguish suspected cancer or diverticular disease. Signs of bowel wall thickening, increased soft tissue density in the pericolic fat, and soft tissue masses related to diverticulitis are helpful for confirming the diagnosis (Figure 27-8), but a perforated carcinoma may exhibit the same changes on CT.[174,238] Some investigators have confirmed the value of CT in identifying intra-abdominal abscess and phlegmon, bladder wall thickening and edema, and extracolonic extension, as well as relatively subtle features suggestive of diverticulitis.[238] However, the decision for or against surgical intervention in a patient with a mass in whom colonoscopy and CT do not give a clear diagnosis will be based on clinical grounds. Even when surgery is undertaken, especially in the acute circumstance, it may not be possible to distinguish tumor from a diverticular phlegmon.

Padidar and colleagues compared the CT scans of 69 patients with proven acute diverticulitis with 29 patients with carcinoma of the sigmoid.[218] When they analyzed the radiologic signs of fluid at the base of the mesentery and engorgement of the sigmoid vessels, they reported sensitivity, specificity, and positive predictive values for each sign of 36%; 90% and 89%; and 29%, 100%, and 100%, respectively. They concluded that these features could be helpful in distinguishing the two pathologies. Goh and coworkers compared quantitative CT perfusion measurements with conventional morphologic appearances in three groups of patients: sigmoid cancer (20), acute diverticulitis (20), and inactive diverticular disease (20).[108] They found that the former were more accurate in differentiating cancer from diverticular disease, with blood flow and blood volume having a sensitivity of 80% and a specificity of 70% to 75%.

Irritable Bowel Syndrome

Many patients with diverticula have symptoms that are indicative of IBS. IBS itself is estimated to affect up to one-fourth of the population of Western countries. Unfortunately, the condition is not well understood (see Chapter 4). Many people with diverticular disease do not have symptoms specifically related

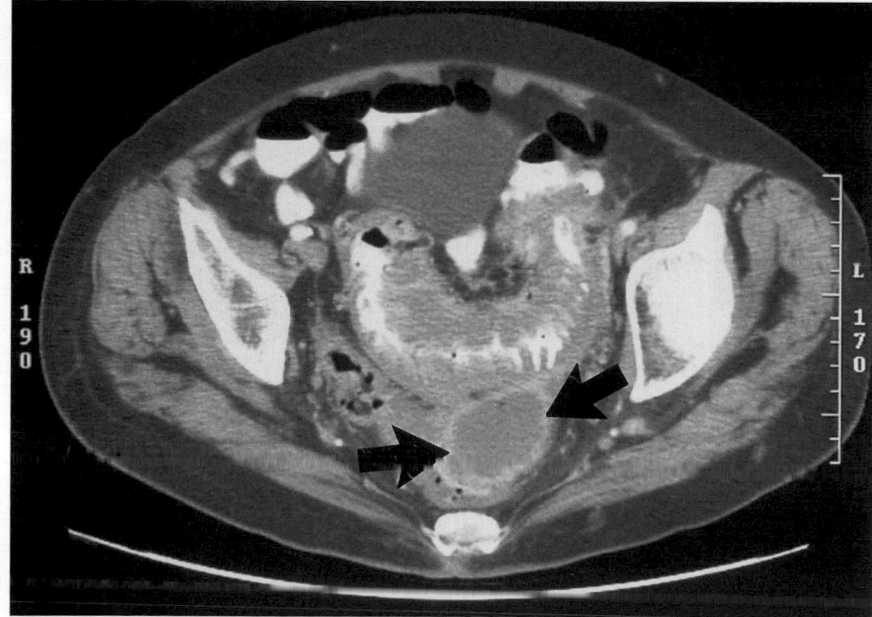

FIGURE 27-8. Computed tomography demonstrating classic findings of acute sigmoid diverticulitis with bowel wall thickening, extensive diverticular outpouchings, narrowing of the lumen, and an abscess (*arrows*).

to the condition. This implies that surgical extirpation of the affected bowel will not necessarily relieve the patient's symptoms. Breen and colleagues found that no inflammation was present in 28% of surgical specimens removed for diverticular disease.[43] These individuals probably had an IBS.

Patients with IBS comprise the vast majority of patients seen by gastroenterologists. The condition is also the single most common reason for referral to major medical clinics. In England, one-fifth of a sample from the general population had experienced abdominal pain more than six times in 1 year.[172] Approximately one-fourth of a similar sample in the United States reported abdominal pain more than six times in the year. IBS is not a precursor of diverticulosis as demonstrated by longitudinal study.[179] Furthermore, there is no evidence that the symptoms of IBS are affected by the presence of diverticula.[216,285,286,307]

The diagnosis of IBS is by exclusion, but the history can sometimes be helpful in suggesting its presence. The diagnostic criteria have been updated according to the Rome III criteria in 2006 as follows:

Recurrent abdominal pain or discomfort at least 3 days per month during the previous 3 months that is associated with two or more of the following[176]:

Relieved by defecation
Onset associated with a change in stool frequency
Onset associated with a change in stool form or appearance

Supporting symptoms include the following:

Altered stool frequency
Altered stool form
Altered stool passage (straining and/or urgency)
Mucorrhea
Abdominal bloating or subjective distension

Still, there may be difficulty in determining whether symptoms are due to diverticular disease or to IBS, and the extent of the diverticula may not be helpful. Severe diverticular-like symptoms may occur in the absence of diverticula as reported in a study of 88 patients with IBS in whom diverticula were present in only 24%.[126] Ritchie found that a high proportion

of patients with IBS had a lower threshold for pain when the colon was distended with a balloon, similar to that observed in individuals who had diverticular disease.[254] Leukocytosis and signs of peritoneal irritation do not occur in IBS, but abdominal tenderness and even the suggestion of a mass in the left lower quadrant may be evident.

In a review, Bergamaschi has discussed the question of interradiologist variation in the diagnostic distinction between diverticulitis and diverticulosis by contrast enema or ultrasound.[34] The sensitivity and specificity of the latter drops off significantly when the results of round-the-clock ultrasound are compared with those of dedicated practitioners. Contrast studies and endoscopy may reveal no abnormality, but many patients are found to have coincidental diverticula with or without evidence of "bowel spasm."

With respect to the apparent difference between the sexes in the results of surgery, men are less likely to have functional bowel complaints. Hence, misinterpretation of symptoms is less of a problem, and the correlation with radiologic and clinical findings is usually self-evident. Thörn and colleagues showed that individuals with functional symptoms or symptoms suggestive of an irritable bowel before surgery predicted a less successful result from surgery.[308]

Inflammatory Bowel Disease

Inflammatory bowel disease can demonstrate signs, symptoms, and findings that may mimic diverticulitis. These include segmental colitis, Crohn's disease, and ulcerative colitis. Ischemic colitis may also mimic acute diverticulitis.

Segmental Colitis

In recent years, the condition of segmental colitis associated with diverticula (SCAD) has been recognized (Figure 27-9). This uncommon condition is an inflammation localized to the sigmoid colon and in the presence of diverticula. Freeman identified 24 patients over a follow-up period of 2 to 16 years who were found to have diverticular disease with symptoms of bleeding, diarrhea, and abdominal pain.[98] Eighty percent

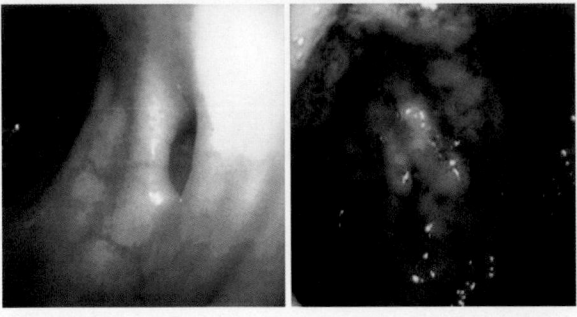

FIGURE 27-9. Colonoscopic appearance of segmental colitis associated with diverticula (SCAD). (From Jani N, Finkelstein S, Blumberg D, et al. Segmental colitis associated with diverticulosis. *Dig Dis Sci.* 2002;47(5):1175–1181.)

responded to 5-aminosalicylic acid medication, but spontaneous remissions also occurred. The condition was not related to neoplasia.

In a systemic review, Mulhall and colleagues identified 18 articles out of a total of 478 that were deemed to be eligible for evaluation.[205] Most of the 478 were not relevant to inflammatory bowel disease, most were retrospective, and one-third were case reports. The 18 articles included 227 patients of average age of 63.7 ± 5.2 years. Sixty-one percent were male. Of the 227 patients, 162 (71%) were classified as having diverticular-associated colitis, of whom 142 were managed conservatively and 28 by surgery. Recurrent symptoms developed in 37 (26%) over a 3-year period. In a prospective multicenter study of four units in Italy, Tursi and colleagues reviewed 8,525 colonoscopies.[320] Of these, 6,041 were performed for symptoms. The target population of patients with diverticula was divided into three groups: those with ulcerative colitis (UC) and diverticula, SCAD with segmental inflammation away from the orifices of the diverticula, and acute uncomplicated diverticulitis (AUD) with the inflammation involving the diverticular orifices. The conclusion from this study was that SCAD and UC in the presence of diverticula is uncommon.

Crohn's Disease

It may be difficult to differentiate Crohn's disease from diverticulitis. There are several symptoms, however, that may lead the surgeon to suspect the possibility of the former, especially if the patient complains of diarrhea and rectal bleeding. The presence of an anal lesion is also suggestive (see Chapters 14 and 30). Rectoscopy reveals a normal rectum in diverticulitis, whereas with Crohn's disease the rectum may or may not be spared. At laparotomy, it may still be impossible to distinguish between the two conditions, even if the resected specimen is opened. Usually, however, in diverticulitis the mucosal surface, although edematous, is otherwise normal. Evidence of granularity or ulceration is indicative of inflammatory bowel disease. A frozen-section examination is not advised because it will not affect the type of operation. The presence of granuloma formation does not necessarily indicate Crohn's disease because foreign body giant cells can be seen with diverticulitis as a reaction to pericolonic abscess.[200] Crohn's disease is second only to diverticular disease as a cause of intestinal fistulization into the bladder.[201]

Berman and colleagues reported 25 patients who required colonic resection for "diverticulitis" on a second occasion,

and all eventually proved to have Crohn's disease.[35] In many instances, Crohn's colitis was suspected, but not until after a subsequent resection with histopathologic confirmation. Symptoms and signs of recurrent illness were similar to those present when the patient was initially seen, that is, before the first operation. In these individuals, there was often a history of smoldering illness in contrast to the more episodic nature of the symptoms in patients with diverticulitis. Age was not particularly helpful in distinguishing the two conditions because in the older age group especially Crohn's disease often tends to involve the large rather than the small bowel. The presence of extracolonic manifestations, such as pyoderma or arthritis, unusual technical difficulty in performing the resection, and failure of the colonic inflammation to resolve, should lead the surgeon to suspect Crohn's disease.

Ulcerative Colitis

The distinction between acute diverticulitis and ulcerative colitis should not be difficult. Rectoscopy virtually always reveals proctitis in patients with ulcerative colitis (see Chapter 29). The importance of performing even a limited proctoscopy before embarking on surgery for acute diverticulitis cannot be overestimated. The presence of inflammatory changes in the rectum or a high index of suspicion of inflammatory bowel disease would certainly indicate the need for medical management or an alternative operative approach.

Ischemic Colitis

Ischemic colitis may pose a problem in differential diagnosis. This is particularly true if the ischemic changes include the rectosigmoid. However, patients with disease limited to this area usually present with frequent bowel movements and rectal bleeding. Abdominal pain suggests a more fulminant and extensive manifestation of ischemic colitis. The presence of thumb printing on the plain abdominal film, particularly in the splenic flexure region, suggests ischemia (see Chapter 28).

Other

Acute appendicitis, pelvic inflammatory disease, and urinary tract disease such as infection and nephrolithiasis are important to exclude.

▶ CLINICAL PRESENTATIONS

Acute Diverticulitis

Acute diverticulitis is a common emergency. In most patients, it is mild and may even be treated as an outpatient with antibiotics. Imaging is not usually contributory in such individuals. If the condition does not settle or worsen, imaging can then be carried out. Many patients, however, will require admission to hospital owing to the severity of the clinical condition. It is now accepted that in patients with general or localized physical signs, or where there is a suspicion of a septic complication, a CT scan is indicated as soon as can reasonably be obtained. In acute diverticulitis, there is thickening of the wall of the sigmoid colon in most cases (>4 mm is taken as indicative), with evidence of inflammation (which may be extraluminal such as fat

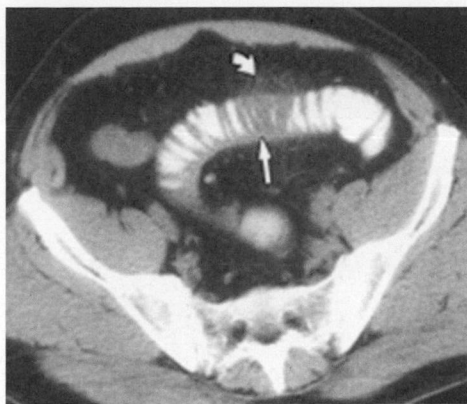

FIGURE 27-10. Acute diverticulitis. A 41-year-old man with acute diverticulitis of sigmoid colon. Axial CT scan obtained with colonic contrast material and 5-mm collimation shows inflammatory wall thickening (*straight arrow*) and fat stranding (*curved arrow*). (From Kircher MF, Rhea JT, Kihiczak D, et al. Frequency, sensitivity, and specificity of individual signs of diverticulitis on thin-section helical CT with colonic contrast material: experience with 312 cases. *AJR Am J Roentgenol.* 2002;178(6):1313–1318.)

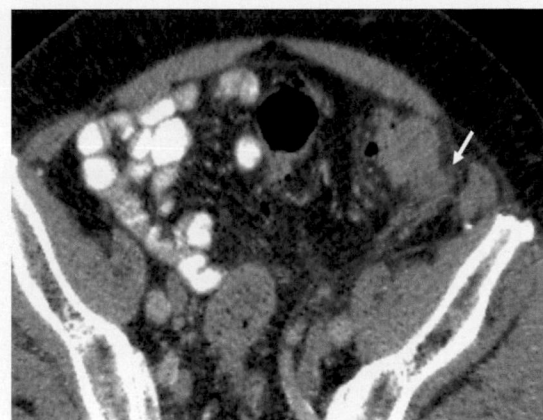

FIGURE 27-11. Computed tomography showing acute diverticulitis with paracolic abscess formation (*arrow*).

stranding [Figure 27-10]). It will also demonstrate whether local paracolic or pelvic abscess formation has occurred (Figure 27-11), or whether there is evidence of extraluminal gas or liquid suggesting peritonitis (Figure 27-12).

Acute diverticulitis can either be an uncomplicated inflammation of the sigmoid colon without perforation, local or free, or it may be associated with perforation which if contained will be manifested as a local abscess, or if free, as peritonitis. Peritonitis may be purulent or fecal.

Complicated diverticulitis has been classified by Hinchey and colleagues[129] as follows (Figure 27-13)

Stage I—Pericolic abscess or phlegmon
Stage II—Pelvic, intra-abdominal, or retroperitoneal abscess
Stage III—Generalized purulent peritonitis
Stage IV—Generalized fecal peritonitis

Clinical Presentation
History
Patients with acute diverticulitis complain primarily of abdominal pain. There may be a prior history of such complaints or of "diverticulitis" or "diverticular disease." John and colleagues, in reporting a series of 100 patients seen as an emergency with a suspected diagnosis of diverticular disease, found that 54 had had a past history of similar abdominal pain.[147] The pain is usually located in the left lower quadrant and tends to be constant rather than colicky in nature. It may radiate to the back, left flank, groin, and leg, although these features may also be seen with an irritable bowel. The duration and severity of symptoms are quite variable, depending on whether the patient has a localized or a diffuse process. Nausea and vomiting are uncommon unless there is some element of intestinal obstruction. A change in bowel habit is frequently observed. Additionally, there may be an absence of bowel movements, or the patient may be experiencing diarrhea.

E. JOHN HINCHEY (1934–PRESENT)

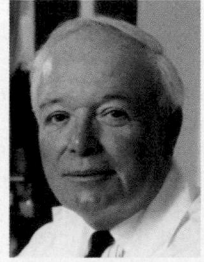

John Hinchey was born in Ontario, Canada. He attended King George School and the Belleville Collegiate Institute prior to enrolling in the Queen's University Medical School in Kingston, graduating in 1959. He served his internship and surgical residency at the Montreal General Hospital. From 1962 to 1966, he was involved in research both at the University Surgical Clinic and in the Department of Surgery at McGill University in Montreal. He went on to achieve his master of sciences and became a fellow of both the Royal College of Surgeons of Canada and the American College of Surgeons. Although serving as an assistant surgeon at the Montreal General Hospital, he began to explore the concept of different approaches to the management of complicated diverticulitis based on the severity of the presentation. However, he credits the famous Australian colon and rectal surgeon, E.S.R. Hughes for initiating the concept 10 years earlier. His ultimate concept of staging evolved over a number of years, culminating in the paper in which he described his four stages. Hinchey has held teaching appointments in the department of anatomy and physiology and ultimately rose to become professor of surgery and director of the Division of General Surgery at Montreal General Hospital/McGill University. Among his many recognitions, he has received the honor of John R. Markle Scholar in Academic Medicine. He is a member of numerous surgical societies, including the American Surgical Association, and served as president of both the Canadian Association of Clinical Surgeons and the Canadian Association of General Surgeons. He has also served as chairman of the Examining Board for General Surgery of the Royal College of Physicians and Surgeons of Canada. Upon achieving emeritus status in 1999, he became director of the Surgical Scientist Program at McGill.

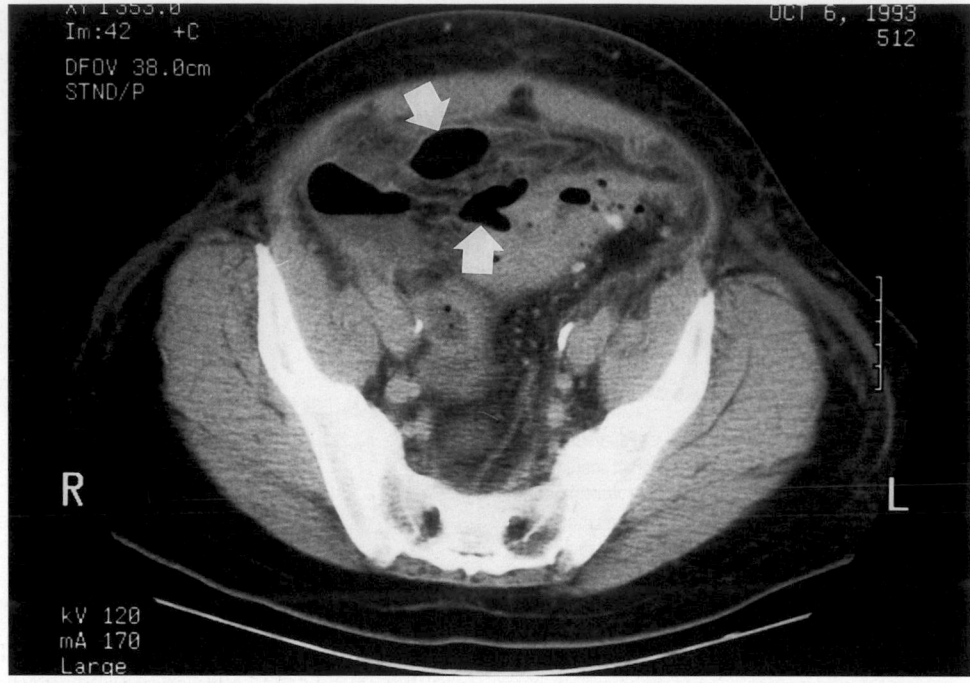

FIGURE 27-12. Computed tomography demonstrates perforated diverticulitis with extraluminal gas (*arrows*).

Individuals with acute diverticular disease often mention urinary symptoms (dysuria, urgency, frequency, nocturia), which may be attributable to irritation by the inflammatory mass on the wall of the bladder. A urinary tract infection may imply communication with the bowel (see later). Passage of gas in the urine or per vaginam is diagnostic of a fistula (see also later). Fever is also commonly observed in those with acute diverticulitis. This is usually of a low grade, but if peritonitis develops or if an abscess is present, the temperature can be considerably elevated or even depressed in patients with septic shock.

Rectal bleeding has been thought to be part of the symptom complex of diverticulosis, but there is confusion on this issue. Massive lower gastrointestinal bleeding in the presence of diverticular disease can be caused by a vascular malformation rather than diverticulosis, but patients with diverticular disease may also bleed from a diverticulum.[40] This aspect of the presentation is discussed in Chapter 28.

Physical Examination
Physical examination will vary according to the severity of the condition. The patient may be systemically well with mild tenderness localized to the left iliac fossa. The white blood cell count may be normal or mildly raised. The C-reactive protein (CRP) level is a more sensitive indication of inflammation and may well be raised when the white blood cell count is normal. In a series of 100 patients admitted as an emergency with a clinical diagnosis of diverticular disease, the CRP was 281 mg/L in those with complicated and 54 mg/L in those with uncomplicated disease.[147] In contrast, the patient may be grossly septic, either with peritonitis or with localized abscess. In such a person, tenderness will be marked, with guarding and rigidity if there is peritonitis. Bowel sounds may be absent. In short, the clinical features of an acute abdominal catastrophe may be evident. Tenderness and a mass in the pelvis from a sigmoid phlegmon or abscess may be noted on rectal or vaginal examination. Also,

an abdominal mass may be felt. Extraperitoneal infection can present with back, buttock, and hip and leg pain; a positive psoas sign; a lower extremity abscess; perineal and scrotal pain and swelling; and subcutaneous, mediastinal, and cervical emphysema.[245] Perforation below the peritoneal reflection can lead to a buttock abscess and a consequent anorectal fistula (see Chapters 13 and 14).[78] Pathways of extraperitoneal pelvic abscess spread to the gluteal area are through the suprapiriformis and infrapiriformis fossae, to the external genitalia via the obturator canal, and to the ischiorectal fossa through the pelvic floor (Figure 27-14).

Imaging
Data are available on the accuracy of water-soluble contrast enema (CE), CT, ultrasonography (US), and MRI in diagnosing acute diverticulitis. Plain x-ray of the chest and abdomen may show free gas and may reveal nonspecific features in up to 50% of patients with diverticulitis and is, therefore, considered inadequate in giving sufficient information in most cases.[190] In a useful systematic review, Liljegren and colleagues carried out a search of the literature for articles dealing with imaging of acute diverticular disease with the particular purpose of assessing their quality.[175] They found 49 of which only 20 were found to pass the test of quality. Of the 29 excluded, 14 were reviews, 6 did not use a reference standard, 8 gave no information on specificity, and 1 was duplicated. Of the 20 included articles, there was 1 (ultrasound compared with CT) with level 1b evidence,[240] 3 (ultrasound 2, magnetic resonance 1) with 2b level,[5,326,343] with the remaining being level 4.

Computed Tomography
Computed tomography began to be used for the diagnosis and assessment of acute diverticulitis in the 1980s.[21,27,123,165] Labs and colleagues evaluated 42 patients suspected of having diverticulitis, of whom 22 were found to have a complication and 20 without a complication.[165] Of the 22 patients, 10 had an abscess and 12 a colovesical fistula. The abscesses were

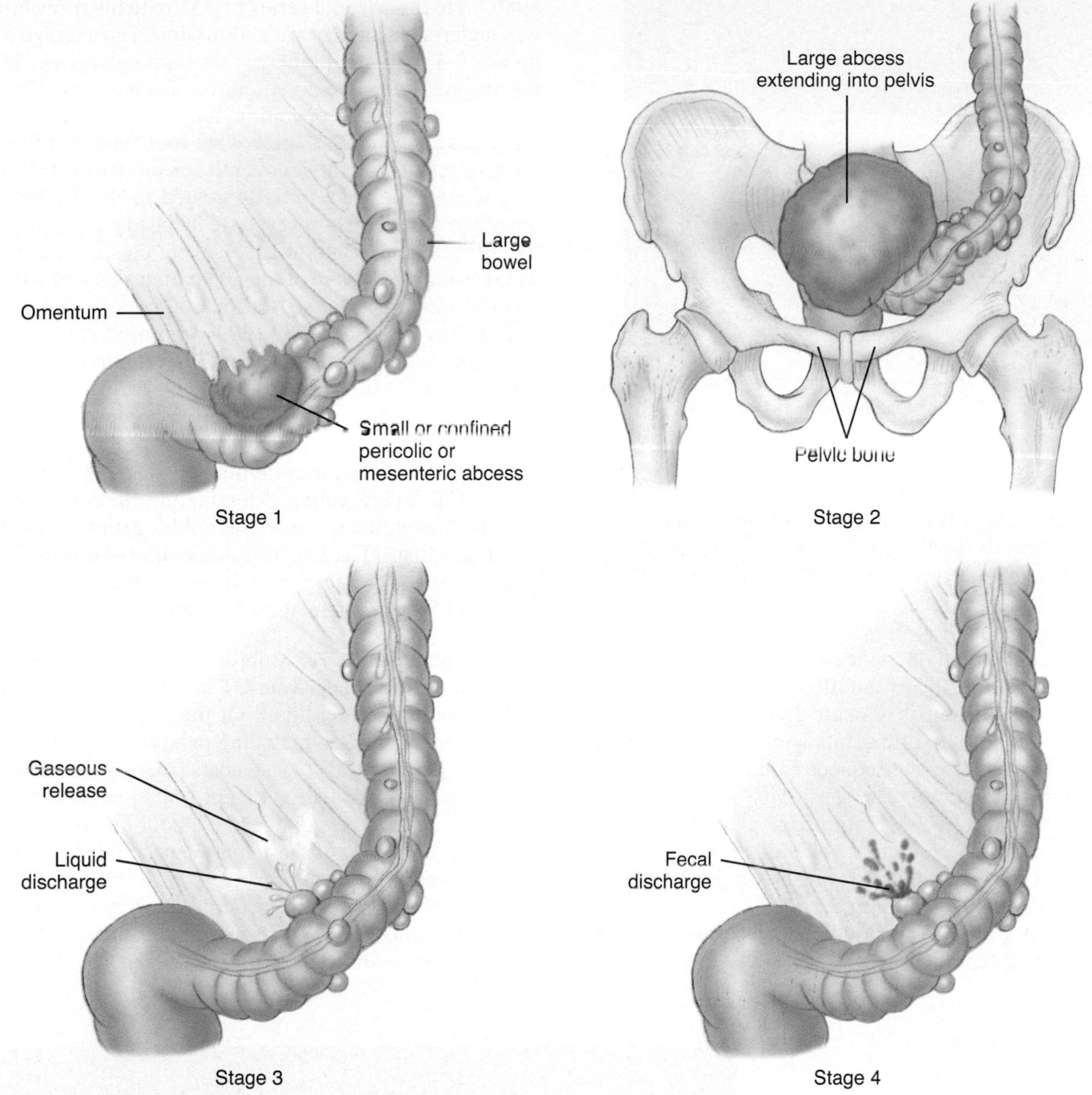

Omentum

Large
bowel

Small or confined
pericolic or
mesenteric abcess

Stage 1

Large abcess
extending into pelvis

Pelvic bone

Stage 2

Gaseous
release

Liquid
discharge

Stage 3

Fecal
discharge

Stage 4

FIGURE 27-13. Hinchey classification of complicated acute diverticulitis.

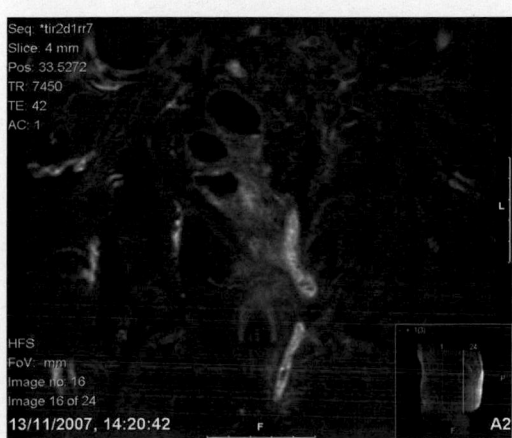

FIGURE 27-14. Magnetic resonance scan of fistula from sigmoid colon to the perineum in a patient with diverticular disease.

correctly identified in all cases by the presence of diverticula, a segmentally thickened colon, and an extravisceral fluid collection. An example of acute diverticulitis with abscess formation is shown in Figure 27-8. Only 25% of those studied by contrast enema were thought to have abscesses. Of the 12 patients with a colovesical fistula, this was confirmed by CT through the identification of air in the bladder, thickened colon adjacent to an area of thickened bladder, and the presence of colonic diverticula. Contrast enema identified only three of eight cases with fistula in whom it was performed. Raval and coworkers recommended that CT be performed with the administration of a rectal contrast medium in order to demonstrate the presence or absence as well as the origin of the colonic inflammation (Figure 27-15), to assess pericolic extent, and to confirm the presence or absence of a colovesical fistula (Figure 27-16).[244]

Hansen and colleagues, in a retrospective study of 243 patients with acute diverticulitis, reported that the sensitivity

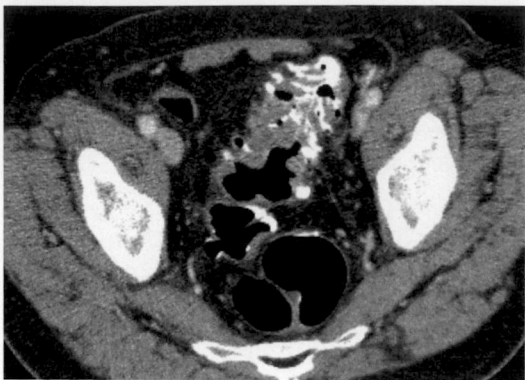

FIGURE 27-15. *CT* with contrast in the lumen demonstrates configuration of severe diverticular hypertrophy but no associated inflammatory changes or thickening.

of CT was 97.5%, with an overall accuracy of 97.1%.[123] A similar sensitivity (98%) was reported by Ambrosetti and colleagues among 470 patients.[16] Pradel and coworkers reported a level 1b evidence prospective study of 64 patients with acute diverticulitis in whom the diagnosis was confirmed subsequently in 33, with 24 patients being diagnosed with another disease.[240] Seven failed to have their diagnosis established. The diagnosis of acute diverticular disease was confirmed on follow-up of patients with typical clinical features, supplemented by subsequent pathology where available and by colonoscopy. The sensitivity and specificity of CT was 85% and 84%, with a positive predictive value of 81% and a negative predictive value of 88%. CT has also been thought to be particularly valuable in the diagnosis of right-sided diverticulitis (Figure 27-17).[70]

In a recent article, Ambrosetti reviewed his experience based on a long-term prospective study that commenced in 1986.[15] He described a series of 355 patients in whom a CT was undertaken shortly after admission. The average follow-up was 9.5 years. He points out the high sensitivity of CT for the diagnosis of acute diverticulitis. There were 132 patients who needed an early operation, and CT correctly diagnosed them in 123 instances. There were four false and five false-positive results, giving an overall sensitivity of 97%. Of the 79 patients who were initially treated medically but subsequently required early surgery, 42 had had a CT scan. Thirty-two (76%) were found to have severe changes on the scan, whereas only 74 (24%) of the 303 patients having successful medical treatment did so. Of the 106 patients found on CT to have severe disease, 32 (30%) required early operation compared with 10 (4%) of the 239 patients with moderate CT changes.

CT was also found to be predictive of complications in the long term. In a subgroup of 118 patients followed more than 9.5 years, the greatest complication rate (54% at 5 years) was in CT-severe young patients, and the lowest (19% at 5 years) was in the CT-moderate older patients. Ambrosetti concluded that CT is sensitive at the time of original presentation and is a predictor of failure of medical treatment as well as of long-term, recurrent complications.[15]

CT as a Predictor of Outcome. Ambrosetti and colleagues reported 107 patients who underwent CT scanning after an initial attack of acute diverticulitis.[21] Of these, 24 (22%) continued to have complications, including persistent diverticulitis (9), recurrent diverticulitis (7), stenosis (6), residual abscess (1), and colovesical fistula (1). Eight (44%) of the 18 patients younger than 50 years of age had a poor outcome compared with only 16 (18%) of the remaining 89. Of the 76 patients who showed mild changes on CT, 12 (16%) subsequently experienced a complication compared with 11 (48%) of the 23 patients whose CT showed evidence of persistent abscess formation or localized gas. In a further report of 542 patients

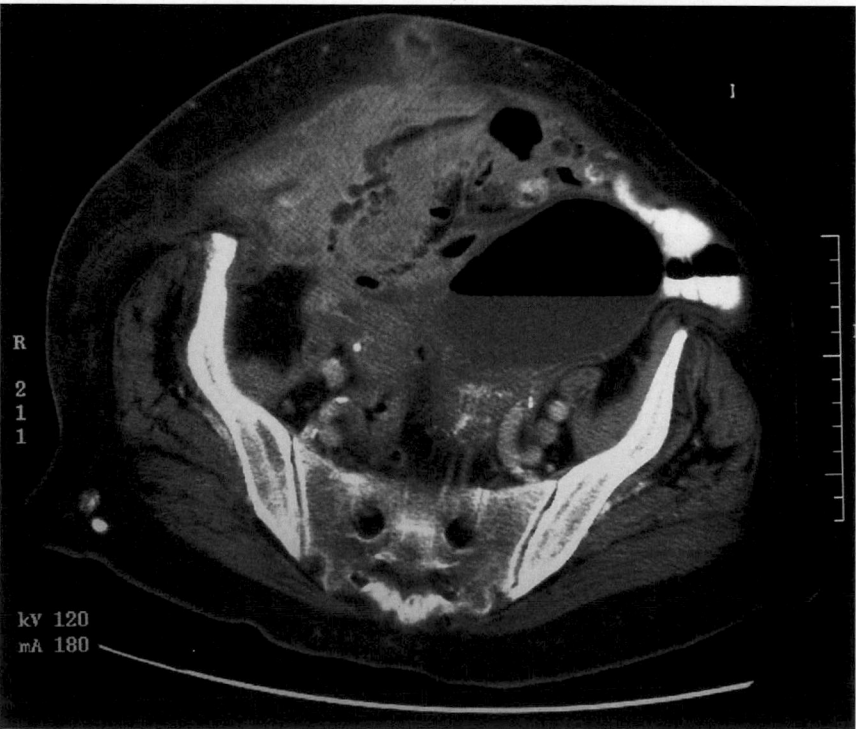

FIGURE 27-16. Computed tomography demonstrates an abnormal sigmoid colon with multiple diverticula and with a large amount of air within the bladder consistent with a colovesical fistula.

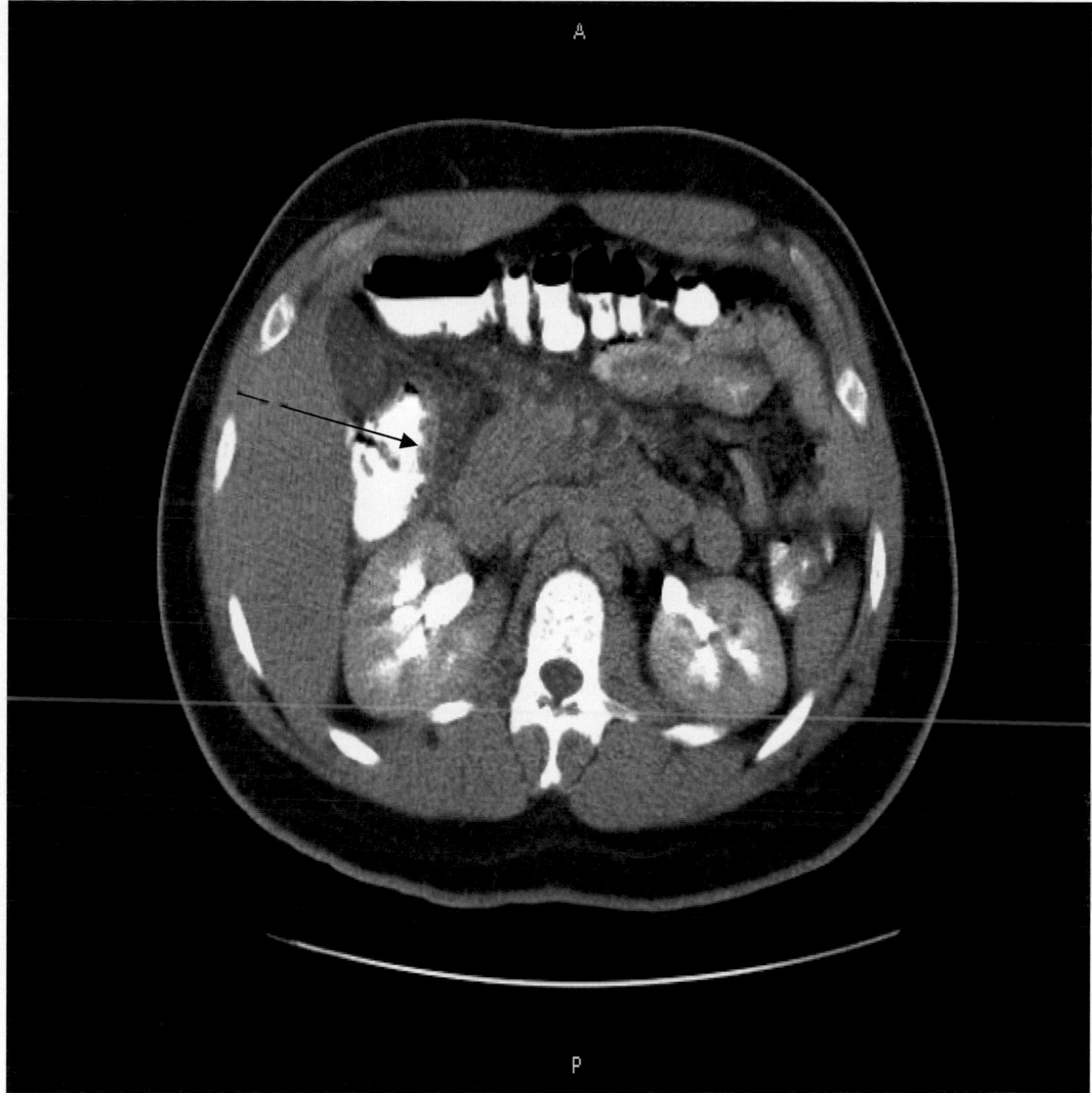

FIGURE 27-17. Right colon diverticulitis. Computed tomography demonstrates eccentric inflammation on the medial wall of the proximal ascending colon, with wall thickening (*arrow*) and with mucosal preservation consistent with diverticulitis. (Courtesy of Avraham Belizon, MD.)

who had the criteria for acute diverticular disease, the same authors reported that 26% of patients with severe findings on CT that had been carried out within 72 hours of admission failed medical treatment. This compared with only 4% in whom the CT findings were moderate. They confirmed that patients with severe CT findings were more likely to have recurrent symptoms than those with moderate changes (36% vs. 17%).[16] These differences were statistically significant.

CT Compared with Other Imaging Modalities

WATER-SOLUBLE CONTRAST ENEMA. Ambrosetti and colleagues compared CT with contrast enema in two publications[16,19]: the first included 420 patients and the second 470, who had both examinations. The results are qualitatively similar. This is

not surprising because the second study was an expansion of the patients accrued in the first. The results of the second report are given next. Those attending between 1986 and 1997 underwent a CT and water-soluble CE within 72 hours of admission. Those with peritonitis were operated on immediately and were, therefore, excluded from the study. Of the 470 patients who had had both examinations, 69 were found to have an abscess on CT, but only 20 of these were seen on CE. The overall diagnostic sensitivity of CT and CE was 98% and 92%, a small but statistically significant difference. Severe disease was detected by CT in 26% compared with 9% by CE. It was possible to stratify severity by CT (see previously) into severe and moderate, which were related to failure of medical treatment (26% vs. 19%) and the chance

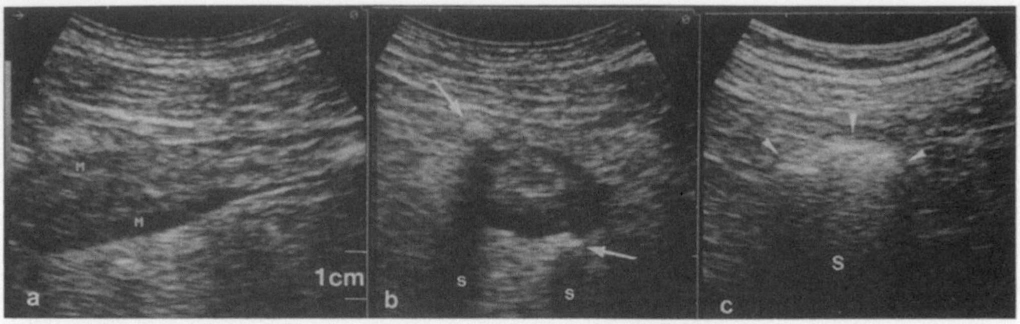

FIGURE 27-18. Sigmoid diverticulitis. Ultrasound examination. **A:** Longitudinal view of the affected segment showing varying degrees of mural thickening and luminal narrowing. M, hypoechoic muscularis externa. **B:** Transverse view. *Arrows* point to an adjacent echogenic diverticula casting sound shadows (S). **C:** Transverse section of normal sigmoid colon showing less than 3-mm wall thickness (*arrowheads*). Reverberation artifacts and sound shadowing (S) are due to highly reflective luminal gas. (Courtesy of Schwerk WB, Schwarz S, Rothmund M. Sonography in acute colonic diverticulitis. A prospective study. *Dis Colon Rectum.* 1992;35(11):1077–1084.)

of a subsequent poor outcome (36% vs. 17%). The authors concluded that CT was better than CE and that CT had the advantage of predicting the outcome more accurately.

Hansen and colleagues obtained a similar result, reporting a sensitivity of 97.5% for CT and 71.6% for CE in diagnosing acute diverticulitis.[123]

ABDOMINAL ULTRASOUND. A prospective study was undertaken by Pradel and colleagues in 1997 in which 64 patients with a clinical diagnosis of acute diverticulitis and who underwent CT and US were assessed by a blinded observer.[240] Subsequent follow-up including colonoscopy and histologic examination of the resected specimen confirmed the condition in 33. There was no significant difference (CT vs. US) in the sensitivity (91% vs. 85%), specificity (77% vs. 84%), positive predictive value (PPV) (81% vs. 85%), and negative predictive value (NPV) (88% vs. 84%). CT and US identified abscess formation in 6 patients, and CT demonstrated an abscess in 3; this was not shown on US. The authors concluded that there was little difference between the studies.

Other reports of ultrasound have supported this finding. Verbanck and colleagues carried out a level 2b evidence prospective study of 123 patients with a clinical diagnosis of acute diverticulitis.[326] Of these, the diagnosis was subsequently confirmed in 52. The sensitivity, specificity, PPV, and NPV were 84.6%, 80.3%, 76.0%, and 87.7%, respectively. They found that hypoechoic bowel wall with a thickness of more than 4 mm was present in 44 of the 52 patients and was therefore a useful radiologic sign indicating acute diverticulitis when clinical suspicion was present. Zielke and colleagues, in a prospective observational level 2b evidence study of 57 consecutive patients, used length and thickening of the bowel wall as criteria for inflammation and involvement.[343] The diagnosis of acute diverticular disease was made by US in 48, giving an accuracy of 84%, with 9 false negatives and 3 nondiagnostic results. Schwerk and colleagues carried out high resolution ultrasound in 130 patients who presented with "abdominal complaints."[280] Of these, 52 (40%) were ultimately confirmed as having diverticulitis. Clinical examination had shown the diagnosis to be "highly suspected," "possible or equivocal," or "very unlikely" in 19 (36.5%), 24 (46.2%), and 9 (17.3%), respectively. Ultrasound was highly accurate, with a sensitivity, specificity, PPV, and NPV of 98.1%, 97.5%, 96.2%, and 98.5%, respectively. The signs of particular value were

a hypoechoic thickened wall and a "target-like" appearance of the bowel in cross section. This latter finding is felt to be due to inflammatory changes and muscular thickening of the bowel wall (Figure 27-18). Of the 13 patients with abscess formation, this was correctly identified in 12, 7 of which were successfully drained percutaneously. A hemispheric mass, the "dome sign," has also been described.[158]

Computed Tomographic Colonography (CTC). Computed tomographic colonography has been compared with conventional colonoscopy in patients with diverticular disease. Lefere and colleagues studied 160 consecutive patients and found that CTC demonstrated wall thickening in 55 (36%), diverticula in 52%, and fecoliths in 39%.[171] The results were similar to that of colonoscopy. In a similar study, Hjern and colleagues, in comparing CTC with colonoscopy in 50 patients by blinded evaluation of the images, demonstrated diverticular disease in 96% and 90%, respectively.[130] The rate of agreement between them was good ($k = 0.64$). Gollub and coworkers performed CTC on 150 patients and found that mucosal thickening in diverticular disease was related to decreased sigmoid distensibility.[109] These results suggested that CTC may be useful in selected cases in whom colonoscopy is either not possible or too dangerous. Flor and associates also found good sensitivity and specificity for CTC (Figure 27-19).[94]

Magnetic Resonance Colonography

Ajaj and colleagues investigated magnetic resonance colonography (MRC) in a prospective level 2b study using dark-lumen MRC in 40 patients presenting with suspected diverticulitis.[5] T1-weighted images were taken after an aqueous enema and gadolinium-based contrast. Bowel wall thickening and pericolic reaction, including mesenteric infiltration indicating diverticular disease, were seen in 23 patients. The remaining 17 were classified as not having diverticular disease, 4 of whom were judged to be false negatives. Of the 23 positive patients, there were 3 false positives due to carcinoma. There is clearly the need to exercise caution in interpreting the images, but the authors concluded that MRC is a useful investigation, particularly when colonoscopy is either not possible or not indicated as a consequence of severe inflammation. MRC has the additional advantage of being able to demonstrate other colonic pathology.

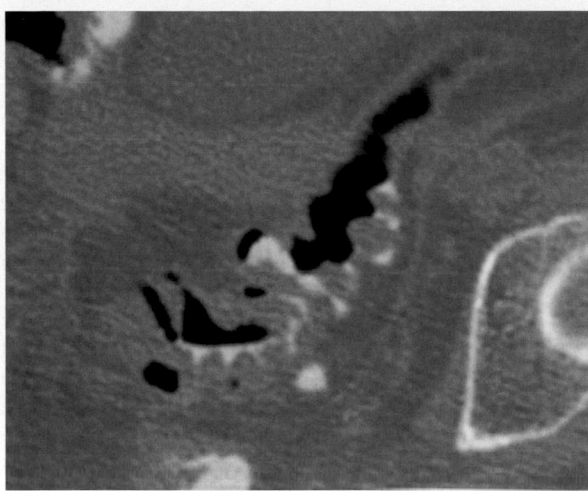

FIGURE 27-19. Computed tomographic colonography (CTC). Example of a patient with severe diverticular disease. Axial prone CTC image shows diffuse wall thickening of the sigmoid colon with deformation and lumen narrowing. (Courtesy of Flor N, Rigamonti P, Leo G, et al. Technical quality of CT colonography in relation with diverticular disease. *Eur J Radiol.* 2012;81(3):e250–e254.)

In another study, MRI-based colonography was compared with spiral CT in 14 patients.[276] The technique involves the administration of an magnetic resonance (MR) opaque enema. In this study, 56 bowel segments were examined, of which 52 were judged to be of adequate image quality. The authors concluded that MRC was as good as CT without the concern for ionizing radiation. It was conceded, however, that there were differences in the availability of the two methods. An example of an MRC image in diverticular disease is shown in Figure 27-20.

Comment

When the patient is admitted with a suspected diagnosis of acute diverticular disease, the choice of imaging will depend on the severity of the condition. This is based on clinical assessment. Because the purpose is to aid in diagnosis and

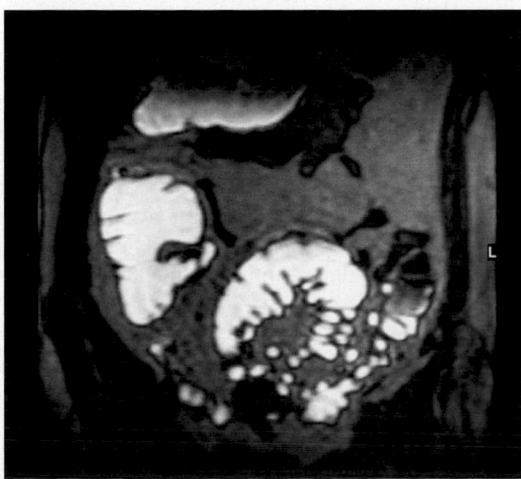

FIGURE 27-20. Magnetic resonance coronal three-dimensional flash image revealing multiple diverticula within an elongated sigmoid colon. (Courtesy of Schreyer AG, Fürst A, Agha A, et al. Magnetic resonance imaging based colonography for diagnosis and assessment of diverticulosis and diverticulitis. *Int J Colorectal Dis.* 2004;19(5):474–480.)

to assess the severity of the condition, imaging should be used in an intelligent manner. Thus, if the clinical diagnosis is one of mild diverticulitis, then it is reasonable to treat with antibiotics without any imaging. As will be outlined in the following section, when medical management is considered, many such patients can be treated as an outpatient with the expectation of rapid resolution of symptoms. To submit such individuals to a CT scan will usually not contribute to decision making and will only incur radiation and expense. It is a little publicized fact that a CT scan of the abdomen and pelvis is equivalent in radiation to 300 to 400 chest x-rays. However, if the patient's condition deteriorates, a CT scan or ultrasound will be necessary.

It is generally believed that CT scan is the diagnostic modality of choice in this condition, but it should be noted that the results of ultrasound are only slightly inferior to CT. However, its ability to detect abscess formation is significantly below that of CT. There is also the value that CT offers in predicting the clinical response to medical treatment and the possibility of long-term complications. Additionally, there is the advantage that the clinician can interpret the images, whereas with ultrasound, someone familiar with the technique is required to inform the clinician of the radio-pathologic situation. There is, however, merit in considering ultrasound in a patient who may require more than one attempt at percutaneous drainage. If a collection is accessible to ultrasound drainage, this may be the better option because there is no radiation hazard with this technique. Clinical discretion always should be used in weighing whether to image and if so what form to use.

► TREATMENT

Acute Diverticulitis (Uncomplicated)

General Statement

In 2009, Etzioni and colleagues published data on the overall burden of diverticulitis in the United States and on the incidence of surgery performed in those admitted with acute diverticulitis.[86] They used the NIS for 1998 and 2005 in order to analyze the outcome of 267,000 admissions for acute diverticulitis and 33,500 elective operations in patients who had had an acute attack. From 1998 to 2004/2005, there was a fall in the proportion of persons who underwent surgery following admission for acute diverticulitis from 17.4% to 14.4%. The prevalence of stoma creation was unchanged at 56.0% and 56.5%. Percutaneous drainage was carried out in only 1.4% of patients in 1998 but rose to 2.5% by 2005. It is evident, therefore, that the vast majority of patients admitted with acute diverticulitis are managed medically. Surgery is indicated for patients with peritonitis, for those with an abscess which does not resolve with antibiotics, or with a minimally invasive drainage procedure (or if it is inaccessible to drainage), and when there is failure to improve more than 24 to 48 hours after initiating medical treatment. The reader is referred to recent reviews on this subject.[120,142–144,177,297]

Risk Factors for Surgery

Age

Age younger than 50 years has been regarded by many to be a risk factor that increases the chance of surgery being required.[2,217,271] Mäkelä and colleagues, in a series of 366 patients followed for more than 10 years, found that males younger than 50 years had more initial operations and more recurrences than other groups.[183] A similar observation was made by Chautems and coworkers in 118 patients followed prospectively.[52] Other articles from the same unit based on the same patient group support the view that patients younger than 50 years were significantly more prone to recurrence and complications after initially successful conservative treatment, whereas older individuals required operation significantly more often during their initial hospitalization.[21,22] Vignati and colleagues reported 40 patients with acute diverticulitis younger than 50 years and who were followed for a minimum of 5 years.[329] Ten underwent immediate surgery. During follow-up, a further 10 of the remaining 30 patients underwent an operation. Although the authors concluded that surgery in this population following a single episode of diverticulitis that resolves was not recommended, the opposite view could be taken from the data. The risk in young patients led Konvolinka and associates to the opinion that any patient younger than 40 years should be considered for surgery even after one attack.[157] Spivak and colleagues evaluated 63 patients younger than 45 years who had been treated for a presumptive diagnosis of acute diverticulitis.[289] Two-thirds responded to antibiotics and bowel rest, whereas the remainder required an emergency operation. At surgery, 20% were found to have appendicitis (which they point out must always be considered in the differential diagnosis). However, others conclude that young patients do not have a more virulent form of the disease nor is the risk of recurrence greater than in older patients. Biondo and coworkers divided 327 patients presenting with acute diverticulitis into two groups.[38] This included 72 younger than 50 years of age and 255 older than 50 years. In those treated medically, recurrence occurred in 25.5% and 22.3% in each group, respectively. Operative mortality for elective resection was 0% and 2.2% and for emergency surgery, 0% and 34.0%. The authors concluded that the disease was not more aggressive in younger patients.

Guzzo and Hyman reported the outcome of 762 patients presenting with sigmoid diverticulitis at one institution over an 11-year period.[116] Of these, 238 (31%) underwent immediate surgery. The risk of this operation was no different in patients older than or younger than 50 years of age. During follow-up, however, elective surgery was carried out in 40% of those younger than 50 years compared with 26% of those older than 50. Of the 196 patients younger than 50 years who were treated medically, only 1 (0.5%) developed a late perforation. Owing to the infrequency of serious later complications, the authors concluded that elective surgery in young patients having had an acute episode of diverticulitis is not warranted.

Comment. Many of the studies estimating the effect of age on outcome are small and lack definitions of what is severe and nonsevere disease. Moreover, there may have been a misdiagnosis of diverticular disease in some cases. The available data give little evidence to support a different management strategy in younger individuals.

Sex

There is less information on sex than on age, although the data of Mäkelä and colleagues suggest that males may be at higher risk of complications and are more likely to require surgery.[183] Epidemiologically, however, more admissions and more operations appear to involve women.[150] There is evidence, moreover, to suggest that males may be more prone to hemorrhage than are females,[188] and younger males with diverticulitis may have more severe CT changes than females.[121]

Drugs

Steroids and NSAIDs are the most consistently identified risk factor for diverticular perforation. These agents account for one-fifth of all cases. It has been suggested that mucosal blood flow falls, owing to the inhibitory effect of NSAIDs on prostaglandin. In a retrospective study of 192 patients with diverticular disease, Corder reported odds ratios for sepsis outside the colon of 13.2 (95% CI, 1.81–96.5) for steroid use and 4.85 (95% CI, 1.58–14.8) for nonsteroidal medication.[65] Campbell and Steele reported that 24 (48%) of 50 patients with complicated disease were taking NSAIDs compared with 18% of a randomly selected group of 50 emergency admissions and 20% of 50 patients with uncomplicated diverticular disease.[50] Others have made a similar observation.[107]

Nash and colleagues investigated the associated factors among 58 patients presenting with perforated diverticular disease over a 2-year period from a population of 531,241. This represented an annual incidence of 4/100,000 population. The incidents of NSAID and opiate consumption were 29% and 26%, respectively. The authors speculated on the possible causative roles of these drugs. Certainly, if this association be accurate, the use of these agents should be a source of concern.[124,197] In another study, the medication taken by 54 patients who had perforated diverticular disease was compared with 183 patients who had verified nonperforated diverticular disease. The odds ratios for NSAIDs, opiates, and steroids were 3.56, 4.51, and 28.28, respectively.[236]

A prospective study of 92 patients with diverticular disease followed over a 3-year period revealed that perforation occurred in 19 of the 31 patients taking NSAIDs compared with 8 of 61 who were not.[337] Further evidence for an association with opiates comes from a study of 899 patients with perforation presenting over a 15-year period (1990 to 2005).[138] These were compared with 8,980 matched controls. Odds ratios for opiate and steroid ingestion were 2.16 and 2.74, respectively. There was no increased risk with calcium antagonists or aspirin. Statins were associated with a reduced risk (OR = 0.44).

NSAIDs also appear to increase the chance of hemorrhage.[313]

The Immunocompromised Patient

Patients on long-term steroid therapy (e.g., for rheumatoid arthritis), those who are immunocompromised, who have renal failure, or who have undergone organ transplantation are prone to a variety of colonic complications, including colonic dilatation, intestinal obstruction, ischemic colitis, necrotizing enterocolitis, ulceration, hemorrhage, and perforated diverticulitis.[4,36,54,117,140,149,155,156,195,250,269] The manifestation of free perforation (Figures 27-21 through 27-23) is much more likely to occur in renal transplant recipients, whereas mesenteric abscess or walled-off perforation is more commonly found in individuals with diverticular disease who have not undergone transplantation. The use of immunosuppressive agents including steroids is believed to be the agent responsible. These drugs can therefore have catastrophic consequences. Even when a person does not manifest systemic signs and symptoms, surgery should be performed early and should always include a resection. These patients must have the focus of sepsis removed; diversion and drainage

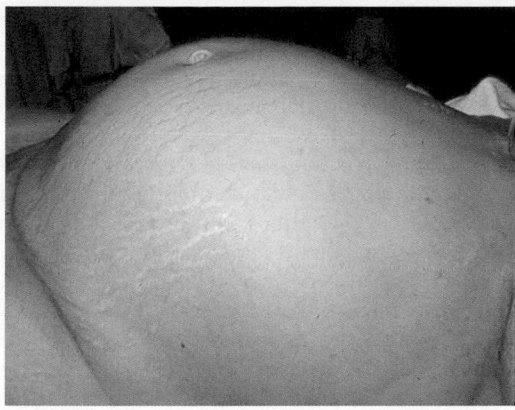

FIGURE 27-21. Free colonic perforation with pneumoperitoneum producing profound abdominal distension in an immunocompromised patient.

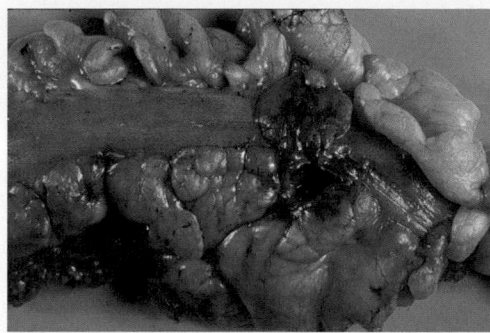

FIGURE 27-23. Perforated sigmoid colon in an immunosuppressed patient. Note the lack of inflammatory response.

simply are not sufficient in this circumstance. Nonoperative treatment is highly unlikely to carry the patient through the hospitalization to discharge. Because of diminished host resistance, perforation or abscess will not resolve with conservative therapy. Such an approach will delay needed surgical intervention.[10,186,234]

Of 1,401 consecutive patients who underwent renal transplantation between 1951 and 1995 at the Brigham and Women's Hospital in Boston, 30 experienced colonic

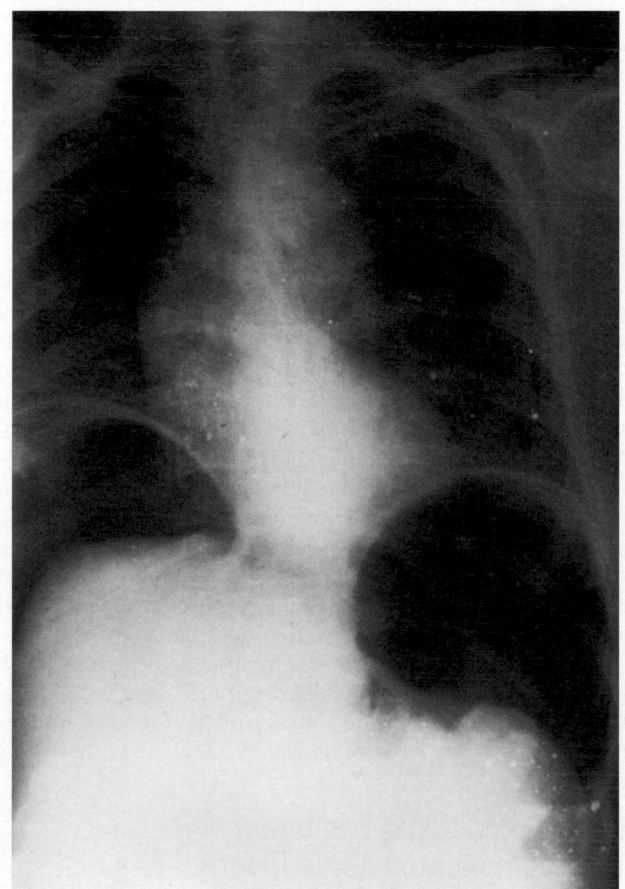

FIGURE 27-22. Upright abdominal roentgenogram reveals gas under both hemidiaphragms, a consequence of perforated diverticulitis.

perforation (34 episodes).[794] In those operated on within 24 hours, the mortality was 22%. This was compared with 47% when this interval was longer. Mortality was related to the intensity of the immunosuppression. Twenty-eight percent of the perforations occurred within the first month, and 47% were seen within 3 months. The masking effects of corticosteroids on symptoms and signs need to be considered when evaluating such individuals. A recent review of the colorectal complications of patients with renal failure deals in particular with diverticular disease.[232]

An increased incidence of colon perforation has also been observed in individuals who have undergone lung transplantation.[30] Since the inception of the lung transplant program at the University of Colorado, 60 procedures had been performed by 1996, with 4 patients suffering spontaneous colonic perforation (7%). Moreover, bowel perforation has been demonstrated to be a frequent cause of mortality after pediatric orthotopic liver transplantation. In the series from the University of California at Los Angeles, 24 bowel perforations occurred in 246 recipients (10%).[282] Most involved the small bowel, predominantly at the Roux-en-Y limb, but 8 involved the transverse colon or terminal ileum.

Starnes and colleagues reported 25 patients with colonic diverticulitis complicating renal failure.[292] Most described acute abdominal pain. The overall mortality was 28%, with no correlation between survival rate and the type of operation performed. Koneru and coworkers noted that 6 of 7 patients (86%) survived when surgery was performed within 24 hours of perforation, whereas only 25% survived when further delay was permitted.[156]

► MEDICAL TREATMENT

The management of acute diverticulitis will depend on the severity of the condition. Clinical assessment will indicate whether the patient is mildly ill or whether local signs indicating peritoneal irritation are severe enough to require admission. Factors such as prior episodes and whether the patient is immunocompromised should be taken into account. The presence or absence of tachycardia, fever, the degree of local tenderness in the left iliac fossa, the white blood cell count, and CRP level will all help in this assessment. If one is in doubt, a CT scan should be requested. The duration and nature of symptoms have an important bearing on the outcome of the disease. Parks noted that one-half of the patients with diverticular disease of the colon were in good health until less than 1 month before hospitalization, and three-fourths had symptoms for less than 1 year.[228] Individuals with some of the most serious complications were essentially asymptomatic until just before admission. One may, therefore, postulate based on the patient's history what the likelihood of resolution will be with medical management.

Antibiotics

Antibiotics alone or in combination should cover aerobic and anaerobic organisms, such as *Bacteroides*, *Clostridium*, *Escherichia coli*, *Klebsiella*, *Proteus*, *Streptococcus*, and *Enterobacter*. In a detailed review, Jacobs sets out the present understanding of best medical treatment.[142] Antibiotics are the mainstay of treatment with the usual regimen of administration for 7 to 10 days. Various combinations are recommended including metronidazole and quinolone such as ciprofloxacin, metronidazole and trimethoprim, amoxicillin-clavulanate for oral administration and metronidazole with a quinolone or cephalosporin, beta-lactam with a beta-lactamase inhibitor, or a carbapenem for intravenous treatment.

Outpatient Management

Those who present with left iliac fossa pain and tenderness in the absence of systemic signs and symptoms may be initially treated on an outpatient basis, provided the patient's social circumstances permit. The home environment should be adequate, and the patient should have the support of a relative or friend. The patient should be able to maintain oral hydration and should not have a condition associated with immunosuppression. In addition, the diverticulitis must not be complicated.

For outpatient treatment, most physicians feel that there is no need for water and food restriction, but a low-residue diet is recommended by some during the acute phase of the illness. It may be preferable to place the bowel at relative rest until such time as the inflammatory process has resolved. In the opinion of some physicians, outpatient treatment should consist of an even more restricted diet, allowing clear liquids only. There is, however, no evidence base to support any of these regimens.

Alonso and colleagues reported a series of 96 patients with CT-confirmed uncomplicated diverticulitis who were assessed for an outpatient treatment.[13] Twenty-six had at least one risk factor and were admitted. Seventy were treated as an outpatient with amoxicillin-clavulanate acid or ciprofloxacin with metronidazole and reviewed at 4 to 7 days. Of these, only 2 required subsequent admission for intravenous antibiotics, thus resolving the acute episode. The remaining 68 all recovered with outpatient treatment. The criteria for admission included the inability to take liquids by mouth, lack of home support, and comorbidities including those with immunosuppression.

In general, if the symptoms continue to improve, elective evaluation is undertaken when the acute process has resolved. If the patient's symptoms fail to improve, inpatient therapy is recommended.

Inpatient Management

Where the patient's condition does not appear to be severe but the decision to admit has been taken, it is probably reasonable to treat with antibiotics and observe. For someone who has more severe abdominal signs and symptoms, has a pyrexia, is immunocompromised, or appears systemically ill, a CT scan should be performed. Medical management includes the usual supportive measures. No oral intake is advised unless the patient's symptoms fail to suggest the need for imminent operation. Under such circumstances, clear liquids are permitted. It is usually unnecessary to employ a nasogastric tube unless intestinal obstruction or vomiting is evident. In the inpatient setting, antibiotics are administered systemically. As the symptoms improve, a progressive diet is instituted, supplemented by a stool softener. There is no good evidence that anticholinergic drugs are effective.[12,297] With aggressive medical management, the patient's symptoms should improve considerably within 24 to 48 hours.

Schechter and colleagues conducted a survey of fellows of the ASCRS to document medical treatment preferences for patients with uncomplicated acute diverticulitis.[273] There were 373 responders. The most common single antibiotic regimens were either a second-generation cephalosporin (27%) or ampicillin/sulbactam (16%). The most frequently employed combination was ciprofloxacin/metronidazole (28%). Upon discharge, 74% prescribed oral antibiotics for 7 to 10 days. Interestingly, dietary recommendations included low residue (68%), regular (21%), and high residue (10%). Clearly, there is an enormous variation in the medical management of diverticulitis among colon and rectal surgeons in the United States.

In a randomized controlled trial, oral and intravenous ciprofloxacin and metronidazole were compared in 41 and 38 patients admitted with left iliac fossa pain and tenderness, with or without fever or leukocytosis.[252] Randomization took place in the emergency room as soon as the diagnosis of uncomplicated diverticulitis had been made on clinical grounds, supported by plain radiology only. Thus, the patients did not have a CT scan. For the first 24 hours, in the oral group intake was allowed, whereas in the intravenous group it was not. Daily clinical assessment of tenderness, white cell count, C-reactive protein (CRP), and estimated sedimentation rate (ESR) was carried out. Complete resolution of symptoms occurred in both groups, and the severity of tenderness on the third day was the same. CRP was found to be the best monitor of progress.

The duration of antibiotic treatment, whether 4 or 7 days, was compared in a multicenter randomized controlled trial.[277] One hundred and twenty-three patients with acute diverticulitis confirmed by CT attending 11 hospitals received ertapenem on admission. On day 4, patients who were not free of symptoms were removed from the study (n = 17), leaving 106 who were then randomized to stop the antibiotic (n = 50) or to continue for a further 3 days to a total of 7 days (n = 56). There was no difference between the groups, and at 1 month 95% of patients had been followed, with no difference in outcome. At 1 year, there was again no difference in the two groups, although 9% of patients overall had developed a recurrence of diverticulitis.

There is some interest in the treatment of patients with SCAD by the anti-inflammatory drug, mesalazine. The evidence for improvement presumably of the mucosal inflammatory element has been reviewed by Floch and others.[93,315]

Results of Medical Treatment for Uncomplicated Acute Diverticulitis

Unfortunately, many reports of results in the literature comingle patients with uncomplicated with complicated diverticulitis. Despite this problem, it is clear that the great majority of individuals resolve their complaints with medical treatment. This result is related to the initial severity of the condition. Response rates of more than 95% to 70% have been reported in many publications.[13,227,252,257,277,291] One retrospective study did, however, separate these two groups.[84] Of 502 patients admitted with acute diverticulitis over a 6-year period, 337 were uncomplicated, and 165 were complicated. Over a follow-up period of 101 months (range, 60 to 124), 73 (22%) in the former group experienced a recurrent attack (one attack, 60 [18.8%]; 15 [4.5%], two or more attacks). Only 5% developed complicated disease. During the initial admission, the continued presence of abscess formation and extracolonic contrast material or gas is indicative of failure of medical treatment. Moreover, the risk for secondary complications after initial successful management of acute diverticulitis is high.[18]

Acute Diverticulitis (Complicated)

Local Perforation, Hinchey Stage I and II
Phlegmon or Abscess

The most common complication of acute diverticulitis is a walled-off perforation leading to abscess formation (Figure 27-24). The acute inflammatory reaction usually involves the sigmoid colon and its mesentery. Signs and symptoms are most often confined to the left lower quadrant of the abdomen. Varying degrees of peritoneal irritation may be manifested. The abscess may sometimes be found at some distance from the sigmoid colon as shown in Figure 27-25, where it lies in the rectovesical space.

Abscess formation has been reported in approximately 10% to 20% of patients diagnosed with acute diverticulitis. In one study of 181 patients with proven acute diverticulitis, 31 (17%) were found to have an abscess on CT.[284] As discussed previously, CT is the imaging modality of choice, although ultrasonography also has a high sensitivity and specificity. Radiologic evaluation with water-soluble contrast may reveal tracking of the material into other areas.

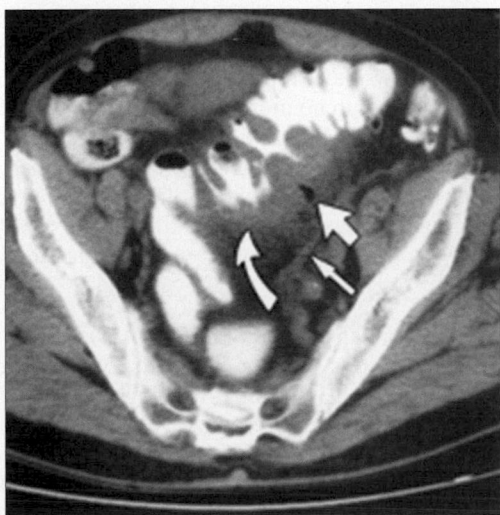

FIGURE 27-24. Computed tomography of a contained perforation in a man with acute diverticulitis. Asymmetric inflammatory wall thickening (*curved arrow*) superimposed on muscular wall hypertrophy (*straight wide arrow*), diverticula, fat stranding, and fascial thickening (*straight thin arrow*). Note contained perforation with formation of phlegmon and extraluminal air (*thick arrow*). No free intraperitoneal extravasation of colonic contrast material is seen.

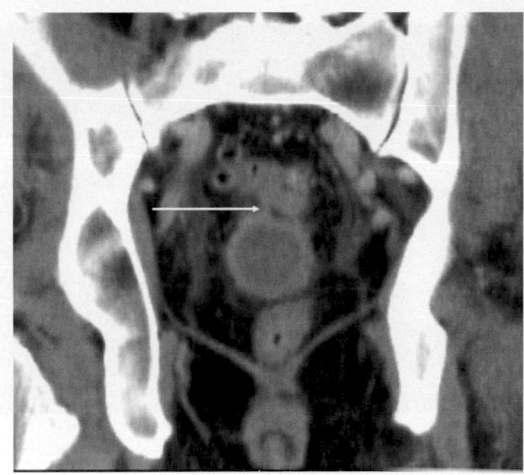

FIGURE 27-25. Pelvic abscess. Computed tomography shows abscess in the rectovesical space with communication to the sigmoid colon.

Medical Treatment of Abscess

Many patients with Hinchey stage I and II disease will respond to medical treatment. The results of prospective studies in which patients were followed from admission up to several years have shown that abscesses smaller than 4 cm are likely to resolve on antibiotics alone.[17,20,284] Ambrosetti and coworkers suggested that mesocolic abscesses can usually be managed without drainage.[20] In a retrospective chart review of 114 patients with intra-abdominal abscess due to diverticulitis, Kumar and colleagues found that 61 (54%) responded to antibiotics alone and 50 (44%) required percutaneous drainage. Abscesses of a diameter of 4 cm were likely to resolve with antibiotics alone, whereas a diameter of 6.5 cm or more and the presence of fever were risk factors that require drainage. In another study, Siewert and colleagues reviewed 181 patients with a CT-proven diagnosis of diverticulitis.[284] Of these, 31 (17%) had an abscess. Twenty-two of these were smaller than 3 cm. All abscesses of this size resolved by antibiotic treatment alone. In the 8 patients with an abscess greater than 3 cm, 4 resolved with antibiotics alone, and the remaining 4 required CT-guided percutaneous drainage.

This information should assist the clinician in deciding on whether referral for percutaneous drainage is necessary. Clearly, one should follow the patient carefully during the first few hours and days after initiating antibiotics, especially if there is evidence of no improvement or deterioration. A repeat CT scan with further clinical evaluation is indicated under these circumstances.

Computed Tomography–Guided Percutaneous Drainage. Patients who fail to respond despite vigorous medical management or who are found on the basis of ultrasonography or CT to have a localized abscess should be considered for CT-guided percutaneous drainage.[85,112,203,210,260,272,339] Success depends on the ability to find a safe, direct route to the abscess cavity (Figure 27-26).

Brolin and associates suggested that patients with persistent leukocytosis or fever at 4 days after drainage should be reevaluated by CT or ultrasonography and considered for either repeated drainage (if appropriate) or laparotomy.[46] Stabile and coworkers reported no complications among 19 patients who underwent drainage, but 2 had persistent fever and leukocytosis.[290] Nine were found to have a colonic

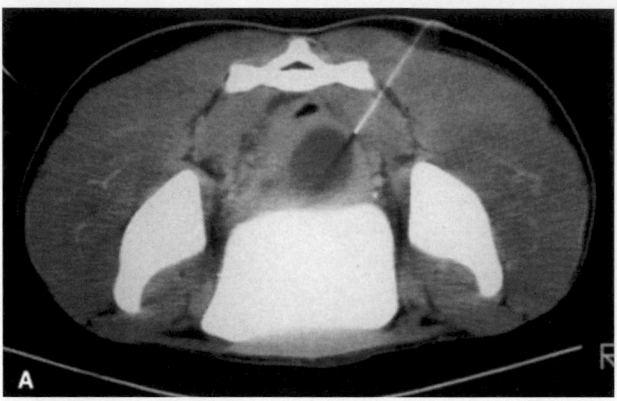
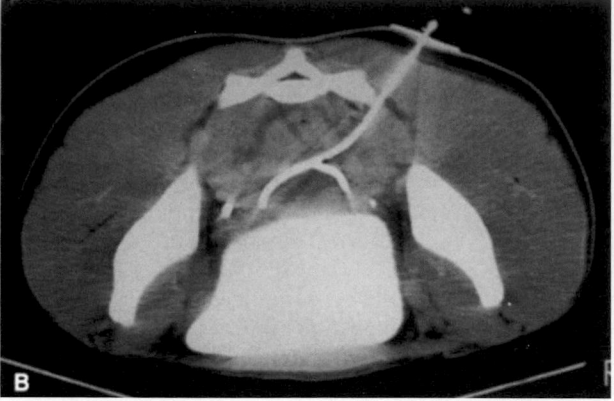

FIGURE 27-26. Pelvic abscess as a consequence of perforated diverticulitis. **A:** Computed tomography–guided needle aspiration through a transgluteal approach confirms the location of the abscess cavity. **B:** A catheter is inserted with the drainage complete; note the absence of gas.

fistula on sonogram, but these patients were able to undergo a subsequent elective, one-stage colectomy.

Surgical resection has been advised after stabilization of the patient through drainage. For example, Mueller and colleagues reported that 14 of 24 patients who underwent such a drainage procedure proceeded to a single-stage resection within 10 days.[203] Today, however, many advise that resection be reserved for the patient who did not settle or if recurrence of the abscess or other complication occurred.

Septic Thrombophlebitis

Rarely, inflammatory changes in the colon can result in a septic thrombophlebitis involving the mesenteric veins that drain the area.[77] This can lead to the demonstration of gas in the mesenteric and ultimately within the portal venous system as seen with CT imaging. The etiology is uncertain, but the possibility of gas-forming organisms entering the circulation is a reasonable theory. This complication is obviously an independent factor that mandates bowel resection.

Free Perforation—Hinchey Stage III and IV
Free perforation with generalized peritonitis is an uncommon but grave complication of diverticulitis, although it accounts for more than one-half of emergency operations for this condition.[64] When it occurs, it can have catastrophic consequences. Patients are critically ill and often demonstrate the signs and symptoms of septicemia. The history may be one of the sudden onset of abdominal pain, usually in the lower abdomen, progressing to generalized involvement. In cases with free perforation, marked abdominal distension may be noted, caused by a pneumoperitoneum (see Figure 27-21). Abdominal rigidity is usually observed. An upright film of the abdomen or a lateral decubitus x-ray film will reveal the presence of free gas (see Figure 27-22). It has been suggested that the amount of gas present on the x-ray will help the surgeon to determine whether it is a colonic or a gastroduodenal perforation; the more gas present, the greater the likelihood of a colonic perforation. This may be a useful distinguishing feature in determining where the incision should be made. CT may also demonstrate a perforation or free gas in the peritoneal cavity (see Figure 27-12). The perforation may be contained by adhesion of the colon to surrounding structures (Figure 27-27), or it may track along tissue plains to the exterior (Figures 27-28 and 27-29).

Purulent Peritonitis (Hinchey Stage III)
Laparoscopic Irrigation Followed by Resection
Up until a few years ago, purulent peritonitis caused by perforation of a diverticulum was treated by open surgery and resection with or without primary anastomosis. Since the late 1990s, reports of laparoscopic treatment have been published. Rizk and colleagues reported 10 patients with perforation (two fecal) who underwent "copious" (15 L) laparoscopic irrigation.[255] There was no mortality, and 9 had a laparoscopic colectomy 3 to 4 months later. In another report using the same approach, 18 patients with peritonitis were treated by this technique.[89] There was no mortality or wound complication. Fourteen patients underwent a laparoscopic resection 3.5 months later.

Franklin and associates, who had originally reported their experience in 1997, published their long-term results of 40 patients with Hinchey II (5), III (32), and IV (3) stage disease in 2008.[97] There was no mortality. Twenty-four patients underwent subsequent resection. Taylor and colleagues reported 14 patients treated in the same manner, 3 of whom did not improve and were operated on.[301] Eleven recovered, of whom 8 underwent resection at 6 weeks, 7 by laparoscopy. A stoma was avoided in all of these individuals. Bretagnol and coworkers reported 24 patients with purulent or fecal peritonitis with no mortality and a morbidity of 8%.[44] Two required subsequent radiologic drainage of a pelvic abscess. Resection was performed in all patients laparoscopically, with a conversion to open rate of 16%. Mutter and colleagues reported 10 cases with a good outcome.[207] A useful commentary on this approach was given by Santaniello and Bergamaschi.[265]

Laparoscopic Irrigation without Subsequent Resection
In all of the previous reports, resection was carried out in most patients at an interval following the laparoscopic lavage. Myers and colleagues, however, may have taken the concept a step further by their report of a multicenter prospective study involving 1,257 admissions for acute diverticulitis, of whom 100 underwent laparoscopic lavage for perforated disease.[208] Eight with fecal peritonitis (Hinchey stage IV) received immediate open surgical treatment, but 92 were followed after laparoscopic lavage. Of these, 2 had a subsequent operation for pelvic abscess, but during a median follow-up period of 30 months (12 to 84), only 2 presented with diverticulitis. It may be possible, therefore,

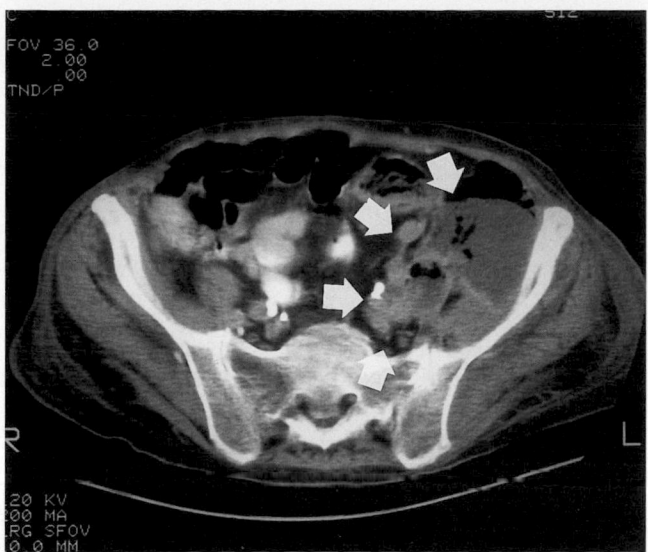 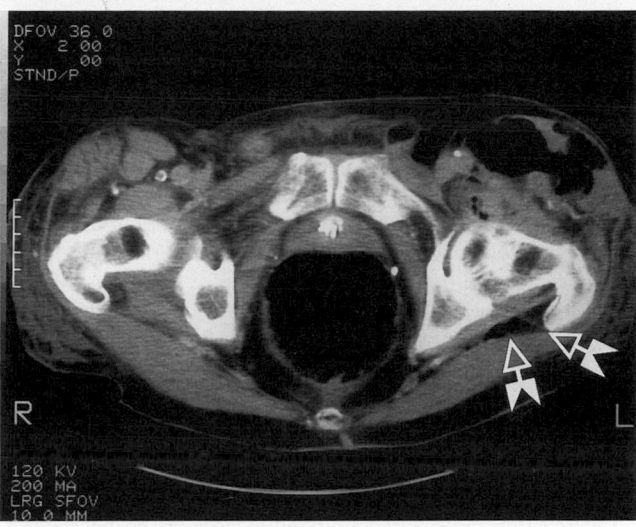

FIGURE 27-27. Perforated diverticulitis. Computed tomography demonstrates **(A)** a large fluid collection with gas involving the iliopsoas muscle (*arrows*), representing a large abscess. **B:** Extension of the abscess seen **(A)** into the left groin. Note the gas in the buttock (*arrows*).

that delayed resection is not a requisite for the majority of patients presenting with purulent peritonitis,[44] although there is insufficient evidence at present to make such a firm recommendation.[96]

This subject is reviewed by Alamili and colleagues and Toorenvliet and associates.[6,311] The latter group reported two prospective cohort studies and nine retrospective series and case reports. Hinchey stage III formed 77% of the 231 patients. Sepsis was successfully controlled in 95.7%, and only 4 of the 231 patients required a stoma. The mortality rate was 1.7%.

These data indicate that with careful individualization patients with purulent peritonitis can be managed with the minimum of surgical trauma, with a resultant low mortality and morbidity, a low incidence of a stoma, and possibly a low need for subsequent surgical resection. When resection becomes necessary, however, a laparoscopic approach can be used if the surgeon is comfortable with this technique (see Chapter 19). This technique may prove to be a major advance in the management of purulent peritonitis from perforated diverticulitis.

Fecal Peritonitis (Hinchey Stage IV)

Fecal peritonitis is less common than purulent. There is no controversy at this time that fecal peritonitis should be treated by resection of the source of the perforation. Whether to perform a primary anastomosis, however, without diversion is questionable. The argument between these techniques often fails to consider the general factors of age of the patient, American Society of Anesthesiologist (ASA) grade, comorbidities, and the actual severity of sepsis. In reports in which these alternatives are discussed, these factors are difficult to quantify, and, in fact, sometimes no attempt is made to do so.

Choice of Operation

There are a number of operations available for the treatment of acute sigmoid diverticulitis. All have potential advantages and disadvantages, depending on the presentation, the operative findings, and the technical capabilities of the surgeon.

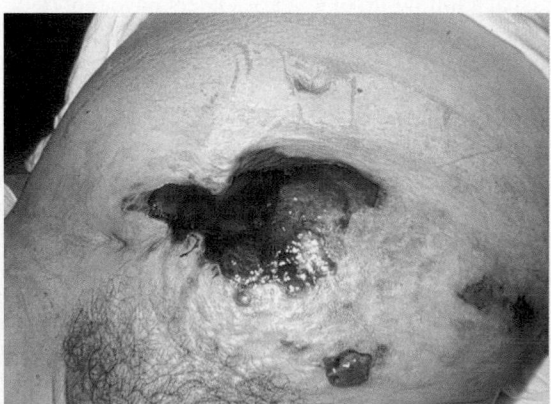

FIGURE 27-28. Gangrene of the abdominal wall from perforation of sigmoid diverticulitis.

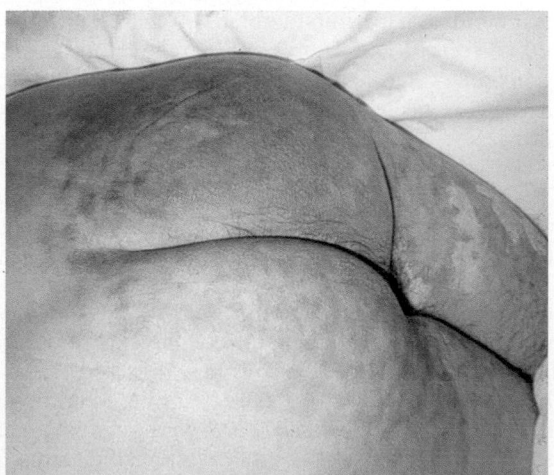

FIGURE 27-29. Right buttock induration with underlying abscess, a consequence of perforated diverticulitis.

Hartmann's Procedure versus Oversewing and Defunctioning Stoma.
Although the Hartmann's operation is probably the most
commonly performed procedure for acute sigmoid diverticulitis today, there is very little literature on randomization or comparison with other methods. However, Kronborg
reported a randomized trial of suturing with defunctioning
stoma compared with resection in 62 patients accrued more
than 14 years and operated on by 27 surgeons.[164] There
was no difference in the mortality of patients with Hinchey
stage IV disease. However, the small numbers and long duration of accrual detract from the value of this trial. Zeitoun
and colleagues reported the results of a randomized, controlled trial of 105 patients admitted to 17 hospitals in France
over a period that extended for up to 7 years.[342]

Hartmann's Procedure versus Resection with Primary Anastomosis. The
technique of removing the acutely inflamed colon is worthy
of comment. When entering the peritoneal cavity, the surgeon is often confronted with what appears to be a large,
fixed, "unresectable" mass. However, one should not be
overwhelmed by first appearances. The acute inflammatory
reaction can often be dealt with by careful blunt dissection
without fear of injuring vital retroperitoneal structures such
as a ureter. Attempts at such mobilization at a later time may
be impossible without sharp scissors dissection. In the latter circumstances, the ureter is much more likely to be injured. If one begins the dissection by gently passing the left
hand lateral to the inflammatory mass and easing the bowel
away from the parietal peritoneum, one may be pleasantly
surprised at how readily the mass seems to come free. An
occasional fibrous band may be snipped with the scissors,
but virtually the entire dissection is carried out bluntly with
the tips of the fingers, either pushing to identify the plane of
dissection or pinching adherent areas.

Abcarian and Pearl make the point that the operation
should be commenced proximal to the inflamed segment,
dividing the bowel with a linear stapler at this location and
developing the plane over Gerota's fascia.[1] A proximal-
to-distal dissection is then undertaken, with the ureter
identified at the cephalad aspect of the mobilization. When
the bowel is delivered into the abdominal cavity, the surgeon
can usually identify 1 or 2 cm of distal rectosigmoid that
seems to be free of inflammatory reaction (Figure 27-30).
This is an important point, because it is this sparing of the
rectosigmoid that permits a relatively safe anastomosis,
should one elect to perform it at this time. However, if the
surgeon prefers Hartmann's operation, the bowel is resected,
a colostomy is created, and the rectal stump is closed. Stump
closure can be effected by conventional suture technique or
more commonly by using a stapler.

The evolution of the surgical technique for perforated
diverticulitis has been reviewed by Vermeulen and Lange.[328]
In their assessment of current practice on behalf of the
ASCRS, Wong and coworkers concluded that a three-stage
resection was no longer to be recommended.[339] In a review
by Salem and Flum, the general conclusion from various
studies is that resection with primary anastomosis is not
inferior to Hartmann's procedure.[261] Ninety-eight studies
published between 1957 and 2003 were analyzed. There
were 1,051 patients from 54 studies who had a Hartmann's
operation and 569 who underwent a resection with primary
anastomosis from 50 studies. The respective mortality was
18.6% and 9.9%, and wound complications occurred in 29%

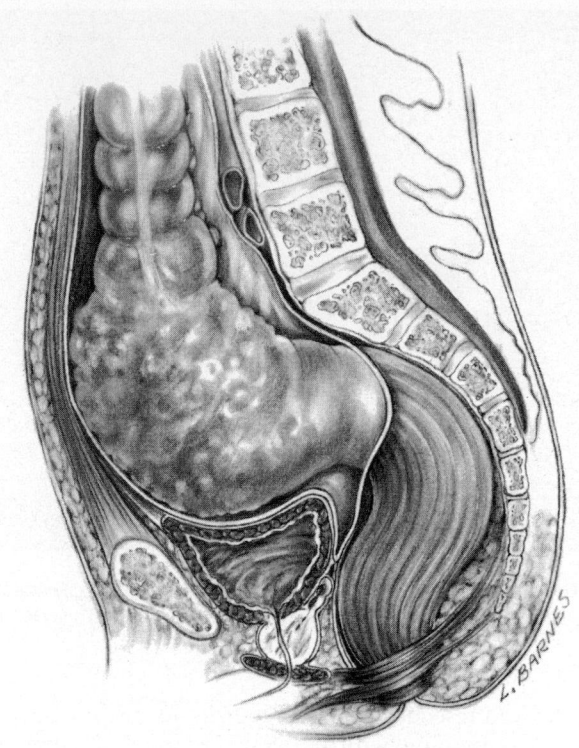

FIGURE 27-30. Sigmoid diverticulitis. The mass usually terminates distally
in relatively normal, uninflamed bowel, just above the peritoneal reflection.

and 9.6%. The anastomotic leakage rate after primary anastomosis was 9.6%.

In another systematic review, Constantinides and colleagues identified 15 of 24 articles in which 547 patients
who underwent resection with primary anastomosis were
compared with 416 having Hartmann's procedure.[63] Thirteen
of the studies were retrospective. The overall mortality was
4.9% versus 15.1%, but in studies matched for the severity
of peritonitis, the mortality rates were no different (14.1%
and 14.4%). This is likely to be true with respect to quality
of life because it is all too frequent that Hartmann's procedure is not reversed. For example, Maggard and associates
reported on 11,582 admissions for diverticular disease in the
State of California, of whom 2,808 (24%) underwent surgery.[180] Hartmann's operation was performed on 41.7%, and
of the 1,176 Hartmann's patients, 35% had not undergone
reversal at a follow-up of 4 years. Others have reported similar findings.[274] However, in a review of 6,619 patients from
12 studies reporting the results of surgery for peritonitis due
to perforated diverticular disease, Constantinides and colleagues noted a subsequent closure rate of 73%.

In an important analysis of 65 patients having undergone Hartmann's procedure and 46 a resection with primary
anastomosis, Zingg and colleagues showed that there were
differences in the composition of the two groups, including the age of patients, POSSUM score (Physiologic and
Operative Severity Score for the enUmeration of Mortality
and Morbidity), and the prevalence of immunosuppressive
medication.[344] The odds ratio of 3.25 (95% CI, 1.26–8.43)
for Hartmann's operation compared with anastomosis
was not significantly different after correction for age and
score. However, the incidence of anastomotic leakage
was 28%. The authors interpreted these data to show that

Hartmann's procedure is safer for patients who are older and/ or have associated morbidities. In another prospective study, Regenet and coworkers reported a mortality after primary anastomosis and Hartmann's procedure of 11% and 12%, respectively for 27 and 33 patients who underwent emergency surgery for Hinchey stage III and IV peritonitis.[247]

It is evident, as previously stated, that when resection with primary anastomosis is compared with Hartmann's procedure without randomization, there is the confounding factor of selection bias; in other words one must conclude that the worse the presentation, the more likely the patient will undergo Hartmann's operation. Binda and associates reported the results of a multicenter study in which 90 patients with perforated diverticular disease associated with fecal peritonitis were randomized to resection with primary anastomosis and loop ileostomy (34) versus Hartmann's procedure (56).[37] The mortality rates were not statistically different, although there was a correlation between procedure type and organ dysfunction. Similar proportions (65% vs. 60%) underwent subsequent closure of the stoma with no mortality and no significant difference in morbidity.

Richter and associates adopted a policy of primary resection with anastomosis without a defunctioning stoma.[251] They reported 34 patients accrued over a 2-year period and followed prospectively. The mortality was 11%, with the relative risk of death, 3.75 for renal failure, and 3.25 for immunosuppression.

Outcome of Surgery for Complicated Diverticular Disease

A national study conducted from data on patients undergoing surgery for complicated diverticular disease submitted by 42 hospitals in the United Kingdom over a 12-month period from January to December 2003 identified 539 patients.[64] The definition of complicated diverticular disease was based on clinical, radiologic, or intraoperative identification of phlegmon, abscess, enteric fistula, perforation, bleeding, or obstruction. Because the study set out to assess the results of surgery, the 92 patients who did not have an operation were excluded from the analysis, and a further 123 were excluded because there was no information on the POSSUM score. There were, therefore, 324 patients on whom a nonelective procedure was performed in 165 (50.9%). The breakdown of pathology was phlegmon, 56; abscess, 76; perforation, 103; fistula, 82; and obstruction, 45. There were 35 (10.8%) individuals older than 80 years; the mean ages of males and females were 58.5 and 68.6 years, with age ranges of 25 to 89 years and 25 to 93 years, respectively. The overall mortality was 10.8%. High POSSUM scores predicted poorly, with a mortality of 21.9%, but this was much more accurate for the modifications of this scoring system using P-POSSUM (Portsmouth-POSSUM) and CR-POSSUM (CR = Colorectal). With these systems, mortality predictions of 10.5% and 10.0%, respectively, were noted. The operations performed included Hartmann's procedure in 108 (33.3%) and resection with a primary anastomosis in 174 (53%). It is not surprising that of the 165 patients undergoing emergency treatment, 103 (62%) were found to have a perforation.

In another study, Vermeulen and colleagues followed 340 patients undergoing surgery for perforated diverticular disease in five hospitals in the Rotterdam, Netherlands region over a 5-year period.[327] Ninety died in hospital leaving 250 operative survivors. At a follow-up of 59 months (1 to 210), another 90 patients had died, giving an overall 5-year survival in the 340 patients of 53%. Thirty-three percent of the 340 patients were older than 75 years of age, 40% were ASA grade III or more, and 58% had general peritonitis. The mortality of those with fecal peritonitis (Hinchey stage IV) was 48% (54 patients). Patients who had undergone a primary resection with primary anastomosis had a better prognosis than those who had Hartmann's procedure, but those in the latter group were older and their ASA grades higher, indicating treatment bias. The survival of Hartmann's patients was lower than in the general age-matched Dutch population, whereas that of primary anastomosis was not significantly different.

Elective Resection after Resolution of Acute Diverticulitis

In their major study of diverticulitis in the United States, Etzioni and colleagues reported that the number of elective operations after an attack of diverticulitis rose from 15,300 in 1998 to 21,300 in 2004/2005.[86] This increase was seen in the age groups 18 to 44 years (73%) and 45 to 64 years (54%). The average age of the patients in 2 years fell from 59.4 to 57.1 years. The rate in those aged 65 to 74 years increased slightly and in those older than 75 years, it fell. Based on an analysis of the chances of recurrence after one or two attacks of diverticulitis and the potential morbidity and mortality for the patient, the document "Practice Parameters for Sigmoid Diverticulitis" was produced by the ASCRS in 1995,[256] with a revision in 2000[339] and with an update again in 2006.[242] The most recent recommendation stipulated that "after one documented attack, successfully treated, there is no reason to consider elective resection unless unusual circumstances are present, such as immunosuppression or perhaps age younger than 45 years." The document further states as follows: "after two documented attacks, successfully treated, a recommendation should be made for elective colon resection unless other comorbid conditions constitute inordinate risk for elective operation." These statements were based on an analysis of risk obtained from the literature at the time. A similar view was held by the working party of the American College of Gastroenterology, which initially reported their conclusions in 1999 and then again in 2004.[296,297] The presence of immunosuppression was regarded by many to be an indication for elective surgery after an acute attack.[234,296,297,321] Where there was uncertainty whether a cancer might be present was another, although uncommon, indication.

Evidence in Favor of Interval Resection

The need for elective resection after a second attack has been inferred from two studies in particular. In an article of only four pages in length, Parks and Connell in 1970 reported the outcome of 455 patients followed for 1 to 16 years who had been admitted to hospital with "diverticular disease."[230] This must have been acute diverticulitis because the patients were all treated with antibiotics. Of these, 317 (70%) were treated medically. Seventy-eight (24.6%) had a second attack (50% within 1 year; 90% within 5 years), and 20 (6.3%) a third attack. Surgery was required in 20, leaving 297 patients who never had surgery. At the final assessment, there were 209 patients who had been managed medically exclusively, of whom 121 (58%) were symptom-free. Of the 88 with symptoms, these were severe in only 11 (5.3%). The mortality in this group was less than 2%. Of the 138 having initial surgery, only 36 required a resection (29 one-stage; 7 Hartmann's). The others underwent a colostomy and drainage (68), laparotomy without resection (22), and drainage of abscess (11). There were 10 postoperative deaths among all of these surgical categories.

Farmakis and coworkers reported the natural history of complicated diverticular disease based on a questionnaire sent to 300 patients.[90] Of 120 responders, 10 had died of recurrent complicated diverticular disease. Of the remaining 110, 40 were still symptomatic. These data were generally taken to support the recommendation for elective resection to prevent persistent symptoms and potentially lethal complications. However, deficiencies in the last study include its multicenter nature (30 units), the method of assessment, and the occurrence of morbidity and mortality unrelated to diverticular disease.

In a series of publications, Ambrosetti and colleagues studied the long-term outcome of patients admitted with CT-proven acute diverticulitis or abscess (Hinchey stages I and II).[22] In 226 with acute diverticulitis, 66 underwent early operation. These included 59 (33%) of 179 patients older than 50 years of age and 7 of 47 patients younger than 50 years. Of the 160 patients who had not undergone early surgery, recurrence or complications during follow-up occurred in 16 of 120 patients older than 50 years and in 11 of 40 younger than 50. The authors concluded that age younger than 50 was a risk factor for further episodes of disease. Eight years later (2002), the same authors reported a series of 144 patients who had been admitted with CT-proven diverticulitis between 1986 and 1991 and who had resolved on medical treatment.[52] Of these, 118 were followed for a median of 9.5 years. Eighty had no further complication, but 38 did. The risk of a complication was highest in patients younger than 50 years with severe disease on an initial CT scan (54% at 5 years), and the lowest in patients older than 50 years with mild disease on CT (19% at 5 years). These data show a fairly high rate of recurrence even in the clinical group with lowest risk.

In the important subgroup of patients with Hinchey stage I and II disease on the initial admission, Ambrosetti and colleagues followed 140 patients admitted with CT-verified diverticulitis.[20] Of these, 22 had an abscess, of whom 13 underwent early surgery. Of the remaining 9 patients, 8 were asymptomatic at 24 months. By 2005, the number of individuals admitted with acute diverticulitis had increased to 465 over an 11-year period (1986 to 1997). Of these, 76 had Hinchey stage I and II disease (45 stage I and 28 stage II). Immediate surgery was carried out in 7 (15%) and 11 (39%), respectively. During the subsequent follow-up, no surgery had been required in 22 (58%) of 38 stage I patients and in 8 (47%) of 17 stage II patients. Over the entire period of follow-up, 50% of Hinchey stage I and 71% of Hinchey stage II patients had undergone surgery. These data indicate, as might be expected, that the presence of an abscess, whether pericolic or pelvic, is a risk factor for requiring subsequent surgery, and that this risk is probably increased by young age.

In a retrospective single institution study of 363 patients admitted between 1985 and 1991, the clinical diagnosis was facilitated by ultrasound (130 patients), contrast enema (255 patients), and CT (50 patients).[202] Of these, 252 (69%) were treated conservatively. Telephone interviews were carried out in 1996 and 2002, at median follow-up periods of 86 months (5 to 127) and 161 months (130 to 196). At the first follow-up, 85 patients had died, with apparently 1 death due to bleeding diverticular disease. Of the remaining 167 patients, 78 developed recurrent symptoms, and 13 required surgery. At the second follow-up now involving 85 patients, there had been 1 death due to perforated diverticular disease, 31 (37%) were symptomatic, and 12 patients had required interim surgery. Despite the retrospective nature of this study and the somewhat unreliable method of follow-up, these data show that recurrent symptoms occur frequently and that surgery is required in approximately 10% of patients.

Mäkelä and colleagues followed 260 patients treated for diverticulitis between 1981 and 2002.[182] The long-term outcome was assessed by a questionnaire that was returned in a satisfactory manner by 171 (70%) patients. These were divided into three groups: no operation, operation for recurrence, and immediate operation for perforation. In those in the first group, the requirement of hospitalization for left lower abdominal pain, fever, and the need for antibiotics and for NSAIDs was more common than in the groups having surgery. This became more evident in patients admitted to hospital for recurrent symptoms for the second time. The authors recommended surgery in this circumstance.

Evidence against Interval Resection

Janes and colleagues attempted to answer this important question.[143] They reviewed the natural history of diverticulitis over time from a study of the literature. Data from seven reports included series ranging in number from 132 to 455 patients followed from 1 to 16 years.[168,227] The diagnosis was made by using CT in four studies. In the seven studies, which included a total of 2,321 patients with uncomplicated diverticulitis, the frequency of early operation ranged from 25% to 31%. Follow-up of the remaining patients over a range of 1 to 16 years showed the incidence of a recurrent attack to be between 8.6% and 29%, but the incidence of a second operation was much lower—between 0% and 10%.[18,22,38,118,183,227] Even in those with complicated diverticulitis, the data available showed rates of recurrence ranging from 2% per year[267] to 8% over 19 months.[21] This was shown to be 32.5% in a series of 120 patients accrued prospectively in 30 centers followed for 5 years.[90,314] In this last series, an assessment was made by a questionnaire. Many patients were elderly, with a high comorbidity reflected in mortality and unsuitability for major surgery. In a prospective study of 232 patients admitted with acute diverticulitis between 1990 and 2004, 38 (16.4%) underwent surgery during the admission.[281] There was 1 death. This left 191 who were followed by a review in 2005. Of these, 35 (18.3%) underwent subsequent resection (26 elective; 9 emergency) with 1 death. Janes and coworkers drew the conclusion that the chance of surgery after a second attack was low and was associated with a low mortality in the total patient group. This was felt to be less than the potential mortality and morbidity from elective surgery for diverticular disease. Supporting this conclusion was the data from the publication of Bokey and associates in their publication of 47 patients who underwent a sigmoid colon resection for diverticular disease and 106 for carcinoma.[39]

It is a well-known fact that 90% of patients who die with perforation have no prior history of diverticulitis.[26] The incidence of known diverticular disease in several series of patients who underwent emergency surgery is 2%, 12%, and 26% over a follow-up of 10, 8, and 5 years.[178,212,288] This suggests that recurrence is not a common reason for operation. In a series of 693 patients with diverticular disease followed for 10 years, Alexander and colleagues reported that 93 (14%) required surgery.[10] This was due primarily to complications such as abscess (36), bleeding (18), perforation (10), obstruction (10), and fistula (5), but only 7 patients underwent surgery for recurrent symptoms. In fact, this last number is similar to the 8 who required surgery to exclude a carcinoma. In summary, Janes and associates demonstrated that in many reports the incidence of surgery for recurrence after an initial attack was low.[143] Only a small proportion of patients who underwent surgery had prior symptoms of diverticular disease. Thus, when compared with an appreciable mortality and morbidity for elective resection, their view is that the risk of severe complications and death is less in those not having an interval resection following a second attack. The question is under current review by the ASCRS. The Association of Coloproctology of Great Britain and Ireland, in their recent position statement, does not advocate routine resection after two attacks.

Commentary

At the moment, the balance of opinion appears to be against a recommendation for surgery after a second attack. This may be a reasonable view based on the current evidence, taking death as the main end point for comparison between resection and continued observation or medical care. It does not, however, take the severity of symptoms into account. Yet some patients will continue to suffer symptoms when surgery might have helped to relieve them. This question is similar to the consideration of surgery in patients with uncomplicated, symptomatic diverticular disease (see next). The question is being currently addressed by a randomized clinical trial in the Netherlands.[322]

Fistulization

Fistula formation is a well-recognized complication of diverticular disease, but it is rare, having been estimated to occur in 2% of patients.[341] It has a chronic presentation and is, therefore, clinically distinct from an acute inflammation. The condition arises from the formation of adhesions through phlegmonous disease or a locally walled-off perforation between the affected colon and the viscus in question. This slowly is then followed by fistula formation as a consequence of the penetrating process. The complication is often insidious, and there often may not been a history of a previous acute episode.

Colovesical Fistula

Colovesical fistula is the most common form of colonic fistula in men (Figures 27-31 and 27-32). In the experience of Colcock and Stahmann, colovesical fistula accounted for one-half of all fistulas secondary to this disease.[57] The second most common fistula in this series was colocutaneous, followed by colovaginal, coloenteric, and other unusual manifestations (e.g., coloureteric [Figure 27-33], colouterine, and even the fallopian tube).[119] In the experience of Kovalcik and associates among the 55 patients found to have colovesical fistula, diverticulitis was the cause in 30 cases (55%).[161]

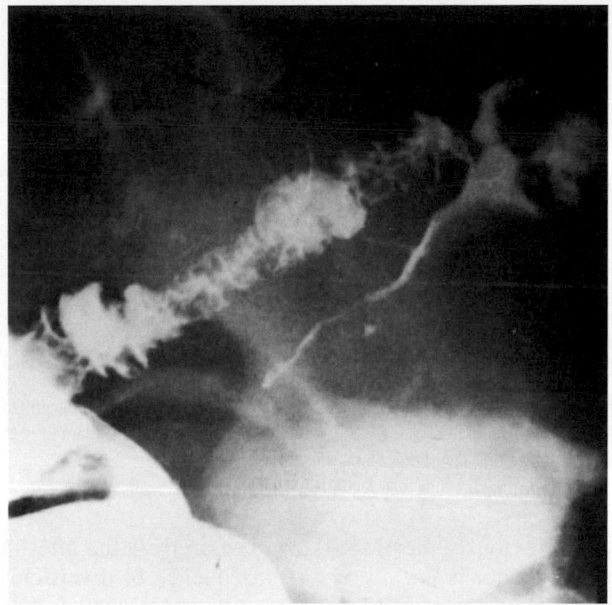

FIGURE 27-31. Colovesical fistula. Diverticular perforation with track entering the bladder.

Other less frequent causes included malignant tumors from several organs, nonspecific inflammatory bowel disease (in particular, Crohn's disease), and the sequelae of radiation therapy. Rarely, injury to the urinary tract or kidney, nephrolithiasis, chronic suppurative processes, tuberculosis, and tumors of the kidney can lead to an enteric communication.[151]

Hool and coworkers reviewed more than 2,300 patients with diverticular disease, 80 of whom required operative treatment.[134] Four coloenteric fistulas were noted, an incidence of 5%. In a subsequent publication from the same unit, Pheils and colleagues noted that 25% of 80 patients for whom elective resection was performed had a fistula, a very high incidence.[235] In the series of Orebaugh and associates, 10% of the 144 patients who underwent resection for diverticular disease (elective and emergency operation) had a colonic fistula.[214] Woods and colleagues reported a series of 84 fistulas, of which 65% were colovesical and 25% were colovaginal.[340] Twelve of the 24 female patients with a colovesical and 19 of the 23 with a colovaginal fistula had undergone a prior hysterectomy.

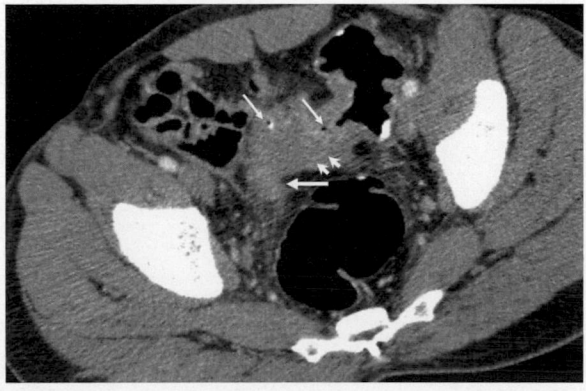

FIGURE 27-32. Colovesical fistula secondary to diverticulitis. Gas pockets within the thickened wall of the sigmoid colon point to a benign cause.

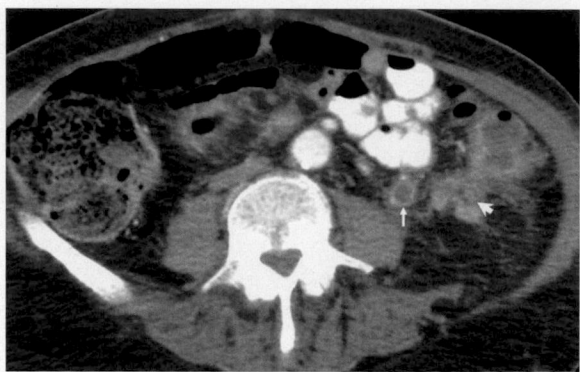

FIGURE 27-33. Coloureteric fistula. CT scan demonstrates pericolic inflammatory mass associated with a coloureteric fistula. Note dilated, inflamed ureter (*narrow arrow*) and diverticular inflammation (*broad arrow*).

As previously mentioned, fistulization from the intestine to the bladder is not always a consequence of diverticular disease. In a series of 51 patients, it was the cause in 41%, but Crohn's disease accounted for 17% and carcinoma for 16%.[201] Of the eight carcinomas, only four were diagnosed preoperatively. The diagnosis of a fistula was not made preoperatively in 20% of the patients.

Colovesical Fistula

In the experience of Kovalcik and colleagues, 69% of patients presented with symptoms related to the urinary tract.[161] Pneumaturia was the most frequent, followed by urinary frequency, dysuria, fecaluria, and hematuria. Complaints unrelated to the urinary tract included lower abdominal pain and fever, although fewer than one-fourth of the patients experienced these symptoms. Passage of urine through the rectum is exceedingly rare and is probably the result of concomitant bladder outflow obstruction.

The studies employed to evaluate patients suspected of having a colovesical fistula include urinalysis, urine culture, the poppy seed test, barium enema, cystoscopy, cystography, CT, and endoscopy.[243] Plain x-ray or CT scan will often show intravesical gas, which confirms the existence of an intestinal fistula (see Figure 27-16). Sarr and coworkers demonstrated the pathognomonic finding of air within the bladder in 20 of 23 patients by CT, although the site of the fistula could not be shown by this means.[268] In terms of a specific abnormality found, however, CT is the most accurate diagnostic tool for confirming that a communication exists between the urinary and gastrointestinal tracts.[23,145,324] Another benefit of CT is the detection of ureteric involvement, particularly by extrinsic compression (see Chapter 24).[211] Some believe that cystoscopy is most likely to identify the fistula,[194] but this is usually inferred by the visualization of an inflammatory reaction in the bladder mucosa rather than actual observation of an opening. Although colonoscopy and sigmoidoscopy may be helpful in evaluating the presence or absence of diverticular or inflammatory bowel disease as well as malignancy, it has a low sensitivity and specificity.[193]

In a recent report of 49 patients (2009) with colovesical fistula, the diagnostic accuracy of various investigations was as follows: poppy seed test (94.6%), CT (61%), MRI (60%), cystogram (16.7%), contrast enema (35%), cystoscopy (10.2%), and colonoscopy (8.5%).[193] This information shows that high resolution imaging has a low sensitivity. It also demonstrates that the simple, inexpensive poppy seed test is by far the most accurate diagnostic study for demonstrating that there is indeed a urinary tract communication. Although it cannot pinpoint its location, it certainly can be regarded as the objective verification of the patient's subjective statement of pneumaturia or fecaluria. Despite all radiologic and endoscopic attempts at diagnosis, it may not be possible to identify a fistula with certainty. An operation can still be recommended, however, based on clinical suspicion by the presence of symptoms of pneumaturia and fecaluria, without the requirement for such confirmation.

Surgical Technique

Characteristically, at laparotomy the sigmoid colon is found to be tethered in the pelvis, fixed to the bladder wall, or to the vagina or uterus in females (Figure 27-34). Usually, the fistula can be divided by blunt dissection, pinching the area between the colon and the bladder or vagina (Figure 27-35). Occasionally, when a long-standing fistula causes extensive fibrosis, sharp dissection and division of the communication are required. It is not necessary to close a vaginal or bladder defect because it will heal once the fistula has been dealt with (Figure 27-36). Excision of a portion of the

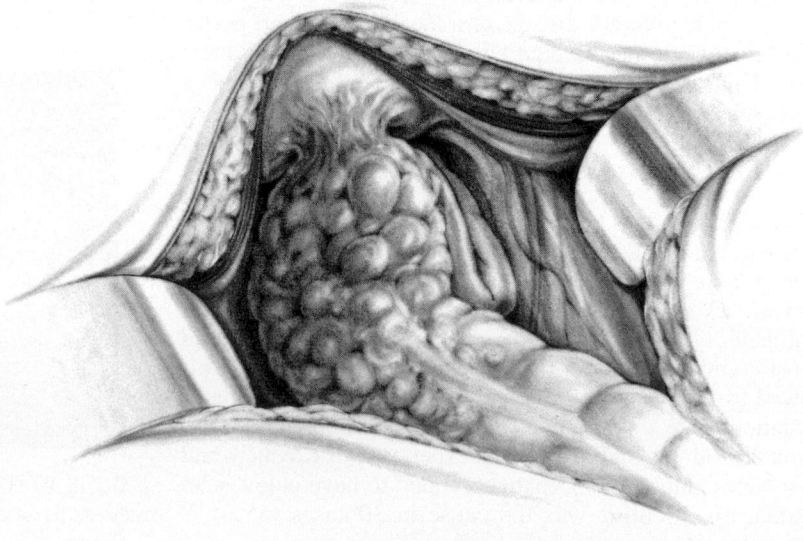

FIGURE 27-34. Artist's conception of a colovesical fistula secondary to diverticulitis. A sigmoidal mass is fixed in the pelvis to the bladder.

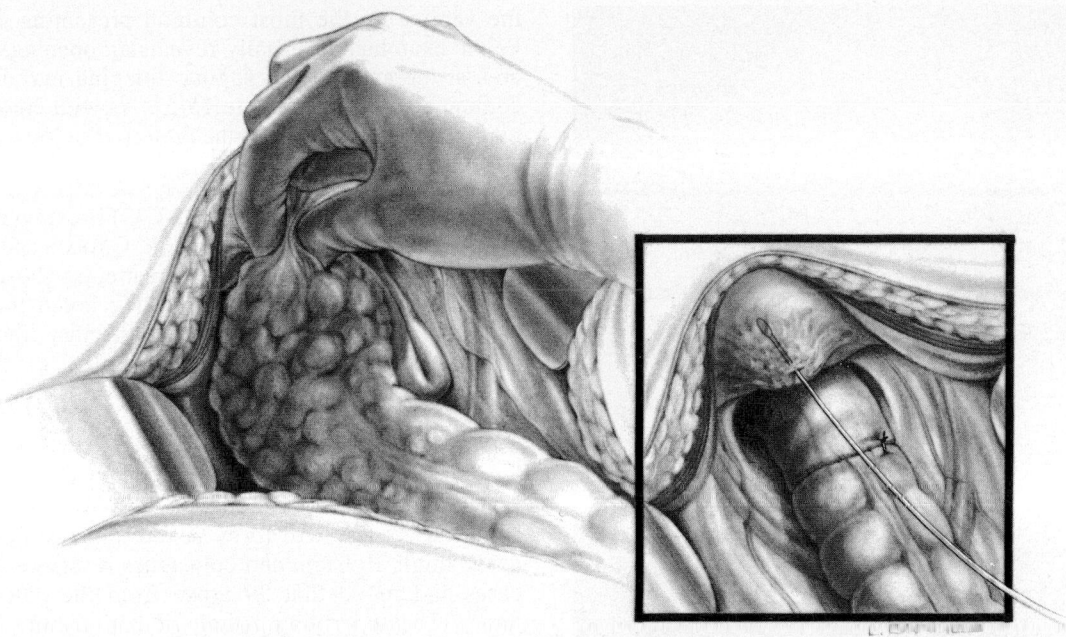

FIGURE 27-35. Using a pinching technique, one can separate the colon mass from the bladder. This minimizes the risk for bladder injury and avoids potential ureteral compromise if bowel fixation is posterior. Occasionally, the fibrosis is too dense for this maneuver, and sharp dissection is required. An opening in the bladder can be confirmed by inserting a probe (*inset*).

bladder wall, formally closing the organ in an area where there is no fibrosis, is unnecessary unless the diagnosis of cancer has not been excluded (Figure 27-36, *inset*). The urethral catheter should be left in place for 1 week and then removed after a cystogram has shown no evidence of a leak (Figure 27-37). The bowel is resected and a primary anastomosis is performed to the upper rectum. Fecal diversion is not advised.

Results

Woods and colleagues reported the Cleveland Clinic experience with internal fistulas.[340] There were 3 deaths (3.5%), a 21% incidence of wound infections, 1 enterocutaneous fistula, and a 5% incidence of anastomotic leaks. Other studies demonstrate the relative safety of one-stage resection.[194,243,264,299] Di Carlo and coworkers conducted a historical cohort study of patients who underwent surgery for

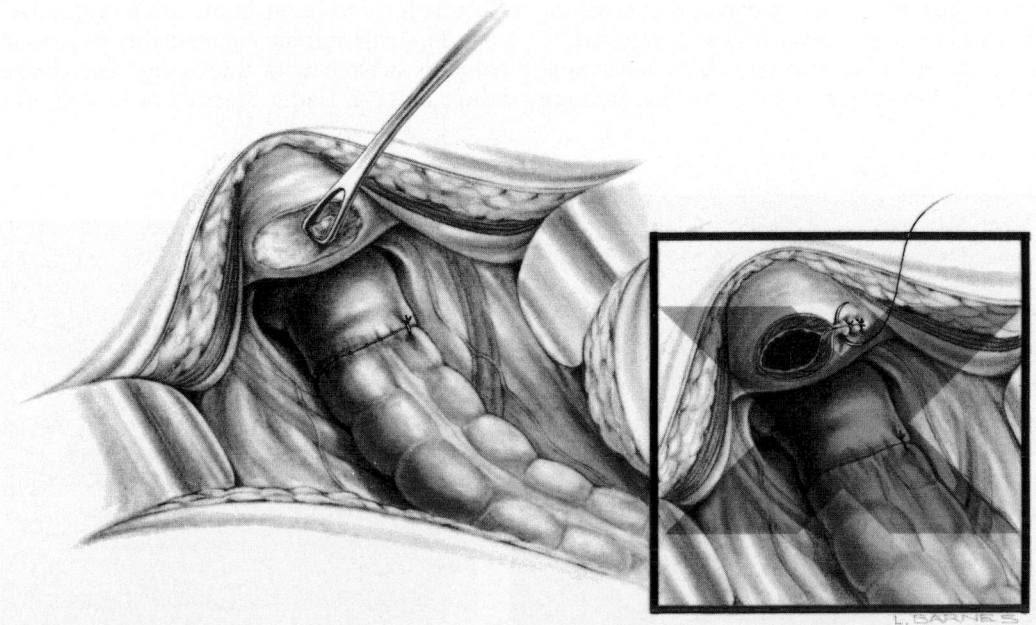

FIGURE 27-36. Curettage of granulation tissue may be all that is necessary for the bladder side of the fistula. The surgeon may wish to place one or two sutures to close the hole, but this is not a requisite because catheter drainage inevitably results in healing. Formal bladder wall excision and closure are unnecessary and meddlesome (*inset*).

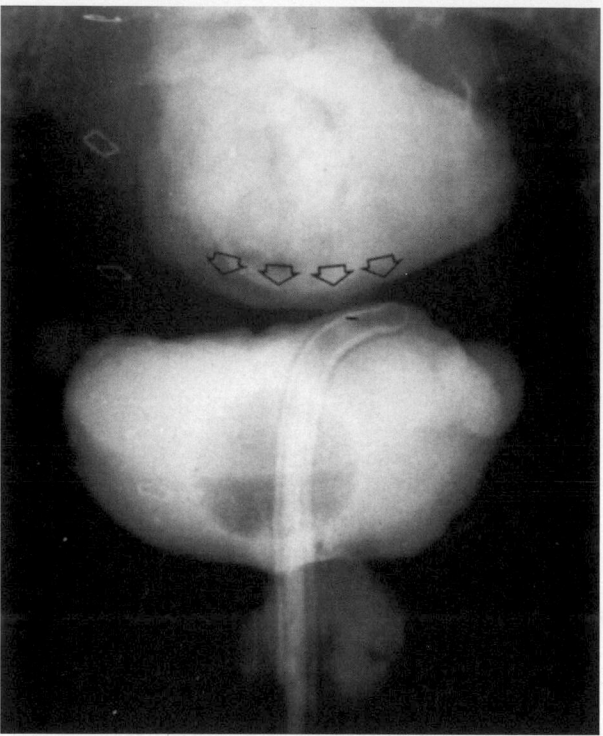

FIGURE 27-37. Bladder extravasation. Precipitous removal of the catheter resulted in leakage from a prior bladder fistula site (*arrows*).

fistula complicating diverticulitis and compared the results of general surgeons with that of colon and rectal surgeons.[74] They concluded that specialization in colon and rectal surgery contributed to an improved outcome, with a lower frequency of fecal diversion, a shorter hospital stay, and a lower complication rate.

Colovaginal Fistula

Colovaginal fistula may be a late consequence of acute diverticulitis after resolution, but such a history is very rare.[246] It virtually never occurs in the absence of a hysterectomy. Discharge of feces, blood, pus, mucus, or gas through the vagina are the most common presenting complaints. Pelvic examination usually reveals an opening or granular area at the apex of the vagina. Imaging may identify the communication (see Figure 15-5). As with colovesical fistula, one-stage resection is the preferred surgical approach.[60]

Ureterocolic Fistula

Ureterocolic fistula (see Figure 27-33) is extremely rare and is usually caused by urinary calculi. Cirocco and colleagues reviewed the literature of those patients whose condition was caused by diverticulitis.[55] They noted that urologic symptoms predominate, especially urinary tract infection (100%), fecaluria (75%), and abdominal (75%) or flank (50%) pain.

Colocutaneous Fistula

Rarely, a fistula can develop from the colon to the skin. If it is not fully communicating with the skin surface, a localized abscess will form. A rare presentation is spread to the thigh. Rotstein and colleagues reviewed 46 reported cases and found that 39 arose from the colon and rectum.[259] The underlying pathologic abnormality is usually a retroperitoneal perforation by diverticulitis or tumor. The external opening is usually in the abdominal wall, but pus may track to the thigh or the perineum where it may be mistaken for the opening of an anal fistula (see Figures 27-27 and 27-29). One should be suspicious of the possibility of a colonic origin if culture of a thigh abscess reveals enteric organisms.

In a series of 93 patients with colocutaneous associated with diverticular disease, Fazio and colleagues found the majority to have developed after surgery for the condition, only 5 being spontaneous.[91] Recurrence following surgery was due to Crohn's disease in 10, and there were 5 carcinomas.

Stricture Formation

Obstruction

Obstruction can occur in diverticular disease for two reasons. First, the chronic inflammatory process in the sigmoid colon associated with thickening and contraction of the bowel wall can lead to stenosis or stricture (Figure 27-38).

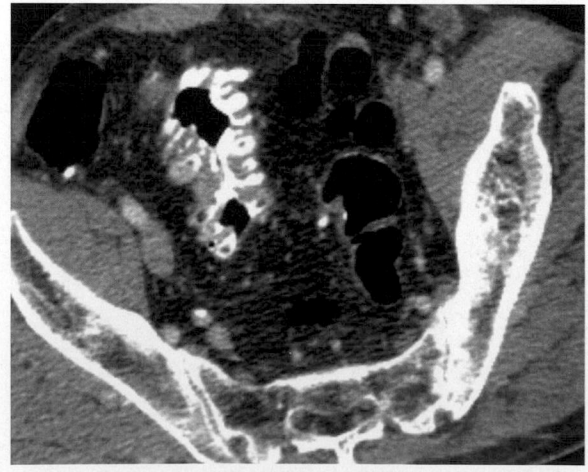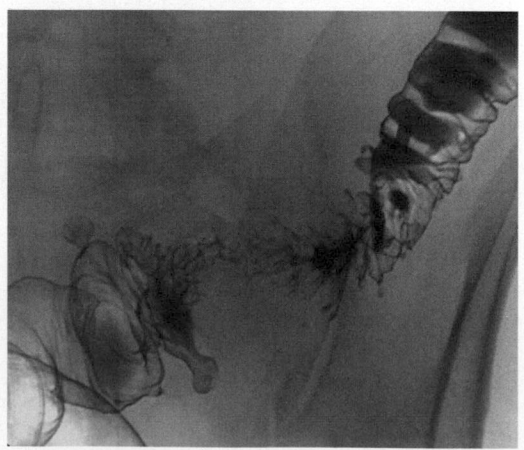

FIGURE 27-38. Computed tomogram **(A)** and contrast enema **(B)** showing stricture formation in the sigmoid colon. The presence of diverticula throughout the stricture with preservation of the mucosa distinguishes diverticular disease from carcinoma.

Symptoms may become exacerbated during an episode of acute diverticulitis, but the stricture can also be responsible for chronic large bowel obstruction. Second, small bowel obstruction can result from adhesion of a loop of the small bowel to an inflamed sigmoid colon. These presentations usually improve as inflammation subsides with effective treatment. Failure to do so should prompt surgical consultation. Recurrent episodes of diverticulitis, sometimes subclinical, can initiate progressive fibrosis and stricturing of the colonic wall without evidence of persistent inflammation. Ultimately, complete obstruction may occur, requiring surgery. Strictures may also present in an insidious manner with nonspecific complaints rather than an acute obstruction. Obstruction due to diverticular disease accounts for about 10% of patients presenting with large bowel obstruction.[113]

Management of Stricture

Generally, a stricture of uncertain cause is identified on colonoscopy, CT, or barium enema. The important issue is to distinguish between a diverticular stricture and a stenosing neoplasm. An attempt should be made to do so by colonoscopy, but it may not always be possible to advance the instrument into the sigmoid colon owing to angulation, narrowing, and tortuosity of the bowel. Conventional CT or CT quantitative perfusion measurement technology has been discussed earlier in this chapter.[108] Where the diagnosis is not certain, surgery is indicated by en bloc resection, adopting the principles of cancer surgery in the event that a neoplasm is actually present.

A trial of endoscopic treatment with balloon dilation can be attempted in patients in whom a neoplasm is judged to be reasonably excluded, but there is always a danger of perforation. Colonic stenting has also been used. Davidson and Sweeney report a single case in whom this was successful,[72] and Tamim and coworkers identified 3 out of an entire series of 11 patients in whom stenting was attempted.[300] Two of these went on to have a subsequent primary resection without a stoma and one refused surgery. In a larger study in which 96 patients underwent stenting, there were 8 with a benign stricture.[192] Only 3 of these gained any benefit, and there was an appreciable morbidity. The authors concluded that they were unable to recommend this technique for diverticular disease.

Most patients with evidence of obstruction will require surgical resection. When this is acute, it will usually be possible to carry out a resection with primary anastomosis. Unless the quality of the colon proximally is poor or profoundly dilated, this can often be done without a defunctioning stoma. An on-table lavage may be useful in clearing the colon of feces (see Chapter 23). If the patient is in poor condition and not deemed a candidate for an anastomosis, a Hartmann's procedure should be performed.

Hemorrhage

Hemorrhage is an important complication of diverticular disease. The bleeding is often voluminous and can be life threatening. The diagnosis can be difficult to make because colonoscopy is often hampered by the presence of blood in the lumen. CT angiogram will demonstrate blood in the lumen (Figure 27-39). It is important to distinguish diverticular bleeding from that of angiodysplasia. The reader is referred to Chapter 28 for a discussion of this subject.

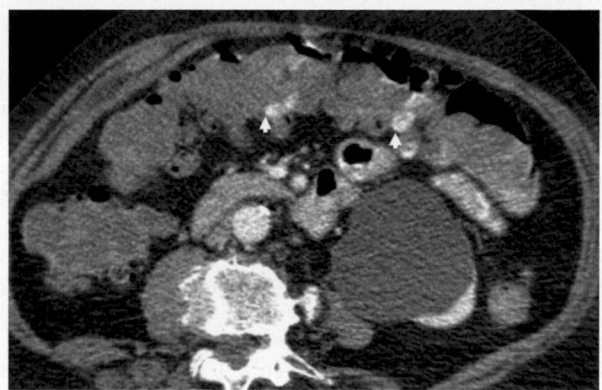

FIGURE 27-39. Blood in the lumen of the transverse colon in an acute diverticular bleed demonstrated on computed tomographic mesenteric angiogram.

▶ SYMPTOMATIC UNCOMPLICATED DIVERTICULAR DISEASE

Natural History

The decision whether to intervene surgically in a patient with uncomplicated sigmoid diverticulosis is a matter of controversy and is always a cause of debate and conflict between internists and surgeons. Clearly, the mere presence of diverticular disease is not a sufficient justification for recommending an operation. In the absence of complications, diverticulosis is unlikely to be the source of symptoms, such as bloating, cramping, abdominal pain, or constipation. However, the antecedent history of a complication of diverticulitis somewhat simplifies the operative recommendation, but many patients who may benefit from resection do not have such a prior history. Conversely, some may be at risk of having an unnecessary operation.

In a useful study on this subject, 163 patients with symptomatic diverticular disease without any inflammatory component were followed for a median of 5.5 years (range, 4.2 to 6.7).[262] The presence of diverticula had been established by colonoscopy (106), flexible sigmoidoscopy (57), or barium enema (31). Nineteen were lost to follow-up, 19 had died of unrelated causes, and 25 were excluded (cancer, 3; hemorrhoids, 11; and polyps, 11). During the course of follow-up, 2 patients had experienced an acute attack and 1 patient underwent surgery for symptoms. The remaining 116 (97%) had either no complaints or mild symptoms at 66 months. The authors concluded that this clinical group of patients was at low risk for complications or surgery, and in most patients the disease took a mild course.

Medical Treatment

The mainstay of medical treatment is fiber. In recent years, however, other options have been investigated. These include the poorly absorbed antibacterial agent, rifaximin, mesalazine, and probiotics. Useful information on this subject is provided in special articles by Korzenik[159] and Rocco.[258]

Fiber

Fiber has been shown to be an effective treatment of many symptomatic patients with uncomplicated diverticular disease.[45,81,139,220,221] In a review by Aldoori and colleagues, the authors consider the evidence that a fruit and vegetable-rich fiber diet with a low fat and red meat content reduces the risk of diverticular disease.[7]

The outer covering of any cereal grain, the bran, is a particularly rich source of fiber. Certain vegetables and fruits are also relatively high in fiber, whereas milk and milk products, chicken, fish, meat, eggs, fats, and beverages have none. Many people believe that by eating a salad each day they should be achieving an adequate fiber intake. However, a whole head of lettuce is not quite equivalent to one serving (one-third of a cup) of a bran cereal. Despite the availability of high fiber foods, most people find them either unpalatable or intolerably repetitive. An alternate approach is to take a proprietary preparation in so-called bulk laxative form. These are derived from the outer covering of the psyllium grain or from sterculia- and ispaghula-derived hydrophilic colloids. Over-the-counter preparations include Konsyl, Citrucel, FiberCon, Fiberall, and Metamucil, among many others. A daily whole grain cereal or bran bread may become rather monotonous, but most people have a glass of juice in the morning. By adding one of the preparations to this or a glass of water, once or twice daily, an effective dietary fiber supplement can be achieved.

Brodribb carried out a randomized trial of fiber in a small group of 18 patients followed for a short period of 3 months.[45] "Significantly greater symptomatic relief was obtained by those on a high fiber regimen than by those in the control group." Unfortunately, the period of the study was too short for the results to be meaningful. Hodgson also found that methylcellulose was better than placebo in improving symptoms of patients with uncomplicated diverticular disease.[132] Ornstein and colleagues conducted a randomized trial of crisp bread and ispaghula husk against placebo in 58 patients with uncomplicated diverticular disease. The patients were reviewed at the short interval of 4 months. There was no difference in the pain score, bowel symptoms, and total symptom score, although constipation improved. The authors ascribed this to a nonspecific effect of fiber on stool frequency.[215]

Drugs
Rifaximin
Cyclic administration of the broad spectrum antibacterial agent, rifaximin, has been used in the treatment of patients with symptomatic diverticular disease based on the finding that there is bacterial overgrowth in the vicinity of diverticula.[325] Papi and colleagues conducted a trial of rifaximin in which 168 patients with symptomatic, uncomplicated diverticular disease were randomized to receive rifaximin (400 mg, 7 days per month) and fiber (glucomannan, 4 g/day) and fiber with placebo.[225] At 12 months, 68.9% in the former group were symptom-free or had only mild symptoms compared with only 39.5% in the latter group.[226] Colecchia and coworkers also conducted a controlled trial of 307 patients randomized to rifaximin (400 mg twice daily for 7 days a month) plus fiber (20 g/day) versus fiber (20 g/day) alone.[59] A symptom score was used to assess the effect of treatment. This included five variables (pain, bloating, tenesmus, diarrhea, and abdominal tenderness), each scored from 0 (absent) to 3 (severe, interfering with normal activities). At 24 months, the score was reduced in both groups, but more so in those taking rifaximin with fiber (6.4 to 1.0; 6.2 to 2.4). In still another prospective multicenter open trial, 968 patients with symptomatic, uncomplicated diverticular

disease were "randomized" to fiber (glucomannan 4 g/day) with rifaximin (400 mg twice daily for 7 days per month) and to fiber alone.[169] At 12 months, 56.5% and 29.2% were symptom-free, and 1.34% and 3.22% had experienced an attack of acute diverticulitis, both differences being statistically significant. The analysis was not carried out on an intention to treat basis, and 10% of patients were unable to complete the trial. In a short-term trial, D'Incà and associates randomized 64 patients with uncomplicated, symptomatic diverticular disease, all of whom were given bran (20 g/day) to two groups, including rifaximin (1,200 mg daily for 2 weeks) and placebo for 2 weeks.[76] At assessment at 1 month, the symptom scores before and after were 7.1 and 4.1 and 6.8 and 6.1, respectively, a significant difference.

Mesalazine
The use of mesalazine was first tested by Tursi and colleagues.[316] Subsequently, Brandimarte and Tursi reported 90 consecutive patients with symptomatic diverticular disease who were given rifaximin (800 mg daily) with added mesalazine, 2.4 g/day for 10 days, followed by 1.6 g/day for 8 weeks.[42] At assessment, 81% had become asymptomatic. Di Mario and colleagues conducted a randomized controlled trial of rifaximin against mesalazine in 170 patients with symptomatic diverticular disease.[75] The were four groups: rifaximin, 200 mg twice daily (39 patients); rifaximin, 400 mg twice daily for 10 days per month (43); mesalazine, 400 mg twice daily (40); and mesalazine, 800 mg twice daily for 10 days per month (48). A global symptomatic score including assessment of 11 symptoms with a maximum of 33 points was used. There were no withdrawals. At 3 months, the symptom score had fallen in the higher dose rifaximin group (9.8–5.9) and in both of the mesalazine groups (11.0–6.7 and 8.8–4.9). In a subsequent paper from the same unit, Comparato and colleagues reported the results of the trial, now expanded to 268 patients followed for 1 year.[61] There were 24 withdrawals, and the results at 12 months were analyzed on an intention to treat basis. The symptom score did not fall in the low-dose rifaximin group. In the higher dose rifaximin group, it fell from 9.16 to 5.64, which was less than in either of the mesalazine groups (10.18–3.67 and 9.48–2.44). The authors concluded that mesalazine was effective in reducing symptoms. These studies did not give details of the randomization process, and there was no indication that assessment was blinded. In an open-label prospective study, Tursi and colleagues divided 40 patients with recurrent symptomatic, not inflammatory diverticular disease in order to take mesalazine, either daily (1.6 g/day) or in a cyclic manner (1.6 g/day for 10 days per month).[318] At 24 months, 6 patients had withdrawn for various reasons, and in the remaining 34, 70% on continuous mesalazine were symptom-free, compared with 45% on cyclic treatment, suggesting that the former method of administration is preferable.

Calcium Channel Blockers
Calcium channel blockers reduce intracolonic pressure and may be associated with a lower incidence of perforation in those with diverticular disease. Thus, in a series of 54 patients who previously had perforated diverticular disease, when compared with 183 patients with verified nonperforated diverticular disease, the odds ratio for calcium channel blocker consumption was 0.14, whereas those for NSAIDs, opiates, and steroids were 3.56, 4.51, and 28.28, respectively.[236] In a

study of 120 patients admitted to hospital with perforated diverticular disease over a 5-year period, comparison of medication was made with patients having cataract surgery and with basal cell carcinoma. Calcium channel blocker consumption in the diverticular patients was 6.7%, 14.2% in cataract patients, and 25.8% in patients with basal cell carcinoma. Despite these observations, there was no difference in other cardiovascular medication taken by the patients in the three groups.[198] In a larger study, however, calcium channel blockers were not associated with a lower incidence.[138]

Opiates, Nonsteroidal Anti-inflammatory Drugs, Steroids

These drugs are associated with perforated diverticular disease and should be stopped in individuals with diverticular disease if this is at all possible (see earlier).

Probiotics

Fric and Zavoral studied 15 patients with uncomplicated diverticular disease (of whom 7 had a previous attack of acute diverticulitis) using a symptom scoring system after two periods of treatment for a week by an antimicrobial.[100] After the second treatment, the patients were then given a nonpathogenic E. coli strain for an average period of 5 weeks. They found little response to the antimicrobial treatment, but there was a significant reduction of the scores for pain, irregular bowel habit, bloating, and flatus. Symptomatic remission was far longer in the probiotic (14 months) group than in the antimicrobial (2.5 months) group. In sequential reports, Tursi and colleagues added Lactobacillus casei (16 billion organisms per day) to two regimens of mesalazine treatment (800 mg/day and 1.6 g/day) for 10 days per month.[317,319] There were 75 patients enrolled, of whom 71 managed to comply with the treatment for 24 months. At that time, 66 (83%) were symptom-free with proportions in the probiotic groups of more than 90%. Unfortunately due to the mixed treatments, the study does not permit an assessment of probiotic effects alone.

Surgery for Symptomatic Uncomplicated Diverticular Disease

How does one advise surgery for a patient with chronic symptomatic disease? Although imaging will give an objective assessment of the morphologic severity of the disease, provided the clinician is certain that there is no cancer present, this must be based on the clinical picture. This includes the severity of the symptoms and the degree which they are influencing the patient's quality of life. Even if radiologic evaluation reveals narrowing, deformity, or partial obstruction, one can never be certain that symptoms will resolve following resection unless there is evidence of the presence of acute disease. It is well accepted that in those with diverticula who also have symptoms, functional bowel disease may actually be the cause. For example, despite a low operative complication rate in 88 patients who underwent elective resection for uncomplicated disease, persistent symptoms were still present in 86%.[249] Furthermore, the fact remains that those with recognized irritable bowel symptoms have a poorer outcome following surgery.[308]

There is, however, a relatively small group of patients who have troublesome symptoms significantly detracting from one's quality of life and in whom the balance of clinical judgment may be in favor of diverticula being the cause as opposed to an IBS. This is a difficult area to opine upon, an issue for which only clinical judgment can be the arbiter.

Surgical Technique

The principles of surgery include removal of the entire sigmoid colon and rectosigmoid junction. Where an anastomosis is performed, this should be made between nonthickened colon and the upper rectum (Figure 27-40). The operation is, therefore, essentially a high anterior resection, leaving sigmoid colon risks recurrence. Preservation of the inferior mesenteric artery might minimize the risk of anastomotic leakage,

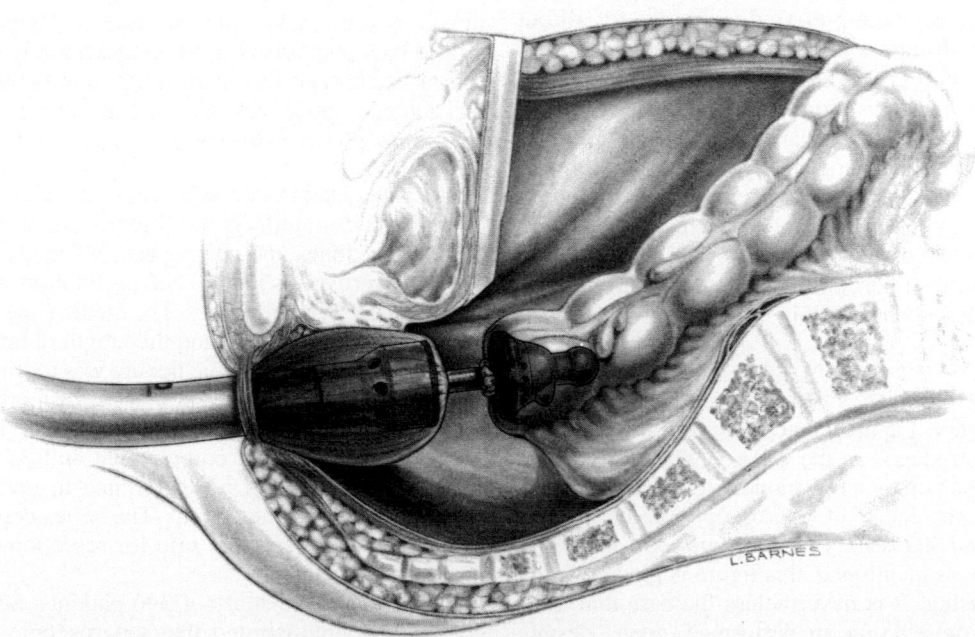

FIGURE 27-40. Circular stapled technique for reestablishing continuity following creation of a Hartmann's pouch or following resection with primary anastomosis. As illustrated, the anastomosis should be created in the rectum (where there are no taenia).

sexual dysfunction from intraoperative nerve injury, and optimize functional results. Mobilization of the splenic flexure should be left to the discretion of the operating surgeon, but some surgeons prefer to accomplish this routinely through laparoscopic mobilization prior to proceeding with an open operation. Involvement of the tissue surrounding the sigmoid colon by the inflammatory process is variable. It is almost always possible to identify the ureters intraoperatively, and the pelvic dissection can be limited to the upper rectum.

There are certainly instances of complicated diverticulitis in which the extent and degree of inflammatory changes warrant the use of ureteral stents and/or the creation of a colorectal anastomosis in the more distal rectum. In such cases, a difficult, prolonged dissection with significant blood loss may also justify the creation of a proximal diverting stoma. With respect to the required extent of resection, it is not necessary or prudent to remove the entire colonic segment bearing diverticula. This may actually be impossible to accomplish in some cases without performing a total colectomy because of the extent and density of diverticula throughout the colon. However, care should be taken to prevent inclusion of any diverticula into a stapled colorectal anastomosis. These difficulties reflect an important surgical principle. Therefore, particular attention must be paid at this point in the operation. The need for adequate blood supply and the avoidance of tension on the anastomosis needs no explanation or amplification. These expressed concerns should apply equally to open or laparoscopic surgery.

The technical details of elective resection for diverticulitis are essentially the same as that for carcinoma of the sigmoid colon, with minor differences. If the diagnosis is in doubt, the operation should be carried out as if a carcinoma were present. The reader is referred to the illustrations and narrative in Chapter 23 for the surgical approach to management.

Laparoscopic Surgery

Since the last edition of this book, there has been a major move toward laparoscopic surgery to the extent that it is now for many surgeons the preferred technique for all but Hinchey stage IV disease and in those for whom a trial of laparoscopic resection proves impracticable. This approach will continue to increase as more surgeons become trained and experienced in this field. Laparoscopic resection should be as safe and as effective as open surgery. It can be applied to most patients with complicated diverticulitis, including those with stricture and fistula. At the moment there is clearly a reluctance to apply it to fecal peritonitis, but given what has happened with purulent peritonitis, it would be surprising if it were not ultimately considered in the most severe cases.

Technique

The reader is also referred to Chapter 19 for the principles of laparoscopic surgery. Laparoscopic resection for colorectal pathology was introduced in the early 1990s and within a short time was taken up by a few pioneering specialist units. Now 20 years on, the uptake of laparoscopic surgery by surgeons in the United States and Europe is approximately 20% to 30%, although, as mentioned, this figure is gradually and constantly increasing. It is nevertheless the case that most procedures at the present time are performed "open," despite the fact that diverticular disease is a benign condition, and that there have been technical advances in the general approach and instrumentation as well as training.

It is clear that laparoscopy can be applied to diverticular disease safely, with a low mortality and a morbidity at least not greater than with open surgery. It is essential, however, that the surgeon be properly trained and that mentoring is continued until the surgeon is fully confident and able to deal with unexpected situations in a safe manner. Conversion rates differ between surgeons and surgical units. To some extent, this is due to the severity of the pathology, as is the case with diverticular disease, but it will also be surgeon-dependent. Estimations of the number of cases a trainee requires before becoming proficient in colorectal laparoscopic surgery will depend on the environment in which the trainee is working. For example, in ileoanal pouch surgery, the learning curve requirement is approximately 26 procedures, but all of these should be carried out under supervision.[302]

In theory, it is possible to perform all operations at least in part, laparoscopically. Various techniques may be employed. These include total laparoscopic resection in which the dissection and anastomosis are carried out entirely intracorporally through small 5- or 12-mm operating ports introduced through trocar incisions. In laparoscopic-assisted surgery, laparoscopic mobilization is combined with open removal of the specimen. An open anastomosis is then accomplished through a small abdominal incision. Hand-assisted laparoscopic surgery involves dissection using laparoscopic instruments, and the hand is inserted into the peritoneal cavity through a specially designed hand port.

Mobilization of the left colon may be carried out in a classic lateral to medial manner, but most laparoscopic surgeons prefer a medial to lateral approach. This allows early identification of the inferior mesenteric artery and the retroperitoneal structures (ureter and gonadal vessels). Division of the inferior mesenteric artery is carried out by the stapler, and the left colon is then further mobilized to the splenic flexure. As with open surgery, it is important to ensure that the dissection is taken sufficiently proximal to pliable nonthickened colon, which will be subsequently used in the anastomosis. Mobilization of the splenic flexure is usually recommended. Distally, the dissection is taken beyond the rectosigmoid junction as judged by a point distal to the coalescence of the taenia coli. The anastomosis is then performed entirely by an intracorporeal double-stapling technique or manually through a small incision through which the specimen has already been removed.

Single Series Laparoscopic Studies. A large series of 500 patients (305 females) undergoing laparoscopic resection was reported by Jones and colleagues.[148] The indication was recurrent diverticulitis in 77% and perforation and fistulization in 10% and 9%, respectively. The median operation time was 120 minutes (45 to 285), and the length of hospital stay was 4 days (2 to 33). The splenic flexure was routinely mobilized. There was one 30-day death, and major morbidity occurred in 55 (11%). Conversion was required in 14 patients (2.8%). This included 5.3% in complicated and 2.1% for uncomplicated disease, with no difference in operating time of complications in either group. The series demonstrated that laparoscopic surgery was safe for resection of diverticular disease of any type.

In a prospective study of 396 patients, Schwandner and colleagues demonstrated that laparoscopic surgery could be used for any patient requiring surgery for diverticular disease, although they excluded those with free perforation or fistula.[279] Thus, patients with Hinchey stage I and II disease, chronic recurrent diverticulitis, and stenosis were included. The rates of conversion (6.8%), anastomotic leakage (1.6%), and all major complications (7.6%) were low. The length of stay was 11.8 (4 to 71) days. These results indicate that laparoscopic surgery can be applied to complicated diverticular disease with a high degree of safety.

When the results of laparoscopic sigmoid resection (LSR) for diverticular disease (n = 363) and noninflammatory conditions such as sigmoidocele or cancer (n = 313) were compared, there was no difference in the outcome. Therefore, the rates of major complications (7.4% vs. 7.9%), minor complications (11.5% vs. 14.5%), reoperation (8.6% vs. 9.3%), and mortality (0.6% vs. 0.7%) were not statistically different.[278] In a small, randomized trial of laparoscopic-assisted versus laparoscopic-facilitated sigmoid colectomy, there was no difference in the outcome between groups of 22 and 23 patients.[233]

Conversion. Reported conversion rates to an open procedure have ranged from less than 10% to more than 30%. Hassan and colleagues, in a series of 125 patients who underwent laparoscopic-assisted or hand-assisted resection for diverticular disease, reported that 33 (26%) required conversion.[125] The only independent variable relating to conversion was prior surgery and not whether the disease was complicated or uncomplicated. Probably not surprisingly converted patients experienced more complications (44% vs. 24%), but there was no difference in morbidity in those who had complicated and uncomplicated disease (39% vs. 24%).

The French Society of Laparoscopic Surgeons conducted a multicenter prospective observational study of 179 patients having a resection for diverticular disease accrued over a 13-month period.[41] The indication was acute diverticulitis in 123 and complicated disease in 47. Conversion was necessary in 25 (13.9%), mostly due to obesity or to adhesions. This resulted in an increased hospital stay from 9 to 13 days. Cole and coworkers showed in a study of 170 patients having a laparoscopic resection for diverticular disease that conversion (19 patients) was related to whether the patient had three or more previous attacks (2.6% vs. 25%) and also whether or not an abscess was present (8% vs. 23%).[58]

Conversion appears to be more common in patients with diverticular disease than with other pathologies. Of 143 patients who underwent laparoscopic surgery for any indication, 16 of the 28 conversions were in individuals with diverticular disease.[32] In addition, the authors found that conversion was far more likely for left than for right-sided resections (86% vs. 14%), and that conversion beyond 30 minutes into the operation was associated with a higher morbidity. The lengths of stay for laparoscopic, open, and converted procedures were 6, 8, and 12 days. A similar result was reported by the Laparoscopic Colorectal Surgery Study Group in which 1,118 patients were recruited into a multicenter study over a 3-year period.[154] The overall conversion rate was 4.2%, but this differed from 2.8% in patients with mild disease to 18.2% in those with complicated disease. There was also a difference in the complication rate in patients having surgery for perforation, fistula, or bleeding (29%) and those without these features (14.8%). The report of the Norfolk Surgical Group Laparoscopic Surgical Registry of 69 patients having surgery for diverticular disease also noted different rates of conversion between uncomplicated and complicated disease (14% vs. 69%).[323]

Conversion may be less if one employs hand-assisted laparoscopy. Chang and associates reported conversion in 13% of 85 patients having standard laparoscopic resection.[51] This compared with no instance among 66 patients operated on by the hand-assisted technique.

Laparoscopic Compared with Open Resection. Purkayastha and colleagues undertook a review with meta-analysis of 12 nonrandomized studies encompassing 19,608 patients.[241] Ninety-four plus percent were accounted for by one study of 18,444 patients.[115] Removing or including the large study did not make any difference in the results. Laparoscopic surgery was associated with reduced complications (expressed as OR using open as the reference) in the following categories: infective (OR = 0.61), pulmonary (OR = 0.4), gastrointestinal (OR = 0.75), and cardiovascular (OR = 0.28). The operating time was longer, and the length of hospital stay was shorter with laparoscopic surgery. Blood loss was less.

Guller and colleagues used the 1998, 1999, and 2000 NISs, adopting the *ICD-9-CM* procedure codes of the *International Classification of Disease, Ninth Edition, Clinical Modification* to identify patients who underwent laparoscopic and open resection of diverticular disease.[115] There found 18,444 patients, including 17,735 open and 709 laparoscopic operations. Length of stay was 9.37 versus 7.47 days, and gastrointestinal and overall complications were less in the laparoscopic patients.

In another retrospective comparison of laparoscopic and open sigmoid resection (OSR) for diverticular disease, Dwivedi and coworkers reported 66 laparoscopic and 88 open procedures.[79] Respective figures for blood loss (143 vs. 314 mL), first introduction of liquids by mouth (2.9 vs. 4.9 days), length of hospital stay (4.8 vs. 8.8 days), anastomotic leakage (1.5% vs. 3.4%), and operating time (212 vs. 143 minutes) all show the value of the former, with the exception of the longer operating time.

Alves and colleagues reported a comparison of open and laparoscopic elective resection of diverticular disease in a prospective national multicenter study in France, conducted over a 4-month period in 2002.[14] Eighty-one centers were involved, including 46 that performed laparoscopic and 67 open surgery. There were 332 patients, 163 laparoscopic and 169 open. One patient (in the open group) died. Morbidity (16% vs. 31%), readmission rates (8% vs. 12%), and length of hospital stay (5 vs. 15 days) favored the laparoscopic group, and morbidity was still higher in the open group after correction for age and ASA status.

A randomized, controlled, blinded trial was carried out by Klarenbeek and colleagues in 104 patients who underwent either LSR (n = 52) or OSR (n = 52).[153] The surgery was performed 3 or more months following the last acute attack. "Sigmoid diverticulitis" was diagnosed by CT and/or barium enema or colonoscopy. Patients with perforation, prior colorectal resection, or previous laparotomy except for a gynecologic indication were excluded. The study was blinded because the assessors were not aware of the patient group, and the abdomen was covered during the admission. The covering was removed at the time of discharge. The operating time was longer and blood loss was less in the LSR group. The conversion rate was 19%, and the operative mortality was 1%. Major complications were less frequent in the LSR group (9.6% vs. 25%), there was less postoperative pain with less analgesic requirement ($P < .29$), and the length of hospital stay was 5 versus 7 days ($P < .46$). The high conversion rate is likely to be due to operative findings, which included patients with locally severe diverticular disease.

Similar results were obtained in another randomized, controlled trial in which the laparoscopic and open groups were blinded by a dressing held in place for 4 days.[106] One hundred and thirteen patients were randomized to laparoscopic (54) and open (59) surgery. The operation times were 165 and 110 minutes, the intervals to first bowel action were 76 and 105 hours, the mean pain scores were 4 and 5, and the lengths of hospital stay were 5 and 7 days.

Other Indications

A laparoscopic approach to Hartmann's procedure has been described in seven patients with Hinchey stage III and IV disease (unspecified).[3] There was no conversion nor mortality, and return of bowel function occurred in 3.7 days.

Those with a colovesical fistula can also be treated by laparoscopic means, although operating time and conversion rates may be higher than that for patients having laparoscopic resection for acute diverticulitis. Bartus and colleagues reported a series of 36 patients with a fistula, whom they compared to 149 operated on for acute diverticulitis without fistula.[28] The operating time (220 vs. 171 minutes), conversion rate (25% vs. 5%), and length of hospital stay (6.2 vs. 4.4 days) were greater in the presence of a fistula.

Results of Elective Surgery

In an early report of elective surgery in 100 consecutive patients, there were no operative deaths, and symptoms were ameliorated in 94%, leaving 6% with pain affecting quality of life.[43] Factors associated with a favorable result included male sex, preoperative symptoms of less than 1 year's duration, abdominal pain localized to the left lower quadrant, and radiologic evidence of "diverticulitis" rather than "diverticulosis." The presence of inflammation in the resected specimen was related to a good clinical result. All patients with evidence of acute or chronic inflammation in the resected specimen even after an elective procedure were improved.[32] Preoperative factors associated with more frequent postoperative complaints included the presence of bowel symptoms for more than 1 year and abdominal pain not localized to the left lower quadrant.

Resection for diverticular disease is associated with a higher complication rate than is essentially the same operation for cancer, although the operative mortality is less.[39,87] Incisional hernia is much more frequently observed, 10% in the experience of Breen and coworkers.[43]

With careful selection of patients most likely to benefit from resection, excellent long-term results may be anticipated. Wolff and associates reviewed the Mayo Clinic experience with 505 elective resections for sigmoid diverticular disease between 1971 and 1976.[338] When the barium enema studies of 61 of these patients were reviewed between 5 and 9 years after resection, only 9 (14.7%) showed progression of diverticula, and this was believed to be minimal in all cases. However, in 7 patients (11.4%), signs and symptoms of recurrent diverticulitis developed. Although the authors believed that there was no benefit in resecting all of the diverticula-bearing colon, the results are somewhat disturbing. Because they described the operation as a "sigmoid resection," the explanation for their less than optimal results could be that the anastomosis was not placed into the rectum and that a zone of increased pressure was permitted to remain distal to the anastomosis. A later study from the same institution confirmed this observation. Recurrent diverticulitis developed in 12.5% of the patients in whom the sigmoid colon had been used for the distal anastomosis but in only 6.7% of those in whom the rectum had been used ($P = .03$).[269] Reoperation was required in 3.4% of the patients in whom the sigmoid colon had been used as the distal anastomotic site and in 2.2% of those in whom the rectum had been used ($P < .05$).[33] The Cleveland Clinic Florida group concluded based on their 236 patients that colorectal (rather than colosigmoid) anastomosis was the single most important predictor of lower recurrence rates after elective resection for uncomplicated diverticulitis.[305]

The Mayo Clinic group analyzed 930 patients with diverticular disease over a 10-year period.[135] The authors described what they called "smoldering diverticular disease" in 5%. These are individuals with chronic, debilitating, left lower quadrant abdominal pain as the only symptom, with no documented history of fever, elevated white cell count, or radiologic evidence of diverticulitis. These patients were found to have complete resolution of symptoms in 76%, with 88% being pain free.

Other Operations

Myotomy and Taeniamyotomy

In the 1950s and 1960s, Reilly advocated myotomy aimed to decrease intracolonic pressure and one which carried less trauma than open resection.[248] The primary indication for the procedure was long-standing, uncomplicated diverticular disease that did not respond to standard medical measures. Such patients comprised 75% of his 104 cases. The remainder were those who exhibited complications of sigmoid diverticulitis and who underwent elective myotomy following resolution of the acute process, sometimes after colostomy and drainage. There was a significant morbidity from leakage, and the operation is now of historical interest only. Hodgson and colleagues proposed transverse taeniamyotomy.[131,133] The two antimesenteric taeniae were transversely incised at 2-cm intervals from the rectosigmoid junction proximally to the normal colon. A later report from Hodgson's group implied less enthusiasm for the technique.[186] This also is of historical interest only.

▶ GIANT COLONIC DIVERTICULUM

Giant colonic diverticulum is quite rare, with only 150 cases reported in the past 40 years.[11,103,128,152,163,184,191,270,309,334] The condition was originally described by Hughes and Greene and by Gabriel.[102,137] Choong and Frizelle believed that this condition should be defined by any diverticulum larger than 4 cm.[53] In their review of the literature, they classified 103 reported cases as type I, a pseudodiverticulum (87%), and type II (13%), a true diverticulum. Toiber-Levy and colleagues found the mean age to be 65 years with an equal sex distribution. The sigmoid colon was involved in 90% of cases.

The most accepted theory for the formation of a giant diverticulum is a contained perforation of a colonic diverticulum. All described cases originated from the antimesenteric border of the colon, with the lesion representing a pseudodiverticulum with or without intact mucosa that becomes progressively enlarged. Still more rarely, a giant diverticulum may be encountered in which all layers of the bowel wall are found; a giant true diverticulum.[204,293,309]

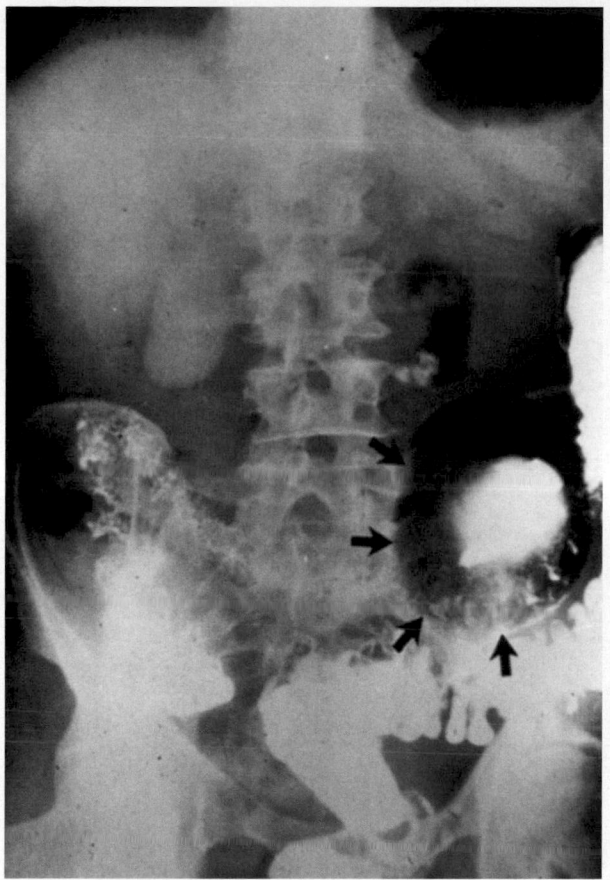

FIGURE 27-41. Giant sigmoid diverticulum. Barium fills part of the cavity; gas is also evident within the lumen (*arrows*).

Most patients complain of abdominal pain or the presence of a lump.[173] A plain abdominal x-ray film may reveal a gas-filled mass of considerable size. Differential diagnosis includes congenital duplication of the colon, colonic volvulus, emphysematous cholecystitis, infected pancreatic pseudocyst, pneumatosis cystoides intestinalis, giant duodenal diverticulum, intestinal obstruction, intra-abdominal lipoma, and intra-abdominal abscess.[104] Barium enema examination will show the lesion filled with contrast material (Figure 27-41). CT scan will show feces filling the diverticulum (Figure 27-42).[196]

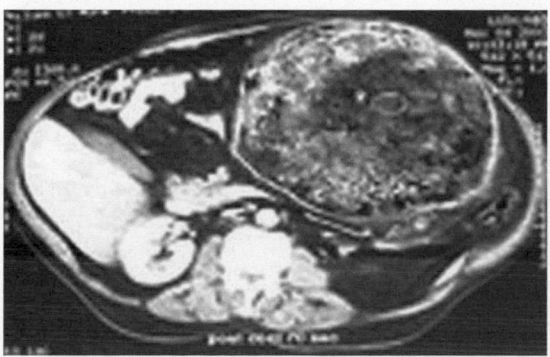

FIGURE 27-42. Giant colonic diverticulum. CT scan of the abdomen and pelvis with oral and intravenous contrast reveals a giant diverticulum arising from the sigmoid colon, mainly containing fecal matter.

Treatment

Resection of the diverticulum with the sigmoid colon is advised (Figure 27-43), although there have been a few reports of diverticulectomy alone.[11,53,173,295] This is not advised, however, because removal of the source of the complication, namely the sigmoid colon, is important.

▶ DIVERTICULAR DISEASE OF THE RIGHT COLON

Diverticulitis of the cecum was first described by Potier in 1912.[239] Although the disease is uncommon in the West, many reports and reviews have been published over the years, mainly of the condition in the Eastern world.

Epidemiology

In a review of the literature from 1950 to 2001, Nakaji and colleagues noted that right-sided disease accounts for 70% of cases in Japan.[209] There was evidence of an increased incidence particularly in urban areas.[141] Adoption of a Western diet may influence the prevalence of diverticular disease, but the site at which diverticula tend to occur is probably determined more by race or by genetic predisposition than environment.[170] Munakata and colleagues are quoted by Nakaji and associates to have demonstrated an inverse relationship between fiber consumption and the incidence of right-sided diverticular disease in Japan from the analysis of 10-year birth cohorts (1905 to 1955).[209] The age of the patients is generally less than those who harbor left-sided disease.[110,160]

Pathophysiology

Diverticula that involve the right colon may be solitary or multiple, but they should be distinguished from right-sided diverticula that exist concurrently with extensive diverticulosis throughout the colon. The former type of diverticulum traditionally has been thought to be congenital, and most were believed to be true diverticula, that is, containing all layers of the intestine. However, Murayama and colleagues measured the thickness of the right colon muscle in right-sided diverticular disease together with the number of haustra in the right colon.[206] They suggested that the etiology is the same as that of left-sided diverticular disease, abnormal thickening of the muscle in the wall of the colon. A solitary diverticulum has a shorter and wider neck than do multiple diverticula.[167] As with left-sided disease, there is an increased intraluminal pressure, and in addition the complications are similar to those that occur in left-sided diverticular disease. However, in support of the theory of a congenital origin, proponents have observed that the condition tends to occur at a much earlier age than does left-sided colitis.

Diagnosis

The main diagnostic difficulty is to distinguish the condition from other causes of acute presentation on the right side of the abdomen. This includes acute appendicitis, chronic cholecystitis, mesenteric adenitis, ischemic colitis, pelvic inflammatory disease, pancreatitis, Meckel's diverticulitis, pyelonephritis, and sigmoid diverticulitis (with a redundant sigmoid loop). With modern imaging technology, the diagnosis will have become easier, but the rarity of the

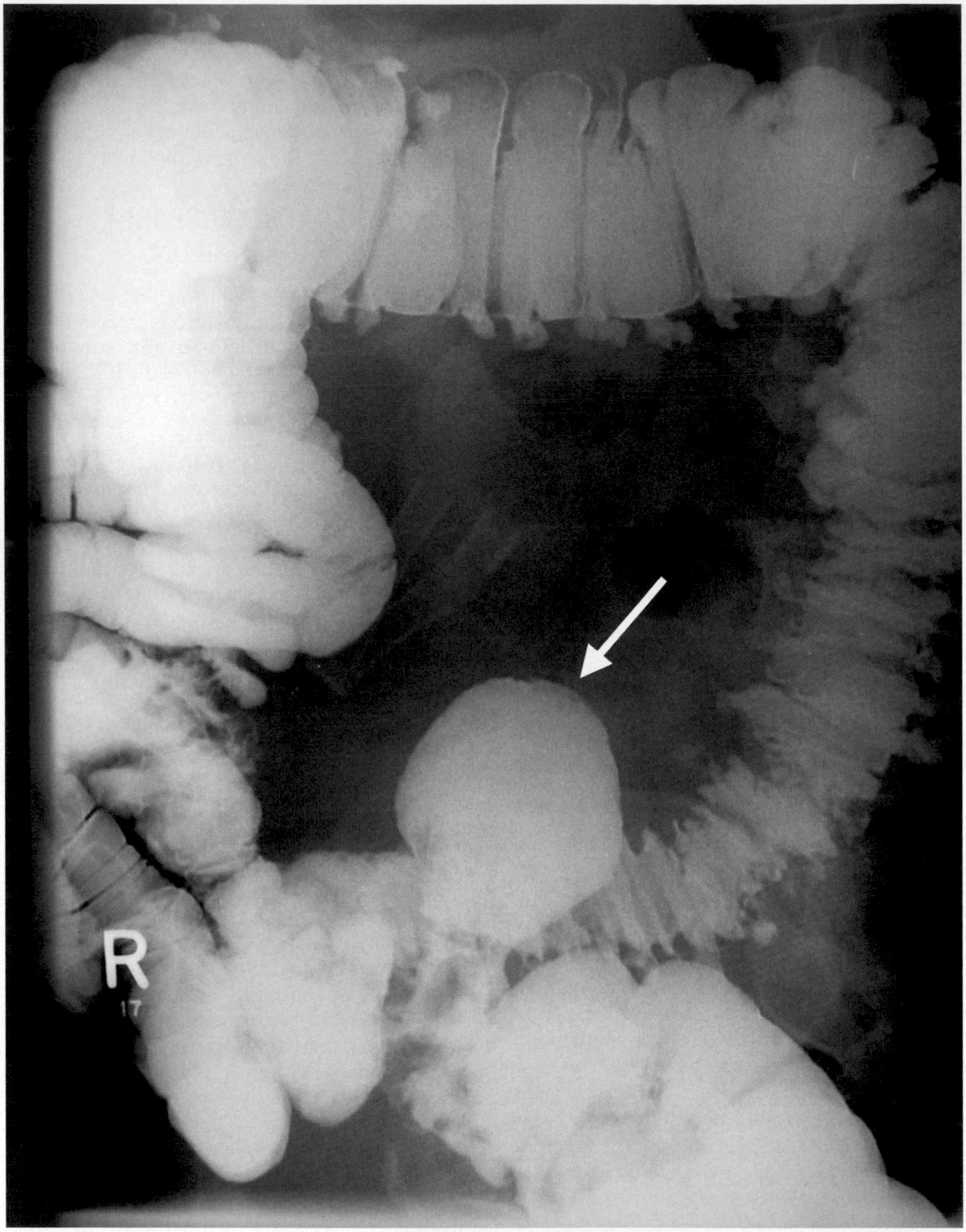

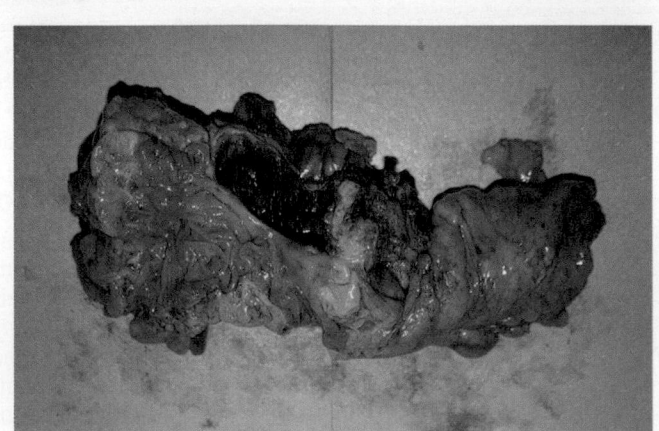

FIGURE 27-43. Giant sigmoid diverticulum.
A: Barium enema study with diverticulum (*arrow*).
B: Resected specimen.

condition is such that the disease may not even be considered. But it should certainly be in the mind of the clinician when treating a patient of Eastern origin.

Clinical Features

The symptoms and signs of right-sided diverticulitis mimic those of appendicitis. Patients may complain of epigastric pain, nausea, and vomiting, with migration of the pain into the right iliac fossa. Depending on whether the process is localized or diffuse, low-grade fever, moderate tenderness, guarding, and rebound may be noted. The leukocyte count is usually elevated. A presentation with major lower gastrointestinal bleeding may be more common in right than in left-sided diverticular disease.

Investigations

For some patients, a clinical diagnosis of appendicitis will be made, and on this basis alone surgery may be advised. There is an increasing tendency, however, for imaging to be requested in a patient with an acute abdomen. CT or abdominal sonography is likely to show a right-sided septic process in most cases, although the precise diagnosis may not always be evident. A paracolic mass or a fistula is highly suggestive of the presence of cecal diverticulitis (see Figure 27-17). In a small early series of 7 patients with diverticulitis of the cecum and ascending colon, there was thickening of the bowel wall, pericolonic inflammation, and associated abscess formation in 5.[70]

Treatment

A limited surgical approach would include simple excision of the involved diverticulum and closure of the bowel, but because the inflammatory mass usually involves much of the cecum or right colon, resection is usually required. Moreover, partial colectomy is probably advisable whenever an inflammatory mass is present because of the difficulty in distinguishing the lesion from a perforating carcinoma.

The literature contains several small case series in which the results of surgery indicate that right hemicolectomy is the most prevalent operation. Of 11 patients who underwent surgery for cecal diverticulitis during a 10-year period, the average age was 49 years, considerably younger than the average age for patients with left-sided diverticulitis.[160] Nine underwent resection, and 8 had a primary anastomosis; 2 had a diverticulectomy. No death or anastomotic leakage was reported. In another report of 14 patients with diverticulitis, all had an inflammatory mass medial and posterior to the ascending colon, with perforation and abscess in 8.[110] There was no case of free perforation. All patients underwent resection with ileocolic anastomosis, without mortality or leakage. McFee and colleagues reported 18 patients with right-sided diverticulitis with an average age of 46 years.[189] All but 1 underwent resection with primary anastomosis. There were no deaths.

At the time of surgery, it may be difficult to distinguish the condition from acute appendicitis or even from sigmoid diverticulitis. In the latter situation, it is imperative to identify the source of the inflammation. The preoperative diagnosis is rarely correct, so a high index of suspicion must be maintained, particularly in those who have undergone prior appendectomy or when rectal bleeding accompanies the abdominal signs and symptoms. In a series of 30 cases,

Sardi and colleagues found that even at the time of surgery, the diagnosis was correct in fewer than 60%.[266]

More recently, Fang and coworkers reported from Taiwan 85 patients with a confirmed diagnosis treated over a 5-year period.[88] Of these, 18 were treated conservatively, 3 of whom developed a subsequent recurrence and had a right hemicolectomy. Of the 67 who underwent surgery, 24 had an appendicectomy. Of these, 7 experienced a further episode of diverticulitis leading to hemicolectomy in three cases. Overall, 34 had a right hemicolectomy and 9 a diverticulectomy. The authors emphasize the variation between mild and severe disease and the difficulty in differentiating between appendicitis and inflammation of a cecal diverticulum. In severe cases, an aggressive approach was recommended. In reporting the largest series from the United States, a right hemicolectomy was carried out initially in 39 (70%), diverticulectomy in 7 (14%), and appendectomy in 3 patients (all of whom required a subsequent right hemicolectomy for recurrence).[166]

It appears, then, that the disease may not be recognized preoperatively. There is also general agreement that resection with primary anastomosis is almost always the preferred treatment, with the anticipation of a low mortality rate.

▶ DIVERTICULAR DISEASE OF THE TRANSVERSE COLON

Reports of acute diverticulitis of the transverse colon are extremely rare.[187,237,283,306] Peck and Villar identified 27 cases and added 3 of their own.[233] The mean age in the collected series was 53 years, and most of the patients (83%) were women. As with right colon diverticulitis, individuals tend to be younger and are most commonly thought to have acute appendicitis or cholecystitis. Other differential diagnostic concerns include perforated colon cancer, ischemic colitis, and Crohn's disease.

Evaluation by means of CT has identified the following findings based on the four cases reported by Jasper and colleagues.[146] These include stranding within the adjacent mesenteric fat, asymmetric wall thickening, and the presence of extraluminal gas or fluid (Figure 27-44). These observations are not dissimilar to that observed in right-sided or sigmoid diverticulitis. Contrast enema is the study most likely to be diagnostic through the identification of mucosal preservation, but the correct diagnosis is usually made at the time of operation. Even then, the condition may be confused with carcinoma of the colon. As with sigmoid diverticulitis in those who are unresponsive to bowel rest and antibiotics, resection is the preferred treatment.

▶ DIVERTICULAR DISEASE OF THE RECTUM

Rectal diverticular disease is a very rare condition, with only a handful of case reports having been published.[122] In the review by Piercy and colleagues, two theories for the low incidence in this area were proposed: the low pressure in the rectum and a reduced peristaltic activity.[237] In contrast to the pseudodiverticula of sigmoid disease, rectal diverticula involve all layers of the bowel wall. Because of the usual absence of symptoms, no treatment is advised. However, inspissated fecal material leading to ischiorectal

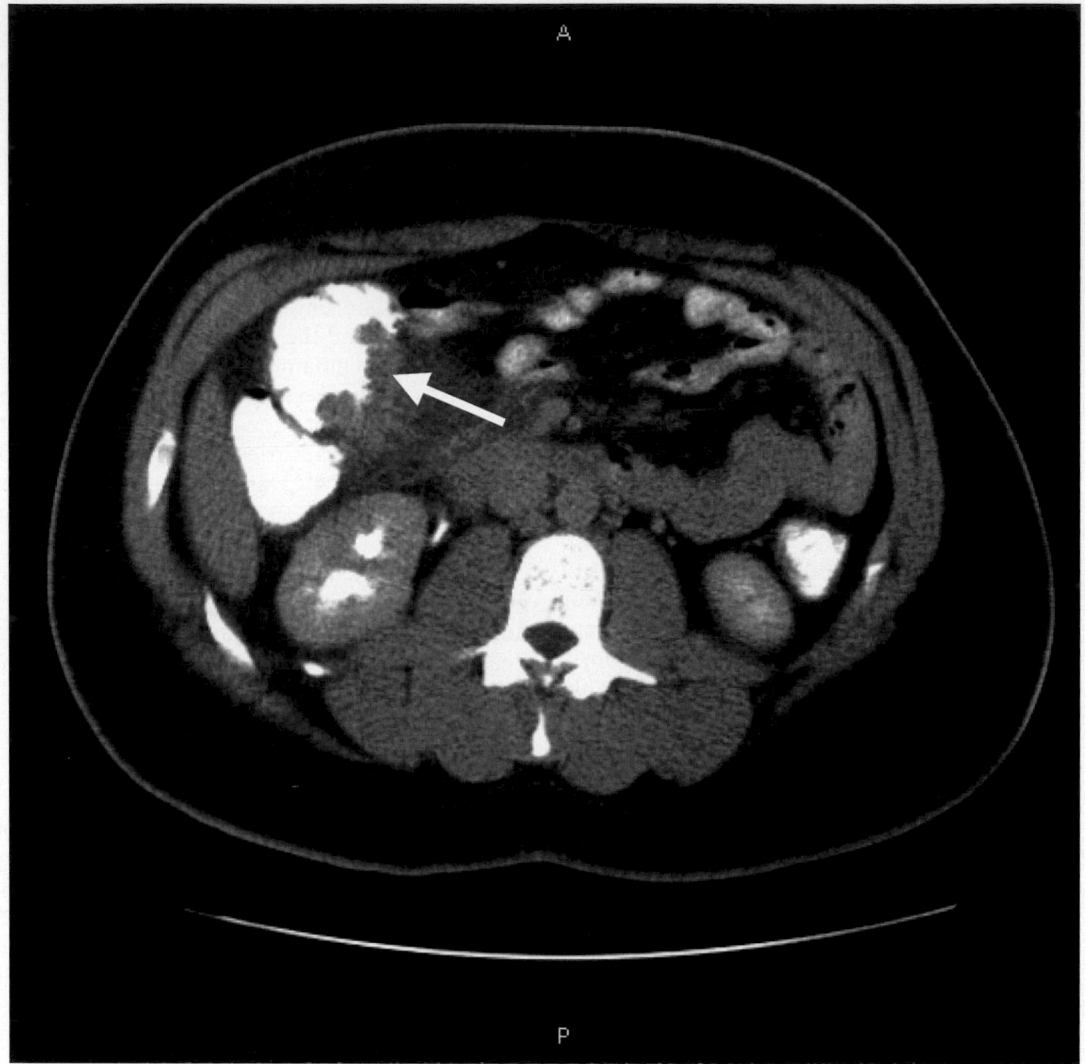

FIGURE 27-44. Diverticulitis of the proximal transverse colon. Computed tomography demonstrates eccentric inflammation on the inferior aspect of the bowel (*arrow*) with the suggestion of an inflammatory mass. (Courtesy of Avraham Belizon, MD.)

abscess formation with subsequent extrasphincteric fistula following incision and drainage has been observed. Another reported complication is rectal prolapse from an inverted diverticulum.[83]

► DIVERTICULAR DISEASE OF THE SMALL BOWEL

Diverticular disease, excluding Meckel's diverticulum, can occur anywhere in the small intestine but is quite uncommon. Most patients are asymptomatic, with the outpouching discovered incidentally during an abdominal exploration or seen in a small bowel series that had been performed for another indication. However, occasionally an individual may develop symptoms related to its presence. Small bowel diverticula may present with such complications as malabsorption, hemorrhage, obstruction, abscess, and fistula formation.[114] Complaints may include abdominal pain, nausea, bloating, vomiting, flatulence, weight loss, and diarrhea. Bleeding is usually the result of erosion of a mesenteric vessel and may be diagnosed by angiography (see Chapter 28). Bowel obstruction may be a consequence of adhesions,

stricture, volvulus, intussusception, or the presence of an enterolith. When inflammation ensues, the presentation is indistinguishable from that of peptic ulcer disease, colon diverticulitis, or appendicitis.[114] If the patient fails to respond to conservative measures, such as bowel rest, nasogastric tube, and antibiotics, or if someone presents with signs and symptoms of perforation, laparotomy with resection is advised.

References

1. Abcarian H, Pearl RK. A safe technique for resection of perforated sigmoid diverticulitis. *Dis Colon Rectum.* 1990;33(10):905–906.
2. Acosta JA, Grebenc ML, Doberneck RC, et al. Colonic diverticular disease in patients 40 years old or younger. *Am Surg.* 1992;58(10): 605–607.
3. Agaba EA, Zaidi RM, Ramzy P, et al. Laparoscopic Hartmann's procedure: a viable option for treatment of acutely perforated diverticulitis. *Surg Endosc.* 2009;23(7):1483–1486.
4. Aguilo JJ, Zincke H, Woods JE, et al. Intestinal perforation due to fecal impaction after renal transplantation. *J Urol.* 1976;116(2):153–155.
5. Ajaj W, Ruehem SG, Lauenstein T, et al. Dark-lumen magnetic resonance colonography in patients with suspected sigmoid diverticulitis: a feasibility study. *Eur Radiol.* 2005;15(11):2316–2322.
6. Alamili A, Gögenur I, Rosenberg J. Acute complicated diverticulitis managed by laparoscopic lavage. *Dis Col Rectum.* 2009;52(7):1345–1349.

7.   Aldoori W, Ryan-Harshman M. Preventing diverticular disease. Review of recent evidence on high-fibre diets. *Can Fam Physician.* 2002;48: 1632–1637.

8.   Aldoori WH, Giovannucci EL, Rimm EB, et al. A prospective study of alcohol, smoking, caffeine, and the risk of symptomatic diverticular disease in men. *Ann Epidemiol.* 1995;5(3):221–228.

9.   Aldoori WH, Giovannucci EL, Rimm EB, et al. Prospective study of physical activity and the risk of symptomatic diverticular disease in men. *Gut.* 1995;36(2):276–282.

10.   Alexander J, Karl RC, Skinner DB. Results of changing trends in the surgical management of complications of diverticular disease. *Surgery.* 1983;94(4):683–690.

11.   Al-Jurf AS, Foucar E. Uncommon features of giant colonic diverticula. *Dis Colon Rectum.* 1983;26(12):808–813.

12.   Almy TP, Howell DA. Medical progress. Diverticular disease of the colon. *N Engl J Med.* 1980;302(6):324–331.

13.   Alonso S, Pera M, Parés D, et al. Outpatient treatment of patients with uncomplicated acute diverticulitis. *Colorectal Dis.* 2009;12(10 online): e278–e282.

14.   Alves A, Panis Y, Slim K, et al. French multicentre prospective observational study of laparoscopic versus open colectomy for sigmoid diverticular disease. *Br J Surg.* 2005;92(12):1520–1525.

15.   Ambrosetti P. Acute diverticulitis of the left colon: value of the initial CT and timing of elective colectomy. *J Gastrointest Surg.* 2008;12(8): 1318–1320.

16.   Ambrosetti P, Becker C, Terrier F. Colonic diverticulitis: impact of imaging on surgical management—a prospective study of 542 patients. *Eur Radiol.* 2002;12(5):1145–1149.

17.   Ambrosetti P, Chautems R, Soravia C, et al. Long-term outcome of mesocolic and pelvic diverticular abscesses of the left colon: a prospective study of 73 cases. *Dis Colon Rectum.* 2005;48(4):787–791.

18.   Ambrosetti P, Grossholz M, Becker C, et al. Computed tomography in acute left colonic diverticulitis. *Br J Surg.* 1997;84(4):532–534.

19.   Ambrosetti P, Jenny A, Becker C, et al. Acute left colonic diverticulitis—compared performance of computed tomography and water-soluble contrast enema: prospective evaluation of 420 patients. *Dis Colon Rectum.* 2000;43(10):1363–1367.

20.   Ambrosetti P, Robert J, Witzig JA, et al. Incidence, outcome, and proposed management of isolated abscesses complicating acute left-sided colonic diverticulitis. A prospective study of 140 patients. *Dis Colon Rectum.* 1992;35(11):1072–1076.

21.   Ambrosetti P, Robert J, Witzig JA, et al. Prognostic factors from computed tomography in acute left colonic diverticulitis. *Br J Surg.* 1992;79(2):117–119.

22.   Ambrosetti P, Robert JH, Witzig JA, et al. Acute left colonic diverticulitis: a prospective analysis of 226 consecutive cases. *Surgery.* 1994;115(5):546–550.

23.   Anderson GA, Goldman IL, Mulligan GW. 3-dimensional computerized tomographic reconstruction of colovesical fistulas. *J Urol.* 1997;158(3 pt 1):795–797.

24.   Arfwidsson S, Knock NG, Lehmann L, et al. Pathogenesis of multiple diverticula of the sigmoid colon in diverticular disease. *Acta Chir Scand Suppl.* 1964;63(suppl 342):1–68.

25.   Arnott I, Paterson H, Nicholls RJ, et al. A doubling of admissions due to diverticular disease in Scottish hospitals, in the last 14 years. *Gut.* 2011;60(suppl 1):A7.

26.   Bahadursingh AM, Virgo KS, Kaminski DL, et al. Spectrum of disease and outcome of complicated diverticular disease. *Am J Surg.* 2003;186(6):696–701.

27.   Balthazar EJ, Megibow A, Schinella RA, et al. Limitations in the CT diagnosis of acute diverticulitis: comparison of CT, contrast enema, and pathologic findings in 16 patients. *AJR Am J Roentgenol.* 1990;154(2):281–285.

28.   Bartus CM, Lipof T, Sarwar CM, et al. Colovesical fistula: not a contraindication to elective laparoscopic colectomy. *Dis Colon Rectum.* 2005;48(2):233–236.

29.   Bassotti G, Battaglia E, Spinozzi F, et al. Twenty-four hour recordings of colonic motility in patients with diverticular disease: evidence for abnormal motility and propulsive activity. *Dis Colon Rectum.* 2001;44(12): 1814–1820.

30.   Beaver TM, Fullerton DA, Zamora MR, et al. Colon perforation after lung transplantation. *Ann Thorac Surg.* 1996;62(3):839–843.

31.   Beer E. Some pathological and clinical aspects of acquired (false) diverticula of the intestine. *Am J Med Sci.* 1904;128:135–145.

32.   Belizon A, Sardinha CT, Sher ME. Converted laparoscopic colectomy: what are the consequences? *Surg Endosc.* 2006;20(6):947–951.

33.   Benn PL, Wolff BG, Ilstrup DM. Level of anastomosis and recurrent colonic diverticulitis. *Am J Surg.* 1986;151(2):269–271.

34.   Bergamaschi R. Uncomplicated diverticulitis of the sigmoid: old challenges. *Scand J Gastroenterol.* 1997;32(12):1187–1189.

35.   Berman IR, Corman ML, Coller JA, et al. Late onset Crohn's disease in patients with colonic diverticulitis. *Dis Colon Rectum.* 1979;22(8):524–529.

36.   Bernstein WC, Nivatvongs S, Tallent MB. Colonic and rectal complications of kidney transplantation in man. *Dis Colon Rectum.* 1973;16(4):255–263.

37.   Binda GA, Karas JR, Serventi A, et al. Primary anastomosis vs. Hartmann for perforated diverticulitis with fecal peritonitis: a randomized controlled trial [abstract]. *Dis Colon Rectum.* 2011;54.

38.   Biondo S, Parés D, Martí Ragué J, et al. Acute colonic diverticulitis in patients under 50 years of age. *Br J Surg.* 2002;89(9):1137–1141.

39.   Bokey EL, Chapius PH, Pheils MT. Elective resection for diverticular disease and carcinoma. Comparison of postoperative morbidity and mortality. *Dis Colon Rectum.* 1981;24(3):181–182.

40.   Bokhari M, Vernava AM, Ure T, et al. Diverticular hemorrhage in the elderly—is it well tolerated? *Dis Colon Rectum.* 1996;39(2):191–195.

41.   Bouillot JL, Berthou JC, Champault G, et al. Elective laparoscopic colonic resection for diverticular disease: results of a multicenter study in 179 patients. *Surg Endosc.* 2002;16(9):1320–1323.

42.   Brandimarte G, Tursi A, Rifaximin plus mesalazine followed by mesalazine alone is highly effective in obtaining remission of symptomatic uncomplicated diverticular disease. *Med Sci Monit.* 2004;10(5):PI70–PI73.

43.   Breen RE, Corman ML, Robertson WG, et al. Are we really operating on diverticulitis? *Dis Colon Rectum.* 1986;29(3):174–176.

44.   Bretagnol F, Pautrat K, Mor C, et al. Emergency laparoscopic management of perforated sigmoid diverticulitis: a promising alternative to more radical procedures. *J Am Coll Surg.* 2008;206(4):654–657.

45.   Brodribb AJ. Treatment of symptomatic diverticular disease with a high-fibre diet. *Lancet.* 1977;1(8013):664–666.

46.   Brolin RE, Flancbaum L, Ercoli FR, et al. Limitations of percutaneous catheter drainage of abdominal abscesses. *Surg Gynecol Obstet.* 1991;173(3):203–210.

47.   Brook I, Frazier EH. Aerobic and anaerobic microbiology in intra-abdominal infections associated with diverticulitis. *J Med Microbiol.* 2000;49(9):827–830.

48.   Burkitt DP, Walker AR, Painter NS. Effect of dietary fibre on stools and transit times, and its role in the causation of disease. *Lancet.* 1972;2(7792):1408–1412.

49.   Burkitt DP, Walker AR, Painter NS. Dietary fiber and disease. *JAMA.* 1974;229(8):1068–1074.

50.   Campbell K, Steele RJ. Non-steroidal anti-inflammatory drugs and complicated diverticular disease: a case-control study. *Br J Surg.* 1991;78(2):190–191.

51.   Chang YJ, Marcello PW, Rusin LC, et al. Hand-assisted laparoscopic sigmoid colectomy: helping hand or hindrance? *Surg Endosc.* 2005;19(5):656–661.

52.   Chautems RC, Ambrosetti P, Ludwig A, et al. Long-term follow-up after first acute episode of sigmoid diverticulitis: is surgery mandatory? A prospective study of 118 patients. *Dis Colon Rectum.* 2002;45(7): 962–966.

53.   Choong CK, Frizelle FA. Giant colonic diverticulum: report of four cases and review of the literature. *Dis Colon Rectum.* 1998;41(9): 1178–1185.

54.   Church JM, Fazio VW, Braun WE, et al. Perforation of the colon in renal homograft recipients. A report of 11 cases and a review of the literature. *Ann Surg.* 1986;203(1):69–76.

55.   Cirocco WC, Priolo SR, Golub RW. Spontaneous ureterocolic fistula: a rare complication of colonic diverticular disease. *Am Surg.* 1994;60(11):832–835.

56.   Cohn KH, Weimar JA, Fani K, et al. Adenocarcinoma arising within a colonic diverticulum: report of two cases and review of the literature. *Surgery.* 1993;113(2):223–226.

57.   Colcock BP, Stahmann FD. Fistulas complicating diverticular disease of the sigmoid colon. *Ann Surg.* 1972;175(6):838–846.

58.   Cole K, Fassler S, Suryadevara S, et al. Increasing the number of attacks increases the conversion rate in laparoscopic diverticulitis surgery. *Surg Endosc.* 2009;23(5):1088–1092.

59.   Colecchia A, Vestito A, Pasqui F, et al. Efficacy of long term cyclic administration of the poorly absorbed antibiotic Rifaximin in symptomatic, uncomplicated colonic diverticular disease. *World J Gastroenterol.* 2007;13(2):264–269.

60.   Colonna JO II, Kang J, Giuliano AE, et al. One-stage repair of colovaginal fistula complicating acute diverticulitis. *Am Surg.* 1990;56(12):788–791.

61.   Comparato G, Fanigliulo L, Cavallaro LG, et al. Prevention of complications and symptomatic recurrences in diverticular disease with mesalazine: a 12-month follow-up. *Dig Dis Sci.* 2007;52(11):2934–2941.

62. Connell AM. Applied physiology of the colon: factors relevant to diverticular disease. *Clin Gastroenterol.* 1975;4(1):23–36.

63. Constantinides VA, Tekkis PP, Athanasiou T, et al. Primary resection with anastomosis vs. Hartmann's procedure in nonelective surgery for acute colonic diverticulitis: a systematic review. *Dis Colon Rectum.* 2006;49(7):966–981.

64. Constantinides VA, Tekkis PP, Senapati A, et al. Comparison of POSSUM scoring systems and the surgical risk scale in patients undergoing surgery for complicated diverticular disease. *Dis Colon Rectum.* 2006;49(9):1322–1331.

65. Corder A. Steroids, non-steroidal anti-inflammatory drugs, and serious septic complications of diverticular disease. *Br Med J (Clin Res Ed).* 1987;295(6608):1238.

66. Corman ML. Colovesical fistula complicating diverticulitis in brothers. *Dis Colon Rectum.* 1999;42(11):1511.

67. Cortesini C, Pantalone D. Usefulness of colonic motility study in identifying patients at risk for complicated diverticular disease. *Dis Colon Rectum.* 1991;34(4):339–342.

68. Cranston D, McWhinnie D, Collin J. Dietary fibre and gastrointestinal disease. *Br J Surg.* 1988;75(6):508–512.

69. Criado FJ, Wilson TH Jr. Technique for reestablishing continuity after the Hartmann operation. *Am Surg.* 1981;47(8):366–367.

70. Crist DW, Fishman EK, Scatarige JC, et al. Acute diverticulitis of the cecum and ascending colon diagnosed by computed tomography. *Surg Gynecol Obstet.* 1988;166(2):99–102.

71. Cruveilhier J. *Traite d'Anatomie Pathologique Generale.* Vol 1. Paris, France: Bailliere; 1849.

72. Davidson R, Sweeney WB. Endoluminal stenting for benign colonic obstruction. *Surg Endosc.* 1998;12(4):353–354.

73. Dean AC, Newell JP. Colonoscopy in the differential diagnosis of carcinoma from diverticulitis of the sigmoid colon. *Br J Surg.* 1973;60(8):633–635.

74. Di Carlo A, Andtbacka RH, Shrier I, et al. The value of specialization—is there an outcome difference in the management of fistulas complicating diverticulitis? *Dis Colon Rectum.* 2001;44(10):1456–1463.

75. Di Mario F, Aragona G, Leandro G, et al. Efficacy of mesalazine in the treatment of symptomatic diverticular disease. *Dig Dis Sci.* 2005;50(3):581–586.

76. D'Incà R, Pomerri F, Vettorato MG, et al. Interaction between rifaximin and dietary fibre in patients with diverticular disease. *Aliment Pharmacol Ther.* 2007;25(7):771–779.

77. Draghetti MJ, Salvo AF. Gas in the mesenteric veins as a nonfatal complication of diverticulitis: report of a case. *Dis Colon Rectum.* 1999;42(11):1497–1498.

78. Duffy F, Lowell JA, Tahan SR, et al. Rectal diverticulitis complicated by perforation and obstruction. *Contemp Surg.* 1994;44:111.

79. Dwivedi A, Chahin F, Agrawal S, et al. Laparoscopic colectomy vs. open colectomy for sigmoid diverticular disease. *Dis Colon Rectum.* 2002;45(10):1309–1315.

80. Eastwood MA, Smith AN, Brydon WG, et al. Colonic function in patients with diverticular disease. *Lancet.* 1978;1(8075):1181–1182.

81. Eastwood MA, Smith AN, Brydon WG. Comparison of bran, ispaghula, and lactulose on colon function in diverticular disease. *Gut.* 1978;19(12):1144–1147.

82. Eastwood MA, Watters DA, Smith AN. Diverticular disease—is it a motility disorder? *Clin Gastroenterol.* 1982;11(3):545–561.

83. Edwards VH, Chen MY, Ott DJ, et al. Rectal diverticulum appearing as a prolapsed rectum. *J Clin Gastroenterol.* 1994;18(3):254–255.

84. Eglinton T, Nguyen T, Raniga S, et al. Patterns of recurrence in patients with acute diverticulitis. *Br J Surg.* 2010;97(6):952–957.

85. Ercoli FR, Milgrim LM, Nosher JL, et al. Percutaneous catheter drainage of abscesses associated with enteric fistulae. *Am Surg.* 1988;54(1):45–49.

86. Etzioni DA, Mack TM, Beart RW Jr, et al. Diverticulitis in the United States: 1998–2005: changing patterns of disease and treatment. *Ann Surg.* 2009;249(2):210–217.

87. Failes D, Killingback M, Stuart M, et al. Elective resection for diverticular disease. *Aust N Z J Surg.* 1979;49(1):66–72.

88. Fang JF, Chen RJ, Lin BC, et al. Aggressive resection is indicated for cecal diverticulitis. *Am J Surg.* 2003;185(2):135–140.

89. Faranda C, Barrat C, Catheline JM, et al. Two-stage laparoscopic management of generalized peritonitis due to perforated sigmoid diverticula: eighteen cases. *Surg Laparosc Endosc Percutan Tech.* 2000;10(3):135–138.

90. Farmakis N, Tudor RG, Keighley MR. The 5-year natural history of complicated diverticular disease. *Br J Surg.* 1994;81(5):733–735.

91. Fazio VW, Church JM, Jagelman DG, et al. Colocutaneous fistulas complicating diverticulitis. *Dis Colon Rectum.* 1987;30(2):89–94.

92. Finney JMT. Diverticulitis and its surgical treatment. *Proc Interstate Post-Grad Med Assembly North Am.* 1928;55:57–65.

93. Floch MH. A hypothesis: is diverticulitis a type of inflammatory bowel disease? *J Clin Gastroenterol.* 2005;40(suppl):S121–S125.

94. Flor N, Rigamonti P, Di Leo G, et al. Technical quality of CT colonography in relation with diverticular disease. *Eur J Radiol.* 2012;81(3):e250–e254.

95. Forde KA. Colonoscopy in complicated diverticular disease. *Gastrointest Endosc.* 1977;23(4):192–193.

96. Fozard JB, Armitage NC, Schofield JB, et al. ACPGBI position statement on elective resection for diverticulitis. *Colorectal Dis.* 2011;13(suppl 3):1–11.

97. Franklin ME Jr, Portillo G, Treviño JM, et al. Long-term experience with the laparoscopic approach to perforated diverticulitis plus generalized peritonitis. *World J Surg.* 2008;32(7):1507–1511.

98. Freeman HJ. Natural history and long-term clinical behavior of segmental colitis associated with diverticulosis (SCAD syndrome). *Dig Dis Sci.* 2008;53(9):2452–2457.

99. Freischlag J, Bennion RS, Thompson JE Jr. Complications of diverticular disease of the colon in young people. *Dis Colon Rectum.* 1986;29(10):639–643.

100. Fric P, Zavoral M. The effect of non-pathogenic *Escherichia coli* in symptomatic uncomplicated diverticular disease of the colon. *Eur J Gastroenterol Hepatol.* 2003;15(3):313–315.

101. Frieden JH, Morgenstern L. Sigmoid diverticulitis in identical twins. *Dig Dis Sci.* 1985;30(2):182–183.

102. Gabriel W. Diverticulitis of the pelvic colon with large solitary diverticulum. *Proc R Soc Med.* 1953;46:416.

103. Gallagher JJ, Welch JP. Giant diverticula of the sigmoid colon: a review of differential diagnosis and operative management. *Arch Surg.* 1979;114(9):1079–1083.

104. Garner OJ Jr, Bolin JA, LeSage MA, et al. Acute solitary cecal diverticulitis. *Am Surg.* 1973;39(12):700–705.

105. Gear JS, Ware A, Fursdon P, et al. Symptomless diverticular disease and intake of dietary fibre. *Lancet.* 1979;1(8115):511–514.

106. Gervaz P, Inan I, Perneger T, et al. A prospective, randomized, single-blind comparison of laparoscopic versus open sigmoid colectomy for diverticulitis. *Ann Surg.* 2010;252(1):3–8.

107. Goh H, Bourne R. Non-steroidal anti-inflammatory drugs and perforated diverticular disease: as case-control study. *Ann R Coll Surg Engl.* 2002;84(2):93–96.

108. Goh V, Halligan S, Taylor SA, et al. Differentiation between diverticulitis and colorectal cancer: quantitative CT perfusion measurements versus morphologic criteria—initial experience. *Radiology.* 2007;242(2):456–462.

109. Gollub MJ, Jhaveri S, Schwartz E, et al. CT colonography features of sigmoid diverticular disease. *Clin Imaging.* 2005;29(3):200–206.

110. Gouge TH, Coppa GF, Eng K, et al. Management of diverticulitis of the ascending colon. 10 years' experience. *Am J Surg.* 1983;145(3):387–391.

111. Graser E. Das falsche Darmdivertikel. *Arch klin Chir.* 1899;59:63–67.

112. Greco RS, Kamath C, Nosher JL. Percutaneous drainage of peridiverticular abscess followed by primary sigmoidectomy. *Dis Colon Rectum.* 1982;25(1):53–55.

113. Greenlee HB, Pienkos EJ, Vanderbilt PC, et al. Proceedings: acute large bowel obstruction. Comparison of county, Veterans Administration, and community hospital populations. *Arch Surg.* 1974;108(4):47–46.

114. Gross SA, Katz S. Small bowel diverticulosis: an overlooked entity. *Curr Treat Options Gastroenterol.* 2003;6(1):3–11.

115. Guller U, Jain N, Hervey S, et al. Laparoscopic vs. open colectomy: outcomes comparison based on large nationwide databases. *Arch Surg.* 2003;138(11):1179–1186.

116. Guzzo J, Hyman N. Diverticulitis in young patients: is resection after a single attack always warranted? *Dis Colon Rectum.* 2004;47(7):1187–1190; discussion 1190–1181.

117. Hadjiyannakis EJ, Evans DB, Smellie WA, et al. Gastrointestinal complications after renal transplantation. *Lancet.* 1971;22(7728):781–785.

118. Haglund U, Hellberg R, Johns;agen C, et al. Complicated diverticular disease of the sigmoid colon. An analysis of short and long term outcome in 392 patients. *Ann Chir Gynaecol.* 1979;68(2):41–46.

119. Hain JM, Sherick DG, Cleary RK. Salpingocolonic fistula secondary to diverticulitis. *Am Surg.* 1996;62(12):984–986.

120. Hall J, Hammerich K, Roberts P. New paradigms in the management of diverticular disease. *Curr Probl Surg.* 2010;47(9):680–735.

121. Hall JF, Roberts PL, Ricciardi R, et al. Colonic diverticulitis: does age predict severity of disease on CT imaging? *Dis Colon Rectum.* 2010;53(2):121–125.

122. Halpert RD, Crnkovich FM, Schreiber MH. Rectal diverticulosis: a case report and review of the literature. *Gastrointest Radiol.* 1989;14(3):274–276.

123. Hansen O, Graupe F, Stock W. [Diagnosis of diverticulitis in routine practice: progress due to pelvic CT?]. *Langenbecks Arch Chir Suppl Kongressbd.* 1998;115:170–173.

124. Hart AR, Kennedy HJ, Stebbings WS, et al. How frequently do large bowel diverticula perforate? An incidence and cross-sectional study. *Eur J Gastroenterol Hepatol.* 2000;12(6):661–665.

125. Hassan I, Cima RR, Larson DW, et al. The impact of uncomplicated and complicated diverticulitis on laparoscopic surgery conversion rates and patient outcomes. *Surg Endosc.* 2007;21(10):1690–1694.

126. Havia T, Manner R. The irritable colon syndrome. A follow-up study with special reference to the development of diverticula. *Acta Chir Scand.* 1971;137(6):569–572.

127. Heaton KW. Diet and diverticulosis—new leads. *Gut.* 1985;26(6): 541–543.

128. Heimann T, Aufses AH Jr. Giant sigmoid diverticula. *Dis Colon Rectum.* 1981;24(6):468–470.

129. Hinchey EJ, Schaal PG, Richards GK. Treatment of perforated diverticular disease of the colon. *Adv Surg.* 1978;12:85–109.

130. Hjern F, Jonas E, Holmström B, et al. CT colonography versus colonoscopy in the follow-up of patients after diverticulitis—a prospective, comparative study. *Clin Radiol.* 2007;62(7):645–650.

131. Hodgson J. Transverse taeniomyotomy for diverticular disease. *Dis Colon Rectum.* 1973;16(4):283–289.

132. Hodgson WJ. The placebo effect. Is it important in diverticular disease? *Am J Gastroenterol.* 1977;67(2):157–162.

133. Hodgson WJ, Schanzer H, Bakare S, et al. Transverse taeniamyotomy in localized acute diverticulitis. *Am J Gastroenterol.* 1979;71(1):61–67.

134. Hool GJ, Bokey EL, Pheils MT. Diverticular colo-enteric fistulae. *Aust N Z J Surg.* 1981;51(4):358–359.

135. Horgan AF, McConnell EJ, Wolff BG, et al. Atypical diverticular disease: surgical results. *Dis Colon Rectum.* 2001;44(9):1315–1318.

136. Hughes LE. Postmortem survey of diverticular disease of the colon: II. The muscular abnormality of the sigmoid colon. *Gut.* 1969;10(5): 344–351.

137. Hughes WL, Greene RC. Solitary air cyst of the peritoneal cavity. *AMA Arch Surg.* 1953;67(6):931–936.

138. Humes DJ, Fleming KM, Spiller RC, et al. Concurrent drug use and the risk of perforated colonic diverticular disease: a population-based case-control study. *Gut.* 2011;60(2):219–224.

139. Hyland JM, Taylor I. Does a high fibre diet prevent the complications of diverticular disease? *Br J Surg.* 1980;67(2):77–79.

140. Indudhara R, Kochhar R, Mehta SK, et al. Acute colitis in renal transplant recipients. *Am J Gastroenterol.* 1990;85(8):964–968.

141. Inoue M. The epidemiologic and clinical features of diverticular disease of the colon [in Japanese]. *J Jpn Soc Coloproctol.* 1992;45: 904–913.

142. Jacobs DO. Clinical practice. Diverticulitis. *N Engl J Med.* 2007;357(20):2057–2066.

143. Janes S, Meagher A, Frizelle FA. Elective surgery after acute diverticulitis. *Br J Surg.* 2005;92(2):133–142.

144. Janes SE, Meagher A, Frizelle FA. Management of diverticulitis. *Br Med J.* 2006;332(7536):271–275.

145. Jarrett TW, Vaughan ED Jr. Accuracy of computerized tomography in the diagnosis of colovesical fistula secondary to diverticular disease. *J Urol.* 1995;153(1):44–46.

146. Jasper DR, Weinstock LB, Balfe DM, et al. Transverse colon diverticulitis: successful nonoperative management in four patients. Report of four cases. *Dis Colon Rectum.* 1999;42(7):955–958.

147. John SK, Teo NB, Forster AL. A prospective study of acute admissions in a surgical unit due to diverticular disease. *Dig Surg.* 2007;24(3): 186–190.

148. Jones OM, Stevenson AR, Clark D, et al. Laparoscopic resection for diverticular disase: follow-up of 500 consecutive patients. *Ann Surg.* 2008;248(6):1092–1097.

149. Julien PJ, Goldberg HI, Margulis AR, et al. Gastrointestinal complications following renal transplantation. *Radiology.* 1975;117(1): 37–43.

150. Kang JY, Hoare J, Tinto A, et al. Diverticular disease of the colon—on the rise: a study of hospital admissions in England between 1989/1990 and 1999/2000. *Aliment Pharmacol Ther.* 2003;17(9):1189–1195.

151. Karamchandani MC, Riether R, Sheets J, et al. Nephrocolic fistula. *Dis Colon Rectum.* 1986;29(11):747–749.

152. Kempczinski RF, Ferrucci JT Jr. Giant sigmoid diverticula: a review. *Ann Surg.* 1974;180(6):864–867.

153. Klarenbeek BR, Veenhof AA, Bergamaschi R, et al. Laparoscopic sigmoid resection for diverticulitis decreases major morbidity rates: a randomized control trial: short-term results of the Sigma Trial. *Ann Surg.* 2009;249(1):39–44.

154. Köckerling F, Schneider C, Reymond MA, et al. Laparoscopic resection of sigmoid diverticulitis. Results of a multicenter study. Laparoscopic Colorectal Surgery Study Group. *Surg Endosc.* 1999;13(6):5 67–571.

155. Koep LJ, Peters TG, Starzl TE. Major colonic complications of hepatic transplantation. *Dis Colon Rectum.* 1979;22(4):218–220.

156. Koneru B, Selby R, O'Hair DP, et al. Nonobstructing colonic dilatation and colon perforations following renal transplantation. *Arch Surg.* 1990;125(5):610–613.

157. Konvolinka CW. Acute diverticulitis under age forty. *Am J Surg.* 1994;167(6):562–565.

158. Kori T, Nemoto M, Maeda M, et al. Sonographic features of acute colonic diverticulitis: the "dome sign." *J Clin Ultrasound.* 2000;28(7): 340–346.

159. Korzenik JR. Case closed? Diverticulitis: epidemiology and fiber. *J Clin Gastroenterol.* 2006;40(suppl 3):S112–S116.

160. Kovalcik PJ, Sustarsic DL. Cecal diverticulitis. *Am Surg.* 1981;47(2): 72–73.

161. Kovalcik PJ, Veidenheimer MC, Corman ML, et al. Colovesical fistula. 1976;19(5):425–427.

162. Kozak LJ, DeFrances CJ, Hall MJ. National hospital discharge survey: 2004 annual summary with detailed diagnosis and procedure data. *Vital Health Stat.* 2006;13(162):1–209.

163. Krishnan S, Hitti IF, Arya Y, et al. Giant sigmoid diverticulum. *Surg Rounds.* 1987;10:124–126.

164. Kronborg O. Treatment of perforated sigmoid diverticulitis: a prospective randomized trial. *Br J Surg.* 1993;80(4):505–507.

165. Labs JD, Sarr MG, Fishman EK, et al. Complications of acute diverticulitis of the colon: improved early diagnosis with computerized tomography. *Am J Surg.* 1988;155(2):331–336.

166. Lane JS, Sarkar R, Schmit PJ, et al. Surgical approach to cecal diverticulitis. *J Am Coll Surg.* 1999;188(6):629–634.

167. Langdon A. Solitary diverticulitis of the right colon. *Can J Surg.* 1982;25(5):579–581.

168. Larson DM, Masters SS, Spiro HM. Medical and surgical therapy in diverticular disease: a comparative study. *Gastroenterology.* 1976;71(5):734–737.

169. Latella G, Pimpo MT, Sottili S, et al. Rifaximin improves symptoms of acquired uncomplicated diverticular disease of the colon. *Int J Colorectal Dis.* 2003;18(1):55–62.

170. Lee YS. Diverticular disease of the large bowel in Singapore. An autopsy survey. *Dis Colon Rectum.* 1986;29(5):330–335.

171. Lefere P, Gryspeerdt S, Baekelandt M, et al. Diverticular disease in CT colonography. *Eur Radiol.* 2003;13(suppl 4):L62–L74.

172. Lennard-Jones JE. Functional gastrointestinal disorders. *N Engl J Med.* 1983;308(8):431–435.

173. Levi DM, Levi JU, Rogers AI, et al. Giant colonic diverticulum: an unusual manifestation of a common disease. *Am J Gastroenterol.* 1993;88(1):139–142.

174. Lieberman JM, Haaga JR. Computed tomography of diverticulitis. *J Comput Assist Tomogr.* 1983;7(3):431–433.

175. Liljegren G, Chabok A, Wickbom M, et al. Acute colonic diverticulitis: a systematic review of diagnostic accuracy. *Colorectal Dis.* 2007;9(6):480–488.

176. Longstreth GF, Thompson WG, Chey WD, et al. Functional bowel disorders. *Gastroenterology.* 2006;130(5):1480–1491.

177. Lopez DE, Brown CV. Diverticulitis: the most common colon emergency for the acute care surgeon. *Scand J Surg.* 2010;99(2):86–89.

178. Lorimer JW. Is prophylactic resection valid as an indication for elective surgery in diverticular disease? *Can J Surg.* 1997;40(6):445–448.

179. Lumsden K, Chaudhary NA, Truelove SC. The irritable colon syndrome. *Clin Radiol.* 1963;14:54–63.

180. Maggard MA, Zingmond D, O'Connell JB, et al. What proportion of patients with an ostomy (for diverticulitis) get reversed? *Am Surg.* 2004;70(10):928–931.

181. Mäkelä J, Kiviniemi H, Laitinen S. Prevalence of perforated sigmoid diverticulitis is increasing. *Dis Colon Rectum.* 2002;45(7):955–961.

182. Mäkelä J, Kiviniemi HO, Laitinen ST. Elective surgery for recurrent diverticulitis. *Hepatogastroenterology.* 2007;54(77):1412–1416.

183. Mäkelä J, Vuolio S, Kiviniemi H, et al. Natural history of diverticular disease: when to operate? *Dis Colon Rectum.* 1998;41(12):1523–1528.

184. Maresca L, Maresca C, Erickson E. Giant sigmoid diverticulum: report of a case. *Dis Colon Rectum.* 1981;24(3):191–195.

185. Max MH, Knutson CO. Colonoscopy in patients with inflammatory colonic strictures. *Surgery*. 1978;84(4):551–556.

186. Mayefsky E, Sicular A, Hodgson WJ. Recurrent diverticulitis after conservative surgery. *Mt Sinai J Med*. 1979;46(6):556–558.

187. McClure ET, Welch JP. Acute diverticulitis of the transverse colon with perforation: report of three cases and review of the literature. *Arch Surg*. 1979;114(9):1068–1071.

188. McConnell EJ, Tessier DJ, Wolff BG. Population based incidence of complicated diverticular disease of the sigmoid colon based on gender and age. *Dis Colon Rectum*. 2003;46(8):1110–1114.

189. McFee AS, Sutton PG, Ramos R. Diverticulitis of the right colon. *Dis Colon Rectum*. 1982;25(3):254–256.

190. McKee RF, Deignan RW, Krukowski ZH. Radiological investigation in acute diverticulitis. *Br J Surg*. 1993;80(5):560–565.

191. McNutt R, Schmitt D, Schulte W. Giant colonic diverticula—three distinct entities. Report of a case. *Dis Colon Rectum*. 1988;31(8): 624–628.

192. Meisner S, Hensler M, Knop FK, et al. Self-expanding metal stents for colon obstruction: experiences from 104 procedures in a single center. *Dis Colon Rectum*. 2004;47(4):444–450.

193. Melchior S, Cudovic D, Jones J, et al. Diagnosis and surgical management of colovesical fistulas due to sigmoid diverticulitis. *J Urol*. 2009;182(3):978–982.

194. Mileski WJ, Joehl RJ, Rege RV, et al. One-stage resection and anastomosis in the management of colovesical fistula. *Am J Surg*. 1987;153(1):75–79.

195. Misra MK, Pinkus GS, Birtch AG, et al. Major colonic disease complicating renal transplantation. *Surgery*. 1973;73(6):942–948.

196. Mohammad AI, Ben-Nakhi AM, Khoursheed M. Giant sigmoid diverticulum: a case report. *Med Princ Pract*. 2009;18(1):70–72.

197. Morris CR, Harvey IM, Stebbings WS, et al. Anti-inflammatory drugs, analgesics and the risk of perforated colonic diverticular disease. *Br J Surg*. 2003;90(10):1267–1272.

198. Morris CR, Harvey IM, Stebbings WS, et al. Do calcium channel blockers and antimuscarinics protect against perforated colonic diverticular disease? A case control study. *Gut*. 2003;52(12):1734–1737.

199. Morson BC. Pathology of diverticular disease of the colon. *Clin Gastroenterol*. 1975;4(1):37–52.

200. Morson BC. Diverticular disease of the colon. *Acta Chir Belg*. 1979;78(6):369–376.

201. Moss RL, Ryan JA Jr. Management of enterovesical fistulas. *Am J Surg*. 1990;159(5):514–517.

202. Mueller MH, Glatzle J, Kasparek MS, et al. Long-term outcome of conservative treatment in patients with diverticulitis of the sigmoid colon. *Eur J Gastroenterol Hepatol*. 2005;17(6):649–654.

203. Mueller PR, Saini S, Wittenburg J, et al. Sigmoid diverticular abscesses: percutaneous drainage as an adjunct to surgical resection in 24 cases. *Radiology*. 1987;164(2):321–325.

204. Muhletaler CA, Berger JL, Robinette CL Jr. Pathogenesis of giant colonic diverticula. *Gastrointest Radiol*. 1981;6(3):217–222.

205. Mulhall AM, Mahid SS, Petras RE, et al. Diverticular disease associated with inflammatory bowel disease-like colitis: a systematic review. *Dis Colon Rectum*. 2009;52(6):1072–1079.

206. Murayama N, Baba S, Kodaira S. An aetiological study of diverticulosis of the right colon. *Aust N Z J Surg*. 1981;51(5):420–425.

207. Mutter D, Bouras G, Forgione A, et al. Two-stage totally minimally invasive approach for acute complicated diverticulitis. *Colorectal Dis*. 2006;8(6):501–505.

208. Myers E, Hurley M, O'Sullivan GC, et al. Laparoscopic peritoneal lavage for generalized peritonitis due to perforated diverticulitis. *Br J Surg*. 2008;95(1):97–101.

209. Nakaji S, Danjo K, Munakata A, et al. Comparison of etiology of right-sided diverticula in Japan with that of left-sided diverticula in the West. *Int J Colorectal Dis*. 2002;17(6):365–373.

210. Neff CC, van Sonnenberg E, Casola G, et al. Diverticular abscesses: percutaneous drainage. *Radiology*. 1987;163:15–18.

211. Ney C, Cruz FS Jr, Carvajal S, et al. Ureteral involvement secondary to diverticulitis of the colon. *Surg Gynecol Obstet*. 1986;163(3):215–218.

212. Nylamo E. Diverticulitis of the colon: role of surgery in preventing complications. *Ann Chir Gynaecol*. 1990;79(3):139–142.

213. Ogunbiyi OA. Diverticular disease of the colon in Ibadan, Nigeria. *Afr J Med Med Sci*. 1989;18(4):241–244.

214. Orebaugh JE, MaCris JA, Lee JF. Surgical treatment of diverticular disease of the colon. *Am Surg*. 1978;44(11):712–715.

215. Ornstein MH, Littlewood ER, Baird IM, et al. Are fibre supplements really necessary in diverticular disease of the colon? A controlled clinical trial. *Br Med J*. 1981;282(6273):1353–1356.

216. Otte JJ, Larsen L, Andersen JR. Irritable bowel syndrome and symptomatic diverticular disease—different diseases? *Am J Gastroenterol*. 1986;81(7):529–531.

217. Ouriel K, Schwartz SI. Diverticular disease in the young patient. *Surg Gynecol Obstet*. 1983;156(1):1–5.

218. Padidar AM, Jeffrey RB Jr, Mindelzun RE, et al. Differentiating sigmoid diverticulitis from carcinoma on CT scans: mesenteric inflammation suggests diverticulitis. *Am J Roentgenol*. 1994;163(1):81–83.

219. Painter NS. Diverticular disease of the colon—a disease of this century. *Lancet*. 1969;2(7620):586–588.

220. Painter NS. The treatment of uncomplicated diverticular disease of the colon with a high fibre diet. *Acta Chir Belg*. 1979;78(6):359–368.

221. Painter NS. Diverticular disease of the colon. The first of the Western diseases shown to be due to a deficiency of dietary fibre. *South Afr Med J*. 1982;61(26):1016–1020.

222. Painter NS, Burkitt DP. Diverticular disease of the colon: a deficiency disease of Western civilization. *Br Med J*. 1971;2(5759):450–454.

223. Painter NS, Burkitt DP. Diverticular disease of the colon, a 20th century problem. *Clin Gastroenterol*. 1975;4(1):3–21.

224. Papagrigoriadis S, Macey L, Bourantas N, et al. Smoking may be associated with complications in diverticular disease. *Br J Surg*. 1999;86(7):923–926.

225. Papi C, Ciaco A, Koch M, et al. Efficacy of rifaximin on symptoms of uncomplicated diverticular disease of the colon. A pilot multicentre open trial. Diverticular Disease Study Group. *Ital J Gastroenterol*. 1992;24(8):452–456.

226. Papi C, Ciaco A, Koch M, et al. Efficacy of rifaximin in the treatment of symptomatic diverticular disease of the colon. A multicentre double-blind placebo-controlled trial. *Aliment Pharmacol Ther*. 1995;9(1):33–39.

227. Parks TG. Natural history of diverticular disease of the colon. A review of 521 cases. *Br Med J*. 1969;4(5684):639–642.

228. Parks TG. Natural history of diverticular disease of the colon. *Clin Gastroenterol*. 1975;4:53–69.

229. Parks TG. The clinical significance of diverticular disease of the colon. *Practitioner*. 1982;226(1366):643–648.

230. Parks TG, Connell AM. The outcome in 455 patients admitted for treatment of diverticular disease of the colon. *Br J Surg*. 1970;57(10): 775–778.

231. Parks TG, Connell AM, Gough AD, et al. Limitations of radiology in the differentiation of diverticulitis and diverticulosis of the colon. *Br Med J*. 1970;2(5702):136–138.

232. Parnaby C, Barrow EJ, Edirimanne SB, et al. Colorectal complications of end-stage renal failure and renal transplantation: a review [published online ahead of print November 4, 2010]. *Colorectal Dis*. doi:10.1111/j.1463-1318.2010.02491.x.

233. Peck MD, Villar HV. Perforated diverticulitis of the transverse colon. *West J Med*. 1987;147(1):81–84.

234. Perkins JD, Shield CF III, Chang FC, et al. Acute diverticulitis. Comparison of treatment in immunocompromised and nonimmunocompromised patients. *Am J Surg*. 1984;148(6):745–748.

235. Pheils MT, Chapuis PH, Bokey EL, et al. Diverticular disease: a retrospective study of surgical management 1970–1980. *Aust N Z J Surg*. 1982;52(1):53–56.

236. Piekarek K, Israelsson LA. Perforated colonic diverticular disease: the importance of NSAIDs, opioids, corticosteroids, and calcium channel blockers. *Int J Colorectal Dis*. 2008;23(12):1193–1197.

237. Piercy KT, Timaran C, Akin H. Rectal diverticula: report of a case and review of the literature. *Dis Colon Rectum*. 2002;45(8): 1116–1117.

238. Pillari G, Greenspan B, Vernace FM, et al. Computed tomography of diverticulitis. *Gastrointest Radiol*. 1984;9(3):263–268.

239. Potier F. Diverticulite et appendicite. *Bull Mem Soc Anat (Paris)*. 1912;137:29–31.

240. Pradel JA, Adell JF, Taourel P, et al. Acute colonic diverticulitis: prospective comparative evaluation with US and CT. *Radiology*. 1997;205(2):503–512.

241. Purkayastha S, Constantinides VA, Tekkis PP, et al. Laparoscopic vs. open surgery for diverticular disease: a meta-analysis of nonrandomized studies. *Dis Colon Rectum*. 2006;49(4):446–463.

242. Rafferty J, Shellito P, Hyman NH, et al. Practice parameters for sigmoid diverticulitis. *Dis Colon Rectum*. 2006;49(7):939–944.

243. Rao PN, Knox R, Barnard RJ, et al. Management of colovesical fistula. *Br J Surg*. 1987;74(5):362–363.

244. Raval B, Lamki N, St Ville E. Role of computed tomography in diverticulitis. *J Comput Tomogr*. 1987;11(2):144–150.

245. Ravo B, Khan SA, Ger R, et al. Unusual extraperitoneal presentations of diverticulitis. *Am J Gastroenterol*. 1985;80(5):346–351.

246. Reeves KO, Young RL, Gordon AN. Sigmoidovaginal fistula secondary to diverticular disease: a report of three cases. *J Reprod Med.* 1988;33(3):313–316.

247. Regenet N, Pessaux P, Hennekinne S, et al. Primary anastomosis after intraoperative colonic lavage vs. Hartmann's procedure in generalized peritonitis complicating diverticular disease of the colon. *Int J Colorectal Dis.* 2003;18(6):503–507.

248. Reilly M. Sigmoid myotomy [Abridged]. *Proc R Soc Med.* 1964;57(7):556–557.

249. Rennie JA, Charnock MC, Wellwood JM, et al. Results of resection for diverticular disease and its complications. *Proc R Soc Med.* 1975;68(9):575.

250. Rice RP, Thompson WM. Colon complications following renal transplantation. In: Greenbaum EI, ed. *Radiographic Atlas of Colon Disease.* Chicago, IL: Year Book; 1980:89.

251. Richter S, Lindemann W, Kollmar O, et al. One-stage sigmoid colon resection for perforated sigmoid diverticulitis (Hinchey stages III and IV). *World J Surg.* 2006;30(6):1027–1032.

252. Ridgway PF, Latif A, Shabbir J, et al. Randomized controlled trial of oral vs intravenous therapy for the clinically diagnosed acute uncomplicated diverticulitis. *Colorectal Dis.* 2009;11(9):941–946.

253. Rink AD, John-Enzenauer K, Haaf F, et al. Laparoscopic-assisted or laparoscopic-facilitated sigmoidectomy for diverticular disease? A prospective randomized trial on postoperative pain and analgesic consumption. *Dis Colon Rectum.* 2009;52(10):1738–1745.

254. Ritchie J. Pain from distension of the pelvic colon by inflating a balloon in the irritable colon syndrome. *Gut.* 1973;14(2):125–132.

255. Rizk N, Barrat C, Faranda C, et al. [Laparoscopic treatment of generalized peritonitis with diverticular perforation of the sigmoid colon. Report of 10 cases]. *Chirurgie.* 1998;123(4):358–362.

256. Roberts P, Abel M, Rosen L, et al. Practice parameters for sigmoid diverticulitis. The Standards Task Force American Society of Colon and Rectal Surgeons. *Dis Colon Rectum.* 1995;38(2):126–132.

257. Roberts PL, Veidenheimer MC. Current management of diverticulitis. *Adv Surg.* 1994;27:189–208.

258. Rocco A, Compare D, Caruso F, et al. Treatment options for uncomplicated diverticular disease of the colon. *J Clin Gastroenterol.* 2009;43(9):803–808.

259. Rotstein OD, Pruett TL, Simmons RL. Thigh abscess. An uncommon presentation of intraabdominal sepsis. *Am J Surg.* 1986;151(3):414–418.

260. Saini S, Mueller PR, Wittenberg J. Percutaneous drainage of diverticular abscess. An adjunct to surgical therapy. *Arch Surg.* 1986;121(4):475–478.

261. Salem L, Flum DR. Primary anastomosis or Hartmann's procedure for patients with diverticular peritonitis? A systematic review. *Dis Colon Rectum.* 2004;47(11):1953–1964.

262. Salem TA, Molloy RG, O'Dwyer PJ. Prospective, five-year follow-up study of patients with symptomatic uncomplicated diverticular disease. *Dis Colon Rectum.* 2007;50(9):1460–1464.

263. Sandler RS, Everhart JE, Donowitz M, et al. The burden of selected digestive diseases in the United States. *Gastroenterology.* 2002;122(5):1500–1511.

264. Sankary HN, Eugene JH, Juler JL. Colovesical fistula: a comparison of the morbidity associated with staged surgical procedures. *Contemp Surg.* 1988;32:28–31.

265. Santaniello M, Bergamaschi R. Perforated diverticulitis: should the method of surgical access to the abdomen determine treatment? *Colorectal Dis.* 2007;9(6):494–495.

266. Sardi A, Gokli A, Singer JA. Diverticular disease of the cecum and ascending colon. A review of 881 cases. *Am Surg.* 1987;53(1):41–45.

267. Sarin S, Boulos PB. Long-term outcome of patients presenting with acute complications of diverticular disease. *Ann R Coll Surg Engl.* 1994;76(2):117–120.

268. Sarr MG, Fishman EK, Goldman SM, et al. Enterovesical fistula. *Surg Gynecol Obstet.* 1987;164(1):41–48.

269. Sawyerr OI, Garvin PJ, Codd JE, et al. Colorectal complications of renal allograft transplantation. *Arch Surg.* 1978;113(1):84–86.

270. Scerpella PR, Bodensteiner JA. Giant sigmoid diverticula. Report of two cases. *Arch Surg.* 1989;124(10):1244–1246.

271. Schauer PR, Ramos R, Ghiatas AA, et al. Virulent diverticular disease in young obese men. *Am J Surg.* 1992;164(5):443–448.

272. Schechter S, Eisenstat TE, Oliver GC, et al. Computerized tomographic scan-guided drainage of intra-abdominal abscesses. Preoperative and postoperative modalities in colon and rectal surgery. *Dis Colon Rectum.* 1994;37(10):984–988.

273. Schechter S, Mulvey J, Eisenstat TE. Management of uncomplicated acute diverticulitis: results of a survey. *Dis Colon Rectum.* 1999;42(4):470–475.

274. Schilling MK, Maurer CA, Kollmar O, et al. Primary vs. secondary anastomosis after sigmoid colon resection for perforated diverticulitis (Hinchey Stage III and IV): a prospective outcome and cost analysis. *Dis Colon Rectum.* 2001;44(5):699–703.

275. Schoetz DJ Jr. Diverticular disease of the colon: a century-old problem. *Dis Colon Rectum.* 1999;42(6):703–709.

276. Schreyer AG, Fürst A, Agha A, et al. Magnetic resonance imaging based colonography for diagnosis and assessment of diverticulosis and diverticulitis. *Int J Colorectal Dis.* 2004;19(5):474–480.

277. Schug-Pass C, Geers P, Hügel O, et al. Prospective randomized trial comparing short-term antibiotic therapy versus standard therapy for acute uncomplicated sigmoid diverticulitis. *Int J Colorectal Dis.* 2010;25(6):751–759.

278. Schwandner O, Farke S, Bruch HP. Laparoscopic colectomy for diverticulitis is not associated with increased morbidity when compared with non-diverticular disease. *Int J Colorectal Dis.* 2005;20(2):165–172.

279. Schwandner O, Farke S, Fischer F, et al. Laparoscopic colectomy for recurrent and complicated diverticulitis: a prospective study of 396 patients. *Langenbecks Arch Surg.* 2004;389(2):97–103.

280. Schwerk WB, Schwarz S, Rothmund M. Sonography in acute colonic diverticulitis. A prospective study. *Dis Colon Rectum.* 1992;35(11):1077–1084.

281. Shaikh S, Krukowski ZH. Outcome of a conservative policy for managing acute sigmoid diverticulitis. *Br J Surg.* 2007;94(7):876–879.

282. Shaked A, Vargas J, Csete ME, et al. Diagnosis and treatment of bowel perforation following pediatric orthotopic liver transplantation. *Arch Surg.* 1993;128(9):994–998.

283. Shperber Y, Halevy A, Oland J, et al. Perforated diverticulitis of the transverse colon. *Dis Colon Rectum.* 1986;29(7):466–468.

284. Siewert B, Tye G, Kruskal J, et al. Impact of CT-guided drainage in the treatment of diverticular abscesses: size matters. *AJR Am J Roentgenol.* 2006;186(3):680–686.

285. Sim G, Scobie BA. Large bowel diseases in New Zealand based on 1118 air contrast enemas. *N Z Med J.* 1982;95(715):611–613.

286. Simpson J, Scholefield JH, Spiller RC. Origin of symptoms in diverticular disease. *Br J Surg.* 2003;90(8):899–908.

287. Slack WW. The anatomy, pathology, and some clinical features of diverticulitis of the colon. *Br J Surg.* 1962;50:185–190.

288. Somasekar K, Foster ME, Haray PN. The natural history of diverticular disease: is there a role for elective colectomy? *J R Coll Surg Edinb.* 2002;47(2):481–484.

289. Spivak H, Weinrauch S, Harvey JC, et al. Acute colonic diverticulitis in the young. *Dis Colon Rectum.* 1997;40(5):570–574.

290. Stabile BE, Puccio E, van Sonnenberg E, et al. Preoperative percutaneous drainage of diverticular abscesses. *Am J Surg.* 1990;159(1):99–104.

291. The Standards Task Force. The American Society of Colon and Rectal Surgeons. Practice parameters for sigmoid diverticulitis—supporting documentation. *Dis Colon Rectum.* 1995;38:126–132.

292. Starnes HJ Jr, Lazarus JM, Vineyard G. Surgery for diverticulitis in renal failure. *Dis Colon Rectum.* 1985;28(11):827–831.

293. Steenvoorde P, Vogelaar FJ, Oskam J, et al. Giant colonic diverticula. Review of diagnostic and therapeutic options. *Dig Surg.* 2004;21(1):1–6.

294. Stelzner M, Vlahakos DV, Milford EL, et al. Colonic perforations after renal transplantation. *J Am Coll Surg.* 1997;184(1):63–69.

295. Stephenson BM, Wheeler MH. Unpredictable course of 'minimal' diverticular disease. *Br J Surg.* 1994;81(7):1050.

296. Stollman NH, Raskin JB. Diagnosis and management of diverticular disease of the colon in adults. Ad Hoc Practice Parameters Committee of the American College of Gastroenterology. *Am J Gastroenterol.* 1999;94(11):3110–3121.

297. Stollman NH, Raskin JB. Diverticular disease of the colon. *Lancet.* 2004;363(9409):631–639.

298. Stumpf M, Cao W, Klinge U, et al. Increased distribution of collagen type III and reduced expression of matrix metalloproteinase 1 in patients with diverticular disease. *Int J Colorectal Dis.* 2001;16(5):271–275.

299. Suits GS, Knoepp LF. A community experience with enterovesical fistulas. *Am Surg.* 1985;51(9):523–528.

300. Tamim WZ, Ghellai A, Counihan TC, et al. Experience with endoluminal colonic wall stents for the management of large bowel obstruction for benign and malignant disease. *Arch Surg.* 2000;135(4):434–438.

301. Taylor CJ, Layani L, Ghusn MA, et al. Perforated diverticulitis managed by laparoscopic lavage. *Aust N Z J Surg.* 2006;76(11):962–965.

302. Tekkis PP, Senagore AJ, Delaney CP, et al. Evaluation of the learning curve in laparoscopic colorectal surgery: comparison of right-sided and left-sided resections. *Ann Surg.* 2005;242(1):83–91.

303. Telling W. Acquired diverticula of the sigmoid flexure, considered especially in relation to secondary pathological processes and their clinical symptoms. *Lancet.* 1908;171(4413):843–850, 928–931.

304. Telling WH, Gruner OC. Acquired diverticula, diverticulitis, and peridiverticulitis of the large intestine. *Br J Surg.* 1917;4:468–530.

305. Thaler K, Baig MK, Berho M, et al. Determinants of recurrence after sigmoid resection for uncomplicated diverticulitis. *Dis Colon Rectum.* 2003;48(3):385–388.

306. Thompson G, Fox PF. Perforated solitary diverticulum of the transverse colon: case report. *Am J Surg.* 1944;66:280.

307. Thompson WG, Patel DG, Tao H, et al. Does uncomplicated diverticular disease produce symptoms? *Dig Dis Sci.* 1982;27(7):605–608.

308. Thörn M, Graf W, Stefànsson T, et al. Clinical and functional results after elective colonic resection in 75 consecutive patients with diverticular disease. *Am J Surg.* 2002;183(1):7–11.

309. Toiber-Levy M, Golffier-Rosete C, Martínez-Munive A, et al. Giant sigmoid diverticulum: case report and review of the literature. *Gastroenterol Clin Biol.* 2008;32(6–7):581–584.

310. Tønnesen H, Engholm G, Møller H. Association between alcoholism and diverticulitis. *Br J Surg.* 1999;86(8):1067–1068.

311. Toorenvliet BR, Swank H, Schoones JW, et al. Laparoscopic peritoneal lavage for perforated colonic diverticulitis: a systematic review. *Colorectal Dis.* 2010;12(9):862–867.

312. Trowell HC, Burkitt DP. Diverticular disease in urban Kenyans. *Br Med J.* 1979;1(6180):1795.

313. Tsuruoka N, Iwakiri R, Hara M, et al. NSAIDs are a significant risk factor for colonic diverticular hemorrhage in elder patients: evaluation by a case-control study. *J Gastroenterol Hepatol.* 2011;26(6):1047–1052. doi:10.1111/j.1440-1746.2010.06610.x.

314. Tudor RG, Faramakis N, Keighley MR. National audit of complicated diverticular disease: analysis of index cases. *Br J Surg.* 1994;81(5):730–732.

315. Tursi A. Mesalazine for diverticular disease of the colon—a new role for an old drug. *Expert Opin Pharmacother.* 2005;6(1):69–74.

316. Tursi A, Brandimarte G, Daffinà R. Long-term treatment with mesalazine and rifaximin versus rifaximin alone for patients with recurrent attacks of acute diverticulitis of the colon. *Dig Liver Dis.* 2002;34(7):510–515.

317. Tursi A, Brandimarte G, Giorgetti GM, et al. Mesalazine and/or *Lactobacillus casei* in preventing recurrence of symptomatic uncomplicated diverticular disease of the colon: a prospective, randomized, open-label study. *J Clin Gastroenterol.* 2006;40(4):312–316.

318. Tursi A, Brandimarte G, Giorgetti GM, et al. Continuous versus cyclic mesalazine therapy for patients affected by recurrent symptomatic uncomplicated diverticular disease of the colon. *Dig Dis Sci.* 2007;52(3):671–674.

319. Tursi A, Brandimarte G, Giorgetti GM, et al. Mesalazine and/or *Lactobacillus casei* in maintaining long-term remission of symptomatic uncomplicated diverticular disease of the colon. *Hepatogastroenterology.* 2008;55(84):916–920.

320. Tursi A, Elisei W, Giorgetti GM, et al. Inflammatory manifestations at colonoscopy in patients with colonic diverticular disease. *Aliment Pharmacol Ther.* 2011;33(3):358–365. doi:10.1111/j.1365-2036.2010.04530.x.

321. Tyau ES, Prystowsky JB, Joehl RJ, et al. Acute diverticulitis. A complicated problem in the immunocompromised patient. *Arch Surg.* 1991;126(7):855–858.

322. van de Wall BJ, Draaisma WA, Consten EC, et al. DIRECT trial. Diverticulitis recurrences or continuing symptoms: operative versus conservative treatment. A multicenter randomised clinical trial. *BMC Surg.* 2010;10:25. doi:10.1186/1471-2482-10-25.

323. Vargas HD, Ramirez RT, Hoffman GC, et al. Defining the role of laparoscopic-assisted sigmoid colectomy for diverticulitis. *Dis Colon Rectum.* 2000;43(12):1726–1731.

324. Vasilevsky CA, Belliveau P, Trudel JL. Fistulas complicating diverticulitis. *Int J Colorectal Dis.* 1998;13(2):57–60.

325. Ventrucci M, Ferrieri A, Bergami R, et al. Evaluation of the effect of rifaximin in colon diverticular disease by means of lactulose hydrogen breath test. *Curr Med Res Opin.* 1994;13(4):202–206.

326. Verbanck J, Lambrecht S, Rutgeerts L, et al. Can sonography diagnose acute colonic diverticulitis in patients with acute intestinal inflammation? A prospective study. *J Clin Ultrasound.* 1989;17(9): 661–666.

327. Vermeulen J, Gosselink MP, Hop WC, et al. Long-term survival after perforated diverticulitis. *Colorectal Dis.* 2011;13(2):203–209.

328. Vermeulen J, Lange JF. Treatment of perforated diverticulitis with generalized peritonitis: past, present, and future. *World J Surg.* 2010;34(3):587–593.

329. Vignati PV, Welch JP, Cohen JL. Long-term management of diverticulitis in young patients. *Dis Colon Rectum.* 1995;38(6):627–629.

330. Walker AR, Segal I. Epidemiology of noninfective intestinal diseases in various ethnic groups in South Africa. *Isr J Med Sci.* 1979;15(4): 309–313.

331. Watters DA, Smith AN. Strength of the colon wall in diverticular disease. *Br J Surg.* 1990;77(3):257–259.

332. Weinreich J, Andersen D. Intraluminal pressure in the sigmoid colon. II. Patients with sigmoid diverticula and related conditions. *Scand J Gastroenterol.* 1976;11(6):581–586.

333. Wess L, Eastwood MA, Wess TJ, et al. Cross linking of collagen is increased in colonic diverticulosis. *Gut.* 1995;37(1):91–94.

334. Wetstein L, Camera A, Trillo RA, et al. Giant sigmoidal diverticulum: report of a case and review of the literature. *Dis Colon Rectum.* 1978;21(2):110–112.

335. Whiteway J, Morson BC. Elastosis in diverticular disease of the sigmoid colon. *Gut.* 1985;26(3):258–266.

336. Williams C. Diverticular disease and strictures. In: Hunt RH, Waye JD, eds. *Colonoscopy: Techniques, Clinical Practice and Colour Atlas.* London, United Kingdom: Chapman & Hall; 1981.

337. Wilson RG, Smith AN, Macintyre IM. Complications of diverticular disease and non-steroidal anti-inflammatory drugs: a prospective study. *Br J Surg.* 1990;77(10):1103–1104.

338. Wolff BG, Ready RL, MacCarty RL, et al. Influence of sigmoidal resection on progression of diverticular disease of the colon. *Dis Colon Rectum.* 1984;27(10):645–647.

339. Wong WD, Wexner SD, Lowry A, et al. Practice parameters for the treatment of sigmoid diverticulitis—supporting documentation. *Dis Colon Rectum.* 2000;43(3):290–297.

340. Woods RJ, Lavery IC, Fazio VW, et al. Internal fistulas in diverticular disease. *Dis Colon Rectum.* 1988;31(8):591–596.

341. Young-Fadok RM, Roberts PL, Spencer MP, et al. Colonic diverticular disease. *Curr Probl Surg.* 2000;37(7):457–514.

342. Zeitoun G, Laurent A, Rouffet F, et al. Multicentre, randomized clinical trial of primary versus secondary sigmoid resection in generalized peritonitis complicating sigmoid diverticulitis. *Br J Surg.* 2000;87(10): 1366–1374.

343. Zielke A, Hasse C, Nies C, et al. Prospective evaluation of ultrasonography in acute colonic diverticulitis. *Br J Surg.* 1997;84(3): 385–388.

344. Zingg U, Pasternak I, Dietrich M, et al. Primary anastomosis vs Hartmann's procedure in patients undergoing emergency left colectomy for perforated diverticulitis. *Colorectal Dis.* 2010;12(1):54–60.

28

Vascular Diseases: Hemorrhage, Mesenteric Occlusive and Nonocclusive Disease, Ischemia, Radiation Enteritis, and Volvulus

Jonathan E. Efron

The only weapon with which the unconscious patient can immediately retaliate on the incompetent surgeon is hemorrhage.

—WILLIAM STEWART HALSTED

▶ HEMORRHAGE

Gastrointestinal (GI) bleeding can be due to numerous causes. It is self-evident that conditions such as colorectal cancer, inflammatory bowel disease, hemorrhoids, infectious colitides, ischemia, radiation, Meckel's diverticulum, and virtually every disease that affects the mucosa of the intestinal tract can be associated, at some time, with bleeding.[215,279] Lower GI tract hemorrhage as a consequence of renal transplantation, presumably due to immunosuppression, has also been reported.[347] Uncommon conditions that can produce massive bleeding are coagulopathy, Osler-Weber-Rendu telangiectasia, Dieulafoy's disease, blue rubber bleb nevus syndrome, Behçet's disease, aortoduodenal fistula, rupture of a splenic artery aneurysm, microaneurysm of the superior hemorrhoidal artery, rupture of a pancreatic pseudocyst into the colon, and angiosarcoma.[30,56,77,197,202,219,279,308] A rare cause of *lower* GI hemorrhage is variceal bleeding. This may be due to a congenital vascular abnormality, portal hypertension, obstruction of mesenteric venous circulation, splenic vein thrombosis, or a cardiac anomaly.[175,382] Those with AIDS can present with GI tract hemorrhage from a number of causes: colitis from cytomegalovirus, herpes simplex, or bacteria; lymphoma; idiopathic proctocolitis; and Kaposi's sarcoma.[77] For our purposes, five specific conditions will be discussed in this section: diverticulosis, angiodysplasia, colorectal varices, Dieulafoy's lesion, and Meckel's diverticulum. Regardless of the cause of bleeding, a systematic approach to diagnosis and management is required to care for the patient adequately. This includes initial workup and stabilization of the patient, followed by diagnostic studies to identify the source of bleeding, and finally intervention to stop the bleeding. Colonoscopy and angiography are used for both localization and intervention.

Initial Presentation

Patients who present with lower GI hemorrhage must be evaluated in a timely fashion and are approached much as one would approach a trauma patient at risk for hemorrhage. Initial assessment includes establishing that the patient is hemodynamically stable. However, whether someone is stable or not, the team first establishing contact should ensure there is adequate intravenous (IV) access with two large bore IV catheters as well as obtaining blood for routine analysis and for a type and crossmatch. Blood products must be available in cases of significant bleeding and/or hemodynamic instability. If the patient is unstable, rapid interventions are required, including massive resuscitation and transfusions. Usually, however, the individual's condition is relatively stable, thus permitting time for evaluation.

Strate and colleagues performed a risk analysis of multiple factors that were thought to be predictive of severe bleeding.[344] Severe bleeding was defined as persistent bleeding during the first 24 hours of admission requiring transfusion of two or more units of packed red blood cells or a decrease in the hematocrit of 20% or more. Also included were patients who rebled after 24 hours of admission and who required transfusion at that time, had a further drop of hematocrit of 20% or more, or those readmitted one week after discharge with a lower GI bleed. The following factors were found to correlate with severe lower GI bleeding: a pulse rate greater than 100 beats per minute on admission, a systolic blood pressure less than 155 mm Hg, the presence of syncope, nontender abdominal examination, bleeding per rectum during the first 4 hours of evaluation, the use of aspirin, and two or more active comorbid conditions.[344] The authors then created a validated scale, assigning each of these risk factors a unit of one. Low-risk patients were those

with no risk factors and were assigned a score of 0, moderate risk patients had a score between 1 and 3, and high-risk patients were those with greater than three factors (i.e., having a score of 4 or more). Those with higher scores have been shown to have a greater risk of requiring blood transfusions, needing surgery, recurrent hemorrhage, or mortality.[345]

Other clinical outcomes have been used in order to examine the results following lower GI bleeding episodes. Das and coworkers created an artificial neural network and multiple logistic regression models to predict poor outcomes in patients experiencing a lower GI hemorrhage.[96] They defined poor outcome as those requiring therapeutic intervention, experiencing rebleeding, or death. Hemodynamic instability, persistent bleeding, and the existence of comorbidities were found to be persistent predictors of poor outcomes.[96]

Strate and Naumann propose the following risk factors for poor outcome in lower intestinal bleeding[343]:

Hemodynamic instability (hypotension, tachycardia, orthostasis, syncope)
Ongoing bleeding (blood at presentation or within 4 hours of presentation)
Older age
Comorbid illness
Bleeding while hospitalized for another process
Anticoagulation or antiplatelet medication
History of diverticular disease or angiogenesis
Nursing home resident
Nontender abdominal exam
Hematocrit less than 35%
Abnormal creatinine
Abnormal white blood cell count

Evaluation of Hemorrhage

The importance of obtaining an accurate history cannot be overemphasized. For example, knowledge of prior abdominal aorta surgery may be critical (Figure 28-1). However, patients usually present with no antecedent history and they frequently have no abdominal pain. Blood from the rectum

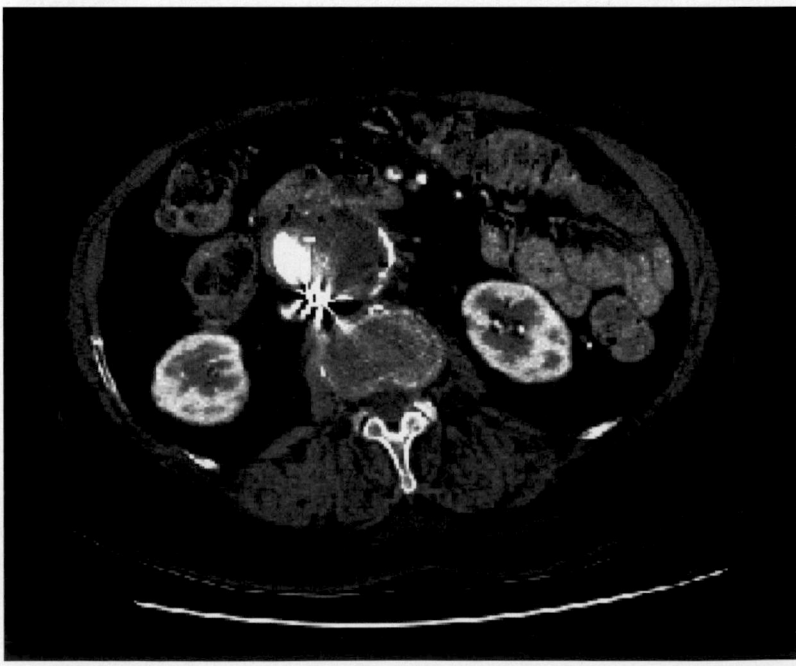

FIGURE 28-1. Aortoduodenal fistula. CT reveals bubbles of air within a mural thrombus. Patient underwent prior reconstruction for an abdominal aortic aneurysm. Note the overlying duodenum. (Courtesy of Allison Burkett, MD.)

may be bright red or maroon and may contain clots. In addition to a detailed medical and surgical history, identifying risk factors for bleeding is essential in the history, such as the patient's use of anticoagulants or antiplatelet drugs. Inflammatory conditions or other vasculitides are important to determine. One must also be wary and cognizant of an individual's consumption of herbal agents because many of these products have anticoagulant properties.

Physical examination of the bleeding patient is usually unrewarding. Even before one can begin investigations, the opportunity for identifying the source of bleeding may be lost because spontaneous cessation is not uncommon. The therapeutic effect of the administration of an enema before endoscopic examination or of a barium enema study is well recognized,[4] but this may be simply coincidental. McGuire undertook a study to ascertain the course of bleeding in 78 individuals who were admitted for a total of 106 times for this complaint, with no specific cause other than colonic diverticula. Bleeding stopped spontaneously in 75% of episodes and in 99% of patients requiring fewer than four units per day of transfusion.

One should, obviously, perform a digital rectal examination and a limited rigid sigmoidoscopy with anoscopy as the initial examination. However, the yield from these diagnostic procedures is less than 10%.[12,86,292] Still, if the source is found, appropriate therapy can be implemented. The treating physician must remember that bleeding suggestive of a lower GI source may actually be originating from the upper GI tract. The simple expediency of the placement of a nasogastric tube can eliminate the stomach as a potential source, especially if clear bile is returned. If the aspirate is positive, one should then proceed with upper GI endoscopy. A recent study by Laine and Shah demonstrated that 15% of patients who present with significant hematochezia had an upper GI source identified on endoscopy.[194] An organized approach to the evaluation of the patient with hemorrhage of presumed lower GI origin is suggested. An algorithm is presented in Figure 28-2, which provides an overview for carrying out the proper sequence of investigations in the bleeding patient. The approach to the bleeding patient—after initial assessment is complete and the patient is believed to have a lower GI source for bleeding—is to proceed with colonoscopic or radiologic investigation.

Colonoscopy

Colonoscopy has been identified by some to be the first-line approach to diagnosing and intervening in lower GI bleeding.[111,405] It identifies a definitive source of bleeding 40% to 90% of the time,[19,144,181,336,346] and a generalized diagnosis for the bleeding 90% to 100% of the time. Zuckerman and Prakash performed an extensive meta-analysis of 13 studies examining colonoscopy in lower GI bleeding.[406] They found a 1.3% complication rate in the 1,561 patients analyzed, thus indicating the procedure can be safely completed in the bleeding patient. Complications included congestive heart failure and worsening of the bleeding, but the rate of perforation was very low (0.3%). These low complication rates, along with high reported yields, make colonoscopy an enticing diagnostic and treatment modality for lower GI bleeding.

There are, however, certain prerequisites for colonoscopy performed during an active lower GI bleed, which include hemodynamic stability and the ability to perform a rapid bowel preparation on the patient. The oral preparation is performed over 4 to 5 hours and is often facilitated by placing a nasogastric tube in the patient. Polyethylene glycol (PEG) solution is delivered via the nasogastric tube over the next 4 hours. Rapid, high-volume preparations may lead to electrolyte abnormalities as well as significant fluid shifts that result in possible congestive heart failure. Aspiration pneumonia is another concern with a rapid prep through a nasogastric tube. Although these risks are rare, those patients undergoing rapid preparation for colonoscopy for suspected lower GI bleeding should receive the prep in a monitored setting in order to prevent or to recognize these potentially fatal complications. Adequate bowel preparation is essential for completing the colonoscopy. Ohyama and associates compared their early results for urgent colonoscopy when oral preparation was not performed with those after they initiated preparation with PEG solution and found significant improvement in their ability to complete the colonoscopy.[258] Others have confirmed these results, with completion rates ranging from 55% to 70% in those with unprepped colons.[81,352] Currently, if colonoscopy is to be attempted for diagnosis and managing lower GI bleeding, *oral preparation is required.*

The colonoscopy should be performed 1 to 2 hours after the preparation is complete, although controversy exists as

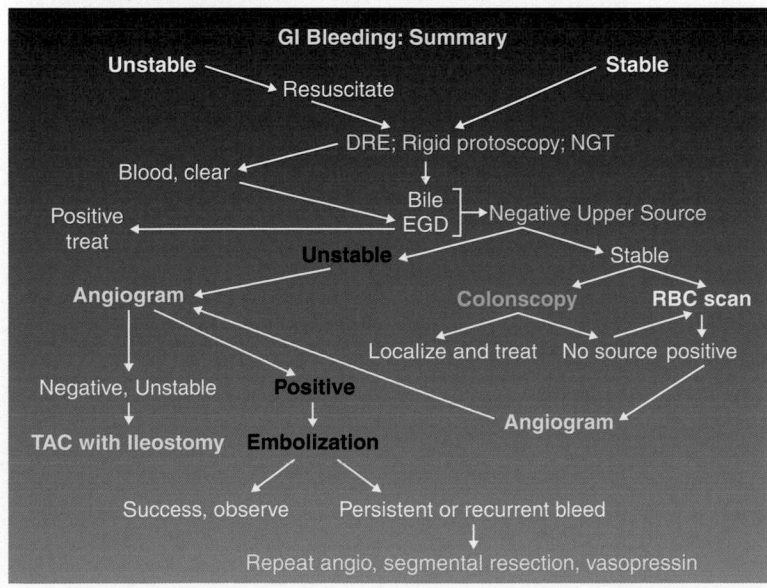

FIGURE 28-2. Algorithm for the management of acute gastrointestinal bleeding. DRE, digital rectal exam; NGT, nasogastric tube; EGD, esophagogastroduodenoscopy; RBC, red blood cell; TAC, total abdominal colectomy.

to the precise timing of colonoscopy for a suspected lower GI bleed. Jensen and colleagues found that colonoscopy performed 6 to 12 hours after admission resulted in significantly lower rebleed or surgery rates.[346] Successful endoscopic intervention was seen in 29% of patients if instrumented within 12 hours of admission. This falls to 13% if one waits between 12 and 24 hours and drops to 4% if one waits longer. Predictors of rebleeding included active bleeding, a visible vessel, and adherent clot.[181] The rebleeding rate in this study after intervention was 0%, and as one would expect this rate has been difficult to reproduce. Overall early rebleeding ranges from 0% to 24%, depending on the therapy used to terminate the bleeding, and late rebleeding rates that range from 0% to 17% have been documented.[343]

One of the key benefits of colonoscopy is that, in addition to being a diagnostic test, it is a therapeutic technique, if there is a skilled endoscopist available to stop active bleeding. Methods of controlling hemorrhage include injection, catheterization, banding, and clipping. The method used for hemostasis is often dependent on the comfort level of the endoscopist and the nature of the specific lesion that is bleeding. As mentioned previously, the overall complication rate, including perforation, is very low with colonoscopy for lower GI bleeding, so when a bleeding source is identified on endoscopy, every attempt should be made to control hemorrhage. If rebleeding occurs after an initially successful intervention, repeat endoscopy with intervention should be initiated. When attempting an intervention, having the patient in a well-controlled setting with adequate equipment is vital. If the patient is actively bleeding, having an anesthesia team to monitor and resuscitate the patient is recommended. Multichannel colonoscopies are required to facilitate active irrigation, suction, and simultaneous intervention to treat the bleeding site. The use of carbon dioxide insufflation may help decrease postprocedure distention.

Thermal ablation of lesions may be attempted by using a heater probe and bipolar or monopolar electrocautery. Argon plasma beam coagulation may also be used to ablate arteriovenous malformations or vessels. When using cautery, the endoscopist should generally use lower settings (10 to 20 W), with short bursts and minimal pressure.[144,181] Electrocautery should be avoided in the right colon, especially within the cecum. The few reported cases of perforation are related to intervention in the right colon.[315]

When one encounters active bleeding from a vessel, an arteriovenous malformation (AVM), or a diverticulum, the endoscopist should attempt injection with epinephrine solution in four quadrants around the bleeding site in order to induce spasm and clotting of the bleeding vessel. A 1 to 10,000 or a 1 to 20,000 dilution of the epinephrine is employed, with 1 to 2 mL injected in each quadrant. Following induction of spasm of the vessel, definitive treatment of the bleeding site can be attempted. Injection of epinephrine alone has a rebleeding rate of approximately 15%.[264,286] Some authors have advocated placement of endoclips as a safer option than electrocautery, although minimal data exists to support that statement.[168,331] When hemodynamically stable, endoscopy with intervention is a viable option for management of lower GI bleeding.

Etiology

Diverticulosis

Classically, massive lower GI bleeding has been generally attributed to diverticular disease, usually without any evidence of diverticulitis.[133,253,391] As discussed in Chapter 27,

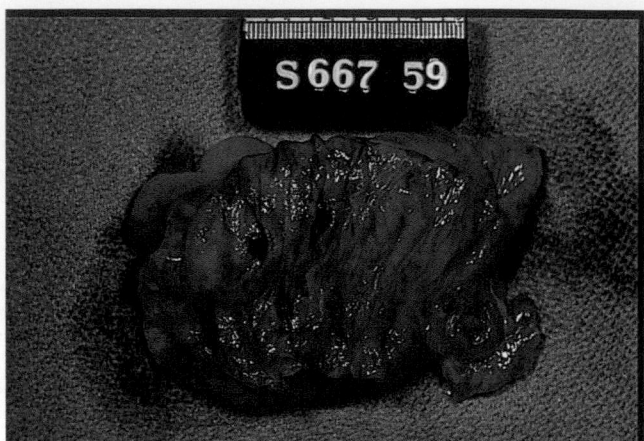

FIGURE 28-3. Portion of sigmoid colon removed for massive lower intestinal hemorrhage that was presumed due to diverticulosis reveals clot in several diverticula.

diverticular disease occurs where tunnels formed by the blood vessels weaken the muscle. Theoretically, the vasa rectum, through its proximity with the diverticulum, can rupture either at the apex or at the neck as the vessel proceeds into the submucosa of the colon (Figure 28-3). Baer demonstrated that 20 of 22 patients had a pathologically proved ruptured vasa rectum within a diverticulum as the source of lower GI hemorrhage (Figure 28-4).[28]

The problem, however, is that most lower GI hemorrhage comes from the right side of the colon, where there are few or

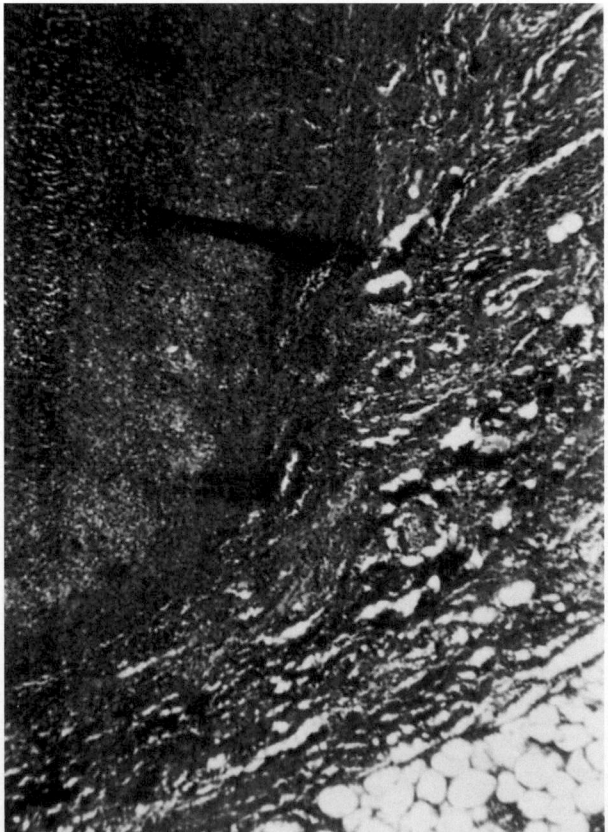

FIGURE 28-4. Diverticulum lined by hemorrhagic granulation tissue in a patient who had massive lower gastrointestinal hemorrhage. (Original magnification × 260; courtesy of Rudolf Garret, MD.)

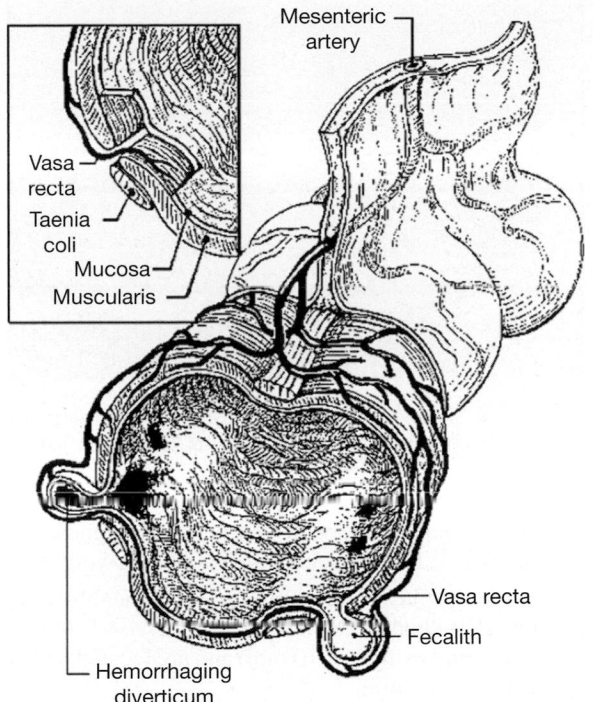

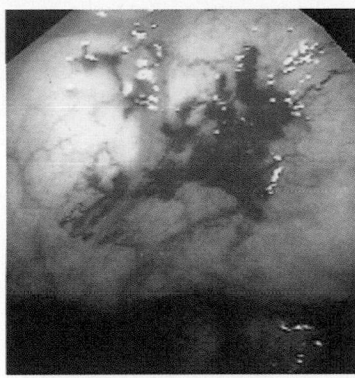

FIGURE 28-6. An angiodysplastic lesion seen on colonoscopy is characteristically a focal, submucosal, vascular ectasia.

FIGURE 28-5. Cross-sectional drawing of the colon showing principal points of diverticular formation between mesenteric and anti-mesenteric teniae. (From Beck DE, Opelka FG. Diverticular disease. In: Beck DE, ed. Handbook of Colorectal Surgery. 2nd ed. New York, NY: Marcel Dekker; 2003: 241–258. Reprinted with permission.)

no diverticula. Evidence suggests that unexplained vigorous lower intestinal bleeding, even in the presence of known diverticulosis, is most likely due to an arteriovenous malformation (vascular ectasia, angiodysplasia).[8,38,39,339] With the availability of angiography and scintigraphy and the ability to identify preoperatively the site of bleeding, arteriovenous malformations have not uncommonly been observed in areas where diverticulosis is present.

Angiodysplasia or Vascular Ectasia

The contemporary attitude is that lower GI bleeding originates from a vascular malformation. Because vascular ectasia is more commonly seen in the right colon and that is the most common site for lower GI hemorrhage, one can inferentially presume that this is the case.[29,50,147,156,238,335,342,355] However, Höchter and colleagues challenged this theory when they reported 59 patients with angiodysplasia to have a more uniform bowel distribution.[167] The sites of the lesions were as follows: cecum, 37%; ascending colon, 17%; transverse colon, 7%; descending colon, 7%; sigmoid, 18%; and rectum, 14%.[167]

Bleeding associated with ectasia is usually less severe than that from diverticular hemorrhage. It tends to be intermittent and is probably due to venous encroachment of the mucosa as compared with the ruptured vasa rectum of a bleeding diverticulum (Figure 28-5).

The etiology of the condition remains somewhat problematic. Boley and associates suggest that the vascular lesions are degenerative, from an acquired and progressive dilatation of previously normal blood vessels, the result of the aging process.[50,53] They propose that muscular contraction or increased intraluminal pressure produces obstruction of the perforating veins.[271] These submucosal structures become dilated and tortuous, with an associated arteriovenous communication (Figure 28-6). Others suggest a congenital etiology; some proposing an association with Meckel's diverticulum,[166] but this only serves to cause confusion. It is perhaps wiser to accept the concept that angiodysplasia is an acquired condition that should be distinguished from the blood vessel tumor, hemangioma (see Chapter 26).

SCOTT J. BOLEY (1927–PRESENT)

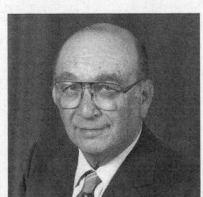

Scott Boley was born in Brooklyn, New York, June 1, 1927. He attended the Wesleyan University in Connecticut and graduated from Jefferson Medical College in 1949. Following 11 years in private practice, he made a commitment to an academic career at the Albert Einstein College of Medicine and the Montefiore Medical Center and is currently professor of surgery and pediatrics. Boley has made numerous contributions to the field of colorectal surgery in particular. For example, he provided the initial description of the entity of noniatrogenic, noncatastrophic colonic ischemia (ischemic colitis) in 1963; he elucidated the cause of small bowel ulcers resulting from enteric-coated potassium diuretic tablets (1965); and he described the endorectal pull-through operation with primary anastomosis for Hirschsprung's disease (1964). He was the first to identify the nature and etiology of vascular ectasia (angiodysplasia) of the colon (1977) and advocated an aggressive approach to the management of acute mesenteric ischemia through the use of early angiography and intra-arterial vasodilators. He also described the right colon patch endorectal pull-through operation for total aganglionosis of the colon. Boley has published more than 250 articles and book chapters and has edited several books and monographs. He continues in active teaching and consulting as of this writing.

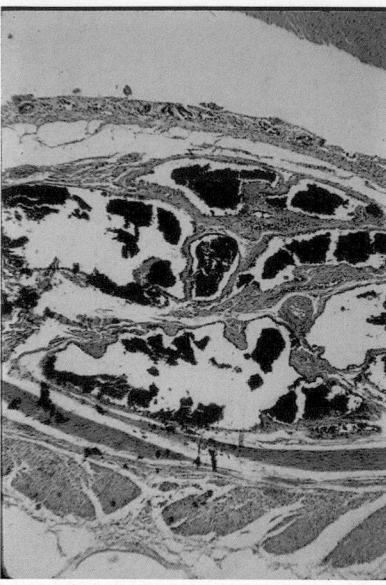

FIGURE 28-7. Angiodysplasia of the cecum. Note the irregular veins and arteries. (Original magnification × 120; courtesy of Rudolf Garret, MD.)

Pathologically, angiodysplastic lesions appear to be ectasias or dilatations of vascular structures. They represent collections of thin-walled, dilated vessels (either capillaries or veins) usually lying in the submucosa (Figures 28-7 and 28-8). Rarely, the condition may be associated with vascular malformations elsewhere in the GI tract (e.g., Osler-Weber-Rendu disease) (Figure 28-9).

There does not appear to be any gender predilection for vascular ectasias. However, two-thirds of the patients of Boley and Brandt were older than 70 years old.[50] Richardson and associates reported 39 patients with bleeding due to vascular malformations of the intestine.[291] There seemed to be a bimodal age distribution, with younger patients having no associated disease, whereas older people often had a cardiac lesion (especially aortic stenosis [see later] and severe atherosclerotic disease). The most common site of bleeding was the cecum, with resection controlling the hemorrhage in the vast majority of patients. However, bleeding can occur from angioplastic lesions in more than one area of the colon.[335] Foutch and colleagues

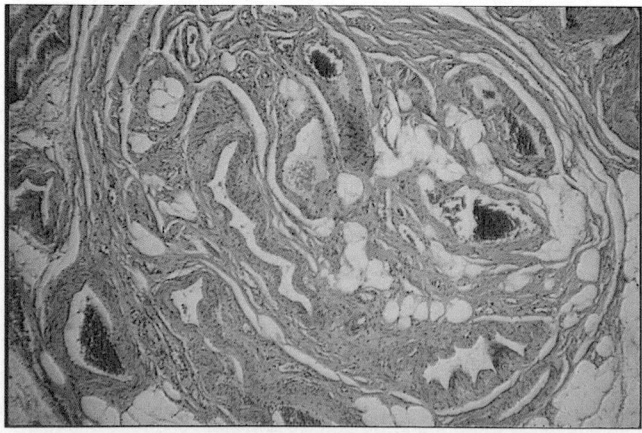

FIGURE 28-8. Vascular malformation showing thick-walled veins and arteries in an irregular distribution. (Original magnification × 250; courtesy of Rudolf Garret, MD.)

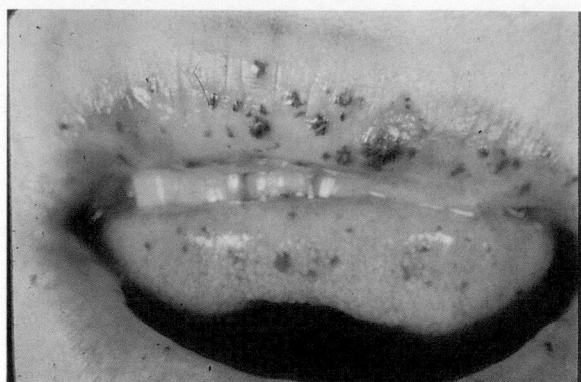

FIGURE 28-9. Telangiectasis of the lips in a patient with hereditary malformations and gastrointestinal hemorrhage. (Courtesy of Rudolf Garret, MD.)

reviewed their experience with 964 patients diagnosed with angiodysplasia.[122] They concluded with the following:

Colonic angiodysplasia is uncommon among healthy asymptomatic individuals (0.83%).

Lesions are usually small (<10 mm) and are located proximal to the hepatic flexure.

The natural history is benign, with the risk of bleeding over a 3-year period nonexistent.

Most opine that endoscopic treatment for nonbleeding lesions is unnecessary.

Relationship to Calcific Aortic Stenosis

Love identified the syndrome of calcific aortic stenosis and GI hemorrhage, suggesting treatment of the bleeding by aortic valve replacement.[212] Shbeeb and colleagues reviewed Love's experience and confirmed the association of calcific aortic stenosis and obscure GI bleeding in the elderly.[325] These authors and others believe that this operation not only corrects the cardiac hemodynamic instability but also stops the GI hemorrhage.[73,145]

A mechanism for the association and the ameliorative response to cardiac surgery is not clear. It may be a consumption phenomenon or a qualitative alteration of platelet function produced by the roughened stenotic valve in the area of greatest pressure and velocity of the bloodstream.[212] This subtle coagulation defect combined with a thin-walled vascular lesion may tend to promote the hemorrhage. Another contributing factor may be the abnormal arterial inflow pulse wave.[145] A coagulation panel, including platelet function, should be part of the preoperative assessment of any patient suspected of bleeding from angiodysplasia.[335] One should be aware of this relationship so that earlier diagnosis may spare these patients from multiple hospitalizations and transfusions.

Dieulafoy's Lesion

Dieulafoy's lesion, also known as Dieulafoy's malformation, was originally described by Paul Georges Dieulafoy in 1898 as a gastric, submucosal aneurysm.[107] Significant, and often recurrent, hemorrhage occurs from a pinpoint nonulcerated arterial lesion, usually high in the gastric fundus. However, the condition has also been described as an unusual cause of small bowel hemorrhage and even rarely the source of bleeding in the colon, rectum, and anal canal.[233]

The lesion has characteristically been described as a solitary, protuberant, serpiginous, and abnormally wide artery

PAUL GEORGES DIEULAFOY (1839–1911)

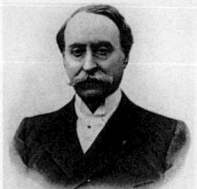

Paul Dieulafoy was born in Toulouse, France, November 18, 1839. He studied in Paris and received his doctorate there in 1869. He ultimately became professor of medicine and chief of medical services at the Hôtel-Dieu in Paris. Dieulafoy has been recognized as an innovative investigator and a keen observer who did seminal work on typhoid, Bright's disease, and appendicitis. Among his eponymously associated contributions were his *apparatus*—a suction pump to evacuate fluid from the chest cavity; his *erosion*—an erosion or ulcer-complicating pneumonia and causing upper gastrointestinal hemorrhage; his *pancreatic crisis*—symptoms of acute abdomen at the onset of hemorrhagic pancreatitis; his *triad*—a hypersensitivity of the skin, tenderness, and muscular contraction at McBurney's point in acute appendicitis; and, of course, his *lesion* or vascular malformation of the stomach. He wrote a manual on pathology and was elected president of the French Académie de Médecin in 1910. Dieulafoy died August 16, 1911, in Paris.

located in the submucosa that has the appearance of a submucosal tumor in an otherwise normal mucosa.[233] Endoscopic criteria for diagnosis include a less than 3-mm mucosal defect in combination with any of the following[25]:

- A protruding 1- to 2-mm blood vessel
- Active arterial bleeding
- Fresh adherent clot with a narrow point of attachment
- Inactive lesion with associated intraluminal blood suggestive of recent hemorrhage

Microscopically, there is usually noted to be a thick-walled vessel without an associated inflammatory reaction.

Treatment may involve intra-arterial vasopressin (see Evaluation of Hemorrhage), sclerotherapy, oversewing (if within reach of rectal instrumentation), or resection.

Meckel's Diverticulum

Meckel's diverticulum is generally acknowledged to be the most prevalent congenital anomaly of the GI tract.[221] Johann Meckel was not the first to recognize this entity, however. Fabricus Hildanus had reported this in 1598 as an unusual diverticulum of the small intestine, but it was Meckel who in 1809 published a meticulous description of its anatomy and embryonic origin.[230] The condition is present in 1% to 2% of autopsies. It represents a diverticulum of the ileum derived from the unobliterated yolk stalk—that is, the remnant of the vitelline duct. Generally, it is found more commonly in males in the ratio of 2:1. In almost 90% of cases, the diverticulum arises on the antimesenteric border. When the remnant persists, it may result in a variety of intra-abdominal complications.

The rule of 2's is the classical description of this anomaly. It is located about 2 ft from the end of the small intestine, is often about 2 in. in length, occurs in about 2% of the population, is twice as common in males, and can contain two types of ectopic tissue—stomach or pancreas.

In the adult, the diverticulum is usually 1.5 to 2 in. long and occurs approximately 2 ft from the ileocecal valve (Figure 28-10). However, the distance is quite variable. The diverticulum contains all layers of the bowel wall, but in some cases it may harbor heterotopic, gastric, pancreatic, biliary, or even colonic tissues (Figure 28-11).[61] The two most frequently observed complications are intestinal

JOHANN FRIEDRICH MECKEL (1781–1833)

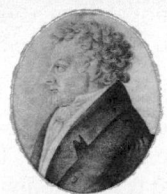

Johann Meckel was born October 17, 1781, in Halle, Prussia. He is known as the Younger, having been born into a family of prominent physicians. His father, Philipp Friedrich Theodore Meckel, was professor of anatomy and surgical obstetrics at the University of Halle, and his grandfather, Johann Friedrich Meckel (the Elder), had occupied the same prestigious chair. Meckel's younger brother, August Albrecht Meckel, also inherited the family's academic attributes and became professor of anatomy and forensic medicine at the University of Bonn in 1821. The younger Meckel, however, as a child had an outspoken aversion to medicine in general and anatomy in particular, perhaps as a consequence of his having to help his father perform dissections. Despite this he ultimately became one of the greatest anatomists of his time. He began his medical studies at Halle and in 1801 moved to the University of Göttingen to expand his interest in comparative anatomy. He received his medical degree the following year in Halle. After several years of travel and study throughout Europe, he ultimately collaborated with the brilliant French anatomist, Cuvier, and translated Cuvier's five-volume work into German, a task that he completed in 1810. Returning to his native Halle in 1806, he found that Napoleon himself had been using his home as temporary headquarters, an intrusion that may have aided in preserving the valuable anatomic collection of the Meckel family. In 1808, he was appointed professor of normal and pathological anatomy, surgery, and obstetrics at Halle. Meckel attracted large numbers to his lectures at Halle, which was then the center of comparative anatomy in Germany. Among his lasting contributions was the study of the abnormalities occurring during embryologic development. Meckel's *teratology* was the first comprehensive description of birth defects. Johann Meckel died October 31, 1833, in Halle. (Photograph courtesy of the Anatomical Institute of the University of Halle).

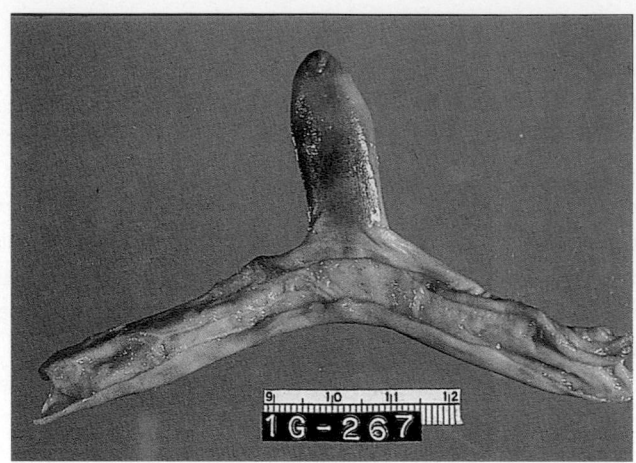
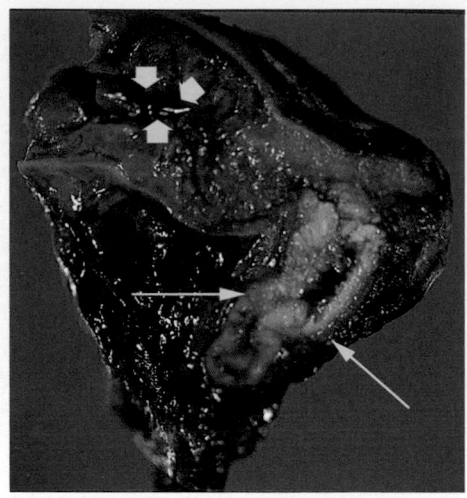

FIGURE 28-10. Meckel's diverticulum. **A:** Typical long, sausagelike resected specimen. **B:** Macroscopic appearance of the opened diverticulum revealing a thick, heterotopic mucosa (*closed arrows*) with an ulcer (*open arrows*) in the otherwise normal bowel. (Reproduced with permission from Lewin KJ, Riddell RH, Weinstein WM. *Gastrointestinal Pathology and Its Clinical Implications.* New York, NY: Igaku-Shoin; 1992.)

obstruction and hemorrhage (Figure 28-12). So-called Meckel's diverticulitis is a third presentation. Intussusception in young children may lead to intestinal obstruction and/or rectal bleeding. Serious hemorrhage from the rectum from a Meckel's diverticulum is usually due to peptic ulceration. This occurs most frequently in children between the ages of 10 and 15, but it is not unusual to observe this presentation in adults. The blood is usually dark red as opposed to the tarry stool of an upper GI source for the hemorrhage or bright red rectal bleeding from a more distal location.

Vane and colleagues reported 217 children with vitelline duct anomalies.[371] Forty-eight presented with rectal bleeding, and at the time of surgery all were found to have ectopic gastric mucosa. Yamaguchi and coworkers identified ectopic gastric mucosa in only 9.1% of their 596 cases.[398] In the experience of Mackey and Dineen, 25% of the individuals who were symptomatic presented with lower GI bleeding.[221] Those who were younger than 40 years were most likely to have symptoms develop.

Diagnostic Studies
Kusumoto and colleagues compared the various modalities of evaluation of bleeding from Meckel's diverticulum in 138 individuals.[192] All underwent any one or more of three examinations: [99m]Tc scintigraphy, angiography, and barium enema study. Thirty-eight percent of patients had positive angiography. Forty-seven percent were diagnosed as having a Meckel's diverticulum on barium study, but scintigraphy had a diagnostic accuracy rate of 83%. The authors concluded that ^{99m}Tc-pertechnetate scintigraphy is the preferred test for evaluating bleeding when Meckel's diverticulum is suspected.[192] Schwartz and Lewis opined, however, that there is a relatively high false-positive and false-negative rate with scintigraphic imaging.[320] Based on their findings, it was suggested that the scanning be supplemented with small bowel infusion or arteriography or both to improve preoperative evaluation in adult patients when this diagnosis is entertained.

Treatment
Excision of Meckel's diverticulum can usually be accomplished by simple diverticulectomy, although a small bowel resection may be necessary, particularly if the base of the diverticulum is quite broad. Closure can be effected by conventional suturing or by any number of techniques using the stapling devices. A laparoscopically assisted approach to Meckel's diverticulectomy has also been described.[24]

Incidental Removal
What is the natural history of Meckel's diverticulum? Should it be removed incidentally when identified?

Soltero and Bill studied 202 cases over a 15-year period in an attempt to answer this question.[338] Using the population averages and the number of cases in each age group (assuming a 2% incidence of Meckel's diverticulum in the general population), they calculated the rates per year of a complication developing from a Meckel's diverticulum using life-table techniques. They concluded that a Meckel's diverticulum has a 4.2% likelihood of causing symptoms during a lifetime, decreasing to zero with old age. They also concluded that it would be necessary to remove approximately 800 asymptomatic Meckel's diverticula in order to save one patient's life from the complications of their presence. The obvious recommendation was that the removal of an asymptomatic Meckel's diverticulum is rarely, if ever, justified.

Colorectal Varices
Since originally described in 1954, fewer than 100 cases of colonic varices have been reported in the literature.[378] This rare cause of lower intestinal hemorrhage is almost always associated with cirrhosis, with resultant portal hypertension, or portal venous obstruction.[174] The condition has been reported in approximately 2.5% of those undergoing sclerotherapy for esophageal varices.[123] As few as 3.6% and as many as 56% of cirrhotic patients have been demonstrated to have concomitant rectal varices. Parenthetically, it must be remembered that hemorrhoids are not rectal varices, and this misnomer should never be applied to that condition.

Another presentation of variceal bleeding that is of interest to the colon and rectal surgeon is also a consequence of portal hypertension—that of stomal and parastomal varices, especially in an individual with sclerosing cholangitis and biliary cirrhosis as an extraintestinal manifestation of inflammatory bowel disease (see Chapters 29 and 31).[158]

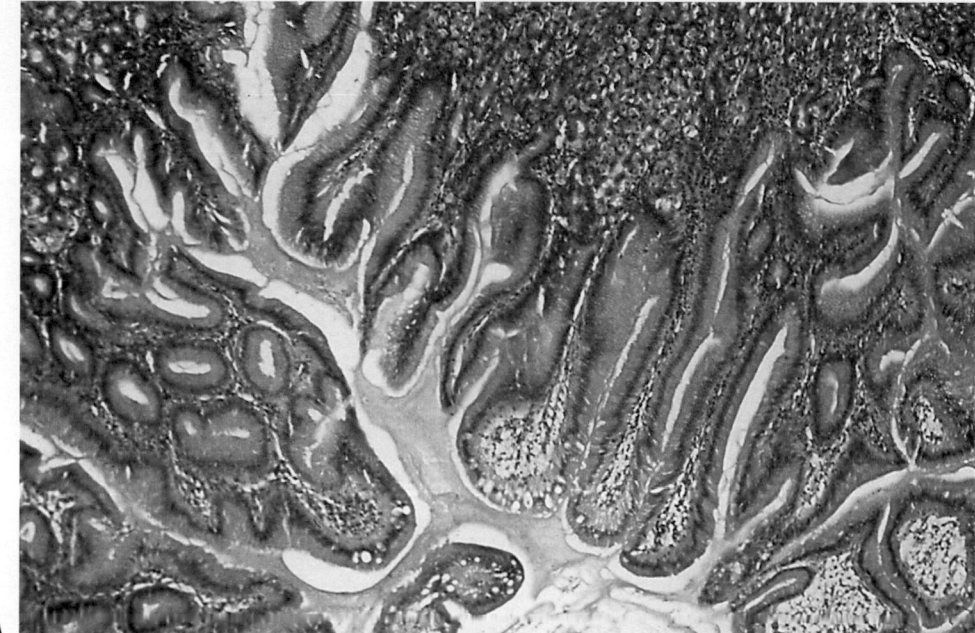

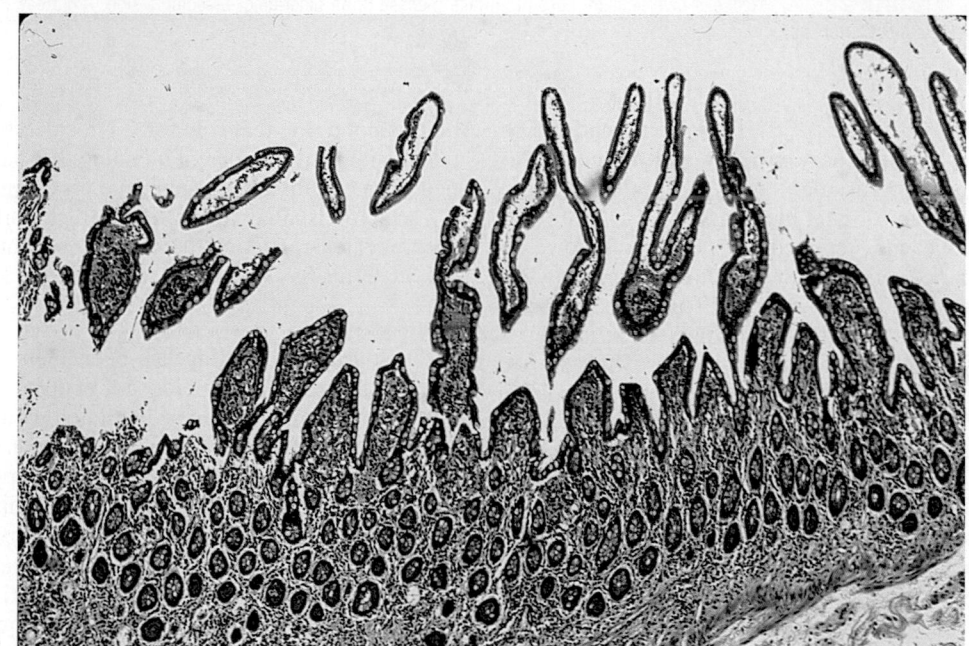

FIGURE 28-11. Meckel's diverticulum demonstrating the appearance of typical small bowel mucosa **(A)** and gastric heterotopia **(B)**. In the latter situation, the mucosa has the appearance of gastric fundus with gastric glands. Occasional goblet cells are present. (Courtesy of Matthew Curran, MD.)

A still rarer cause of colonic varices is the so-called familial or idiopathic variety.[174] The condition may present at any age, including the first decade of life. To conclude that this disease truly represents idiopathic colonic varices, liver disease and portal venous obstruction must be excluded.

Contrast-enhanced, three-dimensional magnetic resonance angiography has been recommended as uniquely helpful for visualizing ectopic varices, that is, colorectal and stomal varices.[158]

Management

Generally, if the bleeding occurs in the group of patients whose colonic varices are secondary to liver disease, treatment parallels that of the management of bleeding esophageal varices from portal hypertension.[326] Conversely, in those individuals whose colonic varices are attributed to a congenital etiology, favorable prognosis has been associated with colonic resection.[378] Transanal application of the circular stapling instrument for the treatment of bleeding rectal varices has also been described.[49]

Diagnosis of Lower Gastrointestinal Bleeding

Colonoscopy

Therapeutic Colonoscopy

Specifically for the treatment of angiodysplastic lesions; sclerotherapy; electrocoagulation; and, more recently, endoscopic GI laser therapy have been successfully employed

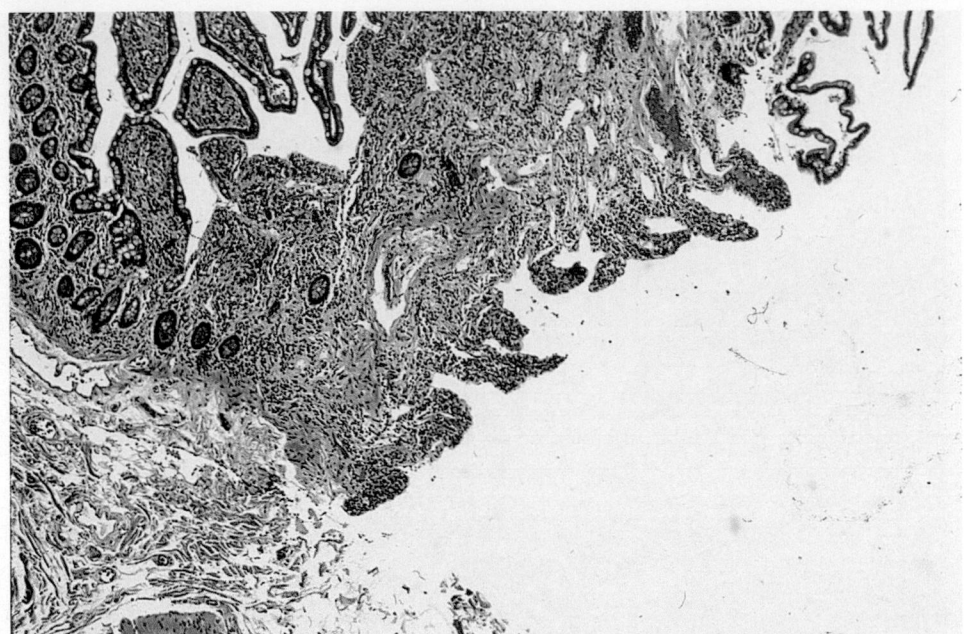

FIGURE 28-12. Meckel's diverticulum. Loss of surface mucosa in an ulcerating, bleeding lesion. (Courtesy of Matthew Curran, MD.)

(see Chapter 5).[50,65,151,167,171,275,318,366] The recommended technique is to treat the periphery initially and the center last in order to reduce the vascular supply to the lesion and to diminish the potential for later bleeding.[50]

Trudel and colleagues reported 71 patients with lower GI bleeding secondary to arteriovenous malformations, of whom 80% were diagnosed by colonoscopy.[366] The mean number of prior hemorrhages was 6.1. Of the 28 individuals treated by endoscopic coagulation, bleeding ceased in approximately two-thirds. A surgical procedure controlled the recurrent bleeding in six of seven cases where electrocoagulation had failed. Therapeutic colonoscopy has been reviewed earlier in this chapter.

Computed Tomographic Colonography

Computed tomographic (CT) colonography is an alternative imaging modality that could, in theory, be effectively used before colonoscopy in selected patients.[358] The use of computed tomography as a diagnostic test for patients with GI hemorrhage has become a viable option since the development of multidetector row CT scans. This technique significantly decreases the time required for scanning, allowing for effective arterial phase imaging, and thereby permitting its use in cases of significant lower GI bleeding. Drawbacks to the technique include a high IV contrast load, with the potential risk of nephrotoxicity as well as the amount of radiation delivered during the scan. Like nuclear medicine scanning, the test is purely diagnostic; it does not have the option for intervention.

Yoon and colleagues performed a randomized, prospective trial to examine the feasibility of multidetector CT scanning for GI hemorrhage.[399] Positive scans were reported in 84% of their patients. They also documented two episodes of renal insufficiency (11%) afterward, both patients having had preexisting diabetic nephropathy. Others have warned of the high contrast load required if progressing to mesenteric angiogram after CT angiography.[178] When comparing multidirectional CT scans to nuclear scintigraphy, nuclear scintigraphy had a higher rate of detection (25% vs. 46%).[403]

At this point, the real role for CT localization may be in patients with active recurrent bleeding that has not been identified. One certain advantage of the procedure is the ability of CT scan to visualize the entire GI tract, perhaps with greater accuracy in localization than nuclear scanning or angiogram, although this has not been documented in the literature.

Angiography

If the source of bleeding has been identified by means of rectal examination, sigmoidoscopy, upper GI endoscopy, or colonoscopy, therapy can be instituted. Unfortunately, in patients who bleed massively from the colon and are unstable, these studies are usually not helpful except to eliminate another cause. The next investigative procedure that should be performed is either selective angiography or radionuclide scan. Unless angiography is not available at the hospital, the patient should not be taken to the operating room without this radiologic investigation. Abbas and coworkers identified instability as the patient having a blood pressure of less than 90 mm Hg and having received five units of packed red blood cells in 24 hours.[2] This combination is predictive of identifying the source of bleeding by means of angiography. With both hypotension and the requirement for transfusion, they identified a bleeding site in 85% of their patients. However, when the patients were stable, the authors' yield was only 15%. Clearly, the rate of bleeding determines the success of angiography in identifying the source. Steer and Silen demonstrated a required bleeding rate of 0.5 cc to 1 cc/minute in order to demonstrate a positive angiogram.[341] The standard sensitivity that most publications suggest in order to identify the source of blood loss by means of angiography is 0.5 mL/minute. This is probably an unrealistically low estimate because it is based on the results of studies performed on the animal model. Bowel gas, the presence of fluid within the lumen, body habitus, and other variables may make it impossible for one to identify extravasation unless the rate of bleeding is as much as 5 mL/minute (300 mL/hour). The

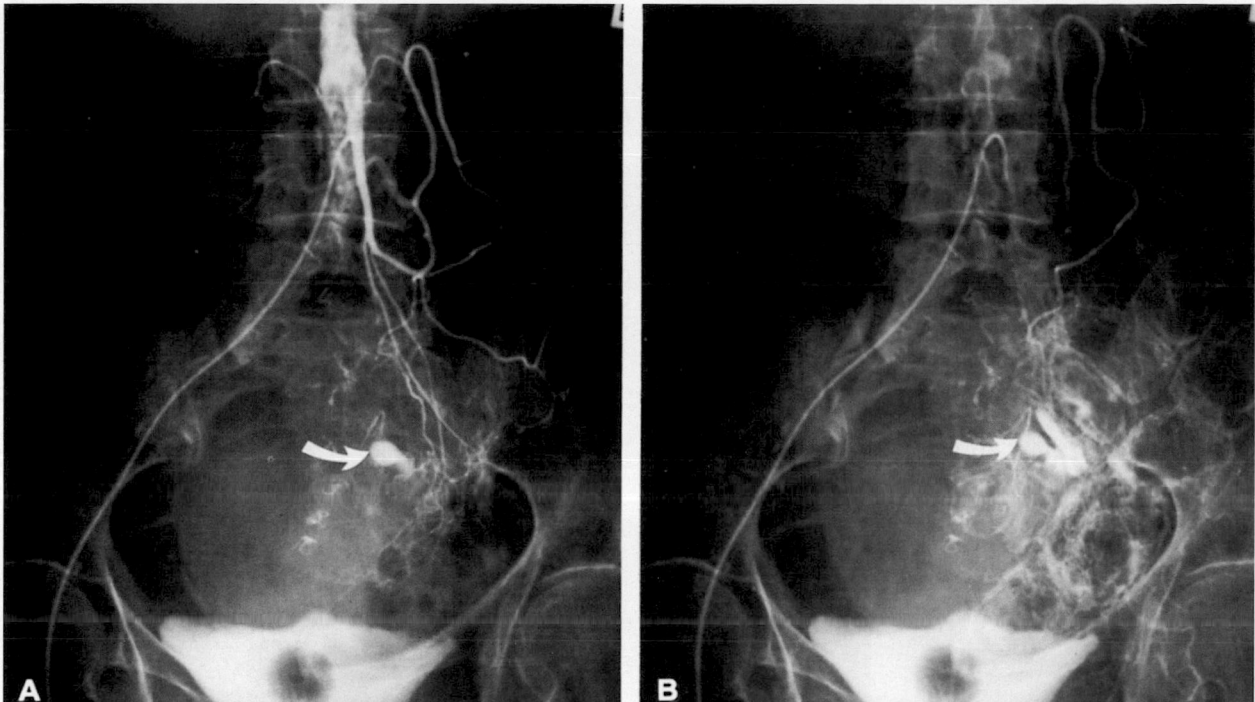

FIGURE 28-13. Bleeding from diverticulum. Early **(A)** and late **(B)** arterial phases of an inferior mesenteric arteriogram demonstrate an active bleeding site in the distal transverse colon (*arrow*).

literature varies widely in the reported success rates of localization with angiography—that is, from 25% to 70%.

Direct selective catheterization of the celiac, superior mesenteric, and inferior mesenteric arteries is accomplished by way of the groin using a modified Seldinger technique.[323] In suspected lower GI bleeding, the superior mesenteric artery is injected first because of the higher incidence of colonic

bleeding from the right side.[138] If the site of the bleeding is not found, the inferior mesenteric artery is studied. Finally, if no source is identified, a celiac injection should be made. As mentioned, on rare occasions upper GI bleeding may seem to be of colonic origin. Radiographic abnormalities include extravasation (Figures 28-13 and 28-14), arteriovenous malformation (Figure 28-15), a delayed emptying vein, and an

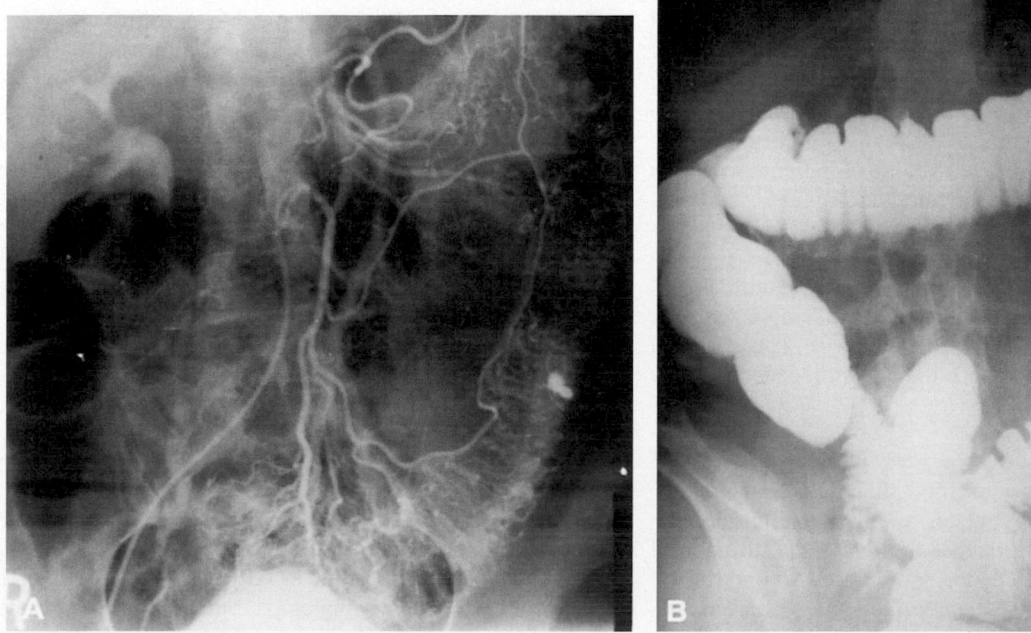

FIGURE 28-14. Bleeding from diverticulum. **A:** Angiogram demonstrates extravasation in upper sigmoid. **B:** Site of bleeding corresponds to larger diverticulum on barium enema.

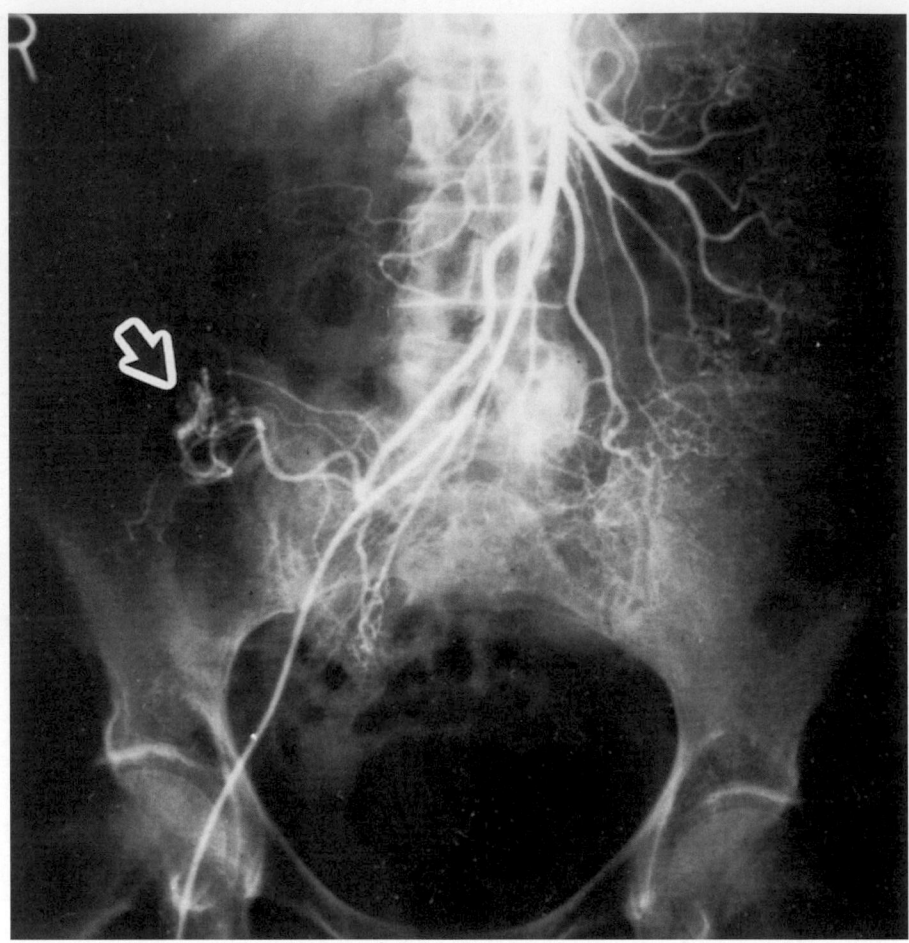

FIGURE 28-15. Arteriovenous malformation "vascular tuft" (*arrow*) demonstrated by SMA injection. (Courtesy of Brian R. Schnier, MD.)

early-filling vein (Figure 28-16). The cecal branch of the ileocolic artery usually is the most likely site for a vascular malformation. The characteristic angiographic signs of angiodysplasia were described by Boley and colleagues and include a dense, slowly emptying vein (92%), a vascular tuft (68%), and an early-filling vein (56%).[54] Extravasation of the contrast material is the least frequently observed finding (8%). Many reports testify to the success of identifying a bleeding site by angiography. For example, Allison and colleagues ascertained the source in 87% of patients in whom the study was undertaken as an emergency, and 74%, if performed electively.[10]

Injection of the major blood vessel in the resected specimen with silicon rubber compound and clearing with methyl salicylate is one means for possibly identifying a vascular tuft or dilated blood vessels (Figure 28-17). The potential value of this technique is to permit the pathologist to identify the lesion macroscopically.

Therapeutic Angiography

If the bleeding point is identified, it may be possible to control the hemorrhage by means of either an embolization technique (Figures 28-18 and 28-19) or by the infusion of Pitressin (vasopressin). Vasopressin causes contraction of smooth muscle, especially the capillaries, small arterioles, and venules, with less effect on the smooth musculature of the larger veins. Many papers have been published that deal with the efficacy of vasopressin in the treatment of

GI hemorrhage.[40,56,112,285,367] But the use of vasopressin has several disadvantages. The drug itself has a number of side effects, including decreased cardiac output, hypertension, and arrhythmias.[138] Because many of these patients are elderly or perhaps have an unstable cardiovascular condition, it is important to carefully monitor the intake and output. Vasopressin has a profound antidiuretic effect. Additionally, there are potential concerns related to prolonged catheter use: embolism, hemorrhage around the puncture site, hematoma, and limitation of activity. An arterial pump is needed to administer the drug, and the position of the catheter has to be checked daily by means of a portable x-ray unit.

Embolization has been reported to be an acceptable alternative to infusing a vasoconstrictive substance.[97,101,139,214,226,235,296,297,337] In the experience of DeBarros and coworkers, all 27 patients who had an angiographically visualized source for colonic hemorrhage underwent successful embolization.[97] Six patients rebled (22%), 5 of whom required surgery. Two demonstrated ischemia (7.4%), 1 of whom required an operation.

Overall advancement in angiography with superselective embolization has allowed greater success and fewer complications in treating lower GI bleeding. Superselective embolization refers to using coaxial microcatheters to selectively cannulate and embolize distal arterial branches. Strate and Naumann compiled 20 studies that used superselective embolization techniques and found a total of 338 patients

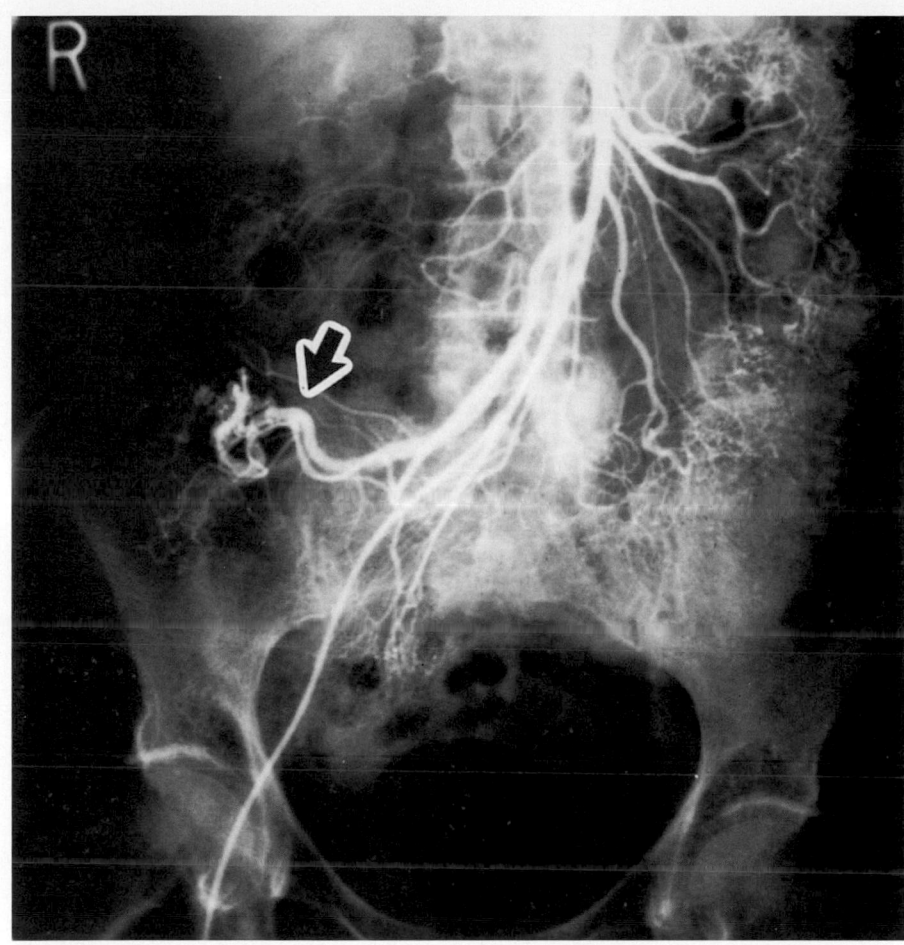

FIGURE 28-16. Early filling vein (*arrow*) draining from the arteriovenous malformation shown in Figure 28-14. (Courtesy of Brian R. Schnier, MD.)

out of 539 that could be embolized. Ninety-six percent achieved immediate hemostasis, with a rebleeding rate of 22%. Seventeen percent of these patients experienced major complications that resulted in surgery or death.[343] Some studies have suggested that diverticular hemorrhage managed with embolization has a lower rebleeding rate and greater initial success rate than embolization performed for other causes of bleeding.[2,185,273]

Currently, three agents are used for embolization: microcoils, polyvinyl alcohol particles, and Gelfoam. None has been shown to have a greater efficacy than another, but currently Gelfoam is rarely used. A potential benefit of alcohol particles is the ability to inject these proximal to a bleeding site when manipulating the microcatheters into the correct position is not possible.

Transcatheter embolization will inevitably lead, in some patients, to postembolic colonic ischemia and possibly even to infarction.[297] Infarction of the embolized segment is the most common complication seen. However, contrast-related injuries such as allergic reaction or nephrotoxicity are also seen as procedure-related issues, as are vessel thrombosis or dissections and hematoma formation. Theoretically, the same segment of ischemic bowel would require removal, a procedure that might be performed under less urgent circumstances than hemorrhage. The incidence of ischemic complications may be reduced by using the least number of emboli required to control the hemorrhage.[297] Not every patient is suitable, nor is every lesion amenable to such

therapy. However, for those deemed appropriate and who achieve a satisfactory response, operative intervention may be avoided or at least delayed so that it can be undertaken at an elective time.

Nuclear Medicine Techniques
Technetium Sulfur Colloid Scintigraphy
Localizing the site of acute GI hemorrhage has been performed using technetium sulfur colloid scintigraphy (^{99m}Tc).[218,260,275,319,330,381] The imaging agent used for conventional liver scans is injected into the venous circulation, and with the abdomen of the patient under the gamma camera, a radionuclide angiogram is obtained. The principle of the study is that the labeled colloid is rapidly cleared from the bloodstream by the reticuloendothelial system, but an active site of bleeding appears as a "hot spot" because the extravasated isotope is no longer recirculating and cannot be cleared by the system.[330,381] The use of technetium sulfur colloid as a scanning method has been supplanted by tagged red blood cells scan.

Tagged Red Blood Cells
Another alternative is the use of technetium (^{99m}Tc) tagged red blood cells.[392,393] This technique permits identification of a bleeding point due to hemorrhage of a lesser magnitude. In contrast to technetium sulfur colloid scintigraphy, the labeled red cells are not cleared rapidly and are available to produce a positive scan through repeated periods of imaging, even if

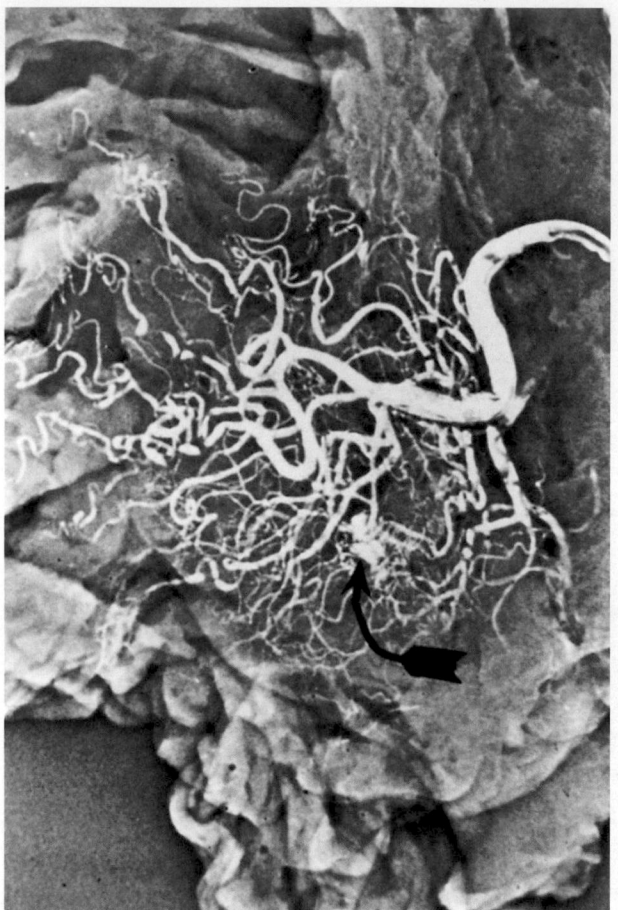

FIGURE 28-17. Angiodysplastic lesion (*arrow*) in an injected specimen following resection for cecal arteriovenous malformation.

the extravasation occurs over a number of days. Retention of this blood-pool radiotracer in the vascular compartment permits this possibility (Figures 28-20 and 28-21). The disadvantage, of course, is that the radioactivity persists for a relatively long time. But the technique can be successful in detecting the presence of continuing hemorrhage, with transfusion requirements as little as 500 mL within 24 hours or 0.05 to 0.1 mL/minute.[393]

Bunker and colleagues, in their initial study, confirmed the site of bleeding in 10 of 11 patients by this method.[69] A later report of 100 individuals demonstrated clear superiority of ^{99m}Tc red blood cells over that of ^{99m}Tc sulfur colloid, with a sensitivity of 93%, a specificity of 95%, and an overall accuracy of 94% in detecting and localizing GI hemorrhage.[70] In 32 patients with documented hemorrhage reported by Winzelberg and colleagues, 29 had positive scintiscans (sensitivity, 91%; 5% false negatives).[392] The data of others support the concept of increasing application.[252] Baum has suggested that as radionuclide scans are more widely employed, angiography will eventually be performed only in those patients with positive scans.[37] Conversely, Bentley and Richardson noted that tagged scans accurately localized the site of bleeding in only 52% of cases and offered the opinion that it is a poor technique for identifying the source.[43] They further questioned its use as a screening tool before angiography. Others also have expressed concern about the scan's ability to accurately localize the site of bleeding. Hunter and Pezim found that performing a surgical procedure that relies exclusively on this technique for localization will "produce an undesirable result in at least 42% of patients."[172] More recent studies have demonstrated accuracy rates between 35% and 100%, with an average of 66%.[64,94,153,200,206,259,403] When a positive result was found, the location of bleeding was confirmed by angiogram,

STANLEY BAUM (1929–PRESENT)

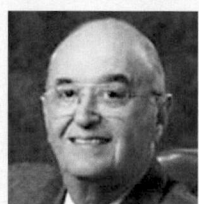

Stanley Baum was born in New York City, December 26, 1929. He received his medical degree in 1957 from the Faculty of Medicine at the University of Utrecht in Holland and completed an internship at Kings County Hospital Medical Center in New York City and a radiology residency at the University of Pennsylvania in Philadelphia. He became a National Cancer Institute trainee before completing a fellowship in cardiovascular radiology at Stanford University Medical Center. Following a brief time on the faculty at Stanford, he returned to the University of Pennsylvania and advanced to the rank of professor of radiology. In 1971, he moved to Harvard as professor of radiology and chief of cardiovascular radiology at Massachusetts General Hospital. In 1975, he returned to the University of Pennsylvania as professor and chairman of the Department of Radiology. Baum held that post for more than 20 years, during which time he became the Eugene P. Pendergrass Professor of Radiology. He contributed to early MRI development and made a significant impact on angiography by describing the roles of vasoconstrictors in controlling gastrointestinal hemorrhage and of angiography in assessing vascular bleeding. He was one of the first interventional radiologists in the United States and was the founder and first president of the Society of Cardiovascular and Interventional Radiology. He was also one of the first diagnostic radiologists elected to the Institute of Medicine. Despite these monumental achievements, some of Baum's most important work came after he stepped down as chairman. He was a founding member of the Academy of Radiology Research (ARR) and was ARR president when the bill to establish the National Institute of Biomedical Imaging and Bioengineering was introduced in the U.S. Senate. Among his numerous awards and honors are the Cannon Medal from the Society of Gastrointestinal Radiologists, and gold medals from the Association of University Radiologists, American Roentgen Ray Society, and Society of Cardiovascular and Interventional Radiology. In 2002, the University of Pennsylvania established the Stanley Baum Professorship in the Department of Radiology. (With appreciation to Arie Pelta, MD.)

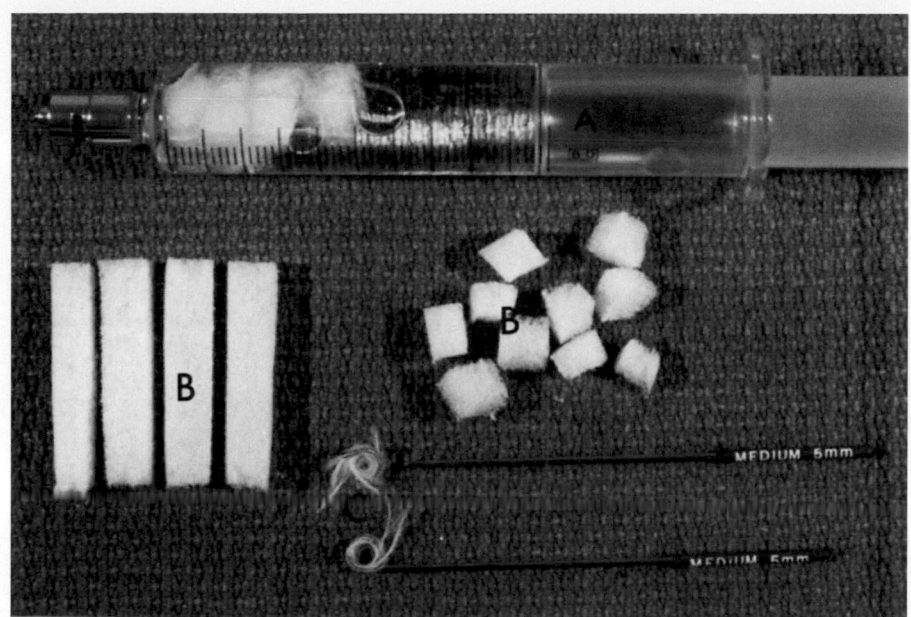

FIGURE 28-18. Thromboembolic devices. A: Syringe with Gelfoam. B: Gelfoam. C: Gianturco coils for occluding medium-sized vessels. (Courtesy of John G. Mardiat, MD.)

colonoscopy, or surgery. Improved sensitivity in localization is seen if scans are positive within 2 hours of injection.[110]

The role of nuclear scintigraphy in the workup of the bleeding patient is still controversial. Tagged red blood cell scans are very sensitive at identifying the presence of bleeding but are not reliable for accurate localization. Although the scans are safe, they provide no ability to intervene and play a purely diagnostic role. There are authors who have advocated its use as a screening tool before angiography in order to confirm active bleeding prior to subjecting a patient to the risks of angiography. Gunderman and associates demonstrated an increased yield for angiography (from 22% to 53%) when patients were previously screened with a tagged red blood cell scan.[150] However, this observation has not been born out in other studies.[43,379] Some interventional radiologists claim the tagged blood scan helps one to localize the angiogram and decreases contrast load. Indeed, in some centers it may be difficult to obtain an angiogram without a prior tagged red blood cell scan. Moreover, there is some debate about using nuclear scintigraphy as an isolated test in order to allow a segmental colectomy in an actively bleeding patient. Suzman and coworkers examined 224 patients who underwent tagged red blood cell bleeding scans over a 5-year period.[350] Fifty-one percent had positive scans, with 42.9% localizing to a specific segment. Fifty patients required surgery, and of those, 38 had undergone scintigraphy, 37 of whom were accurately localized. No patients who underwent segmental resection rebled, but many underwent preoperative localization with another technique, most commonly colonoscopy. Only 18% of the patients in this study underwent angiography, but angiography did not improve localization.

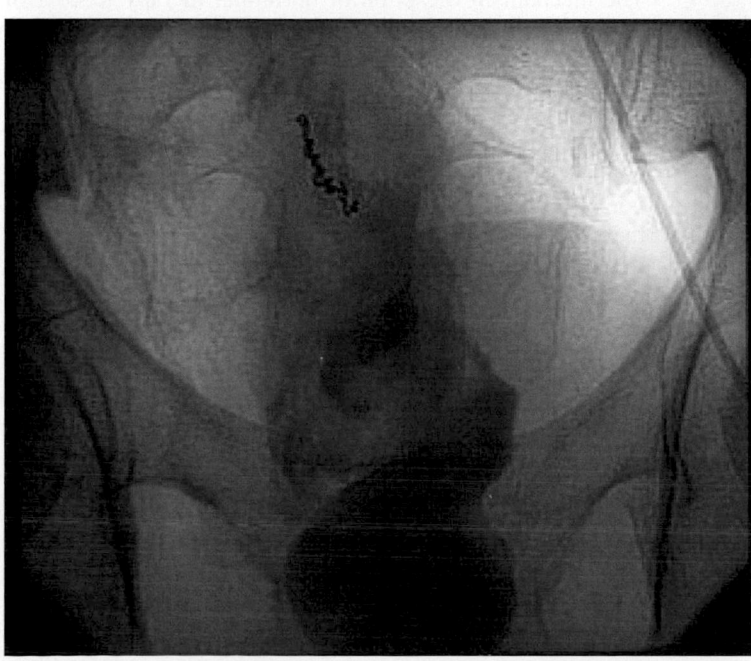

FIGURE 28-19. Embolization with Gianturco coil. Note the position of the coil in the upper pelvis.

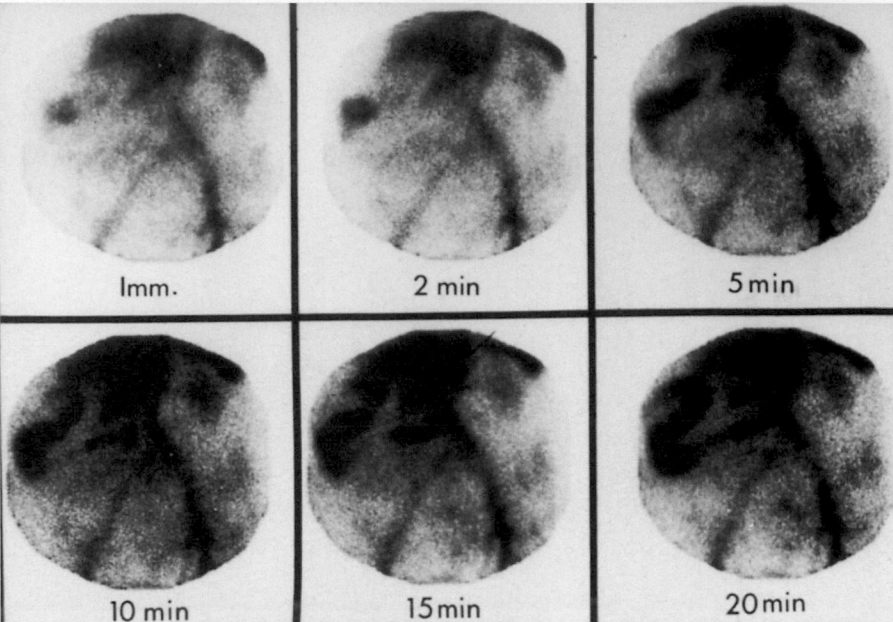

FIGURE 28-20. Scintiscan with ^{99m}Tc-labeled red blood cells. The bleeding site in the ascending colon is seen shortly following injection. The uptake from that site increases in intensity and moves along the bowel. Hemorrhage originated in the hepatic flexure. (Courtesy of Kenneth A. McKusick, MD.)

Opinion

There is no clear consensus at this time, but the overall accuracy rate of nuclear scintigraphy in the literature (66%) makes one wary of performing a limited resection without undertaking other preoperative tests. At this time, radionucleotide scintigraphy should be used as a screening test prior to angiography or applied to those patients where localization has not been possible in an individual with persistent or recurrent bleeding.

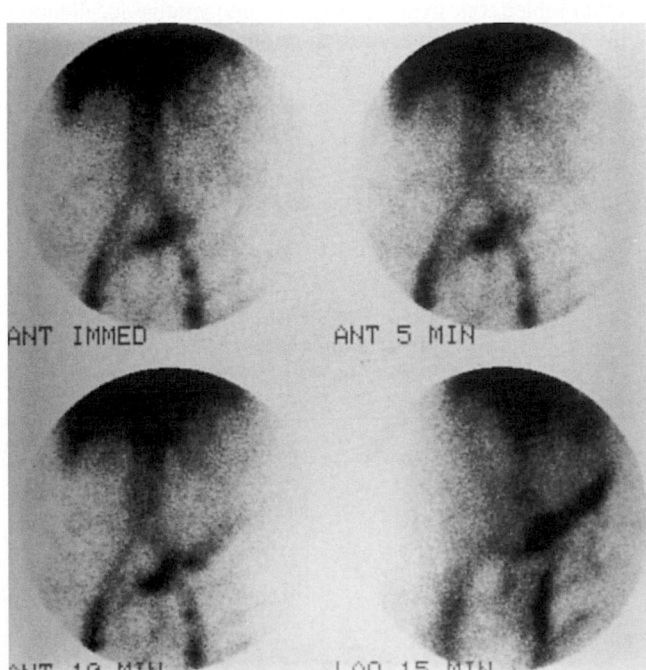

FIGURE 28-21. Labeled red blood cell study reveals prompt extravascular site of bleeding localized just below the bifurcation of the aorta. This is seen to progress transversely to the left upper quadrant. Later views showed the tracer to move down along the left side. This was interpreted to be bleeding that originated in the mid-transverse colon.

I concur that ^{99m}Tc-labeled red blood cell scintigraphy is of primary benefit in directing the patient's diagnostic rather than therapeutic management.[250]

Treatment

As implied from the foregoing, if the bleeding point is identified by means of angiography, tagged red blood cell scan, endoscopy, or barium enema examination, appropriate therapy can be instituted: medical management, a local procedure, or resection, depending on the nature of the lesion and the patient's clinical course.

Estrogen–Progesterone Therapy

A number of papers have appeared that indicate estrogen–progesterone therapy may be effective in controlling severe, recurrent bleeding from GI vascular malformations.[143,244,290,370] The mechanism of action of hormonal therapy to control bleeding with this condition is not clearly understood. Theories include an effect on coagulation, induction of stasis in the mesenteric microcirculation, and improvement in the integrity of the vascular endothelial lining.[244] Side effects are of some concern and include thromboembolic disease, an increased risk for the development of malignancies, nausea, vomiting, loss of libido, and gynecomastia. Still, hormonal therapy should be considered in situations when prolonged, obscure GI bleeding thought to be due to angiodysplasia cannot adequately be managed by other means.[244]

Richardson and Lordon present the typical patient who may be a candidate for this approach.[290] They describe three individuals with chronic renal failure who had GI bleeding caused by angiodysplasia that responded to this treatment.

Obscure Bleeding

Thomas suggests the use of the expression "obscure bleeding" to describe the following situations:

- The cause exists but has been difficult to diagnose or has been overlooked.
- Bleeding results from multisystem disease.
- Investigations have failed to localize the site of hemorrhage.[361]

The reality is, however, that it is only through an organized, algorithmic approach that one may hope to identify and treat the source of GI bleeding. The small bowel, in particular, has been the most difficult area to assess, an area of special concern in an individual with obscure bleeding or bleeding from an unknown source. In the elective situation, a small bowel series, enteroclysis, or capsule endoscopy imaging (see Chapter 5) must be considered.

Obscure bleeding is approached through a variety of new techniques. Most of these patients have already undergone multiple esophagogastroduodenoscopies and colonoscopies. Both tagged red blood cell scans and angiography should be performed, but these are the patients where localization is not possible. Push enteroscopy, video capsule endoscopy, and double-balloon endoscopy are all viable options to help isolate the bleeding source prior to surgery.

Push Enteroscopy. Push enteroscopy refers to the passage of an endoscope into the jejunum via an oral approach without the use of balloons to help advance the scope. Reported success in identifying a source of bleeding in obscure instances ranges from 24% to 56%.[39,227,323] The yield is higher (41% vs. 26%) if there is an active bleeding at the time of the procedure.[196]

Capsule Endoscopy (see also Chapter 5). Capsule endoscopy uses a video capsule to identify lesions within the small intestine. It is diagnostic, not therapeutic. Triester and associates performed a meta-analysis examining the accuracy of capsule endoscopy as compared with other diagnostic techniques.[365] They found capsule endoscopy identified potential bleeding sources at a higher rate than other modalities (23% to 67% yields). If positive findings are identified on video capsule endoscopy, referral for intervention with either surgical resection or double-balloon endoscopy is warranted.

Double-Balloon Endoscopy. Double-balloon endoscopy uses either a single- or double-balloon system in order to pass an enteroscope through the small intestine. It can be performed via either antegrade or retrograde approach. It allows not only for diagnosis but also for therapeutic intervention when lesions are identified. This may include injection, electrocauterization, or clipping. Tattooing marks the areas in the small intestine for possible future surgical resection. The reported positive yield rates for the procedure vary from 43% to 81%, with a similar percentage range of patients having a successful intervention for the bleeding site.[76,232,247,400,401] The procedure appears to be safe, with a minimal complication rate. Zhong and colleagues reported 378 patients who underwent double-balloon endoscopy over 2 years. The most common side effect was mild-to-moderate discomfort, and no perforations occurred. The authors preferentially performed the procedure with conscious sedation, but general anesthesia was used for 42 individuals.

Operative Management

Resection

What is the proper treatment if the patient continues to bleed and the source has not been identified? In the past, individuals were submitted to exploratory laparotomy in the hope that a lesion could be found at the operating table. Multiple enterotomies were undertaken to identify the proximal limit of the bleeding and to perform operative colonoscopy. In someone at high risk, such a prolonged operative procedure exposes the patient to increased mortality as well as to the possibility of

additional morbidity from infection. Alternatively, blind left colectomy has historically been advocated, and later, right colectomy. Most surgeons today, however, believe that subtotal colectomy is the preferred procedure when the source of bleeding has not been identified preoperatively or intraoperatively.

Operative Colonoscopy and Enteroscopy

Another option for operatively identifying the source of bleeding involves a combination of laparotomy and colonoscopy through the application of a two-team approach.[44] A rapid, intraoperative cleansing of the bowel may be effected through a small cecostomy if this is felt advisable.[321] This is analogous to the technique of on-table lavage (see Chapter 23). The abdominal surgeon can assist the colonoscopist in the passage of the instrument to make one final attempt to identify a discrete bleeding point.[376] If one is seen, it may be dealt with through the instrument or it may be effectively treated by a less than total abdominal colectomy.

Intraoperative enteroscopy can be accomplished with the colonoscope passed per orum, guiding the instrument through the duodenum and into the small bowel. Segmental visualization can be accomplished, occluding the bowel at intervals to avoid overdistention.[102] The endoscopic appearance can be supplemented by simultaneous viewing from the serosal aspect of the transilluminated bowel.

Desa and colleagues identified the source in 10 of 12 cases of obscure bleeding by the method of operative enteroscopy.[102] These individuals had previously undergone multiple surgical procedures as well as the usual specialized testing. Flickinger and associates found that this technique influenced the operation in 93% of cases.[120] When an angiodysplastic lesion is identified, one can treat it by electrocoagulation, laser photoablation, or suturing.[1]

Operative Arteriography

Intraoperative localization of vascular ectasias may be accomplished by placing the bowel to be examined on a sterile cassette cover.[294] The segmental arterial branch feeding the area is isolated and injected with methylglucamine diatrizoate (Renografin 76). With the bowel exhibiting pallor and contracting, the film is exposed to identify the lesion. I have had no experience with this technique but would consider its applicability only for small bowel lesions. This method, though, has the potential advantage of a therapeutic option.

McDonald and associates described the use of highly selective angiographic catheter placement combined with intraoperative methylene blue dye injection to precisely identify the source of hemorrhage in three patients who had a small bowel source of bleeding confirmed.[229] At operation, 0.5 mL of methylene blue dye (50 mg/mL) was injected into the catheter, which resulted in immediate demarcation of the small intestine over a length of approximately 20 cm with a brilliant blue color. This enabled the surgeons to resect a limited amount of small intestine.

Results of Surgery

Smith and colleagues identified 24 patients with lower GI hemorrhage due to angiodysplasia, 17 of whom required surgery.[335] With the bleeding point found preoperatively, no patient rebled following either a limited resection or a subtotal colectomy. But coagulopathy, specifically platelet disorders, contributed to a high mortality rate. Boley and Brandt accept a 20% rebleeding rate after right hemicolectomy for angiographically demonstrated ectasias and believe that the risk of subtotal colectomy is greater than the risk of rebleeding.[50] Bender and colleagues reported a mortality of 27% following total colectomy and opined that the procedure under these circumstances is associated with excessive morbidity and mortality.[42] Whether this is a valid criticism of the surgery or a reflection of multiple blood transfusions, age, and other factors was not analyzed. Irrespective of the type of surgery, Leitman and associates found that those who failed transcatheter treatment had a mortality of 36%.[202] Parkes and coworkers reviewed the records of 31 patients who underwent colon resection to determine the most effective surgical treatment for massive lower GI bleeding.[268] The rebleeding rate for subtotal colectomy with a mean follow-up of 1 year was nil. With a segmental resection, even with a positive angiogram, the rebleeding rate was 14%, and if the angiogram was negative, a segmental resection was associated with a rebleeding rate of 42%. This last group of patients had the highest complication rate in the series (83%). This same group of patients also had an extremely high mortality rate (57%).

Comment

Fortunately, with the diagnostic studies available, the surgeon should rarely have to resort to blind resection. It is axiomatic that if a lesion is clearly demonstrated on angiography and cannot be controlled by minimally invasive means, a limited resection is appropriate. However, if there is not complete certainty about the source of the bleeding, the few minutes necessary to remove the remainder of the bowel should add very little risk. Furthermore, in the absence of blood in the small bowel, the maneuvers associated with operative colonoscopy and operative angiography truly prolong the surgical time with its attendant risks and have the potential hazards of contamination with the former technique and toxicity with the latter. Finally, ensuring proper examination of the anus and rectum prior to subtotal colectomy is essential in order to definitively determine that the bleeding site is not within this area.

► MESENTERIC OCCLUSIVE AND NONOCCLUSIVE DISEASE

The gut receives 20% of resting and 35% of postprandial cardiac output, of which 70% supplies the mucosa.[55] In the fasting state, only one in five mesenteric capillaries is open. The bowel, as one can see, has therefore a remarkably resistant ability to withstand ischemia.[55] However, if the blood pressure falls below 70 mm Hg, intestinal perfusion may be compromised. Below 40 mm Hg this mechanism fails, and the bowel becomes progressively more ischemic, with anaerobic metabolism replacing aerobic.[55] The nature and rapidity of the ischemic process are affected by the collateral circulation and by disorders of splanchnic autoregulation.

Major occlusive disease is usually caused by mesenteric vascular obstruction as a consequence of atheroma, thrombus, or embolus. Other etiologies include dissecting aneurysm, arteritis, sepsis, intestinal obstruction, and trauma. Acute mesenteric ischemia usually occurs in patients older than 50 years of age, particularly in those with arteriosclerotic heart disease or valvular involvement.[51] The characteristic person is an elderly man with prior heart disease and symptoms related to peripheral atherosclerosis.[333] Hypercoagulable conditions and the use of oral contraceptives may also precipitate intestinal vascular thromboses, often involving the venous circulation. Other factors that predispose to ischemia include long-standing congestive heart failure, the prolonged use of diuretics, cardiac arrhythmias, recent myocardial infarction, hypovolemia,

hypotension, burns, pancreatitis, and GI hemorrhage.[51,52] Most patients, in fact, who develop ischemic changes of the small and large bowel do not have a demonstrably significant vascular lesion but have so-called nonocclusive vascular disease. Debus and colleagues classify acute mesenteric events into four categories[98]: T acute mesenteric embolus (50% of cases), acute mesenteric thrombus (25%), nonocclusive disease (20%), and mesenteric vein thrombosis (less than 10%).[36]

Signs and Symptoms

The most frequent symptoms of mesenteric occlusion are abdominal pain and rectal bleeding (up to 98%). An early characteristic feature is the disparity between the severity of the pain and the paucity of significant abdominal findings.[51] In other words, the pain is generally out of proportion to the physical findings. Signs and symptoms of peritonitis rapidly ensue in the presence of intestinal infarction. Hypothermia is not uncommonly observed.[333] Other complaints include back pain, nausea, vomiting, and diarrhea. In patients with so-called abdominal angina, abdominal pain is also evident, usually developing 15 to 20 minutes following the ingestion of food.[124] Pain is characteristically epigastric or periumbilical, and weight loss and malnutrition may ensue.

Laboratory and Radiologic Studies

Laboratory investigations usually reveal an elevated white blood cell count and evidence of hemoconcentration—nonspecific abnormalities to be sure, but consistent with the diagnosis of mesenteric ischemia. Metabolic acidosis frequently is noted in patients with intestinal infarction. This is due to tissue hypoxia, persistent hypotension, and the release of vasoactive materials. Determination of arterial blood gases confirms the base deficit and should serve to alert the physician as to the severity of the illness. Plain films of the abdomen may demonstrate thickened bowel loops; a ground-glass appearance from ascites; the classic "thumbprinting"; and gas in the bowel wall, portal vein, or peritoneal cavity (Figure 28-22). However, one-fourth of

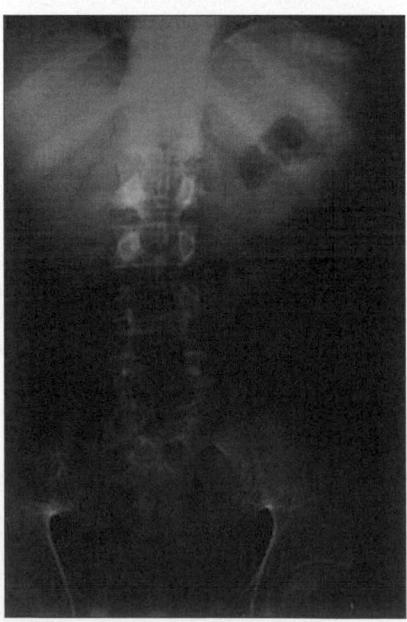

FIGURE 28-22. Plain film of the abdomen. Note thickened and ulcerated transverse colon, ground glass appearance from ascites, and "thumbprinting."

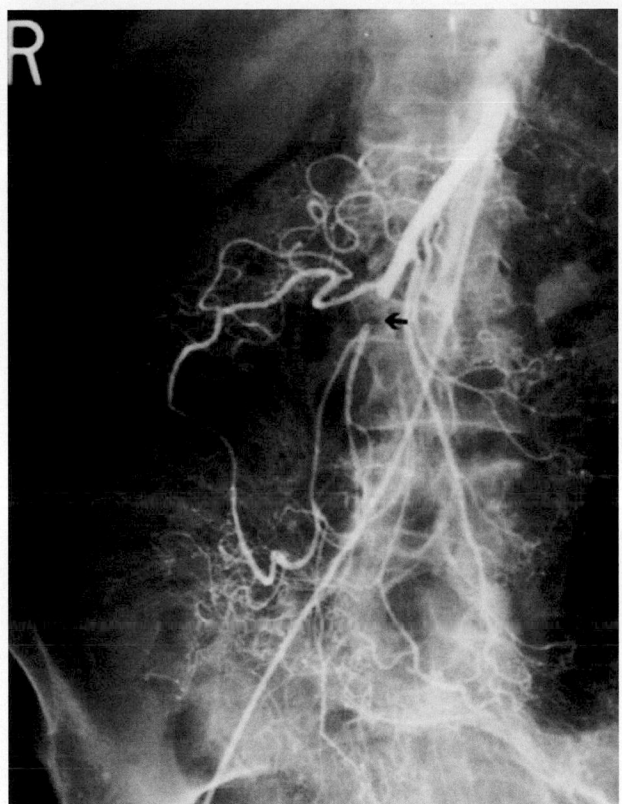

FIGURE 28-23. Superior mesenteric artery embolism (*arrow*). Note the collateral circulation through the meandering vessel.

patients with mesenteric infarction have a normal plain film of the abdomen.

Although a wide range of investigations is available for the assessment of mesenteric ischemia, with the exception of angiography and computed tomography (CT), none is particularly helpful.[55] With the widespread utilization and advances in multidetector computed tomography (MDCT) in conjunction with CT angiography, MDCT with angiography has replaced standard angiography as the procedure of choice for diagnosing mesenteric ischemia.[27,126,169] The sensitivity of detecting bowel ischemia with MDCT has reached 82%.[190]

Findings on CT scan consistent with mesenteric ischemia include bowel wall thickening, intestinal attenuation and enhancement, dilatation, pneumatosis, portal vein gas, and fat stranding and ascites.[380] All of these findings are relatively nonspecific with the exception of portal vein gas. The vascular findings on CT include abrupt termination of a vessel from embolic obstruction of an artery (Figure 28-23). Proximal obstruction is often required for adequate visualization. Venous thrombosis manifests visually as rounded or tubular low-attenuation focus of thrombus, with increased vein caliber in the affected vein.

Evaluation and Treatment Protocol

The clinical pathway for patients with suspected mesenteric ischemia is dependent on the presence of peritonitis on physical exam. Peritonitis with signs of severe sepsis requires immediate laparotomy. If the patient is stable, but he or she has peritonitis, consideration for CT angiography should be given because the results may help guide the planned operation. Irrespective of the findings of the CT scan, however,

one should proceed to the operating room. If ischemia is suspected but no signs of peritonitis are present, then CT angiography followed by either laparotomy or interventional angiography (depending on findings) should be performed.

If dead bowel is encountered in the operating room, the amount of intestine that should be removed is always a subject of concern. Visual appreciation of bowel injury based on capillary bleeding, color, and contractility is often misleading and commonly induces the surgeon to remove more than is necessary.[68] A number of investigators have compared clinical judgment with other methods of determining intestinal viability. Clinical judgment was associated with a relatively high sensitivity, specificity, and overall accuracy, but had a low predictive value.[316] Bowel was incorrectly assessed to be nonviable in 46% of patients in one series, leading to sacrificing more bowel than necessary. In an experimental study, Brolin and colleagues compared five methods for assessing intestinal viability: threshold stimulus level (TSL), the minimal electrical current necessary to produce a smooth muscle contractile response; intestinal color; peristalsis; Doppler ultrasound; and histologically evaluated resection margin.[60] The bowel color, the presence of peristalsis, and the histologic findings failed to correlate with the intestinal survival rate. Conversely, blood flow measured by Doppler ultrasound and the myoelectric parameters established through an electronic contractility meter were directly related to viability. Bulkley and coworkers compared clinical judgment at the time of the operation with Doppler ultrasound and with the use of fluorescein to determine bowel viability in a prospective, controlled study of patients with intestinal ischemia.[60] The fluorescein method was shown to be superior to the Doppler method.

Another option at the time of initial exploration is to resect frankly gangrenous intestine, leaving the questionable bowel in place with planned re-exploration, or second look procedure in 24 to 48 hours (Figure 28-24). Fluorescein may then be used to help determine viability, depending on the appearance of the intestine. An algorithm for the management of mesenteric ischemia is illustrated in Figure 28-25.

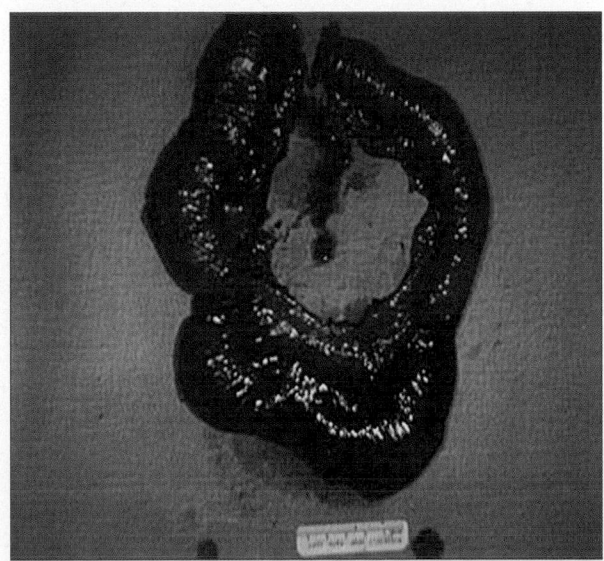

FIGURE 28-24. A resected segment of small bowel showing infarction from prolonged hypotension due to nonocclusive vascular disease. (Courtesy of Rudolf Garret, MD.)

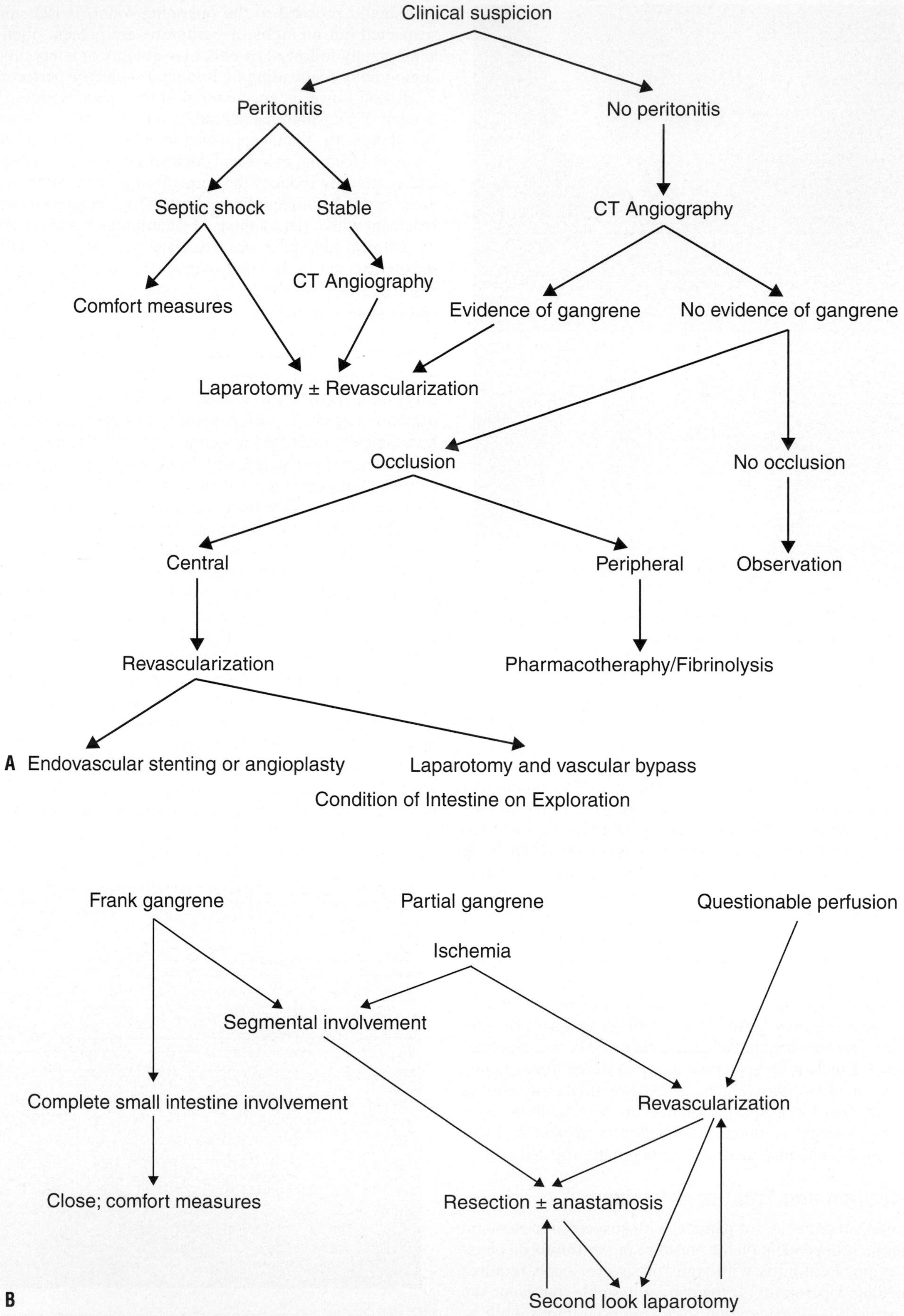

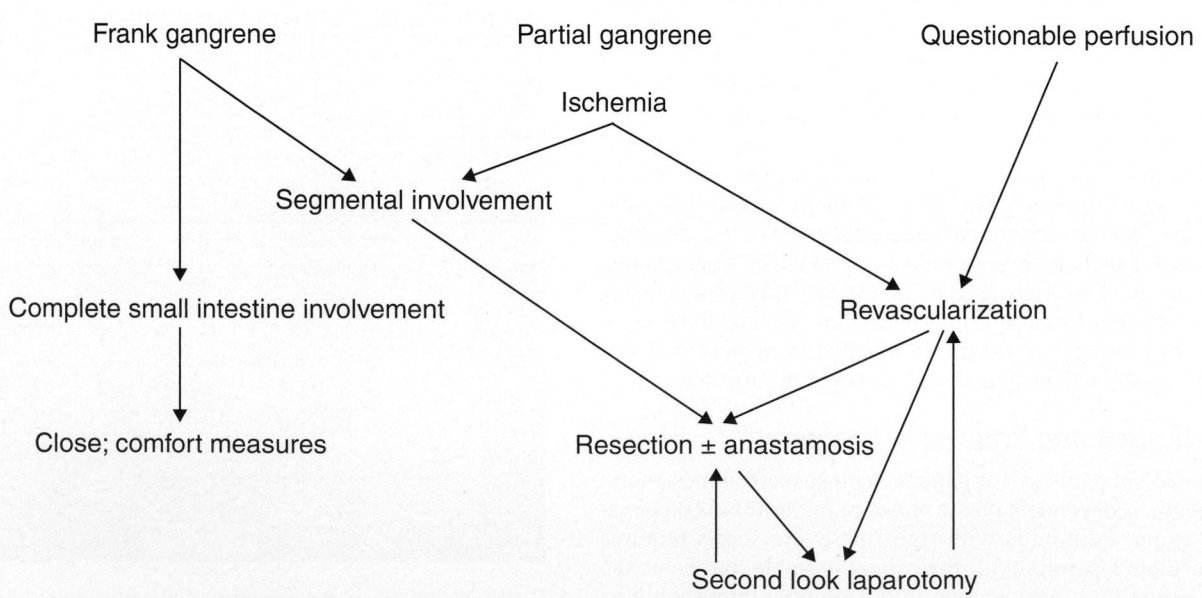

FIGURE 28-25. **A:** Algorithm for the diagnosis and initial management of acute mesenteric ischemia. **B:** Algorithm for the intraoperative management of acute mesenteric ischemia. (Adapted from Debus ES, Müller-Hülsbeck S, Kölbel T, et al. Intestinal ischemia. *Int J Colorect Dis.* 2011;26(9):1087–1097. doi:10.1007/s00384-011-1196-6.)

Results

Boley and colleagues reported their experience with 47 patients with intestinal ischemia due to superior mesenteric artery emboli.[52] The overall mortality was 66%. Those with infarction of more than 50% of the small intestine did especially poorly (17 of 19 such patients died). A survival rate of 55% was obtained in patients managed according to the preceding protocol, whereas only 20% of those treated by traditional methods survived. The best results were obtained in patients who were diagnosed within 24 hours of the onset of pain.

Clavien and colleagues reported their experience of 81 individuals with mesenteric infarction documented by angiography.[85] Almost one-half were felt to have an inoperable situation and were treated by supportive care only. Of those who underwent a laparotomy, 45% survived. Because of the high frequency of progressive infarction following resection (32%), the authors recommend preoperative perfusion of the superior mesenteric artery with vasodilators and postoperative anticoagulation. Sitges-Serra and coworkers identified 44 individuals who underwent massive small bowel resection (mean length of remaining bowel, 60 cm), noting a 46% mortality.[333] Levy and associates reported an overall mortality in 62 surgically treated patients of 40%.[205] They emphasize the importance of establishing double stomas whenever the viability of the remaining bowel is equivocal. Endean and coworkers assessed the University of Kentucky experience in 170 patients with acute intestinal ischemia.[114] Nonthrombotic patients represented 60%; thrombotic, 34%; and indeterminate, 6%. The survival rate for arterial embolism was 41% and for thrombosis, 38%. These results are indicative of an improvement when compared with earlier reports.

Park and colleagues examined the Mayo Clinic experience in 58 patients. Most presented with pain, and all patients underwent laparotomy. Forty-seven underwent revascularization, and 23 had second-look procedures. Thirty-one patients received a bowel resection at the first laparotomy, with 11 patients requiring further resections at the second exploration. Their 30-day mortality was 32%, with patients having nonocclusive mesenteric ischemia having a significantly higher mortality rate (80%). Only an age less than 60 years and a bowel resection were associated with improved survival.[267]

Schoots and associates analyzed the published data on survival following mesenteric ischemia over the past four decades.[317] Forty-five observational studies contained 3,692 patients. They offered the following conclusions:

- Prognosis with acute mesenteric venous occlusion is better (see later).
- Prognosis after mesenteric artery embolism is better than following thrombosis or nonocclusive ischemia.
- The mortality rate following surgical treatment of arterial embolism and venous thrombosis (54% and 32%, respectively) is less than that after surgery for arterial thrombosis and nonocclusive ischemia (77% and 73%, respectively).
- The overall survival has improved during this time.

Venous Mesenteric Ischemia

Venous thrombosis is a rare cause of mesenteric infarction, but the diagnosis is notoriously difficult to make because of the vague presenting signs and symptoms. It accounts for 3% to 15% of all cases of acute mesenteric ischemia.[162] Causes may be primary, such as those conditions that increase viscosity of the blood or its tendency to coagulate (e.g., splenectomy, polycythemia rubra vera, sickle cell disease, platelet disorders, myeloproliferative disease, the use of contraceptive pills, pregnancy, carcinomatosis).[55] A new disease entity—idiopathic mesenteric phlebosclerosis (i.e., nonthrombotic stenosis or occlusion of the mesenteric veins)—has been described.[176] Secondary causes (60%) include portal hypertension, intra-abdominal sepsis, pancreatitis, intra-abdominal neoplasms, inflammatory bowel disease, abdominal trauma, and various gastroenteritides. The condition is usually confined to a limited segment of the bowel and therefore carries with it a better prognosis than that of arterial occlusive or nonocclusive disease. Clavien and colleagues used contrast-enhanced CT to identify a triad of findings in this condition: hypodensity in the trunk of the superior mesenteric vein, thickening of the intestinal wall and valvulae conniventes localized in a jejunoileal segment, and considerable peritoneal fluid.[84] CT scan with IV contrast is the preferred diagnostic test for mesenteric venous thrombosis.[162]

Optimal treatment in those patients with reversible damage is anticoagulation. In those with evidence of gangrene or peritonitis, exploration with resection of gangrenous bowel is required. Intravenous heparin should be administered prior to the operation if the diagnosis is known or in the operating room immediately upon making the diagnosis. In a large retrospective review of 3,700 patients who were treated for mesenteric ischemia, mesenteric venous thrombosis patients were found to have a mortality rate of 44%, as compared with 66% to 89% for those with arterial occlusion.[317] Short-term mortality rates are correlated with the presence or absence of intestinal infarction. The key to a successful outcome involves a high index of suspicion and early diagnosis, and then timely management with anticoagulation.

▶ ISCHEMIC COLITIS

Ischemic colitis is a term coined by Marston and associates to describe a syndrome due to occlusive or nonocclusive vascular disease as it affects the large bowel.[225] It is a very common disorder, being the most common form of intestinal ischemia and responsible for 1 in 2,000 patient admissions.[113] It is a condition that usually is found in the aging population, with an increased incidence in women,[269] although the disease has been associated with hemorrhagic shock even in young patients.[72] Abel and Russell reported that approximately 60% were 70 years of age or older; 78% were women.[3] Ischemic colitis can be a consequence of various resective procedures on the bowel, of operations performed on the aorta (see later), and of embolization for the treatment of colonic hemorrhage.[297] A number of conditions, some of which are included within this chapter, produce their pathologic manifestations at least, in part, on an ischemic basis. These include arteriosclerosis, emboli, myocardial infarction, vasculitis, colorectal neoplasms, portal hypertension, strangulated hernia, volvulus, diabetes mellitus, hypertension, chronic renal failure, periarteritis nodosa, systemic lupus erythematosus, rheumatoid arthritis, polycythemia vera, scleroderma, hemodialysis, anaphylactoid shock, strict dieting, methamphetamine abuse, and many others.[44,51,108,299,327,364] Frequent hypotensive episodes in response to fluid removal and an associated low-flow state are probably responsible for this complication in individuals undergoing hemodialysis.[177] In the experience of Longo and colleagues, ischemic colitis commonly occurred during an unrelated hospital admission and following surgery.[209]

The blood supply to the colon is contributed through the meandering artery or anastomosis of Riolan (the vascular communication between the superior and inferior mesenteric arteries; see Chapter 1 and Biography). The reduction of splanchnic blood flow through this vessel appears to have its greatest vulnerability in two watershed areas: Sudeck's* point and Griffiths'† point (see Chapter 1 and Biography).[146,348] However, a number of factors, such as large and small vessel arterial disease, perfusion pressure, plasma viscosity, and adequacy of collateral circulation, may combine to produce even total colonic ischemia.[385] Although these focal points of ischemia are important anatomic landmarks, Glauser and colleagues reviewed their findings of 49 patients with ischemic colitis who were diagnosed with endoscopy and found the condition equally distributed throughout the colon.[136]

Classification, Symptoms, Findings, and Diagnosis

Ischemic colitis has been classified based on its three general manifestations:

- Gangrenous
- Strictured
- Transient or reversible

In the experience of West and colleagues, of 27 patients who had colonic ischemia, 12 had reversible or transient colitis, and 13 developed a stricture or gangrene that required surgery.[389] The sigmoid colon was the most frequent area of symptomatic stricture.

If gangrene of the colon develops, the patient may complain of severe abdominal pain, nausea, and vomiting. Bowel movements may be absent, or bloody diarrhea may be noted. Passage of a large bowel cast as a consequence of the ischemia has been described.[21] Physical examination will reveal evidence of peritonitis if the bowel is involved by transmural disease, and certainly if there is a perforation. Upright abdominal x-ray may demonstrate free gas under the diaphragm. Flexible endoscopy demonstrates areas of mucosal destruction identified by black necrotic mucosa interspaced with pallid, gray-green, nonperfused mucosa.

The development of an ischemic stricture probably is a consequence of an initial extensive inflammatory process, but not to the point of bowel perforation. This is a very rare manifestation of the ischemic process. Patients may have minimal symptoms, or nausea, vomiting, and abdominal distention may develop. Barium enema may reveal a lesion difficult to distinguish from that of carcinoma (Figure 28-26). According to Brandt and colleagues, approximately one-third

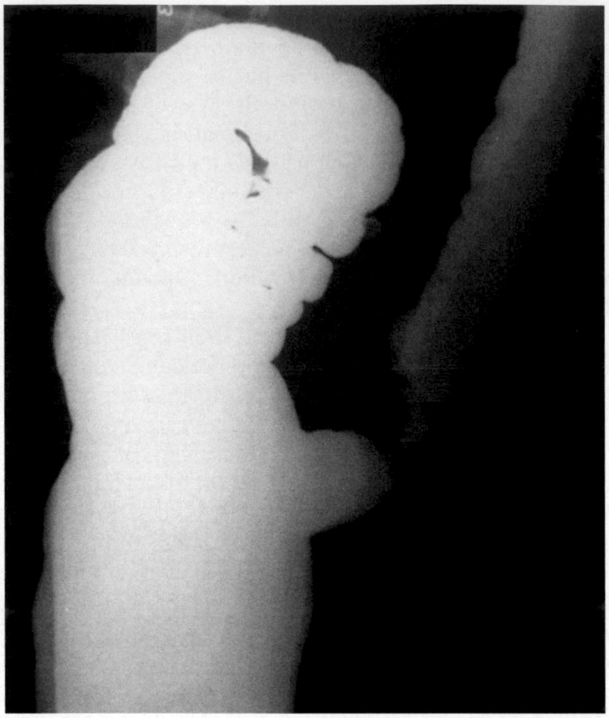

FIGURE 28-26. Ischemic stricture. Barium enema demonstrates profound narrowing at the level of the sigmoid-descending colon junction in an elderly, asymptomatic woman. Intact mucosa suggests a diagnosis other than carcinoma. Biopsy identified only chronic inflammatory cells.

of patients present with a colonic stricture or "chronic colitis."[57] Often, the ischemic nature of the radiologic finding is not readily apparent, although colonoscopy and biopsy will inevitably fail to identify malignant cells. One can consider reevaluation at a later time, but if the patient has a symptomatic stricture and the diagnosis cannot be established with certainty, resection is indicated.

In patients who have reversible or transient ischemic disease, rectal bleeding may be the only complaint. Abdominal pain and tenderness on the left side are usually minimal or may not even be evident. Colonoscopic examination almost always will reveal rectal sparing, with inflammatory changes commencing usually at a level of approximately 15 cm (Figure 28-27). More florid manifestations of inflammatory changes in the mucosa from ischemic colonic disease can be seen in the colonoscopic appearance in Figure 28-27E. It would be essentially impossible to distinguish the changes observed here from those of nonspecific inflammatory bowel disease. The rectum is rarely involved in the ischemic process because of its abundant collateral blood supply,[249] although ischemic proctitis has been reported to be caused by adventitial fibromuscular dysplasia of the superior rectal artery and by myointimal hyperplasia of the mesenteric veins.[283,310] However, if the rectum is involved (see later), serious consideration should be given to another etiology (e.g., ulcerative colitis, antibiotic-associated colitis, or an infectious colitis). It may be very difficult to distinguish the condition from nonspecific inflammatory bowel disease, except that the age of the patient and the history are often helpful. Other endoscopic changes include pallor of the mucosa and hemorrhagic areas. The latter are more likely to be appreciated early in the evolution of the

---

*Sudeck's (critical) point: the region in the colon between the blood supply from the colic artery (i.e., the last sigmoid artery) and that from the superior hemorrhoidal artery.

†Griffiths' point: the potentially vulnerable area in the region of the splenic flexure, which, under some circumstances, may have an inadequate blood supply in the area served by the middle colic artery and the ascending branch of the left colic artery.

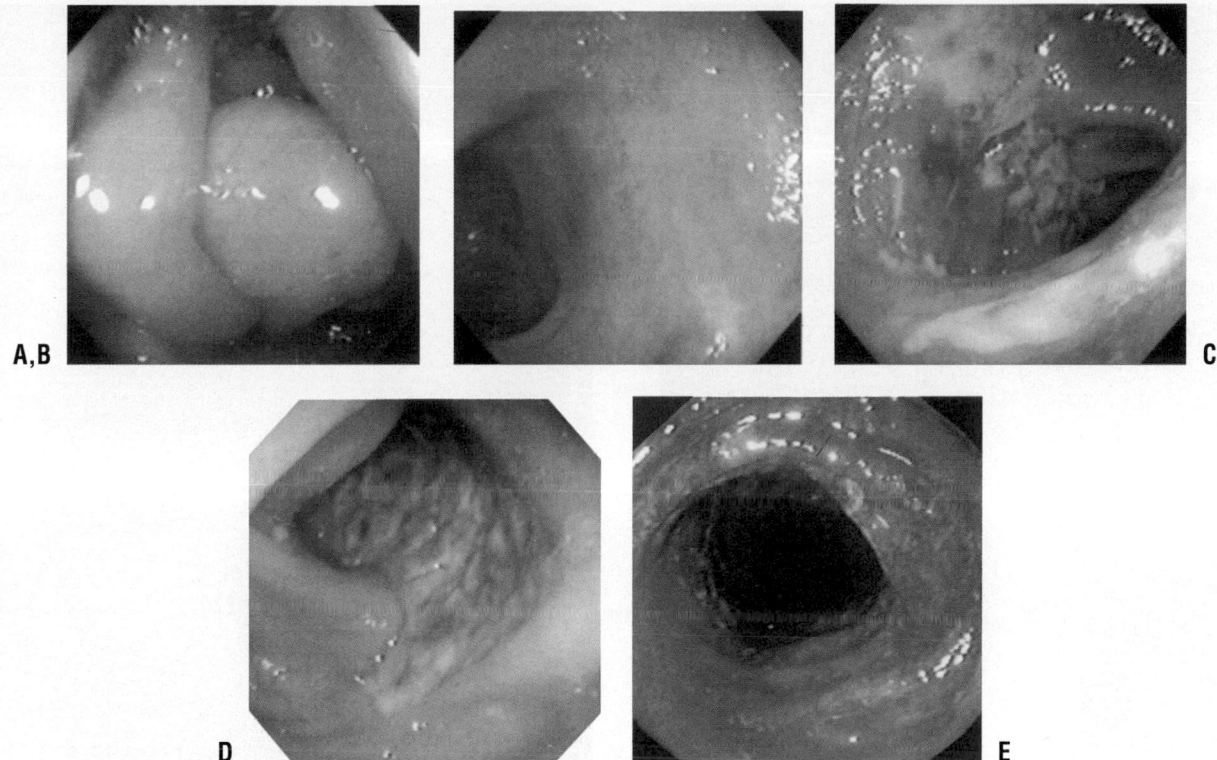

FIGURE 28-27. Colonoscopy reveals all of the characteristic changes of ischemic colitis in the region of the sigmoid colon of the same patient. **A:** Edema. **B:** Hyperemia. **C:** Contact bleeding. **D:** Mucosal pallor and necrosis. **E:** Hemorrhagic, ulcerated mucosa. The condition is difficult to differentiate from inflammatory bowel disease.

inflammatory reaction. Although helpful in distinguishing ischemic colitis from other inflammatory etiologies, the decision to proceed with endoscopy should be made with care. Insufflation and distention may lead to intestinal pressures above 30 mm Hg, further inhibiting colonic blood flow and amplifying the ischemia.[209]

A plain film of the abdomen may reveal characteristic "thumbprinting," usually in the region of the splenic flexure. Depending on the severity of the process, dilated loops of small and large bowel may be seen. In more advanced cases, one may note the presence of gas in the wall of the colon. Barium enema examination characteristically shows thumbprinting, edema of the bowel wall, and narrowing primarily in the areas of the splenic flexure, the distal transverse colon, and the descending colon (Figures 28-28 and 28-29). But with a patient who has a suspected bowel infarction, barium enema is contraindicated (Figure 28-30). An arteriogram may reveal helpful information even if only a flush study of the aorta is carried out (Figure 28-31). Occlusion of one of the major vessels or branches should lead the surgeon to suspect the cause of the patient's symptoms. Because of the risk of worsening ischemia and possible perforation, colonoscopy should be performed to confirm the diagnosis in those patients in whom there is doubt.

Pathologic changes of the colon may reveal disease limited to the mucosa and submucosa (Figure 28-32) because the rich blood supply makes this area more sensitive to ischemic changes. The muscularis propria is relatively resistant to the effects of decreased perfusion, but transmural involvement can occur (Figure 28-33).

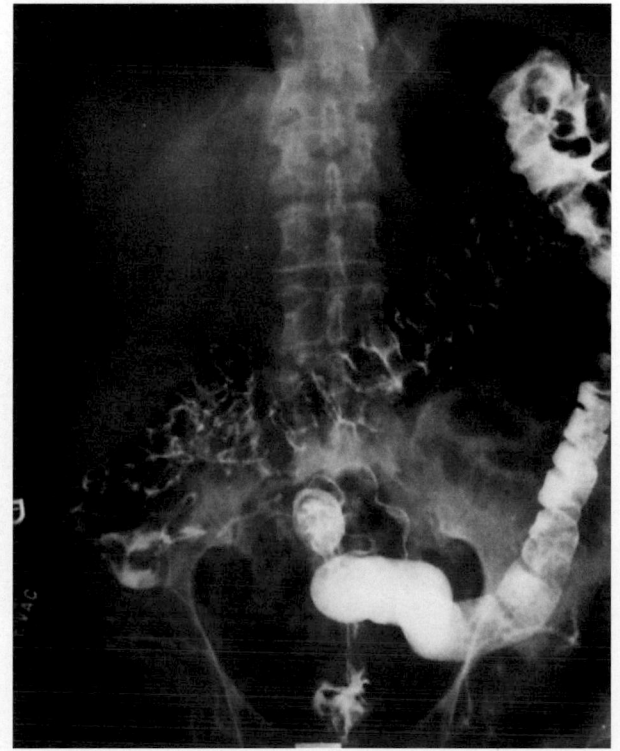

FIGURE 28-28. Ischemic colitis. Postevacuation barium enema showing characteristic thumbprinting from cecum to proximal descending colon.

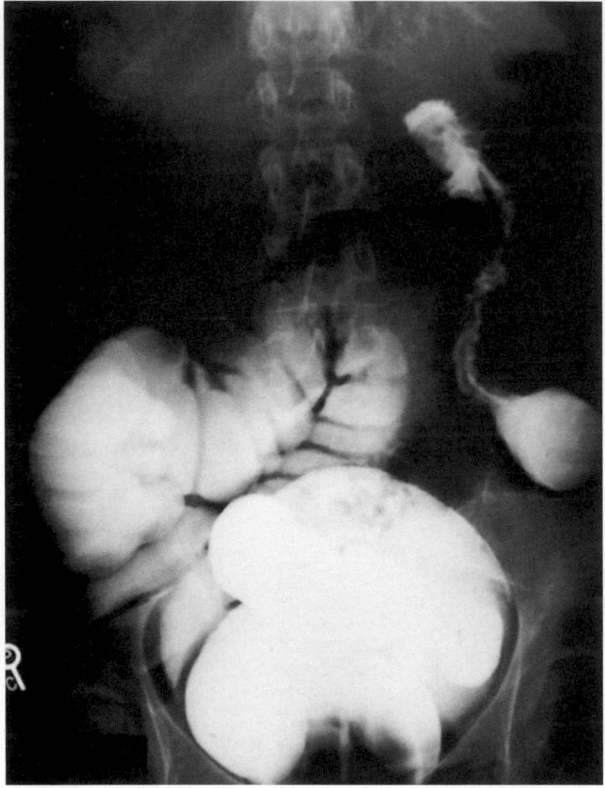

FIGURE 28-29. Ischemic colitis. Barium enema reveals thumbprinting of the splenic flexure and edema and spasm of the descending colon. Note the preservation of mucosa.

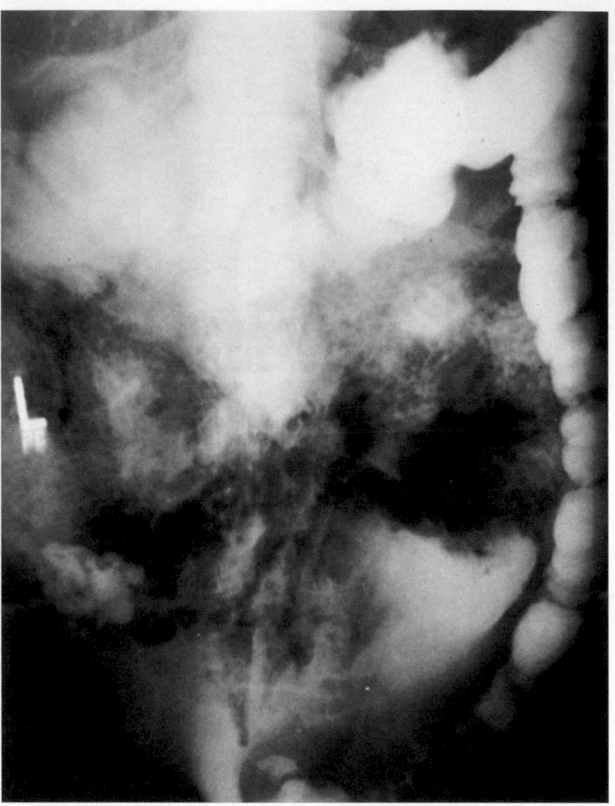

FIGURE 28-30. Ischemic colitis. Transverse colon perforation. Note the extravasation of barium into the peritoneal cavity. (The marker is on the wrong side.)

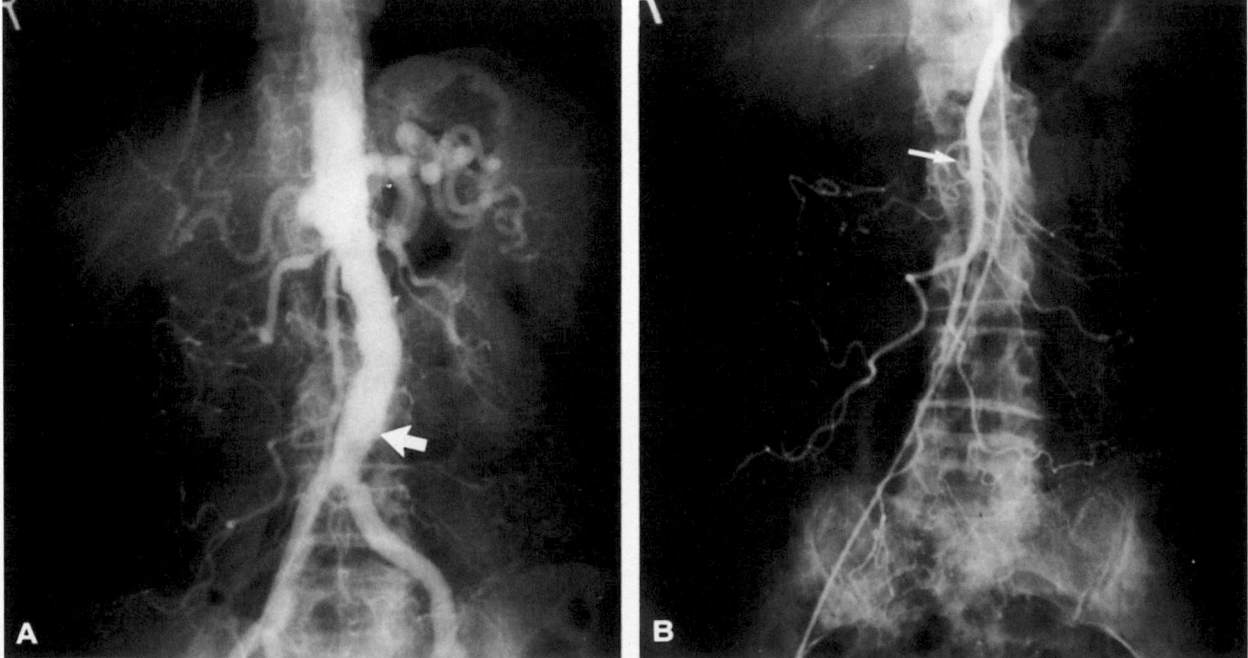

FIGURE 28-31. Ischemic colitis. **A:** Aortogram shows occluded inferior mesenteric artery (*arrow*). **B:** Superior mesenteric angiogram demonstrates occlusion of the middle colic artery (*arrow*).

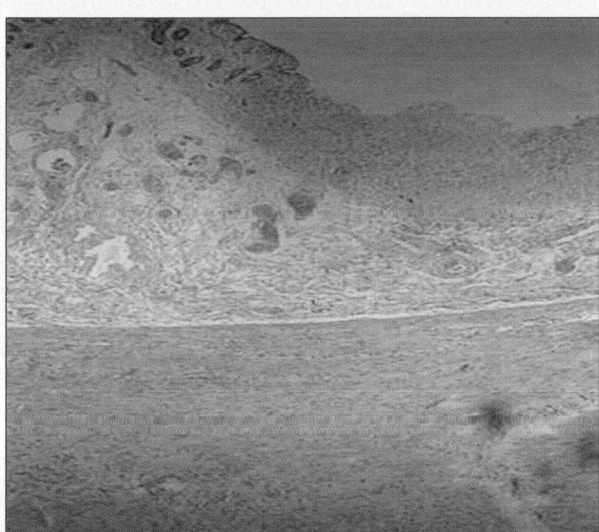 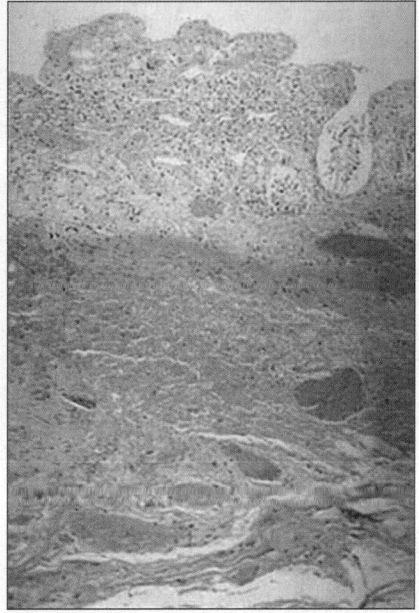

FIGURE 28-32. Ischemic colitis. **A:** Superficial necrosis and ulceration of mucosa with congested submucosal blood vessels. Muscularis propria is viable. (Original magnification × 100.) **B:** Necrosis of full thickness of mucosa with retention of ghost outline of epithelium. (Original magnification × 260.)

Management

Medical management includes intravenous fluid replacement, broad-spectrum antibiotic therapy, and the usual supportive measures.[390] In most cases of colonic ischemia, signs and symptoms subside within a day or two, with resolution of the submucosal or intramural hemorrhage.[130] Surgical intervention is indicated for signs and symptoms of peritonitis and for obstruction. Paterno and colleagues, in an attempt to define ischemic colitis patients who progress to surgical intervention, reviewed their experience with 253 such individuals. On multivariate analysis, only intraperitoneal fluid on CT scan and the absence of blood per rectum predicted a need for surgery.[272]

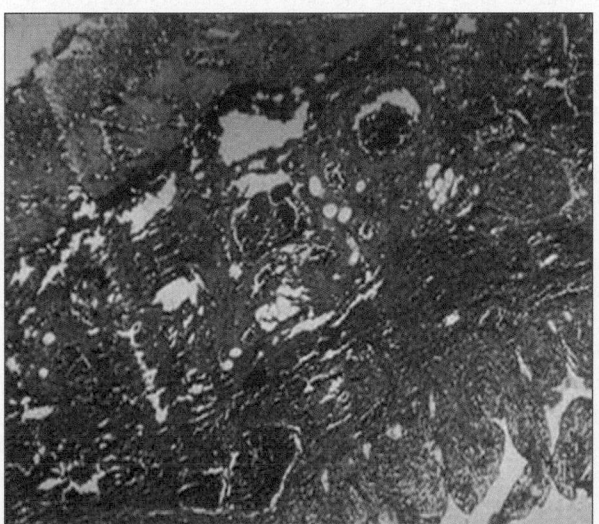

FIGURE 28-33. Ischemic colitis. Necrosis of full thickness of bowel wall. Note hemorrhage and dilated blood vessels. (Original magnification × 80; courtesy of Rudolf Garret, MD.)

The intraoperative diagnosis of the degree of colonic ischemia is often difficult to determine. Care must be taken at the time of resection to ensure adequacy of the blood supply. Partial colectomy for primary colonic ischemia is generally a poor alternative, but if undertaken should always be accompanied by fecal diversion, unless the quality of life with an ileostomy is felt to be unacceptable for that individual. Subtotal or total colectomy is the preferred approach if an anastomosis is contemplated, but even with a total colectomy, resection with an ileostomy is undoubtedly safer.

Results

There are no meaningful statistics concerning the comparative results of the surgical options. In a recent review of 160 patients who underwent elective versus emergency surgery in individuals older than the age of 80, Kurian and colleagues found a 60% 6-month mortality rate in those who required a colon resection for ischemic colitis.[191] Guttormson and Bubrick evaluated 39 individuals with this condition, confirming a close association between ischemic colitis and a number of systemic diseases.[154] The overall mortality rate was 53% for those treated both surgically and nonsurgically. Parish and coworkers observed an increased proportion of postoperative patients with this disease than had been previously noted, an indication, perhaps, that fewer spontaneous cases required hospitalization.[266] Their operative mortality was 62%, whereas those who did not require surgical intervention had a mortality of only 14%. Because of the high incidence of associated cardiovascular disease, the authors emphasize the importance of early diagnosis, as well as careful monitoring, to improve the survival figures. Longo and associates identified 47 patients with nonocclusive ischemia of the large intestine over a 7-year period at Yale University School of Medicine.[208] Almost half of the patients had right colon involvement. Fifteen of 16 were successfully treated nonoperatively by means of bowel rest and antibiotics, but 1 died. The remainder required bowel resection, of which almost one-half had their intestinal continuity reestablished. There was a 29% operative mortality. Others have observed that the right colon appears to be the most severely affected area in this condition. Landreneau and Fry expressed an opinion about the possibility of a "mesenteric steal" from more proximal branches of the superior mesenteric arterial circulation during periods of compromised perfusion as the reason for this distribution.[195] It is evident that if operative intervention is required for ischemic colitis, it is associated with a very high mortality rate, probably because many patients are elderly and have multisystem diseases.[209,231]

Montoro and colleagues reported on the outcome of an open prospective trial evaluating the natural history of colonic ischemia in patients treated in 24 separate Spanish hospitals. This was accomplished through the Workgroup for the Study of Ischemic Colitis of the Spanish Gastroenterological Association.[237] They identified a total of 364 patients during the study period. Of the 364, only 24.2% were clinically suspected of having ischemic colitis. The majority had reversible or transient ischemia (69.8%), but 9.9% had gangrenous colitis, and 17.9% had chronic segmental colitis. Forty-seven patients progressed to either surgery or they expired. On multivariate analysis, predictors of these unfavorable outcomes included abdominal pain without rectal bleeding, nonbloody diarrhea, and peritonitis. Right-sided ischemia also led more frequently to either surgery or to death. The overall mortality rate was 7.7%.

Ischemic Colitis and Surgery of the Abdominal Aorta

Ischemic colitis may develop following resection of an abdominal aortic aneurysm.[58,121,157,187,198,387] The incidence of this complication has been variously reported to be from less than 1% to more than 25%. The higher rates are usually associated with other factors, such as the prolonged hypotension that often accompanies the management of ruptured aneurysm. The changes may be reversible or, as with ischemic colitis not associated with aneurysmectomy, may subsequently lead to stricture, gangrene, or perforation. The combination of intra-abdominal sepsis with a prosthetic vascular graft is potentially catastrophic. With a mortality rate of 75%, this complication may account for as many as one-fourth of the deaths following operations performed on the aorta.[319]

Diagnosis and Prevention

Recommendations for preventing this complication at the time of surgery have included reimplantation of the inferior mesenteric artery if it is large, measurement of the stump pressure, Doppler ultrasound, indirect measurement of pH in the wall of the sigmoid colon, and preservation of the first branch of the vessel.[118,312,319] Unfortunately, inferior mesenteric artery reimplantation does not guarantee colon viability in aortic surgery, implying that other issues, such as intraoperative hypotension, may be an important factor.[236]

Rectal bleeding within the first 72 hours following aneurysmectomy is a characteristic symptom that mandates investigation. Forde and colleagues suggest that colonoscopy is a particularly useful technique for establishing the diagnosis of ischemic colitis in the postoperative period.[121] The findings are similar to those previously described: the rectum and distal sigmoid colon are often spared, with more proximal mucosal ulceration apparent. Dark blue or black nodular areas are suggestive of possible gangrene. The serum D-lactate level has also been shown to have predictive value as an early marker of bowel ischemia after ruptured abdominal aortic aneurysm repair.[278]

Ernst and associates undertook a prospective study on 50 patients to determine the incidence of this complication.[115] Colonoscopic examination was performed within 4 days of operation; three patients had evidence of ischemia (6%). Arteriographic evaluation of collateral circulation by the superior mesenteric artery revealed that colon ischemia did not develop when the collateral blood supply was identified. These authors suggest that despite the relative rarity of clinically significant colitis following aortic reconstruction, colonoscopy may be of value for early detection of possible ischemic changes so that therapy might, if necessary, be initiated sooner. In a study of postoperative colonoscopy following abdominal aortic reconstruction, Hagihara and colleagues determined that 11 of 163 patients who underwent reconstruction of the abdominal aorta demonstrated ischemic changes (7%).[157] These authors implied that the incidence might have been even higher if all patients surviving resection of ruptured abdominal aneurysms had undergone postoperative colonoscopy. In another prospective study by Welch and associates (Manchester Royal Infirmary), colonic ischemia was identified *histologically* in biopsies from 16 of 53 patients (30%) who underwent elective infrarenal aortic surgery.[386] In a retrospective review by Brewster and colleagues from the Massachusetts General Hospital, 0.9% of patients had overt ischemia.[58]

Kim and colleagues analyzed the risk factors for the development of ischemia of the colon following abdominal aortic resection for aneurysm.[187] Prolonged cross-clamp time, hypoxemia, rupture of the aneurysm, hypotension, and arrhythmia occurred with significantly greater frequency among the patients with ischemia than among control subjects. Schiedler and coworkers compared intramural pH measured through a silicone balloon placed in the lumen of the sigmoid colon, with risk factor analysis and inferior mesenteric artery stump pressures as predictors of ischemic colitis in 34 patients undergoing elective or emergency operations on the abdominal aorta.[312] Logistic regression analysis demonstrated that aortic aneurysm, age, and stenosis of the superior mesenteric artery were the only risk factors that bore a statistical relationship to the development of ischemic colitis.[312]

Champagne and colleagues followed 88 patients who underwent emergency repair of a ruptured aortic aneurysm.[78] Of these, 72 patients lived past 24 hours. They performed colonoscopy in 62 of the 72 and documented ischemia in 36%. Nine underwent exploration and resection because of grade 3 ischemic changes seen on endoscopy. Those with ischemia had a 50% mortality. Increased fluid requirements, elevated lactate levels, and immature white blood cells were associated with ischemia.

Treatment

When colonic ischemia occurs as a consequence of surgery on the abdominal aorta, a high index of suspicion is required, and treatment must be initiated promptly and aggressively. As implied from the foregoing, when the condition is recognized intraoperatively, the problem can be handled in one of two ways. One option is to remove the inferior mesenteric artery from its origin, along with a cuff of aorta, and to reimplant it into the aortic prosthesis.[198] One can also consider the possibility of vascular reconstruction by means

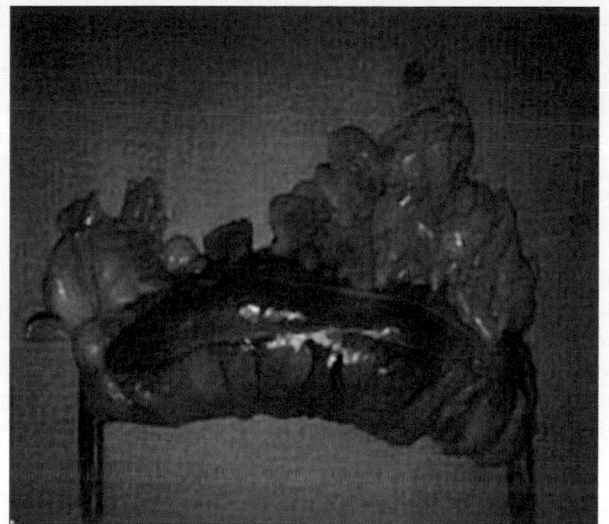

FIGURE 28-34. Polyarteritis nodosa. Blood vessel showing fibrinoid necrosis of the wall with surrounding exudate and superficial ulceration of overlying mucosa. (Original magnification × 120; courtesy of Rudolf Garret, MD.)

of endarterectomy and angioplasty. The other obvious alternative is to resect the diseased segment of bowel when the lack of viability becomes apparent (Figure 28-34).

Brewster and colleagues reviewed the experience with intestinal ischemia complicating abdominal aortic surgery at the Massachusetts General Hospital.[58] Of more than 2,000 patients who underwent abdominal aortic reconstruction, 1.1% had overt intestinal ischemia documented by reoperation or by endoscopic findings. In the group of five individuals recognized to have colonic ischemia during surgery, three with a patent inferior mesenteric artery (IMA) on preoperative angiography underwent IMA reimplantation. Another underwent sigmoid resection with colostomy, and the fifth underwent repair of the marginal artery. All those in this category did well. Of the 14 patients with the diagnosis of ischemia made after the vascular procedure, one-half were managed nonoperatively. Three recovered without complication, and four developed colonic stricture. Half required resection for this complication. The remainder underwent resection for transmural infarction. The mortality rate on these individuals was 57%. Therefore, looking at the entire group, if reoperation was required, the mortality rate was 50%.[58]

It would, therefore, seem self-evident that every effort to determine the adequacy of the circulation to the colon during operations on the aorta should remain the primary goal.

With the advent of endovascular aortic repair, the morbidity and mortality from abdominal aortic aneurysm seems to have decreased. There is evidence to support a lower risk of colonic ischemia with this minimally invasive procedure. Champagne and colleagues examined the outcomes of 44 patients who underwent endovascular repair of ruptured abdominal aortic aneurysms.[79] Thirty-nine survived beyond 24 hours. Thirty-six underwent sigmoidoscopy, and 23% were found to have bowel ischemia. Three of these patients required exploration with resection. Given the high incidence of ischemia in either open or endovascular repair of ruptured abdominal aortic aneurysms, an argument may be made for mandatory flexible sigmoidoscopy in all ruptured aneurysm patients who undergo emergency surgery.

Ischemic Proctitis

As discussed earlier, generally, the rectum is spared from ischemia because of the collateral blood supply. Fewer than 50 cases have been reported that extended to the level of the dentate line. The implication of this manifestation in such a distal location is inadequate collateral circulation.

Diagnosis is usually made by the characteristic appearance on proctosigmoidoscopy. In four of six patients identified with acute ischemic proctitis by Nelson and colleagues, surgical interruption of splanchnic blood flow due to aortoiliac disease was the primary precipitating event.[248] When ischemia of the rectum occurs, the symptoms and pathologic changes are identical to that which has been described for the colon. Treatment usually involves correction of the underlying problem and expectant management, but a single case of hemorrhagic proctitis as a consequence of ischemia was satisfactorily treated with the topical installation of 4% formalin.[75] Rarely does ischemia of the rectum proceed to gangrene, but when it does occur, it requires proctectomy with end colostomy.

Ischemic Colitis: Collagen Vascular Diseases

The collagen vascular diseases represent a collection of conditions that are believed to be due to pathologic alterations in the immune system. They can occur in any organ and may be associated with varied GI complaints. The conditions can affect the blood supply to the colon and produce ischemic changes either isolated to this organ or as part of the systemic process. These diseases included polyarteritis nodosa, cryoglobulinemia, Henoch–Schönlein purpura, Behçet's syndrome, systemic lupus erythematosus, polymyositis, and scleroderma (Figure 28-35).[217,218,263,288] Colonic ischemia in the setting of collagen vascular diseases is usually caused by a vasculitis or, less commonly, thrombosis.[142] Deposition of immune complexes in blood vessel walls is the most widely accepted pathogenic mechanism. This can lead to hemorrhage,

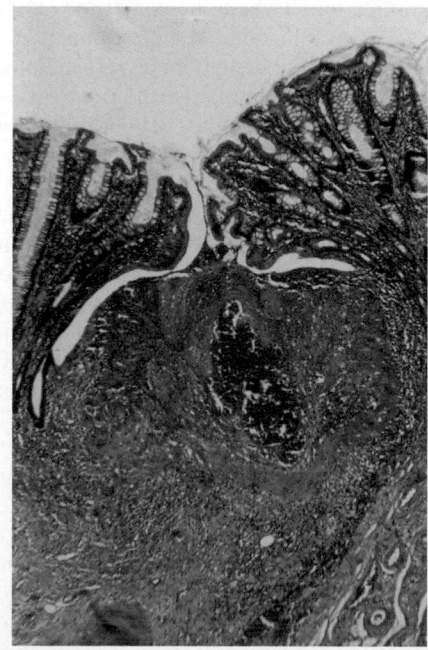

FIGURE 28-35. Sigmoid colon-resected specimen showing gangrene as a consequence of impaired blood supply via the inferior mesenteric artery following abdominal aortic aneurysmectomy.

infarction with perforation, or problems with functional colonic disorders such as inertia (see Chapter 20).[207]

Medical management is usually the primary therapy, but on occasion a patient will require surgical intervention for hemorrhage, obstruction, necrosis, or perforation.

If surgery does become necessary for acute abdominal complications of polyarteritis nodosa, the prognosis is grim. Zizic and colleagues noted no survivors because of involvement by extensive segments of gangrenous bowel.[404] Approximately one-half of the patients with systemic lupus erythematosus who developed an acute abdomen died.

When GI manifestations are complications of *Behçet's disease*, the prognosis is poor.[56] Patients may present with mesenteric ischemia and infarction because of large-vessel disease or with mucosal disease as a result of small-vessel involvement. The condition usually affects the right side of the colon. Hence, it must be differentiated from Crohn's disease. Iida and colleagues studied the postoperative course of intestinal Behçet's disease in nine individuals.[173] Eighty percent developed recurrence of intestinal ulcers. In most instances, these were at or near the anastomotic site. But the mainstay of therapy is medical: corticosteroids, immunosuppressants, and anti-inflammatory medications.

▶ RADIATION ENTERITIS

You have to operate your way in and then operate your way out.

—RUPERT B. TURNBULL
(commenting on surgery after radiation)

Radiation injuries to the GI tract are among the most difficult management problems facing the surgeon. It is not uncommon for the patient to suffer the deleterious effects of ionizing radiation long after the primary disease process for which the radiation was employed had been cured. Radiation is indeed a two-edged sword. Because of the serious consequences and the late complications (which are sometimes lethal), many surgeons have been reluctant to employ this modality if another alternative is felt to be reasonably efficacious.

Radiation damage is cumulative and progressive. A finite amount of radiation is tolerable, beyond which additional radiotherapy at any time following the initial treatment may precipitate complications. Certain conditions such as diabetes mellitus, hypertension, and previous abdominal surgery are believed to predispose the bowel to radiation injury.[20] Other factors that increase the risk include infection, single portal therapy, overlapping portals of therapy, poorly calibrated or uncalibrated dosimeters, inadequate vaginal packing during implants, the presence of intra-abdominal adhesions (by fixing loops of bowel), concomitant chemotherapy, and overlooking signals of distress or masking them by overmedication.[298,357]

It has been estimated that 50% of all cancer patients will receive radiotherapy at some stage during their illness.[116] That figure today may be conservative, in light of the increased application of neoadjuvant and adjuvant chemoradiation therapy. The incidence of radiation enteritis may be increasing according to the experience of Galland and Spencer at the Hammersmith Hospital.[129] This, they believe, can be attributed to the combination of internal and external treatment and to the technique of "afterloading." Virtually, all who undergo radiation to the abdomen will develop early

symptoms of radiation injury to the bowel, and 5% to 20% will have long-term sequelae of radiation enteritis.[90,116,242]

Patients receiving more than 50 Gy are most likely to develop this complication. All individuals are not equally susceptible to intestinal radiation injury, however. For example, children are more likely to have complications associated with radiation enteritis,[109] and people with light complexions are more sensitive than those with dark.[314]

Historically, cervical cancer has been the most commonly radiated lesion and thus is associated with the most radiation complications. Schmitz and colleagues reported that the original diseases in their 37 patients with radiation injuries were cervical carcinoma in 29 and endometrial carcinoma in 8.[314] Other primary diseases for which radiation therapy may subsequently produce problems include carcinoma of the endometrium, carcinoma of the bladder, carcinoma of the rectum or rectosigmoid, prostatic cancer, ovarian cancer, and carcinoma of the anal canal (Figure 28-36). In a review by Hayne and coworkers based on a literature search (MEDLINE), more than three-fourths of patients receiving pelvic radiotherapy experienced acute anorectal symptoms and up to one-fifth suffer from late-phase radiation proctitis.[164] Approximately 5% develop other complications, such as fistula, stricture, and fecal incontinence.

Marks and Mohiudden reported that the most common area of injury was the ileum, followed by the rectum, rectosigmoid, cecum, sigmoid colon, and jejunum.[224] The most common lesion noted in the Cleveland Clinic experience was proctitis; other complications included ulceration, stricture, and fistula to the vagina, bladder, or both.[199] Others have reported that although the small bowel is more sensitive to irradiation, the most common site of injury is the rectum, owing to its fixity in the pelvis.[20,357] Because lymphoid tissue is extremely sensitive to the effects of radiation and there is a high concentration of lymphoid tissue in Peyer's patches, the explanation becomes evident for the frequency of terminal ileal damage despite its relative mobility.[357]

The use of neoadjuvant therapy for rectal cancer is now well established. Preoperative timing of radiation therapy provides similar reduction in local recurrence rates but less toxicity as compared with postoperative therapy. Sauer and coworkers published the results of the German Rectal Cancer Study Group trial comparing preoperative to postoperative chemoradiation therapy. They clearly found a significant reduction in acute (27% vs. 40%) and long-term (14% vs. 24%) toxicity.[309] The use of multidirectional, sharply

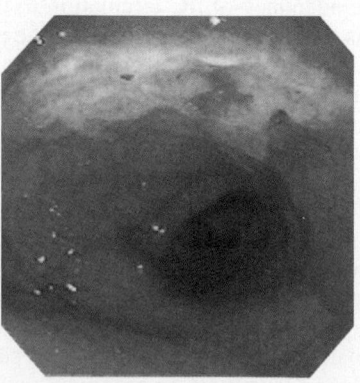

FIGURE 28-36. Endoscopy reveals a whitish area of scar surrounded by erythematous mucosa with evident stenosis characteristic of radiation proctitis.

collimated, high-energy photon and electron beams allows concentration of the radiation to the tumor rather than to normal structures.[89] The treatment is facilitated by highly accurate computer-assisted dosimetric tumor localization systems, by individualized custom-blocking and visceral displacement techniques, and by progressively reducing the radiation field size during the treatment course.[89,293] Early onset of symptoms such as cramping or diarrhea and an objective confirmation of radiation changes on endoscopy or biopsy should alert the therapist to consider modification of the treatment plan by reducing the dose, increasing fractionation over longer periods, or temporarily interrupting the therapy.[242]

A newer technique of delivering intensity modulated radiotherapy (IMRT) has been shown to reduce acute bowel toxicity in patients being treated for rectal cancer. Samuelian and colleagues used IMRT to treat 31 rectal cancer patients and compared that to 61 patients treated with three-field conventional radiotherapy. The IMRT patients had significantly less grade 2 or greater lower GI toxicity as compared with the conventional treatment method (32% vs. 66%).[306]

With respect to prevention, the various techniques of administration of the radiation have already been mentioned. In addition, a number of substances may be given prophylactically that act as radioprotective agents. An elemental diet given during the course of the treatment has been demonstrated to be beneficial, but the mechanism of this action is unclear.[129] Wiseman and colleagues, in an experimental study on rats, documented the prevention of histologic changes with the use of an elemental diet, vitamin A, and sodium meclofenamate.[394] With respect to prevention in the patient being considered for postoperative radiation therapy, the surgeon should attempt to exclude the small intestine from the pelvis before closure of the abdomen (see Chapter 24).[103,104,293,349] Valle and colleagues have reported good success with isolating the small intestine from the pelvis after pelvic exenteration with the use of implantable mammary prostheses. They noted no postoperative complications related to the implantation in 28 patients who underwent postoperative irradiation. No patients suffered from radiation enteritis.[369]

Symptoms

The symptoms of radiation injury depend on whether one is dealing with the acute process, usually occurring during the course of the treatment, or the result of therapy—weeks, months, or even years later. Nausea, vomiting, diarrhea, and cramping abdominal pain are seen in 75% of patients who undergo radiotherapy.[20] Because of complications of radiation to the small intestine, malabsorption, partial intestinal obstruction, and severe diarrhea may lead to malnutrition and fluid and electrolyte imbalance. Complete bowel obstruction may supervene. Depending on the site and type of radiation injury, patients may develop signs and symptoms of urinary fistula, vaginal fistula, anorectal ulcer, and many other manifestations (Figure 28-37).

One must also be wary of the asymptomatic individual who has undergone radiation therapy and who requires an operation for another complaint. There is a serious risk of injuring previously irradiated bowel (see later). Even with the surgeon taking great care, the patient may develop a perforation while convalescing from an operation such as a lysis of adhesions.[127]

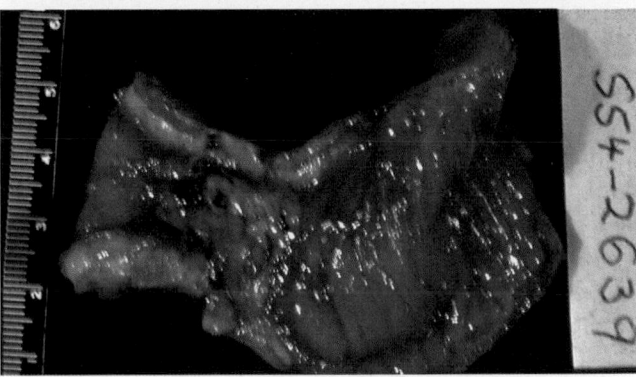

FIGURE 28-37. Rectal resection that was required for bleeding and pain. Note virtually circumferential necrotic ulcer within the specimen.

Evaluation

For disease involving the rectum or rectosigmoid, proctoscopic examination may reveal loss of vessel pattern, edema, contact bleeding, and telangiectasis. Changes may mimic that of nonspecific inflammatory bowel disease, but the history and the presence of telangiectasis usually help prevent any diagnostic confusion. Ulceration and granularity may be noted. Later changes may include thickening of the rectal wall, stricture, or fistula into the vagina or into the bladder. Colonoscopy has been used for studying patients with presumed radiation colitis, particularly for bleeding and for inspection of a colonic stricture.[289] Endoscopic evidence of injury includes pallor of the mucosa, prominent submucosal telangiectatic vessels, friability, erythema, and granularity. Perianal excoriation, erythema, and ulceration may be seen, especially when radiation is given for an anal cancer. Pain and drainage are prominent symptoms in these individuals (Figure 28-38).

Radiologic studies performed during the course of therapy will usually not be helpful in identifying specific radiation changes. Increased irritability and motility of the small bowel are usually noted, and there may be some associated spasticity in the colon.[298] Months or years after the treatment, however, profound radiologic changes may be apparent on contrast study of the intestinal tract. Commonly involved areas include the sigmoid colon, rectum, and terminal ileum (Figure 28-39). Angiographic studies may reveal arterial

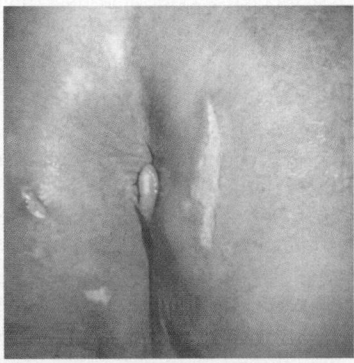

FIGURE 28-38. Erythema and linear ulcerations of the buttocks are evident in this patient who is undergoing radiation therapy for a carcinoma of the anal canal. Part of the lesion is apparent protruding from the anal verge.

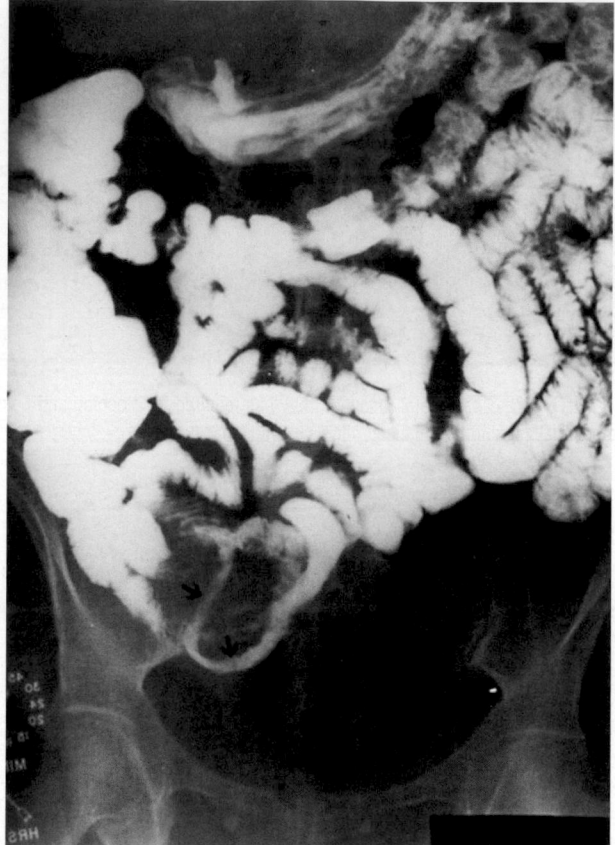

FIGURE 28-39. Radiation enteritis. Terminal ileal radiation changes include rigidity and edema of the bowel wall, apparent mass between loops (*arrows*), and destruction of the mucosal pattern.

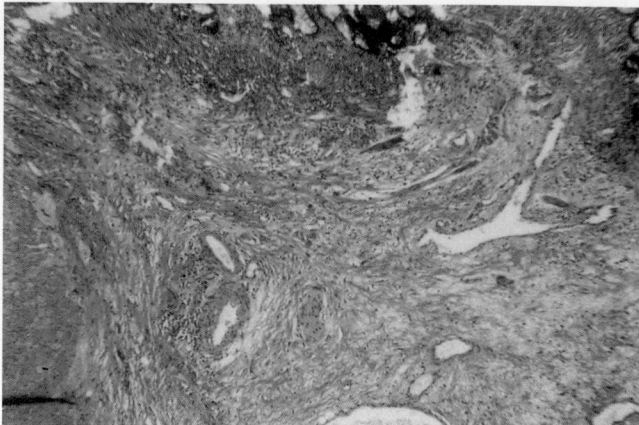

FIGURE 28-40. Radiation colitis. Subacute changes include fibrosis of the submucosa, sclerosis of blood vessels, and perivascular mononuclear cell infiltrate. (Original magnification × 240; courtesy of Rudolf Garret, MD.)

and venous irregularity, beading and focal obstruction of the bowel wall vasculature, and crowding of vessels because of foreshortening of the intestine.[298]

Evaluation of the small intestine may be performed via radiologic investigations such as CT scan, CT enterography, or a small bowel follow-through. More recently, MRI enterography has also been advocated for the diagnosis of radiation enteritis. Findings include an abnormal loop of small intestine in the region of the known radiation field, often with stricturing and proximal dilatation.[91] Kim and colleagues have described a pilot study of the use of capsule endoscopy for the diagnosis of radiation enteritis. They identified radiation enteritis in five of nine patients suspected. Erythematous, congested mucosa was the most frequently seen abnormality.[186]

Pathophysiology

Three phases of radiation effects have been identified: (1) acute, primarily affecting the mucosa; (2) subacute, with predominant effects in the submucosa; and (3) chronic, generally affecting all layers of the bowel wall.[224] Acute radiation enteritis is due to destruction of the rapidly dividing cells at the base of the crypts of the GI mucosa.[116] Destruction of cells that rapidly turn over and obliteration of blood vessels, combined with a fibroblastic response, are the events that produce the less acute and chronic manifestations.[74] Impaired regeneration of the irradiated mucosal epithelium may contribute to the erosions or ulcers, but progressive fibrosis and vascular lesions leading to ischemia are the most important factors.[46]

Depending on the phase, the changes may vary from colitis with capillary dilatation, hemorrhage, edema, and inflammatory cell infiltration in the acute situation to an ischemia from an obliterative endarteritis and fibrosis in the chronic (Figures 28-40 through 28-42). The normal submucosal space may be altered by the deposition of dense hyaline material lacking the normal fibrillar structure of collagen.[189]

Recent studies in microbiology have been revealing with respect to the pathogenesis of radiation enteritis. By means of a literature search, Nguyen and colleagues attempted to identify factors that affect the disease process.[251] They observed that long-term complications are characterized by excessive stimulation of transforming growth factor (TGF-β1). They further suggest that interferon gamma (IFN-γ) inhibits the effects of TGF-β1 and may be ultimately clinically applicable in a treatment program for patients with radiation enteritis.

Surgical Treatment

Before operation, it is important to evaluate the entire intestinal tract for the presence of associated radiation-induced abnormalities and for the possibility of recurrent primary disease. Upper GI x-ray, barium enema, and complete

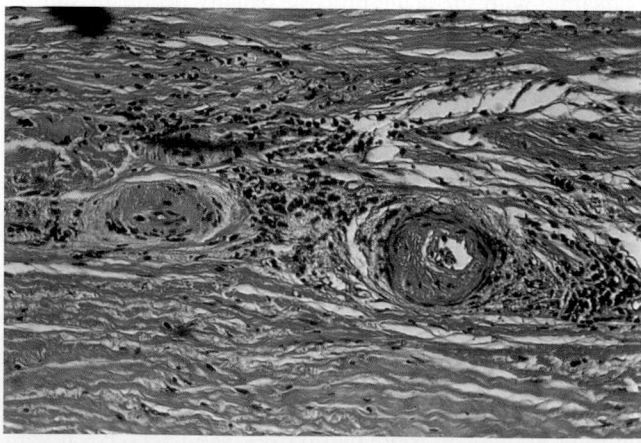

FIGURE 28-41. Radiation colitis. Chronic changes comprise fibrosis, dilatation of the lymphatics, and virtual obliteration of the blood vessels. (Original magnification × 280; courtesy of Rudolf Garret, MD.)

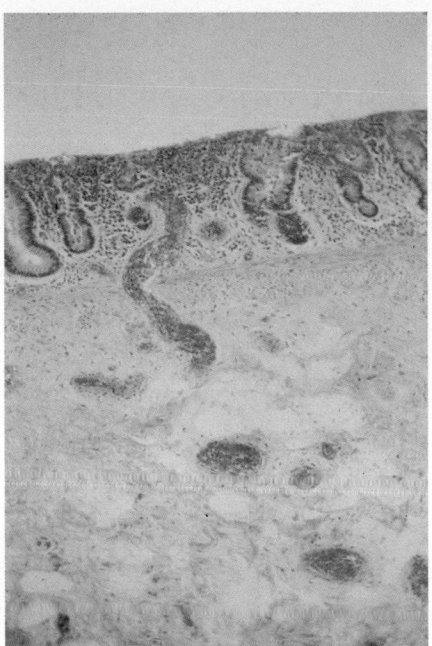

FIGURE 28-42. Radiation proctitis. Atrophy of the mucosa with fibrosis and telangiectasis of the submucosa. (Original magnification × 170.)

endoscopic examinations are necessary. Evaluation of the urinary tract is particularly important because of the high incidence of associated damage to the outflow tracts. The presence of ureteral obstruction necessitates cystoscopy and retrograde pyelography. Additionally, if a resection is attempted, it is helpful to have ureteral catheters inserted at the time of operation. The presence of ureteral catheters does not, of course, guarantee that injury will be avoided, but it is reassuring to be able to palpate the catheters and know the locations of these important structures.

The most frequent indications for surgical intervention in a patient with radiation injury are the presence of a fistula and intestinal obstruction. Fistulization may occur to the vagina, bladder, skin, and other areas of the intestinal tract. Obstructive symptoms also often require surgical treatment.

The choice of procedure will depend on the level of the injury, the patient's prognosis, and the extent of radiation damage as determined at the time of exploration. There are five available options in the surgical management of radiation enteritis: primary closure (of a fistula), resection, bypass, exclusion, and diversionary stoma (ileostomy or colostomy) (Figure 28-43). A sixth alternative may be considered, that of strictureplasty. This has been described by the Cleveland Clinic Ohio Group in five patients with obstructing, diffuse radiation enteritis.[105] The technique is illustrated in Chapter 30. It is generally agreed, however, that operations for radiation enteritis should be avoided except when complications develop. In fact, radiation enteropathy may be characterized by long, symptom-free intervals.[240] Morgenstern stressed a number of general principles that he thought should be employed, if possible, in the management of these patients; they are as follows[240]:

Avoid operation.
Achieve optimal preoperative nutritional status.
Use long intestinal tubes.
Use standard mechanical and antibiotic bowel preparation and postoperative systemic antibiotics.

Employ resection rather than bypass.
Resect rather than close fistulas.
Limit the amount of adhesiolysis.
Use meticulous anastomotic technique.
Identify the anastomosis with a radiopaque marker.
Delay postoperative oral alimentation; use prolonged long-tube decompression.
Avoid irradiated bowel for stomas.

Results

Characteristically, there is a tendency to underestimate the amount of damage produced by the radiation when examination of the serosal surface of the intestine is performed. If one is to anticipate a favorable result of the operation, all radiation-injured tissue must be adequately excised and an anastomosis effected in relatively normal bowel. Morgenstern and colleagues recommend, based on their experience with 52 patients, if an anastomosis seems like it should be required in the region of the terminal ileum, that it be performed in the colon in order to avoid a pelvic suture line.[241,242] Others have reported a lower incidence of leak with ileoileal anastomoses than with ileocolic, but it is impossible to evaluate the significance of this observation with small numbers of patients and with various clinical presentations.[163] Anastomotic leak rates are reported as high as 65%, with mortality rates in excess of 50%, but there is general agreement today that if resection is performed, an ileocolonic anastomosis is preferred.[128,160]

Zhu and colleagues reported on their experience managing 156 patients with chronic radiation enteritis: 112 had intestinal obstruction, 42 suffered fistulizing complications, and 2 had free perforations. Thirty-six patients had associated urinary tract complications, 15 with radiation cystitis, 11 with ureteral obstruction, and 10 with enterovesical fistulas. The authors advocated resection and anastomosis for small intestinal disease, whereas rectosigmoid disease should be treated with diversion. Overall morbidity was 26.7%, with a 2% anastomotic leak rate. Five patients ended up with short bowel syndrome due to extensive resection of the damaged intestine. The authors also transitioned from midline incisions to a transverse subumbilical incision in order to avoid incisions in the lower abdominal wall that are included in the radiation field. With this change, they noted a significant reduction in wound complications.[402]

Bypass operations often fail to relieve symptoms or are associated with recurrent problems.[128] Smith and DeCosse observed that 92% of individuals who harbored an enteric fistula and who underwent an exclusion procedure, without an extensive resection of small bowel, were successfully treated.[334] This compared with a success rate for resection of 67% and for bypass of 69%. Aitken and Elliot reported three patients who successfully underwent sigmoid exclusion for colovesical and colovaginal fistula.[6] The involved sigmoid colon was isolated on its mesentery, the ends closed, and a colorectal or coloanal anastomosis performed. By this technique, a permanent stoma and a urinary conduit could be avoided.

Schmitt and Symmonds reported 93 patients with small bowel radiation enteritis.[313] More than two-thirds underwent intestinal resection, and 20 underwent bypass procedures. Adhesions were lysed in 8 patients. Factors used to select the appropriate operative procedure included age and general medical condition; the location, extent, and degree of the radiation changes; and whether the procedure was carried out on an elective or an emergency basis. Anastomotic dehiscence occurred in 10 patients, and there were six

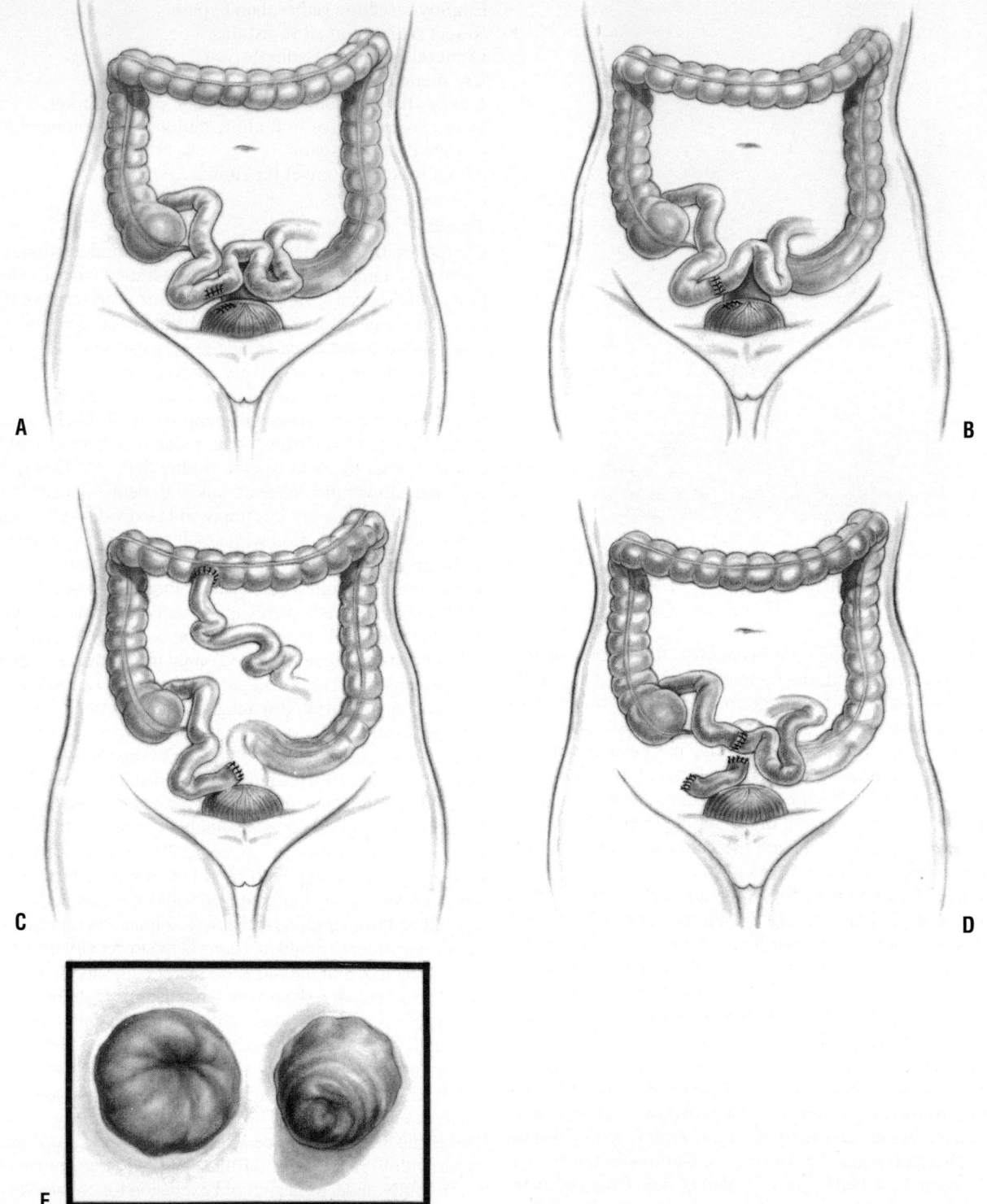

FIGURE 28-43. Options in the surgical management of radiation enteritis with vesical fistulous. **A:** Closure of fistulous communication. **B:** Resection. **C:** Bypass. **D:** Exclusion. **E:** Colostomy or ileostomy.

operative deaths. Cram and associates reviewed their experience with 89 patients with radiation injury to the bowel, of whom 31 required surgical intervention.[90] These authors tended to perform a resection or a bypass for small bowel disease and a colostomy for large bowel involvement. Although they conceded that the "conservative" approach to large bowel radiation injury is not universally accepted, they felt that the high rates of morbidity and mortality associated with resection, and the requirement for possibly multiple procedures, impelled them to adopt this particular approach.

Wellwood and Jackson reported their experience with 38 patients with intestinal complications after radiotherapy, noting a mortality rate of 37%.[388] These authors advise formation of a combined surgical–radiotherapy clinic to monitor and investigate those at risk. They also suggested that prompt radiologic investigation of the intestinal tract be performed if symptoms suggestive of radiation damage are elicited. Tests for malabsorption should also be performed. A number of papers attest to the high morbidity associated with surgical intervention and the need for liberal implementation of a diversionary stoma.[92,161,188,213,234]

Lefevre and associates presented their experience with 107 patients who underwent surgery for chronic radiation enteritis. They documented a significant morbidity rate of 74.8%. They related that reoperation rates at 1 and 3 years of follow-up were 37% and 54%, respectively. The only factor found to diminish the risk of reoperation was ileocecal resection at the first operation. They concluded, therefore, that adhesiolysis or bypass play little role in the management of chronic radiation enteritis, and resection of damaged bowel is of primary importance for long-term recovery.[201]

Home parenteral nutrition has been advocated for the treatment of patients with severe radiation enteritis.[199] Five individuals were reported from the Cleveland Clinic who would have been unable to survive their severe state of malnutrition without this treatment. They were not considered candidates for surgical intervention because of extensive disease and their malnutrition. One patient died of recurrent carcinoma after 14 months, and another died as a result of a pharmaceutical error after 30 months. The other three remained free of morbidity (attributed to the parenteral nutrition) at the time of the follow-up report.

▶ RADIATION PROCTITIS

Because of its fixed position, the rectum is particularly vulnerable to the effects of radiation. Ulcerative proctitis secondary to radiation-induced injury may produce symptoms of rectal bleeding, abdominal pain, diarrhea, passage of mucus, rectal pain, incontinence, and tenesmus.[183] Stricture, obstruction, and fistula formation into the bladder, urethra, or vagina are potential consequences of chronic radiation injury (Figure 28-44). It is an extremely troublesome condition to treat.

Manometric studies confirm a significant reduction in the rectal volume at sensory threshold, suggesting that this reduction and poor compliance are responsible for the frequency and urgency (Figure 28-45).[374] Dysfunction of the internal anal sphincter from damage to the myenteric plexus can contribute further to the symptoms caused by abnormalities of rectal function.[375]

Treatment

Management is usually directed to dietary measures, the addition of "slowing" medications for diarrhea, bulk agents, stool softeners, iron replacement if anemia is a concern, and antispasmodics. Oral vitamin A therapy, 8,000 IU twice daily, has been successfully employed in one instance for an individual in the healing of a postradiation anal ulcer.[203]

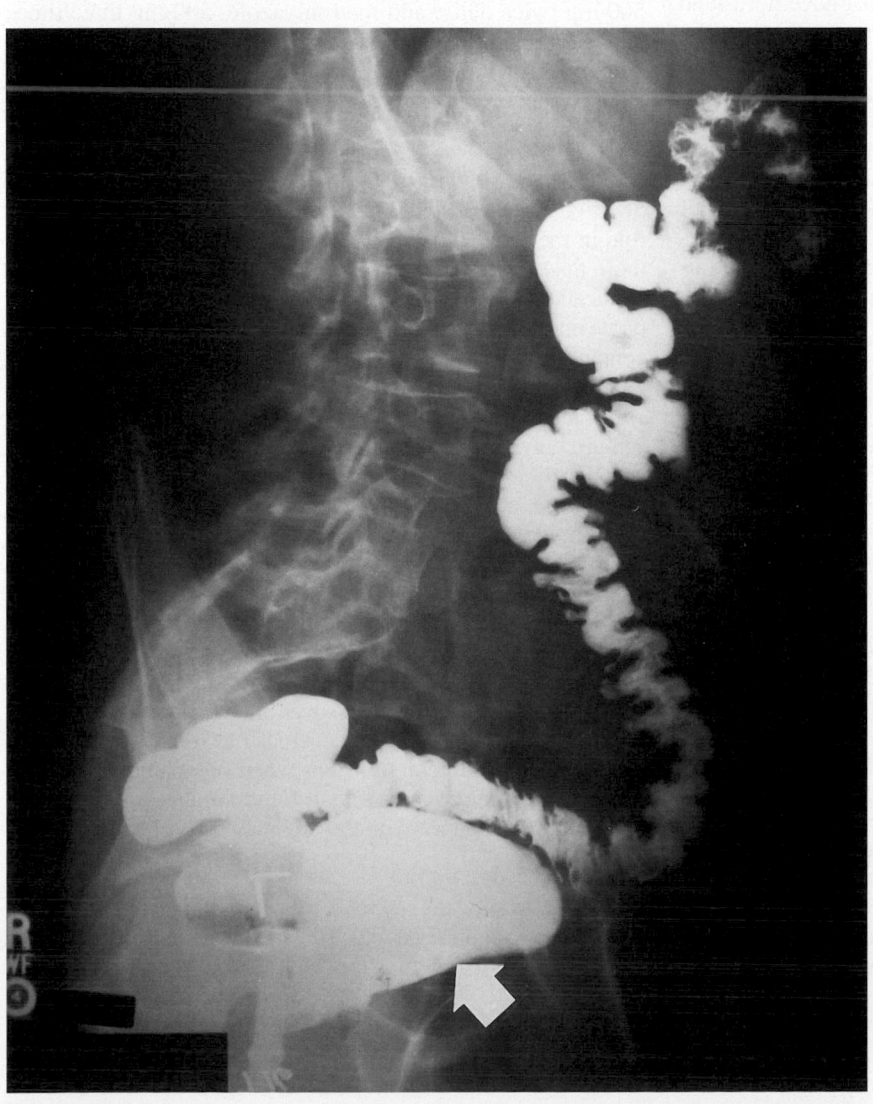

FIGURE 28-44. Rectovesical fistula. Barium enema demonstrates contrast material filling the bladder (*arrow*) from a fistula located in the distal rectum. Patient had undergone intensive radiation therapy for prostatic cancer.

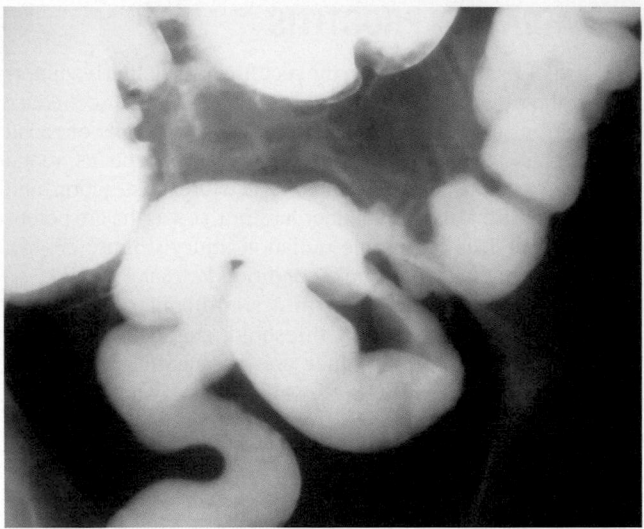

FIGURE 28-45. Barium enema study reveals rigid, nondistensible rectum in a patient with radiation proctitis.

The primary complaint that often demands attention, if not concern, is rectal bleeding. Retention enemas containing hydrocortisone have been recommended, but I have not found them particularly helpful. Approximately one-third of the patients treated by Allen-Mersh and colleagues with a similar regimen had their symptoms resolve within a period of 2 years.[9] Many individuals need only be reassured that they are not harboring a recurrent tumor and that bleeding may be a symptom with which they can and should live in peace.

A number of other topical approaches to the control of symptoms associated with radiation proctitis have been offered, including sulfasalazine, tranexamic acid, and sucralfate enemas, but the efficacy of these approaches has not been well documented.

Formalin

Topical formalin has been used successfully for a number of years to control intractable hemorrhagic cystitis. In recent years, a number of publications have appeared that suggest that rectal bleeding may be controlled by the topical administration of this agent.[216,265,299,302,324] One approach consists of irrigation with a total of 2 L of 3.6% formalin solution for 15 minutes, followed by irrigation with sodium chloride solution.[299] Great care must be taken if using this technique not to allow the formalin to migrate up into the descending and transverse colon as this may result in a significant colitis. Performing the irrigation in the lithotomy or left lateral position helps prevent proximal migration. Another technique that is more controlled consists of the application of gauze soaked in 4% formalin, laid in contact with the hemorrhagic surface until the bleeding ceases.[324] Success was reported in 7 of 8 patients by this initial application according to Seow-Choen and colleagues.[324] Saclarides and associates instilled 500 mL of a 4% formalin solution in 50 mL aliquots in 16 patients.[302] Each aliquot was kept in contact with the rectal mucosa for approximately 30 seconds. Success was identified in 75%, but four developed significant postoperative anal pain. Parikh and coworkers reported 36 patients treated for bleeding from radiation proctitis with topical application of a cotton pledget soaked in 4% formalin.[265] There were no complications, with 88% noting improvement or cessation of symptoms. Others report equally satisfactory results.[216]

Chattopadhyay and colleagues reported on their experience with 23 patients.[80] This prospective trial had a median follow-up of 13 months. Fifteen treated with 4% topical formalin stopped bleeding with the first application, 6 patients stopped after two treatments, and the final 2 patients required three. Bleeding did not recur during the follow-up period, and stool frequency decreased. Wong and associates found in 77 patients that the onset of bleeding was on average 24 months after therapy. Most of their patients responded to 4% formalin therapy (72.5%), whereas 18.2% required surgery for intractable bleeding, intestinal obstruction, or intra-abdominal sepsis.[396] Haas and coworkers treated 100 patients with 10% buffered formalin solution using a 16-in. cotton tip applicator, which was applied through a proctoscope in the office.[155] The mean follow-up was 18 months. An average of 3.5 formalin applications was needed to stop the bleeding in 93% of the patients. Eight patients rebled, and 3 complained of anal pain.

Tap Water Irrigation and Antibiotics

Sahakitrungruang and colleagues have described a new approach to managing hemorrhagic proctitis from radiation injury.[303] They treated 12 patients with daily 1 L low-pressure tap water enemas given via an 18 French Foley catheter for 8 weeks. These individuals were also given oral ciprofloxacin, 500 mg twice daily, and metronidazole, 500 mg three times daily, for 1 week. Five had previously undergone formalin therapy. They noted significant improvements in bleeding, stool frequency, urgency, and diarrhea. No patient required transfusion, and 11 of the 12 were satisfied with the treatment.

Short-Chain Fatty Acids

Short-chain fatty acids have been described as having a pivotal role in the regulation of mucosal proliferation and providing more than half the energy requirements of the mucosa.[377] The application of this concept through the rectal instillation of butyrate enemas for radiation proctitis would seem to be a logical conclusion. Vernia and associates (Milan, Italy) undertook a randomized, crossover, double-blind study involving 20 patients with radiation proctitis through the use of a 3-week course of sodium butyrate enemas (80 mmol/L).[377] A statistically significant benefit was achieved with respect to symptoms, endoscopic appearance, and histology. Pinto and colleagues (Lisbon, Portugal) opined, also in a prospective, randomized, double-blind, controlled trial, that short-chain fatty acid enemas can accelerate the process of healing, but treatment must be continuous to obtain a sustained and complete response.[277] Still, at 6 months, no differences in the two groups were observed. However, Talley and coworkers (Sydney, Australia), in a randomized, double-blind, placebo-controlled, crossover pilot trial with the use of a 2-week course of butyric acid enemas (40 mmol) twice a day, failed to demonstrate any benefit when compared with a placebo.[354] The enemas are difficult to obtain and foul smelling. Therefore, compliance with therapy may be problematic.

Laser Photocoagulation

Those who failed to respond to noninvasive or minimally invasive treatment can be offered the possibility of laser therapy to control symptoms of bleeding caused by radiation proctitis.[7,45,66,67,256,353,362] The procedure can be performed via the flexible sigmoidoscope. Both the argon laser and the Nd:YAG laser have proved effective, but Buchi recommends the former because it has a superficial penetration and is selectively absorbed by hemoglobin, thereby effectively coagulating the mucosal vascular lesions without injuring the underlying submucosa or bowel wall.[66]

Taïeb and coworkers (Grenoble, France) successfully managed 11 such individuals who failed to respond to less invasive measures (mean follow-up, 19 months).[353] Tjandra and Sengupta also noted significant reduction in the severity and frequency of the bleeding in their 12 patients (median follow-up, 11 months).[362] Dent and associates (Canberra, Australia) undertook a prospective Rectal Bleeding Quality of Life Scale patient-completed questionnaire in those who underwent laser or formalin therapy for radiation-induced rectal bleeding.[100] They found a significant improvement with respect to the quality of life reported by these individuals.

Swan and associates reported on 50 patients treated with argon plasma coagulation for chronic radiation proctitis. The majority had grade B or C proctitis and required on average of 1.36 treatments to induce bleeding cessation. Ninety-six percent ceased bleeding after one endoscopy treatment with coagulation. Their short-term complication rate was 34%. One patient experienced a long-term complication (asymptomatic rectal stricture).[351] Karamanolis and colleagues found that 89.5% of the 56 patients treated with argon plasma coagulation were still in remission at 17.9 months.[184] Argon plasma coagulation seems to have satisfactory outcomes, but what appears to be higher short-term complication rates than formalin instillation therapy. Therefore, consideration should be given to using formalin as a first-line therapy for hemorrhagic proctitis as a consequence of radiation.

Hyperbaric Oxygen

Another option that has been offered in the approach to the management of radiation proctitis as well as radiation colitis is hyperbaric oxygenation. Nakada and colleagues employed this therapy, which consisted of 100% oxygen inhalation at two absolute atmospheric pressures, 90 minutes daily for 30 days.[246] Although the treatment succeeded in alleviating the hemorrhage problem and reversed the endoscopic changes, it is difficult to know whether such an occurrence would have taken place in the absence of this treatment. Others, however, have reported successful healing of anal ulcers that resisted conservative treatment.[41]

Operative Approaches

Fistula formation between the urethra and the rectum is of heightened concern as well as a complex management issue in men who are treated with either external beam radiation, brachytherapy (seed implantation), or a combination of both for prostate cancer. The defect that may occur can be quite large, sometimes greater than 2 cm in diameter, with necrosis of the anterior rectal wall and prostate (Figure 28-46). Operative approaches to these fistulas depend on the size of the defect, the patient's degree of pain, and the function of both the anal and urethral sphincters. These defects may be approached from either the abdomen or the perineum. A number of operations for the management of radiation injuries to the rectum have been suggested. These include closure of a fistula by transrectal, transvaginal, transperineal, and transcoccygeal approaches (see Chapters 14 and 24); and resection with restoration of continuity by the abdominosacral procedure, by abdominoanal pull-through, and by coloendoanal anastomosis.[59,117]

Cuthbertson suggests that pull-through resection with delayed anastomosis is the optimal procedure, but his experience

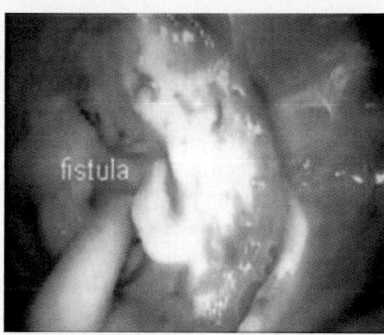

FIGURE 28-46. Endoscopic view through the sigmoidoscope in a patient with a large rectourethral fistula. The urinary catheter can be readily visualized from within the rectum.

is limited to that of 4 patients.[93] Jao and colleagues reported 720 patients from the Mayo Clinic with radiation-induced proctitis, 8.6% of whom required surgical intervention.[180] These 62 individuals underwent a total of 143 operations with eight operative deaths (13%). The morbidity rate was lower after colostomy alone (44%) than after a more aggressive resection (80%). An upper abdominal stoma was felt to be safer than a sigmoid colostomy. A more recent review of the Mayo Clinic experience in treating 51 patients who developed rectourethral fistulas after radiation therapy for prostate cancer was performed by Chrouser and colleagues.[82] The average diameter of the fistulas was 3.2 cm. Conservative management failed to cure any of the patients, with symptomatic relief obtained only by fecal and urinary diversion.

Anseline and colleagues reported the Cleveland Clinic experience of 104 patients with radiation injuries to the rectum as a result of therapy for gynecologic or urologic malignancy.[20] Fifty were treated surgically, and 54 were treated conservatively. The authors concluded that diversion was the safest form of treatment for rectovaginal fistula, rectal stricture, and proctitis that had been unresponsive to medical measures. High rates of morbidity and mortality were recorded in those who underwent resection.

Marks recommends a combined abdominotranssacral reconstruction for the radiation-injured rectum (see Chapter 24).[223] He emphasizes the importance of excising all radiation-injured tissue, performing an anastomosis in normal bowel, mobilizing the splenic flexure, use of ureteral catheters, and obligatory implementation of a diversionary procedure. The author also suggests avoiding retention sutures if at all possible, and instead using delayed primary wound closure or permitting the skin to heal by second intention. He and Mohiudden reviewed their experience with more than 100 patients and noted a very low morbidity and mortality rate, considerably at variance with virtually all other published data.[224] There was not a single instance of a failed intraperitoneal anastomosis, and only 4 of 52 abdominotranssacral anastomoses developed a complication.[224] Lucarotti and colleagues recommend using a coloanal J-reservoir to permit a safer anastomosis with optimal functional results (see Chapter 24).[213]

Cooke and de Moor reported 37 patients with radiation damage to the rectum, 28 of whom had rectovaginal fistulas.[87] Treatment involved resection with restoration of continuity by means of coloanal anastomosis. They noted technical success in all but two individuals with no mortality. Although some patients had impairment of fecal continence, the overwhelming result was favorable. Continued success was evident in a later presentation from the same institution with 59 patients.[88] Faucheron and coworkers (Paris, France) prefer Soave's procedure, having performed this operation in 30 patients with radiation-induced rectal lesions.[117] Others prefer mucosal proctectomy and coloanal anastomosis for radiation stricture, fistula, bleeding, and pain.[9,63,131,255,373]

Lopez and colleagues used a segment of nonirradiated colon for repair of postirradiation rectal stricture.[210] The normal proximal bowel was turned down and anastomosed to the side of the rectum below the site of the injury, creating an end-to-side anastomosis. A proximal anastomosis was effected between the upper colon and the apex of the *U* of the distally rotated bowel. The authors reported successful application of this technique in one patient. A number of papers have been published that attest to the high morbidity of surgery in these individuals as well as to what should be a low threshold on the part of the surgeon for performing fecal diversion.[92,161,188,234]

The perineal approach should be reserved for patients in whom the defect is manageable and are thought to have adequate urinary continence. Dissection is initiated in the perineum and the fistula is divided. Both sides are repaired. This often requires rectal advancement, and then an interposition graft of gracilis muscle, buccal mucosa, or both is placed. Samplaski and colleagues reported on the Cleveland Clinic experience when using the gracilis muscle for rectourethral fistula repair.[305] Eight of their 13 patients had radiation therapy as the cause of the fistula. All had suprapubic catheters in place as well as proximal fecal diversion. Five of the 13 repairs were not successful. Of those deemed a success, 75% had some degree of urinary incontinence, and 3 reported fecal incontinence. Three developed bladder neck contractures.

Vanni and associates reported the Lahey Clinic experience of 74 patients treated with a transperineal repair of the fistulas with a gracilis muscle interposition, with or without a buccal mucosal graft urethral patch.[372] They compared 35 radiated patients to 35 nonradiated individuals. The mean follow-up was 20 months. They found that 100% of the nonradiated fistulas closed, whereas 84% of the radiated patients had achieved closure. All of the radiated patients were able to undergo reversal of the fecal diversion, whereas 31% of the radiated patients required a permanent stoma.

Comment

Intestinal complications of radiation therapy present difficult management problems. My own attitude is to attempt resection for those who are symptomatic when the disease involves primarily the small intestine. Rectal disease with either stricture or fistula formation is more controversial. Care must be taken to identify patients who have the capacity to have adequate functional outcomes if a sphincter-sparing procedure is performed. My tendency is to limit resective sphincter-saving operations to those individuals whose prognosis for long-term survival is good. The surgeon should remember that it is not only the successful application of surgical technique for reestablishing intestinal continuity that is important, but also the subsequent functional results are extremely relevant. The fact is, with a low anastomosis in this group of patients (who often have injury to the sphincter muscle with attendant impairment for bowel control), the functional result may be far less salutary than is a colostomy or ileostomy. Recent advances with gracilis muscle interposition with or without a buccal mucosal flap are promising, but again, those patients with large defects

and severe pain are generally not good candidates, and proximal fecal and urinary diversion may be required. It is important to recognize that fecal diversion without excision of the primary process may not relieve pain symptoms. Therefore, if the patient is in otherwise reasonably good health, the surgeon may wish to consider pelvic exenteration.

▶ VOLVULUS

Sigmoid Volvulus

Sigmoid volvulus is a relatively rare condition that has been recognized since antiquity. Ballantyne noted that the authors of the Ebers Papyrus from ancient Egypt wrote that either the volvulus spontaneously reduced or the sigmoid colon rotted.[33] Detorsion was recognized even then as the requirement for ameliorating the condition. Whether this can be accomplished by medical or by surgical means has been the subject of a considerable body of literature.

In the United States, sigmoid volvulus is a relatively rare cause of intestinal obstruction, whereas in other areas of the world it is the single most common etiology. Ballantyne reported that 30% of intestinal obstructions were caused by sigmoid volvulus in Pakistan, 25% in Brazil, 20% in India, 17% in Poland, and 16% in Russia.[34] High altitude is said to play an important role, but the reason for this is unknown. For example, 230 cases were reported from the Andes region of Bolivia.[23] In the United States, however, the incidence is only approximately 5%. The overall distribution of volvulus at various sites indicates that the sigmoid colon is by far the most commonly involved location (1,400 cases) as compared with the cecum (400 cases), transverse colon (35 cases), and the splenic flexure (4 cases) according to a 1982 publication.[34]

In Ballantyne's report, two different age patterns appear.[34] In countries where sigmoid volvulus is relatively prevalent, the disease is usually seen in middle-aged men. However, in English-speaking countries, the average age is considerably older, and the condition is as likely to occur in either gender. Tegegne has proposed that the differing bowel habits between males and females in developing countries may lead to better regularity in women with worsening constipation in men as they delay defecation for other commitments. Therefore, this leads to irregular emptying in men and fecal overload and an increase in sigmoid volvulus.[359]

Pathogenesis

The pathogenesis of sigmoid volvulus is obscure. Most patients are elderly and have a high incidence of associated medical or psychiatric problems.[17] In this group, chronic constipation is thought to be an important factor.

The condition is associated with an extremely redundant colon, a finding that may be seen in a number of illnesses, such as Chagas' disease, Parkinson's disease, paralytic conditions, ischemic colitis, ulcer disease, and many others.[34] Neurologic problems in particular are frequently seen in association with volvulus. In fact, the high incidence of the condition in institutionalized patients may be more a reflection of the associated neurologic disease than of the fact that the patient happens to reside in such a facility.

An interesting observation is that volvulus is second only to adhesions as the most common cause of intestinal obstruction in *pregnancy*, presumably because a redundant colon is predisposed to torsion and twisting as the uterus raises out of the pelvis.[34,159,211] When volvulus occurs in pregnancy, mortality rates are high. The possibility of volvulus must be considered early in pregnant patients who present with constipation, increased distention, and abdominal pain in order to minimize the risks associated with delay in diagnosis.

Mobilization of the colon coincident with other surgical procedures can predispose to the development of volvulus. For example, this complication may occur following a sling procedure for *rectal prolapse* that is performed without a resection wherein the sigmoid colon may be quite redundant, with fixation at either end of the redundancy (see Chapter 21).

The higher incidence of volvulus in Eastern Europe, India, and Africa is thought to be related to a high-residue diet. The anatomic conditions that predispose to sigmoid volvulus—a long, mobile sigmoid loop with close approximation of the afferent and efferent limbs, creating a short base of mesentery around which axis the volvulus occurs—is found in both Eastern and Western groups of patients.[311] A genetic predisposition has been identified within families and within certain tribes.[254,311]

Signs and Symptoms

Patients with sigmoid volvulus usually present with the characteristic signs and symptoms of colonic obstruction. These include absence of bowel movements, failure to pass flatus, crampy abdominal pain, nausea, and vomiting. Almog and colleagues reported a case of secretory diarrhea and hypokalemia due to intermittent sigmoid volvulus.[11]

Physical examination usually reveals a distended abdomen. Minimal to mild tenderness may be noted, but signs of peritoneal irritation are usually absent unless viability of the bowel is compromised. Rectal examination characteristically demonstrates an empty ampulla. Raveenthiran and coworkers classified the clinical manifestations into two groups: typical and atypical.[287] A typical presentation is acute or fulminant. A sudden onset of severe pain and early vomiting is quite the norm. An indolent presentation, however, represents a slowly progressive onset, with less pain and delayed vomiting. Of course, a recurrent presentation is characterized by return of symptoms and findings after spontaneous or therapeutic detorsion.

Investigations

The plain abdominal x-ray will usually reveal a markedly dilated sigmoid colon and proximal bowel, with relatively minimal gas noted in the rectum (Figure 28-47). Agrez and Cameron reviewed the radiologic findings in 20 patients diagnosed as having a sigmoid volvulus.[5] The standard radiographic feature was that of a distended ahaustral sigmoid loop, the so-called bent inner tube appearance. In analyzing the plain films of 18 individuals found to have sigmoid volvulus, an enlarged ahaustral loop was seen in 11 of them. In the remaining it was not possible to differentiate the distended loop from that of the transverse colon.

Contrast enema examination may demonstrate complete retrograde obstruction at the level of the torsion or may reveal an area of narrowing with proximal dilatation if the obstruction is incomplete or recently reduced (Figure 28-48).

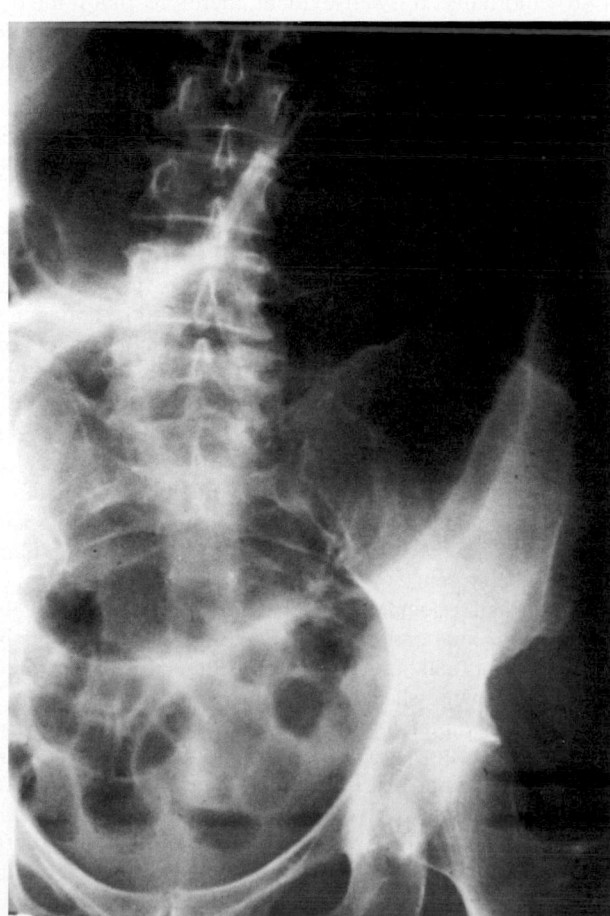

FIGURE 28-47. Sigmoid volvulus. Plain abdominal film reveals massive dilatation of the sigmoid and the so-called bent inner tube appearance. (Courtesy of Hector P. Rodriguez, MD.)

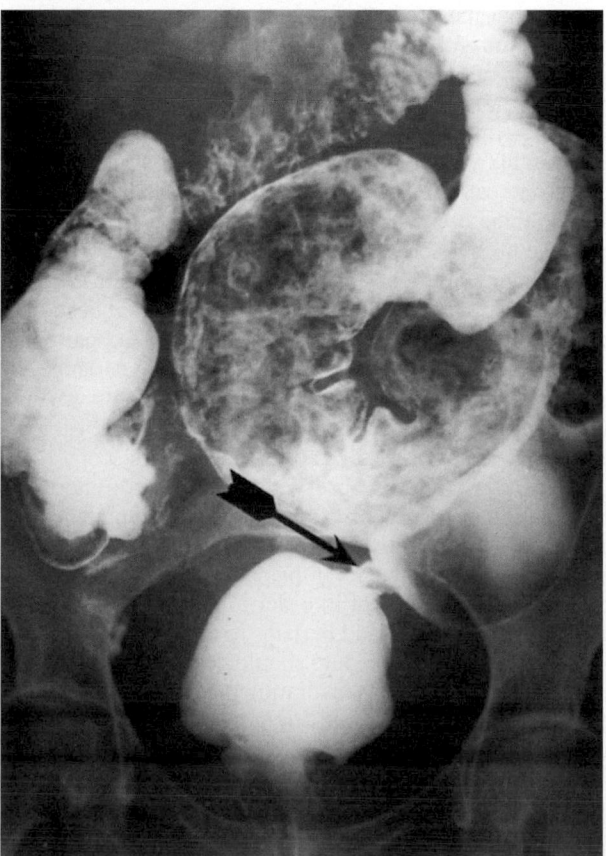

FIGURE 28-48. Sigmoid volvulus. Barium enema reveals a dilated sigmoid loop with a "corkscrew" appearance of the narrowed segment (*arrow*) at the rectosigmoid junction. (Courtesy of Hector P. Rodriguez, MD.)

In the experience of Agrez and Cameron, 10 patients were submitted to barium enema study.[5] In three, there was a probable torsion point; four were definitely diagnostic (e.g., "bird's beak sign" or mucosal spiral pattern), and three had markedly redundant sigmoid loops. None of the barium enema examinations relieved the volvulus.

Endoscopy can be both diagnostic and therapeutic and is discussed below.

Treatment

Ballantyne reviewed the evolution of nonoperative and operative treatment of sigmoid volvulus since the original description from Egyptian antiquity.[33] Suppositories, clysters, enemas, reduction by external manipulation, and a rectal tube have all had their advocates. It was not until the 20th century, however, when laparotomy was employed for the treatment of this condition.

Nonoperative Treatment

Initial management depends on whether the surgeon believes that the bowel is viable or nonviable. In the former circumstance, attempt at reduction should be made by means of proctosigmoidoscopy and insertion of a rectal tube. If the volvulus can be reduced, an explosive discharge of gas and feces will occur. The rectal tube should be left in place, either taped or, ideally, sutured to the buttock for about 48 hours to avoid the possibility of immediate recurrence.

Flexible sigmoidoscopy and colonoscopy have also been successfully employed in the treatment of sigmoid volvulus.[22,134,281,307,340] These techniques have the advantage of permitting evaluation of the viability of a greater area of colonic mucosa, but the procedure must be performed with limited manipulation and especially limited air to minimize the risk of perforation of the distended and edematous bowel.[261] The endoscopist must ensure that he or she enters both the distal point of obstruction and the proximal lumen, thereby fully reducing the volvulus. Intraluminal stenting to prevent early recurrence can be accomplished through the use of flexible plastic tubing or a blunt-ended guidewire.[281,397] An attempt at colonoscopic reduction may be considered if proctosigmoidoscopic manipulation has been unsuccessful. Salim combined percutaneous deflation of the dilated bowel to successfully employ sigmoidoscopic decompression in 20 patients.[304] Tan and colleagues reviewed their 9-year experience with sigmoid volvulus. Ninety percent of the patients were successfully managed with sigmoidoscopic decompression with only one perforation (1.5%) at the time of endoscopy.[356]

If necrotic bowel is observed at the time of endoscopic examination, the surgeon should prepare the patient for an exploratory laparotomy. Proctosigmoidoscopic examination should be undertaken even if the patient has signs and symptoms of nonviable bowel in order to attempt to confirm the extent of involvement and perhaps to establish the diagnosis with certainty. The procedure should be performed, however, with great care to avoid perforating the bowel. The principle of evaluation of the rectum is a requisite before surgery for suspected colorectal pathology because there is no definitive way for one to evaluate the extraperitoneal rectum at the time of laparotomy.

In reviewing almost 600 patients, Ballantyne found that proctosigmoidoscopy and rectal tube insertion were successful in reducing the sigmoid volvulus in 40% of cases, proctosigmoidoscopy alone in 19%, barium enema in 5.4%, and other modalities in approximately 6%.[34] Seventy percent of patients were successfully reduced by some means in the 19 series reviewed by that author. More recent studies generally indicate that if the bowel is viable, one may anticipate successful reduction of the volvulus approximately 90% of the time. Arigbabu and colleagues decompressed 83 consecutive patients with viable bowel by means of colonoscopy.[22] In the U.S. Department of Veterans Affairs database, Grossman and coworkers found that 81% of the 189 patients underwent successful endoscopic decompression,[148] and Chung and associates (Singapore) noted success in 28 of their 29 patients.[83]

Recurrence Following Reduction

Although nonsurgical reduction of the volvulus allows one to avoid an emergency operation, the recurrence rate is very high. In a combined series of 149 patients who were followed after successful reduction, 43% developed a recurrence.[33] There was a mortality rate in excess of 10% in this group. Brothers and colleagues reported that 57% of patients initially treated by endoscopic decompression developed a recurrence.[62] Chung's group found that 12 of their 14 patients who refused operation developed recurrent volvulus at a median of 2.8 months later,[83] whereas the Veterans Administration study noted a 23% recurrence rate.[148] Tan and coworkers examined 71 patients with sigmoid volvulus.[356] Fifty-three (74.6%) had successful reduction, 7 of whom went on to have elective surgery. Forty-six did not undergo operation, and 60.9% (28) of these individuals developed recurrent volvulus. Emergency surgery was associated with a 17.6% mortality. It is self-evident, therefore, that if the patient can possibly undergo an elective operation, this should optimally be performed during the same hospitalization after the bowel and the patient have been adequately prepared.

Operative Management

If one has been unsuccessful in reducing the volvulus, laparotomy is indicated, assuming that the patient can tolerate a laparotomy. The choice of procedure depends on whether the viability of the bowel is compromised. Possible surgical alternatives include resection and anastomosis (total or partial colectomy with or without a proximal colostomy), Hartmann's resection, exteriorization resection, detorsion alone, detorsion with colopexy, and most recently, percutaneous colostomy and percutaneous endoscopic sigmoidopexy.[95,276] Gurel and colleagues used the technique of intraoperative on-table lavage to perform resection and primary anastomosis of the obstructed bowel (see Chapter 24).[152] Others have employed a fixation technique, with or without mesh implantation.[165] Chung and coworkers opine that subtotal colectomy is the preferred approach in the presence of a megacolon or megarectum.[83]

Daniels and associates (Chichester, England) selectively used percutaneous endoscopic colostomy for 14 patients in whom conventional surgery was considered unsafe or inappropriate following successful endoscopic decompression.[95] The procedure is analogous to that of percutaneous endoscopic gastrostomy (PEG). The procedure was carried out under intravenous sedation with a local anesthetic. There were no deaths, but the volvulus recurred in three of eight patients when the tube was removed. Pinedo and Kirberg successfully performed percutaneous colonoscopic sigmoidopexy with the use of T-fasteners for the fixation in two individuals considered unfit for surgery.[276]

Gordon-Weeks and colleagues describe a technique of laparoscopic-assisted endoscopic sigmoidopexy for this condition.[141] They decompress the volvulus endoscopically and then laparoscopically lyse adhesions and approximate the sigmoid colon to the anterior abdominal wall. They place two percutaneous endoscopic colostomy tubes. These tubes fix the sigmoid in place and after 4 to 6 weeks the tubes are removed. In six patients with 10-month follow-up, they reported no leaks or recurrent volvulus. Mullen and associates published a case report on the use of percutaneous endoscopic colostomy for sigmoid volvulus without laparoscopic assistance.[245]

Obviously, if the colon is demonstrated to be nonviable, a resection is indicated. This is undertaken for the same reason and in the same manner that one would perform a resection of a perforated colon for any other condition (diverticulitis, carcinoma). The objective is to remove the focus of sepsis. Whether to perform an anastomosis, a Hartmann's procedure, or one of the other surgical options available is a judgment that each individual surgeon must make. The pros and cons of the different operative approaches are discussed in Chapter 27.

Results
Ballantyne reviewed the experience of 25 American series that included more than 600 patients.[33] Delayed elective resection with primary anastomosis was associated with the lowest mortality rate (8%). Operative mortality, however, in those who underwent resection on an emergency basis was extremely high (at least 25%), irrespective of the method of treatment. When one combines the American experience with that of other countries, it becomes clear that the prognosis of patients with sigmoid volvulus falls into two groups: those with viable bowel and those whose bowel is nonviable. Those with viable bowel had an overall 12.3% operative mortality as compared with an operative mortality of 53% in those with nonviable bowel.[33] The only study to date that has attempted to identify predictors of mortality in patients undergoing surgery for sigmoid volvulus was undertaken by Bac and colleagues.[26] After performing a multivariate analysis, they identified advanced age, delay in admission, and the presence of cardiovascular disease as predictors of mortality.

Ballantyne reported his personal experience of 12 patients with sigmoid volvulus.[32] The two patients who underwent emergency resection both expired, whereas mortality following elective resection was 25%. Pasch and Adams noted a 57% mortality for emergency resection and a 20% mortality rate for elective resection.[270] Bak and Boley, however, reported only a 6% mortality rate for elective resection.[31] Others have found that reduction alone is associated with a lower mortality than resection, but at the cost of a higher incidence of recurrence.[384]

Ryan reported 66 patients with sigmoid volvulus.[301] Emergency operation was required in almost one-half and was associated with a 22% operative mortality rate. The mortality rate with viable colon was twice as high when resection was carried out as when detorsion alone was performed. Because of this observation, Ryan recommends performing only detorsion unless gangrene or perforation require resection. In the report from the Veterans Affairs Medical Centers, the mortality rate was 24% for emergency operations and 6% for elective procedures.[148] Most papers confirm four factors contributing to an adverse outcome: older age, emergency surgery, nonviable bowel, and a history of prior volvulus.[132,135,193,274,368]

Anderson and Lee reported 134 patients with sigmoid volvulus.[15] Rectal decompression was effective in 85%. The best results in individuals who had a nonviable colon were obtained with a Hartmann's resection, although the number in this group was small. Because of the general success of

a resective procedure when viable bowel was found, these authors do not advise detorsion alone. However, they had a limited experience with this approach.

Morrissey and Deitch noted that little attention has been focused on the recurrence rate of sigmoid volvulus following surgical therapy.[243] The authors point out the importance of an associated megacolon with obstruction secondary to the volvulus. Surprisingly, the overall recurrence rate was 36% higher than most would anticipate. This rate varied only slightly according to the operative procedure performed. The authors recommend that a subtotal colectomy should be considered the surgical procedure of choice in those individuals operated on for sigmoid volvulus who have an associated megacolon.[243]

Bhatnagar and Sharma (India) performed an extraperitoneal colostomy (without resection) in 84 patients with nongangrenous sigmoid volvulus.[48] The operative mortality was 9%. There were no recurrences in the 76 patients available for follow-up (median, 6 years).

Comment
My own preference is to perform a limited resection with or without a primary anastomosis, depending on the patient's condition and whether the operation is undertaken on an elective or an emergency basis, and whether the bowel is viable or nonviable. I do not consider detorsion or sigmoidopexy adequate long-term therapy. Certainly when concomitant megacolon is identified with a volvulus, subtotal colectomy should be considered, if the patient will tolerate the somewhat longer procedure. Given the high morbidity and mortality rate seen with surgical management of sigmoid volvulus, continued development of less invasive procedures that do not require general anesthesia or resection is warranted.

Sigmoid Volvulus in Children
Sigmoid volvulus has been infrequently reported in children, with fewer than 93 cases having been published in the English language.[228,287] Extremely rarely, the condition has been identified in association with Hirschsprung's disease or with imperforate anus.[179] Volvulus in children is difficult to diagnose, the course tends to be fulminant, passage of a rectal tube or endoscope may be difficult or impossible, and early operative intervention is more often advised than in adults.[322] Hydrostatic reduction is recommended over endoscopic detorsion because it has a lower rate of perforation.[204]

Ileosigmoid Knotting
Ileosigmoid knotting is unusual in Western countries but is relatively common in Africa, Asia, and the Middle East. The condition is initiated by a loop of ileum wrapping around the base of a redundant sigmoid colon.[13] This generates a closed loop obstruction that requires emergency surgery. The manifestation may be a variant of intestinal malrotation and midgut volvulus.[106] According to Alver and colleagues, as of 1993 the collected series represents 68 patients, constituting 8.8% of 773 cases of sigmoid volvulus.[13] The authors classified the condition into four types according to the active component initiating the knot formation and the direction of rotatory movement. Approximately three-fourths of the patients developed gangrene of the bowel (Figure 28-49). Following resection the mortality rate was 30.9% in this series. Machado reviewed the literature of 280 cases and reported the mortality rate as ranging between 0% and 48%.[220] Mortality is related to the duration of the symptoms

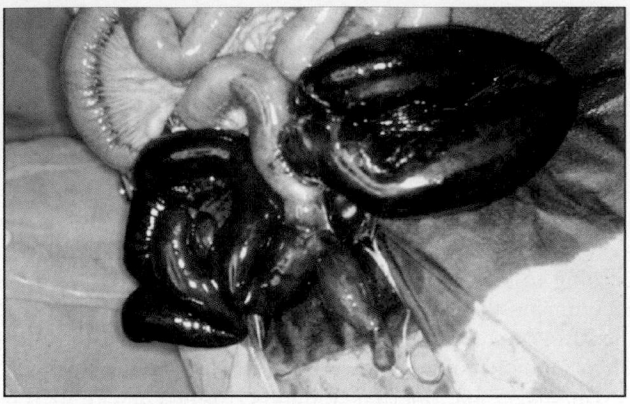

FIGURE 28-49. Gangrenous ileum and sigmoid colon from ileosigmoid knot. (From Machado NO. Ileosigmoid knot: a case report and literature review of 280 cases. *Ann Saudi Med.* 2009;29(5):402–406, with permission.)

and the presence of gangrene and septic shock. When reviewing current literature, gangrene is present 73% to 79% of the time.

Cecal Volvulus

Cecal volvulus is less common than volvulus of the sigmoid colon, representing approximately 25% to 30% of patients with this condition. There is less correlation with geographic location than with sigmoid volvulus, although the two presentations have been known to occur simultaneously.[332] The sine qua non for developing this manifestation is a failure of fusion of the parietal peritoneum to the cecum and ascending colon. Abnormal mobility of the cecum and ascending colon has been estimated to occur in 10% to 20% of the population (Figure 28-50).[295] This predisposes the bowel to twist on its axis (Figure 28-51), to rotate and twist, or to fold upward

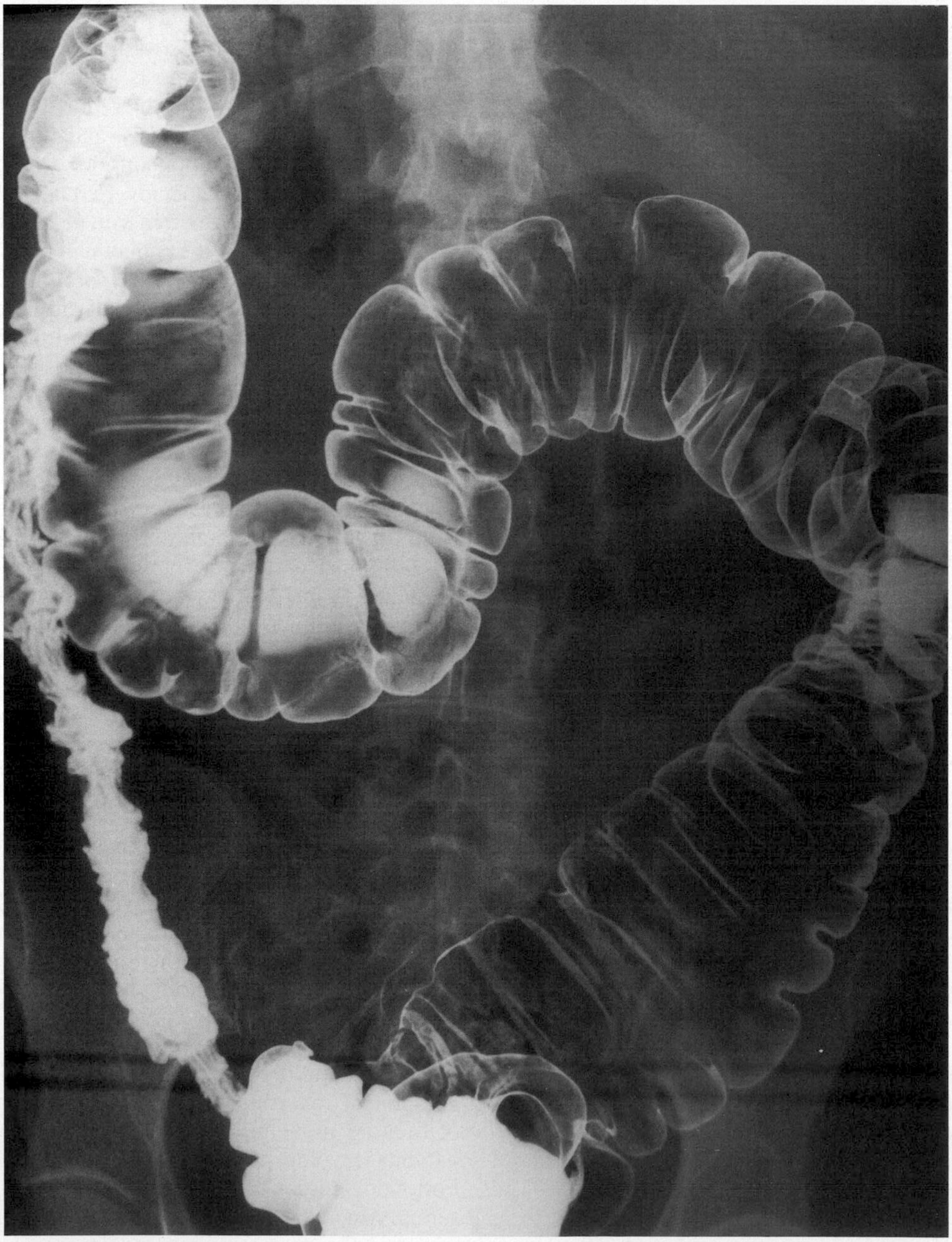

FIGURE 28-50. The mobile cecum and right colon are readily evident on this air-contrast barium enema.

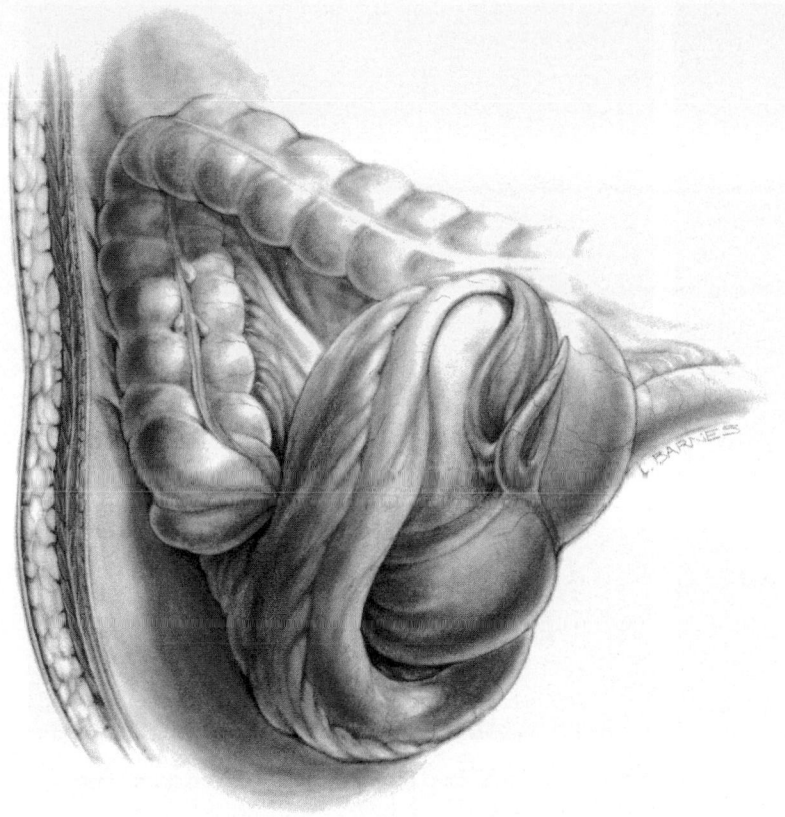

FIGURE 28-51. Cecal volvulus manifested by twisting of the bowel, a consequence of lack of fixation and redundancy.

(cecal bascule) (Figure 28-52). The resultant vascular compromise leads to gangrene and to perforation.

Volvulus of the cecum occurs more frequently in younger patients than does volvulus of the sigmoid. Precipitating causes include distal obstruction, meteorism occurring from unpressurized air travel, pregnancy, prior abdominal operations (adhesions), congenital bands, violent coughing, intermittent positive-pressure breathing, mesenteric adenitis, prolonged constipation, distal obstructing lesion, and colonic atony (adynamic ileus).[119,140,280] An association with jogging has been reported.[282] The simultaneous occurrence of volvulus of the cecum and sigmoid colon has also been documented.[239]

Signs and Symptoms
Abdominal pain is usually the predominant complaint and may be relatively low grade and colicky in nature. Frequently present is abdominal distention, which may be asymmetric, with a mass in the hypogastrium or on the right side. Bowel sounds are usually obstructive. Some patients have more chronic manifestations, with intermittent cramping abdominal pain and distention that usually resolves spontaneously.

Radiologic Studies
Radiologic investigation usually reveals characteristic findings. The cecum and ascending colon can be found in any part of the abdomen, but the most common displacement is into the epigastrium and to the left upper quadrant.[119] An obliquely oriented cecum and ascending colon may be identified extending across the abdominal cavity (Figure 28-53). Classic x-ray findings include a "coffee bean" shape and visible mucosal folds at the site of obstruction (Figure 28-54).[140] Usually, no gas can be seen distal to the point of obstruction. Multiple gas–fluid levels may

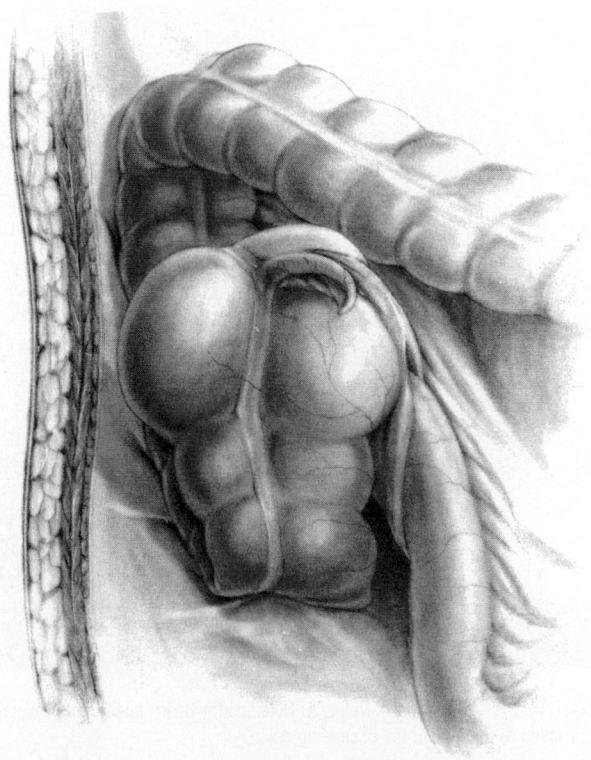

FIGURE 28-52. Cecal bascule. This is a type of volvulus-producing obstruction from a folding of the bowel on itself.

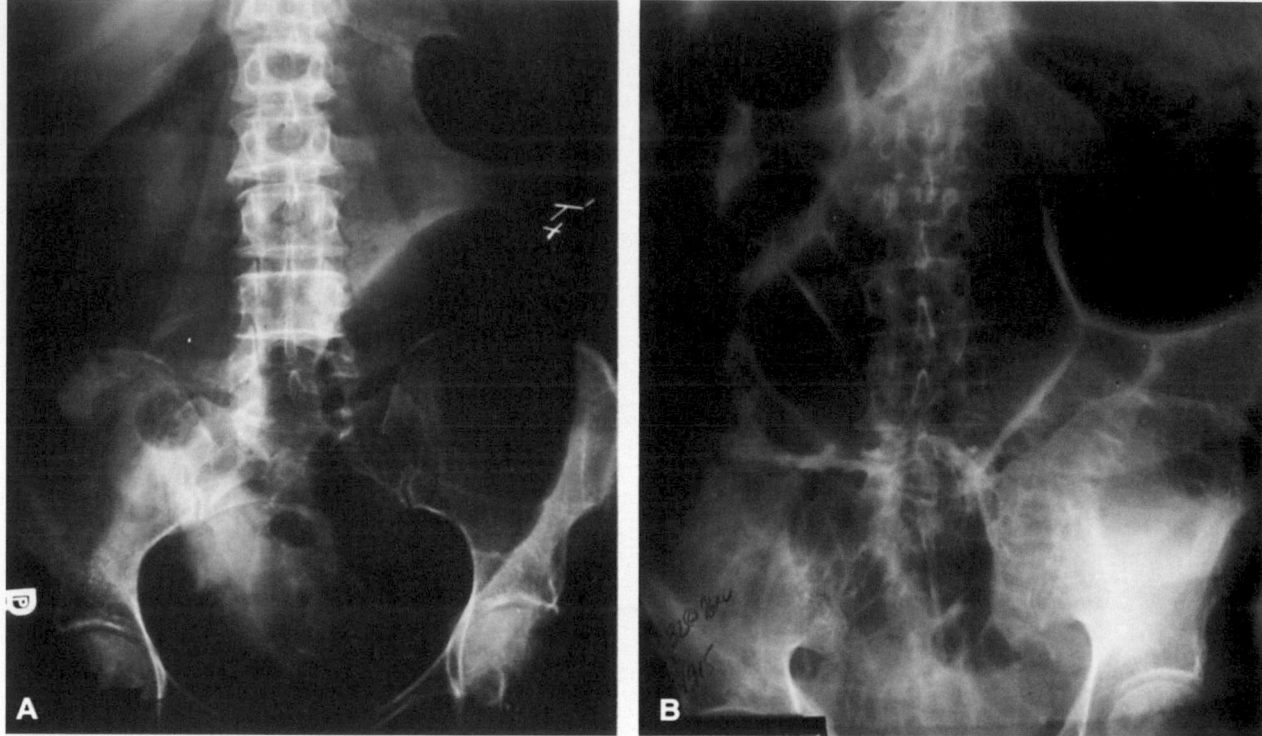

FIGURE 28-53. Cecal bascule. Plane abdominal film demonstrates markedly dilated loop of large bowel projecting to the left upper quadrant. There is no gas in the remainder of the colon. **A:** Without small bowel obstruction. **B:** With small bowel obstruction.

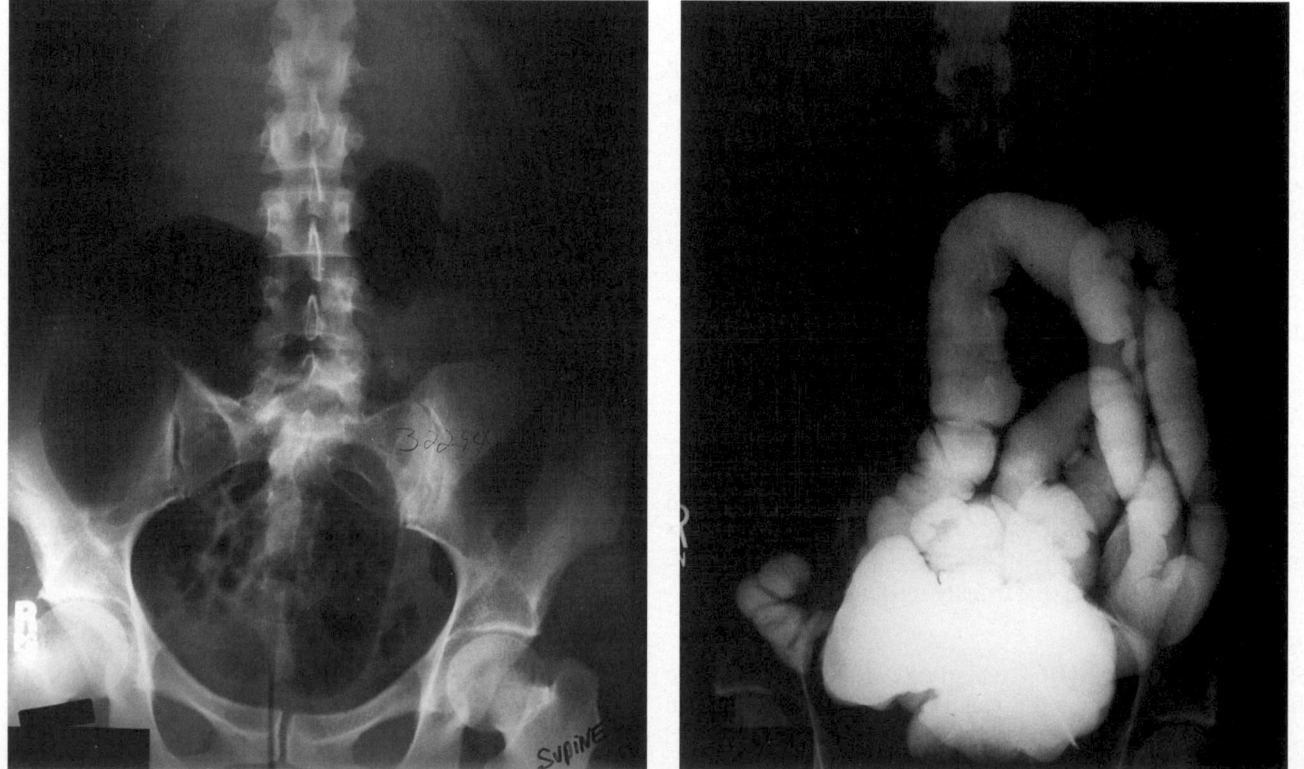

FIGURE 28-54. Cecal volvulus. **A:** Note "coffee bean" appearance on plain abdominal x-ray. **B:** Barium enema shows markedly redundant colon with retrograde obstruction to the flow in the ascending colon.

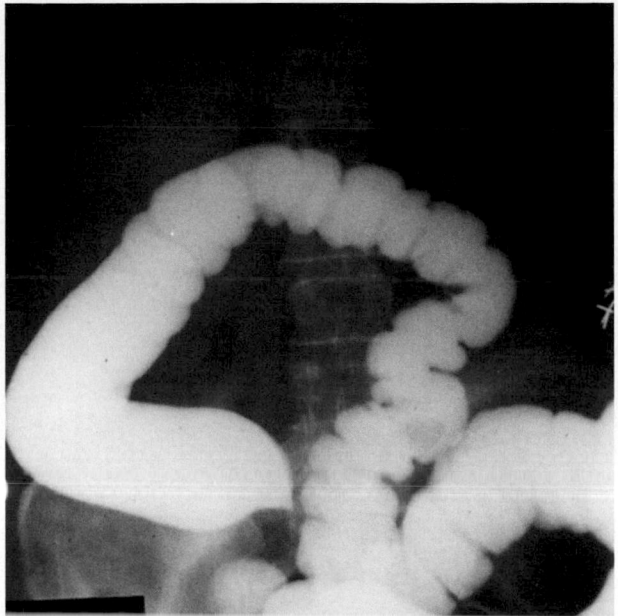

FIGURE 28-55. Cecal volvulus. Barium enema demonstrates obstruction in the proximal ascending colon with "bird's beak" deformity. (Courtesy of Hewitt R. Lang, MD.)

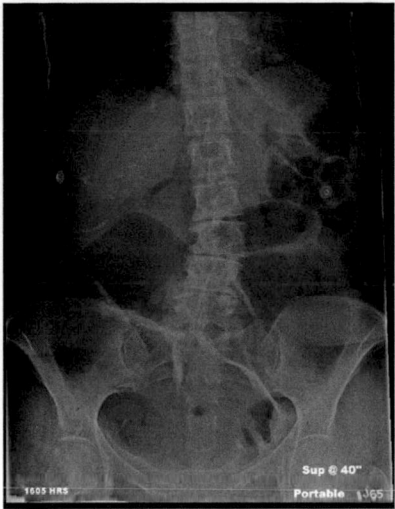

FIGURE 28-56. Plain radiograph of a cecal volvulus with organoaxial torsion.

be noted in the small intestine. Barium enema may reveal the classic bird's beak deformity due to obstruction in the region of the cecum (Figure 28-55). When an organo axial twist occurs, the x-ray shows colonic distention in the left upper and middle abdomen (Figure 28-56).

Treatment

As with the management of sigmoid volvulus, colonoscopy has been successfully employed to reduce volvulus of the cecum. It is important to recognize, however, that unless the procedure is initiated early, persistent efforts are very likely to be more harmful than helpful.[16] Friedman and colleagues failed to reduce the cecal volvulus of any of their 10 patients by this means.[125] In reviewing the literature, Madiba and

Thomson found that endoscopic decompression is often not achievable.[222] Indeed, attempted endoscopic reduction of a cecal bascule may lead to reformation because the point of folding may act as a one-way valve, thereby exacerbating distention and risking perforation of the cecum from insufflation.

Choices of surgical procedures for cecal volvulus without perforation or gangrene include detorsion (with or without appendectomy—Figure 28-57), cecopexy, cecostomy (or a combination of the two), and resection (Figures 28-58, 28-59, and 28-60). Ryan and colleagues suggest another option, that of cecopexy, with the placement of a long (Baker) tube via the rectum to decompress the bowel.[300] This has the theoretical advantages of providing postoperative colonic decompression, minimizing pressure from a full colon on the cecopexy suture line, and avoiding contamination. Laparoscopic cecopexy by placement of anchoring sutures has also been reported.[47,328] Obviously, if the viability of the bowel is compromised or if perforation is present, resection is required.

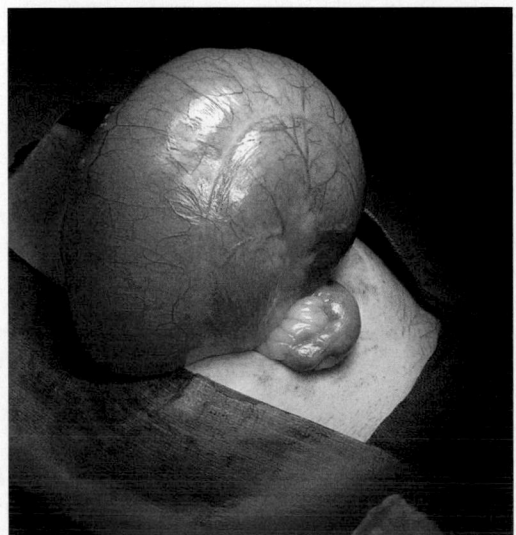
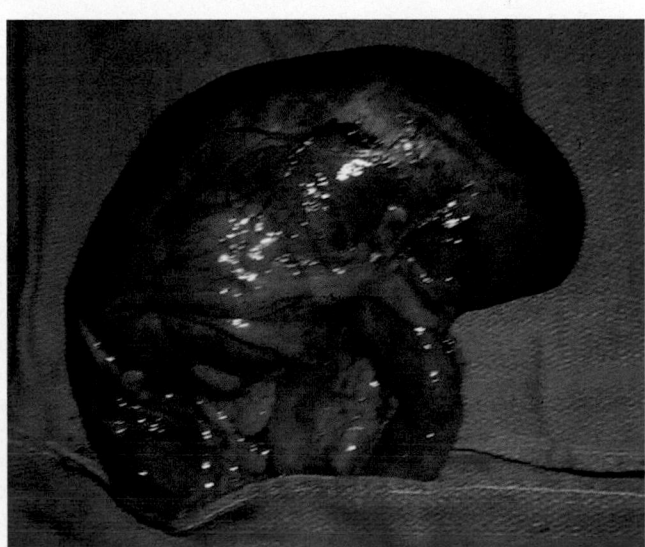

FIGURE 28-57. **A:** Intraoperative view of a cecal volvulus with demonstrably viable bowel. (Courtesy of Scott Fields, MD.) **B:** Operative view of typical cecal bascule.

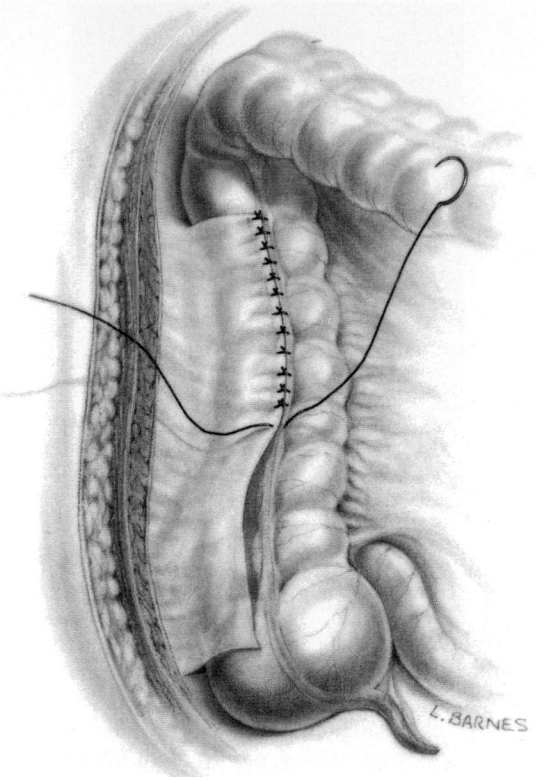

FIGURE 28-58. Cecopexy. An improved method for anchoring the colon is to employ a lateral peritoneal flap. (Adapted from Rogers RL, Harford FJ. Mobile cecum syndrome. *Dis Colon Rectum.* 1984;27(6):399–402.)

Results

Detorsion alone or with appendectomy is generally felt to be associated with a high recurrence rate and is not advocated in any of the contemporary articles on the subject.[71] Interpretation of the results of the other surgical alternatives is

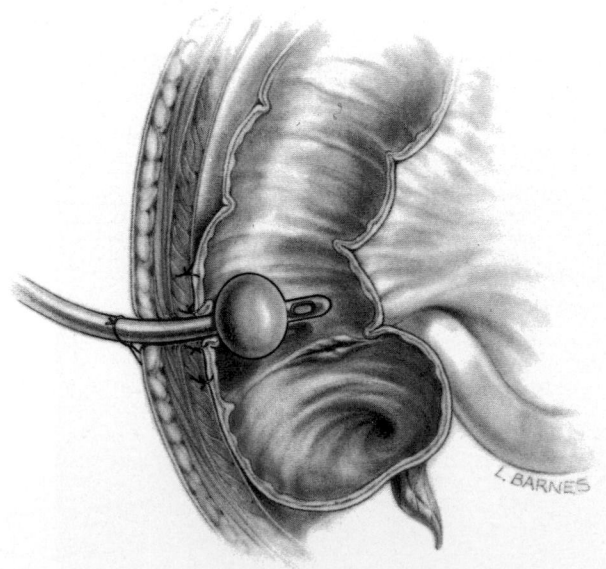

FIGURE 28-59. Tube cecostomy. Cecum is pulled to abdominal wall and anchored with several sutures.

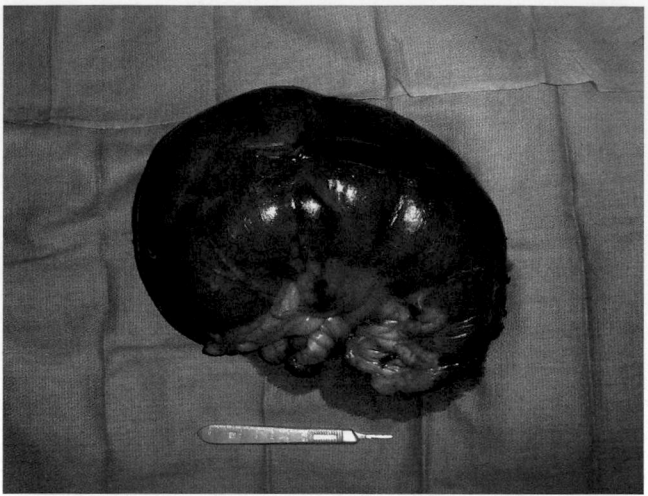

FIGURE 28-60. Resected specimen shown in Figure 28-57A.

somewhat difficult because most papers address mortality and recurrence, but not morbidity.

O'Mara and colleagues reported 50 patients who underwent surgery for cecal volvulus.[257] A variety of operations were performed in the 41 individuals who had no evidence of gangrenous bowel at the time. Four underwent tube cecostomy, with one death. Seven patients underwent resection and primary anastomosis, with no deaths, and 12 underwent detorsion alone, with two operative deaths. Cecopexy was performed on 18 patients, with no deaths. Nine had a gangrenous cecum at the time of surgery; of these individuals, there were three operative deaths (33%). Most series note a high mortality rate in the presence of gangrenous bowel (33% to 55%).[14,15,35]

Cecopexy has the advantage of avoiding potential contamination in unprepared bowel, but the question of recurrence must be addressed. Howard and Catto reported 16 patients with cecal volvulus, 14 of whom underwent a nonresective procedure.[170] In a follow-up averaging 5.6 years, no recurrence was demonstrable. These authors concluded that a resectional operation for viable bowel was unnecessary. Conversely, Todd and Forde, in a review of a number of series, noted that the recurrence rate for cecopexy alone was approximately 28%.[363] There were no recurrences following tube cecostomy, as well as no recurrences following resection, in their search of the literature. These authors, therefore, advocate tube cecostomy as the procedure of choice because it is less hazardous than resection. Depending on whom one reads, an advocate for detorsion alone, cecopexy alone, cecostomy alone, or resection can usually be found in contemporary publications.[284,360]

Anderson and Lee reported 41 cases of acute cecal volvulus.[15] They emphasize that prompt surgery is imperative. Cecopexy was associated with a 25% recurrence rate, but cecopexy with cecostomy was effective in preventing recurrence of symptoms. In the experience of Anderson and Welch with 49 patients having viable bowel, cecopexy alone was followed by a recurrence in 20%, whereas there were no recurrences when cecopexy with cecostomy was performed.[17] The effectiveness of this procedure seems to be due to decompression or venting of the dilated segment, together with fixation in two planes at 90 degrees to each other.[14]

Madiba and Thomson concluded in their review of the subject that resection and anastomosis is the favored option for both gangrenous and viable bowel.[222] The decision of whether to restore intestinal continuity at the time is obviously a matter of surgical judgment. Ostergaard and Halvorsen's outcomes demonstrated higher mortalities from cecostomy (66.6%) and detorsion (14.2%) versus cecal resection (7.2%). Their findings support cecal resection.[262]

Opinion

I have had very few opportunities to perform operations for cecal volvulus. It is evident from the preceding discussion, however, that there is a relatively safe and effective method for the management of the condition when the bowel is viable—cecostomy and cecopexy. But tube cecostomy can be associated with serious potential complications. So I am still inclined to perform resection of the cecum or right colon, a procedure that has been demonstrably successful in individuals requiring an emergency operation for other pathologic entities. Cecopexy whether performed laparoscopically or through an open technique has demonstrated high recurrence rates and should, therefore, be avoided.

Volvulus of the Transverse Colon

The transverse colon is the area of the colon in which volvulus least frequently occurs, representing less than 10% of all volvuli.[395] Usually, supporting tissues and attachments such as gastrocolic omentum, lienocolic, and phrenicocolic ligaments are congenitally absent or may have been surgically removed.[137,393] Another predisposing factor may be an asthenic habitus that permits close approximation of the flexure attachments.[149] As with cecal volvulus, the condition may be associated with distal obstructing lesions, chronic constipation, prior abdominal surgery, or pregnancy. Anderson and colleagues identified 59 cases in the literature and added 7 of their own.[16] The condition is usually not diagnosed preoperatively. The radiologic findings are not truly characteristic except for the demonstration of obvious colonic dilatation. Gangrene was noted in approximately 16% of the patients from the reported series. Without gangrene, surgical mortality is reported to be 6%.[125]

In reviewing the literature, Anderson and associates noted that simple colopexy was followed by a high incidence of recurrence.[16] They, therefore, suggest that at least the transverse colon be resected. This is usually accomplished by means of an extended right hemicolectomy or a partial left colectomy, depending on the presentation. Successful decompression by means of the colonoscope has been described.[182]

Volvulus and Pregnancy

As previously mentioned, one of the predisposing factors for the development of volvuli of all types is pregnancy. Intestinal obstruction during pregnancy is extremely rare, with a reported incidence of one to three per 100,000 pregnancies.[159] However, in this group of patients, 25% of obstructions are caused by volvulus, almost the same incidence as that produced by adhesions.[159,280] The enlarging uterus is believed to create pressure on any redundant or abnormally mobile bowel. Because of the risk not only to the mother, but also to the fetus, urgent surgical intervention is demanded. The diagnosis must always be kept in mind in pregnant patients who present with bowel obstruction. Delay in diagnosis leads to a high mortality rate in these unfortunate women.

References

1. Aalders GJ, Baeten CG, Loffeld RJ. Suturing angiodysplastic lesions of the small intestine. *Surg Gynecol Obstet.* 1991;173(4):323–324.
2. Abbas SM, Bissett IP, Holden A, et al. Clinical variables associated with positive angiographic localization of lower gastrointestinal bleeding. *ANZ J Surg.* 2005;75(11):953–957.
3. Abel ME, Russell TR. Ischemic colitis. Comparison of surgical and nonoperative management. *Dis Colon Rectum.* 1983;26(2):113–115.
4. Adams JT. The barium enema as treatment for massive diverticular bleeding. *Dis Colon Rectum.* 1974;17(4):439–441.
5. Agrez M, Cameron D. Radiology of sigmoid volvulus. *Dis Colon Rectum.* 1981;24(7):510–514.
6. Aitken RJ, Elliot MS. Sigmoid exclusion: a new technique in the management of radiation-induced fistula. *Br J Surg.* 1985;72(9):731–732.
7. Alexander TJ, Dwyer RM. Endoscopic Nd: YAG laser treatment of severe radiation injury of the lower gastrointestinal tract: long-term follow-up. *Gastrointest Endosc.* 1988;34(5):407–411.
8. Alfidi RJ, Esselstyn CD, Tarar R, et al. Recognition and angio-surgical detection of arteriovenous malformations of the bowel. *Ann Surg.* 1971;174(4):573–582.
9. Allen-Mersh TG, Wilson EJ, Hope-Stone HF, et al. The management of late radiation-induced rectal injury after treatment of carcinoma of the uterus. *Surg Gynecol Obstet.* 1987;164(6):521–524.
10. Allison DJ, Hemingway AP, Cunningham DA. Angiography in gastrointestinal bleeding. *Lancet.* 1982;2(8288):30–33.
11. Almog Y, Dranitzki-Elhahlel M, Lax E, et al. Sigmoid volvulus presenting as chronic secretory diarrhea responsive to octreotide. *Am J Gastroenterol.* 1992;87(1):148–150.
12. Al Qahtani AR, Satin R, Stern J, et al. Investigative modalities for massive lower gastrointestinal bleeding. *World J Surg.* 2002;26(5):620–625.
13. Alver O, Oren D, Tireli M, et al. Ileosigmoid knotting in Turkey. Review of 68 cases. *Dis Colon Rectum.* 1993;36(12):1139–1147.
14. Anderson JR, Lee D. Acute caecal volvulus. *Br J Surg.* 1980;67(1):39–41.
15. Anderson JR, Lee D. The management of acute sigmoid volvulus. *Br J Surg.* 1981;68(2):117–120.
16. Anderson JR, Lee D, Taylor TV, et al. Volvulus of the transverse colon. *Br J Surg.* 1981;68(3):179–181.
17. Anderson JR, Welch GH. Acute volvulus of the right colon: an analysis of 69 patients. *World J Surg.* 1986;10(2):336–342.
18. Anderson MJ Sr, Okike N, Spencer RJ. The colonoscope in cecal volvulus: report of three cases. *Dis Colon Rectum.* 1978;21(1):71–74.
19. Angtuaco TL, Reddy SK, Drapkin S, et al. The utility of urgent colonoscopy in the evaluation of acute lower gastrointestinal tract bleeding: a 2-year experience from a single center. *Am J Gastroenterol.* 2001;96(6):1782–1785.
20. Anseline PF, Lavery IC, Fazio VW, et al. Radiation injury of the rectum: evaluation of surgical treatment. *Ann Surg.* 1981;194(5):716–724.
21. Ardigo GJ, Longstreth GF, Weston LA, et al. Passage of a large bowel cast caused by acute ischemia: report of two cases. *Dis Colon Rectum.* 1998;41(6):793–796.
22. Arigbabu AO, Badejo OA, Akinola DO. Colonoscopy in the emergency treatment of colonic volvulus in Nigeria. *Dis Colon Rectum.* 1985;28(11):795–798.
23. Asbun HJ, Castellanos H, Balderrama B, et al. Sigmoid volvulus in the high altitude of the Andes. Review of 230 cases. *Dis Colon Rectum.* 1992;35(4):350–353.
24. Attwood SE, McGrath J, Hill AD, et al. Laparoscopic approach to Meckel's diverticulectomy. *Br J Surg.* 1992;79(3):211.
25. Azimuddin K, Stasik JJ, Rosen L, et al. Dieulafoy's lesion of the anal canal: a new clinical entity. Report of two cases. *Dis Colon Rectum.* 2000;43(3):423–426.
26. Bac B, Aldemir M, Taçyildiz I, et al. Predicting factors for mortality in sigmoid volvulus. *Dicle Tip Dergisi.* 2004;31(2):9–15.
27. Baden JG, Racy DJ, Grist TM. Contrast-enhanced three-dimensional magnetic resonance angiography of the mesenteric vasculature. *Br J Surg.* 1999;10(3):369–375.
28. Baer JW. Pathogenesis of bleeding colonic diverticulosis: new concepts. *CRC Crit Rev Diagn Imaging.* 1978;11(1):1–20.
29. Baer JW. Vascular ectasias. In: Greenbaum EI, ed. *Radiographic Atlas of Colon Disease.* Chicago, IL: Year Book; 1980:623.
30. Baig MK, Lewis M, Stebbing JF, et al. Multiple microaneurysms of the superior hemorrhoidal artery: unusual recurrent massive rectal bleeding: report of a case. *Dis Colon Rectum.* 2003;46(7):978–980.
31. Bak MP, Boley SJ. Sigmoid volvulus in elderly patients. *Am J Surg.* 1986;151(1):71–75.

32. Ballantyne GH. Sigmoid volvulus: high mortality in county hospital patients. *Dis Colon Rectum.* 1981;24(7):515–520.

33. Ballantyne GH. Review of sigmoid volvulus: history and results of treatment. *Dis Colon Rectum.* 1982;25(5):494–501.

34. Ballantyne GH. Review of sigmoid volvulus. Clinical patterns and pathogenesis. *Dis Colon Rectum.* 1982;25(8):823–830.

35. Ballantyne GH, Brandner MD, Beart RW Jr, et al. Volvulus of the colon. Incidence and mortality. *Ann Surg.* 1985;202(1):83–92.

36. Bassiouny HS. Nonoculsive mesenteric ischemia. *Surg Clin North Am.* 1997;77(2):319–326.

37. Baum S. Angiography and the gastrointestinal bleeder. *Radiology.* 1982;143(2):569–572.

38. Baum S, Athanasoulis CA, Waltman AC. Angiographic diagnosis and control of large-bowel bleeding. *Dis Colon Rectum.* 1974;17(4):447–453.

39. Baum S, Athanasoulis CA, Waltman AC, et al. Angiodysplasia of the right colon: a cause of gastrointestinal bleeding. *AJR Am J Roentgenol.* 1977;129(5):789–794.

40. Baum S, Rösch J, Dotter CT, et al. Selective mesenteric arterial infusions in the management of massive diverticular hemorrhage. *N Engl J Med.* 1973;288(24):1269–1272.

41. Bem J, Bem S, Singh A. Use of hyperbaric oxygen chamber in the management of radiation-related complications of the anorectal region: report of two cases and review of the literature. *Dis Colon Rectum.* 2000;43(10):1435–1438.

42. Bender JS, Wiencek RG, Bouwman DL. Morbidity and mortality following total abdominal colectomy for massive lower gastrointestinal bleeding. *Am Surg.* 1991;57(8):536–540.

43. Bentley DE, Richardson JD. The role of tagged red blood cell imaging in the localization of gastrointestinal bleeding. *Arch Surg.* 1991;126(7):821–824.

44. Berken CA. Nd:YAG laser therapy for gastrointestinal bleeding due to radiation colitis. *Am J Gastroenterol.* 1985;80(9):730–731.

45. Berry AR, Campbell WB, Kettlewell MG. Management of major colonic haemorrhage. *Br J Surg.* 1988;75(7):637–640.

46. Berthrong M. Pathologic changes secondary to radiation. *World J Surg.* 1986;10(2):155–170.

47. Bhandarkar DS, Morgan WP. Laparoscopic caecopexy for caecal volvulus. *Br J Surg.* 1995;82(3):323.

48. Bhatnagar BN, Sharma CL. Nonresective alternative for the cure of nongangrenous sigmoid volvulus. *Dis Colon Rectum.* 1998;41(3):381–388.

49. Biswas S, George ML, Leather AJ. Stapled anopexy in the treatment of anal varices: report of a case. *Dis Colon Rectum.* 2003;46(9):1284–1285.

50. Boley SJ, Brandt LJ. Vascular ectasias of the colon—1986. *Dig Dis Sci.* 1986;31(9 suppl):26S–42S.

51. Boley SJ, Brandt LJ, Veith FJ. Ischemic disorders of the intestine. *Curr Probl Surg.* 1978;15(4):1–85.

52. Boley SJ, Feinstein FR, Sammartano R, et al. New concepts in the management of emboli of the superior mesenteric artery. *Surg Gynecol Obstet.* 1981;153(4):561–569.

53. Boley SJ, Sammartano R, Adams A, et al. On the nature and etiology of vascular ectasias of the colon. Degenerative lesions of aging. *Gastroenterology.* 1977;72(4 pt 1):650–660.

54. Boley SJ, Sprayregen S, Sammartano RJ, et al. The pathophysiologic basis for the angiographic signs of vascular ectasias of the colon. *Radiology.* 1974;125(3):615–621.

55. Bradbury AW, Brittenden J, McBride K, et al. Mesenteric ischaemia: a multidisciplinary approach. *Br J Surg.* 1995;82(11):1446–1459.

56. Bradbury AW, Milne AA, Murie JA. Surgical aspects of Behçet's disease. *Br J Surg.* 1994;81(12):1712–1721.

57. Brandt LJ, Katz HJ, Wolf EL, et al. Simulation of colonic carcinoma by ischemia. *Gastroenterology.* 1985;88(5 pt 1):1137–1142.

58. Brewster DC, Franklin DP, Cambria RP, et al. Intestinal ischemia complicating abdominal aortic surgery. *Surgery.* 1991;109(4):447–454.

59. Bricker EM, Kraybill WG, Lopez MJ. Functional results after postirradiation rectal reconstruction. *World J Surg.* 1986;10(2):249–258.

60. Brolin RE, Semmlow JL, Sehonanda A, et al. Comparison of five methods of assessment of intestinal viability. *Surg Gynecol Obstet.* 1989;168(1):6–12.

61. Brookes VS. Meckel's diverticulum in children: a report of 43 cases. *Br J Surg.* 1954;42(171):57–68.

62. Brothers TE, Strodel WE, Eckhauser FE. Endoscopy in colonic volvulus. *Ann Surg.* 1987;206(1):1–4.

63. Browning GG, Varma JS, Smith AN, et al. Late results of mucosal proctectomy and colo-anal sleeve anastomosis for chronic irradiation rectal injury. *Br J Surg.* 1987;74(1):31–34.

64. Brunnler T, Klebl F, Mundorff S, et al. Significance of scintigraphy for the localisation of obscure gastrointestinal bleedings. *World J Gastroenterol.* 2008;14(32):5015–5019.

65. Buchi KN. Endoscopic gastrointestinal laser therapy. *West J Med.* 1985;143(6):751–757.

66. Buchi KN. Radiation proctitis: therapy and prognosis. *JAMA.* 1991;265(9):1180.

67. Buchi KN, Dixon JA. Argon laser treatment of hemorrhagic radiation proctitis. *Gastrointest Endosc.* 1987;33(1):27–30.

68. Bulkley GB, Zuidema GD, Hamilton SR, et al. Intraoperative determination of small intestinal viability following ischemic injury: a prospective, controlled trial of two adjuvant methods (Doppler and fluorescein) compared with standard clinical judgment. *Ann Surg.* 1981;193(5):628–637.

69. Bunker SR, Brown JM, McAuley RJ, et al. Detection of gastrointestinal bleeding sites. Use of in vitro technetium Tc 99m-labeled RBCs. *JAMA.* 1982;247(6):789–792.

70. Bunker SR, Lull RJ, Tanasescu DE, et al. Scintigraphy of gastrointestinal hemorrhage: superiority of 99mTc red blood cells over 99mTc sulfur colloid. *AJR Am J Roentgenol.* 1984;143(3):543–548.

71. Burke JB, Ballantyne GH. Cecal volvulus. Low mortality at a city hospital. *Dis Colon Rectum.* 1984;27(11):737–740.

72. Byrd RL, Cunningham MW, Goldman LI. Nonocclusive ischemic colitis secondary to hemorrhagic shock. *Dis Colon Rectum.* 1987;30(2):116–118.

73. Cappell MS, Lebwohl O. Cessation of recurrent bleeding from gastrointestinal angiodysplasias after aortic valve replacement. *Ann Intern Med.* 1986;105(1):54–57.

74. Carr ND, Pullen BR, Hasleton PS, et al. Microvascular studies in human radiation bowel disease. *Gut.* 1984;25(5):448–454.

75. Cataldo PA, Zarka MA. Formalin instillation for ischemic proctitis with unrelenting hemorrhage: report of a case. *Dis Colon Rectum.* 2000;43(2):261–263.

76. Cazzato IA, Cammarota G, Nista EC, et al. Diagnostic and therapeutic impact of double-balloon enteroscopy (DBE) in a series of 100 patients with suspected small bowel diseases. *Dig Liver Dis.* 2007;30(5):483–487.

77. Cello JP, Wilcox CM. Evaluation and treatment of gastrointestinal tract hemorrhage in patients with AIDS. *Gastroenterol Clin North Am.* 1988;17(3):639–648.

78. Champagne BJ, Darling RC III, Daneshmand M, et al. Outcomes of aggressive surveillance colonoscopy in ruptures abdominal aortic aneurysm. *J Vasc Surg.* 2004;39(4):792–796.

79. Champagne BJ, Lee EC, Valerian B, et al. Incidence of colonic ischemia after repair of ruptured abdominal aortic aneurysm with endograft. *J Am Coll Surg.* 2007;204(4):597–602.

80. Chattopadhyay G, Ray D, Chakravartty S, et al. Formalin instillation for uncontrolled radiation induced haemorrhagic proctitis. *Trop Gastroenterol.* 2010;31(4):291–294.

81. Chaudhry V, Hyser MJ, Gracias VH, et al. Colonoscopy: the initial test for acute lower gastrointestinal bleeding. *Am Surg.* 1998;64(8):723–728.

82. Chrouser KL, Leibovich BC, Sweat SD, et al. Urinary fistulas following external radiation or permanent brachytherapy for the treatment of prostate cancer. *J Urol.* 2005;173(6):1953–1957.

83. Chung YF, Eu KW, Nyam DC, et al. Minimizing recurrence after sigmoid volvulus. *Br J Surg.* 1999;86(2):231–233.

84. Clavien PA, Huber O, Rohner A. Venous mesenteric ischaemia: conservative or surgical treatment? *Lancet.* 1989;2(8653):48.

85. Clavien PA, Muller C, Harder F. Treatment of mesenteric infarction. *Br J Surg.* 1987;74(6):500–503.

86. Colacchio TA, Forde KA, Patsos TJ, et al. Impact of modern diagnostic methods on the management of active rectal bleeding. Ten year experience. *Am J Surg.* 1982;143(5):607–610.

87. Cooke SA, de Moor NG. The surgical treatment of the radiation-damaged rectum. *Br J Surg.* 1981;68(7):488–492.

88. Cooke SA, Wellsted MD. The radiation-damaged rectum: resection with coloanal anastomosis using the endoanal technique. *World J Surg.* 1986;10(2):220–227.

89. Cox JD, Byhardt RW, Wilson JF, et al. Complications of radiation therapy and factors in their prevention. *World J Surg.* 1986;10(2):171–188.

90. Cram AE, Pearlman NW, Jochimsen PR. Surgical management of complications of radiation-injured gut. *Am J Surg.* 1977;133(5):551–553.

91. Cronin CG, Lohan DG, Browne AM, et al. MR enterography in the evaluation of small bowel dilation. *Clin Radiol.* 2009;64(10):1026–1034.

92. Cross MJ, Frazee RC. Surgical treatment of radiation enteritis. *Am Surg.* 1992;58(2):132–135.

93. Cuthbertson AM. Resection and pull-through for rectovaginal fistula. *World J Surg.* 1986;10(2):228–236.

94. Czymek R, Kempf A, Roblick UJ, et al. Surgical treatment concepts for acute lower gastrointestinal bleeding. *J Gastrointest Surg.* 2008;12(12):2212–2220.

95. Daniels IR, Lamparelli MJ, Chave H, et al. Recurrent sigmoid volvulus treated by percutaneous endoscopic colostomy. *Br J Surg.* 2000;87(10):1419.

96. Das A, Ben-Menachem T, Cooper GS, et al. Prediction of outcome in acute lower-gastrointestinal haemorrhage based on an artificial neural network: internal and external validation of a predictive model. *Lancet.* 2003;362(9392):1261–1266.

97. DeBarros J, Rosas L, Cohen J, et al. The changing paradigm for the treatment of colonic hemorrhage: superselective angiographic embolization. *Dis Colon Rectum.* 2002;45(6):802–808.

98. Debus ES, Müller-Hülsbeck S, Kolbel T, et al. Intestinal ischemia. *Int J Colorectal Dis.* 2011;26(9):1087–1097. doi:10.1007/s00384-011-1196-6.

99. de Leusse A, Vahedi K, Edery J, et al. Capsule endoscopy or push enteroscopy for first-line exploration of obscure gastrointestinal bleeding? *Gastroenterology.* 2007;132(3):855–862.

100. Dent OF, Galt E, Chapuis PH, et al. Quality of life in patients undergoing treatment for chronic radiation-induced rectal bleeding. *Br J Surg.* 1998;85(9):1251–1254.

101. Derodra JK, Reidy JF, Jourdan MH. Embolization of superior haemorrhoidal artery in the management of life-threatening rectal bleeding. *Br J Surg.* 1992;79(7):704–705.

102. Desa LA, Ohri SK, Hutton KA, et al. Role of intraoperative enteroscopy in obscure gastrointestinal bleeding of small bowel origin. *Br J Surg.* 1991;78(2):192–195.

103. Devereux DF. Protection from radiation-associated small bowel injury with the aid of an absorbable mesh. *Semin Surg Oncol.* 1986;2(1):17–23.

104. Devereux DF, Thompson D, Sandhaus L, et al. Protection from radiation enteritis by an absorbable polyglycolic acid mesh sling. *Surgery.* 1987;101(2):123–129.

105. Dietz DW, Remzi FH, Fazio VW. Strictureplasty for obstructing small-bowel lesions in diffuse radiation enteritis—successful outcome in five patients. *Dis Colon Rectum.* 2001;44(12):1772–1777.

106. Dietz DW, Walsh RM, Grundfest-Broniatowski S, et al. Intestinal malrotation: a rare but important cause of bowel obstruction in adults. *Dis Colon Rectum.* 2002;45(10):1381–1386.

107. Dieulafoy G. Exulceratio simplex. *Bull Acad Med.* 1898;49:49–84.

108. Dirkx CA, Gerscovich EO. Sonographic findings in methamphetamine-induced ischemic colitis. *J Clin Ultrasound.* 1998;26(9):479–482.

109. Donaldson SS, Jundt S, Ricour C, et al. Radiation enteritis in children. A retrospective review, clinicopathologic correlation, and dietary management. *Cancer.* 1975;35(4):1167–1178.

110. Dusold R, Burke K, Carpentier W, et al. The accuracy of technetium-99m-labeled red cell scintigraphy in localizing gastrointestinal bleeding. *Am J Gastroenterol.* 1994;89(3):345–348.

111. Eisen GM, Dominitz JA, Faigel DO, et al. An annotated algorithmic approach to acute lower gastrointestinal bleeding. *Gastrointest Endosc.* 2001;53(7):859–863.

112. Eisenberg H, Laufer I, Skillman J. Arteriographic diagnosis and management of suspected colonic diverticular hemorrhage. *Gastroenterology.* 1973;64(6):1091–1100.

113. Elder K, Lashner BA, Al Solaiman F. Clinical approach to colonic ischemia. *Cleve Clin J Med.* 2009;76(7):410–409.

114. Endean ED, Barnes SL, Kwolek CJ, et al. Surgical management of thrombotic acute intestinal ischemia. *Ann Surg.* 2001;233(6):801–808.

115. Ernst CB, Hagihara PF, Daugherty ME, et al. Ischemic colitis incidence following abdominal aortic reconstruction: a prospective study. *Surgery.* 1976;80(4):417–421.

116. Fabri PJ. Intestinal ischemia in radiation enteritis. In: Cooperman M, ed. *Intestinal Ischemia.* Mount Kisco, NY: Futura Publishing; 1983:315.

117. Faucheron JL, Rosso R, Tiret E, et al. Soave's procedure: the final sphincter-saving solution for iatrogenic rectal lesions. *Br J Surg.* 1998;85(7):962–964.

118. Fiddian-Green RG, Amelin PM, Herrmann JB, et al. Prediction of the development of sigmoid ischemia on the day of aortic operations. Indirect measurements of intramural pH in the colon. *Arch Surg.* 1986;121(6):654–660.

119. Figiel LS, Figiel SJ. Volvulus of the cecum and right colon. In: Greenbaum EI, ed. *Radiographic Atlas of Colon Disease.* Chicago, IL: Year Book; 1980:637.

120. Flickinger EG, Stanforth AC, Sinar DR, et al. Intraoperative video panendoscopy for diagnosing sites of chronic intestinal bleeding. *Am J Surg.* 1989;157(1):137–144.

121. Forde KA, Lebwohl O, Wolff M, et al. Reversible ischemic colitis—correlation of colonoscopic and pathologic changes. *Am J Gastroenterol.* 1979;72(2):182–185.

122. Foutch PG, Rex DK, Lieberman DA. Prevalence and natural history of colonic angiodysplasia among healthy asymptomatic people. *Am J Gastroenterol.* 1995;90(4):564–567.

123. Foutch PG, Sirak MV Jr. Colonic variceal haemorrhage after endoscopic infection sclerosis of oesophageal varices: a report of three cases. *Am J Gastroenterol.* 1984;79(10):756–760.

124. Friedman G, Sloan WC. Ischemic enteropathy. *Surg Clin North Am.* 1972;52(4):1001–1012.

125. Friedman JD, Odland MD, Bubrick MP. Experience with colonic volvulus. *Dis Colon Rectum.* 1989;32(5):409–416.

126. Furukawa A, Kanasaki S, Kono N, et al. CT diagnosis of acute mesenteric ischemia from various causes. *AJR Am J Roentgenol.* 2009;192(2):408–416.

127. Galland RB, Spencer J. Spontaneous postoperative perforation of previously asymptomatic irradiated bowel. *Br J Surg.* 1985;72(4):285.

128. Galland RB, Spencer J. Surgical management of radiation enteritis. *Surgery.* 1986;99(2):133–139.

129. Galland RB, Spencer J. Natural history and surgical management of radiation enteritis. *Br J Surg.* 1987;74(8):742–747.

130. Gandhi SK, Hanson MM, Vernava AM, et al. Ischemic colitis. *Dis Colon Rectum.* 1996;39(1):88–100.

131. Gazet JC. Parks' coloanal pull-through anastomosis for severe, complicated radiation proctitis. *Dis Colon Rectum.* 1985;28(2):110–114.

132. Geer DA, Arnaud G, Beitler A, et al. Colonic volvulus. The Army Medical Center experience 1983–1987. *Am Surg.* 1991;57(5):295–300.

133. Gennaro AR, Rosemond GP. Colonic diverticula and hemorrhage. *Dis Colon Rectum.* 1973;16(5):409–415.

134. Ghazi A, Shinya H, Wolfe WI. Treatment of volvulus of the colon by colonoscopy. *Ann Surg.* 1976;183(3):263–265.

135. Gibney EJ. Volvulus of the sigmoid colon. *Surg Gynecol Obstet.* 1991;173(3):243–255.

136. Glauser PM, Wermuth P, Cathomas G, et al. Ischemic colitis: clinical presentation, localization in relation to risk factors, and long-term results. *World J Surg.* 2011;35(11):2549–2554. doi:10.1007/s00268-011-1205-5.

137. Goldberg M, Lernau OZ, Mogle P, et al. Volvulus of the splenic flexure of the colon. *Am J Gastroenterol.* 1984;79(9):693–694.

138. Goldberger LE. Diverticular disease of the colon: angiography in diverticular hemorrhage. In: Greenbaum EI, ed. *Radiographic Atlas of Colon Disease.* Chicago, IL: Year Book, 1980:113.

139. Goldberger LE, Bookstein JJ. Transcatheter embolization for treatment of diverticular hemorrhage. *Radiology.* 1977;122(3):613–617.

140. Goosenberg EB, Greenfield SM, Kasama RK. Cecal volvulus update. *Contemp Gastroenterol.* 1991;4:11.

141. Gordon-Weeks AN, Lorenzi B, Lim J, et al. Laparoscopic-assisted endoscopic sigmoidopexy: a new surgical option for sigmoid volvulus. *Dis Colon Rectum.* 2011;54(5):645–647.

142. Gorfine SR. The colon in collagen vascular disease. Paper presented at: The annual meeting American College of Surgeons; September 10, 1996; San Francisco, CA.

143. Granieri R, Mazzula JP, Yarborough GW. Estrogen-progesterone therapy for recurrent gastrointestinal bleeding secondary to gastrointestinal angiodysplasia. *Am J Gastroenterol.* 1988;83(5):556–558.

144. Green BT, Rockey DC, Portwood G, et al. Urgent colonoscopy for evaluation and management of acute lower gastrointestinal hemorrhage: a randomized controlled trial. *Am J Gastroenterol.* 2005;100(11):2395–2402.

145. Greenstein RJ, McElhinney AJ, Reuben D, et al. Colonic vascular ectasias and aortic stenosis: coincidence or causal relationship? *Am J Surg.* 1986;151(3):347–351.

146. Griffiths JD. Surgical anatomy of the blood supply of the distal colon. *Ann R Coll Surg Engl.* 1956;19(4):241–256.

147. Groff WL. Angiodysplasia of the colon. *Dis Colon Rectum.* 1983;26(1):64–67.

148. Grossmann EM, Longo WE, Stratton MD, et al. Sigmoid volvulus in Department of Veterans Affairs Medical Centers. *Dis Colon Rectum.* 2000;43(3):414–418.

149. Gumbs MA, Kashan F, Shumofsky E, et al. Volvulus of the transverse colon. Reports of cases and review of the literature. *Dis Colon Rectum.* 1983;26(12):825–828.

150. Gunderman R, Leef JA, Lipton MJ, et al. Diagnostic imaging and the outcome of acute lower gastrointestinal bleeding. *Acad Radiol.* 1998;5(suppl 2):S303–S305.

151. Gupta N, Longo WE, Vernava AM III. Angiodysplasia of the lower gastrointestinal tract: an entity readily diagnosed by colonoscopy and primarily managed nonoperatively. *Dis Colon Rectum.* 1995;38(9):979–982.

152. Gurel M, Alic B, Bac B, et al. Intraoperative colonic irrigation in the treatment of acute sigmoid volvulus. *Br J Surg.* 1989;76(9):957–958.

153. Gutierrez C, Mariano M, Vander Laan T, et al. The use of technetium-labeled erythrocyte scintigraphy in the evaluation and treatment of lower gastrointestinal hemorrhage. *Am Surg*. 1998;64(10):989–992.

154. Guttormson NL, Bubrick MP. Mortality from ischemic colitis. *Dis Colon Rectum*. 1989;32(6):469–472.

155. Haas EM, Bailey HR, Farragher I. Application of 10 percent formalin for the treatment of radiation-induced hemorrhagic proctitis. *Dis Colon Rectum*. 2007;50(2):213–217.

156. Hagihara PF, Chuang VP, Griffen WO Jr. Arteriovenous malformations of the colon. *Am J Surg*. 1977;133(6):681–687.

157. Hagihara PF, Ernst CB, Griffen WO Jr. Incidence of ischemic colitis following abdominal aortic reconstruction. *Surg Gynecol Obstet*. 1979;149(4):571–573.

158. Handschin AE, Weber M, Weishaupt D, et al. Contrast-enhanced three-dimensional magnetic resonance angiography for visualization of ectopic varices. *Dis Colon Rectum*. 2002;45(11):1541–1544.

159. Harer WB Jr, Harer WB Sr. Volvulus complicating pregnancy and puerperium: report of three cases and review of literature. *Obstet Gynecol*. 1958;12(4):399–406.

160. Harling H, Balslev I. Radical surgical approach to radiation injury of the small bowel. *Dis Colon Rectum*. 1986;29(6):371–373.

161. Harling H, Balslev I. Long-term prognosis of patients with severe radiation enteritis. *Am J Surg*. 1988;155(3):517–519.

162. Harnik IG, Brandt LJ. Mesenteric venous thrombosis. *Vasc Med*. 2010;15(5):407–418.

163. Hatcher PA, Thomson HJ, Ludgate SN, et al. Surgical aspects of intestinal injury due to pelvic radiotherapy. *Ann Surg*. 1985;201(4):470–475.

164. Hayne D, Vaizey CJ, Boulos PB. Anorectal injury following pelvic radiotherapy. *Br J Surg*. 2001;88(8):1037–1048.

165. Hellman AA, Cramer WO. Mesh fixation of the mesentery for treatment of volvulus and recurrent stomal prolapse. *Surg Gynecol Obstet*. 1988;167(3):249–250.

166. Hemingway AP, Allison DJ. Angiodysplasia and Meckel's diverticulum: a congenital association? *Br J Surg*. 1982;69(8):493–496.

167. Höchter W, Weingart J, Kühner W, et al. Angiodysplasia in the colon and rectum. Endoscopic morphology, localisation and frequency. *Endoscopy*. 1985;17(5):182–185.

168. Hokama A, Uehara T, Nakayoshi T, et al. Utility of endoscopic hemoclipping for colonic diverticular bleeding. *Am J Gastroenterol*. 1997;92(3):543–546.

169. Horton KM, Fishman EK. Multidetector CT angiography in the diagnosis of mesenteric ischemia. *Radiol Clin North Am*. 2007;45(2):275–288.

170. Howard RS, Catto J. Cecal volvulus. A case for nonresectional therapy. *Arch Surg*. 1980;115(3):273–277.

171. Hunter JG, Bowers JH, Burt RW, et al. Lasers in endoscopic gastrointestinal surgery. *Am J Surg*. 1984;148(6):736–741.

172. Hunter JM, Pezim ME. Limited value of technetium 99m-labeled red cell scintigraphy in localization of lower gastrointestinal bleeding. *Am J Surg*. 1990;159(5):504–506.

173. Iida M, Kobayashi H, Matsumoto T, et al. Postoperative recurrence in patients with intestinal Behçet's disease. *Dis Colon Rectum*. 1994; 37(1):16–21.

174. Iredale JP, Ridings P, McGinn FP, et al. Familial and idiopathic colonic varices: an unusual cause of lower gastrointestinal haemorrhage. *Gut*. 1992;33(9):1285–1288.

175. Isbister WH, Pease CW, Delahunt B. Colonic varices. Report of a case. *Dis Colon Rectum*. 1989;32(6):524–527.

176. Iwashita A, Yao T, Schlemper RJ, et al. Mesenteric phlebosclerosis: a new disease entity causing ischemic colitis. *Dis Colon Rectum*. 2003;46(2):209–220.

177. Jablonski M, Putzki H, Heymann H. Necrosis of the ascending colon in chronic hemodialysis patients. Report of three cases. *Dis Colon Rectum*. 1987;30(8):623–625.

178. Jaeckle T, Stuber G, Hoffmann MH, et al. Acute gastrointestinal bleeding: value of MDCT. *Abdom Imaging*. 2008;33(3):285–293.

179. Janik JS, Humphrey R, Nagaraj HS. Sigmoid volvulus in a neonate with imperforate anus. *J Pediatr Surg*. 1983;18(5):636–638.

180. Jao SW, Beart RW Jr, Gunderson LL. Surgical treatment of radiation injuries of the colon and rectum. *Am J Surg*. 1986;151(2):272–277.

181. Jensen DM, Machicado GA, Jutabha R, et al. Urgent colonoscopy for the diagnosis and treatment of severe diverticular hemorrhage. *N Engl J Med*. 2000;342(2):78–82.

182. Joergensen K, Kronborg O. The colonoscope in volvulus of the transverse colon. *Dis Colon Rectum*. 1980;23(5):357–358.

183. Johnston MJ, Robertson GM, Frizelle FA. Management of late complications of pelvic radiation in the rectum and anus: a review. *Dis Colon Rectum*. 2003;46(2):247–259.

184. Karamanolis G, Triantafyllou K, Tsiamoulos Z, et al. Argon plasma coagulation has long lasting therapeutic effect in patients with chronic radiation proctitis. *Endoscopy*. 2009;41(6):529–531.

185. Khanna A, Ognibene SJ, Koniaris LG. Embolization as first-line therapy for diverticulosis-related massive lower gastrointestinal bleeding: evidence from a meta-analysis. *J Gastrointest Surg*. 2005;9(3):343–352.

186. Kim HM, Kim YJ, Kim HJ, et al. A pilot study of capsule endoscopy for the diagnosis of radiation enteritis. *Hepatogastroenterology*. 2011;58(106):459–464.

187. Kim MW, Hundahl SA, Dang CR, et al. Ischemic colitis after aortic aneurysmectomy. *Am J Surg*. 1983;145(3):392–394.

188. Kimose HH, Fischer L, Spjeldnaes N, et al. Late radiation injury of the colon and rectum. Surgical management and outcome. *Dis Colon Rectum*. 1989;32(8):684–689.

189. Kinsella TJ, Bloomer WD. Tolerance of the intestine to radiation therapy. *Surg Gynecol Obstet*. 1980;151(2):273–284.

190. Klein HM, Lensing R, Klosterhalfen B, et al. Diagnostic imaging of mesenteric infarction. *Radiology*. 1995;197(1):79–82.

191. Kurian A, Suryadevara S, Ramaraju D, et al. In-hopsital and 6 month mortality rates after open elective vs open emergent colectomy in patients older than 80 years. *Dis Colon Rectum*. 2011;54(4):467–471.

192. Kusumoto H, Yoshida M, Takahashi I, et al. Complications and diagnosis of Meckel's diverticulum in 776 patients. *Am J Surg*. 1992;164(4):382–383.

193. Kuzu MA, Aşlar AK, Soran A, et al. Emergent resection for acute sigmoid volvulus: results of 106 consecutive cases. *Dis Colon Rectum*. 2002;45(8):1085–1090.

194. Laine L, Shah A. Randomized trial of urgent vs. elective colonoscopy in patients hospitalized with lower GI bleeding. *Am J Gastroenterol*. 2010;105:2636–2641.

195. Landreneau RJ, Fry WJ. The right colon as a target organ of nonocclusive mesenteric ischemia. Case report and review of the literature. *Arch Surg*. 1990;125(5):591–594.

196. Lara LF, Bloomfeld RS, Pineau BC. The rate of lesions found within reach of esophagogastroduodenoscopy during push enteroscopy depends on the type of obscure gastrointestinal bleeding. *Endoscopy*. 2005;37(8):745–750.

197. Lau WY, Yuen WK, Chu KW, et al. Obscure bleeding in the gastrointestinal tract originating in the small intestine. *Surg Gynecol Obstet*. 1992;174(2):119–124.

198. Launer DP, Miscall BG, Beil AR Jr. Colorectal infarction following resection of abdominal aortic aneurysms. *Dis Colon Rectum*. 1978;21(8):613–617.

199. Lavery IC, Steiger E, Fazio VW. Home parenteral nutrition in management of patients with severe radiation enteritis. *Dis Colon Rectum*. 1980;23(2):91–93.

200. Lee J, Lai MW, Chen CC, et al. Red blood cell scintigraphy in children with acute massive gastrointestinal bleeding. *Pediatr Int*. 2008;50(2):199–203.

201. Lefevre JH, Amiot A, Joly F, et al. Risk of recurrence after surgery for chronic radiation enteritis. *Br J Surg*. 2011;98(12):1792–1797. doi:10.1002/bjs.7655.

202. Leitman IM, Paull DE, Shires GT III. Evaluation and management of massive lower gastrointestinal hemorrhage. *Ann Surg*. 1989;209(2):175–180.

203. Levitsky J, Hong JJ, Jani AB, et al. Oral vitamin a therapy for a patient with a severely symptomatic postradiation anal ulceration: report of a case. *Dis Colon Rectum*. 2003;46(5):679–682.

204. Levsky JM, Den EI, DuBrow RA, et al. CT findings of sigmoid volvulus. *AJR Am J Roentgenol*. 2010;194(1):136–143.

205. Levy PJ, Krausz MM, Manny J. Acute mesenteric ischemia: improved results—a retrospective analysis of ninety-two patients. *Surgery*. 1990;107(4):372–380.

206. Levy R, Barto W, Gani J. Retrospective study of the utility of nuclear scintigraphic-labelled red cell scanning for lower gastrointestinal bleeding. *ANZ J Surg*. 2003;73(4):205–209.

207. Lindsey I, Farmer CR, Cunningham IG. Subtotal colectomy and cecosigmoid anastomosis for colonic systemic sclerosis: report of a case and review of the literature. *Dis Colon Rectum*. 2003;46(12):1706–1711.

208. Longo WE, Ballantyne GH, Gusberg RJ. Ischemic colitis: patterns and prognosis. *Dis Colon Rectum*. 1992;35(8):726–730.

209. Longo WE, Ward D, Vernava AM III, et al. Outcome of patients with total colonic ischemia. *Dis Colon Rectum*. 1997;40(12):1448–1454.

210. Lopez MJ, Kraybill WG, Johnston WD, et al. Postirradiation reconstruction of the rectum in a male. *Surg Gynecol Obstet*. 1982;155(1):67–71.

211. Lord SA, Boswell WC, Hungerpiller JC. Sigmoid volvulus in pregnancy. *Am Surg*. 1996;62(5):380–382.

212. Love JW. The syndrome of calcific aortic stenosis and gastrointestinal bleeding: resolution following aortic valve replacement. *J Thorac Cardiovasc Surg*. 1982;83(5):779–783.

213. Lucarotti ME, Mountford RA, Bartolo DC. Surgical management of intestinal radiation injury. *Dis Colon Rectum*. 1991;34(10):865–869.

214. Luchtefeld MA, Senagore AJ, Szomstein M, et al. Evaluation of transarterial embolization for lower gastrointestinal bleeding. *Dis Colon Rectum*. 2000;43(4):532–534.

215. Lüdtke FE, Mende V, Köhler H, et al. Incidence and frequency or complications and management of Meckel's diverticulum. *Surg Gynecol Obstet*. 1989;169(6):537–542.

216. Luna-Pérez P, Rodríguez-Ramírez SE. Formalin instillation for refractory radiation-induced hemorrhagic proctitis. *J Surg Oncol*. 2002;80(1):41–44.

217. Luzar MJ. Connective tissue diseases. In: Cooperman M, ed. *Intestinal Ischemia*. Mount Kisco, NY: Futura Publishing; 1983:391.

218. Luzar MJ. Systemic vasculitis. In: Cooperman M, ed. *Intestinal Ischemia*. Mount Kisco, NY: Futura Publishing; 1983:355.

219. Ma CK, Padda H, Pace EH, et al. Submucosal arterial malformation of the colon with massive hemorrhage. Report of a case. *Dis Colon Rectum*. 1989;32(2):149–152.

220. Machado NO. Ileosigmoid knot: a case report and literature review of 280 cases. *Ann Saudi Med*. 2009;29(5):402–406.

221. Mackey WC, Dineen P. A fifty year experience with Meckel's diverticulum. *Surg Gynecol Obstet*. 1983;156(1):56–64.

222. Madiba TE, Thomson SR. The management of cecal volvulus. *Dis Colon Rectum*. 2002;45(2):264–267.

223. Marks G. Combined abdominotranssacral reconstruction of the radiation-injured rectum. *Am J Surg*. 1976;131(1):54–59.

224. Marks G, Mohiudden M. The surgical management of the radiation-injured intestine. *Surg Clin North Am*. 1983;63(1):81–96.

225. Marston A, Pheils MT, Thomas ML, et al. Ischaemic colitis. *Gut*. 1966;7(1):1–15.

226. Matolo NM, Link DP. Selective embolization for control of gastrointestinal hemorrhage. *Am J Surg*. 1979;138(6):840–844.

227. May A, Nachbar L, Schneider M, et al. Prospective comparison of push enteroscopy and push-and-pull enteroscopy in patients with suspected small-bowel bleeding. *Am J Gastroenterol*. 2006;101(9):2016–2024.

228. McCalla TH, Arensman RM, Falterman KW. Sigmoid volvulus in children. *Am Surg*. 1985;51(9):514–519.

229. McDonald ML, Farnell MB, Stanson AW, et al. Preoperative highly selective catheter localization of occult small-intestinal hemorrhage with methylene blue dye. *Arch Surg*. 1995;130(1):106–108.

230. Meckel JF. Ueber die Divertikel am Darmkanal. *Arch die Physiol*. 1809;9:421–453.

231. Medina C, Vilaseca J, Videla S, et al. Outcome of patients with ischemic colitis: review of fifty-three cases. *Dis Colon Rectum*. 2004;47(2):180–184.

232. Mehdizadeh S, Ross A, Gerson L, et al. What is the learning curve associated with double-balloon enteroscopy? Technical details and early experience in 6 U.S. tertiary care centers. *Gastrointest Endosc*. 2006;64(5):740–750.

233. Metyas SK, Mithani VK, Tempera P. Dieulafoy's lesion, a rare cause of lower gastrointestinal hemorrhage. *Hosp Physician*. 2001;37(9):41–45.

234. Miholic J, Schwarz C, Moeschl P. Surgical therapy of radiation-induced lesions of the colon and rectum. *Am J Surg*. 1988;155(6):761–764.

235. Miller MD, Johnsrude IS, Jackson DC. Improved technique for transcatheter embolization of arteries. *AJR Am J Roentgenol*. 1978;180(1):183–184.

236. Mitchell KM, Valentine RJ. Inferior mesenteric artery reimplantation does not guarantee colon viability in aortic surgery. *J Am Coll Surg*. 2002;194(2):151–155.

237. Montoro MA, Brandt LJ, Santolaria S, et al. Clinical patterns and outcomes of ischemic colitis: results of the Working Group for the Study of Ischemic Colitis in Spain (CIE Study). *Scand J Gastroenterol*. 2001;46(2):236–246.

238. Moore JD, Thompson NW, Appleman HD, et al. Arteriovenous malformations of the gastrointestinal tract. *Arch Surg*. 1976;111(4):381–389.

239. Moore JH, Cintron JR, Duarte B, et al. Synchronous cecal and sigmoid volvulus. Report of a case. *Dis Colon Rectum*. 1992;35(8):803–805.

240. Morgenstern L. Surgical aspects of radiation enteropathy. *Surg Rounds*. 1985;8:60–67.

241. Morgenstern L, Hart M, Lugo D, et al. Changing aspects of radiation enteropathy. *Arch Surg*. 1985;120(11):1225–1228.

242. Morgenstern L, Thompson R, Friedman NB. The modern enigma of radiation enteropathy: sequelae and solutions. *Am J Surg*. 1977;134(1):166–172.

243. Morrissey TB, Deitch EA. Recurrence of sigmoid volvulus after surgical intervention. *Am Surg*. 1994;60(5):329–331.

244. Moshkowitz M, Arber N, Amir N, et al. Success of estrogen-progesterone therapy in long-standing bleeding gastrointestinal angiodysplasia. Report of a case. *Dis Colon Rectum*. 1993;36(2):194–196.

245. Mullen R, Church NI, Yalamarthi S. Volvulus of the sigmoid colon treated by percutaneous endoscopic colostomy. *Surg Laparoscopic Endosc Percutan Tech*. 2009;19(2):e64–e66.

246. Nakada T, Kubota Y, Sasagawa I, et al. Therapeutic experience of hyperbaric oxygenation in radiation colitis. Report of a case. *Dis Colon Rectum*. 1993;36(10):962–965.

247. Nakamura M, Niwa Y, Ohmiya N, et al. Preliminary comparison of capsule endoscopy and double-balloon enteroscopy in patients with suspected small-bowel bleeding. *Endoscopy*. 2006;38(1):59–66.

248. Nelson RL, Briley S, Schuler JJ, et al. Acute ischemia proctitis. Report of six cases. *Dis Colon Rectum*. 1992;35(4):375–380.

249. Nelson RL, Schuler JJ. Ischemic proctitis. *Surg Gynecol Obstet*. 1982;154(1):27–33.

250. Ng DA, Opelka FG, Beck DE, et al. Predictive value of technetium Tc 99m-labeled red blood cell scintigraphy for positive angiogram in massive lower gastrointestinal hemorrhage. *Dis Colon Rectum*. 1997;40(4):471–477.

251. Nguyen NP, Antoine JE, Dutta S, et al. Current concepts in radiation enteritis and implications for future clinical trials. *Cancer*. 2002;95(5):1151–1163.

252. Nicholson ML, Neoptolemos JP, Sharp JF, et al. Localization of lower gastrointestinal bleeding using in vivo technetium-99m-labelled red blood cell scintigraphy. *Br J Surg*. 1989;76(4):358–361.

253. Noer RJ, Hamilton JE, Williams DJ, et al. Rectal hemorrhage: moderate and severe. *Ann Surg*. 1962;155:794–805.

254. Northeast AD, Dennison AR, Lee EG. Sigmoid volvulus: new thoughts on the epidemiology. *Dis Colon Rectum*. 1984;27(4):260–261.

255. Nowacki MP, Szawlowski AW, Borkowski A. Parks' coloanal sleeve anastomosis for treatment of postirradiation rectovaginal fistula. *Dis Colon Rectum*. 1986;29(12):817–820.

256. O'Connor JJ. Argon laser treatment of radiation enteritis. *Arch Surg*. 1989;124:749.

257. O'Mara CS, Wilson TH Jr, Stonesifer GL, et al. Cecal volvulus: analysis of 50 patients with long-term follow-up. *Ann Surg*. 1979;189(6):724–731.

258. Ohyama Y, Sakurai Y, Ito M, et al. Analysis of urgent colonoscopy for lower gastrointestinal tract bleeding. *Digestion*. 2000;61(3):189–192.

259. Olds GD, Cooper GS, Chak A, et al. The yield of bleeding scans in acute lower gastrointestinal hemorrhage. *J Clin Gastroenterol*. 2005;39(4):273–277.

260. Orchard JL, Mehta R, Khan AH. The use of colonoscopy in the treatment of colonic volvulus: three cases and review of the literature. *Am J Gastroenterol*. 1984;79(11):864–867.

261. Orecchia PM, Hensley EK, McDonald PT, et al. Localization of lower gastrointestinal hemorrhage. Experience with red blood cells labeled in vitro with technetium Tc 99m. *Arch Surg*. 1985;120(5):621–624.

262. Ostergaard E, Halvorsen JF. Volvulus of the caecum. An evaluation of various surgical procedures. *Acta Chir Scand*. 1990:156(9):629–631.

263. Papa MZ, Shiloni E, McDonald HD. Total colon necrosis. A catastrophic complication of systemic lupus erythematosus. *Dis Colon Rectum*. 1986;29(9):576–578.

264. Pardoll P, Neubrand S. Injection control of colonic hemorrhage with hypertonic saline-epinephrine injection. *Am J Gastroenterol*. 1989;84:1193.

265. Parikh S, Hughes C, Salvati EP, et al. Treatment of hemorrhagic radiation proctitis with 4 percent formalin. *Dis Colon Rectum*. 2003;46(5):596–600.

266. Parish KL, Chapman WC, Williams LF Jr. Ischemic colitis. An ever-changing spectrum? *Am Surg*. 1991;57(2):118–121.

267. Park WM, Gloviczki P, Cherry KJ Jr, et al. Contemporary management of acute mesenteric ischemia: factors associated with survival. *J Vasc Surg*. 2002;35(3):445–452.

268. Parkes BM, Obeid FN, Sorensen VJ, et al. The management of massive lower gastrointestinal bleeding. *Am Surg*. 1993;59(10):676–678.

269. Parks TG. Ischaemic disease of the colon. *Coloproctology*. 1980;4:213.

270. Pasch AR, Adams JT. Acute volvulus of the sigmoid colon: current management. *Cont Surg*. 1985;26:65–68.

271. Patel A, Boley SJ. Vascular ectasias of the colon. *Surg Rounds*. 1990;7:25.

272. Paterno F, McGillicuddy EA, Schuster KM, et al. Ischemic colitis: risk factors for eventual surgery. *Am J Surg*. 2010;200(5):646–650.

273. Pennoyer WP, Vignati PV, Cohen JL. Mesenteric angiography for lower gastrointestinal hemorrhage: are there predictors for a positive study? *Dis Colon Rectum*. 1997;40(9):1014–1018.

274. Peoples JB, McCafferty JC, Scher KS. Operative therapy for sigmoid volvulus. Identification of risk factors affecting outcome. *Dis Colon Rectum*. 1990;33(8):643–646.

275. Petrini JL Jr. Endoscopic therapy for gastrointestinal bleeding. *Postgrad Med*. 1988;84(2):239–245.

276. Pinedo G, Kirberg A. Percutaneous endoscopic sigmoidopexy in sigmoid volvulus with T-fasteners: report of two cases. *Dis Colon Rectum*. 2001;44(12):1867–1869.

277. Pinto A, Fidalgo P, Cravo M, et al. Short chain fatty acids are effective in short-term treatment of chronic radiation proctitis: randomized, double-blind, controlled trial. *Dis Colon Rectum.* 1999;42(6):788–795.

278. Poeze M, Froon AHM, Greve JW, et al. D-lactate as an early marker of intestinal ischaemia after ruptured abdominal aortic aneurysm repair. *Br J Surg.* 1998;85(9):1221–1224.

279. Potter GD, Sellin JH. Lower gastrointestinal bleeding. *Gastroenterol Clin North Am.* 1988;17(2):341–356.

280. Pratt AT, Donaldson RC, Evertson LR, et al. Cecal volvulus in pregnancy. *Obstet Gynecol.* 1981;57(6 suppl):37S–40S.

281. Procaccino J, Labow SB. Transcolonoscopic decompression of sigmoid volvulus. *Dis Colon Rectum.* 1989;32(4):349–350.

282. Pruett TL, Wilkins ME, Gamble WG. Cecal volvulus: a different twist for the serious runner. *N Engl J Med.* 1985;312(19):1262–1263.

283. Quirke P, Campbell I, Talbot IC. Ischaemic proctitis and adventitial fibromuscular dysplasia of the superior rectal artery. *Br J Surg.* 1984;71(1):33–38.

284. Rabinovici R, Simansky DA, Kaplan O, et al. Cecal volvulus. *Dis Colon Rectum.* 1990;33(9):765–769.

285. Ramanath HK, Hinshaw JR. Management and mismanagement of bleeding colonic diverticula. *Arch Surg.* 1971;103(2):311–314.

286. Ramirez FC, Johnson DA, Zierer ST, et al. Successful endoscopic hemostasis of bleeding colonic diverticula with epinephrine injection. *Gastrointest Endosc.* 1996;43(2 pt 1):167–170.

287. Raveenthiran V, Madiba TE, Atamanalp SS, et al. Volvulus of the sigmoid colon. *Colorectal Dis.* 2010;12(7 online):e1–e17.

288. Regan PT, Weiland LH, Geall MG. Scleroderma and intestinal perforation. *Am J Gastroenterol.* 1977;68(6):566–571.

289. Reichelderfer M, Morrissey JF. Colonoscopy in radiation colitis. *Gastrointest Endosc.* 1980;26(2):41–43.

290. Richardson JD, Lordon RE. Gastrointestinal bleeding caused by angiodysplasia: a difficult problem in patients with chronic renal failure receiving hemodialysis therapy. *Am Surg.* 1993;59(10):636–638.

291. Richardson JD, Mas MH, Flint LM Jr, et al. Bleeding vascular malformations of the intestine. *Surgery.* 1978;84(3):430–436.

292. Richter JM, Christensen MR, Kaplan LM, et al. Effectiveness of current technology in the diagnosis and management of lower gastrointestinal hemorrhage. *Gastrointest Endosc.* 1995;41(2):93–98.

293. Ritter EF, Lee CG, Tyler D, et al. Advances in prevention of radiation damage to visceral and solid organs in patients requiring radiation therapy of the trunk. *J Surg Oncol.* 1997;64(2):109–114.

294. Robertson HD, Gathright JB Jr. The technique of intraoperative segmental artery arteriography to localize vascular ectasias. *Dis Colon Rectum.* 1985;28(4):274–276.

295. Rogers RL, Harford FJ. Mobile cecum syndrome. *Dis Colon Rectum.* 1984;27(6):399–402.

296. Rösch J, Dotter CT, Brown MJ. Selective arterial embolization. A new method for control of acute gastrointestinal bleeding. *Radiology.* 1972;102(2):303–306.

297. Rosenkrantz H, Bookstein JJ, Rosen RJ, et al. Postembolic colonic infarction. *Radiology.* 1982;142(1):47–51.

298. Roswit B. Radiation injury of the colon and rectum. In: Greenbaum EI, ed. *Radiographic Atlas of Colon Disease.* Chicago, IL: Year Book; 1980:461.

299. Rubinstein E, Ibsen T, Rasmussen RB, et al. Formalin treatment of radiation-induced hemorrhagic proctitis. *Am J Gastroenterol.* 1986;81(1):44–45.

300. Ryan JA Jr, Johnson MG, Baker JW. Operative treatment of cecal volvulus combining cecopexy with intestinal tube decompression. *Surg Gynecol Obstet.* 1985;160(1):84–86.

301. Ryan P. Sigmoid volvulus with and without megacolon. *Dis Colon Rectum.* 1982;25(7):673–679.

302. Saclarides TJ, King DG, Franklin JL, et al. Formalin instillation for refractory radiation-induced hemorrhagic proctitis. Report of 16 patients. *Dis Colon Rectum.* 1996;39(2):196–199.

303. Sahakitrungruang C, Thum-Umnuaysuk S, Patiwonqgpaisarn A, et al. A novel treatment for haemorrhagic proctitis using colonic irrigation and oral antibiotic administration. *Colorectal Dis.* 2011;13(5):e79–e82. doi:10.1111/j.1463-1318.2010.02527.x.

304. Salim AS. Management of acute volvulus of the sigmoid colon: a new approach by percutaneous deflation and colopexy. *World J Surg.* 1991;15(1):68–72.

305. Samplaski MK, Wood HM, Lane BR, et al. Functional and quality-of-life outcomes in patients undergoing transperineal repair with gracilis muscle interposition for complex rectourethral fistula. *Urology.* 2011;77(3):736–741.

306. Samuelian JM, Callister MD, Ashman JB, et al. Reduced acute toxicity in patients treated with intensity-modulated radiotherapy for rectal cancer [published online ahead of print April 6, 2011]. *Int J Radiation Oncol Biol Phys.*

307. Sanner CJ, Saltzman DA. Detorsion of sigmoid volvulus by colonoscopy. *Gastrointest Endosc.* 1977;23(4):212–213.

308. Santos JC Jr, Feres O, Rocha JJ, et al. Massive lower gastrointestinal hemorrhage caused by pseudocyst of the pancreas ruptured into the colon. Report of two cases. *Dis Colon Rectum.* 1992;35(1):75–77.

309. Sauer R, Becker H, Hohenberger, et al. Preoperative versus postoperative chemoradiotherapy for rectal cancer. *N Engl J Med.* 2004;351(17):1731–1740.

310. Savoie LM, Abrams AV. Refractory proctosigmoiditis caused by myointimal hyperplasia of mesenteric veins: report of a case. *Dis Colon Rectum.* 1999;42(8):1093–1096.

311. Schagen van Leeuwen JH. Sigmoid volvulus in a West African population. *Dis Colon Rectum.* 1985;28(10):712–716.

312. Schiedler MG, Cutler BS, Fiddian-Green RG. Sigmoid intramural pH for prediction of ischemic colitis during aortic surgery. A comparison with risk factors and inferior mesenteric artery stump pressures. *Arch Surg.* 1987;122(8):881–886.

313. Schmitt EH III, Symmonds RE. Surgical treatment of radiation induced injuries of the intestine. *Surg Gynecol Obstet.* 1981;153(6):896–900.

314. Schmitz RL, Chao JH, Bartolome JS Jr. Intestinal injuries incidental to irradiation of carcinoma of the cervix of the uterus. *Surg Gynecol Obstet.* 1974;138(1):29–32.

315. Schmulewitz N, Fisher DA, Rockey DC. Early colonoscopy for acute lower GI bleeding predicts shorter hospital stay: a retrospective study of experience in a single center. *Gastrointest Endosc.* 2003;58(6):841–846.

316. Schneider TA, Longo WE, Ure T, et al. Mesenteric ischemia. Acute arterial syndromes. *Dis Colon Rectum.* 1994;37(11):1163–1174.

317. Schoots IG, Koffeman GI, Legemate DA, et al. Systematic review of survival after acute mesenteric ischaemia according to disease aetiology. *Br J Surg.* 2004;91(1):17–27.

318. Schrock TR. Colonoscopic diagnosis and treatment of lower gastrointestinal bleeding. *Surg Clin North Am.* 1989;69(6):1309–1325.

319. Schroeder T, Christoffersen JK, Andersen J, et al. Ischemic colitis complicating reconstruction of the abdominal aorta. *Surg Gynecol Obstet.* 1985;160(4):299–303.

320. Schwartz MJ, Lewis JH. Meckel's diverticulum: pitfalls in scintigraphic detection in the adult. *Am J Gastroenterol.* 1984;79(8):611–618.

321. Scott HJ, Lane IF, Glynn MJ, et al. Colonic haemorrhage: a technique for rapid intraoperative bowel preparation and colonoscopy. *Br J Surg.* 1986;73(5):390–391.

322. Seger DL, Middleton D. Childhood sigmoid volvulus. *Ann Emerg Med.* 1984;13(2):133–135.

323. Seldinger SI. Catheter replacement of needle in percutaneous arteriography. A new technique. *Acta Radiol.* 1953;39(5):368–376.

324. Seow-Choen F, Goh HS, Eu KW, et al. A simple and effective treatment for hemorrhagic radiation proctitis using formalin. *Dis Colon Rectum.* 1993;36(2):135–138.

325. Shbeeb I, Prager E, Love J. The aortic valve. Colonic axis. *Dis Colon Rectum.* 1984;27(1):38–41.

326. Shibata D, Brophy DP, Gordon FD, et al. Transjugular intrahepatic portosystemic shunt for treatment of bleeding ectopic varices with portal hypertension. *Dis Colon Rectum.* 1999;42(12):1581–1585.

327. Shibata M, Nakamuta H, Abe S, et al. Ischemic colitis caused by strict dieting in an 18-year-old female: report of a case. *Dis Colon Rectum.* 2002;45(3):425–428.

328. Shoop SA, Sackier JM. Laparoscopic cecopexy for cecal volvulus. Case report and a review of the literature. *Surg Endosc.* 1993;7(5):450–454.

329. Sidhu R, McAlindon ME, Kapur K, et al. Push enteroscopy in the era of capsule endoscopy. *J Clin Gastroenterol.* 2008;42(1):54–58.

330. Simpson AJ, Previti FW. Technetium sulfur colloid scintigraphy in the detection of lower gastrointestinal tract bleeding. *Surg Gynecol Obstet.* 1982;155(1):33–36.

331. Simpson PW, Nguyen MH, Lim JK, et al. Use of endoclips in the treatment of massive colonic diverticular bleeding. *Gastrointest Endosc.* 2004;59(3):433–437.

332. Singh G, Gupta SK, Gupta S. Simultaneous occurrence of sigmoid and cecal volvulus. *Dis Colon Rectum.* 1985;28(2):115–116.

333. Sitges-Serra A, Mas X, Roqueta F, et al. Mesenteric infarction: an analysis of 83 patients with prognostic studies in 44 cases undergoing a massive small-bowel resection. *Br J Surg.* 1988;75(6):544–548.

334. Smith DH, DeCosse JJ. Radiation damage to the small intestine. *World J Surg.* 1986;10(2):189–194.

335. Smith GF, Ellyson JH, Parks SN, et al. Angiodysplasia of the colon. A review of 17 cases. *Arch Surg.* 1984;119(5):532–536.

336. Smoot RL, Gostout CJ, Rajan E, et al. Is early colonoscopy after admission for acute diverticular bleeding needed? *Am J Gastroenterol.* 2003;98(9):1996–1999.

337. Sniderman KW, Franklin J Jr, Sos TA. Successful transcatheter Gelfoam embolization of a bleeding cecal vascular ectasia. *AJR Am J Roentgenol.* 1978;131(1):157–159.

338. Soltero MJ, Bill AH. The natural history of Meckel's diverticulum and its relation to incidental removal. A study of 202 cases of diseased Meckel's Diverticulum found in King County, Washington, over a fifteen year period. *Am J Surg.* 1976;132(2):168–173.

339. Spencer J. Lower gastrointestinal bleeding. *Br J Surg.* 1989;76(1):3–4.

340. Starling JR. Initial treatment of sigmoid volvulus by colonoscopy. *Ann Surg.* 1979;190(1):36–39.

341. Steer ML, Silen W. Diagnostic procedures in gastrointestinal hemorrhage. *N Engl J Med.* 1983;309(11):646–650.

342. Stewart WB, Gathright JB Jr, Ray JE. Vascular ectasias of the colon. *Surg Gynecol Obstet.* 1979;148(5):670–674.

343. Strate LL, Naumann CR. The role of colonoscopy and radiological procedures in the management of acute lower intestinal bleeding. *Clinical Gastroenterol Hepatol.* 2010;8(4):333–343.

344. Strate LL, Oray EJ, Syngal S. Early predictors of severity in acute lower intestinal tract bleeding. *Arch Intern Med.* 2003;163(7):838–843.

345. Strate LL, Saltzman JR, Ookubo R et al. Validation of a clinical prediction rule for severe acute lower intestinal bleeding. *Am J Gastroenterol.* 2005;100(8):1821–1827.

346. Strate LL, Syngal S. Timing of colonoscopy: impact on length of hospital stay in patients with acute lower intestinal bleeding. *Am J Gastroenterol.* 2003;98(2):317–322.

347. Stylianos S, Forde KA, Benvenisty AI, et al. Lower gastrointestinal hemorrhage in renal transplant recipients. *Arch Surg.* 1988;123(6):739–744.

348. Sudek P. Über die Gefässversorgung des Mastdarmes in Hinsicht auf die operative Gangrän. *Münch Med Wochenschr.* 1907;54:1314–1317.

349. Sugarbaker PH. Intrapelvic prosthesis to prevent injury of the small intestine with high dosage pelvic irradiation. *Surg Gynecol Obstet.* 1983;157(3):269–271.

350. Suzman MS, Talmor M, Jennis R, et al. Accurate localization and surgical management of active lower gastrointestinal hemorrhage with technetium-labeled erythrocyte scintigraphy. *Ann Surg.* 1996;224(1):29–36.

351. Swan MP, Moore GT, Sievert W, et al. Efficacy and safety of single-session argon plasma coagulation in the management of chronic radiation proctitis. *Gastrointest Endosc.* 2010;72(1):150–154.

352. Tada M, Shimizu S, Kawai K. Emergency colonoscopy for the diagnosis of lower intestinal bleeding. *Gastroenterol Jpn.* 1991;6(suppl 3):121–124.

353. Taïeb S, Rolachon A, Cenni JC, et al. Effective use of argon plasma coagulation in the treatment of severe radiation proctitis. *Dis Colon Rectum.* 2001;44(12):1766–1771.

354. Talley NA, Chen F, King D, et al. Short-chain fatty acids in the treatment of radiation proctitis: a randomized, double-blind, placebo-controlled, cross-over pilot trial. *Dis Colon Rectum.* 1997;40(9):1046–1050.

355. Talman EA, Dixon DS, Gutierrez FE. Role of arteriography in rectal hemorrhage due to arteriovenous malformations and diverticulosis. *Ann Surg.* 1979;190(2):203–213.

356. Tan KK, Chong CS, Sim R. Management of acute sigmoid volvulus: an institution's experience over 9 years. *World J Surg.* 2010;34(8):1943–1948.

357. Tannenbaum GA, Forde KA. Radiation enteritis and colitis: general considerations in medical and surgical management. *Surg Rounds.* 1986;9:42.

358. Taylor SA, Halligan S, Vance M, et al. Use of multidetector-row computer tomographic colonography before flexible sigmoidoscopy in the investigation of rectal bleeding. *Br J Surg.* 2003;90(9):1163–1164.

359. Tegegne A. Cultural bowel paterns and sex difference in sigmoid volvulus morbidity in an Ethiopian hospital. *Trop Geogr Med.* 1995;47(5):212–215.

360. Tejler G, Jiborn H. Volvulus of the cecum. Report of 26 cases and review of the literature. *Dis Colon Rectum.* 1988;31(6):445–449.

361. Thomas MG. Obscure lower gastrointestinal tract bleeding. *Br J Surg.* 1999;86(5):579–580.

362. Tjandra JJ, Sengupta S. Argon plasma coagulation is an effective treatment for refractory hemorrhagic radiation proctitis. *Dis Colon Rectum.* 2001;44(12):1759–1765.

363. Todd GJ, Forde KA. Volvulus of the cecum: choice of operation. *Am J Surg.* 1979;138(5):632–634.

364. Travis S, Davies DR, Creamer B. Acute colorectal ischaemia after anaphylactoid shock. *Gut.* 1991;32(4):443–446.

365. Triester SL, Leighton JA, Leontiadis GI, et al. A meta-analysis of the yield of capsule endoscopy compared to other diagnostic modalities in patients with obscure gastrointestinal bleeding. *Am J Gastroenterol.* 2005;100(11):2407–2418.

366. Trudel JL, Fazio VW, Sivak MV. Colonoscopic diagnosis and treatment of arteriovenous malformations in chronic lower gastrointestinal bleeding. Clinical accuracy and efficacy. *Dis Colon Rectum.* 1988;31(2):107–110.

367. Udén P, Jiborn H, Jonsson K. Influence of selective mesenteric arteriography on the outcome of emergency surgery for massive, lower gastrointestinal hemorrhage. A 15-year experience. *Dis Colon Rectum.* 1986;29(9):561–566.

368. Udezue NO. Sigmoid volvulus in Kaduna, Nigeria. *Dis Colon Rectum.* 1990;33(8):647–649.

369. Valle M, Federici O, Ialongo P, et al. Prevention of complications following pelvic exenteration with the use of mammary implants in the pelvic cavity: technique and results of 28 cases. *J Surg Oncol.* 2011;103(1):34–38.

370. van Cutsem E, Rutgeerts P, Vantrappen G. Treatment of bleeding gastrointestinal vascular malformations with oestrogen-progesterone. *Lancet.* 1990;335(8695):953–955.

371. Vane DW, West KW, Grosfeld JL. Vitelline duct anomalies. Experience with 217 childhood cases. *Arch Surg.* 1987;122(5):542–547.

372. Vanni AJ, Buckley JC, Zinman LN. Management of surgical and radiation induced rectourethral fistulas with an interposition muscle flap and selective buccal mucosal onlay graft. *J Urol.* 2010;184(6):2400–2404.

373. Varma JS, Smith AN. Anorectal function following colo-anal sleeve anastomosis for chronic radiation injury to the rectum. *Br J Surg.* 1986;73(4):285–289.

374. Varma JS, Smith AN, Busuttil A. Correlation of clinical and manometric abnormalities of rectal function following chronic radiation injury. *Br J Surg.* 1985;72(11):875–878.

375. Varma JS, Smith AN, Busuttil A. Function of the anal sphincters after chronic radiation injury. *Gut.* 1986;27(5):528–533.

376. Veidenheimer MC, Corman ML, Coller JA. Colonic hemorrhage. *Surg Clin North Am.* 1978;58(3):581–590.

377. Vernia P, Fracasso PL, Casale V, et al. Topical butyrate for acute radiation proctitis: randomised, crossover trial. *Lancet.* 2000;356(9237):1232–1235.

378. Villarreal HA, Marts BC, Longo WE, et al. Congenital colonic varices in the adult. Report of a case. *Dis Colon Rectum.* 1995;38(9):990–992.

379. Voelle GR, Bunch G, Britt LG. Use of technetium-labeled red blood cell scintigraphy in the detection and management of gastrointestinal hemorrhage. *Surgery.* 1991;110(4):799–804.

380. Wasnik A, Kaza RK, Al-Hawary MM, et al. Multidetector CT imaging in mesenteric ischemia—pearls and pitfalls. *Emerg Radiol.* 2011;18(2):145–156. doi:10.1007/s10140-010-0921-8.

381. Waxman AD. Nuclear medicine techniques in the evaluation of gastrointestinal bleeding. *Curr Concepts Diagn Nucl Imaging.* 1985;2:13.

382. Weingart J, Höchter W, Ottenjann R. Varices of the entire colon—an unusual cause of recurrent intestinal bleeding. *Endoscopy.* 1982;14(2):69–70.

383. Welch GH, Anderson JR. Volvulus of the splenic flexure of the colon. *Dis Colon Rectum.* 1985;28(8):592–593.

384. Welch GH, Anderson JR. Acute volvulus of the sigmoid colon. *World J Surg.* 1987;11(2):258–262.

385. Welch GH, Shearer MG, Imrie CW, et al. Total colonic ischemia. *Dis Colon Rectum.* 1986;29(6):410–412.

386. Welch M, Baguneid MS, McMahon RF, et al. Histological study of colonic ischaemia after aortic surgery. *Br J Surg.* 1998;85(8):1095–1098.

387. Welling RE, Roedersheimer LR, Arbaugh JJ, et al. Ischemic colitis following repair of ruptured abdominal aortic aneurysm. *Arch Surg.* 1985;120(12):1368–1370.

388. Wellwood JM, Jackson BT. The intestinal complications of radiotherapy. *Br J Surg.* 1973;60(10):814–818.

389. West BR, Ray JE, Gathright JB Jr. Comparison of transient ischemic colitis with that requiring surgical treatment. *Surg Gynecol Obstet.* 1980;151(3):366–368.

390. Williams LF Jr, Wittenberg J. Ischemic colitis: an useful clinical diagnosis, but is it ischemic? *Ann Surg.* 1975;182(4):439–448.

391. Williams RA, Wilson SE. Current management of massive lower gastrointestinal bleeding. *Int Surg.* 1980;65(2):157–163.

392. Winzelberg GG, Froelich JW, McKusick KA, et al. Radionuclide localization of lower gastrointestinal hemorrhage. *Radiology.* 1981;139(2):465–469.

393. Winzelberg GG, McKusick KA, Waltman AC, et al. Evaluation of gastrointestinal bleeding by red blood cells labeled in vivo with technetium-99m. *J Nucl Med.* 1979;20(10):1080–1086.

394. Wiseman JS, Senagore AJ, Chaudry IH. Methods to prevent colonic injury in pelvic radiation. *Dis Colon Rectum.* 1994;37(11):1090–1094.

395. Wolf EL, Frager D, Beneventano TC. Volvulus of the transverse colon. *Am J Gastroenterol.* 1984;79(10):797–798.

396. Wong MT, Lim JF, Ho KS, et al. Radiation proctitis: a decade's experience. *Singapore Med J.* 2010;51(4):315–319.

397. Wyman A, Zeiderman MR. Maintaining decompression of sigmoid volvulus. *Surg Gynecol Obstet.* 1989;169(3):265.

398. Yamaguchi M, Takeuchi S, Awazu S. Meckel's diverticulum. Investigation of 600 patients in Japanese literature. *Am J Surg*. 1978;136(2):247–249.

399. Yoon W, Jeong YY, Shin SS, et al. Acute massive gastrointestinal bleeding: detection and localization with arterial phase multi-detector row helical CT. *Radiology*. 2006;239(1):160–167.

400. Zhi FC, Yue H, Jiang B, et al. Diagnostic value of double blloon enteroscopy for small-intestine disease: experience from China. *Gastrointest Endosc*. 2007;66(3 suppl):S19–S21.

401. Zhong J, Ma T, Zhang C, et al. A retrospective study of the application on double-balloon enteroscopy in 378 patients with suspected small-bowel disease. *Endoscopy*. 2007;39(3):208–215.

402. Zhu W, Gong J, Li Y, et al. A retrospective study of surgical treatment of chronic radiation enteritis [published online ahead of print September 19, 2011]. *J Surg Oncol*. doi:10.1002/jso.22099.

403. Zink SI, Ohki SK, Stein B, et al. Noninvasive evaluation of active lower gastrointestinal bleeding: comparison between contrast-enhanced MDCT and 99mTc-labeled RBC scintigraphy. *AJR Am J Roentgenol*. 2008;191(4):1107–1114.

404. Zizic TM, Classen JN, Stevens MB. Acute abdominal complications of systemic lupus erythematosus and polyarteritis nodosa. *Am J Med*. 1982;73(4):525–531.

405. Zuccaro G Jr. Management of the adult patient with acute lower gastrointestinal bleeding American College of Gastroenterology. Practice Parameters Committee. *Am J Gastroenterol*. 1998;93(8): 1202–1208.

406. Zuckerman GR, Prakash C. Acute lower intestinal bleeding: part I: clinical presentation and diagnosis. *Gastrointest Endosc*. 1998;48(6): 606–617.

Ulcerative Colitis

Victor W. Fazio

Five things are proper to the duty of a Chirurgian;
To take away that which is superfluous;
To restore to their places such things as are displaced;
To separate those things which are joined together;
To join those that are separated; and
To supply the defects of nature.
— AMBROISE PARÉ: *Works*, Book I, Chapter 2

The expression *nonspecific inflammatory bowel disease* (IBD) is used to describe two conditions of unknown etiology: ulcerative colitis (UC) and Crohn's disease (CD). With respect to the differential diagnosis, the two diseases often have similar characteristics. The symptoms are frequently quite alike, radiologic investigation may pose confusion in differentiation, and even pathologic evaluation may reveal overlapping features, with an indeterminate colitis reported in as many as 15% of patients. Some have even reported that both conditions can coexist in the same individual.[773] Because of the often diverse approaches to management and the fact that a vulnerable age group is frequently affected (young persons in their late teens and early 20s), these diseases are among the most challenging confronting the physician today. Ulcerative colitis is discussed in this chapter; Crohn's disease and indeterminate colitis are presented in Chapter 30.

► HISTORICAL PERSPECTIVE

It is difficult to know whether ulcerative colitis was truly recognized as a disease prior to the 19th century. Infectious and noninfectious diarrheas have existed since antiquity, but most of the descriptions are of a clinical syndrome—diarrhea and rectal bleeding, the so-called bloody flux. Samuel Wilks is generally credited with coining the term *ulcerative colitis*.[775] In a letter to the editor of the *Medical Times and Gazette* published in 1859, he described the postmortem appearance of the intestine. Subsequently, the surgeon general of the Union Army after the Civil War referred to the disease, ulcerative colitis, and included photomicrographs of the condition.[216] Other detailed descriptions followed,[776] and by the early 20th century, more than 300 case reports of ulcerative colitis had been collected for presentation to the Royal Society of Medicine.[216]

► EPIDEMIOLOGY (INCIDENCE, PREVALENCE) AND ETIOLOGY

As suggested, the nonspecific IBDs, especially Crohn's disease, have become pervasive worldwide, and the two conditions have thus emerged as one of the most important biomedical problems of our time.[352] Unfortunately, our understanding of their pathogenesis still remains obscure.

Evaluation of the epidemiology of the two conditions is made difficult by the plethora of diarrheal states found throughout the world that may be infectious or parasitic in nature and that present with symptoms not unlike those of nonspecific IBD.[352] Furthermore, because of international failure to classify the two diseases as distinct from the numerous specific inflammatory bowel problems, our

SAMUEL WILKS (1842–1911)

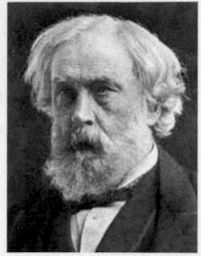

Samuel Wilks was born in 1824 in Camberwell, London. After attending the Aldenham School and the University College School, he served as an apprentice to a general practitioner in Newington. In 1842, he began his long affiliation with Guy's Hospital. He became a member of the Royal College of Surgeons in 1847.

His most important contributions to medicine and research were in the description of ulcerative colitis. In 1859, he suggested that idiopathic colitis should be considered a different entity from that of specific epidemic dysentery. He also first described Crohn's disease in the postmortem autopsy of a 42-year-old woman. In that report he states, "In the small intestine nothing remarkable was observed until the lower end of the ileum was reached, when at about three feet from its termination in the caecum, the mucous membrane commenced to exhibit an inflammatory response. In the caecum, inflammation of the most acute and violent character was observed . . . the bare muscular coat was seen beneath. The muscular coat itself in the caecum was likewise infiltrated with this exudation . . . and there is no doubt that through this part of the intestine some transudation had occurred which had set up the peritonitis. No actual perforation was discoverable." In addition to these observations, Wilks made contributions to Addison's, Bright's, and Hodgkin's diseases, each of which had been previously described by Guy's Hospital physicians. Wilks received numerous honors, including that of appointment as a physician-extraordinary to Queen Victoria as well as an honorary baronetcy. He also served as the president of the Pathological Society (1881–1883) and the president of the Royal College of Physicians (1896–1899). He died in 1911 at the age of 87 after suffering from a stroke. (From Banerjee A. Sir Samuel Wilks: a founding father of clinical science. *J R Soc Med.* 1991;84:44, with permission and with thanks to Michael Polcino, MD.)

ability to obtain meaningful data is compromised. Most of the information, therefore, has been accumulated from Western countries, where the diseases are relatively prevalent. In the United States, however, IBD is not a reportable condition.

Available evidence suggests considerable variation in the incidence rates—common in developed countries and unusual in Asia, Africa, and South America. Because a true surveillance of prevalence requires an exhaustive clinical, endoscopic, and radiologic evaluation of all members of a sample population, the true prevalence is based on inference rather than analysis of well-established data.[487] There even appears to be a seasonal variation, not only of onset, but also of relapse.[624] A statistically significant increase has been observed in the months of August to January.

The incidence of ulcerative colitis and Crohn's disease in England, United States, and Scandinavia is reported to be at least 4 to 6 cases per 100,000 white adults per year, with prevalence rates of between 40 and 100 cases per 100,000.[353] Most studies have demonstrated an increased incidence of Crohn's disease over the past 25 years.[56,67,147,378,472,501,551] The condition is more common in whites, among Jewish people, and among those of Western origin (especially northern Europe and the northern part of eastern Europe).[353] Other countries such as South American nations, the former Soviet Union, and Japan have a much lower incidence and prevalence. More recent reports suggest that UC affects approximately 500,000 individuals in the United States, with an incidence of approximately 12 per 100,000 population per year.[324,325,437,438,536] Moreover, UC posts a considerable health care burden. The disease accounts for more than a quarter million physician visits annually with 30,000 hospitalizations and is also associated with loss of more than a million workdays per year.[694] The direct health care costs are astoundingly high, exceeding $4 billion annually, which includes estimated hospital costs of more than $960 million and drug costs of $680 million.

As with carcinoma of the colon, the prevalence of IBD in many industrialized countries and the development of the conditions among those from low-risk populations who emigrate to higher risk areas suggest an environmental cause.

Investigative efforts to identify the etiologic agent responsible for the nonspecific IBDs have thus far been unsuccessful. IBD that appears nonspecific in nature has been found in hamsters, horses, swine, and the canine population, but an experimental animal model for induction or transmission of the disease still eludes investigators. The three primary areas of investigation that continue to be pursued actively are genetics, immunology, and infection.

Genetics

Several studies have shown the existence of family aggregations with the disease, implying that genetic factors also must play a role.[5,119,148,351,354,384,769] For example, there is a high degree of concordance in monozygotic twins.[599] Although ulcerative colitis and Crohn's disease are not classic genetic disorders, the occurrence of IBD in family members born in widely separated areas or living apart for long periods, along with the increased incidence among Jews and the tendency toward familial aggregation of cases with ankylosing spondylitis in Crohn's disease, suggest a genetically mediated mechanism in the causation of the conditions.[148,353,566] Roth and colleagues, in a study of Ashkenazi Jews with IBD, calculated the true lifetime risk for the development of IBD in relatives to be 8.9% for offspring, 8.8% for siblings, and 3.5% for parents.[634] Although the possibility of a common environment may contribute to the increased risk of IBD, the shared genetic pool is much more likely to be the primary factor. A familial occurrence has been noted in 17.5% of more than 600 patients with IBD.[688] In a report from the Cleveland Clinic, Farmer and colleagues evaluated the family histories of more than 800 patients with an onset of IBD before the age of 21.[148] Twenty-nine percent of those with ulcerative colitis had a positive history, and 35% of those with Crohn's disease had a positive family history for IBD.

The first IBD susceptibility locus was found on chromosome 16 and identified as IBD1. This is apparently a purely Crohn's locus, however. Most of the current studies seem to demonstrate a consistent association with various genetic mutations and Crohn's disease, but not that of ulcerative colitis.

Satsangi and colleagues propose that the ethnic, familial, twin, disease association, and genetic marker studies of IBD are best explained by the concept that the conditions represent multifactorial diseases.[660] Environmental and genetic factors contribute to disease susceptibility. They conclude that it is possible for different susceptibility genes to underlie phenotypic differences between Crohn's disease and ulcerative colitis, leading to diverse manifestations of the two conditions as well as varied degrees of severity. Mendeloff believes that there is a deficiency in the investigation of these diseases because the mortality is low and the genetic determinants are multiple.[487] He suggests that in the future it will be necessary to develop a better fundamental means of acquiring and recording data, and that at least for the immediate present a concerted effort should be made to identify those families in which multiple cases of IBD exist and to investigate these people thoroughly. This would include genetic, psychological, and metabolic studies.

Autoimmunity

The idea of circulating antiepithelial antibodies combining with antigens on the intestinal cell surface and damaging the cells seems a reasonable theory to explain the etiology of IBD. This is the concept of autoimmunity. Snook clearly defines the criteria for the classification of a disease as autoimmune.[692] According to him, such a condition ". . . requires the demonstration of autoreactive lymphocytes or autoantibodies, or both, which are specific for the disease concerned, present in all cases, and most important, capable of reproducing the disease on syngeneic transfer."[692] However, despite the demonstration of anticolon antibodies in both blood and tissue of patients with IBD, current evidence seems to militate against the likelihood that these play a primary pathogenetic role in the two conditions.[642]

Immune complex mediation of IBD has been thought by some to be a responsible factor, but studies have failed to corroborate a significantly increased frequency or concentration of these complexes regardless of disease activity.[642] Other immunologic mechanisms that have been investigated include abnormality and variability of circulating lymphocytes, lymphocyte cytotoxicity, defective cell-mediated immunity, immediate hypersensitivity, leukocyte chemotaxic impairment, and immunoregulatory cellular imbalance.[353,642] At the level of the immune response, a genetic influence is suggested by the association of ulcerative colitis with HLA-DR2 and by the occurrence of various autoantibodies in the unaffected relatives of patients with ulcerative colitis.[677] Furthermore, studies of monozygotic twins have indicated that the altered mucosal production of immunoglobulin G1 (IgG1) and IgG2 in ulcerative colitis may be genetically determined.[677] James and colleagues suggest that the presence of circulating antigen-nonspecific suppressor T cells in patients with Crohn's disease in its early stages is the result of an immunoregulatory abnormality of antigen-specific helper and suppressor T cells.[305] A useful concept of the pathogenesis for IBD may involve an interaction between host responses, immunologic genetic influences, and external agents, but no definitive proof has yet been forthcoming.

Infection

With respect to infectious agents, ulcerative colitis in particular has been attributed to bacterial causes for more than 60 years. In 1928, Bargen reported that the condition was caused by a transmissible diplococcus.[30] He prepared a vaccine from this organism, an approach that was believed to be a valuable part of the treatment of the condition. In the article that introduced the technique of skin-grafted ileostomy for the surgical management of ulcerative colitis (see Chapter 31), Dragstedt and colleagues were persuaded that "bacterium necrophorum, together with other factors . . . plays an etiologic role in the disease."[140] Crohn's disease specifically was often confused with tuberculosis. This observation led Crohn and coworkers to suggest that the disease might be caused by a mycobacterial agent.[114] Subsequent studies have failed to demonstrate conclusively an association with an infective agent, and, in fact, the incidence of IBD correlates inversely

J. ARNOLD BARGEN (1894–1976)

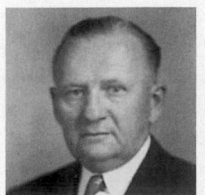

Bargen was born at Mountain Lake, Minnesota. He attended Carleton College in Northfield, Minnesota, and received a BS degree from the University of Chicago in 1918. Following graduation from Rush Medical College, he completed an internship and a 1-year postgraduate fellowship in medicine at St. Luke's Hospital. He then joined the Mayo Clinic as an assistant in medicine and became a part of the clinic staff in 1926. He became head of a section of medicine in 1942, and in 1956 he undertook the chairmanship of four sections of medicine primarily concerned with gastroenterology. Bargen gained a national reputation for his work in diseases of the stomach and colon and was the author or coauthor of four books as well as hundreds of published articles in these fields. Additionally, he served on the editorial board of the journal *Gastroenterology* and was a member or officer of numerous prestigious medical societies, including the American Gastroenterological Association, of which he was president, and the sections of gastroenterology of the American Medical Association and the World Congress of Gastroenterology, of which he was chairman. Bargen was one of the first to recognize the association of ulcerative colitis with carcinoma (1928),[29] but his early affirmation of the concept of a bacterial etiology for this condition was never corroborated. Following his retirement from the Mayo Clinic, he headed the department of gastroenterology at the Scott-White Clinic. He died in Sun City, Arizona, at the age of 82. (Photograph courtesy of the Mayo Clinic.)

with that of the infectious dysenteries.[353] An exception is that of cytomegalovirus infection, which has been shown to complicate ulcerative colitis in immunocompromised patients, such as individuals with AIDS.[761]

The concept of a microbial infection as the offending agent has been resurrected with the recognition of newer bacterial causes of enteritis and colitis (especially *Campylobacter jejuni* and *Clostridium difficile*).[63,380,534,739] Although several studies suggest the possibility of these two organisms contributing to relapse of IBD, Gurian and colleagues, in examination of stool specimens from 32 patients who had exacerbation of IBD, revealed no *Clostridium difficile* cytotoxin and negative cultures for *Campylobacter jejuni*.[235] Other bacteriologic agents (*Shigella*, *Salmonella*, *Streptococcus faecalis*, *Pseudomonas* variant, *Chlamydia*, *Mycobacterium*, and many others) have been proposed, but their role has not been confirmed.[89,203,242,730] More recently, it has been suggested that probiotics play an important role in preventing overgrowth of potentially pathogenic bacteria and in maintaining the integrity of the gut mucosal barrier.[756] Therefore, there may be a role for such agents in the treatment of IBD (see Medical Management).

There has been considerable interest in a possible viral etiology of ulcerative colitis and Crohn's disease. Transmission of granulomatous lesions has been successfully carried out in experimental animals.[98,135,722] Tissue culture and electron microscopic investigation have also suggested that a viral agent is present in tissue from patients with IBD.[14,204,774] However, considerable controversy continues concerning the specificity of these findings. Whether the evidence is sufficiently compelling to permit accurate identification of viral particles on electron microscopic examination of affected tissue remains unresolved.[642,787]

Diet

Dietary factors, especially cow's milk, have been implicated as possible causative agents for the development of IBD. Early studies seemed to demonstrate an elevated milk protein antibody level in patients with ulcerative colitis in comparison with a control population. Subsequent studies in which milk was excluded from the diet failed to demonstrate an improvement in the clinical response, and later studies with milk and milk products failed to demonstrate any correlation. Other factors that have been under investigation include chemical food additives, mercury ingestion, inadequate fiber, excess intake of refined sugar, and even the increased consumption of corn flakes.[471,642] Generally, articles dealing with diet and IBD are conflicting, confusing, and frequently unreliable. One can safely state that there is no clear consensus to suggest that dietary factors play a role in the etiology of either ulcerative colitis or Crohn's disease.

Oxidative Metabolism

Recent evidence suggests that abnormal oxidative metabolism may be of significance in the activity of IBD. Increased attention has been placed on the role of free radicals in both normal metabolism and defense against disease.[687] A free radical is defined as any species capable of independent existence that contains one or more unpaired electrons, an unpaired electron being defined as one that is alone in an orbital.[687] It appears that reactive oxygen metabolites are produced in excess in active IBD. The effects of specific anti-inflammatory antioxidants, such as aminosalicylates, are compatible with the proposition that free radicals play a major role in the pathogenesis of IBD.[687]

Stool

Studies of the role of the fecal stream in causing an exacerbation of symptoms in Crohn's colitis have yielded confusing results. For example, Harper and colleagues evaluated the effects of introducing small bowel effluent and a sterile ultrafiltrate of the effluent into the defunctionalized colon after a loop ileostomy had been created.[254] There was little response to the ultrafiltrate challenge, but there was a definite clinical exacerbation following introduction of the effluent. Conversely, Korelitz and colleagues reported that diverting the fecal stream had an adverse effect on the clinical course in four patients.[368] Following reestablishment of intestinal continuity, the bowel returned to normal.

Smoking

Two distinct patterns of cigarette smoking seem to be relevant in patients with IBD; those with ulcerative colitis are much less likely to smoke than those with Crohn's disease. Additionally, cigarette smoking has been found to have a negative correlation with ulcerative colitis.[77,122,255,310,737,759] In some cases, complete remission of symptoms was obtained through the use of nicotine-laced chewing gum. In other cases, exacerbation of the disease was noted when patients ceased smoking. Conversely, Crohn's disease is more common in smokers than in those who have never smoked.[330,737,759] The increased risk seems to be more apparent in women and may also be associated with a greater likelihood of recurrence.[714]

Oral Contraceptives

Both ulcerative colitis and Crohn's disease have been found to be more common among women using oral contraceptives than in those who do not.[759] A possible vascular (ischemic) basis for this observation has been suggested. There is no information to date on the effect of stopping the contraceptive pill on the activity of IBD.

Psychological Factors

The psychological aspects and the possible psychosomatic factors contributing to the onset and exacerbation of IBD, and of ulcerative colitis in particular, have been a subject of considerable debate since publication of the original article by Murray in 1930.[522] Karush and colleagues, in a book on *Psychotherapy in Chronic Ulcerative Colitis*, state that susceptibility to the problem develops in colitic patients through "disruption and distortion of the relationship to the parents and to other significant persons as early as the second year of life."[328] They further contend that this results in exaggerated emotional manifestations, egocentricity, dependency conflicts, and poor mechanisms for coping with the stresses of life.[328] Frequent anxiety or depression, in the opinion of the authors, is also characteristic, and this predisposition, they believe, explains the relatively high incidence of schizophrenia in patients with ulcerative colitis. In their study of precipitating emotional factors, the authors reported that a well-defined event of powerful emotional impact preceded the onset of the disease by a few days or weeks. Subsequent recurrences were also heralded by such events.

Although many articles have been published to support this description of the susceptible personality, opponents of the psychosomatic theory point out that the concept is based on either anecdotal or uncontrolled studies.[642] Several publications have compared patients with ulcerative colitis with normal subjects and those with other illnesses and have found no evidence of an increased frequency of psychiatric illness.[49,141,267,488] Furthermore, those with ulcerative colitis who had a psychiatric illness did not appear to have more serious gastrointestinal involvement, nor did severity of the ulcerative colitis predict a more frequent or more severe psychiatric disorder.[267] Bercovitz noted that there are no long-term, prospective psychological studies available of any large group of people.[51] North and colleagues reviewed all known English-language articles at the time (138 studies) on the association between psychiatric factors and ulcerative colitis and found that most contained serious flaws in research design (e.g., absence of control subjects and lack of diagnostic criteria).[547] In the seven publications that truly represented meaningful, systematic, investigative efforts, no association was identified. Cunnien concluded that patients with ulcerative colitis have no universal unique personality characteristics and no documented increase in psychiatric illness when compared with medically ill and population controls.[117] He further observed that no demonstrable emotional precipitating factors have been uniformly identified, no symbolic emotional conflicts have been documented in controlled studies, and psychotherapy has not been effective in altering the disease course.

Comment

Serious illness during an extremely vulnerable period of emotional development, the need for hospitalization and psychotropic medications (e.g., corticosteroids), or the fear of surgery (especially the "mutilation" of an ileostomy) may induce considerable stress. In fact, it would be the remarkable patient indeed who was not emotionally troubled by the consequences of such illness. The importance of providing emotional support to the patient cannot be overestimated. Psychotherapy has been demonstrated to be of value, but an internist or a surgeon who understands the role of emotional conflicts and anxieties either as a cause or a result of the patient's illness can provide such counsel.

Appendectomy

As has been suggested, the current concept of the etiology of IBD in most patients is that the condition may be triggered by genetic predisposition to a variety of environmental factors. The association of one of these factors, appendectomy, has been the subject of numerous investigations. Koutroubakis and colleagues undertook a meta-analysis of 17 case-controlled studies and found that appendectomy was inversely associated with the development of ulcerative colitis ($P < .0001$).[372] The role of the appendix in the development of mucosal immunity is currently the subject of intensive study.

Age, Sex, and Race

Ulcerative colitis and Crohn's disease occur at any age but are most commonly seen in persons younger than the age of 30 years. The incidence is highest among teenagers, but a small secondary peak in the incidence of the two conditions

occurs late in the sixth decade.[353] In most series, both sexes are equally affected. Farmer and colleagues noted, in a study covering 20 years ending in 1974, that 838 patients were 20 years old or younger at the time of diagnosis at the Cleveland Clinic.[148] Thirteen percent with ulcerative colitis and 5% with Crohn's disease were younger than 11 years of age. Approximately one-third of the patients in each group were between the ages of 11 and 15. There were 316 patients with ulcerative colitis, with a male-to-female ratio of almost 1:1, and 522 patients with Crohn's disease, 57% of whom were male. In Goligher's experience, approximately one-half of the patients were between 20 and 39 years of age when the disease was diagnosed, with a 4:3 predominance of female over male patients.[212] With Crohn's disease, Goligher reported that in his own personal series, female patients predominated in a 3:2 ratio.[214] There seemed to be a tendency for the disease to develop later than ulcerative colitis does, 70% of patients being between the ages of 20 and 49 years.

In the Lahey Clinic experience of 151 patients who underwent proctocolectomy, the mean age at surgery for both ulcerative colitis and Crohn's disease was 36 years.[108] Fifty-six percent of patients with ulcerative colitis were men, whereas 57% who had Crohn's colitis were women.

Goldman and colleagues suggest that Crohn's disease in black patients may be more common than is generally appreciated.[207] This group represented 11% of the patients in their experience during a 10-year period. The authors noted that extraintestinal manifestations developed in all patients. Furthermore, the disease generally appeared to be associated with more severe complications than had been observed in whites.

▶ DIFFERENTIAL DIAGNOSIS: ULCERATIVE COLITIS VERSUS CROHN'S DISEASE

Ulcerative colitis and Crohn's disease can usually be distinguished based on the clinical course, symptomatology, manifestations, and endoscopic findings. Ulcerative colitis is a disease characterized by exacerbations and remissions. In contrast, the individual with Crohn's disease has less clear-cut periods of flare-up and remission; the disease often tends to run a more smoldering course. Frequently, the patient is really not well and yet is not sufficiently ill to warrant hospitalization. Table 29-1 summarizes a number of the characteristic features that may help to differentiate between the two conditions.

Rectal bleeding is virtually a sine qua non for the diagnosis of ulcerative colitis. A physician might seriously question the accuracy of the diagnosis in the absence of this symptom. Bleeding is much less frequently seen in Crohn's colitis; in fact, 25% of patients with Crohn's disease never manifest bleeding. This should not be surprising because ulcerative colitis is an inflammatory disease of the mucosa, whereas with Crohn's colitis, ulceration may be minimal. However, in rare instances, massive lower gastrointestinal bleeding may be associated with Crohn's disease.[477]

Ulcerative colitis is confined to the colon and rectum; Crohn's disease can occur anywhere in the digestive tract, from the mouth to the anus. Anorectal disease in particular (fissures, abscesses, and fistulas) is more commonly noted in patients with Crohn's disease than in those with ulcerative colitis (see Chapters 12, 13, and 14). The diagnosis is often suspected on examination of the perianal skin (see Figure 14-51).

TABLE 29-1 Features of Nonspecific Inflammatory Bowel Disease

	ULCERATIVE COLITIS	CROHN'S DISEASE
Course	Exacerbations and remissions	Smoldering
Bleeding	Virtually always	Uncommon
Abdominal pain	Uncommon	Common
Perianal disease	Rare	Up to 40%
Fistulas	Never	Occasional
Abdominal mass	Never	Occasional
Carcinoma	Increased association	Increased, but less than in ulcerative colitis
Extraintestinal manifestations	Not unusual	Not unusual
Radiologic and Endoscopic		
Distribution	In continuity with rectum	Skip areas often observed
	Uniform distribution	Often eccentric
	Rectal involvement always	Often rectal sparing
Small bowel	Spared (backwash only)	Often involved
Stricture	Rare, virtually always malignant	Frequent, virtually always benign
Mucosa	Contact bleeding, granularity, superficial ulcers, pseudopolyps	Longitudinal ulcers, fissuring, cobblestone appearance
Microscopic		
Extent	Mucosa and submucosa	Transmural
Granulomas	Never	Common
Dysplasia	Yes	Yes
Lymph nodes	Reactive	With granulomas
Crypt abscesses	Present	Present
Mucus production	Decreased	Increased

Proctosigmoidoscopic examination may be of value in differentiating between the two conditions (see later discussion). The rectum is always diseased during attacks of ulcerative colitis. Characteristic changes include contact bleeding, granularity, and ulceration. In Crohn's colitis, 40% of the patients have sparing of the rectum, irrespective of anal or perianal involvement. However, when the rectum is involved by Crohn's disease, differentiation between the two may be quite difficult.

Extracolonic manifestations had been presumed to be found only with ulcerative colitis, but it is now recognized that these can be observed in both conditions. They are discussed in Chapter 30.

It may not be possible to differentiate between the two diseases either by radiologic or clinical means. In approximately 10% to 15% of cases, distinction cannot be made even pathologically; these patients are thus placed into the so-called indeterminate category (see Chapter 30). The appropriateness of using the ileal pouch-anal operation as an alternative in this group of patients is also discussed in Chapter 30.

Physical Examination

Physical examination is usually unrewarding in patients with ulcerative colitis who do not have fulminant disease. Abdominal tenderness is usually absent, and there is no abdominal distension. No masses are palpable. However, in the acutely ill person, abdominal distension may be associated with toxic megacolon. Diffuse tenderness may be apparent, and if perforation has ensued, all the usual signs and symptoms of an intra-abdominal catastrophe may be noted.

Endoscopic Examination

Proctosigmoidoscopy, flexible sigmoidoscopy, and colonoscopy are important tools for evaluating the bowel and for confirming the presence or absence of IBD. Proctosigmoidoscopic examination is particularly useful in differentiating Crohn's disease from ulcerative colitis; the rectum is always diseased during attacks of ulcerative colitis. The earliest manifestation of inflammation is the loss of a normal vessel pattern, the result of edema of the bowel wall. Contact bleeding, granularity, and ulceration are more obvious signs of inflammatory disease. The rectum is spared in 40% of patients with Crohn's colitis, irrespective of anal or perianal involvement. However, when the rectum is involved by this condition, differentiation between the two diseases may be quite difficult.

In individuals with distal disease (i.e., ulcerative proctitis or proctosigmoiditis), complete endoscopic examination by means of the colonoscope is unnecessary at the time of presentation. The extent of disease can usually be determined with the rigid instrument or the flexible sigmoidoscope. The presence of diffuse, confluent, symmetric disease from the

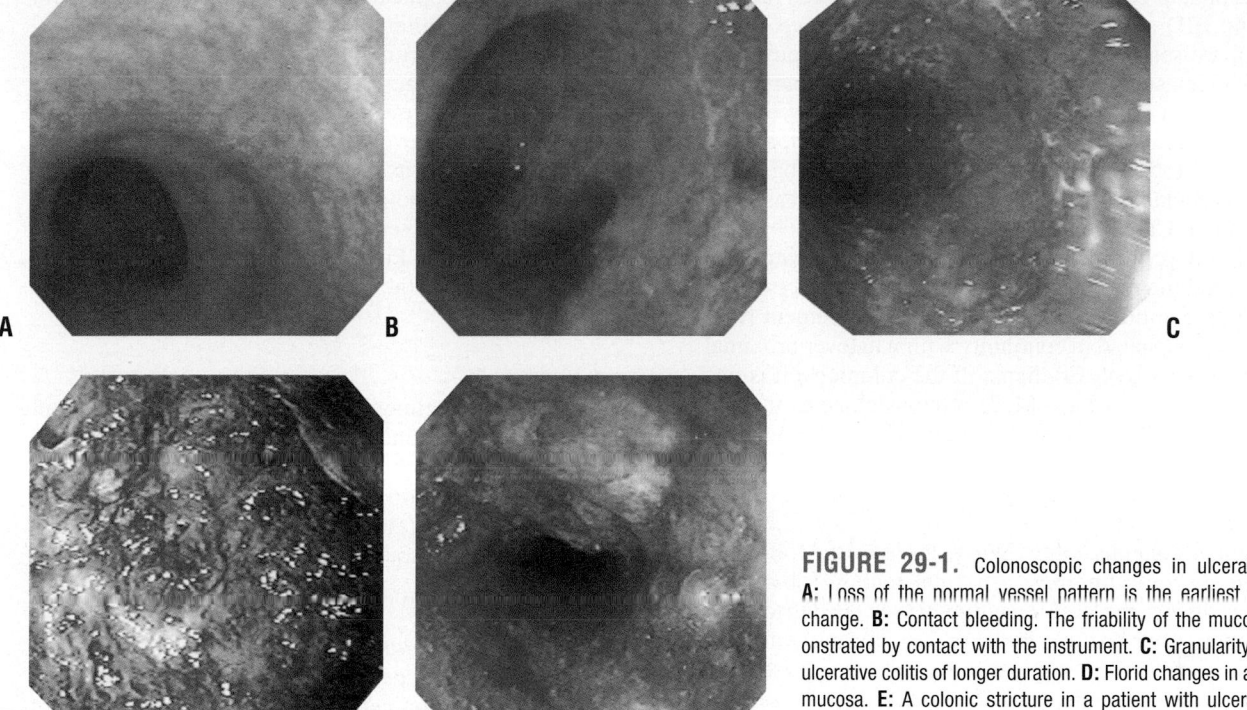

FIGURE 29-1. Colonoscopic changes in ulcerative colitis. **A:** Loss of the normal vessel pattern is the earliest endoscopic change. **B:** Contact bleeding. The friability of the mucosa is demonstrated by contact with the instrument. **C:** Granularity appears in ulcerative colitis of longer duration. **D:** Florid changes in an ulcerated mucosa. **E:** A colonic stricture in a patient with ulcerative colitis proved on biopsy to be malignant.

dentate line cephalad to the limit of the inflammatory reaction is consistent with ulcerative proctitis or proctosigmoiditis, depending on the extent of involvement (Figure 29-1). In individuals with *treated* ulcerative colitis, the finding of rectal sparing or patchiness should not necessarily alter the diagnosis to Crohn's disease.[54] If the patient's symptoms are appropriate to the endoscopic findings, treatment can be initiated without further contrast study or colonoscopy. Conversely, if the patient's disease extends beyond the limit of the endoscopic procedure performed, it will be necessary at some point to undertake total colonic evaluation.

Colonoscopy has replaced barium enema examination for the evaluation of IBD. Generally, endoscopic examination will identify more proximal inflammatory changes than will the radiologic study. Furthermore, histologic examination of random biopsy specimens will often reveal more proximal disease than was suspected by endoscopic examination.[146,783] Das and colleagues reported 31 patients with idiopathic proctitis who underwent colonoscopy while they were asymptomatic.[118] Multiple biopsy samples were taken from throughout the colon and rectum. Although the obvious disease appeared limited to the distal 20 cm, microscopic abnormalities were seen commonly in more proximal locations. The authors postulated that the clinical course would be more consistent with distal disease when this indeed could be confirmed by biopsy, whereas more proximal involvement usually implied that the disease would be refractory to conventional management (e.g., topical steroids). A corollary to this observation is to perform biopsies distal to obvious inflammatory changes if the rectum appears to be spared because one may discover that the rectum is not truly normal. This may cause the physician to reassess the accuracy of a diagnosis of Crohn's disease based on what was initially thought to be a lack of rectal involvement.

The place of colonoscopy in the evaluation and follow-up of IBD has been extensively reviewed by many authors. Teague and Waye recommend colonoscopy for five indications: differential diagnosis, resolution of radiographic abnormalities (e.g., filling defects and strictures), preoperative and postoperative evaluation in Crohn's disease, examination of stomas, and screening for premalignant and malignant changes.[727]

Preparation

Often, colonoscopy can be performed without prior bowel cleansing in patients with mild-to-active IBD, with essentially the same comprehensive evaluation achieved as when a full preparation is used.[34] In the patient who has a history of IBD, the preparation for colonoscopy includes a modified diet. Clear liquids are suggested for 24 hours. Vigorous cleansing enemas such as those that may be used in the evaluation of a noninflamed colon are contraindicated. For someone with a relatively active colitis, no laxative is suggested. In more severe cases, a clear liquid diet as the sole modality for bowel preparation is probably the safer alternative. If the colitis is minimal or relatively inactive, a reduced dose of a laxative is suggested, although it is probably wiser to use a balanced electrolyte solution (e.g., CoLyte, GoLytely, MoviPrep).

Appearance

Ulcerative colitis and Crohn's disease are usually recognized endoscopically by excluding IBD due to specific cause, such as amebic colitis, ischemic colitis, pseudomembranous colitis, and so forth. The most common differential diagnostic problems are related to the numerous and varied infectious colitides (see Chapter 33). Other sources of confusion include radiation changes, the so-called solitary ulcer syndrome, and, of course, the differentiation between the two nonspecific IBD conditions, themselves—ulcerative colitis and Crohn's disease.[727] Biopsy may be helpful because histologic changes suggestive of Crohn's disease in particular may be apparent. Up to 20% of such patients may exhibit granulomas (see Figure 30-2). In patients with ulcerative colitis, rectal biopsy is extremely important for recognizing dysplasia, especially in those with long-standing disease (see Relationship to Carcinoma).

Waye has described a number of colonoscopic features in the differential diagnosis of IBD.[765] He suggests that patients with ulcerative colitis always have rectal involvement from the anal verge cephalad in continuity with whatever proximal involvement is present. Erythema of the colonic wall is one of the early manifestations. More obvious changes include granularity, friability, bleeding, edema with interhaustral septal thickening and blunting, ulceration, mucosal bridging, the presence of pseudopolyps, and the superimposition of carcinoma.

With granulomatous colitis, Waye observed the following major colonoscopic findings: a normal rectum (obviously this is not always the case), asymmetry or eccentricity of involvement, cobblestone appearance, normal vasculature (because friability is not usually encountered except in advanced disease), edema of the bowel wall (as seen in ulcerative colitis), normal mucosa intervening between areas of ulceration, serpiginous or rake ulcers (these may course for several centimeters), pseudopolyps (as in ulcerative colitis), and skip areas (lack of continuity of involvement).[765] He adds another observation, the presence of amyloidosis in the biopsy specimen.

Pera and colleagues undertook a prospective study by means of colonoscopy in 357 patients in order to obtain the best predictive information that would enable the authors to differentiate between the two conditions.[584] An "endoscopic score" was calculated by means of "likelihood ratios." Errors were more frequently noted when severe inflammation was encountered. The most useful endoscopic features in the differential diagnosis were discontinuous involvement, anal lesions, and cobblestone appearance of the mucosa for Crohn's disease, and erosions or microulcers and granularity for ulcerative colitis.[584]

Myren and colleagues performed routine and random histologic evaluation by means of colonoscopic biopsy in patients with and without IBD.[524] In 110 individuals, 278 biopsy specimens were obtained at different levels of the colon. Clinical information, including colonoscopic diagnosis, was available to the pathologist at the initial routine examination. Later, the sections were examined blindly and independently by two pathologists. Agreement was obtained in only two-thirds of the patients. The authors concluded that the limiting factor in making reliable diagnoses was the small size of the tissue specimens available. Also, discrepancies may have been caused by the fact that biopsy specimens were not always representative of the process in the colonic mucosa.

Farmer and colleagues reviewed 100 patients who underwent colonoscopy for distal ulcerative colitis.[148] They classified their patients into two groups: those whose disease was confined to the distal 25 cm and those whose mucosal changes extended above that level but not beyond the splenic flexure. Because flexible sigmoidoscopy or colonoscopy is not as accurate in defining disease in the rectum, whether it

is inflammatory or neoplastic, there was a 5% disagreement about the presence of inflammation in that area of the bowel. Certainly, the rigid instrument is far more useful in evaluating the rectum than the colonoscope. Biopsy specimens were taken at multiple levels, and the retrospective review was performed during several years. It was determined that patients whose disease was initially limited to the rectum and sigmoid colon had a good prognosis—only 10% progressed to more extensive involvement. However, 25% of patients experienced recurrence. Prognosis was similar whether the disease was confined to the lower 25 cm or was distal to the splenic flexure.

Comment

Additional biopsy specimens for the evaluation of a patient with IBD should be obtained from an area that appears macroscopically, at least, to be relatively uninvolved. The true extent of the inflammation as well as the significance of the presence of granulomas (granulomas may be seen in patients with ulcerative colitis underlying an ulcer) can then be interpreted properly.

Colonoscopy versus Barium Enema

In general, colonoscopy permits identification of segmental involvement and microulceration better than does barium enema. However, radiographic studies yield more information about haustra, especially in the right colon.[193] One must remember, however, that the procedure is contraindicated in patients with acute exacerbation of the colitis and certainly in those who have a toxic megacolon. Myren and colleagues performed colonoscopic evaluation in 40 patients and compared the results with that of conventional barium enema.[523] Colonoscopic diagnosis and biopsy results were corroborating in 80% of the patients, whereas colonoscopic evaluation and radiologic survey revealed agreement in only 55%. The area in which radiology seemed to have an advantage was the decreased haustration that was more apparent by x-ray techniques. Erosions, mucosal edema, and vascular injection were not detected by barium enema. Others have confirmed the merits of colonoscopy in the evaluation of patients with nonspecific IBD.[185,723,766,777]

Radiographic Features

Plain Films

In any evaluation of a patient with IBD, the importance of a plain x-ray film of the abdomen (KUB) should not be underestimated. Without submitting patients to the rigors of a contrast study or colonoscopy, particularly when they may be acutely ill, the physician can obtain valuable information about the extent of disease (Figure 29-2).

The importance of a plain film of the abdomen is further increased in those who have toxic dilatation, a condition usually seen in the transverse colon (Figure 29-3). When the radiographic appearance of toxic dilatation is noted, a barium enema examination or colonoscopy is contraindicated due to the risk of iatrogenic perforation, but serial abdominal films are clinically extremely valuable. The effectiveness of medical therapy can be evaluated by determining the increase or decrease in the degree of dilatation. The abdominal examination should not be relied on exclusively because the patient may frequently be confused or even obtunded. However, the degree of dilatation may not necessarily be predictive of

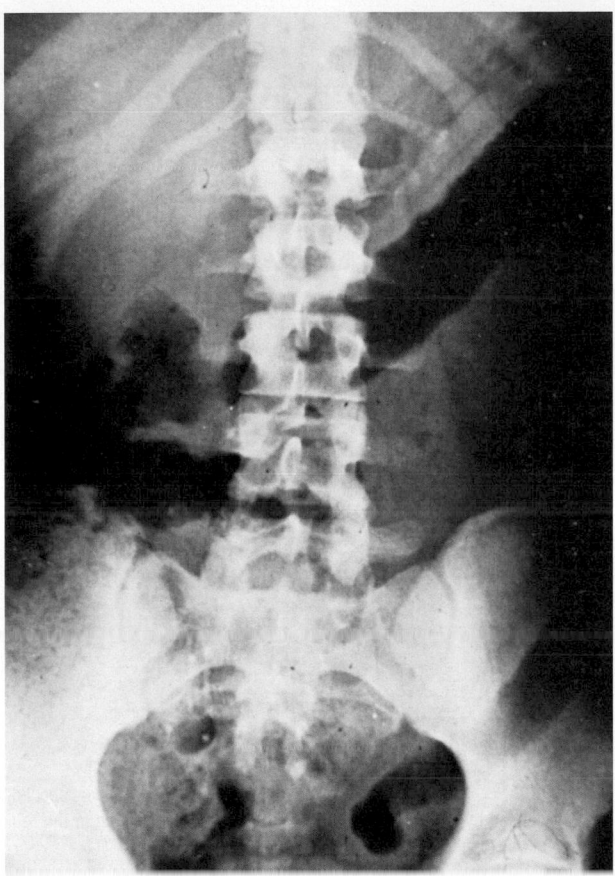

FIGURE 29-2. Ulcerative colitis. This plain abdominal film of an acutely ill patient reveals some thickening of the colonic wall, especially in the region of the sigmoid where it overlies the iliac crest, and loss of haustral markings throughout the left colon and transverse colon to the region of the hepatic flexure. Subsequent barium enema study demonstrated disease extending exactly to the point seen on the plain film. (From Corman ML, Veidenheimer MC, Nugent FW, et al. *Diseases of the Anus, Rectum and Colon. Part II: Nonspecific Inflammatory Bowel Disease.* New York, NY: Medcom; 1976.)

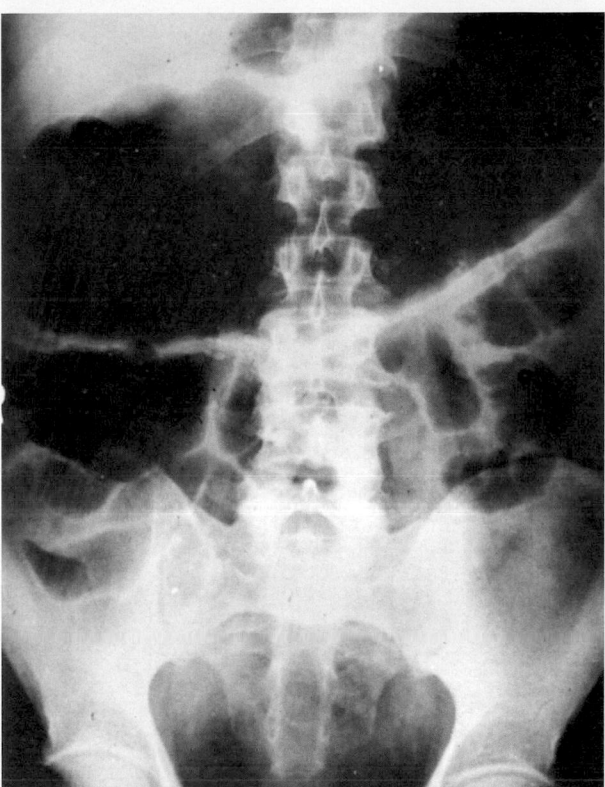

FIGURE 29-3. Ulcerative colitis. This plain abdominal x-ray film reveals marked dilatation of the transverse colon (toxic megacolon). The extent of dilatation may not necessarily be predictive of the need for urgent surgery. However, pneumoperitoneum, sometimes missed by the presence of free gas trapped by the omentum at the inferior border of the transverse colon, is an indication for urgent surgery. (From Corman ML, Veidenheimer MC, Nugent FW, et al. *Diseases of the Anus, Rectum and Colon. Part II: Nonspecific Inflammatory Bowel Disease.* New York, NY: Medcom; 1976.)

the need for surgery. Furthermore, the high dose of steroids often used in the treatment of toxic megacolon may mask abdominal signs.

Barium Enema

The radiologic findings during the acute phase of ulcerative colitis include edema, ulceration, and changes in colonic motility. Edema may be apparent even on the plain film of the abdomen, such as is seen in Figure 29-3. Initially, ulceration may be minimal and difficult to identify. As the disease becomes fulminant, the ulceration becomes more obvious and may take on a "collar button" appearance (Figure 29-4). Edema and inflammation of the mucosa may result in the radiologic appearance that has been called "thumbprinting," a phenomenon characteristically observed in patients with ischemic colitis (Figure 29-5).

When the disease enters a more chronic phase, other features are characteristic on the barium enema examination. These include fibrosis, which results in shortening of the bowel, depression of the flexures, pseudopolyposis, and stricture formation. The bowel wall is less distensible, and the motility pattern is disturbed. Diffuse, confluent, symmetric

disease, beginning with the anorectal junction, are the hallmarks of the radiologic manifestations of chronic ulcerative colitis (Figures 29-6 and 29-7). The presence of polypoid lesions throughout the entire colon may confuse the uninitiated with the radiologic picture seen in familial polyposis (Figure 29-8). Both diseases commonly present with rectal bleeding and diarrhea. In ulcerative colitis, however, foreshortening of the bowel may be evident, particularly at the flexures, and if the outline of the colon is carefully examined, numerous discrete ulcerations can usually be appreciated (Figure 29-9).

Benign strictures are extremely uncommon in ulcerative colitis. In fact, a stricture in this condition should be considered malignant until proved otherwise (see Relationship to Carcinoma).[385] Radiologic examination will usually reveal a smoothly outlined, concentric lumen with tapering margins (Figure 29-10). Areas of spasm are frequently seen in ulcerative colitis and may be difficult to differentiate from stricture. The administration of propantheline (10 mg of Pro-Banthine intravenously) or glucagon (2 mg intramuscularly) may eliminate the stricture caused by such spasm. If the lumen is concentric and the margins are smooth, the lesion may be benign. Conversely, if the lumen is eccentric and the margins are irregular, a carcinoma must be suspected.[462]

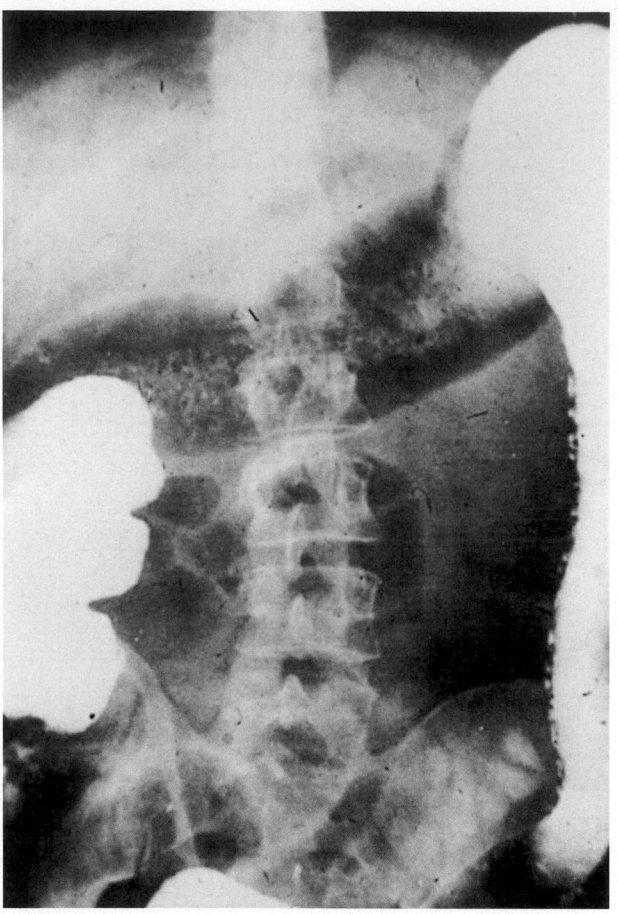

FIGURE 29-4. Acute ulcerative colitis. Note the loss of haustral markings up to and including the mid-ascending colon and numerous discrete ulcerations deep in the submucosa along the descending colon. (From Corman ML, Veidenheimer MC, Nugent FW, et al. *Diseases of the Anus, Rectum and Colon. Part II: Nonspecific Inflammatory Bowel Disease.* New York, NY: Medcom; 1976.)

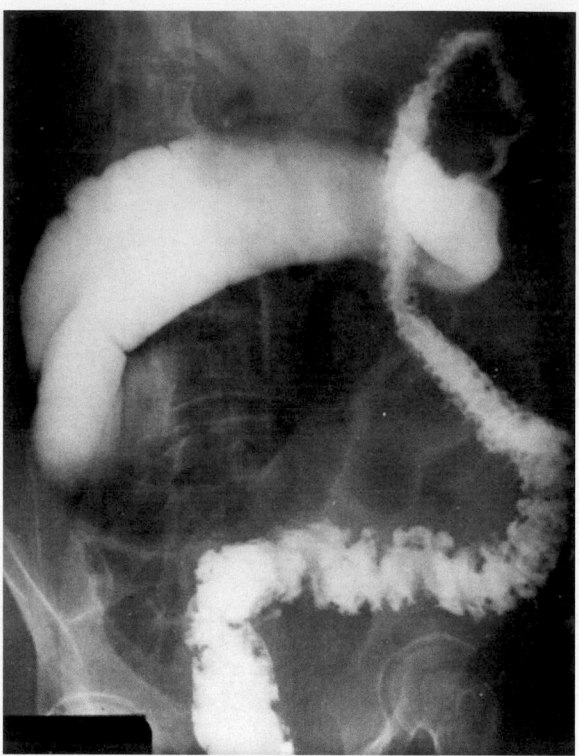

FIGURE 29-5. Edema of the bowel wall in acute ulcerative colitis; flocculation of barium caused by mucus (fuzzy appearance) and thumbprinting in the region of the splenic flexure.

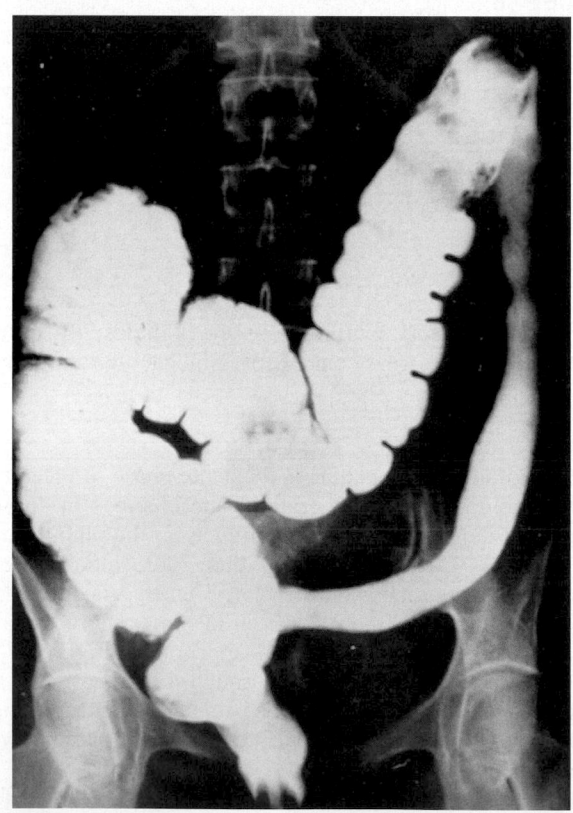

FIGURE 29-6. Chronic ulcerative colitis. Typical changes of left-sided disease include loss of haustral pattern, shortening of the sigmoid, and narrowing of the entire descending and sigmoid colon. (From Corman ML, Veidenheimer MC, Nugent FW, et al. *Diseases of the Anus, Rectum and Colon. Part II: Nonspecific Inflammatory Bowel Disease.* New York, NY: Medcom; 1976.)

Another radiologic finding sometimes observed in patients with ulcerative colitis is "backwash ileitis." This is a very poor term because it implies that the ulcerative colitis has somehow regurgitated through the ileocecal valve to cause the disease in the distal ileum. Marshak and Lindner were able to demonstrate the presence of this phenomenon in approximately 10% of patients with ulcerative colitis whom they had studied.[462] The changes may vary from lack of distensibility, as the head of pressure is increased when the barium is inserted, to ileal dilatation, narrowing, rigidity, and changes that may mimic those of regional enteritis (Figure 29-11). The clinical and therapeutic implications of backwash ileitis are uncertain. There is, however, evidence to suggest higher rates of sclerosing cholangitis in those with this manifestation. Moreover, this observation does not affect the outcome of restorative proctocolectomy in a negative fashion.

Portal venous gas has been reported to be a benign, albeit unusual, consequence of air-contrast barium enema in patients with IBD. Although the implication of such an observation when made in other patients is that antibiotic treatment is required, it may not be necessary if the patient is without bacteremic symptoms.[331]

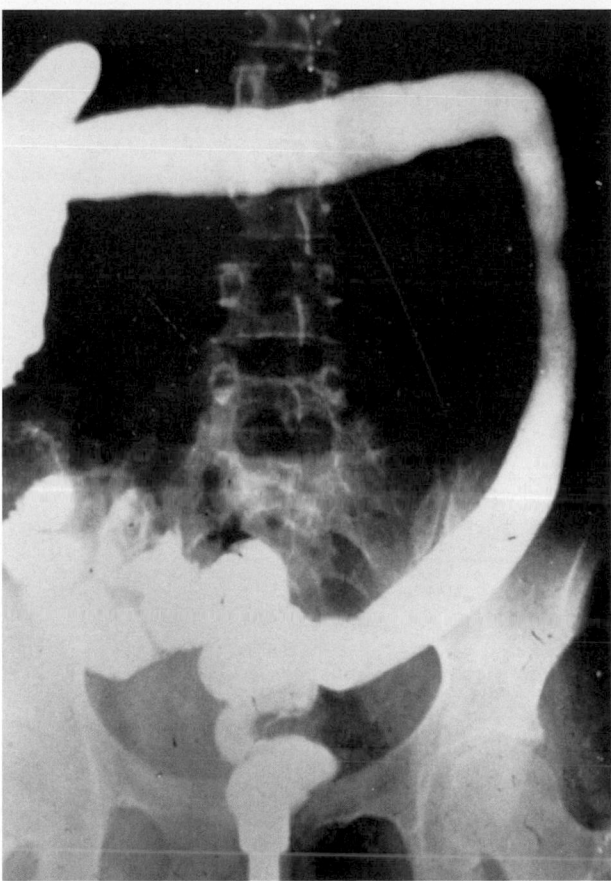

FIGURE 29-7. Chronic ulcerative colitis: a classic example of diffuse, symmetric, confluent disease. Characteristically, the left side is more involved than the right. Note that there is more foreshortening of the splenic flexure than of the hepatic flexure, and there is a suggestion of haustra on the right but not on the left. (From Corman ML, Veidenheimer MC, Nugent FW, et al. *Diseases of the Anus, Rectum and Colon. Part II: Nonspecific Inflammatory Bowel Disease.* New York, NY: Medcom; 1976.)

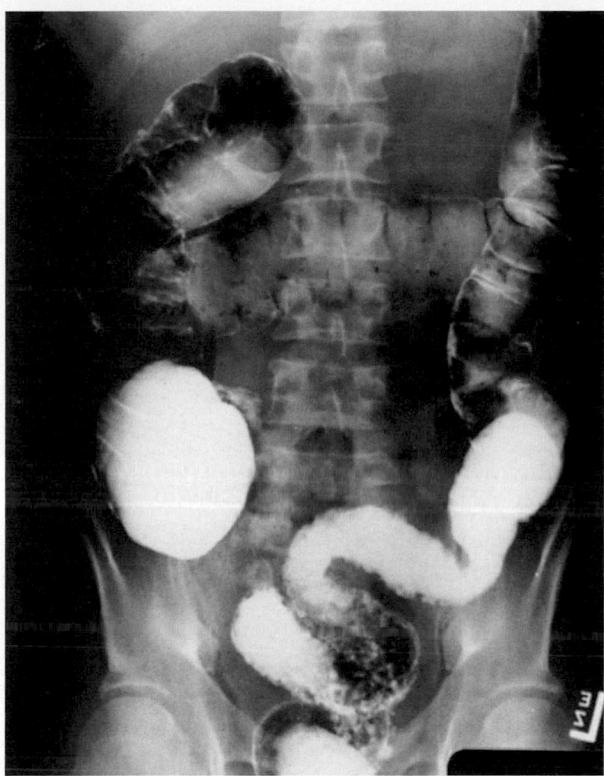

FIGURE 29-8. Ulcerative colitis. This barium enema study reveals extensive pseudopolyposis, especially in the region of the sigmoid colon. Close examination also reveals ulceration, so there should be no confusion with familial polyposis.

Computed Tomography

The advent of computed tomography (CT) has permitted direct visualization of the entire thickness of the bowel wall and mesentery, and determination of the presence or absence of fluid, fistula, or abscess.[440] With the exception of its unique application to abscess drainage, the role of this study in the diagnosis and management of patients with IBD is controversial. One thing is certain, however; CT is of no value in assessing the extent of mucosal disease. Its advantages over contrast enema are primarily in delineating the presence and severity of pericolonic inflammation and in evaluating other organ disease. Although the place of CT in IBD is still a matter of conjecture, it is unlikely to prove to be of benefit in patients with ulcerative colitis. Because Crohn's disease is a transmural process, one may anticipate a greater application with this condition.

Ultrasonography

Hata and colleagues performed ultrasonographic examinations in individuals with ulcerative colitis and Crohn's disease and in 50 patients with no bowel disease.[259] Crohn's disease and ulcerative colitis could be detected by ultrasonography with a sensitivity of 86% and 89%, respectively. The primary benefit appeared to be in the demonstration of thickening of the bowel wall. However, because the study is less invasive than other alternatives and can be done without preparation, it may be used

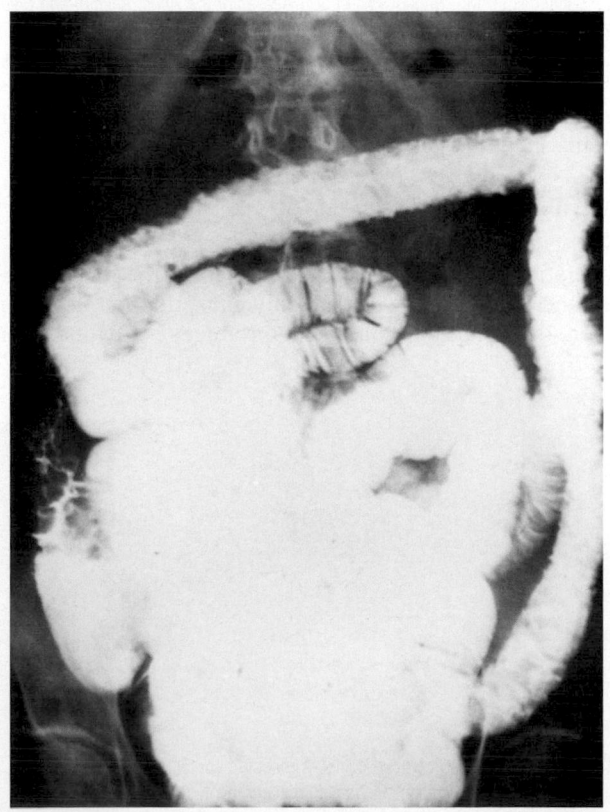

FIGURE 29-9. Ulcerative colitis. Extensive pseudopolyposis with foreshortening of the bowel. Note that the colon is outlined by ulcerations. (From Corman ML, Veidenheimer MC, Nugent FW, et al. *Diseases of the Anus, Rectum and Colon. Part II: Nonspecific Inflammatory Bowel Disease.* New York, NY: Medcom; 1976.)

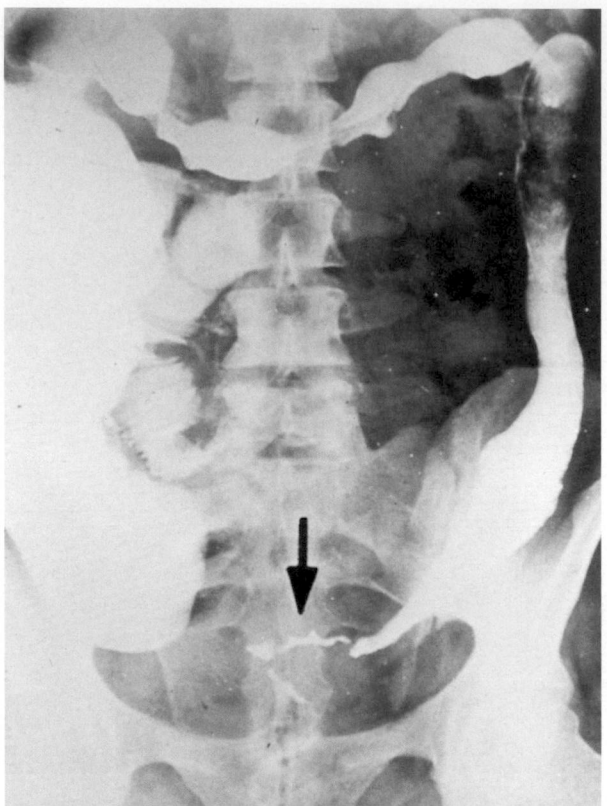

FIGURE 29-10. Ulcerative colitis with stricture. Inflammatory changes are noted to the hepatic flexure, with stricture in the distal sigmoid (*arrow*). The patient subsequently underwent resection, and the lesion was found to be benign. (From Corman ML, Veidenheimer MC, Nugent FW, et al. *Diseases of the Anus, Rectum and Colon. Part II: Nonspecific Inflammatory Bowel Disease.* New York, NY: Medcom; 1976.)

to reduce the frequency of repeated colonoscopic or barium enema studies in patients already known to harbor IBD.[259]

Pathology

Macroscopic Appearance

Ulcerative colitis is a disease confined to the mucosa and submucosa of the bowel. The only exception to this occurs when transmural involvement produces so-called toxic

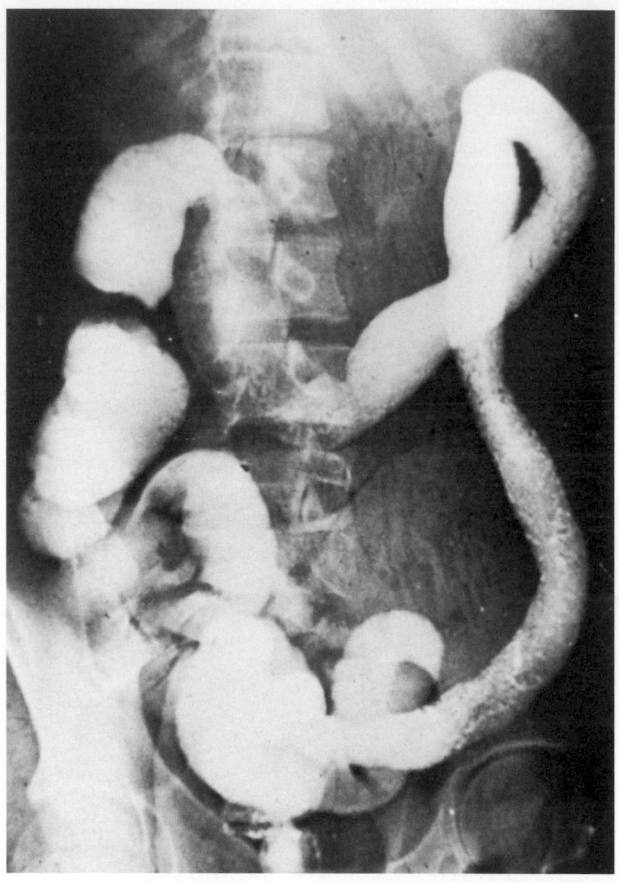

FIGURE 29-11. Extensive ulcerative colitis with loss of haustral markings and destruction of the normal mucosa throughout. Dilatation of the terminal ileum may be evidence of "backwash ileitis." However, if signs of ileal inflammation extend beyond 10 cm, the diagnosis of Crohn's disease is more likely. (From Corman ML, Veidenheimer MC, Nugent FW, et al. *Diseases of the Anus, Rectum and Colon. Part II: Nonspecific Inflammatory Bowel Disease.* New York, NY: Medcom; 1976.)

megacolon. The bowel wall is not thickened, no granulomas are present (except a foreign body giant cell reaction may occasionally be seen in an area of acute inflammation), and there are no skip areas. The rectum is always involved, and the disease extends proximally for varying distances, but

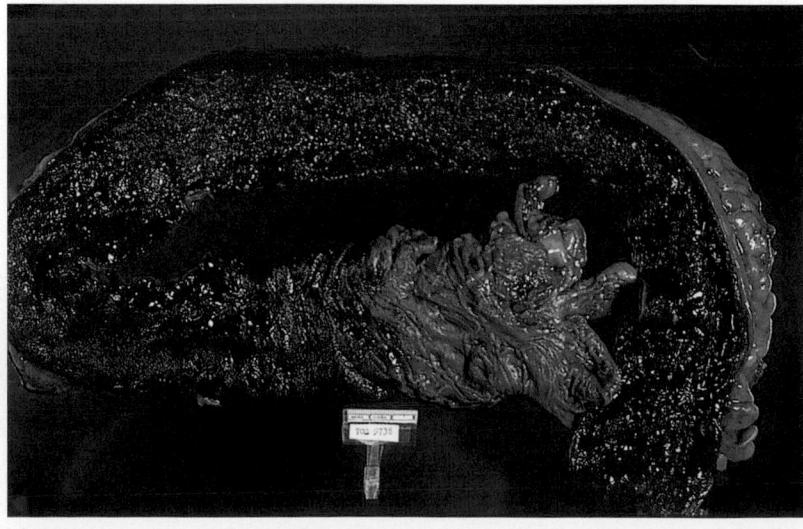

FIGURE 29-12. Ulcerative colitis. A resected specimen (rectum removed separately) shows continuity of involvement from the sigmoid to the mid-ascending colon. Loss of mucosa, deep ulceration, and extensive granularity are evident. (From Corman ML, Veidenheimer MC, Nugent FW, et al. *Diseases of the Anus, Rectum and Colon. Part II: Nonspecific Inflammatory Bowel Disease.* New York, NY: Medcom; 1976.)

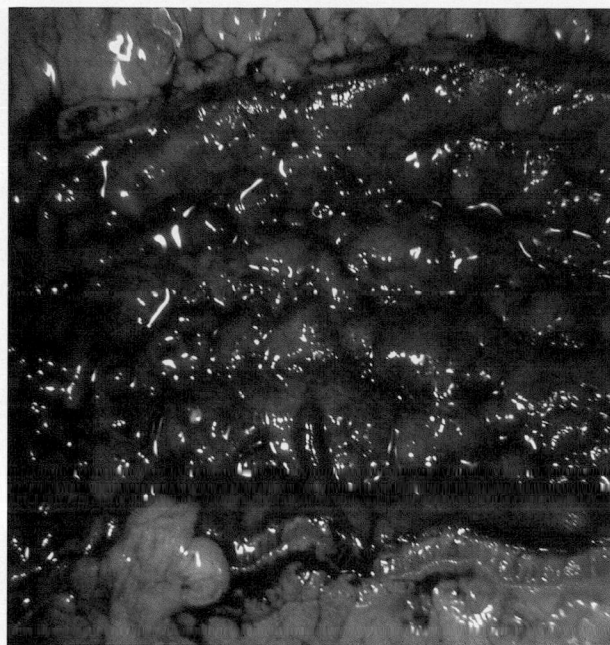

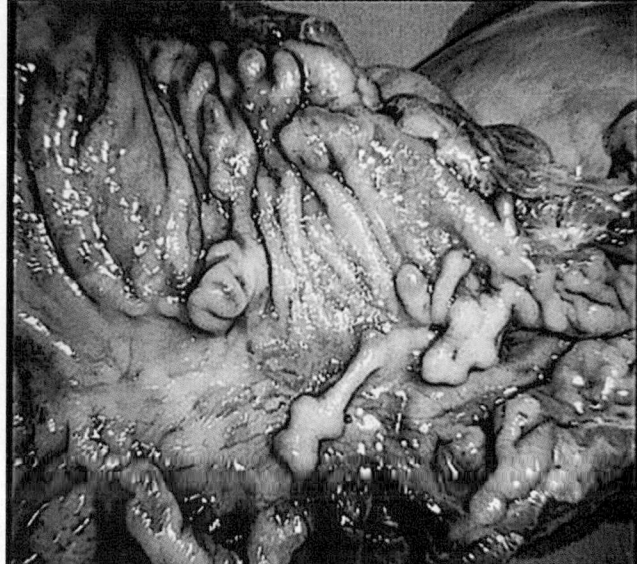

FIGURE 29-15. Ulcerative colitis. Islands of heaped-up mucosa and inflammatory polyps (pseudopolyps). (From Corman ML, Veidenheimer MC, Nugent FW, et al. *Diseases of the Anus, Rectum and Colon. Part II: Nonspecific Inflammatory Bowel Disease.* New York, NY: Medcom; 1976.)

FIGURE 29-13. Ulcerative colitis. Longitudinal furrows of denuded mucosa alternate with islands of heaped-up mucosa, demonstrating how loss of mucosal integrity contributes to fluid and electrolyte depletion. (From Corman ML, Veidenheimer MC, Nugent FW, et al. *Diseases of the Anus, Rectum and Colon. Part II: Nonspecific Inflammatory Bowel Disease.* New York, NY: Medcom; 1976.)

always with continuity of involvement to the proximal extent of the disease process (Figure 29-12). Characteristically, ulcerative colitis tends to involve the bowel more severely in a distal location than proximally. Despite extensive inflammatory reaction, the bowel wall retains its normal thickness (Figure 29-12). The results of the confluence of numerous ulcers are the longitudinal furrows of denuded mucosa that alternate with islands of heaped-up mucosa, the so-called pseudopolyps (Figures 29-13 through 29-15). Pseudopolyps are inflammatory polyps, not neoplastic lesions. These are seen during a quiescent phase of ulcerative colitis and are a later manifestation of this condition. They may be confused

with familial polyposis (see Chapter 22), but the absence of normal mucosa between these polyps suggests the correct diagnosis.

The entire colon, including the cecum and appendix, may be involved (Figure 29-16). Characteristically, however, the disease does not affect the ileum. In fact, if the small bowel is involved for more than a few centimeters, the diagnosis is not ulcerative colitis. One exception to this is the so-called backwash ileitis seen occasionally when the entire colon is affected. This reversible condition, which may be demonstrated radiographically as edematous, thickened mucosal folds, is a nonspecific inflammatory reaction resulting from proximity of the ileum to the diseased colon.

The entire mucosa may be denuded in patients with long-standing, chronic ulcerative colitis (Figure 29-17). Under

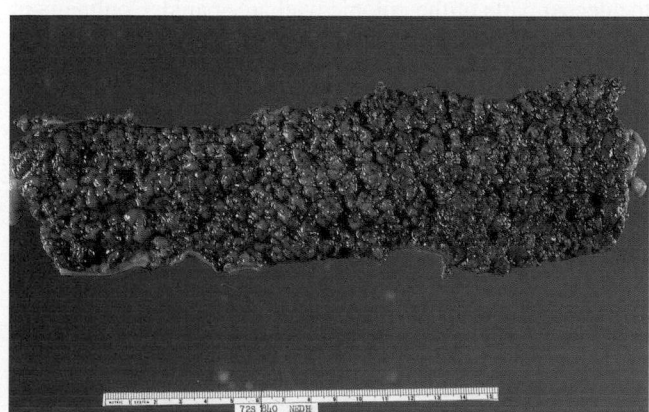

FIGURE 29-14. Extensive pseudopolyps in active ulcerative colitis. Note the relative uniformity of the polyps in comparison with the varied sizes seen in familial polyposis (see Chapter 22). (From Corman ML, Veidenheimer MC, Nugent FW, et al. *Diseases of the Anus, Rectum and Colon. Part II: Nonspecific Inflammatory Bowel Disease.* New York, NY: Medcom; 1976.)

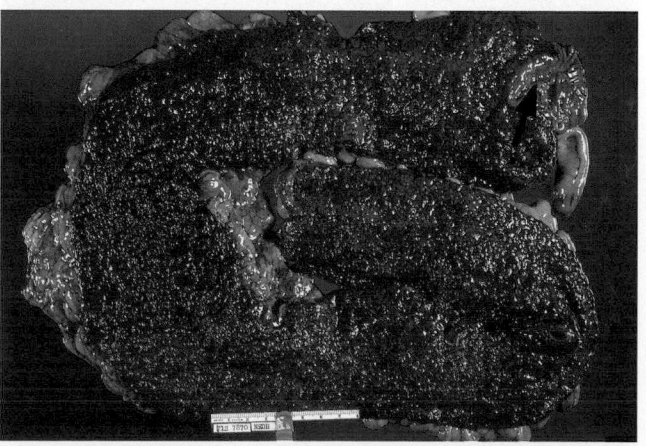

FIGURE 29-16. Ulcerative colitis. The entire colon is involved by inflammatory change, with sparing of the ileum (*arrow*). (From Corman ML, Veidenheimer MC, Nugent FW, et al. *Diseases of the Anus, Rectum and Colon. Part II: Nonspecific Inflammatory Bowel Disease.* New York, NY: Medcom; 1976.)

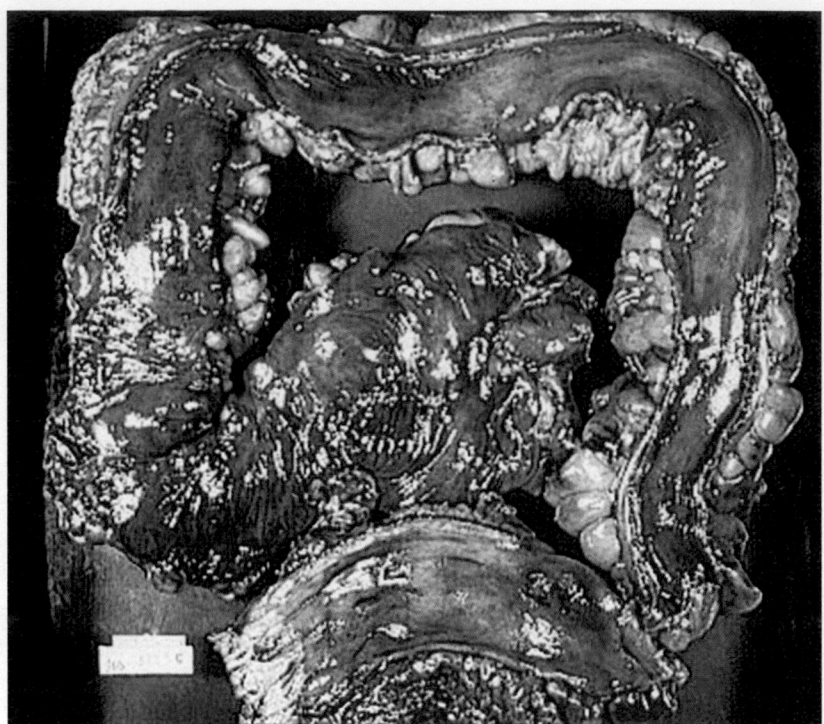

FIGURE 29-17. Ulcerative colitis. Complete desquamation of colonic mucosa. Note the normal bowel wall thickness. (From Corman ML, Veidenheimer MC, Nugent FW, et al. *Diseases of the Anus, Rectum and Colon. Part II: Nonspecific Inflammatory Bowel Disease.* New York, NY: Medcom; 1976.)

these circumstances, the physician may be lulled into a false sense of security because the patient's symptoms are often minimal. It is unlikely that someone will experience discharge of mucus, diarrhea, or bleeding if no inflamed mucosa is present. It is this individual who is particularly susceptible to the development of carcinoma (see Relationship to Carcinoma).

Toxic megacolon is a condition in which an acute inflammatory reaction extends throughout the entire thickness of the bowel wall to the serosa. Gangrene and perforation can result (Figure 29-18). This is the only manifestation of ulcerative colitis that is not limited to the mucosa and submucosa. The term is a poor one because it is not the colon that is toxic; it is obviously the patient.

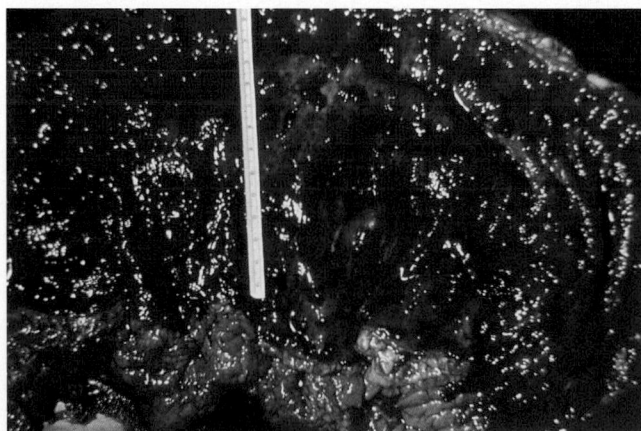

FIGURE 29-18. Ulcerative colitis. Portion of a resected transverse colon showing increased circumference of the bowel. There is practically no mucosa remaining, and circular muscle is exposed in some areas. (From Corman ML, Veidenheimer MC, Nugent FW, et al. *Diseases of the Anus, Rectum and Colon. Part II: Nonspecific Inflammatory Bowel Disease.* New York, NY: Medcom; 1976.)

Histologic Appearance

Ulcerative colitis is characterized histologically by an intense inflammation of the mucosa and submucosa, in addition to the presence of multiple crypt abscesses. Too much emphasis, however, should not be placed on the significance of crypt abscesses. Acute, self-limited colitis (in which cultures are negative) as well as infectious colitides (see Chapter 33) often have overlapping histopathologic features and must be distinguished from ulcerative colitis.[268,282] Marked vascular engorgement accounts for the propensity to rectal bleeding (Figure 29-19). There is an obvious decrease in production of mucus by the crypt epithelial cells (Figure 29-20). The decrease may be explained by injury to these cells.[352] Conversely, increased secretion of mucus is seen in patients with Crohn's disease.

If the bowel is cut longitudinally, it becomes apparent that the deeper parts of the colonic wall are spared. Confinement of the disease to the mucosa and submucosa is the most characteristic finding in ulcerative colitis (Figure 29-21). Abscesses may enlarge to undermine the mucosa, which may then be shed into the bowel lumen, leaving an ulcer behind. When multiple ulcers form, the remaining nonulcerated mucosa extends above the muscularis as polypoid projections, resulting in the well-known pseudopolyps of ulcerative colitis (Figures 29-22 and 29-23). If ulceration continues, the entire mucosa may become denuded, and broad areas of the submucosa may be exposed to the fecal stream.

In toxic megacolon, there is full-thickness involvement of the bowel, necrosis, and friability, the histologic manifestation of which is shown in Figure 29-24.

Lymphoid hyperplasia involving the mucosa and submucosa occurs in up to 25% of patients with ulcerative colitis. This may be present beneath an area of relative inactivity (Figure 29-25).

Seldenrijk and colleagues prospectively performed blind evaluations of multiple colonic mucosal biopsy specimens

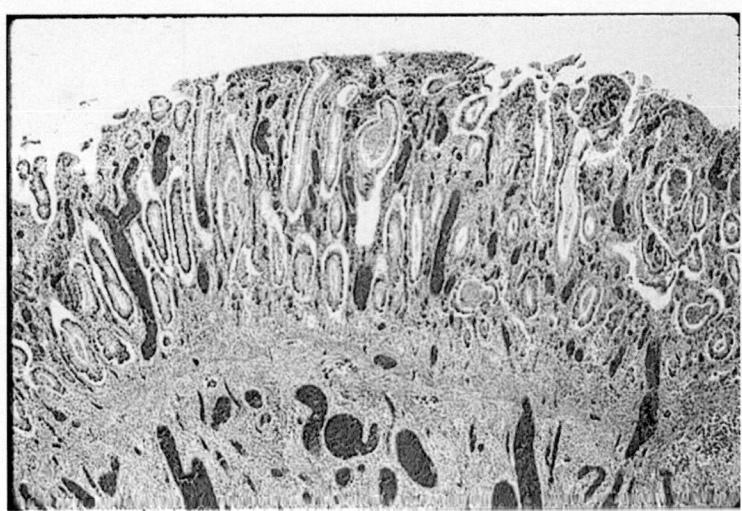

FIGURE 29-19. Ulcerative colitis. Intense inflammation of the mucosa with multiple crypt abscesses. (Original magnification × 80; from Corman ML, Veidenheimer MC, Nugent FW, et al. *Diseases of the Anus, Rectum and Colon. Part II: Nonspecific Inflammatory Bowel Disease.* New York, NY: Medcom; 1976.)

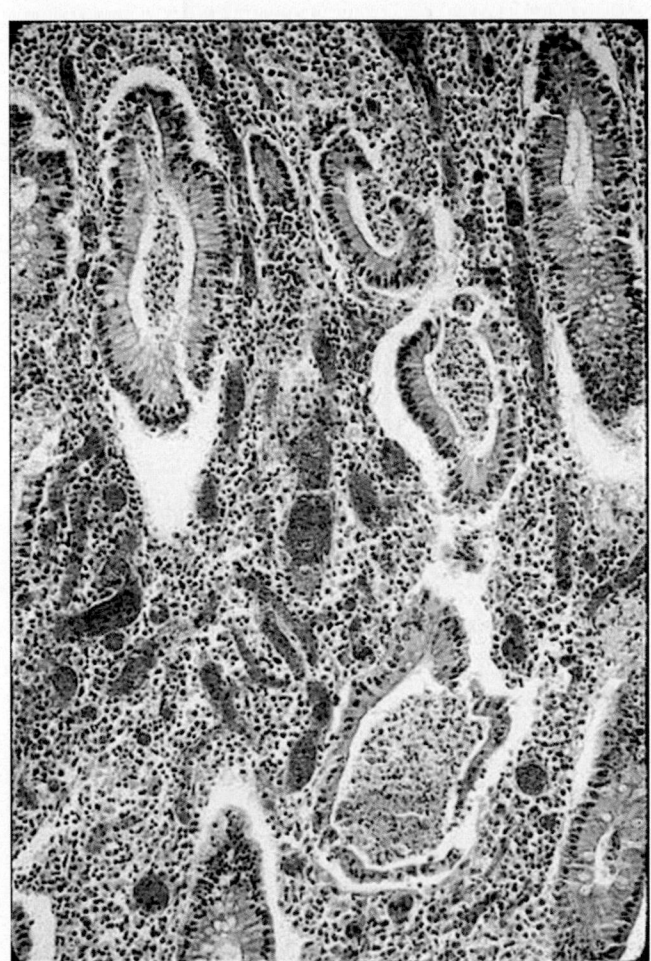

FIGURE 29-20. Ulcerative colitis. Crypt abscesses with degeneration of crypt epithelium and communication between the crypt lumina and lamina propria. Note vascular engorgement and decrease in mucus production by crypt epithelial cells. (Original magnification × 280; from Corman ML, Veidenheimer MC, Nugent FW, et al. *Diseases of the Anus, Rectum and Colon. Part II: Nonspecific Inflammatory Bowel Disease.* New York, NY: Medcom; 1976.)

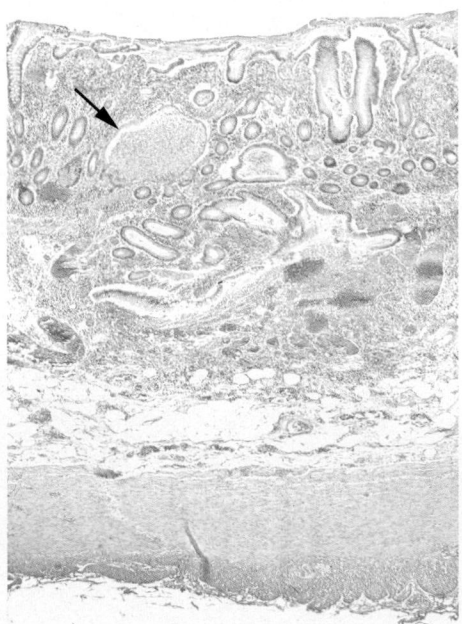

FIGURE 29-21. Ulcerative colitis. Marked inflammation of the mucosa and submucosa. Note the large crypt abscess (*arrow*) that has penetrated into the submucosa and has been lined partially by epithelial cells growing down into the abscess cavity. (Original magnification × 80; from Corman ML, Veidenheimer MC, Nugent FW, et al. *Diseases of the Anus, Rectum and Colon. Part II: Nonspecific Inflammatory Bowel Disease.* New York, NY: Medcom; 1976.)

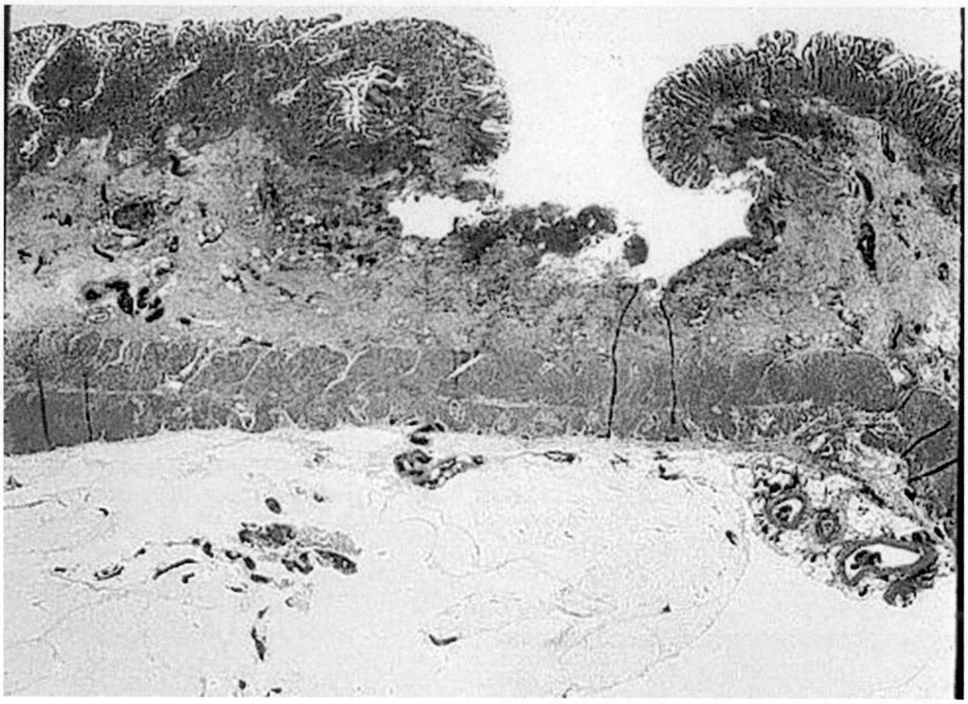

FIGURE 29-22. Ulcerative colitis. An enlarged abscess undermines the mucosa, leaving an ulcer. (Original magnification × 80; from Corman ML, Veidenheimer MC, Nugent FW, et al. *Diseases of the Anus, Rectum and Colon. Part II: Nonspecific Inflammatory Bowel Disease.* New York, NY: Medcom; 1976.)

in individuals with ulcerative colitis and Crohn's disease to identify reproducible histologic features that could be used to distinguish between the two conditions.[672] Three features—an excess of histiocytes in combination with a villous or irregular aspect of the mucosal surface and granulomas—had a high predictive value.

Watanabe and coworkers studied rectal biopsy specimens from patients with ulcerative colitis undergoing colonoscopic examinations for the presence of substance P–containing nerve fibers.[763] It is well known that the bowel is rich in peptidergic innervation, which contributes to the mucosal immune responses. Because substance P has stimulatory effects on various immunocytes in inflammatory diseases, its increased presence paralleling increased disease activity suggests that alterations play an important role in the pathogenesis of ulcerative colitis.[763]

Antineutrophil Cytoplasmic Antibody Determination
Various studies have shown that antineutrophil cytoplasmic antibodies (ANCAs) with a perinuclear staining pattern

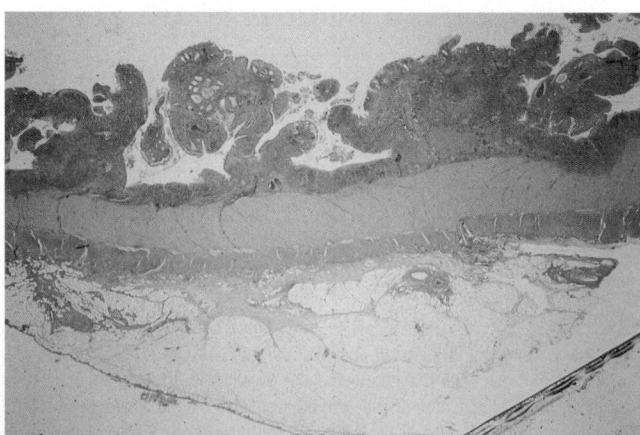

FIGURE 29-23. Ulcerative colitis. Confluence of ulcers results in pseudopolyps. (Original magnification × 80; from Corman ML, Veidenheimer MC, Nugent FW, et al. *Diseases of the Anus, Rectum and Colon. Part II: Nonspecific Inflammatory Bowel Disease.* New York, NY: Medcom; 1976.)

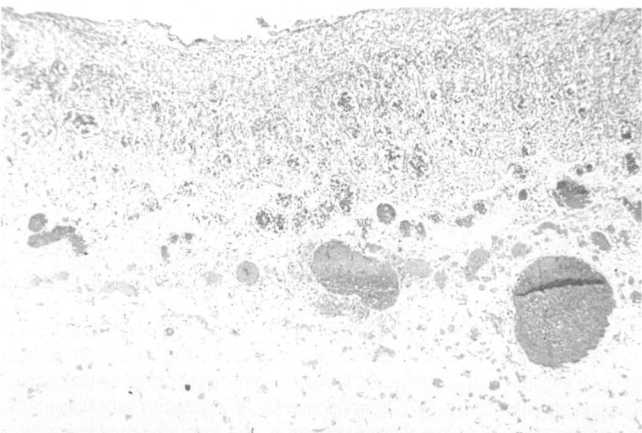

FIGURE 29-24. Ulcerative colitis. Toxic megacolon. Note the loss of epithelium, transmural necrosis, and hemorrhage. (Original magnification × 80; from Corman ML, Veidenheimer MC, Nugent FW, et al. *Diseases of the Anus, Rectum and Colon. Part II: Nonspecific Inflammatory Bowel Disease.* New York, NY: Medcom; 1976.)

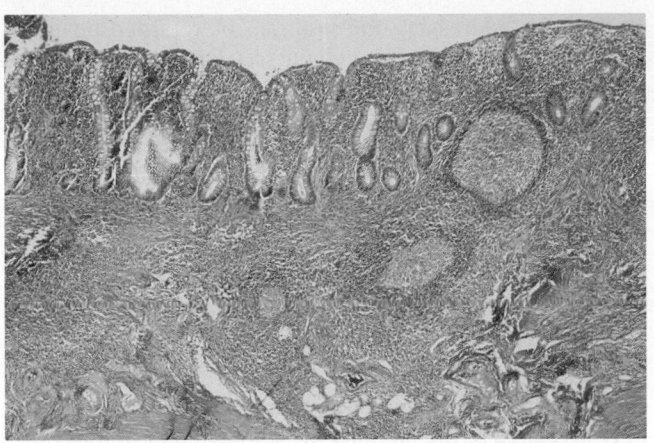

FIGURE 29-25. Lymphoid hyperplasia. Although mucosal disease is relatively inactive, lymphoid hyperplasia is pronounced. (Original magnification × 80; from Corman ML, Veidenheimer MC, Nugent FW, et al. *Diseases of the Anus, Rectum and Colon. Part II: Nonspecific Inflammatory Bowel Disease.* New York, NY: Medcom; 1976.)

(pANCA) are present in up to 86% of patients with ulcerative colitis.[655] Theoretically, this autoimmunity may represent a possible pathogenetic mechanism for the development of ulcerative colitis. A set of marker antibodies is available for the screening and differential diagnosis of ulcerative colitis and Crohn's disease (Prometheus Laboratories, Inc., San Diego, CA). Proven applications of this technology include the following:

- as an adjunct to clinical and tissue pathology in the differential diagnosis of IBD
- confirmation of the correct diagnosis before surgery
- identification of those patients with left-sided ulcerative colitis that may be resistant to treatment
- identification of those patients prone to the development of pouchitis following ileal pouch-anal anastomosis

Although the data provided by the Los Angeles group is persuasive, the reality is that pANCA testing is not commonly used in our practice, except where inflammation is additive to other proven features. Such knowledge might suggest an alternative operative approach.

Breath Pentane Analysis
As previously mentioned, neutrophils, macrophages, and other cells are capable of producing free oxygen radicals that can stimulate lipid peroxidation, especially during periods of active inflammation.[366] To assess the degree of inflammation in IBD, Kokoszka and colleagues quantitatively determined breath pentane and alkane generated by peroxidation of cellular fatty acids.[366] Individuals underwent indium-labeled granulocyte nuclear imaging to assess the presence and location of inflammation. The production of pentane, the product of the peroxidation of polyunsaturated fatty acids, can be quantified by measuring the content of exhaled breath. The investigators concluded that pentane analysis may be correlated with IBD activity.[366]

Leukocyte Scan
Abdominal scintigraphy by means of autologous-labeled leukocytes has been used to assess activity in IBD.

Indium 111 (^{111}In) and technetium 99m (^{99m}Tc) have been the most helpful in this regard. Ståhlberg and colleagues undertook an evaluation using scintigraphy with ^{99m}Tc-labeled leukocytes to assess disease extent and activity in acute colitis.[573] With colonoscopy as the reference method, the maximum extent of colitis was correctly assessed by the scan in two-thirds of patients, but rectal involvement was not perceived in 19%. The intensity of inflammatory activity correlated significantly with the colonoscopic assessment. The authors concluded that the noninvasive nature of this particular approach makes it a reasonable alternative to other investigations of the extent and activity of IBD.

▶ SIGNS, SYMPTOMS, AND PRESENTATIONS

Patients with ulcerative colitis and Crohn's disease may present with very minimal symptoms and moderate complaints, or they may have fulminant manifestations. There is a considerable overlap in the symptomatology of the two conditions, but there are some differences in the presentation between the two. Rectal bleeding is always seen in patients with ulcerative colitis at some time during the course of the illness. It can be safely said that if the patient does not bleed, the diagnosis is not ulcerative colitis. Individuals with Crohn's disease also may bleed, but this is not as frequent a manifestation and may not be as severe. Abdominal pain may be mild or absent in patients with ulcerative colitis, but it is rarely severe except possibly when toxic megacolon supervenes. However, patients with Crohn's disease frequently have abdominal pain.[229] An abdominal mass is occasionally found on physical examination in a patient with Crohn's disease, but it is never seen in a patient with ulcerative colitis, except rarely if carcinoma supervenes.

The presence of diarrhea and the passage of mucus are frequently observed in both conditions and do not serve as distinguishing characteristics. Diarrhea may be manifested as two or three loose stools a day or may be as severe as 20 or more bowel movements within a 24-hour period. Often, patients with ulcerative colitis are more troubled by the frequency of the bowel movements than are those with Crohn's disease. This is, perhaps, because distal disease tends to be associated with more urgency and, in some cases, tenesmus. Patients with Crohn's disease may have rectal sparing and are less likely to experience urgency.

Anal disease is much more commonly seen in Crohn's colitis than in ulcerative colitis. The presence of anal pain, swelling, and discharge may be a presenting feature of the former condition and may be the only abnormality observed on examination and subsequent investigation (see Chapters 14 and 30).

Fever is usually not a concern in patients with ulcerative colitis unless the patient is severely ill (toxic megacolon or toxic colitis). However, in patients with Crohn's disease, a pyrexia is not uncommonly noted and is usually caused by an intra-abdominal abscess or undrained septic focus. Nausea and vomiting are not frequently seen in either condition unless there is evidence of intestinal obstruction. Anorexia, weight loss, anemia, and general debility are associated with relatively long-standing or fulminant disease.

Disease in the Older Adult

The development of IBD in the older adult population has been a source of some confusion. Many older patients who have signs and symptoms suggestive of IBD are thought to have ischemic colitis. Conversely, patients thought to have IBD subsequently have been proved to have ischemia as the cause of their symptoms. Brandt and colleagues reviewed 81 patients with colitis whose symptoms began after the age of 50 years.[68] In this retrospective review, one-half of patients classified as having nonspecific IBD were really thought to have had ischemic colitis. In older persons, ulcerative colitis may have a sudden and fulminating onset progressing to a fatal outcome.

Disease in Children and Adolescents

Data from Edinburgh suggest that the rising incidence of IBD in young people is entirely a consequence of Crohn's disease, a condition now more common than ulcerative colitis in this age group.[670,671] When the condition occurs in children, there may be a more rapid onset and progression than when the disease occurs in young adults. Symptoms are the same as in adults, but toxic megacolon, bowel perforation, and massive hemorrhage are not uncommon sequelae. These youngsters often become chronically ill, have impaired growth and decreased mental acuity, and are less developed physically than their healthy peers (Figure 29-26).[120,121,499,728,747] Growth failure, especially, is the result of prolonged inadequate caloric intake.[343] It is because of these concerns that implementation of an elemental diet and parenteral nutrition are often part of the management of patients in this age group (see Medical Management).[343,658] However, to be maximally effective, therapy must be initiated before puberty.[343] Furthermore, unless medical treatment can achieve a sustained remission, operative intervention may be the only appropriate

method for addressing the problem of retarded development (see Surgical Management).[137] Particular emphasis should be placed on the assessment of growth and development as well as psychological support for both patient and family.[65,633,658] Close cooperation between the physician and the surgeon is perhaps even more than usually appropriate in the management of these vulnerable individuals.[626]

Disease in Pregnancy

Because IBD is common in patients of childbearing age, the possibility of becoming pregnant is often an issue in medical and surgical care. However, pregnancy is not that frequent an event in patients with IBD. The reason probably is related to the fact that these patients may suffer any number of hormonal imbalances as a result of acute and chronic illness, often severely impairing their ability to become pregnant.

However, ulcerative colitis and Crohn's disease do not adversely affect fertility, nor do they necessarily impede the progress of a pregnancy or the delivery of a normal, term infant. According to Zetzel, pregnancy in association with a preexisting colitis or complicated by the development of IBD is attended by the same prospect of a full-term delivery of a healthy child as is pregnancy in a healthy woman.[792] However, Schade and colleagues found a significantly greater incidence of low birth weight (less than 2,500 g) in infants of mothers with ulcerative colitis than in a control population.[662] Baird and colleagues found no evidence of an increased risk for pregnancy loss, but the likelihood of preterm birth was significantly greater.[21]

Levy and colleagues reviewed the *clinical course* of ulcerative colitis with respect to 60 pregnancies in 31 patients.[411] Twenty percent were improved, 18% deteriorated, and 62% demonstrated no change during the course of pregnancy. Fourteen percent of the pregnancies were ended by spontaneous abortion and two by artificial abortions. One premature birth was noted in 50 full-term deliveries. All the births produced healthy children. The authors concluded that pregnancy does not seem to exacerbate preexisting ulcerative colitis, nor does colitis interfere with the outcome of the pregnancy.

Crohn and colleagues reported 74 pregnancies in 47 women whose colitis was inactive at the time of conception.[115] All subsequent therapeutic and spontaneous abortions (including one stillbirth) occurred in patients in whom the colitis became activated. There was no difference in the incidence of abortion in patients who conceived during an active phase of colitis in comparison with those who conceived during an inactive phase. These observations have been confirmed by others.[124]

What happens to the colitis in patients who are pregnant? Zetzel reviewed a number of reported series and found it helpful to group the patients into several categories.[792] Only 30% of patients who became pregnant during a quiescent phase of the colitis had an exacerbation of their disease, but a recrudescence developed in 60% when the pregnancy occurred during an active phase of the illness. In patients whose colitis developed initially during pregnancy or in the postpartum period, a particularly severe result was noted, with more than 60% having worsening of their symptoms. Khosla and colleagues noted that the infertility rate of patients with Crohn's disease was similar to that seen in the

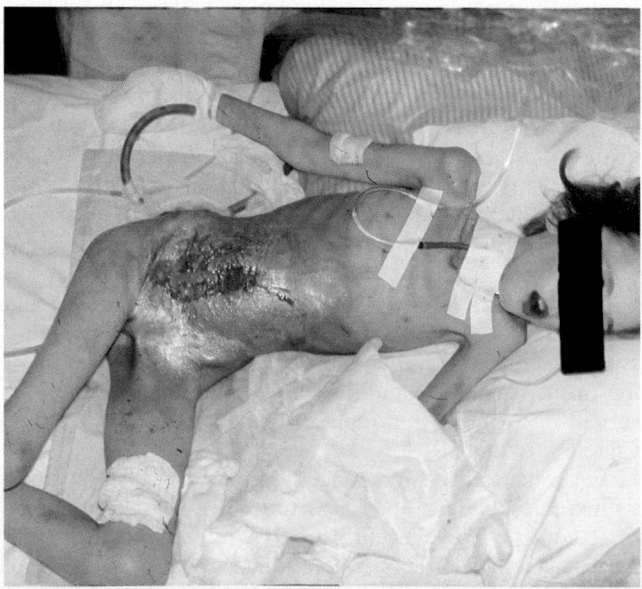

FIGURE 29-26. Crohn's disease. Severe wasting in a 17-year-old girl, who looks much younger. Note the external abdominal wall fistula. (From Corman ML, Veidenheimer MC, Nugent FW, et al. *Diseases of the Anus, Rectum and Colon. Part II: Nonspecific Inflammatory Bowel Disease.* New York, NY: Medcom; 1976.)

general population (12%).[346] Those whose condition was in remission at the time of conception had a normal pregnancy, with the disease remaining quiescent in most individuals. However, active disease at the time of conception tended to inhibit remission despite therapy.[346] In studies specifically in women with Crohn's disease, pregnancy entailed no increased risk for exacerbation of the bowel inflammation.[540,784] However, an increased risk for premature delivery and spontaneous abortion has been observed in those with active disease or in whom resection is required.

In the counseling of a colitis patient who is contemplating pregnancy, there is no justification for suggesting that attempts at conception be avoided, except when the possibility of teratogenic effects of a medication exists (e.g., the use of metronidazole [Flagyl]). Certainly, immunosuppressive treatment should be avoided in a patient wishing to conceive.

Concerns are also expressed about the safety of drug therapy in men, which could damage sperm and theoretically be associated with teratogenicity. Infertility in men is commonly associated with sulfasalazine administration. Sperm analysis may be helpful in determining whether a problem in conception can be attributed to this cause.

As mentioned, women who have a quiescent form of the disease are unlikely to experience problems with pregnancy and delivery. Conversely, if the patient is experiencing an exacerbation of the colitis, the illness itself may preclude the possibility of pregnancy. If the disease is more than moderately active, Zetzel counsels a temporary waiting period and introduction of appropriate medical therapy to secure a remission.[797] However, even in this situation, the chances of a normal pregnancy and delivery approximate 50%.[792] Contraception need be considered only in those women whose disease is so severe that surgery is imminent.[791] Certainly, if the prospective parents wish to have a child, no benefit may be expected from a therapeutic abortion. Even in the severely ill pregnant woman, there is no evidence to suggest that the pregnancy cannot be brought to a successful conclusion with the birth of a healthy child.

If surgery becomes necessary during pregnancy, the method of treatment should be identical to that of a patient who is not pregnant. In other words, drug management (steroids, sulfasalazine) is not contraindicated. It has also been determined that azathioprine is safe and that termination of the pregnancy is not mandatory for those who conceive while taking the drug.[6] Similarly, if an operation becomes necessary, the procedure should be performed as if the patient were not pregnant, although one should probably defer the implementation of a major reconstructive procedure (see Surgical Management). Closer to term, the enlarged uterus may preclude the possibility of performing even a conventional proctectomy; a staged operation, sparing the rectum, is therefore appropriate.

A high fetal and maternal mortality has been reported if surgical intervention becomes necessary for fulminant colitis.[476,575] Bohe and colleagues noted two cases of fulminant disease during pregnancy that required subtotal colectomy and ileostomy in one, and proctocolectomy in the other.[61] These operations were undertaken in the 32nd and 33rd week of pregnancy, respectively. I have performed surgery in two women during pregnancy: one patient underwent a proctocolectomy at 3 months, and the other underwent a total abdominal colectomy and ileostomy at 5 months. Both proceeded to uneventful conclusions of their pregnancy and delivered normal, healthy infants. In my opinion, it is not in the interest of the mother or the fetus to delay surgery until the pregnancy can be terminated with a viable child. In other words, I do not advocate waiting until the 32nd to perform a cesarean section while the mother is forced to postpone needed surgery.

Lindhagen and colleagues assessed the fertility and outcome of pregnancy in 78 women who had previously undergone resection for Crohn's disease.[426] Neither the number of live births nor the frequency of abortions differed from that which would be expected in the general population. The major factor, again, appeared to be that the disease was in remission or, as in the aforementioned reference, removed.

Successful childbirth has been reported following *restorative proctocolectomy* with pelvic ileal reservoir (see later discussion in that section).[490,532,590] Twenty-eight patients carried 37 pregnancies to term after *continent (Kock) ileostomy*, according to a report from Göteborg, Sweden.[562] Problems encountered were an increased urge to empty the reservoir, especially in the last trimester, and some difficulties with intubation. In most patients, a vaginal delivery was successful, with cesarean section reserved for obstetric indications.

If pregnancy develops following *proctocolectomy* and *ileostomy*, the question arises whether the prospective mother should undergo a cesarean section or deliver vaginally. My own feeling is that if the pregnant woman has an adequate pelvis for a normal vaginal delivery, this should be attempted. A cesarean section is not mandatory simply because the patient has an ileostomy, but if an episiotomy is performed, there may be a delay in healing of the perineal wound. However, it has been my experience that the obstetrician almost invariably will opt for a cesarean section. A national registry of ostomates is being maintained; a 1985 United States published survey indicated that about 1,000 had become pregnant.[217] Parenthetically, prolapse of a loop or end colostomy is sometimes seen, especially in the last trimester. This usually will resolve spontaneously following delivery.

Extraintestinal Manifestations

Extraintestinal manifestations were at one time thought to be primarily associated with Crohn's disease, but with several exceptions, they can be found in both conditions. These are discussed in Chapter 30.

▶ COURSE AND PROGNOSIS

As with many diseases, the prognosis for ulcerative colitis today is very different from that of half a century ago. Generally, this is attributed to improved medications, advances in surgical technique, and associated support during major abdominal surgery. Nordenholtz and colleagues examined the causes of death in patients with Crohn's disease and ulcerative colitis through an analysis of death certificates in Rochester, New York.[544] Of the total of 1,358 patients with IBD followed from 1973 to 1989, 130 (59 with ulcerative colitis and 71 with Crohn's disease) were found to have recorded death certificates. Sixty-eight percent of patients with Crohn's disease and 78% of those with ulcerative colitis died of causes unrelated to their IBD.[544] Deaths caused by Crohn's disease decreased from 44% in the first 8-year period to 6%

in the second. Colorectal cancer caused 14% of the deaths in patients with ulcerative colitis, three times more often than in persons with Crohn's disease. Excluding cancer, only two deaths were directly attributable to ulcerative colitis, both occurring within the first 2 years after diagnosis.[544]

With respect to course and prognosis, Langholz and associates at the University of Copenhagen examined 1,161 patients during a 25-year period.[381] The distribution of disease activity was remarkably constant each year, with about 50% of individuals in clinical remission. After 10 years, the colectomy rate was 24%. With 25 years of follow-up, the cumulative probability of a relapsing course was 90%.[381] The probability of maintaining working capacity up to 10 years was approximately 93%. The authors concluded that although ulcerative colitis is a troublesome condition, most patients can manage their lives with little interference.

Maunder conducted a MEDLINE search for articles relating to ulcerative colitis and Crohn's disease published since 1981 to determine the quality of life.[468] Health-related quality of life is a quantitative measurement of the subjective perception of the state of one's health, including emotional and social aspects. The investigators determined that the articles published indicated a trend toward a higher quality of life during the period from 1984 to 1987 in comparison with the period from 1981 to 1984. Although one can certainly question the validity of such an investigative effort, it appears that the previous comment concerning the general improvement in our ability to treat these two conditions is supported.

► RELATIONSHIP TO CARCINOMA

Carcinoma of the colon arising in a patient with ulcerative colitis was initially described by Crohn and Rosenberg in 1925. Since that time, numerous cases have been reported, so that there is uniform agreement with respect to the association between chronic ulcerative colitis and the subsequent development of adenocarcinoma. Primary malignant lymphoma complicating ulcerative colitis, although extremely rare, is nevertheless also thought to be associated with ulcerative colitis.[1] Unfortunately, the true incidence of carcinoma is often a matter of conjecture, depending on the referral nature of the institution from which the report emanates. For example, some population-based studies have shown a lower incidence of colorectal cancer than that reported from major medical centers.[200,601]

Predisposing Factors and Incidence

Various factors predispose a colitic patient to colon cancer. These include total colonic or pancolonic disease; prolonged duration of the illness (the earliest reported case is in a patient with the disease of 7 years' duration); continuous active disease, as opposed to intermittent symptoms; and possibly the severity of disease. An early age of onset probably poses no increased cancer risk save for the fact that cancer risk often parallels duration. The cumulative risk for cancer increases with the duration of colitis, reaching 25% to 30% at 25 years, 35% at 30 years, 45% at 35 years, and 65% at 40 years.[560] The data also indicates a greater risk in patients with a family history of colon cancer and in those with primary sclerosing cholangitis. Sugita and colleagues observed a strong correlation between the age of onset of ulcerative colitis and the age

of onset of cancer, a correlation found both in patients with extensive disease and in those with illness affecting the left side.[712] However, colitis and cancers developed in patients with left-sided colitis about a decade later than in those with extensive disease, although the mean duration of the colitis before the development of cancer was virtually the same in both groups (approximately 21 years), irrespective of the age at onset of the disease.[712] The incidence of cancer in patients with ulcerative colitis has been variously reported to be between 2% and 5%. Öhman reported the overall incidence to be 2.7%.[560] Johnson and coworkers noted long-term findings in more than 1,400 patients with ulcerative colitis and found that colorectal cancer developed in 63 (4.4%).[313] No statistically significant difference was observed in the probability of carcinoma of the colon and rectum developing following proctitis in comparison with total colitis. Patients with left-sided disease seemed to fare considerably better with respect to risk for the development of colorectal cancer. Greenstein reported that neoplasms developed in 11.2% of 267 patients with ulcerative colitis.[226] Colorectal cancers developed in 13% of patients with universal colitis, and malignant change developed in 5% with left-sided colitis. Cancer tended to develop in patients with left-sided disease at least a decade later than in those with universal colitis. The median duration from onset of colitis to diagnosis of cancer was 20 years for those with universal colitis and 32 years for individuals with left-sided colitis.[226] Cancer did not develop in any patient with left-sided colitis before the 23rd year of disease. In a review of more than 1,200 patients seen at the Cleveland Clinic, the cumulative risk for colorectal cancer was significantly higher in those with extensive colitis than with left-sided disease.[504] Ekbom and colleagues reviewed more than 3,000 patients with ulcerative colitis and noted that the absolute risk for the development of colorectal cancer 35 years after diagnosis was 30%.[145]

In patients who undergo resective surgery for ulcerative colitis, the incidence of associated cancer is considerably higher. Van Heerden and Beart reported the Mayo Clinic experience with 726 patients who underwent surgical exploration for chronic ulcerative colitis between the years 1961 and 1975.[754] Seventy patients (9.6%) were found to have a carcinoma of the colon. These individuals represented 1.4% of all patients in whom chronic ulcerative colitis was diagnosed during the period of study.

Generally, the incidence of carcinoma is the same in both sexes. This is not surprising in light of the fact that ulcerative colitis affects each in approximately equal numbers. Welch and Hedberg reported a bimodal distribution of the incidence—one peak in the fourth decade and the other in the seventh.[768]

An increased risk of the development of colon carcinoma also appears to be evident in Crohn's disease, especially of the small bowel.[53] This is discussed in Chapter 30.

Characteristics

The distribution of tumors in patients having ulcerative colitis and carcinoma was reported by Öhman to demonstrate multicentricity much more commonly than in those having colorectal cancer without IBD.[560] He also noted that 28% of patients had lesions of the transverse colon. Similarly, only 28% of patients had cancers involving the rectum and rectosigmoid, whereas patients with lesions of the sigmoid colon comprised 17% of the series. Conversely, Riddell and

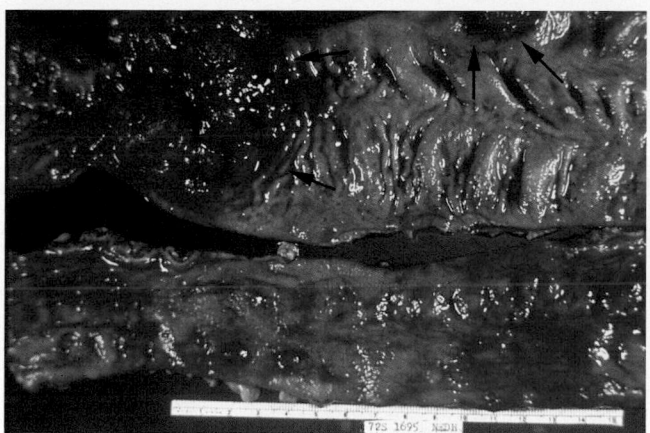

FIGURE 29-27. Carcinomas in ulcerative colitis (*arrows*). (From Corman ML, Veidenheimer MC, Nugent FW, et al. *Diseases of the Anus, Rectum and Colon. Part II: Nonspecific Inflammatory Bowel Disease.* New York, NY: Medcom; 1976.)

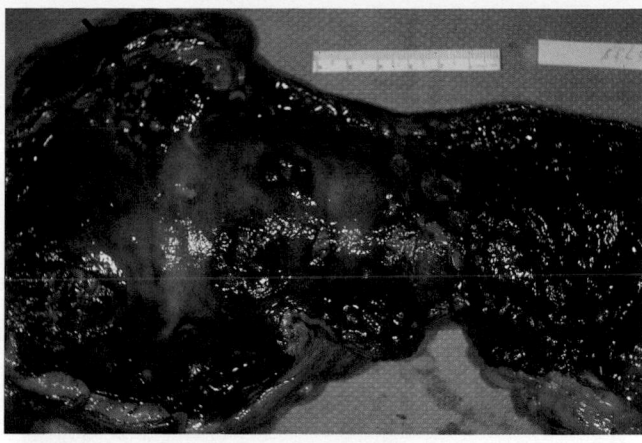

FIGURE 29-29. Ulcerative colitis with ulcerating carcinoma (*arrow*) in the hepatic flexure. (From Corman ML, Veidenheimer MC, Nugent FW, et al. *Diseases of the Anus, Rectum and Colon. Part II: Nonspecific Inflammatory Bowel Disease.* New York, NY: Medcom; 1976.)

colleagues reported that the rectum was the most common site of involvement and that this was more noticeable in men than in women.[623] In their study, more than 40% of the cancers were found in the rectum, and approximately 25% of patients had multiple tumors. It is certainly clear that multicentricity of the cancers is a frequently reported phenomenon (Figure 29-27).

Another characteristic of colorectal cancer with ulcerative colitis is that very often the cancer tends to be infiltrative and scirrhous. Visible tumor involving the mucosa may not be observed even by careful endoscopic examination (Figure 29-28). Although such is the most common clinical presentation of cancer in this disease, it can also appear as a typical ulcerating or polypoid appearance (Figure 29-29).

Another pathologic feature of carcinoma arising in ulcerative colitis is the tendency of the lesion to be highly aggressive and poorly differentiated. More than half

of young patients with ulcerative colitis and colorectal cancers have colloid carcinomas with histologically apparent mucus-secreting tumors of the signet-ring cell type[696] (Figure 29-30; see also Figure 23-22). The fact that there may be few or no symptoms tends to lull both patient and physician into a false sense of security. Witness the situation illustrated in Figure 29-17, in which the mucosa has been completely denuded. When no mucosa is present, bleeding does not occur and mucous discharge is no longer evident. This may cause the physician and the patient to believe the medical measures that have been implemented are effectively controlling the disease. It is in just this kind of circumstance, a patient with long-standing ulcerative colitis, that a carcinoma can supervene. As suggested, physical examination, barium enema, and even endoscopic evaluation may fail to identify the lesion. But when stricture occurs, the patient

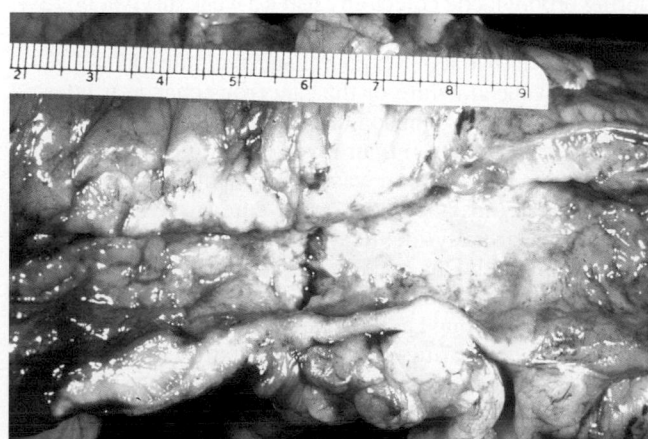

FIGURE 29-28. Carcinoma of the sigmoid in ulcerative colitis. Note the characteristic infiltration of the bowel wall, with an appearance resembling that of the linitis plastica type of carcinoma seen in the stomach. (From Corman ML, Veidenheimer MC, Nugent FW, et al. *Diseases of the Anus, Rectum and Colon. Part II: Nonspecific Inflammatory Bowel Disease.* New York, NY: Medcom; 1976.)

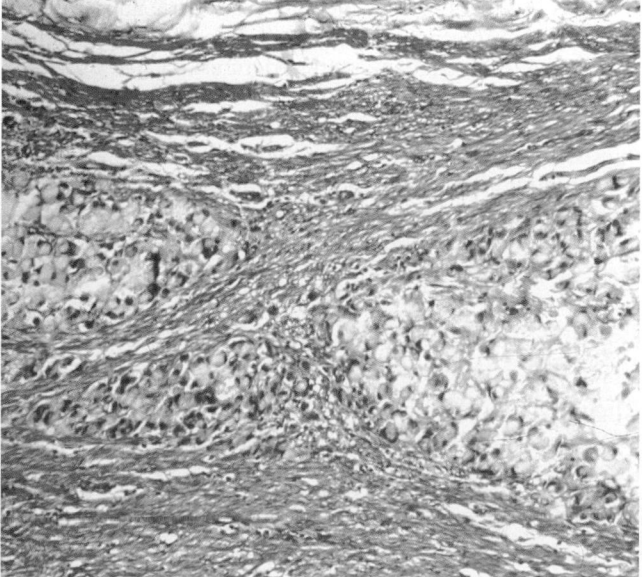

FIGURE 29-30. Signet-ring cell carcinoma infiltration of the muscularis propria in a patient with ulcerative colitis. (Original magnification × 600.)

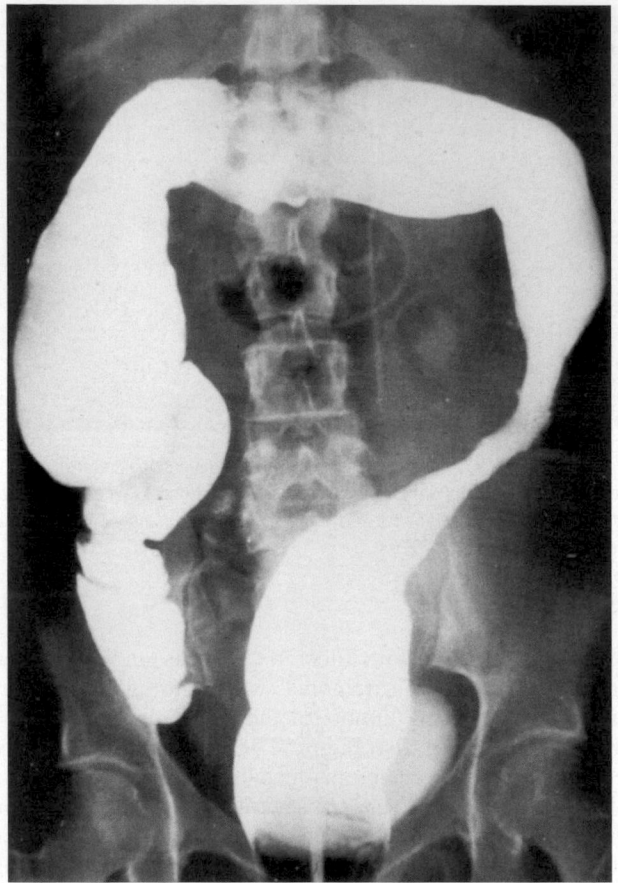

FIGURE 29-31. Stricture in ulcerative colitis. Foreshortening of the lower descending and sigmoid colon with stricture. Laparotomy revealed extensive carcinoma, hepatic metastases, and two additional unsuspected primary cancers in the resected specimen. (From Corman ML, Veidenheimer MC, Nugent FW, et al. *Diseases of the Anus, Rectum and Colon. Part II: Nonspecific Inflammatory Bowel Disease.* New York, NY: Medcom; 1976.)

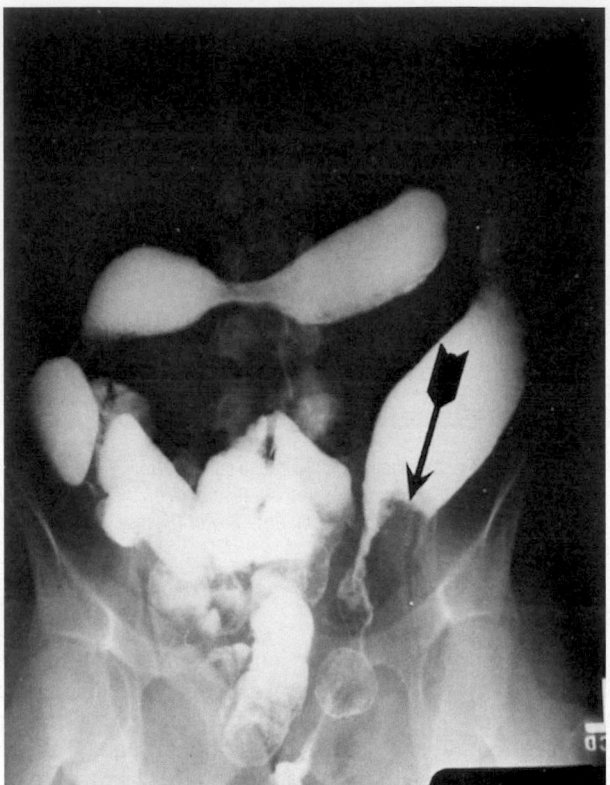

FIGURE 29-32. Carcinoma in ulcerative colitis. Note the loss of haustrations, marked shortening, and sigmoid stricture. The tumor extends cephalad from the stricture to appear as a polypoid filling defect (*arrow*).

must be presumed to have a carcinoma until it can be proved otherwise (Figures 29-31 through 29-33). The presence of a stricture in a patient with ulcerative colitis is an indication for operative intervention. Lashner and colleagues demonstrated that of 15 patients with strictures, 11 had dysplasia and 2 were found to have cancer on colonoscopy/biopsy.[385] An additional 4 patients were found to have carcinomas at the stricture site at the time of colectomy.

Carpeting with "pseudopolyps" makes interpretation of biopsies very difficult. One can make a good case for definitive proctocolectomy and ileo-pouch anal surgery under these circumstances.

Results of Surgery for Cancer Complicating Ulcerative Colitis

Ritchie and colleagues reviewed the St. Mark's Hospital (Harrow, United Kingdom) experience of carcinoma complicating ulcerative colitis between the years 1947 and 1980; 67 patients with carcinoma were identified.[627] In comparison with those who underwent surgery for carcinoma of the colon and rectum in the same time period, it was felt that the colitic group had a higher proportion of inoperable and high-grade tumors, but the prognosis was found to be very similar in patients with and without colitis for the same stage

of lesion. In the Mayo Clinic series, 40% of patients with carcinoma in chronic ulcerative colitis had a Dukes' A or B growth, in comparison with a 63% incidence if carcinoma arose in the absence of the disease.[754] Conversely, 60% with carcinoma and ulcerative colitis had Dukes' C and D lesions, in comparison with 37% who had carcinoma alone. The mean age of their patients at the onset of the colitis was 26 years, with a duration of disease of 17 years before the development of malignancy; 23% exhibited multicentric tumors. Those whose carcinoma was identified incidentally during prophylactic colectomy had a 5-year survival of 72%, whereas those with clinical or radiographic evidence suggestive of cancer had a much poorer survival rate (35%).

The advanced nature of the cancerous change is attested to by the report of Johnson and colleagues.[313] Only 57% of their patients underwent curative resection, and the overall survival rate in this group was 61%. In Öhman's experience, two-thirds of those operated on for cure survived 5 years, a percentage virtually identical to the 69% of noncolitic patients.[560] All with Dukes' A lesions survived 5 years. Lavery and colleagues reviewed the Cleveland Clinic experience with 79 patients found to have carcinoma arising in ulcerative colitis.[388] In comparing their survival statistics with those of patients with noncolitic cancer, they too noted no statistically significant difference in survival rates for the same stage of invasion. The poorer results were a consequence of the fact that a higher percentage of patients presented with more advanced or incurable disease at the time of surgery. All reports confirm that the prognosis for colitis-associated colorectal cancers, as for noncolitic cancers, is directly related to the degree of invasion (i.e., Dukes' stage).[102,711]

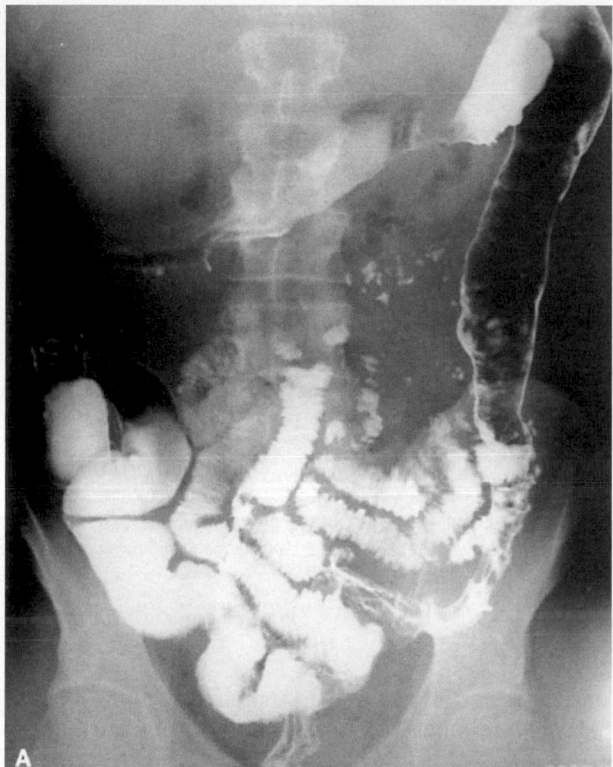
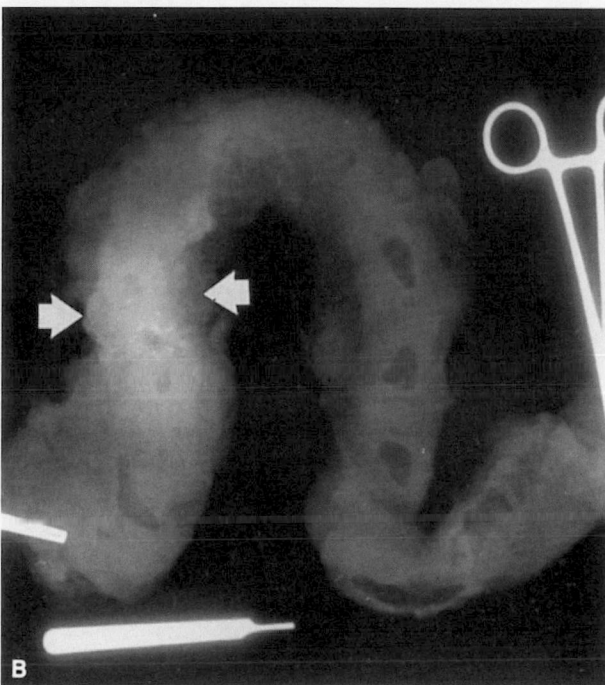

FIGURE 29-33. Carcinoma in ulcerative colitis involving the entire colon. **A:** Barium enema study shows a long stricture in the proximal transverse colon, which proved to be malignant. The short stricture in the distal transverse colon was benign. Note also the dilated terminal ileum, a characteristic of backwash ileitis. **B:** On x ray film, resected specimen shows calcification (*arrows*) in the wall at the site of the stricture. This is seen with signet-ring malignant tumors and mucinous adenocarcinomas and is believed to be caused by inspissated mucin.

Dysplasia

In 1967, Morson and Pang described a phenomenon they called dysplasia, a frequent and widespread histologic change in patients with carcinoma complicating ulcerative colitis.[512] They suggested that biopsy of the rectum could detect this premalignant situation and possibly dictate the requirement for surgical intervention.

This appeared to be a singular advance in the management of patients with long-standing disease. Before the introduction of the concept of dysplasia, "prophylactic" proctocolectomy was advocated to protect patients from the development of malignancy. This was justified on the basis that although the patient might be asymptomatic, the cancer could be far advanced when discovered. Many individuals with few or no complaints related to the gastrointestinal tract were submitted to surgery because of this understandable concern. With the promulgation of this concept, one ideally can seek to identify those patients who on biopsy and histologic examination are found to harbor this dysplastic phenomenon.

Definition and Interpretation

Dysplasia may be interpreted to be mild, moderate, or severe, but the significance of these distinctions has become less important. Clearly, however, the correct interpretation of the biopsy results rests on the talent and experience of the pathologist. It is imperative, therefore, to have available someone who is not only competent but also interested in this particular aspect of colon pathology.

The criteria for diagnosing dysplasia are problematic and vary from institution to institution. Dysplasia includes adenomatous and villous changes in the mucosa, irregular budding tubules beneath the muscularis mucosae, and cellular alterations consisting of a reduced number of goblet cells and the presence of hyperchromatic nuclei, stratified nucleoli, and coarse chromatin[352,638] (Figures 29-34 through 29-36). The following criteria have been proposed by Nugent and colleagues[549]:

Mild dysplasia

- Preservation of crypt architecture
- Nuclear stratification, but not reaching the luminal surface
- Nuclear crowding and hyperchromasia
- Mitoses in upper portion of crypt
- Usually, moderate diminution of goblet cell mucin

Moderate dysplasia

- Distortion of crypt architecture with branching and lateral buds
- Nuclear abnormalities as in mild dysplasia, but stratification reaching luminal surface
- Usually, depletion of goblet cell mucin

Marked dysplasia

- More marked distortion of crypt architecture, frequently with villous configuration of surface epithelium
- Nuclear abnormalities as in moderate dysplasia, but with loss of polarity frequently present
- Frequently, presence of "back-to-back" glands

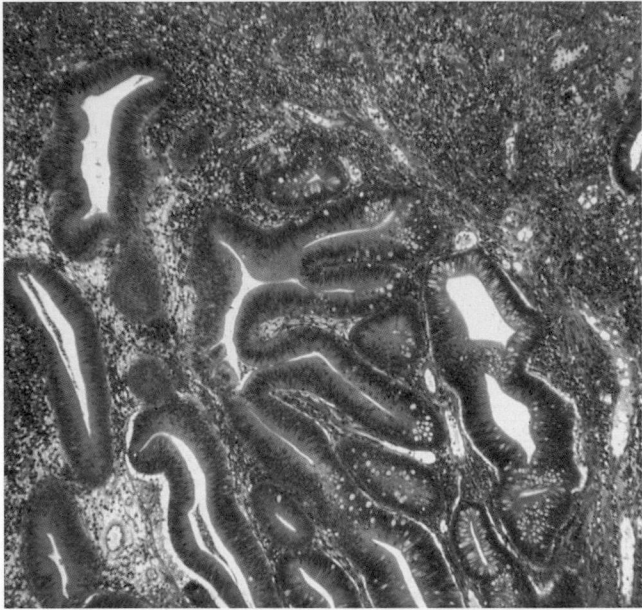

FIGURE 29-34. Moderate dysplasia in a patient with ulcerative colitis. Note the loss of polarity and decreased mucus production. (Original magnification × 80; courtesy of Rudolf Garret, MD.)

The last category includes all abnormalities short of invasive carcinoma and encompasses what some might designate as carcinoma in situ.

Results of Evaluation for Dysplasia

Nugent and colleagues initially reviewed the clinical and histologic data in a retrospective fashion of 23 patients with known colon carcinoma and chronic ulcerative colitis.[549] All but one were found to have dysplasia at a remote site from the cancer. Based on this experience, the authors enrolled 151 patients with more than 7 years of ulcerative colitis in an annual colonoscopy/biopsy surveillance program.[548] The number of specimens taken ranged from 3 to 10. Initial biopsies were positive for high-grade dysplasia in 4 patients, 3 of whom were found to harbor a carcinoma at the time of colectomy. Of 12 with low-grade dysplasia or high-grade dysplasia on initial biopsy, 11 had undergone colectomy; five cancers were found. Of 10 patients in whom dysplasia

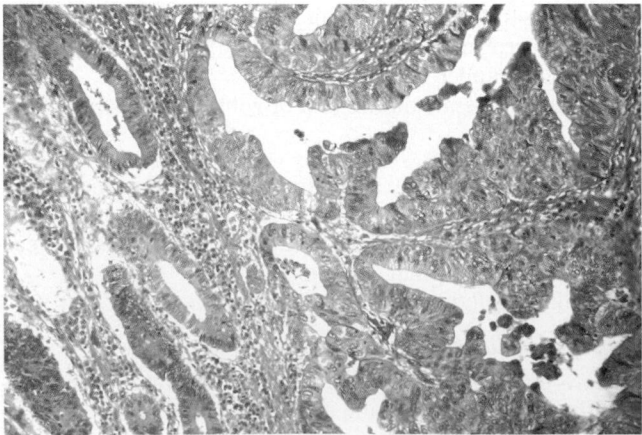

FIGURE 29-35. Moderate dysplasia in ulcerative colitis. Loss of polarity and proliferation of epithelial cells. (Original magnification × 260; courtesy of Rudolf Garret, MD.)

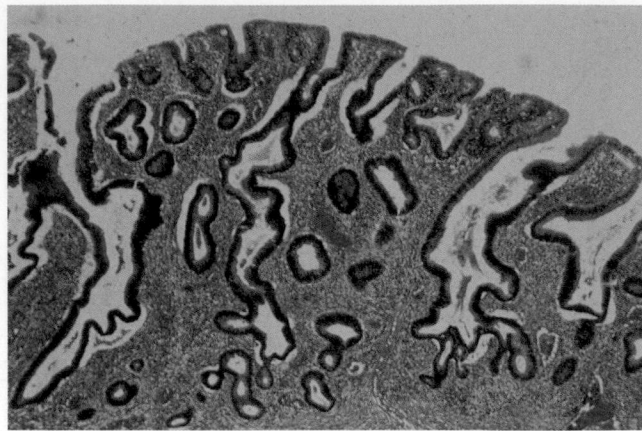

FIGURE 29-36. Severe dysplasia. Atypical hyperplasia with irregularly shaped crypts lined by crowded cells with hyperchromatic nuclei. (Original magnification × 80; from Corman ML, Veidenheimer MC, Nugent FW, et al. *Diseases of the Anus, Rectum and Colon. Part II: Nonspecific Inflammatory Bowel Disease.* New York, NY: Medcom; 1976.)

developed on follow-up, 9 underwent colectomy, and only 1 cancer was found. Carcinoma did not develop in any patient with left-sided disease. A later experience from the same group revealed that carcinoma subsequently developed in none of the 148 patients whose biopsy findings remained negative for dysplasia throughout the study.[550] In a still later review from the same institution, carcinoma associated with ulcerative colitis developed in 41 patients, 19 of whom were under colonoscopic surveillance and 22 of whom were not.[90] It seems then that carcinoma was detected at a significantly earlier Dukes' stage in the surveillance group. The 5-year survival rate was 77.2% for those surveyed, but only 36.3% for the no-surveillance group. The authors concluded that colonoscopic surveillance reduces colorectal carcinoma-related mortality by permitting the detection of carcinoma at an earlier Dukes' stage.[90]

Dickinson and colleagues surveyed 43 patients with long-standing ulcerative colitis extending proximal to the splenic flexure.[133] Dysplasia was found in nine patients in one or more biopsy specimens (severe in two, moderate in one, and mild in six). The two patients with severe dysplasia were subsequently found to harbor carcinomas.

Blackstone and colleagues performed colonoscopy on 112 patients with long-standing ulcerative colitis during a 4-year period.[58] In 12 patients, the procedure revealed a polypoid mass that on biopsy exhibited dysplasia. Seven of these patients were subsequently found to have dysplasia in the absence of a polypoid excrescence (i.e., a flat mucosa), and only one carcinoma was found later. The authors thought the identification of a single polypoid mass to be highly significant for the presence of concurrent invasive cancer. As such, this was strong evidence to support the need for colectomy.

Löfberg and colleagues studied 72 patients with total ulcerative colitis in a 15-year surveillance program.[431] The cumulative risk for the development of at least low-grade dysplasia was found to be 14% after 25 years of disease. Others also recommend the use of surveillance colonoscopy in following patients with high-risk ulcerative colitis.[73,395,454,632,785] Furthermore, Lindberg and associates demonstrated in their 20-year surveillance program of 143 patients with ulcerative colitis that primary sclerosing cholangitis (see Chapter 30) is an independent risk factor for the development of dysplasia or cancer, especially in the proximal colon.[424]

Dysplasia Surveillance Limitations and Concerns

Although the increased risk for the development of colorectal cancer in individuals with long-standing ulcerative colitis is well-known and accepted, in recent years in particular there has been increased concern about the utility of surveillance colonoscopy.[116] For example, Jonsson and colleagues undertook a prospective study of 131 patients with ulcerative colitis and concluded that the surveillance program was resource-consuming, questioning the cost-to-benefit ratio.[318] Of greater concern, however, is the validity of the concept. Taylor and coworkers, reporting from the Mayo Clinic, evaluated the reliability of this premise by means of multiple random biopsies on resected specimens of patients with chronic ulcerative colitis, with and without cancer.[724] Using a standard technique of multiple random biopsies (see later discussion), they used ordinary colonoscopic biopsy forceps to obtain four biopsy specimens from mucosa that was not macroscopically suggestive of dysplasia or cancer in eight defined regions of each of 100 colon specimens obtained. Although an overall association between the presence of cancer and high-grade dysplasia was detected, the sensitivity and specificity to detect concomitant carcinoma were both 0.74. Their findings prompt concern that reliance on random biopsies obtained during colonoscopic surveillance may be inappropriate.[724]

Gorfine and associates reviewed 590 specimens for the presence of dysplasia and found that 77 (13.1%) contained at least one focus.[219] Cancers were significantly more common in those specimens with dysplastic changes than in those without such changes (33/77 vs. 5/513; $P < .001$). Colonoscopically diagnosed dysplasia as a marker for synchronous cancer had a sensitivity of 81% and a specificity of 79%. The authors concluded that the concept of dysplasia is an unreliable marker for the detection of synchronous carcinoma, but when *any degree is discovered* colectomy is indicated.

Bernstein and coworkers summarized 10 prospective studies to ascertain whether colonoscopic surveillance is the appropriate alternative to prophylactic colectomy.[55] First of all, the risk for progression to dysplasia was found to be only 2.4% for individuals whose initial evaluation was negative. Therefore, surveillance might perhaps be less frequently applied for those patients. Of a greater concern, however, is the fact that 32% of the patients with high-grade dysplasia were found to have invasive cancer. For this group, at least, the surveillance program failed to prevent the development of malignancy. However, when an unsuspected cancer is found at the time of surgery performed for dysplasia, it tends to be at a lower TNM stage than the cancer in patients in whom the diagnosis is made prior to surgery. In order for reasoned decisions to be made, therefore, it has been advised that patients be informed about the limitations of colonoscopic surveillance so that they can rationally take part in their management.[51] Unfortunately, a highly malignant carcinoma was reported to have developed in a patient without prior dysplasia or DNA aneuploidy who was enrolled in a colonoscopic surveillance program.[436]

An opposing viewpoint concerning the value of surveillance for dysplasia has been expressed by Collins and colleagues.[100] It is their contention that no compelling evidence proves that such follow-up evaluation is beneficial. Others have also expressed reservations.[383,400–402,602,622] This is especially true with respect to the significance of low-grade dysplasia. In the experience of Befrits and coworkers (Stockholm, Sweden), no progression to high-grade dysplasia was observed during 10 years of follow-up in 60 patients, leading to the conclusion that colectomy in cases with single or even repeated low-grade dysplasia is not justified.[46] Others opine that clinicians have to take not one but two giant leaps of faith to reject the null hypothesis and recommend surgery for low-grade dysplasia.[423] But today, most gastroenterologists are of the opinion that, because dysplasia implies concomitant neoplasia, individuals with even low-grade dysplasia should be counseled to undergo colectomy.[750]

The cost-effectiveness of surveillance colonoscopy has become a hotly debated issue, and as of this writing, accord with respect to the appropriate frequency of such examinations is still an unattained ideal (see the following section).[181,238] There is no controversy, however, with respect to those individuals who harbor a dysplasia-associated lesion or mass (DALM). These patients require colectomy.[46,423] This includes any benign neoplasm (tubular adenoma, villous adenoma) that arises in a segment of inflammatory disease.

Surveillance Program

In a surveillance program, evaluation is advised for those who have had a minimum of 7 years of total or subtotal colonic disease. These persons are then submitted to total colonoscopy with biopsy of any demonstrable lesion. As suggested, the biopsy of a specific, elevated lesion will yield a much higher incidence of dysplasia. Multiple random biopsy samples should be taken throughout the colon. Although traditionally 10 such biopsies have been advised, in recent years some have suggested sampling 30 to 40 specimens. The examination should be performed every other year or more often if dysplasia is identified. Whether one wishes to wait a year and repeat the study once dysplasia, irrespective of degree, has been identified is a subject of controversy (see earlier). It must be remembered, however, that colonoscopy in ulcerative colitis is not necessarily a benign procedure, and performing multiple biopsies may invite complications (Figure 29-37). Therefore, an experienced endoscopist should be selected to examine these patients. Preferably, biopsy specimens should be obtained in areas free from obvious inflammation.[548]

Comment

It is certainly true that cost-benefit analysis has not been determined, that incurable cancer may still supervene, that patient compliance is problematic, and that willingness of patients to commit themselves to a resection if the biopsy reveals dysplasia is doubtful. However, the alternative course is even less agreeable. Barium enema examination is useful only to demonstrate the macroscopic anatomy of the colon: loss of haustrations, shortening, and possible stricture. It is unlikely that this study will reveal a carcinoma earlier than will endoscopic examination with biopsy. Prophylactic colectomy after 8 to 10 years is one option; denial

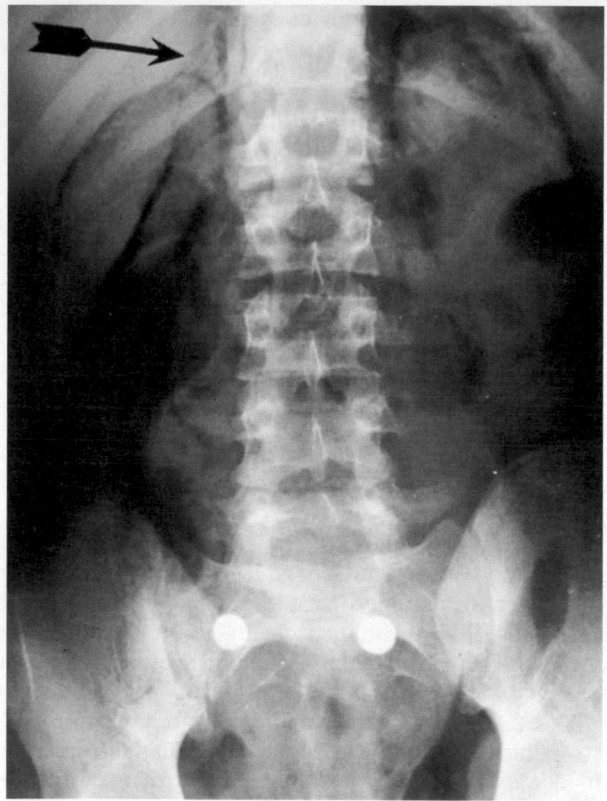

FIGURE 29-37. Retroperitoneal gas from a colon perforated during colonoscopic biopsy for dysplasia in a 19-year-old patient with ulcerative colitis. The renal outlines are clearly evident, as is the right adrenal gland (*arrow*).

is another. However, until a better alternative is available, one should continue to recommend the protocol as outlined, with the performance of flexible sigmoidoscopy in alternate years.

Aneuploidy

Another method for identifying precancerous changes is flow cytometry. Several studies have demonstrated that DNA aneuploidy correlates with the presence of dysplasia and, therefore, a high risk for developing cancer.[286,425,432,485,637,715] Suzuki and colleagues showed that 77% of dysplastic tissue demonstrated aneuploidy or polyploidy, whereas 94% of specimens of nondysplastic tissue exhibited diploidy.[715] Löfberg and colleagues found that 20% of 59 patients with long-standing total ulcerative colitis harbored an aneuploid DNA pattern on colonoscopy/biopsy, and that this correlated with the presence of dysplasia.[431] The frequency of aneuploidy is higher in patients with disease longer than 10 years and with a greater extent of involvement.[286]

As mentioned, one of the problems with the concept of dysplasia alone is interobserver and intraobserver variability.[432] Sampling error as well as total reliance on histologic information has its own inherent limitations. In the experience of Rubin and coworkers, a significant correlation between aneuploidy and severity of histologic abnormality was found in patients at high risk for cancer (negative, indefinite, dysplasia, or cancer).[637] In a prospective study from their institution of 25 high-risk individuals without

dysplasia, 20% were found to have aneuploidy, and all of these patients progressed to dysplasia within 2.5 years. Conversely, all 19 individuals who failed to demonstrate aneuploidy did not progress to either aneuploidy or dysplasia within the limits of the study (up to 9 years). The authors concluded that patients who demonstrate aneuploidy should be submitted to more extensive and frequent colonoscopic surveillance, whereas those who do not require less frequent investigations.[637] Löfberg and colleagues confirmed that nuclear DNA content appears to be an earlier phenomenon than dysplasia in the malignant transformation of the colorectal mucosa, and that the use of flow cytometry in surveillance programs might be of particular value for selecting individuals at an increased risk for the development of cancer.[432]

In summary, flow cytometry may be usefully applied to complement histologic examination when dysplasia is suspected.[408,485] However, there is no evidence to support the use of DNA aneuploidy as the sole indication for prophylactic cancer surgery in patients with ulcerative colitis.[425]

Treatment of Carcinoma

If a carcinoma is identified in the rectum of a patient with ulcerative colitis, proctocolectomy is the treatment of choice. No attempt should be made to preserve the rectal mucosa. Alternative operations may, however, include the continent ileostomy (Kock) and the ileoanal anastomosis with intervening pouch, provided that sphincter preservation does not compromise adequate tumor margins, and the risk for the requirement of postoperative radiation therapy is remote (see Surgical Management).

▶ MEDICAL MANAGEMENT

I have asked two respected colleagues, Udayakumar Navaneethan and Bo Shen, at the Center for Victor W. Fazio, Inflammatory Bowel Disease, Digestive disease Institute, Cleveland Clinic Foundation, Cleveland, Ohio, to help me update this section. *(VWF)*

Introduction

Approximately 4% to 9% of UC patients will require colectomy within the first year of diagnosis[381,517], whereas the risk of colectomy following that is 1% per year afterward.[382] The vast majority of UC patients will require medical therapy throughout their life. Therefore, understanding of the appropriate use of these agents and their adverse effects is important for the physician caring for these individuals. In recent years, the medical management of UC has changed significantly. In particular, the advent and approval of anti-tumor necrosis factor-α (TNF-α) agents like infliximab in the management of moderate-to-severe UC has expanded the role of medical therapy in this condition.[381,382,517]

The general principles in medical therapy for UC patients are improvement of quality of life, induction and maintenance of remission and mucosal healing, avoidance of complications and colectomy, and decreasing the likelihood of the development of cancer. Estimated lifetime risk of a severe exacerbation of UC requiring hospitalization is approximately 15%.[144] Patients with extensive disease (macroscopic disease proximal to the splenic flexure) are more likely to develop acute severe colitis.

A number of agents have been shown to have clinical benefit for induction and maintenance therapy for mild-to-moderate UC. However, the challenge lies with the management of severe UC, which does not respond to corticosteroid therapy. A recent study showed that there was a 7% absolute reduction in the risk of colectomy in the infliximab versus placebo group (10% vs. 17%, respectively) over a 54-week follow-up period.[656] Whether the use of infliximab decreases the risk of colectomy in the long run is not known. This section will address various medications used in the treatment of UC.

5-Aminosalicylates

Sulfasalazine and 5-aminosalicylate (5-ASA) remain the first-line therapy for the induction of remission in patients with mild-to-moderate active UC.[82,713] Oral 5-ASAs come in a wide range of formulations with different release characteristics.[418,420] Sulfasalazine, a 5-ASA bound to sulfapyridine by an azo bond, is the initial form found to be effective in the treatment of UC.[132,603] Because the 5-ASA portion of the agent is the therapeutically active compound, several oral preparations of 5-ASA have subsequently been developed. However, sulfasalazine appears to have comparable efficacy with the newer ASA formulations.[541] The type and dosage of 5-ASA therapy are determined by location, severity of disease, cost and insurance coverage, as well as patient preference. Most ASA agents have comparable pharmacokinetics in terms of systemic absorption, urinary excretion, and fecal excretion of active ingredient. Meta-analyses showed that topical 5-ASA agents delivered rectally appeared to be superior to placebo or topical corticosteroids for the induction of remission in distal UC.[392,463,611] However, concomitant topical application of 5-ASA and corticosteroid agents was shown to be superior to topical 5-ASA alone. Topical 5-ASA appears to be at least as effective as oral 5-ASA in maintaining remission for distal UC. 5-ASA appears to be more effective than placebo across all dosage ranges with a trend toward a dose-response effect. Patients with active proctitis or distal colitis can be treated with either topical (enemas or suppositories) and/or oral 5-ASAs. However, controlled trials have shown that rectal therapies have a more rapid effect than oral treatment. Combination therapy with oral and topical 5-ASAs may achieve a higher remission rate than either rectal 5-ASA or oral 5-ASA alone for distal UC. In one study, patients treated with both topical and oral 5-ASAs had a remission rate of 89%, compared with 69% for topical 5-ASA alone and 46% for oral 5-ASA alone.[644] In patients with left-sided disease or extensive mild-to-moderate active UC, oral 5-ASAs may be used along with topical 5-ASAs.

The available oral 5-ASA agents appear to be equally effective in producing response rates of 40% to 75% after 4 to 8 weeks of treatment.[515] In those with active UC, delayed-release oral mesalamine (Asacol HD; Proctor and Gamble Pharmaceutical, Cincinnati, OH) in doses of 2.4 g/day demonstrated a comparable efficacy (51% vs. 56%) versus 4.8 g/day. However, a dose of 4.8 g/day was more effective in moderate disease (57% vs. 72%).[245] A formulation of ASA using a MultiMatrix (MMX) release system (Lialda; Shire US, Wayne, PA), which, in addition to being pH dependent (breaking down at pH ≥7, normally in the terminal ileum, slowly releases 5-ASA throughout the entire colon), has been studied. Clinical remission rates in active mild-to-moderate UC were 37.2% and 35.1% in the 2.4 and 4.8 g/day groups, respectively, after 8 weeks of treatment, compared with 17.5% in the placebo group.[323,419,653] These once daily doses provide an opportunity to improve patient adherence. Of note, combination therapy with oral and rectal mesalamines may be superior to oral or rectal therapy alone in patients with extensive colitis.[464] With regard to maintenance, oral mesalamine has been shown to decrease relapse rates to 23% to 37% at 12 months compared with 50% to 65% in patients receiving placebo.[515,713]

In a subsequent trial, the efficacy of maintenance therapy of MMX was evaluated over a 12-month period (1.2 g/day vs. 2.4 g/day). Remission rates were similar—64.4% with 1.2 g and 68.5% with 2.4 g/day.[322] Another oral mesalamine formulation was developed with the trade name Apriso (Salofalk Granu-Stix, Dr. Falk Pharma, Buckinghamshire, United Kingdom), which has mesalamine granules that have both a gastric acid–resistant enteric coating (which dissolves at pH >6) that delays release. It also has a retarding polymer matrix in the granule core that extends release throughout the colon. This is similar to Lialda. Clinical trials showed that Apriso can be administered once daily and was shown to be as effective and safe in mild-to-moderate UC, with a three times a day dosing schedule.[373,374,595] Finally, several observational studies and a meta-analysis have shown a potential protective effect of 5-ASA therapy on the development of UC-associated colorectal cancer and dysplasia at doses >1.2 g/day.[409,757]

Corticosteroids

Oral corticosteroids can be used for both left-sided and extensive colitis. In patients with proctitis or left-sided disease, topical corticosteroids in the form of foams and enemas are commonly used. In a meta-analysis of topical therapy for active distal UC, topical hydrocortisone appears to be less effective than topical 5-ASAs in inducing remission, whereas rectal application of hydrocortisone or budesonide may be superior to placebo. Topical hydrocortisone may be considered as an alterative agent in patients who fail topical 5-ASA therapy.[304,399]

In patients with extensive colitis, moderate-to-severe colitis, or refractory disease, oral and topical 5-ASA therapy and oral corticosteroids may be used as induction therapy. However, parenteral corticosteroids are often required in patients with severe colitis.[154] Response to oral corticosteroid therapy is expected to be within 10 to 14 days, but oral corticosteroid agents should be tapered and should not be used for maintenance therapy because of side effects.[740] In fact, one of the common mistakes in managing UC is the use of corticosteroids for long-term maintenance. On the other hand, the requirement for oral or parenteral corticosteroids has been considered a prognostic factor. In UC patients requiring corticosteroids, approximately one-third underwent colectomy within 12 months.[535]

To minimize systemic toxicity, topically active corticosteroid formulations have been tried in UC. Budesonide is an oral glucocorticoid with high first-pass metabolism and, thus, has limited systemic toxicity. In a study evaluating oral budesonide in patients with extensive and left-sided mild-to-moderate UC, comparable efficacy to that of prednisolone in inducing remission was observed. However, improvement in endoscopic and histologic scores was superior in the prednisolone group.[433] Therefore, oral budesonide has not been routinely used in treating UC.

Azathioprine and 6-Mercaptopurine

6-Mercaptopurine (6-MP) and its prodrug, azathioprine (AZA), are antimetabolites that inhibit purine synthesis. Therapeutically, effective doses of AZA are 2.0 to 3.0 mg/kg/day and of 6-MP are 1.0 to 1.5 mg/kg/day. Their therapeutic effect may take up to 17 weeks.[578] The dosage of 6-MP and AZA may be directed by measuring thiopurine S-methyltransferase (TPMT) activity. Low to intermediate levels of TPMT are associated with the risk of leukopenia.[57] Thus, patients with normal TPMT activity may receive standard doses of AZA or 6-MP. Patients with intermediate activity can receive 50% of the standard dose. Those who have no TPMT activity should not be treated with these agents.[693]

6-MP and AZA are mainly used as steroid-sparing drugs for maintenance therapy in UC. It has been shown that patients with UC in remission on AZA ≥6 months, but later crossed over to placebo, had a higher rate of relapse at 1 year (59%) than those who continued AZA (36%).[261] 6-MP/AZA typically works in UC patients whose disease activity responds to corticosteroid therapy.[2,13,198,430] 6-MP/AZA should not be used as an induction agent and perhaps not for maintenance therapy in patients who fail induction therapy with corticosteroids.

6-MP/AZA use may impact the disease course of UC. For example, there appears to be fewer colectomies undertaken in those maintained on AZA.[13,430] A prospective study evaluating the efficacy of AZA in maintaining remission in patients with acute severe UC after successful induction with corticosteroids found decreased rates of relapse (10% vs. 55%) and severe relapse (0% vs. 36%) when compared with a historical cohort that did not receive AZA after steroid-induced remission.[327] Controlled trials also have demonstrated therapeutic benefit of AZA plus sulfasalazine versus sulfasalazine alone in individuals with newly diagnosed UC.[735] A similar ability to maintain remission with less toxicity in AZA alone than AZA plus olsalazine was demonstrated in patients with steroid-dependent UC.[455] In a meta-analysis of 6-MP/AZA compared with either placebo or 5-ASAs, the mean efficacy (pooled data) was 60% (95% confidence interval [CI], 51%–69%) in the 6-MP/AZA group and 37% (95% CI, 28%–47%) in the control group. When only compared to placebo, 6-MP/AZA was found to be beneficial in maintaining remission (odds ratio [OR] = 2.59; 95% CI, 1.26–5.30).[202] The results of the meta-analysis support the efficacy of thiopurines in the maintenance of remission. Accordingly, the American Gastroenterological Association's guidelines recommended that patients with steroid-dependent UC should be treated with 6-MP/AZA, based on the grade A evidence (homogeneous randomized controlled trials or well-designed cohort studies).[415]

Cyclosporine

Cyclosporine A (CSA), an immunosuppressant that inhibits T-lymphocyte function, has been used in severe corticoste-

roid-refractory UC.[421] In a double-blind, placebo-controlled trial of 20 patients who had failed intravenous corticosteroid therapy, 82% responded to CSA, whereas 0% responded to placebo. Of the 9 patients in the placebo group who did not respond initially, 55% did well after crossed over to open-label CSA. However, 3/11 in the cyclosporine group versus 4/9 in the placebo group required colectomy within 1 month.[421] Subsequently, four additional controlled trials of CSA in patients with severe UC were reported. The studies identified a response rate of approximately 80%.[131,514,716,753] In a study of 30 patients who were randomized to either CSA or methylprednisolone, 64% who received CSA and 53% who received corticosteroids achieved clinical remission within 8 days. At 1 year, 78% of patients in the CSA group were in remission as opposed to only 37% in the corticosteroid group. After 1 year, 7/9 responders in the CSA group were still in remission. This compared with 4/8 in the corticosteroid group ($P > .05$); colectomy rates were similar.[131,685]

Long-term response rates in patients treated with CSA have also been evaluated. In a study of 42 patients with severe steroid-refractory UC treated with intravenous CSA who were followed over a 5-year period, 45% were able to avoid colectomy. This represented a higher rate in those who initially responded to CSA and in those concomitantly on AZA or 6-MP (49% vs. 17%).[682] A study comparing quality of life (QOL) in patients who underwent colectomy versus those who were managed with CSA found that the latter individuals scored well or better than their surgical counterparts.[96] In a retrospective single-center study of 86 patients treated with CSA, 25% of initial responders required colectomy at a mean interval of 178 days, and analysis showed that of all patients treated with CSA, 55% would avoid colectomy at 3 years.[15] The dose used in many of the studies is 4 mg/kg per 24 h, with a goal trough serum level of 300 to 400 ng/mL. However, some studies suggest that a lower dose of CSA may be as effective.[514,608] Intravenous CSA is effective in the induction of remission in patients with severe, steroid-refractory UC. However, the efficacy of durable treatment response is limited to those who were "naive" to AZA/6-MP before treatment. All patients require AZA/6-MP for maintenance of remission after induction with CSA.

Antitumor Necrosis Factor Agents

TNF inhibitors have increasingly been used for the treatment of moderate-to-severe UC. Infliximab (IFX), a chimeric monoclonal immunoglobulin G1 antibody to TNF-α, was the first drug of the category approved by the U.S. Food and Drug Administration (FDA) for the treatment of UC. IFX has been studied in several small open-labeled trials in steroid-refractory and steroid-dependent UC.[87,88,222,329,710] Subsequently, a double-blind, placebo-controlled study of IFX was terminated prematurely due to slow enrollment, but it showed a 50% response rate at 2 weeks in those previously refractory to intravenous corticosteroids.[659] Two additional placebo-controlled studies of steroid-refractory disease found favorable results that led to large subsequent studies.[307,596]

The Active Ulcerative Colitis Trials (ACT 1 and 2), which enrolled patients with moderate-to-severe active UC treated with corticosteroids and/or 6-MP/AZA (ACT 1) or with UC refractory to at least one standard therapy (ACT 2), are the landmark studies evaluating the efficacy of IFX.[640] In ACT 1, the clinical response to IFX at 8 weeks was 69% for 5 mg/kg dosing and 61% for 10 mg/kg dosing versus 37% in the placebo group ($P < .001$), and similar response rates were found at 8 weeks in ACT 2. In both studies, patients who received IFX were more likely to have a clinical response at week 30, and in ACT 1, more patients who received IFX had a clinical response at week 54. Endoscopic remission, which has been of interest as an end point, was also seen in more than 50% of the IFX-treated groups in ACT 1 at 30 and 54 weeks. Subsequently, a follow-up study was done to evaluate health-related QOL in patients treated with IFX to see whether improved clinical response translated to improvement in QOL. Substantially improved QOL was sustained through 1 year with maintenance therapy.[162] However, the influence on the risk of colectomy was not evaluated until recently. In a published follow-up of ACT 1 and 2 studies evaluating colectomy rates, the cumulative incidence of colectomy in patients treated with IFX through 54 weeks was 10%.[656] This compared with 17% for the patients in the placebo group. However, those enrolled in the study had moderate-to-severe UC who had not received intravenous corticosteroid within 2 weeks and were judged unlikely to require colectomy within 12 weeks. Hence, the reduction in risk cannot be entirely attributed to IFX.[656]

Previous studies have addressed the risk of colectomy in patients with severe UC. In a small pilot study of 11 patients hospitalized with severe steroid-refractory disease, 50% receiving IFX responded.[659] This compared with no response in patients in the placebo group, but the numbers were too small to detect a statistically significant benefit. In a study of 45 severe UC in-patients at risk for colectomy, a decreased rate of colectomy at 3 months was demonstrated in those who received one dose of IFX (29% vs. 67%, $P = .017$).[307]

The risk of colectomy in the long run was evaluated in a study of 314 UC patients from Italy.[12] Fifty-two (16.5%) had severe UC. Fifteen of the 52 patients (29%) did not respond to a median of 7 days of intravenous corticosteroids. Of these, 4 underwent urgent colectomy, and 11 received IFX. A clinical response was observed in all IFX-treated patients. In the long term, another 6 patients underwent elective colectomy. The overall colectomy rate following acute flare-up was 19%. The long-term colectomy risk was comparable in IFX-treated patients (18%) and in steroid-responsive patients (11%). However, those treated with IFX had a shorter colectomy-free disease course than the individuals who responded to intravenous corticosteroids. The authors speculated that steroid-refractory patients who achieve remission with IFX have a more severe disease than steroid-responsive patients.[12]

Adalimumab (ADA) is a fully humanized IgG1 monoclonal antibody to TNF. Although adalimumab was initially studied in CD, a pilot study subsequently reported its efficacy in UC. More recently, it was studied for the induction of clinical remission in anti-TNF naive patients with moderately to severely active UC.[613] In the multicenter, randomized, double-blind, placebo-controlled study in North America and Europe, patients with a Mayo score of ≥6 points and endoscopic subscore of ≥2 points despite treatment with corticosteroids and/or immunosuppressants were enrolled. These were randomized to subcutaneous treatment with ADA 160/80 (160 mg at week 0, 80 mg at week 2, 40 mg at weeks 4 and 6) or placebo group. At week 8, 18.5% of patients in the ADA 160/80 group were in remission. This compared with 9.2% in the placebo group ($P = .031$). Serious adverse events occurred in 7.6% and 4.0% of patients in the placebo and ADA 160/80 groups, respectively. ADA 160/80 appeared to be safe and modestly effective for induction of clinical remission in patients with moderately to severely active UC who failed treatment with corticosteroids and/or immunosuppressants.[613]

Adverse Effects of Medications

Medications used in the treatment of IBD are associated with a number of adverse effects. Sulfasalazine consists of sulfapyridine linked to 5-ASA (mesalamine, mesalazine) via an azo bond. However, its use is limited by high rates of intolerance among patients. Side effects can include headache, abdominal pain, nausea, vomiting, skin rash, fever, hepatitis, hematologic abnormalities, folate deficiency, pancreatitis, systemic lupus erythematosus, and reduction in sperm counts.[446] Sulfapyridine, a sulfonamide moiety, has been suggested to be responsible for hypersensitivity reactions. Sulfasalazine-induced hepatotoxicity manifests as elevation of aminotransferases; hyperbilirubinemia; and less commonly, fever, hepatomegaly, lymphadenopathy, and granulomatous liver disease.[529] Hepatotoxicity may also be a part of hypersensitivity reactions.[529]

Similarly, thiopurines are known to be associated with liver toxicity.[529] *Hepatotoxicity* usually manifests itself by elevation in aminotransferases, accompanied by flulike symptoms. In some patients, it can present as an isolated cholestatic enzyme elevation. Abnormal liver function tests (LFTs) usually return to normal after discontinuance of the agents.[529] 6-MP/AZA-induced hepatotoxicity occasionally may be idiosyncratic in nature, with rare presentations, such as veno-occlusive disease (VOD).[152] *Acute pancreatitis* is also reported with 6-MP/AZA use in IBD. Pancreatitis is an early idiosyncratic adverse reaction after initiation of treatment, usually occurring within 3 to 4 weeks of therapy. Pancreatitis is considered to be idiosyncratic and dose independent.[459]

The use of anti-TNF agents is associated with a number of adverse effects, including activation of tuberculosis, infusion reactions, hypersensitivity reactions, and the development of *lymphoma*.[683] Hepatosplenic T-cell lymphoma has been described in IBD patients treated with anti-TNF drugs, including infliximab and adalimumab, particularly in combination with immunomodulators.[529] Reports from the manufacturer-maintained TREAT (The Crohn's Therapy Resource, Evaluation, and Assessment Tool) Registry with voluntary reporting system, however, suggest that serious infection from IFX-treated CD patients appeared to be associated with concurrent use of corticosteroids or narcotic analgesics.[417]

The risk of postoperative complications in UC patients treated with IFX before colectomy has been studied.[509,673] After adjusting for age, high-dose corticosteroids, AZA, and severity of colitis, infliximab use was significantly associated with infectious complications in a multivariate analysis (OR = 2.7).[673] In the study from our institution, preoperative IFX use was also found to be associated with an increased risk for three-stage restorative proctocolectomy instead of the traditional two-stage procedure as well as an increased risk of postoperative infectious complications.[509]

A multicenter study from Europe evaluated the safety of IFX in 52 patients with steroid-refractory UC who did not respond to CSA.[85] Fifteen (29%) required colectomy within a median of 5 weeks. The rate of adverse events was 25% (six infections, three infusional reactions, one leukopenia, one bowel perforation, one fever, and one peripheral neuropathy). One death occurred in a 40-year-old man (pneumonia) who underwent surgery 10 days after the first IFX infusion.[85] Therefore, it appears that pushing medical therapy to the limit may be costly in terms of severe adverse effects prior to and following colectomy.

The disease, UC, itself, appears to have no adverse effects on fertility in women nor in men.[306,525] However, a variety of medications used in the management of IBD may affect fertility. Among the medications, sulfasalazine has been shown to be associated with male infertility and abnormalities in sperm count, motility, and morphology.[738] An association between sulfasalazine use in the parent and congenital malformations in the progeny has also been described.[508] 6-MP and AZA do not appear to reduce semen quality in men with IBD.[127] IFX treatment in men may decrease sperm motility and morphology.[448] Safety of anti-TNF agent use during pregnancy is still controversial and is discussed separately.

▶ MANAGEMENT OF INFLAMMATORY BOWEL DISEASE DURING PREGNANCY

The management of IBD during pregnancy is of great concern to patients and to the physicians caring for them. Overall, most medications used for the treatment of IBD are not associated with significant adverse effects. The FDA classification of drugs offers a guide to the use of medications during pregnancy (Table 29-2).

5-Aminosalicylates

All aminosalicylates (sulfasalazine, mesalamines, balsalazide) are pregnancy category B, except olsalazine, which is pregnancy category C. Multiple studies have demonstrated the safety of aminosalicylates in pregnancy. However, because of the antifolate effects, pregnant women are advocates to take folic acid, 2 mg daily, in the prenatal period and throughout pregnancy. Breastfeeding is also considered low risk with sulfasalazine, except for rare diarrhea in infants.

Corticosteroids

Corticosteroids are pregnancy category C drugs. A case-control study of corticosteroid use during the first trimester of pregnancy noted an increased risk of oral clefts in the newborn.[630] This was confirmed by a large case-control study and a meta-analysis that reported a summary for case-control studies that examined the risk of oral clefts (3.35; 95% CI, 1.97–5.69).[574] However, a subsequent study did not confirm this finding.[234] Overall, the use of corticosteroids poses a small risk to the developing infant, but the mother needs to be informed of both the benefits and the risks of therapy.

Methotrexate

Methotrexate, a pregnancy category X drug, is clearly teratogenic and should not be used in women considering conception. Methotrexate is a folic acid antagonist, and its use during the critical period of organogenesis (6 to

FDA CATEGORY	DEFINITION
TABLE 29-2 U.S. Food and Drug Administration (FDA) Data on Fetal Risk	
A	Adequate and well-controlled human studies have failed to demonstrate a risk to the fetus in the first trimester of pregnancy (and there is no evidence of risk in later trimesters).
B	Animal reproduction studies have failed to demonstrate a risk to the fetus and there are no adequate and well-controlled studies in pregnant women or animal studies have shown an adverse effect, but adequate and well-controlled studies in pregnant women have failed to demonstrate a risk to the fetus in any trimester.
C	Animal reproduction studies have shown an adverse effect on the fetus and there are no adequate and well-controlled studies in humans, but potential benefits may warrant use of the drug in pregnant women despite potential risks.
D	There is positive evidence of human fetal risk based on adverse reaction data from investigational studies in humans, but potential benefits may warrant use of the drug in pregnant women despite potential risks.
X	Studies in animals or humans have demonstrated fetal abnormalities and/or there is positive evidence of human fetal risk based on adverse reaction data from investigational experience, and the risks involved in use of the drug in pregnant women clearly outweigh potential benefits.

8 weeks postconception) is associated with multiple congenital anomalies.[70] Methotrexate may persist in tissues for long periods, and it is suggested that patients wait at least 6 months from the discontinuation of the drug before attempting conception.

Azathioprine/6-Mercaptopurine

6-MP and AZA are pregnancy category D drugs. Animal studies have demonstrated teratogenicity with increased frequencies of cleft palate, open-eye, and skeletal anomalies seen in mice exposed to AZA. The largest evidence on safety comes from transplantation studies where rates of anomalies ranged from 0.0% to 11.8%.[593] In IBD, multiple clinical case series have not noted an increase in congenital anomalies.[344,513] One epidemiologic study did report a higher incidence of fetal loss in women with IBD with prior treatment on 6-MP compared with those who never had 6-MP exposure.[795] However, a nationwide cohort study found that women with CD exposed to corticosteroids and AZA/6-MP were more likely to have preterm birth (12.3% and 25.0%, respectively), compared with non-IBD controls (6.5%).[546] Congenital anomalies were also more prevalent among AZA/6-MP–exposed cases compared with the reference group (15.4% vs. 5.7%), with an odds ratio of 2.9 (95% CI, 0.9–8.9).[103] Finally, the largest single-center study to date studied 189 women who were exposed to AZA during pregnancy and compared them with 230 women who did not take any teratogenic medications during pregnancy.[574] The rate of major malformations did not differ between groups.[208] The rate was 3.5% for AZA and 3.0% for the control group ($P = .775$; OR = 1.17). Thus, the conflicting reports in the literature suggest that the decision on the use of 6-MP/AZA during pregnancy should be based on a case-by-case basis.

Cyclosporine and Tacrolimus

Cyclosporine is a pregnancy category C drug. A meta-analysis of 15 studies of pregnancy outcomes after cyclosporine therapy reported a total of 410 patients with data on major malformations.[27] The rate was 4.1%, which is not different from the general population. In the setting of severe, corticosteroid-refractory UC, cyclosporine may be an option rather than surgery if operation poses substantial risk to the mother and fetus.

Infliximab

IFX, a pregnancy category B drug, is an IgG1 antibody, which does not cross the placenta in the first trimester, but very efficiently crosses in the second and third trimesters.[681] Although this protects the infant from exposure during the crucial period of organogenesis, it is present in the infant for several months from birth.

Current evidence suggests that INF is low risk in pregnancy. The two largest studies are from the TREAT Registry[416] and the INF Safety Database.[332] The TREAT Registry is a prospective registry of patients with CD. Of more than 6,200 patients enrolled, 168 pregnancies were reported, 117 with IFX exposure. The rates of spontaneous abortion (10.0% vs. 6.7%) and neonatal complications (6.9% vs. 10.0%) were not significantly different between IFX-treated and IFX-untreated patients, respectively.[416] The INF Safety Database is a retrospective data collection instrument. The expected versus observed outcomes among women exposed to INF were not different from those of the general population.[332]

IFX crosses the placenta and is detectable in the infant for several months after birth. However, IFX has not been detected in breast milk.[449] Anti-TNFs should be continued through conception and the first and second trimesters on schedule. If the patient is in remission, the last dose of IFX needs to be given at week 30 of gestation and then immediately after delivery.[447] The last dose of ADA needs to be given at approximately week 32 of gestation and then immediately after delivery. If the mother flares during this time period, options include giving a dose of anti-TNF or using steroids to manage the patient until delivery.

Adalimumab

Adalimumab (ADA), a pregnancy category B drug, is FDA approved for induction and maintenance of remission in CD. The safety of it in UC patients has not been studied as yet.

MEDICAL MANAGEMENT OF SEVERE ULCERATIVE COLITIS

The definition of severe ulcerative colitis invariably involves more than six bloody stools daily, pain, cramping, toxicity with fever, anemia, tachycardia, and elevated erythrocyte sedimentation rate. This manifestation always requires admission to the hospital for intravenous therapy and observation for the serious complications of megacolon and perforation.

Management

Patients with acute, fulminant, "toxic" megacolon may present with very minimal symptoms or may be critically ill. High fever, tachycardia, and abdominal pain are frequently noted. However, clinical signs and symptoms may be masked by the patient's medications, especially steroids. One must keep in mind the possibility of perforation, even in the absence of colonic dilatation. In the experience of Greenstein and colleagues, classic physical signs of peritonitis were absent in six of seven patients with free perforation.[228]

The usual supportive measures—intravenous fluid replacement, and blood, colloid, and steroid therapy—should be supplemented with broad-spectrum antibiotic coverage. The single most important guide in the management of a patient with acute toxic dilatation is the assessment obtained with plain abdominal x-ray studies. With serial abdominal films, the effectiveness of medical management can be evaluated (see Figure 29-2). If the dilatation decreases, one may be reasonably assured that surgery can be deferred. Conversely, if colonic dilatation progresses or fails to improve during the period of maximum therapy, surgical intervention is advised.

Any medications that "slow" gastrointestinal activity, such as anticholinergics or opiates, are discontinued. A nasogastric tube is suggested, although some physicians prefer a long tube (e.g., Miller–Abbott) in the expectation of decompressing the colon. Placing the patient on the abdomen for a few minutes every 2 or 3 hours may help to distribute the gas, moving it into the rectum. Rectal tubes have also been advocated, but these are potentially dangerous in that they can cause a perforation of the sigmoid colon. Barium enema examination and colonoscopy are contraindicated; in fact, barium enema study has been reported to precipitate toxic megacolon. A case of successful decompression by means of colonoscopy has been reported in a patient who refused surgical intervention.[26]

The clinical course and ultimate outcome of toxic megacolon has been well documented by numerous investigators. A high incidence of recurrent toxic dilatation and perforation and the requirement for emergency or urgent operation have been reported.[224,270] This is in contrast to the group of patients with severe, acute colitis without dilatation, who can usually be effectively managed by nonsurgical means.[510] In the series reported by our group from the Cleveland Clinic, only 7 of 115 patients (6%) were successfully managed medically, and 5 of these came to colectomy in later years.[155]

For those who fail intravenous corticosteroid therapy, intravenous cyclosporine may be a reasonable approach (see earlier discussion), especially in those who refuse surgery. These usually are "first-episode" patients, those lacking a history of chronic debilitation or individuals whose comorbid conditions create a formidable surgical risk.

The cyclosporine experience has had a mixed response, with an initial 82% success rate, but falling to 59% at 6 months.[421] A review of more than 20 uncontrolled studies in 1998 demonstrated a 68% response in avoiding colectomy, but the long-term response was only 42%.[460] An international survey of practitioners (flawed perhaps in that two-thirds of responders had experience with fewer than five patients) reported "good" results in 29.5%, "acceptable" with recurrence in 58.6%, and "poor" in 14%.[495]

The University of Chicago study was most favorable, with 72% of initial responders avoiding colectomy after 5 years.[97] The important observation here was the value of concomitant 6-MP or AZA therapy. Of the patients receiving cyclosporine and given these drugs, 80% avoided colectomy and maintained their initial response. Further analysis of a 5-year follow-up of 42 cyclosporine-treated patients at the University of Chicago initially receiving from one to four courses of intravenous cyclosporine revealed that 18 (43%) retained their colons after a median of 6.7 years.[92] It is interesting to note that only 1 of 8 patients receiving more than one course of cyclosporine avoided colectomy. These investigators concluded that short-term cyclosporine followed by 6-MP/AZA permits more than 50% of steroid-resistant patients to avoid colectomy. However, re-treatment with cyclosporine is rarely successful.[92]

Some reports confirm the efficacy of cyclosporine in the management of severe colitis.[298,474] Although many initial responders subsequently relapse, a substantial minority remain in long-term remission.[474] Moreover, there appears to be no increased incidence of perioperative complications associated with its use, provided the treatment is for a defined period, and needed surgery is not delayed.[298] It is, however, doubtful if cyclosporine can be considered in the realm of a truly long-term, effective therapy.[608]

The following are the guidelines of the American College of Gastroenterology with respect to managing severe ulcerative colitis:

- Hospitalization
- Intravenous corticosteroids, 300 mg/day hydrocortisone, 48 mg/day methylprednisolone, or adrenocorticotropic hormone, for 7 to 10 days, if refractory to maximum doses of oral prednisone, 5-ASAs, and topical agents or if presenting with toxicity
- If no improvement after 7 to 10 days, administer intravenous cyclosporine, 4 mg/kg/day, or refer for surgery
- Adding 6-MP enhances long-term remission

Parenteral Nutrition

Neither an elemental diet nor total parenteral nutrition decreases the inflammation associated with ulcerative colitis.[244] However, evidence suggests that patients frequently are hospitalized with varying states of malnutrition. As a consequence, hyperalimentation, either parenteral or oral, has been recommended in a supportive role for patients with IBD. Specifically, elemental diets and total parenteral nutrition with bowel rest improved the symptoms, inflammatory sequelae, and nutritional status in individuals with Crohn's disease more readily than in those with ulcerative colitis (see Chapter 30). It has been demonstrated by some authors that patients who have lost more than 20% of their usual weight before undergoing abdominal surgery have higher rates of morbidity and mortality than those who have not exhibited weight loss. Conversely,

in a study by Higgens and colleagues, preoperative weight loss did not adversely affect the postoperative outcome in those undergoing elective resection.[280] There is extensive, often confusing literature on nutritional data, diet, and intravenous hyperalimentation.[94,192,263,317,370,405,406,618]

With IBD, the rationale for implementing intravenous hyperalimentation is that the bowel is "put to rest." If this were attempted without supplementary intravenous caloric intake, the patient's nutritional status would rapidly deteriorate. Intravenous hyperalimentation, therefore, permits the patient with IBD to be managed with bowel rest while simultaneously providing adequate amino acids and calories for anabolism.[134,256] If surgery is believed to be inevitable, however, the Veterans Administration Cooperative Study of 395 malnourished patients revealed that total parenteral nutrition should be limited to those who are severely malnourished unless there are other specific indications for this treatment.[760]

Comment

My own attitude is to use total parenteral nutrition only in those patients for whom surgery should be avoided or in whom the nutritional status is so poor that one may anticipate a very high rate of morbidity and mortality. The concept of short-term intravenous hyperalimentation in preparation for bowel surgery may have certain theoretical advantages, but expeditiously performed surgery should allow an earlier commencement of oral intake, a much preferred method of supplying calories. Furthermore, one cannot dispute the facts that intravenous hyperalimentation is costly and not without morbidity.

Other Agents and Approaches to the Management of the Ulcerative Colitis Patient

Sucralfate Enema

Sucralfate, a basic aluminum salt of sucrose octasulfate, has been demonstrated to be an effective drug in the management of peptic ulcer disease. It achieves its therapeutic effectiveness by adhering to mucosal surfaces, increasing prostaglandin levels, increasing mucosal blood flow, and stimulating secretion of mucus. In experimental studies of chemically produced colitis in rats, encouraging results were observed.[789] Kochhar and colleagues noted clinical and sigmoidoscopic improvement in most of their patients, but the study was quite preliminary and uncontrolled.[358] Further trials are awaited.

Butyrate Enema

Short-chain fatty acid irrigation has been demonstrated to be of benefit in the management of individuals with so-called diversion colitis (see Chapter 33). Scheppach and colleagues demonstrated the effect of butyrate enemas on the colonic mucosa in 10 individuals with distal ulcerative colitis who had been unresponsive to or intolerant of standard therapy for 2 months.[663] They showed that butyrate, as an end product of bacterial fermentation in the large bowel, profoundly affects the colonic epithelium in ulcerative colitis. A statistically significant decreased frequency of bowel action was observed, in addition to a marked reduction in bleeding. The authors concluded that butyrate deficiency may actually play a role in the pathogenesis of distal ulcerative colitis and recommended the use of butyrate irrigation as part of a treatment protocol.[663]

Probiotics

Theoretically beneficial bacteria, such as *Lactobacillus acidophilus* and *Bifidobacterium bifidum*, are called probiotics. They are present in fermented dairy foods, especially live culture yogurt, and have been used as a folk remedy for hundreds of years. Probiotic bacteria have been espoused to alter the intestinal microflora, inhibit the growth of harmful bacteria, promote good digestion, improve immune function, and increase resistance to infection. They are important in recolonizing the bowel during and after antibiotic use.

Most physicians associate lactobacilli with *L. acidophilus*, the most popular species in this group of probiotic bacteria. However, other *Lactobacillus* species may be beneficial as well. For example, *Lactobacillus rhamnosus* and *Lactobacillus plantarum* appear to be involved in the production of short-chain fatty acids, as well as the amino acids arginine, cysteine, and glutamine. One probiotic, *Saccharomyces boulardii*, has been shown to prevent diarrhea in several clinical trials.

Probiotics have gained increasing popularity when used to replace or supplant the flora in IBD with so-called kinder and gentler species that may prevent an overgrowth of pathogenic bacteria and maintain the integrity of the mucosal barrier. The Italian experience with VSL#3, a mixture of four strains of lactobacilli, three strains of bifidobacteria, and one *Streptococcus salivarius* subspecies, thermophilus, appeared to assist 15 of 20 patients into remission after 12 months.[758] Furthermore, VSL#3 was successful in treating 30 patients with active mild-to-moderate ulcerative colitis treated for 6 weeks. Nineteen achieved remission (63%) and seven responded (23%). Four had no response, and one patient worsened. No adverse events were reported. This very promising result awaits clinical trials if the marketing process of VSL#3 does not preclude such an attempt.[163] A Japanese study reported a reduction in the number of exacerbations for 3 of 11 patients with ulcerative colitis (27%) treated with a preparation of *Bifidobacterium*-enhanced fermented milk, compared with 9 of 10 patients with ulcerative colitis who were given a placebo.[300]

Nicotine

In addition to what follows here, the reader should also refer to Smoking earlier in this chapter.

As the search for the cause of IBD continues, the association between cigarette smoking and a more favorable clinical course in ulcerative colitis remains the sole epidemiologic feature that distinguishes it from Crohn's disease.[243] Pullan and colleagues reported the results of a randomized, double-blind, controlled trial of transdermal nicotine in patients with active ulcerative colitis.[598] Seventy-two patients were managed with either nicotine patches or placebo patches for a period of 6 weeks. A statistically significant improvement with respect to remission was demonstrated in the treated group in comparison with the placebo group. The most common complaints attributed to the nicotine included nausea, lightheadedness, headache, and sleep disturbance.[598] The authors concluded that the addition of transdermal nicotine to conventional maintenance therapy improved symptoms in persons with active ulcerative colitis.

Nicotine, in two uncontrolled and six controlled trials, appeared to benefit 75% of ex-smokers but did not benefit nonsmokers. Low dosage with gradual escalation was needed for induction of remission, but low-dose transdermal nicotine was not effective for maintenance of remission.

The anticipated side effects of tachycardia, increased blood pressure, nausea, and lightheadedness were noted but appeared less frequently when given as nicotine tartrate in rectal enema with a similar 73% response rate. The fears of nicotine addiction, cardiovascular compromise, cancer, and osteoporosis have not been borne out, but drug interactions have been recorded.

Clearly, ulcerative colitis affects nonsmokers. Ex-smokers and some nonsmokers may enter remission with resumption of nicotine, but side effects and intolerance are common.[165,652] Others question the validity of the effect of nicotine because its slight physiologic effects may have improved patients expectations of benefit and altered their reporting of symptoms.[243] The mechanism for the effect of nicotine is unknown.

Antidiarrheal Agents

The addition of "slowing" medications may be appropriate for the patient having frequent bowel movements out of proportion to the degree of inflammatory involvement of the rectum. Products such as diphenoxylate (Lomotil), loperamide (Imodium), codeine, and deodorized tincture of opium, individually or in combination, can be quite helpful. If an individual harbors an active colitis, slowing medications should be avoided because they can precipitate a toxic megacolon.[266] In patients who have ileal disease or who have undergone ileal resection, cholestyramine (Questran) also causes a reduction in diarrhea by adsorbing and combining with bile acids in the intestine to form an insoluble compound that is excreted in the feces.[302]

Dietary Measures

Additional medical measures include dietary restrictions. This usually involves the omission of all foods that tend to produce increased frequency of bowel movements (e.g., fruits; milk products, especially if the patient has lactose intolerance; and fibers). However, there can be no hard-and-fast rule about complete restriction of these products for every patient. Some individuals may be more tolerant than others. For example, the addition of a bulk agent, such as one of the psyllium-containing products, may be of benefit in giving some form to the stool.

Counseling

The possible value of psychiatric counseling has been discussed earlier. Although the disease may not be of psychogenic origin, there is sufficient evidence to suggest that stress and emotions may play a role in exacerbation or remission of the condition. In addition to the medication and dietary measures presented, it is often helpful to supplement these conventional medical approaches with psychotherapy and other supportive care.

Maintenance of Remission

Therapy must be individualized to the patient's dose-response experience, the extent of the disease, prior relapse history, and whether therapy or "no therapy" has been of value previously. Clearly, most patients will benefit from some form of maintenance treatment. The concept of inducing a *complete remission* must be emphasized before considering changing or reducing an effective treatment program to a maintenance schedule. Prematurely tapering steroids prior to achieving complete remission is a frequent error, but of equal importance is the fact that steroids are ineffective in maintaining remission. Their value is in short-term use or in induction therapy.[244]

The mainstay in this effort is 5-ASA. If left untreated, 80% of patients will relapse. Numerous studies have shown that treated patients will remain in remission longer than those given a placebo.[144,496,505] A multicenter trial comparing oral, topical, and oral with topical mesalamine in maintaining remission in distal ulcerative colitis showed equal efficacy of all three therapies in the prevention of relapse.[281]

Common Errors in Management

Sachar, at the Mount Sinai School of Medicine, presented a personal essay on common errors in the management of IBD which is worthy of reproducing here. They are as follows:

Over-Treating the Irritable Bowel Component

Recall that IBD patients have the same risk (15%) of having symptoms due to an irritable bowel as those individuals without inflammation. Bloating, gas, fullness, and so forth, are not, in and of themselves, indications for one to reach for the steroid bottle.

Under-Treating with Aminosalicylates

Since the efficacy of these agents is dose-related, more may be lost than gained in an effort to give a lower dosage. One should also consider the value of topical treatment for distal disease and encourage the patient to use an enema or suppository once or twice a week to maintain remission.

Over-Treating with Steroids

These drugs are, simply stated, *overused*. Steroids are neither safe nor effective for:

- repeated or frequent relapses
- prolonged, fruitless attempts at tapering
- maintenance of remission

Under-Treating with Antimetabolites

This problem is manifested in three ways:

1. delaying introduction
2. underdosing
3. early suspension or discontinuance

Misusing Infliximab

Sachar summarizes the failings in the use of this agent as follows:

- giving it to people who do not need it
- giving it to people who cannot benefit from it (bowel obstruction and internal fistulas)
- failure to have an exit strategy (the need to administer antimetabolites concomitantly)

Misusing Cyclosporine

Using this drug requires a satisfactory answer to three questions:

1. Does one have the luxury of time, such as with fulminating or hemorrhagic disease?
2. Is the colon really worth saving?
3. Where does one go after its use? This drug must be used as a bridge to other, safer regimens.

Misunderstanding Toxic Colitis

When the syndrome of toxic colitis (not toxic megacolon) persists beyond a few days, an immediate decision must be made either to try cyclosporine or infliximab, or to proceed directly to colectomy.

Choosing the Wrong Goals of Therapy

Coming from an internationally recognized gastroenterologist, Sachar's thoughts on this subject are worth quoting verbatim, even though in this text primarily for surgeons, he would be truly preaching to the choir:

> We too readily accept as a criterion of success the ability to keep our patients from surgery. Somehow the internist tends to view surgery as a "last resort" or as an indication of "failure" of medical therapy. In adopting such an attitude, we render our patients a terrible disservice. The object of treatment should not be simply "the avoidance of surgery," but rather to make our patients well. To be sure, if we can accomplish this purpose with our panoply of pills, powders, and potions, well and good. But if we can restore patients to good health and well-being more swiftly, safely, and surely with surgery, then we should not hesitate to do so. Making people better is, after all, the name of the game.

And it is obviously the name of the game for every one of us—internist, gastroenterologist, and surgeon.

Conclusions

Kornbluth and colleagues conducted a MEDLINE literature search, using the term *severe ulcerative colitis*, to determine the efficacy of current medical therapies.[371] They identified seven studies that comprised 319 treatment episodes in 306 patients. Clinical remission was achieved on average in 62%, whereas 38% came to early colectomy. Remission was maintained in 38% to 71% of patients who achieved success during an acute management episode.[371] The authors concluded that although current medical treatment has improved the outlook for severe ulcerative colitis, one cannot predict with certainty the likelihood of response to any specific therapy based on the clinical features or prior presentations of the disease.[371]

The cornucopia of medications available to clinicians can be overwhelming in deciding which therapy or therapies is appropriate. The key is to design an individualized program geared to that patient's specific needs. There is no "one size" or even "one dose" that fits all. The practitioner must evaluate the patient's response to treatment with each visit, weighing the risks of drug toxicity, cancer surveillance, long-term debility, and surgical candidacy.

▶ SURGICAL MANAGEMENT

Indications

The indications for surgery in ulcerative colitis include toxic megacolon, toxic colitis, perforation, hemorrhage, intolerable extracolonic manifestations, and the concern for malignancy. In addition, because proctocolectomy is curative, resection may be advised for intractable symptoms, even in the absence of a complication. This is the most common indication for surgery today. Conversely, operative treatment for Crohn's disease is advised primarily for complications.

Emergency Surgery

Perforation usually occurs in the patient who exhibits toxic dilatation of the colon and in whom delay in proceeding to surgery has occurred. Diagnosis can usually be made quite readily based on physical examination and a lateral decubitus film of the abdomen. A walled-off perforation may become evident at the time of laparotomy and may be converted to a free perforation as the bowel is mobilized. Although it is well recognized that ulcerative colitis can be associated with toxic megacolon and perforation, Crohn's disease can be as well. These complications tend to occur early in the course of the illness, before thickening of the bowel wall develops.

Hemorrhage

Hemorrhage is occasionally an indication for surgery in ulcerative colitis, but it is very unusual in Crohn's disease (Figure 29-38). Usually, even massive hemorrhage can be controlled by medical means. It should be remembered, however, that a subtotal or total colectomy without proctectomy may not succeed in arresting the bleeding if that is the indication for surgery. It may be necessary to perform a proctectomy in the immediate postoperative period in order to control hemorrhage. In a report from the Mount Sinai Medical Center, there was a 12% risk for continued rectal hemorrhage when subtotal colectomy had been performed for this indication.[628] Pesce and Ceccarino have used rectal washouts with adrenaline chloride in saline solution at 4° to 6° C with some success in controlling bleeding.[589]

Intractability

Intractability is by far the most common indication for surgery in ulcerative colitis. These patients usually harbor total or nearly total colonic disease. Even those individuals with lesser involvement may come to elective surgery, especially in the older age group (more than 60 years). These people seem to tolerate their bowel problems less satisfactorily. It has been said that, ideally, one should be sick enough for long enough to "earn" an ileostomy—that is, a person should feel that the physical and psychological burden of caring for a stoma is indeed justified. Today, with the available alternative of a sphincter-saving approach, there may be a tendency to intervene surgically sooner. Irrespective of the choice of

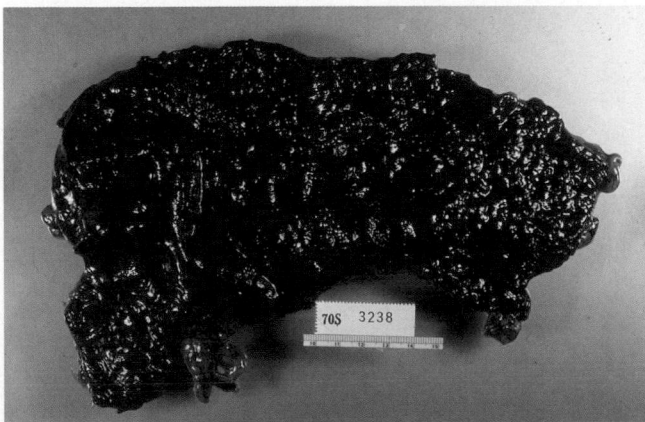

FIGURE 29-38. Ulcerative colitis. A blood clot in the cecum of a patient who underwent emergency proctocolectomy for hemorrhage. (From Corman ML, Veidenheimer MC, Nugent FW, et al. *Diseases of the Anus, Rectum and Colon. Part II: Nonspecific Inflammatory Bowel Disease.* New York, NY: Medcom; 1976.)

operation, there is no justification for deferring an operation until a patient is virtually moribund or has been reduced to a skeletal appearance. Regrettably, referral to the surgeon after such procrastination results in the physician's self-fulfilling prophesy: high morbidity and mortality.

Malignancy

The presence of cancer or the risk for malignant change as an indication for surgery has been previously discussed. Colonoscopic monitoring is still the preferred alternative, with operation reserved for those patients found to have dysplasia. It has been almost 25 years since cancer prevention as an indication for colectomy has been replaced by a cancer surveillance program.[398]

Extracolonic Manifestations

Other indications for surgery include growth retardation and extraintestinal manifestations, such as pyoderma gangrenosum, erythema nodosum, liver function abnormalities, eye complications, and joint disturbances (see Chapter 30).

Preparation of the Patient

Preparation of the patient for elective surgery is not significantly different whether the procedure is resection for IBD or surgery for cancer. It is a wise idea, however, to limit the amount of laxative administered. In fact, if a patient is troubled by diarrhea, a preoperative cathartic should be avoided. On the morning of surgery, an enema may be carefully administered until the returns are clear. This is the only mechanical preparation advised for patients with severe bowel frequency problems. Those who are to undergo small bowel resection for Crohn's disease do not require a mechanical preparation unless the possibility of colonic resection also exists. Intravenous antibiotics are administered as described in Chapter 23.

Because most individuals who are to undergo an operation for IBD have been on steroids for varying periods of time, it is imperative that adequate perioperative "coverage" be maintained to prevent the complications of adrenal insufficiency. Unless the person had been on short-term prednisone therapy many months before the operation, steroid protection should be afforded even if corticosteroids were withdrawn up to 2 years previously. The following protocol is one of many that would be considered acceptable:

- Evening before surgery, 9:00 p.m.: cortisone acetate, 100 mg intramuscularly
- Day of surgery, 6:00 a.m.: cortisone acetate, 100 mg intramuscularly
- Day of surgery, postoperatively: cortisone acetate, 100 mg intramuscularly, three times daily
- First postoperative day: cortisone acetate, 100 mg intramuscularly, three times daily (a tapering schedule is advised after the third postoperative day, depending on the condition of the patient)

A regimen including intravenous hydrocortisone must be appropriately undertaken to minimize the risk for inadequate replacement of the suppressed pituitary-adrenal response. This method requires either continuous infusion or administration every 4 hours. Adequate blood levels are more difficult to maintain if doses are given less often.

In an emergency situation, it is obviously impossible to prepare the bowel adequately, particularly for the complications of toxic colitis or megacolon. Preoperative preparation includes the correction of any fluid and electrolyte abnormalities, blood replacement as necessary, the placement of a nasogastric tube,

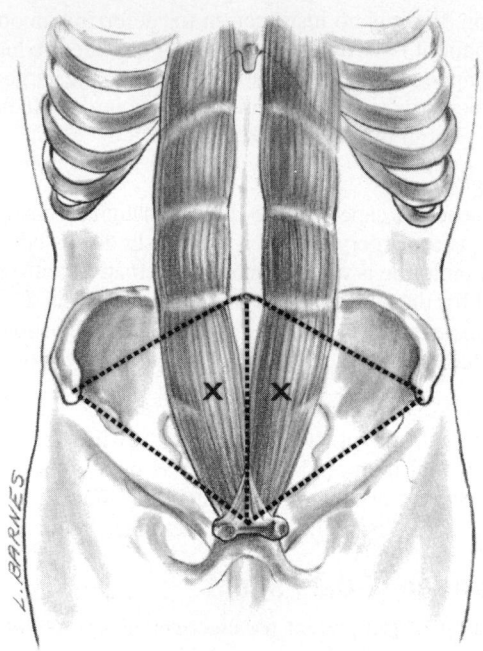

FIGURE 29-39. When a site for ileostomy is chosen, scars, bony prominences, and the umbilicus must be avoided.

the insertion of a Foley catheter (adequate urine output must be established), and the usual large-bore intravenous lines and monitors required for a very ill and potentially unstable patient.

In the elective situation, besides the ample literature available for the patient, it is always helpful to have an ostomate pay a visit. Someone who has achieved success, is of the same sex and age, and ideally of a similar socioeconomic status is preferred. If the surgeon is unable to suggest such a person, the local ostomy association will provide this counsel at no cost. I have always found my patients to be most appreciative of this input. The services of a wound care or an enterostomal therapist are a great asset in preparing the patient, even if one anticipates employing a stoma on a temporary basis only.

Preoperative stoma marking should be accomplished for everyone who is to undergo surgery for IBD, and it is absolutely imperative if an ileostomy is contemplated. Although preoperative marking is strongly advised for those who are to undergo abdominoperineal resection for cancer, the consequences of a poorly placed stoma are not as profound as they are in patients who are to have an ileostomy. It must be remembered that to the patient the stoma is the most important feature of the operation. An improperly located stoma, one that does not permit convenient management, may cause a patient to become significantly disabled and reclusive. The surgeon should put as much effort into creating a satisfactory stoma, in terms of both preoperative location and technique of construction, as to securing adequate hemostasis. The techniques of stomal construction are discussed in Chapter 31, as are the complications of ileostomy and colostomy.

The optimal site is selected with the patient sitting, supine, and standing. It should be away from bony promontories, scars, and the umbilicus. In the elective situation, it may be helpful rarely to have the patient wear the appliance for a day to be certain that the location is satisfactory (e.g., not interfering with the belt line). Often, one should mark two sites in the hypogastrium, one on each side; should it be impossible to create the stoma in one position, an alternative will then be available. The ileostomy should be brought through the split thickness of the rectus muscle (Figure 29-39). My own preference is to mark the site with a scratch from a hypodermic needle (Figure 29-40). Using a pen or India ink is

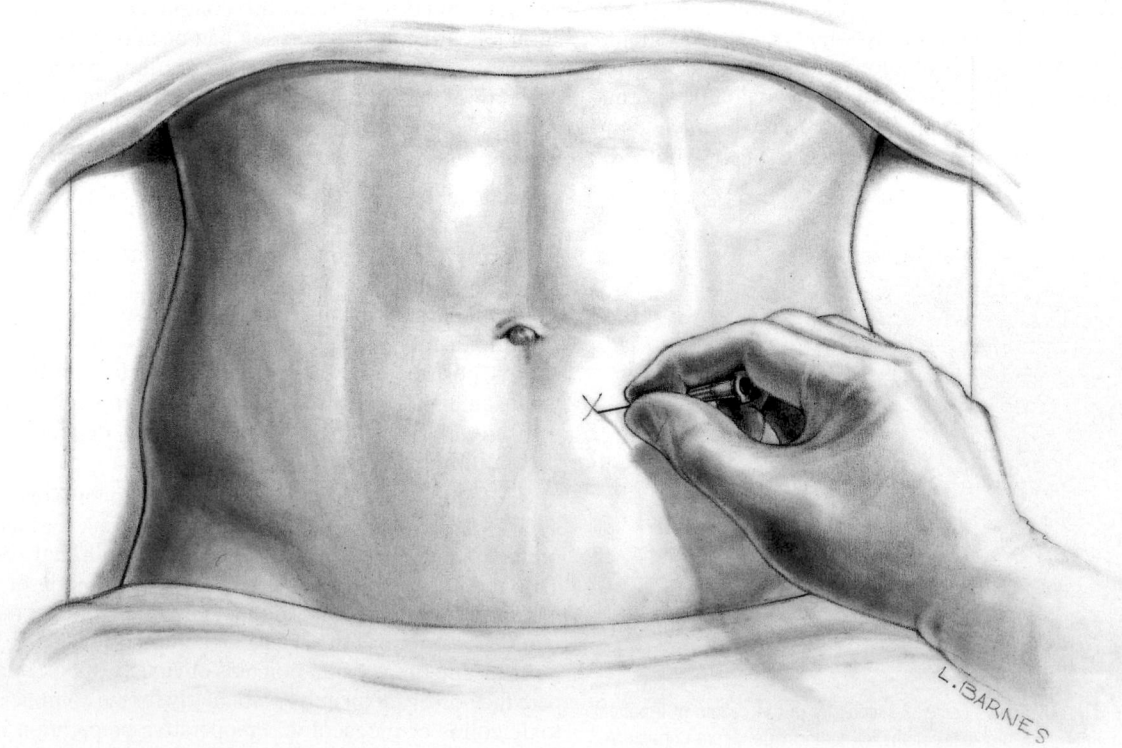

FIGURE 29-40. Stomal marking by scratching the skin with a hypodermic needle. This is easily visualized for 48 to 72 hours.

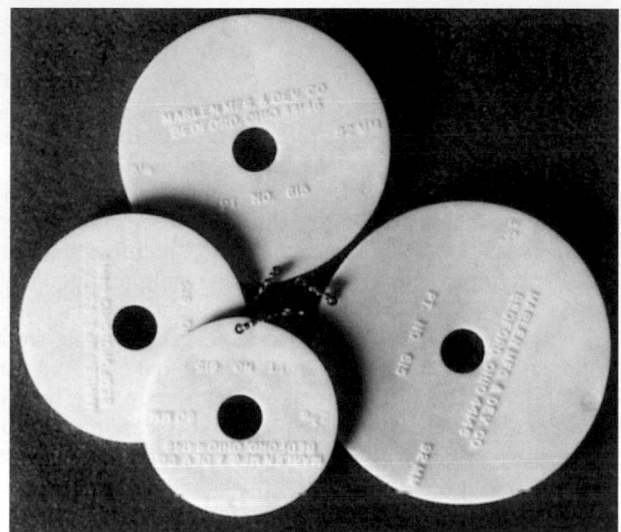

FIGURE 29-41. Variable-diameter faceplate templates for stomal marking. (Courtesy of Marlen Manufacturing and Development Co., Bedford, OH.)

not a good idea. Even the best of dyes cannot be maintained with most skin preparations. It is not necessary to tattoo the scratch because if the patient does not require a stoma, or it must be placed in another location, the tattoo will remain permanently. The scratch itself can easily be identified for several days until it heals.

In an emergency situation, it may not be possible to mark the site adequately preoperatively, particularly if a perforation precipitates the need for surgical intervention. Even under these circumstances, however, an effort should be made to mark the site on the operating table with the patient in the flexed position. Attempts to do this during the operation, with the abdominal wall open, will often result in the stoma being in a less-than-satisfactory location. Before the incision is made, a site may be selected with some degree of assurance through the use of a flange that corresponds to the diameter of the faceplate of an appliance (Figure 29-41). Although the patient under these circumstances can be examined in the supine position only, it is a better alternative than a mere guess. The flange can be sterilized, so that one can still benefit from an intelligent effort to locate the optimal site even when the requirement for an ileostomy has not been anticipated.

The Operations

Alternatives

There are five basic operations for the surgical treatment of ulcerative colitis:

- proctocolectomy and conventional ileostomy
- total or subtotal colectomy with rectal preservation (ileorectal anastomosis, mucous fistula, or closure of rectal stump)
- proctocolectomy with reservoir ileostomy (Kock, Barnett)
- total abdominal proctocolectomy with ileoanal (reservoir-anal) anastomosis and intervening pouch (Parks, Utsunomiya, Peck)

In patients with toxic megacolon, a sixth option is a diverting loop ileostomy with a decompressive skin-level (blowhole) colostomy.

Incision and Exploration

The issue of the nature of the incision has become a heated subject, in light of the development of the minimally invasive approach to bowel resection, including some of the most complicated colorectal operations (see Chapter 19). Although I no longer feel strongly, I have opined that the incision for all colon resections, including operations for IBD, always should be in the midline. The reasons for this have been discussed previously and include rapid and facile entry into the peritoneal cavity, good exposure of all areas within the abdomen, and, most importantly, accessibility of both sides of the abdomen for possible stomal placement. If a paramedian incision is used, that side of the abdomen is excluded for possible location of an ileostomy. This may not seem very important at the time of the procedure, particularly if the surgeon contemplates locating the stoma on the opposite side, but if the ileostomy ever requires relocation, unless the scar is flat, it may be extremely difficult to find a satisfactory alternative site. Placing the stoma in a pararectus location is considered inappropriate (see Chapter 31).

Generally, if a total abdominal colectomy or proctocolectomy is contemplated, the incision is made in the hypogastrium with supraumbilical extension for varying distances. Incision to the level of the xiphoid may be required if splenic flexure mobilization is difficult. In patients with long-standing ulcerative colitis, however, when foreshortening of the bowel may be present, one should begin the incision in the hypogastrium, ascertain the height of the flexures, and extend the incision cephalad if further exposure is required. When operating for toxic megacolon, it is imperative that one have adequate exposure to avoid possible injury to the colon or spleen.

Some surgeons employ a Maylard incision (suprapubic, transverse, muscle-dividing) for many colon procedures, including restorative proctocolectomy as a so-called minilaparotomy. Generally, exposure is adequate and favorably "competes" with minimally invasive surgery on the issues of cosmetics and comfort. If additional exposure is required, the incision may be extended laterally and cephalad on either side to the costal margins, if necessary. Furthermore, any stoma is quite some distance from the incision. In a study by Brown and coworkers, wherein laparoscopic-assisted surgery was compared with minilaparotomy by means of a suprapubic incision in restorative proctocolectomies, there was no difference in postoperative recovery.[75] The only advantage was the slightly smaller wound with laparoscopy.

Exploration of the abdomen will usually reveal the extent of pathology in patients with Crohn's disease because this is a transmural inflammatory process and the serosa is virtually always involved. However, in patients with ulcerative colitis, one may be singularly unimpressed with the extent of disease as it appears from the serosal aspect. The surgeon may appreciate only tortuosity of the vessels, pallor on the serosal aspect, and, of course, in the case of long-standing, chronic ulcerative colitis, bowel shortening.

When operating for ulcerative colitis, one should have a preconceived plan of the surgery that is to be performed. That is to say, almost irrespective of the operative findings, the entire colon should be removed. Whether one wishes to contemplate a more esoteric operation is a decision that should be made preoperatively. One must depend on the preoperative evaluation, history, endoscopic findings, and radiologic studies—not on the operative findings—to determine the extent of resection for ulcerative colitis. Conversely, in patients with Crohn's disease, it is not uncommon to discover that involvement is more extensive than might have been appreciated by preoperative evaluation. In both conditions, one must inspect the entire small bowel for the possibility of other lesions. The small intestine should be carefully examined even in patients with presumed ulcerative colitis because occasionally one may discover a lesion in the proximal bowel consistent with Crohn's disease. Obviously, this might compel the surgeon to perform a different operation.

Proctocolectomy with Ileostomy

Proctocolectomy with ileostomy is the conventional operative approach to the treatment of patients with ulcerative colitis and for most individuals with granulomatous colitis in which the rectum or anus is involved. However, it is interesting to note that there have been very few reports on the management of IBD by this operation in the past 30 years. This phenomenon is initially attributed to the development of the continent, reservoir ileostomy (Kock) and then to restorative proctocolectomy. Currently, the overwhelming number of publications on surgery for ulcerative colitis address the techniques, complications, and results of the various pouch-anal alternatives (see later discussion). However, proctocolectomy and conventional ileostomy should be considered the benchmark procedure with which all other operations must be compared. This approach has been established as relatively safe, curative, and permits the patient to live a virtually normal lifestyle.

The operation has evolved in a sequential way, beginning initially with appendicostomy as a decompressive procedure, then ileostomy, and then staged operations to effect removal of the colon and rectum.[74,83,84,105,379,450,480] During the era of staged procedures, which included staged thyroidectomy, esophageal diverticulectomy, abdominoperineal resection, and pancreatectomy, it was considered perfectly reasonable to perform four operations before completely extirpating the bowel for ulcerative colitis (ileostomy, right hemicolectomy, left hemicolectomy, and then abdominoperineal resection). With advances in anesthesia, blood transfusion, and antibiotics, as well as improved surgical techniques, the staged procedure was reduced to two operations (total abdominal colectomy followed by proctectomy) and inevitably to one-stage total proctocolectomy.[72,112,191,209]

The technique of proctocolectomy essentially combines the operations previously discussed in Chapters 23 and 24: total abdominal colectomy with proctectomy, using either the classic Miles approach or the perineolithotomy position (synchronous combined). There are some minor differences, however, that are important to consider. First, this is not a cancer operation. Hence, it is not necessary to remove a large area of mesentery containing the lymphatic structures. Furthermore, it is not appropriate for the surgeon to excise the parietal peritoneum widely, as one often does for carcinoma of the rectum. The peritoneal cut may be made directly on the bowel wall, thereby expediting and facilitating the dissection. However, the operation can and should be one that takes into account risk factors for cancer (which may be occult) and where a radical colectomy should then be performed.

Another difference in surgical technique when removing the colon and rectum for IBD, as opposed to removing them for cancer, is rectal mobilization. Because of the potential for injury to sympathetic and parasympathetic nerves, it has been suggested that the posterior rectal dissection for this disease be performed between the rectal wall and the mesentery, or at least through the mesorectum. This maneuver is more likely to avoid injury to the presacral nerves, the sympathetic innervation to the pelvic viscera. However, the dissection is tedious and often conducive to hemorrhage. Furthermore, the technique fails to protect the parasympathetic innervation, which is usually of greater concern, especially in men. Erection is a parasympathetically mediated response that is transmitted through the nervi erigentes. These nerves arise from the second, third, and fourth sacral roots. Parasympathetic nerve injury can result in impotence, whereas injury to the presacral (sympathetic) nerves interferes with ejaculation. The presacral nerves originate from the thoracic and lumbar segments of the spinal cord and can be identified if the surgeon makes a modicum of effort to do so. Because there is a ready plane of dissection between the investing fascia of the mesentery of the rectum and the sacrum, I prefer to visualize the presacral nerves directly, displace them posteriorly, and proceed in this plane, in the same manner one does with proctectomy for carcinoma. To accomplish this safely, it is important to begin the dissection sharply with a scissors or electrocautery in the hollow of the sacrum rather than to initiate mobilization of the rectum from the promontory bluntly by means of the hand. After the dissection has proceeded well below the sacral promontory, it is then reasonable to complete the mobilization by blunt dissection, but I still prefer to use sharp dissection as far as it can be technically achieved. With a proper retractor and an able assistant, one can directly visualize the entire posterior dissection to the level of the levators most of the time.

An organized approach to the operation minimizes morbidity and mortality. Having ascertained the extent of the disease, the surgeon proceeds with mobilization of the sigmoid colon and rectum. At this time, the perineal surgeon commences that part of the operation. After completion of the proctectomy, the rectum is delivered to the abdominal operator and wrapped in a towel or placed in a bag, and the rest of the colectomy is completed while the perineal surgeon closes the bottom end wound. Alternatively, the abdominal surgeon may elect to perform a total colectomy initially, calling the perineal surgeon in at the appropriate stage of the operation to complete the proctectomy.

If two teams are not available, the patient may be placed either in the perineolithotomy or in the supine position on the operating table, and the total abdominal colectomy is carried out. The rectum is divided and the abdomen closed, the ileostomy created, and the perineal dissection undertaken with the patient either in the left lateral position or in the lithotomy position.

In contradistinction to what may be done in a proctectomy for carcinoma, the floor of the pelvis is not reconstituted. If one closes the floor with parietal peritoneum, a diaphragm-like effect is created. This results in a dead space that predisposes to the subsequent development of an abscess, perineal sinus, and delayed healing. One must endeavor, in essence, to lower the pelvic floor. Because it is not necessary to excise the levator muscle widely as is often done for cancer, it is always possible to reapproximate this and the external sphincter. It is the external sphincter and levators, then, that form the floor of the pelvis in patients who undergo proctectomy for IBD.

The perineal dissection is undertaken in a manner somewhat different from that for carcinoma. The technique that I prefer is the intersphincteric dissection advocated by Lyttle and Parks[441] (Figure 29-42). This permits a much smaller

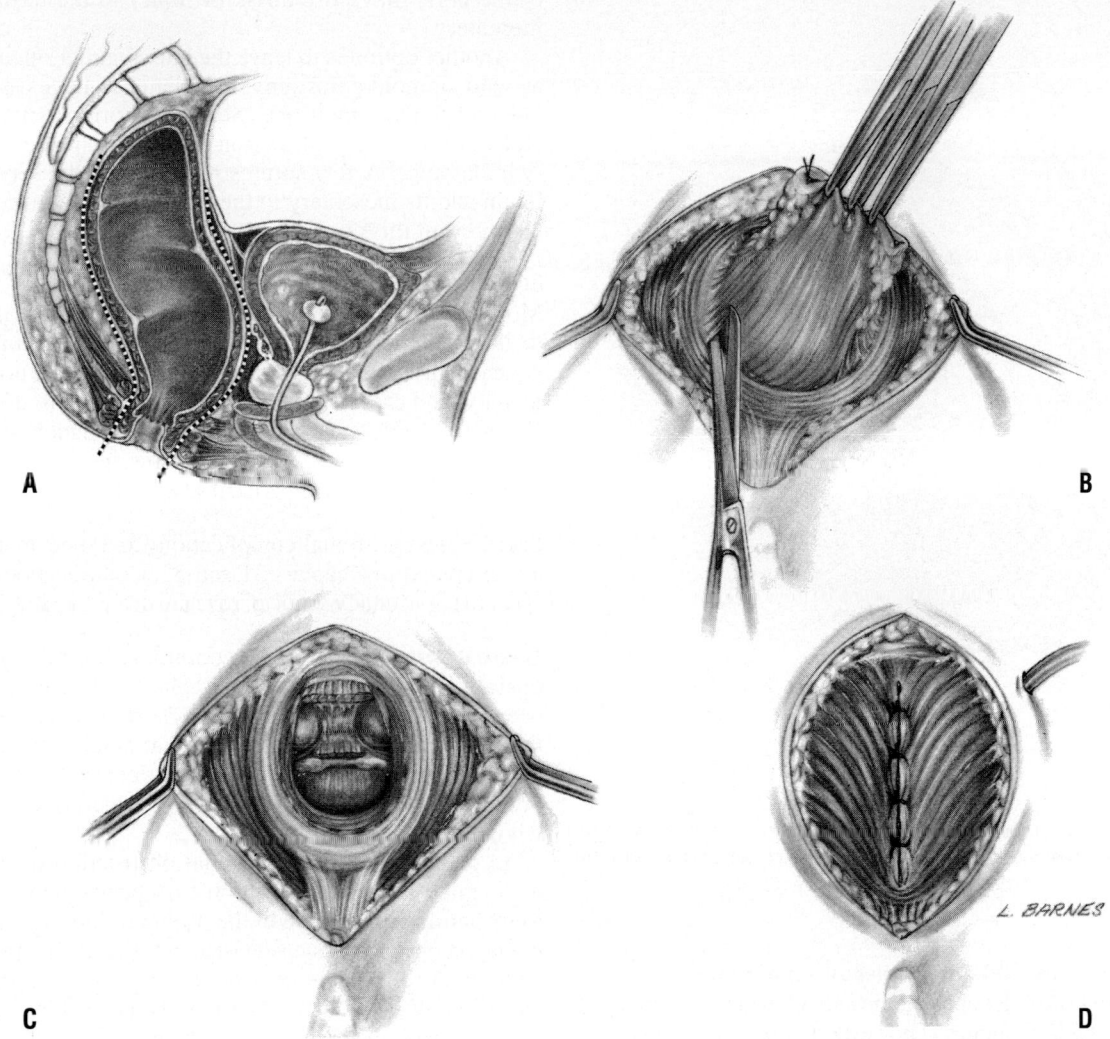

FIGURE 29-42. Technique of intersphincteric proctectomy. **A:** Outline of the area removed. **B:** Dissection proceeds in the intersphincteric plane. **C:** Intact external sphincter and levatores following rectal removal. **D:** Closure of levatores with drainage.

perineal wound. The procedure is carried out in the intersphincteric plane, between the internal and external anal sphincters. When the levator ani muscle is encountered, it is divided close to the rectum. The dissection is completed anteriorly in a manner identical to that for carcinoma of the rectum. A Silastic (Jackson-Pratt) drain is placed into the pelvis, brought out through a stab wound in the buttock, and connected to continuous suction (Figure 29-42D; Figure 29-43). Alternatively, a suprapubic suction drain can be employed. The levator ani muscle and external sphincter are then approximated and the skin closed. The drain is usually removed at 72 hours, depending on the amount collected.

Another method for performing an intersphincteric proctectomy is an endoanal mucosal stripping, such as can be undertaken in conjunction with the ileal pouch-anal procedure (see later discussion).[153] This leaves yet a smaller wound, but the operation may be associated with delayed healing, is tedious to accomplish, and has the theoretical disadvantage of incomplete removal of the mucosa, thereby posing a potential risk for cancer and persistent perineal sinus.[272,568]

Resection of the distal small bowel is sometimes necessary when proctocolectomy is undertaken for Crohn's disease, depending on whether the intestine is involved by the inflammatory process. Conversely, the small intestine is spared when the operation is performed for ulcerative colitis. Every effort should be made to preserve the full length of the small bowel. A contrary view is that resection of the distal 2 to 3 cm of ileum does not add to absorption difficulties but may be helpful to the pathologist in the event that occult Crohn's disease is identified. This might influence the postoperative follow-up of the patient. Still, even modest resection of the distal ileum may lead to malabsorption of nutrients as well as to loss of water and electrolytes.[531]

The distal small bowel may be divided with crushing clamps and delivered through the abdominal opening in a manner similar to that described for colostomy after abdominoperineal resection. Another option is to use a gastrointestinal anastomosis (GIA) stapling device, a Zachary Cope enterostomy clamp, or even paired umbilical clamps.[241] In creating the ileostomy for patients with ulcerative colitis, one may perform an extraperitoneal or an intraperitoneal approach. The former technique permits total obliteration of the paraileostomy gutter, thereby avoiding the potential for herniation. It also facilitates subsequent entrance into the

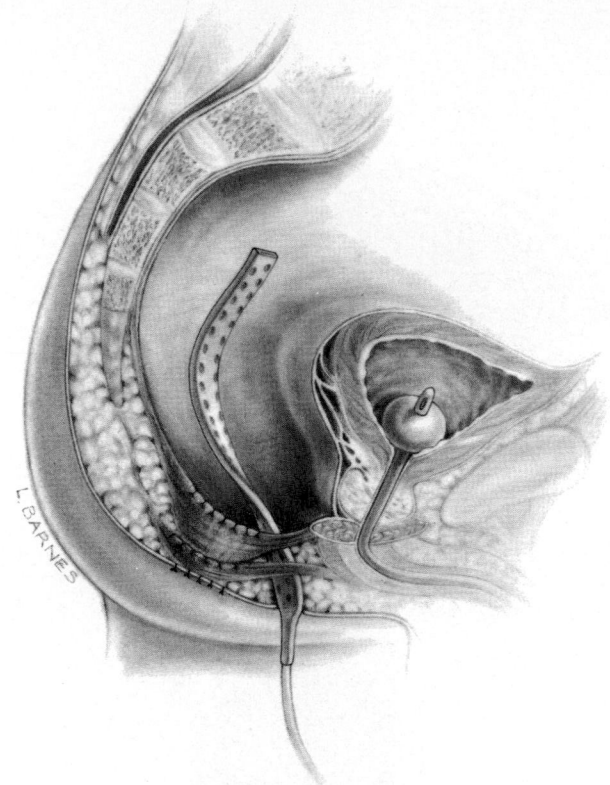

FIGURE 29-43. Lateral view of pelvis following proctectomy for ulcerative colitis. The peritoneal floor is open; the levatores, external sphincter, and skin are closed, and a drain is placed into the pelvis through a stab wound.

abdominal cavity without the risk of injuring the mesentery to the small bowel. Kocher clamps are placed on the cut edge of the parietal peritoneum. The peritoneum is then gently elevated and stripped off the abdominal wall to the point where the ileostomy site is located. An abdominal wall opening is then created, and the end of the ileum is delivered through the defect (Figure 29-44A). The cut edge of the mesentery is then secured to the peritoneum that has been mobilized (Figure 29-44B). Following closure of the abdomen, the ileostomy is matured (see Figures 31-47 through 31-49).

An intraperitoneal ileostomy is the commonly used alternative for most surgeons but is particularly recommended in patients who undergo proctocolectomy for granulomatous colitis, in those who have already had a portion of the terminal ileum removed, and in those for whom "stripping" of the parietal peritoneum is technically impossible. The technique for creation of an intraperitoneal ileostomy and obliteration of the lateral space is illustrated in Figure 29-45. As suggested, the disadvantages are the technical difficulties associated with complete obliteration of the right lateral gutter (the inferior aspect of the distal ileum does not lend itself to closure in a satisfactory fashion), and entrance into the abdominal cavity from the right upper quadrant is impeded. This cautionary note is best illustrated by the example of the patient who undergoes a cholecystectomy several years after intraperitoneal obliteration of the lateral gutter. The surgeon usually elects a subcostal approach to avoid the stoma, but when the peritoneal cavity is entered, the mesentery to the small intestine may be divided, with resultant necrosis of the ileostomy. Even with a laparoscopic approach, placement

of the ports may pose a risk of injury to the terminal ileal mesentery.

Another option is to leave the lateral gutter open because, as with sigmoid colostomy, it is better to have a very large opening than a small one. Some anchoring is nonetheless still required to avoid torsion of the distal ileum on itself (windlassing). A few sutures placed from the serosa of the ileum and its mesentery to the parietal peritoneum will usually prevent this complication (Figure 29-46).

Complications

Most complications following proctocolectomy are not unique to the operation: wound infection, intra-abdominal sepsis, wound dehiscence, ureteral and splenic injury, and urinary, pulmonary, and cardiovascular problems. These are discussed in Chapters 23 and 24. Complications attributed more specifically to this operation include stomal problems, intestinal obstruction, sexual dysfunction, and perineal wound difficulties.

Stomal Problems. Stomal complications and their management are discussed in Chapters 31 and 32. Complications with respect to recurrent Crohn's disease are discussed in Chapter 30.

Intestinal Obstruction. This is a common complication of all operations in which a stoma is placed. The incidence has been reported to be as high as 25%, most occurring within the first year. Turnbull reported that small bowel obstruction developed in 6% of 261 patients who underwent proctocolectomy and ileostomy for ulcerative colitis and who underwent laparotomy.[748]

In patients in whom intestinal obstruction develops following ileostomy, consideration must be given to a paraileostomy hernia as the cause of the problem. Initial conservative management includes nasogastric intubation and possibly an attempt to relieve the obstruction by irrigating the stoma. Occasionally, the obstruction may be caused by inspissated fecal material or undigested food. As long as the patient is passing flatus, it is usually possible to delay surgical intervention. Success of stomal irrigation can be augmented by the use of an intravenous narcotic and repeated saline irrigations, leaving the irrigating tube or Foley catheter draining into a pouch for up to 24 hours, depending on the circumstances. However, if a complete intestinal obstruction is present, early operation may be imperative. The cause of the problem is often a simple adhesion, but if a paraileostomy hernia with entrapment of the small intestine is the cause, the small bowel must be reduced and the defect closed.

Ileal Necrosis. The presence of a nonviable stoma is usually a consequence of torsion. Obviously, if the stoma itself is necrotic, the preoperative diagnosis is self-evident and resection of the stoma and nonviable bowel is necessary. However, if the blood supply to the ileostomy is preserved, the surgeon may be tempted to resect the nonviable bowel and perform an anastomosis a few centimeters from the end of the ileostomy. Such a concept is a dangerous undertaking. Unless the area of nonviability is at least 25 cm from the ileostomy, no anastomotic attempt should be made. The stoma should be resected in continuity with the nonviable bowel and a new ileostomy created. This usually requires relocation to the left lower quadrant. Even though this means sacrificing additional intestine, the risk for an anastomotic leak is so great that preservation of this small segment is not justified.

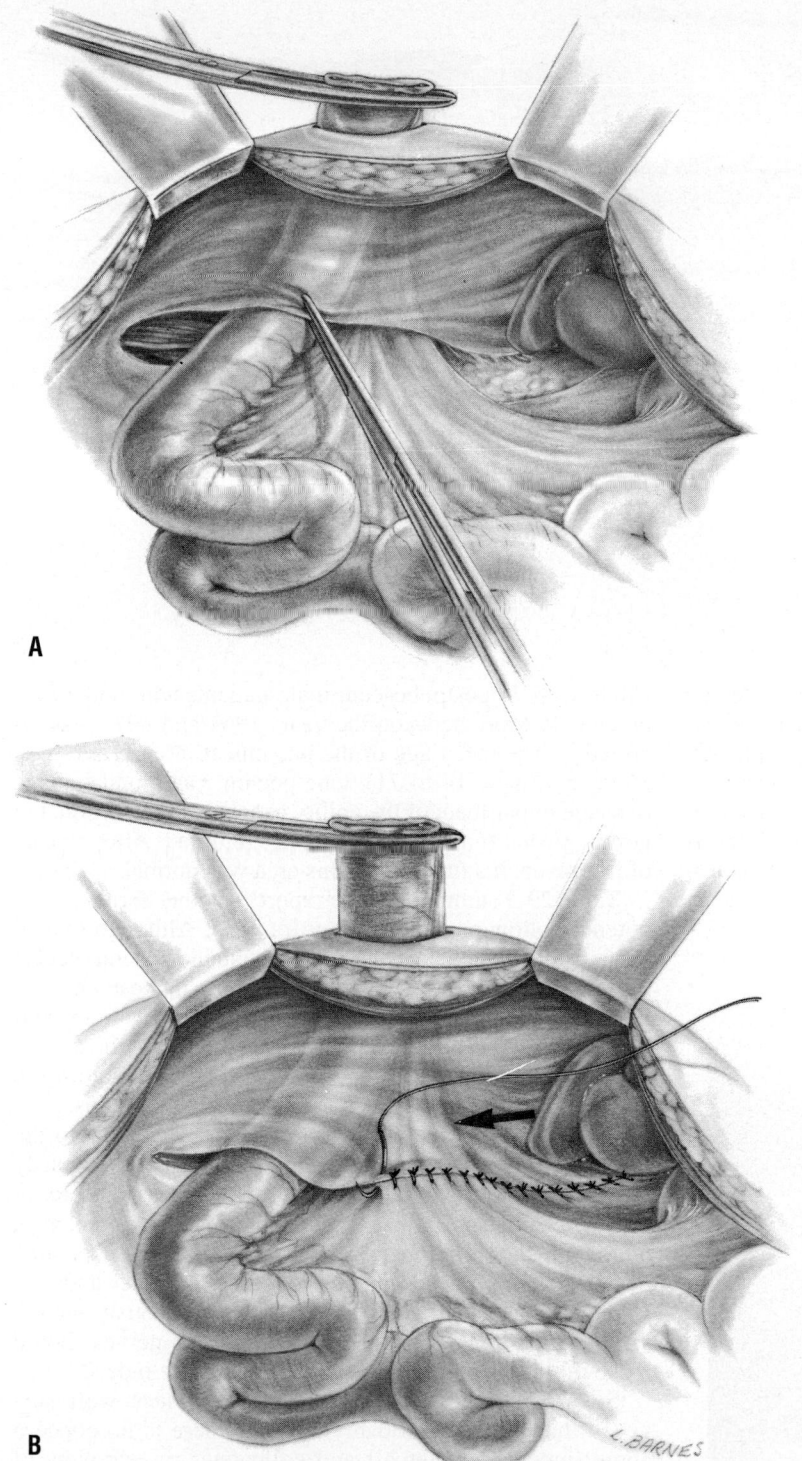

FIGURE 29-44. Extraperitoneal ileostomy. **A:** Mobilized peritoneum from the abdominal wall, with delivery of the terminal ileum through the ileostomy site and closure of the mesenteric defect. **B:** The peritoneum overlies the cut edge of the mesentery (*arrow*). In current practice, this is rarely performed.

Sexual Dysfunction. Sexual dysfunction (retrograde ejaculation and impotence) is well recognized as an unfortunate sequela of proctectomy. It is this complication that causes some surgeons to be unwilling to remove the rectum at the time of the initial procedure, preferring to perform proctectomy at a later date, when it is hoped that the patient will have achieved all procreative ambitions. It is doubtful, however, that a young man in his 30s, with perhaps a sufficient number of children, is particularly grateful for sexual dysfunction at his age any more than he might have been 10 years previously. I believe that there is good evidence

that intra-mesorectal dissection is a safer method with respect to preserving male sexual function.

To delay operation, however, is not without consequences. The patient must contend with another major operation, with its implications of time lost from work, family hardship, and changes in lifestyle. Many patients who feel well are reluctant to submit to an operation that will make them, at least for a time, unwell. Some are lost to follow-up, and some refuse operation. Finally, the risk for malignancy developing is a very real concern. Many surgeons have witnessed the tragedy of incurable carcinoma arising in the long

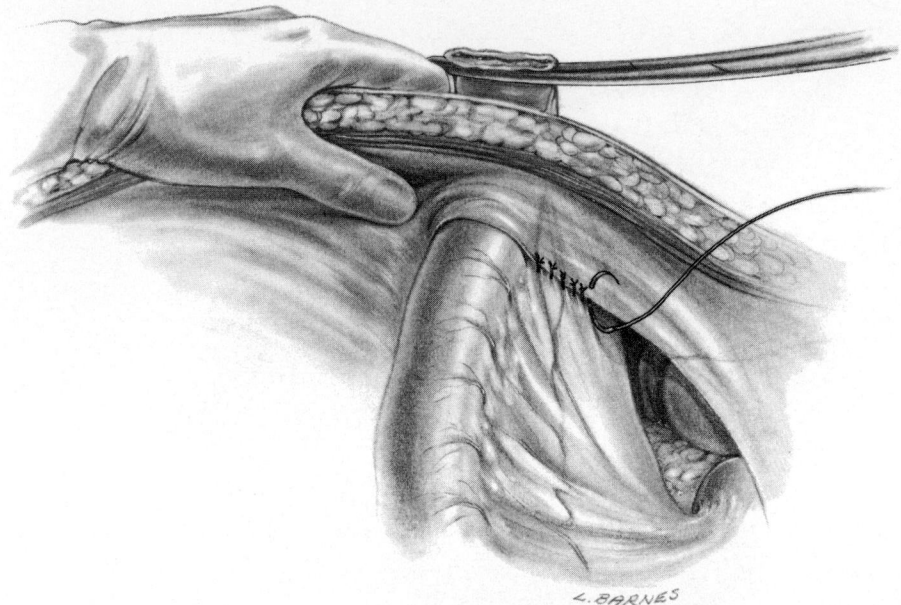

FIGURE 29-45. Intraperitoneal fixation. The falciform ligament is the limit of closure cephalad. The cut edge of the mesentery is sutured to the parietal peritoneum.

forgotten, retained rectum. The concern about the potential risk for malignancy in the retained rectum have become secondary issues in recent years, however, as the pouch-anal procedure is undertaken ideally as a primary procedure.

Impotence after abdominoperineal resection for carcinoma of the rectum is not an uncommon problem, but one questions whether preservation of the rectum in IBD is justified solely because of this risk. Experience at the Lahey Clinic with 76 postpubescent male patients who underwent proctocolectomy between the years 1964 and 1973 was reported.[107] The mean age of the patients at proctectomy was 36 years (range, 14 to 71). One person was found to have transient impairment of the ability to achieve an erection, but normal sexual function subsequently returned. After 6 years of follow-up, his function in this area was normal.

Table 29-3 summarizes the reports of other series on impotence following proctectomy for IBD. Although that of Watts and colleagues found a high incidence of impotence, patients in their series were older than those in most others.[764] In fact, five of seven patients with impotence were in their late 50s or 60s. When this series is excluded from the overall figures, the rate of impotence is 2.7%. The vast majority in all series who are impotent are in the older age groups.

Retrograde ejaculation occurs because of injury to the sympathetic nerves, a complication that has been variously reported to develop in up to 10% of male patients. More recent statistics suggest that, as with the problem of impotence, the complication is much less frequent in younger people. Fewer than 1% of the patients reported by Bauer and colleagues exhibited this difficulty.[35] As previously stated, visualization and avoidance of the presacral nerves should make this complication a very rare occurrence indeed.

Sexual function in women has been less well surveyed than in men, probably because there is no concern about impotence. Metcalf and colleagues, in a review of 100 women who underwent proctocolectomy (with either a Kock pouch or an ileoanal anastomosis), noted that the majority experienced enhanced sexual function.[492] This was attributed to improved health. Those with a pouch had a significantly higher incidence of dyspareunia than those with an ileoanal anastomosis, presumably because of scarring or deformity associated with complete proctectomy (see later discussion).

Other concerns about sexual dysfunction are related primarily to the concept of an ileostomy itself—the need for an external appliance and the possibility of leakage—and its impact on sexuality and body image.[25] These aspects are discussed in Chapters 31 and 32.

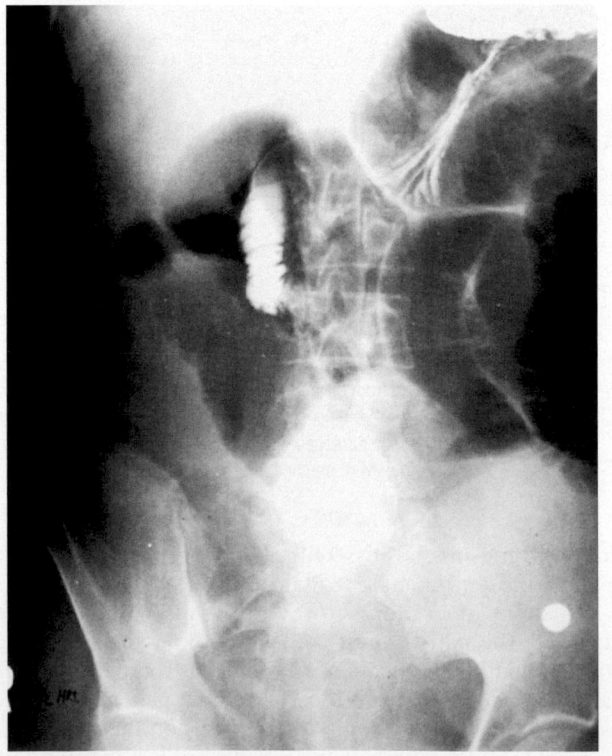

FIGURE 29-46. Small bowel obstruction secondary to torsion of the ileum on its mesentery. Barium study reveals complete obstruction proximal to the ileostomy.

TABLE 29-3 Impotence after Proctectomy for Inflammatory Bowel Disease

| REFERENCE | NUMBER OF PATIENTS | IMPOTENCE | |
		NUMBER	PERCENTAGE
Bacon et al.[19]	39	1	2.8
Burnham et al.[79]	118	6	5.1
Donovan and O'Hara[136]	21	1	4.8
May[470]	17	3	6.1
Stahlgren and Ferguson[699]	25	0	0.0
Van Prohaska and Siderius[755]	79	0	0.0
Watts et al.[764]	41	7	17.1
Corman et al.[107]	76	0	0.0
Total of reported series	446	18	4.0

From Corman ML, Veidenheimer MC, Coller JA. Impotence after proctectomy for inflammatory disease of the bowel. *Dis Colon Rectum.* 1978;21:418.

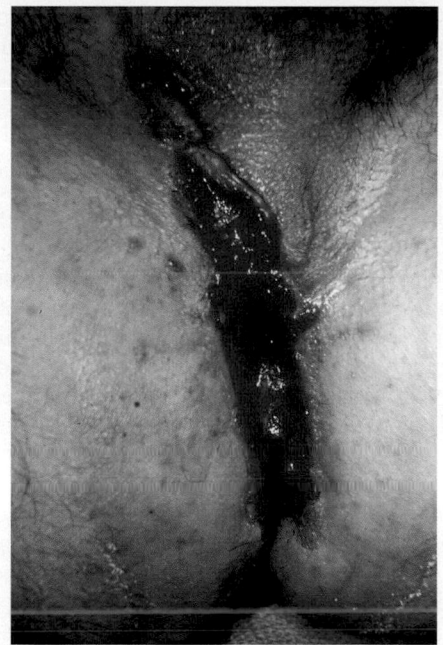

FIGURE 29-47. Persistent perineal sinus following proctectomy for inflammatory bowel disease. A chronic, indolent draining wound.

colitis were not healed, but the wounds of more than one-third of the patients with Crohn's colitis had not healed.

Some authors have demonstrated that packing the perineal wound is associated with delayed healing.[303,636] In a retrospective review from our institution (the Cleveland Clinic), a highly significant difference was appreciated between packing versus levator closure with transabdominal drainage—31% were unhealed at 1 year or required further surgery in the former group, whereas only 9% were unhealed in the latter

Comment. In my opinion, impotence appears to be less the result of the type of operative approach than of the age of the patient. It seems difficult to believe that careful attention to dissection close to the bowel wall is the reason for a low incidence of impotence, whereas the "radical" operation for cancer produces a high incidence. Although one cannot gainsay meticulous surgical technique, preoperative libido is probably a more important factor. A report from the Mayo Clinic seems to concur with this opinion.[786]

Persistent Perineal Sinus. Persistent perineal sinus is one of the most troubling sequelae of proctectomy for IBD (Figures 29-47 and 29-48). The Lahey Clinic group reviewed their experience with 160 patients who underwent proctectomy for this condition.[108] The mean ages of the patients with ulcerative colitis and with Crohn's disease were the same (36 years). The sex incidence was also the same, but more men than women were given a diagnosis of ulcerative colitis and more women than men were diagnosed with Crohn's colitis. The perineal wounds in 75% of patients with ulcerative colitis were healed by the end of the follow-up period without reoperation, whereas only 51% of wounds in those with Crohn's colitis were healed. By the end of the follow-up study, the wounds of only 11% of patients with ulcerative

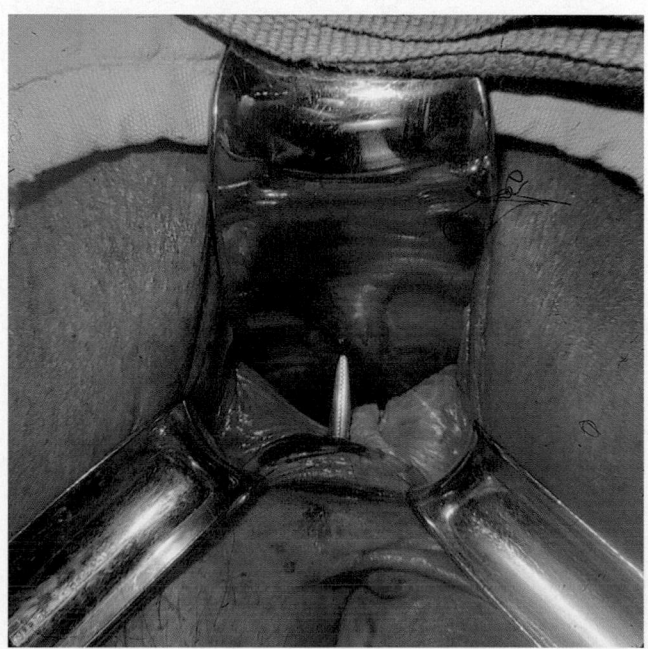

FIGURE 29-48. Perineovaginal fistula following proctectomy. Treatment requires fistulotomy. Pregnancy is unlikely to occur in this situation.

group.[553] Others have confirmed the value of intersphincteric proctectomy in reducing the incidence of delayed perineal wound healing.[35,394,790] Cripps and colleagues even suggest that a proctectomy can be undertaken by preserving the internal sphincter, stripping out only the mucosa, thus leading to more rapid and improved perineal wound healing.[113]

Other factors may be associated with the development of this complication. In the Lahey Clinic's, age was thought to be a relevant consideration. All patients with ulcerative colitis who were older than 50 years of age and all with Crohn's colitis who were older than 60 years of age had healed perineal wounds. With respect to sex, women with ulcerative colitis were more likely to have the perineal wound heal per primum (97.5%), whereas only 82% of men achieved such healing. However, no statistically significant difference in rates of healing was seen when sex distributions in patients with Crohn's disease were compared. Evaluation of the presence or absence of a stoma before proctectomy revealed that in patients with ulcerative colitis, diversion implied an excellent chance for healing. Interestingly, the opposite was true for those with Crohn's colitis.

Perineal disease, specifically fistula-in-ano (present at the time of proctectomy), was not a statistically significant factor in nonhealing at the Lahey Clinic, although the numbers were small. Unless there is active infection in the tract, the rates of nonhealing were almost the same in patients with ulcerative colitis and in those with Crohn's colitis when a fistula was present. However, in the absence of a perianal fistula, a patient with Crohn's colitis did not heal as well as one with ulcerative colitis. These factors are summarized in Table 29-4.

The number of prior operations; extent of disease; the emergent, urgent, or elective nature of the surgical procedure; contamination of the wound; presence or absence and duration of steroid therapy; level of serum albumin; and nutritional state of the patient were all analyzed and found to have no significant role in prolonging perineal wound healing.

A few studies have been summarized in Table 29-5, which serve to indicate the magnitude of the problem. In a report of 112 patients who underwent proctectomy for Crohn's disease, healing was delayed longer than 1 year in almost 20%.[661]

The failure of perineal wounds to heal readily has stimulated considerable discussion and has served as an impetus for the development of a number of operative approaches to deal with the problem.[10,71,294,451,625,639,649,680] Once a perineal sinus has developed, vigorous curettage, creating a pyramidal defect, should be undertaken at 6-month intervals until healing is achieved. Other methods that have been advocated include a gracilis or inferior gluteal myocutaneous flap,[20,66,641] semimembranosus muscle graft,[452] rectus abdominis flap,[689,788] use of an omental graft,[639] skin grafting,[10] and the application of a fibrin adhesive.[7,350] In a report from the General Hospital of Birmingham, England, 13 patients were submitted to treatment by means of this sealant, but only 5 were completely healed at the time of publication.[7]

TABLE 29-4 Healing after Proctectomy

	Ulcerative Colitis			Crohn's Colitis		
	Healed	Not Healed	Percentage Healed	Healed	Not Healed	Percentage Healed
Age in Years						
<20	10	4	71.4	0	2	0.0
20–29	17	2	89.5	14	7	66.7
30–39	21	2	91.3	9	5	64.3
40–49	15	2	88.2	8	5	61.6
50–59	9	0	100.0	6	2	75.0
60–69	7	0	100.0	2	0	100.0
>69	1	0	100.0	1	0	100.0
Sex						
Men	41	9	82.0	17	9	65.4
Women	39	1	97.5	23	12	65.7
Stoma						
Yes	50	1	98.0	25	18	58.1
No	30	9	76.9	15	3	83.3
Fistula						
Yes	4	2	66.7	25	16	61.0
No	76	8	90.5	15	5	75.0

From Corman ML, Veidenheimer MC, Coller JA, et al. Perineal wound healing after proctectomy for inflammatory bowel disease. *Dis Colon Rectum.* 1978;21:155.

TABLE 29-5 Perineal Wound Healing: Summary of Literature

Author, Year	Diagnosis	Healed, Months	Number Healed	Number Not Healed	Percentage Healed
Hughes, 1965[289]	Ulcerative colitis	Not stated	58	13	81.7
Watts et al., 1966[764]	Ulcerative colitis	6	70	23	75.3
Jalan et al., 1969[303]	Ulcerative colitis	6	48	58	45.3
	Crohn's colitis	12	67	39	63.2
Roy et al., 1970[636]	Ulcerative colitis	3	Not stated	Not stated	81.6
	Crohn's colitis	3	Not stated	Not stated	76.3
Oates and Williams, 1970[556]	Both	Not stated	41	12	77.4
de Dombal et al., 1971[123]	Crohn's colitis	6	39	29	57.4
Ritchie, 1971[625]	Ulcerative colitis	6	121	101	54.5
	Crohn's colitis	6	4	15	21.1
Broader et al., 1974[71]	Ulcerative colitis	6	33	8	80.5
	Crohn's colitis	12	11	2	84.6
Irvin and Goligher, 1975[299]	Ulcerative colitis	6	23	10	69.7
	Crohn's colitis	6	12	7	63.2
Corman et al., 1978[108]	Crohn's colitis	6	17	44	27.9
	Ulcerative colitis	6	40	50	44.4

From Corman ML, Veidenheimer MC, Coller JA, et al. Perineal wound healing after proctectomy for inflammatory bowel disease. *Dis Colon Rectum.* 1978;21:155.

Perineal Pain and Phantom Sensations. Phantom sensations of the "need to have a bowel movement" are not unusual after proctectomy. This difficulty is analogous to that which may occur following amputation of an extremity. The cerebral pathway still exists, so that an indeterminate stimulus to the perineum or pelvis may trigger this perception. Treatment is reassurance.

A more troublesome complaint is perineal pain. In contrast to pain that develops following proctectomy for rectal cancer, such pain is obviously not caused by recurrent malignancy, and it is possible to reassure the patient accordingly. Usually, the discomfort can be attributed to a neuroma. If the usual supportive measures (heat, rest, foam rubber cushion, antispasmotics, and nonnarcotic analgesic medications) fail to relieve the symptoms, one should consider excising the perineal fat pad. Almost invariably, the pathologist (if asked) will cooperate and succeed in identifying a neuroma, but the clinical significance and long-term benefits are problematic. Relief can be immediate, but recurrence may develop, presumably because the nerve regenerates. Fortunately, if this occurs, the pain is usually not as severe as initially reported.

Results of Conventional Proctocolectomy and Ileostomy
Proctocolectomy and ileostomy today can be carried out with minimal morbidity and mortality. Mavroudis and Schrock reported an operative mortality of 2% in 100 patients who underwent total abdominal colectomy, proctectomy, or both.[469] In the experience of Goligher, 10 operative deaths were noted in 113 patients who underwent proctocolectomy and ileostomy for Crohn's disease, a rate of 9%.[210] In his personal experience in the management of 504 patients with ulcerative colitis, there were 34 operative deaths, an operative mortality of 6.7%.[213] Elective, urgent, and emergency operations revealed a mortality rate of 3.0%, 10.7%, and almost 25.0%, respectively. Other reports suggest that the overall operative mortality for proctocolectomy and ileostomy is between 7% and 10%.

Ileostomy-Colostomy for the Treatment of Toxic Megacolon
Toxic megacolon has become a progressively rare manifestation of ulcerative colitis over the past 20 years. Because of the high mortality rate associated with the surgical treatment of toxic megacolon by colectomy (in some series, in excess of 30%), Turnbull and colleagues (Cleveland Clinic) in 1971 advocated what was considered a lesser risk procedure.[749] This consisted of a diversionary loop ileostomy and two decompressive colostomies, one in the transverse colon and the other in the sigmoid. The colostomies were created at the skin level and were designed to vent the dilated colon as a blowhole. The major impetus for suggesting this operative approach was to avoid inadvertent fecal soiling

of the peritoneal cavity when a walled-off perforation had been liberated by mobilization of the bowel. This usually occurs in the region of the splenic flexure, an area that is predisposed to bowel wall necrosis. Considerable contamination can result when the dilated colon is decompressed through this inadvertent opening. It was the opinion of our group that diversion and decompression avoided this very serious consequence. This technique has also been successfully used in two women with toxic ulcerative colitis who were pregnant.[467]

The technique consists of making a small midline incision and identifying a loop of distal ileum. This is brought out through a previously marked site in the right lower quadrant, usually over a small rod (Figure 29-49). Ideally, the proximal limb is placed inferiorly and the distal limb superiorly, so that subsequent colon resection will not necessitate a change in the fixation of the distal ileum. Exploration of the right upper quadrant of the abdomen identifies the point of maximal dilatation of the transverse colon, and a small incision is made in the skin, fascia, and rectus muscle. If the sigmoid colon is dilated, it too can be decompressed by making a small incision in the left iliac fossa, permitting the bowel to bulge into the incision. In our later reports, however, this second blowhole has rarely been thought to be necessary. The abdomen is then closed, and the loop ileostomy is matured, emphasizing the proximal limb (see Figures 31-67 through 31-69).

Attention is then turned to the dilated transverse colon. Seromuscular sutures are placed into the colon and the peritoneum and rectus fascia with interrupted fine catgut. A second row of seromuscular sutures is placed between the bowel and the subcutaneous fat. The colon is then opened and the contents evacuated. With successful decompression, sutures may now be placed between the cut edge of the bowel and the skin. The same procedure can be used for the sigmoid colon if an opening is necessary in this area.

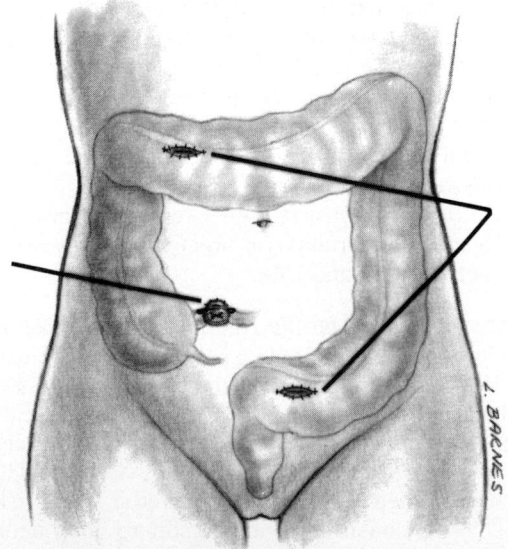

FIGURE 29-49. Diverting ileostomy and decompression colostomies for toxic megacolon. (Adapted from Turnbull RB Jr, Hawk WA, Weakley FL. Surgical treatment of toxic megacolon: ileostomy and colostomy to prepare patients for colectomy. *Am J Surg.* 1971;122:325.)

Although I, too, am relatively supportive of the occasional use of this particular approach, especially in those who are pregnant, there are several potential disadvantages.[155] These include the necessity for further major abdominal surgery and possible continued bleeding if hemorrhage was a presenting problem (approximately one-fourth of these patients will continue to bleed postoperatively). Also, if a septic focus persists, earlier surgical intervention than was first anticipated may be required.

Our group points out that the procedure should not be performed in cases of free perforation but only when obvious acute colonic dilatation exists without peritonitis. Moreover, in a later publication we note that in carefully selected, hemodynamically stable patients with fulminant colitis and without megacolon, restorative proctocolectomy with ileal pouch-anal anastomosis can be safely performed (see later discussion).[793]

Results

I and my colleagues reported the Cleveland Clinic experience of 115 patients seen from 1961 to 1967 with toxic megacolon.[155] Only 7 were discharged following medical management. Of interest is the fact that 5 of the 7 required subsequent colectomy. Subtotal colectomy with ileostomy was performed in 26 patients and decompression and diversion in the remaining 83. The mortality rate following subtotal colectomy was 11.5%. Three patients died after decompression and diversion, a mortality rate of 3.6%. However, 2 additional patients succumbed following elective colectomy, bringing the overall mortality to 6% for the decompression and diversion group. Among the 17 patients found to have free perforations, 5 deaths were reported, a mortality rate of almost 30%.

I am reluctant to draw dogmatic conclusions about the value of diversion and decompression. The mortality rate appears to be lower when patients are treated by this technique, but the series is uncontrolled, and it appears that many of the patients who were treated initially by colectomy actually had free perforations, thus constituting a much higher risk group.

Heppell and colleagues reviewed their experience with 65 patients who were treated for toxic megacolon.[270] The mortality rate following surgery was 27% when colectomy was undertaken for a free or sealed perforation. When toxic megacolon was associated with massive hemorrhage, the mortality was 33%. In the experience of Greenstein and Aufses, the incidence of perforation in toxic megacolon was three times greater for patients with ulcerative colitis than for those with Crohn's colitis.[227] In the absence of toxic megacolon, however, Crohn's disease was as likely to be associated with a perforation as was ulcerative colitis. Interestingly, mortality rates were lower if the perforation occurred in a patient with Crohn's disease.

Comment (MLC)

I am able to restrain my enthusiasm for the decompression and diversion technique in the treatment of toxic megacolon, primarily for the reasons alluded to by Dr. Fazio. It is a troublesome concept to commit the patient to at least one other operation when the procedure can be accomplished in one stage, removing the source of sepsis and liberating the patient from contending with at least two abdominal orifices. Fecal drainage from upper and lower abdominal wounds may be a justifiable, albeit unaesthetic, experience if one is convinced that it is the only lifesaving measure available. However, I believe that an expeditious, well-conceived resection can accomplish the optimal goal. To deal with a sealed perforation, it is suggested that the transverse colon be decompressed by simple needle aspiration before the splenic flexure is "attacked." Another alternative is to mobilize the sigmoid, descending, and transverse colon; to divide the bowel at the point of planned resection; and to exteriorize the segment, so that minimal contamination will result if a sealed perforation is encountered. Finally, there is a certain impracticality when one advises a blowhole colostomy for decompression. In my experience, attempting to suture a profoundly dilated, possibly necrotic transverse colon is more than a frustrating experience; it is impossible. Passing a suture into the bowel, itself, is likely to cause a perforation. The procedure is like attempting to sew wet toilet paper. In an admittedly small personal experience of patients with toxic megacolon, I have applied resection as the modality of therapy, with no deaths.

Total Colectomy with Rectal Preservation

Total abdominal colectomy with ileorectal or ileosigmoid anastomosis for ulcerative colitis has been advocated by a number of authors, but it has been especially championed by Aylett.[16-18] At the Gordon Hospital in London, Aylett developed an interest in the surgical management of IBD. As discussed previously, the standard surgical treatment was removal of the diseased bowel and the creation of a permanent stoma. Aylett thought that the rectum could usually be retained and a stoma avoided. The surgical establishment was outraged by his practice. Critics claimed that the patient would have intractable diarrhea and the risk of cancer developing in the retained bowel. Aylett was pilloried in the medical press and at national meetings. Heated debates ensued, but Aylett consistently showed good results. Although he recognized that cancer was indeed a risk, he believed that

with regular follow-up it could be identified and adequately treated. The surgical establishment failed to match Aylett's results, and it was suggested that with his charisma and charm he was able to seduce his patients into minimizing their problems after surgery. In the beginning of the 21st century, we are seeing his concept applied to selected patients with ulcerative colitis. This is especially true if the rectum is relatively spared and when an individual is motivated and cooperative. Those in the older age group may be selectively and preferentially treated by this operation.

The technical aspect of total colectomy is identical to the surgical approach described in Chapter 23. Laparoscopic total colectomy has also been advocated as a safe option in the elective case or even in acute, nonfulminant colitis (see Chapter 19).[456] One must always recognize the possibility that the diagnosis may be somewhat in question. Still, if the patient subsequently is proved to have Crohn's disease, selection of this procedure might actually have been preferable. Nonetheless, the relative merit of the ileorectal anastomosis for ulcerative colitis has diminished considerably, having been virtually replaced by the ileal pouch anal procedures (see later discussion).

Alternatives to an ileorectal anastomosis are either to close the rectum or to bring out the rectosigmoid as a mucous fistula. My own preference is to close the rectal stump so that the patient will not have to contend with the profuse mucus discharge and blood that is frequently associated with a second opening on the abdominal wall. Many patients find this drainage to be more cumbersome to manage than the stoma, itself. There is the risk, however, of the stump blowing out and leaking contents into the peritoneal cavity. This is especially true when the residual bowel is severely inflamed. A reasonable compromise under the circumstances is to close the bowel in the subcutaneous tissue. If a leak occurs, it can usually be addressed by simple incision and drainage on the abdominal wall. Carter and colleagues comment that

STANLEY O. AYLETT (1911–2003)

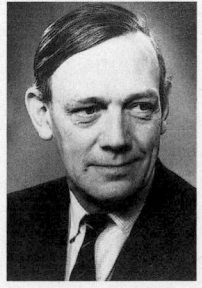

Stanley Aylett, the second son of a building contractor, was born in Islington, England, on July 8, 1911. He was educated at King's College, London. In 1929, he accepted a scholarship at King's College Hospital, at which institution he received a number of awards—including the prizes for anatomy, physiology, midwifery and gynecology, surgery, and surgical pathology. In 1932, he received a bachelor of science degree in physiology with first-class honors. In 1936, he was admitted to fellowship in the Royal College of Surgeons. Aylett joined the Royal Army Medical Corps during World War II and became attached to a casualty clearing station in France, treating the wounded. He was evacuated with the British Expeditionary Force from the beaches at Dunkerque. Subsequently, he served in forward field surgical units in North Africa. In 1944, he returned to England to train and command a field surgical unit in preparation

for the impending invasion of Europe. He landed on D-Day plus three, attached to various casualty clearing stations, and was assigned to the relief of the Sandbostel concentration camp. He was awarded the Croix d'Honneur for services rendered to French prisoners at this camp, and in 1945 he was made a member of the Order of the British Empire for his indefatigable contributions to the care of the sick and wounded. From 1947 until his retirement, he was a consultant surgeon on the staff of the Gordon Hospital. In 1960, he was awarded a Hunterian professorship from the Royal College of Surgeons for his historic presentation on ileorectal anastomosis for ulcerative colitis. Aylett wrote numerous articles on many aspects of colon and rectal surgery, especially surgery for ulcerative colitis. In addition, he is the author of two books, *Surgery of the Rectum and Colon* and *Surgeon at War*. Many awards and honors had been bestowed on him by his colleagues all over the world, including an honorary fellowship in the American Society of Colon and Rectal Surgeons. Stanley Aylett died on January 7, 2003.

exteriorization of the *closed rectal stump* is preferred to an open mucous fistula or a standard Hartmann closure.[81] It is associated with fewer pelvic septic complications, facilitates subsequent pelvic dissection, and is not associated with an increased activity in the retained rectum.

Another option is to perform a total abdominal procto-colectomy, removing the entire diseased bowel to the level of the levators. This then eliminates the requirement for rectal dissection at the time of the second procedure—that is, reservoir-anal anastomosis. This approach is probably not a good alternative in the emergency situation, however, when the patient is septic. One prefers not to open the extraperitoneal planes under these circumstances. Regardless, one should always divide the superior hemorrhoidal vessels in order to permit ready access to the presacral space at the subsequent operation.

Talbot and colleagues reviewed the St. Mark's Hospital experience with so-called conservative proctocolectomy.[720] This is the modification about which I just wrote, in which total abdominal proctocolectomy is performed with anal preservation. Besides the advantages of preserving the sphincters and facilitating the second operation, it does provide the opportunity to obtain a complete pathologic specimen for analysis, an important issue if Crohn's disease cannot be excluded or when there is concern for concomitant malignancy. Performing pelvic radiation in the presence of a pouch is not ideal.

Results

What is the risk for the development of cancer in the retained rectum? Aylett reported the single largest experience with ileorectal anastomosis for ulcerative colitis.[16–18] More than 400 patients underwent this operation, only 8% of whom had to undergo conversion to an ileostomy. Twelve subsequently underwent proctectomy because of carcinoma in the retained rectum.

Johnson and colleagues reported their experience with rectal preservation in patients with ulcerative colitis.[312] Of the 172 individuals who underwent subtotal colectomy and mucous fistula, more than one-half subsequently required rectal excision. In 27% the rectum remained as a mucous fistula. An additional 101 patients underwent an initial primary ileorectal anastomosis. Of the 273 at risk for rectal cancer, a malignant lesion subsequently developed in 10 (3.6%). Unfortunately, more than one-half had disseminated disease at the time of rectal removal, and there were no Dukes' A lesions. The authors estimated that the cumulative probability of a cancer developing in the rectum following subtotal colectomy was 17% at 27 years from the onset of disease. Although the experience of the authors was reasonably favorable, careful endoscopic follow-up is a requisite. Others have also expressed their concern about the retained rectum after colectomy for ulcerative colitis.[369,375,389,473]

Grundfest and colleagues reviewed our experience with 89 patients who underwent total abdominal colectomy and ileorectal anastomosis for ulcerative colitis.[232] Twenty-one percent required subsequent proctectomy, with the overall incidence of carcinoma being 4.8%. The cumulative risk for the development of a rectal cancer was 12.9% (±8.3%) after 25 years, considerably less than when the colon is left intact. We caution that preexisting colonic cancer with severe dysplasia is a relative contraindication to rectal preservation and

also strongly recommend frequent proctosigmoidoscopy and rectal biopsy to look for dysplasia.

Khubchandani and coworkers performed a prospective study to evaluate dysplasia in 34 patients who had previously undergone colectomy and ileorectal anastomosis for IBD.[348] One patient with 23 years of disease demonstrated severe dysplasia, and subsequent proctectomy revealed carcinoma in situ. The authors recommended multiple biopsy examinations of the rectum, ideally from relatively free areas, every 6 months. If a biopsy demonstrates severe dysplasia, a repeated examination is suggested 3 months later. If sequential biopsy demonstrates severe dysplasia, excision of the rectum is recommended.

Evaluation of the rectum by means of proctosigmoidoscopy or flexible sigmoidoscopy can usually be performed relatively easily in a patient whose rectum is in continuity with the intestinal tract. However, if someone has a mucous fistula or an oversewn rectal stump, it may be impossible to pass an instrument in the disused rectum after a time. These individuals are at great risk for the development of malignancy. If continuity has not been reestablished within 2 years following colectomy, serious consideration should be given to removing the rectum. However, even after a considerable period of time following ileostomy, a restorative proctectomy may be offered.

It is difficult to comment on the relative merits of proctocolectomy and total colectomy with rectal preservation with respect to morbidity and mortality. For example, in most series, experience with the latter operation suggests a much higher mortality, but these patients are often submitted to an emergency operation.[396] Farnell and colleagues reported the Mayo Clinic experience with rectal preservation in nonspecific IBD.[149] Sixty-three patients with ulcerative colitis underwent colectomy and ileorectal or ileosigmoid anastomosis. Follow-up was a minimum of 5 years, up to a maximum of 17 years. Preoperative proctoscopic examination revealed a normal rectum in slightly more than one-half of the patients. Moderate disease was present in 38%. During this interval, carcinoma did not develop in the residual rectum in any patient. The requirement for subsequent proctectomy was quite similar for those with ulcerative colitis and those with Crohn's disease (24% vs. 29%, respectively). The quality of life was believed to be satisfactory in more than one-half of the patients with ulcerative colitis, but only approximately one-third of the patients with Crohn's disease were content. Early age of onset of ulcerative colitis was demonstrated to be a poor prognostic factor for subsequent rectal preservation. Conversely, patients in whom the disease developed later in life were more likely to avoid a subsequent proctectomy. Interestingly enough, the presence of moderate rectal mucosal disease did not increase the likelihood of subsequent proctectomy.

Hawley evaluated the St. Mark's Hospital experience with 125 ulcerative colitis patients who underwent colectomy and ileorectal anastomosis.[260] Subsequent excision was required in 33 (26%). A reduction in frequency of bowel movements to 6 or fewer within 24 hours was noted in 83%. Oakley and colleagues reported our experience of 159 patients with this operation.[554,555] Subsequent proctectomy became necessary for 55%, and rectal cancer developed in 9. Leijonmarck and colleagues found that 16% of their 43 patients experienced complications, with a 4% operative mortality.[397] Forty-three percent had their ileorectal anastomosis functioning at follow-up (mean observation time, 13 years). The functional outcome was better than that quoted in the literature for the pouch-anal procedures (see later discussion). Löfberg and colleagues reviewed the 46 patients who underwent this operation in Stockholm County.[434] Twenty-two (49%) subsequently underwent proctectomy for intractable symptoms and 3 (7%) for dysplasia. All of the remaining patients had no evidence of dysplasia, carcinoma, or DNA aneuploidy. Others have also been relatively enthusiastic in recommending ileorectal anastomosis for selected patients with IBD, but the importance of cancer surveillance must be emphasized.[290,311,316,347,390]

With ileorectal anastomosis for ulcerative colitis, the possibility of carcinoma arising in the residual rectum is a source of great concern. If the patient truly understands this risk and is willing to submit to frequent follow-up examinations, I believe that ileorectal anastomosis should be considered for those in whom the rectum is not severely involved by inflammatory disease. However, if concern for possible development of carcinoma is sufficiently great, conventional proctocolectomy or a pouch-anal procedure should be offered.

Limited Resection

Other operations for ulcerative colitis that attempt to maintain intestinal continuity by a limited resection are poor alternatives. Segmental resection of the sigmoid colon, right colon, and so forth will result uniformly in a 100% recurrence rate that will necessitate further resection. The only exception to the admonition against this is the patient who has severe proctitis or proctosigmoiditis. In an individual incapacitated as a consequence of urgency, tenesmus, incontinence, or bleeding, an abdominoperineal resection might be considered. It is understood, however, that palliation of symptoms may not necessarily preclude the possibility of subsequent proximal disease recurrence.

Varma and colleagues reported four patients with symptomatic left-sided ulcerative colitis who were treated by resection, mucosal proctectomy, and coloanal anastomosis.[756]

Within 1 year, recurrence developed in all, and three of them required proctocolectomy.

Ileoanal Anastomosis

Total colectomy and proctectomy, but with preservation of the anal canal and sphincter muscles, was described by Ravitch and Sabiston in 1947.[606,607] The procedure fell into disrepute primarily because of the difficulties associated with frequent bowel movements and fecal incontinence. In 1977, Martin and colleagues described a procedure in children whereby the entire colon was removed in the usual manner, but the mucosa was stripped from its rectal muscular sleeve and an anastomosis effected between the ileum and the anal canal.[466] By this means, intestinal continuity was reestablished, and all the potential disease-bearing area was extirpated. This procedure is theoretically suitable for patients with ulcerative colitis and those with familial polyposis and is a popular option in the pediatric population. However, patients with Crohn's disease should not be considered for this alternative.

Operative Technique

Total colectomy is undertaken in the usual manner, and the bowel is resected in the most distal rectum. It was initially suggested that a mucosal stripping be performed and commenced at the level of the sacral promontory in order to preserve a long muscular sleeve (Figure 29-50). The dissection is facilitated, according to Utsunomiya and colleagues, by the use of a balloon catheter as a rectal internal stent (Figure 29-50C).[751] Theoretically, it was believed that by preserving this sleeve, the anastomosis would be protected. However, the development of complications such as "sleeve abscess," as well as the tedious dissection required, have convinced virtually all surgeons to abandon this particular approach. In current practice, one endeavors to amputate the rectum as low as is possible, removing any residual mucosa transanally. The procedure may be facilitated by infiltrating the submucosa with a dilute epinephrine solution. Because separation of the rectal mucosa may be difficult to accomplish in some patients, either because

---

MARK M. RAVITCH (1910–1989)

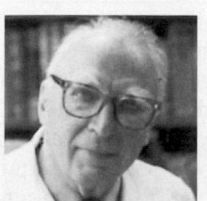

Mark Ravitch was born in New York City, of Russian immigrant parents. He attended the University of Oklahoma and achieved a BA degree in zoology in 1930. He spent 13 years at Johns Hopkins, first as a medical student and later as an intern and surgical resident. It was there that his extraordinary productivity in research and writing developed. He remained on the staff until 1952, at which time he assumed the position of director of surgery at the Mount Sinai Hospital in New York. He returned to Johns Hopkins, attaining the rank of professor of surgery and surgeon-in-chief at the Baltimore City Hospitals; then, in 1969, he assumed a professorship of surgery at the University of Pittsburgh. Ravitch's analysis of intussusception in infants and children led to the development of a nonoperative treatment for the disease—the use of hydrostatic pressure reduction through barium enema. In addition to the concept of ileoanal anastomosis, he suggested the technique of mucosal stripping to limit the likelihood of recurrent disease. Another of his outstanding contributions to colon and rectal surgery was the introduction and development of mechanical stapling devices in the United States. This came about as a result of his excursions to the Soviet Union; his fluency in the Russian language was in no small measure responsible for his success. Ravitch was the author or coauthor of more than 450 articles and editorials, as well as 100 chapters in texts. The list of his honors and contributions encompasses a curriculum vitae of 51 pages. He died of complications related to carcinoma of the colon and prostate. (Photograph courtesy of the Department of Surgery, Montefiore Hospital, Pittsburgh, PA.)

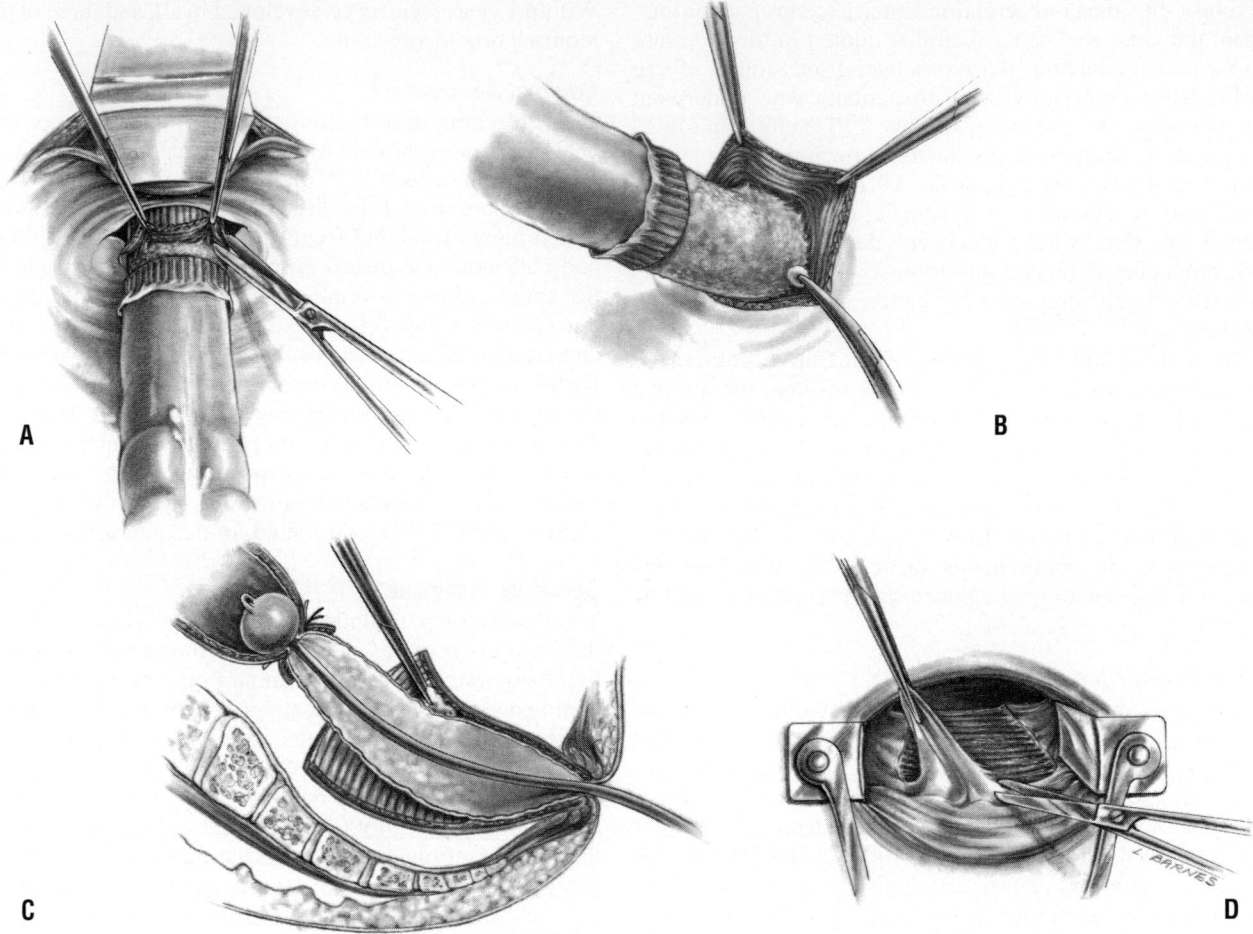

FIGURE 29-50. Classic rectal mucosal stripping. **A:** Beginning at the top of the rectum, **(B)** completed from above, and **(C)** facilitated by internal stent. **D:** By perineal route.

of friability or scarring, some surgeons advocate ultrasonic fragmentation and aspiration.[264,265] Others prefer to evert the anorectal remnant, exposing the mucosa and excising the stump from the dentate line to the cut edge of the rectum[215] (Figure 29-51). Other options for performing rectal mucosectomy are illustrated in Figures 29-52 and 29-53. Another preferred alternative is to employ one of the modifications of the double-stapling technique (see later discussion).

The ileal anastomosis is effected at the level of the dentate line using paired Gelpi retractors or an anal retractor (e.g., Parks, Lone Star) for exposure. Interrupted 3–0 long-term absorbable sutures are suggested to anchor the end of the ileum to the anal canal and underlying internal sphincter (Figure 29-54). A loop ileostomy is virtually always advised (see Figures 31-67 through 31-69).

Results

Very little current data are available for a straight ileoanal anastomosis because the modification that incorporates an intervening pouch has made this operation practically obsolete except in children (see later discussion).[104,569,729] Utsunomiya and colleagues reported a few patients who underwent the procedure, but in the same article, they describe a technique with an intervening pouch.[751] It is difficult to interpret the results because of the multiplicity of techniques used.

Beart and colleagues reported the Mayo Clinic experience with 50 patients who underwent total abdominal colectomy, excision of the rectal mucosa, and ileoanal anastomosis.[38] Forty-one were operated on for chronic ulcerative colitis; familial polyposis was the diagnosis in 7 patients, and Crohn's disease in 2. The authors emphasized the importance of meticulous hemostasis, preservation of the anoderm, careful stripping of all the rectal mucosa, and avoidance of tension on the suture line. A number of these patients had an intervening reservoir. Forty-two individuals had reestablishment of intestinal continuity by closure of the ileostomy, and no deaths occurred in the series. Two had anastomotic strictures requiring conversion to an ileostomy. Nine additional patients were dissatisfied because of intolerable stool frequency and were converted to either a continent ileostomy (Kock pouch—see later discussion) or a conventional ileostomy. In the remaining 30 individuals, stool frequency averaged 8 per day, and most required slowing medications.

Heppell and coworkers reviewed 12 of these patients at least 4 months after the procedure by means of physiologic studies.[271] Anal sphincter resting pressure and squeeze pressure of those who underwent this operation were similar to that of healthy controls, although the rectal inhibitory reflex was absent. The greater the capacity of the new rectum, the

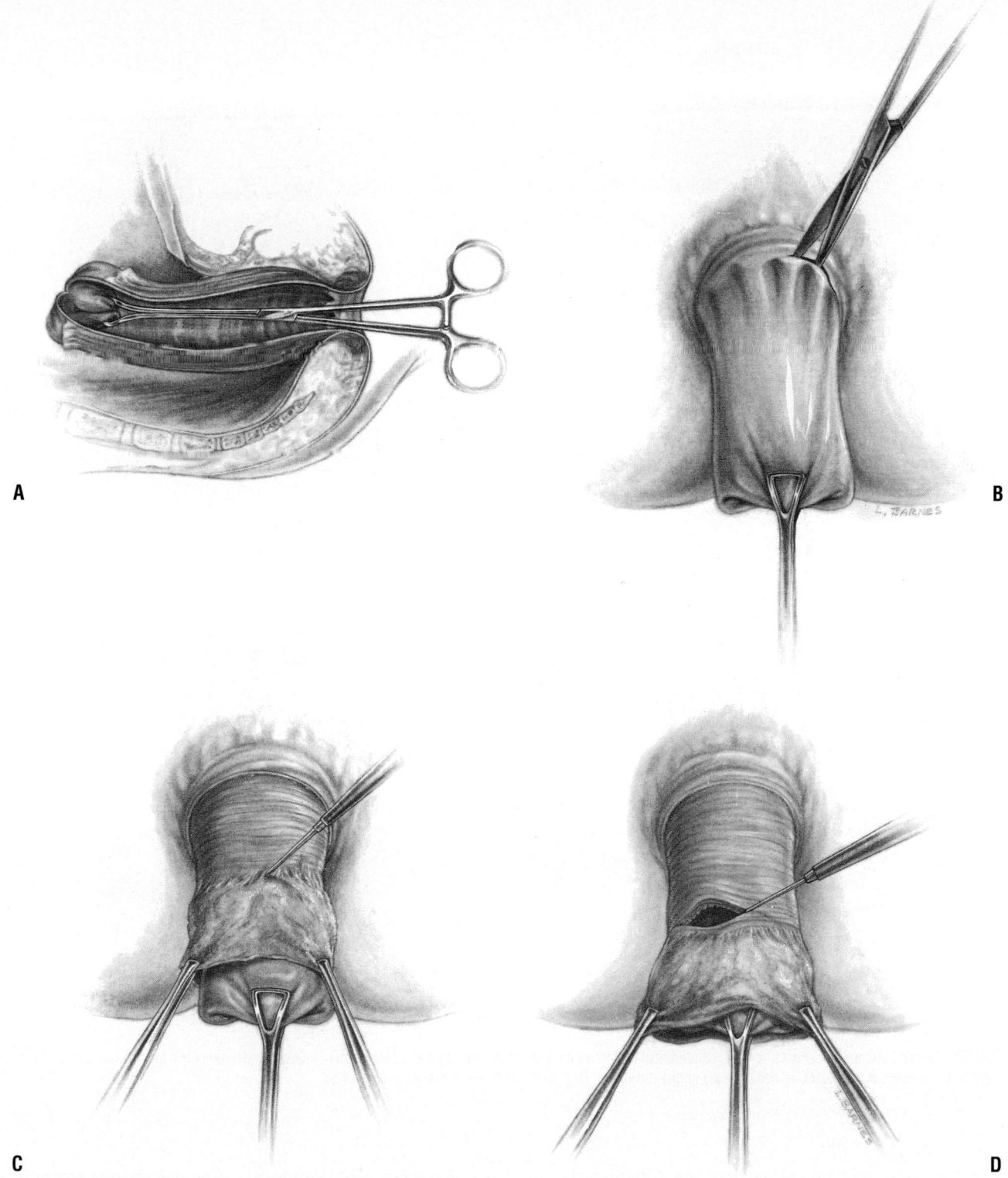

A

B

C

D

FIGURE 29-51. Technique of eversion mucosectomy. **A:** The rectal stump is everted by placing a clamp on the proximal end. **B:** Mucosal stripping is begun from the dentate line. **C:** Mucosa is stripped using diathermy cautery or by scissors dissection. **D:** The mucosa and redundant muscular sleeve are excised.

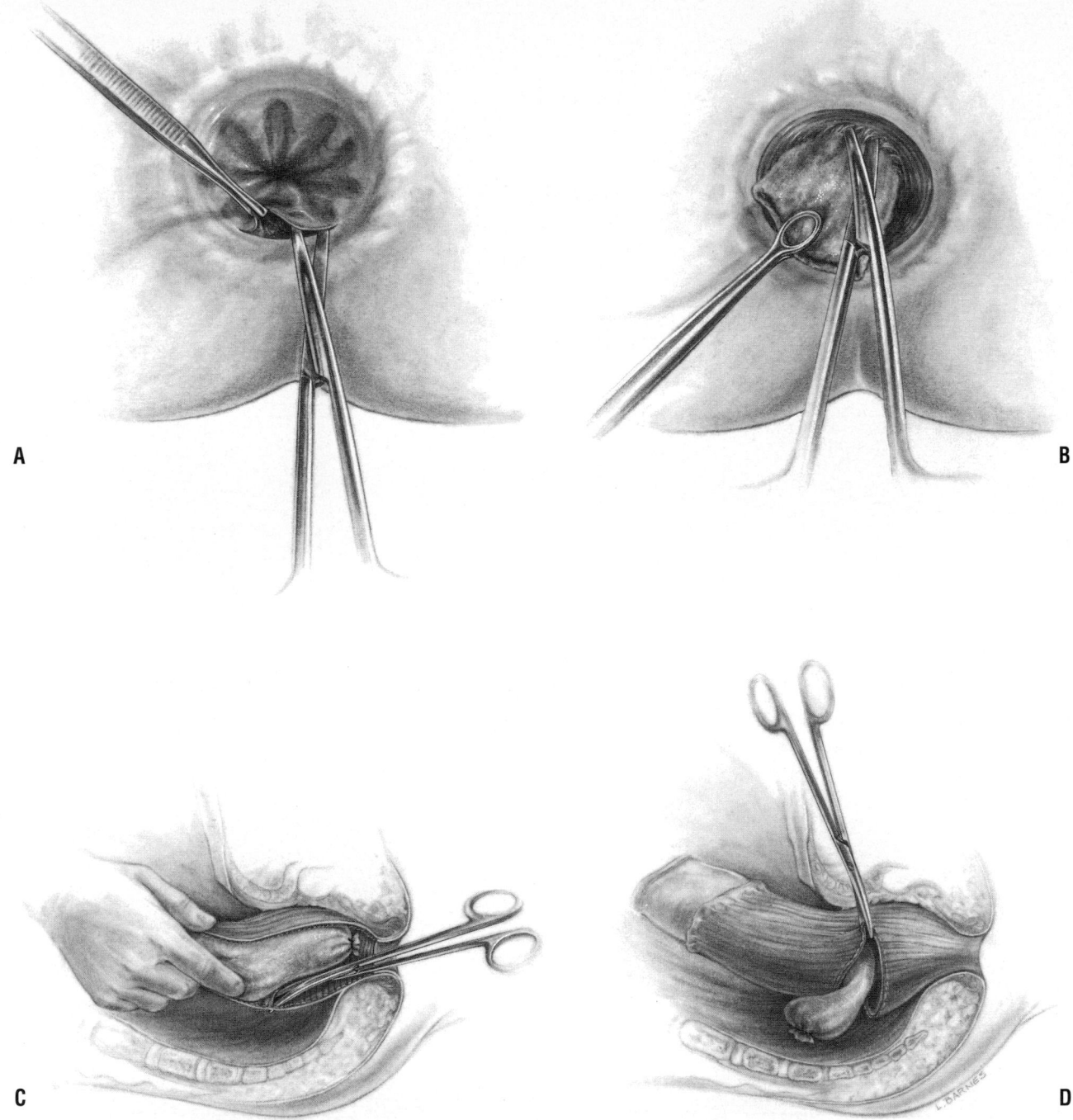

FIGURE 29-52. Rectal mucosectomy. **A:** Circumferential incision at the level of the dentate line. **B:** Elevation of mucosa and submucosa from the underlying internal sphincter. **C:** Division of the muscular sleeve by the perineal surgeon. **D:** Bowel and stripped mucosa are resected.

fewer the number of bowel movements. Although the operation did indeed preserve the anal sphincter, the decreased capacity and lack of compliance of the distal bowel impaired continence.

Coran reported the procedure in 36 children and adults with ulcerative colitis and familial polyposis.[103] Four patients were subsequently converted to an ileostomy. The median stool frequency was 7 per 24 hours. This was interpreted by the author to be an encouraging result. A later report of 100 patients (79 with ulcerative colitis) revealed comparable functional results (7.7 within 24 hours).[104] Interestingly, there

was no statistically significant difference in stool frequency when the ages of the patients were compared. Five required conversion to a conventional ileostomy. Morgan and colleagues evaluated 60 individuals with ulcerative colitis and multiple polyposis who had undergone endoanal anastomosis following total proctocolectomy.[511] Stool frequency after 3 years of follow-up was in excess of 8 per 24 hours. Data in children from the Mayo Clinic demonstrate that clinical results with respect to stool frequency and especially nighttime soiling are better with a J-pouch than with a straight ileoanal anastomosis.[569,729]

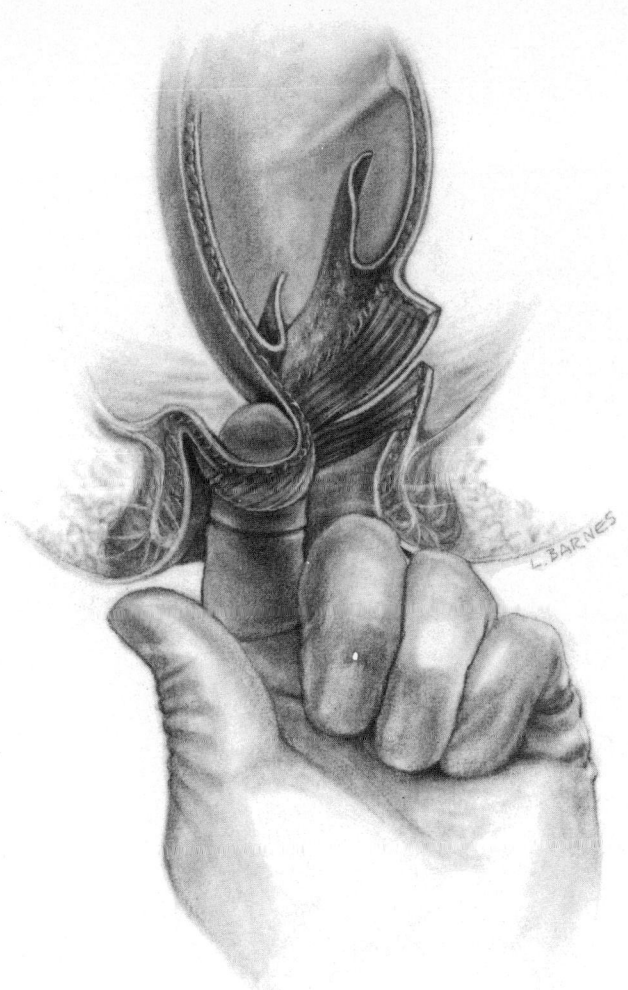

FIGURE 29-53. Rectal mucosectomy. Lateral rectal attachments are divided by the perineal surgeon.

Nelson and associates describe converting the straight ileoanal procedure to a reservoir by means of a long, side-to-side ileal anastomosis, somewhat like that described by Fonkalsrud (see later).[533] The distal ileum is folded over itself so that the point of division reaches down into the pelvis. The authors reported a favorable experience with three patients.

Continent Ileostomy or Kock Pouch Procedure

It is self-evident that many patients are dissatisfied with the encumbrance and emotional burden of wearing an ileostomy appliance. In 1969, Kock described a method of creating a reservoir from the terminal ileum and subsequently modified it to create an intestinal obstruction by means of an intussuscepted portion of distal ileum, the so-called nipple valve.[359–361] Because no appliance is required, the stoma can be placed quite low on the abdominal wall and essentially flush with the skin. The procedure had been enthusiastically received, but in recent years, it has been applied primarily in those for whom pouch-anal operations have failed or are inappropriate, or for the rare individual who had previously undergone proctocolectomy and conventional ileostomy and wishes to have the stoma revised.

Technique

Traditional. There are two basic techniques that may be employed for constructing the reservoir. One is analogous to the S-shaped reservoir, such as is described for the Parks procedure (see later). This method uses approximately 10 cm of ileum for each segment (three in all to create the pouch). An additional 18 to 20 cm is required to create the nipple valve and the conduit.

The Kock technique involves preparation of approximately a 50-cm segment of terminal ileum. A 30-cm segment is used to create the pouch and the remainder to make the valve and the external conduit. Figures 29-55 through 29-63 illustrate the procedure for preparing the continent (reservoir) ileostomy. An alternative to the conventional suturing method is to staple the pouch. This approach is illustrated in Figures 29-64 through 29-66. Before the ileostomy is "matured," the competence of the nipple valve should be tested by occluding the afferent limb with a rubber-shod clamp. A catheter is then inserted through the nipple valve into the reservoir, and the pouch is inflated with air. If the air fails to escape following catheter removal, one may assume that the valve is competent. The catheter is then replaced into the reservoir, and the air should dissipate. The completed reservoir is shown in Figure 29-67.

Modifications. The major problem with the Kock procedure is to maintain the position of the nipple. Slippage is attributed to traction forces on the mesentery of the nipple during filling of the reservoir.[143] Modifications have been proposed to ad-

(text continues on page 1238)

NILS G. KOCK (1924–PRESENT)

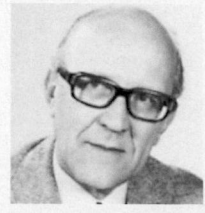

Nils Kock was born in Jacobstad, Finland. Following military service with the Finnish army during World War II, he entered the University of Helsinki Medical School, graduating in 1951. He began his surgical residency in Finland and then spent 5 years in surgical training at the University of Göteborg in Sweden, the institution with which he remained affiliated for his entire professional career. In 1959, he earned a PhD from the University of Göteborg and assumed the position of assistant professor of surgery. A series of promotions followed that culminated in his appointment in 1974 as a professor of surgery at Göteborg and chairman of the department of surgery of Sahlgren Hospital. In 1969, Kock published an article based on extensive laboratory and clinical work: a method for achieving fecal "continence" by means of an intra-abdominal reservoir. For this he attained what many surgeons consider the pinnacle of success—an operation is eponymously associated with his name. In retirement, he maintained a busy animal laboratory, developing techniques for dealing with a host of problems—including that of bowel and urinary conduits.

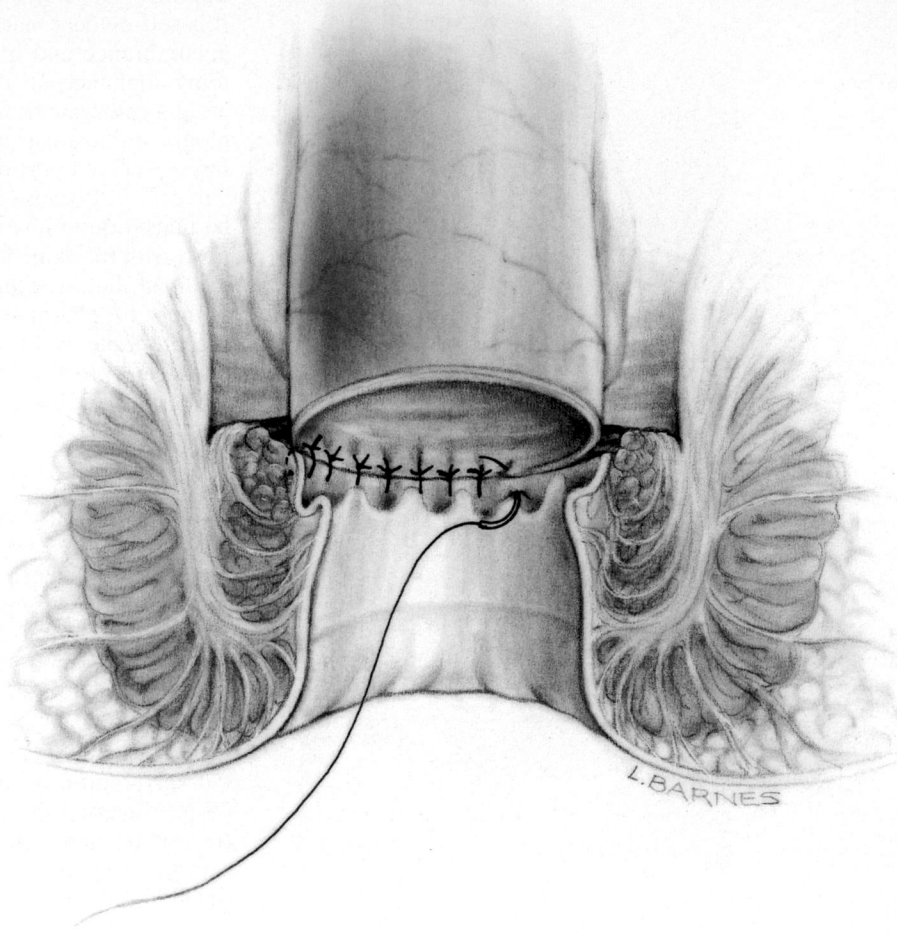

FIGURE 29-54. Endoanal, hand-sewn anastomotic technique. Paired Gelpi, Lone Star, or Parks retractors facilitate the exposure.

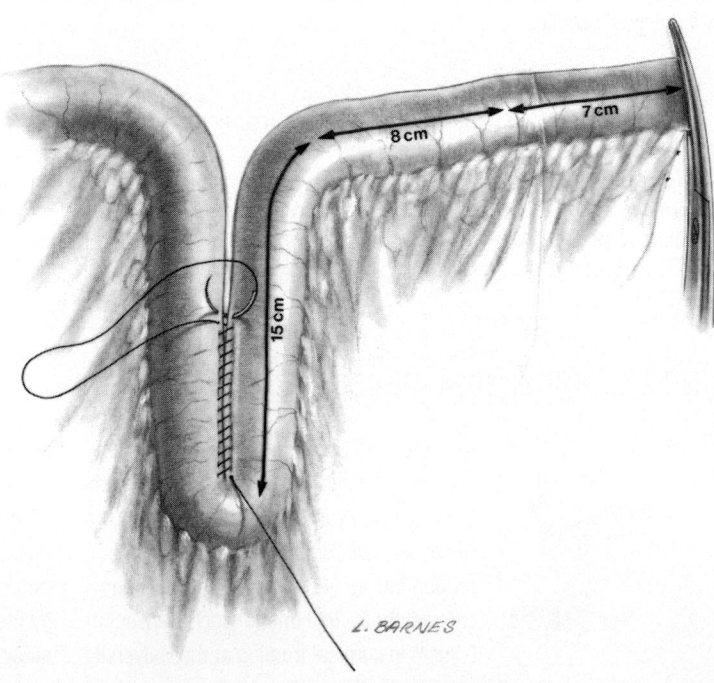

FIGURE 29-55. Continent ileostomy. Apposition of the bowel.

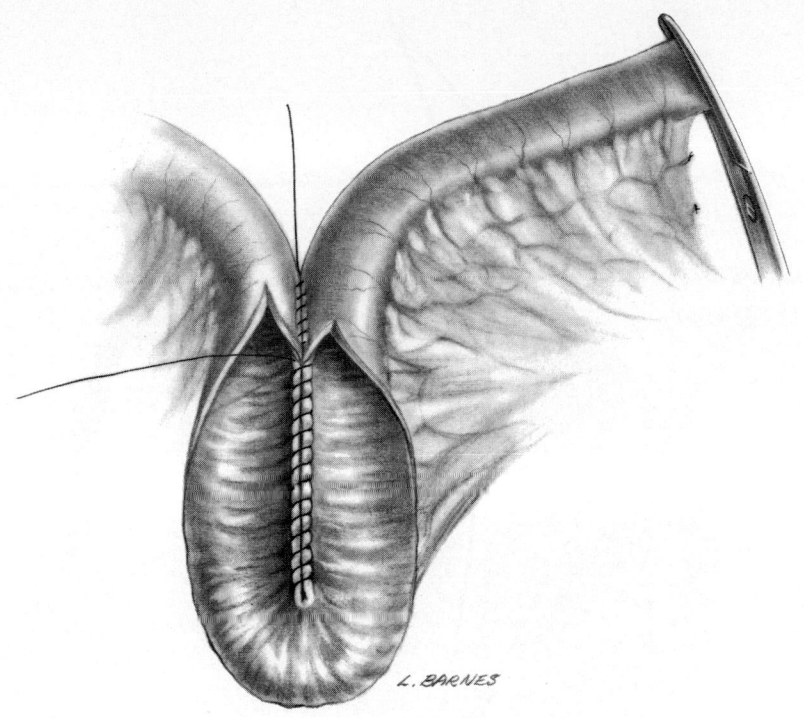

FIGURE 29-56. Continent ileostomy. Bowel opened and posterior row completed.

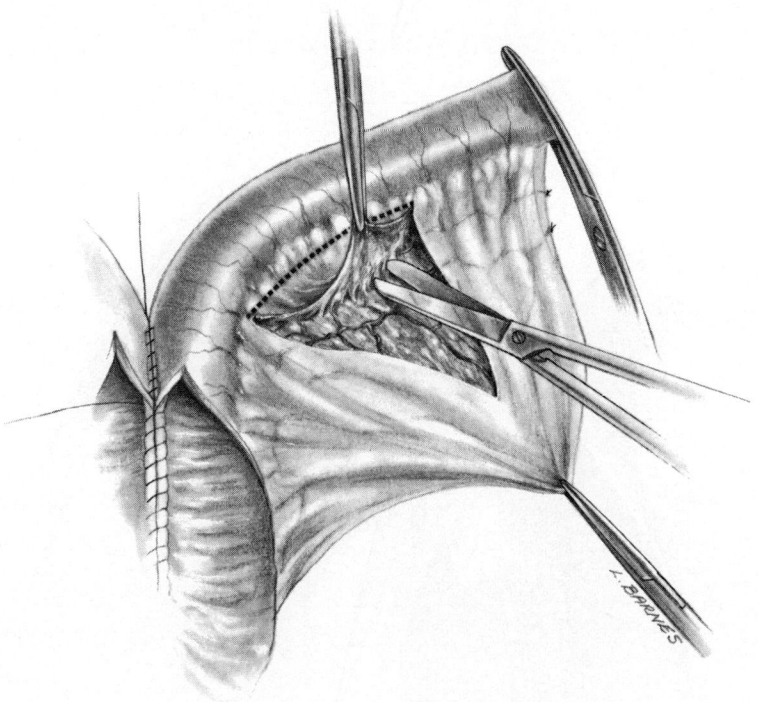

FIGURE 29-57. Continent ileostomy. Excision of peritoneal leaves and defatting of mesentery.

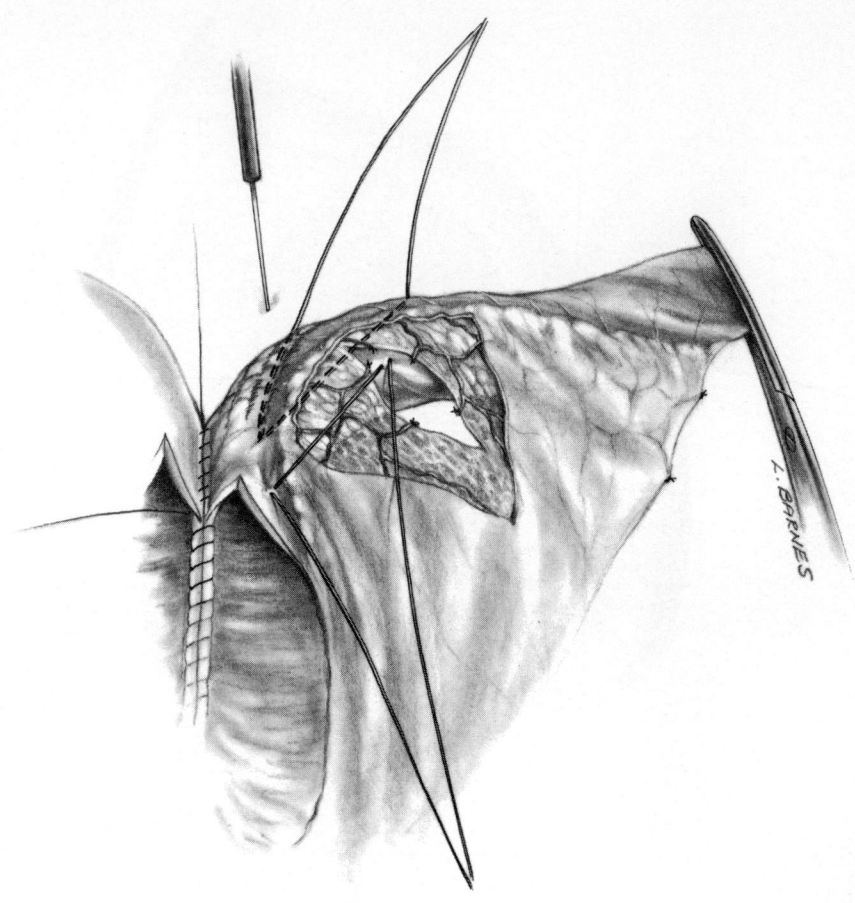

FIGURE 29-58. Continent ileostomy. Cauterization or stripping of the ileal serosa and placement of sutures to rotate the mesentery 90 degrees.

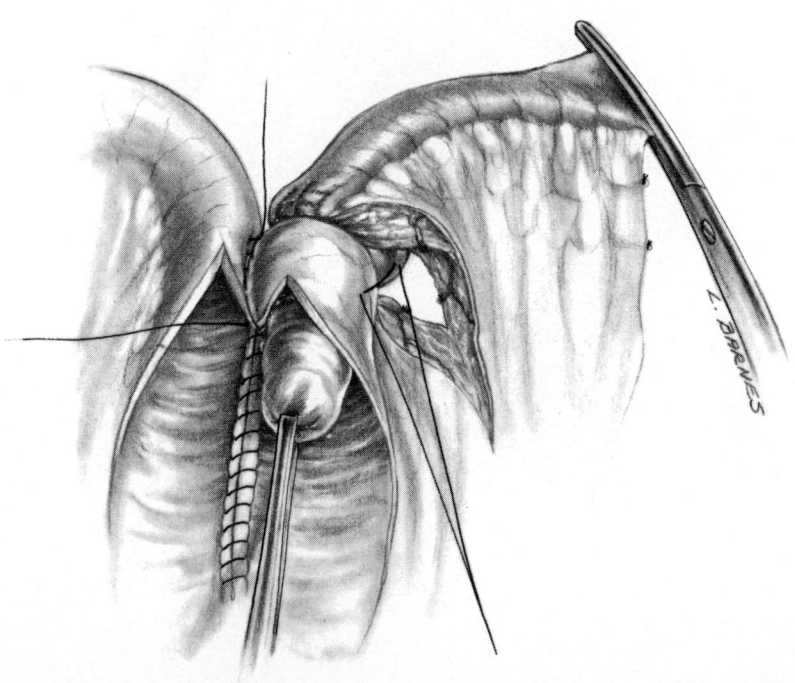

FIGURE 29-59. Continent ileostomy. A nipple is created and sutures are secured.

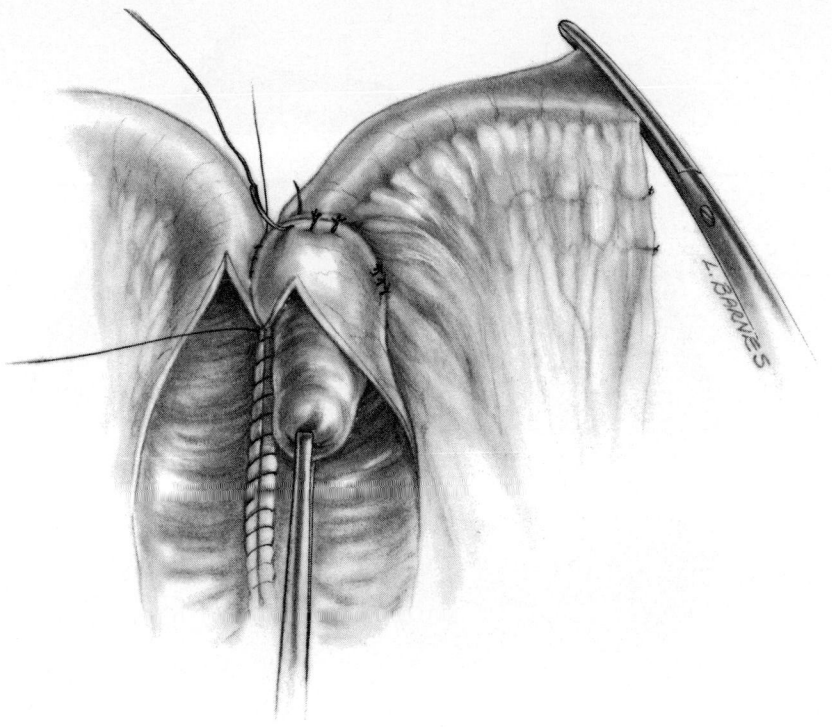

FIGURE 29-60. Continent ileostomy. Silk sutures are placed from conduit to reservoir.

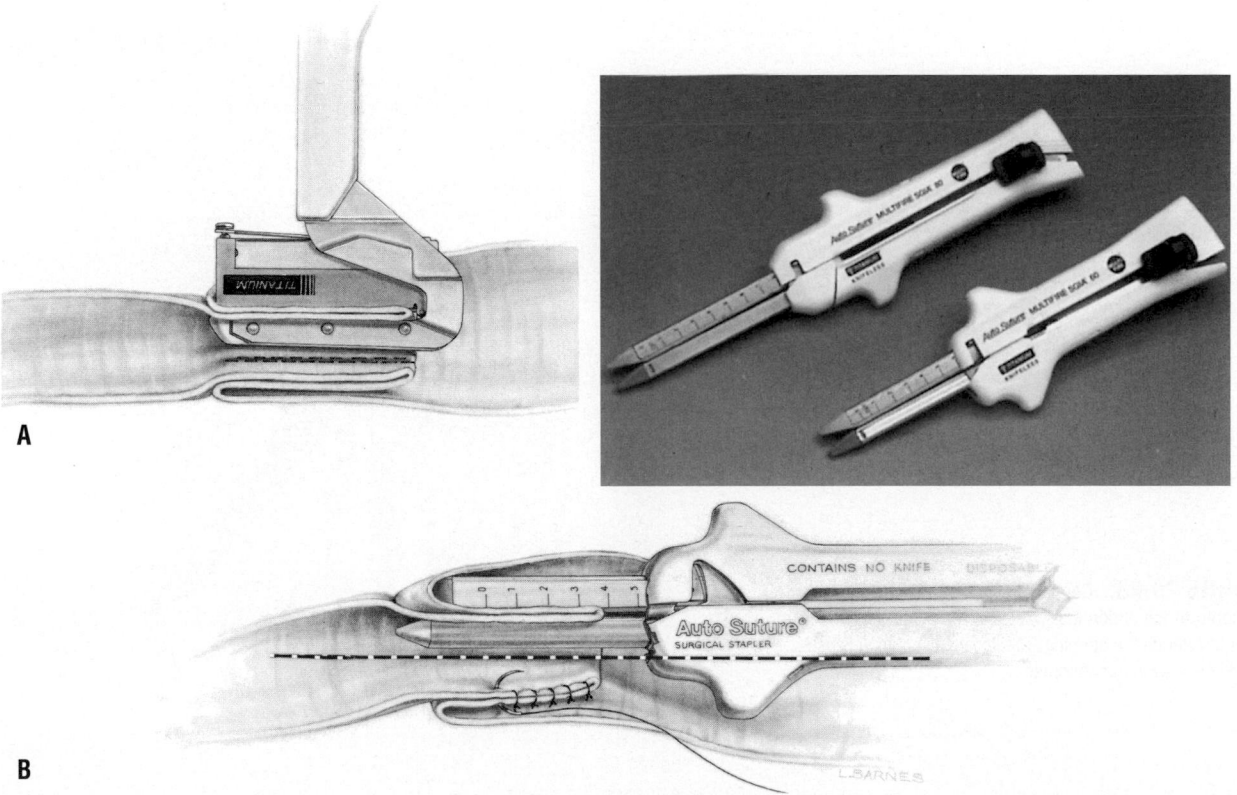

A

B

FIGURE 29-61. Continent ileostomy. **A:** Application of the linear stapler to three areas in the nipple valve to prevent desussception. **B:** Alternatively, one may use an SGIA-60 stapler (without the blade) or simple sutures. The instruments without the knife are available in two sizes (*inset*). (Courtesy of United States Surgical Corp., Norwalk, CT.)

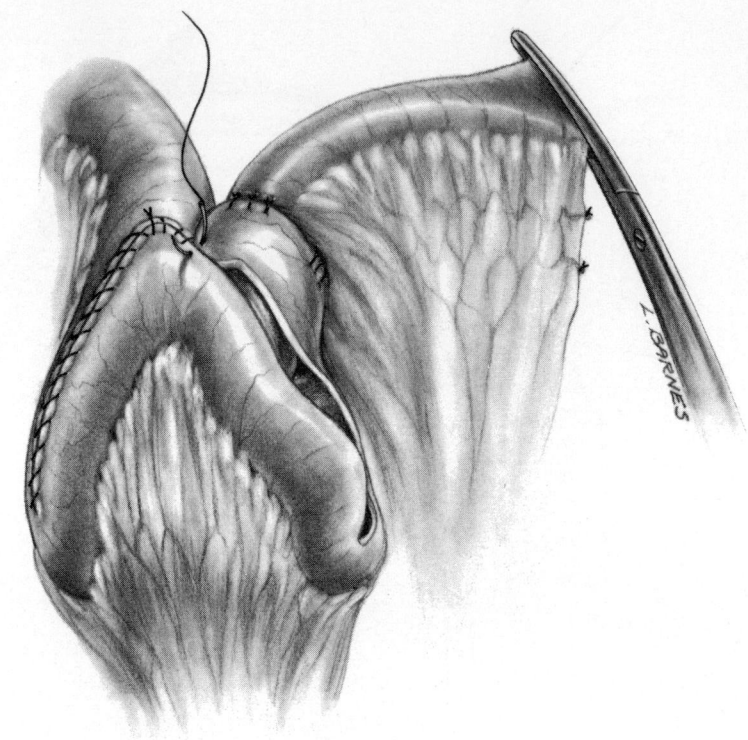

FIGURE 29-62. Continent ileostomy. The reservoir is closed by folding over.

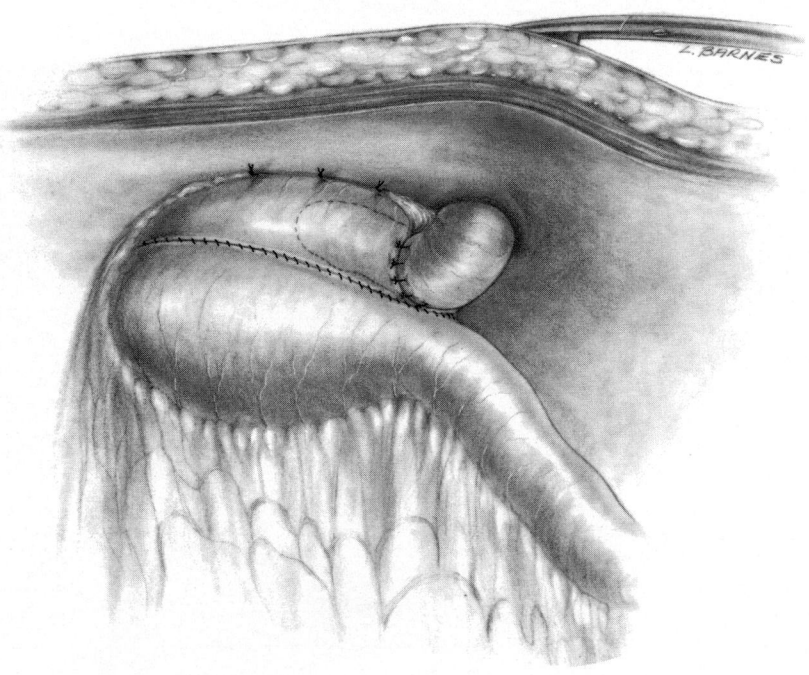

FIGURE 29-63. Continent ileostomy. The reservoir is anchored to the abdominal wall after the conduit has been brought through the opening. The ileostomy opening is usually placed low in the abdomen.

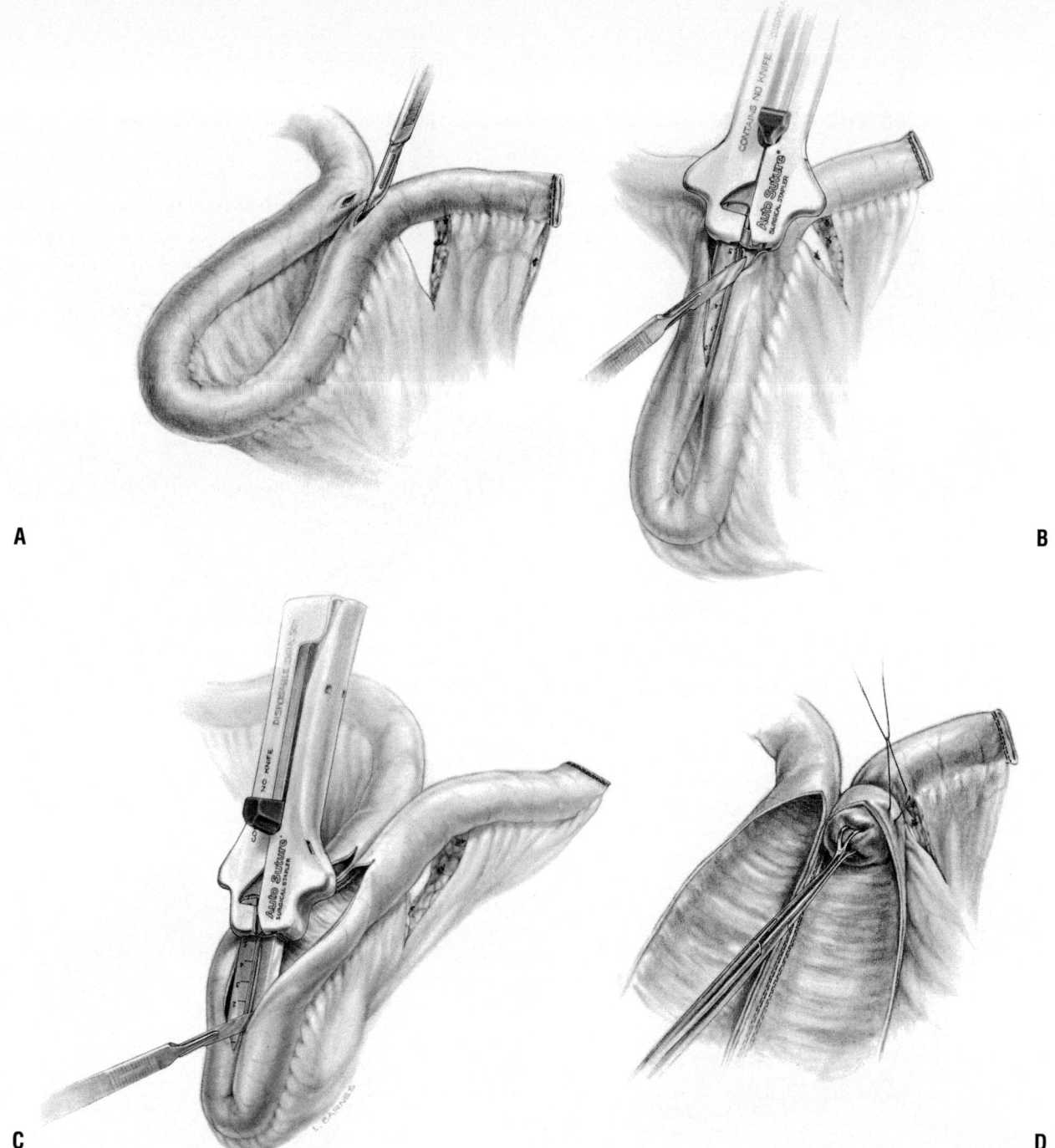

A

B

C

D

FIGURE 29-64. Stapled continent ileostomy (Kock). **A:** Two enterotomies are created. **B:** Insertion of SGIA stapler (without the knife blade). Bowel is incised on the instrument. **C:** Second passage of SGIA stapler with incision of the bowel (third insertion may be required). **D:** Distal ileum is intussuscepted.

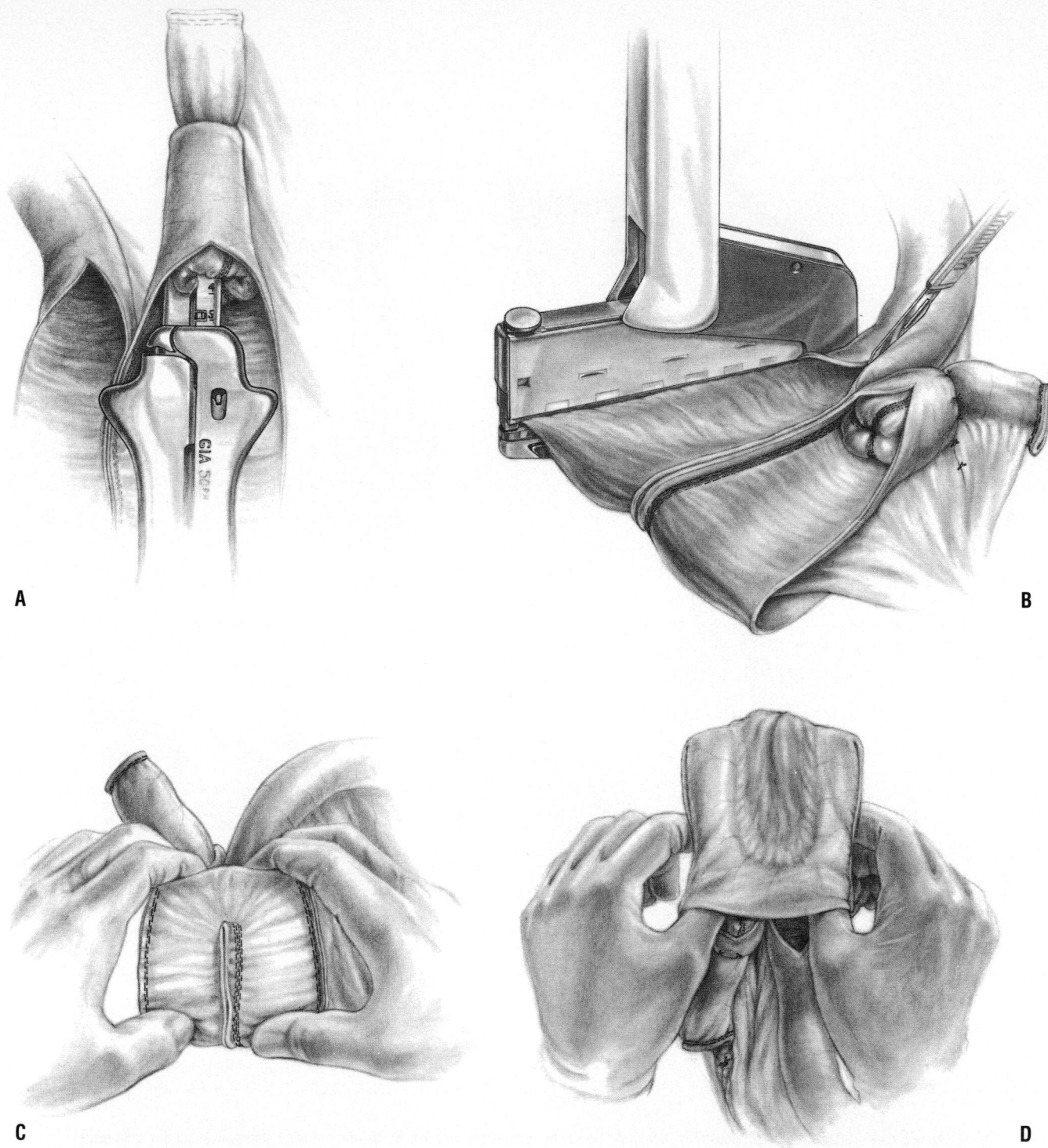

A

B

C

D

FIGURE 29-65. Stapled continent ileostomy (Kock). **A:** Nipple valve stapled. **B:** Long linear stapler (TA-90) secures opposing walls of the bowel. Staple lines are within the pouch. **C,D:** Pouch is reinverted.

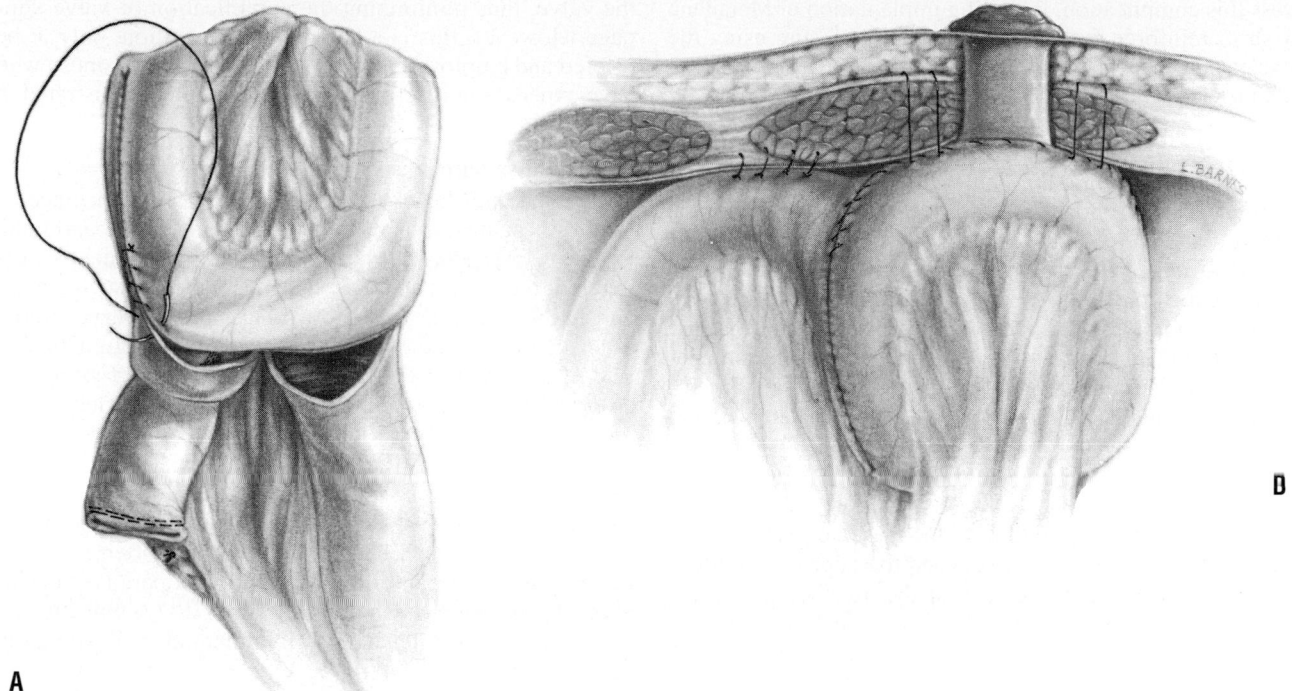

A

B

FIGURE 29-66. Stapled continent ileostomy (Kock). **A:** Manual suture closure of defect. **B:** Completed pouch.

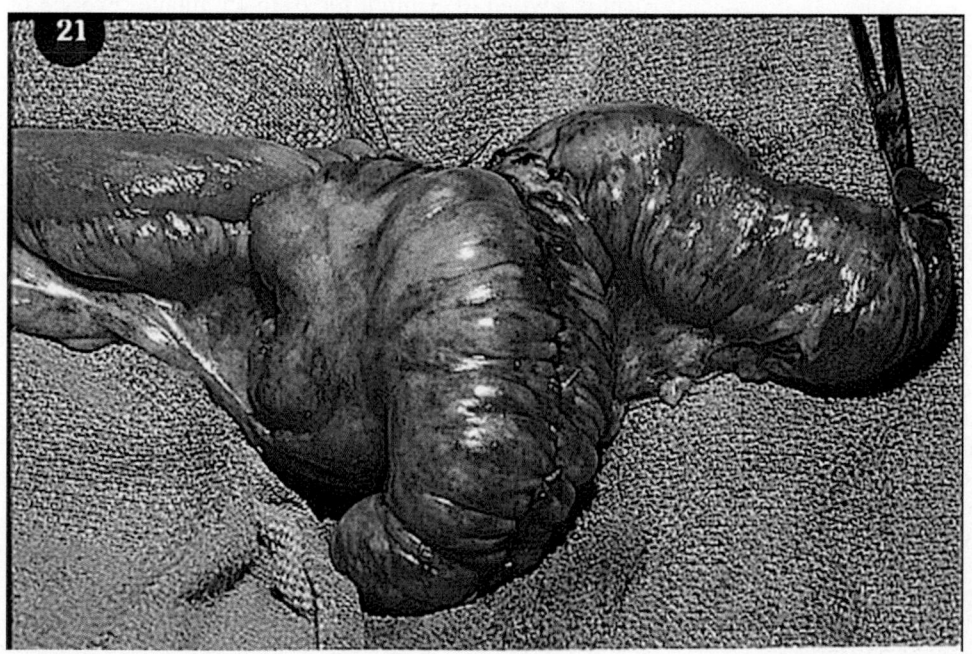

FIGURE 29-67. Continent ileostomy. Completed reservoir and nipple.

dress this complication, including implantation of Mersilene mesh to reinforce the nipple,[36] magnetic closure using the Maclet device,[651] stripping of the serosa, and even creation of a protecting loop ileostomy above the reservoir.[292] Bokey and I have suggested the use of a fascial sling threaded through the mesentery.[62] Gerber and colleagues and others recommend encircling the ileal outlet with a 1-cm strip of Marlex mesh or Teflon (passed through the mesentery of the reservoir and outlet), although this can cause other problems (e.g., a fistula).[199,718,730] However, this technique as well as the use of Marlex or Teflon mesh have largely been abandoned due to erosion into the pouch or valve itself, thus requiring a complex salvage operation.[159] A combination of triangular stripping of the mesenteric fat, serosal scarification, and rotation of the nipple valve segments has been demonstrably safe and quite effective for preventing nipple desusception according to some surgeons.[295] Harford suggests the use of the Cavitational Ultrasonic Surgical Aspirator (CUSA; Valleylab Inc., Boulder, CO) to strip the mesentery and remove the fat.[248] Ecker and coworkers used the approach of ultrasonic mucosectomy in the area of the attached mesentery of the nipple and posterior wall of the pouch.[143] Additionally, two continuous sutures of nylon are employed through all the layers of the bowel on both sides of the main mesenteric vessels. We also have described another technique that our group now prefers.[159] This involves anchoring the nipple valve to the anterior pouch wall by stapling. A 2-cm transverse enterotomy is made in the anterior pouch wall just below the point where the intussuscepted nipple lies. The valve is then aligned with the anterior pouch wall away from the primary anterior suture line, and a single application of the linear stapler is used to anchor the nipple valve to the anterior pouch wall. The anvil of the stapler is brought through the transverse enterotomy from outside the pouch to pass along the inside of the nipple valve, thereby effecting a stapled anchorage.[159] The anterior pouch wall and the enterotomy are then closed.

The current preferred technique for reducing valve prolapse is that of re-stapling if the antimesenteric aspect of the valve (without knife) to the pouch itself, at the line of the anterior suture of the pouch.[159]

Barnett. Barnett undertook a modification for preventing desusception that uses an adjacent segment of intestine to encircle the base of the valve as a "collar," a maneuver analogous to that of a Nissen gastric fundoplication.[32] The lumen of the intestinal collar communicates with the pouch itself, allowing gas and fecal contents to enter. This acts to buttress the nipple valve and conduit, providing a greater degree of security against leakage. The technique is briefly described in Figure 29-68. This unique operation has, however, fallen into disrepute because of the high complication rate.

T-Pouch. Because of the high revision rate for valve failure and the oft requirement for frequent operations, even when applied to urologic conduits, another type of pouch was developed in 1998 by Stein and associates as a neobladder (University of Southern California), the T-pouch.[702] It does not rely on an intussuscepted valve, which means it cannot come apart. Kaiser and colleagues, in their preliminary report involving six patients, described their technique with this design as a continent ileostomy.[321]

The main value of the T-pouch is that when performed meticulously, there is no conventional intussusception of

the valve, thus minimizing the complication of valve slippage. However, this is a complicated operation, only to be offered and employed in highly selected cases by those who have expertise in its creation. The procedure is illustrated in Figure 29-69.

Postoperative Care

Before leaving the operating room, the surgeon places a heavy silk suture around a Silastic catheter (Weber and Judd, Rochester, MN) that has been inserted into the pouch. This is secured to the skin, and a dressing is applied in such a manner that the catheter exits upward and gently curves into a drainage tube, and then into a drainable bag (Figure 29-70). The straight exit of the catheter minimizes the risk for necrosis of the conduit should the catheter be under tension on one side. The dressing is left in place for 72 hours before the stoma is examined. An alternative is to use a Marlen continent ileostomy drainage system (Figure 29-71). The catheter can also be held in place by passing it through one of the perforations in a latex band, the type that is often used as a leg strap for a urine or bile bag.[237] The postoperative appearance of the patient is shown in Figure 29-72. Our method of dressing at the Cleveland Clinic method is illustrated in Figure 32-3.

Usually, there will be only serosanguineous drainage for the first several days, but eventually this becomes bile-stained and then feculent. The patient is then started on a progressive schedule of oral intake, although a low-residue diet is suggested to avoid plugging of the catheter. The drainage tube remains in place for 3 weeks, after which the patient is advised to clamp it for 10 to 15 minutes every 3 or 4 hours. During the night, it is left to drain continuously. After 1 month, intermittent catheterization is advised, initially every 3 or 4 hours, and usually once during the night. After approximately 1 week of this regimen, nightly intubations are omitted and the interval for catheterization during the day is extended. Ultimately, the patient develops a time frequency based on convenience and the feeling of fullness that compels one to drain the reservoir. However, because radiologic studies reveal that reflux into the afferent limb increases with sensations of fullness and abdominal pressure, the patient should probably empty the reservoir at regular intervals.[52]

Some continent ileostomy catheters are shown in Figure 29-73. Occasionally, formed fecal material and high-residue items (e.g., popcorn, mushrooms) require irrigation by means of a syringe, but this is usually unnecessary. A simple dressing is placed over the flush stoma, or one of the commercially available security pouches may be used.

Complications

Anastomotic Leak. The greatest concern in the postoperative period is the possibility of leakage from one of the reservoir suture lines. Obviously, this can be of catastrophic consequence, requiring emergency surgical intervention. Initially, this complication was reported very commonly. The reduced incidence can be attributed to the improved techniques of reservoir construction and the careful selection of patients who undergo this procedure.

If surgical intervention becomes necessary in the immediate postoperative period for presumed suture line leakage, every attempt should be made to preserve the ileal reservoir. This can usually be accomplished by a diverting proximal loop ileostomy and appropriate surgical drainage with or

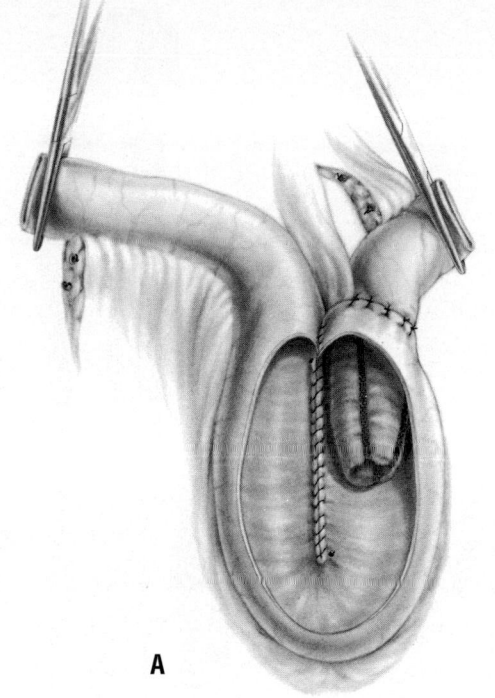

A

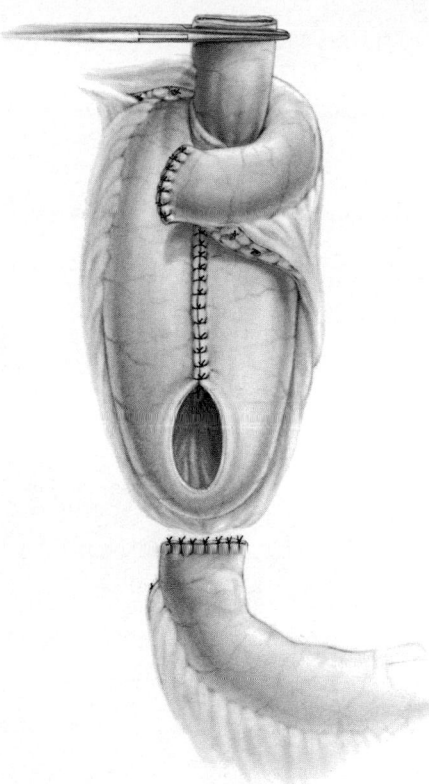

B

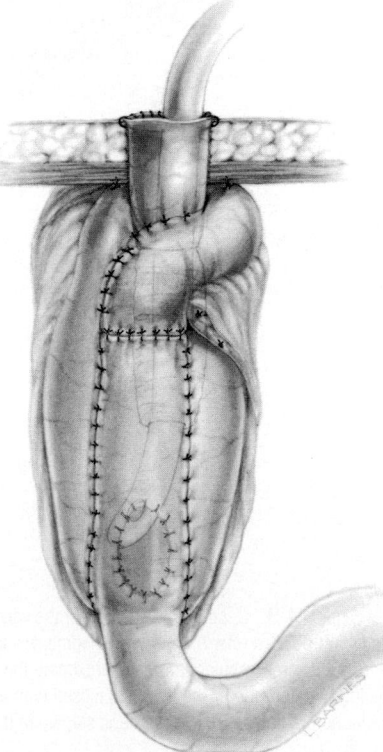

C

FIGURE 29-68. Barnett continent reservoir ileostomy. **A:** The "valve" and reservoir are created in the usual way, but the proximal ileum is divided approximately 8 cm from the pouch. Note defect in the mesentery. **B:** The intestinal segment is passed through the defect and around the exit conduit. It is then sutured back into the reservoir or alternatively anastomosed to it by using the circular stapler. The lumen of the intestinal "collar" communicates with the pouch to create an effect analogous to that of the "Nissen" fundoplication of the stomach. **C:** The proximal small bowel is then anastomosed to the reservoir. Theoretically, as the pouch fills, the "collar" tenses with intestinal contents, and a greater degree of continence is achieved.

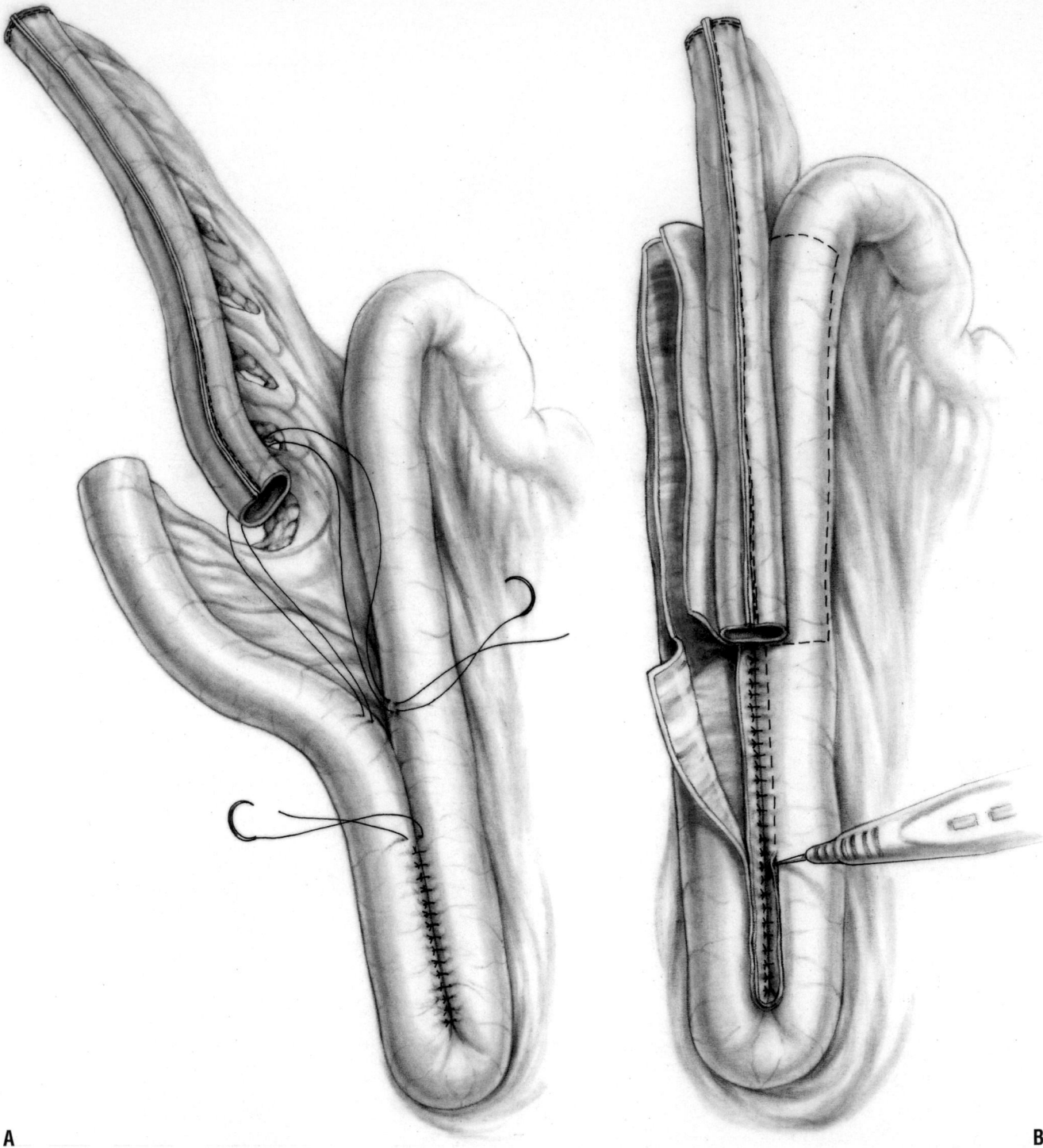

A **B**

FIGURE 29-69. T-pouch. **A:** Creation of the valve's back wall. The vascular arcades of the valve segment are preserved, but in between, the avascular mesenteric windows are opened (*inset*). The whole segment is tapered on its antimesenteric side by means of a multifire gastrointestinal anastomosis (GIA) instrument. A series of interrupted seromuscular sutures approximate the serosa of the two adjacent segments of the U by passing through the previously opened avascular windows. The remaining base portion of the ileal U is closed with a running suture. **B:** Preparation of the valve segment. The two limbs of the bowel U are opened along the seromuscular suture line on their mesenteric side up to the inner valve ostium, and then extending laterally to the antimesenteric border to provide wide flaps. *(continued)*

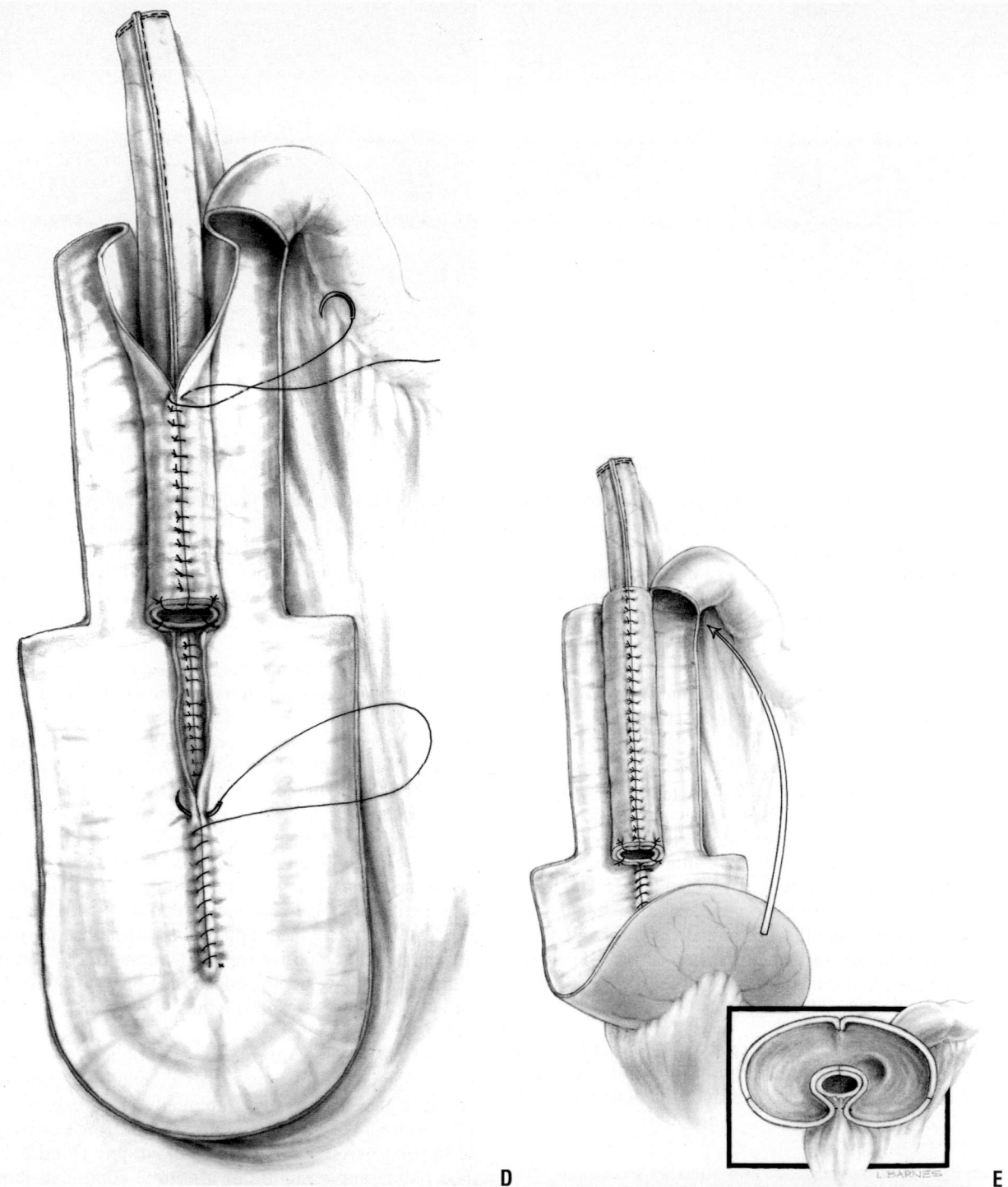

C   D   E

FIGURE 29-69. *(continued)* **C:** Completion of the antireflux valve. The two flaps are brought over the interposed ileal segment to create the antireflux mechanism. The inner valve ostium is matured with interrupted sutures, and running sutures are used to accomplish a mucosal continuity between the two bowel areas. **D:** Formation of the pouch reservoir. The ileal U is folded in half and its apex is approximated to the base of the pouch where the valve originates. The pouch construction is completed by closing both sides with running sutures. **E:** Cross section through completed T-pouch demonstrates the antireflux mechanism, with the isolated valve segment and maintained blood supply lying within a serosa-lined tunnel of the pouch reservoir that results in a flap-valve mechanism. (After Kaiser AM, Stein JP, Beart RW Jr. T-Pouch: a new valve design for a continent ileostomy. *Dis Colon Rectum.* 2002;45:411.)

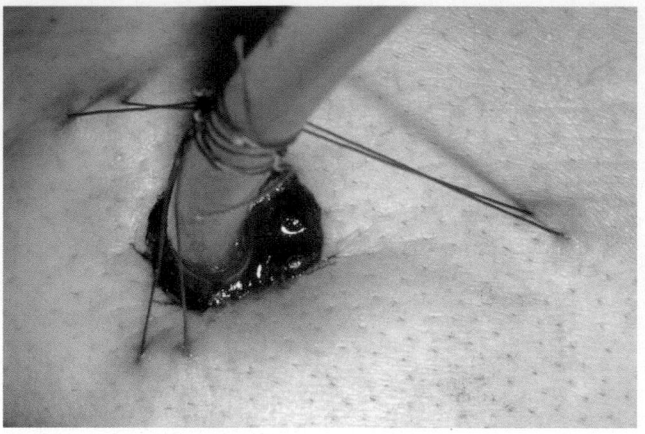

FIGURE 29-70. Continent ileostomy reservoir catheter sutured into position.

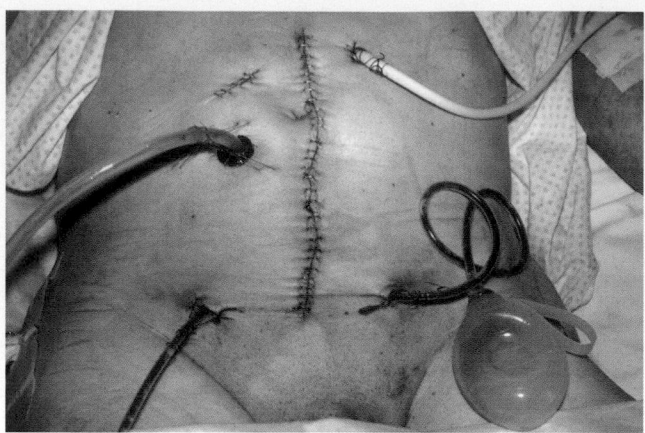

FIGURE 29-72. Immediate postoperative appearance of stoma with abdominal drains.

without closure of the leak. Subsequent radiologic investigation may reveal that the fistula spontaneously closed even without repair. If incontinence of the pouch is due to a valve fistula, in essence bypassing the continence mechanism, then direct repair can be performed by separation of the valve down to the fistula from the pouch wall or from the defect, itself. Then a four-layer fistula repair can be accomplished.

However, if it appears that the reservoir is beyond salvation, it must be resected and a neoileostomy created. If the patient has undergone a procedure for what subsequently proves to be Crohn's disease, a suture line leak has an ominous prognosis indeed. Under such circumstances, it is probably the wiser course to remove the pouch and to create a new ileostomy.

Late complications of the continent ileostomy procedure are numerous and include fecal incontinence resulting from reduction of the nipple valve, ileitis ("pouchitis"), recurrent Crohn's disease, catheter perforation, pouch fistula, detachment of the pouch from the abdominal wall, volvulus of the reservoir, urolithiasis, obstruction from inspissated material, stomal stenosis, and intestinal obstruction from a lost catheter (Figures 29-74 and 29-75).

Nipple Valve Complications—Slippage and Incontinence, Outlet Obstruction, Fistula. The complication associated with reduction of the nipple valve and resultant incontinence is the

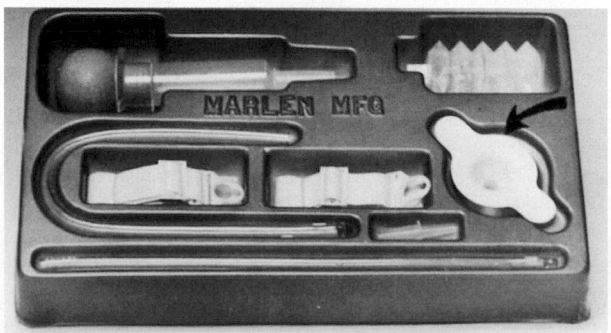

FIGURE 29-71. The continent ostomy set includes catheters, lubricant, belts, irrigating syringe, and a device for immediate postoperative support of the catheter (*arrow*). (Courtesy of Marlen Manufacturing and Development Co., Bedford, OH.)

most troublesome and most frequently observed late management problem (Figure 29-76). Difficulty with intubation of the reservoir is suggestive of desusception. The kinking of the intra-abdominal portion of the distal ileum may in itself create a partial small bowel obstruction. Usually, however, under these circumstances, the patient is incontinent but not obstructed.

Physiologic studies of the nipple valve and pouch reveal that electric and motor patterns of the undistended ileum are similar with both types of ileostomy, but the anatomic and motor properties of the pouch allow it to accept far larger intraluminal volumes both during fasting and after feeding.[4] Pressure studies on the pouch, nipple valve, and outlet demonstrate the presence of a high-pressure zone in the nipple valve relative to the pouch.[545] Distension of the pouch with air causes a tonic contraction that travels from the pouch along the intestinal layers of the intussuscepted nipple valve and the outlet.[545] It is postulated that this is the mechanism for desusception of the nipple valve, a complication that may possibly be avoided by frequent intubation of the pouch. Other studies have demonstrated the functions of the mucosa and smooth muscle of the continent ileal pouch to be similar to that of normal ileum.[187]

The diagnosis of nipple valve slippage can usually be made clinically. However, it is valuable to confirm the position of the nipple radiographically. This can be accomplished by a barium study through the stoma or by means of upper gastrointestinal roentgenography (Figure 29-77). The radiographic feature of a normal continent ileostomy on a plain abdominal film is the presence of a lobulated, gas-filled structure in the middle or right lower abdomen. With contrast material, the terminal, invaginated ileal segment resembles an inverted nipple protruding into the pouch.[507,672] Retrograde barium examination can reveal the size of the reservoir, the effluent can be measured, and the adequacy of the emptying confirmed. Other complications of continent ileostomy may also be confirmed radiographically (e.g., small bowel obstruction, anastomotic leakage, intra-abdominal abscess, fistula formation, failure of the reservoir to dilate, and the presence of recurrent Crohn's disease).[507,731]

Obstruction at the level of the reservoir is usually caused by reduction of the nipple valve and kinking of the conduit.

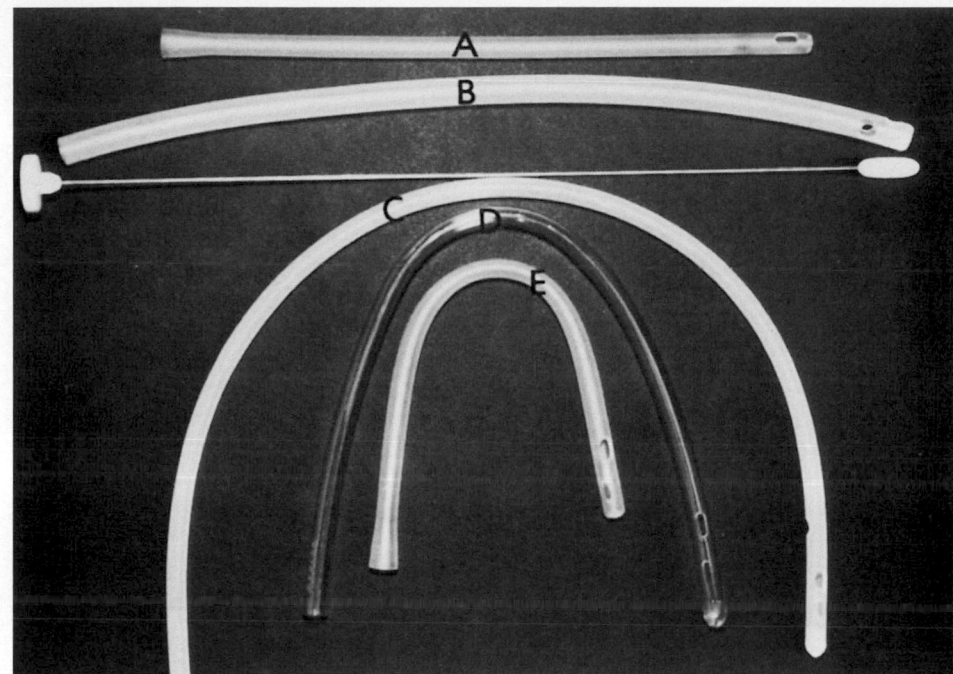

FIGURE 29-73. Continent ileostomy catheters. **A:** Medena, straight (Göteborg, Sweden). **B:** Heyer-Schulte, with introducer (Goleta, CA). **C:** Waters (Rochester, MN). **D:** Marlen (Bedford, OH). **E:** Medena, curved.

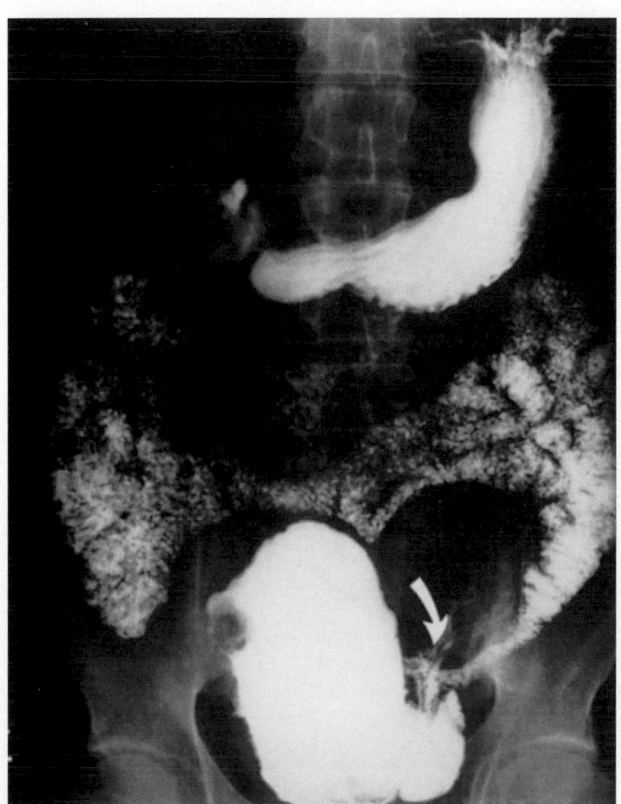

FIGURE 29-74. Continent ileostomy with leakage from pouch (*arrow*). Nipple valve can be clearly seen.

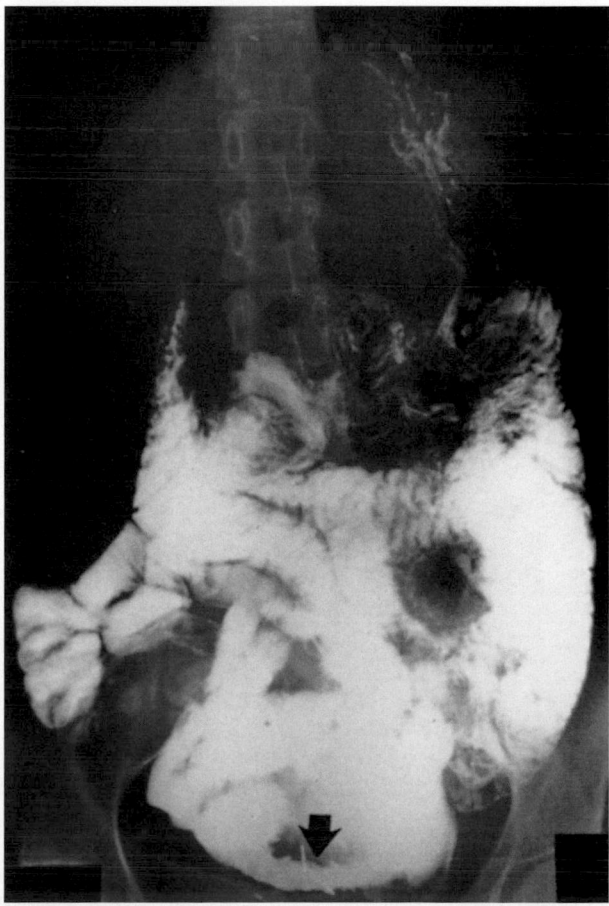

FIGURE 29-75. Recurrent Crohn's disease in terminal ileum (*arrow*) following continent ileostomy.

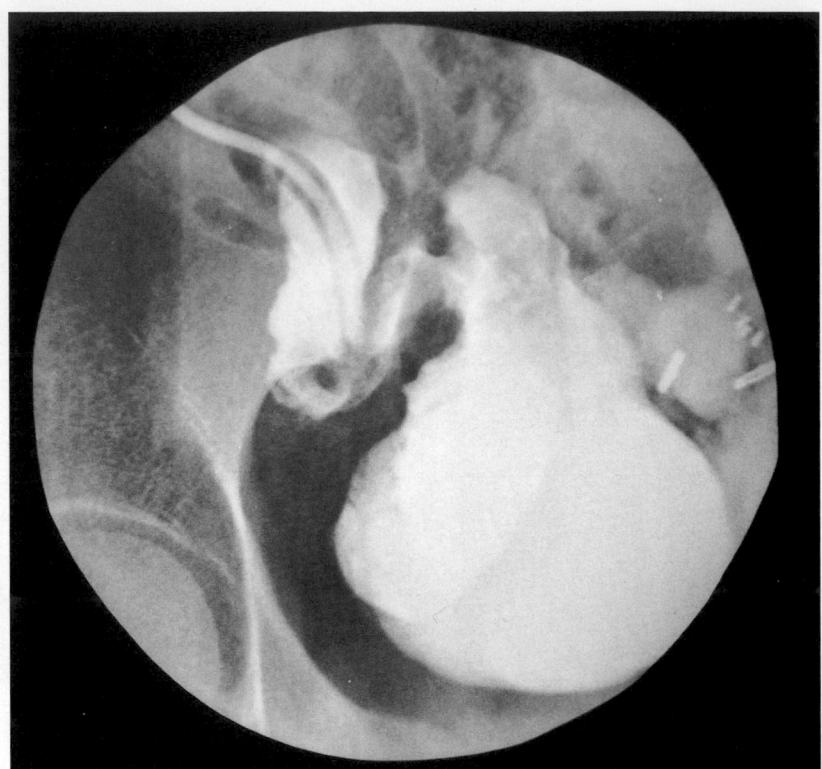

FIGURE 29-76. Desusscepted nipple can be readily appreciated on this "pouchogram." Acute angulation precludes catheterization even if there is no leakage.

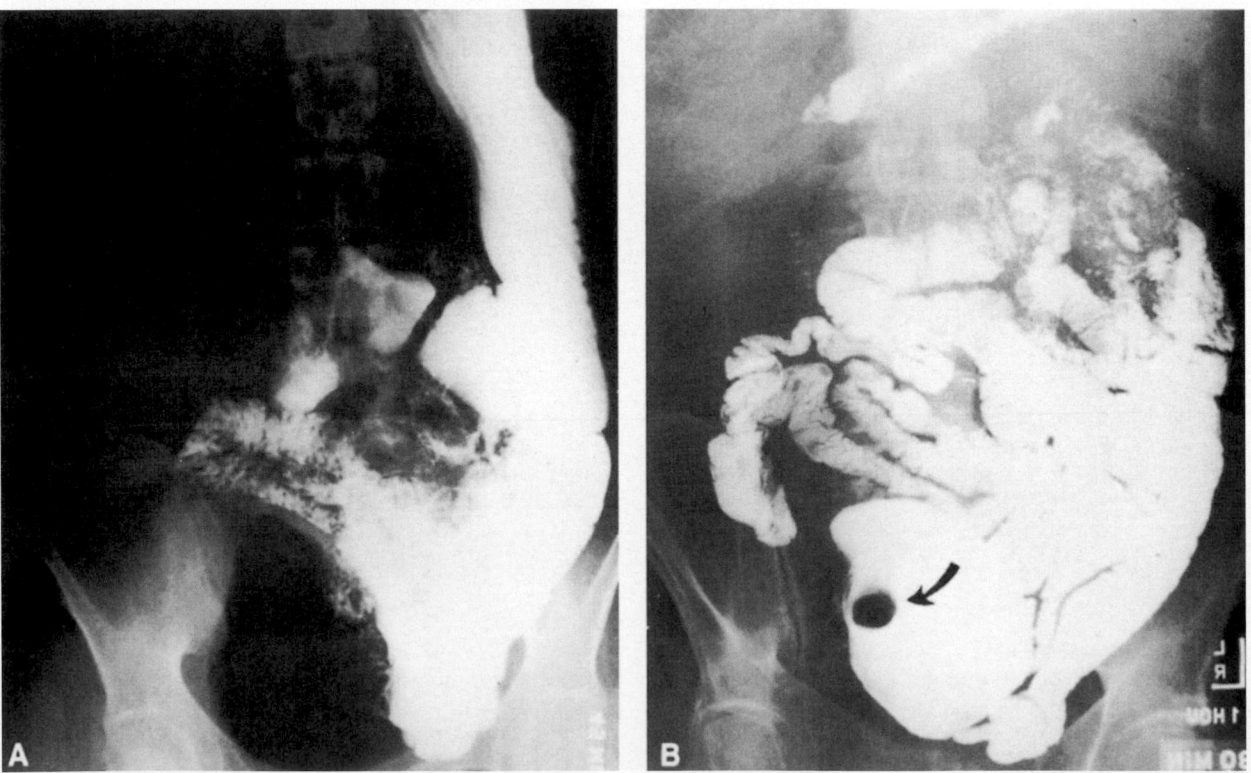

FIGURE 29-77. Continent ileostomy. Small bowel series. **A:** Normal pouch filling the pelvis on the right side. **B:** Normal reservoir and nipple valve (*arrow*).

Outlet obstruction has also been described as a consequence of an implanted sling that had penetrated through the nipple valve into the reservoir.[355] Revision is required to relieve these problems. Although the purpose of the operation, of course, is to create an intestinal obstruction, one of the distinct disadvantages is the need to have a catheter readily available. If a patient loses it and is unable to obtain one conveniently (e.g., while on a camping trip), a serious problem ensues. Relief of the obstruction cannot be obtained unless proper equipment is available. Patients who enjoy outings away from civilization are well advised to secure the catheter on their person with great care.

Nipple Valve Revision. Reconstruction of the nipple may be accomplished by performing an enterotomy in the reservoir, reintussuscepting the distal ileum, and resecuring it. However, it may not be possible to accomplish this maneuver because of necrosis of the ileum, inadequate length of the conduit, or bowel injury during the process of mobilization. Under these circumstances, a new nipple may be created without sacrificing the reservoir. This is achieved by using the afferent limb, oversewing the old efferent conduit opening, and performing an anastomosis of the proximal ileum to another part of the reservoir (Figure 29-78). This is the method usually required to convert a reservoir-ileoanal anastomosis (Parks) to a continent ileostomy (Kock). In the former operation, there is usually none or an insufficient length of terminal ileum remaining (that had been anastomosed to the anal canal) to create a nipple valve and conduit. By oversewing the efferent end and using the proximal bowel to create a new nipple and conduit, the reservoir can be maintained. Conversely, if the sphincter muscles have been preserved, it may be possible to convert a Kock pouch to a reservoir-anal anastomosis. Hultén and colleagues suggest that if a short mesentery precludes the possibility of constructing a pelvic pouch, a temporary continent ileostomy can be performed with the expectation that the expanded reservoir may subsequently permit conversion.[293]

Gottlieb and Handelsman describe a number of outflow tract problems associated with the Kock pouch, offering various approaches to management.[223] Noninvasive means for maintaining continence after the valve has desuscepted include insertion of various balloon tubes, such as an endotracheal tube (Figure 29-79). Unfortunately, it may not be possible to intubate the reservoir in the situation portrayed in Figure 29-79A.

Pouchitis. Pouch ileitis or pouchitis occurs at some time in 7% to 43% of patients with a continent ileostomy.[64,156] Manifestations include a flulike syndrome, fever, diarrhea, bleeding, abdominal pain, generalized toxicity, and severe ileitis. Increased ileostomy output requiring more frequent intubation is a common presentation. The condition is believed to be caused by a change in the flora of the pouch, particularly an overgrowth of anaerobic organisms. Interestingly, this complication is quite rare in patients who undergo the procedure for familial polyposis. Contrast enema study is usually not helpful, although thickening of the mucosal folds may be apparent. Endoscopic examination will usually reveal contact bleeding, friability, and an erythematous, ulcerated mucosa. Oral metronidazole (Flagyl) is the recommended treatment.[482] Additionally, many of these patients respond rapidly to steroids. Continuous drainage of the reservoir may

have an ameliorative effect, but in the rare situation, removal of the pouch may be necessary. Recurrence is not uncommon, and under these circumstances, consideration should be given to the possibility of Crohn's disease. The condition is also seen in those who have undergone restorative proctocolectomy with an ileal reservoir (see further discussion of pouchitis in that section).

Other Complications. Other unusual complications of the reservoir and nipple valve have been reported. These include the development of an enormous ileal pouch (the result of chronic outlet obstruction)[258,762] and *volvulus* with obstruction leading to perforation.[3] A case of invasive *adenocarcinoma* in a reservoir that had been in place for 17 years has also been reported,[110] but Hultén and coworkers found no incident of high-grade dysplasia or invasive carcinoma after a mean follow up of 30 years in 40 patients, leading them to conclude that it is very unlikely for invasive carcinoma to be a complication of this surgery.[296]

Hemorrhage from the nipple valve or reservoir has also been reported. This may be caused by trauma during insertion of the catheter (perforation of the pouch can actually occur), but it is usually associated with nonspecific inflammation of the mucosa—in other words, pouchitis.

Detachment of the pouch from the anterior abdominal wall has been reported to produce angulation of the efferent limb and difficulty intubating the pouch.[767] Operative correction is required.

Urolithiasis is a well-known associated complication in patients who have undergone conventional ileostomy. Stern and colleagues evaluated the problem in patients who had undergone Kock ileostomies and compared them with nine matched patients who had undergone the conventional operation.[705] Both ileostomy groups demonstrated reduced urinary volume, with the Kock procedure group having the lower volume. There was no significant reduction in urinary pH or elevation in urine uric acid concentration in the continent ileostomy group. The results seemed to imply no additional risk for uric acid stone formation in pouch patients.

Malabsorption has been suggested as a possible concern because of intestinal stasis and bacterial overgrowth. Kelly and colleagues studied the nature and frequency of malabsorption in 42 pouch patients and in 19 who had undergone conventional ileostomy.[340] Almost one-third with the reservoir were found to have excess fecal volumes accompanied by increased fecal loss of electrolytes, nitrogen, and fat, and by decreased vitamin B_{12} uptake. The remaining patients had fecal and urinary outputs similar to that of patients with conventional ileostomies. Gadacz and coworkers performed absorptive studies and motor function analysis of the pouch in eight patients.[187] The pouch absorbed vitamin B_{12} that was instilled together with intrinsic factor. Other studies of patients who had documented malabsorption or symptoms of a malfunctioning pouch revealed that the number of jejunal and ileal anaerobic bacteria decreased during treatment with metronidazole, implicating overgrowth of anaerobic bacterial flora in the pathogenesis of the syndrome.[341]

Kay and colleagues determined bile acid and neutral steroid excretion in 15 patients: 5 with conventional ileostomy, 5 with continent ileostomy, and 5 with continent ileostomy and an ileal resection.[333] Bile acid excretion rates were significantly increased in those with a continent ileostomy and an ileal resection. Also, continent ileostomy was associated with a

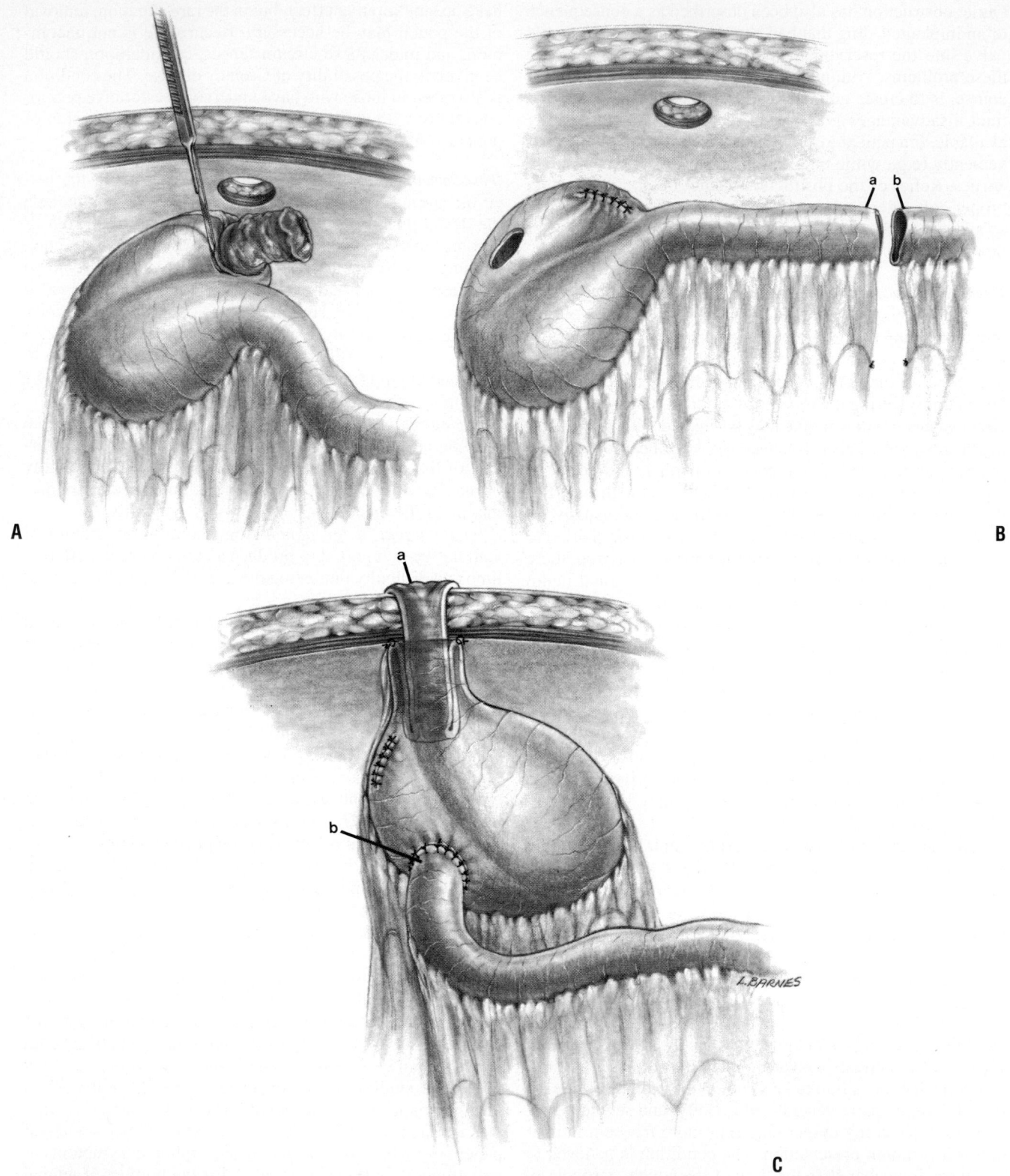

FIGURE 29-78. Construction of a new nipple valve. **A:** Resection of the old conduit. **B:** Division of the proximal (afferent) limb for the creation of a new nipple. **C:** Final position of reservoir and conduit.

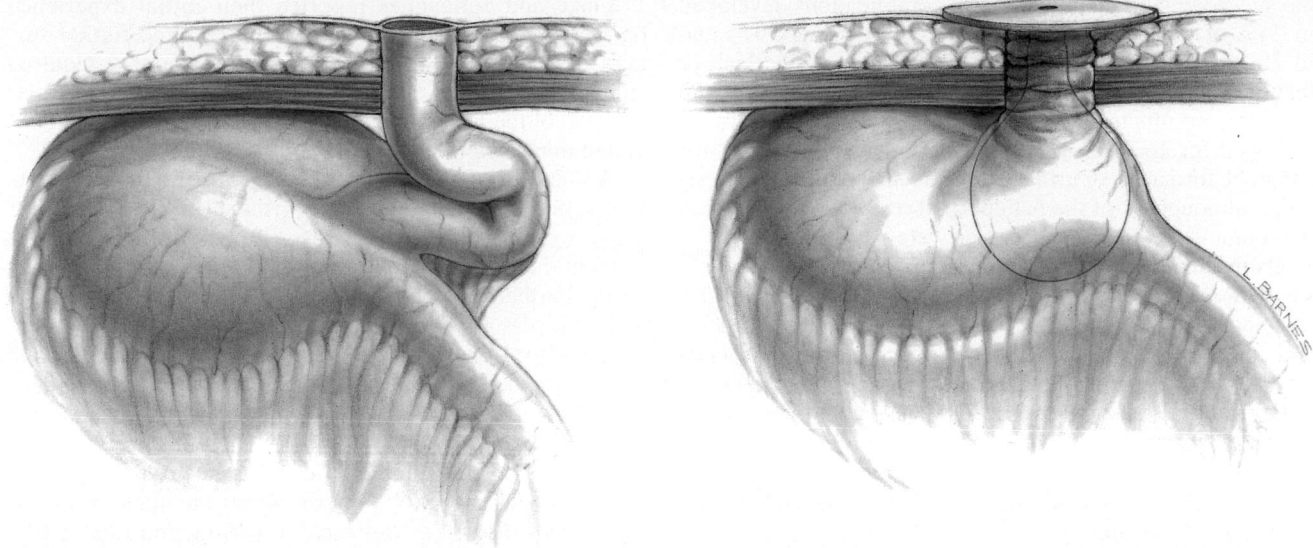

FIGURE 29-79. **A:** Desusscepted nipple valve. **B:** This is treated by the insertion of a balloon plug.

significantly increased percentage of water content and a reduction in the pH of the ileal effluent. Multiple cholesterol stones in the pouch of a patient have been observed (Figure 29-80).

Results

Cranley reviewed the development of the operation and reported that anastomotic leaks occurred in 8.8% of cases.[111] In the experience of Goligher with 62 reservoir operations, leakage occurred in 7, with the development of diffuse peritonitis in 3 and of a localized abscess in 4.[211] An additional two patients required a proximal loop ileostomy for presumed leakage, although no defect in the reservoir could be identified at the time of surgery. Goligher humbly commented that his complications seemed to be observed more frequently than those of other surgeons.

The report by Kock and colleagues in 1981 revealed seven deaths in 314 patients (2.2%).[363] All the operative deaths occurred prior to 1975, with no deaths recorded in

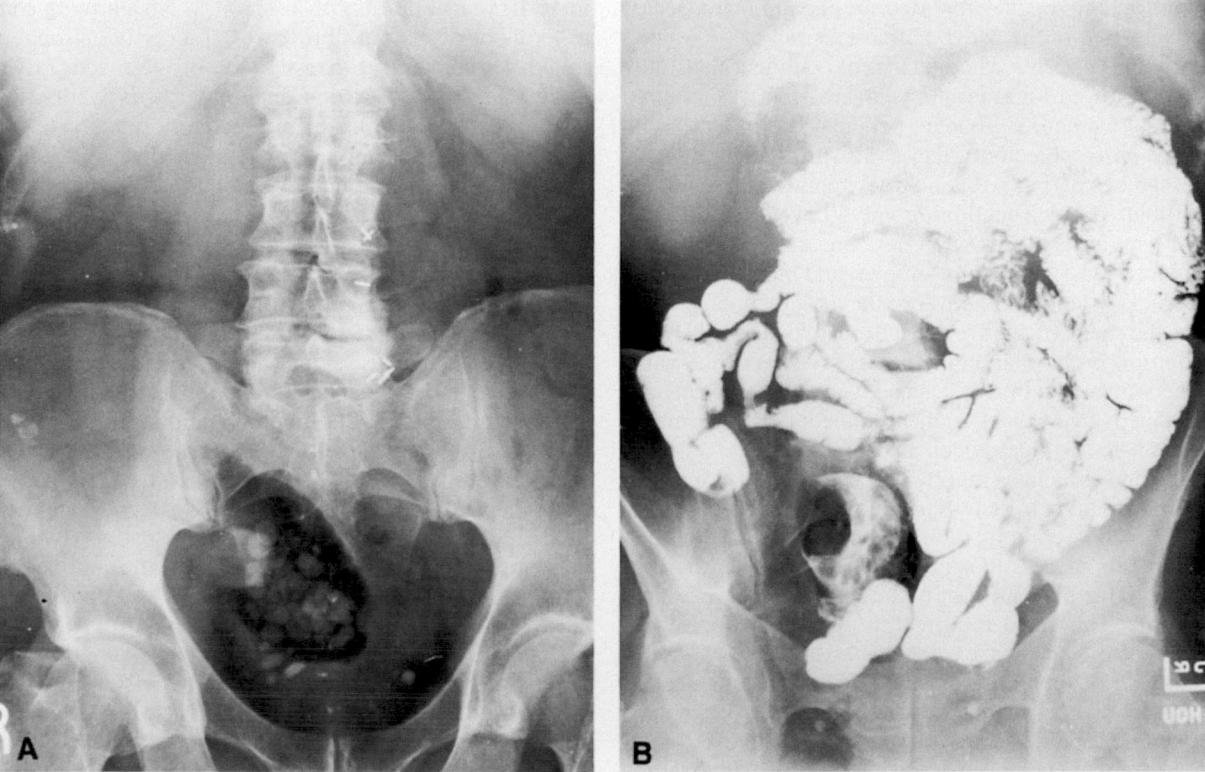

FIGURE 29-80. Continent ileostomy. **A:** Plane abdominal film reveals radiopaque objects in the reservoir (note air shadow). **B:** A small bowel series confirms the presence of "stones" in the pouch.

the succeeding 152 patients. Early complications developed in 24% of those operated on between 1967 and 1974 and in 7% of patients in the later period. Anastomotic leak or fistula occurred in 19 in the earlier group, but in only 1 from the later. Results in 36 patients from Kock's unit who were followed for 16 to 20 years revealed no increased risk for gallstone formation or urinary stone development.[561] Interestingly, although 11 of the patients had reservoirs constructed without a valve, 92% of the series were continent.

Palmu and Sivula reported an experience of 51 patients.[571] There were two perforations of the reservoir (one death), four fecal fistulas, and eight intestinal obstructions. Gelernt and colleagues evaluated their experience of 54 patients and noted a fecal fistula in 6, with hemorrhage from the ileal reservoir in 5.[195] In a study by Halvorsen and coworkers, of the 36 patients who underwent a reservoir ileostomy, 3 died of septic complications.[240] Of the 150 individuals reported from the Mayo Clinic, 16 required excision of the pouch, but only 1 because of a fistula.[37]

Schrock reported a 15% incidence of immediate postoperative complications in 39 patients.[667] Factors that contributed to the complications included older age (greater than 40 years), obesity, and the presence of Crohn's disease. By far, the most common problem was spontaneous reduction of the nipple valve, usually occurring within 3 months. This was observed by the author in one-third of his patients. A much higher incidence of nipple valve failure was noted in those who underwent a secondary operation rather than a primary procedure (proctocolectomy and continent ileostomy at the same time). Forty-six percent of secondarily operated patients had nipple failures, in comparison with 13% of primary surgery patients. Increased weight gain may have been a contributing factor because the patients were generally well and had a much more fatty mesentery when operated on the second time.

Dozois and colleagues reported the factors that affected the revision rate in the Mayo Clinic experience.[139] Among the nearly 300 patients who underwent continent ileostomy and were followed for at least 1 year, revision was required less often in women, in younger patients, and in those with a primary proctocolectomy and continent ileostomy. This was the same experience that Schrock reported. The authors advised that if a malfunctioning valve develops, it ideally should be revised rather than a new one created. Revision was believed to be technically simpler, and the long-term results were comparable. However, if the malfunctioning valve assumes the shape of an inverted ice cream cone—where the distal portion is quite large, then local revision of the valve is not recommended. I favor, instead, valve excision and creation of a neovalve from a segment immediately proximal to the pouch with neo-ileal-pouch anastomosis.

Gerber and associates reported a 19% incidence of nipple valve slippage in their first 48 patients.[199] In the next 48, the incidence of this complication was only 4%. The authors attributed their success to stapling the valve rather than suturing and to the placement of a Marlex mesh sleeve around the conduit. They also reported success in patients with Crohn's colitis, but their experience with ileocolitis, even with removal of the entire diseased bowel, was associated with a prohibitively high incidence of postoperative complications (see Chapter 30). Others suggest that the Kock continent ileostomy may be considered in patients with Crohn's disease, provided that there has been no evidence of recurrence for 5 years.[59]

Flake and colleagues reported their initial experience on 11 patients, three-fourths of whom required further surgery.[169] Four underwent a new Kock ileostomy, 2 required stomal revision, and 2 underwent revision of the valve with removal of the reservoir. Subsequently, 2 patients were converted to a conventional ileostomy.

At the Mayo Clinic, the results from the first 149 patients were compared with those from the last 150 patients.[138] There were no operative deaths. Fifteen pouches were excised in the early group, as opposed to only five in the later group. Furthermore, the requirement for revision of the valve at 1 year was 43% in the early group but only 22% in the later group. Long-term follow-up demonstrated complete continence in 60% of the patients in the early group and 75% in the later group.

The initial experience of Kock and colleagues revealed a 50% incidence of nipple valve complications necessitating revisional surgery.[363] With the newer modifications, their subsequent report demonstrated a malfunction rate of 6%. Putting aside the confusion regarding the definition of a steep learning curve, suffice it to state it is evident that there is indeed a considerable experience required with this operation before one can feel somewhat comfortable.

Approximately one-third of the patients of Palmu and Sivula required revision for nipple insufficiency, but Gelernt and colleagues, in an experience of 54 patients, stated that no nipple revision had ever been required.[195,571] Only 3 patients reported some degree of incontinence. Halvorsen and coworkers noted "disinvagination" of the nipple in more than one-third of their patients.[240] Telander and coworkers reported a 20% requirement for revision of the nipple valve in those younger than 19 years of age who underwent this procedure.[728]

Nilsson and associates performed morphologic and histochemical studies on the continent ileostomy reservoir for up to 10 years after its construction.[543] No alarming changes in terms of dysplasia, fibrosis, or progressive atrophy were found. Histochemical investigation of the mucosa revealed largely unchanged, strong enzymatic activity involved in both oxidative metabolism and secretory functions.[543]

Several studies have been published on the long-term results of this operation. Järvinen and colleagues evaluated 76 such patients 9 years following surgery.[309] Late complications occurred in 54 (72%): 2 (2.7%) pouch-related deaths, 30 (41.0%) nipple desusceptions, 22 (30.0%) cases of pouchitis, and 12 (16.0%) cases of stomal stricture. Additional complications included ventral hernia, nipple valve fistula, intra-abdominal abscess, and foreign body in the reservoir. Two-thirds of the patients required reoperation and revision. However, despite the high complication rate, a good functional result was achieved in 83%, and only four reservoirs were removed. This study and those of others confirm a high level of patient satisfaction even though the complication rate is high. In our experience, 97% of patients would undergo revisional surgery rather than have the continent ileostomy removed.[481] Of 152 patients alive with a pouch from the Cleveland Clinic, 91% were continent.[156]

Lepistö and Järvinen reported their experience with 96 continent ileostomy patients from Helsinki, Finland.[403] Twenty-four percent required conversion to a conventional stoma. Fifty-nine percent underwent valve reconstruction. When compared with restorative proctocolectomy, there was an overall statistically significantly lower success rate ($P < .01$).

Barnett reported 71 patients who underwent his particular modification, 54 of whom were revised from a conventional ileostomy.[33] The overall operative revision rate for valve and pouch problems was 7%. Mullen and colleagues reviewed a multicenter experience with the Barnett continent intestinal reservoir, involving 510 patients with ulcerative colitis or familial polyposis.[520] Follow-up time ranged from 1 to 5 years, with 92% still maintaining the reservoir. Replacement with a conventional ileostomy was required for 6.5%. This excision rate is certainly no worse than those of other series using more conventional approaches to creating the Kock pouch. Excluding pouch removal, the reoperation rate for major pouch-related complications was 12.8%.[520] Their pouch fistula problems and other surgery-related complications are higher than have generally been reported with the standard operation.

Comment

Most observers who are experienced with the continent ileostomy believe that the operation offers a reasonably satisfactory alternative to the conventional procedure.[37,156,211,394,542] The encumbrance of an appliance, the occasional "accidents" with appliance management, the unaesthetic proboscis on the abdominal wall, sexual inhibition, and psychological embarrassment have stimulated many patients to seek an alternative procedure. Unfortunately, however, the operation is no panacea. Despite the many improvements in surgical technique, the procedure is still fraught with numerous complications. The Kock pouch is also not for everyone. It is, in my opinion, contraindicated for patients with Crohn's disease, and the results in older people and those who are somewhat obese are quite poor. However, for those in whom a continent ileostomy has been performed and a Crohn's stricture has been subsequently identified at the entrance to the pouch, success has been realized by means of a strictureplasty of the short segment (see Chapter 30).

The patient should request this operation. It must not be "sold" by the surgeon. However, the quality of life for individuals who have elected the continent ileostomy is unquestionably improved in the vast majority of cases. But as previously stated, this discussion appears to be somewhat academic, because with the exception of conversion of a failed restorative proctocolectomy, the operation has been virtually replaced by the pouch-anal procedure.

Restorative Proctocolectomy (Total Proctocolectomy and Ileoanal Anastomosis with Intervening Pouch [Parks Procedure]; Pouch-Anal Procedure; Ileal Pouch-Anal Procedure)

As previously discussed, total abdominal proctocolectomy with ileoanal anastomosis is associated with frequent bowel movements, urgency, and fecal incontinence in a high percentage of cases. To address this problem, the application of an intervening pouch with an ileoanal anastomosis was described in experimental animals as early as 1933 by Valiente and Bacon and in 1964 by Peck and Hallenbeck.[581,752] With the success of the ileal reservoir as developed by Kock (see previous discussion), Parks and Nicholls in 1978 reported an operation combining the application of an ileal pouch that eliminated propulsive activity and acted as a storage organ with preservation of the entire sphincter mechanism.[572] Others also proposed similar operations.[167,579] The procedure has also been reported, with various modifications, as a means of restoring intestinal activity after conventional proctocolectomy, sometimes after many years.[106,577] In the past 30 years, the preponderance of publications on the surgical management of ulcerative colitis have addressed variations on this procedure, the morbidity, the physiologic effects, and the functional results.

Several controversial issues with respect to this operation are known and are important to discuss. They include the following and will be addressed in this section:

- the type of pouch (J, S, W, Q, and T)
- mucosectomy versus double-stapling
- loop ileostomy versus no protective stoma
- the significance of dysplasia and the risk of malignancy

ALAN GUYATT PARKS (1920–1982)

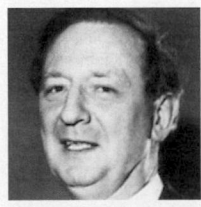

Alan Parks, after attending Epsom College, proceeded to Brasenose, Oxford, and received his bachelor of arts degree in 1943. That same year, he was awarded a Rockefeller fellowship to attend Johns Hopkins University to complete his medical training and medical internship. He returned to Guy's Hospital, London, and in 1949 passed the examination for fellowship in the Royal College of Surgeons. After a period in the National Service in the Far East, Parks came back to Guy's to continue his research on the anatomy of the anal canal. Numerous publications followed, which provide an extraordinary testament to his dedication as a scientist and his ability as a creative writer. Parks was appointed consultant surgeon to the staff of St. Mark's Hospital in 1959 and to the London Hospital the same year. His practice attracted many surgeons from throughout the world who came to train and observe. In 1954, Parks was made a master of surgery for his work leading to a special operation for hemorrhoids (see Chapter 11). Through the years, the name of Alan Parks has been associated with innovation in the field of colon and rectal surgery. His contributions include the development of a number of surgical instruments, studies on the etiology and classification of anal fistula (see Chapter 14) and on the physiology and anatomy of the pelvic floor, the treatment of anal incontinence (see Chapter 16), and the application of the ileal reservoir with ileoanal anastomosis in the surgical management of ulcerative colitis and familial polyposis. Parks' honors have been numerous: presidency of the section of proctology of the Royal Society of Medicine, fellowship in the Royal College of Physicians, and honorary fellowships awarded by the American, Australasian, Canadian, Edinburgh, and Glasgow Colleges of Surgeons. His achievements were further recognized when he was granted a knighthood by the British Government.

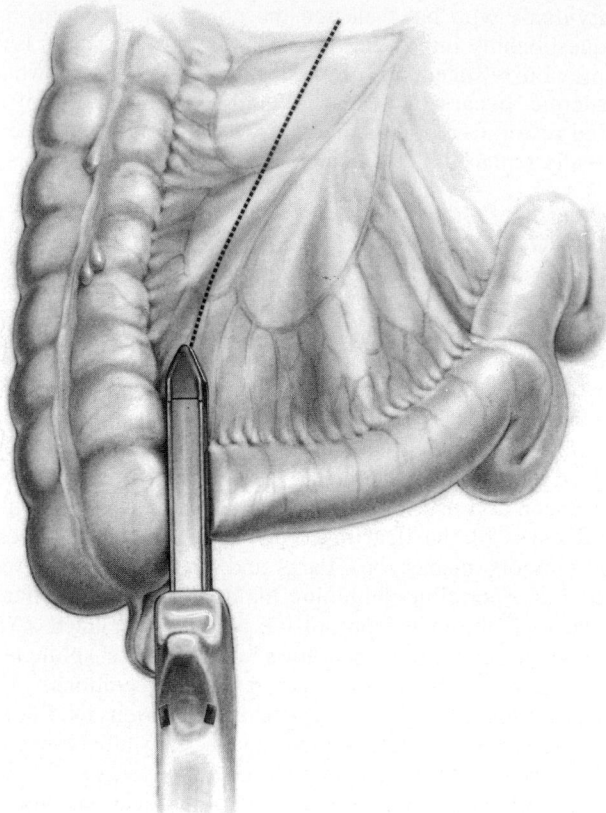

FIGURE 29-81. Ileum is divided as close to the cecum as possible. (Adapted from Burnstein MJ, Schoetz DJ Jr, Coller JA, et al. Technique of mesenteric lengthening in ileal reservoir-anal anastomosis. *Dis Colon Rectum.* 1987;30:863.)

S-Pouch

The patient is placed in the perineolithotomy position as if for an abdominoperineal resection. Following completion of the colectomy and excision of the rectum as far distally as is possible (see previous section), an ileal reservoir is created. The distal ileum is transected with the stapler as close to the cecum as is possible (Figure 29-81).

Tension on the ileal mesentery is a potential problem because the bowel must be brought virtually to the perianal skin. Complete mobilization of the mesentery up to the level of the duodenum is imperative (Figure 29-82). The ileal artery may be divided to achieve additional length, and the parietal peritoneum of the distal ileum may be incised (Figure 29-83). Some believe that complete dissection of the root of the mesentery is a poor lengthening technique and that division of the ileocecal artery is the safest and most effective method for obtaining maximum length.[86] Goes and colleagues recommend preservation of the marginal vascular arcade of the right side of the colon to permit ligation of more mesenteric vessels and to increase the mesenteric length[206] (Figure 29-84). In a series of cadaver studies, Smith and coworkers observed that if the tip of the conduit (or pouch) reaches 6 cm below the pubic symphysis, the dentate line will be satisfactorily reached.[691] Martel and colleagues found that in fresh cadavers, the increase in mesenteric length was greater after dividing the superior mesenteric pedicle (mean, 6.5 cm) as compared with the ileocolic pedicle (mean, 3.0 cm), but if a pouch-anal anastomosis is to be performed, a short segment of terminal ileum must be removed.[465] Regardless of the lengthening technique, the most dependent part of the terminal ileum for effecting the anastomosis should be selected, not a specific, measured distance from the cut end of the ileum.

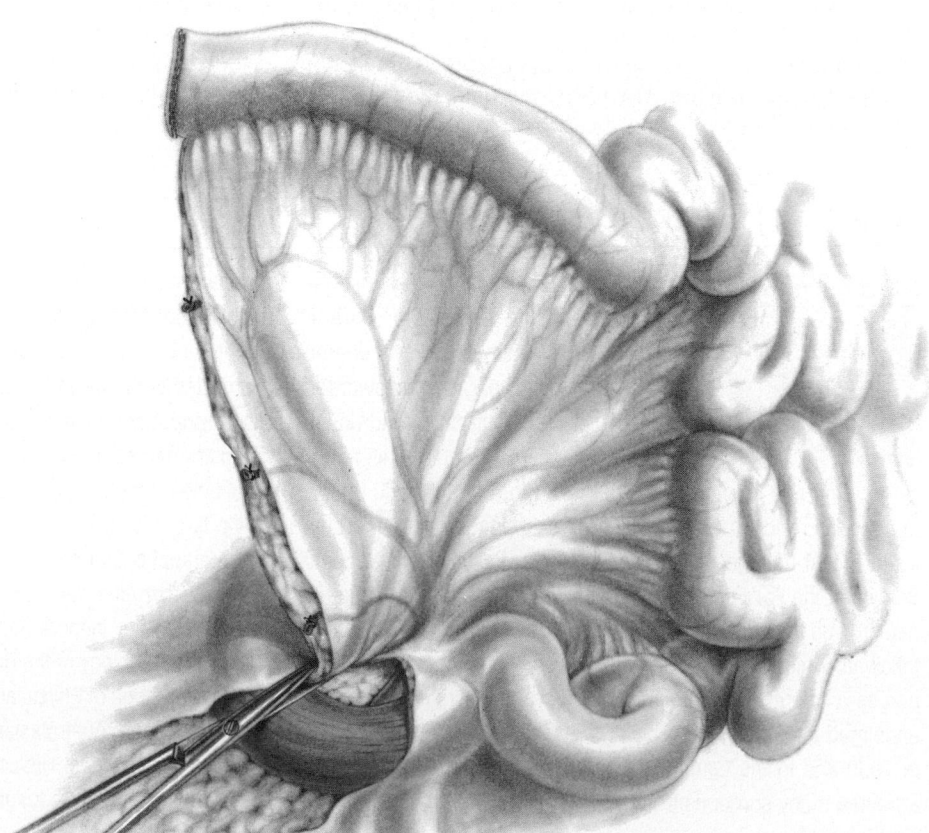

FIGURE 29-82. Dissection is carried out to the root of the mesentery. (Adapted from Burnstein MJ, Schoetz DJ Jr, Coller JA, et al. Technique of mesenteric lengthening in ileal reservoir-anal anastomosis. *Dis Colon Rectum.* 1987;30:863.)

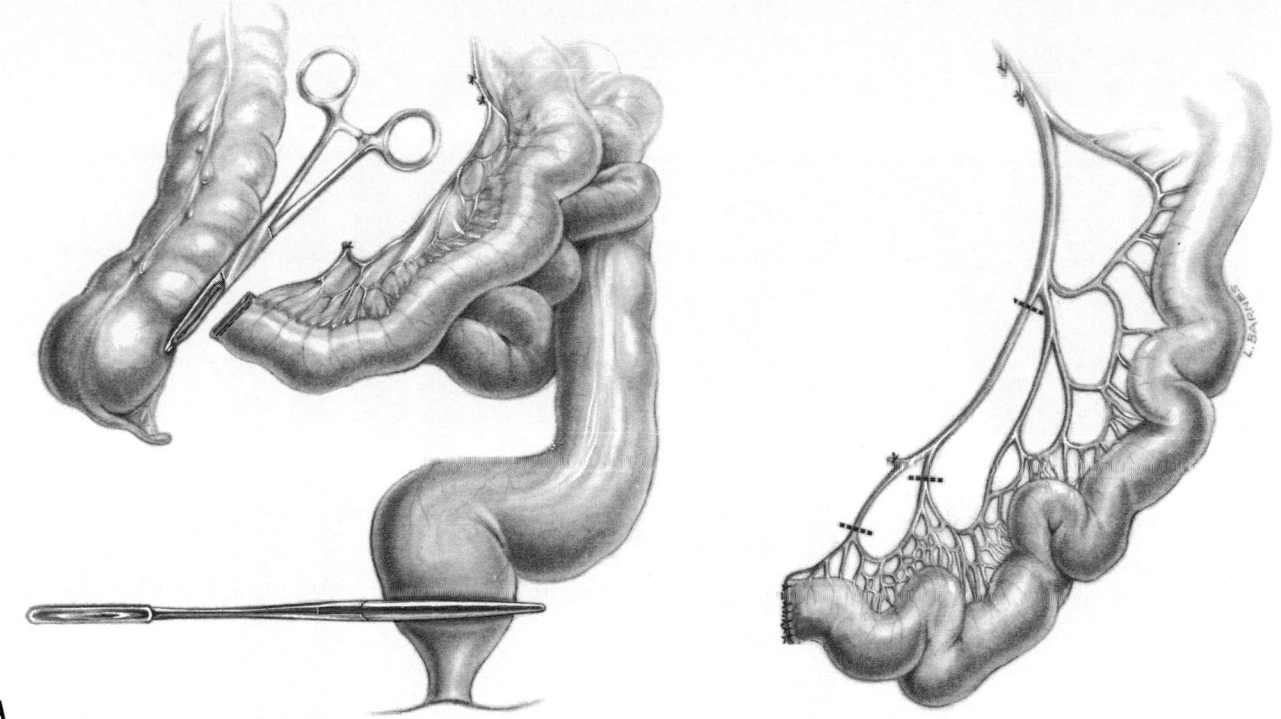

FIGURE 29-83. Preservation of the ileal blood supply. **A:** Transection of the distal ileum as close to the cecum as possible. **B:** Preservation of the blood supply by careful dissection with the aid of transillumination. The *dashed lines* indicate possible sites of division in order to obtain additional length.

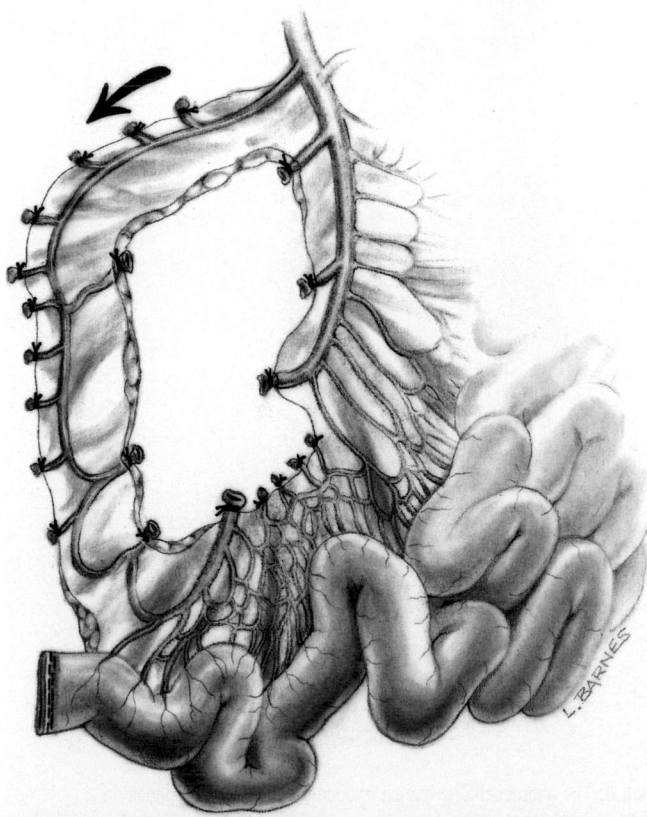

FIGURE 29-84. Schematic representation of the mesenteric vascular arcade with preservation of the blood supply that supplied the right colon. (After Goes RN, Nguyen P, Huang D, et al. Lengthening of the mesentery using the marginal vascular arcade of the right colon as the blood supply to the ileal pouch. *Dis Colon Rectum.* 1995;38:893.)

Parks and Nicholls suggested that an S-type reservoir be created[572] (Figure 29-85). In this modification, the terminal 50 cm of ileum is measured and then folded twice to give three segments of bowel, the proximal two of which are 15 cm long and the distal segment 20 cm long (Figure 29-85A). A 5-cm length of ileum projects beyond the pouch, which is the area to be used for the anastomosis. The ileum is opened on its antimesenteric border (Figure 29-85B), and the adjacent loops are sutured (Figure 29-85C). An interrupted technique may be used, but a continuous suture of 3–0 long-term absorbable material is more expeditious. The two outer edges are then folded across to complete the pouch, with the closure effected using the same suture material (Figure 29-85D).

Another alternative for pouch construction is to employ a stapling technique (see later discussion). This is a much more rapid approach, but it has the theoretical disadvantage of more tissue inversion, and therefore decreased reservoir capacity.[704]

As previously mentioned, the anastomosis is performed via the transanal approach by using an anal retractor (e.g., Parks), paired Gelpi retractors placed at right angles, or a self-retaining Lone Star retractor (Figure 29-86).[629,643] In contrast to earlier suggestions, most surgeons today make no attempt to preserve a muscular sleeve (see Ileoanal Anastomosis, Operative Technique).[284] The full thickness of the ileum is sutured to the anal canal at the level of the dentate line, incorporating the underlying internal anal sphincter muscle (see Figure 29-54). Alternatively, an anastomosis can be performed in the anal canal by using the circular stapling device, with or without a double-stapling approach, but care must be taken to avoid placing the staple line too low (see later discussion).[262,580,778]

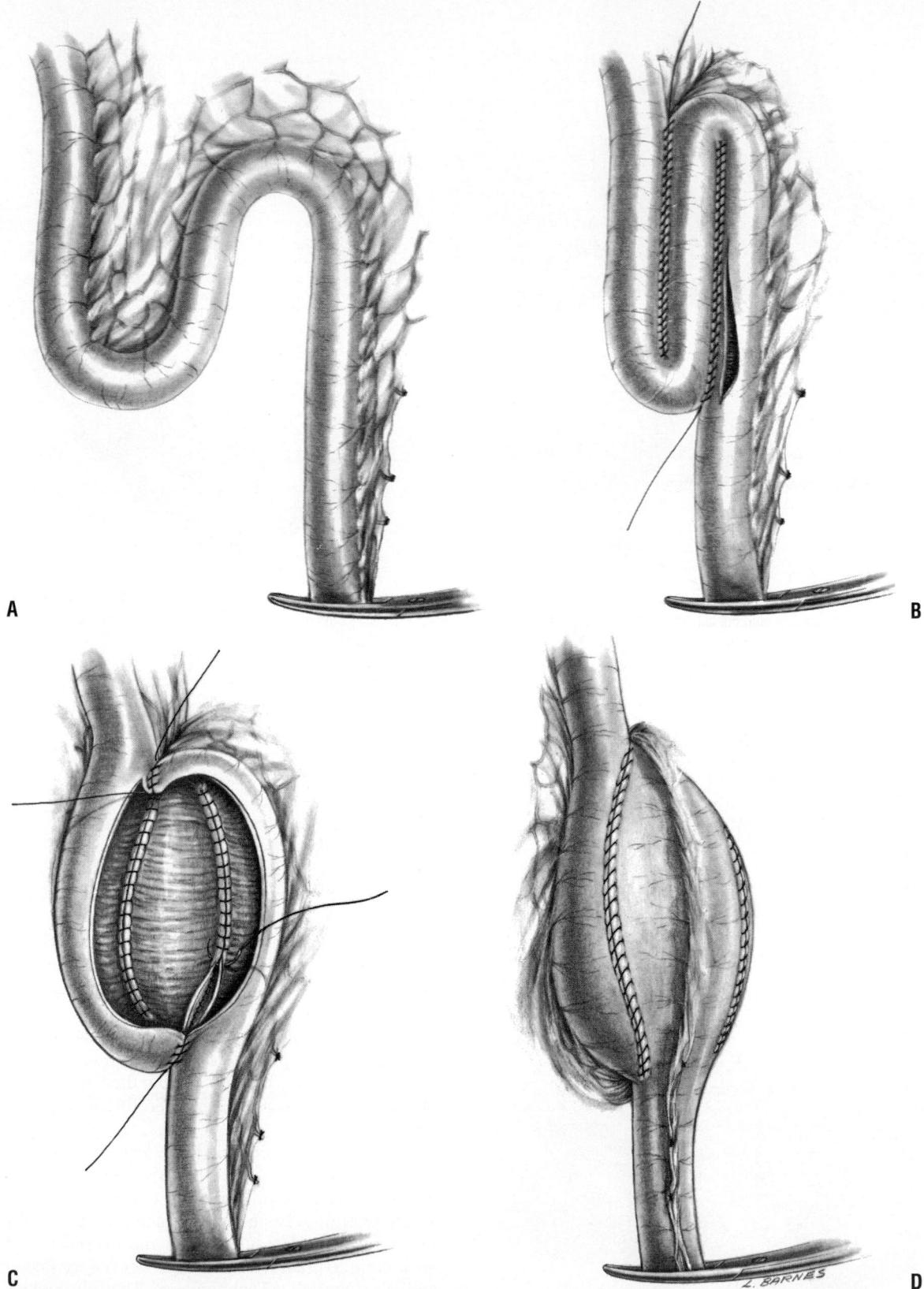

FIGURE 29-85. S-type (Parks) ileal reservoir. **A:** The bowel is aligned. **B:** The antimesenteric aspect is opened after serosal apposition. **C:** Suturing of the adjacent walls. **D:** The reservoir is completed for a planned ileoanal anastomosis. However, as illustrated, the efferent limb is excessively long. Unless the exit conduit is reduced to a 2- to 3-cm length, obstructed defecation will ensue. This figure simulates the S-pouch configuration before the distal limb has been appropriately amputated.

Ambroze and colleagues (Mayo Clinic) have emphasized that retention of the omentum reduces the incidence of sepsis without affecting the frequency of postoperative bowel obstruction.[9] With respect to drains, Parks and coworkers advised draining the pelvis through the intersphincteric plane, but some surgeons prefer either no drain or a suprapubic suction drain.[573] An alternative would be to place the drain in the pelvis and bring it out through the levators and buttock. My personal preference is to use a closed-suction drain, placed in the pelvis and brought out through a stab wound in the left lower quadrant. It is removed when the drainage is less than 100 mL in 24 hours.

Comment. It has been said that the S-pouch can permit an anastomosis lower in the pelvis than that of a J-pouch. In other words, it may be used in the circumstance when the application of a J-pouch cannot permit restoration of intestinal continuity. Such occasions must be rare indeed, however. When an S-pouch is considered in the face of reach difficulties, another alternative includes (after pouch construction) suture of the pouch to the upper surface of the levators. Reoperation after 6 to 12 months will commonly permit a delayed anastomosis because the superior mesenteric vessels will have stretched to accommodate the prior "reach" difficulty. This is analogous to what occurs after redo ileo-pouch-anal anastomosis (IPAA) for fistula complications. There are problems unique to the S-pouch, most especially emptying difficulties if the efferent limb is too long (see Complications of the Pouch Procedures). The ease of construction of the J-reservoir and the comparable results with respect to bowel function (see next section) cause most surgeons to use the following technique.

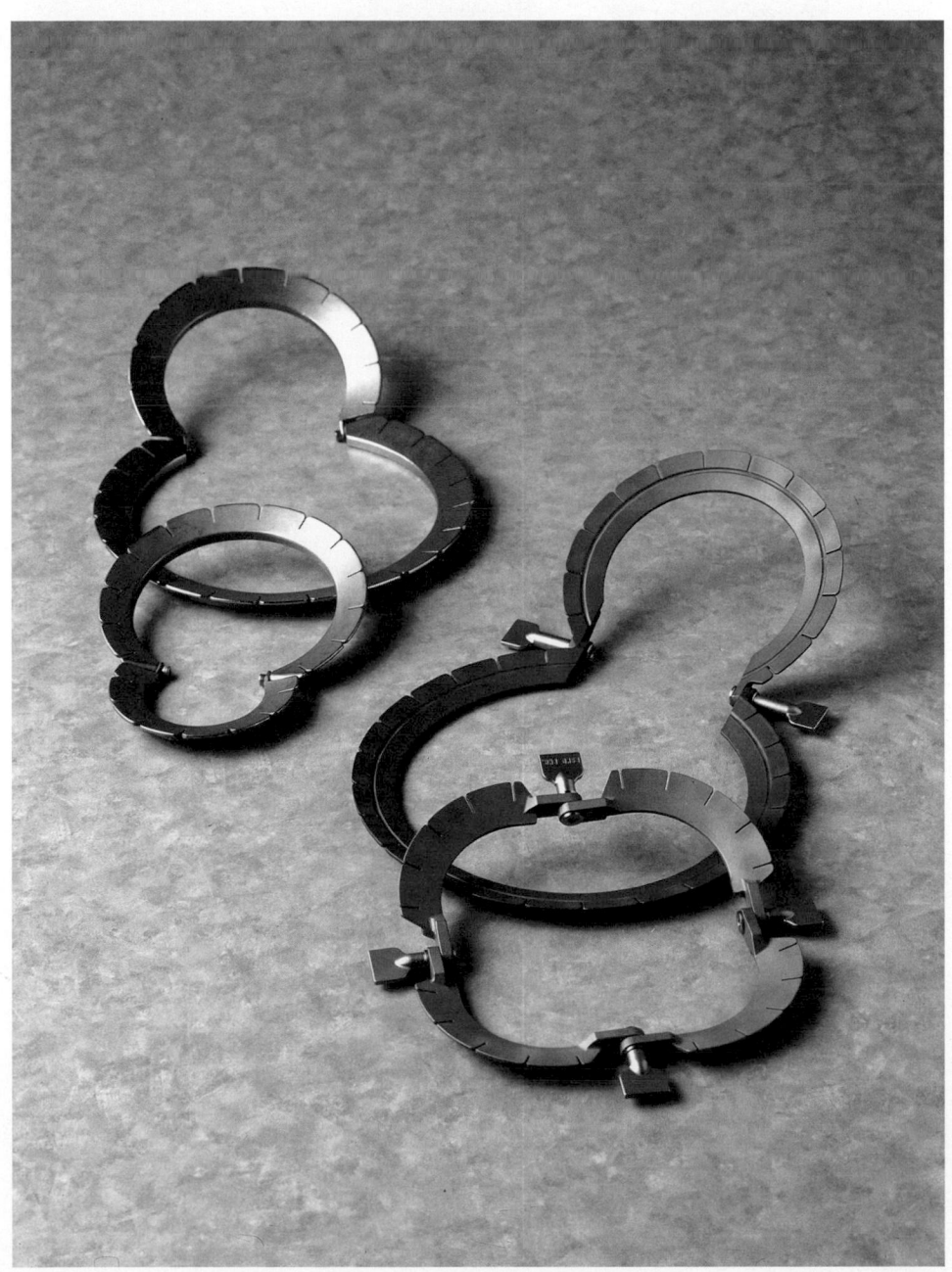

A

FIGURE 29-86. Endoanal anastomosis can be facilitated by means of the Lone Star retractor. Another alternative is to place effacement sutures around the circumference of the anal verge. **A:** Reusable metal retractor rings (foreground—lightweight aluminum; background—stainless steel). *(continued)*

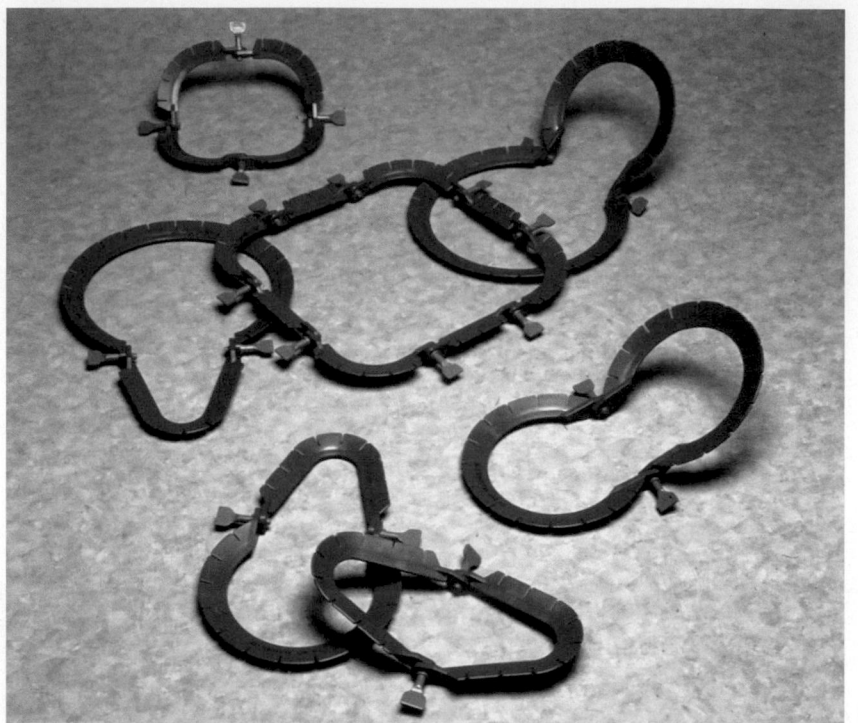

B

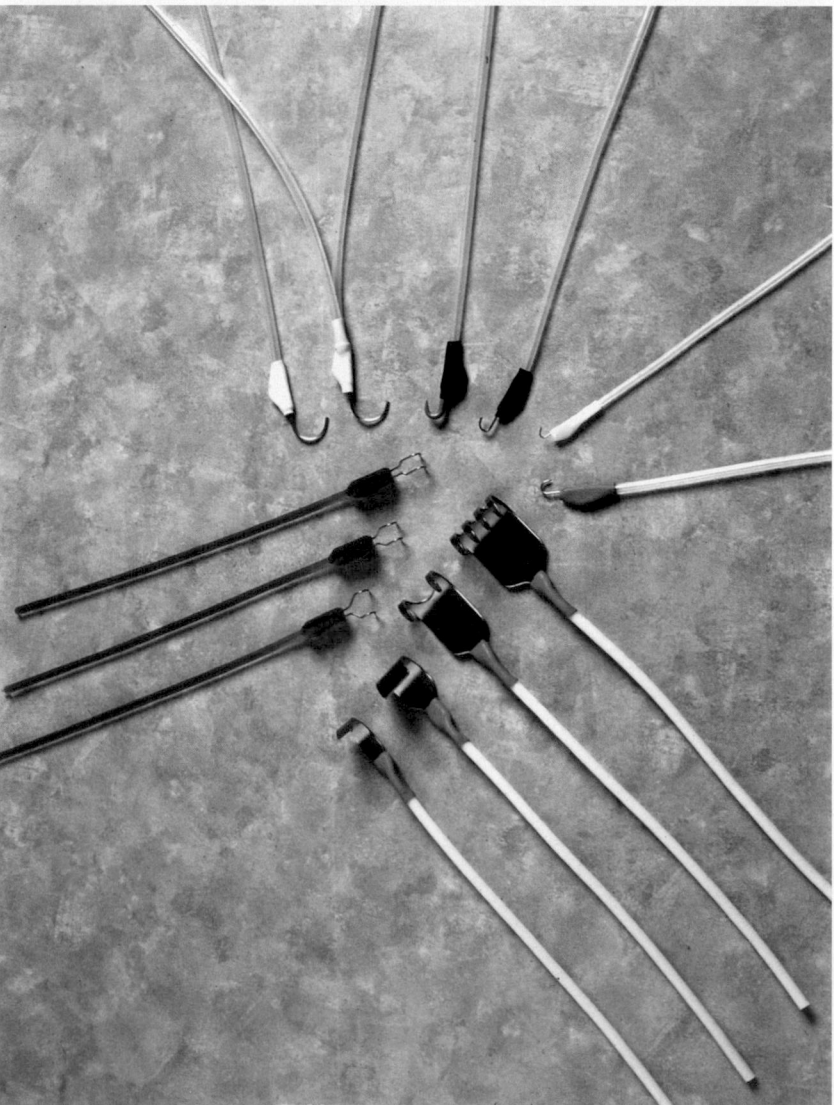

FIGURE 29-86. *(continued)* **B:** Single-use retractor rings. **C:** Various elastic stay hooks. (Courtesy of Lone Star Medical Products, Inc., Houston, TX.)

C

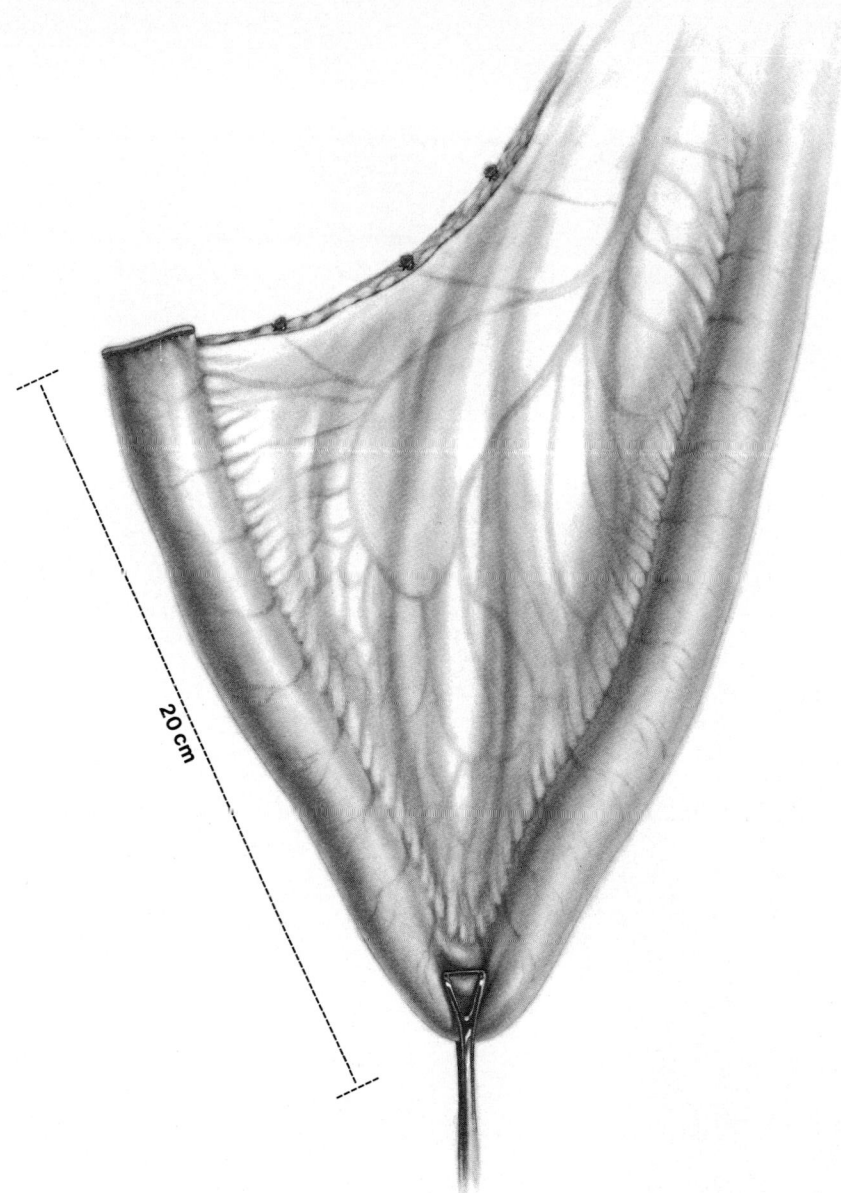

FIGURE 29-87. Maximum length of J-pouch is usually achieved with the apex approximately 20 cm proximal to the ileocecal valve. Other alternatives to alleviating reach problems include serial incisions between the vasa recta. This can be facilitated by a subperitoneal saline injection. (Adapted from Burnstein MJ, Schoetz DJ Jr, Coller JA, et al. Technique of mesenteric lengthening in ileal reservoir-anal anastomosis. *Dis Colon Rectum.* 1987;30:863.)

J-Pouch

Another option, the so-called J-pouch, was initially suggested by Utsunomiya and colleagues.[751] This type of pouch is prepared by selecting the point at which the ileal loop reaches the lowest level in the pelvis, usually about 20 to 30 cm from the end of the ileum (Figure 29-87). The length of the pouch is variable but generally is approximately 20 cm.

As previously noted, one of the critical concerns in the performance of the reservoir-anal techniques is the creation of an anastomosis that is free of tension. Burnstein and colleagues at the Lahey Clinic have outlined a series of steps that they believe offer the optimal approach to mesenteric lengthening.[80] This consists of division of the terminal ileum as close to the cecum as is possible (see Figure 29-81), mobilization of the mesentery of the small bowel to the third portion of the duodenum (see Figure 29-82), and selection of the apex of the J-reservoir with the objective of its extension 6 cm beyond the pubic symphysis (Figure 29-87).[80] Mesenteric lengthening can be achieved through a number of possible maneuvers. In the first instance, care should be taken to divide the mesentery as close to the right colon as possible to preserve the branches of the ileocolic artery. If incisions along the mesenteric peritoneum produce inadequate length and a window must be created, blood supply to the pouch can still be preserved (Figure 29-88).

Apposition of the loop can be performed by using a continuous double-layer suture technique, thereby creating a long, side-to-side anastomosis (Figure 29-89). Most surgeons today prefer to employ the GIA stapling device or equivalent to create the reservoir. An early approach was to use the conventional 5-cm instrument, inserting it by means of enterotomies 5 cm proximal to the point selected as the apex of the pouch (Figure 29-90A). The GIA stapler is then inserted

(text continues on page 1259)

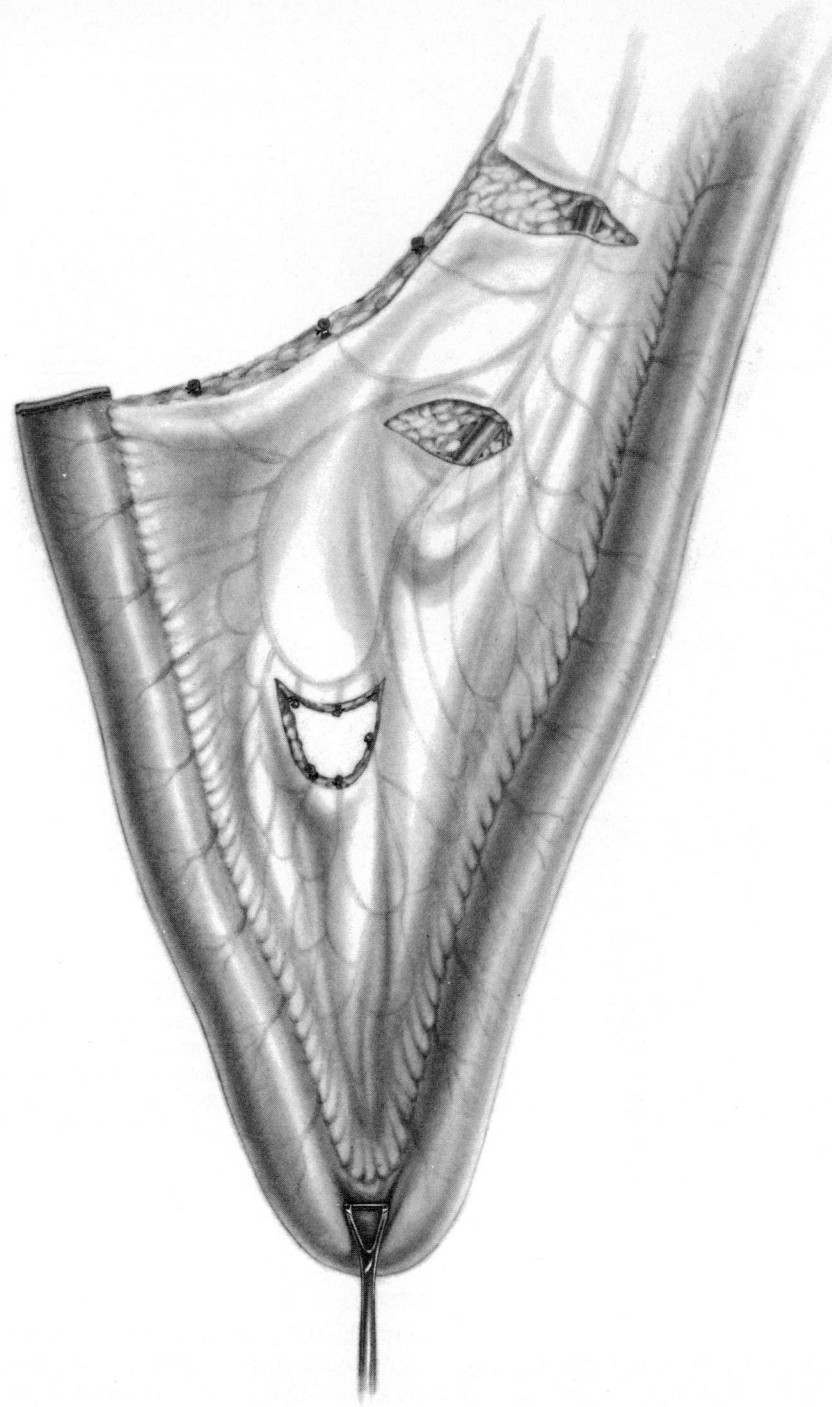

FIGURE 29-88. Incising the peritoneum of the mesentery and creating a window aid in achieving increased length. (Adapted from Burnstein MJ, Schoetz DJ Jr, Coller JA, et al. Technique of mesenteric lengthening in ileal reservoir-anal anastomosis. *Dis Colon Rectum*. 1987;30:863.)

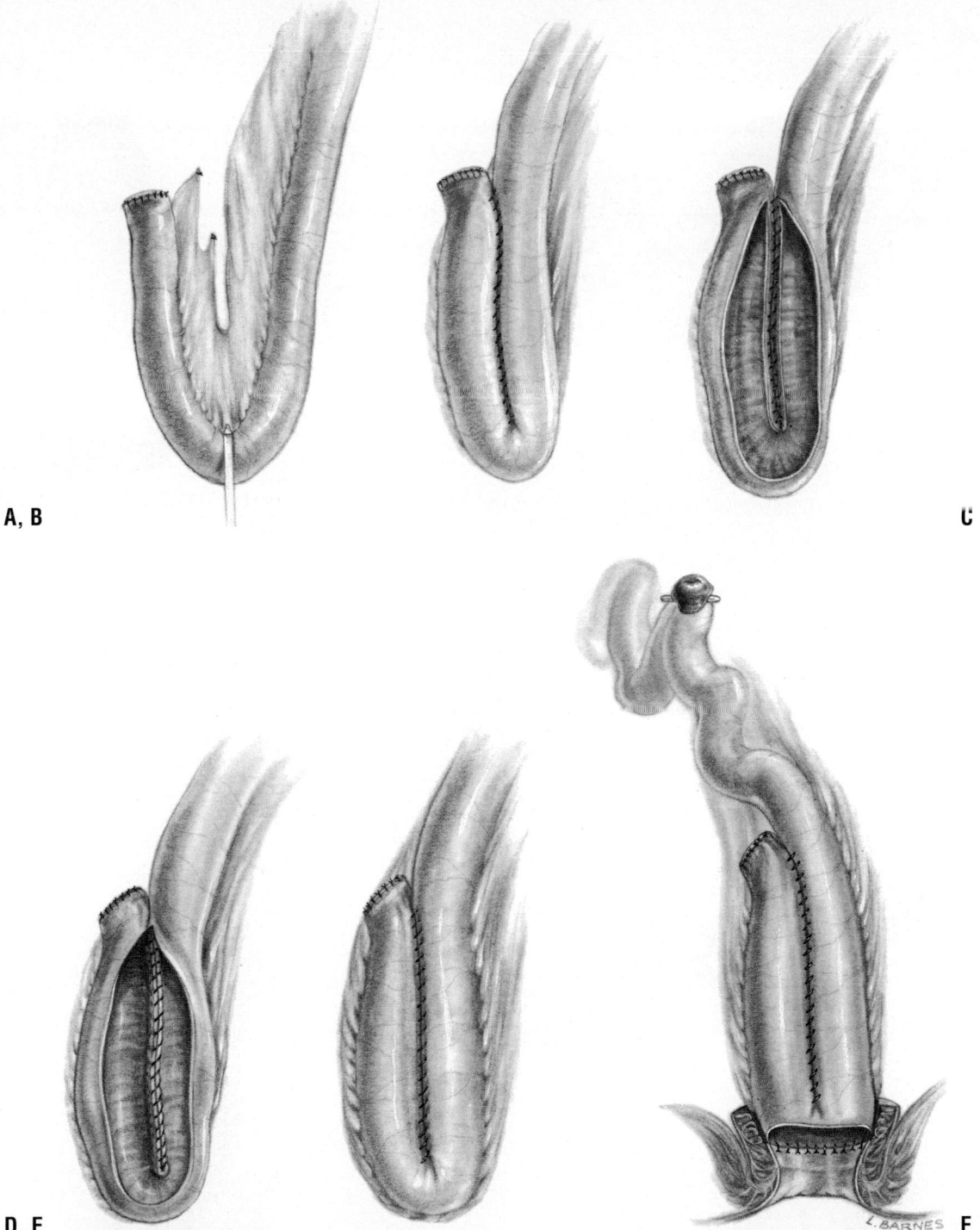

A, B

C

D, E

F

FIGURE 29-89. Pouch-anal procedure (J-type). **A:** Limbs identified with distal ileum closed. **B:** Seromuscular apposition. **C:** Long enterotomy. **D:** Closure of posterior wall. **E:** Closure of anterior wall. **F:** Completed anastomosis of pouch to anus with protecting loop ileostomy.

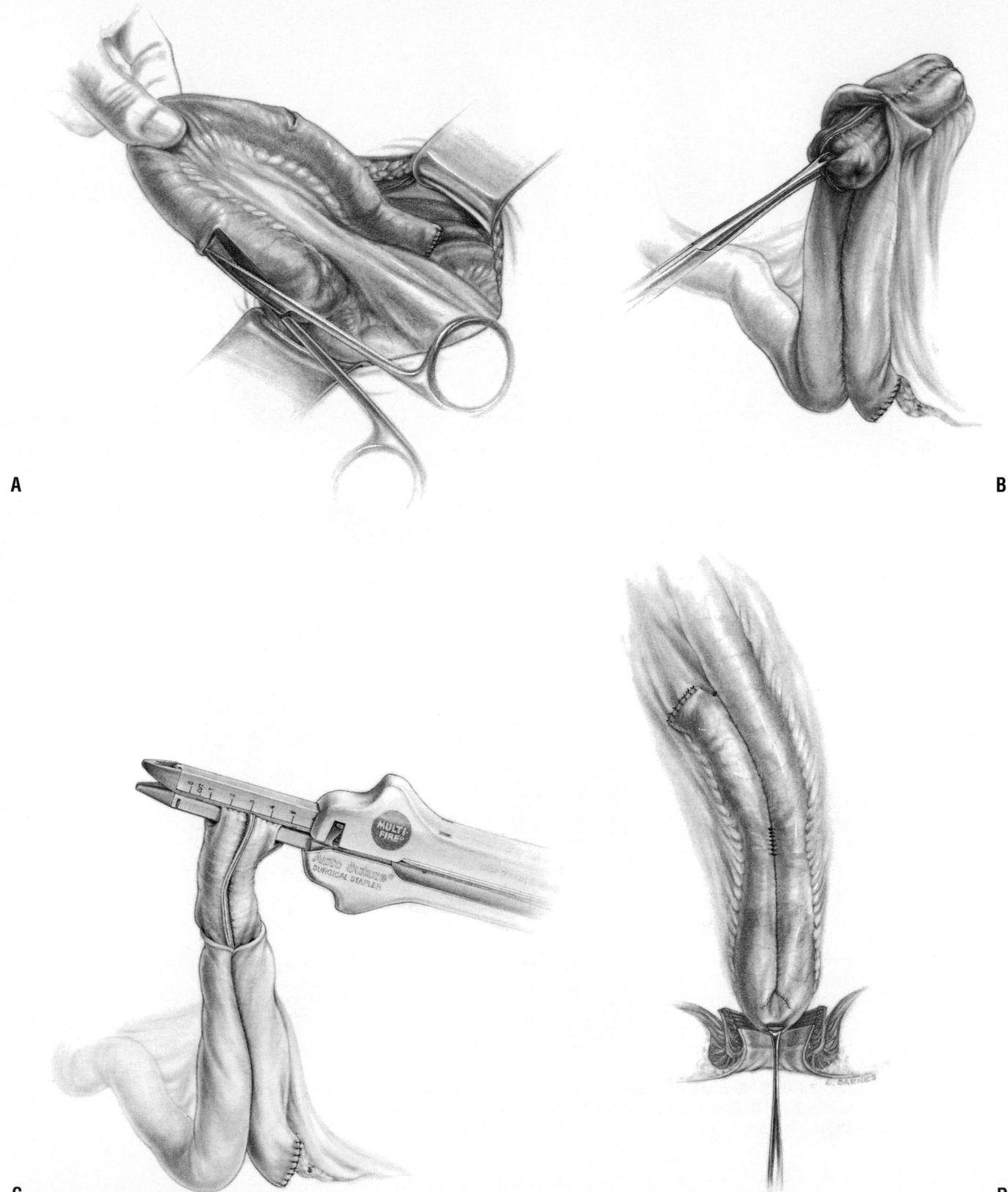

A

B

C

D

FIGURE 29-90. Stapled J-pouch procedure. **A:** Two enterotomies are created and the GIA instrument is inserted in each limb in both directions. **B:** Apical septum is inverted. **C:** Septum is divided by GIA instrument. **D:** Enterotomy is closed longitudinally and anastomosis of pouch to anus is effected.

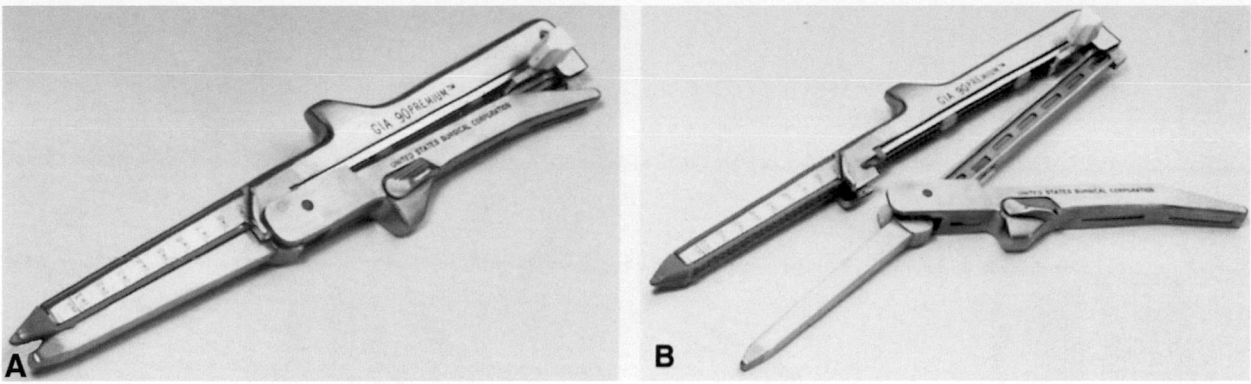

FIGURE 29-91. Long (9-cm) GIA stapler. **A:** Closed position. **B:** Open position. (Courtesy of Covidien, Inc., Norwalk, CT.)

toward the apex and fired. The pouch is turned around and two additional staple cartridges are fired in the opposite direction through the same enterotomies. With a total of three staple cartridges fired, a 15-cm pouch is created. The terminal septum must be inverted and divided either sharply or by another passage of the stapler (Figure 29-90B,C). The enterotomies are closed longitudinally, and the apex of the pouch is delivered to the anal area (Figure 29-90D). A small

enterotomy is made in the pouch, and an anastomosis is effected between the full thickness of bowel and the anal canal in the manner described previously.

Current stapling instruments permit a simpler pouch construction, such as a long (9-cm) GIA (Figure 29-91). The stapler can be inserted in the middle of each limb (Figure 29-92) or optimally through the apex. Care must be taken to pull the mesentery away from the bowel to avoid

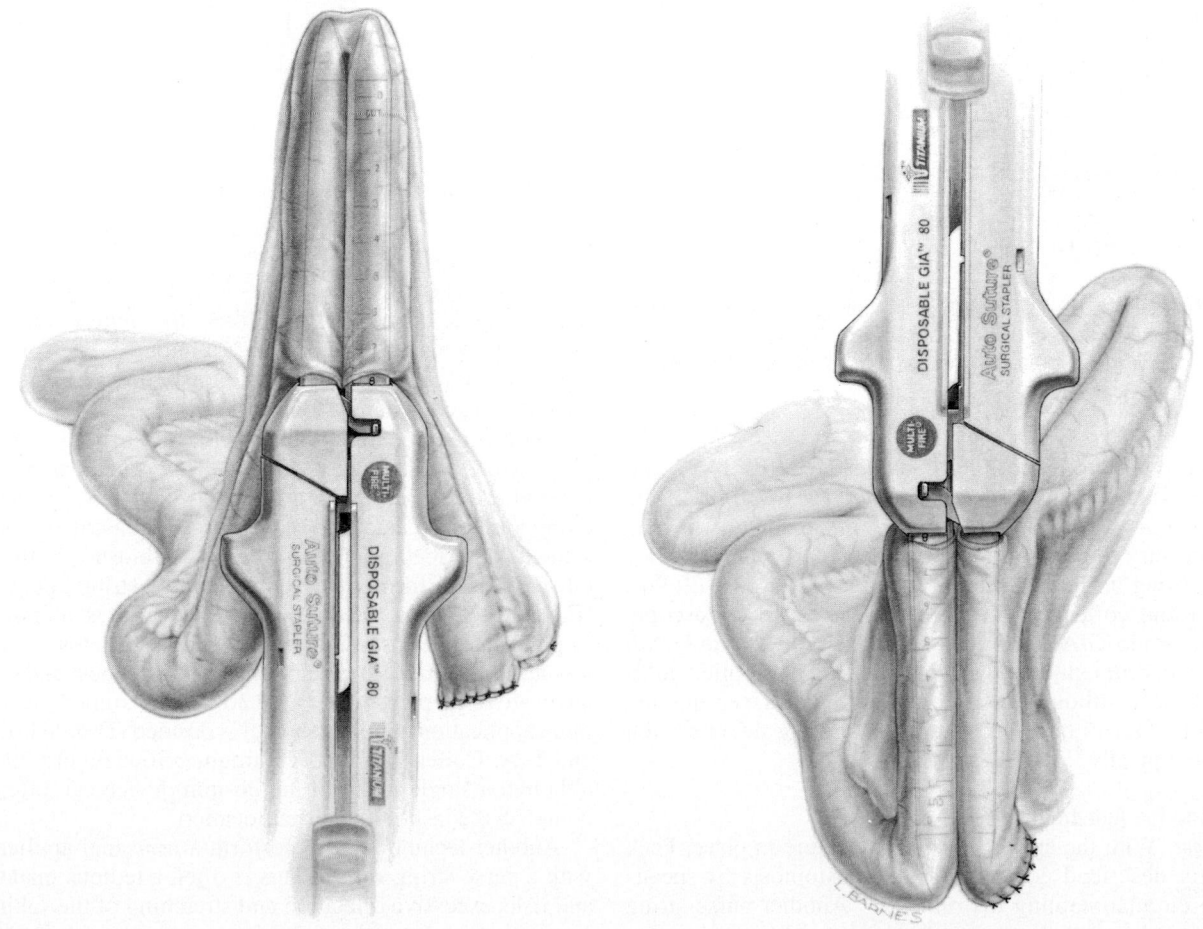

A   **B**

FIGURE 29-92. Construction of J-pouch with long (8-cm) GIA stapler. **A:** Enterotomies with passage toward apex. **B:** Passage cephalad in direction of ileal closure.

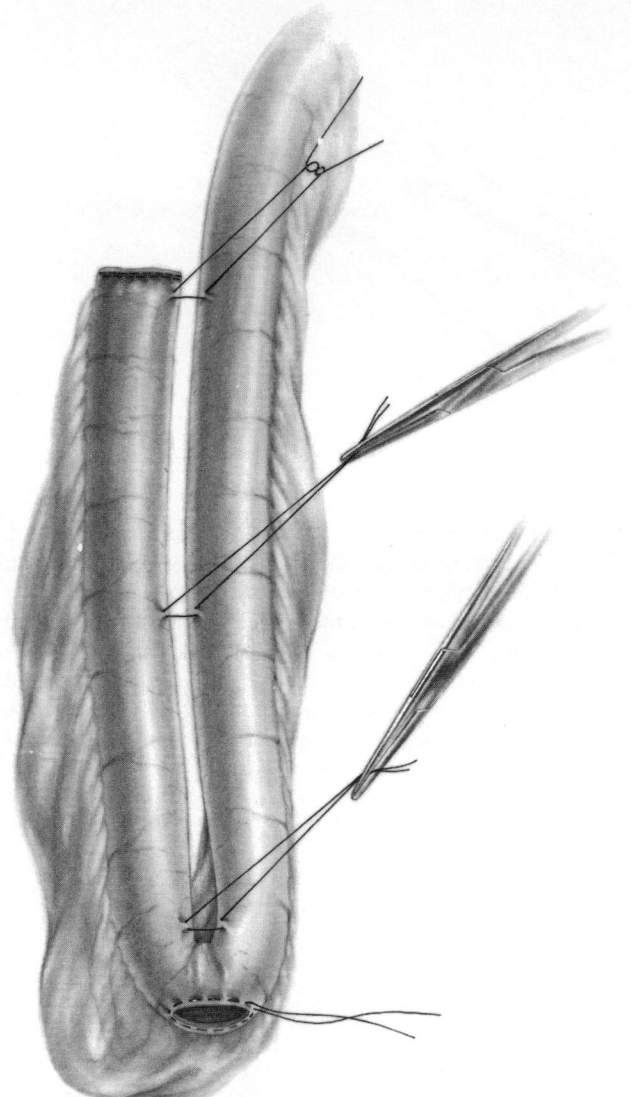

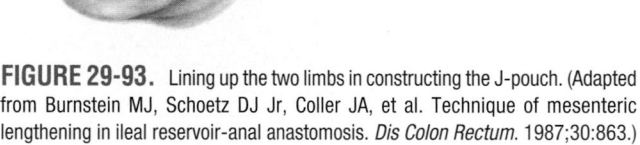

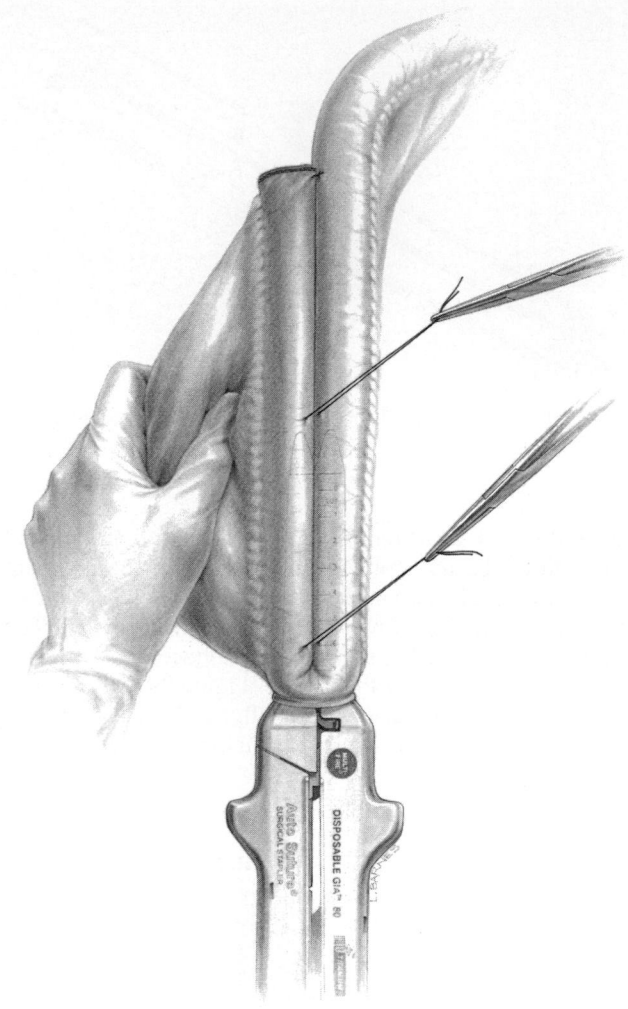

FIGURE 29-94. Tension on bowel mesentery prevents injury from stapler.

FIGURE 29-93. Lining up the two limbs in constructing the J-pouch. (Adapted from Burnstein MJ, Schoetz DJ Jr, Coller JA, et al. Technique of mesenteric lengthening in ileal reservoir-anal anastomosis. *Dis Colon Rectum.* 1987;30:863.)

its incorporation in the line of staples (Figures 29-93 and 29-94). This opening can then be used for insertion of the proximal anvil (Figure 29-95). With this technique, it may be necessary to pass the instrument cephalad once or twice more, using an intussuscepting maneuver (Figure 29-96). Nduka and colleagues suggest the use of an endoscopic stapler (Endo-GIA) to create the J-reservoir.[530] The length of this instrument allows the device to be applied multiple times without the problem of intussuscepting the intestine. Others have suggested performing the operation laparoscopically.[377,615]

Effecting the Anastomosis

Technique. With the apical purse-string suture in place, Peck initially described completing the anastomosis by means of the circular stapling instrument.[580] Another purse-string suture is placed at the top of the anal canal, incorporating the internal sphincter. The sutures are then secured, and the instrument is fired (Figure 29-97). By means of this alterna-

tive, Peck and others are more likely to abjure a protecting ileostomy (see later discussion).[580] Of course, one can use a suture technique, as has been previously described, to complete the pouch-anal anastomosis.

Another method for completing the anastomosis is to employ the double-stapling technique. This is analogous to the method used for effecting a low anastomosis for cancer of the rectum (see Chapter 24). The pouch construction is the same as described previously, but linear closure of the rectal stump is performed instead of a purse-string being used (Figure 29-98). Not uncommonly, however, it is not possible to place the linear stapling device sufficiently low onto the rectal stump. Under these circumstances, Schoetz and Coller advocate serial placement of the 30-mm instrument in two or three applications until the bowel is divided (D. J. Schoetz Jr and J. A. Coller, personal communication; Figure 29-99), although a single firing of the 30-mm device can often accomplish the task in this distal location.

Another technique is to perform a transanal application with a purse-string suture. This is often a tedious maneuver and risks excessive dilatation and stretching of the sphincter mechanism. A possible option is to perform eversion of the rectum to accomplish reestablishment of intestinal continuity and to facilitate a mucosectomy if one wishes to consider

Results).[314,356,580,664,674] However, there is legitimate concern about leaving behind residual viable epithelium, and there is valid objection to unnecessary manipulation of the sphincter mechanism. How to reconcile the two mutually exclusive intentions has precipitated considerable debate. It is self-evident that the more one maneuvers and stretches the anal canal, the more likely one is to impact adversely on bowel control.

Some have criticized the double-stapling technique as inadequate for removing the rectal mucosa. The fear of the possibility of malignancy arising in the remaining glandular epithelium as well as the concern for symptoms from residual inflammation is quite real (see next section). Deen and colleagues opine that high anal transection and pouch-anal anastomosis should be the preferred option in restorative proctocolectomy because a dentate line anastomosis may not fully eliminate columnar epithelium.[125] Moreover, Thompson-Fawcett and coworkers have demonstrated that the anal transitional zone is shorter than most people have recognized, and that after double-stapled restorative proctocolectomy there remains a 1.5- to 2.0-cm cuff of diseased columnar epithelium, an important consideration for long-term follow-up.[733] Preservation of the anal transitional zone may actually preserve disease.[8] A particular concern arises if restorative proctocolectomy is performed with preservation of the anal transition zone in individuals who harbor high-grade dysplasia or carcinoma (see Dysplasia and Malignancy).[794] Some of the criticism may be addressed if one understands that there is further distal rectum removed in the tissue ring when the circular stapler is applied, but there has now developed a considerable literature on the problems associated with residual, viable epithelium.

Mucosectomy (Yes or No!)
Keighley evaluated the functional results following J-pouch construction by comparing endoanal mucosectomy and abdominal mucosectomy.[334] He noted a statistically significant decrease in resting anal canal pressure after the endoanal procedure, but this was not observed with the abdominal approach. The author attributed the increased incidence of soiling with the former technique to the prolonged duration and extent of anal retraction that is required. Gemlo and coworkers conclude that avoidance of mucosectomy does not influence stool frequency but does significantly improve fecal continence and, in their opinion, introduces an undetectable morbidity associated with the retained rectal mucosa.[196] Becker and associates found that the loss of resting pressure of the internal anal sphincter could be correlated with the extent of smooth muscle resection during rectal mucosectomy, and that these factors correlate with increased stool frequency and a greater likelihood of nocturnal stool leakage (see Bowel Frequency and Continence).[43] Others have concluded that a stapled pouch-anal anastomosis, preserving the mucosa of the anal transitional zone, confers no apparent early advantage in terms of decreased stool frequency or fewer episodes of fecal incontinence compared with hand-sewn anastomosis, excising the mucosa.[612] However, they observed that the stapled group had higher resting pressures and less nighttime incontinence.[612]

Dysplasia and Malignancy
One of the concerns expressed when one performs restorative proctocolectomy is the risk for the development of carcinoma

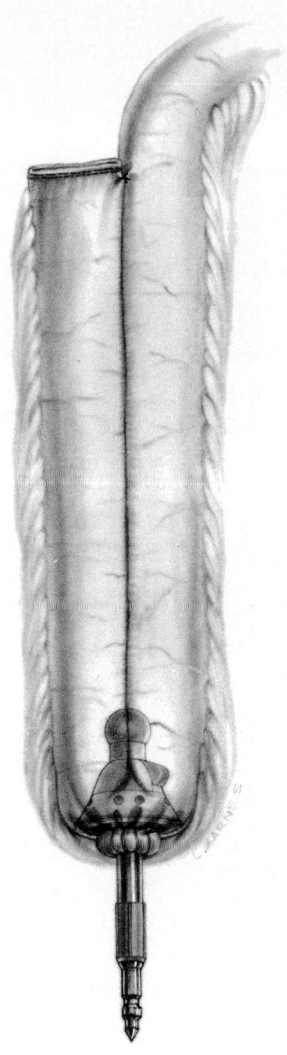

FIGURE 29-95. Anvil head is placed in the apex of the reservoir at the site of insertion of the long GIA stapler. The purse-string suture is then secured.

this[516] (Figure 29-100). By using this approach, Régimbeau and colleagues were able to perform a hand-sewn anal anastomosis on the dentate line, thereby avoiding an incomplete mucosectomy.[610] Another technique has been described by means of stapling a drain to the rectal stump and then pulling it through to evert the rectum.[669] The problem, as alluded to earlier, is that eversion is not associated with as good a functional outcome when compared with a stapled anastomosis prepared without eversion.[500,779]

The stapling technique has permitted relatively effortless pouch construction and anastomosis. As such, it is preferred by the overwhelming majority of surgeons.[126,291,356,695,794] But there are consequences! Figure 29-101 demonstrates the radiographic appearance of a satisfactorily completed J-pouch.

Where to Place the Anastomosis
Where to place the anastomosis is a matter of controversy. Although there is some difference of opinion, most agree that a reservoir anastomosis at the level of the dentate line is associated with suboptimal functional results compared with an anastomosis at the top of the anal canal (see

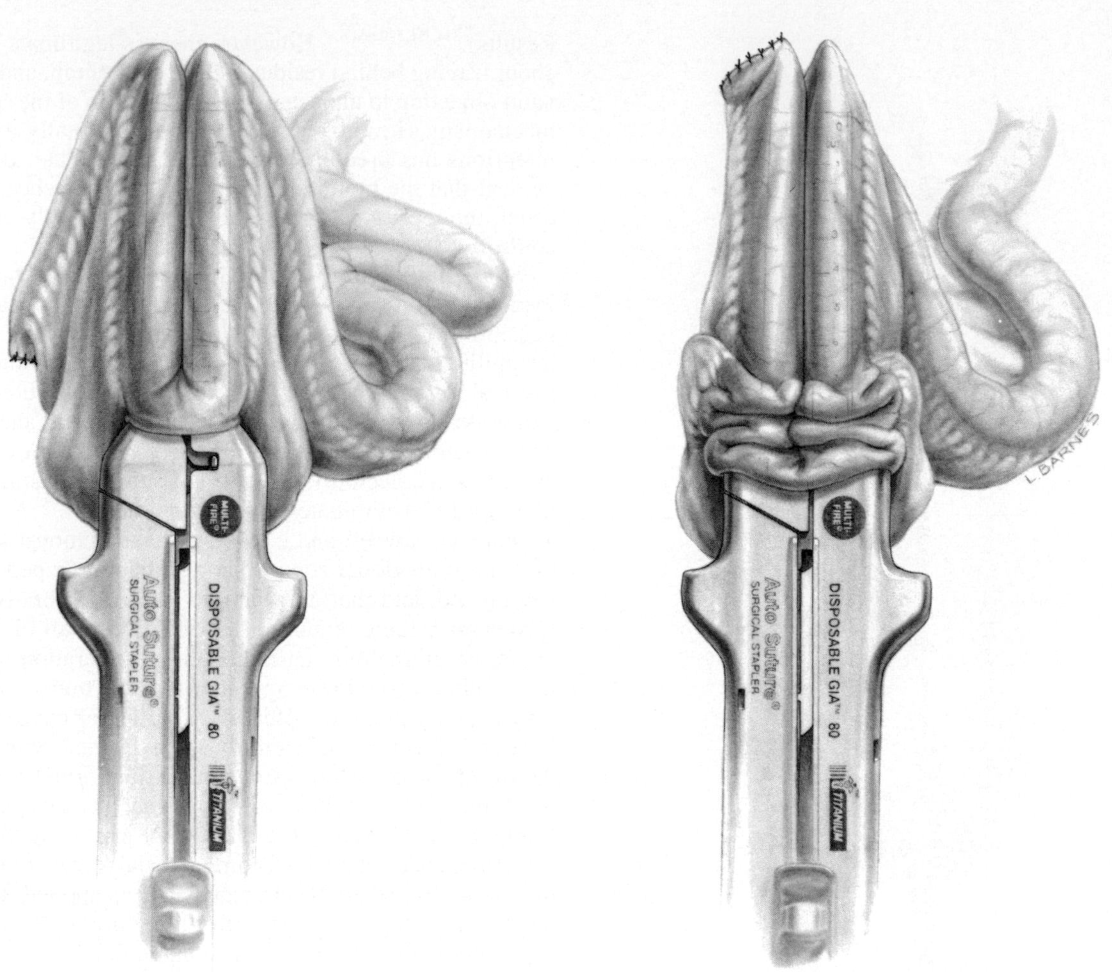

A

B

FIGURE 29-96. Construction of J-pouch with long (8-cm) GIA stapler. **A:** Apex entry. **B:** Intussusception after single firing of instrument from apical position.

if there is residual rectal mucosa present. Stern and colleagues reported the first such experience, a patient who had undergone a "classic" mucosectomy.[706] Since then, several cases have been described.[28,48,387,600,635] Ståhlberg and coworkers opine that this risk may be greater in individuals with concomitant sclerosing cholangitis.[698] Invasive adenocarcinoma has also been described in the pouch, itself,[50,301] but it is unclear whether these arose from the ileal mucosa or from residual rectal epithelium. Heppell and coworkers obtained pathologic specimens of the ileoanal anastomoses from eight patients who required takedown.[272] Reepithelialization of the rectal sleeve did not occur, although a few isolated rectal mucosal cells were seen. In a similar study of 29 patients, O'Connell and coworkers found that the rectal muscle cuff was bound to ileal serosa by dense fibrous tissue.[558] Active rectal mucosal disease, dysplasia, or reepithelialization was not observed.

With less attention to mucosectomy and with no attempt to preserve a muscular sleeve, the concern for the subsequent development of malignancy should be minimal. However, Löfberg and colleagues identified a patient who underwent an S-pouch procedure and who was found 4 years later to harbor low-grade dysplasia and DNA aneuploidy on random biopsy.[435] In an evaluation from the Cleveland Clinic (Florida) of 109 patients who underwent restorative proctocolectomy with nonmucosectomy

and a double-stapled reservoir anastomosis, the risk for malignant transformation in the strip of retained anorectal mucosa was found to be slight and did not increase appreciably in the first few years after operation.[247] According to a further report from our unit, if there is symptomatic proctitis from the residual mucosa, delayed mucosectomy via a perineal approach can be successfully accomplished, provided that the stapled anastomosis is within 3 or 4 cm of the dentate line.[160]

The principle discussed earlier in this chapter concerning the significance of *dysplasia* in ulcerative colitis has been applied to surveillance of those individuals who have undergone restorative proctocolectomy. Coull and coworkers, at the Glasgow Royal Infirmary, analyzed 135 patients by means of cuff surveillance biopsy.[109] There was no evidence of either dysplasia or carcinoma in any of the patients. They concluded that cuff surveillance in the first decade after this operation, in the absence of dysplasia or carcinoma in the original colectomy specimen, is unnecessary. Others confirm the rarity of such changes, but there appears to be a consensus among those most familiar with this operation that an *annual surveillance program* is suggested for all individuals who have undergone restorative proctocolectomy.[567,617,732] However, as with the Kock pouch, routine biopsy of the reservoir itself does not appear to be indicated.[274]

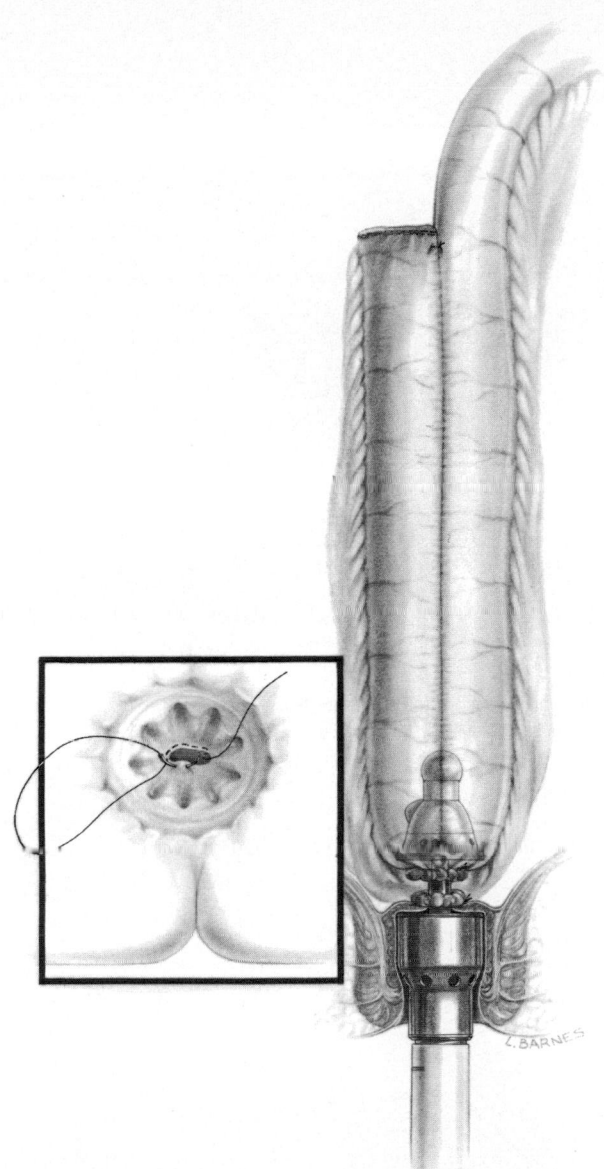

FIGURE 29-97. Pouch-anal anastomosis by means of circular stapler. Insertion of purse-string suture in the anal canal (*inset*).

Two reports of patients in whom a lymphoma developed in the pouch following this operation have been described.[184,552]

Appropriateness of Restorative Proctocolectomy with Concomitant Cancer

With respect to whether restorative proctocolectomy is appropriate for patients found to harbor a carcinoma with ulcerative colitis or polyposis, Wiltz and colleagues suggest that it is probably prudent to delay the pouch construction until a later date because of the potential difficulty of intraoperative staging and the possible requirement for adjuvant therapy.[781] Radiation of the ileal reservoir is poorly tolerated and will inevitably be associated with suboptimal functional results. It would seem self-evident that these individuals should undergo complete mucosectomy and be followed closely.

Management of Residual Symptomatic Mucosa or Dysplasia

If a patient develops bothersome symptoms of rectal bleeding from residual rectal epithelium or is found to harbor

dysplasia, mucosectomy with pouch advancement is indicated. This can usually be accomplished without adversely affecting bowel function (continence and frequency) but may not be easy to accomplish because of scarring. At the very least, the mucosa can and should be ablated. Close follow-up surveillance is, of course, required.

Lateral Ileal Pouch

Fonkalsrud has been an advocate of another type of ileoanal-pouch, the lateral ileal reservoir.[172–174] This is accomplished by dividing and oversewing the proximal end of the ileum approximately 25 to 30 cm above the peritoneal reflection. In the opinion of the author, an ileal reservoir of 14 to 16 cm in length appears to provide optimal function.[703] A temporary end ileostomy is then used for diversion (Figure 29-102A). A lateral reservoir is constructed over the entire length of the original segment at a subsequent operation (Figure 29-102B). Fonkalsrud's approach seems to be used essentially by him alone and has never achieved the popularity of the other alternatives. In fact, Fonkalsrud ultimately adopted the less controversial J-pouch technique prior to his retirement.

W-Pouch

One of the concerns about the S-reservoir is the fact that many patients require catheterization of the pouch to effect evacuation. Conversely, the J-pouch, although eliminating the requirement for catheterization, has been thought to be associated with increased stool frequency because of a smaller reservoir capacity (see later discussion). To address these problems, another modification has been proposed, the so-called quadruple-loop or W-reservoir.[539] The terminal 50 cm of small bowel are folded into four loops, each 12 cm long, forming a W-shaped configuration (Figure 29-103). The W-pouch can also be constructed with the stapling instruments (Figure 29-104). Like the J-pouch, the reservoir itself may be anastomosed to the anal canal.

Pouch with "Nipple"

Harms and colleagues have suggested a modification whereby the apex of the second loop is positioned 3 to 4 cm short of the apex of the first to create a "nipple" on the end of the pouch, making the area for the anastomosis somewhat narrower.[253] Peck adopts an isoperistaltic nipple valve with the J-pouch in the hope of (1) preventing reflux, (2) effecting more complete emptying of the reservoir, (3) minimizing perianal irritation, and (4) slowing intestinal transit[590] (Figure 29-105). There have been no further data on this approach since its initial publication.

Ileal Kock Pouch

Kock and colleagues reported the application of the standard, double-folded ileal reservoir (Kock pouch) as a pouch-anal alternative.[362] Six patients underwent interposition of the pouch between the ileum and the anus following colectomy and mucosal proctectomy. After the ileostomy was closed, the range of bowel evacuations was three to five per 24-hour period. The large reservoir capacity and the low pressure were believed to explain the excellent functional results. Further experience with this approach seems warranted but has not been evident in the literature.

Concomitant Ileostomy

Irrespective of the type of pouch undertaken, a loop ileostomy is usually advised to protect the anastomosis[345]

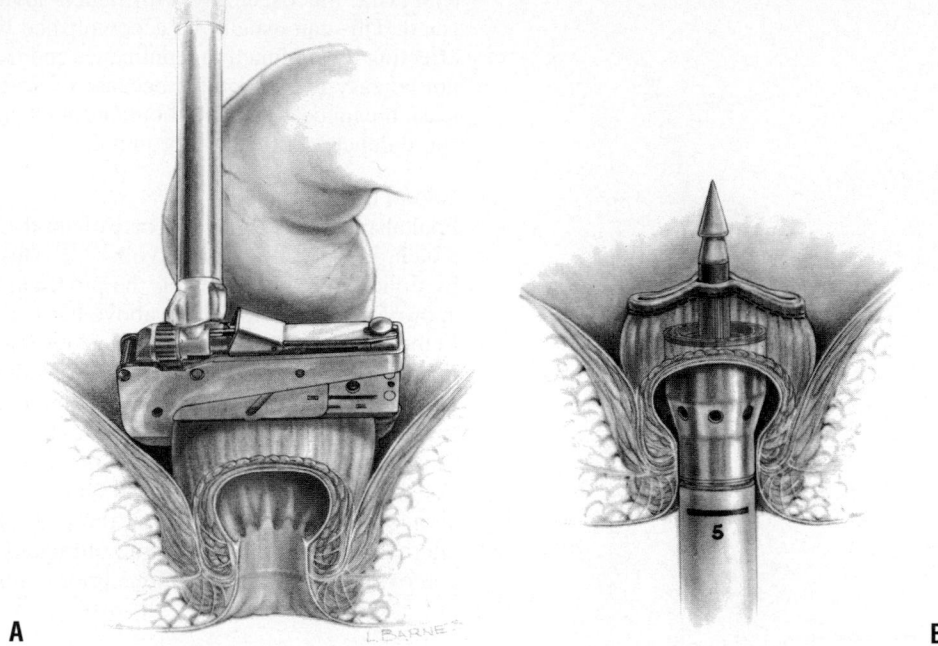

A   **B**

FIGURE 29-98. Pouch-anal anastomosis by double-stapling technique. **A:** Roticulator facilitates linear closure of rectal remnant. **B:** The trocar tip of the circular, end-to-end (CEEA) instrument effects anastomosis to the reservoir. (Courtesy of Covidien, Inc., Norwalk, CT.)

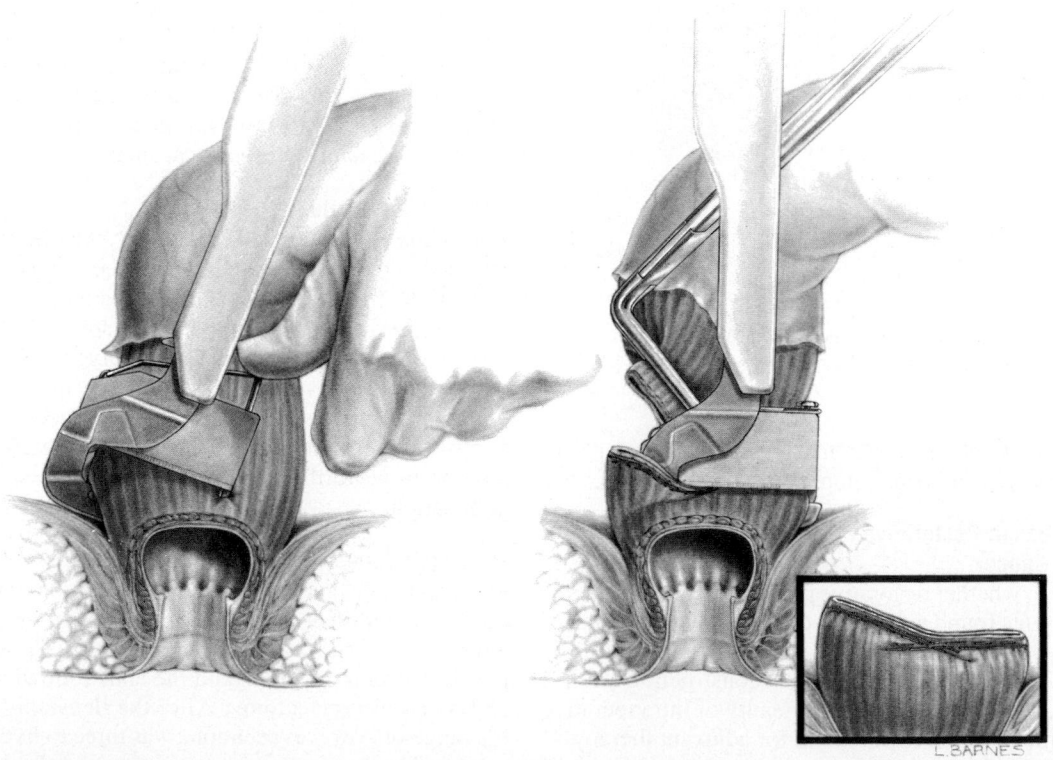

A   **B**

FIGURE 29-99. An alternative method of accomplishing pouch-anal anastomosis by double-stapling technique with narrow pelvis. **A:** Linear stapler (30 mm) is applied across a portion of the rectum. Note that the pin must be pressed through the bowel wall for the instrument to fire. **B:** Overlapping staple lines are created with a second application of the 30-mm linear stapler. The anastomosis is then completed in the manner described in Figure 29-98.

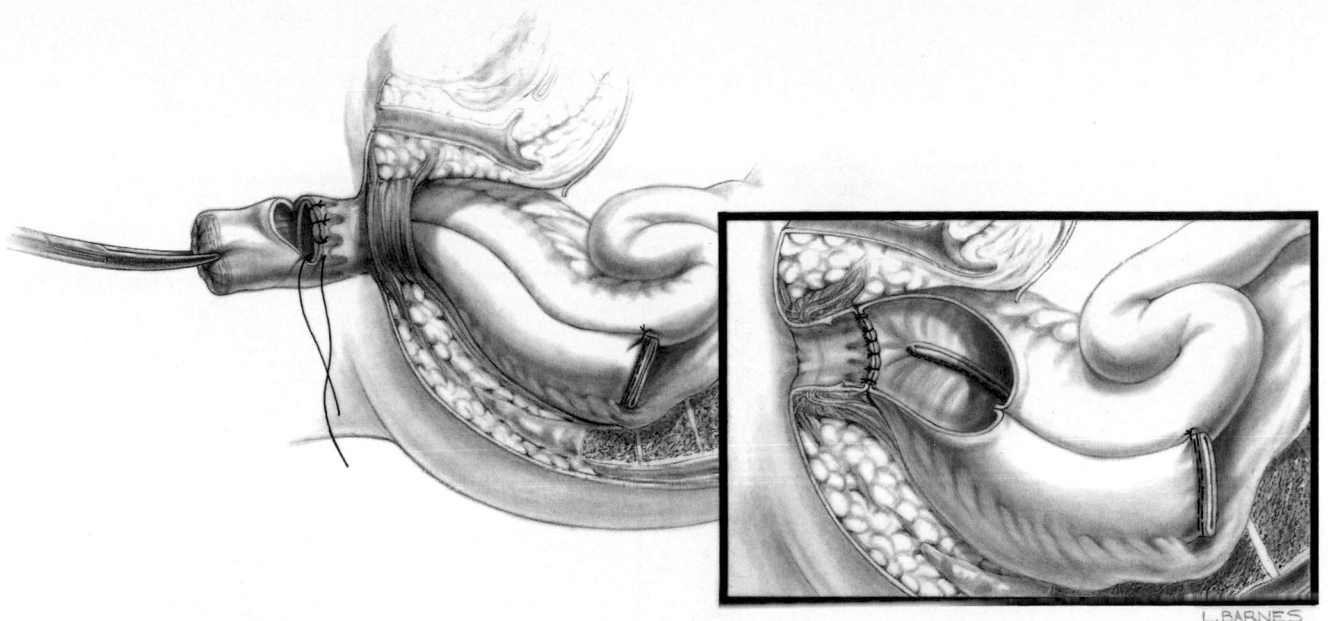

FIGURE 29-100. J-pouch "Swenson" procedure. **A:** The rectum is transected by quadrants just above the dentate line, allowing the ileal J-pouch anastomosis to be undertaken in a controlled manner. **B:** Completed anastomosis. (After Motta JC, Ricketts RR. The J-pouch Swenson procedure for ulcerative colitis and familial polyposis. *Am Surg.* 1992;58:613.)

(Figure 29-106; see Figures 31-67 through 31-69), but some surgeons have selectively performed the procedure without a diversionary stoma.[467] The construction and closure of an ileostomy is not without morbidity (see Chapter 31) and may actually increase the risk for postoperative bowel obstruction. Winslet and colleagues observed that formation and closure of a loop ileostomy were associated with 41% and 30% complication rates, respectively, in a prospective evaluation of 34 patients.[782] Others have reported a statistically significant reduction in total hospital stay, reduced complication rates, fewer episodes of intestinal obstruction, and a shorter operating time in individuals not submitted to ileostomy at the time of pouch construction.[221,230,277,287,308,518,519,646]

Galandiuk and coworkers related the Mayo Clinic experience of 37 patients who underwent an ileal J-pouch procedure without ileostomy.[190] When they were compared

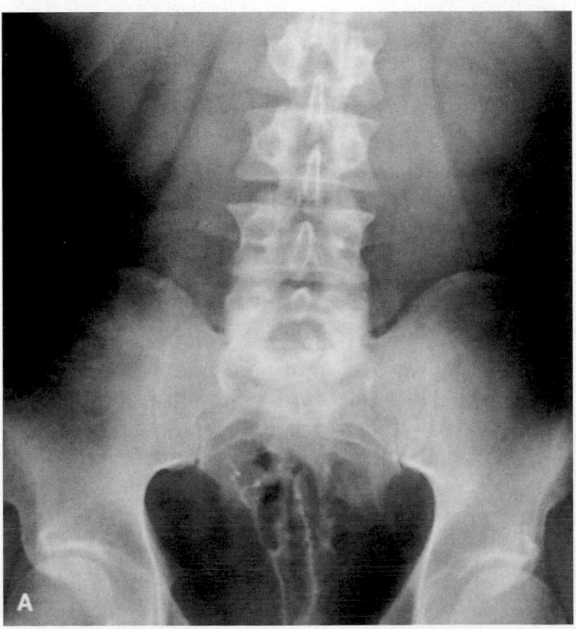 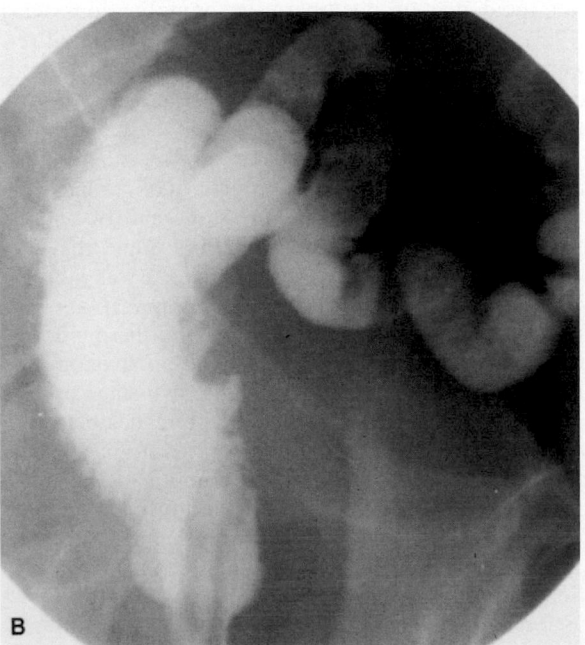

FIGURE 29-101. J-pouch anal anastomosis by stapling technique. **A:** Plain abdominal film demonstrates double line of staples forming the reservoir. **B:** Barium study before ileostomy closure reveals an intact pouch.

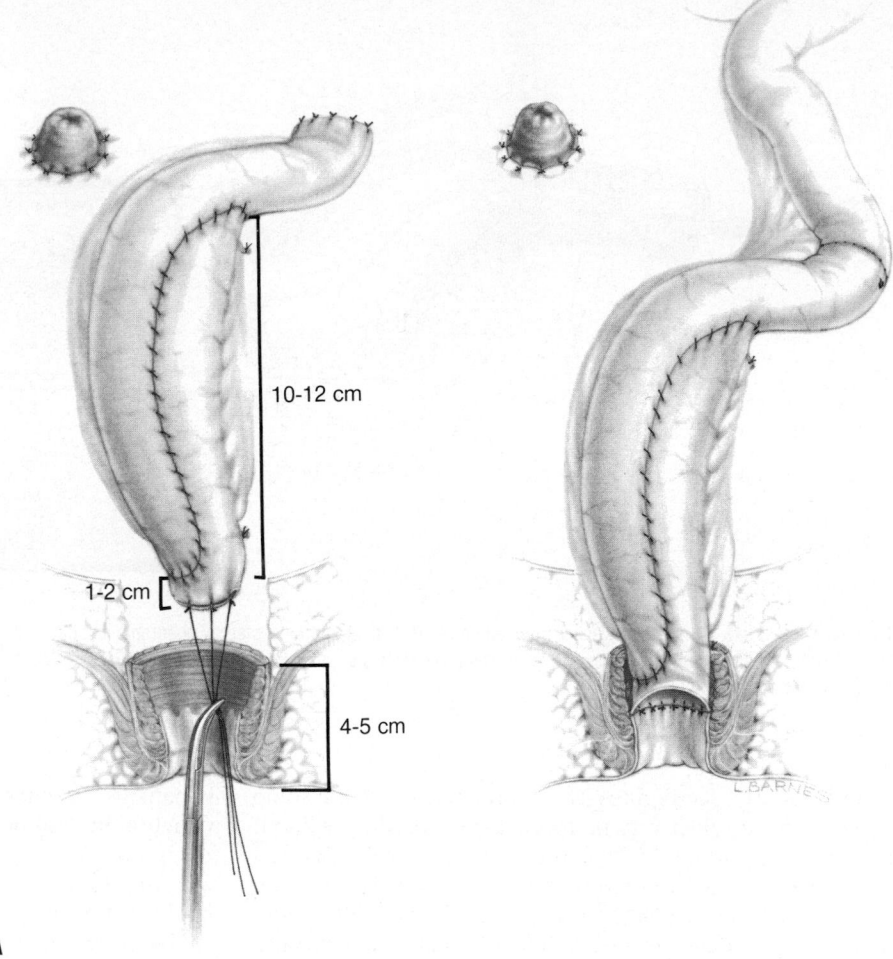

FIGURE 29-102. Lateral ileal reservoir (Fonkalsrud). **A:** Ileal reservoir is created using a side-to-side technique, either by hand-sewing or with the long GIA instrument. **B:** The ileal spout is drawn through the rectal muscle cuff to the anus, and the ileoanal anastomosis is effected. Note that Fonkalsrud prefers to use an end ileostomy. (Adapted from Fonkalsrud EW, Phillips JD. Reconstruction of malfunctioning ileoanal pouch procedures as an alternative to permanent ileostomy. *Am J Surg.* 1990;160:245.)

A

B

with a matched group of patients having a protecting stoma, a higher incidence of postoperative complications was noted (22% vs. 11%). However, subsequent functional results were comparable. According to the authors, suggested criteria for considering this option are absolute lack of tension on the anastomosis, good blood supply to the terminal ileum, good general health, and absence of recent steroids. Similarly, Heuschen and coworkers undertook a matched-pair control study in which the one-stage and two-stage operations were compared.[277] The authors found that the proportion of patients *without* complications was significantly higher, and the frequency of late complications was significantly lower in the one-stage group. Furthermore, the percentage of individuals who developed an anastomotic stricture was significantly higher with the two-stage operation. There were no other significant differences between the two groups with respect to a number of variables: early complications, pouch-related septic complications, pouchitis, duration of surgery, blood loss, and median hospital stay. The critical recommendation in this nonprospective study is "*if there is a choice* [italics, mine] . . . the one stage operation is clearly superior."

Launer and Sackier offer another method for avoiding a protecting ileostomy with this operation, that of the intraluminal bypass tube (Coloshield; Figure 29-107).[386] The authors reported no anastomotic complications or morbidity

related to the bypass tube in eight patients, but the device is not available in the United States.

Several reports have expressed caution with respect to the failure to employ temporary ileostomy when a reservoir-anal procedure is performed. Williamson and associates observed that life-threatening complications were more common among patients who did not have a defunctioning ileostomy.[780] Others observe that restorative proctocolectomy without diversion is not as safe as when it is performed with an ileostomy, especially in persons taking in excess of 20 mg of prednisone per day.[736]

Opinion

Caution would seem to dictate that an ileostomy is a requisite if there is the suggestion of tension on the suture line or if the procedure is performed for fulminant disease. A host of the usual relative contraindications should be considered (e.g., nutritional status, high-dose steroids). If I elect to abjure fecal diversion concomitant with a restorative proctocolectomy, it should have been a technically flawless and uncomplicated operation, with a perfect anastomosis, with no steroid side effects, and with the patient in a good nutritional state. I recognize that there are a number of qualified surgeons who would not be as restrictive. However, I have sufficient chevrons on my sleeve to categorically state that if I do not have to deal with the consequences of another anastomotic leak for

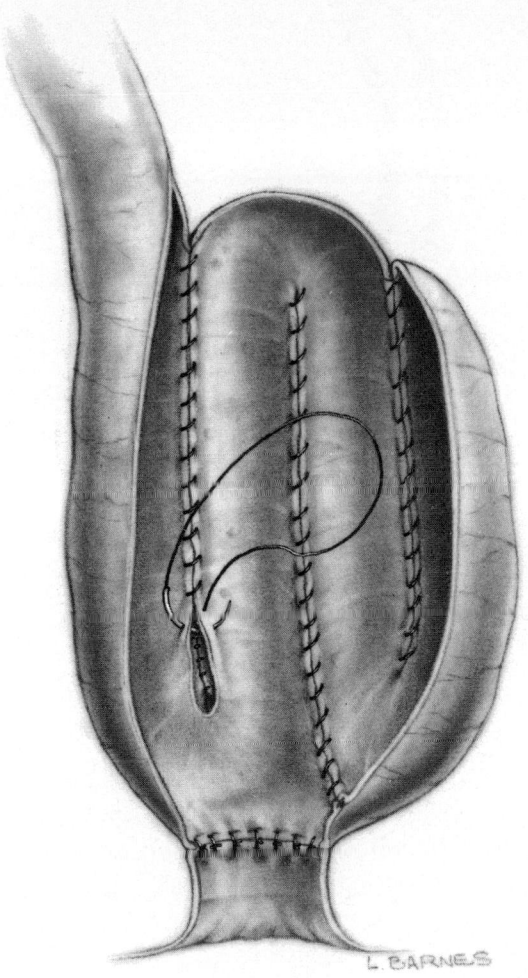

FIGURE 29-103. Quadruple reservoir—hand-sewn.

the remainder of my operating days, I will not be chagrined. One needs to remember, however, that a defunctionalized, stapled anastomosis tends to stricture. My own preference, therefore, is to perform gentle, finger dilatation on a biweekly basis until the stoma has been closed.

Laparoscopic Approach

There is no denying the fact that highly qualified, respected surgeons are applying minimally invasive principles to this operation (see Chapter 19). Many use the technique primarily for taking down the flexures and performing a hypogastric transverse incision for the resection, pouch creation and anastomosis, but some surgeons complete virtually the entire procedure by laparoscopic means. As discussed earlier in this chapter, the concept of minilaparotomy has addressed all of the issues for me that theoretically allow any advantage to laparoscopy (except for flexure mobilization). The functional outcome and the quality of life of laparoscopic-assisted restorative proctocolectomy is not different from that of the conventionally performed surgery.[142]

Postoperative Management

Following one-stage surgery or closure of the ileostomy, patients inevitably are troubled by frequent bowel movements and perhaps problems with continence. It is, therefore, important to prepare the patient emotionally for these consequences and to offer management alternatives. As with ostomates, a wound care or an enterostomal therapist is an invaluable resource for counseling patients.[246] Certain food may increase or decrease stool output and frequency. Those that have been demonstrated to exacerbate gastrointestinal disturbances are apple juice, raw fruits, raw vegetables, popcorn, seeds, nuts, beans, corn, beer, caffeine, chocolate, milk and milk products, and spicy foods. The diet may be supplemented by one of the liquid nutrition products (e.g., Ensure). Ample fluid intake is strongly encouraged to avoid dehydration. Dehydration requiring readmission to the hospital occurred in 20% of the patients in the University of Toronto experience.[164] Supplementary medication in the form of slowing agents is often helpful (e.g., loperamide [Imodium], diphenoxylate [Lomotil], deodorized tincture of opium, paregoric, and codeine). A bulking agent, such as one containing psyllium, may be added, and cholestyramine (Questran) may be ameliorative for some individuals, even without a colon. Topical agents for perianal irritation may be required. An aggressive approach to the medical management of these patients is necessary in order to give them confidence until time permits bowel function to become relatively stabilized.

Complications of the Pouch Procedures

Despite the magnitude of the operation, operative mortality has been remarkably low—virtually anecdotal.[594] In a review from the Mayo Clinic involving 1,603 patients who underwent proctocolectomy with pouch-anal reconstruction, three deaths occurred postoperatively (0.2%).[367] Pulmonary embolism, perforated gastric ulcer, and subarachnoid hemorrhage were the reasons. Late deaths occurred in 29 patients (1.8%).[367] These were primarily related to malignancy and to extracolonic manifestations of underlying or unrelated coexisting diseases and events.[367] However, all published reports recognize that ileoanal-reservoir operations are associated with a high frequency of complications, often well in excess of 50%. These include pouchitis, anal stenosis, intestinal obstruction, "cuff abscess," stomal problems, ileus, fistulas, sepsis, hemorrhage, ischemia, bowel management problems, and others.[180,336,461,483,587,594,772] Generally, complications are more frequent in the early experience with the operation than in the later. Despite what may appear to be indomitable problems, every effort should be made to preserve the pouch. The success with various salvage operations has been reported by a number of investigators (see later discussion).[179,189,533,666,734]

Perforation. With the techniques currently applied for creation of the reservoir, perforation of the pouch itself has become relatively unusual. The rate from Cohen's group at the Toronto General Hospital has been constant at approximately 4%, but the requirement for reservoir excision as a consequence of this complication has decreased as experience has been gained.[99,170] Other centers report rates of 1% to 2%. Perforation of the terminal ileal appendage of the J-pouch has also been noted[591] (Figure 29-108). To avoid this complication, it is probably wise to secure the distal ileum to the reservoir or to amputate any terminal ileal appendage after pouch construction. Parenthetically, perforation of the pouch as a consequence of blunt trauma to the abdomen has also been noted,[288] and one instance has been recorded of a perforation in a woman at 27 weeks' gestation, which was believed to be due to adhesions from the posterior wall of the uterus to the pouch.[11]

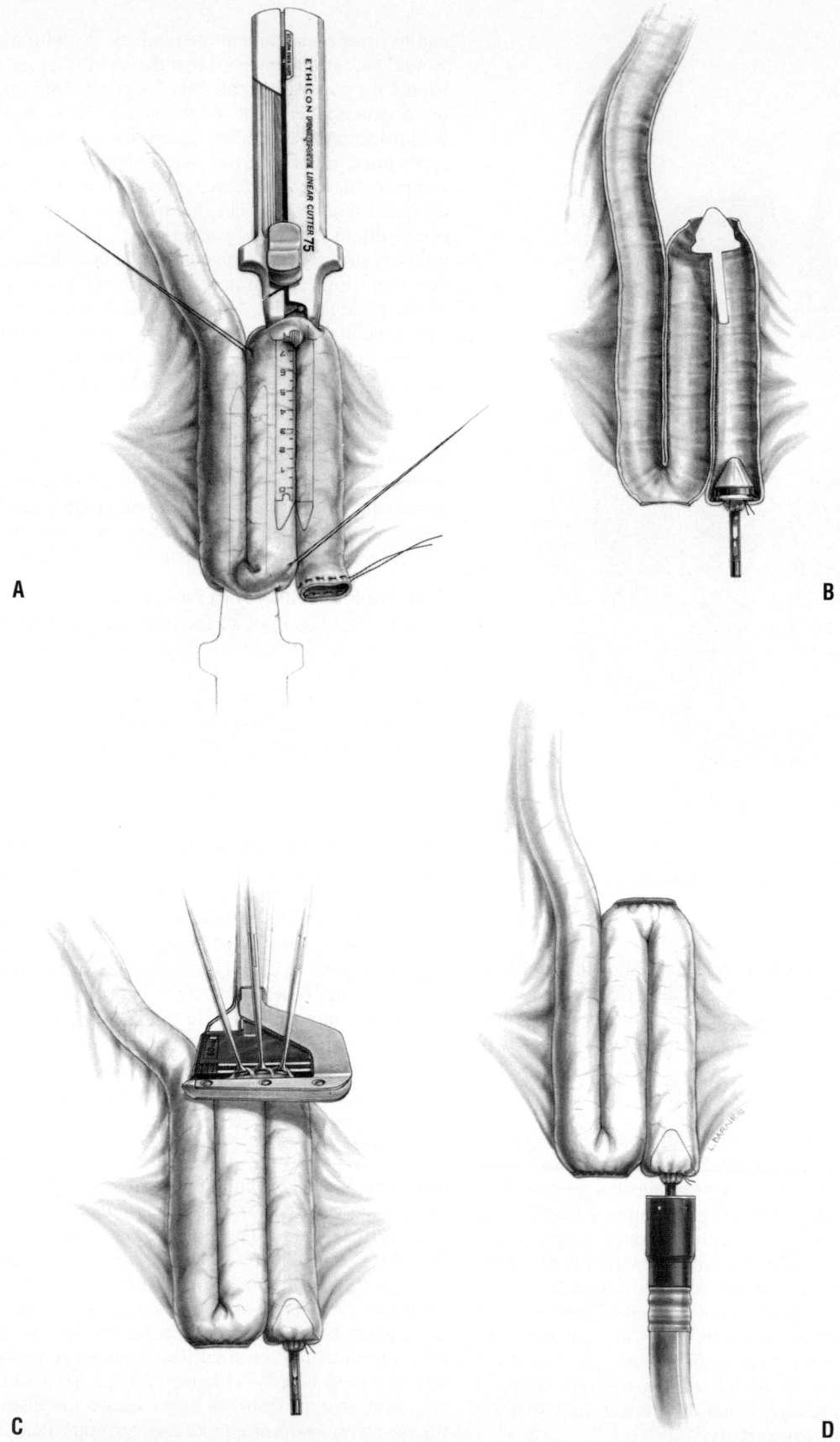

FIGURE 29-104. S-reservoir anal anastomosis by stapling method. **A:** Long GIA stapler is passed twice (in opposite directions). **B:** The detachable anvil head is passed through one of the GIA stapler openings into the most distal limb. Alternatively, linear closure of the other areas can be effected and the proximal limb used. **C:** Linear stapler closure is completed. **D:** The anastomosis to the anal area (not shown) is accomplished in the usual way.

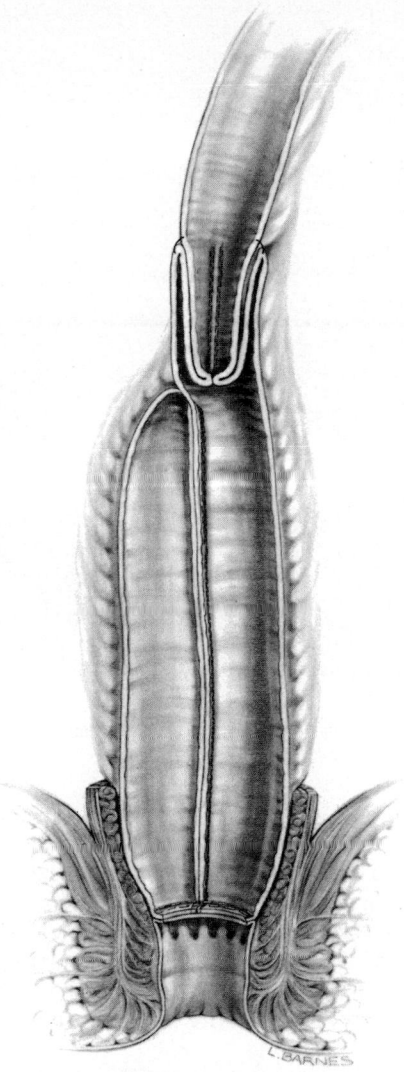

FIGURE 29-105. J-pouch anal procedure with isoperistaltic valve, as suggested by Peck.

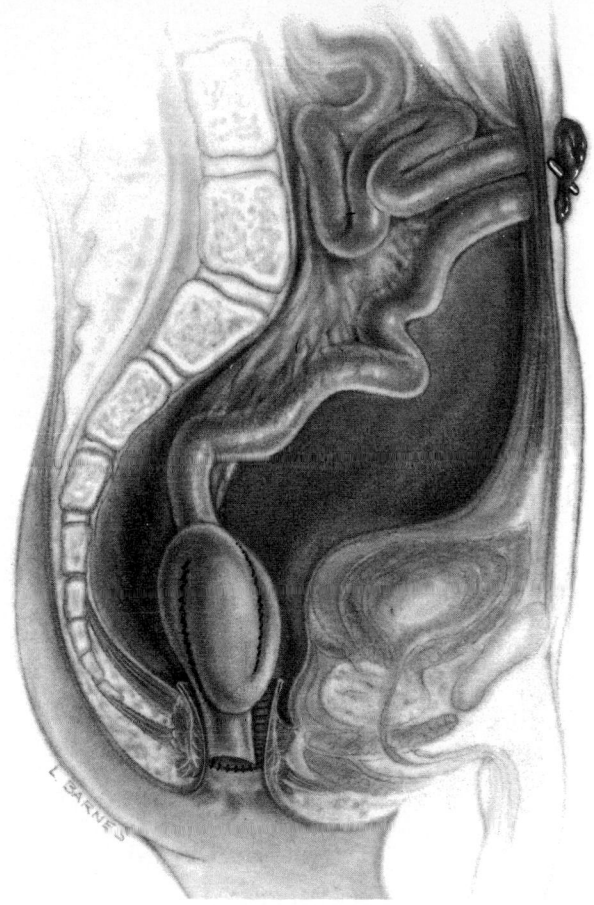

FIGURE 29-106. Final position of pouch-ileoanal anastomosis (S-type) with protecting loop ileostomy.

Anastomotic Leak. Anastomotic leak is inevitably caused by one or more of the usual suspects (tension on the suture line, ischemia, pelvic hematoma, or sepsis) and is often associated with the subsequent development of an anal stricture. It is because of the risk for this complication that a protecting ileostomy is usually advised. Fleshman and colleagues reported a 10% anal anastomotic leak rate in 179 patients.[170] The Mayo Clinic group revealed that radiologic or clinical leaks from the pouch or ileoanal anastomosis occurred in 14%.[726] However, because most centers have adopted a stapling technique, very little has been reported with respect to this particular complication in recent years. Whether this is because of the application of an ileostomy by most surgeons or the failure to pursue appropriate investigation of patients within the first few weeks after operation is not known. Still, according to the University of Toronto group, although the leak rate has remained relatively stable, leaks following a stapled anastomosis seem to have a better prognosis than those that occur following hand-sewn anastomosis.[443]

It is generally agreed that the major causes for pouch failure are poor functional results, pelvic sepsis, and unsuspected

Crohn's disease, as opposed to the other complications, including pouchitis and anastomotic leak.[197]

Cuff Abscess. Pelvic abscess was observed in 11% of patients in the earlier Mayo Clinic series.[493] As mentioned previously, Ambroze and colleagues favor preservation of the omentum to limit the risk for septic complications.[9] Keighley and colleagues observed a significant association between satisfactory functional results and pelvic sepsis.[336] Cuff abscess, specifically, results from the creation of a long muscular sleeve, was a frequently recognized problem when this technique was popularized. Because all surgeons now seem to avoid the creation of a muscular sleeve, this complication has disappeared, at least from the literature.

Intestinal Obstruction. Intestinal obstruction is one of the most frequently encountered problems after this operation. In the experience of Fleshman and colleagues, it developed in 19% of patients,[170] whereas McMullen and coworkers noted a 16% incidence.[483] Initial reports from the Mayo Clinic revealed that small bowel obstruction was noted in 22%, almost one-half of whom required surgical intervention.[493,582] A later assessment found the incidence to be 17%.[183] The obstruction may be caused by adhesions, internal hernia, reservoir angulation, or outlet problems, or it may be related to the loop ileostomy.[170,175,176]

As has been discussed in Chapter 23, the frequency of abdominal adhesions leading to intestinal obstruction

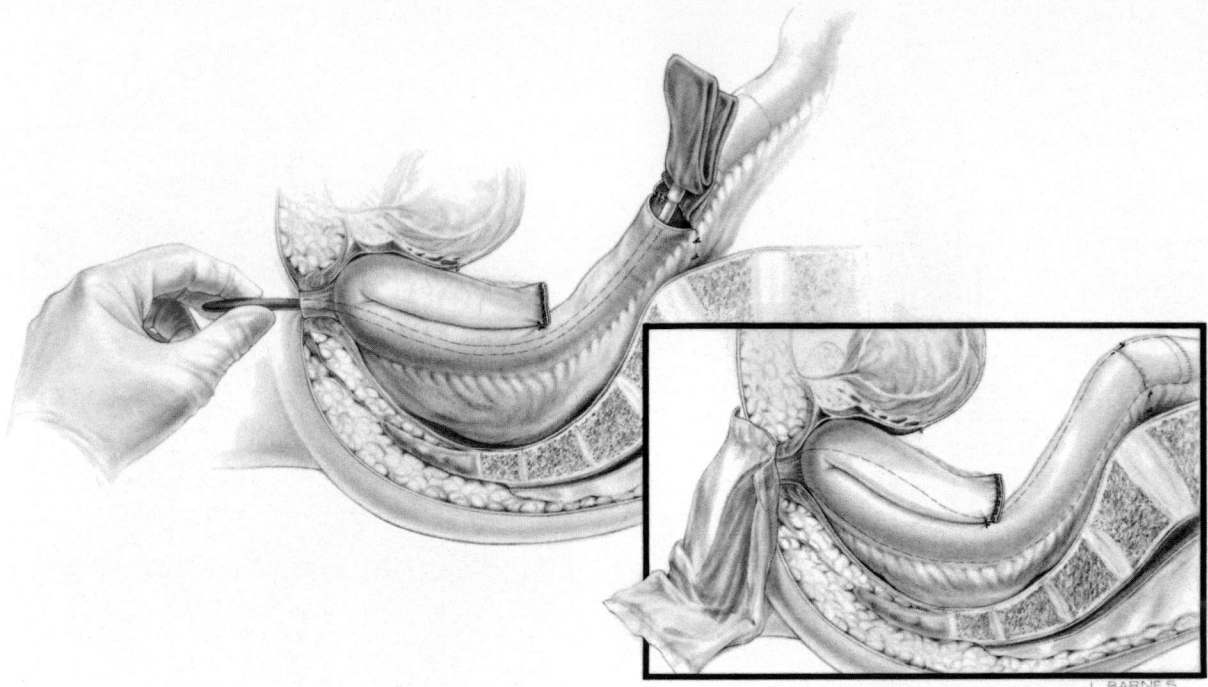

FIGURE 29-107. Ileal J-pouch anal anastomosis using the Coloshield to avoid a temporary ileostomy. (Adapted from Launer DP, Sackier JM. Pouch-anal anastomosis without diverting ileostomy. *Dis Colon Rectum.* 1991;34:193.)

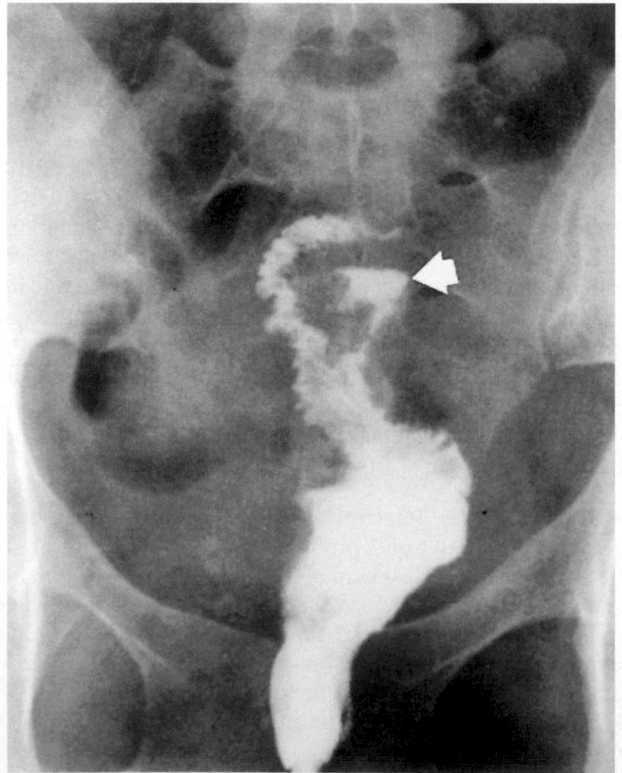

FIGURE 29-108. Pouch leakage. The distal pouch-anal anastomosis is intact. However, contrast is collecting adjacent to the proximal staple line (*arrow*). This proved to be caused by breakdown of the closed end of the reservoir.

precipitated a prospective, randomized trial with the use of a sodium hyaluronate-based bioresorbable membrane.[41] By means of direct, standardized peritoneal visualization before closure of the ileostomy, this membrane was demonstrated to be safe, and it also significantly reduced the incidence, extent, and severity of postoperative abdominal adhesions.[41]

In the experience of the Lahey Clinic surgeons, the most common point of obstruction was at closure of the ileostomy (52%).[458] The authors caution that the ileostomy should not be rotated to facilitate emptying because this seems to predispose to subsequent obstruction in a number of patients. In another report from the same institution, small bowel obstruction was often attributed to acute angulation of the afferent limb at the pouch inlet.[609] The authors offered the suggestion that bypass of the obstructed segment from the distal ileum to the pouch was not only possible but also constituted safe and effective management.

At least three cases of duodenal obstruction resulting from arteriomesenteric obstruction (superior mesenteric artery syndrome) have been reported.[23,91,205]

Stomal Complications. Ileostomy complications, such as stomal retraction, high ileostomy output, and parastomal hernia, are at least as frequent as the problems encountered relative to the pouch or the anastomosis. Stomal management problems are discussed in Chapters 31 and 32. In a report from the Mayo Clinic of 180 patients who underwent temporary ileostomy, transient bowel obstruction developed in 13% following takedown of the stoma.[491] More than one-half had problems with appliance management with retraction being seen in 16%. Other complications included prolapse, fistula, and abscess; ileostomy dysfunction alone was noted in 9%.[493] As discussed earlier, there have been suggestions by some experienced surgeons that a temporary ileostomy can be avoided in selected patients.[494] However, it has been demonstrated that patients with incomplete fecal diversion have a significantly higher incidence of pouch-anal anastomotic complications (44%) than those who have had complete diversion (14%).[491]

Pouch-Anal Sinus. Anastomotic breakdown usually occurs posteriorly and may ultimately lead to a sinus. If this is recognized prior to ileostomy closure, continued diversion is suggested. Otherwise, there is a risk of developing a pelvic abscess. But there comes a time when one must make a decision as to how to proceed. Probably it is wiser to create a larger opening and curette out the tract in order to permit adequate drainage. Removing a part of the back wall of the reservoir may be indicated in order to accomplish this adequately. Conversely, if the patient develops pelvic sepsis following ileostomy closure or if a stoma had not been performed in the first instance, an ileostomy must be established.

Swain and Ellis report successful treatment of pouch-anal anastomotic sinuses with fibrin glue.[717]

Pouch-Vaginal Fistula and Pouch-Perineal Fistula. Fistula between the pouch and the vagina is an uncommon complication following the pouch-anal operations, but is significantly more frequently observed when the operation is performed for ulcerative colitis than for familial adenomatous polyposis.[278] Although there is no clear documentation for the cause, it is likely due to trauma during the anterior dissection, either at the time of mobilization of the rectum through the abdomen or when a transanal dissection is undertaken. It is suspected that in the latter situation, a woman with an ectopic anus (anterior displacement) is most vulnerable (see Chapter 16). Another consideration is the possibility that the patient has Crohn's disease.

Wexner and colleagues reviewed the experience from a number of centers (304 women) and noted an incidence of 6.9% with this complication.[771] The group from the University of Minnesota noted fistulas from the ileoanal reservoir to the perianal skin in 5%, and fistulas from the reservoir or anastomotic line to other sites in an additional 4%.[772]

Treatment options are essentially those that have been previously described for the management of this condition when it is not associated with a pouch procedure (see Chapters 15 and 16). These include transanal, transabdominal, and transvaginal closure; endoanal advancement flap; seton division; fecal diversion; and gracilis muscle interposition.[78,218,335,461,771] Most surgeons prefer endovaginal or endoileal flap advancement.[563] It is probably prudent, however, to consider temporary ileostomy concomitant with any repair.

Our group achieved success in the treatment of fistulas from pelvic pouches in more than 60% of our patients.[570,676] However, we observed that multiple procedures may be needed for a successful outcome, and ultimately 32% had their pouches excised. Heuschen and colleagues found that the incidence of requiring permanent defunctioning or excision of the pouch in 131 patients with septic complications was 23.7% and 6.1%, respectively.[275] Moreover, the estimated 3-, 5-, and 10-year rate of pouch failure in those with septic complications was 9.6%, 31.1%, and 39.2%, respectively. In the Lahey Clinic experience, pouches

complicated by fistulas not associated with Crohn's disease could be salvaged with temporary rediversion.[171] Others observe that the prognosis appears to be worse when pouch-vaginal fistula occurs after ileostomy closure.[231] Late presentation of a vaginal fistula is more frequently associated with Crohn's disease and is unlikely to result in pouch salvage.[194,393,576,676]

Impairment of bowel control following conventional fistula surgery in women is the rule rather than the exception. The likelihood of keeping one's ileoanal reservoir with this complication is therefore problematic.

Epidural Abscess. Murr and Metcalf have described recurrent epidural abscesses from an enteroepidural fistula arising from a J-pouch.[521]

Anal (Anastomotic) Stricture. Considerable variation is evident in the reported incidence of anastomotic stricture following restorative proctocolectomy. This may be attributed to whether a hand-sewn or a stapled technique was employed and whether the procedure was undertaken in one or two stages. Furthermore, most papers do not stratify strictures in the absence of sepsis, sinus, or fistula from that which is seen as a consequence of septic complications. In the experience of the Mayo Clinic group, strictures were observed in 213 of 1,884 patients (11.2%), somewhat less than in their earlier reports.[491,597] This group found that nonfibrotic strictures responded well to anal dilatation, whereas fibrotic strictures were more likely due to septic problems and required more extensive revision and perhaps salvage pouch surgery. Anastomotic stricture occurred in approximately 8% of patients in the Toronto experience.[170] Overweight males and those with blood loss in excess of 1,000 mL have been found to have an increased incidence.[170] According to Fleshman and colleagues, the presence of an anal stricture was the most significant factor contributing to a less-than-satisfactory functional result.[170]

Treatment consists usually of dilatation, but persistent symptoms may require an anoplasty (see Chapter 11) or a pouch advancement and neoileoanal anastomosis.[158] In the experience of the group from the General Infirmary in Leeds, England, the eventual clinical, functional outcome after dilatation of a stricture (39 patients) was as good as the outcome in the 63 patients in whom a stricture did not develop.[412]

Pouchitis. *Pouchitis*, a term coined by Kock to describe the reservoir ileitis seen with the continent ileostomy, is a well-recognized complication of all pouch procedures and is seen about as frequently as that of small bowel obstruction (see earlier discussion). The condition is usually manifested by increased output of liquid stool, sometimes with blood; a low-grade fever; weakness; and malaise. Endoscopic findings include a granular, easily traumatized, edematous mucosa with ulceration and histologic presence of polymorphonuclear leukocyte infiltration with ulceration. This is superimposed on the expected chronic inflammatory cell presence with crypt hyperplasia and villous atrophy.[657] Solitary pouch ulceration has also been described.[170,182,665]

In the Mayo Clinic experience with 734 patients followed for a mean of 41 months, pouchitis developed in 31% of those with ulcerative colitis and 6% with familial polyposis.[439] In the experience of Becker and Raymond, pouchitis was the most common late complication (18%).[45] The Minnesota group noted an incidence of 27%.[772] Ståhlberg and coworkers noted that the risk for pouchitis was highest during the initial 6-month period following pelvic pouch construction.[697] This leveled off after 2 years but was still considerable at 4 years (51%). However, only 2 patients (1.3%) had their pouches removed because of this complication in the experience of this group.[697] Others have also demonstrated that the incidence is approximately 50%, with two-thirds of patients having multiple episodes.[297]

The most commonly used comparative diagnostic instrument is the Pouchitis Disease Activity Index, but it has been primarily a research tool. Still, it is helpful in developing an algorithm for diagnosis, classification, and management of this condition.[276] The index was created in 1994 by Sandborn and associates of the Mayo Clinic group.[657] It is an 18-point instrument that consists of three principal component scores: symptoms, endoscopy, and histology (Table 29-6).

TABLE 29-6 Pouchitis Disease Activity Index

CRITERIA	SCORE
Clinical	
Stool frequency	
Usual postoperative stool frequency	0
1–2 stools per day > postoperative usual	1
3 or more stools per day > postoperative usual	2
Rectal bleeding	
None or rare	0
Present daily	1
Fecal urgency or abdominal cramps	
None	0
Occasional	1
Usual	2
Fever (temperature >37.8° C)	
Absent	0
Present	1
Endoscopic Inflammation	
Edema	1
Granularity	1
Friability	1
Loss of vascular pattern	1
Mucous exudates	1
Ulceration	1
Acute Histologic Inflammation	
Polymorphic nuclear leukocyte infiltration	
Mild	1
Moderate + crypt abscess	2
Severe + crypt abscess	3
Ulceration per low-power field (mean)	
>25%	1
25%–50%	2
>50%	3

From Sandborn WJ, Tremaine WJ, Batts KP, et al. Pouchitis after ileal pouch anal anastomosis: a pouchitis disease activity index. *Mayo Clin Proc.* 1994;69:409.

The severity of the pouchitis has also been measured using another scoring system, the Heidelberg Pouchitis Activity Score.[276] A modified, somewhat simplified index has seen suggested by our group.[679]

ETIOLOGY AND ASSOCIATED CONDITIONS. Pouchitis is believed to be caused by stasis of feces in the pouch with overgrowth of anaerobic organisms. There is the general impression that pouchitis occurs rarely when the various reservoir procedures have been performed for familial polyposis.[444] It has, therefore, been suggested that the likely etiology is related somehow to that of ulcerative colitis.[668]

Gustavsson and colleagues assessed whether the presence of backwash ileitis predisposed to the subsequent development of this problem.[236] Because pouchitis subsequently developed in 13% of patients with backwash ileitis and 16% without ileitis, the authors concluded that there was no relationship. The Mayo Clinic group reported that patients with preoperative and postoperative extraintestinal manifestations had significantly higher rates of pouchitis than did those without such manifestations.[439]

The etiology of the condition has been investigated at a number of centers. Levin and colleagues support a role for mucosal ischemia and production of oxygen free radicals.[407] They employed allopurinol, a xanthine oxidase inhibitor, and found that this agent either terminated an episode of acute pouchitis or prevented pouchitis from recurring in 50% of their patients.[407] Others have observed that smokers have significantly fewer episodes of pouchitis when compared with nonsmokers and former smokers.[489] Finally, the finding that perinuclear antineutrophil cytoplasmic antibodies (pANCAs) occur more frequently in patients with chronic pouchitis suggests the possibility that this antibody may mark a genetically distinct subset of patients with ulcerative colitis who are predisposed to the subsequent development of pouchitis.[654] *C. difficile* infection as a cause of refractory pouchitis has also been reported.[453]

The Lahey Clinic group has recognized two apparently distinct patterns of presentation based on the clinical course: those with two or fewer episodes and those with more than two.[604] Those in the former group responded generally to anti-anaerobic organism therapy, whereas only 25% in the latter group did so. The authors also identified a subset of patients with so-called short-segment pouchitis. They attributed this to retained rectal mucosa and have treated the problem successfully with topical steroid preparations.

MANAGEMENT. Therapy is medical, provided that mechanical outlet obstruction has been ruled out. Treatment usually consists of oral metronidazole, the mainstay of antibiotic therapy,[445] or enemas containing steroids or salicylate derivatives, but recurrence is not uncommon (see earlier discussion). Recourse to ciprofloxacin and amoxicillin/clavulanic acid has been successful if metronidazole's side effects become troublesome or if the drug is no longer effective.[657] A small, randomized trial from our institution revealed a greater reduction of the Pouchitis Disease Activity Index in 6 patients on ciprofloxacin, 500 mg twice daily over 2 weeks, when compared with 9 patients on metronidazole (20 mg/kg).[684] The latter group demonstrated a 33% adverse event rate (emesis, dysgeusia, and peripheral neuropathy). In contrast, dual therapy of active pouchitis with ciprofloxacin and metronidazole over 4 weeks resulted in an 82% remission rate (36 of 44 patients) with 8 additional patients improved.[503]

Other agents include anti-inflammatory drugs, such as 5-ASA and sulfasalazine; immunomodulators, such as budesonide/hydrocortisone enemas and AZA/6-MP/oral steroid combinations; probiotics (VSL#3[201] and lactobacillus GG); nutritional supplements (e.g., glutamine); and butyrate suppositories.

Recurrent or intractable disease should alert the physician to the possibility of Crohn's disease involvement. What recourse is available to those patients who are found to have Crohn's disease after ileoanal pouch surgery? The initial Mayo series with *infliximab* showed a response in six of seven patients after failure of conventional therapy.[619] This experience has been expanded at the Mayo Clinic to 29 patients with Crohn's disease of the pouch, 69% of whom had perianal pouch-vaginal fistulas.[101,620] Half of the patients had a long-term response but required maintenance infliximab therapy. There is no effective surgical salvage for pouchitis.[744]

Skin Irritation. Severe perianal skin irritation is reported to occur in up to 10% of patients. This may be attributed to frequent bowel action and incontinence. Bowel management programs, including bulking agents and diphenoxylate hydrochloride (Lomotil) or loperamide (Imodium), have usually been advised. Topical application of 5% cholestyramine ointment in polyethylene glycol base has been reported to be helpful.[506] There is concern that patients with presumed ulcerative colitis and significant perianal disease may in fact have Crohn's disease.[621] However, a pelvic pouch procedure still may be an acceptable surgical alternative in those patients known to have ulcerative colitis but with perianal disease because the overall pouch failure rate has not been demonstrated to be significantly increased.[621]

Recurrent Disease. The development of Crohn's disease following restorative proctocolectomy or Kock pouch implies an initial error in diagnosis (see earlier discussion). The concern about the performance of reservoir procedures for Crohn's disease has been previously discussed and is further addressed in Chapter 30 (see also Management, earlier).

Evacuation Problems (Outlet Obstruction). Failure to evacuate adequately is usually associated with a long efferent limb, a particular concern with the S-pouch procedure (Figure 29-109; see Results).[422] It is because of this complication that every effort should be made to place the reservoir as close to the anal canal as is reasonably possible. Silvis and colleagues recommend dynamic defecography for determining which reparative approach is most appropriate in those who have problems with impaired evacuation.[686]

Treatment of this complication requires takedown of the anastomosis and shortening of the efferent limb. In the experience from the group at St. Mark's Hospital, combined abdominal-anal salvage surgery for outlet mechanical obstruction was successful in avoiding an ileostomy in 13 of 16 patients, and significantly improved pouch function in 12 of 15.[273]

Impotence and Infertility. As with conventional proctocolectomy and ileostomy, impotence does not seem to be a critical issue (unless you are the patient who experiences this complication), primarily because of the young age of most individuals. In the experience of Lindsey and colleagues, the impotence rate was 3.8%, all in the 50- to 70-year age group.[429] As expected, there was no statistically significant difference in

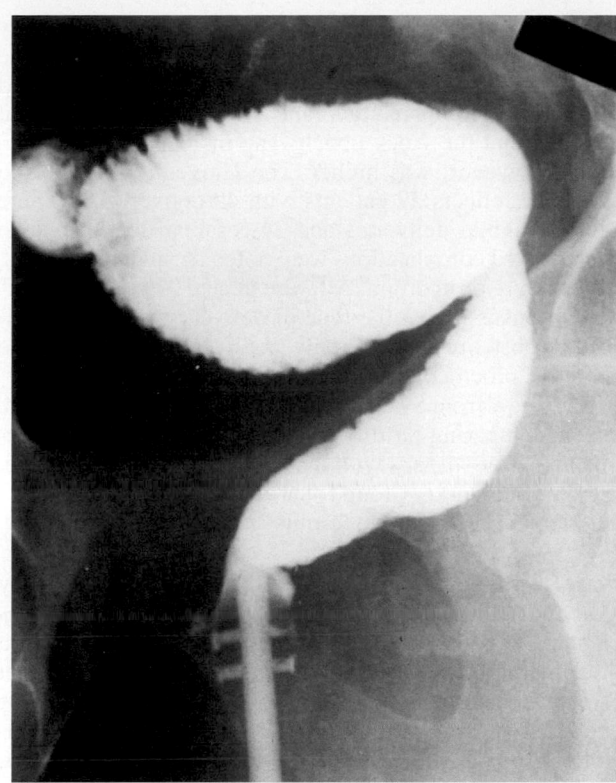

FIGURE 29-109. Long efferent limb of pouch-ileoanal procedure predisposes to difficulties in evacuation. Pouchogram demonstrated part of the reservoir to be inferior to the pouch outlet.

the rate of complete or partial impotence between close rectal and so-called mesorectal dissection. None of the patients experienced difficulty with ejaculation. However, in the Mayo Clinic experience, 9% of men were found to have retrograde ejaculation.[342] No impairment of bladder function was identified in patients of either sex. In a double-blind, placebo-controlled trial, Lindsey and coworkers found that sildenafil (Viagra) satisfactorily improved erectile dysfunction in 79% of those so afflicted.[428]

Other Complications. The usual complications experienced with any major abdominal procedure have been reported following the various pouch-anal procedures. These include adrenal insufficiency, hepatitis, pneumothorax, gastrointestinal bleeding, pancreatitis, cholecystitis, deep vein thrombosis, mesenteric vein thrombosis, and brachial palsy, as well as, of course, wound infection.[168,772] Whether the incidence is higher in comparison with other gastrointestinal operations is problematic.

Pregnancy, Delivery, and Fertility. Successful childbirth has been reported following restorative proctocolectomy with pelvic ileal reservoir.[490,532,590] According to the Mayo Clinic experience, 20 women had had at least one successful pregnancy and delivery following an ileal pouch-anal procedure by 1989.[532] Neither vaginal delivery nor cesarean section affected pouch functional outcome, but the frequency of nocturnal stools increased during the pregnancy and for 3 months thereafter. A later report of 43 women who had a successful pregnancy and delivery following ileal pouch-anal anastomosis at the Mayo Clinic was reviewed.[320] Stool frequency, incontinence, and pad usage were significantly increased during pregnancy, but postpartum function was the same as before pregnancy. The incidence of pouch-related complications compared favorably with that of conventional ileostomy and the Kock pouch. The incidence of cesarean section, however, was higher. The University of Toronto experience reflects 29 patients with 49 deliveries.[605] There were 25 vaginal deliveries and 24 cesarean sections. Two pouch-related complications were noted during pregnancies, and four were postpartum. All were treated "conservatively." The consensus is that the type of delivery should be influenced by obstetric concerns only, not by issues relative to the restorative proctocolectomy.[320,605]

In a review from Sweden and Denmark of 258 consecutive women, comparing fertility prior to restorative proctocolectomy and after surgery with that of the national population, Olsen and coworkers found that there was a considerable reduction in postoperative fertility.[564]

Salvage Surgery. Complications of restorative proctocolectomy are frequent and varied with the consequences of poor function and a diminished quality of life.[796] Ideally, the preferred initial methods of dealing with problems, such as outlet obstruction, fistula, stricture, and so forth, are those that are nonoperative or require limited surgery. When these methods fail, salvage surgery must be considered. There are, in essence, five options:

- perineal operation (e.g., pouch advancement)
- remove, repair, and preserve the pouch, restoring continuity
- resect the pouch and redo the restorative proctocolectomy
- remove and preserve the pouch, and convert to a continent ileostomy
- resect the pouch, and convert to a conventional or continent ileostomy

Obviously, resecting the pouch is not exactly "salvage surgery." It salvages the patient, to be sure, but not the reservoir. A moderate literature on the experience has developed from a number of centers with respect to the results of salvage surgery. Tan and coworkers noted that of nine patients who had their pouches removed and were converted to an end ileostomy, all experienced a higher stomal output, as would be expected, but the other measured parameters (systemic symptoms, functional, social and emotional impairment) did not differ significantly from that of individuals who had initially undergone a conventional proctocolectomy and ileostomy.[721] Behrens and associates converted 42 failed operations to the Barnett modification of a Kock pouch.[47] All but two have a functioning continent ileostomy.

Tulchinsky and colleagues (St. Mark's Hospital) successfully performed major revisional surgery for symptomatic *retained rectal stump* in 15 of 22 patients, noting that the results were worse than in those who underwent first-time restorative proctocolectomy.[746] Without doubt, poor function after pelvic pouch surgery offsets any advantage in body image when compared with a well-functioning ileostomy.[576,745]

The Cleveland Clinic (Florida) group identified 32 patients who underwent reoperative ileoanal pouch surgery.[796] Pouch salvage was attempted in 25 and pouch excision in 10 (3 patients were included in both groups). Five patients (20%) had pouch reconstruction; one was successful. The overall success rate of pouch salvage was 84% (all methods), with approximately two-thirds of patients having acceptable

function. Of interest is the fact that 4 of the 10 patients who underwent pouch excision were ultimately diagnosed with Crohn's disease.[796]

Gorfine and colleagues reported 51 patients who developed sinus or fistula tracts.[220] Eighty-nine salvage operations were performed. One-third required pouch excision, 9.8% had persistent fistulas and remained diverted, and 15.7% had persistent fistulas and were not diverted. The pouch was retained in 56.9%.

Our group identified 101 patients who underwent repeat restorative proctocolectomy.[22] Indications were as follows:

- chronic anastomotic fistula—27
- perineal or pouch-vaginal fistula—47
- anastomotic stricture—22
- dysfunction/long efferent limb of S-pouch—36

Some patients had more than one indication for reconstruction. Of these, 82% have a functioning pouch (median follow-up, 32 months). Thirteen percent underwent pouch excision. They note that although pouch failure occurs more commonly after a second attempt, patient satisfaction and quality of life remained high. The University of Toronto experience (2002) comprises 63 reconstructive procedures in 57 patients.[442] Forty-two (73.6%) maintained a functioning pouch with a mean follow-up of 60 months. More than 80% rated their physical and psychological health as being good to excellent. In a review of the literature on this subject, Tulchinsky and associates noted that failure of the surgery occurs indefinitely during the follow-up to a cumulative rate of about 15% at 10 to 15 years, with sepsis accounting for more than 50%.[744] Abdominal salvage surgery is successful in 20% to more than 80% of the reports, but the variable length of follow-up is probably responsible for this marked discrepancy in their opinion. The Mayo Clinic group has shown that increased experience decreases the risk of pouch-related complications and that with time the functional results remain stable, but the failure rate increases.[484]

Results
Physiologic Studies and Laboratory Evaluation
Anal Manometry; Rectoanal Inhibitory Reflex (RAIR); Determination of Reservoir Capacity; Compliance. Sharp and colleagues do not believe that clinical estimation of sphincter resting tone is a good predictor of postoperative function and advise manometric evaluation.[678] They found a significant decrease in the resting and maximal contraction pressures postoperatively. Grant and colleagues studied anal manometry in S-pouch patients with long rectal cuffs and with short cuffs, matching them for age, sex, and stool frequency.[225] Although functional results and manometric findings were similar, no patient demonstrated a normal rectoanal inhibitory reflex. Postoperative complications were significantly greater in those with long rectal cuffs.

The rectoanal inhibitory reflex is recognized as an important contributor to fecal continence through sampling and discrimination of contents. Preservation of the rectoanal inhibitory reflex has been shown to correlate with a decrease in the incidence of nocturnal soiling after restorative proctocolectomy.[650]

In a study of 34 patients with a J-pouch or with a straight ileoanal anastomosis, Beart and colleagues reported that both groups had satisfactory anal sphincter resting pressures and neorectal capacities, and that all could discriminate stool from gas.[39] It was their opinion that with normal sphincter function, continence correlates with reservoir capacity and compliance as well as with the frequency and strength of intrinsic bowel contractions. Others have demonstrated that the integrity of the sphincter mechanism can be satisfactorily maintained following ileoanal-reservoir operations.[588]

Our group used manometry to investigate the effects of ileal pouch-anal (n = 134) and ileal pouch-coloanal (n = 16) anastomosis on resting anal canal pressures in 150 patients.[93] Manometric measurements were taken preoperatively and 6 weeks following ileostomy closure. We reported a mean fall in pressure of 25 mm Hg for both ileal pouch-anal and ileal pouch-coloanal anastomoses, with no difference between hand-sewn or stapled techniques. However, analysis revealed a significant relationship between preoperative pressure and change in pressure. We also found that patients with high preoperative pressures are at risk for precipitous fall after surgery and, as a consequence, may have a suboptimal result. Paradoxically, patients with low preoperative pressures may actually demonstrate an increase in pressure following surgery. Those who are continent preoperatively are likely to remain continent postoperatively. Therefore, we stress that individuals with low preoperative resting pressures should not be denied an anastomosis to the anus based on this study alone. In our subsequent report in which 1,439 patients had their data collected prospectively, there was a statistically significant association between seepage and degree of incontinence with quality of health, quality of life, energy level, and level of satisfaction with surgery.[239] Perioperative anal sphincter resting pressures greater than 40 mm Hg were associated with significantly better function and quality of life. Our conclusion was that a low preoperative resting pressure does not preclude a successful outcome.[239]

To study motor determinants of incontinence after ileal pouch-anal anastomosis, Ferrara and colleagues placed microtransducer catheters in eight continent and eight incontinent patients 15 months following surgery to record 24-hour ambulatory motor activity.[166] The investigators found that incontinent patients had lower resting pressures, extended anal canal relaxation, higher amplitude high-pressure waves, and a nonresponsive anal canal, all indicating a reversal of the anal canal pressure gradient. The authors concluded that incontinence is most likely a consequence of several factors, including a weak and less responsive anal canal, strong pouch motor activity, and dysfunctional coordination between pouch and anal canal.

Becker and coworkers assessed functional results by means of radiography and manometry.[40,42] The mean maximal anal sphincter resting pressure decreased from 87.1 mm Hg preoperatively to 68.1 mm Hg 8 weeks following surgery, but at 1 year it rose to 72.3 mm Hg. The change in sphincter pressure with voluntary squeeze was greater 8 weeks after the procedure than before the operation. Keighley and associates and others have confirmed that median resting anal canal pressure and maximum squeeze pressure are significantly lower in pouch patients when compared with a control population.[69,339,427] However, better results can be achieved with respect to voluntary control if the surgeon limits the potential for injury to the internal sphincter by avoiding anal dilatation and mucosectomy.[391,743] As has been discussed earlier, this must be balanced with the concern for residual mucosa predisposing to the development of dysplasia and carcinoma.[349]

Wexner and colleagues prospectively analyzed 15 patients who underwent construction of a reservoir anastomosis by the double-stapling technique.[770] There was no significant difference between preoperative values and those obtained 1 year following surgery when mean and maximal squeeze pressures were compared, although the length of the high-pressure zone decreased.

Nasmyth and colleagues as well as others found that the frequency of defecation was inversely correlated to both the capacity and the compliance of the pouch.[526,565] Patients who could postpone defecation for more than 30 minutes had higher anal squeeze pressures and emptied their pouches more completely than those who experienced leakage. The best clinical results were associated with a high anal pressure and with a large volume, high compliance, and complete emptying of the pouch. Harms and associates failed to demonstrate a difference in the mean pressure at normal evacuation volume between S- and W-reservoirs 2 and 12 months postoperatively.[252] Scott and Phillips noted that a low pouch compliance prior to ileostomy closure was associated with an increased frequency of nocturnal stooling, but anal canal length, anal sphincter squeeze pressure, and pouch capacity failed to predict functional outcome.[668] Steens and coworkers found no difference in pouch compliance and sensitivity in patients with uniform pouch design who had normal versus high stool frequency.[700] However, *postprandial pouch tone* was increased significantly in those with a high stool frequency. In another report from the same group, compliance was found to increase significantly during the first year after surgery to values of that in the range of rectal compliance.[701]

Holdsworth and colleagues used continuous ambulatory manometry to evaluate the function of the internal anal sphincter in 35 patients who underwent restorative proctocolectomy and 19 normal healthy volunteers.[285] Of the 35 individuals who underwent restorative proctocolectomy, 13 underwent mucosal proctectomy with endoanal ileoanal anastomosis and 22 patients had an end-to-end ileoanal anastomosis. The authors found that whereas only 38% of the patients who underwent mucosal proctectomy with sutured endoanal anastomosis showed evidence of basal internal sphincter activity, all patients with a stapled end-to-end anastomosis and all control subjects showed this baseline activity. The authors concluded that these data suggest mucosal proctectomy and endoanal anastomosis result in damage to the internal anal sphincter. In contrast, restorative proctectomy with stapled, end-to-end anastomosis was demonstrated to preserve internal anal sphincter function.

Jorge and coworkers used manometry and a questionnaire-based incontinence score to investigate the recovery of anal sphincter function after the double-stapled ileoanal reservoir procedure in 22 patients older than 50 years of age.[319] Manometric measurements were taken preoperatively and postoperatively (before and after ileostomy closure). Results were compared with those of a group of 50 patients with a median age of 32 years. The authors reported that no differences were found relative to preoperative pressures or clinical outcome. However, mean and high resting pressures were significantly lower in the over-50 group when they were examined before ileostomy closure. Although impairment of the internal anal sphincter was more severe after ileoanal reservoir, function had completely recovered after ileostomy closure. The authors concluded that the effect of the ileoanal reservoir on anal sphincters in persons older than the age of 50 years is similar to that noted in younger patients.

Electromyography. Stryker and colleagues used electromyography (EMG) to evaluate the external anal sphincter in 27 patients.[708] Abnormal motor unit potentials were identified in 9 patients, a finding that usually correlates with poor bowel control. All patients older than the age of 40 years had abnormal EMG results.

Farouk and coworkers employed preoperative and postoperative EMG and manometry in 66 patients to determine the role of the internal anal sphincter in the return of continence following restorative proctocolectomy.[150] At 18 months' follow-up, neither EMG measurements nor resting anal pressure measurements of internal anal sphincter function had fully returned to preoperative values. However, the authors concluded that recovery of internal sphincter EMG activity and resting anal pressure is progressive and associated with a gradual decrease in stool frequency. Eleven patients reported leakage in the follow-up period, with nocturnal incontinence the primary complaint, a problem that the authors attribute to poor pouch compliance during filling.

Motility. Pescatori studied electric and motor activity of the terminal ileum in seven patients who underwent this operation.[585] Recordings were carried out with an intraluminal probe, and observations were also made of the electric activity of the rectal sleeve and sphincter muscle. He observed that most of the electric and motor properties of the terminal ileum are retained after surgery, but that pouch motility is reduced. Others have found that jejunoileal motility is not greatly altered by the procedure.[707]

Patients who have poor functional results—incontinence and stool frequency—often have rapid pouch filling and an inability to evacuate completely.[709] O'Connell and colleagues evaluated ileal pouch motility in 23 patients 2 years following the operation by means of an intraluminal bag and pressure-sensitive catheters.[557] Pouch emptying was determined scintigraphically and by stool collection. The authors observed that ileal pouch motility and stool output were major determinants of stool frequency.

Kusunoki and colleagues attempted to determine the mechanism of anal canal motility with the use of various neuroreceptor agents.[376] Their results suggest that the neorectum has hybrid characteristics of both rectum and ileum.

Pouchography and Scintigraphy. Tsao and coworkers studied 463 patients undergoing a pouchogram (Gastrografin) enema before ileostomy closure following ileal pouch-anal anastomosis.[741] The purpose of their investigation was to determine the usefulness of a pouchogram in detecting complications and predicting clinical outcome. Normal pouchograms were reported in 389 (84%) patients, whereas pouchograms of 74 (16%) patients revealed pouch leaks and other abnormal findings. The authors found that abnormal pouchograms identified patients needing surgical intervention before closure as well as those patients who would likely benefit from a delay in ileostomy closure. In addition, the authors reported that abnormal pouchograms were associated with an overall long-term failure rate of 23%, in comparison with a 6% long-term failure rate for patients with normal findings. They concluded that pouchograms have a long-term clinical predictive value.

Pescatori and colleagues further evaluated 34 patients who underwent restorative proctocolectomy with an S-pouch by "evacuation pouchography."[586] The purpose was to determine why some patients could evacuate spontaneously and others had to insert a catheter several times a day to empty the pouch. The 50% who were able to have a spontaneous evacuation had a significantly shorter distal segment (mean, 8 ± 3 cm) than those who had to use a catheter to empty the pouch (mean distal segment length, 11 ± 4 cm). The authors believed that the longer the distal segment, the more likely it was to be angulated. Short segments were demonstrated to fill on straining, in contrast with the longer segments, which often failed to fill under such circumstances.

Heppell and coworkers compared the functional results of J-reservoirs and S-reservoirs by means of a radionuclide enema, measuring emptying following instillation of a semisolid medium labeled with 1.0 mCi of technetium-99m (^{99m}Tc)-sulfur colloid.[269] Ileal pouch counts were determined by using a scintillation camera and computer before and after spontaneous evacuation. Functional results were found to be similar in the two groups, but those who emptied less than 30% were improved by intermittent intubation. The authors believed that a semisolid radionuclide enema could be usefully applied to identify those who would benefit from such intubation.

Barkel and colleagues (Mayo Clinic) used a scintigraphic technique to determine whether the anorectal angle is preserved after ileal pouch-anal anastomosis.[31] They found that changes in the anorectal angle during defecation and during squeeze were similar to that of controls, but that the pelvic floor movements were impaired. Kmiot and coworkers assessed evacuation by means of videoproctography and observed anal stricture to be the only factor consistently associated with poor pouch emptying.[357]

Anal Sensation. Keighley and coworkers assessed anal sensation in control subjects and in patients with ulcerative colitis by means of a constant-current stimulator following restorative proctocolectomy.[337] Excision of the anal transition zone did not eliminate the ability to discriminate and therefore did not increase the risk for control problems following this procedure. Conversely, Holdsworth and Johnston, in assessing the rectoanal inhibitory reflex and the ability of the patient to discriminate between flatus and feces, found that anal sensation and discriminatory function were significantly better without mucosal proctectomy.[283] Others have demonstrated improved sensation to be associated with preservation of the anal transition zone, but correlation with the actual functional results was not obtained.[502]

Bacteriology. O'Connell and colleagues studied the enteric bacteriology of 20 patients in an attempt to relate changes in the functional results of the operation.[559] They observed that jejunal bacterial overgrowth was associated with an increased stool output, azotorrhea, and a poor clinical result. Pouch ileitis did not appear to be caused simply by pouch stasis and bacterial overgrowth within the pouch.

Absorption. One of the concerns that has been expressed with respect to the various pouch-anal alternatives is the problem of absorptive capacity and consequent nutritional disturbance. Nasmyth and associates assessed bile acid absorption by using selenium-66 (^{66}Se) taurohomocholate and noted no statistically significant difference between patients with a conventional ileostomy and those with a pouch-anal procedure.[527] However, bacterial metabolism of primary conjugated bile acids was greater in those with a pouch. Others have observed that almost all postcolectomy patients have supersaturated bile with cholesterol crystals, findings that are usually seen in persons with cholesterol gallstones.[257]

Bowel Frequency and Continence
Interpretation of the results and the relative merits of the varied approaches to the assessment of ileoanal pouch function is obviously quite difficult. For example, one is not always certain how much or if any slowing medications are employed to achieve the median frequency of bowel action that is reported. The four characteristics generally evaluated include spontaneity of defecation, ability to defer defecation, continence, and stool frequency.[410] In the prior edition, the experience of the largest published series was summarized, and I have maintained this information. Moreover, I have supplemented the results in table fashion that incorporates the important literature since 2005.

St. Mark's Hospital. Parks and colleagues reported their early experience of 21 patients from St. Mark's Hospital with the S-pouch, 17 of whom had ulcerative colitis and 4 with polyposis.[573] All were observed to be completely continent of feces during the day, but 1 patient was incontinent at night. The average frequency of bowel evacuation was approximately four times in 24 hours. Approximately one-half of the patients needed a catheter to facilitate defecation. Two required medications to reduce the frequency of bowel actions. A later report from the same center, comprising 55 patients, revealed a mean daily stool frequency of 3.7 (20% required antidiarrheal medications).[537] Spontaneous defecation occurred in 40%, whereas 53% used a catheter to aid evacuation. Continence was "normal" in approximately two-thirds, and minor leakage was reported by 29%, with 5.4% noting soiling. Setti-Carraro and coworkers, reporting from the same institution, reviewed the first 10 years of experience with restorative proctocolectomy.[675] Long-term function was assessed in 80 patients, with a mean follow-up of 99.3 months after ileostomy closure. There were 24 patients with an S-pouch, 24 with a J-pouch, 31 with a W-pouch, and 1 with a pelvic Kock pouch. Sixty-six patients did not use a catheter, with an average diurnal minimum and maximum frequency of 3.8 and 4.9, respectively. Overall, the average minimum 24-hour frequency in these 66 patients was 4.1 and the maximum was 5.7. Forty-nine patients were completely continent. Of the remaining 31, 30 had minor mucous or fecal leaks. In a related study from the same center, Melville and colleagues showed that during a 15-year period (1976 through 1990), the number of elective surgeries for ulcerative colitis increased.[486]

Nicholls and Pezim compared three different designs of reservoirs in 104 patients (triple loop, double loop, and quadruple loop).[539] Frequency of defecation was significantly greater with the double loop and was associated with a much higher incidence of nighttime evacuation. All patients with double- or quadruple-loop reservoirs defecated spontaneously, whereas only 41% with triple-loop pouches did so. The authors concluded that a quadruple reservoir directly connected to the anal canal preserved spontaneous

evacuation and was comparable with the triple loop in preserving adequate retentive ability. A report from the same unit involving functional assessment of 51 patients with the four-loop, W-reservoir revealed the frequency of defecation per day to be 3.3 (range, 1 to 8).[538] Nighttime evacuation occurred in 14%. Harms and colleagues noted a 24-hour stool frequency of 4.8 at 1 year with this type of pouch.[250]

Utsunomiya (Japan). Utsunomiya and colleagues reported their early experience with the J-pouch.[751] They believed that this type of pouch is superior because the reservoir is located in the lowest part of the pelvic area, similar to the normal rectal ampulla.

Mayo Clinic. Taylor and colleagues reported the initial Mayo Clinic experience with 74 patients who underwent ileal pouch-anal anastomosis with a J-reservoir.[725] In comparing their patients with those who underwent a straight ileoanal anastomosis, the authors noted that stool frequency with the pouch was less (mean, 7 per 24 hours, compared with 11 stools per 24 hours in the straight ileoanal group). Major nocturnal incontinence was also less in the pouch group (0% vs. 20%). A later report of 157 patients assessed at least 60 days after ileostomy closure following the J-pouch procedure revealed that all evacuated the neorectum spontaneously.[493,582] Stool frequency was on average 6.0 daily and 1.2 nightly. Seepage was noted in 25% during the day and in 47% at night. Women had more spotting than men, and patients older than 50 years had more stools per day than those 50 years or younger.[582] McIntyre and colleagues published a more recent report from the same institution.[479] They compared functional results 1 year and 10 years after ileal pouch-anal anastomosis for chronic ulcerative colitis.[479] Sixty-one consecutive subjects were identified who underwent a J-pouch procedure, and functional results were recorded 1 year and 10 years following ileostomy closure. At both follow-up times, the median stool frequency was 7 in a 24-hour period. At the 10-year follow-up, 70% had excellent daytime control, 23% had occasional soiling, and 7% reported poor control. Nighttime incontinence was a problem for 23 patients at 1 year, with only 5 reporting improvement at 10 years. Overall, 52% complained of nighttime soiling at the 10-year mark.

Köhler and coworkers, also from the Mayo Clinic, employed a written questionnaire assessing bowel habits, overall quality of life, and several performance-related activities to examine the long-term functional results of persons undergoing an ileal J-pouch–anal anastomosis.[364] A group of patients who had undergone cholecystectomy served as the control group. The authors reported that the ileoanal patients had a median of six stools per day and that 68% of the 240 participating individuals experienced episodes of fecal spotting. Bowel habits remained steady during the 8-year follow-up. Overall, 90% of ileoanal patients reported an excellent overall quality of life, with results closely paralleling those of the control group.

The Mayo Clinic experience with restorative proctocolectomy is commanding. Of the 1,386 patients who were reported in 2000 (median length of follow-up, 8 years), they found that functional outcomes were comparable between men and women, and daytime and nocturnal incontinence was more frequently observed in older individuals.[151]

Cleveland Clinic (Ohio). A nonrandomized report from our institution compared the J-pouch with the S-pouch as performed by the same surgeon.[742] There was no statistically significant difference between the two with respect to the mean maximum resting and squeeze pressures and the maximum tolerated volume. However, a significant difference was noted in mean compliance, the incidence of daytime and nocturnal leakage, and the frequency of bowel action, the S-pouch being superior. In another report from our group, we retrospectively reviewed 1,005 patients who underwent ileal pouch-anal anastomoses from 1983 to 1993.[161] The J-pouch design was performed in two-thirds, with one-third having undergone an S-pouch. Two-thirds of patients had stapled anastomoses, whereas the anastomoses of one-third were hand-sewn. Among the 812 patients who underwent the operation for ulcerative colitis, the median frequency of bowel movements per 24-hour period was 6 (range, 1 to 20). Nighttime seepage was reported in 29%, and 17% experienced day and night seepage. Forty-seven percent sometimes used antidiarrheal medications, and 15% indicated constant use.

More recent papers from the Cleveland Clinic now involve data from almost 2,000 patients. Pouch failure requiring pouch excision or permanent ileostomy was noted in 4.1%.[129] Fourteen percent experienced social, sexual, or work restrictions, and the functional outcome was not as good in older patients.[128] However, our compatriots at the Cleveland Clinic (Florida) note while anorectal function is transiently impaired after restorative proctocolectomy, that impairment is not an age-related phenomenon.[719] Risk factors that have been found to be independent predictors of pouch survival included patient diagnosis, prior anal pathology, abnormal anal manometry, patient comorbidity, pouch-perineal or pouch vaginal fistula, pelvic sepsis, anastomotic stricture, and separation.[157]

Lahey Clinic. Marcello and colleagues prospectively assessed long-term results in 460 patients between 1980 and 1991.[457] A J-pouch was constructed in 94%. With a follow-up greater than 60 months after ileostomy closure, the mean number of bowel movements per 24-hour period was 5.8. After 5 years, 50% of patients did not have nightly bowel movements, and 75% passed flatus independently. After 1 year, the frequency of seepage was 10%, occurring on average 3 days per week. The authors reported that the rate of use of medications regulating gut function remained between 39% and 44% during the follow-up period.

Fonkalsrud (University of California, Los Angeles). Fonkalsrud reported his initial experience with the lateral ileal reservoir in 21 patients (mean age, approximately 17 years) with ulcerative colitis or polyposis.[172–174] He initially thought that the results of the procedure were superior to the results obtained with an S-pouch. A mean of 4 continent bowel movements per 24 hours was achieved within 4 weeks in patients with lateral reservoirs. A later update comprised a total of 83 patients.[698] Late obstruction of the ileal reservoir developed in 19. In 9 patients, the obstruction was caused by a long rectal muscular cuff and a longer distance from the lower end of the reservoir to the anus than is optimal. He recommended that the length be from 10 to 15 cm for children and from 18 to 22 cm for adults. It was also suggested that the pouch be no farther than 5 cm from the ileoanal anastomosis. A still later report involving 127 patients who underwent a lateral reservoir revealed a significantly lower morbidity in comparison with that of patients undergoing the other pouch alternatives.[177] As mentioned earlier, Fonkalsrud is the only surgeon who has extensive experience with this approach. He has also reviewed the long-term results after colectomy and ileoanal pull-through procedure in 116 children 18 years of age or younger.[178] Ninety-four had ulcerative colitis, 17 had familial polyposis coli, and 5 had Hirschsprung's disease. Sixty-two patients had a lateral pouch, 47 a J-pouch, and 7 a straight pull-through. An average of 5.6 bowel movements per 24 hours was found at 3 months, which decreased to 3.9 at 6 months. By 3 months, fewer than 10% of patients experienced daytime soiling, whereas nocturnal soiling was present in 18% at 3 months. However, at the 6-month mark, the incidence had fallen to 6%. Prior to his retirement, Fonkalsrud recommended a J-pouch because of the ease of construction and paucity of long-term complications. He reserved the lateral pouch for patients with a short ileal mesentery and inadequate length for a J-pouch to extend to the anus without tension.

Other Investigators. Becker and Raymond reported their experience with 100 patients who underwent the J-pouch procedure.[45] Stool frequency at 1, 3, 6, 12, and 24 months was 7.5, 6.5, 6.2, 5.4, and 5.4, respectively. No patient was incontinent during the day. By 1 year, 25% noted nocturnal leakage. In contrast to other investigators, the authors did not believe that age was a factor in determining stool frequency. Smith noted that 14 of his 19 patients had 6 or fewer bowel movements per day.[690] Bodzin and colleagues reported that their 19 patients had 3 to 9 bowel movements per day, and nearly all wore a sanitary pad for unpredictable leakage.[60]

Nasmyth and coworkers noted no significant differences between the S-pouches and J-pouches with respect to continence or frequency of defecation at 6 months.[528] However, at 1 year, those with the S-reservoir had a lower stool frequency than those with a J-pouch. Conversely, McHugh and colleagues found that patients with S-pouches appeared to have better early functional results, but no differences were appreciated at 1 year following ileostomy closure.[478]

Reissman and colleagues studied the functional results of the double-stapled ileoanal reservoir in 124 patients at a mean follow-up of 24 months.[614] They reported a mean of 5.4 (range, 2 to 13) bowel movements during the day and a mean of 1.2 (range, 0 to 4) at night. Ninety-five percent of patients reported perfect or almost perfect continence during the day, and 92% during the night. The same authors studied the functional results of the double-stapled ileoanal reservoir in patients older than 60 years of age. They found this operation to be safe and the functional and physiologic results to be comparable with those in younger patients.[616] Keighley and colleagues compared the stapled J-pouch with the sutured W-pouch, observing that the functional results were identical.[338] They concluded that the excessive time required to construct the W-reservoir would not seem to be justified.

A plethora of articles on the functional results of the pouch-anal procedures can be found.[44,76,95,130,186,188,233,251, 326,365,396,404,414,475,497,498,562,592,631,645,647] The general consensus is that this operation, with its various modifications, offers the best quality of life when compared with the alternatives. Tables 29-7 and 29-8 summarize the experiences from a number of institutions that address the issues of bowel frequency and bowel control following restorative proctocolectomy through the year 2003. Table 29-9 illustrates the results from a number of centers since that time to this current writing.

TABLE 29-7 Bowel Frequency following Pouch-Anal Procedures

INSTITUTION	YEAR	NUMBER OF PATIENTS	PRIMARY POUCH	DAILY EVACUATIONS		
				TOTAL (MEAN)	NIGHT (MEAN)	DAY (MEAN)
Mayo Clinic[479]	1994	1,400	J	6	0–1	5–6
St. Mark's Hospital[675]	1994	110	J, S	6	0–1	5
Cleveland Clinic[161]	1995	521	J	6	NS	NS
Cleveland Clinic (FL)[614]	1995	107	J	6.6	1.2	5.4
University of Wisconsin[249]	1992	109	W	4.9	NS	NS
Lahey Clinic[457]	1993	382	J	7	1	6
University of Chicago[498]	1993	50	J	6	NS	NS
Radcliffe Hospital[631]	1997	177	J	5	0–1	4.5
Uppsala, Sweden[326]	2000	155	J	NS	5 (74%)	NS
University of Minnesota[76]	2002	136	J	7	5	2
University of Chicago[497]	2003	234	J	8.5	2.5	6

NS, not stated.

TABLE 29-8 Bowel Control following Pouch-Anal Procedures

INSTITUTION	YEAR	NUMBER OF PATIENTS	PRIMARY POUCH	EXCELLENT OR GOOD (%)	IMPAIRED (%)
Mayo Clinic[479]	1994	1,400	J	48	52
St. Mark's Hospital[675]	1994	110	J, S	45	55
Cleveland Clinic[161]	1995	521	J	71	29
Cleveland Clinic (FL)[614]	1995	107	J	87	13
University of Wisconsin[249]	1992	109	W	61	39
Lahey Clinic[457]	1993	382	J	90	10
University of Chicago[498]	1993	50	J	54	46
Uppsala, Sweden[326]	2000	155	J	76	24
University of Minnesota[76]	2002	136	J	83	17
University of Chicago[497]	2003	234	J	70	30

TABLE 29-9 Results of Restorative Proctocolectomy

YEAR	AUTHORS	INSTITUTION	TOTAL PROCTOCOLECTOMIES REPORTED	COMPLICATIONS	STOOL EVACUATION
1987–2011	Pellino et al.[a]	Second University of Naples, Naples, Italy	241 for UC, FAP, CA (1 S-pouch, 121 W-pouch, 119 J-pouch); 23 (9.5%) without ileostomy	Pelvic sepsis 7.7% and 13% with and without ileostomy, respectively; failure 5% and 4.3%	
1987–2002	Selvaggi et al.[b]	Second University of Naples, Naples, Italy	118 for UC	Early pelvic sepsis 9 (7.69%), 6 required salvage procedures; worse long-term functional results, stool frequency, continence	1- and 5-year follow-up: mean frequency per day 4.6 4.8; incontinence during day 17 and 22, during night 33 and 39
1999–2003	Ikeuchi et al.[c]	Hyogo College of Medicine, Hyogo, Japan	245 IPAA with mucosectomy, 150 no diverting ileostomy	Without ileostomy 48 (32%), with ileostomy 33 (35.9%) with complications	
2002–2007	Fichera et al.[d]	University of Chicago Medical Center, Chicago, IL	179 (73 laparoscopic and 106 open)	Complication rates same	Overall 68.4% patients fully continent at 1 year; average BM 6.8 ± 2.8/day for lap and 6.3 ± 1.7 for open
1995–2003	Swenson et al.[e]	The Penn State College of Medicine, The Milton S. Hershey Medical Center, Hershey, PA	23 two-stage modified procedure (no ileostomy) and 31 three-stage procedure	No differences in complication rates, statistically significantly lower cost of hospital stay in two-stage procedure	Average number BM/day two-stage vs. three-stage 7.5 vs. 6.1 ($P = .0465$), occasional seepage (%) 17.6 vs. 11.8 ($P = .6282$), incontinence 0.00 vs. 0.03 ($P = .3600$)
1983–2001	Remzi et al.[f]	Cleveland Clinic Foundation, Cleveland, OH	1,725 patients with diverting ileostomy, 277 patients without; the rate of previous subtotal colectomy is higher (48% vs. 33%, $P < .001$) in the non-ileostomy group	No differences in septic complications (%) 6.5 vs. 5.4 ($P = .51$); higher rate of hemorrhage (3.7% vs. 1.1%, $P < .001$) and anastomotic stricture (20.4% vs. 9.4%, $P < .001$) in the non-ileostomy group	No major differences in quality of life and functional results between the groups at the interval of 3 months, 1 year, 3 years, 5 years, and 10 years
2000–2007	Joyce et al.[g]	Cleveland Clinic Foundation, Cleveland, OH	835 patients undergoing IPAA; 715 (86%) with diverting ileostomy, 120 (14%) without ileostomy; 41% had preceding STC with end ileostomy	No significant difference in complications; total costs 25% greater in the ileostomy group ($P < .001$)	

(Continued)

TABLE 29-9 Results of Restorative Proctocolectomy *(Continued)*

YEAR	AUTHORS	INSTITUTION	TOTAL PROCTOCOLECTOMIES REPORTED	COMPLICATIONS	STOOL EVACUATION
1990–2005	Lovegrove et al.[h]	Cleveland Clinic Foundation, Cleveland, OH; North West London Hospitals NHS Trust, London, United Kingdom	3,733 patients; 3,196 (85.6%) with proximal diversion; UC indication for RPC in 2,304 (61.7%), J-pouch in 2,657 (71.2%), S-pouch in 459 (12.3%), W-pouch in 441 (11.8%)	Incidences of anastomotic leak, pelvic sepsis, fistulation, and pouch failure did not differ significantly between the 2 groups, but a 2-day increase in the median length of hospital stay in the ileostomy group ($P < .01$); incidence of postoperative hemorrhage (4.0% vs. 2.0%, $P = .03$), anastomotic stricture (18.2% vs. 9.1%, $P < .001$), SBO (19.0% vs. 10.8%, $P < .001$) in the ileostomy vs. non-ileostomy group were statistically significant	
2009–2010	Gash et al.[i]	Frenchay Hospital, Bristol, United Kingdom	10 patients; intracorporeal anastomosis 8 (80%), hand-sewn 2 (20%); diverting loop ileostomy at the SILS site	1 patient with emphysema around the ileostomy site; no deaths or readmissions	At 1-year follow-up 9 report continence, 1 with occasional daily soiling; median BM/day 4 (2–8)
2008–2010	Pedraza et al.[j]	Colorectal Surgical Associates, LTD, LLP Houston, TX	5 patients	No major complications; the mean hospital stay 5.6 days	

UC, ulcerative colitis; FAP, familial adenomatous polyposis; STC, slow-transit constipation; SBO, small bowel obstruction; SILS, single-incision laparoscopic surgery.

[a]Pellino G, Sciaudone G, Canonico S, et al. Role of ileostomy in restorative proctocolectomy. *World J Gastroenterol.* 2012;18:1703.

[b]Selvaggi F, Sciaudone G, Limongelli P, et al. The effect of pelvic septic complications on function and quality of life after ileal pouch-anal anastomosis: a single center experience. *Am Surg.* 2010;76:428.

[c]Ikeuchi H, Nakano H, Uchino M, et al. Safety of one-stage restorative proctocolectomy for ulcerative colitis. *Dis Colon Rectum.* 2005;48:1550.

[d]Fichera A, Silvestri MT, Hurst RD, et al. Laparoscopic restorative proctocolectomy with ileal pouch anal anastomosis: a comprehensive observational study on long-term functional results. *J Gastrointest Surg.* 2009;13:526.

[e]Swenson BR, Hollenbeak CS, Poritz LS, et al. Modified two-stage ileal pouch-anal anastomosis: equivalent outcomes with less resource utilization. *Dis Colon Rectum.* 2005;48:256.

[f]Remzi FH, Fazio VW, Gorgun E, et al. The outcome after restorative proctocolectomy with or without defunctioning ileostomy. *Dis Colon Rectum.* 2006;49:470.

[g]Joyce MR, Kiran RP, Remzi FH, et al. In a select group of patients meeting strict clinical criteria and undergoing ileal pouch-anal anastomosis, the omission of a diverting ileostomy offers cost savings to the hospital. *Dis Colon Rectum.* 2010;53:905.

[h]Lovegrove RE, Tilney HS, Remzi FH, et al. To divert or not to divert: a retrospective analysis of variables that influence ileostomy omission in ileal pouch surgery. *Arch Surg.* 2011;146:82.

[i]Gash KJ, Goede AC, Kaldowski B, et al. Single incision laparoscopic (SILS) restorative proctocolectomy with ileal pouch-anal anastomosis. *Surg Endosc.* 2011;25:3877.

[j]Pedraza R, Patel CB, Ramos-Valadez DI, et al. Robotic-assisted laparoscopic surgery for restorative proctocolectomy with ileal J pouch-anal anastomosis. *Minim Invasive Ther Allied Technol.* 2011;20:234.

Comparison of Reservoir Designs

Much effort has been directed to comparing the functional outcome of patients who have undergone restorative proctocolectomy with creation of a variety of pelvic ileal reservoirs. Although the choice of reservoir is largely a function of the surgeon's personal preference, options are available, including the duplicated-J, triplicated-S, quadruplicated-W, and lateral, as well as modified versions of these.[648] Lewis and colleagues investigated the factors that are important in the creation of an ideal pelvic pouch for achievement of perfect anal continence.[413] The authors found four factors that correlate significantly with an optimal functional result. These are maximum resting anal pressure, sensory threshold in the upper and middle anal canal, compliance of the ileal reservoir, and the presence of a pouch-anal inhibitory reflex. They concluded that the quality of anal continence depends on a compliant ileal reservoir and a strong, sensitive anal sphincter.[413] Various studies have been conducted to investigate the advantages and drawbacks of each design.

Harms and coworkers examined the appropriateness of the W-reservoir in the treatment of ulcerative colitis and familial polyposis in 109 individuals.[249] Stool frequency over a 24-hour period decreased from 7.3 at 2 months to 4.9 at 12 months of follow-up. Ninety-six percent reported continence during the day at 12 months, whereas 10% experienced episodes of nighttime seepage. In addition, compliance increased from 12.7 mL/mm Hg to 14.3 mL/mm Hg between 2 and 12 months of follow-up. The authors concluded that W-ileal reservoirs exhibit optimal function and compliance properties when compared with lower capacity designs.

Johnston and colleagues performed a prospective, randomized trial to elucidate what influence pelvic pouch design has on functional outcome.[315] Sixty patients received either a J- or a W-reservoir, constructed with either 30 or 40 cm of ileum. The authors found that median bowel frequency in 24 hours did not differ significantly in patients with J-reservoirs from that of patients with W-pouches. Similarly, the size (30 or 40 cm) of the reservoir did not produce a significant difference in bowel frequency. The authors concluded that their findings support the use of a small, duplicated ileal reservoir, which is simple to construct by means of linear stapling techniques. Others have confirmed this finding.[279]

Commentary on Restorative Proctocolectomy

The ileal reservoir with endoanal anastomosis has become relatively standardized, at least with respect to the value of the procedure in the surgical management of individuals with ulcerative colitis and the polyposis syndromes. There is no question that most patients are satisfied with the functional results and to some extent serve as their own controls (because most have a protecting ileostomy for a time). However, these so-called control patients may have a less-than-satisfactory loop ileostomy. Moreover, it is more proximally located than a conventional end stoma, and the effluent is therefore more liquid. Furthermore, despite meticulous attention to creating a loop ileostomy, surgeons often find that a consistently salutary stoma is an unachievable ideal. That said, however, a report from the Mayo Clinic compares the quality of life after conventional (Brooke) ileostomy with that after the pouch-anal procedure.[583] After adjusting for age, diagnosis, and reoperation rate, logistic regression analysis of performance scores in seven different categories were used to discriminate between operations. The authors concluded that patients experience significant advantages with respect to their daily activities and quality of life with the pouch-anal procedure in comparison with the standard end ileostomy.

One must also consider the obvious fact that despite many surgeons' increased experience with the technique, the procedure continues to have a high morbidity, albeit much lower than the initial reports indicated. Mortality, however, is quite low, primarily because an ileostomy is usually accomplished until the restorative anastomoses have healed.

Analysis of the numerous reports in the literature reveals a considerable variability in operative technique between surgeons and institutions. Furthermore, with rare exception, the failure to randomize patients also inhibits accurate assessment of the relative merits and risks of the plethora of approaches. Still, a number of appropriate conclusions may be drawn. Before the surgeon agrees to undertake this procedure as an alternative to conventional ileostomy, the patient should be highly motivated to accept the consequences: frequent bowel movements (a minimum of four to six stools per day and the possible requirement for intubation if an S-pouch is elected) as well as the risk for soilage and incontinence. It may take upward of 1 year for a patient to achieve reasonable stability with respect to bowel function and frequency.

A number of factors may make restorative proctocolectomy technically difficult or impossible to accomplish. For example, obesity tends to be associated with a shortened mesentery which may preclude the possibility of bringing the ileum down to effect an anastomosis. One may not be able to position the reservoir in the pelvis if there is considerable fat or if there is narrowing of the inlet. Some surgeons believe that the terminal ileum reaches the dentate line more readily with the S-pouch than when the J-reservoir is used. The patient must, therefore, understand that technical factors or unanticipated pathology may necessitate an alternative surgical approach.

Because of the risk of recurrence, this operation should not be performed in patients with Crohn's disease in my opinion (see Chapter 30). Toxic megacolon is also a contraindication for embarking on this procedure at the time of emergency intervention. The wiser course in the latter situation is to perform a total colectomy and conventional ileostomy with rectal preservation, returning later to perform the restorative procedure. Older age is in itself not a contraindication, but most agree that because the aging process has a pejorative effect on sphincter muscle function, the procedure should probably be limited to patients younger than 70 years, although this is by no means a requirement.

With respect to the type of pouch, a trade-off seems to have evolved: the possible requirement of intubation with the S-pouch versus the theoretically lowered capacity (and therefore increased frequency of defecation) of the J-reservoir. Conversely, many reports suggest that the size of the reservoir may be of limited importance.

Preoperative physiologic studies that evaluate anal squeeze pressure or at least subjectively assess the effectiveness of the sphincter mechanism should be considered before an ileal reservoir anastomosis is performed. The real questions are whether preoperative physiologic studies help to predict the functional results following restorative proctocolectomy or even affect the decision-making process. Still, older patients, and those with a poor resting tone or suboptimal maximum squeeze pressure, might be forewarned that continence could be less than satisfactory.

We have more than reached the point wherein restorative proctocolectomy deserves complete legitimacy for the surgical management of ulcerative colitis. Soldiers on active duty, for example, can anticipate continuation of their military careers after such surgery.[24] Until relatively recently, I had been concerned that the complexity of the operation mandated that it be performed only by surgeons with a sufficiently large number of patients in order to gain adequate experience with the technique. However, with the stapled J-pouch and the application of the double-stapling technique for effecting the anastomosis, the technical aspects of the surgery are relatively well standardized and can be performed by most general surgeons. Yet, the admonition concerning who should perform these restorative procedures has validity. The major problem now is not so much the surgical technique (although this is critically important) as is the requirement for an obsessive, competently applied, follow-up program, as well as the obvious commitment of the surgeon to such a regimen. In my opinion, it is unconscionable for a surgeon to embark on this or any other procedure unless he or she is prepared to adequately communicate the risks and alternatives and to have the knowledge and commitment to appropriately treat the myriad complications and consequences. It appears today, then, that conventional ileostomy will be used primarily for patients with Crohn's disease, for older patients or those doomed to be incontinent, for those with failed pouch procedures, and for those who are not motivated to assume the potential burdens of the pouch alternative.

References

1. Abulafi AM, Fiddian RV. Malignant lymphoma in ulcerative colitis. *Dis Colon Rectum.* 1990;33:615.
2. Adler DJ, Korelitz BI. The therapeutic efficacy of 6 mercaptopurine in refractory ulcerative colitis. *Am J Gastroenterol.* 1990;85:717.
3. Agrez MV, Dozois RR, Beahrs OH. Volvulus of the Kock pouch with obstruction and perforation: a case report. *Aust N Z J Surg.* 1981;51:311.
4. Akwari OE, Kelly KA, Phillips SF. Myoelectric and motor patterns of continent pouch and conventional ileostomy. *Surg Gynecol Obstet.* 1980;150:363.
5. Almy TP, Sherlock P. Genetic aspects of ulcerative colitis and regional enteritis. *Gastroenterology.* 1966;51:757.
6. Alstead EM, Ritchie JK, Lennard-Jones JE, et al. Safety of azathioprine in pregnancy in inflammatory bowel disease. *Gastroenterology.* 1990;99:443.
7. Ambrose NS, Alexander-Williams J. Appraisal of a tissue glue in the treatment of persistent perineal sinus. *Br J Surg.* 1988;75:484.
8. Ambroze WL, Pemberton JH, Dozois RR, et al. The histological pattern and pathological involvement of the anal transition zone in patients with ulcerative colitis. *Gastroenterology.* 1993;104:514.
9. Ambroze WL Jr, Wolff BG, Kelly KA, et al. Let sleeping dogs lie: role of the omentum in the ileal pouch-anal anastomosis procedure. *Dis Colon Rectum.* 1991;34:563.
10. Anderson R, Turnbull RB Jr. Grafting the unhealed perineal wound after coloproctectomy for Crohn's disease. *Arch Surg.* 1976;111:335.
11. Aouthmany A, Horattas MC. Ileal pouch perforation in pregnancy: report of a case and review of the literature. *Dis Colon Rectum.* 2004;47:243.
12. Aratari A, Papi C, Clemente V, et al. Colectomy rate in acute severe ulcerative colitis in the infliximab era. *Dig Liver Dis.* 2008;40:821.
13. Ardizzone S, Molteni P, Imbesi V, et al. Azathioprine in steroid-resistant and steroid-dependent ulcerative colitis. *J Clin Gastroenterol.* 1997;25:330.
14. Aronson MD, Phillips CA, Beeken WL, et al. Isolation and characterization of a viral agent from intestinal tissue of patients with Crohn's disease and other intestinal disorders. *Prog Med Virol.* 1975;21:165.
15. Arts J, D'Haens G, Zeegers M, et al. Long-term outcome of treatment with intravenous cyclosporin in patients with severe ulcerative colitis. *Inflamm Bowel Dis.* 2004;10:73.
16. Aylett SO. Diffuse ulcerative colitis and its treatment by ileorectal anastomosis. *Ann R Coll Surg Engl.* 1960;27:260.
17. Aylett SO. Three hundred cases of diffuse ulcerative colitis treated by total colectomy and ileo-rectal anastomosis. *Br Med J.* 1966;1:1001.
18. Aylett SO. Rectal conservation in the surgical treatment of ulcerative colitis. *Arch Fr Mal App Dig.* 1974;63:585.
19. Bacon HE, Bralow SP, Berkley JL. Rehabilitation and long-term survival after colectomy for ulcerative colitis. *JAMA.* 1960;172:324.
20. Baek SM, Greenstein A, McElhinney AJ, et al. The gracilis myocutaneous flap for persistent perineal sinus after proctocolectomy. *Surg Gynecol Obstet.* 1981;153:713.
21. Baird DD, Narendranathan M, Sandler RS. Increased risk of preterm birth for women with inflammatory bowel disease. *Gastroenterology.* 1990;99:987.
22. Baixauli J, Delaney CP, Wu JS, et al. Functional outcome and quality of life after repeat ileal pouch-anal anastomosis for complications of ileoanal surgery. *Dis Colon Rectum.* 2004;47:2.
23. Ballantyne GH, Graham SM, Hammers L, et al. Superior mesenteric artery syndrome following ileal J-pouch anal anastomosis: an iatrogenic cause of early postoperative obstruction. *Dis Colon Rectum.* 1987;30:472.
24. Bamberger PK, Otchy DP. Ileoanal pouch in the active duty population: effect on military career. *Dis Colon Rectum.* 1997;40:60.
25. Bambrick M, Fazio VW, Hull TL, et al. Sexual function following restorative proctocolectomy in women. *Dis Colon Rectum.* 1996;39:610.
26. Banez AV, Yamanishi F, Crans CA. Endoscopic colonic decompression of toxic megacolon, placement of colonic tube, and steroid colon clysis. *Am J Gastroenterol.* 1987;82:692.
27. Bar Oz B, Hackman R, Einarson T, et al. Pregnancy outcome after cyclosporine therapy during pregnancy: a meta-analysis. *Transplantation.* 2001;71:1051.
28. Baratsis S, Hadjidimitriou F, Christodoulou M, et al. Adenocarcinoma in the anal canal after ileal pouch-anal anastomosis for ulcerative colitis using a double stapling technique: report of a case. *Dis Colon Rectum.* 2002;45:687.
29. Bargen JA. Chronic ulcerative colitis associated with malignant disease. *Arch Surg.* 1928;17:561.
30. Bargen JA. Chronic ulcerative colitis: bacteriologic studies and specific therapy. *Trans Am Proctol Soc.* 1928;28:93.
31. Barkel DC, Pemberton JH, Pezim ME, et al. Scintigraphic assessment of the anorectal angle in health and after ileal pouch anal anastomosis. *Ann Surg.* 1988;208:42.
32. Barnett WO. New approaches for continent ostomy construction. *J Miss State Med Assoc.* 1987;28:1.
33. Barnett WO. Current experiences with the continent intestinal reservoir. *Surg Gynecol Obstet.* 1989;168:1.
34. Bat L, Pines A, Ron E, et al. Colonoscopy without prior preparation in mild to moderate active ulcerative colitis. *J Clin Gastroenterol.* 1991;13:46.
35. Bauer JJ, Gelernt IM, Salk BA, et al. Proctectomy for inflammatory bowel disease. *Am J Surg.* 1986;151:157.
36. Bayer I, Feller N, Chaimoff CH. A new approach to the nipple in Kock's reservoir ileostomy using Mersilene mesh. *Dis Colon Rectum.* 1981;24:428.
37. Beart RW Jr, Beahrs OH, Kelly KA, et al. Continent ileostomy: a viable alternative. *Mayo Clin Proc.* 1979;54:643.
38. Beart RW Jr, Dozois RR, Kelly KA. Ileoanal anastomosis in the adult. *Surg Gynecol Obstet.* 1982;154:826.
39. Beart RW Jr, Dozois RR, Wolff BG, et al. Mechanisms of rectal continence: lessons from the ileoanal procedure. *Am J Surg.* 1985;149:31.
40. Becker JM. Anal sphincter function after colectomy, mucosal proctectomy, and endorectal ileoanal pull-through. *Arch Surg.* 1984;119:526.
41. Becker JM, Dayton MT, Fazio VW, et al. Prevention of postoperative abdominal adhesions by a sodium hyaluronate-based bioresorbable membrane: a prospective, randomized, double-blind multicenter study. *J Am Coll Surg.* 1996;183:297.
42. Becker JM, Hillard AE, Mann FA, et al. Functional assessment after colectomy, mucosal proctectomy and endorectal ileoanal pull-through. *World J Surg.* 1985;9:598.
43. Becker JM, LaMorte W, St. Marie G, et al. Extent of smooth muscle resection during mucosectomy and ileal pouch-anal anastomosis affects anorectal physiology and functional outcome. *Dis Colon Rectum.* 1997;40:653.
44. Becker JM, McGrath KM, Meagher MP, et al. Late functional adaptation after colectomy, mucosal proctectomy, and ileal pouch-anal anastomosis. *Surgery.* 1991;110:718.
45. Becker JM, Raymond JL. Ileal pouch-anal anastomosis: a single surgeon's experience with 100 consecutive cases. *Ann Surg.* 1986;204:375.
46. Befrits R, Ljung T, Jaramillo E, et al. Low-grade dysplasia in extensive, long-standing inflammatory bowel disease. A follow-up study. *Dis Colon Rectum.* 2002;45:615.
47. Behrens DT, Paris M, Luttrell JN. Conversion of failed ileal pouch-anal anastomosis to continent ileostomy. *Dis Colon Rectum.* 1999;42:490.
48. Bell SW, Parry B, Neill M. Adenocarcinoma in the anal transitional zone after ileal pouch for ulcerative colitis: report of a case. *Dis Colon Rectum.* 2003;46:1134.
49. Bellini M, Tansella M. Obsessional scores and subjective general psychiatric complaints of patients with duodenal ulcer or ulcerative colitis. *Psychol Med.* 1976;6:461.
50. Bentrem DJ, Wang KL, Stryker SJ. Adenocarcinoma in an ileal pouch occurring 14 years after restorative proctocolectomy. *Dis Colon Rectum.* 2003;46:544.
51. Bercovitz ZT. Etiology and pathogenesis. In: Bercovitz ZT, Kirsner JB, Lindner AE, et al, eds. *Ulcerative and Granulomatous Colitis.* Springfield, IL: Charles C Thomas; 1973:180.
52. Berglund B, Asztély M, Kock NG, et al. Reflux from the continent ileostomy reservoir: a radiologic evaluation combined with pressure recording. *Dis Colon Rectum.* 1985;28:502.
53. Bernstein CN, Blanchard JF, Kliewer E, et al. Cancer risk in patients with inflammatory bowel disease. *Cancer.* 2001;91:854.

54. Bernstein CN, Shanahan F, Anton PA, et al. Patchiness of mucosal inflammation in treated ulcerative colitis: a prospective study. *Gastrointest Endosc*. 1995;42:232.

55. Bernstein CN, Shanahan F, Weinstein WM. Are we telling patients the truth about surveillance colonoscopy in ulcerative colitis? *Lancet*. 1994;343:71.

56. Binder V, Both H, Hansen PK, et al. Incidence and prevalence of ulcerative colitis and Crohn's disease in the county of Copenhagen, 1962 to 1978. *Gastroenterology*. 1982;83:563.

57. Black AJ, McLeod HL, Capell HA, et al. Thiopurine methyltransferase genotype predicts therapy-limiting severe toxicity from azathioprine. *Ann Intern Med*. 1998;129:716.

58. Blackstone MO, Riddell RH, Rogers BHG, et al. Dysplasia-associated lesion or mass (DALM) detected by colonoscopy in long-standing ulcerative colitis: an indication for colectomy. *Gastroenterology*. 1981;80:366.

59. Bloom RJ, Larsen CP, Watt R, et al. A reappraisal of the Kock continent ileostomy in patients with Crohn's disease. *Surg Gynecol Obstet*. 1986;162:105.

60. Bodzin JH, Kestenberg W, Kaufmann R, et al. Mucosal proctectomy and ileoanal pull-through technique and functional results in 23 consecutive patients. *Am Surg*. 1987;53:363.

61. Bohe MG, Ekelund GR, Genell SN, et al. Surgery for fulminating colitis during pregnancy. *Dis Colon Rectum*. 1983;26:119.

62. Bokey LE, Fazio VW. The mesenteric sling technique. A new method of constructing an intestinal nipple valve for the continent ileostomy. *Cleve Clin Q*. 1978;45:231.

63. Bolton RP, Sherrif RJ, Read AE. *Clostridium difficile*-associated diarrhoea: a role in inflammatory bowel disease? *Lancet*. 1980;1:383.

64. Bonello JC, Thow GB, Manson RR. Mucosal enteritis: a complication of the continent ileostomy. *Dis Colon Rectum*. 1981;24:37.

65. Booth IW, Harries JT. Inflammatory bowel disease in childhood. *Gut*. 1984;25:188.

66. Bostwick J III, Moore J, McGarity WC. Inferior gluteal musculocutaneous flap for the obliteration of acute and chronic proctocolectomy defects. *Surg Gynecol Obstet*. 1988;166:169.

67. Brahme F. Crohn's disease in a defined population. *Gastroenterology*. 1975;69:342.

68. Brandt L, Boley S, Goldberg L, et al. Colitis in the elderly. *Am J Gastroenterol*. 1981;76:239.

69. Braun J, Treutner KH, Harder M, et al. Anal sphincter function after intersphincteric resection and ileal pouch-anal anastomosis. *Dis Colon Rectum*. 1991;34:8.

70. Briggs GG, Freeman RK, Yaffe SJ. *Drugs in Pregnancy and Lactation: A Reference Guide to Fetal and Neonatal Risk*. 7th ed. Philadelphia, PA: Lippincott Williams & Wilkins; 2005.

71. Broader JH, Masselink BA, Oates GD, et al. Management of the pelvic space after proctectomy. *Br J Surg*. 1974;61:94.

72. Brooke BN. The outcome of surgery for ulcerative colitis. *Lancet*. 1956;2:532.

73. Broström O, Löfberg R, Öst A, et al. Cancer surveillance of patients with long-standing ulcerative colitis: a clinical, endoscopical, and histological study. *Gut*. 1986;27:1408.

74. Brown JY. Value of complete physiological rest of large bowel in ulcerative and obstructive lesions. *Surg Gynecol Obstet*. 1913;16:610.

75. Brown SR, Eu KW, Seow-Choen F. Consecutive series of laparoscopic-assisted vs. minilaparotomy restorative proctocolectomies. *Dis Colon Rectum*. 2001;44:397.

76. Bullard KM, Madoff RD, Gemlo BT. Is ileoanal pouch function stable with time? Results of a prospective audit. *Dis Colon Rectum*. 2002;45:299.

77. Bures J, Fixa B, Komárková O, et al. Nonsmoking: a feature of ulcerative colitis. *Br Med J*. 1982;285:440.

78. Burke D, van Laarhoven CJHM, Herbst F, et al. Transvaginal repair of pouch-vaginal fistula. *Br J Surg*. 2001;88:241.

79. Burnham WR, Lennard-Jones JE, Brooke BN. The incidence and nature of sexual problems among married ileostomists [abstract]. *Gut*. 1976;17:391.

80. Burnstein MJ, Schoetz DJ Jr, Coller JA, et al. Technique of mesenteric lengthening in ileal reservoir-anal anastomosis. *Dis Colon Rectum*. 1987;30:863.

81. Carter FM, McLeod RS, Cohen Z. Subtotal colectomy for ulcerative colitis: complications related to the rectal remnant. *Dis Colon Rectum*. 1991;34:1005.

82. Carter MJ, Lobo AJ, Travis SP. Guidelines for the management of inflammatory bowel disease in adults. *Gut*. 2004;53(suppl 5):V1.

83. Cattell RB. The surgical treatment of ulcerative colitis. *JAMA*. 1935;104:104.

84. Cave HW. The surgical management of chronic intractable ulcerative colitis. *Am J Surg*. 1939;46:79.

85. Chaparro M, Burgueno P, Flores E, et al. Efficacy and safety of infliximab rescue therapy after cyclosporine failure in patients with steroid-refractory ulcerative colitis: a multicenter study. *Gastroenterology*. 2010;38:S688.

86. Cherqui D, Valleur P, Perniceni T, et al. Inferior reach of ileal reservoir in ileoanal anastomosis: experimental anatomic and angiographic study. *Dis Colon Rectum*. 1987;30:365.

87. Chey WY. Infliximab for patients with refractory ulcerative colitis. *Inflamm Bowel Dis*. 2001;7(suppl 1):S30.

88. Chey WY, Hussain A, Ryan C, et al. Infliximab for refractory ulcerative colitis. *Am J Gastroenterol*. 2001;96:2373.

89. Chiodini RJ, Van Kruiningen HJ, Thayer WR, et al. Possible role of mycobacteria in inflammatory bowel disease. I: An unclassified *Mycobacterium* species isolated from patients with Crohn's disease. *Dig Dis Sci*. 1984;29:1073.

90. Choi PM, Nugent FW, Schoetz DJ Jr, et al. Colonoscopic surveillance reduces mortality from colorectal cancer in ulcerative colitis. *Gastroenterology*. 1993;105:418.

91. Christie PM, Schroeder D, Hill GL. Persisting superior mesenteric artery syndrome following ileo-anal J-pouch construction. *Br J Surg*. 1988;75:1036.

92. Chung PY, Cohen RD, Kirschner BS, et al. Intravenous cyclosporin in ulcerative colitis: long-term follow-up of the University of Chicago experience. Paper presented at: The American College of Gastroenterology; October 15, 2003.

93. Church JM, Saad R, Schroeder T, et al. Predicting the functional result of anastomoses to the anus: the paradox of preoperative anal resting pressure. *Dis Colon Rectum*. 1993;36:895.

94. Clark ML. Role of nutrition in inflammatory bowel disease: an overview. *Gut*. 1986;27:72.

95. Coffey JC, Winter DC, Neary P, et al. Quality of life after ileal pouch-anal anastomosis: an evaluation of diet and other factors using the Cleveland global quality of life instrument. *Dis Colon Rectum*. 2002;45:30.

96. Cohen RD, Brodsky AL, Hanauer SB. A comparison of the quality of life in patients with severe ulcerative colitis after total colectomy versus medical treatment with intravenous cyclosporin. *Inflamm Bowel Dis*. 1999;5:1.

97. Cohen RD, Stern R, Hanauer SB. Intravenous cyclosporin in ulcerative colitis: a five-year experience. *Am J Gastroenterol*. 1999;94:1587.

98. Cohen Z, Cook MG, Festenstein H. The transmission of human Crohn's disease in inbred strains of mice [abstract]. *Ann R Coll Phys Surg Can*. 1978;2:51.

99. Cohen Z, McLeod RS, Stephen W, et al. Continuing evolution of the pelvic pouch procedure. *Ann Surg*. 1992;216:506.

100. Collins RH Jr, Feldman M, Fordtran JS. Colon cancer, dysplasia, and surveillance in patients with ulcerative colitis: a critical review. *N Engl J Med*. 1987;316:1654.

101. Columbel JF, Ricart E, Loftus EV, et al. Management of Crohn's disease (CD) of the ileoanal pouch with infliximab. *Gastroenterology*. 2003;124(suppl 1):A519.

102. Connell WR, Talbot IC, Harpaz N, et al. Clinicopathological characteristics of colorectal carcinoma complicating ulcerative colitis. *Gut*. 1994;35:1419.

103. Coran AG. The ileal endorectal pull-through procedure. *Surg Rounds*. 1982:40.

104. Coran AG. A personal experience with 100 consecutive total colectomies and straight ileoanal endorectal pull-throughs for benign disease of the colon and rectum in children and adults. *Ann Surg*. 1990;212:242.

105. Corbett RS. Discussion on the surgical treatment of idiopathic ulcerative colitis and its surgical sequelae. *Proc R Soc Med*. 1940;33:647.

106. Corman ML. Total anal reconstruction to restore intestinal continuity after conventional proctocolectomy: report of a case. *Colorectal Dis*. 2003;5:595.

107. Corman ML, Veidenheimer MC, Coller JA. Impotence after proctectomy for inflammatory disease of the bowel. *Dis Colon Rectum*. 1978;21:418.

108. Corman ML, Veidenheimer MC, Coller JA, et al. Perineal wound healing after proctectomy for inflammatory bowel disease. *Dis Colon Rectum*. 1978;21:155.

109. Coull DB, Lee FD, Henderson AP, et al. Risk of dysplasia in the columnar cuff after stapled restorative proctocolectomy. *Br J Surg*. 2003;90:72.

110. Cox CL, Butts DR, Roberts MP, et al. Development of invasive adenocarcinoma in a long-standing Kock continent ileostomy: report of a case. *Dis Colon Rectum*. 1997;40:500.

111. Cranley B. The Kock reservoir ileostomy: a review of its development, problems and role in modern surgical practice. *Br J Surg*. 1983;70:94.

112. Crile G Jr, Thomas CY Jr. Treatment of acute toxic ulcerative colitis by ileostomy and simultaneous colectomy. *Gastroenterology*. 1951;19:58.

113. Cripps NPJ, Senapati A, Thompson MR. Improved perineal healing after internal sphincter-preserving proctectomy in ulcerative colitis. *Br J Surg.* 1999;86:1344.

114. Crohn BB, Ginzburg L, Oppenheimer GD. Regional ileitis: a pathologic and clinical entity. *JAMA.* 1932;99:1323.

115. Crohn BB, Yarnis H, Walter RI, et al. Ulcerative colitis as affected by pregnancy. *N Y State J Med.* 1956;56:2651.

116. Crowson TD, Ferrante WF, Gathright JB Jr. Colonoscopy: inefficacy for early carcinoma detection in patients with ulcerative colitis. *JAMA.* 1976;236:2651.

117. Cunnien AJ. Psychiatric aspects of chronic ulcerative colitis. *Semin Colon Rectal Surg.* 1990;1:158.

118. Das KM, Morecki R, Nair P, et al. Idiopathic proctitis: I. The morphology of proximal colonic mucosa and its clinical significance. *Am J Dig Dis.* 1977;22:524.

119. Dassei PM. A familial pattern in inflammatory disease of the bowel (Crohn's disease and ulcerative colitis). *Dis Colon Rectum.* 1977;20:669.

120. Daum F, Alperstein G. Inflammatory bowel disease in children and adolescents. *Pediatr Gastroenterol.* 1982;6:26.

121. Davidson M. Juvenile ulcerative colitis. *N Engl J Med.* 1967;277:1408.

122. de Castella H. Non-smoking: a feature of ulcerative colitis. *Br Med J.* 1982;284:1706.

123. de Dombal FT, Burton I, Goligher JC. The early and late results of surgical treatment for Crohn's disease. *Br J Surg.* 1971;58:805.

124. de Dombal FT, Watts JM, Watkinson G, et al. Ulcerative colitis and pregnancy. *Lancet.* 1965;2:599.

125. Deen KI, Hubscher S, Bain I, et al. Histological assessment of the distal doughnut in patients undergoing stapled restorative proctocolectomy with high or low anal transection. *Br J Surg.* 1994;81:900.

126. Deen KI, Williams JG, Grant EA, et al. Randomized trial to determine the optimum level of pouch-anal anastomosis in stapled restorative procto-colectomy. *Dis Colon Rectum.* 1995;38:133.

127. Dejaco CMC, Reinisch W. Azathioprine treatment and male fertility in inflammatory bowel disease. *Gastroenterology.* 2001;121:1048.

128. Delaney CP, Dadvand B, Remzi FH, et al. Functional outcome, quality of life, and complications after ileal pouch-anal anastomosis in selected septuagenarians. *Dis Colon Rectum.* 2002;45:890.

129. Delaney CP, Fazio VW, Remzi FH, et al. Prospective, age-related analysis of surgical results, functional outcome, and quality of life after ileal pouch-anal anastomosis. *Ann Surg.* 2003;238:221.

130. de Silva HJ, de Angelis CP, Soper N, et al. Clinical and functional outcome after restorative proctocolectomy. *Br J Surg.* 1991;78:1039.

131. D'Haens G, Lemmens L, Geboes K, et al. Intravenous cyclosporine versus intravenous glucocorticosteroids as a single therapy for severe attacks of ulcerative colitis. *Gastroenterology.* 2001;120:1323.

132. Dick AP, Grayson MJ, Carpenter RG, et al. Controlled trial of sulphasalazine in the treatment of ulcerative colitis. *Gut.* 1964;5:437.

133. Dickinson RJ, Dixon MF, Axon ATR. Colonoscopy and the detection of dysplasia in patients with long-standing ulcerative colitis. *Lancet.* 1980;2:620.

134. Diehl JT, Steiger E, Hooley R. The role of intravenous hyperalimen-tation in intestinal diseases. *Surg Clin North Am.* 1983;63:11.

135. Donnelly BJ, Delaney PV, Healy TM. Evidence for a transmissible factor in Crohn's disease. *Gut.* 1977;18:360.

136. Donovan MJ, O'Hara ET. Sexual function following surgery for ulcerative colitis. *N Engl J Med.* 1960;262:719.

137. Doyle PJ, McKay AJ, Browne MK. Failure to thrive in adolescence due to inflammatory bowel disease. *Practitioner.* 1979;222:253.

138. Dozois RR, Kelly KA, Beart RW Jr, et al. Improved results with continent ileostomy. *Ann Surg.* 1980;192:319.

139. Dozois RR, Kelly KA, Ilstrup D, et al. Factors affecting revision rate after continent ileostomy. *Arch Surg.* 1981;116:610.

140. Dragstedt LR, Dack GM, Kirsner JB. Chronic ulcerative colitis: a summary of evidence implicating bacterium necrophorum as an etiologic agent. *Ann Surg.* 1941;114:653.

141. Drossman DA. Psychosocial factors in inflammatory bowel disease. *Pract Gastroenterol.* 1992;16:24N.

142. Dunker MS, Bemelman WA, Slors JFM, et al. Functional outcome, quality of life, body image, and cosmesis in patients after laparoscopic-assisted and conventional restorative proctocolectomy. *Dis Colon Rectum.* 2001;44:1800.

143. Ecker KW, Hildebrandt U, Haberer M, et al. Biomechanical stabiliza-tion of the nipple valve in continent ileostomy. *Br J Surg.* 1996;83:1582.

144. Edwards F, Truelove SC. The course and prognosis of ulcerative coli-tis. Part I: short-term prognosis. *Gut.* 1963;4:299.

145. Ekbom A, Helmick C, Zack M, et al. Ulcerative colitis and colorectal cancer: a population-based study. *N Engl J Med.* 1990;323:1228.

146. Emmanouilidis A, Manoussos O, Nicolaou A, et al. Colonoscopy in ulcerative colitis. *Am J Proctol Gastroenterol Colon Rectal Surg.* 1983;34:5.

147. Evans JG, Acheson ED. An epidemiological study of ulcerative coli-tis and regional enteritis in the Oxford area. *Gut.* 1965;6:311.

148. Farmer RG, Michener WM, Mortimer EA. Studies of family history among patients with inflammatory bowel disease. *Clin Gastroenterol.* 1980;9:271.

149. Farnell MB, Van Heerden JA, Beart RW Jr, et al. Rectal preservation in nonspecific inflammatory disease of the colon. *Ann Surg.* 1980;192:249.

150. Farouk R, Duthie GS, Bartolo DCC. Recovery of the internal anal sphincter and continence after restorative proctocolectomy. *Br J Surg.* 1994;81:1065.

151. Farouk R, Pemberton JH, Wolff BG, et al. Functional outcomes after ileal pouch-anal anastomosis for chronic ulcerative colitis. *Ann Surg.* 2000;231:919.

152. Farrell GC. *Drug-Induced Liver Disease.* Singapore: Churchill Livingstone; 1994.

153. Fasth S, Öresland T, Ahrén C, et al. Mucosal proctectomy and ileostomy as an alternative to conventional proctectomy. *Dis Colon Rectum.* 1985;28:31.

154. Faubion WA Jr, Loftus EV Jr, Harmsen WS, et al. The natural history of corticosteroid therapy for inflammatory bowel disease: a population-based study. *Gastroenterology.* 2001;121:255.

155. Fazio VW. Toxic megacolon in ulcerative colitis and Crohn's colitis. *Clin Gastroenterol.* 1980;9:389.

156. Fazio VW, Church JM. Complications and function of the continent ileostomy at the Cleveland Clinic. *World J Surg.* 1988;12:148.

157. Fazio VW, Tekkis PP, Remzi F, et al. Quantification of risk for pouch failure after ileal pouch anal anastomosis surgery. *Ann Surg.* 2003;238:605.

158. Fazio VW, Tjandra JJ. Pouch advancement and neoileoanal anastomosis for anastomotic stricture and anovaginal fistula complicating restorative proctocolectomy. *Br J Surg.* 1992;79:694.

159. Fazio VW, Tjandra JJ. Technique for nipple valve fixation to prevent valve slippage in continent ileostomy. *Dis Colon Rectum.* 1992;35:1177.

160. Fazio VW, Tjandra JJ. Transanal mucosectomy: ileal pouch advancement for anorectal dysplasia or inflammation after restorative proctocolectomy. *Dis Colon Rectum.* 1994;37:1008.

161. Fazio VW, Ziv Y, Church JM, et al. Ileal pouch-anal anastomoses: complications and function in 1005 patients. *Ann Surg.* 1995;222:120.

162. Feagan BG, Reinisch W, Rutgeerts P, et al. The effects of infliximab therapy on health-related quality of life in ulcerative colitis patients. *Am J Gastroenterol.* 2007;102:794.

163. Fedorak RN, Gionchetti P, Campieti M, et al. VSL#3 probiotic mixture induces remission in patients with active ulcerative colitis. *Gastro-enterology.* 2003;124:A377(M1582).

164. Feinberg SM, McLeod RS, Cohen Z. Complications of loop ileostomy. *Am J Surg.* 1987;153:102.

165. Fergani H, Fardy J. Smoking and inflammatory bowel disease: an effect of disease or disease location: a meta-analysis. *Gastroenterology.* 2002;122:A604.

166. Ferrara A, Pemberton JH, Grotz RL, et al. Motor determinants of incontinence after ileal pouch-anal anastomosis. *Br J Surg.* 1994;81:285.

167. Ferrari BT, Fonkalsrud EW. Endorectal ileal pullthrough operation with ileal reservoir after total colectomy. *Am J Surg.* 1978;136:113.

168. Fichera A, Cicchiello LA, Mendelson DS, et al. Superior mesenteric vein thrombosis after colectomy for inflammatory bowel disease: a not uncommon cause of postoperative acute abdominal pain. *Dis Colon Rectum.* 2003;46:643.

169. Flake WK, Altman MS, Cartmill AM, et al. Problems encountered with the Kock ileostomy. *Am J Surg.* 1979;138:851.

170. Fleshman JW, Cohen Z, McLeod RS, et al. The ileal reservoir and ileoanal anastomosis procedure: factors affecting technical and functional outcome. *Dis Colon Rectum.* 1988;31:10.

171. Foley EF, Schoetz DJ Jr, Roberts PL, et al. Rediversion after ileal pouch-anal anastomosis: causes of failures and predictors of subsequent pouch salvage. *Dis Colon Rectum.* 1995;38:793.

172. Fonkalsrud EW. Total colectomy and endorectal ileal pullthrough with internal ileal reservoir for ulcerative colitis. *Surg Gynecol Obstet.* 1980;150:1.

173. Fonkalsrud EW. Endorectal ileal pullthrough with lateral ileal reservoir for benign colorectal disease. *Ann Surg.* 1981;194:761.

174. Fonkalsrud EW. Endorectal pullthrough with ileal reservoir for ulcerative colitis and polyposis. *Am J Surg.* 1982;144:81.

175. Fonkalsrud EW. Endorectal ileoanal anastomosis with isoperistaltic ileal reservoir after colectomy and mucosal proctectomy. *Ann Surg.* 1984;199:151.

176. Fonkalsrud EW. Endorectal ileal pullthrough with isoperistaltic ileal reservoir for colitis and polyposis. *Ann Surg.* 1985;202:145.

177. Fonkalsrud EW. Update on clinical experience with different surgical techniques on the endorectal pullthrough operation for colitis and polyposis. *Surg Gynecol Obstet.* 1987;165:309.

178. Fonkalsrud EW. Long-term results after colectomy and ileoanal pull-through procedure in children. *Arch Surg.* 1996;131:881.

179. Fonkalsrud EW, Phillips JD. Reconstruction of malfunctioning ileoanal pouch procedures as an alternative to permanent ileostomy. *Am J Surg.* 1990;160:245.

180. Fonkalsrud EW, Stelzner M, McDonald N. Experience with the endorectal ileal pullthrough with lateral reservoir for ulcerative colitis and polyposis. *Arch Surg.* 1988;123:1053.

181. Fozard JBJ, Dixon MF. Colonoscopic surveillance in ulcerative colitis—dysplasia through the looking glass. *Gut.* 1989;30:285.

182. Franceschi D, Chen PF, Yuh JN. Solitary J-pouch ulcer causing pouchitis-like syndrome. *Dis Colon Rectum.* 1986;29:515.

183. Francois Y, Dozois RR, Kelly KA, et al. Small intestinal obstruction complicating ileal pouch-anal anastomosis. *Ann Surg.* 1989;209:46.

184. Frizzi JD, Rivera DE, Harris JA, et al. Lymphoma arising in an S-pouch after total proctocolectomy for ulcerative colitis: report of a case. *Dis Colon Rectum.* 2000;43:540.

185. Frühmorgen P. Diagnosis of inflammatory disease of the colon by colonoscopy. *Acta Gastroenterol Belg.* 1974;37:154.

186. Fujita S, Kusunoki M, Shoji Y, et al. Quality of life after total proctocolectomy and ileal J-pouch-anal anastomosis. *Dis Colon Rectum.* 1992;35:1030.

187. Gadacz TR, Kelly KA, Phillips SF. The continent ileal pouch: absorptive and motor features. *Gastroenterology.* 1977;72:1287.

188. Galandiuk S, Pemberton JH, Tsao J, et al. Delayed ileal pouch-anal anastomosis: complications and functional results. *Dis Colon Rectum.* 1991;34:755.

189. Galandiuk S, Scott NA, Dozois RR, et al. Ileal pouch-anal anastomosis. *Ann Surg.* 1990;212:446.

190. Galandiuk S, Wolff BG, Dozois RR, et al. Ileal pouch-anal anastomosis without ileostomy. *Dis Colon Rectum.* 1991;34:870.

191. Gardner C, Miller GG. Total colectomy for ulcerative colitis. *Arch Surg.* 1951;63:370.

192. Gassull MA, Abad A, Cabré E, et al. Enteral nutrition in inflammatory bowel disease. *Gut.* 1986;27:76.

193. Geboes K, Vantrappen G. The value of colonoscopy in the diagnosis of Crohn's disease. *Gastrointest Endosc.* 1975;22:18.

194. Gecim IE, Wolff BG, Pemberton JH, et al. Does technique of anastomosis play any role in developing late perianal abscess or fistula? *Dis Colon Rectum.* 2000;43:1241.

195. Gelernt IM, Bauer JJ, Kreel I. The reservoir ileostomy: early experience with 54 patients. *Ann Surg.* 1977;185:179.

196. Gemlo BT, Belmonte C, Wiltz O, et al. Functional assessment of ileal pouch-anal anastomotic techniques. *Am J Surg.* 1995;169:137.

197. Gemlo BT, Wong WD, Rothenberger DA, et al. Ileal pouch-anal anastomosis: patterns of failure. *Arch Surg.* 1992;127:784.

198. George J, Present DH, Pou R, et al. The long term outcome of ulcerative colitis treated with 6-mercaptopurine. *Am J Gastroenterol.* 1996;91:1711.

199. Gerber A, Apt MK, Craig PH. The Kock continent ileostomy. *Surg Gynecol Obstet.* 1983;156:345.

200. Gilat T, Fireman Z, Grossman A, et al. Colorectal cancer in patients with ulcerative colitis: a population study in central Israel. *Gastroenterology.* 1988;94:870.

201. Gionchetti P, Rizzello F, Venturi A, et al. Oral bacteriotherapy as maintenance treatment in patients with chronic pouchitis: a double-blind, placebo-controlled trial. *Gastroenterology.* 2000;119:305.

202. Gisbert JP, Linares PM, McNicholl AG, et al. Meta-analysis: the efficacy of azathioprine and mercaptopurine in ulcerative colitis. *Aliment Pharmacol Ther.* 2009;30:126.

203. Gitnick GL. Is Crohn's disease a mycobacterial disease after all? *Dig Dis Sci.* 1984;29:1086.

204. Gitnick GL, Rosen VJ, Arthur MH, et al. Evidence for the isolation of a new virus from ulcerative proctitis patients: comparison with virus derived from Crohn's disease. *Dig Dis Sci.* 1979;24:609.

205. Goes RN, Coy CSR, Amaral CA, et al. Superior mesenteric artery syndrome as a complication of ileal pouch-anal anastomosis: report of a case. *Dis Colon Rectum.* 1995;38:543.

206. Goes RN, Nguyen P, Huang D, et al. Lengthening of the mesentery using the marginal vascular arcade of the right colon as the blood supply to the ileal pouch. *Dis Colon Rectum.* 1995;38:893.

207. Goldman CD, Kodner IJ, Fry RD, et al. Clinical and operative experience with non-Caucasian patients with Crohn's disease. *Dis Colon Rectum.* 1986;29:317.

208. Goldstein LH, Dolinsky G, Greenberg R, et al. Pregnancy outcome of women exposed to azathioprine during pregnancy. *Birth Defects Res A Clin Mol Teratol.* 2007;79:696.

209. Goligher JC. Primary excisional surgery in treatment of ulcerative colitis. *Ann R Coll Surg Engl.* 1954;15:316.

210. Goligher JC. Inflammatory disease of the bowel: results of resection for Crohn's disease. *Dis Colon Rectum.* 1976;19:584.

211. Goligher JC. Continent ileostomy: commentary. *World J Surg.* 1980;4:147.

212. Goligher JC. *Surgery of the Anus, Rectum and Colon.* 4th ed. London, United Kingdom: Bailliére Tindall; 1980:689.

213. Goligher JC. *Surgery of the Anus, Rectum and Colon.* 4th ed. London, United Kingdom: Bailliére Tindall; 1980:793.

214. Goligher JC. *Surgery of the Anus, Rectum and Colon.* 4th ed. London, United Kingdom: Bailliére Tindall; 1980:828.

215. Goligher JC. Eversion technique for distal mucosal proctectomy in ulcerative colitis: a preliminary report. *Br J Surg.* 1984;71:26.

216. Goligher JC, de Dombal FT, Watts J McK, et al. *Ulcerative Colitis.* London, United Kingdom: Bailliére, Tindall and Cassell; 1968:2.

217. Gopal KA, Amshel AL, Shonberg IL, et al. Ostomy and pregnancy. *Dis Colon Rectum.* 1985;28:912.

218. Gorenstein L, Boyd JB, Ross TM. Gracilis muscle repair of rectovaginal fistula after restorative proctocolectomy: report of two cases. *Dis Colon Rectum.* 1988;31:730.

219. Gorfine SR, Bauer JJ, Harris MT, et al. Dysplasia complicating chronic ulcerative colitis. *Dis Colon Rectum.* 2000;43:1575.

220. Gorfine SR, Fichera A, Harris MT, et al. Long-term results of salvage surgery for septic complications after restorative proctocolectomy: does fecal diversion improve outcome? *Dis Colon Rectum.* 2003;46:1339.

221. Gorfine SR, Gelernt IM, Bauer JJ, et al. Restorative proctocolectomy without diverting ileostomy. *Dis Colon Rectum.* 1995;38:188.

222. Gormet JM, Couve S, Hassani Z, et al. Infliximab for refractory ulcerative colitis or indeterminate colitis: an open label multicentre study. *Aliment Pharmacol Ther.* 2003;18:175.

223. Gottlieb LM, Handelsman JC. Treatment of outflow tract problems associated with continent ileostomy (Kock pouch): report of six cases. *Dis Colon Rectum.* 1991;34:936.

224. Grant CS, Dozois RR. Toxic megacolon: ultimate fate of patients after successful medical management. *Am J Surg.* 1984;147:106.

225. Grant D, Cohen Z, McHugh S, et al. Restorative proctocolectomy: clinical results and manometric findings with long and short rectal cuffs. *Dis Colon Rectum.* 1986;29:27.

226. Greenstein AJ. Cancer in inflammatory bowel disease. *Surg Rounds.* 1982:44.

227. Greenstein AJ, Aufses AH Jr. Differences in pathogenesis, incidence and outcome of perforation in inflammatory bowel disease. *Surg Gynecol Obstet.* 1985;160:63.

228. Greenstein AJ, Barth JA, Sachar DB, et al. Free colonic perforation without dilatation in ulcerative colitis. *Am J Surg.* 1986;152:272.

229. Greenstein AJ, Mann D, Heimann T, et al. Spontaneous free perforation and perforated abscess in 30 patients with Crohn's disease. *Ann Surg.* 1987;205:72.

230. Grobier SP, Hosie KB, Keighley MRB. Randomized trial of loop ileostomy in restorative proctocolectomy. *Br J Surg.* 1992;79:903.

231. Groom JS, Nicholls RJ, Hawley PR, et al. Pouch-vaginal fistula. *Br J Surg.* 1993;80:936.

232. Grundfest SF, Fazio V, Weiss RA, et al. The risk of cancer following colectomy and ileorectal anastomosis for extensive mucosal ulcerative colitis. *Ann Surg.* 1981;193:9.

233. Guillemot F, Leroy J, Boniface M, et al. Functional assessment of coloanal anastomosis with reservoir and excision of the anal transition zone. *Dis Colon Rectum.* 1991;34:967.

234. Gur C, Diav-Citrin O, Shechtman S, et al. Pregnancy outcome after first trimester exposure to corticosteroids: a prospective controlled study. *Reprod Toxicol.* 2004;18:93.

235. Gurian L, Klein K, Ward TT. Role of *Clostridium difficile* and *Campylobacter jejuni* in relapses of inflammatory bowel disease. *West J Med.* 1983;138:359.

236. Gustavsson S, Weiland LH, Kelly KA. Relationship of backwash ileitis to ileal pouchitis after ileal pouch-anal anastomosis. *Dis Colon Rectum.* 1987;30:25.

237. Gutierrez P, Stahlgren LH. A technique for catheter fixation for continent ileostomy. *Surg Gynecol Obstet.* 1983;156:808.

238. Gyde S. Screening for colorectal cancer in ulcerative colitis: dubious benefits and high costs. *Gut.* 1990;31:1089.

239. Halverson AL, Hull TL, Remzi F, et al. Perioperative resting pressure predicts long-term postoperative function after ileal pouch-anal anastomosis. *J Gastrointest Surg.* 2002;6:316.

240. Halvorsen JF, Heimann P, Hoel R, et al. The continent reservoir ileostomy: review of a collective series of 36 patients from three surgical departments. *Surgery*. 1978;83:252.

241. Ham RJ, Ball A. A convenient alternative to the Zachary Cope enterostomy clamp. *Ann R Coll Surg Engl*. 1985;67:82.

242. Hampson SJ, McFadden JJ, Hermon-Taylor J. Mycobacteria and Crohn's disease. *Gut*. 1988;29:1017.

243. Hanauer SB. Nicotine for colitis—the smoke has not yet cleared. *N Engl J Med*. 1994;330:856.

244. Hanauer SB. Inflammatory bowel disease. *N Engl J Med*. 1996;334:841.

245. Hanauer SB, Sandborn WJ, Dallaire C, et al. Delayed-release oral mesalamine 4.8 g/day (800 mg tablets) compared to 2.4 g/day (400 mg tablets) for the treatment of mildly to moderately active ulcerative colitis: the ASCEND I trial. *Can J Gastroenterol*. 2007;21:827.

246. Hanson PA. Diet for control of an ileoanal reservoir. *Ostomy Wound Manage*. 1990;28:24.

247. Haray PN, Amarnath B, Weiss EG, et al. Low malignant potential of the double-stapled ileal pouch-anal anastomosis. *Br J Surg*. 1996;83:1406.

248. Harford FJ Jr. Use of the ultrasonic aspirator to strip the mesentery in construction of the continent ileostomy. *Dis Colon Rectum*. 1987;30:736.

249. Harms BA, Andersen AB, Starling JR. The W ileal reservoir: long-term assessment after proctocolectomy for ulcerative colitis and familial polyposis. *Surgery*. 1992;112:638.

250. Harms BA, Hamilton JW, Yamamoto DT, et al. Quadruple-loop (W) ileal pouch reconstruction after proctocolectomy. *Surgery*. 1987;102:561.

251. Harms BA, Myers GA, Rosenfeld DJ, et al. Management of fulminant ulcerative colitis by primary restorative proctocolectomy. *Dis Colon Rectum*. 1994;37:971.

252. Harms BA, Pahl AC, Starling JR. Comparison of clinical and compliance characteristics between S and W ileal reservoirs. *Am J Surg*. 1990;159:34.

253. Harms BA, Pellett JR, Starling JR. Modified quadruple-loop (W) ileal reservoir for restorative proctocolectomy. *Surgery*. 1987;101:234.

254. Harper PH, Lee ECG, Kettlewell MGW, et al. Role of the faecal stream in the maintenance of Crohn's colitis. *Gut*. 1985;26:279.

255. Harries AD, Baird A, Rhodes J. Non-smoking: a feature of ulcerative colitis. *Br Med J*. 1982;284:706.

256. Harries AD, Danis VA, Heatley RV. Influence of nutritional status on immune functions in patients with Crohn's disease. *Gut*. 1984;25:465.

257. Harvey PRC, McLeod RS, Cohen Z, et al. Effect of colectomy on bile consumption, cholesterol crystal formation, and gallstones in patients with ulcerative colitis. *Ann Surg*. 1991;214:396.

258. Hashimoto L, Seidner D, Steiger E, et al. Recurrent small bowel obstruction secondary to a dilated Kock pouch: a case report. *Am Surg*. 1995;61:334.

259. Hata J, Haruma K, Suenaga K, et al. Ultrasonographic assessment of inflammatory bowel disease. *Am J Gastroenterol*. 1992;87:443.

260. Hawley PR. Ileorectal anastomosis. *Br J Surg*. 1985;72(suppl):S75.

261. Hawthorne AB, Logan RF, Hawkey CJ, et al. Randomised controlled trial of azathioprine withdrawal in ulcerative colitis. *BMJ*. 1992;305:20.

262. Heald RJ, Allen DR. Stapled ileo-anal anastomosis: a technique to avoid mucosal proctectomy in the ileal pouch operation. *Br J Surg*. 1986;73:571.

263. Heimann TM, Greenstein AJ, Mechanic L, et al. Early complications following surgical treatment for Crohn's disease. *Ann Surg*. 1985;201:494.

264. Heimann TM, Kurtz RJ, Aufses AH Jr. Ultrasonic fragmentation: a new technique for mucosal proctectomy. *Arch Surg*. 1985;120:1200.

265. Heimann TM, Slater G, Kurtz RJ, et al. Ultrasonic mucosal proctectomy in patients with ulcerative colitis. *Ann Surg*. 1989;210:787.

266. Heit HA. Use of antidiarrheals in ulcerative colitis [letter and reply]. *Gastroenterology*. 1988;94:1520.

267. Helzer JE, Stillings WA, Chammas S, et al. A controlled study of the association between ulcerative colitis and psychiatric diagnosis. *Dig Dis Sci*. 1982;27:513.

268. Hensley GT. Interpretation of colonic mucosal biopsy in IBD: potential pitfalls. *Pract Gastroenterol*. 1987;11(3):15.

269. Heppell J, Belliveau P, Taillefer R, et al. Quantitative assessment of pelvic ileal reservoir emptying with a semisolid radionuclide enema: a correlation with clinical outcome. *Dis Colon Rectum*. 1987;30:81.

270. Heppell J, Farkouh E, Dubé S, et al. Toxic megacolon: an analysis of 70 cases. *Dis Colon Rectum*. 1986;29:789.

271. Heppell J, Kelly KA, Phillips SF, et al. Physiologic aspects of continence after colectomy, mucosal proctectomy, and endorectal ileo-anal anastomosis. *Ann Surg*. 1982;195:435.

272. Heppell J, Weiland LH, Perrault J, et al. Fate of the rectal mucosa after rectal mucosectomy and ileoanal anastomosis. *Dis Colon Rectum*. 1983;26:768.

273. Herbst F, Sielezneff I, Nicholls RJ. Salvage surgery for ileal pouch outlet obstruction. *Br J Surg*. 1996;83:368.

274. Herline AJ, Meisinger LL, Rusin LC, et al. Is routine pouch surveillance for dysplasia indicated for ileoanal pouches? *Dis Colon Rectum*. 2003;46:156.

275. Heuschen UA, Allemeyer EH, Hinz U, et al. Outcome after septic complications in J pouch procedures. *Br J Surg*. 2002;89:194.

276. Heuschen UA, Autschbach F, Allemeyer EH, et al. Long-term follow-up after ileoanal pouch procedure: algorithm for diagnosis, classification, and management of pouchitis. *Dis Colon Rectum*. 2001;44:487.

277. Heuschen UA, Hinz U, Allemeyer EH, et al. One- or two-stage procedure for restorative proctocolectomy: rationale for a surgical strategy in ulcerative colitis. *Ann Surg*. 2001;234:788.

278. Heuschen UA, Hinz U, Allemeyer EH, et al. Risk factors for ileoanal J pouch-related septic complications in ulcerative colitis and familial adenomatous polyposis. *Ann Surg*. 2002;235:207.

279. Hewett PJ, Stitz R, Hewett MK. Comparison of the functional results of restorative proctocolectomy for ulcerative colitis between the J and W configuration ileal pouches with sutured ileoanal anastomosis. *Dis Colon Rectum*. 1995;38:567.

280. Higgens CS, Keighley MRB, Allan RN. Impact of preoperative weight loss and body composition changes on postoperative outcome in surgery for inflammatory bowel disease. *Gut*. 1984;25:732.

281. Hinojosa J, Aad A, Panes J, et al. Multicenter, randomized trial comparing oral, topic and oral plus topic mesalazine in prevention of relapse in distal ulcerative colitis (DUC) [abstract]. *Gastroenterology*. 2001;120.A12.

282. Holdsworth CD. Acute self-limited colitis [editorial]. *Br Med J*. 1984;289:270.

283. Holdsworth PJ, Johnston D. Anal sensation after restorative proctocolectomy for ulcerative colitis. *Br J Surg*. 1988;75:993.

284. Holdsworth PJ, Johnston D. Use of the end-to-end anastomosis without mucosal stripping diminishes morbidity and time in hospital after restorative proctocolectomy. *Br J Surg*. 1988;75:1232.

285. Holdsworth PJ, Sagar PM, Lewis WG, et al. Internal anal sphincter activity after restorative proctocolectomy for ulcerative colitis: a study using continuous ambulatory manometry. *Dis Colon Rectum*. 1994;37:32.

286. Holzmann K, Klump B, Borchard F, et al. Flow cytometric and histologic evaluation in a large cohort of patients with ulcerative colitis: correlation with clinical characteristics and impact on surveillance. *Dis Colon Rectum*. 2001;44:1446.

287. Hosie KB, Grobler SP, Keighley MRB. Temporary loop ileostomy following restorative proctocolectomy. *Br J Surg*. 1992;79:33.

288. Hsu TC. Traumatic perforation of ileal pouch: report of a case. *Dis Colon Rectum*. 1989;32:64.

289. Hughes ESR. The treatment of ulcerative colitis. *Ann R Coll Surg Engl*. 1965;37:191.

290. Hughes ESR, McDermott FT, Masterton JP. Ileorectal anastomosis for inflammatory bowel disease: 15-year follow-up. *Dis Colon Rectum*. 1979;22:399.

291. Hughes JP, Bauer AR Jr, Bauer CM. Stapling techniques for easy construction of an ileal J-pouch. *Am J Surg*. 1988;155:783.

292. Hultén L, Fasth S. Loop ileostomy for protection of the newly constructed ileostomy reservoir. *Br J Surg*. 1981;68:11.

293. Hultén L, Fasth S, Nordgren S, et al. Kock's pouch converted to a pelvic pouch: report of a case. *Dis Colon Rectum*. 1988;31:457.

294. Hultén L, Kewenter J, Knutsson U, et al. Primary closure of perineal wound after proctocolectomy or rectal excision. *Acta Chir Scand*. 1971;137:467.

295. Hultén L, Svaninger G. Facts about the Kock continent ileostomy. *Dis Colon Rectum*. 1984;27:553.

296. Hultén L, Willén R, Nilsson O, et al. Mucosal assessment for dysplasia and cancer in the ileal pouch mucosa in patients operated on for ulcerative colitis: a 30-year follow-up study. *Dis Colon Rectum*. 2002;45:448.

297. Hurst RD, Molinari M, Chung TP, et al. Prospective study of the incidence, timing, and treatment of pouchitis in 104 consecutive patients after restorative proctocolectomy. *Arch Surg*. 1996;131:497.

298. Hyde GM, Jewell DP, Kettlewell MGW, et al. Cyclosporin for severe ulcerative colitis does not increase the rate of perioperative complications. *Dis Colon Rectum*. 2001;44:1436.

299. Irvin TT, Goligher JC. A controlled clinical trial of three different methods of perineal wound management following excision of the rectum. *Br J Surg*. 1975;62:287.

300. Ishikawa A, Lamoke A, Umesaki Y, et al. Randomized controlled trial of the effect of bifidobacterium-fermented milk on ulcerative colitis [abstract]. *Gastroenterology*. 2000;128:A778.

301. Iwama T, Kamikawa J, Higuchi T, et al. Development of invasive adenocarcinoma in a long-standing diverted J-pouch for ulcerative colitis: report of a case. *Dis Colon Rectum*. 2000;43:101.

302. Jacobsen O, Hojgaard L, Moller EH, et al. Effect of enterocoated cholestyramine on bowel habit after ileal resection: a double-blind crossover study. *Br Med J.* 1985;290:1315.

303. Jalan KN, Smith AN, Ruckley CV, et al. Perineal wound healing in ulcerative colitis. *Br J Surg.* 1969;56:749.

304. James SL, Irving PM, Gearry RB, et al. Management of distal ulcerative colitis: frequently asked questions analysis. *Intern Med J.* 2008;38:114.

305. James SP, Strober W, Quinn TC, et al. Crohn's disease: new concepts of pathogenesis and current approaches to treatment. *Dig Dis Sci.* 1987;32:1297.

306. Järnerot G. Fertility, sterility, and pregnancy in chronic inflammatory bowel disease. *Scand J Gastroenterol.* 1982;17:1.

307. Järnerot G, Hertervig E, Friis-Liby I, et al. Infliximab as rescue therapy in severe to moderately severe ulcerative colitis: a randomized, placebo-controlled study. *Gastroenterology.* 2005;128:1805.

308. Jörvinen HJ, Luukkonen P. Comparison of restorative proctocolectomy with and without covering ileostomy in ulcerative colitis. *Br J Surg.* 1991;78:199.

309. Järvinen HJ, Mäkitie A, Sivula A. Long-term results of continent ileostomy. *Int J Colorectal Dis.* 1986;1:40.

310. Jick H, Walker AM. Cigarette smoking and ulcerative colitis. *N Engl J Med.* 1983;308:261.

311. Johnson WR, Hughes ESR, McDermott FT, et al. The outcome of patients with ulcerative colitis managed by subtotal colectomy. *Surg Gynecol Obstet.* 1986;162:421.

312. Johnson WR, McDermott FT, Hughes ESR, et al. The risk of rectal carcinoma following colectomy in ulcerative colitis. *Dis Colon Rectum.* 1983;26:44.

313. Johnson WR, McDermott FT, Hughes ESR, et al. Carcinoma of the colon and rectum in inflammatory disease of the intestine. *Surg Gynecol Obstet.* 1983;156:193.

314. Johnston D, Holdsworth PJ, Nasmyth DG, et al. Preservation of the entire anal canal in conservative proctocolectomy for ulcerative colitis: a pilot study comparing end-to-end ileo-anal anastomosis without mucosal resection with mucosal proctectomy and endo-anal anastomosis. *Br J Surg.* 1987;74:940.

315. Johnston D, Williamson MER, Lewis WG, et al. Prospective controlled trial of duplicated (J) versus quadruplicated (W) pelvic ileal reservoirs in restorative proctocolectomy for ulcerative colitis. *Gut.* 1996;39:242.

316. Jones PF, Bevan PG, Hawley PR. Ileostomy or ileorectal anastomosis for ulcerative colitis. *Br Med J.* 1978;1:1459.

317. Jones VA, Dickinson RJ, Workman E, et al. Crohn's disease: maintenance of remission by diet. *Lancet.* 1985;2:177.

318. Jonsson B, Åhsgren L, Andersson LO, et al. Colorectal cancer surveillance in patients with ulcerative colitis. *Br J Surg.* 1994;81:689.

319. Jorge JMN, Wesner SD, James K, et al. Recovery of anal sphincter function after the ileoanal reservoir procedure in patients over the age of 50. *Dis Colon Rectum.* 1994;37:1002.

320. Juhasz ES, Fozard B, Dozois RR, et al. Ileal pouch-anal anastomosis function following childbirth: an extended evaluation. *Dis Colon Rectum.* 1995;38:159.

321. Kaiser AM, Stein JP, Beart RW Jr. T-pouch: a new valve design for a continent ileostomy. *Dis Colon Rectum.* 2002;45:411.

322. Kamm MA, Lichtenstein GR, Sandborn WJ, et al. Randomised trial of once- or twice-daily MMX mesalazine for maintenance of remission in ulcerative colitis. *Gut.* 2008;57:893.

323. Kamm MA, Sandborn WJ, Gassull M, et al. Once-daily, high concentration MMX mesalamine in active ulcerative colitis. *Gastroenterology.* 2007;132:66, quiz 432–433.

324. Kappelman MD, Rifas-Shiman SL, Kleinman K, et al. The prevalence and geographic distribution of Crohn's disease and ulcerative colitis in the United States. *Clin Gastroenterol Hepatol.* 2007;5:1424.

325. Kappelman MD, Rifas-Shiman SL, Porter C, et al. Direct health care costs of Crohn's disease and ulcerative colitis in US children and adults. *Gastroenterology.* 2008;135:1907.

326. Karlbom U, Raab Y, Ejerblad S, et al. Factors influencing the functional outcome of restorative proctocolectomy in ulcerative colitis. *Br J Surg.* 2000;87:1401.

327. Karoui S, Djebbi S, Belkhodja A, et al. Maintenance therapy by azathioprine after successful treatment by intravenous corticosteroid in acute severe colitis. An open prospective study. *Tunis Med.* 2008; 86:322.

328. Karush A, Daniels GE, Flood C, et al. *Psychotherapy in Chronic Ulcerative Colitis.* Philadelphia, PA: WB Saunders; 1977:148.

329. Kaser A, Mairinger T, Vogel W, et al. Infliximab in severe steroid refractory ulcerative colitis: a pilot study. *Wien Klin Wochenschr.* 2001; 113:930.

330. Katschinski B, Logan RFA, Edmond M, et al. Smoking and sugar intake are separate but interactive risk factors in Crohn's disease. *Gut.* 1988;29:1202.

331. Katz BH, Schwartz SS, Vender RJ. Portal venous gas following a barium enema in a patient with Crohn's colitis: a benign finding. *Dis Colon Rectum.* 1986;29:49.

332. Katz JA, Antoni C, Keenan GF, et al. Outcome of pregnancy in women receiving infliximab for the treatment of Crohn's disease and rheumatoid arthritis. *Am J Gastroenterol.* 2004;99:2385.

333. Kay RM, Cohen Z, Siu KP, et al. Ileal excretion and bacterial modification of bile acids and cholesterol in patients with continent ileostomy. *Gut.* 1979;21:128.

334. Keighley MRB. Abdominal mucosectomy reduces the incidence of soiling and sphincter damage after restorative proctocolectomy and J-pouch. *Dis Colon Rectum.* 1987;30:386.

335. Keighley MRB, Grobler SP. Fistula complicating restorative proctocolectomy. *Br J Surg.* 1993;80:1065.

336. Keighley MRB, Winslet MC, Flinn R, et al. Multivariate analysis of factors influencing the results of restorative proctocolectomy. *Br J Surg.* 1989;76:740.

337. Keighley MRB, Winslet MC, Yoshioka K, et al. Discrimination is not impaired by excision of the anal transition zone after restorative proctocolectomy. *Br J Surg.* 1987;74:1118.

338. Keighley MRB, Yoshioka K, Kmiot W. Prospective randomized trial to compare the stapled double-lumen pouch and the sutured quadruple pouch for restorative proctocolectomy. *Br J Surg.* 1988;75:1008.

339. Keighley MRB, Yoshioka K, Kmiot W, et al. Physiological parameters influencing function in restorative proctocolectomy and ileo-pouch-anal anastomosis. *Br J Surg.* 1988;75:997.

340. Kelly DG, Branon ME, Phillips SF, et al. Diarrhoea after continent ileostomy. *Gut.* 1980;21:711.

341. Kelly DG, Phillips SF, Kelly KA, et al. Dysfunction of the continent ileostomy: clinical features and bacteriology. *Gut.* 1983;24:193.

342. Kelly KA. Ileal pouch-anal anastomosis after proctocolectomy. *Surg Rounds.* 1985;8:48.

343. Kelts DG, Grand RJ, Shen G, et al. Nutritional basis of growth failure in children and adolescents with Crohn's disease. *Gastroenterology.* 1979;76:720.

344. Khan ZH, Mayberry JF, Spiers N, et al. Retrospective case series analysis of patients with inflammatory bowel disease on azathioprine. A district general hospital experience. *Digestion.* 2000;62:249.

345. Khoo REH, Cohen MM, Chapman GM, et al. Loop ileostomy for temporary fecal diversion. *Am J Surg.* 1994;167:519.

346. Khosla R, Willoughby CP, Jewell DP. Crohn's disease and pregnancy. *Gut.* 1984;25:52.

347. Khubchandani IT, Sandfort MR, Rosen L, et al. Current status of ileorectal anastomosis for inflammatory bowel disease. *Dis Colon Rectum.* 1989;32:400.

348. Khubchandani IT, Stasik JJ Jr, Nedwich A. Prospective surveillance by rectal biopsy following ileorectal anastomosis for inflammatory disease. *Dis Colon Rectum.* 1982;25:343.

349. King DW, Lubowski DZ, Cook TA. Anal canal mucosa in restorative proctocolectomy for ulcerative colitis. *Br J Surg.* 1989;78:970.

350. Kirkegaard P, Madsen PV. Perineal sinus after removal of the rectum: occlusion with fibrin adhesive. *Am J Surg.* 1983;145:791.

351. Kirsner JB. Genetic aspects of inflammatory bowel disease. *Clin Gastroenterol.* 1973;2:557.

352. Kirsner JB, Shorter RG. Recent developments in "nonspecific" inflammatory bowel disease, part I. *N Engl J Med.* 1982;306:775.

353. Kirsner JB, Shorter RG. Recent developments in nonspecific inflammatory bowel disease, part II. *N Engl J Med.* 1982;306:837.

354. Kirsner JB, Spencer JA. Family occurrences of ulcerative colitis, regional enteritis, and ileocolitis. *Ann Intern Med.* 1963;59:133.

355. Klingler PJ, Neuhauser B, Peer R, et al. Nipple complication caused by a mesenteric GORE-TEX® sling reinforcement in a Kock ileal reservoir: report of a case. *Dis Colon Rectum.* 2001;44:128.

356. Kmiot WA, Keighley MRB. Totally stapled abdominal restorative proctocolectomy. *Br J Surg.* 1989;76:961.

357. Kmiot WA, Yoshioka K, Pinho M, et al. Videoproctographic assessment after restorative proctocolectomy. *Dis Colon Rectum.* 1990;33:566.

358. Kochhar R, Mehta SK, Aggarwal R, et al. Sucralfate enema in ulcerative rectosigmoid lesions. *Dis Colon Rectum.* 1990;33:49.

359. Kock NG. Intra-abdominal "reservoir" in patients with permanent ileostomy: preliminary observations on a procedure resulting in fecal "continence" in five ileostomy patients. *Arch Surg.* 1969;99:223.

360. Kock NG, Darle N, Hultén L, et al. Ileostomy. *Curr Probl Surg.* 1977;14:1.

361. Kock NG, Darle N, Kewenter J, et al. The quality of life after procto-colectomy and ileostomy: a study of patients with conventional ileostomies converted to continent ileostomies. *Dis Colon Rectum.* 1974;17:287.

362. Kock NG, Hultén L, Myrvold HE. Ileoanal anastomosis with interposition of the ileal "Kock pouch"—preliminary results. *Dis Colon Rectum.* 1989;32:1050.

363. Kock NG, Myrvold HE, Nilsson LO, et al. Continent ileostomy: an account of 314 patients. *Acta Chir Scand.* 1981;147:67.

364. Köhler LW, Pemberton JH, Hodge DO, et al. Long-term functional results and quality of life after ileal pouch-anal anastomosis and cholecystectomy. *World J Surg.* 1992;16:1126.

365. Köhler LW, Pemberton JH, Zinmeister AR, et al. Quality of life after proctocolectomy: a comparison of Brooke ileostomy, Kock pouch, and ileal pouch-anal anastomosis. *Gastroenterology.* 1991;101:679.

366. Kokoszka J, Nelson RL, Swedler WI, et al. Determination of inflammatory bowel disease activity by breath pentane analysis. *Dis Colon Rectum.* 1993;36:597.

367. Kollmorgen CF, Nivatvongs S, Dean PA, et al. Long-term causes of death following ileal pouch-anal anastomosis. *Dis Colon Rectum.* 1996;39:525.

368. Korelitz BI, Cheskin LJ, Sohn N, et al. Proctitis after fecal diversion in Crohn's disease and its elimination with reanastomosis: implications for surgical management. Report of four cases. *Gastroenterology.* 1984;87:710.

369. Korelitz BI, Dyck WP, Klion FM. Fate of the rectum and distal colon after subtotal colectomy for ulcerative colitis. *Gut.* 1969;10:198.

370. Koretz RL. Nutritional support: how much for how much? *Gut.* 1986;27:85.

371. Kornbluth A, Marion JF, Salomon P, et al. How effective is current medical therapy for severe ulcerative and Crohn's colitis? An analytic review of selected trials. *J Clin Gastroenterol.* 1995;20:280.

372. Koutroubakis IE, Vlachonikolis IG, Kouroumalis EA. Role of appendicitis and appendectomy in the pathogenesis of ulcerative colitis: a critical review. *Inflamm Bowel Dis.* 2002;8:277.

373. Kruis W, Jonaitis L, Pokrotnieks J, et al. Once daily 3 g mesalamine is the optimal dose for maintaining clinical remission in ulcerative colitis: a double-blind, double-dummy, randomized, controlled, dose-ranging study. *Gastroenterology.* 2008;134(suppl 1):A489.

374. Kruis W, Kiudelis G, Racz I, et al. Once daily versus three times daily mesalazine granules in active ulcerative colitis: a double-blind, double-dummy, randomised, non-inferiority trial. *Gut.* 2009;58:233.

375. Kurtz LM, Flint GW, Platt N, et al. Carcinoma in the retained rectum after colectomy for ulcerative colitis. *Dis Colon Rectum.* 1980;23:346.

376. Kusunoki M, Shoji Y, Fujita S, et al. Characteristics of anal canal motility after ileoanal anastomosis. *Surg Gynecol Obstet.* 1992;174:22.

377. Ky AJ, Sonoda T, Milsom JW. One-stage laparoscopic restorative proctocolectomy: an alternative to the conventional approach. *Dis Colon Rectum.* 2002;45:207.

378. Kyle J. An epidemiological study of Crohn's disease in northeast Scotland. *Gastroenterology.* 1971;61:826.

379. Lahey FH. Ulcerative colitis. *N Y State J Med.* 1941;41:475.

380. La Mont JT, Trnka YM. Therapeutic implications of *Clostridium difficile* toxin during relapse of chronic inflammatory bowel disease. *Lancet.* 1980;1:381.

381. Langholz E, Munkholm P, Davidsen M, et al. Course of ulcerative colitis: analysis of changes in disease activity over years. *Gastroenterology.* 1994;107:3.

382. Langholz E, Munkholm P, Davidsen M, et al. Changes in extent of ulcerative colitis: a study on the course and prognostic factors. *Scand J Gastroenterol.* 1996;31:260.

383. Lashner BA. Recommendations for colorectal cancer screening in ulcerative colitis: a review of research from a single university-based surveillance program. *Am J Gastroenterol.* 1992;87:168.

384. Lashner BA, Evans AA, Kirsner JB, et al. Prevalence and incidence of inflammatory bowel disease in family members. *Gastroenterology.* 1986;91:1396.

385. Lashner BA, Turner BC, Bostwick DG, et al. Dysplasia and cancer complicating strictures in ulcerative colitis. *Dig Dis Sci.* 1990;35:349.

386. Launer DP, Sackier JM. Pouch-anal anastomosis without diverting ileostomy. *Dis Colon Rectum.* 1991;34:993.

387. Laureti S, Ugolini F, D'Errico A, et al. Adenocarcinoma below ileoanal anastomosis for ulcerative colitis: report of a case and review of the literature. *Dis Colon Rectum.* 2002;45:418.

388. Lavery IC, Chiulli RA, Jagelman DG, et al. Survival with carcinoma arising in mucosal ulcerative colitis. *Ann Surg.* 1982;195:508.

389. Lavery IC, Jagelman DG. Cancer in the excluded rectum following surgery for inflammatory bowel disease. *Dis Colon Rectum.* 1982;25:522.

390. Lavery IC, Michener WM, Jagelman DG. Ileorectal anastomosis for inflammatory bowel disease in children and adolescents. *Surg Gynecol Obstet.* 1983;157:553.

391. Lavery IC, Tuckson WB, Easley KA. Internal anal sphincter after total abdominal colectomy and stapled ileal pouch-anal anastomosis without mucosal proctectomy. *Dis Colon Rectum.* 1989;32:950.

392. Lee FI, Jewell DP, Mani V, et al. A randomised trial comparing mesalazine and prednisolone foam enemas in patients with acute distal ulcerative colitis. *Gut.* 1996;38:229.

393. Lee PY, Fazio VW, Church JM, et al. Vaginal fistula following restorative proctocolectomy. *Dis Colon Rectum.* 1997;40:752.

394. Leicester RJ, Ritchie JK, Wadsworth J, et al. Sexual function and perineal wound healing after intersphincteric excision of the rectum for inflammatory bowel disease. *Dis Colon Rectum.* 1984;27:244.

395. Leidenius M, Kellokumpu I, Husa A, et al. Dysplasia and carcinoma in long-standing ulcerative colitis: an endoscopic and histological surveillance programme. *Gut.* 1991;32:1521.

396. Leijonmarck CE, Broström O, Monsen U, et al. Surgical treatment of ulcerative colitis in Stockholm County, 1955 to 1984. *Dis Colon Rectum.* 1989;32:918.

397. Leijonmarck CE, Löfberg R, Öst A, et al. Long-term results of ileorectal anastomosis in ulcerative colitis in Stockholm County. *Dis Colon Rectum.* 1990;33:195.

398. Leijonmarck CE, Persson PG, Hellers G. Factors affecting colectomy rate in ulcerative colitis: an epidemiologic study. *Gut.* 1990;31:329.

399. Lemann M, Galian A, Rutgeerts P, et al. Comparison of budesonide and 5-aminosalicylic acid enemas in active distal ulcerative colitis. *Aliment Pharmacol Ther.* 1995;9:557.

400. Lennard-Jones JE. Cancer risk in ulcerative colitis: surveillance or surgery. *Br J Surg.* 1985;72(suppl):S84.

401. Lennard-Jones JE. Compliance, cost, and common sense limit cancer control in colitis. *Gut.* 1986;27:1403.

402. Lennard-Jones JE, Melville DM, Morson BC, et al. Precancer and cancer in extensive ulcerative colitis: findings among 401 patients over 22 years. *Gut.* 1990;31:800.

403. Lepistö AH, Järvinen HJ. Durability of Kock continent ileostomy. *Dis Colon Rectum.* 2003;46:925.

404. Lepistö AH, Luukkonen P, Järvinen HJ. Cumulative failure rate of ileal pouch-anal anastomosis and quality of life after failure. *Dis Colon Rectum.* 2002;45:1289.

405. Levenstein S, Prantera C, Luzi C, et al. Low residue or normal diet in Crohn's disease: a prospective controlled study in Italian patients. *Gut.* 1985;26:989.

406. Levi AJ. Diet in the management of Crohn's disease. *Gut.* 1985; 26:985.

407. Levin KE, Pemberton JH, Phillips SF, et al. Role of oxygen free radicals in the etiology of pouchitis. *Dis Colon Rectum.* 1992;35:452.

408. Levine DS, Rabinovitch PS, Haggitt RC, et al. Distribution of aneuploid cell populations in ulcerative colitis with dysplasia or cancer. *Gastroenterology.* 1991;101:1198.

409. Levine JS, Burakoff R. Chemoprophylaxis of colorectal cancer in inflammatory bowel disease: current concepts. *Inflamm Bowel Dis.* 2007;13:1293.

410. Levitt MD, Lewis AAM. Determinants of ileoanal pouch function. *Gut.* 1991;32:126.

411. Levy N, Roisman I, Teodor I. Ulcerative colitis in pregnancy in Israel. *Dis Colon Rectum.* 1981;24:351.

412. Lewis WG, Kuzu A, Sagar PM, et al. Stricture at the pouch-anal anastomosis after restorative proctocolectomy. *Dis Colon Rectum.* 1994;37:120.

413. Lewis WG, Miller AS, Williamson MER, et al. The perfect pelvic pouch—what makes the difference? *Gut.* 1995;37:552.

414. Lewis WG, Sagar PM, Holdsworth PJ, et al. Restorative proctocolectomy with end-to-end pouch-anal anastomosis in patients over the age of 50. *Gut.* 1993;34:948.

415. Lichtenstein GR, Abreu MT, Cohen R, et al. American Gastroenterological Association Institute technical review on corticosteroids, immunomodulators, and infliximab in inflammatory bowel disease. *Gastroenterology.* 2006;130:940.

416. Lichtenstein G, Cohen RD, Feagan BG, et al. Safety of infliximab in Crohn's disease: data from the 5000-patient TREAT Registry [abstract]. *Gastroenterology.* 2004;126(suppl 4):A54.

417. Lichtenstein GR, Feagan B, Cohen RD, et al. Risk factors for serious infections in patients receiving infliximab and other Crohn's disease therapies: TREAT registry data. *Gastroenterology.* 2010;38:S475.

418. Lichtenstein GR, Kamm MA. Review article: 5-aminosalicylate formulations for the treatment of ulcerative colitis—methods of comparing release rates and delivery of 5-aminosalicylate to the colonic mucosa. *Aliment Pharmacol Ther.* 2008;28:663.

419. Lichtenstein GR, Kamm MA, Boddu P, et al. Effect of once- or twice daily MMX mesalamine (SPD476) for the induction of remission of mild to moderately active ulcerative colitis. *Clin Gastroenterol Hepatol.* 2007;5:95.

420. Lichtenstein GR, Kamm MA, Sandborn WJ, et al. MMX mesalazine for the induction of remission of mild-to-moderately active ulcerative colitis: efficacy and tolerability in specific patient subpopulations. *Aliment Pharmacol Ther.* 2008;27:1094.

421. Lichtiger S, Present DH, Kornbluth A, et al. Cyclosporine in severe ulcerative colitis refractory to steroid therapy. *N Engl J Med.* 1994;330:1841.

422. Liljeqvist L, Lindquist K. A reconstructive operation on malfunctioning S-shaped pelvic reservoirs. *Dis Colon Rectum.* 1985;28:506.

423. Lim CH, Axon ATR. Low-grade dysplasia: nonsurgical treatment. *Inflamm Bowel Dis.* 2003;9:270.

424. Lindberg BU, Broomé U, Persson B. Proximal colorectal dysplasia or cancer in ulcerative colitis. The impact of primary sclerosing cholangitis and sulfasalazine. Results from a 20-year surveillance study. *Dis Colon Rectum.* 2001;44:77.

425. Lindberg JÖ, Stenling RB, Rutegard JN. DNA aneuploidy as a marker of premalignancy in surveillance of patients with ulcerative colitis. *Br J Surg.* 1999;86:947.

426. Lindhagen T, Bohe M, Ekelund G, et al. Fertility and outcome of pregnancy in patients operated on for Crohn's disease. *Int J Colorectal Dis.* 1986;1:25.

427. Lindquist K. Anal manometry with microtransducer technique before and after restorative proctocolectomy. *Dis Colon Rectum.* 1990;33:91.

428. Lindsey I, George B, Kettlewell M, et al. Randomized, double-blind, placebo-controlled trial of sildenafil (Viagra®) for erectile dysfunction after rectal excision for cancer and inflammatory bowel disease. *Dis Colon Rectum.* 2002;45:727.

429. Lindsey I, George B, Kettlewell M, et al. Impotence after mesorectal and close rectal dissection for inflammatory bowel disease. *Dis Colon Rectum.* 2001;44:831.

430. Lobo AJ, Foster PN, Burke DA, et al. The role of azathioprine in the management of ulcerative colitis. *Dis Colon Rectum.* 1990;33:374.

431. Löfberg R, Broström O, Karlén P, et al. Colonoscopic surveillance in long-standing total ulcerative colitis—a 15-year follow-up study. *Gastroenterology.* 1990;99:1021.

432. Löfberg R, Broström O, Karlén P, et al. DNA aneuploidy in ulcerative colitis: reproducibility, topographic distribution, and relation to dysplasia. *Gastroenterology.* 1992;102:1149.

433. Löfberg R, Danielsson A, Suhr O, et al. Oral budesonide versus prednisolone in patients with active extensive and left sided ulcerative colitis. *Gastroenterology.* 1996;110:1713.

434. Löfberg R, Leijonmarck CE, Broström O, et al. Mucosal dysplasia and DNA content in ulcerative colitis patients with ileorectal anastomosis. *Dis Colon Rectum.* 1991;34:566.

435. Löfberg R, Liljeqvist L, Lindquist K, et al. Dysplasia and DNA aneuploidy in a pelvic pouch. *Dis Colon Rectum.* 1991;34:280.

436. Löfberg R, Lindquist K, Veress B, et al. Highly malignant carcinoma in chronic ulcerative colitis without preceding dysplasia or DNA aneuploidy: report of a case. *Dis Colon Rectum.* 1992;35:82.

437. Loftus CG, Loftus EV Jr, Harmsen WS, et al. Update on the incidence and prevalence of Crohn's disease and ulcerative colitis in Olmsted County, Minnesota, 1940–2000. *Inflamm Bowel Dis.* 2007;13:254.

438. Loftus EV Jr, Silverstein MD, Sandborn WJ, et al. Ulcerative colitis in Olmsted County, Minnesota, 1940–1993: incidence, prevalence, and survival. *Gut.* 2000;46:336.

439. Lohmuller JL, Pemberton JH, Dozois RR, et al. Pouchitis and extraintestinal manifestations of inflammatory bowel disease after ileal pouch-anal anastomosis. *Ann Surg.* 1990;211:622.

440. Lubat E, Balthazar EJ. The current role of computerized tomography in inflammatory disease of the bowel. *Am J Gastroenterol.* 1988;83:107.

441. Lyttle JA, Parks AG. Intersphincteric excision of the rectum. *Br J Surg.* 1977;64:413.

442. MacLean AR, O'Connor B, Parkes R, et al. Reconstructive surgery for failed ileal pouch-anal anastomosis: a viable surgical option with acceptable results. *Dis Colon Rectum.* 2002;45:880.

443. MacRae HM, McLeod RS, Cohen Z, et al. Risk factors for pelvic pouch failure. *Dis Colon Rectum.* 1997;40:257.

444. Madden MV, Farthing MJG, Nicholls RJ. Inflammation in ileal reservoirs: "pouchitis." *Gut.* 1990;31:247.

445. Madden MV, McIntyre AS, Nicholls RJ. Double blind crossover trial of metronidazole vs. placebo in chronic unremitting pouchitis. *Dig Dis Sci.* 1994;39:1193.

446. Mahadevan U. Medical treatment of ulcerative colitis. *Clin Colon Rectal Surg.* 2004;17:7.

447. Mahadevan U. Pregnancy and inflammatory bowel disease. *Med Clin North Am.* 2010;94:53.

448. Mahadevan U, Terdiman JP, Aron J, et al. Infliximab and semen quality in men with inflammatory bowel disease. *Inflamm Bowel Dis.* 2005;11:395.

449. Mahadevan U, Terdiman J, Church J, et al. Infliximab levels in infants born to women with inflammatory bowel disease [abstract]. *Gastroenterol.* 2007;132(4 suppl 2):A144.

450. Maingot R. Terminal ileostomy in ulcerative colitis. *Lancet.* 1942; 2:121.

451. Manjoney DL, Koplewitz MJ, Abrams JS. Factors influencing perineal wound healing. *Am J Surg.* 1983;145:183.

452. Mann CV, Springall R. Use of a muscle graft for unhealed perineal sinus. *Br J Surg.* 1986;73:1000.

453. Mann SD, Pitt J, Springall RG, et al. *Clostridium difficile* infection—an unusual cause of refractory pouchitis: report of a case. *Dis Colon Rectum.* 2003;46:267.

454. Manning AP, Bulgim OR, Dixon MF, et al. Screening by colonoscopy for colonic epithelial dysplasia in inflammatory bowel disease. *Gut.* 1987;28:1489.

455. Mantzaris GJ, Sfakianakis M, Archavlis E, et al. A prospective randomized observer-blind 2-year trial of azathioprine monotherapy versus azathioprine and olsalazine for the maintenance of remission of steroid-dependent ulcerative colitis. *Am J Gastroenterol.* 2004;99:1122.

456. Marcello PW, Milsom JW, Wong SK, et al. Laparoscopic total colectomy for acute colitis: a case-control study. *Dis Colon Rectum.* 2001;44:1441.

457. Marcello PW, Roberts PL, Schoetz DJ Jr, et al. Long-term results of the ileoanal pouch procedure. *Arch Surg.* 1993;128:500.

458. Marcello PW, Roberts PL, Schoetz DJ Jr, et al. Obstruction after ileal pouch-anal anastomosis: a preventable complication? *Dis Colon Rectum.* 1993;36:1105.

459. Mardini HE. Azathioprine-induced pancreatitis in Crohn's disease: a smoking gun or guilt by association. *Aliment Pharmacol Ther.* 2005;21:195.

460. Marion JF, Present DH. Modern medical management of acute severe ulcerative colitis. *Eur J Gastroenterol Hepatol.* 1997;9:831.

461. Markham NI, Watson GM, Lock MR. Rectovaginal fistulae after ileoanal pouches. *Lancet.* 1991;337:1295.

462. Marshak RH, Lindner AE. Radiologic diagnosis of chronic ulcerative colitis and Crohn's disease of the colon. In: Kirsner JB, Shorter RG, eds. *Inflammatory Bowel Disease*. Philadelphia, PA: Lea & Febiger; 1975:241.

463. Marshall JK, Irvine EJ. Putting rectal 5-aminosalicylic acid in its place: the role in distal ulcerative colitis. *Am J Gastroenterol.* 2000;95:1628.

464. Marteau P, Probert CS, Lindgren S, et al. Combined oral and enema treatment with Pentasa (mesalazine) is superior to oral therapy alone in patients with extensive mild/moderate active ulcerative colitis: a randomised, double blind, placebo controlled study. *Gut.* 2005;54:960.

465. Martel P, Blanc P, Bothereau H, et al. Comparative anatomical study of division of the ileocolic pedicle or the superior mesenteric pedicle for mesenteric lengthening. *Br J Surg.* 2002;89:775.

466. Martin LW, LeCoultre C, Schubert WK. Total colectomy and mucosal proctectomy with preservation of continence in ulcerative colitis. *Ann Surg.* 1977;186:477.

467. Matikainen M, Santavirta J, Hiltunen KM. Ileoanal anastomosis without covering ileostomy. *Dis Colon Rectum.* 1990;33:384.

468. Maunder RG, Cohen Z, McLeod RS, et al. Effect of intervention in inflammatory bowel disease on health-related quality of life: a critical review. *Dis Colon Rectum.* 1995;38:1147.

469. Mavroudis C, Schrock TR. The dilemma of preservation of the rectum: retention of the rectum in colectomy for inflammatory disease of the bowel. *Dis Colon Rectum.* 1977;20:644.

470. May RE. Sexual dysfunction following rectal excision for ulcerative colitis. *Br J Surg.* 1966;53:29.

471. Mayberry JF, Rhodes J. Epidemiological aspects of Crohn's disease: a review of the literature. *Gut.* 1984;25:886.

472. Mayberry JF, Rhodes J, Hughes LE. Incidence of Crohn's disease in Cardiff between 1934 and 1977. *Gut.* 1979;20:602.

473. Mayo CW, Fly OA Jr, Connelly ME. Fate of the remaining segment after subtotal colectomy for ulcerative colitis. *Ann Surg.* 1956;144:753.

474. McCormack G, McCormick PA, Hyland JM, et al. Cyclosporin therapy in severe ulcerative colitis: is it worth the effort? *Dis Colon Rectum.* 2002;45:1200.

475. McCourtney JS, Finlay IG. Totally stapled restorative proctocolectomy. *Br J Surg.* 1997;84:808.

476. McEwan HP. Ulcerative colitis in pregnancy. *Proc R Soc Med.* 1972;65:279.

477. McGarrity TJ, Manasse JS, Koch KL, et al. Crohn's disease and massive lower gastrointestinal bleeding: angiographic appearance and two case reports. *Am J Gastroenterol.* 1987;82:1096.

478. McHugh SM, Diamant NE, McLeod R, et al. S-pouches versus J-pouches. A comparison of functional outcomes. *Dis Colon Rectum.* 1987;30:671.

479. McIntyre PB, Pemberton JH, Wolff BG, et al. Comparing functional results 1 year and 10 years after ileal pouch-anal anastomosis for chronic ulcerative colitis. *Dis Colon Rectum.* 1994;37:303.

480. McKittrick LS, Miller RH. Idiopathic ulcerative colitis: a review of 149 cases with particular reference to the value of, and indications for, surgical treatment. *Ann Surg.* 1935;102:656.

481. McLeod RS, Fazio VW. Quality of life with the continent ileostomy. *World J Surg.* 1984;8:90.

482. McLeod RS, Taylor DW, Cohen Z, et al. Single patient randomised clinical trial: use in determining optimum treatment for patient with inflammation of Kock continent ileostomy reservoir. *Lancet.* 1986; 1:726.

483. McMullen K, Hicks TC, Ray JE, et al. Complications associated with ileal pouch-anal anastomosis. *World J Surg.* 1991;15:763.

484. Meagher AP, Farouk R, Dozois RR, et al. J ileal pouch-anal anastomosis for chronic ulcerative colitis: complications and long-term outcome in 1310 patients. *Br J Surg.* 1998;85:800.

485. Melville DM, Jass JR, Shepherd NA, et al. Dysplasia and deoxyribonucleic acid aneuploidy in the assessment of precancerous changes in chronic ulcerative colitis. *Gastroenterology.* 1988;95:668.

486. Melville DM, Ritchie JK, Nicholls RJ, et al. Surgery for ulcerative colitis in the era of the pouch: the St Mark's Hospital experience. *Gut.* 1994;35:1076.

487. Mendeloff AI. The epidemiology of idiopathic inflammatory bowel disease. In: Kirsner JB, Shorter RG, eds. *Inflammatory Bowel Disease.* 2nd ed. Philadelphia, PA: Lea & Febiger; 1980:5.

488. Mendeloff AI, Monk M, Siegel CI, et al. Illness experience and life stresses in patients with irritable colon and ulcerative colitis: an epidemiologic study of ulcerative colitis and regional enteritis in Baltimore, 1960–1964. *N Engl J Med.* 1970;282:14.

489. Merrett MN, Mortensen N, Kettlewell M, et al. Smoking may prevent pouchitis in patients with restorative proctocolectomy for ulcerative colitis. *Gut.* 1996;38:362.

490. Metcalf AM, Dozois RR, Beart RW Jr, et al. Pregnancy following ileal pouch-anal anastomosis. *Dis Colon Rectum.* 1985;28:859.

491. Metcalf AM, Dozois RR, Beart RW Jr, et al. Temporary ileostomy for ileal pouch-anal anastomosis: function and complications. *Dis Colon Rectum.* 1986;29:300.

492. Metcalf AM, Dozois RR, Kelly KA. Sexual function in women after proctocolectomy. *Ann Surg.* 1986;204:624.

493. Metcalf AM, Dozois RR, Kelly KA, et al. Ileal "J" pouch-anal anastomosis: clinical outcome. *Ann Surg.* 1985;202:735.

494. Metcalf AM, Dozois RR, Kelly KA, et al. Ileal pouch-anal anastomosis without temporary diverting ileostomy. *Dis Colon Rectum.* 1986;29:33.

495. Meuwissen SGM, Ewe K, Gassull MA, et al. I.O.I.B.D. questionnaire on the clinical use of azathioprine, 6-mercaptopurine, cyclosporin and methotrexate in the treatment of I.B.D. [abstract]. *Gut.* 1996;39:A242.

496. Meyers S, Janowitz HD. The "natural history" of ulcerative colitis: an analysis of the placebo response. *J Clin Gastroenterol.* 1989;11:33.

497. Michelassi F, Lee J, Rubin M, et al. Long-term functional results after ileal pouch anal restorative proctocolectomy for ulcerative colitis: a prospective observational study. *Ann Surg.* 2003;238:433.

498. Michelassi F, Stella M, Block GE. Prospective assessment of functional results after ileal J pouch-anal restorative proctocolectomy. *Arch Surg.* 1993;128:889.

499. Michener WM. Ulcerative colitis in children. *Pediatr Clin North Am.* 1967;94:159.

500. Miller AS, Lewis WG, Williamson MER, et al. Does eversion of the anorectum during restorative proctocolectomy influence functional outcome? *Dis Colon Rectum.* 1996;39:489.

501. Miller DS, Keighley AC, Langman MJS. Changing patterns in epidemiology of Crohn's disease. *Lancet.* 1974;2:691.

502. Miller R, Bartolo DCC, Orrom WJ, et al. Improvement of anal sensation with preservation of the anal transition zone after ileoanal anastomosis for ulcerative colitis. *Dis Colon Rectum.* 1990;33:414.

503. Mimura T, Rizzello F, Gionchetti P, et al. Four-week treatment of metronidazole and ciprofloxacin markedly decreases refractory pouchitis and improves the quality of life [abstract]. *Gastroenterology.* 2001;120:A453.

504. Mir-Madjlessi SH, Farmer RG, Easley KA, et al. Colorectal and extracolonic malignancy in ulcerative colitis. *Cancer.* 1986;58:1569.

505. Misciewicz JJ, Lennard-Jones JE, Connell AM, et al. Controlled trial of sulfasalazine in maintenance therapy for ulcerative colitis. *Lancet.* 1965;1:185.

506. Moller P, Lohmann M, Brynitz S. Cholestyramine ointment in the treatment of perianal skin irritation following ileoanal anastomosis. *Dis Colon Rectum.* 1987;30:106.

507. Montagne JP, Kressel HY, Moss AA, et al. Radiologic evaluation of the continent (Kock) ileostomy. *Radiology.* 1978;127:325.

508. Moody GA, Probert C, Jayanthi V, et al. The effects of chronic ill health and treatment with sulphasalazine amongst men and women with inflammatory bowel disease in Leicestershire. *Int J Colorectal Dis.* 1997;12:220.

509. Mor IJ, Vogel JD, da Luz Moreira A, et al. Infliximab in ulcerative colitis is associated with an increased risk of postoperative complications after restorative proctocolectomy. *Dis Colon Rectum.* 2008;51:1202.

510. Morel P, Hawker PC, Allan RN, et al. Management of acute colitis in inflammatory bowel disease. *World J Surg.* 1986;10:814.

511. Morgan RA, Manning PB, Coran AG. Experience with the straight endorectal pullthrough for the management of ulcerative colitis and familial polyposis in children and adults. *Ann Surg.* 1987;206:595.

512. Morson BC, Pang LSC. Rectal biopsy as an aid to cancer control in ulcerative colitis. *Gut.* 1967;8:423.

513. Moskovitz DN, Bodian C, Chapman ML, et al. The effect on the fetus of medications used to treat pregnant inflammatory bowel-disease patients. *Am J Gastroenterol.* 2004;99:656.

514. Moskovitz DN, Van Assche G, Maenhout B, et al. Incidence of colectomy during long term follow up after cyclosporin-induced remission of severe ulcerative colitis. *Clin Gastroenterol Hepatol.* 2006;4:760.

515. Moss AC, Peppercorn MA. The risks and the benefits of mesalazine as a treatment for ulcerative colitis. *Expert Opin Drug Saf.* 2007;6:99.

516. Motta JC, Ricketts RR. The J-pouch Swenson procedure for ulcerative colitis and familial polyposis. *Am Surg.* 1992;58:613.

517. Moum B, Vatn MH, Ekbom A, et al. Incidence of inflammatory bowel disease in southeastern Norway: evaluation of methods after 1 year of registration. Southeastern Norway IBD Study Group of Gastroenterologists. *Digestion.* 1995;56:377.

518. Mowschenson PM, Critchlow JF. Outcome of early surgical complications following ileoanal pouch operation without diverting ileostomy. *Am J Surg.* 1995;169:143.

519. Mowschenson PM, Critchlow JF, Rosenberg SJ, et al. Factors favoring continence, the avoidance of a diverting ileostomy and small intestinal conservation in the ileoanal pouch operation. *Surg Gynecol Obstet.* 1993;177:17.

520. Mullen P, Behrens D, Chalmers T, et al. Barnett continent intestinal reservoir: multicenter experience with an alternative to the Brooke ileostomy. *Dis Colon Rectum.* 1995;38:573.

521. Murr MM, Metcalf AM. Spinal epidural abscess complicating an ileal J-pouch-anal anastomosis. *Dis Colon Rectum.* 1993;36:293.

522. Murray CB. Psychogenic factors in the etiology of ulcerative colitis and bloody diarrhea. *Am J Med Sci.* 1930;180:239.

523. Myren J, Eie H, Serck-Hanssen A. The diagnosis of colitis by colonoscopy with biopsy and x-ray examination. A blind comparative study. *Scand J Gastroenterol.* 1976;11:141.

524. Myren J, Serck-Hanssen A, Solberg L. Routine and blind histological diagnosis on colonoscopic biopsies compared to clinical-colonoscopic observations in patients without and with colitis. *Scand J Gastroenterol.* 1976;11:135.

525. Narendranathan M, Sandler RS, Suchindran CM, et al. Male infertility in inflammatory bowel disease. *J Clin Gastroenterol.* 1989;11:403.

526. Nasmyth DG, Johnston D, Godwin PGR, et al. Factors influencing bowel function after ileal pouch-anal anastomosis. *Br J Surg.* 1986; 73:469.

527. Nasmyth DG, Johnston D, Williams NS, et al. Changes in the absorption of bile acids after total colectomy in patients with an ileostomy or pouch-anal anastomosis. *Dis Colon Rectum.* 1989;32:230.

528. Nasmyth DG, Williams NS, Johnston D. Comparison of the function of triplicated and duplicated pelvic ileal reservoirs after mucosal proctectomy and ileo-anal anastomosis for ulcerative colitis and adenomatous polyposis. *Br J Surg.* 1986;73:361.

529. Navaneethan U, Shen B. Hepatopancreatobiliary manifestations and complications associated with inflammatory bowel disease [published online ahead of print March 2, 2010]. *Inflamm Bowel Dis.*

530. Nduka CC, Menzies-Gow N, Darzi A. Simple ileal J-pouch construction using an endoscopic stapler. *Dis Colon Rectum.* 1995;38:98.

531. Neal DE, Williams NS, Barker MCJ, et al. The effect of resection of the distal ileum on gastric emptying, small bowel transit and absorption after proctocolectomy. *Br J Surg.* 1984;71:666.

532. Nelson H, Dozois RR, Kelly KA, et al. The effect of pregnancy and delivery on the ileal-pouch-anal anastomosis functions. *Dis Colon Rectum*. 1989;32:384.

533. Nelson RL, Prasad ML, Pearl RK, et al. Inverted U-pouch construction for restoration of function in patients with failed straight ileoanal pull-throughs. *Dis Colon Rectum*. 1991;34:1040.

534. Newman A, Lambert JR. *Campylobacter jejuni* causing flare-up in inflammatory bowel disease [letter]. *Lancet*. 1980;2:919.

535. Ng SC, Kamm MA. Therapeutic strategies for the management of ulcerative colitis. *Inflamm Bowel Dis*. 2009;15:935.

536. Nguyen GC, Tuskey A, Dassopoulos T, et al. Rising hospitalization rates for inflammatory bowel disease in the United States between 1998 and 2004. *Inflamm Bowel Dis*. 2007;13:1529.

537. Nicholls J, Pescatori M, Motson RW, et al. Restorative proctocolectomy with a three-loop ileal reservoir for ulcerative colitis and familial adenomatous polyposis. *Ann Surg*. 1984;199:383.

538. Nicholls RJ, Lubowski DZ. Restorative proctocolectomy: the four loop (W) reservoir. *Br J Surg*. 1987;74:564.

539. Nicholls RJ, Pezim ME. Restorative proctocolectomy with ileal reservoir for ulcerative colitis and familial adenomatous polyposis: a comparison of three reservoir designs. *Br J Surg*. 1985;72:470.

540. Nielsen OH, Andreasson B, Bondesen S, et al. Pregnancy in Crohn's disease. *Scand J Gastroenterol*. 1984;19:724.

541. Nikfar S, Rahimi R, Rezaie A, et al. A meta-analysis of the efficacy of sulfasalazine in comparison with 5-aminosalicylates in the induction of improvement and maintenance of remission in patients with ulcerative colitis. *Dig Dis Sci*. 2009;54:1157.

542. Nilsson LO, Kock NG, Kylberg F, et al. Sexual adjustment in ileostomy patients before and after conversion to continent ileostomy. *Dis Colon Rectum*. 1981;24:287.

543. Nilsson LO, Kock NG, Lindgren I, et al. Morphological and histochemical changes in the mucosa of the continent ileostomy reservoir 6–10 years after its construction. *Scand J Gastroenterol*. 1980;15:737.

544. Nordenholtz KE, Stowe SP, Stormont JM, et al. The cause of death in inflammatory bowel disease: a comparison of death certificates and hospital charts in Rochester, New York. *Am J Gastroenterol*. 1995;90:927.

545. Nordgren S, Cohen Z, Greig PD, et al. Pressure studies on the continent reservoir ileostomy. *Surg Gynecol Obstet*. 1982;155:646.

546. Norgard B, Pedersen L, Christensen LA, et al. Therapeutic drug use in women with Crohn's disease and birth outcomes: a Danish nationwide cohort study. *Am J Gastroenterol*. 2007;102:1406.

547. North CS, Clouse RE, Spitznagel EL, et al. The relation of ulcerative colitis to psychiatric factors: a review of findings and methods. *Am J Psychiatry*.1990;147:974.

548. Nugent FW, Haggitt RC. Results of a long-term prospective surveillance program for dysplasia in ulcerative colitis. *Gastroenterology*. 1984;86:1197.

549. Nugent FW, Haggitt RC, Colcher H, et al. Malignant potential of chronic ulcerative colitis. *Gastroenterology*. 1979;76:1.

550. Nugent FW, Haggitt RD, Gilpin PA. Cancer surveillance in ulcerative colitis. *Gastroenterology*. 1991;100:1241.

551. Nunes GC, Ahlquist RE. Increasing incidence of Crohn's disease. *Am J Surg*. 1983;145:578.

552. Nyam DCNK, Wolff BG, Dozois RR, et al. Does the presence of a pre-ileostomy closure asymptomatic pouch-anastomotic sinus tract affect the success of ileal pouch-anal anastomosis? *J Gastrointest Surg*. 1997;1:274.

553. Oakley JR, Fazio VW, Jagelman DG, et al. Management of the perineal wound after rectal excision for ulcerative colitis. *Dis Colon Rectum*. 1985;28:885.

554. Oakley JR, Jagelman DG, Fazio VW, et al. Complications and quality of life after ileorectal anastomosis for ulcerative colitis. *Am J Surg*. 1985;149:23.

555. Oakley JR, Lavery IC, Fazio VW, et al. The fate of the rectal stump after subtotal colectomy for ulcerative colitis. *Dis Colon Rectum*. 1985;28:394.

556. Oates GD, Williams JA. Primary closure of the perineal wound in excision of the rectum. *Proc R Soc Med*. 1970;63(suppl):128.

557. O'Connell PR, Pemberton JH, Brown ML, et al. Determinants of stool frequency after ileal pouch-anal anastomosis. *Am J Surg*. 1987;153:157.

558. O'Connell PR, Pemberton JH, Weiland LH, et al. Does rectal mucosa regenerate after ileoanal anastomosis? *Dis Colon Rectum*. 1987;30:1.

559. O'Connell PR, Rankin DR, Weiland LH, et al. Enteric bacteriology, absorption, morphology and emptying after ileal pouch-anal anastomosis. *Br J Surg*. 1986;73:909.

560. Öhman U. Colorectal carcinoma in patients with ulcerative colitis. *Am J Surg*. 1982;344.

561. Öjerskog B, Kock NG, Nilsson LO, et al. Long-term follow-up of patients with continent ileostomies. *Dis Colon Rectum*. 1990;33:184.

562. Öjerskog B, Kock NG, Philipson BM, et al. Pregnancy and delivery in patients with a continent ileostomy. *Surg Gynecol Obstet*. 1988;167:61.

563. O'Kelly TJ, Merrett M, Mortensen NJ, et al. Pouch-vaginal fistula after restorative proctocolectomy: aetiology and management. *Br J Surg*. 1994;81:1374.

564. Olsen KØ, Joelsson M, Laurberg S, et al. Fertility after ileal pouch-anal anastomosis in women with ulcerative colitis. *Br J Surg*. 1999;86:493.

565. Öresland T, Fasth S, Nordgren S, et al. Pouch size: the important functional determinant after restorative proctocolectomy. *Br J Surg*. 1990;77:265.

566. Orholm M, Munkholm P, Langholz E, et al. Familial occurrence of inflammatory bowel disease. *N Engl J Med*. 1991;324:84.

567. O'Riordain MG, Fazio VW, Lavery IC, et al. Incidence and natural history of dysplasia of the anal transitional zone after ileal pouch-anal anastomosis. *Dis Colon Rectum*. 2000;43:1660.

568. Orkin BA, Soper NJ, Kelly KA, et al. Influence of sleep on anal sphincteric pressure in health and after ileal pouch-anal anastomosis. *Dis Colon Rectum*. 1992;35:137.

569. Orkin BA, Telander RL, Wolff BG, et al. The surgical management of children with ulcerative colitis: the old versus the new. *Dis Colon Rectum*. 1990;33:947.

570. Ozuner G, Hull T, Lee P, et al. What happens to a pelvic pouch when a fistula develops? *Dis Colon Rectum*. 1997;40:543.

571. Palmu A, Sivula A. Kock's continent ileostomy: results of 51 operations and experiences with correction of nipple-valve insufficiency. *Br J Surg*. 1978;65:645.

572. Parks AG, Nicholls RJ. Proctocolectomy without ileostomy for ulcerative colitis. *Br Med J*. 1978;2:85.

573. Parks AG, Nicholls RJ, Belliveau P. Proctocolectomy with ileal reservoir and anal anastomosis. *Br J Surg*. 1980;67:533.

574. Park-Wyllie L, Mazzotta P, Pastuszak A, et al. Birth defects after maternal exposure to corticosteroids: prospective cohort study and meta-analysis of epidemiological studies. *Teratology*. 2000;62:385.

575. Patterson M, Eytinge EJ. Chronic ulcerative colitis and pregnancy. *N Engl J Med*. 1952;246:691.

576. Paye F, Penna C, Chiche L, et al. Pouch-related fistula following restorative proctocolectomy. *Br J Surg*. 1996;83:1574.

577. Pearl RK, Nelson RL, Prasad ML, et al. Ileoanal anastomosis 24 years after total proctocolectomy for ulcerative colitis. *Dis Colon Rectum*. 1985;28:180.

578. Pearson DC, May GR, Fick GH, et al. Azathioprine and 6-mercaptopurine in Crohn's disease. A meta-analysis. *Ann Intern Med*. 1995;123:132.

579. Peck DA. Rectal mucosal replacement. *Ann Surg*. 1980;191:294.

580. Peck DA. Stapled ileal reservoir to anal anastomosis. *Surg Gynecol Obstet*. 1988;166:562.

581. Peck DA, Hallenbeck GA. Fecal continence in the dog after replacement of rectal mucosa with ileal mucosa. *Surg Gynecol Obstet*. 1964;119:1312.

582. Pemberton JH, Kelly KA, Beart RW Jr, et al. Ileal pouch-anal anastomosis for chronic ulcerative colitis: long-term results. *Ann Surg*. 1987;206:504.

583. Pemberton JH, Philips SF, Ready RR, et al. Quality of life after Brooke ileostomy and ileal pouch-anal anastomosis. *Ann Surg*. 1989;209:620.

584. Pera A, Bellando P, Caldera D, et al. Colonoscopy in inflammatory bowel disease: diagnostic accuracy and proposal of an endoscopic score. *Gastroenterology*. 1987;92:181.

585. Pescatori M. Myoelectric and motor activity of the terminal ileum after pelvic pouch for ulcerative colitis. *Dis Colon Rectum*. 1985;28:246.

586. Pescatori M, Manhire A, Bartram CI. Evacuation pouchography in the evaluation of ileoanal reservoir function. *Dis Colon Rectum*. 1983;26:365.

587. Pescatori M, Mattana C, Castagneto M. Clinical and functional results after restorative proctocolectomy. *Br J Surg*. 1988;75:321.

588. Pescatori M, Parks AG. The sphincteric and sensory components of preserved continence after ileoanal reservoir. *Surg Gynecol Obstet*. 1984;158:517.

589. Pesce G, Ceccarino R. Treatment of severe hemorrhage from a defunctionalized rectum with adrenaline chloride in ulcerative colitis. *Dis Colon Rectum*. 1991;34:1139.

590. Pezim ME. Successful childbirth after restorative proctocolectomy with pelvic ileal reservoir. *Br J Surg*. 1984;71:292.

591. Pezim ME, Taylor BA, Davis CJ, et al. Perforation of terminal ileal appendage of J-pelvic ileal reservoir. *Dis Colon Rectum*. 1987;30:161.

592. Phillips RKS. Pelvic pouches. *Br J Surg*. 1991;78:1025.

593. Polifka JE, Friedman JM. Teratogen update: azathioprine and 6-mercaptopurine. *Teratology*. 2002;65:240.

594. Poppen B, Svenberg T, Bark T, et al. Colectomy-proctomucosectomy with S-pouch: operative procedures, complications, and functional outcome in 69 consecutive patients. *Dis Colon Rectum.* 1992;35:40.

595. *Prescribing Information for Apriso (Extended Release Mesalamine).* Morrisville, NC: Salix Pharmaceuticals, Inc; 2009.

596. Probert CS, Hearing SD, Schreiber S, et al. Infliximab in moderately severe glucocorticoid resistant ulcerative colitis: a randomised controlled trial. *Gut.* 2003;52:998.

597. Prudhomme M, Dozois RR, Godlewski G, et al. Anal canal strictures after ileal pouch-anal anastomosis. *Dis Colon Rectum.* 2003;46:20.

598. Pullan RD, Rhodes J, Ganesh S, et al. Transdermal nicotine for active ulcerative colitis. *N Engl J Med.* 1994;330:811.

599. Purrmann J, Bertrams J, Borchard F, et al. Monozygotic triplets with Crohn's disease of the colon. *Gastroenterology.* 1986;91:1553.

600. Puthu D, Rajan N, Rao R, et al. Carcinoma of the rectal pouch following restorative proctocolectomy. *Dis Colon Rectum.* 1992;35:257.

601. Ransohoff DF. Colon cancer in ulcerative colitis. *Gastroenterology.* 1988;94:1089.

602. Ransohoff DF, Riddell RH, Levin B. Ulcerative colitis and colonic cancer: problems in assessing the diagnostic usefulness of mucosal dysplasia. *Dis Colon Rectum.* 1985;28:383.

603. Rao SS, Dundas SA, Holdsworth CD, et al. Olsalazine or sulphasalazine in first attacks of ulcerative colitis? A double blind study. *Gut.* 1989;30:675.

604. Rauh SM, Schoetz DJ Jr, Roberts PL, et al. Pouchitis—is it a waste-basket diagnosis? *Dis Colon Rectum.* 1991;34:685.

605. Ravid A, Richard CS, Spencer LM, et al. Pregnancy, delivery, and pouch function after ileal pouch-anal anastomosis for ulcerative colitis. *Dis Colon Rectum.* 2002;45:1283.

606. Ravitch MM. Anal ileostomy with sphincter preservation in patients requiring total colectomy for benign conditions. *Surgery.* 1948;24:170.

607. Ravitch MM, Sabiston DC Jr. Anal ileostomy with preservation of the sphincter: a proposed operation in patients requiring total colectomy for benign lesions. *Surg Gynecol Obstet.* 1947;84:1095.

608. Rayner CK, McCormack G, Emmanuel AV, et al. Long-term results of low-dose intravenous ciclosporin for acute severe ulcerative colitis. *Aliment Pharmacol Ther.* 2003;18:303.

609. Read TE, Schoetz DJ Jr, Marcello PW, et al. Afferent limb obstruction complicating ileal pouch-anal anastomosis. *Dis Colon Rectum.* 1997;40:566.

610. Régimbeau JM, Panis Y, Pocard M, et al. Handsewn ileal pouch-anal anastomosis on the dentate line after total proctectomy: technique to avoid incomplete mucosectomy and the need for long-term follow-up of the anal transition zone. *Dis Colon Rectum.* 2001;44:43.

611. Regueiro M, Loftus EV Jr, Steinhart AH, et al. Medical management of left-sided ulcerative colitis and ulcerative proctitis: critical evaluation of therapeutic trials. *Inflamm Bowel Dis.* 2006;12:979.

612. Reilly WT, Pemberton JH, Wolff BG, et al. Randomized prospective trial comparing ileal pouch-anal anastomosis performed by excising the anal mucosa to ileal pouch-anal anastomosis performed by preserving the anal mucosa. *Ann Surg.* 1997;225:666.

613. Reinisch W, Sandborn WJ, Hommes DW, et al. Adalimumab for induction of clinical remission in moderately to severely active ulcerative colitis: results of a randomised controlled trial [published online ahead of print January 5, 2011]. *Gut.*

614. Reissman P, Piccirillo M, Ulrich A, et al. Functional results of the double-stapled ileoanal reservoir. *J Am Coll Surg.* 1995;181:444.

615. Reissman P, Salky BA, Pfeifer J, et al. Laparoscopic surgery in the management of inflammatory bowel disease. *Am J Surg.* 1996;171:47.

616. Reissman P, Teoh TA, Weiss EG, et al. Functional outcome of the double-stapled ileoanal reservoir in patients more than 60 years of age. *Am J Surg.* 1996;62:178.

617. Remzi FH, Fazio VW, Delaney CP, et al. Dysplasia of the anal transitional zone after ileal pouch-anal anastomosis: results of prospective evaluation after a minimum of ten years. *Dis Colon Rectum.* 2003;46:6.

618. Rhodes J, Rose J. Does food affect acute inflammatory bowel disease? The role of parenteral nutrition, elemental and exclusion diets. *Gut.* 1986;27:471.

619. Ricart E, Panaccione R, Loftus EV, et al. Successful management of Crohn's disease of the ileoanal pouch with infliximab: a case report of seven patients. *Am J Gastroenterol.* 1998;94:2648.

620. Ricart E, Panaccione R, Loftus EV, et al. Successful management of Crohn's disease of the ileoanal pouch with infliximab. *Gastroenterology.* 1999;117:429.

621. Richard CS, Cohen Z, Stern HS, et al. Outcome of the pelvic pouch procedure in patients with prior perianal disease. *Dis Colon Rectum.* 1997;40:647.

622. Riddell RH. Dysplasia and cancer in inflammatory bowel disease. *Br J Surg.* 1985;72(suppl):S83.

623. Riddell RH, Shove DC, Ritchie JK, et al. Precancer in ulcerative colitis. In: Morson BC, ed. *The Pathogenesis of Colorectal Cancer.* Philadelphia, PA: WB Saunders; 1978:95.

624. Riley SA, Mani V, Goodman MJ, et al. Why do patients with ulcerative colitis relapse? *Gut.* 1990;31:179.

625. Ritchie JK. Ileostomy and excisional surgery for chronic inflammatory disease of the colon: a survey of one hospital region. *Gut.* 1971;12:528.

626. Ritchie JK. Crohn's disease in young people. *Br J Surg.* 1985;72 (suppl):S90.

627. Ritchie JK, Hawley PR, Lennard-Jones JE. Prognosis of carcinoma in ulcerative colitis. *Gut.* 1981;22:752.

628. Robert JH, Sachar DB, Aufses AH Jr, et al. Management of severe hemorrhage in ulcerative colitis. *Am J Surg.* 1990;159:550.

629. Roberts PL, Schoetz DJ Jr, Murray JJ, et al. Use of new retractor to facilitate mucosal proctectomy. *Dis Colon Rectum.* 1990;33:1063.

630. Rodriguez-Pinilla E, Martinez-Frias ML. Corticosteroids during pregnancy and oral clefts: a case-control study. *Teratology.* 1998;58:2.

631. Romanos J, Samarasekera DN, Stebbing JF, et al. Outcome of 200 restorative proctocolectomy operations: the John Radcliffe Hospital experience. *Br J Surg.* 1997;84:814.

632. Rosenstock E, Farmer RG, Petras R, et al. Surveillance for colonic carcinoma in ulcerative colitis. *Gastroenterology.* 1985;89:1342.

633. Rosenthal SR, Snyder JD, Hendricks KM, et al. Growth failure and inflammatory bowel disease: approach to treatment of a complicated adolescent problem. *Pediatrics.* 1983;72:481.

634. Roth MP, Petersen GM, McElree C, et al. Familial empiric risk estimates of inflammatory bowel disease in Ashkenazi Jews. *Gastroenterology.* 1989;96:1016.

635. Rotholtz NA, Pikarsky AJ, Singh JJ, et al. Adenocarcinoma arising from along the rectal stump after double-stapled ileorectal J-pouch in a patient with ulcerative colitis: the need to perform a distal anastomosis. *Dis Colon Rectum.* 2001;44:1214.

636. Roy PH, Sauer WG, Beahrs OH, et al. Experience with ileostomies: evaluation of long-term rehabilitation in 497 patients. *Am J Surg.* 1970;119:77.

637. Rubin CE, Haggitt RC, Burmer GC, et al. DNA aneuploidy in colonic biopsies predicts future development of dysplasia in ulcerative colitis. *Gastroenterology.* 1992;103:1611.

638. Rubio CA, Johansson C, Slezak P, et al. Villous dysplasia: an ominous histologic sign in colitic patients. *Dis Colon Rectum.* 1984;27:283.

639. Ruckley CV, Smith AN, Balfour TW. Perineal closure by omental graft. *Surg Gynecol Obstet.* 1970;131:300.

640. Rutgeerts P, Sandborn WJ, Feagan BG, et al. Infliximab for induction and maintenance therapy for ulcerative colitis. *N Engl J Med.* 2005;353:2462.

641. Ryan JA Jr. Gracilis muscle flap for the persistent perineal sinus of inflammatory bowel disease. *Am J Surg.* 1984;148:64.

642. Sachar DB, Auslander MO, Walfish JS. Aetiological theories of inflammatory bowel disease. *Clin Gastroenterol.* 1980;9:231.

643. Sachs T, Applebaum H, Touran T. An effective self-retaining retractor for anorectal procedures. *J Pediatr Surg.* 1991;26:90.

644. Safdi M, DeMicco M, Sninsky C, et al. A double-blind comparison of oral versus rectal mesalamine versus combination therapy in the treatment of distal ulcerative colitis. *Am J Gastroenterol.* 1997;92:1867–1871.

645. Sagar PM, Holdsworth PJ, Godwin PGR, et al. Comparison of triplicated (S) and quadruplicated (W) pelvic ileal reservoirs: studies on manovolumetry, fecal bacteriology, fecal volatile fatty acids, mucosal morphology, and functional results. *Gastroenterology.* 1992;102:520.

646. Sagar PM, Lewis W, Holdsworth PJ, et al. One-stage restorative proctocolectomy without temporary defunctioning ileostomy. *Dis Colon Rectum.* 1992;35:582.

647. Sagar PM, Lewis W, Holdsworth PJ, et al. Quality of life after restorative proctocolectomy with a pelvic ileal reservoir compares favorably with that of patients with medically treated colitis. *Dis Colon Rectum.* 1993;36:584.

648. Sagar PM, Taylor BA. Pelvic ileal reservoirs: the options. *Br J Surg.* 1994;81:325.

649. Saha SK, Robinson AF. A study of perineal wound healing after abdominoperineal resection. *Br J Surg.* 1976;63:555.

650. Saigusa N, Belin BM, Choi HJ, et al. Recovery of the rectoanal inhibitory reflex after restorative proctocolectomy: does it correlate with nocturnal continence? *Dis Colon Rectum.* 2003;46:168.

651. Salmon R, Bloch P, Loygue J. Magnetic closure of a reservoir ileostomy. *Dis Colon Rectum.* 1980;23:242.

652. Sandborn WJ. Nicotine therapy for ulcerative colitis: a review of rationale, mechanisms, pharmacology, and clinical results. *Am J Gastroenterol.* 1995;90:220.

653. Sandborn WJ, Kamm MA, Lichtenstein GR, et al. MMX Multi Matrix System mesalazine for the induction of remission in patients with mild-to-moderate ulcerative colitis: a combined analysis of two randomized, double-blind, placebo-controlled trials. *Aliment Pharmacol Ther*. 2007;26:205.

654. Sandborn WJ, Landers CJ, Tremaine WJ, et al. Antineutrophil cytoplasmic antibody correlates with chronic pouchitis after ileal pouch-anal anastomosis. *Am J Gastroenterol*. 1995;90:740.

655. Sandborn WJ, Landers CJ, Tremaine WJ, et al. Association of antineutrophil cytoplasmic antibodies with resistance to treatment of left-sided ulcerative colitis: results of a pilot study. *Mayo Clin Proc*. 1996;71:431.

656. Sandborn WJ, Rutgeerts P, Feagan BG, et al. Colectomy rate comparison after treatment of ulcerative colitis with placebo or infliximab. *Gastroenterology*. 2009;137:1250.

657. Sandborn WJ, Tremaine WJ, Batts KP, et al. Pouchitis after ileal pouch anal anastomosis. a pouchitis disease activity index. *Mayo Clin Proc*. 1994;69:409.

658. Sanderson IR, Walker-Smith JA. Crohn's disease in childhood. *Br J Surg*. 1985;72(suppl):S87.

659. Sands BE, Tremaine WJ, Sandborn WJ, et al. Infliximab in the treatment of severe, steroid-refractory ulcerative colitis: a pilot study. *Inflamm Bowel Dis*. 2001;7:83.

660. Satsangi J, Jewell DP, Rosenberg WMC, et al. Genetics of inflammatory bowel disease. *Gut*. 1994;35:696.

661. Scammell BE, Keighley MRB. Delayed perineal wound healing after proctectomy for Crohn's colitis. *Br J Surg*. 1986;73:150.

662. Schade RR, Van Thiel DH, Gavaler JS. Chronic idiopathic ulcerative colitis: pregnancy and fetal outcome. *Dig Dis Sci*. 1984;29:614.

663. Scheppach W, Sommer H, Kirchner T, et al. Effect of butyrate enemas on the colonic mucosa in distal ulcerative colitis. *Gastroenterology*. 1992;103:51.

664. Schmitt SL, Wexner SD, Lucas FV, et al. Retained mucosa after double-stapled ileal reservoir and ileoanal anastomosis. *Dis Colon Rectum*. 1992;35:1051.

665. Schoetz DJ Jr, Coller JA, Veidenheimer MC. Ileoanal reservoir for ulcerative colitis and familial polyposis. *Arch Surg*. 1986;121:404.

666. Schoetz DJ Jr, Coller JA, Veidenheimer MC. Can the pouch be saved? *Dis Colon Rectum*. 1988;31:671.

667. Schrock TR. Complications of continent ileostomy. *Am J Surg*. 1979;138:162.

668. Scott AD, Phillips RKS. Ileitis and pouchitis after colectomy for ulcerative colitis. *Br J Surg*. 1989;76:668.

669. Scotté M, Téniére P, Planet M, et al. Eversion of the rectum: a simplified technical approach to ileoanal anastomosis. *Dis Colon Rectum*. 1995;38:96.

670. Sedgwick DM, Barton JR, Hamer-Hodges DW, et al. Population-based study of surgery in juvenile-onset Crohn's disease. *Br J Surg*. 1991;78:171.

671. Sedgwick DM, Barton JR, Hamer-Hodges DW, et al. Population-based study of surgery in juvenile-onset ulcerative colitis. *Br J Surg*. 1991;78:176.

672. Seldenrijk CA, Morson BC, Meuwissen SGM, et al. Histopathological evaluation of colonic mucosal biopsy specimens in chronic inflammatory bowel disease: diagnostic implications. *Gut*. 1991;32:1514.

673. Selvasekar CR, Cima RR, Larson DW, et al. Effect of infliximab on short-term complications in patients undergoing operation for chronic ulcerative colitis. *J Am Coll Surg*. 2007;204:956.

674. Seow-Choen F, Tsunoda A, Nicholls RJ. Prospective randomized trial comparing anal function after hand-sewn ileoanal anastomosis with mucosectomy versus stapled ileoanal anastomosis without mucosectomy in restorative proctocolectomy. *Br J Surg*. 1991;78:430.

675. Setti-Carraro P, Ritchie JK, Wilkinson KH, et al. The first 10 years' experience of restorative proctocolectomy for ulcerative colitis. *Gut*. 1994;35:1070.

676. Shah NS, Remzi F, Massmann A, et al. Management and treatment outcome of pouch-vaginal fistulas following restorative proctocolectomy. *Dis Colon Rectum*. 2003;46:911.

677. Shanahan F. Pathogenesis of ulcerative colitis. *Lancet*. 1993;342:407.

678. Sharp FR, Bell GA, Seal AM, et al. Investigations of the anal sphincter before and after restorative proctocolectomy. *Am J Surg*. 1987;153:469.

679. Shen B, Achkar JP, Connor JT, et al. Modified pouchitis disease activity index: a simplified approach to the diagnosis of pouchitis. *Dis Colon Rectum*. 2003;46:748.

680. Silen W, Glotzer DJ. The prevention and treatment of the persistent perineal sinus. *Surgery*. 1974;75:535.

681. Simister NE. Placental transport of immunoglobulin G. *Vaccine*. 2003;21:3365.

682. Shah SB, Parekh NK, Hanauer SB, et al. Intravenous cyclosporine in severe steroid-refractory ulcerative colitis: long term follow-up [abstract 1041]. *Gastroenterology*. 2008.

683. Shale M, Kanfer E, Panaccione R, et al. Hepatosplenic T cell lymphoma in inflammatory bowel disease. *Gut*. 2008;57:1639.

684. Shen B, Achkar JP, Lashner BA, et al. A randomized clinical trial of ciprofloxacin and metronidazole to treat acute pouchitis. *Inflamm Bowel Dis*. 2001;7:301.

685. Shibolet O, Regushevskaya E, Brezis M, et al. Cyclosporine A for induction of remission in severe ulcerative colitis. *Cochrane Database Syst Rev*. 2005;(1):CD004277.

686. Silvis R, Delemarre JBVM, Gooszen HG. Surgical treatment and role of dynamic defecography in impaired evacuation after ileal pouch-anal anastomosis: technical solutions to a difficult problem. *Dis Colon Rectum*. 1997;40:84.

687. Simmonds NJ, Rampton DS. Inflammatory bowel disease: a radical view. *Gut*. 1993;34:865.

688. Singer HC, Anderson JGD, Frischer H, et al. Familial aspects of inflammatory bowel disease. *Gastroenterology*. 1971;61:423.

689. Skene AI, Gault DT, Woodhouse CRJ, et al. Perineal, vulval and vaginoperineal reconstruction using rectus abdominis myocutaneous flap. *Br J Surg*. 1990;77:635.

690. Smith LE. A review of 21 rectal mucosectomy and ileal pouch pull-through procedures. *Am Surg*. 1986;52:182.

691. Smith L, Friend WG, Medwell SJ. The superior mesenteric artery: the critical factor in the pouch pull-through procedure. *Dis Colon Rectum*. 1984;27:741.

692. Snook J. Are the inflammatory bowel diseases autoimmune disorders? *Gut*. 1990;31:961.

693. Snow JL, Gibson LE. A pharmacogenetic basis for the safe and effective use of azathioprine and other thiopurine drugs in dermatologic patients. *J Am Acad Dermatol*. 1995;32:114.

694. Sonnenberg A, Chang J. Time trends of physician visits for Crohn's disease and ulcerative colitis in the United States, 1960–2006. *Inflamm Bowel Dis*. 2008;14:249.

695. Soper NJ, Becker JM. A stapled technique for construction of ileal J pouches. *Surg Gynecol Obstet*. 1988;166:557.

696. Stahl D, Tyler G, Fischer JE. Inflammatory bowel disease—relationship to carcinoma. In: *Current Problems in Cancer*. Chicago, IL: Year Book Medical Publishers; 1981:5.

697. Ståhlberg D, Gullberg K, Liljeqvist L, et al. Pouchitis following pelvic pouch operation for ulcerative colitis. *Dis Colon Rectum*. 1996;39:1012.

698. Ståhlberg D, Veress B, Tribukait B, et al. Atrophy and neoplastic transformation of the ileal pouch mucosa in patients with ulcerative colitis and primary sclerosing cholangitis: a case control study. *Dis Colon Rectum*. 2003;46:770.

699. Stahlgren LH, Ferguson LK. Effects of abdominoperineal resection on sexual function in 60 patients with ulcerative colitis. *Arch Surg*. 1959;78:604.

700. Steens J, Bemelman WA, Meijerink WJHJ, et al. Ileoanal pouch function is related to postprandial pouch tone. *Br J Surg*. 2001;88:1492.

701. Steens J, Penning C, Brussee J, et al. Prospective evaluation of ileoanal pouch characteristics measured by barostat. *Dis Colon Rectum*. 2002;45:1295.

702. Stein JP, Lieskovsky G, Ginsberg DA, et al. The T-pouch: an orthotopic ileal neobladder incorporating a serosal lined ileal antireflux technique. *J Urol*. 1998;159:1836.

703. Stelzner M, Fonkalsrud EW. Significance of reservoir length in the endorectal ileal pullthrough with ileal reservoir. *Arch Surg*. 1988;123:1265.

704. Stern H, Bernstein M, Killam S, et al. A stapled S-shaped ileoanal reservoir. *Dis Colon Rectum*. 1987;30:214.

705. Stern H, Cohen Z, Wilson DR, et al. Urolithiasis risk factors in continent reservoir ileostomy patients. *Dis Colon Rectum*. 1980;23:556.

706. Stern H, Walfisch S, Mullen B, et al. Cancer in ileoanal reservoir: a new late complication? *Gut*. 1990;31:473.

707. Stryker SJ, Borody TJ, Phillips SF, et al. Motility of the small intestine after proctocolectomy and ileal pouch-anal anastomosis. *Ann Surg*. 1985;201:351.

708. Stryker SJ, Daube JR, Kelly KA, et al. Anal sphincter electromyography after colectomy, mucosal rectectomy, and ileoanal anastomosis. *Arch Surg*. 1985;120:713.

709. Stryker SJ, Phillips SF, Dozois RR, et al. Anal and neorectal function after ileal pouch-anal anastomosis. *Ann Surg*. 1986;203:55.

710. Su C, Salzberg BA, Lewis JD, et al. Efficacy of anti-tumor necrosis factor therapy in patients with ulcerative colitis. *Am J Gastroenterol*. 2002;97:2577.

711. Sugita A, Greenstein AJ, Ribeiro MB, et al. Survival with colorectal cancer in ulcerative colitis: a study of 102 cases. *Ann Surg.* 1993;218:189.

712. Sugita A, Sachar DB, Bodian C, et al. Colorectal cancer in ulcerative colitis. Influence of anatomical extent and age at onset on colitis-cancer survival. *Gut.* 1991;32:167.

713. Sutherland L, Macdonald JK. Oral 5-aminosalicylic acid for induction of remission in ulcerative colitis. *Cochrane Database Syst Rev.* 2006:CD000543.

714. Sutherland LR, Ramcharan S, Bryant H, et al. Effect of cigarette smoking on recurrence of Crohn's disease. *Gastroenterology.* 1990;98:1123.

715. Suzuki K, Muto T, Masaki T, et al. Microspectrophotometric DNA analysis in ulcerative colitis with special reference to its application in diagnosis of carcinoma and dysplasia. *Gut.* 1990;31:1266.

716. Svavoni F, Bonassi U, Bagnolo F, et al. Effectiveness of cyclosporine in the treatment of refractory ulcerative colitis. *Gastroenterology.* 1998;114:A1096.

717. Swain BT, Ellis CN. Fibrin glue treatment of low rectal and pouch-anal anastomotic sinuses. *Dis Colon Rectum.* 2004;47:253.

718. Taha AM, Shah RS. A modified technique for Kock ileostomy. *Surg Gynecol Obstet.* 1986;163:376.

719. Takao Y, Gilliland R, Nogueras JJ, et al. Is age relevant to functional outcome after restorative proctocolectomy for ulcerative colitis? Prospective assessment of 122 cases. *Ann Surg.* 1998;227:187.

720. Talbot RW, Ritchie JK, Northover JMA. Conservative proctocolectomy: a dubious option in ulcerative colitis. *Br J Surg.* 1989;76:738.

721. Tan HT, Morton D, Connolly AB, et al. Quality of life after pouch excision. *Br J Surg.* 1998;85:749.

722. Taub RN, Sachar D, Janowitz HD, et al. Induction of granulomas in mice by inoculation of tissue homogenates from patients with inflammatory bowel disease and sarcoidosis. *Ann N Y Acad Sci.* 1976;278:560.

723. Tawile NT, Priest RJ, Schuman BM. Colonoscopy in inflammatory bowel disease. *Gastrointest Endosc.* 1975;22:11.

724. Taylor BA, Pemberton JH, Carpenter HA, et al. Dysplasia in chronic ulcerative colitis: implications for colonoscopic surveillance. *Dis Colon Rectum.* 1992;35:950.

725. Taylor BM, Beart RW Jr, Dozois RR, et al. Straight ileoanal anastomosis versus ileal pouch anal anastomosis after colectomy and mucosal proctectomy. *Arch Surg.* 1983;118:696.

726. Taylor BM, Beart RW Jr, Dozois RR, et al. The endorectal ileal pouch-anal anastomosis. *Dis Colon Rectum.* 1984;27:347.

727. Teague RH, Waye JD. Inflammatory bowel disease. In: Hunt RH, Waye JD, eds. *Colonoscopy: Techniques, Clinical Practice and Colour Atlas.* London, United Kingdom: Chapman & Hall; 1981:343.

728. Telander RL, Smith SL, Marcinek HM, et al. Surgical treatment of ulcerative colitis in children. *Surgery.* 1981;90:787.

729. Telander RL, Spencer M, Perrault J, et al. Long-term follow-up of the ileoanal anastomosis in children and young adults. *Surgery.* 1990;108:717.

730. Thayer WR, Coutu JA, Chiodini RJ, et al. Possible role of mycobacteria in inflammatory bowel disease. II. Mycobacterial antibodies in Crohn's disease. *Dig Dis Sci.* 1984;29:1080.

731. Thompson JS, Williams SM. Fistula following continent ileostomy. *Dis Colon Rectum.* 1984;27:193.

732. Thompson-Fawcett MW, Rust NA, Warren BF, et al. Aneuploidy and columnar cuff surveillance after stapled ileal pouch-anal anastomosis in ulcerative colitis. *Dis Colon Rectum.* 2000;43:408.

733. Thompson-Fawcett MW, Warren BF, Mortensen NJ. A new look at the anal transitional zone with reference to restorative proctocolectomy and the columnar cuff. *Br J Surg.* 1998;85:1517.

734. Thomson WHF, O'Kelly TJ. Ileal salvage from failed pouches. *Br J Surg.* 1988;75:1227.

735. Timmer A, McDonald JW, Macdonald JK. Azathioprine and 6-mercaptopurine for maintenance of remission in ulcerative colitis. *Cochrane Database Syst Rev.* 2007;(1):CD000478.

736. Tjandra JJ, Fazio VW, Milsom JW, et al. Omission of temporary diversion in restorative proctocolectomy: is it safe? *Dis Colon Rectum.* 1993;36:1007.

737. Tobin MV, Logan RFA, Langman MJS, et al. Cigarette smoking and inflammatory bowel disease. *Gastroenterology.* 1987;93:316.

738. Toovey S, Hudson E, Hendry WF, et al. Sulphasalazine and male infertility: reversibility and possible mechanism. *Gut.* 1981;22:445.

739. Trnka YM, LaMont JT. Association of *Clostridium difficile* toxin with symptomatic relapse of chronic inflammatory bowel disease. *Gastroenterology.* 1981;80:693.

740. Truelove SC, Willoughby CP, Lee EG, et al. Further experience in the treatment of severe attacks of ulcerative colitis. *Lancet.* 1978;2:1086.

741. Tsao JI, Galandiuk S, Pemberton JH. Pouchogram: predictor of clinical outcome following ileal pouch-anal anastomosis. *Dis Colon Rectum.* 1992;35:547.

742. Tuckson WB, Fazio VW. Functional comparison between double and triple ileal loop pouches. *Dis Colon Rectum.* 1991;34:17.

743. Tuckson WB, Lavery I, Fazio V, et al. Manometric and functional comparison of ileal pouch-anal anastomosis with and without anal manipulation. *Am J Surg.* 1991;161:90.

744. Tulchinsky H, Cohen CRG, Nicholls RJ. Salvage surgery after restorative proctocolectomy. *Br J Surg.* 2003;90:909.

745. Tulchinsky H, Hawley PR, Nicholls J. Long-term failure after restorative proctocolectomy for ulcerative colitis. *Ann Surg.* 2003;238:229.

746. Tulchinsky H, McCourtney JS, Subba Rao KV, et al. Salvage abdominal surgery in patients with a retained rectal stump after restorative proctocolectomy and stapled anastomosis. *Br J Surg.* 2001;88:1602.

747. Tumen HJ, Valdes-Dapena A, Haddad H. Indications for surgical intervention in ulcerative colitis in children. *Am J Dis Child.* 1968;116:641.

748. Turnbull RB Jr. The surgical approach to the treatment of inflammatory bowel disease (IBD): a personal view of techniques and prognosis. In: Kirsner JB, Shorter RG, eds. *Inflammatory Bowel Disease.* Philadelphia, PA: Lea & Febiger; 1975:338.

749. Turnbull RB Jr, Hawk WA, Weakley FL. Surgical treatment of toxic megacolon. Ileostomy and colostomy to prepare patients for colectomy. *Am J Surg.* 1971;122:325.

750. Ullman TA. Patients with low-grade dysplasia should be advised to undergo colectomy. *Inflamm Bowel Dis.* 2003;9:267.

751. Utsunomiya J, Iwama T, Imajo M, et al. Total colectomy, mucosal proctectomy, and ileoanal anastomosis. *Dis Colon Rectum.* 1980;23:459.

752. Valiente MA, Bacon HE. Construction of pouch using "pantaloon" technique for pull-through of ileum following total colectomy: report of experimental work and results. *Am J Surg.* 1955;90:742.

753. Van Assche G, D'Haens G, Noman M, et al. Randomized double-blind comparison of 4 mg/kg/day versus 2 mg/kg/day intravenous cyclosporine in severe ulcerative colitis. *Gastroenterology.* 2003;125:1025.

754. Van Heerden JA, Beart RW Jr. Carcinoma of the colon and rectum complicating chronic ulcerative colitis. *Dis Colon Rectum.* 1980;23:155.

755. Van Prohaska J, Siderius NJ. The surgical rehabilitation of patients with chronic ulcerative colitis. *Am J Surg.* 1962;103:42.

756. Varma JS, Browning GGP, Smith AN, et al. Mucosal proctectomy and colo-anal anastomosis for distal ulcerative proctocolitis. *Br J Surg.* 1987;74:381.

757. Velayos FS, Terdiman JP, Walsh JM. Effect of 5-aminosalicylate use on colorectal cancer and dysplasia risk: a systematic review and metaanalysis of observational studies. *Am J Gastroenterol.* 2005;100:1345.

758. Venturi A, Gionchetti P, Rizzello F, et al. Impact on the composition of the faecal flora by a new probiotic preparation: preliminary data on maintenance treatment of patients with ulcerative colitis. *Aliment Pharmacol Ther.* 1999;13:1103.

759. Vessey M, Jewell D, Smith A, et al. Chronic inflammatory bowel disease, cigarette smoking, and use of oral contraceptives: findings in a large cohort study of women of childbearing age. *Br Med J.* 1986;292:1101.

760. The Veterans Affairs Total Parenteral Nutrition Cooperative Study Group. Perioperative total parenteral nutrition in surgical patients. *N Engl J Med.* 1991;325:525.

761. Wada Y, Matsui T, Matake H, et al. Intractable ulcerative colitis caused by cytomegalovirus infection. A prospective study on prevalence, diagnosis and treatment. *Dis Colon Rectum.* 2003;46(suppl):S59.

762. Wapnick S, Grosberg S, Farman J, et al. Volvulus of the Kock reservoir. *Dis Colon Rectum.* 1979;22:55.

763. Watanabe T, Kubota Y, Muto T. Substance P-containing nerve fibers in rectal mucosa of ulcerative colitis. *Dis Colon Rectum.* 1997;40:718.

764. Watts JM, de Dombal FT, Goligher JC. Long-term complications and prognosis following major surgery for ulcerative colitis. *Br J Surg.* 1966;53:1014.

765. Waye JD. The role of colonoscopy in the differential diagnosis of inflammatory bowel disease. *Gastrointest Endosc.* 1977;23:150.

766. Waye JD. Endoscopy in inflammatory bowel disease. *Clin Gastroenterol.* 1980;9:279.

767. Weinstein M, Rubin RJ, Salvati EP. Detachment of the continent ileostomy pouch from the anterior abdominal wall: report of two unusual cases. *Dis Colon Rectum.* 1976;19:705.

768. Welch CE, Hedberg SE. Colonic cancer in ulcerative colitis and idiopathic colonic cancer. *JAMA.* 1965;191:815.

769. Weterman IT, Peña AS. Familial incidence of Crohn's disease in the Netherlands and a review of the literature. *Gastroenterology.* 1984;86:449.

770. Wexner SD, James K, Jagelman DG. The double-stapled ileal reservoir and ileoanal anastomosis: a prospective review of sphincter function and clinical outcome. *Dis Colon Rectum.* 1991;34:487.

771. Wexner SD, Rothenberger DA, Jensen L, et al. Ileal pouch vaginal fistulas: incidence, etiology, and management. *Dis Colon Rectum.* 1989;32:460.

772. Wexner SD, Wong WD, Rothenberger DA, et al. The ileoanal reservoir. *Am J Surg.* 1990;159:178.

773. White CL III, Hamilton SR, Diamond MP, et al. Crohn's disease and ulcerative colitis in the same patient. *Gut.* 1983;24:857.

774. Whorwell PJ, Phillips CA, Beeken WL, et al. Isolation of reovirus-like agents from patients with Crohn's disease. *Lancet.* 1977;1:1169.

775. Wilks S. The morbid appearances in the intestines of Miss Bankes. *Med Times Gaz.* 1859;2:264.

776. Wilks S, Moxon W. *Lectures on Pathological Anatomy.* 2nd ed. London, United Kingdom: J & A Churchill; 1875:408,672.

777. Williams CB, Waye JD. Colonoscopy in inflammatory bowel disease. *Clin Gastroenterol.* 1978;7:701.

778. Williams NS, Marzouk DEMM, Hallan RI, et al. Function after ileal pouch and stapled pouch-anal anastomosis for ulcerative colitis. *Br J Surg.* 1989;76:1168.

779. Williamson MER, Lewis WG, Miller AS, et al. Clinical and physiological evaluation of anorectal eversion during restorative proctocolectomy. *Br J Surg.* 1995;82:1391.

780. Williamson MER, Lewis WG, Sagar PM, et al. One-stage restorative proctocolectomy without temporary ileostomy for ulcerative colitis: a note of caution. *Dis Colon Rectum.* 1997;40:1019.

781. Wiltz O, Hashmi HF, Schoetz DJ Jr, et al. Carcinoma and the ileal pouch-anal anastomosis. *Dis Colon Rectum.* 1991;34:805.

782. Winslet MC, Barsoum G, Pringle W, et al. Loop ileostomy after ileal pouch-anal anastomosis—is it necessary? *Dis Colon Rectum.* 1991; 34:267.

783. Wolff WI, Shinya H, Geffen A, et al. Comparison of colonoscopy and the contrast enema in 500 patients with colorectal disease. *Am J Surg.* 1975;129:181.

784. Woolfson K, Cohen Z, McLeod RS. Crohn's disease and pregnancy. *Dis Colon Rectum.* 1990;33:869.

785. Woolrich AJ, DaSilva MD, Korelitz BI. Surveillance in the routine management of ulcerative colitis: the predictive value of low-grade dysplasia. *Gastroenterology.* 1992;103:431.

786. Yeager ES, Van Heerden JA. Sexual dysfunction following procto-colectomy and abdominoperineal resection. *Ann Surg.* 1980;191:169.

787. Yoshimura HH, Estes MK, Graham DY. Search for evidence of a viral aetiology for inflammatory bowel disease. *Gut.* 1984;25:347.

788. Young MRA, Small JO, Leonard AG, et al. Rectus abdominis flap for persistent perineal sinus. *Br J Surg.* 1988;75:1228.

789. Zahavi I, Avidor I, Marcus H, et al. Effect of sucralfate on experimental colitis in the rat. *Dis Colon Rectum.* 1989;32:95.

790. Zeitels JR, Fiddian-Green RG, Dent TL. Intersphincteric proctectomy. *Surgery.* 1984;96:617.

791. Zeldis JB. Pregnancy and inflammatory bowel disease. *West J Med.* 1989;151:168.

792. Zetzel L. Fertility, pregnancy, and idiopathic inflammatory bowel disease. In: Kirsner JB, Shorter RG, eds. *Inflammatory Bowel Disease.* Philadelphia, PA: Lea & Febiger; 1975:146.

793. Ziv Y, Fazio VW, Church JM, et al. Safety of urgent restorative proctocolectomy with ileal pouch-anal anastomosis for fulminant colitis. *Dis Colon Rectum.* 1995;38:345.

794. Ziv Y, Fazio VW, Church JM, et al. Stapled ileal pouch-anal anastomoses are safer than hand-sewn anastomoses in patients with ulcerative colitis. *Am J Surg.* 1996;171:320.

795. Zlatanic J, Korelitz BI, Rajapakse R, et al. Complications of pregnancy and child development after cessation of treatment with 6-mercaptopurine for inflammatory bowel disease. *J Clin Gastroenterol.* 2003;36:303.

796. Zmora O, Efron JE, Nogueras JJ, et al. Reoperative abdominal and perineal surgery in ileoanal pouch patients. *Dis Colon Rectum.* 2001; 44:1310.

30

Crohn's Disease and Indeterminate Colitis

Victor W. Fazio

The knife cannot always have fresh fields for conquest; and although methods of practice may be modified and varied, and even improved to some extent, it must be within a certain limit.

SIR JOHN ERICHSEN, *Lancet.* 1873;2:489

► CROHN'S DISEASE

Crohn's disease of the bowel was initially described by Crohn, Ginzburg, and Oppenheimer in 1932, at which time they noted a transmural inflammatory condition of the terminal ileum.[96] The authors apparently listed their names in alphabetical order for the purpose of publication. It would certainly appear that if one is concerned about eponymous immortality, it is helpful to have a name occurring early in the alphabet. Interestingly, many of the cases were based on the large patient experience of Berg.[340] Had Dr. Berg wished to include his name on the paper, the condition today would probably be termed *Berg's disease*. Ginzburg reflected on the myths and misunderstandings concerning the evolution of the concept of Crohn's disease in his interesting paper "The Road to Regional Enteritis."[180] A number of publications followed from the experience of Crohn and his associates, confirming the location in the small bowel, but also noting that in a number of cases the colon was to some extent involved.

Another interesting historical footnote was suggested by Goligher[189] that Crohn's disease was actually initially described in 1907 by Lord Moynihan when Moynihan presented his experience with six patients who harbored benign lesions that mimicked carcinoma.[368] In 1913, Dalziel reported an obscure tuberculosis-like condition that he called "chronic interstitial enteritis" but which must have been Crohn's disease.[99] In 1923, Moschowitz and Wilensky described four patients with a granulomatous disease of the intestine and the amelioration of the condition by intestinal bypass.[366]

In 1951, Marshak noted the radiologic findings of what he felt was granulomatous disease of the *colon*, a clinical entity distinct from that of ulcerative colitis.[340] This view was not generally accepted until 1959, when Morson and Lockhart-Mummery described the characteristic pathologic features of granulomatous colitis.[364] It can be appreciated, therefore, that our concepts of disease involvement in this area are scarcely one-half century old.

Incidence, Epidemiology, Etiology, and Pathogenesis

The incidence, epidemiology, and theories concerning the etiology and pathogenesis of both Crohn's disease and ulcerative colitis are discussed in Chapter 29. Inflammatory bowel disease (IBD) remains a complex polygenic disorder interacting with environmental factors that trigger abnormal responses in genetically susceptible individuals.[394] The incidence of IBD development in identical twins is 60% in Crohn's but only 15% in ulcerative colitis.[483] Subclinical intestinal inflammation has also been documented in symptomatic first-degree relatives of Crohn's disease patients.

It is interesting to note that *Mycobacterium paratuberculosis* DNA has been found in Crohn's diseased tissue.[482] The concept of a bacterial cause for IBD has been discussed in Chapter 29, an issue that has generally been refuted. In one study, however, *M. paratuberculosis* was identified in 65% of specimens in individuals with Crohn's disease but in only

(text continues on page 1300)

BURRILL BERNARD CROHN (1884–1983)

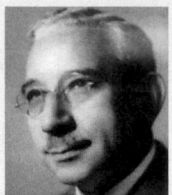

Burrill Crohn was born in New York City, June 13, 1884. He graduated from the City College of New York in 1902 and received his medical degree from Columbia University College of Physicians and Surgeons in 1907. Crohn began his internship at Mount Sinai Hospital, the institution with which he was affiliated for his entire professional life. In 1920, he was named the first head of the department of gastroenterology. Henry Janowitz wrote that the "eponym [of Crohn's disease] is deserved not because of a fortuitous alphabetical listing, but because for many years Crohn alone called attention to this enigmatic inflammation of the bowel, by carefully collecting cases and by publishing his clinical observations." Janowitz further stated that although not displeased with the honor and the name recognition, Crohn was always modest with respect to his role in the original description. Crohn himself expressed the feeling that the name *Crohn's disease* was inappropriate despite its virtually universal use, preferring instead the term *regional enteritis*. In 1956, when President Dwight D. Eisenhower required surgery for ileitis, it was Crohn who was called to the White House to act as spokesman to explain the disease and the prognosis to the American people. Crohn authored three texts and more than 100 scientific papers. Among his numerous awards were the Townsend Harris Medal by the City College of New York, the Julius Friedenthal Medal of the American Gastroenterological Association, and the Mount Sinai Hospital's Jacobi Medal. He was also elected president of the American Gastroenterological Association. Crohn died in New Milford, Connecticut, at the age of 99.

LEON GINZBURG (1899–1988)

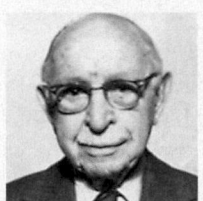

Leon Ginzburg was born in Bayonne, New Jersey. He completed his undergraduate studies at Columbia University in 1920 and went on to accomplish his surgical training at the Mount Sinai Hospital. Following a tour of the major European institutions, he returned to become A. A. Berg's House Surgeon at Mount Sinai. For the ensuing 5 years, he was an adjunct on Berg's ward service and his assistant in the private practice of surgery. The association with Mount Sinai lasted for 40 years, with Ginzburg achieving the rank of clinical professor. From 1947 to 1967, he was director of surgery at the Beth Israel Hospital, as the medical center was then known. The recognition of ileitis was accomplished by examining surgically excised specimens, which led in 1927 to his first description. There was a well-recognized controversy between Ginzburg and Crohn concerning each individual's respective role in the early observations. As both physicians neared their 90s, Ginzburg compared the discovery of regional ileitis to the controversy over the naming of the United States after Amerigo Vespucci rather than after Christopher Columbus. He likened the former map maker to Crohn, who spent considerable time and effort traveling, lecturing, and spreading knowledge about the disease, while he credited himself with the original description. Leon Ginzburg was active in practice at Beth Israel Medical Center until his death in 1988 at the age of 89. (With special appreciation to Lester Rosen, MD.)

GORDON DAVID OPPENHEIMER (1900–1974)

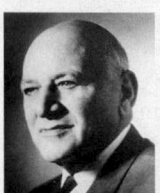

Gordon Oppenheimer was born on June 30, 1900, in New York City and received his baccalaureate from Columbia College in 1919, and his medical degree from Columbia College of Physicians and Surgeons in 1922. He then became a house officer at the Mount Sinai Hospital, eventually entering the pathology laboratory where he collaborated with Ginzburg in his work on the study of inflammatory lesions of the terminal ileum. Oppenheimer ultimately became a urologist, rising to the position of Chief of Urology at Mount Sinai Hospital, a post he occupied from 1947 to 1963. He authored 69 papers, including a monograph he published with Leon Ginzburg, *Urological Complications of Regional Ileitis*. In addition to his responsibilities as chairman of the department and director of the residency program, Oppenheimer found time to serve for 14 years as a medical officer with the New York City Fire Department. During World War II, he acted as Second in Command of the General Surgical Service at Mount Sinai Hospital. He is remembered as a kind, gentle, and humble man, an especially humane physician who was much sought after as a consultant urologist. He died of cardiac failure, December 9, 1974, at the age of 74.

ALBERT ASHTON BERG (1872–1950)

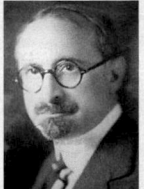

It might seem incongruous that I have elected to include A. A. Berg as an individual to be recognized with a biographic sketch in this text. But he represents for me a special person—someone who could afford the "luxury of integrity." Berg declined to add his name to the alphabetical listing of coauthors because, even though the publication was based on his surgical patients, he did not contribute to the writing. He was born in New York City, August 10, 1872, and attended City College of New York, graduating from the College of Physicians and Surgeons at Columbia University in 1894. After his surgical training at the Mount Sinai Hospital, he joined the staff. In his early years, he was an assistant to Arpad Gerster, the man who introduced Listerian principles to the United States. Berg developed an enormous clinical practice, arguably the largest in the city of New York, having been recognized as a phenomenal technician. He is credited with having performed the first gastrectomy for ulcer disease in the United States. In 1930, he published his experiences with more than 500 patients on the morbidity and mortality of subtotal gastrectomy in the management of gastric and duodenal ulcer. In 1905, he published a text, *Surgical Diagnosis: A Manual for Students and Practitioners*. In 1934, when he retired from the teaching service at Mount Sinai, the hospital published *The Surgical Technique of Dr. A.A. Berg: A Tribute to Forty Years' Service at the Mt. Sinai Hospital*. The chapters were written by his students, including contributions on the small bowel and colon by Leon Ginzburg. Along with his brother (an internist), he amassed a library of 50,000 rare volumes of English and American literature, bequeathing the collection to New York University, Mount Sinai Hospital, and the New York Public Library. Today there exists at Mount Sinai a Berg Laboratory Building and an Institute for Research, and at the New York Public Library, a Berg Room, where the collection is housed. Albert Berg died following kidney surgery on July 1, 1950, at the age of 77.

BERKELEY GEORGE ANDREW MOYNIHAN (1865–1936)

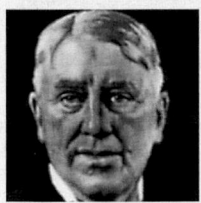

Berkeley Moynihan was born on the island of Malta, the only son of a distinguished army captain. He received his premedical education at the Royal Naval School and his medical training at the Leeds Medical School (1885) and at the University of London (1887). In 1893, he was awarded a gold medal in the examination for master of surgery. In 1895, he married the daughter of T. R. Jessop, the man who preceded him as surgeon to the Leeds General Infirmary. Moynihan was a masterful surgeon, particularly for surgery of the abdomen. He served as professor of surgery from 1902, becoming emeritus professor in 1926. In 1905, he published his outstanding book, *Abdominal Operations*, which ran through four editions. Among his numerous contributions and distinctions were founder and editor of the *British Journal of Surgery*, president of the Royal College of Surgeons, Hunterian Professor, and successively, knight, baronet, and baron.

THOMAS KENNEDY DALZIEL (1861–1924)

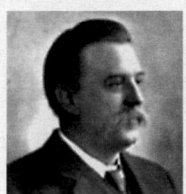

T. Kennedy Dalziel (pronounced "dee-yell") was born in Scotland at Merkland, Penpont, Dumfriesshire. He received his early education at a private school in Dumfries and studied medicine at Edinburgh University, graduating in 1883. He continued his medical studies in Berlin and Vienna, where he specialized in experimental surgery and pathology. In 1885, he began his practice in Glasgow, and in 1889, he joined the staff of the Royal Hospital for Sick Children. For his services in World War I to the Advisory Council of the Royal Army Medical Corps, the king conferred on him the honor of knighthood. His successes and the public position he attained were the result of an unusual combination of qualities—charm, kindliness, extraordinary teaching skills, and marvelous manipulative dexterity. He was considered the best technical surgeon in the West of Scotland. His contributions to the medical literature were considerable, dealing primarily with that of abdominal surgery.

RICHARD H. MARSHAK (1912–1982)

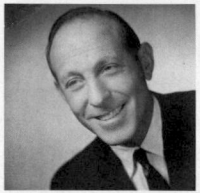

Richard Marshak received his MD with honors from the University of Louisville in 1937. After completing residencies in pathology and radiology, Marshak was invited by Burrill Crohn at Mount Sinai Hospital to join his private practice as a consulting radiologist. Consequently, Marshak saw hundreds of patients with gastrointestinal disorders. His unique forte consisted of correlating the pathologic findings of the gastrointestinal tract with the radiologic features. He, along with Bernard Wolf, elucidated the radiologic changes in esophagitis, hiatal hernia, and inflammatory bowel disease. Wolf's collaborations, over a period of many years with Richard Marshak and Mansho Khilnani, on the physiologic and anatomic details of the esophagus and gastrointestinal tract and on the various aspects of inflammatory bowel disease, were unique. Much of what we take for granted today was first articulated during this era by these three men. Bernard Wolf, chairman of the department of radiology presented the Jacobi Medallion of the Alumni Association to Richard Marshak in 1972. Dick, as he was called, was the first president of the Society of Gastrointestinal Radiologists (SGR) and helped found the Health Insurance Plan. Before it became such a hot button, current topic, he pressed for the availability of medicine to everyone. He was the recipient of the Townsend Harris medal, given by the Alumni Association of the City College for outstanding achievements. He also received the Gold Medal Award from the Radiological Society of North America for distinction as an author, scholar, teacher, and scientist. Marshak was past president of the New York Academy of Gastroenterology, the New York Roentgen Society, and the American College of Gastroenterology. A dominant figure in radiology for more than 30 years, Richard H. Marshak belongs to a group of Mount Sinai physicians who are remembered equally for their scientific achievements and for their colorful personalities. Marshak finished his career as clinical professor of radiology at the Mount Sinai School of Medicine, continuing to work steadily until his death in 1982. As a founding member and the first president of the former Society of Gastrointestinal Radiologists, Marshak is recognized for his spirit of leadership and dedication to the SGR. An annual award given in his memory, the Richard H. Marshak International Lecture is presented to a member of the Society of Abdominal Radiology who represents the organization at the International Education Conference held annually in a country that cannot support education in the field of abdominal radiology. An annual contribution of $4,000 is received from the Marshak Fund in support of this award.

When the ravages of diabetes resulted in Marshak's almost complete loss of vision, with the assistance of his long-time associate, Daniel Maklansky, himself a gifted radiologist and teacher, Marshak continued to give lectures, describing in detail slides he could barely see. Richard Marshak died of a heart attack at Lenox Hill Hospital, December 20, 1982, at the age of 70. He died just before the publication of the last in a series of books he had written on gastrointestinal diseases. (Photograph courtesy of the Mount Sinai Archives.)

4.3% of those with ulcerative colitis.[482] The control tissues were found to have this DNA element in 12.5%. It was concluded that these observations are consistent with an etiologic role for *M. paratuberculosis* in Crohn's disease. A statistically significant association between the onset of Crohn's disease and prior antibiotic use has been demonstrated.[75] This suggests that a change in the bacterial environment within the intestinal tract in a susceptible host may be responsible for triggering the disease in some patients. Smokers are also overrepresented in Crohn's patients and underrepresented in ulcerative colitis, and they have an increased risk of recurrence after surgery when compared with nonsmokers.[598,603]

Another observation involves the identification of genes associated with IBD. Pokorny and associates identified a genetic and clinical association between the DNA repair gene, *MLH1*, and both ulcerative colitis and Crohn's disease (see Chapter 29).[412] Most exciting is the identification of the *NOD2* gene (now renamed *CARD15*) as the IBD1 gene in the pericentromeric region of chromosome 16 which signals the opening of a vast arena of genetic research to provide a basic understanding of IBD.[217,251,389] *NOD2* is involved in the activation of nuclear factor-kappa B (NF-κB) transcription factor that plays a significant role in Crohn's disease. *NOD2* encodes a protein homologous to plant disease resistance genes that are involved in the immune response to infectious organisms, particularly the leucine-rich region that binds to bacterial lipopolysaccharides. Ten percent of Crohn's patients have a frameshift mutation (via a cytosine insertion) that fails to induce NF-κB in the presence of bacterial lipopolysaccharide, suggesting a common link to the failure of immune response to bacterial components and thereby possibly explaining the role of antibiotics or the value of probiotics in the therapy of Crohn's. Certainly, Crohn's disease appears to be influenced by a wide range of genetic and environmental factors.[522]

Signs, Symptoms, and Presentations

Patients with Crohn's disease may present with very minimal symptoms and moderate complaints, or they may have fulminant manifestations. The considerable overlap in the presentations of ulcerative colitis and Crohn's disease is addressed in Chapter 29. For example, individuals with Crohn's disease may bleed, but this is not as frequent a presentation and may not be as severe.[349] However, life-threatening hemorrhage has been reported.[85] Abdominal pain may be mild or absent in patients with ulcerative colitis, but those with Crohn's disease frequently complain of pain. This may be colicky in nature and may be associated with intestinal obstruction, or it may be continual and related to the presence of a septic process within the abdomen. An abdominal mass is not uncommonly found on physical examination in a patient with Crohn's disease, but it is never seen in a patient with ulcerative colitis.

Diarrhea is usually a more troublesome concern in patients with ulcerative colitis. This may be because distal disease tends to be associated with more urgency, and in some cases, tenesmus. Patients with Crohn's disease may have rectal sparing and are less likely to experience this urgency. Conversely, with rectal involvement, Crohn's patients experience symptoms similar to those with ulcerative colitis. It is important to consider also the possibility of opportunistic infections and concomitant neoplasms, including cytomegaloviral infection and Kaposi's sarcoma, especially in individuals with prolonged immunosuppressive therapy for this disease (see later, Medical Management).[89]

Anal disease is much more commonly seen in patients with Crohn's colitis than in those with ulcerative colitis. The presence of anal pain, swelling, and discharge may be a presenting feature of the former condition and may be the only abnormality observed on examination and on subsequent investigation. In the experience of the Lahey Clinic group with anal complications in patients with Crohn's disease, 22% of 1,098 were so afflicted.[585] Anal fissure was diagnosed in 29% of patients who had anal manifestations; a fistula was found in 28%, an abscess in 23%, and multiple presentations in 20%. Crohn's colitis was much more frequently associated with an anal lesion than was Crohn's disease of the small bowel (52% vs. 14%). Within 1 year following the anal manifestation, Crohn's disease presented elsewhere in 59% of patients. All the remaining developed gastrointestinal disease within 5 years. In the St. Mark's Hospital experience, 34% of patients with small bowel Crohn's disease had anal lesions, whereas 58% of those with colon disease were found to have anal involvement.[321] Of 126 consecutive patients with perianal Crohn's disease seen regularly in one outpatient clinic, 48% were diagnosed as having an abscess.[532]

A high level of suspicion should exist if the examiner notes characteristic edematous tags, blue discoloration of the skin, an eccentrically located fissure, a broad-based ulcer, a rigid or strictured canal, or an anal fistula, especially if the patient reports gastrointestinal symptoms. A clinical classification of perianal Crohn's disease has been proposed by Hughes.[248] The reader is referred to Chapters 13 and 14 for a discussion of the management of anal complications.

Fever is usually not a concern in patients with ulcerative colitis unless the patient is severely ill (e.g., toxic megacolon). However, in those with Crohn's disease, a pyrexia is not uncommonly noted and is usually due to the presence of an intra-abdominal abscess or undrained septic focus. Nausea and vomiting are not frequently noted in either condition unless there is evidence of intestinal obstruction. Anorexia, weight loss, anemia, and general debility are associated with relatively long-standing or fulminant disease.

Disease in Children and Adolescents
When the condition occurs in children, there may be a more rapid onset and progression than when the disease occurs in young adults. These youngsters often become chronically ill, have growth impairment, have decreased mental acuity, and are less developed physically than their healthy peers (see Figure 29-26). It is because of these concerns that implementation of either an elemental diet or parenteral nutrition is an especially important part of the management in this age group (see Medical Management).[267,481] However, in order to be maximally effective, therapy must be initiated before puberty.[267] Furthermore, unless medical treatment can achieve a sustained remission, operative intervention may be the only effective means for addressing the problem of retarded development (see later).[119]

Elliott and colleagues reported the prognosis of 57 patients with Crohn's disease of the large bowel seen within 6 months of the onset of symptoms during 1969 to 1978 and followed until 1984 at St. Mark's Hospital.[133] The cumulative probability of an operation was 35% at 5 years and 39% at 10 years. They concluded that about one-half of all such patients can be treated successfully without abdominal surgery. However, children and adolescents with colonic disease are much more likely to require resection, often after a relatively short period of illness.[171,432] Growth retardation as an indication for surgery may be one of the reasons for this difference.

As with adults, the efficacy of surgery for Crohn's disease in children seems to depend mainly on disease location and perhaps the choice of surgical procedure itself.[101] Assessment of growth and development, psychological support for both the patient and the family, and close cooperation between the physician and the surgeon are important concepts in the management of these young people.[449,455,481]

Disease in Pregnancy
For a discussion of disease in pregnancy, see Chapter 29.

Physical Examination
In contrast to individuals with ulcerative colitis, even in the absence of toxic megacolon, a patient with Crohn's disease may demonstrate obvious findings on physical examination. As mentioned, although it is true that anorectal disease can occur with ulcerative colitis, it is much more common in those with Crohn's disease. The diagnosis is often suspected on examination of the perianal skin (see Figure 14-51). Simple inspection will often show the edematous tags, fissures, abscess, or fistulas characteristically seen in this condition. The anal canal may be stenotic, fibrotic, and thickened on digital examination. If an anal fissure is apparent, severe pain is noted (Figure 30-1).

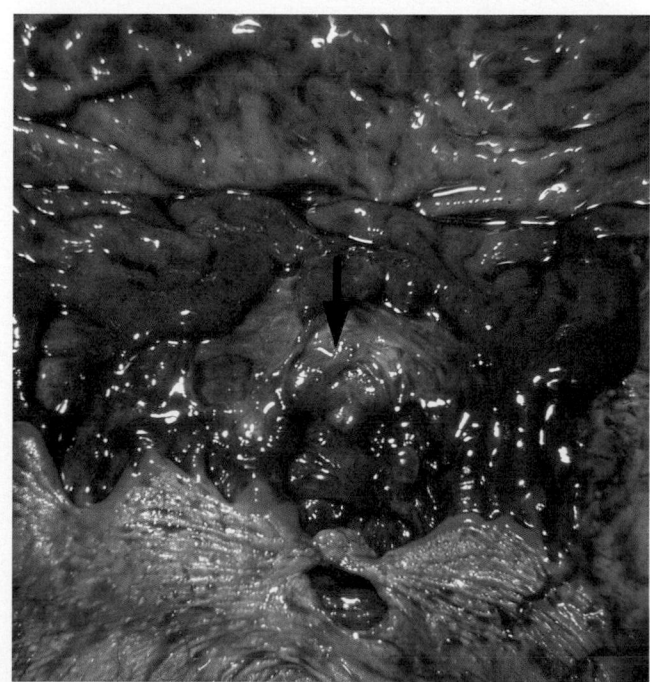

FIGURE 30-1. Crohn's disease. Proctectomy specimen with a broad-based anal fissure (*arrow*). Just distal to the dentate line, an external opening of a fistula is evident. (From Corman ML, Veidenheimer MC, Nugent FW, et al. *Diseases of the Anus, Rectum and Colon. Part II: Non-specific Inflammatory Bowel Disease.* New York, NY: Medcom; 1976.)

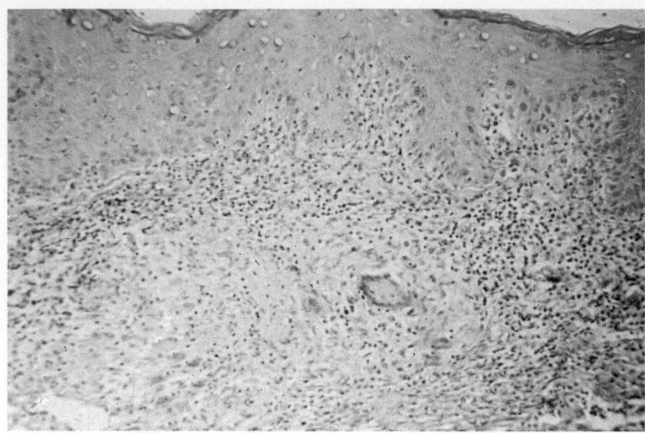

FIGURE 30-2. This section from a macroscopically normal anus reveals a submucosal granuloma. The patient subsequently proved to have Crohn's disease. (Original magnification × 80; from Corman ML, Veidenheimer MC, Nugent FW, et al. *Diseases of the Anus, Rectum and Colon. Part II: Non-specific Inflammatory Bowel Disease.* New York, NY: Medcom; 1976.)

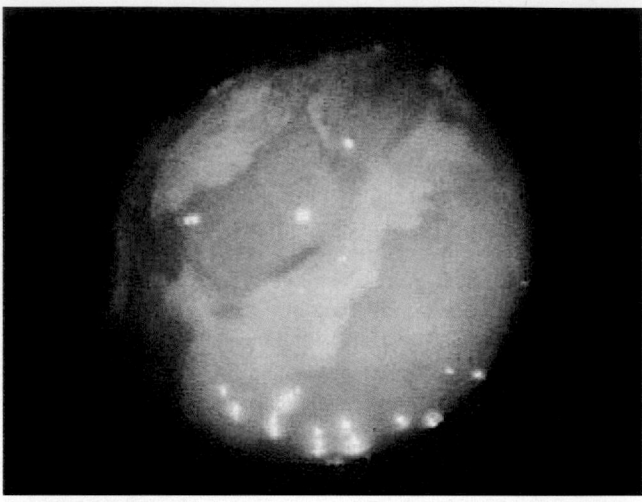

FIGURE 30-3. Colon in Crohn's colitis demonstrates deep linear ulcerations with pus—rake ulcers.

Pelvic examination in a woman may reveal a rectovaginal fistula, and bimanual examination may show the presence of a pelvic mass. A biopsy of a sinus tract or an abscess cavity may demonstrate the granulomas characteristic of Crohn's colitis (Figure 30-2).

Abdominal findings are more common in patients with Crohn's disease than in those with ulcerative colitis. A mass may be felt in the right iliac fossa, a common observation when regional enteritis involves the terminal ileum. A large, mesenteric abscess can often be palpated. Crohn's colitis, however, usually is not associated with clinically demonstrable abdominal abnormalities.

Endoscopic Examination

Proctosigmoidoscopic examination is often helpful in differentiating between ulcerative colitis and Crohn's disease. The rectum is always diseased during attacks of ulcerative colitis, whereas with Crohn's colitis, 40% of patients have sparing of the rectum, irrespective of anal or perianal involvement (see Chapter 29). But when the rectum is involved by Crohn's disease, differentiation between the two may be quite difficult.

A corollary to this observation is to perform biopsies distal to obvious inflammatory changes if the rectum appears to be spared because one may discover that the rectum is not truly normal. This may cause the physician to reassess the accuracy of a diagnosis of Crohn's disease for what was initially thought to be lack of rectal involvement. Biopsy may be helpful because histologic changes suggestive of Crohn's disease in particular may be apparent. Up to 20% of such patients may exhibit granulomata.

The place of colonoscopy in the evaluation and follow-up of IBD has been extensively reviewed by many authors. Teague and Waye recommend colonoscopy for five indications: differential diagnosis, resolution of radiographic abnormalities (e.g., filling defects and strictures), preoperative and postoperative evaluation in Crohn's disease, examination of stomas, and screening for premalignant and malignant changes.[546] With granulomatous colitis, Waye observed the following major colonoscopic findings: a normal rectum (obviously this is not always the case), asymmetry or

eccentricity of involvement, cobblestone appearance, normal vasculature, edema of the bowel wall (as seen in ulcerative colitis), normal mucosa intervening between areas of ulceration, serpiginous ulcers (these may course for several centimeters), pseudopolyps (as in ulcerative colitis), and skip areas (lack of continuity of involvement).[330] He adds another observation, the presence of amyloidosis in the biopsy specimen. An endoscopic index for determining the severity of colonic Crohn's disease has also been proposed.[344] Figure 30-3 illustrates the characteristic longitudinal ulcerations seen in Crohn's disease.

Unfortunately, there are frequent difficulties in the interpretation of the biopsies obtained by means of proctosigmoidoscopy or colonoscopy. In a prospective study that Geboes and Vantrappen performed over an 18-month period, 71 colonoscopies were undertaken on 59 patients with Crohn's disease.[172] In comparison with barium enema examination, the segmental nature of the involvement was more apparent by means of colonoscopy. Microulceration was also more evident than by radiologic means. Radiographs yielded more information about the haustra, especially in the right colon. Colonoscopy permitted a histologic diagnosis in 24% of patients, but granulomas were found in only 19 of 321 specimens (6%). In more than one-fourth, the entire colon could not be examined, and no complications occurred. Hogan and colleagues observed that inconsistencies are often noted between macroscopic observations by the endoscopist and histologic interpretation of the biopsy specimen by the pathologist.[242] They felt that the reason for this problem is the overlapping of the histologic features of the two conditions, ulcerative colitis and Crohn's disease.

Changes in patients with ulcerative colitis are truly nonspecific, unless atypia or frank carcinoma supervenes. The most useful lesion found on colonoscopic mucosal biopsy of patients with Crohn's disease is a granuloma. The limiting factor in establishing the correct diagnosis by means of biopsy, however, is the small size of the specimen. Hence, the physician or surgeon, having the benefit of clinical evaluation and the history, is often in the better position to make the correct diagnosis.

Distribution

The primary locations of the disease have been categorized by Bernell and coworkers as follows[38]:

- Orojejunal (oral to the ligament of Treitz)
- Small bowel (excluding terminal 30 cm of ileum)
- Ileocecal (distal 30 cm of ileum with or without cecal involvement)
- Continuous ileocolic (continuous ileocolic involvement)
- Discontinuous ileocolic (both small and large bowel involvement, but without continuous inflammation in the ileocecal region)
- Colorectal (confined to the colon or rectum or both only)

Radiographic Features

As previously mentioned, Crohn's disease can occur anywhere in the alimentary tract. The disease tends to be segmental and asymmetric. Radiologic findings include skip lesions, contour defects, longitudinal ulcers, transverse fissures, eccentric involvement, pseudodiverticula, narrowing or stricture formation, pseudopolypoid changes that may be cobblestone-like, sinus tracts, and fistulas.[341]

A plain film of the abdomen may be quite useful in the early stages of Crohn's colitis. Although toxic megacolon is much less common in Crohn's disease than it is in ulcerative colitis, acute toxic dilatation may occur before any firm cicatrix has formed in the bowel wall (Figure 30-4).

Colon

The postevacuation film is most useful in identifying numerous discrete ulcers (Figure 30-5). Small ulcerations may combine to produce large, longitudinal ulcers (Figure 30-6), and when the longitudinal ulcers combine with transverse fissures, they produce the cobblestone appearance seen radiologically (Figure 30-7). Intramural fistulas can result from the coalescing of the numerous longitudinal ulcers, which in turn may produce a double-lumen appearance (Figure 30-8). Ulcerations may penetrate beyond the contour of the bowel and present as numerous long spicules or as sinus tracts (Figure 30-9). These deep fissures may be confused with diverticula, but with experience the physician should be readily able to differentiate them. If one examines the whole-mount specimen shown in Figure 30-42, one can appreciate how such a radiologic picture can evolve.

Although the standard barium enema examination has been routinely employed in the past for evaluating IBD, contemporary evidence suggests that the air-contrast technique is preferred. Radiologists have prided themselves on their ability to identify somewhat unusual radiographic features of IBD. These include mucosal bridging and aphthoid ulcers.[44,216,477,513] Although these findings are helpful in the evaluation of patients with IBD, their ready documentation by means of colonoscopy would diminish the value of the radiologic observation.

Superficial mucosal abnormalities are not uncommonly seen in the distal part of the ileum, and concern is often

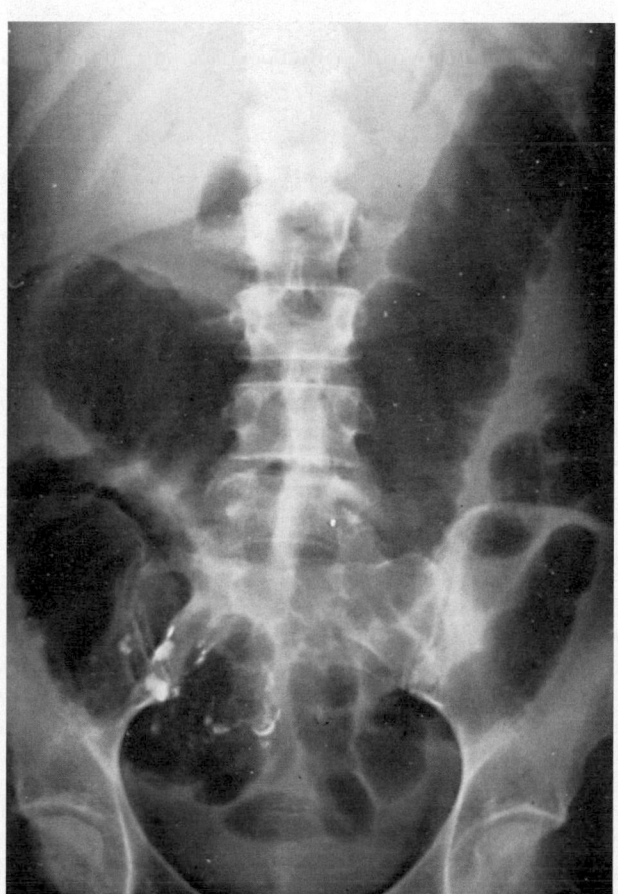

FIGURE 30-4. Crohn's colitis. This plain abdominal film demonstrates marked colonic dilatation. Toxic megacolon may be recognized during the initial attack, before fibrosis and thickening develop. (From Corman ML, Veidenheimer MC, Nugent FW, et al. *Diseases of the Anus, Rectum and Colon. Part II: Non-specific Inflammatory Bowel Disease.* New York, NY: Medcom; 1976.)

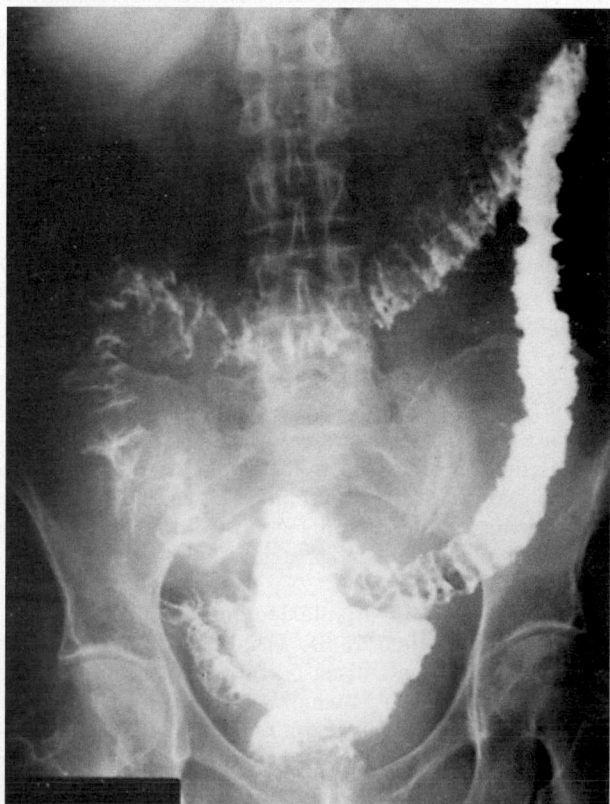

FIGURE 30-5. Crohn's colitis. Extensive loss of the normal mucosal pattern with multiple tiny marginal ulcers along the left colon border. Deeper ulcers are evident on the inferior margin of the distal transverse colon.

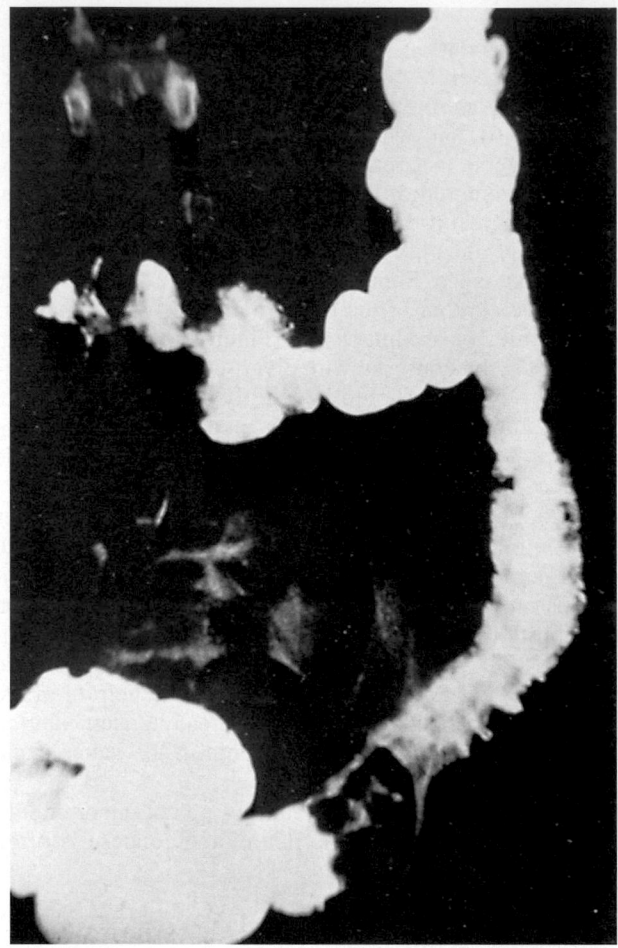

FIGURE 30-6. Crohn's colitis. Extensive longitudinal and transverse ulcers are evident in the descending and sigmoid colon. (From Corman ML, Veidenheimer MC, Nugent FW, et al. *Diseases of the Anus, Rectum and Colon. Part II: Non-specific Inflammatory Bowel Disease.* New York, NY: Medcom; 1976.)

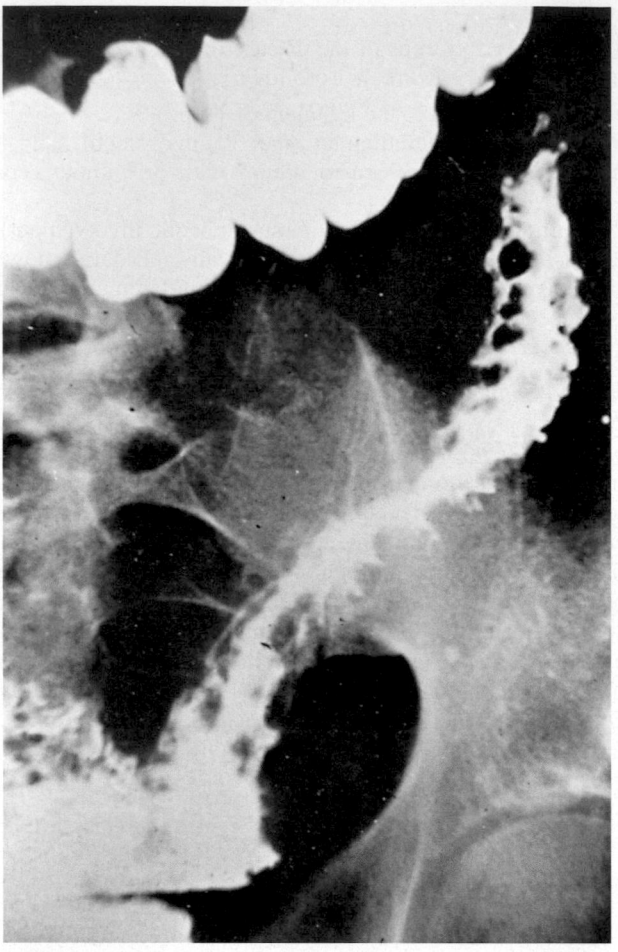

FIGURE 30-7. Crohn's colitis. Coarse cobblestoning of the left colon with intramural fistula traversing longitudinally along the bowel wall. (From Corman ML, Veidenheimer MC, Nugent FW, et al. *Diseases of the Anus, Rectum and Colon. Part II: Non-specific Inflammatory Bowel Disease.* New York, NY: Medcom; 1976.)

expressed as to the likelihood of such a patient developing clinically recognizable Crohn's disease. Ekberg and colleagues identified mucosal abnormalities in the distal ileum of 21 patients by means of air-contrast enemas.[131] From 4 to 7 years later, neither Crohn's disease nor any other progressive condition of the small bowel developed.

Figure 30-10 demonstrates a number of the classical changes that one may see in the radiographic appearance of Crohn's colitis. These include segmental distribution with sparing of the rectum, stenosis, thickening of the bowel wall, ulceration, and a suggestion of a double-lumen appearance.

Strictures are of variable lengths and may be quite extensive indeed (Figures 30-11 and 30-12). When a stricture occurs in Crohn's disease, it does not imply a malignant association, such as when it is seen in a patient with ulcerative colitis. However, individuals with Crohn's disease have been shown to have an increased risk for the development of malignancy (see Relationship to Carcinoma). Differential diagnosis between a Crohn's stricture and that of a carcinoma is usually not difficult. Close inspection often reveals that the bowel in adjacent areas is

ulcerated (Figure 30-13). Contrast this x-ray with that of Figure 30-14. Although a scirrhous carcinoma must always be considered in the differential diagnosis, the lack of associated ulceration or inflammatory changes elsewhere in the colon usually clarifies the dilemma. Still, one must be wary of the possibility (see Figure 30-12).

A most difficult problem is to differentiate radiographically Crohn's disease from tuberculosis (see Chapter 33). When the condition is confined to the ileocecal region, it is virtually impossible to distinguish between the two diseases.

Barium enema has been used to evaluate the *anal canal* in patients with Crohn's disease.[120] Although direct visual examination is more accurate, there are characteristic changes that may be identified by means of careful radiologic examination of the area. The hallmark of a radiologically normal anal canal is the presence of straight, smooth lines of barium between the folds, whereas an abnormal anal canal may show distortion of the folds, ulcers, fissures, sinus tracts, and fistulas.[120] However, if one requires the assistance of a radiologist to make the diagnosis of anal Crohn's disease, that physician must be considered diagnostically destitute.

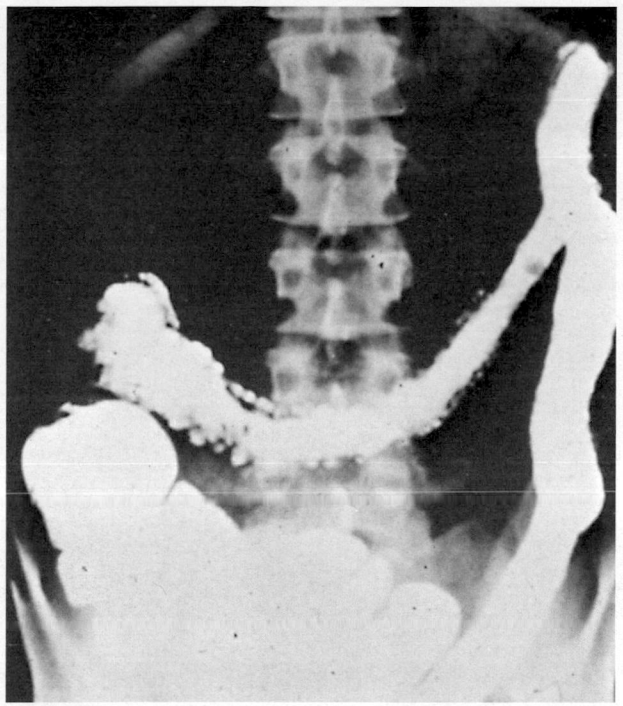

FIGURE 30-8. Crohn's colitis. Longitudinal intramural fistulas are evident in the proximal transverse colon and splenic flexure. (From Corman ML, Veidenheimer MC, Nugent FW, et al. *Diseases of the Anus, Rectum and Colon. Part II: Non-specific Inflammatory Bowel Disease.* New York, NY: Medcom; 1976.)

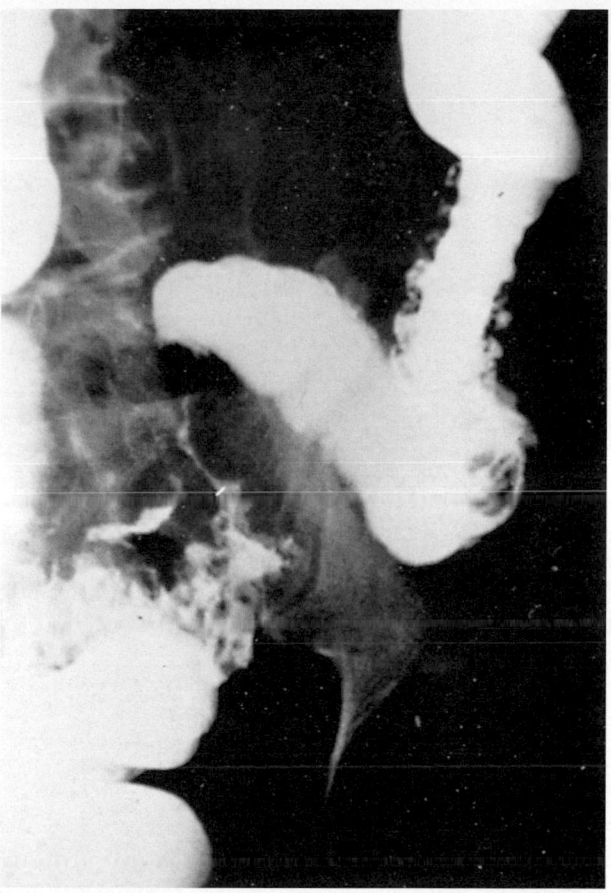

FIGURE 30-10. Crohn's colitis. Typical segmental involvement with a normal rectum, markedly stenotic lower sigmoid, relatively normal midsigmoid area, and then a further area of involvement of the upper sigmoid just distal to an uninvolved descending colon. Thickening of the bowel wall is seen in the upper sigmoid. (From Corman ML, Veidenheimer MC, Nugent FW, et al. *Diseases of the Anus, Rectum and Colon. Part II: Non-specific Inflammatory Bowel Disease.* New York, NY: Medcom; 1976.)

Small Bowel

Upper gastrointestinal and small bowel x-ray films are quite helpful for evaluating IBD in this area of the alimentary tract, especially because there is no truly adequate nonoperative endoscopic examination of the small intestine, except for the very distal ileum, putting aside capsule endoscopy. Radiologically, evaluation of the terminal

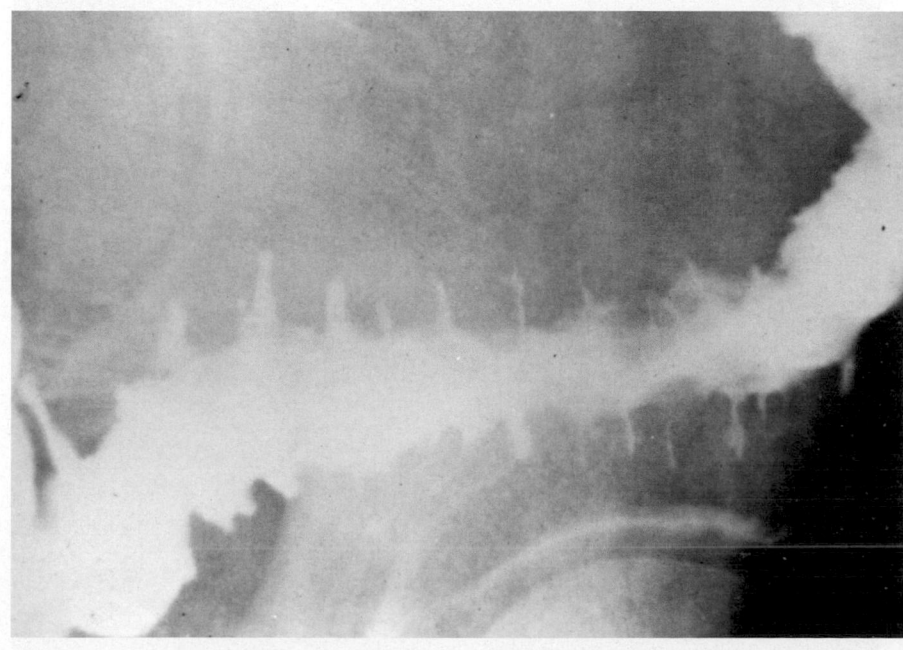

FIGURE 30-9. Crohn's colitis. Deep fissuring of the bowel wall in the sigmoid colon giving a thornlike appearance. (From Corman ML, Veidenheimer MC, Nugent FW, et al. *Diseases of the Anus, Rectum and Colon. Part II: Non-specific Inflammatory Bowel Disease.* New York, NY: Medcom; 1976.)

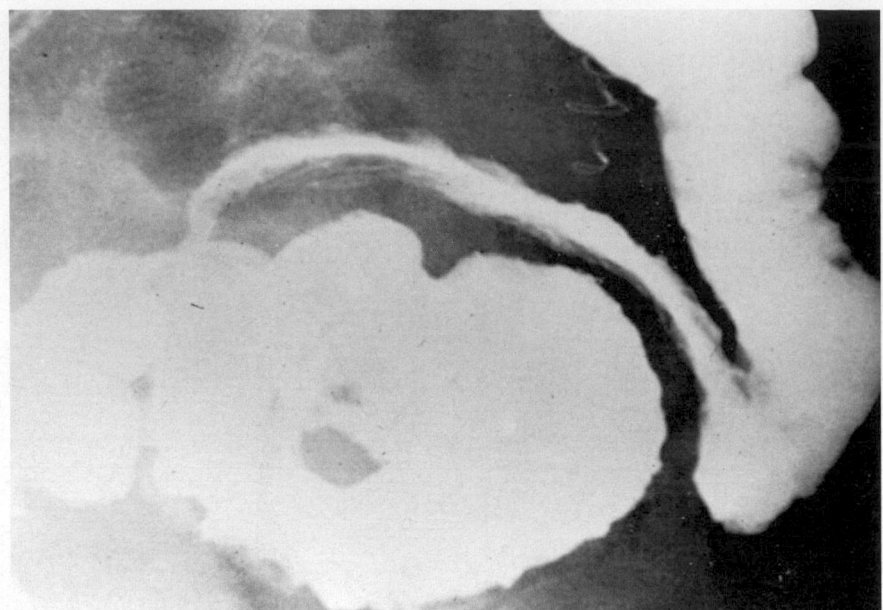

FIGURE 30-11. Crohn's colitis. Long sigmoid stricture with ulceration distally. (From Corman ML, Veidenheimer MC, Nugent FW, et al. *Diseases of the Anus, Rectum and Colon. Part II: Non-specific Inflammatory Bowel Disease.* New York, NY: Medcom; 1976.)

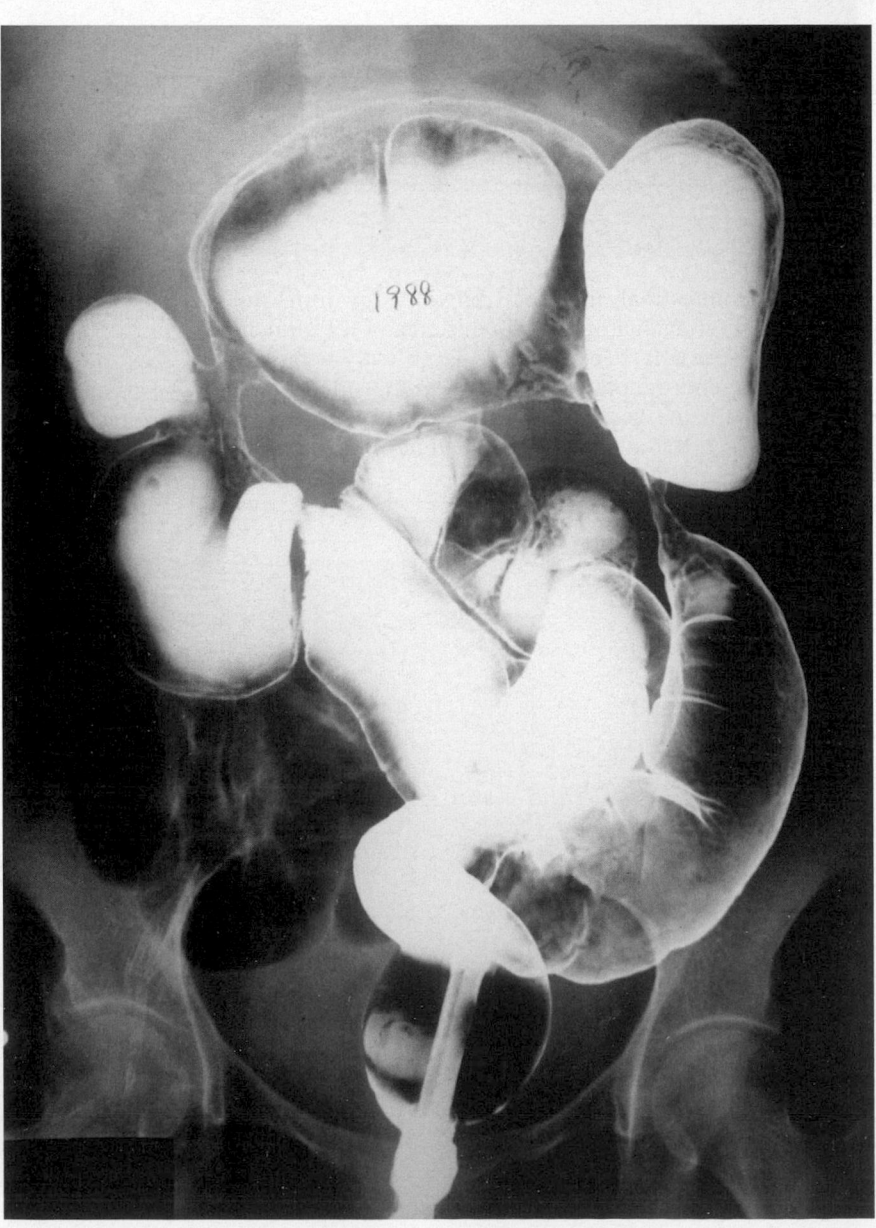

FIGURE 30-12. Air-contrast barium enema reveals multiple strictures in the colon in an individual with Crohn's disease. At the time of surgery, these all proved to be benign.

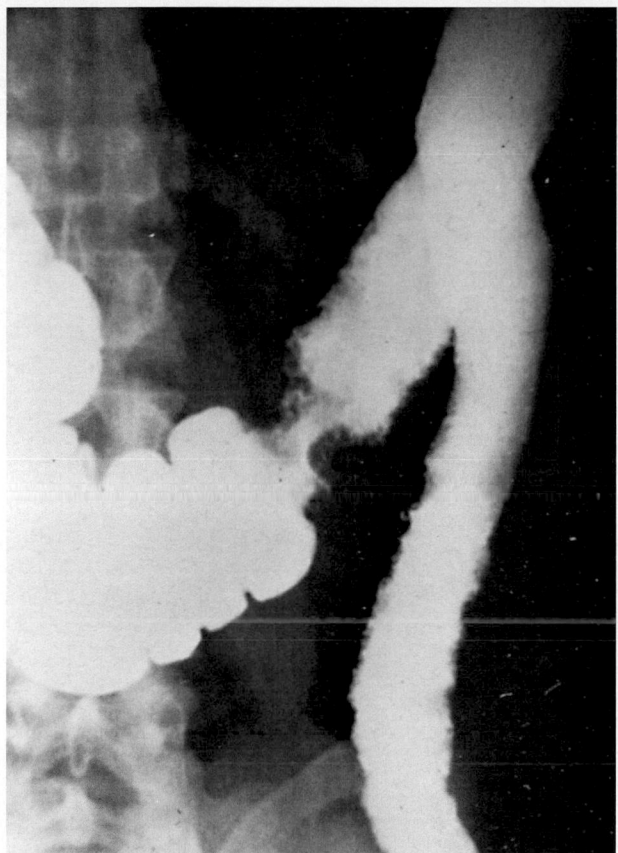

FIGURE 30-13. Crohn's colitis with transverse colon stricture, an "apple core" lesion suggestive of carcinoma. Note, however, that the distal bowel is ulcerated. (From Corman ML, Veidenheimer MC, Nugent FW, et al. *Diseases of the Anus, Rectum and Colon. Part II: Non-specific Inflammatory Bowel Disease.* New York, NY: Medcom; 1976.)

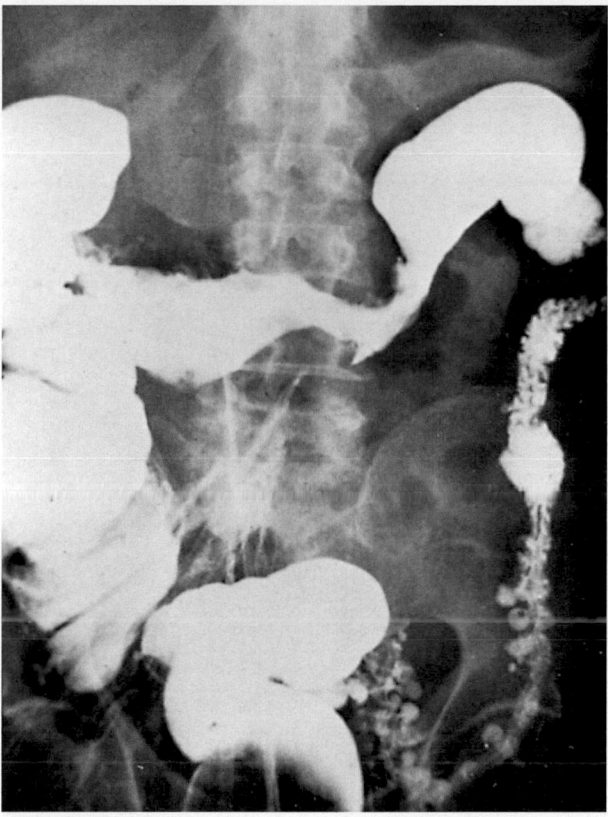

FIGURE 30-14. Scirrhous carcinoma of the transverse colon. Contrast the absence of adjacent mucosal abnormality with the previous figure. (From Corman ML, Veidenheimer MC, Nugent FW, et al. *Diseases of the Anus, Rectum and Colon. Part II: Non-specific Inflammatory Bowel Disease.* New York, NY: Medcom; 1976.)

ileum is best obtained by reflux on barium enema examination, but unfortunately, as many as 20% of patients will not demonstrate this phenomenon. Alternatively, a small bowel follow-through study or an enteroclysis with good spot films can be used.

Increasingly, CT enterography has become utilized for demonstrating luminal disease, extent of involvement, points of obstruction, and extraintestinal complications. This study will also show the degree of mural thickening, the presence of fistula, as well as sepsis/abscess. It may show the site of target organ involvement, such as duodenum, sigmoid, and ileocolic fistula. This serves as a guide to the endoscopist as well. In the case of ileosigmoid fistula, this may be confirmed endoscopically by the appearance of a granulomatous nodule, wherein the sigmoid and rectum are otherwise normal. This may, in the case of a rare entity, ileorectal fistula, have a bearing on the surgical strategy—such as the need for mobilization of the rectum when segmental rectal resection may be required. Crohn's disease of the terminal ileum has a characteristic appearance. Thickening of the bowel wall narrows the lumen, resulting in a degree of obstruction in some patients. This is the most frequent cause of abdominal pain in individuals with Crohn's disease. The radiologic appearance of the terminal ileum has been described as having a "string sign" (Figure 30-15). Involvement of the terminal ileum may be seen as an isolated finding or may be

associated with multiple diseased areas throughout the small intestine (Figure 30-16). In contrast to radiologic evaluation of the colon for Crohn's disease, it is virtually impossible to differentiate a benign from a malignant stricture in the small intestine (Figure 30-17). As with carcinoma of the small bowel in an individual without Crohn's disease, the prognosis is extremely poor.

Fistulous complications are frequently seen in patients with Crohn's disease. Communication between the ileum and colon is not uncommon (Figure 30-18), but other types of fistulas have been observed, including coloduodenal (Figures 30-19 and 30-20), and those to pelvic organs (Figure 30-21).

Ultrasound

Ultrasound examination is of quite limited value in patients with IBD because of the presence of considerable artifact associated with the loops of bowel. The presence of air or fluid in the intestine and adhesed loops may simulate a septic focus. That stated, Sonnenberg and colleagues performed a prospective clinical trial comparing 51 patients with Crohn's disease with 124 controlled subjects by means of grayscale ultrasound.[528] Diagnosis by ultrasound reflected primarily the thickening of the gastrointestinal wall itself, perceived as a characteristic "target" appearance. The study demonstrated that there were very few false negatives. The occasional false-positive phenomenon was usually attributed to the presence of a gastrointestinal tumor.

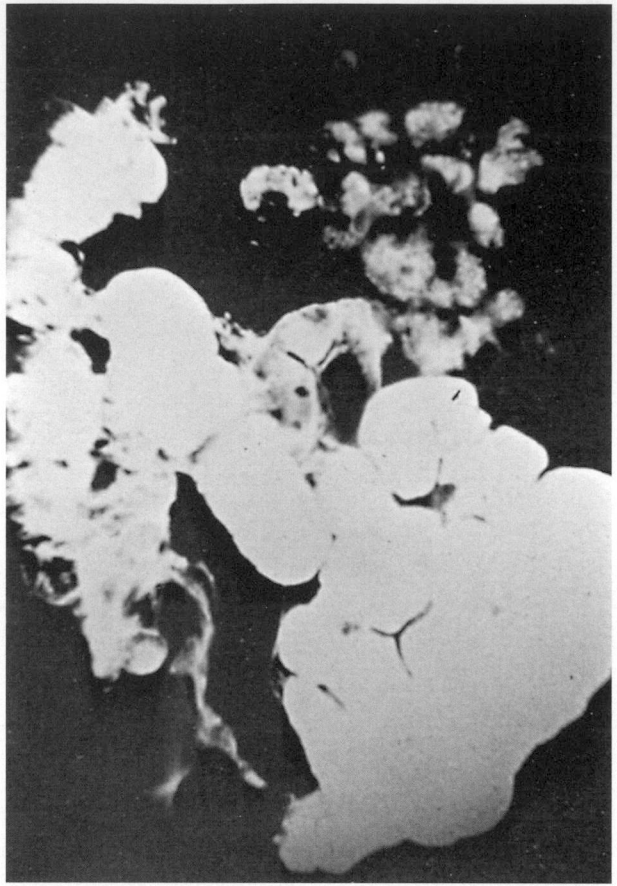

FIGURE 30-15. Distal ileal Crohn's disease. Edema and thickening of the bowel wall produce the characteristic "string sign." (From Corman ML, Veidenheimer MC, Nugent FW, et al. *Diseases of the Anus, Rectum and Colon. Part II: Non-specific Inflammatory Bowel Disease.* New York, NY: Medcom; 1976.)

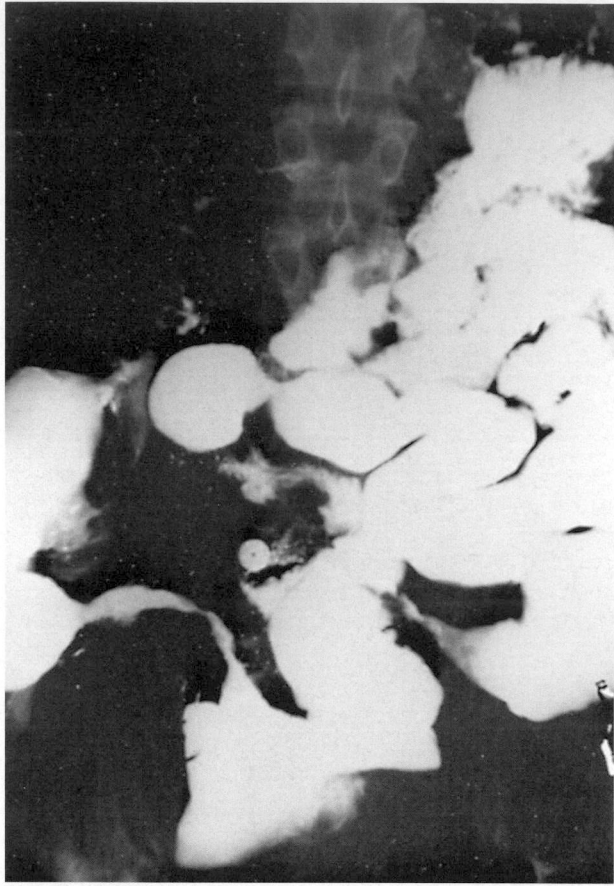

FIGURE 30-16. Small bowel Crohn's disease. Terminal ileal disease in addition to multiple skip areas. (From Corman ML, Veidenheimer MC, Nugent FW, et al. *Diseases of the Anus, Rectum and Colon. Part II: Non-specific Inflammatory Bowel Disease.* New York, NY: Medcom; 1976.)

van Outryve and coworkers studied transrectal ultrasound in individuals with Crohn's disease and in control subjects.[571] The authors observed that the procedure sharply delineates the rectal wall and may detect unsuspected abscesses and fistulas in the pararectal and para-anal tissues (see Chapters 5 and 7). Abdominal ultrasound may also allow for accurate measurement of mural thickness. In the case of multiple small bowel strictures, this may impact on surgical decision making. For example, one is more likely to favor resection of a stricture if the wall thickness is 9 mm or more. Strictureplasty, if performed under this circumstance, leads to early recurrence (see later).

Computed Tomography

Computed tomography (CT) is able to demonstrate thickening of the colon, nodularity, adenopathy, and intra-abdominal abscess (Figure 30-22). The presence of any fistula, especially an enterocutaneous communication, is often demonstrable by means of CT scan with oral or rectal contrast. In most cases, however, adequate evaluation of intra-abdominal pathology can be obtained by means of endoscopic examination and by standard contrast techniques.

Yousem and colleagues studied CT scans of 200 consecutive patients with Crohn's disease in order to determine the frequency and patterns of perirectal and perianal involvement.[609] They observed inflammation of fat planes (73%), bowel wall thickening (30%), fistulas or sinus tracts (22%), and abscesses (14%). Because more than one-third had abnormal CT manifestations below the symphysis pubis, the authors emphasize the importance of scanning sequences to the perineum in individuals with Crohn's disease.

Gore and colleagues attempted to provide the perspective of CT criteria in the evaluation of ulcerative, granulomatous and indeterminate colitis.[191] Unfortunately, features were often overlapping, and CT did not alter the original diagnosis in any patient.

Capsule Endoscopy

The application of capsule endoscopy for evaluating the small bowel has been discussed in Chapter 5. Several studies have been published that attest to its value in assessing the small bowel in individuals with Crohn's disease.[132,162,236] However, although it may be useful for identifying an occult source of bleeding, the reality is that the overwhelming majority of patients can have their disease identified by simpler, less expensive means. Furthermore, there is a real risk of precipitating a small bowel obstruction if the capsule cannot pass a strictured area. Still, in a limited number of individuals, capsule endoscopy may be a useful diagnostic tool for this condition.

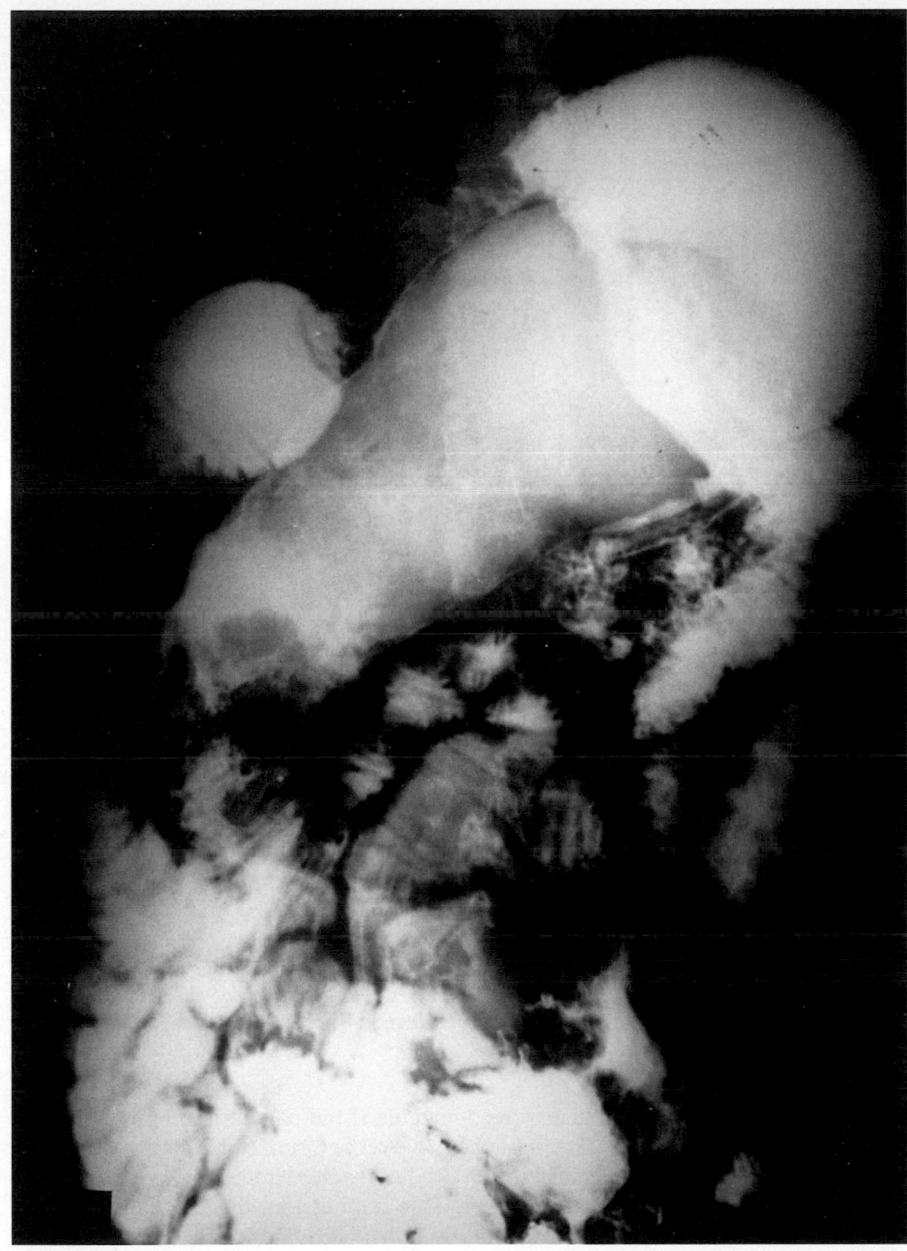

FIGURE 30-17. Small bowel series demonstrates proximal obstruction secondary to a stricture that proved to be malignant. Additional benign strictures from Crohn's disease are also evident on this radiologic study.

Angiography

Another method for identifying the site of small bowel bleeding in an individual with Crohn's disease has been described, that of the combined use of preoperative angiography and highly selective methylene blue injection.[441] It was felt that this technique may aid the surgeon in the preoperative and intraoperative localization of occult bleeding sites in this condition.

The Significance of Special Laboratory Studies

A number of specialized laboratory studies have been advised, primarily for evaluation of Crohn's disease. Some have suggested the use of an indium-labeled leukocyte scan to distinguish patients for whom medical therapy may be preferable from those who may be optimally treated by surgery.[518] For example, in active Crohn's disease, labeled leukocytes are excreted into the bowel lumen from the inflamed mucosa. Patients with positive scans, therefore, have higher values of indices of disease activity. In a study by Slaton and colleagues, a negative indium leukocyte scan suggested a fibrotic ileal stricture and the advisability of surgical intervention.[518] As an anatomic indicator of acute granulocytic infiltration of the intestinal mucosa and submucosa, Nelson and colleagues found that this scan had a 97% rate of sensitivity and a 100% specificity.[376] The study may be best applied in individuals with fulminant disease, especially those who cannot safely be put through the rigors of endoscopy or barium contrast radiologic evaluation.

Brignola and colleagues studied various laboratory indices to determine whether any had predictive value for recurrence of Crohn's disease.[58] There was a significant correlation with recurrence and alteration of acid

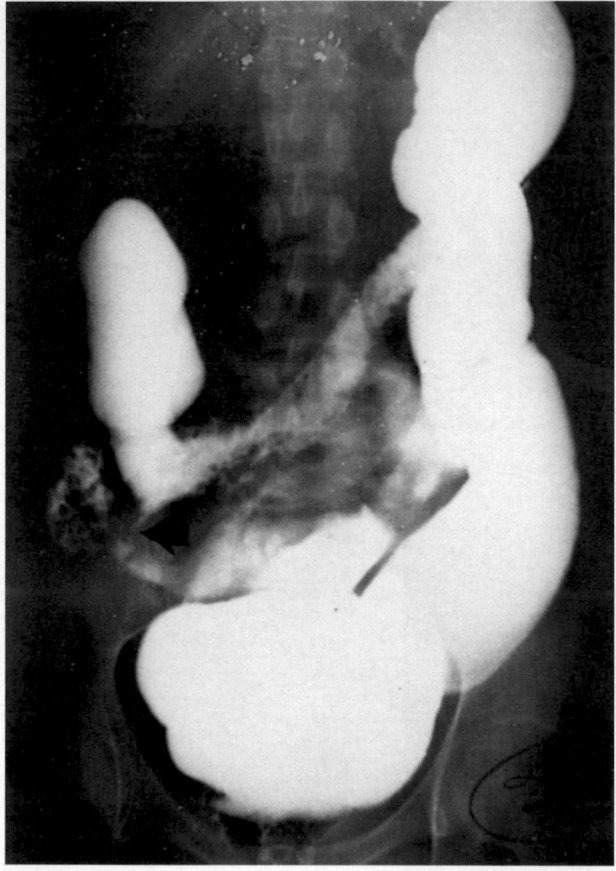

FIGURE 30-18. Ileocolic fistula (*arrow*). Extensive transverse colon disease with fistulous communication to the ileum. (From Corman ML, Veidenheimer MC, Nugent FW, et al. *Diseases of the Anus, Rectum and Colon. Part II: Non-specific Inflammatory Bowel Disease.* New York, NY: Medcom; 1976.)

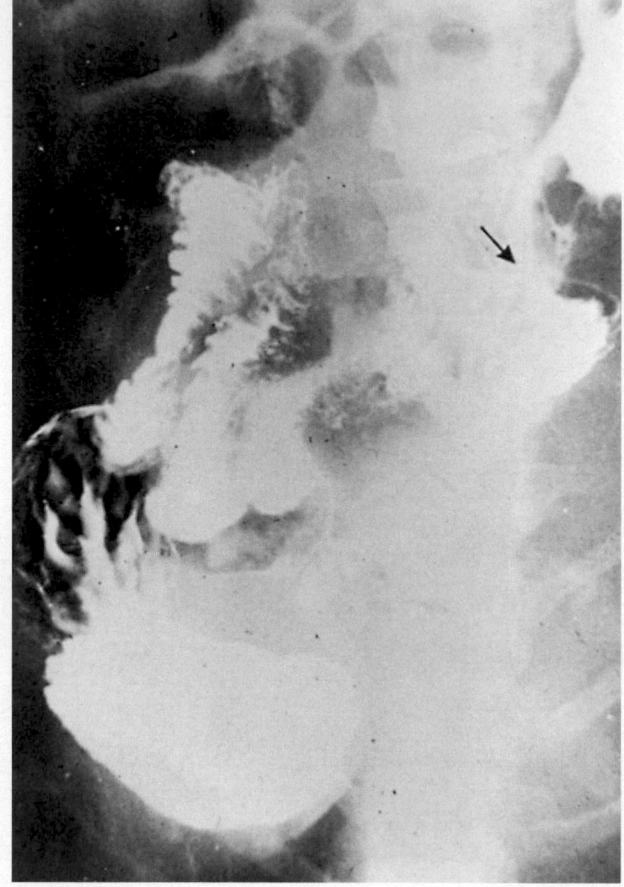

FIGURE 30-19. An upper gastrointestinal series demonstrates fistula (*arrow*) between the duodenum and the ascending colon. (From Corman ML, Veidenheimer MC, Nugent FW, et al. *Diseases of the Anus, Rectum and Colon. Part II: Non-specific Inflammatory Bowel Disease.* New York, NY: Medcom; 1976.)

1-glycoprotein, 2-globulin, and erythrocyte sedimentation rate in comparison with the patients who remained in remission. Also, it has been demonstrated that patients with Crohn's disease requiring operative treatment often have a severe peripheral lymphopenia.[233] Mahida and colleagues have been able to detect interleukin-6 in seven out of eight peripheral and mesenteric samples from patients with Crohn's disease.[331] Heimann and Aufses showed that individuals who developed recurrences had significantly lower preoperative lymphocyte counts than those who were free of disease 3 years following resection.[232] As more information becomes available, it is possible that these and other studies will help the physician and surgeon determine which patients are at increased risk and perhaps influence the timing and the type of therapy.

Pathology

Macroscopic Appearance

Crohn's disease may have protean clinical and pathologic manifestations. The condition can be confined to the colon alone or may involve only the anal canal. Fistulas, segmental involvement, rectal sparing, perianal disease, and abscess formation are all characteristic of granulomatous colitis. Some of the earliest changes in the serosal aspect of the small intestine involved by Crohn's disease may be

immediately recognizable if the patient is submitted to surgery. The intraoperative recognition of Crohn's disease can also be inferred by the corkscrew appearance of vessels on the serosal aspect. This implies that this segment has been subjected to intermittent obstruction. The serosal vessels elongate as the bowel distends proximal to a stricture, and

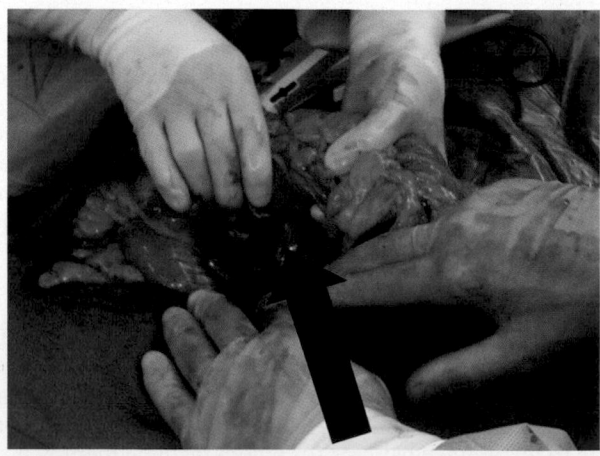

FIGURE 30-20. Coloduodenal fistula. At operation, fistula between the two structures is clearly demonstrated (*arrow*).

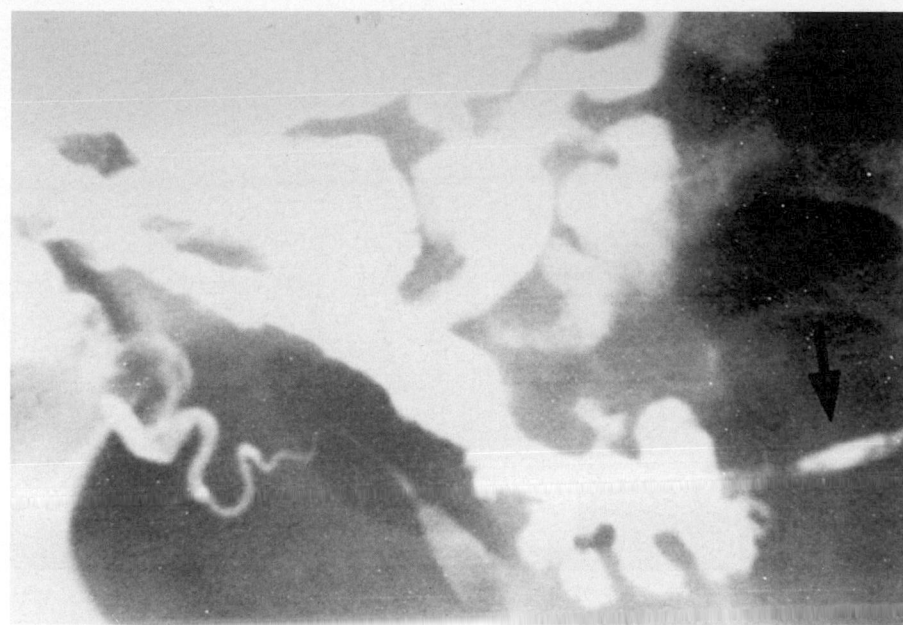

FIGURE 30-21. A fistula between the colon and the fallopian tube is an unusual complication of Crohn's colitis. Note that a second fistula passes into an abscess and out to the skin (*arrow*). (From Corman ML, Veidenheimer MC, Nugent FW, et al. *Diseases of the Anus, Rectum and Colon. Part II: Non-specific Inflammatory Bowel Disease.* New York, NY: Medcom; 1976.)

when the intermittent dilatation contracts, these stretched vessels assume a corkscrew appearance. Other points suggesting involved small bowel are mesenteric marginal thickening, which corresponds to the longitudinal ulcers of Crohn's disease in the small bowel.

Subserosal extension of fat around the surface of the bowel ("fat wrapping") and a prominent vascular pattern in the serosa are characteristic of the disease (Figure 30-23). The serosal surface may be granular and bleed easily on any intraoperative abrasion. It has been demonstrated that fat wrapping correlates best with transmural inflammation and represents part of the connective tissue changes that accompany intestinal Crohn's disease.[504]

The disease frequently affects the bowel in a segmental fashion. This may produce extensive skip areas (Figures 30-24 and 30-25), limited involvement to an area of the bowel (Figure 30-26), or even a focal, isolated stricture (Figure 30-27).

Classically, Crohn's colitis involves the intestine in an asymmetric fashion. Areas of the bowel may demonstrate disease on the mucosal aspect with sparing of adjacent sites, leaving islands of somewhat edematous but otherwise non-ulcerated mucosa (Figures 30-28 through 30-30). Ulceration in an irregular fashion with large areas of uninvolved mucosa interspersed between broad, twisting lesions is quite

(text continues on page 1314)

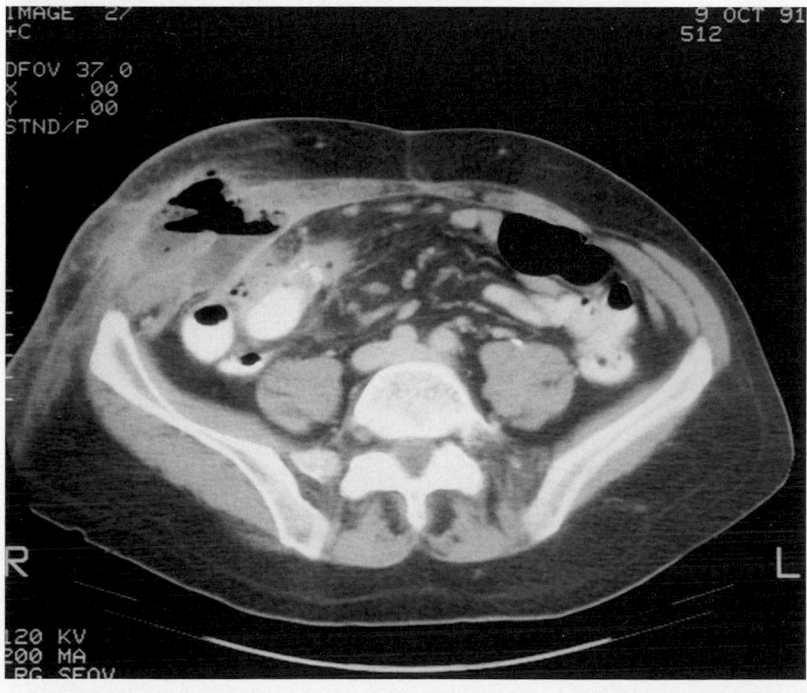

FIGURE 30-22. Computed tomography demonstrates abdominal wall abscess on the right side. This was secondary to a perforating ileocolic Crohn's inflammation.

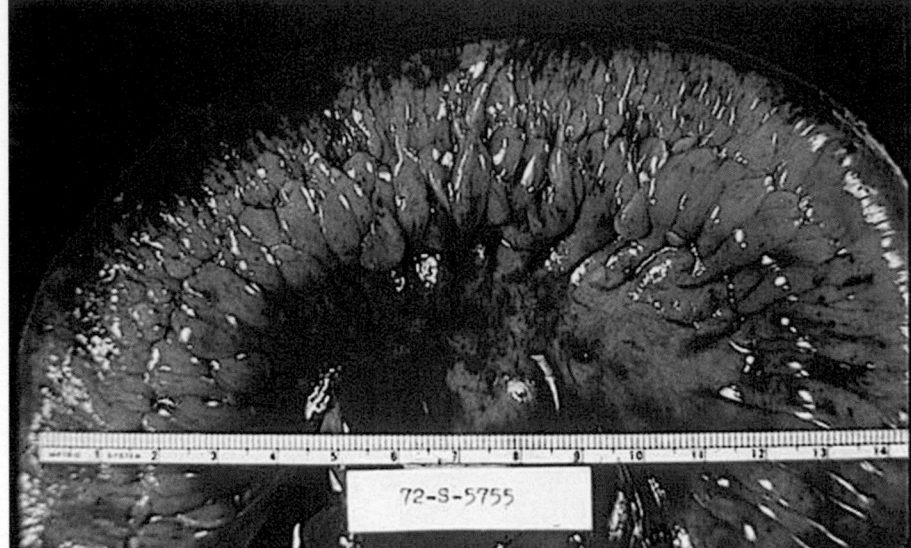

FIGURE 30-23. Ileal Crohn's disease. Subserosal inflammation and "fat wrapping" are evident. (From Corman ML, Veidenheimer MC, Nugent FW, et al. *Diseases of the Anus, Rectum and Colon. Part II: Non-specific Inflammatory Bowel Disease*. New York, NY: Medcom; 1976.)

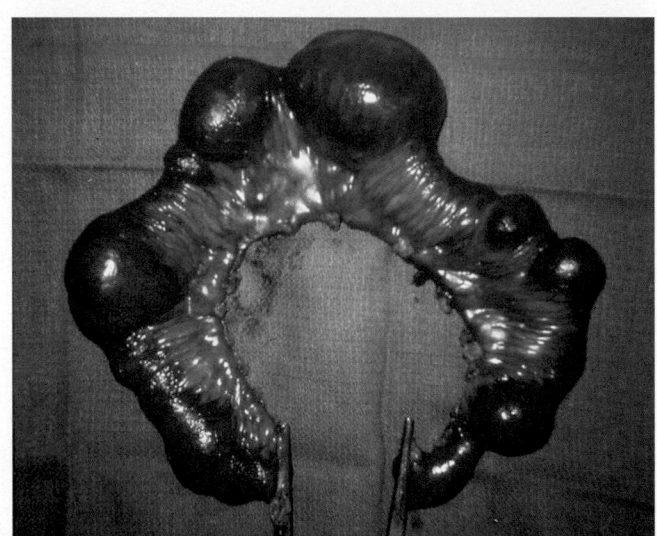

FIGURE 30-24. Crohn's disease. Segmental constrictions of small bowel with dilated bowel between each stenotic area. (From Corman ML, Veidenheimer MC, Nugent FW, et al. *Diseases of the Anus, Rectum and Colon. Part II: Non-specific Inflammatory Bowel Disease*. New York, NY: Medcom; 1976.)

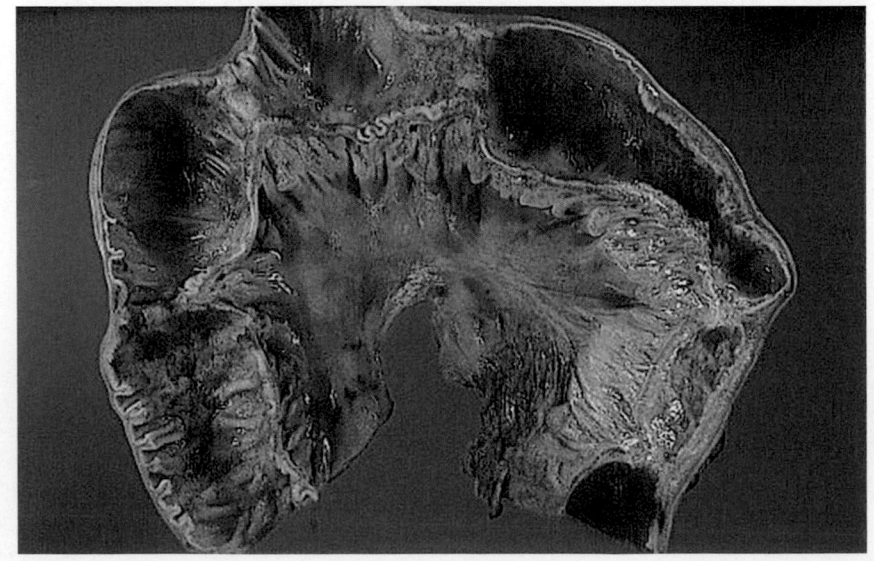

FIGURE 30-25. Crohn's disease. This opened specimen from Figure 30-24 reveals the segmental nature of the disease. Thickening of the mesentery is a prominent feature. (From Corman ML, Veidenheimer MC, Nugent FW, et al. *Diseases of the Anus, Rectum and Colon. Part II: Non-specific Inflammatory Bowel Disease*. New York, NY: Medcom; 1976.)

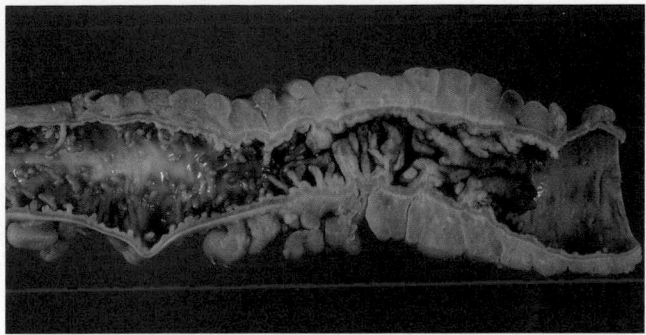

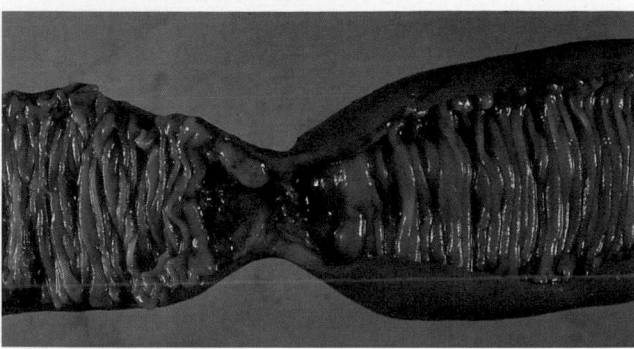

FIGURE 30-26. Crohn's colitis. Segmental involvement of the sigmoid with marked narrowing of the midportion. Thickening of all layers of bowel is evident. At each end, the bowel is less involved and more distensible. (From Corman ML, Veidenheimer MC, Nugent FW, et al. *Diseases of the Anus, Rectum and Colon. Part II: Non-specific Inflammatory Bowel Disease.* New York, NY: Medcom; 1976.)

FIGURE 30-27. Crohn's disease. Short segment of constriction. Note edematous mucosa and evidence of bowel dilatation on the right side, produced by partial obstruction. (From Corman ML, Veidenheimer MC, Nugent FW, et al. *Diseases of the Anus, Rectum and Colon. Part II: Non-specific Inflammatory Bowel Disease.* New York, NY: Medcom; 1976.)

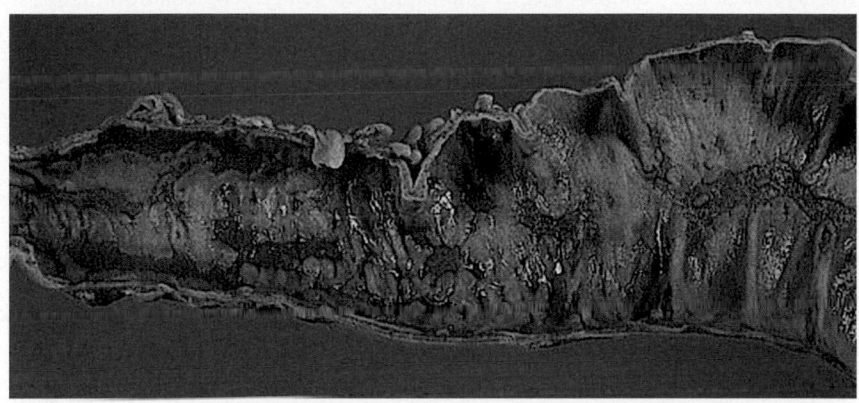

FIGURE 30-28. Crohn's colitis. Irregularly ulcerated mucosa with sparing between ulcers. (From Corman ML, Veidenheimer MC, Nugent FW, et al. *Diseases of the Anus, Rectum and Colon. Part II: Non-specific Inflammatory Bowel Disease.* New York, NY: Medcom; 1976.)

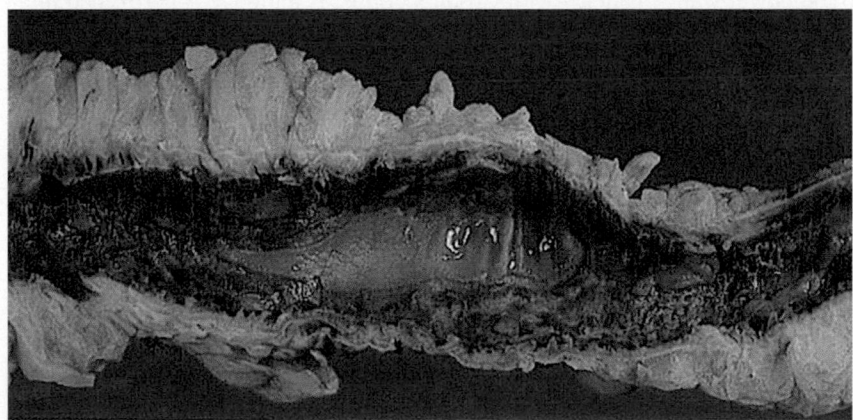

FIGURE 30-29. Crohn's colitis. An island of normal mucosa lies in the middle of the specimen, with largely denuded, ulcerated mucosa on either side. (From Corman ML, Veidenheimer MC, Nugent FW, et al. *Diseases of the Anus, Rectum and Colon. Part II: Non-specific Inflammatory Bowel Disease.* New York, NY: Medcom; 1976.)

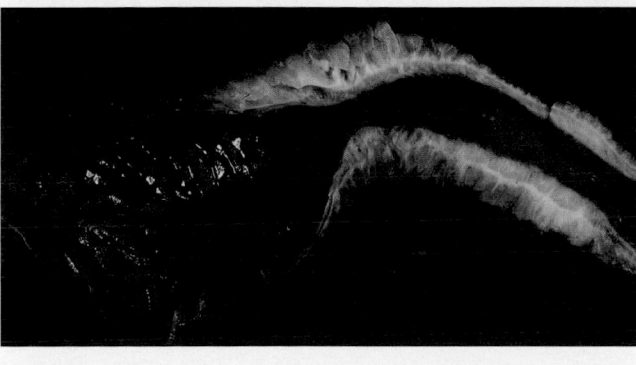

FIGURE 30-30. Crohn's colitis. Severe stenosis on the right and ulceration surrounded by normal mucosa on the left, a typical feature of this disease. (From Corman ML, Veidenheimer MC, Nugent FW, et al. *Diseases of the Anus, Rectum and Colon. Part II: Non-specific Inflammatory Bowel Disease.* New York, NY: Medcom; 1976.)

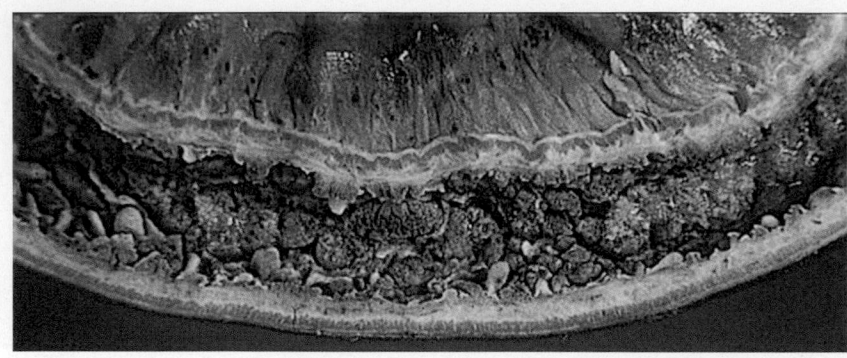

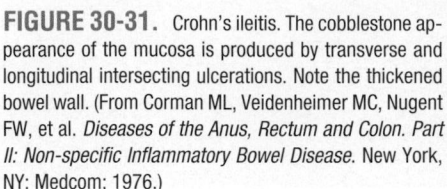

FIGURE 30-31. Crohn's ileitis. The cobblestone appearance of the mucosa is produced by transverse and longitudinal intersecting ulcerations. Note the thickened bowel wall. (From Corman ML, Veidenheimer MC, Nugent FW, et al. *Diseases of the Anus, Rectum and Colon. Part II: Non-specific Inflammatory Bowel Disease.* New York, NY: Medcom; 1976.)

characteristic. The relative sparing between ulcers is not seen in ulcerative colitis. Another characteristic feature of the macroscopic appearance of Crohn's disease is the thickening of the bowel wall. Involvement through all the layers, along with the cobblestone appearance of the mucosa, has been described as "stones in a running brook" (Figure 30-31).

Crohn's colitis frequently involves the colon and ileum in continuity. Conversely, cecal ulceration can be seen with primarily ileal disease (Figure 30-32). Occasionally, the ileal disease may terminate abruptly at the ileocecal valve, sparing the large bowel (Figure 30-33). Thickening of the bowel wall may produce sufficient narrowing to precipitate intestinal obstruction or to impede the passage of swallowed seeds or nuts (Figure 30-34). Gallstone ileus has even been reported to produce obstruction at a point of stenosis caused by Crohn's disease.[499]

A common manifestation of Crohn's disease is fistula formation. Fistulas may occur into any adjacent organ, such as the small or large bowel, bladder, vagina, uterus, ureter, or skin. Burrowing of the fissures deep into the bowel wall predisposes to fistula formation. Fistulas occur more commonly in the mesocolic aspect of the bowel than on the antimesocolic border (Figure 30-35).

Although nodal adenopathy is frequently present, the location of enlarged, paraileal lymph nodes is a reasonably accurate way of identifying the proximal extent of disease without the need of verifying this by entering the bowel.

Occasionally, diffuse mucosal disease may produce a pseudopolypoid pattern similar to that of chronic ulcerative colitis. Giant pseudopolyps may actually mimic neoplasms endoscopically and radiographically. The condition is most likely the result of fusion of numerous fingerlike pseudopolyps.[207] A number of reports and reviews of this manifestation have been published.[113,207,263]

Histologic Appearance

The three primary histopathologic findings in patients with Crohn's colitis are transmural inflammation and fibrosis, granulomas, and narrow, deeply penetrating ulcers or "fissures" (Figure 30-36). The mucosal inflammation of Crohn's disease differs from that of ulcerative colitis in that typically there are fewer crypt abscesses, there is less congestion, and there is better preservation of the goblet cell population (Figure 30-37).

Granulomas may occur in any part of the bowel wall and are usually identified in approximately two-thirds of all patients with Crohn's colitis. If a biopsy is performed in an attempt to differentiate between the two inflammatory conditions, the material should be obtained from a noninflamed area if possible (Figure 30-38). A granuloma, albeit a foreign body type, may actually be seen even with ulcerative colitis in an area of acute inflammation. Multiple biopsy specimens are suggested because submucosal lesions tend to be very small (microgranulomas).[289] The microscopic appearance of

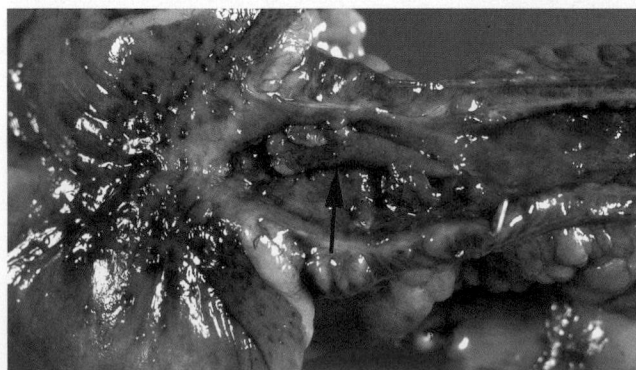

FIGURE 30-32. Crohn's disease. Cecal ulceration and ileal disease with involvement of the ileocecal valve. Note the large ileal mucosal tag (*arrow*). (From Corman ML, Veidenheimer MC, Nugent FW, et al. *Diseases of the Anus, Rectum and Colon. Part II: Non-specific Inflammatory Bowel Disease.* New York, NY: Medcom; 1976.)

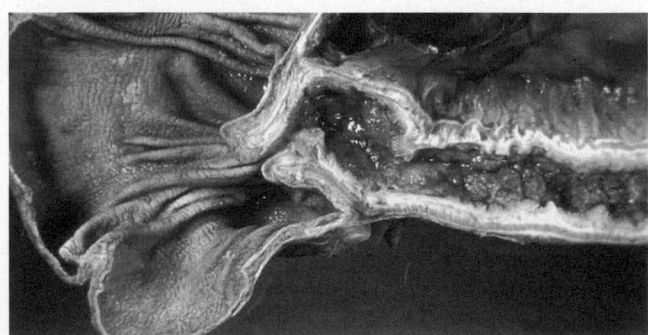

FIGURE 30-33. Crohn's ileitis. Ileal involvement with sparing of the large bowel. Note the abrupt cessation of the disease at the ileocecal valve. (From Corman ML, Veidenheimer MC, Nugent FW, et al. *Diseases of the Anus, Rectum and Colon. Part II: Non-specific Inflammatory Bowel Disease.* New York, NY: Medcom; 1976.)

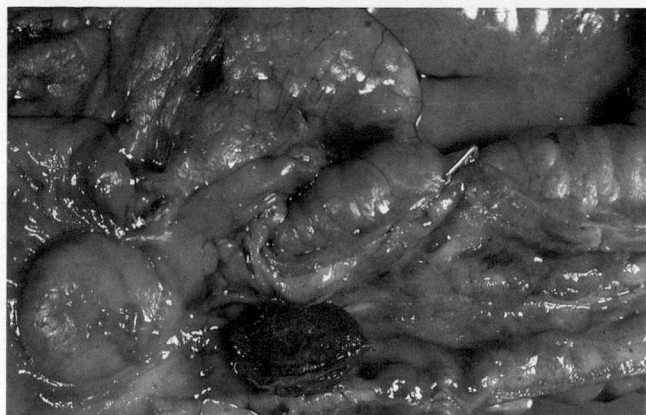

FIGURE 30-34. Crohn's ileitis. This unusual specimen demonstrates a prune pit trapped in a narrowed segment of terminal ileum, precipitating intestinal obstruction. (From Corman ML, Veidenheimer MC, Nugent FW, et al. *Diseases of the Anus, Rectum and Colon. Part II: Non-specific Inflammatory Bowel Disease.* New York, NY: Medcom; 1976.)

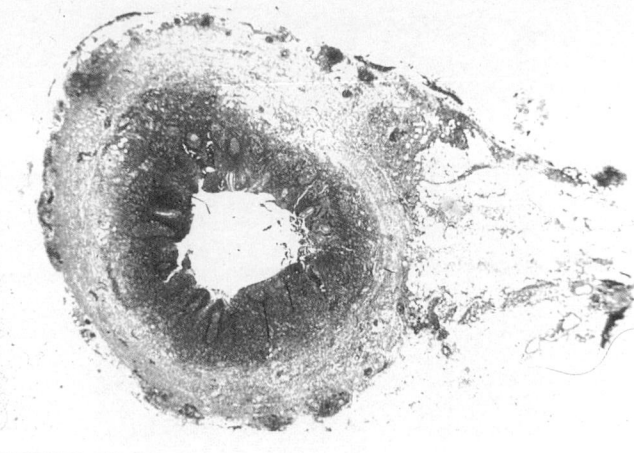

FIGURE 30-36. Crohn's disease of the appendix. Cross section demonstrates inflammatory changes at all levels: mucosa, muscularis, and serosa. (Original magnification × 80; from Corman ML, Veidenheimer MC, Nugent FW, et al. *Diseases of the Anus, Rectum and Colon. Part II: Non-specific Inflammatory Bowel Disease.* New York, NY: Medcom; 1976.)

the granuloma is not diagnostic, and the possibility of an infectious agent should always be considered (Figure 30-39). Granulomas can also occur in the liver (Figure 30-40) and in the omentum (Figure 30-41) as well as in other sites.

Narrow, deeply penetrating ulcers or fissures are the third characteristic feature of Crohn's disease. The fissures may penetrate through the inner circular layer of the muscularis and are visible on the radiographs after a barium enema as spicules. A sinus tract present in the fat adjacent to the bowel wall indicates that one of the fissures has penetrated through the wall (Figure 30-42). When this occurs, a sinus may burrow into another organ to produce a fistula.

Information about the pathology of IBD has been further gleaned by means of *electron microscopy*. Early epithelial changes can be identified using this modality in areas that appear to be uninvolved. These include necrosis of individual columnar epithelial cells; budding of the tips of microvilli; thickening, shortening, irregularity, and fusion of intestinal

villi; numerous Paneth's cells; hyperplasia of goblet cells; and augmented mucous secretion.[271] Other studies such as tissue-enzyme analysis, jejunal-surface pH, and differences in sodium flux and mucosal potential imply that the disease often is far more extensive than is recognized by other, more conventional means, and certainly much more extensive than is usually apparent at the time of surgery.

Another observation is the increased secretion of mucus by the bowel in Crohn's disease as compared with decreased colonic mucus in ulcerative colitis. The decrease may be explained by destruction of the epithelial cells.[271] A number of biochemical changes have also been observed.

Extraintestinal Manifestations

For convenience and in order to avoid duplication, I have elected to place the discussion of extraintestinal manifestations in this chapter. Moreover, because so many of the

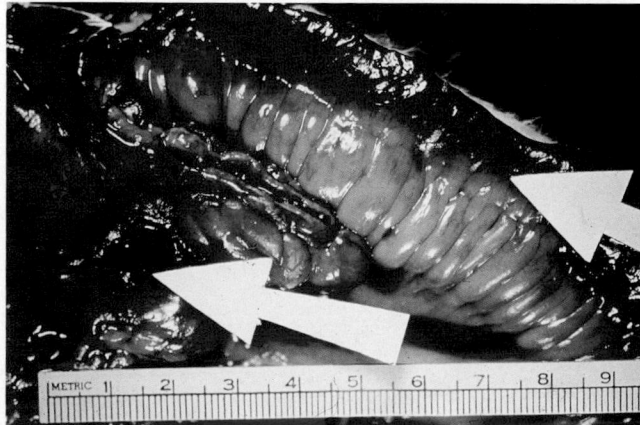

FIGURE 30-35. Crohn's disease. A fistula (*arrow*) has passed through the mesocolon and into an adjacent structure at some distance from the point of origin in the bowel. The characteristic small bowel fat wrapping is marked at right (*arrowhead*). (From Corman ML, Veidenheimer MC, Nugent FW, et al. *Diseases of the Anus, Rectum and Colon. Part II: Non-specific Inflammatory Bowel Disease.* New York, NY: Medcom; 1976.)

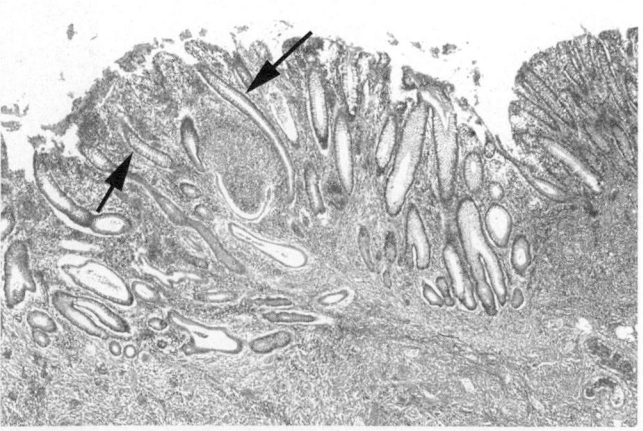

FIGURE 30-37. Crohn's disease. Note the crypts (*arrows*) on either side of the crypt abscess contain an almost normal complement of goblet cells. (Original magnification × 80; from Corman ML, Veidenheimer MC, Nugent FW, et al. *Diseases of the Anus, Rectum and Colon. Part II: Non-specific Inflammatory Bowel Disease.* New York, NY: Medcom; 1976.)

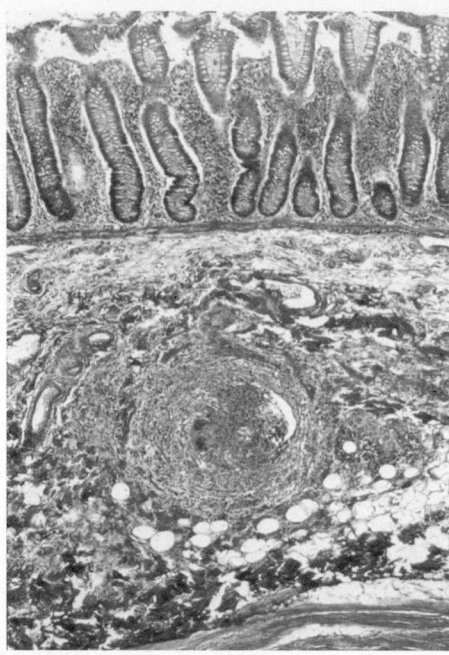

FIGURE 30-38. Crohn's disease. Submucosal granuloma. Note that the overlying mucosa has inflammatory cells in the lamina propria but no crypt abscess or ulceration. (Original magnification × 80; from Corman ML, Veidenheimer MC, Nugent FW, et al. *Diseases of the Anus, Rectum and Colon. Part II: Non-specific Inflammatory Bowel Disease.* New York, NY: Medcom; 1976.)

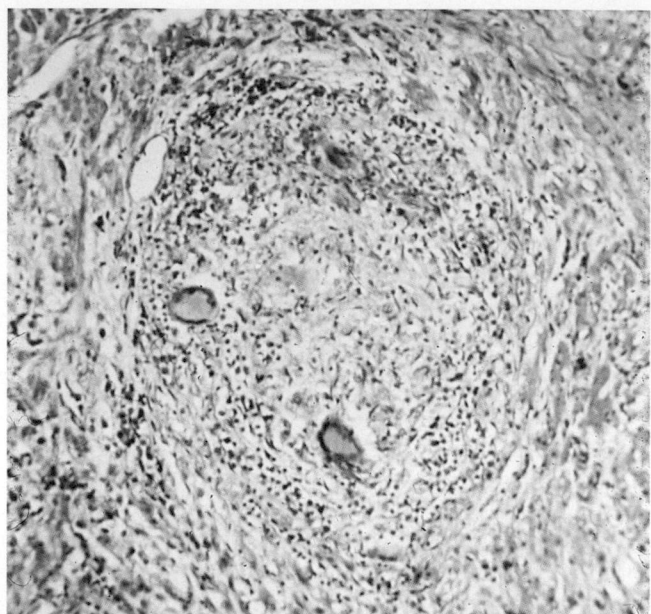

FIGURE 30-39. Crohn's disease. Granuloma within muscularis propria. (Original magnification × 280; from Corman ML, Veidenheimer MC, Nugent FW, et al. *Diseases of the Anus, Rectum and Colon. Part II: Non-specific Inflammatory Bowel Disease.* New York, NY: Medcom; 1976.)

manifestations in other areas of the body are exclusively seen in Crohn's disease, the discussion is placed here, although many such problems may be seen in both ulcerative colitis and Crohn's disease. Increasing evidence supports the statement that inflammatory disease of the intestine is a systemic problem rather than one localized to the small or large bowel. In a population-based study from Sweden of 1,274 patients with ulcerative colitis, the overall prevalence of extracolonic diagnoses was 21%.[363] As discussed in Chapter 29, many etiologic concepts have been considered, but regardless of the sequence of pathologic changes in the colon, there is little

question about the presence of related events, at times profound, in distant areas of the body. The joints, skin, liver, kidneys, eyes, mouth, blood, nervous system, and, of course, other areas of the alimentary tract may be sites of lesions that, at least in the extraintestinal manifestations, often seem dependent on the presence of diseased bowel. So broad indeed is the spectrum of Crohn's disease that specialists in dentistry, otorhinolaryngology, ophthalmology, and dermatology must be prepared to recognize its manifestations.

Oral Manifestations
Oral lesions were first identified in Crohn's disease by Dudeney and Todd in 1969.[121] Since then, a number of papers

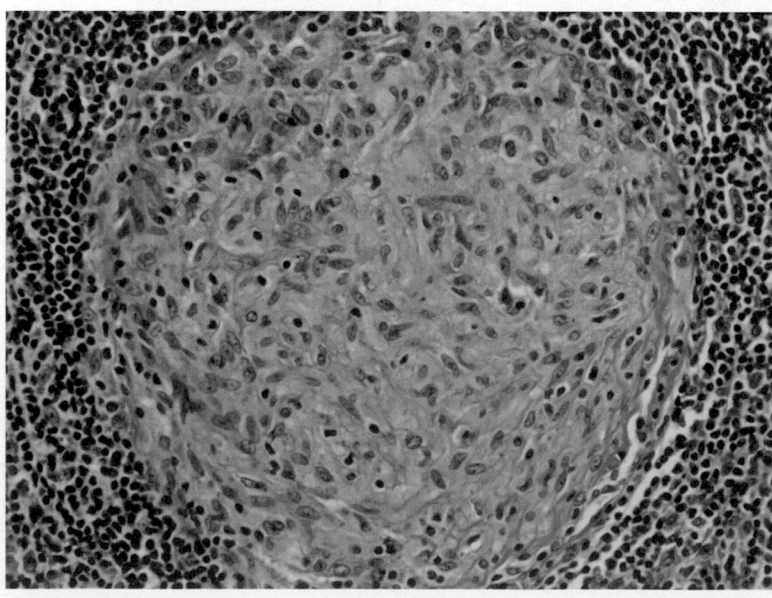

FIGURE 30-40. Crohn's disease. Granuloma of the liver in a patient with Crohn's colitis. (Original magnification × 260.)

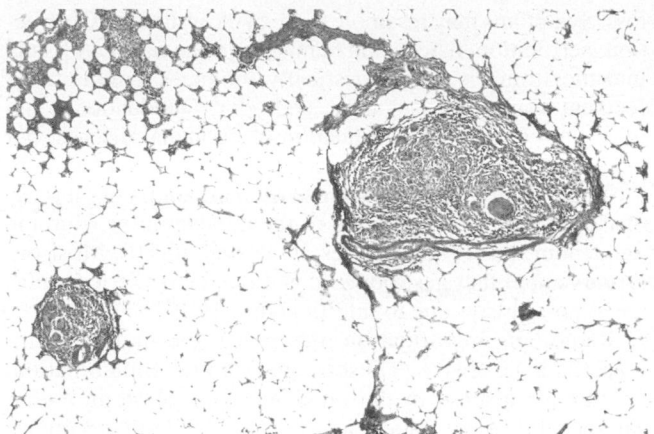

FIGURE 30-41. Crohn's colitis. Two omental granulomas are seen in a patient with Crohn's colitis. (Original magnification × 00, from Corman ML, Veidenheimer MC, Nugent FW, et al. *Diseases of the Anus, Rectum and Colon. Part II: Non-specific Inflammatory Bowel Disease.* New York, NY: Medcom; 1976.)

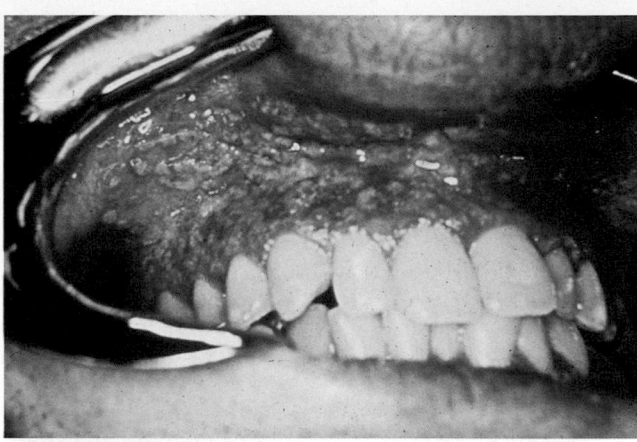

FIGURE 30-43. Pyostomatitis vegetans. Involvement of the gingival mucosa by papillary projections. (From Corman ML, Veidenheimer MC, Nugent FW, et al. *Diseases of the Anus, Rectum and Colon. Part II: Non-specific Inflammatory Bowel Disease.* New York, NY: Medcom; 1976.)

have been published on the subject.[42,47,521,574] Inflammatory changes in the mouth may even be the initial site of involvement.[87] Basu and Asquith reviewed the oral manifestations of IBD, describing a number of lesions.[33] These included recurrent aphthous ulcers, pyoderma gangrenosum, pyostomatitis vegetans, hemorrhagic ulceration, glossitis, macroglossia, and moniliasis. The authors reported that the incidence is not as uncommon as one might expect, with up to 20% having been described as having oral lesions. The most frequently affected areas and their respective appearances are the buccal mucosa (a cobblestone pattern), the vestibule (linear, hyperplastic folds), and the lips (diffusely swollen and indurated).[43]

Aphthous ulcers usually parallel the course or activity of the IBD: the more active the disease, the more likely one is to develop this complication. Biopsy usually shows a chronic inflammatory reaction.

Pyostomatitis vegetans is an unusual manifestation of IBD. Papillary projections of mucous membrane can be seen separated by small areas of ulceration (Figure 30-43). Biopsy

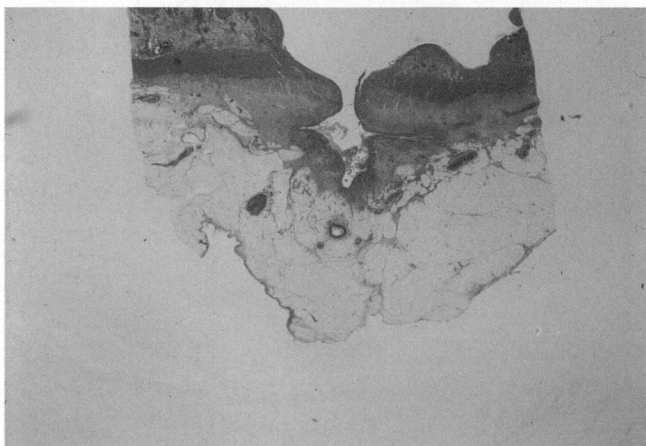

FIGURE 30-42. Crohn's disease: a whole-mount specimen demonstrates a fissure extending through the colon wall and into the pericolonic fat. This is the origin of a fistula. (From Corman ML, Veidenheimer MC, Nugent FW, et al. *Diseases of the Anus, Rectum and Colon. Part II: Non-specific Inflammatory Bowel Disease.* New York, NY: Medcom; 1976.)

may reveal suprabasal separation of the oral epithelium and infiltration with eosinophils.

The recognition of the specific oral granuloma is important because it may be the first manifestation of Crohn's disease.[521] Scully and colleagues reported 19 patients with clinical evidence of oral Crohn's disease but no intestinal symptoms.[498] More than one-third were demonstrated either on rectal biopsy or by contrast gastrointestinal x-ray films to have IBD, even in the absence of symptoms.

Treatment

Because the lesions are resistant to local therapy, general measures for soothing the oral discomfort are advised. The symptoms and clinical findings of oral problems are often ameliorated with appropriate treatment of the intestinal disease.

Esophageal Involvement

Patients with Crohn's disease of the esophagus will present with symptoms not unlike those associated with other lesions of that organ, such as carcinoma. Substernal discomfort, dysphagia, epigastric pain, weight loss, nausea, and vomiting are all part of the clinical spectrum. Other gastrointestinal symptoms are usually due to the presence of disease elsewhere in the alimentary tract.[126,174,231] It must be remembered that dysphagia and the demonstration of an esophageal ulcer or esophagitis in a patient with known Crohn's disease can be due to reflux esophagitis, certain drugs or corrosive agents, pressure from a nasogastric tube, infectious agents, sarcoidosis, or Behçet's disease.[380] In point of fact, many published reports of esophageal Crohn's disease cannot be supported by critical review.

Physical examination is usually unrewarding with respect to esophageal involvement. Diagnosis is usually made by a high index of suspicion and radiologic investigation, which obviously would include a barium swallow (Figure 30-44). This study may reveal thickened mucosal folds, multiple ulcerations, or, most commonly, a stricture. This last finding makes differentiation from carcinoma quite difficult, except that the presence of disease elsewhere or the relatively young age of the patient should lead one to suspect an inflammatory process.

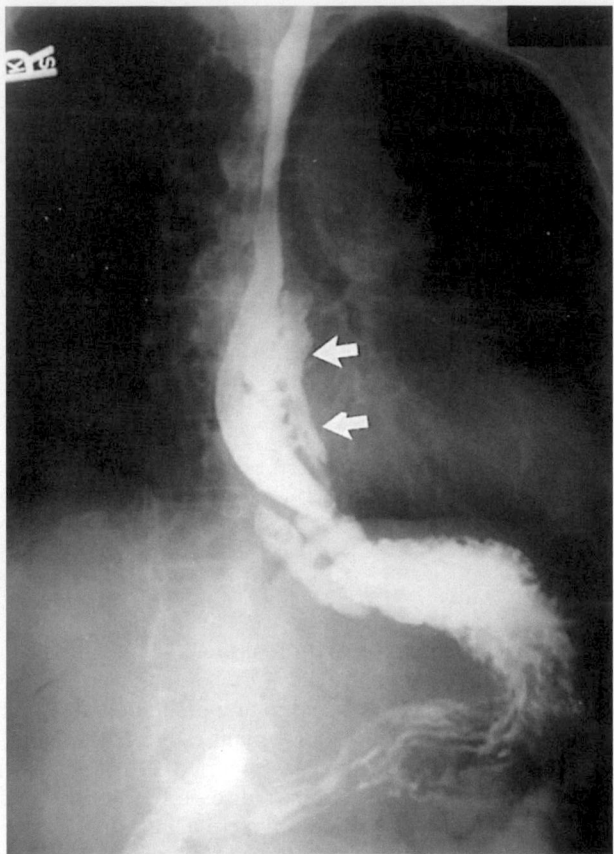

FIGURE 30-44. Esophageal Crohn's disease in patient with known, extensive small bowel involvement. Large ulcerating lesion involving the distal third of the esophagus extending to the gastroesophageal junction, with possible involvement of the cardia. There are irregular superior and inferior margins and a suggestion of two intramural tracts or double-lumen appearance (*arrows*).

Endoscopic examination will usually reveal hyperemia with possibly either an ulcerated mucosa or the presence of an inflammatory stricture. Biopsies usually show an inflammatory reaction, but the absence of granulomata does not exclude the diagnosis of Crohn's disease.[126]

Treatment usually consists of the standard medical management appropriate for Crohn's disease of the small or large bowel (see Chapter 29 and Medical Management). Resection is rarely indicated.

Gastroduodenal Crohn's Disease

Crohn's disease involving the stomach and duodenum may not be as rare as originally suspected. Since the original description in 1937 by Gottlieb and Alpert of the condition in the duodenum, a number of cases have been reported.[192] In 1981, Korelitz and colleagues performed random endoscopic biopsies of the stomach and duodenal mucosa in patients with Crohn's disease, frequently demonstrating the presence of microscopic alterations consistent with this inflammatory process in the upper gastrointestinal tract.[282] Clinically, evident IBD of the gastroduodenal area is believed to occur in approximately 2% or 3% of all patients with Crohn's disease. The condition can occur without involvement elsewhere in the gastrointestinal tract, but this is extremely uncommon.

Patients usually present with epigastric abdominal symptoms exacerbated by eating—nausea, vomiting, and weight loss. Symptoms may resemble those of ulcer disease. Obstruction, perforation, fistula, and hemorrhage can occur. A fistula into the stomach characteristically produces symptoms of feculent vomiting, eructation, and odor. Duodenocolic fistula is a recognized complication of duodenal disease, but in evaluation of patients with this finding, it is important to ascertain whether the fistula arose from inflammatory disease of the intestinal tract outside of the duodenum or from the duodenum, itself (see Figures 30-19 and 30-20). Most observers agree that gastroenteric and duodenoenteric fistulas are almost always due to intestinal disease.

Radiologic investigation may reveal the findings summarized by Cohen.[91] These include antral inflammation, contiguous disease in the duodenum, cobblestone mucosal appearance with thickened folds, reduced distensibility or stricture, and ulceration (Figure 30-45). Barium enema examination is the preferred study for identifying a fistula between the upper gastrointestinal tract and the colon.

Endoscopic examination may reveal ulceration, cobblestoning, or stricture. As with esophageal disease, the absence of granulomata does not necessarily mean that the patient does not have Crohn's. Nugent and Roy found granulomas in 37 of 76 individuals (49%).[385]

Treatment usually consists of antacids and proton pump inhibitors or H_2 receptor blockers (an antiulcer program), the medical regimens discussed later, hyperalimentation, and possibly surgical intervention. The primary indications for operation are the presence of a fistula and obstruction (see later). If hemorrhage cannot be controlled by medical means, either resectional surgery or oversewing the bleeding

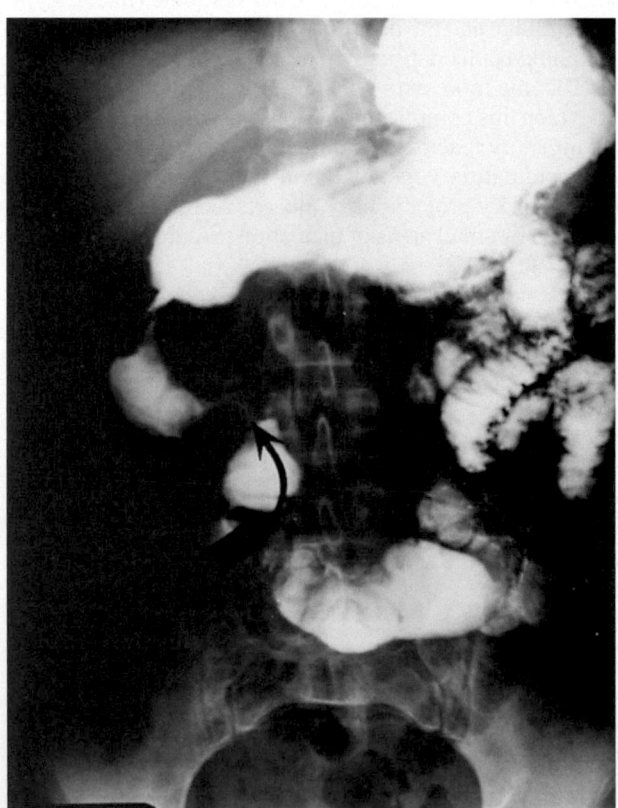

FIGURE 30-45. Duodenal Crohn's disease. This film from an upper GI series demonstrates stricture of the second portion of the duodenum with a fistula from the third portion to the small bowel (*arrow*).

point is the treatment of choice. Usually, however, surgery for primary gastroduodenal Crohn's disease can be avoided.

Management of Duodenal Stricture

The most commonly performed operative procedure for duodenal Crohn's disease is gastrojejunostomy, but complications such as bile reflux gastritis, stomal ulceration, blind loop syndrome, and the potential need for a vagotomy are real concerns. Strictureplasty has also been applied for duodenal disease, but in the findings of the Birmingham, England, group, it is associated with a high incidence of postoperative complications, the need for reoperative surgery, and the likelihood of restricture.[601] However, our group undertook duodenal strictureplasty on 13 patients and found that it is a safe and effective operation that should be considered when technically feasible.[596]

A number of cases and reviews have been published on the evaluation and management of the condition as it affects this area.[93,100,140,164,255,470,592] Nugent and colleagues reported 18 patients from the Lahey Clinic who were relieved of obstruction by means of gastrojejunostomy.[384] This was their preferred treatment for those with this complication. The authors did not advise vagotomy because of the risk of diarrhea and the fact that there was no difference in results between the vagotomized and nonvagotomized groups. A later report from the same institution involved 25 patients who required operation.[371] That study revealed that one-third who underwent bypass required reoperation, usually for marginal ulceration or for gastroduodenal obstruction. Although the authors did not feel that the addition of vagotomy protected against the subsequent development of marginal ulceration, they recommend in their latest report that a vagotomy be performed. Shepherd and Alexander-Williams have lent additional support to the concept of vagus nerve interruption when they reported a patient who developed a stomal ulcer 8 weeks following gastroenterostomy without vagotomy.[505]

Management of Gastric and Duodenal Fistulas

When a fistula develops as a consequence of intestinal disease, simple closure of the stomach or duodenum is all that is usually required, along with resection of the involved bowel segment. Gastric fistulas are always due to disease in the intestine. Treatment of the gastric opening is wedge excision. Occasionally, the opening in the duodenum may occur in an area that is difficult to close, such as adjacent to the pancreas. In this situation and when a large defect is created, an omental or jejunal patch, or the creation of a duodenojejunostomy may be necessary. Lee and Schraut reported one death due to a duodenal leakage in 11 patients with fistulas.[300] Greenstein and colleagues noted only nine instances of gastric fistula in a review of 1,480 individuals with Crohn's disease.[200]

Results

Ross and associates reviewed the long-term results of surgery for duodenal Crohn's disease that had been initially reported by Farmer and colleagues at our institution.[140,457] Of the 11 patients, 7 required a total of 10 further operations; the mean follow-up was approximately 14 years. Indications for subsequent surgery included marginal ulceration, recurrence producing obstruction at the enteroenterostomy, and duodenal fistula. Eight of the 11 also required surgery for Crohn's disease elsewhere in the intestinal tract. The authors concluded that bypass surgery alone was unsatisfactory in the long term and suggested that vagotomy be added at the

time of operation. Functional results were felt to be better, particularly if reoperative surgery were done in an expeditious and timely manner.

The Lahey Clinic experience now comprises 89 patients.[385] Their investigators conclude that irrespective of medical or surgical treatment, duodenal Crohn's disease follows a more benign course than when it affects the small bowel or colon.

Pancreatic Manifestations

Pancreatitis or pancreatic insufficiency has occasionally been reported with IBD, but this had been felt to be coincidental. One must be aware, however, of the risk of pancreatitis that may be associated with the administration of mercaptopurine (Purinethol). Seyrig and colleagues identified six patients who were thought to have a nonfortuitous association.[500] They noted the following, possibly important, clinical distinctions:

- Abdominal pain was absent or moderate and probably due to bowel involvement.
- Pancreatic calcifications were absent.
- Those patients with pancreatic insufficiency had essentially normal pancreatograms.
- More information will be necessary before one can establish with certainty whether pancreatic disease is truly an extraintestinal manifestation of IBD.

Hepatobiliary Disease

Liver function studies and liver biopsy often demonstrate abnormal results in both ulcerative colitis and Crohn's disease patients. Cohen and associates performed a prospective study of liver function in 50 consecutive patients with regional enteritis.[90] Thirty percent had abnormal results, most commonly an elevation of the serum alkaline phosphatase, but none had significant liver disease. Fifteen patients of the 19 who underwent liver biopsy had evidence of chronic pericholangitis. Others reported an even higher associated incidence of liver abnormalities.[103,118] The reasons for the association between hepatobiliary disease and IBD are not known, but a number of studies have postulated that recurrent cholangitis is due to a portal bacteremia from the interrupted intestinal mucosa, in addition to a probable genetic predisposition.[83] Hepatoportal venous gas has been seen in patients with known Crohn's disease.[12]

Gallbladder

Cholelithiasis has been reported in up to one-third of patients with IBD, especially in those with Crohn's ileitis.[90] The explanation for this association is believed to involve the enterohepatic circulation. Disease or resection of the terminal ileum leads to loss or malabsorption of bile acids. Because the solubility of cholesterol depends on bile acids, excessive loss may precipitate this substance. This, in turn, may result in stone formation. Another explanation may be the colonization of the terminal ileum by anaerobic bacteria that deconjugate the bile acids to less well-absorbed substances. It is not clear, however, that there is a higher incidence of gallstones in patients with Crohn's disease than in individuals with ulcerative colitis. Lorusso and colleagues demonstrated an increased risk of gallstones in both conditions, but it was highest in those with Crohn's disease involving the distal ileum.[326] Because of the high prevalence of cholelithiasis in the population, gallbladder imaging has been recommended preoperatively and in the follow-up of IBD patients.[290]

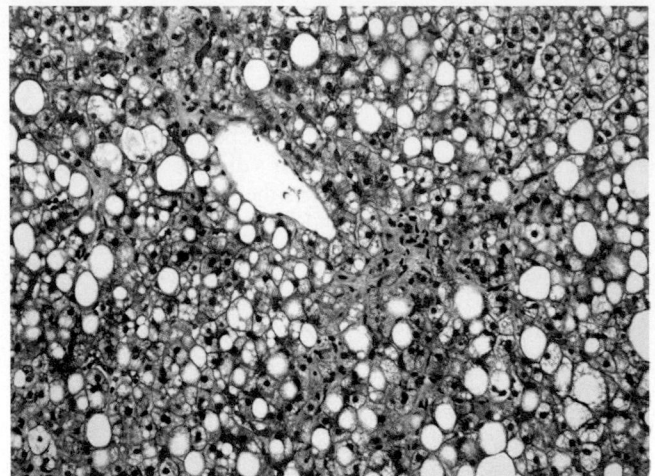

FIGURE 30-46. Fatty degeneration of the liver. Note the fat globules in the liver parenchyma. (Original magnification × 260, Trichrome stain.)

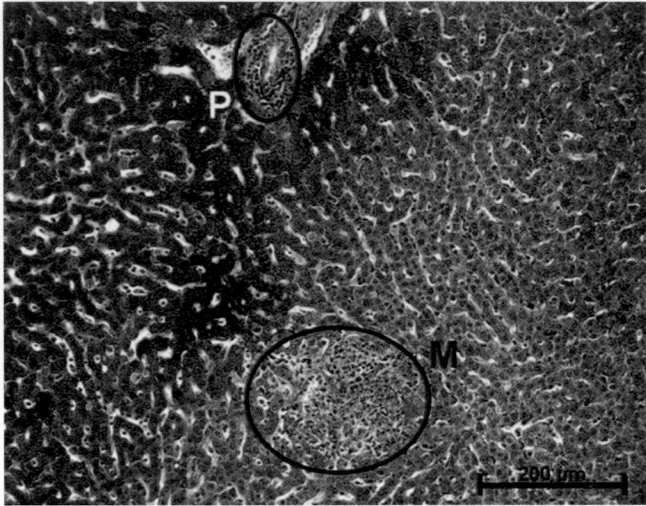

FIGURE 30-47. Pericholangitis. An inflammatory infiltrate within the portal areas surrounds the bile ducts and may result in cirrhosis through a process of progressive fibrosis. Section of the liver, showing microgranuloma (M) as well as pericholangitis (P) (Original magnification × 260; courtesy of Tufts OpenCourseWare, Tufts University.)

A different perspective was expressed by Chew and colleagues.[82] They retrospectively studied 134 of their patients who had undergone ileocolic resection for Crohn's disease by means of a questionnaire, using a control group matched for age and gender. There was no significant difference between the groups with respect to prevalence of cholecystectomy. However, those who had more than 30 cm of ileum removed were more likely to have undergone a cholecystectomy. The investigators concluded that synchronous prophylactic cholecystectomy with ileocolic resection cannot be justified based on their data.[82]

Fatty Degeneration

Fatty degeneration is probably the most frequently encountered microscopic abnormality (Figure 30-46). The incidence has been reported to be as high as 80% and to be due to the relatively poor nutritional state of many colitic patients.[83] Occasionally, a granuloma may be seen (see Figure 30-47). Treatment is directed toward correction of the malnutrition.

Pericholangitis

Another common histologic manifestation of liver disease is pericholangitis (Figure 30-47). A more accurate term is *portal triaditis* because of involvement of bile ductules, portal venules, lymphatics, and hepatic parenchyma.[83] The condition may present with jaundice, abdominal pain, fever, and pruritus. Many patients, however, are asymptomatic. Bacterial infection and an autoimmune process have been implicated as possible causative factors. There is no specific treatment for this condition.

Hepatitis

Chronic active hepatitis occurs in only 1% of patients with IBD. Conversely, the incidence of IBD in patients with chronic active hepatitis varies from 4% to 30%.[83] Patients have been reported to improve following removal of diseased bowel.

Sclerosing Cholangitis

One of the most serious, albeit rare, consequences of IBD that occurs as a complication of both ulcerative colitis and Crohn's disease is primary sclerosing cholangitis. Olsson and associates diagnosed this condition in 3.7% of indi-

viduals with ulcerative colitis.[391] LaRusso and colleagues reported that 70% of their patients with primary sclerosing cholangitis had IBD.[295] Broomé and coworkers determined in their evaluation of 76 patients with primary sclerosing cholangitis that histologic changes within the bowel itself may be observed and may actually precede development of clinical symptoms by as much as 7 years.[60] The importance of identifying such individuals cannot be overestimated. It has been suggested that even the preclinical manifestations of IBD may subject that individual to an increased risk for the development of malignancy.

Primary sclerosing cholangitis has been much more common in patients with ulcerative colitis than in those with Crohn's disease. The cause is unknown, but toxins, infectious agents, altered immunity, and a genetic predisposition have been suggested.[295] To establish this diagnosis, there must be no prior history of biliary surgery or gallstones, no diffuse involvement of the extrahepatic biliary ducts, and the absence of subsequent development of cholangiocarcinoma.[576] Symptoms include right upper quadrant abdominal pain, vomiting, jaundice, and pruritus. Laboratory studies demonstrate the usual changes suggestive of an obstructive jaundice. Cholangiogram reveals a strictured bile duct (Figure 30-48). In contrast to other extraintestinal manifestations of IBD, when the sclerosing cholangitis has been established, removal of the diseased colon *does not reverse the condition*. The condition is a progressive disease that leads to liver damage and, eventually, liver failure. Liver transplant is the only known cure for primary sclerosing cholangitis, but transplant is typically reserved only for those with severe liver disease. Researchers continue looking into treatments to slow or reverse bile duct damage caused by primary sclerosing cholangitis. But until an effective protocol is found, treatment is directed toward reducing signs and symptoms. Medications and management include a choleretic, such as ursodeoxycholic acid, periodic MR studies of the liver, and as needed endoscopic retrograde cholangiopancreatography (ERCP) with dilation of strictures. Endoscopic dilation of dominant strictures, with

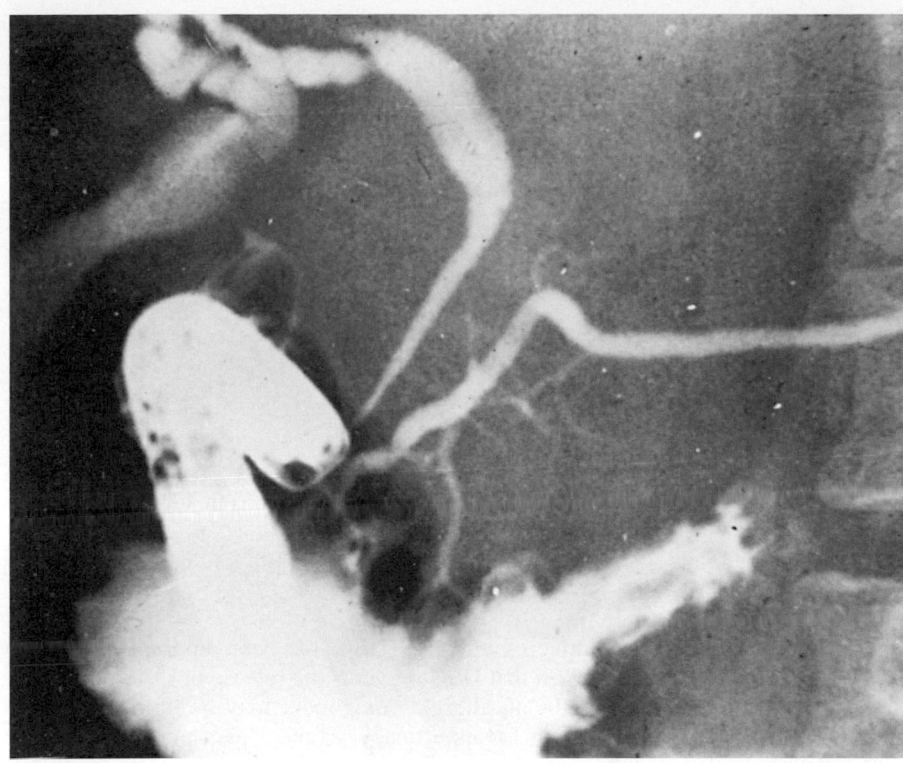

FIGURE 30-48. Sclerosing cholangitis. Endoscopic retrograde cholangiopancreatography (ERCP) demonstrates narrowing of the distal common bile duct with complete obstruction at the level of the common hepatic duct. (From Corman ML, Veidenheimer MC, Nugent FW, et al. *Diseases of the Anus, Rectum and Colon. Part II: Non specific Inflammatory Bowel Disease.* New York, NY: Medcom; 1976.)

or without stenting, has been shown to alleviate cholestasis and to improve laboratory test results. Monitoring with liver function tests is advisable.

Shaked and coworkers reported their experience with 36 patients who underwent orthotopic liver transplantation for primary sclerosing cholangitis, using immunosuppression with cyclosporine, azathioprine (AZA), and steroids.[502] Of these individuals, 29 were known to have chronic ulcerative colitis. The investigators demonstrated that liver replacement and immunosuppression in those suffering from sclerosing cholangitis and ulcerative colitis do not alter the course of the colonic disease. Bleday and colleagues have demonstrated that there appears to be a group of patients who have undergone liver transplant who rapidly develop colorectal malignancy.[49] These individuals require frequent, long-term surveillance following transplant. This suggests that the immunosuppressive agents employed for managing patients who have undergone orthotopic liver transplantation may have a pejorative effect on the colon through increased predisposition for the development of malignancy. But there is no evidence to suggest an association between sclerosing cholangitis itself and colorectal carcinoma in patients with IBD.[382] However, a number of cases of carcinoma of the gallbladder have been described in individuals with sclerosing cholangitis and ulcerative colitis.[119]

Interestingly, despite massive immunosuppression associated with transplanting small intestine, histologically confirmed recurrent Crohn's disease has been demonstrated in the transplanted bowel.[539]

Cangemi and colleagues prospectively compared the progression of clinical, biochemical, cholangiographic, and hepatic histologic features in 45 patients with both primary sclerosing cholangitis and ulcerative colitis, 20 of whom underwent proctocolectomy and 25 of whom had not.[72] No beneficial effect was seen as a consequence of the operation. Because of the profoundly serious consequences of progressive cholangitis, a case may be made for "prophylactic" removal of the inflammatory bowel process if early changes in the biliary tract are observed. This has been suggested even when the gastrointestinal manifestations are quite minimal, but there is no evidence to support implementation of this concept. Still, if surgical treatment is needed for the IBD itself, those with well-controlled primary sclerosing cholangitis can undergo such operations as restorative proctocolectomy safely (for ulcerative colitis).[415]

Cirrhosis

Although cirrhosis is an uncommon complication of IBD, it has, in the past at least, been felt to cause 10% of deaths.[83] When it occurs it is usually a consequence of sclerosing cholangitis. Patients may develop the characteristic stigmata of portal hypertension, including bleeding esophageal varices, and ileostomy hemorrhage (see Chapter 31).

Carcinoma of the Bile Duct

Carcinoma of the bile duct arising in a patient with ulcerative colitis is a rare complication. The association was originally described by Parker and Kendall in 1954.[402] In 1974, Ritchie and colleagues identified 67 cases.[450] The condition is more common in men and is usually seen in patients who have had a prolonged history of colitis. Patients give a history of typical biliary obstruction with painless jaundice, weight loss, and pruritic symptoms. Diagnosis is usually confirmed by ultrasound demonstration of dilated intrahepatic ducts and by endoscopic retrograde cholangiography. Prognosis is poor, with biliary diversion the usual surgical approach.[587]

Cutaneous Manifestations
Pyoderma Gangrenosum

Pyoderma gangrenosum is a condition found exclusively in individuals with IBD but is fortunately uncommon,

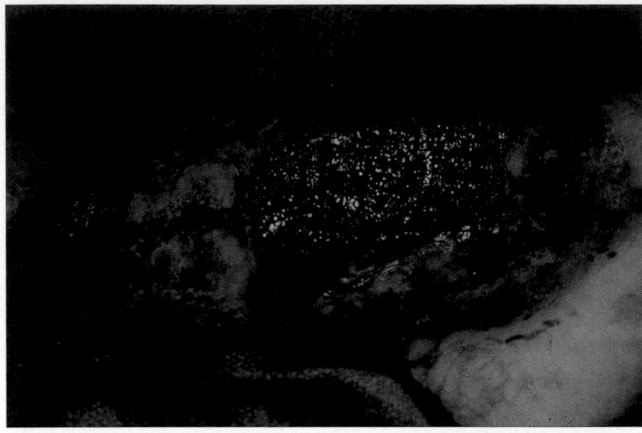

FIGURE 30-49. Pyoderma gangrenosum. Irregularly outlined, sharply defined ulceration with edematous edges and pyodermatous base in a patient with ulcerative colitis. (Courtesy of Rudolf Garret, MD.)

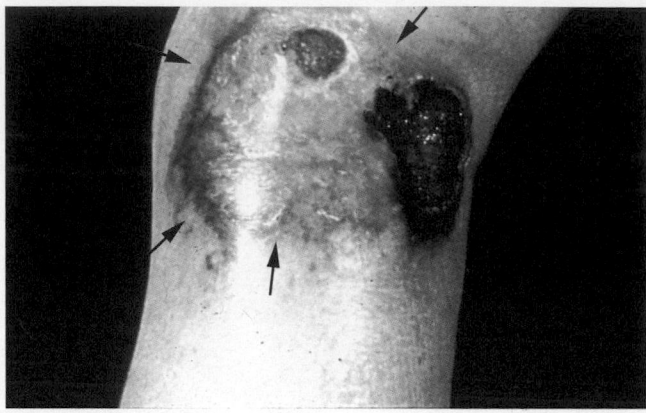

FIGURE 30-51. Pyoderma gangrenosum. In this photograph taken 1 month following a proctocolectomy, a much smaller ulcer is evident. Compare this with the original lesion (outlined by *arrows*). (From Corman ML, Veidenheimer MC, Nugent FW, et al. *Diseases of the Anus, Rectum and Colon. Part II: Non-specific Inflammatory Bowel Disease.* New York, NY: Medcom; 1976.)

occurring in no more than 2% of patients.[362] Schoetz and associates identified 8 of 961 with Crohn's disease (an incidence of 0.8%).[495] The vast majority of patients have active intestinal disease at the time the pyoderma develops, although in rare cases the skin lesions may antedate apparent bowel involvement.[362] Clinically, the lesion appears as a spreading, undermining ulceration that has a characteristic violaceous border (Figures 30-49 and 30-50). It is usually found on the extremities, the most common location being the anterior tibial area.[419] However, the ulcers can occur on the trunk, buttocks, and other places. Usually, there are only one or two lesions, but these can be of considerable size.

Biopsy shows no definite characteristics that would identify the ulcer as being specific for a complication associated with IBD. A vasculitis has been suggested as a possible etiology.

Treatment consists of administration of systemic steroids and occasionally intralesional steroids, and, of course, the management of the colitis.[186] Successful response to topical

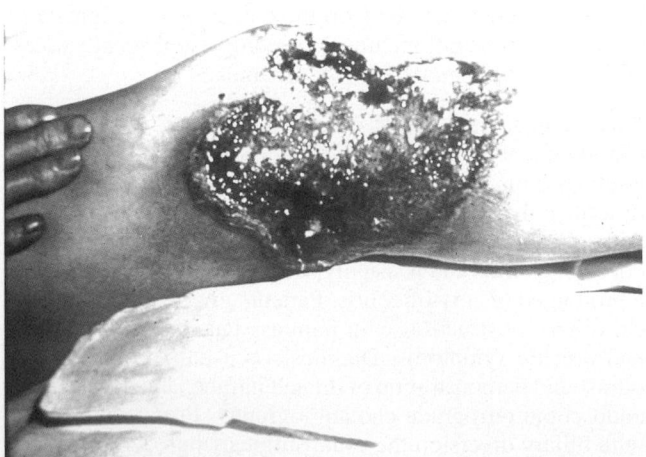

FIGURE 30-50. Pyoderma gangrenosum. An undermined ulcer with a violaceous border. (From Corman ML, Veidenheimer MC, Nugent FW, et al. *Diseases of the Anus, Rectum and Colon. Part II: Non-specific Inflammatory Bowel Disease.* New York, NY: Medcom; 1976.)

disodium cromoglycate (DSG) has been reported.[77] Because it is known that DSG prevents the release of histamine from mast cells, an allergic component may be involved in the mechanism for its efficacy. Topical measures also should include appropriate antibiotics if culture suggests the value of such treatment or if lymphangitis or cellulitis is present. As with so many other extraintestinal manifestations, the course of the pyoderma parallels the clinical progress of the intestinal disease.

Rarely does the skin condition assume such significance that colectomy must be performed for this indication alone. A total colectomy with preservation of the rectum may result in incomplete healing of the pyoderma, but the residual skin problem can fail to clear until proctectomy is subsequently performed (Figure 30-51).

A variant of this manifestation is *parastomal gangrenosum*, a paraileostomy ulceration/fistula. In this condition, there are multiple cutaneous defects surrounding the stoma. These may drain pus and are exquisitely painful. One can probe the external openings, but there is no evident fistulous communication. These are characteristically subcutaneous and may lead to overlying skin necrosis. There is usually a communication at the mucocutaneous attachment of the stoma. This is different from that of pyoderma in that this condition usually appears away from the mucocutaneous junction.

Treatment of parastomal gangrenosum involves unroofing of these extensions. In severe cases, this may lead to circumferential excision of skin, leaving a defect that may make pouch security impossible. The defect in the subcutaneous tissue harbors exuberant granulation tissue, which is curetted down to the base of the ulcer. Pouching is accomplished by using a nonseal appliance. Application of layered cotton dressings soaked in Domeboro's solution is used over the defect. A Perry model no. 51 sleeve is then applied to the ostomy (see Chapter 32). This is kept in place with straps applied to belt hooks. The dressing is changed daily. Defect closure by secondary intention may be accomplished in 4 to 6 weeks. For lesser degrees of parastomal ulceration, a Telfa dressing is applied. The stoma is then pouched with daily changes. Stomal relocation is rarely required.

Polyarteritis Nodosa

Polyarteritis nodosa is a rare cutaneous manifestation of Crohn's disease. Kahn and colleagues reviewed 11 cases in the literature and added one of their own.[316] The presence of erythematous, tender nodules in the extremities should lead one to suspect the diagnosis. Biopsy or excision may reveal an arteritis with luminal narrowing by fibrinous thrombus.

The relationship of the cutaneous manifestation to systemic polyarteritis nodosa is controversial, but in the case reported by the authors, when subsequent resection of the bowel was carried out, there was no evidence of such an arteritis. The condition should be distinguished from other cutaneous manifestations, such as those in the following discussion.

Erythema Nodosum

Erythema nodosum is another cutaneous manifestation that is relatively uncommonly seen with IBD with up to 5% of patients reported to be afflicted.[259] In a report from our institution, 90% had active bowel disease at the time skin lesions developed.[362] In their experience, erythema nodosum typically occurred as a single episode and lasted for several days, associated with active bowel disease and joint symptoms. Tender, subcutaneous nodules are usually seen on the pretibial aspects of the legs. As with other extracolonic manifestations, the clinical course usually parallels that of the intestinal disease.

Psoriasis

There appears to be an increased risk for the development of psoriasis in patients with IBD.[250,454] In a report by Yates and colleagues, the prevalence of psoriasis in Crohn's disease (11.2%) and in ulcerative colitis (5.7%) was significantly greater than that of the control group (1.5%).[607] The increased association of the two conditions as well as the higher rate of psoriasis in first-degree relatives of Crohn's patients implies the possibility of a genetic link.[299]

Cutaneous Crohn's Disease

Crohn's disease of the skin can develop with the characteristic histologic feature of the bowel condition—specifically, granulomatous inflammation of the dermis. When this occurs other than by direct extension from the gastrointestinal tract, it has been given what one may consider to be a poor but now accepted term, *metastatic cutaneous Crohn's disease*. Fewer than 50 cases have been reported.[210,311,516,541,564] The condition has a variable macroscopic appearance, including ulceration, erythema, and nodularity. Biopsy is required to establish the diagnosis, with differentiation from sarcoidosis a potential problem, because the two diseases have similar cutaneous findings.[350] Treatment by means of intralesional steroid therapy has been attempted with usually transient improvement. Therapeutic benefit has also been achieved with oral metronidazole (Flagyl).[52,496]

Arthritis and Rheumatologic Conditions

Depending on the interpretation of what truly constitutes arthritic or rheumatologic conditions associated with IBD, there are perhaps as many as four clinical patterns: first, a peripheral joint synovitis that is closely related to the activity of the bowel disease (15% to 20% of patients); second, ankylosing spondylitis (3% to 6%), in which the relationship with the bowel disorder is less clearly defined; third, a bilateral symmetric sacroiliitis (5% to 15%); and a fourth

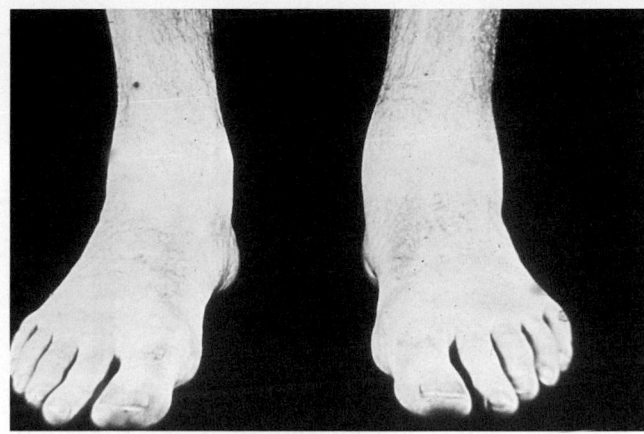

FIGURE 30-52. Colitic arthritis. Bilateral ankle swelling is evident, the left ankle greater than the right, in a patient with ulcerative colitis. (From Corman ML, Veidenheimer MC, Nugent FW, et al. *Diseases of the Anus, Rectum and Colon. Part II: Non-specific Inflammatory Bowel Disease.* New York, NY: Medcom; 1976.)

category, which includes rheumatic complications, such as granulomas of bones and joints, clubbing, periostitis, osteomalacia, osteoporosis, septic arthritis, and complications of corticosteroid therapy.[193,378]

Colitic Arthritis

Colitic arthritis or enteropathic arthritis is the most common joint manifestation of IBD and is seen more frequently with Crohn's disease than with ulcerative colitis. The large joints are primarily involved (knees, ankles, elbows, and wrists). They may be swollen, warm, and red (Figure 30-52). The appearance may not be dissimilar to that of rheumatoid arthritis, but it is nondeforming and seronegative: that is, rheumatoid factor is absent from the blood. Although any joint may be attacked, small joints are less frequently affected (Figure 30-53).

Symptoms of the arthritis usually develop after the IBD has been diagnosed and tend to parallel the course of the intestinal disease. The inflammation is usually adequately controlled by means of anti-inflammatory agents or by the use of steroids. The arthritis completely resolves after colectomy.

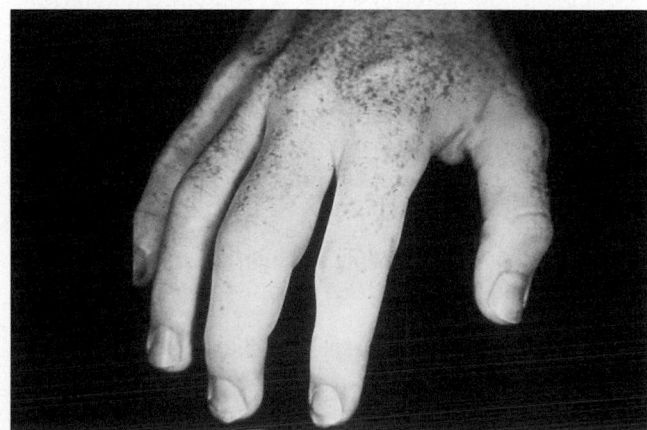

FIGURE 30-53. Colitic arthritis. Proximal interphalangeal joint involvement in a 20-year-old man with acute ulcerative colitis. (From Corman ML, Veidenheimer MC, Nugent FW, et al. *Diseases of the Anus, Rectum and Colon. Part II: Non-specific Inflammatory Bowel Disease.* New York, NY: Medcom; 1976.)

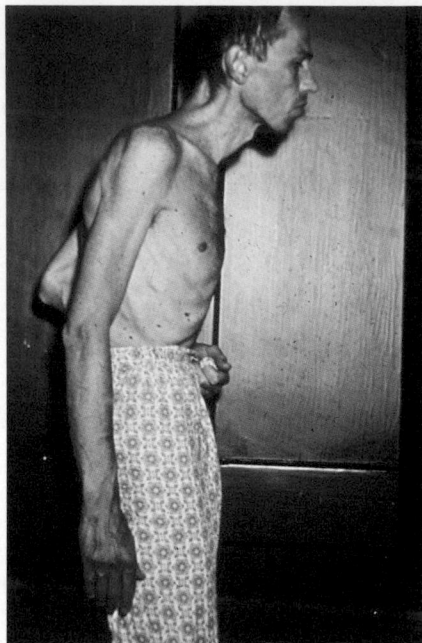

FIGURE 30-54. Rheumatoid spondylitis. Note the kyphosis in this patient with chronic ulcerative colitis. (From Corman ML, Veidenheimer MC, Nugent FW, et al. *Diseases of the Anus, Rectum and Colon. Part II: Non-specific Inflammatory Bowel Disease.* New York, NY: Medcom; 1976.)

Rheumatoid Spondylitis

As stated, other joint disorders that may be encountered are severe arthralgias and rheumatoid spondylitis.[1,193,256,348,613] The incidence of rheumatoid spondylitis is considerably higher in patients with IBD than in the general population, with estimates ranging in excess of 20 times. The well-known gender incidence (4:1 ratio of men to women) is reversed when rheumatoid spondylitis complicates IBD. A genetic association between the two diseases has been demonstrated. In contradistinction to most other extracolonic manifestations, spondylitis does not parallel the activity of the bowel disease. The incidence is similar in Crohn's disease and ulcerative colitis.

The patient initially develops pain in the lumbosacral region, but the discomfort may rapidly progress to involve the thoracic and cervical spine. As ankylosis progresses, the patient exhibits the characteristic dorsal kyphosis (Figure 30-54). Interestingly, isolated asymptomatic sacroiliitis occurs more often than does spinal involvement (4% to 18%).[193]

Treatment consists of physiotherapy, anti-inflammatory agents, and steroids. Colectomy is not indicated for the treatment of the arthritic manifestations.

Hypertrophic Osteoarthropathy or Finger Clubbing

Finger clubbing has also been reported in association with IBD. It may regress after resection of the involved bowel segment and usually correlates with disease activity.[161]

Polymyositis

Polymyositis has been reported on rare occasions to be a condition associated with IBD, especially ulcerative colitis.[84] As with other unusual extraintestinal manifestations, one must always be concerned about the possibility that the condition may be simply coincidental. Still, because of the possible

autoimmune etiology of the two diseases, a causal link may be considered plausible.

Bronchopulmonary Disease

Pulmonary manifestations have been said to be associated with IBD, including bronchiectasis, granulomatous lung disease, interstitial fibrosis, and sulfasalazine pneumonitis.[14,305] Storch and coworkers reported more than 400 instances, categorizing the cases by disease mechanism into drug-induced disease, anatomic disease, overlap syndromes, autoimmune disease, physiologic consequences of IBD, pulmonary function test abnormalities, and nonspecific lung disease.[537] The authors conclude that manifestations of IBD in the lung vary and often present a confounding diagnostic problem, necessitating a complex workup.[537] Investigation of respiratory factors in patients with Crohn's disease free of clinical pulmonary symptoms and with normal chest roentgenograms was studied by Bonniere and colleagues.[54] This included serum angiotensin-converting enzyme, pulmonary function tests, bronchoalveolar lavage, and pulmonary scanning. Results suggest that most patients with Crohn's disease have a much higher frequency of latent lung abnormalities than would be expected in a control population.

Ocular Manifestations

Ocular disease including orbital congestion, uveitis, conjunctivitis, iritis, and keratitis are found in up to 10% of patients with IBD. The most common ocular lesion is episcleritis, an inflammation overlying the sclera, under the conjunctiva. A thickened, deep red appearance is usually noted in one segment of the eye (Figure 30-55). Burning, itching, and pain are the primary symptoms, but the patient often seeks medical attention because of the appearance. Steroids and anti-inflammatory agents are the treatments of choice. Episcleritis is often associated with exacerbations of the underlying IBD but is unrelated to extent or severity.[14] Because of the complications that may lead to a chorioretinitis, ophthalmologic consultation is advised.

Uveitis usually produces ocular pain, blurred vision, and headache and may occur whether the underlying disease is symptomatic or in remission.[14] The diagnosis is established by slit lamp examination. Treatment consists of pupillary dilatation to relieve spasm, an eye patch, and the application of topical corticosteroids.

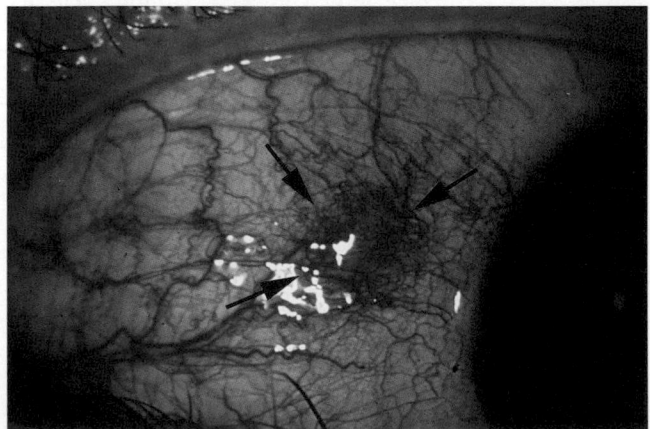

FIGURE 30-55. Episcleritis. Note the nodular, focal, erythematous lesion (*arrows*). (From Corman ML, Veidenheimer MC, Nugent FW, et al. *Diseases of the Anus, Rectum and Colon. Part II: Non-specific Inflammatory Bowel Disease.* New York, NY: Medcom; 1976.)

Amyloidosis

Secondary amyloidosis was initially described in 1949 by Cohen and Fishman in a patient with IBD and is still a rare reported finding.[88] When recognized, it occurs almost exclusively with Crohn's disease. The diagnosis has been made usually at postmortem examination, although confirmation has been established in a few patients who presented with renal failure and who underwent renal biopsy.[14] In the absence of kidney dysfunction, a search for secondary amyloidosis is probably not justified.[327] The application of rectal biopsy for establishing the diagnosis is discussed in Chapter 26. Regression of proteinuria and other manifestations of renal as well as hepatic dysfunction has been reported following bowel resection.[128,163,181]

Urologic Complications

Urologic complications are commonly seen in association with IBD. These include chronic interstitial nephritis, chronic pyelonephritis, acute tubular necrosis, urinary fistulas, ureteral obstruction, and nephrolithiasis.

Ureteral Obstruction

Ureteral obstruction is much more frequently identified in association with Crohn's disease than with ulcerative colitis (Figure 30-56). This is due to periureteric fibrosis. The incidence has been reported to be as high as 50% in this

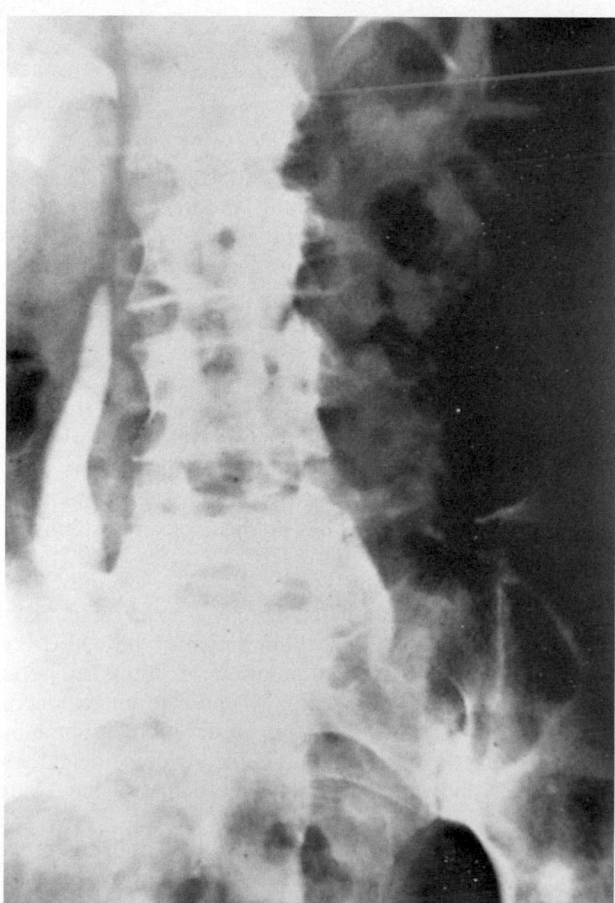

FIGURE 30-56. Ureteral obstruction in a patient with distal ileitis and pelvic abscess. Note the dilated right collecting system and the right ureter. (From Corman ML, Veidenheimer MC, Nugent FW, et al. *Diseases of the Anus, Rectum and Colon. Part II: Non-specific Inflammatory Bowel Disease.* New York, NY: Medcom; 1976.)

group of patients. An inflammatory mass involving the terminal ileum and occasionally the sigmoid colon can produce extrinsic compression of the distal ureters, with the right more frequently involved than the left. The result is hydroureter, hydronephrosis, and possibly, caliectasis. Symptoms related to the urinary tract may be minimal and, if present, may actually be due to compression of the bladder by an inflammatory mass rather than to the obstruction of a ureter. Flank pain is suggestive of ureteral obstruction.

Treatment involves removal of the mass that is causing the compression. In the past, ureterolysis had been advocated, but this risks ureteric ischemia. Complete resolution may be expected, assuming that the obstruction has not produced irreversible renal damage. Indeed, in some cases, drainage of the accompanying abscess alone will be sufficient to relieve the obstruction. Preoperative identification of ureteral dilatation should warn the surgeon that a meticulous dissection may be required to avoid ureteral injury (see Chapter 24). The preoperative placement of ureteral catheters should be considered.

Nephrolithiasis and Bladder Calculi

Nephrolithiasis and bladder calculi are seen in at least 5% of individuals with IBD. Following proctocolectomy and ileostomy, patients are still at risk for the development of nephrolithiasis. Many factors contribute to the development of calculi in chronic IBD: decreased urine volume, increased crystalloid concentration, urinary electrolyte and pH changes, and recurrent urinary tract infections. The more acid urine favors precipitation of urates, and, as a result, uric acid calculi are more common in patients with IBD than in the "normal" population of stone formers. Intestinal absorption of oxylate is increased when ileal disease is present, and this is a further reason for formation of stones. Figure 30-57 demonstrates numerous bladder calculi that developed in a 60-year-old man who had extensive Crohn's disease of the small intestine for more than 20 years.

Bambach and associates reported that 10% of patients who underwent resection for IBD gave a history of urinary stone formation after surgery.[29] Ileostomy patients were demonstrated to have a significantly lowered urinary pH and volume and a higher concentration of calcium, oxylate, and uric acid. The authors advise close follow-up of patients with ileostomies and with small bowel resections in particular, in order to assess fecal losses and urinary composition. Ideally, patients who are at an increased risk for the formation of urinary stones could then be identified.

An adequate urinary volume should be maintained by encouraging the patient to consume sufficient water to increase urinary volume without increasing ileostomy output, by alkalinization in selected patients, by a diet low in oxylate and fat, and by "slowing" medications to reduce the ileostomy volume.[29]

Psoas Abscess

Psoas abscess has long been recognized as a complication of Crohn's disease, but it has also been found, albeit rarely, with ulcerative colitis.[4,572] The condition is secondary to posterior perforation of the diseased organ. In our experience, 73% of individuals presenting with this manifestation had regional enteritis.[431] When seen as a consequence of Crohn's disease, it may be the result of a fistula or abscess from the terminal ileum on the right side or of disease of the jejunum or sigmoid on the left.[308] Pain in the iliac fossa, abdomen,

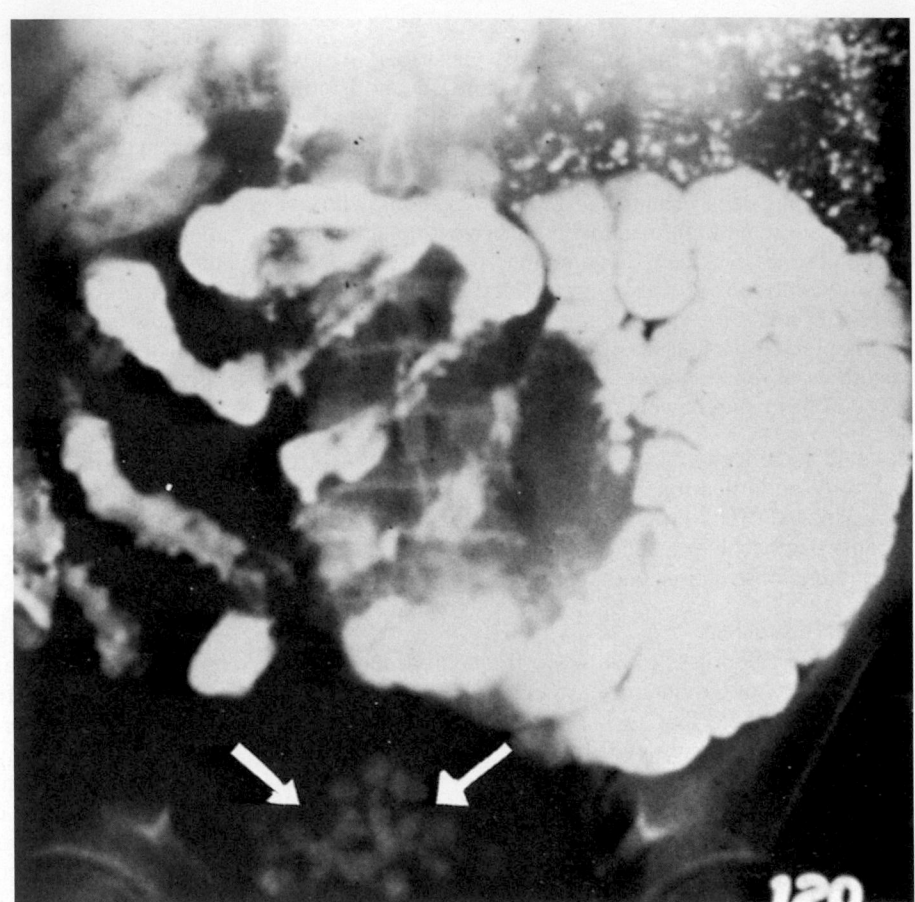

FIGURE 30-57. Bladder calculi (*arrows*) in a patient with long-standing Crohn's disease. (From Corman ML, Veidenheimer MC, Nugent FW, et al. *Diseases of the Anus, Rectum and Colon. Part II: Non-specific Inflammatory Bowel Disease.* New York, NY: Medcom; 1976.)

groin, or hip is the usual symptom. Chills and fever, abdominal or flank mass, and an associated cutaneous fistula may be apparent.

In the past, a limited open drainage (a so-called finger laparotomy) was done. Currently, CT-guided abscess drainage is favored. After sepsis has resolved, usually within 6 weeks, then laparotomy and resection of the source—namely, ileocolic resection or, in certain cases, sigmoid resection—may be done.

Operating on a psoas abscess may require an extensive dissection. There may even be a horseshoe appearance with extension up one or both retroperitoneal gutters. Curettage of the retroperitoneal tract is carried out with great care. For tracts extending into the deep pelvis, curettage may provoke alarming hemorrhage from disruption of pelvic branches of the iliac vessels. The tract is then drained through a lateral incision. Following resection of the diseased bowel segment, omentum is placed between the curetted abscess tract and the anastomosis in order to minimize the risk of reperforation. Extension of the septic process with establishment of a spinal extradural abscess requiring emergency laminectomy has been reported.[6]

Cardiac Complications

Cardiac complications in association with IBD are extremely unusual, with pericarditis being the most frequently described. Ballinger and Farthing postulate that heart block may, in some individuals, be a complication of ulcerative colitis and not a coincidental association.[28] Others opine that IBD may be considered an independent risk factor for the development of bacterial endocarditis.[288] Therefore, endocarditis prophylaxis should be considered, according to some investigators, even in the absence of predisposing primary cardiac factors for the development of bacterial endocarditis.[288]

Other Manifestations

A number of other conditions have been suggested to be associated with nonspecific IBD. Evidence of Crohn's disease has been found in voluntary muscle, the larynx, and the ovary. Whether these and other manifestations such as hyperthyroidism, hyperparathyroidism, and hematologic problems are coincidental has not been clearly established.

Relationship to Carcinoma

For many years, it was felt that there was no increased risk for the development of carcinoma in patients who had Crohn's disease. However, an accumulation of published reports beginning in the 1960s seems to indicate an exponential increase in the frequency of this observation.[461] Some have suggested that the observations are merely coincidental. Most investigators, however, accept the thesis that such a relationship does indeed exist.[15,41,57,94,178,195,214,284,293,444,486,529,606] This association is not equivalent to that which has been observed in long-standing, chronic ulcerative colitis, however.

In 1980, Zinkin and Brandwein identified 43 patients with adenocarcinoma arising in a segment of Crohn's colitis and added one of their own.[612] Hawker and associates reviewed the literature on Crohn's disease of the small intestine and identified 61 cases, including their own experience.[230] There were 41 tumors of the ileum, 18 of the jejunum, 1 in the duodenum and ileum, and 1 in the ileum and colon. Eighteen occurred in bypassed intestinal loops. More recently, Rubio and colleagues found 174 small and large bowel cancers occurring in Crohn's disease in their literature review. Stahl and coworkers identified 22 patients with malignancies at the Lahey Clinic.[529] The median age at diagnosis of Crohn's disease was 37 years and at diagnosis of carcinoma was 54 years.

It is very difficult to assess the true incidence of Crohn's disease and carcinoma in the small intestine because small bowel carcinoma is such a rare condition. However, the association appears genuine and is based on several observations. There is a different distribution of small bowel cancer in Crohn's disease when compared with cancer of the small intestine that occurs in the absence of this inflammatory condition. In Crohn's disease, two thirds of the small bowel cancers occur in the ileum, whereas no more than 30% develop in this area when it is not involved by disease.[230] In the large intestine, Crohn's disease with cancer is usually found on the right side of the colon, as compared with the usual more distal bowel involvement in the general population. In a study from Birmingham, England, Gyde and colleagues demonstrated a significant excess of tumors in both the upper and lower gastrointestinal tract in patients with Crohn's disease.[213] They further demonstrated that the whole tract may be at an increased risk and that this risk is not confined to areas of obvious inflammatory involvement. Additional features of carcinoma in Crohn's disease include multifocal lesions and metachronous intestinal and extraintestinal cancers. Patients who develop carcinoma in Crohn's disease are usually relatively young, and more than one-half with colonic cancer are younger than the age of 40 years.[520] A long duration of illness also appears to be an underlying factor, and there is perhaps a tenfold greater risk of developing colon cancer in this circumstance than in the general population.[447]

The likelihood of the development of carcinoma is greatly enhanced in patients who have undergone intestinal bypass.[202,214,230] This is particularly true when chronic inflammatory disease persists for many years. Lavery and Jagelman identified two cases of carcinoma that developed in the out-of-circuit rectum after subtotal colectomy and ileostomy for Crohn's disease.[296] The mortality rate from patients who develop cancer in excluded bowel is extremely high (>80%), probably because recognition is very late in the progression of the disease.[195] Even without an exclusion or bypass procedure having been performed, survival is poor with small bowel cancer. In the experience of Michelassi and coworkers, the mean survival rate was only 6 months compared with 65 months for those with large bowel cancer.[359] The observation of new signs and symptoms after a prolonged period of quiescence, particularly with long-standing disease, and especially if the patient had previously undergone an exclusion or bypass procedure, should be vigorously evaluated for the possible presence of a malignancy.

This change in symptoms after a period of quiescence is of critical concern also with respect to prior strictureplasty (see later). Ribeiro and colleagues recommend that all strictures be widely opened and carefully examined prior to strictureplasty, with frozen-section biopsies of all suspicious areas.[444] Although the risk of adenocarcinoma developing at the site of a strictureplasty is quite remote, several such instances have been reported.[257,336]

Anal Crohn's disease also appears to be associated with an increased risk for the development of anal carcinoma.[57,293,517,524] Malignant changes may be inapparent, especially when the tumor arises in a fistula. Pain, stricture, and induration often preclude the performance of an adequate examination.[293] Deterioration of an individual's perianal symptoms and clinical findings warrants investigation and possible biopsy.[57] There also seems to be a relationship with intestinal–cutaneous fistulas, although there is always the question of whether the fistula may be secondary to an underlying malignancy in the intestine.[86] Whether the anal or abdominal fistula causes malignant change to occur by "irritation" or by a stimulus to mucosal regeneration is a matter for conjecture.

Although carcinoma arising at the stomal site in patients with polyposis or ulcerative colitis has been described (see Chapter 31), it was only recently that the complication has been reported in Crohn's disease.[301] In both of the cases, dysplasia was identified in adjacent tissue.

Specific symptoms suggestive of malignancy are rarely identified. However, the important issue, as stated, is that any change, especially following a period of quiescence, demands investigation. Cancer should also be considered when complete obstruction fails to resolve with adequate decompression.[444]

Dysplasia

As with carcinoma in ulcerative colitis, radiologic diagnosis of malignant change in patients with Crohn's disease is virtually impossible. Endoscopic examination likewise is of very little benefit in establishing the diagnosis. However, dysplasia, if present, probably is as significant a finding as it is with ulcerative colitis.[185,214,408] The dysplasia that is recognized is essentially identical to that described in patients with ulcerative colitis (see Chapter 29).[179,279,445,447,460,461] Unfortunately, with the exception of the very distal ileum, the small intestine does not lend itself to investigation by means of biopsy, especially if the segment is excluded. It is probably a reasonable precaution to recall all patients who have undergone a bypass or an exclusion procedure and evaluate them for resection.

Korelitz and colleagues analyzed 356 patients with Crohn's disease by means of rectal biopsy in order to study epithelial dysplasia.[279] Eighteen (5%) exhibited this finding, including those with a normal-appearing mucosa. Colorectal carcinoma was found in 11% of these individuals. Four patients developed carcinoma who did not have dysplasia on rectal biopsy. Löfberg and colleagues evaluated 24 patients with long-standing colonic Crohn's disease by means of colonoscopic biopsy at 10 predetermined sites.[322] Although none had definite dysplasia, three demonstrated DNA aneuploidy, one of whom subsequently developed a carcinoma. The authors believe that dysplasia is rare in Crohn's disease but that DNA aneuploidy needs to be carefully assessed. Obviously, further studies are needed. Richards and associates suggest that surveillance of the colon should commence after 10 years of disease.[447] How frequently this should be undertaken is still not determined, but the issues and concerns expressed in Chapter 29 should be well heeded.

Comment

As was discussed in Chapter 29, the concept of surveillance to identify dysplasia before malignancy supervenes has been subjected to a more critical analysis in recent years. The same should be true for the concept in the management of patients with Crohn's disease. A statement made by Sachar is worth quoting completely because it reflects my own views on this subject.

> The most rationale position, therefore, in view of the equivalent risks, might be to adopt equivalent policies for the two diseases. In other words, debate the pros and cons of surveillance programs to your heart's content; but in the end, whatever you choose to do for your patients with ulcerative colitis, do no differently for those with Crohn's colitis of similar duration and extent.[473]

Other Malignancies

The issue of extraintestinal malignancies with IBD is a matter of some controversy. Whether the association is valid or merely coincidental is still unresolved. Concomitant malignant melanoma and lymphoma have been suggested to be more than mere coincidence, perhaps related to immunosuppression from the disease itself or from medical treatment.[148,152,199,203]

Medical Management

The reader is directed to Chapter 29 *for a comprehensive discussion of the medical management of ulcerative colitis.*

The management of Crohn's disease is dependent on the assessment of the disease location, the severity, the exclusion of abscess, and the elimination of extraluminal factors, such as cigarette smoking, nonsteroidal anti-inflammatory drugs, *Clostridium difficile*, acute self-limited infections, or irritable bowel-like symptoms that might better respond to conventional therapy.[220] Confounding factors, of course, include undetected but coexistent carcinoma and AIDS. Dietary problems referable to sorbitol or lactose may obscure the initial concern that this is actually Crohn's disease. Approaches to the management of patients include lifestyle, diet, and pharmaceuticals, each of which may independently aid in the management of the asymptomatic individual with Crohn's disease.[241] The therapeutic goals are to induce a clinical remission, to maintain that remission, and to prevent postoperative relapse.

The plethora of information regarding pathogenetic mechanisms in the understanding of Crohn's disease has led to a number of imaginative and innovative treatment approaches. Kornbluth and colleagues undertook a study to determine the efficacy of various medical therapies in the treatment of severe IBD based on a MEDLINE computer-assisted literature search.[283] They determined that clinical remission was achieved on average in 65% of individuals with Crohn's disease. They concluded that current medical therapy for severe Crohn's colitis seems to spare many patients early colectomy. The Crohn's Disease Activity Index (CDAI), which consists of the clinical variables correlated with the physician's assessment of the patient's well-being, although validated, has been criticized because of its subjectivity and interobserver variability.[218]

Mild-to-Moderate Disease

In mild-to-moderate disease, the initial drug of choice is 5-ASA in a form targeted to the inflammatory site, using higher doses than that which is required for ulcerative colitis. It is anticipated that there will be a 40% to 60% response rate.[515] Metronidazole and ciprofloxacin regimens can produce results similar to those of 5-ASA, particularly in Crohn's ileocolitis and in perianal disease.[421,540] However, these observations have been challenged for induction of remission with either high-dose 5-ASA or antibiotics and certainly are not as impressive as those with immunomodulator therapy.[222]

Moderate-to-Severe Disease

Moderate-to-severe disease almost always requires steroids initially, but only for short-term use. No long-term benefit has been proven. However, there is an 80% relapse rate when steroids are terminated prematurely. The concern, of course, is that 35% of patients may become steroid-dependent in 1 year, but 20% remain in remission.[369] There is no value in low-dose steroids in preventing relapse.

Severe Disease

In severe Crohn's disease, patients are admitted into the hospital and treated with intravenous medications only (Figure 30-58). There have been no unequivocal data that intravenous cyclosporine has a therapeutic advantage over intravenous corticosteroids, nor has a sustained benefit been demonstrated in Crohn's disease.[153] This has been particularly true with the low dose and the oral route. Drainage of abscess is, of course, mandatory.

Maintenance of Remission

In maintaining remission, the maintenance dose of 5-ASA is the inductive dose—that is, the dose that prevents relapse or recurrence after surgery. However, it may be less effective if steroids, 6-mercaptopurine (6-MP), or AZA induced that remission. If steroids did induce the remission, there is a better

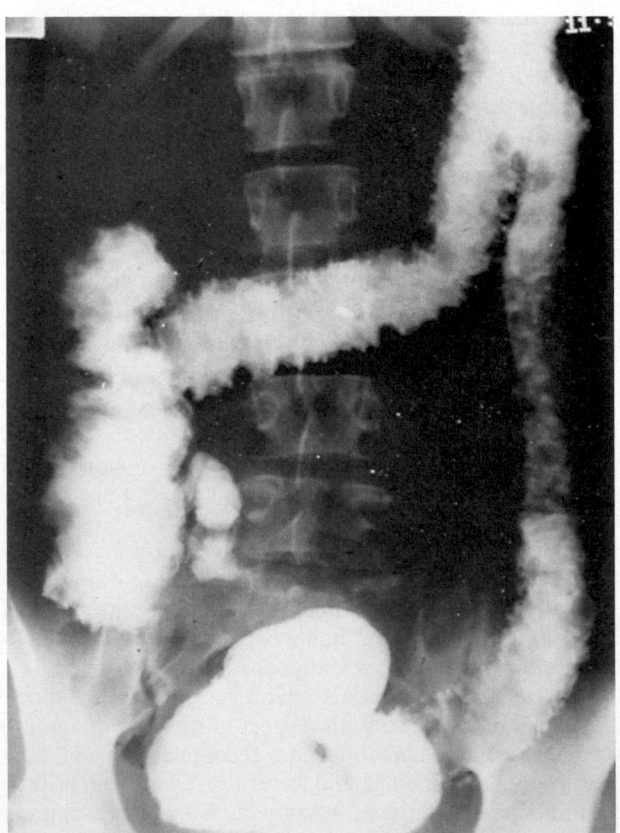

FIGURE 30-58. Fulminant acute Crohn's colitis. Barium enema reveals total colonic ulceration and bowel wall edema.

chance of maintaining that remission with 6-MP and AZA (or possibly methotrexate) than with continued use of 5-ASA.[220]

Postoperative Recurrence

The maintenance of remission following resection for Crohn's disease continues to be a topic of concern among internists, gastroenterologists, and surgeons. Symptomatic relapses occur at a rate of 40% to 70% in most series within 2 years following operation.[175] Endoscopic recurrence actually increases that rate to 80%. In the natural course of the disease, the inflammatory process may tend to extend distally, but rarely proximally. However, once the patient undergoes surgery, proximal involvement is more likely to develop, usually at and just above the anastomosis.

Korelitz believed that sulfasalazine is more effective in preventing recurrence in Crohn's disease than it is with ulcerative colitis.[275] However, the initial enthusiasm for the value of 5-ASA in reducing the likelihood of postoperative recurrence has not been supported by later investigations.[59] The European Cooperative Crohn's Disease Study showed no significant reduction in the clinical relapse rate.[318] Yet a meta-analysis of the 5-ASA experience did show an effect on reducing recurrence postoperatively.[2]

There is, however, value to the postoperative use of immunomodulators and some short-term improvement with metronidazole if side effects can be tolerated.[278] Further study of 55 postoperative Crohn's patients randomized to 6-MP or control showed *no* difference in time to relapse, but the postoperative endoscopic score of disease activity was significantly lower in the 6-MP patients.[48]

Aminosalicylates

The primary drugs that have been traditionally employed for the treatment of Crohn's disease are sulfasalazine and steroids (see Chapter 29). Aminosalicylates can delay recurrence, but concern has been expressed about the clinical efficacy of 5-ASA and antibiotics in Crohn's disease.[222] For example, sulfasalazine has been shown to have a minimal effect on inducing remission in active Crohn's disease when compared with a placebo.[538] Moreover, convincing evidence is lacking that mesalamine is effective for treatment of active Crohn's disease. Gendre and colleagues employed a placebo-controlled study with the use of oral mesalamine (Pentasa) for maintenance therapy and found a statistically significant difference in the maintenance of quiescence in the treated group.[175] Likewise, Brignola and coworkers performed a controlled study with mesalamine and found a statistically significant difference in the incidence of endoscopic lesions and severity in the treated group compared with the placebo.[59] A similar favorable result was observed in individuals who were treated with oral 5-ASA (Asacol).[422]

Sandborn and Feagan suggest an alternative treatment algorithm as a result of their analysis of randomized controlled trials for mild-to-moderate Crohn's disease.[480] Their evidence-based conclusions are as follows:

1. Colonic disease.
2. Sulfasalazine for colonic Crohn's induction of remission with budesonide 9 mg/day for ileal or right disease.
3. Conventional steroids for more severe disease activity, budesonide failures, and patients allergic to or intolerant of sulfasalazine.

Mesalamine has limited value in preventing relapse after a medically induced remission, especially if it has been steroid-induced, or in maintaining remission postoperatively.[69,318] The question of mesalamine's role in preventing postoperative recurrence of Crohn's disease has been revisited by Caprilli and coworkers who found no clinically significant advantage between 84 patients receiving 4.0 g/day (12%) versus 81 patients given 2.4 g/day (14%).[74]

Steroids

A dramatic response is often observed when intravenous steroids are administered. A mass may rapidly disappear, or a patient's acute abdominal symptoms may resolve. The natural history of corticosteroid use in IBD was reviewed in 173 patients treated in Olmstead County, Minnesota, a community-based experience rather than a study of patients referred to a tertiary medical center.[146] Of 74 individuals (43%) treated with corticosteroids, 43 (58%) entered complete remission, 19 (26%) had a partial remission, and 12 (16%) had no response. At 1 year, however, only 24 (32%) still had a prolonged response, yet 21 (28%) were steroid dependent, and 38 required surgery (38%). Thus, of 84% initial responders, only 32% maintained that response free of steroids and without surgery. It should be noted that only 38% of Crohn's patients in this population needed steroids, thus speaking for mild disease. A second lesson learned was that the need for steroids in this group suggested a poorer prognosis and a higher likelihood that surgery would be required.

A double-blind study of the effectiveness of sulfasalazine compared with 6-methylprednisolone in patients with Crohn's disease revealed that the addition of the former drug offered no advantage.[333]

Budesonide (Entocort) in ileocolonic Crohn's disease produced a 45% improvement in 8 weeks in the Canadian experience, with no significant long-term steroid side effects, and with a remission rate at 8 weeks comparable to that of prednisone, with less adrenal suppression.[71] Both prednisone and budesonide induced remission in approximately 60% of patients, with fewer side effects with budesonide in the Italian and Israeli experience.[31,70,395,469] Short-term use of budesonide appeared superior to that of mesalamine (5-ASA) in preventing relapse at 1 year in steroid-dependent patients who were intolerant to AZA/6-MP.[176]

Budesonide may be a reasonable alternative as replacement therapy in glucocorticoid-dependent patients. Cortot and colleagues described 118 individuals with inactive Crohn's disease who were randomized to budesonide, 6 mg, or placebo, while tapering prednisolone.[95] At 13 weeks, 68% of budesonide patients were in remission versus 35% of placebo patients. There was a demonstrable reduction of glucocorticoid side effects—that is, moon face, acne, insomnia, and mood swings—in both the budesonide and the placebo groups.

In a meta-analysis, budesonide was less likely to induce remission in active Crohn's disease than conventional corticosteroids but was better than mesalamine or placebo over 8 weeks and with fewer steroid adverse events.[396] There appears to be a role for budesonide as pulse therapy for quickly inducing a remission for a Crohn's flare and using it as bridge therapy until AZA/6-MP can "kick in."

Antibiotics (Metronidazole [Flagyl] and Ciprofloxacin [Cipro])

Metronidazole was initially introduced for the treatment of *Trichomonas vaginalis* infections but was subsequently demonstrated to be a very effective antibiotic against anaerobic organisms. It was also found to have activity against gram-positive and gram-negative bacteria. The drug is a substituted imidazole that is rapidly absorbed orally and rectally and can be given intravenously to the acutely ill patient. A number of theories suggesting the mechanism of its action have been proposed: immunosuppression, an effect on wound healing, stimulation of leukocyte chemotaxis, and, of course, its antimicrobial effect.

A controlled clinical trial from Sweden compared the efficacy of metronidazole with sulfasalazine in the treatment of patients with active Crohn's disease.[453,566] Seventy-eight participated in the study during two 4-month periods. Metronidazole was demonstrated to be slightly more effective than sulfasalazine. Although metronidazole may be beneficial for some patients with intestinal disease, some have shown that it does not appear to have therapeutic potential for preventing relapse of Crohn's disease.[18] In other studies, metronidazole appears to be of modest value in preventing postoperative recurrence or maintaining remission, but it is limited by bacterial resistance and drug intolerance, particularly the neuropathic side effects and lack of response at the 3-year mark.[56,468] When it has been added to ciprofloxacin, there has been an improvement through the reduction of the CDAI. Forty-five percent of patients went into remission in both the Italians' and the Canadians' experiences, with better results noted with colonic or ileocolonic disease as opposed to ileal disease alone.[194,424] Patients undergoing prolonged treatment need to be closely monitored for the development of peripheral neuropathy.[125]

Prolonged antibiotic therapy (i.e., 6 months) appears to be of value in cipro-treated patients by reducing their CDAI compared with placebo.[25] It is not surprising because many clinicians maintain patients on antibiotics for years with ileocolonic Crohn's.

Conclusions regarding clinical trials of antibiotics support a role for metronidazole–imidazoles, cipro, and possibly clarithromycin in Crohn's colitis and ileocolitis, and less so for ileitis. Better data are still needed with respect to efficacy, recognition of the toxicity of metronidazole, and the expense of other medications.

Metronidazole has been suggested as being particularly useful in the management of *anal* and *perianal Crohn's disease* (see Chapters 13 and 14).[42,56,130] Bernstein and associates demonstrated that drainage, erythema, and induration diminished dramatically in all 21 patients so treated, with complete healing obtained in more than one-half of those who were maintained on therapy.[42] Eisenberg compared surgery alone in the management of complicated anal Crohn's disease with surgery plus metronidazole.[130] The patients were randomly allocated, but it was not a double-blind study. An intravenous loading dose of 15 mg/kg (usually 1 g) was given, with maintenance therapy of 500 mg intravenously every 6 hours for 5 days. Outpatient treatment was continued at the dosage of 250 mg, three times daily, for 4 weeks or until complete healing occurred. Twelve of 14 patients (86%) receiving metronidazole treatment had a satisfactory response—complete healing of anorectal–perineal disease without relapse during a follow-up period of 1 to 5 years. In the control group, 11 of 17 patients (65%) treated by surgery alone had satisfactory healing.

In a follow-up study of long-term administration of metronidazole, Brandt and colleagues evaluated whether the drug could be reduced or stopped in these patients without creating an exacerbation.[56] They reported that dosage reduction was associated with recurrent disease activity in all patients but that healing occurred promptly when the full dose of metronidazole was reinstituted.

It appears, then, that definitive anal surgery can be undertaken even in the presence of anal Crohn's disease with some reasonable expectation of success if supplementary metronidazole therapy is administered.

Antituberculous Chemotherapy

As has been discussed in Chapter 29 concerning etiology, Crohn's disease had been thought to resemble tuberculosis in many respects, and multiple attempts to isolate microbacteria have been made, albeit unsuccessfully. A controlled trial of antituberculous chemotherapy was performed through the Department of Gastroenterology at the University of Wales at Cardiff.[542] In a double-blind, randomized program involving rifampin, isoniazid, and ethambutol, or placebo, no tangible benefit from these agents was identified.[542]

Immunosuppressive Agents
Azathioprine and 6-Mercaptopurine

Because of the supposition that IBD is an autoimmune condition, treatment with immunosuppressive drugs has been recommended.[277,425,591] The two agents that have been used extensively are 6-MP and its analog, AZA. Although immunosuppressive drugs have been shown to be effective in both ulcerative colitis and Crohn's disease, and with few exceptions the complications have been reversible, many physicians, perhaps inappropriately, fear to employ this modality in the management of their patients.

Korelitz uses immunosuppressive drugs when other treatment modalities fail, when there is no indication for operative intervention, and as an option offered to the patient as an alternative to surgery.[276] Present and colleagues performed a double-blind study on 83 patients and noted a 67% response with 6-MP as compared with a modest 8% improvement with a placebo.[425]

Azathioprine and 6-mercaptopurine have been successful in maintaining remission, with a 5% recurrence rate using azathioprine versus a 41% rate of recurrence with placebo at 1 year.[388] Long-term follow-up in the 6-MP experience in 120 patients revealed that those on 6-MP had a relapse of 47% at 5 years, whereas those who discontinued 6-MP had a 97% relapse rate. This was higher in younger patients who had discontinued the drug for "other reasons than a relapse."[270] The question, "Why do patients stop AZA and what happens to them?" was answered in a study of 266 patients.[117] Twenty-five percent discontinued the AZA for blood count abnormalities, and of those who stopped, 60% needed surgery or became steroid-dependent.

The use of 6-MP and AZA as medical therapy for enterovesical fistula seems to have been supported by the Mount Sinai Hospital experience with 31 patients.[582] Wheeler and colleagues demonstrated a 58% clinical response to 5-ASA, antibiotics, and AZA. The fistulas closed in 13 of 31 patients (42%), with two-thirds medically successfully managed over 8 years.

There appears to be no greater risk of malignancy with 6-MP or AZA in the experience involving 626 patients treated for a mean of 27 months and mean follow-up of 13.7 years in the United Kingdom.[165] Their overall rates of colorectal cancer or dysplasia was 0.4% at 10 years, 1.3% at 20 years, 9.0% at 30 years, and 15.5% at 40 years. The study from the Lenox Hill Hospital in New York involving 410 patients followed between 1980 and 1999 revealed that 6-MP and AZA are safe drugs for long-term use.[575] However, there is concern regarding the predisposition to lymphoma with long-term use of 6-MP in some series.[144,345]

Ewe and colleagues performed a randomized, prospective study comparing AZA in combination with prednisolone versus prednisolone alone in the treatment of active Crohn's disease.[139] They found that the combination regimen was superior to that of treatment with prednisolone alone, in that more frequent remissions were observed and with lower doses of prednisolone.[139] Most studies have demonstrated efficacy in approximately two-thirds of patients. The drugs are not felt to be effective in the treatment of fulminant disease but should be used in those individuals who can tolerate the relatively slow response to treatment (commonly, at least 6 months). They have been recommended for the treatment of perianal disease, small bowel obstruction (when surgery is contraindicated), and fistula complications, and for the management of children.[790] In the experience of Lecomte and colleagues (Paris, France), one-third of patients with perianal lesions improved.[297] Prophylaxis after two surgical resections is another possible indication.

Complications include bone marrow suppression, liver abnormalities (including liver necrosis), pancreatitis, and hair loss. Present and colleagues assessed the toxicity of 6-MP in 396 patients (276 with Crohn's disease).[427] Pancreatitis was seen in 3.3%, bone marrow depression in 2%, and allergic reactions in 2%. All were reversible. Markowitz and colleagues identified no serious complications with treatment of 36 adolescents by means of 6-MP in dosages of 1.5 mg/kg to a maximum of 75 mg/day.[338] Follow-up after 1 year demonstrated continued remission in 77%. Others have also confirmed the effectiveness and relative safety of these drugs.[387] The steroid-sparing effects are felt to be of particular benefit in this group of patients.

Methotrexate

In addition to the preceding, methotrexate (MTX), a folic acid antagonist, has been used in the treatment of IBD. In an open-label pilot study, Kozarek and colleagues used this drug in ulcerative colitis and Crohn's disease patients who had failed conventional medical therapy.[287] Preliminary results were encouraging. Feagan and colleagues, with the North American Crohn's Study Group Investigators, conducted a double-blind, placebo-controlled multicenter study of weekly injections of MTX in patients who had chronically active Crohn's disease despite a minimum of 3 months of prednisone therapy.[155] They were randomly assigned to treatment with methotrexate or a placebo for a period of 16 weeks. A statistically significant improvement was observed in the methotrexate group with respect to symptoms and the reduction of requirement for prednisone.[155]

Forty-one of 49 French patients entered clinical remission and were then maintained on MTX for a median of 18 months.[306] Relapse rates were 29% at 1 year, 41% at 2 years, and 48% at 3 years, with a greater relapse rate in women and in ileocolitis patients. A randomized, 16-week, single-blind comparison of 15 or 25 mg of MTX in 32 Crohn's patients at the Mayo Clinic showed the same efficacy of remission (17%) and response rate (45%) with both

doses.[129] The experience in 76 refractory Crohn's patients at the University of Chicago resulted in 63% improvement at 9 weeks.[78] In another study, an impressive 65% of MTX-treated patients (26/40), as the only therapy, remained in remission from 16 to 24 weeks, compared with 39% of the controls.[154] There appears to be a role for MTX in maintaining remission *if* MTX induced that remission. Its success in causing remission may be facilitated by the concomitant use of corticosteroids.

Cyclosporine

Cyclosporine, a drug that has been widely used in organ transplantation, has been subjected to extensive evaluation in the management of Crohn's disease. The cyclosporine story, however, has not been favorable. In one study, a 52% relapse rate occurred during its acute use.[303] However, in a randomly assigned, placebo-controlled, double-blind study of a group of patients who were resistant to or intolerant of steroids, Brynskov and colleagues found a significant improvement in the CDAI.[62] Elson suggested that the rapidity of response may give it some role in the acutely ill individual.[135]

Cyclosporine's value with perianal Crohn's disease seems more impressive, with 10 of 14 patients (71%) achieving relief of fistulous drainage.[304] Hanauer and Smith employed cyclosporine in the management of five patients with chronic draining fistulas that had been unresponsive to prior surgery, steroids, antibiotics, total parenteral nutrition (TPN), and other immunosuppressives.[221] All fistulas responded to this infusion through decreased drainage and with improvement of both inflammatory reaction and patient comfort. However, cyclosporine has not been shown to be of value for maintaining remission, and its toxicity precludes its long-term use.

Biologics (Antibody Therapy)

In the late 1990s, the first in a new class of treatment options emerged for application to Crohn's disease. Referred to as biologic response modifiers or biologics, these drugs reduce inflammation and can also bring about remission as well as maintain remission. They are indicated for use when someone has moderate-to-severe Crohn's disease and has not responded adequately to other Crohn's disease alternatives. Four biologics are U.S. Food and Drug Administration (FDA) approved for this condition. Three block a protein, tumor necrosis factor (TNF), that is involved in inflammation. These are often called anti-TNF drugs or TNF inhibitors. They include Cimzia (certolizumab), Humira (adalimumab), and Remicade (infliximab). The fourth medication, Tysabri (natalizumab), is an integrin receptor antagonist. Because they suppress the immune system, all biologics carry an increased risk of infection. In rare instances, lymphoma has been reported. Tysabri increases the risk of a rare but potentially fatal brain infection, progressive multifocal leukoencephalopathy (PML). The drug also can cause allergic reactions and liver disease.

TNF-α has been shown to have an important role in the pathogenesis of Crohn's disease. Stack and coworkers performed a double-blind, placebo-controlled study, using a genetically engineered human antibody to TNF-α, CDP571, to determine whether disease activity could be modified.[528] A significant fall in the median CDAI was identified in the treatment group. These data suggest that antibody neutralization of TNF-α is a potentially effective strategy in the management of Crohn's disease.

In a short-term study using a single infusion of a chimeric monoclonal antibody to TNF, 65% of the patients improved versus 17% with the placebo.[544] Clinical remission was achieved at 4 weeks in 33% of the patients treated versus 4% of those treated with a placebo. A majority maintained that response at 12 weeks. Additional experience demonstrated that fistulas closed in 62% of the patients versus 26% in the placebo group.[426] In another report, however, despite the fact that infliximab (Remicade) was associated with a 61% complete or partial response rate, the drug did not supplant the requirement for surgery.[416] Seventy-three percent either ultimately needed surgery or had persistent fistulas, although the drug was much more effective in controlling perianal disease. Others have found that selective seton placement, combined with infliximab infusion and maintenance immunosuppressives, resulted in complete healing of two-thirds of perianal fistulas.[560]

The continued experience with anti-TNF has shown that there is considerable endoscopic healing in resistant, active Crohn's disease. In the Amsterdam report involving 108 patients, 65% showed improvement when treated with infliximab.[110] The clinical postmarketing experience with more than 170,000 patients so managed appears to mirror the results achieved in the initial trials. Two-thirds of patients responded, and one-third entered remission.

The first 100 patients treated at Beth Israel Hospital in Boston and Brown University with infliximab demonstrated a 60% response rate, and 36% went into remission.[143] The mean time to response was 6.5 days, but the mean duration of response was only 12 weeks. The Mayo Clinic's experience with the first 100 patients was compartmentalized into those with complete, partial, or no response and by disease activity.[446] Inflammatory Crohn's patients had the best response (52.5%), whereas fistula patients had a 34.6% complete response. Fistulas healed completely in 46% and partially in 23%, with a mean duration of response of 10 weeks.

Short-term infliximab has been shown to be well tolerated, but the incidence of serious adverse events (serum sickness, sepsis, autoimmune phenomena, and opportunistic infections) requires careful surveillance.[92] Additionally, caution is required in individuals with stricture.[108,561,579] A decreased (i.e., worsened) response occurred in 57 stricture patients compared with the nonstricture population in a University of Pennsylvania report.[501] Yet infliximab itself has not been shown to cause intestinal stricture or obstruction.[313]

Rectovaginal fistula in Crohn's disease represents one of the most challenging problems. Remarkably, five of six such patients responded to a three-infusion regimen and four continued to improve with an 8-week infusion cycle while on immunomodulators.[463] Four of six became asymptomatic, with a range of remission from 4 to 7 weeks. Another report involved 28 patients with rectovaginal fistula.[484] A 57% response rate was noted with a three-dose induction regimen. Although fistulas appear to respond to treatment longer than for those with luminal disease following three doses of infliximab, evaluation by MRI or endorectal sonography may still demonstrate clinically inapparent abscesses or persistent fistulas.[5,34,568] A parameter that may predict responsiveness to infliximab is endoscopic healing, which significantly correlates with a more prolonged time to relapse.[465] Results of responses to an IBD questionnaire reveal that infliximab significantly improved the quality of life in those with active disease, thereby increasing ability to work and to participate in leisure activities while decreasing feelings of fatigue, depression, and anger.[312]

Because of the increased risk of tuberculosis in patients given infliximab, it is now advised that patients be skin tested and a chest x-ray be obtained.[367] Any evidence of active TB mandates treatment before initiating infliximab therapy.

Enteric-Coated Fish Oil

Belluzzi and associates performed a 1-year, double-blind, placebo-controlled study to investigate the effects of a fish oil preparation on the maintenance of remission in 78 patients with Crohn's disease.[35] A statistically significant difference was achieved with the use of this preparation when compared with the placebo group with respect to reduction of relapses. The anti-inflammatory effect of fish oil has been well documented to reduce production of a number of agents, such as leukotriene B_4 and thromboxane A_2, which have been observed in the inflamed intestinal mucosa of patients with Crohn's disease. Inhibition of the synthesis of cytokines and TNF has also been demonstrated with fish oil.

Withdrawal of Smoking

Smoking has been shown to have a pejorative effect on the clinical course of individuals with Crohn's disease. Lindberg and associates demonstrated a statistically significantly increased risk of the requirement for surgery in those who smoke more than one-half pack of cigarettes a day.[316] Irrespective of how the course of Crohn's disease is analyzed, it is much less favorable for those who smoke, especially if they are heavy smokers. As part of the therapeutic regimen, therefore, patients with Crohn's disease should be dissuaded from smoking.[316]

Oral contraceptives together with smoking are additive risk factors for relapse in Crohn's disease, with some 40% of patients relapsing with unfavorable outcomes. Prior smoking, however, has not been shown to be an increased risk, but prior oral contraceptives were used more frequently in relapsed patients in one study.[556]

Nutritional Therapy
Parenteral Hyperalimentation

As discussed in Chapter 29, hyperalimentation, either parenteral (TPN) or oral (enteral), has been recommended in a supportive role for patients with Crohn's disease.[228,235,260,309,310,508] The rationale is to replenish nutritional deficits, to allow bowel rest for healing and "repair," and to provide perioperative support for healing in an attempt to reduce morbidity and mortality.[508] We reported the Cleveland Clinic's experience of 81 courses of TPN in the treatment of Crohn's disease.[149] Two groups of patients were treated, one by definitive therapy and a second for adjunctive treatment. Indications in the former group included diffuse small intestinal disease, short bowel syndrome, acute ileitis or colitis (in which there was inadequate response to alternative medical treatment), poor nutrition, and enteric fistulas. A subsequent report revealed 23 patients in the primary therapy group.[224] A remission occurred in approximately two-thirds, while the remaining 8 patients required an operation during the hospitalization. In the adjunctive group, 58 patients were treated, of whom almost one-fourth entered remission, obviating the need for surgical intervention during that hospitalization. These patients, in fact, satisfied the criteria for primary therapy, although this was not the design in that group of patients.

The course of treatment ranged from 10 to 264 days. The average treatment course was almost 3 weeks.

Of the 21 patients with Crohn's disease who were treated with TPN as primary therapy, there were only 4 (19%) who did not eventually require surgery. Three of the five patients with ulcerative colitis who were so treated responded well enough to medical therapy to have deferred surgery for an average of 2 years. We concluded that there appeared to be no lasting benefit for hyperalimentation as a primary method of therapy for patients with IBD, particularly for those with Crohn's disease. However, if the purpose of the treatment is to defer surgical intervention so that it can be pursued on an elective basis, hyperalimentation should be considered.

Shiloni and Freund studied the effect of TPN on 19 patients suffering from active Crohn's disease.[509] Although only approximately one-third did not require surgery during the follow-up (up to 3 years), the authors felt that the treatment was highly effective as supportive therapy, enabling a patient to undergo uneventful major surgery. Others have recommended preoperative TPN for at least 5 days in patients with IBD who have severe protein depletion.[452] However, McIntyre and colleagues, in a controlled trial of 47 severe, acute colitis patients, noted that bowel rest did not affect the outcome.[352] An extensive review by Payne-James and Silk can be summarized by the statement, "Evidence at present indicates that TPN in Crohn's disease should be restricted to a supportive role, rather than employed as primary therapy."[405] In a more general sense, a cooperative Veterans Administration study of 395 malnourished patients who required laparotomy or noncardiac thoracotomy concluded that the use of preoperative TPN should be limited to those who are severely malnourished.[573]

Home Parenteral Nutrition

One additional application of parenteral nutrition needs to be addressed—home parenteral nutrition (HPN)—for the patient who has a short bowel syndrome, a potential consequence of multiple or extensive resections for Crohn's disease.[123,206,302,346,531] In 1966, the first hospitalized patient in the United States received parenteral nutrition, and in 1968, the first patient was discharged on HPN.[122] In the years that followed, there was rapid growth in the use of HPN nationwide.[530] In 1976, reimbursement became available under Medicare through the prosthetic device benefit act and soon thereafter by private insurance companies.[245] In 1983, the Oley Foundation was established as an organization whose focus was to share information and support for HPN and enteral nutrition consumers (http://www.oley.org). In 1984, a voluntary patient registry was developed to track the longitudinal outcomes of a cohort of home patients in the United States and Canada. The registry, called OASIS (Oley–A.S.P.E.N. Information System), was a joint effort of the Oley Foundation and the American Society for Parenteral and Enteral Nutrition (A.S.P.E.N.) and existed from 1985 to 1992.[247] The prevalence of HPN during that time was 238 patients per million people in the United States.[246] Currently, in the United States, little is known about the annual use of HPN. Medicare, a large payer for HPN, does not generate specific public access reports on this patient population. A national HPN registry, Sustain, LLC, was developed by the A.S.P.E.N. to capture data on this patient population.[209] Registries have also been created in the Canada, New Zealand-Australia, Spain, and Ireland.[535]

It is suggested that the reader communicate his or her interest to Peggi Guenter, PhD, RN, Senior Director of Clinical Practice, Advocacy, and Research Affairs, American Society for Parenteral and Enteral Nutrition (peggig@aspen.nutr.org; [610] 649-7994; http://www.nutritioncare.org).

Almost all patients who require rehospitalization do so because of problems with the catheter, and in our experience, mortality is usually due to the underlying disease process rather than to the therapy.[531] Dudrick and colleagues have accumulated more than 100 patient-years' experience with home TPN.[123] Catheter-related sepsis occurred seven times, equivalent to one episode per three catheter-years. Our group has also accumulated more than 100 years of patient experience.[169] Greater than one-half had at least one or more hyperalimentation-related complications—catheter sepsis, blocked or damaged catheters, and dehydration or electrolyte imbalance. Analysis seems to indicate that the only valued nutritional parameters in monitoring patient well-being are body weight and serum albumin.[535] Although this therapeutic modality is extremely tedious for the patient, it does permit an improvement in the quality of life.

Oral or Enteral Nutrition

The place of an elemental diet in the management of Crohn's disease has been evaluated. Teahon and colleagues reported success in inducing remission in 85% of 113 patients.[547] Some suggest that the remission rate may be comparable to that achieved with steroids.[16,392] Failure to tolerate the diet is, of course, one potential problem. Lochs and associates showed that enteral nutrition was less effective than a combination of 6-MP and sulfasalazine in treating active Crohn's disease.[319] Obviously, if the patient fulfills the same criteria for treatment as those selected for ambulatory hyperalimentation, it would seem that the preferred alternative is oral management, if indeed it can be adequately achieved.

However, drug therapy remains the primary approach, with no good evidence to suggest that nutritional therapy alone alters the clinical course of Crohn's disease or of ulcerative colitis.[406,562] TPN may play an adjunctive role in achieving remission in steroid-refractory Crohn's disease individuals who are unable to maintain the enteral route. There is little difference in efficacy with the type of TPN or enteral support regarding healing of fistulas or delaying surgery, and there is no superiority of elemental diets over so-called polymeric diets.

Comment

I state again, as I did in Chapter 29, that I do not defer needed surgery in order to employ TPN. The concept of short-term intravenous hyperalimentation may have certain theoretical advantages, but an expeditiously performed operation should allow an earlier resumption of oral intake, a much preferred method of administrating calories. If the patient is severely malnourished and can be placed in a more favorable nutritional state by such treatment, I obviously would have no objections. But there is no question in my mind that hyperalimentation, as the sole modality of therapy, cannot be justified.

Somatostatin

Somatostatin, a tetradecapeptide growth hormone release inhibiting factor, has been found to have a powerful inhibitory action on gastrointestinal endocrine and exocrine secretions.[115,274,383] As a consequence of its ability to profoundly decrease the volume and the enzyme content of the gastro-intestinal tract, the drug has been used in the management of intestinal fistulas. It therefore has particular merit for the treatment of patients with Crohn's disease, especially those individuals who have fistula complications.[527] Continuous intravenous infusion of somatostatin (250 μg/hour) has been demonstrated to result in reduced output and, in some cases, spontaneous fistula closure.[173] The synthetic analog, SMS 901–225 (Sandostatin), has been developed to provide a longer half-life with less influence on insulin secretion.[383] It has also been shown to prolong gastrointestinal transit time and to improve water and electrolyte absorption. The drug is supplied in 1-mL ampules containing 100 μg and is administered subcutaneously at a dose of 1 mL every 8 hours. I have had considerable success with a limited number of fistula patients who have been submitted to this treatment.

Probiotics

Probiotics are microbial supplements presumed to antagonize the effect of more noxious or pathogenic gut microorganisms. These microbial "cocktails" include *Lactobacillus* bifidobacteria, *Streptococcus salivarius*, and enterococci, as well as yeasts, such as sacchomonocytes, *Aspergillus*, or *Torulopsis*.[332]

The presumption is that the "good bugs" will replace the "bad bugs." These good bugs then will produce nutrients essential to gut integrity, prevent overgrowth of the more pathogenic organisms, stimulate the intestinal immune systems, and eliminate intestinal toxins. However, the experience in Crohn's is more limited than that which has been reported for ulcerative colitis (see Chapter 29). The discouraging news of the failure of *Lactobacillus* GG to prevent endoscopic recurrence or reduce the severity of recurrent lesions has dampened the initial enthusiasm.[423]

Growth Hormone, Glutamine, and Diet

There have been several papers from the Brigham and Women's Hospital of Harvard Medical School by Wilmore and colleagues that report a new method of treatment for individuals with short bowel syndrome through the administration of growth hormone, glutamine, and a specialized diet.[66,67,588] With this regimen, the investigators were able to reduce parenteral nutrition requirements in 80% of the more than 125 patients they treated. Furthermore, more than 40% were relieved of the TPN requirement completely. The theory concerning the efficacy of treatment is based on the fact that intestinal growth and adaptation are mediated in part by factors extrinsic to the gastrointestinal tract, such as growth hormone and thyroxine.[66] Furthermore, the amino acid glutamine is a primary energy source for the gastrointestinal tract by exerting trophic effects on the bowel and through stimulation of nutrient absorption.[66,67] The authors emphasize that such a bowel rehabilitation program offers patients a reduction in risk that is normally associated with TPN while improving an individual's lifestyle.[588]

Conclusion—Medical Management

The task of caring for the patient with Crohn's disease can be daunting. There is no "one size fits all" therapy. Each individual's condition and treatment response is unique. The challenge for the clinician is to continually remain informed as to the varied and evolving options in order to find the "right fit" for that person.

Operative Management

Indications

Operative treatment for Crohn's disease is advised primarily for complications (abscess, fistula, perforation, obstruction; see Figure 29-26) because surgical intervention may not cure the patient. Severe inanition, extraintestinal manifestations, and the presence or risk of malignancy are uncommon indications for surgery in this condition. It is well established that ulcerative colitis can produce toxic megacolon and perforation, but it is important to recognize that early in the course of the illness, Crohn's disease can also.[65]

Free perforation of the small bowel in Crohn's disease has been reported to occur in fewer than 1% of hospitalized patients.[197,198] *Hemorrhage* is rarely an indication for surgery with Crohn's disease, although the approach to surgical intervention tends to be somewhat more conservative than that with ulcerative colitis. Because the latter condition can be cured with resection, there is less tendency to procrastinate if hemorrhage is profuse. A more circumspect attitude generally pervades with Crohn's disease. Robert and colleagues identified 21 patients from the Mount Sinai Hospital who were admitted with severe lower intestinal hemorrhage.[451] Their data suggested that removal of diseased bowel with the initial episode of hemorrhage was probably the better option because 30% who were treated conservatively subsequently bled massively.

The presence of an *abscess* or *fistula* virtually excludes the diagnosis of ulcerative colitis. Internal and external fistulas associated with Crohn's disease are usually indications for surgical intervention.[182,187,197,254,292,569] As previously stated, TPN may succeed in effecting temporary closure, and the place of somatostatin has likewise been addressed.[173] However, patients almost invariably develop symptoms severe enough to justify surgical intervention. In the experience of Greenstein and colleagues, 36 of 38 patients (95%) eventually required operation.[204] Glass and colleagues suggest that an internal fistula is not an absolute indication for surgery and that severity of the symptoms should dictate the treatment.[183,184] Even if the fistula involves the bladder, the authors believe that urinary tract infection may respond to antibiotics, and spontaneous closure may occur, although this surely must represent a minority opinion.

Greenstein and coworkers identified 770 patients who underwent intestinal surgery for Crohn's disease during a 24-year period.[197] They felt that the disease presents essentially in two clinical patterns: perforating and nonperforating. Operations for perforating indications were followed by the requirement for reoperation approximately twice as often as those patients who underwent surgery for the other indication.

Abscess formation is usually a consequence of fistula in Crohn's disease.[201,533] Greenstein and associates reported that 20% of 230 patients with Crohn's colitis and ileocolitis underwent surgery for intra-abdominal abscess.[201] The most frequent site of origin was the terminal ileum, with the abscess located in the right lower quadrant.

Stricture is a common feature of Crohn's disease and a frequent indication for surgery. A number of reports suggest that abnormalities of collagen metabolism may be important in the pathogenesis of both fistulas and strictures and, in fact, may predate gross pathologic changes.[7]

Appendiceal Crohn's Disease

Crohn's disease confined to the appendix is a very unusual entity. In 1990, Ruiz and colleagues identified 85 cases limited to the appendix in the literature.[464] The disease was found most commonly in the second and third decades. The signs and symptoms mimicked those of acute appendicitis, with 27% having a palpable mass. The authors suggest that a protracted preoperative history of symptoms should alert the surgeon to this possibility. Lindhagen and associates identified 50 cases and added 12 of their own.[317] The indications for surgery in their patients were appendicitis in 8, appendiceal abscess in 2, suspected pyosalpinx in 1, and ovarian cyst in 1. All but two of the eight appendicitis patients underwent appendectomy, whereas the others underwent a more extensive resection. There was no incident of subsequent fecal fistula. With a median follow-up of almost 14 years and with no further manifestation of the disease, the authors concluded that when Crohn's disease is confined to the appendix, the prognosis is very favorable.

Acute Ileitis Masquerading as Acute Appendicitis

Occasionally, a patient is submitted to a laparotomy for presumed appendicitis and found to have distal ileal Crohn's disease (acute ileitis). There is some controversy about the appropriate management under these circumstances, the critical issue being whether one removes the appendix.[286,343,514] Simonowitz and associates reviewed the records of 20 patients who underwent incidental appendectomy and made the following recommendations: if the patient has abdominal pain for less than 1 week, appendectomy is followed by minimal complications.[514] For those who have symptoms longer than this period, incidental appendectomy is followed by an 83% incidence of fistula or sinus tract arising *not from the* appendiceal stump but from the terminal ileum. Most surgeons agree that the fistula arises from the ileum unless the cecum is involved with the disease. Weston and associates, reporting from the Lahey Clinic Medical Center, identified 36 patients who had laparotomy for presumed appendicitis and who were found to have Crohn's disease of the terminal ileum.[581] After initial ileocolic resection, one-half required no further resection, with a mean follow-up of more than 12 years. Conversely, 92% of those who did not undergo resection required ileocolic resection for intractability or complications of Crohn's disease. The authors concluded that most patients who are found to have Crohn's disease at laparotomy for appendicitis require an early ileocolic resection.[581] They opine that perhaps the traditional concept of nonresectional surgery for these individuals should be reevaluated.

My own preference is to perform an appendectomy if I am convinced that the cecum is normal. It simplifies the differential diagnosis in the subsequent evaluation of abdominal pain. In reality, however, right lower quadrant abdominal pain with the finding of peritoneal signs not related to the known Crohn's disease must be virtually unheard of.[435] And if it does occur, it is very likely to be associated with a long delay before one initiates surgical treatment.

The surgeon should exercise caution if terminal ileitis is identified at the time of operation for what was presumed to be acute appendicitis. It may be easier to advise than to perform, but the surgeon should not attempt to "break up" adhesions to the abdominal wall under these circumstances because of the risk of precipitating an abscess or a fecal fistula.

One must always be aware of the differential diagnosis in the presence of terminal ileitis. A self-limited process due to *Yersinia enterocolitica* should be considered, as should the diagnosis of *Campylobacter* (see Chapter 33).

Anal Manifestations

Anorectal abscess and anal fistula are frequent complications of Crohn's disease, especially when the condition involves the colon or rectum. If the disease is confined to the small intestine, however, anal manifestations are less common. In the absence of other areas of involvement, anorectal disease itself is rarely an indication for surgical intervention outside of the anus and perineum (Figure 30-59). However, in those patients with fecal incontinence or in whom a rectovaginal or anovaginal fistula develops, radical surgery may be indicated for these complications alone.[238] Under these circumstances, a permanent ileostomy or colostomy is usually required, but a temporary diversionary procedure may permit the surgeon to perform a reconstruction on selected patients. Linares and colleagues evaluated 44 patients with anorectal strictures complicating Crohn's disease to determine the natural history and outcome of surgical treatment.[314] Almost all had demonstrable proctitis. Approximately one-half required either a proctectomy or a diversion, whereas the remainder could be managed by means of periodic dilatations.

Definitive surgery has been recommended and has been successfully performed in patients with anal fistulas in Crohn's disease (see Chapter 14).[8,160,167,240,339] The success that these authors have had is, I am certain, due to careful patient selection. One must make the distinction between anal Crohn's disease and a fistula-in-ano arising in the patient who has IBD without anal involvement. In this latter group, definitive anal surgery may be undertaken with reasonable expectation of healing. This is particularly true if the involved bowel segment either has been resected or is quiescent. Conversely, healing of wounds in a patient with anal Crohn's disease or with active disease elsewhere in the gastrointestinal tract will often lead to chronic, draining, indolent, painful ulcers, which create more problems in management than did the original complaint (see Figure 14-52). To assess adequately the extent of disease, examination under anesthesia may be required. Endoscopic and/or radiologic evaluation of the entire gastrointestinal tract is a requisite before one considers definitive surgery in a patient with known or suspected anal Crohn's disease.

In a report from the Mayo Clinic of 86 patients with anorectal involvement, only those whose active proximal disease was removed benefited from conservative management.[595] On the

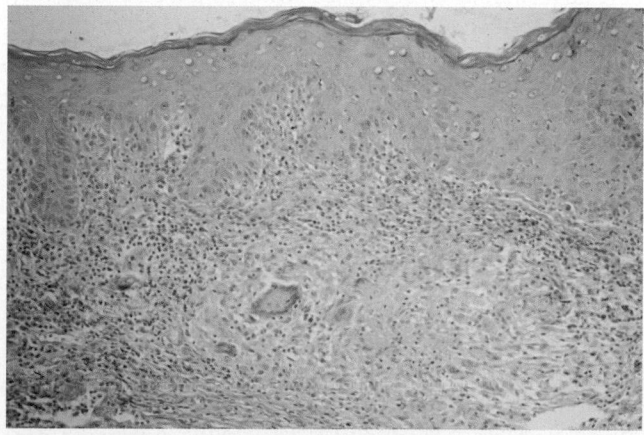

FIGURE 30-59. Anal Crohn's disease. This in anal biopsy from a patient with Crohn's colitis reveals a submucosal granuloma. Anal and rectal granulomas may occur in the absence of clinical disease in these sites.

basis of experience with 109 patients with perianal disease, Alexander-Williams and Buchmann recommend a conservative policy.[10] It is self-evident that the optimal form of therapy for anal Crohn's is medical management (see earlier) and simple drainage of an abscess when it occurs (see Chapters 13 and 14).[429] Long-term catheter or seton drainage may offer the best palliation for recurrent suppuration (see Figures 14-53 through 14-55). Treatment by local depot methylprednisolone injection (Depomedrone, 40 to 80 mg) has been attempted with some success in alleviating severe anal pain.[249]

Preparation of the Patient

For a discussion of preparing the patient, see Chapter 29.

Operative Approaches

Regardless of the choice of operation and irrespective of how radical the extirpation, surgery for Crohn's disease is primarily palliative, not curative. Therefore, operative intervention is recommended essentially for the complications that have been previously discussed. For individuals requiring surgery for disease involving the colon and rectum, proctocolectomy with ileostomy is considered the optimal operation, although preservation of the rectum may be contemplated if this area is relatively spared and/or compliant. When Crohn's disease affects other segments of the gastrointestinal tract, the choice of operation will depend on the location and the extent of disease. Most surgeons are of the opinion that restorative proctocolectomy and the continent ileostomy are contraindicated in individuals with granulomatous colitis, but some are selectively applying these alternatives (see later).

General Principles of Intraoperative Evaluation and Decision Making

Exploration of the abdomen will usually reveal the extent of pathology in those with Crohn's disease because this is a transmural inflammatory process and the serosa is virtually always involved. In fact, it is not uncommon to discover that the disease is more extensive than can be appreciated by preoperative evaluation. Conversely, with ulcerative colitis, one is usually unimpressed with the severity of inflammation as perceived from the serosal aspect.

The small intestine should be carefully examined, and the areas of disease identified and marked with sutures, if necessary. This is a particularly important principle if more than one segment is surgically treated. Measurement of the length of residual normal and diseased bowel (if left behind) is very helpful if further surgery is to be considered later.

Some surgeons had at one time thought it prudent to remove enlarged lymph nodes, believing that the nodes harbor a factor that predisposes the individual to recurrent disease. There is no evidence to suggest that this is the case, and the surgeon is not advised to pursue a more radical excision in an effort to eliminate this tissue.

An intra-abdominal abscess is not uncommonly encountered during the course of a laparotomy for Crohn's disease. Obviously, one would have preferred to have had the abscess drained preoperatively by means of a CT-guided approach. However, when an abscess is encountered at surgery, this does not necessarily mean that a stoma must be performed. Generally, the procedure should be undertaken as planned. In the St. Mark's Hospital experience of 28 patients who were found to have an abscess at surgery, only 4 required a stoma, but the complication rate was 43%.[258] Risk factors for intra-abdominal sepsis after surgery for Crohn's disease include preoperative low albumin level, steroid use, and the presence of an abscess or fistula.[600]

In patients with Crohn's disease, retroperitoneal inflammation may pose some risk for ureteral injury during mobilization of the right colon or the rectosigmoid. Care should be taken during this maneuver to identify the ureter and to keep it out of harm's way (see Chapter 24). Similarly, the duodenum is vulnerable to injury, particularly if transmural involvement by Crohn's disease causes fixation of the bowel to the second and third portions. Careful dissection between these structures must be performed by dropping the duodenum posteriorly until it is well out of the area of dissection. Shortening and thickening of the mesentery of the right colon and proximal transverse colon also predisposes the duodenum to possible injury. By clamping the blood vessels on one side only, dividing the mesentery on the bowel side, one is less likely to incorporate the side wall of the duodenum. Back-bleeding can then be addressed with the bowel delivered away from the area of potential injury. This maneuver is analogous to that which one may perform when dividing the lateral ligaments of the rectum.

When duodenal involvement occurs, either as primary disease (rare) or by secondary involvement from more distal Crohn's disease, a Kocher maneuver should be performed (Figure 30-60). Special care must be taken because the affected duodenum is often fibrotic. In the case of a fistula, the duodenum may need to be resected, but this is rarely necessary. Gastrojejunostomy is the preferred alternative, usually by freshening of the edges of the duodenal defect and by closing it, as with a strictureplasty (see later). However, there exists data on the value of performing a gastroduodenostomy, wherein normal intestinal flow is preserved. Here, the defect in the duodenum is closed by the strictureplasty technique. Where this is not feasible, then duodenal closure by duodenojejunostomy is accomplished with mucosa-to-mucosal anastomosis.

Because of the often very thick bowel mesentery, suturing generally requires stout (no. 1 chromic catgut or no. 1 Vicryl). If the vascular pedicle appears too large, one should incise the peritoneum in order to allow for seating of the suture more securely without encompassing as much fatty tissue. One may even employ a finger fracture technique in the dissection of the small and large bowel mesentery, similar to

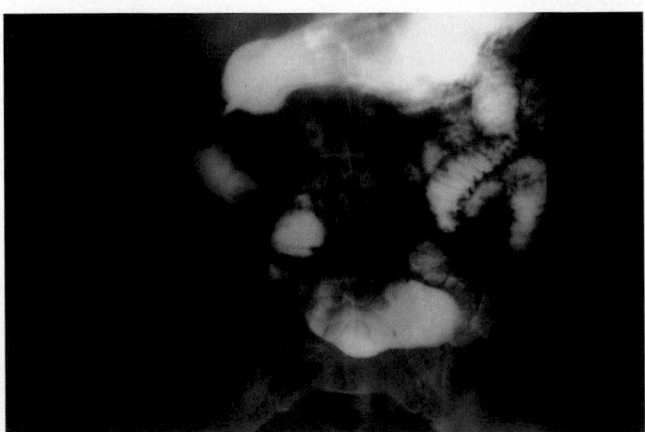

FIGURE 30-60. Duodenal Crohn's disease. Upper gastrointestinal series demonstrates long duodenal stricture as a consequence of primary disease in this area.

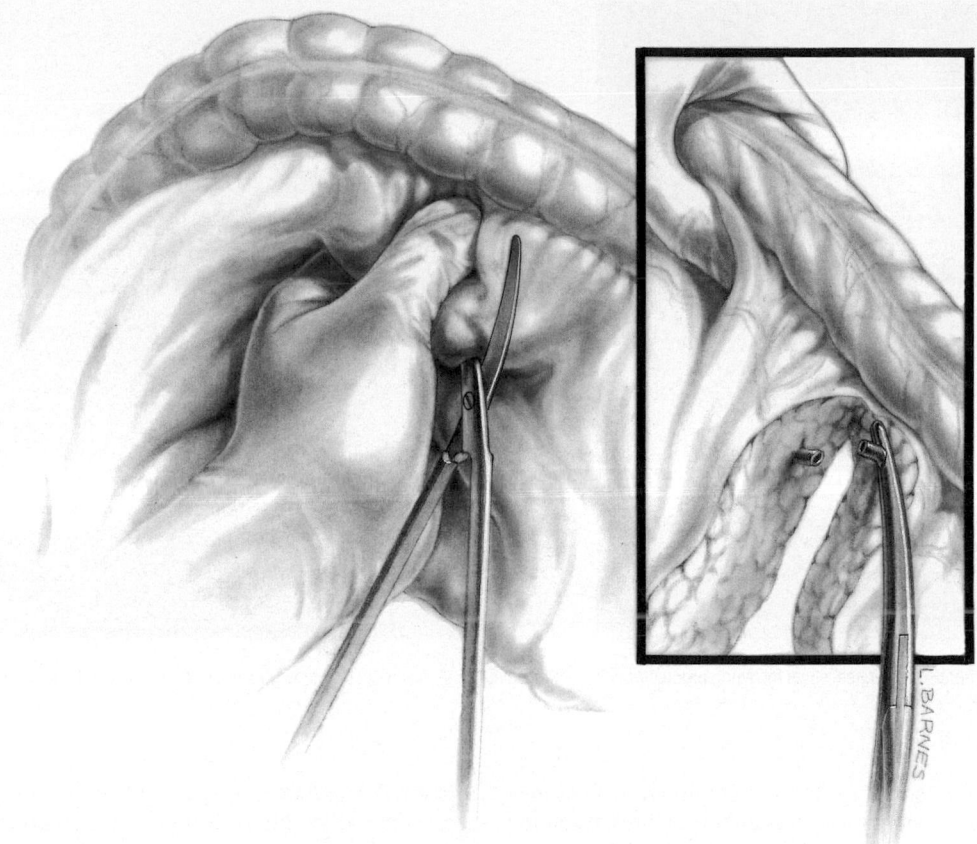

FIGURE 30-61. Division of thickened mesentery in a patient with Crohn's disease by finger fracture technique. *Inset:* Illustrates identification of the individual vessel for clamping.

that described for hepatic resection, identifying the vessels after the mesentery has been separated (Figure 30-61).[102]

Proctocolectomy

Proctocolectomy with ileostomy is the conventional operative approach for the treatment of ulcerative colitis and for most patients with Crohn's colitis in which the rectum or anus is involved. The technique is described in detail in the preceding chapter. Resection of the distal small bowel is sometimes necessary when proctocolectomy is undertaken for Crohn's disease, depending on whether the small bowel is involved by the inflammatory process. Even modest resection of the distal ileum may lead to rapid small bowel transit and malabsorption of nutrients, as well as water and electrolyte loss.[375] The surgeon should not remove any normal small bowel and should limit the resection of ileum to the minimum length necessary for extirpation of macroscopic disease (see Management of Small Bowel Crohn's Disease). An exception to this dictum, however, is that 1 to 2 cm of terminal ileum may be resected with advantage when there is doubt on the diagnosis (Crohn's disease of the terminal ileum or indeterminate colitis). Here, histology of the terminal ileum may be assessed with minimal risk of induction of short bowel syndrome and minimal risk of compromising the reach problem associated with construction of an ileal pouch and anastomosing it to the anal canal. The clinician may find that if occult Crohn's disease is present, subsequent treatment may be influenced.

An intraperitoneal ileostomy is the recommended technique for stomal creation in a patient with Crohn's colitis, in those who have already had a portion of the terminal ileum removed, and in those for whom "stripping" of the parietal peritoneum is technically impossible. The technique for creating an intraperitoneal ileostomy and obliteration of the lateral space is illustrated in Figure 29-45. The relative disadvantages of this procedure when compared with the extraperitoneal approach are mitigated by the occasional requirement for revision as a consequence of recurrent disease. This is easier to accomplish with an intraperitoneal ileostomy.

Complications. Most complications of proctocolectomy are not specific for this operation and are discussed in Chapters 23, 24, and 29. However, proctocolectomy for Crohn's disease is associated with a high incidence of complications, especially delayed perineal wound healing.[597,599] Sexual dysfunction, intestinal obstruction, and perineal difficulties are addressed in Chapter 29 (see Figure 29-47 and Figure 30-62).

STOMAL PROBLEMS. Stomal problems and their management are discussed in Chapters 31 and 32. A special concern is recurrence in the ileum or in the ileostomy following proctocolectomy for Crohn's disease (Figure 30-63). Although proctocolectomy is usually curative when Crohn's colitis is confined to the colon, rectum, and anus, between 10% and 20% of patients will develop a proximal recurrence, usually

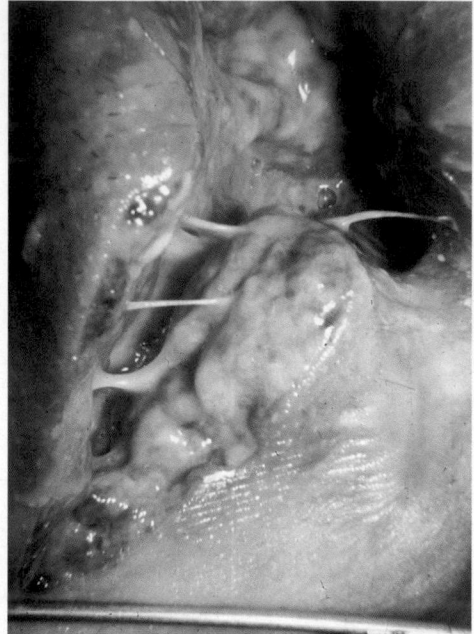
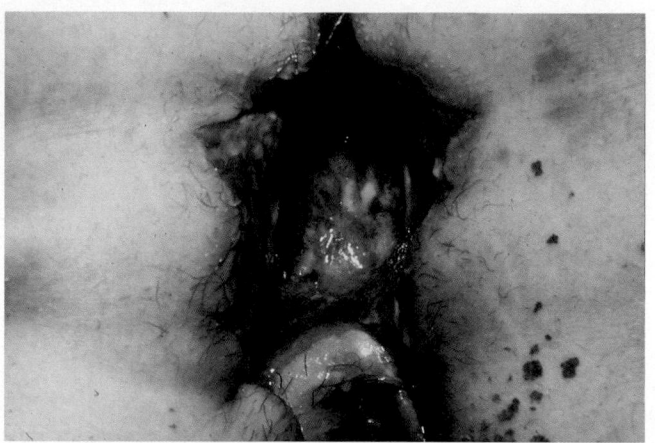

FIGURE 30-62. Persistent perineal sinus following proctectomy for Crohn's disease. **A:** Necrotic, purulent, open wound. **B:** Open, indolent perineal wound 9 months following proctectomy.

at or just above the ileostomy. The development of a paraileostomy abscess in a patient who has undergone resection for Crohn's disease implies recurrence until proved otherwise. Evaluation may include endoscopic examination of the ileostomy, radiologic investigation by means of a barium enema through the stoma, or both (Figure 30-64).

Treatment almost always requires resection of the involved ileum and ileostomy with relocation of the stoma to another site. In the acute situation, it may be possible to drain the abscess by inserting a clamp at the mucocutaneous junction and liberating the pus. This, then, can be incorporated in the ileostomy appliance with a drain left in the cavity. Alternatively, if the abscess "points" at some distance from the ileostomy, drainage should be effected outside of the faceplate of the appliance. Every attempt should be made to avoid draining the abscess directly under the faceplate because such a maneuver will inevitably make management of the ileostomy effluent most difficult.

RECURRENT CROHN'S DISEASE. Recurrent Crohn's disease can develop at any time following resection for the condition, even as early as a few days postoperatively. For example, occasionally one must reoperate on patients who underwent proctocolectomy and ileostomy whose entire small bowel was felt to be normal at the time of resection. Because of acute peritoneal signs, the

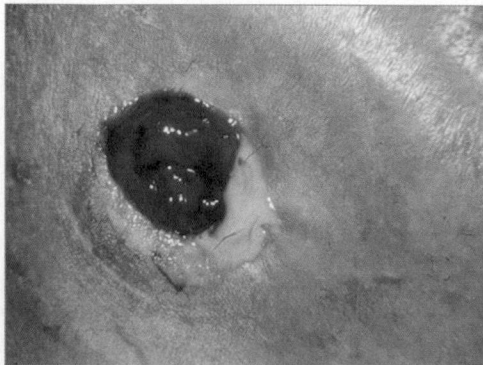

FIGURE 30-63. Paraileostomy abscess following proctocolectomy and ileostomy for Crohn's disease. The patient was demonstrated to have terminal ileal recurrence.

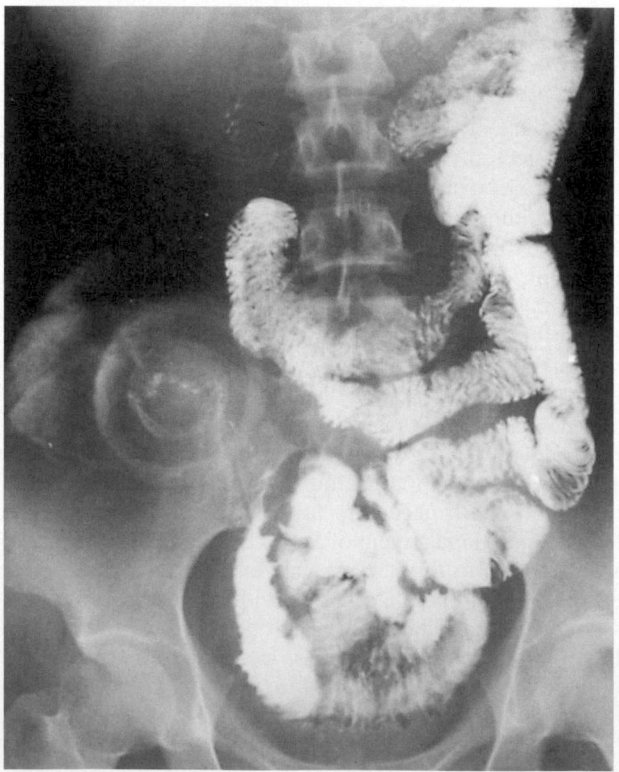

FIGURE 30-64. Recurrent Crohn's disease in distal ileum following proctocolectomy and ileostomy.

patients may require submission to re-exploration within 1 week of the surgery and can be found to have fulminant IBD involving extensive areas of the ileum and jejunum.

Results. In the experience of Goligher, 10 operative deaths were noted in 113 patients who underwent this operation for Crohn's disease, a rate of 9%.[188] Today this would be considered an unacceptably high rate. In the experience of the Birmingham, England, group, the operative mortality was 2% in 103 patients who underwent this procedure.[599] Today proctocolectomy and ileostomy can be carried out with minimal morbidity and mortality.

Recurrence following proctocolectomy for Crohn's disease, when the disease had initially been confined to the colon, has been reported to be between 10% and 25%, depending on the length of the follow-up.[22,188,281,532,599] Of Goligher's 162 patients treated by ileostomy and colectomy or proctocolectomy and followed for a mean of 15 years, 14.8% developed a recurrence.[190] Scammell and colleagues reported a cumulative reoperation rate at 5 and 10 years of 19% and 24%, respectively.[488] Male patients had a significantly higher incidence of recurrence than females in one study.[599] The prognosis appears to be better if total proctocolectomy is performed as compared with restoration of intestinal continuity.[386] The recurrence rates following restorative surgery in the small and large bowel are discussed later.

Ileostomy

Although ileostomy (without resection) for the management of toxic megacolon in patients with ulcerative colitis is generally recognized, it may also be usefully applied to those whose disease fails to respond to medical therapy or who have specific problems (e.g., perianal sepsis).[127,145] Zelas and Jagelman reported loop ileostomy as the sole initial procedure in 79 patients who were severely debilitated with Crohn's colitis, 91% of whom improved.[611] Definitive resection was then undertaken at a later stage without an operative death. They recommended loop ileostomy in certain severely ill patients with this disease. Likewise, Harper and associates discussed the value of ileostomy alone for IBD.[227] In 102 patients with Crohn's colitis, there was an immediate clinical improvement in 95, with sustained remission of symptoms for considerable lengths of time. It was possible to restore intestinal continuity subsequently in a number of patients who might otherwise have been treated by proctocolectomy. Winslet and colleagues found that 70% of their 44 patients who underwent fecal diversion for colonic Crohn's disease maintained a sustained period of remission.[589] Furthermore, diversion was associated with a significant reduction of steroid requirements and a significant improvement in the blood count as well as the serum albumin. They concluded with a statement that restoration of intestinal continuity for these individuals is quite problematic. Others have found that fecal diversion alone is associated with acute rapid clinical remission in the majority of patients with Crohn's colitis and severe perianal disease, but sustained benefit occurs less often.[127]

In the experience of Greenstein and Aufses, the incidence of perforation in toxic megacolon was three times higher for ulcerative colitis patients than for those with Crohn's colitis.[196] Without toxic megacolon, however, Crohn's disease was as likely to be associated with a perforation as was ulcerative colitis. Interestingly, mortality rates were better if the perforation occurred in a patient with Crohn's disease.

Harper and colleagues found that instillation of ileostomy effluent into the efferent limb of a divided or loop ileostomy may cause exacerbation of the IBD.[226] Others have attempted to use this information to determine selectively which patients could have the stoma closed without resection, but the results correlate poorly.[145,590]

The indications and technique for ileostomy with and without so-called blowhole colostomy are discussed in Chapter 29.

Colectomy with Ileorectal Anastomosis

For patients with colonic Crohn's disease and rectal sparing, colectomy and ileorectal anastomosis constitute the optimal procedure. This operation offers the best functional results for an individual who wishes to maintain intestinal continuity. Whether one is an appropriate candidate depends on the presence (or absence) of the following favorable criteria:

- Rectal sparing or relative rectal sparing
- Compliant rectum
- Absence of anal or perianal disease
- Normal, intact small bowel
- Absence of extraintestinal manifestations
- Individual motivated to avoid a stoma
- Individual motivated to be followed up closely
- Older age (?)

The technique is described in Chapter 23.

Results. Interpretation of the results of colonic resection is often difficult because some authors combine limited, segmental resection of the colon with that of total colectomy.[22,324] Farnell and colleagues reported the Mayo Clinic experience with rectal preservation in nonspecific IBD.[142] Eighty patients with Crohn's disease underwent colectomy and ileorectal or ileosigmoid anastomosis. Follow-up was a minimum of 5 years up to a maximum of 17 years. The rectum was felt to be uninvolved in 70%, and moderate disease was present in 19%. During this interval, no patient developed carcinoma in the residual rectum. The requirement for subsequent proctectomy was quite similar for both ulcerative colitis and Crohn's disease patients (24% vs. 29%, respectively). Whereas the quality of life was felt to be satisfactory in more than one-half of the patients with ulcerative colitis, only one-third of those with Crohn's disease were content.

Buchmann and colleagues reported 105 patients treated with colectomy and ileorectal anastomosis for Crohn's disease.[63] The mean follow-up was approximately 7.5 years. The presence or absence of ileal disease or perianal disease at the time of the anastomosis did not affect the prognosis, but patients with sigmoidoscopic evidence of inflammatory disease in the rectum appeared to do less well. The need for reoperation due to recurrence was calculated actuarially to be 50% after 16 to 20 years. The authors felt that the anastomotic procedure as described was a reasonable alternative for most patients with Crohn's colitis who do not have severe involvement of the rectum.

From the same unit, Keighley and associates performed balloon distention of the rectum and barium enema examination to assess rectal capacity.[266] They determined that a severely contracted rectum was associated with the need for a stoma in 6 of 7 patients, compared with only 2 of 13 patients who did not have radiologic signs of narrowing. A later study with a longer follow-up confirms the predictive value of maximum tolerated volume with respect to function of an ileorectal anastomosis.[578]

Ambrose and colleagues evaluated 63 patients with Crohn's disease treated by colectomy and ileorectal anastomosis.[19] At 10 years, the cumulative reoperation rate was 48%, and the cumulative recurrence rate was 64%. Even after resection for proximal recurrence, intestinal continuity could often be preserved. With a mean follow-up time of 10 years, two-thirds of the patients had an intact anastomosis. Goligher followed 45 patients treated by colectomy and ileorectal anastomosis for a mean period of 15 years and noted a recurrence rate of 71%.[190] Nineteen (42%) proceeded to rectal excision and ileostomy.

Mortensen and colleagues evaluated 18 patients who underwent emergency colectomy, 17 of whom were initially spared excision of the rectum, with subsequent proctectomy required in 10 individuals.[365] This result suggested to the authors that acute colonic Crohn's disease requiring surgery is less likely than ulcerative colitis to be amenable to restorative surgery despite a policy of rectal preservation.

In our experience, 131 patients underwent ileorectal anastomosis for Crohn's colitis.[325] After a mean follow-up of 9.5 years, 61% retained a functioning anastomosis, with 61% being free of disease. The mean stool frequency was 4.7 per day. Cattan and colleagues (Paris, France) noted that 63% of their 144 patients who underwent total colectomy had a functional ileorectal anastomosis 10 years following surgery.[76] Moreover, they observed that absence of extraintestinal manifestations and prophylactic treatment with 5-ASA were felt to be important facts associated with long-term rectal preservation. Others confirm that total colon resection without proctectomy can, in selected individuals with limited rectal disease, delay or avoid the necessity of a permanent stoma.[51,81,136,325,404,420]

Comment. Ileorectal anastomosis for Crohn's colitis is the procedure of choice when the rectum is relatively spared and when the patient does not have significant anal disease. With the passage of time, approximately one-third will develop symptoms severe enough to require either proctectomy or diversion. Even those who must undergo a second procedure can be relatively well served by temporarily avoiding an ileostomy. The problem, of course, is to select the appropriate patients, an exceedingly difficult task. One is often surprised at the degree of inflammatory reaction a patient may harbor in the rectum or indeed in the anal region and still have for a time a relatively salutary result following a restorative operation. However, patients who demonstrate pelvic sepsis, an intra-abdominal abscess, or a fistula to the rectum should probably undergo a diverting loop ileostomy to protect the anastomosis. This is obviously a surgical decision, and each patient must be treated on an individual basis. Preoperative decision making can be facilitated by a determination of rectal capacity and compliance. These physiologic studies are discussed in Chapters 5 and 7.

Those who are troubled by frequent bowel movements can often be helped by the addition of a bulk agent containing psyllium, as well as slowing medications such as codeine, deodorized tincture of opium, and diphenoxylate or loperamide. If resection of the distal ileum were performed, cholestyramine (Questran) may be helpful in controlling diarrhea.

Segmental Colon Resection

With Crohn's disease, restoration of intestinal continuity is certainly a viable option under many circumstances, depending on the location and the extent of involvement. Because the condition can occur anywhere in the gastrointestinal tract, it is difficult to discuss the operative choices as they pertain solely to the colon and rectum. However, it is probably appropriate to perform one of only three sphincter-saving operations for colonic disease: right hemicolectomy (for ileocolonic and right-sided involvement), total or subtotal colectomy (for disease involving at least one-half of the colon), and sigmoid colectomy or anterior resection (in the unusual situation when the disease is limited to this area). One may add abdominoperineal resection with sigmoid colostomy as another limited-resectional option for patients whose disease is limited to the anorectum and in whom the complications were unable to be controlled by local measures or fecal diversion alone.

Results. Results of segmental resection suggest that recurrence rates and requirement for reoperation are similar to that of total colectomy with restoration of continuity. Olaison and associates noted that lesions appear endoscopically soon after ileocolic resection, implicating new inflammation rather than residual disease or incomplete anastomotic healing.[390] Their data further suggest that despite clinical remission after complete extirpation of disease, the bowel is "permanently inflamed" in this condition. Longo and colleagues reported a recurrence rate of 62% in those treated by segmental resection and 67% managed by total colectomy.[324] In spite of these suboptimal statistics, more than 80% of patients were able to preserve bowel continuity. Andrews and coworkers noted cumulative reoperation rates at 5 and 10 years after right hemicolectomy to be 26% and 46%, respectively; after total colectomy and ileorectal anastomosis, it was 46% and 60%.[22] Allan and associates, reporting a very limited experience with segmental colon resection (colo-colonic anastomosis), implied that there is no difference in complication and recurrence rates when the procedure is compared with total colectomy and ileorectal anastomosis.[13] I question the validity of their observations, and I counsel against any anastomotic procedure in the colon except those previously mentioned. Still, Andersson and coworkers (Linköping, Sweden) opine that resection with colo-colic anastomosis should be considered in limited Crohn's colitis.[21] However, their numbers were few, and in the absence of a prospective study, I shall continue to stand by my opinion.

The perioperative morbidity associated with the performance of intestinal anastomoses in this condition has been prospectively reviewed in 429 patients from the University of Heidelberg.[302] Postoperative complications and mortality were observed in 9.7% and 0.5%, respectively. Besides the presence of sepsis at the time of operation, long-term corticosteroid therapy was the only variable found to significantly affect morbidity. No statistically significant association was observed with respect to age, gender, duration of disease, prior surgery, nutritional status, extent of disease, type, number and location of anastomoses, or presence of disease at the margin of resection.[417]

An interesting technical variation designed to reduce the incidence of recurrent disease was suggested by the Mayo Clinic group.[370] They performed a case-control comparative analysis of 138 patients, half of whom underwent conventional sutured end-to-end anastomosis; the other half received a wide-lumen stapled (side-to-side, function end-to-end) anastomosis. They found that the cumulative reoperation rate for anastomotic recurrence was significantly lower ($P = .017$) for the wide-lumen anastomosis group. It would therefore seem prudent to perform as large an anastomosis as is reasonable when the patient undergoes a colectomy for this indication.

Laparoscopic Resection

As with virtually all operations on the intestinal tract, laparoscopic techniques have been applied for resection in patients with Crohn's disease. The hypothetical and actual advantages such as earlier return of bowel function, reduced length of stay, less discomfort, faster recovery of pulmonary function, and more cosmetic incisions have been discussed elsewhere in this book (see Chapter 19). The greater benefit of this approach for this condition is the likelihood of the requirement for reoperation. Conversely, the disadvantage of the lack of tactile ability (unless a hand port is used), in an operation wherein careful inspection and even palpation of the entire small bowel must be performed, requires consideration. A further concern is that without tactile ability, occult bowel strictures may be missed. One must also be mindful that surgery for Crohn's disease may optimally involve hand dissection and specifically a finger fracture technique. A low threshold for conversion to an open operation should be maintained.

There is a rapidly expanding literature on the experience of laparoscopic resection for this condition.[22,36,124,138,229,329,361,494,577] Preliminary results suggest comparable recurrence rates. There may even be a reduced incidence of small bowel obstruction, a critically important issue in differential diagnosis and therapy with these patients.[36] Still, this can be a technically demanding approach—it is not for the novice laparoscopist, especially in the presence of a phlegmon, fistula, or abscess.[138]

Resection with Exclusion of Rectum (Hartmann Procedure)

As previously suggested, resection of the colon without reestablishment of intestinal continuity is a reasonable option in the management of Crohn's colitis. Guillem and colleagues reviewed the Lahey Clinic experience of such surgery to determine the factors relating to the fate of the rectal segment.[211] At a median follow-up time of 6 years, 70% had developed disease in the excluded rectum. Approximately one-half of the total series had undergone proctectomy by 2.4 years. Nineteen percent retained the rectum with disease. Neither initial involvement of the terminal ileum nor endoscopic inflammatory changes seen in the rectum predicted eventual disease of the excluded rectal segment. However, initial perianal disease was predictive of persistent rectal segment involvement, often requiring subsequent proctectomy. The authors suggest that early completion proctectomy or primary total proctocolectomy should be seriously considered in this group of patients. Harling and associates observed a 5-year cumulative ileal resection rate with an out-of-circuit rectum of 29%.[225] The 10-year risk of subsequent proctectomy was 50%.

Sher and associates noted that a Hartmann resection affords excellent palliation in individuals with severe anorectal disease.[506] Although none of their 25 patients subsequently underwent reestablishment of intestinal continuity, the authors felt that the problem of an unhealed perineal wound can be averted when elective resection is undertaken with quiescent anorectal and perianal disease.

Management of Small Bowel Crohn's Disease

The indications for surgery for regional enteritis include inanition, intra-abdominal sepsis, intestinal obstruction, fistulas, urologic complications, and extraintestinal manifestations. In the Lahey Clinic's reported experience with the long-term follow-up of small intestinal Crohn's disease, the most common indication for surgical treatment was chronic obstruction (35%), followed by internal fistulas (30%), intractability (22%), and abscess formation (11%).[536] Types of operation include limited small bowel resection, multiple small bowel resections (with enteroenterostomy and/or diversion), bypass, strictureplasty, balloon dilatation, and resection of small bowel in continuity with cecum, or right colon, or most or all of the colon, and rectum.

Acute Ileitis

As previously discussed, occasionally a patient is submitted to laparotomy with a presumed diagnosis of acute appendicitis. The appendix may be safely removed if there is no evidence of cecal disease. Conversely, if the cecum appears to be involved by the inflammatory process, appendectomy may result in a fecal fistula. Laparotomy alone may lead to a fistula through handling of the diseased bowel, presumably from disrupting microperforations of the distal ileum.[147] In any event, resection of the ileum is not advised under these circumstances. In an extensive review of the incidence of progression of regional enteritis involving only the distal ileum, Gump and associates reported that fewer than 10% of patients developed subsequent identifiable ileitis.[212]

Small Bowel Resection

When an operation is indicated for other than acute ileitis, resection of the involved segment is usually performed. The choice of operative procedure depends on the intra-abdominal findings, including the length of segment or segments involved, the location within the intestinal tract, whether there is concomitant colonic involvement, the presence of a fistula or abscess, whether bowel had been resected previously, how much one is removing, and how much would remain. It is not usually difficult to identify the area of involvement because of the macroscopic appearance of the serosal surface of the bowel—fat wrapping, inflammatory changes, stricture, and so on. Still, it is discouraging to note that in a study by Lescut and coworkers, 65% of patients operated on for Crohn's disease had lesions of the small intestine undetected by the surgeon but which were identified by means of perioperative endoscopy of the whole small bowel.[307] It appears then that recurrence may not truly represent recurrence in every instance but may represent persistent disease.

Small bowel resection is usually a rather straightforward procedure, an operation that is familiar to all general surgeons. A special concern is the often remarkable thickness of the mesentery. It is sometimes helpful to simply divide the mesentery without the use of clamps, maintaining pressure on the blood supply with the fingers, and then performing suture ligation of the cut ends of the vessels (see Figure 30-61). This will certainly expedite what can be a tedious dissection, one that can lead to significant blood loss and a large mesenteric hematoma. The finger fracture technique has been mentioned earlier.[102] Transillumination of the mesentery is another method for identifying the blood supply to the bowel (Figure 30-65). It is a particularly useful method when creating an ileostomy or performing a pouch procedure. To ensure adequacy of the blood supply to the area, the overhead light is lowered or, preferably, a portable lamp is used. (Goligher took great pride

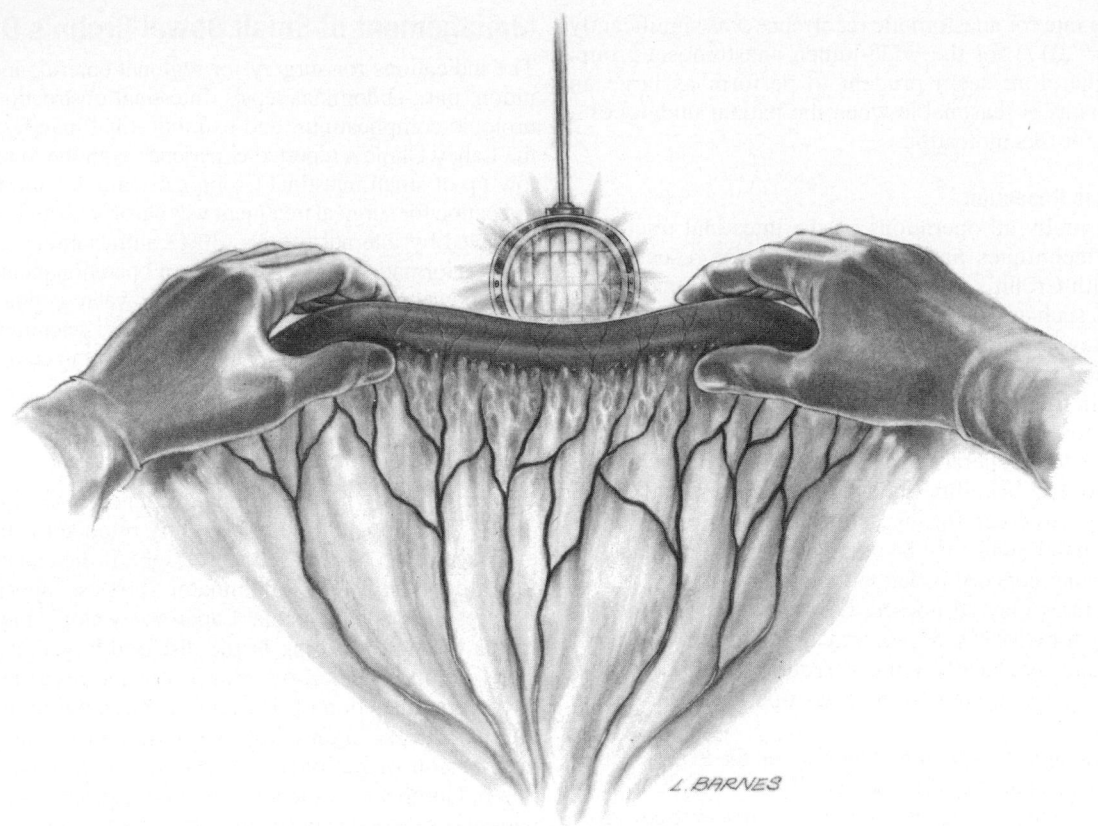

FIGURE 30-65. Transillumination is a useful technique for identifying the mesenteric blood supply. When tailoring the distal ileum in preparation for an ileostomy or the creation of a pouch, this approach can be invaluable.

in mounting a Rolls-Royce headlamp on a pole in the operating room. The concept was that if you could see the backcountry road surface on a foggy night in Yorkshire, this light should permit you to visualize the blood supply to the small bowel.)

The intestine is elevated to reveal the vascular structures. If one uses a sharply pointed forceps and paired straight clamps, the mesentery can be divided much more expeditiously than with the familiar curved clamp "poke-through and hunt for the opening" method (Figure 30-66). Although it has been said that the small bowel can be safely reapproximated with chewing gum and baling wire, an interrupted single-layer technique or stapling method is suggested (Figures 30-67 through 30-69).

Resection is usually undertaken leaving a minimum normal bowel margin of 5 or 6 cm. If multiple "skip" areas are present, one endeavors to remove or bypass only the most constricting portions that may be causing the symptoms. If two segments are involved in relative proximity (e.g., <30 cm), it is probably safer to perform an en bloc resection of both segments rather than to perform two anastomoses. Another option is that of combination strictureplasty (see the following section). In the situation where small bowel preservation is critical and where two or more medium length strictures are close together, the enterotomy may be made sufficiently long as to encompass both strictures.

Smedh and colleagues have suggested an innovative concept to prevent coloileal reflux after ileocecal resection.[519] They believe that reflux of intestinal contents may be responsible for recurrence at and just proximal to the anastomosis. The technique is shown in Figure 30-70.

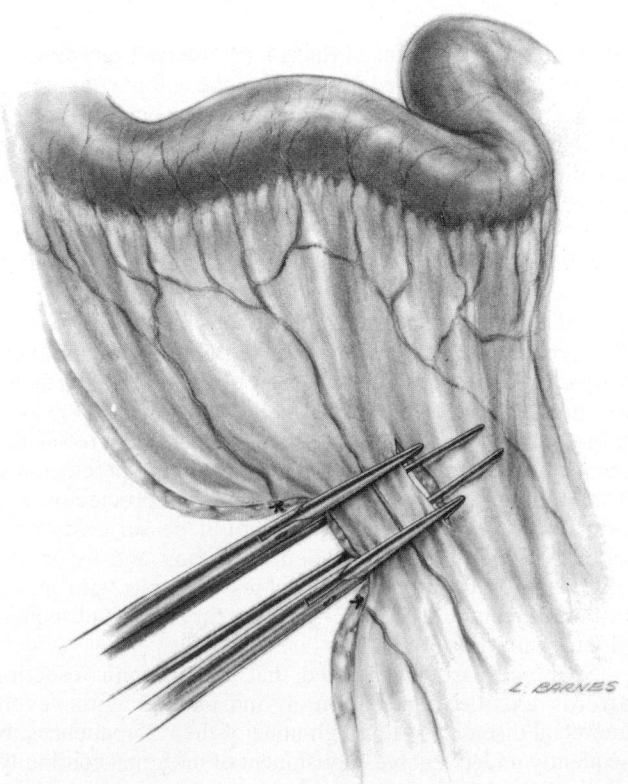

FIGURE 30-66. Small bowel resection using sharply pointed forceps and paired straight clamps.

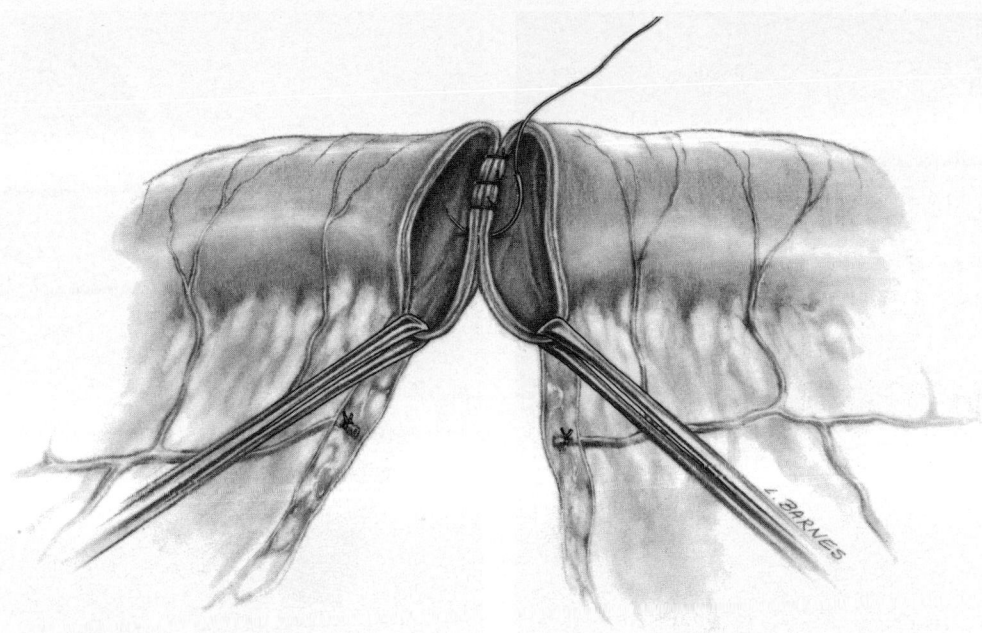

FIGURE 30-67. Small bowel resection. Anastomosis by conventional, interrupted, inverting, single-layer suture.

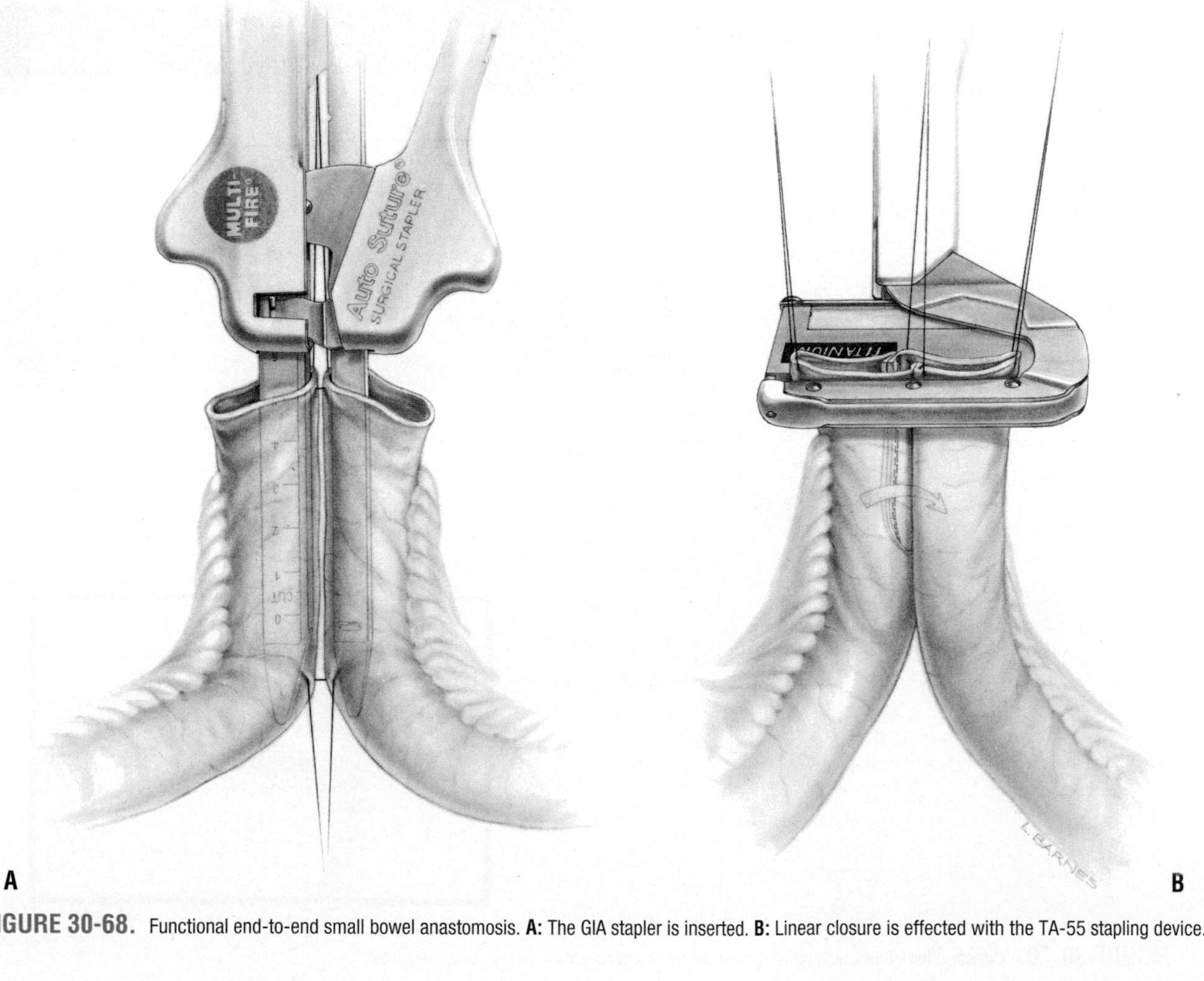

A

B

FIGURE 30-68. Functional end-to-end small bowel anastomosis. **A:** The GIA stapler is inserted. **B:** Linear closure is effected with the TA-55 stapling device.

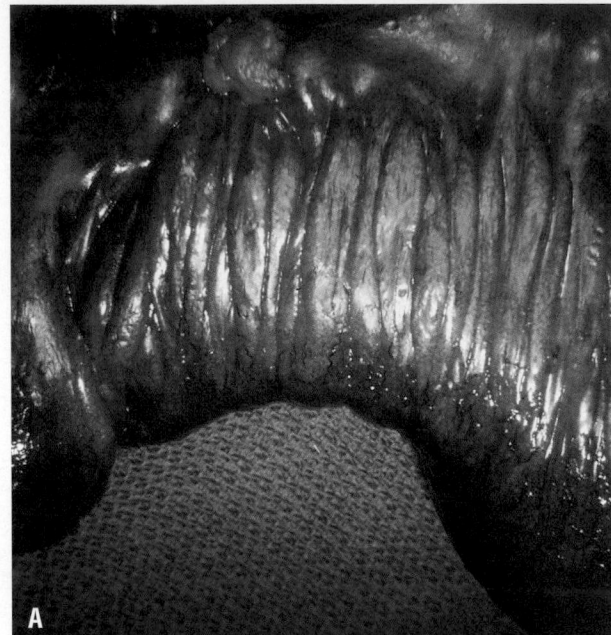

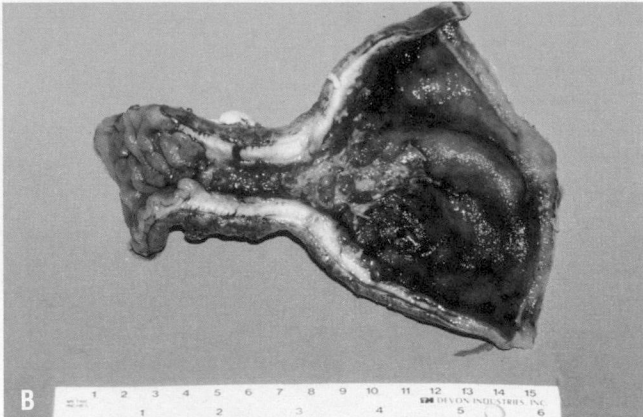

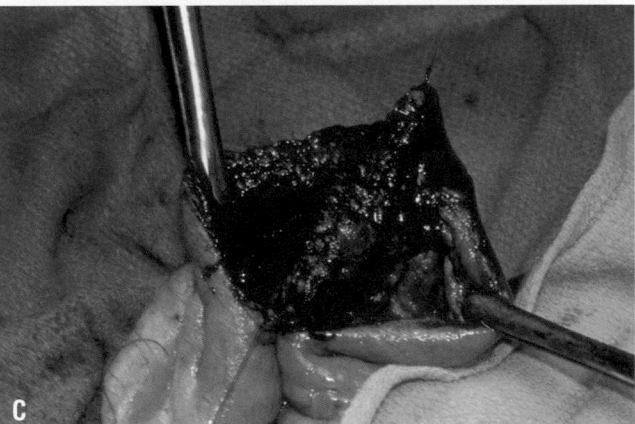

FIGURE 30-69. Small bowel resection for Crohn's disease. Note fat wrapping. **A:** Resected specimen showing thickened bowel with proximal dilatation **(B).** Posterior layer of anastomosis completed **(C).**

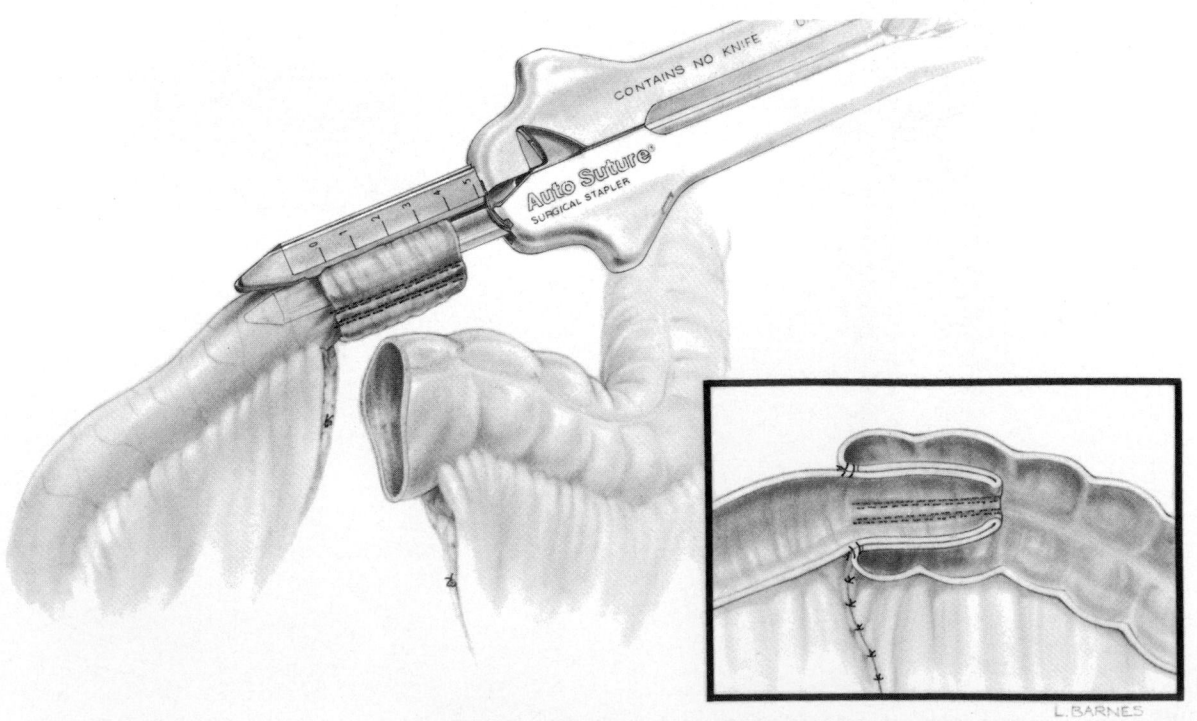

FIGURE 30-70. Construction of ileocecal nipple anastomosis as advocated by Smedh and associates.[519]

The authors observed that there was a suggestion of radiologically demonstrable preserved nipple function and remission of disease when compared with patients who underwent conventional anastomosis and those who had no visible nipple on follow-up examination. Further information on this concept is warranted.

Strictureplasty

Radical excision of the small bowel in an attempt to remove all obvious disease may result in profound disturbances in fluid and electrolytes as well as severe malnutrition (Figure 30-71). In recent years, strictureplasty has been suggested as an alternative in this situation (Figure 30-72).[9,55,64,112,148,151,330,397,399,545,555,558,559,596] The procedure was originally advocated by Katariya and colleagues for the treatment of tubercular strictures but was successfully applied to the management of extensive Crohn's disease by Lee and Papaioannou.[262,298] The primary indications are the presence of multiple, relatively short strictures and the need to conserve intestinal length because of extensive disease or prior resection. The procedures advocated for pyloroplasty (either Heineke-Mikulicz for short strictures or Finney for long ones) may be used (Figures 30-72 to 30-74). An interrupted single-layer technique is less likely to cause luminal narrowing, and patching the suture line to the serosa of the adjacent bowel may help prevent leakage.[551] Taschieri and coworkers offer a number of bowel-sparing techniques for the management of long strictures due to Crohn's disease (Figures 30-75 to 30-77).[545] As with all operations designed to coapt intestine, a stapler modification may also be used, but the presence of thickened bowel may preclude the application

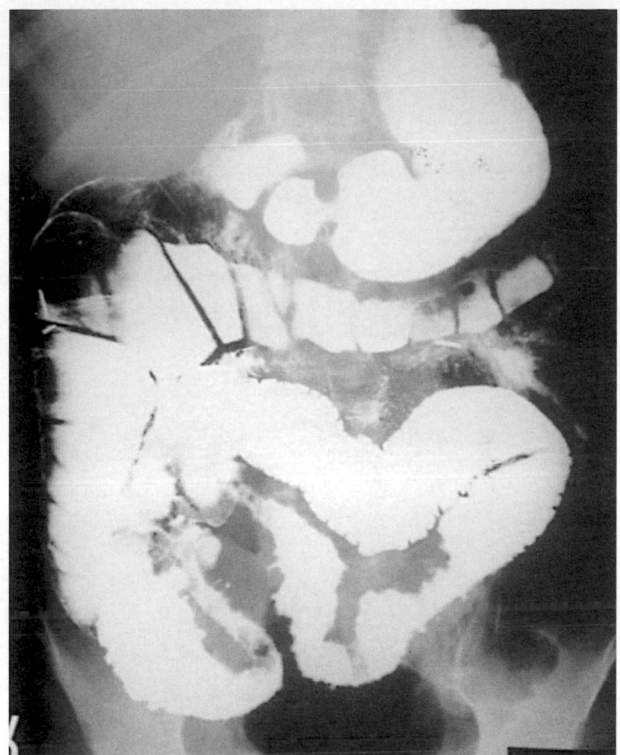

FIGURE 30-71. Upper gastrointestinal small bowel series demonstrates only a limited amount of small bowel remaining in an individual who had previously undergone several resections. Note that the small intestine which remains is extensively involved by recurrent Crohn's disease. Parenthetically, the colon appears spared.

EMANOEL CECIL GRUEBER LEE (1933–1986)

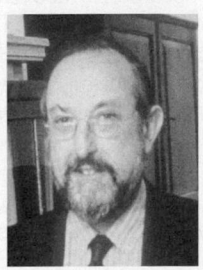

Emanoel Lee was born in Johannesburg, South Africa, the son of a physician. He was educated at Parktown High School and studied medicine at the University of the Witwatersrand, where he graduated with his MB, ChB degree in 1955. Following junior faculty appointments in South Africa, Lee traveled to England and completed his surgical training at St. George's Hospital in London. He transferred to Oxford in 1968, initially as a first assistant, later becoming a clinical reader for the Nuffield Department of Surgery. In 1972, he earned his ChM from the University of the Witwatersrand. He was appointed consultant surgeon at Oxford and held a Hunterian Professorship at the Royal College of Surgeons in 1975. In addition to his distinguished surgical career, Lee was a devoted historian with a passion for South African history. In 1985, he published his first book, *To the Bitter End: A Photographic History of the Boer War, 1899–1902*. His artistic contributions were extraordinary and included numerous paintings and sculptures. He was known for his charisma, and he had a huge circle of friends in the United Kingdom and throughout

the world. His clinical interests were mainly in gastroenterology at the same unit being formed at Oxford by another icon, Sidney Truelove. Lee was known primarily for his introduction of bowel-sparing strictureplasty in patients with extensive Crohn's disease. It was during a sabbatical trip to India that Lee became interested in this operation. An Indian surgeon, Katarya, practiced small bowel conservation surgery for multiple tuberculous strictures of the small bowel. Lee reasoned there were close parallels with that of strictures due to Crohn's disease. Upon his return to Oxford, he related his observations to Sidney Truelove. Truelove in turn became enthusiastic about this possibility as a reasonable alternative to multiple resections when medical treatment had failed. In 1982, Lee published his experience with nine individuals treated by a variety of strictureplasty techniques, noting that long-term results were promising. To this day, variations of his technique including isoperistaltic side-to-side and combination strictureplasties are commonly used for the surgical treatment of Crohn's disease. Lee continued his surgical career at Oxford until his early, sudden death on January 25, 1986, at the age of 52. (Courtesy of Obituary. *Br Med J.* 1986;292:835 and Brett T. Phillips, MD.)

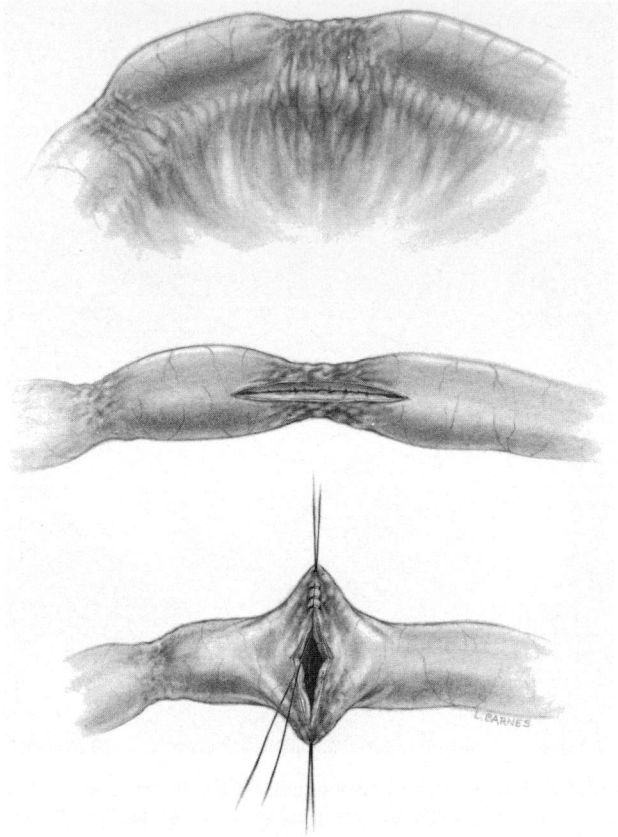

FIGURE 30-72. Strictureplasty for Crohn's disease. Short stricture treated by the technique analogous to Heineke-Mikulicz pyloroplasty. Longitudinal enterotomy is closed transversely using interrupted no. 3–0 long-term absorbable sutures.

of this instrument (Figures 30-74 and 30-78).[64,107,265] Kendall and colleagues suggest the use of a 2-cm bougie to identify all areas of significant narrowing.[268] Alexander-Williams prefers to use a Foley catheter,[9] whereas García-Granero and coworkers recommend a 2.5 cm medical plastic sphere.[170] One may combine strictureplasty with limited small bowel resection and bypass, all within the same individual, depending on the operative findings (Figure 30-79).

One of the concerns that has been expressed is the possibility of performing strictureplasty in the presence of cancer arising in Crohn's disease. It is therefore prudent to perform a small biopsy of the full thickness of the bowel before completing the procedure, obtaining frozen sections to confirm the absence of malignant change. We also recommend that the site(s) of the strictureplasty(ies) be marked with a titanium clip for subsequent radiologic and possible operative localization.

Results

Alexander-Williams reviewed 146 procedures performed on 57 patients without a death.[9] There were four anastomotic leaks, and eight required reoperation 6 months to 3 years later. Kendall and colleagues treated seven patients by a total of 45 strictureplasties.[268] Two developed enterocutaneous fistulas; recurrent symptoms were noted in six, four of whom required surgery.

Our group has reported what is inarguably the world's largest experience with strictureplasty.[398] The latest publication involves 162 patients who underwent a total of 698 strictureplasties (Heineke-Mikulicz, 617; Finney, 81). The mean number performed for each individual was three. There were no deaths. The cumulative 5-year incidence of reoperation for recurrence was 28%, with a mean follow-up of 42 months. Symptoms of obstruction were relieved in 98% of the patients. Reoperative rates were comparable to that of resection.[398] For patients treated by strictureplasty alone, the cumulative reoperation rate at 5 years was 31%, whereas for those who underwent concomitant bowel resection it was 27%. In another report from the Cleveland Clinic with longer follow-up, we concluded that strictureplasty is a safe and durable alternative to resection for diffuse Crohn's jejunoileitis, but those with a short duration of disease and reduced interval since the last surgery are at an increased risk of accelerated recurrence.[112]

Saylan and colleagues studied the need for reoperation following this procedure.[487] The results were also not significantly different from those individuals treated by resection. Others have confirmed the comparative safety and effectiveness of this operation.[9,55,64,104,399,545,558] Moreover, there is ample radiologic, endoscopic, histopathologic, and operative evidence that active Crohn's disease regresses at the site of the strictureplasty, especially when a large anastomosis (i.e., Finney type) has been performed.[356,555,559] For example, with the use of abdominal ultrasound, Maconi and colleagues found that the thickening of diseased bowel wall may improve after conservative surgery, a favorable prognostic factor.[330]

We have also performed strictureplasty for recurrent disease at the ileocolic anastomosis.[557] In 22 individuals so treated, there was no mortality or major septic complication. This method is therefore recommended to preserve small bowel length and as a reasonable alternative to re-resection.[557]

Balloon Dilatation

Another alternative to the management of colonic strictures is balloon dilatation. This technique has been performed successfully via the colonoscope with the use of the Riglex TTS dilating balloons.[377] Williams and Palmer have undertaken the procedure in seven patients without complication.[584] Two were unsuccessful, but five exhibited sustained improvement for up to 2 years. Alexander-Williams has used operative balloon dilatation of strictures between 20 and 25 mm in diameter, whereas Neufeld and colleagues noted that endoscopic application of the electrosurgical sphincterotome can be applied to fibrotic strictures.[11,377]

Management of Enteric Fistulas

Approximately 30% of patients with Crohn's disease will develop a fistula; one-third of these will be external. An external fistula may be the manifestation by which the patient presents initially, but it is obviously much more commonly recognized as a postoperative complication. The nonsurgical approach to this problem has been discussed previously (see Medical Management). Hill and colleagues reported the principles of surgical and metabolic management in accordance with a standard protocol[239]:

- Drainage of the septic process
- Correction of any metabolic deficits
- Identification of anatomy and the pathologic process
- Resection of the origin of the fistula and closure of the target organ defect

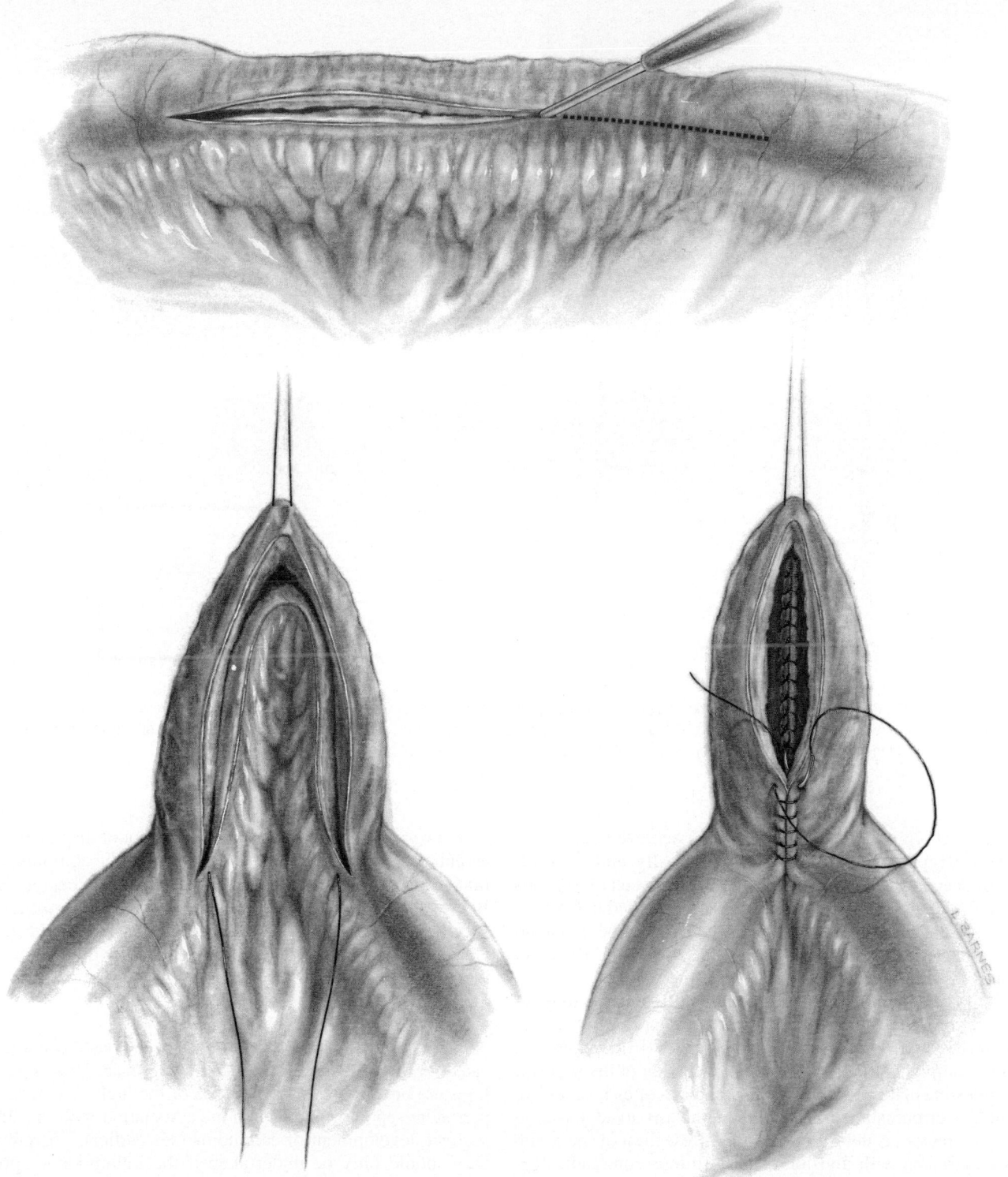

FIGURE 30-73. Strictureplasty for Crohn's disease. Long stricture treated by equivalent of Finney "pyloroplasty" technique. A long antimesenteric incision is made over the stricture site and carried into the normal bowel.

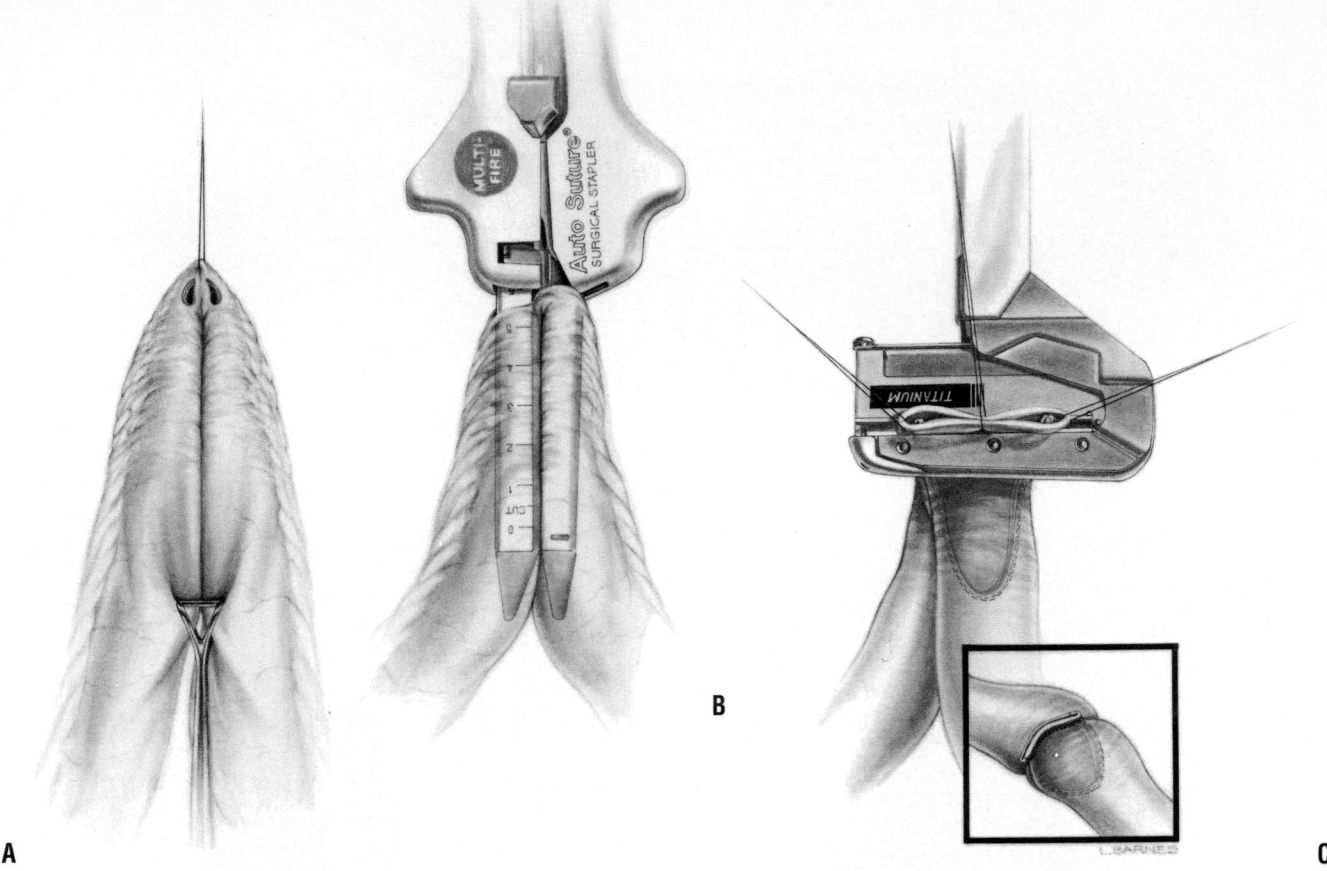

FIGURE 30-74. Stapled strictureplasty for Crohn's disease. **A:** The midpoint of the stricture becomes the apex; the bowel is held in position by means of a suture or a Babcock clamp. Two small enterotomies are created. **B:** The two limbs of the stapler are inserted and fired. The stapler instrument size may be changed to accommodate the length of the stricture. **C:** The linear stapler is fired. A biopsy specimen may be obtained by trimming the residual tissue (*inset*).

In a group of 85 patients, 69 (82%) achieved successful closure (approximately one-half surgically and one-half spontaneously). The authors distinguish between two groups of individuals: those whose fistulas are unrelated to Crohn's disease and those with known residual IBD. They contend that enterocutaneous fistulas arising from diseased small intestine all require surgery.

When an enteroenteric fistula is identified, it is important to try to ascertain whether the bowel is primarily or secondarily involved by Crohn's disease (Figure 30-80). For example, in the latter situation, resection of the segment of intestine that is not actually diseased can often be avoided. Such a circumstance arises when the involved terminal ileum creates an ileosigmoid fistula. Resection of the ileum is undertaken with division of the fistulous communication to the sigmoid colon. Whether resection of the sigmoid is appropriate depends on the degree of inflammatory reaction; if the opening can simply be sutured, no resection is advised.

Saint-Marc and colleagues reviewed their experience with 74 patients who harbored 100 internal fistulas.[476] Closure of the defect of the so-called victim organ was achieved by resection in 41 instances and sutured in 59. In the Mayo Clinic experience involving 90 patients with ileosigmoid fistula secondary to Crohn's disease, repair rather than resection did not increase the risk of complications, provided that standard surgical principles were applied.[608] Others confirm that the procedure can be accomplished with minimal morbidity and mortality.[357]

If a *vesical fistula* develops, management of the bladder is essentially the same as that described when the communication is a consequence of radiation injury (see Chapter 28). Because there is no disease affecting the bladder itself, no specific measures aside from urinary drainage are indicated. Cystoscopy is the most accurate investigative procedure for identifying such a fistula.[354]

Bypass or Exclusion

A bypass or exclusion procedure has in the past been advocated for distal ileal and cecal Crohn's disease. These operations are open to criticism because of the high incidence of persistent septic problems and the association with the subsequent development of carcinoma (see earlier). Therefore, they should only be undertaken if the inflammatory process cannot be removed for technical reasons or because of comorbid conditions.

One exception to the caution of applying bypass is in patients with duodenal Crohn's. A gastroenterostomy is often advised in this circumstance, but a strictureplasty should definitely be considered (see earlier discussion).

Continent or Kock Ileostomy

As stated earlier, the application of the continent ileostomy in the management of Crohn's colitis is contraindicated. The technique is described in Chapter 29. Myrvold and Kock reported 52 patients with Crohn's disease who underwent

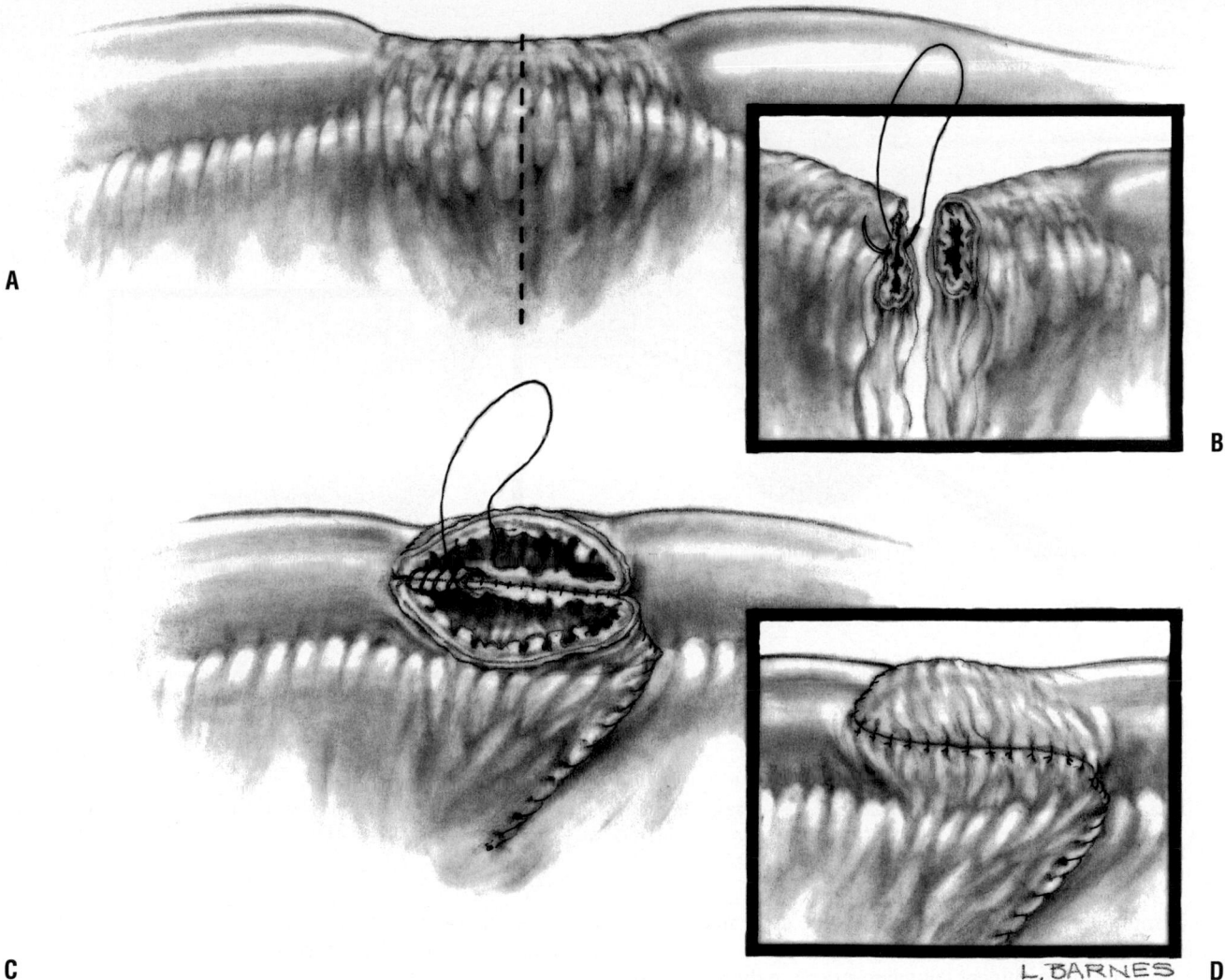

FIGURE 30-75. Crohn's stricture. **A:** Severe narrowing of a long segment of small bowel. **B:** The bowel is transected. **C:** Suturing of the two ends by means of a two-layer, hand-sewn running suture. Approximation of the two segments in a parallel fashion. **D:** Completion of side-to-side ileal-ileal anastomosis. The original lumen has been doubled, thus sparing half the length of the intestine. (After Taschieri AM, Cristaldi M, Elli M, et al. Description of new bowel-sparing techniques for long strictures of Crohn's disease. *Am J Surg.* 1997;173:509.)

continent ileostomy.[374] Most were performed in the mistaken belief that the patient had ulcerative colitis. Recurrence in the reservoir and/or distal ileum occurred in 53%. Although the functional results were in general reasonably satisfactory, the incidence of postoperative and late complications was significantly higher than that which was observed in those who underwent the procedure for ulcerative colitis.

There are "courageous surgeons" (I prefer the phrase "courageous patients"), however, who believe that the procedure can be applied selectively to some individuals with this disease. The usual circumstance is the patient who underwent proctocolectomy and conventional ileostomy a number of years previously, with no evidence of recurrence in the interim. With this scenario, one may be willing to accept the risks of high morbidity and recurrent disease, and with appropriate patient consent proceed to a continent ileostomy. However, one must remember the issues and concerns expressed earlier in this chapter. I refer to the support for the concept of creating a large anastomosis or a wide-open strictureplasty. By producing a distal obstruction, one changes

the environment to the extent that it is quite likely that the risk of recurrence will be considerably increased.

Bloom and colleagues reported the clinical course of seven patients who were submitted to this procedure.[50] All were women, with a mean disease-free interval before conversion of nearly 8 years (minimum, 5 years). The postoperative complication rate and revision rate of 28% was comparable to that which is observed when the operation is performed for ulcerative colitis or multiple polyposis (see Chapter 29). No patient underwent conversion to a conventional ileostomy. Gerber and associates also reported success in patients with Crohn's colitis, but their experience with ileocolitis, even with removal of the entire diseased bowel, was associated with a prohibitively high incidence of postoperative complications.[177] Handelsman and coworkers reported their experience from the Johns Hopkins University Hospital with eight patients diagnosed with Crohn's disease or colitis of indeterminate origin who underwent a continent ileostomy.[223] All required removal of the pouch or continued medical management for recurrent disease. In their opinion

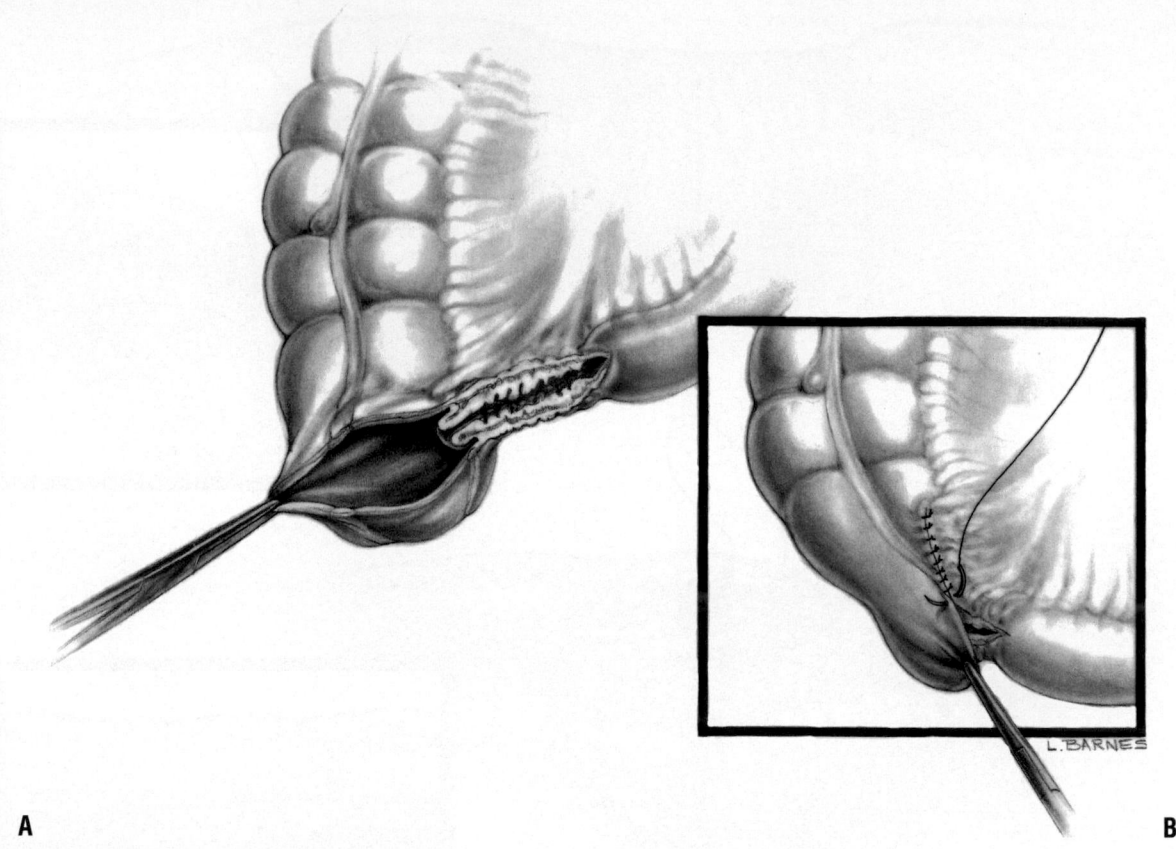

A

B

FIGURE 30-76. Terminal ileal Crohn's disease. **A:** Severe disease with extensive narrowing at the level of the ileocecal valve. **B:** Side-to-side ileocolic anastomosis. (After Taschieri AM, Cristaldi M, Elli M, et al. Description of new bowel-sparing techniques for long strictures of Crohn's disease. *Am J Surg.* 1997;173:509.)

and in mine, Crohn's disease is an absolute contraindication for performing this operation.

Barnett used a continent jejunal reservoir in three patients with colonic Crohn's disease, theorizing that there should be a reduced risk of recurrence in a pouch constructed at such a proximal level.[32] The new pouch and valve are transplanted and anastomosed to the terminal ileum. This concept proved to be disastrous for all concerned.

Restorative Proctocolectomy (Ileo-Pouch Anal Procedure)
The experience with the restorative proctocolectomy in this condition is based primarily on those who underwent the

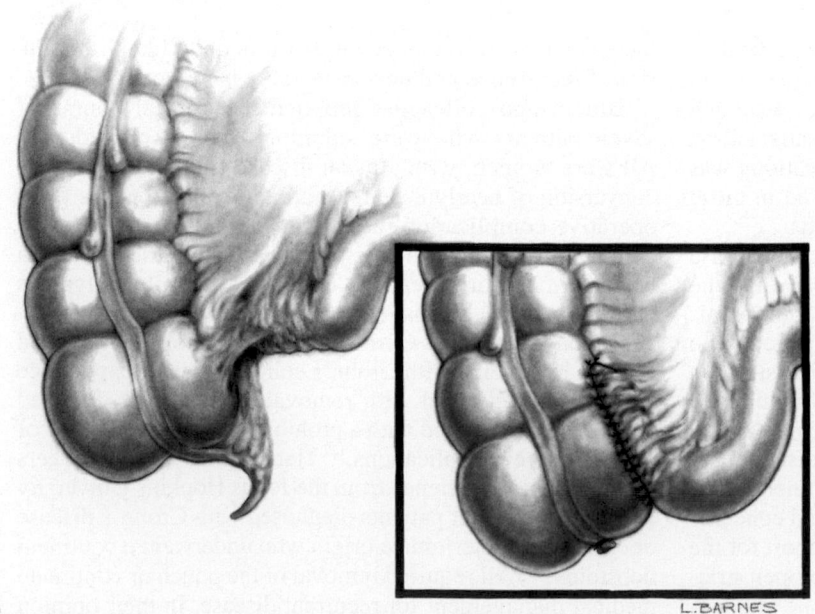

A

B

FIGURE 30-77. A: Marked narrowing of the terminal ileum with associated narrowing at the level of the ileocecal valve. **B:** Side-to-side ileocolic anastomosis. (After Taschieri AM, Cristaldi M, Elli M, et al. Description of new bowel-sparing techniques for long strictures of Crohn's disease. *Am J Surg.* 1997;173:509.)

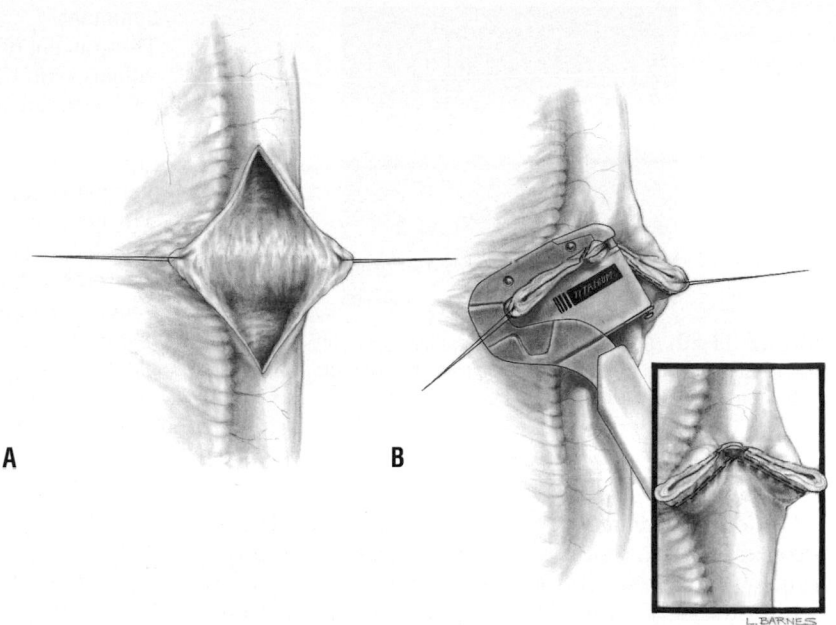

FIGURE 30-78. Stapled strictureplasty. **A:** The bowel is opened in a longitudinal fashion. **B,C:** Using a linear stapler and overlapping staple lines, the strictureplasty is performed.

operation for presumed ulcerative colitis only to discover after pathologic assessment of the surgical specimen that the diagnosis was in error. Another group of patients who have undergone this procedure are those who subsequently developed Crohn's disease even though retrospective analysis of the specimen fails to confirm the diagnosis. The third and smallest group represents those known to have Crohn's dis-

ease confined to the colon and rectum, with no small bowel or anal involvement.

Results following Restorative Proctocolectomy

Results according to our experience suggest that there are two distinct categories of patients: those with preoperative stigmata of Crohn's disease and those whose Crohn's

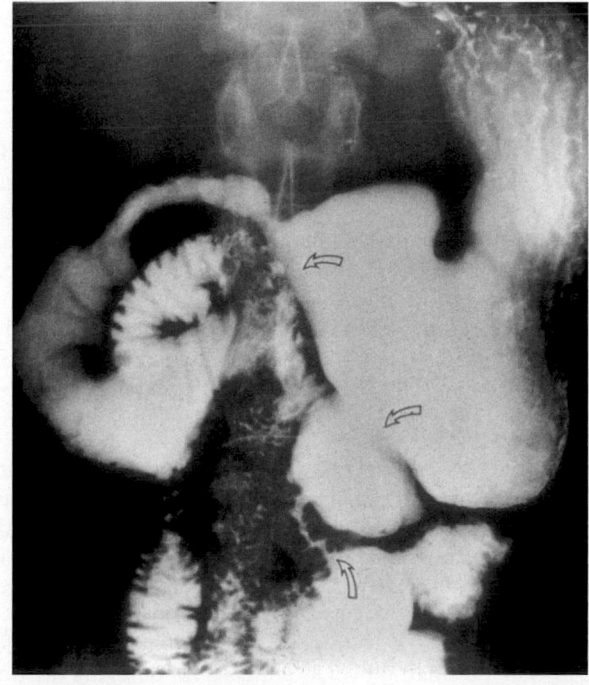

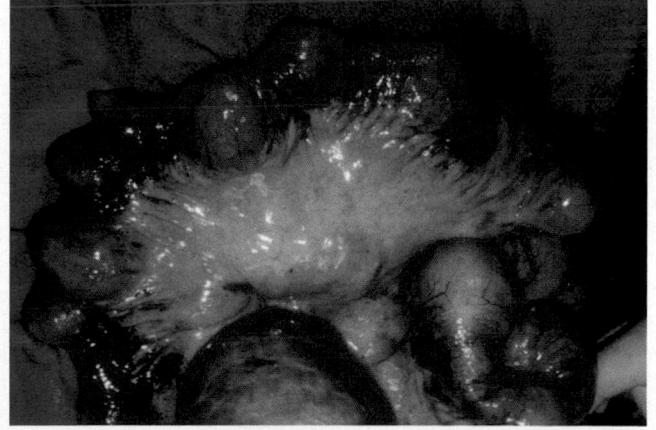

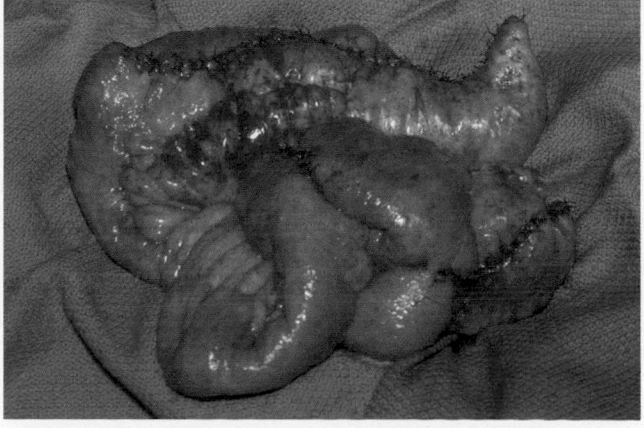

FIGURE 30-79. Extensive small bowel Crohn's disease. Small bowel follow-through demonstrates strictures (*arrows*) virtually throughout the intestinal tract. Intraoperative appearance of the small bowel in the small patient (**B**). Completion of multiple strictureplasties (**C**).

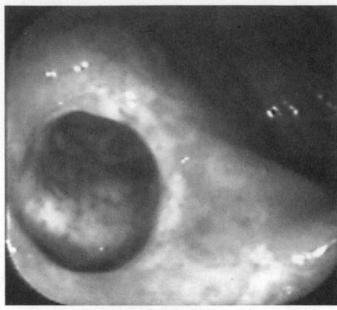

FIGURE 30-80. Colonoscopy demonstrates the opening of a fistula into the small intestine with acute and chronic inflammatory reaction. The proximal lumen of the colon can be seen in the upper right.

disease was not suspected but only discovered based on the histologic evaluation.[252] Patients in whom there is any preoperative suggestion of Crohn's disease, clinically or pathologically, had very poor results following this operation. Conversely, in the short term at least, if the clinical diagnosis of ulcerative colitis seems assured, early results following restorative proctocolectomy are significantly better with postoperative, histologically proven Crohn's disease than when Crohn's disease is suspected preoperatively. In a preliminary report, 15 of 16 patients in the former group maintained their pouches, compared with only 1 of 9 in the latter in our experience.[252]

Based on the poor results observed in most of the nine patients found to have Crohn's disease postoperatively, the Toronto General Hospital Group counsel that the pelvic pouch procedure should not knowingly be performed in these individuals.[106] A total of 37 patients were identified in the Mayo Clinic experience who inadvertently underwent restorative proctocolectomy and were subsequently proven to have Crohn's disease.[475] Approximately one-third developed complex fistulas. Recurrent Crohn's disease developed in 100%. However, after a mean of 10 years (range, 3 to 14 years), the pouch remained in place in 20 individuals, but in 7 a diversion was performed. The overall failure rate was interpreted to be 45%.[475] In the report of Regimbeau and coworkers (Clichy, France), 41 patients with Crohn's disease underwent ileal pouch anastomotic surgery.[438] In 26, the diagnosis was established preoperatively or in the pathologic report, whereas 15 subsequently developed Crohn's disease–related complications. Twenty patients were followed for more than 10 years. The rates of Crohn's disease–related complications and pouch excision were 35% and 10%, respectively. These results led the investigators to conclude that it is reasonable to propose restorative proctocolectomy in selected patients with limited colorectal Crohn's disease.

The Birmingham, United Kingdom, group performed restorative proctocolectomy in 23 patients with Crohn's disease, 12 of whom had disease evidence at the time of the operation.[372] At a mean follow-up of 10.2 years, almost 50% underwent pouch excision. In a comparison with ileoproctostomy, the investigators concluded that restorative proctocolectomy was inferior, but the functional results of those with a successful outcome were comparable. Others confirm that the short- to medium-term functional results are acceptable if the pouch can be retained.[208]

Comment

The concept of offering restorative proctocolectomy to individuals with Crohn's disease in which the small bowel and anal areas are spared is based on the understanding that any operation for this condition will not guarantee cure, and even proctocolectomy and ileostomy in such a patient is associated with a recurrence rate of approximately 20%. Therefore, why not consider restoration of intestinal continuity and provide such a person with the benefits of that operation? Now that one has longer term follow-up, it appears that the rate of pouch excision may be only slightly greater than when the operation is performed for ulcerative colitis in these selected patients. Members of the panel at a meeting of the American Society of Colon and Rectal Surgeons in 1990 opined that they would refuse to perform reservoir procedures in patients with Crohn's disease, even when the disease has been limited to the colon, and despite no evidence of small bowel recurrence with long-term follow-up.[458] Clearly, that attitude can no longer be considered the standard of care. Many of these same individuals have altered their position, but there is no disagreement that the patient must have a full and complete understanding of the risks associated with this alternative.

Recurrence

A number of factors have been at some time suggested to contribute to an increased risk for recurrence after resection: site of involvement, age at onset of disease, age at first resection, gender, prior resection, extent of resection, presence or absence of gross/microscopic disease at resection margin, presence of perianal disease, immunologic factors (T-cell and total lymphocyte counts), blood transfusion, choice of operation, pathologic variables, and probably others.[586]

Following the Patient

The protocol for following the patient who has undergone resection in order to identify early recurrence has never been clearly established nor is it without controversy. A variety of approaches include regular follow-up visits, periodic endoscopic evaluation, and radiologic and laboratory investigations, as well as issues involving long-term drug therapy. The fecal excretion of 1-antitrypsin has been felt to be a reliable marker of intestinal protein loss. It has therefore been evaluated for its efficacy as an early indicator for recurrence in Crohn's disease.[53] Boirivant and colleagues believe that it is indeed a sensitive, noninvasive, inexpensive marker for those who undergo regular supervision after surgery.[53]

Stoma versus Anastomosis

Ileostomy itself seems to be associated with a significantly lower early recurrence risk than those individuals who have undergone colon anastomoses.[234] Others suggest that the fecal stream and reflux of colonic contents are important factors in determining the pattern of recurrence.[68] However, more recently surgeons have been exploring the concept of a wide side-to-side anastomosis of the ileum to the colon and also in the small bowel as a means for delaying the time interval for recurrence.[593] Prospective, randomized trials are currently being conducted on this variation in technique.

Trnka and colleagues reviewed 113 patients with Crohn's disease whose initial procedure involved an anastomosis.[563] The recurrence rate was 29% at 5 years, 52% at 10 years, and 84% at 25 years. There was no relationship between the incidence of recurrence and the age of the patient, the gender, the duration of disease, the presence or absence of granulomas, the length of the resected specimen, and the presence or absence of disease at the proximal resection margin. Patients with colon disease who underwent an anastomosis had a much higher incidence of recurrence than those who had small bowel involvement.

Location

Our institution has been associated with more papers, with greater numbers of patients, than any other. Results of a study involving 615 consecutive patients revealed the following primary clinical patterns: ileocolic, 41.0%; small intestine, 28.6%; colon, 27.0%; anorectal, 3.4%.[152] At 10 years, more than 90% of patients with ileocolitis underwent surgery, and nearly 70% of patients with ileal or colonic disease required operation. Those with ileocolic disease had the highest rate of recurrence requiring another operation (53%), compared with 45% for colonic and 44% for small intestinal patterns.[152] We conclude with the following main characteristics of patients with Crohn's disease:

- Most undergo surgery at some point.
- Reoperation is always a possibility.
- Prognosis with respect to recurrence differs based on the initial pattern of presentation.[152]

We reviewed the Cleveland Clinic experience with 592 patients followed for a mean of 13 years.[583] Those with ileocolic disease had the highest rate of recurrence: 53%, compared with 45% for colonic and 44% for small intestinal involvement. The estimated median time for recurrence was similar for all three groups, but the presence of an internal fistula or perianal disease was associated with an increased risk. Lock and colleagues reported our experience of 127 patients with Crohn's disease of the large bowel who underwent excisional surgery.[320] Initial involvement of the terminal ileum as well as the large bowel was associated with a significantly higher incidence of overall recurrence and earlier postoperative recurrence when compared with patients who had ileal sparing.

Another report from the same institution analyzed perforating and nonperforating Crohn's disease to see if these two expressions are reflected in a difference in the incidence of subsequent recurrence.[347] No such relationship was observed. This view was disputed by the experience at Mount Sinai Hospital in New York City, in which recurrence is more likely to occur with the perforating phenotype of Crohn's disease. Chardavoyne and colleagues reviewed the records of 187 patients who underwent resection for Crohn's disease.[79] Age, gender, age at onset of the disease and at time of resection, family history, presence of granulomata, and microscopic involvement at the line of resection did not affect the rate of recurrence. Patients with predominantly large bowel disease were found to have a higher rate of re-resection (45%) than those with small intestinal involvement (32%). Lind and colleagues noted that the cumulative reoperation rate at 10 years was 71% for ileocolonic disease, 47% for colonic, and 58% for small bowel.[315] The crude reoperation rate for patients who had one resection in the experience of Valiulis and Currie was 37%.[567] Frikker and Segall reported that patients with small bowel disease had a better prognosis than did individuals with ileocolic involvement.[166]

In the experience of the group from Huddinge, Sweden, the cumulative 10-year risk of a symptomatic recurrence was 58% after colectomy and ileorectal anastomosis and 47% after segmental colonic resection.[40] Their resection rates for ileocecal disease were 61%, 77%, and 83% at 1, 5, and 10 years, respectively.[39] They conclude that three of four patients with Crohn's disease will undergo a bowel resection, half of whom will ultimately relapse.[38]

Homan and Dineen compared the results of resection, bypass, and exclusion for ileocecal Crohn's disease.[243] In a total of 161 patients, resection was performed in 115, bypass with exclusion in 25, and bypass alone in 21. Recurrence rates were 25% for resection, 63% for bypass with exclusion, and 75% for bypass alone. With 15 years of follow-up, bypass was seen to be associated with a 94% recurrence rate. The authors concluded that resection can be performed with morbidity and mortality equivalent to either of the bypass procedures and that the recurrence rate following resection is significantly lower than that for either bypass or exclusion. Others confirm that bypass and diversion procedures increase the likelihood of the need for further surgery.[134]

In the Lahey Clinic experience of resection for small bowel disease, 85% underwent excision of the terminal ileum and cecum with an anastomosis performed between the distal ileum and the ascending colon.[536] No frozen-section biopsies of the proximal margin were performed, and subsequent histologic examination revealed two instances (3%) in which the surgeon did not suspect involvement. Recurrent Crohn's disease developed after the initial bowel resection in 51 patients (69%). Of these, 28 (55%) required a second operation. Of these individuals, 18 had further recurrence of the disease, but in none did additional operative intervention prevent subsequent recurrence. Some patients even required a third and fourth procedure because of disease-related complications. In other words, no patient was cured if he or she required a third operation (Figure 30-81). Table 30-1 summarizes the pertinent literature on the subject of bowel resection and recurrence since 2003.

Margin

A number of studies have demonstrated that the risk of recurrence is unaffected by the width of the macroscopically normal margin of resection.[150,593] Furthermore, recurrence rates are generally felt not to be increased when microscopic Crohn's disease is present at the resection margins, although there is difference of opinion. Some have opined that the presence of granulomas is associated with a statistically significant increased risk of recurrence.[23] There appears to be a close correlation between the duration of postoperative recurrence and the extent of presurgical disease.[109] Others confirm that disease extent has prognostic value with respect to the risk of symptomatic recurrence, whereas the length of resection margins does not appear to influence this risk.[433] All these papers reaffirm the importance of a conservative approach to resection margin in individuals with Crohn's disease.[418]

Adloff and colleagues reviewed 58 patients who underwent resection for Crohn's disease and found no statistically significant difference in recurrence rates between individuals with and without involved margins.[3] Wolff and associates reported the Mayo Clinic experience of more than 700 patients who underwent surgery for Crohn's disease with an anastomosis.[594] Those who were demonstrated to have microscopic involvement of the resection margin were

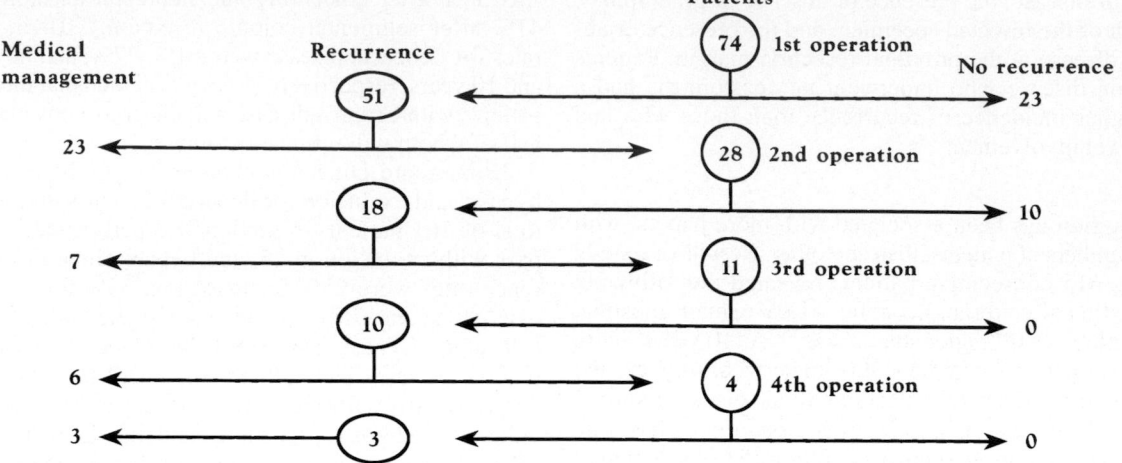

FIGURE 30-81. Pattern of recurrence in patients who underwent resection for small bowel Crohn's disease. (Adapted from Stone W, Veidenheimer MC, Corman ML, et al. The dilemma of Crohn's disease: long-term follow-up of Crohn's disease of the small intestine. *Dis Colon Rectum.* 1977;20:372.)

found to have a recurrence rate of more than 90% within the follow-up period of 8 years. Those patients who did not have such involvement had a 55% incidence of recurrence at 10 years. The authors concluded that clear margins should be obtained in resections for Crohn's disease if this is at all possible. Conversely, others have demonstrated that microscopic involvement does not seem to increase the rate of recurrence.[237,285]

Hamilton and coworkers analyzed 79 patients who underwent resection and ileocolonic anastomosis.[215] In approximately one-half, the margin was determined by frozen section, and in the other group by visual inspection alone. In spite of negative initial microscopic evaluation, one-third was demonstrated to have involvement on final section. There was no statistically significant difference in the outcome of the two groups. The authors' findings support the concept of visual examination of the margins of resection, especially because one is usually able to preserve additional bowel by this approach. I believe that this is the correct position for a surgeon to take.

Rutgeerts and colleagues performed endoscopy and biopsy on 114 patients who underwent "curative" resection of the terminal ileum and part of the colon.[466] The recurrence rate within 1 year of the operation was 72%. A later report from the same group revealed that the endoscopic recurrence rate had increased to 85% at 3 years.[467] When patients were stratified for preoperative disease activity, the severity of lesions found at endoscopy remained a strong predictive factor for symptomatic recurrence.

Blood Transfusion

Because blood transfusion has been demonstrated to suppress the immune system, Peters and colleagues reviewed the records of 79 patients to determine whether perioperative blood transfusion affects recurrence rates.[407] A decreased rate of recurrence in those who received multiple transfusions was noted. However, an opposite conclusion was reached in a review of 197 patients from St. Mark's Hospital; there appeared to be no such association.[497] Although no one is suggesting a prospective clinical trial for obvious reasons, it would be ideal if this issue could be resolved.

Recurrent "Diverticulitis"

Patients who require re-resection after a procedure for what was initially thought to have been sigmoid diverticulitis should be presumed to have Crohn's colitis until proved otherwise. A high index of suspicion should be apparent if the illness is characterized by the requirement for multiple operations, if a diversionary procedure fails to control the distal disease, or if one of the following is noted: anorectal disease, rectal bleeding, or fistula. In the Lahey Clinic experience with 25 patients requiring resection for "diverticulitis" a second time, all pathologic specimens were diagnosed as Crohn's disease.[37]

Mortality

Probert and colleagues studied the mortality among 610 people with Crohn's disease that were identified in a population-based study from 1972 to 1989.[430] The overall mortality was not increased. Nordgren and associates studied the long-term follow-up in 136 patients from Göteborg, Sweden.[381] In a follow-up of 16.6 years, 18 patients had died, 3 from Crohn's disease. In our series of 592 patients observed for a mean of 13 years, 12.7% died from all causes, but 6.0% of the deaths were directly related to Crohn's disease.[141] General opinion is that Crohn's disease does not significantly increase long-term mortality, a factor that needs to be conveyed to actuaries, insurers, and those individuals who advise employers.[430]

Surgical Management of Short Bowel Syndrome

For the sake of completeness, it is worth mentioning that there are surgical approaches to the treatment of patients with the short bowel syndrome. Some are considered somewhat experimental, such as intestinal transplantation and the growing of new intestinal mucosa by means of serosal patching.[86,360,553,554] Other options include intestinal tapering and lengthening, creating of intestinal valves and sphincters, constructing antiperistaltic intestinal segments, intestinal pacing, and implementation of recirculating intestinal loops.[413] It is not within the purview of this text to detail all the potential options. Thompson has very nicely outlined the range of possibilities and appends a useful bibliography from which the reader may begin his or her exploration.[552]

(text continues on page 1384)

continued

TABLE 30-1 Multi-institutional Results of Surgical Treatment of Crohn's Disease

YEAR	INSTITUTION	REFERENCE	TYPE OF STUDY	INTERVENTION	NO. OF PARTICIPANTS	LENGTH OF FOLLOW-UP	RESULTS	P VALUE	CONCLUSION	RISK FACTORS	MORBIDITY	MORTALITY
2003	Angers University Hospital, France	36	Retrospective	Open vs. lap	Open: 53 Lap: 39	5 years	Recurrence in open resection 29.1% vs. lap 27.7%	$P = .9104$	Compared recurrence confirmed by histology between open vs. laparoscopic ileocolic resection for CD at 5 years	Smoking matched per group	SBO: open 35.4% vs. lap 11.1% ($P = .02$)	0
2003	Department of Surgical Sciences, San Camillo Hospital, Italy	549	Nonrandomized prospective	Hand-sewn vs. stapled anastomosis	Hand-sewn: 30 Stapled: 76		Recurrence in hand-sewn 16.7% vs. stapled 2.6%	?	Recurrence after ileocolic resection for CD with hand-sewn anastomosis vs. stapled. Time to follow-up unknown		Hand-sewn: 3 complications Stapled: 1 complication	Hand-sewn: 1 postoperative death
2003	University of Padova, Italy	489	Retrospective cohort	Bowel resection for obstructing CD	N = 120	Mean follow-up: 83 + 72 months	Patients younger than 30 25% recurrence rate at 5 years vs. older than 30 0%	$P \leq .01$	Younger age, SB disease and anastomosis, emergency conditions, and postoperative complications increase the risk of recurrence for stenosing CD	Age <30, postoperative complications, type of resection, SB anastomosis, hand-sewn anastomosis	NA	NA
							Postoperative complications recurrence 34% vs. uneventful postoperative course 21%	$P = .02$				
							Recurrence after ileocolonic resection at 5-year follow-up: 13% vs. SB 30% vs. colonic 58%	SB, $P < .01$ Colonic, $P = .04$				
							Small bowel anastomosis 40% vs. ileocolonic anastomosis 17%	$P = .01$				
							Stapled anastomosis 9% vs. hand-sewn 28%	$P = .02$				

TABLE 30-1 Multi-institutional Results of Surgical Treatment of Crohn's Disease (continued)

YEAR	INSTITUTION	REFERENCE	TYPE OF STUDY	INTERVENTION	NO. OF PARTICIPANTS	LENGTH OF FOLLOW-UP	RESULTS	P VALUE	CONCLUSION	RISK FACTORS	MORBIDITY	MORTALITY
2004	Stanford University, CA	472	Survey	Quit smoking	N = 584: 267 responses (46%)		Smokers no. of reoperations 1: RIR 1.32; 95% CI, 1.10–1.60 2: RIR 1.55; 95% CI, 1.09–2.20 3: RIR 1.77; 95% CI, 1.02–3.06 Nonsmokers no. of reoperations 1: RIR 0.25; 95% CI, 0.15–0.41 2: RIR 0.30; 95% CI, 0.16–0.57 3: RIR 0.27; 95% CI, 0.15–0.47	NA	Reduced risk of reoperation for CD after quitting smoking	NA	Reoperations: see results	NA
2004	IBD Centre and Department of Surgery, Yokkaichi Social Insurance Hospital, Japan	604	Prospective, blind cohort	After operation, all patients received Pentasa	N = 36: 20 in remission, 16 relapses	1 year	IL-1, IL-6, and TNF-α median levels at enrollment were higher for relapsing group, but IL-6 was the only significant independent risk factor for relapse	$P = .03$	IL-6 in ileal mucosa after ileal or ileocecal resection for CD is an independent predictor for future relapse at 1-year follow-up	RF for relapse: younger age at operation, shorter disease duration before operation, fistulating disease	NA	None
2004	Ospedale Luigi Sacco, Italy	479	Prospective observational	Nonconventional strictureplasties (NCSP)	N = 102 (1993–2002)	10 years	10-year clinical and surgical recurrence rates: 43% and 27% Recurrence at NCSP site: 0.8%	NA	Perioperative and long-term results of NCSP are comparable to conservative and resective surgery as reported in literature	NA	Complication rate: 5.7%	None

continued

| 2004 | University of Padova, Italy | 490 | Prospective observational | Stapled side-to-side anastomosis vs. stapled end-to-side or hand-sewn side-to-side | N = 84: 12 stapled S-S, 36 stapled E-S, 36 hand-sewn S-S | ? | No difference between 3 groups in early postoperative period. Stapled S-S had better symptom-free survival than stapled E-S (*P* = .04). S-S stapled and hand-sewn had lower reoperation rates for recurrence than stapled E-S (*P* = .01 and *P* = .05) | Longer follow-up showed lower incidence of reoperation recurrence in stapled and hand-sewn side-to-side anastomosis compared to stapled end-to-side anastomosis | NA | NA | NA | NA |
| 2004 | University of Chicago | 219 | RCT double-blind | 6-MP and mesalamine to placebo | N = 131 s/p resection and ileocolonic anastomosis | 24 months | Clinical recurrence rates for 6-MP, mesalamine, and placebo at 24 months: 50% (95% CI, 34%–68%) 58% (95% CI, 41%–75%) 77% (95% CI, 61%–91%) Endoscopic recurrence rates for 6-MP, mesalamine, and placebo: 43% (95% CI, 28%–63%) 63% (95% CI, 47%–79%) 64% (95% CI, 46%–81%) Radiographic recurrence rates for 6-MP, mesalamine, and placebo: 33% (95% CI, 19%–54%) 46% (95% CI, 29%–66%) 49% (95% CI, 30%–72%) | 6-MP was more effective than placebo at preventing clinical and endoscopic recurrence over 2 years (*P* < .05) | NA | NA |

TABLE 30-1 Multi-institutional Results of Surgical Treatment of Crohn's Disease *(continued)*

YEAR	INSTITUTION	REFERENCE	TYPE OF STUDY	INTERVENTION	NO. OF PARTICIPANTS	LENGTH OF FOLLOW-UP	RESULTS	P VALUE	CONCLUSION	RISK FACTORS	MORBIDITY	MORTALITY
2004	Polo Universitario, Italy	24	RCT	AZA or mesalamine	N = 142	24 months	Clinical relapse was comparable after conservative surgery for azathioprine and mesalamine group: OR, 2.04; 95% CI, 0.89–4.67 OR, 1.79; 95% CI, 0.80–3.97 Azathioprine was more effective than mesalamine in preventing relapse for patients with prior intestinal resections (OR, 4.83; 95% CI, 1.47–15.8)		No difference between azathioprine and mesalamine in preventing surgical and clinical recurrence after conservative surgery. However, azathioprine was more effective in preventing relapse in patients with previous resections	NA	More patients withdrew resection from side effects of azathioprine (22% vs. 8%; P = .04)	NA
2004	Sacco University, Italy	401	Prospective	Bowel wall thickness measured s/p CD surgery	N = 127	Median follow-up: 41 months	90% CD recurrence for unchanged/worsened bowel wall thickness vs. 33% improved bowel wall thickness at 12 months >6 mm wall thickness at 12 months HR for recurrence: 6.5 (95% CI, 2.8–15.4)		Systemic ultrasound follow-up may be a tool to identify patient at high risk for recurrence	Smoking, perianal disease, previous surgery, total bowel length resection >50 cm	NA	NA
2004	Queen Elizabeth Hospital, United Kingdom	503	Retrospective	Comparison of long strictureplasty (LS) vs. short strictureplasty (SS) for CD	N = 62	Median follow-up: 121 months (7–253)	3-, 5-, and 10-year disease-free rates for LS and SS 3-year: 80.4% and 62.1% 5-year: 55.2% and 49.8% 10-year: 49.1% and 33.5%		Long strictureplasty (>20 cm) is safe and produces equivalent results to short strictureplasty	NA	LS: 2 abscesses SS: 1 leak, 1 abscess	None

Year		Institution	Study type	Intervention	N	Follow-up	Results	P value	Conclusion		Complications	
2005	261	University of Chicago	Retrospective data review	Smoking vs. nonsmoking	N = 59	250 weeks	Clinical relapse following surgery for CD for smokers 69% vs. nonsmokers 23% Time to clinical relapse in smokers 130 weeks vs. 234 weeks nonsmokers	P = .02 P < .001	Smoking is associated with clinical recurrence in CD, and time to recurrence is shorter in smokers	NA	NA	NA	NA
2005	543	General Infirmary at Leeds, United Kingdom	Prospective observational	Infliximab	N = 21	Median follow-up: 20 months (12–52)	Perianal CD fistula rx with seton and infliximab rx: 11/21 continued with weekly maintenance rx 10/21 (47%) complete response 11/21 (53%) with partial response No failed rx	NA	The combination of seton drainage and infliximab is an effective treatment for CD perianal fistulas	NA	4 adverse reactions to infliximab: 2 mild allergies, 1 rash, 1 joint pain	NA
2005	158	University of Chicago	Prospective cohort	Surgically treated Crohn's colitis	N = 179: 55 segmental colectomy, 49 total abdominal colectomy, 75 total proctocolectomy	Median follow-up: segmental colectomy: 61 months total colectomy: 25 months proctocolectomy: 14 months	31 patients with surgical recurrence: 19 (38.8%) in segmental colectomy (SC), 8 (22.9%) in TAC, 4 (3.3%) in total proctocolectomy (TP) SC had shorter time to first recurrence than TP (P = .014); SC had greater risk of recurrence than TP (P = .006)	NA	TP is associated with lower morbidity risk recurrence, and longer time to recurrence	NA	Postoperative complications: SC: 9.3% TAC: 6.1% TP: 7.9% (P = .84)	None

continued

TABLE 30-1 Multi-institutional Results of Surgical Treatment of Crohn's Disease *(continued)*

YEAR	INSTITUTION	REFERENCE	TYPE OF STUDY	INTERVENTION	NO. OF PARTICIPANTS	LENGTH OF FOLLOW-UP	RESULTS	P VALUE	CONCLUSION	RISK FACTORS	MORBIDITY	MORTALITY
2005	University Hospital Gasthuis-berg, Belgium	471	RCT	Ornidazole	N = 80	1 year	Clinical recurrence rate at 1 year from 15 of 40 (37.5%) patients in the placebo group to 3 of 38 (7.9%) patients in the ornidazole group	Fisher exact test, 8.03; $P =$ .0046; OR, 0.14; 95% CI, 0.037–0.546	Ornidazole (1 g/day) is effective in preventing recurrence after il-eocolonic resection for CD	NA	SE of drug = w/d from study: 1 abnl LFTs, 5 n/v;1 pares-thesia, 1 polyneu-ropathy, 1 disease activity, 2 compli-ance	None
							Endoscopic recurrence at 12 months from 26 of 33 (79.0%) in the placebo group to 15 of 28 (53.6%) in the ornidazole group	χ^2, 4.37; $P =$ .037; OR, 0.31; 95% CI, 0.10–0.94				
2005	Chikushi Hospital, Fukuoka University, Japan	168	Retrospective	Strictureplasty (SP)	N = 103 (average of 2.3 SP per person)	Mean follow-up: 80.3 months	5- and 10-year reop-eration rate was 45.0% and 61.9%, respectively		Strictureplasty is safe and useful for preserving the intestine in the sur-gical treatment of Crohn's disease if strictures are care-fully selected	NA	4 with sepsis from leak, fistula or abscess (2 requir-ing reop-eration), 2 ileus, 1 stenosis	None
							45 patients (43.7%) required further operation for recur-rence, of whom 21 patients (20.4%) had recurrence at the site of stricture-plasty, which was restricture in 14 patients and per-forating disease in 7 patients					

Year	N	Institution	Study type	Intervention	Sample	Follow-up	Results	P value	Conclusion	Risk factor	Complications	Conflict
2005	264	Queen Elizabeth Hospital, United Kingdom	Retrospective cohort	Jejunal resection for CD	n = 28 for jejunal CD, matched with n = 84 ileocecal CD for control group	Median follow-up: 19 years	3-year recurrence rate requiring reoperation: jejunal CD, 43%; ileocecal disease, 22% (P = 03) 5 years: jejunal CD, 50%; ileocecal disease, 30% (P = 05) 10 years jejunal CD, 61%; ileocecal, 51% (P = 3)		Presence of jejunal CD associated with higher rate of early disease recurrence compared to ileocecal disease	Jejunal CD	NA	None
2005	550	Cleveland Clinic Florida	Retrospective analysis	Lap (LR) vs. open ileocecal resection (OR)	37 patients: 21 lap, 16 open	Mean follow-up: 42.6 + 25.8 months	Recurrence LR: 7/21 (33%) OR: 7/16 (44%)	P value nonsignificant	No difference in recurrence between open vs. lap ileocecal resection for CD	NA	Incisional hernia: LR: 1/21 (5%) OR: 2/16 (13%)	None
2005	414	Academic Medical Centre, The Netherlands	Retrospective cohort	Segmental colon resection for CD (no ileocecal resection)	91 patients	Median follow-up: 8.3 years	30 patients (33%): at least one re-resection. For recurrence after colonic resection: Woman: OR, 12.52; 95% CI, 2.38–65.84 Perianal disease: OR, 13.94; 95% CI, 3.02–64.27	NA	Recurrence is more frequent in women and those with history of perianal disease	Women/history of perianal disease	NA	NA
2005	456	Mount Sinai, NY	Meta-analysis	Lap vs. open surgery for CD	16 studies: 1 RCT, 13 retrospective, 2 prospective	17–60 months	Lap resection requires more operating time (25.8 minutes; 95% CI 6.4–47.2 minutes), but decreased time of postoperative ileus (−2.62 days; 95% CI −3.62 to −1.62)	NA	Laparoscopic surgery for CD is safe and associated with a shorter hospital stay than open resection	NA	Lap resection decreased complications (OR, 0.62; 95% CI, 0.42–0.91)	NA

continued

TABLE 30-1 Multi-institutional Results of Surgical Treatment of Crohn's Disease *(continued)*

YEAR	INSTITUTION	REFERENCE	TYPE OF STUDY	INTERVENTION	NO. OF PARTICIPANTS	LENGTH OF FOLLOW-UP	RESULTS	*P* VALUE	CONCLUSION	RISK FACTORS	MORBIDITY	MORTALITY
2005	Hospital Clinic, Spain	17	Prospective cohort	*NOD2/CARD15* gene testing	170 patients	7.4 ± 6.1 years	Initial surgery was more frequent for patients with *NOD2/CARD15* variants and earlier time to surgery. 70/170 required initial surgery. Postoperative recurrence was more frequent with *NOD2/CARD15* variant (OR, 3.29; 95% CI, 1.13–9.56)	NA	*NOD2/CARD15* variant patients have an earlier time to initial surgery as well as higher risk of recurrence	NA	NA	NA
2005	Kyushu University, Japan	137	Retrospective analysis	Enteral nutrition (EN) >1,200 kcal/day vs. non-EN	40 patients requiring surgery for CD with intraoperative enteroscopy; 24 EN vs. 16 non-EN	6–83 months	Postoperative recurrence was high in patients with cobblestone appearance (*P* = .006), EN reduced postoperative recurrence (*P* = .017)	NA	Enteral nutrition prevents postoperative recurrence of CD	Cobblestone appearance at intraoperative endoscopy	NA	NA
2005	Chaim Sheba Medical Center, Israel	27	Retrospective analysis	Surgery for CD	86	Mean follow-up: 42 months	26/86 (30%) with postoperative recurrence. Smoking (OR, 3.69; 95% CI, 2.06–11.52) and perforating disease (OR, 4.09; 95% CI, 1.31–12.65) are associated with risk of recurrence	NA	Risk of recurrence in CD related to smoking and perforating disease	Smoking/ perforating disease	NA	NA

2006	459	Retrospective review	Strictureplasty for active CD	14 patients (mean strictureplasty, 5.2)	Median follow-up: 41 months (11–87)	All patients s/p strictureplasty and resection and >70% of patients with strictureplasty alone were intervention free at 41 months and 70 months	NA	Strictureplasty in active disease strictures is well tolerated and has similar recurrence/complication rates when compared with limited resections in patients with similar disease profiles	NA	1/14 leak requiring reoperation and resection	None
St. George's Hospital, United Kingdom											
2006	328	Retrospective analysis	Lap vs. open ileocolic resection	113: 63 lap, 50 open	Lap mean follow-up: 62.9 months; open mean follow-up: 81.8 months	Surgical recurrence lap 9.5% vs. open 24.0% ($P = .18$); median time to recurrence lap 59.7 months vs. open 61.6 months	NA	Long-term recurrence rates between both groups are similar. No difference in postoperative complications as well	NA	Lap 19% vs. open 34% ($P = .098$); wound infections/ileus, intra-abdominal abscess, hernia	None
Washington University, MO											
2006	342	RCT double-blind	Lactobacillus s/p intestinal resection for CD	98: 48 in Lactobacillus (LA) group	6 months	Endoscopic recurrence 30/47 in placebo; 21/43 in LA group	$P = .15$	No difference in endoscopic recurrence for patients who received Lactobacillus after intestinal resection for CD	NA	NA	NA
Hôpital Européen Georges Pompidou, France											
2006	548	Meta-analysis	Segmental colon resection vs. total/subtotal colectomy	6 studies (1984–2002) 488 patients: 223 IRA, 265 SC	NA	No significant difference between IRA and SC. Time to recurrence was longer in IRA by 4.4 years (95% CI, 3.1–5.8; $P < .001$)	NA	Segmental colectomy resulted in earlier recurrence than total/subtotal colectomy. No difference in recurrence rates	NA	No difference in postoperative complications: OR, 1.4; 95% CI, 0.16–12.74	NA
Imperial College London, United Kingdom											
2006	156	Prospective cohort	Ileocolonic resection	59 patients with CD and 21 control patients	3 months for all, 1 year for 32 patients	Myenteric plexitis in 32/59 patients (54%). Endoscopic recurrence rates at 3 months 75% vs. 41% (OR, 4.36; 95% CI, 1.44–13.23; $P = .003$)	NA	Patients with myenteric plexitis had higher endoscopic recurrence rates and earlier recurrence	Myenteric plexitis	NA	NA
University Hospital of Gasthuisberg, Belgium											

continued

TABLE 30-1 Multi-institutional Results of Surgical Treatment of Crohn's Disease (*continued*)

YEAR	INSTITUTION	REFERENCE	TYPE OF STUDY	INTERVENTION	NO. OF PARTICIPANTS	LENGTH OF FOLLOW-UP	RESULTS	P VALUE	CONCLUSION	RISK FACTORS	MORBIDITY	MORTALITY
							Patients with myenteric plexitis recurrence rate at 1 year 93% vs. 59% (OR, 9.8: 95% CI, 1.04–92.70; $P = .041$)					
2006	Linköping University Hospital, Sweden	373	Prospective cohort	AZA	14 controls, 28 in treatment group	Median follow-up: 84.7 months	CDAI in AZA group 93 vs. 184 for control ($P = .01$); time to clinical relapse 53 vs. 24 months ($P < .05$)		AZA decreased CD symptoms postsurgery and delayed clinical recurrence	NA	NA	NA
2006	Ullevål University Hospital, Norway	294	Retrospective analysis	Intestinal resection for CD	53 patients (1954–2002; mean resection, 2.7)	Median follow-up: 26.5 years	111/144 resections were performed during first three operations. From first to third operation, there was an increase in penetrating disease from 15% to 39% ($P = .046$); decrease in stricturing disease from 72% to 44% ($P = .048$); decrease in ileocolic disease from 45% to 5% ($P = .003$)		A higher percentage of patients requiring multiple surgeries for CD had penetrating CD	Penetrating disease	11.3% required re-operation for ileus, anastomotic bleeding, bowel perforation, and abdominal pain	1 from rectosigmoid perforation

Year	Institution	N	Study type	Intervention	Patients	Follow-up	Results	P value	Conclusions			
2006	University of Chicago	157	Retrospective analysis	Operative rx for CD	78 patients (134 operative interventions)	Median: 41 months (1–161)	78 patients with 149 sites of disease; 134/149 required intervention, CD recurrence in 79 sites at mean of 46.4 months; recurrence at small bowel anastomotic line 17/29 (59%); at proximal limb for small bowel and colon 29/35 (83%) Fewer recurrence at strictureplasty than at recurrence site 22/49 (45%) vs. 57/85 (70%)	$P < .01$ $P < .05$	Site of original operation is the most common site of recurrence. Small bowel is a more common site of recurrence	Small bowel anastomosis	NA	NA
2007	Erasme University Hospital, Belgium	570	RCT	*Lactobacillus* (LA1)	70 patients: LA1 group 34, LA2 36	12 weeks	Mean endoscopic score LA1, 1.5; placebo, 1.22 ($P = .48$) Severe recurrence in LA1, 21%; placebo, 15% ($P = .33$)		*Lactobacillus* failed to prevent early endoscopic recurrence at 12 weeks	NA	NA	NA
2007	Rambam Health Care Campus, Israel	80	RCT	Synbiotic	30 patients: 20 in rx group, 10 placebo	24 months (9 patients completed study)	No difference in endoscopic and clinical recurrence between groups		Synbiotic 2000 had no effect on postoperative recurrence of patients with CD	NA	1 postoperative complication in placebo group	None
2007	Cornell University, NY	358	Prospective observational	Side-to-side isoperistaltic strictureplasty in CD	184 patients from 6 centers in the United States, Italy, and Japan	Variable	41/184 required reoperation for recurrent disease, with average time to recurrence of 35 months; cumulative reoperation-free 5-year survival of 77%		This procedure has low morbidity, mortality associated with it	NA	2% GI bleed, 1% suture line dehiscence, 1% bowel obstruction	1 from PE

continued

TABLE 30-1 Multi-institutional Results of Surgical Treatment of Crohn's Disease (continued)

YEAR	INSTITUTION	REFERENCE	TYPE OF STUDY	INTERVENTION	NO. OF PARTICIPANTS	LENGTH OF FOLLOW-UP	RESULTS	P VALUE	CONCLUSION	RISK FACTORS	MORBIDITY	MORTALITY
2007	University of Heidelberg, Germany	580	Retrospective analysis	Ileocecal resection	100	Median follow-up: 6 years 10 months	Recurrence rates at 5 and 9 years: 28.7% and 56.4% Relaparotomy RR = 5.88 (1.86–18.57; $P = .0006$)		Relaparotomy in same hospital stay was an independent predictor of recurrence	Relaparotomy	16.3% morbidity rate: 4.3% leak; 10% postoperative wound infection	None
2007	University of Padova, Italy	492	Prospective observational	s/p ileocolonic resection	63 patients	Median follow-up after resection: 40.5 months	Lactoferrin was higher in patients who had CD in other parts of bowel in addition to IC region and in patients with clinical recurrence. Calprotectin levels correlated significantly with CRP levels. CRP, calprotectin levels, and clinical recurrence predicted lactoferrin levels		Expression of inflammatory markers after ileocecal resection for CD may be sign of ongoing intestinal inflammation	NA	NA	NA
2007	University of Padova, Italy	493	Retrospective	Lap vs. open, stapled vs. hand-sewn for ileocolic resection	141 patients: 56 stapled S-S, 37 stapled E-S, 48 hand-sewn S-S	Median follow-up: 39 months	Hand-sewn S-S had lower recurrence rate than stapled E-S ($P < .05$). Anastomosis type, surgical complications, and age at CD onset are significant predictors of reoperation for CD recurrence		Side-to-side anastomosis seems to delay reoperation. Postoperative complications and young age at onset of disease may be signs of aggressive CD that may benefit from prophylactic therapy	Stapled E-S anastomosis, surgical complications at index resection, and younger age at CD onset	Surgical complications Stapled S-S: 5% Stapled E-S: 8% Hand-sewn S-S: 6%	None

2007	York Hospital, United Kingdom	291	Retrospective cohort	Intestinal resection for CD	98 patients	36 months	49% developed recurrence. Trends toward fewer early recurrences were seen in patients with colonic disease (33% vs. 56%; $P = .068$) Smokers: recurrence 60% vs. 43% ($P = .269$)	NA	Symptomatic postoperative recurrence of CD remains unpredictable. Smoking was not a significant predictor of early recurrent disease	NA	NA	NA
2007	St. Vincent's University Hospital, Ireland	97	Retrospective analysis	Ileocecal resection for CD	139 patients (from 1980 to 2000)	?	52% developed disease recurrence. Median time to recurrence was 7 years. 35% required repeat surgery with median time to surgery at 7.2 years	Granulomas	Long-term outcomes for ileoceca resection in CD are excellent with 48% remaining symptom free	NA	NA	NA
2007	Imperial College London, United Kingdom	511	Meta-analysis	Conventional end-to-end anastomosis vs. other configurations after resection for CD	8 studies: 2 RCTs, 1 nonrandomized prospective, 5 retrospective	661 patients: 712 anastomoses: 383 HS E-E; 329 others	Anastomotic leak rate in hand-sewn vs. other OR, 4.37; $P = .02$); S-S anastomosis had shorter hospital stay (mean difference, 2.81; $P = .007$)	NA	End-to-end anastomosis is associated with increased leak rate, but not an increase in recurrence rate when compared to side-to-side anastomosis	E-E anastomosis postoperative complications (OR, 2.64; $P < .001$)	NA	NA
2007	The Cleveland Clinic Foundation, OH	602	Meta-analysis	Strictureplasty	1,112 patients underwent 3,259 strictureplasties (H-M, Finney, side-to-side isoperistaltic)	94% site of strictureplasty: ileum/jejunum; surgical recurrence, 23%; 5-year recurrence rate, 28%. In 90%, recurrence occurred at nonstrictureplasty site	Strictureplasty is safe and effective	NA	4% septic complications: leak, fistula, abscess	NA	NA	NA

continued

TABLE 30-1 Multi-institutional Results of Surgical Treatment of Crohn's Disease *(continued)*

YEAR	INSTITUTION	REFERENCE	TYPE OF STUDY	INTERVENTION	NO. OF PARTICIPANTS	LENGTH OF FOLLOW-UP	RESULTS	P VALUE	CONCLUSION	RISK FACTORS	MORBIDITY	MORTALITY
2007	The Cleveland Clinic Foundation, OH	98	Retrospective cohort	Lap vs. open colectomy for CD	27 lap cases vs. 27 open cases	Follow-up in lap, 12 months (median); open, 40 months	Median operation times were longer for lap 240 minutes vs. open 150 minutes (*P* < .01). Overall length of stay less in lap group vs. open group (*P* = .02); recurrence similar between groups (lap, 11 patients; open, 9 patients)		There was no difference in recurrence of CD after lap and open colectomy for CD. Lap colectomy is safe and may be beneficial for decreased overall length of stay in hospital	NA	No difference between lap vs. open for postoperative morbidity	None
2007	University Hospital, Italy	526	Prospective nonrandomized trial	Infliximab/MTX vs. mesalamine	7 patients in rx group vs. 16 patients in control group	2 years	No endoscopic or clinical recurrence in rx group with infliximab after 2 years. In control group, only 4/16 (25%) were disease free 2 years after surgery		Limited study to show the effect of infliximab because it is not randomized and not a large enough study	NA	No adverse SE due to medication	NA
2007	Imperial College London, United Kingdom	437	Meta-analysis	Strictureplasty vs. resection for SB CD	7 studies (from 1980 to 2006) 688 CD patients: 311 strictureplasty alone, 377 bowel resection with or without strictureplasty	NA	Surgical recurrence after strictureplasty alone (OR, 1.36; 95% CI, 0.96–1.93; *P* = .09); resection—longer recurrence-free survival (HR, 1.08; 95% CI, 1.02–1.15; *P* = .01)		Surgical recurrence is higher following strictureplasty alone	NA	Strictureplasty alone vs. SB resection postoperative complication: OR, 0.6; 95% CI, 0.31–1.16; *P* = .13	NA

continued

Year	Institution	n	Study type	Topic	Patients	Follow-up	Results	P value	Conclusion			
2007	Wisconsin Medical College	46	Retrospective review	Surgery for CD	65 patients requiring 2 or more operations for CD		32/65 required reoperation within 2 years. Residual strictures and technical error accounted for 20% of procedures; ineffective medical therapy was identified in 64%, whereas severe disease despite medical therapy was a contributing factor in 14%		Identifying strictures and improved medical therapy may help improve reoperation rates	Poor medical therapy, technical error	NA	NA
2007	University of Chicago	159	Prospective nonrandomized observational	Lap vs. open for ileocolonic CD	146 patients: lap 59, open 87	Median follow-up: 19 months	In lap group, patients were younger, had lower BMI, and had shorter length of stay. No recurrence at the time of follow-up	$P = .001$, .008	In selected patients, laparoscopy leads to faster recovery without compromising remission	NA	1 anastomotic leak per group	None
2008	Imperial College London, United Kingdom	512	Meta-analysis	Surgery for perforating vs. nonperforating CD	13 studies (from 1988 to 2005) 3,044 patients: 1,337 PD; 1,707 NP		Recurrence was higher in P group (HR, 1.5; $P = .002$); at reoperation, concordance was found in those representing with perforating disease (OR, 5.93; $P < .001$)		Indication for reoperation remains the same as the primary operation. Perforating CD may also be associated with higher recurrence rate	Perforating disease	NA	NA
2008	Università di Tor Vergata, Italy	510	Prospective observational	Lap vs. open for ileocolonic CD	28 patients: 15 lap, 13 open	1 year	Lap group had longer operating time, lower need for pain killers postoperative, faster passage of flatus to stool, and shorter recovery period. No difference in recurrence ($P = .63$)	$P = .003$, .05, .004, .007	Laparoscopic surgery is safe with a shorter recovery	NA	No major intraoperative complications in either group	None

TABLE 30-1 Multi-institutional Results of Surgical Treatment of Crohn's Disease *(continued)*

YEAR	INSTITUTION	REFERENCE	TYPE OF STUDY	INTERVENTION	NO. OF PARTICIPANTS	LENGTH OF FOLLOW-UP	RESULTS	P VALUE	CONCLUSION	RISK FACTORS	MORBIDITY	MORTALITY
2008	Hospital Universitari Germans Trias i Pujol, Spain	116	Prospective observational	AZA	56 patients after curative resection for CD	5 years	Of 22 patients with EPR, 23% suffered a complete PR during follow-up, cumulative probability of endoscopic PR was 44%, 53%, 69%, and 82% at 1, 2, 3, and 5 years, respectively		Early postoperative use of AZA seems to delay EPR development in comparison to historical series or placebo groups in randomized controlled trials	None	NA	NA
2008	Ematologia II Ospedale V. Cervello, Italy	442	Prospective cohort	Surgery for CD	110 patients	7 years	32/110 required reoperation. Stricturing and penetrating pattern were predictors of surgery (HR, 1.7; 95% CI, 1.0–2.8; HR, 3.2; 95% CI, 1.8–5.5, respectively). Smoking habit at diagnosis (HR, 3.6; 95% CI, 1.4–9.1) was predictive of surgical recurrence		Smoking predicts recurrence after surgery	Penetrating disease, stricturing disease, smoking	NA	NA
2008	Università "Tor Vergata" Roma, Italy	45	Prospective observational	Lap vs. open for ileocolonic CD	22 patients: 10 lap, 12 open	1 year	Endoscopic recurrence at 1 year, 21/22 patients; laparoscopy 9 of 10 (90%) vs. laparotomy 12 of 12 (100%). All patients remained in clinical remission at 12 months on mesalamine		No difference in recurrence between open vs. lap ileocecal resection for CD	NA	NA	NA

2008	Washington University of Medicine, MO	565	Retrospective analysis	Ileocolonic resection for CD	176 patients	A family history of inflammatory bowel disease (HR, 2.24; 95% CI, 1.16–4.30; $P = .016$), smoking at time of initial ileocolic resection (HR, 2.08; 95% CI, 1.11–3.91; $P = .023$) was associated with an increased risk of a second ileocolic resection, whereas postoperative prescription of immunomodulators (HR, 0.40; 95% CI, 0.18–0.88; $P = .022$) was associated with a decreased risk of a second ileocolic resection	Family history and smoking are predictors of surgical CD recurrence, whereas postoperative medical therapy decreased the risk of surgical recurrence in CD	Family history, smoking	NA	NA
2008	University of Pennsylvania	403	Meta-analysis	Surgery for CD	12 studies	Median follow-up: 52 weeks	Prior steroid therapy was the only factor found to be associated with maintaining remission ($P = .04$). The pooled placebo endoscopic recurrence rate was 58% (95% CI, 51%–65%; range, 36%–80%) during a median follow-up of 52 weeks (range, 12–156 weeks), with significant heterogeneity noted ($P = .0003$)	Placebo rates in PC-RCTs evaluating postoperative clinical and endoscopic recurrence demonstrate significant variability, which is influenced by specific study characteristics	Prior surgery, penetrating CD	NA	NA

continued

TABLE 30-1 Multi-institutional Results of Surgical Treatment of Crohn's Disease *(continued)*

YEAR	INSTITUTION	REFERENCE	TYPE OF STUDY	INTERVENTION	NO. OF PARTICIPANTS	LENGTH OF FOLLOW-UP	RESULTS	P VALUE	CONCLUSION	RISK FACTORS	MORBIDITY	MORTALITY
							Prior surgery, concomitant small bowel and colonic disease, fistulizing phenotype, or prior immunomodulator therapy influenced endoscopic recurrence (*P* < .05)					
2009	Department of Gastroenterology-Hepatology, The Netherlands	355	Retrospective	Surgery for CD	87 patients		The T allele at TIMP-1 SNP +372 T/C was found to be associated with an increased risk for surgical recurrence. Higher levels of TIMP-1, TIMP-2, and MMP-9 in noninflamed CD tissue, but not in inflamed tissue, and negative smoking status independently protected against diagnostic and/or surgical recurrence		The TIMP-1 SNP +372 T allele with an increased risk of recurrence is in line with our previous results demonstrating increased CD susceptibility and low TIMP-1 protein expression associated with this allele. High TIMP and MMP-9 levels in noninflamed tissue are predictive of a favorable disease recurrence in CD. The contribution of MMP-9 and TIMPs to disease recurrence appears not to be mediated by smoking status	T allele at TIMP-1 SNP +372 T/C, smoking	NA	NA

Year	N	Location	Study	Topic	Sample	Duration	Findings	Complications	Recurrence risk	IASC	Deaths
2008	253	University of Regensburg, Germany	Retrospective	Surgery for CD	282 patients underwent 331 intestinal resections		The incidence of the postoperative IASC is predominantly determined by preoperative disease severity. IASC have a detrimental influence on the long-term outcome following intestinal resections in patients with Crohn's disease, leading to increased number of repeat resection surgery	Articular disease manifestation ($P = .03$), duration of symptoms leading to surgery ($P = .09$), and weight loss ($P = .03$) were associated with occurrence of postoperative complications	Increased risk of surgical recurrence postoperative IASC ($P = .0002$) and previous bowel resections ($P = .002$)	IASCs occurred after 46 operations (16%)	4 patients died (1.2%)
2008	111	Department of Gastroenterology, Leuven University Hospitals, Belgium	RCT	AZA/metronidazole vs. metronidazole alone	81 patients: 40 in AZA, 41 in metronidazole	12 months	Endoscopic recurrence 14/32 (43.7%) AZA patients and 20/29 (69.0%) placebo patients at 12 months postsurgery ($P = .048$). At month 12, 7 of 32 patients had no endoscopic lesions in the AZA group vs. 1 of 29 in the placebo group ($P = .037$)	AZA with metronidazole decreased endoscopic recurrence rates postoperatively for CD	NA	NA	NA
2008	443	Università di Palermo, Italy	Meta-analysis	Recurrence outcome postsurgery for CD in placebo arm	Studies from 1990 to 2006		Placebo relapse rate was 23.7% (95% CI, 13–35; range, 0–78), significant heterogeneity among studies ($P < .0001$)	There is significant heterogeneity among placebo rates in postoperative CD. No single-design variable was identified that explained the heterogeneity in placebo outcomes for clinical or endoscopic recurrence	NA	NA	NA

continued

TABLE 30-1 Multi-institutional Results of Surgical Treatment of Crohn's Disease *(continued)*

YEAR	INSTITUTION	REFERENCE	TYPE OF STUDY	INTERVENTION	NO. OF PARTICIPANTS	LENGTH OF FOLLOW-UP	RESULTS	P VALUE	CONCLUSION	RISK FACTORS	MORBIDITY	MORTALITY
2008	Cleveland Clinic Ohio	534	Randomized trial	Lap vs. open ileocolectomy	56 patients: 27 lap, 29 open	Mean follow-up: 10.5 years	8 patients for each group underwent initial reoperative (26% LC vs. 28% OC; $P = .89$). OC patients requiring operation during follow-up were significantly more likely than LC to require multiple operations ($P = .006$)		Long-term data from this prospective randomized trial confirm that LC is at least comparable to OC in the treatment of ileocolic CD	NA	1 patient with incisional hernia repair after LC (4%) vs. 4 patients (14%) after OC ($P = .61$). 2 patients in the LC group adhesiolysis vs. none after OC ($P = .23$)	1 patient died, cause unrelated to CD
2008	Imperial College London, United Kingdom	436	Meta-analysis	None	16 studies: N = 2,962; smokers = 1,393; nonsmokers = 1,425	5 and 10 years	OR = 2.15 for smokers compared to nonsmokers	$P < .001$	Patients with CD who smoke have 2.5 times increased risk of surgical recurrence and 2 times increased risk of clinical risk compared to nonsmokers	Smoking	NA	NA
2009	University of Pittsburgh, PA	439	RCT	Infliximab vs. placebo	24	1 year	Rx group: 1/11 (9.1%) Placebo group: 11/13 (84.6%)	$P = .0006$	Proportion of CD patients with endoscopic recurrence after ileal resection at 1 year	Smoking	NA	0
2009	University of Padova, Italy	491	Prospective	None	N = 20 (1999–2005)	?	TGF-β1 production in healthy bowels has direct correlation to clinical CD recurrence	$P = .04$	High levels of TGF-β1 in healthy bowels of patient undergoing ileocolic resection for CD are associated with earlier clinical disease recurrence	NA	NA	NA

continued

Year		Institution	Study type	Intervention	N		Results	P value	Conclusion			Adverse	
							Higher TGF-β1 mRNA transcripts in healthy intestines associated with higher cumulative experience	P = .02					
2009	393	Università Tor Vergata di Roma, Italy	Retrospective	None	N = 537	?	Frequency of recurrence was higher in patients with ileocolonic resection than in those with other types of resections OR = 2.56 for surgical recurrence for smokers at 10-year follow-up	P < .0001; P < .001	Postoperative recurrence is observed in high proportion of CD after resection other than ileocolonic	RF comparable for both groups: smoking, appendectomy, family history	NA		NA
2009	114	Beth Israel Deaconess Boston, MA	Meta-analysis	Use of medical therapy post-operatively	23 RCT studies	NA	Nitroimidazole antibiotics CR: RR, 0.23; 95% CI, 0.09–0.57; NNT = 4; ER: RR, 0.44; 95% CI, 0.26–0.74; NNT = 4. Mesalamine CR: RR, 0.76; 95% CI, 0.62–0.94; NNT = 12; ER: RR, 0.50; 95% CI, 0.29–0.84; NNT = 8. AZA/6-MP CR: RR, 0.59; 95% CI, 0.38–0.92; NNT = 7; ER: RR, 0.64; 95% CI, 0.44–0.92; NNT = 4	NA	Nitroimidazole antibiotics, mesalamine, and immunosuppressive therapy with AZA/6-MP are superior to placebo for the prevention of postoperative recurrence of CD	NA	NA	Adverse reaction of nitroimidazole antibiotics: RR, 2.39; 95% CI, 1.5–3.7	NA

TABLE 30-1 Multi-institutional Results of Surgical Treatment of Crohn's Disease (continued)

YEAR	INSTITUTION	REFERENCE	TYPE OF STUDY	INTERVENTION	NO. OF PARTICIPANTS	LENGTH OF FOLLOW-UP	RESULTS	PVALUE	CONCLUSION	RISK FACTORS	MORBIDITY	MORTALITY
2009	Saint-Antoine Hospital, France	523	Retrospective data review	Ileocolonic or ileal resection for CD	N = 164 patients (from 1995 to 2006)	2 years	Early clinical recurrence in 28.1%	NA	Submucosal plexitis is associated with early clinical recurrence	Active smoking: HR, 1.94; 95% CI, 1.06–3.60; P = .033 Submucosal plexitis: HR, 1.87; 95% CI, 1.00–3.46; P = .48	NA	NA
2009	Universitaire de Lille, France	409	Meta-analysis	AZA/6-MP	4 RCTs: 3 AZA, 1 6-MP; N = 433	1 year	AZA/6-MP were more effective at preventing clinical recurrence at 1 year: mean difference, 8; 95% CI, 1%–15%; NNT = 13	P = .021	Purine analogs are more effective than placebo in preventing clinical and endoscopic recurrence in CD but have more adverse events leading to drug withdrawal	None	Rate of adverse events leading to drug withdrawal 17.2% vs. 9.8% (P = .021)	NA
2009	University of Toronto, Canada	353	RCT	Stapled side-to-side anastomosis vs. hand-sewn end-to-end	N = 139	12 months	Endoscopic recurrence: 42.5% in end-to-end hand-sewn and 37.9% in stapled side-to-side (−4.6%; 95% CI, −21.0 to 11.9)	P = .55	No difference in rate of recurrence between types of anastomoses after ileocolic resection for CD	Mean duration of disease, number of previous resections, compliance with postoperative maintenance therapy	Complications: E-E anastomosis, 24%; S-S anastomosis 20%, p.79 (leaks/abscess)	NA
2009	Mount Sinai Medical Center, NY	205	Retrospective observational cohort	Strictureplasties for CD strictures	N = 88 patients, 339 strictureplasties	5 and 10 years	Reoperation for CD recurrence. 5-year reoperation rates: 14% ≤ 8 strictures, 31% > 8 strictures	P = .01	Number of strictures and strictureplasties are associated with CD recurrence	Number of strictures and strictureplasties	9 complications: 2 abscesses, 3 ileus, 4 wound infections	NA

Year	Ref	Institution	Study design	Intervention	Sample	Follow-up	Results	P value	Comment	Risk factors	Morbidity	Mortality
							5-year reoperation rates: 14% ≤ 4 strictureplasties compared with 33% > 4 strictureplasties	$P < .01$	NA	NA	NA	
2009	605	Yokkaichi Social Insurance Hospital, Japan	Prospective nonrandomized	Infliximab rx after endoscopic recurrence 6 months postoperative	N = 26: 10 mesalamine, 8 infliximab, 8 azathioprine	6 months	Clinical recurrence (CDAI ≥ 150): 0 in infliximab group, 3 (38%) azathioprine group, 7 (70%) mesalamine group / Endoscopic inflammation was improved: 75% infliximab group, 38% azathioprine, 0% mesalamine	$P = .01$ / $P = .006$	Infliximab rx shows suppressive effects on clinical and endoscopic disease activity. Infliximab also decreased inflammatory cytokine levels at 6-month follow-up when compared to baseline, and at 6 months when compared to mesalamine and azathioprine	NA	NA	NA
2009	474	Mount Sinai University Hospital, NY	Retrospective cohort	Ileocolonic resection	N = 34: 12 with stricturing disease, 22 with penetrating disease	Up to 25 years	3-year time point indicated early recurrence. 0/12 had recurrence at 3 years for stricturing disease. 12/22 (55%) had recurrence at 3 years	$P = .002$	There is a strong association between penetrating CD and postoperative recurrence	Penetrating disease	NA	NA
2009	379	Melbourne University, Australia; Imperial College London, United Kingdom	Retrospective cohort	Ileocolonic resection between the years 2002 and 2005	N = 99: 57 females, 42 males	Mean: 32 months (12–48)	Clinical recurrence rate after index ileocolonic resection was 28% at 1 year and surgical recurrence rate was 5%		Postoperative recurrence of CD was high in short term	Previous surgery	2 anastomotic leaks, 1 intra-abdominal abscess	1 death, 2/2 hypovolemic shock

continued

TABLE 30-1 Multi-institutional Results of Surgical Treatment of Crohn's Disease (continued)

YEAR	INSTITUTION	REFERENCE	TYPE OF STUDY	INTERVENTION	NO. OF PARTICIPANTS	LENGTH OF FOLLOW-UP	RESULTS	PVALUE	CONCLUSION	RISK FACTORS	MORBIDITY	MORTALITY
2009	University Hospital of Heidelberg, Germany	323	Retrospective cohort		n = 147 with anorectal or rectovaginal fistulas	5 years	At 5 years, complex fistulas had a trend toward higher recurrence rate (45.6%) after surgery than submucosal fistulas (18.8%) No recurrence after surgery for submucosal fistulas at 13 months	P = .079	There is a trend toward higher recurrence rates of CD after surgical repair of complex fistulas	NA	NA	NA
2009	Guangxi Medical University, China	73	Meta-analysis	Medical rx p surgical resection for CD	14 studies, N = 1,497	NA	Clinical recurrence with medical treatment: RR, 0.74; 95% CI, 0.64–0.87	P = .000	Medical treatment decreases risk of clinical postoperative recurrence in patients with CD	NA	NA	NA
2009	Luigi Sacco University Hospital, Italy; University College of London, United Kingdom	478	Prospective cohort	Conservative surgery for SB CD	n = 393 patients, 865 jejunoileal segments underwent 318 SBRs and 367 strictureplasties	5.2 years ± 3.25 SD	Young age: HR, 2.4; 95% CI, 1.0–5.4; P = .03 Upper jejunal location: HR, 2.5; 95% CI, 1.3–4.7; P = .004 Stricturing: HR, 2.2; 95% CI, 1.1–4.1; P = .01 SB thickening at 12 months: HR, 4.5; 95% CI, 2.3–8.6; P = .000		Young patients with extended and stricturing disease and bowel thickening 12 months after surgery are at high risk for recurrence after surgery	Younger age, extended SB disease, strictures, SB thickening at 12 months	Complication rate, 5.6%: anastomotic leak 15/22; hemoperitoneum, PE, postoperative ileus	None
2010	Multicentre trial (21 from Austria, Czech Republic, Germany, and Israel)	440	Double-blind RCT	AZA vs. mesalazine	N = 78 with CD s/p IC resection with known endoscopic recurrence	1 year	Treatment failure: Azathioprine (22%) Mesalazine (10.8%)	P = .19	Azathioprine group had higher rate of treatment failure, 2/2 stopping rx because of adverse reaction. However, that group had less clinical recurrence	NA	Adverse reaction to azathioprine: pancreatitis, leukopenia, vomiting, glomerulonephritis	NA

continued

Year	Center	No.	Design	Question	N	Follow-up	Outcome	P value	Comments	Predictor	
							Clinical recurrence: Azathioprine (0%) Mesalazine (10.8%)	P = .031		NA	NA
							Drug discontinuation 2/2 adverse reaction: Azathioprine (22%) Mesalazine (0%)	P = .023			
2010	University of Udine, Italy; University of Manchester, United Kingdom	525	Prospective cohort	Stopping infliximab	N = 12	1 year	10/12 patients recurred once infliximab stopped at 3-year time point	NA	Patients were observed postsurgically for 3 years on infliximab and 1 year after once infliximab was discontinued. No recurrence at the time infliximab was stopped. Follow-up after 1 year led to endoscopic recurrence. Mucosa integrity maintained on low-dose infliximab	3/12 smokers	NA
							Negative association between infliximab dose and CRP/FC	P = .0001			
2010	Mayo Clinic, Rochester, MN	334	Retrospective record review	Laparoscopic primary ileocolic CD	n = 89	Median follow-up: 3.5 years (1.8 months to 11 years)	Presence of granuloma: HR, 2.89; 95% CI, 1.26–6.64	P = .01	5–/109 (61%) recurrence at 13.1 months (median). Analysis of clinical factors age, type of anastomosis, medically refractory disease, smoking, +granulomas, postoperative prophylaxis) showed that presence of granulomas was the only significant predictor of recurrence. No significant difference in recurrence for those receiving postoperative prophylaxis	Presence of granuloma in resected specimen	NA

TABLE 30-1 Multi-institutional Results of Surgical Treatment of Crohn's Disease (continued)

YEAR	INSTITUTION	REFERENCE	TYPE OF STUDY	INTERVENTION	NO. OF PARTICIPANTS	LENGTH OF FOLLOW-UP	RESULTS	PVALUE	CONCLUSION	RISK FACTORS	MORBIDITY	MORTALITY
2010	University of Vienna, Austria	400	Retrospective	Postoperative exposure to thiopurines	N = 326	3–265 months	SR 151/326 (46.3%) median time of 71 months (3–265); reduction of SR reduced with AZA/6-MP postoperatively for ≥ 36 months compared with < 36 months or without postoperative rx of AZA/6-MP	P = .004	Long-term maintenance rx (AZA/6-MP ≥ 36 months) reduces the risk of surgical recurrence. Smoking is a risk factor for surgical recurrence	Smoking: HR, 1.6; 95% CI, 1.14–2.40; P = .008	NA	NA
2011	Cleveland Clinic Florida	411	Retrospective	Laparoscopy for recurrent CD compared with primary laparoscopy	N = 130 (2001–2008): group 1, primary laparoscopy; group 2, reoperative lap	?	G1, 80 patients; G2, 50 patients G2 with longer period of disease (15.5 vs. 8.9 years; P = .0002) Immunosuppressive rx: G1, 83%; G2, 84% Conversion rates: G1, 18.7% vs. G2, 32% (P = .09)	NA	No difference between lap-assisted resection for recurrent CD when compared to primary laparoscopy, when comparing length of surgery, blood loss, conversion to open, and postoperative complications	NA	Anastomotic leak: G1, 5%; G2, 2% (P = .65) Abdominal abscess: G1, 3.75%; G2, 8.00% (P = .56) Reoperation rates: G1, 10%; G2, 6% (P = .53)	None
2011	General Infirmary at Leeds, United Kingdom	30	Retrospective data review	Laparoscopic resection for recurrent CD	N = 27 (2005–2009)	NA	All patients had recurrent CD at ileocolic anastomosis. Median operative time was 110 minutes (70–170 minutes) with conversion rate of 2/27. Length of stay was 4 days (2–7 days) with return to full activity of 3.5 weeks (2–7 weeks)	NA	Laparoscopic resection of recurrent ileocolic CD is safe and feasible	NA	NA	NA

Year	Institution	Study type	Topic	N	Follow-up	Results	P	Conclusion	RF for conversion to open	Morbidity	
2010	University of Paris, France	Retrospective data review	Laparoscopic resection for recurrent CD	n = 62 reoperations in 57 patients for CD recurrence (1998–2008)	NA	29 laparoscopic (LG), 33 open (OG) Intraoperative intestinal injury: LG, 5; OG, 0 (P = .01) Difference in mean operating time and use of stoma between the OG and LG group was nonsignificant	NA	Morbidity rate is similar when comparing open to lap approach for reoperation for CD. Laparoscopy is feasible for reoperation especially for nonfistulizing disease	fistulizing disease (P = .02) and intraoperative intestinal injury (P < .001)	Morbidity rate: LG, 38% OG, 30%	None
2011	Asahikawa Medical University, Japan	Retrospective	Kono-S anastomosis	N = 142 patients: 69 in exp group S (2003–2009); 73 in comparison group C (1993–2003)	Median follow-up exp: 42 months (7–82); control: 52 (1–120)	Median endoscopic recurrence score in group S 2.6 vs. 3.4 in group C Lesser problem of anastomotic surgical recurrence in group S at 5 years (0% vs. 15%; P = .0013)	P = .008	Kono-S anastomosis appears to be effective in preventing anastomotic surgical recurrence in CD	NA	Group C: 3 anastomotic leaks, surgical site infection, intra-abdominal abscess, ileus Group S: 3 surgical site infections	None
2011	Miyazaki University School of Medicine, Japan	Prospective observational	Infliximab after seton placement anal fistula in CD	20 patients (from 2002 to 2009)	31.8 ± 4.2 months	After induction therapy, complete response (CR) in 8/20 patients, partial response (PR) in 9/20, disease progress in 3/20. After maintenance therapy, CR in 13/17 patients	NA	Seton drainage and infliximab therapy is effective in patients with perianal CD	NA	NA	NA

continued

TABLE 30-1 Multi-institutional Results of Surgical Treatment of Crohn's Disease *(continued)*

YEAR	INSTITUTION	REFERENCE	TYPE OF STUDY	INTERVENTION	NO. OF PARTICIPANTS	LENGTH OF FOLLOW-UP	RESULTS	P VALUE	CONCLUSION	RISK FACTORS	MORBIDITY	MORTALITY
2011	Cleveland Clinic Ohio	269	Prospective cohort		69 patients: 45 females, 24 males	Median time: 38 months (3.3–236.0)	Median time to reoperation = 38 months. Early reoperation (< 38 months): 1. Stricturing disease 2. Penetrating disease 3. Postoperative complications from previous surgery	1. OR, 12.1; 95% CI, 1.8–80.9 2. OR, 9.9; 95% CI, 1.40–67.9 3. OR, 12.1; 95% CI, 1.2–126.6	Early recurrence of CD requiring reoperation is associated with specific disease and potentially modifiable operation such as postoperative complications	NA	NA	NA
2011	Hôpital Saint-Louis, France	20	Retrospective cohort	Total proctocolectomy with definitive ileostomy	N = 55	Median follow-up: 5.4 years	Clinical recurrence at 1, 5, and 8 years: 4%, 27%, 39% Clinical recurrence rate was higher with penetrating disease: RR, 1.7; 95% CI, 1.5–19.0 Reoperation for CD recurrence at 1, 5, and 8 years: 0%, 10%, 18%	P = .05	Recurrence after total proctocolectomy with definitive ileostomy for CD is not uncommon	NA	NA	NA

Year	Ref	Institution	Study type	Intervention	N	Follow-up	Postoperative course	Conclusion	Risk factors	Complications	
2011	337	Filippo Neri Hospital, Italy	Retrospective cohort	Ileocecal resection	N = 212	Median follow-up: 117 months	Postoperative course without clinical recurrence at 30, 60, 90, and 120 months: 78.2%, 69.4%, 58.0%, 50.6%; without surgical recurrence: 97.0%, 96.4%, 85.6%, 72.0%; early surgery (within 3 years of diagnosis) was associated with longer postoperative course without recurrence	Early surgery should be considered for isolated ileocecal disease	Late surgery > 3 years from diagnosis	NA	NA
2011	448	University of Toronto, Canada	Retrospective cohort	Colectomy/ileorectal anastomosis	N = 81 (1982–2010)	5 and 10 years	At 5 and 10 years, percentage with functioning ileorectal anastomosis are as follows: 87.0% (95% CI, 75.5–93.3) 72.2% (95% CI, 55.8–83.4)	Reoperation rate and/or proctectomy rate is 30% after colectomy and ileorectal anastomosis for Crohn's colitis	Smoking proctectomy: HR, 3.93; 95% CI, 1.46–10.55 Reoperative: HR, 2.12; 95% CI, 0.96–4.72	Overall anastomotic leak rate: 7.4%	NA
2012	485	University of Genoa, Italy	Case series	Adalimumab	6 patients s/p ileocecal resection	3 years	No recurrence in any of the patients. Disease-free for ≈3 years after surgery on clinical, radiologic, and endoscopic/histologic grounds (CDAI ≤ 110 in all occasions)	These are the first cases, to our knowledge, in which adalimumab has been successfully used to prevent the postsurgical recurrence of CD. Need for clinical trial	NA	NA	NA

AZA, azathioprine; BMI, body mass index; CD, Crohn's disease; CDAI, Crohn's Disease Activity Index; CI, confidence interval; CR, clinical recurrence; CRP, C-reactive protein; E-E, end-to-end; E-S, end-to-side; EPR, endoscopic postoperative recurrence; ER, endoscopic recurrence; FC, fecal calprotectin; H-M, Heineke-Mikulicz; HS, hand-sewn; HR, hazard ratio; IL, interleukin; IRA, ileorectal anastomosis; IC, ileocolonic; IASC, intra-abdominal septic complication; LC, laparoscopic; MTX, methotrexate; NA, not applicable; NNT, number needed to treat; OR, odds ratio; OC, open ileocolectomy; PC-RCTs, placebo in randomized clinical trials; PR, postoperative recurrence; RCT, randomized controlled trial; RF, risk factor; RIR, relative incidence rate; RR, risk ratio; SB, small bowel; SBO, small bowel obstruction; SBR, small bowel resection; SC, segmental colectomy; 6-MP, 6-mercaptopurine; SNP, single-nucleotide polymorphism; SR, surgical recurrence; S-S, side-to-side; TGF, transforming growth factor; TIMP, tissue inhibitors of metalloproteinases; TNF, tumor necrosis factor.

▶ INDETERMINATE COLITIS

The differential diagnosis between ulcerative colitis and Crohn's colitis can usually be made based on clinical, radiologic, endoscopic, and pathologic criteria. However, up to 15% of patients develop nonspecific IBD of a type that cannot clearly be labeled as one or the other, often because of overlapping features. These individuals therefore have been classified as having an indeterminate colitis.

Indeterminate colitis is essentially a pathologic diagnosis; that is to say, there are often equivocal or contradictory histologic observations. In a review from St. Mark's Hospital of 30 such cases, nearly all patients had undergone urgent surgery.[428] As a consequence, these individuals had histologic features of incipient or established fulminant disease. This clinical presentation is probably the reason for the confusing histologic picture because the pathology of Crohn's disease and that of ulcerative colitis in the acute phase have much in common.[428] There is insufficient opportunity—clinically, radiologically, or endoscopically—to clarify the nature of the disease. It follows, then, that the disease activity affects the evaluation of morphologic features and that, given the opportunity, repeat evaluation during a quiescent phase may clarify any confusion.

The diagnosis of Crohn's colitis is made by either the clinician (preoperatively or intraoperatively) or the pathologist. It is the latter who is responsible for creating the diagnosis of indeterminate colitis. Typical features in patients otherwise thought to have ulcerative colitis include "intermittent" ulceration, relative rectal sparing, preservation of goblet cell population, and deep fissuring. Absence of granulomas in certain patients with presumed Crohn's disease also may place the patient in an indeterminate category. Lee and colleagues suggest the additional criteria of extensive mucosal and submucosal ulceration separated by normal colonic mucosa, nonaggregate full-thickness inflammation, increased vascularity in the base of the ulceration, and absence of both crypt abscesses and transmural lymphoid aggregates.[301]

Surgical Options

If the accuracy of the clinical (endoscopic, radiologic) and pathologic diagnosis is problematic, the surgeon would be wise to stage the procedure and not to embark on restorative proctocolectomy. Unfortunately, this admonition is only helpful when there is indeed a heightened suspicion as to the potential for error in diagnosis. By definition, patients with indeterminate colitis never have the diagnosis truly clarified, or Crohn's disease is demonstrated in the resected specimen, or Crohn's disease develops subsequently. One may also consider performing a total abdominal proctocolectomy, leaving only the anus and sphincters. This important technical consideration, resecting the rectum as low as is possible, facilitates the subsequent procedure—either completion proctectomy or a restorative operation. A particularly compelling caution against performing restorative proctocolectomy is the presence of an anal fistula or perineal disease.

Results of Restorative Proctocolectomy

Pezim and colleagues reviewed the Mayo Clinic experience with 25 patients who underwent restorative proctocolectomy for indeterminate colitis.[410] There were no significant differences in complication rates, pouch function, incidence of "pouchitis," or requirement for pouch excision, when comparing these individuals with those who underwent the operation for ulcerative colitis. However, the experience from the Lahey Clinic was quite different.[272] In a retrospective review of 18 patients so identified, 50% experienced complications. This compares with a complication rate of only 3% when the procedure was performed for ulcerative colitis. Furthermore, the requirement for subsequent ileostomy was much greater in individuals with indeterminate colitis. In another paper from the same institution, the authors suggest that pouchitis will usually respond to metronidazole and is less likely to recur if the patient truly harbored ulcerative colitis initially.[434] Conversely, individuals with indeterminate colitis were less likely to respond to metronidazole, required sulfasalazine and/or steroids, and had more frequent exacerbations. In a still later paper from the Lahey Clinic Medical Center, now involving 42 patients with indeterminate colitis, the preceding concerns still persisted—that is, increased risk of pouch-related complications, eventual pouch failure, and the discovery of Crohn's disease subsequently.[335]

Our experience at the Cleveland Clinic with indeterminate colitis consists of 115 individuals.[105] Functional results and the incidence of some complications were comparable to that of the ulcerative colitis patients. The incidence of pouch failure was identical also, 3.4%. However, indeterminate colitis patients were more likely to develop minor perineal fistulas, pelvic abscess, and, of course, Crohn's disease.

A report from the Mayo Clinic involved 71 patients who underwent ileal pouch-anal anastomosis for what proved to be indeterminate colitis.[351] At a mean of nearly 5 years following surgery, failure occurred more frequently in those with indeterminate colitis than in those diagnosed with ulcerative colitis. Still, more than 80% were felt to have long-term functional results identical to those of patients with ulcerative colitis.[351] In a later report from the same institution involving 82 patients, with a median follow-up of 83 months, the investigators concluded that those who underwent restorative proctocolectomy who did not subsequently develop Crohn's disease had nearly identical results as those who underwent the surgery for ulcerative colitis.[610] Conversely, those who developed Crohn's disease had significantly poorer results. The experience of Atkinson and colleagues was similar.[26] In their 16 patients diagnosed with indeterminate colitis, the success rate for restorative proctocolectomy was 81%, compared with 95% for ulcerative colitis. Others opine that it is reasonable to offer restorative proctocolectomy to those with indeterminate colitis despite the increased incidence of fistulas.[462] Until further data become available, utilization of the pouch procedure in these individuals requires circumspection.

▶ CONCLUSION

The results of surgery for Crohn's disease are less than satisfactory. The concept that repeated resections will ultimately cure the patient is obviously erroneous. It is evident that as additional operations are required, the likelihood of recurrence is actually increased. One must therefore limit surgical intervention to those patients who have complications severe enough to justify an operation. Long-standing disease is not yet a surgical indication, as it classically has been for ulcerative colitis. Because it is not clear what the actual prognostic validity of the concept of dysplasia is in patients with Crohn's colitis and because the incidence of malignant change is low, long duration of disease is not itself an indication for surgical intervention. However, recent opinions suggest that when dysplastic changes are identified, resection should be advised. Bypass procedures and exclusion operations should not be performed except under unusual circumstances. If carried out, definitive resection should be undertaken at the earliest possible time. Strictureplasty should be applied for those in whom a resection would result in the potential for significant disability. Creating a large anastomosis whenever one is performed is probably prudent, even without level 1 evidence to support the concept. Because important endoscopic lesions may be present without clinical symptoms, periodic colonoscopy should be part of the follow-up evaluation of all patients who have undergone an anastomosis in the colon for Crohn's disease.

The future is very hopeful. There are a number of new and exciting nonoperative treatments. It is hoped that within the next few years successful medical management can be anticipated and that surgery for this condition will be relegated to that of a historical curiosity.

References

1. Acheson ED. An association between ulcerative colitis, regional enteritis, and ankylosing spondylitis. *Q J Med*. 1960;29:489.
2. Achkar JP, Hanauer SB. Medical therapy to reduce post-operative Crohn's disease recurrence. *Am J Gastroenterol*. 2000;95:1139.
3. Adloff M, Arnaud JP, Ollier JC. Does the histologic appearance at the margin of resection affect the postoperative recurrence of Crohn's disease? *Am Surg*. 1987;53:543.
4. Agha FP, Woolsey EJ, Amendola MA. Psoas abscess in inflammatory bowel disease. *Am J Gastroenterol*. 1985;80:924.
5. Agnholt J, Dahlerup J, Lyhne-Nielsen S, et al. Treatment of fistulizing Crohn's disease with infliximab: one year follow by MR scan, ultrasound and clinical examination. *Gastroenterology*. 2002;122:A612.
6. Aitken RJ, Wright JP, Bok A, et al. Crohn's disease precipitating a spinal extradural abscess and paraplegia. *Br J Surg*. 1986;73:1004.
7. Alexander AC, Irving MH. Accumulation and pepsin solubility of collagens in the bowel of patients with Crohn's disease. *Dis Colon Rectum*. 1990;33:956.
8. Alexander-Williams J. Perianal Crohn's disease. *World J Surg*. 1980;4:203.
9. Alexander-Williams J. The technique of intestinal strictureplasty. *Int J Colorect Dis*. 1986;1:54.
10. Alexander-Williams J, Buchmann P. Perianal Crohn's disease. *World J Surg*. 1980;4:203.
11. Alexander-Williams J, Haynes IG. Conservative operations for Crohn's disease of the small bowel. *World J Surg*. 1985;9:945.
12. Al-Jahdali H, Thompson WG, Matzinger FR. Non-fatal portal pyaemia complicating Crohn's disease of the terminal ileum. *Gut*. 1994;35:560.
13. Allan A, Andrews H, Hilton CJ, et al. Segmental colonic resection is an appropriate operation for skip lesions due to Crohn's disease in the colon. *World J Surg*. 1989;13:611.
14. Allan RN. Extra-intestinal manifestations of inflammatory bowel disease. *Clin Gastroenterol*. 1983;12:617.
15. Allen DC, Hughes DF, Calvert CH. Carcinoma in Crohn's disease of the colon. *Dis Colon Rectum*. 1986;29:760.
16. Alum Jones V. Comparison of total parenteral nutrition and elemental diet in induction of remission of Crohn's disease. *Dig Dis Sci*. 1986;32:100.
17. Alvarez-Lobos M, Arostequi JI, Sans M, et al. Crohn's disease patients carrying NOD2/Card15 gene variants have an increased and early need for first surgery due to stricturing disease and higher rate of surgical recurrence. *Ann Surg*. 2005;242:693.
18. Ambrose NS, Allan RN, Keighley MRB, et al. Antibiotic therapy for treatment in relapse of intestinal Crohn's disease: a prospective randomized study. *Dis Colon Rectum*. 1985;28:81.
19. Ambrose NS, Keighley MRB, Alexander-Williams J, et al. Clinical impact of colectomy and ileorectal anastomosis in the management of Crohn's disease. *Gut*. 1984;25:223.
20. Amiot A, Gornet JM, Baudry C, et al. Crohn's disease recurrence after total proctocolectomy with definitive ileostomy. *Dig Liver Dis*. 2011;43:698.
21. Andersson P, Olaison G, Hallbök O, et al. Segmental resection or subtotal colectomy in Crohn's colitis? *Dis Colon Rectum*. 2002;45:47.
22. Andrews HA, Lewis P, Allan RN. Prognosis after surgery for colonic Crohn's disease. *Br J Surg*. 1989;76:1184.
23. Anscline PF, Wlodarczyk J, Murugasu R. Presence of granulomas is associated with recurrence after surgery for Crohn's disease: experience of a surgical unit. *Br J Surg*. 1997;84:78.
24. Ardizzone S, Maconi G, Sampietro GM, et al. Azathioprine and mesalamine for prevention of relapse after conservative surgery for Crohn's disease. *Gastroenterology*. 2004;127:730.
25. Arnold GL, Beaves MR, Pryjdun VO, et al. Preliminary study of ciprofloxacin in active Crohn's disease. *Inflamm Bowel Dis*. 2002;8:10.
26. Atkinson KG, Owen DA, Wankling G. Restorative proctocolectomy and indeterminate colitis. *Am J Surg*. 1994;167:516.
27. Avidan B, Sakhini E, Lahat A, et al. Risk factors regarding the need for a second operation in patients with Crohn's disease. *Digestion*. 2005;72:248.
28. Ballinger A, Farthing MJG. Ulcerative colitis complicated by Wenckebach arteriovenascular block. *Gut*. 1992;33:1427.
29. Bambach CP, Robertson WG, Peacock M, et al. Effect of intestinal surgery on the risk of urinary stone formation. *Gut*. 1981;22:257.
30. Bandyopadhyay D, Sagar PM, Mirnezami A, et al. Laparoscopic resection for recurrent Crohn's disease: safety, feasibility, and short-term outcomes. *Colorectal Dis*. 2011;13:161.
31. Bar-Meir S, Chowers Y, Lavy A, et al. Budesonide vs. prednisone in the treatment of active Crohn's disease. *Gastroenterology*. 1998;115:835.
32. Barnett WO. The continent jejunal reservoir in Crohn's colitis. *J Miss State Med Assoc*. 1986;27:119.
33. Basu MK, Asquith P. Oral manifestations of inflammatory bowel disease. *Clin Gastroenterol*. 1980;9:307.
34. Bell SJ, Halligan S, Windsor A, et al. Value of MRI in assessing the response of fistulating Crohn's disease to treatment with infliximab. *Gastroenterology*. 2002;122:A617.
35. Belluzzi A, Brignola C, Campieri M, et al. Effect of an enteric-coated fish-oil preparation on relapses in Crohn's disease. *N Engl J Med*. 1996;334:1557.
36. Bergamaschi R, Pessaux P, Arnaud JP. Comparison of conventional and laparoscopic ileocolic resection for Crohn's disease. *Dis Colon Rectum*. 2003;46:1129.
37. Berman IR, Corman ML, Coller JA, et al. Late onset Crohn's disease in patients with colonic diverticulitis. *Dis Colon Rectum*. 1979;22:524.
38. Bernell O, Lapidus A, Hellers G. Risk factors for surgery and postoperative recurrence in Crohn's disease. *Ann Surg*. 2000;231:38.
39. Bernell O, Lapidus A, Hellers G. Risk factors for surgery and recurrence in 907 patients with primary ileocaecal Crohn's disease. *Br J Surg*. 2000;87:1697.
40. Bernell O, Lapidus A, Hellers G. Recurrence after colectomy in Crohn's colitis. *Dis Colon Rectum*. 2001;44:647.
41. Bernstein CN, Blanchard JF, Kliewer E, et al. Cancer risk in patients with inflammatory bowel disease: a population-based study. *Cancer*. 2001;91:854.
42. Bernstein LH, Frank MS, Brandt LJ, et al. Healing of perineal Crohn's disease with metronidazole. *Gastroenterology*. 1980;79:357.
43. Bernstein ML, McDonald JS. Oral lesions in Crohn's disease: report of two cases and update of the literature. *Oral Surg*. 1978;46:234.
44. Beubige EJ, Bagless TM, Milligan FD. Mucosal bridging in Crohn's disease of the colon. *Gastrointest Endosc*. 1975;21:189.
45. Biancone L, Sica GS, Calabrese E, et al. Frequency and pattern of endoscopic recurrence in Crohn's disease patients with ileocolonic resection using a laparoscopic versus laparotomic approach: a prospective longitudinal study. *Am J Gastroenterol*. 2008;103:809.
46. Binion DG, Theriot KR, Shidham S, et al. Clinical factors contributing to rapid reoperation for Crohn's disease patients undergoing resection and/or strictureplasty. *J Gastrointest Surg*. 2007;11:1692.
47. Bishop RP, Brewster AC, Antonioli DA. Crohn's disease of the mouth. *Gastroenterology*. 1972;62:302.
48. Blank A, Korelitz BI. Efficacy of 6-MP in prevention of endoscopic recurrence at anastomotic site after ileo-colic resection for Crohn's disease. *Am J Gastroenterol*. 2002;97:S255.
49. Bleday R, Lee E, Jessurun J, et al. Increased risk of early colorectal neoplasms after hepatic transplant in patients with inflammatory bowel disease. *Dis Colon Rectum*. 1993;36:908.
50. Bloom RJ, Larsen CP, Watt R, et al. A reappraisal of the Kock continent ileostomy in patients with Crohn's disease. *Surg Gynecol Obstet*. 1986;162:105.
51. Bodzin JH, Klein SN, Priest SG. Ileoproctostomy is preferred over ileoanal pull-through in patients with indeterminate colitis. *Am Surg*. 1995;61:590.

52. Boerr LA, Bai JC, Olivares L, et al. Cutaneous metastatic Crohn's disease: treatment with metronidazole. *Am J Gastroenterol.* 1987;82:1326.

53. Boirivant M, Pallone F, Ciaco A, et al. Usefulness of fecal á₁-antitrypsin clearance and fecal concentration as early indicator of postoperative asymptomatic recurrence in Crohn's disease. *Dig Dis Sci.* 1991;36:347.

54. Bonniere P, Wallaert B, Cortot A, et al. Latent pulmonary involvement in Crohn's disease: biological, functional, bronchoalveolar lavage and scintigraphic studies. *Gut.* 1986;27:919.

55. Borley NR, Mortensen NJ, Chaudry MA, et al. Recurrence after abdominal surgery for Crohn's disease. *Dis Colon Rectum.* 2002;45:377.

56. Brandt LJ, Bernstein LH, Boley SJ, et al. Metronidazole therapy for perineal Crohn's disease: a follow-up study. *Gastroenterology.* 1982;83:383.

57. Brenner A, Lavery I, Church J, et al. Perianal Crohn's disease and associated carcinoma. *Dis Colon Rectum.* 2001;44:A27.

58. Brignola C, Campieri M, Bazzocchi G, et al. A laboratory index for predicting relapse in asymptomatic patients with Crohn's disease. *Gastroenterology.* 1986;91:1490.

59. Brignola C, Cottone M, Pera A, et al. Mesalamine in the prevention of endoscopic recurrence after intestinal resection for Crohn's disease. *Gastroenterology.* 1995;108:345.

60. Broomé U, Löfberg R, Lundqvist K, et al. Subclinical time span of inflammatory bowel disease in patients with primary sclerosing cholangitis. *Dis Colon Rectum.* 1995;38:1301.

61. Brouquet A, Bretagnol F, Soprani A, et al. A laparoscopic approach to iterative ileocolonic resection for the recurrence of Crohn's disease. *Surg Endosc.* 2010;24:879.

62. Brynskov J, Freund L, Rasmussen SN, et al. A placebo-controlled, double-blind, randomized trial of cyclosporine therapy in active chronic Crohn's disease. *N Engl J Med.* 1989;321:845.

63. Buchmann P, Weterman IT, Keighley MRB, et al. The prognosis of ileorectal anastomosis in Crohn's disease. *Br J Surg.* 1981;68:7.

64. Bufo AJ, Feldman S, Daniels GA, et al. Stapled strictureplasty for Crohn's disease: a new technique. *Dis Colon Rectum.* 1995;38:664.

65. Bundred NJ, Dixon JM, Lumsden AB, et al. Free perforation in Crohn's colitis: a ten-year review. *Dis Colon Rectum.* 1985;28:35.

66. Byrne TA, Morrissey TB, Nattakom TV, et al. Growth hormone, glutamine, and a modified diet enhance nutrient absorption in patients with severe short bowel syndrome. *J Parenteral Enteral Nutr.* 1995;19:296.

67. Byrne TA, Persinger RL, Young LS, et al. A new treatment for patients with short-bowel syndrome: growth hormone, glutamine, and a modified diet. *Ann Surg.* 1995;222:243.

68. Cameron JL, Hamilton SR, Coleman J, et al. Patterns of ileal recurrence in Crohn's disease: a prospective randomized study. *Ann Surg.* 1992;215:546.

69. Camma C, Giuta M, Rosselli M, et al. Mesalamine in the maintenance and treatment of Crohn's disease: a meta-analysis adjusted for confounding variables. *Gastroenterology.* 1997;113:1465.

70. Campieri M, Ferguson A, Doe W, et al. Oral budesonide is as effective as oral prednisone in active Crohn's disease. The global budesonide study group. *Gut.* 1997;41:209.

71. Canadian Inflammatory Bowel Disease Study Group. Oral budesonide in active Crohn's disease: interim report of a placebo-controlled randomized trial. *Gastroenterology.* 1993;104:A175.

72. Cangemi JR, Wiesner RH, Beaver SJ, et al. Effect of proctocolectomy for chronic ulcerative colitis on the natural history of primary sclerosing cholangitis. *Gastroenterology.* 1989;96:790.

73. Cao Y, Gao F, Liao C. Meta-analysis of medical treatment and placebo treatment for preventing postoperative recurrence in Crohn's disease. *Int J Colorectal Dis.* 2009;24:509.

74. Caprilli R, Areoli A, Capurso L, et al. Oral mesalamine (5-aminosalicylic acid; Asacol) for the prevention of post-operative recurrence of Crohn's disease. *Aliment Pharmacol Ther.* 1994;8:35.

75. Card T, Logan RFA, Rodrigues LC, et al. Antibiotic use and the development of Crohn's disease. *Gut.* 2004;53:246.

76. Cattan P, Bonhomme N, Panis Y, et al. Fate of the rectum in patients undergoing total colectomy for Crohn's disease. *Br J Surg.* 2002;89:454.

77. Cave DR, Burakoff R. Pyoderma gangrenosum associated with ulcerative colitis: treatment with disodium cromoglycate. *Am J Gastroenterol.* 1987;82:802.

78. Chang RY, Hanauer SB, Cohen RD, et al. Parenteral methotrexate in refractory Crohn's disease. *Aliment Pharmacol Ther.* 2001;15:15.

79. Chardavoyne R, Flint GW, Pollack S, et al. Factors affecting recurrence following resection for Crohn's disease. *Dis Colon Rectum.* 1986;29:495.

80. Chermesh I, Tamir A, Reshef R, et al. Failure of Synbiotic 2000 to prevent postoperative recurrence of Crohn's disease. *Dig Dis Sci.* 2007;52:385.

81. Chevalier JM, Jones DJ, Ratelle R, et al. Colectomy and ileorectal anastomosis in patients with Crohn's disease. *Br J Surg.* 1994;81:1379.

82. Chew SSB, Douglas PR, Newstead GL, et al. Cholecystectomy in patients with Crohn's ileitis. *Dis Colon Rectum.* 2003;46:1484.

83. Christophi C, Hughes ER. Hepatobiliary disorders in inflammatory bowel disease. *Surg Gynecol Obstet.* 1985;160:187.

84. Chugh S, Dilawari JB, Sawhney IMS, et al. Polymyositis associated with ulcerative colitis. *Gut.* 1993;34:567.

85. Cirocco WC, Reilly JC, Rusin LC. Life-threatening hemorrhage and exsanguination from Crohn's disease. *Dis Colon Rectum.* 1995;38:85.

86. Clark CLI, Lear PA, Wood S, et al. Potential candidates for small bowel transplantation. *Br J Surg.* 1992;79:676.

87. Coenen C, Börsch G, Müller K-M, et al. Oral inflammatory changes as an initial manifestation of Crohn's disease antedating abdominal diagnosis. *Dis Colon Rectum.* 1988;31:548.

88. Cohen H, Fishman AP. Regional enteritis and amyloidosis. *Gastroenterology.* 1949;12:502.

89. Cohen RL, Tepper RE, Urmacher C, et al. Kaposi's sarcoma and cytomegaloviral ileocolitis complicating long-standing Crohn's disease in an HIV-negative patient. *Am J Gastroenterol.* 2001;96:3029.

90. Cohen S, Kaplan M, Gottlieb L, et al. Liver disease and gallstones in regional enteritis. *Gastroenterology.* 1971;60:237.

91. Cohen WN. Gastric involvement in Crohn's disease. *Am J Roentgenol.* 1967;101:425.

92. Colombel JF, Loftus EV Jr, Tremaine WJ, et al. The safety profile of infliximab for Crohn's disease in clinical practice: the Mayo Clinic experience in 500 patients. *Gastroenterology.* 2004;126:19.

93. Comfort MW, Weber HM, Baggenstoss AH, et al. Nonspecific granulomatous inflammation of the stomach and duodenum: its relation to regional enteritis. *Am J Med Sci.* 1950;220:616.

94. Connell WR, Sheffield JP, Kamm MA, et al. Lower gastrointestinal malignancy in Crohn's disease. *Gut.* 1994;35:347.

95. Cortot A, Colombel JF, Rutgeerts P, et al. Switch from systemic steroids to budesonide in steroid dependent patients with inactive Crohn's disease. *Gut.* 2001;48:186.

96. Crohn BB, Ginzburg L, Oppenheimer GD. Regional ileitis: a pathologic and clinical entity. *JAMA.* 1932;99:1323.

97. Cullen G, O'toole A, Keegan D, et al. Long-term clinical results of ileocecal resection for Crohn's disease. *Inflamm Bowel Dis.* 2007;13:1369.

98. Da Luz M, Stocchi K, Remzi FH, et al. Laparoscopic surgery for patients with Crohn's colitis: a case-matched study. *J Gastrointest Surg.* 2007;11:1529.

99. Dalziel TK. Chronic interstitial enteritis. *Br Med J.* 1913;2:1068.

100. Danzi JT, Farmer RG, Sullivan BH Jr, et al. Endoscopic features of gastroduodenal Crohn's disease. *Gastroenterology.* 1976;70:9.

101. Davies G, Evans CM, Shand WS, et al. Surgery for Crohn's disease in childhood: influence of site of disease and operative procedure on outcome. *Br J Surg.* 1990;77:891.

102. Decker GAG, Schein M. The finger fracture technique in the fat laden mesentery. *Surg Gynecol Obstet.* 1988;166:369.

103. de Dombal FT, Goldie W, Watts J, et al. Hepatic histological changes in ulcerative colitis: a series of 58 consecutive operative liver biopsies. *Scand J Gastroenterol.* 1966;1:220.

104. Dehn TCB, Kettlewell MGW, Mortensen NJ, et al. Ten-year experience of strictureplasty for obstructive Crohn's disease. *Br J Surg.* 1989;76:339.

105. Delaney CP, Remzi FH, Gramlich T, et al. Equivalent function, quality of life and pouch survival rates after ileal pouch-anal anastomosis for indeterminate and ulcerative colitis. *Ann Surg.* 2002;236:43.

106. Deutsch AA, McLeod RS, Cullen J, et al. The results of the pelvic pouch procedure in patients with Crohn's disease. *Dis Colon Rectum.* 1991;34:475.

107. Deutsch AA, Stern HS. Stapler strictureplasty for Crohn's disease. *Surg Gynecol Obstet.* 1989;169:458.

108. Devang NP, Saeian K, Kim J, et al. Symptomatic luminal strictures underlies infliximab non-response in Crohn's disease. *Gastroenterology.* 2002:A100 (A777).

109. D'Haens GR, Gasparaitis AE, Hanauer SB. Duration of recurrent ileitis after ileocolonic resection correlates with presurgical extent of Crohn's disease. *Gut.* 1995;36:715.

110. D'Haens GR, van Deventer SJH, Van Hogezand R, et al. Anti-TNFa monoclonal antibody (cA2) produces endoscopic healing in patients with treatment-resistant, active Crohn's disease. *Am J Gastroenterol.* 1998;114:A964.

111. D'Haens GR, Vermeire S, Van Assche G, et al. Therapy of metronidazole with azathioprine to prevent postoperative recurrence of Crohn's disease: a controlled randomized trial. *Gastroenterology.* 2008;135:1123.

112. Dietz DW, Fazio VW, Laureti S, et al. Strictureplasty in diffuse Crohn's jejunoileitis: safe and durable. *Dis Colon Rectum.* 2002;45:764.

113. Di Febo G, Gizzi G, Cappelo IP. Unusual case of colonic sub-obstruction by giant pseudopolyposis in Crohn's colitis. *Endoscopy*. 1981;13:90.

114. Doherty G, Bennett G, Patil S, et al. Interventions for prevention of post-operative recurrence of Crohn's disease. *Cochrane Database Syst Rev*. 2009;(4):CD006873.

115. Dollinger HC, Raptis S, Pfeiffer EF. Effects of somatostatin on exocrine and endocrine pancreatic function stimulated by intestinal hormones in man. *Horm Metab Res*. 1976;8:74.

116. Domènech E, Mañosa M, Bernal I, et al. Impact of azathioprine on the prevention of postoperative Crohn's disease recurrence: results of a prospective, observational, long-term follow-up study. *Inflamm Bowel Dis*. 2008;14:508.

117. Donnelly MT, Davies DR, Carter MJ, et al. Why do patients with inflammatory bowel disease stop azathioprine and what happens to them? *Am J Gastroenterol*. 1998;114:A968.

118. Dordal E, Glagov S, Kirsner JB. Hepatic lesions in chronic inflammatory bowel disease. *Gastroenterology*. 1967;52:239.

119. Dorudi S, Chapman RW, Kettlewell MGW. Carcinoma of the gallbladder in ulcerative colitis and primary sclerosing cholangitis. *Dis Colon Rectum*. 1991;34:827.

120. DuBrow RA, Frank PH. Barium evaluation of anal canal in patients with inflammatory bowel disease. *AJR*. 1983;140:1151.

121. Dudeney TP, Todd IP. Crohn's disease of the mouth. *Proc R Soc Med*. 1969;62:1237.

122. Dudrick SJ. Rhoads Lecture: a 45-year obsession and passionate pursuit of optimal nutrition support: puppies, pediatrics, surgery, geriatrics, home TPN, A.S.P.E.N., et cetera. *JPEN J Parenter Enteral Nutr*. 2005;29:272.

123. Dudrick SJ, O'Donnell JJ, Englert DM, et al. 100 patient-years of ambulatory home: total parenteral nutrition. *Ann Surg*. 1984;199:770.

124. Duepree HJ, Senagore AJ, Delaney CP, et al. Advantages of laparoscopic resection for ileocecal Crohn's disease. *Dis Colon Rectum*. 2002;45:605.

125. Duffy LF, Daum F, Fisher SE, et al. Peripheral neuropathy in Crohn's disease patients treated with metronidazole. *Gastroenterology*. 1985;88:681.

126. Dyer NH, Cook PL, Kemp-Harper RA. Oesophageal stricture associated with Crohn's disease. *Gut*. 1969;10:549.

127. Edwards CM, George BD, Jewell DP, et al. Role of a defunctioning stoma in the management of large bowel Crohn's disease. *Br J Surg*. 2000;87:1063.

128. Edwards P, Cooper DA, Turner J, et al. Resolution of amyloidosis (AA type) complicating chronic ulcerative colitis. *Gastroenterology*. 1988;95:810.

129. Egan LJ, Sandborn WJ, Tremaine WJ, et al. A randomized dose-response and pharmacokinetic study of methotrexate for refractory inflammatory Crohn's disease and ulcerative colitis. *Aliment Pharmacol Ther*. 1999;13:1597.

130. Eisenberg HW. Combined metronidazole and surgery in the management of complicated Crohn's disease. *Contemp Surg*. 1982;21:95.

131. Ekberg O, Baath L, Sjöström B, et al. Are superficial lesions of the distal part of the ileum early indicators of Crohn's disease in adult patients with abdominal pain? A clinical and radiologic long term investigation. *Gut*. 1984;25:341.

132. Eliakim R, Fischer D, Suissa L, et al. Wireless capsule video endoscopy is a superior diagnostic tool in comparison to barium follow-through and computerized tomography in patients with suspected Crohn's disease. *Eur J Gastroenterol Hepatol*. 2003;15:363.

133. Elliott PR, Ritchie JK, Lennard-Jones JE. Prognosis of colonic Crohn's disease. *BMJ*. 1985;291:178.

134. Ellis L, Calhoun P, Kaiser DL, et al. Postoperative recurrence in Crohn's disease: the effect of the initial length of bowel resection and operative procedure. *Ann Surg*. 1984;199:340.

135. Elson CO. Cyclosporine in Crohn's disease—low doses won't do it. *Gastroenterology*. 1990;98:1383.

136. Elton C, Makin G, Hitos K, et al. Mortality, morbidity and functional outcome after ileorectal anastomosis. *Br J Surg*. 2003;90:59.

137. Esaki M, Matsumoto T, Hizawa K, et al. Preventive effect of nutritional therapy against postoperative recurrence of Crohn disease, with reference to findings determined by intra-operative enteroscopy. *Scand J Gastroenterol*. 2005;40:1431.

138. Evans J, Poritz L, MacRae H. Influence of experience on laparoscopic ileocolic resection for Crohn's disease. *Dis Colon Rectum*. 2002;45:1595.

139. Ewe K, Press AG, Singe CC, et al. Azathioprine combined with prednisone or monotherapy with prednisone in active Crohn's disease. *Gastroenterology*. 1993;105:367.

140. Farmer RG, Hawk WA, Turnbull RB Jr. Crohn's disease of the duodenum (transmural duodenitis): clinical manifestations: report of 11 cases. *Am J Dig Dis*. 1972;17:191.

141. Farmer RG, Whelan G, Fazio VW. Long-term follow-up of patients with Crohn's disease. Relationship between the clinical pattern and prognosis. *Gastroenterology*. 1985;88:1818.

142. Farnell MB, Van Heerden JA, Beart RW Jr, et al. Rectal preservation in nonspecific inflammatory disease of the colon. *Ann Surg*. 1980;192:249.

143. Farrell FJ, Shah SA, Lodhavia PJ, et al. Infliximab therapy in 100 Crohn's disease patients: adverse events and clinical efficacy. *Am J Gastroenterol*. 2000;95:3490.

144. Farrell RJ, Ang Y, Kileen P, et al. Increased incidence of non-Hodgkin's lymphoma in inflammatory bowel disease patients or immunosuppressive therapy but overall risk is low. *Gut*. 2000;47:514.

145. Fasoli R, Kettlewell MGW, Mortensen N, et al. Response to faecal challenge in defunctioned colonic Crohn's disease: prediction of long-term course. *Br J Surg*. 1990;77:616.

146. Faubion WA Jr, Loftus EV Jr, Harmsen WS, et al. The natural history of corticosteroid therapy for inflammatory bowel disease: a population-based study. *Gastroenterology*. 2001;121:255.

147. Fazio VW. Regional enteritis (Crohn's disease): indications for surgery and operative strategy. *Surg Clin North Am*. 1983;63:27.

148. Fazio VW, Galandiuk S, Jagelman DG, et al. Strictureplasty for Crohn's disease. *Ann Surg*. 1989;210:621.

149. Fazio VW, Kodner I, Jagelman DG, et al. Inflammatory disease of the bowel: parenteral nutrition as primary or adjunctive treatment (symposium). *Dis Colon Rectum*. 1976;19:574.

150. Fazio VW, Marchetti F, Church JM, et al. Effect of resection margins on the recurrence of Crohn's disease in the small bowel: a randomized controlled trial. *Ann Surg*. 1996;224:563.

151. Fazio VW, Tjandra JJ, Lavery IC, et al. Long-term follow-up of strictureplasty in Crohn's disease. *Dis Colon Rectum*. 1993;36:355.

152. Fazio VW, Wu JS. Surgical therapy for Crohn's disease of the colon and rectum. *Surg Clin North Am*. 1997;77:197.

153. Feagan BG. Cyclosporine has no proven role as therapy in Crohn's disease. *Inflamm Bowel Dis*. 1995;1:335.

154. Feagan BG, Fedorak RN, Irvine EJ, et al. A comparison of methotrexate with placebo for the maintenance of remission in Crohn's disease. *New Engl J Med*. 2000;342:1627.

155. Feagan BG, Rochon J, Fedorak RN, et al. Methotrexate for the treatment of Crohn's disease. *N Engl J Med*. 1995;332:292.

156. Ferrante M, de Hertogh G, Hlavaty T, et al. The value of myenteric plexitis to predict early postoperative Crohn's disease recurrence. *Gastroenterology*. 2006;130:1596.

157. Fichera A, Lovadina S, Rubin M, et al. Patterns and operative treatment of recurrent Crohn's disease: a prospective longitudinal study. *Surgery*. 2006;140:649.

158. Fichera A, McCormack R, Rubin MA, et al. Long-term outcome of surgically treated Crohn's colitis: a prospective study. *Dis Colon Rectum*. 2005;48:963.

159. Fichera A, Peng SL, Elisseou NM, et al. Laparoscopy or conventional open surgery for patients with ileocolonic Crohn's disease? A prospective study. *Surgery*. 2007;142:566.

160. Fielding JF. Perianal lesions in Crohn's disease. *J R Coll Surg Edinb*. 1972;17:32.

161. Fielding JF, Cooke WT. Finger clubbing in regional enteritis. *Gut*. 1971;12:442.

162. Fireman Z, Mahajna E, Broide E, et al. Diagnosing small bowel Crohn's disease with wireless capsule endoscopy. *Gut*. 2003;52:390.

163. Fitchen JH. Amyloidosis and granulomatous colitis: regression after surgical removal of the involved bowel. *N Engl J Med*. 1975;292:352.

164. Fitzgibbons TJ, Green G, Silberman H, et al. Management of Crohn's disease involving the duodenum, including duodenal cutaneous fistula. *Arch Surg*. 1980;115:1022.

165. Fraser AG, Orchard TR, Robinson EM, et al. Long-term risk of malignancy after treatment of inflammatory bowel disease with azathioprine. *Aliment Pharmacol Ther*. 2002;16:1225.

166. Frikker MJ, Segall MM. The resectional reoperation rate for Crohn's disease in a general community hospital. *Dis Colon Rectum*. 1983;26:305.

167. Fry RD, Shemesh EI, Kodner IJ, et al. Techniques and results in the management of anal and perianal Crohn's disease. *Surg Gynecol Obstet*. 1989;168:42.

168. Futami K, Arima S. Role of strictureplasty in surgical treatment of Crohn's disease. *J Gastroenterol*. 2005;40(suppl 16):35.

169. Galandiuk S, O'Neill M, McDonald P, et al. A century of home parenteral nutrition for Crohn's disease. *Am J Surg*. 1990;159:540.

170. García-Granero E, Esclápez P, García-Armengol J, et al. Simple technique for the intraoperative detection of Crohn's strictures with a calibration sphere. *Dis Colon Rectum*. 2000;43:1168.

171. Gazzard B. Long term prognosis of Crohn's disease with onset in childhood and adolescence. *Gut.* 1984;25:325.

172. Geboes K, Vantrappen G. The value of colonoscopy in the diagnosis of Crohn's disease. *Gastrointest Endosc.* 1975;22:18.

173. Geerdsen JP, Pedersen VM, Kjaergard HK. Small bowel fistulas treated with somatostatin: preliminary results. *Surgery.* 1986;100:811.

174. Gelfand MD, Krone CL. Dysphagia and esophageal ulceration in Crohn's disease. *Gastroenterology.* 1968;55:510.

175. Gendre JP, Mary JY, Florent C, et al. Oral mesalamine (pentasa) as maintenance treatment in Crohn's disease: a multicenter placebo-controlled study. *Gastroenterology.* 1993;104:435.

176. Gerassimos J, Mantzaris GJ, Petraki K, et al. Budesonide is superior to mesalazine in maintaining disease remission for patients with steroid-dependent Crohn's disease. *Gastroenterology.* 2000;118:780 (A4174).

177. Gerber A, Apt MK, Craig PH. The Kock continent ileostomy. *Surg Gynecol Obstet.* 1983;156:345.

178. Gillen CD, Andrews HA, Prior P, et al. Crohn's disease and colorectal cancer. *Gut.* 1994;35:651.

179. Gillen CD, Walmsley RS, Prior P, et al. Ulcerative colitis and Crohn's disease: a comparison of the colorectal cancer risk in extensive colitis. *Gut.* 1994;35:1590.

180. Ginzburg L. The road to regional enteritis. *Mt Sinai J Med.* 1974;41:272.

181. Gitkind MJ, Wright SC. Amyloidosis complicating inflammatory bowel disease: a case report and review of the literature. *Dig Dis Sci.* 1990;35:906.

182. Givel JC, Hawker P, Allan RN, et al. Enterovaginal fistulas associated with Crohn's disease. *Surg Gynecol Obstet.* 1982;155:494.

183. Glass RE. The management of internal fistulae in Crohn's disease. *Br J Surg.* 1985;72:S93.

184. Glass RE, Ritchie JK, Lennard-Jones JE, et al. Internal fistulas in Crohn's disease. *Dis Colon Rectum.* 1985;28:557.

185. Glotzer DJ. The risk of cancer in Crohn's disease. *Gastroenterology.* 1985;89:438.

186. Goldstein F, Krain R, Thornton JJ. Intralesional steroid therapy of pyoderma gangrenosum. *J Clin Gastroenterol.* 1985;7:499.

187. Goldwasser B, Mazor A, Wiznitzer T. Enteroduodenal fistulas in Crohn's disease. *Dis Colon Rectum.* 1981;24:485.

188. Goligher JC. Inflammatory disease of the bowel: results of resection for Crohn's disease (symposium). *Dis Colon Rectum.* 1976;19:584.

189. Goligher JC. *Surgery of the Anus, Rectum and Colon.* 5th ed. London, United Kingdom: Balliére Tindall; 1984:971.

190. Goligher JC. The long-term results of excisional surgery for primary and recurrent Crohn's disease of the large intestine. *Dis Colon Rectum.* 1985;28:51.

191. Gore RM, Marn CS, Kirby DF, et al. CT findings in ulcerative, granulomatous, and indeterminate colitis. *AJR.* 1984;143:279.

192. Gottlieb C, Alpert S. Regional jejunitis. *AJR.* 1937;38:881.

193. Gravallese EM, Kantrowitz FG. Arthritic manifestations of inflammatory bowel disease. *Am J Gastroenterol.* 1988;83:703.

194. Greenbloom SL, Steinhart AH, Greenberg GR, et al. Ciprofloxacin and metronidazole: combination antibiotic therapy for ileocolonic Crohn's disease. *Gastroenterology.* 1995;108:A827.

195. Greenstein AJ. Cancer in inflammatory bowel disease. *Surg Rounds.* 1982:44.

196. Greenstein AJ, Aufses AH Jr. Differences in pathogenesis, incidence and outcome of perforation in inflammatory bowel disease. *Surg Gynecol Obstet.* 1985;160:63.

197. Greenstein AJ, Lachman P, Sachar DB, et al. Perforating and non-perforating indications for repeated operations in Crohn's disease: evidence for two clinical forms. *Gut.* 1988;29:588.

198. Greenstein AJ, Mann D, Sachar DB, et al. Free perforation in Crohn's disease: I. A survey of 99 cases. *Am J Gastroenterol.* 1985;80:682.

199. Greenstein AJ, Mullin GE, Strauchen JA, et al. Lymphoma in inflammatory bowel disease. *Cancer.* 1992;69:1119.

200. Greenstein AJ, Present DH, Sachar DB, et al. Gastric fistulas in Crohn's disease: report of a case. *Dis Colon Rectum.* 1989;32:888.

201. Greenstein AJ, Sachar DB, Greenstein RJ, et al. Intraabdominal abscess in Crohn's (ileo) colitis. *Am J Surg.* 1982;143:727.

202. Greenstein AJ, Sachar DB, Pucillo A, et al. Cancer in Crohn's disease after diversionary surgery: a report of seven carcinomas occurring in excluded bowel. *Am J Surg.* 1978;135:86.

203. Greenstein AJ, Sachar DB, Shafir M, et al. Malignant melanoma in inflammatory bowel disease. *Am J Gastroenterol.* 1992;87:317.

204. Greenstein AJ, Sachar DB, Tzakis A, et al. Course of enterovesical fistulas in Crohn's disease. *Am J Surg.* 1984;147:178.

205. Greenstein AJ, Zhang LP, Miller AT, et al. Relationship of the number of Crohn's strictures and strictureplasties to postoperative recurrence. *J Am Coll Surg.* 2009;208:1065.

206. Grundfest S, Steiger E. Home parenteral nutrition. *JAMA.* 1980; 244:1701.

207. Grüner OPN, Refsum S, Fausa O, et al. Giant pseudopolyposis causing colonic obstruction: report of a case seemingly associated with Crohn's disease of the colon. *Scand J Gastroenterol.* 1978;13:65.

208. Grobler SP, Hosie KB, Affie E, et al. Outcome of restorative proctocolectomy when the diagnosis is suggestive of Crohn's disease. *Gut.* 1993;34:1384.

209. Guenter P, Robinson L, DiMaria-Ghalili R, et al. Development of Sustain™ A.S.P.E.N.'s national patient registry for nutrition care [published online ahead of print January 26, 2012]. *JPEN J Parenter Enteral Nutr.*

210. Guest GD, Fink RLW. Metastatic Crohn's disease. *Dis Colon Rectum.* 2000;43:1764.

211. Guillem JG, Roberts PL, Murray JJ, et al. Factors predictive of persistent or recurrent Crohn's disease in excluded rectal segment. *Dis Colon Rectum.* 1992;35:768.

212. Gump FE, Lepore M, Barker HG. A revised concept of acute regional enteritis. *Ann Surg.* 1967;166:942.

213. Gyde SN, Prior P, Macartney JC, et al. Malignancy in Crohn's disease. *Gut.* 1980;21:1024.

214. Hamilton SR. Colorectal carcinoma in patients with Crohn's disease. *Gastroenterology.* 1985;89:398.

215. Hamilton SR, Reese J, Pennington L, et al. The role of resection margin frozen section in the surgical management of Crohn's disease. *Surg Gynecol Obstet.* 1985;160:57.

216. Hammerman AM, Shatz BA, Susman N. Radiographic characteristics of colonic "mucosal bridges": sequelae of inflammatory bowel disease. *Radiology.* 1978;47:611.

217. Hampe J, Cuthbert A, Crouchrer PJ, et al. Association between insertion mutation in NOD2 gene and Crohn's disease in German and British populations. *Lancet.* 2001;357:1925.

218. Hanauer SB. Inflammatory bowel disease. *N Engl J Med.* 1996; 334:841.

219. Hanauer SB, Korelitz BI, Rutgeerts P, et al. Postoperative maintenance of Crohn's disease remission with 6-mercaptopurine, mesalamine, or placebo: a 2-yr trial. *Gastroenterology.* 2004;127:723.

220. Hanauer SB, Meyers S. Management of Crohn's disease in adults. *Am J Gastroenterol.* 1997;92:559.

221. Hanauer SB, Smith MB. Rapid closure of Crohn's disease fistulas with continuous intravenous cyclosporin A. *Am J Gastroenterol.* 1993;88:646.

222. Hanauer SB, Stromberg V. Efficacy of oral Pentasa 4 gm in treatment of active Crohn's disease: a meta-analysis double-blind placebo controlled trial. *Gastroenterology.* 2001;120(suppl 1):A453.

223. Handelsman JC, Gottlieb LM, Hamilton SR. Crohn's disease as a contraindication to Kock pouch (continent ileostomy). *Dis Colon Rectum.* 1993;36:840.

224. Harford FJ Jr, Fazio VW. Total parenteral nutrition as primary therapy for inflammatory disease of the bowel. *Dis Colon Rectum.* 1978;21:555.

225. Harling H, Hegnj J, Rasmussen TN, et al. Fate of the rectum after colectomy and ileostomy for Crohn's colitis. *Dis Colon Rectum.* 1991;34:931.

226. Harper PH, Lee ECG, Kettlewell MGW, et al. Role of the faecal stream in the maintenance of Crohn's colitis. *Gut.* 1985;26:279.

227. Harper PH, Truelove SC, Lee ECG, et al. Split ileostomy and ileocolostomy for Crohn's disease of the colon and ulcerative colitis: a 20 year survey. *Gut.* 1983;24:106.

228. Harries AD, Danis VA, Heatley RV. Influence of nutritional status on immune functions in patients with Crohn's disease. *Gut.* 1984;25:465.

229. Hasegawa H, Watanabe M, Nishibori H, et al. Laparoscopic surgery for recurrent Crohn's disease. *Br J Surg.* 2003;90:970.

230. Hawker PC, Gyde SN, Thompson H, et al. Adenocarcinoma of the small intestine complicating Crohn's disease. *Gut.* 1982;23:188.

231. Heffernon EW, Kepkay PH. Segmental esophagitis gastritis and enteritis. *Gastroenterology.* 1954;26:83.

232. Heimann TM, Aufses AH Jr. The role of peripheral lymphocytes in the prediction of recurrence in Crohn's disease. *Surg Gynecol Obstet.* 1985;160:295.

233. Heimann TM, Bolnick K, Aufses AH Jr. Prognostic significance of severe preoperative lymphopenia in patients with Crohn's disease. *Ann Surg.* 1986;203:132.

234. Heimann TM, Greenstein AJ, Lewis B, et al. Prediction of early symptomatic recurrence after intestinal resection in Crohn's disease. *Ann Surg.* 1993;218:294.

235. Heimann TM, Greenstein AJ, Mechanic L, et al. Early complications following surgical treatment for Crohn's disease. *Ann Surg.* 1985;201:494.

236. Herrerías JM, Caunedo A, Rodríguez-Téllez M, et al. Capsule endoscopy in patients with suspected Crohn's disease and negative endoscopy. *Endoscopy.* 2003;35:564.

237. Heuman R, Boeryd B, Bolin T, et al. The influence of disease at the margin of resection on the outcome of Crohn's disease. *Br J Surg.* 1983;70:519.

238. Heyen F, Winslet MC, Andrews H, et al. Vaginal fistulas in Crohn's disease. *Dis Colon Rectum.* 1989;32:379.

239. Hill GL, Bourchier RG, Witney GB. Surgical and metabolic management of patients with external fistulas of the small intestine associated with Crohn's disease. *World J Surg.* 1988;12:191.

240. Hobbis JH, Schofield PF. Management of perianal Crohn's disease. *J R Soc Med.* 1982;75:414.

241. Hodgson HH. Keeping Crohn's disease quiet. *N Engl J Med.* 1996; 334:1599.

242. Hogan WJ, Hensley GT, Geenen JE. Endoscopic evaluation of inflammatory bowel disease. *Med Clin North Am.* 1980;64:1083.

243. Homan WP, Dineen P. Comparison of the results of resection, bypass, and bypass with exclusion for ileocecal Crohn's disease. *Ann Surg.* 1978;187:530.

244. Hotokezaka M, Ikeda T, Uchiyama S. Results of seton drainage and infliximab infusion for complex anal Crohn's disease. *Hepatogastroenterology.* 2011;58:1189.

245. Howard L. A global perspective of home parenteral and enteral nutrition. *Nutrition.* 2000;16.625.

246. Howard L, Amernt C, Fleming CR, et al. Current use and clinical outcome of home parenteral and enteral nutrition therapies in the United States. *Gastroenterology.* 1995;109:355.

247. Howard L, Heaphey L, Fleming CR, et al. Four years of North American registry home parenteral nutrition outcome data and their implications for patient management. *JPEN J Parenter Enteral Nutr.* 1991;15:384.

248. Hughes LE. A clinical classification of perianal Crohn's disease. *Dis Colon Rectum.* 1992;35:928.

249. Hughes LE, Donaldson DR, Williams JG, et al. Local depot methylprednisolone injection for painful anal Crohn's disease. *Gastroenterology.* 1988;94:709.

250. Hughes S, Williams SE, Turnberg LA. Crohn's disease and psoriasis. *N Engl J Med.* 1983;308:101.

251. Hugot JP, Charmaillard M, Zonali H, et al. Association of NOD2 leucine rich repeat variants with susceptibility to Crohn's disease. *Nature.* 2001;411:599.

252. Hyman NH, Fazio VW, Tuckson WB, et al. Consequences of ileal pouch-anal anastomosis for Crohn's colitis. *Dis Colon Rectum.* 1991;34:653.

253. Iesalnieks I, Kilger A, Glass H, et al. Intraabdominal septic complications following bowel resection for Crohn's disease: detrimental influence on long-term outcome. *Int J Colorectal Dis.* 2008;23:1167.

254. Irving M. Assessment and management of external fistulas in Crohn's disease. *Br J Surg.* 1983;70:233.

255. Jacobson IM, Schapiro RH, Warshaw AL. Gastric and duodenal fistulas in Crohn's disease. *Gastroenterology.* 1985;89:1347.

256. Jalan KN, Prescott RJ, Walker RJ, et al. Arthropathy, ankylosing spondylitis, and clubbing of fingers in ulcerative colitis. *Gut.* 1970;11:748.

257. Jaskowiak NT, Michelassi F. Adenocarcinoma at a strictureplasty site in Crohn's disease: report of a case. *Dis Colon Rectum.* 2001;44:284.

258. Jawhari A, Kamm MA, Ong C, et al. Intra-abdominal and pelvic abscess in Crohn's disease: results of non-invasive and surgical management. *Br J Surg.* 1998;85:367.

259. Johnson ML, Wilson HT. Skin lesions in ulcerative colitis. *Gut.* 1969;10:255.

260. Jones VA, Dickinson RJ, Workman E, et al. Crohn's disease: maintenance of remission by diet. *Lancet.* 1985;2:177.

261. Kane SV, Flicker M, Katz-Nelson F. Tobacco use is associated with accelerated clinical recurrence of Crohn's disease after surgically induced remission. *J Clin Gastroenterol.* 2005;39:32.

262. Katariya RN, Sood S, Rao PG, et al. Stricture-plasty for tubercular strictures of the gastro-intestinal tract. *Br J Surg.* 1977;64:496.

263. Katz S, Rosenberg RF, Katzka I. Giant pseudopolyps in Crohn's colitis. *Am J Gastroenterol.* 1981;76:267.

264. Keh C, Shatari T, Yamamoto T, et al. Jejunal Crohn's disease is associated with a higher postoperative recurrence rate than ileocaecal Crohn's disease. *Colorectal Dis.* 2005;7:366.

265. Keighley MRB. Stapled strictureplasty for Crohn's disease. *Dis Colon Rectum.* 1991;34:945.

266. Keighley MRB, Buchmann P, Lee JR. Assessment of anorectal function in selection of patients for ileorectal anastomosis in Crohn's colitis. *Gut.* 1982;23:102.

267. Kelts DG, Grand RJ, Shen G, et al. Nutritional basis of growth failure in children and adolescents with Crohn's disease. *Gastroenterology.* 1979;76:720.

268. Kendall GPN, Hawley PR, Nicholls RJ, et al. Strictureplasty: a good operation for small bowel Crohn's disease? *Dis Colon Rectum.* 1986;29:312.

269. Khoury W, Strong SA, Fazio VW, et al. Factors associated with operative recurrence early after resection for Crohn's disease. *J Gastrointest Surg.* 2011;15:1354.

270. Kim PS, Zlatanic J, Gleim GM, et al. Long-term follow-up of 6MP-treated Crohn's disease patients. *Am J Gastroenterol.* 1997;92:A310 (1661).

271. Kirsner JB, Shorter RG. Recent developments in "nonspecific" inflammatory bowel disease, part I. *N Engl J Med.* 1982;306:775.

272. Koltun WA, Schoetz DJ Jr, Roberts PL, et al. Indeterminate colitis predisposes to perineal complications after ileal pouch-anal anastomosis. *Dis Colon Rectum.* 1991;34:857.

273. Kono T, Ebisawa Y, Okamoto K, et al. A new antimesenteric functional end-to-end handsewn anastomosis: surgical prevention of anastomotic recurrence in Crohn's disease. *Dis Colon Rectum.* 2011;54:586.

274. Konturek SJ. Somatostatin and the gastrointestinal secretions. *Scand J Gastroenterol.* 1976;11:1.

275. Korelitz BI. Therapy of inflammatory bowel disease, including use of immunosuppressive agents. *Clin Gastroenterol.* 1980;9:331.

276. Korelitz BI. The treatment of ulcerative colitis with "immunosuppressive" drugs. *Am J Gastroenterol.* 1981;76:297.

277. Korelitz BI, Glass JL, Wisch N. Long-term immunosuppressive therapy of ulcerative colitis. *Am J Dig Dis.* 1973;18:317.

278. Korelitz BI, Hanauer S, Rutgeerts P, et al. Post-operative prophylaxis with 6MP, 5-ASA or placebo in Crohn's disease: a 2-year multicenter trial [abstract]. *Gastroenterology.* 1998;114:A1011.

279. Korelitz BI, Lauwers GY, Sommers SC. Rectal mucosal dysplasia in Crohn's disease. *Gut.* 1990;31:1382.

280. Korelitz BI, Present DH. Favorable effect of 6-mercaptopurine on fistulae of Crohn's disease. *Dig Dis Sci.* 1985;30:58.

281. Korelitz BI, Present DH, Alpert LI, et al. Recurrent regional ileitis after ileostomy and colectomy for granulomatous colitis. *N Engl J Med.* 1972;287:110.

282. Korelitz BI, Waye JD, Kreuning J, et al. Crohn's disease in endoscopic biopsies of the gastric antrum and duodenum. *Am J Gastroenterol.* 1981;76:103.

283. Kornbluth A, Marion JF, Salomon P, et al. How effective is current medical therapy for severe ulcerative and Crohn's colitis? An analytic review of selected trials. *J Clin Gastroenterol.* 1995;20:280.

284. Kotanagi H, Kon H, Iida M, et al. Adenocarcinoma at the site of ileoanal anastomosis in Crohn's disease. Report of a case. *Dis Colon Rectum.* 2001;44:1210.

285. Kotanagi H, Kramer K, Fazio VW, et al. Do microscopic abnormalities at resection margins correlate with increased anastomotic recurrence in Crohn's disease? A prospective analysis of 100 cases. *Dis Colon Rectum.* 1991;34:909.

286. Kovalcik P, Simstein L, Weiss M, et al. The dilemma of Crohn's disease: Crohn's disease and appendectomy. *Dis Colon Rectum.* 1977;20:377.

287. Kozarek RA, Patterson DJ, Gelfand MD. Methotrexate induces clinical and histologic remission in patients with refractory inflammatory bowel disease. *Ann Intern Med.* 1989;110:353.

288. Kreuzpaintner G, Horstkotte D, Heyll A, et al. Increased risk of bacterial endocarditis in inflammatory bowel disease. *Am J Med.* 1992;92:391.

289. Kuramoto S, Oohara T, Ihara O, et al. Granulomas of the gut in Crohn's disease: a step sectioning study. *Dis Colon Rectum.* 1987;30:6.

290. Kurchin A, Ray JE, Bluth EI, et al. Cholelithiasis in ileostomy patients. *Dis Colon Rectum.* 1984;27:585.

291. Kurer MA, Stamou KM, Wilson TR, et al. Early symptomatic recurrence after intestinal resection in Crohn's disease is unpredictable. *Colorectal Dis.* 2007;9:567.

292. Kurtz RS, Heimann TM, Aufses AH. The management of intestinal fistulas. *Am J Gastroenterol.* 1981;76:377.

293. Ko A, Sohn N, Weinstein MA, et al. Carcinoma arising in anorectal fistulas of Crohn's disease. *Dis Colon Rectum.* 1998;41:992.

294. Landsend E, Johnson E, Johannessen JO, et al. Long-term outcome after intestinal resection for Crohn's disease. *Scand J Gastroenterol.* 2006;41:1204.

295. LaRusso NF, Wiesner RH, Ludwig J, et al. Primary sclerosing cholangitis. *N Engl J Med.* 1984;310:899.

296. Lavery IC, Jagelman DG. Cancer in the excluded rectum following surgery for inflammatory bowel disease. *Dis Colon Rectum.* 1982;25:522.

297. Lecomte T, Contou JF, Beaugerie L, et al. Predictive factors of response of perianal Crohn's disease to azathioprine or 6-mercaptopurine. *Dis Colon Rectum.* 2003;46:1469.

298. Lee ECG, Papaioannou N. Minimal surgery for chronic obstruction in patients with extensive or universal Crohn's disease. *Ann R Coll Surg Engl.* 1982;64:229.

299. Lee FI, Bellary SV, Francis C. Increased occurrence of psoriasis in patients with Crohn's disease and their relatives. *Am J Gastroenterol.* 1990;85:962.

300. Lee KKW, Schraut WH. Diagnosis and treatment of duodenoenteric fistulas complicating Crohn's disease. *Arch Surg*. 1989;124:712.

301. Lee KS, Medline A, Shockey S. Indeterminate colitis in the spectrum of inflammatory bowel disease. *Arch Pathol Lab Med*. 1979;103:173.

302. Lees CD, Steiger E, Hooley RA, et al. Home parenteral nutrition. *Acta Chir Scand*. 1981;507:113.

303. Lemann M, Gerard de La Valussiere F, Bouhnik Y, et al. Intravenous cyclosporine for refractory attacks of Crohn's disease (CD): long-term follow-up of patients. *Am J Gastroenterol*. 1998;114:A1020.

304. Lemann M, Gerard de La Valussiere F, Carbonnel F, et al. Intravenous cyclosporine for perianal Crohn's disease (CD). *Gastroenterology*. 1998;114:A1020.

305. Lemann M, Messing B, D'Agay F, et al. Crohn's disease with respiratory tract involvement. *Gut*. 1987;28:1669.

306. Lemann M, Zenjari T, Bouhnik Y, et al. Methotrexate in Crohn's disease: long-term efficacy and toxicity. *Am J Gastroenterol*. 2000;95:1619.

307. Lescut D, Vanco D, Bonniére P, et al. Perioperative endoscopy of the whole small bowel in Crohn's disease. *Gut*. 1993;34:647.

308. Leu SY, Leonard MB, Beart RW Jr, et al. Psoas abscess: changing patterns of diagnosis and etiology. *Dis Colon Rectum*. 1986;29:694.

309. Levenstein S, Prantera C, Luzi C, et al. Low residue or normal diet in Crohn's disease: a prospective controlled study in Italian patients. *Gut*. 1985;26:989.

310. Levi AJ. Diet in the management of Crohn's disease. *Gut*. 1985;26:985.

311. Levine N, Bangert J. Cutaneous granulomatosis in Crohn's disease. *Arch Dermatol*. 1982;118:1006.

312. Lichtenstein GR, Bala M, Han C, et al. Infliximab improves quality of life in patients with Crohn's disease. *Inflamm Bowel Dis*. 2002;8:237.

313. Lichtenstein GR, Olson A, Bao W, et al. Infliximab treatment does not result in an increased risk of intestinal strictures or obstruction in Crohn's disease patients: Accent l Study Results. *Am J Gastroenterol*. 2002;97:S255.

314. Linares L, Moreira LF, Andrews H, et al. Natural history and treatment of anorectal strictures complicating Crohn's disease. *Br J Surg*. 1988;75:653.

315. Lind E, Fausa O, Gjone E, et al. Crohn's disease: treatment and outcome. *Scand J Gastroenterol*. 1985;20:1014.

316. Lindberg E, Järnerot G, Huitfeldt B. Smoking in Crohn's disease: effect on localisation and clinical course. *Gut*. 1992;33:779.

317. Lindhagen T, Ekelund G, Leandoer L, et al. Crohn's disease confined to the appendix. *Dis Colon Rectum*. 1982;25:805.

318. Lochs H, Mayer M, Fleig WE, et al. Prophylaxis of post-operative relapse in Crohn's disease with mesalamine. *Gastroenterology*. 2000;118:264.

319. Lochs H, Steinhardt HJ, Klaus-Wentz B, et al. Comparison of enteral nutrition and drug treatment in active Crohn's disease. *Gastroenterology*. 1991;101:881.

320. Lock MR, Fazio VW, Farmer RG, et al. Proximal recurrence and the fate of the rectum following excisional surgery for Crohn's disease of the large bowel. *Ann Surg*. 1981;194:754.

321. Lockhart-Mummery HE. Anal lesions in Crohn's disease. *Br J Surg*. 1985;72:S95.

322. Löfberg R, Broström O, Karlén P, et al. Carcinoma and DNA aneuploidy in Crohn's colitis—a histological and flow cytometric study. *Gut*. 1991;32:900.

323. Loffler T, Welsch T, Muhl S, et al. Long-term success rate after surgical treatment of anorectal and rectovaginal fistulas in Crohn's disease. *Int J Colorectal Dis*. 2009;24:521.

324. Longo WE, Ballantyne GH, Cahow E. Treatment of Crohn's colitis. *Arch Surg*. 1988;123:588.

325. Longo WE, Oakley JR, Lavery IC, et al. Outcome of ileorectal anastomosis for Crohn's disease. *Dis Colon Rectum*. 1992;35:1066.

326. Lorusso D, Leo S, Mossa A, et al. Cholelithiasis in inflammatory bowel disease: a case-control study. *Dis Colon Rectum*. 1990;33:791.

327. Lowdell CP, Shousha S, Parkins RA. The incidence of amyloidosis complicating inflammatory bowel disease: a prospective survey of 177 patients. *Dis Colon Rectum*. 1986;29:351.

328. Lowney JK, Dietz DW, Birnbaum EH, et al. Is there any difference in recurrence rates in laparoscopic ileocolic resection for Crohn's disease compared with conventional surgery? A long-term, follow-up study. *Dis Colon Rectum*. 2006;49:58.

329. Ludwig KA, Milsom JW, Church JM, et al. Preliminary experience with laparoscopic intestinal surgery for Crohn's disease. *Am J Surg*. 1996;171:52.

330. Maconi G, Sampietro GM, Cristaldi M, et al. Preoperative characteristics and postoperative behavior of bowel wall on risk of recurrence after conservative surgery in Crohn's disease: a prospective study. *Ann Surg*. 2001;233:345.

331. Mahida YR, Kurlac L, Gallagher A, et al. High circulating concentrations of interleukin-6 in active Crohn's disease but not ulcerative colitis. *Gut*. 1991;32:1531.

332. Makowiec F, Jehle EC, Becker HD, et al. Perianal abscess in Crohn's disease. *Dis Colon Rectum*. 1997;40:443.

333. Malchow H, Ewe K, Brandes JW, et al. European cooperative Crohn's disease study (ECCDS): results of drug treatment. *Gastroenterology*. 1984;86:249.

334. Malireddy K, Larson DW, Sandborn WJ, et al. Recurrence and impact of postoperative prophylaxis in laparoscopically treated primary ileocolic Crohn disease. *Arch Surg*. 2010;145:42.

335. Marcello PW, Schoetz DJ Jr, Roberts PL, et al. Evolutionary changes in the pathologic diagnosis after the ileoanal pouch procedure. *Dis Colon Rectum*. 1997;40:263.

336. Marchetti F, Fazio VW, Ozuner G. Adenocarcinoma arising from a strictureplasty site in Crohn's disease. *Dis Colon Rectum*. 1996;39:1315.

337. Margagnoni G, Aratari A, Mangone M. Natural history of ileo-caecal Crohn's disease after surgical resection. A long term study. *Minerva Gastroenterol Dietol*. 2011;57:335.

338. Markowitz J, Rosa J, Grancher K, et al. Long-term 6mercaptopurine treatment in adolescents with Crohn's disease. *Gastroenterology*. 1990;99:1347.

339. Marks CG, Ritchie JK, Lockhart-Mummery HE. Anal fistulas in Crohn's disease. *Br J Surg*. 1981;68:525.

340. Marshak RH, Lindner AE. Chronic inflammatory disease of the colon: historical perspective. In: Bercovitz ZT, Kirsner JB, Lindner AE, et al, eds. *Ulcerative and Granulomatous Colitis*. Springfield, MO: Charles C Thomas; 1973:xvii.

341. Marshak RH, Lindner AE. Radiologic diagnosis of chronic ulcerative colitis and Crohn's disease of the colon. In: Kirsner JB, Shorter RG, eds. *Inflammatory Bowel Disease*. Philadelphia, PA: Lea & Febiger; 1975:241.

342. Marteau P, Lemann M, Seksik P, et al. Ineffectiveness of *Lactobacillus johnsonii* LA1 for prophylaxis of postoperative recurrence in Crohn's disease: a randomized, double blind, placebo controlled GETAID trial. *Gut*. 2006;55:842.

343. Marx FW Jr. Incidental appendectomy with regional enteritis. *Arch Surg*. 1964;88:546.

344. Mary JY, Modigliani R. Development and validation of an endoscopic index of severity for Crohn's disease: a prospective multicentre study. *Gut*. 1989;30:983.

345. Massell SC, Hanauer SB. Increased association of lymphoma and inflammatory bowel disease. *Gastroenterology*. 2000;118:A119.

346. Matuchansky C. Parenteral nutrition in inflammatory bowel disease. *Gut*. 1986;27:81.

347. McDonald PJ, Fazio VW, Farmer RG, et al. Perforating and nonperforating Crohn's disease: an unpredictable guide to recurrence after surgery. *Dis Colon Rectum*. 1989;32:117.

348. McEwen C, Di Tata D, Lingg C, et al. Ankylosing spondylitis and spondylitis accompanying ulcerative colitis, regional enteritis, psoriasis and Reiter's disease: a comparative study. *Arthritis Rheum*. 1971;14:291.

349. McGarrity TJ, Manasse JS, Koch KL, et al. Crohn's disease and massive lower gastrointestinal bleeding: angiographic appearance and two case reports. *Am J Gastroenterol*. 1987;82:1096.

350. McGillis ST, Huntley AC. Metastatic Crohn's disease. *West J Med*. 1989;151:203.

351. McIntyre PB, Pemberton JH, Wolff BG, et al. Indeterminate colitis: long-term outcome in patients after ileal pouch-anal anastomosis. *Dis Colon Rectum*. 1995;38:51.

352. McIntyre PB, Powell-Tuck J, Wood SR, et al. Controlled trial of bowel rest in the treatment of severe acute colitis. *Gut*. 1986;27:481.

353. McLeod RS, Wolff BG, Ross S, et al. Recurrence of Crohn's disease after ileocolic resection is not affected by anastomotic type: results of a multicenter, randomized, controlled trial. *Dis Colon Rectum*. 2009;52:919.

354. McNamara MJ, Fazio VW, Lavery IC, et al. Surgical treatment of enterovesical fistulas in Crohn's disease. *Dis Colon Rectum*. 1990;33:272.

355. Meijer MJ, Mieremet-Ooms MA, Sier CF, et al. Matrix metalloproteinases and their tissue inhibitors as prognostic indicators for diagnostic and surgical recurrence in Crohn's disease. *Inflamm Bowel Dis*. 2009;15:84.

356. Michelassi F, Hurst RD, Melis M, et al. Side-to-side isoperistaltic stricureplasty in extensive Crohn's disease: a prospective longitudinal study. *Ann Surg*. 2000;232:401.

357. Michelassi F, Stella M, Balestracci T, et al. Incidence, diagnosis, and treatment of enteric and colorectal fistulae in patients with Crohn's disease. *Ann Surg*. 1993;218:660.

358. Michelassi F, Taschieri A, Tonelli F, et al. An international, multicenter, prospective, observational study of the side-to-side isoperistaltic strictureplasty in Crohn's disease. *Dis Colon Rectum*. 2007;50:277.

359. Michelassi F, Testa G, Pomidor WJ, et al. Adenocarcinoma complicating Crohn's disease. *Dis Colon Rectum.* 1993;36:654.

360. Middleton SJ, Pollard S, Friend PJ, et al. Adult small intestinal transplantation in England and Wales. *Br J Surg.* 2003;90:723.

361. Milsom JW, Hammerhofer KA, Böhm B, et al. Prospective, randomized trial comparing laparoscopic vs. conventional surgery for refractory ileocolic disease. *Dis Colon Rectum.* 2001;44:1.

362. Mir-Madjlessi SH, Taylor JS, Farmer RG. Clinical course and evolution of erythema nodosum and pyoderma gangrenosum in chronic ulcerative colitis: a study of 42 patients. *Am J Gastroenterol.* 1985;80:615.

363. Monsén U, Sorstad J, Hellers G, et al. Extracolonic diagnoses in ulcerative colitis: an epidemiological study. *Am J Gastroenterol.* 1990;85:711.

364. Morson BC, Lockhart-Mummery HE. Crohn's disease of the colon. *Gastroenterologia.* 1959;92:168.

365. Mortensen NJ, Ritchie JK, Hawley PR, et al. Surgery for acute Crohn's colitis: results and long term follow-up. *Br J Surg.* 1984;71:783.

366. Moschowitz E, Wilensky AO. Non-specific granulomata of the intestine. *Am J Med Sci.* 1923;166:48.

367. Mow WS, Abreu MT, Papadakis KA, et al. High incidence of anergy limits the usefulness of PPD screening for tuberculosis prior to Remicade in inflammatory bowel disease. *Gastroenterology* 2002;122:A100.

368. Moynihan BGA. The mimicry of malignant disease in the large intestine. *Edinburgh Med J.* 1907;21:228.

369. Munkholm P, Langholz E, Davidsen M, et al. Frequency of glucocorticoid resistance and dependency in Crohn's disease. *Gut.* 1994;35:360.

370. Muñoz-Juárez M, Yamamoto T, Wolff BG, et al. Wide lumen stapled anastomosis vs. conventional end-to-end anastomosis in the treatment of Crohn's disease. *Dis Colon Rectum.* 2001;44:20.

371. Murray JJ, Schoetz DJ Jr, Nugent FW, et al. Surgical management of Crohn's disease involving the duodenum. *Am J Surg.* 1984;147:58.

372. Mylonakis E, Allan RN, Keighley MRB. How does pouch construction for a final diagnosis of Crohn's disease compare with ileoproctostomy for established Crohn's proctocolitis? *Dis Colon Rectum.* 2001;44:1137.

373. Myrelid P, Svarm S, Andersson P, et al. Azathioprine as a postoperative prophylaxis reduces symptoms in aggressive Crohn's disease. *Scand J Gastroenterol* 2006;41:1190.

374. Myrvold HE, Kock NG. Continent ileostomy in patients with Crohn's disease. *Gastroenterology.* 1981;80:1237.

375. Neal DE, Williams NS, Barker MCJ, et al. The effect of resection of the distal ileum on gastric emptying, small bowel transit and absorption after proctocolectomy. *Br J Surg.* 1984;71:666.

376. Nelson RL, Subramanian K, Gasparaitis A, et al. Indium 111-labeled granulocyte scan in the diagnosis and management of acute inflammatory bowel disease. *Dis Colon Rectum.* 1990;33:451.

377. Neufeld DM, Shemesh EI, Kodner IJ, et al. Endoscopic management of anastomotic colon strictures with electrocautery and balloon dilation. *Gastrointest Endosc.* 1987;33:24.

378. Neumann V, Wright V. Arthritis associated with bowel disease. *Clin Gastroenterol.* 1983;12:767.

379. Ng SC, Lied GA, Arebi N, et al. Clinical and surgical recurrence of Crohn's disease after ileocolonic resection in a specialized unit. *Euro J Gastroenterol Hepatol.* 2009;21:551.

380. Niv Y. Esophageal involvement in Crohn's disease. *Am J Gastroenterol.* 1988;83:205.

381. Nordgren SR, Fasth SB, Öresland TO, et al. Long-term follow-up in Crohn's disease: mortality, morbidity, and functional status. In: Schölmerich J, Goebell H, Kruis W, et al, eds. *Inflammatory Bowel Disease: Pathophysiology as Basis of Treatment.* Dordrecht, The Netherlands: Kluwer Academic Publishers; 1992:334.

382. Nuako KW, Ahlquist DA, Sandborn WJ, et al. Primary sclerosing cholangitis and colorectal carcinoma in patients with chronic ulcerative colitis. *Cancer.* 1998;82:822.

383. Nubiola P, Badia JM, Martinez-Rodenas F, et al. Treatment of 27 postoperative enterocutaneous fistulas with the long half-life somatostatin analogue SMS 201–995. *Ann Surg.* 1989;210:56.

384. Nugent FW, Richmond M, Park SK. Crohn's disease of the duodenum. *Gut.* 1977;18:115.

385. Nugent FW, Roy MA. Duodenal Crohn's disease: an analysis of 89 cases. *Am J Gastroenterol.* 1989;84:249.

386. Nugent FW, Veidenheimer MC, Meissner WA, et al. Prognosis after colonic resection for Crohn's disease of the colon. *Gastroenterology.* 1973;65:398.

387. O'Brien JJ, Bayless TM, Bayless JA. Use of azathioprine or 6-mercaptopurine in the treatment of Crohn's disease. *Gastroenterology.* 1991;101:39.

388. O'Donaghue DP, Dawson AM, Powell-Tuck J, et al. Double-blind withdrawal trial of azathioprine as maintenance treatment for Crohn's disease. *Lancet.* 1978;2:955.

389. Ogura Y, Bonen DK, Inohara N, et al. A frameshift mutation in NOD2 associated with susceptibility to Crohn's disease. *Nature.* 2001;411:603.

390. Olaison G, Smedh K, Sjödahl R. Natural course of Crohn's disease after ileocolic resection: endoscopically visualized ileal ulcers preceding symptoms. *Gut.* 1992;33:331.

391. Olsson R, Danielsson A, Järnerot G, et al. Prevalence of primary sclerosing cholangitis in patients with ulcerative colitis. *Gastroenterology.* 1991;100:1319.

392. O'Morain C, Segal AW, Levi AJ. Elemental diet as primary treatment of acute Crohn's disease: a controlled trial. *BMJ.* 1984;288:1859.

393. Onali S, Petruzziello C, Calabrese E, et al. Frequency, pattern, and risk factors of postoperative recurrence of Crohn's disease after resection different from ileo-colonic. *J Gastrointest Surg.* 2009;13:246.

394. Orholm M, Binder V, Sorensen TL, et al. Concordance of inflammatory bowel disease among Danish twins. Results of a nationwide study. *Scand J Gastroenterol.* 2000;35:1075.

395. Ostergaard-Thomsen O, Cortot A, Lewell D, et al. A comparison of budesonide and mesalamine for active Crohn's disease. *N Engl J Med.* 1998;339:370.

396. Otley A, Thomson AB, Modigiliani R, et al. Budesonide for the induction of remission in Crohn's disease: meta-analysis of randomized controlled trials. *Gastroenterology.* 2003;124:A378.

397. Ozuner G, Fazio VW, Lavery IC, et al. How safe is strictureplasty in the management of Crohn's disease? *Am J Surg.* 1996;171:57.

398. Ozuner G, Fazio VW, Lavery IC, et al. Reoperative rates for Crohn's disease following strictureplasty. *Dis Colon Rectum.* 1996;39:1199.

399. Pace BW, Bank S, Wise L. Strictureplasty: an alternative in the surgical treatment of Crohn's disease. *Arch Surg.* 1984;119:861.

400. Papay P, Reinisch W, Ho E, et al. The impacts of thiopurines on the risk of surgical recurrence in patients with Crohn's disease after the first intestinal surgery. *Am J Gastroenterol.* 2010;105:1158.

401. Parente F, Sampietro GM, Molteni M, et al. Behavior of the bowel wall during the first year after surgery is a strong predictor of symptomatic recurrence of Crohn's disease: a prospective study. *Aliment Pharmacol Ther.* 2004;20:959.

402. Parker RGF, Kendall EJC. Liver in ulcerative colitis. *BMJ* 1954; 2:1030.

403. Pascua M, Su C, Lewis JD, et al. Meta-analysis: factors predicting post-operative recurrence with placebo therapy in patients with Crohn's disease. *Aliment Pharmacol Ther.* 2008;28:545.

404. Pastore RLO, Wolff BG, Hodge D. Total abdominal colectomy and ileorectal anastomosis for inflammatory bowel disease. *Dis Colon Rectum.* 1997;40:1455.

405. Payne-James JJ, Silk DBA. Total parenteral nutrition as primary treatment in Crohn's disease—RIP? *Gut.* 1988;29:1304.

406. Pearson M, Teahor K, Levi AJ, et al. Food intolerance and Crohn's disease. *Gut.* 1993;34:783.

407. Peters WR, Fry RD, Fleshman JW, et al. Multiple blood transfusions reduce the recurrence rate of Crohn's disease. *Dis Colon Rectum.* 1989;32:749.

408. Petras RE, Mir-Madjlessi SH, Farmer RG. Crohn's disease and intestinal carcinoma: a report of 11 cases with emphasis on associated epithelial dysplasia. *Gastroenterology.* 1987;93:1307.

409. Peyrin-Biroulet L, Deltenre P, Ardizzone S, et al. Azathioprine and 6-mercaptopurine for the prevention of postoperative recurrence in Crohn's disease: a meta-analysis. *Am J Gastroenterol.* 2009;104:2089.

410. Pezim ME, Pemberton JH, Beart RW Jr, et al. Outcome of "indeterminant" colitis following ileal pouch anal anastomosis. *Dis Colon Rectum.* 1989;32:653.

411. Pinto RA, Shawki S, Narita K, et al. Laparoscopy for recurrent Crohn's disease: how do the results compare with the results for primary Crohn's disease? *Colorectal Dis.* 2011;13:302.

412. Pokorny RM, Hofmeister A, Galandiuk S, et al. Crohn's disease and ulcerative colitis are associated with the DNA repair gene MLH1. *Ann Surg.* 1997;225:718.

413. Pokorny WJ, Fowler CL. Isoperistaltic intestinal lengthening for short bowel syndrome. *Surg Gynecol Obstet.* 1991;172:39.

414. Polle SW, Slors JF, Weverling GJ, et al. Recurrence after segmental resection for colonic Crohn's disease. *Br J Surg.* 2005;92:1143.

415. Poritz LS, Koltun WA. Surgical management of ulcerative colitis in the presence of primary sclerosing cholangitis. *Dis Colon Rectum.* 2003;46:173.

416. Poritz LS, Rowe WA, Kolyun WA. Remicade does not abolish the need for surgery in fistulizing Crohn's disease. *Dis Colon Rectum.* 2002;45:771.

417. Post S, Betzler M, von Ditfurth B, et al. Risks of intestinal anastomoses in Crohn's disease. *Ann Surg.* 1991;213:37.

418. Post S, Herfarth C, Böhm E, et al. The impact of disease pattern, surgical management, and individual surgeons on the risk for relaparotomy for recurrent Crohn's disease. *Ann Surg.* 1996;223:253.

419. Powell FC, Schroeter AL, Su WPD, et al. Pyoderma gangrenosum: a review of 86 patients. *Q J Med*. 1985;55:173.

420. Prabhakar LP, Laramee C, Nelson H, et al. Avoiding a stoma: role for segmental or abdominal colectomy in Crohn's colitis. *Dis Colon Rectum*. 1997;40:71.

421. Prantera C, Kohn A, Zannari F, et al. Metronidazole plus ciprofloxacin in the treatment of active refractory Crohn's disease: results of an open study. *J Clin Gastroenterol*. 1994;19:79.

422. Prantera C, Pallone F, Brunetti G, et al. Oral 5-aminosalicylic acid (Asacol) in the maintenance treatment of Crohn's disease. *Gastroenterology*. 1992;103:363.

423. Prantera C, Scrihano ML, Falasco G, et al. Ineffectiveness of probiotics in preventing recurrence after "curative" resection for Crohn's disease: a randomized controlled trial with *Lactobacillus* GG. *Gut*. 2002;51:405.

424. Prantera C, Zannoni F, Scriband ML, et al. An antibiotic regimen for the treatment of active Crohn's disease: a randomized controlled clinical trial of metronidazole plus ciprofloxacin. *Am J Gastroenterol*. 1996;91:A328.

425. Present DH, Korelitz BI, Wisch N, et al. Treatment of Crohn's disease with 6-mercaptopurine: a long-term randomized, double-blind study. *N Engl J Med*. 1980;302:981.

426. Present DH, Mayer L, van Deventer SJH. Anti-TNF alpha chimeric antibody (cA2) is effective in the treatment of fistulae of Crohn's disease: a multi-center, randomized, double-blind, placebo-controlled study. *Am J Gastroenterol*. 1997;92:A648 (1746).

427. Present DH, Meltzer SJ, Krumholz MP, et al. 6-mercaptopurine in the management of inflammatory bowel disease: short- and long-term toxicity. *Ann Intern Med*. 1989;111:641.

428. Price AB. Overlap in the spectrum of non-specific inflammatory bowel disease-colitis indeterminate. *J Clin Pathol*. 1978;31:567.

429. Pritchard TJ, Schoetz DJ, Roberts PL, et al. Perirectal abscess in Crohn's disease: drainage and outcome. *Dis Colon Rectum*. 1990;33:933.

430. Probert CSJ, Jayanthi V, Wicks ACB, et al. Mortality from Crohn's disease in Leicestershire, 1972–1989: an epidemiological community based study. *Gut*. 1992;33:1226.

431. Procaccino JA, Lavery IA, Fazio VW, et al. Psoas abscess: difficulties encountered. *Dis Colon Rectum*. 1991;34:784.

432. Puntis J, McNeish AS, Allan RN. Long term prognosis of Crohn's disease with onset in childhood and adolescence. *Gastroenterology*. 1984;25:329.

433. Raab Y, Bergström R, Ejerblad S, et al. Factors influencing recurrence in Crohn's disease: an analysis of a consecutive series of 353 patients treated with primary surgery. *Dis Colon Rectum*. 1996;39:918.

434. Rauh SM, Schoetz DJ Jr, Roberts PL, et al. Pouchitis: is it a wastebasket diagnosis? *Dis Colon Rectum*. 1991;34:685.

435. Rawlinson J, Hughes RG. Acute suppurative appendicitis: a rare associate of Crohn's disease. *Dis Colon Rectum*. 1985;28:608.

436. Reese GE, Nanidis T, Borysiewicz C, et al. The effect of smoking after surgery for Crohn's disease: a meta-analysis of observational studies. *Int J Colorectal Dis*. 2008;23:1213.

437. Reese GE, Purkayastha S, Tilney HS, et al. Strictureplasty vs resection in small bowel Crohn's disease: an evaluation of short-term outcomes and recurrence. *Colorectal Dis*. 2007;9:686.

438. Regimbeau JM, Panis Y, Pocard M, et al. Long-term results of ileal pouch-anal anastomosis for colorectal Crohn's disease. *Dis Colon Rectum*. 2001;44:769.

439. Reguerio M, Schraut W, Baidoo L, et al. Infliximab prevents Crohn's disease recurrence after ileal resection. *Gastroenterology*. 2009;136:441.

440. Reinisch W, Angelberger S, Petritsch W, et al. Azathioprine versus mesalazine for prevention of postoperative clinical recurrence in patients with Crohn's disease with endoscopic recurrence: efficacy and safety results of a randomized, double-blind, double-dummy, multicentre trial. *Gut*. 2010;59:752.

441. Remzi FH, Dietz DW, Unal E, et al. Combined use of preoperative provocative angiography and highly selective methylene blue injection to localize an occult small-bowel bleeding site in a patient with Crohn's disease: report of a case. *Dis Colon Rectum*. 2003;46:260.

442. Renda MC, Orlando A, Civitavecchia G, et al. The role of CARD15 mutations and smoking in the course of Crohn's disease in a Mediterranean area. *Am J Gastroenterol*. 2008;103:649.

443. Renna S, Cammà C, Modesto I, et al. Meta-analysis of the placebo rates of clinical relapse and severe endoscopic recurrence in postoperative Crohn's disease. *Gastroenterology*. 2008;135:1500.

444. Ribeiro MB, Greenstein AJ, Heimann TM, et al. Adenocarcinoma of the small intestine in Crohn's disease. *Surg Gynecol Obstet*. 1991;173:343.

445. Ribeiro MB, Greenstein AJ, Sachar DB, et al. Colorectal adenocarcinoma in Crohn's disease. *Ann Surg*. 1996;223:186.

446. Ricart E, Panaccione R, Loftus EV, et al. Infliximab for Crohn's disease in clinical practice at the Mayo Clinic: the first 100 patients. *Gastroenterology*. 2000;118:568 (A2967).

447. Richards ME, Rickert RR, Nance FC. Crohn's disease associated carcinoma: a poorly recognized complication of inflammatory bowel disease. *Ann Surg*. 1989;209:764.

448. Riordan JM, O'Connor BI, Huang H, et al. Long-term outcome of colectomy and ileorectal anastomosis for Crohn's colitis. *Dis Colon Rectum*. 2011;54:1347.

449. Ritchie JK. Crohn's disease in young people. *Br J Surg*. 1985;72:S90.

450. Ritchie JK, Allan RN, Macartney J, et al. Biliary tract carcinoma associated with ulcerative colitis. *Q J Med*. 1974;43:263.

451. Robert JR, Sachar DB, Greenstein AJ. Severe gastrointestinal hemorrhage in Crohn's disease. *Ann Surg*. 1991;213:207.

452. Rombeau JL, Barot LR, Williamson CE, et al. Preoperative total parenteral nutrition and surgical outcome in patients with inflammatory bowel disease. *Am J Surg*. 1982;143:139.

453. Rosén A, Ursing B, Alm T, et al. A comparative study of metronidazole and sulfasalazine for active Crohn's disease: the cooperative Crohn's disease study in Sweden. I. Design and methodologic considerations. *Gastroenterology*. 1982;83:541.

454. Rosenberg EW, Spitzer RE, Marley, et al. Inflammatory bowel disease, psoriasis, and complement. *N Engl J Med*. 1982;307:685.

455. Rosenthal SR, Snyder JD, Hendricks KM, et al. Growth failure and inflammatory bowel disease: approach to treatment of a complicated adolescent problem. *Pediatrics*. 1983;72:481.

456. Rosman AS, Melis M, Fichera A. Metaanalysis of trials comparing laparoscopic and open surgery for Crohn's disease. *Surg Endosc*. 2005;19:1549.

457. Ross TM, Fazio VW, Farmer RG. Long-term results of surgical treatment for Crohn's disease of the duodenum. *Ann Surg*. 1983;197:399.

458. Rothenberger DA (moderator), Fazio VW, Cohen Z, et al. Symposium on ileoanal anastomosis in Crohn's disease: is it feasible? Paper presented at: 89th Convention of the American Society of Colon and Rectal Surgeons; April 29 to May 4, 1990; St. Louis, MO.

459. Roy P, Kumar D. Strictureplasty for active Crohn's disease. *Int J Colorectal Dis*. 2006;21:427.

460. Rubio CA, Befrits R. Colorectal adenocarcinoma in Crohn's disease: a retrospective histologic study. *Dis Colon Rectum*. 1997;40:1072.

461. Rubio CA, Befritz R, Poppen B, et al. Crohn's disease and adenocarcinoma of the intestinal tract. *Dis Colon Rectum*. 1991;34:174.

462. Rudolph WG, Uthoff SMS, McAuliffe TL, et al. Indeterminate colitis: the real story. *Dis Colon Rectum*. 2002;45:1528.

463. Rusche M, O'Brian J. Infliximab in the management of recto-vaginal fistulous Crohn's disease. *Am J Gastroenterol*. 2001;95:S306.

464. Ruiz V, Unger SW, Morgan J, et al. Crohn's disease of the appendix. *Surgery*. 1990;107:113.

465. Rutgeerts P, Colombel JF, van Deventer S, et al. Endoscopic healing induced by infliximab maintenance therapy correlates with long-term clinical response in patients with active Crohn's disease. Results of endoscopic substudy of Accent I. *Am J Gastroenterol*. 2002;97:S260.

466. Rutgeerts P, Geboes K, Vantrappen G, et al. Natural history of recurrent Crohn's disease at the ileocolonic anastomosis after curative surgery. *Gut*. 1984;25:665.

467. Rutgeerts P, Geboes K, Vantrappen G, et al. Predictability of the postoperative course of Crohn's disease. *Gastroenterology*. 1990;99:956.

468. Rutgeerts P, Hiele M, Gelives K, et al. Controlled trial of metronidazole treatment for prevention of Crohn's recurrence after ileal resection. *Gastroenterology*. 1995;108:1617.

469. Rutgeerts P, Lofberg R, Melchow H, et al. Budesonide versus prednisone for the treatment of active ileocecal Crohn's disease: a European, multi-center trial. *Gastroenterology*. 1993;104:A772.

470. Rutgeerts P, Onette E, Vantrappen G, et al. Crohn's disease of the stomach and duodenum: a clinical study with emphasis on the value of endoscopy and endoscopic biopsies. *Endoscopy*. 1980;12:288.

471. Rutgeerts P, Van Assche G, Vermeire S, et al. Ornidazole for prophylaxis of postoperative Crohn's disease recurrence: a randomized, double-blind placebo-controlled trial. *Gastroenterology*. 2005;128:856.

472. Ryan WR, Allan RN, Yamamoto T, et al. Crohn's disease patients who quit smoking have a reduced risk of reoperation for recurrence. *Am J Surg*. 2004;187:219.

473. Sachar DB. Cancer in Crohn's disease: dispelling the myths. *Gut*. 1994;35:1507.

474. Sachar DB, Lemmer E, Ibrahim C, et al. Recurrence patterns after first resection for stricturing or penetrating Crohn's disease. *Inflamm Bowel Dis*. 2009;15:1071.

475. Sagar PM, Dozois RR, Wolff BG. Long-term results of ileal pouch-anal anastomosis in patients with Crohn's disease. *Dis Colon Rectum*. 1996;39:893.

476. Saint-Marc O, Tiret E, Vaillant JC, et al. Surgical management of internal fistulas in Crohn's disease. *J Am Coll Surg*. 1996;183:97.

477. Samach M, Train J. Demonstration of mucosal bridging in Crohn's colitis. *Am J Gastroenterol.* 1980;74:50.

478. Sampietro GM, Corsi F, Maconi G, et al. Prospective study of long-term results and prognostic factors after conservative surgery for small bowel Crohn's disease. *Clin Gastroenterol Hepatol.* 2009;7:183.

479. Sampietro GM, Cristaldi M, Maconi G, et al. A prospective, longitudinal study of nonconventional strictureplasty in Crohn's disease. *J Am Coll Surg.* 2004;199:8.

480. Sandborn WJ, Feagan BG. Review article: mild to moderate Crohn's disease: defining the basis for a new treatment algorithm. *Aliment Pharmacol Ther.* 2003;18:263.

481. Sanderson IR, Walker-Smith JA. Crohn's disease in childhood. *Br J Surg.* 1985;72:S87.

482. Sanderson JD, Moss MT, Tizard MLV, et al. *Mycobacterium paratuberculosis* DNA in Crohn's disease tissue. *Gut.* 1992;33:890.

483. Sands BE. Therapy of inflammatory bowel disease. *Gastroenterology.* 2000;118(suppl 1):S68.

484. Sands BE, Blank M, Masters P, et al. Long-term treatment of rectovaginal fistulas in Crohn's disease: response to infliximab in the Accent II trial. *Gastroenterology.* 2003;124:A380.

485. Savarino E, Dulbecco P, Bodini G, et al. Prevention of postoperative recurrence of Crohn's disease by adalimumab: a case series. *Eur J Gastroenterol Hepatol.* 2012;24:468.

486. Savoca PE, Ballantyne GH, Cahow CE. Gastrointestinal malignancies in Crohn's disease: a 20-year experience. *Dis Colon Rectum.* 1990;33:7.

487. Saylan J, Wilson DAL, Allan A, et al. Recurrence after strictureplasty or resection for Crohn's disease. *Br J Surg.* 1989;76:335.

488. Scammell BE, Andrews H, Allan RN. Results of proctocolectomy of Crohn's disease. *Br J Surg.* 1987;74:671.

489. Scarpa M, Angriman I, Barollo M, et al. Risk factors of recurrence of stenosis in Crohn's disease. *Acta Biomed.* 2003;74(suppl 2):80.

490. Scarpa M, Angriman I, Barollo M, et al. Role of stapled and hand-sewn anastomoses in recurrence of Crohn's disease. *Hepatogastroenterology.* 2004;51:1053.

491. Scarpa M, Bortolami M, Morgan SL, et al. TGF-beta 1 and IGF-production and recurrence of Crohn's disease after ileocolonic resection. *J Surg Res.* 2009;152:26.

492. Scarpa M, D'Inca R, Basso D, et al. Fecal lactoferrin and calprotectin after ileocolonic resection for Crohn's disease. *Dis Colon Rectum.* 2007;50:861.

493. Scarpa M, Ruffolo C, Bertin E, et al. Surgical predictors of recurrence of Crohn's disease after ileocolonic resection. *Int J Colorectal Dis.* 2007;22:1061.

494. Schmidt CM, Talamini MA, Kaufman HS, et al. Laparoscopic surgery for Crohn's disease: reasons for conversion. *Ann Surg.* 2001;233:733.

495. Schoetz DJ Jr, Coller JA, Veidenheimer MC. Pyoderma gangrenosum and Crohn's disease: eight cases and a review of the literature. *Dis Colon Rectum.* 1983;26:155.

496. Schulman D, Beck LS, Roberts IM, et al. Crohn's disease of the vulva. *Am J Gastroenterol.* 1987;82:1328.

497. Scott ADN, Ritchie JK, Phillips RKS. Blood transfusion and recurrent Crohn's disease. *Br J Surg.* 1991;78:455.

498. Scully C, Cochran KM, Russell RI, et al. Crohn's disease of the mouth: an indicator of intestinal involvement. *Gut.* 1982;23:198.

499. Senofsky GM, Stabile BE. Gallstone ileus associated with Crohn's disease. *Surgery.* 1990;108:114.

500. Seyrig JA, Jian R, Modigliani R, et al. Idiopathic pancreatitis associated with inflammatory bowel disease. *Dig Dis Sci.* 1985;30:1121.

501. Shah SA, Fefferman DS, Farrell RJ, et al. Efficacy and safety of infliximab in 221 Crohn's disease patients. *Am J Gastroenterol.* 2000;95:2640 (A787).

502. Shaked A, Colonna JO, Goldstein L, et al. The interrelation between sclerosing cholangitis and ulcerative colitis in patients undergoing liver transplantation. *Ann Surg.* 1992;215:598.

503. Shatari T, Clark MA, Yamamoto T, et al. Long strictureplasty is as safe and effective as short strictureplasty in small bowel Crohn's disease. *Colorectal Dis.* 2004;6:438.

504. Sheehan AL, Warren BF, Gear MWL, et al. Fat-wrapping in Crohn's disease: pathological basis and relevance to surgical practice. *Br J Surg.* 1992;79:955.

505. Shepherd AFI, Alexander-Williams J. Stomal ulcer complicating bypass for duodenal Crohn's disease. *World J Surg.* 1986;10:146.

506. Sher ME, Bauer JJ, Gorphine S, et al. Low Hartmann procedure for severe anorectal Crohn's disease. *Dis Colon Rectum.* 1992;35.

507. Sherlock DJ, Suarez V, Gray JG. Stomal adenocarcinoma in Crohn's disease. *Gut.* 1990;31:1329.

508. Shiloni E, Coronado E, Freund HR. Role of total parenteral nutrition in the treatment of Crohn's disease. *Am J Surg.* 1989;157:180.

509. Shiloni E, Freund HR. Total parenteral nutrition in Crohn's disease: is it a primary or supportive mode of therapy? *Dis Colon Rectum.* 1983;26:275.

510. Sica GS, Iaculli E, Benavoli D, et al. Laparoscopic versus open ileocolonic resection in Crohn's disease: short- and long-term results from a prospective longitudinal study. *J Gastrointest Surg.* 2008;12:1094.

511. Simillis C, Purkayastha S, Yamamoto T, et al. A meta-analysis comparing conventional end-to-end anastomosis vs. other anastomotic configurations after resection in Crohn's disease. *Dis Colon Rectum.* 2007;50:1647.

512. Simillis C, Yamamoto T, Reese GE, et al. A meta-analysis comparing incidence of recurrence and indication for reoperation after surgery for perforating versus nonperforating Crohn's disease. *Am J Gastroenterol.* 2008;103:196.

513. Simkins KC. Aphthoid ulcers in Crohn's colitis. *Clin Radiol.* 1977;28:601.

514. Simonowitz DA, Rusch VW, Stevenson JK. Natural history of incidental appendectomy in patients with Crohn's disease who required subsequent bowel resection. *Am J Surg.* 1982;143:171.

515. Singleton JW, Hanauer SB, Gitnick GL, et al. Mesalamine capsules for the treatment of active Crohn's disease: results of a 16-week trial. *Gastroenterology.* 1993;104:1293.

516. Slaney G, Muller S, Clay J, et al. Crohn's disease involving the penis. *Gut.* 1986;27:329.

517. Slater G, Greenstein A, Aufses AH Jr. Anal carcinoma in patients with Crohn's disease. *Ann Surg.* 1984;199:348.

518. Slaton GD, Navab F, Boyd CM, et al. Role of delayed indium-111 labeled leukocyte scan in the management of Crohn's disease. *Am J Gastroenterol.* 1985;80:790.

519. Smedh K, Olaison G, Sjödahl R. Ileocolic nipple valve anastomosis for preventing recurrence of surgically treated Crohn's disease: long-term follow-up in six patients. *Dis Colon Rectum.* 1990;33:987.

520. Smith TR, Conradi H, Bernstein R, et al. Adenocarcinoma arising in Crohn's disease: report of two cases. *Dis Colon Rectum.* 1980;23:498.

521. Snyder MB, Cawson RA. Oral changes in Crohn's disease. *J Oral Surg.* 1976;34:59.

522. Sofaer J. Crohn's disease: the genetic contribution. *Gut.* 1993;34:869.

523. Sokol H, Polin V, Lavergne-Slove A, et al. Plexitis as a predictive factor of early postoperative clinical recurrence in Crohn's disease. *Gut.* 2009;58:1218.

524. Somerville KW, Langman MJS, Da Cruz DJ, et al. Malignant transformation of anal skin tags in Crohn's disease. *Gut.* 1984;25:1124.

525. Sorrentino D, Paviotti A, Terrosu G, et al. Low-dose maintenance therapy with infliximab prevents postsurgical recurrence of Crohn's disease. *Clin Gastroenterol Hepatol.* 2010;8:591.

526. Sorrentino D, Terrosu G, Avellini C, et al. Infliximab with low-dose methotrexate for prevention of postsurgical recurrence of ileocolonic Crohn's disease. *Arch Int Med.* 2007;167:1804.

527. Spiliotis J, Briand D, Gouttebel MC, et al. Treatment of fistulas of the gastrointestinal tract with total parenteral nutrition and octeotide in patients with carcinoma. *Surg Gynecol Obstet.* 1993;176:575.

528. Stack WA, Mann SD, Roy AJ, et al. Randomised controlled trial of CDP571 antibody to tumour necrosis factor-á in Crohn's disease. *Lancet.* 1997;349:521.

529. Stahl TJ, Schoetz DJ Jr, Roberts PL, et al. Crohn's disease and carcinoma: increasing justification for surveillance? *Dis Colon Rectum.* 1992;35:850.

530. Steiger E, Ireton-Jones C. The evolution of home parenteral nutrition in the United States. *Nutr Clin Pract.* 1991;16:236.

531. Steiger E, Srp F. Morbidity and mortality related to home parenteral nutrition in patients with gut failure. *Am J Surg.* 1983;145:102.

532. Steinberg DM, Allan RN, Thompson H, et al. Excisional surgery with ileostomy for Crohn's colitis with particular reference to factors affecting recurrence. *Gut.* 1974;15:845.

533. Steinberg DM, Cooke WT, Alexander-Williams J. Abscess and fistulae in Crohn's disease. *Gut.* 1973;14:865.

534. Stocchi L, Milsom JW, Fazio VW. Long-term outcomes of laparoscopic versus open ileocolic resection for Crohn's disease: follow-up of a prospective randomized trial. *Surgery.* 2008;144:622.

535. Stokes MA, Irving MH. How do patients with Crohn's disease fare on home parenteral nutrition? *Dis Colon Rectum.* 1988;31:454.

536. Stone W, Veidenheimer MC, Corman ML, et al. The dilemma of Crohn's disease: long-term follow-up of Crohn's disease of the small intestine. *Dis Colon Rectum.* 1977;20:372.

537. Storch I, Sachar D, Katz S. Pulmonary manifestations of inflammatory bowel disease. *Inflamm Bowel Dis.* 2003;9:104.

538. Summers RW, Switz DM, Sessions JT Jr, et al. National Cooperative Crohn's Disease Study: results of drug treatment. *Gastroenterology.* 1979;77:847.

539. Sustento-Reodica N, Ruiz P, Rogers A, et al. Recurrent Crohn's disease in transplanted bowel. *Lancet.* 1997;349:688.

540. Sutherland L, Singleton J, Sessions J, et al. Double-blind, placebo-controlled trial of metronidazole in Crohn's disease. *Gut.* 1991;32:1071.

541. Sutphen JL, Cooper PH, Mackel SE, et al. Metastatic cutaneous Crohn's disease. *Gastroenterology*. 1984;86:941.
542. Swift GL, Srivastava ED, Stone R, et al. Controlled trial of anti-tuberculous chemotherapy for two years in Crohn's disease. *Gut*. 1994;35:363.
543. Talbot C, Sagar PM, Johnston MJ, et al. Infliximab in the surgical management of complex fistulating anal Crohn's disease. *Colorectal Dis*. 2005;7:164.
544. Targan SR, Hanauer SB, van Deventer SJH, et al. A short-term study of chimeric monoclonal antibody cA2 to tumor necrosis factor alpha for Crohn's disease. Crohn's Disease cA2 Study Group. *N Engl J Med*. 1997;337:1029.
545. Taschieri AM, Cristaldi M, Elli M, et al. Description of new bowel-sparing techniques for long strictures of Crohn's disease. *Am J Surg*. 1997;173:509.
546. Teague RH, Waye JD. Inflammatory bowel disease. In: Hunt RH, Waye JD, eds. *Colonoscopy: Techniques, Clinical Practice and Colour Atlas*. London, United Kingdom: Chapman & Hall; 1981:343.
547. Teahon K, Bjarnson I, Pearson M, et al. Ten years' experience with an elemental diet in the management of Crohn's disease. *Gut*. 1990;31:1133.
548. Tekkis PP, Purkayastha S, Lanitis S, et al. A comparison of segmental vs subtotal/total colectomy for Crohn's disease: a meta-analysis. *Colorectal Dis*. 2006;8:82.
549. Tersigni R, Alessandroni L, Barreca M, et al. Does stapled functional end-to-end anastomosis affect recurrence of Crohn's disease after ileocolonic resection? *Hepatogastroenterology*. 2003;50:1422.
550. Thaler L, Dinnewitzer A, Oberwalder M, et al. Assessment of long-term quality of life after laparoscopic and open surgery for Crohn's disease. *Colorectal Dis*. 2005;7:375.
551. Thompson JS. Strategies for preserving intestinal length in the short-bowel syndrome. *Dis Colon Rectum*. 1987;30:208.
552. Thompson JS. The current status of surgical therapy for the short bowel syndrome. *Contemp Surg*. 1988;33:27.
553. Thompson JS. Surgical management of short bowel syndrome. *Surgery*. 1993;113:4.
554. Thompson S, Langnas AN, Pinch LW, et al. Surgical approach to short-bowel syndrome: experience in a population of 160 patients. *Ann Surg*. 1995;222:600.
555. Tichansky D, Cagir B, Yoo E, et al. Strictureplasty for Crohn's disease: meta-analysis. *Dis Colon Rectum*. 2000;43:911.
556. Timmer A, Sutherland L, Martin F. Oral contraceptive use and smoking are risk factors for relapse in Crohn's disease. *Gastroenterology*. 1998;114:1143.
557. Tjandra JJ, Fazio VW. Strictureplasty for ileocolic anastomotic strictures in Crohn's disease. *Dis Colon Rectum*. 1993;36:1099.
558. Tjandra JJ, Fazio VW. Strictureplasty without concomitant resection for small bowel obstruction in Crohn's disease. *Br J Surg*. 1994;81:561.
559. Tonelli F, Fedi M, Paroli GM, et al. Indications and results of side-to-side isoperistaltic strictureplasty in Crohn's disease. *Dis Colon Rectum*. 2004;47:494.
560. Topstad DR, Panaccione R, Heine JA, et al. Combined seton placement, infliximab infusion, and maintenance immunosuppressives improve healing rate in fistulizing anorectal Crohn's disease: a single center experience. *Dis Colon Rectum*. 2003;46:577.
561. Toy LS, Scherl EJ, Kornbluth A, et al. Complete bowel obstruction following initial response to infliximab therapy for Crohn's disease: a series of a newly described complication. *Gastroenterology*. 2000;118:569 (A2974).
562. Tremaine WJ. Maintenance therapy in IBD. *Inflamm Bowel Dis*. 1998;44:292.
563. Trnka YM, Glotzer DJ, Kasdon EJ, et al. The long-term outcome of restorative operation in Crohn's disease: influence of location, prognostic factors and surgical guidelines. *Ann Surg*. 1982;196:345.
564. Tweedie JH, McCann BG. Metastatic Crohn's disease of thigh and forearm. *Gut*. 1984;25:213.
565. Unkart JT, Anderson L, Li E, et al. Risk factors for surgical recurrence after ileocolic resection of Crohn's disease. *Dis Colon Rectum*. 2008;51:1211.
566. Ursing B, Alm T, Bárány F, et al. A comparative study of metronidazole and sulfasalazine for active Crohn's disease: the cooperative Crohn's disease study in Sweden. II. Result. *Gastroenterology*. 1982;83:550.
567. Valiulis A, Currie DJ. A surgical experience with Crohn's disease. *Surg Gynecol Obstet*. 1987;164:27.
568. van Bodegraven AA, Sloots CEJ, Felt-Bersma RJF, et al. Endosonographic evidence of persistence of Crohn's disease-associated fistulas after infliximab treatment, irrespective of clinical response. *Dis Colon Rectum*. 2002;45:39.
569. van Dongen LM, Lubbers EJC. Fistulas of the bladder in Crohn's disease. *Surg Gynecol Obstet*. 1984;158:308.
570. Van Gossum A, Dewit O, Louis E, et al. Multicenter randomized-controlled clinical trial of probiotics (*Lactobacillus johnsonii*, LA1) on early endoscopic recurrence of Crohn's disease after ileo-caecal resection. *Inflamm Bowel Dis*. 2007;13:135.
571. van Outryve MJ, Pelckmans PA, Michielsen PP, et al. Value of transrectal ultrasonography in Crohn's disease. *Gastroenterology*. 1991;101:1171.
572. Van Patter WN, Bargen JA, Dockerty MB, et al. Regional enteritis. *Gastroenterology*. 1954;26:347.
573. The Veteran Affairs Total Parenteral Nutrition Cooperative Study Group. Perioperative total parenteral nutrition in surgical patients. *N Engl J Med*. 1991;325:525.
574. Ward CS, Dunphy EP, Jagoe WS, et al. Crohn's disease limited to the mouth and anus. *J Clin Gastroenterol*. 1985;7:516.
575. Warman JI, Korelitz BI, Fleisher MR, et al. Cumulative experience with short and long-term toxicity in 6-mercaptopurine in the treatment of Crohn's disease and ulcerative colitis. *J Clin Gastroenterol*. 2003;37:220.
576. Warren KW, Athanassiades S, Monge JI. Primary sclerosing cholangitis. *Am J Surg*. 1966;3:23.
577. Watanabe M, Hasegawa H, Yamamoto S, et al. Successful application of laparoscopic surgery to the treatment of Crohn's disease with fistulas. *Dis Colon Rectum*. 2002;45:1057.
578. Weaver RM, Keighley MRB. Measurement of rectal capacity in the assessment of patients for colectomy and ileorectal anastomosis in Crohn's colitis. *Dis Colon Rectum*. 1986;29:443.
579. Weinberg AM, Lewis JD, Su C, et al. Response to infliximab in Crohn's disease: do strictures make a difference? *Am J Gastroenterol*. 2001;96:S312.
580. Welsch T, Hinz U, Loffler T, et al. Early re-laparotomy for post-operative complications is a significant risk factor for recurrence after ileocaecal resection for Crohn's disease. *Int J Colorectal Dis*. 2007;22:1043.
581. Weston LA, Roberts PL, Schoetz DJ Jr, et al. Ileocolic resection for acute presentation of Crohn's disease in the ileum. *Dis Colon Rectum*. 1996;39:841.
582. Wheeler SC, Marion JF, Present DH. Medical therapy, not surgery, is the appropriate first line treatment for Crohn's enterovesical fistula. *Am J Gastroenterol*. 1998;114:A1113.
583. Whelan G, Farmer RG, Fazio VW, et al. Recurrence after surgery in Crohn's disease: relationship to location of disease (clinical pattern) and surgical indication. *Gastroenterology*. 1985;88:1826.
584. Williams AJK, Palmer KR. Endoscopic balloon dilatation as a therapeutic option in the management of intestinal strictures resulting from Crohn's disease. *Br J Surg*. 1991;78:453.
585. Williams DR, Coller JA, Corman ML, et al. Anal complications in Crohn's disease. *Dis Colon Rectum*. 1981;24:22.
586. Williams JG, Wong WD, Rothenberger DA, et al. Recurrence of Crohn's disease after resection. *Br J Surg*. 1991;78:10.
587. Williams SM, Harned RK. Bile duct carcinoma associated with chronic ulcerative colitis. *Dis Colon Rectum*. 1981;24:42.
588. Wilmore DW, Lacey JM, Soultanakis RP, et al. Factors predicting a successful outcome after pharmacologic bowel compensation. *Ann Surg*. 1997;226:288.
589. Winslet MC, Andrews H, Allan RN, et al. Fecal diversion in the management of Crohn's disease of the colon. *Dis Colon Rectum*. 1993;36:757.
590. Winslet MC, Keighley MRB. Faecal challenge as a predictor of the effect of restoring intestinal continuity in defunctionalized Crohn's colitis. *Gut*. 1988;29:1475.
591. Wisch N, Korelitz BI. Immunosuppressive therapy for ulcerative colitis, ileitis, and granulomatous colitis. *Surg Clin North Am*. 1972;52:961.
592. Wise L, Kyriakos M, McCown A, et al. Crohn's disease of the duodenum: a report and analysis of eleven new cases. *Am J Surg*. 1971;121:184.
593. Wolff BG. Resection margins in Crohn's disease. *Br J Surg*. 2001;88:771.
594. Wolff BG, Beart RW Jr, Frydenberg HB, et al. The importance of disease-free margins in resection for Crohn's disease. *Dis Colon Rectum*. 1983;26:239.
595. Wolff BG, Culp CE, Beart RW Jr, et al. Anorectal Crohn's disease: a long-term prospective. *Dis Colon Rectum*. 1985;28:709.
596. Worsey MJ, Hull T, Ryland L, et al. Strictureplasty is an effective option in the operative management of duodenal Crohn's disease. *Dis Colon Rectum*. 1999;42:596.
597. Yamamoto T, Allan RN, Keighley MRB. Persistent perineal sinus after proctocolectomy for Crohn's disease. *Dis Colon Rectum*. 1999;42:96.
598. Yamamoto T, Allan RN, Keighley MRB. Smoking is a predictive factor for outcome after colectomy and ileorectal anastomosis in patients with Crohn's disease. *Br J Surg*. 1999;86:1069.
599. Yamamoto T, Allan RN, Keighley MRB. Audit of single-stage proctocolectomy for Crohn's disease: postoperative complications and recurrence. *Dis Colon Rectum*. 2000;43:249.
600. Yamamoto T, Allan RN, Keighley MRB. Risk factors for intra-abdominal sepsis after surgery in Crohn's disease. *Dis Colon Rectum*. 2000;43:1141.

601. Yamamoto T, Bain IM, Connolly AB, et al. Outcome of stricture-plasty for duodenal Crohn's disease. *Br J Surg*. 1999;86:259.

602. Yamamoto T, Fazio VW, Tekkis PP. Safety and efficacy of stric-tureplasty for Crohn's disease: a systematic review and meta-analysis. *Dis Colon Rectum*. 2007;50:1968.

603. Yamamoto T, Keighley MRB. Smoking and disease recurrence after operation for Crohn's disease. *Br J Surg*. 2000;78:398.

604. Yamamoto T, Umegae S, Kitagawa T, et al. Mucosal cytokine pro-duction during remission after resection for Crohn's disease and its relation-ship to future relapse. *Aliment Pharmacol Ther*. 2004;19:671.

605. Yamamoto T, Umegau S, Matsumoto K. Impact of infliximab therapy after early endoscopic recurrence following ileocolonic resection of Crohn's disease: a prospective pilot study. *Inflamm Bowel Dis*. 2009;15:1460.

606. Yamazaki Y, Ribeiro MB, Sachar DB, et al. Malignant colorectal strictures in Crohn's disease. *Am J Gastroenterol*. 1991;86:882.

607. Yates VM, Watkinson G, Kelman A. Further evidence for an associa-tion between psoriasis, Crohn's disease and ulcerative colitis. *Br J Derma-tol*. 1982;106:323.

608. Young-Fadok TM, Wolff BG, Meagher A, et al. Surgical management of ileosigmoid fistulas in Crohn's disease. *Dis Colon Rectum*. 1997;40:558.

609. Yousem DM, Fishman EK, Jones B. Crohn disease: perirectal and perianal findings at CT. *Radiology*. 1988;167:331.

610. Yu CS, Pemberton JH, Larson D. Ileal pouch-anal anastomosis in patients with indeterminate colitis. *Dis Colon Rectum*. 2000;43:1487.

611. Zelas P, Jagelman DG. Loop ileostomy in the management of Crohn's colitis in the debilitated patient. *Ann Surg*. 1980;191:164.

612. Zinkin LD, Brandwein C. Adenocarcinoma in Crohn's colitis. *Dis Colon Rectum*. 1980;23:115.

613. Zvaifler NJ, Martel W. Spondylitis in chronic ulcerative colitis. *Arthritis Rheum*. 1960;3:76.

31
Intestinal Stomas

Marvin L. Corman

Th' incurable cut off, the rest reforme.
—BEN JONSON, *Cynthia's Revels 5.11*

The purpose of this chapter is to amplify on the methods of creating a satisfactory stoma, the means of closure, the results with these procedures, and the complications and their management.

▶ PREPARING THE PATIENT

Overcoming ignorance and fear is often the most important issue that must be addressed by the surgeon in preparing an individual for a stoma. Some patients have had unpleasant associations with ostomies through experiences and jeremiads of family and friends. Myths and misunderstandings further prejudice the patient. The surgeon must confront someone's fear of the disease itself, the potential for complications, and, indeed, possible mortality. These issues must be addressed as part of a comprehensive rehabilitative program. It is usually very helpful to provide literature concerning the nature of the surgery and the reasonableness of living with a colostomy or an ileostomy (see also the following chapter). In addition, it is often helpful to have an individual of similar age, gender, and socioeconomic position serve to acquaint a patient with the concept of living and functioning normally with a stoma. Whenever possible, the wound/ostomy, continence (WOC) nurse should be involved with the preoperative counseling, not necessarily to provide detailed stomal care at that time, but to supply information about the wide variety of ostomy products available.[1] Bass and colleagues evaluated their stoma registry, consisting of 1,790 patients, for early and late complications with respect to whether they underwent stomal marking (see later) and education by the WOC nurse.[17] The difference in the total number of complications between the two groups was found to be statistically significant, confirming that preoperative evaluation by a WOC nurse, marking of the skin site, and providing patient education contribute to reduction of adverse outcomes. Nugent and coworkers (Southampton, United Kingdom) concluded in their questionnaire involving 391 patients that "improved preoperative assessment and counseling with longer follow-up by the stoma department would be helpful in the management of these patients and probably would contribute to improvement in the quality of their lives."[174] Moreover, in a report by Chaudhri and colleagues, stoma education was found to be more effective if undertaken in the preoperative setting.[43] They noted, "It results in shorter times to stoma proficiency and earlier discharge from the hospital. It also reduces stoma-related interventions in the community and has no adverse effects on patient well-being."

Stomal Marking

The location of the stoma has a direct bearing on subsequent ostomy management. Establishment of the stomal site prior to surgery is usually the responsibility of the surgeon, but in many instances may be delegated to a trained WOC nurse (Figure 31-1). Proper location of the colostomy or ileostomy can often prevent complications, such as prolapse, hernia, and skin problems.[53,115]

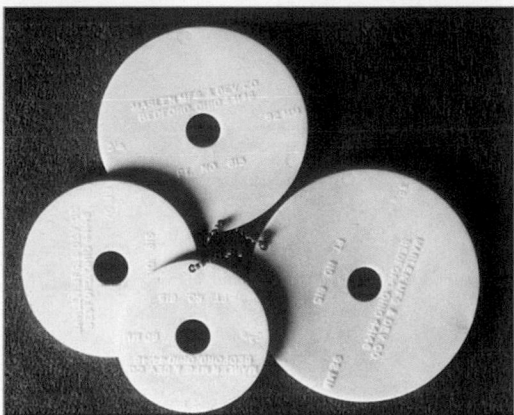

FIGURE 31-1. Four different sized templates of faceplates used by WOC nurses for marking the optimal stomal site.

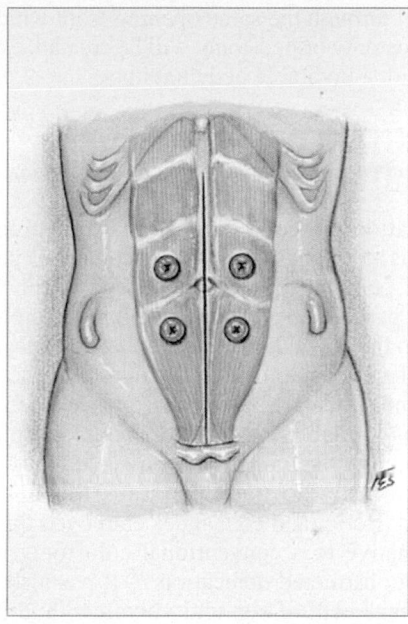

FIGURE 31-2. The stoma should be brought through the split rectus muscle irrespective of the quadrant in which it is located. The upper quadrants may be required for a small bowel stoma or when scars and obesity preclude the use of the lower abdomen.

The groin, the waistline, the costal margins, the umbilicus, skin folds, and scars frequently interfere with appliance management. It is advisable to leave a 5-cm margin of smooth skin around the stoma. The stoma should always be placed at the summit of the infraumbilical bulge and within the rectus muscle. When the site is being marked, it is helpful to have the patient lie in the supine position and tense the abdominal muscles. This allows one to feel the lateral border of the rectus muscle. A triangle is formed by drawing an imaginary line from the umbilicus to the pubis, one from the umbilicus to the anterosuperior iliac spine, and another from the pubis to the anterosuperior iliac spine (the inguinal ligament; see Figure 29-39). The stoma usually should be in the center. The faceplate should be taped over the site and the patient should stand, sit, and bend with the faceplate in place. Slight adjustments may be required because of interference from skin creases and adiposity.

Another factor to consider is the patient's preference for clothing style, especially where the belt is worn, because stomas ideally should be placed below the waist and preferably below the belt line. Should an individual require two stomas, the new opening must be placed either above or below the existing one. Occasionally, it may be necessary to keep a faceplate in place for 24 hours to ensure the patient's subsequent comfort and ease of movement. This is especially true when the abdomen contains multiple scars. My own preference is simply to scratch a mark onto the proposed location (see Figure 29-40). The use of a pen is not advised because such markings are often obliterated during the abdominal preparation.

If a site is not selected until the patient is in the operating room, what is perceived to be an ideal location may subsequently present a difficult management problem. The outer margin of the faceplate may appear at the waistline or in the groin, or the stoma may be found on the undersurface of the infraumbilical bulge, making it impossible for the patient to fit the skin barrier properly and to center the pouch. At the very least, a flange can be used that corresponds to the diameter of the faceplate of an appliance in order to identify the site and to give some degree of assurance.

The aforementioned considerations are applicable to all intestinal stomas—ileostomy, sigmoid colostomy, transverse colostomy, and urinary conduit (Figure 31-2). However, it is unfortunate that what we surgeons strive for may be difficult to achieve—namely, preoperative determination of the proper site for the stoma. Because patients are commonly admitted the day of surgery in the United States, preoperative counseling and stomal location often are relegated to a secondary role because of other, important concerns, such as anesthetic clearance, operative consent, site verification, confirmation of the presence of a myriad of legal and medical paperwork on the chart—the list seems endless. This is why every effort should be made to accomplish this task at a time when one is not attempting to respond to the demands and concerns that are inherent to the preoperative preparation process.

▶ LAPAROSCOPIC-ASSISTED STOMAL CREATION

One of the indications for performing minimally invasive surgery, that is, laparoscopic bowel surgery, is the creation and closure of intestinal stomas (see Chapter 19). A number of papers have been published that attest to the fact that this approach is well tolerated and can be performed safely and effectively.[76,104,113,147,173,200,228,232,272] Obvious advantages include the avoidance of a laparotomy while still maintaining the ability to precisely identify and orient the pertinent bowel segment. The approach to performing these techniques is discussed in Chapter 19.

▶ COLONOSCOPIC-ASSISTED STOMAL CREATION

Another minimally invasive approach to the creation of a colostomy that has been proffered is to insert a colonoscope in order to identify the site in the colon that could permit (by means of transillumination) the appropriate site for creating the stoma.[150,170] Of course, one may still do the entire stomal construction through the same opening from which the subsequent colostomy or ileostomy will be created, especially in someone with a favorable body habitus.

► PERCUTANEOUS ENDOSCOPIC COLOSTOMY

A modification of colonoscopic-assisted colostomy or cecostomy is analogous to that of percutaneous gastrostomy and that of percutaneous endoscopic colostomy. A colonoscope is passed, and a percutaneous colostomy tube is inserted into the bowel lumen. One must be concerned about the risk of fecal contamination or rupture of the thin colon wall, a potentially catastrophic consequence when there is no ready means available to limit the amount of spillage. Furthermore, with this minimally invasive alternative, the fecal stream is not truly diverted; therefore, this application is very limited. Heriot and colleagues employed this approach as an alternative to a conventional colostomy in a single patient with obstructed defecation.[106] It has also been used for the management of sigmoid volvulus[58] and for colonic pseudoobstruction.[33,185]

► SIGMOID COLOSTOMY

The most common indication for performing a *permanent* sigmoid colostomy is carcinoma of the rectum. Other possible indications for either a permanent or a temporary stoma include diverticulitis, Crohn's disease, congenital anomalies, anal incontinence, and colorectal trauma. Certainly, the most frequent reason for performing a sigmoid colostomy today is the Hartmann's procedure for sigmoid diverticulitis, although the stoma is generally intended to be temporary.

The historical aspects of the evolution of colostomy are discussed in Chapters 23 and 24. See also comprehensive reviews on the subject by Cromar,[56] Dinnick,[59] and McGarity.[154] The technique for creating a satisfactory end-sigmoid colostomy has been described previously as it pertains to the abdominoperineal resection for carcinoma of the rectum (see Figures 24-68 through 24-70). As has been repeatedly emphasized, it is important that the colon be brought through the split rectus muscle and sutured to the skin without tension. Ideally, redundant colon should be excised in order to permit a satisfactory irrigation should the patient so elect and to minimize bowel symptoms. If the surgeon elects to perform a paramedian incision, then he or she must create the stoma either in a pararectus location or bring the colostomy through the wound. Neither of these methods is appropriate unless there literally is no other place to put it. A pararectus colostomy predisposes to peristomal hernia (see later).

A "flush" colostomy can be performed with reasonable safety because the colostomy effluent is noncorrosive, but such a technique is not advised. With the patient's possible weight gain, the stoma may retract. This makes appliance management more difficult. Hence, the stoma should be permitted to pout slightly, but not to the extent of a conventional ileostomy (Figure 31-3). When the colostomy has been created, a transparent drainable bag is placed before the patient leaves the operating room (see Figure 32-5). This permits visualization of the stoma during the immediate postoperative period, and the viability

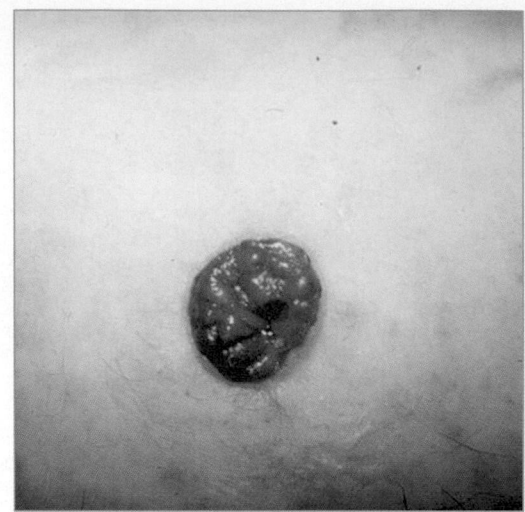

FIGURE 31-3. Normal-appearing end-sigmoid colostomy.

of the bowel can be determined on a continual basis. Usually, when the colostomy begins to function (after 2 or 3 days), the bag is removed and the stoma and skin are carefully inspected.

Complications

The principles of proper stomal construction have already been outlined. The bowel must be drawn through the abdominal wall without tension; it should be brought through the split rectus muscle; it must be sutured primarily to the skin; and the viability of the end of the colon must be clearly demonstrated.[249] Although no method guarantees that subsequent complications will be avoided, attention to the said principles will minimize the risks. But the fact of the matter is that most colostomy complications are preventable.

Ischemia and Stomal Necrosis

Ischemia and stomal necrosis are obviously due to inadequate blood supply. This is more likely to develop if the ascending branch of the left colic artery is not preserved, a consequence of high ligation of the inferior mesenteric artery (on the aorta). Another possible source for compromise of the blood supply occurs if the meandering artery of Drummond has been divided or if collateral circulation from the middle colic vessels is inadequate.

Recognition of stomal ischemia should not be difficult. If the mucosa looks blue, it probably is ischemic. Occasionally, after a difficult abdominoperineal resection, one may be less compulsive in creating the colostomy or perhaps somewhat less concerned about the possible nonviability of the stoma. It is better to reopen the abdomen to free a further length in order to effect a satisfactory stoma at the time of the resection than to have to return the patient to the operating room several days or weeks later. Many surgeons prefer to always take down the splenic flexure when a left-sided colostomy is planned in order to create adequate bowel length, preserve blood supply, and avoid tension. Splenic flexure mobilization is one of the major benefits of combining laparoscopy with an open operation (see Chapter 19). The philosophy expressed by the

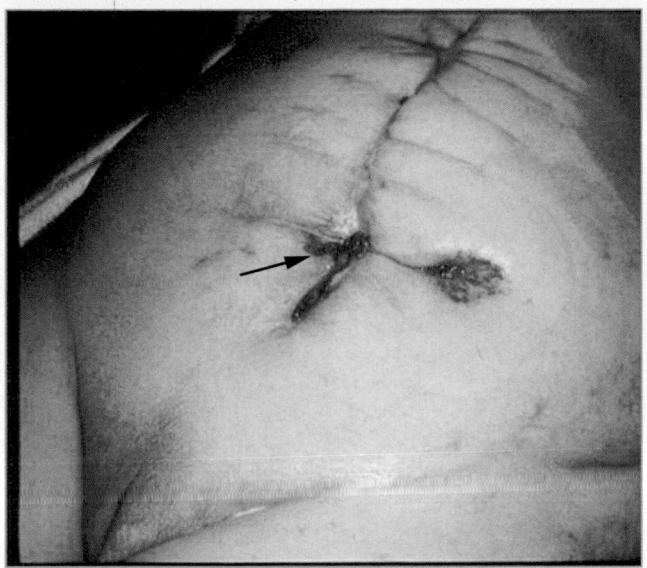

FIGURE 31-4. Sigmoid colostomy. Retraction with feces draining entirely from the abdominal wound (*arrow*).

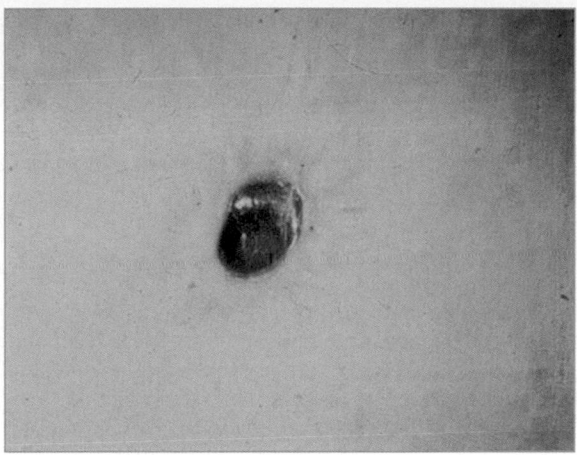

FIGURE 31-5. Retracted sigmoid colostomy. Only granulation tissue is evident.

statement, "It looks a bit dark, but it will probably be all right," is delusional. If the stoma is nonviable, the bowel may retract into the peritoneal cavity. Peritonitis can ensue and necessitate emergency surgical intervention. Equally concerning is the situation illustrated in Figure 31-4. The sigmoid colostomy has retracted, and the stool presents in the lower portion of the abdominal incision, tracking subcutaneously from the original opening in the rectus fascia. In a less ominous consequence, the stoma may separate from the skin at the area of nonviability, with a resultant stricture (Figure 31-5).

Management

Many patients are able to cope reasonably well even with a severely stenotic colostomy. Formed stool may be able to pass without difficulty, and appliance management is rarely a problem. However, if the individual cannot cope with symptoms associated with the retraction or stenosis, revision is required. Dilatation alone of a skin-level stenosis is not recommended because it usually re-strictures. The trauma from manipulation may also cause hemorrhage and further inflammatory reaction and may actually worsen the condition.

A laparotomy with colostomy resection and the creation of a new stoma are necessary if adequate length cannot be established by a limited approach. However, an attempt should be made to circumcise the colostomy, to free up the bowel, and to re-suture it. The technique is illustrated in Figure 31-6. The application of the circular

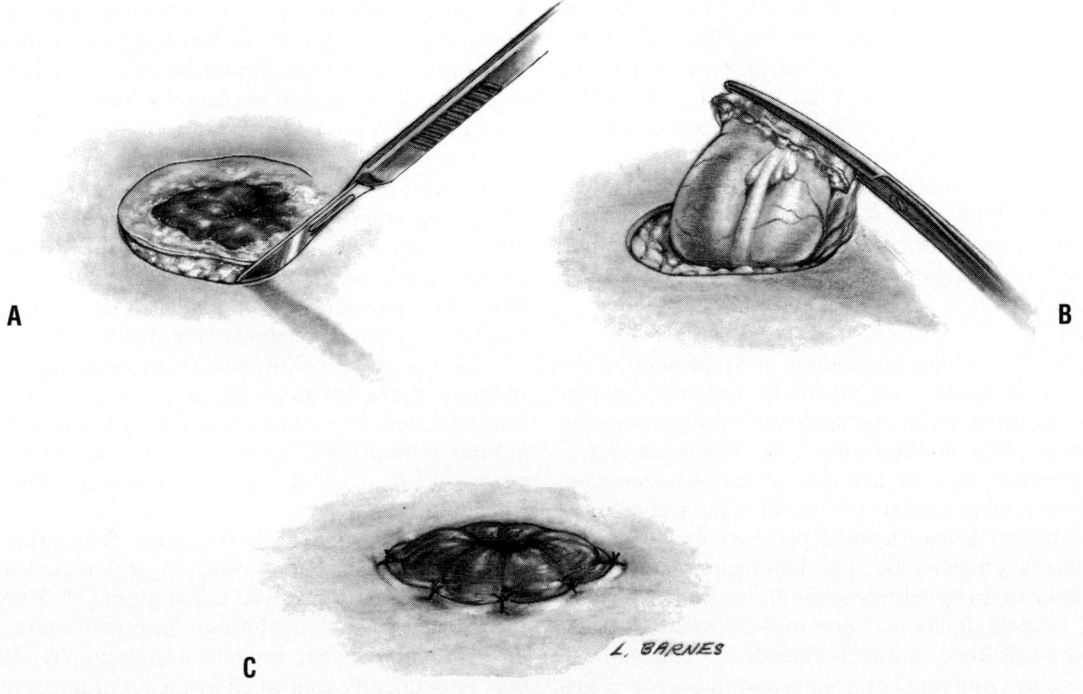

L. BARNES

FIGURE 31-6. Revision of retracted or stenotic colostomy. **A:** Skin is incised. **B:** Bowel is mobilized. **C:** New stoma is matured.

stapler for resection of a colostomy stricture has also been suggested.[193]

Rarely, the stenosis occurs at the fascial level. This is usually due to an inadequate opening in the fascia itself or to vascular compromise. Treatment usually requires mobilization of the bowel, enlargement of the opening in the fascia, and re-suturing of the colon.

Results

Only a limited number of papers have been published in recent years. Park and coworkers reporting the Cook County Hospital experience noted that 34% of 553 responding patients had stomal complications (stenosis, 2%) and emphasized the importance of preoperative stoma site marking.[178] Allen-Mersh and Thomson reviewed their experience with the surgical treatment of colostomy complications, identifying 65 patients who underwent revision due to stenosis.[9] This represented 53% of the operative stomal problems. Local excision of the scar tissue at the mucocutaneous junction was associated with a 61% success rate for relief of their symptoms.

Paracolostomy Abscess and Perforation

Paracolostomy abscess is an unusual postoperative complication. It should be a particularly unlikely event if the stoma is placed outside of the abdominal incision. The problem is more likely to be seen after an ileostomy when sutures may be placed too deeply and penetrate the bowel lumen at the time of eversion (see later). Another possible cause of a parastomal abscess in a patient who has undergone an ileostomy is recurrent Crohn's disease.

If the colostomy retracts and there is fecal contamination in the subcutaneous tissue, an abscess can result. However, by far the most common reason for paracolostomy abscess is the performance of an improper irrigation technique (see later and Chapter 32). Either the irrigating fluid or the device used for insertion into the stoma may perforate the bowel.

Symptoms include an unrewarding irrigation, which is often associated with immediate abdominal pain.[117] Obvious sepsis may supervene with evidence of cellulitis of the abdominal wall. If the process dissects into the peritoneal cavity or had started within the abdomen, it can lead to generalized peritonitis. Predisposing factors for the development of this complication include the presence of a pericolostomy hernia, alcoholism, psychological disturbance (e.g., self-mutilation), and, of course, carelessness. A case of burn and stricture of the ostomy has been reported due to the accidental insertion of boiling water for irrigation.[84]

Management

Treatment usually requires laparotomy and relocation of the colostomy, but Reynolds and colleagues reported satisfactory management by means of adequate surgical drainage and intravenous hyperalimentation or an elemental diet.[196] In their experience, no proximal diversion was undertaken. However, in my own experience with this complication, usually in patients who develop a bowel perforation secondary to irrigation, this is a major septic problem requiring an urgent operation and extensive debridement, drainage, stomal relocation, and, in some situations, a proximal colostomy or ileostomy. Gomez and Rosenthal recommended a semisynthetic biologic dressing (Biobrane) as a skin substitute when colostomy perforation caused massive abdominal wall tissue loss.[92]

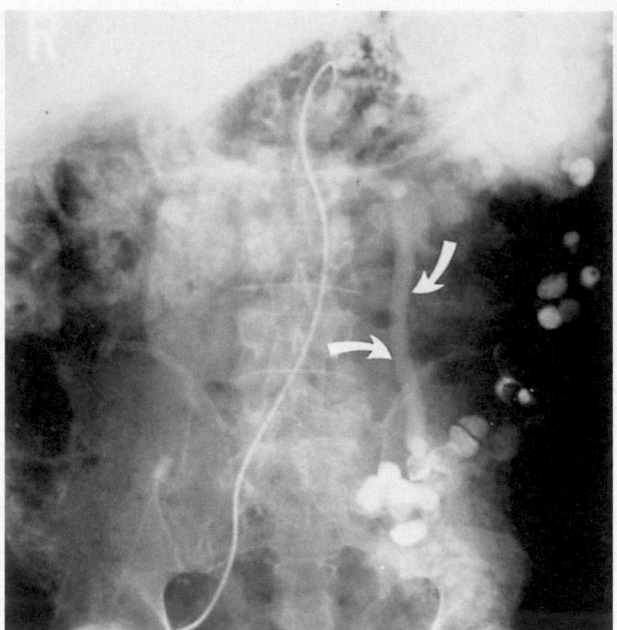

FIGURE 31-7. Hemorrhage from colostomy in patient with portal hypertension. Angiogram demonstrates delayed emptying of inferior mesenteric vein (*arrows*).

Results

Isa and Quan reviewed the Memorial Sloan-Kettering experience with colostomy perforation.[117] This was observed 10 times in a 10-year period ending in 1975, almost historical data at this date. In nine cases, the cause of the perforation was irrigation of the colostomy, and in one instance a barium enema examination. Barium enema perforation can usually be avoided by the use of a cone tip (see Figure 5-17B) or other device.[212] As previously discussed, the use of a balloon catheter should be vigorously condemned.

Hemorrhage

Colostomy hemorrhage is extremely unusual in the immediate postoperative period. However, in the event of underlying portal hypertension from cirrhosis secondary to alcohol ingestion or sclerosing cholangitis, the mucosa of the exposed bowel is predisposed to the possibility of considerable bleeding (Figure 31-7). This rare complication is more commonly seen in someone with an ileostomy, usually because of the association between inflammatory bowel disease (IBD), sclerosing cholangitis, and portal hypertension (see Figure 31-65). Roberts and colleagues identified 12 patients from the Lahey Clinic who had bleeding from stomal varices; all but one had ulcerative colitis.[198]

The bleeding originates from enterostomal varices located at the level of the mucocutaneous junction, a consequence of communication with the high-pressure venous network of the superior and inferior mesenteric veins.[50,198] Erosion of the varix or trauma can exacerbate the hemorrhage.

Handschin and coworkers (Zurich, Switzerland) reported a man with portal hypertension and recurrent bleeding from varices in a sigmoid colon stoma.[101] They localized the bleeding source through contrast-enhanced three-dimensional magnetic resonance angiography. The bleeding was subsequently controlled by means of the implantation of a transjugular intrahepatic shunt.

Treatment

Direct pressure is usually the initial approach. Other alternatives such as suture ligation of the bleeding areas, beta blockade, and injection sclerotherapy (by means of polidocanol, phenol [5%] in almond oil, or tetradecyl sulfate) have all been tried with varying degrees of success.[70,107,166] Goldstein and colleagues concluded in their review that control of major stomal hemorrhage by local measures is often ineffective and that portosystemic shunting may be required.[90]

Beck and associates performed mucocutaneous disconnections in 9 of their 11 patients who failed with one or more of the lesser options.[20] The dissection is carried down to the level of the fascia, and the varix is divided and ligated. With a follow-up of up to 4.6 years, two individuals required reoperation for hemorrhage. The alternative approach employed by this group was stomal relocation (two patients, one failure).

Prolapse

An end colostomy prolapse is an uncommon complication and is especially unusual following abdominoperineal re section. Chandler and Evans identified only 2 patients of 217 who underwent the procedure (less than 1%).[42] The problem occurs much more frequently in those who have undergone a loop colostomy (see later) than in those with an end stoma. The etiology of the problem may be an oversized opening in the abdominal wall, a redundant sigmoid loop leading to the stoma, sudden increased abdominal pressure (e.g., straining or coughing), or a rigid appliance worn with a tight belt.[135] The condition is frequently associated with a paracolostomy hernia. Adequate fixation of the mesentery and bowel to the peritoneum has been suggested as a means for preventing this complication, but I do not agree with this view. Sometimes those who develop end-sigmoid colostomy "prolapse" have a stoma that was initially created too long (Figure 31-8). This technical error, in combination with several other predisposing factors, such as the presence of a redundant loop of sigmoid colon, an asthenic patient, or an individual with chronic obstructive lung disease, tends to create the problem.

Treatment

In the absence of an associated hernia, treatment of a prolapse usually does not require a laparotomy. If the prolapse occurs relatively soon after it has been constructed, the colostomy is circumcised at the mucocutaneous junction and the bowel liberated, resected, and re-sutured (Figure 31-9). If the prolapse occurs several months after the initial operation, the incision should be made *into the mucosa* rather than into the skin (Figure 31-10A). The blood supply from the adjacent skin will be sufficient to maintain viability of the stoma, and an anastomosis is actually effected between the distal colon and the residual mucosa (Figure 31-10C). This technical detail is an important concept to remember because if the skin is incised, too large an opening will be created when the stoma is subsequently matured (Figure 31-10D). It is important to liberate as much intra-abdominal colon as possible and to resect it in order to avoid recurrent prolapse. With a particularly mobile colon, one may actually ultimately be creating an end-transverse colostomy in the left iliac fossa.

Abulafi and colleagues offer a unique approach to the management of colostomy prolapse, a modification of the

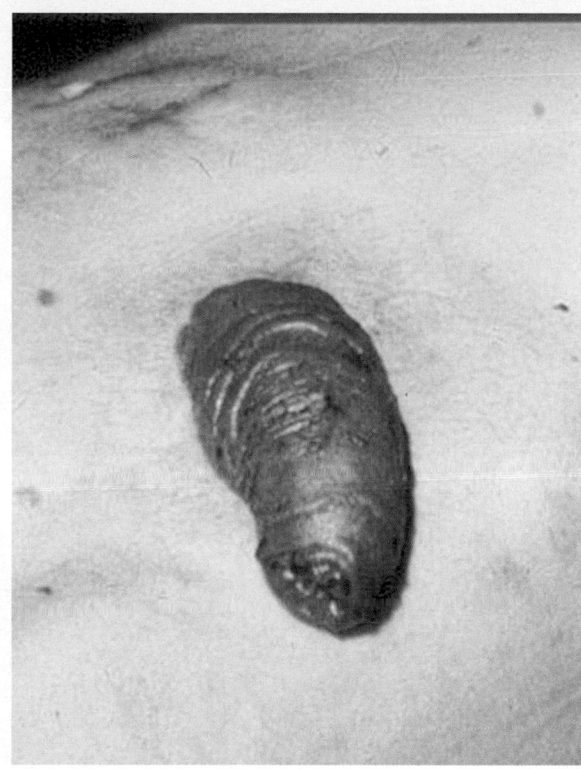

FIGURE 31-8. This sigmoid colostomy prolapse developed 1 month following operation after a bout of coughing. At the time of the initial procedure, considerable redundant sigmoid colon had been permitted to remain.

Delorme procedure (see Chapter 21).[5] The submucosa is infiltrated with a dilute adrenaline solution, and a mucosal incision is made 10 to 15 mm from the mucocutaneous junction (Figure 31-11A). Following separation of the mucosa for the full length of the prolapse, six to eight plicating sutures are placed in the muscular wall from the mucocutaneous junction to the apex (Figure 31-11B,C). The redundant mucosa is excised and the mucosa re-sutured (Figure 31-11D).

Acute stomal prolapse is uncommon and requires immediate attention to reduce it. This is usually accomplished by gentle pressure such as has been described in the chapter on rectal prolapse (see Chapter 21). As with osmotic therapy through the use of sugar applied to the prolapse, the same treatment has been demonstrated to be effective for acute, irreducible stomal prolapse.[72]

Rarely, sigmoid colostomy prolapse may produce compromise of the blood supply to the bowel and gangrene of the stoma (Figure 31-12). Depending on the level of involvement, resection of the necrotic bowel may be accomplished without a laparotomy, or alternatively an intra-abdominal procedure may be required. If a prolapse is associated with a paracolostomy hernia, relocation of the stoma may be necessary (see the following section).

Results

The previously mentioned report of Allen-Mersh and Thomson identified 16 individuals who underwent surgery for colostomy prolapse.[9] This represented 13% of the stomal complications requiring operation. Local fixation procedures failed to prevent recurrent prolapse in two-thirds.

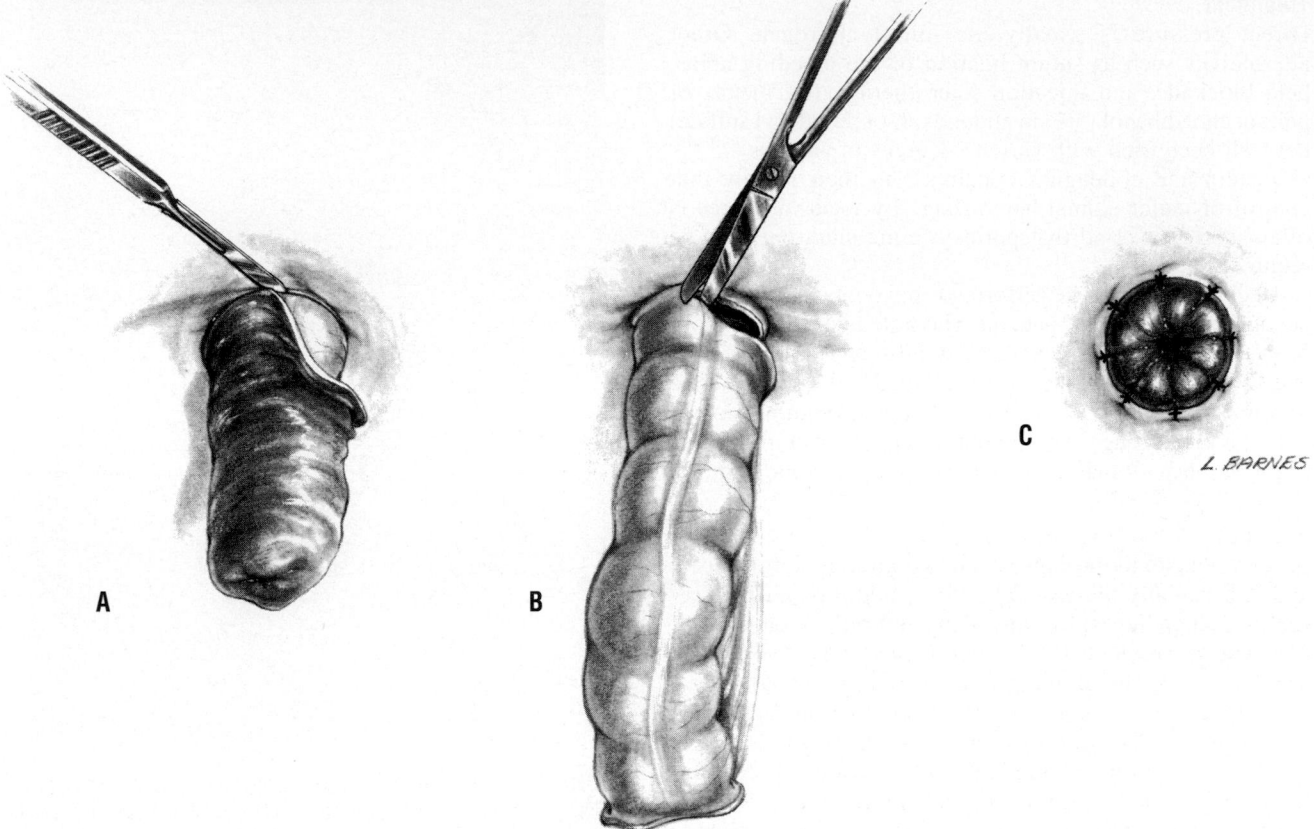

FIGURE 31-9. Revision of sigmoid colostomy prolapse that might take place relatively soon after surgery. **A:** Incision at the mucocutaneous junction. **B:** Delivery and resection of redundant bowel. **C:** Colostomy matured in the usual manner.

Parastomal Hernia

Parastomal hernia is the most common late complication of abdominoperineal resection. Between 87,000 and 135,000 intestinal stomas (ileostomy and colostomy) are created each year. It is estimated that one-half of these will be permanent stomas, of which 30% to 50% (i.e., 20,000 to 35,000) will then develop parastomal hernias. In a prospective audit of individuals attending a routine outpatient clinic at the Alfred Hospital in Melbourne, Australia, 90 consecutive patients were assessed for the presence of a parastomal hernia.[183] One-third were found to harbor this complication. As mentioned earlier, the usual reason for development of this problem has been felt to be the placement of the stoma in a pararectus location. Sjödahl and colleagues studied the location of the stoma in relation to the rectus abdominis muscle, noting that

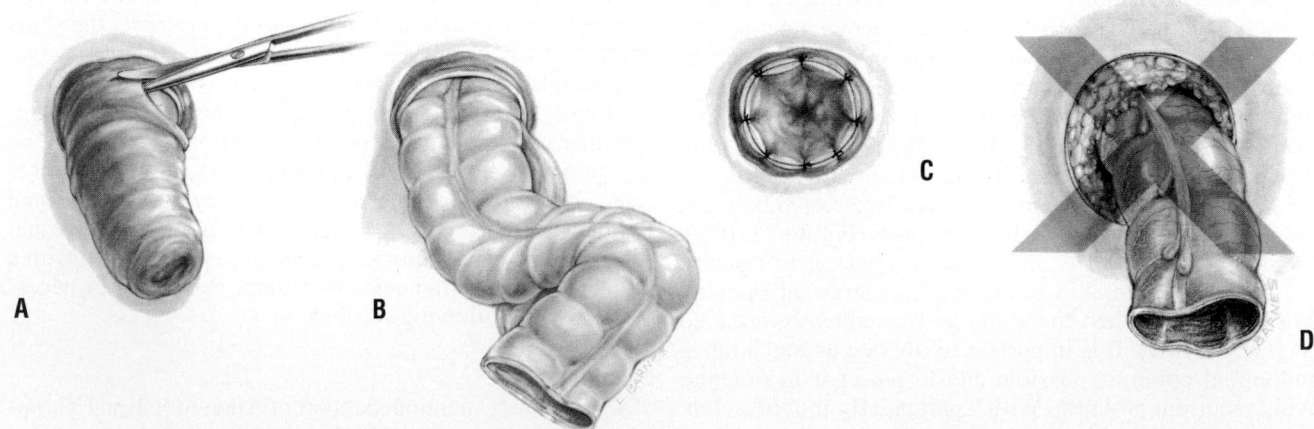

FIGURE 31-10. Revision of prolapsed sigmoid colostomy (after several months). **A:** Incision into mucosa itself rather than at mucocutaneous junction. **B:** The redundant bowel is exteriorized and resected. **C:** Final maturation is obtained by mucosa-to-mucosa suturing. **D:** Incorrect incision in the skin creates too-large an opening.

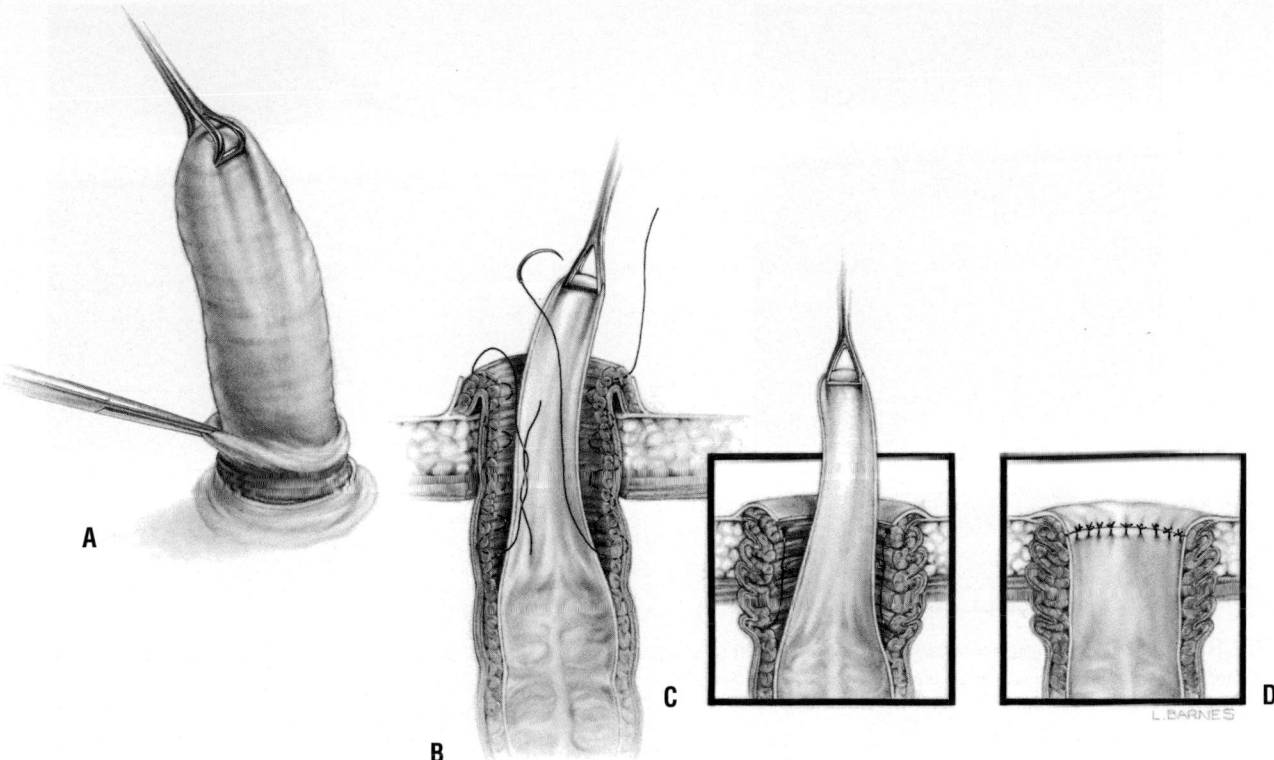

FIGURE 31-11. Repair of colostomy prolapse by Delorme modification. **A:** Incision into the mucosa is made proximal to the mucocutaneous junction. **B:** Plicating sutures of an absorbable material are taken in the muscularis from the apex to the most distal point. **C:** The sutures are then tied and the redundant mucosa excised. **D:** Mucosa-to-mucosa apposition takes place with interrupted, simple, absorbable sutures.

the prevalence of parastomal hernia was 2.8% in those brought through the muscle and 21.6% in those placed laterally, a highly significant difference.[221] The St. Mark's Hospital group studied the long-term complication rate of end-sigmoid colostomy and found that the crude and actuarially corrected risks of paracolostomy complications in 203 patients at 13 years were 51.2% and 58.1%, respectively.[145] They concluded that siting the stoma through the rectus muscle did not reduce the risk of hernia. However, an extraperitoneal course was associated with a significantly lower risk of herniation when compared with a transperitoneal course. The authors opined that parastomal hernia is technically avoidable.[145] Other possible causes of paracolostomy hernia include locating the stoma in the incision itself and the creation of too large an opening in the abdominal wall (Figures 31-13 through 31-15). Some surgeons are sufficiently nihilistic that they believe

FIGURE 31-12. Gangrene at the end of a prolapsed colostomy. Obviously, a resection is mandated.

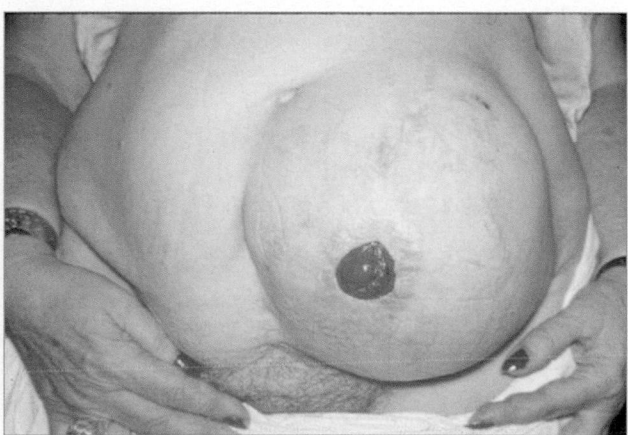

FIGURE 31-13. Massive paracolostomy hernia. Note that the stoma had been brought through the left paramedian incision.

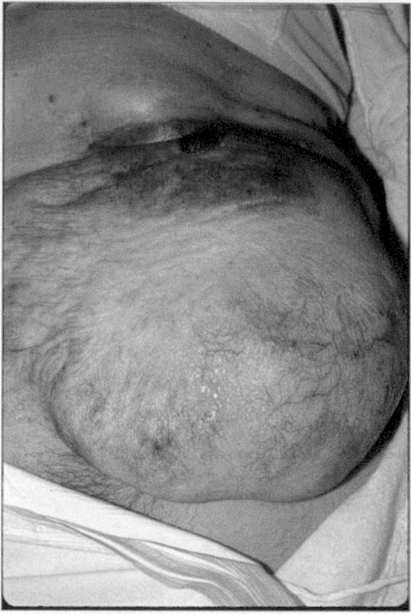

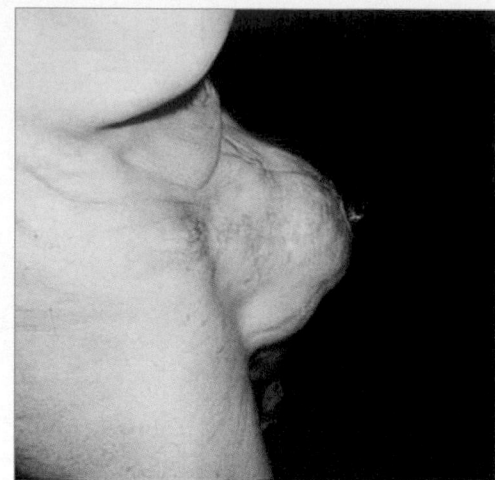

FIGURE 31-15. Typical paracolostomy hernia with the stoma at the center of the defect.

FIGURE 31-14. Paracolostomy hernia. Atrophic skin is the only covering of the abdominal cavity. The stoma is at the proximal aspect of the defect.

this complication is inevitable if the patient survives long enough—a theory impossible to dispute. Certainly, weight gain, the effects of the aging process, other systemic diseases, nutritional problems, and many other factors may predispose to the development of this problem. Symptoms may be only those related to esthetic concerns expressed as the unsightly bulging. Other complaints include problems with appliance management (leakage, soiling, and detachment), pain, and rarely obstructive symptoms (due to bowel incarceration adjacent to the stoma). The diagnosis is usually self-evident, but computed tomography (CT) is felt by some to be a valuable tool in determining the true incidence of parastomal hernias. It will also aid in diagnosing occult parastomal hernias.[46]

Treatment

The choices of operative approaches to the repair of a peristomal hernia are usually dictated by its size. Relatively

small defects may be repaired by direct suture, circumcising the colostomy, closing the abdominal wall, and re-maturing the stoma (Figure 31-16). This technique, suggested by Thorlakson,[243] may be employed with two caveats: if the colostomy has been created in the proper location, that is, through the split rectus muscle, and if there is only a small defect. If a small hernia is present in conjunction with an improperly located stoma, the colostomy should probably be relocated. Such relocation can sometimes be accomplished by an intraperitoneal tunnel method, closing the defect at the original site (Figure 31-17). If the rectus location is still available, this is the optimal site. If not considered appropriate, one has three options for potential placement: use the opposite side of the abdomen, place the stoma at the umbilicus, or employ a mesh replacement by one of a number of approaches.

The use of the umbilical site is not a unique concept. Some surgeons prefer to create the colostomy in the umbilicus initially. Raza and colleagues evaluated 101 patients in whom they performed such a stoma.[194] They strongly supported the concept of this location because of their low incidence of complications: only four patients required

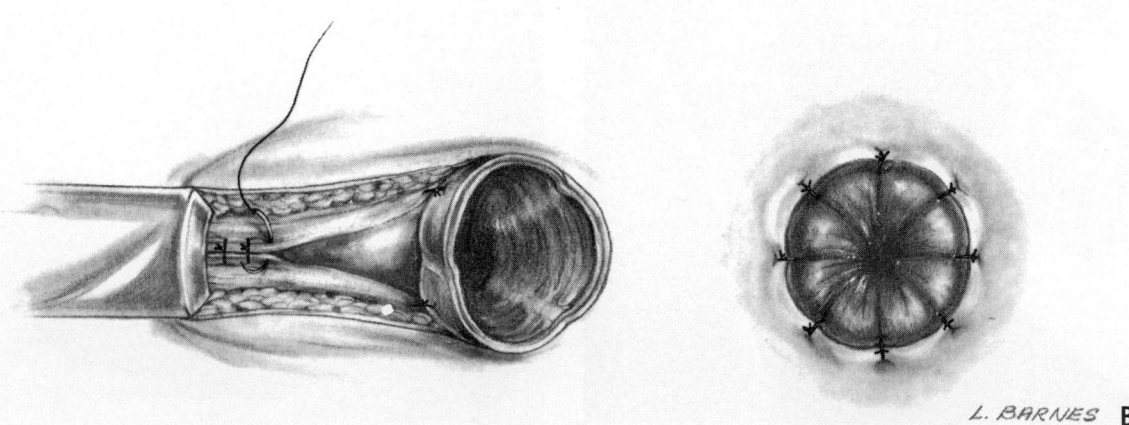

A   L. BARNES B

FIGURE 31-16. Paracolostomy hernia repair for a small defect at the correctly located site. **A:** Direct repair with fascial closure (note serosa to fascia sutures). **B:** Mucocutaneous sutures are placed in the usual way.

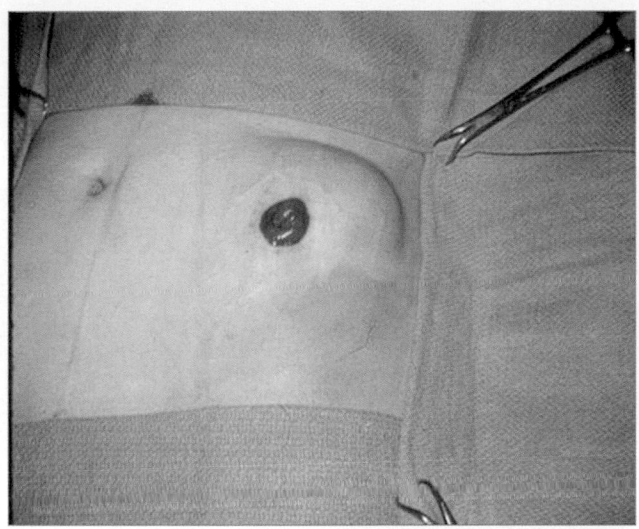
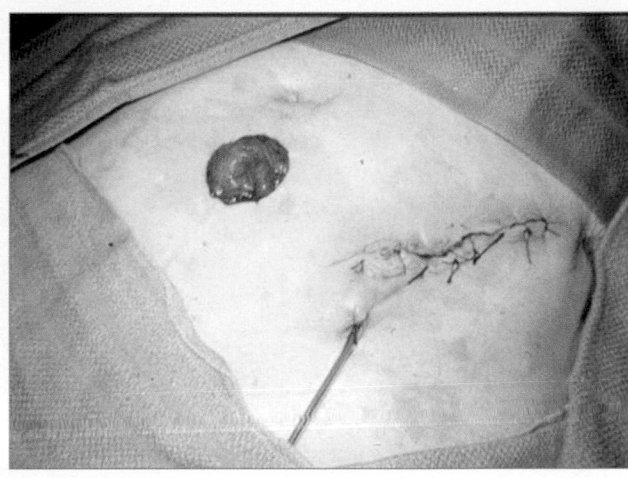

A

B

FIGURE 31-17. Paracolostomy hernia repair for small defects in the pararectus location. **A:** The stoma has been relocated after intraperitoneal tunneling and the defect repaired. **B:** The wound can be closed secondarily, not necessarily by the primary closure and drainage method, which is shown.

reoperation. There were no parastomal hernias and no prolapses in their experience. If an umbilical colostomy is created, the technique of construction is essentially the same, but it is important to remove all of the skin that tends to turn inward. Turnbull (see Biography) commented that this is why the Almighty created the umbilicus—namely, as a backup resource for the placement of a stoma. It is generally preferred to use the patient's own tissue for repair if one can achieve a successful result, but reconstruction of larger hernias requires insertion of prosthetic material. This may be accomplished either by the open method or laparoscopically.[2,37,124,165,192,205,230,237]

In repairing the hernia, some surgeons prefer to maintain the stoma at the original location, using the mesh around the colostomy as an onlay, an inlay, or an underlay (sublay) repair. The last technique is my personal preference. Others bring the bowel through the middle of the material, the "keyhole" method (Figure 31-18). In my opinion, relocating the stoma elsewhere is preferable if it can be accomplished (Figure 31-19). In the Sugarbaker modification, an underlay mesh is placed with the stoma exiting at the lateral border of the mesh.[231] Overlap is achieved with the mesh lying on the distal few centimeters of the stoma. Figure 31-20 demonstrates various techniques for mesh implantation, including that of a minimally invasive approach (see later). Tekkis and colleagues use a Thorlakson method at the site of the stoma, incorporating an incomplete circumferential mesh.[237]

There is always the possibility of infection and persistent drainage if a nonabsorbable prosthetic material is placed in a contaminated field, but this is uncommon and usually not a concern. A number of products are available for implantation. Sepramesh (a polypropylene composite) has the advantage of limiting adhesion formation to the implant. Others advocate porcine dermal collagen (Permacol) and other bioprosthetic meshes to perhaps minimize the risk of persistent infection but at the cost of (again "perhaps") an increased recurrence rate.[64,116,244] Other choices include polyvinylidene fluoride (PVDF—Tecaflon),[24] polytetrafluo-

roethylene (PTFE),[141,227] polypropylene (Marlex, Surgipro, Surumesh),[110] and Gore-tex.

Moisidis and coworkers simulated the "stresses" imposed on Marlex mesh and found that the hole tends to enlarge and to become distorted.[165] They suggest that the cut margins should be reinforced with a polypropylene purse-string suture in order to stabilize the opening. Hofstetter and coworkers describe a technique using PTFE mesh in 13 patients, wherein the stoma is fully mobilized, but the mucocutaneous anastomosis is not disrupted.[112] The abdominal wall repair is reinforced with a 10-cm × 12-cm sheet, with the mesh incised and wrapped around the bowel. The hole that is created in the mesh is described as having an eight-pointed, star-shaped configuration.

Laparoscopic Approach. In recent years, there has been an interest in effecting repair by means of a laparoscopic technique.[27,186,257] Laparoscopic hernia repair is considered by some to be a less invasive procedure that may be used for incisional hernia, as well as parastomal hernia. The technique involves access from a site not involving the stoma or scars (see principles discussed in Chapter 19). The procedure generally requires three trocar sites: one for the endoscope and the others for the dissection. During a laparoscopic incisional hernia repair, the hernial sac is pushed inside the abdominal cavity. The defect is covered with a mesh graft placed in an underlay fashion.

There are two types of laparoscopic parastomal techniques: one through the mesh or keyhole approach (similar to that shown in Figure 31-18) and the second, the so-called Sugarbaker modification. In keyhole repairs, the parastomal hernia is fixed with an intraperitoneal mesh, with the creation of an opening to allow the intestine through. In the "Sugarbaker" or "modified Sugarbaker" repair, the mesh is also placed intraperitoneally but without creating an opening. The mesh covers the defect and surrounds the bowel as in the previously discussed open technique. Transfacial sutures are recommended to be placed along the side of the stoma.

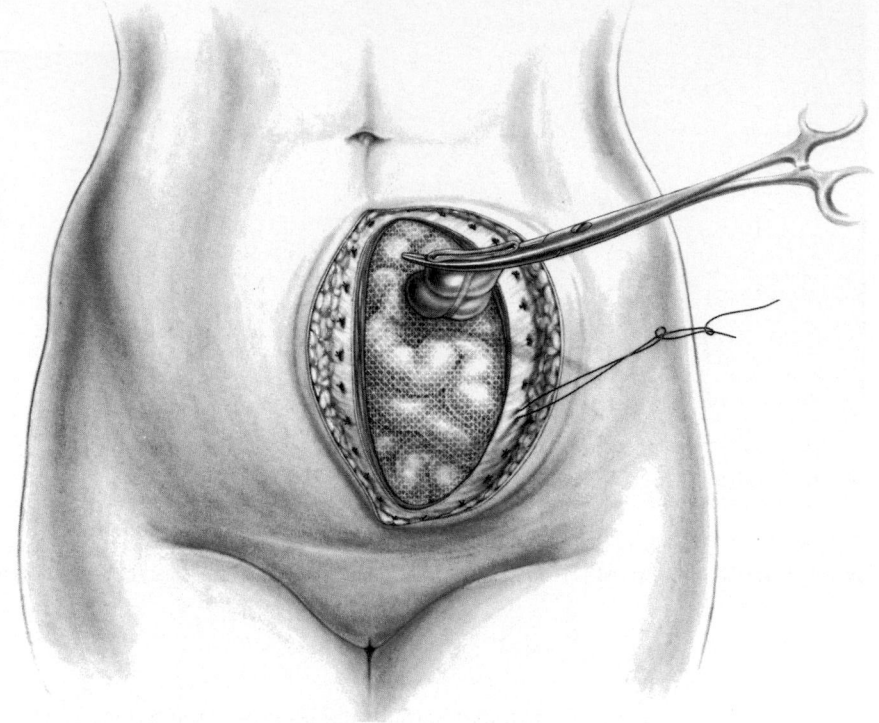

A

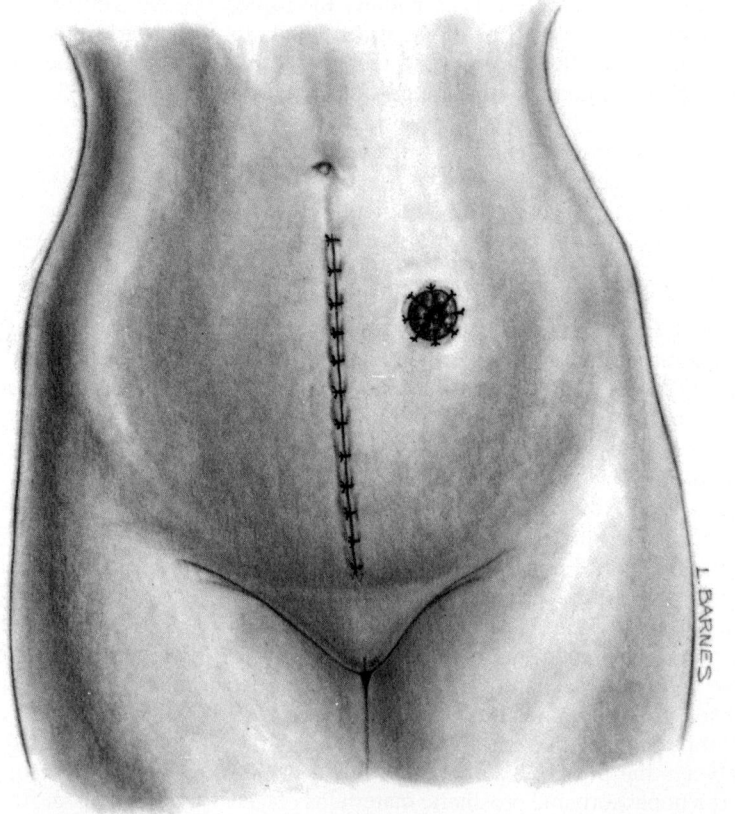

B

FIGURE 31-18. Underlay repair (the author's preference) of a large parastomal hernial defect with mesh, without relocating stoma. **A:** The stoma is brought through the mesh, and the mesh is anchored to the fascia with monofilament nonabsorbable sutures by an interrupted mattress technique placed through the abdominal wall muscle and fascia. **B:** Stoma is matured at the original location.

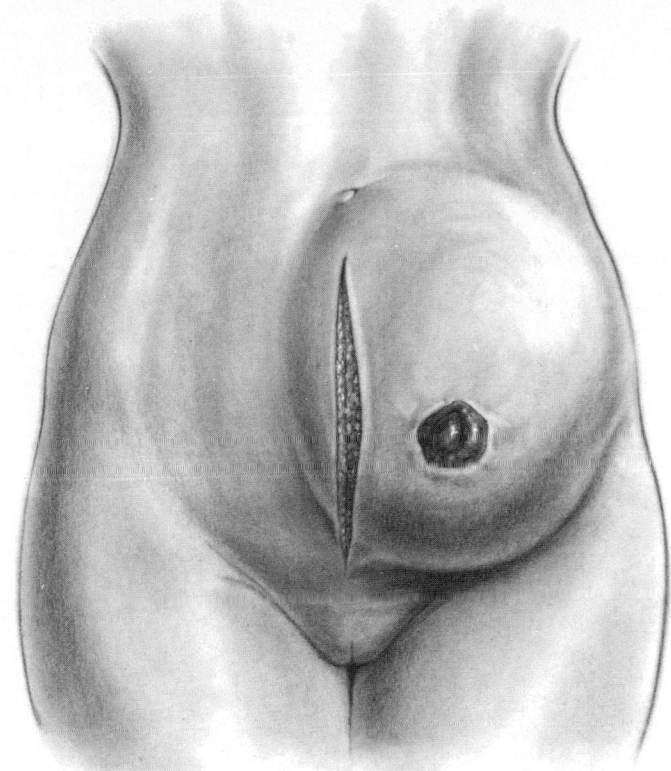

A

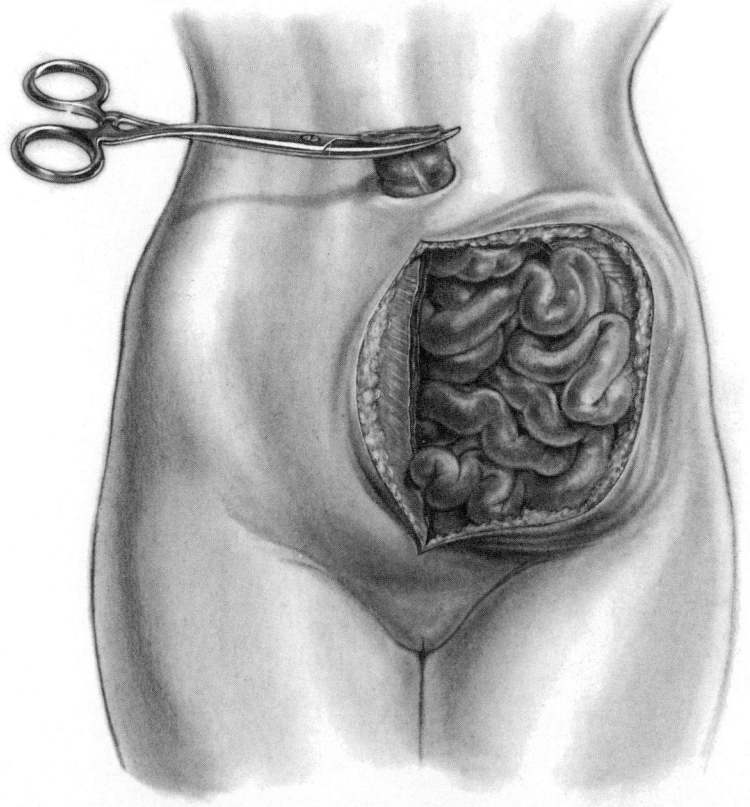

B

FIGURE 31-19. Underlay repair of large parastomal hernial defect with mesh, transplanting stoma. **A:** Incision. **B:** Relocation of stoma to the umbilicus. *(continued)*

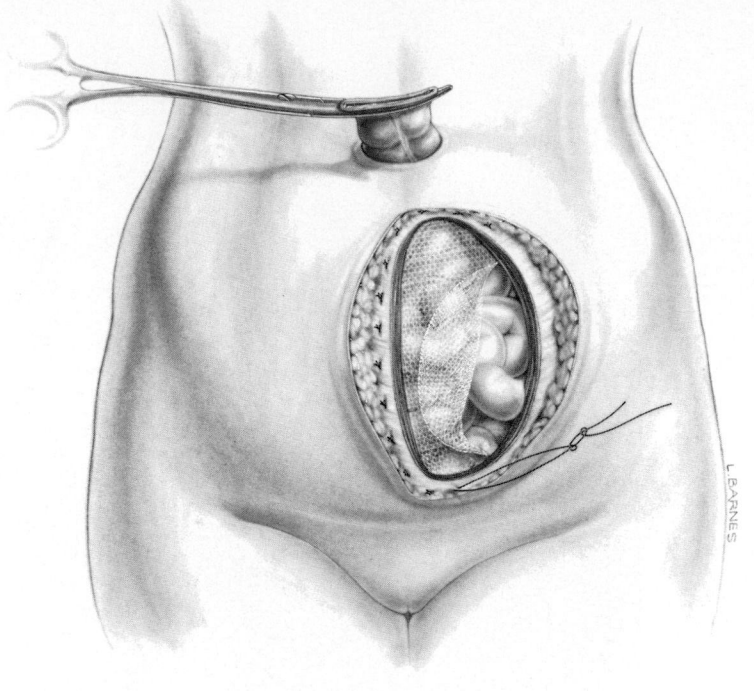

C

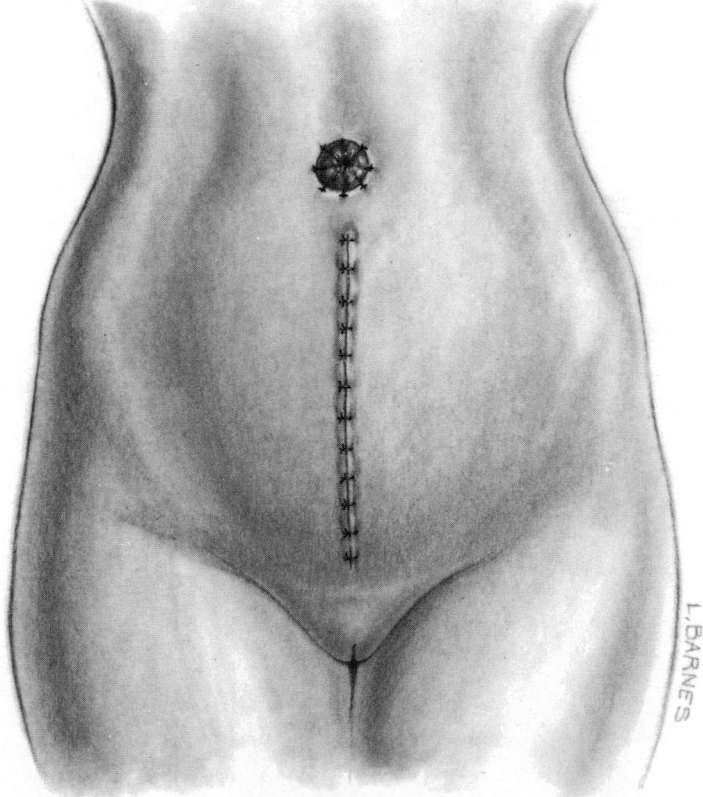

FIGURE 31-19. *(continued)* **C:** Placement of mesh, anchoring it to the undersurface of the abdominal wall with interrupted, monofilament, nonabsorbable sutures. **D:** Wound closure and maturation of stoma.

D

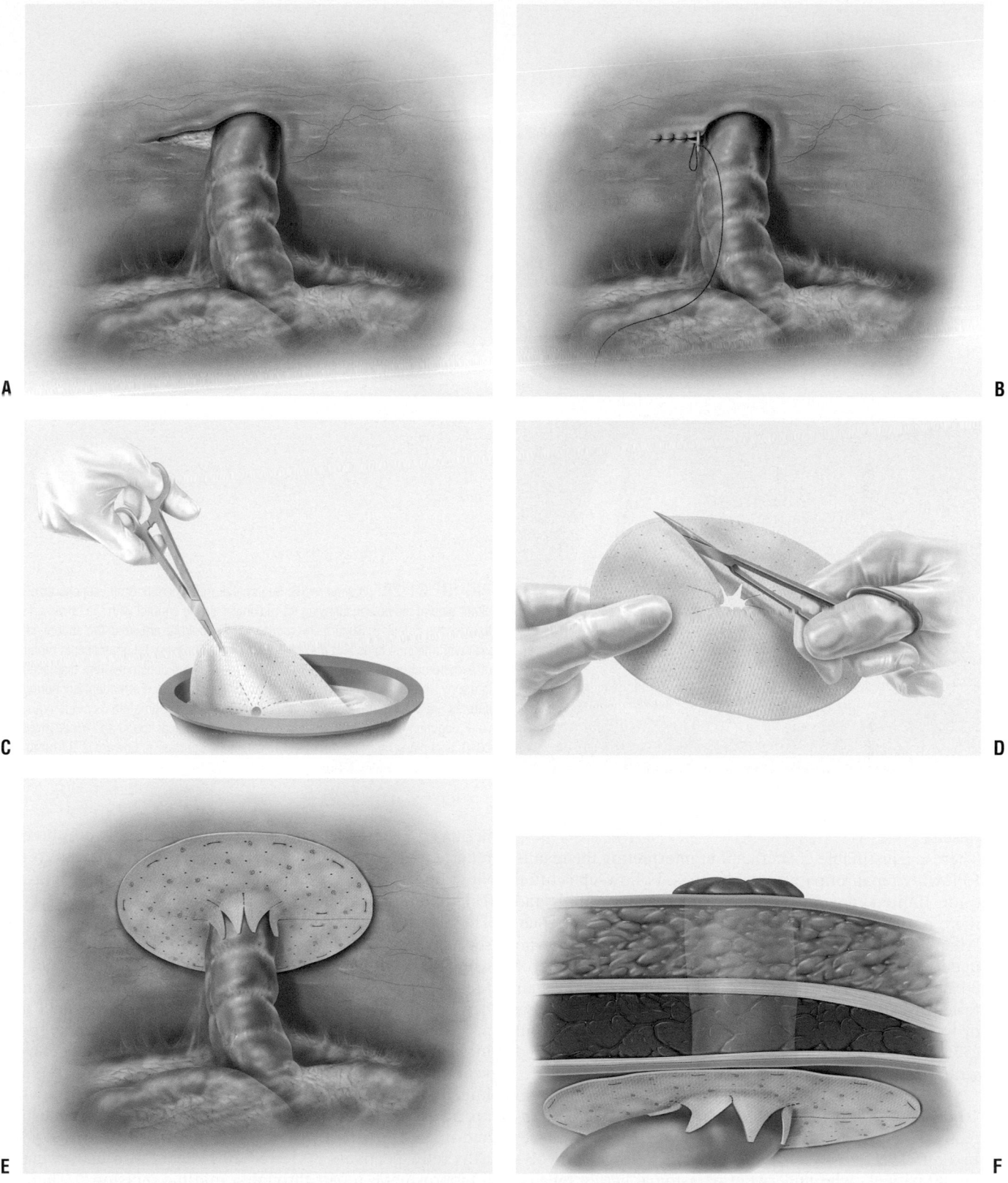

FIGURE 31-20. Techniques for parastomal hernia repairs using Biodesign Parastomal Reinforcement Graft. **A:** Hernial defect is identified. **B:** Suture closure of defect to proper anatomy (if possible). **C:** Hydration of graft less than 1 minute in room temperature, sterile lactated Ringer's solution, or sterile saline. **D:** Cutting the graft to facilitate placement. The graft is designed to fit various bowel diameters in a keyhole fashion. **E:** The graft is sutured or tacked into position as an underlay. Alernatives include an overlay and sublay. **F:** Final position. *(continued)*

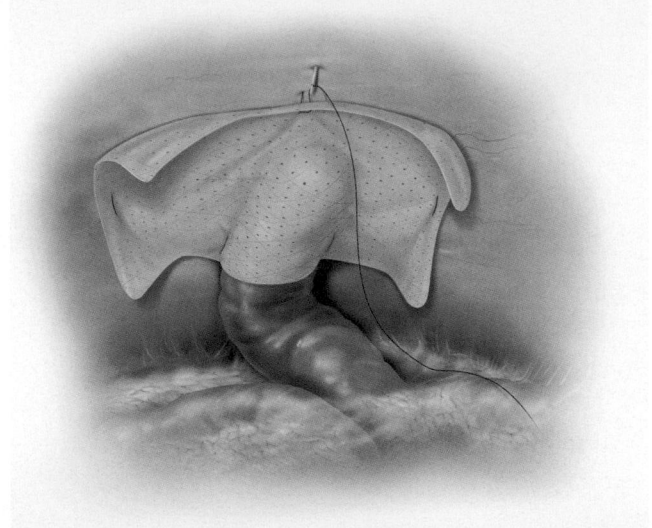

G

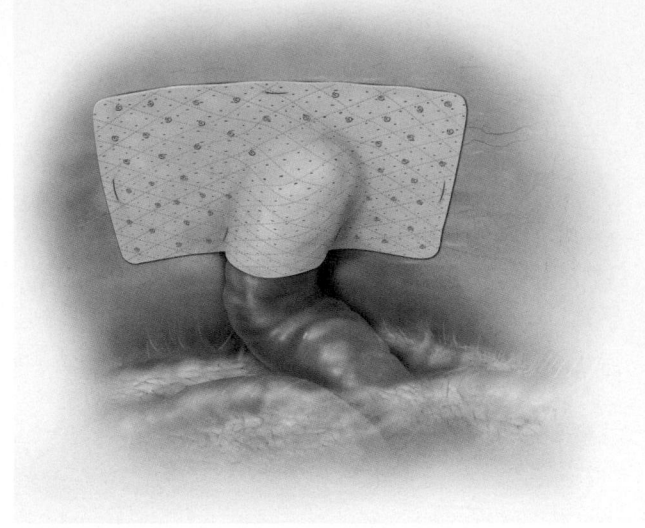

H

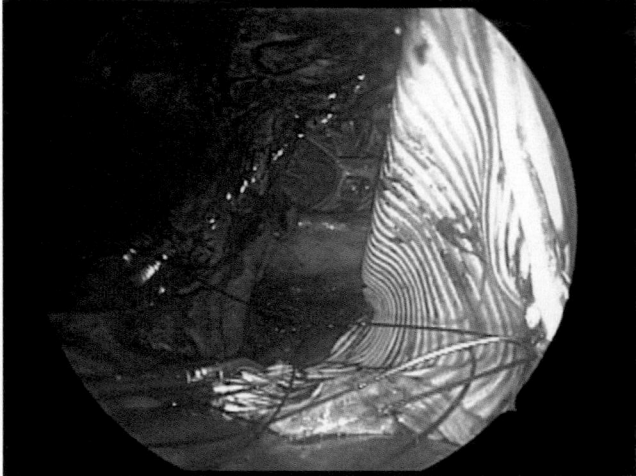

I

FIGURE 31-20. *(continued)* **G:** Sugarbaker modification. Graft is anchored on either side of the bowel, allowing for maximum tissue contact with the bowel and to close the defect. **H:** Sugarbaker (*cont.*). Graft should be affixed to the abdominal wall with minimal folds and maximum contact with tissue. **I:** Laparoscopic repair of parastomal hernia with the use of PTFE mesh. Note ileostomy limb displaced inferiorly, the defect, and beginning of mesh implantation. Permanent anchoring sutures are placed at the periphery of the mesh at approximately 6 cm intervals. (*A–F*, copyright 2011, Lisa Clark, courtesy of Cook Medical, Inc. *G and H*, copyright 2010, Lisa Clark, courtesy of Cook Medical, Inc. *I*, Courtesy of Edward C. Borrazzo, MD and Neil H. Hyman, MD.)

Results

There is a justifiable concern about interpreting the results following repair of parastomal hernias. Follow-up is often quite limited, the series generally are very small, and there is a nonexistent randomized, controlled experience. Allen-Mersh and Thomson identified 42 individuals who underwent repair of paracolostomy hernia, an incidence of 34% of all operative stomal complications.[9] Local repair failed in 47%, but re-siting the stoma to the umbilicus or to the right side of the abdomen was more successful (57%). Re-siting to the same (left) side was associated with a failure rate of 86%.

Alexandre and Bouillot used a Dacron prosthesis in 10 patients with pericolostomy hernia.[8] There were no infections and no mortality, but there was one recurrence. In a retrospective review by Rubin and colleagues involving 80 patients who underwent parastomal hernia repairs, the investigators concluded that stomal relocation is superior to that of direct fascial repair.[207] Furthermore, for those that recur, they found that the use of prosthetic material is the most successful method for effecting cure. Cheung and associates retrospectively reviewed their 43 patients who underwent repair of parastomal hernia.[44] The overall recurrence rate was 40%. Stelzner and coworkers reviewed 20 patients who underwent PTFE repair for large stomal

hernias.[227] There were no infections, and there were three recurrences (mean follow-up, 3.5 years). In a literature review on the use of mesh repairs for parastomal hernias, Tekkis and colleagues were able to identify 72 cases.[237] The overall failure rate due to recurrence or mesh-related sepsis was 8.3%. Carne and colleagues conducted a search using the Medline database and concluded that no technical factors related to construction have been shown to prevent herniation.[39] However, Jänes and coworkers undertook a prospective clinical trial in which 54 individuals undergoing permanent colostomy were randomized to have a conventional stoma or a mesh placed in a sublay position.[118] No infection or fistula was observed. At the 12-month follow-up, parastomal hernia was present in 8 of 18 without a mesh and none of 16 patients in whom the mesh was used.[118] Ellis retrospectively reviewed 20 patients who underwent a bioprosthetic repair through a midline incision.[64] There were no infections, but two recurrences were noted at a median follow-up of 18 months (range, 12 to 54). Berger and Bientzle undertook laparoscopic repair of 66 patients with parastomal hernias with "promising results."[24]

Unfortunately, many of colostomy patients are elderly or represent a high risk for a major abdominal operation, and relocation and mesh implant indeed comprise a major procedure. There may be no recourse for some except to use some form of abdominal support. Fortunately, many individuals are relatively asymptomatic[180]; hence, operative intervention is not necessarily a requisite.

Prophylactic Mesh Insertion. A number of publications have appeared in recent years on the insertion of a mesh at the time of stomal construction, both open and laparoscopic, on a prophylactic basis to "strengthen the colostomy outlet" and to prevent a subsequent parastomal hernia.[19,86,118,143,146,148,255] Bayer and coworkers reported 43 patients with no evidence of hernia after a 4-year follow-up by means of the prophylactic placement of polypropylene mesh.[19] Gögenur and coworkers also placed polypropylene mesh in an onlay position at the primary operation in 25 patients.[86] At a median follow-up of 1 year, no infections or early complications were noted (there was one unrelated death). Two patients developed parastomal hernias, one at 6 and the other at 12 months.

Recurrent Disease

Recurrence of the primary condition may develop at the site of the stoma. This is usually seen in patients who have undergone abdominoperineal resection or a diversionary colostomy for IBD (ulcerative colitis or Crohn's disease). The mucosa appears edematous and friable, bleeds easily, and may be granular or ulcerated. Medical management of IBD may resolve the inflammation and ameliorate the patient's complaints. However, because of diarrhea and the inability to maintain an appliance satisfactorily, a more extensive bowel resection and possible ileostomy may be required (see Ileostomy Complications).

Recurrent malignancy may occur at the site of the colostomy and is a rare and potentially fatal complication (Figure 31-21). This may be due to tumor implantation at the time of the resection or to an inadequate margin of resection. Another possibility is that it may actually represent a second

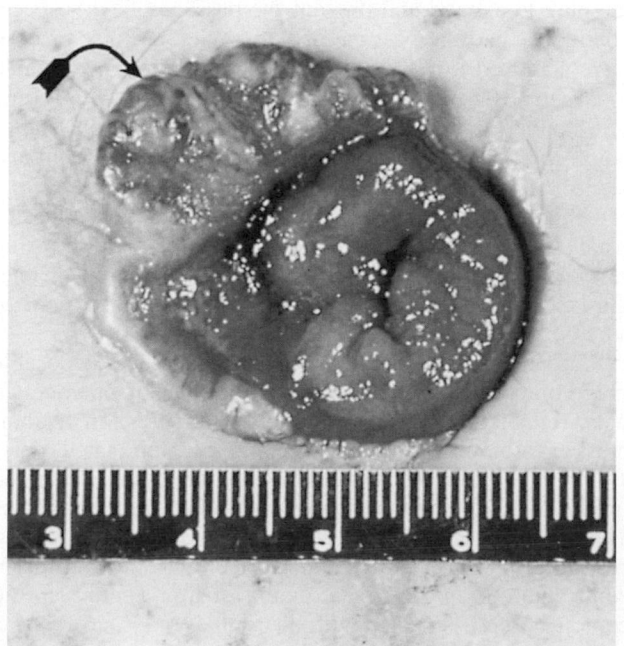

FIGURE 31-21. Recurrent carcinoma adjacent to the stoma (*arrow*). (Courtesy of Rudolf Garret, MD.)

TABLE 31-1 Complications of Terminal Colostomy (251 Patients)

COMPLICATION	NUMBER OF CASES	PERCENT OF SERIES
Infection	34	14
Mucocutaneous separation	24	10
Pericolostomy hernia	36	14
Prolapse	12	5
Recession (retraction)	1	0.4
Stenosis	9	4
Fistula	1	0.4

Adapted from Whittaker M, Goligher JC. A comparison of the results of extraperitoneal and intraperitoneal techniques for construction of terminal iliac colostomies. *Dis Colon Rectum.* 1976;19(4):342–344.

primary lesion. For example, epidermoid carcinoma of the parastomal skin has also been reported.[83] Radical resection of the involved area including part of the abdominal wall with relocation of the stoma is the recommended treatment.

Results of Colostomy Creation

Whittaker and Goligher reviewed their experience with colostomy following abdominoperineal resection of the rectum in 251 patients who survived for at least 2 years.[263] Upon comparison of extraperitoneal and intraperitoneal colostomy, it appeared that the complication rate was higher with the latter technique (see Figures 29-44 and 29-45 as applied to ileostomy, but the principle is the same). The difference, however, was not statistically significant. Table 31-1 demonstrates the results of this study. It can be appreciated that colostomy construction is associated with a high incidence of complications. Almost 50% of the patients in this series (those who survived for at least 2 years) developed a stomal problem. One can only conjecture that had the patients been followed for a longer period, the complication rate would be higher.

Porter and colleagues reviewed their experience with 130 end colostomies, followed for an average of 35 months.[187] There were 69 complications in 55 patients (44%). These included 11 strictures, 9 wound infections, 14 hernias, 9 small bowel obstructions, 4 prolapses, 2 abscesses, and 1 parastomal fistula. Mealy and associates reviewed 120 patients who underwent colostomy both on an elective and an emergency basis.[157] Colostomy-related morbidity included stenosis, retraction, prolapse, and hernia formation. These were observed in 19.2% of their 120 patients. There was no difference in incidence between the emergency and elective groups.

Marks and Ritchie reviewed their experience with complications following abdominoperineal resection for carcinoma of the rectum during the period 1968 through 1972 at St. Mark's Hospital.[149] Of the 227 patients who formed the basis of this study, three died in the postoperative period. By far, the most common stomal problem encountered was hernia, which occurred in 23 patients, approximately 10%. It was felt that the cumulative risk of developing a paracolostomy hernia in the sixth postoperative year was approximately 33%. The authors believed that extraperitoneal colostomy seemed to offer some protection against herniation. The other reported complications included retraction, stenosis, abscess, and prolapse. The cumulative incidence of all these stomal complications was approximately 7%. This report and others confirm that most colostomy hernias seem to develop in the first few years.[136]

Quality of life is an important area for assessment following colostomy, but there are few publications on this subject. Baxter and coworkers have developed a Stoma Quality of Life Scale to better analyze the results of this procedure.[18] They were able to demonstrate that this instrument correlated well in those with improved versus those with worsened quality of life.

Alternative Techniques for Sigmoid Colostomy Creation and Management

Maturation by Stapling

In addition to the conventional maturation technique for creating a sigmoid colostomy, the circular stapling device has been advocated for performing end colostomies.[45,134,195] This permits a geometrically perfect opening that can be theoretically calibrated to be optimal size for a particular bowel diameter.

Technique

Instead of a disk of skin being excised from the abdominal wall, a small opening is created just large enough to pass the center rod without the anvil. A purse string is created of the distal colon in the usual manner and the anvil inserted into the bowel. The cartridge and anvil are approximated, and the instrument is fired. One tissue "doughnut" consists of the skin, and the other is made up of the bowel. In effect, it is a colocutaneous anastomosis by means of the circular stapling device.

Another application of a stapler is the use of ordinary skin staples for maturing the stoma.[11] They are then removed on the 10th postoperative day.

Opinion

Although the former procedure does have some theoretical appeal, it would certainly make the subcutaneous dissection and rectus splitting much more tedious. Furthermore, it is more likely that the inferior epigastric vessels will be injured during the course of the dissection. Moreover, as previously discussed, the factors that predispose to the subsequent development of stoma complications are related to ischemia, tension, improper location, and size of the abdominal wall opening—issues that are not avoided merely by creating a perfectly circular skin aperture.

As for the use of skin staplers to mature the stoma, one may reasonably ask what the advantage is when an additional effort must be made to remove them.

Continent Colostomy

The search for continence in a colostomy has stimulated many attempts to control bowel movements by means of prosthetic devices. Tenney and colleagues reviewed the various approaches that have been attempted or proposed.[238] The authors considered the concepts according to four categories: external devices, surgical technique alone, surgical technique with passive implanted devices, and surgical technique with active implanted devices. There has been and continues to be considerable interest in developing a device for controlling bowel movements, whether for anal incontinence (see Chapter 16) or for ostomates. Initial publications are uniformly enthusiastic, but sometimes for inapparent reasons the product disappears from the literature and from the manufacturer's inventory.

Kock Continent Colostomy

Kock and associates proposed a method, analogous to that of the continent ileostomy, through the use of the descending colon to create a nipple valve.[130] In five patients, the end sigmoidostomy was provided with such a valve, but evacuation by irrigation through a catheter was laborious, and the procedure has since been abandoned.[131] Some success was noted, however, with a continent cecostomy (see later).

Inflatable Cuff

A simple inflatable cuff has been attempted by the Mayo Clinic group, using the cuff end of a tracheostomy tube. The procedure was performed initially in animals and then in patients who had failed nipple valves following a Kock continent ileostomy. It was also considered for patients with conventional ileostomies who had not undergone a reservoir procedure. There appears to have been no further communication about this approach.

Colostomy Plug

In 1986, Burcharth and colleagues reported the use of a colostomy plug (Conseal; Coloplast, Inc., Tampa, FL) on 53 patients.[35] The device is a two-piece system consisting of an adhesive baseplate and a disposable plug attachable to the plate (Figure 31-22). It is packed and compressed in a water-soluble film that disintegrates after insertion, allowing the plug to expand and prevent the passage of feces. Fecal continence and the passage of flatus without noise or odor were achieved in 90% of individuals.[35] Patients were able to effectively use the device for a median application time of 8 hours. Potential advantages include the elimination of noise, the filtering of odor, the elimination of a pouch, and the lack of obtrusiveness.

Clague and Heald used this device in 100 individuals.[47] Analysis of patient evaluations indicated that the plug restored continence and improved lifestyle in more than one-third of the ostomates who used it. Others have also reported a favorable experience with this device.[48,224]

Cerdán and colleagues describe a one-piece disposable plug composed of a soft, flexible cylinder of open-celled polyurethane foam.[41] The device is supplied in a compressed form, enclosed in a water-soluble, lubricated, polyvinyl alcohol film. This is analogous to the plug illustrated in Figure 16-22 for the management of anal incontinence. The authors used the device in 20 patients with sigmoid colostomies. All but three found it comfortable and that it contributed to an improved quality of life. There were no complications associated with its use.

The use of a new continence device (Vitala) for colostomy patients was reported by Maxwell and colleagues.[151] The appliance uses a pillow-shaped sealing element of

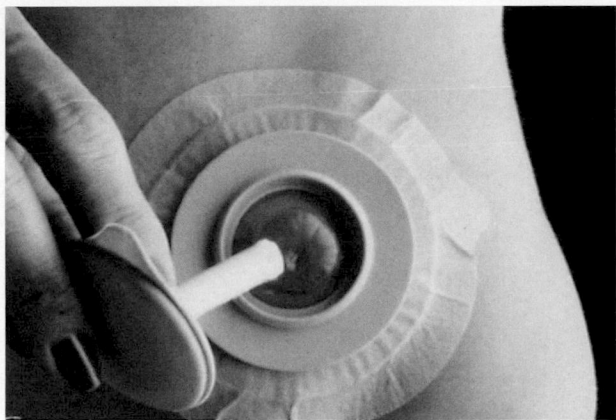

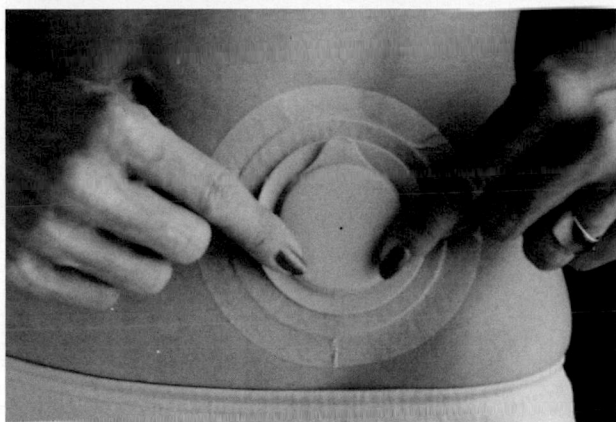

FIGURE 31-22. Conseal continent colostomy system. (Courtesy of Coloplast, Inc.)

thin, plastic film (the Air Seal), which contains a soft foam that expands slowly, conforming to the shape of the stoma (Figure 31-23). A valve in the Air Seal allows it to inflate quickly and deflate slowly when external pressure is applied. Flatus can be released, and an in-built waste bag is deployed to capture any stool. In a preliminary study with 26 patients, the authors concluded that Vitala provides an important option for colostomy continence.[151]

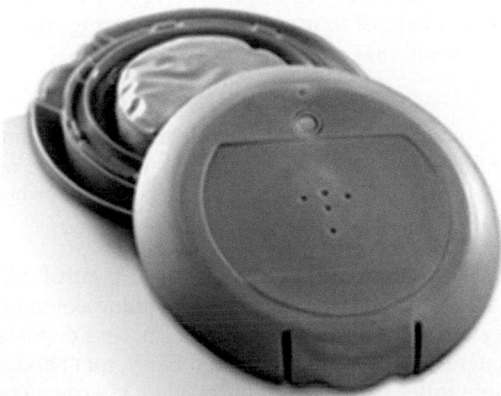

FIGURE 31-23. Vitala continence control device functions by sealing against the stoma to prevent the release of stool while permitting the gas to vent through an integrated deodorizing filter. (Courtesy ConvaTec, Skillman, NJ.)

Artificial Sphincter

Szinicz described an implantable hydraulic sphincter prosthesis that consists of a compressible driving and control system together with a sleeve that is implanted around the bowel.[234] The sleeve is connected to the compliance chamber by means of a connecting tube. The author reported his experience in animal experiments and in seven patients. Heiblum and Cordoba implanted an inflatable plastic balloon in the subcutaneous tissue around the stoma in order to achieve fecal continence.[103] The connecting tube was tunneled subcutaneously from the balloon and brought out through a small wound at some distance from the stoma. The authors reported their experience in six patients, all but one of whom underwent the prosthesis insertion secondarily. Complete continence to feces and gas was obtained. One device had to be removed because it eroded the skin, and subcutaneous infection was a problem in three individuals. Here again, these approaches seem to have fallen off the surgical map.

Muscle Transplantation

Intestinal smooth muscle has been used to construct a continent colostomy.[213] Freely transplanted, this is tailored as a 10- to 15-cm long segment of large intestinal muscle (usually the sigmoid), devoid of mucosa and mesenteric fat. The seromuscular sleeve is incised longitudinally through one of the taeniae, soaked in an antibiotic solution, and sutured to the serosa of the bowel approximately 2 or 3 cm proximal to the site for the creation of the stoma. Sutures are placed so that the transplant is imbricated. This creates a length of about 6 cm, which in effect increases the muscular mass. The author emphasizes that, after securing one edge of the graft, the muscle must be stretched maximally, and the graft wrapped around the bowel and secured. The mesenteric vessels are incorporated by the graft.

Schmidt reported his experience with this technique in more than 500 patients, 231 of whom underwent surgery in his own unit.[213] Approximately 80% did not require an appliance, there was no mortality, and only five required removal of the surgical implant. Apparently, the transplants are nourished by means of secondary vascularization, and an irrigation technique facilitates defecation. In most patients who underwent the procedure secondarily, "nearly all viewed their postoperative situation as markedly improved."

Kostov and coworkers used a modified smooth muscle "sphincteroplasty" for increasing intraluminal pressure in the colon proximal to the stoma in 72 rectal cancer patients.[132] Their technique involves resection and transplantation of a 4-cm long portion of sigmoid colon muscularis. This is then passed around the colon through a defect in the mesentery, fixing it to the taenia. The procedure is combined with colonic irrigation to produce some level of bowel control and regularity. In an experience involving 72 patients, the weekly spontaneous stools were felt to be three to five times less frequent than in controls.

It seems that these publications have accrued a remarkably large number of patients, but unfortunately the surgeons as individuals or as groups who are interested in this problem seem to represent essentially that of lone experience.

Magnetic Colostomy

In 1975, Feustel and Hennig of Erlangen, Germany, described a device to create continence in patients who underwent conventional sigmoid colostomy: a magnetic ring implant.[68]

A ring of samarium cobalt encased in plastic is buried in the subcutaneous tissue around the colon. The colostomy is matured in the usual manner and, when the wound has completely healed (usually several weeks later), an external cap containing a ring magnet in the top and a core magnet in the center pin is inserted to create a plug.

Results of the magnetic continent colostomy device were initially quite favorable, although subsequent results have been less optimistic.[91] Khubchandani and associates reported their experience in 14 patients, one-half of whom had good results.[129] There was no morbidity attributable to insertion of the ring, and there was no incident of wound infection. However, other problems developed, including the triggering of security monitors at airports, disturbances of television reception if one is sitting close, malfunctioning of wrist watches, and adherence of the patient to anything metallic (e.g., a kitchen sink). Alexander-Williams and associates reviewed their experience with 61 patients: 55 primary and 6 secondary implants.[7] One individual died, possibly as a consequence of sepsis at the site of the implant. Twelve (20%) required removal of the ring because of failure of healing or late skin necrosis. Approximately one-half of the remaining patients were not using the magnetic cap at all at the time of the review. The reason for this failure was the fact that the device did not afford complete continence. Of the 21 patients who used the cap regularly, 15 were continent. In these authors' experience, therefore, only one-fourth of the patients who underwent the operation were completely continent.

Kewenter reported 21 patients who underwent magnetic colostomy, all but three of whom had the procedure performed at the time of the primary resection.[127] Three died soon after operation (unrelated to the surgery). Eight were considered a success in that the cap was used under all circumstances, and two patients were considered partial successes. If one groups these two categories together, excluding the patients who expired, the rate of success with the procedure in Kewenter's experience was 44%.

Comment

It appears that implantation of the magnetic stoma device is not a very forgiving technique. It requires meticulous dissection and careful patient selection. Complete control is successful in no more than 50% of patients. The matter now, however, is academic because the device has been taken from the market and is no longer available. As a consequence, I no longer include a description of the operative technique or the illustrations in this text, but I do wish to recommend to the reader and to the future investigator that the concept of an implanted device for creating a continent colostomy should not be resurrected. The following is another.

Implantable Ring and Balloon Plug

In 1983, Prager described a device for control of feces following abdominoperineal resection and sigmoid colostomy.[188] It is composed of two parts: a silicone ring, which is produced in three different internal diameters with a flange on the upper surface reinforced with Dacron mesh, and a silicone balloon, which is made in varying lengths. The balloon is inflated and deflated by means of a 30-mL syringe. The ring is implanted within the peritoneal cavity and sewn onto the undersurface of the abdominal wall where the opening has been made for the stoma to be delivered. The abdominal

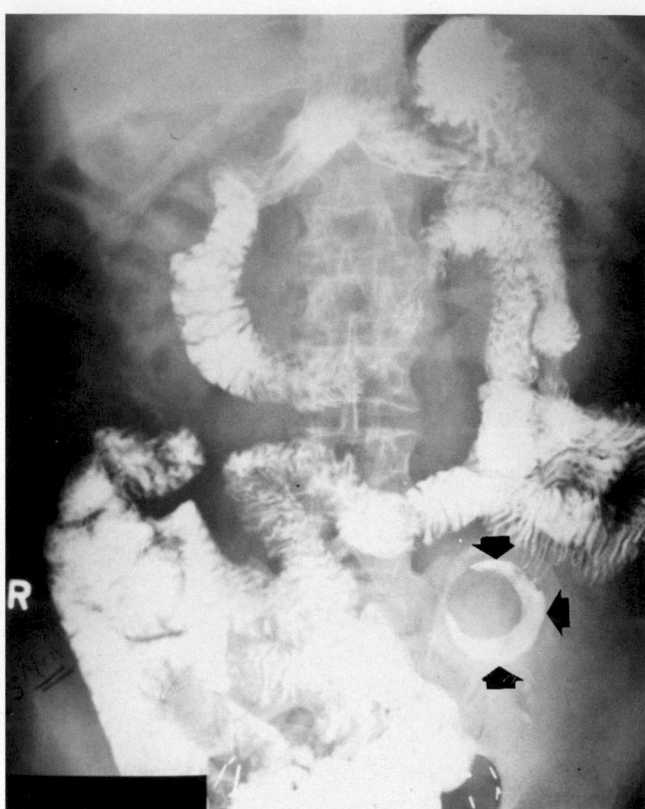

FIGURE 31-24. Small bowel barium study demonstrates a halo of extravasated contrast material (*arrows*) at the site of the implantable ring. It is because of this complication that the implantable ring and balloon plug are no longer considered appropriate for patients with a sigmoid colostomy.

incision is then closed, and the colostomy matured in the usual manner. Beginning approximately 1 week after the operation, the patient begins to use the plug.

Results

A multicenter study was undertaken to evaluate the safety and efficacy of the device.[189] Seventy-four patients underwent insertion of the ring.[189] Three were removed because of encapsulation of the ring. This is a complication common to all medical-grade implantable silicon and appears to be an insoluble dilemma. Two patients had the rings removed because of bowel necrosis or fistulization (Figure 31-24). Many individuals elected not to use the plug, preferring instead to employ a conventional appliance or irrigation.

Comment

As with the magnetic ring colostomy device, the implantable ring and balloon plug are no longer available because of the complications of erosion and necrosis of the stoma or bowel.

Colostomy Irrigation

Colostomy irrigation is a method of bowel control offered to selected patients with sigmoid or descending colon colostomies (see also the following chapter). Success depends on personal interest, bowel habits before surgery, manual dexterity, available toilet facilities, and lifestyle. Gawron suggests the following selection criteria for colostomy irrigation[81]:

- Permanent descending or sigmoid colostomy
- Physically and mentally capable of performing self-care

- Motivated to learn the procedure and adhere to a schedule
- No prior history of IBD, radiation therapy (to the abdomen or pelvis), or other major intestinal resection
- A history of regular bowel pattern or constipation
- Availability of bathroom facilities, including running water

Irrigation techniques are often taught on the fifth or sixth postoperative day, and for some individuals, a few months following the operation. Again, because of cost-containment and the possibility of delaying discharge, some patients may require instruction a few weeks later.

Most individuals tend to return to the bowel habits they had prior to operation, usually within 6 to 12 weeks after surgery. In other words, if one defecated every morning after breakfast, the colostomy will probably function on that schedule. Under these circumstances, irrigating may be unnecessary, and such patients can frequently avoid an appliance for the rest of the day or merely use a small dressing. A closed-ended "security pouch" can also be employed.

Conversely, if a patient had irregular bowel function preoperatively, the colostomy will probably act irregularly postoperatively. Such a person may be more content by irrigating. However, under no circumstances should one insist that the stoma be irrigated. It may be advisable to learn the technique, but the decision whether to actually use irrigation should be personal.

Method

A nipple, cone, or catheter is inserted into the stoma. The cone tip is now being used more frequently for colostomy irrigation than the catheter, not only because there is less risk of perforating the bowel but also because it provides a dam to prevent backflow. If a catheter is selected, it should be inserted no farther than 3 in. A rubber nipple with a hole enlarged to accommodate the catheter tip can act as a flange and temporary dam while fluid is running in. Several companies manufacture irrigation kits (Figure 31-25).

The colon does not need to be washed out; the bowel is merely stimulated with the irrigant to produce evacuation. The bottom of the bag for irrigation is usually placed at shoulder height when the patient is seated. However, the height of the bag should be adjusted to permit a steady flow into the stoma.[71] An alternative technique has been suggested by Schwemmle and coworkers; a specially constructed basin is used at stoma level when the patient is standing.[215] Obviously, this requires a unique plumbing arrangement in the patient's bathroom.

Tepid water (750 to 1,000 mL) is slowly instilled over a 5- to 10-minute period. After waiting approximately 1 minute, the patient removes the cone, and the water and stool are permitted to pass through the irrigation sleeve into the toilet bowl. Most of the returns are usually collected within 15 minutes. The collecting sleeve can then be closed while one tends to other activities. After about 45 minutes, the irrigant usually will have been expelled. With time, the patient may require irrigations only every 48 hours or even every 72 hours. Some, however, may never be able to irrigate satisfactorily and may require a pouch all of the time. Under these circumstances, it is difficult to justify the time and effort expended to perform this task.

Results

Meyerhoff and colleagues performed a randomized study, comparing the effects of irrigating with different volumes: 250, 500, and 1,000 mL.[159] A double-isotope technique was

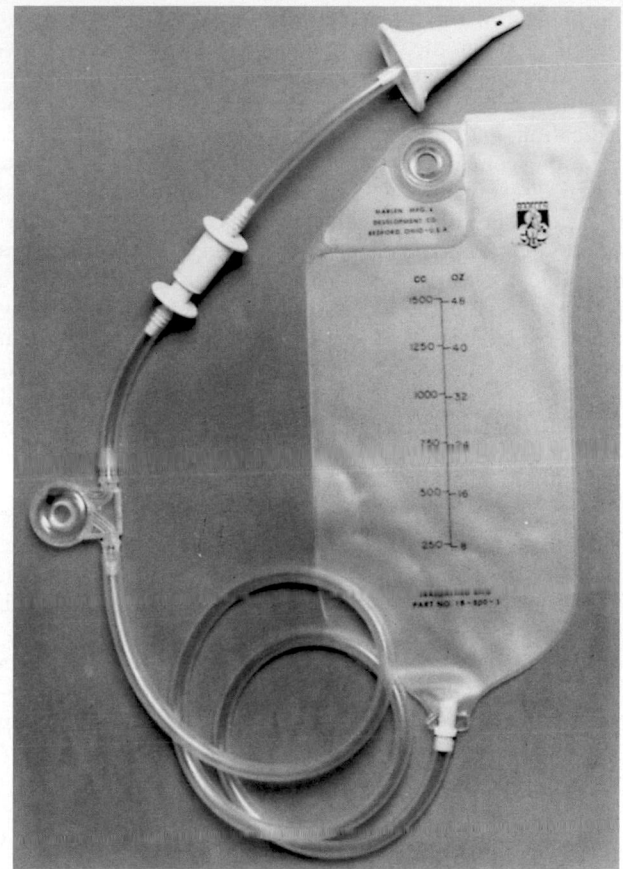

FIGURE 31-25. Colostomy irrigating system. This unit has a soft-tipped cone. (Courtesy of Marlen Manufacturing and Development Co., Bedford, OH.)

developed to evaluate colonic emptying of irrigation fluid and feces. This was accomplished through radioactive labeling of the fecal contents by the ingestion of 10 MBq ^{69}Cr-EDTA 24 hours before scintigraphic investigation. The authors discovered that the general recommendation of 1,000 mL is not optimal for all patients. In many instances, a volume of 500 mL was preferred because of reduced inflow time, complete colonic emptying of more consistent fecal contents, and minimal retention of irrigant. It appears, therefore, that one should experiment with different irrigation volumes in order to determine the most efficacious program for the individual.

Watt categorized those patients who probably are not candidates for controlling bowel elimination by irrigation as follows: those with irritable bowel syndrome, individuals who underwent irradiation therapy and sustained radiation enteritis, and the terminally ill. Stomal management problems such as hernia and stenosis, poor eyesight, impaired dexterity, fear of the irrigation procedure, and resentment of the time necessary militate against irrigating.[260]

Terranova and colleagues evaluated irrigation and compared the technique with natural evacuation in 340 patients.[239] They concluded that because of the feeling of security gained by relative continence, cleanliness, and the avoidance of an appliance, the vast majority of patients preferred irrigating. Williams and Johnston performed a prospective randomized study using colostomy irrigation and natural evacuation in 30 selected patients.[266]

The mean time spent managing the stoma was 45 minutes per day in the spontaneous group versus 53 minutes when irrigation was performed. Because of reduction of odor and flatus, the lack of requirement for medication, and the ability of many to avoid an appliance, irrigation seemed to offer an improved lifestyle. In a questionnaire response of 223 patients from the Mayo Clinic, 60% were "continent" with irrigation, 22% were "incontinent" with irrigation, and 18% had discontinued the technique for various reasons.[119] Doran and Hardcastle performed a controlled trial of colostomy management by natural evacuation, by irrigation, and by means of a foam enema.[61] By evaluating 20 patients who used each technique for 2 months, the authors concluded that almost all felt that irrigation or the foam enema improved their quality of life. Furthermore, they opted to continue with irrigation on completion of the study.

The St. Mark's Hospital group attempted to shorten the time it takes to complete a satisfactory irrigation through the use of glyceryl trinitrate solution.[175] They demonstrated that this agent, through the induction of gastrointestinal smooth muscle relaxation, accelerates stool expulsion. In a study involving 15 colostomy patients, each with more than 3 years of experience with irrigation, a significant reduction in colostomy irrigating time was noted when compared with tap water. However, there was a very high incidence of cramping and headaches with the glyceryl trinitrate solution.

Venturini and colleagues evaluated colostomy irrigation in the elderly, noting that age is no restriction on the ability to achieve successful irrigation and to improve the quality of life.[254]

▶ TRANSVERSE COLOSTOMY

The history of colostomy can be found in Chapters 23 and 24. The first documented transverse colon stoma was performed by Fine in 1797 in Geneva.[69] He successfully decompressed an obstruction from carcinoma of the rectum by drawing out a loop of bowel and securing the mesentery to the skin. Maydl (1888) was the first to suggest an external apparatus to accomplish stomal support for minimizing retraction and for facilitating spur formation.[152] However, it was not until 1951 that Patey advised that a transverse colostomy should be opened and matured at the time of the initial procedure.[179]

Numerous alternatives have been offered to accomplish adequate diversion, such as a deep retention suture with retained polyethylene sleeve, the application of a skin bridge, suturing of the fascia between the leaves of the mesentery, and various support devices (goose quill, harelip pin, rods,

KARL MAYDL (1853–1903)

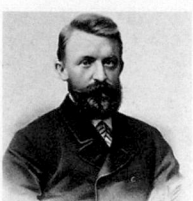

Karl Maydl was born March 10, 1853, in Rokitnic, Czechoslovakia and entered medical school in Prague. He undertook his doctoral thesis in 1876 and began his surgical residency under the direction of Heine. Following a teaching position at Innsbruck and Vienna, he attended the Military Medical School in Belgrade, and in 1886 became a surgical professor and chief of the surgical unit of the General Ambulance in Vienna. In 1891, Maydl became head of surgery at the University of Prague where he had great impact on Czechoslovakian surgery. The so-called Maydl technique concerned visceral ectopy, and his artificial anus method was a well-recognized and important achievement. He is the individual who perfected the concept of a loop colostomy, accomplished initially through the use of gauze passed through the mesocolon, but he also suggested that a rod may be created using rubber (vulcanite) or a goose feather. He was also one of the first to perform a laminectomy and to remove a tumor of the central nervous system. Karl Maydl died August 8, 1903, in Dobřichovice, Czechoslovakia. (Biography courtesy of Oliver Pfaar, MD.)

DAVID HOWARD PATEY (1899–1977)

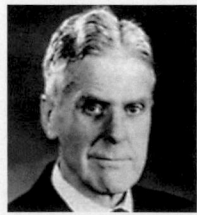

David Patey was born in Monmouthshire, Wales, the eldest of three children. In 1916, he entered Middlesex Hospital Medical School for his preclinical and clinical work, an institution with which he maintained affiliation for the remainder of his life. Following interruption for military service during World War I, he returned to Middlesex and won the hospital's highest undergraduate award. He passed the final MB at London University in 1923 with the gold medal and with honors in surgery and in obstetrics and gynecology. In 1930, after a period as a research fellow in the department of anatomy, Patey was appointed to the staff of the Middlesex Hospital. That same year he won the Jacksonian Prize of the Royal College of Surgeons and was Streatfield Scholar of the Royal College of Physicians. The following year he was named Hunterian Professor, receiving the honor again in 1964. Patey was recognized for his work and publications primarily on salivary gland tumors, breast cancer, and, interestingly, pilonidal sinus. Perhaps his most important contribution was founding the Surgical Research Society of Great Britain, for which he later became president. A true scholar with a fluent knowledge of Russian and French, Patey was recognized for his unshakable integrity, unassuming modesty, and clear thinking. He died in his 78th year. (Photograph courtesy of Professor Michael Hobsley, David Patey Professor, Department of Surgery, University College and Middlesex School of Medicine, London, United Kingdom.)

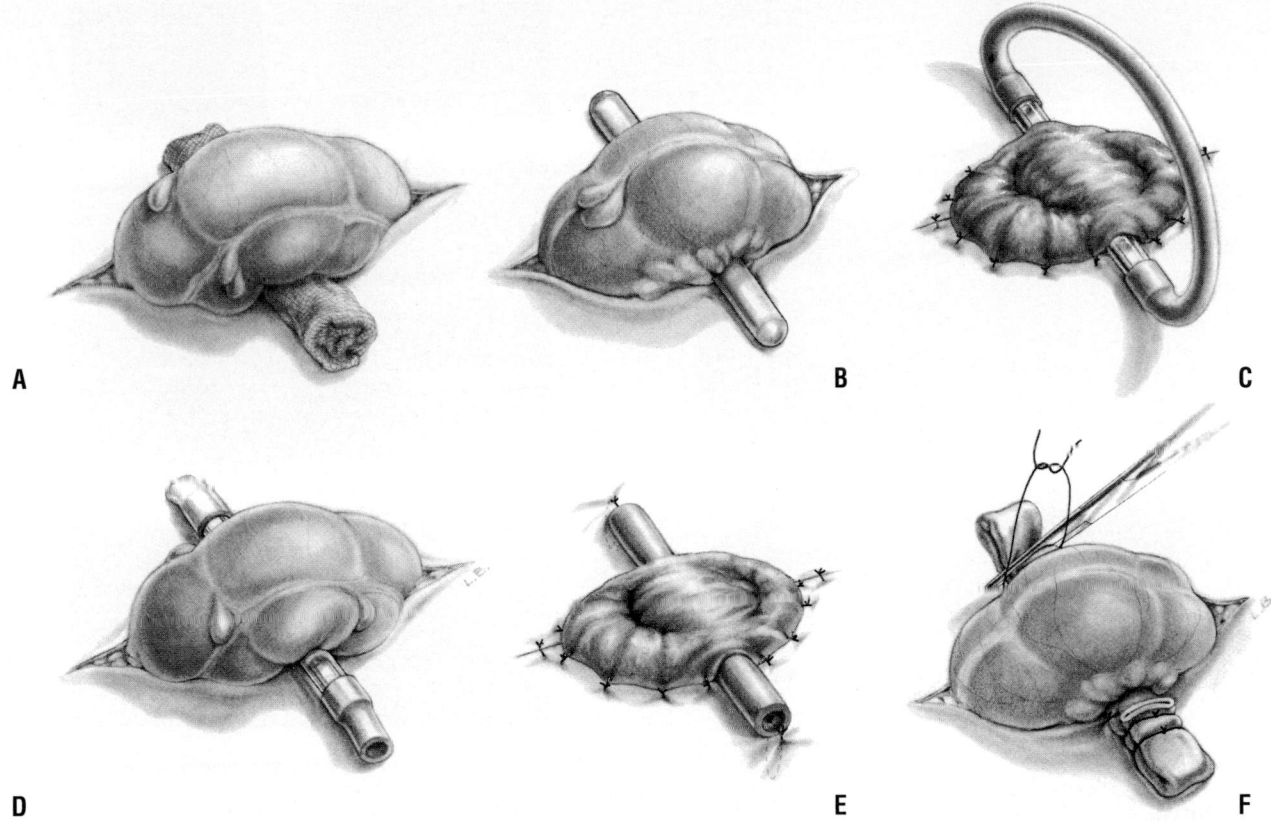

FIGURE 31-26. Alternatives for securing the loop of colon. **A:** Rolled gauze. **B:** Glass rod. **C:** Glass rod with rubber loop. **D:** Glass rod with rubber sleeves. **E:** Rubber tubing. **F:** Folded tubing or drain. (From Corman JM, Odenheimer DB. Securing the loop—historic review of the methods used for creating a loop colostomy. *Dis Colon Rectum.* 1991;34(11):1014–1021.)

tubes, drains, and catheters) from the ingenious to the absurd (Figure 31-26).[14,25,34,71,88,120,137,202,256] One may elect to simply use a no. 14 French red rubber catheter to support the spur of the loop, and sew a no. 24 French catheter onto each end. Any tubing or drain has the advantage of flexibility, thereby permitting relative ease in changing the appliance.

Alternatively, one may employ a commercially available system such as that made by Hollister (Figure 31-27) or by ConvaTec (Figure 31-28).[52] For further reading on the history of transverse colostomy, the reader is referred to Corman and Odenheimer's review of the evolution of methods used for creating a loop colostomy.[51]

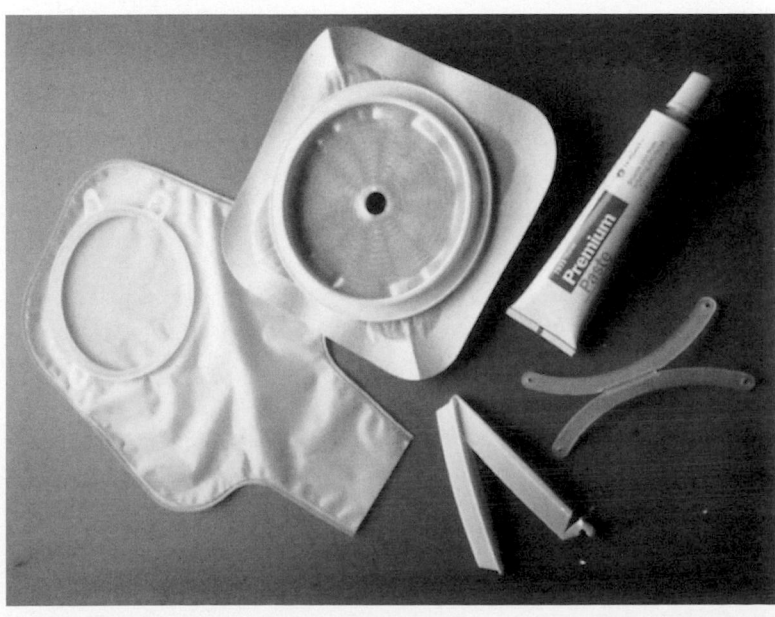

FIGURE 31-27. Two-piece loop ostomy system with bridge. (Courtesy of Hollister, Inc., Libertyville, IL.)

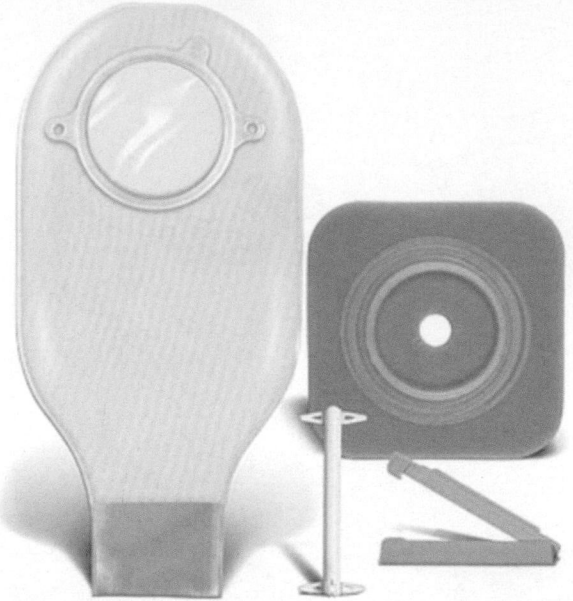

FIGURE 31-28. Gentle Touch loop ostomy system. (Courtesy of ConvaTec, Skillman, NJ.)

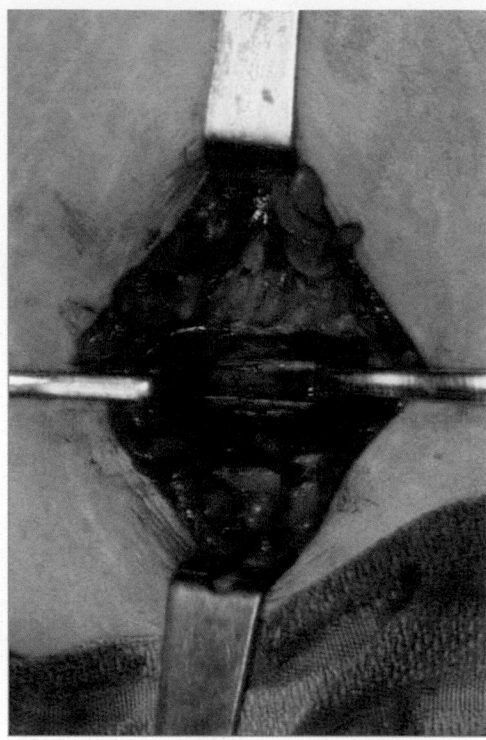

FIGURE 31-29. Creation of a transverse colostomy. The rectus muscle is split.

Indications

Transverse colostomy is a procedure employed on a temporary basis for a number of indications, especially by general surgeons: obstructing or perforating lesions of the left colon, trauma, anastomotic leak, congenital anomalies, fecal incontinence, and to protect the anastomosis.

Technique

Loop Colostomy

If a transverse colostomy is undertaken in an emergency situation, it should be accompanied by a full exploratory laparotomy, identifying the nature of the pathology. However, one is generally loathe even to perform a transverse colostomy with the expectation that it will be permanent for several reasons. First, if it is maintained for a sufficient time, it will inevitably prolapse. Because of the mobility of the transverse colon, it is the efferent limb that does this, assuming that the procedure was a loop right transverse colostomy. By placing the opening in the left transverse colon, the splenic flexure tethers the bowel and limits the risk of this complication, but then one must be deal with the possibility of prolapse of the afferent limb. Still, the surgeon may limit the concern for pouch leakage, a real problem with transverse colostomies when an afferent limb prolapse occurs. With efferent limb prolapse, the proximal limb retracts and leakage ensues. Another reason for performing the colostomy in the distal transverse colon is that the stool is theoretically somewhat more formed than it would be in a more proximal location. But transverse colostomies have other disadvantages—the odor of the stool and the looseness. And as implied, appliance management is cumbersome. It is for these reasons that colon and rectal surgeons have virtually abandoned transverse colostomy for temporary diversion in favor of loop ileostomy (see later).

As with sigmoid colostomy and ileostomy, the transverse colostomy should be brought through the split rectus muscle (Figure 31-29). The omentum is freed from the colon for a sufficient distance to permit exteriorization without tension. A tape or Penrose drain is passed through the leaves of the mesentery and the bowel delivered through the abdominal wound. A rod or bridge is passed through the same plane as the drain (Figures 31-26, 31-30, and 31-31).[216] The colostomy is then "matured" by opening it longitudinally and suturing the bowel edge to the skin (Figure 31-32). An appliance is

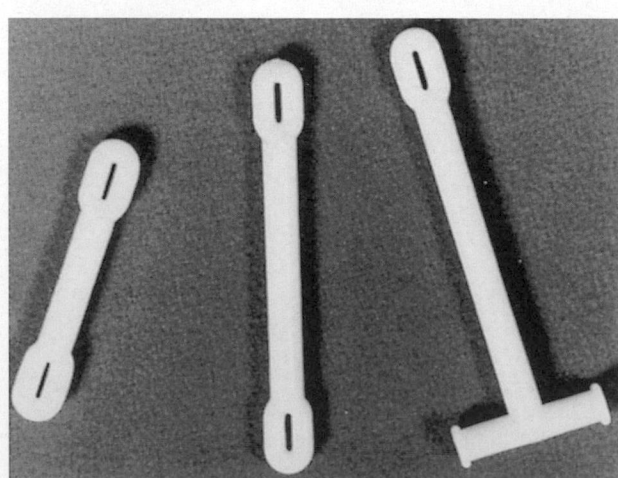

FIGURE 31-30. Marlen plastic loop ostomy rods. (Courtesy of Marlen Manufacturing and Development Co., Bedford, OH.)

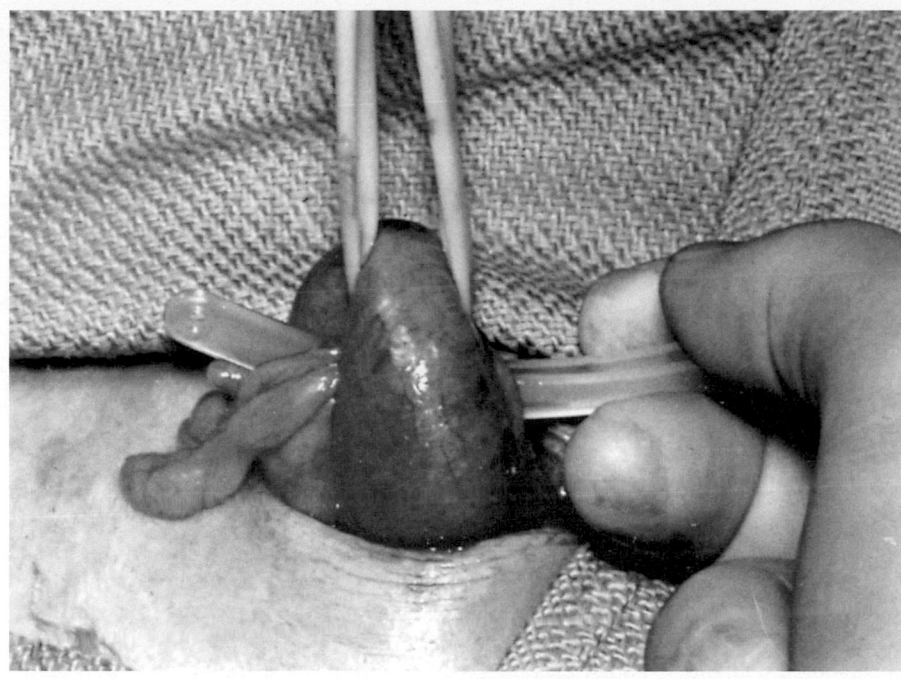

FIGURE 31-31. Creation of a transverse colostomy. A Hollister bridge is passed through the mesentery. Traction on the Penrose drain delivers the bowel.

then used (Figure 31-33). A number of authors have expressed concern about the difficulty in managing an appliance with a rod in place. Some suggest the interposition of a tongue shaped skin flap, whereas others offer a subcutaneous modification of a bridging approach (Figure 31-34).[14,22]

Adequacy of Diversion

A properly constructed loop transverse colostomy should be fully diverting, relatively easy to manage, and not unduly offensive (Figure 31-35). Stool does not have eyes. It cannot enter the bag, look around, and disappear into the distal limb. There is no such event as the fecal jumping distance.

Conversely, if the proximal limb retracts, stool may flow into the distal bowel.

The bridge or rod can be removed as soon as sufficient edema is present to maintain exteriorization of the colon. It is not necessary to leave the rod or tube in place for an arbitrary 1 week, as has been sometimes advised, because very often the rod itself will cause an element of obstruction that impedes the patient's recovery. Conversely, if the colostomy seems to be functioning well with the rod in place, and very little edema is evident, the bridge may be maintained for a longer period.

Rombeau and colleagues performed a barium swallow in 25 patients following loop transverse colostomy.[203]

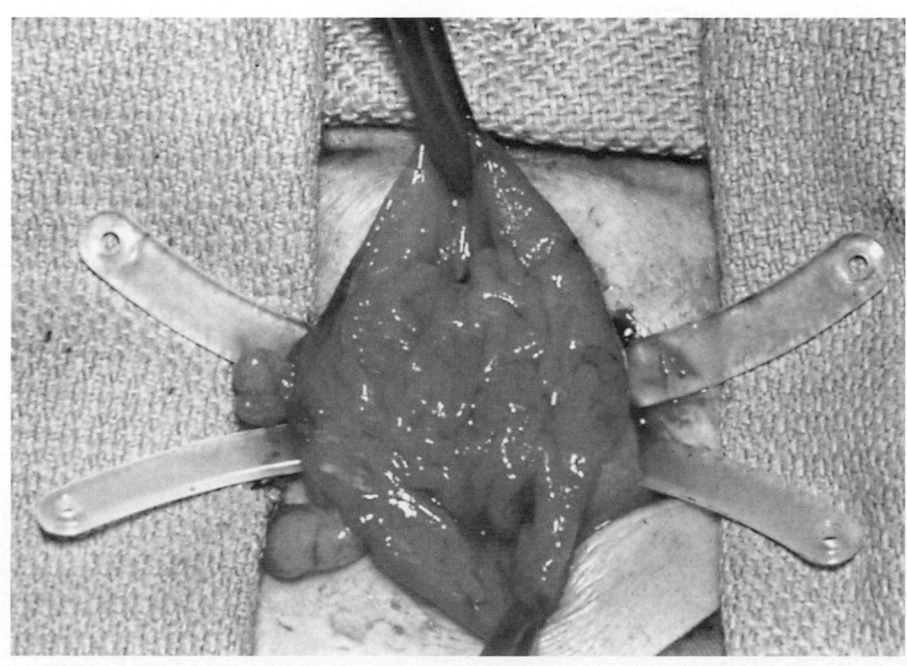

FIGURE 31-32. Creation of a transverse colostomy. Colostomy is matured.

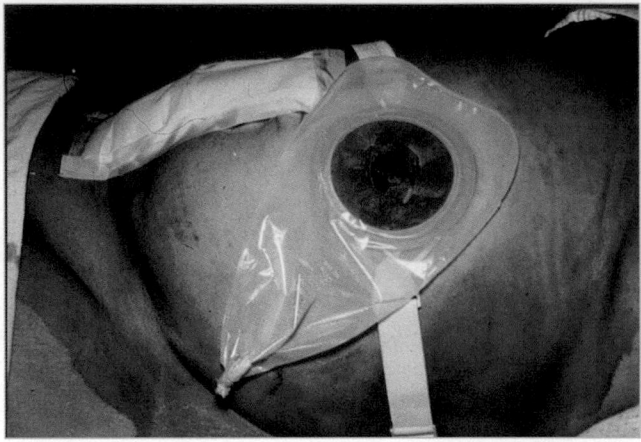

FIGURE 31-33. Creation of a transverse colostomy. Appliance is secured.

Follow-up films were obtained up to 4 days later, and barium was not visible in the distal colon in any of the patients. This same study performed *4 weeks* following diverting colostomy failed to show barium in the distal colon segment. Others attest to the adequacy of diversion if a loop colostomy is properly constructed.[168] However, although intra-abdominal or skin-level colostomies without a bridge, rod, drain, or tube may succeed in venting the colon adequately, they are not truly diverting.[65,233]

Fontes and colleagues identified three factors that are usually responsible for the failure of loop colostomies to be fully diverting[73]:

• Retraction
• Reduction of a prolapsed loop colostomy (invariably associated with retraction)
• Improper technique

Divided Colostomy

The theoretical concern about inadequate diversion can be addressed by "stapling" the distal end[169,208] or by dividing the colon, creating an end-transverse colostomy, and performing a side-to-side colon anastomosis of the distal segment.[139] This last method, an alternative to the concept of a "double-barreled" stoma, is time consuming to create and may require a laparotomy to close.

The so-called end-loop colostomy is another option. The proximal limb and the antimesenteric corner of the distal limb are drawn through the abdominal wall following stapled division of the bowel.[190,220,250] In an obese patient, it is sometimes impossible to deliver the transverse colon out as a loop. Accordingly, the bowel is divided and the distal end oversewn. The colostomy is then created using the end of the transverse colon, maturing it in a similar manner to that

A   **B**

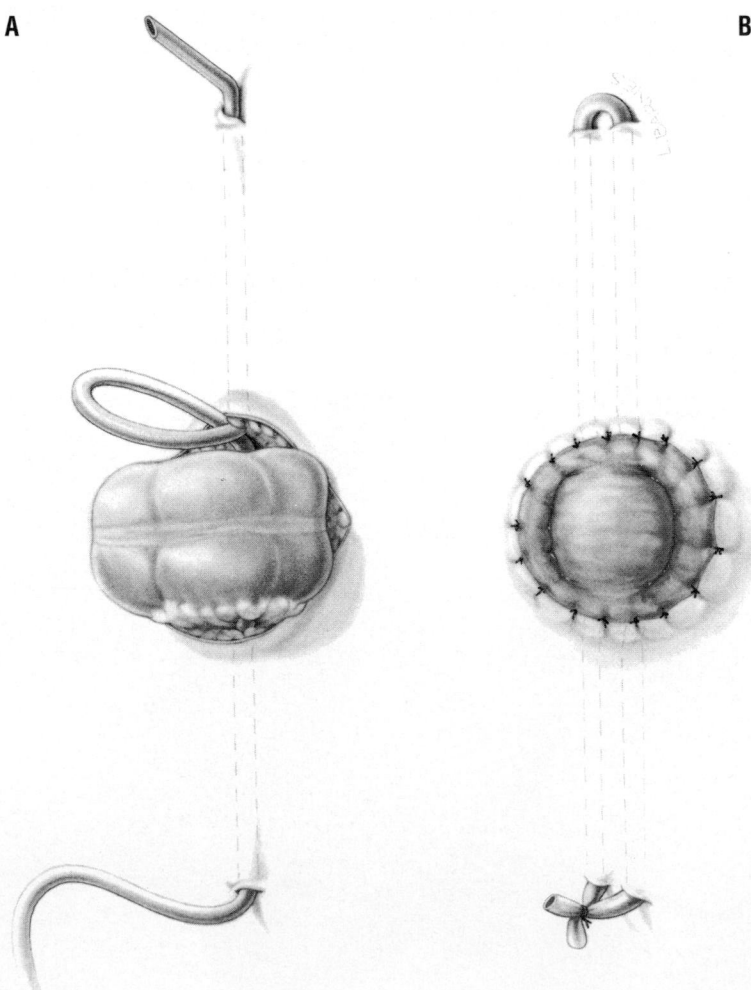

FIGURE 31-34. Technique of colostomy bridging by means of a plastic tubing and trocar. **A:** The catheter is secured quite laterally. **B:** The stoma is matured in the usual way. (Adapted from Bergren CT, Laws HL. Modified technique of colostomy bridging. *Surg Gynecol Obstet.* 1990;170(5):453–454.)

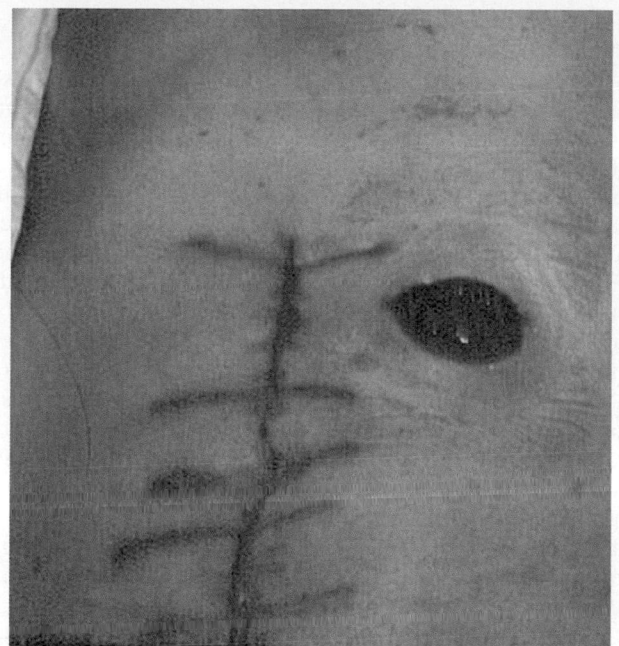

FIGURE 31-35. Loop transverse colostomy. The patient is shown 1 month following perforated diverticulitis with a well-functioning, fully diverting, left-sided stoma.

of a conventional sigmoid colostomy (Figure 31-36). Another alternative in an obese individual is to perform a loop ileostomy (see later).

Results of Loop Colostomy Construction

Numerous modifications have been proposed to simplify the creation of a loop colostomy stoma, to facilitate appliance management, and to expedite closure with a decreased morbidity.[14,34,65,108,139,172,202,203,208,233] My associates and I reviewed our experience with complications of colostomy construction and closure.[163] In 162 patients who underwent a loop colostomy, 12 (7.4%) developed a prolapse,

6 (3.7%) were noted to have retracted stomas, and 4 (2.5%) had abscesses. In the series, almost 14% developed a complication related to the colostomy construction alone. This does not, of course, take into consideration the morbidity associated with closure of a colostomy (see Colostomy Closure section).

Embarking upon a transverse colostomy cannot be considered a whimsical undertaking. As with loop ileostomy to "protect" a distal anastomosis, one must be able to justify the indications for this procedure and to ensure that it is not being performed because it makes the surgeon "feel better." Abrams and colleagues reported an overall complication rate of 41% in 248 patients who underwent a colostomy.[4] A hospital death rate of 24% was also noted. However, many of the patients had other serious illnesses, so that one cannot blame the colostomy exclusively for the high rates of morbidity and mortality. Wara and coworkers reviewed 250 patients who underwent transverse colostomy for fecal diversion, with a morbidity rate of 28%.[258] The two most important factors affecting the morbidity were emergency procedures and colostomies in infants. The overall incidence of specific colostomy complications was 26% in adults and 50% in children. Excluding infection, the most common complication was prolapse, followed by retraction, peristomal hernia, and stomal necrosis. Miles and Greene noted a complication rate related to stomal construction of 11% in almost 200 patients, and Smit and Walt reported almost a 10% incidence of complications related to creation of the stoma.[161,223]

The methods for preventing complications of transverse colostomy are quite similar to that of sigmoid colostomy. The size of the opening must be adequate in order to avoid edema, stricture, and obstruction. As repeatedly emphasized, ideally, the appropriate site should be selected before the operation, but this is not always possible if the colostomy construction was unanticipated. If the colostomy is created with the bowel under tension, it is likely to retract or to necrose (Figure 31-37). But a more common complication is colostomy prolapse,

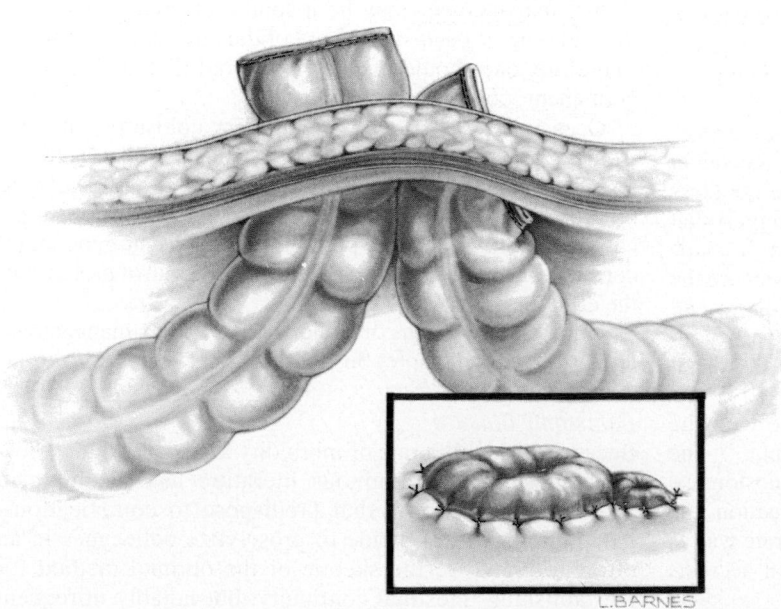

L.BARNES

FIGURE 31-36. Divided colostomy (end-loop colostomy). The functioning end is matured and the distal end de-emphasized.

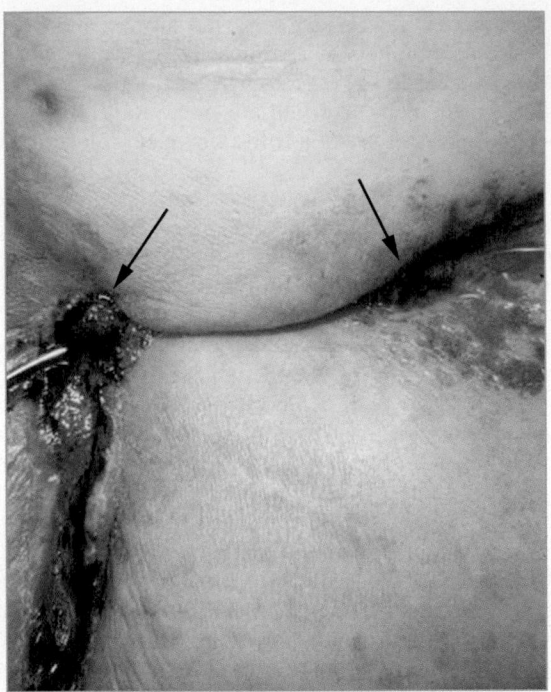

FIGURE 31-37. Retracted transverse loop colostomy, the result of mesenteric tension in an obese patient. Only two fecal fistulas remain (*arrows*). Metal probe can be seen in one granulating tract.

almost inevitably of the efferent (nonfunctioning) limb (see earlier discussion and Figure 31-38). If a colostomy is brought through the abdominal incision, it will always prolapse (Figure 31-39).

Chandler and Evans reported that 40% of adult loop colostomies involving the right side of the transverse colon prolapsed, a statistically significant increased incidence exceeding the rate for loop colostomies in more distal sites.[42] They further observed that the presence of obstruction at the time the colostomy was created seemed to predispose to the subsequent development of prolapse. Thirty-eight percent of all stomas originally made for obstruction prolapsed, compared with only 7% of those placed in unobstructed bowel. The proposed mechanism for this appeared to be a disproportion between the size of the fascial defect and the smaller diameter of the bowel following decompression.

Schofield and colleagues recommend rotating the colostomy 90 degrees so that the proximal end is in a dependent position.[214] The authors contend that not only is the stool less likely to flow into the distal loop, but also they suggest that this method avoids colostomy prolapse and hernia. It is difficult for me to understand why this would be so because the predisposing factors for these complications are still present. Furthermore, as previously mentioned, with a properly constructed standard loop colostomy, overflow into the distal limb should not occur.

Unti and colleagues reported their experience with the end-loop colostomy as performed on 135 patients.[250] The authors also included 70 ileocolostomies and 24 ileostomies, so it is impossible to state what the exact complication rate is with the colon alone. The overall complication rate was as follows: leakage (3.5%), retraction (3.5%), partial necrosis (2.6%), and peristomal sepsis (1.8%).

Quality of Life/Sexual Function (see later discussion)
Treatment of Loop Colostomy Prolapse

A number of methods have been devised to treat colostomy prolapse. Zinkin and Rosin modified the technique originally described by Mayo and have adapted it to an office procedure.[153,273] A smooth-backed button is placed on the abdominal wall, and a nonabsorbable suture is passed through the buttonhole, skin, fascia, and intestine. A finger in the lumen of the intestine helps to reduce the prolapse and to direct the entrance of the needle through the bowel. The result is to fix the reduced intestine firmly against the anterior abdominal wall, preventing further intussusception.

Krasna uses a purse-string suture to narrow the colostomy orifice, whereas Colmer and Foxx describe an external prolapse control device that consists of attaching the base of a Gellhorn pessary to the faceplate of a colostomy appliance.[49,133] The device is held in place by a colostomy bag belt. Because the "cork" is not completely obstructing, the stool passes around it, but the prolapse remains reduced.

Another option for treating prolapse is to circumcise the distal limb, divide the bowel, oversew it, and re-suture the end colostomy stoma (Figure 31-40). This can often be accomplished with a local anesthetic.

Opinion

Winkler and Volpe advise that loop transverse colostomy is a holdover from the past and that it is all too often permanent rather than temporary.[268] They suggest that all colostomies should be created as end stomas. Although their proposal emphasizes the magnitude of the problem, I prefer a loop stoma because of the relative ease of subsequent closure, but I hate loop transverse colostomy.

Fortunately, most patients who have undergone a transverse colostomy are inconvenienced for a relatively short period. When the colostomy is performed for terminal disease, however, many individuals live long enough to develop severe management problems with the stoma. This is particularly true when abdominal distention as a result of liver enlargement or ascites produces a parastomal hernia or an irreducible prolapse. In fact, the problems associated with stomal management may be a source of greater disability than all other aspects of the care of the terminally ill patient. Therefore, one should endeavor to avoid if at all possible a permanent loop transverse colostomy.

Occasionally, a so-called temporary colostomy may inevitably become permanent. This is usually because a distal anastomosis has failed to heal or the patient has developed other serious medical problems that preclude further surgical intervention. If such a problem arises, the surgeon might consider one of the methods described to control prolapse of the efferent limb.

Other issues such as diversion colitis and its management are discussed in Chapter 33.[97]

Colostomy Closure

Because of the high rate of morbidity associated with colostomy closure, a voluminous literature has accumulated addressing the factors that predispose to complications. Attempts have been made to proselytize colleagues in an effort to convince the skeptic of the optimal method for reestablishing intestinal continuity, but notably infrequent

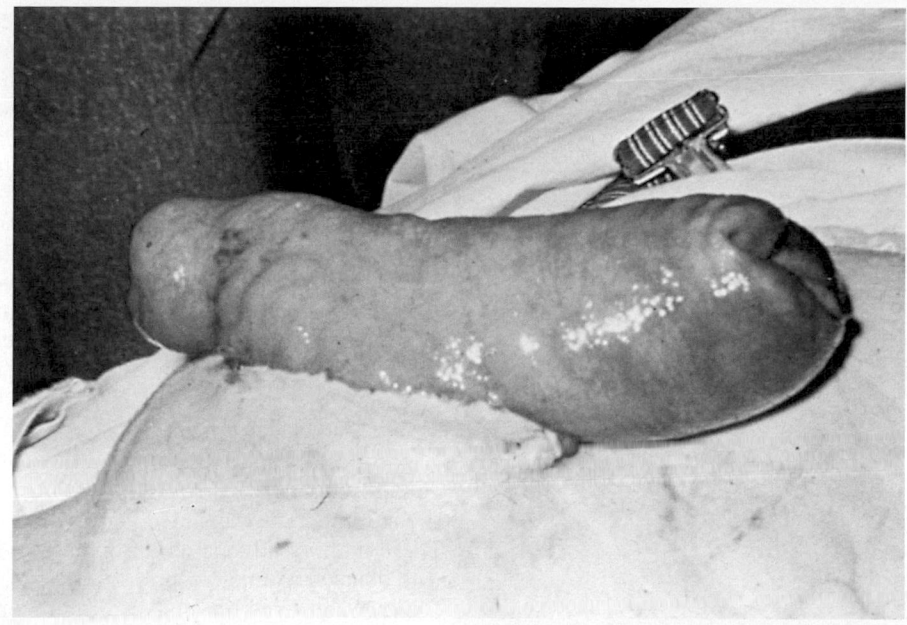

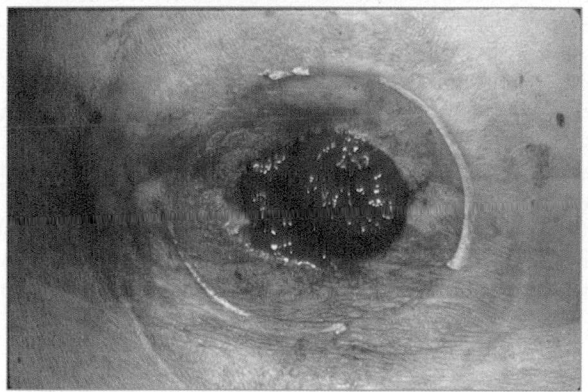

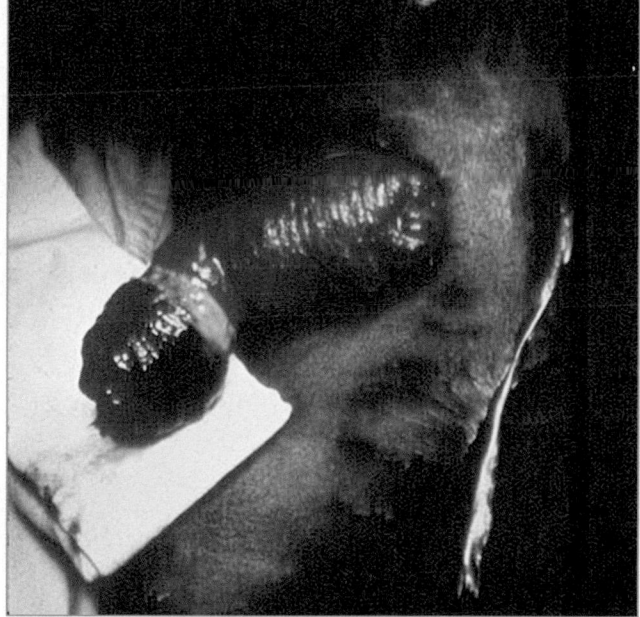

FIGURE 31-38. Loop transverse colostomy with prolapse **(A)**. Note retracted afferent limb with prolapsing distal limb **(B)**. Skin changes are indicative of leakage. Ischemia leading to gangrene of a prolapsed efferent limb **(C)**.

are controlled studies. Controversy still exists over the relative merits of intra-abdominal versus extra-abdominal closure, closure with resection versus closure without resection, and primary wound closure versus delayed.

Technique

The patient is placed on a full bowel preparation as if for colon resection. Irrigation of both limbs of the colostomy and of the rectum is performed the morning of surgery until the returns are clear. Antibiotics are administered in the operating room prior to initiating the surgery, that is, the same protocol employed for bowel resection.

The colostomy is circumcised by means of a diathermy cautery, leaving an attached cuff of skin (Figure 31-41A). No attempt is made to pack the lumen with sterile dressings or to suture the edges closed. Four Kocher clamps are placed on the skin around the colostomy, and four triple hooks (Lahey clamps) are placed on the surrounding skin

to act as retractors (Figure 31-41B). The Kocher clamps are held by the surgeon and serve as a handle while the assistant uses the hooks as retractors. The peritoneal cavity is entered, clamps are placed on the fascia, and the bowel is liberated (Figure 31-41C).

With the colostomy now separated from the abdominal wall, the skin and any remaining fibrous tissue are excised (Figure 31-42A). Closure of the anterior wall of the bowel is then effected in a transverse fashion with interrupted long-term absorbable sutures in the same manner that the anterior row of a colon anastomosis is completed (Figure 31-42B). Alternatively, if edema and fibrosis prevent safe closure, the bowel is resected and an anastomosis performed as with any colon resection. The fascia is then approximated with interrupted, heavy, long-term absorbable sutures (Figure 31-42C). An alternative, simpler approach is to effect closure by means of a stapling technique (Figure 31-43).

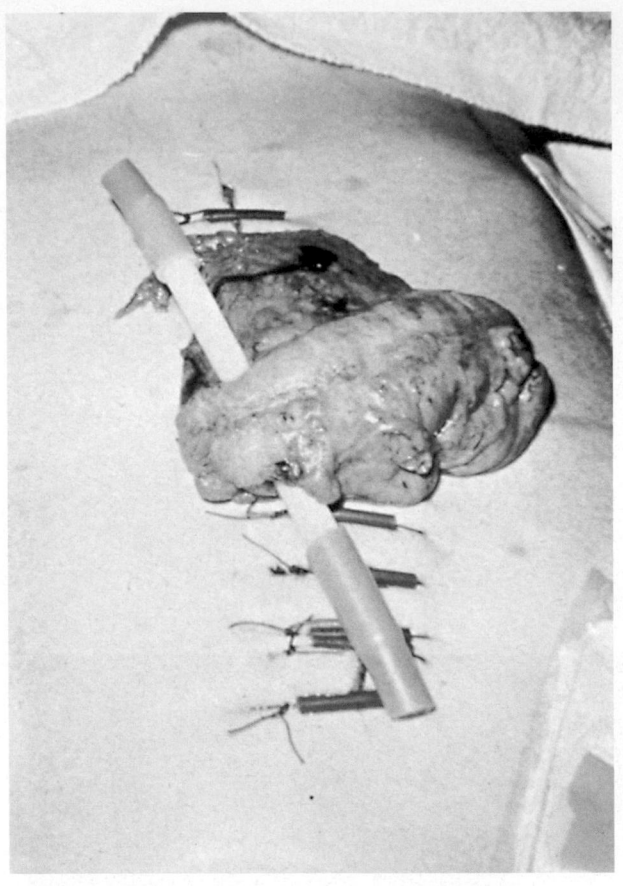

FIGURE 31-39. Prolapsed loop colostomy. This developed soon after the operation, a consequence of bringing the colon through the abdominal incision.

Because of the high risk of infection, the wound is left open for delayed primary closure. This is accomplished by placing skin sutures in loosely and securing them onto a tongue depressor (Figure 31-44A). The wound is packed either with iodoform gauze or a Betadine-soaked sponge and is secondarily closed 3 or 4 days later (Figure 31-44B). The incision is closed completely by pulling on the tongue depressor, and the assistant merely cuts each suture in turn while the surgeon ties it. With this technique, no anesthetic is required, and the tension produced by individually pulling and tying the sutures is avoided.

Postoperatively, the patient is maintained on intravenous fluids with advancement of the diet as tolerated. No nasogastric tube is advised.

Results

Yajko and colleagues reported a 28% incidence of complications associated with colostomy closure in 100 patients.[271] Wound infection was noted in 10% and fecal fistula in 4%. These authors advocated an open, two-layer anastomosis with delayed wound closure.

Beck and Conklin analyzed the records of 77 Vietnam War casualties who underwent loop colostomy closure.[21] The postoperative complication rate was 9% with simple loop closure as compared with 24% with resection and anastomosis. These authors felt that closure without resection was technically easier and associated with a lower morbidity than resection of the stoma with reanastomosis.

Wara and associates noted a morbidity rate of 57% (a leakage rate of 10%) and a mortality rate of 1.7% in 105 patients.[258] There was a significantly increased incidence of fecal fistula and incisional hernia when closure was performed as a single procedure subsequent to a definitive

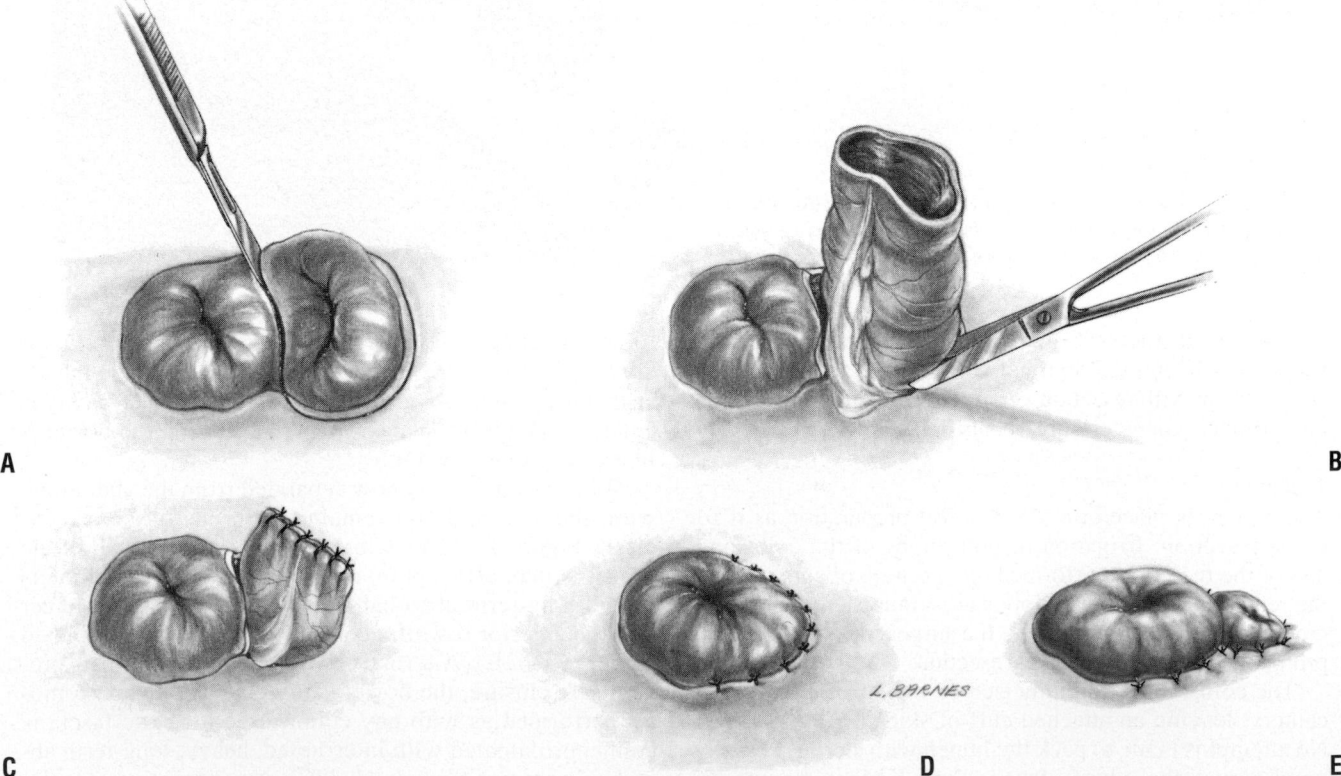

FIGURE 31-40. Surgical treatment of loop colostomy prolapse. **A:** The distal mucosal rim is circumcised. **B:** The bowel is divided. **C:** The distal bowel is oversewn or stapled. **D:** Final maturation as an end stoma. **E:** Alternatively, the distal end can be opened as previously described.

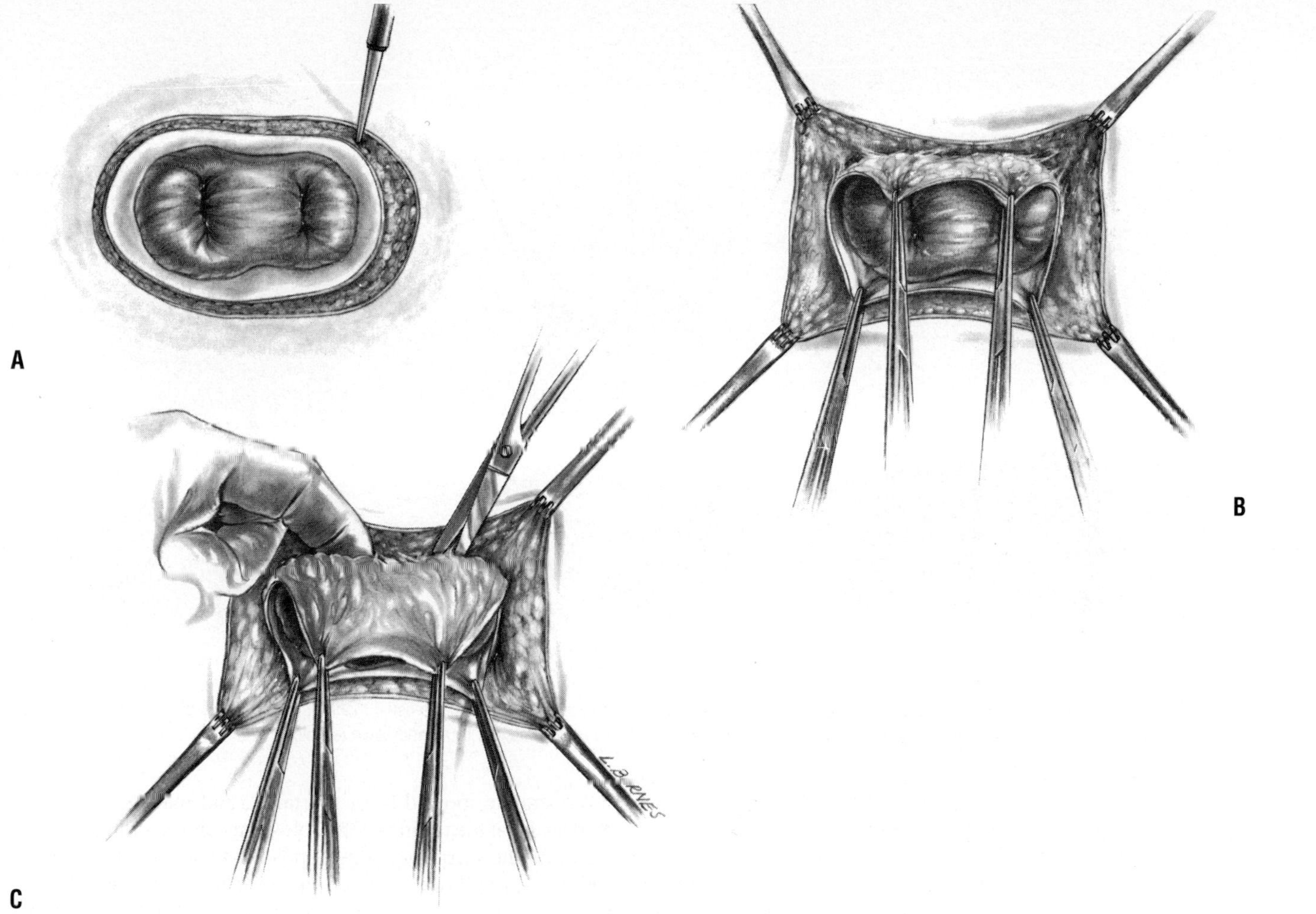

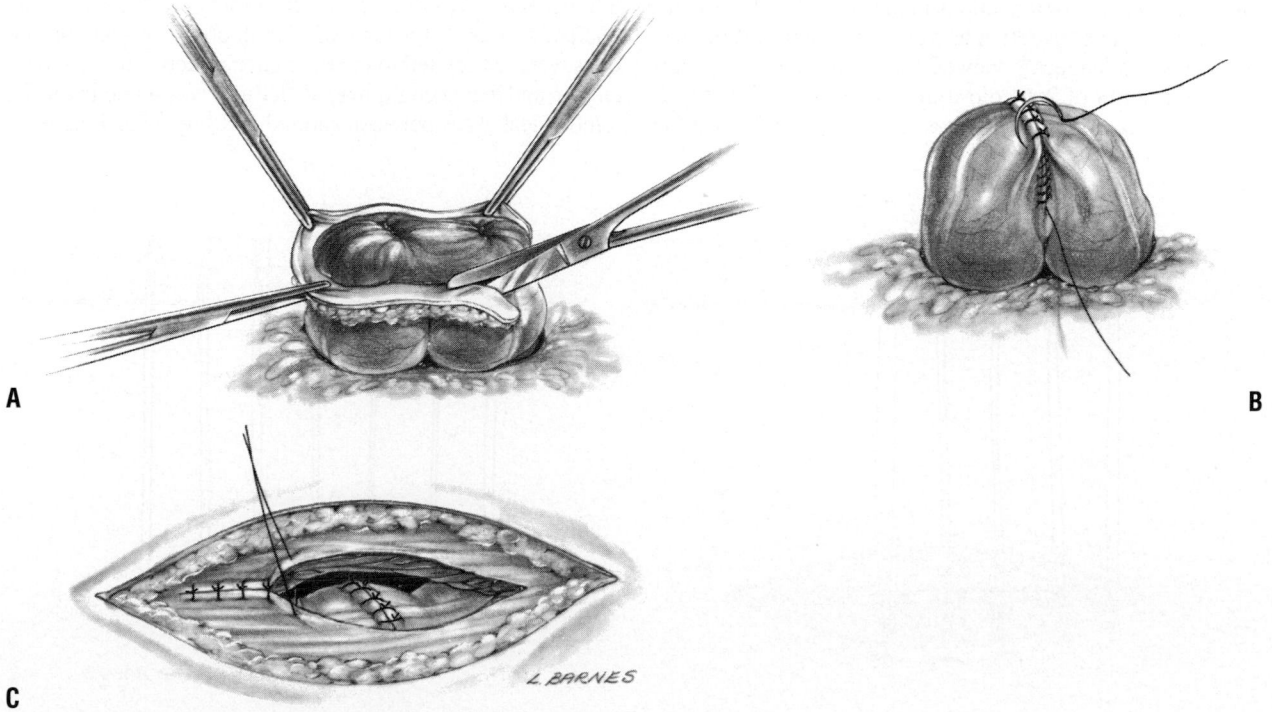

FIGURE 31-41. Technique of loop colostomy closure. **A:** The colostomy is circumcised. **B:** Kocher clamps on the skin around the stoma serve as a handle, and triple hooks are used as retractors. **C:** The peritoneal cavity is entered, and the colostomy is dissected from the abdominal incision.

FIGURE 31-42. Technique of loop colostomy closure. **A:** Excision of the skin and eschar. **B:** The anterior bowel wall is closed transversely. **C:** The fascia is closed.

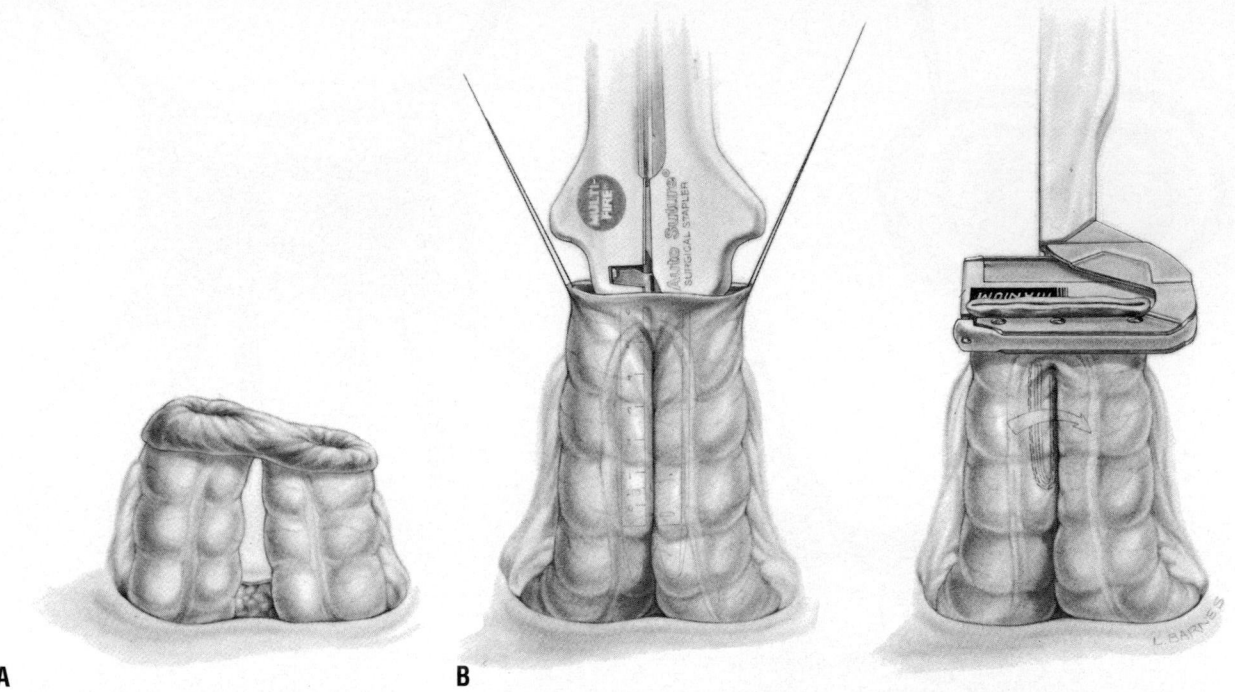

A   **B**   **C**

FIGURE 31-43. Closure of loop colostomy by stapling technique. **A:** The colostomy is circumcised in the usual manner. **B:** The GIA stapler effects a functional end-to-end anastomosis. **C:** Closure of the bowel is accomplished with the linear stapler as illustrated or by a hand-sewn technique.

resection. They believed that the difference might be explained by better accessibility when the colostomy was performed at the same time as the resection.

Smit and Walt reported a complication rate of 30% in 167 patients who underwent colostomy closure.[223] Wound infection was seen in more than 17%. These authors felt that the optimal period for closure was from 2 to 3 months after colostomy construction. They further noted that there was a higher incidence of complications in patients who did not undergo a full bowel preparation or who were not on antibiotics.

Todd and colleagues reviewed their experience in a retrospective fashion of 206 colostomy closures.[246] They found that the method employed did not significantly influence the postoperative morbidity or mortality, and that there was no evidence that the timing of the colostomy closure was a critical factor for the subsequent development of anastomotic complications. Varnell and Pemberton found that the time interval between colostomy creation and closure did not affect morbidity, nor did intraoperative wound management, the use of systemic antibiotics alone, and the location of the loop colostomy.[252] Their morbidity rate was 44%. Aston and Everett also felt that early closure of a loop colostomy could be undertaken relatively safely.[12] Pittman and Smith observed that complications were not related to the time interval between creation and closure and that no significant difference was found in the anastomotic leak rates between sutured and stapled techniques.[184]

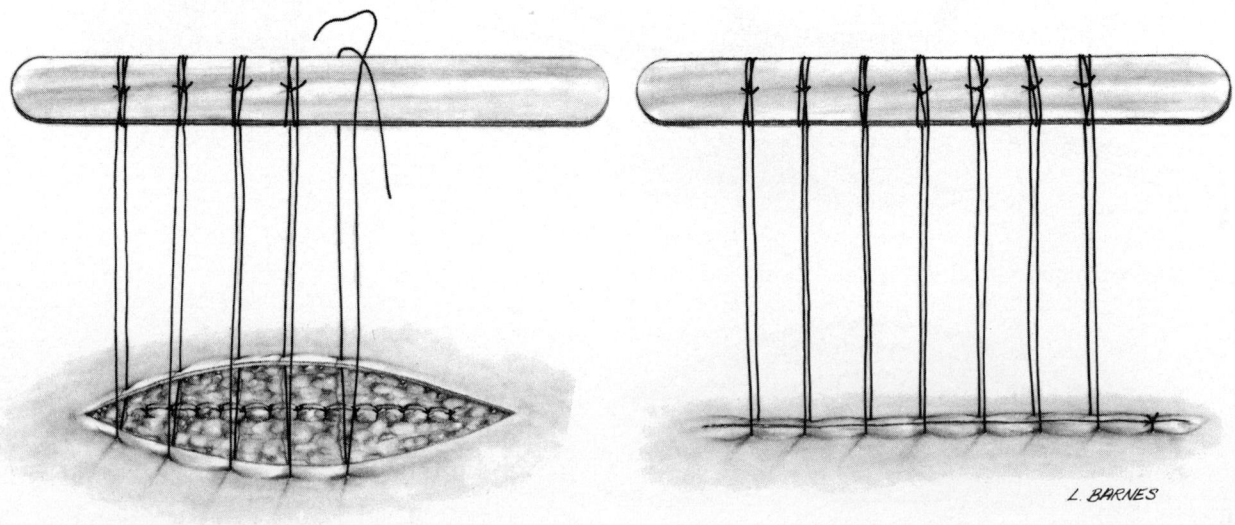

A   **B**

FIGURE 31-44. Delayed wound closure. **A:** Sutures are placed and taped onto a tongue depressor. **B:** The wound is pulled closed and the sutures tied.

TABLE 31-2 Interval between Colostomy and Closure

INTERVAL (MONTHS)	NUMBER OF PATIENTS	NUMBER WITH COMPLICATIONS	PERCENT WITH COMPLICATIONS
0–3	41	21	51.2
4–6	35	12	34.3
7–12	26	9	34.6
>12	16	3	18.8
Total	118	45	—

From Mirelman D, Corman ML, Veidenheimer MC, et al. Colostomies: indications and contraindications: Lahey Clinic experience, 1963–1974. *Dis Colon Rectum.* 1978;21(3):172–176.

Conversely, Freund and colleagues felt that the two major factors determining subsequent complications were timing and method of closure.[75] Simple closure was associated with fewer complications than resection, and colostomies closed sooner than 12 weeks after their construction had twice the incidence of complications than those which were closed after that time. Oluwole and associates also concur that colostomy closure 3 months following construction is preferred.[177] Other factors associated with a lower incidence of complications in their experience included mechanical and antibiotic bowel preparation, intraperitoneal closure, resection of the anastomosis, and delayed (secondary) skin closure. Rosen and Friedman, however, noted that the incidence of wound infection was not significantly improved by the use of systemic or nonabsorbable intestinal antibiotics.[204] Furthermore, intraperitoneal drainage alone or in combination with subcutaneous drainage resulted in the highest rate of wound infection in their experience.

Billings and colleagues suggest that the high rate of morbidity associated with colostomy closure may be attributable to an inadequate blood supply.[28] They recommend that consideration be given to performing weekly laser Doppler flowmetry of the stoma until an optimal blood flow is achieved.

Berne and associates performed a prospective randomized study of three different methods of wound closure: primary, primary with subcutaneous drainage, and delayed primary.[26] No statistically significant difference in frequency of wound infections was demonstrated (overall wound infection rate, 4.8%). Banerjee uses a purse-string closure of the skin that permits drainage of hematoma or exudate through the gap.[16]

Rickwood and coworkers reported a study of 100 consecutive colostomy closures in infants and children; they used a resection technique with intraperitoneal closure.[197] Wound infection was noted in 43 patients, a fecal fistula in 5, and other major complications in 8 instances. The overall morbidity, therefore, was in excess of 50%.

In addition to the studies already referred to, 11 selected reports from the literature on the results of colostomy closure revealed a mean morbidity rate of 24% (range, 14% to 38%).[10,30,60,78,105,109,162,164,187,210,262]

We reviewed our experience with colostomy closure at the Lahey Clinic from 1963 to 1974.[163] The results were most unsatisfactory, perhaps because much of the period covered during the study antedated contemporary techniques. The combined early and late morbidity was 49%, with wound infections found in about 25%. A fecal fistula occurred in 9.3%. Closure of the colostomy without resection was associated with the lowest incidence of complications (6.8%) when compared with other types of closure. Superficial subcutaneous drains did not prevent wound infections, and patients with intra-abdominal drains had an even higher incidence. Analysis of the intervals between creation and closure of the colostomies demonstrated that individuals whose stomas were closed within 3 months after creation had a morbidity rate of more than 50% (Table 31-2). This decreased to approximately 34% for closure after at least a 4-month interval.

Late complications occurred in 28 patients, with incisional hernia, suture sinus, and intestinal obstruction being the most frequently seen (Table 31-3). As previously mentioned, with a complication rate such has been reported in most series, particularly with respect to closure of the colostomy, the

TABLE 31-3 Late Complications of Colostomy Closure

COMPLICATION	NUMBER OF PATIENTS	PERCENT OF SERIES
Incisional hernia	19	16.4
Suture sinus	3	2.6
Intestinal obstruction	2	1.7
More than one of the above	4	3.7
Total	28	24.4

From Mirelman D, Corman ML, Veidenheimer MC, et al. Colostomies: indications and contraindications: Lahey Clinic experience, 1963–1974. *Dis Colon Rectum.* 1978;21(3):172–176.

surgeon should be circumspect in the initial selection of patients for a diversionary procedure.

One must recognize that the results of many published studies would not tolerate the scrupulous assessment of statistical analysis and that indeed the picture is not as discouraging as the literature often implies. Subjectively at least, most surgeons have noted a decreased incidence of complications in all aspects of bowel surgery, including that of colostomy closure. For example, Foster and colleagues compared the first and second 4-year periods of colostomy closure in their evaluation of 113 patients.[74] Improvement was noted in the rate of wound infection (24% vs. 51%) and in the frequency of anastomotic leak (10% vs. 30%).

Two reports demonstrate a remarkably low incidence of problems associated with colostomy closure. Salley and colleagues reported a complication rate of 7.8% in 166 patients operated on from 1974 to 1981.[209] The infection rate was extremely low—only 2.4%. The authors attributed their success to a vigorous mechanical bowel preparation and the use of luminal and parenteral antibiotics. With respect to operative technique, the bowel was sutured both by resection and by simple closure, and the wounds were closed by four different methods. Garnjobst and associates reviewed their experience of 125 consecutive colostomy closures, noting a complication rate of 5.6% in the early phase, and a later complication rate of 4% (primarily due to incisional hernia).[79] The authors credited their low rates of morbidity to simple closure rather than to resection of the bowel (no local complications in 63 patients), antibiotic wound irrigation, and primary wound closure.

Comment

If, after reading the aforementioned outlined review, the surgeon is not confused about the optimal means for avoiding complications following colostomy closure, one should be greatly surprised. If a thread of consistency can be extracted from the data, it is that early closure of the colostomy is associated with a higher rate of morbidity and that resection of the bowel, in the experience of most surgeons, is more hazardous than simple closure. Wound infection is by far the most common complication. Delayed wound closure should obviate that concern, however.

▶ CECOSTOMY

The procedure of cecostomy could be removed from our surgical armamentarium with very little consequence to the quality of health care delivery. In fact, because the operation is used for the wrong indications, it probably is responsible for adverse results more often than it ameliorates a condition. The procedure has been advocated to "protect" a left-sided anastomosis, in the treatment of large bowel obstruction, for cecal perforation, and in the management of cecal volvulus.[23,89,111,241,270] In my opinion, the only possible valid indications for performing cecostomy are cecal volvulus (see Chapter 28) and colonic ileus (Ogilvie's syndrome; see Chapter 20). But even with these conditions, the applicability is extremely limited.

A cecostomy is a decompressive procedure and, as such, produces essentially a venting of the bowel. *It does not divert the fecal stream.* Therefore, if a diversion is required, a loop ileostomy (see later) or transverse colostomy (see earlier) should be considered. In a study by Thomson and coworkers, 226 patients underwent restorative rectal resection with on-table lavage and tube cecostomy.[242] Clinical anastomotic

leak rates occurred in 25 patients (11.1%). The authors concluded that not only does tube cecostomy fail to protect an anastomosis, but also complications are common and may indeed be life threatening under the circumstances.

A loop ileostomy is an eminently satisfactory procedure and a preferable alternative not only for diversion, but also for permitting reasonable appliance management. Cecostomy virtually always commits the patient to continued hospitalization until such time as the opening is surgically closed. An exception to this is if a so-called tube cecostomy is employed (see Figure 28-59). Other problems may still develop, however. For example, the tube may obstruct, or the cecum may become detached from the abdominal wall, leading to an intra-abdominal abscess or even generalized peritonitis. Ultimately, the fistula may still require surgical closure.

With the limited indications mentioned, cecostomy should optimally be accomplished by the exteriorization technique. If it is to be performed as a "blind" procedure for acute cecal dilatation, a small incision is made in the right lower quadrant in a manner similar to the approach used for appendectomy. However, instead of the muscle being split, the external and internal oblique and transversus abdominis are divided. The peritoneum is exposed and carefully incised. The cecum will tend to pout into the open wound, but if it is so distended that it cannot be delivered through the incision, it can be decompressed by needle or trocar aspiration. The seromuscular surface of the cecum is sutured to the abdominal wall with interrupted long-term absorbable sutures (Figure 31-45). After the peritoneal cavity is walled off in this manner, the cecum is opened and the cut edge of the bowel is sutured to the full thickness of the skin in a manner similar to that used when one matures a conventional colostomy.

Even when this technique is applied properly, appliance management can be extremely cumbersome. The effluent is corrosive and liquid. But because the cecostomy does not truly divert, drainage may actually be quite minimal. It may consist mostly of gas, hence its primary benefit for decompressing an acutely dilated cecum. At least with the procedure mentioned, the cecum is unlikely to become detached or to retract into the peritoneal cavity, leading to a possibly life-threatening situation.

The paucity of recent literature on the subject is a testament to its lack of applicability and to its replacement by alternative diversionary procedures.

Continent Cecostomy

Kock and colleagues performed a continent cecostomy on 30 patients by isolating the cecum from the remainder of the colon and providing the distal end with an intussuscepted valve constructed from an isolated segment of ileum.[131] Eight were later given continent ileostomies, two were converted to conventional sigmoid colostomies, and one had continuity reestablished. The complication rate was 23%, with two-thirds of the patients requiring revision of the intussuscepted valve. When comparing the functional results of continent cecostomy with that of continent ileostomy, it becomes obvious that the latter is superior.

▶ ILEOSTOMY

An ileostomy is usually advised for IBD (ulcerative colitis or Crohn's disease). Other indications include familial polyposis, carcinomatosis, trauma, and congenital anomalies.

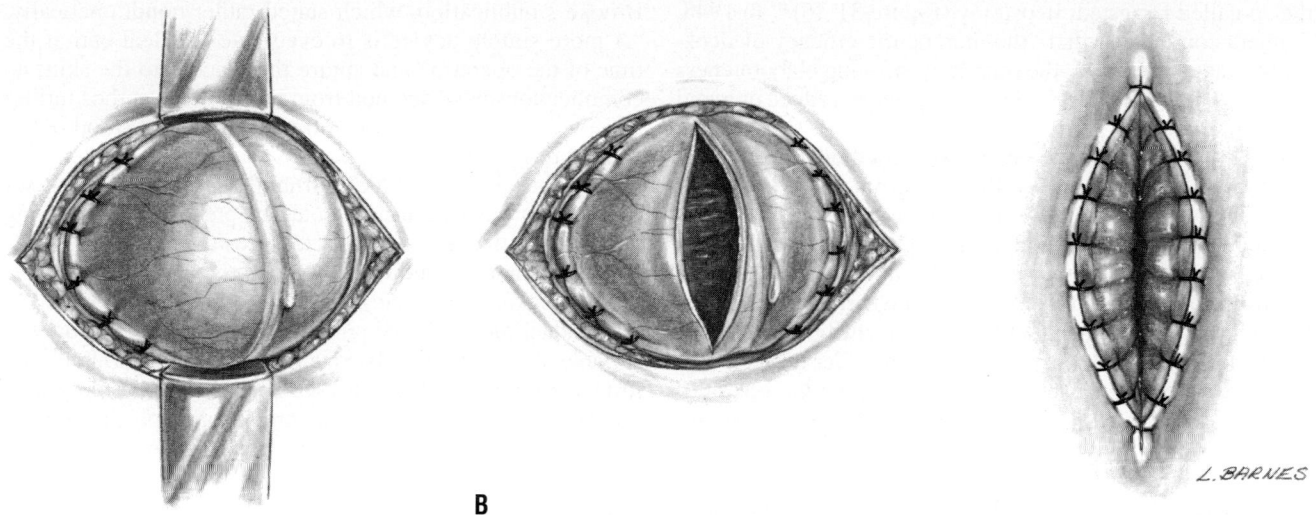

A **B** L.BARNES **C**

FIGURE 31-45. Technique of cecostomy. **A:** Obliteration of the peritoneal opening by suture of the bowel wall to the fascia. **B:** Opening of the cecum. **C:** Primary maturation to the skin.

Ideally, the patient should be well informed about the need for an ileostomy before the operation is required. It is usually of great benefit to acquaint the patient with someone of comparable age, gender, and socioeconomic status who has an ileostomy and is well adjusted to it, so that the individual can be assured of a normal lifestyle. Unfortunately, some patients do not receive adequate preoperative counseling, either because the physician fails to mention the possibility of an ileostomy during the course of treatment of the relevant condition or because the patient requires urgent surgical intervention, such as may be necessary for hemorrhage, toxic megacolon, perforation, or sepsis. Under these circumstances, the patient may always believe that the operation was performed too precipitously and that, perhaps with more vigorous medical management, surgery might have been avoided or at least deferred until a later time.

As has been previously discussed, preoperative consideration of the placement of the stoma is very important. The patient may actually wear the appliance prior to the operation

and note areas where subsequent appliance management may become difficult: an area of skin folds, the waistline, and the usual position of pants or belt. The surgeon should not delay the determination of the site of the stoma until the patient is on the operating table because abdominal skin folds may not be apparent when someone is lying down

Historic Perspective

Prior to the 1940s, for a patient to be confronted with an ileostomy was a traumatic event indeed. For ulcerative colitis, the colectomy itself was a high-risk procedure, often performed in stages—an initial ileostomy, then a right hemicolectomy, followed by a left hemicolectomy. The fourth stage was the proctectomy. There were no appliances as we now appreciate them, so the ileum was brought out several inches to drain with a decompression tube inserted. This technique is generally attributed to Cattell.[40] In 1941, grafting of skin onto the end of the ileum was suggested in order for the corrosive effluent to be able to pass into some kind of appliance,

RICHARD B. CATTELL (1900–1964)

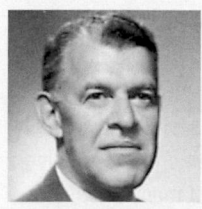

Richard Cattell was born in Martin's Ferry, Ohio. At the age of 17, he served in France as a private in a U.S. Army Evacuation Hospital. After the war, he received his A.B. from Mount Union College in Alliance, Ohio and graduated from Harvard Medical School in 1925. Following internship at St. Luke's Hospital in New York, he joined the Lahey Clinic in 1927, demonstrating his surgical skills in many fields. Like Lahey, he acquired special experience and competence in surgery of the thyroid. He also became particularly interested in surgery of the biliary tract and pancreas and was considered the world authority on reconstruction of biliary stricture. Upon the death of Lahey in 1953, he succeeded as director of the Lahey Clinic. Cattell was largely responsible for developing the Ciné Clinics film program, one of the most popular features of the Annual Clinical Congress of the American College of Surgeons. One of the first films produced (1950) was his performance of an abdominoperineal resection. Those who worked with him remember the smooth, unhurried grace of movement, which was the outstanding characteristic of his surgical technique. His Miles resection was called "the hour of charm." Cattell became a member of the Board of Governors of the American College of Surgeons, and he received numerous honors and recognitions throughout the world. His vast clinical experience has been documented in a total of 252 publications. Cattell died in Boston 2 years after failing health compelled him to retire from professional activities. (Photograph courtesy of Fabian Bachrach.)

the so-called Dragstedt ileostomy (Figure 31-46).[62] In 1948, Sanders commented that "the therapeutic efficacy of ileostomy is antagonized by the morale-destroying elaborateness and messiness of the dressing care needed to reduce or avoid skin excoriation."[211] He felt that the Dragstedt skin-grafted ileostomy was the most satisfactory method for addressing these shortcomings. In 1951, Warren and McKittrick of Boston coined the term "ileostomy dysfunction" to describe functional obstruction of the stoma.[259] In an evaluation based on 240 ileostomy patients, the authors recognized a syndrome of watery discharge, abdominal cramps, and hypovolemia as signs of intestinal obstruction attributed to edema of the noneverted, nonmatured stoma. In order to overcome what they thought was contracting scar when the serosa of the ileum is exposed to the air, they recommended longitudinal incisions through the indurated seromuscular layers, performing this operation more than 100 times.[259] In 1952, a signal advance was made in ileostomy construction through Brooke's publication, which stated rather nondramatically, "A more simple device is to evaginate the ileal end at the time of the operation and suture the mucosa to the skin; no complications have accrued from this."[31] This author further observed that the ileostomy did not retract, but stood out in conical form; furthermore, prolapse was not encountered.

At about the same time, Turnbull suggested that the so-called ileostomy dysfunction could be prevented by covering the serosa of the newly constructed ileostomy with mucosa.[248] He advised a technique whereby the seromuscular coat of the distal one-half of the exteriorized ileostomy is removed, and the residual mucosal tube pulled down over the ileostomy as a viable sliding graft. Subsequently, Crile and Turnbull confirmed Warren and McKittrick's concept of ileostomy dysfunction, a violation of the basic surgical principle of exposing an unprotected surface.[55] This exposure leads to serositis with fibrinopurulent exudate by the third or fourth postoperative day; in essence, peritonitis of the protruding segment. It is based on

LESTER R. DRAGSTEDT (1893–1975)

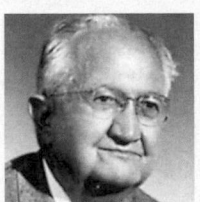

Lester Dragstedt was born in Anaconda, Montana, the son of Swedish immigrant parents. His entire college and professional education was obtained at the University of Chicago where he received the BS degree in 1915, a master's degree in physiology in 1916, a PhD in physiology in 1920, and the MD degree in 1921. His first academic appointment was as a physiologist at the State University of Iowa. In 1925, Dragstedt was recruited by Dallas B. Phemister to help design the new University Hospital research facilities on the campus of the University of Chicago. Following completion of this responsibility, Phemister appointed Dragstedt to serve as associate professor of surgery, stating, "I can teach surgery to a physiologist; I am interested in teaching physiology to surgeons." In 1947, Dragstedt succeeded Phemister as chair, a post he occupied until his retirement in 1959. Dragstedt was particularly recognized for his contributions as physiologist–surgeon to the treatment of diseases of the pancreas, parathyroids, and especially diseases of the stomach. In 1943, he performed a transthoracic vagotomy on a patient with a duodenal ulcer, an individual who refused to accept the standard operation, subtotal gastrectomy. Dragstedt was the originator of the skin-grafted ileostomy in the treatment of ulcerative colitis. He described a complete "take" of the split-thickness graft in four patients, although he perceived that the "resulting ileostomy looked somewhat like a penis." Dragstedt's competence as a basic scientist was illustrated by his election to the National Academy of Sciences. Following his Chicago retirement, he became again a full-time physiologist with appointments as research professor at the University of Florida College of Medicine. Active until the end, he died at his summer home on Elk Lake, Michigan.

BRYAN NICHOLAS BROOKE (1915–1998)

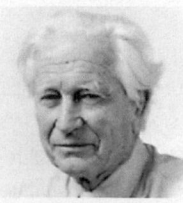

Bryan Nicholas Brooke was born in Croydon, Surrey, Feburary 21, 1915. He graduated from Cambridge and St. Bartholomew's Hospital in 1940, achieving his FRCS in 1942 and masters in surgery in 1944. After military service in World War II, he was appointed senior lecturer in Aberdeen in 1946 and reader in surgery at the University of Birmingham in 1947. It was there that he developed the concept of an everting ileostomy. In 1963, he was offered the chair in surgery at St. George's Hospital in London, a position he occupied until 1976. Many of Brooke's important writings were in the field of colon and rectal surgery, including that of ulcerative colitis and Crohn's disease. As a consequence of his unique contributions to the development of improved surgical techniques for stomal construction, he was motivated to become founder and president of the Ileostomy Association of Great Britain and Ireland, a post he held for 26 years. A recipient of many awards, he was recognized by Corpus Christi College of Cambridge University through the Copeman Medal for scientific research. Additionally, he received the A.B. Graham award of the American Proctologic Society in 1961 and was an honorary fellow of many international organizations. Brooke has been described as an individual with a great zest for life, coupled with a wonderful sense of humor. He held numerous one-man exhibitions of his paintings, many of which currently reside at prominent public institutions throughout the world. On retiring, one of his favorite activities was writing, and he became honorary associate editor of the journal, *World Medicine*. Bryan Brooke died in Surrey on September 18, 1998.

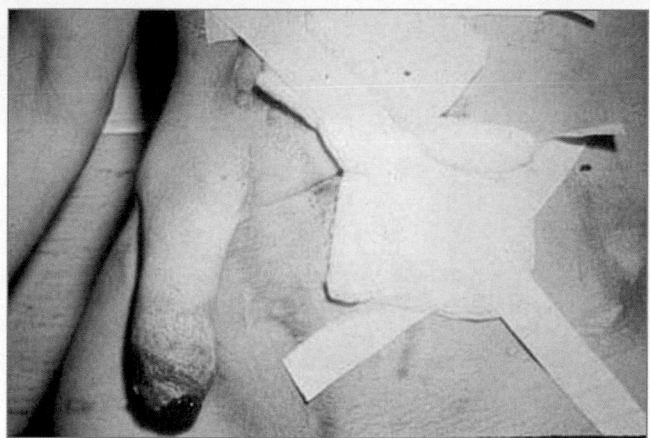

FIGURE 31-46. Dragstedt skin grafted ileostomy created before the development of effective adhesives and the current maturation techniques. (From Corman ML, Veidenheimer MC, Coller JA. Ileostomy complications: prevention and treatment. *Contemp Surg.* 1976;8:36.)

the writings of Brooke, Crile, and Turnbull that our current concepts of primary ileostomy maturation have developed.

Principles and Concerns

Despite advances in operative technique, the creation of a satisfactory ileal stoma and the proper management of ileostomy complications are often unachieved ideals. This is not difficult to comprehend for a number of reasons.

First, most busy general surgeons perform perhaps only two or three ileostomies in a given year. Second, when the procedure is performed on an emergency basis, the surgeon's main concern is saving the patient's life, and sufficient care may not be given to creating the stoma. For example, during a colectomy and ileostomy for toxic megacolon, the colon must be removed as expeditiously as possible. In addition, the patient's cardiac, renal, and pulmonary functions may be severely compromised. With these pressing concerns, the surgeon may not be as meticulous as he or she should be in performing the ileostomy.

Another reason for difficulties with ileostomy management may be the surgeon's lack of familiarity with techniques for properly locating and maturing the stoma. Besides problems with the appliance itself, the primary causes of encumbrance following an ileostomy are improper placement and incorrect construction of the stoma.

Unfortunately, a mystique surrounds stomal management. Surgeons who can successfully treat gangrene of the abdominal wall are confounded by a peristomal dermatitis. In the past, patients themselves had to search for answers amidst ignorance and superstition. It was because of this lack of support that ostomy associations were formed. Today, patients with stoma problems are most often referred to these groups. Individuals who are wound/ostomy, continence nurses and caregivers (see the following chapter) meet the needs of such individuals, but the person's own physician can assist greatly by learning how to apply a few, simple principles.

Technique

A disk of skin is excised from a previously marked site on the abdominal wall. Because a subcuticular technique is used instead of sutures through full-thickness skin, it is helpful to cut the skin obliquely, such as shown in Figure 24-68A. This emphasizes the subcuticular aspect for easy suturing. The ileum is brought through the split rectus muscle, protruding for a distance of approximately 4 or 5 cm. There is no reason to create a stoma that when everted is longer than 2 cm because the appliances that are now available are so satisfactory that a phallus-like ileostomy is truly unnecessary. Following extraperitoneal or intraperitoneal fixation (see Figures 29-44 and 29-45), the mesentery to the distal ileum is trimmed (Figure 31-47).

Turnbull and Weakley have advised passing an absorbable suture around the mesentery at skin level and excising the mesenteric fat from the distal ileum to overcome the bowing effect (Figure 31-47).[249] The submucosal vascular supply can nourish at least 6 cm of ileum after the mesentery has been divided. Although this may be a safe maneuver in patients with ulcerative colitis, those with Crohn's disease who may have a thickened mesentery or in whom the bowel is partially obstructed may not tolerate mesenteric stripping

RUPERT BEACH TURNBULL (1913–1981)

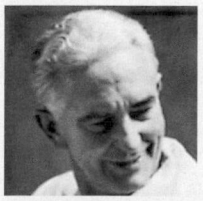

Rupert Turnbull was born in Pasadena, California. An outstanding athlete, he represented the United States in the 1932 Olympics in Italy, and won the cup for outboard hydroplane racing. He attended Pomona College, graduating in 1936, and achieved his medical degree from McGill University in 1940. During World War II, he served in the South Pacific as a field surgeon and then in China as hospital commander. Following the war, he elected to continue his surgical training at the Cleveland Clinic and ultimately joined the staff. Turnbull began to develop an interest in colon and rectal surgery, especially after he "inherited" the ostomy patients of his late chief, Tom Jones. Many of his earlier writings in particular were on stomal problems and their management. He serendipitously discovered the value of karaya as a skin protector and codesigned the first postoperative pouch for ostomy patients. Through his encouragement, the nursing specialty of enterostomal therapy was initiated. In 1962, during a convention held in Cleveland, Turnbull was a principal in founding the United Ostomy Association. Turnbull contributed extensively to the literature, primarily in the treatment of inflammatory bowel disease and cancer. With his colleague, Frank L. Weakley, he wrote the definitive *Atlas of Intestinal Stomas*. Turnbull achieved numerous honors and distinctions throughout his career. He is remembered as a master surgeon and an innovative thinker. (Photo courtesy of the Cleveland Clinic.)

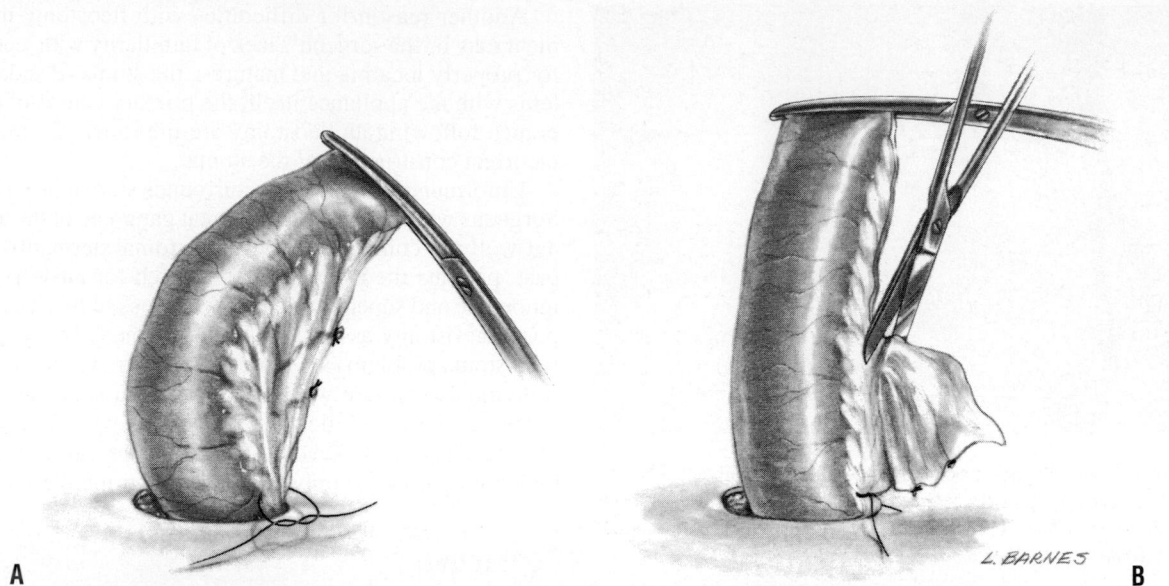

FIGURE 31-47. Maturation of ileostomy stoma by excising the mesentery. **A:** Ligation of the mesentery at the skin level. **B:** Trimming of the mesentery to remove the "chordee." (Adapted from Turnbull RB, Weakley FL. *Atlas of Intestinal Stomas.* St. Louis, MO: Mosby; 1967.)

for such a length. One should exercise caution in carrying out this maneuver under such circumstances. At this point, any redundant ileum can be amputated, leading to a final ileostomy length of approximately 2 cm.

Three sutures are then placed, one on the antimesenteric aspect and one each on either side of the mesentery (Figure 31-48). A triangulation technique is recommended. This consists of a full-thickness suturing of the end of the bowel, the seromuscular aspect of the ileum (at the skin level), and the subcuticular skin. The seromuscular bite aids in the subsequent eversion of the bowel. Some surgeons criticize this method because of the risk of possible fistula formation should the suture be placed too deeply. Obviously, care is required if one is to perform this maneuver properly

and avoid this complication. Babcock clamps placed within the bowel lumen and at the end facilitate eversion. With proper length and appropriate eversion, the stoma is primarily matured with interrupted absorbable sutures (Figure 31-49).

Complications: Prevention and Treatment

Complications following an ileostomy may be due to a technical error on the part of the surgeon, such as improper location or a faulty maturation technique. Second, disease may be a cause for subsequent stomal problems. Third, the patient, either through inadequate education, neglect, or misuse, can precipitate stomal problems that may actually necessitate surgical intervention.

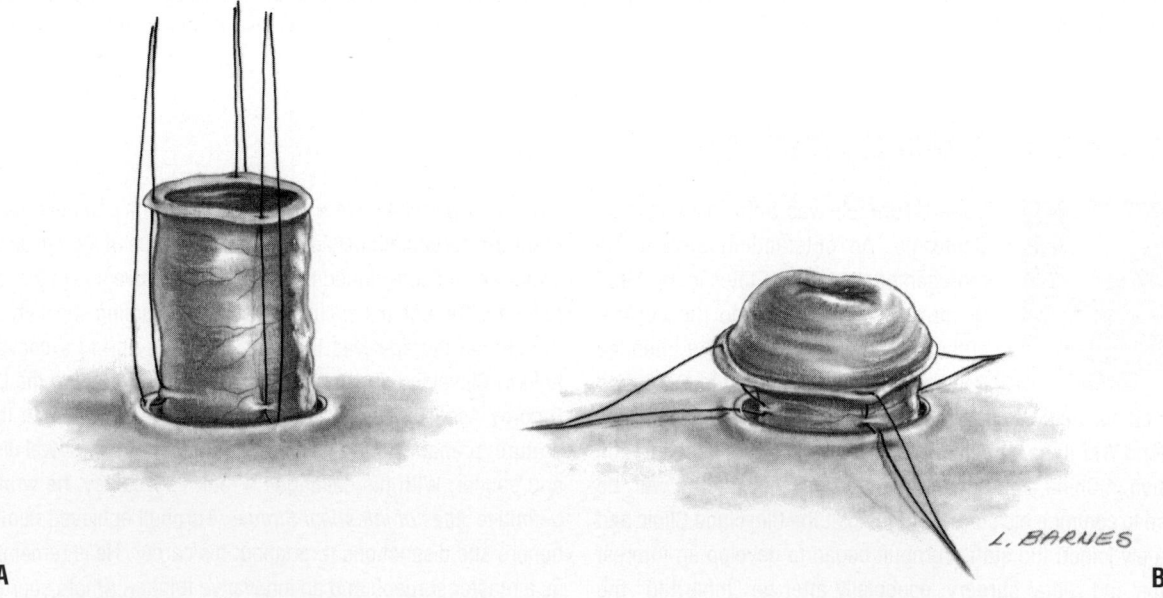

FIGURE 31-48. Maturation of ileostomy stoma. **A:** Three sutures are placed, incorporating the seromuscular layer to facilitate eversion. **B:** The sutures are secured, everting the bowel.

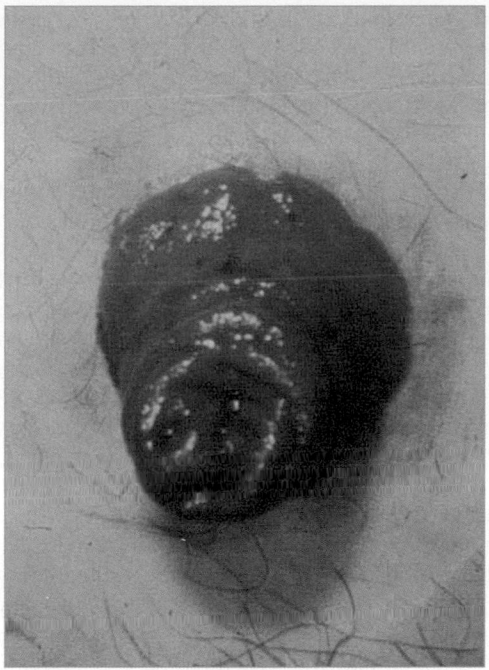

FIGURE 31-49. Normal ileostomy of optimal length.

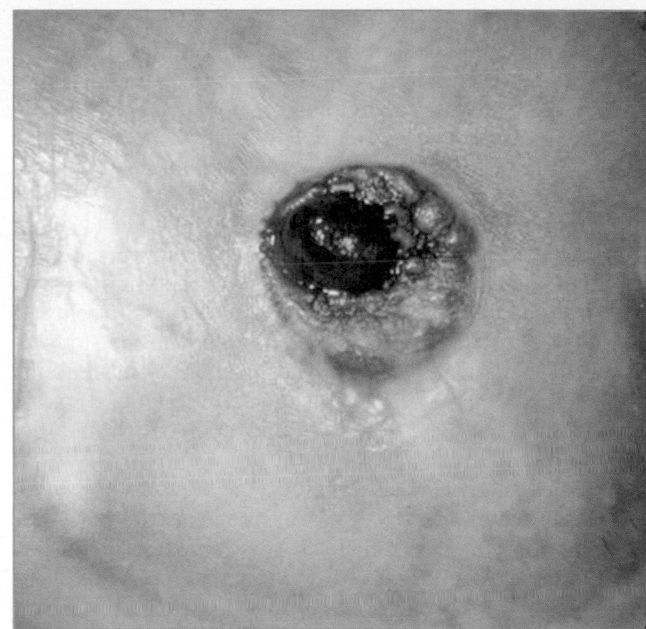

FIGURE 31-51. Retracted ileostomy from ischemia and tension with stricture due to inadequate length and adequate blood supply of the initially created stoma. (From Corman ML, Veidenheimer MC, Coller JA. Ileostomy complications: prevention and treatment. *Contemp Surg.* 1976;8:36.)

Complications due to Improper Maturation Technique
Stenosis and Retraction

Stenosis and retraction are the most common indications for revising an ileostomy in our experience.[87] My colleagues and I noted that 30% of revisions were performed for these reasons. Speakman and associates estimated an incidence of 18.5% from the literature.[225] As has been mentioned with respect to colostomy, the primary causes are inadequate initial stomal length, vascular compromise, and improper skin excision (Figures 31-50 and 31-51). With respect to the issue of blood supply, the attitude that the stoma may be a little purple or perhaps a bit blue, but it will probably be all right, is usually an unrealized prophecy. It is far preferable to reopen the abdomen and create an adequate length of viable bowel, prolonging the

operation for whatever time is necessary, than to return on a subsequent occasion or to relegate the patient to a disability because of difficulty in managing the appliance. In addition to these factors, weight gain may also be responsible (Figure 31-52). It is not inconceivable that a patient can triple his or her weight within a period of 1 year following proctocolectomy.

Handelsman and Fishbein recommend that retraction or prolapse can be prevented by placing a ribbon of fascia obtained from the abdominal wall through the mesentery adjacent to the bowel between the vessels.[100] It is neither wrapped around the intestine nor sutured to it. The authors believe that this technique will secure the position of the ileostomy without risking a possible fistula from suturing the bowel wall. I personally doubt the need for such a procedure.

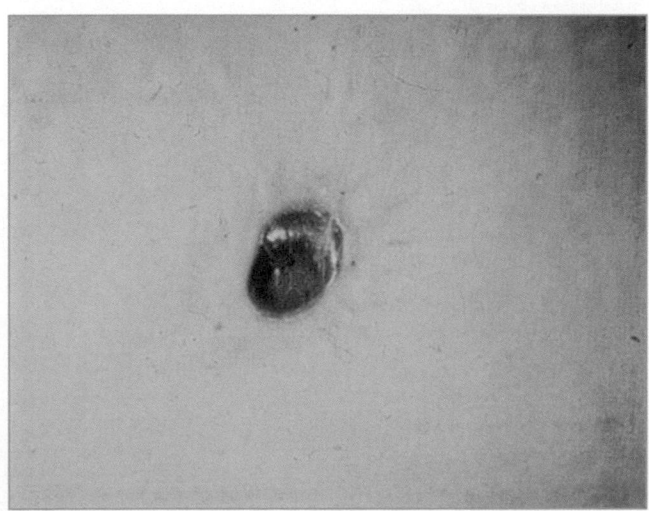

FIGURE 31-50. Stenotic ileostomy due to inadequate skin excision and necrosis of the end of the ileum.

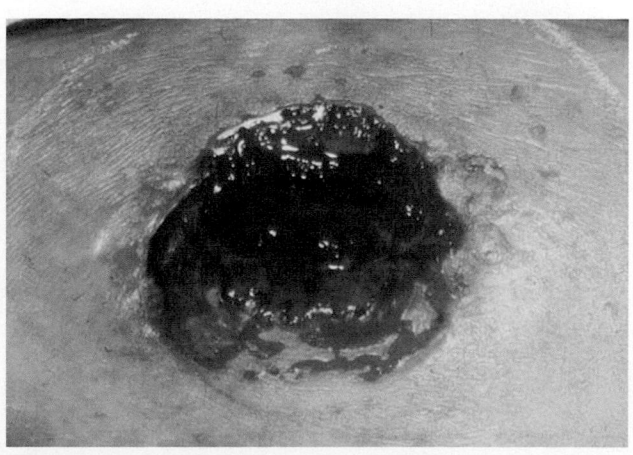

FIGURE 31-52. Retracted ileostomy with skin excoriation secondary to weight gain. (From Corman ML, Veidenheimer MC, Coller JA. Ileostomy complications: prevention and treatment. *Contemp Surg.* 1976;8:36.)

Treatment. Ideally, revision of a stenosis or retraction may be accomplished without a formal abdominal operation. Unfortunately, retraction is a complication that may sometimes require an open laparotomy or a laparoscopic revision in order to obtain the desired length of ileum necessary to create a satisfactory stoma. Therefore, it is prudent to warn the patient that this may be an eventuality.

Correction of the retraction or stenosis requires (1) excision of sufficient skin to create a proper-sized opening and (2) mobilization of the bowel as much as is necessary to prepare a stoma of adequate length. Intraperitoneal freeing of the ileum is carried out as far as possible, and the stoma is matured in the usual manner. Truedson and Press suggest the implantation of three strips of polyglactin 910 (Vicryl) mesh, longitudinally fixed to the serosa prior to eversion, in order to prevent subsequent retraction.[247]

Winslet and colleagues describe a method of stabilization to prevent recurrence of retraction by means of a GIA stapling device without the blade.[269] This can be accomplished without an anesthetic, but only if the retraction is not of the fixed type. That is, the ileostomy protrudes for an appropriate length but intermittently falls back to produce a flush or retracted stoma. Three rows of the stapler are fired the length of the ileostomy. One may also elect to use a linear stapler for the same purpose, thereby facilitating the maintenance of the everted position. The authors comment that initially the stoma is unsightly, but after 6 weeks the staples are no longer evident. Speakman and associates reported the St. Mark's Hospital experience with this method in 10 patients.[225] There were four failures requiring additional surgery (40%: two re-retractions, one sepsis, and one abscess).

A particularly difficult problem arises when an individual subsequently becomes obese and the stoma disappears into the fat. This can be addressed by performing a panniculectomy and abdominoplasty, with relocation of the stoma into the new, flattened abdominal wall. Such an operative undertaking does not necessarily require the expertise of a plastic surgeon. As a matter of fact, plastic surgeons are often reluctant to embark upon a major reconstruction when there is risk of contamination from stool or the presence of a stoma. However, we who muck around in the bowels all day have no such fear. Besides, the principles of skin flap elevation and advancement are quite familiar to colon and rectal surgeons (see Anoplasty section, Chapter 11). One does not require advanced reconstructive surgical credentialing to perform this relatively straightforward operation. Figure 31-53 illustrates the technique for accomplishing a revision under these circumstances. Evans and colleagues performed abdominal wall recontouring and stomal revision on eight patients using a similar technique.[66] All experienced improvement in appliance management and body image.

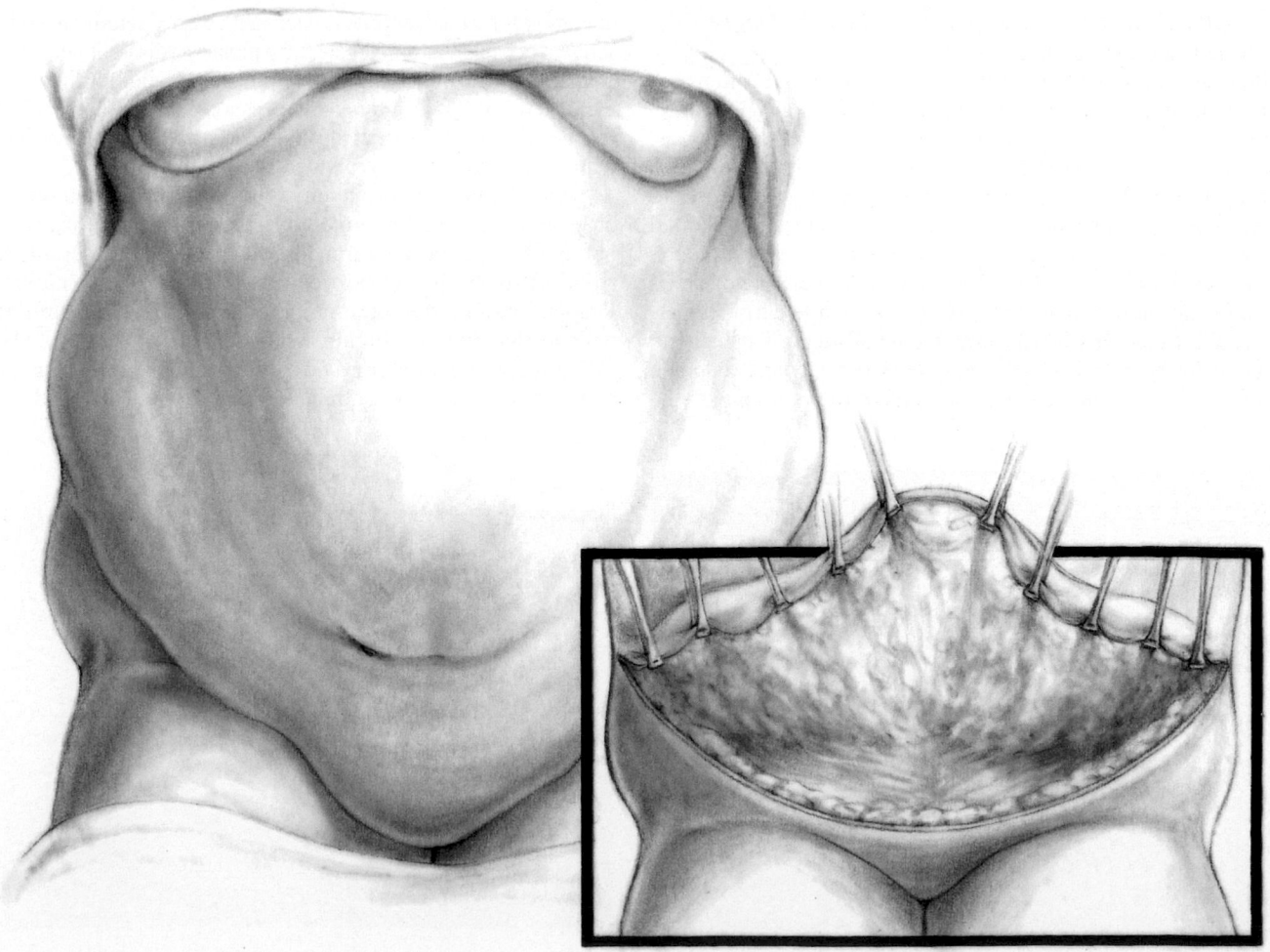

A

B

FIGURE 31-53. Technique for revision of an ileostomy due to weight gain (panniculectomy and abdominoplasty). **A:** Ileostomy is retracted into fold of panniculus. **B:** Long, transverse, suprapubic incision deepened to expose the fascia. *(continued)*

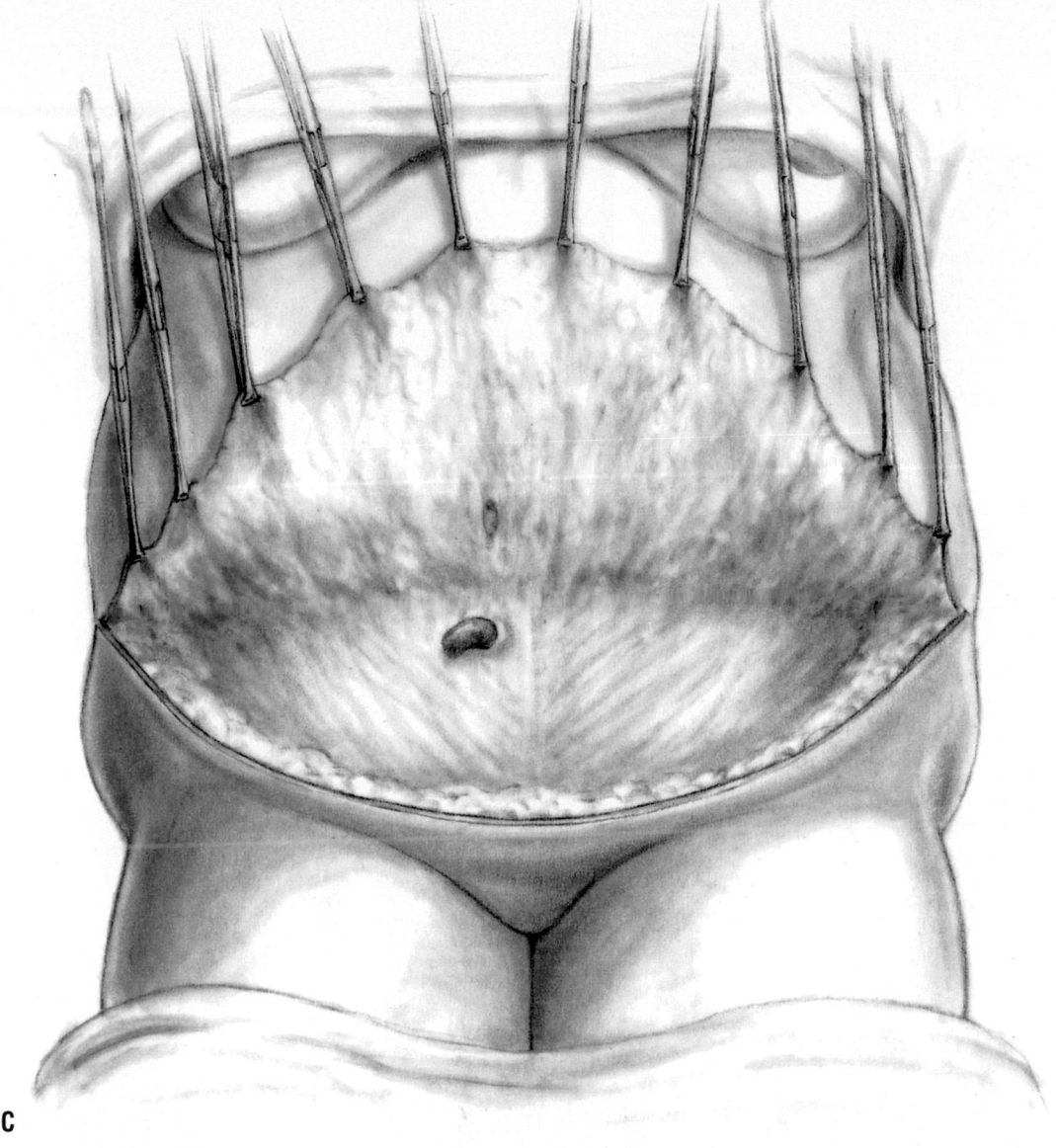

FIGURE 31-53. *(continued)* **C:** The skin and subcutaneous tissue are elevated to the costal margin, detaching the stoma.

Prolapse

Prolapse may be of two types: fixed (irreducible) or sliding. In my experience, the fixed type always occurs without any prior history of stomal revision. Conversely, the sliding type is seen with the second or later revision. This implies inadequate abdominal fixation and indicates that mobilizing an ileostomy when performing a revision predisposes to subsequent problems with the sliding type of prolapse (Figure 31-54). Prolapse is usually not associated with skin problems if it is of the fixed type, but if it retracts and becomes flush, leakage can occur. Too long a stoma is prone to trauma from contact with the appliance and may lead to psychological problems as well (Figure 31-55).

Treatment. If the stomal protrusion is not a true prolapse, but simply an ileostomy that was created too long initially, treatment is relatively simple. The ileal mucosa is incised, preserving the mucocutaneous junction, and the stoma is inverted (Figure 31-56). Redundant ileum is resected, and the stoma is matured in the usual manner. This maneuver is identical to that shown earlier for colostomy prolapse, remembering that the incision must be made into the bowel itself, not into the skin. This will maintain the proper-sized opening in the abdominal wall.

One should not attempt to perform an intra-abdominal dissection in order to avoid disrupting the intraperitoneal fixation. Occasionally, however, with a sliding type of prolapse, so much small bowel is delivered that some form of intraperitoneal fixation is prudent. Reduction of the ileum is usually technically difficult to accomplish and may result in recurrence of the prolapse, but resection of a long segment of intestine is not justified. Intraperitoneal fixation may necessitate a laparotomy/laparoscopy to manage the complication adequately. Alternatively, one may consider the linear stapling method of fixation mentioned in the previous section.

Fistula

Fistula is not an uncommon reason for ileostomy revision in that 15% are performed for this indication. The most frequent cause of fistula is recurrent Crohn's disease. Erosion of the

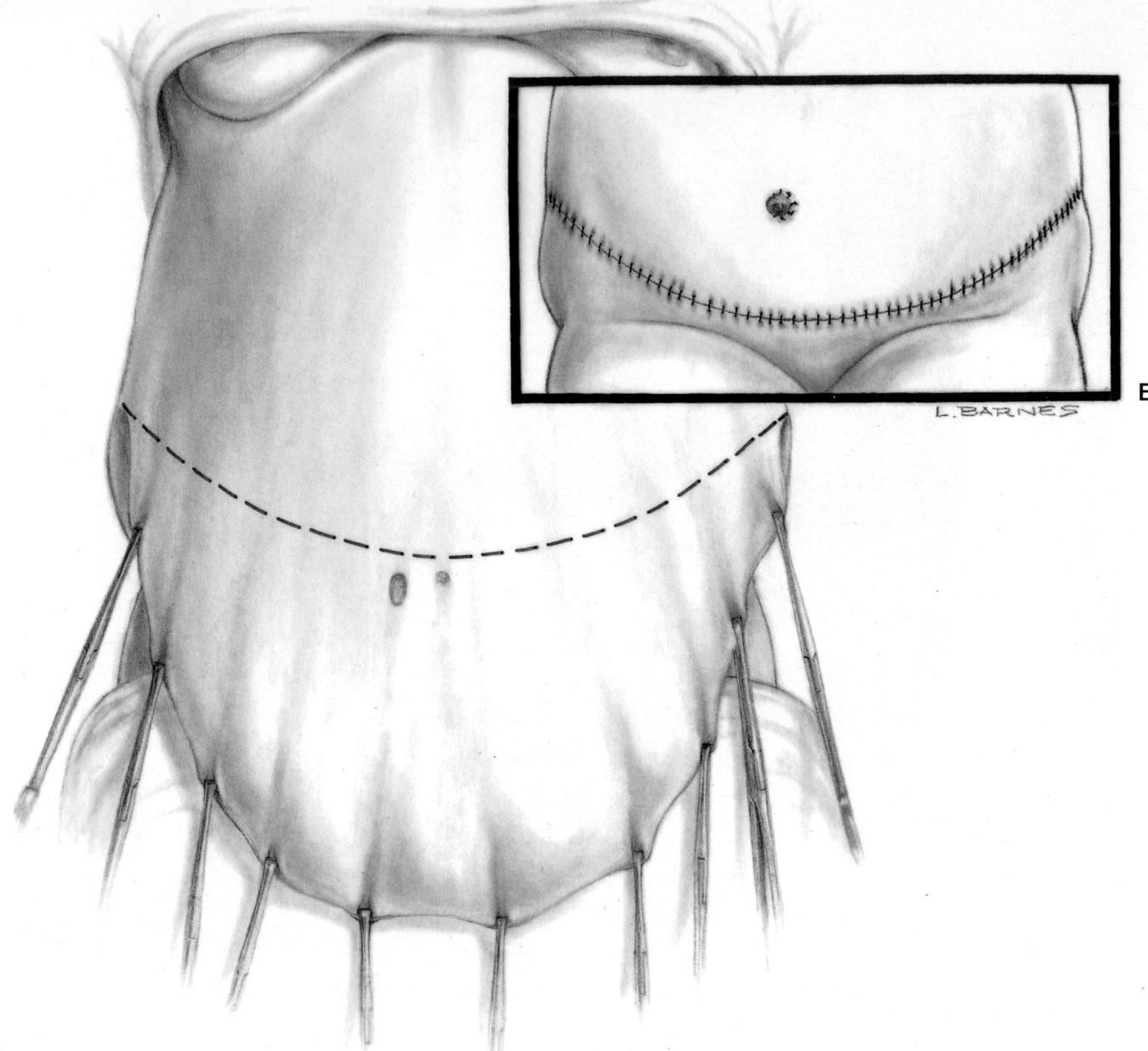

D

E

FIGURE 31-53. *(continued)* E: The new opening is created for the ileostomy, and the stoma is matured in the usual way. Closed-suction, subcutaneous drains (not shown) are advised. If a hernia is present, mesh may be used for the repair. If further intestinal length or relocation of the stoma is necessary, the abdomen may be opened.

stoma by the faceplate of an appliance or from deep placement of a suture are other possible etiologies (Figure 31-57). Symptoms may be associated with the underlying disease, but inability to maintain an appliance without leakage and skin irritation is initially the overriding concern. This complication presents a much more difficult management problem than does prolapse. Closure of the fistula may be attempted if no inflammatory disease is present, but subsequent breakdown is quite likely. If the fistula is resected, a laparotomy may be required in order to obtain sufficient length of ileum for adequate maturation.

Greatorex suggested a simplified method for closing a fistula, the insertion of a pipe cleaner soaked in 6% aqueous phenol.[95] Immediate cessation of leakage with subsequent healing occurred in two of three patients.

Greenstein and colleagues identified 15 of 214 patients with an ileostomy constructed for Crohn's disease and in whom a paraileostomy fistula developed.[96] In every case, this was due to recurrent disease. All required resection and reconstruction of the stoma.

If the skin at the original stomal site has been injured by the ileal effluent or if additional small bowel must be resected, the stoma should be created in an alternative location, usually in the left lower quadrant.

Seeding
Seeding of viable ileal mucosa can develop along the suture line if subcuticular sutures for maturation are not employed (Figure 31-58). Such seeding can lead to persistent secretion and, consequently, to problems in fitting the appliance.

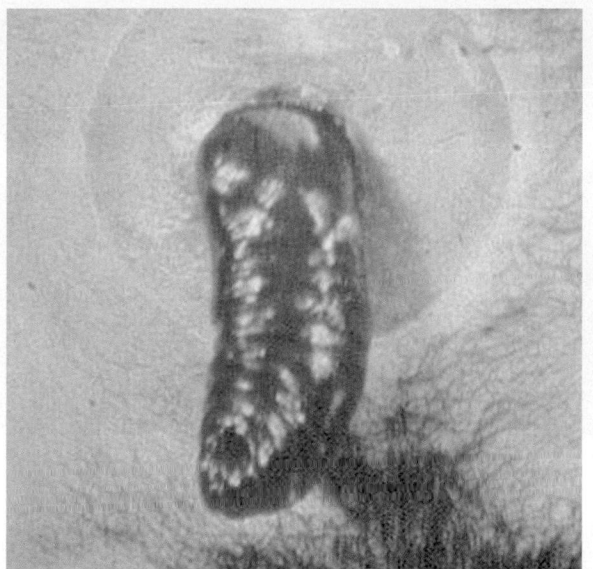

FIGURE 31-54. Ileostomy "prolapse" in this patient was due to creating too-long a stoma initially.

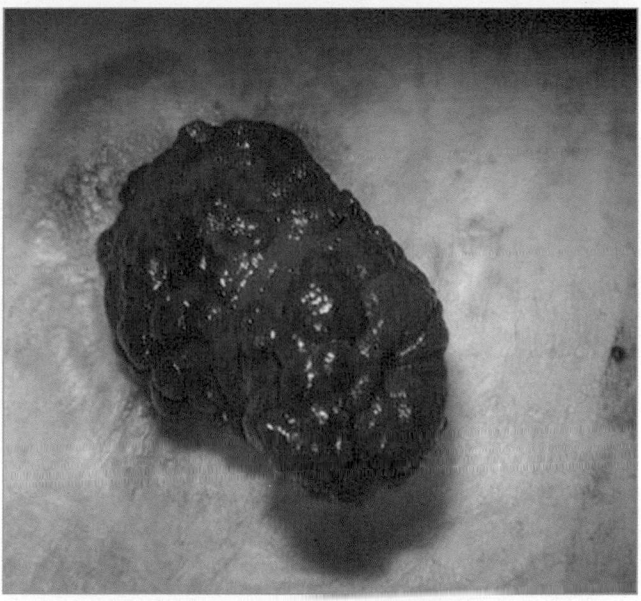

FIGURE 31-55. A prolapsed ileostomy causing irritative trauma from the appliance. This produces the so-called pseudoepitheliomatous hyperplasia. Pseudoepitheliomatous hyperplasia is a benign condition, characterized by hyperplasia of the epidermis or mucosa. It may be present in a number of conditions characterized by prolonged inflammation and/or chronic infection, as well as in association with many cutaneous neoplasms.

Management. For what might seem to be a rather trivial concern, treatment is quite difficult. Attempts at cauterizing of the ectopically located mucosa are fruitless. The only effective management is excision, and even with this procedure, the viable ileal mucosal cells may grow again to the surface from a deeply implanted location. A plastic surgical procedure, rotating a skin flap to cover the defect, may be attempted successfully, but more often relocation of the stoma may be required.

This is a totally preventable complication if one uses a subcuticular suturing technique.

Complications due to Improper Placement

The aforementioned complications are generally due to errors in ileostomy maturation technique. Another potential cause of difficulty after stomal construction is the initial improper location of the stoma. As discussed previously, the site chosen should be free of eschar, especially if the scar is irregular rather than flat. The stoma should not be near any

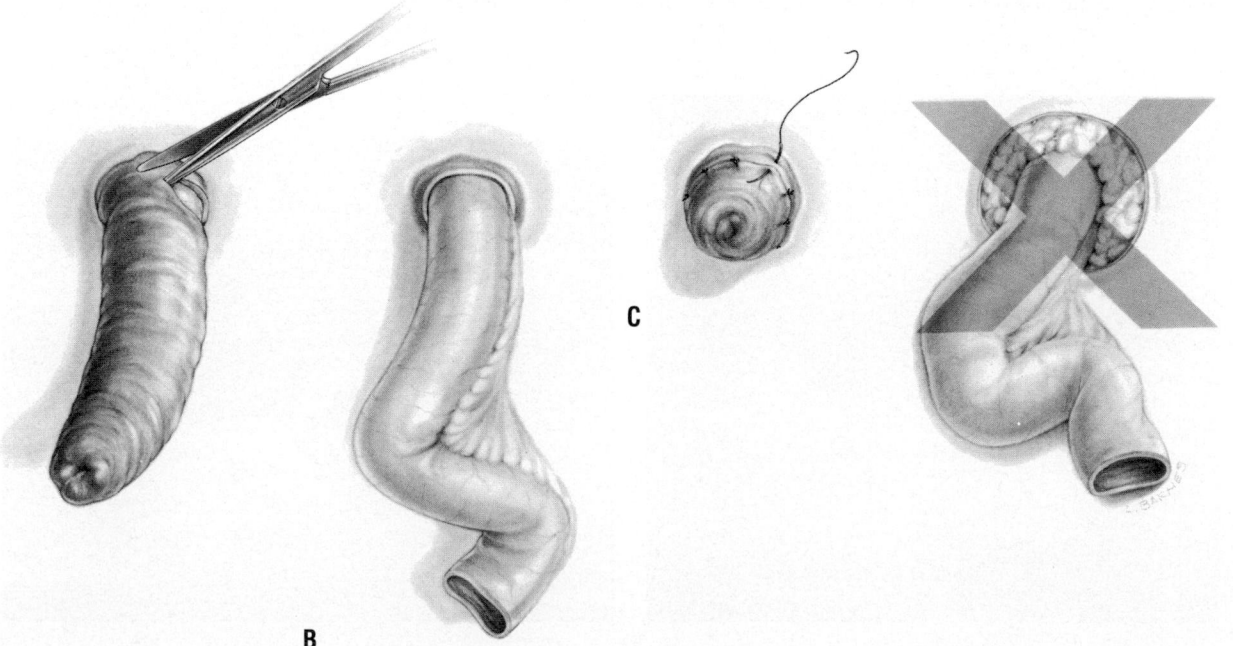

A   **B**   **C**   **D**

FIGURE 31-56. Revision of ileostomy prolapse. **A:** Incision is made into the ileostomy, not at the mucocutaneous junction. A large skin opening should be avoided. **B:** The redundant bowel is delivered. **C:** The ileostomy is then "matured" in the usual way. **D:** A large defect would be produced if the incision had initially been made in the skin.

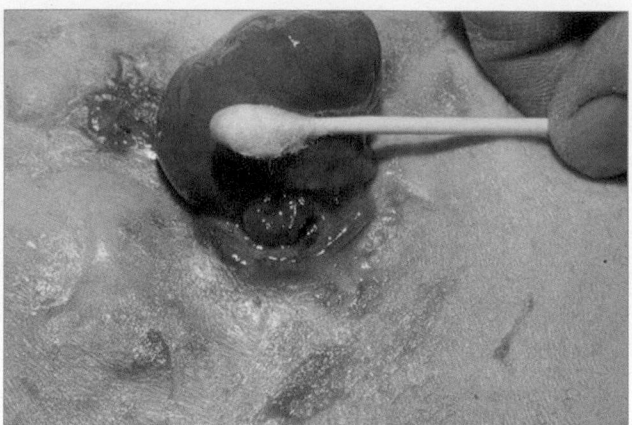

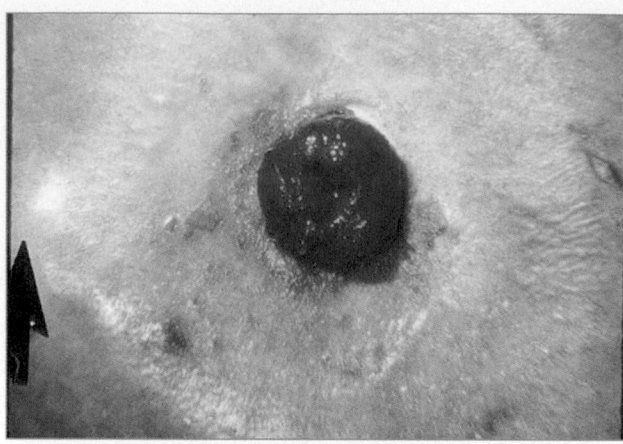

FIGURE 31-57. Ileostomy fistula presumed secondary to a deeply placed seromuscular anchoring suture. (From Corman ML, Veidenheimer MC, Coller JA. Ileostomy complications: prevention and treatment. *Contemp Surg.* 1976;8:36.)

FIGURE 31-59. Positioning the stoma too close to the iliac crest causes an inability to maintain the appliance. Note the parastomal dermatitis. *Arrow* indicates the anterior superior iliac spine. (From Corman ML, Veidenheimer MC, Coller JA. Ileostomy complications: prevention and treatment. *Contemp Surg.* 1976;8:36.)

bony promontory, such as the iliac crest (Figure 31-59) or the rib margin (Figure 31-60), and should be placed in such a way that the intestine can be pulled through the split rectus muscle. Failure to do so often results in parastomal herniation (Figure 31-61). Bringing the stoma through the incision is contraindicated, not only because of the risk of hernia, but also because of the difficulties in maintaining an appliance and the delay in wound healing created by spilling of the effluent onto the skin (Figure 31-62). The stoma must be placed in an area where the patient can care for it properly and wear the appliance with confidence and without the fear of leakage (Figure 31-63).

Treatment

If the stoma is improperly located and appliance management is unsatisfactory, relocation is necessary. This usually involves a laparotomy with its attendant morbidity,

although it may be possible to perform a revision and relocation of the stoma by a tunneling method, without a complete abdominal exploration, as was discussed earlier with respect to colostomy revision.[236] With this technique, as usual, the site selection should be carefully determined preoperatively. The ileal stoma is mobilized by a circumstomal incision into the peritoneal cavity. The distal segment is delivered if possible and resected. The bowel is returned to the peritoneal cavity after closure of the distal end. Long sutures are left outside the abdomen should retrieval be necessary. By blunt dissection from the original abdominal wall opening, a space is created to tunnel the distal ileum to the new site. A disk of skin is excised, the rectus is split, and the peritoneal cavity is entered at the new location. The ileum is pulled through by means of the long sutures that had been left attached, and the new stoma is constructed.

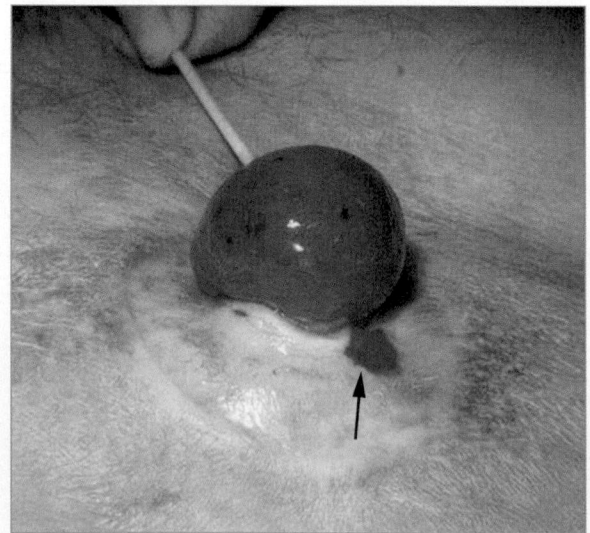

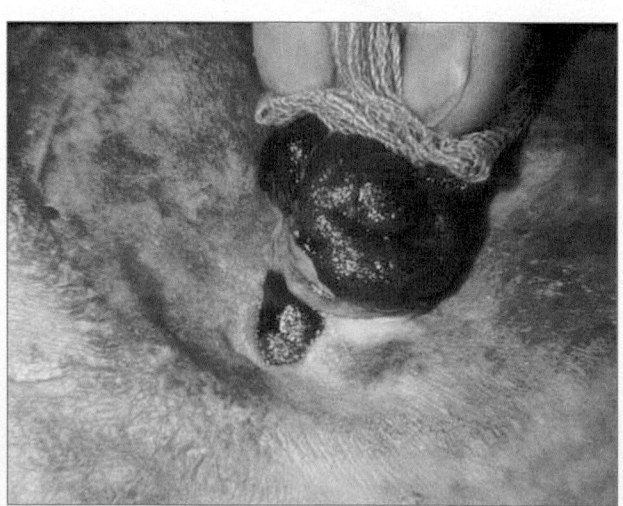

A

B

FIGURE 31-58. **A:** Mucosal "seeding" (*arrow*) due to improper suturing of the ileum to the subcuticular skin. **B:** Another example of mucosal seeding leading to inability to maintain the appliance. Note the severe skin changes. (From Corman ML, Veidenheimer MC, Coller JA. Ileostomy complications: prevention and treatment. *Contemp Surg.* 1976;8:36.)

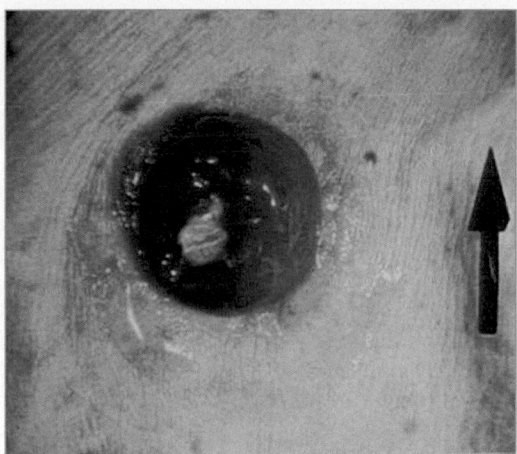

FIGURE 31-60. Ileostomy too close to the rib margin (*arrow*). (From Corman ML, Veidenheimer MC, Coller JA. Ileostomy complications: prevention and treatment. *Contemp Surg.* 1976;8:36.)

Comment

Although one can avoid a larger incision by this technique, I do not believe that it is a quantum advance in the treatment of ileostomy complications requiring revision. However, through the incorporation of laparoscopic techniques, relocation without a full laparotomy is indeed feasible. Regardless, stomal location errors are inevitably preventable problems.

Paraileostomy Hernia

Paraileostomy hernia seems to be a less frequent observation, judging, at least, from personal experience. Perhaps this is because the stoma is more likely to be temporary but more probably because the consequences of an ill-placed stoma are more concerning. Therefore, greater attention may be paid by the surgeon (and the patient) to potential problems. Williams and colleagues reviewed 46 patients who had undergone an end ileostomy for ulcerative colitis or Crohn's disease for evidence of paraileostomy hernia.[265] This complication was observed in 13 individuals (28%). The authors found that computed tomography was helpful in confirming the presence of a defect.

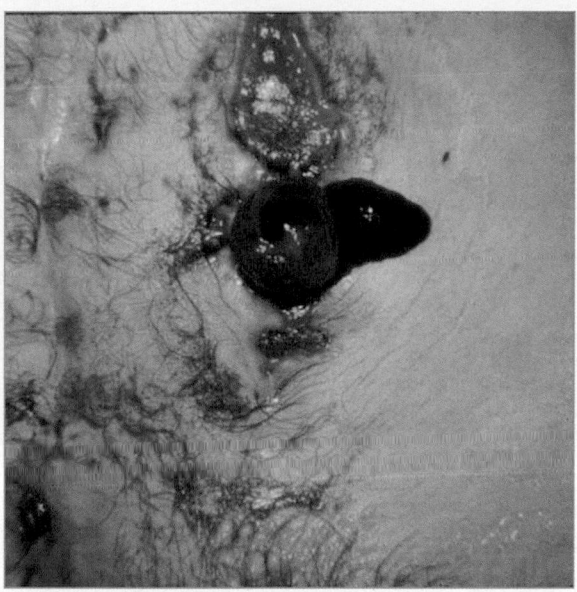

FIGURE 31-62. Open, indolent, draining incision due to the fact that the ileostomy was brought through the wound.

Treatment. As with paracolostomy hernia, this complication is usually due to an error in the location of the stoma. Repair is effected in a similar manner to that which has been previously described for colostomy hernia with or without mesh (see Figures 31-16 through 31-20 above).[80] Unfortunately, most such complications usually require relocation of the ileostomy.

Even in the absence of a parastomal hernia, additional pouch support may be achieved by the use of a belt, especially during lifting or exercise (Figure 31-64). For nonsurgical management of a hernia, the device is available up to 9-in. wide.

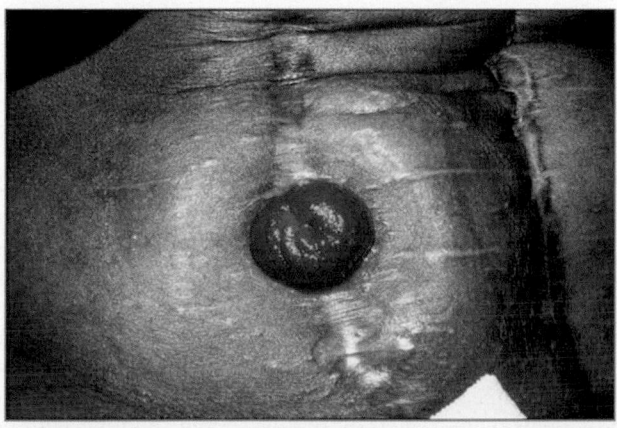

FIGURE 31-61. Ileostomy brought through an abdominal incision creates difficulty in appliance management. Note hernia.

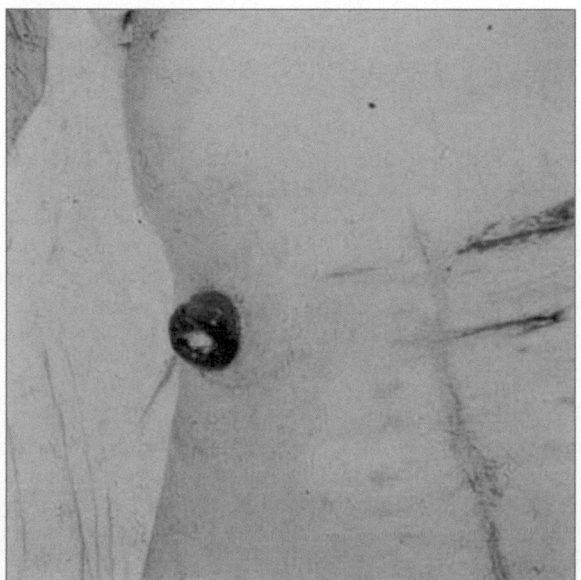

FIGURE 31-63. Appliance management is a challenge when the stoma is placed on the hip. (From Corman ML, Veidenheimer MC, Coller JA. Ileostomy complications: prevention and treatment. *Contemp Surg.* 1976;8:36.)

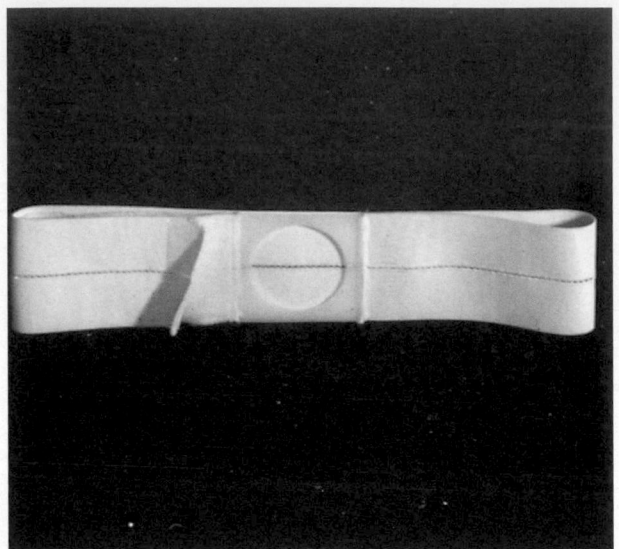

FIGURE 31-64. Support belt for ostomy. (Courtesy of Nu-Hope Laboratories, Inc.)

Other Complications

Recurrent Crohn's Disease and Other Manifestations of Inflammatory Bowel Disease at the Ileostomy

It is self-evident that Crohn's disease can recur in the stoma or in the small bowel proximal to the ileostomy (see Figure 30-63). Management of this problem is discussed in Chapter 30. Additionally, paraileostomy skin ulceration may be a consequence of IBD. Pyoderma gangrenosum is an associated condition with IBD (see Chapter 30). The variable clinical outcomes of parastomal pyoderma gangrenosum may be related to the activity of the underlying IBD and, in fact, may not be successfully treated until the residual disease has been extirpated (see Chapter 30).[245] A vigorous program involving a wound care/enterostomal therapist is usually required (see Chapter 32). Any disseminated skin condition when it occurs adjacent to or near the stoma can present severe management problems. For example, pemphigus vulgaris has been reported to cause severe skin management problems in a patient who harbored a stoma (see Chapter 9).[102] A case of bullous pemphigoid at the ostomy site has also been reported.[251]

Last and colleagues reported 17 patients with Crohn's disease who developed parastomal ulcers.[138] Conservative management included debridement, curettage, unroofing, and pouching of the stoma with Telfa strips placed in the ulcer base with a conventional appliance or a Perry model no. 51 device. Most were healed by 3 months. When medical therapy fails, surgical revision with possible relocation is necessary, either open or laparoscopic.[155] Rotation or advancement skin grafts have also been employed with some success.

Infectious Enteritides

Campylobacter jejuni has been reported to cause profound ulceration of the stoma in association with an acute ileitis.[158] This case report emphasizes the importance of obtaining a stool culture in the evaluation of a patient with suspected recurrent IBD.

Carcinoma at the Ileostomy

Inflammatory Bowel Disease. A number of instances of carcinoma arising in an ileostomy following proctocolectomy have been reported, possibly due to seeding viable tumor cells at the time of the original procedure, but more likely a consequence of a late-developing dysplastic phenomenon.[22,29,57,77,122,199,219,222,253] Sherlock and colleagues have reported the first two instances of stomal adenocarcinoma in Crohn's disease.[218] Most publications note that this complication develops many years following the construction of the stoma.[77]

The most common presenting signs and symptoms include bleeding, ulceration, and the presence of a friable mass at the ileostomy site.[253]

The pathogenesis is largely speculative, but Roberts and colleagues observed that with one exception, all individuals in their study had antecedent backwash ileitis or dysplasia.[199] Although this cannot be considered a preventable complication, particular attention should be given to the application of proper cancer technique if a tumor is present at the time of stomal construction. Certainly, if the tumor appears to have seeded the abdomen or has breached the seromuscular surface of the bowel wall, perhaps at least a change of gloves should be in order at the time of the maturation of the ileostomy. Treatment requires en bloc resection of the stoma, adjacent mesentery, and abdominal wall, and the creation of a new ileostomy.[68] Screening of asymptomatic patients with ileostomies of long standing by means of biopsy, looking for dysplastic or neoplastic changes, may be appropriate.[68,218,222]

A case of primary squamous cell carcinoma of a skin-grafted ileostomy has been described,[176] as has squamous cell carcinoma of the peristomal skin.[38]

Familial Adenomatous Polyposis

As discussed in Chapter 22, familial adenomatous polyposis (FAP) may be associated with tumors and tumorlike conditions throughout the gastrointestinal tract. Although most lesions in the small bowel are areas of lymphoid hyperplasia, Nakahara and colleagues found adenomas to be present in 20% of the ileums studied.[171] Such tumors may be evident on the stoma. Adenocarcinoma has also been reported.[82] In light of the fact that the potential for malignant change has not been clearly defined, careful follow-up with ileoscopy and biopsy is recommended.

Hemorrhage

Patients who have undergone an ileostomy for chronic ulcerative colitis or Crohn's disease may develop cirrhosis and portal hypertension. The problem is relatively common in those with sclerosing cholangitis. These individuals have the potential for shunts developing within adhesions between the ileal (portal) veins and the anterior abdominal wall (systemic) veins.[181] This may lead to ileostomy hemorrhage from parastomal varices (Figure 31-65).[50,198] Of interest is the fact that colectomy probably limits the likelihood of the development of encephalopathy.

Sclerotherapy may be expected to afford only temporary benefit (see earlier discussion with respect to colostomy). Successful shunting directed at relieving the portal hypertension should prevent subsequent hemorrhage, but the procedure may accelerate liver failure.[181]

Adson and Fulton identified 19 cirrhotic patients who bled repeatedly from the mucocutaneous junction of the ileal or colonic stomas and added three of their own.[6] These individuals were treated by portosystemic shunting with no evidence of recurrent bleeding. The authors advised ileostomy revision to control hemorrhage, but when stomal and

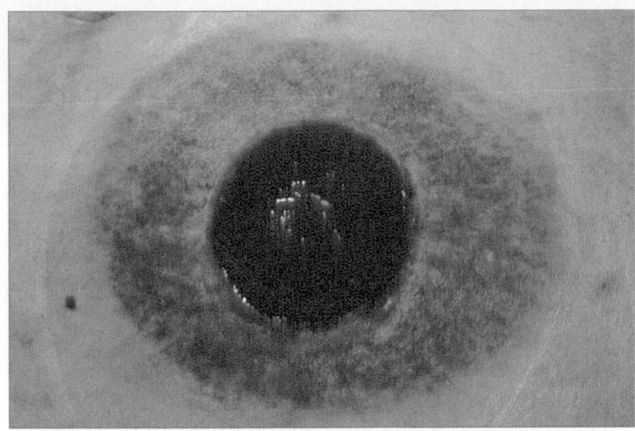

FIGURE 31-65. Parastomal varices in a patient with portal hypertension

esophageal varix bleeding coexist, a portosystemic shunt procedure was felt to be justified. Others also have concluded that a shunt procedure offers the best opportunity for controlling the bleeding.[50,198] Liver transplantation may be the preferred option in selected patients.

Trauma

Trauma to the ileostomy can be accidental or deliberate (Figure 31-66). Wilkinson and Humphreys reported a patient who suffered a laceration of the ileostomy as a result of a seat belt injury.[264] Following satisfactory repair, the individual was admitted to another hospital at a later time with total avulsion of his stoma as a result of direct trauma during a brawl. Although these types of injuries are not necessarily preventable and although one should create the stoma of sufficient prominence to satisfactorily maintain an appliance, a longer length not only is unsightly but also increases susceptibility to trauma.

Results of Ileostomy Creation

As recently as 40 years ago, the complication rate for the creation of an ileostomy alone approached 100%. In 1981, Morowitz and Kirsner observed that at least one-fourth of their patients required ileostomy revision.[167] Reoperation for bowel obstruction was performed in more than 10%,

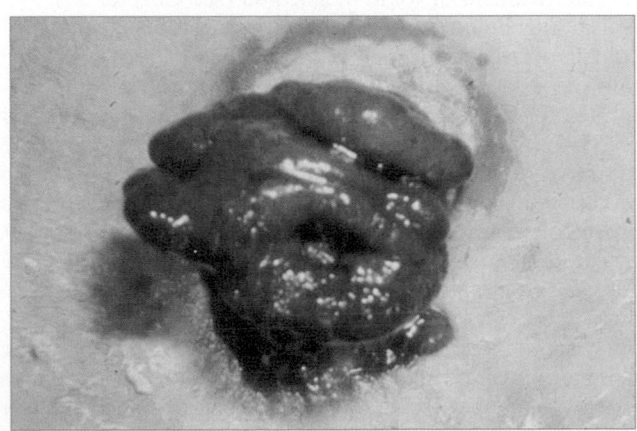

FIGURE 31-66. Macerated ileostomy with multiple fistulas in a psychotic patient who attempted to "destroy" the stoma.

TABLE 31-4 Reasons for Ileostomy Revision

COMPLICATION	NUMBER	PERCENT
Stenosis	20	23.8
Fistula	12	14.2
Prolapse	10	11.9
Retraction	10	11.9
Recurrent disease	8	9.5
Small bowel obstruction	8	9.5
Poor placement	5	6.0
Stomal bleeding	3	3.6
Dermatitis	2	2.4
Necrosis	2	2.4
Stomal pain	2	2.4
Paraileostomy hernia	1	1.2
Paraileostomy abscess	1	1.2
Total	84	100.0

From Goldblatt MS, Corman ML, Haggitt RC, et al. Ileostomy complications requiring revision: Lahey Clinic experience, 1964–1973. *Dis Colon Rectum.* 1977;20(3):209–214.

and diarrhea and nephrolithiasis were frequent problems. Medication was necessary for 20%.

It has been now almost 40 years since my colleagues and I reviewed our experience with ileostomy complications requiring revision during a 10-year period, ending in 1973.[76] Eighty-four revisions were performed on 50 individuals. The reasons for revision are summarized in Table 31-4. Thirty-one patients underwent only one revision, and subsequent stomal operations were required in 19. Nine of these underwent a third revision, four a fourth, and two a fifth. Ileostomy complications requiring revision were more frequent in those who had Crohn's disease.[76] Roy and coworkers noted that 9.7% of their patients with ulcerative colitis needed revisions, as compared with 26.5% with Crohn's disease.[206] Steinberg and coworkers found a similar incidence.[226] Leong and associates reported the St. Mark's Hospital experience with ileostomy complications, actuarially analyzing 150 permanent stomas constructed over a 10-year period.[142] By 20 years, the incidence of stomal complications approached 76% in those with ulcerative colitis and 59% in those with Crohn's disease. These differences were statistically significant and essentially the opposite ratio of that reported in the three papers mentioned previously. Revisional rates were also higher in individuals with ulcerative colitis. The four most common complications were skin problems (cumulative probability, 34%), intestinal obstruction (23%), retraction (17%), and parastomal herniation (16%).[142] Interestingly, the incidence of parastomal herniation was not reduced by siting through the rectus muscle (21%) when compared with those that were created outside of the muscle (7%). Although the differences were not statistically significant, they are certainly opposite from what one would have predicted and which I have repeatedly advised throughout this chapter. Since the publication of the last edition of this text, there seems to be a paucity of literature on the incidence of complications of ileostomy. Perhaps it is because we, as surgeons, are doing a better job of minimizing the risks. What appears to have increased, however, are the publications dedicated to improving the complication rates associated with *closing* the ileostomy.

Ileostomy in the Elderly

Advanced age does not appear to be a contraindication to ileostomy. My colleagues and I reviewed our experience with ileostomy in patients aged more than 60 years.[3] The median age was 64 at the time of surgery, and there was no mortality. All accepted and managed their stomas in much the same manner as younger people; no specialized nursing care was necessary. Four of 10 required ileostomy revisions. Although this was a small series, the incidence is not significantly greater than in younger people. Stryker and coworkers surveyed 67 patients older than 60 from the Mayo Clinic.[229] They found that although lifestyle did not appear to be altered more in the elderly than in younger individuals, older patients experienced a greater frequency of appliance management difficulties.

▶ CONTINENT ILEOSTOMY DEVICE

Pemberton and colleagues have described the Mayo Clinic use of a continent ileostomy device in four individuals with conventional ileostomies.[182] The apparatus consists of a modified endotracheal tube. Through the application of intermittent balloon inflation, an obstruction is created, dilatation of the ileum is produced, and a simulated reservoir results. The authors concluded that chronic intermittent occlusion with an indwelling stomal device achieves enteric continence without impairing intestinal function. However, no subsequent reports have been forthcoming.

▶ PATIENT EVALUATION OF RESULTS: LIFESTYLE AND SEXUAL FUNCTION

Morowitz and Kirsner reported their experience using a questionnaire of almost 2,000 patients who had undergone ileostomy for ulcerative colitis.[167] Satisfaction with the ileostomy was certainly improved when compared with preoperative status. This was substantiated by the dramatic decrease in the number of colitis patients under the care of a physician after the operation. Furthermore, the ileostomy seemed to have an ameliorative effect on marital status and there appeared to be no significant adverse effect on childbearing. A relatively low number of unemployed persons was noted in their experience. Conversely, Halevy and colleagues reported a survey from the Israel Ostomy Association and found a low rate of rehabilitation as measured by failure to return to previous occupation and problems with sexual and social adjustment.[99]

Many studies have addressed the psychological and sexual aspects of patients who have undergone an operation resulting in an ileostomy or colostomy.[32,36,85,94,156,201] Problems expressed include impotence, dyspareunia, decreased physical attractiveness, concern for odor, fear of injuring the stoma, fear of leakage, and fear of rejection by the sexual partner. In a survey performed by McLeod and coworkers of 322 ileostomies from the Cleveland Clinic, 22% reported psychological problems because of "poor body image," and 12% noted sterility or impotence.[156] Skin irritation (49%), offensive noise and odor (42%), and detection of the appliance (29%) were some of the problems encountered.[156] Awad and associates conducted a postal questionnaire of 113 patients with a permanent ileostomy.[13] They analyzed the quality of life as well as the psychological morbidity, including whether the patient would prefer to have an ileoanal pouch. A total of 93% of the respondents were content with the ileostomy and appeared to have a normal lifestyle. Moreover, approximately 87% stated that they would keep the ileostomy rather than be submitted to a major operation for reestablishment of intestinal continuity. Significant psychological morbidity was observed in only 5% of patients.[13]

These reviews uniformly suggest that the surgeon and/or wound care/enterostomal therapist should discuss these concerns with patients prior to performing permanent ostomy surgery. Brouillette and colleagues observed that many problems were resolved by the patients themselves, but the authors strongly advocate that an understanding surgeon as well as a knowledgeable wound care/enterostomal therapist and site visitor can create a climate in which the patient can feel at ease in asking for guidance on sexual matters (see Chapter 32).[32] There is no gainsaying the fact that stomal surgery has a profound influence on a patient's daily life.[94] If there are ostomy management problems, the data imply that the patient will have some degree of psychosexual dysfunction.

▶ LOOP ILEOSTOMY

Loop ileostomy was originally described by Turnbull and Weakley as a procedure to divert the fecal stream primarily for the treatment of toxic megacolon (see Chapter 29).[249] It is also a technique that is effective for the management of colonic obstruction (much preferred than a cecostomy) and to protect an ileorectal anastomosis, especially when performed for IBD, and an anastomosis following low anterior resection (as an alternative to transverse colostomy). In more recent years, it has been almost routinely applied in order to protect an ileoanal anastomosis concomitant with restorative proctocolectomy.

An indication for loop ileostomy that is not sufficiently appreciated as an option is when an end ileal stoma is technically difficult to create, the so-called end-loop ileostomy. Such a problem arises with obese patients, in whom the mesentery may be shortened and thickened, and it can also be encountered when the distal ileum has been previously resected.[54] In the latter situation, the blood supply often enters radially, with little collateral circulation between the arcade vessels.

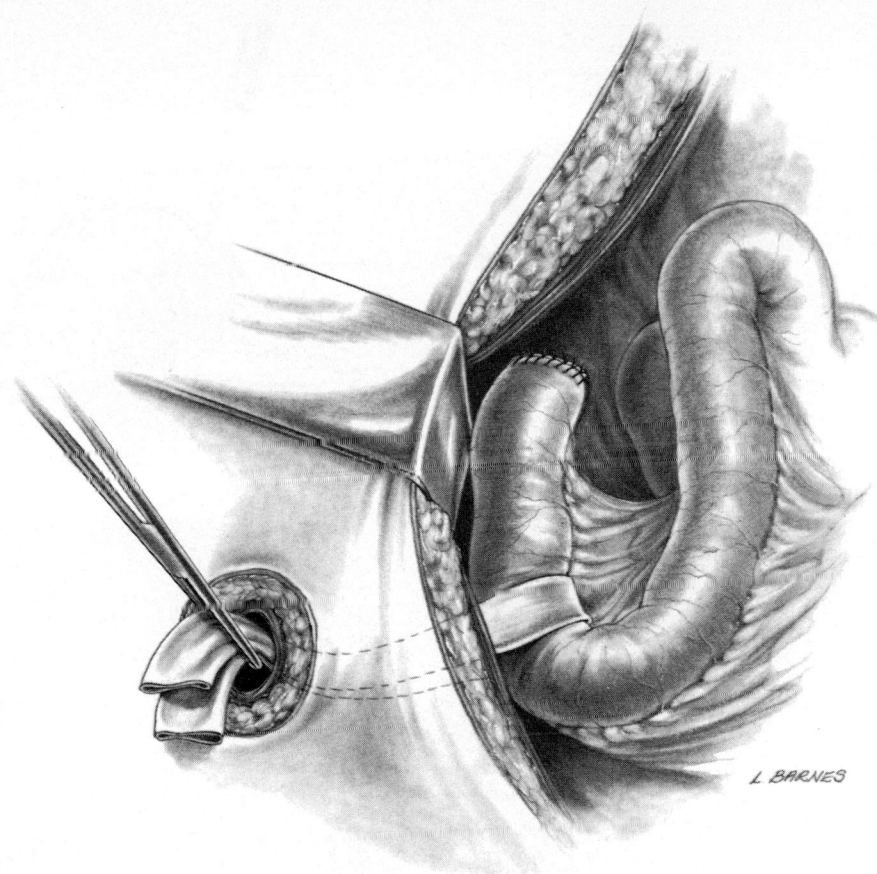

FIGURE 31-67. Loop ileostomy. The distal ileum is closed and the loop prepared for exteriorization.

Every surgeon has been confronted with the problem of insufficient bowel length for creating an adequate stoma. This necessitates trimming the mesentery, which in turn may result in devascularization of the distal ileum. When the devitalized bowel is excised, a satisfactory length again becomes unavailable, and the mesenteric vessels are again divided with the same viability problem. Finally, the surgeon may compromise and accept a less-than-optimal stomal protrusion or construct an ileostomy of sufficient length but of questionable viability. This problem can be avoided by using a loop ileostomy.

Construction Technique

After the colectomy has been performed, the distal end of the small intestine is oversewn. A disk of skin is excised in the same manner and at the same location as if for a conventional ileostomy. A point is selected 10 cm proximal to the closed ileum (a more proximal site is chosen in a grossly obese patient), and a narrow Penrose drain, vessel loop, or Robinson catheter is placed around the intestine. The loop of small bowel is brought through the split rectus muscle (Figure 31-67). A rod or catheter supports the loop, and the bowel is opened at the level of the skin on the distal, nonfunctioning side. The stoma is created by eversion with interrupted mucosubcuticular sutures of fine absorbable sutures (Figure 31-68). Eversion may be facilitated by means of Babcock clamps. The technique that has been illustrated is an alternative to an end stoma, but it is essentially the same approach if used in continuity with the distal ileum

and the colon or following restorative proctocolectomy. It is extremely useful to place Seprafilm around the small bowel (or colon, especially if the stoma is anticipated to be temporary) before it is passed through the abdominal wall (Figure 31-69). This greatly facilitates the subsequent takedown of the stoma. Moreover, the use of this material has been shown to facilitate early closure.[235]

The rod or catheter is usually removed in 3 to 5 days. Eventually, the distal end completely retracts, and the general appearance and the functional results are virtually identical to that obtained by conventional end ileostomy (Figure 31-70).

Prasad and colleagues believe that the small bowel can be transected, the mesentery incised, and the proximal and distal ends brought out together, with the distal segment de-emphasized.[191] This is analogous to that of the previously mentioned end-loop colostomy (see Figure 31-36 above). Although this may often be accomplished with safety, there is the potential risk of compromise to the blood supply. The procedure has also been described laparoscopically (see Chapter 19).[121,128]

Results

The place of loop ileostomy on a temporary basis as associated with restorative proctocolectomy has been discussed in Chapter 29. As was mentioned, there are indeed complications associated with the creation of the ileostomy itself, and they must be considered when a temporary stoma of this nature is considered. Senapati and colleagues reviewed the experience from the St. Mark's Hospital with 296 patients over a 15-year period.[217] Ileostomy-related complications prior to

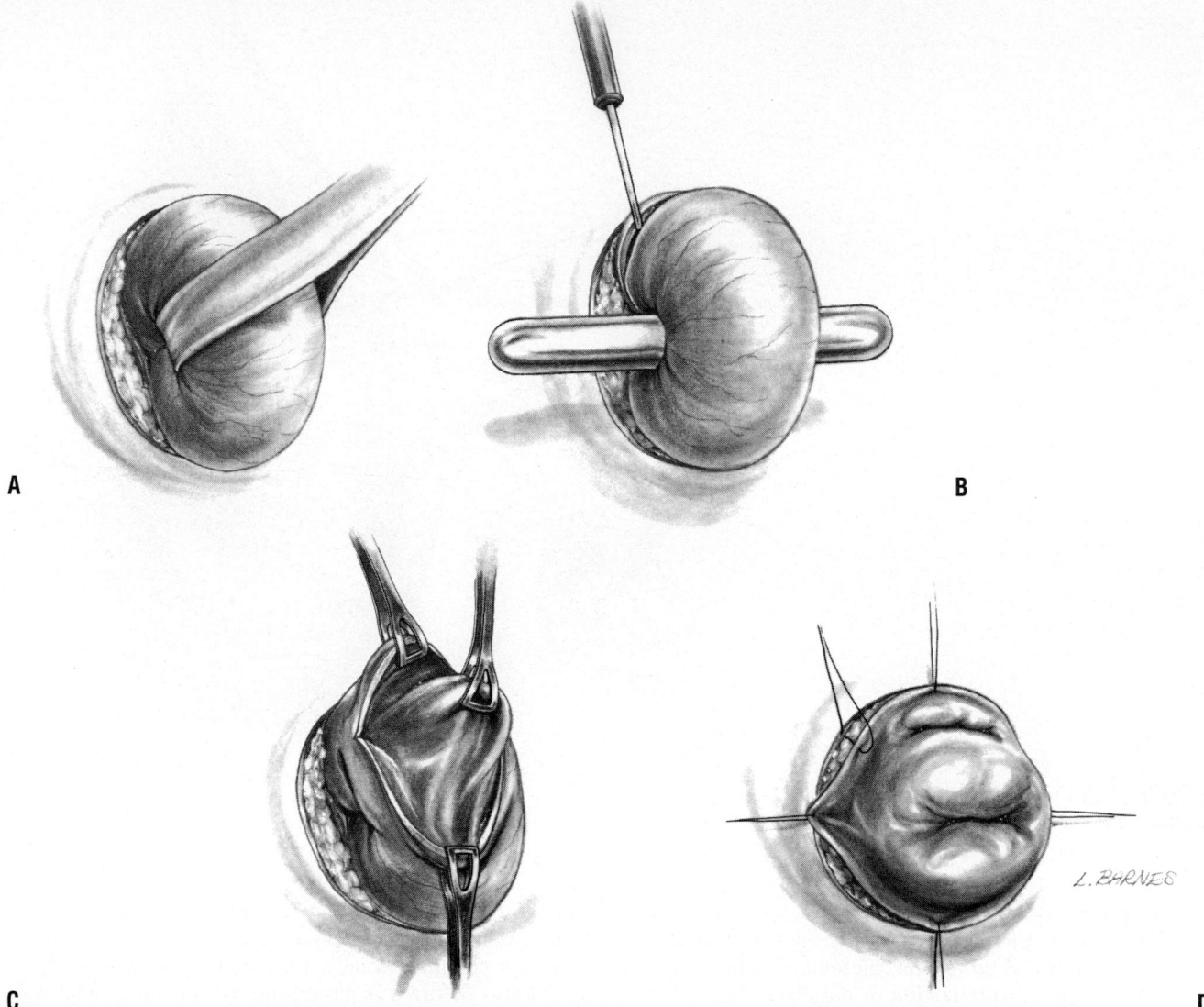

FIGURE 31-68. Loop ileostomy. **A:** Exteriorization. **B:** The distal limb is incised from mesentery to mesentery at skin level. Care must be taken to make certain which side is **proximal. C: Eversion. D:** Maturation. The rod has been omitted for simplicity of illustration.

closure occurred in 5.7%. Laparotomy for obstruction was required in 2.4%, retraction requiring revision occurred in 1%, and a peristomal abscess occurred in one patient (0.3%). Appliance management problems were seen in 2.4%. These are actually fewer complications than have been reported from other series.

Wexner and associates reported the Cleveland Clinic (Florida) experience in a prospective fashion on 83 consecutive patients who required temporary loop ileostomy for anastomoses associated with various operative procedures.[261] Four developed dehydration and electrolyte abnormalities secondary to high stomal output. One stoma retracted following rod removal. Specifically, there was no instance of stomal ischemia, hemorrhage, prolapse, or mortality.[261] Thalheimer and colleagues quantified the morbidity of temporary loop ileostomy following colorectal cancer resection in 120 patients.[240] During the 8-year study, 13.3% experienced stoma-related complications.

Williams and colleagues performed a prospective trial of patients who were undergoing colorectal surgery, randomly allocating 24 to a loop colostomy and 23 to a loop ileostomy.[267] Although both procedures adequately diverted the fecal stream, loop ileostomy was associated with significantly less odor, required fewer appliance changes, and had a lower incidence of complications when closed. Similarly, Edwards and associates (Basingstoke, United Kingdom) performed a prospective, randomized trial of the two diversion methods concomitant with low colorectal and coloanal anastomoses.[63] The higher frequency of herniation with colostomy supported their preference for loop ileostomy. Others—including me—also advocate loop ileostomy as being superior to transverse colostomy for temporary fecal diversion.[67]

A contrary view has been expressed by Law and coworkers (Hong Kong) who randomized patients following low anterior resection to loop ileostomy or loop transverse colostomy.[140] Intestinal obstruction and ileus were more common after loop ileostomy. They, therefore, recommend loop transverse colostomy as the preferred method of proximal diversion following this operation. In another randomized study of these two alternatives applied to those

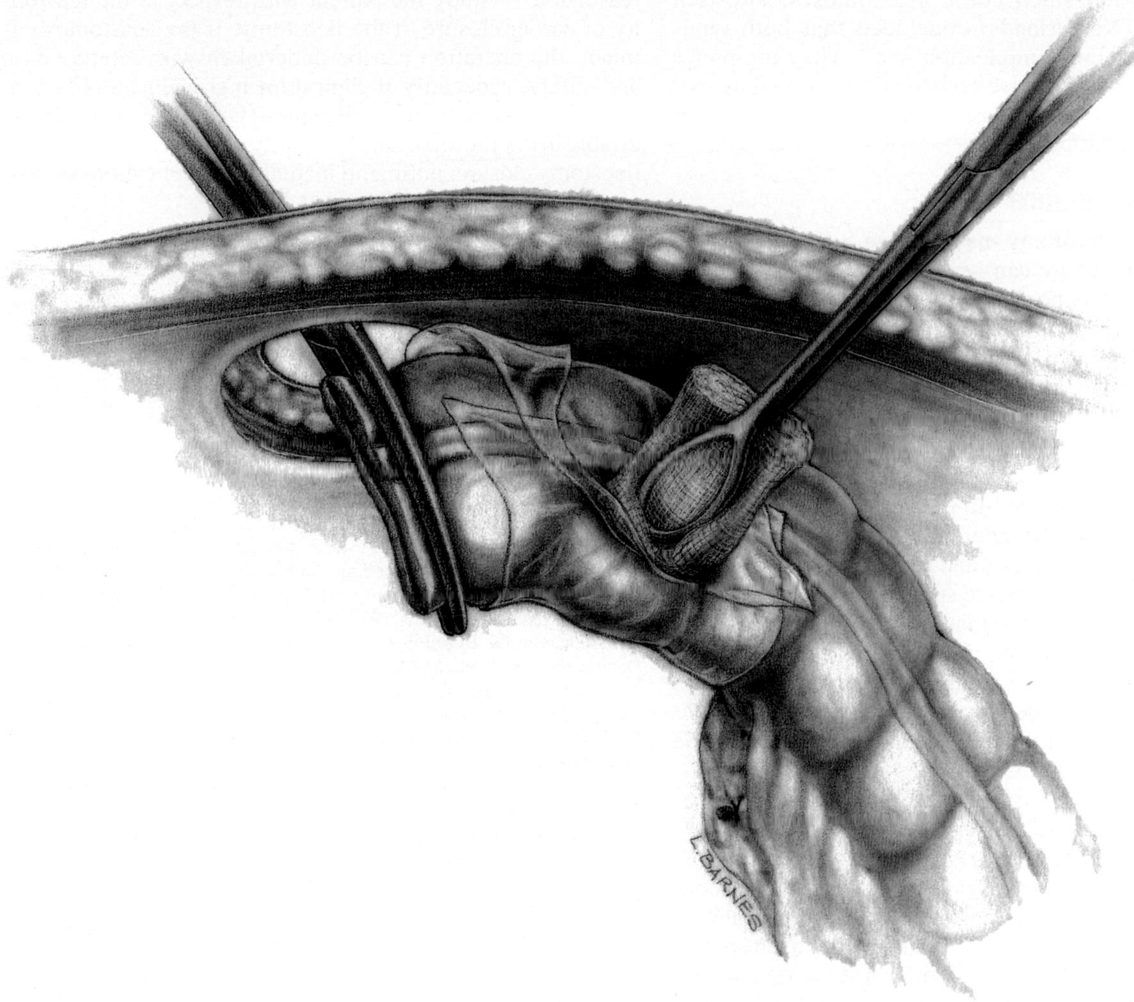

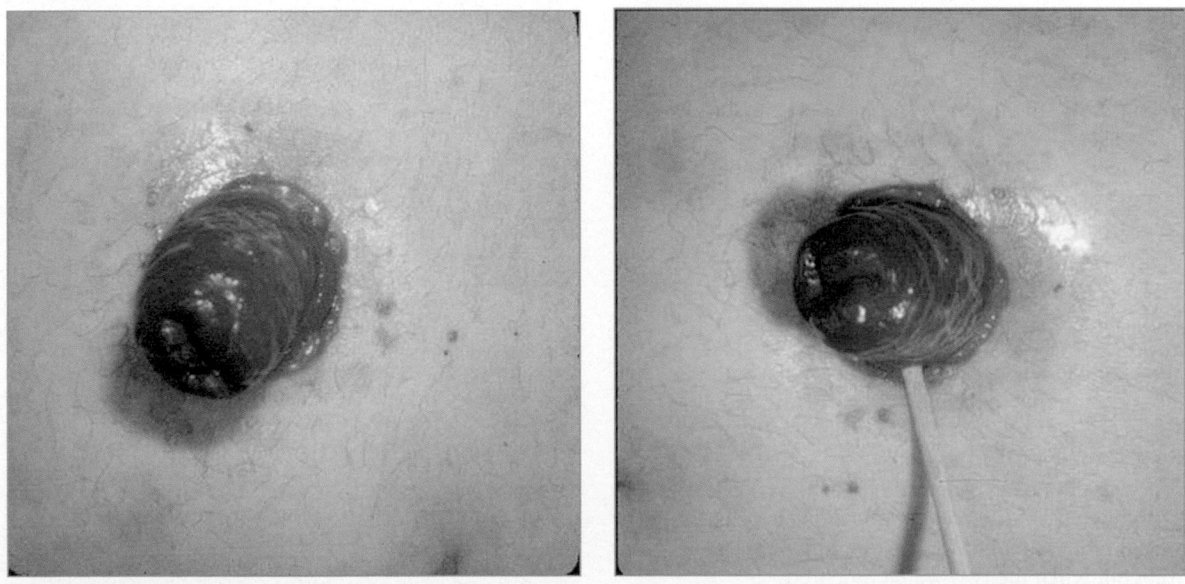

FIGURE 31-69. Wrapping the stoma with Seprafilm (Genzyme Corporation, Cambridge, MA), in this case a colostomy, prior to delivering it through the opening in the abdominal wall. This facilitates subsequent takedown.

FIGURE 31-70. Loop ileostomy several weeks following construction. **A:** On inspection, simulates an end stoma. **B:** A cotton tip applicator disappears into the distal limb inferiorly.

who underwent left-sided colon anastomoses, Gooszen and colleagues (Netherlands) concluded that both types of stomas have a high complication rate.[93] They too prefer transverse colostomy because construction, as well as closure of a loop ileostomy, was associated with more frequent and more serious complications.

Technique for Closure

Closure of a loop ileostomy may involve a resection or no resection. The procedure can be undertaken without a full laparotomy, circumcising the ileostomy as if for a revision. The proximal and distal bowel is mobilized, and the intestine is either resected or the skin and mucosa are debrided prior to simple closure. A conventional single-layer, interrupted anastomosis may be performed, and the bowel is returned to the peritoneal cavity. Along with others, I prefer, whenever possible, to employ a stapling technique, performing a side-to-side (functional end-to-end) anastomosis with the GIA stapler.[126] This has the theoretical advantage of creating a much larger luminal diameter and is generally simple to accomplish. Closure with the linear stapler completes the anastomosis in a manner similar to that described in Figure 31-43 (as applied to loop colostomy). However, resection and/or a sutured anastomosis may be necessary when there is bowel thickening or edema or when intraperitoneal adhesions limit one's ability to deliver an adequate length in order to use the side-to-side stapling instrument.

A number of skin closure techniques have been described.[125,144,160] A delayed primary closure as discussed earlier essentially eliminates the possibility of wound infection. Some have recommended irrigating with a solution containing an antibiotic. Others have shown in a randomized, double-blind, placebo-controlled trial that a collagen sponge soaked in gentamicin failed to demonstrate a statistically significant reduction in wound infection rate (40 patients in each group).[98]

Results

As mentioned earlier, the Cleveland Clinic (Florida) experience was reported by Wexner and colleagues in a prospective study involving 83 consecutive patients who underwent loop ileostomy for various indications.[261] Of the 67 who had reestablishment of intestinal continuity, three required a full laparotomy. A side-to-side stapled anastomosis was effected in approximately three-quarters of the patients. All skin wounds were left open, and the mean hospital stay was 5 days. Two developed anastomotic leaks that spontaneously healed without reoperation. One wound infection was observed, but with the skin wounds left open, this should be a rare complication indeed. Thalheimer and associates observed three anastomotic leaks after ileostomy closure in their 120 patients (2.5%) with two deaths.[240] Minor complications overall were noted in 16.7%, with neoadjuvant or adjuvant therapy associated with a 25.5% incidence. However, if no such therapy had been delivered, the incidence was 9.2%. Hull and associates evaluated the Cleveland Clinic's (Ohio) experience with hand-sewn versus stapled loop ileostomy closure.[114] This was undertaken in a randomized, prospective fashion. The procedure was performed in a statistically significantly shorter time in the stapled group, but the incidence of complications was similar and infrequent when the two were compared.[114]

When a patient is readmitted to the hospital for a problem related to the stoma or with intestinal obstruction, it is reasonable to study the patient with respect to the feasibility of earlier closure of the ileostomy. If the anastomosis is intact, the operation can be undertaken with relative ease and safety, especially if Seprafilm had been initially employed.[15,235] Kalady and colleagues (Duke University) have established a protocol for 23-hour hospitalization after loop ileostomy closure, noting no increased complications or hospital readmissions in 28 patients.[123]

References

1. Abcarian H, Pearl RK. Stomas. *Surg Clin North Am.* 1988;68(6): 1205–1305.
2. Abdu RA. Repair of paracolostomy hernias with Marlex mesh. *Dis Colon Rectum.* 1982;25(6):529–531.
3. Abrams AV, Corman ML, Veidenheimer MC. Ileostomy in the elderly. *Dis Colon Rectum.* 1975;18(2):115–117.
4. Abrams BL, Alsikafi FH, Waterman NG. Colostomy: a new look at morbidity and mortality. *Am Surg.* 1979;45(7):462–464.
5. Abulafi AM, Sherman IW, Fiddian RV. Délorme operation for prolapsed colostomy. *Br J Surg.* 1989;76(12):1321–1322.
6. Adson MA, Fulton RE. The ileal stoma and portal hypertension: an uncommon site of variceal bleeding. *Arch Surg.* 1977;112(4):501–504.
7. Alexander-Williams J, Amery AH, Devlin HB, et al. Magnetic continent colostomy device. *Br Med J.* 1977;1(6071):1269–1270.
8. Alexandre JH, Bouillot JL. Paracolostomal hernia: repair with use of a Dacron prosthesis. *World J Surg.* 1993;17(5):680–682.
9. Allen-Mersh TG, Thomson JP. Surgical treatment of colostomy complications. *Br J Surg.* 1988;75(5):416–418.
10. Anderson E, Carey LC, Cooperman M. Colostomy closure: a simple procedure? *Dis Colon Rectum.* 1979;22(7):466–468.
11. Antrum RM, Price JJ. Use of skin staples for fashioning colostomies. *Br J Surg.* 1988;75(8):736.
12. Aston CM, Everett WG. Comparison of early and late closure of transverse loop colostomies. *Ann R Coll Surg Engl.* 1984;66(5):331–333.
13. Awad RW, el-Gohary TM, Skilton JS, et al. Life quality and psychological morbidity with an ileostomy. *Br J Surg.* 1993;80(2):252–253.
14. Baker FS. The "rodless" loop colostomy. *Dis Colon Rectum.* 1975;18(6):528.
15. Bakx R, Busch OR, van Geldere D, et al. Feasibility of early closure of loop ileostomies: a pilot study. *Dis Colon Rectum.* 2003;46(12): 1680–1684.
16. Banerjee A. Pursestring skin closure after stoma reversal. *Dis Colon Rectum.* 1997;40(8):993–994.
17. Bass EM, Del Pino A, Tan A, et al. Does preoperative stoma marking and education by the enterostomal therapist affect outcome? *Dis Colon Rectum.* 1997;40(4):440–442.
18. Baxter NN, Novotny PJ, Jacobson T, et al. A stoma quality of life scale. *Dis Colon Rectum.* 2006;49(2):205–212.
19. Bayer I, Kyzer S, Chaimoff CH. A new approach to primary strengthening of colostomy with Marlex mesh to prevent paracolostomy hernia. *Surg Gynecol Obstet.* 1986;163(6):579–580.
20. Beck DE, Fazio VW, Grundfest-Broniatowski S. Surgical management of bleeding stomal varices. *Dis Colon Rectum.* 1988;31(5):343–346.
21. Beck PH, Conklin HB. Closure of colostomy. *Ann Surg.* 1975;181(6): 795–798.
22. Bedetti CD, DeRisio VJ. Primary adenocarcinoma arising at an ileostomy site. An unusual complication after colectomy for ulcerative colitis. *Dis Colon Rectum.* 1986;29(9):572–575.
23. Benacci JC, Wolff BG. Cecostomy. Therapeutic indications and results. *Dis Colon Rectum.* 1995;38(5):530–534.
24. Berger D, Bientzle M. Laparoscopic repair of parastomal hernias: a single surgeon's experience in 66 patients. *Dis Colon Rectum.* 2007;50(10):1668–1673.
25. Bergren CT, Laws HL. Modified technique of colostomy bridging. *Surg Gynecol Obstet.* 1990;170(5):453–454.
26. Berne TV, Griffith CN, Hill J, et al. Colostomy wound closure. *Arch Surg.* 1985;120(8):957–959.
27. Bickel A, Shinkarevsky E, Eitan A. Laparoscopic repair of paracolostomy hernia. *J Laparoendosc Adv Surg Tech.* 1999;9(4):353–355.
28. Billings PJ, Leaper DJ. Laser Doppler velocimetry and the measurement of colostomy blood flow. *Dis Colon Rectum.* 1987;30(5):376–380.
29. Blake DP, Scheithauer BW, van Heerden JA. Metastasis to a Brooke ileostomy—an unusual cause of stomal dysfunction. *Dis Colon Rectum.* 1981;24(8):644–646.

30. Bozzetti F, Nava M, Bufalino R, et al. Early local complications following colostomy closure in cancer patients. *Dis Colon Rectum*. 1983;26(1):25–29.

31. Brooke BN. The management of an ileostomy including its complications. *Lancet*. 1952;2(6725):102–104.

32. Brouillette JN, Pryor E, Fox TA Jr. Evaluation of sexual dysfunction in the female following rectal resection and intestinal stoma. *Dis Colon Rectum*. 1981;24(2):96–102.

33. Brown S, Holloway B, Hosie K. Percutaneous endoscopic colostomy: an alternative treatment of acute colonic pseudo-obstruction. *Colorectal Dis*. 2000;2:367.

34. Browning GG, Parks AG. A method and the results of loop colostomy. *Dis Colon Rectum*. 1983;26(4):223–226.

35. Burcharth F, Ballan A, Kylberg F, et al. The colostomy plug: a new disposable device for a continent colostomy. *Lancet*. 1986;2(8515):1062–1063.

36. Burnham WR, Lennard-Jones JE, Brooke BN. Sexual problems among married ileostomists. Survey conducted by the Ileostomy Association of Great Britain and Ireland. *Gut*. 1977;18(8):673–677.

37. Byers JM, Steinberg JB, Postier RG. Repair of parastomal hernias using polypropylene mesh. *Arch Surg*. 1992;127(10):1246–1247.

38. Carne PW, Farmer KC. Squamous-cell carcinoma developing in an ileostomy stoma: report of a case. *Dis Colon Rectum*. 2001,44(4):594.

39. Carne PW, Robertson GM, Frizelle FA. Parastomal hernia. *Br J Surg*. 2003;90(7):784–793.

40. Cattell RB. A new type of ileostomy for chronic ulcerative colitis. *Surg Clin North Am*. 1939;19:629.

41. Cerdán FJ, Díez M, Campo I, et al. Continent colostomy by means of a new one-piece disposable device. Preliminary report. *Dis Colon Rectum*. 1991;34(10):886–890.

42. Chandler JG, Evans BP. Colostomy prolapse. *Surgery*. 1978;84(5):577–582.

43. Chaudhri S, Brown L, Hassan I, et al. Preoperative intensive, community-based vs. traditional stoma education: a randomized, controlled trial. *Dis Colon Rectum*. 2005;48(3):504–509.

44. Cheung MT, Chia NH, Chiu WY. Surgical treatment of parastomal hernia complicating sigmoid colostomies. *Dis Colon Rectum*. 2001;44(2):266–270.

45. Chung RS. End colostomy and Brooke's ileostomy constructed by surgical stapler. *Surg Gynecol Obstet*. 1986;162(1):62–64.

46. Cingi A, Cakir T, Sever A, et al. Enterostomy site hernias: a clinical and computerized tomographic evaluation. *Dis Colon Rectum*. 2006;49(10):1559–1563.

47. Clague MB, Heald RJ. Achievement of stomal continence in one-third of colostomies by use of a new disposable plug. *Surg Gynecol Obstet*. 1990;170(5):390–394.

48. Codina Cazador AC, Piñol M, Marti Rague J, et al. Multicentre study of a continent colostomy plug. *Br J Surg*. 1993;80(7):930–932.

49. Colmer ML, Foxx MJ. A device for the control of colostomy prolapse. *Surg Gynecol Obstet*. 1981;152(6):827–828.

50. Conte JV, Arcomano TA, Naficy MA, et al. Treatment of bleeding stomal varices. Report of a case and review of the literature. *Dis Colon Rectum*. 1990;33(4):308–314.

51. Corman JM, Odenheimer DB. Securing the loop—historic review of the methods used for creating a loop colostomy. *Dis Colon Rectum*. 1991;34(11):1014–1021.

52. Corman ML, Veidenheimer MC, Coller JA. An appliance for management of the diverting loop colostomy. *Arch Surg*. 1974;108(5):742–743.

53. Corman ML, Veidenheimer MC, Coller JA. Ileostomy complications: prevention and treatment. *Contemp Surg*. 1976;8:36.

54. Corman ML, Veidenheimer MC, Coller JA. Loop ileostomy as an alternative to end stoma. *Surg Gynecol Obstet*. 1979;149(4):585–586.

55. Crile G Jr, Turnbull RB Jr. The mechanism and prevention of ileostomy dysfunction. *Ann Surg*. 1954;140(4):459–466.

56. Cromar CD. The evolution of colostomy. *Dis Colon Rectum*. 1968;11:256,367,423.

57. Cuesta MA, Donner R. Adenocarcinoma arising at an ileostomy site: report of a case. *Cancer*. 1976;37(2):949–952.

58. Daniels I, Lamparelli MJ, Chave H, et al. Recurrent sigmoid volvulus treated by percutaneous endoscopic colostomy. *Br J Surg*. 2000;87(10):1419.

59. Dinnick T. The origins and evolution of colostomy. *Br J Surg*. 1934–1935;22:142.

60. Dolan PA, Caldwell FT, Thompson CH, et al. Problems of colostomy closure. *Am J Surg*. 1979;137(2):188–191.

61. Doran J, Hardcastle JD. A controlled trial of colostomy management by natural evacuation, irrigation, and foam enema. *Br J Surg*. 1981;68(10):731–733.

62. Dragstedt LR, Dack GM, Kirsner JB. Chronic ulcerative colitis: a summary of evidence implicating *Bacterium necrophorum* as an etiologic agent. *Ann Surg*. 1941;114(4):653–662.

63. Edwards DP, Leppington-Clarke A, Sexton R, et al. Stoma-related complications are more frequent after transverse colostomy than loop ileostomy: a prospective randomized clinical trial. *Br J Surg*. 2001;88(3):360–363.

64. Ellis CN. Short-term outcomes with the use of bioprosthetics for the management of parastomal hernia. *Dis Colon Rectum*. 2010;53(3):279–283.

65. Eng K, Localio A. Simplified complementary transverse colostomy for low colorectal anastomosis. *Surg Gynecol Obstet*. 1981;153(5):735.

66. Evans JP, Brown MH, Wilkes GH, et al. Revising the troublesome stoma: combines abdominal wall recontouring and revision of stomas. *Dis Colon Rectum*. 2003;46(1):122–126.

67. Fasth S, Hultén L. Loop ileostomy: a superior diverting stoma in colorectal surgery. *World J Surg*. 1984;8(3):401–407.

68. Feustel H, Hennig G. Kontinent kolostomie durch magnetverschluss [Colostomy continence achieved with an implanted circular magnet]. *Dtsch Med Wochenschr*. 1975;100(19):1063–1064.

69. Fine P. *Am de la Soc de Montpelier*. 1797;6:34.

70. Finemore RG. Repeated haemorrhage from a terminal colostomy due to mucocutaneous varices with coexisting hepatic metastatic rectal adenocarcinoma: a case report. *Br J Surg*. 1979;66(11):806.

71. Fitzgibbons RJ Jr, Schmitz GD, Bailey RT Jr. A simple technique for constructing a loop enterostomy which allows immediate placement of an ostomy appliance. *Surg Gynecol Obstet*. 1987;164(1):78–80.

72. Fligelstone LJ, Wanendeya N, Palmer BV. Osmotic therapy for acute irreducible stoma prolapse. *Br J Surg*. 1997;84(3):390.

73. Fontes B, Fontes W, Utiyama EM, et al. The efficacy of loop colostomy for complete fecal diversion. *Dis Colon Rectum*. 1988;31(4):298–302.

74. Foster ME, Leaper DJ, Williamson RC. Changing patterns in colostomy closure: the Bristol experience 1975–1982. *Br J Surg*. 1985;72(2):142–145.

75. Freund HR, Raniel J, Muggia-Sulam M. Factors affecting the morbidity of colostomy closure: a retrospective study. *Dis Colon Rectum*. 1982;25(7):712–715.

76. Fuhrman GM, Ota DM. Laparoscopic intestinal stomas. *Dis Colon Rectum*. 1994;37(5):444–449.

77. Gadacz TR, McFadden DW, Gabrielson EW, et al. Adenocarcinoma of the ileostomy: the latent risk of cancer after colectomy for ulcerative colitis and familial polyposis. *Surgery*. 1990;107(6):698–703.

78. Garber HI, Morris DM, Eisenstat TE, et al. Factors influencing the morbidity of colostomy closure. *Dis Colon Rectum*. 1982;25(5):464–470.

79. Garnjobst W, Leaverton GH, Sullivan ES. Safety of colostomy closure. *Am J Surg*. 1978;136(1):85–89.

80. Garnjobst W, Sullivan ES. Repair of paraileostomy hernia with polypropylene mesh reinforcement. *Dis Colon Rectum*. 1984;27(4):268–269.

81. Gawron CL. Colostomy irrigations: mechanism guidelines. *Ostomy Wound Manage*. 1990;28:56–61.

82. Gilson TP, Sollenberger LL. Adenocarcinoma of an ileostomy in a patient with familial adenomatous polyposis. Report of a case. *Dis Colon Rectum*. 1992;35(3):261–265.

83. Gazzard BS, Januzzi JL. Paracolostomy carcinoma. *Am J Proctol Gastroenterol Colon Rectal Surg*. 1984;35:9.

84. Giunchi F, Cacciaguerra G, Drudi G. Burn and stricture of the ostomy due to colostomy irrigation. Report of a case. *Dis Colon Rectum*. 1985;28(11):873–874.

85. Gloeckner MR, Starling JR. Providing sexual information to ostomy patients. *Dis Colon Rectum*. 1982;25(6):575–579.

86. Gögenur I, Mortensen J, Harvald T, et al. Prevention of parastomal hernia by placement of a polypropylene mesh at the primary operation. *Dis Colon Rectum*. 2006;49(8):1131–1135.

87. Goldblatt MS, Corman ML, Haggitt RC, et al. Ileostomy complications requiring revision: Lahey Clinic experience, 1964–1973. *Dis Colon Rectum*. 1977;20(3):209–214.

88. Goldstein S, Sohn N, Weinstein MA, et al. Simplified loop ostomy fixation using rubber tubing. *Surg Gynecol Obstet*. 1984;158(4):375–376.

89. Goldstein SD, Salvati EP, Rubin RJ, et al. Tube cecostomy with cecal extraperitonealization in the management of obstructing left sided carcinoma of the large intestine. *Surg Gynecol Obstet*. 1986;162(4):379–380.

90. Goldstein WZ, Edoga J, Crystal R. Management of colostomal hemorrhage resulting from portal hypertension. *Dis Colon Rectum*. 1980;23(2):86–90.

91. Goligher JC, Lee PW, McMahon MJ, et al. The Erlangen magnetic colostomy control device: technique of use and results in 22 patients. *Br J Surg*. 1977;64(7):501–507.

92. Gomez ER, Rosenthal D. Management of a subcutaneous colostomy perforation. The role a new synthetic skin. *Dis Colon Rectum*. 1984;27(10):651–653.

93. Gooszen AW, Geelkerken RH, Hermans J, et al. Temporary decompression after colorectal surgery: randomized comparison of loop ileostomy and loop colostomy. *Br J Surg*. 1998;85(1):76–79.

94.   Gooszen AW, Geelkerken RH, Hermans J, et al. Quality of life with a temporary stoma: ileostomy vs. colostomy. *Dis Colon Rectum.* 2000;43(5):650–655.

95.   Greatorex RA. Simple method of closing a para-ileostomy fistula. *Br J Surg.* 1988;75(6):543.

96.   Greenstein AJ, Dicker A, Meyers S, et al. Periileostomy fistulae in Crohn's disease. *Ann Surg.* 1983;197(2):179–182.

97.   Guillemot F, Colombel JF, Neut C, et al. Treatment of diversion colitis by short-chain fatty acids. Prospective and double-blind study. *Dis Colon Rectum.* 1991;34(10):861–864.

98.   Haase O, Raue W, Böhm B, et al. Subcutaneous gentamycin implant to reduce wound infections after loop-ileostomy closure: a randomized, double-blind, placebo-controlled trial. *Dis Colon Rectum.* 2005;48(11):2025–2031.

99.   Halevy A, Adam Y, Eshchar J. Ileostomates in Israel. *Dis Colon Rectum.* 1977;20(6):482–485.

100. Handelsman JC, Fishbein RH. Stabilization of ileostomy position with fascia. *Surgery.* 1983;93(1 pt 1):88–90.

101. Handschin AE, Weber M, Weinhaupt D, et al. Contrast-enhanced three-dimensional magnetic resonance angiography for visualization of ectopic varices. *Dis Colon Rectum.* 2002;45(11):1541–1544.

102. Harries K, Owen C, Mills C, et al. Acute stomal "contact" dermatitis or pemphigus. *Br J Surg.* 1997;84(5):685.

103. Heiblum M, Cordoba A. An artificial sphincter: a preliminary report. *Dis Colon Rectum.* 1978;21(8):562–566.

104. Hellinger MD, Martinez SA, Parra-Davila E, et al. Gasless laparoscopic-assisted intestinal stoma creation through a single incision. *Dis Colon Rectum.* 1999;42(9):1228–1231.

105. Henry MM, Everett WG. Loop colostomy closure. *Br J Surg.* 1979;66(4):275–277.

106. Heriot AG, Tilney HS, Simson JN. The application of percutaneous endoscopic colostomy to the management of obstructed defecation. *Dis Colon Rectum.* 2002;45(5):700–702.

107. Hesterberg R, Stahlknecht CD, Röher HD. Sclerotherapy for massive enterostomy bleeding resulting from portal hypertension. *Dis Colon Rectum.* 1986;29(4):275–277.

108. Hines JR. A method of transverse loop colostomy. *Surg Gynecol Obstet.* 1975;141(3):426–428.

109. Hines JR, Harris GD. Colostomy and colostomy closure. *Surg Clin North Am.* 1983;57:1379.

110. Hiranyakas A, Ho YH. Laparoscopic parastomal hernia repair. *Dis Colon Rectum.* 2010;53(9):1334–1336.

111. Hoffmann J, Jensen HE. Tube cecostomy and staged resection for obstructing carcinoma of the colon. *Dis Colon Rectum.* 1984;27(1):24–32.

112. Hofstetter WL, Vukasin P, Ortega AE, et al. New technique for mesh repair of paracolostomy hernias. *Dis Colon Rectum.* 1998;41(8):1054–1055.

113. Hollyoak MA, Lumley J, Stitz RW. Laparoscopic stoma formation for faecal diversion. *Br J Surg.* 1998;85(2):226–228.

114. Hull TL, Kobe I, Fazio VW. Comparison of handsewn with stapled loop ileostomy closures. *Dis Colon Rectum.* 1996;39(10):1086–1089.

115. Hunt N, Corman ML. Enterostomal therapy. *Contemp Educ.* 1982:79.

116. Inan I, Gervaz P, Hagen M, et al. Multimedia article. Laparoscopic repair of parastomal hernia using a porcine dermal collagen (Permacol) implant. *Dis Colon Rectum.* 2007;50(9):1465.

117. Isa S, Quan SH. Colostomy perforation. *Dis Colon Rectum.* 1978;21(2):92–93.

118. Jänes A, Cengiz Y, Israelsson LA. Randomized clinical trial of the use of a prosthetic mesh to prevent parastomal hernia. *Br J Surg.* 2004;91:280.

119. Jao SW, Beart RW Jr, Wendorf LJ, et al. Irrigation management of sigmoid colostomy. *Arch Surg.* 1985;120(8):916–917.

120. Jarpa S. Transverse or sigmoid loop colostomy fixed by skin flaps. *Surg Gynecol Obstet.* 1986;163(4):372–374.

121. Jess P, Christiansen J. Laparoscopic loop ileostomy for fecal diversion. *Dis Colon Rectum.* 1994;37(7):721–722.

122. Johnson WR, McDermott FT, Pihl E, et al. Adenocarcinoma of an ileostomy in a patient with ulcerative colitis. *Dis Colon Rectum.* 1980;23(5):351–352.

123. Kalady MF, Fields RC, Klein S, et al. Loop ileostomy closure at an ambulatory surgery facility: a safe and cost-effective alternative to routine hospitalization. *Dis Colon Rectum.* 2003;46(4):486–490.

124. Kald A, Landin S, Masreliez C, et al. Mesh repair of parastomal hernias: new aspects of the Onlay technique. *Tech Coloproctol.* 2001;5(3):169–171.

125. Keating J, Kelly EW, Hunt I. Save the skin and improve the scar: a simple tecnique to minimize the scar from a temporary stoma. *Dis Colon Rectum.* 2003;46(10):1428–1429.

126. Kestenberg A, Becker JM. A new technique of loop ileostomy closure after endorectal ileoanal anastomosis. *Surgery.* 1985;98(1):109–111.

127. Kewenter J. Continent colostomy with the aid of a magnetic closing system: a preliminary report. *Dis Colon Rectum.* 1978;21(1):46–51.

128. Khoo RE, Montrey J, Cohen MM. Laparoscopic loop ileostomy for temporary fecal diversion. *Dis Colon Rectum.* 1993;36(10):966–968.

129. Khubchandani IT, Trimpi HD, Sheets JA, et al. The magnetic stoma device: a continent colostomy. *Dis Colon Rectum.* 1981;24(5):344–350.

130. Kock NG, Geroulanos S, Hahnloser P, et al. Continent colostomy: an experimental study in dogs. *Dis Colon Rectum.* 1974;17(6):727–734.

131. Kock NG, Myrvold HE, Philipson BM, et al. Continent cecostomy. An account of 30 patients. *Dis Colon Rectum.* 1985;28(10):705–708.

132. Kostov DV, Temelkov TD, Dragnev NA, et al. Smooth muscle sphincteroplasty in colostomy. *Dis Colon Rectum.* 2004;47(4):486–493.

133. Krasna IH. A simple purse string suture technique for treatment of colostomy prolapse and intussusception. *J Pediatr Surg.* 1979;14(6):801–802.

134. Krause R, Freund HR, Fischer JE. A new technique for performing end enterostomies using a stapling device. *Am J Surg.* 1979;138(3):461–462.

135. Kretschmer KP. *The Intestinal Stomas: Indications, Operative Methods, Care, Rehabilitation.* Philadelphia, PA: WB Saunders; 1978.

136. Kronborg O, Kramhöft J, Backer O, et al. Late complications following operations for cancer of the rectum and anus. *Dis Colon Rectum.* 1974;17(6):750–753.

137. Lafreniere R, Ketcham AS. The Penrose drain: a safe, atraumatic colostomy bridge. *Am J Surg.* 1985;149(2):288–291.

138. Last M, Fazio V, Lavery I, et al. Conservative management of para-ileostomy ulcers in patients with Crohn's disease. *Dis Colon Rectum.* 1984;27(12):779–786.

139. Lau JT. Proximal end transverse colostomy in children. A method to avoid colostomy prolapse in Hirschsprung's disease. *Dis Colon Rectum.* 1983;26(4):221–222.

140. Law WL, Chu KW, Choi HK. Randomized clinical trial comparing loop ileostomy and loop transverse colostomy for faecal diversion following total mesorectal excision. *Br J Surg.* 2002;89(6):704–708.

141. LeBlanc KA, Bellanger DE. Laparoscopic repair of paraostomy hernias: early results. *J Am Coll Surg.* 2002;194(2):232–239.

142. Leong AP, Londono-Schimmer EE, Phillips RK. Life-table analysis of stomal complications following ileostomy. *Br J Surg.* 1994;81(5):727–729.

143. Light HG. A secure end colostomy technique. *Surg Gynecol Obstet.* 1992;174(1):67–68.

144. Lim JT, Shedda SM, Hayes IP. "Gunsight" skin incision and closure technique for stoma reversal. *Dis Colon Rectum.* 2010;53(11):1569–1575.

145. Londono-Schimmer EE, Leong AP, Phillips RK. Life table analysis of stomal complications following colostomy. *Dis Colon Rectum.* 1994;37(9):916–920.

146. López-Cano M, Lozoya-Trujillo R, Espin-Basany E. Prosthetic mesh in parastomal hernia prevention. A laparoscopic approach. *Dis Colon Rectum.* 2009;52(5):1006–1007.

147. Ludwig KA, Milsom JW, Garcia-Ruiz A, et al. Laparoscopic techniques for fecal diversion. *Dis Colon Rectum.* 1996;39(3):285–288.

148. Marimuthu K, Vijayasekar C, Ghosh D, et al. Prevention of parastomal hernia using preperitoneal mesh: a prospective observational study. *Colorectal Dis.* 2006;8(8):672–675.

149. Marks CG, Ritchie JK. The complications of synchronous combined excision for adenocarcinoma of the rectum at St. Mark's Hospital. *Br J Surg.* 1975;62(11):901–905.

150. Mattingly M, Wasvary H, Sacksner J, et al. Minimally invasive, endoscopically assisted colostomy can be performed without general anesthesia or laparotomy. *Dis Colon Rectum.* 2003;46(2):271–273.

151. Maxwell TR, Taylor D, Durnal AM, et al. Safety and efficacy of a novel continence device in colostomy patients. *Dis Colon Rectum.* 2010;53(10):1422–1431.

152. Maydl K. Zur technik der kolostomie. *Centralbl Chir.* 1888;24:433.

153. Mayo CW. Button colopexy for prolapse of colon through colonic stoma. *Mayo Clin Proc.* 1939;14:439.

154. McGarity WC. The evolution of continence following total colectomy. *Am J Surg.* 1992;58(1):1–16.

155. McGarity WC, Robertson DB, McKeown PP, et al. Pyoderma gangrenosum at the parastomal site in patients with Crohn's disease. *Arch Surg.* 1984;119(10):1186–1188.

156. McLeod RS, Lavery IC, Leatherman JR, et al. Patient evaluation of the conventional ileostomy. *Dis Colon Rectum.* 1985;28(3):152–154.

157. Mealy K, O'Broin E, Donohue J, et al. Reversible colostomy—what is the outcome? *Dis Colon Rectum.* 1996;39(11):1227–1231.

158. Meuwissen SG, Bakker PJ, Rietra PJ. Acute ulceration of ileal stoma due to *Campylobacter fetus* subspecies *jejuni*. *Br Med J (Clin Res Ed)*. 1981;282(6273):1362.

159. Meyerhoff HH, Andersen B, Nielsen SL. Colostomy irrigation: a clinical and scintigraphic comparison between three different irrigation volumes. *Br J Surg*. 1990;77(10):1185–1186.

160. Milanchi S, Nasseri Y, Kidner T, et al. Wound infection after ileostomy closure can be eliminated by circumferential subcuticular wound approximation. *Dis Colon Rectum*. 2009;52(3):469–474.

161. Miles RM, Greene RS. Review of colostomy in a community hospital. *Am Surg*. 1983;49(4):182–186.

162. Mileski WJ, Rege RV, Joehl RJ, et al. Rates of morbidity and mortality after closure of loop and end colostomy. *Surg Gynecol Obstet*. 1990;171(1):17–21.

163. Mirelman D, Corman ML, Veidenheimer MC, et al. Colostomies: indications and contraindications. Lahey Clinic experience, 1963–1974. *Dis Colon Rectum*. 1978;21(3):172–176.

164. Mitchell WH, Kovalcik PJ, Cross GH. Complications of colostomy closure. *Dis Colon Rectum*. 1978;21(3):180–182.

165. Moisidis E, Curtiskis JI, Brooke-Cowden GL. Improving the reinforcement of parastomal tissues with Marlex mesh: laboratory study identifying solutions to stomal aperture distortion. *Dis Colon Rectum*. 2000;43(1):55–60.

166. Morgan TR, Feldshon SD, Tripp MR. Recurrent stomal variceal bleeding. Successful treatment using injection sclerotherapy. *Dis Colon Rectum*. 1986;29(4):269–270.

167. Morowitz DA, Kirsner JB. Ileostomy in ulcerative colitis. A questionnaire study of 1,803 patients. *Am J Surg*. 1981;141(3):370–375.

168. Morris DM, Rayburn D. Loop colostomies are totally diverting in adults. *Am J Surg*. 1991;161(6):668–671.

169. Moseson MD, Labow SB, Hoexter B. Technique for totally diverting loop transverse colostomy. *Dis Colon Rectum*. 1983;26(3):195.

170. Mukherjee A, Parikh VA, Aguilar PS. Colonoscopic-assisted colostomy—an alternative to laparotomy: report of two cases. *Dis Colon Rectum*. 1998;41(11):1458–1460.

171. Nakahara S, Itoh H, Iida M, et al. Ileal adenomas in familial polyposis coli. Differences before and after colectomy. *Dis Colon Rectum*. 1985;28(11):875–877.

172. Narasimharao KL, Chatterjee H. A new technique of prolapse-free transverse colostomy. *Surg Gynecol Obstet*. 1984;158(3):283.

173. Nguyen HM, Causey MW, Steele SR, et al. Single-port laparoscopic diverting sigmoid colostomy. *Dis Colon Rectum*. 2011;54(12):1585–1588.

174. Nugent KP, Daniels P, Stewart B, et al. Quality of life in stoma patients. *Dis Colon Rectum*. 1999;42(12):1569–1574.

175. O'Bichere A, Bossom C, Gangoli S, et al. Chemical colostomy irrigation with glyceryl trinitrate solution. *Dis Colon Rectum*. 2001;44(9):1324–1327.

176. O'Connell PR, Dozois RR, Irons GB, et al. Squamous cell carcinoma occurring in a skin-grafted ileostomy stoma. Report of a case. *Dis Colon Rectum*. 1987;30(6):475–478.

177. Oluwole SF, Freeham HP, Davis K. Morbidity of closure of colostomy. *Dis Colon Rectum*. 1982;25:422.

178. Park JJ, Del Pino A, Orsay CP, et al. Stoma complications: the Cook County Hospital experience. *Dis Colon Rectum*. 1999;42(12):1575–1580.

179. Patey DH. Primary epithelial apposition in colostomy. *Proc R Soc Med*. 1951;44(6):423–424.

180. Pearl RK. Parastomal hernia. *World J Surg*. 1989;13(5):569–572.

181. Peck JJ, Boyden AM. Exigent ileostomy hemorrhage. A complication of proctocolectomy in patients with chronic ulcerative colitis and primary sclerosing cholangitis. *Am J Surg*. 1985;150(1):153–158.

182. Pemberton JH, van Heerden JA, Beart RW Jr, et al. A continent ileostomy device. *Ann Surg*. 1983;197(5):618–626.

183. Pilgrim CH, McIntyre R, Bailey M. Prospective audit of parastomal hernia: prevalence and associated comorbidities. *Dis Colon Rectum*. 2010;53(1):71–76.

184. Pittman DM, Smith LE. Complications of colostomy closure. *Dis Colon Rectum*. 1985;28(11):836–843.

185. Ponsky JL, Aszodi A, Perse D. Percutaneous endoscopic cecostomy: a new approach to nonobstructive colonic dilation. *Gastrointest Endosc*. 1986;32(2):108–111.

186. Porcheron J, Payan B, Balique JG. Mesh repair of parastomal hernia by laparoscopy. *Surg Endosc*. 1998;12(10):1281.

187. Porter JA, Salvati EP, Rubin RJ, et al. Complications of colostomies. *Dis Colon Rectum*. 1989;32(4):299–303.

188. Prager E. The continent colostomy. *Dis Colon Rectum*. 1984;27(4):235–237.

189. Prager E, Gall F. A new method of stoma control. *Contemp Surg*. 1985;26:81.

190. Prasad ML, Pearl RK, Abcarian H. End-loop colostomy. *Surg Gynecol Obstet*. 1984;158(4):380–382.

191. Prasad ML, Pearl RK, Orsay CP, et al. Rodless ileostomy. A modified loop ileostomy. *Dis Colon Rectum*. 1984;27(4):270–271.

192. Prian GW, Sawyer RB, Sawyer KC. Repair of peristomal colostomy hernias. *Am J Surg*. 1975;130(6):694–696.

193. Ramia JM, Ibarra A, Alcalde J. Resection of an end-colostomy stricture with a circular stapling device. *Br J Surg*. 1996;83(11):1581.

194. Raza SD, Portin BA, Bernhoft WH. Umbilical colostomy: a better intestinal stoma. *Dis Colon Rectum*. 1977;20(3):223–230.

195. Resnick S. New method of bowel stoma formation. *Am J Surg*. 1986;152(5):545–548.

196. Reynolds HM Jr, Frazier TG, Copeland EM III. Treatment of paracolostomy abscess without proximal diverting colostomy: report of two cases. *Dis Colon Rectum*. 1976;19(5):458–459.

197. Rickwood AM, Hemalatha V, Brooman P. Closure of colostomy in infants and children. *Br J Surg*. 1979;66(4):273–274.

198. Roberts PL, Martin FM, Schoetz DJ Jr, et al. Bleeding stomal varices. The role of local treatment. *Dis Colon Rectum*. 1990;33(7):547–549.

199. Roberts PL, Veidenheimer MC, Cassidy S, et al. Adenocarcinoma arising in an ileostomy. *Arch Surg*. 1989;124(4):497–499.

200. Roe AM, Barlow AP, Durdey P, et al. Indications for laparoscopic formation of intestinal stomas. *Surg Laparosc Endosc*. 1994;4(5):345–347.

201. Rolstad BS, Wilson W, Rothenberger DA. Sexual concerns in the patient with an ileostomy. *Dis Colon Rectum*. 1983;26(3):170–171.

202. Rombeau JL, Turnbull RB Jr. Hidden-loop colostomy. *Dis Colon Rectum*. 1978;21(3):177–179.

203. Rombeau JL, Wilk PJ, Turnbull RB Jr, et al. Total fecal diversion by the temporary skin-level loop transverse colostomy. *Dis Colon Rectum*. 1978;21(4):223–226.

204. Rosen L, Friedman IH. Morbidity and mortality following intraperitoneal closure of transverse loop colostomy. *Dis Colon Rectum*. 1980;23(7):508–512.

205. Rosin JD, Bonardi RA. Paracolostomy hernia repair with Marlex mesh: a new technique. *Dis Colon Rectum*. 1977;20(4):299–302.

206. Roy PH, Saver WG, Beahrs OH, et al. Experience with ileostomies. Evaluation of long-term rehabilitation in 497 patients. *Am J Surg*. 1970;119(1):77–86.

207. Rubin MS, Schoetz DJ Jr, Matthews JB. Parastomal hernia. Is stoma relocation superior to fascial repair? *Arch Surg*. 1994;129(4):413–418.

208. Sachatello CR, Maull KI. Rapid totally diverting loop sigmoid colostomy with noncontaminating rectal irrigation. *Am J Surg*. 1977;134(2):300.

209. Salley RK, Bucher RM, Rodning CB. Colostomy closure. Morbidity reduction employing a semi-standardized protocol. *Dis Colon Rectum*. 1983;26(5):319–322.

210. Samhouri F, Grodsinsky C. The morbidity and mortality of colostomy closure. *Dis Colon Rectum*. 1979;22(5):312–314.

211. Sanders GB. Experiences with the Dragstedt skin-covered ileostomy. *Arch Surg*. 1948;57(4):487–496.

212. Sarashina H, Ozaki A, Fukao K, et al. A new device for barium-enema examination following colostomy. *Radiology*. 1979;133(1):241–242.

213. Schmidt E. The continent colostomy. *World J Surg*. 1982;6(6):805–809.

214. Schofield PF, Cade D, Lambert M. Dependent proximal loop colostomy: does it defunction the distal colon? *Br J Surg*. 1980;67(3):201–202.

215. Schwemmle K, Kunze HH, Padberg W. Management of the colostomy. *World J Surg*. 1982;6(5):554–559.

216. Senapati A, Nicholls RJ. Formation of a loop stoma. *Br J Surg*. 1991;78(1):23.

217. Senapati A, Nicholls RJ, Ritchie JK, et al. Temporary loop ileostomy for restorative proctocolectomy. *Br J Surg*. 1993;80(5):628–630.

218. Sherlock DJ, Suarez V, Gray JG. Stomal adenocarcinoma in Crohn's disease. *Gut*. 1990;31(11):1329–1332.

219. Sigler L, Jedd FL. Adenocarcinoma of the ileostomy occurring after colectomy for ulcerative colitis: report of a case. *Dis Colon Rectum*. 1969;12(1):45–48.

220. Sigurdson E, Myers E, Stern H. A modification of the transverse loop colostomy. *Dis Colon Rectum*. 1986;29(1):65–66.

221. Sjödahl R, Anderberg B, Bolin T. Parastomal hernia in relation to site of the abdominal stoma. *Br J Surg*. 1988;75(4):339–341.

222. Smart PJ, Sastry S, Wells S. Primary mucinous adenocarcinoma developing in an ileostomy stoma. *Gut*. 1988;29(11):1607–1612.

223. Smit R, Walt AJ. The morbidity and cost of the temporary colostomy. *Dis Colon Rectum*. 1978;21(5):558–561.

224. Soliani P, Carbognani P, Piccolo P, et al. Colostomy plug devices: a possible new approach to the problem of incontinence. *Dis Colon Rectum*. 1992;35(10):969–974.

225. Speakman CT, Parker MC, Northover JMA. Outcome of stapled revision of retracted ileostomy. *Br J Surg.* 1991;78(8):935–936.

226. Steinberg DM, Allan RN, Brooke BN, et al. Sequelae of colectomy and ileostomy: comparison between Crohn's colitis and ulcerative colitis. *Gastroenterology.* 1975;68(1):33–39.

227. Stelzner S, Hellmich G, Ludwig K. Repair of paracolostomy hernias with a prosthetic mesh in the intraperitoneal onlay position: modified Sugarbaker technique. *Dis Colon Rectum.* 2004;47(2):185–191.

228. Stephenson ER Jr, Ilahi O, Koltun WA. Stoma creation through the stoma site: a rapid, safe technique. *Dis Colon Rectum.* 1997;40(1):112–115.

229. Stryker SJ, Pemberton JH, Zinsmeister AR. Long-term results of ileostomy in older patients. *Dis Colon Rectum.* 1985;28(11):844–846.

230. Sugarbaker PH. Prosthetic mesh repair of large hernias at the site of colonic stomas. *Surg Gynecol Obstet.* 1980;150(4):576–578.

231. Sugarbaker PH. Peritoneal approach to prosthetic mesh repair of paraostomy hernias. *Ann Surg.* 1985;201(3):344–346.

232. Swain BT, Ellis CN Jr. Laparoscopy-assisted loop ileostomy: an acceptable option for temporary fecal diversion after anorectal surgery. *Dis Colon Rectum.* 2002;45(5):705–707.

233. Sykes FR. Transcutaneous defunctioning colostomy. *Br J Surg.* 1979;66(7):505–506.

234. Szinicz G. A new implantable sphincter prosthesis for artificial anus. *Int J Artif Organs.* 1980;3(6):358–362.

235. Tang CL, Seow-Choen F, Fook-Chong S, et al. Bioresorbable adhesion barrier facilitates early closure of the defunctioning ileostomy after rectal excision: a prospective, randomized trial. *Dis Colon Rectum.* 2003;46(9):1200–1207.

236. Taylor RL Jr, Rombeau JL, Turnbull RB Jr. Transperitoneal relocation of the ileal stoma without formal laparotomy. *Surg Gynecol Obstet.* 1978;146(6):953–958.

237. Tekkis PP, Kocher HM, Payne JG. Parastomal hernia repair: modified Thorlakson technique, reinforced by polypropylene mesh. *Dis Colon Rectum.* 1999;42(11):1505–1508.

238. Tenney JB, Graney MJ. The quest for continence: a morphologic survey of approaches to a continent colostomy. *Dis Colon Rectum.* 1978;21(7):522–533.

239. Terranova O, Sandei F, Rebuffat C, et al. Irrigation vs. natural evacuation of left colostomy: a comparative study of 340 patients. *Dis Colon Rectum.* 1979;22(1):31–34.

240. Thalheimer A, Bueter M, Kortuem M, et al. Morbidity of temporary loop ileostomy in patients with colorectal cancer. *Dis Colon Rectum.* 2006;49(7):1011–1017.

241. Thomson JPS. Caecostomy and colostomy. Part I: surgical procedures and complications. *Clin Gastroenterol.* 1982;11:285.

242. Thomson WH, White S, O'Leary DP. Tube caecostomy to protect rectal anastomoses. *Br J Surg.* 1998;85(11):1533–1534.

243. Thorlakson RH. Technique of repair of herniations associated with colonic stomas. *Surg Gynecol Obstet.* 1965;120:347–350.

244. Timucin T, Cima RR, Larson DW, et al. The use of human acellular dermal matrix for parastomal hernia repair in patients with inflammatory bowel disease: a novel technique to repair fascial defects. *Dis Colon Rectum.* 2009;52:349.

245. Tjandra JJ, Hughes LE. Parastomal pyoderma gangrenosum in inflammatory bowel disease. *Dis Colon Rectum.* 1994;37(9):938–942.

246. Todd GJ, Kutcher LM, Markowitz AM. Factors influencing the complications of colostomy closure. *Am J Surg.* 1979;137(6):749–751.

247. Truedson H, Press V. A new method of stomal reconstruction in patients with retraction of conventional ileostomy. *Surg Gynecol Obstet.* 1986;162(1):60–61.

248. Turnbull RB Jr. Management of ileostomy. *Am J Surg.* 1953;86(5):617–624.

249. Turnbull RB, Weakley FL. *Atlas of Intestinal Stomas.* St. Louis, MO: CV Mosby; 1967:207.

250. Unti JA, Abcarian H, Pearl RK, et al. Rodless end-loop stomas. Seven-year experience. *Dis Colon Rectum.* 1991;34(11):999–1004.

251. Vande Maele DM, Reilly JC. Bullous pemphigoid at colostomy site: report of a case. *Dis Colon Rectum.* 1997;40(3):370–371.

252. Varnell J, Pemberton LB. Risk factors in colostomy closure. *Surgery.* 1981;89(6):683–686.

253. Vasilevsky CA, Gordon PH. Adenocarcinoma arising at the ileocutaneous junction occurring after proctocolectomy for ulcerative colitis. *Br J Surg.* 1986;73(5):378.

254. Venturini M, Bertelli G, Forno G, et al. Colostomy irrigation in the elderly. Effective recovery regardless of age. *Dis Colon Rectum.* 1990;33(12):1031–1033.

255. Vijayasekar C, Marimuthu K, Jadhav V, et al. Parastomal hernia: is prevention better than cure? Use of preperitoneal polypropylene mesh at the time of stoma formation. *Tech Coloproctol.* 2008;12(4):309–313.

256. Vogel SL, Maher JW. An improved method for construction of loop colostomy. *Surg Gynecol Obstet.* 1986;162(4):377–378.

257. Voitk A. Simple technique for laparoscopic paracolostomy hernia repair. *Dis Colon Rectum.* 2000;43(10):1451–1453.

258. Wara P, Sorensen K, Berg V. Proximal fecal diversion: review of ten years' experience. *Dis Colon Rectum.* 1981;24(2):114–119.

259. Warren R, McKittrick LS. Ileostomy for ulcerative colitis: technique, complications, and management. *Surg Gynecol Obstet.* 1951;93(5):555–567.

260. Watt RC. Colostomy irrigation: yes or no? *Am J Nurs.* 1977;77(3):442–444.

261. Wexner SD, Taranow DA, Johansen OB, et al. Loop ileostomy is a safe option for fecal diversion. *Dis Colon Rectum.* 1993;36(4):349–354.

262. Wheeler MH, Barker J. Closure of colostomy: a safe procedure? *Dis Colon Rectum.* 1977;20(1):29–32.

263. Whittaker M, Goligher JC. A comparison of the results of extraperitoneal and intraperitoneal techniques for construction of terminal iliac colostomies. *Dis Colon Rectum.* 1976;19(4):342–344.

264. Wilkinson AJ, Humphreys WG. Seat-belt injury to ileostomy. *Br Med J.* 1978;1(6122):1249–1250.

265. Williams JG, Etherington R, Hayward MW, et al. Paraileostomy hernia: a clinical and radiological study. *Br J Surg.* 1990;77(12):1355–1357.

266. Williams NS, Johnston D. Prospective controlled trial comparing colostomy irrigation with "spontaneous-action" method. *Br Med J.* 1980;281(6233):107–109.

267. Williams NS, Nasmyth DG, Jones D, et al. De-functioning stomas: a prospective controlled trial comparing loop ileostomy with loop transverse colostomy. *Br J Surg.* 1986;73(7):566–570.

268. Winkler MJ, Volpe PA. Loop transverse colostomy. The case against. *Dis Colon Rectum.* 1982;25(4):321–326.

269. Winslet MC, Alexander-Williams J, Keighley MR. Ileostomy revision with a GIA stapler under intravenous sedation. *Br J Surg.* 1990;77(6):647.

270. Yagüe S. A new technique for temporary transparietocecal ileal diversion in the prevention of anastomotic leakage in colonic operations. *Surg Gynecol Obstet.* 1986;162(4):381–382.

271. Yajko RD, Norton LW, Bioemendal L, et al. Morbidity of colostomy closure. *Am J Surg.* 1976;132(3):304–306.

272. Zaghiyan KN, Murrell Z, Fleshner PR. Scarless single-incision laparoscopic loop ileostomy: a novel technique. *Dis Colon Rectum.* 2011;54(12):1542–1546.

273. Zinkin LD, Rosin JD. Button colopexy for colostomy prolapse. *Surg Gynecol Obstet.* 1981;152(1):89–90.

32

Wound, Ostomy, and Continence Nursing

Paula Erwin-Toth

It is necessary hoe hym that is sycke to have
two or three good keepers.

—ANDREW BOORDE (1490–1549):
The Dyetary of Helth XL

The care of the patient who will undergo or who has undergone ostomy surgery involves close cooperation among the surgeon; the wound/ostomy, continence (WOC) nurse; and the patient in order to achieve optimal rehabilitation. Parenthetically, the nursing specialty of "enterostomal therapy" has been replaced by the title, "wound, ostomy, and continence nursing." As discussed in Chapter 31, the technique for fashioning an ostomy falls within the purview of the surgeon. However, much of the physical, emotional, and educational aspects of the rehabilitation process usually fall within the domain of the WOC nurse.[6,14] Still, if a WOC nurse is not available, responsibility for stoma assessment, fitting, and rehabilitation still properly rests with the surgeon.[6]

▶ PREOPERATIVE CARE

As stated in Chapter 31, optimal postoperative stomal management begins with preoperative preparation.[8] The patient and family members ideally should receive comprehensive information concerning overall ostomy rehabilitation, plans, and management. This includes activity, diet, clothing, and sexual concerns. The patient should be reassured that self-care may, at first, seem awkward, but all can be mastered by almost any patient at any age in a relatively short time.[8] Contact with an ostomy visitor may be especially beneficial. A confident, fully rehabilitated ostomy/site visitor can provide hope and improve morale for the apprehensive patient.

As discussed in Chapter 31, the site should ideally fall below the umbilicus in the left or right lower quadrant, on the superior aspect of the infraumbilical fat mound, and should lie within the surface marking of the rectus sheath (see Figures 29-39 and 29-40).[7,14] It is important to avoid scars, creases, and bony prominences in order to provide a smooth pouching surface postoperatively (Figure 32-1). It is also imperative for the individual to see the site. To accomplish this, the patient is evaluated while he or she is supine, sitting, and standing because positional changes can materially alter the abdominal configuration (Figure 32-2). A patient with a protuberant abdomen or someone requiring long-term use of a wheelchair may be better served with a stoma located in the upper abdomen.[7] It is axiomatic that self-care will be rendered difficult or impossible if the patient is unable to see the stoma. Although stoma site selection is truly the responsibility of the surgeon, it is appropriate and reasonable to delegate this task to a WOC nurse.[14] Preoperatively, using a surgical marking pen or a fine-gauge needle (see Figure 29-40) provides a guide to the ideal location so that intraoperative guessing is eliminated. Even those patients who undergo emergency or temporary stomas should optimally have preoperative stomal marking.[7,14]

Independence in ostomy care requires integration of the stoma into the patient's everyday life. In addition to site selection, stoma construction itself can have a profound influence on the effectiveness of a pouching system (see Chapters 29 and 31). A budded stoma in a preselected location offers the best chance for successful ostomy management. A patient who is offered a comprehensive preoperative educational program is much more likely to

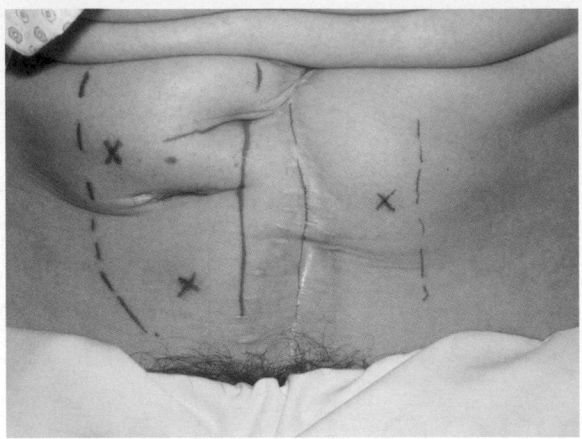

FIGURE 32-1. Selection of potential stomal sites is particularly difficult in this obese patient with a left paramedian incision. Note the deep scar from a prior stoma in the right lower quadrant. The *dashed lines* represent the outer border of the rectus muscles. The optimal site for this individual is the one marked on the left side.

be an active participant in postoperative activities. Even those individuals in whom there is only the possibility of a stoma or in whom the stoma is to be temporary should be marked and offered counseling preoperatively by the surgeon and/or the WOC nurse.[8] National guidelines for enterostomal patient education have been established by the Standards Development Committee of the United Ostomy Association, with the assistance of Prospect Associates.[2]

STOMAL FUNCTION AND CARE

Fecal and urinary diversion may be performed in patients for a variety of clinical indications and situations. A brief overview of these various stomas follows.

Gastrointestinal Stomas

Jejunostomy

Jejunostomy function usually begins within the first 48 hours after surgery. If the stoma was created laparoscopically, function will usually commence earlier. Initially, the effluent is watery, clear, and dark green. Because the volume of output may approach 2,400 mL in 24 hours, the patient must be monitored closely for electrolyte imbalance. Because the absorption of nutrients, fluids, and electrolytes may be deficient in a patient with a jejunostomy, total parenteral nutrition or fluid/electrolyte support may be required.[14] In order to minimize the inconvenience associated with the need for frequent pouch emptying, connection to gravity drainage is advisable.

Ileostomy

An ileostomy generally begins to function within the first 48 to 72 hours after surgery, although those undergoing laparoscopic construction may evidence an effluent within 24 hours. The initial appearance may be viscous and green, but such an output does not necessarily indicate the return of peristalsis. Rather, it may represent the elimination of secretions that have collected in the distal small bowel. Once peristalsis has returned, the patient may enter a period of high-volume output known as the adaptation phase. Output during this time may exceed 1,000 mL/day, frequently

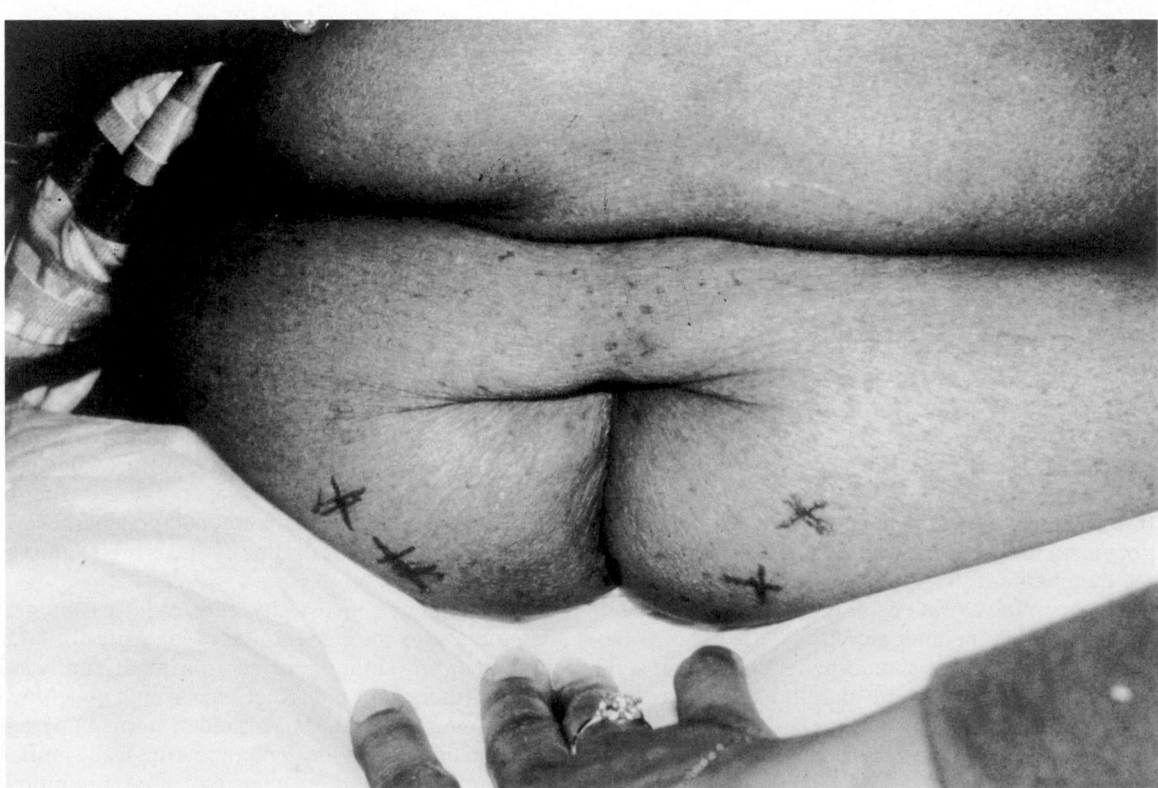

FIGURE 32-2. Site selection was inappropriately marked on both sides with the patient supine. The *X*'s in the superior aspect were elected because the inferior ones would have fallen below the fat bulge.

reaching 1,500 to 1,800 mL/day. The physiologic basis for this high-output phase is the loss of the colonic absorptive surface, coupled, theoretically, with the loss of the ileocecal valve. During this period, the patient should be monitored for signs and symptoms of fluid and electrolyte imbalance.

A loop ileostomy–supporting rod is removed by the third to fifth postoperative day, depending on the amount of edema of the stoma itself. The greater the swelling, the earlier the rod may be removed. The less tissue reaction present, the longer the rod should be maintained. Edema itself tends to prevent the stoma from retracting, and the rod may actually intensify and prolong the duration of the edematous reaction. Patients with a loop ileostomy proximal to a pelvic pouch will experience a higher output and have an increased risk for fluid and electrolyte management problems. Readmission may be necessary for these individuals, and early stomal closure may be required for this indication. As with jejunostomy, connection of the pouch to gravity drainage will prevent overdistension of the appliance. If the stool thickens but output remains high, use of anesthesia tubing and a plastic bottle can be adapted. This is especially convenient if one uses a two-piece pouching system. While ambulating, the patient can wear a standard pouch and closure clamp, but a second pouch secured to the gravity drainage system can be attached while one is resting.

Over a period of days to weeks, the proximal small bowel increases fluid absorption. Gradually, the volume of output decreases and the stool thickens to toothpaste-like consistency. Initially, the output from an ileostomy can vary from 500 to 1,500 mL in a 24-hour period. But, after adaptation, the average output decreases to between 500 and 800 mL/day.[14]

Continent Ileostomy

Since the advent of the pelvic pouch procedure (see Chapter 29), the continent ileostomy today is primarily performed for the indications of an elective conversion in those with a permanent, conventional (Brooke) ileostomy; for those with a failed reservoir-anal procedure; and for patients with anal incontinence. One of the important concerns is to stabilize the defunctioning drainage catheter that is placed in the pouch (see Figures 29-70 and 29-72). This may be achieved through a variety of methods, including a stomal plate, ostomy appliance belt, or a baby nipple (Figure 32-3). A sterile gauze dressing around the stoma will absorb mucous and moisture as well as afford protection.[9,18]

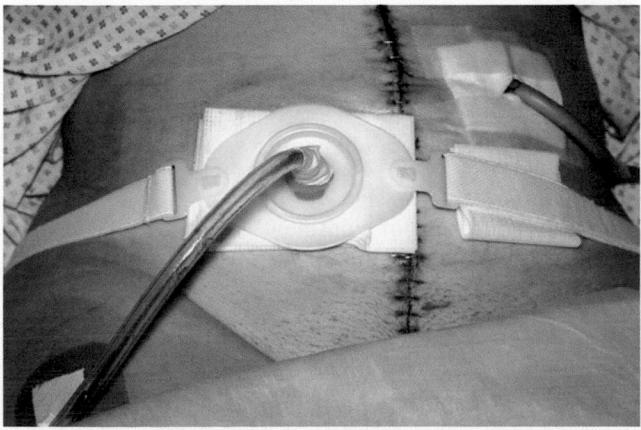

FIGURE 32-3. Continent ileostomy stoma plate. Baby bottle nipple anchors catheter device after removal of tripod sutures.

To minimize tube blockage, gentle irrigation with 20 to 30 mL of normal saline is recommended, commencing in the recovery unit and continuing every 2 to 3 hours for the next few days.[9,18] Intervals between irrigations can be increased based on how well the tube is draining. It is extremely important to avoid overdistension of the pouch for the first few weeks following surgery in order to limit the likelihood of desussception. A bedside drainage bag or leg bag must be used to maintain constant drainage.

Colostomy

The initial output from a colostomy varies depending on the location of the stoma within the colon. Because the colon absorbs all but approximately 100 mL of the 1,000 mL of contents that passes through the ileocecal valve daily, the output from distal colonic stomas has a thicker consistency and smaller volume than that of proximal colonic stomas.

Cecostomy

A cecostomy usually begins to function by the third postoperative day. The output may be projectile (because of close proximity to the ileocecal valve), and it is initially liquid. The place of cecostomy in colon and rectal surgery has been discussed in the previous chapter and in Chapter 20. A cecostomy may be either skin level or tubal (see Figures 28-59 and 31-45). As has already been discussed in this text, the location, output characteristics, and construction combine to make this a difficult stoma with which to deal. The tube cecostomy poses a special management problem because stool tends to flow both through and around the tube. Furthermore, tube cecostomies are also associated with a greater risk of intra-abdominal spillage.

Transverse Colostomy

A transverse colostomy usually begins to function on postoperative day 3 or 4. Output, which varies from pasty to soft, usually occurs after meals and at intervals throughout the day. For a loop colostomy, a supporting device (e.g., rod or bridge) placed during surgery is removed 3 to 5 days later (see Chapter 31). Corman and Odenheimer have described numerous methods for creating a loop colostomy in order to maintain stomal support.[5]

Descending/Sigmoid Colostomy

A descending or sigmoid colostomy requires the longest time to regain normal function, perhaps not until postoperative day 5. After this period, one logically should be concerned with issues that may cause delay in colonic function—ileus, administration of narcotics, obstruction, and so on. One may consider the option of stimulating colonic evacuation by means of a no. 20 French Foley catheter gently advanced into the stoma. A warmed solution of 500 mL of normal saline can be instilled via gravity drainage and allowed to return.[6,8,14] This procedure initiates a reflex contraction, stimulating peristalsis and providing relief of gaseous distention. Because many patients with a colostomy are discharged as early as the fourth postoperative day, self-care instruction may not be adequate because of the lack of output. Another alternative is to use a stool substitute placed in the pouch to assist in teaching pouch-emptying techniques. Instruction is continued following hospital discharge in the patient's home or in the outpatient department.

Once normal bowel function has returned, the output from a descending or sigmoid colostomy usually is a soft, formed stool. Elimination patterns generally are the same as that experienced by the patient before he or she became ill. Colostomy irrigation with a cone may also be performed as a management option to avoid an appliance in selected patients or in preparation for diagnostic testing (Figure 31-25). The technique for colostomy irrigation has been discussed in Chapter 31. However, instructions for the patient appear here in Tables 32-1 and 32-2.

Urinary Stomas

Vesicostomy

Drainage is provided by a Foley catheter placed in the anterior dome of the bladder. Should pouching be requested, the suprapubic location may make obtaining a secure seal problematic. Shaving the pubic hair is helpful in order to facilitate pouch adherence and removal.

Ureterostomy

Creation of unilateral or bilateral ureteral openings to the skin is uncommonly employed. The flush or retracted stoma associated with ureterostomies can pose a real pouching challenge. If the stoma is located in the flank, self-care may be impossible. Therefore, a family member or other home caregiver should be instructed on how to manage this ostomy.[8]

Nephrostomy

Generally, nephrostomies are managed by means of a sterile closed drainage system. A skin barrier wafer is usually placed on the skin around the tube to protect the skin and to anchor the tube to prevent accidental dislodgement.[8]

TABLE 32-1 Colostomy Irrigation with a Cone

1. Apply the irrigation sleeve securely around the stoma to prevent leakage.
2. Close the shutoff valve. Fill the irrigation bag with 500–100 mL of tepid water and hang the irrigation bag on a hook.
3. Remove air from the tubing by opening the shutoff valve until the water runs out of the cone. Close the shutoff valve and lubricate the end of the cone with water-soluble lubricant.
4. Sit up straight on a chair or toilet with irrigating sleeve just touching the water level in the toilet bowl.
5. Open the shutoff valve until the water flows slowly. Insert the lubricated cone into the stoma until the water enters without leakage. Increase the flow rate as tolerated. If a cramp develops, stop or decrease the water flow until the cramp passes and then resume the water flow.
6. When the 500–1,000 mL of water has entered the colon, remove the cone and close the top of the irrigation sleeve. The bottom of the irrigation sleeve should remain in the toilet bowl for no less than *15 minutes*. By then, the majority of the stool and water will have returned.
7. Rinse the inside of the irrigation sleeve with water to remove the waste material. Remove the irrigation sleeve from the bowl. Dry and clip the bottom of the irrigation sleeve to the top of the sleeve. It may take up to *45 minutes* for the rest of the water and stool to return.

TABLE 32-2 Colostomy Irrigation Helpful Hints

Spray the inside of the irrigation sleeve with any liquid soap or detergent prior to administering the enema so that the stool will drain easily, the sleeve will clean faster, and less odor will be retained.

During the enema, if you experience

CRAMPING:

May indicate constipation; recall firmness of prior evacuation.

- Slow or stop the flow of water, relax and deep breathe.
- Recheck the rate of water flow; flow rate should be approximately 10 minutes for 1,000 mL of water; 5–7 minutes for 500 mL.
- Check the height of enema bag; it should be approximately 12–20 in. (30–50 cm) above the shoulder level when one is seated.

SLUGGISH/NO RETURNS:

May indicate constipation; recall firmness of prior evacuation.

- Look at diet; may need to increase bulk, such as bran, fresh fruits, and vegetables.

May indicate dehydration; increase oral fluid intake to *8* glasses of liquid per day.

- Increase physical activity.

After the enema, if one experiences

SPILLAGE:

May indicate constipation; recall firmness of prior evacuation.

- Look at the volume of water inserted during the enema; most individuals require 1,000 mL.
- Do not use more than 1,000 mL without physician's permission.
- Check that the enema solution does not escape around the cone or shield.

EXCESSIVE GAS OR FLATUS:

- Avoid gas-forming foods.
- Eat regular meals; chew food well.
- Avoid air swallowing, that is, mouth breathing, gum chewing, smoking, straws, carbonated beverages, alcohol.

Conduits

Ileal, jejunal, and colonic conduits are frequently employed methods for effecting urinary diversion. Preoperative stoma sighting and construction of a properly budded stoma will improve the potential for obtaining a secure pouch seal.

Continent Urinary Diversion

A variety of forms of continent urinary diversion are performed. Preoperative and postoperative management techniques for these types of diversion are similar to that of continent ileostomy.

The ileocecal reservoir, commonly known as an Indiana pouch, uses a variety of tubes and drains. Drainage of the newly created urinary reservoir is accomplished by means of a cecostomy tube, bilateral urinary stents, and a catheter placed into the plicated exit conduit (Figure 32-4).[1,9,18] Depending on the surgeon's preference, gentle irrigation of

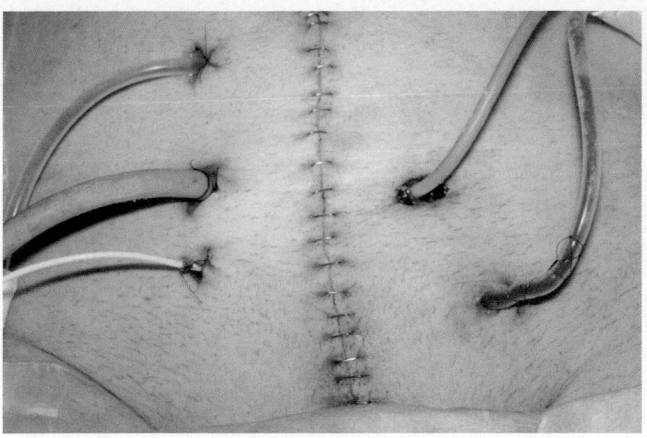

FIGURE 32-4. Multiple drains including ostomy tube in a patient who underwent a continent urostomy (ileoocecal reservoir), a so-called Indiana pouch.

the cecostomy tube with 20 to 30 mL of normal saline is performed every 2 to 3 hours.[9] As with the continent ileostomy, the goal is to maintain the patency of the catheter and to prevent overdistension of the newly created reservoir. It is not uncommon to cap the catheter into the exit conduit to avoid disruption of the newly plicated ileal segment.

Stabilization of the tubes and drains can be achieved by a variety of tube anchoring devices. Use of constant drainage by means of a bedside drainage bag or leg bag is recommended for the first few weeks after surgery.[9,18]

▶ OSTOMY MANAGEMENT

Immediate Postoperative Period

Proper application of a pouching system should begin in the operating room. The appliance is fixed to clean, dry skin in order to protect the incision and the peristomal skin and to contain stomal discharge. Although it is true that most fecal stomas will not begin to function for a few days, mucosal secretions are ideally collected with a pouch. Conversely, urinary stomas will function immediately unless anastomotic disruption of the urinary-bowel connection has occurred. Pouch application coupled with connection to gravity drainage is indicated for urinary stomas.

A variety of one-piece or two-piece, disposable, odor-proof, pouching systems may be used (Figure 32-5 and Table 32-3). By using a disposable measuring guide and by sizing the aperture of the pouch within 1/8 in. (3 mm) of the base of the stomal mucosa, one can protect the peristomal skin and prevent mucosal trauma (Figure 32-6). Removal of the release paper and gentle pressure on the abdomen following pouch application will enhance pouch adherence. A transparent, drainable pouch will permit the clinician to assess stoma viability as well as output. A closure clamp or tubing device is then securely applied (Figure 32-7).

A healthy, viable stoma appears moist, beefy red, and often edematous. However, a continent ileostomy stoma may have a darker, bruised appearance due to mesenteric venous compression. Some individuals with a history of using senna-containing laxatives may demonstrate melanosis coli

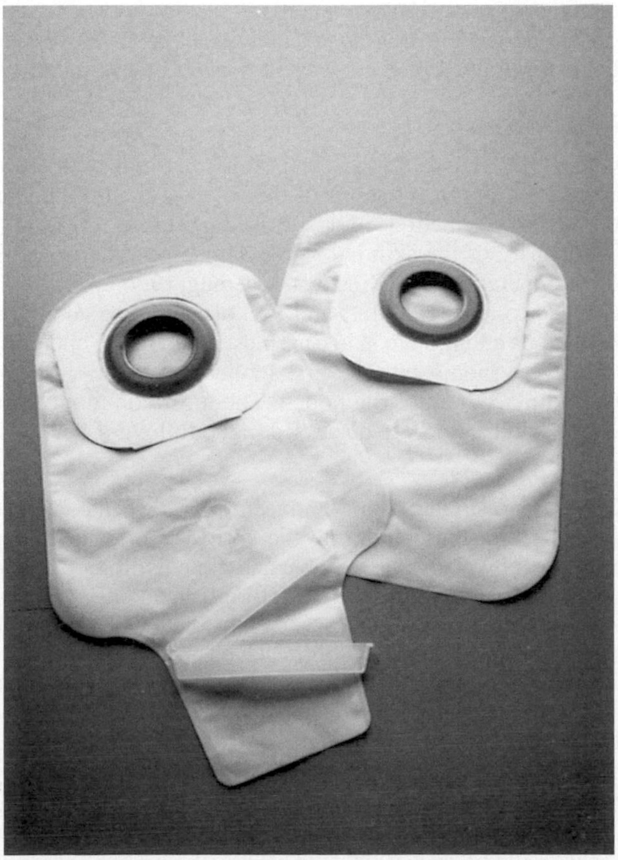

FIGURE 32-5. Drainable and closed pouches with karaya seal and adhesive. (Courtesy of Hollister, Inc.)

TABLE 32-3 Pouching Systems

TYPE	FEATURES/VARIETIES
One-piece drainable, closed-end urostomy	Flexible, semiflexible, firm, with or without skin barrier attached. Flat and with convexity ranging from shallow to very deep precut and cut to fit.
Two-piece	With or without adhesive tape collar. Precut and cut-to-fit varieties. Built-in convexity or option of convex insert. Adult/pediatric sizes. Pouch removable without disturbing flange. Clear and opaque pouches. Variety of size and shapes of pouches, irrigation sleeves, and stoma caps. Belt hooks for optional belt use. Provides sense of security especially for very active ostomates.
Pouching tips	Peel off all backing paper. Size properly—decrease aperture as stoma edema decreases. Assess need for convexity. Close pouch properly. Be alert for candidiasis. Snap on pouch securely to flange in two-piece system.

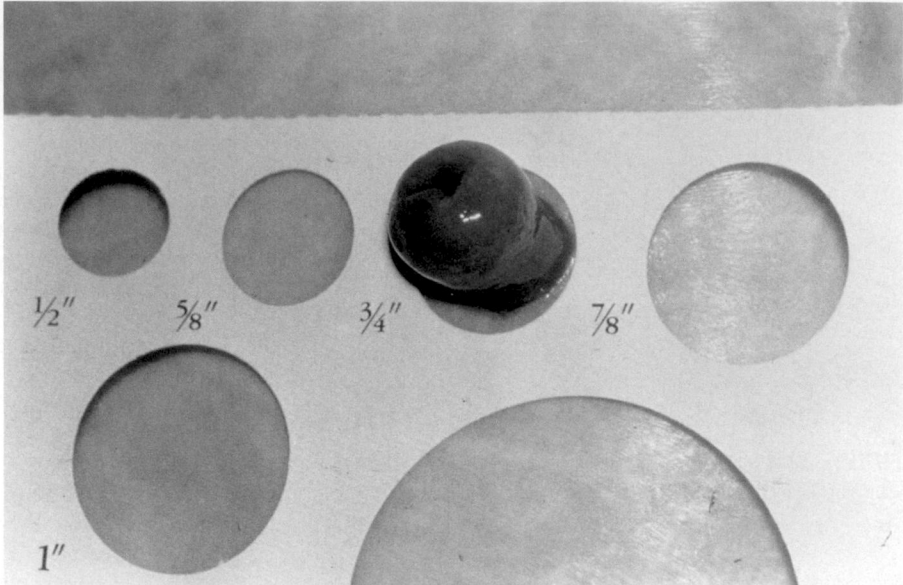

FIGURE 32-6. Disposable measuring guide permits use of properly sized faceplate.

in the mucosa of their colostomy. This stoma may appear moist and gray to brown or even black in appearance due to staining of the bowel mucosa (see Figure 20-1A).

Assessment of the mucosa is evaluated with each pouch change. Viability and function can be evaluated daily by the surgeon, by the WOC nurse, and by each shift of the nursing staff.

Principles of Fitting

In order to provide some appreciation for the alternative methods of managing ostomies, it is important to have an understanding of ostomy collection devices. It is not important for a surgeon to be familiar with every company and every product in the field. It is merely necessary to be aware of the general principles for using the various devices and to have, perhaps, one or two alternatives from which to choose should the need arise.

Three primary parts—skin barrier, faceplate, and pouch—are necessary for an effective collecting system, but there are a variety of additional accessories.[11] The newer generation of appliances incorporates these parts into a single disposable or reusable system.

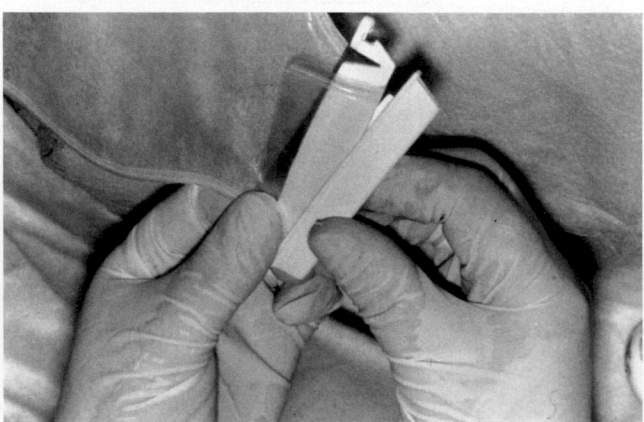

FIGURE 32-7. Applying closure clamp to drainable pouch.

Skin Protective Agent

A skin sealant, such as Skin Prep (Smith and Nephew), provides a clear film that coats the skin. Generally, protective agents are used when tapelike products (e.g., double-faced disks) or cement contact the skin in order to limit the likelihood of irritation. They also augment adherence of an appliance and facilitate adhesive removal from reusable faceplates.[19] These protective agents are available as gels, sprays, wipes, paint-on solutions, or pastes. Distinction must be made between a skin barrier and a protecting agent; individuals with ileostomies should never use a protective agent in place of a skin barrier.

Skin Barrier

A skin barrier is an adherent porous material that offers protection from the contents of the colon or ileum (e.g., karaya or carboxymethylcellulose-based products). Preserving the integrity of the skin is of great concern in the immediate postoperative period. Moist, weeping, oily, eroded skin will lead to leakage, odor, and loss of appliance adhesion. Meticulous attention to skin care must begin in the operating or recovery rooms with the first application of the skin barrier and placement of the pouch. The most commonly employed skin barriers are discussed in the following sections.

Karaya Products

Karaya is a resin that forms a protective base when combined with glycerin, thus inhibiting the corrosive effects of ileal contents. It is relatively insoluble and quite hydroscopic. It is refined and marketed in different forms, including powders, washers, wafers, and blankets, and mixed with natural clays. It is also manufactured in paste form, which provides an excellent means for filling in crevices created by abdominal folds near the stoma. Karaya stretches, and when it is used as a washer, it should measure about 1/4 in. smaller than the base of the stoma in order to fit it snugly. Specially prepared hole-cutter tools are available from several ostomy manufacturers (Figure 32-8).

Karaya is nonallergenic, although the ingredients in some products may cause some sensitivity. If this is a problem, a change to a karaya product manufactured by another company may be all that is required.

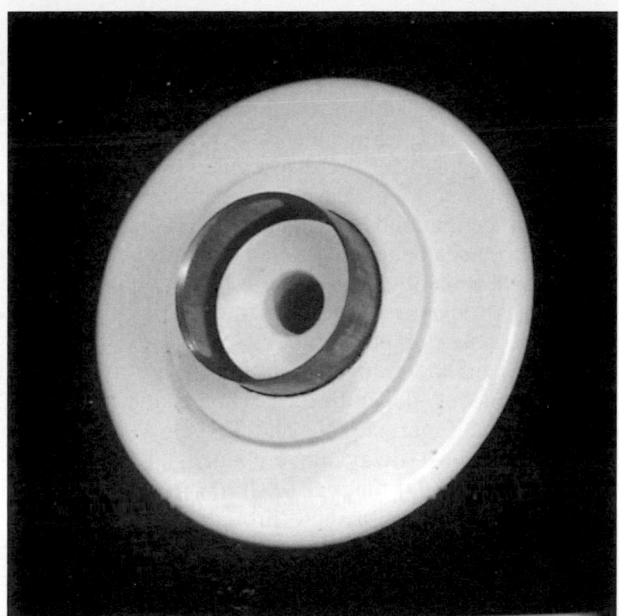

FIGURE 32-8. Hole cutter tool. A steel blade is mounted in a plastic handle. This can be prepared by request for various diameters. (Courtesy of Nu-Hope Laboratories.)

One disadvantage of karaya products is the tendency to break down in the presence of urine. Therefore, they should never be used with urinary diversions. Karaya melts easily in heat or even when the patient has an elevated temperature. Thus, for ostomates who live in warm climates, a different skin barrier should be used (e.g., Stomahesive or Hollihesive). Generally, the use of karaya is advised less often than the products subsequently discussed.

Colly-Seel
Colly-Seel is another, more solid form of karaya. Natural clays have been added, which cause it to be less vulnerable to heat; thus, it is a suitable barrier for both urinary and ileostomy effluents. Colly-Seel is available in varying thicknesses as well as in washer, wafer, and sheet form. It does not stretch, and so the inner diameter should be cut approximately the same size or 1/16 in. larger than the diameter of the stomal base. It must be moistened slightly before application. Colly-Seel is sometimes recommended for a patient with a soft or flabby abdominal wall or when considerable scarring is present. However, it is used less often today, having been replaced by more flexible products. It should be placed on the abdomen while it is still sticky.

Gelatin–Pectin Skin Barriers
Generally, the gelatin–pectin skin barriers have an advantage over the karaya products because they are more water resistant and therefore permit a longer interval between appliance changes.[19]

Stomahesive (ConvaTec)
Stomahesive is composed of gelatin, pectin, carboxymethylcellulose sodium, and polyisobutylene. It is nonallergenic and looks like a piece of American cheese. Its shiny surface is affixed to the appliance, and the sticky side is secured to the skin. It should be cut to fit around the stoma, leaving a 2- or 3-mm clearance, and it may be used as a washer or as a whole wafer. The product is also available in a powder or a paste, which many WOC nurses and patients prefer to karaya. Stomahesive can be applied directly onto denuded skin and provides an excellent means for filling in crevices created by abdominal folds near the stoma.

A skin barrier such as Stomahesive is appropriate for intestinal as well as urinary tract diversions and should be placed on the skin immediately after the operation. The inner diameter should be cut to fit around the base of the stoma. The outer aspect should be rounded and made slightly smaller than the adhesive portion of a soft-backed disposable clear pouch. The skin must be completely dry before applying Stomahesive or any other skin barrier.

Durahesive (ConvaTec)
Durahesive is similar to Stomahesive, but it has specific hydrophilic properties that absorb fluid from the effluent. This causes the product to swell or "turtleneck" around the stoma. It is a particularly advantageous barrier for urinary ostomies. It has been reported that some patients may achieve up to 14 days of use without leakage when this product is employed.

Hollihesive
Hollihesive is similar in composition to Stomahesive, except that it is a bit more flexible and stickier to the touch. It, too, is available as a paste. Another product from the same manufacturer is called Premium Barrier. It is allegedly more resistant to breakdown.

Reliaseal (Bard)
Reliaseal is similar in composition to Stomahesive. It is available in a round or oval disk with precut inner diameter sizes at 1/8-in. intervals. It has two adhesive sides, one covered with white paper and the other with blue. The white paper is peeled off and that side is placed directly on the skin; then the blue paper covering is removed, and that side is placed directly on the faceplate of the pouch. "Blue to the sky" is a helpful memory device to teach patients how to use this barrier. Reliaseal is also an effective washer for an ileal conduit. When using Stomahesive or Reliaseal, many patients choose to add a small karaya or Stomahesive washer before applying the barrier for an added peristomal seal.

Other Barriers
For many years, United was one of the well-established and well-recognized ostomy manufacturing companies. More recently, United was purchased by Smith and Nephew with selected items from their line sold to Torbot manufacturing. Some of the former United products, therefore, are no longer available. Smith and Nephew's Soft-Guard XL is very pliable and is resistant to breakdown. Coloplast manufactures Comfeel, and Nu-Hope has skin barrier wafers, precut round and oval washers, and paste strips for flexibility. Eakin Cohesive Seals can be used as an ostomy seal or an external packing agent around stomas. They are moldable, pectin-based rings that absorb moisture and act as a physical and waterproof barrier. They are marketed in the United States by ConvaTec.

Faceplate (aka Stomaplate)
The faceplate or mounting area is that part of the appliance that supports the pouch and attaches it to the body.[11] It may

be made of rubber, metal, paper, adhesive, or plastic. It can be flexible or hard; convex, flat, or concave. Due to the popularity of disposable pouching systems, the selection of stomaplates is limited. Companies that still produce a selection include Torbot, Marlen, and Permatype.

Adhesives

Adhesives are of two types: liquids (cements) and disks. Adhesive cements are generally made of acrylic or rubber but are usually unnecessary.[19] If used, they should be applied lightly and evenly as a single coat to the skin or to the barrier. Those who seem to prefer this method usually have had their appliance for many years. Cement is occasionally recommended for a patient with a difficult abdominal contour or in whom a satisfactory seal cannot be established by another means. Many of the cements are latex based; therefore, caution must be exercised in their use.

The most popular method of adhering a reusable appliance is by a double-faced adhesive cloth disk. This must exactly measure the inner diameter of the faceplate. Before a new disk is applied, the faceplate should be cleansed of any residual adhesive.

Pouch

There are numerous disposable and reusable pouch systems available (Table 32-3 and Figures 32-9 through 32-12). Selection will depend on a variety of physical and psychosocial factors affecting the patient. The pouch can be made of synthetic material or of rubber. Some disposal pouches come with an adhesive or microporous tape backing and, in some instances, with a soft plastic faceplate and belt tabs (see Figures 32-5 and 32-9). A number of such commonly used products include the Hollister, ConvaTec, Marlen, Coloplast, and Nu-Hope pouches. They are lightweight, easy to apply, and very effective choices for the firm abdomen that does not require a more rigid faceplate for peristomal support. In addition, no assembly is required.

Two-piece disposable appliances have become quite popular. They consist of a skin barrier with a plastic ring (see Figure 32-10). A pouch with a ring snaps or sticks onto the barrier ring. Variations on this concept are made by ConvaTec, Hollister, United, and Coloplast.

The disadvantages of the disposable system include the possibility of a shorter wearing time, increased cost, and limitation to certain body configurations. A faceplate with a firm base provides better peristomal support, particularly in a patient with a "flabby" abdomen. A disposal pouch always requires a skin barrier to enhance the wearing time and to provide adequate skin protection.

Reusable or "permanent" appliances are available in one or two pieces, depending on whether the faceplate is detachable (see Figures 32-11 and 32-12). A faceplate for any appliance must always have a means of securing it to the body regardless of the type of skin barrier used. Attachment is usually accomplished through the use of precut, double-faced adhesive seals or disks. The inner diameter of an adhesive disk must exactly equal the inner diameter of the faceplate.

A one-piece appliance may be preferred by patients with arthritis affecting the hands, those who have poor eyesight or who are blind, active youngsters who need a secure pouch construction with ease of application, those with a neurologic deficit, and those with flush stomas. Disposable one-piece equipment often is available precut, so that one merely peels off the protective paper and affixes the appliance (e.g., ConvaTec, Active Life, and Hollister FirstChoice). However, the selection of a one-piece appliance may also be simply personal preference.

The main advantages of the two-piece system are cost-effectiveness and durability. An elastic ring around the neck of the pouch holds the appliance to the faceplate. The attachment of a double-faced adhesive disk to the back of the faceplate is the same as that with the one-piece appliance. Generally, the firmer the abdomen, the softer and flatter the

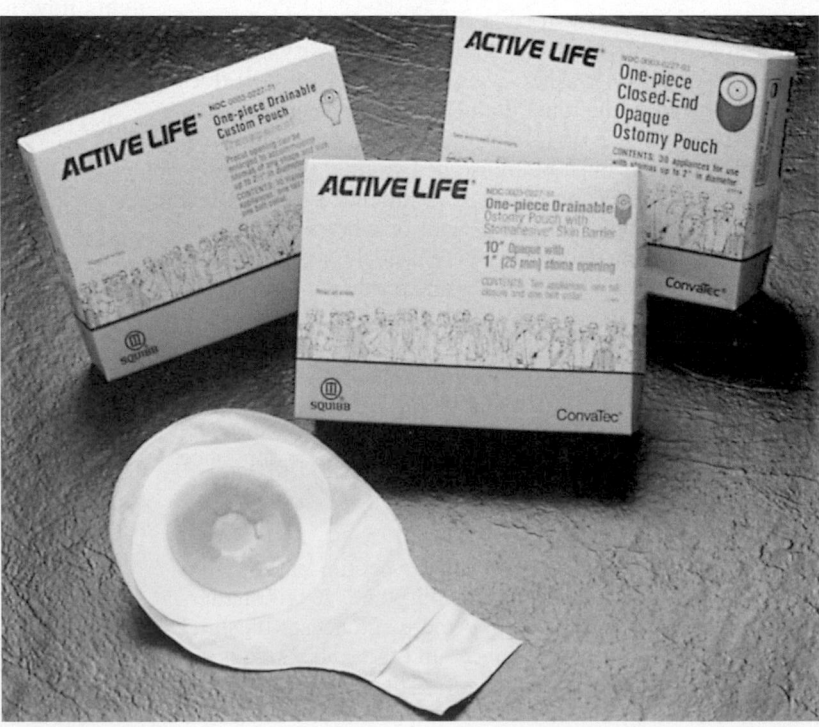

FIGURE 32-9. Drainable and closed-end pouches. Sur-Fit Natura system with Stomahesive wafer and flange. (Courtesy of ConvaTec.)

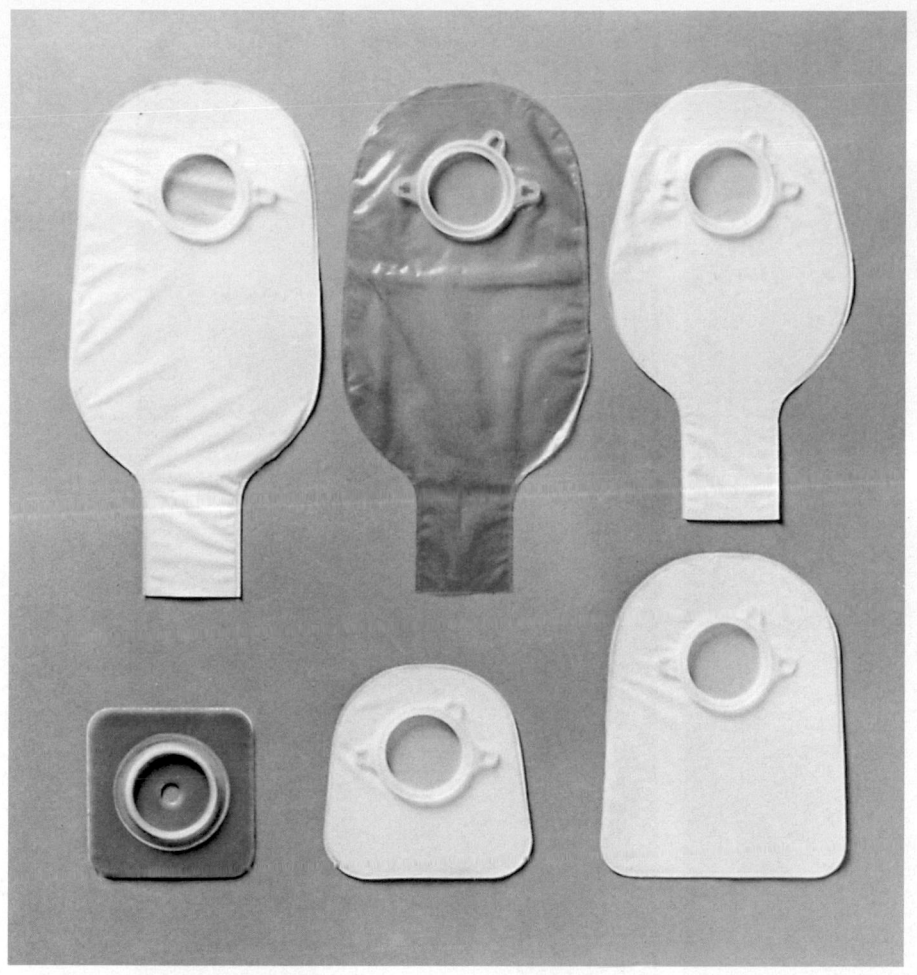

FIGURE 32-10. Drainable and closed-end pouches. Sur-Fit Natura system with Stomahesive wafer and flange. (Courtesy of ConvaTec.)

faceplate should be. For example, a pregnant woman will require a soft, flat faceplate, but a corpulent person will need a firm, convex one to lend sufficient peristomal support in order to prevent undermining of the seal. Most patients, with the exception of those who are very slender or who have firm abdomens, will need a slightly convex faceplate. In addition to the reusable system, many individuals maintain a supply of disposable pouches for an "emergency," for rapid change, or for camping and traveling. Although it is valuable for everyone to be aware of the availability of both systems, the overwhelming majority of patients select disposable equipment.

Even though commercially manufactured equipment is preferred, an adequate "homemade" appliance can be constructed if one has limited financial resources or if there is lack of access to manufactured products.[17] Meier and Tarpley, working in Ogbomoso, Nigeria, write of an appliance made from a tin can, a piece of rubber from an inner tube, household twine, and disposable plastic bags.[16]

Belt and Tape

Many patients feel secure when wearing a belt, but this device is not meant to hold the appliance in place. It is intended merely to support the weight of the pouch. Belts may ride up on the hip and cause detachment of the appliance, which may then lead to stomal injury. Some patients wear the belt too tightly and cause deep marks on the skin or even ulceration. With few exceptions (e.g., active children or problem stomas where revision is not advisable), the use of belts should be discouraged.

An alternative to a belt, such as framing the faceplate or adhesive area with paper tape, is much the preferred approach. For swimming or bathing, many types of waterproof tapes are available.

Appliance Management

Establishment of the optimum frequency for a pouch change requires individual adjustment and experimentation. In the immediate postoperative period, the pouch is changed more frequently than is required at a later time in order to permit stomal assessment and to provide instruction in self-care procedures. After discharge, the patient is encouraged to gradually extend the interval between pouch changes until optimum frequency can be determined. This frequency then becomes the basis for routine pouch changes. The patient is also taught to recognize the signs of undermining and impending leakage (i.e., itching or burning of the peristomal skin, odor noted when the pouch is closed, or visible meltdown of the skin barrier) and to change the pouch promptly whenever any of these signs are present. The goal is to change the pouch before leakage or skin irritation occurs.

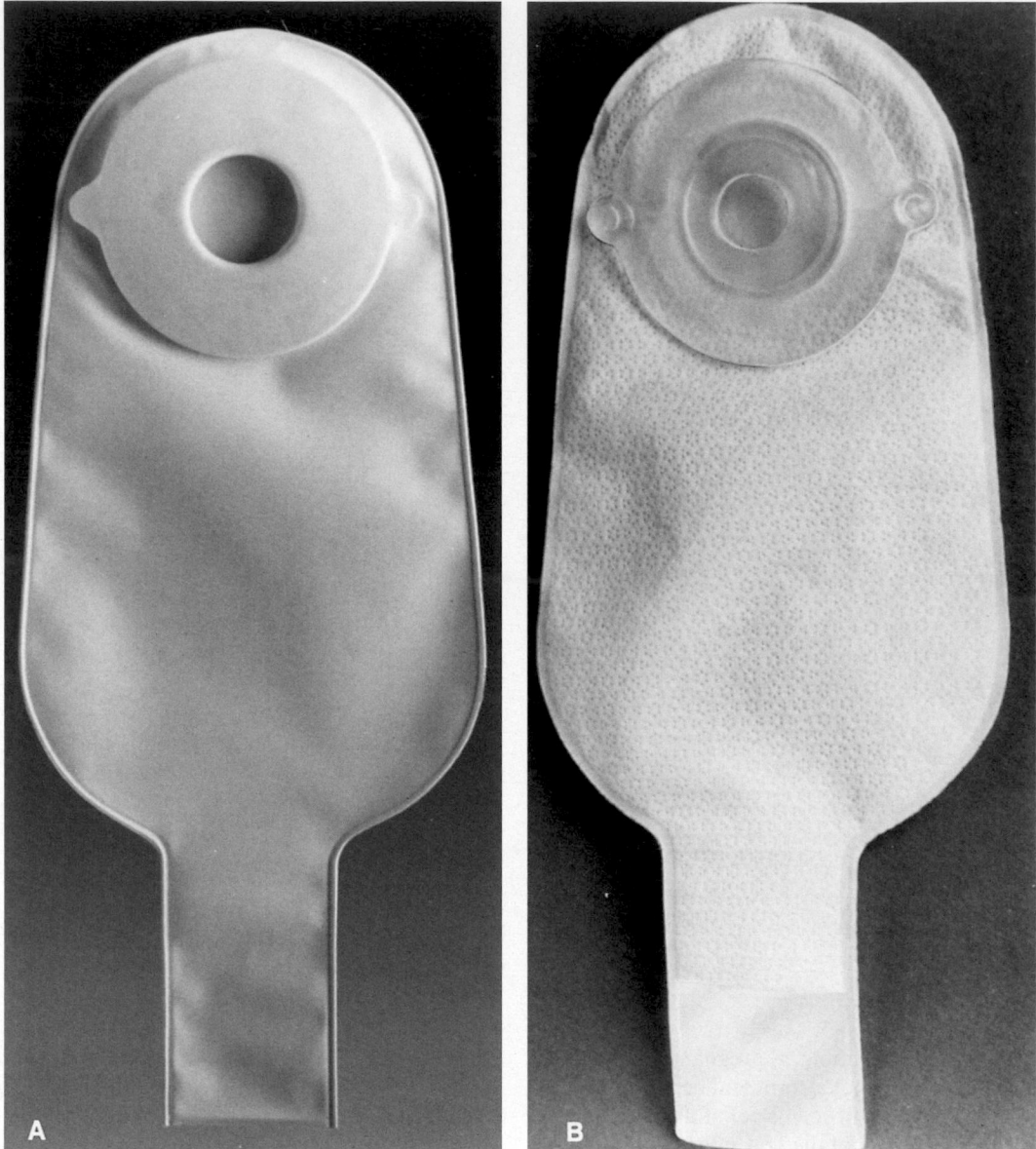

FIGURE 32-11. Reusable ileostomy appliances. **A:** One-piece standard appliance ("odor ban"). **B:** One-piece lightweight ("solo") limited reusable appliance. (Courtesy of Marlen Manufacturing and Development Co.)

There is no correct frequency for pouch change. The goal is to establish a routine schedule that prevents leakage and provides the individual with control. The stoma that is appropriately sited and well constructed usually can be managed with a pouch change every 5 to 7 days. The presence of a rigid rod will require the use of a flexible barrier that will mold over the rod. Use of a barrier under a rod is usually not recommended due to potential stoma damage from pressure or from traumatic removal.

The selection criteria for a pouching system include the type of effluent and the size, shape, and location of the stoma. Contour of the patient's abdomen and any special psychomotor challenges are also considerations. Patients with ileostomies, jejunostomies, and urostomies are often optimally managed with extended-wear barriers that do not readily erode in a high-output, liquid environment.[6,8]

Initially, cut-to-fit barriers are preferred in order to adapt to decreasing stomal edema. After 6 to 8 weeks, the patient may elect to use a presized pouch if the stoma size has stabilized. Individuals with oval stomas may still be best served with cut-to-fit systems. Some pouches can be custom cut at the factory to accommodate a special need.[8]

As mentioned, patients who have a soft abdomen, with a flush or retracted stoma, may require a semiflexible system or one with shallow to medium convexity. A budded stoma, which is preferable from a fitting standpoint, may be pouched with a flat or semiflexible system or may require shallow convexity. Convexity, which can make a significant contribution to preventing leakage, adds varying degrees of pressure around the base of the stoma to aid in securing a seal.

Shallow convexity can be achieved through a convex insert, either added to or built into a one- or two-piece pouching

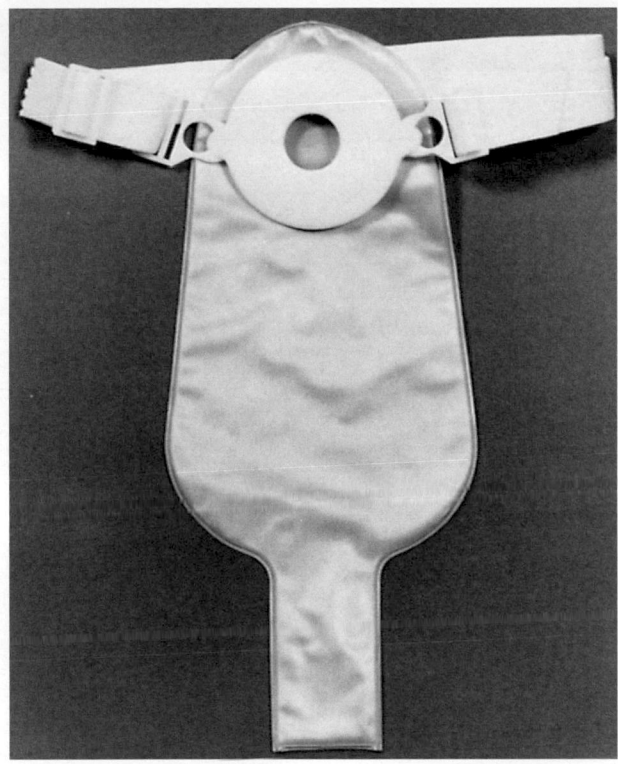

FIGURE 32-12. Example of two-piece, precut flat pouch.

system. A patient with a very soft abdomen may require a firm system with deep to very deep convexity (Figure 32-13).[6,8] The WOC nurse can determine the amount of convexity needed by assessing the presence and depth of skin creases, as well as by applying gentle pressure around the base of the flush stoma, to determine how much pressure is required to help the stoma bud out. Even deep convex systems can be modified to increase convexity by the addition of a skin barrier washer (Figure 32-14). Accessories such as skin barrier pastes, powders, and belts, applied with gentle tension, can all improve pouching success (see previous discussion and Tables 32-4 and 32-5). In the presence of severe peristomal skin erosion, modifications of pouching equipment systems

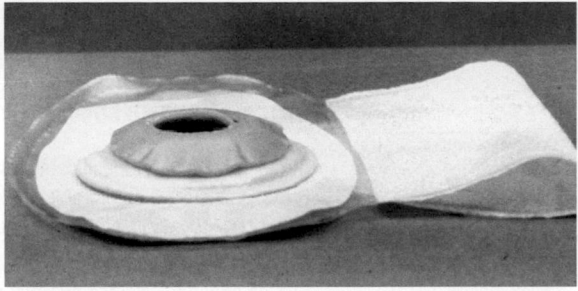

FIGURE 32-14. One-piece, precut, deep convex pouch with skin barrier washer added to deepen convexity.

can be made to create a nonadherent system. This approach is not highly secure, but the advantages are ready access to the stoma site and containment of the effluent.

The major difference between an ileostomy and a colostomy appliance is that some form of protective ring must be used around the ileostomy stoma because of the corrosive nature of the effluent. During the first 6 to 8 days after surgery, a disposable, soft-backed pouch will be required in addition to an appropriate skin barrier. By the seventh or

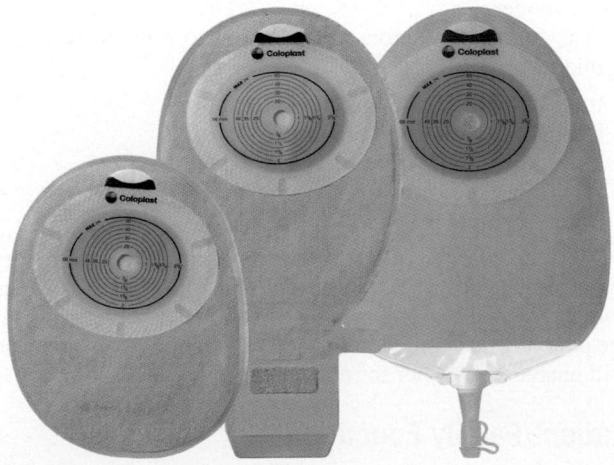

FIGURE 32-13. Examples of one-piece Coloplast systems. (Courtesy of Coloplast USA, Minneapolis, MN.)

TABLE 32-4 Skin Products

PRODUCT	FORM	COMPOSITION
Skin sealants	Wipes, sprays, gels, liquids	Contain plasticized ethyl cellulose and alcohol. Some are water soluble.
Skin barriers	Wafers, rings, washers, paste, strips, powders	May be made from karaya gum, pectin, carboxymethyl cellulose, gelatin, copolymers.
Skin adhesives/ cement	Liquids, sprays, tubes	Silicone or latex based.
Skin solvents	Wipes, liquids	Primary ingredient: trichlorethane, a liquid petroleum.
Skin cleansers	Liquids, wipes, sprays, foams	May contain water, lanolin, urea, propylene glycol, fragrance, and artificial colors. Rinsing may be required to remove residue of cleanser before pouching.
Skin lotions	Wipes, creams	May contain lanolin, fragrance, water. Some contain topical steroids and antifungal ingredients. Apply sparingly and remove residue before applying pouching system.

TABLE 32-5 Accessories

TYPES	DESCRIPTION AND COMMENTS
Belts	Some are company specific, others interchangeable. Sizes: small, medium, large, extra large, and pediatric. Support belts 2–6 in. with or without prolapse support can be special ordered to accommodate specific needs.
Convex inserts	Can be added to selected two-piece systems. Some systems can accommodate two inserts for additional convexity. Insert should be 1/8 in. larger than stoma.
Bedside drainage system for urinary stomas	Can be secured to bed frame, mattress, or put on floor. Available as bags or bottles. Can be attached to pouch with use of adapter.
Pouch covers	Prevent allergic rash of skin to pouch. Provide moisture barriers between pouch/skin. Custom fit or already made. Adult and pediatric sizes. May enhance feelings of attractiveness.
Underwear/swimwear	Provide support to pouching system. Adult and pediatric sizes. May enhance feelings of attractiveness.
Closure clamps	Available from numerous manufacturers. Some not interchangeable from one manufacturer to another.
Stoma guide strips	Made from rice paper. Can be inserted in opening of pouching system to aid patient when centering during application. Strip will dissolve when moistened.
Tapes	Most are hypoallergenic. May be waterproof. Available in many sizes and types from variety of manufacturers.

eighth day, the stoma should be remeasured because the edema will usually have resolved, although it usually takes from 4 to 6 weeks for the stoma to shrink to its smallest size. Therefore, the size of the opening will require changes during this initial period.

Figure 32-15 outlines the procedure for application of a conventional reusable appliance. With a well-positioned stoma of adequate length, a properly applied reusable pouch should remain in place without leakage and without skin injury for 4 to 7 days. One may also shower or bathe with the pouch in place.

When removing the pouch, if a protective skin shield was used, the appliance may be pulled directly away from the skin. However, if adhesive cement has been employed, it may be necessary to drip a solvent with a pipette between the skin and the faceplate as it is lifted off. Adhesive remover wipes are also available. All of the solvent should then be thoroughly washed off the skin.

Before limitations imposed on hospitals and physicians concerning acceptable duration of hospital stay for a given illness, the patient was able to remain until adequate appliance training had been achieved. However, because of so-called cost-containment, individuals are now sent home much sooner.

The following factors are essential to a properly fitting appliance:

- It must not leak contents nor cause odor.
- It must not cause skin or stomal irritation.
- It must be comfortable for all levels of activity.
- It must not require a wardrobe change.
- It must be unobtrusive.

With knowledge of a few basic principles, a satisfactory management protocol can be developed. What may seem complex in the beginning will be routine in a brief time as the patient gains confidence that the system will not leak and will enable him or her to return to productive activity.

Patient/Family Education

Ideally, the timing of instruction should be based on learner readiness. However, as mentioned, shorter hospital lengths of stay often accelerate the teaching process, but unfortunately,

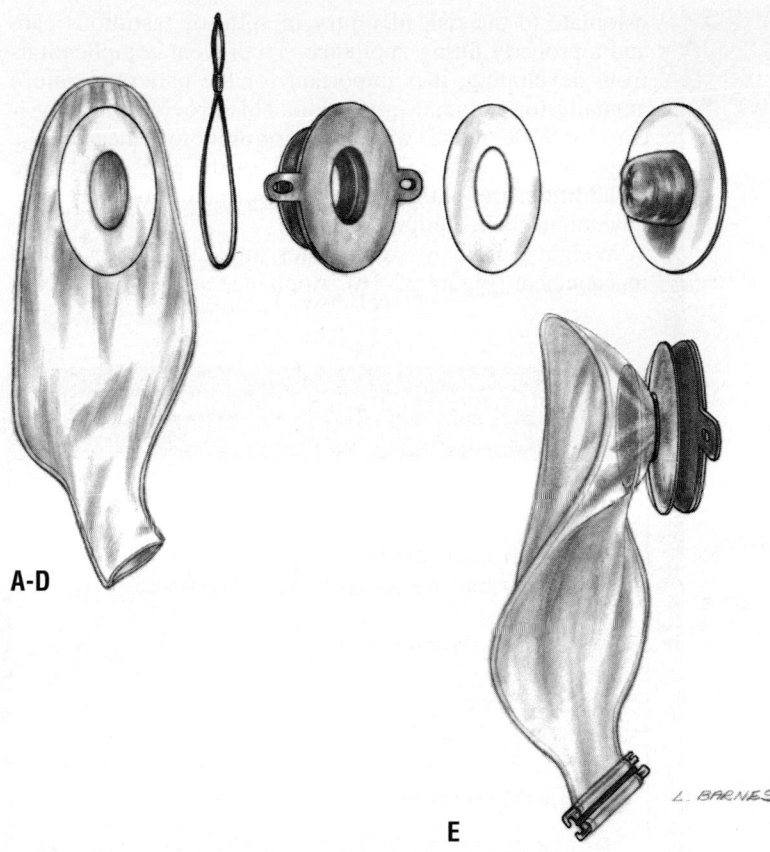

A-D

E

L. BARNES

FIGURE 32-15. Application of a reusable appliance. **A,B:** Mount the faceplate on the pouch (if using a two-piece appliance) and apply the elastic O-ring. **C:** Apply the double-faced adhesive to the back of the faceplate. **D:** After the skin is prepared, place the skin protector around the stoma. **E:** After exposure of the other side of the adhesive disk, the appliance is seated with the aid of a guide strip.

learning may not be enhanced.[8,20] Support from family, friends, and home care nurses will ease the transition to home self-care. It is important that these support services build on the patient's previous knowledge in order to avoid fostering dependence.[15] Lessons should be conducted when the patient is alert and rested. Early in morning, right after breakfast, is the optimal time for effective teaching.

If the patient's activity tolerance and space permit, self-care lessons should be conducted in the bathroom. This encourages the patient and the family to relate ostomy care to toilet activities, rather than to a medical, nursing procedure.[8]

Ostomy self-care instructions ideally take place at least 3 to 4 consecutive days prior to discharge. The first lesson may consist of a detailed demonstration of the entire pouch-changing procedure. The patient is instructed on pouch emptying, the use of the closure clamp or spout, and ostomy system removal. Soiled pouches should be placed in a plastic bag or similar container and disposed of promptly. Examples of patient instruction sheets distributed at the Cleveland Clinic are reproduced in Tables 32-6 and 32-7.

The peristomal skin is cleansed using a nonoily cleanser or nonlotion, nondeodorant soap, and then rinsed and patted dry. Use of lotions or ointments on the peristomal skin is discouraged because these products may prevent the ability of the skin barrier or adhesive to adhere to the skin. If hair growth in the peristomal area is a problem, it can be removed with an electric razor or scissors. Use of a disposable blade is discouraged because it may result in stripping the epithelial surface of the skin and in predisposing the patient to folliculitis.[8,13] The skin should be cleansed from the outside in toward the stoma because this will prevent mucus and effluent from resoiling the skin. Because the stoma is highly vascular, slight bleeding during cleansing is not unusual.[8,13] For reasons of cost, patients are encouraged to use washcloths or soft paper towels at home instead of the gauze commonly used in hospitals. After discharge, many individuals elect to shower before or after they have removed their pouches. It is important to remind patients that it is not necessary to remove the pouch every time they bathe. Those with colostomies or ileostomies will wish to time their pouch changes to coincide with intestinal activity. Because urinary stomas function at will, the timing of the pouch change and showering is best undertaken prior to ingestion of liquids.

Patients and families need to be supplied with a discharge folder that includes step-by-step written instructions specific for their type of ostomy and pouching system, along with stock numbers and ordering information; a list of dealers and manufacturers; referral phone numbers; and discharge instructions (Table 32-8). Information related to the advantages of wearing a medical condition identification tag is advisable. If the patient is ever in an accident or unconscious, the nature of the ostomy can be communicated to emergency medical personnel. This is especially important for patients with continent diversions or pelvic pouches.

Prior to discharge those with *continent diversions* are instructed in catheter irrigation, stoma and skin care, and management of leg and bedside drainage bags. Once the internal reservoir is safely healed, intubation instruction is generally conducted in the outpatient department or office by the WOC nurse 3 to 4 weeks following discharge. A patch or gauze is then applied over the stoma to absorb mucous.[9,18] Frequency of intubation is initially every 2 hours for the first week, increasing the interval by 1 hour the following weeks. Eventually, most patients will intubate approximately every

TABLE 32-6 How to Change Your Disposable, One-piece, Cut-to-Fit Pouch with Attached Skin Barrier

Gather the following supplies:

Washcloths or paper towels
Nonoily soap (Ivory and Dial are recommended brands)
Scissors
Plastic bag or newspaper
New pouch
Accessory products

Prepare the new pouch:

Trace the pattern (sized to fit within 1/8 in. of stoma) on the cover paper of the skin barrier.
Cut out the skin barrier. Be careful not to cut through the front of the pouch.
Remove the covers from the skin barrier and the adhesive surface of the pouch.
Set the pouch aside, sticky side up.

Remove the worn pouch:

Holding the pouch upright, remove the clip from the end of the pouch.
Empty the waste from the pouch into the toilet.
Remove the worn pouch by:
• Applying light pressure on the skin with one hand.
• Gently pulling the pouch from the skin with the other hand.
• Wrap the worn pouch in newspaper or place in a plastic bag and discard.

Cleanse the skin around the stoma:

Wash the area around the stoma with nonoily soap and warm water.
Rinse the area thoroughly with warm water.
Pat the skin dry with a washcloth or paper towel.

Apply the new pouch:

Center the pouch opening over the stoma and press into place.
Smooth the sticky surface of the pouch onto the skin.
Hold the pouch firmly in place for a few moments.

Close the pouch end securely

Fasten the pouch end securely with the clip.

---

ostomate to the risk of injury in spite of fastidious care and a properly fitting appliance. To prevent complications from developing, it is important for the patient to return annually for a stomal inspection. This provides the physician (or WOC nurse) with an opportunity to remeasure the stoma and to evaluate the integrity of the peristomal skin. In addition, the patient can be informed about any new developments in equipment.

Weight gain or loss has major implications for stomal management (Figure 32-16). Appliance size and convexity

TABLE 32-7 How to Change Your Disposable, Two-piece Pouch with Cut-to-Fit

Gather the following supplies:

Washcloths or paper towels
Nonoily soap (Ivory and Dial are recommended brands)
Scissors
Plastic bag or newspaper
New pouch
Skin barrier flange
Accessory products

Prepare the new pouch:

Trace the pattern (sized to fit within 1/4 in. of stoma) on the cover paper of the skin barrier flange.
Cut out the skin barrier flange.
Remove the cover papers from the skin barrier and the adhesive surface of the flange.
Set the skin barrier flange aside, sticky side up.
Set the pouch next to the flange.

Remove the worn pouch:

Holding the pouch upright, remove the clip from the end of the pouch.
Empty the waste from the pouch into the toilet.
Remove the worn pouch and skin barrier by:
• Applying light pressure on the skin with one hand.
• Gently pulling the pouch from the skin with the other hand.
• Wrap the worn pouch in newspaper or place in a plastic bag and discard.

Cleanse the skin around the stoma:

Wash the area around the stoma with nonoily soap and warm water.
Rinse the area thoroughly with warm water.
Pat the skin dry with a washcloth or paper towel.

Apply the prepared pouch:

Center the skin barrier flange opening over the stoma and press into place.
Smooth the sticky surface of the skin barrier flange onto the skin.
Snap the pouch securely onto the skin barrier flange.
Hold the pouch firmly in place for a few moments.

Close the pouch end securely:

Fasten the pouch end securely with the clip.

---

4 hours. During the night, they are advised to set an alarm or connect the catheter to constant drainage. Prevention of overdistension of the pouch must be emphasized.

Prevention and Treatment of Skin Irritation

As previously discussed, the corrosive effluent from an ileostomy demands careful appliance management. Additionally, mechanical irritation, allergic and nonallergic dermatitis, and various infections may predispose the

TABLE 32-8 Colostomy Manufacturers and Products

COMPANY	PRODUCTS	COMPANY	PRODUCTS
CR Bard, Inc. 111 Spring Street Murray Hill, NJ 07974	Disposable pouches; ReliaSeal; skin care cream and cleanser	Nu-Hope Laboratories, Inc. 12640 Branford St. Pacoima, CA 91331	Appliances; adhesive foam pads; accessories; support belts; appliance covers; hole cutter tool; skin barriers
Blanchard Ostomy Products 1510 Raymond Ave. Glendale, CA 91201	Karaya wafers and powder; pouches; faceplates; accessories	Palex Medical, Inc. 8807 Northwest 23rd St. Miami, FL 33172	Ostomy products
Chattem, Inc. 1715 W. 38th Street Chattanooga, TN 37409	Nullo deodorant	Parthenon Co., Inc. 3311 W. 2400 South Salt Lake City, UT 84119	Devrom chewable tablets
Coloplast Corp. 1955 West Oak Circle Marietta, GA 30062	Disposable appliances; two-piece system; conseal continent colostomy system; Comfeel; skin creams and ointments; Peri-Wash	Perma-Type Co., Inc. 83 Northwest Drive Farmington Industrial Park Plainville, CT 06062	Reusable appliances; accessories; Fresh Tabs (deodorant)
ConvaTec Squibb P.O. Box 5254 Princeton, NJ 08543–5254 http://www.convatec.com	Sur-Fit system; DuoDERM; Kenalog spray; Mycostatin powder; Stomahesive; Durahesive; Active life; pediatric pouches	HW Rutzen and Son 345 W Irving Park Road Chicago, IL 60618	Reusable appliances; accessories
Cymed Ostomy Co. 1440C Fourth St. Berkeley, CA 94710 http://www.cymed-ostomy.com	Disposable appliances	Rystan Co., Inc. 47 Center Street, P.O. Box 214 Little Falls, NJ 07424	Derifil tablets and powder
Hollister, Inc. 2000 Hollister Drive Libertyville, IL 60048 http://www.hollister.com	Disposable appliances; Hollihesive; irrigation equipment; karaya paste; Skin Gel; incontinence devices; accessories	Schilling and Morris Marketing, Ltd. 215 Tremond St. Rochester, NY 14614	Ostobon deodorant
Incutech, Inc. 307-A, S. Westgate Drive Greensboro, NC 27407	Disposable pouches; skin barriers; skin lotion; irrigation equipment accessories	Richard C. Shelton Co. 1525 Wayne Avenue Dayton, OH 45409	Osto-Zyme (spray deodorant)
Marlen Manufacturing and Development Co. 5150 Richmond Road Bedford, OH 44146	Reusable appliances; accessories; stoma paper guide strips; loop ostomy rods; irrigation equipment; stoma location disks	Smith and Nephew United, Inc. P.O. Box 1970 Largo, FL 34649	Appliances; accessories; adhesive foam pads; Banish; Skin Prep; irrigation educational material and teaching aids; Soft-Guard XL skin barrier
Mason Laboratories, Inc. P.O. Box 334 Horsham, PA 19044	Colly-Seel; Skin Tac; appliances; M-9 deodorant drops	Torbot Co. 1185 Jefferson Blvd. Warwick, RI 12886	Reusable appliances; accessories; rigid faceplates
Mentor Corporation 600 Pine Avenue Santa Barbara, CA 93117	Appliances; accessories; irrigation equipment; Stomapaper guide strips; Skin Shields	VPI—A Cook Group Co. P.O. Box 266 Spencer, IN 47460	Nonadhesive ostomy systems
3M Medical Products 3M Center St. Paul, MN 55101	Double-faced adhesives; adhesive foam pads; micropore paper tape; Stomaseal		

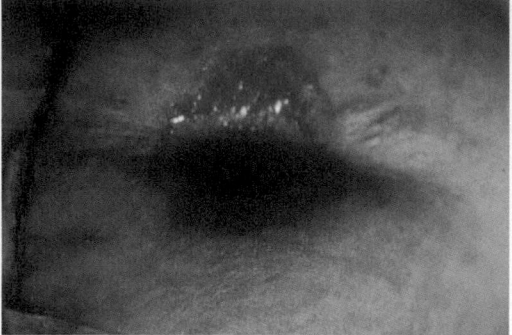

FIGURE 32-16. Weight gain and poor colostomy location in a skin fold result in a stoma that cannot be managed by conventional means. Note dermatitis inferior to the retracted ostomy opening.

may require a change (Figure 32-17), and skin sensitivity may develop to products even after many years of use (Figures 32-18 and 32-19). A number of skin complications and treatments are discussed in Table 32-9.

Mild Irritation

Even mild skin irritation must be treated promptly to prevent serious consequences. Mild or moderate dermatitis may be

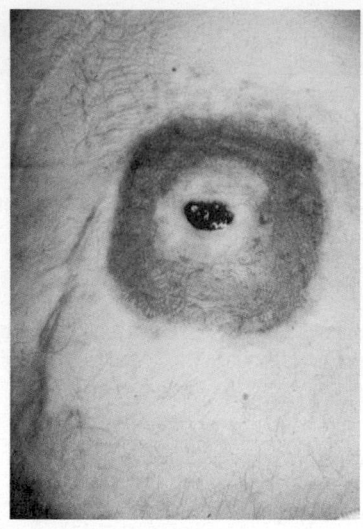

FIGURE 32-18. Pericolostomy dermatitis from an allergy to adhesive. Note the halo of protected skin around the stoma from the karaya ring.

managed by gently washing the peristomal skin with warm water. Standard soaps should not be used; several companies make special ones for ostomy care only (e.g., Coloplast). The area should be permitted to dry thoroughly. A hair dryer (on the coolest setting) held approximately 1 ft away from the skin can be used. Karaya or Stomahesive powder should be dusted on the area, and the excess brushed off. After a skin protective agent is applied and permitted to dry, a skin barrier is used with a clean appliance.

Severe Irritation

Severe irritation may be caused by improper fitting of the faceplate, leakage, allergy to the adhesive product, or yeast

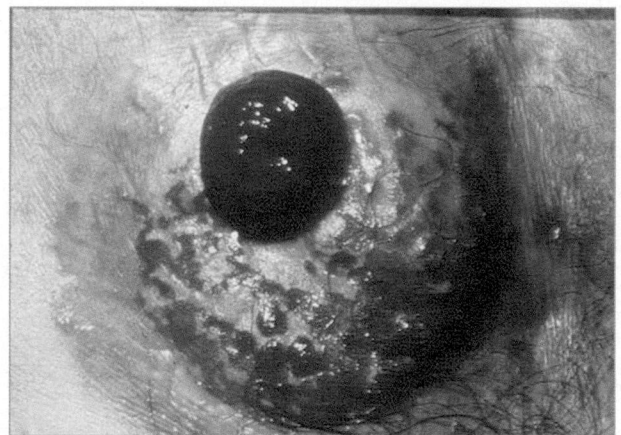

A

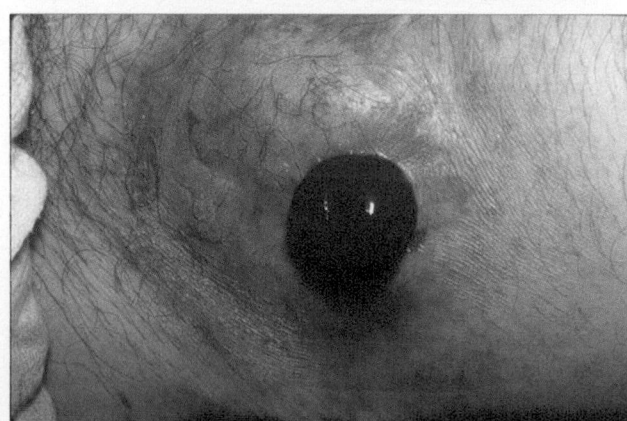

B

FIGURE 32-17. Improper fitting faceplate. **A:** Severe peristomal dermatitis from the faceplate being too large. **B:** Resolution following use of a proper-fitting appliance. (From Corman ML, Veidenheimer MC, Coller JA. Ileostomy complications: prevention and treatment. *Contemp Surg.* 1976;8:36.)

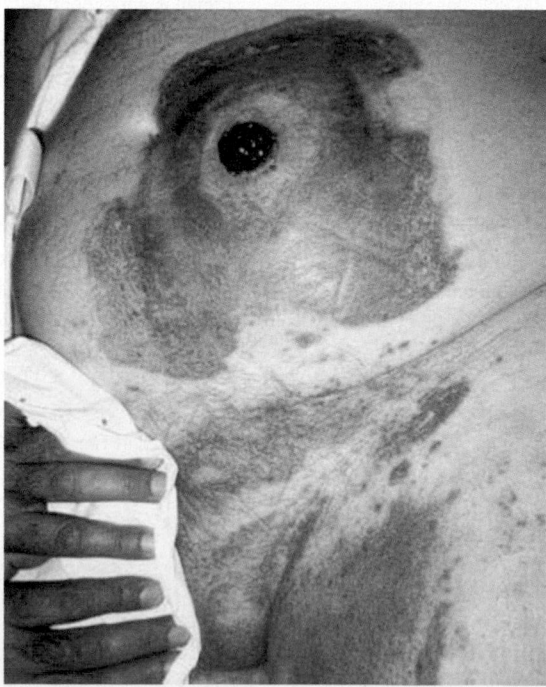

FIGURE 32-19. Severe allergy to adhesive and to the pouch itself. The bag hung in the groin, hence the inflammation in that area. Skin testing with a piece of pouch plastic yielded a positive response.

TABLE 32-9 Important Peristomal Skin Conditions

CONDITION	CHARACTERISTICS	TREATMENT
Allergic contact dermatitis (Figures 32-18 and 32-19)	Allergic response generated by patient sensitivity to a particular product. Skin appears erythematous, edematous, eroded, weepy, or bleeding. Generally corresponds to the exposed area.	Remove the allergen, avoid other irritants, protect the skin. Patch test with other products as needed.
Candidiasis (Figure 32-23)	Warm, moist environment creates milieu for proliferation of *Candida albicans*. Generally diffuse erythematous papules. Can form plaques with characteristic advancing border and satellite lesions. Severe pruritus common.	Topical antifungal powder. Assess pouching system for leakage or undermining of seal.
Caput medusa (peristomal varices) (Figures 31-65 and 32-24)	In patients with portal hypertension, the pressure at the portal systemic shunt in the mucocutaneous junction increases, creating venous engorgement. With trauma, profuse bleeding can occur.	Direct pressure or use of hemostatic agents (e.g., silver nitrate). Cautery or surgical ligation may be necessary. Careful pouch removal. Avoid aggressive skin barriers and skin sealants. If stoma is relocated, varices will eventually recur around the new stoma.
Folliculitis (Figure 32-25)	Traumatic removal of hair during pouch changes results in inflammation and infection of hair follicles. Lesions are painful and moist.	Topical antimicrobial powder, cover large lesions with nonadherent gauze. Once healed, patient should carefully shave the area. Use of adhesive remover and skin sealant is advised.
Irritant dermatitis (Figure 32-26)	Chemical destruction of the skin caused by topical products or leakage. Area appears erythematous, moist, and painful. May be localized to a specific area of pouch undermining or leakage.	Review patient's product usage and techniques to determine cause Correct as needed.
Mechanical trauma (Figures 32-22 and 32-27)	External item or force causing damage to the stoma and/or skin from pressure, laceration, friction, or shear.	Assess equipment and pouching technique. Modify equipment and accessories to prevent reinjury.
Peristomal ulcer or abscess (Figure 32-28)	Presents with one or more open, painful lesions surrounded by a halo of erythema. Not uncommon in patients with active Crohn's disease in distal bowel.	Unroofing of ulcer by surgeon. Management depends on size Options include nonadherent gauze, hydrogel, astringent solution, or hydrocolloid wafer. A nonadherent pouching system can be fashioned with a one-piece pouch with belt tabs and an extra gasket.
Pseudoverrucous lesions (Figures 31-55 and 32-29)	Overgrowth of tissue caused by overexposure to moisture. Appears as raised, moist lesions with wartlike appearance. Lesions are often painful.	Assess equipment for proper aperture and fit. Resize as needed. In severe cases, sharp debridement may be required.
Pyoderma gangrenosum (Figure 32-30)	Associated with IBD, arthritis, leukemia, polycythemia vera, and multiple myeloma. Red open lesions become raised with irregular purplish margins.	Systemic treatment of underlying disease, local ulcer treatment. Curettage is generally not advised. Topical therapy and pouching same as with abscess.
Radiation injury	Red, thinned skin. Easily traumatized by removal of skin adhesives.	Gently cleanse skin with cool water. Select pouching system with barrier that is easy to remove. Be cautious in use of solvents or skin sealants due to frequent sensitivities.
Parastomal abscess (Figure 30-63)	Mucocutaneous sepsis. Infected parastomal hematoma. Occult fistula. Extraperitoneal perforated colostomy. Recurrent Crohn's disease	Incision and drainage. May be done well lateral to stoma so skin barrier can still be applied or drainage catheter can be used at site of mucocutaneous separation and incorporated to pouch.

IBD, inflammatory bowel disease.

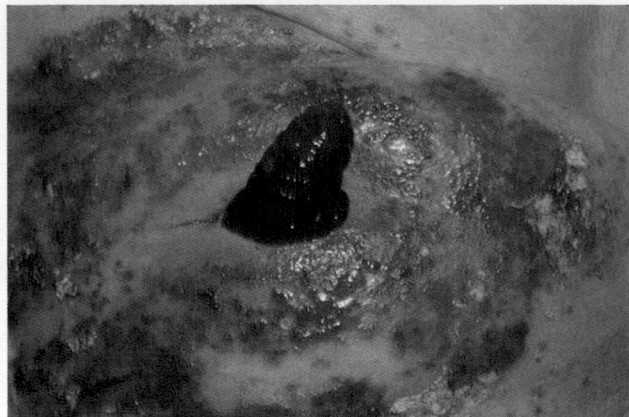

FIGURE 32-20. Severe dermatitis with a yeast infection in a patient whose appliance management was poor, with frequent leakage.

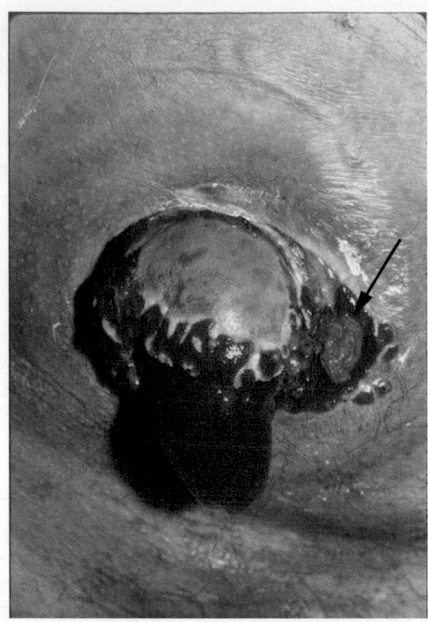

FIGURE 32-22. Fecal fistula (*arrow*) secondary to erosion from an improperly fitted appliance.

infection (Figures 32-19 through 32-22). After drying, a skin protective agent is applied, followed by a skin barrier and a clean pouch. Occasionally, a small piece of nonadherent gauze or wound dressing may be placed over a draining area to prevent undermining of the skin barrier and to allow absorption to take place. This appliance may require daily changing until the problem resolves.

Yeast and Fungal Infections
Problems with yeast or fungal infections often occur during warm weather or whenever moisture accumulates under the appliance (Figure 32-23). The area should be cleansed and dried gently, and a small amount of topical steroid spray may be applied on the affected area. However, the use of a topical steroid spray is not generally advisable for a fungal infection. The response to a topical antifungal agent alone is generally effective. After the excess is wiped off, the area should be dusted lightly with an antifungal powder and the excess brushed off. The skin barrier should follow and then the pouch. Depending on the severity of the infection, this unit may be left in place for 48 hours and the process repeated once or twice more if necessary.

Diet
Dietary modifications in patients with fecal and urinary diversions may be advisable. Generally, a low residue diet

is suggested for the first 6 to 8 weeks following surgery. Patients with ileostomies may find it difficult to tolerate poorly digested foods, such as corn, nuts, and raw fruits and vegetables. These products may result in a food bolus obstruction at the ileostomy. Certain foods such as applesauce, rice, and bananas can decrease bowel frequency. Conversely, caffeine, fiber, spicy foods, and raw fruits and vegetables may increase function. Individuals with continent ileostomies will need to keep the stool fairly liquid in order to allow passage of the effluent through the catheter. Six or 8 oz of prune juice daily may adequately thin the stool for this purpose. All patients with small bowel stomas are advised to avoid the use of laxatives.

After the initial postoperative period, individuals with urostomies have no dietary restrictions. However, patients may find that fish and asparagus can cause a strong, offensive odor. Use of ascorbic acid, cranberry supplements, and prophylactic antibiotic therapy is controversial. When concerned, a patient should be referred to a urologist.

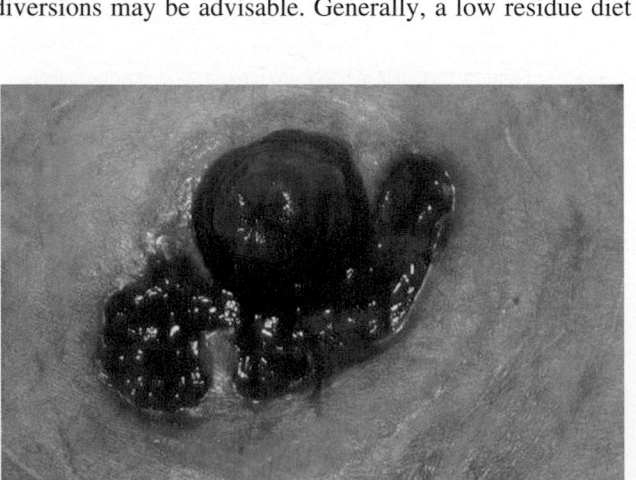

FIGURE 32-21. Ulcerating areas around an ileostomy are due to a neglected leakage problem.

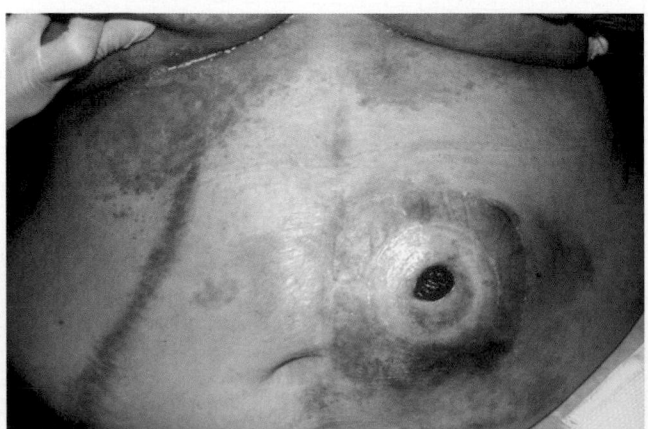

FIGURE 32-23. Candidiasis. Peristomal involvement is seen as well as involvement beneath the breast.

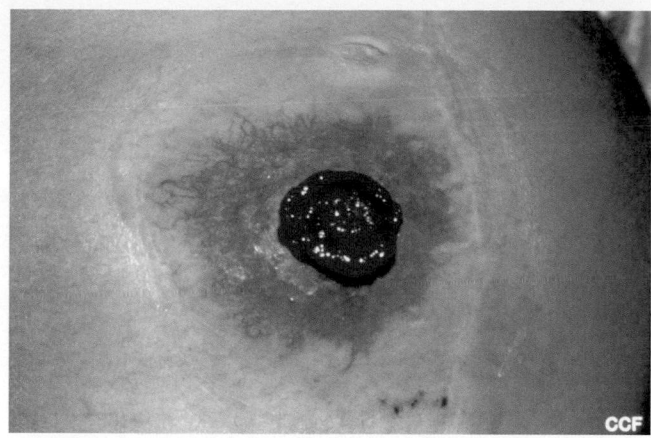

FIGURE 32-24. Caput medusa.

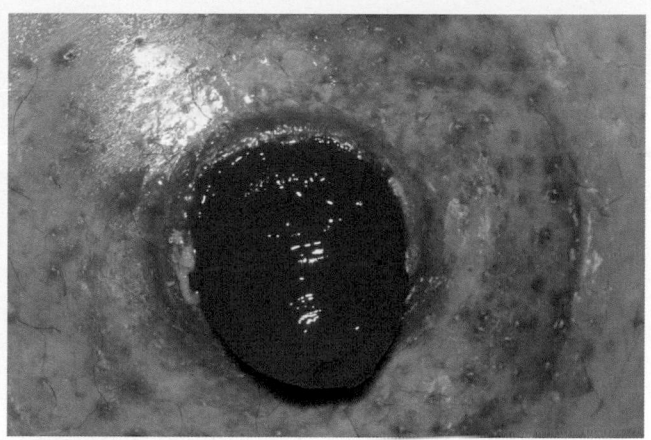

FIGURE 32-25. Folliculitis

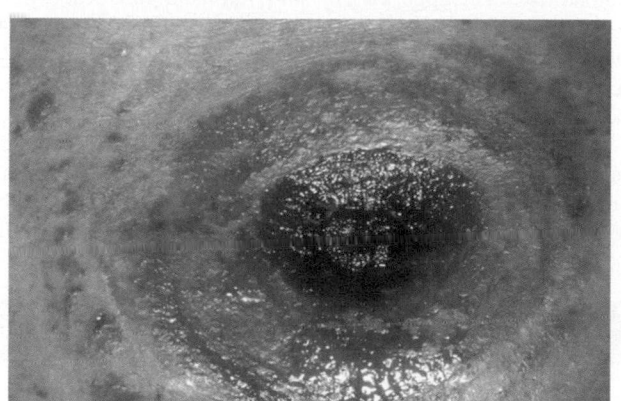

FIGURE 32-26. Ileostomy with chemical destruction of skin.

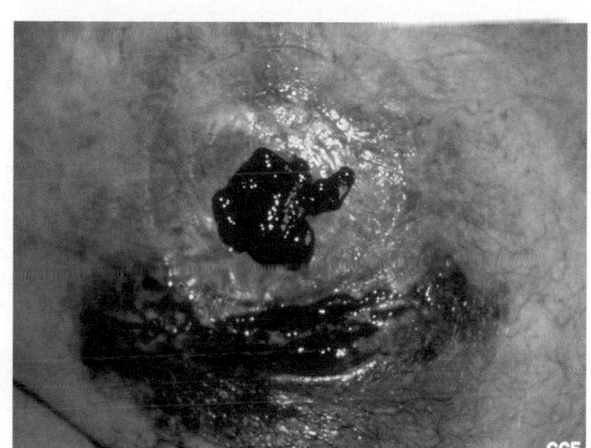

FIGURE 32-27. Mechanical trauma. Stomal laceration.

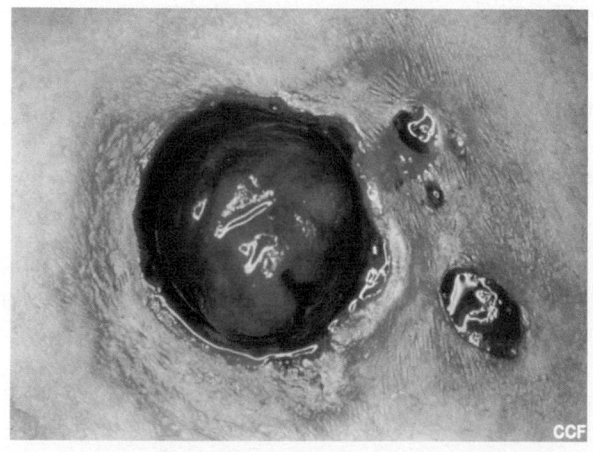

A

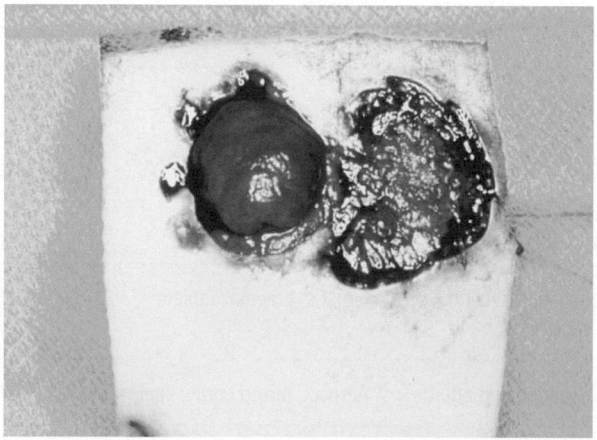

B

FIGURE 32-28. **A:** Peristomal ulcer. **B:** Peristomal ulcer after unroofing.

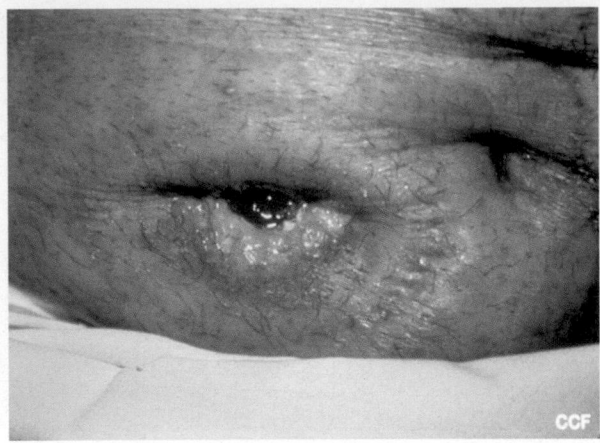

FIGURE 32-29. Pseudoverrucous lesions (formerly known as pseudoepithe-liomatous hyperplasia).

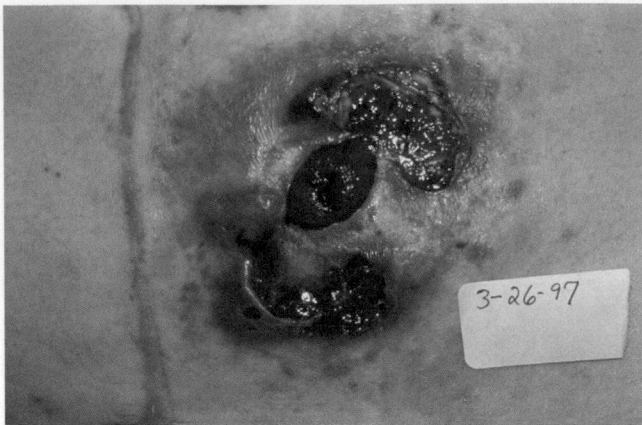

FIGURE 32-30. Peristomal pyoderma gangrenosum.

Odor Control

Diet and personal hygiene probably are the most effective means for decreasing odor.[4] Gazzard and associates studied 50 ileostomy patients and 50 colostomy patients in an attempt to ascertain which foods upset stomal function.[12] Only a small variety of foodstuffs produced symptoms in a significant number of patients. Individuals with colostomies found flatulence to be more of a problem than odor, particularly after eating vegetables or fruit. Items in this study that tended to be associated with an increased odor differed for ileostomy patients when compared with those who had a colostomy. Fish, eggs, cheese, and onions, in that order, were a greater problem for ileostomy patients, and green vegetables were the primary agents in patients with a colostomy. Yogurt, buttermilk, and parsley have been said to decrease odor in colostomy patients.[4]

A number of products are available that help to reduce odor (Table 32-10). Liquid deodorants are generally more successful than tablets for use in pouches because tablets do not dissolve quickly enough. Recommended items

TABLE 32-10 Products to Control Odor

INTERNAL	FORM	SIDE EFFECTS
Activated charcoal	Capsules	Large dose can interfere with absorption of vitamins. Darkens stool.
Chlorophyllin copper complex	Tablets	Absorbs some gas. Turns stool dark green.
Bismuth subgallate	Tablets	Can cause toxicity if taken in large doses.
Bismuth subcarbonate	Tablets	Constipation.

EXTERNAL	FORM	DESCRIPTION
Pouch-deodorizing agents	Liquids, powder, tablets	May contain a combination of water, zinc ricinoleate, propylene glycol. Some contain silver nitrate, organic acids, urea, and fragrance.
Air-deodorizing agents	Aerosol, pump spray, liquids, solids	May contain water, ethanol, fragrance, and artificial colors.
Pouch-cleaning/ deodorizing agents		Used to clean and deodorize reusable stoma plates and pouches. May contain water, detergent, surfactants, liquid petroleum. Must rinse well.
Gas filters	Stick to one- to two-piece drainable pouches	Charcoal filter incorporated to deodorize gas. Some plastic pouches may not permit a secure seal of the adhesive. Not suitable for use with watery effluent.

include Super Banish (Smith and Nephew), OAD (Coloplast), M-9 (Hollister), Dignity, Osto-Zyme, and Nil-Odor. Approximately six drops are placed inside the pouch after each emptying.

If these are not adequate for control, several oral preparations are very effective. Derifil (chlorophyllin), one to three tablets daily taken orally, has been demonstrated to be an effective agent for eliminating or reducing odors of fecal and urinary drainage. Devrom (bismuth subgallate), a chewable tablet taken one half hour before meals, two or three times daily, is also an effective odor-reduction agent. It also tends to thicken and darken the stool. Bismuth subcarbonate has a similar effect. Some patients may experience difficulty tolerating certain oral products.

Sexual Concerns

A patient may express concerns about sexuality during his or her hospitalization. In collaboration with the surgeon, the WOC nurse should address this topic as part of the patient's preoperative and postoperative counseling. Issues about reproduction, sexual function, and interpersonal relationships are common. Teenagers may be especially reluctant to talk about dating, sex, and reproduction in front of their families. Women with pelvic pouches or perineal incisions often experience vaginal dryness. Use of a water-soluble lubricant during sexual intercourse may, therefore, be indicated.[3] Support for gay or lesbian patients with ostomies can be obtained from the gay/lesbian support group (GLO) of the United Ostomy Associations of America (UOAA). Initially, most individuals are often more concerned with the practical aspects of managing their ostomies than with psychosexual concerns. It is for this reason that postdischarge follow-up by a WOC nurse is beneficial.

Discharge Planning

Discharge planning should begin at the time of admission to the hospital.[10] Active communication among the surgeon, nurse providing ostomy care, staff nurses, social worker, case manager, discharge planner, and the patient and family will ease the transition to life at home.[6,8,10] If placement in a subacute unit or extended care facility is contemplated, the nurse or social worker will contact the institution to promote continuity of care.[21] If a home care referral is initiated, contact between the hospital-based nurse providing ostomy care and the staff nurse at the home care agency is essential. For an especially complex pouching system, it is helpful for the hospital nurse and the home care or extended care facility nurse to make a joint visit prior to the patient's discharge from the hospital.[21] Long-term follow-up will be based on the patient's underlying condition. It is recommended that the WOC nurse or surgeon evaluate the stoma, pouching, skin, and overall rehabilitation at least once a year.

Activity

Once recuperation from surgery is complete, patients should be encouraged to enjoy a full and active life. Heavy lifting and contact sports are best avoided because of the risk for hernia or stomal trauma. Otherwise, there are no physical restrictions associated with fecal or urinary diversions.

Additional Considerations

Insurance coverage is an important concern. In the United States, patients with Medicare are afforded protection included under "prosthetic devices." This will provide coverage for much of the appliance expense. The usual cost for equipment is $700 to $1,200 a year.

As part of a comprehensive rehabilitative planning program, it is helpful to provide other resources for information. The local chapter of the American Cancer Society and the UOAA make available a number of booklets and brochures that the patient will usually find quite helpful (see the following).

▶ ADDITIONAL INFORMATION RESOURCES

American Cancer Society
250 Williams Street, NW
Atlanta, GA 30303
Phone: (800) 227-2345
TTY: (866) 228-4327
EIN: 13 1788491

For information and support for people with cancer, also contact the local chapter of the American Cancer Society.

The Cleveland Clinic
Wound, Ostomy and Continence/Enterostomal Therapy Nursing
9500 Euclid Ave. NA40
Cleveland, OH 44195
Phone: (216) 444-6677 or (800) 223-2273, ext. 46677
Fax: (216) 445-6343

For WOC/ET nursing support and advice regarding pouch management or adjustment difficulties.

Crohn's and Colitis Foundation of America
444 Park Ave. South
New York, NY 10016
Phone: (212) 685-3440
http://www.ccfa.org

For information on and support for people with Crohn's disease or ulcerative colitis.

Patient Education Press
417 Cleveland Ave.
Plainfield, NJ 07060

For the following publications: *Ostomy Care for Children, Colostomy Care, Ileostomy Care, Urinary Diversion,* and *Ostomy Dietary Guidelines.*

United Ostomy Association of America
P.O. Box 512
Northfield MN 55057-0512
http://www.uoaa.org

WOCN Society National Office
15000 Commerce Parkway, Suite C
Mt. Laurel, NJ 08054
Phone (Toll Free): (888) 224-WOCN (9626)

Other Publications

Broadwell DC, Jackson BS, eds. *Principles of Ostomy Care.* St. Louis, MO: Mosby; 1982.
Cox BG, Wentworth AE. *The Ileal Pouch Procedure.* Rochester, MN: Mayo Comprehensive Cancer Center; 1977.

Hampton B, ed. *Ostomies and Continent Diversions.* St. Louis, MO: Mosby–Year Book; 1992.

Hill GL. *Ileostomy: Surgery, Physiology, and Management.* New York, NY: Grune and Stratton; 1976.

Jeter KF. *These Special Children.* Palo Alto, CA: Bull Publishing; 1982.

Journal of Enterostomal Therapy. Official publication of the International Association for Enterostomal Therapists, published quarterly by Mosby (St. Louis).

Mullen BD, McGinn DA. *The Ostomy Book: Living Comfortably with Colostomies, Ileostomies, and Urostomies.* Palo Alto, CA: Bull Publishing; 1980.

Ostomy Quarterly. A publication of the United Ostomy Association, published quarterly.

Steiner-Grossman P, Banks PA, Present DH, eds. *People Not Patients: A Source Book for Living with Inflammatory Bowel Disease.* New York, NY: National Foundation for Ileitis and Colitis; 1985.

Walker FC, ed. *Modern Stoma Care.* London, United Kingdom: Churchill-Livingstone; 1976.

References

1. Ahlering TE, Weinberg AC, Razor B. Modified Indiana pouch. *J Urol.* 1991;145(6):1156–1158.

2. Aukett LK, Bonsaint R, Corbin C, et al. National guidelines for enterostomal patient education. *Dis Colon Rectum.* 1994;37(6):559–563.

3. Bambrick M, Fazio VW, Hull TL, et al. Sexual function following restorative proctocolectomy in women. *Dis Colon Rectum.* 1996;39(6):610–614.

4. Boston A, Litman L, Rush A, et al. Controlling colostomy odor. *Am J Nurs.* 1977;77(3):444.

5. Corman JM, Odenheimer DB. Securing the loop—historic review of the methods used for creating a loop colostomy. *Dis Colon Rectum.* 1991;34(11):1014–1021.

6. Erwin-Toth P. Advances in enterostomal therapy. *Perspect Colon Rectal Surg.* 1995;8:227.

7. Erwin-Toth P, Barrett P. Stoma site marking: a primer. *Ostomy Wound Manage.* 1997;43(4):18–22.

8. Erwin-Toth P, Doughty D. Principles and procedures of stomal management. In: Hampton B, Bryant R, eds. *Ostomies and Continent Diversions: Nursing Management.* St. Louis, MO: Mosby; 1992.

9. Erwin-Toth P, Floruta C. Nursing management of continent ostomy diversions. *Progressions.* 1993;5:3.

10. Ewing G. The nursing preparation of stoma patients for self-care. *J Adv Nurs.* 1989;14(5):411–420.

11. Felice P. The many parts of ostomy collection systems: what are your options? *Ostomy Wound Manage.* 1985;9:31.

12. Gazzard BG, Saunders B, Dawson AM. Diets and stoma function. *Br J Surg.* 1978;65(9):642–644.

13. Kodner I. Stoma complications. In: Fazio V, ed. *Current Therapy in Colon and Rectal Surgery.* Philadelphia, PA: BC Decker; 1990.

14. Lavery IC, Erwin-Toth P. Stoma therapy. In: Cataldo PA, MacKeigan JM, eds. *Intestinal Stomas: Principles, Techniques, and Management.* 2nd ed. St. Louis, MO: Quality Medical Publishing; 1993:65–90.

15. Lewis C. *Aging: The Health Care Challenge.* Philadelphia, PA: FA Davis; 1990.

16. Meier DE, Tarpley JL. Improvisation in the developing world. *Surg Gynecol Obstet.* 1991;173(5):404–406.

17. Rodriguez R, Wiener I. A home made colostomy bag. *Surg Gynecol Obstet.* 1986;163(3):277.

18. Rolstad BS, Hoyman K. Continent diversions and reservoirs, ostomies and continent diversions. *Nurse Manager.* 1992;145:55.

19. Rothstein MS. Prevention and treatment of peristomal skin problems. *Ostomy Wound Manage.* 1985;9:6.

20. Ruzicki DA. Realistically meeting the educational needs of hospitalized acute and short-stay patients. *Nurs Clin North Am.* 1989;24(3):629–637.

21. Zarle NC. Continuity of care. Balancing care of elders between health care settings. *Nurs Clin North Am.* 1989;24(3):697–705.

33

Miscellaneous Colitides

Marvin L. Corman and Albert O. Kwon

This chapter addresses a number of inflammatory conditions of the bowel that, in general, are either infectious or noninfectious. The two conditions that have been discussed in previous chapters, ulcerative colitis and Crohn's disease, have been excluded. The common denominator for all of these diseases is an association with the symptom of diarrhea. The great majority of colitides are infectious in nature and are frequently the result of ingestion of contaminated food or water. Enteric diseases can also be sexually transmitted, especially through anal intercourse. This is a particular issue in immunosuppressed and HIV patients (see Chapter 10).

Although diarrheal disease is still one of the leading causes of morbidity and mortality, especially among children in the developing world, it is not an insignificant source of morbidity in Western countries due to the ubiquitous nature of travel and immigration. In the United States, adults experience an average of 4 episodes per year, and children experience 7 to 15 episodes by age 5.[218] Certainly, in elderly individuals or those who are immunocompromised, the potential for mortality is increased. Although it is indeed true that most diarrheal conditions are self-limiting, the surgeon must always be alert to the fact that even an acute onset of diarrheal disease may be the initial presentation of an underlying disorder that mandates thorough gastrointestinal investigation.[317]

▶ NONINFECTIOUS COLITIDES

I am poured out like water, and all my bones are out of joint; my heart is like wax; it is melted in the midst of my bowels.

—PSALM 22:14

Eosinophilic Gastroenteritis (Eosinophilic Colitis)

Primary eosinophilic gastroenteritis is a disorder that selectively affects the gastrointestinal tract. First described in 1937 by Kaisjer, it is characterized by an eosinophil-predominant chronic inflammatory process of unknown etiology. The eosinophilia is present not only in the peripheral blood but also in the intestinal tissue.[276] However, it has been reported that up to 23% of individuals do not present with peripheral eosinophilia.[223] With approximately 75% of affected individuals found to have an allergic or atopic history, such an association has been suggested, but it has yet to be proven.[219,223] However, it is known that the expansion and tissue distribution of eosinophils are regulated by IL-5 and eotaxin 1.[263] Furthermore, eosinophilic gastroenteritis has strong genetic and allergic components and presents immunopathogenic features similar to those of other allergic disorders, such as asthma.

Eosinophilic gastroenteritis can potentially affect any portion of the gastrointestinal tract. This can lead to eosinophilic esophagitis, eosinophilic gastritis, eosinophilic gastroenteritis, and eosinophilic colitis. The gastric antrum and the proximal small intestine are most frequently involved, whereas the colon is a rare location for the condition. Perianal disease has also been reported.[176] Eosinophilic colitis has a bimodal distribution, primarily affecting neonates and young adults.

The three major clinical patterns have been described based on the level of eosinophilic infiltration within the intestinal wall. The extent of disease corresponds to the clinical signs and symptoms of eosinophilic colitis. Primary mucosal disease is associated with enteric protein loss, diarrhea, and malabsorption. Predominant muscle layer disease is characterized by obstructive symptoms as well as bowel thickening and may result in volvulus, intussusception, or perforation. Primary subserosal disease classically presents with eosinophilic ascites.[35,171,223,235] The most common presenting symptoms are abdominal pain and change in bowel habits. Nausea, vomiting, weight loss, and rectal bleeding are also frequently noted.

Tissue eosinophilia is a common feature of eosinophilic gastroenteritis. Although eosinophiles are recognized manifestation in numerous gastrointestinal conditions, especially Crohn's disease and ulcerative colitis, there is no comparison with the massive infiltration present in eosinophilic gastroenteritis and colitis.[219] When the condition occurs in the colon, it may radiologically mimic tuberculosis, amebiasis, or Crohn's disease.[276] Based on the few cases reported thus far, the proximal colon seems to have a greater predilection for involvement. Colonoscopic evaluation may reveal changes from erythema and friability, to granularity and narrowing.[235] Tedesco and colleagues suggested that eosinophilic ileocolitis may be more common than originally thought, and postulated that biopsy and counting of high-power microscopic fields for eosinophils may be a useful means for distinguishing eosinophilic colitis from that of Crohn's disease (Figure 33-1).[302] Eosinophilic colitis is largely a diagnosis of exclusion. In addition to inflammatory bowel disease (IBD), the differential diagnosis should include infectious colitides, such as helminthiasis and amebiasis (see later), systemic hypereosinophilia syndrome, milk protein colitis, vasculitis, and allergic gastroenteropathy.[35] Evaluation of IgE levels may help in determining the possibility of allergen involvement. Moreover, immunohistochemical analysis of intestinal eosinophil activation in patients with eosinophilic gastroenteritis suggests that the eosinophil cationic protein stored in eosinophil granules and secreted by activated eosinophils may be a tissue marker for eosinophilic gastroenteritis.[28] However, the combination of histologic and clinical patterns is the mainstay for the diagnosis of inflammatory conditions of the colon.[47] Although diagnostic criteria have been established for eosinophilic esophagitis, there has yet to be a consensus reached for eosinophilic colitis. Many investigators have used 20 eosinophils per high power field as being diagnostic. It is important to note, however, that the amount of eosinophils present varies depending on the location within the colon, ranging significantly above and below the aforementioned threshold.[223]

Prognosis is generally good, with clinical, hematologic, roentgenographic, and histologic improvement occurring spontaneously (usually in children) or with corticosteroid therapy.[125] Commonly, symptoms will resolve within 2 weeks on steroid treatment. However, recurrence is not infrequent. Novel therapeutic approaches to the management of eosinophilic gastroenteritis are currently being assessed, including treatment with newer antihistamines, leukotriene receptor antagonists, and monoclonal antibodies, such as anti–IL-5 (mepolizumab) and anti-IgE (omalizumab).[108,223] However, resection of the involved bowel may be required for unremitting symptoms or to exclude another diagnosis.[219]

Microscopic Colitis: Lymphocytic Colitis and Collagenous Colitis

Microscopic colitis is an inflammatory condition that was initially described in 1976 by Lindström and colleagues.[183] It is characterized by chronic, watery diarrhea and grossly normal appearing colonic mucosa on endoscopic examination, with inflammation evident only on microscopic examination. Terminology for the disease has evolved as further investigation has allowed the disease to be more well defined. At present, it is widely accepted that microscopic colitis consists of two subtypes: lymphocytic colitis and collagenous colitis. Although the clinical manifestations are similar, the subtypes can be differentiated based on the presence of intraepithelial lymphocytosis and subepithelial collagen deposition, respectively.[274]

The actual incidence of microscopic colitis is unknown because it is a poorly reported condition. A study from Sweden by Olesen and colleagues[224] noted an increasing incidence of microscopic colitis over the past decades from 1.8 per 100,000 to 6 per 100,000 inhabitants. The authors concluded that the incidence of microscopic colitis is higher than previously described and is as common as Crohn's disease in Örebro, Sweden. Microscopic colitis was diagnosed in 10% of patients with nonbloody diarrhea and up to 20% of those individuals who were older than age 70 years. There is no association of microscopic colitis with an increased risk of colorectal cancer.[186] The incidence of microscopic colitis within the United States was recently investigated in a population-based study in Olmsted County, Minnesota. Over the duration of the study, investigators also reported an increasing incidence from 1.1 to 19.6 cases per 100,000 person-years. A positive association with older age was noted as well.[234] In a Canadian population-based study conducted by Williams and colleagues, the authors found that individuals aged 65 and older were five times more likely to have the disease, and an increased risk was found in women for both subtypes of microscopic colitis.[324]

A definitive cause of microscopic colitis has yet to be determined. Reports in the literature have described a correlation between the disease and certain medications,

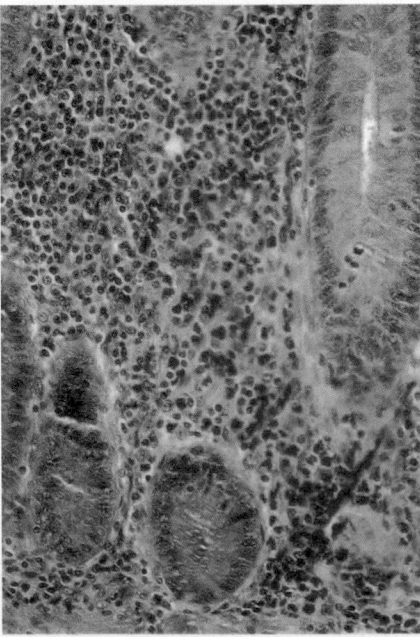

FIGURE 33-1. Eosinophilic enteritis. Intense inflammatory infiltration by eosinophils is seen within the mucosa and submucosa of the small bowel. (Original magnification × 330.)

such as nonsteroidal anti-inflammatory drugs (NSAIDs). However, no causal relationship has been established.[299] With respect to disease associations, links to autoimmunity are widely accepted, and an increased prevalence of microscopic colitis among patients with celiac disease has been described.[57,224] Moreover, Koskela and colleagues recently determined that HLA DR3-DQ2 (already linked to celiac disease) and TNF2 allele carriage (associated with autoimmunity) were also associated with both subtypes of microscopic colitis.[170]

The clinical course of this disease is benign, with spontaneous remission of symptoms occurring within a few years of onset. Watery diarrhea may persist over weekly or monthly intervals in association with fecal incontinence. Anemia, increased erythrocyte sedimentation rate, hypokalemia, and hypoalbuminemia are common findings. Microscopic colitis is often misdiagnosed as irritable bowel syndrome (IBS). However, its incidence in older individuals as well as the absence of abdominal discomfort as a significant complaint are distinguishing features.[274] Endoscopic examination and radiologic studies have demonstrated a normal appearing mucosa in the majority of individuals. However, edema, friability, pinpoint mucosal hemorrhages, and hyperemia have been occasionally seen.[248] Definitive diagnosis is based on histologic evaluation of colonic biopsies. Although microscopic colitis is a diffuse disease, it is recommended that one avoid rectal biopsies because the subepithelial collagen layer tends to be thicker in the rectum.[274] Both subtypes demonstrate damage to the epithelial cells, such as flattening and depletion along with a predominantly mononuclear inflammation of the lamina propria and preservation of crypt architecture. The inflammation is found to be remarkably uniform, indicative of a total colitis. As mentioned, additional histologic features distinguish lymphocytic colitis from collagenous colitis. Lymphocytic colitis is characterized by greater than 20 intraepithelial lymphocytes per 100 surface epithelial cells (Figure 33-2), whereas a thickened subepithelial collagen layer is typical in collagenous colitis (Figure 33-3).[89] The thickening of the subepithelial collagen layer may be a response to chronic

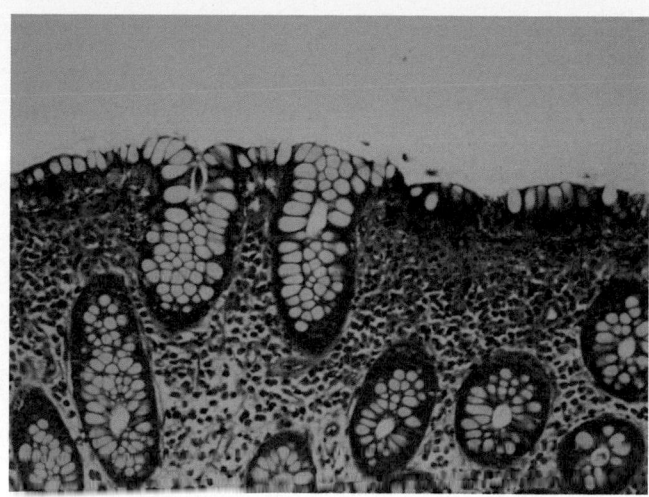

FIGURE 33-3. Collagenous colitis. Note the deposit of collagen in the upper lamina propria underneath the slightly denuded superficial epithelium. Trichrome-stained section highlights the subepithelial collagen (*blue* in color). (Magnification × 200.)

inflammation or a local abnormality of collagen synthesis.[289] It has been postulated that the disease may be attributable to reduced cell turnover, allowing fibrocytes to remain longer in the mature phase, hence producing more collagen and a thicker collagen plate.[158] Another subtype, although rare, has been described by Sandmeier and Bouzourene.[211] This type is characterized by the presence of subepithelial multinucleated giant cells, which the authors consider an important diagnostic criterion in the differential diagnosis of granulomatous infections and Crohn's disease. Moreover, it seems that this atypical subtype of microscopic colitis has a more favorable prognosis and a better response to corticosteroid therapy.

Recommended treatments have included nonspecific antidiarrheal agents, such as loperamide, bismuth subsalicylate, sulfasalazine, mesalamine, bile acid–binding agents (e.g., cholestyramine), budesonide, prednisone, and in refractory cases, immunosuppressive drugs.[118,274] In the Swedish experience, prednisolone was most effective, with a response rate of 82%. However, the required dose was often quite high, and the effect was not maintained following withdrawal of the medication. The response rates for antibiotics, cholestyramine, and loperamide were 63%, 59%, and 71%, respectively. Conversely, spontaneous resolution may occur.[32] Reported success rates with sulfasalazine and mesalamine are lower (40% to 50%).[274] A publication by the Cochrane database concerned a review of five randomized trials. It identified three treatment options for collagenous colitis. Budesonide was found to be an effective agent for the management of this disease; however, there was weak evidence to support the value of bismuth subsalicylate and prednisolone.[58] More recently, several randomized, double-blinded, placebo-controlled trials have demonstrated the efficacy of oral budesonide in both subtypes of microscopic colitis. Two trials involved the administration of budesonide, 6 mg daily, as maintenance treatment over 6 months in patients with collagenous colitis. The response rates in the treatment groups as compared with the placebo groups were 74.0% and 76.5% compared to 35% and 12%, respectively.[33,201] A third trial reported a response rate of 86% versus 48% placebo in patients with lymphocytic colitis who were given budesonide, 9 mg daily, for a 6-week duration.

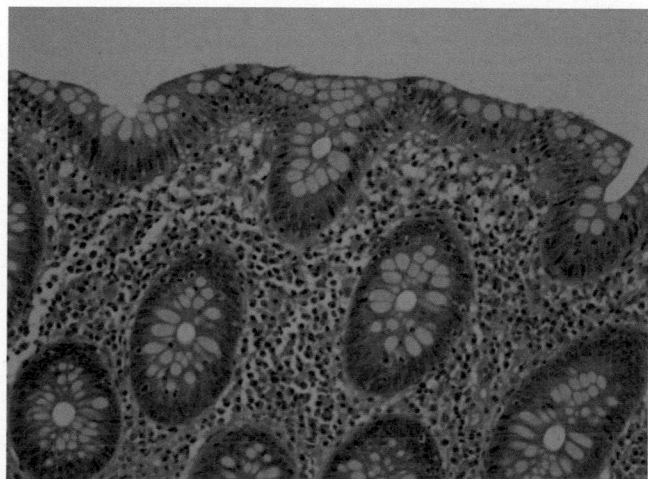

FIGURE 33-2. Microscopic colitis (lymphocytic colitis). Heavy lymphocytic infiltration confined to the mucosa and filling the lamina propria. There is a decrease in glandular mucus content as well as cryptoglandular distortion, but there is no suggestion of crypt abscess. (Original magnification × 400.)

Clinical relapses were noted but were treatable with repeated administration of budesonide.[202]

Rare refractory cases may benefit from operative management, but the role of surgery in this condition is extremely limited.[126] Fecal diversion, subtotal colectomy,[190] and restorative proctocolectomy with ileo-pouch anal anastomosis have all been suggested as therapeutic options.[313]

Neutropenic Enterocolitis (Ileocecal Syndrome or Typhlitis)

Neutropenic enterocolitis also known as ileocecal syndrome or typhlitis is a syndrome associated with bowel wall necrosis that was initially recognized in pediatric leukemic patients.[69] With the development of effective chemotherapeutic agents, this clinical entity has become increasingly prevalent in the adult population. It can occur during treatment of hematologic malignancies, especially leukemia, lymphoma, and aplastic anemia.[172] Those chemotherapeutic agents associated with neutropenic enterocolitis include paclitaxel, gemcitabine, cytosine, arabinoside, vincristine, doxorubicin, cyclophosphamide, 5-fluorouracil, leucovorin, and daunorubicin.[69] Neutropenic enterocolitis has also been reported as a complication of other therapeutic modalities, such as antithyroid therapy,[60] and chemotherapy for lung, breast, ovarian, and colon cancer,[69,101] or as the presenting complication of acute lymphoblastic leukemia.[244] It has also been described as a complication of cyclic neutropenia, a rare benign hematologic disorder.[222] Profound neutropenia secondary to chemotherapy has been considered the hallmark of the disease and the major etiologic factor in its development.[213] This is a condition characterized by regular oscillations in blood neutrophil counts, in which sporadic disappearance of these cells from the circulation occurs. Involvement of the process is most commonly seen in the cecum, possibly due to its distensibility and limited blood supply.[85] Other frequent sites include the terminal ileum and right colon, possibly because of the higher concentration of lymphatic tissue in these areas.

Patients exhibit symptoms of diarrhea, abdominal pain, sepsis, and findings typical of acute appendicitis. Even when the pain is localized to the right lower quadrant, the rapidity of the appearance of toxicity, with tachycardia, fever, and delirium, can be extremely dramatic. Koea and Shaw reported three individuals with leukemia who presented with fever, abdominal pain, and signs of peritonitis localized to the right iliac fossa.[166] Each patient was found to have a nonviable cecum.

The pathogenesis of the disease involves disruption of the intestinal mucosa in a neutropenic state compounded by damage secondary to chemotherapy. The disruption of gut mucosal integrity allows for the invasion of pathogenic bacteria leading to the release of endotoxins and to the development of necrosis and hemorrhage (Figure 33-4). A wide spectrum of bacteria have been identified in surgical specimens, such as clostridial species, gram-negative rods, gram-positive cocci, and *Candida* species.[69] The diagnosis is based on clinical presentation and a low neutrophil count. The presence of radiologic abnormalities, however, is essential with CT and ultrasound imaging serving as the studies of choice (Figure 33-5).[85] Kirkpatrick and Greenberg described pneumatosis intestinalis as the most common computed tomographic observation suggestive of neutropenic

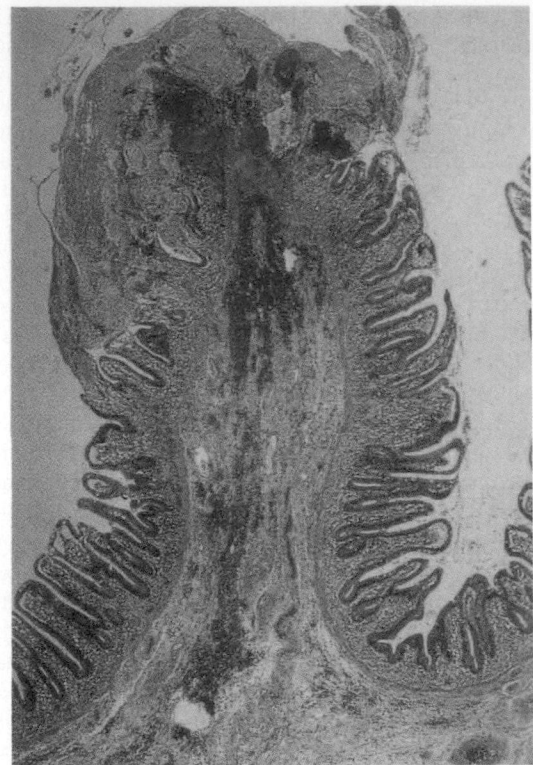

FIGURE 33-4. Neutropenic enterocolitis (typhlitis). Crypts of this mucosal fold are intensely inflamed and necrotic in an individual on chemotherapy. (Original magnification × 380.)

enterocolitis (21% of patients).[160] Bowel wall thickening, mesenteric stranding, bowel dilatation, mucosal enhancing, and ascites are also frequently reported.[160] In patients who are hemodynamically unstable, ultrasound should be considered as an alternative diagnostic modality given its ease of use and ability to quickly detect bowel wall thickening as well as rapidly eliminating other possible diagnoses, such as appendicitis and pancreatitis.[69] One prospective study evaluating the use of ultrasound in leukemic patients postchemotherapy found that bowel wall thickening greater than

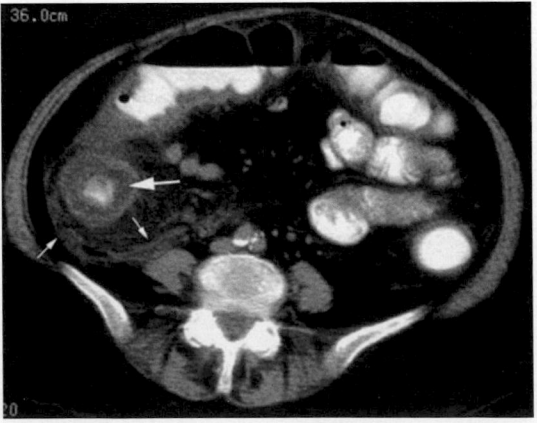

FIGURE 33-5. Computed tomography showing typhlitis. Marked low-attenuation cecal wall thickening (*large arrow*) with moderate pericolonic inflammatory stranding (*small arrows*). Note thickening of transverse colon wall posteriorly.

4 mm was present only in those who symptomatically satisfied the criteria for neutropenic enterocolitis. As such, some advocate that the diagnostic criteria for neutropenic enterocolitis should include the presence of bowel wall thickening identified on CT scan or ultrasound (greater than 4 mm on transverse scan over greater than 30 mm on longitudinal scan), in addition to the clinical presentation of fever and abdominal pain.[85]

Given high mortality rates, the management of neutropenic enterocolitis has been traditionally aggressive, with a low threshold for surgical intervention. However, because an increasing number of cases successfully treated with medical therapy alone have been reported, there has been a shift in the treatment paradigm. Intensive support with close monitoring, fluid resuscitation, bowel rest, and broad-spectrum antibiotics are key components to conservative management. Antibiotic treatment may be initiated with single drug regimens, such as piperacillin-tazobactam, or with dual agents, such as a beta-lactam antipseudomonal drug paired with an aminoglycoside. Coverage should be targeted at gram-positive and gram-negative bacteria, as well as pseudomonas, clostridial, and fungal species. Moreover, the use of recombinant granulocyte colony-stimulating factor (G-CSF) has been administered to help normalize white blood cell levels and consequently to lead to clinical improvement. Its efficacy, however, is not well established and is currently recommended for only the sickest of patients.[69]

Surgical intervention should be considered in those individuals with persistent gastrointestinal bleeding, free intra-abdominal perforation, clinical worsening, or to exclude other acute abdominal disease processes. Resection is necessary with perforated or necrotic bowel; however, in the setting of neutropenia, a primary bowel anastomosis is not recommended. Rather, resection with diversion is the preferred alternative.[85]

Diversion Colitis, Disuse Colitis, and Starvation Colitis

Diverting the fecal stream and defunctionalizing the bowel can produce a noninfectious colitis, an observation made by Glotzer and colleagues in 1981.[113] Generally, patients are asymptomatic, although mucus discharge and bleeding may be noted. Fenton and Siegel have shown that 70% of their ostomy patients had gross or microscopic findings of diversion colitis despite the absence of symptoms.[100] Roe and colleagues reported that all of their 12 patients who had undergone a Hartmann's procedure demonstrated histologic abnormalities consistent with diversion colitis by 3 months.[253] An association of microcarcinoids with diversion colitis has also been reported.[122] This occurrence has been attributed to neurogenic hyperplasia, which represents proliferation of a separate, neuron-associated, extraglandular population of endocrine cells.[120]

Proctosigmoidoscopic findings are essentially that of a mild inflammatory bowel disease suggestive of ulcerative colitis. Microscopic alterations, however, tend to be rather focal and include crypt abscesses, epithelial cell degeneration, acute and chronic inflammation in the lamina propria, and regenerative changes in the crypts (Figure 33-6).[113] The crypt cell production rate has been determined to be less than half that of controls. Additionally, crypt length and width are lower.[10] However, the histologic picture with the condition

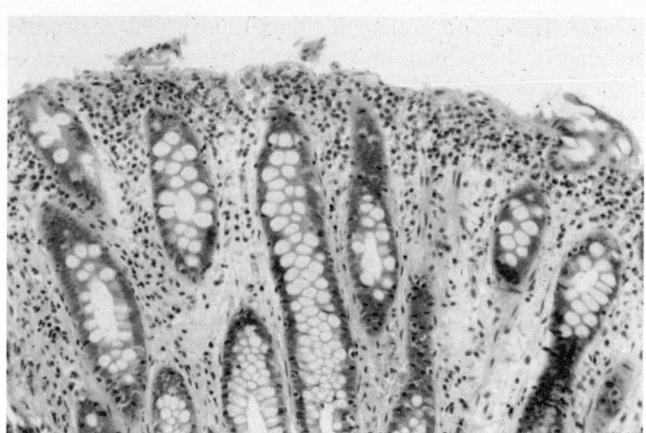

FIGURE 33-6. Diversion colitis. A 37 year old woman underwent a Hartmann's resection for perforated diverticulitis. Because of the complaint of mucus discharge, a biopsy was taken. Edematous colonic mucosa with focal surface erosion is seen, in addition to a mild increase of chronic inflammatory cells in the lamina propria and into the glandular epithelium. The changes are consistent with diversion colitis. (Original magnification × 280.)

is quite variable. Pathologic evaluation of more severely diseased, resected specimens may demonstrate diffuse nodularity caused by lymphoid hyperplasia and an inflammatory process confined to the mucosa and submucosa.[214]

The mucosa of the intestinal tract is unique in that it draws nutrients not only from the vasculature, but also from the bowel lumen.[254] It is not difficult to appreciate how this entity can develop when examining the radiologic picture shown in Figure 33-7. Nutrition of the colonic epithelial cells is mainly from short-chain fatty acids produced by bacterial fermentation in the colonic lumen.[254] Deficiency in these substances initially leads to mucosal hypoplasia and subsequently to a more typical picture of nonspecific inflammatory bowel

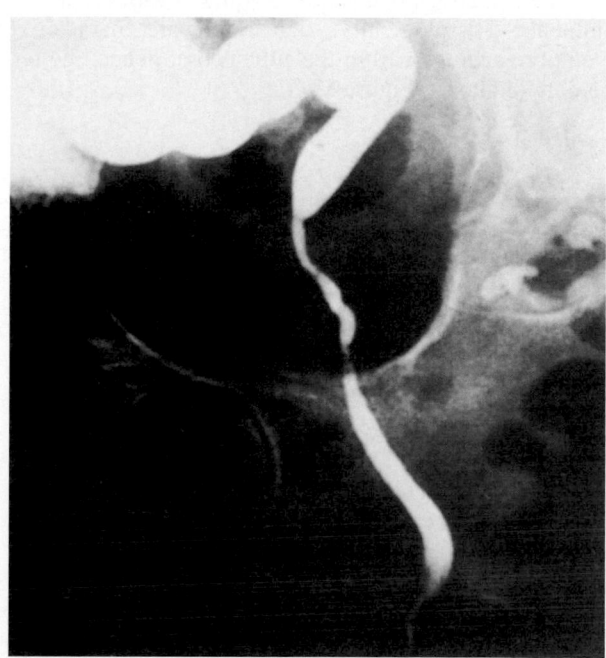

FIGURE 33-7. Barium study reveals an atrophic rectum, a consequence of disuse for many years following the creation of a colostomy.

disease. Harig and colleagues have shown that negligible amounts of short-chain fatty acids can be identified in a segment of excluded rectosigmoid.[129] They further demonstrated that installation of a solution containing short-chain fatty acids twice daily resulted in the disappearance of symptoms and in the inflammatory changes observed at endoscopy within a period of 6 weeks. Short-chain fatty acids have also been used for the management of diversion colitis in children.[156] Others have shown that the condition may be successfully treated with the use of 5-aminosalicylic acid enemas.[307] However, the only curative approach is stoma reversal or rectal excision.

The affected bowel rapidly returns to a normal appearance following reestablishment of intestinal continuity. Orsay prospectively evaluated 34 patients who were scheduled to undergo colostomy closure and who were demonstrated to have diversion colitis.[225] There was no increased infection rate or any other complications following colostomy closure.

Iatrogenic Chemical Colitis (Pseudolipomatosis)

Chemical colitis is a rare clinical entity that can be induced by iatrogenic means with contaminated endoscopes or with intentional or accidental administration of corrosive enemas. Iatrogenic chemical colitis was first described in the 1960s and has been reported in the literature in numerous case reports and series.[281] Although disinfectant solutions are known to be caustic to the intestinal mucosa, controversy exists as to the exact causative agent. The main disinfectants implicated are glutaraldehyde, peracetic acid, and hydrogen peroxide (a breakdown product of peracetic acid when it is combined with water). The residual presence of such chemicals on endoscopic equipment may be the result of malfunction of automated disinfecting devices or lack of staff education in proper cleansing techniques.

Injury to the colon typically becomes manifest at the time of endoscopy with the classic "snow white sign," multiple areas of elevated whitish yellow plaques of variable size and confluence. Histologically, such lesions are characterized by empty vacuoles within the submucosa; hence, the term pseudolipomatosis (Figure 33-8).[145,210]

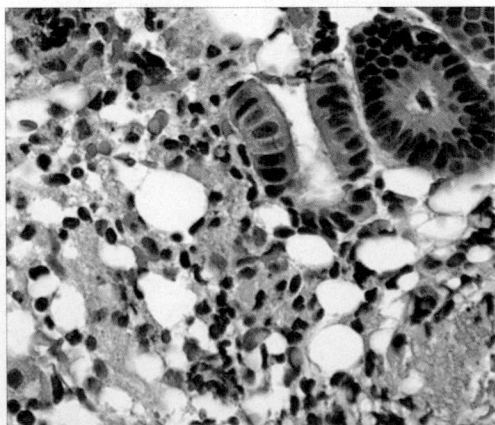

FIGURE 33-8. Iatrogenic chemical colitis (pseudolipomatosis). Colonic mucosa demonstrating spaces devoid of epithelial lining in the lamina propria. Note the similarity to pneumatosis coli (see Figure 26-106). Note also the absence of nuclei. These are empty spaces, not lipocytes. (Original magnification × 560.)

Signs and symptoms range from no clinical sequelae to fever, abdominal pain, and bloody diarrhea within 48 hours of endoscopic examination. Radiologic findings on CT scan after glutaraldehyde-induced colitis may demonstrate a "target sign" of circumferential colonic wall thickening. Resolution is usually seen with bowel rest and conservative treatment. Empiric antibiotics and steroids may be administered, but no evidence of their efficacy has been reported.[281]

Corrosive Colitis

Oral administration of a host of corrosives is a well-recognized entity for which surgical intervention is often required. Less well recognized, however, is the installation of various toxic or corrosive materials by means of an enema. Cappell and Simon reviewed the literature on the reported intra-rectally administered toxic agents and found that the most common was hydrogen peroxide.[45] Other agents included detergent enemas, herbal medicines, acetic acid, ethyl alcohol, sodium hydroxide, and hydrofluoric acid. Pikarsky and colleagues presented a case of severe formalin-induced colitis 5 days after rectal instillation of formalin for radiation proctitis.[238] Drugs such as ergotamine can also be associated with inflammatory reaction and toxicity. Toxic exposure may result from conventional medical therapy, unconventional medical therapy, radiographic examination, colonoscopic examination (see previous discussion), deliberate self-mutilation, or accidental self-administration.[45]

Rectal bleeding, diarrhea, and abdominal pain are frequent symptoms. Endoscopic examination usually reveals nonspecific changes consistent with inflammatory bowel disease, including erythema, ulceration, granularity, friability, and purulent exudate. A history of medication use or exposure to toxic agents is obviously helpful.

Treatment is generally supportive care, although emergency laparotomy and bowel resection may be required for fulminant acute colitis, stricture, or perforation (see also Chapter 17).

Nonsteroidal Anti-inflammatory Drug Colopathy

Adverse effects of NSAIDs on the upper gastrointestinal tract and small intestine are well recognized.[84] Since the initial description of NSAID-induced colonic injury by Debenham,[86] a growing number of reports have associated the use of NSAIDs and salicylates with colonic complications. However, the true incidence of NSAID colopathy is unknown. A study from Jersey (United Kingdom) estimated that approximately 1:1,200 NSAID users may develop colitis.[112] Recognized colonic complications secondary to NSAID use include the development of primary macroscopic colitis, worsening of inflammatory bowel disease, collagenous colitis, gastrointestinal bleeding, and increased complications in association with diverticular disease.[16]

The clinical presentation of NSAID-induced colitis is based on the development of an acute, nonspecific inflammatory process involving the colonic mucosa.[94] With long-term NSAID use, it may progress to chronic disease characterized by the presence of fibrosis and strictures.[2] Symptoms include bloody diarrhea, sporadic melanotic stool leading to iron-deficiency anemia, weight loss, fatigue, anorexia, and even death. The pathogenesis of NSAID-induced colitis may be related to the inhibition of prostaglandin synthesis.[84]

In addition to the oral route, NSAID-induced suppository toxicity has been recognized.

Colonoscopy may demonstrate diffuse inflammation, with erosions or ulcerations. The presence of diaphragmatic-like strictures or webs, most commonly in the right colon, has been described as a pathognomonic sign of NSAID-induced colitis.[149] However, the most common finding is a solitary or limited number of cecal ulcerations, or they may be scattered throughout the colon and rectum.[241] The condition may be difficult to differentiate from that of ulcerative colitis in its early presentation.

NSAID ingestion should certainly be considered in the differential diagnosis of colitis. The use of NSAIDs in the form of suppositories may induce rectal bleeding and proctitis due to the high concentration of the drug in direct contact with the rectal mucosa.[111,180] Moreover, the severity of rectal symptoms may be dose dependent. It has been estimated that up to 30% of patients using NSAID-containing suppositories may develop rectal symptoms such as pain, inflammation, bleeding, ulcerations, and stricture.[84]

One would certainly expect an ameliorative response of the bowel to the discontinuation of the medication. Additionally, the use of sulfasalazine and metronidazole has proven to be somewhat beneficial.[95] Surgical treatment is reserved for cases of life-threatening complications or refractory colitis.

Toxic Epidermal Necrolysis

Toxic epidermal necrolysis is a rare and severe reaction to certain drugs that results in full-thickness epidermal skin necrosis.[48] Other mucosal surfaces have been implicated, including the large bowel. The most common drugs associated with this condition include sulfonamides, penicillin, NSAIDs (see previous discussion), phenytoin anticonvulsants, and barbiturates.[48]

Symptoms include abdominal pain and bloody diarrhea, usually concomitant with the development of the skin lesions. Several cases of colonic necrosis complicating this condition have been reported.[48]

▶ INFECTIOUS COLITIDES

Tis now the very witching time of night,
when churchyards yawn and hell itself
breathes out contagion to this world.
—WILLIAM SHAKESPEARE: *Hamlet*, III, 2

The gastrointestinal tract is susceptible to infection by a host of organisms, including bacteria, viruses, fungi, and parasites. The upper intestine tends to be attacked by organisms that produce toxins (e.g., *Vibrio cholerae*), whereas in general, colonic infection is associated with organisms that produce dysentery (e.g., *Shigella*). In the former situation, infection tends to leave the mucosa uninvolved, whereas in the latter, the intestinal mucosa is often ulcerated or destroyed. Upper intestinal organisms tend to produce diarrhea with severe dehydration. However, there is usually no septicemia. Those that affect the large bowel often produce severe abdominal pain, tenesmus, and signs and symptoms of generalized infection (e.g., malaise, pyrexia). A rapid onset is often due to the presence of a toxin produced by a bacterium rather than to the bacterium itself. This type of syndrome is occasionally associated with certain restaurant foods. Gorbach stated that the incubation period from a toxin is so brief that the symptoms occur either when one is paying the check or when on the way to the parking lot.[119]

Most episodic diarrheas are caused by an infection acquired by ingesting fecally contaminated food or beverages. *Escherichia coli* is the most common pathogen, although many other bacteria, viruses, and protozoa have been implicated.[74] The "immunologically naive" traveler to developing areas is the individual most susceptible to the bacterial and protozoal indigenous organisms.[124] Prevention can be best described by the adage, "cook it, boil it, peel it, or forget it."[124]

Traveler's Diarrhea Prophylaxis

The main nonantibiotic agent for prophylaxis against traveler's diarrhea is bismuth subsalicylate, which has been shown to decrease incidence rates from 40% to 14%. The Centers for Disease Control and Prevention recommend avoidance of prophylactic antibiotics for the average traveler due to concerns for possible adverse drug reactions. For those who are immunosuppressed or at high risk, prophylaxis with fluoroquinolones is the current recommendation. Although the majority of diarrheal illnesses represent little more than a self-limited nuisance, oral rehydration along with antibiotic treatment is recommended for severe cases. Fluoroquinolones such as levofloxacin are considered first-line therapy with azithromycin as an alternative in cases of drug resistance.[75]

Comprehensive microbiologic testing and thorough gastrointestinal studies for every individual with the complaint of diarrhea are both impractical and costly.[130,329] As enteric infections frequently present with vague, nonspecific signs and symptoms, it is imperative that the clinician obtain a thorough history considering recent travel and other possible sources of exposure to infectious agents. Generally, for the younger patient, no investigations, except perhaps a rigid or flexible sigmoidoscopy and biopsy, are necessary if weight is stable and the stool is free of occult blood.[130] Nonetheless, a few individuals will require a more extensive evaluation, a decision that must rest with the physician's clinical judgment.

In this section, the various enteric infections of potential interest to the surgeon are discussed with respect to epidemiology, clinical presentation, diagnosis, therapy, and prevention.

▶ BACTERIAL INFECTIONS

Clostridium difficile Colitis, Pseudomembranous Colitis, and Antibiotic-Associated Colitis

The first reported case of pseudomembranous colitis actually antedated the antibiotic era and is generally attributed to Finney of Johns Hopkins.[102] His patient developed bloody diarrhea, perhaps as a consequence of enema feedings following a gastric procedure. The discussants of his paper presented what were than a "who's who" of American medicine prior to the turn of the 20th century—Halsted, Osler, Thayer, and Flexner.

Epidemiology, Etiology, and Incidence

Clostridium difficile is a gram-positive, anaerobic, spore-forming bacillus, first described in 1935 as a component

JOHN MILLER TURPIN FINNEY (1863–1942)

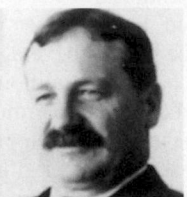

Finney was born in Natchez, Mississippi, the son and grandson of Presbyterian ministers. He was raised in Bel Air, Maryland, where his father assumed a church position. Finney attended Princeton University, receiving his bachelor's degree in 1884, and completed his medical education at Harvard Medical School in 1889. Following his graduation, he interned at the Massachusetts General Hospital before being appointed to a faculty position at the Johns Hopkins Medical School where he remained of his entire career. He was well respected within the Baltimore community as a distinguished citizen and surgeon. He served as head of the surgical dispensary and ultimately held the position of professor of clinical surgery and surgeon-in-chief. Finney was highly sought after and asked to assume the presidency of Princeton University and chairman of the Department of Surgery at Harvard, both of which he declined. Devoted to surgery, Finney developed one of the largest practices in the United States while playing a pivotal role in establishing the Johns Hopkins' Surgical Residency Training Program. When the American College of Surgeons was formed in 1913, Finney was named its first president. He also went on to serve as president of the American Surgical Association. During World War I, Finney was recruited as director of a base hospital in France. He ultimately became chief consultant in surgery to the U.S. Army and was ultimately awarded the Distinguished Service Medal and the French Legion of Honor. Although he retired in 1933, Finney remained active on various academic boards, devoting much of his time to charitable work as chairman of the Baltimore Chapter of the American Red Cross. (Photo courtesy of the Alan Mason Chesney Medical Archives of the Johns Hopkins Medical Institutions, Baltimore, MD.)

of normal newborn fecal flora.[127] However, the role of C. difficile in the pathogenesis of antibiotic-associated colitis was not reported until the late 1970s.[295] The rising incidence of C. difficile colitis in hospitalized patients has become a matter of concern among physicians, especially surgeons. Recent reports have shown that 20% to 25% of hospitalized individuals will acquire C. difficile. Moreover, one-third of these patients will develop diarrhea.[123] In a prospective analysis from the Department of Surgery at the New York Hospital–Cornell University Medical Center, the incidence of diarrhea in surgery patients was 6.1%, and the incidence of C. difficile–associated diarrhea was found to be 2%.[192] C. difficile colitis is now the most frequent cause of nosocomial infectious diarrhea, with an estimated half a million cases annually in nursing homes and hospitals in the United States.[265] Generally, this has been attributed to a heightened awareness of the condition, better diagnostic methods, more widespread use of broad-spectrum antibiotics, and the increasing number of elderly or immunocompromised patients.[36,184,192] During the past 10 years, researchers have identified highly virulent strains of C. difficile, NAP1/BI/027 and PCR ribotype 078, which have caused severe disease in the United States and in Europe.[221]

Any patient who develops diarrhea either during or after receiving antibiotic therapy must be considered at risk for this complication until proven otherwise, although it is certainly possible that colitis may not be associated with antibiotic therapy.[90] Antibiotic-associated diarrhea is often mild and self-limited, demonstrating rapid improvement with discontinuance or change of the antibiotic. Although almost one-third of cases of antibiotic-associated diarrhea are due to C. difficile, 2% to 3% are secondary to other infectious organisms, such as Clostridium perfringens, Staphylococcus aureus, and Candida albicans.[136] C. difficile–associated diarrhea may commence within 48 hours after the administration of the drug. However, the condition can develop after 6 to 10 weeks following stoppage of the antibiotic, an observation noted in 25% to 40% of patients.[123]

The pathophysiology of C. difficile colitis is related to the breakdown of normal colonic microflora, followed by colonization with C. difficile and the production of invasive toxins leading to mucosal inflammation. Contamination occurs via the oral–fecal route. C. difficile produces two toxins in the intestinal lumen, known as A (enterotoxin) and B (cytotoxin), which adhere to the surface of the epithelial layer and produce an inflammatory reaction. Toxin A causes actin disaggregation and intracellular release of calcium. Toxin B is a necrotizing enterotoxin, significantly more potent than toxin A. Both toxins, however, cause colonic mucosal damage and diarrhea. Nonetheless, C. difficile rarely produces colonic injury by direct invasion of the mucosa.[97] The severity of comorbid conditions and low serum levels of IgG antibody to toxin A have been related to a higher probability of acquiring symptomatic C. difficile colitis.[173]

Relatively rare in comparison to hospital rates, the reported incidence of community-associated C. difficile infection ranges from 6.9 to 46 cases per 100,000 person-years in the United States.[221] Two to three percent of healthy individuals are asymptomatic carriers. However, more than 80% of neonates and up to 70% of infants and young children harbor C. difficile in fecal flora without any intestinal manifestations.[123,126] It has been noted in recent years that the incidence of infection in populations previously considered low risk, such as children and pregnant women, has increased. Contaminated food, soil, and water have been considered as potential sources for community infection. However, no conclusive evidence has been demonstrated as of yet.[265]

The most common antibiotics associated with C. difficile colitis are cephalosporin, clindamycin, ampicillin, and amoxicillin. However, virtually all antibiotics, including metronidazole and even vancomycin (perhaps doubtful), have been suggested to cause this syndrome. In the Mayo Clinic experience, 70% of their cases were associated with a cephalosporin.[297] The significance of this observation is somewhat diminished by the fact that this is the class of antibiotics most often administered in hospitals.[261] In addition to antibiotics, C. difficile colitis has also been reported in patients receiving antineoplastic agents, such as cisplatin, doxorubicin, methotrexate, teicoplanin,

TABLE 33-1 Practice Guidelines for Prevention and Control of *Clostridium difficile* Infection (CDI)
• Gloves and gowns must be worn upon entry to a room of a patient with CDI.
• Practice of hand hygiene should be emphasized.
• With an outbreak or an increased CDI rate, wash hands with soap (or antimicrobial soap) and water after caring for or contacting patients with CDI.
• Provide patients with CDI a private room with contact precautions. If single rooms are unavailable, cohort patients, providing a dedicated commode for each patient.
• Contact precautions are necessary for the entire duration of diarrhea.
• It is not necessary or effective to routinely identify or treat asymptomatic carriers for infection control purposes.

and tacrolimus.[215] The condition has also been reported as a complication of sulfasalazine therapy in a patient with inflammatory bowel disease.[239] The occurrence of this particular complication poses a considerable challenge in the differential diagnosis because the symptoms of the two diseases are very similar.

Those who appear to be at increased risk are individuals who are somewhat immunocompromised (e.g., with cystic fibrosis, neurologic disease, liver or renal disease, malnutrition, diabetes mellitus, hematologic disorders).[261,206] Other factors associated with an increased risk of infection include advanced age, malignancy, chronic pulmonary disease, prolonged hospitalization (more than 4 weeks), nursing home residents, transfer from another hospital, antibiotic course of more than 7 days, treatment with more than one antibiotic, immunosuppressive medication, chemotherapy, antiperistaltic medications, antacid therapy, an intensive care unit location, non–single room accommodation, and those conditions in which the intestinal motility is altered.[36] With respect to pathogenesis and prevention, a number of authors have emphasized that education of the hospital staff is mandatory if one is to reduce the incidence of this common and costly colitis.[167] For example, McFarland and colleagues found that the infection is frequently transmitted among hospitalized patients and that the organism is often present on the hands of hospital personnel caring for these individuals.[194] The Society for Healthcare Epidemiology of America (SHEA) and the Infectious Diseases Society of America (IDSA) have published updated clinical practice guidelines for the prevention and control of *C. difficile* infection (Table 33-1).[70]

Clinical Manifestations

The clinical presentation of *C. difficile* colitis varies from the asymptomatic carrier to a fulminant illness that may result in death. Approximately 20,000 people die annually in the United States from *C. difficile* infection.[265] Mild disease presents with diarrhea, crampy abdominal pain, and diffuse patchy, nonspecific colitis on endoscopic examination. Moderate cases are often associated with fever, nausea, anorexia, abdominal distention, and cramps, in addition to profuse diarrhea. Those patients with severe *C. difficile* colitis appear toxic, dehydrated, and with signs of peritonitis on physical examination. These individuals in particular may go on to manifest a fulminant colitis, develop a colonic perforation, and succumb to the complications of their disease.

Evaluation

The initial assessment of a patient with possible *C. difficile*–associated diarrhea and colitis includes a complete history and physical examination as well as laboratory evaluation of electrolytes, white blood cell count, nutritional status,

and stool testing to rule out other sources of diarrhea. Dehydration, electrolyte imbalance, leukocytosis, and hypoalbuminemia may often accompany severe disease. Stool examination reveals the presence of leukocytes in one-half of the cases. The hemoccult test may be positive in severe colitis, but grossly bloody diarrhea is unusual.

The most sensitive test for diagnosing *C. difficile* infection is stool culture (Figure 33-9). Despite a long turnaround time, stool culture in combination with toxigenic culture is the current diagnostic standard. With a lack of a single test with adequate sensitivity and specificity, the development of two- or three-step testing has emerged. The SHEA-IDSA clinical practice guidelines recommend the initial use of an enzyme immunoassay (EIA) of glutamate dehydrogenase (GDH) followed by either cell cytoxicity assay or toxigenic culture of GDH-positive stool as confirmation. Another alternative that may prove to be sensitive and specific with a rapid testing time is the PCR assay. Several PCR-based assays are currently available. However, further investigation is necessary to promote its routine use.[70]

Endoscopic evaluation will demonstrate edema and mucosal inflammation. Pseudomembranes are present in 14% to 25% of patients with mild disease and 87% of those with severe colitis.[122] The disease often involves the entire colon. Therefore, colonoscopy is preferable to that of flexible sigmoidoscopy because 10% of patients present with pseudomembranes beyond the reach of the sigmoidoscope (Figure 33-10). Seppälä and associates also stressed the importance of colonoscopy in the diagnosis of this condition.[280] In a review of 16 patients with histologically proven antibiotic-associated pseudomembranous colitis, only 31% were confirmed by sigmoidoscopy, as compared with 85% in whom colonoscopy was performed. Others have noted

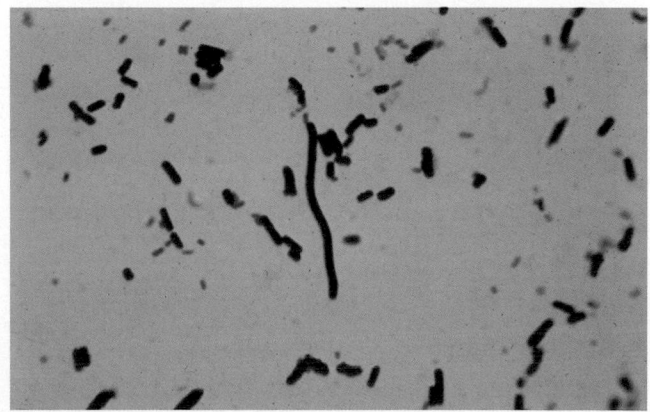

FIGURE 33-9. *Clostridium difficile.* Gram stain of stool reveals gram-positive rods. (Original magnification × 800.)

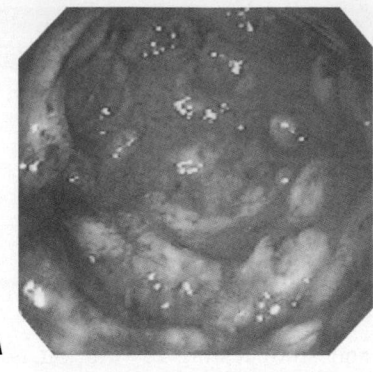 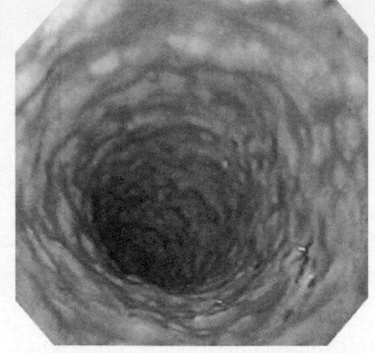

FIGURE 33-10. **A,B:** Colonoscopy clearly demonstrates the patterns of yellow and yellow-white adherent plaques in pseudomembranous colitis.

the importance of total colonoscopy as the preferred means for establishing the diagnosis, particularly because there is not uncommonly right-sided involvement and a relatively normal distal bowel.[40,82,266,270,301] Tedesco showed that five of six patients with tissue culture evidence of a clostridial toxin in the stool had either a normal or merely an edematous distal rectal mucosa.[301] Thus, proctosigmoidoscopy would have failed to identify the abnormality.

Biopsy of the lesion is not mandatory for confirming the diagnosis. However, if there is any question as to the etiology of the inflammatory change, tissue should be obtained (Figures 33-11 and 33-12). Histopathologic examination of the pseudomembranous plaque shows a mix of mucinous fibrinous exudate and polymorphonuclear neutrophils.

Radiographic imaging studies may reveal a paralytic ileus and pancolonic dilatation. Differential diagnosis must include Ogilvie's syndrome (colonic ileus), ischemia, and volvulus.[305] Pneumoperitoneum due to colonic perforation in severe or toxic colitis can also be found on plain abdominal radiography. Computerized tomography may show a diffusely thickened and edematous colonic wall.[215] Barium enema examination may demonstrate "thumbprinting," which is due to bowel wall edema. In more advanced stages, severe ulceration may be present (Figure 33-13). The procedure, however, is contraindicated in the acutely ill patient because of the risk of precipitating toxic megacolon or a perforation.[72,99,286]

Treatment

Despite the high mortality rate in critically ill individuals, most patients with mild *C. difficile* colitis will recover even without specific treatment. Adequate antibiotic therapy with metronidazole or vancomycin leads to symptomatic improvement in the overwhelming majority within the first 24 to 72 hours, with complete resolution in 1 or 2 weeks.

Treatment of *C. difficile* colitis includes cessation of the causative antibiotic. Adequate fluid and electrolyte replacement is also essential to overall patient management. Asymptomatic carriers do not require treatment. Conversely, fulminant colitis frequently requires intensive care monitoring and emergency surgery. More than 95% of patients respond to therapy with oral or intravenous metronidazole or oral vancomycin.[123,215] Metronidazole is the treatment of choice for mild-to-moderate disease, leading to a 99.9% reduction in organisms. It provides a 95% to 100% response rate and is more cost effective than vancomycin.[123] The recommended dose is 500 mg orally three times daily, for a total of 10 to 14 days.[70] The intravenous route is used in patients who are intolerant of oral intake.

Vancomycin is equally as effective as metronidazole when taken orally because the poor intestinal absorption promotes a high luminal concentration. Its mechanism of action is the inhibition of bacterial wall synthesis. In addition to the high cost, the major disadvantage of this drug is the emergence of vancomycin-resistant enterococci. Furthermore, unlike metronidazole,

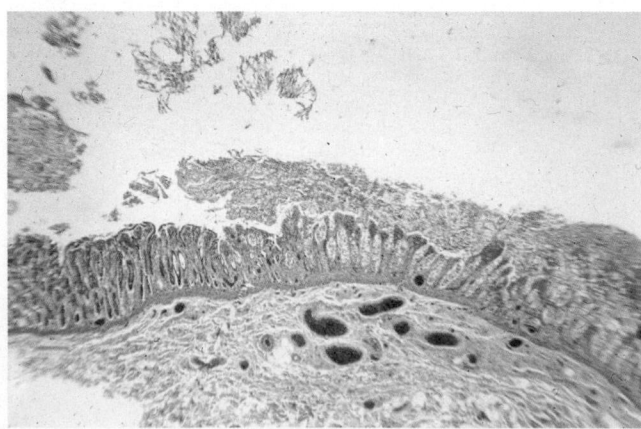 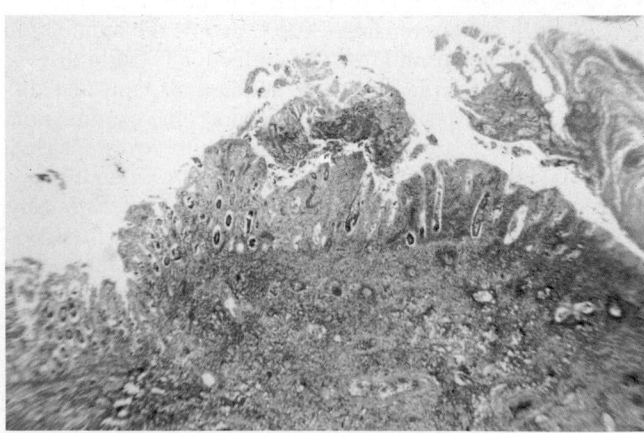

FIGURE 33-11. Pseudomembranous colitis. Superficial necrosis with acute inflammatory mucosal exudate. (Original magnification × 80.)

FIGURE 33-12. Pseudomembranous colitis. Total necrosis of the mucosa with inflammatory exudate in the submucosa. (Original magnification × 80.)

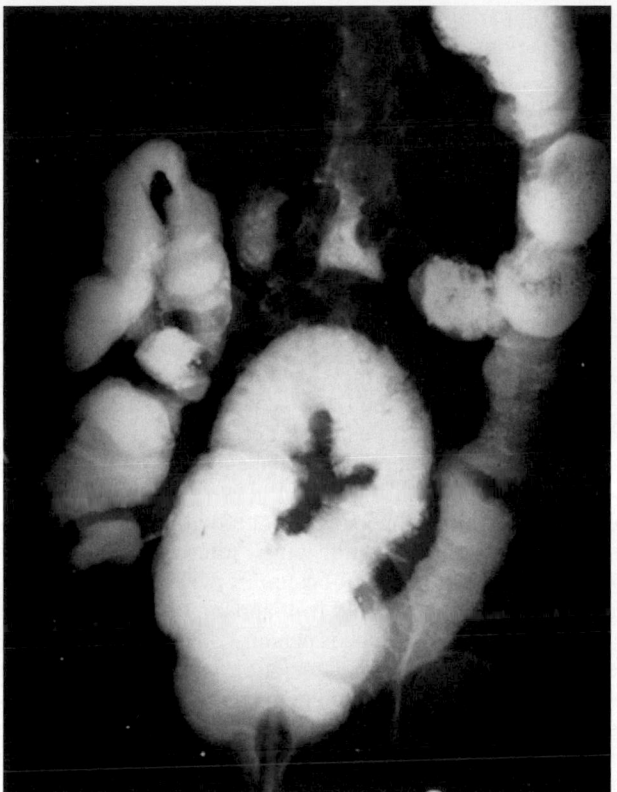

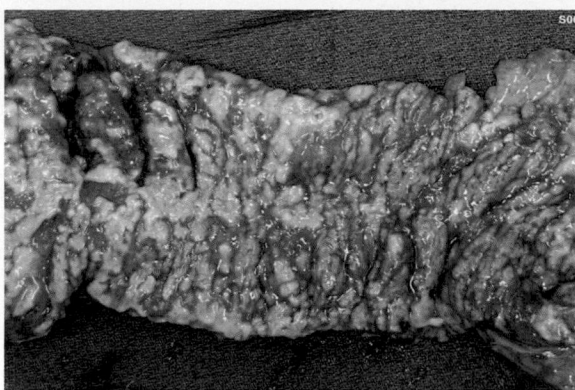

FIGURE 33-14. Pseudomembranous colitis. Opened partial specimen from total colectomy demonstrates the classic mucosal findings of this disease.

FIGURE 33-13. Pseudomembranous colitis. Barium enema demonstrates extensive ulceration. Note the collar button appearance of the ulcers extending into the bowel wall.

intravenous vancomycin is not excreted into the gastrointestinal tract. Vancomycin is considered the treatment of choice for an initial episode of severe *C. difficile* infection.[70] The recommended dose is 125 mg, orally, four times daily for 10 to 14 days and 40 mg/kg/day, divided three or four times a day for 7 to 10 days in pediatric patients.[123] Vancomycin enemas can be used in patients with *C. difficile* proctosigmoiditis or in those who have undergone emergency subtotal colectomy with an end ileostomy. Under these circumstances, with a diseased rectum, topical vancomycin is a very good treatment option.

Anion exchange resins such as cholestyramine (Questran) will bind to the *C. difficile* toxin, forming a nonabsorbable complex with bile acids in the intestinal lumen. Cholestyramine will also bind to vancomycin. Therefore, both medications should not be used in combination. This drug is less efficacious than metronidazole or vancomycin, but it may have a role in patients with relapsing disease. The suggested dose is 4 g orally, three times daily for 10 to 14 days.[97,123] Because *C. difficile* is a transferable enteric pathogen, stool precautions for the duration of the illness are advised.[17]

Medications that slow peristalsis should be avoided because elimination of the toxin is inhibited.[99] In fact, some have suggested that reduced colonic motility as seen with colonic obstruction, sepsis, uremia, generalized debilitating conditions, burns, and other illnesses may contribute to the development of pseudomembranous colitis.[66]

Colectomy is generally performed in patients who develop megacolon, an acute abdomen, perforation, and septic shock. In patients who are severely ill, close monitoring of serum lactate levels as well as white blood cell counts may be useful in determining the need for surgical intervention. Significantly higher perioperative mortality is associated with a serum lactate level of 5 mmol/L or greater and a white blood cell count of 50,000 cells/μL.[70] The most frequent indication for operative intervention is perforation, although pseudomembranous colitis may be a terminal complication in patients with a malignancy. Figures 33-14 and 33-15 demonstrate the appearance of the mucosa in such individuals. Acute abdominal signs and symptoms may, in fact, be the

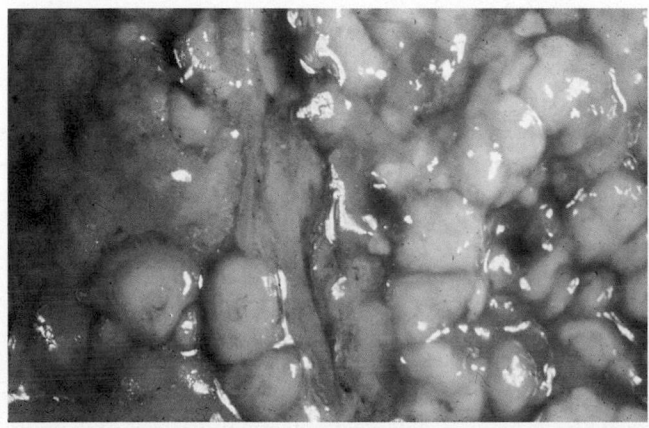

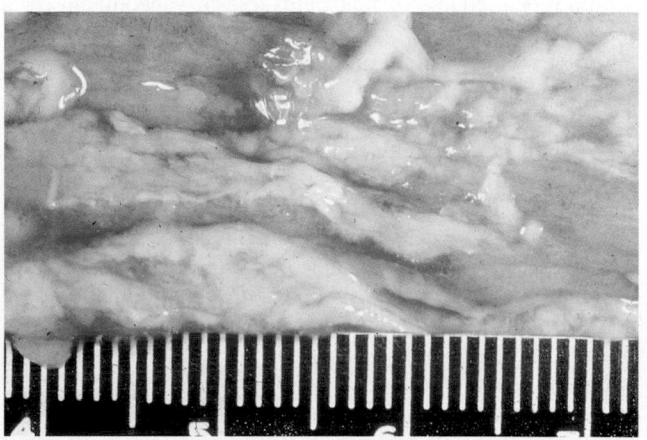

FIGURE 33-15. Pseudomembranous colitis. **A,B:** Whitish plaques of pseudomembranes cannot be wiped off. The patient expired of acute leukemia.

initial presenting manifestations.[305] Total colectomy with ileostomy, preserving the rectum, is the preferred treatment for a perforation or for fulminant disease.[184,197,211,212,308] It must be remembered that at laparotomy, the external colonic appearance may be deceptively normal. This finding should not influence the surgical procedure—that is, total colectomy.[184] With sepsis or a dilated bowel, and in the absence of necrosis or perforation, an ileostomy alone may be adequate surgical management. However, there are no meaningful statistics concerning the relative merits of this option.

Lipsett and colleagues reported an overall mortality rate in their series of 38%, with a 100% mortality in those who underwent partial colectomy and a 14% mortality for those who underwent subtotal colectomy.[184] Others report a high mortality rate for this disease, especially if a less than subtotal colectomy is performed.[197,212,308]

Recurrence

One of the concerns with this disease is the possibility of relapse following treatment, a frequency that has been reported to be from 10% to 30%.[123] This often occurs within 1 to 3 weeks following completed therapy and is likely due to the original *C. difficile* strain. However, a new strain may be found, especially if the patient remains in the same high-risk environment. The number of relapses increases exponentially after the second episode to greater than 65%.[123] Walters and colleagues reported a relapse of antibiotic-associated colitis while the patient was maintained on vancomycin therapy.[316] Eight of 15 individuals so treated demonstrated a clinical relapse after therapy was discontinued. These results suggest that stool evaluation should be performed during and after treatment to indicate whether the antibiotic therapy should be maintained or reinstituted or that alternative therapeutic approaches be considered.

Recurrence due to antibiotic resistance has yet to be proven, but it seems that persistent *C. difficile* spores in the colon may lead ultimately to clinical disease. It has also been proposed that the absence of *Bacteroides* species predisposes to recrudescence. Attempts have been made to identify risk factors for recurrence, including those with prior *C. difficile* infection, chronic renal failure, prolonged antibiotic therapy, patients with community-acquired *C. difficile*, significant leukocytosis, and particular strains of *C. difficile*.[98,215]

Management in this situation is quite challenging, with no uniform treatment having been accepted. The first relapse after successful treatment of *C. difficile* colitis may be treated with a repeat course of metronidazole or vancomycin for a total of 10 to 14 days.[215] This regimen is effective in 95% of cases. However, a small number of patients will go on to develop multiple episodes of recurrence. Metronidazole is not recommended beyond the first recurrence, however, because of possible neurotoxicity. Vancomycin may be used for multiple recurrences in a prolonged tapering or pulse regimen.[70] In a recent case series, a regimen of oral rifaximin, 400 mg, twice a day for 2 weeks immediately after a course of vancomycin led to a cure rate of 86% in patients with multiple recurrences.[141] *Saccharomyces boulardii*, in combination with standard antibiotic therapy, is also an option for refractory disease, but this is not available in the United States and is yet to proven as an effective therapy.[70,123,140]

Another treatment alternative is fecal transplantation via colonoscopy. It has reportedly been effective in small studies, but the results of the first randomized controlled study comparing fecal transplantation with antibiotic therapy in patients with recurrent *C. difficile* infection are still pending.[15,255,311] Other treatment modalities such as immunoglobulin therapy and the use of monoclonal antibodies directed against *C. difficile* toxins require further investigation. Research and development of *C. difficile* toxoid and DNA vaccines are currently ongoing as well.[221]

Campylobacter Enteritis

Campylobacter jejuni and *Campylobacter coli* are the leading causes of infectious enterocolitis worldwide. In fact, *Campylobacter* has become one of the major causes of infectious diarrhea in the United States, with a reported 13 laboratory-confirmed cases per 100,000 annually.[53] Within the United States, it is noted to occur most commonly in children younger than the age of 4. Internationally, infection is typically sporadic in poor developing countries as well as in military personnel stationed abroad.[159] The organism is a curved or "gull wing" microaerophilic, grampositive rod. Transmission occurs by way of the fecal–oral route through contaminated fruit and water or by direct contact with infected animals or persons.[30] Epidemiologic studies have demonstrated an association with the handling and consumption of poultry and beef. The risk of contamination is higher with raw meats, especially at barbecues. This is believed to be due to the ready transfer of the bacteria to other foods and then to the mouth.[42] This bacterium is also found in shellfish and dairy products and has also been diagnosed in hospitalized patients. *Campylobacter* is vulnerable to temperature extremes as well as to oxygen in atmospheric concentrations. In contrast to that of *Salmonella*, *Campylobacter* does not survive in pelleted meals, egg powder, and spices.

Symptoms and findings may be difficult to differentiate from those of other diseases affecting the intestinal tract, particularly nonspecific inflammatory bowel disease.[246] In fact, *Campylobacter* enteritis must be considered in the differential diagnosis of any patient who presents with rectal bleeding and diarrhea. Abdominal pain, fever, nausea, and vomiting may also be associated complaints. Toxic megacolon, necessitating total colectomy, has been reported.[9]

Proctosigmoidoscopic examination usually reveals an edematous, inflamed mucosa. Histologic examination of biopsy specimens is nonspecific. A double-contrast barium enema may demonstrate aphthoid ulcers and a stippled appearance.[304]

A high index of suspicion must be maintained if one is to establish the diagnosis and to initiate therapy promptly. Examination of the fecal specimen within 2 hours of passage by dark-field or phase-contrast microscopy may identify the organism.[30] The presence of polymorphonuclear leukocytes in the fecal stream is not uncommon but is not pathognomonic for the condition.

Infection with *C. jejuni* may lead to various postinfectious sequelae, including reactive arthritis, Reiter's syndrome, Guillain–Barré syndrome, IBS, and IBD.[23] The incidence of IBS- and IBD-associated cases ranges from 4% to 32%. Research has demonstrated a consistent association between length of clinical illness (greater than 1 week) and the development of postinfectious IBS. Debate still remains, however, over the mechanism of disease as well as the question of whether infection with *Campylobacter* leads to IBS and IBD or whether patients with such intestinal diseases are simply predisposed to the bacterial infection.[159]

In the majority of patients, symptomatic infection is usually self-limited and does not require antibiotic therapy, but relapses are frequent. In severe cases, those associated with fever, bloody diarrhea, and cramping, hospitalization and fluid and electrolyte replacement may be necessary. Although the mainstay of treatment has been fluoroquinolones, antibiotic resistance has increased rapidly with a reported prevalence of 26% in 2007. Consequently, single dose administration of azithromycin has been recommended as an effective alternative.[159] Appropriate stool precautions (particularly for hospitalized patients) are indicated, with proper disposal of contaminated linens and washing of hands. With respect to prevention, avoiding raw meats, particularly poultry, is recommended.

Currently, research is focusing on the identification and eradication of bacterial reservoirs. Additionally, molecular studies, leading to a better understanding of Campylobacter-associated diseases, are being conducted in order to improve prevention techniques and to offer alternative therapeutic approaches.[182] The development of vaccines against *C. jejuni* has posed a significant challenge due to its microbiologic characteristics. Presently, phase I/II human trials are being conducted with preclinical experiments demonstrating promising data on a capsular conjugate vaccine.[159]

Yersinia Enterocolitis

Yersinia enterocolitica is a relatively recently recognized cause of enteric infection. *Yersinia* enterocolitis is of particular interest to the surgeon because of its prevalence and its occasional confusion with regional enteritis. A former name for the causative organism was *Pasteurella pseudotuberculosis*, again implying confusion with another bacterial infection that tends to involve the ileocecal region. Epidemics due to contamination of food, water, and milk have been reported.[29] *Y. enterocolitica* most commonly affects infants, young children, and young adults.

The disease is caused by a facultative anaerobic, gram-negative coccoid bacillus resembling nonlactose-fermenting *E. coli*.[78,312] It grows optimally in cold temperatures. The diagnosis is established by isolation of the bacteria from stool, blood, fluids, or tissue. However, *Y. enterocolitica* culture is not standard in most clinical laboratories and must be specifically requested.[312] Biotyping and serotyping according to O antigens have been the most helpful of the epidemiologic techniques.[78]

After a median incubation period of 4 days, the organism may produce signs and symptoms of an acute enterocolitis. This may be accompanied by pharyngitis as a consequence of invasion of epithelial cells and the penetration of the intestinal mucosa, as well as the presence of the lymphoid-abundant tonsils.[306] Bloody diarrhea is frequently observed in addition to abdominal pain.[268] Joint pain may also be a manifestation of this disease. Drainage of the bacteria into regional lymph nodes accounts for the systemic complications. Mesenteric lymphadenitis may develop from colonization of Peyer's patches communicating directly with mesenteric lymph nodes. A syndrome simulating appendicitis is seen in 40% of patients—that is, fever, leukocytosis, right lower quadrant abdominal tenderness, and pain.[78,268] However, a small number of patients with *Y. enterocolitica* will actually develop true appendicitis as a manifestation of the disease.[283] The condition may produce generalized septicemia and "metastatic" abscesses in other organs. It can also present as a colonic abscess or as toxic megacolon.[272,296]

Sometimes the disease may pursue a chronic course for many weeks, particularly if not treated with appropriate antibiotics. Postinfection manifestations include erythema nodosum and reactive arthritis.[78] Predisposing factors to the development of the infection follow:

- cirrhosis
- hemochromatosis
- acute iron poisoning
- transfusion-dependent blood dyscrasias
- immunosuppression
- diabetes mellitus
- malnutrition[78]

Results of radiologic examination were evaluated in a review by Vantrappen and colleagues.[312] A coarse, irregular, nodular mucosal pattern was seen in the terminal ileum; ulcerations were also noted. In contrast to Crohn's disease, infection of the terminal ileum is usually confined to the mucosa and submucosa, and the characteristic "string sign" is absent. Endoscopic examination demonstrates signs of inflammatory disease in approximately one half of the patients. Findings are nonspecific and variable, including aphthoid lesions within the cecum, as well as small round elevations in the terminal ileum with or without exudate.[155]

Recommended treatment includes antipseudomonal aminoglycosides, trimethoprim/sulfamethoxazole, ceftizoxime, or ceftriaxone, but antimicrobial therapy has not been proven essential or necessarily efficacious in the uncomplicated situation.[78] However, when systemic illness supervenes or when the patient is immunocompromised, doxycycline or trimethoprim/sulfamethoxazole is advisable. *Y. enterocolitica* is generally resistant to penicillin and first generation cephalosporins. Sporadic resistance to macrolides and fluoroquinolones has been reported as well.[155]

Prevention of yersiniosis includes adequate treatment and handling of raw poultry, beef, and pork as potential sources of infection. Consumption of raw milk should be avoided and hand washing after using the toilet or diaper changes as well as after handling pets and animals is mandatory.[220]

Salmonellosis: Enteric Fever and Nontyphoidal Salmonellosis

Enteric Fever

Enteric fever is caused by *Salmonella enterica*, an anaerobic gram-negative bacillus, which includes serotypes *S. typhi* and *S. paratyphi*. It is transmitted via fecal–oral transmission among humans, its only reservoir, and occurs largely in areas with poor sanitation and contaminated water supplies. Its incidence in the United States has decreased significantly due to improvements in sanitary conditions, and it has mainly become a travelers' disease within developed countries. However, it still remains a considerable disease burden in developing countries worldwide, particularly in the Indian subcontinent and Southeast Asia.[76] According to the World Health Organization (WHO), it is estimated that approximately 21 million people are affected annually; infection is associated with a 1% mortality rate.[81] In recent years, the incidence of enteric fever caused by *S. paratyphi* A has increased substantially in Asia. This poses a significant health concern because the current available vaccines do not protect against *S. paratyphi*.[200]

The diagnosis of enteric fever based on clinical presentation is challenging, as the disease causes a constellation of signs and symptoms that may easily mimic other febrile illnesses, bacterial or viral infections. A number of laboratory tests are available but are lacking in sensitivity and specificity. Within industrialized countries, blood culture is used frequently (an 80% sensitivity). Newer serologic tests have been developed based on enzyme-linked immunosorbent assays (ELISAs) and nucleic acid analysis, as well as multiplex PCR to detect both *S. typhi* and *S. paratyphi*. However, their successful clinical application remains to be seen.[200]

Completion of the *S. enterica* serovar typhi genome sequence has led researchers to new avenues of investigation into the biology of this pathogen. *S. typhi* produces extensive epithelial invasion along the small bowel and colon without destruction of the intestinal mucosa.[193] The bacteria breach the mucosa and submucosa in areas of an inflammatory reaction, and an endotoxin is produced upon autolysis of the bacterial cell. If the organism enters the bloodstream, severe septicemia may result. Characteristics of this illness include fever, headache, delirium, splenic enlargement, abdominal pain, maculopapular rash, and leukopenia.[208] Generalized hyperplasia of the entire reticuloendothelial system occurs, particularly in the Peyer's patches of the ileum and solitary lymph follicles of the cecum.[208]

Of interest to the surgeon is the fact that acute cholecystitis may occur, which may progress to gangrene and perforation. Toxic megacolon and intestinal perforation can also complicate the disease, and on rare occasion, massive lower gastrointestinal hemorrhage can develop.[110,115,208,252,323] The process is usually limited to the terminal 70 cm of ileum and proximal colon.

Abdominal examination may reveal mild tenderness or signs suggestive of generalized peritonitis if a perforation has ensued. Obviously, a laparotomy is required if perforation supervenes. The choice of operation, however, is open to some debate. Meier and colleagues reported their operative experience from Nigeria with 108 consecutive patients who developed perforated typhoid enteritis.[199] Multiple perforations were found in 19%. Debridement of the perforations with closure was effected in 93% of these individuals, with an operative mortality of 32%. In an experience from Ghana involving 195 patients, the overall mortality rate of 31% was worsened by extremes of age, generalized peritonitis, lower white blood cell count, increased numbers of perforations, and the presence of a postoperative enterocutaneous fistula.[205] However, the mortality rate was reduced to 8% if patients received a combination antibiotic regimen that included chloramphenicol, gentamicin, and metronidazole. If the surgeon has the benefit of Western surgical facilities, resection and/or diversion usually offers better results.

Medical management includes the use of parenteral or enteral nutrition and antibiotics. These traditionally consisted of ampicillin, chloramphenicol, or trimethoprim/sulfamethoxazole. However, the development of plasma-mediated resistance as well as chromosomal mutations has led to increasing drug resistance.[76] More recently, nalidixic acid resistant *S. typhi* and *S. paratyphi* (NARST) has forced clinicians to look beyond the once effective oral fluoroquinolones. Consequently, the present recommendation is the use of third-generation cephalosporins or alternatively, azithromycin. Further investigation is ongoing with combination antibiotic regimens as well as fourth-generation fluoroquinolones. As mentioned previously, prevention is available with vaccination, which is recommended to those who intend to travel to endemic areas. However, vaccination against *S. paratyphi*, a major pathogen

in many of these areas, is not available. Newer vaccines against *S. typhi* and a live attenuated oral vaccine against *S. paratyphi* are currently being investigated.[200]

Nontyphoidal Salmonellosis

Nontyphoidal salmonellosis (NTS) is a major cause of diarrheal disease in the United States and worldwide, particularly in Africa. It is the leading cause of foodborne illness in the United States, with 1.4 million cases reported annually. More than 2,500 serotypes have been implicated. However, the most commonly identified serotypes include *S. typhimurium*, *S. enteritidis*, and *S. Newport*.[80] In developing regions, such as Africa, invasive NTS has become a growing concern because it causes invasive diarrheal illness in both adults and children. Those who are immunosuppressed due to HIV/AIDS are at particular risk for developing severe NTS.[121] Transmission may occur through several sources. Within industrialized countries, it occurs mainly through contaminated food sources. In the United States, contaminated eggs were identified as a major cause of NTS from the 1970s to the 1990s. Contaminated peanut butter was implicated for the first time in 2007, with more than 600 individuals afflicted with gastrointestinal and urinary symptoms.[80] Other modes of transmission such as direct human contact and nosocomial spread are more commonly identified in developing countries.

Diarrheal disease occurs as the organisms penetrate through the distal ileum and proximal colon. Severe illness may result with spread to the mesenteric lymph nodes, visceral organs, and bloodstream. The severity of disease is directly associated with the quantity of organisms ingested. The most common manifestation of NTS is gastroenteritis. This is characterized by nausea, vomiting, abdominal discomfort, and nonbloody diarrhea. Symptoms typically occur within 48 hours of exposure. The usual course results in clinical resolution within 3 to 7 days. However, chronic carrier states occur in approximately 0.5% of cases and represent a significant public health concern. The most frequent complication associated with NTS is bacteremia. Individuals who are more susceptible to such systemic involvement include infants, the elderly, and those who are immunosuppressed.[80]

The diagnosis of NTS requires isolation of the organism. Often, however, diagnosis must be made based on clinical presentation because it can take as long as 1 week for stool culture results to return. It is also important to note that culture sensitivity diminishes with time and with antibiotic therapy.[227] For most cases, NTS is self-limited and does not require initiation of antibiotic therapy. However, for individuals who are at risk for severe NTS, administration of antibiotics, such as fluoroquinolones, azithromycin, or trimethoprim-sulfamethoxazole, should be considered. Systemic illness due to *Salmonella* requires a 1- to 2-week intravenous administration of both a fluoroquinolone and a third-generation cephalosporin because of the concern for antibiotic resistance. Once drug sensitivity results are obtained, appropriate adjustments should be made to the treatment regimen. Antibiotics recommended for individuals who become chronic carriers include amoxicillin, 1 g three times per day for 3 months; trimethoprim-sulfamethoxazole, one double-strength tablet (160 mg/800 mg) twice per day for 3 months; or ciprofloxacin, 750 mg twice per day for 1 month.

Surgical intervention may become necessary in those individuals who develop endovascular complications or in those with localized infection requiring debridement. Preventative measures to limit the incidence of NTS include implementation of good hand hygiene practices, avoidance of consumption of raw or undercooked eggs and meat products, and adequate washing of vegetables and fruits. Additionally, the judicious use of antibiotics in the agricultural setting, as well as in treating patients with NTS, is essential to limiting drug resistance.[80]

Tuberculosis

Tuberculosis involving the intestinal tract may be due to either *Mycobacterium tuberculosis* or *Mycobacterium bovis*. In the former situation, the disease is primary to the lungs and is carried to the intestinal tract by swallowing of sputum. The latter organism produces the infection in association with swallowing nonpasteurized milk. This condition is extremely unusual in most Western countries because pasteurization of milk is standardized. According to the WHO, tuberculosis infection afflicts approximately one-third of the population across the globe, with the majority of new cases occurring in Southeast Asia. The estimated mortality rate internationally is 19 per 100,000 persons.[327] Within the United States, tuberculosis disproportionately affects the Asian immigrant population, with a rate of infection 10 times that of U.S. born individuals.[52] Additionally, among those with HIV/AIDS, tuberculosis represents a significant disease burden. It is the leading cause of mortality in this population.[327]

Compared with immunocompetent patients, the proportion with extrapulmonary tuberculosis is much higher in those with HIV/AIDS—approximately 50% in the latter group—hence, the increased frequency of published reports of intestinal tuberculosis in these individuals.[128] Of those with extrapulmonary tuberculosis (EPTB), 11% to 16% have abdominal tuberculosis, the sixth most common EPTB site. This is classified as tuberculosis affecting the intestine, peritoneum, lymph nodes, and/or solid visceral organs.[87,154] Fewer than 200 cases of abdominal tuberculosis were reported in the United States from 1950 to 1980, but the incidence, especially in urban areas, has been increasing steadily.[7,135] When the disease does affect the intestinal tract, it is usually caused by the pulmonary strain and most commonly is localized to the ileocecal region (for discussion of anorectal tuberculosis, see Chapter 9). The reasons for this distribution are believed to be the presence of an abundant lymphoid tissue in the area, an increased physiologic stasis, and an increased rate of absorption in the proximal bowel.[146] Although the condition is most commonly seen in the proximal colon and ileum, segmental bowel involvement has occasionally been observed.[39]

Symptoms and Findings

The presenting signs and symptoms of abdominal tuberculosis are commonly nonspecific, making diagnosis difficult. The most common presenting complaints are abdominal pain, weight loss, and fever. Tuberculosis affecting the ileocecal region typically is manifested as abdominal pain, with blood per rectum and change in bowel habits. Differential diagnosis includes Crohn's disease, malignancy, and infection.[87] Approximately 10% of intestinal tuberculosis occurs in the colon and may be confused with malignancy or inflammatory bowel disease.[87] Bowel obstruction, intestinal perforation, or acute abdomen are also possible presentations of intestinal tuberculosis.[38,298] Tuberculous peritonitis, however, usually presents as an acute abdomen that mimics appendicitis. The condition is seen mainly in young children or adolescents.[1] Ascites, with abdominal pain and distention, may be the first indication of this complication. In the experience of Lisehora and colleagues from the Tripler Army Medical Center in Honolulu, Hawaii, most individuals presented with a chronic wasting illness, mild abdominal pain, and fever.[185]

Physical examination may reveal the presence of a mass, usually in the right lower quadrant. In the rare situation when tuberculosis involves the rectum or anus, a stricture or fistula may be apparent. Depending on whether the lesion produces ulceration or stricture, it can simulate carcinoma. In fact, in the absence of a pulmonary lesion, it is not unlikely that the surgeon could perform a cancer operation for this disease.[157]

Evaluation

The diagnosis requires a high index of suspicion. Obviously, when a pulmonary lesion is present, intestinal tuberculosis should be considered. The presence of concomitant pulmonary tuberculosis is variable with rates reported as high as 29%.[154,228] Acid-fast bacilli will rarely be identified in the stool (Figure 33-16). Although a positive tuberculin test result may be useful, it does not establish the diagnosis with certainty.

Radiologic investigation is helpful but not necessarily diagnostic of the condition. A plain abdominal x-ray film in a patient with intestinal obstruction secondary to a stricture or mass may reveal the absence of gas shadows in the right iliac fossa or distortion of the cecum and ascending colon by a mass.[59] Free perforation with pneumoperitoneum is extremely rare. Barium enema study may reveal retrograde obstruction, stricture, or a "conical cecum." The terminal ileum may be normal, dilated, ulcerated, or strictured. Han and colleagues reviewed double-contrast barium enema examinations in 25 patients in an attempt to identify characteristic findings of tuberculous colitis.[128] They found that involvement was asymmetric in 12, with skip lesions noted in 13. They concluded that ulcers aligned in a transverse or circumferential pattern, involvement at the right colon, and deformity of the ileocecal valve suggest a diagnosis of tuberculous colitis.[128]

The most useful imaging studies include ultrasonography, computed tomographic (CT) scan, positron emission tomography (PET), and MRI. Findings may consist of enlarged para-aortic lymph nodes, ascites, asymmetric bowel thickening, an inflammatory mass, a narrowed terminal ileum

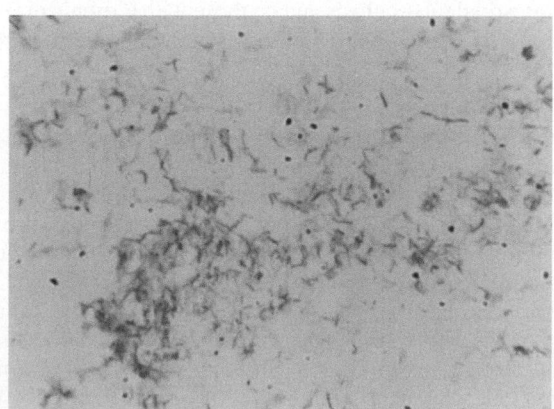

FIGURE 33-16. Pleomorphic red-staining bacilli that are acid-fast because they retain carbol fuchsin and resist decolorization with acid alcohol. (Original magnification × 1,060.)

with a thickened ileocecal valve, lymphatic infiltration seen as a "white bowel" sign, and bowel surrounded by fluid noted as a "sliced bread" sign.[87] A nonspecific ultrasonic finding, the "pseudokidney sign," has also been identified in association with ileal tuberculosis.[31] This is a pattern that consists of a strong echogenic center surrounded by a sonolucent rim, the common factor being bowel wall thickening. The most common CT findings reported in a study conducted by Tan and colleagues were bowel thickening, mesenteric lymphadenopathy, and ascites.[298] Yilmaz and coworkers also identified nonspecific CT changes in abdominal tuberculosis, such as ascites, intraperitoneal and extraperitoneal lymphadenopathy, ileocecal wall thickening, and thickening and calcifications on peritoneal surfaces.[328] However, these findings can only be relevant if abdominal tuberculosis is suspected, a consideration that usually involves high-risk populations.

Definitive diagnosis of tuberculosis is dependent on obtaining tissue for histologic examination and identification of acid-fast bacilli. Options for biopsy include laparoscopy, laparotomy, colonoscopy, percutaneous biopsy, and fine needle aspiration.[87] Allowing for adequate sampling and direct visualization with less perioperative morbidity when compared with laparotomy, laparoscopy is considered an effective method of diagnosing abdominal tuberculosis.[298] Bhargava and colleagues reported laparoscopic findings in 38 cases of peritoneal tuberculosis.[27] They classified the laparoscopic appearances according to three types: thickened peritoneum with miliary; yellowish white tubercles, with or without adhesions (n = 25); thickened peritoneum only, with or without adhesions (n = 8); and a fibroadhesive pattern (n = 5); visual diagnosis was accurate in 95% of patients. The authors concluded that although target biopsy is an effective method of obtaining an early diagnosis of peritoneal tuberculosis, they believe that chemotherapy may be initiated based on the visual laparoscopic appearance alone.[27]

The distinction between tuberculosis and Crohn's disease may not be possible radiologically or endoscopically, although colonoscopy with biopsy has been suggested as a useful tool.[39,105,133,169] Kochhar and colleagues were able to use colonoscopic fine needle aspiration cytology in two patients in order to identify acid-fast bacilli and establish the diagnosis of ileocecal tuberculosis.[165] Gan and associates have suggested the use of polymerase chain reaction (PCR) in the differential diagnosis of Crohn's disease and intestinal tuberculosis.[107] PCR was performed on endoscopic biopsy samples of patients with intestinal tuberculosis and on those with Crohn's disease. Positivity rates of 64.1% and 0%, respectively, were reported.

Histopathology

Generally, the macroscopic appearance of the cecum is indistinguishable from that of Crohn's disease, but the diagnosis may be established by histologic examination.[228] According to Radhakrishnan and colleagues, the yield of biopsy-proven granulomas in tuberculous lesions was 100%, although acid-fast bacilli could not be recovered.[247]

Examination of the resected specimen may reveal thickening of the bowel wall, mucosal ulceration, localized segmental disease, or skip lesions. The mucosal appearance may demonstrate characteristic transverse ulcers (Figure 33-17). The classical histologic criteria include the presence of submucosal or serosal Langhans giant cells and the presence of caseous necrosis (Figure 33-18). The organism may be demonstrated in the specimen or may be grown by guinea pig culture.

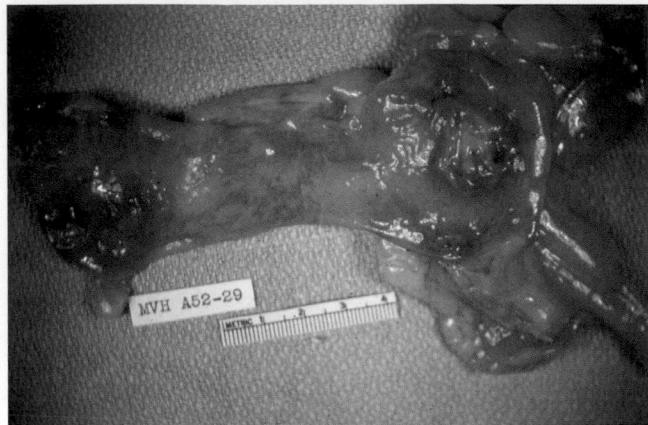

FIGURE 33-17. Cecal tuberculosis. Note the transverse ulcer on the right side of the specimen. (Courtesy of Rudolf Garret, MD.)

Treatment

Conventional antituberculous agents are recommended in the uncomplicated case. Approximately one-half of the patients with colonic or ileocolonic tuberculosis may be adequately treated with medical therapy alone.[83] The current standard for treatment of abdominal tuberculosis consists of rifampin, isoniazid, pyrazinamide, and ethambutol (RIPE) for a 2-month duration, followed by rifampin and isoniazid for 4 to 7 additional months. Because successful treatment is dependent on consistent administration of the aforementioned medications, directly observed treatment short course (DOTS) is frequently implemented to ensure compliance. Of particular concern in patients who are HIV positive is the possibility of drug interaction. It has been suggested that rifabutin is an appropriate substitute for rifampin, whereas nucleoside-only medications should be prescribed as part of the antiretroviral regimen.[87]

During treatment, the patient must be carefully monitored because all of the drugs can produce hepatic dysfunction, although this is relatively uncommon.[275] Patients with ulcerating lesions are more likely to respond to medical management than are those with the hypertrophic form of the disease. Anand and colleagues undertook a prospective clinical trial of 39 patients with bowel obstruction and evidence of intesti-

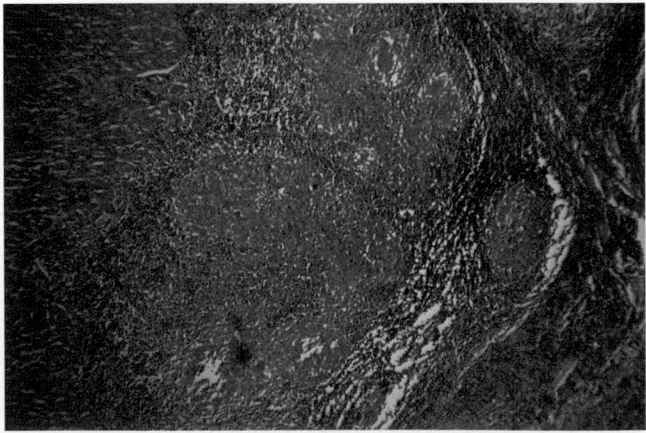

FIGURE 33-18. Tuberculous granulomas (note caseous necrosis) in a mesenteric lymph node. (Original magnification × 180; courtesy of Rudolf Garret, MD.)

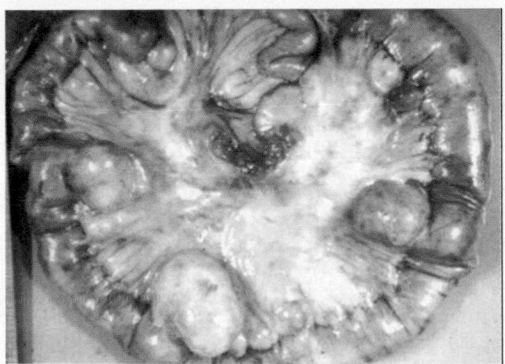

FIGURE 33-19. Tuberculosis of the small bowel. Resected specimen demonstrates typical caseating masses of the adjacent mesentery. (Courtesy of T. Cristina Sardinha, MD.)

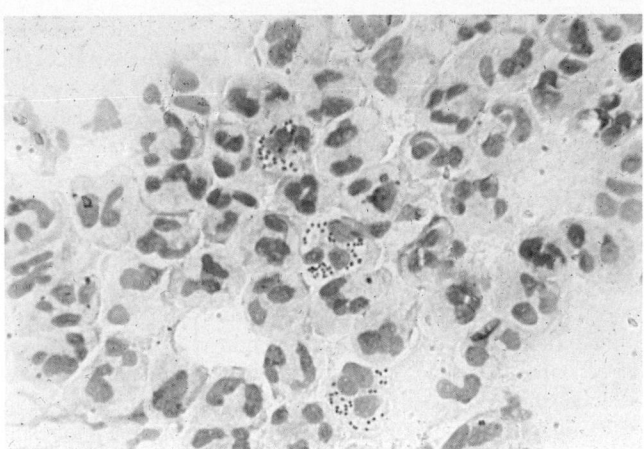

FIGURE 33 20. Gonorrhea. Smear reveals gram-negative intracellular diplococci in the cytoplasm of polymorphonuclear cells. (Original magnification × 1,000.)

nal stricture secondary to tuberculosis.[8] All were treated with conventional antituberculous drugs (streptomycin, rifampin, and isoniazid); only three were unresponsive and underwent surgery. Complete resolution of the radiologic abnormality was noted in 70%.[8]

As has been implied, abdominal tuberculosis can be cured medically if recognized early, but the nonspecific presentation that is often observed tends to delay the diagnosis in many instances.[163]

Surgical treatment should be conservative and limited to those patients with symptomatic localized disease (Figure 33-19).[135] Obviously, if the distinction cannot be made between tuberculosis and carcinoma by endoscopic means, a resection is indicated. Tubercular involvement of the rectum, although uncommon, is an important cause of rectal stricture in India.[243] Even in this area, response to antitubercular chemotherapy is quite good, and surgery is seldom required for these individuals.

Gonococcal Proctitis

Gonorrhea is a common sexually transmitted acute infectious disease of the mucous membranes affecting the urethra, vagina, and cervix. Rectal gonorrhea, however, has been relatively recently recognized. Most physicians, in fact, did not appreciate the concept of rectal coitus in men prior to Kinsey's report in 1948, which discussed the widespread incidence of male homosexuality.[226]

The disease is caused by the bacterium, *Neisseria gonorrhoeae* (the gonococcus), a gram-negative diplococcus. Characteristically, the organism appears on smears as intracellular gram-negative diplococci (Figure 33-20). In order to confirm the presence of the organism by culture, rectal swabs are inoculated on a selective chocolate agar (Thayer Martin) and sent to the laboratory without delay, where they are placed in a carbon dioxide jar and incubated.

In men, the disease is most commonly associated with the homosexual population and is transmitted by anal intercourse (see Chapter 10). However, in women the disease is usually transferred to the rectum by discharge from the vagina, presumably when the rectal mucosa is everted during defecation.[50] Usually, only the lower rectum is involved.

Asymptomatic gonococcal proctitis has been proven to be a misconception. However, the incidence has been declining due to better patient education with respect to safe sex practices. Symptoms usually start 5 to 7 days after exposure

and include pruritus, mucous or pus-like discharge, rectal bleeding, diarrhea, and concerns referable to either gonorrhea or syphilis in other sites. Disseminated disease may occur (septicemia), as well as pericarditis, endocarditis, meningitis, perihepatitis, and gonococcal arthritis. Characteristically, the arthritis produces an acute purulent effusion of a single joint.[50]

Proctosigmoidoscopic examination usually reveals edematous, friable mucosa with occasional areas of ulceration. Biopsy may show degeneration of the epithelium, capillary engorgement, and infiltration with inflammatory cells.[226] However, in many individuals no identifiable lesion will be noted.

Quinn and colleagues reviewed their experience with anorectal infections in 52 homosexual men.[245] They reported that the Gram stain of the rectal exudate was insensitive for the diagnosis of rectal gonorrhea, with up to 50% of missed culture-positive cases. The authors further observed that due to the reportedly high prevalence of asymptomatic anorectal gonorrhea and the frequency of mixed infections, the isolation of the organism from a homosexual male with anorectal symptoms did not prove that the gonococcus was responsible for the symptoms. Lebedeff and Hochman showed, in a study of 1,262 patients who had rectal symptoms, that 554 had culture-proven rectal gonorrhea.[175] Of the individuals who had demonstrated organisms, 82% were symptomatic, one-fourth had a history of contact, and 10% had a history of a prior positive culture. Of those who reported symptoms, 71% complained of mucus in the stool and 62% reported rectal discomfort.

Janda and associates studied the prevalence and pathogenicity of *Neisseria* in 815 homosexual men.[139] Interestingly, *Neisseria meningitidis* was isolated from more patients than *N. gonorrhoeae*. When the organism occurred in the rectum, it was usually not associated with clinical illness.

Stansfield evaluated anorectal gonorrhea in women.[291] In a retrospective assessment of 159 patients who had undergone proctosigmoidoscopy, 127 (80%) had known contacts with infected patients. One-half of these individuals harbored the organism. Of these, the vast majority had the organism in the rectum as well as in the urethra and cervix; only four (6.3%) had the organism confined to the rectum. Gram stain smears demonstrated positive results in less than one-half of the patients with rectal gonorrhea.

DNA assays are currently used for the diagnosis of urogenital gonococcal infection; however, this has not been extensively studied for gonococcal proctitis. Lewis and co-workers reported 100% sensitivity for detecting gonococcal proctitis through the application of the PACE-2 DNA probe assay (Gen-Probe, San Diego, CA) in a population where the prevalence of gonococcal proctitis was 4.7%.[181]

Treatment

Management of *N. gonorrhoeae* proctitis consists of single-dose regimens of drugs effective against β-lactamase–producing strains. The CDC recommends either a single dose of ceftriaxone, 125 mg, intramuscularly, which cures 99.1% of uncomplicated anorectal and urogenital gonorrhea or a single dose of cefixime 400 mg.[51,278] Other effective therapeutic options include single oral dose fluoroquinolones, such as ciprofloxacin (500 mg) or ofloxacin (400 mg). This has been shown to result in cure rates of 99.8% and 98.4%, respectively.[209] If concurrent *Chlamydia trachomatis* infection has not been excluded, additional antibiotics against *C. trachomatis* should also be administered because the incidence of coinfection is high. It is also important to identify and initiate treatment in those who have had sexual contact with an infected individual. The importance of close follow-up examination with culture in order to assess the adequacy of the therapy cannot be overestimated.

Syphilis of the Rectum (Syphilitic Proctitis)

Syphilis of the anal canal and perianal skin is a well-recognized clinical entity (see Chapter 9), but the manifestation of syphilitic proctitis is less familiar to most physicians. The condition occurs almost exclusively in homosexual males.

Symptoms include mucus discharge, bleeding, tenesmus, and change in bowel habits. During the first stage of the disease, a single painless ulcer with raised borders is often found at the site of sexual contact. This is known as a sore or chancre. In addition, enlarged, firm, and rubbery inguinal lymph nodes can also be palpable. In the second phase, syphilitic anal and rectal wartlike growths are seen. The late or third stage of the disease manifests with cardiovascular and neurologic involvement.[288]

Anorectal lesions have been divided into four categories[4]:

- anal ulceration
- rectal ulceration
- granulomatous (hyperplastic)
- miscellaneous (fixed, tumorlike)

Endoscopic examination may reveal a mass or an ulcerating lesion that is suggestive of carcinoma.[18] However, biopsies fail to reveal tumor.

Although the diagnosis can be confirmed by means of dark-field examination of the exudate (see Figure 9-45), disclosing the presence of the treponemal organisms, this does require a high index of suspicion.[4] Treatment is that which has been described in Chapter 9.

Shigellosis

Shigellosis, also known as bacillary dysentery, is an infectious enterocolitis characterized by inflammatory diarrhea. It is caused by one of four species of the genus, *Shigella*. These include *Shigella dysenteriae*, *Shigella flexneri*, *Shigella boydii*, and *Shigella sonnei*. This nonspore-forming, gram-negative rod is divided into 40 serotypes (Figure 33-21). According to the WHO, shigellosis is a worldwide endemic disease that affects 163.2 million people in developing countries and 1.5 million in industrialized countries. Estimated

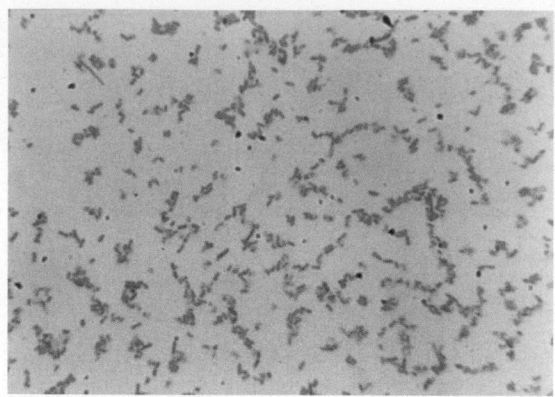

FIGURE 33-21. *Shigella.* Gram-negative bacilli, which, on biochemical and serologic testing, reveal *Shigella.* (Original magnification × 1,060.)

yearly mortality is 650,000 worldwide.[232,321] Within the United States, the most common serotype encountered is *S. sonnei*, which accounts for approximately 80% of bacillary dysentery. In contrast, *S. dysenteriae* and *S. flexneri* are largely responsible for disease within developing countries. *Shigella* is easily spread via fecal–oral or oral–anal transmission, with ingestion of only a small number of bacteria necessary to cause clinical disease. Contaminated water and milk are also major sources of infectious transmission. Settings in which *Shigella* are commonly found within industrialized nations include day care centers and nursery schools, as well as among homosexual males.[232]

Shigellosis is a communicable disease during the acute infectious phase, and although the infectious agent is in the stool, this may last up to 4 weeks. The incubation period varies between several hours to more than 1 week. Shigellosis may present acutely with fever, diarrhea, nausea, vomiting, abdominal cramps, rectal burning, and severe dehydration. Diarrhea may progress from watery to bloody and mucoid with invasion of the Shiga toxin within the colonic epithelium. Severe colitis is associated with fever, and the patient may actually seek emergency care due to severe toxemia.[131] Nonetheless, asymptomatic infections can occur. This illness is frequently self-limited, averaging 4 to 7 days in adults and 1 to 3 days in children. Although the symptoms are usually related to the mucosal manifestation, intestinal obstruction, perforation, and toxic megacolon have been reported.[22,232] In the experience of Bennish and colleagues, 9% of those treated in Bangladesh developed obstruction, one-third of whom died.[22]

The severity of the disease depends on the *Shigella* serotype as well as the patient's age and nutritional status. Infection caused by *S. dysenteriae* is often severe and associated with a high fatality rate, as opposed to *S. sonnei* that usually presents with a short clinical course and has a low fatality rate. Two-thirds of cases and most deaths are in children younger than 10 years of age.

Shigellosis is another disease that is virtually epidemic in the male homosexual population and in those individuals with AIDS (see Chapter 10). Bovée and colleagues demonstrated that *S. sonnei* is the usual infective agent in homosexual patients.[34] In the experience of Heller with this population, the clinical presentation may be one of subacute or chronic abdominal distress without fever and/or diarrhea.[131] Alternatively, the organism may persist in the stool of untreated patients for prolonged periods in a "carrier state."[131] Obviously, this presents an epidemiologic problem. The author states that unlike the heterosexual population in which the need for antibiotic therapy may not be indicated, all homosexual men with *Shigella* cultures should be treated.

Shigella most frequently affects the rectum and sigmoid colon. Colonoscopy may reveal the typical changes of a proctitis, with edema, friability, and ulceration along with aphthoid erosions and grayish white mucopurulent material.[232] The appearance may be indistinguishable from that of nonspecific inflammatory bowel disease. The most satisfactory means for establishing the diagnosis is culture obtained by swabbing any ulcerating lesion during endoscopy; alternatively, mucus or fecal material may be used for culture.[83] Because the organism is somewhat labile, the plates should be inoculated as soon as possible.

Treatment

As suggested, because of the usually self-limited nature of the condition, supportive measures may be the only treatment required, although some believe that all patients should undergo antibiotic therapy irrespective of the severity of symptoms.

A Cochrane review of randomized controlled trials evaluating the use of antibiotics for *Shigella* dysentery found no superior antibiotic when comparing drug classes. Certain drugs such as ampicillin, cotrimoxazole, nalidixic acid, ciprofloxacin, pivmecillinam, ceftriaxone, and azithromycin were noted to be effective for variable periods within specific parts of the world.[64] With antibiotic resistance across the globe, antibiotic susceptibility testing is becoming increasingly necessary in order to effectively treat the disease.

As with other infectious colitides, it is important to re-evaluate the stool to be certain that the bacterium has been eliminated. Moreover, preventative measures should also be employed to investigate food, water, and milk supplies. Specific attention must be given to hand washing after toilet use

Brucellosis

Brucellosis is a zoonosis, that is, a disease transmitted from animals to humans. There are six main species of *Brucella*, named after the animal source or feature of the infection. Four of the species cause infection in humans; these are *Brucella suis* (from pigs, highly infective), *Brucella melitensis* (from sheep with the highest pathogenicity), *Brucella abortus* (from cattle), and *Brucella canis* (from dogs). *Brucella* is an aerobic gram-negative coccobacilli. The disease is caused by the ingestion of unpasteurized milk, direct contact with an infected animal, or inhalation of aerosols. However, the most common routes of contamination in the United States are via needle-stick, conjunctival exposure through eye splash, and inhalation.[189,292] It is the most common bacterial zoonosis worldwide with an annual incidence of approximately 500 million cases even as brucellosis is largely underdiagnosed and underreported. However, the potential for chronic infection and its ease of transmission through aerosols and inhalation makes *Brucella* species a category B bioterrorism agent. *Brucella* spreads through the lymphatic system and can affect any organ in the body. It presents a diagnostic challenge because its presentation is so variable and nonspecific that it has been termed one of the "great imitators." Obtaining a comprehensive clinical and epidemiologic history with possible exposure to infected dairy products or animals is crucial to arriving at the diagnosis. As with all bacterial infections, blood culture is the gold standard for diagnosis. Several serologic tests are available including the Rose Bengal test as a screening tool and the serum agglutination test for confirmation.[104]

Gastrointestinal manifestations of brucellosis are uncommon with few reports in the literature. Rarely, brucellosis can cause a severe colitis.[142,292] It has been suspected that mesenteric lymphadenitis and Peyer's patches ulcerations are potential mechanisms for abdominal pain and the bloody diarrhea seen in patients with ileocolitis.[191] The symptoms and endoscopic findings are essentially the same as that for other inflammatory bowel conditions.

The WHO recommends an oral combination of doxycycline, 200 mg, with rifampin, 600 to 900 mg, daily for at least a 6-week course. An alternative treatment option substitutes streptomycin, 15 mg/kg, for rifampin during the first 2 to 3 weeks of therapy. High treatment failure rates have been observed, and the optimal drug combination has yet to be determined.[104]

Actinomycosis

Actinomycosis is a suppurative, granulomatous disease that tends to form draining sinus tracts, discharging granules (see Figure 9-32 and Chapter 9 for the discussion of perirectal actinomycosis). The organism, *Actinomyces israelii*, an anaerobic, gram-positive bacterium, is a normal inhabitant of the mouth, lungs, and intestinal tract.[303] *Actinomyces* causes abdomino-pelvic disease 20% of the time.[310] When the disease involves the colon or rectum, it usually presents with an abdominal mass, a fistula, or a sinus (Figure 33-22). Stenosis

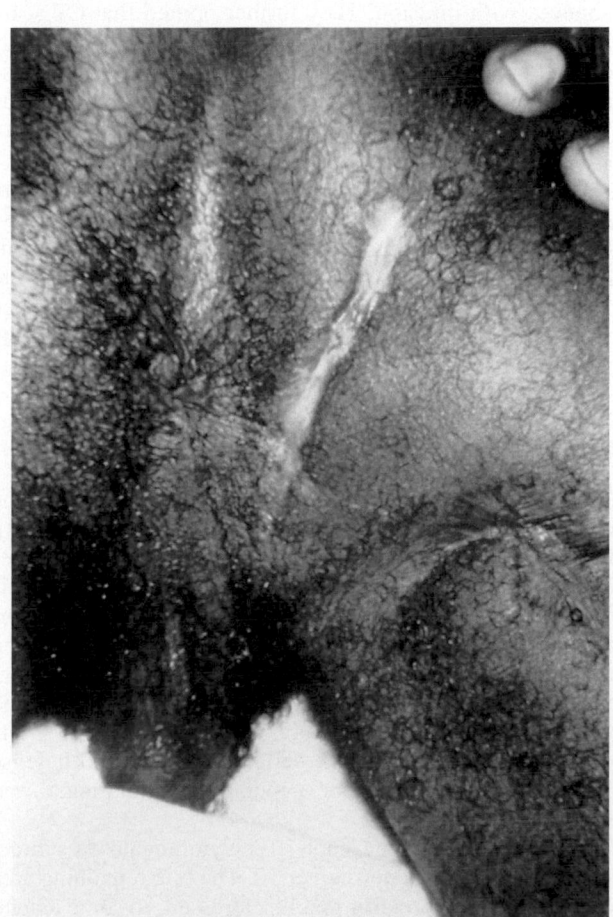

FIGURE 33-22. Actinomycotic fistula. (Courtesy of Daniel Rosenthal, MD.)

may result due to mass effect or associated inflammation. Although ileocecal involvement is the most common intestinal manifestation, rectal stricture has also been reported.[250] Several cases of actinomycosis mimicking carcinoma have been reported. Moreover, it has been noted that the correct diagnosis has been made in fewer than 10% of cases prior to surgical resection.[71,178,269,303] The high incidence of misdiagnosis is attributed to its variable, subacute, and uncommon presentation.

Weese and Smith reviewed their experience of 57 patients who were subsequently proven to have this condition.[320] In only four instances was the disease diagnosed correctly on admission. Udagawa and associates reported 2 patients with primary actinomycotic infections involving the colon and rectum.[309] The diagnosis was established by histologic examination and by bacteriologic culture. In one individual, the presence of an abdominal mass was noted by the patient herself. Back pain, weight loss, and night sweats were also prominent complaints. Barium enema examination revealed segmental involvement of the descending colon by a stricture, and resection was undertaken. In the second patient, proctologic examination revealed a mass in the perianal area. This is a much more frequent finding in those who present with actinomycosis and is more likely to lead one to suspect the diagnosis.[303]

Cintron and colleagues confirmed that radiologic studies have not generally been useful in the preoperative assessment.[67] However, CT, in their experience, seemed to be quite helpful, demonstrating a solid mass with focal areas of attenuation or a cystic mass with a thickened wall that enhances with infusion. They further opined that CT scanning in conjunction with fine needle aspiration may not only be diagnostic but also therapeutic.[67] Given the nonspecific nature of the disease, actinomycosis is usually diagnosed by specimen examination for the presence of sulfur granules or by culture.[310]

The treatment of actinomycosis consists of abscess drainage and high doses of penicillin. Tetracycline, erythromycin, or clindamycin may be options, especially in patients allergic to penicillin. Antibiotics should be taken for 6 to 12 months to prevent relapse.[196] For actinomycosis confined to the colon, resection is the optimal treatment, in addition to that of antibiotic therapy.

▶ VIRAL INFECTIONS

Viral infections that specifically attack the rectum or colon are extremely rare. However, there are three areas that merit attention in a book on colon and rectal surgery: AIDS, herpes simplex proctitis, and cytomegalovirus infection.[285,288] HIV is important to address because so many of the complications and manifestations of the disease affect the anus, rectum, and colon. The reason for this is the fact that the gastrointestinal tract is the largest lymphoid organ in the body, and as such is an enormous potential reservoir for HIV.[287] The adverse consequences on the cellular and humoral defense mechanisms lead to a plethora of viral, bacterial, fungal, and protozoal infestations.

AIDS is discussed in Chapter 10. Cytomegalovirus infection is also discussed in Chapter 10. The one remaining area is herpes simplex proctitis that is addressed, to some extent, in Chapter 9. The following discussion, however, is limited to that of the inflammatory change in the rectum.

Herpes Simplex Proctitis

Herpes simplex virus (HSV) proctitis typically occurs in two patient populations: (1) those who are immunosuppressed from bone marrow or solid organ transplantation or from HIV/AIDS and (2) sexually active male homosexuals. Prophylaxis with antivirals has reduced the incidence of HSV proctitis in solid organ transplant patients by 73%. However, in men who have sex with men, it has been stated to be the most common cause of nongonococcal proctitis.[174] Klausner and colleagues reported a 16% incidence among homosexual men.[161] For both affected groups, HSV proctitis is more likely the result of reactivation rather than primary disease. However, in those who are not immunocompromised, HSV proctitis is usually a result of primary infection.[174] HSV-2 is the most common type of herpes virus that causes proctitis, but HSV-1 can also produce genital infections and proctitis. Anorectal herpes can be acquired via anal intercourse or anal–oral sex.

Herpes proctitis appears to be a distinctive condition that can often be clinically distinguished from other infectious proctitides. Initially, the infection may involve the perianal skin and anal canal and progress into the rectum. Herpes infections in AIDS patients may also develop an ulcerative proctitis, which remains confined to the rectum.[73] In a report by Goodell and associates, the virus was detected in approximately 20% of 102 male homosexuals who presented with anorectal pain, discharge, tenesmus, or rectal bleeding, as compared with 3 of 75 homosexual men without intestinal symptoms.[117] The likelihood of having a proctitis that is due to the herpes virus is greater if the patient has tenesmus, anorectal pain, constipation, and perianal ulceration. Difficulty in urinating, S4–S5 dysesthesias, sacral paresthesias, temporary impotence, and diffuse ulceration of the distal rectal mucosa also suggest the nature of the condition. Anorectal incontinence may also occur during the acute phase, with resolution after treatment of the HSV infection.[143] Intestinal perforation associated with intestinal herpes simplex infection in an immunocompromised patient has been reported.[319]

Examination of the perianal area reveals typical herpetic vesicles, pustules, and ulcerations. The most severe cases present with edema and erythema that can be confused with a yeast infection. Digital examination and anoscopy are very painful.

Sigmoidoscopic examination reveals an acute proctitis. The mucosa is often edematous, friable, and ulcerated. The infection is usually confined to the rectum in immunocompetent individuals and rarely extends beyond 15 cm.[257] A high index of suspicion as to the etiology may be based on the fact that an individual is a homosexually active male. Viral culture is considered the gold standard for diagnosing HSV. Currently, there are also several FDA-approved HSV type-specific antibody tests available.[315] The management of HSV proctitis is primarily focused on symptomatic relief with the use of oral analgesics as well as sitz baths. Oral antivirals such as acyclovir, valacyclovir, and famciclovir have been shown to decrease viral shedding and shorten the symptomatic period.[315] An evaluation of oral acyclovir therapy (400 mg, five times daily for 10 days) in the treatment of proctitis was undertaken by Rompalo and colleagues.[258,259] In one analysis of 24 patients in a double-blind, placebo-controlled study, a significant decrease in mean viral shedding time, duration of anal pain, rectal discomfort, and tenesmus was appreciated in the treated group. In another trial from the same institution, it was demonstrated that daily administration of 2 g of oral acyclovir for 10 days alleviated some of the clinical signs of herpes simplex rectal infection.[258] In still another report from the same institution, individuals with acute proctitis were submitted to an empirical regimen of penicillin and probenecid, followed by doxycycline.[260] Because 25% failed to respond, the authors recommended appropriate pretreatment diagnostic tests and the empirical regimen for the initial management of acute proctitis in homosexual men with no clinical evidence of AIDS or AIDS-related complex.[260]

The CDC recommendations for the treatment of HSV proctitis are the same as those for genital HSV. Patients presenting with their first clinical episode may be treated with one of three oral antivirals: acyclovir, 400 mg, three times daily for a course of 10 days; valacyclovir, 1g, twice daily for 7 to 10 days; or famciclovir, 250 mg, three times daily for 7 to 10 days.[54]

Severe infection in AIDS patients, regardless of the site, should be treated with intravenous acyclovir at 5 to 10 mg/kg every 8 hours until clinical resolution, followed by oral antiviral therapy. Suppressive therapy is recommended to decrease relapses. Schacker and coworkers reported, in a prospective, placebo-controlled, crossover trial of oral famciclovir (500 mg twice daily) versus placebo for a total of 8 weeks, a significant reduction in HSV infection symptoms.[273] In addition, there was a significant reduction in HSV shedding among symptomatic and asymptomatic HIV-positive patients. This regimen also decreased the percentage of genital lesions from 13.8% to 4.9%. All recurrent anogenital lesions were due to HSV-2. Current CDC guidelines for suppressive therapy in AIDS patients are oral acyclovir, 400 to 800 mg, twice daily three times a day; oral famciclovir, 500 mg, twice daily; or oral valacyclovir, 500 mg, twice daily.[54]

► FUNGAL INFECTIONS

Candidiasis (Moniliasis)

Severe fungal infections of the gastrointestinal tract are extremely rare in the healthy person. However, fungemia can be lethal in debilitated and immunosuppressed individuals. For example, diffuse fungal infections are the common causes of death in those with terminal cancer. Asymptomatic oropharyngeal colonization can be found in 30% to 55% of healthy adults, and Candida species may be present in 40% to 65% of normal fecal flora.[134] Candida species are the most common fungal pathogens causing mucosal and systemic infections. Associated risk factors include parenteral hyperalimentation, granulocytopenia, indwelling catheters, prolonged use of broad-spectrum antibiotics, malignancy, recent trauma or major gastrointestinal surgery, prolonged hospitalization, burns, and HIV/AIDS. All of the aforementioned factors may lead to immunosuppression and are also associated with increased candidal colonization of mucocutaneous surfaces.

The most frequent segment of the gastrointestinal tract affected by Candida is the oropharynx and esophagus, followed by the stomach and small bowel. The frequency of large bowel infection by Candida is approximately 20%.[134] Symptoms of gastrointestinal candidiasis include epigastric or abdominal pain, nausea, vomiting, fever, and the presence of an abdominal mass. Internal fistulas may develop. Candida peritonitis may occur as a consequence of gastrointestinal surgery, perforated viscus, or peritoneal dialysis. Fifteen percent of patients with Candida peritonitis will develop candidemia.

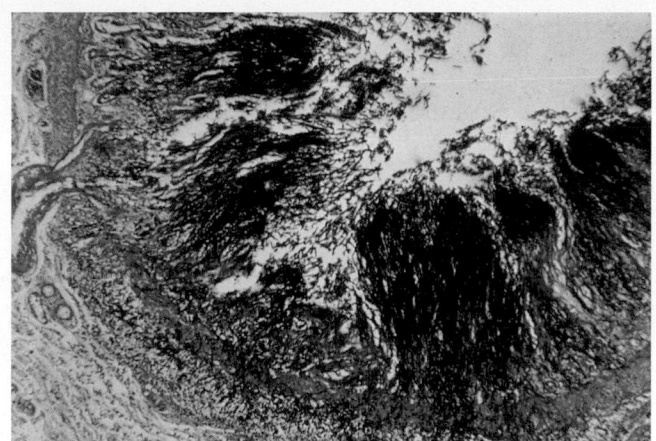

FIGURE 33-23. Intestinal candidiasis (moniliasis). Postmortem biopsy demonstrates characteristic pseudohyphae replacing mucosa. (Original magnification × 180; courtesy of Rudolf Garret, MD.)

The diagnosis of Candida infection is based on clinical suspicion, culture, and endoscopic findings. Because approximately 20% to 25% of the population is colonized by Candida species, culture alone should not be the sole diagnostic criterion.[132] Endoscopic examination reveals small, creamy-white, curd-like patches on the mucosal surface. In addition, the mucosa also appears edematous and inflamed. Biopsies should be taken for histologic identification of yeast cells, hyphae, or pseudohyphae (Figure 33-23). Infection of the perianal skin is discussed in Chapter 9.

More than 100 different species of Candida have been described. However, only a few are clinically significant, including Candida albicans (50% to 60%), Candida glabrata (15% to 20%), Candida parapsilosis (10% to 20%), Candida tropicalis (6% to 12%), Candida krusei (1% to 3%), Candida lusitaniae (less than 5%), and Candida dubliniensis (primarily in HIV patients).[18]

Treatment

First-line therapy for nonneutropenic individuals with candidemia consists of either fluconazole or one of the echocandins (caspofungin, micafungin, or anidulafungin) for a course of at least 2 weeks. Amphotericin B is an alternative treatment in the presence of intolerance or limited availability.[233] Prophylactic antifungal therapy is recommended for high-risk patients, such as those undergoing bone marrow or solid organ transplants, and recurrent symptomatic candidiasis in HIV patients.

Histoplasmosis

Histoplasmosis is caused by the dimorphic fungus, Histoplasma capsulatum, which is found in soil contaminated by bird and bat droppings and transmitted by inhalation of spores. It is endemic to the Midwest and the Mississippi River Valley, with a reported incidence of 500,000 cases annually.[217] Histoplasmosis is usually a subclinical infection in otherwise healthy individuals, but in immunocompromised persons (e.g., those with AIDS), disseminated disease is common.[68,77] It has been reported that 95% of HIV-positive patients infected with H. capsulatum develop widespread infection. Although the lung is by far the most common organ involved, the condition may affect the entire gastrointestinal tract; in HIV-negative patients, the terminal ileum is the most frequently affected site, whereas in HIV-positive patients, the colon is the most common location. Typical symptoms associated with gastrointestinal histoplasmosis in AIDS patients include fever, diarrhea, weight loss, and abdominal pain. Morbidity and mortality is associated with hemorrhage, stricture, bowel obstruction, and perforation.[11] The condition may sometimes be confused with colon carcinoma.[3,153,279] Isolated colonic histoplasmosis in immunosuppressed patient has also been reported.[138]

Endoscopic examination may reveal skip areas of inflammation, with plaques, ulcers, and pseudopolyps that can mimic malignancy or inflammatory disease.[11] Although biopsy may demonstrate the characteristic intracellular oval budding yeasts within the mucosa, serologic complement-fixation titers of 1:8 or greater are suggestive of the disease. Fungal culture of biopsy specimens will also confirm the diagnosis. If pathologic changes are correlated with the roentgenographic features, six patterns of gastrointestinal involvement have been described by Lee and Lin[177]:

- malabsorptive (edema, diffuse inflammatory infiltrates)
- ulcerative
- polypoid (nodular hyperplasia of lymphoid follicles)
- granulomatous (diffuse infiltrates)
- tumefactive (large granulomas)
- compressive (enlarged lymph nodes)

Common physical findings are peripheral lymphadenopathy and hepatosplenomegaly.[44]

Treatment

Most healthy individuals with a normal immune system do not require treatment for histoplasmosis because in the majority of cases, the disease will subside within a few weeks without long-term sequelae. However, more severe cases require treatment with amphotericin B. Itraconazole is effective in treating localized and nonmeningeal disease and is also used for long-term therapy in order to prevent relapse, especially in HIV and immunosuppressed patients.[282] Diversion or resection of strictures may be indicated, in addition to aggressive long-term amphotericin B therapy for those afflicted with AIDS.[120]

▶ PARASITIC INFECTIONS

Parasitic infections involve organisms whose survival is dependent on another host organism. Morbidity is secondary to the parasitic load, its infiltration into various organs, and the emission of toxic waste as it resides in the human. Humans can acquire parasites either by fecal–oral transmission or through skin contact. The distribution of disease is concentrated mainly in developing countries as poor sanitation frequently leads to ingestion of contaminated water and food. The spread of parasitic infections to developed countries is largely the result of travel and immigration. Although parasitic infections may be asymptomatic in an otherwise healthy individual, those with immunocompromised states are particularly at risk for chronic, debilitating manifestations of disease.

The diagnosis of parasitic infections may be elusive, especially within developed countries, due to its uncommon presentation and similarity with clinical features of other microbial and nonmicrobial diseases. Parasites that reside in the intestinal tract may be identified by examination of stool specimens as well as blood assays. Although advances in pharmacotherapy have led to the development of antimicrobial medications with variable efficacy rates, prevention through education and improved sanitation is essential to controlling this international health care problem. Although parasites can cause multiorgan disease, this section seeks to highlight the pertinent aspects of certain parasitic infections with particular attention to their gastrointestinal manifestations.

Amebiasis

Amebiasis refers to an infection with *Entamoeba histolytica*. Amebiasis occurs worldwide with its prevalence concentrated mainly in subtropical and tropical regions. It has been estimated that 500 million people are infected with *Entamoeba* across the globe; 90% are infected with the avirulent *E. dispar*, whereas the remaining 10% are infected with *E. histolytica*.[262] Amebiasis has been cited as the most frequent parasitic condition encountered by surgeons in the United States.[91]

An outbreak of amebiasis was reported to have occurred in a chiropractic clinic in patients who received colonic irrigation therapy.[137] But the largest reservoir for *E. histolytica* infection is the male homosexual population.[41,195] In a report by Allason-Jones and colleagues, 20% of men attending a clinic in London for the treatment of sexually transmitted diseases were infected with *E. histolytica*.[6]

Amebiasis is transmitted via the fecal–oral route. The risk factors for transmission of the disease in industrialized countries include recent travel to or from endemic areas, residents from mental institutions, and sexually active homosexual males (now primarily infected by *E. dispar*).

Pathogenesis

E. histolytica is a nonflagellated protozoan that exists in the colon as either a trophozoite, the invasive form of the parasite (Figure 33-24), or as a cyst, the infective form. The cytoplasm of the organism usually is quite granular owing to ingestion of many bacteria, red blood cells, and other cellular debris (Figure 33-25). Transmission occurs either through water or food contaminated by carriers of the cysts. The swallowed cysts pass into the small intestine where the trophozoites are released. These burrow into the mucosa and result in the characteristic flask-shaped ulcer (Figure 33-26). Ulcers are usually identified in the cecum and ascending colon, but the process may be diffuse throughout the bowel. It is rare for the small intestine to be involved.

Symptoms and Findings

Clinical signs and symptoms typically arise after an incubation period of 7 to 21 days.[147] Symptoms of amebiasis can range from asymptomatic illness to acute and fulminant infection. Acute intestinal amebiasis is often ushered in abruptly by cramping abdominal pain, tenesmus, and bloody stools.[300] The most common complaint is diarrhea, which may be bloody and contain mucus. Bowel movements can be frequent, in excess of 10 per day. The most severe presentation of amebic colitis is fulminant necrotizing colitis. This is associated with a greater than 50% mortality rate and is more common in children, pregnant women, and patients on corticosteroids or who are immunosuppressed.[147] Amebiasis can also cause peritonitis, toxic megacolon, and extraintestinal manifestations, such

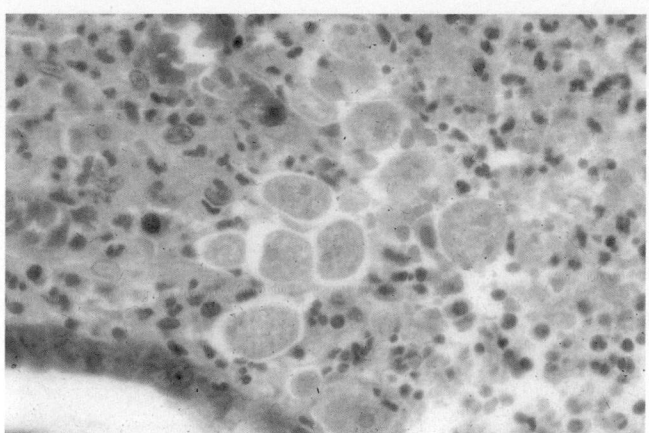

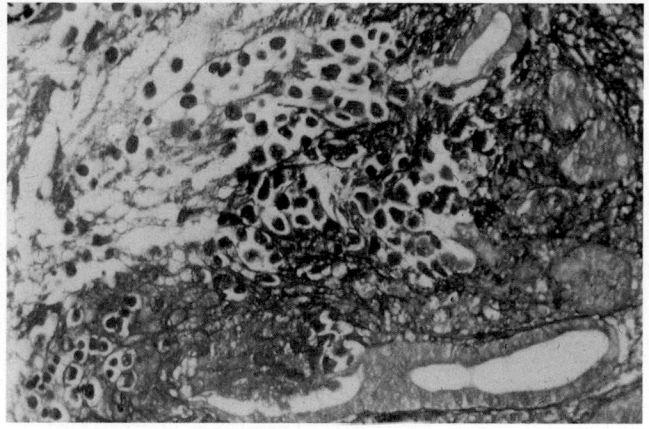

FIGURE 33-24. **A:** *Entamoeba histolytica.* Trophozoites in a colon ulcer **B:** PAS stain demonstrates parasites. (Original magnification × 280; courtesy of Rudolf Garrot, MD.)

as cutaneous amebiasis, ameboma, liver abscess, brain abscess, empyema, and pericarditis, as well as brain and skin involvement (see Chapter 9).

Liver abscess is the most common extraintestinal manifestation of amebiasis. Patients usually present with fever, right upper quadrant pain, hepatomegaly, weight loss, and abnormal liver function tests. Most of the time, this disease complication occurs in young male, Hispanic immigrants.[147] Misra and colleagues reported symptomatic colonic involvement in more than half of patients who presented with amebic liver abscess.[203]

Diagnosis

A key element in the diagnosis of amebiasis is the identification of the *Entamoeba* species as *E. histolytica*. Diagnosis is frequently made through a combination of stool examination, serology, and endoscopic evaluation, especially by microscopic examination of fresh stool specimens for the trophozoites. It is recommended that three stool specimens be examined over a period of 10 days because the presence of cysts and trophozoites in feces can be variable. The detection rate with this method of collection is between 85% and 95%.[103] It is important that stool examination be undertaken before any barium investigation, the use of mineral oil, or

treatment with broad-spectrum antibiotics. Such interventions may impede one's ability to identify the protozoan.[83]

Unfortunately, microscopic examination alone cannot differentiate *E. histolytica* from *E. dispar* and *E. moshkovskii*. Options for further identification include serologic testing for antibodies or antigens, as well as biopsy and molecular assays. The most commonly used assay worldwide is ELISA. This test is effective in diagnosing asymptomatic and symptomatic patients as well as those with amebic liver abscesses. It is 97.9% sensitive and 94.8% specific in detecting antibodies to *E. histolytica* in patients with liver abscess. The use of antigen-based ELISA is more applicable within developing countries where amebiasis is endemic and where evaluation is restricted by cost. Molecular assays such as PCR provide approximately 100 times more sensitivity than ELISA. However, their use in routine diagnosis is currently limited.[103]

Sigmoidoscopic examination is a valuable method for diagnosis because ulcerations are visible in the rectum in up to 85% of the cases.[144] However, because the disease occurs more frequently in a proximal location than it does distally, a negative proctosigmoidoscopy does not rule out the diagnosis. Colonoscopy has been felt to be a useful technique for this reason (Figure 33-27).[247] Crowson and Hines reported

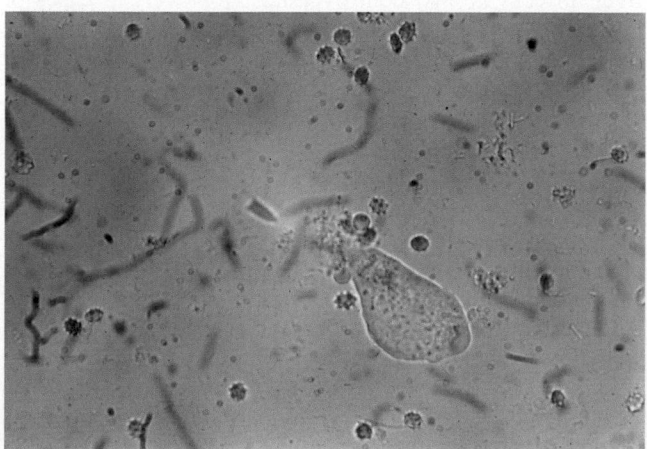

FIGURE 33-25. *E. histolytica* ingesting red blood cells. (Wet preparation, original magnification × 360; courtesy of Rudolf Garret, MD.)

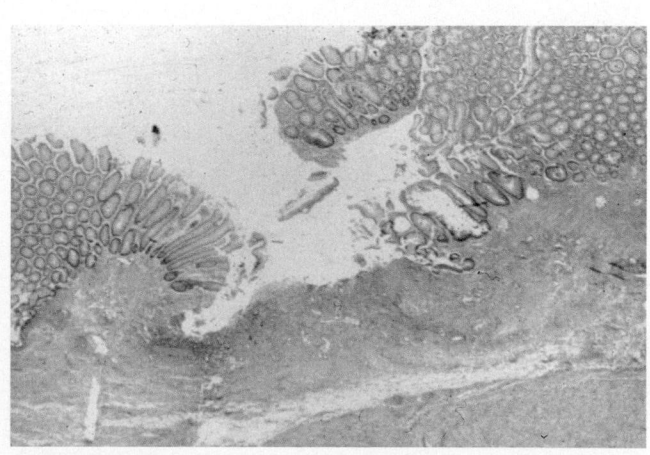

FIGURE 33-26. Amebic ulcer. Note the characteristic flask shape. (Original magnification × 80.)

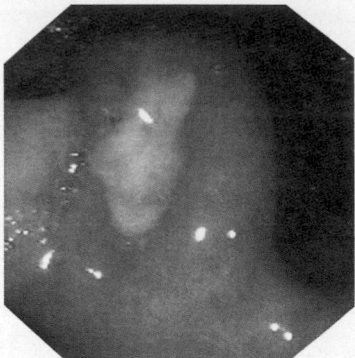

FIGURE 33-27. Colonoscopy demonstrates an exudative amebic ulcer that appears flask shaped even in this projection. Overhanging mucosa and undermining margins are present. Microscopic examination of the stool was positive for the trophozoites.

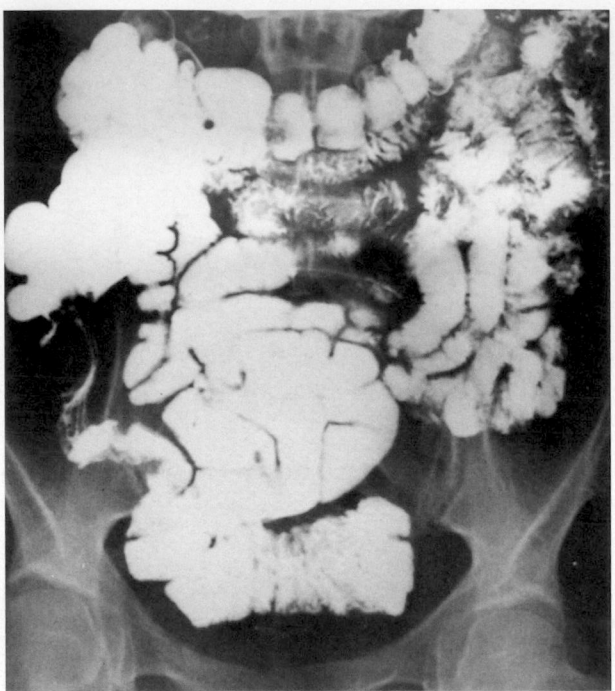

FIGURE 33-29. Cecal ameboma. Barium enema demonstrates extrinsic compression of the cecum and terminal ileum with marked narrowing. The mucosa appears intact.

identification of the disease by means of colonoscopy in an individual whose sigmoidoscopy was normal.[79] In the two patients of Rozen and colleagues, the symptom of rectal bleeding caused the authors to perform multiple colonoscopic biopsies that identified the nature of the condition.[264] Although the histologic appearance is usually indistinguishable from nonspecific inflammatory bowel disease, the overhanging mucosa; undermining margins; or flask shape, along with the appropriate history, suggest amebic colitis (Figure 33-28).

Occasionally, a granulomatous reaction may lead to the formation of a mass, the so-called *ameboma*. When this clinical picture is present, it may be difficult to differentiate it from Crohn's colitis or carcinoma. Amebomas can be found in 1.5% of patients with amebiasis[294] and has been reported to involve the rectum.[256]

Barium enema examination may reveal a multitude of changes in a patient with amebic colitis. As mentioned, toxic dilatation can occur, a contraindication to the performance of the study. Characteristic changes include the so-called collar button ulcer, a cobblestone appearance, thumbprinting, and signs of nonspecific inflammatory bowel disease. Amebiasis is almost always multifocal, so that a careful search of the entire colon for other areas of infection is an important aspect of diagnosis.[229] The presence of a stricture or tumorlike ameboma may confuse the interpretation (Figure 33-29).

Management

In order to prevent tissue invasion and reduce the spread of infection, the WHO recommends that all documented cases of *E. histolytica* be treated regardless of symptoms. Luminal amebicides such as paromomycin or diloxanide furoate are effective in eradicating intestinal cysts and treating asymptomatic disease. Management of intestinal and extraintestinal disease requires the additional use of a tissue amebicide, such as metronidazole, which is absorbed in the bloodstream and eliminates tissue trophozoites. A 5- to 10-day course of metronidazole, 750 mg, three times daily is the most common treatment in the United States. It is also effective in treating amebic liver abscesses.[242]

Surgical drainage of uncomplicated liver abscess should be avoided. The role of percutaneous drainage of amebic liver abscess is also controversial. However, in cases of large liver abscess, percutaneous aspiration may decrease the length of hospitalization and improve the overall clinical status of the patient.[83,143,290]

If the patient requires surgical intervention for hemorrhage or for perforation, resection of the involved bowel must be performed. Indications include the following:

- Free extraperitoneal perforation, impending perforation, or perforation during antiamebic chemotherapy
- Failure of perforation with a localized abscess to respond to antiamebic drugs
- Persistence of or the development of abdominal distention and abdominal tenderness in patients undergoing treatment
- Persistence of severe diarrhea after 5 days of chemotherapy
- Symptoms of postamebic colitis with unremitting anemia and hypoproteinemia[91]

Total colectomy may be required if multiple areas of perforation are identified. Due to the high risk of anastomotic

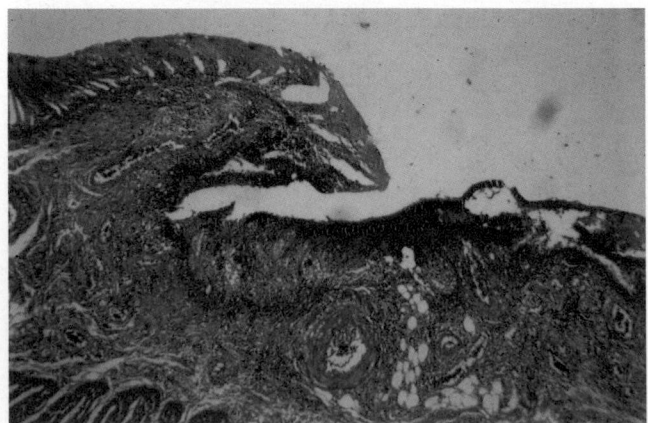

FIGURE 33-28. Amebic ulcer. Note the undermined margin. (Original magnification × 180; courtesy of Rudolf Garret, MD.)

leak, some suggest exteriorization, or at least, a concomitant diversionary procedure.[14,284] Luvuno advises that an ileostomy be performed in addition to colonic lavage rather than risk opening a walled-off perforation and further contaminating the abdominal cavity.[187] Even in patients for whom an operation is considered, aggressive medical treatment is recommended because it may obviate the need for surgery or improve the likelihood of survival following resection in this high-risk situation.[65,230]

Balantidiasis

Balantidiasis is caused by a protozoan, *Balantidium coli*, the largest protozoan parasite to infect humans and the only ciliated protozoan known to infect humans.[63] Locomotion is by means of longitudinal rows of cilia that cover the body and propel it forward with a spiral motion.[162] It is believed that the worldwide prevalence is approximately 1%. However, infections are more frequent in Latin America, Southeast Asia, and New Guinea, mainly where the water supply is contaminated with porcine or human feces. Exposure to pigs is a significant risk factor as they are the known primary reservoir for *B. coli*.[63]

Infection is acquired through the ingestion of infective cysts. The cyst then passes into the small intestine where it excysts, and the trophozoite then migrates into the colon where it penetrates the intestinal epithelium.[63] Ulcerations are produced, similar to those seen with amebic colitis.[83,162] In fact, it is not uncommon for the two conditions to coexist. The trophozoite resides in the intestinal lumen, can measure up to 200 μm in length, and may occasionally be seen with the naked eye (Figure 33-30). Transformation into cysts occurs either within the large intestine or once the parasite is passed in the feces.

Infection with *B. coli* may result in asymptomatic disease, with humans serving as reservoirs; chronic disease characterized by nonbloody diarrhea, vomiting, and abdominal pain; or severe disease, with bloody mucoid diarrhea associated with dehydration, weight loss, and tenesmus. Fatality has been associated with balantidiasis due to hemorrhage, intestinal perforation, and sepsis.[277] Immunosuppressed and HIV patients may develop more profound manifestations of *B. coli* infection.[55,161]

Diagnosis of balantidiasis requires a high degree of clinical suspicion because it is a rare entity within developed countries. It should be considered as part of the differential diagnosis in those with a history of travel to endemic areas who experience the aforementioned symptoms. The diagnosis can be made by examining wet smears of fresh diarrheal stool samples or through scrapings from mucosal ulcers. The trophozoite can be recognized by its large size, short ciliary covering, and a spiraling motility. Colonoscopic evaluation with biopsies from the periphery of the ulcers will aid in the diagnosis of balantidiasis.[116] Endoscopic findings can mimic amebiasis. An additional method for confirmation is to obtain the trophozoites by means of duodenal aspiration or by the use of a recoverable nylon yarn swallowed in a weighted capsule.[162]

A number of drugs are effective in the treatment of balantidiasis. Primary options include tetracyclines (500 mg, four times daily for 10 days) and metronidazole (typically 750 mg, three times daily for 5 days). A 20-day course of iodoquinol is also considered effective therapy.[277] Follow-up with a repeat stool test is required to ensure eradication of the parasite. Treatment should be directed toward the asymptomatic carrier, as well as to the patient with acute or chronic illness, in order to eliminate the organism and to prevent its spread.[83]

Cryptosporidiosis

Human cryptosporidiosis is caused by *Cryptosporidium parvum* and *Cryptosporidium hominis* and is often a self-limited diarrheal infection in healthy individuals, mostly children. However, the disease has been recognized as an important

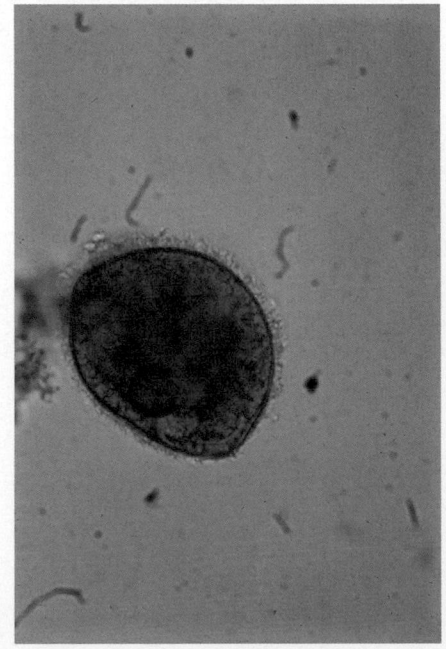
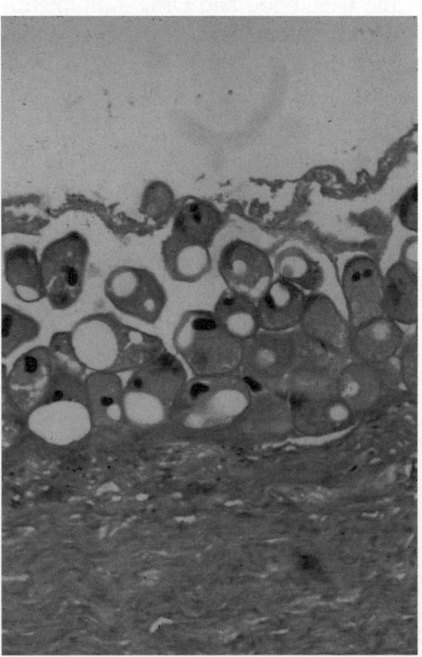

FIGURE 33-30. *Balantidium coli.* **A:** Trophozoite. Note the cilia. **B:** Surface of the colonic mucosa replaced by trophozoites of *B. coli.* (Original magnification × 280; courtesy of Rudolf Garret, MD.)

opportunistic infection in immunocompromised patients, particularly those with T-cell deficiencies.[56] The main source of endemic cryptosporidiosis is human-to-human fecal–oral transmission, which is a concern in the nosocomial and day care setting. Additionally, animal-to-human (especially cats) and waterborne transmission is also common.[300] C. parvum is the most frequent pathogen in HIV-positive patients who have symptoms of diarrhea. In fact, the diagnosis of AIDS can be made if the infection lasts longer than 3 weeks.[109] Nonetheless, the prevalence of cryptosporidiosis has decreased significantly since the introduction of highly active antiretroviral therapy (HAART) in the management of HIV/AIDS.

The gastrointestinal tract is predominantly affected, with the production of severe, watery, debilitating, chronic diarrhea. Malabsorption, wasting, and weight loss may be evident. Systemic manifestations such as fever, loss of appetite, malaise, nausea, and vomiting may also be present, but abdominal pain is unusual. Immunocompetent individuals typically experience such symptoms to varying degrees over a period of days to weeks with spontaneous resolution. Immunocompromised patients, however, in addition to significant gastrointestinal disease also experience extraintestinal symptoms such as pancreatitis, cholecystitis, and biliary infection.[56]

Cryptosporidiosis should be considered in all patients with chronic diarrhea, especially in those who are immunocompromised or have HIV/AIDS. The risk of C. parvum diarrhea in AIDS patients is higher when the CD4 count is 200 cells/mm^3 or fewer.[326] Testing for Cryptosporidium is not routinely performed on standard ova and parasites examination and must be specifically requested. Diagnosis can be made by tinctorial, fluorescent, immunofluorescent, or modified acid-fast staining of stool specimens as well as enzyme immunoassays (Figure 33-31). As oocysts may elude detection even in the symptomatic patient, it is recommended to examine at least three stool samples to increase diagnostic yield.[56]

Treatment of cryptosporidiosis in otherwise healthy individuals mainly requires supportive measures, including fluid and electrolyte supplementation. One drug currently available and approved by the U.S. Food and Drug Administration for use in HIV-negative patients with cryptosporidiosis is nitazoxanide. The range of cure rates in this population varies widely from 67% to 93%. It is also the only medication effective in the treatment of children. Other alternatives include paromomycin and azithromycin.[231]

The treatment of immunocompromised patients involves optimizing CD4$^+$ counts with HAART along with the use of antimotility agents and antiparasitic medications. Specifically, protease inhibitor–based HAART has been shown to reduce morbidity through both immune reconstitution and direct inhibition of the parasites by protease inhibitors. The application of nitazoxanide alone for use in HIV/AIDS patients is limited with studies showing a lack of efficacy. However, longer treatment course with higher dosages has been shown to be effective in HIV/AIDS patients with higher CD4$^+$ counts. The current treatment recommendation is concomitant use of antiretrovirals and antiparasitic medications for a synergistic effect against Cryptosporidium until resolution of symptoms, elimination of the parasite from stool, and an increase in CD4$^+$ count to more than 100 cells/mm^3.[231]

Giardiasis

Giardiasis is a disease caused by a flagellated protozoan, *Giardia lamblia*. It is a worldwide condition, with the vast majority of patients being asymptomatic. Hikers and backpackers drinking untreated water from mountain lakes and streams, where animals serve as a reservoir for the parasite, are at risk. It is probably the most common intestinal protozoan in the United States. Estimates based on the Centers for Disease Control and Prevention state that surveillance data indicate an incidence of 2.5 million cases of giardiasis yearly.[106] The carrier rate is 30% to 60% among children in day care centers, institutionalized individuals, and Native Americans living on reservations.[237] This disease, however, is much more prevalent in developing countries.

As with balantidiasis, the protozoan exists both as a cyst and as a trophozoite. Infection results from ingestion of the cyst, which excysts in the small intestine. The ingestion of 25 cysts will lead to a 100% infection rate.[237] This may lead to a variety of histologic changes, ranging from minimal

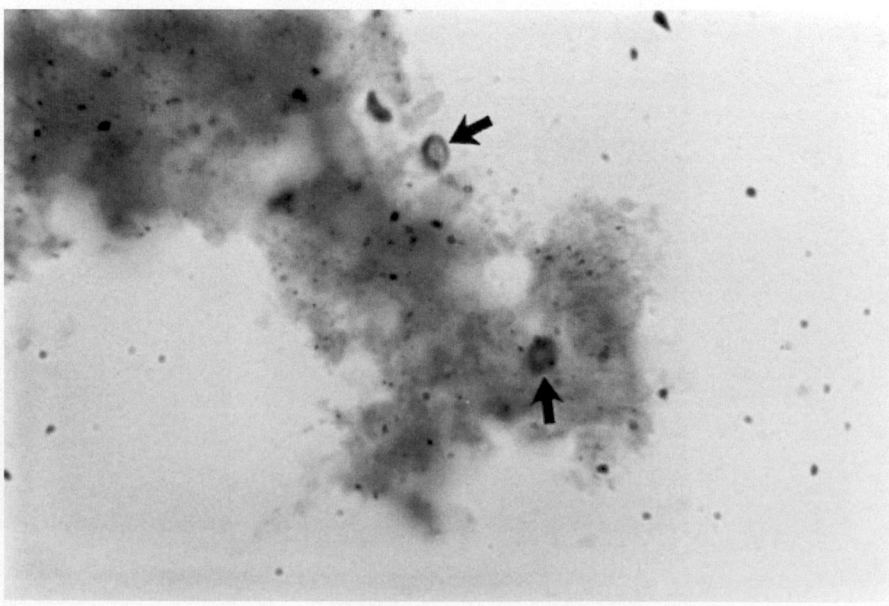

FIGURE 33-31. Cryptosporidiosis. Small, round- to oval-shaped forms usually seen by acid-fast stain or fluorescent staining techniques. (Original magnification × 1,000.)

cellular infiltration of the lamina propria, reduction in the height and the number of villi, loss of the brush border, and an increase in epithelial cell mitosis.[300]

Symptoms

Giardiasis causes explosive, watery diarrhea associated with abdominal cramps and foul flatus. Symptoms typically appear within 1 to 2 weeks from infection. The mechanism for the diarrhea is poorly understood. Vomiting, fever, malaise, weight loss, and dehydration may also be experienced. The symptoms usually last 3 to 4 days before evolving into a subacute phase. However, the majority of patients will present with a more insidious onset of recurrent or resistant symptoms. Diarrhea may alternate with soft stool or even constipation. Because giardiasis is not a form of dysentery, stool does not contain blood or pus.

Giardiasis can also present with upper intestinal manifestations exacerbated by eating. These include epigastric pain, nausea, early satiety, bloating, sulfurous belching, substernal burning, and acid indigestion. Such symptoms can be confused with gastroesophageal reflux or peptic ulcer disease. Chronic disease in adults causes a long-standing malabsorption syndrome and, in children, a failure to thrive. Although on rare occasions the disease can pursue a fulminating course, most infected individuals are asymptomatic carriers.

Diagnosis

The diagnosis of giardiasis as with other parasitic infections involves stool examination. Loose stool contains only the trophozoites, but in formed stool there may be cysts as well (Figure 33-32).[162] The trophozoites disintegrate rapidly and may be undetectable unless fresh, semiformed to formed stool is examined. Therefore, if not immediately examined, the stool sample should be preserved in polyvinyl, in alcohol, or in a formalin preparation. Rectal biopsy may also be helpful in identifying the organism. A negative stool examination, however, does not exclude the diagnosis. Sensitivity increases to 90% with three stool specimens. Therefore, at least three stool samples taken at 2-day intervals should be tested. Stool cultures are not useful because the organism does not reliably grow in the patient's stool samples.

Diagnosis by stool antigen testing with the use of immunofluorescent antibody (IFA) or enzyme-linked immunosorbent assay (ELISA) is the most sensitive and specific method of detecting *G. lamblia*. However, it is important to note that sole reliance on antigen testing precludes evaluation of possible simultaneous bacterial or parasitic infections. Proctosigmoidoscopic examination may reveal changes impossible to differentiate from those of amebiasis. The diagnosis can also be made by examination of scrapings of the base of the ulcer for the trophozoites.[83]

Treatment

Three drugs are available as first-line therapy against *G. lambia*. Metronidazole, although not FDA-approved, is the most frequently used medication for giardiasis in the United States, with 85% to 95% efficacy. The suggested dose is 250 mg, orally, three times daily for 5 to 7 days (the pediatric dose is 5 mg/kg three times daily for 5 to 7 days). Tinidazole administered as a single 2-g dose is reportedly 90% effective. Additionally, nitazoxanide 500 mg twice daily for 3 days is a third option with comparable efficacy.[306] Paromomycin (25 to 30 mg/kg three times daily for 7 to 10 days) may be considered for severe infection in pregnant women.

The treatment of patients with refractory giardiasis is not well established, but combination therapy may be required, especially in HIV/AIDS patients. The association of quinacrine and metronidazole has been reported to be an effective option for this patient population.[62,216] Treatment of the asymptomatic carrier is somewhat controversial, but prudence would seem to dictate that both the asymptomatic person and the acute or chronically ill patient should undergo therapy in order to prevent spread of the disease. There is no chemoprophylactic agent available. However, patient education, especially directed to hikers and travelers, to avoid ingestion

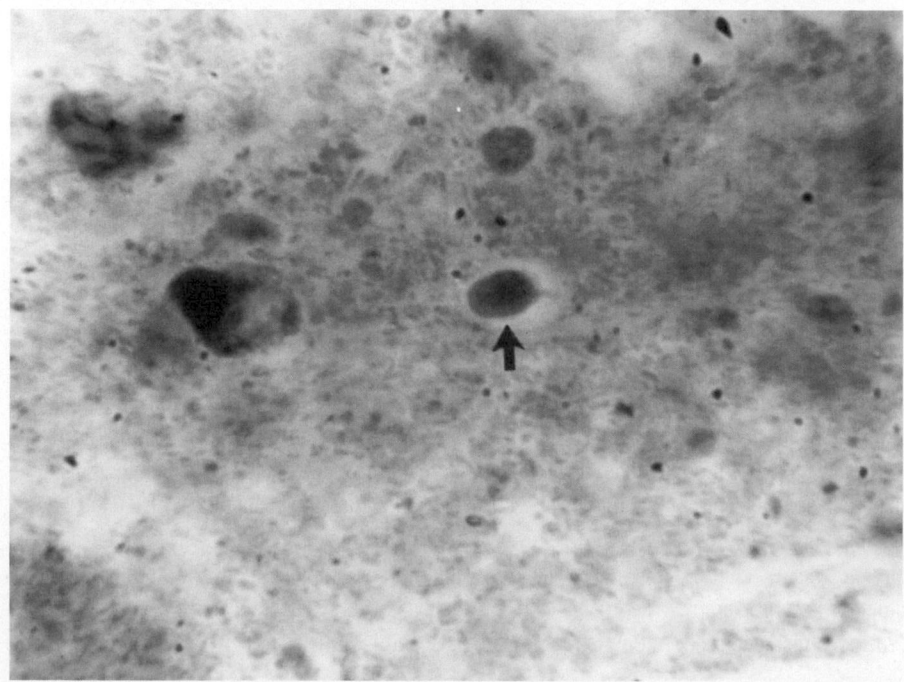

FIGURE 33-32. Giardiasis. Oval-shaped parasite demonstrating retraction from cyst wall. Two nuclei can be appreciated. (Original magnification × 1,000.)

of potentially contaminated water, as well as strict personal hygiene and hand washing, will help to control the disease. In addition, patients should be advised to avoid oral–anal and oral–genital sex.

Trypanosomiasis (Chagas Disease)

The disease caused by the flagellate protozoan, *Trypanosoma cruzi*, was first reported in 1909 by the Brazilian physician, Carlos Chagas. Chagas disease is frequently transmitted by triatomines known as "kissing bugs" because of their nocturnal habits and because they frequently bite the individual in the face while sleeping.[19,46] The trypanosomes are deposited when the bug defecates while taking a blood meal. Phagocytosis of the invading organisms is performed by histiocytes in the skin, fat, and muscle; this is the so-called leishmanial form of the disease. Rupture of the cell causes escape of a large number of the trypanosomal forms into the circulation (Figure 33-33). Transmission is also

known to occur through blood transfusions, which has lead to compulsory blood screening within developing countries as well as within the United States.[293] Vertical transmissions through birth and through organ transplantation have also been reported.[330]

Chagas disease is endemic in developing countries, especially in Central and South America. It represents a huge burden of disease, with an estimated 8 million infected and more than 100 million individuals at risk for infection in Latin America. Spread to developed countries such as the United States has become a growing concern because immigration has resulted in an estimated 300,000 cases within the United States. The magnitude of disease worldwide, however, has significantly improved in recent years due to vector control programs, as well as the implementation of mandatory blood screening.[249]

Gastrointestinal manifestations occur from 2 to 20 years or more following initial infection.[207] The release of the toxin destroys the submucosal and myenteric plexi, with the colon

CARLOS J. R. CHAGAS (1879–1933)

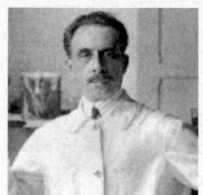

Carlos Chagas was born in the town of Oliveira, Brazil, to an upper-class family of coffee growers. Chagas did not follow his mother's dream of his becoming a mining engineer, choosing instead to pursue a medical career. He firmly believed that the growth and evolution of Brazil depended on the eradication of endemic diseases, such as yellow fever, smallpox, syphilis, malaria, and bubonic plague. Chagas went on to write his thesis at the Oswaldo Cruz Institute under the guidance of the renowned parasitologist Oswaldo Cruz. However, he refused Cruz's invitation to continue his work on malarial research and entered the practice of family medicine. Chagas, being of an inquisitive mind, was innovative and experimental. He studied parasites and insects in their natural habitat and evaluated epidemics in order to broaden his background. In 1908, Chagas set up a simple laboratory to study a disease that was taking the lives of immigrant railroad workers in central Brazil. By 1909, he not only identified the insect carrying the flagellate that transmitted the disease, but also described the complete cycle of the *Trypanosoma cruzi*, which he named after his mentor. Through his extensive investigations, Chagas reported the acute clinical presentation as well as the diverse chronic manifestations of the disease that bears his name. Unfortunately, following his death in 1933, very few additional contributions have been made in the study of Chagas disease. (Courtesy of T. Cristina Sardinha, MD.)

OSWALDO GONÇALVES CRUZ (1872–1917)

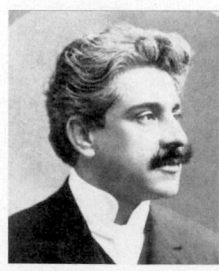

Oswaldo Cruz was born in Paraitinga (São Paulo) Brazil. At the age of 15, he began his medical studies at the Faculty of Medicine of Rio de Janeiro, and in 1892 he graduated with a thesis on water as the vehicle for the propagation of microbes. Inspired by the work of Louis Pasteur, he went to Paris to specialize in bacteriology at the Pasteur Institute from 1896 through 1899, under the renowned professor, Émile Roux. He returned to Brazil in 1899 and organized the control of the bubonic plague in the city of Santos (São Paulo), demonstrating that the epidemic was not possible to control without the adequate serum antidote. Because the importation took a long time for the serum to get to the country, he was recruited to create what would become the Federal Institute for Serum Therapy where the drug was then locally produced. Cruz became recognized as a scientist, an epidemiologist, and a specialist in sanitation. He was the coordinator for the campaigns for eradication of yellow fever and smallpox in the city of Rio de Janeiro, as well as in the states of northern Brazil (Para and Amazonas). He received the highest award of the International Congress of Hygiene and Demography at the Berlin meeting (1907). In 1909, when another Brazilian scientist, Carlos Chagas, identified the protozoan that caused the disease, Chagas gave it the name, *Trypanosoma cruzi*, honoring Oswaldo Cruz. In 1913, Cruz was elected a member of the Brazilian Academy of Arts and Letters, and in 1915, due to health problems, he resigned from the directorship of the Oswaldo Cruz Institute, moving to Petrópolis, a small city in the mountains near Rio. In 1916, he was elected mayor of that city and outlined an extensive urbanization project, which he would not see implemented. On the morning of February 11, 1917, at only 44 years of age, he died of kidney failure. (Courtesy of Renato A. Bonardi, MD.)

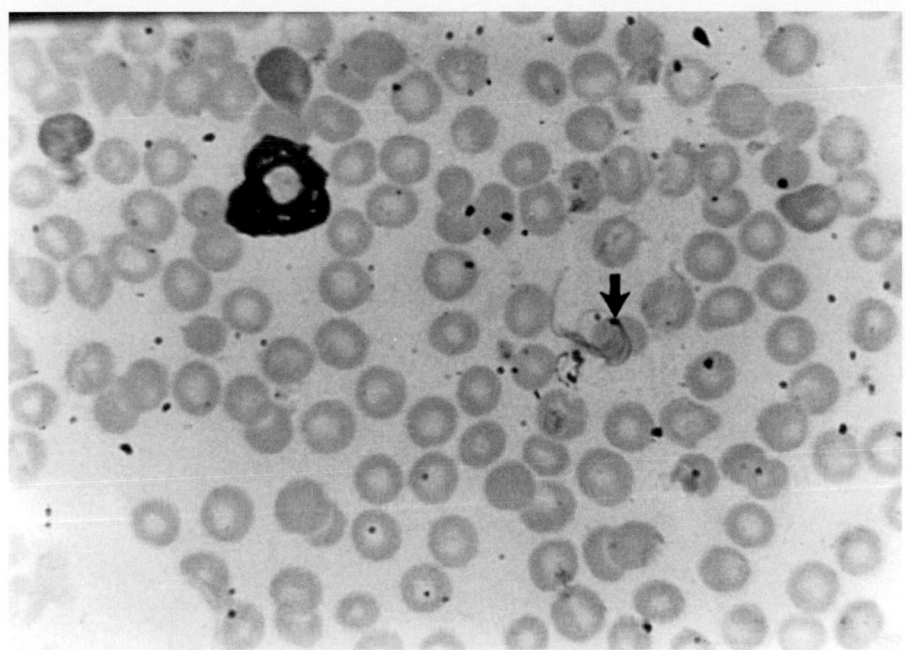

FIGURE 33-33. Trypanosomiasis. C-shaped configuration found in human blood. Organism has prominent terminal kinetoplast. Intercellular location is typical of trypanosomes. (Original magnification × 1,000.)

and the esophagus most frequently involved, although the stomach, small bowel, bladder, and ureters can be affected. Involvement of the myocardium and central nervous system can also develop. In the intestine, the parasympathetic intramural denervation is dispersed irregularly, but the manifestations are primarily in the esophagus and the colon, especially the sigmoid. The bowel presents a functional peristaltic alteration leading to progressive dilatation and elongation of the affected segment, which slows down the transit time. The patient may become severely constipated as the bowel becomes progressively dilated because of the neurologic abnormality and the presence of inspissated feces (Figure 33-34). Although obstipation may necessitate the use of frequent enemas, often the patient compensates and is able to lead a fairly normal existence.[207] Volvulus, however, is a potential complication (Figures 33-35 and 33-36). In those individuals with chagasic megacolon, clinical signs and symptoms include severe pain and progressive abdominal distention, accompanied by fever, severe toxemia, and shock.[164]

The diagnosis of Chagas disease is based on clinical presentation and immunologic tests such as indirect hemagglutination, immunofluorescence, and enzyme immunosorbent assay. PCR has also been described as a diagnostic modality, as well as hemoculture.[46]

Radiologic examination may reveal an enormously dilated and elongated colon (Figure 33-37). In contradistinction to other forms of megacolon, the distribution may be segmental (Figure 33-38).[207]

Patients with achalasia caused by the disease may undergo treatment with pneumatic dilatation of the esophagus or possibly esophagomyotomy.[83] Resection of the aperistaltic esophagus or colon may be necessary if symptoms warrant (Figure 33-39). A variety of procedures have been proposed, including Duhamel–Haddad, sigmoidectomy, low anterior resection, left hemicolectomy, and subtotal colectomy. The rectal wall is also often thickened and hypertrophied in addition to the dilatation in the proximal rectum. This may result in difficulty with a stapled anastomosis and lead to an increased recurrence rate. Therefore, one is advised to perform a low anterior resection with distal colorectal anastomosis.[46] Total colectomy with ileostomy is suggested if toxic megacolon is the indication for the operation.

Currently, there is no effective treatment to eradicate Chagas disease. Surgical resection of the affected segment of bowel is the mainstay of therapy. Drugs such as benznidazole and nifurtimox have been successfully used in patients

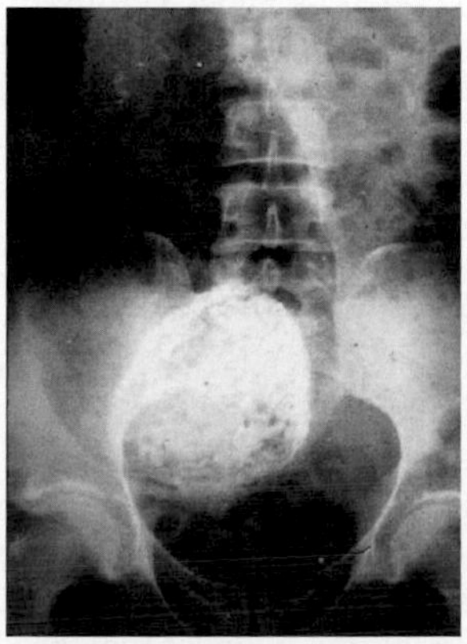

FIGURE 33-34. Abdominal x-ray showing fecaloma in a patient with Chagas disease. (Courtesy of T. Cristina Sardinha, MD.)

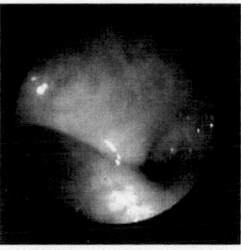

FIGURE 33-35. Proctosigmoidoscopic appearance of classic narrowing as a consequence of a sigmoid volvulus in a patient with Chagas disease. (Courtesy of T. Cristina Sardinha, MD.)

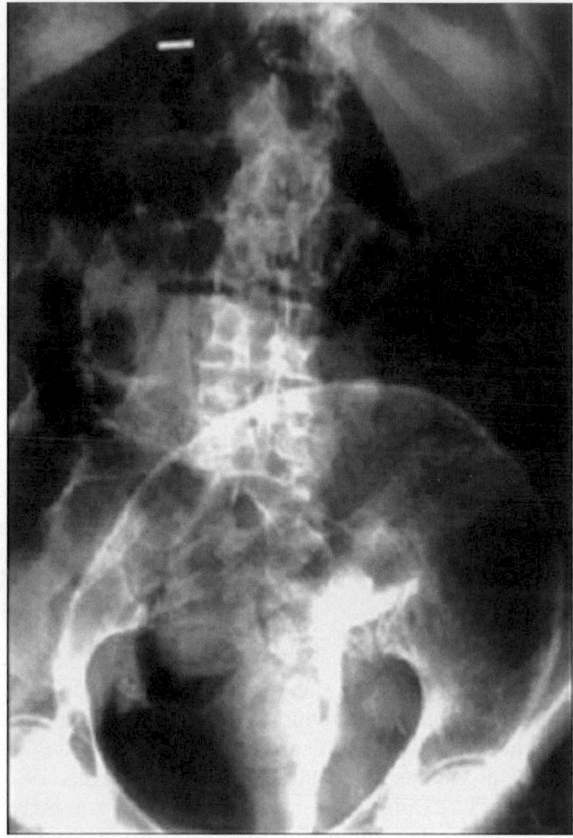

FIGURE 33-36. Plain abdominal x-ray showing sigmoid volvulus in a patient with Chagas disease. (Courtesy of T. Cristina Sardinha, MD.)

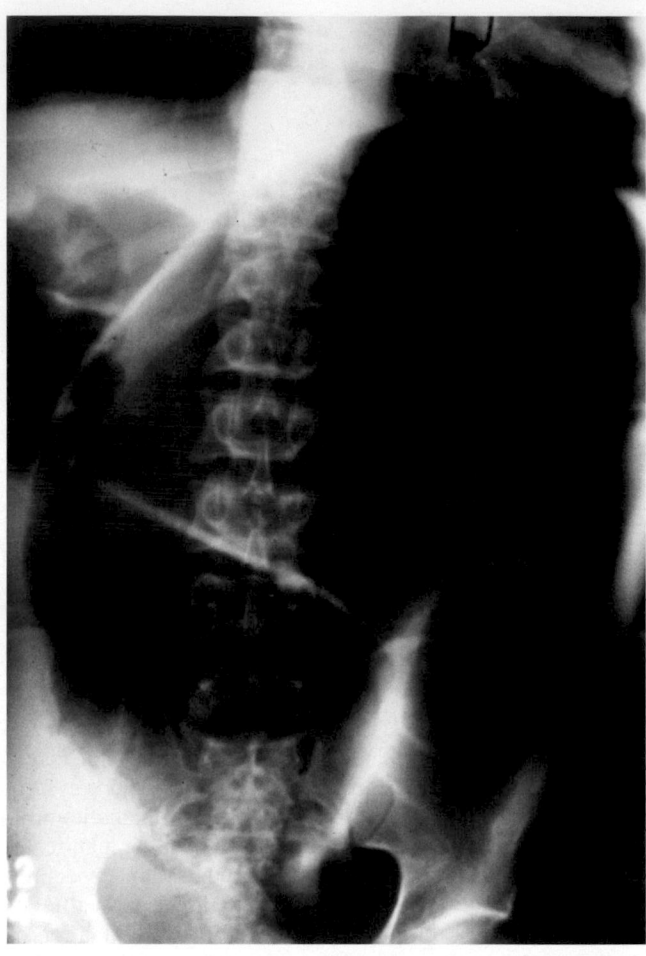

FIGURE 33-37. Chagasic megacolon. Plain abdominal x-ray reveals typical profound colonic dilatation.

with early presentation. However, once the neurologic and anatomical damage has been established, there is no possibility for cure.[46]

Schistosomiasis (Bilharziosis)

Schistosomiasis is a worldwide condition affecting more than 200 million people. The disease is caused by a trematode, a blood fluke that is seen in three forms: *Schistosoma mansoni*, *Schistosoma japonicum*, and *Schistosoma haematobium*. A snail host is required to complete the life cycle. The disease is frequently seen in tropical and subtropical climates.

Pathogenesis

The life cycle of the organism is of some interest. The infection is acquired by exposure to contaminated water containing the cercarial form (Figure 33-40).[83] The cercaria invades the skin, loses its tail, and enters the host's subcutaneous veins. From there, it spreads to the heart and lungs and may produce a transient pneumonitis. Ultimately reaching the portal circulation, it grows, feeds, and differentiates into a male or a female form (Figure 33-41). Following fertilization, the worms migrate together into the terminal mesenteric venules. There, the female deposits the fertilized eggs. The egg secretes a lytic substance that permits it to migrate through the surrounding tissue, into the intestinal lumen, and into the stool.[83]

The three forms of the infestation are differentiated based on the appearance of the *Schistosoma* ova (Figures 33-42 and 33-43). The *S. mansoni* ovum has a prominent lateral spine, the *S. haematobium* has a projecting terminal spine, and the *S. japonicum* has no definite spine. *S. japonicum* preferentially invades the superior mesenteric veins, thus involving the small intestine and ascending colon; *S. mansoni* usually invades the inferior mesenteric veins, perforating through the descending colon; and *S. haematobium* tends to invade the bladder vessels, thus producing symptoms in the bladder, pelvic organs, and rectum.[83]

Signs and Symptoms

Symptoms are initially related to the cercarial dermatitis. This is a pruritic rash due to the cercaria penetrating the skin (see Chapter 9). The most common acute symptoms are fever, lethargy, and myalgia. Other complaints include cough, headache, lower abdominal pain, diarrhea, and anorexia. Usually, the patient reports recent exposure to fresh water. Chronic manifestations of the disease depend on which type is responsible for the infection. Bessa and associates reported 40 patients with colonic schistosomiasis due to *S. mansoni*, a common health problem in Egypt.[25] The primary complaint was severe diarrhea; three developed intestinal obstruction due to rectal or sigmoid stricture. Three-fourths of the patients had a palpable mass.

Children are particularly susceptible to acute dysentery.[83,168] Fibrosis and thickening may result, and polyp formation may also occur. Other complications include intussusception and rectal prolapse. Portal involvement may produce granulomas, hepatosplenomegaly, and portal hypertension. Central nervous system complications can also develop.

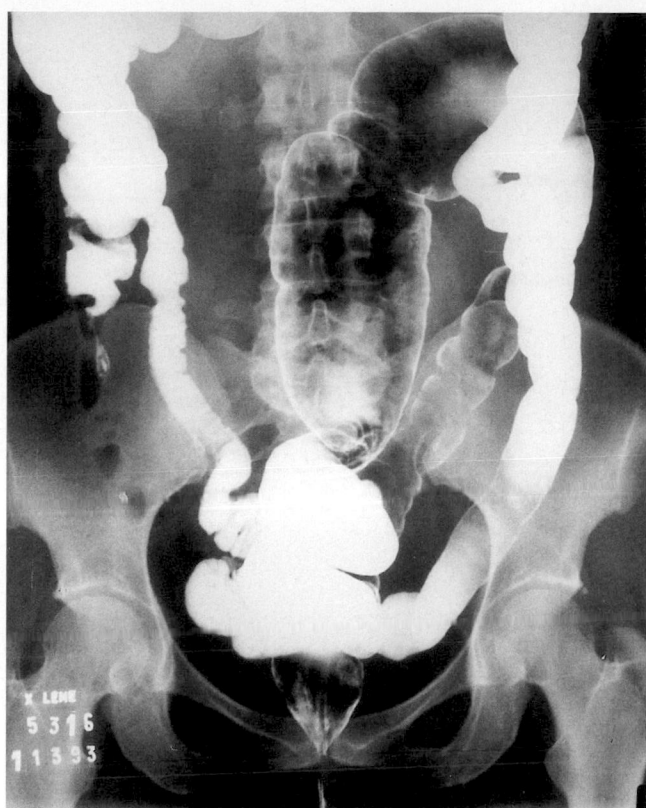

FIGURE 33-38. Chagas disease. Barium enema demonstrates segmental nature of the dilated colon.

Diagnosis

The diagnosis is usually made by identification of the ova in fresh stool specimens. Rectal biopsy frequently reveals the presence of eggs in the mucosa or submucosa (Figures 33-44 and 33-45). The diagnosis may also be made by means of a wet preparation; the biopsy specimen is compressed between two cover slips and examined for the ova (Figure 33-46). Urinary excretion of the eggs (usually *S. hematobium*) is more frequently found between 10 a.m. and 2 p.m. The urine or stool quantitative evaluation of the eggs suggests the severity of the infection.[168] Fewer than 100 eggs per gram is a mild infection; more than 400 eggs per gram is considered a heavy infection. The acute infection is often associated with an eosinophilia.

Serologic evaluation is a useful epidemiologic tool. However, it cannot differentiate active from inactive infection. The Falcon assay screening test/enzyme-linked immunosorbent assay (FAST-ELISA) and confirmatory enzyme-linked immunoelectrotransfer blot (EITB) tests are highly sensitive and specific for all species of schistosoma.[188] Colonoscopy with biopsy has been demonstrated to confirm the diagnosis, especially when ova are present.[247]

Patients with an acute schistosomal colitis may present with ova within the lamina propria as well as submucosa along with neutrophilic granulocytes and eosinophils. Those with chronic schistosomal colitis may demonstrate calcified ova associated with submucosal plasma cells and lymphocytes. A classic finding associated with schistosomiasis on colonoscopy is the presence of gray-yellow or yellowish white nodules. However, such nodules are not typically

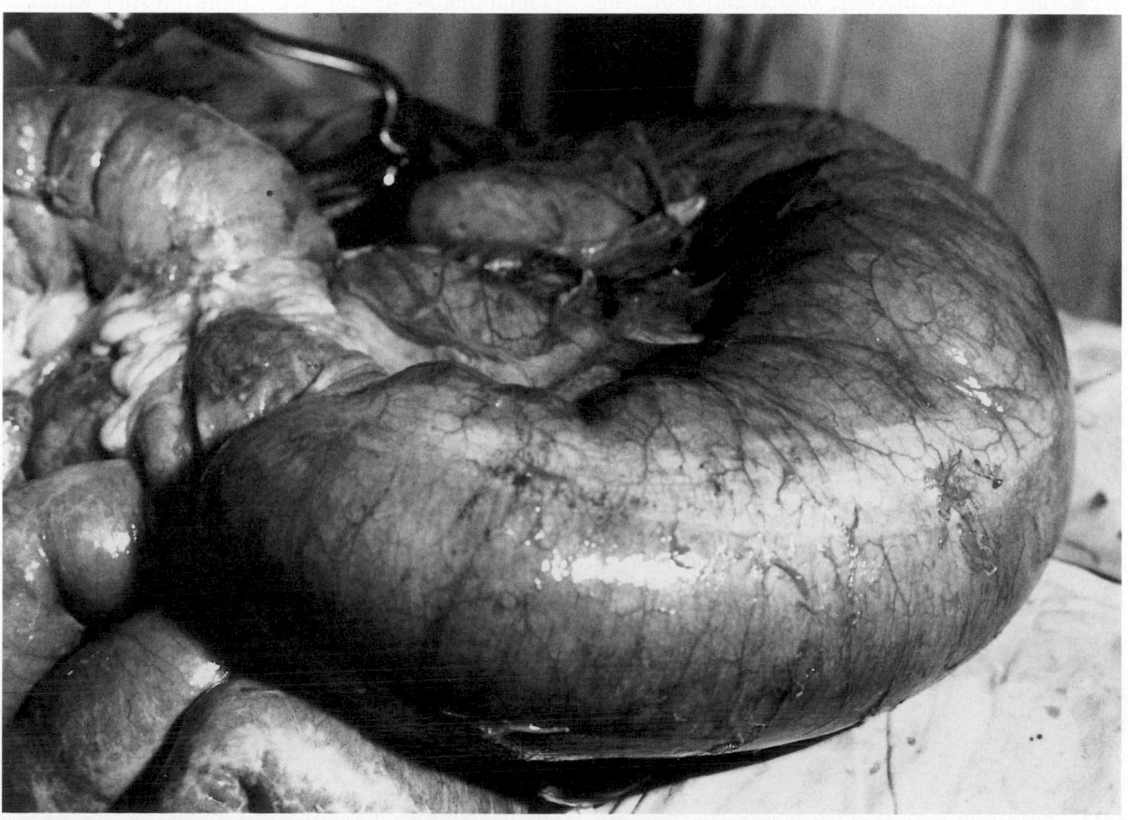

FIGURE 33-39. Resection of profoundly dilated Chagasic colon. (Courtesy of Fernando Jorge de Souza, MD.)

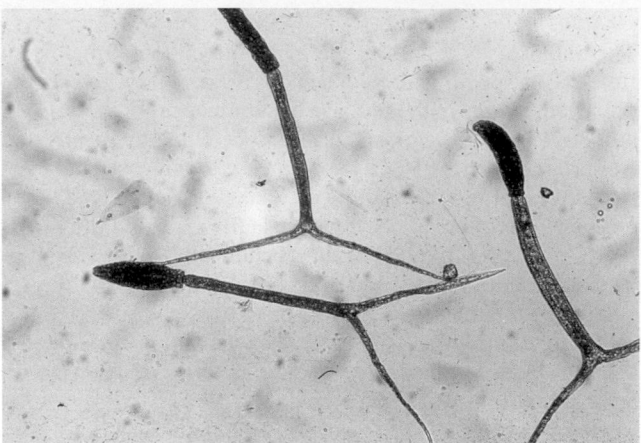

FIGURE 33-40. *Schistosoma*, fork-tailed cercaria. (Courtesy of Rudolf Garret, MD.)

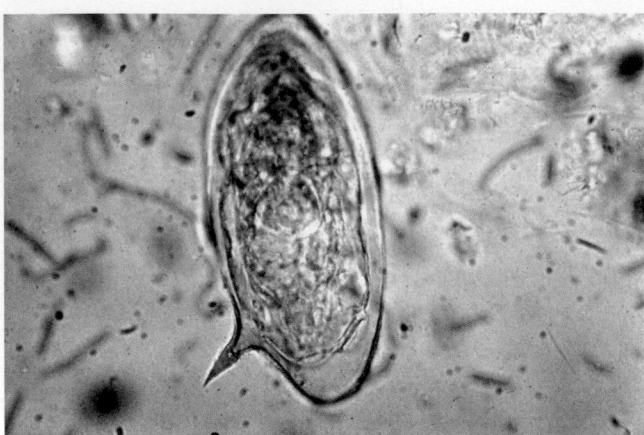

FIGURE 33-42. *S. mansoni* ovum. Note the lateral spine. (Courtesy of Rudolf Garret, MD.)

seen.[43] Polyps are not uncommon, and because large or pedunculated ones tend not to regress but to cause persistent bleeding, colonoscopy–polypectomy is recommended.[24,206] However, one must expect that additional polyps will regrow because the mucosa does not revert to normal. Rectocolic and urinary tract calcifications, as seen on radiologic studies, are felt to be associated with a clinically latent or mild form of schistosomiasis.[93]

Treatment

The treatment of schistosomiasis involves the use of a single chemotherapeutic drug. Oral praziquantel, 40 to 60 mg/kg, in divided doses over 1 day is the drug of choice, with an 80% to 90% success rate of reducing egg burden and achieving parasitic cure.[188] It is generally well tolerated with few side effects. The issue of drug resistance has been investigated, but no clinically significant resistance has been documented to date.[188] The use of artemisinins and trioxolanes are now being studied as possible alternatives.[21]

Treatment of the colonic complications involves a variety of resective and diversionary procedures. Anastomosis without a colostomy appears to be associated with a prohibitively high incidence of leakage.[25]

Relationship to Carcinoma

The risk of cancer in patients with schistosomiasis is well known, especially in those infected with *S. haematobium*. The malignancy with this type often occurs in the urinary bladder. This concern is especially evident in the Middle East and parts of Africa where there is a high incidence of schistosomiasis.[20] Patients with long-standing schistosomal colitis are at an increased risk for the development of colon and rectal carcinoma, although this applies primarily to *S. japonicum*.[150,206] The pathogenesis is yet to be fully understood but is possibly related to chronic inflammatory changes induced by the trematode. Chen and colleagues reported a retrospective study of 60 patients with schistosomal granulomatous disease of the large intestine without obvious evidence of carcinoma and noted that 36 had mild-to-severe

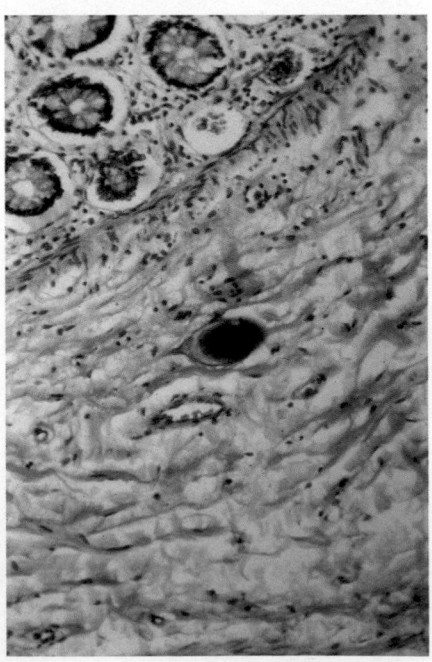

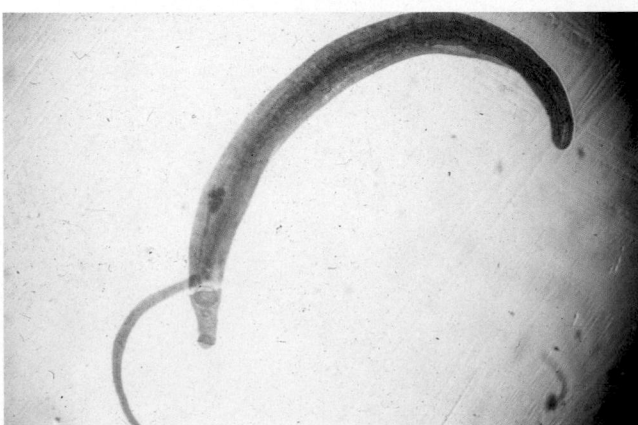

FIGURE 33-41. *Schistosoma mansoni*, adult male and female. The female occupies the male's genital groove. (Courtesy of Rudolf Garret, MD.)

FIGURE 33-43. *S. haematobium* in the rectal wall. Note the terminal spine. (Original magnification × 180; courtesy of Rudolf Garret, MD.)

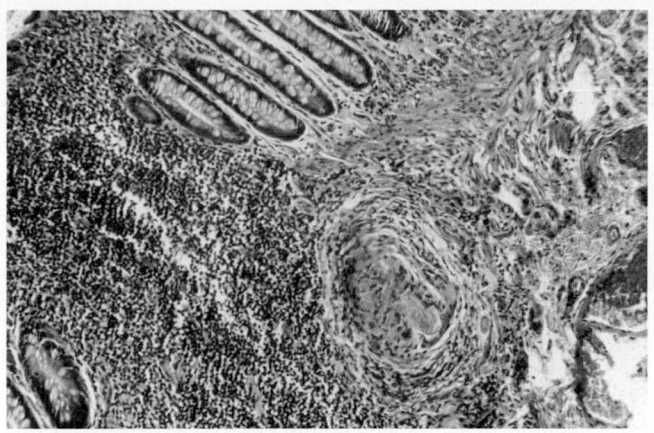

FIGURE 33-44. *S. mansoni* in the wall of the rectum. (Original magnification × 240; courtesy of Rudolf Garret, MD.)

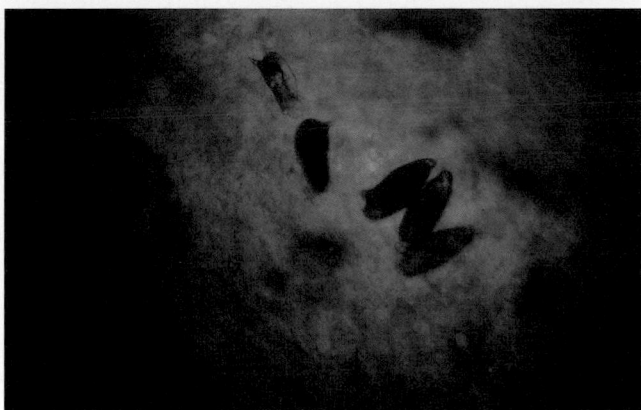

FIGURE 33-46. *S. mansoni* ova, wet preparation. (Courtesy of Rudolf Garret, MD.)

dysplasia.[61] The authors regarded the changes as presumptive evidence for the premalignant potential of schistosomal colitis and felt that the findings were analogous to those observed in patients with long-standing chronic ulcerative colitis. In a study of 352 colon cancer patients, Mei and colleagues found 14.3% with a history of schistosomiasis.[198] Moreover, in a retrospective study conducted by Cao and colleagues, 8 of 46 patients infected with schistosomiasis were found to have colon cancer, and 2 of 46 demonstrated high-grade intraepithelial neoplastic changes.[43] Investigation into the relationship between schistosomiasis and colorectal carcinoma is currently ongoing.

Relationship to Portal Hypertension

Cirrhosis with portal hypertension may produce massive hemorrhage from varices that requires emergency therapy. The initial management includes endoscopic ligation or sclerosis of the bleeding variceal vein.[26] However, failure of endoscopic control requires the placement of a transjugular intrahepatic portosystemic shunt. Long-term management of portal hypertension includes repeated endoscopic treatment, long-term β-blockers,[267] surgical shunt, and liver transplantation. The use of octreotide has also been reported as an effective measure for the management of bleeding.[92]

An approach has been suggested that involves cannulation of the portal vein, followed by trapping of the adult worms in a filter system (Figure 33-47). Administration of antimony potassium tartrate, an extremely toxic drug, has been demonstrated to increase the yield of the worms removed by stimulating migration into the portal circulation.

Ascariasis

Ascariasis is the most common intestinal helminth infection worldwide. The disease is estimated to affect 25% of the world's population.[236] The condition is endemic in tropical and subtropical areas where poor sanitation and hygiene are prevalent, but epidemics have been reported in Europe and even in small, focal areas of the United States. It is estimated that approximately 4 million people in the United States are

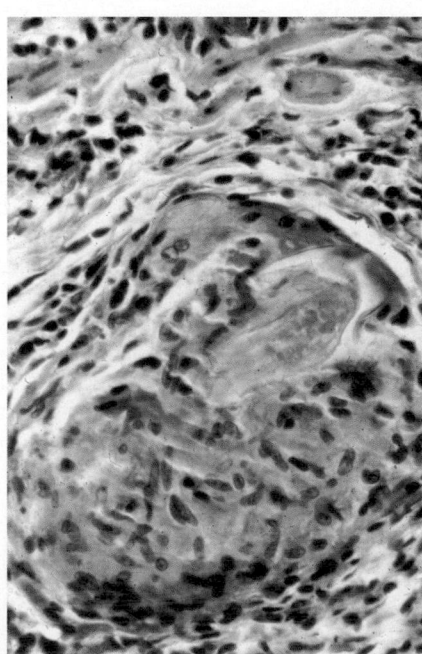

FIGURE 33-45. *S. mansoni* in the wall of the rectum surrounded by epithelioid cells. (Original magnification × 600; courtesy of Rudolf Garret, MD.)

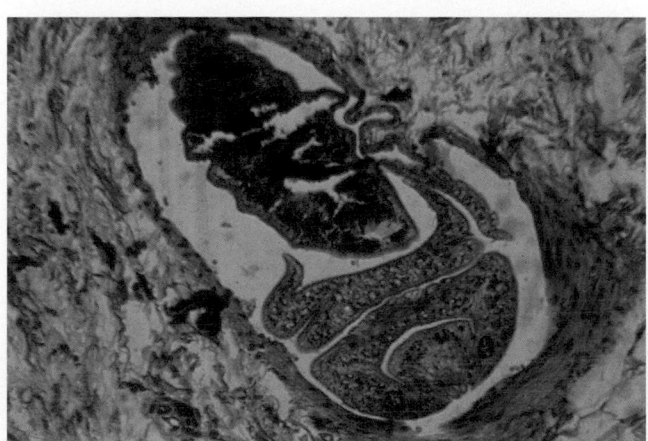

FIGURE 33-47. *S. mansoni* adult in a mesenteric vein. (Original magnification × 133; courtesy of Rudolf Garret, MD.)

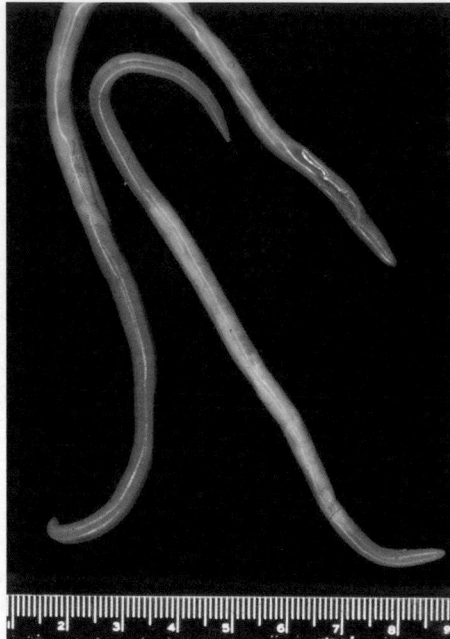

FIGURE 33-48. *Ascaris lumbricoides*, adult worms. (Courtesy of Rudolf Garret, MD.)

infected with *Ascaris lumbricoides* (Figure 33-48). Children are more frequently infected than adults and harbor heavier parasitic loads.[262]

Pathophysiology

Infection occurs from ingestion of the eggs in contaminated food and drink (Figure 33-49). Following ingestion, the larvae emerge from the ovum and migrate through the wall of the small intestine into the portal venous system, passing through the liver and into the lungs.[37] Ultimately, the larvae migrate through the capillaries, into the alveoli and the bronchioles, and are coughed up and swallowed. Once in the small intestine, they develop into the adult worm.

Symptoms and Signs

Most individuals infected with *A. lumbricoides* are asymptomatic. Early symptoms (4 to 16 days after ingestion of the

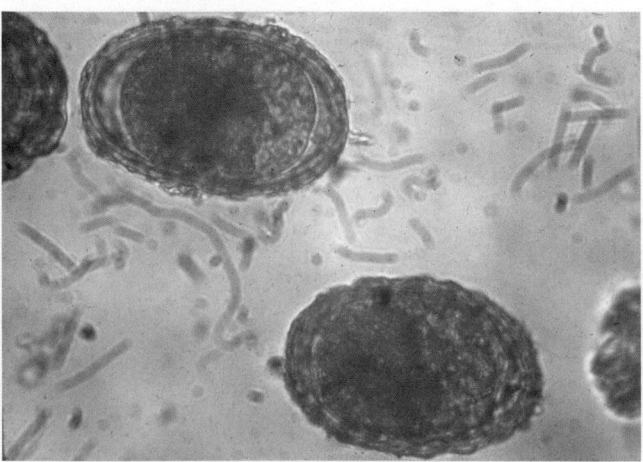

FIGURE 33-49. *A. lumbricoides*, ova. (Courtesy of Rudolf Garret, MD.)

egg) are related to the tissue migratory phase and include fever, cough, and wheezing. During the late phase (6 to 8 weeks after contamination), patients present with gastrointestinal symptoms resulting from mechanical irritation of the adult parasite. Vague abdominal complaints such as cramping, nausea, and vomiting are common. The migration of the worm can lead to pancreatitis, cholecystitis, biliary obstruction, bowel obstruction, and even appendicitis. The patient occasionally eliminates the parasite through the anus or through the mouth and nose, a particularly unpleasant event in children.[148,236] Bowel perforation is unlikely to be due to this condition, unless there is an associated ulceration of the intestine such as is seen with amebiasis or typhoid.[88] Small bowel volvulus can also occur.[321] Additionally, allergic reactions (asthma, urticaria, and conjunctivitis) may be the result of absorption of toxins from the worm.[37]

Physical examination may reveal minimal signs, but obviously in the presence of intestinal obstruction, abdominal distention, and diffuse tenderness may be noted. Occasionally, perforation can ensue, and the patient will present with signs of peritonitis.

Diagnosis

The diagnosis of ascariasis is made by locating the eggs, larvae, or adult worms. It typically takes approximately 2 months from the time of infection before the eggs appear in the stool. The worms may also be recovered from the sputum and occasionally from emesis.[37] Laboratory studies are usually of no value because the only significant abnormality is the presence of an eosinophilia.

Small bowel x-ray films may reveal the presence of the worms in the distal ileum. Characteristically, the gastrointestinal tract of the worm may be identified because it is filled with the contrast material (Figure 33-50). Ultrasonography has been found to be useful in the diagnosis of intestinal obstruction from ascariasis. Characteristic sonographic features of railway track sign and bull's-eye appearance are helpful in making the diagnosis.[318]

Treatment

The treatment of ascariasis consists of a single-dose regimen of mebendazole (500 mg), albendazole (400 mg), or pyrantel pamoate (10 mg/kg).[151] Follow-up is suggested to confirm cure.

If an operation is required and perforation has not occurred, it is best to attempt manipulation of the worms through the ileum into the cecum rather than to open the bowel. Resection is advised if required, as opposed to enterotomy and extraction of the worms (Figure 33-51). The instillation of intraluminal vermifuge intraoperatively has been reported to minimize the risk of postoperative worm migration through suture lines and anastomoses.[322] Early clinical diagnosis together with prompt surgery for obstruction are important in reducing a high mortality rate in this potentially devastating condition.[5,318]

Strongyloidiasis

Strongyloidiasis is a parasitic disease often seen in tropical climates and caused by another roundworm, *Strongyloides stercoralis*. The condition usually occurs in the small bowel, but the colon may occasionally be the site of involvement. Somewhat similar to hookworm, the larvae penetrate the skin and are carried by way of the circulation

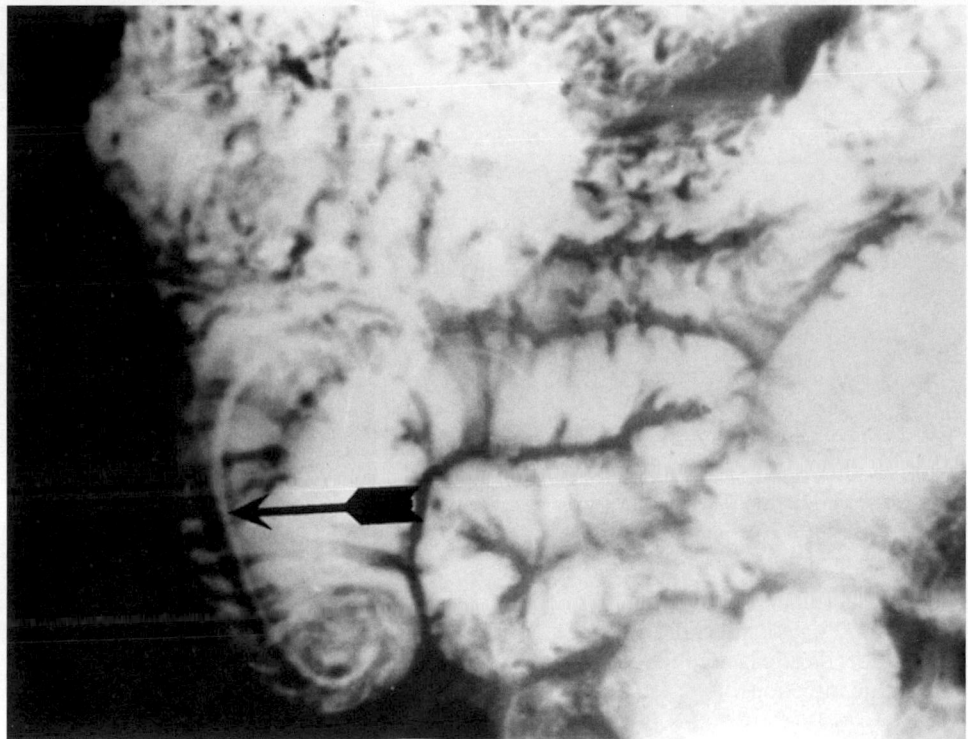

FIGURE 33-50. Ascariasis. Small bowel x-ray demonstrates *Ascaris*. The gastrointestinal tract of the worm can be identified (*arrow*).

to the lungs. They then rupture into the alveoli and develop into adolescent worms.[37] The swallowed female invades the small intestinal mucosa where it remains, depositing eggs (Figure 33-52). A unique feature of *S. stercoralis* is its ability to reproduce asexually, leading to autoinfection and chronic parasitism.

Symptoms referable to the intestinal tract may be minimal, or the patient may complain of diarrhea, nausea, vomiting, and abdominal pain. Rectal pain and tenesmus have been reported in association with involvement in that area, and proctitis may be present on sigmoidoscopy.[251] This clinical syndrome of hyperinfection is particularly devastating in immunocompromised patients with the most significant risk factors being use of glucocorticoids and infection with human T-lymphotropic virus type 1. Gastrointestinal symptoms are variable and may be associated with ileus and small bowel obstruction.[152]

The diagnosis is established by examination of duodenal secretions; suction biopsy of the duodenum is a poor way of finding the parasite.[37] Additionally, strongyloidiasis can be diagnosed by finding the larvae in the feces; this is the only intestinal nematode from which larvae rather than eggs are identified in the stool. Serologic testing is available and sensitive although not specific for strongyloidiasis.[152]

In the severe form of the disease, mortality is usually due to dehydration and electrolyte imbalance; the result of vomiting and diarrhea.[49] Strongyloidiasis can be effectively

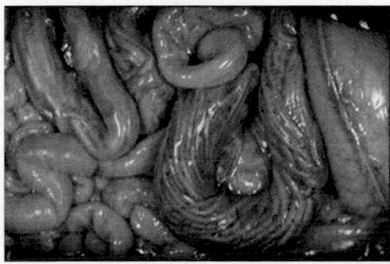

FIGURE 33-51. Loop of small bowel containing innumerable, large round worms. (Courtesy of T. Cristina Sardinha, MD.)

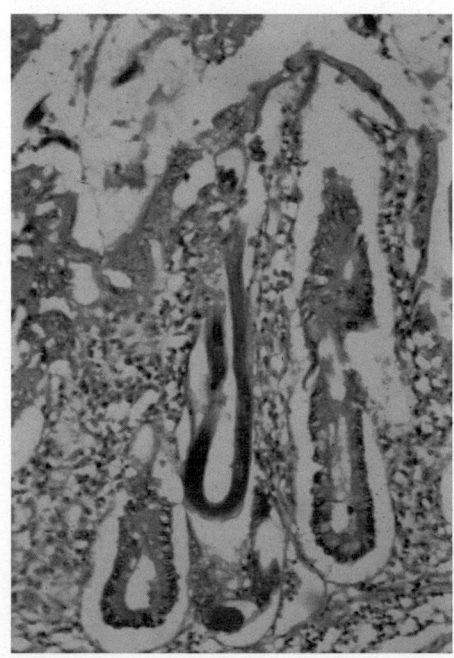

FIGURE 33-52. *Strongyloides stercoralis.* Larvae and eggs in intestinal mucosa. (Original magnification × 280; courtesy of Rudolf Garret, MD.)

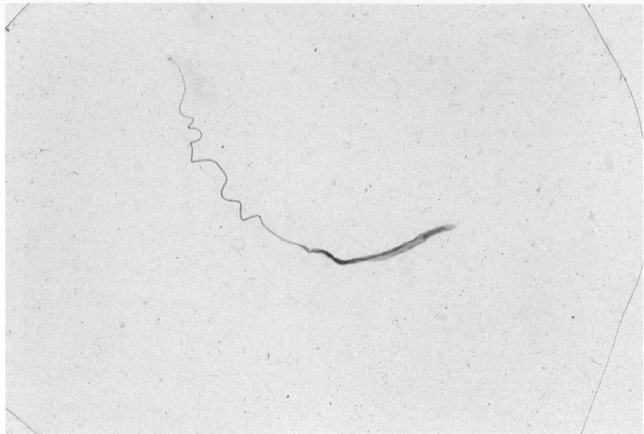

FIGURE 33-53. Adult *Trichuris trichiura*. Note the slender neck, which gives the worm its common name, whipworm. (Courtesy of Rudolf Garret, MD.)

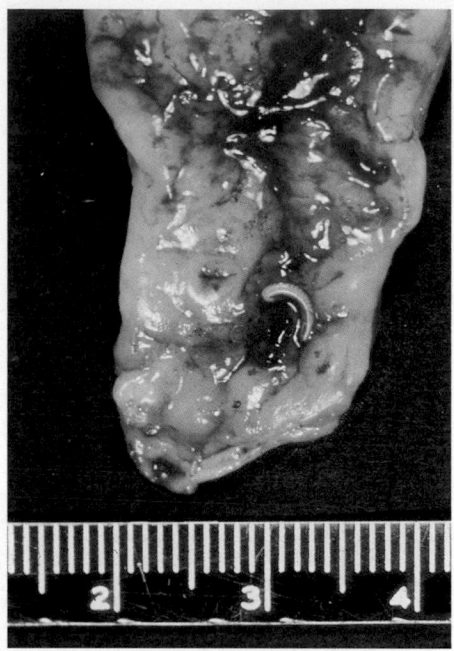

FIGURE 33-55. *T. trichiura* (whipworm) in the lumen of the appendix. (Courtesy of Rudolf Garret, MD.)

treated in the acute and chronic phases with ivermectin (200 μg/kg/day, orally, for 2 days). Albendazole is the second-line therapy, and thiabendazole is used for disseminated illness or mixed helminthic infections.[240]

Trichuriasis

Trichuriasis is caused by the roundworm *Trichuris trichiura*, the so-called whipworm. Its common name is misleading because the whip or tail is actually its head (Figure 33-53). Approximately one-quarter of the world's population, generally in tropical areas, has been infected with *T. trichiura*.[114]

The egg has a characteristic barrel shape with a nonstaining prominence at each end (Figure 33-54). Infection occurs via fecal–oral transmission with ingestion of food or water containing the eggs. The eggs are digested in the intestinal tract, releasing larvae into the small intestine. The larvae

reside in the mucosa for several days, and then relocate to the cecal area where they mature over a period of 2 to 3 months (Figure 33-55).[37]

Patients may be virtually asymptomatic or have moderate or severe infective symptoms, depending on the extent of involvement. Lower abdominal pain, diarrhea, and rectal bleeding may be reported. Nausea, vomiting, flatulence, abdominal distention, headache, and weight loss are also noted.[325]

Appendicitis and rectal prolapse may be a consequence of whipworm infection.[37] A number of worms together, creating blockage of the appendiceal lumen, accounts for the signs and symptoms of appendicitis. Rectal prolapse is thought to result from straining at defecation due to the massive number of worms in the rectum.[325] *T. trichiura* eggs have also been identified in a patient with an anal abscess.[96] Furthermore, the worm has been demonstrated to suck blood from the colon, and it is estimated that 0.005 mL may be lost per day per worm.[325] Consequently, severe infestation may cause anemia. However, significant blood loss in the adult has only rarely been recognized.

The diagnosis is made by the identification of the characteristic eggs in the stool. Egg counts are useful in determining the degree of infection and for evaluating the efficacy of treatment.[325] Barium enema examination may reveal evidence of the worms on air-contrast study.

Treatment with mebendazole (Vermox) has been found to be highly effective against *Trichuris* as well as against other worms.[37] Albendazole is an alternative therapeutic option.

Anisakiasis

The most common nematode worm infection found in humans is *Anisakis simplex*, an intestinal parasite of marine fish and mammals. Anisakiasis is most frequently reported in Japan, a consequence of the consumption of raw or undercooked fish. Cases occurring in the United States are

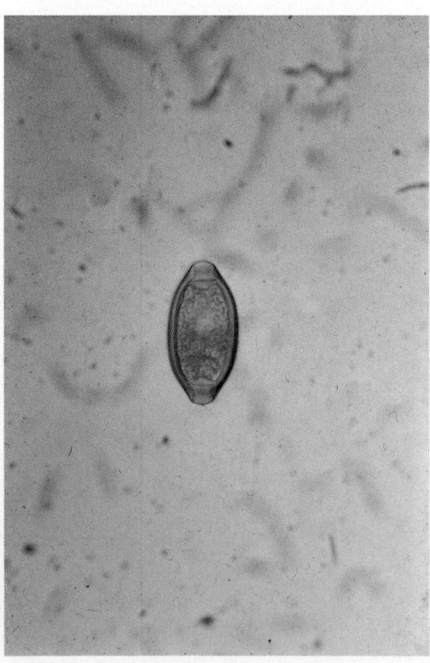

FIGURE 33-54. *T. trichiura* ovum. Note the characteristic barrel shape with a "plug" at either end. (Courtesy of Rudolf Garret, MD.)

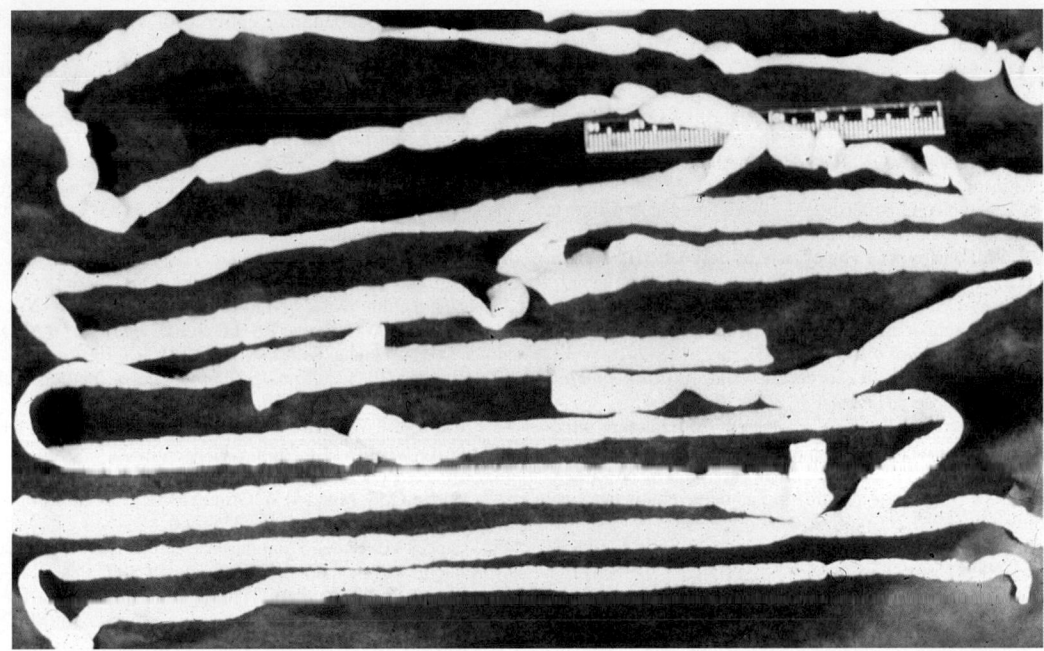

FIGURE 33-56. *Taenia saginata*. Beef tapeworm adult. (Courtesy of Rudolf Garret, MD.)

most commonly attributed to Pacific salmon. Disease can be caused by *A. simplex* in one of two ways: direct larvae penetration into the gastrointestinal mucosa or allergy to chemicals released by the nematode within cooked fish, also termed gastroallergic anisakiasis.

Signs and symptoms of infection typically develop within several hours of ingestion and may include acute abdominal pain, nausea, vomiting, and diarrhea.[13] Findings can mimic those of regional enteritis. Verhamme and Ramboer suggest that a high index of suspicion must be maintained, requiring a carefully obtained history, if one is to avoid emergency laparotomy and bowel resection.[314] Most symptoms of infection with this parasite will resolve spontaneously. However, intussusception has been reported as a rare complication of anisakiasis.[204]

A. simplex has been implicated as a significant cause of hypersensitivity, particularly within the Basque Country in northern Spain. Those exposed may experience both manifestations of infection as well as allergic reactions, ranging from urticaria to severe anaphylaxis. The incidence of allergy to the nematode has become so common that *A. simplex* is now routinely included in allergen testing. The U.S. Food and Drug Administration has set guidelines for deep freezing fish intended for raw consumption as a preventative measure.[12]

Beef Tapeworm (Taenia saginata)

The beef tapeworm, *T. saginata*, is by far the most common taeniid in humans, the definitive hosts. It is found throughout the world, but is particularly common in Africa, South America, and eastern Europe. The adult, an hermaphroditic cestode, can achieve several meters in length over a period of several months (Figure 33-56). *T. saginata* is characterized by a scolex with four suckers.[179] The eggs are spherical in shape and cannot be distinguished from those of the pork tapeworm (Figure 33-57).

Infection with *T. saginata* occurs after consumption of undercooked beef and is typically asymptomatic. Uncommonly, abdominal discomfort, nausea, vomiting, cutaneous sensitivity, headache, and malaise have been reported.[207] Because of the large size of the worm, obstructive symptoms can occasionally develop. The recommended treatment for taeniasis is praziquantel. Prevention of taeniasis includes avoidance of cattle consumption of human feces and proper cooking of beef.

References

1. Addison NV. Abdominal tuberculosis—a disease revived. *Ann R Coll Surg Engl*. 1983;65(2):105–111.
2. Aftab AR, Donnellan F, Zeb F, et al. NSAID-induced colopathy. A case series. *J Gastrointestin Liver Dis*. 2010;19(1):89–91.
3. Aisenberg G, Marcos LA, Ogbaa I. Recurrent histoplasmosis in AIDS mimicking a colonic carcinoma. *Int J STD AIDS*. 2009;20(6):429–430.
4. Akdamar K, Martin RJ, Ichinose H. Syphilitic proctitis. *Am J Dig Dis*. 1977;22(8):701–704.
5. Akgun Y. Intestinal obstruction caused by *Ascaris lumbricoides*. *Dis Colon Rectum*. 1996;39(10):1159–1163.

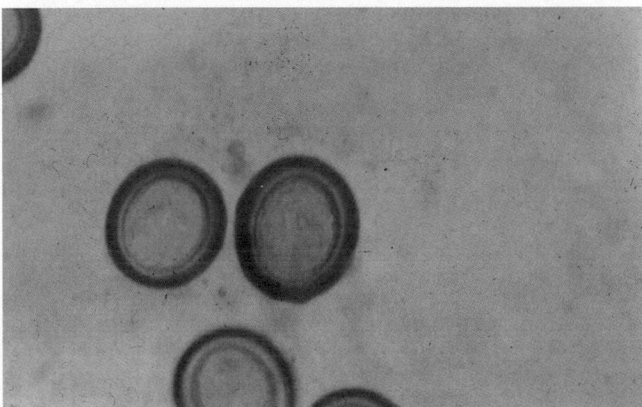

FIGURE 33-57. *T. saginata* eggs. (Courtesy of Rudolf Garret, MD.)

6. Allason-Jones E, Mindel A, Sargeaunt P, et al. *Entamoeba histolytica* as a commensal intestinal parasite in homosexual men. *N Engl J Med.* 1986;315(6):353–356.

7. Almadi MA, Ghosh S, Aljebreen AM. Differentiating intestinal tuberculosis from Crohn's disease: a diagnostic challenge. *Am J Gastroenterol.* 2009;104(4):1003–1012.

8. Anand BS, Nanda R, Sachdev GK. Response of tuberculous stricture to antituberculous treatment. *Gut.* 1988;29(1):62–69.

9. Anderson JB, Tanner AH, Brodribb AJ. Toxic megacolon due to *Campylobacter* colitis. *Int J Colorect Dis.* 1986;1(1):58–59.

10. Appleton GV, Williamson RC. Hypoplasia of defunctioned rectum. *Br J Surg.* 1989;76(8):787–789.

11. Assi M, McKinsey DS, Driks MR, et al. Gastrointestinal histoplasmosis in the acquired immunodeficiency syndrome: report of 18 cases and literature review. *Diagn Microbiol Infect Dis.* 2006;55(3):195–201.

12. Audicana MT, Ansotegui IJ, de Corres LF, et al. *Anisakis simplex:* dangerous—dead and alive? *Trends Parasitol.* 2002;18(1):20–25.

13. Audicana MT, Kennedy MW. *Anisakis simplex:* from obscure infectious worm to inducer of immune hypersensitivity. *Clin Microbiol Rev.* 2008;21(2):360–379.

14. Babb RR, Trollope ML. Acute fulminating amoebic colitis: survival after total colectomy. *Gut.* 1985;26(3):301–303.

15. Bakken JS. Fecal bacteriotherapy for recurrent *Clostridium difficile* infection. *Anaerobe.* 2009;15(6):285–289.

16. Ballinger A. Adverse effects of non-steroidal anti-inflammatory drugs on the colon. *Curr Gastroenterol Rep.* 2008;10(5):485–489.

17. Bartlett JG. Treatment of *Clostridium difficile* colitis. *Gastroenterology.* 1985;89(5):1192–1195.

18. Bassi O, Cosa G, Colavolpe A, et al. Primary syphilis of the rectum—endoscopic and clinical features: report of a case. *Dis Colon Rectum.* 1991;34(11):1024–1026.

19. Beard CB, Pye G, Steurer FJ, et al. Chagas disease in a domestic transmission cycle, southern Texas, USA. http://www.cdc.gov/ncidod/EID/vol9no1/02–0217.htm. 2003. Accessed 2004.

20. Bedwani R, Renganathan E, El Kwhsky F, et al. Schistosomiasis and the risk of bladder cancer in Alexandria, Egypt. *Br J Cancer.* 1998;77(7):1186–1189.

21. Behrman AJ. Emergent management of schistosomiasis. http://emedicine.medscape.com/article/788867-overview. Updated July 27, 2011. Accessed 2010.

22. Bennish ML, Azad AK, Yousefzadeh D. Intestinal obstruction during shigellosis: incidence, clinical features, risk factors, and outcome. *Gastroenterology.* 1991;101(3):626–634.

23. Bereswill S, Kist M. Recent development in *Campylobacter* pathogenesis. *Curr Opin Infect Dis.* 2003;16(5):487–491.

24. Bessa SM, Helmy I, El-Kharadly Y. Colorectal schistosomiasis. Endoscopic polypectomy. *Dis Colon Rectum.* 1983;26(12):772–774.

25. Bessa SM, Helmy I, Mekky F, et al. Colorectal schistosomiasis: clinicopathologic study and management. *Dis Colon Rectum.* 1979;22(6):390–395.

26. Besson I, Ingrand P, Person B, et al. Sclerotherapy with or without octreotide for acute variceal bleeding. *N Engl J Med.* 1995;333(9):555–560.

27. Bhargava DK, Shriniwas, Chopra P, et al. Peritoneal tuberculosis: laparoscopic patterns and its diagnostic accuracy. *Am J Gastroenterol.* 1992;87(1):109–112.

28. Bischoff SC, Mayer J, Nguyen QT, et al. Immunohistological assessment of intestinal eosinophile activation in patients with eosinophilic gastroenteritis and inflammatory bowel disease. *Am J Gastroenterol.* 1999;94(12):3521–3529.

29. Black RE, Jackson RJ, Tsai T, et al. Epidemic *Yersinia enterocolitica* infection due to contaminated chocolate milk. *N Engl J Med.* 1978;298(2):76–79.

30. Blaser MJ, Reller LB. *Campylobacter* enteritis. *N Engl J Med.* 1981;305(24):1444–1452.

31. Bluth EI, McVay LV III, Gathright JB Jr. Ultrasonic characteristics of ileal tuberculosis. *Dis Colon Rectum.* 1985;28(8):613–614.

32. Bohr J, Tysk C, Eriksson S, et al. Collagenous colitis: a retrospective study of clinical presentation and treatment in 163 patients. *Gut.* 1996;39(6):846–851.

33. Bonderup O, Hansen JB, Teglbjaerg PS, et al. Long-term budesonide treatment of collagenous colitis: a randomised, double-blind, placebo-controlled trial. *Gut.* 2009;58(1):68–72.

34. Bovée LP, Peerbooms PG, van den Hoek JA. Shigellosis, a sexually transmitted disease in homosexual men [in Dutch]. *Ned Tijdschr Geneeskd.* 2003;147(49):2438–2439.

35. Box JC, Tucker J, Watne AL, et al. Eosinophilic colitis presenting as a left-sided colocolonic intussusception with secondary large bowel obstruction: an uncommon entity with a rare presentation. *Am Surg.* 1997;63(8):741–743.

36. Bradbury AW, Barrett S. Surgical aspects of *Clostridium difficile* colitis. *Br J Surg.* 1997;84(2):150–159.

37. Brandborg LL. Parasitic diseases. In: Sleisenger MH, Fordtran JS, eds. *Gastrointestinal Disease.* 2nd ed. Philadelphia, PA: WB Saunders; 1978:1154.

38. Brandt MM, Bogner PN, Franklin GA. Intestinal tuberculosis presenting as a bowel obstruction. *Am J Surg.* 2002;183(3):290–291.

39. Breiter JR, Hajjar JJ. Segmental tuberculosis of the colon diagnosed by colonoscopy. *Am J Gastroenterol.* 1981;76(4):369–373.

40. Burbige EJ, Radigan JJ. Antibiotic-associated colitis with normal-appearing rectum. *Dis Colon Rectum.* 1981;24(3):198–200.

41. Burnham WR, Reeve RS, Finch RG. *Entamoeba histolytica* infection in male homosexuals. *Gut.* 1980;21(12):1097–1099.

42. Butzler JP, Oosterom J. *Campylobacter:* pathogenicity and significance in foods. *Int J Food Microbiol.* 1991;12(1):1–8.

43. Cao J, Liu WJ, Xu XY, et al. Endoscopic findings and clinicopathologic characteristics of colonic schistosomiasis: a report of 46 cases. *World J Gastroenterol.* 2010;16(6):723–727.

44. Cappell MS, Mandell W, Grimes MM, et al. Gastrointestinal histoplasmosis. *Dig Dis Sci.* 1988;33(3):353–360.

45. Cappell MS, Simon T. Fulminant acute colitis following a self-administered hydrofluoric acid enema. *Am J Gastroenterol.* 1993;88(1):122–126.

46. Carlier Y, Luquetti AO, Dias JCP, et al. Chagas disease (American trypanosomiasis), 2004. http://www.emedicine.com/MED/topic327.htm. Accessed.

47. Carpenter HA, Talley NJ. The importance of clinicopathological correlation in the diagnosis of inflammatory conditions of the colon: histological patterns with clinical implications. *Am J Gastroenterol.* 2000;95(4):878–896.

48. Carter FM, Mitchell CK. Toxic epidermal necrolysis—an unusual cause of colonic perforation. *Dis Colon Rectum.* 1993;36(8):773–777.

49. Carvalho Filho E. Strongyloidiasis. *Clin Gastroenterol.* 1978;7(1):179–200.

50. Catterall RD. Sexually transmitted diseases of the anus and rectum. *Clin Gastroenterol.* 1975;4(3):659–669.

51. Centers for Disease Control and Prevention. Updated recommended treatment regimens for gonococcal infections and associated conditions—United States, April 2007. Atlanta GA: Author.

52. Centers for Disease Control and Prevention. Trends in tuberculosis—United States, 2008. *MMWR Morb Mortal Wkly Rep.* 2009;58(10):249–253.

53. Centers for Disease Control and Prevention. Preliminary FoodNet data on the incidence of infection with pathogens transmitted commonly through food—10 states, 2009. *MMWR Morb Mortal Wkly Rep.* 2010;59(14):418–422.

54. Centers for Disease Control and Prevention, Workowski KA, Berman SM. Sexually transmitted diseases treatment guidelines, 2006. *MMWR Recomm Rep.* 2006;55(RR-11):1–94.

55. Cermeño JR, Hernández De Cuesta I, Uzcátegui O, et al. *Balantidium coli* in an HIV-infected patient with chronic diarrhea. *AIDS.* 2003;17(6):941–942.

56. Chalmers RM, Davies AP. Minireview: clinical cryptosporidiosis. *Exp Parasitol.* 2010;124(1):138–146.

57. Chande N, Driman DK, Reynolds RP. Collagenous colitis and lymphocytic colitis: patient characteristics and clinical presentation. *Scand J Gastroenterol.* 2005;40(3):343–347.

58. Chande N, McDonald JW, MacDonald JK. Interventions for treating collagenous colitis. *Cochrane Database Syst Rev.* 2004;(1):CD003575.

59. Chawla S. Tuberculosis of the colon. In: Greenbaum EI, ed. *Radiographic Atlas of Colon Disease.* Chicago, IL: Year Book; 1980:557.

60. Chen DF, Chao IM, Huang SH. Neutropenic colitis with cecal perforation during antithyroid therapy. *J Formos Med Assoc.* 2003;102(9):644–646.

61. Chen MC, Chang PY, Chuang CY, et al. Colorectal cancer and schistosomiasis. *Lancet.* 1981;1(8227):971–973.

62. Chester AC, MacMurray FG, Restifo MD, et al. Giardiasis as a chronic disease. *Dig Dis Sci.* 1985;30(3):215–218.

63. Chijide VM, Woeltje KF. Balantidiasis, 2004. http://emedicine.com/med/topic203.htm. Accessed.

64. Christopher PR, David KV, John SM, et al. Antibiotic therapy for Shigella dysentery. *Cochrane Database Syst Rev.* 2010;(8):CD006784.

65. Chun D, Chandrasoma P, Kiyabu M. Fulminant amebic colitis. A morphologic study of four cases. *Dis Colon Rectum.* 1994;37(6):535–539.

66. Church JM, Fazio VW. A role for colonic stasis in the pathogenesis of disease related to *Clostridium difficile. Dis Colon Rectum.* 1986;29(12):804–809.

67. Cintron JR, Del Pino A, Duarte B, et al. Abdominal actinomycosis. *Dis Colon Rectum.* 1996;39(1):105–108.

68. Clarkston WK, Bonacini M, Peterson I. Colitis due to *Histoplasma capsulatum* in the acquired immune deficiency syndrome. *Am J Gastroenterol.* 1991;86(7):913–916.

69. Cloutier RL. Neutropenic enterocolitis. *Hematol Oncol Clin North Am.* 2010;24(3):577–584.

70. Cohen SH, Gerding DN, Johnson S, et al; Infectious Diseases Society of America. Clinical practice guidelines for *Clostridium difficile* infection in adults: 2010 update by the Society for Healthcare Epidemiology of America (SHEA) and the Infectious Diseases Society of America (IDSA). *Infect Control Hosp Epidemiol.* 2010;31(5):431–455.

71. Colovic;aa R, Grubor N, Micev M, et al. Actinomycosis of the caecum simulating carcinoma in a patient with a long-term intrauterine device [in Serbian]. *Srp Arh Celok Lek.* 2009;137(5–6):285–287.

72. Cone JB, Wetzel W. Toxic megacolon secondary to pseudomembranous colitis. *Dis Colon Rectum.* 1982;25(5):478–482.

73. Cone LA, Woodard DR, Potts BE, et al. An update on the acquired immunodeficiency syndrome (AIDS). Associated disorders of the alimentary tract. *Dis Colon Rectum.* 1986;29(1):60–64.

74. Connolly GM, Dryden MS, Shanson DC, et al. Cryptosporidial diarrhoea in AIDS and its treatment. *Gut.* 1988;29(5):593–597.

75. Connor BA. Travelers' diarrhea. Travelers' Health—Yellow Book 2010. http://wwwnc.cdc.gov/travel/yellowbook/2010/chapter-2/travelers-diarrhea.aspx. Accessed 2010.

76. Connor BA, Schwartz E. Typhoid and paratyphoid fevers in travelers. *Lancet Infect Dis.* 2005;5(10):623–628.

77. Couppié P, Sobesky M, Aznar C, et al. Histoplasmosis and acquired immunodeficiency syndrome: a study of prognostic factors. *Clin Infect Dis.* 2004;38(1):134–138.

78. Cover TL, Aber RC. *Yersinia enterocolitica.* *N Engl J Med.* 1989; 321(1):16–24.

79. Crowson TD, Hines C Jr. Amebiasis diagnosed by colonoscopy. *Gastrointest Endosc.* 1978;24(5):254–255.

80. Crum-Cianflone NF. Salmonellosis and the gastrointestinal tract: more than just peanut butter. *Curr Gastroenterol Rep.* 2008;10(4):424–431.

81. Crump JA, Luby SP, Mintz ED. The global burden of typhoid fever. *Bull World Health Organ.* 2004;82(5):346–353.

82. Cumming JA, McCann BG, Ralphs DN. Fulminant pseudomembranous colitis with left hemicolon and rectal sparing. *Br J Surg.* 1988;75(4):341.

83. Curtis KJ, Sleisenger MH. Infectious and parasitic diseases. In: Sleisenger MH, Fordtran JS, eds. *Gastrointestinal Disease.* 2nd ed. Philadelphia, PA: WB Saunders; 1978:1679.

84. Davies NM. Toxicity of nonsteroidal anti-inflammatory drugs in the large intestine. *Dis Colon Rectum.* 1995;38(12):1311–1321.

85. Davila ML. Neutropenic enterocolitis: current issues in diagnosis and management. *Curr Infect Dis Rep.* 2007;9(2):116–120.

86. Debenham GP. Ulcer of the cecum during oxyphenbutazone (tandearil) therapy. *Can Med Assoc J.* 1966;94(22):1182–1184.

87. Donoghue H, Holton J. Intestinal tuberculosis. *Curr Opin Infect Dis.* 2009;22(5):490–496.

88. Efem SE. *Ascaris lumbricoides* and intestinal perforation. *Br J Surg.* 1987;74(7):643–644.

89. Ekrikpo UE, Otegbayo JA, Oluwasola AO. Lymphocytic colitis presenting as difficult diarrhoea in an African woman: a case report and review of the literature. *J Med Case Reports.* 2010;4:31.

90. Ellis ME, Watson BM, Milewski PJ, et al. *Clostridium difficile* colitis unassociated with antibiotic therapy. *Br J Surg.* 1983;70(4):242–243.

91. Ellyson JH, Bezmalinovic Z, Parks SN, et al. Necrotizing amebic colitis: a frequently fatal complication. *Am J Surg.* 1986;152(1):21–26.

92. Erstad BL. Octreotide for acute variceal bleeding. *Ann Pharmacother.* 2001;35(5):618–626.

93. Fataar S, Jacob GS, Bassiony H, et al. Rectocolonic calcification due to schistosomiasis. A clinicoradiologic study. *Dis Colon Rectum.* 1984;27(3):164–167.

94. Faucheron JL. Toxicity of non-steroidal anti-inflammatory drugs in the large bowel. *Eur J Gastroenterol Hepatol.* 1999;11(4):389–392.

95. Faucheron JL, Parc R. Non-steroidal anti-inflammatory drug-induced colitis. *Int J Colorectal Dis.* 1996;11(2):99–101.

96. Feigen GM. Suppurative anal cryptitis associated with *Trichuris trichiura.* Report of a case. *Dis Colon Rectum.* 1987;30(8):620–622.

97. Fekety R. Guidelines for the diagnosis and management of *Clostridium difficile*–associated diarrhea and colitis. American College of Gastroenterology, Practice Parameters Committee. *Am J Gastroenterol.* 1997;92(5):739–750.

98. Fekety R, McFarland LV, Surawicz CM, et al. Recurrent *Clostridium difficile* diarrhea: characteristics of and risk factors for patients in a prospective, randomized, double-blinded trial. *Clin Infect Dis.* 1997;24(3):324–333.

99. Fekety R, Quintiliani R. Current approach to the treatment of antibiotic-associated diarrhea. *Infect Surg.* 1982;1:13.

100. Ferguson CM, Siegel RJ. A prospective evaluation of diversion colitis. *Am Surg.* 1991;57(1):46–49.

101. Ferrazzi E, Toso S, Zanotti M, et al. Typhlitis (neutropenic enterocolitis) after a single dose of vinorelbine. *Cancer Chemother Pharmacol.* 2001;47(3):277–279.

102. Finney JMT. Gastroenterostomy for cicatrizing ulcer of the pylorus. *Johns Hopkins Hosp Bull.* 1893;4:53.

103. Fotedar R, Stark D, Beebe N, et al. Laboratory diagnostic techniques for *Entamoeba* species. *Clin Microbiol Rev.* 2007;20(3):511–532.

104. Franco MP, Mulder M, Gilman RH, et al. Human brucellosis. *Lancet Infect Dis.* 2007;7(12):775–786.

105. Franklin GO, Mohapatra M, Perrillo RP. Colonic tuberculosis diagnosed by colonoscopic biopsy. *Gastroenterology.* 1979;76(2):362–364.

106. Furness BW, Beach MJ, Roberts JM. Giardiasis surveillance—United States, 1992–1997. *MMWR CDC Surveill Summ.* 2000;49(7): 1–13. http://www.cdc.gov/epo/mmwr/preview/mmwrhtml/ss4907a1.htm. Accessed 2004.

107. Gan HT, Chen YQ, Ouyang Q, et al. Differentiation between intestinal tuberculosis and Crohn's disease in endoscopic biopsy specimens by polymerase chain reaction. *Am J Gastroenterol.* 2002;97(6):1446–1451.

108. Garret JK, Jameson SC, Thomson B, et al. Anti-interleukin-5 (mepolizumab) therapy for hypereosinophilic syndromes. *J Allergy Clin Immunol.* 2004;113(1):115–119.

109. Gazzard BG. HIV disease and the gastroenterologist. *Gut.* 1988;29(11):1497–1505.

110. Gill KP, Feeley TM, Keane FB. Toxic megacolon and perforation caused by *Salmonella.* *Br J Surg.* 1989;76(8):796.

111. Gizzi G, Villani V, Brandi G, et al. Ano-rectal lesions in patients taking suppositories containing non-steroidal anti-inflammatory drugs (NSAID). *Endoscopy.* 1990;22(3):146–148.

112. Gleeson MH, Davis AJ. Non-steroidal anti-inflammatory drugs, aspirin and newly diagnosed colitis: a case-control study. *Aliment Pharmacol Ther.* 2003;17(6):817–825.

113. Glotzer DJ, Glick ME, Goldman H. Proctitis and colitis following diversion of the fecal stream. *Gastroenterology.* 1981;80(3):438–441.

114. Goldberg JE. Parasitic colitides. *Clin Colon Rectal Surg.* 2007; 20(1):38–46.

115. González A, Vargas V, Guarner L, et al. Toxic megacolon in typhoid fever. *Arch Intern Med.* 1985;145(11):2120.

116. González de Canales Simón P, del Olmo Martínez L, Cortejoso Hernández A, et al. Colonic balantidiasis [in Spanish]. *Gastroenterol Hepatol.* 2000;23(3):129–131.

117. Goodell SE, Quinn TC, Mkrtichian E, et al. Herpes simplex virus proctitis in homosexual men. Clinical, sigmoidoscopic, and histopathological. *N Engl J Med.* 1983;308(15):868–871.

118. Goosenberg E. Collagenous and lymphocytic colitis 2009. http://emedicine.medscape.com/article/180664-treatment. Accessed 2010.

119. Gorbach SL. Infectious diarrheas. Paper presented at: Annual Meeting of the American Society of Colon and Rectal Surgeons; 1983; Boston, MA.

120. Graham BD, McKinsey DS, Driks MR, et al. Colonic histoplasmosis in acquired immunodeficiency syndrome. Report of two cases. *Dis Colon Rectum.* 1991;34(2):185–190.

121. Graham SM. Nontyphoidal salmonellosis in Africa. *Curr Opin Infect Dis.* 2010;23(5):409–414.

122. Griffiths AP, Dixon MF. Microcarcinoids and diversion colitis in a colon defunctioned for 18 years. Report of a case. *Dis Colon Rectum.* 1992;35(7):685–688.

123. Gronczewski CA, Katz JP. *Clostridium difficile* colitis, 2003. http://www.emedicine.com/med/topic3412.htm. Accessed 2004.

124. Guerrant RL, Bobak DA. Bacterial and protozoal gastroenteritis. *N Engl J Med.* 1991;325(5):327–340.

125. Haberkern CM, Christie DL, Haas JE. Eosinophilic gastroenteritis presenting as ileocolitis. *Gastroenterology.* 1978;74(5 pt 1):896–899.

126. Halaby IA, Rantis PC, Vernava AM III, et al. Collagenous colitis: pathogenesis and management. *Dis Colon Rectum.* 1996;39(5):573–578.

127. Hall IC, O'Toole E. Intestinal flora in newborn infants with a description of a new pathogenic anaerobe, *Bacillus difficilis.* *Am J Dis Child.* 1935;49:390.

128. Han JK, Kim SH, Choi BI, et al. Tuberculous colitis. Findings at double-contrast barium enema examination. *Dis Colon Rectum.* 1996; 39(11):1204–1209.

129. Harig JM, Soergel KH, Komorowski RA, et al. Treatment of diversion colitis with short-chain-fatty acid irrigation. *N Engl J Med.* 1989;320(1):23–28.

130.   Heaton KW. Functional diarrhoea: the acid test. *Br Med J (Clin Res Ed)*. 1985;290(6478):1298–1299.

131.   Heller M. The gay bowel syndrome: a common problem of homosexual patients in the emergency department. *Ann Emerg Med*. 1980;9(9): 487–493.

132.   Henderson SO. Candidiasis, 2002. http://www.emedicine.com/emerg/topic76.htm. Accessed 2004.

133.   Hiatt GA. Miliary tuberculosis with ileocecal involvement diagnosed by colonoscopy. *JAMA*. 1978;240(6):561–562.

134.   Hidalgo JA, Vazquez JA. Candidiasis, 2002. http://www.emedicine.com/med/topic264.htm. Accessed.

135.   Horvath KD, Whelan RL, Weinstein S, et al. Isolated sigmoid tuberculosis. Report of a case. *Dis Colon Rectum*. 1995;38(12):1327–1330.

136.   Hurley BW, Nguyen CC. The spectrum of pseudomembranous enterocolitis and antibiotic-associated diarrhea. *Arch Intern Med*. 2002;162(19):2177–2184.

137.   Istre GR, Kreiss K, Hopkins RS, et al. An outbreak of amebiasis spread by colonic irrigation at a chiropractic clinic. *N Engl J Med*. 1982;307(6):339–342.

138.   Jain S, Koirala J, Castro-Paiva F. Isolated gastrointestinal histoplasmosis: case report and review of the literature. *South Med J*. 2004;97(2): 172–174.

139.   Janda WM, Bohnoff M, Morello JA, et al. Prevalence and site-pathogen studies of *Neisseria meningitidis* and *N. gonorrhoeae* in homosexual men. *JAMA*. 1980;244(18):2060–2064.

140.   Johnson S, Gerding DN. *Clostridium difficile*–associated diarrhea. *Clin Infect Dis*. 1998;26(5):1027–1034.

141.   Johnson S, Schriever C, Galang M, et al. Interruption of recurrent *Clostridium difficile*–associated diarrhea episodes by serial therapy with vancomycin and rifaximin. *Clin Infect Dis*. 2007;44(6):846–848.

142.   Jorens PG, Michielsen PP, Van den Enden EJ, et al. A rare cause of colitis—*Brucella melitensis*. Report of a case. *Dis Colon Rectum*. 1991;34(2):194–196.

143.   Joseph D, Jin H, Ryan C, et al. Resolution of anorectal incontinence in herpes proctitis confirmed by anorectal manometry. *Gastrointest Endosc*. 1997;45(5):429–432.

144.   Juniper K. Amoebiasis. *Clin Gastroenterol*. 1978;7(1):3–29.

145.   Kara M, Turan I, Polat Z, et al. Chemical colitis caused by peracetic acid or hydrogen peroxide: a challenging dilemma. *Endoscopy*. 2010;42(suppl 2):E3–E4.

146.   Kasulke RJ, Anderson WJ, Gupta SK, et al. Primary tuberculous enterocolitis. Report of three cases and review of the literature. *Arch Surg*. 1981;116(1):110–113.

147.   Katz DE, Taylor DN. Parasitic infections of the gastrointestinal tract. *Gastroenterol Clin North Am*. 2001;30(3):797–815.

148.   Katz Y, Varsano D, Siegal B, et al. Intestinal obstruction due to *Ascaris lumbricoides* mimicking intussusception. *Dis Colon Rectum*. 1985;28(4):267–269.

149.   Kaufman HL, Fisher AH, Carroll M, et al. Colonic ulceration associated with nonsteroidal anti-inflammatory drugs. Report of three cases. *Dis Colon Rectum*. 1996;39(6):705–710.

150.   Kaw LL Jr, Punzalan CK, Crisostomo AC, et al. Surgical pathology of colorectal cancer in Filipinos: implications for clinical practice. *J Am Coll Surg*. 2002;195(2):188–195.

151.   Keiser J, Utzinger J. Efficacy of current drugs against soil-transmitted helminth infections: systematic review and meta-analysis. *JAMA*. 2008; 299(16):1937–1948.

152.   Keiser PB, Nutman TB. *Strongyloides stercoralis* in the immunocompromised population. *Clin Microbiol Rev*. 2004;17(1):208–217.

153.   Khalil M, Iwatt AR, Gugnani HC. African histoplasmosis masquerading as carcinoma of the colon. Report of a case and review of literature. *Dis Colon Rectum*. 1989;32(6):518–520.

154.   Khan R, Abid S, Jafri W, et al. Diagnostic dilemma of abdominal tuberculosis in non-HIV patients: an ongoing challenge for physicians. *World J Gastroenterol*. 2006;12(39):6371–6375.

155.   Khan ZZ, Salvaggio MR, Johnston MH, et al. *Yersinia enterocolitica*, 2009. http://emedicine.medscape.com/article/232343-overview. Accessed 2010.

156.   Kiely EM, Ajayi NA, Wheeler RA, et al. Diversion procto-colitis: response to treatment with short-chain fatty acids. *J Pediatr Surg*. 2001;36(10): 1514–1517.

157.   King HC, Voss EC Jr. Tuberculosis of the cecum simulating carcinoma. *Dis Colon Rectum*. 1980;23(1):49–53.

158.   Kingham JG, Levison DA, Morson BC, et al. Collagenous colitis. *Gut*. 1986;27(5):570–577.

159.   Kirkpatrick BD, Tribble DR. Update on human *Campylobacter jejuni* infections. *Curr Opin Gastroenterol*. 2011;27(1):1–7.

160.   Kirkpatrick ID, Greenberg HM. Gastrointestinal complications in the neutropenic patient: characterization and differentiation with abdominal CT. *Radiology*. 2003;226(3):668–674.

161.   Klausner JD, Kohn R, Kent C. Etiology of clinical proctitis among men who have sex with men. *Clin Infect Dis*. 2004;38(2):300–302.

162.   Knight R. Giardiasis, isosporiasis and balantidiasis. *Clin Gastroenterol*. 1978;7(1):31–47.

163.   Ko CY, Schmit PJ, Petrie B, et al. Abdominal tuberculosis: the surgical perspective. *Am Surg*. 1996;62(10):865–868.

164.   Kobayasi S, Mendes EF, Rodrigues MA, et al. Toxic dilatation of the colon in Chagas' disease. *Br J Surg*. 1992;79(11):1202–1203.

165.   Kochhar R, Rajwanshi A, Goenka MK, et al. Colonoscopic fine needle aspiration cytology in the diagnosis of ileocecal tuberculosis. *Am J Gastroenterol*. 1991;86(1):102–104.

166.   Koea JB, Shaw JH. Surgical management of neutropenic enterocolitis. *Br J Surg*. 1989;76(8):821–824.

167.   Kofsky P, Rosen L, Reed J, et al. *Clostridium difficile*—a common and costly colitis. *Dis Colon Rectum*. 1991;34(3):244–248.

168.   Kogulam P, Lucey DR. Schistosomiasis, 2002. http://emedicine.com/med/topic2071.htm. Accessed 2004.

169.   Koo J, Ho J, Ong GB. The value of colonoscopy in the diagnosis of ileo-cecal tuberculosis. *Endoscopy*. 1982;14(2):48–50.

170.   Koskela RM, Karttunen TJ, Niemelä SE, et al. Human leucocyte antigen and TNFalpha polymorphism association in microscopic colitis. *Eur J Gastroenterol Hepatol*. 2008;20(4):276–282.

171.   Kraft SC, Kirsner JB. Immunology in gastroenterology. In: Berk JE, ed. *Bockus Gastroenterology*. 4th ed. Philadelphia, PA: WB Saunders; 1985:4507.

172.   Kunkel JM, Rosenthal D. Management of the ileocecal syndrome. Neutropenic enterocolitis. *Dis Colon Rectum*. 1986;29(3):196–199.

173.   Kyne L, Warny M, Qamar A, et al. Asymptomatic carriage of *Clostridium difficile* and serum levels of IgG antibody against toxin A. *N Engl J Med*. 2000;342(6):390–397.

174.   Lavery EA, Coyle WJ. Herpes simplex virus and the alimentary tract. *Curr Gastroenterol Rep*. 2008;10(4):417–423.

175.   Lebedeff DA, Hochman EB. Rectal gonorrhea in men: diagnosis and treatment. *Ann Intern Med*. 1980;92(4):463–466.

176.   Lee FI, Costello FT, Cowley DJ, et al. Eosinophilic colitis with perianal disease. *Am J Gastroenterol*. 1983;78(3):164–166.

177.   Lee KR, Lin F. The Radiology Corner. Gastrointestinal histoplasmosis, roentgenographic, clinical and pathological correlation. *Am J Gastroenterol*. 1975;63(3):255–265.

178.   Lee YK, Bae JM, Park YJ, et al. Pelvic actinomycosis with hydronephrosis and colon stricture simulating an advanced ovarian cancer. *J Gynecol Oncol*. 2008;19(2):154–156.

179.   Levinson W. Cestodes. In: *Review of Medical Microbiology and Immunology*. 11th ed. New York, NY: McGraw-Hill; 2010:chap 42. http://www.accessmedicine.com/content.aspx?aID=6458115. Accessed 2010.

180.   Levy N, Gasper E. Rectal bleeding and indomethacin suppositories [letter]. *Lancet*. 1975;1(7906):577.

181.   Lewis JS, Fakile O, Foss E, et al. Direct DNA probe assay for *Neisseria gonorrhoeae* in pharyngeal and rectal specimens. *J Clin Microbiol*. 1993;31(10):2783–2785.

182.   Lindmark H, Harbom B, Thebo L, et al. Genetic characterization and antibiotic resistance of *Campylobacter jejuni* isolated from meats, water, and humans in Sweden. *J Clin Microbiol*. 2004;42(2):700–706.

183.   Lindström CG. "Collagenous colitis" with watery diarrhoea—a new entity? *Pathol Eur*. 1976;11(1):87–89.

184.   Lipsett PA, Samantaray DK, Tam ML, et al. Pseudomembranous colitis: a surgical disease? *Surgery*. 1994;116(3):491–496.

185.   Lisehora GB, Peters CC, Lee YT, et al. Tuberculous peritonitis—do not miss it. *Dis Colon Rectum*. 1996;39(4):394–399.

186.   Loftus EV. Microscopic colitis: epidemiology and treatment. *Am J Gastroenterol*. 2003;98(suppl 12):S31–S36.

187.   Luvuno FM. Role of intraoperative prograde colonic lavage and a decompressive loop ileostomy in the management of transmural amoebic colitis. *Br J Surg*. 1990;77(2):156–159.

188.   Mahmoud AAF. Schistosomiasis and other trematode infections. In: Fauci AS, Braunwald E, Kasper DL, et al, eds. *Harrison's Principles of Internal Medicine*. 17th ed. New York, NY: McGraw-Hill; 2008:chap 212. http://www.accessmedicine.com/content.aspx?aID=2896895. Accessed .

189.   Maloney GE Jr. CBRNE brucellosis, 2001. http://www.emedicine.com/emerg/topic883.htm. Accessed 2004.

190.   Marshall JK, Irvine EJ. Lymphocytic and collagenous colitis: medical management. *Curr Treat Options Gastroenterol*. 1999;2(2):127–133.

191.   Mazokopakis EE, Giannakopoulos T, Christias EG. Acute brucellosis as a cause of infective colitis. *Mil Med*. 2008;173(11):1145–1147.

192. McCarter MD, Abularrage C, Velasco FT, et al. Diarrhea and *Clostridium difficile*–associated diarrhea on a surgical service. *Arch Surg.* 1996;131(12):1333–1337.

193. McClelland M, Sanderson KE, Spieth J, et al. Complete genome sequence of *Salmonella enterica* serovar Typhimurium LT2. *Nature.* 2001;413(6858):852–856.

194. McFarland LV, Mulligan ME, Kwok RY, et al. Nosocomial acquisition of *Clostridium difficile* infections. *N Engl J Med.* 1989;320(4):204–210.

195. McMillan A, Gilmour HM, McNeillage G, et al. Amoebiasis in homosexual men. *Gut.* 1984;25(4):356–360.

196. Medical Network Inc. Encyclopedia Index A. Actinomycosis, 2003. http://healthatoz.com/healthatoz/Atoz/ency/actinomycosis.html. Accessed 2004.

197. Medich DS, Lee KK, Simmons RL, et al. Laparotomy for fulminant pseudomembranous colitis. *Arch Surg.* 1992;127(7):847–852.

198. Mei J, Hong HL, Ding YP, et al. Clinicopathologic characteristics of chronic schistosomiasis complicating carcinoma of large intestine. *Zhonghua Xiaohuaneijing Zazhi.* 2004;21:49–50.

199. Meier DE, Imediegwu OO, Tarpley JL. Perforated typhoid enteritis: operative experience with 100 cases. *Am J Surg.* 1989;157(4):423–427.

200. Meltzer E, Schwartz E. Enteric fever: a travel medicine oriented view. *Curr Opin Infect Dis.* 2010;23(5):432–437.

201. Miehlke S, Madisch A, Bethke B, et al. Oral budesonide for maintenance treatment of collagenous colitis: a randomized, double-blind, placebo-controlled trial. *Gastroenterology.* 2008;135(5):1510–1516.

202. Miehlke S, Madisch A, Karimi D, et al. Budesonide is effective in treating lymphocytic colitis: a randomized, double-blind placebo-controlled study. *Gastroenterology.* 2009;136(7):2092–2100.

203. Misra SP, Misra V, Dwivedi M, et al. Factors influencing colonic involvement in patients with amebic liver abscess. *Gastrointest Endosc.* 2004;59(4):512–516.

204. Miura T, Iwaya A, Shimizu T, et al. Intestinal anisakiasis can cause intussusception in adults: an extremely rare condition. *World J Gastroenterol.* 2010;16(14):1804–1807.

205. Mock CN, Amaral J, Visser LE. Improvement in survival from typhoid ileal perforation. Results of 221 operative cases. *Ann Surg.* 1992;215(3):244–249.

206. Mohamed AR, al Karawi M, Yasawy MI. Schistosomal colonic disease. *Gut.* 1990;31(4):439–442.

207. Monroe LS. Gastrointestinal parasites. In: Berk JE, ed. *Bockus Gastroenterology.* 4th ed. Philadelphia, PA: WB Saunders; 1985:4250.

208. Montefusco PP, Geiss AC, Randall S. Typhoid fever and massive intestinal hemorrhage. *Contemp Surg.* 1984;24:61.

209. Moran JS, Levine WC. Drugs of choice for the treatment of uncomplicated gonococcal infections. *Clin Infect Dis.* 1995;20(suppl 1):S47–S65.

210. Morini S, Campo SM, Zullo A, et al. Chemical colitis induced by peracetic acid: further evidence. *Endoscopy.* 2009;41(4):383.

211. Morris JB, Zollinger RM Jr, Stellato TA. Role of surgery in antibiotic-induced pseudomembranous colitis. *Am J Surg.* 1990;160(5):535–539.

212. Morris LL, Villalba MR, Glover JL. Management of pseudomembranous colitis. *Am Surg.* 1994;60(7):548–551.

213. Mower WJ, Hawkins JA, Nelson EW. Neutropenic enterocolitis in adults with acute leukemia. *Arch Surg.* 1986;121(5):571–574.

214. Murray FE, O'Brien M, Birkett DH, et al. Diversion colitis. Pathologic findings in a resected sigmoid colon and rectum. *Gastroenterology.* 1987;93(6):1404–1408.

215. Mylonakis E, Ryan ET, Calderwood SB. *Clostridium difficile*–associated diarrhea: a review. *Arch Intern Med.* 2001;161(4):525–533.

216. Nash TE, Ohl CA, Thomas E, et al. Treatment of patients with refractory giardiasis. *Clin Infect Dis.* 2001;33(1):22–28.

217. Nason Katie S, Maddaus Michael A, Luketich James D. Chest wall, lung, mediastinum, and pleura. In: Brunicardi FC, Andersen DK, Billiar TR, et al, eds. *Schwartz's Principles of Surgery.* 9th ed. New York, NY: McGraw-Hill; 2011:chap 19. http://www.accessmedicine.com/content.aspx?aID=5016069. Accessed 2010.

218. National Digestive Diseases Information Clearinghouse. Diarrhea. http://digestive.niddk.nih.gov/ddiseases/pubs/diarrhea/. Accessed 2010.

219. Naylor AR, Pollet JE. Eosinophilic colitis. *Dis Colon Rectum.* 1985;28(8):615–618.

220. New York City Department of Health and Mental Hygiene Bureau of Communicable Disease. http://www.nyc.gov/html/doh/html/cd/cdyer.html. 2003. Accessed 2004.

221. O'Donoghue C, Kyne L. Update on *Clostridium difficile* infection. *Curr Opin Gastroenterol.* 2011;27(1):38–47.

222. O'Hanrahan T, Dark P, Irving MH. Cyclic neutropenia—unusual cause of acute abdomen. Report of a case. *Dis Colon Rectum.* 1991; 34(12):1125–1127.

223. Okpara N, Aswad B, Baffy G. Eosinophilic colitis. *World J Gastroenterol.* 2009;15(24):2975–2979.

224. Olesen M, Eriksson S, Bohr J, et al. Microscopic colitis: a common diarrhoeal disease. An epidemiological study in Orebro, Sweden, 1993–1998. *Gut.* 2004;53(3):346–350.

225. Orsay CP, Kim DO, Pearl RK, et al. Diversion colitis in patients scheduled for colostomy closure. *Dis Colon Rectum.* 1993;36(4): 366–367.

226. Owen RL. Rectal gonorrhea. In: Sleisenger MH, Fordtran JS, eds. *Gastrointestinal Disease.* 2nd ed. Philadelphia, PA: WB Saunders; 1978:1692.

227. Owens MD, Warren DA. Salmonella infection 2010. http://emedicine.medscape.com/article/785774-overview. Accessed 2010.

228. Palmer KR, Patil DH, Basran GS, et al. Abdominal tuberculosis in urban Britain—a common disease. *Gut.* 1985;26(12):1296–1305.

229. Palmer PES. Amebiasis and tropical diseases of the colon. In: Greenbaum EI, ed. *Radiographic Atlas of Colon Disease.* Chicago, IL: Year Book; 1980:9.

230. Pangan JC. Severe amebic colitis with hemorrhage and perforation. *Contemp Surg.* 1986;28:73.

231. Pantenburg B, Cabada MM, White AC Jr. Treatment of cryptosporidiosis. *Expert Rev Anti Infect Ther.* 2009;7(4):385–391.

232. Papaconstantinou HT, Thomas JS. Bacterial colitis. *Clin Colon Rectal Surg.* 2007;20(1):18–27.

233. Pappas PG, Kauffman CA, Andes D, et al. Clinical practice guidelines for the management of candidiasis: 2009 update by the Infectious Diseases Society of America. *Clin Infect Dis.* 2009;48(5):503–535.

234. Pardi DS, Loftus EV Jr, Smyrk TC, et al. The epidemiology of microscopic colitis: a population based study in Olmsted County, Minnesota. *Gut.* 2007;56(4):504–508.

235. Partyka EK, Sanowski RA, Kozarek RA. Colonoscopic features of eosinophilic gastroenteritis. *Dis Colon Rectum.* 1980;23(5):353–356.

236. Pawlowski ZS. Ascariasis. *Clin Gastroenterol.* 1978;7(1):157–178.

237. Pennardt A. Giardiasis, 2002. http://www.emedicine.com/emerg/topic215.htm. Accessed 2004.

238. Pikarsky AJ, Belin B, Efron J, et al. Complications following formalin installation in the treatment of radiation induced proctitis. *Int J Colorect Dis.* 2000;15(2):96–99.

239. Pokorney BH, Nichols TW Jr. Pseudomembranous colitis. A complication of sulfasalazine therapy in a patient with Crohn's colitis. *Am J Gastroenterol.* 1981;76(4):374–376.

240. Polenakovik H, Polenakovik S. Strongyloidiasis, 2004. http://www.emedicine.com/med/topic2189.htm. Accessed 2004.

241. Price AB. Pathology of drug-associated gastrointestinal disease. *Br J Clin Pharmacol.* 2003;56(5):477–482.

242. Pritt BS, Clark CG. Amebiasis. *Mayo Clin Proc.* 2008;83(10): 1154–1159.

243. Puri AS, Vij JC, Chaudhary A, et al. Diagnosis and outcome of isolated rectal tuberculosis. *Dis Colon Rectum.* 1996;39(10):1126–1129.

244. Quigley MM, Bethel K, Nowacki M, et al. Neutropenic enterocolitis: a rare presenting complication of acute leukemia. *Am J Hematol.* 2001;66(3):213–219.

245. Quinn TC, Corey L, Chaffee RG, et al. The etiology of anorectal infections in homosexual men. *Am J Med.* 1981;71(3):395–406.

246. Quondamcarlo C, Valentini G, Ruggeri M, et al. *Campylobacter jejuni* enterocolitis presenting as inflammatory bowel disease. *Tech Coloproctol.* 2003;7(3):173–177.

247. Radhakrishnan S, Al Nakib B, Shaikh H, et al. The value of colonoscopy in schistosomal, tuberculous, and amebic colitis. Two-year experience. *Dis Colon Rectum.* 1986;29(12):891–895.

248. Rams H, Rogers AI, Ghandur-Mnaymneh L. Collagenous colitis. *Arch Intern Med.* 1987;106(1):108–113.

249. Rassi A Jr, Rassi A, Marin-Neto JA. Chagas disease. *Lancet.* 2010;375(9723):1388–1402.

250. Ratliff DA, Carr N, Cochrane JP. Rectal stricture due to actinomycosis. *Br J Surg.* 1986;73(7):589–590.

251. Reddy KR, Thomas E. Proctitis: an unusual presentation of *Strongyloides stercoralis* infestation. *Am J Proctol Gastroenterol Colon Rectal Surg.* 1983;34:11.

252. Reyes E, Hernández J, González A. Typhoid colitis with massive lower gastrointestinal bleeding. An unexpected behavior of *Salmonella typhi. Dis Colon Rectum.* 1986;29(8): 511–514.

253. Roe AM, Warren BF, Brodribb AJ, et al. Diversion colitis and involution of the defunctioned anorectum. *Gut.* 1993;34(3):382–385.

254. Roediger WE. The starved colon—diminished mucosal nutrition, diminished absorption, and colitis. *Dis Colon Rectum.* 1990;33(10): 858–862.

255. Rohlke F, Surawicz CM, Stollman N. Fecal flora reconstitution for recurrent *Clostridium difficile* infection: results and methodology. *J Clin Gastroenterol.* 2010;44(8):567–570.

256. Rominger JM, Shah AN. Ameboma of the rectum. *Gastrointest Endosc.* 1979;25(2):71–73.

257. Rompalo AM. Diagnosis and treatment of sexually acquired proctitis and proctocolitis: an update. *Clin Infect Dis.* 1999;28(suppl 1):S84–S90.

258. Rompalo AM, Mertz GJ, Davis LG, et al. Oral acyclovir for treatment of first-episode herpes simplex virus proctitis. *JAMA.* 1988;259(19):2879–2881.

259. Rompalo AM, Mertz GJ, Mkrtichian EE, et al. Oral acyclovir vs placebo for treatment of herpes simplex virus proctitis in homosexual men. *Clin Res.* 1985;33:58A.

260. Rompalo AM, Roberts P, Johnson K, et al. Empirical therapy for the management of acute proctitis in homosexual men. *JAMA.* 1988;260(3):348–353.

261. Rosenberg JM, Walker M, Welch JP, et al. *Clostridium difficile* colitis in surgical patients. *Am J Surg.* 1984;147(4):486–491.

262. Rosenthal Philip J. Protozoal & helminthic infections. In: McPhee SJ, Papadakis MA, eds. Current Medical Diagnosis & Treatment 2011. New York, NY: McGraw-Hill; 2011:chap 35. http://www.accessmedicine.com/content.aspx?aID=778110. Accessed.

263. Rothenberg ME. Eosinophilic gastrointestinal disorders (EGID). *J Allergy Clin Immunol.* 2004;113(1):11–28.

264. Rozen P, Baratz M, Rattan J. Rectal bleeding due to amebic colitis diagnosed by multiple endoscopic biopsies: report of two cases. *Dis Colon Rectum.* 1981;24(2):127–129.

265. Rupnik M, Wilcox MH, Gerding DN. *Clostridium difficile* infection: new developments in epidemiology and pathogenesis. *Nat Rev Microbiol.* 2009;7(7):526–536.

266. Russo A, Cirino E, Sanfilippo G, et al. Ampicillin-associated colitis. Case report. *Endoscopy.* 1980;12(2):97–99.

267. Saab S, DeRosa V, Nieto J, et al. Cost and clinical outcomes of primary prophylaxis of variceal bleeding in patients with hepatic cirrhosis: a decision analytic model. *Am J Gastroenterol.* 2003;98(4):763–770.

268. Saebø A, Lassen J. Acute and chronic gastrointestinal manifestations associated with *Yersinia enterocolitica* infection. A Norwegian 10-year follow-up study on 458 hospitalized patients. *Ann Surg.* 1992;215(3):250–255.

269. Saha S, Mukherjee AJ, Agarwal N, et al. Colonic actinomycosis masquerading as perforated colonic carcinoma. *Trop Gastroenterol.* 2007;28(2):74–75.

270. Sakurai Y, Tsuchiya H, Ikegami F, et al. Acute right-sided hemorrhagic colitis associated with oral administration of ampicillin. *Dig Dis Sci.* 1979;24(12):910–915.

271. Sandmeier D, Bouzourene H. Microscopic colitis with giant cells: a rare new histopathologic subtype? *Int J Surg Pathol.* 2004;12(1):45–48.

272. Sanford AH. *Yersinia enterocolitica* abscess of the transverse colon. Report of a case. *Dis Colon Rectum.* 1990;33(11):985–986.

273. Schacker T, Hu HL, Koelle DM, et al. Famciclovir for the suppression of symptomatic and asymptomatic herpes simplex virus reactivation in HIV-infected persons. A double-blind, placebo-controlled trial. *Arch Intern Med.* 1998;128(1):21–28.

274. Schiller LR. Diagnosis and management of microscopic colitis syndrome. *J Clin Gastroenterol.* 2004;38(5 suppl 1):S27–S30.

275. Schofield PF. Abdominal tuberculosis. *Gut.* 1985;26(12):1275–1278.

276. Schulze K, Mitros FA. Eosinophilic gastroenteritis involving the ileocecal area. *Dis Colon Rectum.* 1979;22(1):47–50.

277. Schuster FL, Ramirez-Avila L. Current world status of *Balantidium coli. Clin Microbiol Rev.* 2008;21(4):626–638.

278. Schwebke JR, Whittington W, Rice RJ, et al. Trends in susceptibility of *Neisseria gonorrhoeae* to ceftriaxone from 1985 through 1991. *Antimicrob Agents Chemother.* 1995;39(4):917–920.

279. Sehgal S, Chawla R, Loomba PS, et al. Gastrointestinal histoplasmosis presenting as colonic pseudotumour. *Indian J Med Microbiol.* 2008;26(2):187–189.

280. Seppälä K, Hjelt L, Sipponen P. Colonoscopy in the diagnosis of antibiotic-associated colitis. A prospective study. *Scand J Gastroenterol.* 1981;16(4):465–468.

281. Sheibani S, Gerson LB. Chemical colitis. *J Clin Gastroenterol.* 2008;42(2):115–121.

282. Shelburne SA, Hamill RJ. Mycotic infections. In: McPhee SJ, Papadakis MA, eds. *Current Medical Diagnosis & Treatment 2011.* New York, NY: McGraw-Hill; 2011:chap 36. http://www.accessmedicine.com/content.aspx?aID=19953. Accessed .

283. Shorter NA, Thompson MD, Mooney DP, et al. Surgical aspects of an outbreak of *Yersinia enterocolitis. Pediatr Surg Int.* 1998;13(1):2–5.

284. Shukla VK, Roy SK, Vaidya MP, et al. Fulminant amebic colitis. *Dis Colon Rectum.* 1986;29(6):398–401.

285. Siegal FP, Lopez C, Hammer GS, et al. Severe acquired immunodeficiency in male homosexuals, manifested by chronic perianal ulcerative herpes simplex lesions. *N Engl J Med.* 1981;305(24):1439–1444.

286. Silva J Jr. Update on pseudomembranous colitis. *West J Med.* 1989;151(6):644–648.

287. Smith PD, Quinn TC, Strober W, et al. NIH conference. Gastrointestinal infections in AIDS. *Arch Intern Med.* 1992;116(1):63–77.

288. Soni HC, Hardin E. Proctitis, 2001. http://emedicine.com/aaem/topic368.htm. Accessed 2004.

289. Stampfl DA, Friedman LS. Collagenous colitis: pathophysiologic considerations. *Dig Dis Sci.* 1991;36(6):705–711.

290. Stanley SL Jr. Amoebiasis. *Lancet.* 2003;361(9362):1025–1034.

291. Stansfield VA. Diagnosis and management of anorectal gonorrhoea in women. *Br J Vener Dis.* 1980;56(5):319–321.

292. Stermer E, Levy N, Potasman I, et al. Brucellosis as a cause of severe colitis. *Am J Gastroenterol.* 1991;86(7):917–919.

293. Stimpert KK, Montgomery SP. Physician awareness of Chagas disease, USA. *Emerg Infect Dis.* 2010;16(5):871–872. http://www.cdc.gov/EID/content/16/5/871.htm. Accessed 2010.

294. Stockinger ZT. Colonic ameboma: its appearance on CT: report of a case. *Dis Colon Rectum.* 2004;47(4):527–529.

295. Stoddart B, Wilcox MH. *Clostridium difficile. Curr Opin Infect Dis.* 2002;15(5):513–518.

296. Stuart RC, Leahy AL, Cafferkey MT, et al. *Yersinia enterocolitica* infection and toxic megacolon. *Br J Surg.* 1986;73(7):590.

297. Talbot RW, Walker RC, Beart RW Jr. Changing epidemiology, diagnosis, and treatment of *Clostridium difficile* toxin-associated colitis. *Br J Surg.* 1986;73(6):457–460.

298. Tan KK, Chen K, Sim R. The spectrum of abdominal tuberculosis in a developed country: a single institution's experience over 7 years. *J Gastrointest Surg.* 2009;13(1):142–147.

299. Tangri V, Chande N. Microscopic colitis: an update. *J Clin Gastroenterol.* 2009;43(4):293–296.

300. Tanowitz HB, Weiss LM, Wittner M. Diagnosis and treatment of protozoan diarrheas. *Am J Gastroenterol.* 1988;83(4):339–350.

301. Tedesco FJ. Antibiotic associated pseudomembranous colitis with negative proctosigmoidoscopy examination. *Gastroenterology.* 1979;77(2):295–297.

302. Tedesco FJ, Huckaby CB, Hamby-Allen M, et al. Eosinophilic ileocolitis: expanding spectrum of eosinophilic gastroenteritis. *Dig Dis Sci.* 1981;26(10):943–948.

303. Thompson JR, Watts R Jr, Thompson WC. Actinomycetoma masquerading as an abdominal neoplasm. *Dis Colon Rectum.* 1982;25(4):368–370.

304. Tielbeek AV, Rosenbusch G, Muytjens HL, et al. Roentgenologic changes of the colon in *Campylobacter* infection. *Gastrointest Radiol.* 1985;10(4):358–361.

305. Triadafilopoulos G, Hallston AE. Acute abdomen as the first presentation of pseudomembranous colitis. *Gastroenterology.* 1991;101(3):685–891.

306. Trier JS. Acute diarrheal disorders. In: Greenberger NJ, Blumberg RS, Burakoff R, eds. *Current Diagnosis & Treatment: Gastroenterology, Hepatology, & Endoscopy.* New York, NY: McGraw-Hill; 2009:chap 5. http://www.accessmedicine.com/content.aspx?aID=6200376. Accessed 2010.

307. Tripodi J, Gorcey S, Burakoff R. A case of diversion colitis treated with 5-aminosalicylic acid enemas. *Am J Gastroenterol.* 1992;87(5):645–647.

308. Trudel JL, Deschênes M, Mayrand S, et al. Toxic megacolon complicating pseudomembranous enterocolitis. *Dis Colon Rectum.* 1995;38(10):1033–1038.

309. Udagawa SM, Portin BA, Bernhoft WH. Actinomycosis of the colon and rectum: report of two cases. *Dis Colon Rectum.* 1974;17(5):687–695. http://www.xs4all.nl/~rainmed/bulletin/disdeg-e.html. Accessed 2004.

310. Valko P, Busolini E, Donati N, et al. Severe large bowel obstruction secondary to infection with *Actinomyces israelii. Scand J Infect Dis.* 2006;38(3):231–234.

311. van Nood E, Speelman P, Kuijper EJ, et al. Struggling with recurrent *Clostridium difficile* infections: is donor faeces the solution? *Euro Surveill.* 2009;14(34):pii:19316.

312. Vantrappen G, Ponette E, Geboes K, et al. *Yersinia* enteritis and enterocolitis: gastroenterological aspects. *Gastroenterology.* 1977;72(2):220–227.

313. Varghese L, Galandiuk S, Tremaine WJ, et al. Lymphocytic colitis treated with proctocolectomy and ileal J-pouch-anal anastomosis: report of a case. *Dis Colon Rectum.* 2002;45(1):123–126.

314. Verhamme MA, Ramboer CH. Anisakiasis caused by herring in vinegar: a little known medical problem. *Gut.* 1988;29(6):843–847.

315. Voth ML, Akbari RP. Sexually transmitted proctitides. *Clin Colon Rectal Surg.* 2007;20(1):58–63.

316. Walters BA, Roberts R, Stafford R, et al. Relapse of antibiotic associated colitis: endogenous persistence of *Clostridium difficile* during vancomycin therapy. *Gut.* 1983;24(3):206–212.

317. Wanke CA. Practical approach to diarrheal illness. *Mediguide Infect Dis.* 1997;17:1.

318. Wasadikar PP, Kulkarni AB. Intestinal obstruction due to ascariasis. *Br J Surg.* 1997;84(3):410–412.

319. Wasselle JA, Sedgwick JH, Dawson PJ, et al. Intestinal herpes simplex infection presenting with intestinal perforation. *Am J Gastroenterol.* 1992;87(10):1475–1477.

320. Weese WC, Smith IM. A study of 57 cases of actinomycosis over a 36-year period. A diagnostic "failure" with good prognosis after treatment. *Arch Intern Med.* 1975;135(12):1562–1568.

321. WHO Diarrheal Diseases Steering Committee. Montreaux, Switzerland: World Health Organization, September 10–11, 2003.

322. Wiersma R, Hadley GP. Small bowel volvulus complicating intestinal ascariasis in children. *Br J Surg.* 1988;75(1):86–87.

323. Wig JD, Malik AK, Khanna SK, et al. Massive lower gastrointestinal bleeding in patients with typhoid fever. *Am J Gastroenterol.* 1981;75(6):445–448.

324. Williams JJ, Kaplan GG, Makhija S, et al. Microscopic colitis-defining incidence rates and risk factors: a population-based study. *Clin Gastroenterol Hepatol.* 2008;6(1):35–40.

325. Wolfe MS. Oxyuris, trichostrongylus and trichuris. *Clin Gastroenterol.* 1978;7(1):201–217.

326. Wong B. Parasitic diseases in immunocompromised hosts. *Am J Med.* 1984;76(3):479–486.

327. World Health Organization. WHO tuberculosis fact sheet 2010. http://who.int/mediacentre/factsheets/fs104/en/. Accessed 2010.

328. Yilmaz T, Sever A, Gür S, et al. CT findings of abdominal tuberculosis in 12 patients. *Comput Med Imaging Graph.* 2002;26(5):321–325.

329. Yungbluth PM. Practical approach to the use of the laboratory in infectious enteritis. *Practical Gastroenterol.* 1987;11:35.

330. Zayas CF, Perlino C, Caliendo A, et al. Chagas disease after organ transplantation—United States, 2001. http://www.cdc.gov/mmwr.preview/mmwrhtml/mm5110a3.htm. Accessed 2004.

34

Medicolegal Aspects of Colon and Rectal Surgery

Alan V. Abrams

> *If he [the surgeon] caused loss of life or limb, he lost his hands . . .*
>
> —BABYLONIAN LAW[12]

In the United States, the issue of alleged medical negligence has reached crisis proportions in many jurisdictions. Although no field of medicine is exempt from this concern, colon and rectal surgery has its own, unique areas of potential vulnerability. Practice patterns and self-education demand continuous reevaluation in order to provide the optimal care for our patients while protecting ourselves from the vicissitudes of the legal arena.

Although the penalty for medical malpractice in contemporary society is thankfully less severe than that demanded by Babylonian law, the ordeal of a malpractice suit can exact a heavy emotional, and sometimes financial, toll on the surgeon. While practicing "good medicine" is the best defense against claims of negligence, it is not always sufficient to avoid lawsuits. In fact, malpractice actions commonly arise in situations in which medical management has, by all objective criteria, conformed to the standard of care. Conversely, although many patients incur injuries during the course of treatment, studies have shown that only 1 in 10 individuals who sustain such injuries actually sue. Even in cases in which peer review evaluation concludes that negligence occurred, a patient rarely sues his or her physicians.[11] It is clear that in addition to the quality of care, other factors play a role in determining whether an injured patient will commence a legal action. Consequently, the surgeon must not only understand the law as it applies to medical malpractice but also must be aware of these contributory factors in order to minimize the likelihood of litigation when such an injury occurs.

► HISTORICAL BACKGROUND

The concept of assessing penalty for negligence resulting in injury dates back to Babylonian times, when individuals and sometimes even their families were held directly accountable. Under Hammurabi's code of justice (c. 1750 BC), if a builder constructed a house so poorly that it collapsed and killed the son of the owner, the law allowed for the execution of the builder's son. As judged by the quotation above, physicians were held to a similarly harsh standard. After their Babylonian captivity, the Hebrews adopted many aspects of Babylonian law but limited penalties to the practitioner himself.[11] Greek civilization did not recognize professions as such, so the conceptual basis for professional negligence was lacking. Under the Roman law, however, negligent infliction of personal injury could result in compensation for the patient's medical expenses and lost wages.

Licensing of physicians, which first occurred in the late Middle Ages, marked a major development in the evolution of personal injury law by identifying physicians as a class, separate from the rest of society by virtue of their possessing special knowledge and skill, and holding them responsible in the exercise of that skill.[6]

The first recorded suit for medical malpractice in English common law occurred in 1374. The United States, which adopted English common law, recorded its first case in 1794.[9]

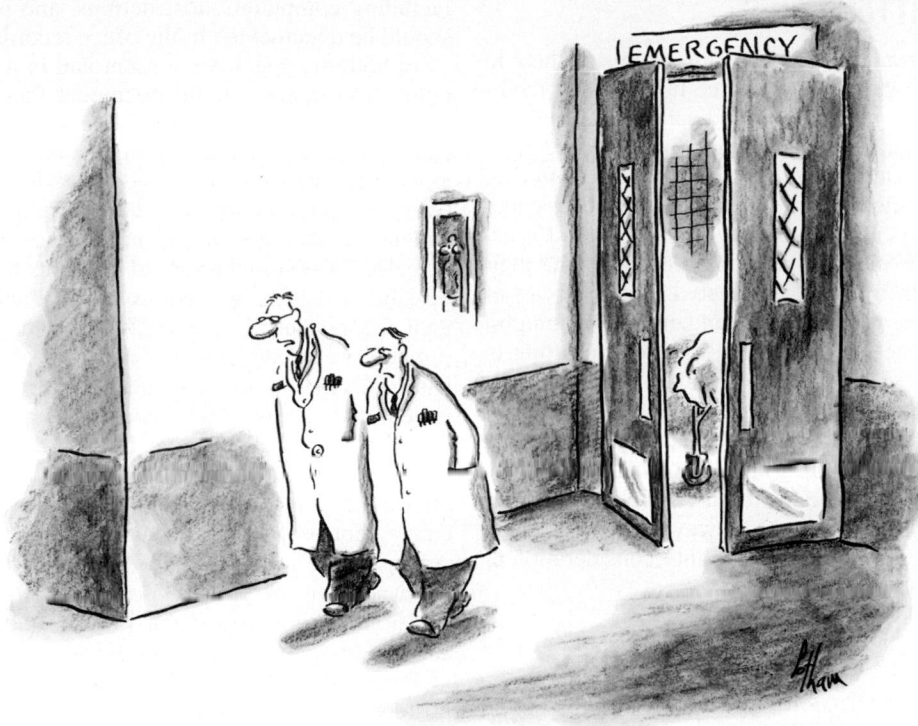

"I don't feel quite as fulfilled when I've saved a lawyer."

▶ THE WRITTEN LAW

Medical malpractice is not a separate branch of law, but rather is a subdivision of personal injury law. In order for the plaintiff (the patient) to prevail over the defendant (the physician) in a suit for malpractice, the law requires that four elements be proven: duty, breach of duty, causation, and damages.

Duty

The surgeon has a responsibility to the patient to conform to the standard of care—that is, to exercise the skill and provide a level of medical care equivalent to that which is generally employed by the profession under similar circumstances. The duty element is usually not at issue in medical malpractice cases because once the physician undertakes care of a patient, a legally binding physician–patient relationship is established, and the physician is obligated to provide competent care. Such a relationship also exists when a physician provides coverage for a colleague or assumes responsibility for a clinic in which indigent patients are treated.[1] The matter may be contested, however, if there is a question whether a valid physician–patient relationship existed.

The physician is also responsible for the actions of his office staff and may be held vicariously liable for care rendered by them, even if the physician had no knowledge of it. Training of personnel and development of proper office policies are thus essential.[2,7]

Breach of Duty

The physician, either by omission or commission, did not conform to the standard of care. The central issue in most malpractice cases is determining what the standard of care should have been in a particular clinical setting, a matter usually argued by expert witnesses for each side. The law does not require that the physician's care be equivalent to the best available nationally or even locally—only that it meet an accepted, usually national standard. If, as is often the case, there is more than one acceptable treatment for a condition, the physician cannot be held liable solely because the treatment mode selected results in an adverse outcome.

Causation

The physician's failure to conform to the standard of care directly caused or contributed to the patient's injury, a matter that is also usually the subject of expert witness testimony.

Damages

As a direct result of the physician's failure to meet the standard of care, the patient suffered an injury that, in a civil court, is compensable by the award of monetary damages. Conversely, if the patient did not sustain an injury, he cannot recover anything, no matter what the level of care.

Unlike a criminal trial, in which the prosecution must prove its case beyond a reasonable doubt, a malpractice suit requires only that the plaintiff prove that his or her version of events is more likely than not, a standard commonly referred to as *proof to a reasonable degree of medical probability (or certainty).* The burden of proof for all of these elements lies with the plaintiff, however, and if proof of any one element is lacking, the plaintiff's complaint of negligence cannot be sustained.

► THE UNWRITTEN LAWS

The most important rule to which a surgeon must adhere to prevent malpractice suits is to practice high-quality medicine. Because of the complexity of medical decision making, the law allows physicians considerable latitude in their practice by defining the standard of care as *what a reasonable*, rather than what the most expert practitioner would do under similar circumstances and conditions. Nevertheless, it is essential that surgeons maintain and continually update their knowledge and skills by conscientiously keeping abreast of the medical literature and regular attendance at meaningful educational conferences. Although most errors resulting in malpractice claims occur during the conduct of routine procedures rather than "index" operations,[10] before undertaking a new or advanced procedure independently, the surgeon should receive adequate training and mentoring by someone competent in performing the technique. Aside from maintaining a high level of competence, however, there are many other factors that a surgeon must take into consideration to reduce the likelihood of being sued.

Patient Selection

One need not have extensive psychiatric training to realize that there are patients who, for a variety of reasons, seek to have surgery when none is indicated. Because the indications for many colorectal procedures (surgery for hemorrhoids, abdominal pain/diverticular disease, and constipation/colonic inertia) are in part subjective, such an issue is not infrequent. If there is any question about an individual's emotional stability or motivation, the surgeon must meticulously evaluate the patient to be certain that objectively verifiable indications for surgery exist; that the patient has realistic expectations about possible outcomes, including negative ones and complications; and that all of the above is documented in the medical record. Second opinions in these situations are also valuable.

Documentation

In combination with high-quality care, good documentation is the surgeon's strongest line of defense in malpractice litigation. Creating a medical record offers surgeons the opportunity to present their version of events contemporaneous with their occurrence. Such documentation has much more credibility in a legal setting than after-the-fact explanations and rationalizations. In a court room, if actions or discussions have not been documented, they are often considered not to have occurred.[5]

Notes must be legible and self-explanatory to readers other than the author. Documentation comprehensible only to the surgeon is inadequate in court, as lawyers, experts, and jurors may be unable to make sense of what the surgeon has written. Legible notes also avoid the possible additional allegation that others participating in the patient's care misunderstood the note and, as a result, committed an error.[5]

Office notes should document not only the medical history, physical findings, and differential diagnosis, but also treatment alternatives, recommendations, and possible complications. Plans for follow-up should document the party to whom the discharge instructions were given, the plan of care, and the need for any additional testing. Missed appointments or other indicators of possible patient noncompliance should be noted. All telephone communications with the patient, including complaints, instructions, and recommendations, should be documented in the office records.

In both the operative consent and in a separate progress note, the surgeon should document that he has informed the patient (or other responsible party) of the purpose and extent of the planned procedure, the benefits and major risks associated with the proposed procedure, and its alternatives. The surgeon need not disclose remote risks unless the patient specifically requests that all known complications be revealed.[3] The surgeon should make the patient aware of the possibility that the procedure may not achieve its intended goal. Guarantees of a successful outcome, whether stated or implied, are to be avoided. The risk of death, brain damage, and paralysis should be included in the consent form of any patient undergoing general anesthesia.

All too many operative reports devote an inordinate amount of attention to descriptions of opening and closing the wound, placing sutures, and firing staplers. Such "cookie cutter" notes offer little legal protection for the surgeon. An operative report should describe not only the technical aspects of the procedure, but also the findings and the decision-making process that flowed from them, leading the surgeon to do what was done.

Progress notes should be written at least daily on recent postoperative or severely ill patients. In addition to the date, the notes should record the time at which they were written. The notes should be factual. Impressions and tentative diagnoses, if included at all, should be clearly labeled as such. Inclusion of vital signs, physical findings, and laboratory and imaging results in the notes not only facilitates reconstruction of events long after they have occurred, but also documents the surgeon's awareness of them and may, at a later date, provide support in explaining why a particular course of action was adopted. Like operative reports, progress notes should describe not only the facts, but also the surgeon's reasoning in making his or her decisions.

Relations with Patient and Family

The surgeon's relationship with the patient and her family is often as important as the quality of care in determining whether an action for malpractice is brought,[3] and the key to that relationship is *communication*. The surgeon must remain accessible and communicative to the patient and to the family at all times, particularly if postoperative complications develop. Although the situation may be frustrating and emotionally draining for the surgeon, he must maintain a professional demeanor and avoid the appearance of antagonism, anger, or hostility.

During the preoperative period, the surgeon should explain the rationale and goals of treatment in terms readily comprehensible to the layperson. If the surgeon encounters an unexpected finding intraoperatively and is considering a significant deviation from the planned procedure, he or she is advised to leave the operating room, with the patient adequately monitored and supervised, to discuss the findings and possible courses of action with the responsible family member or health care proxy.

If significant postoperative complications develop, the surgeon should communicate on a regular, preferably daily, basis with the family to explain the nature of the problems and what is being done to investigate the causes and to treat them. Patients and their families will often accept major complications, and even death, if they believe that the physician is sympathetic to their plight and that of the patient and is doing everything possible to address the situation. Conversely, even the best medical care may not avoid a lawsuit if accompanied by a perceived attitude of indifference or avoidance.

▶ SPECIAL SITUATIONS IN COLON AND RECTAL SURGERY

Although the following guidelines are not intended to be either medically or legally definitive or exhaustive, they are offered in the hope that they may prove useful in managing common conditions that form the basis for much malpractice litigation in the field of colorectal surgery.

Anal Conditions

Hemorrhoids and fissures have two common features: their symptoms can often be ameliorated or cured by nonsurgical means and they are not life threatening. Therefore, surgery should usually not be the first option for either condition. Instead, the surgeon should initially offer the patient a trial of nonoperative management, and only after this has failed should surgery be considered. Exceptions are the excruciatingly painful fissure that significantly impairs the patient's quality of life, and massively prolapsed, thrombosed hemorrhoids, situations in which surgery is often the most expeditious and humane means of alleviating the patient's pain and correcting the underlying pathology. Even in these settings, however, the surgeon should document that he has discussed potential nonoperative management alternatives with the patient, that surgery is recommended because of the severity of the clinical situation, and that the patient understands these considerations and accepts the recommendation.

Informed consent prior to elective anal surgery should include a discussion of the possibility of postoperative impairment of continence and recurrence of symptoms. Exact figures regarding the incidence of these two complications should not be given unless specifically requested by the patient, but he or she must understand that, despite their low incidence, there is a possibility that either may occur postoperatively.

When performing a hemorrhoidectomy, the surgeon should refrain from undertaking a concomitant sphincterotomy unless a fissure is present and the patient has granted informed consent for this additional procedure. Should the surgeon ignore this guideline, any degree of postoperative incontinence experienced by the patient, even if physiologically unrelated to the sphincterotomy, may be attributed to it in a legal proceeding and serve as the basis of a lawsuit on the grounds that the sphincterotomy exceeded the scope of the patient's consent.

Similarly, when performing a sphincterotomy, hemorrhoids, except for sentinel tags and hemorrhoidal tissue adjacent to the fissure that may interfere with healing, should not be removed without the patient's prior approval.

Rectal Bleeding

Failure to conduct a thorough evaluation for rectal bleeding may result in a delayed diagnosis of cancer, which is one of the most common causes of malpractice litigation in colorectal surgery.[4] It is both impractical and unethical to recommend colonoscopy to every patient with rectal bleeding. At a minimum, however, patients with this complaint should have anoscopy or preferably rigid or flexible sigmoidoscopy. If a nonneoplastic source of bleeding is found within the anorectum, the surgeon may offer a course of nonoperative management and should arrange for follow-up, either office visit or telephone call, to document that the bleeding has resolved.

Irrespective of the means for follow-up, the surgeon should instruct the patient to establish contact within a stated period if the bleeding persists and document this recommendation in the record. Failure to adopt this simple measure has often resulted in a weakened defense in lawsuits in which there is a charge of delayed diagnosis of cancer because the patient may deny or not remember ever having been informed of the need for follow-up. Written documentation of the surgeon's admonition avoids the dilemma that a jury may face in having to decide between the word of the patient and that of the surgeon.

If the bleeding persists despite adequate nonoperative or surgical treatment or if no source of bleeding is found on initial endoscopic examination in a patient who, either due to age or some other factor, is at increased risk for colorectal cancer, either a total colonoscopy, or less optimally, flexible sigmoidoscopy with barium enema (or CT colonography), is indicated. Even if benign anorectal disease were the true source of bleeding, a colonic neoplasm may become manifest some time in the future, and the patient may claim delayed diagnosis on the basis of an incomplete evaluation of the colon in the face of ongoing rectal bleeding.

Anastomotic Leak

No matter how experienced or technically adept he or she may be, every surgeon will encounter anastomotic leaks. Because an anastomotic leak is recognized as a risk inherent in colon surgery, its occurrence is not, per se, evidence of substandard care. Instead, malpractice litigation in this setting is usually the result of the surgeon's failure to diagnose and treat the leak in a timely fashion. Because of their frequency and the serious consequences associated with this complication, the possibility of an anastomotic leak should *always* be discussed preoperatively with the patient as part of the informed consent in every individual for whom an anastomosis is contemplated.

Most leaks become clinically apparent between the 5th and 10th postoperative days. Patients usually present with tachycardia, fever, ileus, abdominal pain, and distension, as well as a leukocytosis. Although identical clinical findings may result from processes unrelated to the anastomosis, it is incumbent upon the surgeon, when confronted with this constellation of findings, to promptly establish whether an anastomotic leak exists. Appropriate tools for this purpose are CT scan of the abdomen and pelvis with or without contrast or a low-pressure contrast study of the anastomosis, preferably from below, using water-soluble contrast material.

If an anastomotic leak is diagnosed promptly and managed properly, the most serious sequelae of ongoing sepsis, such as acute respiratory distress syndrome, and renal and hepatic failure can often be avoided. Litigation commonly arises when the surgeon fails to consider the possibility of an anastomotic leak, often resulting in an extended period of untreated fecal peritonitis and its devastating consequences.

Colonoscopic Perforation

Perforation of the colon as the result of diagnostic or therapeutic colonoscopy has much in common with anastomotic leak. It is a risk inherent to the procedure, and this possibility should be mentioned in the informed consent. From a medicolegal perspective, litigation is often the result of delay in diagnosis.

The development of abdominal pain and distension within a few hours of completion of colonoscopy should suggest the possibility of mechanical injury to the colon. These symptoms are often relayed to the physician by the patient or his relative by telephone, since by this time the patient has usually been discharged from the endoscopy unit. If there is any question as to the significance or validity of the complaints, a qualified observer should examine the patient and imaging studies performed to detect the presence of free intraperitoneal gas. Upright chest x-rays and flat plate and upright abdominal films are usually sufficient, but if these studies are inconclusive, a CT scan of the abdomen may reveal small amounts of free air not readily identified on plain films.

Similar symptoms may develop following biopsy, fulguration, or removal of polyps or other lesions, although their onset in these settings may be delayed for a day or more because of the more gradual progression of the transmural injury. Again, direct physical examination and appropriate imaging studies should be undertaken to establish the diagnosis.

As with anastomotic leak, the occurrence of a colonoscopic perforation does not, in itself, constitute malpractice, whereas failure to recognize and treat it does. By giving credence to the patient's complaints, promptly performing the necessary examinations, and instituting the appropriate treatment, the surgeon will conform to good medical practice and provide himself or herself with the best protection against a malpractice claim.

▶ IF YOU'RE SUED

Often the surgeon's first indication that a suit is being considered is receipt of a letter from an attorney requesting the medical record of a patient who has suffered a complication or incurred some other unfavorable outcome. Although receipt of such a request may alarm the surgeon, he must restrain the natural impulse to contact the patient, the family, or the attorney to discuss the case or to inquire what, if any, action may be contemplated. Instead the surgeon should notify his or her liability insurance carrier or other responsible risk manager of the request and then comply with the request, provided that it is accompanied by a valid "release of information" form signed by the patient or designated medical power of attorney or, if the patient is deceased, by the next of kin. In complying with the request, the surgeon should send only a copy of the record, retaining the original. If a hospital chart is involved, it should be secured so that no outside parties have access to it. It is also recommended that the surgeon keep a second copy in a location remote from other office records to avoid the problems that would ensue if the original were to be damaged, lost, or stolen. For example, if the records are lost or misplaced, it may be construed that such was done intentionally and that the surgeon has something to hide. If the patient has been hospitalized, the surgeon should acquire a copy of the entire hospital record, even if the latter is voluminous and expensive to duplicate. These copies of the office and hospital records will serve as "working" documents that can be marked and highlighted by the surgeon and his attorney in preparing the defense. It cannot be emphasized too strongly, however, that the original

documents must not be altered in any way. Such after-the-fact changes, even if reflective of the true course of events, are easily detected and may be subsequently used to impugn the surgeon's integrity. Moreover, if the changes are fabrications, they may serve as the basis for criminal prosecution.

A sensitive situation arises if the patient, having enlisted an attorney to review the medical records, seeks ongoing care from the surgeon. In doing so the patient may be motivated by a genuine desire for treatment, or he or she may be attempting to elicit an expression of guilt or responsibility from the surgeon. If the surgeon is willing to continue treatment, parameters for the scope of physician–patient discussions should be developed with the assistance of the insurance carrier or risk manager. If the surgeon does not wish to continue treating the patient, he or she must follow established ethical and legal guidelines for terminating care. Failure to do so may result in a claim of abandonment.

Some states have enacted "apology laws," under which the physician expresses regret to the patient or family for a medical error that has resulted in injury in the hope that such action will reduce the likelihood of a lawsuit. The validity of this assumption is unproven, and in the majority of states that have enacted apology laws, statements regarding causation and fault contained in the apology may be admitted in court.[2] Furthermore, the apology may provide useful information to the plaintiff's attorney. In general, it is reasonable for the surgeon to demonstrate empathy to the patient and family for an unfavorable outcome without admitting fault or acknowledging the outcome to have been the result of medical error.

In order to initiate a malpractice suit, the patient's attorney must file a complaint in state or federal court. The complaint may be specific as to its allegations, or it may only vaguely stipulate that the surgeon deviated from the standard of care and that an injury or injuries resulted. The plaintiff's attorney must also issue summons to the surgeon, specifying a period in which to file a response to the complaint. Upon receipt of formal notification that a suit has been filed, the surgeon must notify the insurance carrier or risk manager promptly if this has not already been done. Otherwise one risks denial of coverage. The insurance carrier will then appoint an attorney to defend the surgeon. Although reimbursed by the insurance carrier, the defense attorney's primary responsibility is to the surgeon, and if, for any reason, one is dissatisfied with the appointed attorney's performance, he has the right to request that an alternate be provided. Once the attorney–surgeon relationship has been established, the surgeon should fully cooperate with the attorney and actively participate in the defense by supplying documents and conferring with the attorney as requested. The surgeon should, however, refrain from discussing the case with any parties other than the attorney and one's spouse. E-mails and other forms of electronic communication with individuals other than the surgeon's attorney or spouse containing information about the case are not protected and are thus admissible in court. The surgeon must also bear in mind that discussion of the case in a setting accessible to the public, whether a mobile phone or a hospital elevator, may be overheard.[3] In most situations, the defense attorney will also solicit opinions from physicians with appropriate expertise to evaluate the case. To assist in this process, the defendant may suggest the names of experts with whom he or she is familiar but should not include individuals with whom she has a professional, financial, or social relationship.

The next stage in formal proceedings is that of discovery, during which the plaintiff's attorney will issue a set of written questions (interrogatories) about the care rendered and to which the defendant must respond. The interrogatories are likely to be more detailed than the formal complaint with regard to specific claims of negligence and will usually identify the plaintiff's expert witnesses as well as shed light on their opinions. Statements under oath (depositions) will then be taken from the patient, the surgeon, the expert witnesses (in most states), and any other relevant individuals, the purpose of which is to discover what the various parties are prepared to testify about at trial. Finally, in most jurisdictions, unless the case is settled, the action will proceed to trial, which is almost always conducted before a jury or arbitrating tribunal. A jury decision supporting the plaintiff's claim of malpractice or any monetary award regardless of the amount, even if achieved through a pretrial settlement, must be reported to the National Practitioner Data Bank and to state licensing boards.[8]

As the case proceeds through the legal process, the surgeon will be called upon to give testimony in deposition and at trial, proceedings for which he should adopt differing strategies. At deposition, the plaintiff's attorney will attempt to discover what factual testimony the surgeon will give at trial and to evaluate the surgeon's strengths and weaknesses as a witness before a jury. In this situation, the surgeon should answer questions precisely and honestly, but should not volunteer information that is not encompassed within the scope of the question, nor should explanations be offered of the medical technicalities unless specifically requested to do so. Efforts to "educate" the plaintiff's attorney at deposition will only assist that person in preparing his or her case.

In contrast, at trial the surgeon will be attempting to explain and justify to the jury the care that was rendered. In doing so, the surgeon must conform to the testimony given at deposition, but should now feel free to expand on the answers in order to educate the jury and to explain the rationale and justification for one's actions. Despite competing demands for the surgeon's time, he or she should remain in attendance throughout the trial in order to serve as a medical advisor to one's attorney and to avoid giving the jury the impression of indifference as to the outcome. One must understand that the surgeon is "playing on a foreign and unfamiliar ball field" and that the arena adheres to the dictates of the legal profession. This is not one's operating room or office. The code of conduct is, therefore, rigorously prescribed by rules outside of the jurisdiction of the physician. All the more reason to rely on one's attorney.

At both deposition and trial, the surgeon, despite genuine feelings of concern as to the patient's problems, must remain firm in the conviction of the rightness of one's position and should avoid making admissions based on retrospective analysis or in speculating as to what she or he might have done differently in response to "knowing-what-you-know-now" questions. The surgeon can also favorably influence the jury by dressing conservatively without ostentatious jewelry, remaining composed and polite, not losing one's temper, and not appearing arrogant or condescending. In presenting an image of competence, forthrightness, and professionalism, the surgeon will conform to the jury's image of what every patient would like to see in a physician and will thereby maximize the likelihood of a favorable outcome in what is inevitably a stressful and emotionally charged experience. Regardless of the result, the surgeon must endeavor to remember that a medical malpractice lawsuit is the price of "doing business." Although the experience is unequivocally traumatic, it is self-limiting and transient; it shall pass. Still, one may be advised to seek psychiatric or other medical support should the experience appear excessively burdensome.

▶ CONCLUSION

The guidelines contained in this chapter are intended to protect the surgeon from becoming the subject of a malpractice suit. Unfortunately, given the litigious atmosphere in which American surgeons practice, such claims are likely to arise during the course of a surgical career. Adherence to the principles of providing high quality care, documenting discussions and events clearly and comprehensively, and maintaining strong lines of communication with the patient and his or her family, however, will serve as the basis for a strong defense in the event of such an eventuality.

References

1. Bal BS. An introduction to medical malpractice in the United States. *Clin Orthop Relat Res.* 2009;467(2):339–347.
2. Feld AD, Moses RE. Most doctors win: what to do if sued for medical malpractice. *Am J Gastroenterol.* 2009;104(6):1346–1351.
3. Hoffman PJ, Plump JD, Courtney MA. The defense counsel's perspective. *Clin Orthop Relat Res.* 2005;(443):15–25.
4. Kern KA. Medical malpractice involving colon and rectal disease: a 20-year review of United States civil court litigation. *Dis Colon Rectum.* 1993;36(6):531–539.
5. Lyons JM III, Martinez JA, O'Leary JP. Medical malpractice matters: medical record M & Ms. *J Surg Educ.* 2009;66(2):113–117.
6. Moore TA. *Medical Malpractice Discovery and Trial.* 7th ed. New York, NY: Practising Law Institute Press; 2004.
7. Moses RE, Feld AD. Physician liability for errors of nonphysician clinicians: nurse practitioners and physician assistants. *Am J Gastroeneterol.* 2007;102(1):6–9.
8. Nepps ME. The basics of medical malpractice. *Chest.* 2008;134(5):1051–1055.
9. Nora PF, ed. *Professional Liability/Risk Management: A Manual for Surgeons.* Chicago, IL: American College of Surgeons; 1991.
10. Regenbogen SE, Greenberg CC, Studdert DM, et al. Patterns of technical error among surgical malpractice claims: an analysis of strategies to prevent injury to surgical patients. *Ann Surg.* 2007;246(5):705–711.
11. Sloan FA, Githens PB, Clayton EW. *Suing for Medical Malpractice.* Chicago, IL: University of Chicago Press; 1993. Quoted in: Moore TA. *Medical Malpractice Discovery and Trial.* 7th ed. New York, NY: Practising Law Institute Press; 2004.
12. Zane JM. *The Story of Law.* 2nd ed. Indianapolis, IN: Liberty Fund; 1998. Quoted in: Moore TA. *Medical Malpractice Discovery and Trial.* 7th ed. New York, NY: Practising Law Institute Press; 2004.

Index

Biography Index